MATERNITY and PEDIATRIC Nursing

Susan Scott Ricci, ARNP, MSN, MEd, CNE
College of Nursing Faculty
University of Central Florida
Orlando, Florida
Former Nursing Program Director and Faculty
Lake Sumter State College
Leesburg, Florida

Terri Kyle, MSN, CPNP, CNE
Program Chair-Nursing
Herzing University—Orlando
Winter Park, Florida

Susan Carman, MSN, MBA
Professor of Nursing
Most recently, Edison Community College
Fort Myers, Florida

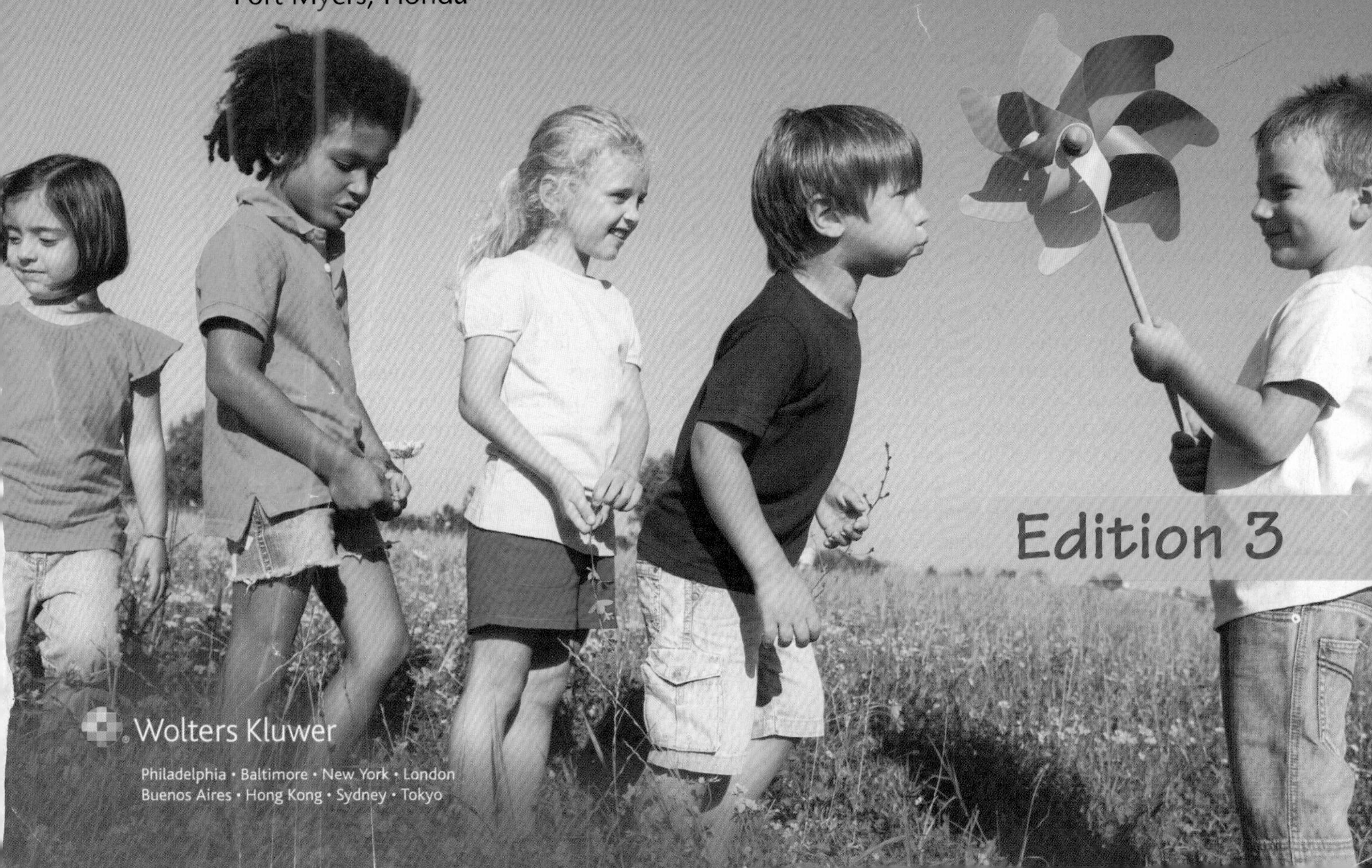

Edition 3

Wolters Kluwer

Philadelphia • Baltimore • New York • London
Buenos Aires • Hong Kong • Sydney • Tokyo

Acquisitions Editor: Natasha McIntyre
Director of Product Development: Jennifer Forestieri
Product Development Editor: Annette Ferran
Editorial Assistant: Dan Reilly
Production Project Manager: Marian Bellus
Design Coordinator: Holly McLaughlin
Illustration Coordinator: Jennifer Clements
Manufacturing Coordinator: Karin Duffield
Prepress Vendor: Aptara, Inc.

3rd Edition

9 8 7 6 5 4 3 2 1

Printed in China

Library of Congress Cataloging-in-Publication Data

Names: Ricci, Susan Scott, author. | Kyle, Terri, author. | Carman, Susan, author.
Title: Maternity and pediatric nursing / Susan Scott Ricci, Terri Kyle, Susan Carman.
Description: Third edition. | Philadelphia : Wolters Kluwer, [2017] | Includes bibliographical references and index.
Identifiers: LCCN 2016030558 | ISBN 9781451194005 (hardback)
Subjects: | MESH: Maternal-Child Nursing | Pediatric Nursing | Women's Health
Classification: LCC RG951 | NLM WY 157.3 | DDC 618.92/00231--dc23
LC record available at https://lccn.loc.gov/2016030558

Care has been taken to confirm the accuracy of the information presented and to describe generally accepted practices. However, the authors, editors, and publisher are not responsible for errors or omissions or for any consequences from application of the information in this book and make no warranty, expressed or implied, with respect to the currency, completeness, or accuracy of the contents of the publication. Application of this information in a particular situation remains the professional responsibility of the practitioner; the clinical treatments described and recommended may not be considered absolute and universal recommendations.

The authors, editors, and publisher have exerted every effort to ensure that drug selection and dosage set forth in this text are in accordance with the current recommendations and practice at the time of publication. However, in view of ongoing research, changes in government regulations, and the constant flow of information relating to drug therapy and drug reactions, the reader is urged to check the package insert for each drug for any change in indications and dosage and for added warnings and precautions. This is particularly important when the recommended agent is a new or infrequently employed drug.

Some drugs and medical devices presented in this publication have Food and Drug Administration (FDA) clearance for limited use in restricted research settings. It is the responsibility of the health care provider to ascertain the FDA status of each drug or device planned for use in his or her clinical practice.

LWW.com

CCS0916

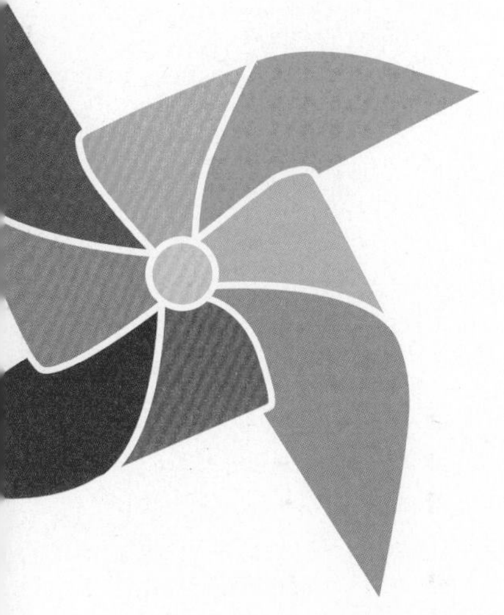

This book is lovingly dedicated to my husband Glenn, who is the wind beneath my wings, and I am thankful for his enduring love, encouragement, and confidence in me. Also to my children, Brian and Jennifer, who have always inspired me throughout their lives. And lastly, to my grandchildren—Leyton, Peyton, Alyssa, Wyatt, Michael, Rylan, and Brody who bring me life's greatest joys.

SUSAN SCOTT RICCI

This text is dedicated to my initial mentor into pediatric nursing, Gayle Maloney. She role-modeled and inspired my passion for excellence in the care of children and families. Thank you to my ever-faithful and consistently dedicated husband John and my amazing and delightful children, Christian and Caitlin.

TERRI KYLE

This book is dedicated to all the children out there and the wonderful nurses who care for them. They inspire me to become a better nurse, educator, and person. This book is also dedicated to my loving and supportive family. My husband Chris without whom I could not have reached this accomplishment. My four beautiful girls, Grace, Ella, Lily, and Maya, who have allowed me to learn firsthand about growth and development and who truly amaze me each and every day. My parents, Lene and Kishor Patel, who always taught me I could do whatever I put my mind to. To Terri Kyle, thank you for this opportunity, your endless support, and your incredible vision.

SUSAN CARMAN

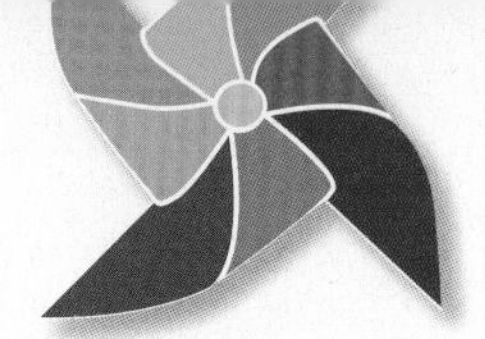

About the Authors

Susan Scott Ricci

Susan Scott Ricci earned a diploma in nursing from the Washington Hospital Center School of Nursing, and went on to receive a BSN and MSN in Maternal—Infant Nursing, from the Catholic University of America in Washington, DC. She also obtained an MEd in Counseling from the University of Southern Mississippi, along with a recent national certification as a nurse educator. She has worked in a variety of women's health care settings, including labor and birth, postpartum, prenatal, and family planning ambulatory care clinics. Susan is a certified women's health care nurse practitioner who has spent 30+ years in nursing education teaching in LPN, ADN, and BSN programs. She is involved in several professional nursing organizations and holds application of knowledge within nursing practice.

Terri Kyle

Terri Kyle earned a Bachelor of Science in Nursing from the University of North Carolina at Chapel Hill and a Master of Science in Nursing from Emory University in Atlanta, Georgia. She is a certified pediatric nurse practitioner, and practicing pediatric nursing for over 30 years, she has had the opportunity to serve children and their families in a variety of diverse settings. Terri also holds the credential of certified nurse educator.

She has experience in inpatient pediatrics, in pediatric and neonatal intensive care units, newborn nursery, specialized pediatric units, and community hospitals. She has worked as a pediatric nurse practitioner in pediatric specialty clinics and primary care. She has been involved in teaching nursing for over 25 years with experience in both graduate and undergraduate education. Terri is a fellow in the National Association of Pediatric Nurse Practitioners and a member of the Sigma Theta Tau International Honor Society of Nursing, the National League for Nursing, and the Society of Pediatric Nurses.

With the limited time allotted to the topic of maternity and pediatric nursing in nursing programs, Terri recognized the need for a textbook that "got to the point." She strongly believes in a concept-based approach for learning nursing—that is, to teach the basics to students in a broad, contextual format so that they can apply that knowledge in a variety of situations. The concept-based approach to nursing education is time efficient for nursing educators and fosters the development of critical thinking skills in student nurses.

Susan Carman

Susan Carman earned a Bachelor of Science in Nursing from the University of Wisconsin-Madison and a Master of Science in Nursing and Master in Business Administration from the University of Colorado-Denver. As a pediatric nurse for over 20 years, Susan has had the opportunity to care for children in a variety of diverse settings and in many of the major children's hospitals throughout the United States. She also has provided volunteer nursing care in a variety of settings including the Dominican Republic and India. She has been involved in teaching nursing for the past 15 years and enjoys watching students transform into competent nurses with strong critical thinking skills. She is a member of Sigma Theta tau and Beta Gamma Sigma.

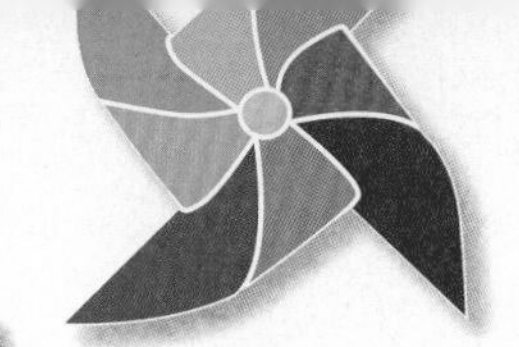

Reviewers to the Third Edition

Dolores Holland, MSN, RN, CNOR
McLennan Community College
Waco, Texas

Terri Kahle, MSN, RNC, CNE
Instructor
Southeast Missouri Hospital College of Nursing and Health Sciences
Cape Girardeau, Missouri

Deborah Raines, PhD, EdS, RN, ANEF
Associate Professor
State University of New York at Buffalo
Buffalo, New York

Leslie S. Reifel, MSN, RN, CPNP, CNE
Associate Professor
Sentara College of Health Sciences
Chesapeake, Virginia

Valerie Taylor-Haslip, PhD, RN, FNP
Associate Professor
Chairperson
Department of Nursing
York College
City University of New York
Jamaica, New York

Diane Tinker, RN, MNSc, CNM
Lead Faculty
Obstetrical Nursing
Brookline College
Phoenix, Arizona

Elaine Webber, MS, RNCS, IBCLC
Assistant Professor
University of Detroit Mercy
Huntington Woods, MI

Barbara Morrison Wilford, DNP, MBA/HCA, CKC, RN
Associate Professor
Allied Health and Nursing
Lorain County Community College
Elyria, Ohio

Preface

Many nursing curricula combine and teach maternity and pediatrics in tandem. This can be viewed as a *natural fit* of two content areas that belong together. Nursing education in general is founded upon the principle of mastering simpler concepts first and incorporating those concepts into the student's knowledge base. The student is then able to progress to problem solving in more complex situations. In today's education climate with reduced class time devoted to specialty courses, it is particularly important for nursing educators to focus on key concepts, rather than attempting to cover everything within a specific topic.

The intent of *Maternity and Pediatric Nursing* is to provide the nurse the basis needed for sound nursing care of women and children. The content in the book will enable the reader to guide women and children toward higher levels of wellness throughout the life cycle. In addition, the focus of the textbook will allow the reader to anticipate, identify, and address common problems and provide timely, evidence-based interventions to reduce long-term sequelae.

This textbook is designed as a practical approach to understanding the health of women and children. The main objective is to help the student build a strong knowledge base and assist with the development of critical thinking skills. Women in our society are becoming empowered to make informed and responsible choices regarding their health and that of their children, but to do so they need the encouragement and support of nurses who care for them. This textbook focuses on women and children throughout their life span, covering a broad scope of topics with emphasis placed upon common issues. Maternity nursing content coverage is comprehensive, yet presented in a concise and straightforward manner. The pediatric nursing content presents the important differences when caring for children compared with caring for adults. A nursing process approach provides relevant information in a concise and nonredundant manner.[1] The content covered in the text arms the student or practicing nurse with essential information to care for women and their families, to assist them to make the right choices safely, intelligently, and with confidence.

[1]Nursing Process Overview contains NANDA-I approved nursing diagnoses. Material related to nursing diagnoses is from Nursing Diagnoses—Definitions and Classification 2015-2017 © 2014, 2012 2009, 2007, 2005, 2003, 2001, 1998, 1996, 1994 NANDA International. Used by arrangement with Wiley-Blackwell Publishing, a company of John Wiley & Sons, Inc. In order to make safe and effective judgments using NANDA-I nursing diagnoses it is essential that nurses refer to the definitions and defining characteristics of the diagnoses listed in this work.

Organization

Each chapter of *Maternity and Pediatric Nursing* focuses on a different aspect of maternity and/or pediatric nursing care. The book is divided into eleven units, beginning with general concepts related to maternity and pediatric nursing care, progressing from women's health, pregnancy and birth, through child health promotion and nursing management of alterations in children's health.

Unit 1: Introduction to Maternity and Pediatric Nursing

Unit 1 helps build a foundation for the student beginning the study of the care of women, infants, and children. This unit explores contemporary issues and trends in maternity and pediatric nursing. Perspectives on women's health and pediatric nursing, core concepts of maternal and pediatric nursing, including, family-centered and atraumatic care, and communication, and community-based nursing are addressed.

Unit 2: Women's Health Throughout the Life Span

Unit 2 introduces the student to selected women's health topics, including structure and function of the reproductive system, common reproductive concerns, sexually transmitted infections, problems of the breast, and benign disorders and cancers of the female reproductive tract. This unit encourages the student to assist women in maintaining their quality of life, reducing their risk of disease, and becoming active partners with their health care professional.

Unit 3: Pregnancy

Unit 3 addresses topics related to normal pregnancy, including fetal development, genetics, and maternal adaptation to pregnancy. Nursing management during normal pregnancy is addressed, encouraging application of basic knowledge to nursing practice. Nursing management includes maternal and fetal assessment throughout pregnancy, interventions to promote self-care and minimize common discomforts, and patient education.

Unit 4: Labor and Birth

Unit 4 begins with an explanation of the normal labor and birth process, including maternal and fetal adaptations. This is followed by content focusing on the nurse's role during normal labor and birth, which includes maternal and fetal assessment, pharmacologic and nonpharmacologic comfort measures and pain management, and specific nursing interventions during each stage of labor and birth.

Unit 5: Postpartum Period

Unit 5 focuses on maternal adaptation during the normal postpartum period. Both physiologic and psychological aspects are explored. Paternal adaptation is also considered. This unit also presents related nursing management, including assessment of physical and emotional status, promoting comfort, assisting with elimination, counseling about sexuality and contraception, promoting nutrition, promoting family adaptation, and preparing for discharge.

Unit 6: The Newborn

Unit 6 covers physiologic and behavioral adaptations of the normal newborn. It also delves into nursing management of the normal newborn, including immediate assessment and specific interventions as well as ongoing assessment, physical examination, and specific interventions during the early newborn period.

Unit 7: Childbearing at Risk

Unit 7 shifts the focus to at-risk pregnancy, childbirth, and postpartum care. Pre-existing conditions of the woman, pregnancy-related complications, at-risk labor, emergencies associated with labor and birth, and medical conditions and complications affecting the postpartum woman are all covered. Treatment and nursing management are presented for each medical condition. This organization allows the student to build on a solid foundation of normal material when studying the at-risk content.

Unit 8: The Newborn at Risk

Unit 8 continues to center on at-risk content. Issues of the newborn with birthweight variations, gestational age variations, congenital conditions, and acquired disorders are explored. Treatment and nursing management are presented for each medical condition. This organization helps cement the student's understanding of the material.

Unit 9: Health Promotion of the Growing Child and Family

Unit 9 provides information related to growth and development expectations of the well child from newborn through adolescence. Although not exhaustive in nature, this unit provides a broad knowledge base related to normal growth and development that the nurse can draw on in any situation. Common concerns related to growth and development and client/family education are included in each age-specific chapter.

Unit 10: Children and Their Families

Unit 10 covers broad concepts that provide the foundation for providing nursing care for children. Rather than reiterating all aspects of nursing care, the unit focuses on specific details needed to provide nursing care for children in general. The content remains focused upon differences in caring for children compared with adults. Topics covered in this unit include atraumatic care, anticipatory guidance and routine well child care (including immunization and safety), health assessment, nursing care of the child in diverse settings, including the hospital and at home, concerns common to special needs children, pediatric variations in medication and intravenous fluid delivery and nutritional support, and pain management in children.

Unit 11: Nursing Care of the Child With a Health Disorder

Unit 11 focuses on children's responses to health disorders. This unit provides comprehensive coverage of illnesses affecting children and is presented according to broad topics of disorders organized with a body systems approach. It also includes infectious, genetic, and mental health disorders as well as pediatric emergencies. Each chapter follows a similar format in order to facilitate presentation of the information as well as reduce repetition. The chapters begin with a nursing process overview for the particular broad topic, presenting differences in children and how the nursing process applies. The approach provides a general framework for addressing disorders within the chapter. Individual disorders are then addressed with attention to specifics related to pathophysiology, nursing assessment, nursing management, and special considerations. Common pediatric disorders are covered in greater depth than less common disorders. The format of the chapters allows for the building of a strong knowledge base and encourages critical thinking. Additionally, the format is nursing process driven and consistent from chapter to chapter, providing a practical and sensible presentation of the information.

Recurring Features

In order to provide the instructor and student with an exciting and user-friendly text, a number of recurring features have been developed.

Key Terms

A list of terms that are considered essential to the chapter's understanding is presented at the beginning of each chapter. Each key term appears in boldface, with the definition included in the text. Key terms may also be accessed on thePoint.

Learning Objectives

Learning Objectives included at the beginning of each chapter guide the student in understanding what is important and why, leading the student to prioritize information for learning. These valuable learning tools also provide opportunities for self-testing or instructor evaluation of student knowledge and ability.

Words of Wisdom

Each chapter opens with inspiring Words of Wisdom (WOW), which offer helpful, timely, or interesting thoughts. These WOW statements set the stage for each chapter and give the student valuable insight into nursing care of women, children, and their families.

Threaded Case Studies

Real-life scenarios present relevant woman, child, and family information that are intended to perfect the student's caregiving skills. Questions about the scenario provide an opportunity for the student to critically evaluate the appropriate course of action.

Evidence-Based Practice

The consistent promotion of evidence-based practice is a key feature of the text. Throughout the chapters, pivotal questions addressed by current research have been incorporated into Evidence-Based Practice displays, which cite studies relevant to chapter content.

Healthy People 2020

Throughout the textbook, relevant *Healthy People 2020* objectives are outlined in box format. The nursing implications or guidance provided in the box serve as a roadmap for improving the health of women, mothers, and children.

Atraumatic Care

These highlights, located throughout the pediatric sections of the book, provide tips for providing atraumatic care to children in particular situations in relation to the topic being discussed.

Thinking About Development

The content featured in these boxes in chapters related to the care of children will encourage student to think critically about special developmental concerns relating to the topic being discussed.

Teaching Guidelines

An important tool for achieving health promotion and disease prevention is health education. Throughout the textbook, Teaching Guidelines raise awareness, provide timely and accurate information, and are designed to ensure the student's preparation for educating women, children, and their families about various issues.

Consider This!

In every chapter the student is asked to *Consider This!* These first-person narratives engage the student in real-life scenarios experienced by their clients. The personal accounts evoke empathy and help the student to perfect caregiving skills. Each box ends with an opportunity for further contemplation, encouraging the student to think critically about the scenario.

Take Note!

The *Take Note!* feature draws the student's attention to points of critical emphasis throughout the chapter. This feature is often used to stress life-threatening or otherwise vitally important information.

Drug Guides

Drug guide tables summarize information about commonly used medications. The actions, indications, and significant nursing implications presented assist the student in providing optimum care to women, children, and their families.

Common Laboratory and Diagnostic Tests

The Common Laboratory and Diagnostic Tests tables in many of the chapters provide the student with a general understanding of how a broad range of disorders is diagnosed. Rather than reading the information repeatedly throughout the narrative, the student is then able to refer to the table as needed.

Common Medical Treatments

The Common Medical Treatments tables in many of the nursing management chapters provide the student with a broad awareness of how a common group of disorders is treated either medically or surgically. The tables serve as a reference point for common medical treatments.

Nursing Care Plans

Nursing Care Plans provide concrete examples of each step of the nursing process and are included in numerous chapters. The Nursing Care Plans summarize issue- or system-related content, thereby minimizing repetition.

Comparison Charts

These charts compare two or more disorders or other easily confused concepts. They serve to provide an explanation that clarifies the concepts for the student.

Nursing Procedures

Step-by-step Nursing Procedures are presented in a clear, concise format to facilitate competent performance of relevant procedures as well as to clarify pediatric variations when appropriate.

Icons

 WATCH AND LEARN

A special icon throughout the book directs students to free video clips locate on thePoint that highlight growth and development, communicating with children, and providing nursing care to the child in the hospital.

 CONCEPTS IN ACTION ANIMATIONS

These unique animations, also located on thePoint bring physiologic and pathophysiologic concepts to life and enhance student comprehension.

Tables, Boxes, Illustrations, and Photographs

Abundant tables and boxes summarize key content throughout the book. Additionally, beautiful illustrations and photographs help the student to visualize the content. These features allow the student to quickly and easily access information.

Key Concepts

At the end of each chapter, Key Concepts provide a quick review of essential chapter elements. These bulleted lists help the student focus on the important aspects of the chapter.

References and helpful Websites

References used in the development of the text are provided at the end of each chapter. These listings enable the student to further explore topics of interest. Many online resources are provided on thePoint as a means for the student to electronically explore relevant content material. These resources can be shared with women, children, and their families to enhance patient education and support.

Chapter Worksheets

Chapter worksheets at the end of each chapter assist the student in reviewing essential concepts. Chapter worksheets include:

- **Multiple Choice Questions**—These review questions are written to test the student's ability to apply chapter material. Questions cover maternal-newborn, women's health, and pediatric content that the student might encounter on the national licensing exam (NCLEX®).
- **Critical Thinking Exercises**—These exercises challenge the student to incorporate new knowledge with previously learned concepts and reach a satisfactory conclusion. They encourage the student to think critically, problem solve, and consider his or her own perspective on given topics.
- **Study Activities**—These interactive activities promote student participation in the learning process. This section encourages increased interaction/learning via clinical, on-line, and community activities.

Teaching–Learning Package

Instructor's Resources

Tools to assist you with teaching your course are available upon adoption of this text on thePoint.

- An **E-Book** on thePoint gives you access to the book's full text and images online.
- A **Test Generator** that features hundreds of questions within a powerful tool to help the instructor create quizzes and tests.
- **PowerPoint presentations** with **Guided Lecture Notes** provide an easy way for you to integrate the textbook with our students' class-room experience, either via slide shows or handouts. Multiple choice and true/false questions are integrated into the presentations to promote class participation and allow you to use i-clicker technology.
- An **Image Bank** lets you use the photographs and illustrations from this textbook in your PowerPoint slides or as you see fit in your course.
- **Case Studies** with related questions (and suggested answers) give students an opportunity to apply their knowledge to a client case similar to one they might encounter in practice.
- **Pre-Lecture Quizzes** (and answers) are quick, knowledge-based assessments that allow you to check students' reading.
- **Discussion Topics** (and suggested answers) can be used as conversation starters or in online discussion boards.
- **Assignments** (and suggested answers) include group, written, clinical, and web assignments.
- Sample **Syllabi** provide guidance for structuring your pediatric nursing courses and are provided for four different course lengths: 4, 6, 8, and 10 weeks.
- **Journal Articles**, updated for the new edition, offer access to current research available in Lippincott Williams & Wilkins journals.

Contact your sales representative or check out LWW.com/Nursing for more details and ordering information.

Student Resources

An exciting set of free resources is available to help students review material and become even more familiar with vital concepts. Students can access all these resources on thePoint using the codes printed in the front of their textbooks.

- **NCLEX-Style Review Questions** for each chapter help students review important concepts and practice for NCLEX. **Over 700 questions** are included, more than twice as many as last edition!
- **Multimedia Resources** appeal to a variety of learning styles. Icons in the text direct readers to relevant videos and animations:
  - **Watch and Learn Videos** highlight growth and development, communicating with children, and providing nursing care to the child in the hospital.
  - **Concepts in Action Animations** bring physiologic and pathophysiologic concepts to life and enhance student comprehension.
- A **Spanish–English Audio Glossary** provides helpful terms and phrases for communicating with patients who speak Spanish.
- **Journal Articles** offer access to current research available in Lippincott Williams & Wilkins journals.

Contents in Brief

Contents

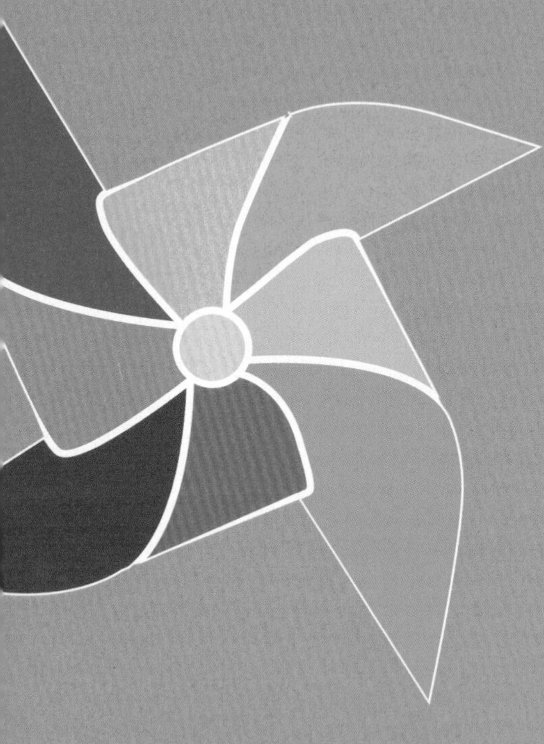

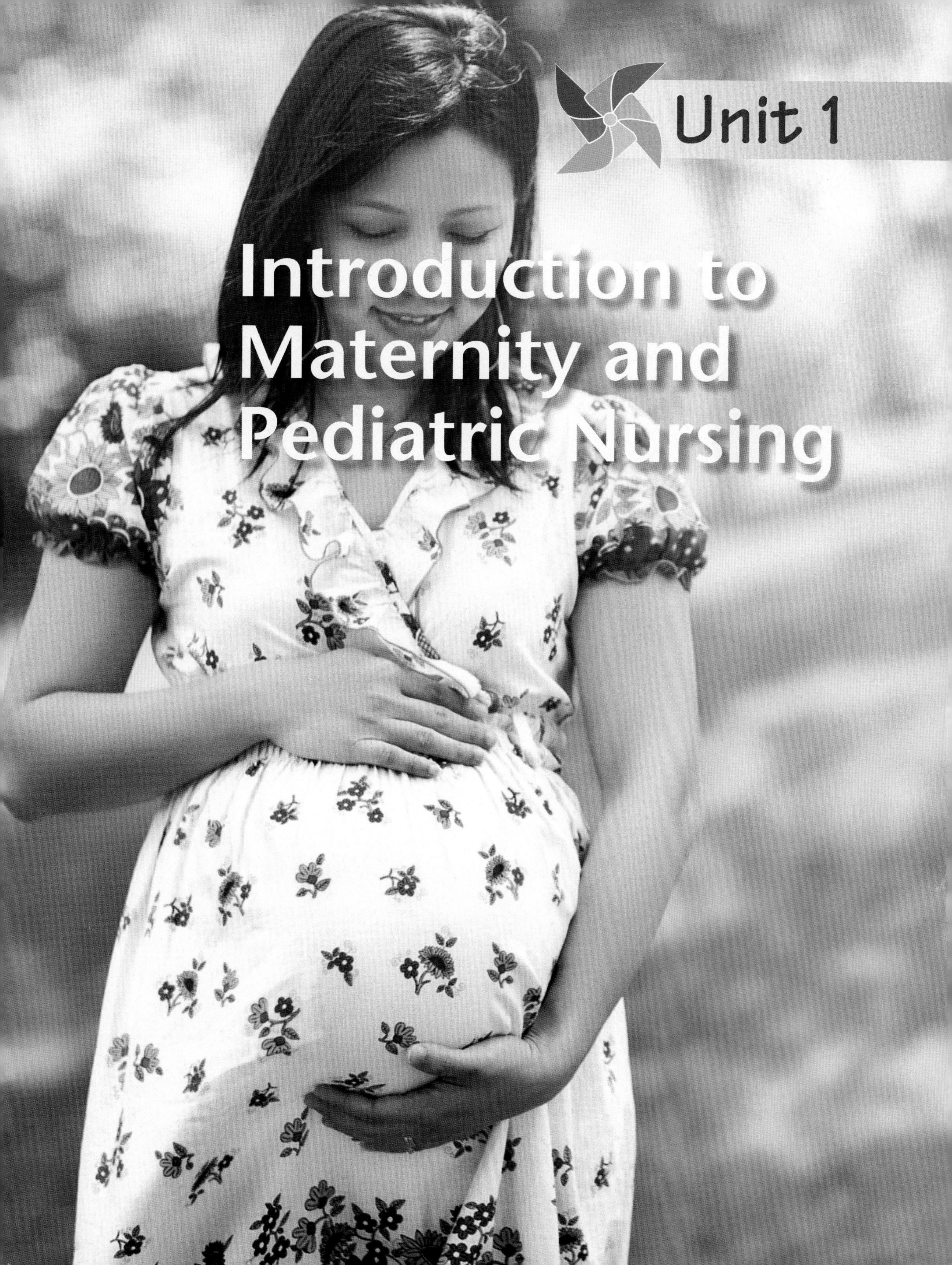

Unit 1

Introduction to Maternity and Pediatric Nursing

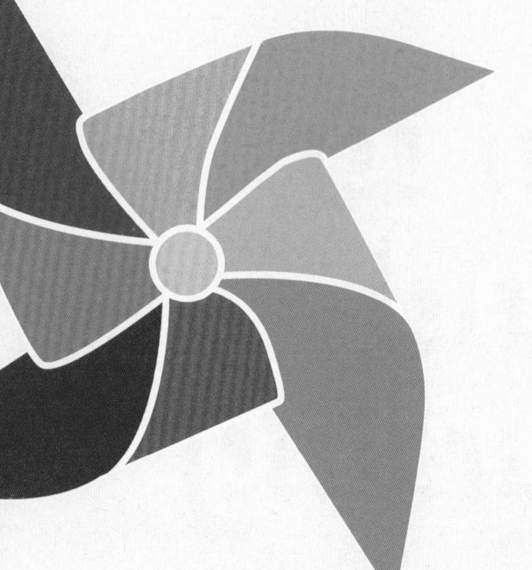

1

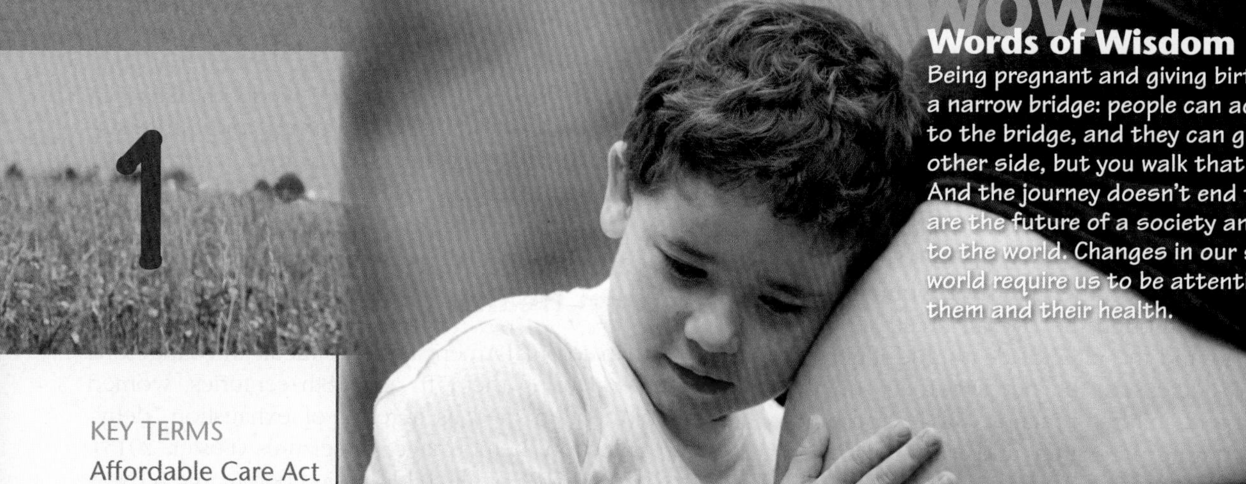
WOW
Words of Wisdom
Being pregnant and giving birth is like crossing a narrow bridge: people can accompany you to the bridge, and they can greet you on the other side, but you walk that bridge alone. And the journey doesn't end there: children are the future of a society and special gifts to the world. Changes in our society and world require us to be attentive to and value them and their health.

KEY TERMS

Affordable Care Act (ACA)
assent
certified nurse midwife (CNM)
child abuse and neglect
childhood mortality rate
cultural competence
discipline
dissent
do not attempt resuscitate (DNAR) orders
doula
emancipated minor
enculturation
ethnocentrism
family structure
fetal mortality rate
foster care
infant mortality rate
maternal–fetal conflict
maternal mortality ratio
mature minor
morbidity
neonatal mortality rate
punishment
resilience
stem cells

Perspectives on Maternal and Child Health Care

Learning Objectives

Upon completion of the chapter, you will be able to:

1. Analyze the key milestones in the history of maternal, newborn, and child health and health care.
2. Outline the evolution of maternal, newborn, and pediatric nursing.
3. Compare the past definitions of health and illness to the current definitions, as well as the measurements used to assess health and illness in children.
4. Assess the factors that affect maternal and child health.
5. Differentiate the structures, roles, and functions of the family and how they affect the health of women and children.
6. Evaluate how society and culture can influence the health of women, children, and families.
7. Appraise the health care barriers affecting women, children, and families.
8. Research the ethical and legal issues that may arise when caring for women, children, and families.

***Sophia Greenly*, a 38-year-old woman pregnant with her third child, comes to the prenatal clinic for a routine follow-up visit. Her mother, Betty, accompanies her because Sophia's husband is out of town. Sophia lives with her husband and two children, ages 4 and 9. She works part-time as a lunch aide in the local elementary school. What factors may play a role in influencing the health of Sophia and her family?**

INTRODUCTION

A person's ability to lead a fulfilling life and to participate fully in society depends largely on his or her health status. This is especially true for women, who commonly are responsible for not only their own health, but also that of others: their children and families. Thus, it is important to concentrate on the health of women, children, and families. Although the overall health of children has improved and the rates of death and illness in some areas have decreased, the need to focus on the health of women and children remains. Habits and practices established during pregnancy and early childhood can have profound effects on a person's health and illness throughout life. As a society, creating a population that cares about women, children, and families and promotes solid health care and lifestyle choices is crucial.

Maternity care is an integrated care process, which consists of different services (prenatal, intranatal, and postnatal), involves different professionals, and covers extended time frames. Maternal and newborn nursing encompasses a wide scope of practice typically associated with childbearing. It includes care of the woman before pregnancy, care of the woman and her fetus during pregnancy, care of the woman after pregnancy, and care of the newborn, usually during the first 6 weeks after birth. The overall goal of maternal and newborn nursing is to promote and maintain optimal health of the woman and her family. Providing quality maternity care includes client satisfaction and achieving best evidence-based outcomes with the fewest interventions. Child health nursing, commonly referred to as pediatric nursing, involves the care of the child from infancy through adolescence. In the United States, the number of children under age 18 years is approximately 73.6 million, accounting for 23.1% of the population (Federal Interagency Forum on Child and Family Statistics [FIFCFS], 2013). The overall goal of pediatric nursing practice is to promote and assist the child in maintaining optimal levels of health, while recognizing the influence of the family on the child's well-being. This goal involves health promotion and disease and injury prevention as well as assisting with care during illness. The common thread in both of these is the care of the family.

This chapter presents a general overview of the health care of women, children, and families and describes the major factors affecting maternal and child health. Nurses need to be knowledgeable about these concepts and factors to ensure that they provide professional care.

HISTORICAL DEVELOPMENT

The health care of women and children has changed over the years due in part to changes in childbirth methods, devastating epidemics, social trends in our country, changes in the health care system, and federal and state regulations. By reviewing historical events, nurses can gain a better understanding of the current and future status of maternal and child health and how maternal and pediatric nursing care has evolved.

The History of Maternal and Newborn Health and Health Care

Childbirth in colonial America was a difficult and dangerous experience. During the 17th and 18th centuries, women giving birth often died as a result of exhaustion, dehydration, infection, hemorrhage, or seizures (Foster, 2015). Approximately 50% of all children died before age 5 (Norman, 2015), compared with the 0.06% **infant mortality rate** of today (Central Intelligence Agency, 2015).

There was a time when nearly every infant that came into this world was attended by a midwife. Centuries ago, "granny midwives" handled the normal birthing process for most women. They learned their skills through an apprenticeship with a more experienced midwife. Physicians usually were called only in extremely difficult cases, and all births took place at home. The rise of obstetrics in the 1800s drove midwifery to the periphery, but within the last century, midwifery has reemerged as an organized profession, appearing everywhere from home births to hospital labor units. Women who labored and gave birth at home were traditionally attended to by relatives and midwives. Having continuous support during childbirth yields better outcomes (see Evidence-Based Practice 1.1).

During the early 1900s, physicians attended about half the births in the United States. Midwives often cared for women who could not afford a doctor. Many women were attracted to hospitals because this showed affluence and they provided pain management, which was not available in home births. In the 1950s, "natural childbirth" practices advocating birth without medication and focusing on relaxation techniques were introduced. These techniques opened the door to childbirth education classes and helped bring the father back into the picture. Both partners could participate by taking an active role in pregnancy, childbirth, and parenting (Fig. 1.1).

Box 1.1 shows a time line of childbirth in America. In many ways, childbirth practices in the United States have come full circle, as we see the return of nurse midwives and **doulas**. Today, childbirth choices are often based on what works best for the mother, child, and family.

The History of Child Health and Child Health Care

In past centuries in the United States, the health of the country was poorer than it is today; mortality rates were high and life expectancy was short. Infectious diseases

EVIDENCE-BASED PRACTICE 1.1 CONTINUOUS SUPPORT FOR WOMEN DURING CHILDBIRTH

STUDY

Throughout history, women have been helping other women in labor by providing emotional support, comfort measures, information, and advocacy. However, in recent years this practice has waned, and facilities frequently adhere to strict specific routines that may leave women feeling "dehumanized." A study was done to assess the effects on mothers and their newborns of continuous, one-to-one intrapartum care in comparison to usual care. The study also evaluated routine practices and policies in the birth environment that might affect a woman's autonomy, freedom of movement, and ability to cope with labor; who the caregiver was, whether or not a staff member of the facility; and when the support began, early or late in labor.

All published and unpublished randomized clinical trials (23) comparing continuous support during labor with usual care were examined involving 15,000 women. One author and one research assistant used standard methods for data collection and analysis and extracted the data independently. Clinical trial authors provided additional information. The researchers used relative risk for categorical data and weighted mean difference for continuous data.

Findings

Women receiving continuous intrapartum support had a greater chance of a spontaneous vaginal delivery (including without forceps or vacuum extraction). They also had a slight decrease in the length of labor and required less analgesia during this time. These women also reported increased satisfaction with their labor and childbirth experience. Overall, the support, when provided by someone other than a facility staff member and initiated early in labor, proved to be more effective.

Nursing Implications

Based on this research, it is clear that women in labor benefit from one-to-one support during labor. Nurses can use the information gained from this study to educate women about the importance of support persons during labor and delivery. Nurses can also act as client advocates in facilities where they work to foster an environment that encourages the use of support persons during the intrapartum period. The focus of nursing needs to be individualized, supportive, and collaborative with the family during their childbearing experience. In short, nurses should place the needs of the mother and her family first in providing a continuum of care.

Although the study found that support is more effective when provided by someone other than a staff member, support from an individual is essential. Assigning the same nurse to provide care to the couple throughout the birthing experience also fosters a one-to-one relationship that helps meet the couple's needs and promotes feelings of security. By meeting the couple's needs, the nurse is enhancing their birthing experience.

Hodnett, E. D., Gates, S., Hofmeyr, G. J., & Sakala, C. (2013). Continuous support for women during childbirth. *Cochrane Database of Systematic Reviews, 7*:CD003766.

were rampant, and unsanitary food sources contributed to illness in children. Devastating epidemics of smallpox, diphtheria, scarlet fever, and measles hit children the hardest. During this period, the prevalent view was that children were a commodity; their role was to increase the population and share in the work to be done. This view changed over the years. Public schools were established and the court system began viewing children as minors. The health of children began to receive more and more attention.

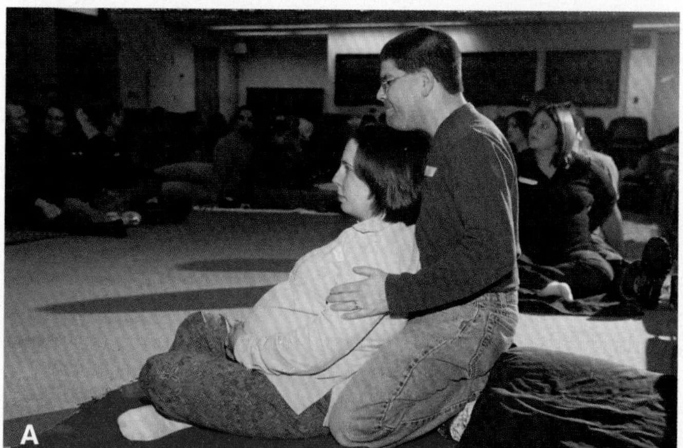

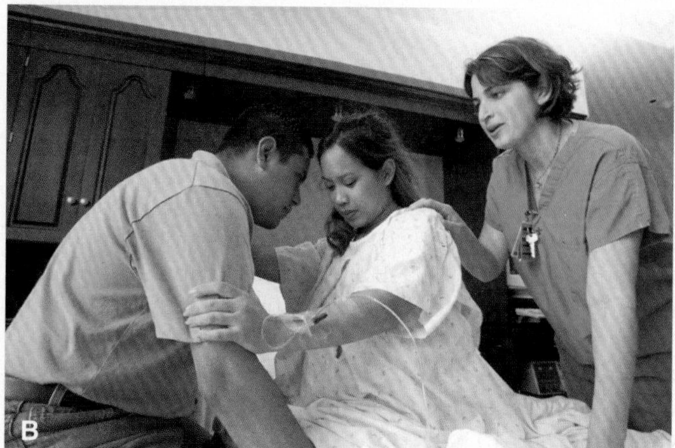

FIGURE 1.1 Today fathers and partners are welcome to take an active role in the pregnancy and childbirth experience. **A.** A couple can participate together in childbirth education classes. (Photo by Gus Freedman.) **B.** Fathers and partners can assist the woman throughout her labor and delivery. (Photo by Joe Mitchell.)

BOX 1.1

CHILDBIRTH IN AMERICA: A TIME LINE

1700s Men did not attend births because it was considered indecent.
Women faced birth not with joy and ecstasy but with fear of death.
Female midwives attended the majority of all births at home.

1800s There is a shift from using midwives to doctors among middle-class women.
The word *obstetrician* was formed from the Latin, meaning "to stand before."
Puerperal (childbed) fever was occurring in epidemic proportions.
Louis Pasteur demonstrated that streptococci were the major cause of puerperal fever that was killing mothers after delivery.
The first cesarean section was performed in Boston in 1894.
The x-ray was developed in 1895 and was used to assess pelvic size for birthing purposes.

1900s Twilight sleep (a heavy dose of narcotics and amnesiacs) was used on women during childbirth in the United States.
The United States was 17th out of 20 nations in infant mortality rates.
Of all women, 50–75% gave birth in hospitals by 1940.
Nurseries were started because mothers could not care for their baby for several days after receiving chloroform gas.
Dr. Grantley Dick-Reed (1933) wrote *Childbirth Without Fear,* which reduced the "fear–tension–pain" cycle women experienced during labor and birth.
Dr. Fernand Lamaze (1984) wrote *Painless Childbirth: The Lamaze Method,* which advocated distraction and relaxation techniques to minimize the perception of pain.
Amniocentesis was first performed to assess fetal growth in 1966.
In the 1970s the cesarean section rate was about 5%. In 2011 it rose to 32%, where it stands currently.
The 1970s and 1980s see a growing trend to return birthing back to the basics—nonmedicated, nonintervening childbirth.
In the late 1900s, freestanding birthing centers—LDRPs—were designed, and the number of home births began to increase.

2000s One in three women undergoes a surgical birth (cesarean).
CNMs once again assist couples at home, in hospitals, or in freestanding facilities with natural childbirths. Research shows that midwives are the safest birth attendants for most women, with lower infant mortality and maternal rates, and fewer invasive interventions such as episiotomies and cesareans.
Childbirth classes of every flavor abound in most communities.
According to the latest available data, the United States ranks 48th in the world in maternal deaths. The maternal mortality ratio is approximately 28 in 100,000 live births.
According to the latest available data, the United States ranks 55th in the world (compared to 224 other countries) in infant mortality rates. The infant mortality rate is approximately 6.17 in 1,000 live births.

Adapted from CIA World Factbook. (2015). *Country comparison: Infant mortality rate.* Retrieved from https://www.cia.gov/library/publications/the-world-factbook/rankorder/2091rank.html; World Bank. (2015c). *Maternal mortality ratio per 100,000 live births.* Retrieved from http://data.worldbank.org/indicator/SH.STA.MMRT; and Cox, K. J., & King, T. L. (2015). Preventing primary cesarean births: Midwifery care. *Clinical Obstetrics and Gynecology, 58*(2), 282–293.

As the end of the 19th century neared, doctors and scientists gained a better understanding of the root causes of illness. This knowledge helped fuel public health efforts such as the campaign for safe milk supply, which lead to pasteurizing milk and to dispensing free milk in some cities (U.S. Department of Health and Human Services [USDHHS], n. d.). Compulsory vaccination programs began during this time. In the late 1800s some states mandated smallpox vaccination as a condition of school attendance. These public health efforts led to a decrease in infant and child deaths (USDHHS, n. d.).

In the late 19th and early 20th centuries, cities became healthier places to live due to urban public health improvements such as sanitation services, treated municipal water, and improvements in hygiene (USDHHS, n. d.). Diseases such as diphtheria, cholera, polio, and yellow fever began to take less of a toll on children (USDHHS, n. d.). The turn of the 20th century brought new knowledge about nutrition, sanitation, bacteriology, pharmacology, medication, and psychology. Penicillin, corticosteroids, and increased numbers of vaccines, which were developed during this time, assisted with the fight against communicable diseases. Thus, by the end of the 20th century, unintentional injuries surpassed disease as the leading cause of death for children greater than 1-year old (Epstein, 2011).

Technologic advances have significantly affected all aspects of health care and led to increased survival rates in children. However, many children who survive illnesses that were previously considered fatal are left with chronic disabilities. For example, before the 1960s, extremely premature infants did not survive because of the immaturity of their lungs. Mechanical ventilation and the use of medications to foster lung development have increased survival rates in premature infants, but survivors are often faced with a myriad of chronic illnesses such as chronic lung disease (bronchopulmonary dysplasia), retinopathy of prematurity, cerebral palsy, or developmental delay. This increased survival has resulted in a significant increase in chronic illness relative to acute illness as a cause of hospitalization and mortality (Kelly, 2010).

In recent years advances in biomedicine have created a trend toward earlier diagnosis and treatment of disorders and diseases. Additionally, genetics have been linked with pathophysiologic processes. For example, female fetuses diagnosed with congenital adrenal hyperplasia, a genetic disorder resulting in a steroid enzyme deficiency leading to disfiguring anatomic abnormalities of sexual characteristics, are able to receive treatment before birth (Mayo Clinic Staff, 2015). In addition, early genetic defect identification allows for appropriate counseling.

In addition to improvement in technology and biomedicine, a number of national and international organizations have been formed in recent years to protect children's rights both in the United States and worldwide. These organizations focus on such issues as violence and abuse, child labor and soldiering, juvenile justice, child immigrants and orphaned children, and abandonment and homelessness—all of which have a negative impact on children's health. A child whose rights are restored and upheld has an improved opportunity for growth, development, education, and health.

The gains in child health have been huge but, unfortunately, these gains are not shared equally among all children. Certain health concerns such as asthma, obesity, poor nutrition, environmental toxin exposure, and learning or behavioral disorders affect poor children at higher rates than affluent and middle-class children (Seith & Isakson, 2011). Unintentional injuries continue to be the leading cause of death in children greater than 1 year, but children's health remains threatened by illnesses and other health-related conditions in the 21st century (Centers for Disease Control and Prevention [CDC]/National Center for Health Statistics [NCHS], 2015). Obesity, environmental toxins, allergies, drug abuse, child abuse and neglect, and mental health problems are among some of the key issues that endanger children's health today.

Evolution of Maternal and Newborn Nursing

The history of maternity nursing is characterized by innovations that became common practice in later years. These innovations include fetal monitoring, mother/baby care, and early postpartum discharge. The driving forces behind changes in care within the social context of the times were scientific/medical developments and families' desires for the best possible childbearing experience.

Prior to World War II, American women moved from home to the hospital for childbirth in part because they were convinced that setting would improve birth outcomes. Hospitals were the major employers of maternity nurses. Early ambulation and rooming-in induced changes in the focus of care for the growing numbers of mothers and infants. Maternity nurses' focus shifted away from carrying out tasks and performing procedures to teaching mothers about self and infant care. Improved staffing patterns within hospitals meant longer hospital stays for the mothers, which allowed maternity nurses to spend more time with mothers for teaching purposes. Maternity nursing has changed dramatically since the Baby Boom era. The natural childbirth movement became a catalyst to bring about a change in nursing practice on the postpartum nursing units.

Other innovations that came later included breastfeeding and rooming-in to facilitate maternal–newborn bonding. Maternity nurses were then able to help the new mothers learn better how to care for their infants, to promote breast-feeding and bonding. The mid-1960s and early 1970s ushered in a consumer revolt which brought back home births, prepared childbirth, birth centers, the father's/partner's involvement in the birthing process, and nurse midwives—which had all but disappeared from the American health system (Stapleton & Rooks, 2015). Maternal–infant bonding became recognized as an essential part of postnatal care, and maternity nurses took a lead role to facilitate it.

With innovations becoming commonplace, maternity nursing practice has become more complex. How maternity nurses approach present-day challenges of increasing technology of birth, looming threats of litigation, and providing care under time and economic restraints is continuing to evolve.

A **certified nurse midwife (CNM)** has postgraduate training in the care of normal pregnancy and delivery and is certified by the American College of Nurse Midwives (ACNM). Midwives are primary care providers for women with a special emphasis on pregnancy, childbirth, and reproductive health. They are committed to providing ethical, individualized, evidence-based care for all women throughout their life cycle (American College of Nurse-Midwives, 2015).

A **doula** is a nonmedical birth companion who provides continuous emotional, physical, and educational support to the woman and family during childbirth and the postpartum period. Doulas do not perform clinical or medical tasks; they are there to comfort and support the mother and to enhance communication between the mother and medical professionals (DONA International, n. d.). Many nurses working in labor and birth areas today are credentialed in their specialty so that they can provide optimal care to the woman and her newborn.

Evolution of Pediatric Nursing

In 1870, the first pediatric professorship for a physician was awarded in the United States to Abraham Jacobi, known as the father of pediatrics. For the first time, the medical community realized the need to provide specialized training and education about children to health care providers. In the early 1900s, Lillian Wald established the Henry Street Settlement House in New York City; this was the start of public health nursing. This facility provided medical and other services to poor families. These services included home nurse visits to teach mothers about health care.

During this time, health care personnel were trained to take care of children in hospitals, but parents of hospitalized children were discouraged from visiting to prevent the spread of infection. Restricting parents from being involved in their child's care was also thought to minimize emotional stress.

Nursing in public schools began in 1902 with the appointment of Lina Rogers as a full-time public school nurse in New York. A professional course in pediatric nursing was started in the early 1900s at Teachers' College of Columbia University.

In the 1960s, changes in the health care delivery system and shifts in the population's health status led to the development of the nurse practitioner role. Loretta Ford was the founder of the first nurse practitioner program. The 1970s brought cost-control systems from the federal government because of rapid escalation of health care expenditures. In addition, the considerable changes in the U.S. health care system in the 1980s have affected pediatric nursing and child health care. The emphasis of care was on quality outcomes and cost containment. Some of these changes brought more advanced practice nurses into the field of pediatrics.

In the 1980s, the Division of Maternal–Child Health Nursing Practice of the American Nurses Association developed maternal–child health standards to provide important guidelines for delivering nursing care.

In the 1990s the Health and Medicine Division published reports pointing out the need to improve quality and safety of the American health care system. This led to an increased focus on improving health care outcomes. As the health care environment continued to increase in complexity and patients hospitalized got sicker, programs were created for nurses to obtain a level of expertise and validate mastery of their skills and knowledge by passing a national standardized examination. Registered nurses and nurse practitioners can be certified in their specialty, such as pediatrics. These certifications show a commitment to lifelong learning and the ability to stay up to date in the rapidly changing health care environment. In recent years, pediatric nursing certifications have become increasingly specialized, such as a certified pediatric hematology/oncology nurse or a certified pediatric emergency nurse.

HEALTH STATUS OF WOMEN AND CHILDREN

At one time, health was defined simply as the absence of disease. Health was measured by monitoring the mortality and morbidity of a group. Over the past century, however, the focus on health has shifted to disease prevention, health promotion, and wellness. The World Health Organization (WHO) (2015b) defines health as "a state of complete physical, mental, and social well-being, and not merely the absence of disease or infirmity." The definition of health is complex. It is not merely the absence of disease or an analysis of mortality and morbidity statistics.

In 1979, the US Surgeon General's Report, *Healthy People,* presented an agenda for the nation that identified the most significant preventable threats to health. With the series of updates that followed, including the present one, *Healthy People 2020,* the United States has a comprehensive health promotion and disease prevention agenda that is working toward improving the quantity and quality of life for all Americans (USDHHS, 2015). Overarching goals are to eliminate preventable disease, disability, injury, and premature death; achieve health equity, eliminate disparities, and improve the health of all groups; create physical and social environments that promote good health; and promote healthy development and behaviors across every stage of life (USDHHS, 2015). The principle behind this report is that setting national objectives and monitoring their progress can motivate action and change. In developing the health objectives, the report incorporates input from public health and prevention experts; federal, state, and local governments; over 2,000 organizations; and the public.

There are specific health topic areas, including women and children's health topics, which serve as a method for evaluation of progress made in public health. These topic areas also serve as focal points to coordinate the national health improvement efforts. For example, one objective under the physical activity topic is to increase the proportion of adolescents who meet current federal physical activity guidelines for aerobic physical activity and for muscle-strengthening activity (USDHHS, 2015). *Healthy People 2020* monitors four foundation health measures to assess the progress toward promoting health, preventing disease and disability, eliminating disparities, and improving quality of life (USDHHS, 2015). (See the *Healthy People 2020* feature for additional information on these health measures.)

Measuring health status is not always a simple process. For example, some women and children with

HEALTHY PEOPLE 2020

Four Foundation Health Measures

1. General Health Status
   - Measures include:
     - Life expectancy
     - Healthy life expectancy
     - Years of potential life lost
     - Physically and mentally unhealthy days
     - Self-assessed health status
     - Limitation of activity
     - Chronic disease prevalence
2. Health-Related Quality of Life and Well-Being
   - Measures include:
     - Physical, mental, and social health-related quality of life
     - Well-being/satisfaction
     - Participation in common activities
3. Determinants of Health (a range of personal, social, economic, and environmental factors that influence health status)
   - Include:
     - Biology
     - Genetics
     - Individual behavior
     - Access to health services
     - The environment in which people are born, live, learn, play, work, and age
4. Disparities
   - Measures include differences in health status based on:
     - Race/ethnicity
     - Gender
     - Physical and mental ability
     - Geography

U.S. Department of Health & Human Services, 2015.

chronic illnesses do not see themselves as "ill" if their disease is under control. A traditional method of measuring health is to examine mortality and morbidity data. This information is collected and analyzed to provide an objective description of the nation's health.

Mortality

Mortality is the incidence or number of people who have died over a specific period. This statistic is presented as rates per 100,000 and is calculated from a sample of death certificates. The National Center for Health Statistics, under the DHHS, collects, analyzes, and disseminates the data on America's mortality rates.

Maternal Mortality

The **maternal mortality ratio** is the annual number of deaths from any cause related to or aggravated by pregnancy or its management (excluding accidental or incidental causes) during pregnancy and childbirth or within 42 days of termination of pregnancy, irrespective of the duration and site of the pregnancy, per 100,000 live births, for a specified year. In the United States, approximately 700 to 800 women die each year during pregnancy or shortly after childbirth. The rate of maternal mortality in the United States has more than doubled in the past few decades. A significant proportion of these deaths are preventable (Maron, 2015).

In the United States, the maternal mortality ratio is mixed depending on ethnic background. African American women suffer maternal mortality ratios far higher than any other ethnic group. The risk of maternal mortality has remained about three to four times higher among Black women when compared to White women during the past six decades. About 42.8 of 100,000 African American mothers die due to childbirth, as compared to much lower rates in Whites (12.5) and Hispanics (8.9) (CDC, 2015f). The federal government has pledged to improve maternal–child care outcomes and thus reduce mortality ratios for women and children by endorsing the *Healthy People 2020,* but the WHO (2015c) data show that the United States ranks 48th in the world for maternal mortality. In fact, maternal mortality ratios are higher than almost all European countries, as well as several countries in Asia and the Middle East. For a country that spends more than any other country on health care and more on childbirth-related care than any other area of hospitalization, US $88 billion a year, this is a shockingly poor return on investment (Lu et al., 2015).

During the past several decades, mortality and morbidity have dramatically decreased as a result of an increased emphasis on hygiene, good nutrition, exercise, and prenatal care for all women. However, women are still experiencing complications at significant rates. The United States is one of the most medically and technologically advanced nations and has the highest per capita spending on health care in the world, but our current mortality rates indicate the need for improvement. For example:

- Approximately 700 to 800 women die each year in the United States as a result of pregnancy or a childbirth complication (CDC, 2015a).
- The United States ranks 48th (in other words, below 47 other countries) in rates of maternal deaths (deaths per 100,000 live births; WHO, 2015a).
- Most pregnancy-related complications are preventable. The leading causes of pregnancy-related mortality are hemorrhage, infection, preeclampsia–eclampsia, obstructed labor, and unsafe abortion (CDC, 2015e).

The maternal mortality and morbidity rates for African American women have been three to four times higher than for Whites (USDHHS, 2015). This major racial disparity has persisted for more than 60 years. Black women have at least double the risk of pregnancy-related death compared with White women. This striking difference in the pregnancy-related mortality ratio is the largest disparity in the area of maternal and child health. Researchers do not entirely understand what accounts for this disparity, but some suspected causes of the higher maternal mortality rates for minority women include low socioeconomic status, limited or no insurance coverage, bias among health care providers (which may foster distrust), and quality of care available in the community. Language and legal barriers may also explain why some immigrant women do not receive good prenatal care. Lack of care during pregnancy is a major factor contributing to a poor outcome. Prenatal care is well known to prevent complications of pregnancy and to support the birth of healthy infants, but not all women receive the same quality and quantity of health care during pregnancy. Pregnancy-related mortality is on the rise in the United States. The *Healthy People 2020* goal for maternal deaths is 11.4 per 100,000 live births (USDHHS, 2015). Black women had higher degrees of hypertension and lower hemoglobin levels on admission and had presented for prenatal care much later, on average, than White women or not at all (Stallings, 2015).

The CDC (2015f) has noted that the disparity in maternal mortality rates between women of color and White women represents one of the largest racial disparities among public health indicators. Eliminating racial and ethnic disparities in maternal–child health care requires enhanced efforts at preventing disease, promoting health, and delivering appropriate and timely care. The CDC has called for more research and monitoring to understand and address racial disparities, along with increased funding for prenatal and postpartum care. Research is needed to identify causes and to design initiatives to reduce these disparities, and the CDC is calling on Congress to expand programs to provide preconception and prenatal care to underserved women.

Fetal Mortality

The **fetal mortality rate** or fetal death rate refers to the spontaneous intrauterine death of a fetus at any time during pregnancy per 1,000 live births. Fetal deaths later in pregnancy (>20 weeks of gestation) are also referred to as stillbirths. Fetal mortality may be attributable to maternal factors (e.g., malnutrition, disease, or preterm cervical dilation) or fetal factors (e.g., chromosomal abnormalities or poor placental attachment).

Fetal mortality is a major, but often overlooked, public health problem. Fetal mortality refers to spontaneous intrauterine death at any time during pregnancy. The fetal mortality rate in the United States is 6.2 per 1,000 live births (CDC, 2015c). *Healthy People 2020's* goal is to reduce it to 5.6 fetal deaths (USDHHS, 2015). Much of the public concern regarding reproductive loss has concentrated on infant mortality, as less is known about fetal mortality. However, the impact of fetal mortality on United States families is considerable, as it provides an overall picture of the quality of maternal health and prenatal care.

Neonatal and Infant Mortality

The **neonatal mortality rate** is the number of infant deaths occurring in the first 28 days of life per 1,000 live births. The United States now ranks 41st in the world in terms of neonatal mortality, the death rate of infants less than 1-month old. The neonatal mortality rate is 4.5 per 1000 live births (World Bank, 2015c). *Healthy People 2020's* goal is to reduce it to 4.1 per 1000 live births (USDHHS, 2015). Each year the deaths of 2 million babies are linked to complications during birth or within the first month. Furthermore, the burden is inequitably carried by the poor. Evidence-based strategies are urgently needed to reduce the burden of intrapartum-related deaths and effective interventions to address these problems must be incorporated into policy decisions (Oza et al., 2015). The reliability of the neonatal mortality estimates depends on accuracy and completeness of reporting and recording of births and deaths. Underreporting and misclassification are common, especially for deaths occurring early on in life.

Perinatal mortality encompasses late and early neonatal mortality and is defined as the number of stillbirths and deaths in the first week of life per 1,000 live births; it is also a useful indicator. The perinatal mortality is the sum of the fetal mortality and the neonatal mortality. Work is ongoing to improve estimates of stillbirth rates, a major component of perinatal mortality (WHO, 2015c).

The infant mortality rate is the number of deaths occurring in the first 12 months of life (Fig. 1.2). It

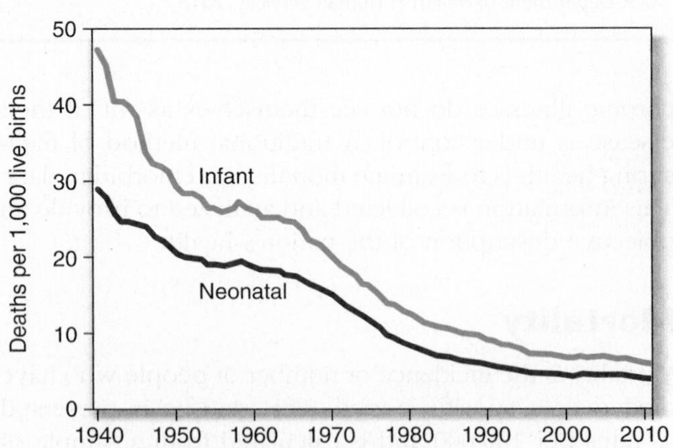

FIGURE 1.2 Infant and neonatal mortality from 1940 to 2011. (Adapted from Kochanek, K. D., Sherry, L., Murphy, S. L., & Xu, J. Q. (2015). Deaths: Final data for 2011. *National Vital Statistics Reports, 63*(3). Hyattsville, MD: National Center for Health Statistics. Retrieved from http://www.cdc.gov/nchs/data/nvsr/nvsr63/nvsr63_03.pdf.)

also is documented as the number of deaths of infants younger than 1 year of age per 1,000 live births. Neonatal mortality and post neonatal mortality (covering the remaining 11 months of the first year of life) are reflected in the infant mortality rate. The infant mortality rate is used as an index of the general health of a country. Generally, this statistic is one of the most significant measures of children's health. The current infant mortality in the United States is 6.17 per 1000 live births (World Bank, 2015b).

The infant mortality rate varies greatly from state to state as well as between ethnic groups. The United States has one of the highest gross national products in the world and is known for its technologic capabilities, but its infant mortality rate is much higher, in some cases double, than most other developed nations (Gissler, 2015). In 2014, the United States ranked 28th in infant mortality rates among industrialized nations (MacDorman et al., 2014). The main causes of early infant death in the United States include problems occurring at birth or shortly thereafter, such as prematurity, low birthweight, congenital and chromosomal anomalies, sudden infant death syndrome (SIDS), respiratory distress syndrome, unintentional injuries, bacterial sepsis, and necrotizing enterocolitis (Osterman et al., 2015).

Take Note!

Non-Hispanic, African American infants have consistently had higher infant mortality rates than other ethnic groups (Bediako, BeLue, & Hillemeier, 2015).

Congenital anomalies remain the leading cause of infant mortality in the United States (Egbe et al., 2015). In addition, low birthweight and prematurity are major indicators of infant health and significant predictors of infant mortality (Griffin et al., 2015). The lower the birthweight, the higher the risk of infant mortality. The percentage of infants born preterm in the United States is increasing, thus the impact of preterm-related causes of infant death has increased. Therefore, the high incidence of low birthweight (<2,500 g) in the United States is a significant reason why its infant mortality rate is higher than that of many other countries (March of Dimes, 2014).

After birth, other health promotion strategies can significantly improve an infant's health and chances of survival. Breast-feeding has been shown to reduce rates of infection in infants and to improve their long-term health. Human milk also reduces the risk for allergic and autoimmune diseases, and the risk of obesity and its complications (Wilson et al., 2016). Emphasizing the importance of placing an infant on his or her back to sleep will reduce the incidence of SIDS. In addition, parents/partners should not share a bed with an infant younger than 12 weeks old and should avoid exposing the infant to tobacco smoke (Adams, Ward, & Garcia, 2015). Encouraging mothers to join support groups to prevent postpartum depression and learn sound child-rearing practices will improve the health of both mothers and their infants.

Childhood Mortality

The **childhood mortality rate** is the number of deaths per 100,000 population in children 1 to 14 years of age. The childhood mortality rate in the United States has decreased significantly since 1980 but disparities by gender, age, race, and ethnicity persist (Child Trends DataBank, 2015a). The current mortality rate for children between ages 1 and 4 years is 25.5 per 100,000, with the leading cause of death being unintentional injuries followed by congenital malformations (CDC/NCHS, 2015). The mortality rate for children of ages 5 to 14 years is 13 per 100,000, with the leading cause being unintentional injuries followed by cancer (CDC/NCHS, 2015). Other causes of childhood mortality include suicide, homicide, diseases of the heart, influenza, and pneumonia.

Even as research continues into the preventable nature of childhood injuries, unintentional injury (e.g., motor vehicle accidents, fires, drowning, bicycle or pedestrian accidents, poisoning, falls) remains a leading cause of mortality and morbidity in children. These injuries have far-reaching consequences for children, families, and society in general. Risk factors associated with childhood injuries include young age, male gender, low socioeconomic status, parents who are unmarried or single, low maternal education level, poor housing, parental drug or alcohol abuse, and low support within the family. These deaths can often be prevented through education about the value of using car seats and seat belts, the dangers of driving under the influence of alcohol and other substances, and the importance of pedestrian and bicycle safety, fire safety, water safety, and home safety.

Take Note!

In the United States, American Indian/Alaska Natives children, followed by African American children, have the highest unintentional injury death rate (Gilchrist, Ballesteros, & Parker, 2012).

Morbidity

Morbidity is the measure of the prevalence of a specific illness in a population at a particular time. It is presented in rates per 1,000 population. Morbidity is often difficult to define and record because the definitions used vary widely. For example, morbidity may be defined as visits to the physician or diagnosis for hospital admission. Also, data may be difficult to obtain. Morbidity statistics are revised less frequently because of the difficulty in defining or obtaining the information.

Women's Health Indicators

Women today face not only diseases of genetic origin but also diseases that arise from poor personal habits. Even though women represent 51% of the population, only recently have researchers and the medical community focused on their special health needs. The USDHHS adopted the Health and Medicine Division's recommendations that eight preventive services for women be included in the defined list of preventive care services provided without cost sharing under the **Affordable Care Act (ACA)** because they give women access to comprehensive preventive services to achieve health and wellness. Unfortunately, many women are unaware about what is covered, and thus don't take advantage of them. The National Women's Law Center (NWLC) has developed resources on well women visits to ensure that women are able to understand and access the preventive services now available to them under the ACA (Waxman & Johnson, 2015). A recent significant study identified an urgent need to improve women's access to health insurance and health care services, place a stronger emphasis on prevention, and invest in more research on women's health (National Women's Law Center, 2010). It identified 26 indicators of women's access to health care services, measuring the degree to which women receive preventive health care and engage in health-promoting activities (Box 1.2). The report card gave the nation an overall grade of "unsatisfactory," and not a single state received a grade of "satisfactory." In the 2010 National Report Card, the nation met three benchmarks since 2007: colorectal cancer screening, annual dental visits, and mammograms. However, the nation missed the other 23 benchmarks. Other substandard findings included the following:

- No state has focused enough attention on preventive measures, such as smoking cessation, exercise, nutrition, and screening for diseases.
- Too many women lack health insurance coverage: nationally, nearly one in five women has no health insurance.
- No state has adequately addressed women's health needs in the areas of reproductive health, mental health, and violence against women.
- Limited research has been done on health conditions that primarily affect women and that affect women differently than men (NWLC, 2010).

BOX 1.2

THE NATIONAL INDICATORS OF WOMEN'S HEALTH

- Lung cancer death rate
- Diabetes
- Heart disease death rate
- Binge drinking
- High school completion
- Poverty
- Wage gap
- Rate of AIDS
- Maternal mortality rate
- Rate of *Chlamydia* infection
- Breast cancer death rate
- Heart disease death rate
- Smoking
- Being overweight
- No physical activity during leisure time
- Eating five fruits and vegetables daily
- Colorectal screening
- Mammograms
- Pap smears
- First-trimester prenatal care
- Access to health insurance

Adapted from National Women's Law Center. (2010). *Making the grade on women's health: A national and state by state report card.* Washington, DC: National Women's Law Center.

Cardiovascular disease (CVD) is the number-one cause of death in women, regardless of racial or ethnic group. More women than men die each year from CVD. More than 500,000 women die annually in the United States of CVD—about one death per minute. More than 8.6 million women die from CVD globally each year (World Heart Federation [WHF], 2015). Women who have a heart attack are more likely than men to die. Heart attacks in women are often more difficult to diagnose than in men because of their vague and varied symptoms. Heart disease is still thought of as a "man's disease," and thus a heart attack may not be considered in the differential diagnosis when a woman presents to the emergency room.

Nurses need to look beyond the obvious "crushing chest pain" textbook symptom that heralds a heart attack in men. Risk factors of heart disease differ between men and women in several other ways—for example, menopause (associated with a significant rise in coronary events); diabetes, high cholesterol levels, and left ventricular hypertrophy; and repeated episodes of weight loss and gain (increased coronary morbidity and mortality) (WHF, 2015). Clinical manifestations of a heart attack observed in women include nausea, dizziness, irregular heartbeat, unusual fatigue, sleep disturbances, indigestion, anxiety, shortness of breath, pain or discomfort in one or both arms, and weakness (Brown, 2015). The prevalence, mortality, lack of warning signs in some women, and decreased awareness within this population make it imperative for nurses to assume an active role in assessing these clients, evaluating risk factors, and advocating for prevention of CVD in all women.

Cancer is a major public health problem in the United States and globally. It is the second leading cause of death among women, and is expected to surpass heart disease as the leading cause of death in the next few years (Siegel, Miller, & Jemal, 2015). Women have a one-in-three lifetime risk of developing cancer, and one out of every four deaths is from cancer (American Cancer Society [ACS], 2015a). Although much attention is focused on cancer of the reproductive system, lung cancer is the number-one killer of women. Lung cancer accounts for about 27% of all cancer deaths. More people die of lung cancer than of colon, breast, and prostate cancers combined. Lung cancer is largely the result of smoking and second-hand smoke. Lung cancer has no early symptoms, making early detection almost impossible. Thus, lung cancer has the lowest survival rate of any cancer; more than 90% of people who get lung cancer die of it (ACS, 2015c).

Breast cancer occurs in one in every seven women in a lifetime. It is estimated that in 2015 about 231,840 new cases of invasive breast cancer will be diagnosed among women in the United States. An estimated 40,290 women are expected to die from the disease in 2015 (ACS, 2015b). White women get breast cancer at a higher rate than African American women, but African American women are more likely to get breast cancer before they reach 40, and are more likely to die from it at any age. This is likely because the cancer is more advanced when it is found in African American women, and because survival at every cancer stage is worse among African American women (ACS, 2015b).

Women living in North America have the highest rate of breast cancer in the world. At this time there are about 2.8 million breast cancer survivors in the United States. It is the most common malignancy in women and second only to lung cancer as a cause of cancer mortality in women (ACS, 2015b). Although a positive family history of breast cancer, aging, and irregularities in the menstrual cycle at an early age are major risk factors, other risk factors include excess weight or obesity, not having children, oral contraceptive use, excessive alcohol consumption, a high-fat diet, sedentary lifestyle, and long-term use of hormone therapy after menopause (ACS, 2015b). Breast cancer rates have dropped recently, possibly due to the decreased use of long-term menopausal hormone therapy that occurred after the Women's Health Initiative (WHI) report was released in 2002 and the Million Women Study in 2003 (Kyvernitakis et al., 2015). However, early detection and treatment continue to offer the best chance for a cure, and reducing the risk of cancer by decreasing avoidable risks continues to be the best preventive plan.

Pregnant women are by no means immune to any of the health issues presented thus far. Many women begin a pregnancy with existing health conditions, including hypertension, obesity, CVD, diabetes, inflammatory processes, autoimmune diseases, anemia, asthma, sexually transmitted infections, depression, or cancer. Although the majority of pregnant women are young and fairly healthy, the incidence of certain chronic health issues in them is increasing secondary to the obesity epidemic in the United States (Cancello, 2015).

Women's health is a complex issue, and no single policy is going to change the overall dismal state ratings. Although progress in science and technology has helped reduce the incidence of, and improve the survival rates for, several diseases, women's health issues continue to have an impact on our society. By eliminating or decreasing some of the risk factors and causes for prevalent diseases and illnesses, society and science could minimize certain chronic health problems. Focusing on the causes and effects of particular illnesses could help resolve many women's health issues of today.

Childhood Morbidity

In general, 56% of children in the United States enjoyed excellent health and 27% had very good health as reported in a summary of health statistics for children in 2011 (Bloom, Cohen, & Freeman, 2012). However, obesity, environmental toxins, allergies, drug abuse, child abuse and neglect, and mental health problems are among some of the key issues that endanger children's health today. Factors that may increase morbidity include homelessness, poverty, low birthweight, chronic health disorders, foreign-born adoption, attendance at daycare centers, and barriers to health care. For example, 21.8% of children live in poverty and have a higher incidence of disease, limited coordination of health services, and limited access to health care, except for visits to the emergency department (DeNavas-Walt, Proctor, & Smith, 2013). The overall poverty rate is 15%, which is the highest poverty rate since 1994 (DeNavas-Walt et al., 2013). However the poverty rate among African Americans and Hispanics is 27.2% and 26%, respectively. These children are particularly at increased risk for illness (DeNavas-Walt et al., 2013).

The most important aspect of morbidity is the degree of disability it produces, which is identified in children as the number of days missed from school or confined to bed. In 2011, more than one quarter of schoolchildren, ages 5 to 17, did not miss any school due to illness or injury. However, approximately 5% missed 11 or more days of school because of injury or illness (Bloom et al., 2012).

Common health problems in children include respiratory disorders such as asthma; gastrointestinal disturbances, which lead to malnutrition and dehydration; and injuries. Asthma is the leading chronic disease in children affecting 14% of children in the United States (Bloom et al., 2012). Another 11% of children have respiratory allergies, 9% suffer from hay fever, 6% from food allergies, and 13% from skin allergies (Bloom et al., 2012). Diseases of the respiratory system, such as asthma and pneumonia, were the major cause of hospitalization for children of ages 1 to 9, while mental health disorders are the leading cause for children 10 to 14 years of age (USDHHS, Health Resources and Services

Administration [HRSA], Maternal and Child Health Bureau [MCHB], 2013). In the United States during 2010, there were 3.5 hospital discharges for every 100 children (age 1 to 21 years) (USDHHS, HRSA, MCHB, 2013). Figure 1.3 shows the major causes of hospitalization by age in the United States.

As more immunizations become available, common childhood communicable diseases affect fewer children. The tracking of the leading topics from *Healthy People 2020* provides some positive information related to improving children's health. Improvements have occurred in child health but morbidity and disability from some conditions, such as asthma, diabetes, attention-deficit/hyperactivity disorder, and obesity, have increased in recent decades. Also, disparities in health status among children in the United States according to race and socioeconomic status demonstrate widening social inequalities.

One trend in the United States is the increasing number of children with mental health disorders and related emotional, social, or behavioral problems. The American Academy of Pediatrics (AAP) estimates that one in five children in the United States have mental health–related problems (American Academy of Pediatrics, n. d.; Office of Adolescent Health, 2015). These problems may limit the child's educational success. They also increase the child's risk for significant mental health problems later in life or emotional problems and possible use of firearms, reckless driving, promiscuous sexual activity, and substance abuse during adolescence.

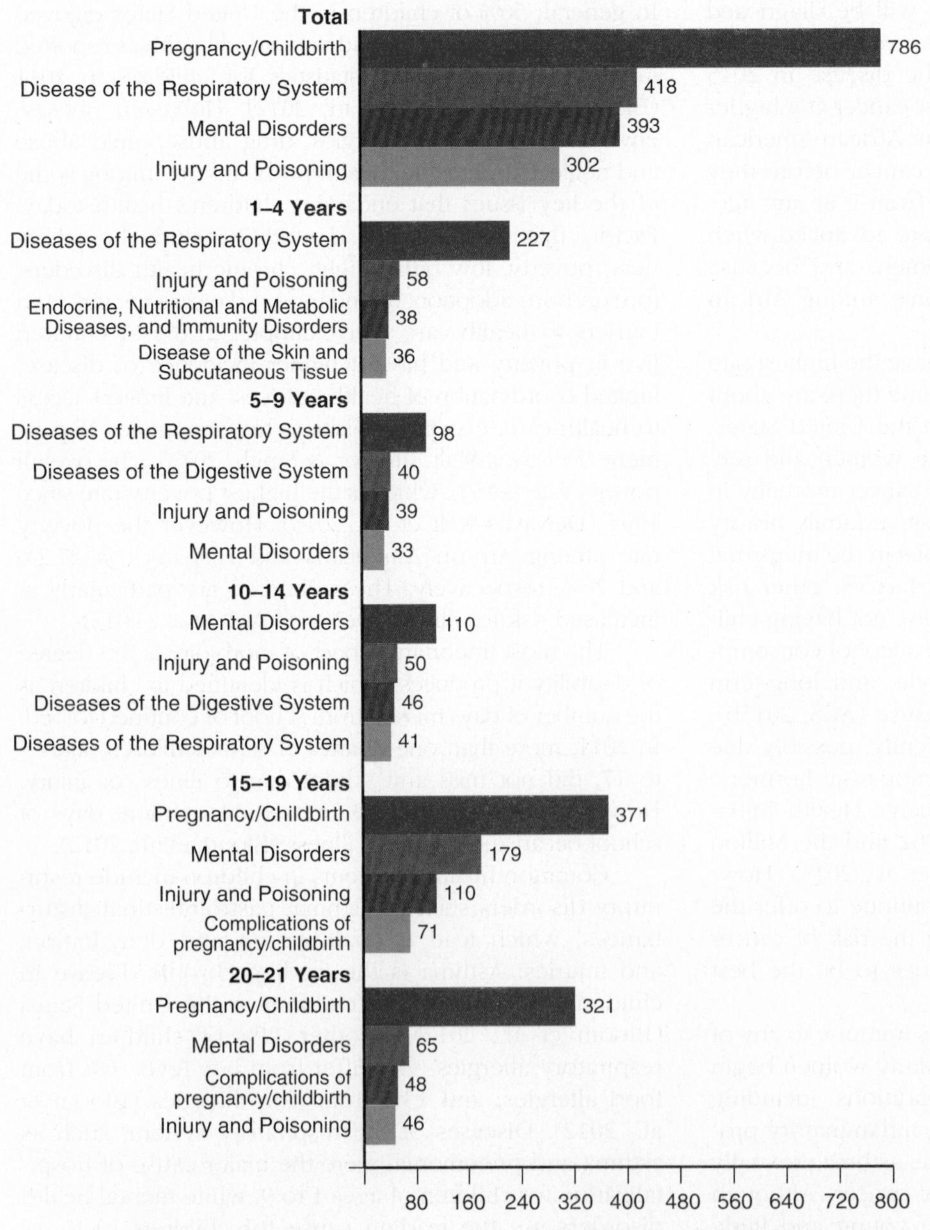

FIGURE 1.3 Causes of hospitalization in children, 2010. (From U.S. Department of Health and Human Services, Health Resources and Services Administration, Maternal and Child Health Bureau. (2013). *Child health USA 2012*. Rockville, MD: U.S. Department of Health and Human Services. Retrieved from http://mchb.hrsa.gov/chusa12/hs/hsc/downloads/img/hHa.gif.)

Overall, these behavioral, social, and educational problems can interfere with children's social and academic development. Often, insurance does not reimburse for these problems, leading to additional concerns such as lack of treatment.

Environmental and psychosocial factors are now an area of concern in children.

These include academic difficulties, complex psychiatric disorders, self-harm and harm to others, use of firearms, hostility at school, substance abuse, HIV/AIDS, and adverse effects of the media.

FACTORS AFFECTING MATERNAL AND CHILD HEALTH

From conception, children are shaped by a myriad of factors, such as genetics and the environment. As members of a family, they are also members of a specific population, community, culture, and society. As they learn and grow, they are affected by multiple, complex, and ever-changing influences around them. For example, dramatic demographic changes in the United States have led to shifts in majority and minority population groups. Globalization has led to an international focus on health. Access to health care and the types of health care available have changed due to modifications in health care delivery and financing. In addition, the United States is still grappling with issues such as immigration, poverty, environmental warming, homelessness, and violence (Alzola & Marino, 2015). The factors affecting maternal and child health discussed in this section include family, genetics, society, culture, health status and lifestyle, access to health care, improvements in diagnosis and treatments, and empowerment of health care consumers.

These factors may affect the person positively, by promoting healthy growth and development, or negatively, by increasing the person's health risks. Nurses, especially those working with women and children, need to understand how these influences affect the quality of nursing care and health outcomes. They must examine the impact of these variables to gain the knowledge and skills needed to plan effective care, thereby achieving the best possible outcomes for women, children, and families.

Family

The family is considered the basic social unit. The U.S. Census Bureau defines a family as a group of two or more persons related by birth, marriage, or adoption and living together (Vespa, Lewis, & Kreider, 2013). Earlier definitions of family emphasize the legal ties or genetic relationships of people living in the same household with specific roles. Given the diversity of families in today's society, however, some believe that family should be defined as whatever the client says it is (Holtzman, 2011; Patterson, 1995) (Fig. 1.4).

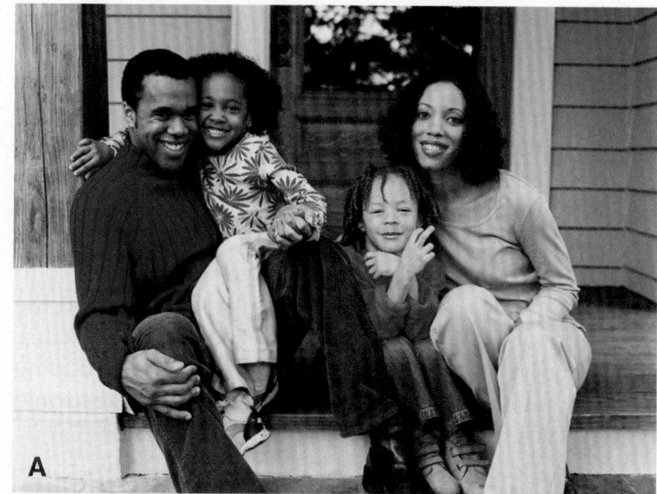

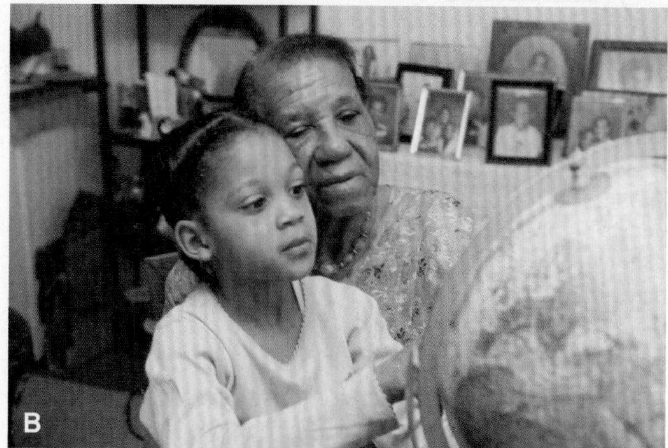

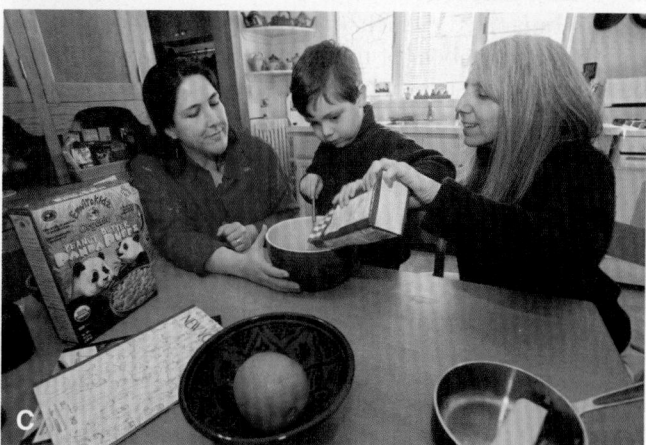

FIGURE 1.4 Nurses must take into account family dynamics when providing health care. There are many different family structures, and they influence the client's needs. **A.** The traditional nuclear family is composed of two parents and their biologic or adopted children. **B.** The extended family includes the nuclear family plus other family members, such as grandparents, aunts, uncles, and cousins. **C.** Gay and lesbian families comprise two people of the same sex sharing a committed relationship with or without children.

The family greatly influences the development and health of its members. For example, children learn health care activities, health beliefs, and health values from their family. The family's structure, the roles assumed by family members, and social changes that affect the family's life can influence the woman's and child's health status. Families are unique; each one has different views and requires distinct methods for support.

Various theories and models have been generated to explain the concept of family. They have influenced the definition of family, the understanding of the structure and function of the family, and the way family coping and adaptation are assessed. Table 1.1 summarizes some of the major theories related to family.

Take Note!

The lifestyle of the parents basically is the lifestyle of the children. For instance, parents who are inactive and eat poorly will have children who do the same, and the problems associated with these unhealthy habits, such as diabetes, obesity, and early heart disease, are showing up earlier in children and adolescents. It is important for parents to serve as role models for proper nutrition and physical activity (through sports, hobbies, or other activities).

Family Structure

Family structure is the composition of people who interact with one another on a regular, recurring basis in socially sanctioned ways. It involves how the family unit is organized, which often influences the relationship of the members of the family. Family members can be gained or lost through events such as divorce, marriage, birth, death, abandonment, and incarceration. All of these events can alter the family structure, leading to roles being redefined or redistributed. Table 1.2 provides examples of the types of family structures found in today's society.

The traditional nuclear family is no longer considered the dominant family structure. From 1980 to 2012, the percentage of children who were living with their own married parents decreased steadily from 77% to 64% (FIFCFS, 2013). By understanding clients' family structure and any changes that may occur, nurses can provide them with support to alleviate or prevent dysfunctional alterations in family coping and adaptation.

Families today face complex challenges as they try to nurture, develop, and socialize their members. Family structure changes such as divorce, blending families, adoption, or **foster care** can have wide-ranging and lifelong effects. These special situations require astute assessment and proactive intervention to minimize the risk to the family.

DIVORCED FAMILY

Divorce is a common reason why the family structure changes. Today, over 40% of marriages end in divorce and many of these marriages include children (Serwint, 2011). Divorce can have a great impact on the child, with chronic and devastating results. Typically, divorce is not a single event. Changes have most likely been occurring in the family for years, and children may have been exposed to turmoil, violence, or changes in structure before the actual divorce. Children feel scared and confused by the threat divorce poses on their security. The initial response of children to divorce depends on their age; problems are most apparent the year after the divorce and diminish over the next couple of years (Kim, 2011). However, regardless of family type, children whose parents had a hostile interparental relationship during the marriage tended to have poorer emotional well-being than children whose parents had a nonhostile relationship (Baxter, Weston, & Lixia, 2011).

Parents need to understand the impact that divorce can have on their children so that they can place the children's interests in the forefront. The loss of a parent through divorce can leave children vulnerable to physical and mental illnesses (American Academy of Child and Adolescent Psychiatry [AACAP], 2012a). However, by appropriately utilizing family strengths and providing care and attention, children can be helped to deal constructively with divorce (AACAP, 2012a). Parents can use the rules in Box 1.3 to help reduce tension and conflict, thereby minimizing the impact of separation and divorce on their children. Health care providers can offer support, guidance, and resources to help make the strain of divorce easier on the entire family.

SINGLE-PARENT FAMILIES

Single-parent families can result from divorce or separation, death of a spouse, an unmarried woman raising her own child, or adoption by an unmarried man or woman. In 2014 approximately 64% of children under age 18 live with two married parents, with 24% living in mother-only households and 4% living with the father only (Child Trends Databank, 2015b). In addition, one in three children born in the United States is to a single mother (Bembry, 2011).

Single-parent families have several concerns that can affect the health of the children. Life in a single-parent household can be stressful for both the adult and the children. The single parent may feel overwhelmed with no one to share the day-to-day responsibilities of juggling the care of the children, maintaining a job, and keeping up with the home and finances. These issues may be compounded by other pressures, such as custody problems, decreased time available to spend with

TABLE 1.1 SUMMARY OF MAJOR THEORIES RELATED TO FAMILY

Theory	Description	Key Components
Friedman's structural functional theory	Emphasizes the social system of family, such as the organization or structure of the family and how the structure relates to the function	Identified five functions of families: • Affective function: meeting the love and belonging needs of each member • Socialization and social placement function: teaching children how to function and assume adult roles in society • Reproductive role: continuing the family and society in general • Economic function: ensuring the family has necessary resources with appropriate allocation • Health care function: involving the provision of physical care to keep family healthy
Duvall's developmental theory	Emphasizes the developmental stages that all families go through, beginning with marriage; the longitudinal career of the family is also known as the family life cycle	Described eight chronologic stages with specific predictable tasks that each family completes: • Marriage: beginning of family • Childbearing stage • Family with preschool children • Family with school-age children • Family with adolescents • Family with young adults • Middle-age parents • Family in later years
Von Bertalanffy: general system theory applied to families	Emphasizes the family as a system with interdependent, interacting parts that endure over time to ensure the survival, continuity, and growth of its components; the family is not the sum of its parts but is characterized by wholeness and unity	Used to define how families interact with and are influenced by the members of their family and society and how to analyze the interrelationships of the members and the impact that change affecting one member will have on other members
Family stress theory	Addresses the way families respond to stress and how the family copes with the stress as a group and how each individual member copes	Described elements of stress as occurring internally within the family (e.g., values, beliefs, structure) that the family can control or change or externally from outside the family (e.g., culture of the surrounding community, genetics, the family's current time or place) over which the family has no control Mobilization of family resources resulting in either a positive response of constructive coping or negative response of a crisis Identified the main determinant of adequate coping based on the meaning of the stressful event to the family and its individual members
Resiliency model of family stress and family adjustment, and adaptation response model	Addresses the way families adapt to stress and can rebound from adversity	Identified the elements of risks and protective factors that aid a family in achieving positive outcomes

Adapted from Friedman, M. M. (1998). *Family nursing: Theory and practice* (4th ed.). Stanford, CT: Appleton & Lange; Duvall, E. (1997). *Marriage and family development* (5th ed.). Philadelphia, PA: J. B. Lippincott; Von Bertalanffy, L. (1968). *General systems theory*. London: Penguin Press; Boss, P. (2001). *Family stress management*. Newbury Park, CA: Sage; and Patterson, J. (2002). Integrating family resilience and family stress theory. *Journal of Marriage and Family, 64*(2), 349–360.

TABLE 1.2 TYPES OF FAMILY STRUCTURES

Structure	Description	Specific Issues
Nuclear family	Husband, wife, and children living in same household	May include natural or adopted children Once considered the traditional family structure; now decreased due to trends in divorce rates or other social situations such as nonmarital childbearing
Binuclear family	Child who is member of two families due to joint custody; parenting is considered a joint venture	Always works better when the interests of the child are put above the parents' needs and desires
Single-parent family	One parent responsible for care of children	May result from death, divorce, desertion, birth outside marriage, or adoption Likely to encounter several challenges because of economic, social, and personal restraints; one person as homemaker, caregiver, and financial provider
Commuter family	Adults in the family living and working apart for professional or financial reasons, often leaving the daily care of children to one parent	Similar to single-parent family, but without as much economic challenge
Step or blended family	Adults with children from previous marriages or from the new marriage	May lead to family conflict due to different expectations for the child and adults; may have different views and practices related to child care and health
Extended family	Nuclear family and grandparents, cousins, aunts, and uncles	Need to determine decision maker as well as primary caretaker of the children May be encouraged and supported by some cultures, such as Hispanic and Asian cultures
Same-sex family (also called homosexual or gay/lesbian family)	Adults of the same sex living together with or without children	May face prejudice against those with different lifestyles
Communal family	Group of people living together to raise children and manage household; unrelated by blood or marriage	May face prejudice against those with different lifestyles Need to determine the decision maker and caretaker of children
Foster family	A temporary family for children who are placed away from their parents to ensure their emotional and physical well-being	May include foster family's children and other foster children in the home Foster children are more likely to have unmet health needs and chronic health problems because they may have been living in a variety of settings (AAP, 2000)
Grandparents-as-parents families	Grandparents raising their grandchildren if parents are unable to do so	May increase the risk for physical, financial, and emotional stress on older adults May lead to confusion and emotional stress for child if biologic parents are in and out of the child's life
Adolescent families	Young parents still mastering the developmental tasks of their own childhood	Teenage girls have greater risk for health problems during pregnancy and delivery of premature infants, leading to risk of subsequent health and developmental problems Probably still need support from their family related to financial, emotional, and school issues

BOX 1.3

RULES FOR DIVORCING PARENTS

1. Tell your children about the divorce and the reasons for the divorce in terms that they can understand. Be sure that you and your spouse are present together when telling the children; tell all the children at the same time.
2. Reassure your children that the divorce is not their fault. Repeat this as often as possible and as necessary.
3. Inform the children well in advance of anyone moving out of the house (except when abuse is present or there are concerns for immediate safety).
4. Clearly inform the children about the family structure after the divorce, such as who will live with whom and where; also discuss visitation clearly and honestly.
5. Do not make your children be or act like adults. Seek support from other adults in your life.
6. Do not discuss money or finances with your children.
7. Minimize unpredictable schedules and maintain routines, rules, and discipline, and be consistent in this area.
8. Never force or allow your children to take sides.
9. Avoid belittling your former spouse when the children can hear. However, do not lie to cover up for irresponsible behavior by the other parent.
10. Never put your children in the middle between you and your ex-spouse.
11. Keep each parent involved in the child's life. Write letters, emails, phone calls, and text messages to continue communication. This shows the child they remain important to you even when they are with the other parent.
12. Communicate directly with the other parent. Avoid making the child your messenger.

Adapted from New, M. (2011). *Helping your child through divorce.* KidsHealth for Parents. Retrieved from http://kidshealth.org/parent/positive/talk/help_child_divorce.html#; and Kemp, G., Smith, M., & Segal, J. (2015). Children and divorce. Retrieved from http://www.helpguide.org/articles/family-divorce/children-and-divorce.htm.

children, continuing conflicts between parents who are separated or divorced, or changes in relationships with extended family members.

Communication and support are essential to the optimal functioning of the single-parent family. The parent and children need to be able to express their feelings and work through the problems together. Single parents must provide greater support for their children. Even though a single parent may feel alone they need to ensure they treat their children as children and not a substitute for a partner. Support and comfort needs to come from outside resources. Community resources can be helpful. Parents Without Partners, for instance, is an international organization that has over 200 chapters in the United States and Canada. Links to these organizations' websites can be found under Web Resources on thePoint.

BLENDED FAMILIES

Before the age of 15, one third of children in the United States are anticipated to live in a stepfamily (Pew Research Center, 2011). Creating a blended family (parents and their stepchildren), even though considered a form of "normal" these days, can be stressful for the parents and children alike. Although it creates a structure and stability and reduces some of the financial stresses of single parenthood, making the transition to a blended family takes time. Children may feel jealous of the stepparent or feel disloyal toward the previous biologic parent. There may be competition or rivalry among the stepchildren. The child may fear that the stepparent is interfering with the child's relationship with the parent or taking away his or her source of love, affection, and attention.

Mutual respect and open, honest communication among all individuals involved are key, and this should include the previous biologic parent when possible. Responsibilities for parenting must be shared, including decisions about expectations, limits, and discipline. The continued role of the previous biologic parent and the role of the stepparent in the child's life are important to address.

ADOPTED FAMILIES

Adoption can occur domestically (through an agency or intermediary such as an attorney in the family's own area or country), or the family may choose to adopt a child from another country. The child may be of a different culture, race, or ethnicity (Fig. 1.5). Most children in need of adoption in the United States and overseas are not infants. In recent years there has been

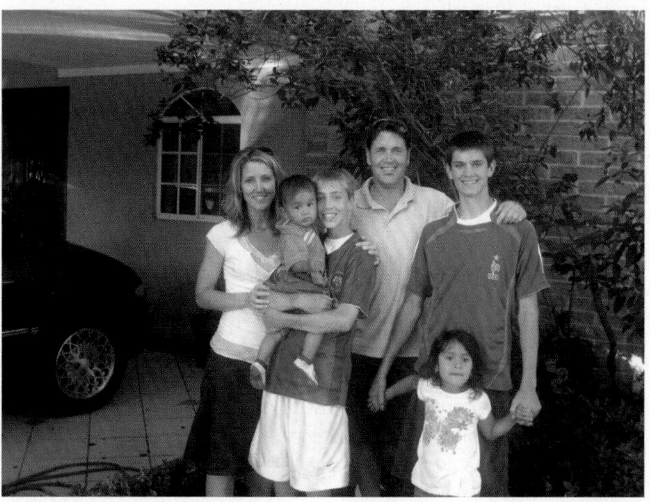

FIGURE 1.5 An adoptive family with children from a different culture.

an increasing number of children adopted from the US child welfare systems and internationally (Simms & Wilson, 2011).

The amount of contact between the child and the birth mother can vary greatly. In a closed adoption there is no contact between the adoptive parents, the adopted child, and the birth mother. In an open adoption there is as much contact among the individuals as desired. Regardless of the method used to adopt a child, adoptive families may be faced with unique issues. Some adopted children have complex medical, developmental, behavioral, educational, and psychological issues (Faver & Alanis, 2012). They may have been exposed to poverty, neglect, infectious diseases, and lack of adequate food, clothing, shelter, and nurturing, placing them at risk for medical problems, physical growth and development delays or abnormalities, and behavioral, cognitive, and emotional problems. The adoptive parents may know about these problems, but in other situations little if any history may be available.

Differences in culture, ethnicity, or race can further influence the adopted child's sense of identity (Faver & Alanis, 2012). Children may be subjected to racism or bigotry. Extended family members may not accept the child as part of the family. Parents need to emphasize that the adopted child is their child and is as much a part of the family as any other member. Parents need to openly recognize racial differences that exist between them and their child. Parents should encourage and assist the child to learn about their heritage, culture, and ethnic group (Jones et al., 2012). Adopted adolescents and adults may feel a need to identify their biologic parents. Children adopted from other countries may travel to the country of their birth, and children adopted domestically may search for biologic relatives. Although this search is an indicator of healthy emotional growth, it can upset the adoptive parents, who may feel rejected.

As the adopted child grows older, he or she may feel the loss of a birth family or may question what he or she did that led to the birth parents' decision to proceed with adoption. Attachment to the adoptive family is important. In order to attach in future relationships children must appropriately grieve past losses. This can be particularly complex and difficult for older children and children previously living in foster care or orphanages.

Take Note!

Adolescents face vast challenges adjusting to adoption at this age because of the added complexity of identity issues facing this age group (Jones et al., 2012).

Clear, open, honest communication and discussion are essential to promote a healthy, strong relationship. Support, guidance, and open communication are key for all parties involved. Open acknowledgment of the adoptive relationship helps to nurture trust, security, and a child's self-esteem as he or she learns to understand what it means to be part of a family through adoption (Jones et al., 2012).

The pediatric nurse needs to be sensitive, understanding, and supportive when interacting with adopted children and their families. "Positive" adoption language should be used. This includes saying "birth parent" when referring to biologic parents instead of "natural" or "real parent" and just parents when talking about adoptive parents (Jones et al., 2012). Also, do not refer to the child as their "adopted child" or other children as "natural child" (Jones et al., 2012). When discussing adoption using terms such as "make an adoption plan" instead of "give away" or "give up for adoption" are preferred (Jones et al., 2012). The nurse also needs to provide reassurance and understanding regarding missing health information and provide appropriate resources and referrals to resources that are knowledgeable about adoption and sensitive to the issues that may arise. Sources of information and support available are the Center for Adoption Support and Education and the North American Council on Adoptable Children, links to which are provided on thePoint.

FOSTER CARE FAMILY

Foster care is a situation in which a child is cared for in an alternative living situation apart from his or her parents or legal guardians. The child may be placed in this living situation due to difficulties in the family situation, such as abuse, neglect, abandonment, or the parents' inability to meet the child's needs, due to illness, substance abuse, or death. The child may be sent to live with relatives (kinship care) or foster parents, who are strangers providing protection and shelter in a state-approved foster home.

There are about 397,122 children in the United States currently living in some form of foster care (U.S. Department of Health and Human Services, Administration for Children & Families, Administration on Children, Youth and Families, Children's Bureau [USDHHS, ACF, ACYF, CB], 2013a). Since 2002 there has been a steady decline in children in foster care (USDHHS, ACF, ACYF, CB, 2013b). The goal of foster care is to provide temporary services until the child can return home to his or her family or be adopted. Unfortunately, children may remain in foster care for several years or longer and may be moved from one foster family to another.

Many children who are placed in foster care have been the victims of abuse or neglect. Children in foster care are more likely to exhibit a wide range of medical, emotional, behavioral, dental, educational, or developmental problems (Bernedo et al., 2012).

However, children are very resilient and most children in foster care are determined to live their lives, but they may struggle with certain issues, including the following:

- Unmet health care needs
- Significant mental health problems, such as depression, social problems, anxiety, and posttraumatic stress disorder due to trauma, loss, and unpredictability
- Behavioral problems such as substance use, problems with the law, and self-destructive behaviors
- Interruptions in developmental stages and developmental delay
- Educational obstacles due to frequent moves and educational difficulties
- Self-blame and feelings of guilt
- Feelings of being unwanted
- Feelings of helplessness and powerlessness
- Insecurity about the future
- Ambivalent feelings related to foster parents; feelings of being disloyal to birth parents (Zlotnick, Tam, & Soman, 2012)

Individual attention to the child in foster care is essential. A multidisciplinary approach to care that includes the birth parents, foster parents, child, health care professionals, and support services is important to meet the child's needs for growth and development. Nurses play a key role in advocating for the child.

Family Roles and Functions

Regardless of the structure of the family, the role of the family in caring for the child includes not only providing physical and emotional care but also imparting the rules and expected behaviors of society through teaching and discipline techniques. These expected behaviors depend on the culture, values, and beliefs of the family and the child's developmental stage and physical and cognitive abilities. Roles and functions are further defined by each family's own traditions and values and the family's set of standards for interaction within and outside the family. For instance, some families may value privacy more than others. These family members may tend to be more self-protective and secretive.

CAREGIVER–CHILD INTERACTION

The caregiver–child interaction is critical to the survival and healthy development of a young child (WHO, 2012; Xu, 2011). Typically, the primary caregivers are the parents. Ideally, parents nurture their children and provide them with an environment in which they can become competent, productive, self-directed members of society. For young children in particular, growth, health, and their very personhood itself depend on the ability of the adults in their life to understand and respond to them (Groark & McCall, 2011; WHO, 2012).

PARENTAL ROLES

Parenting is an enormous responsibility and takes a lot of time as well as physical and mental energy. Parental roles are vast and numerous. Typical parental roles include nurturer/caregiver, financial provider, decision maker, schedule manager, financial manager, problem solver, counselor, teacher, behavior support and manager, and health manager.

CHANGES IN PARENTAL ROLES OVER TIME

Parental roles evolve due to societal and economic changes as well as individual family changes. Traditionally, the role of provider was assigned to the father. However, with increased numbers of women in the workplace and more households with two parents working, today both parents are often the providers as well as the nurturers to the children. Technologic innovations have provided parents with opportunities to work at home, allowing some parents to maintain the provider role while simultaneously fulfilling the nurturer and health manager roles. Fathers are taking on greater responsibilities related to household management and child care. Also, the number of children being raised by their grandparents is increasing (AACAP, 2012b). Moreover, as baby boomers age, parents may find themselves caring for both their children and their aging parents.

Recall Sophia, the pregnant woman described at the beginning of the chapter. Identify the parental roles Sophia would assume. How might these roles be different from those of her mother when she was Sophia's age?

PARENTING STYLES

Beginning in the 1960s with Baumrind, a psychologist, and further research in the 1980s by Maccoby and Martin were the basis of the development of four major parenting styles seen in our society: authoritarian, authoritative, permissive, and uninvolved or rejecting-neglecting (as cited in Cherry, 2015). The styles are defined by the amount of support and control exerted over the child during parenting. Many parents may use more than one parenting style and may fall somewhere in between styles instead of adhering strictly to one style. Also some parents may change parenting styles as the child ages and matures. Whatever the style, sensitive and responsive caregiving is needed to promote appropriate physical, neurophysiologic, and psychological development (Beers, 2011). Nurses need to recognize different parenting styles and provide support to parents by discussing the effects of different parenting models and teaching parenting skills.

AUTHORITARIAN

The *authoritarian* parent expects obedience from the child and discourages the child from questioning the family's rules. The parent provides low support and high control over the child (Cherry, 2015). The rules and standards set forth by the parents are strictly enforced and firm. The parents expect the child to accept the family's beliefs and values and demand respect for these beliefs. The parents are the ultimate authority and allow little, if any, participation by the child in making decisions. Behavior that does not adhere to the family's rules and standards is punished. This parenting style is associated with negative effects on self-esteem, happiness and social skills, increased aggression, and defiance (Cherry, 2015; Hamon & Schrodt, 2012).

AUTHORITATIVE

The *authoritative* or democratic parent shows some respect for the child's opinions. Although parents still have the ultimate authority and expect the child to adhere to the rules, authoritative parents allow children to be different and believe that each child is an individual. They exhibit warmth and consistently, fairly, and firmly enforce the family's rules and standards without emphasizing punishment. This type of parenting is associated with increased independence, happiness, self-confidence, and socially responsible individuals (Cherry, 2015; Piko & Balázs, 2012).

PERMISSIVE

Permissive or laissez-faire parents have little control over the behavior of their children. Rules or standards may be inconsistent, unclear, or nonexistent. Permissive parents allow their children to determine their own standards and rules for behavior. Discipline can be lax, inconsistent, or absent. Parents can be warm, cool, or uninvolved. There are more negative than positive effects associated with this style of parenting. Negative effects include children being impulsive, low happiness, poor school performance, problems with authority, lacking responsibility and independence (Cherry, 2015; Hamon & Schrodt, 2012).

UNINVOLVED OR REJECTING-NEGLECTING

Uninvolved parents are indifferent. They do not provide rules or standards. The child's basic needs are often met but the parent is disconnected from the child's life. In some cases the parents may neglect or reject the child. They can be cold and uninterested in meeting the child's needs. They minimize their interactions and time with the children. This type of parenting is associated with negative effects such as the child lacking interest in school, lacking interest in the future, and lacking emotional and self-control (Cherry, 2015). This type of parenting may also lead to lack of trust, low self-esteem, and anger toward others (Cherry, 2015; Kawabata et al., 2011).

DISCIPLINE

Much of parenting involves increasing desirable behavior and decreasing or eliminating undesirable behavior, a process generally known as **discipline**. There are various opinions in our society about the best or most effective method of discipline. Each child and family is unique. Discipline that works with one child or within one family may not work for another family. Discipline should focus on the development of the child while ensuring to preserve their self-esteem and dignity. It should be based on age-appropriate expectations with clear, consistent guidelines while offering meaningful choices when possible. Discipline involves teaching and it is ongoing, not something that is done just when the child misbehaves.

The AAP (2012a, 2015a) suggests three strategies for effective discipline (see also Teaching Guidelines 1.1):

- Maintaining a positive, supportive, nurturing caregiver–child relationship
- Using positive reinforcement to increase desirable behaviors
- Removing positive reinforcements or using punishment to reduce or eliminate undesirable behaviors

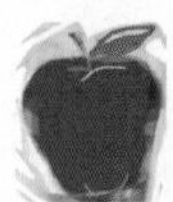

Teaching Guidelines 1.1
PROMOTING EFFECTIVE DISCIPLINE

- Set clear, consistent, and developmentally appropriate expected behaviors; offer choices whenever possible.
- Maintain consistency in responding to behaviors; provide encouragement and affection.
- Role-model appropriate behaviors.
- Provide an age-appropriate explanation of the consequence if the child demonstrates unacceptable behavior.
- Always administer the consequence soon after the unacceptable behavior.
- Keep the consequence appropriate to the age of the child and the situation.
- Stay calm but firm without showing anger when administering the consequence.
- Always praise the child for displaying appropriate behavior (positive reinforcement).
- Set the environment to assist the child in accomplishing the appropriate behavior; remove temptations that may lead to inappropriate behavior.
- Reinforce that the child's behavior was "bad" but the child was not "bad."
- Use extinction to reduce or eliminate reinforcement for an inappropriate behavior (e.g., ignore a temper tantrum).

- When using time-out, use 1 minute per year of the child's age. Do not exceed 5 minutes.
- Maintaining a positive, supportive, nurturing caregiver–child relationship
  - Using positive reinforcement to increase desirable behaviors
  - Using extinction or punishment to reduce or eliminate undesirable behaviors

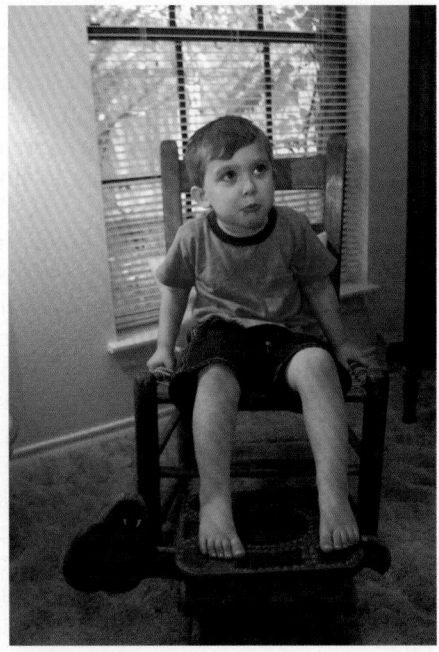

FIGURE 1.6 Although he might not like it, quiet solitude helps the child develop inner control.

POSITIVE REINFORCEMENT

Attention from parents is a very powerful form of positive reinforcement and can help increase desirable behaviors. The key is to focus on the child's appropriate behaviors rather than emphasize the inappropriate ones. Immediate, consistent, and frequent feedback is crucial. This feedback can be in the form of smiles, praise, special attention, or rewards such as extra privileges or a special token or activity. Providing the feedback immediately is important so that the child learns to associate the feedback with the appropriate behavior, thereby reinforcing the behavior.

EXTINCTION

Another form of discipline is extinction, which focuses on reducing or eliminating the positive reinforcement for inappropriate behavior. Examples are ignoring the temper tantrums of a toddler, withholding or removing privileges, and requiring "time-out." Withholding or removing privileges such as TV, music device, computer, or cell phone use is most effective for older children and adolescents. The adolescent may be grounded for a short time or not allowed to drive the car. To be effective, the privilege being withheld or removed must be something that the child values.

Time-out is an extinction discipline method that is most effective with toddlers, preschoolers, and early school-age children. It involves removing the child from the problem area and placing him or her in a neutral, nonthreatening, safe area where no interaction occurs between the child and parents or others for a specifically determined period (Fig. 1.6).

Take Note!

The amount of time that a child spends in time-out is typically 1 minute per year of age. For example, a 3-year-old would spend 3 minutes in time-out (AAP, 2013b).

PUNISHMENT

Discipline is often confused with punishment, but **punishment** involves a negative or unpleasant experience or consequence for doing or not doing something. Although punishment is sometimes a necessary element of discipline, to be an effective tool it must be coupled with rewards for good behavior (AAP, 2012a, 2015a; Flaskerud, 2011).

Punishment may be verbal or corporal. Verbal punishment commonly takes the form of reprimands or scolding (the use of disapproving statements). The statements are intended to change or eliminate the inappropriate behavior. Verbal reprimands can be effective in the short term if they are used sparingly and are focused on the child's specific behavior. If verbal reprimands are used frequently and indiscriminately, they lose their effectiveness, can provoke anxiety in the child, and encourage the child to ignore the parent. Frequent use also may reinforce the behavior by providing the child with attention (AAP, 2012a, 2015a; Flaskerud, 2011).

Corporal punishment involves the use of physical pain as a means to decrease inappropriate behavior. The most common form of corporal punishment is spanking (the use of an open hand to the buttocks or an extremity with the intention of modifying behavior without causing injury) (Flaskerud, 2011). Research shows that many parents have spanked their children at some point, with 90% of parents having spanked their child at least once (AAP, 2012a, 2015a; Larzelere, 2011). Spanking decreases as children age, but is still used as a discipline strategy in adolescents. Over the past two decades a growing body of research has suggested that corporal punishment can cause an increase in behavior problems and have lasting effects into adulthood (Lansford et al., 2012).

Initially, spanking may be effective because of its sudden and shocking nature. However, over time it loses its effectiveness because its shock value declines. Spanking may stop the negative behavior, but it also increases the chance for physical injury, especially for infants and young children, and may lead to altered caregiver–child relationships (AAP, 2012a, 2015a; Flaskerud, 2011). Because the effects of spanking diminish, the intensity of the spanking must be increased to achieve the same effects. Thus, it is important for parents to understand the consequences of its use.

Spanking is a controversial issue. Some argue that it provides children with a model of aggressive behavior as a solution for conflict, that it has been associated with increased aggression in children, and that it can lead to an altered parent–child relationship. Various studies have linked spanking in childhood with physical aggression and violence in childhood and persistent anger in adulthood (AAP, 2013b; Lansford et al., 2012). Because of the negative consequences of spanking, and because it has been shown to be no more effective than other methods for managing inappropriate behavior, the AAP recommends that parents use methods other than spanking to respond to inappropriate behavior (AAP, 2012a, 2015a).

Take Note!

Other forms of discipline, if used incorrectly, can also cause problems for the child and interfere with the caregiver–child relationship. For example, disapproval using tone of voice, facial expression, or gestures can be effective in stopping inappropriate behavior, but if the disapproval comes in the form of verbal statements that attack the child rather than the behavior, negative consequences may occur (AAP, 2012a, 2015a; Flaskerud, 2011).

Genetics

Genetics, the study of heredity and its variations, is a field that has applications to all stages of life and all types of diseases. The child's biologic traits, including gender, race, some behavioral traits, and the presence of certain diseases or illnesses, are directly linked to genetic inheritance. Heredity is the process of transmitting genetic characteristics from parent to offspring.

Gender

Gender is established when the sex chromosomes join. A person's gender can influence many aspects, such as physical characteristics and personal attributes, attitudes, and behaviors. Some diseases or illnesses are more common in one gender; for example, scoliosis is more common in females and color blindness in males (Lewis, 2011).

In addition to the specific biologic and physical traits related to gender are the social effects. The child develops specific gender attitudes and behaviors that are appropriate in his or her own culture. Interactions with family members and peers as well as activities and societal values affect how children perceive themselves as a specific gender (Fig. 1.7).

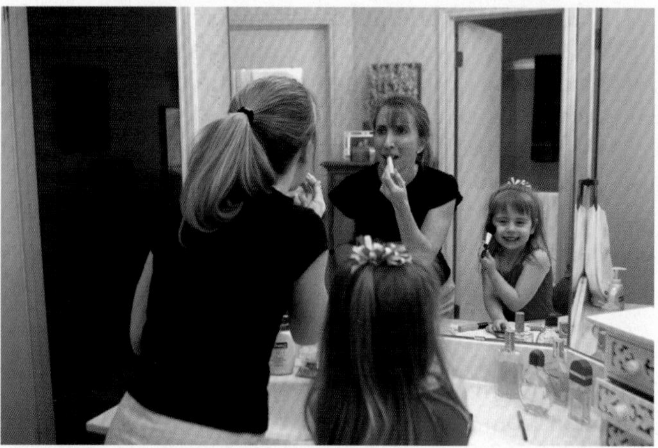

FIGURE 1.7 Interactions with family members and peers as well as activities and societal values affect how children perceive themselves as a certain gender.

Race

Race refers to the physical features that distinguish members of a particular group, such as skin color, bone structure, or blood type. Some of the physical variations may be normal in a particular race but may be considered an identifying characteristic of a disorder in other races. For example, epicanthal folds (the vertical folds of skin that partially or completely cover the inner canthi of the eye) are normal in Asian children but may occur with Down syndrome or renal agenesis in other races. In addition, certain malformations and diseases are found more commonly in specific races. For example, sickle cell anemia occurs more often in African Americans (Long et al., 2011).

Public awareness is important in educating couples at genetic risk about the benefits of screening programs and proactively seeking preconceptual genetic counseling to consider options that could include preimplantation genetic diagnosis (the use of in vitro fertilization technology to screen for unaffected embryos) (Rafi & Kai, 2011). The lack of engagement by ethnic minorities might simply reflect a lack of genetic awareness. Nurses can take the lead in assisting couples to gain that needed awareness to be empowered to make intelligent reproductive decisions.

Temperament

Temperament is the manner in which a child interacts with the environment. The way a child experiences a particular event will be influenced by his or her temperament, and the child's temperament will influence the responses of others, including the parents, to the child. Early on, infants demonstrate differences in their behavior in response to stimuli. These responses are an integral part of the infant's developing personality and individuality. Although a child's temperament is intrinsic and relatively resistant to change, it does stabilize as the child matures (Crawford, Schrock, & Woodruff-Borden, 2011). Knowing a child's temperament can help parents understand and accept the characteristics of the child without feeling responsible for having caused them.

The classic temperament theory proposes nine parameters of temperament: activity level, rhythmicity, approach and withdrawal, adaptability, threshold of responsiveness, intensity of reaction, quality of mood, distractibility, and attention span and persistence (Feigelman, 2011). This theory seeks to identify behavioral characteristics that lead the child to respond to the world in specific ways. Using the nine parameters, children's temperaments may be categorized into three major groups: easy, difficult, and slow to warm up; various temperaments are a combination of these groups (Kiff, Lengua, & Zalewski, 2011; Feigelman, 2011). Easy children are even-tempered and have regular biologic functions, predictable behavior, and a positive attitude toward new experiences. Difficult children are irritable, highly active, and intense; they react to new experiences by withdrawing and are frustrated easily. Children in the slow-to-warm-up category are moody and less active and have more irregular reactions; they react to new experiences with mild but passive resistance and need extra time to adjust to new situations.

A child's temperament may cause problems in the family if it conflicts with that of the parents (e.g., a difficult 2-year-old with slow-to-warm-up parents). If parents want and expect their child to be predictable but that is not the child's style, parents may perceive the child to have problems; this conflict may then affect the child's health. The key is not to label the child but to recognize the strengths and limitations of each group. Understanding a child's temperament can help parents understand a child's characteristics and behaviors and allow parents to adjust their parenting style.

Genetically Linked Diseases

New technologies in molecular biology and biochemistry have led to better understanding of the mechanisms involved in hereditary transmission, including those associated with genetic disorders. These advances are now leading to better diagnostic tests and management options.

Reproductive genetic testing, counseling, and other genetic services can be valuable components in the reproductive health care of women and their families. These services have the potential to increase knowledge about possible pregnancy outcomes that may occur if a woman decides to reproduce; to provide reassurance during pregnancy; and to enhance the developing relationship between the woman, her expected child, and others (Edwards et al., 2015). This awareness can provide each woman with an opportunity to have access to desired genetic services in a way that will improve her control over the circumstances of her reproductive life, her pregnancies, childbearing, and parenting, within a framework that is sensitive to her needs and values. Nurses can be a vital facilitator in this process and to these services.

Two major areas of study in genetics that are important to pediatrics are cytogenetics and the Human Genome Project. Cytogenetics is the study of genetics at the chromosome level. Since the genetic code was deciphered, much has been learned about the chromosomal structure shared by all human organisms. Chromosomal anomalies occur in 0.4% of all live births and are the most prevalent cause of cognitive impairment and congenital anomalies or birth defects (Ferguson-Smith, 2015). Anomalies are even more common among spontaneous abortions and stillbirths. The Human Genome Project was an international research effort involving the localization, isolation, and characterization of human genes and investigation of the function of the gene products and their interaction with one another. It was considered one of the most ambitious and successful international research collaborations in the history of biology. Completion of this project provided scientists with greatly enhanced information about how DNA shapes species development and genetic diseases to aid in developing new ways to identify, treat, cure, or even prevent them. Chapters 10 and 49 offer a more detailed discussion of genetics.

Society

Society has a major impact on the health of women, children, and families. Major components of a society that influence children and their health include social roles, socioeconomic status, the media, and the expanding global nature of society. Each of these areas may influence a person's self-concept, the communities where they live, their choice of lifestyle, and their health. Nurses need to assess these areas and their influence on the child and family so that individualized strategies can be designed and implemented to enhance the positive effects and minimize the negative effects on the child's and family's health.

Social Roles

Society often prescribes specific patterns of behaviors: certain behaviors are permitted and others are prohibited. These social roles are often an important factor in the development of self-concept. Social roles influence a person's ideas about self. Social roles are generally carried out in groups with which the individual has intimate daily contact, such as the family, school, workplace, or peer groups.

Socioeconomic Status

Another dominant influence is a person's socioeconomic status, meaning his or her relative position in society. This includes the family's economic, occupational, and educational levels. Children are raised differently by parents of different educational levels, occupations, and incomes. Low socioeconomic status typically has an adverse influence on an individual's health. Health care costs are continuing to rise, as are health insurance premiums. The family may not be able to afford food, health care, and housing; meals may be unbalanced, erratic, or insufficient. Housing may be overcrowded or have poor sanitation. These families may not understand the importance of preventive care or may simply not be able to afford it. As a result, they may be exposed to health risks such as lead poisoning or may not be immunized against communicable diseases. Studies have documented that children who come from low socioeconomic status are more likely to suffer from acute and chronic conditions experiencing more limitations from these, as well as injuries and mental health conditions (Allin & Stabile, 2012).

Take Note!

A recent research study showed that lower socioeconomic status was associated with increased cortisol levels over time (Chen, Cohen, & Miller, 2010). Cortisol plays a role in psychiatric and physical illnesses; therefore, findings of elevated cortisol levels in children from a low socioeconomic status may help explain why low socioeconomic status is negatively related to health (Chen et al., 2010).

POVERTY

Poverty is a measurement based on the specific monetary income of a family. The poverty threshold is the dollar amount that the U.S. Census Bureau uses to determine whether a family is living in poverty. It is based on the family's size and income (Table 1.3). If the individual's or family's income is below the threshold, then that person or family is said to be living in poverty.

Despite the many global economic gains that have been made during the past century, poverty continues to grow and the gap between rich and poor is widening. Major gaps continue between the economic opportunities and status afforded to women and those offered to men. A disproportionate share of the burden of poverty rests on women's shoulders, and this undermines their health. However, poverty, particularly for women, is more than monetary deficiency. Women continue to lag behind men in control of cash, credit, and collateral. Other forms of impoverishment may include deficiencies in literacy, health care access, education, skills, employment opportunities, mobility, and political representation, as well as pressures on time and energy linked to their responsibilities. These poverty factors may affect a woman's health (Robinson, Stoffel, & Haider, 2015).

TABLE 1.3 2013 US POVERTY GUIDELINES

Size of Family Unit	48 Contiguous States and D.C.	Alaska	Hawaii
1	$11,490	$14,350	$13,230
2	$15,510	$19,380	$17,850
3	$19,530	$24,410	$22,470
4	$23,550	$29,440	$27,090
5	$27,570	$34,470	$31,710

Adapted from U.S. Department of Health and Human Services (2013). *2013 Poverty Guidelines.* Retrieved from http://aspe.hhs.gov/poverty/13poverty.cfm#thresholds; Federal Register, Vol. 78, No. 16, January 24, 2013, pp. 5182–5183.

Over the past decade the number and rate of children living in poverty has risen. According to the Children's Defense Fund (2012), 16.4 million American children live in poverty, with 7.4 million living in extreme poverty. The rate of poverty is closely tied to the overall health of the economy; therefore, in times of recession, a rise is usually seen. Family structure is an important factor associated with poverty rates for children. The poverty rate for married-couple families is much less than that for families headed by a single parent. Of the families living below poverty level, 30.9% were single-mother families with no husband present, 16.4% were single-father families with no wife present, and 6.3% were married couples (Denavas-Walt et al., 2013). Educational level is another important factor: as education increases, unemployment declines and annual income rises. However, a chronic physical or emotional problem in any wage earner may lead to unemployment, and this can cause the family to spiral downward into poverty.

The effects of poverty on children's health can be wide-ranging. The family may be able to afford only substandard housing or a house or apartment in a dangerous neighborhood (e.g., unsanitary conditions, toxins, violence). Poverty may also lead to homelessness.

Basic financial stability enhances the general health and well-being of children, and thus an important negative influence on children's health is poverty. Children living in poverty are more likely to have poor health, be retained in a grade or drop out of school, become teen parents, experience violent crimes, and become poor adults (Da Fonseca, 2012). They have greater rates of death and illness from almost all causes, except suicide and motor vehicle accidents (Da Fonseca, 2012).

HOMELESSNESS

It is impossible to measure homelessness with 100% accuracy. Therefore, looking at trends is important to demonstrate if progress is being made or not. Recent research suggests that homelessness among families is increasing. In a given year, approximately 1.6 million (1 in 45) children are likely to experience homelessness in America (National Center on Family Homelessness [NCFH], 2015). Over 60% of homeless families are ethnic minorities and the typical homeless family is headed by a single mother with two children (NCFH, 2015).

Homelessness occurs in large urban areas and midsize cities as well as suburban and rural areas. The principal causes of homelessness in families are poverty and lack of affordable housing. Other causes include cutbacks in public welfare programs, mental health issues, and traumatic events such as unemployment, illness, or accidents and personal crises such as divorce, domestic violence, or substance abuse. Children may be forced out of their house or choose to run away and become homeless because they have been abused or neglected, lived in foster homes, or were placed in residential treatment or juvenile detention centers.

Homelessness can have a negative impact on health and well-being in numerous ways, including the following:

- Increased mental health issues such as anxiety, depression, or aggressive behavior
- Higher incidence of chronic health problems and trauma-related injuries
- Problems related to nutritional deficiencies, affecting fetal or child growth and development
- Participation in behaviors such as illegal substance use or unprotected sex with multiple partners
- Limited access to health care services such as preventive care, prenatal care, or dental care
- Inability to attend school consistently, because the environment is not conducive to learning; may result in learning problems, socialization issues, or behavioral issues (NCFH, 2015).

Media

Prolonged sitting and watching television or surfing the Internet while pregnant impairs the blood return in the legs and causes swelling. This immobility may also increase the risk of blood clot formation. Nurses can instruct their pregnant clients that it is important to improve circulation to the legs by not crossing them at the knees and to keep the legs moving by rotating the feet at the ankles. Sitting with the feet up with support to the ankles is also helpful. Changing the sitting position and getting up at least every hour is essential to prevent complications.

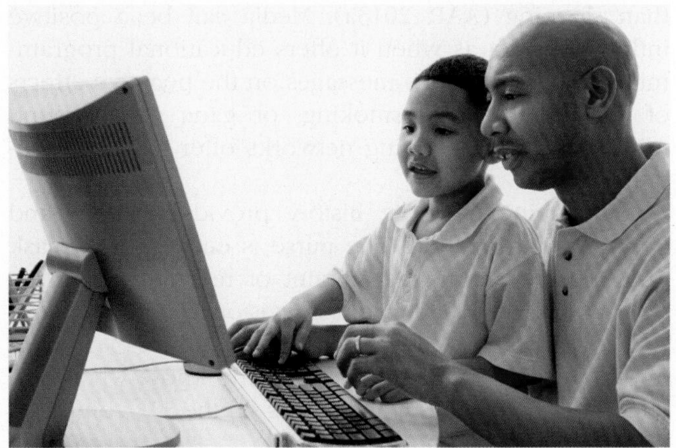

FIGURE 1.8 Computer games can be fun and educational, but the child should be monitored while using the computer and other forms of media to minimize negative effects.

Today's children are inundated with various forms of media, such as television, video and computer games, iPods, iPads, the Internet, social media, such as Facebook, movies, magazines, books, and newspapers (Fig. 1.8). Media has both positive and negative effects on the development of children and much depends on the content to which they are exposed (AAP, 2013a). Some of the images and information are not always in the best interests of children. Children may identify with, and mimic, characters who engage in risk-taking behaviors or lifestyles. Health risk behaviors, such as excessive caloric intake, physical inactivity, smoking, underage drinking, and violent behavior have been linked to media exposure (AAP, 2013a; Strasburger, 2011). Research has established a strong link between media violence and violent, aggressive behavior (Martins & Wilson, 2012). If an image or type of behavior is portrayed as the norm, children may view this as acceptable behavior without examining the potential health risks or other long-term consequences. For example, thinness is portrayed as the body type that is identified with beauty, leading some children to develop unhealthy dieting or other behaviors to develop that body type. For the child who has a body type that does not fit the ideal, depression or self-esteem issues may develop.

Overall, the images children view every day will affect their behavior and possibly their health, and pediatric nurses should take this into account when working with children and their families.

The media's influence relates not only to the content but also to the total viewing time. For example, excessive TV viewing has been linked to obesity, poor cognitive skills, and irregular sleep patterns. Overuse of computer or video games may lead to poor school performance. Media has become a major factor in children's lives with TV remaining the dominant medium (AAP, 2013a). Young children spend more time on media then they do in school. It is the leading activity other than sleeping (AAP, 2013a). Media can be a positive influence, such as when it offers educational programming or public service messages on the negative effects of substance abuse, smoking, or gang involvement. Also, public broadcasting networks offer valuable programming.

Obtaining a media history provides helpful and important information. The nurse is encouraged to ask questions regarding the amount of recreational screen time and if the child has a television or Internet-connected device in their bedroom (AAP, 2013a). It is important for parents to set limits and know what their children are viewing, whether it is on the TV, computer, iPod, tablet, or phone.

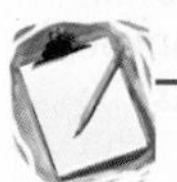

Take Note!

The American Academy of Pediatrics discourages any screen media before the age of 2 (AAP, 2013a).

Widespread access to the Internet has fostered a connection to other areas of the world that would not have been possible in previous years. Children are no longer limited to their immediate surroundings, and they have access to a wealth of information. The Internet can be a valuable resource for parents and children to access information, learn new things, and communicate with friends and family. However, online threats exist that can affect the child's health and safety such as sexual predators, pornography, violence, and racism. Parents need to be alert to these hazards and set up safety guidelines (see Teaching Guidelines 1.2).

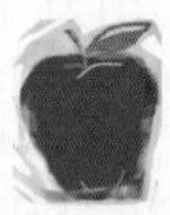

Teaching Guidelines 1.2

PROMOTING SAFE INTERNET USE

- Determine a specific time limit that your child can spend online each day or week. Be consistent in enforcing this time limit.
- Ensure that Internet use does not replace or interfere with homework, friends, or household or school activities.
- Tell your child NEVER to share personal information with anyone online unless you are sure of the person and the child has your permission to do so.
- Urge your child NEVER to share his or her password with anyone, even friends.
- Review Internet sites with your child, and explain what information and websites are appropriate. Use safety and parental controls offered by your Internet service provider.
- Avoid placing the computer in the child's room. Instead, place the computer in a public area of your home, such as the den or kitchen, so that you can monitor your child's use.
- Discuss with your child the need for maintaining safety while using the Internet. Explain potential hazards in terms the child can understand.
- Advise your child to immediately close any sites or stop any communication that makes him or her confused or uncomfortable. Tell your child NEVER to arrange any face-to-face meeting with persons he or she meets online. Urge your child to seek you out if he or she encounters such a situation.
- Teach the child NEVER to open email from any unknown senders.
- Be aware of computer use policies in your child's school.

Global Society

The world is connected in many ways today: people travel from one nation to another easily, new products and immigrants arrive each day, and the Internet makes worldwide communication simple. The United Nations Children's Fund and the WHO lead the world in dealing with the issues of children. Every year about 7.6 million children die around the world, over 21,000 every day (Shah, 2011). Hundreds of thousands of children born in developing countries and their families are moving to more developed nations such as the United States as refugees, immigrants, or international adoptees. These families become part of this nation.

Nurses need to be aware of the impact of worldwide events, such as natural and man-made disasters, on families. Families can be displaced by events such as hurricanes or wars, placing them at increased risk for problems such as infectious diseases, malnutrition, and psychological trauma.

Young children bear the brunt of the global burden of disease but progress has been made in reducing mortality in children less than 5 years old (WHO, 2014). The United Nations Children's Fund (UNICEF) and the World Health Organization (WHO) have identified major problems affecting child growth and development and survival:

- Acute respiratory infections, such as pneumonia
- Malnutrition, including micronutrient deficiency
- HIV/AIDS
- Diarrhea related to lack of clean water and sanitation
- Vaccine-preventable diseases such as measles
- Malaria
- Preterm birth complications
- Poor health care of pregnant and nursing mothers (WHO, 2014; UNICEF, 2015)

These organizations work to propose ways to eradicate these conditions by improving the case management skills of providers with adapted guidelines; improving the health systems with good district health planning and management as well as appropriate supplies, medications, information systems, and referral systems; and improving the family and community practices (WHO, 2012).

Today, families, children, and society as a whole have concerns over world threats and safety. Disasters such as the terrorist attacks of September 11, 2001, the killings at Columbine High School and Sandy Hook Elementary School, and devastating weather events such as Hurricane Katrina can have a significant impact on the well-being of women and children. The increase in stressors such as war, terrorism, school violence, and natural disasters puts women, children, and their families at risk for experiencing mental health difficulties. Children who have experienced these events are at risk for issues such as posttraumatic stress disorder, behavioral problems, depression, anxiety, sleep disturbances, restlessness, irritability, aggression, bullying, physiologic responses such as gastrointestinal symptoms, changes in academic performance, social isolation, and safety and security concerns (American Psychological Association, 2015). Children's coping abilities may be reduced and alterations in growth and development may be seen. Children's reactions depend on age and developmental level and are highly influenced by the emotional state of their caregivers. Nurses must be aware of the effects of world threats on women and children so that they can assess for alterations and intervene to promote security and stability.

Violence

Violence can occur in any setting and can involve any person. Violence against women is a major health concern—it affects thousands of lives and costs the health care system millions of dollars. Violence affects families, women, and children of all ages, ethnic backgrounds, races, educational levels, and socioeconomic levels. Pregnancy is often a time when physical abuse starts or escalates, resulting in poorer outcomes for the mother and the baby. The effects of intimate partner violence (IPV) on maternal health include insufficient or inconsistent prenatal care, poor nutrition, substance abuse, inadequate weight gain, and depression. Adverse neonatal outcomes include low birthweight, preterm birth, and small for gestational age infants (Alhusen et al., 2015). Many of these can lead to maternal or neonatal morbidity or mortality.

There are many opportunities within the current health care system for screening and early intervention during routine prenatal care or during episodic care in a hospital setting. The nurse is responsible for assessing for and following up on any abuse. Due to the potential impact of violence on women, children, and families, it is essential to identify any violent situation via a thorough assessment. All nurses need to include "RADAR" in every client visit (Box 1.4). Nurses serve their clients best not by trying to rescue them, but by helping them build on their strengths and providing support. Essentially, nurses empower their clients to help themselves. Providing referrals to shelters and child advocacy centers and intervening to assist women and children in dealing with this issue are paramount.

BOX 1.4

RADAR

R—Routinely screen every client for abuse.
A—Ask direct, supportive, and nonjudgmental questions.
D—Document all findings.
A—Assess your client's safety.
R—Review options and provide referrals.

INTIMATE PARTNER VIOLENCE

Violence in the home environment, known as intimate partner violence, affects many lives in the United States. The U.S. Bureau of Justice Office on Violence against Women (2015) estimates that over 1 million violent crimes are committed by former spouses, boyfriends, or girlfriends each year; about 85% of the victims are women. This violence is known as intimate partner abuse, family violence, wife beating, battering, marital abuse, or partner abuse, but regardless of the term used, its effects are widespread.

Children exposed to family violence are more likely to be physically, sexually, or emotionally abused themselves (Child Trends, 2013). The federal Child Abuse Prevention and Treatment Act (CAPTA) defines **child abuse and neglect** as "any recent act or failure to act on the part of a parent or caretaker that results in death, serious physical or emotional harm, sexual abuse or exploitation, or an act or failure to act that presents an imminent risk of serious harm to a child" (Child Welfare Information Gateway, 2013).

In 2012, approximately 686,000 cases of child maltreatment occurred in the United States (CDC, 2014b). Of the number of children identified as being maltreated, 78% were victims of neglect, 18% were victims of physical abuse, 9% were victims of sexual abuse, and 11% were victims of other maltreatment, such as emotional or psychological abuse (CDC, 2014b). Approximately 1,640 children died from abuse and neglect in 2012; nearly 70% of those children were less than 3 years of age (CDC, 2014b).

Take Note!

Children of African American and American Indian or Alaska Native descent have higher rates of abuse and neglect (CDC, 2014b).

Children who are exposed to stressors such as domestic violence or who are victims of childhood abuse or neglect are at high risk for short- and long-term problems. These problems manifest differently based on the child's age and developmental ability; the younger the child, and the longer the exposure, the more serious the problems seen. Short-term problems include sleep disturbances, headaches, stomachaches, depression, asthma, enuresis, aggressive behaviors, such as increased peer aggression and bullying, decreased social competencies, withdrawal, avoidance attachment, developmental regression, fears, anxiety, and learning problems. Long-term problems may include poor school performance, truancy, absenteeism, and difficulty with adult relationships and tasks. There is a strong correlation between the number of exposures to adverse events and negative behaviors such as early initiation of smoking, sexual activity, and illicit drug use, adolescent pregnancies, and suicide attempts (CDC, 2014a).

Take Note!

Witnessing and being exposed to violence in childhood results in a higher tolerance, and greater use, of violence as an adult (Child Trends, 2013).

Not all children exposed to violence suffer negative consequences. Children have resilience, and preliminary studies have identified protective factors that can help buffer children from the effects of violence and reduce the risk that the child will develop violent behaviors (Futures Without Violence, 2012). Examples of protective factors include the following:

- Feelings of connectedness or a secure attachment to a nonviolent parent or caregiver
- Strong commitment to school and academic performance
- Involvement in social activities
- Social and community support
- Positive sibling and peer relationships
- Ability to discuss problems with parents or a supportive adult
- Consistent presence of a parent at least once during the day, such as in the morning on awakening, when getting home from school, at dinnertime, or when going to bed
- Positive view of self
- Strong cultural and/or spiritual identity

Thus, interventions need to focus on reducing children's exposure to violence and fostering protective factors.

YOUTH VIOLENCE

Youth violence affects the community as well as the child and family. Studies have shown that youth violence is associated with a disruption in social services, an increase in health care costs, and a decline in property values (CDC, 2015c). Research continues to show that children exposed to violence suffer serious consequences, such as problems with development, behavior, and physical and mental health issues, that last a lifetime (Finkelhor et al., 2013).

VIOLENT CRIMES

Violent crimes include murder, rape, robbery, and aggravated assault. Statistics from the Centers for Disease Control and Prevention (2012) show that for people of ages 10 to 24 years:

- Approximately 4,828 people were murdered in 2011; of those deaths, firearms accounted for 83%.
- More than 707,212 people were treated in emergency departments for injuries due to violence in 2011.
- Homicide remained the leading cause of death for African Americans, the second-leading cause of death for Hispanics, and the third-leading cause of death for American Indians and Alaska Natives.

Suicide is a serious public health problem affecting young people today. Suicide is the third-leading cause of death in people of ages 10 to 14 years, with 56.9% due to firearms and 34.8% due to poisoning (CDC, 2015h). Of these reported suicides, boys (77.9%) were much more likely than girls to die from suicide (CDC, 2015h).

In 2013, a nationwide survey of students in grades 9 to 12 in public and private schools found that 17% reported seriously considering suicide in the previous 12 months (CDC, 2015h).

Take Note!

Cultural variations in youth suicide rates are present; American Indian/Alaskan Natives youths have the highest rate of suicide while Hispanic youth are more likely to report attempting suicide (CDC, 2015h).

SCHOOL VIOLENCE

In recent years, due to several high-profile cases of school shootings, much attention has been directed at school violence and concern for student safety. However, statistically, between 1% and 2% of school-age homicides occur on the way to or from school, at school events, or during school hours (CDC, 2014c). Students are much less likely to be victims of crime at school than away, but some schools continue to have serious crime and violence problems (CDC, 2014c). In a 2013 nationwide survey, 8% of high school students reported being involved in a physical altercation at least once in the previous year (CDC, 2015j). The percentage of youths who reported carrying a weapon (gun, knife, or club) for at least one of the days in the month prior to the survey was about 5% (CDC, 2015j).

Much of school violence involves bullying, which is repeated negative actions that are clearly malicious and unwarranted, by one or more persons directed at a victim. Among 9th to 12th graders, nearly 20% report being a target of bullying (CDC, 2015i). Many cases of bullying go unreported, but bullying can affect school performance and social relationships and have long-lasting traumatic effects such as depression, low self-esteem, anxiety, academic problems and violence later in adolescence and adulthood (CDC, 2015i). School nurses need to be aware of bullying and offer support, guidance, and intervention when necessary to the students and staff.

Safe schools are essential for proper learning, growth and development, development of healthy relationships, and overall health of our children. Violence in schools has a negative effect not only on students but also on the school and the entire community. The continued coordination among schools, law enforcement, social services, and mental health systems and the development of effective programs will help to reduce these risk behaviors.

Community

Community encompasses a broad range of concepts, from the nation where a person lives, to a particular neighborhood or group. The surrounding community affects many aspects of a person's health and general welfare. The quality of life within the community has a great influence on a person's ability to develop and become a functional member of society. Community influences include the school, which is a community in itself, and peer groups. The support and assistance offered to women, children, and families from other areas of the community, such as school programs and community centers, can improve the person's overall health and well-being.

SCHOOLS AND OTHER COMMUNITY CENTERS

Children today start school at an earlier age, spend more time in child care settings, and are involved in various community centers and activities. By age 3 or 4, many children are in a preschool setting for several hours a day. Some children spend more awake time in school and child care settings than in their family home. Thus, schools and child care settings have become major influences on children.

School also provides a means of socialization. School rules about attendance and authority relationships and the system of sanctions and rewards based on achievement help to teach children behavioral expectations that they will need for future employment and relationships in the adult world. Although the primary role of schools has always been academic education, today schools are performing more health-related functions. Schools play an important role in promoting healthy behaviors and educating children about proper exercise, nutrition, safety, sex, drugs, and mental health.

Academic success is linked to healthy behaviors. Academic success is a good indicator of child well-being and is a predictor of adult health outcomes (CDC, 2015a). Academic failure is linked to health risk behaviors such as substance use, violence, and physical inactivity. School health programs have positive impacts on health outcomes and health risk behaviors along with educational outcomes (CDC, 2015a).

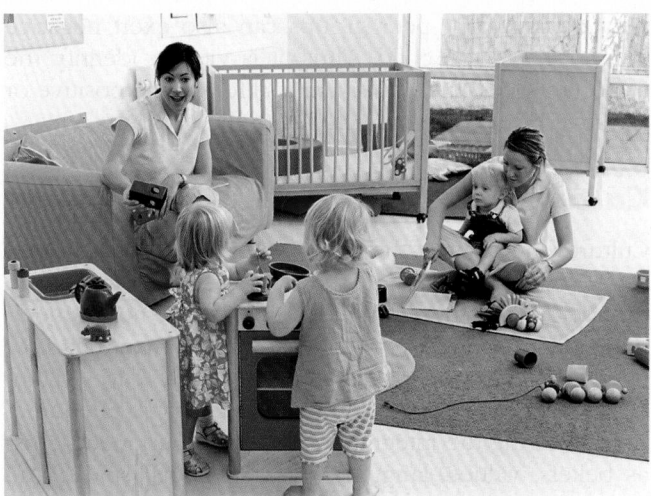

FIGURE 1.9 Daycare centers provide socialization and support for young children.

Because in many families both parents need to work, many children are enrolled in child care and after-school programs. Thus, the socialization process begins earlier and involves a larger percentage of the child's waking hours (Fig. 1.9).

After-school hours are a critical time where children may participate in risky health behaviors if they are not provided with supervised, structured activity where they can learn and grow. Community centers and after-school programs can provide an opportunity for children to learn new skills, have new experiences, and develop relationships with caring adults in a safe and supportive environment.

PEER GROUPS

A child's friends can have a major influence, positive or negative, on his or her growth and development. Peer group relationships often begin early and are a large part of the child's world, particularly with school-age children and adolescents. This influence starts in playgroups in preschool or elementary school. The child is confronted with a variety of values and belief systems from interactions with friends. To be accepted, the child must conform to the specific values and beliefs of the group. When these values and beliefs differ from those of the adults in the child's world, conflicts can occur, possibly separating children from the adults and strengthening their sense of belonging to the peer group.

When the child's friends are successful in school or other activities, the growth and development of the child continues in a healthy and positive way. When these groups demonstrate healthy behaviors, the influence is very positive, but peer groups can also exert negative influences on the child. Thus, it is vital to identify the important peer groups in a child's life and the positive or negative behaviors connected with these groups.

Culture

Culture (the view of the world and implementation of a set of traditions that are used by a specific social group in order to pass these traditions along to the next generation) plays a critical role in shaping a woman, child, or family including their health and health practices (Stanhope & Lancaster, 2011). Culture is a complex phenomenon involving the integration of many components such as beliefs, values, language, time, personal space, and view of the world, all of which shape a person's actions and behavior. Individuals learn these patterns of cultural behaviors from their family and community through a process called **enculturation**, which involves acquiring knowledge and internalizing values (Adams-Leander & Rector, 2014; Yoon et al., 2012).

Culture is learned first in the family, then in school, and then in the community and other social organizations. Culture influences every aspect of development and is reflected in childbearing and child-rearing beliefs and practices designed to promote healthy adaptation (Andrews & Boyle, 2015).

With today's changing demographic patterns, nurses must be able to incorporate cultural knowledge into their interventions so that they can care effectively for culturally diverse women, children, and families. They must be aware of the wide range of cultural traditions, values, and ethics that exist in the United States today. All nurses must establish **cultural competence**, the ability to apply knowledge about a client's culture so that health care interventions can be adapted to meet the needs of the client. Cultural competence refers to the process by which individuals and systems respond respectfully and effectively to people of all cultures, languages, ethnic backgrounds, disabilities, religions, sexual orientation, and other diversity factors in a manner that recognizes, and values the worth of individuals, families, and communities (Oregon Department of Education, 2015).

The nurse should know about various cultural groups, ethnicity, culture-based health practices and how they may affect children, as well as the demographics of the local population. The goal is for the nurse to view culture as a point of congruence rather than a potential source of conflict.

Cultural Groups

A cultural group is a self-defined group of people who share a commonality such as religion, language, nationality, ethnicity, race, or a physical trait. In a society there are typically dominant and minority groups. The dominant group, often the largest group, has the greatest authority to control the values and sanctions of the society (Adams-Leander & Rector, 2014; Kersey-Matusiak, 2012). As a result, the dominant culture may have the largest impact on the individual's health, whereas minority cultural groups may still maintain some of their own traditions and values.

The relationship of culture to health care can become obscured by the use of broad group titles. In reality, there are many distinct cultural groups, and within a group there may be many subcultures. Geographic differences also can occur. For example, the Latin Americans living in New York may be quite different from the Latin Americans living in Florida. Nurses must be aware of these distinct cultural groups so they can provide culturally competent care.

Nurses should also be aware of the traditional health care values and practices that are passed along from one generation to the next. For example, some cultures believe in consulting folk healers, and this belief may have a major influence on children's health (Table 1.4). The nurse must remember that diversity exists within cultures and this is as important as the diversity between cultures. Every person is a unique individual with his or her own beliefs, values, and history. Nurses must avoid stereotyping, which can lead to misconceptions.

Ethnicity

Ethnicity, a term sometimes used synonymously with culture, involves group membership by virtue of common ancestry shared culture and identity. The basic groups are differentiated by their customs, characteristics, language, or similar distinguishing factors. Ethnic groups have their own family structures, languages, food preferences, moral codes, and health care practices. Children learn the accepted mode of behavior by observing and imitating those around them. The influences of culture and ethnicity on women, children, and families are highly variable and dynamic. Probably the most important characteristic of ethnicity is the sense of shared identity felt by members (Nagle & Clancy, 2012).

Children who come from a minority group may experience conflict and difficulties with interactions, including health care providers, because their native customs are different from those of the dominant culture. Many Americans in the dominant culture do not view themselves as belonging to a specific ethnic group, but many minority groups still identify closely with their ethnicity and emphasize their cultural or racial differences (Nagle & Clancy, 2012).

Stereotyping or labeling can result from **ethnocentrism**, a belief that one's own ethnic group is superior to other ethnic groups. This attitude can lead

TABLE 1.4 BELIEFS AND PRACTICES OF SELECTED CULTURAL GROUPS

Cultural Group	Beliefs and Practices Affecting Children's Health
African Americans	Strong extended family relationships; mother as head of household; elder family members valued and respected Food as a symbol of health and wealth View of health as harmony with nature, illness as disruption in harmony Use of folk healing and home remedies common to treat body, mind, and spirit Strong church/religious affiliation Belief in illnesses as natural (due to natural forces that the person hasn't protected self against) and unnatural (due to person or spirit) Individuals vulnerable to external forces
Asian Americans	Strong loyalty to the family, father head of household Family as the center, with members expected to care for one another Preserving family pride and dignity is important Use of complementary modalities with Western health care practices View of life as a cycle, with everything connected to health Health viewed as a balance between the forces of *yang (hot)* and *yin (cold)* resulting in *qi* (pronounced chee), which is a balanced state of harmony Respect for authority emphasized
Arab Americans	Women subordinate to men; young individuals subordinate to older persons Family loyalty is primary Modesty is a core value Disease and illness attributed to the will of Allah Good health associated with eating properly, consuming nutritious foods, and fasting to cure disease Illness due to inadequate diet, shifts in hot and cold, exposure of stomach while sleeping, emotional or spiritual distress, and "evil eye" Cleanliness important for prayer
American Indian/ Alaska Native	High value on family and tribe; respect for elders Family as an extended network providing care for newborns and children Women as the verbal decision makers Celebrations to mark the stages of growth and development Use of food to celebrate life events and in healing and religious ceremonies Health as harmony with nature; illness due to disharmony, evil spirits; purification rituals (immersion in water, sweat lodges) to cleanse the body and spirit and maintain harmony with nature Prefer restoration of physical, mental, and spiritual balance through herbal medicines and healing ceremonies
Hispanics	Family important; father as the source of strength, wisdom, and self-confidence Mother as the caretaker and decision maker for health View of children as persons to continue the family and culture Use of food for celebrations and socialization Health as God's will maintainable with a balance of hot and cold food intake Cope with illness through prayer and faith in God Freedom from pain indicative of good health; pain tolerated stoically due to belief that it is God's will Folk medicine practices and prayers, herbal teas, and poultices for illness treatment

Adapted from Adams-Leander, S. & Rector, C. (2014). Chapter 5: Transcultural nursing in the community. In J. A. Allender, C. Rector, & K. D. Warner (Eds.), *Community & public health nursing. Promoting the public's health* (8th ed., pp. 115–149). Philadelphia, PA: Wolters Kluwer Health/Lippincott Williams & Wilkins.

to a slanted view of the world, and it may hinder the nurse's ability to provide culturally competent care.

Cultural Health Practices

Health practices are often the result of health beliefs derived from a person's culture. For example, do the child and family view health and illness as the result of natural forces, supernatural forces, or the imbalance of forces? Most cultures have remedies that people may use or consider before they seek professional health care. People from some cultures may go to folk healers who they believe can cure certain illnesses. For example, the *curandero* (male) or the *curandera* (female) of the Mexican American community is believed to have healing powers as a gift from God. Asian Americans may consult a practitioner who specializes in traditional Asian therapies such as acupuncture, acupressure, and moxibustion. These folk healers are often very powerful in their community, speak the language, and are very familiar with the culture's spiritual or religious aspects.

If the folk remedies or practices of the folk healers are compatible with the health regimen and support appropriate health practices, these practices and beliefs do no harm; in fact, they may even benefit the child and family. However, use of a folk healer can lead to a delay in beneficial treatment or create other problems. Some traditional health practices may be misinterpreted as being harmful, and some actually are harmful. For example, the Vietnamese practice of coining, which involves rubbing the edge of a coin on an oiled symptomatic body area to rid the body of disease, may be misinterpreted as a sign of physical abuse (Adams-Leander & Rector, 2014). This practice also can lead to burns, bruising, or welt-like lesions on the child's skin if it is done frequently. *Azarcon* and *greta,* powders containing high amounts of lead, are used as a folk remedy in Mexico to treat *empacho,* digestive problems such as diarrhea, and indigestion; and in some cases have resulted in lead toxicity (Adams-Leander & Rector, 2014).

Take Note!

Nurses can help to shape a person's lifelong perceptions of health and health services. An understanding of how the woman's, child's, and family's culture affects their health practices gives the nurse an opportunity to incorporate appropriate and beneficial health practices into the family's cultural milieu, providing sources of strength rather than areas of conflict.

Changing Cultural Demographics

The United States is no longer a melting pot of various cultures and ethnicities but a society with each individual bringing a diversity and richness that enriches the country as a whole. In 2012, 53% of the population is White, 14% is Black or African American, 24% is Hispanic, 5% is Asian, and 5% is non-Hispanic other races (FIFCFS, 2013). The Hispanic population has increased substantially over the past decade (FIFCFS, 2013). It is projected by 2050 that 36% of the US population of children will be Hispanic and 36% will be White, non-Hispanic (FIFCFS, 2013). In addition, the increasing number of intermarriages between individuals from different ethnic origins is producing an increasing number of children who have a heritage that represents more than one cultural group.

Immigration

Employment and economic opportunities, expanded human rights, educational opportunities, and other types of freedoms and opportunities encourage many foreigners to move to the United States. There are a growing number of immigrants with approximately one in five children in the United States being immigrants or members of an immigrant family (Stanton & Behrman, 2011). This includes both children born outside the United States or with at least one foreign-born parent. Some communities welcome the new members, but others do not. Partly due to fears of terrorism, the United States is evaluating, enforcing, and changing many of its immigration laws.

Immigration can affect the health, educational, and social services provided in the United States. It also presents issues related to access to care and the types of care that need to be offered. Immigration imposes stresses on women, children, and families, including the following:

- Depression, grief, or anxiety due to migration and adoption of a new culture
- Separation from support systems
- Inadequate language skills
- Differences in social, professional, and economic status between the country of origin and the United States
- Traumatic events such as war that may have occurred in their homeland (AAP, 2010)

Inability to speak English can hinder an immigrant's educational attainment, economic opportunities, and ability to join the mainstream of society. Twenty-two percent of children living in the United States speak a language other than English at home and 22% of children in immigrant families live in a linguistically isolated home (i.e., no person 14 years or older speaks fluent English) (Kids Count Data Center, 2014a, 2014b). Immigrant parents who do not speak English may have trouble accessing health care and health insurance, enrolling their children in school or becoming involved in school activities, and accessing work or better-paying jobs.

Immigrant families also may arrive in the United States with significant health problems. They may present with diseases that are more common in their country of origin but rarely seen in the United States, such as malaria. The health status of immigrant children may be compromised due to the lack of at-birth and early childhood screenings, which may manifest with problems such as inborn errors of metabolism, lack of preventive care, no immunizations, and no dental care. Due to financial, language, cultural, and other types of barriers that immigrant families sometimes face, they may not receive the necessary preventive care or receive care for minor conditions until they become more serious. Stresses experienced by immigrant children and their families, such as those associated with relocation, separation, and traumatic events, also can have a negative impact on their psychological health.

Spirituality and Religion

Spirituality is a basic human quality involving the belief in something greater than oneself and a faith that affirms life positively. It is a major influence in many people's lives, providing a meaning or purpose to life and a foundation for and source of love, relationships, and service. Spirituality is considered a universal human phenomenon with an assumption of the wholeness of people and their connectedness to a higher being. During life-changing events and crises, such as a serious illness or the birth of a child with a congenital defect, families often turn to spirituality for hope, comfort, and relief.

The word *religion* is often used interchangeably with spirituality in our society. However, spirituality is a more private and individual belief, whereas religion is an organized way of sharing beliefs and practicing worship. Over 90% of Americans believe in God (Bohon, 2011). Therefore, spirituality and religion are an important focus when working with women, children, and their families. A person's reaction to health and illness may be affected by these beliefs. In some religions, illness is seen as a punishment for sin or wrongdoing. Other religions view illness as a test of strength (Adams-Leander & Rector, 2014).

People appreciate the recognition of, and respect for, their beliefs. Therefore, identifying the individual's and family's religious beliefs and customs is important. People may adhere to special dietary restrictions, rituals such as baptism or holy communion, use of amulets or icons, or practices related to dying that can be incorporated into the plan of care. Using open-ended questions and observing for the use of religious articles during assessment can provide clues to the family's beliefs and practices. Visits from spiritual leaders may also be noted. Table 1.5 identifies some of the ways in which tenets of major religious beliefs may affect children's health.

Take Note!

Never make assumptions about a family's religious or spiritual affiliation. Although they may belong to a particular religion, family members may not adhere to all of its beliefs or participate in all aspects of the religion. Be alert for clues that would provide insight into their specific beliefs.

Health Status and Lifestyle

Obviously, the general health status of a person and specific lifestyle can influence a person's health. Health status may be a factor soon after birth. Societal shifts, triggered by a greater focus on education and careers, have resulted in a trend toward delayed childbearing in American women. This timing has increased the incidence of multiple births due to the increased use of in vitro fertilization and other assisted reproductive technologies along with women delaying childbearing until they are older (Crawford & Steiner, 2015). Potential complications of multiple births include prematurity and intrauterine growth retardation, which may lead to chronic health problems in the child. Children with chronic health conditions may also have developmental delays, especially in acquiring skills related to cognition, communication, adaptation, social functioning, and motor functioning. Thus, the beginning health status of a child may affect his or her long-term health and development.

Developmental Level and Disease Distribution

Developmental level has a major impact on a person's health status. In general, the distribution of diseases or illnesses varies with age. For example, adolescents who become pregnant are at a higher risk for certain complications, such as anemia, hypertension, preterm labor, cephalopelvic disproportion, and postpartum hemorrhage. Pregnant adolescents also experience higher rates of intimate partner violence and substance abuse. Moreover, substance abuse can contribute to low birthweight, intrauterine growth restriction, preterm births, newborn addiction, and sepsis (Wong, Ordean, & Kahan, 2011). Women who become pregnant after age 35 are at risk for hypertension, dystocia, and postpartum hemorrhage. Older pregnant women are also more likely to have a pre-existing condition that could complicate the pregnancy. Moreover, fetuses of older pregnant women are at risk for chromosomal abnormalities.

Certain communicable diseases are more commonly associated with certain age groups. Roseola, which is a viral illness resulting in high fevers and rash, is most often seen in infants 6 to 15 months; scarlet fever, a group A streptococci infection, is a disease that primarily affects children between 4 and 8 years of age. The physiologic immaturity of an infant's body systems increases the risk for infection. Ingestion of toxic substances and poisoning are major health concerns for toddlers as they become more mobile and inquisitive. Because preschool and school-age children are generally quite active, they are more prone to injury and accidents. Adolescents are establishing their identity, which may lead them to distance themselves from their family values and traditions for a period of time and conform more with their peers. This journey may lead to risky behaviors, resulting in injuries or other situations that may impair their health.

Nutrition

Nutrition provides the body with the calories and nutrients to sustain life and promote growth, as well

TABLE 1.5 SELECTED RELIGIOUS BELIEFS AFFECTING CHILDREN'S HEALTH

Religion	Beliefs About Health and Illness	Dietary Practices	Beliefs About Birth and Death
Buddhism	Illness from karmic causes (ignorant craving) Illness as an opportunity to develop the soul Ultimate goal of achieving nirvana (state of supreme tranquility, purity, and stability) No restrictions for medications, vaccines, nutritional therapies, or other therapeutic interventions	Moderation in diet encouraged Some sects vegetarian; some branches have strict dietary regulation; therefore, it is important to inquire about client's preferences	No baptism Last rite chanting at bedside soon after death; if there is hope for recovery and continuing the pursuit of enlightenment all means of intervention are encouraged Organ donation acceptable Cremation common
Christian Science	Disease viewed as error of human mind that can be dispelled by spiritual truth Health viewed within a spiritual framework; healing through prayer and spiritual regeneration Possible contact of own healing ministry (Christian Science practitioners) if child is hospitalized General opposition to human interventions with drugs or other therapies except for legally required immunizations Usually do not use blood or blood components, seek transplants or act as donors, seek biopsies or physical examination	No special requirements or restrictions	No baptism or last rites Unlikely to seek medical means to prolong life, use of prayer for recovery. Disposal of body in death left to family to decide
Hindu	Illness due to sins committed in previous life Acceptance of most medical practice/care Nonviolent approach to life	Meat consumption forbidden (especially beef) Some are strict vegetarians	No baptism View of death as a step in an ongoing cycle to reach nirvana Certain prescribed rites after death, such as washing the body by family and restrictions on who touches the body Cremation common
Islam	Belief that God cures but will accept treatment Compulsory prayers at dawn, noon, afternoon, after sunset, and after nightfall	Ingestion of pork and pork products and alcohol forbidden Fasting (by boys from age 7, girls from age 9, and adults) required during Ramadan (ninth month of Islamic year) (exceptions for pregnant/nursing mothers, elderly, or very ill)	No baptism Special party (*Aqeeqa*) to celebrate birth Specific burial rituals (rinsing and washing, wrapping, special prayers, and burial)

TABLE 1.5 SELECTED RELIGIOUS BELIEFS AFFECTING CHILDREN'S HEALTH (continued)

Religion	Beliefs About Health and Illness	Dietary Practices	Beliefs About Birth and Death
Judaism (orthodox and conservative)	Illness as possible reason for violating some dietary restrictions No treatments or procedures on Sabbath (which begins 18 minutes before sunset on Friday and ends 42 minutes after sunset on Saturday) or holy days	Ingestion of blood (such as raw meat) prohibited Kosher dietary laws; highly individualized observance Abstinence from ingestion of pork and predatory fowl and no mixing of milk dishes with meat dishes; ingestion of only fish with fins and scales; no shellfish (strict followers) Fasting during Yom Kippur, and matzo replaces leavened bread during Passover week	No baptism Ritual circumcision of male infants on eighth day of life Ritual of washing body after death; family and close friends remain with the deceased for a period of time No cremation
Mormon (Church of Jesus Christ of Latter-Day Saints)	Belief in divine health via laying on of hands. Medical therapy not prohibited Common use of herbal folk remedies	Ingestion of caffeinated tea, coffee, and alcohol and use of tobacco prohibited Fasting (no food or drink including water) once a month for 24 hours on a designated day, exceptions made (pregnant women, very young or old, and ill)	Baptism at older age (approximately 8 years old); infant blessed by church official after the birth Death believed to be another step in eternal progression Cremation discouraged, but not forbidden
Roman Catholic	Care of sick encouraged Misuse of any substance considered harmful to the body and a sin Eucharist as the food of healing and health	Moderation in diet encouraged Fasting and abstinence from meat and meat products on Ash Wednesday and Good Friday Abstinence on Fridays during Lent, but exceptions made if ill	Infant baptism; sacrament of the sick if prognosis is poor while child is alive; anointing of the sick Burial and treatment of the body with respect and honor Cremation is acceptable in certain circumstances

Adapted from Andrews, M. M., & Boyle, J. (2015). *Transcultural concepts in nursing care* (7th ed.). Philadelphia, PA: Lippincott Williams & Wilkins; Hanson, P. A., & Andrews, M. M. (2012). Chapter 13: Religion, culture and nursing. In M. M. Andrews, & J. S. Boyle (Eds.), *Transcultural concepts in nursing care* (6th ed., pp. 351–402). Philadelphia, PA: Wolters Kluwer Health/ Lippincott Williams & Wilkins.

as the essentials required to maintain health and prevent illness.

Nutritional deficiencies, such as iron-deficiency anemia, or excesses, such as the increasing incidence of childhood obesity, are still common problems in the United States. Effective obesity prevention and treatment interventions targeting children and their families are needed to help curb the obesity epidemic (Seburg et al., 2015). Some factors contributing to poor nutrition include inadequate food intake, nutritionally unsound social and cultural food practices, the easy accessibility of processed and nutritionally inadequate foods, lack of nutrition education in homes and schools, and the presence of illness that interferes with ingestion, digestion, and absorption of food.

During pregnancy, a woman needs additional calories to support fetal growth and development as well as to support her own needs, and an adequate intake of folic acid is important to prevent neural tube defects (Fig. 1.10). For the child, inadequate nutrition is associated with lowered cognitive ability, poor or altered emotional and mental health, increased susceptibility to childhood illnesses, and stunted physical growth (Miller & Scott, 2015). The so-called fast food or junk food that is

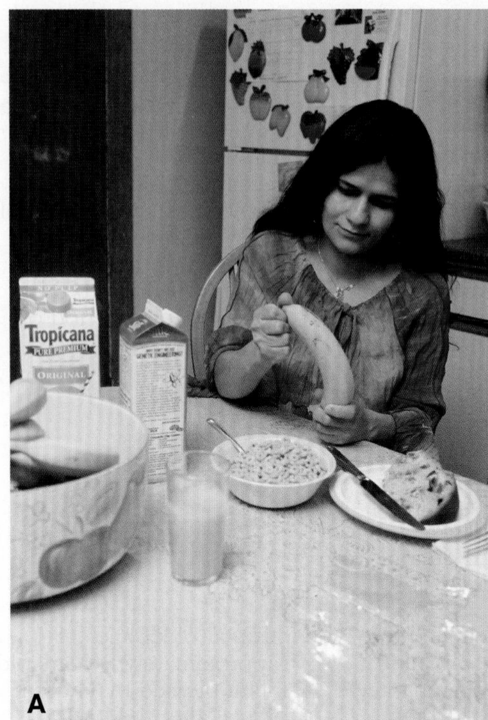

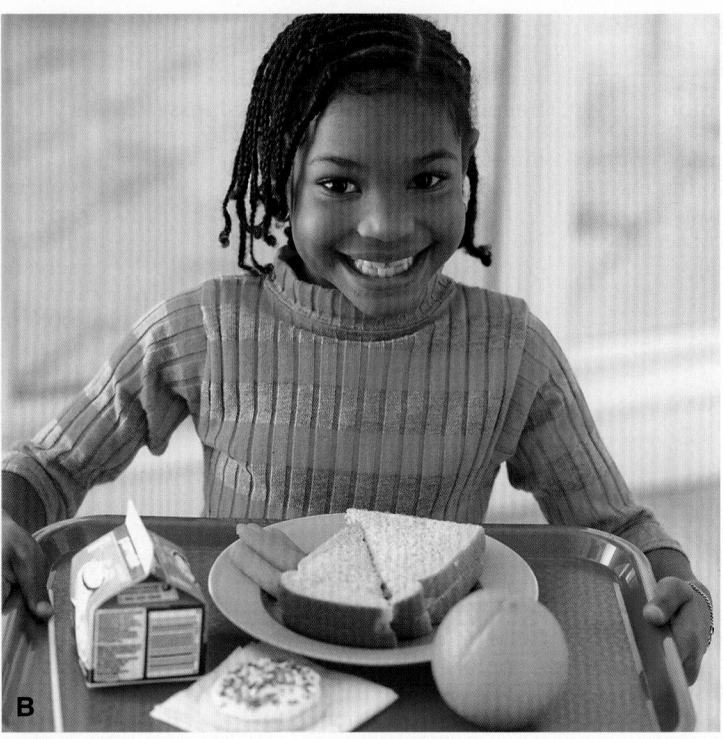

FIGURE 1.10 **A.** This pregnant client is eating a healthy meal to ensure adequate nutrition. **B.** The dietary habits established early in life can have a long-lasting impact on the child's health and quality of life.

prevalent in today's society is a key factor in the epidemic of childhood obesity and increases in the prevalence of childhood type 2 diabetes. Nutrition and its effects on health status are integrated throughout this text.

Lifestyle Choices

Lifestyle choices that affect a person's health include patterns of eating; amount and type of exercise; use of tobacco, drugs, or alcohol; and methods of coping with stress. Most health problems that arise today are due to a person's lifestyle. For children, the lifestyle of the parents basically is the lifestyle of the child. Inactive parents who eat poorly commonly have children with the same habits, which can result in diabetes, obesity, and early heart disease. These typically adult problems are being diagnosed more frequently in children and adolescents today. Parents should first self-evaluate their own dietary and activity habits, make changes where necessary, and then strive to encourage healthy eating habits and an appropriate level of physical activity in the child's life through sports, hobbies such as dancing, or family activities.

Environmental Exposure

Some environmental exposures can jeopardize health. In utero, the child can be affected by poor maternal nutrition, maternal infections, or maternal use of alcohol, tobacco, and drugs. Nurses caring for pregnant women should be aware of the risks to the fetus posed by certain drugs, chemicals, and dietary agents, as well as maternal illnesses. These agents, known as teratogens, may be linked to birth defects in children. Not all drugs or agents are associated with fetal effects, however, and research is necessary to identify the correlations between teratogens and other variables.

The environment continues to affect a child's health after birth. Exposure to air pollution, tobacco, and water or food contaminants can impair a child's health status. Safety hazards in the home or community can contribute to falls, burns, drowning, or other accidents. Exposure to second-hand smoke and other pollutants, such as from radiation or chemicals, is a health hazard for children. Because children are smaller and still developing, environmental exposures can cause them additional health problems. For example, lead exposure is a common preventable poisoning in children, especially children less than 6 years of age. Due to their rapidly developing nervous system, young children are more sensitive to the effects of lead. Sources include lead paint, lead-contaminated dust, and lead contained in soil and water. Lead exposure can result in developmental and behavioral problems ranging from inattentiveness and hyperactivity to permanent brain damage and death, depending on the level of exposure.

Take Note!

A recent study found that residual tobacco smoke and carcinogens remain after a cigarette is extinguished (referred to as third-hand smoke). These toxins cling to the smoker's hair and clothes and can be present on any surface in the house, such as carpet and cushions. Children are particularly susceptible to third-hand smoke since they breathe near, crawl, touch, and mouth contaminated surfaces (Karim et al., 2015).

Stress and Coping

Disasters, such as the terrorist attacks of September 11, 2001, or Hurricane Katrina, can have a significant impact on the well-being of women, children, and families. Stressors such as war, terrorism, school violence, and natural disasters may decrease a person's coping ability (Yahav, 2011) and lead to alterations in growth and development (Masten & Narayan, 2012). Exposure to traumatic events and violence may have long-term effects on an individual's psychosocial development and status. Some children can adapt and respond to the stress, while others do not. The term **resilience** refers to the qualities that enable a person to cope with significant adverse events or stresses and still function competently (Masten & Narayan, 2012).

Exposure to stress is not limited to disasters or traumatic events, however. Stress can also include areas such as inadequate finances, family crises such as divorce, inadequate support systems, illness, or violence. Stress can also be associated with the normal problems associated with growth and development, such as entering a new classroom, learning a new skill, or being teased by a classmate. Similar to disasters and traumatic events, the effects of these stressors can dramatically affect the health status of a woman, child, or family.

Recall Sophia, the 38-year-old pregnant woman who has come to the prenatal clinic for a visit. While talking with the nurse, Sophia mentions that her children are very involved in activities. She says, "My husband is busy at work, so I do most of the running around. Sometimes I feel like the people at the drive-thru know me by name! My husband helps out on the weekends, but during the week, it's all me." What factors may be influencing Sophia's health? How might these factors be influencing the health of the children and the family?

Access to Health Care

The health care system, including the delivery and financing of this system, continues to change and evolve. In the United States, changes in the health care system result from pressures from many directions. These changes reflect shifts in social and economic realities and the results of the biomedical and technologic progress over the past several decades. Every person who seeks health care in any form feels the effects. Access to health care is affected negatively by lack of health insurance. People without health insurance typically cannot afford to seek health care for maintenance and prevention interventions. The "working poor" may not earn enough money to afford health insurance or medical care, and part-time workers do not always receive benefits such as health insurance. In most states, a man and a woman of the same age and health status will be charged different rates for exactly the same individual health insurance policy, a practice called "gender rating." Women continue to pay a much higher health insurance rate for the same coverage versus men in the United States, an inequality that continues today. This causes women more psychological distress than men (Weissman et al., 2015).

Parents with uninsured children often delay care for their children and are less likely to have a usual place of care for their children (FIFCFS, 2013). The percentage of children without health insurance has dropped slightly over the past 2 years to 9.7% in 2011 (FIFCFS, 2013). This decrease is attributed to the stabilization of private employer–based insurance plans and the states' ability to improve enrollment in Medicaid and the State Children's Health Insurance Program (The Kaiser Commission on Medicaid and the Uninsured [KCMU], 2013). Medicaid is a joint federal and state program that provides health insurance to low-income children and their parents. It is state administered and each state has its own set of guidelines. In 1997, Congress passed legislation that led to the creation of the State Children's Health Insurance Program (S-CHIP) (now known as Children's Health Insurance Programs [CHIP]). The purpose of this program is to help insure low-income children who are ineligible for Medicaid, but cannot afford private health insurance. This program is also funded jointly by the federal and state governments, but administered by the individual states. In recent years Medicaid and CHIP have focused on increasing enrollment by increasing outreach, simplifying enrollment procedures, and retaining eligible enrollees. Legislation, such as The Children's Health Insurance Program Reauthorization Act of 2009 (CHIPRA) and the ACA, has helped support this (KCMU, 2012). Despite these efforts, half of uninsured children are eligible for these public programs but not enrolled (Children's Defense Fund, 2012). During the recent economic downturn and recession the uninsured rate for children has actually declined with the majority of the uninsured coming from low-income working families (KCMU, 2013). Medicaid and CHIP provide a good base of coverage for low-income children, but unfortunately eligibility for parents is much more limited.

These programs rely on adequate state and federal funding. Therefore, the continued success of these programs depends on future legislation. Tough economic times along with changes in employer-based health insurance will continue to challenge the nation to ensure adequate health care for all children.

Preventive Care Focus

The emphasis on cost reduction also led to an emphasis on preventive care and services. Anticipatory guidance is vital during each health contact with women, children, and families. Education of the family includes everything from keeping the home safe to preventing illness.

The Continuum of Care Emphasis

A "continuum of care" strategy is cost-effective and provides more efficient and effective services. This continuum extends from acute care settings such as hospitals to outpatient settings such as ambulatory care clinics, primary care offices, rehabilitative units, community care settings, long-term facilities, homes, and even schools. For example, the hospital stay is now integrated into a continuum that allows the client to complete therapy at home, school, or other community settings, while reentering the hospital for short periods for specific treatments or illnesses.

Improvements in Diagnosis and Treatments

Because of the tremendous improvements that have been made in technology and biomedicine, disorders and diseases are being diagnosed and treated earlier. The 1990s witnessed a remarkable and productive connection between genetics and various pathophysiologic processes. For example, female fetuses with congenital adrenal hyperplasia, a genetic disorder resulting in a steroid enzyme deficiency that can lead to disfiguring anatomic abnormalities, are beginning to receive treatment before birth. In addition, many genetic defects are being identified so counseling and treatment may occur early. With these improved diagnoses and treatments, nurses may now be caring for people who have survived situations that once would have been fatal, who are living well beyond their life expectancy for a specific illness, or who are functioning with chronic disabilities (CDC, 2015b). For example, at one time women with congenital heart disease did not live long enough to become pregnant. However, with new surgical techniques to correct the defects, many of these women survive and become pregnant, progressing through their pregnancy without significant problems.

While positive and exciting, these advances and trends also pose new challenges for the health care community. For example, as health care for premature newborns improves and survival rates increase, the incidence of long-term chronic conditions such as respiratory airway dysfunction or developmental delays has also increased. As a result, nurses are faced with caring for clients at all stages along the health–illness continuum, such as well children, those who are occasionally ill, and women, children, and families with chronic and sometimes disabling conditions.

Empowerment of Health Care Consumers

Due to the influence of managed care, the focus on prevention, a more educated population, and technologic advances, individuals and families have taken an increased responsibility for their own health. Health consumers are now better informed, and they want to play a greater role in managing health and illness. Families want information about illnesses and they want to participate in making decisions about treatment options. As client advocates valuing family-centered care, nurses are instrumental in promoting this empowerment. To do this, the nurse should respect the family's views and concerns, address all issues and concerns, consider the family members as important participants, and always include the woman, child, and family in the decision-making process.

BARRIERS TO HEALTH CARE

Women are major consumers of health care services, in many cases arranging not only their own care but also that of family members. Compared with men, women have more health problems, longer life spans, and more significant reproductive health needs (Davis, 2014). Access to care can be jeopardized by lower incomes and greater responsibilities (juggling work and family). Barriers to health care include lack of finances; sociocultural barriers, including lack of transportation, no babysitters, and language; and health care delivery system barriers, including inconvenient clinic hours and poor attitudes by health care workers. These barriers often discourage clients from seeking health care (Patel & Rushefsky, 2015).

Finances

Financial barriers are one of the most important factors that limit care. Childbirth is the leading reason for hospitalization in the United States. For both private insurers and Medicaid, hospital maternity and newborn charges exceed those for any other condition. In US hospitals, vaginal and cesarean deliveries cost approximately $10,000 to $17,000 and $16,000 to $25,000, respectively (Lincoln, 2015). Many women have limited or no health insurance and cannot afford to pay for maternity care. The intent of the ACA is to provide access to health care services for many (Crissman et al., 2015). Although Medicaid covers prenatal care in most states, the paperwork and enrollment process can be so overwhelming that many women do not register.

After a decade of decline, the percentage of children living in low-income families has again been on the rise. In 2011, 45% of children were living in low-income families and 22% were living in poor families (Addy, Engelhardt, & Skinner, 2013). Many children and families do not have insurance, do not have enough insurance to cover services obtained, or cannot pay for services. Nurses need to assess for financial barriers to health care and be aware of resources available to help families overcome these barriers.

Sociocultural Barriers

Lack of transportation and the need for both parents to work also pose barriers to seeking health care. It can be difficult to attend all recommended prenatal health care visits or well-child visits, especially if the woman has other small children who must be taken along on the visit. These challenges can reduce the adherence to scheduled appointments and follow-up. Knowledge barriers (e.g., lack of understanding of the importance of prenatal care or preventive health care), language barriers (e.g., speaking a different language than the health care providers), or spiritual barriers (e.g., religious beliefs discouraging some forms of treatment) also exist.

Health Care Delivery System Barriers

The health care delivery system itself can create barriers, such as the cost containment movement. Fifty-eight percent of employed families with insurance are covered by some type of managed health care plan or health maintenance organization (HMO), but millions of Americans remain uninsured (Douthit et al., 2015). This prospective payment system based on diagnosis-related groups (DRGs) limits the amounts of health care the family may receive. This also includes Medicaid reimbursement. Due to cost-containment efforts, the trend is to discharge clients as soon as possible from the hospital and to deliver care in the home or through community-based services (Riggs & Alexander, 2015). Although overall insurance plans may improve access to preventive services, they may limit access to specialty care—which greatly affects clients with chronic or long-term illnesses.

Clinic hours must meet the needs of the clients, not the health care providers who work there. Evening or weekend hours might be needed to meet the schedules of working clients. Clinic personnel should evaluate the availability and accessibility of the services they offer.

Unfortunately, some health care workers exhibit negative attitudes toward poor or culturally diverse families, and this could deter these clients from seeking health care. Long delays, hurried examinations, and rude comments by staff discourage clients from returning.

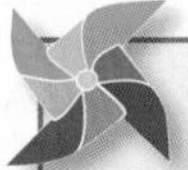

Consider This

I was a 17-year-old pregnant migrant worker needing prenatal care. Although my English wasn't good, I was able to show the receptionist my "big belly" and ask for services. All the receptionist seemed interested in was a social security number and health insurance—neither of which I had. She proceeded to ask me personal questions concerning who the father was and commented on how young I looked. The receptionist then "ordered" me in a loud voice to sit down and wait for an answer by someone in the back, but never contacted anyone that I could see. It seemed to me like all eyes were on me while I found an empty seat in the waiting room. After sitting there quietly for over an hour without any attention or answer, I left.

Thoughts: Why did she leave before receiving any health care service? What must she have been feeling during her wait? Would you come back to this clinic again? Why or why not?

LEGAL AND ETHICAL ISSUES IN MATERNAL AND CHILD HEALTH CARE

Law and ethics are interrelated and affect all of nursing. Professional nurses must understand their scope of practice, standards of care, institutional or agency policies, and state laws. Every nurse is responsible for knowing current information regarding ethics and laws related to their practice. Numerous federal programs have had a major impact on women's and children's health (Table 1.6).

Several areas are of particular importance to the health care of women and children. These include abortion, substance abuse, fetal therapy, maternal–fetal conflict, stem cell research, umbilical cord blood banking, informed consent, client rights, and confidentiality.

Abortion

Abortion was a volatile legal, social, and political issue even before *Roe v. Wade,* the 1973 Supreme Court decision that legalized abortion. Nearly half of pregnancies among American women are unintended, and about 4 in 10 of these are terminated by abortion. Twenty-two

(text continues on page 46)

TABLE 1.6 MILESTONES IN FEDERAL PROGRAMS IN SUPPORT OF THE HEALTH OF WOMEN AND CHILDREN

Date	Action	Impact
1909	First White House Conference on Care of Dependent Children (convened by President Theodore Roosevelt) Prevention of Infant Mortality Association formed	Addressed the poor working and living conditions of many children in the United States Aimed at improving the lives of children The Association played a major role in creating a new registration procedure for all infant births and deaths nationally
1912/1913	U.S. Children's Bureau	Established the first governmental agency to oversee children's health and environmental conditions Purpose is to research and report all issues pertaining to all children's well-being; to assist states and local government in preventing child abuse and neglect
1921	Maternity & Infancy (Sheppard–Towner) Act	Provided grants to states to establish maternal and child health divisions in state health departments
1930	White House Conference on Child Welfare Standards	Produced the Children's Charter, documenting the child's need for health, education, welfare, and protection
1935	The Social Security Act Introduction of vitamin K to newborns	Established federal–state partnership and provided Aid to Dependent Families and Children (ADFC), maternal–child health services, and child welfare services This discovery led to the prevention of hemorrhagic disease in newborns
1938	Initiation of the March of Dimes	Through research, defeated polio and now improves lives through the prevention of birth defects, prematurity, and infant mortality
1946	National School Lunch Program Centers for Disease Control and Prevention established	Provides nutritious, well-balanced lunches to children each day at school for free or at low cost. It also provides meal supplements for children in afterschool care and nutrition programs for homeless children. The CDC is globally recognized as a leading force in public health expertise
1962	National Institute of Child Health and Human Development (NICHD)	Supports and performs research on child, maternal, adult, and family health issues
1964	Head Start Developed	Head Start provides child development programs to pregnant women, families, and children from birth to age 5 with the overarching goal of increasing school readiness for children from low-income families.
1965	Medicaid Program under Title XIX of Social Security Act; special programs such as Child Health Assessment Program	Provided state block grants to reduce financial barriers to health care for the poor and special services to pregnant women, young children, and people with disabilities
1966/1974	Women, Infants, Children (WIC) program	Provided nutritional supplementation and education to low-income families; pregnant, postpartum, and lactating women; and infants and children up to age 5
1968	Expansion of Lunch & Nutrition Act	Provide food for low-income, school-age children year-round along with low-income children in day care and Head Start programs
1969	U.S. Children's Bureau moves to Office of Health, Education, & Welfare (HEW)	Established greater presence for the programs

TABLE 1.6 MILESTONES IN FEDERAL PROGRAMS IN SUPPORT OF THE HEALTH OF WOMEN AND CHILDREN (continued)

Date	Action	Impact
1972	Head Start to Serve Handicapped Children	Congress mandated that at least 10% of the children enrolled in Head Start must be handicapped children.
1975	Education for All Handicapped Children Act (Public Law 94–142) Title XX Social Services	Established federally mandated special education in public schools Provided block grants to day care, emergency shelters, counseling, family planning, and other services for children
1976	Improved Pregnancy Outcome Projects	Raised awareness of the importance of maternal health during pregnancy to reduce infant mortality
1976	The Supplemental Security Income (SSI) Disabled Children's Program	Provided cash to low-income children with disabilities to help their families manage their healthcare costs.
1979	National health objectives for 1990	These early efforts resulted in *Healthy People 2010* and *2020*
1981	Alcohol, Drug Abuse, & Mental Health block grants Healthy Mothers, Healthy Babies Coalition	Began funding services for children and adolescents with mental health issues Raised public awareness of prenatal care, good nutrition, avoidance of drugs, and promotion of breast-feeding
1986	Education of Handicapped Act Amendments (Public Law 99–457)	Established federal funding for states to create statewide, comprehensive, coordinated, and multidisciplinary early-intervention services for handicapped infants and toddlers
1990	Omnibus Budget Reconciliation Act	Extended Medicaid coverage to all children (6 to 18 years) with family income below 133% of poverty level
1990	Bright Futures Initiated	Provided a comprehensive set of child health supervision guidelines for health professionals, families, and communities and train these groups to work toward optimal child health
1991	Healthy Start initiated	Is a community-based program that serves at-risk women to reduce infant mortality during and after their pregnancy
1993	Family & Medical Leave Act (FMLA)	Allowed eligible employees to take up to 12 weeks of unpaid leave from their jobs every year to care for newborns or newly adopted children or children, parents, or spouses who have a serious health condition; employee can return to previous job or a comparable job with the same conditions
1994	Back to Sleep Campaign	A national campaign to prevent sudden infant death syndrome (SIDS) by placing infants on their backs to sleep
1995	Early Head Start Program	Federally funded community-based program for low-income families (infants, toddlers, and pregnant women) that focuses on child development
1997	Children's Health Insurance Program (CHIP) (formerly known as State Children's Health Insurance Program [SCHIP]) (National Conference of State Legislatures, 2015)	Offers federal assistance to state-based health insurance for low-income families that are not eligible for Medicaid but cannot afford private insurance
2000	Children's Health Act	Lead to increased research and treatment of health issues concerning children such as autism, asthma, epilepsy, and oral health
2002	No Child Left Behind Act	To ensure that all children in all classrooms receive research-based curriculum, well-prepared teachers, and a safe learning environment

(continued)

TABLE 1.6 MILESTONES IN FEDERAL PROGRAMS IN SUPPORT OF THE HEALTH OF WOMEN AND CHILDREN (continued)

Date	Action	Impact
2006	Combating Autism Act	Lead to increasing autism awareness by increasing funding for research, surveillance, diagnosis, and treatment
2007	WIC Food Package Revised	Designed to improve nutritional intake of WIC recipients by supporting and promoting long-term breast-feeding and adding fruits and vegetables, whole grains, soy-based foods, and a variety of culturally appropriate foods
2008	Newborn Screening Saving Lives Act	Provided increased funding for newborn screening grants and provided more education and outreach, coordination of follow-up care after screening and evaluation of newborn screening programs effectiveness
2009	Children's Health Insurance Program Reauthorization Act	Expanded the program to cover more uninsured children
2009	American Recovery and Reinvestment Act	Designated money to fund and expand programs such as Head Start, foster care, and the Supplemental Nutrition Assistance Program (Food Stamp Program) as well as creating new jobs and improving services such as community health centers and unemployment benefits during the economic recession
2010	Affordable Care Act (Patient Protection & Affordable Care Act); Health Care & Education Reconciliation Act	Increases coverage by expanding Medicaid, ends pre-existing conditions exclusion for children; holds insurance companies accountable by ending lifetime coverage limits, requiring insurance companies to publicly justify premium increases; decreases healthcare costs; increases choice and enhances quality of care for all Americans by covering all preventative care

Adapted from National Conference of State Legislatures. (2015). *Children's Health Insurance Program (CHIP)*. Retrieved from https://www.healthcare.gov/medicaid-chip/childrens-health-insurance-program/; Yarrow, A. L. (2011). A history of federal child antipoverty and health policy in the United States since 1900. *Child Development Perspectives, 5*(1), 66–72; U.S. Department of Health and Human Services [USDHHS]. (2015). MCH timeline. *Maternal and Child Health Bureau*. Retrieved from http://mchb.hrsa.gov/about/timeline/index.html

percent of all pregnancies (excluding miscarriages) end in abortion (Alan Guttmacher Institute [AGI], 2014). In September 2000, the U.S. Food and Drug Administration approved mifepristone to be marketed in the United States as an alternative to surgical abortion. Medication abortion using mifepristone or a similar medication accounted for 38% of all nonhospital abortions, and about one quarter of abortions before 9 weeks' gestation (AGI, 2014).

Abortion has become a hotly debated political issue that separates people into two camps: pro-choice and pro-life. The pro-choice group supports the right of any woman to make decisions about her reproductive functions based on her own moral and ethical beliefs. The pro-life group feels strongly that abortion is murder and deprives the fetus of the basic right to life. Both sides will continue to debate this very emotional issue for years to come.

Medical and surgical modalities are available to terminate a pregnancy, depending on how far the pregnancy has developed. A surgical intervention can be performed up to 12 weeks' gestation; a medical intervention can be performed up to 9 weeks' gestation (King et al., 2015). All women undergoing abortion need emotional support, a stable environment in which to recover, and nonjudgmental care throughout the experience.

Abortion is a complex issue, and the controversy is not only in the public arena; many nurses struggle with the conflict between their personal convictions and their professional duty. Nurses are taught to be supportive client advocates and to interact with a nonjudgmental attitude under all circumstances even when personal and political views differ from those of their clients.

With all the advances in abortion care, this points toward greater nursing involvement. Although this bodes well for woman-centered care, the burden on nurses is likely to increase incrementally. This may have an adverse effect on the affective attributes or emotions that those nurses possess (McLemore, Levi, & James, 2015).

Nurses need to clarify their personal values and beliefs on this issue and must be able to provide nonbiased care before assuming responsibility for clients who might be in a position to consider abortion. Their decision to care for or refuse to care for such clients affects staff unity, influences staffing decisions, and challenges the ethical concept of duty (McLemore, Kools, & Levi, 2015).

The American Nurses Association's updated Code of Ethics for Nurses upholds the nurse's right to refuse to care for a client undergoing an abortion if the nurse ethically opposes the procedure (ANA, 2016). Nurses need to make their values and beliefs known to their managers before the situation occurs so that alternative staffing arrangements can be made. Open communication and acceptance of the personal beliefs of others can promote a comfortable working environment.

Substance Abuse

Substance abuse for any person is a problem, but when it involves a pregnant woman, substance abuse can cause fetal injury and thus has legal and ethical implications. Substance abuse during pregnancy may cause fetal anomalies, preterm birth, placenta abruption, and central nervous system developmental alterations (Viteri et al., 2015). Many state laws require reporting evidence of prenatal drug exposure, which may lead to charges of negligence and child endangerment against the pregnant woman. It has been found that incarceration, or threat of it, has no effect in reducing cases of alcohol or drug abuse (Malinowska-Semprunch & Rychkova, 2015). This punitive approach to fetal injury raises ethical and legal questions about the degree of governmental control that is appropriate in the interests of child safety. All pregnant women and women of childbearing age should be screened periodically for alcohol, tobacco, and prescription and illicit drug use. Nurses should employ a flexible approach to the care of women who have substance use problems, and they should encourage the use of all available community resources. Nurses should counsel women about the risks of preconception, antepartum, and postpartum substance abuse in a calm, nonjudgmental manner (Galante, French, & Grace, 2015).

Intrauterine Therapy

Progress in prenatal diagnosis can lead to the diagnosis of severe fetal abnormalities for which previously one would anticipate a fatal outcome or the development of severe disability despite optimal postnatal care. Intrauterine therapy can now be offered in these selected cases and also in the treatment of fetal obstructive uropathy, intrauterine transfusions for fetal anemia, spina bifida repair, and stem cell transplantation. Intrauterine therapy is a procedure that involves opening the uterus during pregnancy, performing a surgery, and replacing the fetus in the uterus. Although the risks to the fetus and the mother are both great, fetal therapy may be used to correct anatomic lesions (Yuan, 2015). Some argue that medical technology should not interfere with nature, and thus this intervention should not take place. Others would argue that the surgical intervention improves the child's quality of life. For many people, these are the subjects of debates and intellectual discussions, but for nurses, these procedures may be part of their daily routine.

Nurses play an important supportive role in caring and advocating for clients and their families. As the use of technology grows, situations will surface more frequently that test a nurse's belief system. Encouraging open discussions to address emotional issues and differences of opinion among staff members is healthy and increases tolerance for differing points of view.

Maternal–Fetal Conflict

In maternity nursing, the ethical principles of beneficence and autonomy provide the fundamental framework that guides the management of all pregnant women. As there is the need for consideration of the fetus, autonomy can become a complex issue, which gives rise to what is sometimes called the **maternal–fetal conflict**.

Fetal care becomes problematic when what is required to benefit one member of the dyad will cause an unacceptable harm to the other. When a fetal condition poses no health threat to the mother, caring for the fetal client will always carry some degree of risk to the mother, without direct therapeutic benefit for her. The ethical principles of beneficence ("be of benefit") and nonmaleficence ("do no harm") can come into conflict.

Because the clients are biologically linked, both, or neither, must be treated alike. It would be unethical to recommend fetal therapy as if it were medically indicated for both clients. Still, given a recommendation for fetal therapy, pregnant women, in most cases, will consent to treatment, which promotes fetal health. When pregnant women refuse therapy, health care providers must remember that the ethical injunction against harming one client in order to benefit another is virtually absolute.

The use of court orders to force treatment on pregnant women raises many ethical concerns. Court orders force pregnant women to forfeit their autonomy in ways not required of competent men or nonpregnant women. There is an inconsistency in allowing competent adults to refuse therapy in all cases but pregnancy. The American College of Obstetricians and Gynecologists (ACOG) advocates counseling and education to convince a mother to follow her doctor's advice and condemns the use of coercion on a pregnant woman, as this violates the intent of the informed consent process. Faced with a continuing disagreement with a pregnant woman, a physician should turn to an institutional ethics committee. Resorting to the legal system is almost never justified (Avci, 2015).

Stem Cell Research

Stem cells constitute one of the most promising tools for regenerative medicine. They can grow into any cell type in the body and have been touted as a potential cure for everything from type 1 diabetes to stroke. The goal of stem cell research is a relief of human suffering, which ethically is good. Benefits of stem cell research include therapies for Parkinson disease, regeneration of diseased body tissues, repair of spinal cord injuries, and the growing of needed organs for transplant.

It would seem morally compelling to explore all the sources that might provide us with them, but the ethical concerns surrounding stem cell research vary depending on the origin of the stem cells. Adult stem cells are found in adults, who can replace old cells by reproducing new ones (e.g., blood and liver cells). Bone marrow transplants are examples of the use of adult stem cells in medical therapy. Embryonic stem cells are derived from the inner cell mass of an early embryo. They aren't without controversy; the process of obtaining these cells results in the destruction of the embryo. However, they hold huge promise too (de Miguel-Beriain, 2015).

Some people feel that the destruction of the human embryo constitutes the killing of a human being and reject this practice on religious grounds. Views about when life begins and whether the early embryo is considered a person with moral status are the heart of the ethical deliberations related to embryonic stem cells. Everyone has to decide based on their own personal values and ethical background.

Umbilical Cord Blood Banking

Umbilical cord blood, the remaining blood in the umbilical cord at birth, can be collected and be a source of stem cells for an individual in need of a bone marrow transplant later in life. It can also be used for admission laboratory studies in neonates and also for a transfusion if needed (Carroll & Christensen, 2015). The extraordinary scientific and technologic advance of contemporary medicine constantly leads toward the introduction of new treatments. Umbilical cord blood is a potential vast source of primitive hematopoietic stem and progenitor cells available for clinical application. Cord blood can be used as an alternative source for bone marrow transplantation and its use is developing into a new field of treatment for pediatric and adult clients presenting with hematologic disorders, immunologic defects, and specific genetic diseases (Roura et al., 2015).

Blood from a newborn's umbilical cord, once considered a waste product that was routinely discarded along with the placenta, is now considered to contain potentially life-saving stem cells. Banks were initially developed to store cord blood stem cells from newborns, for a fee, for potential future use by the same child or a family member if the child developed disease later in life. Today, there are public banks that store, for free, stem cells that can be used by anyone needing them, similar to how public blood banks work.

Pregnant women should be aware that stem cells from cord blood cannot currently be used to treat inborn errors of metabolism or other genetic diseases in the same individual from which they were collected because the cord blood would have the same genetic mutation. Cord blood collected from a newborn that later develops childhood leukemia cannot be used to treat that leukemia for much the same reason. Umbilical cord banks are a central component, as umbilical cord tissue providers, in both medical treatment and scientific research with stem cells. But, whereas the creation of umbilical cord banks is seen as successful practice, others perceive it as ethically risky.

The fact that private cord banks offer their services as "biologic insurance" in order to obtain informed consent by promising the parents that the tissue that will be stored to insure the health of their child in the future raises the issue of whether the consent is freely given or given under coercion. Another consideration that must be made in relation to privately owned cord banks involves the ownership of the stored umbilical cord. Conflicts between moral principles and economic interests (many physicians own private blood banks) cause dilemmas in the clinical practice of umbilical cord blood storage and use, especially in privately owned banks (Ballen, Verter, & Kurtzberg, 2015).

Both the ACOG (2012) and AAP (2012) have reaffirmed previously issued statements opposing the use of for-profit banks and criticizing their marketing tactics. Instead, they recommended that parents donate cord blood to public banks, which make it available for free to anyone who needs it. Globally, other organizations have done the same. Private umbilical cord blood banking raises a question of special legal regulation. This practice promises the safe storage of biologic material on the assumption that it may be useful, at a certain moment in future, for its own donor (or for a donor's close family member) for curing serious blood diseases (Kim, Han, & Shin, 2015). Nurses need to provide unbiased education about this topic with all pregnant women and their families to allow informed choices to be made.

Informed Consent

Most care given in a health care setting is covered by the initial consent for treatment signed when the person becomes a client at that office or clinic, or by the consent to treatment signed upon admission to the hospital or other inpatient facility. Certain procedures, however, require a specific process of informed consent. Procedures that require informed consent include major and minor surgery; invasive procedures such as amniocentesis, internal fetal monitoring, lumbar puncture, or bone marrow aspiration; treatments placing the person at higher risk, such as chemotherapy or radiation therapy; procedures or treatments involving research; application of restraints; and photography involving the person.

Generally, only people over the age of majority (18 years of age) can legally provide consent for health care. Because children are minors, the process of consent involves obtaining written permission from a parent or legal guardian. In cases requiring a signature for consent, usually the parent gives consent for care of children less than 18 years of age except in certain situations (see discussion that follows).

Take Note!

Never assume that the adult accompanying the child is the parent or legal guardian. Always clarify the relationship of the accompanying adult.

The informed consent process, which must be done before the procedure or specific care, addresses the legal and ethical requirement of informing the person about the procedure. It originates from the right of the child and family to direct their care and the ethical responsibility of health care providers to involve the child and family in health care decisions. Nurses should involve children and adolescents in the decision-making process to the extent possible, though the parent is still ultimately responsible for giving consent. The physician or advanced practitioner providing or performing the treatment and/or procedure is responsible for informing the child and family about the procedure and obtaining consent by providing a detailed description of the procedure or treatment, the potential risks and benefits, and alternative methods available.

The nurse's responsibility related to informed consent includes the following:

- Ensuring that the consent form is completed with signatures from the client (or parents or legal guardians if the client is a child)
- Serving as a witness to the signature process
- Determining whether the client or parents or legal guardians understand what they are signing by asking them pertinent questions

Box 1.5 describes the key elements of informed consent, although laws vary from state to state.

Nurses must become familiar with state laws as well as the policies and procedures of the health care agency. Treating children without obtaining proper informed consent violates their rights, and the physician and/or facility may be held liable for any damages (Murray, 2012).

BOX 1.5

KEY ELEMENTS OF INFORMED CONSENT

- The decision maker must be of legal age in that state, with full civil rights, and must be competent (have the ability to make the decision).
- Present information that is simple, concise, and appropriate to the level of education and language of the individual responsible for making the decision.
- The decision must be voluntary, and without coercion, force, or influence of duress.
- Have a witness to the process of informed consent.
- Have the witness sign the consent form.

Special Situations to Informed Consent

There are special situations related to informed consent. If the parent is not available, then the person in charge (relative, babysitter, or teacher) may give consent for emergency treatment if that person has a signed form from the parent or legal guardian allowing him or her to do so. During an emergency situation, a verbal consent via the telephone may be obtained. Two witnesses must be listening simultaneously and will sign the consent form, indicating that consent was received via telephone. Health care providers can provide emergency treatment to a child without consent if they have made reasonable attempts to contact the child's parent or legal guardian (AAP, Committee on Pediatric Emergency Medicine, & Committee on Bioethics [CPEMCB], 2011; Wright, 2011). In urgent or emergent situations, appropriate medical care never should be delayed or withheld due to an inability to obtain consent (AAP, CPEMCB, 2011; Wright, 2011). Certain federal laws, such as the Emergency Medical Treatment and Labor Act (EMTALA), require that every client who presents at an emergency department is given a medical examination regardless of informed consent or reimbursement ability (AAP, CPEMCB, 2011; Wright, 2011). Table 1.7 gives further information about other special situations.

Exceptions to Parental Consent Requirement

In some states, a **mature minor** may give consent to certain medical treatment. The health care provider must determine that the adolescent (usually over 14 years of age) is sufficiently mature and intelligent to make the decision for treatment. The provider also considers the complexity of the treatment, its risks and benefits, and whether the treatment is necessary or elective before obtaining consent from a mature minor (AAP, CPEMCB, 2011; Wright, 2011).

TABLE 1.7 SPECIAL CONSIDERATIONS RELATED TO INFORMED CONSENT

Issue	Definition	Nursing Considerations
Child not living with biologic or adoptive parents	Child living: • In foster care • With potential adoptive parent • With a relative	Legally appointed guardian must provide consent Verify authority and include documentation of legally appointed guardian in child's medical record
Parent consent after divorce	Ability to give consent for health care rests with parent who has legal custody by divorce degree	Determine if the parents have joint custody or if there is sole custody by one parent Even the parent with only physical custody may give consent for emergency care May need to seek court involvement if there is joint legal custody but parents disagree on care
Consent for organ donation	For a minor to donate, the parents must be aware of the risks and benefits and must provide emotional support to the child. There should be a close relationship between the donor and recipient, if living-related donation is occurring The minor must agree to donate without coercion in live organ donation	Potential donors should be referred to local organ procurement organization Educate family about policies related to organ donation Legal guardian or parent consents to organ donation (AAP, 2013)
Consent for medical experimentation	Requirements include consent of parents, assent of child, and a perceived benefit to the child (USDHHS, n.d.)	Comply with all federal regulations if federal funds are received (refer to section on assent)

Adapted from American Academy of Pediatrics, Committee on Hospital Care, Section on Surgery, and Section on Critical Care. (2010). Pediatric organ donation and transplantation. *Pediatrics, 125*(4), 822–828; and U.S. Department of Health and Human Services. (n.d.). *Special protections for children as research subjects.* Retrieved from http://www.hhs.gov/ohrp/policy/populations/children.html

State laws vary in relation to the definition of an **emancipated minor** and the types of treatment that may be obtained by an emancipated minor (without parental consent). The nurse must be familiar with the particular state's law. Emancipation may be considered in any of the following situations, depending on the state's laws:

- Membership in a branch of the armed services
- Marriage
- Court-determined emancipation
- Financial independence and living apart from parents
- Pregnancy
- Mother less than 18 years of age

The emancipated minor is considered to have the legal capacity of an adult and may make his or her own health care decisions (AAP, Committee on Bioethics [CB], 2012; Wright, 2011).

Many states do not require consent or notification of parents or legal guardians when providing specific care to minors. Depending on the state law, health care may be provided to minors for certain conditions, in a confidential manner, without including the parents. These types of care may include pregnancy counseling, prenatal care, contraception, testing for and treatment of sexually transmitted infections and communicable diseases (including HIV), substance abuse, and mental illness counseling and treatment (AAP, CB, 2012; Brooke, 2011). These exceptions allow children to seek help in a confidential manner in situations where they might otherwise avoid care if they were required to inform their parents or legal guardian. Again, laws vary by state, so the nurse must be knowledgeable about the laws in the state where he or she is licensed to practice.

Assent

Assent means agreeing to something. In pediatric health care, the term **assent** refers to the child's participation in the decision-making process about health care (AAP, 2012). The age of assent depends on the child's developmental level, maturity, and psychological state. The AAP recommends that children and adolescents be involved in the discussions about their health care and kept informed in an age-appropriate manner (AAP, CB, 2012; Sirbaugh & Diekema, 2011). As a child gets older, assent or dissent should be given more serious consideration. The pediatric client needs to be empowered by health care providers to the extent of their capabilities and as children mature and develop over time they should become the primary decision maker regarding their own health care (AAP, CB, 2012; Sirbaugh & Diekema, 2011). The AAP recommends that if a health care provider asks the child's opinion about the direction of treatment or participation in research, then the child's view and desires should be seriously considered (AAP, CB, 2012; Sirbaugh & Diekema, 2011).

When obtaining assent, first help the child to understand his or her health condition, depending on the child's developmental level. Next, inform the child of the treatment planned and discuss what he or she should expect. Then determine what the child understands about the situation and make sure he or she is not being unduly influenced to make a decision one way or another. Finally, ascertain the child's willingness to participate in the treatment or research (AAP, CB, 2012 Sirbaugh & Diekema, 2011). Assent is a process and should continue throughout the course of treatment or research protocol.

The converse of assent is **dissent** (disagreeing with the treatment plan), and it may be ethically binding (AAP, CB, 2012). If the health care provider is not going to honor the pediatric client's dissent, then the argument can be made that the provider should not ask for the client's assent. In some cases, such as in those of significant morbidity or mortality, dissent may need to be overridden. These cases need to be looked at on an individual basis. If the decision is made to move forward with treatment despite the child's dissent, then this decision must be explained to the child in developmentally appropriate terms.

There has been an increased emphasis on including children in research studies. Children are not little adults but 70% of medicines given to children have only been tested on adults (National Institutes of Health, 2012). In research studies investigators and investigation review boards (IRBs) are responsible for ensuring measures are taken to protect the children in the studies. The nurse caring for these children also has the responsibility to ensure protection at all stages of the research process. Nurses can become members of the IRB; they should also become familiar with studies that have been approved in their work setting to help ensure their pediatric clients are protected.

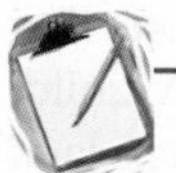

Take Note!

Whenever possible, obtain assent for participation from the child.

Refusal of Medical Treatment

All clients have the right to refuse medical treatment, based on the American Hospital Association's Bill of Rights. Ideally, medical care without informed consent should be used only when the client's life is in danger. Clients may refuse treatment if it conflicts with their religious or cultural beliefs (Brudney & Lantos, 2011). An example would be a Jehovah's Witness. Individuals of this faith have strong beliefs based upon passages from the Bible that are interpreted as prohibiting the "consumption" of blood. Their beliefs prevent them from accepting transfusion of whole blood or its primary components. With recent advances and use of biologic hemostats that aid coagulation and reduce blood loss, major surgery can be performed safely in the Jehovah's Witness who refuses blood transfusion by utilizing these devices (Darwish, 2011). In these cases, it is important to educate the client and family about the importance of the recommended treatment without coercing or forcing the client to agree. Sometimes common ground may be reached between the family's religious or cultural beliefs and the health care team's recommendations. Communication and education are the keys in this situation.

In the case of a child, parental autonomy (the right to decide for or against medical treatment) is a fundamental, constitutionally protected right, but not an absolute one. The general assumption is that parents act in the best interests of their children. Ideally, medical care without informed consent should be given only when the child's life is in danger. In some cases parents may refuse medical treatment for their child. This refusal may arise when treatment conflicts with their religious or cultural beliefs, and the nurse should be aware of some of these common beliefs. Some religions, such as Christian Science, Pentecostal, Church of the First Born, and Followers of Christ, prefer prayer or faith healing over allopathic medicine (Bingham, 2012; Hall, 2013). The Black Muslim culture advocates vegan diets and refuses pork-based medicines or treatments. Hindus may refuse beef-based foods and medicines. People from an Islamic background may refuse the use of any potentially addictive substances such as narcotics or medicines containing alcohol (Leever, 2011). Sometimes common ground may be reached between the family's religious or cultural beliefs and the health care team's recommendations.

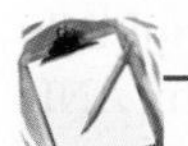

Take Note!

Do not assume what a family's beliefs are based on religious affiliation. Assess each family and child views on an individual basis.

In other cases, parents may refuse treatment if they perceive that their child's quality of life may be significantly impaired by the medical care that is offered. The health care team must appropriately educate the family and communicate with them on a level that they can understand. The child and family should be informed of what to expect with certain tests or treatments. The health care team should make a clinical assessment of the child's and family's understanding of the situation and their reasons for refusing treatment. Active listening may allow the health care provider to address the concerns, fears, or reservations the family may have regarding their child's care.

Refusal of medical care may be considered a form of child neglect. If providing medical treatment may prevent substantial harm and suffering, or save a child's life, health care providers and the judicial system strive to advocate for the child. The state has an overriding interest in the health and welfare of the child and can order that medical treatment to proceed without signed informed consent; this is referred to as *parens patriae* (the state has a right and a duty to protect children). If the parents refuse treatment and the health care team feels the treatment is reasonable and warranted, the case should be referred to the institution's ethics committee. If the issue remains unresolved, or in complex cases, the judicial system may become involved (AAP, 2012).

Advance Directives

The Patient Self-Determination Act of 1990 established the concept of advance directives. Advance directives determine the child's and family's wishes should life-sustaining care become necessary. Parents are generally the surrogate decision makers for children. If the child's interests are not served by prolonged survival, then the physician or advanced practitioner should educate the parents about the extent of the child's illness and potential for ongoing quality of life (Edwards et al., 2012). After discussion with other family members, friends, and spiritual advisors, the parents may make the decision to forego life-sustaining medical treatment, either withdrawing treatment or deciding to withhold further treatment or opt not to resuscitate in the event of cardiopulmonary arrest (McGowan, 2011).

Life-sustaining care may include antibiotics, chemotherapy, dialysis, ventilation, cardiopulmonary resuscitation, and artificial nutrition and hydration. Some families may choose to withdraw these treatments if they are already in place or to not begin them should the need arise. **Do not attempt resuscitation (DNAR)** orders are in place for some children, particularly the terminally ill. Some institutions have started using the term AND (Allow Natural Death). No matter what term is used, these orders should include specific instructions regarding the child's and family's wishes (e.g., some families may desire oxygen but not chest compressions or code medications). When the child is hospitalized, the DNAR order must be documented in the physician orders and updated according to the facility's policy. DNAR orders may also be in place in the home, but only a few states allow emergency medical services to honor a child's DNAR order in the home. Children with DNAR orders may also still be attending school. In that case, the health care professionals involved should meet with the school officials (the board of education and its legal counsel) to discuss how the DNAR request can be upheld in the school setting (McGowan, 2011). The health care provider should help educate the school about the child's condition, potential complications, and health care goals (AAP, Committee on School Health and Committee on Bioethics [CSHCB], 2013). They should work with the school and family on developing an individualized health care plan that will include what to do instead of CPR such as comfort measures (AAP, CSHCB, 2013).

The Baby Doe regulations, which are an amendment to the United States Child Abuse Protection and Treatment Act, provide specific guidelines on how to treat extremely ill, premature, terminally ill, and/or disabled infants regardless of the parents' wishes (Tucker et al., 2011).

Health care providers must continue to work with parents of extremely sick or premature infants to ensure they are accurately informed about the condition of their child and the risks and benefits to treatment. Health care providers must also be aware of federal, state, and hospital policy regarding care of very ill, premature, and/or disabled newborns.

The nurse must be knowledgeable about the laws related to health care of children in the state where he or she practices as well as the policies of the health care institution. The nurse must be sensitive to the various ethical situations that he or she may become involved in and should apply knowledge of laws as well as concepts of ethics to provide appropriate care.

Client Rights

The American Hospital Association first established a Patient's Bill of Rights in 1972 as a way to promote the value and dignity of the client. This information is updated periodically. Most health care agencies and professional organizations have developed some type of document that addresses client rights.

Ensuring that client rights are upheld is a key aspect in the care of any client. For the pregnant woman, two clients must be considered—the pregnant woman and her fetus. The American Foundation for Maternal and Child Health developed the Pregnant Patient's Bill of Rights to address specific concerns and situations involving the health and well-being of the mother and her fetus. In addition, the U.S. Department of Health and Human Services has issued laws related to protecting the welfare of newborns (the Baby Doe law). A child, due to his or her age and developmental level, may lack mature decision-making abilities. Many pediatric institutions have adopted a bill of rights for children's health care specific to that institution. This might include the following rights:

- To be called by name
- To receive compassionate health care in a careful, prompt, and courteous manner

- To know the names of all providers caring for the child
- To have basic needs met and usual schedules or routines honored
- To make choices whenever possible
- To be kept without food or drink when necessary for the shortest time possible
- To be unrestrained if able
- To have parents or other important persons with the child
- To have an interpreter for the child and family when needed
- To object noisily if desired
- To be educated honestly about the child's health care
- To be respected as a person (not having people talk about the child within earshot unless the child knows what is happening)
- For all health care providers, to respect the child's confidentiality about his or her illness at all times (adapted from Children's Hospital Los Angeles, 2012)

Confidentiality

With the establishment of the Health Insurance Portability and Accountability Act (HIPAA) of 1996, the confidentiality of health care information is now mandated by law. The primary intent of the law is to maintain health insurance coverage for workers and their families when they change or lose jobs. Another aspect of the law requires the Department of Health and Human Services to establish national standards for electronic transmission of health information. With the increased use of electronic medical records (EMRs) and electronic billing came the increased possibility that personal health information might be inappropriately distributed. Client confidentiality and privacy must be maintained in the same manner as it is with paper documentation. Nurses can ensure that privacy is maintained when using computerized documentation and EMRs by doing the following:

- Always maintain the security of personal log-in information; nurses should never share it with other health care providers or other persons.
- Always log off when leaving the computer.
- Do not leave client information visible on a monitor screen when the computer/monitor is unattended.
- Use safeguards, such as encryption, when using alternative means of communication such as email.

Exceptions to confidentiality exist. For example, suspicion of physical or sexual abuse and injuries caused by a weapon or criminal act must be reported to the proper authorities. Abuse cases are reported to the appropriate welfare authorities, whereas criminal acts are reported to the police. In addition, if the minor is a threat to self, then information may need to be disclosed to protect the child. The health care provider must also follow public health laws that require reporting certain infectious diseases to the local health department (e.g., tuberculosis, hepatitis, HIV, and other sexually transmitted infections). Finally, there is a duty to warn third parties when a specific threat is made to an identifiable person.

Health care providers must strike a balance between confidentiality and required disclosure. Even if disclosure is required it is recommended that the health care provider attempt to gain consent for the disclosure and when possible inform the minor of the limits to confidentiality and consent prior to the initiation of care (Murray, Calhoun, & Philipsen, 2011).

IMPLICATIONS FOR NURSES

The health care system is intricately woven into the political and social structure of our society, and nurses should understand social, legal, and ethical health care issues so that they can play an active role in meeting the health care needs of women, children, and families. Nurses need to take a proactive role in advocating for and empowering their clients. For example, nurses can help women to increase control over the factors that affect health, thereby improving their health status. A woman may become empowered by developing skills not only to cope with her environment, but also to change it. Nurses also can assume this mentoring role with children and families, thus helping them to improve their overall health status and health outcomes.

Nurses must have a solid knowledge base about the factors affecting maternal and child health and barriers to health care. They can use this information to provide anticipatory guidance, health counseling, and teaching for women, children, and families. It also is useful in identifying high-risk groups so that interventions can be initiated early on, before problems occur.

When caring for women, children, and families, the nurse operates within the framework of the nursing process, which is applicable to all health care settings. Maternal and child health nursing is everchanging as globalization and the exchange of information expands. Nurses must remain up to date about new technologies and treatments and integrate high-quality, evidence-based interventions into the care they provide.

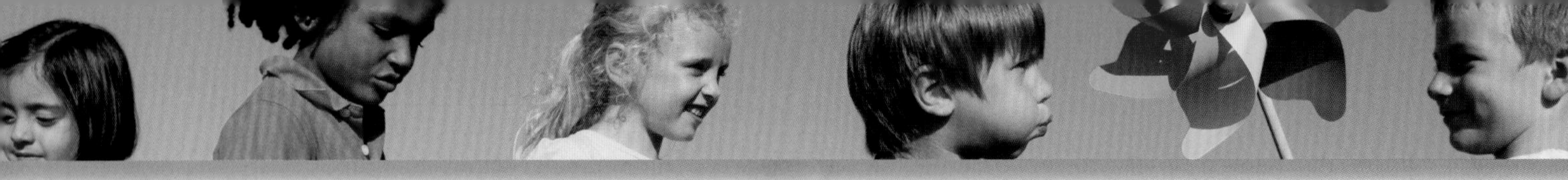

KEY CONCEPTS

- *Healthy People 2020* presents a national set of health goals and objectives for adults and children that focus on health promotion and disease prevention.
- One method to establish the aggregate health status of women, infants, and children is with statistical data, such as mortality and morbidity rates.
- The infant mortality rate is the lowest in the history of the United States, but it is still higher when compared with other industrialized countries. This high rate may be the result of the increase in low-birth-weight infants born in this country.
- The family is considered the basic social unit. The family greatly influences the development and health of its members. Members learn health care activities, health beliefs, and health values from their family.
- Social roles are often an important factor in the development of one's self-concept, which can have a very positive influence on health or present various limitations and problems, possibly resulting in a negative influence on health.
- Culture influences every aspect of development and is reflected in childbearing and child-rearing beliefs and practices designed to promote healthy adaptation.
- Spirituality, a major influence for many individuals, provides a meaning and purpose to life and is a foundation for and a source of love, relationships, and service. Spiritual and religious beliefs and views can provide strength and support to women, children, and their families during times of stress and illness.
- Other factors impacting the health of women and children include health status and lifestyles, improved diagnosis and treatment, and health care consumer empowerment. Finances, transportation, language, culture, and the health care delivery system can provide barriers to health care.
- Advances in science and technology have led to increased ethical dilemmas in health care.
- All clients have the right to refuse medical treatment based on the American Hospital Association's Bill of Rights. For a child, the parents have the legal right to decide for or against medical treatment. Minor children (under the age of 18 years) must have their parents or legal guardians provide consent for health care in most cases.
- In certain states, mature minors and emancipated minors may consent to their own health care and certain health care may be provided to adolescents without parental notification, including contraception, pregnancy counseling, prenatal care, testing and treatment of sexually transmitted infections and communicable diseases (including HIV), substance abuse and mental illness counseling and treatment, and health care required as a result of a crime-related injury.
- The nurse must be knowledgeable about the laws related to health care of women and children in the specific state of nursing practice as well as the specific policies of the health care institution.

REFERENCES AND RECOMMENDED READINGS

Adams, S. M., Ward, C. E., & Garcia, K. L. (2015). Sudden infant death syndrome. *American Family Physician, 91*(11), 778–783.

Adams-Leander, S., & Rector, C. (2014). Chapter 5: Transcultural nursing in the community. In J. A. Allender, C. Rector, & K. D. Warner (Eds.), *Community & public health nursing. Promoting the public's health* (8th ed., pp. 115–149). Philadephia, PA: Wolters Kluwer Health/Lippincott Williams & Wilkins.

Addy, S., Engelhardt, W., & Skinner, C. (2013). *Basic facts about low-income children: Children under 18 years, 2011*. Retrieved from http://www.nccp.org/publications/pdf/text_1074.pdf

Alan Guttmacher Institute. (2014). *Induced abortion in the United States*. Retrieved from http://www.guttmacher.org/pubs/fb_induced_abortion.html

Alhusen, J. L., Ray, E., Sharps, P., & Bullock, L. (2015). Intimate partner violence during pregnancy: Maternal and neonatal outcomes. *Journal of Women's Health, 24*(1), 100–106.

Allin, S., & Stabile, M. (2012). Socioeconomic status and child health: What is the role of health care, health conditions, injuries and maternal health? *Health Economics, Policy, and Law, 7*(2), 227–242.

Alzola, K. J., & Marino, M. (2015). Women's mental health around the world: Education, poverty, discrimination and violence, and political aspects. In *Psychopathology in women* (pp. 3–24). New York, NY: Springer International Publishing.

American Academy of Child and Adolescent Psychiatry. (2012a). *Children and divorce*. Retrieved from http://www.aacap.org/App_Themes/AACAP/docs/facts_for_families/01_children_and_divorce.pdf

American Academy of Child and Adolescent Psychiatry. (2012b). *Facts for families: Grandparents raising grandchildren*. Retrieved from http://www.aacap.org/App_Themes/AACAP/docs/facts_for_families/77_grandparents_raising_grandchildren.pdf

American Academy of Pediatrics. (2012a). *Guidance for effective discipline.* Retrieved from http://pediatrics.aappublications.org/content/101/4/723.full.

American Academy of Pediatrics. (2012b). Policy statement reaffirmed: Cord blood banking for potential future transplant. *Pediatrics, 130*(2), e467–e468.

American Academy of Pediatrics. (2013a). Policy statement: Children, adolescents, and the media. *Pediatrics.* doi: 10.1542/peds.2013-2656.

American Academy of Pediatrics. (2013b). Policy statement: Ethical controversies in organ donation after circulatory death. *Pediatrics, 131*(5), 1021–1026.

American Academy of Pediatrics. (2015a). *Disciplining your child.* Retrieved from http://www.healthychildren.org/english/family-life/family-dynamics/communication-discipline/pages/disciplining-your-child.aspx.

American Academy of Pediatrics. (2015b). *Gender identity development in children.* Retrieved from http://www.healthychildren.org/English/ages-stages/gradeschool/pages/Gender-Identity-and-Gender-Confusion-In-Children.aspx

American Academy of Pediatrics. (2015c). *The internet and your family.* Retrieved from http://www.healthychildren.org/English/family-life/Media/pages/The-Internet-and-Your-Family.aspx

American Academy of Pediatrics. (n. d.). *Promoting children's mental health.* Retrieved from http://www.aap.org/en-us/advocacy-and-policy/federal-advocacy/Pages/mentalhealth.aspx

American Academy of Pediatrics, Committee on Bioethics. (2012). *Informed consent, parental permission, and assent in pediatric practice.* Retrieved from http://pediatrics.aappublications.org/content/95/2/314

American Academy of Pediatrics, Committee on Community Health Services. (2010). Providing care for immigrant, homeless, and migrant children. *Pediatrics, 115*(4), 1095–1100.

American Academy of Pediatrics, Committee on Hospital Care, Section on Surgery, and Section on Critical Care. (2010). Pediatric organ donation and transplantation. *Pediatrics, 125*(4), 822–828.

American Academy of Pediatrics, Committee on Pediatric Emergency Medicine, & Committee on Bioethics. (2011). Consent for emergency medical services for children and adolescents. *Pediatrics, 128*(2), 427–433.

American Academy of Pediatrics, Committee on School Health and Committee on Bioethics. (2013). Policy statement: Honoring do-not-attempt resuscitation requests in school. *Pediatrics, 125*(5), 1073–1077.

American Cancer Society. (2015a). *Cancer facts for women.* Retrieved from http://www.cancer.org/healthy/findcancerearly/womenshealth/cancer-facts-for-women

American Cancer Society. (2015b). *What are the key statistics about breast cancer?* Retrieved from http://www.cancer.org/cancer/breastcancer/detailedguide/breast-cancer-key-statistics

American Cancer Society. (2015c). *What are the key statistics about lung cancer?* Retrieved from http://www.cancer.org/cancer/lungcancer-non-smallcell/detailedguide/non-small-cell-lung-cancer-key-statistics

American College of Nurse-Midwives. (2015). *About midwives.* Retrieved from http://www.midwife.org/About-Midwives

American College of Obstetricians and Gynecologists. (2012). *Committee opinion number 399: Umbilical cord blood banking.* Retrieved from http://www.acog.org/Resources-And-Publications/Committee-Opinions/Committee-on-Obstetric-Practice/Umbilical-Cord-Blood-Banking

American Nurses Association [ANA]. (2016). *Code of ethics for nurses.* Retrieved from: http://www.nursingworld.org/codeofethics

American Psychological Association. (2015). *The impact of terrorism and disasters on children.* Retrieved from http://www.apa.org/about/gr/issues/cyf/disaster.aspx

Andrews, M. M., & Boyle, J. (2015). *Transcultural concepts in nursing care* (7th ed.). Philadelphia, PA: Lippincott Williams & Wilkins.

Avci, E. (2015). Caregivers' role in maternal–fetal conflict. *Narrative Inquiry In Bioethics, 5*(1), 67–76.

Ballen, K. K., Verter, F., & Kurtzberg, J. (2015). Umbilical cord blood donation: Public or private? *Bone Marrow Transplantation, 50*(10), 1271–1278.

Baxter, J., Weston, R., & Lixia, Q. (2011). Family structure, co-parental relationship quality, post-separation paternal involvement and children's emotional well-being. *Journal of Family Studies, 17*(2), 86–109.

Bediako, P. T., BeLue, R., & Hillemeier, M. M. (2015). A comparison of birth outcomes among Black, Hispanic, and Black Hispanic women. *Journal of Racial and Ethnic Health Disparities, 2*(4), 573–582.

Beers, M. (2011). Strategies for intervention: Guiding parents of young children in sensitive caregiving. *Brown University Child & Adolescent Behavior Letter, 27*(12), 1–7.

Bembry, J. (2011). Strengthening fragile families through research and practice. *Journal of Family Social Work, 14*(1), 54–67.

Bernedo, I. M., Salas, M. D., García-Martín, M. A., & Fuentes, M. J. (2012). Teacher assessment of behavior problems in foster care children. *Children & Youth Services Review, 34*(4), 615–621.

Bingham, S. (2012). Refusal of treatment and decision-making capacity. *Nursing Ethics, 19*(1), 167–172.

Bloom B., Cohen R. A., & Freeman G. (2012). Summary of health statistics for U.S. children: National Health Interview Survey, 2011. National Center for Health Statistics. *Vital Health Stat, 10*(254), 1–88.

Bohon, D. (2011). Gallop: More than 90 percent of Americans believe in God. *The Eau Claire Journal.* Retrieved from http://www.eauclairejournal.com/news/story.phtml/8EE8E277/religion/gallup_more_than_90_percent_of_americans_believe_in_god/archive/

Brooke, P. (2011). Legal questions. Informed consent: Take time to ask. *Nursing, 41*(8), 12.

Brown, N. (2015). How the American Heart Association helped change women's heart health. *Circulation: Cardiovascular Quality and Outcomes, 8*(2 suppl 1), S60–S62.

Brudney, D., & Lantos, J. (2011). Agency and authenticity: Which value grounds patient choice? *Theoretical Medicine and Bioethics, 32*(4), 217–227.

Cancello, R. (2015). Obesity and inflammation in pregnancy. In *Metabolic syndrome and complications of pregnancy* (pp. 65–75). New York, NY: Springer International Publishing.

Carroll, P. D., & Christensen, R. D. (2015). New and underutilized uses of umbilical cord blood in neonatal care. *Maternal Health, Neonatology and Perinatology, 1*(1), 16–23.

Ceballos, K., & Dunwoody, M. E. (2015). *Cultural perspectives in childbearing*. Retrieved from http://ce.nurse.com/course/ce263–60/cultural-perspectives-in-childbearing/

Centers for Disease Control and Prevention. (2012). *Youth violence facts at a glance*. Retrieved from http://www.cdc.gov/violenceprevention/pdf/yv-datasheet-a.pdf

Centers for Disease Control and Prevention (CDC) (2014a). *Adverse childhood experiences study: Major findings*. Retrieved from http://www.cdc.gov/violenceprevention/acestudy/findings.html

Centers for Disease Control and Prevention. (2014b). *Child maltreatment facts at a glance*. Retrieved from http://www.cdc.gov/violenceprevention/pdf/childmaltreatment-facts-at-a-glance.pdf

Centers for Disease Control and Prevention. (2014c). *School violence: Data & statistics*. Retrieved from http://www.cdc.gov/violenceprevention/youthviolence/schoolviolence/data_stats.html

Centers for Disease Control and Prevention (2015a). *Adolescent and school health: Health & academics*. Retrieved from http://www.cdc.gov/HealthyYouth/health_and_academics/index.htm

Centers for Disease Control and Prevention. (2015b). *Deaths and mortality*. Retrieved from http://www.cdc.gov/nchs/fastats/deaths.htm

Centers for Disease Control and Prevention. (2015c). *Fetal deaths*. Retrieved from http://www.cdc.gov/nchs/fetal_death.htm

Centers for Disease Control and Prevention. (2015d). *Deaths and Mortality*. Retrieved from http://www.cdc.gov/nchs/fastats/deaths.htm

Centers for Disease Control and Prevention. (2015e). *Pregnancy complications*. Retrieved from http://www.cdc.gov/reproductivehealth/MaternalInfantHealth/PregComplications.htm

Centers for Disease Control and Prevention. (2015f). *Pregnancy Mortality Surveillance System*. Retrieved from http://www.cdc.gov/reproductivehealth/maternalinfanthealth/pmss.html

Centers for Disease Control and Prevention. (2015g). *Pregnancy-related deaths*. Retrieved from http://www.cdc.gov/reproductivehealth/maternalinfanthealth/pregnancy-relatedmortality.htm

Centers for Disease Control and Prevention. (2015h). *Suicide facts at a glance*. Retrieved from http://www.cdc.gov/violenceprevention/pdf/suicide-datasheet-a.pdf

Centers for Disease Control and Prevention. (2015i). *Understanding bullying fact sheet*. Retrieved from http://www.cdc.gov/ViolencePrevention/pdf/Bullying_Factsheet-a.pdf

Centers for Disease Control and Prevention. (2015j). *Understanding school violence fact sheet*. Retrieved from http://www.cdc.gov/violenceprevention/pdf/school_violence_fact_sheet-a.pdf

Centers for Disease Control and Prevention. (2015k). *Understanding youth violence fact sheet*. Retrieved from http://www.cdc.gov/violenceprevention/pdf/yv-factsheet-a.pdf

Centers for Disease Control and Prevention, National Center for Health Statistics. (2015). *Child health*. Retrieved from http://www.cdc.gov/nchs/fastats/child-health.htm

Central Intelligence Agency. (2015). *The CIA world factbook 2015*. Retrieved from https://www.cia.gov/library/publications/the-world-factbook/geos/us.html

CIA World Factbook. (2015). *Country comparison: Infant mortality rate*. Retrieved from https://www.cia.gov/library/publications/the-world-factbook/rankorder/2091rank.html

Chen, E., Cohen, S., & Miller, G. E. (2010). How low socioeconomic status affects 2-year hormonal trajectories in children. *Psychological Science, 21*(1), 31–37.

Cherry, K. (2015). Parenting styles: The four styles of parenting. Retrieved from http://psychology.about.com/od/developmentalpsychology/a/parenting-style.htm

Children's Defense Fund. (2012). *The state of America's children: 2012*. Retrieved from http://www.childrensdefense.org/child-research-data-publications/data/soac-2012-handbook.pdf

Child Trends. (2013). *Children's exposure to violence*. Retrieved from http://www.childtrends.org/?indicators=childrens-exposure-to-violence

Child Trends DataBank. (2015a). *Infant, child, and teen morality*. Retrieved from http://www.childtrends.org/wp-content/uploads/2012/11/63_Child_Mortality.pdf

Child Trends DataBank. (2015b). Family Structure: Indicators on children and youth. Retrieved from http://www.childtrends.org/wp-content/uploads/2015/03/59_Family_Structure.pdf

Children's Hospital Los Angeles. (2012). *Your child's rights*. Retrieved from http://www.chla.org/patient-rights

Child Welfare Information Gateway. (2013). *What is child abuse and neglect? Recognizing the signs and symptoms*. Washington, DC: U.S. Department of Health and Human Services, Children's Bureau.

Cox, K. J., & King, T. L. (2015). Preventing primary cesarean births: Midwifery care. *Clinical Obstetrics and Gynecology, 58*(2), 282–293.

Crawford, N. M., & Steiner, A. Z. (2015). Age-related infertility. *Obstetrics and Gynecology Clinics of North America, 42*(1), 15–25.

Crawford, N. A., Schrock, M., & Woodruff-Borden, J. (2011). Child internalizing symptoms: Contributions of child temperament, maternal negative affect, and family functioning. *Child Psychiatry & Human Development, 42*(1), 53–64.

Crissman, H., Hall, K. S., Patton, E. W., Zochowski, M. K., Davis, M. M., & Dalton, V. K. (2015). US women's intended sources for reproductive health care [23]. *Obstetrics & Gynecology, 125*, 7S.

Da Fonseca, M. A. (2012). The effects of poverty on children's development and oral health. *Pediatric Dentistry, 34*(1), 32–38.

Darwish, A. (2011). Liver transplant in Jehovah's Witnesses patients. *Current Opinion in Organ Transplantation, 16*(3), 326–330.

Davis, K. E. (2014). *Statistical brief #461: Access to health care of adult men and women, ages 18–64*. Retrieved from http://meps.ahrq.gov/mepsweb/data_files/publications/st461/stat461.shtml

de Miguel-Beriain, I. (2015). The ethics of stem cells revisited. *Advanced Drug Delivery Reviews, 82*, 176–180.

DeNavas-Walt, C., Proctor, B. D., & Smith, J. C., U. S. Census Bureau, Current Population Reports, P60–245. (2013). *Income, poverty, and health insurance coverage in the United States*. Washington, DC: U.S. Government Printing Office.

DONA International. (n. d.). *What is a doula*? Retrieved from http://www.dona.org/mothers/index.php

Douthit, N., Kiv, S., Dwolatzky, T., & Biswas, S. (2015). Exposing some important barriers to health care access in the rural USA. *Public Health, 129*(6), 611–620.

Duvall, E. (1997). *Marriage and family development* (5th ed.). Philadelphia, PA: J. B. Lippincott.

Edwards, J. D., Kun, S. S., Graham, R. J., & Keens, T. G. (2012). End-of-life discussions and advanced care planning for children on long-term assisted ventilation with life-limiting conditions. *Journal of Palliative Care, 28*(1), 21–27.

Edwards, J. G., Feldman, G., Goldberg, J., Gregg, A. R., Norton, M. E., Rose, N. C., et al. (2015). Expanded carrier screening in reproductive medicine—Points to consider: A joint statement of the American College of Medical Genetics and Genomics, American College of Obstetricians and Gynecologists, National Society of Genetic Counselors, Perinatal Quality Foundation, and Society for Maternal-Fetal Medicine. *Obstetrics & Gynecology, 125*(3), 653–662.

Egbe, A., Lee, S., Ho, D., Uppu, S., & Srivastava, S. (2015). Racial/ethnic differences in the birth prevalence of congenital anomalies in the United States. *Journal of Perinatal Medicine, 43*(1), 111–117.

Epstein, R. H. (2011). *Get me out: A history of childbirth from the Garden of Eden to the sperm bank.* New York, NY: W.W. Norton & Company.

Faver, C. A., & Alanis, E. (2012). Fostering empathy through stories: A pilot program for special needs adoptive families. *Children & Youth Services Review, 34*(4), 660–665.

Federal Interagency Forum on Child and Family Statistics. (2013). *America's children: Key national indicators of well-being, 2013.* Washington, DC: U.S. Government Printing Office.

Feigelman, S. (2011). Chapter 6: Overview and assessment of variability. In R. M. Kleigman, B. F. Stanton, J. W. St. Geme III, N. F. Schor, & R. E. Behrman (Eds.), *Nelson textbook of pediatrics* (19th ed., pp. 26). Philadelphia, PA: Saunders.

Ferguson-Smith, M. A. (2015). History and evolution of cytogenetics. *Molecular Cytogenetics, 8*(1), 19–27.

Finkelhor, D., Turner, H. A., Shattuck, A., & Hamby, S. L. (2013). Violence, crime, and abuse exposure in a national sample of children and youth: An update. *JAMA Pediatric, 167*(7), 614–621.

Flaskerud, J. H. (2011). Discipline and effective parenting. *Issues in Mental Health Nursing, 32*(1), 82–84.

Foster, I. (2015). *History of midwifery – Home birth through the ages.* Retrieved from http://sistersmidwifery.com/history-of-midwifery-home-birth/

Friedman, M. M. (1998). *Family nursing: Theory and practice* (4th ed.). Stanford, CT: Appleton & Lange.

Futures Without Violence (2012). *Protective factors & resiliency.* Retrieved from http://promising.futureswithoutviolence.org/what-do-kids-need/supporting-parenting/protective-factors-resiliency/

Galante, L., French, C., & Grace, K. B. (2015). Nursing perspectives in managing patients with substance abuse. In *Substance abuse* (pp. 229–248). New York, NY: Springer Publishers.

Gilchrist, J., Ballesteros, M. F., & Parker, E. M. (2012). Vital signs: Unintentional injury deaths among persons aged 0–19 years—United States, 2000–2009. *Morbidity and Mortality Weekly Report (MMWR), 61*(15), 270–276.

Gissler, M. (2015). Successes and challenges in infant mortality. *Acta Paediatrica, 104*, 440–441.

Griffin, I. J., Lee, H. C., Profit, J., & Tancedi, D. J. (2015). The smallest of the small: Short-term outcomes of profoundly growth restricted and profoundly low birth weight preterm infants. *Journal of Perinatology, 35*, 503–510.

Groark, C. J., & McCall, R. B. (2011). Implementing changes in institutions to improve young children's development. *Infant Mental Health Journal, 32*(5), 509–525.

Hall, H. (2013). Faith healing: Religious freedom vs. child protection. Science based medicine. Retrieved from http://www.sciencebasedmedicine.org/faith-healing-religious-freedom-vs-child-protection/

Hamon, J. D., & Schrodt, P. (2012). Do parenting styles moderate the association between family conformity orientation and young adults' mental well-being? *Journal of Family Communication, 12*(2), 151–166.

Hanson, P. A., & Andrews, M. M. (2012). Chapter 13: Religion, culture and nursing. In M. M. Andrews, & J. S. Boyle (Eds.), *Transcultural concepts in nursing care* (6th ed., pp. 351–402). Philadelphia, PA: Wolters Kluwer Health/Lippincott Williams & Wilkins.

Hodnett, E. D., Gates, S., Hofmeyr, G. J., & Sakala, C. (2013). Continuous support for women during childbirth. *Cochrane Database of Systematic Reviews, 7*:CD003766.

Holtzman, M. (2011). Nonmarital unions, family definitions, and custody decision making. *Family Relations, 60*(5), 617–632.

Jones, V. F., Schulte, E. E., Committee on Early Childhood, Council on Foster Care, Adoption, and Kinship Care. (2012). The pediatrician's role in supporting adoptive families. *Pediatrics, 130*(4), e1040–e1049.

Karim, Z. A., Alshbool, F. Z., Vemana, H. P., Adhami, N., Dhall, S., Espinosa, E. V., et al. (2015). Third hand smoke: Impact on hemostasis and thrombogenesis. *Journal of Cardiovascular Pharmacology, 66*(2):177–182.

Kawabata, Y., Alink, L. A., Tseng, W., van IJzendoorn, M. H., & Crick, N. R. (2011). Maternal and paternal parenting styles associated with relational aggression in children and adolescents: A conceptual analysis and meta-analytic review. *Developmental Review, 31*(4), 240–278.

Kelly, M. M. (2010). Prematurity. In P. J. Allen, J. A. Vessey, & N. A. Schapiro (Eds.), *Primary care of the child with a chronic condition* (5th ed.). St. Louis, MO: Mosby.

Kemp, G., Segal, J., & Robinson, L. (2015). *Step-parenting and blended families.* Retrieved from http://www.helpguide.org/family-divorce/step-parenting-blended-families.htm

Kemp, G., Smith, M., & Segal, J. (2015). Children and divorce. Retrieved from http://www.helpguide.org/articles/family-divorce/children-and-divorce.htm

Kersey-Matusiak, G. (2012). Culturally competent care: Are we there yet?. *Nursing, 42*(2), 49–52.

Kids Count Data Center. (2014a). *Children who speak a language other than English at home.* Retrieved from http://datacenter.kidscount.org/data/tables/81-children-who-speak-a-language-other-than-english-at-home#detailed/1/any/false/36,868,867,133,38/any/396,397

Kids Count Data Center. (2014b). *Children living in linguistically isolated households by children in immigrant families.* Retrieved from http://datacenter.kidscount.org/data/tables/129-children-living-in-linguistically-isolated-households-by-children-in-immigrant-families?loc=1&loct=2#detailed/1/any/false/867/78,79/472,473

Kiff, C. J., Lengua, L. J., & Zalewski, M. (2011). Nature and nurturing: Parenting in the context of child temperament. *Clinical Child and Family Psychology Review, 14*(3), 251–301.

Kim, H. (2011). Consequences of parental divorce for child development. *American Sociological Review, 76*(3), 487–511.

Kim, M., Han, S., & Shin, M. (2015). Influencing factors on the cord-blood donation of post-partum women. *Nursing & Health Sciences, 17*, 269–275.

King, T. L., Brucker, M. C., Kriebs, J. M., Fahey, J. O., Grgor, C. L., & Varney, H. (2015). *Varney's midwifery*. (5th ed.). Burlington, MA: Jones & Bartlett Learning.

Kochanek, K. D., Sherry, L., Murphy, S. L., & Xu, J. Q. (2015). Deaths: Final data for 2011. *National Vital Statistics Reports, 63*(3). Hyattsville, MD: National Center for Health Statistics. Retrieved from http://www.cdc.gov/nchs/data/nvsr/nvsr63/nvsr63_03.pdf

Kyvernitakis, I., Kostev, K., Hars, O., Albert, U. S., & Hadji, P. (2015). Discontinuation rates of menopausal hormone therapy among postmenopausal women in the Post-WHI Study era. *Climacteric, 18*(5), 737–742.

Lansford, J. E., Wager, L. B., Bates, J. E., Pettit, G. S., & Dodge, K. A. (2012). Forms of spanking and children's externalizing behaviors. *Family Relations, 61*(2), 224–236.

Larzelere, R. E. (2011). Should there be a law banning spanking of children? *U.S. News Digital Weekly, 3*(36), 17.

Leever, M.G. (2011). Culture competence: Reflection on patient autonomy and patient good. *Nursing Ethics, 18*(4), 560–570.

Lewis, R. (2011). *Human genetics: Concepts and applications* (10th ed.). New York, NY: McGraw-Hill Publishers.

Lincoln, J. (2015). *Which costs more: vaginal or C-section?* Retrieved from http://www.bundoo.com/articles/which-delivery-costs-more-vaginal-or-c-section/

Long, K., Thomas, S., Grubs, R., Gettig, E., & Krishnamurti, L. (2011). Attitudes and beliefs of African-Americans toward genetics, genetic testing, and sickle cell disease education and awareness. *Journal of Genetic Counseling, 20*(6), 572–592.

Lu, M. C., Highsmith, K., de la Cruz, D., & Atrash, H. K. (2015). Putting the "M" back in the maternal and child health bureau: Reducing maternal mortality and morbidity. *Maternal and Child Health Journal, 19*, 1435–1439.

Lyness, D. (2015). *Helping your child through divorce*. Retrieved from http://kidshealth.org/parent/positive/talk/help_child_divorce.html

MacDorman, M. F., Matthews, T. J., Mohangoo, A. D., & Zeitlin, J. (2014). International comparisons of infant mortality and related factors: United States and Europe, 2010. *National Vital Statistics Reports: from the Centers for Disease Control and Prevention, National Center for Health Statistics, National Vital Statistics System, 63*(5), 1–7.

Malinowska-Sempruch, K., & Rychkova, O. (2015). *The impact of drug policy on women*. Retrieved from https://www.opensocietyfoundations.org/reports/impact-drug-policy-women

March of Dimes. (2014). *Low birthweight*. Retrieved from http://www.marchofdimes.org/baby/low-birthweight.aspx

Maron, D. F. (2015.) Has maternal mortality really doubled in the US? *Scientific American*. Retrieved from http://www.scientificamerican.com/article/has-maternal-mortality-really-doubled-in-the-u-s/

Martins, N., & Wilson, B. J. (2012). Social aggression on television and its relationship to children's aggression in the classroom. *Human Communication Research, 38*(1), 48–71.

Masten, A. S., & Narayan, A. J. (2012). Child development in the context of disaster, war, and terrorism: Pathways of risk and resilience. *Annual Review of Psychology, 63*(1), 227–257.

Mayo Clinic Staff. (2015). *Congenital adrenal hyperplasia*. Retrieved from http://www.mayoclinic.org/diseases-conditions/congenital-adrenal-hyperplasia/basics/definition/con-20030910

McClamrock, H. D., Jones, H. W., & Adashi, E. Y. (2012). Ovarian stimulation and intrauterine insemination at the quarter centennial: implications for the multiple births epidemic. *Fertility & Sterility, 97*(4), 802–809.

McGowan, C. (2011). Legal aspects of end-of-life care. *Critical Care Nurse, 31*(5), 64–69.

McLemore, M. R., Kools, S., & Levi, A. J. (2015). Calculus formation: Nurses' decision-making in abortion-related care. *Research in Nursing & Health, 38*, 222–231.

McLemore, M., Levi, A. J., & James, E. A. (2015). Strategies to recruit and retain expert nurses who provide abortion care. *Journal of Obstetric, Gynecologic, & Neonatal Nursing, 44*, S75.

Miao, T., Umemoto, K., Gonda, D., & Hishinuma, E. (2011). Essential elements for community engagement in evidence-based youth violence prevention. *American Journal of Community Psychology, 48*(1/2), 120–132.

Miller, J., & Scott, J. (2015). Newborn and infant (0–12 months). In *Food and Nutrition Throughout Life: A comprehensive overview of food and nutrition in all stages of life, 117*. London, UK: Allen & Unwin Publishers.

Murray, B. (2012). Informed consent: What must a physician disclose to a patient? *American Medical Association Journal of Ethics, 14*(7), 563–566.

Murray, T. L., Calhoun, M., & Philipsen, N. C. (2011). Privacy, confidentiality, HIPAA, and hightech: Implications for the health care practitioner. *Journal for Nurse Practitioners, 7*(9), 747–752.

Nagle, J., & Clancy, M. C. (2012). Constructing a shared public identity in ethno nationally divided societies: Comparing consociational and transformationist perspectives. *Nations & Nationalism, 18*(1), 78–97.

National Center on Family Homelessness. (2015). *What is family homelessness?* Retrieved from http://www.familyhomelessness.org/facts.php?p=tm

National Conference of State Legislatures. (2015). *Children's Health Insurance Program (CHIP)*. Retrieved from http://www.ncsl.org/research/health/childrens-health-insurance-program-overview.aspx

National Institutes of Health. (2012). *Children and clinical studies: Why it's important*. Retrieved from http://www.nhlbi.nih.gov/childrenandclinicalstudies/whydo.php

National Women's Law Center. (2010). *Making the grade on women's health: A national and state by state report card*. Retrieved from http://hrc.nwlc.org/states/national-report-card

Norman, A. (2015). *The complicated birth of midwifery*. Retrieved from http://all-that-is-interesting.com/midwife-history

Office of Adolescent Health. (2015). *Mental Health*. Retrieved from http://www.hhs.gov/ash/oah/adolescent-health-topics/mental-health/home.html

Oregon Department of Education. (2015). *Working definition of cultural competency*. Retrieved from http://www.ode.state.or.us/search/page/?id=656

Osterman, M. J., Kochanek, K. D., MacDorman, M. F., Strobino, D. M., & Guyer, B. (2015). Annual summary of vital statistics: 2012–2013. *Pediatrics, 135*(6), 1115–1125.

Oza, S., Lawn, J. E., Hogan, D. R., Mathers, C., & Cousens, S. N. (2015). Neonatal cause-of-death estimates for the early and late neonatal periods for 194 countries: 2000–2013. *Bulletin of the World Health Organization, 93*(1), 19–28.

Parents without Partners. (n. d.). *Who we are*. Retrieved from http://www.parentswithoutpartners.org/?page=AboutWho

Patel, K., & Rushefsky, M. E. (2015). *Health care in America: Separate and unequal*. New York, NY: Routledge.

Patterson, J. (1995). Promoting resilience in families experiencing stress. *Pediatric Clinics of North America, 42*(1), 47–63.

Patterson, J. (2002). Integrating family resilience and family stress theory. *Journal of Marriage and Family, 64*(2), 349–360.

Pew Research Center. (2011). A portrait of step families. Retrieved from http://www.pewsocialtrends.org/2011/01/13/a-portrait-of-stepfamilies/

Piko, B. B., & Balázs, M. M. (2012). Control or involvement? Relationship between authoritative parenting style and adolescent depressive symptomatology. *European Child & Adolescent Psychiatry, 21*(3), 149–155.

Rafi, I., & Kai, J. (2011). Genetics and ethnicity. *Pulse, 71*(6), 22–23.

Riggs, K. R., & Alexander, G. C. (2015). Cost containment and patient well-being. *Journal of General Internal Medicine, 30*(6), 701–702.

Robinson, N., Stoffel, C., & Haider, S. (2015). Global women's health is more than maternal health: A review of gynecology care needs in low-resource settings. *Obstetrical & Gynecological Survey, 70*(3), 211–222.

Roura, S., Pujal, J. M., Gálvez-Montón, C., & Bayes-Genis, A. (2015). The role and potential of umbilical cord blood in an era of new therapies: A review. *Stem Cell Research & Therapy, 6*(1), 1–11.

Seburg, E. M., Olson-Bullis, B. A., Bredeson, D. M., Hayes, M. G., & Sherwood, N. E. (2015). A review of primary care-based childhood obesity prevention and treatment interventions. *Current Obesity Reports, 4*(2), 157–173.

Seith, D., & Isakson, E. (2011). *Who are America's poor children? Examining health disparities among children in the United States*. New York, NY: National Center for Children in Poverty.

Serwint, J. R. (2011). Chapter 16: Separation, loss & bereavement. In R. M. Kleigman, B. F. Stanton, J. W. St. Geme III, N. F. Schor & R. E. Behrman (Eds.), *Nelson textbook of pediatrics* (19th ed., pp. 45). Philadelphia, PA: Saunders.

Shah, A. (2011). *Today, over 21,000 children died around the world*. Global Issues. Retrieved from http://www.globalissues.org/article/715/today-over-26500-children-died-around-the-world

Siegel, R. L., Miller, K. D., & Jemal, A. (2015). Cancer statistics, 2015. *CA: A Cancer Journal for Clinicians, 65*(1), 5–29.

Simms, M. D., & Wilson, S. L. (2011). Chapter 34: Adoption. In R. M. Kliegman, B. F. Stanton, J. W. St. Geme, N. F. Schor, & R. E. Behrman (Eds.), *Nelson's textbook of pediatrics* (19th ed., pp. 130–134). Philadelphia, PA: Saunders.

Sirbaugh, P. E., & Diekema, D. S. (2011). Policy statement-consent for emergency medical services for children and adolescents. *Pediatrics, 128*(2), 427–433.

Stallings, D. T. (2015). Illness perceptions and health behaviors of black women. *The Journal of Cardiovascular Nursing*. doi: 10.1097/JCN.0000000000000276.

Stanhope, M., & Lancaster, J. (2011). *Public health nursing: Population-centered health care in the community*. (8th ed.). St. Louis, MO: Mosby Elsevier.

Stanton, B. F., & Behrman, R. E. (2011). Chapter 1: Overview of pediatrics. In R. M., Kliegman, B. F., Stanton, J.W. St. Geme III, N. F. Schor, & R. E. Behrman (Eds.), *Nelson's textbook of pediatrics* (19th ed., pp. 1–13). Philadelphia, PA: Saunders.

Stapleton, S., & Rooks, J. P. (2015). Birth centers. UpToDate. Retrieved from http://www.uptodate.com/contents/birth-centers

Strasburger, V. (2011). Children, adolescents, obesity, and the media. *Pediatrics, 128*(1), 201–208.

The Kaiser Commission on Medicaid and the Uninsured. (2012). *The uninsured a primer: key facts about americans without health insurance*. Retrieved from http://kaiserfamilyfoundation.files.wordpress.com/2013/01/7451–08.pdf

The Kaiser Commission on Medicaid and the Uninsured. (2013). *Key facts about the uninsured population*. Retrieved from http://kaiserfamilyfoundation.files.wordpress.com/2013/09/8488-key-facts-about-the-uninsured-population.pdf

Tsai, A. C., Manchester, D. K., & Elias, E. R. (2011). Genetics and dysmorphology. In W. W. Hay, M. J. Levin, J. M. Sondheimer, & R. R. Deterding (Eds.), *Current diagnosis and treatment: Pediatrics* (20th ed.). New York, NY: McGraw-Hill.

Tucker, B., Fager, C., Srinivas, S., & Lorch, S. (2011). Racial and ethnic differences in use of intubation for periviable neonates. *Pediatrics, 127*(5), e1120–e1127.

UNICEF (2015). Our Mission: Working to make the world better for children. Retrieved from http://www.unicefusa.org/mission

U.S. Bureau of Justice Office on Violence against Women. (2015). *Domestic violence*. Retrieved from http://www.ovw.usdoj.gov/domviolence.htm

U. S. Census Bureau. (2011). 2010 census shows nation's Hispanic population grew four times faster than total United States population. Retrieved from https://www.census.gov/newsroom/releases/archives/2010_census/cb11-cn146.html

U. S. Census Bureau. (2013). Current population survey (CPS): Definitions and explanations. Retrieved from http://www.census.gov/cps/about/cpsdef.html

U. S. Census Bureau. (2012). Section 2: Births, deaths, marriages, & divorces: Marriages and divorces. *The 2012 Statistical Abstract*. Retrieved from https://www.census.gov/prod/2011pubs/12statab/vitstat.pdf

U.S. Department of Agriculture, Food and Nutrition Service. (2015). *National school lunch program*. Retrieved from http://www.fns.usda.gov/nslp/national-school-lunch-program-nslp

U. S. Department of Health and Human Services. (n. d.). *Special protections for children as research subjects*. Retrieved from http://www.hhs.gov/ohrp/policy/populations/children.html

U. S. Department of Health and Human Services. (2013). *2013 poverty guidelines.* Retrieved from http://aspe.hhs.gov/poverty/13poverty.cfm#thresholds

U. S. Department of Health and Human Services. (2015). *Healthy People 2020.* Retrieved from http://www.healthypeople.gov/2020/default

U. S. Department of Health and Human Services, Administration for Children & Families, Administration on Children, Youth and Families, Children's Bureau. (2013a). *The AFCARS report.* Retrieved from http://www.acf.hhs.gov/sites/default/files/cb/afcarsreport20.pdf

U. S. Department of Health and Human Services, Administration for Children & Families, Administration on Children, Youth and Families, Children's Bureau. (2013b). *Trends in foster care and adoption.* Retrieved from http://www.acf.hhs.gov/sites/default/files/cb/trends_fostercare_adoption2012.pdf

U. S. Department of Health and Human Services, Health Resources and Services Administration, Maternal and Child Health Bureau. (2013). *Child health USA 2012.* Rockville, MD: U. S. Department of Health and Human Services.

U.S. Department of Health and Human Services, Maternal and Child Health Bureau. (n. d.). *Timeline.* Retrieved from http://mchb.hrsa.gov/about/timeline/index.html

U. S. Department of Health & Human Resources Office of Minority Health. (2015). *Culturally competent nursing care: A cornerstone of caring.* Retrieved from https://ccnm.thinkculturalhealth.hhs.gov/

Vespa, J., Lewis, J. M., & Kreider, R. M. (2013). America's families and living arrangements: 2012, population characteristics. Retrieved from http://www.census.gov/prod/2013pubs/p20–570.pdf

Viteri, O. A., Soto, E. E., Bahado-Singh, R. O., Christensen, C. W., Chauhan, S. P., & Sibai, B. M. (2015). Fetal anomalies and long-term effects associated with substance abuse in pregnancy: A literature review. *American Journal of Perinatology, 32*(5), 405–416.

Von Bertalanffy, L. (1968). General systems theory. London: Penguin Press.

Waxman, J. D., & Johnson, P. A. (2015). Well-woman visits: Guidance and monitoring are key in this turning point for women's health. *Women's Health Issues, 25*(2), 89–90.

Weissman, J., Pratt, L. A., Miller, E. A., & Parker, J. D. (2015). Serious psychological distress among adults: United States, 2009–2013. *NCHS data brief,* (203), 1–8.

Wilson, C. B., Nizet, V., Maldonado, Y., Remington, J. S., & Klein, J. O. (2016). *Remington and Klein's infectious diseases of the fetus and newborn infant.* Philadelphia, PA: Elsevier Health Sciences.

Wong, S., Ordean, A., & Kahan, M. (2011). Substance use in pregnancy. *Journal of Obstetrics and Gynecology Canada, 4,* 367–384.

World Bank. (2015a). *Maternal mortality ratio per 100,000 live births.* Retrieved from http://data.worldbank.org/indicator/SH.STA.MMRT

World Bank. (2015b). *Mortality rate, infant (per 1000 live births).* Retrieved from http://data.worldbank.org/indicator/SP.DYN.IMRT.IN

World Bank. (2015c). *Mortality rate, neonatal (per 1000 live births).* Retrieved from http://data.worldbank.org/indicator/SH.DYN.NMRT

World Health Organization. (2012). Geneva, Switzerland: Author. Retrieved from http://www.unicef.org/earlychildhood/files/3.CCD_-_Participant_Manual.pdf

World Health Organization (WHO). (2014). Children: reducing mortality. Retrieved from http://www.who.int/mediacentre/factsheets/fs178/en/

World Health Organization. (2015a). *Country comparison – maternal mortality rate.* Retrieved from http://www.who.int/gho/maternal_health/countries/usa.pdf?ua=1

World Health Organization. (2015b). *Frequently asked questions.* Retrieved from http://www.who.int/suggestions/faq/en/index.html

World Health Organization. (2015c). *Maternal and perinatal health.* Retrieved from http://www.who.int/maternal_child_adolescent/topics/maternal/maternal_perinatal/en/

World Heart Federation. (2015). Women and CVD. Retrieved from http://www.world-heart-federation.org/what-we-do/awareness/women-and-cvd/

Wright, T. (2011). Consent and children: A practical summary. *Clinical Risk, 17*(5), 192–194.

Xu, Y. (2011). The effects of teaching primary caregivers to conduct formative assessment on caregiver-child social interaction and children's developmental outcomes. *Early Child Development and Care, 181*(4), 549–571.

Yahav, R. (2011). Exposure of children to war and terrorism: A review. *Journal of Child & Adolescent Trauma, 4*(2), 90–108.

Yarrow, A. L. (2011). A history of federal child antipoverty and health policy in the United States since 1900. *Child Development Perspectives, 5*(1), 66–72.

Yoon, E., Hacker, J., Hewitt, A., Abrams, M., & Cleary, S. (2012). Social connectedness, discrimination, and social status as mediators of acculturation/enculturation and well-being. *Journal of Counseling Psychology, 59*(1), 86–96.

Yuan, S. M. (2015). Fetal cardiac interventions. *Pediatrics & Neonatology, 56*(2), 81–87.

Zlotnick, C., Tam, T. W., & Soman, L. A. (2012). Life course outcomes on mental and physical health: The impact of foster care on adulthood. *American Journal of Public Health, 102*(3), 534–540.

CHAPTER WORKSHEET

MULTIPLE-CHOICE QUESTIONS

1. When preparing a presentation for a local woman's group on women's health problems, what would the nurse include as the number-one cause of mortality for women in the United States?
   a. Breast cancer
   b. Childbirth complications
   c. Injury resulting from violence
   d. Heart disease
2. Which factor would most likely be responsible for a pregnant women's failure to receive adequate prenatal care in the United States?
   a. Belief that it is not necessary in a normal pregnancy
   b. Use of denial to cope with pregnancy
   c. Lack of health insurance to cover expenses
   d. Inability to trust traditional medical practices
3. When caring for an adolescent, in which instance must the nurse share information with the parents, no matter which state care is provided in?
   a. Pregnancy counseling
   b. Depression
   c. Contraception
   d. Tuberculosis
4. The following events were milestones in the support of women's and children's health. Place the events in the correct sequence, from oldest to most recent.
   a. Declaration of the Rights of the Child approved
   b. WIC program established
   c. U.S. Children's Bureau established
   d. Sheppard–Towner Act passed
   e. Family and Medical Leave Act passed
   f. Education for All Handicapped Children Act passed
5. The nurse is preparing a class for a group of students about homelessness. Which factors contribute to homelessness? Select all that apply.
   a. Decrease in the number of people living in poverty
   b. Rises in unemployment
   c. Exposure to abuse or neglect
   d. Cutbacks in public welfare programs
   e. Development of community crisis centers

CRITICAL THINKING EXERCISES

1. As a nurse working in a federally funded low-income clinic offering women's health services, you are becoming increasingly frustrated with the number of "no-shows," or appointments missed in your maternity clinic. Some clients come for their initial prenatal intake appointment and never come back. You realize that some just forget their appointments, but most don't even call to notify you. Many of the clients are high risk and thus are jeopardizing their health and the health of their future child.
   a. What changes might be helpful to address this situation?
   b. Outline what you might say at your next staff meeting to address the issue of clients making one clinic visit and then never returning.
   c. What strategies might you use to improve attendance and notification?
   d. Describe what cultural and customer service techniques might be needed.
2. A couple has adopted an 11-month-old infant girl from China and brought her to the health care facility for a checkup. The couple had no contact with the infant's birth parents. The infant spent 7 months in an orphanage before being adopted. Describe the family structure and the issues that may affect this family.
3. You have been asked by the local school district to speak to a group of middle-school children and their parents about Internet safety. Describe the topics that you should address.
4. A 12-year-old is to undergo research treatment for a serious illness. Explain the concept of assent as it relates to this situation.

STUDY ACTIVITIES

1. Research a current policy, bill, or issue being debated on the community, state, or national level that pertains to the health and welfare of women or children. Summarize the major facts and supporting and opposing arguments, and prepare an oral report on your findings.
2. Within your clinical group, debate the following statement: Should access to health care be a right or a privilege?
3. Visit a local community health center that offers services to women and children from various cultures. Interview the staff about any barriers to health care that they have identified. Investigate what the staff has done to minimize these barriers.

BRINGING IT ALL TOGETHER: A CASE STUDY

Maali, a 19-year-old Arab immigrant, presents at the local prenatal clinic accompanied by her husband Labib. The couple and their 18-month-old daughter, Labiba, have lived with relatives since arriving in America 5 months ago. During the prenatal interview, Maali reports that she is 4 months pregnant and is the primary caregiver for their daughter as well as caring for Labib's sister's toddler son while her sister-in-law is at work during the day.

Go to thePoint to find questions to consider about this case.

2

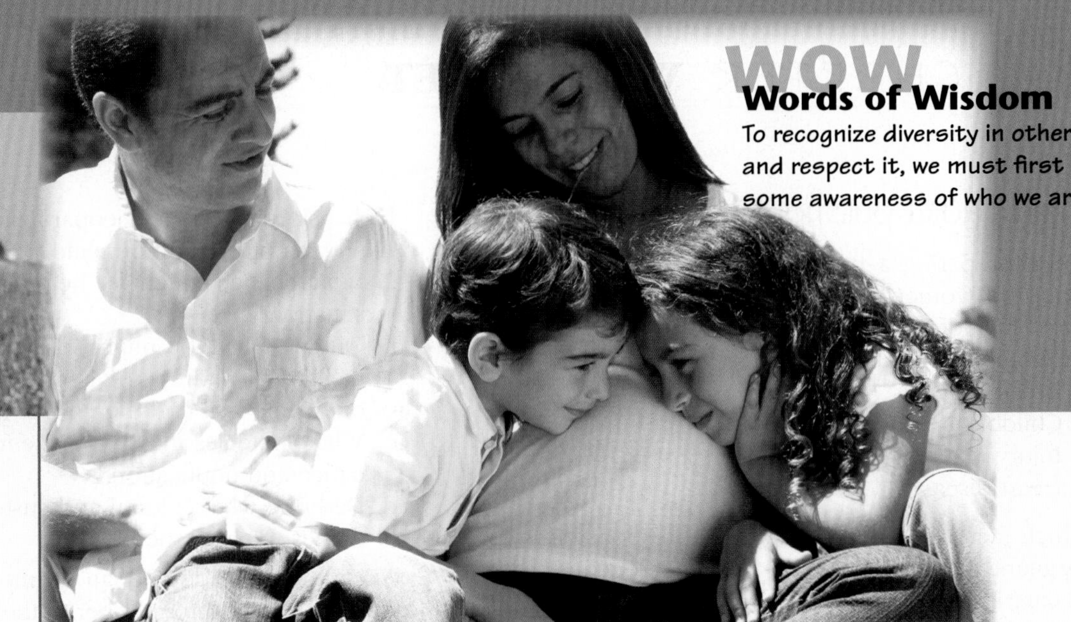

WOW

Words of Wisdom

To recognize diversity in others and respect it, we must first have some awareness of who we are.

Family-Centered Community-Based Care

Learning Objectives

Upon completion of the chapter, you will be able to:

1. Identify the core concepts associated with the nursing management of women, children, and families.
2. Examine the major components and key elements of family-centered care.
3. Explain the different levels of prevention in nursing, providing examples of each.
4. Give examples of cultural issues that may be faced when providing nursing care.
5. Provide culturally competent care to women, children, and families.
6. Outline the various roles and functions assumed by the nurse working with women, children, and families.
7. Demonstrate the ability to use excellent therapeutic communication skills when interacting with women, children, and families.
8. Explain the process of health teaching as it relates to women, children, and families.
9. Examine the importance of discharge planning and case management in providing nursing care.
10. Explain the reasons for the increased emphasis on community-based care.
11. Differentiate community-based nursing from nursing in acute care settings.
12. Identify the variety of settings where community-based care can be provided to women, children, and families.

KEY TERMS

atraumatic care
case management
community
cultural competence
epidemiology
evidence-based nursing practice
family-centered care
health literacy
nonverbal communication
population
verbal communication

***Maria* was home a few days after giving birth to her first child. She had just changed her newborn son and placed him on his stomach for a nap when the community health nurse arrived for a postpartum visit. Because the nurse didn't speak Spanish and Maria didn't speak English, a great deal of gesturing followed. After examining Maria, the nurse then picked up her son and placed him on his back in the crib. How might the nurse have prepared for this home visit? What message did the nurse convey in changing the newborn's position?**

INTRODUCTION

Now more than ever, nurses contribute to nearly every health care experience. Historically, people were born at home, cared for when ill at home, and then died at home surrounded by loved ones. Today, these events from birth to death, and every health care emergency in between, will likely involve the presence of a nurse. Involvement of a knowledgeable, supportive, comforting nurse often leads to a positive health care experience. Skilled nursing practice depends on a solid base of knowledge and clinical expertise delivered in a caring, holistic manner. Nurses, using their knowledge and passion, help meet the health care needs of their clients throughout the life span, whether the client is a pregnant woman, a fetus, a partner, a child, or the parents or family members of a child. Nurses fill a variety of roles in helping clients to live healthier lives by providing direct care, emotional support, comfort, information, advice, advocacy, support, and counseling. Nurses are often "in the trenches" advocating on various issues, drawing attention to the importance of health care for women and children, encouraging a focus on education and prevention, and assisting families who lack resources or access to health care.

Women, children, and families receive a majority of their health care, both well and ill care, in the community setting. During the past several years, the health care delivery system has changed dramatically. Medicare's prospective payment system (PPS) for hospitals, introduced in the United States in 1983, replaced cost reimbursement with a system of fixed rates which created incentives for hospitals to control costs. With a focus on cost containment, people are spending less time in the hospital. Clients are being discharged "sicker and quicker" from their hospital beds (Hansen, 2015). The health care system has moved from reactive treatment strategies in hospitals to a proactive approach in the community. This has resulted in an increasing emphasis on health promotion and illness prevention within the community.

Nurses play an important role in the health and wellness of a community. This is an exciting time for nurses delivering out-of-hospital care. The rising trend of delivering care in or near people's homes and away from acute care facilities will necessitate flexible ways of working and greater integration of community nursing roles (Massey, 2015). They not only meet the health care needs of the individual but also go beyond that to implement interventions that affect the community as a whole. Nurses practice in a variety of settings within a community, such as clinics and physician offices, schools, shelters, churches, health departments, community health centers, and homes. They promote the health of individuals, families, groups, communities, and populations and promote an environment that supports health.

This chapter describes the core concepts of maternal and child health nursing and community and community-based nursing. Nurses need to be knowledgeable about these concepts to ensure that they provide professional care.

CORE CONCEPTS OF MATERNAL AND CHILD HEALTH NURSING

Maternal and child health nursing focuses on providing evidence-based care to the client within the context of the family. This care involves the implementation of an interdisciplinary plan in a collaborative manner to ensure continuity of care that is cost-effective, quality-oriented, and outcome-focused. Nurses provide this care by focusing on the family, using evidence-based practice, working collaboratively, providing atraumatic therapeutic care, communicating effectively, providing education, providing discharge planning and case management, providing advocacy and resource management, providing preventative care, providing culturally competent nursing care, and being knowledgeable about complementary and alternative medicine (CAM).

Family-Centered Care

Family-centered care refers to the collaborative partnership among the individual, family, and caregivers to determine goals, share information, offer support, and formulate plans for health care. It is generally understood to be an approach in which clients and their families are considered integral components of the health care decision-making and delivery processes. It recognizes the client and the family as the source of control and a full partner in their care (Roberts, 2015). It is based on mutual trust and collaboration between women, children, families, and the health care professional. It is a partnership approach of families and their caregivers that recognizes the strength and integrity of the family.

The philosophy of family-centered care recognizes the family as the constant. The health and functioning of the family affect the health of the client and other members of the family. Family members support one another well beyond the health care provider's brief time with them, such as during the childbearing process or during a child's illness.

Family-centered care requires sensitivity to the client's and family's beliefs and those supporting their culture. This involves listening to the family's needs and a shift of the nurse's authoritarian role to the family to empower them to make their own decisions within the context of a supportive environment.

With family-centered care, support and respect for the uniqueness and diversity of families are essential, along with encouragement and enhancement of the family's strengths and competencies. It is important to create opportunities for families to demonstrate their abilities and skills. Families also can acquire new abilities and skills to maintain a sense of control and empowerment in meeting the needs of the client. Family-centered care promotes greater family self-determination, decision-making abilities, control, and self-efficacy, thereby enhancing the client's and family's sense of empowerment. When implementing family-centered care, nurses seek caregiver input. These suggestions and advice are incorporated into the client's plan of care as the nurse counsels and teaches the family appropriate health care interventions. Today, as nurses partner with various experts to provide high-quality and cost-effective care, one expert partnership that nurses can make is with the client's family.

The impact of family-centered care can be seen in the models of care delivery for women and children. From the 1980s to the present, there has been increased access to care for all women (regardless of their ability to pay) and hospital redesigns (labor, delivery, and recovery [LDR] rooms; labor, delivery, recovery, and postpartum [LDRP] spaces) aimed at keeping families together during the childbirth experience and to minimize interruptions in breast-feeding dyads (Ayers, Grassley, & Koprowski, 2015). This impact also can be seen in the care of children. For example, rooming-in and liberal visiting policies allow parents and other family members to participate in the child's care (Fig. 2.1).

Family-centered care works well in all arenas of health care, from preventive care to long-term care. Using a family-centered approach is associated with positive outcomes such as decreased anxiety, improved pain management, shorter recovery times, and enhanced confidence and problem-solving skills. Communication between the health care team and the family is also improved, leading to greater satisfaction for both health care providers and health care consumers (families). It is important for nurses to remain neutral to all they hear and see in order to enhance trust and maintain open communication lines with all family members. Nurses need to remember that clients are an expert of their own health, thus nurses should work within the clients' framework when planning health promotion interventions.

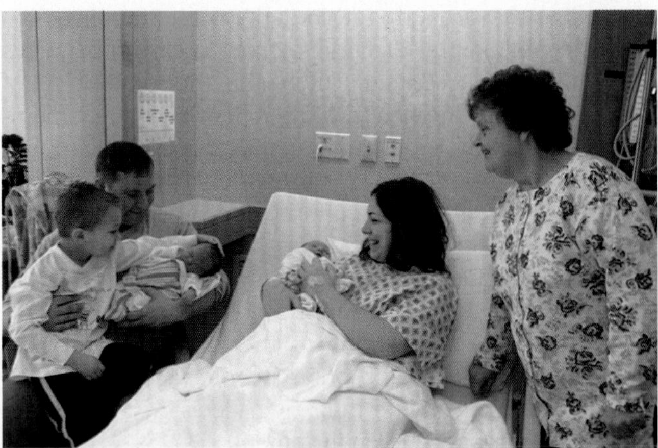

FIGURE 2.1 Providing an opportunity for the parent to interact with the child is an important component of family-centered nursing care.

Evidence-Based Care

Evidence-based nursing practice involves the use of research or evidence in establishing a plan of care and then implementing that care. It is a clinical decision-making approach that involves the integration of the best scientific evidence, client values and preferences, clinical circumstances, and clinical expertise to promote best outcomes (Williamson et al, 2015). It is important that nurses develop the skills and knowledge necessary to ask pertinent clinical questions, search for current best evidence, analyze the evidence, integrate the evidence into practice when appropriate, and evaluate outcomes. Evidence-based practice may lead to a decrease in variations in care while at the same time increasing quality and improving health care.

Scientific research findings help nurses not only stay current in their clinical specialties, but also in their choice of the most effective interventions. Many of the professional organizations Association of Women's Health, Obstetric and Neonatal Nurses (AWHONN, ANA, NLN, etc.) have developed evidence-based clinical practice guidelines for the safest and effective delivery of family-centered nursing care. Nurses should be diligent in seeking out these evidence-based guidelines to ensure excellence in their daily practice. When evidence-based practice (EBP) is delivered in a context of caring and in a supportive organizational culture, the highest quality of care and best client outcomes can be achieved (Bridges, 2015; Makic et al., 2015).

Collaborative Care

Nurses must embrace interprofessional collaborative care because health care reform has transformed health care delivery models that require team work. Nurses must transition from working in a silo to working with interprofessional teams. This transition is needed to provide high-quality, safe, and accountable care to achieve positive client outcomes (Lomax & White, 2015). Modern health care focuses on an interdisciplinary plan of care designed to meet a client's physical, developmental, educational, spiritual, and psychosocial needs. This interdisciplinary collaborative type of care is termed **case management**, a collaborative process involving assessment, planning, implementation, coordination, monitoring, and evaluation. It involves the following components:

- Advocacy, communication, and resource management
- Client-focused comprehensive care across a continuum

- Coordinated care with an interdisciplinary approach (Commission for Case Management Certification, n.d.)

When the nurse effectively functions in the role as a case manager, client and family satisfaction is increased, fragmentation of care is decreased, and outcome measurement for a homogenous group of clients is possible.

Atraumatic Pediatric Care

Children undergo a wide range of interventions, many of which can be traumatic, stressful, and painful. The various settings where the child receives care can be scary and overwhelming to the child and family. The child and family interact with various health care personnel, which leads to an increased potential for anxiety. A major component of the child health nursing philosophy is the importance of providing atraumatic care. **Atraumatic care** refers to the delivery of care that minimizes or eliminates the psychological and physical distress experienced by children and their families in the health care system (Wong, n.d.). The key principles of atraumatic care include the following:

- Preventing or minimizing physical stressors
- Preventing or minimizing separation of the child from the family
- Promoting a sense of control

Nurses must be alert for any situation that has the potential for causing distress and should be able to identify potential stressors. Pediatric nurses should minimize separation of the child from the family, should decrease the child's exposure to stressful situations, and should strive to prevent or minimize pain and injury. The importance of providing atraumatic care to children is integrated throughout this text and discussed in detail in Chapter 30.

Communication

Communication is a way of conveying messages to various people using a common system of symbols, signs, or behaviors. Infants start their first communication soon after birth when they cry to convey the message of discomfort or hunger. Effective therapeutic communication with women, children, and families is essential to the provision of quality nursing care. Client- and family-centered communication increases satisfaction with nursing care and aids in improving knowledge and health care skills (Arnold & Boggs, 2016). The significance of communication revolves around its effectiveness and the climate in which communication occurs. Trust, respect, and empathy are three factors needed to create and foster effective therapeutic communication between people. (See Chapter 30 for specifics on effective communication when working with children.)

Verbal Communication

Communicating through the use of words, either written or spoken, is termed **verbal communication**. Nurses use verbal communication throughout the day when interacting with clients. Good verbal communication skills are necessary when performing nursing assessments and providing child/family teaching. General guidelines for appropriate verbal communication include the following:

- Use open-ended questions that do not restrict the child's or parents' answers.
- Redirect the conversation to maintain focus.
- Use reflection to clarify the parents' feelings.
- Paraphrase the child's or parents' feelings to demonstrate empathy.
- Acknowledge emotions.
- Demonstrate active listening by using the child's or family's own words.

Remember that most parents are laypersons, so avoid using medical jargon. The abbreviations and shortened terms that health care providers use almost without thinking may sound scary or foreign to children and parents. When medical terminology is necessary, provide a definition using developmentally appropriate language (*Healthy People 2020*).

Nonverbal Communication

Nonverbal communication, or body language, includes attending to others and active listening. The nurse should listen to the other person's verbal communication from the beginning of the interaction. When women, children, and parents feel they are being heard, trust and rapport are established. Guidelines for appropriate nonverbal communication include the following:

- Relax; maintain an open posture, with the arms uncrossed.

HEALTHY PEOPLE 2020

Objective	Significance
Increase the proportion of persons who report that their health care providers have satisfactory communication skills. (Developmental) Improve the health literacy of the population.	• Assess health learning needs of children and their families. • Plan health care education in collaboration with children and their families. • Provide health education at each client encounter. • Assess for poor health literacy skills

Healthy People Objectives retrieved from http://www.healthypeople.gov.

- Sit opposite the family and lean forward slightly.
- Maintain eye contact.
- Nod your head to demonstrate interest.
- Note the child's or parent's posture, eye contact, and facial expressions.

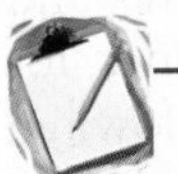

Take Note!

People of all ages desire to be listened to without interruption (Gupta, Mehta, & Sagar, 2015).

Active listening is critical to the communication process. Listening may uncover fears or concerns that the nurse may not have discovered through questioning.

Paying attention while children and parents talk is a powerful communication tool. By not listening, the nurse may miss critical information and the family may be reluctant to share further. When interacting with the child and family, determine whether the messages sent by the child's or parents' verbal and nonverbal communication are congruent.

Recall Maria, who recently was discharged from the hospital with her newborn son. How did the nurse communicate with Maria? Did the nurse's actions during the visit promote the development of trust between Maria and the nurse? What might have been done differently to foster trust?

Communicating Across Cultures

Understanding and respecting the client's and family's culture helps foster good communication and improves child and family education about health care. Culture, religion, and spirituality are intertwined concepts that affect the client's and family's communication styles, health status, and health beliefs. It is important to be aware of the family's background, lifestyle, and health care practices to meet their information needs.

Learning about the practices of various cultures is just the beginning; the nurse must assess each family's individual beliefs and practices, not generalize. The best way to assess the family's cultural practices is to ask and then listen. Determine the language spoken at home and observe the use of eye contact and other physical contact. Demonstrate a caring, nonjudgmental attitude and sensitivity to the client's and family's cultural diversity.

Working with an Interpreter

Attempting to communicate with a family who does not speak English can be one of the most frustrating situations in which health care providers find themselves. In this situation, trained interpreters are an invaluable aid and an essential component of client and family education. Whether working with an interpreter in person or over the phone, it is important to coordinate efforts so that both the family and the interpreter understand the information to be communicated. Working as a team, the nurse questions or informs and the interpreter conveys the information completely and accurately (see Healthy People, 2020). Well-trained translators can also help prevent cultural missteps and can help guide the health care provider to provide information in a more culturally accepted manner (Levetown and the Committee on Bioethics, 2011). Box 2.1 presents tips for working with an interpreter to maximize teaching efforts.

HEALTHY PEOPLE 2020

Objective	Significance
Increase the proportion of local health departments that have established culturally appropriate and linguistically competent community health promotion and disease prevention programs.	• Work with professionals and individuals from various cultures to develop materials and programs for health promotion that are culturally competent. • Ensure teaching materials are provided in the appropriate language.

Healthy People Objectives retrieved from http://www.healthypeople.gov.

Several helpful resources and websites are listed on thePoint, including Language Line, which offers telephone interpreters who speak 150 languages, and The Center for Applied Linguistics, Northwest Translators and Interpreters Society, among others.

On the second visit to Maria's home, the nurse brought a Spanish-speaking interpreter who explained the reason for the "back to sleep" position and demonstrated to Maria several other useful positions for feeding and holding. Maria was smiling when the nurse left and asking when she would be back. What made the difference in their relationship the second visit? What interventions demonstrate culturally competent care?

Communicating With Deaf or Hearing-Impaired Clients and Families

Nearly one in five Americans has hearing loss, and for those over the age of 65, the ratio climbs to one in three (Berg & Serpanos, 2016). Health care providers are under a duty to provide auxiliary aids and services to

BOX 2.1

TIPS FOR WORKING WITH AN INTERPRETER

- **Help the interpreter prepare and understand what needs to be done ahead of time.** A few minutes of preparation may save a lot of time and help communication flow more smoothly in the long run.
- **Introduce yourself to both parties.** It is the key to easy communication across the language barrier.
- **Physically place yourselves so that you are facing your client, and your client is facing you.** Place the interpreter physically close to both of you, but not in a position that breaks the line of sight between you and your client.
- **Begin with a minute or two of light conversation to establish a rhythm before getting into the business at hand.** This establishes the quantity of speech in the conversation.
- **Remember, the interpreter is the "communication bridge" and not the "content expert."** The nurse's presence at teaching sessions is vital.
- **Establish a rapport with the interpreter.**
- **Be patient. The interpreter's timing may not match that of others involved.** It often takes longer to say in some languages what has already been said in English; therefore, plan for more time than you normally would.
- **Speak slowly and clearly.** Avoid jargon. Use short sentences and be concise. Avoid interrupting the interpreter.
- **Pause every few sentences so the interpreter can translate your information.** After 30 seconds of speaking, stop and let the interpreter express the information. Talk directly to the family, not the interpreter.
- **Give the family and the interpreter a break.** Sessions that last longer than 20 or 30 minutes are too much for anyone's attention span and concentration.
- **Express the information in two or three different ways if needed.** There may be cultural barriers as well as language and dialect differences that interfere with understanding. Interpreters may often know the correct communication protocols for the family.
- **Use an interpreter to help ensure the family can read and understand translated written materials.** The interpreter can also help answer questions and evaluate learning.
- **Avoid side conversations during sessions.** These can be uncomfortable for the family and jeopardize client–provider relationships and trust.
- **Remember, just because someone speaks another language doesn't mean that he or she will make a good interpreter.** An interpreter who has no medical background may not understand or interpret correctly, no matter how good his or her language skills are.
- **Do not use children as interpreters.** Doing so can affect family relationships, proper understanding, and compliance with health care issues.

Adapted from American Speech-Language Hearing Association. (2015). *Tips for working with an interpreter.* Retrieved from http://www.asha.org/practice/multicultural/issues/interpret.htm; and Refugee Health Technical Assistance Center. (2011). *Best practices for communicating through an interpreter.* Retrieved from http://refugeehealthta.org/access-to-care/language-access/best-practices-communicating-through-an-interpreter/

establish effective communication with their clients. Providing assistance to the hearing impaired in health care settings is critically important because, without assistance through auxiliary aids and services, health service providers run the risk of not understanding the client's symptoms, misdiagnosing the client's health problem, and prescribing inadequate or even harmful treatment (Smith, 2015).

Hearing-impaired pregnant women are often neglected mostly due to a lack of understanding of how best to care for women with different communication needs. Nurses have a key role in exchanging information and taking the time to understand their needs in order to act as an advocate and help them to overcome the barriers that can be created by deafness. In order to fulfill this role, nurses need to have an understanding of the problems faced by women with hearing impairment and their partners when accessing maternity services (Jackson, 2011).

For the hearing-impaired, determine the method of communication used: lip reading, American Sign Language (ASL), another method, or some combination. If the nurse is not proficient in ASL and the client or family uses it, then an ASL interpreter must be available if another adult family member is not present for translation. According to federal law (Americans With Disabilities Act), deaf clients and deaf family members must be given the ability to communicate effectively with health care providers (Burkey, 2015).

Education

Due to shortened hospital stays and decreased admissions, providing client and family education is a key role for nurses. Many times teaching begins in the primary care setting and then continues in the community setting, especially the home. In the community-based setting, client teaching is often focused on assisting the client and family to achieve independence.

Regardless of the type of setting, nurses are in a unique position to help clients and families manage their own health care needs. Clients and families need to be knowledgeable about areas such as their condition, the health care management plan, and when and how to contact health care providers. With the limited time available in all health care arenas, nurses must focus on teaching goals and begin teaching at the earliest opportunity. Education and planning care are essential components of quality client care (Peter et al., 2015).

Client education occurs when nurses share information, knowledge, and skills with clients and families, thus empowering them to take responsibility for their health care. Through client education, clients and families can overcome feelings of powerlessness and helplessness and gain the confidence and capability to be active members in their plan of care.

HEALTHY PEOPLE 2020

Objective	Significance
Increase the proportion of persons appropriately counseled about health behaviors. (Developmental) Increase the proportion of health care organizations that provide client and family education; increase the proportion of clients who report that they are satisfied with the client education they receive from their health care organization.	• Assess health learning needs of women, children, and their families. • Plan health care education in collaboration with clients and their families. • Provide health education at each client encounter.

Healthy People Objectives retrieved from http://www.healthypeople.gov.

Overall, client and family education allows clients and families to make informed decisions, ensures the presence of basic health care skills, promotes recognition of problem situations, promotes appropriate responses to problems, and allows for questions to be answered. When thorough and structured education begins in the hospital setting, it can carry over into the home setting, which can decrease hospital readmissions. Verification sheets can play an important role in aiding bedside nurses to provide early formal education for clients and families being discharged home with a new device so that safe care can be achieved in the home setting (Hamilton, 2011). Client and family education is a priority and is addressed in *Healthy People 2020.*

Take Note!

To cope effectively with illness, understand and participate in decisions about treatment plans, and maintain and improve health after treatment, clients and their families must have access to the specific knowledge and skills relevant to their conditions (Patient Education Institute, 2013).

Steps of Client and Family Education

The steps of client and family education are similar to the steps of the nursing process. The nurse must assess the client, develop a plan, implement services needed, perform follow-up evaluation, and finally document education. Once the nurse achieves a level of comfort and experience with each of these steps, they all blend together into one harmonious whole that becomes an everyday part of nursing practice. Client education begins with the first client encounter and proceeds through discharge and beyond. Reassessment after each step or change in the process is critical to ensuring success.

ASSESSING TEACHING AND LEARNING NEEDS

Excellent nursing care begins with a thorough assessment of the client. In the same way, client and family education begins with a learning needs assessment that includes the client's and family's learning needs, learning styles and preferences, and potential barriers to learning. Based on the results of the assessment, an individualized plan can be developed to reduce the time and effort required for teaching while maximizing learning for the client and family. Although actual nursing care in pediatrics is given to the child, the educational process is targeted at both the child, when developmentally appropriate, and the adult members of the family. Therefore, it is advisable to conduct a learning needs assessment on both the adult caregivers and the child, when appropriate. Box 2.2 describes the components of a learning needs assessment. This is also a good time to establish rapport with the family, demonstrating your interest in them and your confidence in their ability to learn.

Share the assessment with all members of the interdisciplinary team so that the entire team can support the client's and family's learning. Although assessment generally takes place during the first or second meeting with the client and family, it should also occur with each encounter to check for any changes that may occur.

Malcolm Knowles outlined core learning principles to consider when teaching adults (Knowles, Holton III,

BOX 2.2

COMPONENTS OF LEARNING NEEDS ASSESSMENT

Assess

- Learner characteristics: Find out more about the child and family's life and how the child's illness has affected it. Learn more about the child and family's social, cultural, and spiritual values.
- Learner needs and readiness: Including what they want and need to know and what they know already; readiness and willingness to learn; motivation to learn and emotional concerns; capacity to learn such as physical or cognitive abilities including ability to read and developmental level.
- Learning style: How does the child and family learn best; preferred learning methods.
- Learning barriers: Cultural or language barriers; cognitive or physical disabilities; presence of pain; lack of support network.

Adapted from The Sentinel Watch: Nursing. (2014). *Improve your patient education skills to enhance care.* Retrieved from http://www.americansentinel.edu/blog/2014/12/17/improve-your-patient-education-skills-to-enhance-care/; and The Joint Commission. (2012). *Patient education.* Retrieved from http://www.mghpcs.org/eed_portal/Documents/PatientEd/JC_Standards_PatientEd.pdf

BOX 2.3

SPECIFIC LEARNING PRINCIPLES RELATED TO PARENTS

- **Adults are self-directed.** Adults value independence and want to learn on their own terms. Teaching strategies that include such concepts as role playing, demonstration, and self-evaluation are most helpful. Using this model, nurses can partner with families to ensure that education is interactive and adopt the role of facilitator rather than lecturer.
- **Adults are problem-focused and task-oriented.** Adults learn best when they perceive there is a gap in their knowledge base and want information and skills to fill the gap. Providing a reason to learn can often motivate families that appear slow to comply with their child's care and education.
- **Adults are goal oriented.** Adults learn best at a time when learning meets an immediate need. Presenting information in an organized, sequential, and timely fashion can often help families understand the importance of learning a particular piece of information or task.
- **Adults value past experiences and beliefs.** Adults bring an accumulated wealth of experiences to each health care encounter; this provides a rich base for new learning. Education should take into account a wide range of backgrounds. Appreciating and using individual differences during teaching encounters can help improve compliance and reduce resistance to educational goals.

Knowles, M. S., Holton III, E. F., & Swanson, R. A. (2011). *The adult learner* (7th ed.). Burlington, MA: Elsevier.

& Swanson, 2011). He found that instruction for adults needs to focus more on the process than on the content. Box 2.3 lists adult learner-centered principles.

CULTURAL IMPACT ON ASSESSMENT OF LEARNING NEEDS

In addition to determining the language spoken in the home and use of eye and physical contact, investigate the following during the assessment:

- Who is the person caring for the child at home?
- Who is the authority figure in the family?
- What is the social support structure?
- Are there any special dietary needs and concerns?
- Are any traditional health practices used (e.g., healers, shamans, talismans, folk remedies, and herbs)?
- Are any special clothes or other items used to help maintain health?
- What religious beliefs, ceremonies, and spiritual practices are important?

Learning needs can then be negotiated with the family and met based on the assessment. Issues encountered when teaching immigrant or refugee families might include confusion regarding the use of the English versus the metric scale; preparing formulas and medicines using a "handful" or "pinch" of ingredients rather than specific measurements such as a measuring cup or syringe; access to refrigeration for liquid antibiotics; and breastfeeding practices.

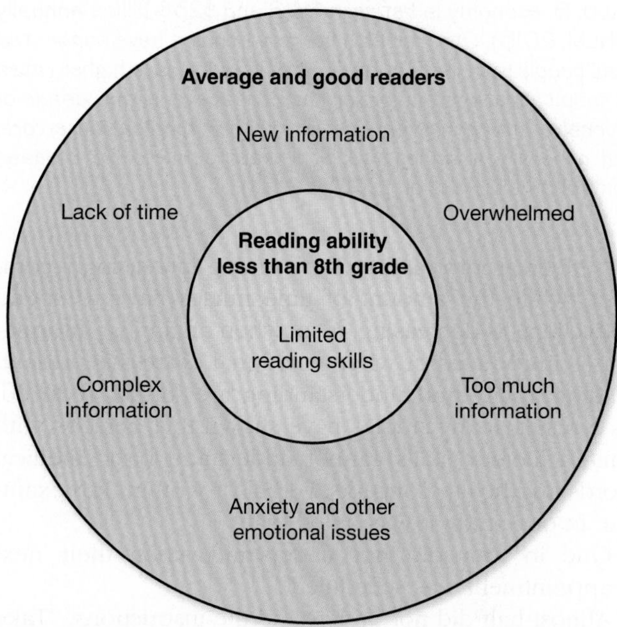

FIGURE 2.2 Factors contributing to poor health literacy.

LITERACY ISSUES

Adequate literacy skills are essential for client and family education, yet many people in America today have marginal reading capabilities. In the United States, 36 million adults cannot read better than the average third grader (ProLiteracy, 2014).

Even people with adequate literacy skills may have difficulty reading, understanding, and applying information to health care situations (Fig. 2.2). **Health literacy** is the ability to read, understand, and use health care information to make appropriate health care decisions and successfully navigate the health care system (Hersh, Salzman, & Snyderman, 2015). It is not simply having the ability to read the health care information, but also includes listening; displaying oral, analytic, and decision-making skills; using electronic technology; and applying these skills to health care situations. The inability to read and comprehend health care information is an enormous problem for many Americans today. Low health literacy affects people of all ages, races, and educational and income levels.

Take Note!

The American Medical Association reports that poor health literacy skills are a stronger predictor of health status than age, income, employment status, education level, or racial or ethnic group (NNLM, 2015). Poor health literacy leads to increased complications and increased mortality (Boodman, 2011). The cost of low health literacy to the U. S. economy is between $106 and $238 billion annually (NNLM, 2015). Other health literacy studies have suggested that people with inadequate health literacy have higher rates of hospitalization and longer hospital stays, higher usage of expensive emergency services, increased medication errors, and generally a higher level of illness (Centers for Disease Control and Prevention [CDC], 2015d).

Medical information is becoming increasingly complex, while the amount of time nurses have to spend with clients is decreasing. Also, when unfamiliar information is introduced or when emotional distress is present, reading ability and understanding are further reduced. As a result, many studies have shown that persons with limited literacy skills cannot understand basic medical words and health concepts, verbal or written. For example, in one study it was noted that:

- One in four did not understand when their next appointment was scheduled.
- Almost half did not understand the instructions, "Take medication on an empty stomach."
- Three quarters misunderstood warnings on medication labels or the rights and responsibilities section of a Medicaid application (Duell et al., 2015).

Take Note!

Recent Federal programs, such as the Affordable Care Act of 2010, the Department of Health and Human Services' National Action Plan to Improve Health Literacy, and the Plain Writing Act of 2010 have been developed to improve health literacy (Koh et al., 2012).

RECOGNIZING POOR HEALTH LITERACY SKILLS

Poor health literacy skills are difficult to recognize: appearance, verbal ability, employment status, and educational level cannot reliably detect persons who do not read well. Also, many people who do not read well go to great lengths to hide their disability; 68% of people with limited literacy skills have never told their spouse and 75% have never told their health care provider (Brega et al., 2015). Poor health literacy affects all segments of the population but certain groups such as the elderly, the poor, members of minority groups, recent immigrants to the United States who do not speak English, and those who are born in the United States but English is a second language are at higher risk (Zambrana et al., 2015).

Red flags that might indicate poor literacy skills include the following:

- Difficulty filling out registration forms, questionnaires, and consent forms; forms are incomplete, incorrect, or inaccurate
- Frequently missed appointments
- Noncompliance and lack of follow-up with treatment regimens
- History of medication errors
- Responses such as, "I forgot my glasses" or "I'll read this when I get home"
- Inability to answer common questions about their treatment or medicines
- Avoiding asking questions for fear of looking "stupid" (Brega et al., 2015)

Nurses need to provide understandable and accessible information to all clients, regardless of their literacy or education levels. This would include avoiding medical jargon, breaking down information or instructions into small concrete steps, limiting the focus of a visit to three key points or tasks, and assessing for comprehension. In addition, printed information should be written at or below a 5th to 6th grade reading level with plenty of visual aids or pictures (Hersh et al., 2015).

PLANNING EDUCATION

Once the assessment is completed, plan mutually agreed-upon, achievable learning goals and objectives. It is important that both the teacher and learner believe the goals can be accomplished. Finding common ground and building a bridge between the client's and family's concerns and what the health care team believes they need to know is a critical part of an education plan. This also is an excellent time to consider which client education materials and resources can be used to maximize learning and retention. No single teaching method will suit every client and family. Individualize educational methods to meet the learning needs and abilities of the audience that is being taught. Ensuring instructional methods are chosen based on educational outcomes is a key to success (Su, Herron, & Osisek, 2011).

A review of recent research on patient education found effective teaching strategies that include computer technology, audiotapes, videos, written materials prepared at an appropriate reading level for the general population, and demonstration (Friedman et al., 2011). Verbal instruction was found to be least effective and should be used along with another teaching method (Friedman et al., 2011). Using multiple teaching strategies, such as using videos, dolls, play therapy, or computer-based instruction along with written material for future reference, are beneficial. Almost 67% of patients had better outcomes when multiple teaching methods were used (Friedman et al., 2011). Visual aids such as pictures and illustrations are very helpful and can assist those with low literacy. Education that is culturally appropriate, presented in a structured manner and specific to the individual has been found to be more effective (Friedman et al., 2011).

Planning client and family education should involve input from the entire interdisciplinary team when appropriate. Through good communication and collaboration, team members can work together to empower the child and family to become knowledgeable and skillful

TABLE 2.1 SIX TECHNIQUES TO IMPROVE LEARNING

Technique	Explanation
Slow down and repeat information often.	Since most of the education in a health care setting is done verbally, repeat important information at least four or five times.
Speak in conversational style using plain, nonmedical language.	When writing directions, write only several words, bullet points, or phrases. Use common, "living-room-type" language containing one or two syllables whenever possible.
Group information and teach it in small amounts using logical steps.	This is especially important when there are large amounts of complex information for the family to learn. Teach for 10 to 15 minutes, give the learner a break, and return later to teach again.
Prioritize information and teach "survival skills" first.	Due to time constraints and multiple demands on the part of staff, coupled with the rapid turnaround times of health care encounters for clients, there never seems to be enough time to teach. Nurses must provide the client and family with the necessary information to meet their immediate needs. This may include information about the following: • The child's medical condition • Treatment information • Why the information is important • Possible problems, adverse effects, or concerns • What to do if problems arise • Who to contact for further help, information, or supplies
Use visuals, such as pictures, videos, and models.	Use visual resources to enhance and reinforce learning when available. Drawing simple pictures and charts or using alternative methods such as color-coding often allows learning to occur for families who are having difficulty grasping information or concepts.
Teach using an interactive, "hands-on" approach.	When the learner uses hands-on practice or participates in care, learning occurs more quickly and easily. Learning first on a doll or model can ease anxiety and bolster self-confidence before actually doing care or procedures on the child.

caregivers. Leaving behind the traditional path of teacher-centered education and providing family-centered education instead requires thought and skill.

PRACTICAL INTERVENTIONS TO ENHANCE LEARNING

The assessed needs and planned learning objectives lead to good teaching interventions. Evaluate these interventions frequently to ensure that the child and family are learning and meeting agreed-upon goals. Table 2.1 presents six techniques that can help improve learning.

HELPING CHILDREN AND FAMILIES WITH POOR HEALTH LITERACY SKILLS

Nurses are in an excellent position to create a "blame-free" environment and offer help. It is entirely appropriate to say to the child or family member, "Many people have a problem reading and remembering the information on this teaching sheet (booklet, manual). Is this ever a problem for you?" For children or family members with low health literacy, the nurse can adjust oral communication techniques and written materials to assist with learning, and should communicate this need to the entire interdisciplinary health care team.

If literacy problems are known or suspected, the nurse can take the following steps to enhance learning:

- Draw pictures or use medical illustrations.
- Use videos.
- Color-code medications or the steps of a procedure.
- Record an audiotape.
- Repeat verbal information often and organize it into small groups.
- Teach a "back-up" family member.

EVALUATING LEARNING

Teaching, even when done well, does not necessarily mean that learning has occurred. Evaluation of learning is critical to ensure that the client and family have actually learned what was taught. In a health care setting, perform an evaluation with each educational encounter and adjust goals and interventions accordingly. The nurse, along with the rest of the interdisciplinary team, is responsible for client and family learning. Help ensure understanding by asking for feedback and offering an opportunity for questions. Also, assessing for signs of confusion, such as increased anxiety, can help evaluate learning. If they have not learned, the health care team ensures that teaching strategies are adjusted so that the client or family does learn.

Take Note!

The ultimate goal of education is a change in behavior on the part of the child and family; this change can occur in their level of knowledge, skill, or both.

Evaluation can occur in several different ways, depending on the topic and the method of teaching. The child or family may:

- Demonstrate a skill, often referred to as return demonstration. Learning can quickly and easily be identified using this method.
- Repeat back or teach back the information using their own words.
- Answer open-ended questions. Open-ended questions provide an opportunity to assess for missing or incorrect information. Open-ended questions are those that cannot be answered with a simple "yes" or "no."

Another option to evaluate learning is to provide a "pretend" scenario for the family, mentally placing them in their own home. Have them verbalize all the steps needed to care for their child, from routine care to handling an emergency situation. They will need to convey information accurately and completely as they walk through the steps necessary to provide care for their child independently at home.

DOCUMENTING EDUCATION FOR THE CHILD AND FAMILY

Documenting child care and education on the medical record is part of every nurse's professional practice and serves four main purposes. First and foremost, the child's medical record serves as a communication tool that the entire interdisciplinary team can use to keep track of what the child and family has learned already and what learning still needs to occur. Next, it serves to testify to the education the family has received if and when legal matters arise. Thirdly, it verifies standards set by The Joint Commission, Centers for Medicare and Medicaid Services (CMS), and other accrediting bodies that hold health care providers accountable for child and family education activities. Finally, it informs third-party payers of goods and services provided for reimbursement purposes.

Documentation of child and family education is imperative. It is the only way to ensure that the family's educational plan and objectives have been completed and that the family is ready for discharge. Documentation of child and family education should include such topics as the following:

- The learning needs assessment
- Information on the client's medical condition and plan of care
- Goals of client education; the date goal is met
- Teaching method used and how it was received by client and family
- Medications, including drug–drug and drug–food interactions
- Modified diets and nutritional needs
- Safe use of medical equipment
- Follow-up care and community resources discussed

Client and family education plays an essential role in promoting safe self-management practice. To ensure that clients and their families attain the required abilities, client and family education needs to be competency based. When developing and applying a competency-based education lesson/program, each nurse must identify essential competencies to be taught, optimal teaching methods, best method to evaluate achievement, and documentation of evidence of learning taken place (King, 2015).

Discharge Planner and Case Manager

Discharge planning involves the development and implementation of a comprehensive plan for the safe discharge of a client from a health care facility and for continuing safe and effective care in the community and at home. Case management focuses on coordinating health care services while balancing quality and cost outcomes. Due to the short length of stays in acute settings and the shift to community settings for clients with complex health needs, discharge planning and case management have become an especially important nursing role in the community (Stanhope & Lancaster, 2015). Often clients requiring community-based care, especially home care, have complex medical needs that require an interdisciplinary team to meet their physical, psychosocial, medical, nursing, developmental, and education needs. The nurse plays an important role in initiating and maintaining the link between team members and the client to ensure that the client and family are receiving comprehensive, coordinated care. (See Chapter 33 for more information on discharge planning and case management for the pediatric population.)

Client Advocate and Resource Manager

Client advocate is another important role of the maternity and pediatric nurse to ensure that the client's and family's needs are being met. Advocacy also helps ensure that the client and family have available resources and appropriate health care services. For example, the pregnant woman on bed rest at home may need help in caring for her other children, maintaining the household, or getting to her appointments. Children with complex medical needs may require financial assistance through Medicaid or Medicaid waivers (state-run programs that use federal and state money to pay for the health care of individuals with certain medical conditions). They may also need assistance in obtaining needed equipment, additional services, and transportation. Nurses need a basic understanding of community, state, and federal resources to ensure that clients and their families have access to those necessary for them. (See Chapter 33 for more information on advocacy and resource management in the pediatric population.)

Preventative Care

The concept of prevention is a key part of maternal and pediatric nursing. The emphasis on health care delivery has moved beyond primary preventive health care (e.g., well-child checkups, routine physical examinations, prenatal care, and treatment of common acute illnesses) and now encompasses secondary and tertiary care.

Primary Prevention

It is the responsibility of all nurses to incorporate health promotion and disease prevention activities into their professional roles. The concept of primary prevention involves preventing the disease or condition before it occurs through health promotion activities, environmental protection, and specific protection against disease or injury. Its focus is on health promotion to reduce the person's vulnerability to any illness by strengthening the person's capacity to withstand physical, emotional, and environmental stressors (Clark, 2014). It encompasses a vast array of areas, including nutrition, good hygiene, sanitation, immunizations, protection from ultraviolet rays, genetic counseling, bicycle helmets, handrails on bathtubs, drug education for school children, adequate shelter, smoking cessation, family planning, and the use of seat belts (Stanhope & Lancaster, 2015). See Figure 2.3 for examples.

Approximately 3,000 children each year in the United States are born with defects of the neural tube – the part of a growing fetus that will become the brain and spinal cord—which can cause severe mental and physical disability or death (CDC, 2015b). Prevention of neural tube defects (NTDs), such as anencephaly and spina bifida, is an example of primary prevention. The use of folic acid supplementation daily for 3 months before and 3 months after conception reduces the risk of first occurrence of an NTD. Women who get enough folic acid have a 50% to 70% reduced risk of having a baby with such a defect (CDC, 2015b). All women of

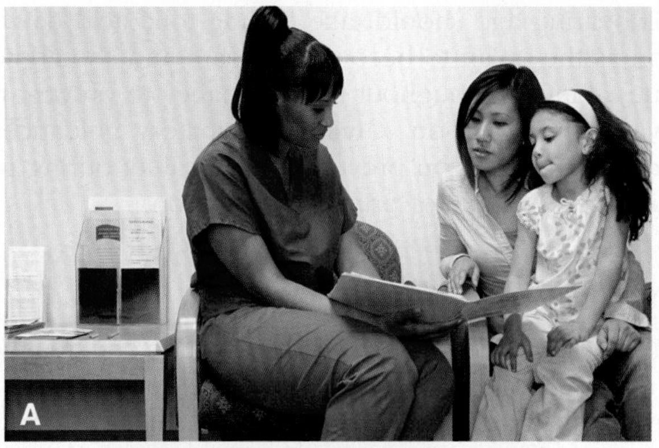

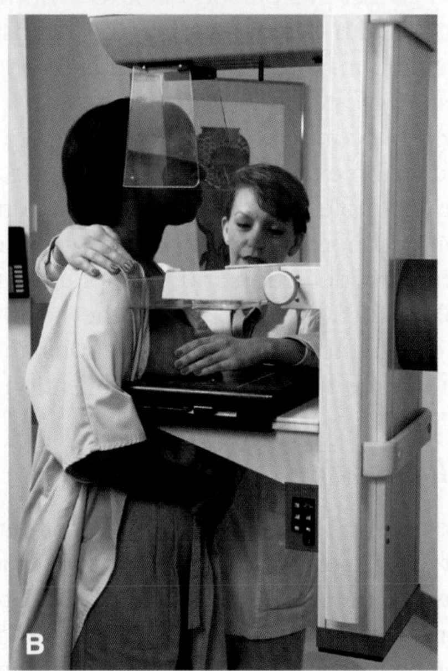

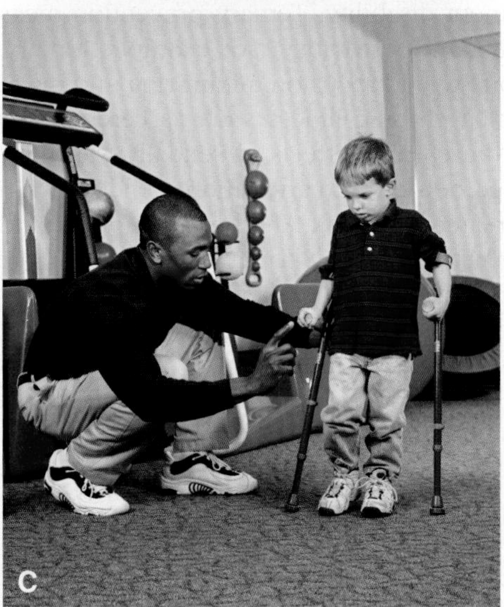

FIGURE 2.3 Levels of prevention. **A.** At the primary prevention level, the nurse provides anticipatory guidance and family teaching. **B.** At the secondary level of prevention, a woman undergoes a mammography screening for early detection of breast problems. **C.** At the tertiary level of prevention, a child with a developmental disability participates in a rehabilitation program.

childbearing age should take 0.4-mg folic acid daily as soon as they plan to become pregnant and should continue taking it throughout the pregnancy to prevent this devastating condition. Giving anticipatory guidance to parents about poison prevention and safety during play is another example of primary prevention.

Secondary Prevention

Secondary prevention is the early detection and treatment of adverse health conditions. This level of prevention is aimed at halting the disease, thus shortening its duration and severity to get the person back to a normal state of functioning. Health screenings are the mainstay of secondary prevention. Pregnancy testing, blood pressure evaluations, cholesterol monitoring, fecal occult blood testing, breast examinations, mammography screening, hearing and vision examinations, and Papanicolaou (Pap) smears are examples of this level of prevention. Such interventions do not prevent the health problem but are intended for early detection and prompt treatment to prevent complications (Smith, 2015). If the health condition cannot be cured and further complications and disability moves in, then the tertiary level of prevention is needed.

Tertiary Prevention

Tertiary prevention is designed to reduce or limit the progression of a permanent, irreversible disease or disability. The purpose of tertiary prevention is to restore individuals to their maximum potential (Klemp, 2015). Tertiary intervention takes place only if the condition results in a permanent disability. Tertiary prevention measures are supportive and restorative. For example, tertiary prevention efforts would focus on minimizing and managing the effects of a chronic illness such as cerebrovascular disease or the chronic effects of sexually transmitted infections (e.g., herpes, human immunodeficiency virus [HIV], and untreated syphilis). Another example would involve working with women who have suffered long-term consequences of violence. Client education is the cornerstone of all disease management programs. The focus of the nurse would be to maximize the woman's strengths through education, to help her recover from the trauma and loss, and to build support systems.

The Nurse's Role in Preventive Care

All health professionals have a special role in health promotion, health protection, and disease prevention. Much of nursing involves prevention, early identification, and prompt treatment of health problems and monitoring for emerging threats that might lead to health problems. Nurses provide health care for women and children at all three levels of prevention. This care often involves advocacy for services to meet their needs.

Culturally Competent Nursing Care

The United States contains an ever-changing mix of cultural groups. The Migration Policy Institute (2015) reports that immigrants accounted for 13% of the total 316 million U.S. residents; adding the U.S.-born children (of all ages) of immigrants means that approximately 80 million people, or one-quarter of the overall U.S. population, is either of the first or second generation. This population is made up of numerous diverse cultural backgrounds arriving from every corner of the world into our country daily.

Take Note!

One million immigrants come to the United States each year, and more than half are of childbearing age. Latin America accounts for more than 50% of immigrants to the United States. By the year 2050, people of African, Asian, and Latino backgrounds will make up one half of our population (Colby & Ortman, 2015).

This growing diversity has significant implications for the health care system. For years nurses have struggled with the issues of providing optimal health care that meets the needs of women, children, and their families from varied cultures and ethnic groups. In addition to displaying competence in technical skills, nurses must also become competent in caring for clients from varied ethnic and racial backgrounds. Adapting to different cultural beliefs and practices requires flexibility and acceptance of others' viewpoints. Nurses must listen to clients and learn about their beliefs about health and wellness. To provide culturally appropriate care to diverse populations, nurses need to know, understand, and respect culturally influenced health behaviors. Chapter 1 provides a more detailed discussion of culture and its impact on the health of women, children, and families.

Nurses must research and understand the cultural characteristics, values, and beliefs of the various people to whom they deliver care so that false assumptions and stereotyping do not lead to insensitive care. Time orientation, personal space, family orientation (patriarchal, matriarchal, or egalitarian), and language are important cultural concepts. Although the location might be different in community-based care, these principles apply to both inpatient and outpatient settings.

Nurses should possess an understanding of the perspectives, traditions, values, practices, and family systems of culturally diverse individuals, families, communities, and populations for whom they provide care, as well as knowledge of the complex variables that affect the achievement of health and well-being (USDHHS Office of Minority Health, n.d.). **Cultural competence** is a dynamic process during which nurses obtain and then apply cultural information. Nurses must look at clients through their own eyes and the eyes of clients and family members. Nurses must develop nonjudgmental acceptance of cultural differences in clients,

BOX 2.4

STEPS TO DEVELOPING CULTURAL COMPETENCE

1. Cultural Self-Awareness
   - Become aware of, appreciate, and become sensitive to the values, beliefs, customs, and behaviors that have shaped one's own culture.
   - Engage in self-exploration beyond one's own culture and "see" clients from different cultures.
   - Health care has a multicultural environment.
   - Cultural diversity is awareness of the presence of differences among clients.
   - Examine personal biases and prejudices toward other cultures.
   - Become aware of differences in personal and clients' backgrounds.
2. Cultural Knowledge
   - Obtain knowledge about various worldviews of different cultures, such as through reading about different cultures, attending continuing education courses on different cultures, accessing websites, and attending cultural diversity conferences.
   - Become familiar with culturally/ethnically diverse groups, worldviews, beliefs, practices, lifestyles, and problem-solving strategies.
3. Cultural Skills
   - Learn how to perform a competent cultural assessment.
   - Assess each client's unique cultural values, beliefs, and practices without depending solely on written facts about specific cultural groups.
   - Embracing ethics empowers mutual respect, equality, and trust.
4. Cultural Encounter
   - Engage in cross-cultural interactions with people from culturally diverse backgrounds, such as attending religious services or ceremonies and participating in important family events.
   - Participate in as many cultural encounters as possible to avoid cultural stereotyping.

Adapted from Burnard, P., & Gill, P. (2015). *Culture, communication and nursing* (2nd ed.). New York, NY: Taylor & Francis Publishers; Harkess, L., & Kaddoura, M. (2015). Culture and cultural competence in nursing education and practice: The state of the art. *Nursing Forum*. doi: 10.1111/nuf.12140; and Darnell, L. K., & Hickson, S. V. (2015). Cultural competent patient-centered nursing care. *Nursing Clinics*, *50*(1), 99–108.

using diversity as a strength that empowers them to achieve mutually acceptable health care goals. Nurses must integrate their client's cultural beliefs and practices into health prescriptions to eliminate or mitigate health disparities and provide client satisfaction. Cultural competence is a dynamic, lifelong learning process. Understanding the process for assessing cultural patterns and factors that influence individual and group differences is critical in preventing overgeneralization and stereotyping (Harkess & Kaddoura, 2015). This cultural awareness allows nurses to see the entire picture and improves the quality of care and health outcomes (Box 2.4). Cultural competence does not appear suddenly; it must be developed through a series of steps.

Consider This

Our medical mission took a team of nurse practitioners into the rural mountains of Guatemala to offer medical services to people who had never had any. One day, a distraught mother brought her 10-year-old daughter to the mission clinic, asking me if there was anything I could do about her daughter's right wrist. She had sustained a fracture a year ago and it had not healed properly. As I looked at the girl's malformed wrist, I asked if it had been splinted to help with alignment, knowing what the answer was going to be. The interpreter enlightened me by saying that this young girl would never marry and have children because of this injury. I appeared puzzled at the interpreter's prediction of this girl's future. It was later explained to me that if the girl couldn't make tortes from corn meal for her husband because of her wrist disability, she would not be worthy of becoming someone's wife and thus would probably live with her parents the rest of her life.

I reminded myself during the week of the medical mission not to impose my cultural values on the women for whom I was caring and to accept their cultural mores without judgment. These silent self-reminders served me well throughout the week, for I was open to learning about their lifestyles and customs.

Thoughts: What must the young girl be feeling at the age of 10, being rejected for a disability that wasn't her fault? What might have happened if I had imposed my value system on this client? How effective would I have been in helping her if she didn't feel accepted? This incident ripped my heart out, for this young girl will be deprived of a fulfilling family life based on a wrist disability. This is just another example of female suppression that happens all over the world—such a tragedy—and yet a part of their culture, on which nurses should not pass judgment.

Barriers to Cultural Competence

Illness is culturally shaped in the sense that how we perceive, experience, and cope with disease is based upon our explanations of sickness. Awareness of how this might be of influence—instead of mere knowledge about the cultural practices or beliefs of specific ethnic groups—and an appreciation of this factor helps nurses deal effectively with cultural issues (Burnard & Gill, 2015). When a health care provider lacks knowledge of a client's cultural practices and beliefs or when the provider's beliefs differ from those of the client, the provider may be unprepared to respond when the client makes unexpected health care decisions. System-related barriers can occur if agencies that have not been designed for cultural diversity want all clients to conform to the established rules and regulations and attempt to fit everyone into the same mold.

Cultural competence does not mean replacing one's own cultural identity with another, ignoring the variability within cultural groups, or even appreciating the cultures being served. Instead, nurses skilled at cultural competence show a respect for difference, an eagerness to learn, and a willingness to accept multiple views of the world. Much of the process of developing cultural competence involves a reexamination of our values and the influence of these values on our beliefs, which affect our attitudes and actions. At the core of both client centeredness and cultural competence is the importance of seeing the client as a unique person (Dauvrin & Lorant, 2015). It is important for all nurses to incorporate the client's traditional healing and health practices with conventional medicine by asking such questions as, Do you have treatment preferences you would like me to include in your care plan? Some clients may prefer certain foods or drinks when they are ill. In addition, during fasting and religious seasons, diets may be different and need to be considered during the process of determining the appropriate course of treatment. Some may have a different idea of what caused the illness. Spirituality, culture, and experience may have a significant role in the client's understanding and treatment of the illness.

Complementary and Alternative Medicine

The federal government formed the National Center for Complementary and Integrative Health (NCCIH) to conduct and support research and education and to provide information on complementary and alternative medicine (CAM) to health care providers and the public. The use of CAM is not unique to a specific ethnic or cultural group: interest in CAM therapies continues to grow nationwide and will affect care of many clients. People from all walks of life and in all areas of the community use CAM. Overall, CAM use is seen more in women than men, and in people with higher educational levels. In the United States, approximately 36% of adults (about 4 in 10) and approximately 12% of children (about 1 in 9) are using some form of CAM. Prayer specifically for health reasons is the most commonly used CAM therapy (NCCIH, 2015a). It is well known that CAM, including homeopathy, acupuncture, phytotherapy, and hydrotherapy, is also being used increasingly by midwives for childbirth (Hall, Griffiths, & McKenna, 2015).

CAM includes diverse practices, products, and health care systems that are not currently considered to be part of conventional medicine (NCCIH, 2015a). *Complementary* medicine is used together with conventional medicine, such as using aromatherapy to reduce discomfort after surgery or to reduce pain during a procedure or during early labor. *Alternative* medicine is used in place of conventional medicine, such as eating a special natural diet to control nausea and vomiting or to treat cancer instead of undergoing surgery, chemotherapy, or radiation that has been recommended by a conventional doctor. *Integrative* medicine combines mainstream medical therapies and CAM therapies for which there is some scientific evidence of safety and effectiveness (NCCIH, 2015a). These include acupuncture, reflexology, therapeutic touch, meditation, yoga, herbal therapies, nutritional supplements, homeopathy, naturopathic medicine, and many more used for the promotion of health and well-being (Holden et al., 2015).

The philosophy of integrative medicine focuses on treating the whole person, not just the disease. The goal is to treat the mind, body, and spirit all at the same time. History has taught us that in science application of the results is never determined by a single study, but by the weight of the evidence. It is right that medicine rests upon a foundation that begins with good clinical observations, case reports, and careful interpretations. Replication across scientists, which is the true hallmark of valid science, establishes whether those clinical observations are important and perhaps applicable. While some of the therapies used are nonconventional, a guiding principle within integrative medicine is to use therapies that have some high-quality evidence to support them (George, 2015). Integrative medicine combines conventional Western medicine with complementary treatments—all in the effort to treat the whole person. The nurse should avoid judgment and encourage the family to research all approaches that are evidence based that support healthy outcomes. Table 2.2 describes selected CAM therapies and treatments.

The theoretic underpinnings of complementary and alternative health practices propose that health and illness are complex interactions of the mind, body, and spirit. It is then surmised that many aspects of clients' health experiences are not subject to traditional scientific methods. This field does not lend itself readily to scientific study or to investigation and therefore is not easily embraced by many hard-core scientists (Ernst, 2015). Much of what is considered to be alternative medicine comes from the Eastern world, folk medicine, and religious and spiritual practices. There is no unifying basic theory for the numerous treatments or modalities, except (as noted previously) that health and illness are considered to be complex interactions among the body, mind, and spirit.

Because of heightened interest in complementary treatments and their widening use, anecdotal efficacy, and growing supporting research evidence, nurses need to be sensitive to and knowledgeable enough to answer many of the questions clients ask and to guide them in a safe, objective way (Ernst, 2015). Nurses have a unique opportunity to provide services that facilitate wholeness. They need to understand all aspects of CAM, including costs, client knowledge, and drug interactions, if they

TABLE 2.2 SELECTED COMPLEMENTARY AND ALTERNATIVE THERAPIES

Therapy	Description
Aromatherapy	Use of essential oils to stimulate the sense of smell for balancing mind, body, and spirit
Homeopathy	Based on the theory of "like treats like"; helps restore the body's natural balance
Acupressure	Restoration of balance by pressing an appropriate point so self-healing capacities can take over
Feng shui (pronounced *fung shway*)	The Chinese art of placement. Objects are positioned in the environment to induce harmony with chi.
Guided imagery	Use of consciously chosen positive and healing images along with deep relaxation to reduce stress and to help people cope
Reflexology	Use of deep massage on identified points of the foot or hand to scan and rebalance body parts that correspond with each point
Therapeutic touch	Balancing of energy by centering, invoking an intention to heal, and moving the hands from the head to the feet several inches from the skin
Herbal medicine	The therapeutic use of plants for healing and treating diseases and conditions
Spiritual healing	Praying, chanting, presence, laying on of hands, rituals, and meditation to assist in healing
Chiropractic therapy	Aimed at removing irritants to the nervous system to restore proper function—spinal manipulation done for musculoskeletal complaints
Massage therapy	Therapeutic stroking or kneading of the body to decrease pain, produce relaxation, and/or to improve circulation to that body part

Adapted from Hall, H. G., Griffiths, D., & McKenna, L. G. (2015). Complementary and alternative medicine: Interaction and communication between midwives and women. *Women and Birth*, *28*(2), 137–142; and National Center for Complementary and Integrative Health. (2015a). *Complementary, alternative, or integrative health: What's in a name?* Retrieved from https://nccih.nih.gov/health/integrative-health

are to promote holistic strategies for clients and families. With all of the enthusiasm in favor of CAM therapies, nurses must not forget their obligation to embrace the principles of evidence-based practice and critical evaluation before being misled into therapies that have no scientific basis to justify their use.

The growing use of complementary and alternative therapies during pregnancy and childbirth could be interpreted as a response by women regarding a need for autonomy and active participation in their health care during this time. Studies show that massage, acupuncture, vitamins, and herbs are the most frequently applied methods during pregnancy. In a recent study, only half of the pregnant women revealed their use of CAM to their health care provider during their prenatal visits (Holden et al., 2015).

Many clients who use complementary or alternative therapies do not reveal this fact to their health care provider. Therefore, one of the nurse's most important roles during the assessment phase of the nursing process is to encourage clients to communicate their use of these therapies to eliminate the possibility of harmful interactions and contraindications with current medical therapies. When assessing clients, ask specific questions about any nonprescription medications they may be taking, including vitamins, minerals, or herbs. Clients should also be asked about any therapies they are taking that have not been ordered by their primary health care provider.

When caring for clients and their families who practice CAM, nurses need to:

- Be culturally sensitive to nontraditional treatments
- Acknowledge and respect different beliefs, attitudes, and lifestyles
- Keep an open mind, remembering that standard medical treatments do not work for all clients
- Accept CAM and integrate it if it brings comfort without harm
- Provide accurate information, not unsubstantiated opinions
- Advise clients how they can best monitor their condition using CAM
- Discourage practices only if they are harmful to the client's health

- Instruct the client to weigh the risks and benefits of CAM use
- Avoid confrontation when asking clients about CAM
- Be reflective, nonjudgmental, and open-minded about CAM.

The use of complementary therapies is widespread, especially by women desiring to alleviate the nausea and vomiting of early pregnancy. Ginger powder or tea, Sea-Bands (acupressure), hypnosis, and vitamin B6 are typically used to treat morning sickness (Tyler & Nagtalon-Ramos, 2015). Although these may not cause any ill effects during the pregnancy, most substances ingested cross the placenta and have the potential to reach the fetus, so nurses should stress to all pregnant women that it is better to be cautious when using CAM.

Women at risk for osteoporosis are seeking alternatives to menopausal hormone therapy since the Women's Health Initiative (WHI) study raised doubts about the benefit of estrogen. Some of the alternative therapies for osteoporosis include soy isoflavones, progesterone cream, magnet therapy, tai chi, and hip protectors (NCCIH, 2015b). In addition, menopausal women may seek CAM therapies for hot flashes. Once again, despite many claims, most of these therapies have not undergone scientific testing and thus could place the woman at risk.

If clients are considering the use of or using CAM therapies, suggest they check with their health care provider before taking any "natural" substance. Offer clients the following instructions:

- Do not take for granted that because a substance is a natural herb or plant product, it is beneficial or harmless.
- Seek medical care when ill.
- Always inform the provider if you are taking herbs or other therapies.
- Be sure that any product package contains a list of all ingredients and amounts of each.
- Be aware that frequent or continual use of large doses of a CAM preparation is not advisable, and harm may result if therapies are mixed (e.g., vitamin E, garlic, and aspirin all have anticoagulant properties).
- Research CAM through resources such as books, websites, and articles (Chang & Chang, 2015).

All nurses, especially nurses working in the community, must educate themselves about the pros and cons of CAM and be prepared to discuss and help their clients make sense of it all. Expanding our consciousness by understanding and respecting diverse cultures and CAM will enable nurses to provide the best treatment for clients and their families receiving community-based care.

COMMUNITY-BASED CARE

Community may be defined as a specific group of people, often living in a defined geographical area, who share common interests, who interact with each other, and who function collectively within a defined social structure to address common concerns (Stanhope & Lancaster, 2015). The common features of a community may be common rights and privileges as members of a certain city or common ties of identity, values, norms, culture, language, or social support. Women are caregivers to children, parents, spouses, and neighbors and provide important social support in these roles. The child's community consists of the family, school, neighborhood, youth organizations, and other peer groups.

A person can be a part of many communities during the course of daily life. Examples might include area of residence (home, apartment, shelter), gender, place of employment (organization or home), language spoken (Spanish, Chinese, English), educational background or student status, culture (Italian, African American, Indian), career (nurse, businesswoman, housewife), place of worship (church or synagogue), and community memberships (garden club, YMCA, support group, school PTA, youth organizations, athletic teams).

A **population** is a group of people who share personal or environmental characteristics. Typically the most common characteristic is geographic location. Populations are made up of human beings within complex social and physical environments. The betterment of human populations remains the goal of community-based nursing care.

In community-based care, the community is the unit of service. The providers of care are concerned not only with the clients who present for service but also with the larger population of potential or at-risk clients.

Community Health Nursing

Community health nursing focuses on preventing illness and improving the health of populations and communities. Population is defined as a group of people who may or may not interact with each other within a defined geographic location (McMurray & Clendon, 2015). Community health nurses work in geographically and culturally diverse settings. They address current and potential health needs of the population or community. They promote and preserve the health of a population and are not limited to particular age groups or diagnoses. Public health nursing is a specialized area of community health nursing.

Epidemiology, the study of the causes, distribution, and control of disease in populations, can help determine the health and health needs of a population and assist in planning health services. Community health nurses perform epidemiologic investigations to help analyze and develop health policy and community health initiatives. Community health initiatives can be focused on the community as a whole or a specific target population with specific needs. *Healthy People 2020: Improving the Health of Americans* (HP 2020) is an example of national health initiatives developed using the epidemiologic process. HP 2020 ensures that health care professionals evaluate the individual as well as the community. It emphasizes the ever-present link between the individual's health and the health of the community (Thomas et al., 2015). HP 2020 identifies two major goals: to increase the quality of life and the life expectancy of individuals of all ages and to decrease health disparities among different populations (U.S. Department of Health and Human Services [USDHHS], 2015a). Relevant HP 2020 objectives are highlighted throughout this text.

The focus of health care initiatives today is on people and their needs, strengthening their abilities to shape their own lives. The emphasis has shifted away from dependence on health professionals toward personal involvement and personal responsibility, and this gives nurses the opportunity to interact with individuals in a variety of self-help roles. Nurses in the community can be the primary force in identifying the challenges and implementing changes in women's and children's health for the future.

Community-Based Nursing

In the past, the only community-based roles for nurses were community health nurses or public health nurses. This is now a subset of what is considered community-based nursing. The health needs of the society and consumer demand brought about community-based and community-focused services. The movement from an illness-oriented "cure" perspective in hospitals to a focus on health promotion and primary health care in community-based settings has dramatically changed employment opportunities for today's nurses.

This shift in emphasis to primary care and outpatient treatment and management will likely continue. As a result, employment growth in a variety of community-based settings can be expected for properly educated nurses.

With the worldwide strategic shift of health care delivery from secondary to primary care settings, more newly qualified nurses are working in primary care, making exposure to the variety of roles available to nurses essential for future workforce development. The idea of nurses being change agents and thriving amidst change may seem overwhelming, but all nurses need to be open to change. The time is now for nurses to be lifelong learners prepared for change in any health care setting (Orr & Davenport, 2015).

The Bureau of Labor Statistics, U.S. Department of Labor, Occupational Employment Statistics (2014) found the following trends in registered nurse (RN) employment settings:

- 61% of RNs work in the hospital setting.
- 26% work outside the hospital setting in community-based settings.
- The number of RNs employed in community-based settings has continued to grow largely due to an increase in nurses working in home health care and managed care organizations.

Shift in Responsibilities from Hospital-Based to Community-Based Nursing

Many nurses find the shift from acute care nursing to a community setting challenging. Community care, especially home care, is a rapidly growing service in the United States. Nurses play an important role in the treatment and care of clients in the community and need to collaborate with acute care nurses to integrate appropriate community interventions along the continuum of care (Lemetti et al., 2015). Community-based care has been shown to be a cost-effective method for providing care. An increase in disposable income and the increased longevity of people with chronic and debilitating health conditions have also contributed to the continued shift of health care to the community and home setting. Technology has advanced, allowing for improved monitoring of clients in community settings and at home as well as allowing complicated procedures to be done at home, such as intravenous administration of antibiotics, telehealth surveillance, and renal dialysis (Farrar, 2015).

Caring for children at home not only improves their physical health but also allows for adequate growth and development within their family. They are in a familiar environment with the comfort and support of family, which leads to improved care and quality of life.

Community-based nursing settings include ambulatory care, home health care, occupational health, school health, and hospice settings (Table 2.3). Clinical practice within the community may also include case management, research, quality improvement, and discharge planning. Nurses with advanced practice and experience may be employed in areas of staff development, program development, and community education.

Community-Based Nursing Interventions

Nursing interventions involve any treatment that the nurse performs to enhance the client's outcome. Nursing practice in the community uses the nursing process and is similar to that in the acute care setting, because assessing, performing procedures, administering medications, coordinating services and equipment, counseling clients and their families, and teaching about care are all part of the care administered by nurses in the community. See Evidence-Based Practice 2.1. Box 2.5 highlights the most common nursing interventions used in community-based nursing practice.

TABLE 2.3 **COMMUNITY-BASED PRACTICE SETTINGS**

Setting	Description
Ambulatory care	Doctor's offices settings Health maintenance organizations (HMOs) Day surgery centers Freestanding urgent care centers Family planning clinics Mobile mammography centers
Home health care services	High-risk pregnancy/neonate care Maternal/child newborn care Skilled nursing care Hospice care
Health Department services	Maternal/child health clinics Family planning clinics Sexually transmitted infection programs Immunization clinics Substance abuse programs Jails and prisons
Long-term care	Skilled nursing facilities Nursing homes Hospices Assisted living
Other community-based settings	Parish nursing programs Summer camps Childbirth education programs School health programs Occupational health programs

EVIDENCE-BASED PRACTICE 2.1 **COMMUNITY-BASED INTERVENTION PACKAGES FOR REDUCING MATERNAL–NEONATAL MORBIDITY AND MORTALITY AND IMPROVING NEONATAL OUTCOMES**

Maternal, infant, and under-five child mortality rates have declined significantly in the past decades, but newborn mortality rates have reduced more slowly. About half of all newborn deaths are preventable by using evidence-based interventions such as tetanus toxoid immunizations to mothers, clean and skilled care at birth, newborn resuscitation, exclusive breast-feeding, clean umbilical cord care, and management of newborn infections. A large portion of these maternal and newborn deaths and diseases can be addressed through community-based packaged interventions.

STUDY

The purpose of this study was to assess the effectiveness of community-based intervention packages in reducing maternal and neonatal morbidity and mortality to improve neonatal outcomes. The authors found 26 randomized and quasi-randomized controlled studies evaluating the impact of community-based intervention packages for the prevention of maternal illnesses and death and in improving newborn health outcomes.

Findings

A statistically significant reduction was observed in maternal morbidity, neonatal mortality, and perinatal mortality as a consequence of implemented community-based interventional care packages. It is found that the value of integrating maternal and newborn care in community settings through a range of interventions impacts the health of this vulnerable population positively.

Nursing Implications

This review highlights the importance of integrating maternal and newborn care in community settings through a range of interventions which can be delivered by community health nurses and health promotion groups. There is sufficient evidence to scale up community-based care. As this study pointed out—maternal–child care can't stop upon discharge from the hospital, it must continue in community health care settings and homes to impact maternal–neonatal outcomes positively. Community health nurses can take a lead role in facilitating this care to improve maternal–child outcomes.

Adapted from Lassi, Z. S., & Bhutta, Z. A. (2015). Community-based intervention packages for reducing maternal and neonatal morbidity and mortality and improving neonatal outcomes. *Cochrane Database of Systematic Reviews*, 3:CD007754. doi: 10.1002/14651858.CD007754.pub3.

BOX 2.5

COMMUNITY-BASED NURSING INTERVENTIONS

- Health screening—detecting unrecognized or preclinical illness among individuals so they can be referred for definitive diagnosis and treatment (e.g., mammogram or Pap smear, well-child vision and hearing checks)
- Health education programs—assisting clients in making health-related decisions about self-care, use of health resources, and social health issues such as smoking bans and motorcycle helmet laws (e.g., childbirth education or breast self-examination, child safety programs, poisoning prevention, youth drug awareness programs)
- Medication administration—preparing, giving, and evaluating the effectiveness of prescription and over-the-counter drugs (e.g., hormone replacement therapy in menopausal women, childhood immunizations)
- Telephone consultation—identifying the problem to be addressed; listening and providing support, information, or instruction; documenting advice/instructions given to concerns raised by caller (e.g., consultation for a mother with a newborn with colic, interaction with a parent whose child has a fever or is vomiting)
- Health system referral—passing along information about the location, services offered, and ways to contact agencies (e.g., referring a woman for a breast prosthesis after a mastectomy, arranging for home tutoring for a child with a long-term illness)
- Instructional—teaching an individual or a group about a medication, disease process, lifestyle changes, community resources, or research findings concerning their environment (e.g., childbirth education class, basic life support classes for parents, child safety education classes)
- Nutritional counseling—demonstrating the direct relationship between nutrition and illness while focusing on the need for diet modification to promote wellness (e.g., Women, Infants, and Children [WIC] program; counselor interviewing a pregnant woman or a child and parents who have anemia; eating disorders program)
- Risk identification—recognizing personal or group characteristics that predispose people to develop a specific health problem, and modifying or eliminating them (e.g., genetic counseling of an older pregnant woman at risk for a Down syndrome infant; genetic screening of family members for cystic fibrosis or Huntington disease)

Adapted from Wright, L. M., & Leahey, M. (2013). *Nurses and families: A guide to family assessment and intervention* (6th ed.). Philadelphia, PA: F.A. Davis Company.

Community-Based Nursing Challenges

Despite the benefits achieved by caring for families in their own homes and communities, challenges also exist. Clients are being discharged from acute care facilities very early in their recovery course and present with more health care needs than in the past. As a result, nursing care and procedures in the home and community are becoming more complex and time-consuming. Consider the example of a woman who developed a systemic infection, a pelvic abscess, and deep vein thrombosis in her leg after a cesarean birth who is being discharged from the hospital. The nurse's primary focus of care in this situation would be to administer heparin and antibiotics intravenously rather than educating her about child care and follow-up appointments. In the past, this woman would have remained hospitalized for treatment, but home infusion therapy is now less costly and allows the client to be discharged sooner.

This demand on the nurse's time may limit the amount of time spent on prevention measures, education, and the family's psychosocial issues. More time may be needed to help families deal with these issues and concerns. With large client caseloads, nurses may find it difficult to spend the time needed while meeting the time restrictions dictated by their health care agencies. Nurses need to plan the tasks to be accomplished (Box 2.6).

Nurses working in the community have fewer resources available to them compared with the acute care setting. Decisions often have to be made in isolation. The nurse must possess excellent assessment skills and the ability to communicate effectively with the family to be successful in carrying out the appropriate plan of care.

Nurses interested in working in community-based settings must be able to apply the nursing process in an environment that is less structured or controlled than that associated with acute care facilities. Nurses must be able to assimilate information well beyond the immediate physical and psychosocial needs of the client in a controlled acute care setting and deal with environmental threats, lifestyle choices, family issues, different cultural patterns, financial burdens, transportation problems, employment hazards, communication barriers, limited resources, and client acceptance and compliance.

Although opportunities for employment in community-based settings are plentiful, many positions require a baccalaureate degree. Previous medical–surgical experience in an acute care setting is typically required by home health agencies because these nurses must function fairly independently within the home environment.

The nurse must also be familiar with and respectful of many different cultures and socioeconomic levels, remaining objective in dealing with such diversity and demonstrating an understanding of and appreciation for cultural differences. Nurses are increasingly working with

BOX 2.6

HOME CARE VISITATION PLANNING

- Review previous interventions to eliminate unsuccessful ones.
  - Check previous home visit narrative to validate interventions.
  - Communicate with previous nurse to ask questions and clarify.
  - Formulate plan of interventions based on data received (e.g., client preference of IV placement or order of fluids).
- Prioritize client needs based on their potential to threaten the client's health status.
  - Use Maslow's hierarchy of needs to set forth a plan of care.
  - Address life-threatening physiologic issues first (e.g., an infectious process would take precedence over anorexia).
- Develop goals that reflect primary, secondary, and tertiary prevention levels.
  - *Primary prevention*—Have the client consume adequate fluid intake to prevent dehydration.
  - *Secondary prevention*—Administer drug therapy as prescribed to contain and treat an existing infectious process.
  - *Tertiary prevention*—Instruct the stroke client how to exercise to minimize disability.
- Bear in mind the client's readiness to accept intervention and education.
  - Ascertain the client's focus and how she sees her needs.
  - Address client issues that might interfere with intervention (e.g., if the client is in pain, attempting to teach her about her care will be lost; her pain must be addressed first before she is ready to learn).
- Consider the timing of the visit to prevent interfering with other client activities.
  - Schedule all visits at convenient times per client if possible (e.g., if the client has a favorite television show to watch, attempt to schedule around that event if at all possible).
  - Reschedule a home visit if a client event comes up suddenly.
- Outline nursing activities to be completed during the scheduled visit.
  - Know the health care agency's policy and procedures for home visits.
  - Consider the time line and other visits scheduled that day.
  - Research evidence-based best practices to use in the home to validate your intervention decisions.
- Obtain necessary materials/supplies before making the visit.
  - Assemble all equipment needed for any procedure in advance.
  - Secure any equipment that might be needed if a problem occurs (e.g., bring additional IV tubing and a catheter to make sure the procedure can be carried out without delay).
- Determine criteria to be used to evaluate the effectiveness of the home visit.
  - Revisit outcome goals to determine the effectiveness of the intervention.
  - Assess the client's health status to validate improvement.
  - Monitor changes in the client's behavior toward health promotion activities and disease prevention (e.g., verify/observe that the client demonstrates correct hand-washing technique after instruction and reinforcement during the home care visit).

Adapted from Stanhope, M., & Lancaster, J. (2015). *Public health nursing: Population-centered health care in the community* (9th ed.). St. Louis, MO: Mosby Elsevier; Iván, A., Perry, J., & Johnson, V. (2015). Pathways to resilience: Enhancing family well-being with a home visitation model. *Feature Articles Exploring Overparenting within the Context of Youth Development Programs, 10*(1), 35–58; and Aston, M., Price, S., Etowa, J., Vukic, A., Young, L., Hart, C., et al. (2015). The power of relationships exploring how public health nurses support mothers and families during postpartum home visits. *Journal of Family Nursing, 21*(1), 11–34.

clients from diverse cultural backgrounds with different cultural values pertaining to their health. Interventions must be individualized to address the cultural, social, and economic diversity among clients in their own environment (Darawsheh & Chard, 2015).

Community-Based Nursing Care Settings for Women and Children

Community-based nursing takes place in a variety of settings, including physician's offices, clinics, health departments, urgent care centers, hospital outpatient centers, schools, camps, churches, shelters, and clients' homes. Nurses provide well care, episodic ill care, and chronic care. They work to promote, preserve, and improve the health of the women, children, and families in these settings.

Due to technologic advances, cost containment, and shortened hospital stays, the home is a common care setting for women, children, and families today. Home care is geared toward the needs of the client and family. Private-duty nursing care is used when more extensive care is needed; it may be delivered hourly (several hours per day) or on a full-time, live-in basis. Periodic nursing visits may be used for intermittent interventions, such as IV antibiotic administration, follow-up with client teaching, and monitoring. The goals of nursing care in the home setting include promoting, restoring, and maintaining the health of the client.

Home care focuses on minimizing the effects of the illness or disability along with providing the client with the means to care for the illness or disability at home. Nurses in the home care setting are direct care providers, educators, advocates, and case managers.

Prenatal Care

Early, adequate prenatal care has long been associated with improved pregnancy outcomes (March of Dimes, 2015). Adequate prenatal care is a comprehensive process in which any problems associated with pregnancy are identified and treated. Basic components of prenatal care are early and continuing risk assessment, health promotion, medical and psychosocial interventions, and follow-up. Within the community setting, several services are available to provide health care for pregnant women (Box 2.7).

Not all women are aware of the community resources available to them. Most public health services are available for consultation, local hospitals have "hotlines" for questions, and public libraries have pregnancy-related resources as well as Internet access. Nurses can be a very helpful link to resources for all women regardless of their economic status.

Technologically advanced care has been shown to improve maternal and child outcomes. Regionalized high-risk care, recommended by the American Academy of Pediatrics in the late 1970s, aimed to promote uniformity nationwide, covering the prenatal care of high-risk pregnancies and high-risk newborns. The advanced technology found in perinatal regional centers and community-based prenatal surveillance programs have resulted in better risk-adjusted mortality rates. Regionalized systems of perinatal care are recommended to ensure that each mother and newborn achieve optimal outcomes. A recent proposed classification system for multiple levels of maternal care pertains to birth centers, basic care (level I), specialty care (level II), subspecialty care (level III), and regional perinatal health care centers (level IV). The goal of regionalized maternal care is for high-risk pregnant women to receive care in facilities that are prepared to provide the required level of specialized care, thereby reducing maternal morbidity and mortality rates (American College of Obstetricians and Gynecologists [ACOG], 2015). For example, fetal monitoring and ultrasound technology have traditionally been used in acute care settings to monitor the progress of many high-risk pregnancies. However, with the increased cost of hospital stays, many services were moved to outpatient facilities and into the home. The intent was to reduce health care costs and to monitor women with complications of pregnancy in the home rather than in the hospital. Examples of services offered in the home setting might include the following:

- Infusion therapy to treat infections or combat dehydration
- Hypertension monitoring for women with gestational hypertension
- Uterine monitoring for mothers who are at high risk for preterm labor
- Fetal monitoring to evaluate fetal well-being
- Portable ultrasound to perform a biophysical profile to assess fetal well-being

BOX 2.7

MATERNAL–CHILD COMMUNITY HEALTH CARE SERVICES

- State public health prenatal clinics provide access to care based on a sliding scale payment schedule or have services paid for by Medicaid.
- Federally funded community clinics typically offer a variety of services, which may include prenatal, pediatric, adult health, and dental services. A sliding scale payment schedule or Medicaid may cover costs.
- Hospital outpatient health care services offer maternal–child health services. Frequently they are associated with a teaching hospital in which medical school students, interns, and OB/GYN residents rotate through the clinic services to care for clients during their education process.
- Private OB/GYN offices are available for women with health insurance seeking care during their pregnancies. Some physicians in private practice will accept Medicaid clients as well as private clients.
- Community free clinics offer maternal–child services in some communities for women with limited economic resources (homeless, unemployed).
- Freestanding birth centers offer prenatal care for low-risk mothers as well as childbirth classes to educate couples regarding the birthing process. Most centers accept private insurance and Medicaid for reimbursement services.
- Midwifery services are available in many communities where midwives provide women's health services. They usually accept a multitude of payment plans from private pay to health insurance to Medicaid for reimbursement purposes.
- WIC provides food, nutrition counseling, and access to health services for low-income women, infants, and children. WIC is a federally funded program and is administered by each state. All people receiving Aid to Families with Dependent Children (AFDC), food stamps, or Medicaid are automatically eligible for WIC. WIC serves 53% of all infants born in the United States up to their fifth birthday (USDA Food and Nutrition Service, 2015).
- Childbirth classes offer pregnant women and their partners a series of educational classes on childbirth preparation. Women attend them during their last trimester of pregnancy. Some classes are free and some have a fee.
- Local La Leche League groups provide mother-to-mother support for breast-feeding, nutrition, and infant care problem-solving strategies. All women who have an interest in breast-feeding are welcome to participate in the meetings, which are typically held in the home of a La Leche member.

Adapted from USDA Food and Nutrition Service. (2015). *Women, Infants and Children (WIC)*. Retrieved from http://www.fns.usda.gov/wic/about-wic-wic-glance; Community Health Network. (2015). *Women's services*. Retrieved from http://www.ecommunity.com/s/womens-services/; and La Leche League International. (2014). *La Leche League mother-to-mother forums*. Retrieved from http://forums.llli.org/

As a result, home care has the potential to produce cost savings compared to inpatient care.

Labor and Birth Care

Pregnancy involves numerous choices: cloth or disposable diapers, breast-feeding or bottle feeding, doctor or midwife, and where to give birth—at a birthing center, at home, or at a hospital. Deciding where to give birth depends on the woman's pregnancy risk status. For the pregnant woman who is at high risk as a result of medical or social factors, the hospital is considered the safest place for birth. Potential complications can be addressed because medical technology, skilled professionals, and neonatal services are available. For low-risk women, a freestanding birthing center or a home birth is an option.

The choice between a birthing center, home birth, or hospital depends on the woman's preferences, her risk status, and her distance from a hospital. Some women choose an all-natural birth with no medications and no medical intervention, whereas others would feel more comfortable in a setting in which medications and trained staff are available if needed. Presenting the facts to women and allowing them to choose in collaboration with their health care provider is the nurse's role. Client safety is paramount, but at the same time nurses must protect the woman's right to select birth options and should promote family-centered care in all maternity settings.

BIRTHING CENTER

A birthing center is a cross between a home birth and a hospital. Birthing centers offer a home-like setting but with close proximity to a hospital in case of complications. Midwives often are the sole care providers typically in freestanding birthing centers, with obstetricians as backups in case of emergencies. Birthing centers usually have fewer restrictions and guidelines for families to follow and allow for more freedom in making decisions about labor. The rates of cesarean birth and the costs are much lower than those of a hospital (Childbirth Connection, 2015). Midwife-led comprehensive care in a birthing center using the same medical guidelines as in standard care in hospitals reduced medical interventions without jeopardizing maternal and infant health. Birthing centers advertise themselves as a natural alternative to a hospital, as well as a place of female empowerment and control (American Association of Birth Centers [AABC], 2015). The normal discharge time after birth is usually measured in hours (4 to 24 hours), not days.

Birthing centers aim to provide a relaxing home environment and promote a culture of normalcy. Currently, we are seeing a rise in the number of birth centers being established, which is essential in the promotion of normality. It is in these birth centers that midwives will learn about normalcy, building the skills needed to support women through labor, rather than managing labor. The current economic climate may result in more efficient use of resources, possibly normalizing birth (AABC, 2015). Birth is considered a normal physiologic process, and most centers use a noninterventional view of labor and birth. The range of services for the expectant family often includes prenatal care, childbirth education, intrapartum care, and postpartum care, including home follow-up and family planning (Fig. 2.4). One of the hallmarks of the freestanding birthing center is that it can provide truly family-centered care by approaching pregnancy and birth as a normal family event and encouraging all family members to participate. Education is often provided by such centers, encouraging families to become informed and self-reliant in the care of themselves and their families (Steinberg & Sackmary, 2015).

Birthing centers provide an alternative for women who are uncomfortable with a home birth but who do not want to give birth in a hospital. Advantages of birthing centers include a noninterventional approach to obstetric care, freedom to eat and move around during labor, ability to give birth in any position, and the right to have any number of family and friends attend the birth. Disadvantages are that some centers have rigid screening criteria, which may eliminate healthy mothers from using birth centers; many have rigid rules concerning transporting the mother to the hospital (e.g., prolonged labor, ruptured membranes); and many have no pediatrician on staff if the newborn has special needs after birth (Childbirth Connection, 2015).

HOME BIRTH

For centuries women have been giving birth to babies in their home. Many feel more comfortable and relaxed when giving birth in their own environment. Women who want no medical interventions and a very family-centered birth often choose to have a home birth. Home births are recommended for pregnant women who are considered to be at low risk for complications during labor and birth (Zielinski, Ackerson, & Low, 2015). Home birth is advantageous because it:

- Is the least expensive
- Allows the woman to experience labor and birth in the privacy, comfort, and familiarity of home while surrounded by loved ones
- Permits the woman to maintain control over every aspect affecting her labor (e.g., positions, attire, support people)
- Minimizes interference and unnecessary interventions, allowing labor to progress normally
- Provides continuous one-on-one care by the midwife throughout the childbirth process
- Promotes the development of a trusting relationship with the nurse midwife (American Pregnancy Association, 2015).

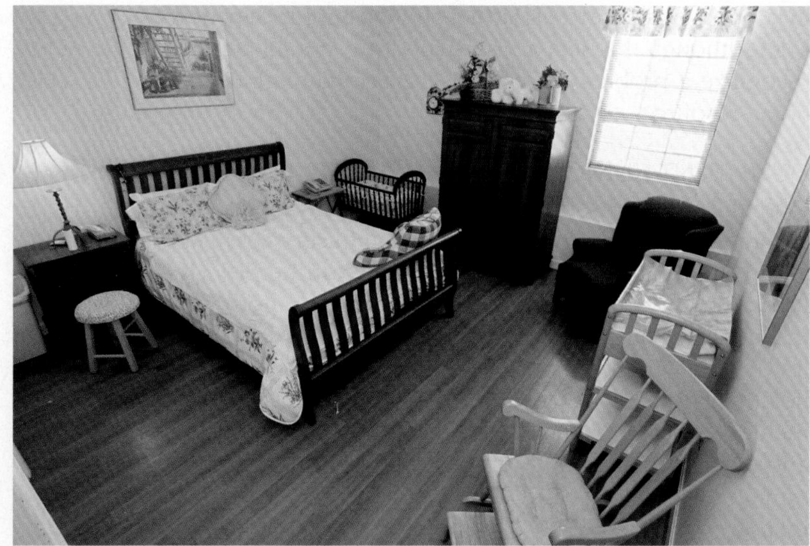

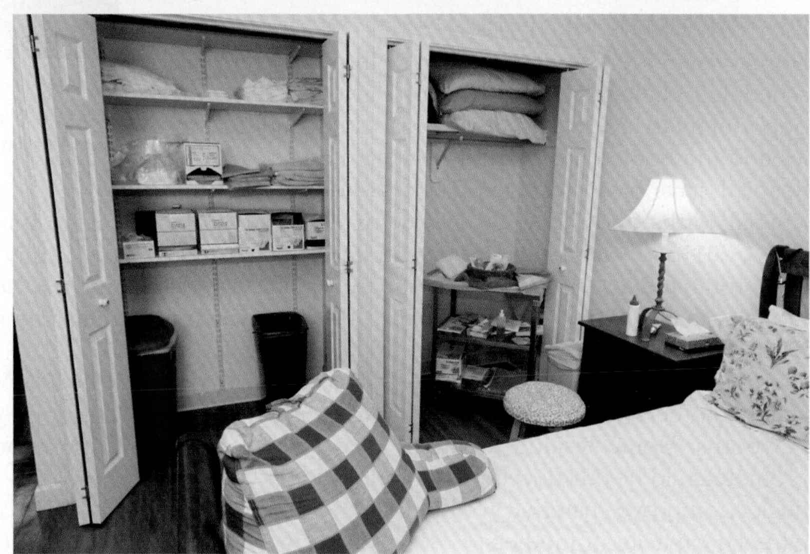

FIGURE 2.4 Birthing centers aim to provide a relaxing home environment and promote a culture of normality while offering a full range of health care services to the expectant family. (Photos by Gus Freedman.)

A home birth has certain disadvantages, however, including the limited availability of pain medication and danger to the mother and baby if an emergency arises (e.g., placenta abruptio, uterine rupture, cord prolapse, or a distressed fetus). Delay in getting to the hospital could jeopardize the life of the child or the mother. A backup plan for a health care provider and nearby hospital on standby must be established should an emergency occur. The available evidence suggests that planned home birth is safe for women who are at low risk of complications and are cared for by appropriately qualified and licensed midwives with access to timely transfer to a hospital if required (Zielinski et al., 2015).

Postpartum and Newborn Care

Recent reforms in health care financing have reduced hospital stays significantly for new mothers. As a result, community-based nurses play a major role in extending care beyond the hospital setting. When new mothers are discharged from the hospital, most are still experiencing perineal discomfort and uterine cramping. They may still have pain from an episiotomy. They are fatigued and may be constipated. They may feel uncertain about feeding and caring for their newborn. These new mothers need to be made aware of community resources such as telephone consultation by nurses, outpatient clinics, home visits, neighborhood mothers' support groups, and online new parent forums.

TELEPHONE CONSULTATION

Many hospitals offer telephone consultation services by their maternity nurses. The discharged mother is given the phone number of the nursing unit on the day of discharge and is instructed to call if she has any questions or concerns. Because the nurses on the unit are familiar with her birth history and the newborn, they are in a good position to assist her in adjusting to her new role. Although this service is usually free, not all families recognize a problem early or use this valuable informational resource.

OUTPATIENT CLINICS

Outpatient clinics offer another community-based site where the childbearing family can obtain services. Usually the mother has received prenatal care before giving birth and thus has established some rapport with the nursing staff there. The clinic staff is usually willing to answer any questions she may have about her health or that of her newborn. Appointments usually include an examination of the mother and newborn and instructions about umbilical cord care, postpartum and infant care, and nutrition for both mother and infant.

POSTPARTUM HOME VISITS

Home visits offer services similar to those offered at a scheduled clinic visit, but they also give the nurse an opportunity to assess the family's adaptation and dynamics and the home environment. During the past decade, hospital stays have averaged 24 to 48 hours or less for vaginal births and 72 to 96 hours for cesarean births (CDC, 2015c). Federal legislation went into effect in 1998 that prohibited insurers from restricting hospital stays for mothers and newborns to less than 2 days for vaginal births or 4 days for cesarean births (CDC, 2015c). These shortened stays have reduced the time available for educating mothers about caring for themselves and their newborns. Home visiting programs in general seek to promote child health/development, prevent child abuse/neglect, improve maternal well-being, and improve the parental capacity of mothers.

Postpartum care in the home environment usually includes the following:

- Monitoring the physical and emotional well-being of the family members (Fig. 2.5)
- Identifying potential or developing complications for the mother and newborn
- Breast care during breast-feeding and engorgement
- Instruction on pelvic floor exercises, nutrition, and self-hygiene care
- Linking the family, as needed, to community social services, housing, and governmental programs
- Bridging the gap between discharge and ambulatory follow-up for mothers and their newborns (King et al., 2015)

SUPPORT GROUPS FOR NEW MOTHERS

Typically these groups are locally led by a facilitator with previous experience in motherhood, breast-feeding, and infant care. Usually they are composed of 6 to 12 mothers who share information on breast-feeding techniques, infant sleeping patterns, child care issues, body image issues, and how to integrate the new baby into the family unit. The support group usually meets weekly and provides an avenue of support for new mothers on the same journey.

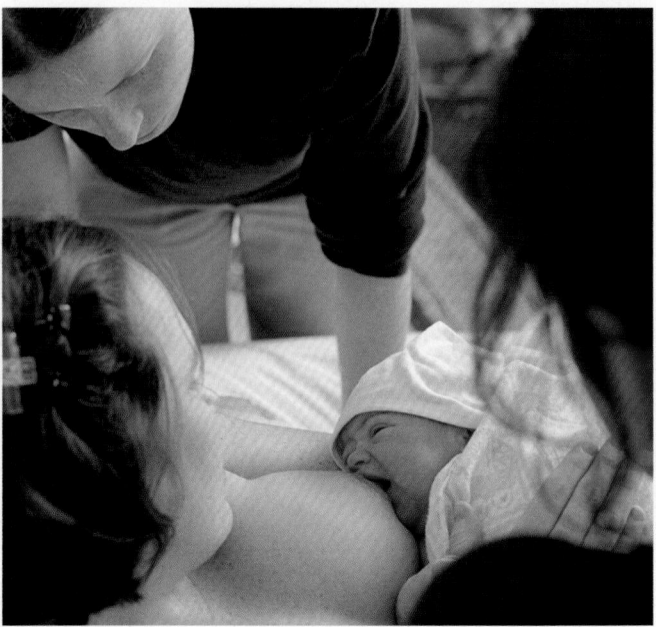

FIGURE 2.5 The nurse makes a postpartum home visit to assess the woman and her newborn. During the visit, the nurse assists the mother with breast-feeding.

ONLINE MOTHERHOOD FORUMS/BLOGS

Support groups in online communities provide an anonymous place to exchange information and advice. Previous research has suggested that these groups offer a safe, nonjudgmental forum for new mothers to share experiences and interact anonymously. They serve as a safe, supportive space in which new mothers can better understand their new role of parenting. They offer a viable form of education for new parents, but caution must be used on advice provided on some websites to new mothers (Makinen & Tuominen, 2015).

HIGH-RISK NEWBORN HOME CARE

With the reduced lengths of stay, high-risk newborns are also being cared for in community settings. High-technology care once was provided only in the hospital. Now, however, the increasing cost of complex care and the influences of managed care have led to the provision of such care at home. Families have become "health care systems" by providing physical, emotional, social, and developmental home care for their technology-dependent infants. Suitable candidates for home care may include preterm infants who continue to need oxygen, low-birthweight infants needing nutritional or hypercaloric formulas or adjunct feeding methods (e.g., tube feedings), or infants with hydrocephalus or cerebral palsy. Home care with prepared caregivers might contribute to earlier detection of significant residual/recurrent problems amenable to therapy (Stewart, 2015). A wide range of equipment may be used, including mechanical ventilation, electronic apnea monitors, home oxygen equipment, intravenous infusions, respiratory nebulizers, phototherapy, and suction equipment.

All family members must work together to provide 24-hour care. The parents must negotiate with insurers for reimbursement for durable medical equipment, must be able to troubleshoot equipment problems, and must be able to manage inventories of supplies and equipment. In addition, they must be able to assess the infant for problems; determine the problem; decide when to call the nurse, pharmacist, or physical therapist; and interpret and implement prescriptions. Technology in the home requires nurses to focus on the family "home care system" to provide total care to the infant.

Nurses can play a key role in assisting families by preparing them for and increasing their confidence in caring for their infants at home. This adaptation begins before discharge from the hospital. Family members are active participants in the transition-to-home plan. Recognition of parental needs and addressing each area in the discharge plan will ease the transition home.

Assessment of the family's preparedness is essential. The following areas should be explored:

- *Parenting education*—assess the family's knowledge of positioning and handling of their infant, nutrition, hygiene, elimination, growth and development, immunizations needed, and recognition of illnesses. Asking questions in a sensitive manner will assist the nurse in identifying knowledge deficiencies, so they can be reinforced in the nurse's teaching plan.
- *Postpartum care*—determine the mother's concerns in areas of body image, weight loss, sleep/rest needs, discomfort, fatigue, and adjustment to her new role. Asking open-ended questions concerning these areas will help the nurse extract more information to include in the teaching plan. Targeting the mother's areas of concern will help the nurse focus on needed education to facilitate the mother's transition into her new role as a parent.
- *Support systems*—assess physical and emotional support for the new mother by asking questions about the availability of her immediate family, other relatives, and significant others to help out. If lacking, referrals may need to be made to community parenting programs, cooperative daycare, or other community resources needed to assist this family. Exploring these vital areas through sensitive questioning hopefully will convey the nurse's concern for the infant and family while obtaining a thorough assessment of the family's learning needs.

Once preparedness has been assessed, the nurse can intervene as necessary. For example, if the caretakers do not think they are prepared to maintain machinery, technology, medication, or developmental therapy, then the nurse can demonstrate the care to the family. The nurse provides instructions and hands-on experience within a supportive environment until the family's confidence increases. The nurse can also assist the family to anticipate the common problems that might occur (e.g., advising them to avoid running out of supplies, to have enough medication or special formula mixture to last throughout the weekend, and to keep backup batteries for powering machines or portable oxygen). The outcome of the preparedness assessment and intervention is that the safety of the infant is established and maintained.

Nursing for families who are using complex home care equipment requires caring for the infant and family members' physical and emotional well-being as well as providing effective solutions to problems they may encounter. Home health nurses need to identify, mobilize, and adapt a myriad of community resources to support the family in giving the best possible care in the home setting. Preparing families for high-tech care before hospital discharge, with home health nurses continuing and reinforcing that focus, will help ease the burden of managing high-tech equipment in the home.

Women's Health Care

A woman's reproductive years span half her lifetime, on average. This is not a static period, but rather one that encompasses several significant stages. As her reproductive goals change, so do a woman's health care needs. Because of these changing needs, comprehensive community-centered care is critical.

Community-based women's health services have received increased emphasis during the past few decades simply because of economics. Women use more health care services than men, they make as many as 90% of health care decisions, and they represent the majority of the population (CDC, 2015a). Women spend 66 cents of every health care dollar, and 7 of the 10 most frequently performed surgeries in the United States are specific to women (Alexander et al., 2014). Examples of community-based women's health care services that can be freestanding or hospital-based include the following:

- Screening centers that offer mammograms, Pap smears, bone density assessments, genetic counseling, ultrasound, breast examinations, complete health risk appraisals, laboratory studies (complete blood count, cholesterol testing, thyroid testing, glucose testing for diabetes, follicle-stimulating hormone [FSH] levels), and electrocardiograms
- Educational centers that provide women's health lectures, instruction on breast self-examinations and Pap smears, and computers for research

- Counseling centers that offer various support groups: genetics, psychotherapy, substance abuse, sexual assault, and domestic violence
- Wellness centers that offer stress reduction techniques, massage therapy, guided imagery, hypnosis, smoking cessation, weight reduction, tai chi, yoga, and women's fitness/exercise classes
- Alternative/wholeness healing centers that provide acupuncture, aromatherapy, biofeedback, therapeutic touch, facials, reflexology, and herbal remedies
- Retail centers that offer specialty equipment for rental and purchase, such as breast prostheses

Women have multiple choices regarding services, settings, and health care providers. In the past most women received health care services from physicians such as obstetricians, gynecologists, and family physicians, but today nurse midwives and nurse practitioners are becoming more prevalent in providing well-women care.

Nurses who work in community-based settings need to be familiar with the many health issues commonly encountered by women within their communities. All nurses who work with women of any age in community-based settings, including the workplace, schools, practitioner offices, and clinics, should possess a thorough understanding of the scope of women's health care and should be prepared to intervene appropriately to prevent problems and to promote health.

Child Health Care

The majority of care for a child occurs in the community setting. The numerous settings may be broad or highly specialized. For example, one setting may provide well-child care as well as illness-related care. Another setting may be limited to providing well-child care; a third setting may be limited to diagnostic evaluation, emergency care, or surgical intervention. Other settings may focus on caring for children with specific conditions or diagnosis, such as diabetes or cancer. See Chapter 33 for specific community-based child health care settings.

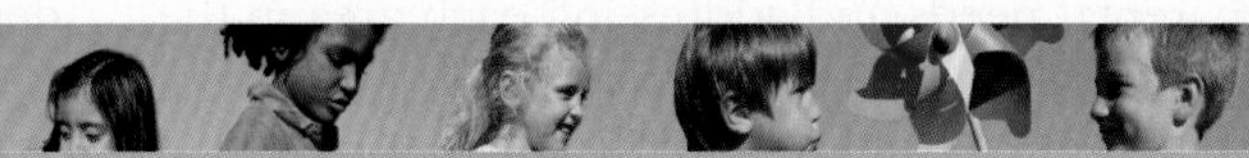

KEY CONCEPTS

- Core concepts of maternal and pediatric nursing include family-centered care, evidence-based practice, collaborative care, atraumatic therapeutic care, communication, education, discharge planning and case management, advocacy and resource management, preventative care, culturally competent care, and being knowledgeable about CAM.
- Family-centered care recognizes the concept of the family as the constant. The health and functioning ability of the family influences and impacts the health of the client and other members of the family. Family-centered care recognizes and respects family strengths and individuality, encourages referrals for family support, and facilitates collaboration. It ensures flexible, accessible, and responsive health care delivery while incorporating developmental needs and implementing policies to provide emotional and financial support to women, children, and their families.
- Open, honest lines of communication are essential for nurses. The use of an interpreter may be necessary to ensure effective communication with women, children, and their families in the community setting. Maintaining confidentiality and privacy are key.
- A family's knowledge related to the client's health or illness is vitally important. Nurses play a major role in educating women, children, and their families. For children, teaching is provided based on the child's developmental level.
- Discharge planning provides a comprehensive plan for the safe discharge of a client from a health care facility and for continuing safe and effective care in the community. Case management focuses on coordinating health care services while balancing quality and cost outcomes. Both contribute to improved transition from the hospital to the community for women, children, their families, and the health care team.
- Advocacy and resource management help ensure that the client and family have the necessary resources and appropriate health care services available to them.
- Health care delivery has moved from acute care settings out into the community, with an emphasis on health promotion and illness prevention (Clark, 2011). Community health nursing focuses on prevention and improvement of the health of populations and communities, addressing current and potential health needs of the population or community, promoting and preserving the health of

a population regardless of a particular age group or diagnosis. Community health nurses perform epidemiologic investigations to help analyze and develop health policy and community health initiatives.

- Community-based nurses focus on providing personal care to individuals and families in the community. They focus on promoting and preserving health as well as preventing disease or injury. They help women, children, and their families cope with illness and disease. Community-based nurses are direct care providers as well as advocators and educators. They focus on minimizing and removing barriers to allow the client to develop to his or her full potential.
- Settings for community-based nursing include physicians' offices, clinics, health departments, urgent care centers, clients' homes, schools, camps, churches, and shelters such as abuse, homeless, and disaster shelters. Nurses provide both well, episodic ill care, and chronic care to women, children, and their families.
- There has been a rise in home health care due to shorter hospital stays and cost containment along with an increase in income and longevity of people with chronic and debilitating health conditions. Technology also has improved, which allows clients to be monitored and to undergo complicated procedures at home.

REFERENCES AND RECOMMENDED READINGS

Alexander, L. L., LaRosa, J. H., Bader, H., & Garfield, S. (2014). *New dimensions in women's health* (6th ed.). Sudbury, MA: Jones and Bartlett Publishers.

Almader-Douglas, D. (2013). *Health literacy*. National Network of Libraries of Medicine. Retrieved from http://nnlm.gov/outreach/consumer/hlthlit.html

American Association of Birth Centers. (2015). *What is a birth center*? Retrieved from http://www.birthcenters.org/?page=bce_what_is_a_bc

American College of Obstetricians & Gynecologists. (2015). Levels of maternal care. *American Journal of Obstetrics and Gynecology, 212*(3), 259–271.

American Pregnancy Association. (2015). *Home birth*. Retrieved from http://americanpregnancy.org/labor-and-birth/home-birth/

American Speech-Language Hearing Association. (2015). *Tips for working with an interpreter.* Retrieved from http://www.asha.org/practice/multicultural/issues/interpret.htm

Arnold, E. C., & Boggs, K. U. (2015). *Interpersonal relationships: Professional communication skills for nurses*. St. Louis, MO: Elsevier Health Sciences.

Arnold, E. C., & Boggs, K. U. (2016). *Interpersonal relationships: Professional communication skills for nurses*. St. Louis, MO: Elsevier Health Sciences.

Arroyave, A., Penaranda, E. K., & Lewis, C. L. (2011). Organizational change: A way to increase colon, breast and cervical cancer screening in primary care practices. *Journal of Community Health, 36*(2), 281–288.

Aston, M., Price, S., Etowa, J., Vukic, A., Young, L., Hart, C., et al. (2015). The power of relationships exploring how public health nurses support mothers and families during postpartum home visits. *Journal of Family Nursing, 21*(1), 11–34.

Ayers, B., Grassley, J., & Koprowski, K. (2015). Pilot study of breastfeeding support on the night shift. *Clinical Lactation, 6*(2), 53–59.

Berg, A. L., & Serpanos, Y. C. (2016). Hearing and aging. *Communication and aging: Creative approaches to improving the quality of life,* (pp.121–156). San Diego, CA: Plural Publishing.

Boodman, S. G. (2011). *Helping patients understand their medical treatment.* Kaiser Health News. Retrieved from http://khn.org/news/health-literacy-understanding-medical-treatment/

Brega, A. G., Barnard, J., Mabachi, N. M., Weiss, B. D., DeWalt, D. A., Brach, C et al. (2015). *AHRQ health literacy universal precautions toolkit* (2nd ed.). AHRQ publication no. 15–0023-EF. Rockville, MD: Agency for Healthcare Research and Quality.

Bridges, E. J. (2015). Research at the bedside: It makes a difference. *American Journal of Critical Care, 24*(4), 283–289.

Bureau of Labor Statistics, U.S. Department of Labor, Occupational Employment Statistics (2014). *Occupational Outlook Handbook, 2014–15 Edition, Registered Nurses.* Retrieved from http://www.bls.gov/ooh/healthcare/registered-nurses.htm

Burkey, J. M. (2015). *The hearing-loss guide: Useful information and advice for patients and families.* New Haven, CT: Yale University Press.

Burnard, P., & Gill, P. (2015). *Culture, communication and nursing* (2nd ed.). New York, NY: Taylor & Francis.

Centers for Disease Control and Prevention. (2015a). *Learn about health literacy.* Retrieved from http://www.cdc.gov/healthliteracy/learn/index.html

Centers for Disease Control and Prevention. (2015b). *Folic acid.* Retrieved from http://www.cdc.gov/ncbddd/folicacid/features/foic-acid-use-ntd.html

Centers for Disease Control and Prevention. (2015c). *Hospital utilization (in non-federal short stay hospitals).* Retrieved from http://www.cdc.gov/nchs/fastats/hospital.htm

Centers for Disease Control and Prevention. (2015d). *Access to health care.* Retrieved from http://www.cdc.gov/nchs/fastats/access-to-health-care.htm

Chang, H. Y., & Chang, H. L. (2015). A review of nurses' knowledge, attitudes, and ability to communicate the risks and benefits of complementary and alternative medicine. *Journal of Clinical Nursing, 24*, 1466–1478.

Childbirth Connection. (2015). *Choosing a place of birth.* Retrieved from http://www.childbirthconnection.org/article.asp?ClickedLink=252&ck=10145&area=27

Clark, C. C. (2011). *Evidence based health promotion for nurses.* Sudbury, MA: Jones & Bartlett Learning.

Clark, C. C., & Paraska, K. K. (2012). *Health promotion for nurses.* Burlington, MA: Jones & Bartlett Learning.

Clark, M. J. (2014). *Community health nursing: Advocating for healthy populations* (6th ed.). Upper Saddle River, NJ: Prentice Hall.

Colby, S. L. & Ortman, J. M. (2015). *Projections of the size and composition of the U. S. population: 2014 to 2060 population estimates and projections.* Retrieved from http://www.census.gov/content/dam/Census/library/publications/2015/demo/p25–1143.pdf?

Commission for Case Management Certification. (n. d.). *Frequently asked questions.* Retrieved from http://ccmcertification.org/certification-faqs

Community Health Network. (2015). *Maternity services.* Retrieved from http://www.ecommunity.com/s/maternity-services/pregnancy-and-childbirth/

Coyne, I., O'Neill, C., Murphy, M., Costello, T., & O'Shea, R. (2011). What does family-centered care mean to nurses and how do they think it could be enhanced in practice. *Journal of Advanced Nursing, 67*(12), 2561–2573.

Darawsheh, W., & Chard, G. (2015). Towards culturally competent professional practice: Exploring the concepts of independence and interdependence. *Social Services Research Group Journal: Research, Policy and Planning, 31*(1), 3–17.

Darnell, L. K., & Hickson, S. V. (2015). Cultural competent patient-centered nursing care. *Nursing Clinics, 50*(1), 99–108.

Dauvrin, M., & Lorant, V. (2015). Leadership and cultural competence of health care professionals: A social network analysis. *Nursing Research, 64*(3), 200–210.

de la Rosa, I., Perry, J., & Johnson, V. (2015). Pathways to resilience: Enhancing family well-being with a home visitation model. *Journal of Youth Development, 10*(1), 35–58.

Duell, P., Bhattacharya, D., Wright, D., & Renzaho, A. (2015). Optimal health literacy measurement instrument for the assessing health literacy in a clinical setting: A systematic review. *Patient Education and Counseling, 98*(11): 1295–1307.

Dykes, D. C., & White III, A. A. (2011). Culturally competent care pedagogy: What works? *Clinical Orthopedics & Related Research, 469*(7), 1813–1816.

Eisler, K. (2011). Executive director's report. Patient and family centered care: What does it mean for RNs? *SRNA Newsbulletin, 13*(1), 4.

Ernst, E. (2015). How nurses can be misled about complementary and alternative medicine. *Journal of Advanced Nursing, 71*(2), 235–236.

Farrar, F. C. (2015). Transforming home health nursing with telehealth technology. *Nursing Clinics of North America, 50*(2), 269–281.

Friedman, A. J., Cosby, R., Boyko, S., Hatto-bauer, J., & Turnbull, G. (2011). Effective teaching strategies and methods of delivery for patient education: A systematic review and practice guideline recommendations. *Journal of Cancer Education, 26*(1), 12–21.

George, M. (2015). Integrative medicine is integral to providing patient-centered care. *Annals of Allergy, Asthma & Immunology, 114*(4), 261–265.

Gupta, D., Mehta, M., & Sagar, R. (2015). Interpersonal skills. In *A practical approach to cognitive behaviour therapy for adolescents* (pp. 91–107). India: Springer Publishers.

Hall, H. G., Griffiths, D., & McKenna, L. G. (2015). Complementary and alternative medicine: Interaction and communication between midwives and women. *Women and Birth, 28*(2), 137–142.

Hamilton, K. (2011). Family education: Development of a formal education process to ensure quality education prior to discharge. *Journal of Pediatric Nursing, 26*(2), e3.

Hansen, L. O. (2015). Passing beyond a wing and a prayer after hospital discharge. *Journal of General Internal Medicine, 30*(4), 390–391.

Harkess, L. & Kaddoura, M. (2015). Culture and cultural competence in nursing education and practice: The state of the art. *Nursing Forum.* doi: 10.1111/nuf.12140

Hersh, L., Salzman, B., & Snyderman, D. (2015). Health literacy in primary care practice. *American Family Physician, 92*(2), 118–124.

Holden, S. C., Gardiner, P., Birdee, G., Davis, R. B., & Yeh, G. Y. (2015). Complementary and alternative medicine use among women during pregnancy and childbearing years. *Birth, 42*(3), 261–269.

Jackson, M. (2011). Deafness and antenatal care: Understanding issues with access. *British Journal of Midwifery, 19*(5), 280–284.

The Joint Commission. (2012). *Patient education.* Retrieved from http://www.mghpcs.org/eed_portal/Documents/PatientEd/JC_Standards_PatientEd.pdf

Kelly, M. M., & Penney, E. D. (2011). Collaboration of hospital case managers and home care liaisons when transitioning patients. *Professional Case Management, 16*(3), 128–138.

King, T. L., Brucker, M. C., Kriebs, J. M., Fahey, J. O., Gegor, C. L., & Varney, H. (2015). *Varney's midwifery* (5th ed.). Burlington, MA: Jones & Bartlett Learning.

King, S. B. (2015). Competency-based education. *JACC: Cardiovascular Interventions, 8*(2), 374–375.

Klemp, J. R. (2015). Breast cancer prevention across the cancer care continuum. *Seminars in Oncology Nursing, 31*(2), 89–99.

Knowles, M. S., Holton III, E. F., & Swanson, R. A. (2011). *The adult learner* (7th ed.). Burlington, MA: Elsevier.

Koh, H. K., Berwick, D. M., Clancy, C. M., Baur, C., Brach, C., Harris, L. M, et al. (2012). New federal policy initiatives to boost health literacy can help the nation move beyond the cycle of costly 'crisis care. *Health Affairs, 31*(2), 434–443.

La Leche League International. (2014). *La Leche League mother-to-mother forums.* Retrieved from http://forums.llli.org/

Lassi, Z. S., & Bhutta, Z. A. (2015). Community-based intervention packages for reducing maternal and neonatal morbidity and mortality and improving neonatal outcomes. *Cochrane Database of Systematic Reviews*, Issue 3, CD007754.

Lemetti, T., Stolt, M., Rickard, N., & Suhonen, R. (2015). Collaboration between hospital and primary care nurses: A literature review. *International Nursing Review, 62*, 248–266.

Levetown, M., American Academy of Pediatrics Committee on Bioethics. (2011). Communicating with children and families: From everyday interactions to skill in conveying distressing information. *Pediatrics, 121*(5), e1441–e1460. doi: 10.1542/peds.2008–0565

Lomax, S. W., & White, D. (2015). Interprofessional collaborative care skills for the frontline nurse. *Nursing Clinics of North America, 50*(1), 59–73.

Makic, M. B., Rauen, C., Jones, K., & Fisk, A. C. (2015). Continuing to challenge practice to be evidence based. *Critical Care Nurse, 35*(2), 39–50.

Makinen, R., & Tuominen, P. (2015). Discussion frames in motherhood blogs: A case study on suburban mom. In *Innovation, finance, and the economy* (pp. 47–67). New York, NY: Springer International Publishing.

March of Dimes. (2015). *Prenatal care*. Retrieved from http://www.marchofdimes.com/pregnancy/prenatalcare.html

Massey, M. T. (2015). New focus on community nurses. *Primary Health Care, 25*(4), 5–6.

McMurray, A., & Clendon, J. (2015). *Community health and wellness: Primary care in practice* (5th ed.). Chatswood, NSW: Elsevier Australia.

Migration Policy Institute. (2015). *Frequently requested statistics on immigrants and immigration in the United States*. Retrieved from http://www.migrationpolicy.org/article/frequently-requested-statistics-immigrants-and-immigration-united-states

National Center for Complementary and Integrative Health. (2015a). *Complementary, alternative, or integrative health: What's in a name?* Retrieved from https://nccih.nih.gov/health/integrative-health

National Center for Complementary and Integrative Health. (2015b). *Osteoporosis*. Retrieved from https://nccih.nih.gov/health/osteoporosis

National Institutes of Health. (2015). *Health literacy*. Retrieved from: http://www.nih.gov/clearcommunication/healthliteracy.htm.

National Network of Libraries of Medicine [NNLM]. (2015). *Health literacy*. Retrieved from http://nnlm.gov/outreach/consumer/hlthlit.html

Orr, P., & Davenport, D. (2015). Embracing change. *Nursing Clinics of North America, 50*(1), 1–18.

Patient Education Institute. (2013). *Benefits of patient education*. Retrieved from http://ww2.patient-education.com/main.asp?p=aboutus&s=bope&fs=aboutus&mode=FULL

Peter, D., Robinson, P., Jordan, M., Lawrence, S., Casey, K., & Salas-Lopez, D. (2015). Reducing readmissions using teach-back: Enhancing patient and family education. *Journal of Nursing Administration, 45*(1), 35–42.

Pierce, D., Pompe-Waltman, J., Stanton, N., & Bland, L. (2011). Congratulations on your new baby: A nursing model for successful family transitions. *JOGNN: Journal of Obstetric, Gynecologic & Neonatal Nursing, 40*, 83.

ProLiteracy. (2014). *Growing demand, dwindling resources*. Retrieved from http://www.proliteracy.org/the-crisis/the-us-crisis

Refugee Health Technical Assistance Center. (2011). *Best practices for communicating through an interpreter*. Retrieved from http://refugeehealthta.org/access-to-care/language-access/best-practices-communicating-through-an-interpreter/

Roberts, B. (2015). Person and family centered care. *Creative Nursing, 21*(1), 63–66.

Schierloh, J. M. (2015). *Adult literacy in America: A first look at the results of the National Adult Literacy Survey*. Retrieved from http://literacy.kent.edu/Oasis/Pubs/nalsrev.htm

Shepperd, S., Doll, H., Angus, R. M., Clarke, M. J., Iliffe, S., Kalra, L., et al. (2011). Hospital at home admission avoidance. *Cochrane Database of Systematic Reviews*, 4:CD007491.

Shorofi, S. (2011). Complementary and alternative medicine (CAM) among hospitalized patients: Reported use of CAM and reasons for use, CAM preferred during hospitalization, and the socio-demographic determinants of CAM users. *Complementary Therapies in Clinical Practice, 17*(4), 199–205.

Smith, L. S. (2015). Tune into safety for hearing-impaired patients. *Nursing, 45*(6), 64–66.

Smith, G. N. (2015). The maternal health clinic: Improving women's cardiovascular health. *Seminars in Perinatology, 39*(4), 316–319.

Stanhope, M., & Lancaster, J. (2015). *Public health nursing: Population-centered health care in the community* (9th ed.). St. Louis, MO: Mosby Elsevier.

Steinberg, M., & Sackmary, B. (2015). Marketing in health services: A review of recent trends in obstetrics. *Proceedings of the 1988 International Conference of Services Marketing* (pp. 306–316). New York, NY: Springer International Publishing.

Stewart, J. (2015). Discharge planning for high risk newborns. UpToDate. Retrieved from http://www.uptodate.com/contents/discharge-planning-for-high-risk-newborns

Su, W., Herron, B., & Osisek, P. (2011). Using a competency-based approach to patient education: Achieving congruence among learning, teaching and evaluation. *Nursing Clinics of North America, 46*(3), 291–298.

The Sentinel Watch: Nursing. (2014). *Improve your patient education skills to enhance care*. Retrieved from http://www.americansentinel.edu/blog/2014/12/17/improve-your-patient-education-skills-to-enhance-care/

Thomas, S. D., Hudgins, J. L., Sutherland, D. E., Ange, B. L., & Mobley, S. C. (2015). Perinatal program evaluations: Methods, impacts, and future goals. *Maternal and Child Health Journal, 19*, 1440–1446.

Tyler, S., & Nagtalon-Ramos, J. (2015). Managing nausea and vomiting of pregnancy. *Women's Healthcare, 3*(2), 7–14.

USDA Food and Nutrition Services. (2015). *Women, Infants and Children (WIC)*. Retrieved from http://www.fns.usda.gov/wic/about-wic-wic-glance

U. S. Department of Health and Human Services. (2015a). *About Healthy People*. Retrieved from http://www.healthypeople.gov/2020/About-Healthy-People

U. S. Department of Health and Human Services. (2015b). *Healthy People 2020*. Retrieved from http://healthypeople.gov/2020/topics-objectives

U. S. Department of Health and Human Services Office of Minority Health. (n. d.). *Culturally competent nursing care: A cornerstone of caring*. Retrieved from https://ccnm.thinkculturalhealth.hhs.gov/

Williamson, K. M., Almaskari, M., Lester, Z., & Maguire, D. (2015). Utilization of evidence-based practice knowledge, attitude, and skill of clinical nurses in the planning of professional development programming. *Journal for Nurses in Professional Development, 31*(2), 73–80.

Wong, D. L. (n. d.). *Innovative approaches for atraumatic cancer care* [PowerPoint slides]. Retrieved from http://www.author stream.com/presentation/Carolina-48857-op077-INNOVATIVE-APPROACHES-ATRAUMATIC-CANCER-

CARE-DEFINITION-SOURCES-PATIENT-FAMILY-STRESSORS-as-Entertainment-ppt-powerpoint/

Wright, L. M. & Leahey, M. (2013). *Nurses and families: A guide to family assessment and intervention* (6th ed.). Philadelphia, PA: F.A. Davis Company.

Zambrana, R. E., Meghea, C., Talley, C., Hammad, A., Lockett, M., & Williams, K. P. (2015). Association between family communication and health literacy among underserved racial/ethnic women. *Journal of Health Care for the Poor and Underserved, 26*(2), 391–405.

Zielinski, R., Ackerson, K., & Low, L. K. (2015). Planned home birth: benefits, risks, and opportunities. *International Journal of Women's Health, 7*, 361–377.

CHAPTER WORKSHEET

MULTIPLE-CHOICE QUESTIONS

1. When caring for children, how should the nurse best incorporate the concept of family-centered care?
   a. Encourage the family to allow the physician to make health care decisions for the child.
   b. Use the concepts of respect, family strengths, diversity, and collaboration with family.
   c. Advise the family to choose a pediatric provider who is on the covered child's health care plan.
   d. Recognize that families undergoing stress related to the child's illness cannot make good decisions.

2. A community-based nurse is involved in secondary prevention activities. Which activities might be included? Select all that apply.
   a. Fecal occult blood testing
   b. Hearing screening
   c. Smoking cessation program
   d. Cholesterol testing
   e. Hygiene program
   f. Pregnancy testing

3. A woman is to undergo a colonoscopy at a freestanding outpatient surgery center. Which would the nurse identify as a major disadvantage associated with this community-based setting?
   a. Increased risk for infection
   b. Increased health care costs
   c. Need to be transferred if overnight stay is required
   d. Increased disruption of family functioning

4. When developing a teaching plan for a child and his parents, which action would the nurse do first?
   a. Decide which procedures and medications the child will be discharged on.
   b. Determine the child's and family's learning needs and styles.
   c. Ask the family if they have ever performed this type of procedure.
   d. Tell the child and family what the goals of the teaching session are.

5. The clinic nurse is concerned about the client's ability to understand the instructions given and the health literacy level of her client. Which of the following can the nurse employ to increase the client's understanding of the instructions?
   a. Draw pictures of the procedure and write down the steps to it.
   b. Instruct the client to call the nurse if they have questions.
   c. Discuss the instructions with an elderly family member in addition to the client.
   d. Question the client about their reading level and educational level.

CRITICAL THINKING EXERCISES

1. A 3-year-old girl from Saudi Arabia has become seriously ill while on a visit to the United States. It is projected that she will require a lengthy hospitalization. Describe the steps the nurse should take to communicate with and provide extensive health care teaching to this child's family.

2. A pregnant woman is discharged home from the hospital after admission due to preterm labor. The woman is to be on complete bed rest and will receive home health care through a local agency to assist her and her family and to monitor her health status. As the home health nurse assigned to this woman, what should your nursing assessment include?

STUDY ACTIVITIES

1. Shadow a nurse working in a community setting, such as a women's health clinic, birthing center, camp, home care, or health department. Identify the role the nurse plays in the health of women, children, and families in the setting and in the community.

2. Arrange for a visit to a community health center that offers services to various cultural groups. Interview the staff about the strategies used to overcome communication barriers and different health care practices for the women and children in these groups.

3. Select one of the websites listed on thePoint and explore the information provided. How could a community-based nurse use this information?

BRINGING IT ALL TOGETHER: A CASE STUDY

Bianca, a 23-year-old Hispanic, is about to give birth to her first child, a daughter that will be named Amelia. Her partner, Alejandro, has been supportive of Bianca during her labor and plans to be present during the delivery but seems uneasy about the prospect of caring for his daughter claiming, "I'm not use to being around little babies." The birthing center focuses on family-centered care and the nurse will plan the care of Bianca and Amelia as well as the support of Alejandro based on that model.

Go to thePoint to find questions to consider about this case.

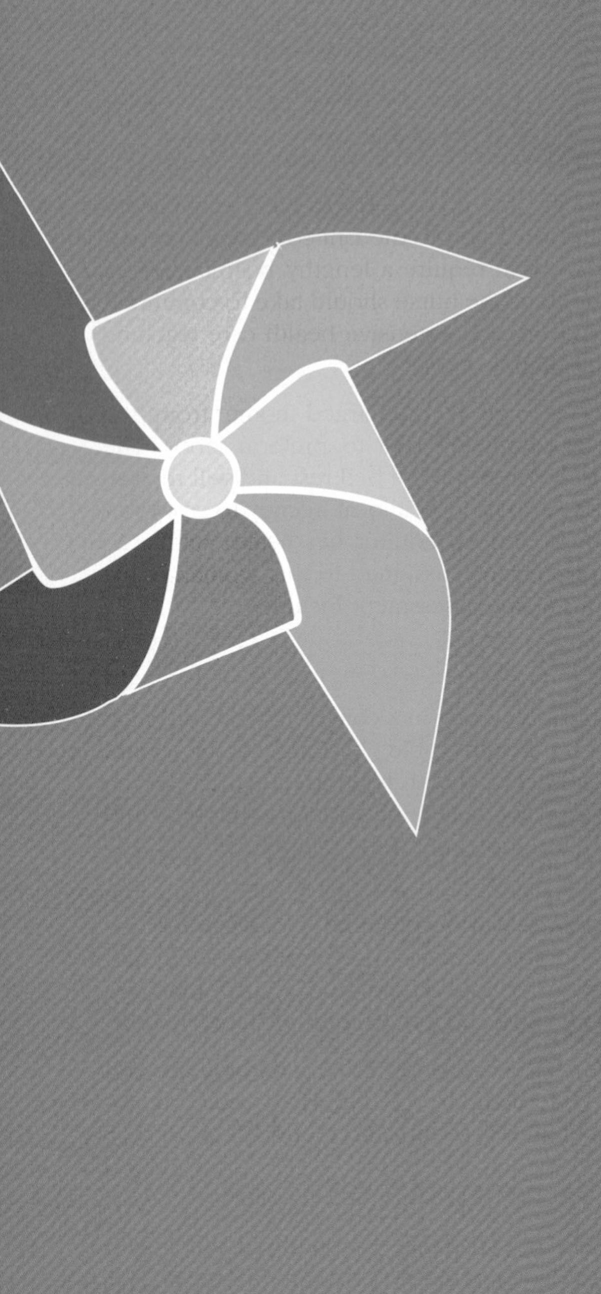

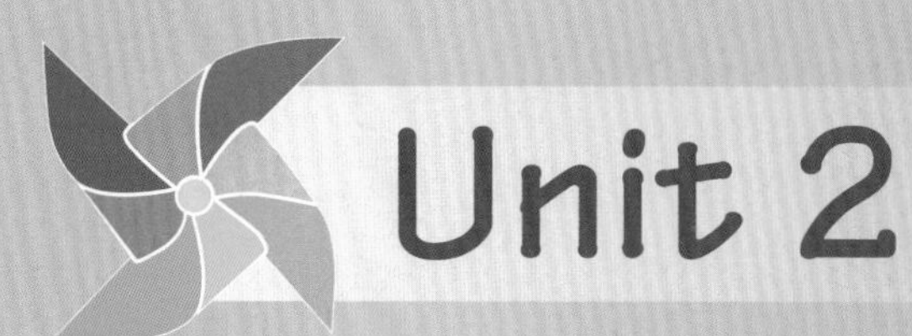

Women's Health Throughout the Life Span

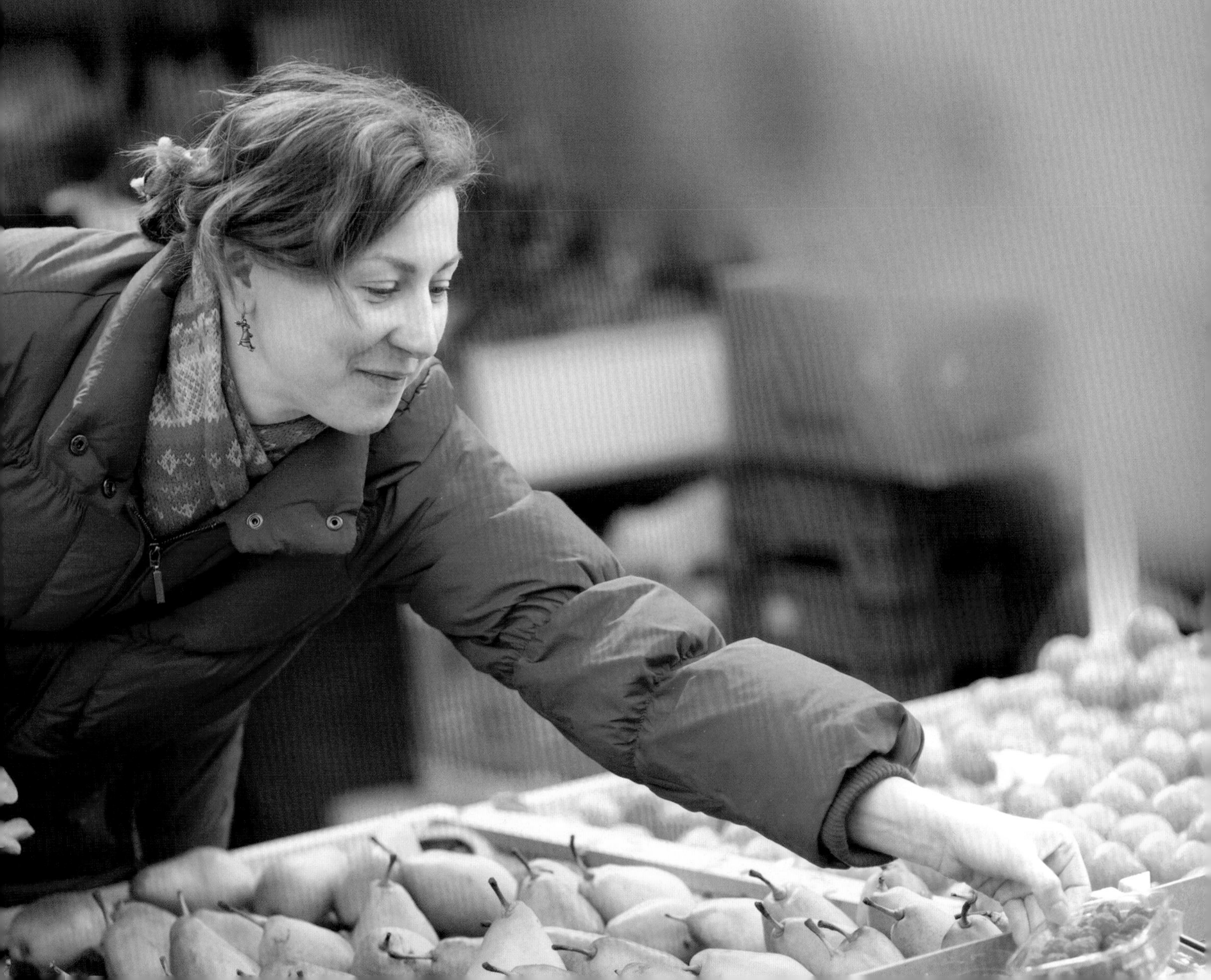

3

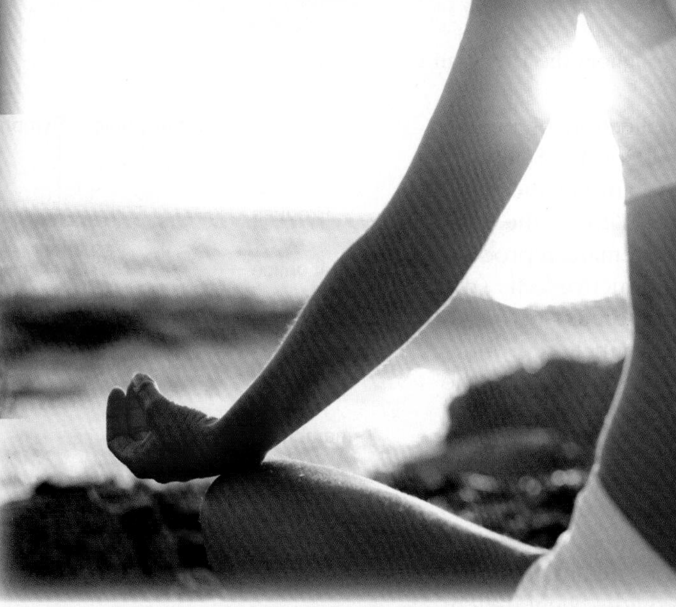

WOW

Words of Wisdom

All nurses should take care of and respect the human body, for it is a wondrous precision machine.

Anatomy and Physiology of the Reproductive System

KEY TERMS

breasts
cervix
endometrium
estrogen
fallopian tubes
follicle-stimulating hormone (FSH)
luteinizing hormone (LH)
menarche
menstruation
ovaries
ovulation
penis
progesterone
testes
uterus
vagina
vulva

Learning Objectives

Upon completion of the chapter, you will be able to:

1. Contrast the structure and function of the major external and internal female genital organs.
2. Outline the phases of the menstrual cycle, the dominant hormones involved, and the changes taking place in each phase.
3. Classify external and internal male reproductive structures and the function of each in hormonal regulation.

***Linda*, 49, started menstruating when she was 12 years old. Her menstrual periods have always been regular, but now she is experiencing irregular, heavier, and longer ones. She wonders if there is something wrong or if this is normal.**

The reproductive system is a collection of organs that function in the production of offspring. Scientists argue that the reproductive system is among the most important systems in the entire body. Without the ability to reproduce, a species dies. The female reproductive system produces the female reproductive cells (the eggs, or ova) and contains an organ (**uterus**) in which development of the fetus takes place; the male reproductive system produces the male reproductive cells (the sperm) and contains an organ (**penis**) that deposits the sperm within the female. Nurses need to have a thorough understanding of the anatomy and physiology of the male and female reproductive systems to be able to assess the health of these systems, to promote reproductive system health, to care for conditions that might affect the reproductive organs, and to provide client teaching concerning the reproductive system. This chapter reviews the female and male reproductive systems and the menstrual cycle as it relates to reproduction.

FEMALE REPRODUCTIVE ANATOMY AND PHYSIOLOGY

The female reproductive system is composed of both external and internal reproductive organs. It consists of the paired ovaries and oviducts, the uterus, the vagina, the external genitalia, and the mammary glands. All of these structures have evolved for the important functions of **ovulation**, fertilization of an ovum by a sperm, support of the developing embryo and fetus, and the birth and care of a newborn.

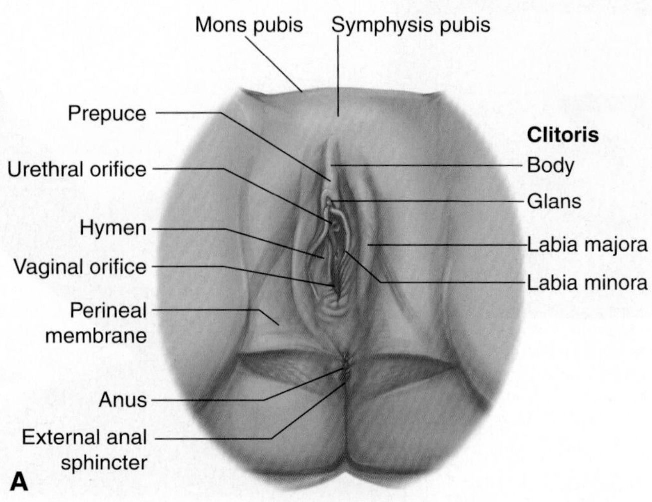

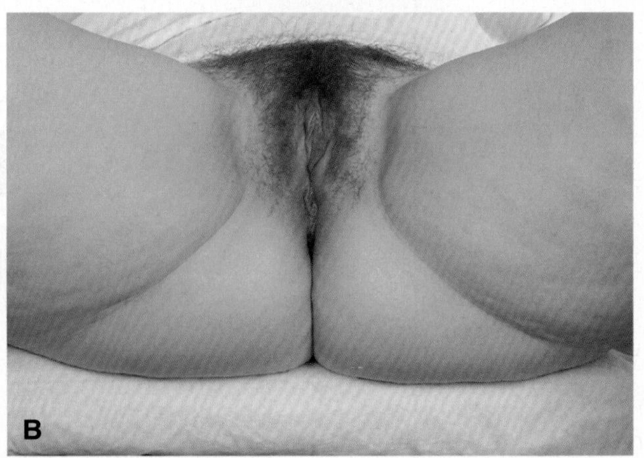

FIGURE 3.1 **A.** The external female reproductive organs. **B.** Normal appearance of external structures. (Photo by B. Proud.)

External Female Reproductive Organs

The external female reproductive organs collectively are called the **vulva** (which means "covering" in Latin). The vulva serves to protect the urethral and vaginal openings and is highly sensitive to touch to increase the female's pleasure during sexual arousal (Patton & Thibodeau, 2016). The structures that make up the vulva include the mons pubis, the labia majora and minora, the clitoris and prepuce, the structures within the vestibule, and the perineum (Fig. 3.1).

Mons Pubis

The mons pubis is the elevated, rounded, fleshy prominence made up of fatty tissue that overlays the symphysis pubis. The skin of this fatty tissue is covered with coarse, curly public hair after puberty. The mons pubis protects the symphysis pubis during sexual intercourse.

Labia

The labia majora (large lips), which are relatively large and fleshy, are comparable to the scrotum in males. The labia majora contain sweat and sebaceous (oil-secreting) glands; after puberty, they are covered with hair. Their function is to protect the vaginal opening and provide cushioning during sexual activity. The labia minora (small lips) are the delicate hairless inner folds of skin; they can be very small or up to 2 in wide. They lie just inside the labia majora and surround the openings to the vagina and urethra. The labia minora grow down from the anterior inner part of the labia majora on each side. These lips surround the vaginal opening and extend upward to form protection around both the clitoris and urethra. They are highly vascular and abundant in nerve supply. They lubricate the vulva, swell in response to stimulation, and are highly sensitive.

Clitoris and Prepuce

The clitoris is a small, cylindrical mass of erectile tissue and nerves. It is highly sensitive and is analogous to the head of the male's penis. Unlike the penis, however, the function of the clitoris is purely erogenous. Most of the components of the clitoris are buried under the skin and connective tissue of the vulva. It is located at the anterior junction of the labia minora. There are folds above and below the clitoris. The joining of the folds above the clitoris forms the prepuce, a hood-like covering over the clitoris; the junction below the clitoris forms the frenulum.

Take Note!

The hood-like covering over the clitoris is the site for female genital mutilation or cutting, which is a cultural ritual still practiced in some countries, including in the United States. It is internationally recognized as a human rights violation against women.

A rich supply of blood vessels gives the clitoris a pink color. Like the penis, the clitoris is very sensitive to touch, stimulation, and temperature and can become erect. For its small size, 9 to 11 cm, it has a generous blood and nerve supply. There are more free nerve endings of sensory reception located on the clitoris than on any other part of the body, and it is, unsurprisingly, the most erotically sensitive part of the genitalia for most females. Its function is sexual stimulation (Pauls, 2015).

Take Note!

The word clitoris is from the Greek word for "key"; in ancient times the clitoris was thought to be the key to a woman's sexuality.

Vestibule

The vestibule is an oval area enclosed by the labia minora laterally. It is inside the labia minora and outside of the hymen and is perforated by six openings. Opening into the vestibule are the urethra from the urinary bladder, the vagina, and two sets of glands. The opening to the vagina is called the introitus, and the half-moon–shaped area behind the opening is called the fourchette. Through tiny ducts beside the introitus, Bartholin glands, when stimulated, secrete mucus that supplies lubrication for intercourse. Skene glands are located on either side of the opening to the urethra. They secrete a small amount of mucus to keep the opening moist and lubricated for the passage of urine (Velkey, Hall, & Robboy, 2015).

The vaginal opening is surrounded by the hymen (maidenhead). The hymen is a tough, elastic, perforated, mucosa-covered tissue across the vaginal introitus. In a virgin, the hymen may completely cover the opening, but it usually encircles the opening like a tight ring. Because the degree of tightness varies among women, the hymen may tear at the first attempt at intercourse, or it may be so soft and pliable that no tearing occurs. In a woman who is not a virgin, the hymen usually appears as small tags of tissue surrounding the vaginal opening, but the presence or absence of the hymen can neither confirm nor rule out sexual experience (Acien & Acien, 2015).

Take Note!

Heavy physical exertion, use of tampons, or injury to the area can alter the appearance of the hymen in girls and women who have not been sexually active.

Perineum

The perineum is the most posterior part of the external female reproductive organs. This external region is located between the vulva and the anus. It is made up of skin, muscle, and fascia. The perineum can become lacerated or incised during childbirth and may need to be repaired with sutures. Incising the perineum area to provide more space for the presenting part is called an episiotomy. Although still a common obstetric procedure, the use of episiotomy has decreased during the past 25 years. The procedure should be applied selectively rather than routinely. An episiotomy can add to postpartum discomfort and perineal trauma and can lead to fecal incontinence (King, et al., 2015).

Internal Female Reproductive Organs

The internal female reproductive organs consist of the vagina, uterus, fallopian tubes, and ovaries (Fig. 3.2). These structures develop and function according to specific hormonal influences that affect fertility and childbearing.

Vagina

The **vagina** is a highly distensible canal situated in front of the rectum and behind the bladder. It is a tubular, fibromuscular organ lined with mucous membrane that lies in a series of transverse folds called rugae. The rugae allow for extreme dilation of the canal during labor and birth. The vagina is a canal that connects the external genitals (vulva) to the cervix. It receives the penis and the sperm ejaculated during sexual intercourse, and it serves as an exit passageway for menstrual blood and for the fetus during childbirth. The front and back walls normally touch each other so that there is no space in the vagina except when it is opened (e.g., during a pelvic examination or intercourse). In the adult, the vaginal cavity is 3 to 4 in long. Muscles that control its diameter surround the lower third of the vagina. The upper two thirds of the vagina lies above these muscles and can be stretched easily. During a woman's reproductive years, the mucosal lining of the vagina has a corrugated appearance and is resistant to bacterial colonization. Before puberty and after menopause (if the woman is not taking estrogen), the mucosa is smooth due to lower levels of estrogen (Farage, Miller, & Maibach, 2015).

The vagina has an acidic environment, which protects it against ascending infections. Antibiotic therapy, douching, perineal hygiene sprays, and deodorants

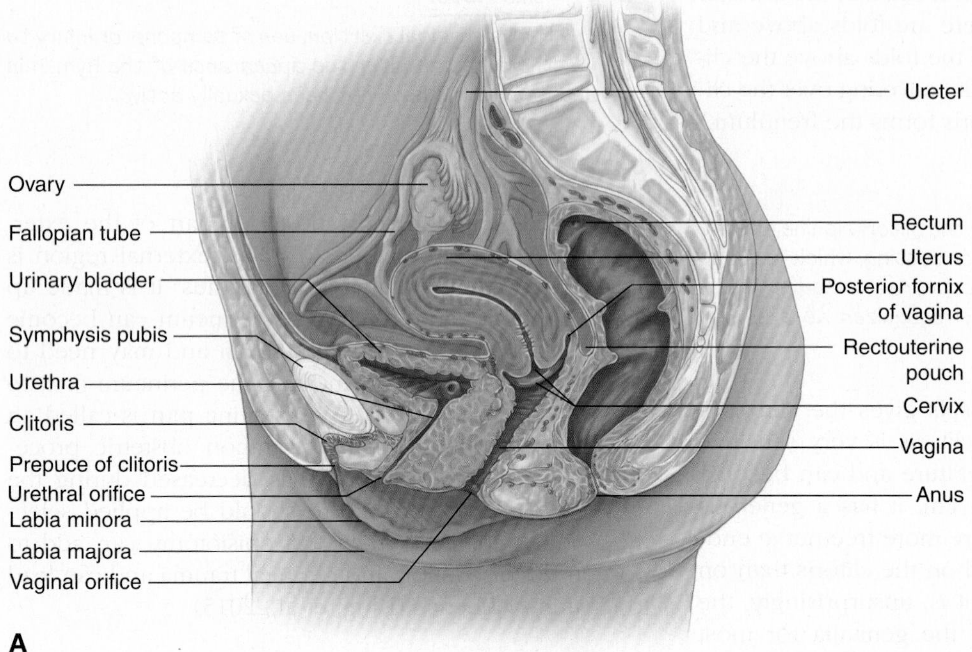

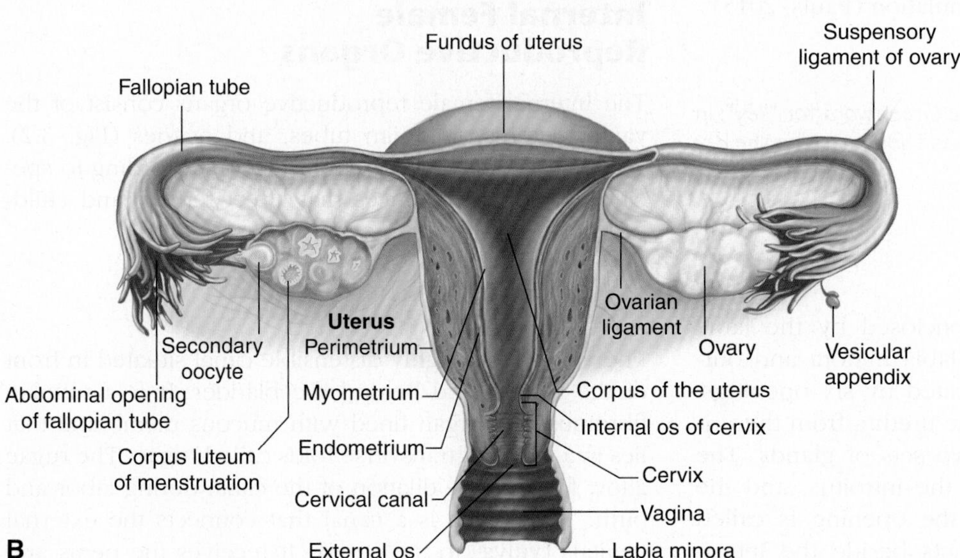

FIGURE 3.2 The internal female reproductive organs. **A.** Lateral view. **B.** Anterior view. (Adapted from Anatomical Chart Company. (2001). *Atlas of human anatomy*. Springhouse, PA: Springhouse.)

upset the acid balance within the vaginal environment and can predispose women to infections.

Uterus

The uterus is an inverted, pear-shaped muscular organ at the top of the vagina. It lies behind the bladder and in front of the rectum and is anchored in position by eight ligaments, although it is not firmly attached or adherent to any part of the skeleton. A full bladder tilts the uterus backward; a distended rectum tilts it forward. The uterus alters its position by gravity or with change of posture, and is the size and shape of an inverted pear. It is the site of menstruation, receiving a fertilized ovum, development of the fetus during pregnancy, and contracting to help in the expulsion of the fetus and placenta. Before the first pregnancy, it measures approximately 3 in long, 2 in wide, and 1 in thick. After a pregnancy, the uterus remains larger than before the pregnancy. After menopause, it becomes smaller and atrophies.

The uterine wall is relatively thick and composed of three layers: the **endometrium** (innermost layer), the myometrium (muscular middle layer), and the perimetrium (outer serosal layer that covers the body of the uterus). The endometrium is the mucosal layer that lines the uterine cavity in nonpregnant women. It varies in thickness from 0.5 to 5 mm and has an abundant supply of glands and blood vessels (Tambouret & Wilbur, 2015).

The myometrium makes up the major portion of the uterus and is composed of smooth muscle linked by connective tissue with numerous elastic fibers. During pregnancy, the upper myometrium undergoes marked hypertrophy, but there is limited change in the cervical muscle content.

Anatomic subdivisions of the uterus include the convex portion above the uterine tubes (the fundus), the central portion (the corpus or body) between the fundus and the cervix, and the cervix, or neck, which opens into the vagina.

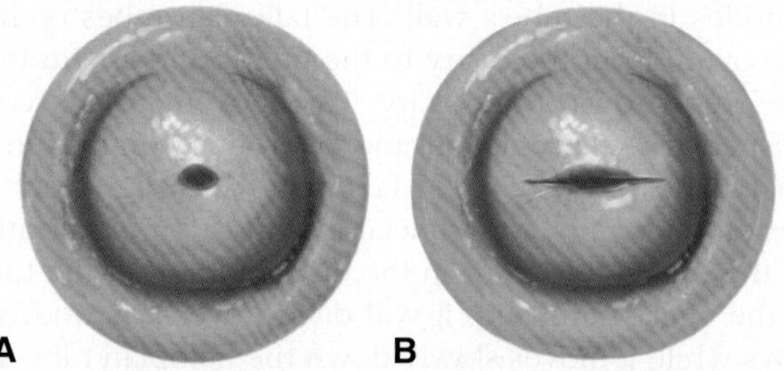

FIGURE 3.4 **A.** Nulliparous cervical os. **B.** Parous cervical os.

CERVIX

The **cervix**, the lower part of the uterus, is sometimes called the neck of the uterus. It opens into the vagina and has a channel that allows sperm to enter the uterus and menstrual discharge to exit. It is composed of fibrous connective tissue. During a pelvic examination, the part of the cervix that protrudes into the upper end of the vagina can be visualized. Like the vagina, this part of the cervix is covered by mucosa, which is smooth, firm, and doughnut shaped, with a visible central opening called the external os (Fig. 3.3). Before childbirth, the external cervical os is a small, regular, oval opening. After childbirth, the opening is converted into a transverse slit that resembles lips (Fig. 3.4). Except during menstruation or ovulation, the cervix is usually a good barrier against bacteria. The cervix has an alkaline environment, which protects the sperm from the acidic environment in the vagina.

The canal or channel of the cervix is lined with mucus-secreting glands. This mucus is thick and impenetrable to sperm until just before the ovaries release an egg (ovulation). At ovulation, the consistency of the mucus changes so that sperm can swim through it, allowing fertilization. At the same time, the mucus-secreting glands of the cervix actually become able to store live sperm for 2 or 3 days. These sperm can later move up through the corpus and into the fallopian tubes to fertilize the egg; thus, intercourse 1 or 2 days before ovulation can lead to pregnancy. Because some women do not ovulate consistently, pregnancy can occur at varying times after the last menstrual period. During pregnancy the cervix is the vital mechanical barrier which resists compressive and tensile loads generated from a growing fetus. The channel in the cervix is too narrow for the fetus to pass through during pregnancy, but during labor it stretches to let the newborn through.

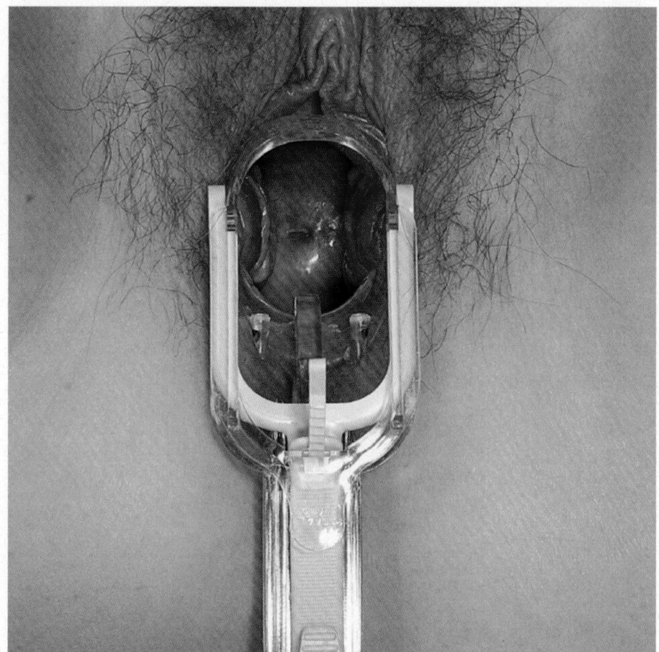

FIGURE 3.3 Appearance of normal cervix. *Note:* This is the cervix of a multipara female. (Photo by B. Proud.)

CORPUS

The corpus, or the main body of the uterus, is a highly muscular organ that enlarges to hold the fetus during pregnancy. The inner lining of the corpus (endometrium) undergoes cyclic changes as a result of the changing levels of hormones secreted by the ovaries: it is thickest during the part of the menstrual cycle in which a fertilized egg would be expected to enter the uterus and is thinnest just after menstruation. If fertilization does not take place during this cycle, most of the endometrium is shed and bleeding occurs, resulting in the monthly period. If fertilization does take place, the embryo attaches to the wall of the uterus, where it becomes embedded in the endometrium (about 1 week after fertilization); this process is called implantation (Patton & Thibodeau, 2015). Menstruation then ceases during the 40 weeks (280 days) of pregnancy. During labor, the muscular walls of the corpus contract to push the baby through the cervix and into the vagina.

Fallopian Tubes

The **fallopian tubes**, also known as oviducts, are hollow, cylindrical structures that extend 2 to 3 in from the upper edges of the uterus toward the ovaries. Each tube is about 7 to 10 cm long (4 in) and approximately 0.7 cm in diameter. The end of each tube flares into a funnel shape, providing a large opening for the egg to fall into when it is released from the ovary. Cilia (beating, hair-like extensions on cells) line the fallopian tube and the muscles in the tube's wall. The fallopian tubes convey the ovum from the ovary to the uterus and sperm from the uterus toward the ovary. This movement is accomplished via ciliary action and peristaltic contraction. If sperm are present in the fallopian tube as a result of sexual intercourse or artificial insemination, fertilization of the ovum can occur in the distal portion of the tube. If the egg is fertilized, it will divide over a period of 4 days while it moves slowly down the fallopian tube and into the uterus, where it implants into the uterine lining.

Ovaries

The **ovaries** are a set of paired glands resembling unshelled almonds that are the organs of gamete production in the female. They are set in the pelvic cavity below and to either side of the umbilicus. They are usually pearl colored, oblong, and have a lumpy surface. They are homologous to the testes. Each mature ovary weighs from 2 to 5 g and is about 4 cm long, 2 cm wide, and 1 cm thick (Jones & Lopez, 2014). The ovaries are not attached to the fallopian tubes but are suspended nearby from several ligaments, which help hold them in position. The development and the release of the ovum and the secretion of the hormones **estrogen** and **progesterone** are the two primary functions of the ovary. The ovaries link the reproductive system to the body's system of endocrine glands, as they produce the ova (eggs) and secrete, in cyclic fashion, the female sex hormones estrogen and progesterone. After an ovum matures, it passes into the fallopian tubes.

Breasts

The two mammary glands, or **breasts**, are accessory organs of the female reproductive system that are specialized to secrete milk following pregnancy. They overlie the pectoralis major muscles and extend from the second to the sixth ribs and from the sternum to the axilla. Each breast has a nipple located near the tip, which is surrounded by a circular area of pigmented skin called the areola. Each breast is composed of approximately nine lobes (the number can range between 4 and 18), which contain glands (alveolar) and a duct (lactiferous) that leads to the nipple and opens to the outside (Fig. 3.5). The lobes are separated by dense connective and adipose tissues, which also help support the weight of the breasts (Kandeel, 2014).

During pregnancy, placental estrogen and progesterone stimulate the development of the mammary glands. Because of this hormonal activity, the breasts may double in size during pregnancy. At the same time, glandular tissue replaces the adipose tissue of the breasts.

Following childbirth and the expulsion of the placenta, levels of placental hormones (progesterone and lactogen) fall rapidly, and the action of prolactin (milk-producing hormone) is no longer inhibited. Prolactin stimulates the production of milk within a few days after childbirth, but in the interim, dark yellow fluid called colostrum is secreted. Colostrum contains more minerals and protein, but less sugar and fat, than mature breast milk. Colostrum secretion may continue for approximately a week after childbirth, with gradual conversion to mature milk. Colostrum is rich in maternal antibodies, especially immunoglobulin A (IgA), which offers protection for the newborn against enteric pathogens.

Female Sexual Response

The sexual response in both females and males is governed primarily by the nervous system rather than by hormones. The sexual response starts in a state of sexual neutrality, and the person's sexual desire is more of a reciprocal response than a spontaneous one (Housman & Odum, 2016). The sexual cycle is usually thought of as having five phases: desire, excitement, plateau, orgasm, and resolution:

1. *Desire:* starts with a desire for sexual intimacy, also known as *libido*

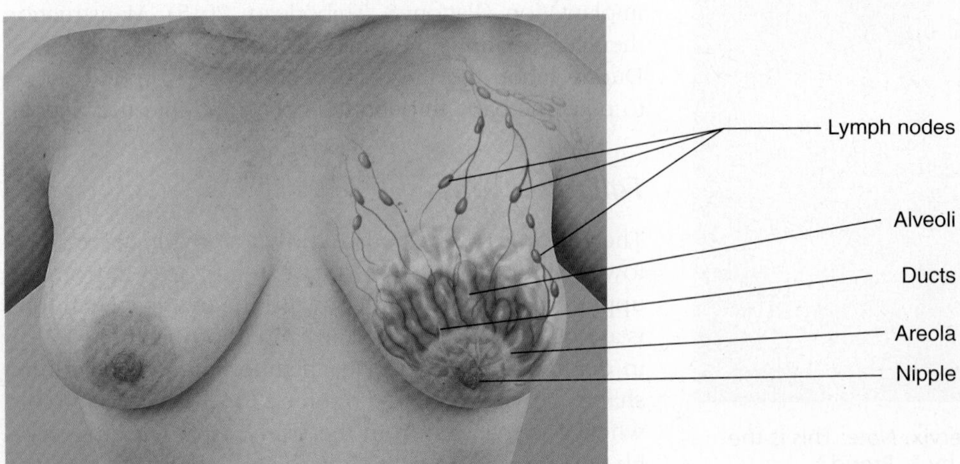

FIGURE 3.5 Anatomy of the breasts. (Photo by B. Proud.)

2. *Excitement:* both men and women have a heightened sexual awareness. When a female is sexually aroused, her brain coordinates a patterned sexual response cycle consisting of increased heart rate, respiratory rate, blood pressure, and general level of excitement (Sherwood, 2016). With sexual stimulation, tissues in the clitoris and breasts and around the vaginal orifice fill with blood and the erectile tissues swell. At the same time, the vagina begins to expand and elongate to accommodate the penis. As part of the whole vasocongestive reaction, the labia majora and minor swell and darken. As sexual stimulation intensifies, the vestibular glands secrete mucus to moisten and lubricate the tissues to facilitate insertion of the penis. Hormones play an integral role in the female sexual response as well. Adequate estrogen and testosterone must be available for the brain to sense incoming arousal stimuli. Research indicates that estrogen preserves the vascular function of female sex organs and affects genital sensation. It also is believed to promote blood flow to these areas during stimulation. Testosterone is needed to stimulate sexual desire in women. Recent research findings also suggest that testosterone therapy improves sexual desire, arousal, orgasm frequency, and satisfaction in women (Davis, 2013).
3. *Plateau:* The heart rate, blood pressure, level of muscle tension, and respiration rate all increase. During this phase, the penile erection intensifies and the vagina constricts around the penis. Continued stimulation of the clitoris and penis with movement leads to the next phase of the sexual response—*orgasmic phase.*
4. *Orgasm:* women experience rhythmic contractions of the pelvic muscles and vaginal walls. In men, ejaculation occurs during the *orgasmic phase* and both sexes experience a peak of sexual pleasure at orgasm. Typically the woman feels warm and relaxed after an orgasm. Within a short time after orgasm, the two physiologic mechanisms that created the sexual response, vasocongestion and muscle contraction, rapidly dissipate. The orgasmic experience varies from person to person and from time to time in the same person. Orgasm is an intense sensation of pleasure achieved by stimulation of erogenous zones. Women do not have a refractory period after each orgasm and can, therefore, experience multiple orgasms. Clitoral sexual response and the female orgasm are not affected by aging (Minkin, 2016). Some orgasms are intense, some are quiet, and some are gentle (Wheatley & Puts, 2015). At the completion of the sexual episode, the brain and body return to an unaroused state, which is termed *sexual resolution.* During this phase, the heart rate, blood pressure, and respirations slow; the muscles relax. Frequently, fatigue sets in for both people.

THE FEMALE REPRODUCTIVE CYCLE

The female reproductive cycle is a complex process that encompasses an intricate series of chemical secretions and reactions to produce the ultimate potential for fertility and birth. The female reproductive cycle is a general term that includes the ovarian cycle, the endometrial (uterine) cycle, the hormonal changes that regulate them, and the cyclical changes in the breasts. The endometrium, ovaries, pituitary gland, and hypothalamus are all involved in the cyclic changes that help to prepare the body for fertilization. Absence of fertilization results in menstruation, the monthly shedding of the uterine lining. **Menstruation** (shedding of the endometrium) marks the beginning and end of the monthly cycle. Menopause is the naturally occurring cessation of menstrual cycles.

The menstrual cycle results from a functional hypothalamic–pituitary–ovarian axis and a precise sequencing of hormones that lead to ovulation. The ovarian cycle, during which ovulation occurs, and the endometrial cycle, during which menstruation occurs, are divided at midcycle by ovulation. Ovulation occurs when the ovum is released from its follicle; after leaving the ovary, the ovum enters the fallopian tube and journeys toward the uterus. If sperm fertilize the ovum during its journey, pregnancy occurs (Fig. 3.6).

Ovarian Cycle

The ovarian cycle is the series of events associated with a developing oocyte (ovum or egg) within the ovaries. Whereas men manufacture sperm daily, often into advanced age, women are born with a single lifetime supply of ova that are released from the ovaries gradually throughout the childbearing years. In the female ovary, 1 million oocytes are present at birth, and about 200,000 to 400,000 follicles are still present at puberty. Typically, a woman ovulates one oocyte per month over an approximately 40-year reproductive life span. This accounts for the loss of 400 to 500 follicles. By age 35 she will have fewer than 100,000 follicles, and, by menopause, her follicular supply will be nearly depleted (Jones & Lopez, 2014). The ovarian cycle begins when the follicular cells (ovum and surrounding cells) swell and the maturation process starts. The maturing follicle at this stage is called a graafian follicle. The ovary raises many follicles monthly, but usually only one follicle matures to reach ovulation. The ovarian cycle consists of three phases: the follicular phase, ovulation, and the luteal phase.

Follicular Phase

This phase is so named because it is when the follicles in the ovary grow and form a mature egg. The goal of

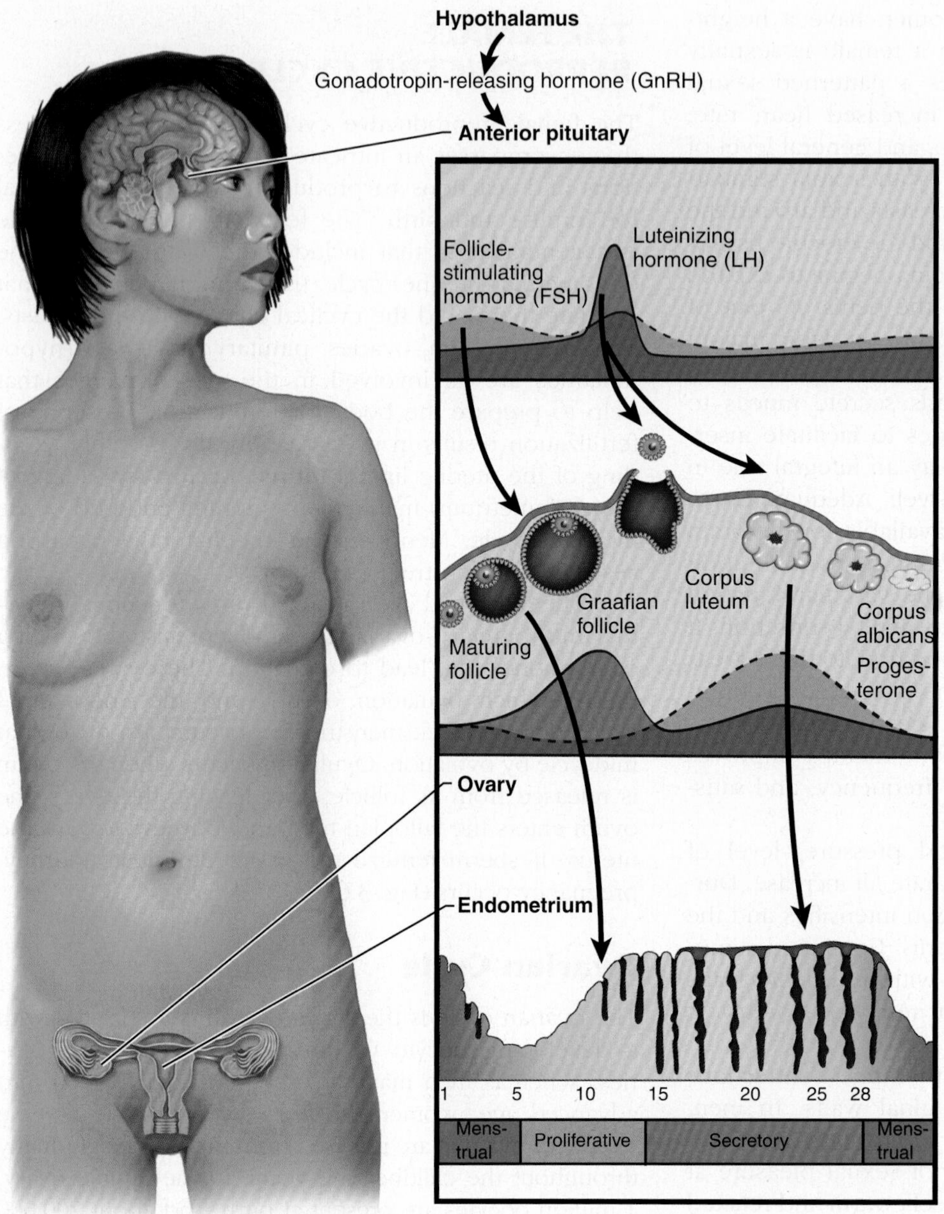

FIGURE 3.6 Menstrual cycle summary based on a 28-day (average) menstrual cycle.

this phase is to produce an ovum for fertilization. This phase starts on day 1 of the menstrual cycle and continues until ovulation, approximately 10 to 14 days later. The follicular phase is not consistent in duration because of the time variations in follicular development. These variations account for the differences in menstrual cycle lengths (Sherwood, 2016). The hypothalamus is the initiator of this phase. Increasing levels of estrogen secreted from the maturing follicular cells and the continued growth of the dominant follicle cell induce proliferation of the endometrium and myometrium. This thickening of the uterine lining supports an implanted ovum if pregnancy occurs.

Prompted by the hypothalamus, the pituitary gland releases **follicle-stimulating hormone (FSH)**, which stimulates the ovary to produce 5 to 20 immature follicles. Each follicle houses an immature oocyte or egg. The follicle that is targeted to mature fully will soon rupture and expel a mature oocyte in the process of ovulation. A surge in **luteinizing hormone (LH)** from the anterior pituitary gland is actually responsible for affecting the final development and subsequent rupture of the mature follicle.

Ovulation

At ovulation, a mature follicle ruptures in response to a surge of LH, releasing a mature oocyte (ovum). No one single event causes ovulation. This usually occurs on day 14 in a 28-day cycle. When ovulation occurs, there is a drop in estrogen. Typically ovulation takes place approximately 10 to 12 hours after the LH peak and 24 to 36 hours after estrogen levels peak (King et al., 2015). The distal ends of the fallopian tubes become active near the time of ovulation and create currents that help carry the ovum into the uterus. The life span of the ovum is only about 24 hours; unless it meets a sperm on its journey within that time, it will die.

During ovulation, the cervix produces thin, clear, stretchy, slippery mucus that is designed to capture the man's sperm, nourish it, and help the sperm travel up through the cervix to meet the ovum for fertilization. Ovulation symptoms also include vaginal spotting, an increase in vaginal discharge giving the woman a "feeling of wetness," an increased libido leading to more desire to be intimate, a slight rise in basal body temperature, and lower abdominal cramping.

The one constant, whether a women's cycle is 28 days or 120 days, is that ovulation takes place 14 days before menstruation (Housman & Odum, 2016).

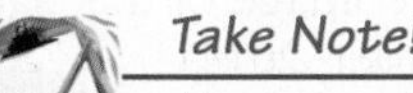

Take Note!

About one in five women can feel a pain on one side of the abdomen around the time the egg is released. This midcycle pain is called mittelschmerz.

Luteal Phase

The luteal phase begins at ovulation and lasts until the menstrual phase of the next cycle. It typically occurs on days 15 through 28 of a 28-day cycle. After the follicle ruptures as it releases the egg, it closes and forms a corpus luteum. The corpus luteum secretes increasing amounts of the hormone progesterone, which interacts with the endometrium to prepare it for implantation. At the beginning of the luteal phase, progesterone induces the endometrial glands to secrete glycogen, mucus, and other substances. These glands become tortuous and have large lumens due to increased secretory activity. The progesterone secreted by the corpus luteum causes the temperature of the body to rise slightly until the start of the next period. A significant increase in temperature, usually 0.5° to 1°F, is generally seen within a day or two after ovulation has occurred; the temperature remains elevated until 3 days before the onset on the next menstruation (Housman & Odum, 2016). This rise in temperature can be plotted on a graph and gives an indication of when ovulation has occurred. In the absence of fertilization, the corpus luteum begins to degenerate and consequently ovarian hormone levels decrease. As estrogen and progesterone levels decrease, the endometrium undergoes involution. In a 28-day cycle, menstruation then begins approximately 14 days after ovulation in the absence of pregnancy. FSH and LH are generally at their lowest levels during the luteal phase and highest during the follicular phase.

Endometrial (Uterine) Cycle

The endometrial (uterine) cycle occurs in response to cyclic hormonal changes. The four phases of the endometrial cycle are the proliferative phase, secretory phase, ischemic phase, and menstrual phase.

Proliferative Phase

The proliferative phase of the endometrial cycle corresponds to the follicular phase of the ovarian cycle. It starts with enlargement of the endometrial glands in response to increasing amounts of estrogen. The blood vessels become dilated and the endometrium increases in thickness dramatically from 0.5 to 5 mm in height and increases eightfold in thickness in preparation for implantation of the fertilized ovum (Oyelowo & Johnson, 2016). Cervical mucus becomes thin, clear, stretchy, and more alkaline, making it more favorable to sperm to enhance the opportunity for fertilization. The proliferative phase starts on about day 5 of the menstrual cycle and lasts to the time of ovulation. This phase depends on estrogen stimulation resulting from ovarian follicles, and this phase coincides with the follicular phase of the ovarian cycle.

Secretory Phase

The secretory phase begins at ovulation to about 3 days before the next menstrual period. Under the influence of progesterone released by the corpus luteum after ovulation, the endometrium becomes thickened and more vascular (growth of the spiral arteries) and glandular (secretion of more glycogen and lipids). These dramatic changes are all in preparation for implantation, if it were to occur. This phase typically lasts from day 15 (after ovulation) to day 28 and coincides with the luteal phase of the ovarian cycle. In the absence of fertilization by day 23 of the menstrual cycle, the corpus luteum begins to degenerate and consequently ovarian hormone levels decrease. As estrogen and progesterone levels decrease, the endometrium undergoes involution.

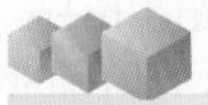

Concept Mastery Alert

Proliferative Versus Secretory Phases of the Uterine Cycle

During the proliferative phase, the ovarian follicles are producing increased amounts of estrogen, and the endometrium prepares for possible fertilization with pronounced growth. The secretory phase begins at time of ovulation. If the ovum is not fertilized, then the corpus luteum degenerates and hormone levels fall, ultimately resulting in menstruation.

Ischemic Phase

If fertilization does not occur, the ischemic phase begins. Estrogen and progesterone levels drop sharply during this phase as the corpus luteum starts to degenerate. Changes in the endometrium occur with spasm of the arterioles, resulting in ischemia of the basal layer. The ischemia leads to shedding of the endometrium down to the basal layer, and menstrual flow begins.

Menstrual Phase

The menstrual phase begins as the spiral arteries rupture secondary to ischemia, releasing blood into the uterus, and the sloughing of the endometrial lining begins. If fertilization does not take place, the corpus luteum degenerates. As a result, both estrogen and progesterone levels fall and the thickened endometrial lining sloughs away from the uterine wall and passes out via the vagina. The beginning of the menstrual flow marks the end of one menstrual cycle and the start of a new one. Most women report menstrual bleeding for an average of 3 to 7 days. The amount of menstrual flow varies, but averages 1 ounce or a range of approximately 2/3 to 2 2/3 ounces in volume per cycle (Thornhill & Gangestad, 2015).

Menstruation

Menstruation is a term derived from the Latin word *mensis,* meaning "month." It is the normal, predictable physiologic process whereby the inner lining of the uterus (endometrium) is expelled by the body. Typically, this occurs monthly. Menstruation has many effects on girls and women, including emotional and self-image issues. In the United States, the average age at **menarche** (the start of menstruation in females) is 12.8 years, with a range between 8 and 18. Genetics is the most important factor in determining the age at which menarche starts, but geographic location, nutrition, weight, general health, nutrition, cultural and social practices, the girl's educational level, attitude, family environment, and beliefs are also important (Krieger et al., 2015).

Pubertal events preceding the first menses have an orderly progression: thelarche, the development of breast buds; adrenarche, the appearance of pubic and then axillary hair, followed by a growth spurt; and menarche (occurring about 2 years after the start of breast development). In healthy pubertal girls, the menstrual period varies in flow heaviness and may remain irregular in occurrence for up to 2 years following menarche. After that time, the regular menstrual cycle should be established. Most women will experience 300 to 400 menstrual cycles within their lifetime (King et al., 2015). Normal, regular menstrual cycles vary in frequency and blood loss (Kandeel, 2014). Irregular menses can be associated with irregular ovulation, polycystic ovary syndrome, type 2 diabetes, weather conditions, stress, disease, and hormonal imbalances (Senie, 2014).

Think back to Linda, who was introduced at the beginning of the chapter. What questions might need to be asked to assess her condition? What laboratory work might be anticipated to validate her heavier flow?

Although menstruation is a normal process, various world cultures have taken a wide variety of attitudes toward it, seeing it as everything from a sacred time to an unclean time. Folk culture surrounding menstrual-related matters has considerable implications for symptom expression and treatment-seeking behavior. Recent research findings imply the need for education to help adolescent girls manage menstrual symptoms and increase awareness of the benefit of treating them. Given that menstrual-related information comes from mothers, family, and social culture, negative attitudes toward their monthly cycles can be formed in young impressionable girls. Nurses, through formal instruction, can help young girls in shaping good menstrual attitudes and a more positive image of this natural physiologic process (Clark & Paraska, 2014).

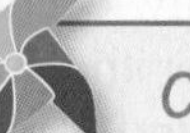

Take Note!

Knowledge about menstruation has increased significantly and attitudes have changed. What was once discussed only behind closed doors is discussed openly today.

Consider This

We had been married 2 years when my husband and I decided to start a family. I began thinking back to my high school biology class and tried to remember about ovulation and what to look for. I also used the Internet to find the answers I was seeking. As I was reading, it all started to come into place. During ovulation, a woman's cervical mucus increases and she experiences a wet sensation for several days midcycle. The mucus also becomes stretchable during this time. In addition, body temperature rises slightly and then falls if no conception takes place. Armed with this knowledge, I began to check my temperature daily before arising and began to monitor the consistency of my cervical mucus. I figured that monitoring these two signs of ovulation could help me discover the best time to conceive. After 6 months of trying without results, I wondered what I was doing wrong. Did I really understand my body's reproductive activity?

Thoughts: What additional suggestions might the nurse offer this woman in her journey to conception? What community resources might be available to assist this couple? How does knowledge of the reproductive system help nurses take care of couples who are trying to become pregnant?

BOX 3.1

SUMMARY OF MENSTRUAL CYCLE HORMONES

- Luteinizing hormone (LH) rises and stimulates the follicle to produce estrogen.
- As estrogen is produced by the follicle, estrogen levels rise, inhibiting the output of LH.
- Ovulation occurs after an LH surge damages the estrogen-producing cells, resulting in a decline in estrogen.
- The LH surge results in establishment of the corpus luteum, which produces estrogen and progesterone.
- Estrogen and progesterone levels rise, suppressing LH output.
- Lack of LH promotes degeneration of the corpus luteum.
- Cessation of the corpus luteum means a decline in estrogen and progesterone output.
- The decline of the ovarian hormones ends their negative effect on the secretion of LH.
- LH is secreted, and the menstrual cycle begins again.

Menstrual Cycle Hormones

The menstrual cycle involves a complex interaction of hormones. The predominant hormones include gonadotropin-releasing hormone (GnRH), FSH, LH, estrogen, progesterone, and prostaglandins. Box 3.1 summarizes menstrual cycle hormones.

Gonadotropin-Releasing Hormone

GnRH is secreted from the hypothalamus in a pulsatile manner throughout the reproductive cycle. It pulsates slowly during the follicular phase and increases during the luteal phase. GnRH induces the release of FSH and LH to assist with ovulation.

Follicle-Stimulating Hormone

FSH is secreted by the anterior pituitary gland and is primarily responsible for the maturation of the ovarian follicle. FSH secretion is highest and most important during the first week of the follicular phase of the reproductive cycle.

Luteinizing Hormone

LH is secreted by the anterior pituitary gland and is required for both the final maturation of preovulatory follicles and luteinization of the ruptured follicle. As a result, estrogen production declines and progesterone secretion continues. Thus, estrogen levels fall a day before ovulation, and progesterone levels begin to rise.

Estrogen

Estrogen is secreted by the ovaries and is crucial for the development and maturation of the follicle. Estrogen is predominant at the end of the proliferative phase, directly preceding ovulation. After ovulation, estrogen levels drop sharply as progesterone dominates. In the endometrial cycle, estrogen induces proliferation of the endometrial glands. Estrogen also causes the uterus to increase in size and weight because of increased glycogen, amino acids, electrolytes, and water. Blood supply is expanded as well.

Progesterone

Progesterone is secreted by the corpus luteum. Progesterone levels increase just before ovulation and peak 5 to 7 days after ovulation. During the luteal phase, progesterone induces swelling and increased secretion of the endometrium. This hormone is often called the hormone of pregnancy because of its calming effect (reduces uterine contractions) on the uterus, allowing pregnancy to be maintained.

Prostaglandins

Prostaglandins are primary mediators of the body's inflammatory processes and are essential for the normal physiologic function of the female reproductive system. They are a closely related group of oxygenated fatty acids that are produced by the endometrium, with a variety of effects throughout the body. Although they have regulatory effects and are sometimes called hormones, prostaglandins are not technically hormones because they are produced by all tissues rather than by special glands (Jones & Lopez, 2014). Prostaglandins increase during follicular maturation and play a key role in ovulation by freeing the ovum inside the graafian follicle. Large amounts of prostaglandins are found in menstrual blood. Current research suggests that the pathogenesis of menstrual cramps/pain is due to prostaglandin F2a (PGF2a), a potent myometrial stimulant and vasoconstrictor, in the secretory endometrium. Elevated prostaglandin levels are found in the endometrial fluid of women with dysmenorrhea (painful menses) and correlates well with their degree of pain. Nonsteroidal anti-inflammatory drugs have been introduced as the primary choice of treatment for menstrual cramps (Nguyen, et al., 2015).

Perimenopause

Perimenopause or menopausal transition and menopause are biologic markers of the transition from young adulthood to middle age. Neither of these is a symptom or disease, but rather a natural maturing of the reproductive system.

During the perimenopausal years (2 to 8 years prior to menopause), women may experience physical changes associated with decreasing estrogen levels, which may include vasomotor symptoms of hot flashes, irregular menstrual cycles, sleep disruptions, forgetfulness, irritability, mood disturbances, weight gain and bloating, irregular menses, headaches, decreased vaginal lubrication, night sweats, fatigue, vaginal atrophy, and depression (McNamara, Batur, & DeSapri, 2015). Vasomotor symptoms (hot flashes and night sweats) are the most common complaints for which women seek treatment. Several therapies can be considered to help manage these complaints. Choosing an appropriate treatment approach for the management of these symptoms requires careful assessment of the risk/benefit ratio of each alternative, as well as individual client preference (Schuiling & Likis, 2016).

Menopause

Menopause is a universal and irreversible part of the overall aging process involving a woman's reproductive system, after which she no longer menstruates. This naturally occurring phase of every woman's life marks the end of her childbearing capacity. The average age of natural menopause—defined as 1 year without a menstrual period—is 50 to 51 years old (Alexander et al., 2014). This period is frequently termed the *climacteric* or *perimenopause,* but mostly recently the *menopausal transition* has been used (Hoyt & Falconi, 2015). As the average life expectancy for women increases, the number of women reaching and living in menopause has escalated. Most women can expect to spend more than one third of their lives beyond menopause. It is usually marked by atrophy of the breasts, uterus, fallopian tubes, and ovaries (Crawford, 2015).

Many women pass through menopause without untoward symptoms. These women remain active and in good health with little interruption of their daily routines. Other women experience vasomotor symptoms, which give rise to sensations of heat, cold, sweating, headache, insomnia, and irritability. A recent study found that women experiencing menopausal symptoms reported significantly lower health-related quality of life and significantly high work impairment when compared to women without menopausal symptoms (Coney, 2015).

Until recently, hormone therapy was the mainstay of menopause pharmacotherapy, but with the recent results of the Women's Health Initiative trial and the Heart and Estrogen Replacement Study (HERS), the use of hormone therapy has become controversial. Many women have turned to nontraditional remedies to manage their menopausal symptoms. Common complementary and alternative medicine (CAM) remedies used for the treatment of menopausal symptoms include black cohosh, dong quai, St John wort, hops, wild yam, ginseng, evening primrose oil, exercise, and acupuncture. Evidence supporting the efficacy and safety of most CAM for relief of menopausal symptoms is limited and most of the reports of efficacy don't support use of them (Wicks & Mahady, 2015). Nurses can play a major role in assisting menopausal women by educating and counseling them about the multitude of options available for disease prevention and treatments for menopausal symptoms during this time of change in their lives. Menopause should be an opportunity for women to strive for a healthy, long life, and nurses can help to make this opportunity a reality. (See Chapter 4 for more information about menopause.)

Recall Linda, who was experiencing changes in her menstrual patterns. Which hormones might be changing, and which systems might they affect? What approach should the nurse take to enlighten Linda about what is happening to her?

MALE REPRODUCTIVE ANATOMY AND PHYSIOLOGY

The male reproductive system, like that of the female, consists of those organs that facilitate reproduction. The male organs are specialized to produce and maintain the male sex cells, or sperm; to transport them, along with supporting fluids, to the female reproductive system; and to secrete the male hormone testosterone. The organs of the male reproductive system include the penis, scrotum, two **testes** (where sperm cells and testosterone are made), and accessory organs (epididymis, vas deferens, seminal vesicles, ejaculatory duct, urethra, bulbourethral glands, and prostate gland).

External Male Reproductive Organs

The penis and the scrotum form the external genitalia in the male (Fig. 3.7).

Penis

The penis is the organ for copulation and serves as the outlet for both sperm and urine. The penis becomes

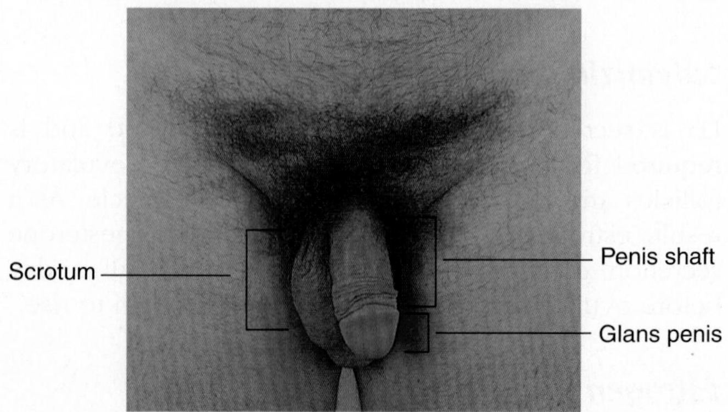

FIGURE 3.7 The external male reproductive organs. (Photo by B. Proud.)

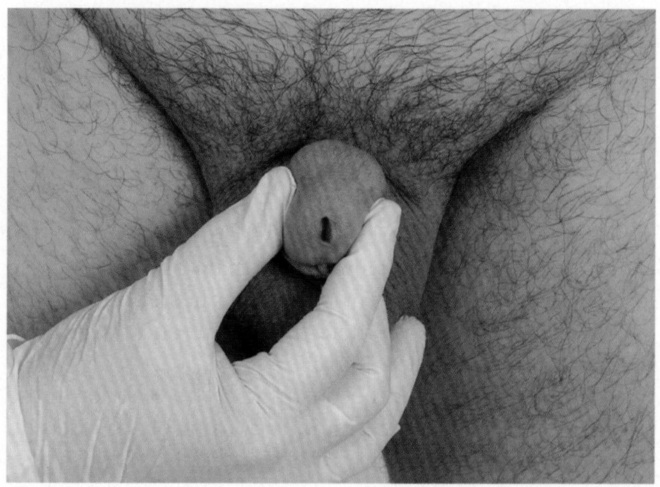

FIGURE 3.8 The urinary meatus. (Photo by B. Proud.)

engorged with blood during sexual arousal and is inserted into the female vagina during intercourse. The skin of the penis is thin, with no hairs. The prepuce (foreskin) is a circular fold of skin that extends over the glans unless it is removed by circumcision shortly after birth. The urinary meatus, located at the tip of the penis, serves as the external opening to the urethra (Fig. 3.8). The penis is composed mostly of erectile tissue. Most of the body of the penis consists of three cylindrical spaces (sinuses) of erectile tissue. The two larger ones, the corpora cavernosa, are side by side. The third sinus, the corpus spongiosum, surrounds the urethra. Erection results when nerve impulses from the autonomic nervous system dilate the arteries of the penis, allowing arterial blood to flow into the erectile tissues of the organ.

Scrotum

The scrotum is the thin-skinned sac that surrounds and protects the testes. The scrotum also acts as a climate-control system for the testes, because they need to be slightly cooler than body temperature to allow normal sperm development. The scrotum is covered with hair starting in puberty. The cremaster muscles in the scrotal wall relax or contract to allow the testes to hang farther from the body to cool or to be pulled closer to the body for warmth or protection (Patton & Thibodeau, 2015). A medial septum divides the scrotum into two chambers, each of which encloses a testis.

Internal Male Reproductive Organs

The internal structures include the testes, the ductal system, and accessory glands (Fig. 3.9).

Testes

The testes are oval bodies in the size of large olives that lie in the scrotum; usually the left testis hangs a little lower than the right one. These two nut-like

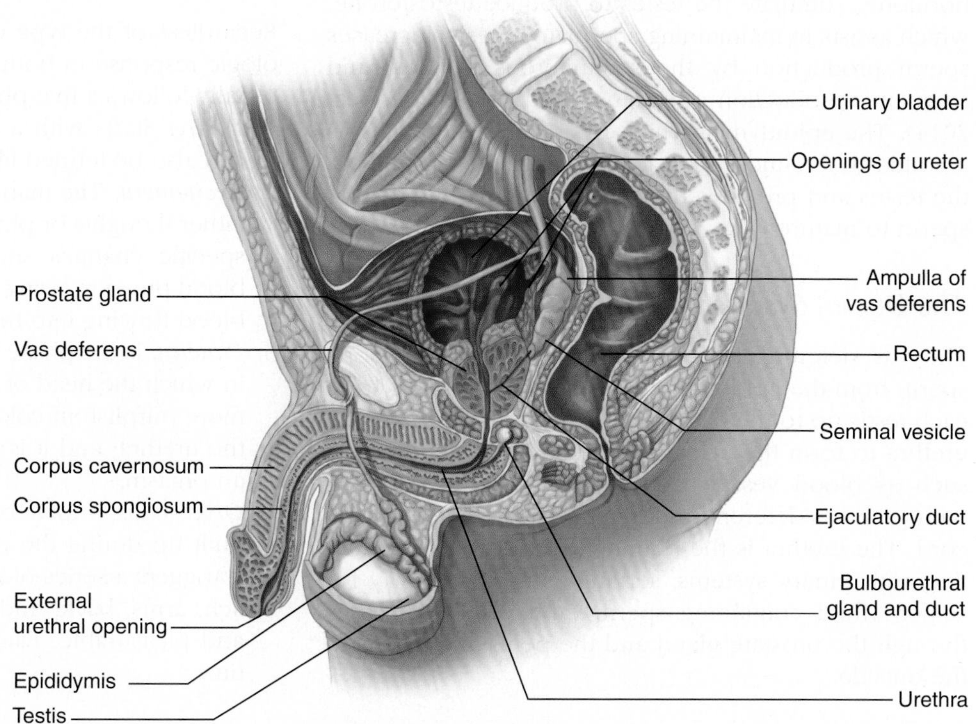

FIGURE 3.9 Lateral view of the internal male reproductive organs. (Adapted from Anatomical Chart Company. (2001). *Atlas of human anatomy*. Springhouse, PA: Springhouse.)

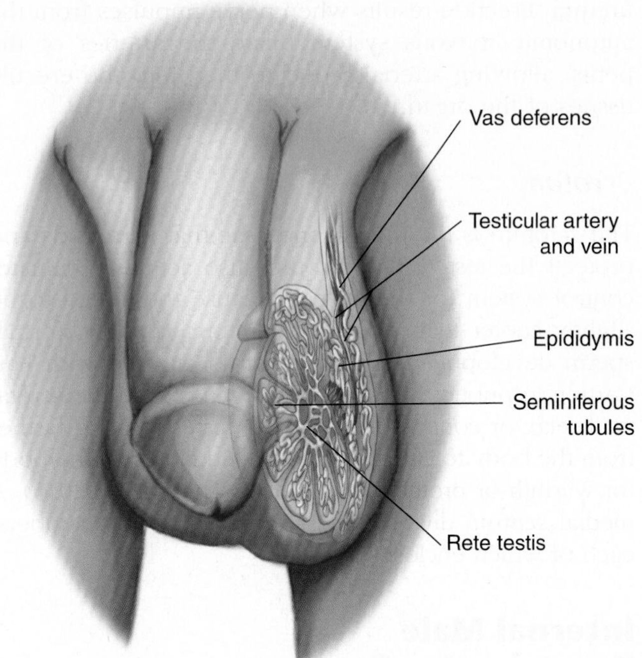

FIGURE 3.10 Internal structures of a testis.

structures are analogous to ovaries in the female and two testes are present in males. The testes have two functions: producing sperm and synthesizing testosterone (the primary male sex hormone). Sperm is produced in the seminiferous tubules of the testes. Similar to the female reproductive system, the anterior pituitary releases the gonadotropins, FSH and LH. These hormones stimulate the testes to produce testosterone, which assists in maintaining spermatogenesis, increases sperm production by the seminiferous tubules, and stimulates production of seminal fluid (Jones & Lopez, 2014). The epididymis, which lies against the testes, is a coiled tube almost 20 ft long. It collects sperm from the testes and provides the space and environment for sperm to mature (Fig. 3.10).

The Ductal System

The vas deferens is a cord-like duct that transports sperm from the epididymis. One such duct travels from each testis up to the back of the prostate and enters the urethra to form the ejaculatory ducts. Other structures, such as blood vessels and nerves, also travel along with each vas deferens and together form the spermatic cord. The urethra is the terminal duct of the reproductive and urinary systems, serving as a passageway for semen (fluid containing sperm) and urine. It passes through the prostate gland and the penis and opens to the outside.

Accessory Glands

The seminal vesicles, which produce nutrient seminal fluid, and the prostate gland, which produces alkaline prostatic fluid, are both connected to the ejaculatory duct leading into the urethra. The paired seminal vesicles are convoluted pouch-like structures lying posterior to, and at the base of, the urinary bladder in front of the rectum. They secrete an alkaline fluid that contains fructose and prostaglandins. The fructose supplies energy to the sperm on its journey to meet the ovum, and the prostaglandins assist in sperm mobility.

The prostate gland lies just under the bladder in the pelvis and surrounds the middle portion of the urethra. Usually the size of a walnut, this gland enlarges with age. The prostate and the seminal vesicles above it produce fluid that nourishes the sperm. This fluid provides most of the volume of semen, the secretion in which sperm are expelled during ejaculation. Other fluid that makes up the semen comes from the vas deferens and from mucous glands in the head of the penis.

The bulbourethral glands (Cowper glands) are two small structures about the size of peas, located inferior to the prostate gland. They are composed of several tubes whose epithelial linings secrete a mucus-like fluid. It is released in response to sexual stimulation and lubricates the head of the penis in preparation for sexual intercourse, in addition, neutralizes the acidity of the urethra to protect sperm during their journey out of the body during ejaculation. Their existence is said to be constant, but they gradually diminish in size with advancing age.

Male Sexual Response

Regardless of the type of sexual stimulation, the physiologic response in both men and women is similar and usually follows a five-phase pattern, as described earlier:

1. *Desire:* Starts with a desire for sexual intimacy. This can also be termed libido.
2. *Excitement:* The man experiences sexual arousal with either thoughts or physical sexual stimuli which cause specific changes such as the heart beating faster, blood pressure rising, the testicles enlarging and more blood flowing into the penis, creating an erection.
3. *Plateau:* is the phase between excitement and orgasm in which the head of the penis enlarges and becomes more purplish in color; the glands secrete semen into the urethra; and it is challenging to stop from having an orgasm.
4. *Orgasm:* is a total body response. The tension that built up during the previous two phases is released. It triggers a series of muscle spasms in the legs, stomach, arms, back, and penis. The feelings are intense and pleasurable. Ejaculation of semen occurs at this time.

5. *Resolution:* The body returns to the physiologic nonstimulated state. The blood flows out of the penis and erection ceases; an overall feeling of relaxation ensues, and the testes and scrotum return to their normal size (Housman & Odum, 2016).

Sexual behavior involves the participation of autonomic and somatic nerves and the integration of numerous spinal sites in the central nervous system (CNS). The penile portion of the process that leads to erections represents only a single component. Penile erections are an integration of complex physiologic processes involving the CNS, peripheral nervous system, and hormonal and vascular systems (Sherwood, 2016). With sexual stimulation, the arteries leading to the penis dilate and increase blood flow into erectile tissues. At the same time, the erectile tissue compresses the veins of the penis, reducing blood flow away from the penis. Blood accumulates, causing the penis to swell and elongate and producing an erection. As in women, the culmination of sexual stimulation is an orgasm, a pleasurable feeling of physiologic and psychological release.

Orgasm is accompanied by emission (movement of sperm from the testes and fluids from the accessory glands) into the urethra, where the sperm and fluids are mixed to form semen. As the urethra fills with semen, the base of the erect penis contracts, this increases pressure. This pressure forces the semen through the urethra to the outside (ejaculation). During ejaculation, the ducts of the testes, epididymis, and vas deferens contract and cause expulsion of sperm into the urethra, where the sperm mixes with the seminal and prostatic fluids. These substances, together with mucus secreted by accessory glands, form the semen, which is discharged from the urethra.

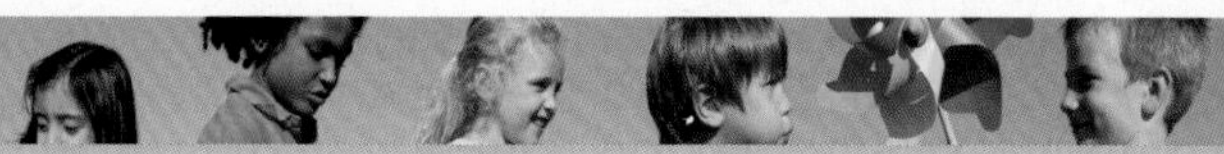

KEY CONCEPTS

- The female reproductive system produces the female reproductive cells (the eggs, or ova) and contains an organ (uterus) where the fetus develops. The male reproductive system produces the male reproductive cells (the sperm) and contains an organ (penis) that deposits the sperm within the female.
- The internal female reproductive organs consist of the vagina, the uterus, the fallopian tubes, and the ovaries. The external female reproductive organs make up the vulva. These include the mons pubis, the labia majora and minora, the clitoris and prepuce, structures within the vestibule, and the perineum.
- The breasts are accessory organs of the female reproductive system that are specialized to secrete milk following pregnancy.
- The main function of the reproductive cycle is to stimulate growth of a follicle to release an egg and prepare a site for implantation if fertilization occurs.
- Menstruation, the monthly shedding of the uterine lining, marks the beginning and end of the cycle if fertilization does not occur.
- The ovarian cycle is the series of events associated with a developing oocyte (ovum or egg) within the ovaries.
- At ovulation, a mature follicle ruptures in response to a surge of luteinizing hormone (LH), releasing a mature oocyte (ovum).
- The endometrial cycle is divided into four phases: the follicular or proliferative phase, the luteal or secretory phase, the ischemic phase, and the menstrual phase.
- The menstrual cycle involves a complex interaction of hormones. The predominant hormones are gonadotropin-releasing hormone (GnRH), follicle-stimulating hormone (FSH), LH, estrogen, progesterone, and prostaglandins.
- The organs of the male reproductive system include the penis, scrotum, two testes (where sperm cells and testosterone are made), and accessory organs (epididymis, vas deferens, seminal vesicles, ejaculatory ducts, urethra, bulbourethral glands, and prostate gland).

REFERENCES AND RECOMMENDED READINGS

Acién, M., & Acién, P. (2015). Normal embryological development of the female genital tract. In *Female genital tract congenital malformations* (pp. 3–14). London, UK: Springer.

Alexander, L. L., LaRosa, J. H., Bader, H., & Garfield, S. (2014). *New dimensions in women's health* (6th ed.). Sudbury, MA: Jones and Bartlett.

Clark, C. C., & Paraska, K. K. (2014). *Health promotion for nurses: A practical guide.* Burlington, MA: Jones & Bartlett Learning.

Coney, P. (2015). Menopause. eMedicine. Retrieved from http://emedicine.medscape.com/article/264088-overview

Crawford, S. L. (2015). What should women expect after stopping hormone therapy?. *Menopause, 22*(4), 367–368.

Davis, S. R. (2013). Androgen therapy in women, beyond libido. *Climacteric, 16*, 18–24.

Farage, M. A., Miller, K. W., & Maibach, H. I. (2015). Postmenopausal vulva and vagina. In *Skin, mucosa and menopause* (pp. 385–395). Heidelberg, Berlin: Springer.

Housman, J., & Odum, M. (2016) *Alters & Schiff's essential concepts for healthy living* (7th ed.). Burlington, MA: Jones & Bartlett Learning.

Hoyt, L. T., & Falconi, A. (2015). Puberty and perimenopause: Reproductive transitions and their implications for women's health. *Social Science & Medicine, 132*, 103–112. doi:10.1016/j.socscimed.2015.03.031

Jones, R. E., & Lopez, K. H. (2014) *Human reproductive biology* (4th ed.). Waltham, MA: Elsevier.

Kandeel, F. (2014). *Female reproductive and sexual medicine.* New York, NY: Springer.

King, T. L., Brucker, M. C., Kriebs, J. M., Fahey, J. O., Gegor, C. L., & Varney, H. (2015). *Varney's midwifery* (5th ed.). Burlington, MA: Jones & Bartlett Learning.

Krieger, N., Kiang, M. V., Kosheleva, A., Waterman, P. D., Chen, J. T., & Beckfield, J. (2015). Age at menarche: 50-year socioeconomic trends among US-born black and white women. *American Journal of Public Health, 105*(2), 388–397.

McNamara, M., Batur, P., & DeSapri, K. T. (2015). Perimenopause. *Annals of Internal Medicine, 162*(3), ITC1–ITC15.

Minkin, M. J. (2016) Sexual health and relationships after age 60. *Matutitas, 83*, 27–32. doi: 10.1016/j.maturitas.2015.10.004

Nguyen, A. M., Humphrey, L., Kitchen, H., Rehman, T., & Norquist, J. M. (2015). A qualitative study to develop a patient-reported outcome for dysmenorrhea. *Quality of Life Research, 24*(1), 181–191.

Oyelowo, T., & Johnson, J. L. (2016). *A guide to women's health* (2nd ed.). Burlington, MA: Jones & Bartlett Learning.

Patton, K.T., & Thibodeau, G. A. (2016) *The Human Body in Health and Disease* (6th ed.). St. Louis, MO: Mosby Elsevier.

Patton, K. T., & Thibodeau, G. A. (2015). *Anatomy & physiology* (9th ed.). St. Louis, MO: Mosby Elsevier.

Pauls, R. N. (2015). Anatomy of the clitoris and the female sexual response. *Clinical Anatomy, 28*(3), 376–384.

Senie, R. T. (2014). *Epidemiology of women's health*. Burlington, MA: Jones & Bartlett Learning.

Schuiling, K. D., & Likis, F. E (2016). *Women's gynecologic health* (3rd ed.). Burlington, MA: Jones and Bartlett Learning.

Sherwood, L. (2016) *Human physiology: From cells to systems* (9th ed.). Boston, MA: Cengage Learning.

Tambouret, R. H., & Wilbur, D. C. (2015). Normal histology and cytology of the endocervix and endometrium. In *Glandular lesions of the uterine cervix* (pp. 25–40). New York, NY: Springer.

Thornhill, R., & Gangestad, S. W. (2015). The functional design and phylogeny of women's sexuality. In *The evolution of sexuality* (pp. 149–184). Springer International Publishing.

Velkey, J. M., Hall, A. H., & Robboy, S. J. (2015). Normal vulva: Embryology, anatomy, and histology. In *Vulvar Pathology* (pp. 3–17). New York, NY: Springer

Wheatley, J. R., & Puts, D. A. (2015). Evolutionary science of female orgasm. In *The evolution of sexuality* (pp. 123–148). Springer International Publishing.

Wicks, S. M., & Mahady, G. B. (2015). Herbal and complementary medicines used for women's health. In *Medicines for women* (pp. 373–399). Springer International Publishing.

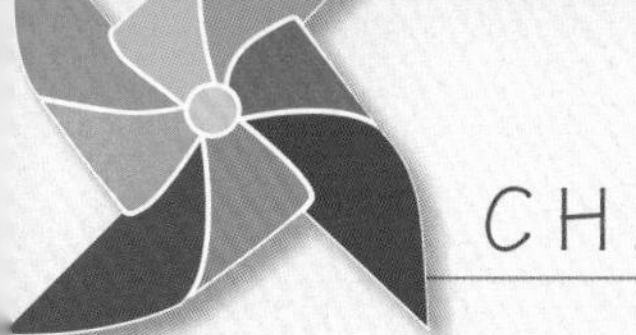

CHAPTER WORKSHEET

MULTIPLE-CHOICE QUESTIONS

1. The predominant anterior pituitary hormones that orchestrate the menstrual cycle include:
   a. Thyroid-stimulating hormone (TSH)
   b. Follicle-stimulating hormone (FSH)
   c. Corticotropin-releasing hormone (CRH)
   d. Gonadotropin-releasing hormone (GnRH)

2. Which glands are located on either side of the female urethra and secrete mucus to keep the opening moist and lubricated for urination?
   a. Cowper's
   b. Bartholin's
   c. Skene's
   d. Seminal

3. What event occurs during the proliferative phase of the menstrual cycle?
   a. Menstrual flow starts
   b. Endometrium thickens
   c. Ovulation occurs
   d. Progesterone secretion peaks

4. Which hormone is produced in high levels to prepare the endometrium for implantation just after ovulation by the corpus luteum?
   a. Estrogen
   b. Prostaglandins
   c. Prolactin
   d. Progesterone

5. Sperm maturation and storage in the male reproductive system occur in the:
   a. Testes
   b. Vas deferens
   c. Epididymis
   d. Seminal vesicles

6. The nurse is preparing to teach a class to a group of middle-aged women regarding the most common vasomotor symptoms experienced during menopause and possible modalities of treatment available. Common vasomotor symptoms would include which of the following?
   a. Chronic fatigue and confusion
   b. Forgetfulness and irritability
   c. Night sweats and hot flashes
   d. Decrease in sexual response and appetite

CRITICAL THINKING EXERCISE

1. The school nurse was asked to speak to a 10th-grade biology class about menstruation. The teacher felt that the students did not understand this monthly event and wanted to dispel some myths about it. After the nurse explains the factors influencing the menses, one girl asks, "Could someone get pregnant if she had sex during her period?"
   a. How should the nurse respond to this question?
   b. What factor regarding the menstrual cycle was not clarified?
   c. What additional topics might this question lead to that might be discussed?

STUDY ACTIVITIES

1. Should sex education be taught in public schools, and if so, what topics should be addressed? Debate the pros and cons of teaching this and then outline which topics should be covered.

2. Respond to the following as a topic sentence: "When I was growing up, talking about sexual matters with my parents was ______________ because ______________ Now the situation is ______________?

3. List the predominant hormones and their function in the menstrual cycle.

4. The ovarian cycle describes the series of events associated with the development of the ______________ within the ovaries.

5. Sperm cells and the male hormone testosterone are made in which of the following structures? Select all that apply.
   a. Vas deferens
   b. Penis
   c. Scrotum
   d. Ejaculatory ducts
   e. Prostate gland
   f. Testes
   g. Seminiferous tubules
   h. Bulbourethral glands

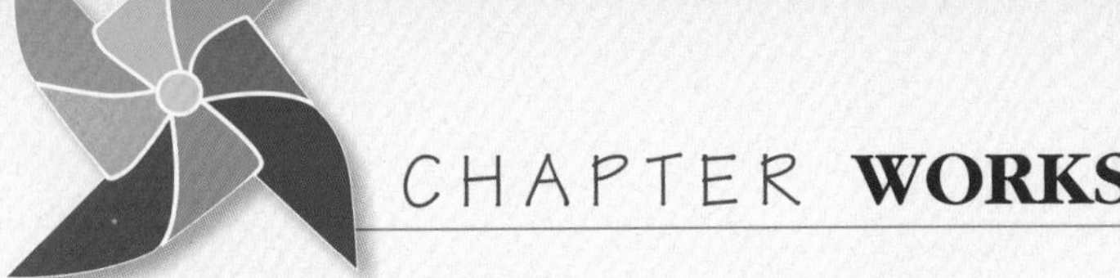

CHAPTER **WORKSHEET**

BRINGING IT ALL TOGETHER: A CASE STUDY

A 53-year-old woman came to see her women's health nurse practitioner for her annual examination. She had a hysterectomy 20 years ago for a prolapsed uterus and has been healthy up until now. She had a long list of symptoms that had been bothering her, but until recently just chalked them up to the aging process. She told the nurse practitioner that she was experiencing insomnia, weight gain around her middle despite not consuming additional calories, painful intercourse and hot flashes that were increasing in frequency throughout the day and night. She had been taking black cohosh for these distressing symptoms for the past several months, but was not getting any relief. She was concerned that something awful was wrong with her since this natural herb was not reducing her symptoms and they seemed to be getting worse.

1. What explanation should be offered to this woman regarding what is causing her distress?
2. What is the current thinking regarding natural herbs in the treatment of menopausal symptoms?
3. What treatment might be suggested for this woman?
4. What is the current principle concerning hormone therapy in the treatment of menopause?

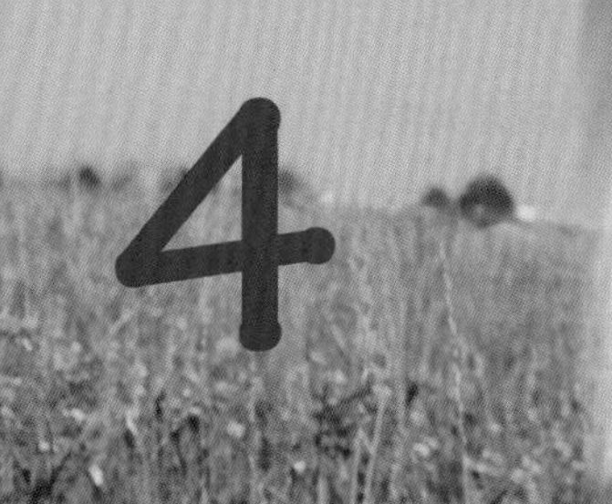

4

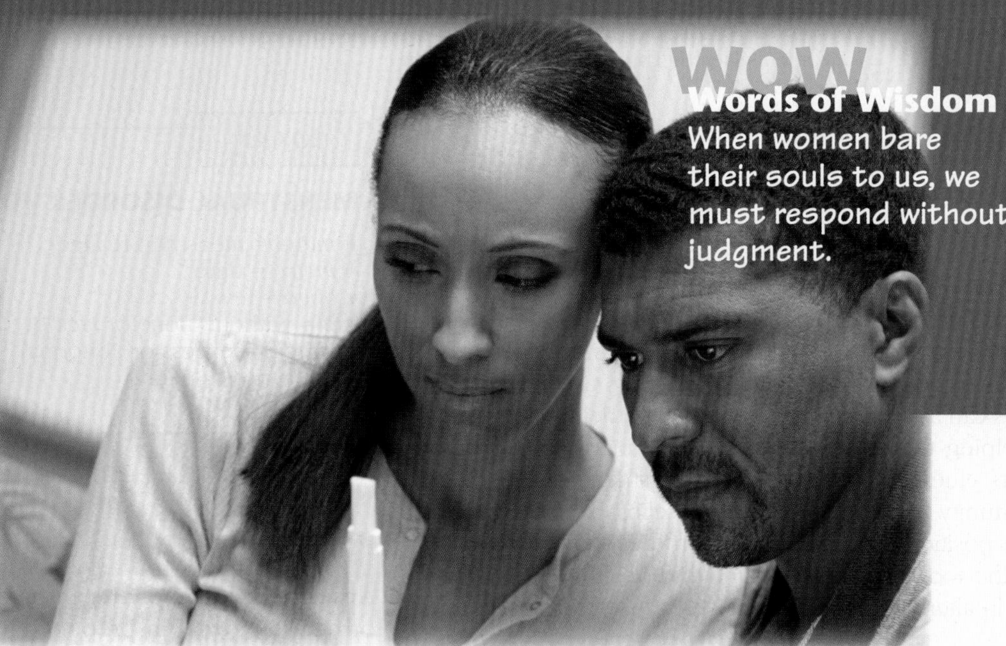

WOW
Words of Wisdom
When women bare their souls to us, we must respond without judgment.

KEY TERMS
abnormal uterine bleeding (AUB)
abortion
amenorrhea
basal body temperature (BBT)
cervical cap
cervical mucus ovulation method
coitus interruptus
condoms
contraception
contraceptive sponge
Depo-Provera
diaphragm
dysmenorrhea
dyspareunia
emergency contraception (EC)
endometriosis
fertility awareness
implant
infertility
intrauterine contraceptive (IUC)
lactational amenorrhea method (LAM)
menopausal transition
oral contraceptives (OCs)
osteoporosis
premenstrual syndrome (PMS)
sexual abstinence
Standard Days Method (SDM)
sterilization
symptothermal method
transdermal patch
tubal ligation
vaginal ring
vasectomy

Common Reproductive Issues

Learning Objectives

Upon completion of the chapter, you will be able to:

1. Examine common reproductive concerns in terms of symptoms, diagnostic tests, and appropriate interventions.
2. Identify risk factors and outline appropriate client education needed in common reproductive disorders.
3. Compare and contrast the various contraceptive methods available and their overall effectiveness.
4. Analyze the physiologic and psychological aspects of menopausal transition.
5. Delineate the nursing management needed for women experiencing common reproductive disorders.

***Izzy*, a 27-year-old, presents to her health care provider complaining of progressive severe pelvic pain associated with her monthly periods. She has to take off work and "dope up" with pills to endure the pain. In addition, she has been trying to conceive for over a year without any luck.**

INTRODUCTION

Good health throughout the life cycle begins with the individual. Women today can expect to live well into their 80s and need to be proactive in maintaining their own quality of life. Women need to take steps to reduce their risk of disease and need to become active partners with their health care professional to identify problems early, when treatment may be most successful (Teaching Guidelines 4.1). Nurses can assist women in maintaining their quality of life by helping them to become more attuned to their body and its clues and can use the assessment period as an opportunity for teaching and counseling. Nurses are in a prime position to offer information that provides women with the tools needed to maintain a healthy lifestyle and assist in altering behaviors that may cause harm or illness.

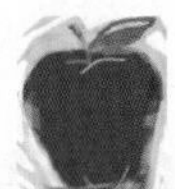

Teaching Guidelines 4.1

TIPS FOR BEING AN ACTIVE PARTNER IN MANAGING YOUR HEALTH

- Become an informed consumer. Read, ask, and search.
- Know your family history and know factors that put you at high risk.
- Maintain a healthy lifestyle and let moderation be your guide.
- Schedule regular medical checkups and screenings for early detection.
- Ask your health care provider for a full explanation of any treatment.
- Seek a second medical opinion if you feel you need more information.
- Know when to seek medical care by being aware of disease symptoms.

Common reproductive issues addressed in this chapter that nurses might encounter in caring for women include menstrual disorders, infertility, contraception, abortion, and the menopausal transition.

MENSTRUAL DISORDERS

Many women sail through their monthly menstrual cycles with little or no concern. With few symptoms to worry about, their menses are like clockwork, starting and stopping at nearly the same times every month. For others, the menstrual cycle causes physical and emotional symptoms that initiate visits to their health care provider for consultation. The following menstruation-related conditions will be discussed in this section: amenorrhea, dysmenorrhea, abnormal uterine bleeding (AUB), premenstrual syndrome (PMS), premenstrual dysphoric disorder (PMDD), and endometriosis. To gain an understanding of menstrual disorders, nurses should know the terms used to describe them (Box 4.1).

BOX 4.1

MENSTRUAL DISORDER VOCABULARY

- *meno* = menstrual related
- *metro* = time
- *oligo* = few
- *a* = without, none or lack of
- *rhagia* = excess or abnormal
- *dys* = not or pain
- *rhea* = flow

Amenorrhea

Amenorrhea simply means absence of menses. Amenorrhea is normal in prepubertal, pregnant, postpartum, and postmenopausal females. The uterus, endometrial lining, ovaries, pituitary, and hypothalamus must function properly and in harmony for a menstrual cycle to occur. The two categories of amenorrhea are primary and secondary amenorrhea. Primary amenorrhea is defined as either the:

1. Absence of menses by age 14, with absence of growth and development of secondary sexual characteristics, or
2. Absence of menses by age 16, with normal development of secondary sexual characteristics (Schuiling & Likis, 2016).

Ninety-eight percent of girls living in the United States menstruate by age 15 (Krieger, Kiang, Kosheleva, et al., 2015). Findings of recent studies indicate that age at menarche has overall declined since the 20th century (King, Brucker, Kriebs, et al., 2015). Once menarche has occurred, cycles may take up to 2 years to become regular, ovulatory cycles. Secondary amenorrhea is the absence of regular menses for three cycles or irregular menses for 6 months in women who have previously menstruated regularly.

Nurses need to consider the causes of amenorrhea as occurring in one of four anatomical areas: outflow area of the uterus and vagina; the ovaries, the pituitary gland, or the central nervous system. Outflow area problems are obstructive in nature and can be found on physical examination, whereas ovarian, pituitary, and central nervous system problems involve disruptions in the hypothalamic–pituitary–ovarian axis that controls the neuroendocrine processes required for a normal menstrual cycle and are generally found through laboratory analysis (King et al., 2015).

Etiology

Primary amenorrhea has multiple causes:

- Extreme weight gain or loss
- Congenital abnormalities of the reproductive system

- Stress from a major life event
- Excessive exercise
- Eating disorders (anorexia nervosa or bulimia)
- Cushing disease
- Polycystic ovary syndrome
- Hypothyroidism
- Turner syndrome—defective development of the gonads (ovary or testes)
- Imperforate hymen
- Chronic illness—diabetes, thyroid disease, depression
- Pregnancy
- Cystic fibrosis
- Congenital heart disease (cyanotic)
- Ovarian or adrenal tumors

Causes of secondary amenorrhea can include:

- Pregnancy
- Breast-feeding
- Emotional stress
- Pituitary, ovarian, or adrenal tumors
- Depression
- Hyperthyroid or hypothyroid conditions
- Malnutrition
- Hyperprolactinemia
- Rapid weight gain or loss
- Chemotherapy or radiation therapy to the pelvic area
- Vigorous exercise, such as long-distance running
- Kidney failure
- Colitis
- Chemotherapy, irradiation
- Use of tranquilizers or antidepressants
- Postpartum pituitary necrosis (Sheehan syndrome)
- Early menopause (Kovanci & Schutt, 2015).

Therapeutic Management

Therapeutic intervention depends on the cause of the amenorrhea. The treatment of primary amenorrhea involves the correction of any underlying disorders and estrogen replacement therapy to stimulate the development of secondary sexual characteristics (Moses, 2015a). If a pituitary tumor is the cause, it might be treated with drug therapy, surgical resection, or radiation therapy. Surgery might be needed to correct any structural abnormalities of the genital tract. Dopamine agonists are effective in treating hyperprolactinemia. In most cases, this treatment restores normal ovarian endocrine function and ovulation (Goswami, 2015). Therapeutic interventions for secondary amenorrhea can include:

- Cyclic progesterone, when the cause is anovulation, or **oral contraceptives** (OCs)
- Bromocriptine to treat hyperprolactinemia
- Nutritional counseling to address anorexia, bulimia, or obesity
- Gonadotropin-releasing hormone (GnRH), when the cause is hypothalamic failure
- Thyroid hormone replacement, when the cause is hypothyroidism (Creatsas & Creatsa, 2015).

Nursing Assessment

Nursing assessment for a young girl or a woman experiencing amenorrhea includes a thorough health history, physical examination, and several laboratory and diagnostic tests of selected hormone levels to help to identify an underlying cause.

HEALTH HISTORY AND PHYSICAL EXAMINATION

A thorough history and physical examination are needed to determine the etiology. The history should include questions about the women's menstrual history; past illnesses; hospitalizations and surgeries; obstetric history; use of prescription and over-the-counter drugs; recent or past lifestyle changes; and history of present illness, with an assessment of anybody changes.

The physical examination should begin with an overall assessment of the woman's nutritional status and general health. A sensitive and gentle approach to the pelvic examination is critical in young women. Height, weight, and body mass index (BMI) should be taken, along with vital signs. Hypothermia, bradycardia, hypotension, and reduced subcutaneous fat may be observed in women with anorexia nervosa. Facial hair and acne might be evidence of androgen excess secondary to a tumor. The presence or absence of axillary and pubic hair may indicate adrenal and ovarian hyposecretion or delayed puberty. A general physical examination may uncover unexpected findings that are indirectly related to amenorrhea. For example, hepatosplenomegaly, which may suggest a chronic systemic disease or an enlarged thyroid gland, might point to a thyroid disorder as well as a reason for amenorrhea (Tharpe, Farley, & Jordan, et al., 2016). Examination of the breasts also deserves careful attention because breast development is a reliable indicator of estrogen production. The Tanner stages of breast development should be noted also. The Tanner stages include:

- Stage I—Papilla elevation only
- Stage II—Breast buds palpable and areolae enlarge ~11 years old
- Stage III—Elevation of breast contour; areolae enlarge ~12 years old
- Stage IV—Areolae forms secondary mound on the breast ~13 years old
- Stage V—Adult breast contour; areola recesses to breast contour (Moses, 2015b)

Information gained from the history and physical examination clearly can exclude certain diagnostic possibilities, but first impressions also can be deceiving and lead to errors in judgment. A methodical, systematic approach to identify the etiology of amenorrhea is best.

LABORATORY AND DIAGNOSTIC TESTS

Common laboratory tests that might be ordered to determine the cause of amenorrhea include:

- Karyotype (might be positive for Turner syndrome)
- Ultrasound to detect ovarian cysts
- Quantitative human chorionic gonadotropin (hCG) test to rule out pregnancy
- Thyroid function studies to determine thyroid disorder
- Prolactin level (an elevated level might indicate a pituitary tumor)
- Follicle-stimulating hormone (FSH) level (an elevated level might indicate ovarian failure)
- Luteinizing hormone (LH) level (an elevated level might indicate gonadal dysfunction)
- 17-ketosteroids (an elevated level might indicate an adrenal tumor) (Pagana, Pagana, & Pagana, 2015).

Nursing Management

Counseling and education are primary interventions and appropriate nursing roles. Address the diverse causes of amenorrhea, the relationship to sexual identity, possible infertility, and the possibility of a tumor or a life-threatening disease. Evidence is mounting that loss of menstrual regularity is a risk factor for later development of osteoporosis and hip fractures, so treatment to restore regular menstrual cycles is essential (Carlson, 2015). In addition, inform the woman about the purpose of each diagnostic test, how it is performed, and when the results will be available to discuss with her. Listening sensitively, interviewing, and presenting treatment options are paramount to gain the woman's cooperation and understanding.

Nutritional counseling is also vital in managing this disorder, especially if the woman has findings suggestive of an eating disorder. The relation between eating disorders and menstrual dysfunction has been identified in research studies. Careful evaluation of menstrual status is warranted for all women with eating disorders. Timely intervention is important because shorter duration of illness is associated with improved outcomes (Golden, Katzman, Sawyer, et al., 2015). Although not all causes can be addressed by making lifestyle changes, emphasize maintaining a healthy lifestyle (Teaching Guidelines 4.2).

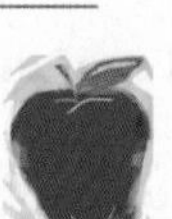

Teaching Guidelines 4.2

TIPS FOR MAINTAINING A HEALTHY LIFESTYLE

- Balance energy expenditure with energy intake to maintain ideal weight range.
- Modify your diet to maintain ideal weight to avoid becoming over weight.
- Avoid excessive use of alcohol and mood-altering or sedative drugs.
- Avoid cigarette smoking to prevent cardiovascular disease and lung cancer.
- Identify areas of emotional stress and seek assistance to resolve them.
- Balance work, recreation, and rest to reduce anxiety and stress in life.
- Maintain a positive outlook regarding the diagnosis and prognosis.
- Participate in ongoing care to monitor any medical conditions.
- Maintain bone density through:
  - Calcium intake (1,200 to 1,600 mg daily)
  - Vitamin D (600 to 1,000 International Units/daily)
  - Weight-bearing exercise (30 min or more daily)
  - Hormone therapy for low risk women

Adapted from Centers for Disease Control and Prevention [CDC] (2015a) *Healthy eating for a healthy weight.* Retrieved from http://www.cdc.gov/healthyweight/healthy_eating/; Housman, J., & Odum, M. (2016) *Alters & Schiff's essential concepts for healthy living* (7th ed.). Burlington, MA: Jones & Bartlett Learning.

Dysmenorrhea

Dysmenorrhea refers to painful menstruation and is a common problem in adolescence. This condition has also been termed *cyclic perimenstrual pain.* Usually pain starts along with the start of bleeding and lasts for 48 to 72 hours (Creatsas & Creatsa, 2015). The term *dysmenorrhea* is derived from the Greek words *dys,* meaning "difficult, painful, or abnormal," and *rrhea,* meaning "flow." Based on results of large epidemiological studies, it is estimated that it may affect more than half of menstruating women. It is the leading cause of absenteeism of work and school and has adverse effects on the quality of life of young women (Joshi, Kural, Agrawal, et al., 2015). Another recent research study linked early smoking (<13 years old) to an increased risk for developing chronic dysmenorrhea (Weinberger, Smith, Allen, et al., 2015). Uterine contractions occur during all periods, but in some women these cramps can be frequent and very intense. It has a major impact on women's quality of life, work productivity, and health care utilization. Dysmenorrhea is classified as primary (spasmodic) or secondary (congestive) (Calis, Popat, Dang, et al., 2015).

Etiology

Primary dysmenorrhea refers to painful menstrual bleedings in the absence of any detectable underlying pathology. It is caused by increased prostaglandin production by the endometrium in an ovulatory cycle. This hormone causes contraction of the uterus, and levels tend to be higher in women with severe menstrual pain than women who experience mild or no menstrual pain. Dysmenorrhea is caused by an excess of prostaglandin production.

These levels are highest during the first 2 days of menses, when symptoms peak (Maurice & Rosenzweig, 2015). This results in increased rhythmic uterine contractions from vasoconstriction of the small vessels of the uterine wall. This condition usually begins within a few years of the onset of ovulatory cycles at menarche.

Secondary dysmenorrhea is painful menstruation due to pelvic or uterine pathology. It may be caused by endometriosis, adenomyosis, fibroids, pelvic infection, an intrauterine system (IUS), cervical stenosis, or congenital uterine or vaginal abnormalities. Adenomyosis involves the ingrowth of the endometrium into the uterine musculature. Endometriosis involves ectopic implantation of endometrial tissue in other parts of the pelvis. It occurs most commonly in the third or fourth decades of life and affects 10% of women of reproductive age. The pain tends to get worse, rather than better, over time (American College of Obstetricians & Gynecologists [ACOG], 2015a). **Endometriosis** is the most common cause of secondary dysmenorrhea and is associated with pain beyond menstruation, dyspareunia, low back pain, heavy or irregular bleeding, bloating, nausea, and vomiting, and infertility (ACOG, 2015a). Treatment is directed toward removing the underlying pathology.

Think back to Izzy from the chapter opener. Is her pelvic pain complaint a common one with women?

Therapeutic Management

The goal of treatment is to provide adequate pain relief to allow the woman to perform her usual activities. Current treatment is mainly based on surgery and ovarian suppressive agents (OCs, progestins, GnRh antagonist, levonorgestrel-releasing intrauterine system [LNG-IUS], and androgenic agents). Hormonal treatments are often associated with unwanted side effects and recurrence of symptoms when stopped. Severe dysmenorrhea can be distressing, adversely affecting social and occupational activities. Treatments vary from over-the-counter remedies to hormonal control. However, for some women satisfactory pain relief is difficult to achieve and increasingly, they seek alternative options. Complementary therapies such as acupuncture (needles are used to stimulate certain points of the body to balance the flow of energy within the body) and acupressure (the use of fingers and hands to stimulate acupoints and maintains the balance of energy) are gaining popularity and the evidence base for their use is growing (Wicks & Mahady, 2015).

Therapeutic intervention is directed toward pain relief and building coping strategies that will promote a productive lifestyle. General measures for management include client education and reassurance. Treatment is supportive and should be guided by individual needs. Treatment measures usually include treating infections if present; suppressing the endometrium if endometriosis is suspected by administering low-dose OCs; administering prostaglandin inhibitors to reduce the pain; administering Depo-Provera to suppress ovulation, which thins the endometrial lining of the uterus with subsequent reduction of fluid contents of the uterus during menses; and initiating lifestyle changes (Schuiling & Likis, 2016). Table 4.1 lists selected treatment options for dysmenorrhea.

Nursing Assessment

As with any gynecologic complaint, a thorough focused history and physical examination are needed to make the diagnosis of primary or secondary dysmenorrhea. In primary dysmenorrhea, the history usually reveals the typical cramping pain with menstruation, and the physical examination is completely normal. In secondary dysmenorrhea, the history discloses cramping pain starting after 25 years old with a pelvic abnormality, a history of infertility, heavy menstrual flow, irregular cycles, and little response to nonsteroidal anti-inflammatory drugs (NSAIDs), OCs, or both (Elnashar, 2015).

HEALTH HISTORY AND CLINICAL MANIFESTATIONS

Note past medical history, including any chronic illnesses and family history of gynecologic concerns. Determine medication and substance use, such as prescription medications, contraceptives, anabolic steroids, tobacco, and marijuana, cocaine, or other illegal drugs. A detailed sexual history is essential to assess for inflammation and scarring (adhesions) secondary to pelvic inflammatory disease (PID). Women with a previous history of PID, sexually transmitted infections (STIs), low consumption of fruits and vegetables, depression, high stress level, multiple sexual partners, or unprotected sex are at increased risk (Tharpe et al., 2016).

During the initial interview, the nurse might ask some of the following questions to assess the woman's history of dysmenorrhea:

- At what age did your menstrual cycles start?
- Have your cycles always been painful, or did the pain start recently?
- When in your cycle do you experience the pain?
- How would you describe the pain you feel?
- Are you sexually active?
- What impact does your cycle have on your physical and social activities?
- When was the first day of your last menstrual cycle?
- Was the flow of your last menstrual cycle a normal amount for you?
- Do your cycles tend to be heavy or last longer than 5 days?
- Are your cycles generally regular and predictable?

TABLE 4.1 TREATMENT OPTIONS FOR DYSMENORRHEA

Therapy Options	Dosage	Comments
Nonsteroidal anti-inflammatory drugs (NSAIDs)		NSAIDS prevent prostaglandin synthesis by inhibiting COX-1 and COX-2 conversion, reducing cramping
Ibuprofen (Advil, Motrin, Midol)	400–800 mg TID	Take with meals Do not take with aspirin
Naproxen (Anaprox, Naprelan, Naprosyn, Aleve)	250–500 mg TID	Avoid alcohol Watch for signs of GI bleeding Same as above
Hormonal contraceptives		Decrease prostaglandin synthesis; second-line treatment
Low-dose oral contraceptives	Taken daily—extended cycle formulas (84 days on, 7 days off)	Take active pills for an extended time to reduce number of monthly cycles
Depo-medroxyprogesterone (DMPA), Depo-Provera	150 mg IM every 12 wks	Within 9–12 mo of DMPA therapy, 75% of women will experience amenorrhea
Levonorgestrel-releasing IUS (Mirena)	Inserted into uterine cavity and may remain for up to 5 yrs	Inhibits ovulation and decreases thickness of endometrium Inhibits uterine contractions and reduces pain from menstrual cramps
Selective estrogen receptor modulators (SERMs)	Used for women not responding to NSAIDs and oral contraceptives; dosage is individualized	Adverse effects include hot flashes, nausea and vomiting, and risk of thromboembolism
Raloxifene hydrochloride (Evista); tamoxifen citrate (Nolvadex)		Research is needed to validate effectiveness, doses, side effects, and contradictions
Complementary therapies Thiamine (vitamin B) Vitamin E (tocopherols) Magnesium Omega-3 fatty acids (fish oil)		Gives sense of control over life
Lifestyle changes Daily exercise Limited salty foods Weight loss Smoking cessation Relaxation techniques		

Adapted from Calis, K. A., Popat, V., Dang, D. K., & Kalantaridou, S. N. (2015). Dysmenorrhea. *eMedicine.* Retrieved from http://emedicine.medscape.com/article/253812-overview; King, T. L., Brucker, M. C., Kriebs, J. M., Fahey, J. O., Gegor, C. L., & Varney, H. (2015) *Varney's midwifery* (5th ed.), Burlington, MA: Jones and Bartlett Learning; Schuiling, K. D. & Likis, F. E. (2016). *Women's gynecologic health.* (3rd ed.) Burlington, MA: Jones & Bartlett Learning.

- What have you done to relieve your discomfort? Is it effective?
- Has there been a progression of symptom severity?
- Do you have any other symptoms?

Assess for clinical manifestations of dysmenorrhea. Affected women experience sharp, intermittent spasms of pain, usually in the suprapubic area. Pain may radiate to the back of the legs or the lower back. Pain usually develops within hours of the start of menstruation and peaks as the flow becomes heaviest during the first day or second day of the cycle (King et al., 2015). Systemic symptoms of nausea, vomiting, diarrhea, fatigue, fever, headache, or dizziness are fairly common. Explore the history for physical symptoms of bloating, water retention, weight gain, headache, muscle aches, abdominal pain, food cravings, or breast tenderness.

PHYSICAL EXAMINATION

The physical examination performed by the health care provider centers on the bimanual pelvic examination. This examination is done during the nonmenstrual phase of the cycle. Explain to the woman how it is to be performed, especially if it is her first pelvic examination. Prepare the woman in the examining room by offering her a cover gown to put on and covering her lap with a privacy sheet on the examination table. Remain in the examining room throughout the examination to assist the health care provider with any procedures or specimens and to offer the woman reassurance.

LABORATORY AND DIAGNOSTIC TESTS

Common diagnostic tests that may be ordered to determine the cause of dysmenorrhea can include:

- Complete blood count to rule out anemia
- Urinalysis to rule out a bladder infection
- Pregnancy test (hCG level) to rule out pregnancy
- Cervical culture to exclude STI
- Erythrocyte sedimentation rate to detect an inflammatory process
- Stool guaiac test to exclude gastrointestinal bleeding or disorders
- Pelvic and/or vaginal ultrasound to detect pelvic masses or cysts
- Diagnostic laparoscopy and/or laparotomy to visualize pathology that may account for the symptoms (Tharpe et al., 2016).

What diagnostic tests might be ordered to diagnose Izzy's pelvic pain?

Nursing Management

Educating the client about the normal events of the menstrual cycle and the etiology of her pain is paramount in achieving a successful outcome. Explaining the normal menstrual cycle will teach the woman the correct terms to use so she can communicate her symptoms more accurately and will help dispel myths. Provide the woman with monthly graphs or charts to record menses, the onset of pain, the timing of medication, relief afforded, and coping strategies used. This involves the woman in her care and provides objective information so that therapy can be modified if necessary.

The nurse should explain in detail the dosing regimen and the side effects of the medication therapy selected. Commonly prescribed drugs include NSAIDs such as ibuprofen (Motrin, Advil) or naproxen (Naprosyn). These drugs alleviate dysmenorrhea symptoms by decreasing intrauterine pressure and inhibiting prostaglandin synthesis, thus reducing pain (Skidmore-Roth, 2015). The primary goal of NSAID therapy of dysmenorrhea is to preempt the production of prostaglandins; thus starting the medication prophylactically and using sufficient doses to maximally suppress prostaglandin production are essential. If pain relief is not achieved in two to four cycles, a low-dose combination OC may be initiated. Client teaching and counseling should include information about how to take pills, side effects, and danger signs to watch for.

Encourage the woman to apply a heating pad or warm compress to alleviate menstrual cramps. Additional lifestyle changes that the woman can make to restore some sense of control and active participation in her care are listed in Teaching Guidelines 4.3.

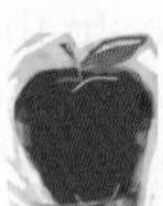

Teaching Guidelines 4.3

TIPS FOR MANAGING DYSMENORRHEA

- Exercise to increase endorphins and suppress prostaglandin release.
- Limit salty foods to prevent fluid retention.
- Increase water consumption to serve as a natural diuretic.
- Increase fiber intake with fruits and vegetables to prevent constipation.
- Use heating pads or warm baths to increase comfort.
- Take warm showers to promote relaxation.
- Sip on warm beverages, such as decaffeinated green tea.
- Keep legs elevated while lying down or lie on side with knees bent.
- Use stress management techniques to reduce emotional stress.
- Practice relaxation techniques to enhance ability to cope with pain.
- Stop smoking and decrease alcohol use which causes vasoconstriction

Adapted from Calis, K. A., Popat, V., Dang, D. K., and Kalantaridou, S. N. (2015). Dysmenorrhea. *EMedicine.* Retrieved from http://emedicine.medscape.com/article/253812-overview; Smith, R. P., & Kaunitz, A. M. (2015). Painful menstrual periods: Beyond the basics. *UpToDate,* Retrieved from http://www.uptodate.com/contents/painful-menstrual-periods-dysmenorrhea-beyond-the-basics; ACOG (2015d) *Dysmenorrhea: Painful periods.* FAQ046. Retrieved from www.acog.org/~/media/For Patients/faq046.ashx

Abnormal Uterine Bleeding

Disturbances of menstrual bleeding manifest in a wide range of presentations. *Abnormal uterine bleeding* is the umbrella term used to describe any deviation from normal menstruation or from a normal menstrual cycle pattern. It can occur in women of any age. The key characteristics are regularity, frequency, volume or heaviness of flow, and duration of flow, but each of these may exhibit considerable variability.

Abnormal uterine bleeding (AUB) is a disorder that occurs most frequently in women at the beginning and end of their reproductive years. AUB is defined as painless endometrial bleeding that is prolonged, excessive, and irregular and not attributed to any underlying structural or systemic disease (Creatsas & Creatsa, 2015). It is frequently associated with anovulatory cycles, which are common for the first year after menarche and is associated with immaturity of the hypothalamic–pituitary–ovarian axis. It also occurs later in life as women approach menopause and experience irregular menstrual cycles.

The pathophysiology of AUB is related to a hormone disturbance. With anovulation, estrogen levels rise as usual in the early phase of the menstrual cycle. In the absence of ovulation, a corpus luteum never forms and progesterone is not produced. The endometrium moves into a hyperproliferative state, ultimately outgrowing its estrogen supply. This leads to irregular sloughing of the endometrium and excessive bleeding (King et al., 2015). If the bleeding is heavy enough and frequent enough, anemia can result. AUB is similar to several other types of uterine bleeding disorders and sometimes overlaps these conditions. They include:

- Menorrhagia (abnormally long, heavy periods, prolonged bleeding)
- Oligomenorrhea (bleeding occurs at intervals of more than 35 days)
- Metrorrhagia (bleeding between periods, irregular bleeding)
- Menometrorrhagia (excessive uterine bleeding at and between menstrual periods)
- Polymenorrhea (too frequent periods)

Etiology

The possible causes of AUB may include:

- Adenomyosis
- Pregnancy
- Hormonal imbalance
- Fibroid tumors (see Chapter 7)
- Endometrial polyps or cancer
- Endometriosis
- IUSs
- Polycystic ovary syndrome
- Morbid obesity
- Adnomyosis
- Steroid therapy
- Hypothyroidism
- Blood dyscrasias/clotting disorder
- Malignancy and hyperplasia
- Uterine polyps

Therapeutic Management

Treatment of AUB depends on the cause of the bleeding, the age of the client, and whether or not she desires future fertility. When known, the underlying cause of the disorder is treated. Otherwise, the goal of treatment is to normalize the bleeding, correct the anemia, prevent or diagnose early cancer, and restore quality of life (Schuiling & Likis, 2016).

Treatment options for AUB include combined OCs, progestogens, NSAIDs, tranexamic acid (antifibrinolytic), GnRH analogs, Danazol, and LNG-IUS (Bitzer, Heikinheimo, Nelson, et al., 2015).

Management of AUB might include medical care with pharmacotherapy or insertion of a hormone-secreting intrauterine system. OCs are used for cycle regulation as well as for contraception. They help prevent the risks associated with prolonged, unopposed estrogen stimulation of the endometrium. NSAIDs and progestin therapy (progesterone-releasing IUS [Mirena] or Depo-Provera) significantly decrease menstrual blood loss (Skidmore-Roth, 2015). The drug categories used in the treatment of AUB are:

- *Estrogens:* cause vasospasm of the uterine arteries to decrease bleeding
- *Progestins:* used to stabilize an estrogen-primed endometrium
- *OCs:* regulate the cycle and suppress the endometrium
- *NSAIDs:* inhibit prostaglandins in ovulatory menstrual cycles
- *Progesterone-releasing IUSs:* suppress endometrial growth
- *Androgens:* create a high-androgen/low-estrogen environment that inhibits endometrial growth
- *Antifibrinolytic drugs:* (tranexamic acid) prevent fibrin degradation to reduce bleeding
- *Iron replacement therapy:* replenish iron stores lost during heavy bleeding

If the client does not respond to medical therapy, surgical intervention might include dilation and curettage (D&C), endometrial ablation, uterine artery embolization, or hysterectomy. Surgery should be considered in women for whom medical treatment has failed, cannot be tolerated, or is contraindicated (Kho & Mathur, 2015). Endometrial ablation is an alternative to hysterectomy, but both would be for the woman no longer desiring fertility as both procedures can cause infertility. Techniques used for ablation include laser, electrosurgery excision procedure, freezing, heated fluid infusion, or thermal balloon ablation. Most women will have reduced menstrual flow following endometrial ablation, and up to half will stop having periods. Younger women are less likely than older women to respond to endometrial ablation. Recent scientific evidence supports that up to one quarter of clients treated with endometrial ablation require repeat ablation or subsequent hysterectomy to stop AUB. Hysterectomy should be considered a last resort for AUB (ACOG, 2015b).

Nursing Assessment

A thorough history should be taken to differentiate between AUB and other conditions that might cause vaginal bleeding, such as pregnancy and pregnancy-related conditions (abruptio placentae, ectopic pregnancy, abortion, or placenta previa); systemic conditions such as Cushing disease, blood dyscrasias, liver disease, renal disease, or thyroid disease; and genital tract pathology such as infections, tumors, or trauma (Schuiling & Likis, 2016).

Assess for clinical manifestations of AUB, which commonly include vaginal bleeding between periods, irregular menstrual cycles (usually less than 28 days between cycles), infertility, mood swings, hot flashes, vaginal tenderness, variable menstrual flow ranging from scanty to profuse, obesity, acne, stress, anorexia, thyroid disease, and diabetes. Signs of polycystic ovary syndrome might be present, because it is associated with unopposed estrogen stimulation, elevated androgen levels, and insulin resistance and is a common cause of anovulation (Tharpe et al., 2016).

Measure orthostatic blood pressure and orthostatic pulse; a drop in pressure or pulse rate may occur with anemia. The health care provider, with the nurse assisting, performs a pelvic examination to identify any structural abnormalities.

Common diagnostic/lab tests that may be ordered to determine the cause of AUB include:

- Complete blood count to detect anemia
- Prothrombin time to detect blood dyscrasias
- Pregnancy test to rule out a spontaneous abortion or ectopic pregnancy
- Thyroid-stimulating hormone level to screen for hypothyroidism
- Transvaginal ultrasound to measure endometrium
- Pelvic ultrasound to view any structural abnormalities
- Endometrial biopsy to check for intrauterine pathology
- D&C for diagnostic evaluation

Nursing Management

Educate the client about normal menstrual cycles and the possible reasons for her abnormal pattern. Inform the woman about treatment options. Do not simply encourage the woman to "live with it." Instruct the client about any prescribed medications and potential side effects. For example, if high-dose estrogens are prescribed, the woman may experience nausea. Teach her to take antiemetics as prescribed and encourage her to eat small, frequent meals to alleviate nausea. Adequate follow-up and evaluation are essential for women who do not respond to medical management. See Nursing Care Plan 4.1: Overview of a Woman with Abnormal Uterine Bleeding (at the end of chapter).

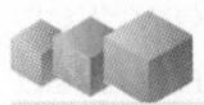

Concept Mastery Alert

Treatments for Premenstrual Syndrome

Possible treatment options for PMS include reduction of caffeine intake, vitamin and mineral supplements, diuretic therapy, and NSAIDs. Medication therapies that have been found to be helpful for clients with PMS are antidepressants and anxiolytics. Other medications that are used are diuretics and NSAIDs.

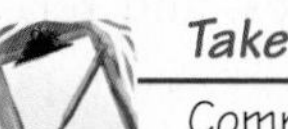

Take Note!

Complications such as infertility can result from lack of ovulation, severe anemia can result secondary to prolonged or heavy menses, depression and embarrassment may be secondary to the irregular and heavy bleeding, and endometrial cancer can occur associated with prolonged buildup of the endometrial lining without menstrual bleeding (Hoyt & Falconi, 2015).

Premenstrual Syndrome

Premenstrual syndrome (PMS) describes a constellation of recurrent symptoms that occur during the luteal phase or last half of the menstrual cycle and resolve with the onset of menstruation. A majority of women in their reproductive years experience a variety of premenstrual symptoms that can alter their behavior and well-being. Women have between 400 and 500 menstrual cycles over their reproductive years, and since premenstrual distress symptoms peak during 4 to 7 days prior to menses, consistently symptomatic women may spend up to 10 years of their lives in a state of compromised physical functioning and/or psychological well-being; thus it would constitute a major health problem for women (Tacani, Ribeiro, Barros Guimarães, et al., 2015). ACOG defines PMS as "the cyclic occurrence of symptoms that are sufficiently severe to interfere with some aspects of life, and that appear with consistent and predictable relationship to menses" (ACOG, 2015c). A woman experiencing PMS may have a wide variety of seemingly unrelated symptoms; for that reason, it is difficult to define and more challenging to diagnose. PMS affects millions of women during their reproductive years. Approximately 80% of women will experience cyclic fluctuations in mood, sleep, and sense of well-being, related to their menstrual cycles (King et al., 2015). The exact cause of PMS is not known. It is thought to be related to the interaction between hormonal events and neurotransmitter function, specifically serotonin. Not all women respond to serotonin reuptake inhibitors (SSRIs; Prozac, Paxil, Zoloft), however, which implies that other mechanisms may be involved (Skidmore-Roth, 2015).

As defined by the American Psychiatric Association, PMDD is a more severe variant of PMS affecting 5 to 8% of premenopausal women. Experts compare the difference between PMS and PMDD to the difference between a mild tension headache and a migraine. Risk factors identified that predispose to PMS/PMDD are age between 25 and 35 years, a psychiatric history, a family history of PMDD, unhealthy living habits, and stressful life events (Santamaria & Lago, 2015). PMDD markedly interferes with work, school, social activities, and relationships with others.

BOX 4.2

TREATMENT OPTIONS FOR PMS AND PMDD

- Lifestyle changes
  - Reduce stress.
  - Exercise three to five times each week.
  - Eat a balanced diet and increase water intake.
  - Decrease caffeine intake.
  - Stop smoking and limit the intake of alcohol.
  - Attend a PMS/women's support group.
- Vitamin and mineral supplements
  - Multivitamin daily
  - Vitamin E, 400 units daily
  - Calcium, 1,200 to 1600 mg daily
  - Magnesium, 200 to 400 mg daily
- Medications
  - NSAIDs taken a week prior to menses
  - Oral contraceptives (low dose)
  - Antidepressants (SSRIs)
  - Anxiolytics (taken during luteal phase)
  - Diuretics to remove excess fluid
  - Progestins
  - Gonadotropin-releasing hormone (GnRH) agonists
  - Danazol (androgen hormone inhibits estrogen production)

Adapted from Walsh, S., Ismaili, E., Naheed, B., et al. (2015). Diagnosis, pathophysiology and management of premenstrual syndrome. *The Obstetrician & Gynaecologist*. doi:10.1111/tog.12180; King, T. L., Brucker, M. C., Kriebs, J. M., Fahey, J. O., Gegor, C. L., & Varney, H. (2015) *Varney's midwifery* (5th ed.). Burlington, MA: Jones & Bartlett Learning; Htay, T. T., and Aung, K. (2015). Premenstrual dysphoric disorder. *eMedicine*. Retrieved from http://emedicine.medscape.com/article/293257-overview

Therapeutic Management

Treatment of PMS is often frustrating for both clients and health care providers. Clinical outcomes can be expected to improve as a result of recent consensus on the diagnostic criteria for PMS and PMDD, data from clinical trials, and the availability of evidence-based clinical guidelines.

The management of PMS or PMDD requires a multidimensional approach because these conditions are not likely to have a single cause, and they appear to affect multiple systems within a woman's body; therefore, they are not likely to be amenable to treatment with a single therapy (Naeimi, 2015). To reduce the negative impact of premenstrual disorders on a woman's life education, along with reassurance and anticipatory guidance, is needed for women to feel they have some control over their condition.

Take Note!

Because there are no diagnostic tests that can reliably determine the existence of PMS or PMDD, the woman herself must decide that she needs help during this time of the month. The woman must embrace multiple therapies and become an active participant in her treatment plan to find the best level of symptom relief.

Therapeutic interventions for PMS and PMDD address the symptoms because the exact cause of this condition is still unknown. Treatments may include vitamin supplements, diet changes, exercise, lifestyle changes, and medications (Box 4.2). Medications used in treating PMDD may include antidepressant and antianxiety drugs, diuretics, anti-inflammatory medications, analgesics, synthetic androgen agents, OCs, or GnRH agonists to regulate menses. Unlike the approach to the treatment of depression, antidepressants need not be given daily but can be effective when used cyclically, only in the luteal phase, or even limited to the duration of the monthly symptoms.

COMPLEMENTARY AND ALTERNATIVE THERAPIES

No single treatment is universally recognized as effective, and many clients often turn to therapeutic approaches outside of conventional medicine. Many women use dietary supplements and herbal remedies for their menstrual health and treating their bleeding disorders, although there has been little research to demonstrate their efficacy. Alternative treatments for treating PMDD include calcium supplementation, vitex agnus castus (chaste tree berry), hypericum perforatum (St John's wort), and cognitive/behavioral/relaxation therapies (Wicks & Mahady, 2015). Some other alternative therapies include the use of yoga, magnesium, vitamin B_6, evening primrose oil, vitex agnus castus, ginkgo biloba, viburnum, dandelion, stinging nettle, burdock, raspberry leaf, and skullcap (Tremellen & Pearce, 2015). Although research has not validated the efficacy of these alternative therapies, it is important for the nurse to be aware of the alternative products that many women choose to use.

Nursing Assessment

Although little consensus exists in the medical literature and among researchers about what constitutes PMS and PMDD, the physical and psychological symptoms are very real. The extent to which the symptoms debilitate or incapacitate a woman is highly variable.

More than 150 symptoms are assigned to PMS, but irritability, food cravings, mood swings, tearfulness, depression, sleep disturbances, headache, back pain, fatigue, bloating, edema of the face, abdominal area, and extremities, tension, and dysphoria (a profound state of unease and anxiety) are the most prominent and consistently described (Tacani et al., 2015). To establish the diagnosis of PMS, elicit a description of cyclic symptoms occurring before the woman's menstrual period. The woman should chart her symptoms daily for two cycles. These data will help demonstrate symptoms clustering around the luteal phase of ovulation, with resolution after bleeding starts. Ask the woman to bring her list of symptoms to the next appointment. Symptoms can be categorized using the following:

- **A**—*anxiety:* difficulty sleeping, tenseness, mood swings, and clumsiness
- **C**—*craving:* cravings for sweets, salty foods, chocolate
- **D**—*depression:* feelings of low self-esteem, anger, easily upset
- **H**—*hydration:* weight gain, abdominal bloating, breast tenderness
- **O**—*other:* hot flashes or cold sweats, nausea, change in bowel habits, aches or pains, dysmenorrhea, acne breakout (Naeimi, 2015).

The ACOG diagnostic criteria for PMS consist of having at least one of the following affective and somatic symptoms during the 5 days before menses in each of the three previous cycles:

- Affective symptoms: depression, angry outbursts, irritability, anxiety
- Somatic symptoms: breast tenderness, abdominal bloating, edema, headache
- Symptoms relieved from days 4 to 13 of the menstrual cycle (ACOG, 2015c).

In PMDD, the main symptoms are mood disorders such as depression, anxiety, tension, and persistent anger or irritability. Physical symptoms such as headache, joint and muscle pain, lack of energy, bloating, and breast tenderness are also present (Htay, 2015). It is estimated that up to 75% of reproductive-age women experience premenstrual symptoms that meet the ACOG criteria for PMS and up to 5% meet the diagnostic criteria for PMDD (Pearlstein, 2015).

According to the American Psychiatric Association, a woman must have at least five of the typical symptoms to be diagnosed with PMDD (Pearlstein, 2015). These must occur during the week before and a few days after the onset of menstruation and must include one or more of the first four symptoms:

- Affective lability: sadness, tearfulness, irritability
- Anxiety and tension
- Persistent or marked anger or irritability
- Depressed mood, feelings of hopelessness
- Difficulty concentrating
- Sleep difficulties
- Increased or decreased appetite
- Increased or decreased sexual desire
- Chronic fatigue
- Headache
- Constipation or diarrhea
- Breast swelling and tenderness (Htay, 2015).

Nursing Management

Educate the client about the management of PMS or PMDD. Advise her that lifestyle changes often result in significant symptom improvement without pharmacotherapy. Encourage women to eat a balanced diet that includes nutrient-rich foods to avoid hypoglycemia and associated mood swings. Encourage all women to participate in aerobic exercise three times a week to promote a sense of well-being, decrease fatigue, and reduce stress. Administer calcium (1,200 to 1,600 mg/day), magnesium (400 to 800 mg/day), and vitamin B_6 (50 to 100 mg/day) as prescribed. In some studies, these nutrients have been shown to decrease the intensity of PMS symptoms. NSAIDs may be useful for painful physical symptoms and spironolactone (Aldactone) may help with bloating and water retention. Herbs such as vitex agnus castus (chaste tree berry), evening primrose, and SAM-e (a dietary supplement used to enhance mood) may be recommended; although not harmful, not all herbs have enough clinical or research evidence to document their safety or efficacy. Nutritional treatments include a diet low in salt, alcohol, caffeine, and sugar (Schuiling & Likis, 2016).

A recent research study proposes calcium (1,600 mg/day) and vitamin D (400 International Units/day) supplementation in adolescents and women in an effort to prevent PMS, but further research using a larger population needs to be conducted to validate this (Santamaria & Lago, 2015).

Explain to your client the relationship between cyclic estrogen fluctuation and changes in levels of serotonin levels, and how the different management strategies help maintain serotonin levels, thus improving symptoms. It is important to rule out other conditions that might cause erratic or dysphoric behavior. If the initial treatment regimen does not work, explain to

EVIDENCE-BASED PRACTICE 4.1

THE EFFECT OF WHEAT GERM EXTRACT ON PREMENSTRUAL SYNDROME SYMPTOMS

STUDY

Premenstrual syndrome is one of the most common disorders in women and impairs work and social relationships. Several treatment modalities have been proposed including herbal medicines. Herbal medicines are among the most common treatments because they are economical, safe, noninvasive, and have fewer side effects than do traditional medicines. Wheat germ contains magnesium, zinc, calcium, selenium, potassium, phosphorus, chromium, and vitamins A, E, C, B12, B6, Niacin, folic acid. Considering the properties of wheat germ, this study aimed to determine the effects of wheat germ extract on the symptoms of premenstrual syndrome.

Findings

This triple blind clinical trial was conducted on 84 women that completed daily records regarding their symptoms for two consecutive months while taking 400 mg capsules of wheat germ extract or placebo three times a day from day 16 until day 5 of the next menstrual cycle. The study found that wheat germ significantly reduced the severity of physical symptoms (64%), psychological symptoms (66%), and general symptoms (65%) when compared to the placebo group within the first month of treatment. No complications were observed in either group.

Nursing Implications

Based on the study results, it seems that using wheat germ extract reduces the severity of general, psychological, and physical symptoms of premenstrual syndrome in women that take it during their midcycle. Given the positive effects of taking B6 and E, calcium, and magnesium in previous studies to reduce the symptoms of PMS, it makes sense that wheat germ which contains all of the compounds listed would help relieve PMS symptoms. Nurses can suggest using nontraditional modalities to women that request them and cite this study's results to validate them.

Adapted from Ataollahi, M., Akbari, S. A., Mojab, F., & Alavi Majd, H. (2015). The effect of wheat germ extract on premenstrual syndrome symptoms. *Iranian Journal of Pharmaceutical Research: IJPR, 14*(1), 159–166.

the woman that she should return for further testing. Behavioral counseling and stress management might help women regain control during these stressful periods. Reassuring the woman that support and help are available through many community resources/support groups can be instrumental in her acceptance of this monthly disorder. Nurses can be a very calming force for many women experiencing PMS or PMDD. A holistic approach, including lifestyle modifications, pharmacotherapy, herbal therapies, and cognitive behavioral therapy, is most beneficial for symptom reduction, improvement in daily functioning, and quality of life. See Evidence-Based Practice 4.1.

Take Note!

Adolescents and women who experience more extensive emotional symptoms with PMS should be evaluated for PMDD, because they may require antidepressant therapy.

Endometriosis

Endometriosis is one of the most common gynecologic diseases, affecting more than 6 million women in the United States, about 10% of the adult women population (Kapoor, Alderman, Hiraoka, et al., 2015). In this condition, for unknown reasons bits of functioning endometrial tissue are located outside of their normal site, the uterine cavity. This endometrial tissue is commonly found attached to the ovaries, fallopian tubes, the outer surface of the uterus, the bowels, the area between the vagina and the rectum (rectovaginal septum), and the pelvic side wall (Fig. 4.1). The places where the tissue attaches are called implants, or lesions. Endometrial tissue found outside the uterus responds to hormones released during the menstrual cycle in the same way as endometrial lining within the uterus.

At the beginning of the menstrual cycle, when the lining of the uterus is shed and menstrual bleeding begins, these abnormally located implants swell and bleed also. In short, the woman with endometriosis experiences several "mini-periods" throughout her abdomen, wherever this endometrial tissue exists. In addition to cyclic bleeding outside the uterus, scarring and adhesion formation throughout the pelvis occur. Symptoms begin as early as adolescence and typically settle after menopause.

Think back to Izzy, with her progressive pelvic pain and infertility concerns. After a pelvic examination, her health care provider suspects she has endometriosis.

Etiology and Risk Factors

It is not currently known why endometrial tissue becomes transplanted and grows in other parts of the body. Several theories exist, but to date none has been scientifically proven. However, several factors that increase a

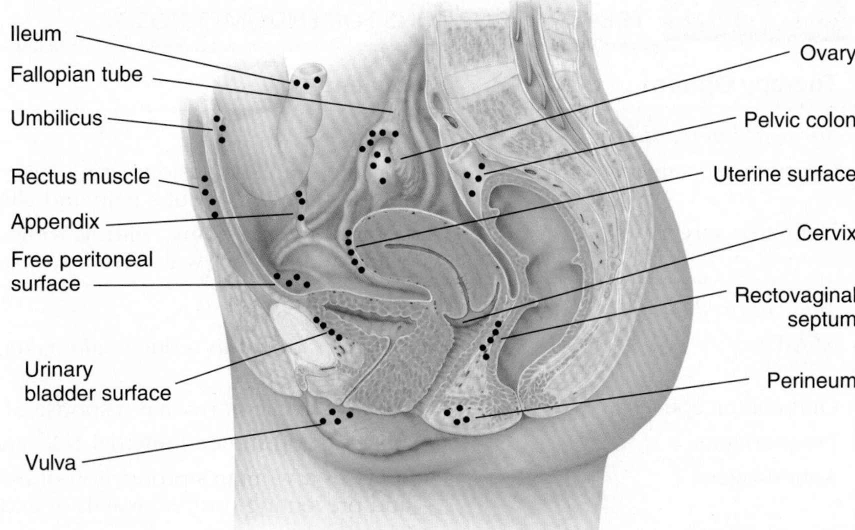

FIGURE 4.1 Common sites of endometriosis formation. (Asset provided by Anatomical Chart Co.)

woman's risk of developing endometriosis have been identified:

- The aging process
- Family history of endometriosis in a first-degree relative
- Short menstrual cycle (less than 28 days)
- Long menstrual flow (more than 1 week)
- High dietary fat consumption
- Young age of menarche (younger than 12)
- Few (one or two) or no pregnancies (Johnston, Reid, & Hunter, 2015).

Therapeutic Management

Therapeutic management of the client with endometriosis needs to take into consideration the following factors: severity of symptoms, desire for fertility, degree of disease, and the client's therapy goals. The aim of therapy is to suppress levels of estrogen and progesterone, which cause the endometrium to grow. Current treatment of endometriosis is mainly based on surgery and ovarian suppressive agents (OCs, progestins, GnRh agonists, and androgenic agents). Approximately only half of women with endometriosis experience pain relief from existing medial or surgical treatments (NICHD, 2015). Treatment can include surgical removal of ectopic endometrial tissue or medications such as NSAIDs, OCs, Depo-Provera, synthetic testosterone, GnRH agonists. Also, alternative therapies may be used, including acupuncture and supplements of vitamins, minerals, and fish oil (Elnashar, 2015). These interventions may control symptoms initially, but many have significant adverse effects and limits on duration of therapy (Table 4.2).

Nursing Assessment

Nurses encounter women with endometriosis in a variety of settings: community health settings, schools, clinics, day surgical centers, and hospitals. Health care professionals must not trivialize or dismiss the concerns of these women, because early recognition is essential to preserve fertility. The diversity of presenting symptoms and a low index of suspicion contribute to women with endometriosis falling through the cracks and not being diagnosed promptly.

HEALTH HISTORY

Obtain a health history and elicit a description of signs and symptoms to determine risk factors. Endometriosis is often asymptomatic, but it can be a severe and debilitating condition. It typically is chronic and progressive. Ask specifically about menarche, history of menstrual problems, details of pregnancies, and difficulties with conception. Assess the client for clinical manifestations, which include:

- Infertility
- Back pain
- Pain before and during menstrual periods
- Pain during or after sexual intercourse
- Painful urination
- Depression
- Fatigue
- Painful bowel movements
- Chronic pelvic pain
- Hypermenorrhea (heavy menses)
- Pelvic adhesions
- Irregular and more frequent menses
- Premenstrual vaginal spotting (Schuiling & Likis, 2016)

The two most common symptoms are infertility and pelvic pain. Endometriosis occurs in 38% of infertile women and in 71% to 87% of women with chronic pelvic pain (Kapoor et al., 2015). About 30% to 40% of women with this condition are infertile, making it one of the top three causes of female infertility (Brown & Farquhar, 2015).

TABLE 4.2 TREATMENT OPTIONS FOR ENDOMETRIOSIS

Therapy Options	Comment
Surgical intervention	
Conservative surgery	Removal of implants/lesions using laser, cautery, or small surgical instruments. This intervention will reduce pain and allows pregnancy to occur in the future
Definitive surgery	Abdominal hysterectomy, with or without bilateral salpingo-oophorectomy. Will eliminate pain but will leave a woman unable to become pregnant in the future
Medication therapy	
NSAIDs	First-line treatment to reduce pain; taken early when premenstrual symptoms are first felt
Oral contraceptives	Suppresses cyclic hormonal response of the endometrial tissue
Progestogens	Used to cast off the endometrial cells and thus destroy them
Antiestrogens	Suppresses a woman's production of estrogen, thus stopping the menstrual cycle and preventing further growth of endometrium
Gonadotropin-releasing hormone analogs (GnRH-a)	Suppresses endometriosis by creating a temporary pseudomenopause

Adapted from Kapoor, D. W., Alderman, E., Hiraoka, M. K., & Davila, G.W. (2015). Endometriosis. *eMedicine.* Retrieved from http://emedicine.medscape.com/article/271899-overview; Elnashar, A. (2015). Emerging treatment of endometriosis. *Middle East Fertility Society Journal.* doi:10.1016/j.mefs.2014.12.002. Retrieved from http://www.sciencedirect.com/science/article/pii/S1110569014200562; King, T. L., Brucker, M. C., Kriebs, J. M., Fahey, J. O., Gegor, C. L., & Varney, H. (2015) *Varney's midwifery* (5th ed.), Burlington, MA: Jones and Bartlett Learning.

What are the two most common symptoms experienced by women with endometriosis? Is Izzy's profile typical? As a nurse, what would be your role in Izzy's continued workup?

PHYSICAL EXAMINATION AND LABORATORY AND DIAGNOSTIC TESTS

The pelvic examination typically correlates with the extent of the endometriosis. The usual finding is nonspecific pelvic tenderness. The hallmark finding is the presence of tender nodular masses on the uterosacral ligaments, the posterior uterus, or the posterior cul-de-sac. The only definitive diagnosis is one made during surgery (Signorile & Baldi, 2015).

After a thorough history and a pelvic examination, the health care provider may suspect endometriosis, but the only certain method of diagnosing it is by seeing it. Pelvic or transvaginal ultrasound is used to assess pelvic organ structures. However, a laparoscopy is needed to diagnose endometriosis. Laparoscopy is the direct visualization of the internal organs with a lighted instrument inserted through an abdominal incision. A tissue biopsy of the suspected implant taken at the same time and examined microscopically confirms the diagnosis.

Nurses can play a role by offering a thorough explanation of the condition and explaining why tests are needed to diagnose endometriosis. The nurse can set up appointments for imaging studies and laparoscopy.

Nursing Management

In addition to the interventions outlined above, the nurse should encourage the client to adopt healthy lifestyle habits with respect to diet, exercise, sleep, and stress management. Referrals to support groups and Internet resources can help the woman to understand this condition and to cope with chronic pain. A number of organizations provide information about the diagnosis and treatment of endometriosis and offer support to women and their families. Nurses are uniquely situated to improve client outcomes by assisting women to make informed treatment decisions. A prompt diagnosis ensures appropriate care (Box 4.3).

INFERTILITY

Infertility is defined as the inability to conceive a child after 1 year of regular sexual intercourse unprotected by contraception (RESOLVE, 2015). Secondary infertility is the inability to conceive after a previous pregnancy. Many people take the ability to conceive and produce a child for granted, but infertility affects more than 6 million Americans, or up to 20% of the reproductive-age population and as many 186 million people worldwide, according to the American Society for Reproductive Medicine (ASRM, 2015). Infertility is a widespread problem that has an emotional, social, and economic impact on couples. Although male infertility contributes to more than half of all causes, infertility remains a woman's social burden. It affects relationships, leads to

BOX 4.3

ORGANIZATIONS AND WEB RESOURCES TO ASSIST THE CLIENT WITH ENDOMETRIOSIS

- American College of Obstetricians and Gynecologists (ACOG)
  http://www.acog.org
  e-mail: resources@acog.org
- American Society of Reproductive Medicine
  http://www.asrm.org
  e-mail: asrm@asrm.org
- Center for Endometriosis Care
  http://www.centerforendo.com
- Endometriosis Association
  http://www.endometriosisassn.org
  http://www.KillerCramps.org
- Endometriosis Association support groups
  e-mail: support@endometriosisassn.org
- National Institute of Child Health and Human Development Information Resource Center
  http://www.nichd.nih.gov
  e-mail: NICHDClearinghouse@mail.nih.gov
- National Women's Health Information Center (U.S. Department of Health and Human Services)
  http://www.4women.gov

tension and anger between partners, and can result in severe sexual dysfunction and breakdown of the relationship. Nurses must recognize infertility and understand its causes and treatment options so that they can help couples understand the possibilities as well as the limitations of current therapies. Nurses have a central role in supporting couples through these stressful treatments. Couples will frequently confide in their nurse and can gain great benefit from a sympathetic and sensible discussion. Recent studies have found that women wish to be treated with respect and dignity and given appropriate information and support. Infertility was once considered a disorder of inconvenience, but it is now classified as a disease in the United States regulatory Americans with Disabilities Act (Turchi, 2015). Women want their distress recognized and they want to feel cared for and to have confidence in health care providers in situations where outcomes are uncertain. The caring aspect of professional nursing is an essential component of meeting the special needs of these couples (Whitman, 2015). Prevention of infertility through education should also be incorporated into any client–nurse interaction.

After completing several diagnostic tests, Izzy is diagnosed with endometriosis. She asks you about her chances of becoming pregnant and becoming pain-free. What treatment options would you explain to Izzy? What information can you give about her future childbearing ability?

Cultural Considerations

Infertility is not only a physiologic problem, but is one that can initiate a life crisis that is experienced with psychologic, familial, social, and cultural consequences. Cross-culturally, the expectation for couples to reproduce is an accepted norm and the inability to conceive may be considered a violation of this cultural norm. In this context, infertility represents a crisis for the couple. The manner in which different cultures, ethnic groups, and religious groups perceive and manage infertility may be very different. For example, many African Americans believe that assisted reproductive techniques are unnatural and that they remove the spiritual or divine nature of creation from conception. For this reason, they may seek spiritual rather than medical assistance when trying to conceive. The Hispanic culture believes that children validate the marriage, so families are typically large. Like the African-American culture, Hispanics are very spiritual and may consider infertility a test of faith and seek spiritual counseling. Disappointing one's spouse is of greater concern to African-American women, whereas avoiding the stigmatization of infertility is of greatest concern to Asian-American women (Inhorn & Patrizio, 2015).

Religion often influences cultural factors and for this reason may also be considered when pursuing treatment for infertility. In the Orthodox Jewish religion procreation is considered to be a "mitzvah," a commandment to have children. However, even Orthodox Jews accept the use of contraceptives to prevent conception when it is not desired. Conservative and Reform Jews put no restrictions on contraception (McFarland & Wehbe-Alamah, 2015). Roman Catholics have a very restrictive view on the use of assisted reproductive technologies since in their view procreation cannot be separated from the relationship between parents. Thus, God wants human life to begin through the "conjugal act" and not artificially. Most religious teachings speak to the significance of procreation, thus infertility can impact the self and relational identities of the couple wishing to become parents. Therefore, the risk is present for both a crisis of identity and of faith (Dombo & Flood, 2015). Nurses must be cognizant of the client's cultural and religious background and how it may dictate which, if any, reproductive treatment options are chosen. Nurses need to include this awareness in their counseling of infertile couples.

Etiology and Risk Factors

Reproduction requires the interaction of the female and the male reproductive tracts, which involves (1) the release of a normal preovulatory oocyte, (2) the production of adequate spermatozoa, (3) the normal transport of the gametes to the ampullary portion of the fallopian tube (where fertilization takes place), and (4) the

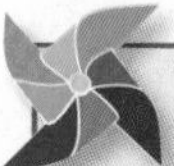

Consider This

We had been married for 3 years and wanted to start a family, but much to our dismay nothing happened after a year of trying. I had some irregular periods and was finally diagnosed with endometriosis and put on Clomid for three cycles. After that time without achieving a pregnancy, I went to a fertility expert. The doctor lasered the misplaced endometriosis tissue, sent carbon dioxide through my tubes to make sure they were patent, and put me back on Clomid, but still with no luck. Finally, 2 years later, we were put on an in vitro fertilization (IVF) waiting list and prayed we would have the money for the procedure when we were chosen. By then I felt a failure as a woman. We then decided that it was more important for us to be parents than it was for me to be pregnant, so we considered adoption. We tried for another year without any results.

We went to the adoption agency to fill out the paperwork for the process to begin. Our blood was taken and we waited for an hour, wondering the whole time why it was taking so long for the results. The nurse finally appeared and handed a piece of paper to me with the word "positive" written on it. I started to cry tears of joy, for a pregnancy had started and our long journey of infertility was finally ending.

Thoughts: For many women the dream of having a child is not easily realized. Infertility can affect self-esteem, disrupt relationships, and result in depression. This couple experienced many years of frustration in trying to have a family. What help can be offered to couples during this time? What can be said to comfort the woman who feels she is a failure?

subsequent transport of the cleaving embryo into the endometrial cavity for implantation and development (Puscheck & Woodward, 2015).

Multiple known and unknown factors affect fertility. Female-factor infertility is detected in about 40% of cases, male-factor infertility in about 40% of cases. The remaining 20% fall into a category of combined (both male and female factors) or unexplained infertility. In women, ovarian dysfunction (40%) and tubal/pelvic pathology (40%) are the primary contributing factors to infertility (ASRM, 2015).

Risk factors for infertility in women include:

- Overweight or underweight (can disrupt hormone function)
- Hormonal imbalances leading to irregular ovulation
- Uterine fibroids
- Tubal blockages
- Cervical stenosis
- Reduced oocyte quality
- Chromosomal abnormalities
- Congenital anomalies of the uterus
- Immune system disorders
- Chronic illnesses such as diabetes, thyroid disease, asthma
- STIs
- Ectopic pregnancy
- Age older than 27
- Endometriosis
- Turner syndrome
- Eating disorders
- History of PID
- Smoking and alcohol consumption
- Multiple miscarriages
- Menstrual abnormalities
- Exposure to chemotherapeutic agents
- Psychological stress (Senie, 2014)

Risk factors for infertility in men include:

- Exposure to toxic substances (lead, mercury, x-rays, chemotherapy)
- Cigarette or marijuana smoke
- Heavy alcohol consumption
- Use of prescription drugs for ulcers or psoriasis
- Exposure of the genitals to high temperatures (hot tubs or saunas)
- Hernia repair
- Obesity is associated with decreased sperm quality
- Cushing syndrome
- Frequent long-distance cycling or running
- STIs
- Undescended testicles (cryptorchidism)
- Mumps after puberty (Puscheck & Woodward, 2015)

Therapeutic Management

As noted earlier, the main causes of infertility are female factor (anovulation, tubal damage, endometriosis, and ovarian failure), male factor (low or absent numbers of motile sperm in the ejaculate, and erectile dysfunction), or unexplained infertility (Jin, 2015). The test results are presented to the couple and different treatment options are suggested. The majority of infertility cases are treated with drugs or surgery. Treatment options include lifestyle changes, such as weight loss, and smoking cessation; taking clomiphene to promote ovulation; hormone injections to promote ovulation; intrauterine insemination; and IVF. Various ovulation-enhancement drugs and timed intercourse might be used for the woman with ovulation problems. The woman should understand a drug's benefits and side effects before consenting to take it. Depending on the type of drug used and the dosage, some women may experience multiple births. If the woman's reproductive organs are damaged, surgery can be done to repair them. Still other couples might opt for the hi-tech approaches of artificial insemination (Fig. 4.2), IVF (Fig. 4.3), and egg donation or they may contract for

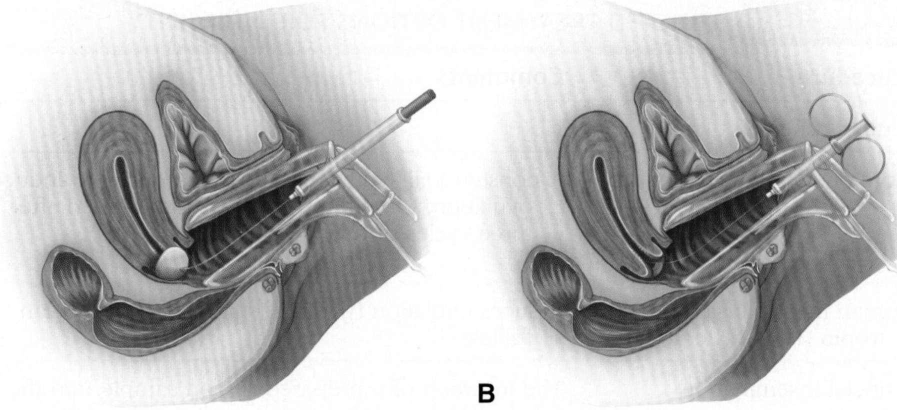

FIGURE 4.2 Artificial insemination. Sperm are deposited next to the cervix (**A**) or injected directly into the uterine cavity (**B**).

a gestational carrier or surrogate (Jin, 2015). Table 4.3 lists selected treatment options for infertility.

Nursing Assessment

Infertile couples are under tremendous pressure and often keep the problem a secret, considering it to be very personal. Couples are often beset by feelings of inadequacy and guilt, and many are subject to pressures from both family and friends. As the problem becomes more chronic, they may begin to blame one another, with consequent marital discord. Seeking help is often a very difficult step for them, and it may take a lot of courage to discuss something about which they feel deeply embarrassed or upset. The nurse working in this specialty setting must be aware of the conflict and problems couples present with and must be very sensitive to their needs.

A full medical history should be taken from both partners, along with a physical examination. The data needed for the infertility evaluation are very sensitive and of a personal nature, so the nurse must use very professional interviewing skills.

Infertility has numerous causes and contributing factors, so it is important to use the process of elimination, determining what problems do not exist to better comprehend the problems that do exist. At the first visit, a plan of investigation is outlined and a complete health history is taken. This first visit forces many couples to confront the reality that their desired pregnancy may not occur naturally. Alleviate some of the anxiety associated with diagnostic testing by explaining the timing and reasons for each test.

Assessing Male Factors

The initial screening evaluation for the male partner should include a reproductive history and a semen analysis. From the male perspective, three things must happen for conception to take place: the number of sperm must be adequate; those sperm must be healthy and mature; and the sperm must be able to penetrate and fertilize the egg. Normal males have more than 20 million sperm per milliliter with greater than 50% motility (World Health Organization [WHO], 2015). Semen analysis is the most

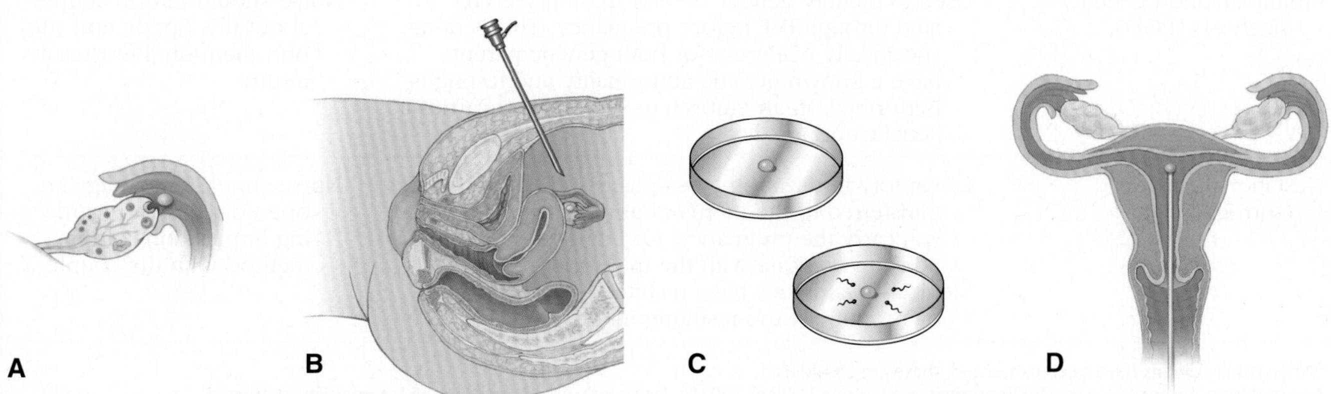

FIGURE 4.3 Steps involved in in vitro fertilization. **A.** Ovulation. **B.** Capture of the ova (done here intra-abdominally). **C.** Fertilization of ova and growth in culture medium. **D.** Insertion of fertilized ova into uterus.

TABLE 4.3 SELECTED TREATMENT OPTIONS FOR INFERTILITY

Procedure	Comments	Nursing Considerations
Fertility drugs		
Clomiphene citrate (Clomid)	A nonsteroidal synthetic antiestrogen used to induce ovulation. Clomid is typically discontinued after three cycles of use	Nurse can advise the couple to have intercourse every other day for 1 wk starting after day 5 of medication
Human menopausal gonadotropin (HMG); Pergonal	Induces ovulation by direct stimulation of ovarian follicle	Same as above
Artificial insemination	The insertion of a prepared semen sample into the cervical os or intrauterine cavity Enables sperm to be deposited closer to improve chances of conception. Husband or donor sperm can be used	Nurse needs to advise couple that the procedure might need to be repeated if not successful the first time
Assisted reproductive technologies[a]		
In vitro fertilization (IVF)	Oocytes are fertilized in the lab and transferred to the uterus Usually indicated for tubal obstruction, endometriosis, pelvic adhesions, and low sperm counts	Nurse advises woman to take medication to stimulate ovulation so the mature ovum can be retrieved by needle aspiration
Gamete intrafallopian transfer (GIFT)	Oocytes and sperm are combined and immediately placed in the fallopian tube so fertilization can occur naturally Requires laparoscopy and general anesthesia, which increases risk	Nurse needs to inform couple of risks and have consent signed
Intracytoplasmic sperm injection (ICSI)	One sperm is injected into the cytoplasm of the oocyte to fertilize it. Indicated for male factor infertility	Nurse needs to inform the male that sperm will be aspirated by a needle through the skin into the epididymis
Donor oocytes or sperm	Eggs or sperm are retrieved from a donor and the eggs are inseminated; resulting embryos are transferred via IVF Recommended for women older than 40 yrs and those with poor-quality eggs	Nurse needs to support couple in their ethical/religious discussions prior to deciding
Preimplantation genetic diagnosis (PGD)	Used to identify genetic defects in embryos created through IVF before pregnancy. This is done specifically when one or both genetic parents have a known genetic abnormality and testing is performed on an embryo to see if it also carries a genetic abnormality	Nurse should inform couple about this option and support them until test results return
Gestational carrier (surrogacy)	Laboratory fertilization takes place and embryos are transferred to the uterus of another woman, who will carry the pregnancy. Or intrauterine insemination can be done with the male sperm Medical–legal issues have resulted over the "true ownership" of the resulting infant	Nurse should encourage an open discussion regarding implications of this method with the couple

[a]When other options have been exhausted, these are considered.

Adapted from American Society for Reproductive Medicine [ASRM]. (2015). Frequently asked questions about infertility. Retrieved from http://www.asrm.org/detail.aspx?id=2322; Jin, J. (2015). Treatments for infertility. *JAMA, 313*(3), 320–320; Puscheck, E. E., & Woodward, T. L. (2015). Infertility. *eMedicine.* Retrieved from http://emedicine.medscape.com/article/274143-overview

important indicator of male fertility. The man should abstain from sexual activity for 24 to 48 hours before giving the sample. For a semen examination, the man is asked to produce a specimen by ejaculating into a specimen container and delivering it to the laboratory for analysis within 1 to 2 hours. When the specimen is brought to the laboratory, it is analyzed for volume, viscosity, number of sperm, sperm viability, motility, and sperm shape. If semen parameters are normal, no further male evaluation is necessary (Puscheck & Woodward, 2015).

A recent study shows that social strain and stress are highest among couples without a clear etiology for their infertility. These findings highlight the clinically significant negative sexual, personal, and social strains of a perceived infertility diagnosis for men (Cavallini, 2015). Nurses need to be very cognizant of this impact on males and address it.

The physical examination routinely includes:

- Assessment for appropriate male sexual characteristics, such as body hair distribution, development of the Adam's apple, and muscle development
- Examination of the penis, scrotum, testicles, epididymis, and vas deferens for abnormalities (e.g., nodules, irregularities, varicocele)
- Assessment for normal development of external genitalia (small testicles)
- Performance of a digital internal examination of the prostate to check for tenderness or swelling (Dohle, 2015)

Assessing Female Factors

The initial assessment of the woman should include a thorough history of factors associated with ovulation and the pelvic organs. Diagnostic tests to determine female infertility may include:

- Assessment of ovarian function
- Ovulation predictor kits used midcycle
- Urinary LH level
- Clomiphene citrate challenge test
- Assessment of pelvic organs
- Papanicolaou (Pap) smear to rule out cervical cancer or inflammation
- Cervical culture to rule out any STIs
- Ultrasound to assess pelvic structures
- Hysterosalpingography to visualize structural defects
- Laparoscopy to visualize pelvic structures and diagnose endometriosis (Dadhich, Ramasamy, & Lipshultz, 2015)

Laboratory and Diagnostic Testing

The diagnostic procedures that should be done during an infertility workup should be guided by the couple's history. They generally proceed from less to more invasive tests.

HOME OVULATION PREDICTOR KITS

Home ovulation predictor kits contain monoclonal antibodies specific for LH and use the ELISA test to determine the amount of LH present in the urine. A significant color change from baseline indicates the LH surge and presumably the most fertile day of the month for the woman.

CLOMIPHENE CITRATE CHALLENGE TEST

The clomiphene citrate challenge test is used to assess a woman's ovarian reserve (ability of her eggs to become fertilized). FSH levels are drawn on cycle day 3 and on cycle day 10 after the woman has taken 100 mg clomiphene citrate on cycle days 5 through 9. If the FSH level is greater than 15, the result is considered abnormal and the likelihood of conception with her own eggs is very low (Schuiling & Likis, 2016).

HYSTEROSALPINGOGRAPHY

Hysterosalpingography is the gold standard in assessing patency (being open and unobstructed) of the fallopian tubes. Fallopian tube obstruction is among the most common causes of female factor infertility. Ultrasonography and magnetic resonance imaging (MRI) are used in this assessment. In hysterosalpingography, 3 to 10 mL of an opaque contrast medium is slowly injected through a catheter into the endocervical canal so that the uterus and tubes can be visualized during fluoroscopy and radiography. If the fallopian tubes are patent, the dye will ascend upward to distend the uterus and the tubes and will spill out into the peritoneal cavity (Hemingway & Trew, 2015) (Fig. 4.4).

LAPAROSCOPY

A laparoscopy is usually performed early in the menstrual cycle. It is not part of the routine infertility evaluation. It is used when abnormalities are found on the ultrasound or the hysterosalpingogram. Because of the added risks of surgery, the need for anesthesia, and operative costs, it is only used when clearly indicated. During the procedure, an endoscope is inserted through

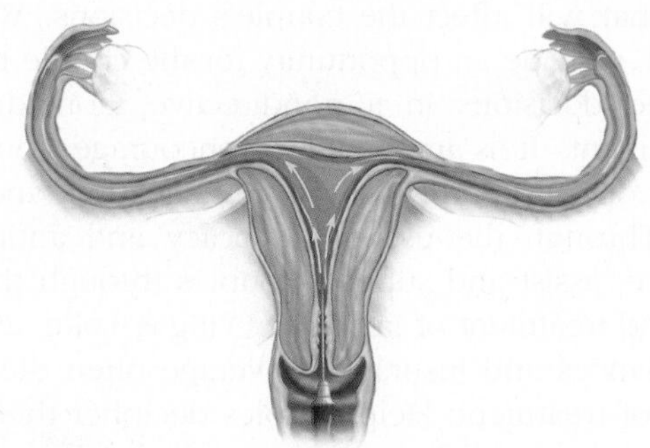

FIGURE 4.4 Insertion of a dye for a hysterosalpingogram. The contrast dye outlines the uterus and fallopian tubes on an x-ray to demonstrate patency.

a small incision in the anterior abdominal wall. Visualization of the peritoneal cavity in an infertile woman may reveal endometriosis, pelvic adhesions, tubal occlusion, fibroids, or polycystic ovaries (Kodaman, 2015).

Nursing Management

Nurses play an important role in the care of infertile couples. They are pivotal educators about preventive health care. A number of potentially modifiable risk factors are associated with the development of impaired fertility in women, and women need to be aware of these risks to institute change. The nurse is most effective when he or she offers care and treatment in a professional manner and regards the couple as valued and respected individuals. The nurse must be respectful of and mindful that many women may seek spiritual help for their infertility issues in addition to traditional medical modalities (King et al., 2015). The nurse's focus must encompass the whole person, not just the results of the various infertility studies. Throughout the entire process, the nurse's role is to provide information, anticipatory guidance, stress management, and counseling. The couple's emotional distress is usually very high, and the nurse must be able to recognize that anxiety and provide emotional support. The nurse may need to refer couples to a reproductive endocrinologist or surgeon, depending on the problem identified.

There is no absolute way to prevent infertility per se because so many factors are involved in conception. Nurses can be instrumental in educating men and women about the factors that contribute to infertility. The nurse can also outline the risks and benefits of treatments so that the couple can make an informed decision. As couples struggle with infertility, they frequently turn to nurses for empathy, counseling, and support. By understanding the struggles and lived experiences of women and couples experiencing infertility, the nurse can tailor his/her approach to better meet their needs so that the pregnancy and birth experience of these women is healing, transformative, and positive.

With advances in genetics and reproductive medicine also come a myriad of ethical, social, and cultural issues that will affect the couple's decisions. With this in mind, provide an opportunity for the couple to make informed decisions in a nondirective, nonjudgmental environment. It is important to encourage couples to remain optimistic throughout investigation and treatment. Through the use of advocacy and anticipatory guidance, assist and support couples through the diagnosis and treatment of infertility (Ying & Loke, 2015).

Finances and insurance coverage often dictate the choice of treatment. Help couples decipher their insurance coverage and help them weigh the costs of various procedures by explaining what each will provide in terms of their infertility problems. Assisting them to make a priority list of diagnostic tests and potential treatment options will help the couple plan their financial strategy.

Many infertile couples are not prepared for the emotional roller coaster of grief and loss that accompanies infertility treatments. Financial concerns and coping as a couple are two major areas of stress when treatment is undertaken. During the course of what may be months or even years of infertility care, it is essential to develop a holistic approach to nursing care. Stress management and anxiety reduction need to be addressed, and referral to a peer support group such as RESOLVE might be in order (Box 4.4).

BOX 4.4

ORGANIZATIONS AND WEB RESOURCES TO ASSIST THE CLIENT WITH INFERTILITY

- RESOLVE: A nationwide network of chapters dedicated to providing education, advocacy, and support for men and women facing infertility. They provide a helpline, medical referral services, and a member-to-member contact system (http://www.resolve.org).
- American Society of Reproductive Medicine (ASRM): Provides fact sheets and other resources on infertility, treatments, insurance, and other issues (http://www.asrm.org).
- International Council on Infertility Information Dissemination (INCIID): Provides information about infertility, support forums, and a directory of infertility specialists (http://www.inciid.org).
- American Fertility Association: Offers education, referrals, research, support, and advocacy for couples dealing with infertility (http://www.americaninfertility.org).
- Bertarelli Foundation—The Human Face of Infertility: Aims to promote and improve understanding of infertility by offering resources (http://www.bertarelli.edu).
- International Consumer Support for Infertility: An international network engaged in advocacy on behalf of infertile couples via fact sheets and information (http://www.icsi.ws).

CONTRACEPTION

Contraception is any method that prevents conception or childbirth, including OCs, sterilization of the female, and the male condom, which are the most popular methods in the United States (Alan Guttmacher Institute, 2015a). Additional types of contraceptives are discussed later in this chapter.

In the United States, there are approximately 68 million women in their childbearing years (between the ages of 15 and 44), and throughout those years a variety of contraceptive methods may be used. Studies have shown that 98% of sexually active women in the United States admit to having used at least one form of contraception; however, despite widespread use of contraceptives, almost half of all pregnancies in the United States are unintended, accounting for a higher unintended pregnancy rate than any other Western county (Centers for Disease Control and Prevention [CDC], 2015a). As outlined in the United Nations Population Fund (UNFPA) *State of the World Population 2014 Report,* over 7 billion people inhabit the earth now and over 80 million people are added to the world each year, more than half of whom are unintended.

In addition to unwanted pregnancies, which can result in abortion, some contraceptives also help prevent transmission of STIs and human immunodeficiency virus (HIV). The UNFPA report also shows that about 50,000 people in the United States become infected with HIV every year. Much of this suffering could be prevented by access to and consistent use of safe, efficient, appropriate, modern contraception for everyone who wants it, as well as proper education regarding benefits and instructions for use (UNFPA, 2015). In addition, climate change (extreme temperature changes and rising ocean levels) will interact with population growth in ways that put additional stress on already weak health systems and will exacerbate vulnerability to the adverse health effects of climate change. The damage done to the environment by modern society is perhaps one of the most inequitable health risks of our time (UNFPA, 2015).

Today, the voluntary control of fertility is of vital importance to modern society. From a global perspective, countries currently face a crisis of rapid population growth that has begun to threaten human survival. At the present rate, the population of the world will double in 40 years; in several of the more socioeconomically disadvantaged countries, populations will double in less than 20 years (UNFPA, 2015).

Types of Contraceptive Methods

Contraceptive methods can be divided into four types: behavioral methods, barrier methods, hormonal methods, and permanent methods. Women must decide which method is appropriate for them to meet their changing contraceptive needs throughout their life cycles. Nurses can educate and assist women during this selection process. This part of the chapter will outline the most common birth control methods available.

In an era when many women wish to delay pregnancy and avoid STIs, choices are difficult. Numerous methods of contraception are available today, and many more will be offered in the near future. The ideal contraceptive method for many women would have the following characteristics: ease of use, safety, effectiveness, minimal side effects, "naturalness," nonhormonal method, and immediate reversibility (Samra-Latif & Wood, 2015). Currently, no one contraceptive method offers everything. Box 4.5 outlines the contraceptive methods available today. Table 4.4 provides a detailed summary of each type, including information on failure rates, advantages, disadvantages, STI protection, and danger signs.

(text continues on page 140)

HEALTHY PEOPLE 2020

Objective	Nursing Significance
FP-1 Increase the proportion of pregnancies that are intended.	Would reduce number of unplanned pregnancies and girls not finishing their education. This would in turn reduce the number of single parents on state financial assistance.
FP-2 Reduce the proportion of females experiencing pregnancy despite use of a reversible contraceptive method.	Awareness of contraceptive methods and accessibility brings about better compliance and prevention of unintended pregnancies.
FP-3 Increase the proportion of publicly funded family planning clinics that offer the full range of FDA-approved methods of contraception, including emergency contraception, on site.	Would increase accessibility to contraception and prevent unintended pregnancies.
FP-7 Increase the proportion of sexually active persons who received reproductive health services.	Accessibility of reproductive resources can offer pregnancy prevention and preventive education.

Healthy People objectives based on data from http://www.healthypeople.gov

BOX 4.5

OUTLINE OF CONTRACEPTIVE METHODS

Reversible Methods

- **Behavioral**
  - Abstinence
  - Fertility awareness–based methods
  - Withdrawal (coitus interruptus)
  - Lactational amenorrhea method (LAM)
- **Barrier**
  - Condom (male and female)
  - Diaphragm
  - Cervical cap
  - Sponge
- **Hormonal**
  - Oral contraceptive
  - Injectable contraceptive
  - Transdermal patch
  - Vaginal ring
  - Implantable contraceptive
  - Intrauterine contraceptive
  - Emergency contraceptive

Permanent Methods

- Tubal ligation or Essure for women
- Vasectomy for men

TABLE 4.4 SUMMARY OF CONTRACEPTIVE METHODS

Type	Description	Failure Rate	Pros	Cons	STI Protection	Danger Signs	Comments
Abstinence	Refrain from sexual activity	None	Costs nothing	Difficult to maintain	100%	None	Must be joint couple decision
Fertility awareness–based methods	Refrain from sex during fertile period	25%	No side effects; acceptable to most religious groups	High failure rate with incorrect use	None	None	Requires high level of couple commitment
Withdrawal (coitus interruptus)	Man withdraws before ejaculation	27%	Involves no devices and is always available	Requires considerable self-control by the man	None	None	Places woman in trusting and dependent role
Lactational amenorrhea method (LAM)	Uses lactational infertility for protection from pregnancy	1–2% chance of pregnancy in first 6 mo	No cost; not coitus linked	Temporary method; effective for only 6 mo after giving birth	None	None	Mother must breast-feed infant on demand without supplementation for 6 mo
Male condom	Thin sheath placed over an erect penis, blocking sperm	15%	Widely available; low cost; physiologically safe	Decreased sensation for man; interferes with sexual spontaneity; breakage risk	Provides protection against STIs	Latex allergy	Couple must be instructed on proper use of condom
Female condom	Polyurethane sheath inserted vaginally to block sperm	21%	Use controlled by woman; eliminates postcoital drainage of semen	Expensive for frequent use; cumbersome; noisy during sex act; for single use only	Provides protection against STIs	Allergy to polyurethane	Couple must be instructed on proper use of condom
Diaphragm with spermicide	Shallow latex cup with spring mechanism in its rim to hold it in place in the vagina	16%	Does not use hormone; considered medically safe; provides some protection against cervical cancer	Requires accurate fitting by health care professional; increase in UTIs	None	Allergy to latex, rubber, polyurethane, or spermicide Report symptoms of toxic shock syndrome May become dislodged in female superior position	Woman must be taught to insert and remove diaphragm correctly

Cervical cap with spermicide	Soft cup-shaped latex device that fits over base of cervix	24%	No use of hormones; provides continuous protection while in place	Requires accurate fitting by health care professional; odor may occur if left in too long	None	Irritation, allergic reaction; abnormal Pap test; risk of toxic shock syndrome	Instructions on insertion and removal must be understood by client
Sponge with spermicide	Disk-shaped polyurethane device containing a spermicide that is activated by wetting it with water	25%	Offers immediate and continuous protection for 24 hrs; OTC	Can fall out of vagina with voiding; is not form fitting in the vagina	None	Irritation, allergic reactions; toxic shock syndrome can occur if sponge left in too long	Caution woman not to leave sponge in beyond 24 hrs
Oral contraceptives (combination)	A pill that suppresses ovulation by combined action of estrogen and progestin	8%	Easy to use; high rate of effectiveness; protection against ovarian and endometrial cancer	User must remember to take pill daily; possible undesirable side effects; high cost for some women; prescription needed	None	Dizziness, nausea, mood changes, high blood pressure, blood clots, heart attacks, strokes	Each woman must be assessed thoroughly to make sure she is not a smoker and does not have a history of thromboembolic disease
Oral contraceptives (progestin-only minipills)	A pill containing only progestin that thickens cervical mucus to prevent sperm from penetrating	8%	No estrogen-related side effects; may be used by lactating women; may be used by women with history of thrombophlebitis	Must be taken with meticulous accuracy; may cause irregular bleeding; less effective than combination pills	None	Irregular bleeding, weight gain, increased incidence of ectopic pregnancy	Women should be screened for history of functional ovarian cysts, previous ectopic pregnancy, and hyperlipidemia prior to giving prescription
Patch (Ortho Evra)	Transdermal patch that releases estrogen and progestin into circulation	8%	Easy system to remember; very effective	May cause skin irritation where it is placed; may fall off and not be noticed and thus provide no protection	None	Less effective in women weighing more than 200 lb	Instruct woman to apply patch every week for 3 wks and then not to wear one during week 4

(continued)

TABLE 4.4 SUMMARY OF CONTRACEPTIVE METHODS (continued)

Type	Description	Failure Rate	Pros	Cons	STI Protection	Danger Signs	Comments
Ring (NuvaRing)	Vaginal contraceptive ring about 2 in in diameter that is inserted into the vagina; releases estrogen and progestin	8%	Easy system to remember; very effective	May cause a vaginal discharge; can be expelled without noticing and not offer protection	None	Similar to oral contraceptives	Instruct woman to use a backup method if ring is expelled and remains out for more than 3 hrs
Depo-Provera injection	An injectable progestin that inhibits ovulation	3%	Long duration of action (3 mo); highly effective; estrogen-free; may be used by smokers; can be used by lactating women	Menstrual irregularities; return visit needed every 12 wks; weight gain, headaches, depression; return to fertility delayed up to 12 mo	None	If depression is a problem, this method may increase the depression	Inform woman that fertility is delayed after stopping the injections
Implant (Nexplanon)	A time-release implant (one rod) of levonorgestrel for 3 yrs	0.05%	Long duration of action; low dose of hormones; reversible; estrogen-free	Irregular bleeding; weight gain; breast tenderness; headaches; difficulty in removal	None	If bleeding is heavy, anemia may occur	Before insertion, assess woman to make sure she is aware that this method will produce about 3 yrs of infertility
Intrauterine contraceptives (IUCs)	A T-shaped device inserted into the uterus that releases copper or progesterone or levonorgestrel	1%	It is immediately and highly effective; allows for sexual spontaneity; can be used during lactation; return to fertility not impaired; requires no motivation by the user after insertion	Insertion requires a skilled professional; menstrual irregularities; prolonged amenorrhea; can be unknowingly expelled; may increase the risk of pelvic infection; user must regularly check string for placement; no protection against STIs; delay of fertility after discontinuing for possibly 6–12 mo	None	Cramps, bleeding, pelvic inflammatory disease; infertility; perforation of the uterus	Instruct woman how to locate string to check monthly for placement

Postcoital emergency contraceptives (ECs)	Combination of levonorgestrel-only pills; combined estrogen and progestin pills; or the copper IUS inserted within 72 hrs after unprotected intercourse	80%	Provides a last chance to prevent a pregnancy	Risk of ectopic pregnancy if EC fails	None	Nausea, vomiting, abdominal pain, fatigue, headache	Inform woman that ECs do not interrupt an established pregnancy, and the sooner they are taken the more effective they are
Permanent sterilization							
Male	Sealing, tying, or cutting the vas deferens	<1%	One-time decision provides permanent sterility; short recovery time; low long-term risks	Procedures are difficult to reverse; initial cost may be high; chance of regret; some pain/discomfort after procedures	None for both	Postoperative complications: pain, bleeding, infection	Counsel both as to permanence of procedure and urge them to think it through prior to signing consent
Female	Fallopian tubes are blocked to prevent conception	<1%					

Adapted from Raymond, E. G., & Cleland, K. (2015). Emergency contraception. *New England Journal of Medicine, 372*(14), 1342–1348; King, T. L., Brucker, M. C., Kriebs, J. M., Fahey, J. O., Gegor, C. L., & Varney, H. (2015). *Varney's midwifery* (5th ed.). Burlington, MA: Jones & Bartlett Learning; Ilic, K. (2015). Emergency contraception. In *Medicines for Women* (pp. 203–225). Springer International Publishing; Samra-Latif, O. M., & Wood, E. (2015). Contraception. *eMedicine*. Retrieved from http://emedicine.medscape.com/article/258507-overview; Schuiling, K.D. & Likis, F.E. (2016). *Women's gynecologic health*. (3rd ed.). Burlington, MA: Jones & Bartlett Learning.

Sexual Abstinence

Sexual abstinence (not having vaginal or anal intercourse) is one of the least expensive forms of contraception and has been used for thousands of years. Basically, pregnancy cannot occur if sperm is kept out of the vagina. It also reduces the risk of contracting HIV/AIDS and other STIs, unless body fluids are exchanged through oral sex; however, some infections, like herpes and human papilloma virus (HPV), can be passed by skin-to-skin contact. Dental dams can be used to prevent transmission, however. There are many pleasurable options for sex play without intercourse ("outercourse"), such as kissing, masturbation, erotic massage, sexual fantasy, sex toys such as vibrators, and oral sex.

Many people have strong feelings about abstinence based on religious and moral beliefs. There are many good and personal reasons to choose abstinence. For some it is a way of life, whereas for others it is a temporary choice. Some people choose sexual abstinence because they want to:

- Wait until they are older
- Wait for a long-term relationship
- Avoid pregnancy or STIs
- Relieve feelings of depression or anxiety
- Follow religious or cultural expectations

Fertility Awareness–Based Methods

Fertility awareness refers to any natural contraceptive method that does not require hormones, pharmaceutical compounds, physical barriers, or surgery to prevent pregnancy. Fertility awareness–based methods (FAMs) use physical signs and symptoms that change with hormone fluctuations throughout a woman's menstrual cycle to predict a woman's fertility. Ovulation occurs on 1 day during each menstrual cycle, and the several days preceding ovulation are when intercourse is most likely to result in pregnancy. Collectively, the potentially fertile days up to and including the day of ovulation are called the "fertile window." Awareness of fertility is a better fertility-producing method than contraceptives. Less than 1% of women in the United States who use contraception employ these methods (King et al., 2015). The unifying theme of FAMs is that a woman can reduce her chance of pregnancy by abstaining from coitus or using barrier methods during times of fertility. These methods require couples to take an active role in preventing pregnancy through their sexual behaviors and women need to have regular menstrual cycles for it to be effective. Couples agree to practice certain techniques, use calculations, and be observant of the "fertile" and the "safe" periods in a monthly menstrual cycle. Using these methods for birth control requires a strong commitment from both partners. The normal physiologic changes caused by hormonal fluctuations during the menstrual cycle can be observed and charted. This information can then be used to avoid or promote pregnancy. Fertility awareness methods rely on the following assumptions:

- A single ovum is released from the ovary 14 days before the next menstrual period. It lives approximately 24 hours.
- Women using this method must have regular menstrual cycles for it to be effective.
- Sperm can live up to 5 days after intercourse. The "unsafe period" during the menstrual cycle is thus approximately 6 days: 3 days before and 3 days after ovulation. Because body changes start to occur before ovulation, the woman can become aware of them and not have intercourse on these days or use another method to prevent pregnancy.
- The exact time of ovulation cannot be determined, so 2 to 3 days are added to the beginning and end to avoid pregnancy.

Techniques used to determine fertility include the cervical mucus ovulation method, the basal body temperature (BBT) method, the symptothermal method, standard day's method, and two-day method (Everett, 2014). Fertility awareness methods are moderately effective but are very unforgiving if not carried out as prescribed. Fertility awareness can be used in combination with coital abstinence or barrier methods during fertile days if pregnancy is not desired.

CERVICAL MUCUS OVULATION METHOD

Cervical mucus is a jellylike vaginal discharge that comes from the cervix. The **cervical mucus ovulation method** is used to assess the character of the cervical mucus. Cervical mucus changes consistently during the menstrual cycle and plays a vital role in fertilization of the egg. Studies conducted by the WHO indicate that 93% of women, regardless of their education level, are capable of identifying and distinguishing fertile and infertile cervical secretions (Planned Parenthood, 2015a). In the days preceding ovulation, fertile cervical mucus helps draw sperm up and into the fallopian tubes, where fertilization usually takes place. It also helps maintain the survival of sperm. As ovulation approaches, the mucus becomes more abundant, clear, slippery, and smooth; it can be stretched between two fingers without breaking. Under the influence of estrogen, this mucus looks like egg whites. It is called *spinnbarkeit* mucus (Fig. 4.5). After ovulation, the cervical mucus becomes thick and dry under the influence of progesterone.

The cervical position can also be assessed to confirm changes in the cervical mucus at ovulation. Near ovulation, the cervix feels soft and is high/deep in the vagina, the os is slightly open, and the cervical mucus is copious

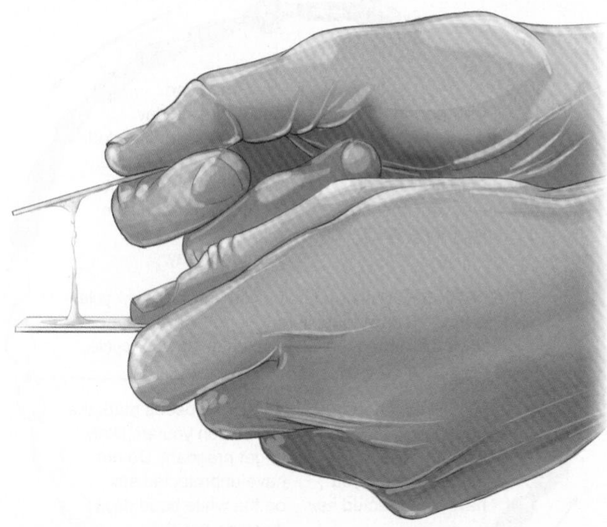

FIGURE 4.5 Spinnbarkeit mucus is cervical mucus that can stretch a distance before breaking.

and slippery (Bieber, Sanfilippo, Horowitz, et al., 2015). This method works because the woman becomes aware of her body changes that accompany ovulation. When she notices them, she abstains from sexual intercourse or uses another method to prevent pregnancy. Each woman is an individual, so each woman's unsafe time of the month is unique and thus must be individually assessed and determined.

BASAL BODY TEMPERATURE METHOD

The **basal body temperature** (BBT) refers to the lowest temperature reached on awakening. The woman takes her temperature orally before rising and records it on a chart. Preovulation temperatures are suppressed by estrogen, whereas postovulation temperatures are increased under the influence of heat-inducing progesterone. Temperatures typically rise within a day or two after ovulation and remain elevated for approximately 2 weeks (at which point bleeding usually begins). If using this method by itself, the woman should avoid unprotected intercourse until the BBT has been elevated for 3 days. Nurses should instruct women using the BBT method that it is important to keep in mind that illness and any drugs, including alcohol, can raise their body temperature and give a false reading. Other fertility awareness methods should be used along with BBT for better results (Fig. 4.6).

SYMPTOTHERMAL METHOD

The **symptothermal method** relies on a combination of techniques to recognize ovulation, including BBT, cervical mucus changes, alterations in the position and firmness of the cervix, and other symptoms of ovulation, such as increased libido, *mittelschmerz* (midcycle, lower abdominal pain at ovulation), pelvic fullness or

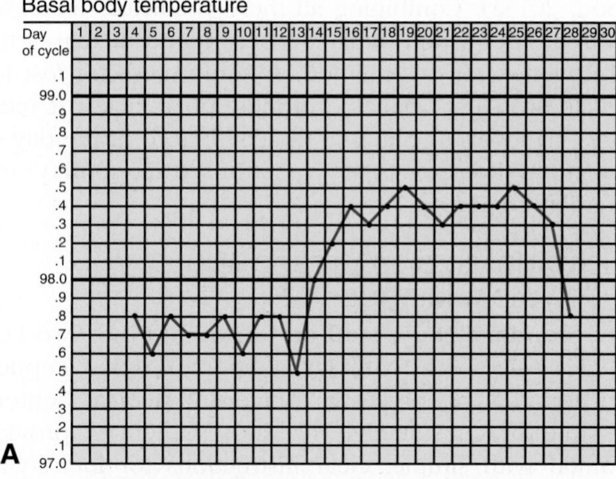

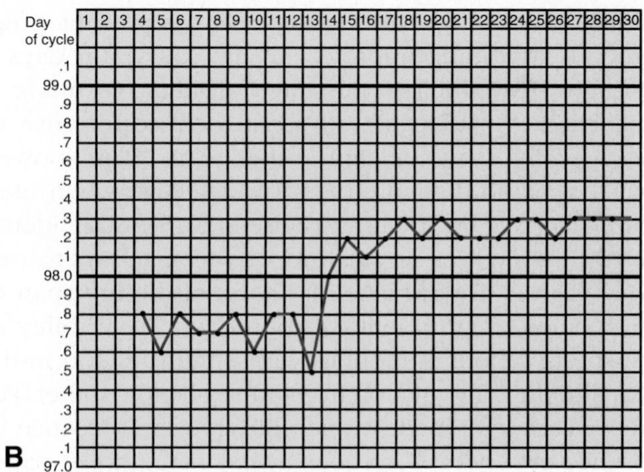

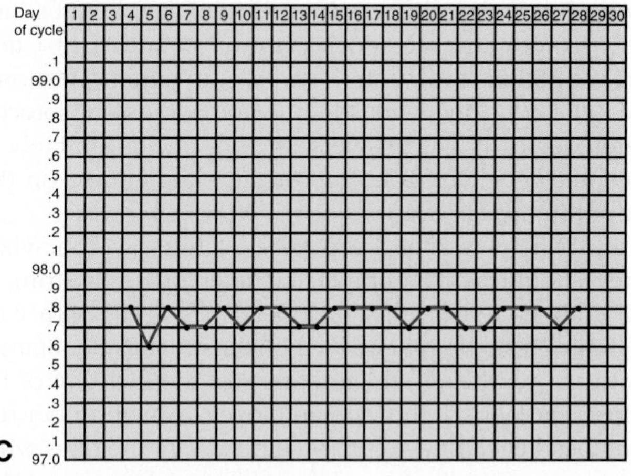

FIGURE 4.6 Basal body temperature graph. **A.** The woman's temperature dips slightly at midpoint in the menstrual cycle, then rises sharply, an indication of ovulation. Toward the end of the cycle (the 24th day), her temperature begins to decline, indicating that progesterone levels are falling and that she did not conceive. **B.** The woman's temperature rises at the midpoint in the cycle and remains at that elevated level past the time of her normal menstrual flow, suggesting that pregnancy has occurred. **C.** There is no preovulatory dip and no rise of temperature anywhere during the cycle. This is the typical pattern of a woman who does not ovulate.

tenderness, and breast tenderness (Planned Parenthood, 2015a). Combining all these predictors increases awareness of when ovulation occurs and increases the effectiveness of this method. A home predictor test for ovulation is also available in most pharmacies. It measures LH levels to pinpoint the day before or the day of ovulation. These tests are widely used for fertility and infertility regimens.

THE STANDARD DAYS METHOD AND THE TWO-DAY METHOD

The **Standard Days Method** (SDM) and the Two-Day Method are both natural methods of contraception developed by Georgetown University Medical Center's Institute for Reproductive Health. Both methods provide women with simple, clear instructions for identifying fertile days. Women with menstrual cycles between 26 and 32 days long can use the SDM to prevent pregnancy by avoiding unprotected intercourse on days 8 through 19 of their cycles. Most SDM users utilize a visual aid—CycleBeads—to assist their correct use of SDM. An international clinical trial of the SDM showed that the method is more than 95% effective when used correctly (Wright, Iqteit, & Hardee, 2015). SDM identifies the 12-day "fertile window" of a woman's menstrual cycle. These 12 days take into account the life span of the women's egg (about 24 hours) and the viability of the sperm (about 5 days) as well as the variation in the actual timing of ovulation from one cycle to another. For the Two-Day Method, women observe the presence or absence of cervical secretions by examining toilet paper or underwear or by monitoring their physical sensations. Every day, the woman asks two simple questions: "Did I note any secretions yesterday?" and "Did I note any secretions today?" If the answer to either question is yes, she considers herself fertile and avoids unprotected intercourse. If the answers are no, she is unlikely to become pregnant from unprotected intercourse on that day (King et al., 2015).

To help women keep track of the days on which they should avoid unprotected intercourse, a string of 32 color-coded beads (CycleBeads) is used, with each bead representing a day of the menstrual cycle. Starting with the red bead, which represents the first day of her menstrual period, the woman moves a small rubber ring one bead each day. The brown beads are the days when pregnancy is unlikely, and the white beads represent her fertile days (Stanford, 2015). This method has been used in underdeveloped countries for women with limited educational resources (Fig. 4.7).

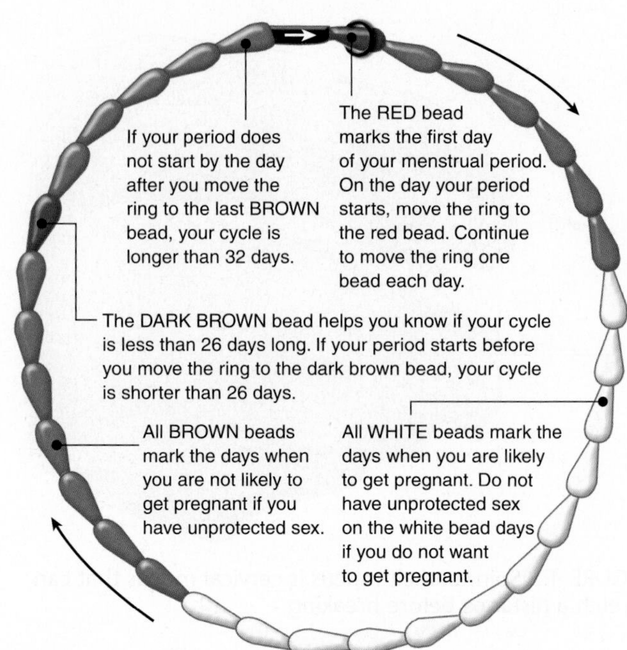

If your period does not start by the day after you move the ring to the last BROWN bead, your cycle is longer than 32 days.
The RED bead marks the first day of your menstrual period. On the day your period starts, move the ring to the red bead. Continue to move the ring one bead each day.
The DARK BROWN bead helps you know if your cycle is less than 26 days long. If your period starts before you move the ring to the dark brown bead, your cycle is shorter than 26 days.
All BROWN beads mark the days when you are not likely to get pregnant if you have unprotected sex.
All WHITE beads mark the days when you are likely to get pregnant. Do not have unprotected sex on the white bead days if you do not want to get pregnant.

FIGURE 4.7 CycleBeads help women use the Standard Days Method.

Withdrawal (Coitus Interruptus)

In **coitus interruptus**, also known as withdrawal, a man controls his ejaculation during sexual intercourse and ejaculates outside the vagina. It is better known colloquially as "pulling out in time" or "being careful." It is one of the oldest and most widely used means of preventing pregnancy in the world and also one of the least effective methods in preventing pregnancy (Creatsas, 2015). The problem with this method is that the first few drops of the true ejaculate contain the greatest concentration of sperm, and if some pre-ejaculatory fluid escapes from the urethra before orgasm, conception may result. This method requires that the woman rely solely on the cooperation and judgment of the man. Nurses might wish to discuss emergency contraceptives be available with this couple or use a more effective method of contraception.

Lactational Amenorrhea Method

The **lactational amenorrhea method** (LAM) is an effective temporary method of contraception used by breast-feeding mothers. It relies on physiologic changes associated with breast-feeding for contraception. Continuous breast-feeding usually can postpone ovulation and thus prevent pregnancy. Breast-feeding stimulates the hormone prolactin, which is necessary for milk production, and also inhibits the release of another hormone, gonadotropin, which is necessary for ovulation.

Breast-feeding as a contraceptive method can be fairly effective for up to 6 months after giving birth only if:

- A woman has not had a period since she gave birth
- Infant is younger than 6 months of age

- The woman breast-feeds her baby at least six times daily on both breasts
- She breast-feeds her baby "on demand" at least every 4 hours
- A woman does not substitute other foods for a breast-milk meal
- Nighttime feedings are provided at least every 6 hours

Also, pumping or manual expression of milk may reduce effectiveness, Do not rely on this method after 6 months (Planned Parenthood, 2015a).

Nurses can help couples to make a decision about family planning options available in the postpartum period by discussing the advantages and disadvantages of each, taking into consideration the demands of the postpartum period. The options they may consider include lactational amenorrhea, combined oral contraception, implants, intrauterine systems, injectable methods, barrier methods, emergency contraception (EC), and sterilization (Hughes, 2015).

Barrier Methods

Barrier contraceptives are forms of birth control that prevent pregnancy by preventing the sperm from reaching the ovum. Mechanical barriers include condoms, diaphragms, cervical caps, and sponges. These devices are placed over the penis or cervix to physically obstruct the passage of sperm through the cervix. Chemical barriers called spermicides may be used along with mechanical barrier devices. They come in creams, jellies, foam, suppositories, and vaginal films. They chemically destroy the sperm in the vagina. These contraceptives are called barrier methods because they not only provide a physical barrier for sperm, but also protect against STIs. Since the HIV/AIDS epidemic started in the early 1980s, these methods have become extremely popular. Progress has been made in society's reaction to condom use as a disease prevention device now and not just as a contraceptive (Haddad, Philpott-Jones, & Schonfeld, 2015).

Many of these barrier methods contain latex. Allergy to latex was first recognized in the late 1970s, and since then it has become a major health concern, with increasing numbers of people affected. According to the American Academy of Allergy, Asthma and Immunology (AAAAI) (2015), 6% of the general population, 10% of health care workers, and 50% of spina bifida clients are sensitive to natural rubber latex. Health care workers in both the medical and dental environments, as well as specific groups of individuals including those with spina bifida, myelodysplasia, and food allergies (banana, kiwi, avocado, and others), are at increased risk of sensitization (Kim, 2015). Teaching Guidelines 4.4 provides tips for individuals with latex allergy.

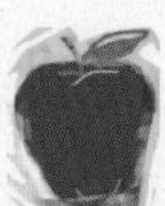

Teaching Guidelines 4.4
TIPS FOR INDIVIDUALS ALLERGIC TO LATEX

Symptoms of latex allergy include:

- Skin rash, itching, hives
- Itching or burning eyes
- Swollen mucous membranes in the genitals
- Shortness of breath, difficulty breathing, wheezing
- Anaphylactic shock
- Use of or contact with latex condoms, cervical caps, and diaphragms is contraindicated for men and women with a latex allergy
- If the female partner is allergic to latex, have the male partner apply a natural condom over the latex one
- If the male partner experiences penile irritation after condom use, try different brands or place the latex condom over a natural condom.
- Use polyurethane condoms rather than latex ones.
- Use female condoms; they are made of polyurethane.
- Switch to another birth control method that is not made with latex, such as oral contraceptives, intrauterine systems, Depo-Provera, fertility awareness, and other nonbarrier methods. However, these methods do not protect against sexually transmitted infections.

Adapted from American Academy of Allergy, Asthma and Immunology [AAAAI]. (2015). Latex allergy: Tips to remember. Retrieved from http://www.aaaai.org/conditions-and-treatments/library/allergy-library/latex-allergy.aspx; Kim, J. S. (2015). Latex allergy. In H. A. Sampson (Ed.), *Allergy and Clinical Immunology*, (pp. 288–293), Chichester, UK: John Wiley & Sons. doi:10.1002/9781118609125.ch32; Occupational Health and Safety Administration [OSHA]. (2015). *Latex allergy.* Retrieved from http://www.osha.gov/SLTC/latexallergy

CONDOMS

Condoms are barrier methods of contraceptives made for both males and females. The male condom is made from latex or polyurethane or natural membrane and may be coated with spermicide. Male condoms are available in many colors, textures, sizes, shapes, and thicknesses. When used correctly, the male condom is put on over an erect penis before it enters the vagina and is worn throughout sexual intercourse (Fig. 4.8). It serves as a barrier to pregnancy by trapping seminal fluid and sperm and offers protection against STIs. Condoms are not perfect barriers, however, because breakage and slippage can occur. Emergency postcoital contraception may need to be sought to prevent a pregnancy. In addition, the nonlatex condoms have a higher risk of pregnancy and STIs than latex condoms (Everett, 2014).

The female condom is a polyurethane pouch inserted into the vagina. It consists of an outer and inner ring that is inserted vaginally and held in place by the pubic bone. Some women complain that the female condom is cumbersome to use and makes noise during intercourse. Female condoms are readily available,

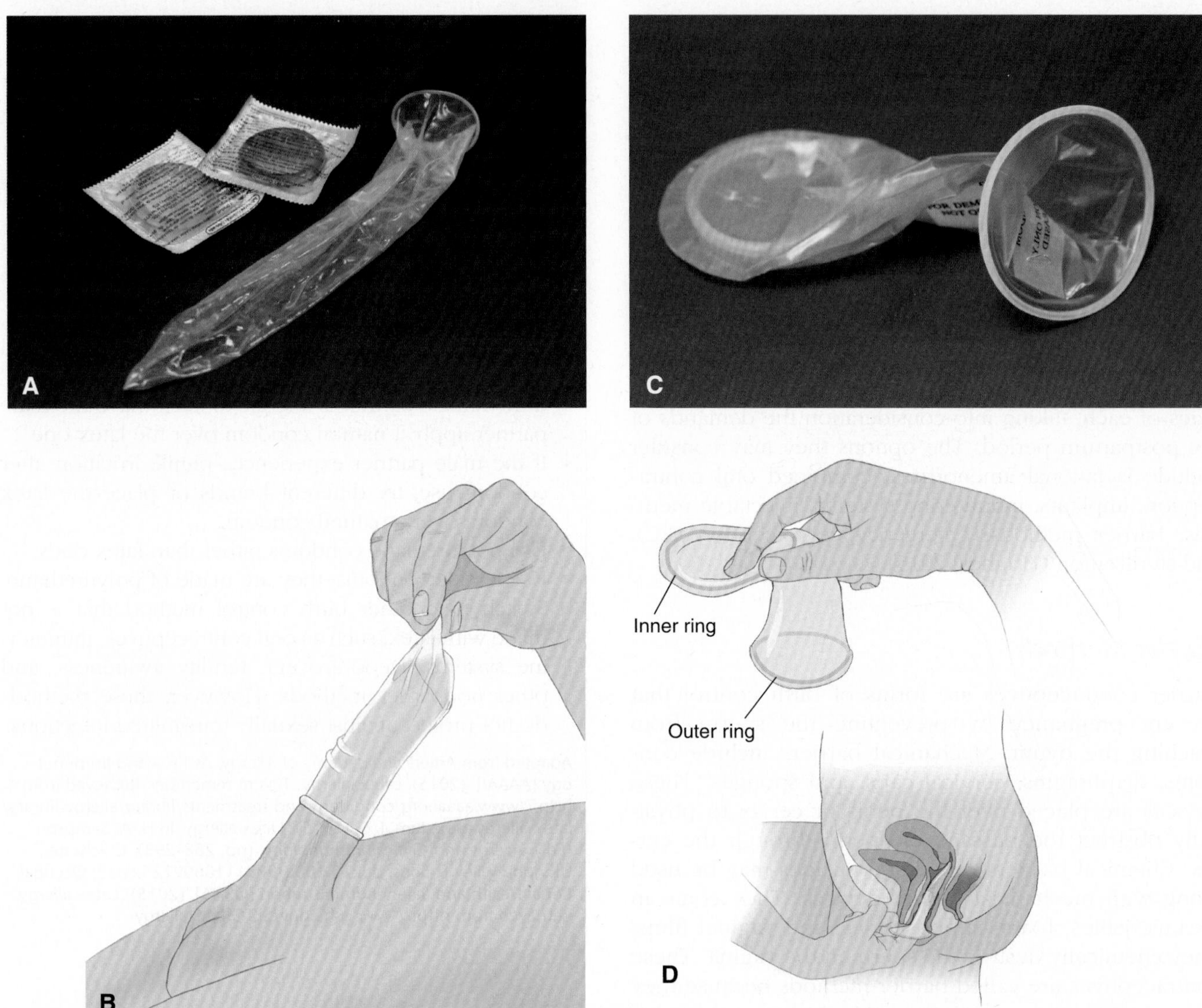

FIGURE 4.8 **A.** Male condom. **B.** Applying a male condom. Leaving space at the tip helps to ensure the condom will not break with ejaculation. **C.** The female condom. **D.** Insertion technique.

are inexpensive, and can be carried inconspicuously by the woman. The female condom was the first woman-controlled method that offered protection against pregnancy and some STIs. Nurses can play a key role in educating clients on how to initiate and maintain use of the female condom, an underused method for HIV/STI and pregnancy prevention in the United States. Providing a brief education session along with free samples would go a long way to promote increased use of this device to prevent STIs transmission as well as pregnancy (Boyd, Perkins, Lawrence, et al., 2015).

DIAPHRAGM

The **diaphragm** is a soft latex dome surrounded by a metal spring. Used in conjunction with a spermicidal jelly or cream, it is inserted into the vagina to cover the cervix (Fig. 4.9). The diaphragm may be inserted up to 4 hours before intercourse but must be left in place for at least 6 hours afterward. Diaphragms are available in a range of sizes and styles. The diaphragm is available only by prescription and must be professionally fitted by a health care provider. Women may need to be refitted with a different-sized diaphragm after pregnancy, abdominal or pelvic surgery, or weight loss or gain of 10 lb or more. As a general rule, diaphragms should be replaced every 1 to 2 years. Recently, a single-sized diaphragm used with contraceptive jelly was introduced and studied for its effectiveness. The single-sized diaphragm was deemed safe and as effective as a standard individually fitted one based on a population sample of >400 women that participated in the research study (Schwartz, Weiner, Lai, et al., 2015). The diaphragm provides both a physical and chemical barrier to sperm (Tharpe et al., 2016).

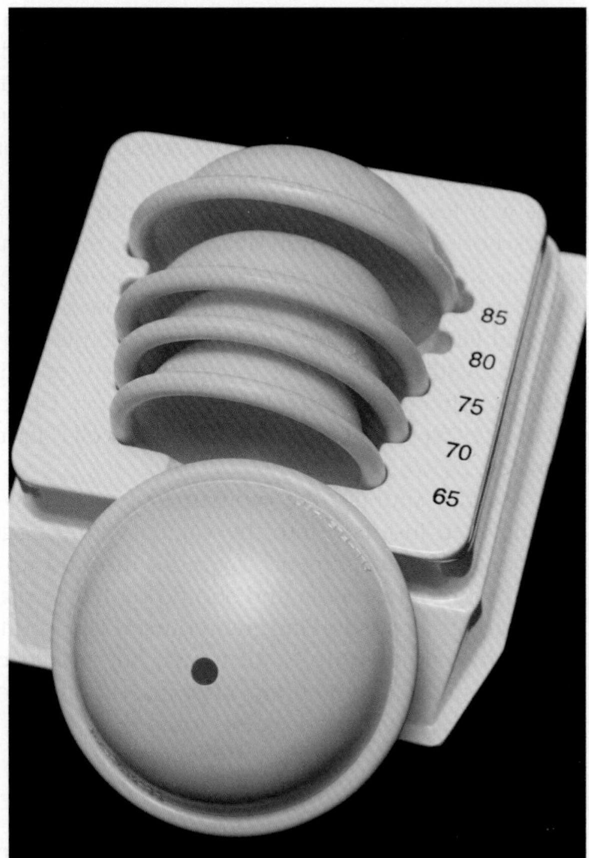

FIGURE 4.9 Sample diaphragm used for measuring.

Diaphragms are user-controlled, nonhormonal methods that are needed only at the time of intercourse, but they are not effective unless used correctly. Women need to receive thorough instruction about diaphragm use and should practice putting one in and taking it out before they leave the health care office (Fig. 4.10).

Results of a 2-year multisite study indicate that the effectiveness rates of the SILCS single-sized, contoured diaphragm, are similar to those of traditional diaphragms, but they also provide a long-term controlled release of the lead candidate anti-HIV microbicide dapivirine. This would make it a new multipurpose prevention device (Schwartz et al., 2015). The biggest difference with this new device is that since it is single size, a pelvic examination to assess the size is not required, and it also releases an anti-HIV microbicide that potentially is capable of preventing HIV transmission. Most women in the study were able to correctly insert, remove, and check correct position of the device by simply using the instructions (Schwartz et al., 2015).

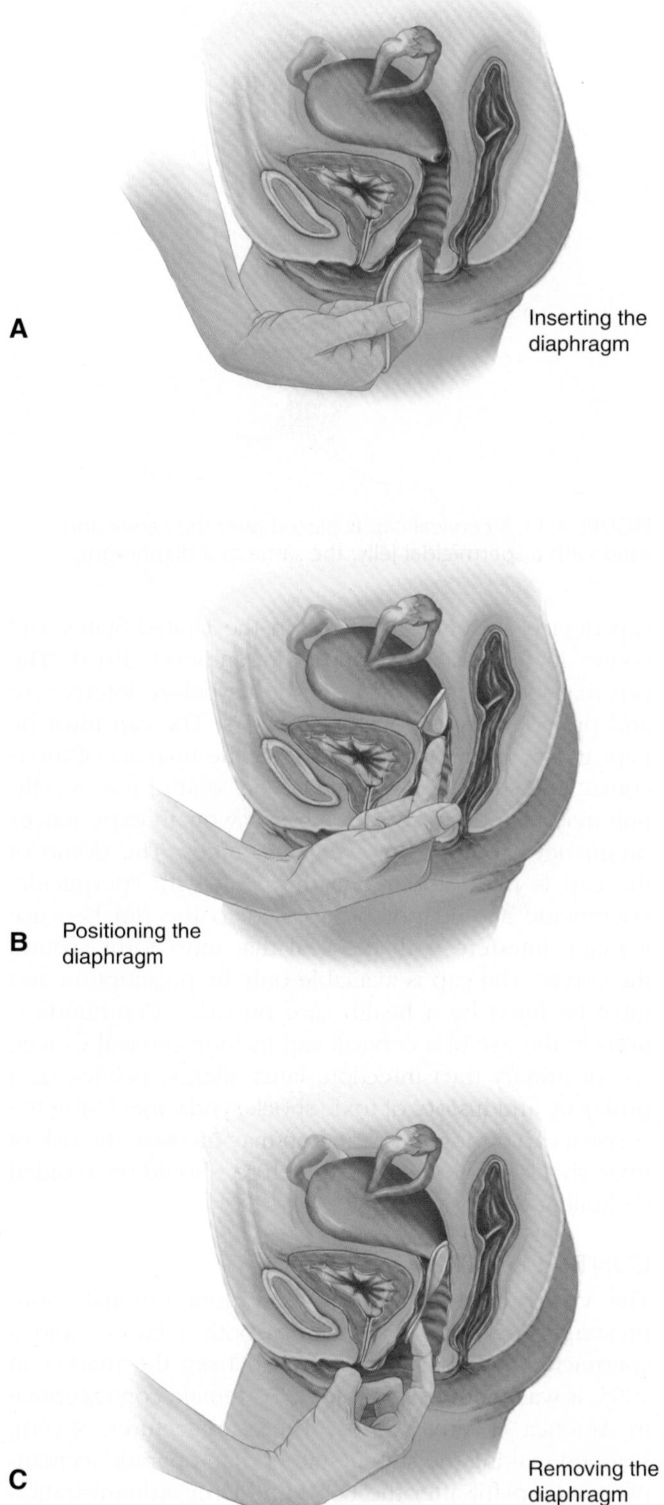

FIGURE 4.10 Application of a diaphragm. **A.** To insert, fold the diaphragm in half, separate the labia with one hand, then insert upward and back into the vagina. **B.** To position, make certain the diaphragm securely covers the cervix. **C.** To remove, hook a finger over the top of the rim and bring the diaphragm down and out.

CERVICAL CAP

The **cervical cap** is smaller than the diaphragm and covers only the cervix; it is held in place by suction. Caps are made from silicone or latex and are used with spermicide (Fig. 4.11). The FemCap is the only cervical

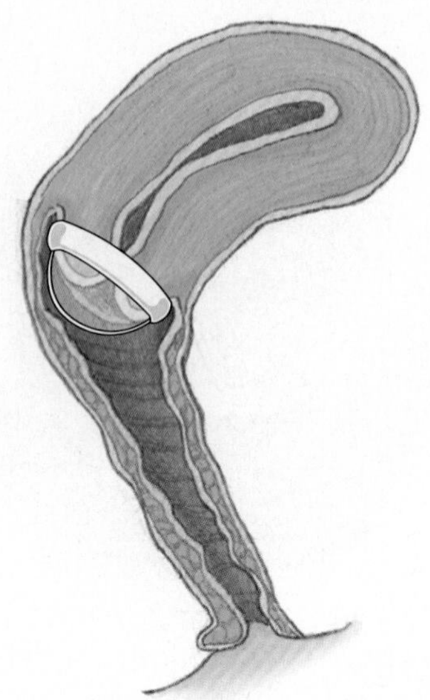

FIGURE 4.11 A cervical cap is placed over the cervix and used with a spermicidal jelly, the same as a diaphragm.

cap device currently available in the United States and comes in three sizes (Planned Parenthood, 2016). The cap may be inserted up to 36 hours before intercourse and provides protection for 48 hours. The cap must be kept in the vagina for 6 hours after the final act of intercourse and should be replaced every year of use. A refitting may also be necessary when a woman experiences pregnancy, abortion, or weight changes. The dome of the cap is filled about one third full with spermicide. Spermicide should not be applied to the rim because it might interfere with the seal that must form around the cervix. The cap is available only by prescription and must be fitted by a health care provider. Contraindications to the use of a cervical cap include cervical cancer, recent urinary tract infection, latex allergy, pelvic-organ prolapse, and history of toxic shock syndrome. Using the cervical cap during menstruation may increase the risk of toxic shock syndrome and, therefore, should be avoided (Schuiling & Likis, 2016).

CONTRACEPTIVE SPONGE

The **contraceptive sponge** is a nonhormonal, nonprescription device that includes both a barrier and a spermicide. When it was removed from the market in 1995, it was the most popular OTC female contraceptive in America (Everett, 2014). The manufacturer, Wyeth, stopped making the sponge rather than upgrade its manufacturing plant after the Food and Drug Administration (FDA) found deficiencies, but the device's effectiveness and safety were never questioned. After receiving reapproval from the FDA in 2009, the contraceptive sponge is once again being marketed to women.

The contraceptive sponge is a soft concave device that prevents pregnancy by covering the cervix and releasing spermicide. The sponge, made of polyurethane saturated with nonoxynol-9 (1,000 mg), releases 125 mg of the spermicide over 24 hours of use. Unlike the diaphragm, the sponge can be used for more than one coital act within 24 hours without the insertion of additional spermicide, and the sponge does not require fitting or a prescription from a health care provider (Zieman, 2015). While it was less effective than several other methods and does not offer protection against STIs, the sponge achieved a wide following among women who appreciated the spontaneity with which it could be used and its easy availability. When compared with the diaphragm in a recent study, the sponge was found to be less effective than the diaphragm in preventing pregnancy. Discontinuation rates were higher at 12 months as well (Sharma & Walmsley, 2015).

To use the sponge, the woman first wets it with water, and then inserts it into the vagina with a finger, using a cord loop attachment. It can be inserted up to 24 hours before intercourse and should be left in place for at least 6 hours following intercourse. The sponge provides protection for up to 12 hours, but should not be left in for more than 30 hours after insertion to avoid the risk of toxic shock syndrome (Moses, 2015c).

Hormonal Methods

Several options are available to women who want long-term but not permanent protection against pregnancy. These methods of contraception work by altering the hormones within a woman's body. They rely on estrogen and progestin or progestin alone to prevent ovulation. When used consistently, these methods are a reliable way to prevent pregnancy. Hormonal methods include OCs, injectables, implants, vaginal rings, and transdermal patches.

ORAL CONTRACEPTIVES

As early as 1937, scientists recognized that the injection of progesterone inhibited ovulation in rabbits and provided contraception. The first hormonal pill, called *Enovid,* was approved by the FDA in May 1960. It contained high levels of estrogen to prevent ovulation. Since that time, it has evolved through gradual lowering of estrogen and is now combined with many different progestins. Breakthrough bleeding was reported in early clinical trials in women, and the role of estrogen in cycle control was launched. This established the rationale for modern-combination OCs that contains both estrogen and progesterone (Stewart & Black, 2015).

Development of hormonal contraception marked a revolutionary step in social change that has improved the lives of women and families worldwide. Since the first OC was introduced, hormonal contraception has undergone various stages of advancement. Today, OC regimens are safer and more tolerable, with equal or improved efficacy, than the early formulations. Incremental decreases in the estrogen dosage helped to alleviate some of the

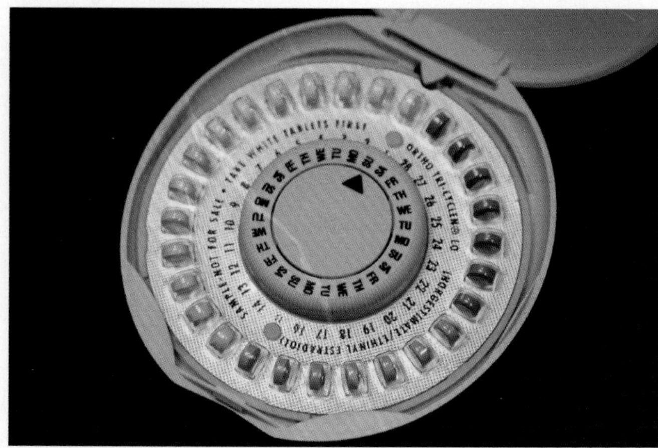

FIGURE 4.12 Oral contraceptive.

unwanted side effects of the pill (Craik & Melvin, 2015). Today, over 30 combination OCs are available in the United States. The most notable change in over 50 years of OC improvement has been the lowering of the estrogen dose to as low as 10 mcg and the introduction of new progestins.

Oral contraception is the most popular method of nonsurgical contraception, used by approximately 25 million women in the United States (Samra-Latif & Wood, 2015) (Fig. 4.12). Unlike the original OCs that women took decades ago, the new low-dose forms carry fewer health risks.

OC, although most commonly prescribed for contraception, has long been used in the management of a wide range of conditions and has many health benefits, such as:

- Reduced incidence of ovarian and endometrial cancer
- Prevention and treatment of endometriosis
- Decreased incidence of acne and hirsutism
- Decreased incidence of ectopic pregnancy
- Decreased incidence of acute PID and possible protection against PID
- Reduced incidence of fibrocystic breast disease
- Decreased perimenopausal symptoms
- Reduced risk of developing uterine fibroids
- Maintenance of bone mineral density (BMD)
- Improvement in asthmatic symptoms
- Delayed onset of multiple sclerosis and arthritis
- Increased menstrual cycle regularity
- Lower incidence of colorectal cancer
- Decreased number of pregnancy-related deaths by preventing pregnancy
- Reduced iron-deficiency anemia by treating menorrhagia
- Reduced incidence of dysmenorrhea (Evans & Sutton, 2015).

OCs work primarily by suppressing ovulation by adding estrogen and progesterone to a woman's body, thus mimicking pregnancy. This hormonal level stifles GnRH, which in turn suppresses FSH and LH and thus inhibits ovulation. Cervical mucus also thickens, which hinders sperm transport into the uterus. Implantation is inhibited by suppression of the maturation of the endometrium and alterations of uterine secretions (Everett, 2014).

The combination pills are prescribed as monophasic pills, which deliver fixed dosages of estrogen and progestin, or as multiphasic ones. Multiphasic pills (e.g., biphasic and triphasic OCs) alter the amount of progestin and estrogen within each cycle. To maintain adequate hormonal levels for contraception and enhance adherence to the regimen, OCs should be taken at the same time daily.

OCs that contains progestin only are sometimes called mini-pills. Progestin-only pills (POPs) have both advantages and disadvantages when compared with combined pills. The pill-taking regimen is simple and fixed; no pill color changes or days without pill-taking occur. These pills are appropriate for women who cannot take estrogen in combined OCs, for example, a woman older than 35 years who smokes cigarettes. They are prescribed for women who cannot take estrogen at all. These OCs work primarily by thickening the cervical mucus to prevent penetration of the sperm and make the endometrium unfavorable for implantation. Progestin-only pills must be taken at a certain time every 24 hours. Breakthrough bleeding and a higher risk of pregnancy have made these OCs less popular than combination OCs (Craik & Melvin, 2015).

Extended OC regimens have been used for the management of menstrual disorders and endometriosis for years but now are attracting wider attention. Surveys asking women about their willingness to reduce their menstrual cycles from 12 to 4 annually were returned with a resounding "yes!" (Zorbas, Economopoulos, & Vlahos, 2015). Research has confirmed that the extended use of active OC pills carries the same safety profile as the conventional 28-day regimens. OCs taken continuously or in long cycles offer benefits with regard to menstrual symptoms and the recurrence of symptoms related to endometriosis (Zieman, 2015). The extended regimen consists of 84 consecutive days of active combination pills, followed by 7 days of placebos. The woman has four withdrawal-bleeding episodes a year. Seasonale and Seasonique, a combination OC, is on the market for women who choose to reduce the number of periods that they have. In 2009, the makers of Seasonique came out with LoSeasonique. LoSeasonique consists of 84 orange tablets containing 0.1 mg levonorgestrel and 0.02 mg ethinyl estradiol and 7 yellow tablets containing 0.01 mg ethinyl estradiol. The risk profile is similar to those of its sister products, Seasonale and Seasonique; however, the risk of unplanned breakthrough bleeding is increased (Samra-Latif & Wood, 2015).

COMPARISON CHART 4.1 ADVANTAGES AND DISADVANTAGES OF ORAL CONTRACEPTIVES

Advantages	Disadvantages
Regulate and shorten menstrual cycle	Offer no protection against STIs
Decrease severe cramping and bleeding	Pose slightly increased risk of breast cancer
Reduce anemia	
Reduce ovarian and colorectal cancer risk	Modest risk for venous thrombosis and pulmonary emboli
Decrease benign breast disease	Increased risk for migraine headaches
Reduce risk of endometrial cancer, colorectal cancer, and ovarian cancer	
Improve acne and reduces incidence of menstrual headaches	Increased risk for myocardial infarction, stroke, and hypertension for women who smoke
Minimize perimenopausal symptoms	May increase risk of depression
Decrease incidence of rheumatoid arthritis	User must remember to take pill daily
Improve PMS symptoms	High cost for some women
Protect against loss of bone density and reduces risk of osteoporosis	

Adapted from Jick, S. (2015). Oral contraceptives and the risk of venous thromboembolism. In *Medicines for women* (pp. 181–201). Springer International Publishing.; Zieman, M. (2015) *Managing contraception on the go* (13th ed.), New York, NY: Ardnet Media; Everett, S. (2014) *Handbook of contraception and sexual health* (3rd ed.), New York, NY: Routledge.

Lybrel was the first FDA-approved OC with 365-day combination dosing. It contains a low combined daily dose of the hormones levonorgestrel and ethinyl estradiol (90 mcg and 20 mcg, respectively). It provides women with more hormonal exposure on a yearly basis (13 additional weeks of hormone intake per year) than conventional cyclic OCs that contain the same strength of synthetic estrogens and similar strength of progestins (Samra-Latif & Wood, 2015). There is no physiologic requirement for cyclic hormonal withdrawal bleeds while taking OCs (Skidmore-Roth, 2015).

A growing body of evidence indicates that an over-the-counter access to OC pills is safe and effective and that women are interested in obtaining pills this way. With half of all pregnancies being unintended—a figure that has remained unchanged for decades—innovation is needed to address this statistic. Although an over-the-counter contraceptive pill may sound revolutionary in the United States, over-the-counter access is already a reality in more than 100 countries and has been for decades. ACOG supports over-the-counter access to contraceptive pills, but numerous social and professional groups oppose it (Foster, Biggs, Phillips, et al., 2015). Even after ACOG's support, women will probably not be seeing an over-the-counter OC product on the local pharmacy shelf any time soon, despite its cost-effectiveness and impact on reduction in unintended pregnancies.

The balance between the benefits and the risks of OCs must be determined for each woman when she is being assessed for this type of contraceptive. It is a highly effective contraceptive when taken properly but can aggravate many medical conditions, especially in women who smoke. Comparison Chart 4.1 lists advantages and disadvantages of OCs. A thorough history and pelvic examination, including a Pap smear, are not required before the medication is prescribed, but a regular medical follow-up is advised. Women should also be counseled that the effectiveness of OCs is decreased when the woman is taking antibiotics; thus, the woman will need to use an alternative or secondary method during this period to prevent pregnancy.

Nurses need to provide OC users with a great deal of education before they leave the health care facility. They need to be able to identify early signs and symptoms that might indicate a problem.

Take Note!

The mnemonic "ACHES" can help women remember the early warning signs that necessitate a return to the health care provider (Box 4.6).

BOX 4.6

EARLY SIGNS OF COMPLICATIONS FOR USERS OF ORAL CONTRACEPTIVES

A = Abdominal pain may indicate liver or gallbladder problems.
C = Chest pain or shortness of breath may indicate a pulmonary embolus.
H = Headaches may indicate hypertension or impending stroke.
E = Eye problems may indicate hypertension or an attack.
S = Severe leg pain may indicate a thromboembolic event.

Adapted from Everett, S. (2014) *Handbook of contraception and sexual health.* (3rd ed.), New York, NY: Routledge.

INJECTABLE CONTRACEPTIVE

Injectable contraception includes progestin-only and combination estrogen and progestin agents that provide safe and highly effective birth control for up to 3 months. Injectable agents are widely available and play an important role in family planning worldwide. They offer a discreet, convenient, reversible, and non–coital-dependent method of birth control.

Depo-Provera is the trade name for an intramuscular injectable of a progesterone-only contraceptive given every 12 weeks which contains 150 mg/1 mL. Depo-subQ Pronera is a lower-dose injectable given subcutaneously delivering 104 mg/0.65 mL every 12 weeks. They are the only injectable agents available in the United States. Depo-Provera works by suppressing ovulation and the production of FSH and LH by the pituitary gland, by increasing the viscosity of cervical mucus and causing endometrial atrophy. A single injection of 150 mg into the buttocks acts like other progestin-only products to prevent pregnancy for 3 months at a time (Fig. 4.13). The primary side effect of Depo-Provera is menstrual cycle disturbance.

Recent clinical studies have raised concerns about whether Depo-Provera reduces BMD. This evidence has prompted the manufacturer and the FDA to issue a warning about the long-term use (>2 years) of Depo-Provera and bone loss (Wolfe & Cansino, 2015). It is not entirely clear if this loss in BMD is reversible because there have not been any long-term prospective studies in current and past users. It is highly recommended that bone density scans be done while on Depo-Provera (U.S. Selected Practice Recommendations for Contraceptive Use, 2014).

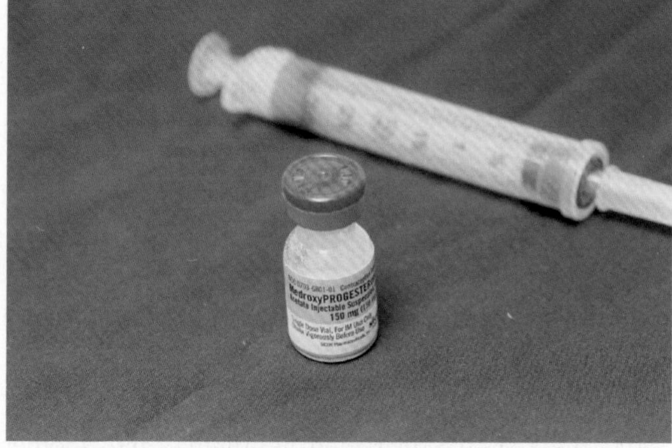

FIGURE 4.13 Injectable contraceptive.

TRANSDERMAL PATCHES

Transdermal delivery of contraceptive hormones avoids hepatic first-pass metabolism, allowing a lower total hormone doses when compared to that of oral products that are metabolized in the liver. A **transdermal patch**, Ortho Evra, is available in the United States. It is a matchbox-sized patch containing hormones that are absorbed through the skin when placed on the lower abdomen, upper outer arm, buttocks, or upper torso (avoiding the breasts). The patch is applied weekly for 3 weeks, followed by a patch-free week during which withdrawal bleeding occurs. The patch delivers continuous levels of progesterone and estrogen. Transdermal absorption allows the drug to enter the bloodstream directly, avoiding rapid inactivation in the liver known as first-pass metabolism. Because estrogen and progesterone are metabolized by liver enzymes, avoiding first-pass metabolism was thought to reduce adverse effects. However, recent evidence suggests that the risk of venous thrombosis and embolism is increased with the patch and the risk of skin burns occurring if undergoing an MRI, but still less than the risk of venous thromboembolism during pregnancy (Nelson, 2015). Additional studies are under way to understand the clinical significance of these latest findings, but in the interim nurses need to focus on ongoing risk assessment and should be prepared to discuss current research findings with clients.

Adherence to the regimen of combination contraceptive patch use has been shown to be significantly greater than adherence with OCs. In addition, research suggests that overweight and obese women with weights exceeding 198 lb should be advised of the potentially decreased effectiveness of the patch and increase incidence of venous thromboembolism and weight gain (Pocius & Dutton, 2015). The patch provides combination hormone therapy with a side-effect profile similar to that of OCs (Fig. 4.14).

VAGINAL RINGS

Approved in 2001 by the FDA, the **vaginal ring** contains both estrogen and progesterone hormones. The contraceptive vaginal ring, NuvaRing, is a flexible, soft, transparent ring that is inserted by the user for a 3-week period of continuous use followed by a ring-free week to allow withdrawal bleeding (Fig. 4.15). Ethinyl estradiol and etonogestrel are rapidly absorbed through the vaginal epithelium and result in a steady serum

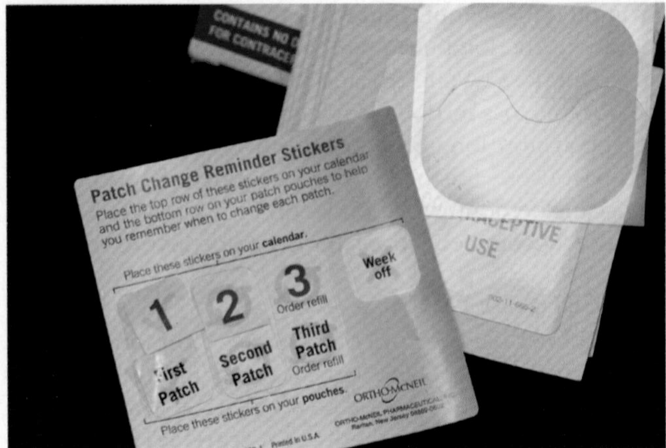

FIGURE 4.14 Transdermal patch.

concentration. Because the hormones are released directly into the vagina, a lower daily dose of hormones is required in comparison with OC doses. Studies have demonstrated that the efficacy and safety of the ring are equivalent to those of OCs. Clients report being highly satisfied with the vaginal ring and report fewer systemic side effects than do OC users. The ring provides effective cycle control as well as symptom relief for women with menorrhagia, dysmenorrhea, and polycystic ovarian syndrome. Reported problems associated with the use of vaginal rings include erosion of vaginal wall, ring expulsion, interference with coitus, unpleasant ring odor, and premature discontinuation due to vaginal discomfort (Khan & Krupanidhi, 2015). The ring can be inserted by the woman and does not have to be fitted. The woman compresses the ring and inserts it into the vagina, behind the pubic bone, as far back as possible, but precise placement is not critical. The hormones are absorbed through the vaginal mucosa. It is left in place for 3 weeks and then removed and discarded. Effectiveness and adverse events are similar to those seen with combination OCs. Clients need to be counseled regarding timely insertion

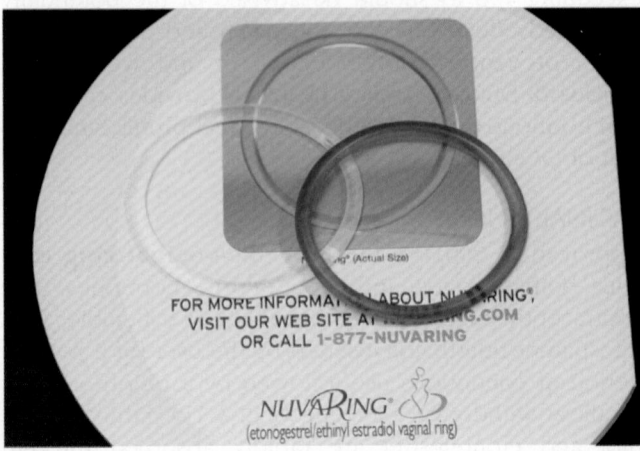

FIGURE 4.15 Vaginal ring.

of the ring and what to do in case of accidental expulsion. Recent studies suggest that a vaginal ring containing etonogestrel and ethinyl estradiol used in an extended regimen is a safe contraceptive method that offers good cycle control and can be an option for women who have gastric intolerance or other side effects when using oral hormonal contraceptives (King et al., 2015).

IMPLANTABLE CONTRACEPTIVES

The **implant** is a subdermal time-release method that delivers synthetic progestin that inhibits ovulation. Once in place, it delivers 3 years of continuous, highly effective contraception. Like progestin-only pills, implants act by inhibiting ovulation and thickening cervical mucus so sperm cannot penetrate. A single-rod progestin implant (Nexplanon) is currently available in the United States. Nexplanon is 4 cm long and 2 mm in diameter, and contains 68 mg of the hormone progestin. The implant is radio-opaque and is over 99% effective (King et al., 2015). The side effects are also similar to those of progestin-only pills: irregular bleeding, headaches, weight gain, breast tenderness, and depression. Fertility is restored quickly after it is removed. Implants require a minor surgical procedure for both insertion and removal. The implants do not offer any protection against STIs.

Hormonal side effects are not exclusive to implants but tend to be a problem with all hormonal contraceptives. Preinsertion counseling by the nurse is essential to prepare the woman for any such side effects. Expert counseling should cover the one-side effect most likely to cause discontinuation: initial irregular bleeding and the possibility of amenorrhea with longer use (Craik & Rowlands, 2015).

INTRAUTERINE CONTRACEPTIVES

Intrauterine contraceptives are classified as either hormonal or nonhormonal. Both types prevent pregnancy via inhibition of sperm mobility and sperm viability and change the speed of transport of the ovum in the fallopian tube. An intrauterine contraceptive (IUC) is a small plastic T-shaped object that is placed inside the uterus to provide contraception (Fig. 4.16). It prevents pregnancy by making the endometrium of the uterus hostile to implantation of a fertilized ovum by causing a nonspecific inflammatory reaction and inhibiting sperm and ovum from meeting (Wildemeersch & Jandi, 2015). The hormonal IUC will make monthly periods lighter, shorter, and less painful, making this a useful method for women with heavy, painful periods. The implants contain either copper or progesterone to enhance their effectiveness. One or two attached strings protrude into the vagina so that the user can check for placement.

Currently three intrauterine contraceptives are available in the United States: the copper ParaGard-TCu-380A, the LNG-IUS marketed as Mirena, and another LNG-IUD marketed as Skyla. The ParaGard-TCu-380A is

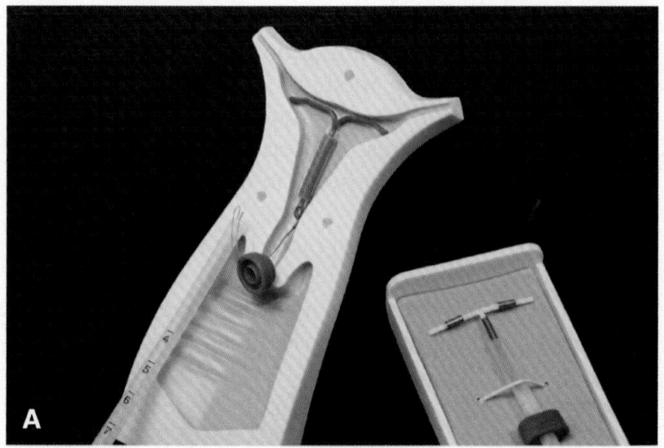

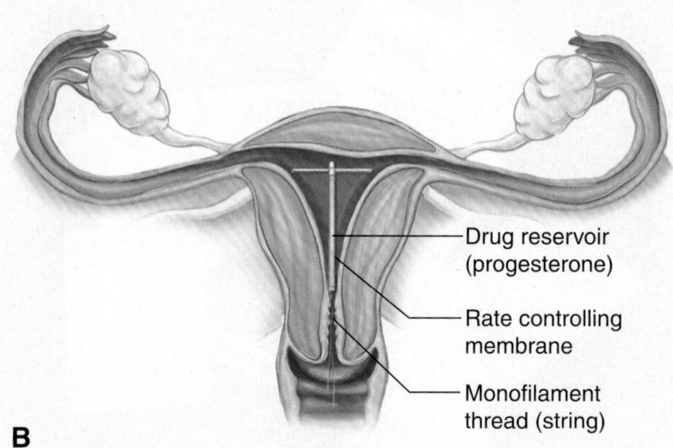

FIGURE 4.16 **A.** Intrauterine contraceptive. **B.** An IUC in place in the uterus.

approved for 10 years of use and is nonhormonal. Its mechanism of action is based on the release of copper ions, which alone are spermicidal. Additionally, the device causes an inflammatory action leading to a hostile uterine environment. The TCu-380A is also approved for use as EC. Mirena provides intrauterine conception for 5 years, but has been shown to be effective for as long as 7 years. Skyla has been approved for 3 years of pregnancy prevention. Both devices release a low dose of progestin causing thinning of the endometrium and thickening of cervical mucus, which inhibits sperm entry into the upper genital tract. Their use results in a major reduction in menstrual flow and dysmenorrhea, suggesting that they are viable alternative to hysterectomy and endometrial ablation in women with menorrhagia (Atkin, Beal, Long-Middleton, et al., 2015). An advantage of these hormonally impregnated intrauterine systems is that they are relatively maintenance-free: users must consciously discontinue using them to become pregnant rather than making a daily decision to avoid conception (Alan Guttmacher Institute, 2015a).

The intrauterine contraceptives provide a safe, highly effective, long-lasting, yet reversible method of contraception. Expanding access to intrauterine contraception is an important measure to reduce the rate of unintended pregnancy in the United States. Nurses should consider including them in their discussion to appropriate candidates, including women who are nulliparous, adolescent, immediately postpartum, or postabortion and those who desire EC, and as an alternative to permanent sterilization. Limitations Barriers to obtaining intrauterine contraception such as requiring cervical cancer screening before insertion, routine testing for gonorrhea and chlamydial infection in low-risk women, or scheduling insertion only during menses are unnecessary. IUC insertion can take place on any day of the menstrual cycle, if absence of pregnancy is confirmed (Cheng & Van Leuven, 2015). Box 4.7 highlights the warning signs of the potential complications of IUCs.

EMERGENCY CONTRACEPTION

Unplanned pregnancy is a major health, economic, and social issue for women. Approximately one third of all unplanned pregnancies end in abortion (CDC, 2015b). Using an emergency contraceptive provides a woman a second chance to prevent an unintended pregnancy. **Emergency contraception** (EC) reduces the risk of pregnancy after unprotected intercourse or contraceptive failure such as condom breakage (Raymond & Cleland, 2015). It is used within 72 hours of unprotected intercourse to prevent pregnancy. The sooner ECs are taken, the more effective they are. They reduce the risk of pregnancy for a single act of unprotected sex by almost 80% (Samra-Latif & Wood, 2015). The methods available in the United States are progestin-only pills, Plan B One-Step (Fig. 4.17), Next Choice, Next Choice One Dose; combined estrogen and progestin pills, or insertion of a copper-releasing intrauterine system up to 7 days after unprotected intercourse. Ulipristal acetate (marketed as Ella) is a selective progesterone receptor modulator that, when taken as a single 30-mg dose, is a new, safe, and effective emergency contraceptive that can be used from the first day and up to 5 days following unprotected intercourse. The older progesterone-only emergency contraceptive, levonorgestrel, is taken as two 0.75-mg

BOX 4.7

WARNINGS FOR INTRAUTERINE SYSTEM USERS OF POTENTIAL COMPLICATIONS

P = Period late, pregnancy, abnormal spotting or bleeding
A = Abdominal pain, pain with intercourse
I = Infection exposure, abnormal vaginal discharge
N = Not feeling well, fever, chills
S = String length shorter or longer or missing

Adapted from King, T. L., Brucker, M. C., Kriebs, J. M., Fahey, J. O., Gegor, C. L., & Varney, H. (2015) *Varney's midwifery* (5th ed.). Burlington, MA: Jones & Bartlett Learning.

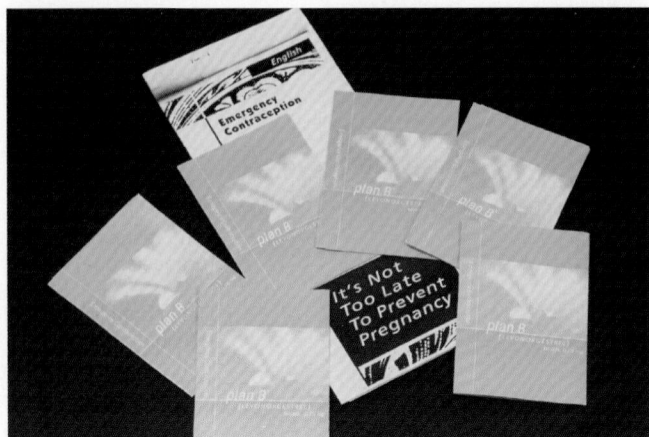

FIGURE 4.17 Emergency contraceptive kit.

pills 12 hours apart (Next Choice; Watson Pharmaceuticals Inc., Morristown, NJ, USA) or as a single 1.5-mg pill (Plan B One-Step; Watson Pharmaceuticals Inc.), and is approved for only 72 hours after unprotected intercourse (Mulligan, 2015).

Access to emergency contraceptives has been controversial for minors. Prior to 2013, the pills were available by prescription only, and even when approved for nonprescription status, access was restricted based on age. In 2013, several judicial courts and the FDA ruled in favor of nonprescription access to EC by all women regardless of age. At this time, the federal government has not appealed these rulings, but many states have placed restrictions on access of EC (Casey & Isaacs, 2015). The only contraindication to the use of any of the four EC methods is a known pregnancy as defined as implantation.

Although access to EC has increased with nonprescription status and approval of Plan B One-Step without age restrictions, many barriers remain in public awareness and unintended pregnancies continue to rise. Because of the lack of awareness of EC and the politics surrounding it, EC is not used as widely as would be warranted by the incidence of unprotected coitus. Nurses need to educate their female clients to bring about increased awareness of this second chance method. Table 4.5 lists recommended oral medication and intrauterine regimens.

Prime points to stress-concerning ECs are:

- ECs do not offer any protection against STIs or future pregnancies.
- ECs should not be used in place of a regular birth control method, because they are less effective.
- ECs may delay the next menses, so evaluation for pregnancy is needed if menses does not occur within 3 weeks after EC use.
- Report any severe abdominal pain to health care provider immediately.
- ECs are regular birth control pills given at a higher dose.
- ECs are contraindicated during pregnancy (Ilic, 2015).

Take Note!

Contrary to popular belief, ECs do not induce abortion and are not related to mifepristone or RU-486, the so-called abortion pill approved by the FDA in 2000.

Mifepristone chemically induces abortion by blocking the body's progesterone receptors, which are necessary for pregnancy maintenance. ECs simply prevent embryo creation and uterine implantation from occurring in the first place. There is no evidence that ECs have any effect on an already implanted ovum. The side effects are nausea and vomiting.

Sterilization

Sterilization is a permanent, safe, and highly effective method of contraception for those who are certain they do not want any or any more, children. Vasectomy is the only highly reliable form of male contraception. Approximately 600,000 tubal occlusions and 200,000 vasectomies are performed in the United States annually

TABLE 4.5 EMERGENCY POSTCOITAL CONTRACEPTION OPTIONS

Product	Dosage (Within 72 hrs)	Comments
Combined estrogen and progestin pills (Yuzpe regimen)	OCs are taken in various formulations to prevent conception	Interfere with the cascade of events that result in ovulation and fertilization
Plan B One-Step	1.5 mg pill taken	Can cause nausea and vomiting
Intrauterine		
Copper-bearing IUS (ParaGard-TCu-380A)	Inserted within 5 days after unprotected sexual episode	Can be left in for long-term contraception (10 yrs)

Adapted from King, TL., Brucker, MC., Kriebs, JM., Fahey, JO., Gegor, CL., & Varney, H. (2015) *Varney's midwifery* (5th ed.). Burlington, MA: Jones & Bartlett Learning; Ilic, K. (2015). Emergency contraception. In *Medicines for Women* (pp. 203–225). Springer International Publishing.

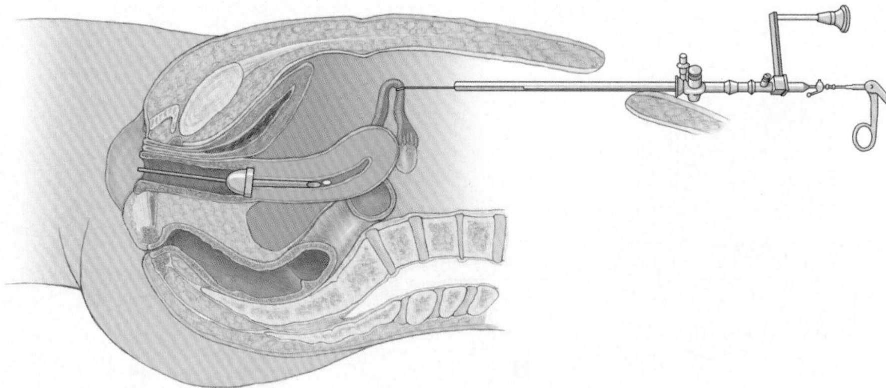

FIGURE 4.18 Laparoscopy for tubal sterilization.

and over 220 million worldwide (Shoupe & Mishell, 2016). It is the most widely used method of family planning in the world in both developed and developing countries. Sterilization refers to surgical procedures intended to render the person infertile. Laparoscopic, abdominal, and hysteroscopic methods of female sterilization are available in the United States, with most of these procedures performed outside the hospital. Sterilization is a safe and effective form of permanent birth control. In the United States, it is still the second most commonly used form of contraception overall and is the most frequently used method among married women and among women over 30 years of age (McKay & Schunmann, 2015). More women than men undergo surgical sterilization. According to the CDC (2015b) approximately 18% of women undergo female sterilization in comparison with 7% of men in the United States. Sterilization should be considered a permanent end to fertility because reversal surgery is difficult, expensive, and not always successful. Because these methods are intended to be irreversible, all couples should be appropriately counseled about the permanency of sterilization and the availability of highly effective, long-acting, reversible methods of contraception before their decision is made.

TUBAL LIGATION

Tubal ligation, the sterilization procedure for women, can be performed postpartum, after an abortion, or as an interval procedure unrelated to pregnancy. Minilaparotomies and laparoscopies are the two most common techniques. In the laparoscopy procedure, the abdomen is filled with carbon dioxide gas so that the abdominal wall balloons away from the tubes provide a view of the fallopian tubes. They are grasped and sealed with a cauterizing instrument or with rings, bands, or clips or cut and tied (Fig. 4.18).

ESSURE

Essure is a nonsurgical, nonhormonal, permanent birth control method that is 99% effective. This method is for women who desire no more children as it is a permanent method of birth control. It offers several advantages over a conventional tubal ligation: general anesthesia and incisions are not needed, thereby increasing safety, lowering costs, and improving access to sterilization. A tiny coil (Essure) is introduced and released into the fallopian tubes through the cervix. The coil promotes tissue growth in the fallopian tubes, and over a period of 3 months, this growth blocks the tubes. The buildup of tissue creates a barrier that keeps sperm from the reaching the ovum, thus preventing conception (Thurkow, 2015). This less-invasive technique uses a hysteroscopy under local anesthesia in an office setting. Sterilization does not occur immediately after this procedure, so women must be educated to use additional contraception for 3 months until permanent tubal occlusion is verified.

VASECTOMY

Male sterilization is accomplished with a surgical procedure known as a **vasectomy**. More than 500,000 men have a vasectomy performed in the United States each year (McFarlane, 2015). It is usually performed under local anesthesia in a urologist's office, and most men can return to work and normal activities in a day or two. The procedure involves making a small incision into the scrotum and cutting the vas deferens, which carries sperm from the testes to the penis (Fig. 4.19). Complications from vasectomy are rare and minor in nature. Immediate risks include infection, hematoma, and pain. After vasectomy, semen no longer contains sperm. This is not immediate, though, and the man must submit semen specimens for analysis 8 to 16 weeks after a vasectomy until two specimens show that no sperm is present. When the specimen shows azoospermia, the man's sterility is confirmed (Whitaker, 2015).

Nursing Management of the Woman Choosing a Contraceptive Method

The choice of a contraceptive method is a very personal one involving many factors. What makes a woman

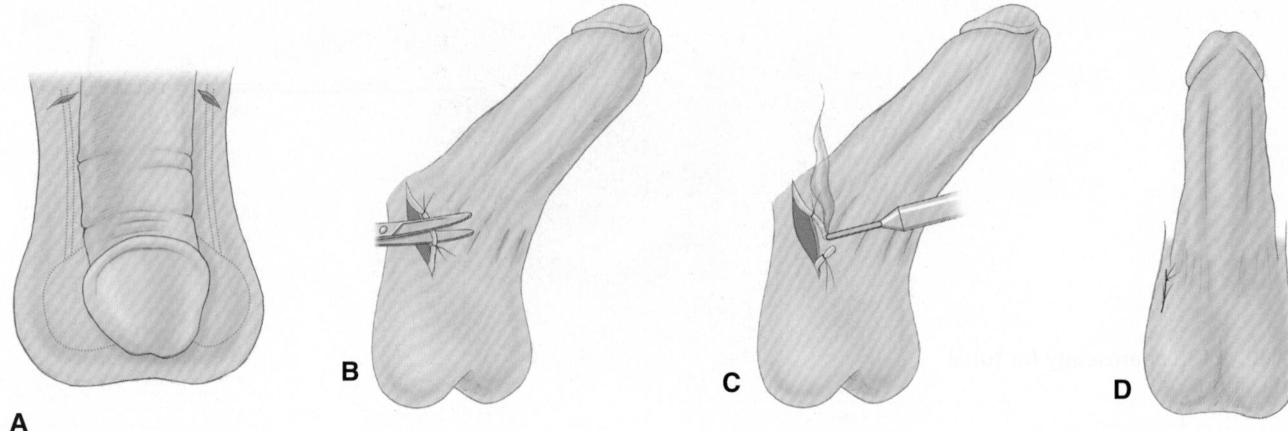

FIGURE 4.19 Vasectomy. **A.** Site of vasectomy incisions. **B.** The vas deferens is cut with surgical scissors. **C.** Cut ends of the vas deferens are cauterized to ensure blockage of the passage of sperm. **D.** Final skin suture.

choose one contraceptive method over another? In making contraceptive choices, couples must balance their sexual lives, their reproductive goals, and each partner's health and safety. The search for a choice that satisfies all three objectives is challenging. A method that works for a sexually active teenage girl may not meet her needs later in life. Several considerations influence a person's choice of contraceptives:

- Motivation
- Cost
- Cultural and religious beliefs (Box 4.8)
- Convenience
- Effectiveness
- Side effects
- Desire for children in the future
- Safety of the method
- Comfort level with sexuality
- Protection from STIs
- Interference with spontaneity

If a contraceptive is to be effective, the woman must understand how it works, must be able to use it correctly and consistently, and must be comfortable and confident with it. If a client cannot adhere to taking a pill daily, consider a method used once a week (transdermal patches), once every 3 weeks (transvaginal ring), or once every 3 months (Depo-Provera injection). Another option may be a progesterone intrauterine contraceptive that lasts 3 to 5 years and reduces menstrual flow significantly.

Regardless of which method is chosen, the client's needs should be paramount in the discussion. The nurse can educate clients about which methods are available and their advantages and disadvantages, efficacy, cost, and safety. Knowledge of contraceptive effectiveness is crucial to making an informed choice. The couple has to comprehend the pros and cons of the contraceptive methods being considered. Choice may be influenced by understanding the likelihood of pregnancy with each method and factors that influence effectiveness. Counseling can help the woman choose a contraceptive method that is efficacious and fits her preferences and lifestyle.

BOX 4.8

SELECTED RELIGIOUS CHOICES FOR FAMILY PLANNING AND ABORTION

- Roman Catholic—Abstinence and natural family planning; no abortion
- Judaism (Orthodox)—Family planning and abortion accepted in first trimester. Conservative and Reform Judaism accept both family planning and abortion
- Islam—Family planning accepted; abortion only for serious reasons
- Protestant Christianity—Firmly in favor of family planning; mixed on abortion
- Buddhism—Long experience with family planning and abortion
- Hinduism—Accept both family planning and abortion
- Native American religions—Accept both family planning and abortion
- Chinese religions—Taoism and Confucianism accept both

Adapted from McFarland, M. R., & Wehbe-Alamah, H. B. (2015) *Leininger's cultural care diversity and universality: A worldwide nursing theory* (3rd ed.), Burlington, MA: Jones & Bartlett Learning; McFarlane, D.R. (2015) *Global population and reproductive health.* Burlington, MA: Jones & Bartlett Learning.

Nursing Assessment

When assessing which contraceptive method might meet the client's needs, the nurse might ask:

- Do your religious beliefs interfere with any methods?
- Will this method interfere with your sexual pleasure?

- Are you aware of the various methods currently available?
- Is cost a major consideration, or does your insurance cover it?
- Does your partner influence which method you choose?
- Are you in a stable, monogamous relationship?
- Have you heard anything troubling about any of the methods?
- How comfortable are you touching your own body?
- What are your future plans for having children?

Although deciding on a contraceptive is a very personal decision between a woman and her partner, nurses can assist in this process by performing a complete health history and physical examination, and by educating the woman and her partner about necessary laboratory and diagnostic testing. Areas of focus during the nursing assessment are as follows:

- Medical history: smoking status, cancer of reproductive tract, diabetes mellitus, migraines, hypertension, thromboembolic disorder, allergies, risk factors for cardiovascular disease (CVD)
- Family history: cancer, CVD, hypertension, stroke, diabetes
- OB/GYN history: menstrual disorders, current contraceptive, previous STIs, PID, vaginitis, sexual activity
- Personal history: use of tampons and female hygiene products, plans for childbearing, comfort with touching herself, number of sexual partners and their involvement in the decision
- Physical examination: height, weight, blood pressure, breast examination, thyroid palpation, pelvic examination
- Diagnostic testing: urinalysis, complete blood count, Pap smear, wet mount to check for STIs, HIV/AIDS tests, lipid profile, glucose level

Figure 4.20 shows an example of a family planning flow record that can be used during the assessment. After collecting the assessment data above, consider the medical factors to help decide if the woman is a candidate for all methods or whether some should be eliminated. For example, if she reports she has multiple sex partners and a history of pelvic infections, she would not be a good candidate for an intrauterine contraceptive. Barrier methods (male or female condoms) of contraception might be recommended to this client to offer protection against STIs.

Nursing Diagnoses

A few nursing diagnoses that might be appropriate based on the nurse's assessment during the decision-making process include:

- Deficient knowledge related to:
  - Methods available
  - Side effects/safety
  - Correct use of method chosen
  - Previous myths believed
- Risk for infection related to:
  - Unprotected sexual intercourse
  - Past history of STIs
  - Methods offering protection

Nursing diagnoses applicable to the contraceptive would be:

- Health-seeking behaviors related to:
  - Perceived need for limiting number of children
  - Overall health relative to contraceptives
- Risk for ineffective health maintenance related to:
  - Not being familiar with the various contraceptive methods
  - Being unaware of high-risk sexual behavior leading to STIs
- Fear related to:
  - Not understanding the correct procedure to use
  - Unintended pregnancy occurring if not used correctly
  - General health concerning the long-term side effects

Nursing Interventions

Contraception is an important issue for all couples, and the method used should be decided by the woman and her partner jointly. Facilitate this process by establishing a trusting relationship with the client and by providing unbiased, accurate information about all methods available. As a nurse, reflect honestly on your feelings about contraceptives while allowing the client's feelings to be paramount. Be aware of the practical issues involved in contraceptive use, and avoid making assumptions, making decisions on the woman's behalf, and making judgments about her and her situation. To do so, it is important to keep up to date on the latest methods available and convey this information to clients. Encourage female clients to take control of their lives by sharing information that allows them to plan their futures.

The following guidelines are helpful in counseling and educating the client or couple about contraceptives:

- Encourage the client/couple to participate in choosing a method.
- Provide client education. The client/couple must become informed users before the method is chosen. Education should be targeted to the client's level so it is understood. Provide step-by-step teaching and an opportunity for practice for certain methods (cervical caps, diaphragms, vaginal rings, and condoms). See Teaching Guidelines 4.5 and Figure 4.21.

FAMILY PLANNING FLOW (VISIT) RECORD

Name:
ID #:
Date of Birth:

	Date:		Date:	
Current Method				
Reason for Visit				
LMP				
SUBJECTIVE DATA	**Pt.**	**Comments**	**Pt.**	**Comments**
Severe headaches				
Depression				
Visual abnormalities				
Dyspnea/chest pain				
Breast changes				
SBE				
Abdominal pain				
Nausea and vomiting				
Dysuria/frequency				
Menstrual irregularities				
Vaginal discharge/infections				
Leg pain				
Surgery, injury, infections, or serious illness since last visit				
Allergic reaction				
Pregnancy plans				
Other				
OBJECTIVE DATA	**Weight**	**B.P.**	**Weight**	**B.P.**
Other				
Lab				
ASSESSMENT				
Check here if assessment continues on progress notes	O		O	
PLAN				
Type of contraceptive given				
COUNSELING/EDUCATION				
Next appointment				
SIGNATURE/TITLE				
SIGNATURE/TITLE				

O = normal ✓= abnormal

FIGURE 4.20 Family planning flow (visit) record.

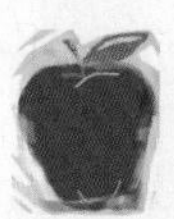

Teaching Guidelines 4.5

TIPS FOR THE USE OF CERVICAL CAPS, DIAPHRAGMS, VAGINAL RINGS, AND CONDOMS

Cervical Cap Insertion/Removal Technique

- It is important to be involved in the fitting process.
- To insert the cap, pinch the sides together, compress the cap dome, insert into the vagina, and place over the cervix.
- Use one finger to feel around the entire circumference to make sure there are no gaps between the cap rim and the cervix.
- After a minute or two, pinch the dome and tug gently to check for evidence of suction. The cap should resist the tug and not slide off easily.
- To remove the cap, press the index finger against the rim and tip the cap slightly to break the suction. Gently pull out the cap.
- The woman should practice inserting and removing the cervical cap three times to validate her proficiency with this device.

Client Teaching and Counseling Regarding the Cervical Cap

- Fill the dome of the cap up about one third full with spermicide cream or jelly. Do not apply spermicide to the rim, since it may interfere with the seal.
- Wait approximately 30 minutes after insertion before engaging in sexual intercourse to be sure that a seal has formed between the rim and the cervix.
- Leave the cervical cap in place for a minimum of 6 hours after sexual intercourse. It can be left in place for up to 48 hours without additional spermicide being added.
- Do not use during menses due to the potential for toxic shock syndrome. Use an alternative method such as condoms during this time.
- Replace the cervical cap after each year of use.
- Inspect the cervical cap prior to insertion for cracks, holes, or tears.
- After using the cervical cap, wash it with soap and water, dry thoroughly, and store in its container.

Diaphragm Insertion/Removal Technique

- Always empty the bladder prior to inserting the diaphragm.
- Inspect diaphragm for holes or tears by holding it up to a light source, or fill it with water and check for a leak.
- Place approximately a tablespoon of spermicidal jelly or cream in the dome and around the rim of the diaphragm.
- The diaphragm can be inserted up to 6 hours prior to intercourse.
- Select the position that is most comfortable for insertion:
  - Squatting
  - Leg up, raising the nondominant leg up on a low stool
  - Reclining position, lying on back in bed
  - Sitting forward on the edge of a chair
- Hold the diaphragm between the thumb and fingers and compress it to form a "figure-eight" shape.
- Insert the diaphragm into the vagina, directing it downward as far as it will go.
- Tuck the front rim of the diaphragm behind the pubic bone so that the rubber hugs the front wall of the vagina.
- Feel for the cervix through the diaphragm to make sure it is properly placed.
- To remove the diaphragm, insert the finger up and over the top side and move slightly to the side, breaking the suction.
- Pull the diaphragm down and out of the vagina.

Client Teaching and Counseling Regarding the Diaphragm

- Avoid the use of oil-based products, such as baby oil, because they may weaken the rubber.
- Wash the diaphragm with soap and water after use and dry thoroughly.
- Place the diaphragm back into the storage case.
- The diaphragm may need to be refitted after weight loss or gain or childbirth.
- Diaphragms should not be used by women with latex allergies.

Vaginal Ring Insertion/Removal Technique and Counseling

- Each ring is used for one menstrual cycle, which consists of 3 weeks of continuous use followed by a ring-free week to allow for menses.
- No fitting is necessary—one size fits all.
- The ring is compressed and inserted into the vagina, behind the pubic bone, as far back as possible.
- Precision placement is not essential.
- Backup contraception is needed for 7 days if the ring is expelled for more than 3 hours during the 3-week period of continuous use.
- The vaginal ring is left in place for 3 weeks, then removed and discarded.
- The vaginal ring is not recommended for women with uterine prolapse or lack of vaginal muscle tone (Schuiling & Likis, 2016).

Male Condom Insertion/Removal Technique and Counseling

- Always keep the condom in its original package until ready to use.
- Store in a cool, dry place.
- Spermicidal condoms should be used if available.
- Check expiration date before using.

- Use a new condom for each sexual act.
- Condom is placed over the erect penis prior to insertion.
- Place condom on the head of the penis and unroll it down the shaft.
- Leave a half-inch of empty space at the end to collect ejaculate.
- Avoid use of oil-based products, because they may cause breakage.
- After intercourse, remove the condom while the penis is still erect.
- Discard condom after use.

Female Condom Insertion/Removal Technique and Counseling

- Practice wearing and inserting prior to first use with sexual intercourse.
- Condom can be inserted up to 8 hours before intercourse.
- Condom is intended for one-time use.
- It can be purchased over the counter—one size fits all.
- Avoid wearing rings to prevent tears; long fingernails can also cause tears.
- Spermicidal lubricant can be used if desired.
- Insert the inner ring high in the vagina, against the cervix.
- Place the outer ring on the outside of the vagina.
- Make sure the erect penis is placed inside the female condom.
- Remove the condom after intercourse. Avoid spilling the ejaculate.

Education and Counseling of Women Using Injectable Contraceptives

- Consume a diet high in calcium and vitamin D to prevent bone mineral loss
- Know the conditions that need to be reported to the health care provider
  - Significant headaches
  - Menorrhagia
  - Depression
  - Severe abdominal pain
- Awareness of any infection present at injection site

- Obtain written informed consents, which are needed for intrauterine contraceptives, implants, abortion, or sterilization. Informed consent implies that the client is making a knowledgeable, voluntary choice; has received complete information about the method, including the risks; and is free to change her mind before using the method or having the procedure (Schuiling & Likis, 2016).
- Discuss contraindications for all selected contraceptives.
- Consider the client's cultural and religious beliefs when providing care.

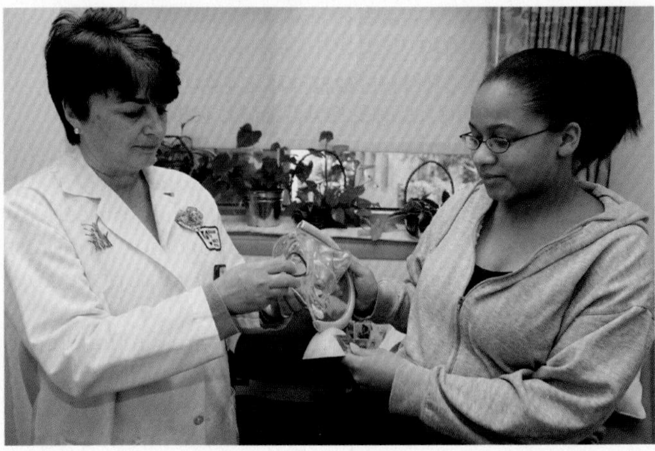

FIGURE 4.21 The nurse demonstrates insertion of a vaginal ring during client teaching.

- Address myths and misperceptions about the methods under consideration in your initial discussion of contraceptives.

It is also important to clear up common misconceptions about contraception and pregnancy. Clearing up misconceptions will permit new learning to take hold and a better client response to whichever methods are explored and ultimately selected. Some common misconceptions include:

- Breast-feeding protects against pregnancy.
- Pregnancy can be avoided if the male partner "pulls out" before he ejaculates.
- Pregnancy cannot occur during menses.
- Douching after sex will prevent pregnancy.
- Pregnancy will not happen during the first sexual experience.
- Taking birth control pills protects against STIs.
- The woman is too old to get pregnant.
- If female orgasm is not reached, conception is not likely.
- Irregular menstruation prevents pregnancy.

When discussing in detail each method of birth control, focus on specific information for each method outlined. Include information such as how this particular method works to prevent pregnancy under normal circumstances of use; the noncontraceptive benefits to overall health; advantages and disadvantages of all methods; the cost involved for each particular method; danger signs that need to be reported to the health care provider; and the required frequency of office visits needed for the particular method.

In addition, outline factors that place the client at risk for method failure. Contraceptives can fail for any of many reasons. Use Table 4.6 to provide client education concerning a few of the reasons for contraceptive failure. Help clients who have chosen abstinence or fertility awareness methods to define the sexual activities in which they do or do not want to participate. This

TABLE 4.6 CONTRACEPTIVE PROBLEMS AND EDUCATIONAL NEEDS

Contraceptive Failure Problem	Client Education Needed
Not following instructions for use of contraceptive correctly	Take pill the same time every day Use condoms properly and check condition before using Make sure diaphragm or cervical cap covers cervix completely Check IUD for placement monthly
Inconsistent use of contraceptive	Contraceptives must be used regularly to achieve maximum effectiveness All it takes is one unprotected act of sexual intercourse to become pregnant Two to 5% of condoms will break or tear during use
Condom broke during sex	Check expiration date Store condoms properly Use only a water-based lubricant Watch for tears caused by long fingernails Use spermicides to decrease possibility of pregnancy Seek emergency postcoital conception
Use of antibiotics or other herbs taken with OCs	Use alternative methods during the antibiotic therapy, plus 7 additional days. Implement on day 1 of taking antibiotics
Belief that you can't get pregnant during menses or that it is safe "just this one-time"	It may be possible to become pregnant on almost any day of the menstrual cycle

helps them set sexual limits or boundaries. Help them to develop communication and negotiation skills that will allow them to be successful. Supporting, encouraging, and respecting a couple's choice of abstinence is vital for nurses.

After clients have chosen a method of contraception, it is important to address the following:

- Emphasize that a second method to use as a backup is always needed.
- Provide both oral and written instructions on the method chosen.
- Discuss the need for STI protection if not using a barrier method.
- Inform the client about the availability of ECs.

Steady progress in contraception research has been achieved over the past several years. Hormonal and nonhormonal contraceptives have improved women's lives by reducing different health conditions that contribute to morbidity. However, the contraceptives available today are not suitable to all users, and the need to expand contraceptive choices still exists. It is hoped that the introduction of newer methods in the near future with additional health benefits will continue to help women and couples meet their family planning needs.

ABORTION

Abortion is defined as the expulsion of an embryo or fetus before it is viable (Alexander, LaRosa, Bader, et al., 2014). Abortion can be a medical or surgical procedure. The purpose of abortion is to terminate a pregnancy. More than 40% of all women will end a pregnancy by abortion at some time in their reproductive lives. Both in the United States and globally, more than one fifth of all known pregnancies end in abortion (McFarlane, 2015). Surgical abortion is the most common procedure performed in the United States (approximately 1.3 million annually) and might be the most common surgical procedure in the world (Alan Guttmacher Institute, 2015b). Both medical and surgical abortions are safe and legal in the United States; an abortion is considered a woman's constitutional right based on the fundamental right to privacy. Eighty-nine percent of abortions occur in the first 12 weeks of pregnancy (Alan Guttmacher Institute, 2015b).

Since the landmark U.S. Supreme Court decision *Roe v. Wade* legalized abortion in 1973, debate has continued over how and when abortions are provided. Every state has laws regulating some aspects of the provision of abortion, and many have passed restrictions such as parental consent or notification requirements, mandated counseling and waiting periods, and limits on funding for abortion. Each state addresses these matters independently, and the laws that are passed or enforced are legislative decisions and a function of the political system. Although opponents of abortion continue to be very much a part of the current debates, recently they have refocused their attention on "regulation legislation" among the states to reduce the number of abortions not medically necessary (Kreitzer, 2015).

Surgical Abortion

Two types of surgical abortion are available: vacuum aspiration or dilation, and evacuation (D&C). Method selection is based on gestational age. It is an ambulatory procedure done under local anesthesia. The cervix is dilated prior to surgery and then the products of conception are removed by suction evacuation. The uterus may gently be scraped by curettage to make sure that it is empty. The entire procedure lasts about 10 minutes. The overall risk of complications is less than 1% for surgical termination (Upadhyay, Desai, Zlidar, et al., 2015). The major risks and complications in the first trimester are infection, retained tissue, or hemorrhage, uterine perforation, retained products of conception, or cervical tear (Udoh, Effa, Oduwole, et al., 2015). For women whose blood is Rh negative, *RhoGAM* is indicated prior to start of either medical or surgical termination.

Medical Abortion

Medical abortions are achieved through administration of medication either vaginally or orally. The administration of medication occurs in the clinic or doctor's office, may require two to four office visits, and costs between $300 and $800 (Planned Parenthood, 2015b). Three drugs are currently used to terminate a pregnancy during the first trimester. The first drug is methotrexate (an antineoplastic agent; Rheumatrex) followed by misoprostol (a prostaglandin agent; Cytotec) given as a vaginal suppository or in oral form 3 to 7 days later. Methotrexate induces abortion because of its toxicity to trophoblastic tissue, the growing embryo. Misoprostol works by causing uterine contractions, which helps to expel the products of conception. This method is 90% to 98% successful in completing an abortion (Patil & Edelman, 2015).

The second drug used to induce first-trimester abortions involves using mifepristone (a progesterone antagonist; Mifeprex, RU-486) followed 48 hours later by misoprostol (a prostaglandin agent), which causes contractions of the uterus and expulsion of the uterine contents. Currently, the most widely used method of medication abortion in the United States is the administration of mifepristone in conjunction with misoprostol. Another frequent method used includes the combination of methotrexate with misoprostol (Schuiling & Likis, 2016). Mifepristone, the generic name for RU-486, is sold under the brand names Mifeprex and Early Option. Mifepristone is an antiprogestin and blocks the action of progesterone, which is necessary for the maintenance of the pregnancy. This method is 95% effective when used within 49 days after the last menstrual cycle (Patil & Edelman, 2015).

Another drug frequently used is misoprostol (Cytotec), which is a prostaglandin analog that softens the cervix and causes uterine contractions, which results in the expulsion of uterine contents. There is no standard protocol for use of misoprostol (Cytotec) alone for termination of early pregnancy, and it is not FDA-approved for this purpose (King et al., 2015). Complications of medical abortions include incomplete expulsion of uterine contents; uterine infection; and heavy bleeding (Ganatra, Guest, & Berer, 2015).

The assessment of the woman with an unintended pregnancy should be performed with cautious sensitivity. It is essential to explore the women's feelings about pregnancy before congratulating or consoling her. The encounter should be guided by the feelings of the client, not by the assumptions and values of the nurse.

Abortion is a very emotional, deeply personal issue. Give support and accurate information. If for personal, religious, or ethical reasons you feel unable to actively participate in the care of a woman undergoing an abortion, you still have the professional responsibility to ensure that the woman receives the nursing care and help she requires. This may necessitate a transfer to another area or a staffing reassignment. Nurses must keep in mind that all women have the right to have access to unbiased, factual information about available reproductive health choices, whether they seek to end or start a pregnancy, from which they can then make informed decisions about their own reproductive health.

MENOPAUSAL TRANSITION

Menopause is a natural process that occurs in all women's lives as part of normal aging. *Meno* is derived from the Greek word for "month," and *pause* is derived from the Greek word for "pause" or "halt." Menopause is the technical term for a point in time at which menses and fertility cease (King et al., 2015). The change of life. The end of fertility. The beginning of freedom. Whatever people call it, menopause is a unique and personal experience for every woman. The term **menopausal transition** refers to the transition from a woman's reproductive phase of her life to her final menstrual period. This period is also referred to as *perimenopause*. It is the end of her menstruation and childbearing capacity. The average age of natural menopause—defined as 1 year without a menstrual period—is 51.4 years old. The average age of natural menopause has remained constant for the last several hundred years despite improvements in nutrition and health care (Alexander et al., 2014). With current female life expectancy at 84 years, this event comes in the middle of a woman's adult life. Many women go through the menopausal transition with few or no symptoms, while some have significant or even disabling symptoms (Kessenich, 2015).

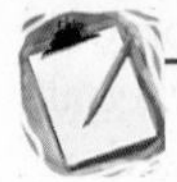

Take Note!

Humans are virtually the only species to outlive their reproductive capacities.

Menopause signals the end of an era for many women. It concludes their ability to reproduce, and some women find advancing age, altered roles, and these physiologic changes to be overwhelming events that may precipitate depression and anxiety (Woods & Mitchell, 2015). Menopause does not happen in isolation. Midlife is often experienced as a time of change and reflection. Change happens in many arenas: children are leaving or returning home, employment pressures intensify as career moves or decisions are required, older adult parents require more care or the death of a parent may have a major impact, and partners are retrenching or undergoing their own midlife crises. Women must negotiate all these changes in addition to menopause. Managing these stressful changes can be very challenging for many women as they make the transition into midlife.

A woman is born with approximately 2 million ova, but only about 400 ever mature fully to be released during the menstrual cycle. The absolute number of ova in the ovary is a major determinant of fertility. Over the course of her premenopausal life there is a steady decline in the number of immature ova (Wood, 2015). No one understands this depletion, but it does not occur in isolation. Maturing ova are surrounded by follicles that produce two major hormones: estrogen, in the form of estradiol, and progesterone. The cyclic maturation of the ovum is directed by the hypothalamus. The hypothalamus triggers a cascade of neurohormones, which act through the pituitary and the ovaries as a pulse generator for reproduction. This hypothalamic–pituitary–ovarian axis begins to break down long before there is any sign that menopause is imminent. Some scientists believe that the pulse generator in the hypothalamus simply degenerates; others speculate that the ovary becomes more resistant to the pituitary hormone FSH and simply shuts down (Schuiling & Likis, 2016). The final act in this well-orchestrated process is amenorrhea.

As menopause approaches, more and more of the menstrual cycles become anovulatory. This period of time, usually 2 to 8 years before cessation of menstruation, is termed *perimenopause* (McNamara, Batur, & DeSapri, 2015). In perimenopause, the ovaries begin to fail, producing irregular and missed periods and an occasional hot flash. When menopause finally appears, viable ova are gone. Estrogen levels plummet by 90%, and estrone, produced in fat cells, replaces estradiol as the body's main form of estrogen. The major hormone produced by the ovaries during the reproductive years is estradiol; the estrogen found in postmenopausal women is estrone. Estradiol is much more biologically active than estrone (Hoyt & Falconi, 2015). In addition, testosterone levels decrease with menopause.

Menopausal transition, with its dramatic decline in estrogen, affects not only the reproductive organs, but also other body systems:

- Brain: hot flashes, disturbed sleep, mood and memory problems
- Cardiovascular: lower levels of HDL and increased risk of CVD
- Skeletal: rapid loss of bone density that increases the risk of osteoporosis
- Breasts: replacement of duct and glandular tissues by fat
- Genitourinary: vaginal dryness, stress incontinence, cystitis
- Gastrointestinal: less absorption of calcium from food, increasing the risk for fractures
- Integumentary: dry, thin skin and decreased collagen levels
- Body shape: more abdominal fat; waist size that swells relative to hips

Therapeutic Management

Menopausal transition should be managed individually. In the past, despite the wide diversity of symptoms and risks, the traditional reaction was to reach for the one-size-fits-all therapy: hormone therapy. Today the medical community is changing its thinking in light of the Women's Health Initiative (WHI) study and the Heart and Estrogen/Progestin Replacement Study Follow-Up (HERS II), which reported that long-term hormone therapy (HT) increased the risks of heart attacks, strokes, and breast cancer; in short, the overall health risks of HT exceeded the benefits (Kyvernitakis, Kostev, Hars, et al., 2015). In addition, HT did not protect against the development of coronary artery disease (CAD), nor did it prevent the progression of CAD, as it was previously touted to do.

A recent research finding examined the timing of HT in relation to CAD in women and it found that the earlier initiation of HT was associated with less CAD in women with natural but not surgical menopause. A Cochrane Review study found that hormone therapy in postmenopausal women overall, had little benefit in CAD prevention, but caused an increase in the risk of stroke and venous thromboembolic events (Boardman Hartley, Eisinga, et al., 2015). As expected, the fallout from this study and others forced practitioners to reevaluate their usual therapies and tailor treatment to each client's history, needs, and risk factors. A current study, however, shows that the incidence of fractures among menopausal transition and postmenopausal women increased significantly in the 3 years after publication of the WHI and HERS II results. This trend followed a decline in the use of hormone therapy, concurrent with an increase in the use of other bone-modifying agents (Bakour & Williamson, 2015). There is considerable evidence that estrogen or hormone therapy reduces the risk of postmenopausal osteoporotic fracture of both the spine and hip (Mirkin, Archer, Pickar, et al., 2015).

A number of treatment options are available, but factors in the client's history should be the driving force when determining therapy. Women need to educate themselves about the latest research findings and collaborate with their health care provider on the right menopause therapy. The following factors should be considered in management:

- The risk/benefit ratio is highest in younger women who begin HT not long after menopause.
- HT is approved for two indications: relief of vasomotor symptoms and prevention of osteoporosis.
- Research suggests that HT may be beneficial for preventing diabetes, improving mood, or avoiding urinary tract problems.
- Using HT long beyond menopause carries increased risks, which, for some women, may be outweighed by the benefits (Bakour & Williamson, 2015).

Many women consider nonhormonal therapies such as bisphosphonates and selective estrogen receptor modulators (SERMs). Consider weight-bearing exercises, calcium, vitamin D, smoking cessation, and avoidance of alcohol to treat or prevent osteoporosis. Annual breast examinations and mammograms are essential. Local estrogen creams can be used for vaginal atrophy. Consider herbal therapies for symptoms, although none have been validated by rigorous research studies (Ismail, Taylor-Swanson, Thomas, et al., 2015).

ACOG recently revised guidelines on treating menopausal symptoms. Their recommendations include systemic HT, with estrogen or estrogen plus progestin, which is the most effective approach for treating vasomotor symptoms; the lowest effective dose for the shortest duration is the best regimen; thromboembolic disease and breast cancer are risks for combined systemic HT; and local estrogen therapy is advised for isolated atrophic vaginal symptoms (2014).

Although numerous symptoms have been attributed to menopause (Box 4.9), some of them are more closely related to the aging process than to estrogen deficiency. A few of the more common menopausal conditions and their management are discussed next.

BOX 4.9

COMMON SYMPTOMS OF MENOPAUSE

- Hot flashes or flushes of the head and neck
- Dryness in the eyes and vagina
- Personality changes
- Anxiety and/or depression
- Loss of libido
- Decreased lubrication
- Weight gain and water retention
- Night sweats
- Atrophic changes—loss of elasticity of vaginal tissues
- Fatigue
- Irritability
- Poor self-esteem
- Insomnia
- Stress incontinence
- Heart palpitations

Adapted from Coney, P. (2015) Menopause. *eMedicine.* Retrieved from http://emedicine.medscape.com/article/264088-overview; Kessenich, C. R. (2015). Inevitable menopause. *Nursing Spectrum.* Retrieved from http://ce.nurse.com/ce232-60/Inevitable-Menopause; Schuiling, K. D., & Likis, F. E. (2016) *Women's gynecologic health* (3rd ed.). Burlington, MA: Jones & Bartlett Learning.

Managing Hot Flashes and Night Sweats

The emergence of hot flashes and night sweats (also known as vasomotor symptoms) coincides with a period in life that is also marked by dynamic changes in hormone and reproductive function that interconnect with the aging process, changes in metabolism, lifestyle behaviors, and overall health (Wood, 2015). Hot flashes and night sweats are classic signs of estrogen deficiency and the predominant complaint of perimenopausal women. A hot flash is a transient and sudden sensation of warmth that spreads over the body, particularly the neck, face, and chest. Hot flashes are caused by vasomotor instability. This instability causes inappropriate peripheral vasodilation of superficial blood vessels, which gives the sensation of heat. Nearly 85% of menopausal women experience them (Alexander et al., 2014). Hot flashes are an early and acute sign of estrogen deficiency. These flashes can be mild or extreme and can last from 2 to 30 minutes and may occur as frequently as every hour to several times per week. On average, women experience hot flashes for a period of 6 months to 2 years, but the symptoms may last up to 10 years or more. Severe vasomotor symptoms can have a significant and detrimental effect on quality of life. Factors that trigger vasomotor symptoms include caffeine and alcohol consumption, intake of hot drinks and spicy foods, hot environment, depression, stress and anxiety (Avis, Crawford, Greendale, et al., 2015).

Many options are available for treating hot flashes. Treatment must be based on symptom severity, the client's medical history, and the client's values and concerns. Although the gold standard in the treatment of hot flashes is estrogen, this is not recommended for all women who have high risk factors in their history.

TRADITIONAL THERAPIES FOR THE MANAGEMENT OF HOT FLASHES

The following are traditional therapies for the management of hot flashes:

- Pharmacologic options
- HT unless contraindicated
- Androgen therapy (potentiates estrogen)
- Estrogen and androgen combinations
- Progestin therapy (Depo-Provera injection every 3 months)
- Clonidine (central alpha-adrenergic agonist) weekly patch
- Neurontin (antiseizure) decreased hot flashes
- Propranolol (beta-adrenergic blocker)
- Brisdelle: FDA-approved nonhormonal medication
- Short-term sleep aids: Ambien, Dalmane
- Gabapentin (Neurontin): antiseizure drug

- SSRIs: venlafaxine (Effexor) and paroxetine (Paxil) have shown promise (King & Brucker, 2016).

COMPLEMENTARY AND ALTERNATIVE THERAPIES FOR MANAGEMENT OF HOT FLASHES

Many women are choosing alternative treatments for managing menopausal symptoms. Bioidentical hormones have the ability to bind to receptors in the human body and function in the same way as a woman's natural hormones. They simulate three estrogens (estradiol, estriol, and estrone), as well as progesterone, testosterone, dehydroepiandrosterone (DHEA), thyroxine, and cortisol. Bioidentical hormones are not, however, natural hormones. The estrogens are derived via a chemical process from soybeans (*Glycine max*) and progesterone from Mexican yam (*dioscorea villosa*). As with conventional hormones, however, bioidentical hormones are available only with a physician's prescription and through a pharmacy. Because of their natural origin, women perceive that alternative treatments are safer. The interest in phytoestrogens came about because of the low prevalence of hot flashes in Asian women, which was attributed to their diet being rich in phytoestrogens. Recent studies have found that black cohosh, multibotanical herbs, and increased soy intake do not reduce the frequency or severity of menopausal hot flashes or night sweats.

Other remedies for easing menopausal symptoms might include red clover, motherwort, ginseng, sarsaparilla root, valerian root, L-tryptophan, calcium-magnesium, and kelp tablets (Ismail et al., 2015). Again, research thus far has been skeptical about their efficacy, but many women report they ease their symptoms and their use has skyrocketed. Although some benefits may accrue from their use, evidence of the efficacy of alternative products in menopause is largely anecdotal. Small, preliminary clinical trials might demonstrate the safety of some of the nonpharmacologic products. Nurses should be aware of the purported action of these agents as well as any adverse effects or drug interactions.

The following are lifestyle changes and CAM therapies for the treatment of hot flashes:

- Lifestyle changes
- Lower room temperature; use fans.
- Wear clothing in layers for easy removal.
- Limit caffeine and alcohol intake.
- Drink 8 to 10 glasses of water daily.
- Stop smoking or cut back.
- Avoid hot drinks and spicy food.
- Take calcium (1,200 to 1,600 mg) and vitamin D (400 to 600 International Units).
- Exercise daily, but not just before bedtime.
- Maintain a healthy weight.
- Identify stressors and learn to manage them.
- Keep a diary to identify triggers of hot flashes.
- Phytoestrogens: isoflavones, ligands, coumetrols
- Black cohosh
- Chamomile: mild sedative to alleviate insomnia
- Unopposed transdermal progesterone
- Compounded bioidentical hormones
- Try relaxation techniques, deep breathing, and meditation
- Acupuncture may reduce the frequency of hot flashes
- Vitamin E: 100 mg daily
- DHEA
- Chaste tree berry (vitex): balances progesterone and estrogen
- Dong quai: acts as a form of phytoestrogen
- Ginseng: purported to improve memory
- St. John's wort: reduces depression and fatigue
- Wild yam: treats menopausal symptoms
- Valerian root: induces sleep and relaxation (Wood, 2015).

Managing Urogenital Changes

Menopausal transition can be a physically and emotionally challenging time for women. In addition to the psychological burden of leaving behind the reproductive phase of life and the stigma of an aging body, sexual difficulties resulting from urogenital changes plague most women but are frequently not addressed. Sexual desire is affected by endocrine and psychosocial factors. Menopausal hormonal changes are relevant to the causes of sexual dysfunction during reproductive aging. The frequency of sexual intercourse declines as women enter midlife. Whereas partner availability and function probably play a role, menopausal symptoms, such as vaginal dryness, are also present (Comhaire & Depypere, 2015).

Vaginal atrophy occurs during menopause because of declining estrogen levels. These changes include thinning of the vaginal walls, an increase in pH, irritation, increased susceptibility to infection, **dyspareunia** (difficult or painful sexual intercourse), loss of lubrication with intercourse, vaginal dryness, and a decrease in sexual desire related to these changes. Decreased estrogen levels can also influence a woman's sexual function as well. Delayed clitoral reaction, decreased vaginal lubrication, diminished circulatory response during sexual stimulation, and reduced contractions during orgasm have all been linked to low estrogen levels (Coney, 2015).

Management of these changes might include the use of estrogen vaginal tablets (Vagifem) or Premarin cream; Estring, an estrogen-releasing vaginal ring that lasts for months; testosterone patches; and over-the-counter moisturizers and lubricants (Astroglide) (King et al., 2015). A positive outlook on sexuality and a supportive partner are also needed to make the sexual experience enjoyable and fulfilling. Nurses can improve the sexual health and quality of life in menopausal women by educating them about their symptoms and offering them choices about managing them.

Take Note!

Sexual health is an important aspect of the human experience. By keeping an open mind, listening to women, and providing evidence-based treatment options, the nurse can help improve quality of life for menopausal women.

Preventing and Managing Osteoporosis

Osteoporosis has been recognized as a significant worldwide public health problem. As the world's population ages, both in the United States and internationally, the prevalence of osteoporosis is expected to increase significantly. **Osteoporosis** is the state of diminished bone density. This disorder is a systemic skeletal disease characterized by low bone mass and microarchitectural deterioration of bone tissue with a consequent increase in bone fragility and susceptibility to fracture (National Osteoporosis Foundation [NOF], 2015a).

According to recent information from NOF (2015a), osteoporosis is a major medical problem that affects 10 million women and 2 million men in the United States. An additional 34 million Americans have low bone mass. Each year, an estimated 1.5 million individuals in the United States experience a fragility fracture secondary to osteoporosis, resulting in an annual cost of $18 billion. By 2025, experts predict that osteoporosis will be responsible for approximately 3 million fractures and $26 billion in costs each year (NOF, 2015a). With the rapidly aging population, the problem of osteoporosis is now reaching epidemic proportions. Seventy-five million baby boomers are entering the stage in their lives when they are most at risk for osteoporosis. One half of all women and one third of all men will sustain a fragility fracture during their lifetimes. Osteoporosis continues to be underdiagnosed and undertreated because it is often not recognized until the first fracture occurs.

Women are greatly affected by osteoporosis after menopause. Osteoporosis is a condition in which bone mass declines to such an extent that fractures occur with minimal trauma. Bone loss begins in the third or fourth decade of a woman's life and accelerates rapidly after menopause (Alexander et al., 2014). This condition puts many women into long-term care, with a resulting loss of independence. Figure 4.22 shows the skeletal changes associated with osteoporosis.

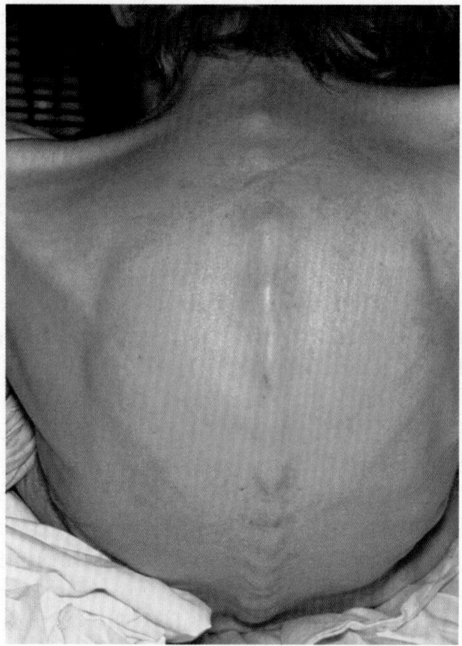

FIGURE 4.22 Skeletal changes associated with osteoporosis. (John Radcliffe Hospital/Photo Researcher Inc.)

Most women with osteoporosis do not know they have the disease until they sustain a fracture, usually of the wrist or hip. Risk factors include:

- Increasing age
- Postmenopausal status without hormone replacement
- Small, thin-boned frame
- Low BMD
- White or Asian with small bone frame
- Impaired eyesight that would increase risk of falling
- Rheumatoid arthritis
- Family history of osteoporosis
- Sedentary lifestyle
- History of treatment with:
  - Antacids with aluminum
  - Heparin
  - Long-term use of steroids >3 months
  - Thyroid replacement drugs
- Smoking and consuming alcohol
- Low calcium and vitamin D intake
- Excessive amounts of caffeine
- Personal history of nontraumatic fracture
- Anorexia nervosa or bulimia (NOF, 2015a)

Currently, no method exists for directly measuring bone mass. Instead a BMD measurement is used. BMD is a two-dimensional measurement of the average content of mineral in a section of bone. BMD evaluations are made at the hip, femoral neck, and spine. There is a significant relationship between BMD and fracture: as BMD is reduced, the risk of fracture increases (Sullivan, Lehman, Thomas, et al., 2015). Screening tests to measure bone density are not good predictors for young women who might be at risk for developing this condition. Dual-energy x-ray absorptiometry (DXA or DEXA) is a screening test that calculates the mineral content of the bone at the spine and hip. It is highly accurate, fast, and relatively inexpensive. The dual-energy x-ray absorptiometry scan (DEXA scan) is the gold standard radiologic method for identifying osteoporosis through measuring BMD (U.S. Preventive Services Task Force, 2015).

Hip fracture is the most devastating of the fragility fractures secondary to osteoporosis. A number of medical, social, and economic consequences follow a hip fracture. Of women older than 50 years, on average, 24% die within the first year after hip fracture (Wang, Chen, Cheng, et al., 2015). The concern surrounding osteoporosis is not the rate of fracture alone but also the potential for lifelong disability secondary to fracture. The incidence of hip fracture is estimated to double by the year 2025 and nearly double again by 2050. For women, this is a projected 240% increase (NOF, 2015a).

The best management for this painful, crippling, and potentially fatal disease is prevention.

Women can modify many risk factors by doing the following:

- Engage in daily weight-bearing exercise, such as walking to increase osteoblast activity.
- Increase calcium and vitamin D intake.
- Avoid smoking and excessive alcohol (more than two drinks per day).
- Discuss bone health with a health care provider.
- When appropriate, have a bone density test and take medication if needed (NOF, 2015b).

Medications that can help in preventing and managing osteoporosis include:

- HT (Premarin)
- SERMs (raloxifene [Evista])
- Calcium and vitamin D supplements (Tums)
- Estrogen agonist/antagonist (SERM) (Evista)
- Bisphosphonates (Actonel, Fosamax, Boniva, or Reclast)
- Parathyroid hormone (Forteo)
- Calcitonin (Miacalcin) (King & Brucker, 2016).

Preventing and Managing Cardiovascular Disease

Despite the dramatic decrease in annual CVD mortality and total cardiovascular mortality for American women each year since 2000, CVD remains the number-one killer of women, accounting for 1 in 3 deaths in the United States. This is likely due to increased rates of obesity, sedentary lifestyle, diabetes, and high cholesterol levels (Chomistek, Chiuve, Eliassen, et al., 2015). More women die from heart disease and stroke than the next five causes of death combined, including breast cancer. Half a million women die annually in the United States of CVD, with strokes accounting for about 20% of the deaths (Alexander et al., 2014). This translates into approximately one death every minute. While men's mortality from CVD has decreased since the 1980s, women's mortality from CVD has climbed. This has resulted in a sex-related CVD mortality gap, with women having higher mortality than men since 1984. Contributing to this female-majority CVD mortality gap is a lack of awareness among women and their physicians of the risk for CVD. Awareness campaigns, such as the Heart Truth and the Red Dress symbol, appear to have improved recognition of CVD risk in women. Further, female-specific guidelines have been developed to prevent and reduce CVD in women. Though the current understanding of the role of menopause in CVD is controversial, studies suggest that menopause does not exacerbate CVD independent of aging, and HT is not effective for secondary prevention of CVD (Hale & Shufelt, 2015).

For the first half of a woman's life, estrogen seems to be a protective substance for the cardiovascular system by smoothing, relaxing, and dilating blood vessels. It even helps boost HDL and lower HDL levels, helping to keep the arteries clean from plaque accumulation. But when estrogen levels plummet as women age and experience menopause, the incidence of CVD increases dramatically. Women are more likely to have atypical cardiovascular symptoms compared with men. This may lead to a delayed or misdiagnosis of CAD and suboptimal treatment. These symptoms may include:

- A—Angina (chest pain)
- B—Breathlessness
- C—Chronic fatigue
- D—Dizziness
- E—Edema of hands and feet
- F—Fluttering of the heart
- G—Gastric upset
- H—Heavy pain in back and shoulders

Menopause is not the only factor that increases a woman's risk for CVD. Lifestyle and medical history factors such as the following play a major role:

- Smoking
- Obesity
- High-fat diet
- Sedentary lifestyle
- High cholesterol levels
- Family history of CVD
- Hypertension
- Apple-shaped body
- Diabetes

Two of the major risk factors for coronary heart disease are hypertension and dyslipidemia. Both are modifiable and can be prevented by lifestyle changes and, if needed, controlled by medication. This is why prevention is essential. In addition, women who experience early menopause lose the protection afforded by endogenous estrogen to the cardiac system and are at greater risk for more extensive atherosclerosis. Major preventive strategies include a healthy diet, increased activity, exercise, smoking cessation, decreased alcohol intake, and weight reduction.

Nurses, particularly those caring for women during their reproductive years, are uniquely positioned to provide education and support for women's long-term cardiovascular health. Raising awareness of heart disease in women is an essential role for nurses. The good news is that CVD is largely preventable. Because CVD is a chronic disease that develops over time, primary prevention lifestyle modification interventions are most effective if initiated before the development of overt disease. Stressing the importance of lifestyle modifications must begin early in life and should be reinforced from the beginning of a young woman's reproductive years through menopause (CDC, 2015b). Nurses are in an ideal position to teach the importance of good nutrition, healthy weight, and daily exercise before CVD becomes clinically evident.

Nursing Assessment

Menopausal transition is a universal and irreversible part of the overall aging process involving a woman's reproductive system. Although not a disease state, menopausal transition does place women at greater risk for the development of many conditions of aging. Nurses can help the woman become aware of her risk for postmenopausal diseases, as well as strategies to prevent them. The nurse can be instrumental in assessing risk factors and planning interventions in collaboration with the client. These might include:

- Screening for osteoporosis, CVD, and cancer risk:
  - Assessment of blood pressure to identify hypertension
  - Blood cholesterol test to identify hyperlipidemia risk
  - Mammogram to find a cancerous lesion
  - Pap smear to identify cervical cancer
  - Pelvic examination to identify endometrial cancer or masses
  - Digital rectal examination to assess for colon cancer
  - Bone density testing as a baseline at menopause to identify osteopenia (low bone mass), which might lead to osteoporosis
- Assessing lifestyle to plan strategies to prevent chronic conditions:
  - Dietary intake of fat, cholesterol, and sodium
  - Weight management
  - Calcium intake
  - Use of tobacco, alcohol, and caffeine
  - Amount and type of daily exercise routines

Nursing Management

There is no "magic bullet" in managing menopause. Nurses can counsel women about their risks and help them to prevent disease and debilitating conditions with specific health maintenance education. Women should make their own decisions, but the nurse should make sure they are armed with the facts to do so intelligently. Nurses can offer a thorough explanation of the menopausal process, including the latest research findings, to help women understand and make decisions about this inevitable event.

If the woman decides to use HT to control her menopausal symptoms, after being thoroughly educated, she will need frequent reassessment. There are no hard-and-fast rules that apply to meeting a woman's individual needs. The nurse can provide realistic expectations of the therapy to reduce the woman's anxiety and concern.

It is also useful to emphasize the value of friends to gain support and share information and resources. Often just talking about emotional difficulties such as the death of a parent or problematic relationships helps solve problems. It also shows the woman that her emotional responses are valid.

Healthy lifestyles and stress management techniques are vital to health and longevity, and it is important to keep these on the client's agenda when discussing menopause (North American Menopause Society, 2015). Evidence-based interventions include lifestyle modifications, risk management therapies, and preventive drug interventions, such as the following:

- Participate actively in maintaining health.
- Exercise regularly to prevent CVD and osteoporosis.
- Take supplemental calcium and eat appropriately to prevent osteoporosis.
- Stop smoking to prevent lung and heart disease.
- Reduce caffeine and alcohol intake to prevent osteoporosis.
- Monitor blood pressure, lipids, and diabetes (drug therapy management).
- Use low-dose aspirin to prevent blood clots.
- Reduce dietary intake of fat, cholesterol, and sodium to prevent CVD.
- Maintain a healthy weight for body frame.
- Perform breast self-examinations for breast awareness.
- Control stress to prevent depression (Worel & Hayman, 2015; Houseman & Odum, 2016).

These life approaches may seem low-tech, but they can stave off menopause-related complications such as CVD, osteoporosis, and depression. These tips for healthy living work well, but the client needs to be motivated to stick with them.

NURSING CARE PLAN 4.1

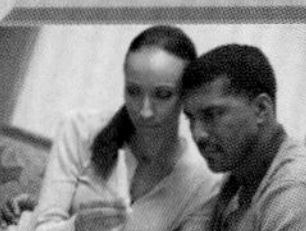

Overview of a Woman with Abnormal Uterine Bleeding

Stacy, a 52-year-old obese woman, comes to her gynecologist with the complaint of heavy erratic bleeding. Her periods were fairly regular until about 4 months ago, and since that time they have been unpredictable, excessive, and prolonged. Stacy reports she is tired all the time, can't sleep, and feels "out of sorts" and anxious. She is fearful she has cancer.

NURSING DIAGNOSIS: Fear related to current signs and symptoms possibly indicating a life-threatening condition

Outcome Identification and Evaluation

The client will acknowledge her fears as evidenced by statements made that fear and anxiety have been lessened after explanation of diagnosis.

Interventions: ***Reducing Fear and Anxiety***

- Distinguish between anxiety and fear to determine appropriate interventions.
- Check complete blood count and assess for possible anemia secondary to excessive bleeding to determine if fatigue is contributing to anxiety and fear. Fatigue occurs because the oxygen-carrying capacity of the blood is reduced.
- Reassure client that symptoms can be managed to help address her current concerns.
- Provide client with factual information and explain what to expect to assist client with identifying fears and help her to cope with her condition.
- Provide symptom management to reduce concerns associated with the cause of bleeding.
- Teach client about early manifestations of fear and anxiety to aid in prompt recognition and to minimize escalation of anxiety.
- Assess client's use of coping strategies in the past and reinforce use of effective ones to help control anxiety and fear.
- Instruct client in relaxation methods, such as deep-breathing exercises and imagery, to provide her with additional methods for controlling anxiety and fear.

NURSING DIAGNOSIS: Deficient knowledge related to menopausal transition and its management

Outcome Identification and Evaluation

The client will demonstrate understanding of her symptoms as evidenced by making health-promoting lifestyle choices, verbalizing appropriate health care practices, and adhering to measures and complying with therapy.

Interventions: ***Providing Client Education***

- Assess client's understanding of menopausal transition and its treatment to provide a baseline for teaching and developing a plan of care.
- Review instructions about prescribed procedures and recommendations for self-care, frequently obtaining feedback from the client to validate adequate understanding of information.
- Outline link between anovulatory cycles and excessive buildup of uterine lining in menopausal transition women to assist client in understanding the etiology of her bleeding.
- Provide written material with pictures to promote learning and help client visualize what is occurring to her body during menopausal transition.
- Inform client about the availability of community resources and make appropriate referrals as needed to provide additional education and support.
- Document details of teaching and learning to allow for continuity of care and further education, if needed.

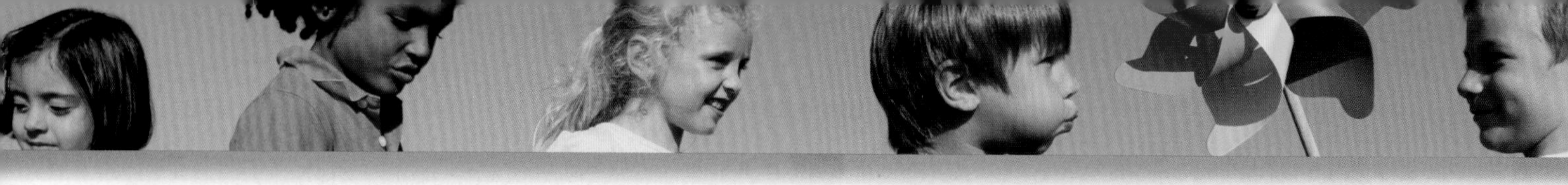

KEY CONCEPTS

- Establishing good health habits and avoiding risky behaviors early in life will prevent chronic conditions later in life.
- PMS has more than 150 symptoms, and at least two different syndromes have been recognized: PMS and PMDD.
- Endometriosis is a condition in which bits of functioning endometrial tissue are located outside their normal site, the uterine cavity.
- Infertility is a widespread problem that has an emotional, social, and economic impact on couples.
- More than half of all unintended pregnancies occur in women who report using some method of birth control during the month of conception.
- Hormonal methods include OCs, injectables, implants, vaginal rings, and transdermal patches.
- Recent studies have shown that the extension of active extended cycle OC pills carries the same safety profile as the conventional 28-day regimens (Shoupe, 2016).
- Currently three intrauterine contraceptives are available in the United States: the copper ParaGard-TCu-380A, the LNG-IUS marketed as Mirena, and another LNG-IUD marketed as Skyla (King et al., 2015).
- OCs, sterilization, and male condoms are the most popular methods of contraception in the United States and worldwide (Alan Guttmacher Institute, 2015a).
- Menopause, with a dramatic decline in estrogen levels, affects not only the reproductive organs but also other body systems.
- Most women with osteoporosis do not know they have the disease until they sustain a fracture, usually of the wrist or hip (NOF, 2015a).
- Half a million women die annually in the United States of CVDs, with strokes accounting for about 20% of the deaths (Alexander et al., 2014).
- Nurses should aim to have a holistic approach to the sexual health of women from menarche through menopause.

REFERENCES AND RECOMMENDED READINGS

Alan Guttmacher Institute. (2015a). Facts on contraceptive use. Retrieved from http://www.guttmacher.org/pubs/fb_contr_use.html

Alan Guttmacher Institute (2015b). Facts on induced abortion in the United States. Retrieved from http://www.guttmacher.org/pubs/fb_induced_abortion.html

Alexander, L. L., LaRosa, J. H., Bader, H., & Garfield, S. (2014). *New dimensions in women's health* (6th ed.). Sudbury, MA: Jones & Bartlett.

American Academy of Allergy, Asthma and Immunology [AAAAI]. (2015). Latex allergy: Tips to remember. Retrieved from http://www.aaaai.org/conditions-and-treatments/library/allergy-library/latex-allergy.aspx

American College of Obstetricians & Gynecologists [ACOG]. (2014a) ACOG Practice bulletin no. 133: benefits and risks of sterilization. (2013). *Obstetrics and Gynecology, 121*(2 Pt 1), 392–404.

American College of Obstetricians & Gynecologists [ACOG]. (2014b) Practice Bulletin #114: Management of menopausal symptoms. *Obstetrics & Gynecology, 123*(1), 202–216.

American College of Obstetricians & Gynecologists [ACOG]. (2015a) *Dysmenorrhea: Painful periods*. Retrieved from https://www.acog.org/-/media/For-Patients/faq046.pdf?dmc=1&ts=20150312T1116116502

American College of Obstetricians & Gynecologists [ACOG]. (2015b) *Management of acute abnormal uterine bleeding with ovarian dysfunction*. Retrieved from http://contemporaryobgyn.modernmedicine.com/contemporary-obgyn/content/tags/abnormal-uterine-bleeding/acog-guidelines-glance-bulletin-aub-o-much?page=full

American College of Obstetricians & Gynecologists [ACOG]. (2015c). *Premenstrual syndrome*. Retrieved from http://www.acog.org/Search.aspx?Keyword=PMS

American College of Obstetricians & Gynecologists [ACOG]. (2015d) *Dysmenorrhea: Painful periods*. FAQ046. Retrieved from www.acog.org/~/media/For Patients/faq046.ashx

American Society for Reproductive Medicine [ASRM]. (2015). Frequently asked questions about infertility. Retrieved from http://www.asrm.org/Patients/faqs.html

Ataollahi, M., Akbari, S. A., Mojab, F., & Alavi Majd, H. (2015). The effect of wheat germ extract on premenstrual syndrome symptoms. *Iranian Journal of Pharmaceutical Research: IJPR, 14*(1), 159–166.

Atkin, K., Beal, M. W., Long-Middleton, E., & Roncari, D. (2015). Long-acting reversible contraceptives for teenagers: Primary care recommendations. *The Nurse Practitioner, 40*(3), 38–46.

Avis, N. E., Crawford, S. L., Greendale, G., Bromberger, J. T., Everson-Rose, S. A., Gold, E. B., et al. (2015). Duration of menopausal vasomotor symptoms over the menopause transition. *JAMA Internal Medicine, 175*(4), 531–539.

Bakour, S. H., & Williamson, J. (2015). Latest evidence on using hormone replacement therapy in the menopause. *Obstetrician & Gynecologist, 17*(1), 20–28.

Bieber, E. J., Sanfilippo, J. S., Horowitz, I. R., & Shafi, M. I. (2015). *Clinical gynecology* (2nd ed.), Cambridge, UK: Cambridge University Press.

Bitzer, J., Heikinheimo, O., Nelson, A. L., Calaf-Alsina, J., & Fraser, I. S. (2015). Medical management of heavy menstrual bleeding: A comprehensive review of the literature. *Obstetrical & Gynecological Survey, 70*(2), 115–130.

Black, D. M., & Rosen, C. J. (2016). Postmenopausal osteoporosis. *New England Journal of Medicine,* 374: 254–262. doi: 10.1056/NEJMcp1513724

Boardman, H. M., Hartley, L., Eisinga, A., Main, C., Roqué i Figuls, M., Bonfill Cosp, X., et al. (2015) Hormone therapy for preventing cardiovascular disease in post-menopausal women. *Cochrane Database of Systematic Reviews, 3,* CD002229.

Boyd, K., Perkins, P., Lawrence, K., Sutherland, J., & Blake, K. (2015). The female condom: Knowledge, image, and power. *Journal of Black Sexuality and Relationships, 1*(3), 97–112.

Brown, J., & Farquhar, C. (2015). An overview of treatments for endometriosis. *JAMA, 313*(3), 296–297.

Calis, K. A., Popat, V., Dang, D. K., & Kalantaridou, S. N. (2015). Dysmenorrhea. *eMedicine.* Retrieved from http://emedicine.medscape.com/article/253812-overview

Carlson, J. L. (2015). The menstrual cycle. In C. M. Gordon & Meryl LeBoff (Eds.), *The Female Athlete Triad: A Clinical Guide* (pp. 29–38). Philadelphia, PA: Springer Publishers.

Casey, F., & Isaacs, C. (2015). Are we getting the word out about emergency contraception? *Contemporary OB/GYN, 60*(2), 18–19.

Cavallini, G. (2015). General therapeutic approach to male infertility. In G. Cavallini & G. Beretta (Eds.), *Clinical Management of Male Infertility* (pp. 33–39). Switzerland: Springer International Publishing.

Centers for Disease Control and Prevention [CDC]. (2015a). *Contraceptive use.* National Center for Health Statistics. Retrieved from http://www.cdc.gov/women/natstat/reprhlth.htm#contraception

Centers for Disease Control and Prevention [CDC]. (2015b). *Healthy eating for a healthy weight.* Retrieved from http://www.cdc.gov/healthyweight/healthy_eating/

Cheng, S. C., & Van Leuven, K. A. (2015). Intrauterine contraception and the facts for college health. *The Journal for Nurse Practitioners, 11*(4), 417–423.

Chomistek, A. K., Chiuve, S. E., Eliassen, A. H., Mukamal, K. J., Willett, W. C., & Rimm, E. B. (2015). Healthy lifestyle in the primordial prevention of cardiovascular disease among young women. *Journal of the American College of Cardiology, 65*(1), 43–51.

Comhaire, F. H., & Depypere, H. T. (2015). Hormones, herbal preparations and nutraceuticals for a better life after the menopause: part I. *Climacteric: The Journal of the International Menopause Society,* 1–6.

Coney, P. (2015) Menopause. *eMedicine.* Retrieved from http://emedicine.medscape.com/article/264088-overview

Craik, J., & Rowlands, S. (2015). Contraceptive devices for women: Implants, intrauterine devices and other products. In *Medicines for women* (pp. 227–270). Switzerland: Springer International Publishing.

Craik, J., & Melvin, L. (2015). Oral contraceptives: Benefits and risks. In M. Harrison-Woolrych (Ed.), *Medicines for women* (pp. 141–180). Switzerland: Springer International Publishing.

Creatsas, G. K. (2015). Prevention of adolescent pregnancies. In A. R. Genazzani & M. Brincat (Eds.), *Frontiers in Gynecological Endocrinology* (pp. 41–45). Switzerland: Springer International Publishing.

Creatsas, G. K., & Creatsa, M. (2015). Disorders of the menstrual cycle during adolescence. In A. R. Genazzani & M. Brincat (Eds.), *Frontiers in Gynecological Endocrinology* (pp. 3–9). Switzerland: Springer International Publishing.

Dadhich, P., Ramasamy, R., & Lipshultz, L. I. (2015). The male infertility office visit. *The Italian Journal of Urology and Nephrology.* Retrieved from http://europepmc.org/abstract/med/25604696

Dohle, G. R. (2015). Male factors in couple's infertility. In V. Mirone (Ed.), *Clinical uro-andrology* (pp. 197–201). Berlin, Heidelberg: Springer Publishers.

Dombo, E. A., & Flood, M. (2015). Spirituality infertility counseling. *Fertility counseling, 11,* (pp.74–85), Cambridge, UK: Cambridge University Press.

Elnashar, A. (2015). Emerging treatment of endometriosis. *Middle East Fertility Society Journal.* doi:10.1016/j.mefs.2014.12.002. Retrieved from http://www.sciencedirect.com/science/article/pii/S1110569014200562

Evans, G., & Sutton, E. L. (2015). Oral contraception. *Medical Clinics of North America, 99*(3), 479–503.

Everett, S. (2014) *Handbook of contraception and sexual health* (3rd ed.). New York, NY: Routledge

Foster, D. G., Biggs, M. A., Phillips, K. A., Grindlay, K., & Grossman, D. (2015). Potential public sector cost-savings from over-the-counter access to oral contraceptives. *Contraception.* doi:http://dx.doi.org/10.1016/j.contraception.2015.01.010

Ganatra, B., Guest, P., & Berer, M. (2015). Expanding access to medical abortion: Challenges and opportunities. *Reproductive Health Matters, 22*(44), 1–3.

Golden, N. H., Katzman, D. K., Sawyer, S. M., Ornstein, R. M., Rome, E. S., Garber, A. K., et al. (2015). Update on the medical management of eating disorders in adolescents. *Journal of Adolescent Health, 56*(4), 370–375.

Goswami, D. (2015). Primary ovarian insufficiency: The paradox of menopause in young women. *MAMC Journal of Medical Sciences, 1*(1), 3.

Haddad, L. B., Philpott-Jones, S., & Schonfeld, T. (2015). Contraception and prevention of HIV transmission: a potential conflict of public health principles. *Journal of Family Planning and Reproductive Health Care, 41*(1), 20–23.

Hale, G. E., & Shufelt, C. L. (2015). Hormone therapy in menopause: An update on cardiovascular disease considerations. *Trends in Cardiovascular Medicine, 25*(6):540–549.

Hemingway, A. P., & Trew, G. H. (2015). Hysterosalpingography. In *Female genital tract congenital malformations* (pp. 49–61). London: Springer Publishers.

Housman, J., & Odum, M. (2016). *Alters & Schiff's essential concepts for healthy living* (7th ed.). Burlington, MA: Jones & Bartlett Learning.

Hoyt, L. T., & Falconi, A. (2015). Puberty and perimenopause: Reproductive transitions and their implications for women's health. *Social Science & Medicine, 132,* 103–112.

Htay, T. T. (2015). Premenstrual dysphoric disorder. *eMedicine.* Retrieved from http://emedicine.medscape.com/article/293257-overview

Hughes, H. (2015). Postpartum contraception. *Journal of Family Health Care, 19*(1), 9–10.

Ilic, K. (2015). Emergency contraception. In M. Harrison-Woolrych (Ed.), *Medicines for Women* (pp. 203–225). Switzerland: Springer International Publishing. doi: 10.1007/978-3-319-12406-3_1

Inhorn, M. C., & Patrizio, P. (2015). Infertility around the globe: New thinking on gender, reproductive technologies and global movements in the 21st century. *Human Reproduction Update*, dmv016. doi:10.1093/humupd/dmv016

Ismail, R., Taylor-Swanson, L., Thomas, A., Schnall, J. G., Cray, L., Mitchell, E. S., et al. (2015). Effects of herbal preparations on symptom clusters during the menopausal transition. *Climacteric, 18*(1), 11–28.

Jick, S. (2015). Oral contraceptives and the risk of venous thromboembolism. In M. Harrison-Woolrych *Medicines for Women* (pp. 181–201). Switzerland: Springer International Publishing.

Jin, J. (2015). JAMA patient page. Treatments for infertility. *Journal of the American Medical Association, 313*(3), 320.

Johnston, J. L., Reid, H., & Hunter, D. (2015). Diagnosing endometriosis in primary care: Clinical update. *British Journal of General Practice, 65*(631), 101–102.

Joshi, T., Kural, M. R., Agrawal, D. P., Noor, N. N., & Patil, A. (2015). Primary dysmenorrheaand its effect on quality of life in young girls. *International Journal of Medical Science and Public Health, 4*(3), 381–385.

Kapoor, D. W., Alderman, E., Hiraoka, M. K., & Davila, G. W. (2015). Endometriosis. *eMedicine*. Retrieved from http://emedicine.medscape.com/article/271899-overview

Khan, A. B., & Krupanidhi, C. S.. (2015). A review on vaginal drug delivery system. *RGUHS Journal of Pharmaceutical Sciences, 4*(4), 142–147.

Kessenich, C. R. (2015). Inevitable menopause. *Nursing Spectrum*. Retrieved from http://ce.nurse.com/ce232–60/Inevitable-Menopause

Kho, C. L., & Mathur, M. (2015). Uterine artery embolization for acute dysfunctional uterine bleeding with failed medical therapy: A novel approach to management. *BMJ Case Reports,* doi:10.1136/bcr-2014-204446

Kim, J. S. (2015) Latex allergy. In H. A. Sampson (Ed.), *Allergy and Clinical Immunology* (pp. 288–293), Chichester, UK: John Wiley & Sons.

King, T. L., & Brucker, M. C. (2016) *Pharmacology for women's health* (2nd ed.). Sudbury, MA: Jones & Bartlett Learning.

King, T. L., Brucker, M. C., Kriebs, J. M., Fahey, J. O., Gegor, C. L., & Varney, H. (2015) *Varney's midwifery* (5th ed.). Burlington, MA: Jones & Bartlett Learning.

Kodaman, P. H. (2015). Current strategies for endometriosis management. *Obstetrics and Gynecology Clinics of North America, 42*(1), 87–101.

Kovanci, E., & Schutt, A. K. (2015). Premature ovarian failure: Clinical presentation and treatment. *Obstetrics and Gynecology Clinics of North America, 42*(1), 153–161.

Kreitzer, R. J. (2015). Politics and morality in state abortion policy. *State Politics & Policy Quarterly, 15*(1), 41–66. doi:10.1177/1532440014561868

Krieger, N., Kiang, M. V., Kosheleva, A., Waterman, P. D., Chen, J. T., & Beckfield, J. (2015). Age at menarche: 50-year socioeconomic trends among US-born Black and White women. *American Journal of Public Health, 105*(2), 388–397.

Kyvernitakis, I., Kostev, K., Hars, O., Albert, U., & Hadji, P. (2015). Discontinuation rates of menopausal hormone therapy among postmenopausal women in the post-WHI Study ERA. *Climacteric: The Journal of the International Menopause Society*, 1–22.

Maurice, J. M., & Rosenzweig, B. A. (2015). Acute gynecologic pelvic pain. In *Common surgical diseases* (pp. 319–322). New York, NY: Springer Publishers.

McFarland, M. R., & Wehbe-Alamah, H. B. (2015). *Leininger's cultural care diversity and universality: A worldwide nursing theory.* (3rd ed.). Burlington, MA: Jones & Bartlett Learning.

McFarlane, D. R. (2015). *Global population and reproductive health*. Burlington, MA: Jones & Bartlett Learning.

McKay, R., & Schunmann, C. (2015). Male and female sterilization. *Obstetrics, Gynecology & Reproductive Medicine*. doi:http://dx.doi.org/10.1016/j.ogrm.2015.02.004

McNamara, M., Batur, P., & DeSapri, K. T. (2015). In the clinic. Perimenopause. *Annals of Internal Medicine, 162*(3), ITC1–ITC15.

Mirkin, S., Archer, D. F., Pickar, J. H., & Komm, B. S. (2015). Recent advances help understand and improve the safety of menopausal therapies. *Menopause (10723714), 22*(3), 351–360.

Moses, S. (2015a) Primary amenorrhea. *Family Practice Notebook.* Retrieved from http://www.fpnotebook.com/gyn/Menses/PrmryAmnrh.htm

Moses, S. (2015b) Female Tanner stage. *Family Practice Notebook.* Retrieved from http://www.fpnotebook.com/endo/exam/fmltnrstg.htm

Moses, S. (2015c) Contraceptive sponge. *Family Practice Notebook.* Retrieved from http://www.fpnotebook.com/gyn/contraception/CntrcptvSpng.htm

Mulligan, K. (2015). Access to emergency contraception and its impact on fertility and sexual behavior. *Health Economics*, doi:10.1002/hec.3163

Naeimi, N. (2015). The prevalence and symptoms of premenstrual syndrome under examination. *Journal of Biosciences and Medicines, 3*, 1–8. doi:10.4236/jbm.2015.31001

National Institute of Child Health and Human Development [NICHD]. (2015). Endometriosis (NIH Pub. No. 02-2413). Retrieved from http://www.nichd.nih.gov/publications/pubs/endometriosis

National Osteoporosis Foundation [NOF]. (2015a). Osteoporosis: Fast facts. Retrieved from http://www.nof.org/osteoporosis/diseasefacts.htm

National Osteoporosis Foundation [NOF]. (2015b). Steps to prevent osteoporosis. Retrieved from http://www.nof.org/prevention/index.htm

Nelson, A. L. (2015). Transdermal contraception methods: Today's patches and new options on the horizon. *Expert Opinion on Pharmacotherapy, 16*(6), 863–873.

North American Menopause Society. (2015). *Staying healthy at menopause and beyond*. Retrieved from http://www.menopause.org/for-women/menopauseflashes/staying-healthy-at-menopause-and-beyond

Occupational Health and Safety Administration. (2015). *Latex allergy*. Retrieved from http://www.osha.gov/SLTC/latexallergy

Pagana, K. D., & Pagana, T. J., & Pagana, T. N. (2015). *Mosby's diagnostic and laboratory test reference* (12th ed.). St. Louis, MO: Elsevier Mosby.

Patil, E., & Edelman, A. (2015). Medical abortion: Use of mifepristone and misoprostol in first and second trimesters of pregnancy. *Current Obstetrics and Gynecology Reports*, 1–10.

Pearlstein, T. (2015) Depressive disorders: Premenstrual dysphoric disorder. In *Psychiatry* (4th ed.). Chichester, UK: John Wiley & Sons.

Planned Parenthood (2015a) *Fertility awareness-based methods.* Retrieved from http://www.plannedparenthood.org/health-topics/birth-control/fertility-awareness-4217.htm

Planned Parenthood (2015b) *The abortion pill.* Retrieved from http://m.plannedparenthood.org/mt/www.plannedparenthood.org/health-topics/abortion/abortion-pill-medication-abortion-4354.asp

Planned Parenthood. (2016). *Cervical cap (FemCap).* Retrieved from https://www.plannedparenthood.org/learn/birth-control/cervical-cap

Pocius, K. D., & Dutton, C. R. (2015). Update on hormonal contraception and obesity. *Current Obstetrics and Gynecology Reports, 4*, 61–68.

Puscheck, E. E., & Woodward, T. L. (2015). Infertility. *eMedicine.* Retrieved from http://emedicine.medscape.com/article/274143-overview

Raymond, E. G., & Cleland, K. (2015). Emergency contraception. *New England Journal of Medicine, 372*(14), 1342–1348.

RESOLVE (National Infertility Association). (2015). What is infertility? Retrieved from http://www.resolve.org/infertility-overview/what-is-infertility

Samra-Latif, O. M., & Wood, E. (2015). Contraception. *eMedicine.* Retrieved from http://emedicine.medscape.com/article/258507-overview

Santamaría, M., & Lago, I. (2015). Premenstrual experience premenstrual syndrome and dysphoric disorder. In M. Saenz-Herrero (Ed.), *Psychopathology in Women* (pp. 423–449). Switzerland: Springer International Publishing.

Schuiling, K. D. & Likis, F. E. (2016). *Women's gynecologic health.* (4th ed.). Burlington, MA: Jones & Bartlett Learning.

Schwartz, J. L., Weiner, D. H., Lai, J. J., Frezieres, R. G., Creinin, M. D., Archer, D. F., et al. (2015). Contraceptive efficacy, safety, fit, and acceptability of a single-size diaphragm developed with end-user input. *Obstetrics & Gynecology, 125*(4), 895–903.

Senie, R. T. (2014). *Epidemiology of Women's Health.* Burlington, MA: Jones & Bartlett Learning.

Sharma, M., & Walmsley, S. (2015), Contraceptive options for HIV-positive women: Making evidence-based, patient-centered decisions. *HIV Medicine.* doi:10.1111/hiv.12221

Shoupe, D., & Mishell, D. R. (2016). *The handbook of contraception: A guide for practical management.* (2nd ed), Switzerland: Springer International Publishing.

Signorile, P. G., & Baldi, A. (2015). New evidence in endometriosis. *The International Journal of Biochemistry & Cell Biology, 60*, 19–22.

Skidmore-Roth, L. (2015). *Mosby's 2015 nursing drug reference* (28th ed.). St. Louis, MO: Elsevier Mosby.

Smith, R. P., & Kaunitz, A. M. (2015). Treatment of primary dysmenorrhea in adult women. *UpToDate.* Retrieved from http://www.uptodate.com/contents/treatment-of-primary-dysmenorrhea-in-adult-women

Stanford, J. B. (2015) Revisiting the fertile window. *Fertility and Sterility*, Available online March 2015. doi:10.1016/j.fertnstert.2015.02.015

Stewart, M., & Black, K. (2015). Choosing a combined oral contraceptive pill. *Australian Prescriber, 38*(1), 6–11.

Sullivan, S. D., Lehman, A., Thomas, F., Johnson, K. C., Jackson, R., Wactawski-Wende, J., et al. (2015). Effects of self-reported age at nonsurgical menopause on time to first fracture and bone mineral density in the Women's Health Initiative Observational Study. *Menopause (New York, N.Y.), 22*(10):1035–1044.

Tacani, P. M., Ribeiro, D. O., Barros Guimarães, B. E., Machado, A. P., & Tacani, R. E. (2015). Characterization of symptoms and edema distribution in premenstrual syndrome. *International Journal of Women's Health, 7*, 7297–7303.

Tharpe, N. L., Farley, C. L., & Jordan, R. G. (2016). *Clinical practice guidelines for midwifery & women's health* (5th ed.). Burlington, MA: Jones & Bartlett Learning.

Tremellen, K., & Pearce, K. (2015). *Nutrition, fertility, and human reproductive function.* Boca Raton, FL: CRC Press Taylor & Francis Group.

Thurkow, A. L. (2015). Hysteroscopic sterilization. In *Minimally invasive gynecological surgery* (pp. 49–59). Berlin, Heidelberg: Springer.

Turchi, P. (2015). Prevalence, definition, and classification of infertility. In G. Cavallini & G. Beretta *Clinical management of male infertility* (pp. 5–11). Switzerland: Springer International Publishing.

Udoh, A., Effa, E. E., Oduwole, O., Okusanya, B. O., Okafo, O., & Iya, J. (2015) Antibiotics for treating septic abortion. *Cochrane Database of Systematic Reviews* 2015, *2*, CD011528.

UNFPA. (2015). The state of the world population 2014 report. Retrieved from http://www.unfpa.org/swp#ref_state-of-world-population-2014

Upadhyay, U. D., Desai, S., Zlidar, V., Weitz, T. A., Grossman, D., Anderson, P., et al. (2015). Incidence of emergency department visits and complications after abortion. *Obstetrics & Gynecology, 125*(1), 175–183.

U.S. Selected Practice Recommendations for Contraceptive Use, 2013. (2014). *MMWR Recommendations & Reports, 62*(5), 1–61.

Wang, Q., Chen, D., Cheng, S. M., Nicholson, P., Alen, M., & Cheng, S. (2015). Growth and aging of proximal femoral bone: a study with women spanning three generations. *Journal of Bone and Mineral Research: The Official Journal of the American Society for Bone and Mineral Research, 30*(3), 528–534.

Walsh, S., Ismaili, E., Naheed, B., & O'Brien, S. (2015). Diagnosis, pathophysiology and management of premenstrual syndrome. *The Obstetrician & Gynaecologist.* doi:10.1111/tog.12180

Weinberger, A. H., Smith, P. H., Allen, S. S., Cosgrove, K. P., Saladin, M. E., Gray, K. M., et al. (2015). Systematic and meta-analytic review of research examining the impact of menstrual cycle phase and ovarian hormones on smoking and cessation. *Nicotine & Tobacco Research, 17*(4), 407–421.

Whitaker, T. (2015). Vasectomy. In A. L. Halverson & D. C. Borgstrom (Eds.), *Advanced Surgical Techniques for Rural Surgeons* (pp. 251–254). New York, NY: Springer.

Whitman, M. (2015). Patient education: What worries the patient most? *Nursing2015; 45*(1), 52–54.

Wicks, S. M., & Mahady, G. B. (2015). Herbal and complementary medicines used for women's health. In M. Harrison-Woolrych (Ed.),*Medicines for women* (pp. 373–399). Switzerland: Springer International Publishing.

Wildemeersch, D., & Jandi, S. (2015). Intrauterine device quo vadis? Why intrauterine device use should be revisited particularly in nulliparous women? *Open Access Journal of Contraception, 6*, 1–12.

Wolfe, K., & Cansino, C. (2015). Injectable contraception: Current practices and future trends. *Current Obstetrics and Gynecology Reports, 4*(1), 26–36.

Wood, D. (2015). Inevitable menopause. *Nurse.Com Nursing Spectrum (Philadelphia Tri-State), 24*(3), 26–31.

Woods, N. F., & Mitchell, E. S. (2015). The menopausal transition and women's health. In M. A. Farage, K. W. Miller, N. F. Woods, & H. I. Maibach (Eds.), *Skin, Mucosa and Menopause: Management of Clinical Issues* (pp. 433–452). Berlin, Heidelberg: Springer.

Worel, J. N., & Hayman, L. L. (2015). Cardiovascular disease prevention in women: Reducing the major threat to women's health. *Journal of Cardiovascular Nursing, 30*(1), 5–7.

World Health Organization [WHO]. (2015). Infertility in developing countries. Reproductive health. Retrieved from http://www.who.int/reproductive-health/infertility/index.htm

Wright, K., Iqteit, H., & Hardee, K. (2015). Standard Days Method of contraception: Evidence on use, implementation, and scale-up. *Working paper.* Washington, DC: Population Council, The Evidence Project.

Ying, L. Y., & Loke, A. Y. (2015). An analysis of the concept of partnership in the couples undergoing infertility treatment. *Journal of Sex & Marital Therapy*. doi:10.1080/0092623X.2015.1010676

Zieman, M. (2015). *Managing contraception on the go* (13th ed.), New York, NY: Ardnet Media.

Zorbas, K. A., Economopoulos, K. P., & Vlahos, N. F. (2015). Continuous versus cyclic oral contraceptives for the treatment of endometriosis: a systematic review. *Archives of Gynecology and Obstetrics*, 1–7. doi:10.1007/s00404-015-3641-1

CHAPTER WORKSHEET

MULTIPLE-CHOICE QUESTIONS

1. A couple is considered infertile after how many months of trying to conceive?
   a. 6 months
   b. 12 months
   c. 18 months
   d. 24 months

2. A couple reports that their condom broke while they were having sexual intercourse last night. What would you advise to prevent pregnancy?
   a. Inject a spermicidal agent into the woman's vagina immediately.
   b. Obtain emergency contraceptives and take them immediately.
   c. Douche with a solution of vinegar and hot water tonight.
   d. Take a strong laxative now and again at bedtime.

3. Which of the following combination contraceptives has been approved for extended continuous use?
   a. Seasonale
   b. Triphasil
   c. Ortho Evra
   d. Mirena

4. Which of the following measures helps prevent osteoporosis?
   a. Supplementing with iron
   b. Sleeping 8 hours nightly
   c. Eating lean meats only
   d. Walking daily

5. Which of the following activities will increase a woman's risk of cardiovascular disease if she is taking oral contraceptives?
   a. Eating a high-fiber diet
   b. Smoking cigarettes
   c. Taking daily multivitamins
   d. Drinking alcohol

6. The nurse is preparing to teach a class to a group of middle-aged women regarding the most common vasomotor symptoms experienced during menopause and possible modalities of treatment available. Which of the following would be a vasomotor symptom experienced by menopausal women?
   a. Weight gain
   b. Bone density
   c. Hot flashes
   d. Heart disease

7. Throughout life, a woman's most proactive activity to promote her health would be to engage in:
   a. Consistent exercise
   b. Socialization with friends
   c. Quality quiet time with herself
   d. Consuming water

8. What comment by a woman would indicate that a diaphragm is not the best contraceptive device for her?
   a. "My husband says it is my job to keep from getting pregnant."
   b. "I have a hard time remembering to take my vitamins daily."
   c. "Hormones cause cancer and I don't want to take them."
   d. "I am not comfortable touching myself down there."

9. The most common cause of menstrual abnormality in a reproductive–age woman is:
   a. Ectopic pregnancy
   b. Coagulopathy
   c. Carcinoma
   d. Anovulation

The correct response is "D" because abnormal uterine bleeding typically occurs when menstrual ovulation doesn't occur within the monthly cycle. Chronic anovulation causes a variety of abnormal bleeding patterns. Response "A" is incorrect because amenorrhea would be present secondary to the pregnancy, although misplaced. Response "B" is incorrect because other symptoms would be present due to a coagulation problem systemically. Response "C" is incorrect since most uterine cancers occur in postmenopausal women, not reproductive–aged women.

CRITICAL THINKING EXERCISE

1. Ms. London, age 25, comes to your family planning clinic requesting to have an intrauterine contraceptive (IUC) inserted because "birth control pills give you cancer." In reviewing her history, you note she has been into the STI clinic three times in the past year with vaginal infections and was hospitalized for PID last month. When you question her about her sexual history, she reports having sex with multiple partners and not always using protection.
   a. Is an IUC the most appropriate method for her? Why or why not?
   b. What myths/misperceptions will you address in your counseling session?
   c. Outline the safer sex discussion you plan to have with her.

CHAPTER WORKSHEET

STUDY ACTIVITIES

1. Develop a teaching plan for an adolescent with premenstrual syndrome and dysmenorrhea.
2. Arrange to shadow a nurse working in family planning for the morning. What questions does the nurse ask to ascertain the kind of family planning method that is right for each woman? What teaching goes along with each method? What follow-up care is needed? Share your findings with your classmates during a clinical conference.
3. Surf the Internet and locate three resources for infertile couples to consult that provide support and resources.
4. Sterilization is the most prevalent method of contraception used by married couples in the United States. Contact a local urologist and gynecologist to learn about the procedure involved and the cost of a male and female sterilization. Which procedure poses less risk to the person and costs less?
5. Take a field trip to a local drugstore to check out the variety and costs of male and female condoms. How many different brands did you find? What was the range of costs?
6. Noncontraceptive benefits of combined oral contraceptives include which of the following? Select all that apply.
   a. Protection against ovarian cancer
   b. Protection against endometrial cancer
   c. Protection against breast cancer
   d. Reduction in incidence of ectopic pregnancy
   e. Prevention of functional ovarian cysts
   f. Reduction in deep venous thrombosis
   g. Reduction in the risk of colorectal cancer

BRINGING IT ALL TOGETHER: A CASE STUDY

L.H. is a 66-year-old White female who presents to the Women's Health Primary Care Clinic for her annual gynecologic examination. She states that she is fairly healthy with no active medical conditions other than hypertension controlled with medication. She is postmenopausal and feels she is doing well, but has a few questions and concerns. Her primary concern is that she is bothered by vaginal dryness and pain with sexual intercourse. Over-the-counter lubricants and moisturizers have not been useful. She never took HT since her hot flashes were not severe, but asks if she should start taking it now to reduce her vaginal dryness.

ASSESSMENT

L.H.'s family history includes an aunt who had breast cancer at the age of 60 and her mother who died of a heart attack at the age of 71. L.H. is a nonsmoker and drinks a glass of wine at dinner daily. Her last DXA bone scan indicated osteopenia and her pelvic examination demonstrated extensive atrophic changes in her vulvovaginal tissue. Her vital signs were within normal range; her weight was 125; her height was 5 feet 2 inches tall. She states she seemed to be taller previously as her slacks seem to be too long and she needs to hem them now.

1. What is this woman's chief complaint today? What is the etiology of it?
2. Any concerns about this woman's history or her family history?
3. Based on her height and weight, is there a health concern here?

L.H. has significant vulvovaginal atrophy that is not responding to OTC lubricants and is not likely to improve with anything other than estrogen therapy. She has an unfavorable family history of cancer and cardiovascular disease. Her bone density results indicate osteoporosis.

PLAN

1. What health issues should the nurse address with this woman after her examination?
2. What health promotion measures are needed to reduce her risk of osteoporosis?
3. What medications might be prescribed for this woman?
4. When would you have this woman return for follow-up care?

The nurse should discuss vaginal estrogen products such as vaginal cream, tablets, and the vaginal ring to address L.H.'s vaginal atrophy. It should be up to the client to decide which form of estrogen she is comfortable with. These therapies provide local, vaginal effects, not systemic effects, which may place her at risk based on her family history.

To build or maintain bone health, the nurse should encourage her to take 1,200 to 1,600 mg of calcium and 600 to 1,000 IU of vitamin D, through diet and/or supplements. She should also be instructed to walk daily with a gradual increase in distance.

L.H. is also a candidate for osteoporosis pharmacotherapy. The risks and benefits should be discussed. The initial drug prescribed might be a bisphosphonate. An annual return appointment is needed with a repeat DXA in 2 years to monitor her response to therapy.

5

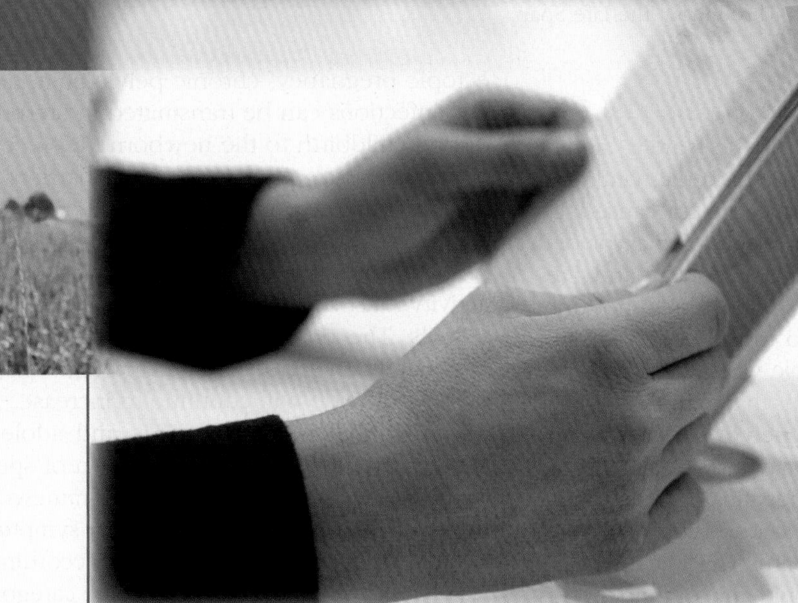

Words of Wisdom
Unconditional self-acceptance in clients is the core to reducing risky behavior and fostering peace of mind.

Sexually Transmitted Infections

KEY TERMS
bacterial vaginosis
cervicitis
chlamydia
genital/vulvovaginal candidiasis
gonorrhea
pelvic inflammatory disease (PID)
sexually transmitted infection (STI)
syphilis
trichomoniasis
vaginitis

Learning Objectives

Upon completion of the chapter, you will be able to:

1. Evaluate the spread and control of sexually transmitted infections.
2. Identify risk factors and outline appropriate client education needed in common sexually transmitted infections.
3. Describe how contraceptives can play a role in the prevention of sexually transmitted infections.
4. Analyze the physiologic and psychological aspects of sexually transmitted infections.
5. Outline the nursing management needed for women with sexually transmitted infections.

***Sandy*, a 19-year-old, couldn't imagine what these "things" were that appeared "down there" in her genital area last week. She was too embarrassed to tell anyone, so she stopped by the college health service today to find out what they were.**

INTRODUCTION

Sexually transmitted infections (STIs) are a significant global health challenge. STIs are bacterial, viral, and parasitic infections of the reproductive tract caused by microorganisms transmitted through vaginal, anal, or oral sexual intercourse (Centers for Disease Control and Prevention [CDC], 2014a). STIs pose a serious threat not only to women's sexual health, but also to the general health and well-being of millions of people worldwide. STIs are responsible for genital tract infections that may lead to later complications in women such as **pelvic inflammatory disease (PID)** or infertility. They may also cause chronic liver diseases and cancer due to hepatitis B virus (HBV) and hepatitis C virus (HCV) infections: genital cancer associated with human papillomavirus (HPV), and AIDS caused by HIV. STIs constitute an epidemic of tremendous magnitude globally with approximately 500 million new cases of curable STIs each year. An estimated 65 million people live with an incurable STI, and another 20 million are infected each year in the United States. STIs cost the U.S. health care system $17 billion annually (CDC, 2014b), and their incidence continues to rise.

STIs are biologically sexist, presenting greater risk and causing more complications among women than among men. Women are diagnosed with two thirds of the estimated 19 million new cases of STIs annually in the United States. After only a single exposure, women are twice as likely as men to acquire infections from pathogens causing **gonorrhea**, **chlamydia** infection, hepatitis B, HPV, and **syphilis** (Oyelowo & Johnson, 2016). STIs may contribute to cervical cancer, infertility, ectopic pregnancy, chronic pelvic pain, and death. Certain infections can be transmitted in utero to the fetus or during childbirth to the newborn (Table 5.1). STIs know no class, racial, ethnic, or social barriers—all individuals are vulnerable if exposed to the infectious organism. Safer-sex practices that include limiting the number of sexual partners and using latex condoms during sexual activity must be recommended to all sexually active individuals. The problem of STIs has still not been tackled adequately on a global scale, and until this is done, numbers worldwide will continue to increase.

A special section on STIs and adolescents is presented next, followed by discussion of specific STIs categorized according to the CDC framework. The CDC groups STIs according to the major symptom manifested (Box 5.1). The CDC classifies STIs according to their clinical symptoms – See Box 5.1 for the categories. A section on preventing STIs is included at the end of the chapter.

SEXUALLY TRANSMITTED INFECTIONS AND ADOLESCENTS

Individuals aged 15 to 24 years represent almost half of all cases of new STIs acquired (CDC, 2014b). Today, 4 in 10 sexually active teen girls have an STI that can cause infertility and even death. Adolescent males make up more than three fourths of HIV diagnosis among 13- to 19-year-olds (U.S. Department of Health and Human Services Office of Adolescent Health, 2015). In the United States, teens who are sexually active experience high rates of STIs, and some groups are at higher risk, including African American, American Indian/Alaska Native,

TABLE 5.1 EFFECTS OF SEXUALLY TRANSMITTED INFECTIONS ON THE FETUS OR NEWBORN

STI	Effects on Fetus or Newborn
Chlamydia	Newborn can be infected during delivery Eye infections (neonatal conjunctivitis), pneumonia, low birth weight, increased risk of premature rupture of the membranes (PROM), preterm birth, and stillbirth
Gonorrhea	Newborn can be infected during delivery. Increased risk of miscarriage, PROM, and preterm birth Rhinitis, vaginitis, urethritis, inflammation of sites of fetal monitoring Gonococcal ophthalmia neonatorum can lead to blindness and sepsis (including arthritis and meningitis)
Herpes type II (genital herpes)	Contamination can occur during birth. Newborn may develop skin or mouth sores Mental retardation, premature birth, low birth weight, blindness, death
Syphilis	Can be passed in utero Can result in fetal or infant death Congenital syphilis symptoms include skin ulcers, rashes, fever, weakened or hoarse cry, swollen liver and spleen, jaundice and anemia, various deformations
Trichomoniasis	Low birth weight, increased risk of PROM, and preterm birth
Venereal warts	May develop warts in throat (laryngeal papillomatosis); uncommon but life-threatening

Adapted from March of Dimes. (2015). *Your top STD questions answered.* Retrieved http://newsmomsneed.marchofdimes.org/?tag=stis

BOX 5.1

CDC CLASSIFICATION OF STIS

- Infections characterized by vaginal discharge
  - Vulvovaginal candidiasis
  - Trichomoniasis
  - Bacterial vaginosis
- Infections characterized by cervicitis
  - Chlamydia
  - Gonorrhea
- Infections characterized by genital ulcers
  - Genital herpes simplex
  - Syphilis
- Pelvic inflammatory disease (PID)
- Human immunodeficiency virus (HIV)
- Human papillomavirus infection (HPV)
- Vaccine-preventable STIs
  - Hepatitis A
  - Hepatitis B
- Ectoparasitic infections
- Pediculosis pubis
- Scabies

and Hispanic youths, youths living in poverty, and those with limited educational attainment (CDC, 2015m).

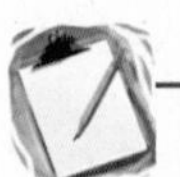

Take Note!

It is estimated that before graduating from high school, 25% of adolescents will contract an STI (Guttmacher Institute, 2014).

Biologic, social, and behavioral factors place teenagers at high risk. Female adolescents are more susceptible to STIs due to their anatomy. During adolescence and young adulthood, women's columnar epithelial cells are especially sensitive to invasion by sexually transmitted organisms, such as chlamydia and gonococci, because they extend out over the vaginal surface of the cervix, where they are unprotected by cervical mucus; these cells recede to a more protected location as women age. Social factors such as poverty, lack of education, social inequality, and limited access to health care services impact the prevalence of STIs in this high-risk population. Adolescent females may perceive that they have limited power over when and where intercourse occurs with their partners. They typically lack negotiating skills and self-confidence needed to successfully negotiate for safer sex practices and thus are exposed to STIs (Petrova & Garcia-Retamero, 2015).

Behaviorally, adolescents and young adults tend to think they are invincible and deny the risks of their behavior. This risky behavior exposes them to STIs and HIV/AIDS. Adolescents frequently have unprotected intercourse, they engage in partnerships of limited duration, and they face many obstacles that prevent them from using the health care system (CDC, 2015o) (*Healthy People 2020*).

Nursing Assessment

Many health care providers fail to assess adolescent sexual behavior and STI risks, to screen for asymptomatic infection during clinic visits, or to counsel adolescents on STI risk reduction. Nurses need to remember that they play a key role in the detection, prevention, and treatment of STIs in adolescents. All states allow adolescents to give consent to confidential STI testing and treatment. Table 5.2 discusses clinical manifestations of common STIs in adolescents.

(text continues on page 182)

***HEALTHY PEOPLE** 2020*

Objective	Significance
Reduce the proportion of adolescents and young adults with *Chlamydia trachomatis* infections.	Provide confidential care to all adolescents.
Reduce gonorrhea.	Assess for sexual behaviors and STI risks during clinic visits; take every opportunity to educate the risks of STIs and risk reduction.
Reduce sustained domestic transmission of primary and secondary syphilis.	Be direct and nonjudgmental and tailor your approach to the client.
(Developmental) Reduce the proportion of females with human papillomavirus (HPV) infection.	Encourage adolescents to postpone initiation of sexual intercourse for as long as possible. For teens who have already had sexual intercourse, encourage abstinence at this point.
Reduce the proportion of young adults with genital herpes infection due to herpes simplex type 2 virus	Encourage adolescents to minimize their lifetime number of sexual partners.
Increase the proportion of sexually active persons aged 15–19 yrs who use condoms to both effectively prevent pregnancy and provide barrier protection against disease.	Educate about the importance of correct and consistent condom use.

Source: U.S. Department of Health and Human Services (2015). *Healthy People 2020*. Retrieved from http://www.healthypeople.gov/2020/topics-objectives

TABLE 5.2 SEXUALLY TRANSMITTED INFECTIONS COMMON IN ADOLESCENTS

Disease	Causative Organism	Transmission Mode	Diagnostic Testing and Recommended Screening for Sexually Active Adolescent
Chlamydia Curable STI Seen frequently among sexually active adolescents and young adults	*Chlamydia trachomatis* (bacteria)	Vaginal, anal, and oral sex and by childbirth	Culture fluid from urethral swabs in males or endocervical swabs for females Noninvasive, non–culture-based testing is available using nucleic acid amplification and testing (NAAT) from urine—single test can test for chlamydia and gonorrhea Conjunctival secretions in neonates Females: screen annually Males: screen high-risk adolescents
Gonorrhea Curable STI Adolescent often coinfected with *Chlamydia trachomatis*	*Neisseria gonorrhoeae* (bacteria)	Vaginal, anal, and oral sex and by childbirth	Gram stain or culture directly for the bacterium or same noninvasive, non–culture-based test, NAAT, as chlamydia Females: screen annually Male: screen high-risk adolescents
Herpes type 2 (genital herpes) Lifelong recurrent viral disease Most people have not been diagnosed There is no cure	Herpes simplex virus 1 and 2 (HSV-1 and HSV-2)	HSV-1 is spread through oral secretions; can be spread to genitals through poor handwashing of infected person or oral-genital contact HSV-2 is spread by having sexual contact (vaginal, oral, or anal) with someone who is shedding the herpes virus either during an outbreak or during a period with no symptoms; can be spread to an infant through childbirth	Visual inspection and symptoms or culture from swabs taken from lesions (success depends stage of lesion—optimum is during vesicular stage) Polymerase chain reaction is more sensitive than culture Serologic tests, such as antibody-based testing (herpes Western blot assay is the most sensitive) Type specific laboratory testing important Routine screening not recommended

Female Symptoms	Male Symptoms	Recommended Treatment
May be asymptomatic Dysuria, urinary frequency. dyspareunia Cervical discharge (mucus or pus) Endocervicitis May lead to pelvic inflammatory disease, ectopic pregnancy, infertility Can cause inflammation of the rectum and conjunctiva Can infect the throat from oral sexual contact with an infected partner	May be asymptomatic Dysuria, urethral itching Penile discharge (mucus or pus) Urethral tingling May lead to epididymitis and sterility Can cause inflammation of the rectum and conjunctiva Can infect the throat from oral sexual contact with an infected partner	Azithromycin (Zithromax) Doxycycline (Vibramycin) Erythromycin (EES) Levofloxacin Ofloxacin (Floxin) Sexual partners need evaluation, testing, and treatment also Abstinence from sexual activity until therapy complete and symptoms no longer present Retesting in 3 months to rule out recurrence
May be asymptomatic or no recognizable symptoms until serious complications such as pelvic inflammatory disease Dysuria Urinary frequency Vaginal discharge (yellow and foul) Dyspareunia Endocervicitis Arthritis May lead to pelvic inflammatory disease, ectopic pregnancy, infertility Symptoms of rectal infection include discharge, anal itching, and occasional painful bowel movements with fresh blood	Most produce symptoms, but can be asymptomatic Dysuria Penile discharge (pus) Arthritis May lead to epididymitis and sterility Symptoms of rectal infection include discharge, anal itching, and occasional painful bowel movements with fresh blood	At this time, due to concerns about N. gonorrhoeae resistance to certain antimicrobials, the CDC currently recommends only one regimen, dual therapy with ceftriaxone and azithromycin Sexual partners need evaluation, testing, and treatment also Abstinence from sexual activity until therapy complete and symptoms no longer present Retesting in 3 months to rule out recurrence
Initial symptoms include itching, tingling, and pain in genital area followed by small pustules and blister-like genital lesions that then crust over and gradually heal. Recurrence episodes are usually milder than the initial episode Dysuria, dyspareunia, and urine retention Fever, headache, malaise, muscle aches	Same as female	Antivirals used to treat first episode, recurrence, and suppression Acyclovir, Valacyclovir, and Famciclovir mainstay in treatment Does not cure; just controls symptoms Counseling important to help adolescent cope and to prevent transmission Sexual partners benefit from evaluation and counseling. If symptomatic, need treatment If asymptomatic, offer testing and education

(continued)

TABLE 5.2 SEXUALLY TRANSMITTED INFECTIONS COMMON IN ADOLESCENTS (continued)

Disease	Causative Organism	Transmission Mode	Diagnostic Testing and Recommended Screening for Sexually Active Adolescent
Syphilis	*Treponema pallidum* (spirochete bacteria)	Sexual contact with an infected person	Serologic testing mainstay for diagnosis Venereal Disease Research Laboratory (VDRL), rapid plasma reagin (RPR), and treponemal tests (e.g., fluorescent treponemal antibody absorbed [FTA-ABS]) can lead to a presumptive diagnosis and are useful for screening. Use of 2 tests required Darkfield examination and direct fluorescent antibody tests of lesion exudate or tissue provide definitive diagnosis of early syphilis New tests are in development such as enzyme immunoassay Screen based on epidemiology and personal risk factors
Trichomoniasis	*Trichomonas vaginalis* (protozoa)	Vaginal intercourse with an infected partner May be picked up from direct genital contact with damp or moist objects, such as towels or wet clothing, or	Highly sensitive and specific testing available and recommended, such as NAAT Microscopic evaluation of vaginal secretions or culture still common but less sensitive
Venereal warts (condylomata acuminata) One of the most common STIs in the United States Could lead to cancers of the cervix, vulva, vagina, anus, or penis No cure; warts can be removed but virus remains	Human papillomavirus	Vaginal, anal, or oral sex with an infected partner	Visual inspection Abnormal pap smear may indicate cervical infection of human papillomavirus (HPV)

Adapted from Centers for Disease Control and Prevention. (2015). *Sexually Transmitted Diseases Treatment Guidelines, 2015. Morbidity and Mortality Weekly Report (MMWR), 64*(3), 1–137. Retrieved from http://www.cdc.gov/std/tg2015/tg-2015-print.pdf; and Grossman, L. C. (2014). Chapter 55: Sexually transmitted infections. In S. Grossman, & C. M. Porth (Eds.), *Porth's Pathophysiology: Concepts of altered health states* (9th ed., pp. 1416–1429). Philadelphia, PA: Wolters Kluwer Health/Lippincott Williams & Wilkins.

Female Symptoms	Male Symptoms	Recommended Treatment
Course of disease divided into stages **Primary infection:** • Chancre on place of entrance of bacteria (usually vulva or vagina but can develop in other parts of the body) **Secondary infection:** • Maculopapular rash (hands and feet) • Sore throat • Lymphadenopathy • Flu-like symptoms **Latent infection:** • No symptoms • Can be infective during first 1–2 years of latency • Many people if not treated will suffer no further signs and symptoms Some people will go on to develop tertiary or late syphilis **Tertiary infections:** • Tumors of skin, bones, and liver • Central nervous system symptoms • Cardiovascular symptoms • Usually not reversible at this stage	Course of disease divided into stages **Primary infection:** • Chancre on place of entrance of bacteria (usually on penis but can develop in other parts of the body) **Secondary, latent, and tertiary infections:** All similar to female symptoms	Benzathine penicillin G injection (if penicillin allergy, doxycycline, tetracycline, or erythromycin) Sexual partners need evaluation and testing
Many women have symptoms but some may be asymptomatic Dysuria Frequency Vaginal discharge (yellow, green, or gray and foul odor) Dyspareunia Irritation or itching of genital area	Most men infected are asymptomatic Dysuria Penile discharge (watery white)	Metronidazole (Flagyl) or tinidazole Sexual partners need evaluation, testing, and treatment also Abstinence recommended until therapy complete
Wart-like lesions that are soft, moist, or flesh colored and appear on the vulva and cervix, and inside and surrounding the vagina and anus Sometimes appear in clusters that resemble cauliflower-like bumps, and are either raised or flat, small or large	Wart-like lesions that are soft, moist, or flesh colored and appear on the scrotum or penis. They sometimes appear in clusters that resemble cauliflower-like bumps, and are either raised or flat, small or large	May disappear without treatment Treatment is aimed at removing the lesions rather than HPV itself No optimal treatment has been identified, but there are several ways to treat depending on size and location Most methods rely on chemical or physical destruction of the lesion: Imiquimod cream 20% Podophyllin antimitotic solution 0.5% Podofilox solution 5% 5-fluorouracil cream Trichloroacetic acid (TCA) Small warts can be removed by: • Freezing (cryosurgery) • Burning (electrocautery) • Laser treatment • Surgical excision Large warts that have not responded to treatment may be removed surgically Vaccination recommended starting around age 12 and may lead to decrease in cancer associated with HPV Abstinence from sexual activity during treatment to promote healing

Nursing Management

Nurses working with adolescents need to convey their willingness to discuss sexual habits. Provide effective guidance that promotes sexual health so that primary and/or repeat infections can be avoided. Adolescents bear disproportionate burdens when it comes to STIs, so nurses need to educate them to protect their client's reproductive futures.

Encourage the client to complete the antibiotic prescription (specific management for each type of STI is discussed further in the chapter).

Prevention of STIs among adolescents is critical. Health care providers have a unique opportunity to provide counseling and education to their clients. Adapt the style, content, and message to the adolescent's developmental level. Identify risk factors and risk behaviors and guide the adolescent to develop specific individualized actions of prevention. The nurse's interaction and conversation with the adolescent needs to be direct and nonjudgmental.

Encourage adolescents to postpone initiation of sexual intercourse for as long as possible, but if they choose to have sexual intercourse, explain the necessity of using barrier methods, such as male and female condoms (Teaching Guidelines 5.1). For teens who have already had sexual intercourse, the clinician can encourage abstinence at this point. If adolescents are sexually active, they should be directed to teen clinics where contraceptive options can be explained. In areas where specialized teen clinics are not available, nurses should feel comfortable discussing sexuality, safety, and contraception with teens. Encourage adolescents to minimize their lifetime number of sexual partners, to use barrier methods consistently and correctly, and to be aware of the connection between drug and alcohol use and the incorrect use of barrier methods. Table 5.3 discusses barriers to condom use and means to overcome them.

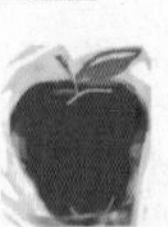

Teaching Guidelines 5.1
PROPER CONDOM USE

- Use latex condoms.
- Use a new condom with each act of vaginal, anal or oral sex. Never reuse a condom.
- Handle condoms with care to prevent damage from sharp objects such as fingernails and teeth.
- Ensure condom has been stored in a cool, dry place away from direct sunlight. Do not store condoms in wallet or automobile or anywhere where they would be exposed to extreme temperatures.
- Do not use a condom if it appears brittle, sticky, or discolored. These are signs of aging.
- Put condom on before any genital contact.
- Put condom on when penis is erect with rolled side out. Ensure it is placed so it will readily unroll.
- Hold the tip of the condom while unrolling. Ensure there is a space at the tip for semen to collect (about ½ in), but make sure no air is trapped in the tip (air bubbles can cause breakage).
- Ensure adequate lubrication during intercourse. If external lubricants are used, use only water-based lubricants such as KY jelly with latex condoms. Oil-based or petroleum-based lubricants, such as body lotion, massage oil, or cooking oil, can weaken latex condoms.
- If you feel the condom break, stop immediately, withdraw, remove broken condom, and replace.
- Withdraw while penis is still erect, and hold condom firmly against base of penis. Remove carefully to ensure no semen spills out. Dispose of properly.

Adapted from CDC (2013). *Condom effectiveness.* Retrieved from http://www.cdc.gov/condomeffectiveness/docs/condomfactsheetinbrief.pdf

Think back to Sandy, who was introduced at the beginning of the chapter. How should the nurse handle Sandy's anxious state? What specific questions should the nurse ask Sandy to determine the source of the possible infection in her genital area?

INFECTIONS CHARACTERIZED BY VAGINAL DISCHARGE

Vaginitis is a generic term that means inflammation and infection of the vagina. There can be hundreds of causes for vaginitis, but more often than not the cause is infection by one of three organisms:

- Candida, a fungus
- Trichomonas, a protozoa
- Gardnerella, a bacterium

The complex balance of microbiologic organisms in the vagina is a key element in the maintenance of health. Subtle shifts in the vaginal environment may allow organisms with pathologic potential to proliferate, causing infectious symptoms.

The nurse's role in managing vaginitis is one of primary prevention and education to limit recurrences of these infections. Primary prevention begins with changing the sexual behaviors that place women at risk for infection. In addition to assessing women for the common signs and symptoms and risk factors, the nurse can help women to avoid vaginitis or to prevent a recurrence by teaching them to take the precautions highlighted in (Teaching Guidelines 5.2).

TABLE 5.3 BARRIERS TO CONDOM USE AND MEANS TO OVERCOME THEM

Perceived Barrier	Intervention Strategy
Decreases sexual pleasure (sensation) Note: Often perceived by those who have never used a condom	• Encourage client to try • Put a drop of water-based lubricant or saliva inside the tip of the condom or on the glans of the penis before putting on the condom • Try a thinner latex condom or a different brand or more lubrication
Decreases spontaneity of sexual activity	• Incorporate condom use into foreplay • Remind client that peace of mind may enhance pleasure for self and partner
Embarrassing, juvenile, "unmanly"	• Remind client that it is "manly" to protect himself and others.
Poor fit (too small or too big, slips off, uncomfortable)	• Smaller and larger condoms are available.
Requires prompt withdrawal after ejaculation	• Reinforce the protective nature of prompt withdrawal and suggest substituting other postcoital sexual activities.
Fear of breakage may lead to less vigorous sexual activity	• With prolonged intercourse, lubricant wears off and the condom begins to rub. Have a water-soluble lubricant available to reapply.
Nonpenetrative sexual activity	• Condoms have been advocated for use during fellatio; unlubricated condoms may prove best for this purpose due to the taste of the lubricant • Other barriers, such as dental dams or an unlubricated condom, can be cut down the middle to form a barrier; these have been advocated for use during certain forms of nonpenetrative sexual activity (e.g., cunnilingus and anolingual sex)
Allergy to latex	• Polyurethane male and female condoms are available • A natural skin condom can be used together with a latex condom to protect the man or woman from contact with latex

Adapted from Public Health Agency of Canada. (2015). *Canadian guidelines on sexually transmitted infections.* Retrieved from http://www.phac-aspc.gc.ca/std-mts/sti-its/

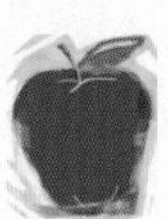

Teaching Guidelines 5.2

PREVENTING VAGINITIS

- Avoid douching to prevent altering the vaginal environment.
- Use condoms to avoid spreading the organism.
- Avoid tights, nylon underpants, and tight clothes.
- Wipe from front to back after using the toilet.
- Avoid powders, bubble baths, and perfumed vaginal sprays.
- Wear clean cotton underpants.
- Change out of wet bathing suits as soon as possible.
- Become familiar with the signs and symptoms of vaginitis.
- Choose to lead a healthy lifestyle.

Genital/Vulvovaginal Candidiasis (VVC)

Genital/VVC is one of the most common causes of vaginal discharge. It is also referred to as yeast, monilia, and a fungal infection. It is not considered an STI because Candida is a normal constituent in the vagina and becomes pathologic only when the vaginal environment becomes altered. An estimated 75% of women will have at least one episode of VVC, and 40% to 50% will have two or more episodes in their lifetime (CDC, 2016).

Therapeutic Management

Treatment of candidiasis includes one of the following medications:

- Miconazole cream or suppository
- Clotrimazole tablet or cream
- Terconazole cream or intravaginal suppository
- Fluconazole oral tablet (CDC, 2015a)

Most of these medications are used intravaginally in the form of a cream, tablet, or suppositories for 3 to 7 days. If fluconazole is prescribed, a 150-mg oral tablet is taken as a single dose.

Topical azole preparations are effective in the treatment of VVC, relieving symptoms and producing negative cultures in 80% to 90% of women who complete therapy (CDC, 2015a). If VVC is not treated effectively during pregnancy, the newborn can develop an oral infection known as thrush during the birth process; that infection must be treated with a local azole preparation after birth.

Nursing Assessment

Assess the client's health history for predisposing factors for VVC, which include:

- Pregnancy
- Use of oral contraceptives with a high estrogen content
- Use of broad-spectrum antibiotics
- Diabetes mellitus
- Obesity
- Use of steroid and immunosuppressive drugs
- HIV infection
- Wearing tight, restrictive clothes and nylon underpants
- Trauma to vaginal mucosa from chemical irritants or douching

Assess the client for clinical manifestations of VVC. Typical symptoms, which can worsen just before menses, include:

- Pruritus
- Vaginal discharge (thick, white, curd-like)
- Vaginal soreness
- Vulvar burning
- Erythema in the vulvovaginal area
- Dyspareunia
- External dysuria

Figure 5.1 shows the typical appearance of VVC.

Speculum examination will reveal white plaques on the vaginal walls. The vaginal pH remains within normal range. Definitive diagnosis is made by a wet smear, which reveals the filamentous hyphae and spores characteristic of a fungus when viewed under a microscope.

Nursing Management

Teach preventive measures to women with frequent VVC infections, including:

- Reduce dietary intake of simple sugars and soda.
- Wear white, 100% cotton underpants.
- Avoid wearing tight pants or exercise clothes with spandex.
- Shower rather than taking tub baths.
- Wash with a mild, unscented soap and dry the genitals gently.
- Avoid the use of bubble baths or scented bath products.
- Wash underwear in unscented laundry detergent and hot water.
- Dry underwear in a hot dryer to kill the yeast that clings to the fabric.
- Remove wet bathing suits promptly.

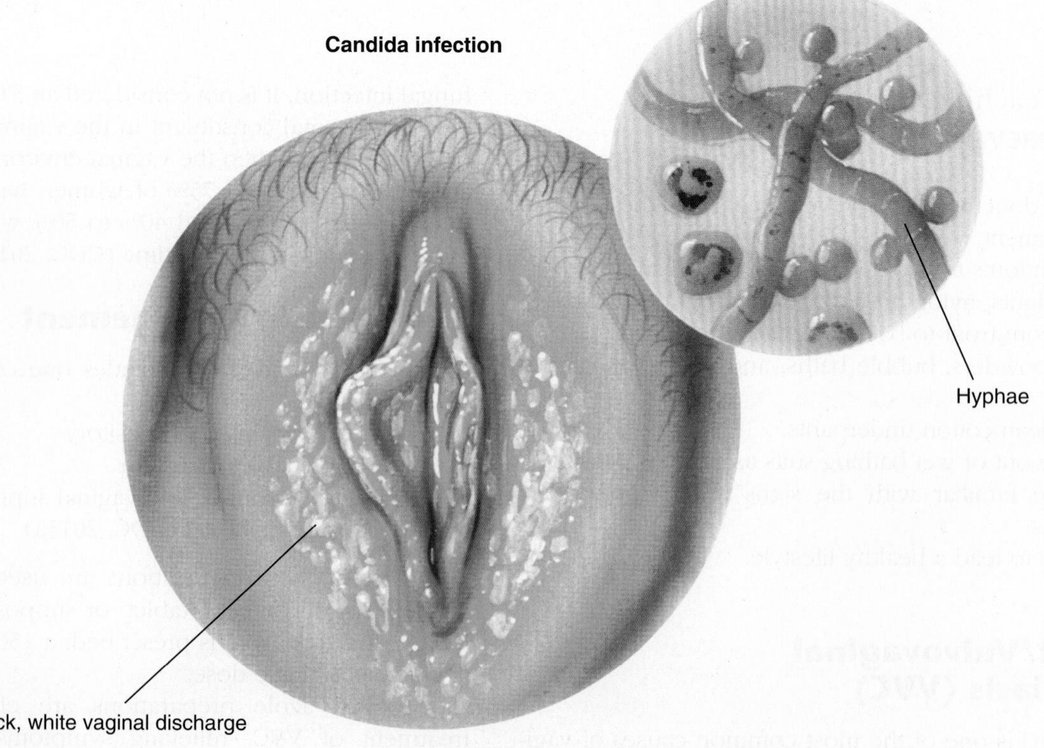

FIGURE 5.1 Vulvovaginal candidiasis. (Asset provided by Anatomical Chart Co.)

- Practice good body hygiene.
- Avoid vaginal sprays/deodorants.
- Avoid wearing pantyhose (or cut out the crotch to allow air circulation).
- Use white, unscented toilet paper and wipe from front to back.
- Avoid douching (which washes away protective vaginal mucus).
- Avoid the use of super-absorbent tampons (use pads instead).

Trichomoniasis

Trichomoniasis is another common vaginal infection that causes a discharge, but is not always sexually transmitted. The organism can live on damp/wet surfaces and poorly cleaned/maintained hot tubs and drains. The woman may be markedly symptomatic or asymptomatic. When symptoms are present, they include vulvar itching and a malodorous foamy vaginal discharge. Men are asymptomatic carriers. Although this infection is localized, there is increasing evidence of preterm birth and postpartum endometritis in women with this vaginitis (CDC, 2015a). The high prevalence of this infection globally and frequency of coinfection with other STIs make trichomoniasis a public health concern. Notably, research finds that an infection with trichomoniasis increases the risk of HIV transmission in both men and women (Smith & Ramos, 2015). *Trichomonas vaginalis* is an ovoid, single-cell protozoan parasite that can be observed under the microscope making a jerky swaying motion.

Therapeutic Management

A single 2-g dose of oral metronidazole or tinidazole for both partners is a common treatment for this infection. Sex partners of women with trichomoniasis should be treated to avoid recurrence of infection.

Nursing Assessment

Assess the client for clinical manifestations of trichomoniasis, which include:

- A heavy yellow/green or gray frothy or bubbly discharge
- Vaginal pruritus and vulvar soreness
- Dyspareunia
- Cervix may bleed on contact
- Dysuria
    - Vaginal odor, described as foul
    - Vaginal or vulvar erythema
- Petechiae on the cervix

Figure 5.2 shows the typical appearance of trichomoniasis.

The diagnosis is confirmed when a motile flagellated trichomonad is visualized under the microscope. In addition, a vaginal pH of greater than 4.5 is a typical finding. FDA-cleared tests for trichomoniasis in women include OSOM Trichomonas Rapid Test (Genzyme Diagnostics, Cambridge, Massachusetts), an immunochromatographic capillary flow dipstick technology, and the Affirm VP III (Becton Dickenson, San Jose, California), a nucleic acid probe test that evaluates for *T. vaginalis, Gardnerella vaginalis,* and *Candida albicans*. Each of these tests,

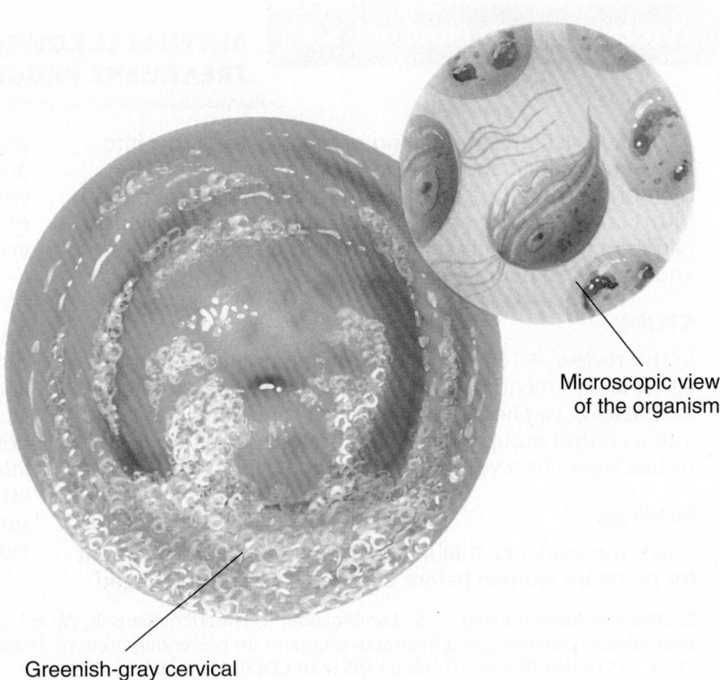

FIGURE 5.2 Trichomoniasis. (Asset provided by Anatomical Chart Co.)

which are performed on vaginal secretions, have a sensitivity of 83% and a specificity of 97%. Both tests are considered point-of-care diagnostics (CDC, 2015a).

Nursing Management

Instruct clients to avoid sexual activity until they and their sex partners are cured (i.e., when therapy has been completed and both partners are symptom-free) and also to avoid consuming alcohol during treatment because mixing the medications and alcohol causes severe nausea and vomiting (CDC, 2015a). In addition, it is important to provide information regarding infection cause and transmission, effects on reproductive organs and future fertility, and the need for partner notification and treatment. Follow-up testing is not indicated if symptoms resolve with treatment. See Evidence-Based Practice 5.1 for interventions for trichomoniasis in pregnancy.

Bacterial Vaginosis

A third common infection of the vagina is **bacterial vaginosis** caused by the gram-negative bacillus *G. vaginalis*. It is the most prevalent cause of vaginal discharge or malodor, but up to 50% of women are asymptomatic. Bacterial vaginosis is a sexually associated infection characterized by alterations in vaginal flora in which lactobacilli in the vagina are replaced with high concentrations of anaerobic bacteria. The cause of the microbial alteration is not fully understood, but is associated with having multiple sex partners, douching, and lack of vaginal lactobacilli. Bacterial vaginosis can increase a woman's susceptibility to other STIs such as HIV, herpes, chlamydia, and gonorrhea (CDC, 2015a). Research suggests that bacterial vaginosis is associated with preterm labor, premature rupture of membranes (PROM), chorioamnionitis, postpartum endometritis, and PID (CDC, 2015a).

Therapeutic Management

Treatment for bacterial vaginosis includes metronidazole (oral or gel) or clindamycin cream. Treatment of the male partner has not been beneficial in preventing recurrence because sexual transmission of bacterial vaginosis has not been proven (CDC, 2015a).

Nursing Assessment

Assess the client for clinical manifestations of bacterial vaginosis. Primary symptoms are a thin, white homogeneous vaginal discharge and a characteristic "stale fish" odor. Figure 5.3 shows the typical appearance of bacterial vaginosis.

To diagnose bacterial vaginosis, three of the four criteria must be met:

- Thin, white homogeneous vaginal discharge
- Vaginal pH 4.5
- Positive "whiff test" (secretion is mixed with a drop of 10% potassium hydroxide on a slide, producing a characteristic stale fishy odor)
- The presence of clue cells on wet-mount examination (CDC, 2015a)

EVIDENCE-BASED PRACTICE 5.1

ANTENATAL LOWER GENITAL TRACT INFECTION SCREENING AND TREATMENT PROGRAMS FOR PREVENTING PRETERM DELIVERY

A genital tract infection during pregnancy can cross into the amniotic fluid and result in prelabor rupture on the membranes and is associated with preterm births. Preterm births are associated with poor infant health, admissions to NICUs in the first weeks of life, prolonged hospital stays, and long-term neurologic disabilities.

STUDY

In this review, 4,155 women were randomly assigned to either an intervention group whereby they were treated for bacterial vaginosis, trichomoniasis, and candidiasis, or into a control group where they received screening but results were not revealed and treatment not instituted.

Findings

There was evidence that infection screening and treatment for pregnant women before 20 weeks' gestation reduced preterm births and low-weight infants. Infection screening and treatment programs are associated with cost savings when used for prevention of preterm births. The numbers of low-weight infants were significantly lower in the intervention group when compared to the control group.

Nursing Implications

A simple infection screening and treatment program done during routine prenatal care may reduce preterm births and preterm low-weight infants. Nurses can apply this study's findings when educating women preconceptually how important prenatal care is and screening for vaginal infections that may be asymptomatic. It is important to establish a link between preterm birth prevention measures to improve maternal–infant outcomes in all pregnant women.

Source: Sangkomkamhang, U. S., Lumbiganon, P., Prasertcharoensuk, W., & Laopaiboon, M. (2015). Antenatal lower genital tract infection screening and treatment programs for preventing preterm delivery. *Cochrane Database of Systematic Reviews 2015, 2:* CD006178. doi: 10.1002/14651858.CD006178.pub3.

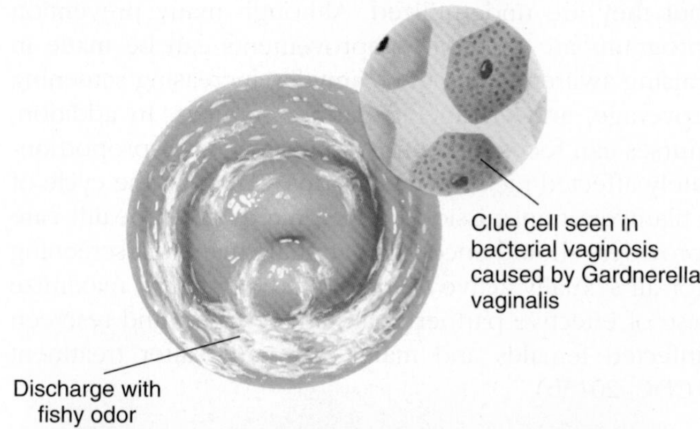

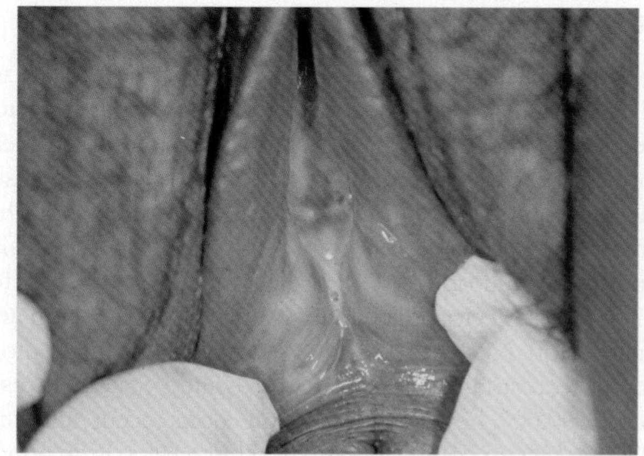

FIGURE 5.3 Bacterial vaginosis. (Illustration provided by Anatomical Chart Co. Photograph from Sweet, R. L., Gibbs, R. S. (2005). *Atlas of infectious diseases of the female genital tract*. Philadelphia, PA: Lippincott Williams & Wilkins.)

Nursing Management

The nurse's role is one of primary prevention and education to limit recurrences of these infections. Primary prevention begins with changing the sexual behaviors that place women at risk for infection. In addition to assessing women for common signs, symptoms, and risk factors, the nurse can help women to avoid vaginitis or to prevent a recurrence by teaching them to take the precautions highlighted in Teaching Guidelines 5.2.

INFECTIONS CHARACTERIZED BY CERVICITIS

Cervicitis is a catchall term that implies the presence of inflammation or infection of the cervix. It is used to describe everything from symptomless erosions to an inflamed cervix that bleeds on contact and produces quantities of purulent discharge containing organisms not ordinarily found in the vagina. Cervicitis is usually caused by gonorrhea or chlamydia, as well as almost any pathogenic bacterial agent and a number of viruses. The treatment of cervicitis involves the appropriate therapy for the specific organism that has caused it.

Chlamydia

Chlamydia is the most commonly reported bacterial STI in the United States. The CDC (2014b) estimates that there are 2.8 million cases in the United States annually; the highest predictor for this infection is age. The highest rates of infection are among those aged 15 to 19 years, mainly because their sexual relations are often unplanned and are sometimes the result of pressure or force, and typically happen before they have the experience and skills to protect themselves. The rates are highest among this group regardless of demographics or location (CDC, 2014a). The young have the most to lose from acquiring STIs, since they will suffer the consequences the longest and might not reach their full reproductive potential. The most common risk factors associated with chlamydia are age less than 25 years, recent change in sexual partner or multiple sexual partners, poor socioeconomic conditions, exchange of sex for money, nonwhite race, single status, and lack of use of barrier contraception. Worldwide, it is likely the most common infectious cause of infertility in women. An estimated 106 million cases of chlamydia occur globally among both men and women each year, so the global burden is substantial (Brunham, 2015).

Asymptomatic infection is common among both men and women. Men primarily develop urethritis. In women, chlamydia is linked with cervicitis, acute urethral syndrome, salpingitis, ectopic pregnancy, PID, and infertility (Qureshi, 2015). Chlamydia causes half of the 1 million recognized cases of PID in the United States each year, and treatment costs run over $701 million yearly. The CDC (2014a) recommends yearly chlamydia testing of all sexually active women aged 25 years or younger, older women with risk factors for chlamydial infections (those who have a new sex partner or multiple sex partners), and all pregnant women.

Chlamydia trachomatis is the bacterium that causes chlamydia. It is an intracellular parasite that cannot produce its own energy and depends on the host for survival. It is often difficult to detect, and this can pose problems for women due to the long-term consequences of untreated infection. Moreover, lack of treatment provides more opportunity for the infection to be transmitted to sexual partners. Newborns delivered to infected mothers may develop conjunctivitis which occurs in 25% to 50% of all newborns. Ophthalmia neonatorum is an acute mucopurulent conjunctivitis occurring in the first month of birth. It is essentially an infection acquired during vaginal delivery. The most frequent infectious agents involved in are Chlamydia trachomatis and Neisseria gonorrhea (Thomas, Bates, & Mathew, 2015).

Therapeutic Management

Antibiotics are usually used in treating this STI. The CDC treatment options for chlamydia include doxycycline

100 mg orally twice a day for 7 days or azithromycin 1 g orally in a single dose. Because of the common coinfection of chlamydia and gonorrhea, a combination regimen of ceftriaxone with doxycycline or azithromycin is prescribed frequently (CDC, 2015a). Additional CDC guidelines for client management include annual screening of all sexually active women aged 20 to 25 years old; screening of all high-risk people; and treatment with antibiotics effective against both gonorrhea and chlamydia for anyone diagnosed with a gonococcal infection (CDC, 2014a). Except in pregnant women, test-of-cure (repeat testing 3 to 4 weeks after completing therapy) is not recommended for women treated with the recommended or alterative regimens, unless therapeutic compliance is in question, symptoms persist, or reinfection is suspected (CDC, 2015a).

Nursing Assessment

Assess the health history for significant risk factors for chlamydia, which may include:

- Being an adolescent
- Having multiple sex partners
- Having a new sex partner
- Engaging in sex without using a barrier contraceptive (condom)
- Using oral contraceptives
- Being pregnant
- Having a history of another STI (King et al., 2015).

Assess the client for clinical manifestations of chlamydia. The majority of women (70% to 80%) are asymptomatic (CDC, 2014a). If the client is symptomatic, clinical manifestations include:

- Mucopurulent vaginal discharge
- Urethritis
- Bartholinitis
- Endometritis
- Salpingitis
- Dysfunctional uterine bleeding

The diagnosis can be made by urine testing or swab specimens collected from the endocervix or vagina. Culture, direct immunofluorescence, enzyme immunoassay (EIA), or nucleic acid amplification methods such as GenProbe or Pace2) are highly sensitive and specific when used on urethral and cervicovaginal swabs. They can also be used with good sensitivity and specificity on first-void urine specimens (Qureshi, 2015). The chain reaction tests are the most sensitive and cost-effective. The CDC (2015b) strongly recommends screening of asymptomatic women at high risk in whom infection would otherwise go undetected.

Chlamydia is an important preventable cause of infertility and other adverse reproductive health outcomes. Effective prevention interventions are available to reduce the burden of chlamydia and its sequelae, but they are underutilized. Although many prevention programs are available, improvements can be made in raising awareness about chlamydia, increasing screening coverage, and enhancing partner services. In addition, nurses can focus their efforts on reaching disproportionately affected racial/ethnic groups. To break the cycle of chlamydia transmission in the United States, health care providers should encourage annual chlamydia screening for all sexually active females aged >25 years, maximize use of effective partner treatment services, and rescreen infected females and males 3 months after treatment (CDC, 2015b).

Gonorrhea

Gonorrhea is a serious, and potentially very severe, bacterial infection. It is the second most commonly reported infection in the United States, and is an urgent problem globally because it is now capable of developing resistance to multiple antibiotic classes. Gonorrhea is highly contagious and is a reportable infection to the health department authorities. Gonorrhea increases the risk for PID, infertility, ectopic pregnancy, and HIV acquisition and transmission (CDC, 2015f). It is rapidly becoming more and more resistant to cure. In the United States, an estimated 800,000 new gonorrhea infections occur annually (CDC, 2015f). In common with all other STIs, it is an equal-opportunity infection—no one is immune to it, regardless of race, creed, gender, age, or sexual preference.

The cause of gonorrhea is an aerobic gram-negative intracellular diplococcus, *Neisseria gonorrhoeae*. The site of infection is the columnar epithelium of the endocervix. Gonorrhea is almost exclusively transmitted by sexual activity. In pregnant women, gonorrhea is associated with chorioamnionitis, premature labor, PROM, and postpartum endometritis (Ross et al., 2015). It can also be transmitted to the newborn in the form of ophthalmia neonatorum during birth by direct contact with gonococcal organisms in the cervix. Ophthalmia neonatorum is highly contagious and if untreated leads to blindness in the newborn.

Therapeutic Management

Gonorrhea can be cured with the right treatment. CDC now recommends dual therapy (i.e., using two drugs as the treatment for gonorrhea). Dual therapy is recommended to prevent drug resistance and is also effective against chlamydia. The treatment of choice for uncomplicated gonococcal infections is azithromycin 1 g orally in a single dose and ceftriaxone 250 mg intramuscular (IM) in a single dose (CDC, 2015a).

Azithromycin orally or doxycycline should accompany all gonococcal treatment regimens if chlamydial infection is not ruled out (CDC, 2015a). Pregnant women with gonorrhea should not be treated with quinolones or tetracyclines. Pregnant women with a positive test for gonorrhea should be treated with the same recommended dual therapy of ceftriaxone with either azithromycin or amoxicillin (CDC, 2015a). To prevent gonococcal ophthalmia neonatorum, a prophylactic agent should be instilled into the eyes of all newborns; this procedure is required by law in most states. Erythromycin or tetracycline ophthalmic ointment in a single application is recommended (King et al., 2015). With use of recommended treatment, follow-up testing to document eradication of gonorrhea is no longer recommended. Instead, rescreening in 2 to 3 months to identify reinfection is suggested (CDC, 2015a).

Nursing Assessment

Assess the client's health history for risk factors, which may include low socioeconomic status, living in an urban area, single status, inconsistent use of barrier contraceptives, age under 20 years old, and multiple sex partners. Assess the client for clinical manifestations of gonorrhea, keeping in mind that between 50% and 90% of women infected with gonorrhea are totally symptom-free (Wong, 2015). Because women are so frequently asymptomatic, they are regarded as a major factor in the spread of gonorrhea. If symptoms are present, they might include:

- Abnormal vaginal discharge
- Dysuria
- Cervicitis
- Enlarged lymph glands locally
- Abnormal vaginal bleeding
- Bartholin abscess
- PID
- Neonatal conjunctivitis in newborns
- Mild sore throat (for pharyngeal gonorrhea)
- Rectal infection (itching, soreness, bleeding, discharge)
- Perihepatitis (King et al., 2015)

Sometimes, a local gonorrhea infection is self-limiting (there is no further spread), but usually the organism ascends upward through the endocervical canal to the endometrium of the uterus, further on to the fallopian tubes, and out into the peritoneal cavity. When the peritoneum and the ovaries become involved, the condition is known as PID. The scarring to the fallopian tubes is permanent. This damage is a major cause of infertility and is a possible contributing factor in ectopic pregnancy (Heller, 2015).

If gonorrhea remains untreated, it can enter the bloodstream and produce a disseminated gonococcal infection. This severe form of infection can invade the joints (arthritis), the heart (endocarditis), the brain (meningitis), and the liver (toxic hepatitis). Figure 5.4 shows the typical appearance of gonorrhea.

The CDC recommends screening for all women at risk for gonorrhea. Pregnant women should be screened at the first prenatal visit and again at 36 weeks of gestation. Nucleic acid hybridization tests (GenProbe) are used for diagnosis. Any woman suspected of having gonorrhea should be tested for chlamydia also because coinfection (45%) is extremely common (CDC, 2015f).

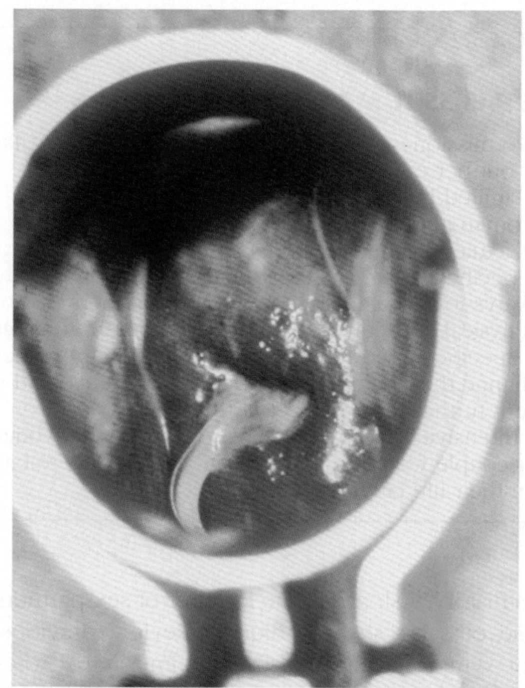

FIGURE 5.4 Gonorrhea. (From Jensen, S. (2015). *Nursing Health Assessment: A Best Practice Approach*, 2nd ed. Philadelphia, PA: Wolters Kluwer.)

Nursing Management of Chlamydia and Gonorrhea

The prevalence of chlamydia and gonorrhea is increasing dramatically, and these infections can have long-term effects on people's lives. Sexual health is an important part of a person's physical and mental health, and nurses have a professional obligation to address it. Be particularly sensitive when addressing STIs because women are often embarrassed or feel guilty. There is still a social stigma attached to STIs, so women need to be reassured about confidentiality.

The nurse's knowledge about chlamydia and gonorrhea should include treatment strategies, referral sources, and preventive measures. It is important to be skilled at client education and counseling and to be comfortable talking with, and advising, women diagnosed with these infections. Provide education about risk factors for these infections. High-risk groups include single women, women younger than 25 years, African American women, women with a history of STIs, those with new or multiple sex partners, those with inconsistent use of barrier contraception, and women living in communities with high infection rates (Wong, 2015). Assessment involves taking a health history that includes a comprehensive

BOX 5.2

THE P-LI-SS-IT MODEL

P – Permission—gives the woman permission to talk about her experience
LI – Limited Information—information given to the woman about STIs
- Factual information to dispel myths about STIs
- Specific measures to prevent transmission
- Ways to reveal information to her partners
- Physical consequences if the infections are untreated

SS – Specific Suggestions—an attempt to help women change their behavior to prevent recurrence and prevent further transmission of the STI
IT – Intensive Therapy—involves referring the woman or couple for appropriate treatment elsewhere based on their life circumstances

sexual history. Ask about the number of sex partners and the use of safer sex techniques. Review previous and current symptoms. Emphasize the importance of seeking treatment and informing sex partners. The four-level P-LI-SS-IT model (Box 5.2) can be used to determine interventions for various women because it can be adapted to the nurse's level of knowledge, skill, and experience. Of utmost importance is the willingness to listen and show interest and respect in a nonjudgmental manner.

In addition to meeting the health needs of women with chlamydia and gonorrhea, the nurse is responsible for educating the public about the increasing incidence of these infections. This information should include high-risk behaviors associated with these infections, signs and symptoms, and the treatment modalities available. Stress that both of these STIs can lead to infertility and long-term sequelae. Teach safer sex practices to people in nonmonogamous relationships. Know the physical and psychosocial responses to these STIs to prevent transmission and the disabling consequences. Nurses must also inform their pregnant clients that they should avoid quinolones or tetracyclines to prevent risks associated with malformation of teeth, bones, and joints in the fetus and possible hepatotoxicity and pancreatitis in the mother (King et al. 2015).

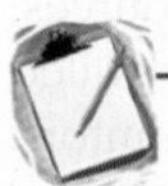

Take Note!

If the epidemic of chlamydia and gonorrhea is to be halted, nurses must take a major front-line role now.

INFECTIONS CHARACTERIZED BY GENITAL ULCERS

In the United States, the majority of young, sexually active clients who have genital ulcers have genital herpes, syphilis, or chancroid. The frequency of each condition differs by geographic area and client population; however, genital herpes is the most prevalent of these diseases. More than one of these diseases can be present in a client who has genital ulcers. All three of these diseases have been associated with an increased risk for HIV infection. Not all genital ulcers are caused by STIs.

Genital Herpes Simplex

Genital herpes is a recurrent, lifelong viral infection that has the potential for transmission throughout the lifespan. The CDC estimates that one out of six people 14 to 49 years old have genital herpes simplex (HSV) infection, with 500 million worldwide new cases annually (CDC, 2015e). Two serotypes of HSV have been identified: HSV-1 and HSV-2. Today, a smaller portion of genital herpes infections are thought to be caused by HSV-1 and the bulk of them by HSV-2. HSV-1 mostly causes the familiar fever blisters or cold sores on the lips, eyes, and face. HSV-2 typically invades the mucous membranes of the genital tract and is known as herpes genitalis. Most people infected with HSV-2 have not been diagnosed.

The herpes simplex virus is transmitted by contact of mucous membranes or breaks in the skin with visible or nonvisible lesions. Most genital herpes infections are transmitted by individuals unaware that they have an infection. Many have mild or unrecognized infections but still shed the herpes virus intermittently. HSV is transmitted primarily by direct contact with an infected individual who is shedding the virus. Kissing, sexual contact, including oral sex, and vaginal birth are means of transmission. The virus replicates at the site of infection, then travels to the dorsal root ganglia and remains latent until stimuli such as fever, stress, ultraviolet radiation, or immunosuppression occurs and reactivates it (Selim et al., 2015).

Having sex with an infected partner places the individual at risk for contracting HSV. After the primary outbreak, the virus remains dormant in the nerve cells for life, resulting in periodic recurrent outbreaks. Recurrent genital herpes outbreaks are triggered by precipitating factors such as emotional stress, menses, and sexual intercourse, but more than half of recurrences occur without a precipitating cause. Immunocompromised women have more frequent and more severe recurrent outbreaks than normal hosts (Silasi et al., 2015).

Living with genital herpes can be difficult due to the erratic, recurrent nature of the infection, the location of the lesions, the unknown causes of the recurrences, and the lack of a cure. Further, the stigma associated with this infection may affect the individual's feelings about herself and her interaction with partners. Potential psychosocial consequences may include emotional distress, isolation, fear of rejection by a partner, fear of transmission of the disease, loss of confidence, and altered interpersonal relationships (Alexander et al., 2014).

Along with the increase in the incidence of genital herpes has been an increase in neonatal herpes simplex viral infections, which are associated with a high incidence of mortality and morbidity. The risk of neonatal infection with a primary maternal outbreak is between 30% and 50%; it is less than 1% with a recurrent maternal infection (CDC, 2015e).

Therapeutic Management

No cure exists, but antiviral drug therapy helps to reduce or suppress symptoms, shedding, and recurrent episodes. Advances in treatment with acyclovir 400 mg orally three times daily for 7 to 10 days, famciclovir 250 mg orally three times daily for 7 to 10 days, and valacyclovir 1 g orally twice daily for 7 to 10 days have resulted in an improved quality of life for those infected with HSV. However, these drugs neither eradicate latent virus nor affect the risk, frequency, or severity of recurrences after the drug is discontinued (CDC, 2015a). Suppressive therapy is recommended for individuals with six or more recurrences per year. The natural course of the disease is for recurrences to be less frequent over time.

The management of genital herpes includes antiviral therapy. The safety of antiviral therapy has not been established during pregnancy. Disclosure of this lifelong viral infection is often a challenge for individuals living with genital herpes. Therapeutic management also includes counseling regarding the natural history of the disease, the risk of sexual and perinatal transmission, and the use of methods to prevent further spread. The following are a few guidelines to delivering information in a time-limited environment: (a) use all available client reading materials; (b) have another knowledgeable staff member in the office who can spend extra time with women who need it; (c) refer clients to good and accurate websites such as the American Social Health Association (www.ashastd.org/hrc); (d) know the phone numbers of herpes support groups in your area; (e) educate the client to abstain from all sexual activity until HSV lesions resolve; (f) use good hand washing technique to prevent spread; (g) educate that there is no cure, and that practicing safe sex (using condoms) with every sex act is essential to prevent transmission; and (h) encourage all clients to inform their current sex partners that they have genital herpes and to inform future partners before initiating a sexual relationship. Finally, many experts recommend a sympathetic, nonjudgmental approach. The nurse can state in clear terms that having herpes does not change the core of the person or make them less worthwhile (Myers et al., 2015).

Nursing Assessment

Assess the client for clinical manifestations of HSV. Clinical manifestations can be divided into the primary episode and recurrent infections. The first or primary episode is usually the most severe, with a prolonged period of viral shedding. Primary HSV is a systemic disease characterized by multiple painful vesicular lesions, mucopurulent discharge, superinfection with candida, fever, chills, malaise, dysuria, headache, genital irritation, inguinal tenderness, and lymphadenopathy. The lesions in the primary herpes episode are frequently located on the vulva, vagina, and perineal areas. The vesicles will open and weep and finally crust over, dry, and disappear without scar formation (Fig. 5.5). This viral shedding process usually takes up to 2 weeks to complete.

Recurrent infection episodes are usually much milder and shorter in duration than the primary one. Tingling, itching, pain, unilateral genital lesions, and a more rapid resolution of lesions are characteristics of recurrent infections. Recurrent herpes is a localized disease characterized by typical HSV lesions at the site of initial viral entry. Recurrent herpes lesions are fewer in number and less painful and resolve more rapidly (King et al., 2015).

Diagnosis of HSV is often based on clinical signs and symptoms and is confirmed by viral culture of fluid from the vesicle. Papanicolaou (Pap) smears are an insensitive and nonspecific diagnostic test for HSV and should not be relied on for diagnosis. The woman should be tested for all common STIs, especially if she has a new sexual partner. Hopefully, the woman would initiate an open conversation with her sexual partner about the risk of transmission and the need for safer sexual practices.

Syphilis

Syphilis is a chronic, multistage, curable bacterial infection caused by the spirochete *Treponema pallidum* that is typically transmitted sexually with an infected partner or congenitally from an infected mother to her fetus. It is a serious systemic disease that can lead to disability and death if untreated. Rates of syphilis in the United States are increasing. Of primary and secondary syphilis cases, 75% occur in men who have sex with men (CDC, 2015k). It continues to be one of the most important STIs both because of its biologic effect on HIV acquisition and transmission and because of its impact on infant health. Because there is no vaccine to prevent syphilis, control is mainly dependent on the identification and treatment of infected individuals and their contacts with penicillin G, the first-line drug for all stages of syphilis (Stamm, 2015).

The spirochete rapidly penetrates intact mucous membranes or microscopic lesions in the skin and within hours enters the lymphatic system and bloodstream to produce a systemic infection long before the appearance of a primary lesion. The site of entry may be vaginal, rectal, or oral (Euerle et al., 2014). The syphilis spirochete can cross the placenta at any time during pregnancy. One out of every 10,000 infants born in the United States

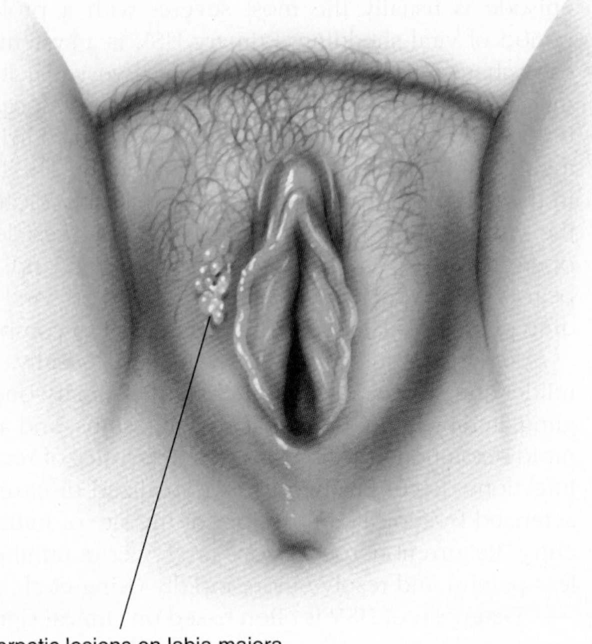

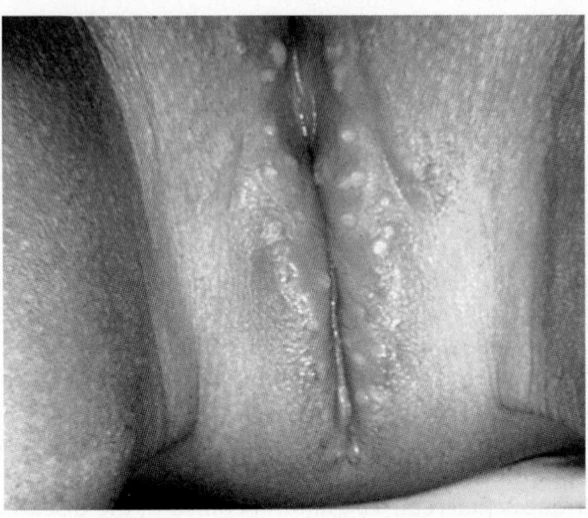

FIGURE 5.5 Genital herpes simplex. (Illustration provided by Anatomical Chart Co. Photograph courtesy of Stephen Ludwig, MD.)

has congenital syphilis (CDC, 2015c). Maternal infection consequences include spontaneous abortion, low birth weight, fetal growth restriction, prematurity, stillbirth, and multisystem failure of the heart, lungs, spleen, liver, and pancreas, as well as structural bone damage and nervous system involvement and mental retardation (Chen et al., 2015). Most newborns born with congenital syphilis are exposed in utero after the fourth month of pregnancy, although syphilis acquired late in the third trimester can also be transmitted to an infant through exposure to an active genital lesion at the time of birth. If untreated, syphilis is a lifelong infection progressing in orderly staging. The five stages of syphilis infection are: (1) primary, (2) secondary, (3) early latent, (4) late latent, and (5) tertiary. The primary, secondary, and early latent stages are considered the most infectious: the estimated risk of per person transmission is 60% (Queenan, Spong, & Lockwood, 2015).

Therapeutic Management

Fortunately, there is effective treatment for syphilis. Benzathine penicillin G, administered by either the IM or intravenous route, is the preferred drug for all stages of syphilis. For pregnant or nonpregnant women with syphilis of less than 1 year's duration, the CDC recommends 2.4 million units of benzathine penicillin G intramuscularly in a single dose. If the syphilis is of longer duration (more than 1 year) or of unknown duration, 2.4 million units of benzathine penicillin G is given intramuscularly once a week for 3 weeks. The preparations used, the dosage, and the length of treatment depend on the stage and clinical manifestations of disease (CDC, 2015a). Other medications, such as doxycycline, are available if the client is allergic to penicillin.

Women should be re-evaluated at 6 and 12 months after treatment for primary or secondary syphilis with additional serologic testing. Women with latent syphilis should be followed clinically and serologically at 6, 12, and 24 months and also tested for HIV (Lawrence et al., 2015).

Nursing Assessment

Assess the client for clinical manifestations of syphilis. Syphilis is divided into four stages: primary, secondary, latency, and tertiary. Primary syphilis is characterized by a chancre (painless ulcer) at the site of bacterial entry that will disappear within 1 to 6 weeks without intervention (Fig. 5.6). Motile spirochetes are present on darkfield examination of ulcer exudate. In addition, painless bilateral adenopathy is present during this highly infectious period. If left untreated, the infection progresses to the secondary stage. Secondary syphilis appears 2 to 6 months after the initial exposure and is manifested by flu-like symptoms and a maculopapular rash of the trunk, palms, and soles. Alopecia and adenopathy are both common during this stage. In addition to rashes, secondary syphilis may present with symptoms of fever, pharyngitis, weight loss, and fatigue (Euerle et al.,

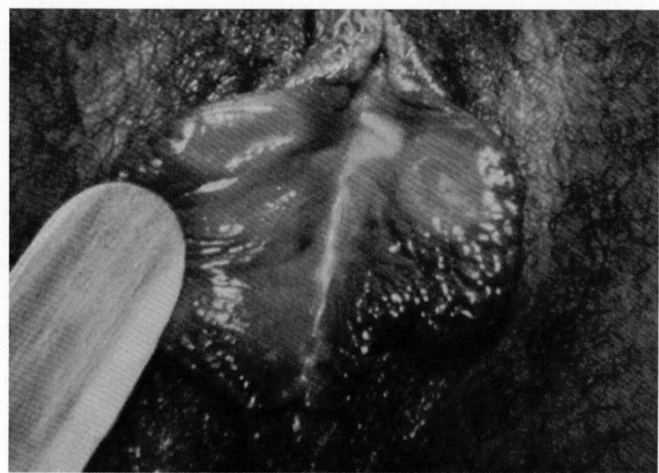

FIGURE 5.6 Chancre of primary syphilis. (From Sweet R. L, Gibbs R. S. (2005). *Atlas of infectious diseases of the female genital tract.* Philadelphia, PA: Lippincott Williams & Wilkins.)

2014). The secondary stage of syphilis lasts about 2 years. Once the secondary stage subsides, the latency period begins. This stage is characterized by the absence of any clinical manifestations of disease, although the serology is positive. This stage can last as long as 20 years. If not treated, tertiary or late syphilis occurs, with life-threatening heart disease and neurologic disease that slowly destroys the heart, eyes, brain, central nervous system, and skin.

Clients with a diagnosis of HIV or another STI should be screened for syphilis, and all pregnant women should be screened at their first prenatal visit. Dark-field microscopic examinations and direct fluorescent antibody tests of lesion exudate or tissue are the definitive methods for diagnosing early syphilis. A presumptive diagnosis can be made by using two serologic tests:

- Nontreponemal tests (Venereal Disease Research Laboratory [VDRL] and rapid plasma reagin [RPR])
- Treponemal tests (fluorescent treponemal antibody absorbed [FTA-ABS] and *T. pallidum* particle agglutination [TP-PA]). Dark-field microscopic examinations and direct fluorescent antibody tests of lesion exudate or tissue are the definitive methods for diagnosing early syphilis (CDC, 2015p).

Nursing Management of Herpes and Syphilis

Genital ulcers from either herpes or syphilis can be devastating to women, and the nurse can be instrumental in helping her through this difficult time. Referral to a support group may be helpful. Address the psychosocial aspects of these STIs with women by discussing appropriate coping skills, acceptance of the lifelong nature of the condition (herpes), and options for treatment and rehabilitation. Teaching Guidelines 5.3 highlights appropriate teaching points for the client with genital ulcers.

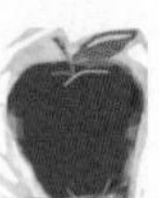

Teaching Guidelines 5.3
CARING FOR GENITAL ULCERS

- Abstain from intercourse during the prodromal period and when lesions are present.
- Wash hands with soap and water after touching lesions to avoid autoinoculation.
- Use comfort measures such as wearing nonconstricting clothes, wearing cotton underwear, urinating in water if urination is painful, taking lukewarm sitz baths, and air-drying lesions with a hair dryer on low heat.
- Avoid extremes of temperature such as ice packs or hot pads to the genital area as well as application of steroid creams, sprays, or gels.
- Use condoms with all new or noninfected partners.
- Inform health care professionals of your condition.

PELVIC INFLAMMATORY DISEASE

PID is an infection-induced inflammation of the female upper reproductive tract. PID rates remain unacceptably high. PID may involve the uterine lining (endometritis), the connective tissue adjacent to the uterus (parametritis), the Fallopian tubes (salpingitis), or the serous membrane that lines part of the abdominal cavity and viscera (peritonitis), or it may manifest as tubo-ovarian abscess (Brunham, Gottlieb, & Paavonen, 2015). PID results from an ascending polymicrobial infection of the upper female reproductive tract, frequently caused by untreated chlamydia or gonorrhea (Fig. 5.7). An estimated 750,000 women are diagnosed annually, resulting in over 250,000 hospitalizations (CDC, 2015n). Complications include

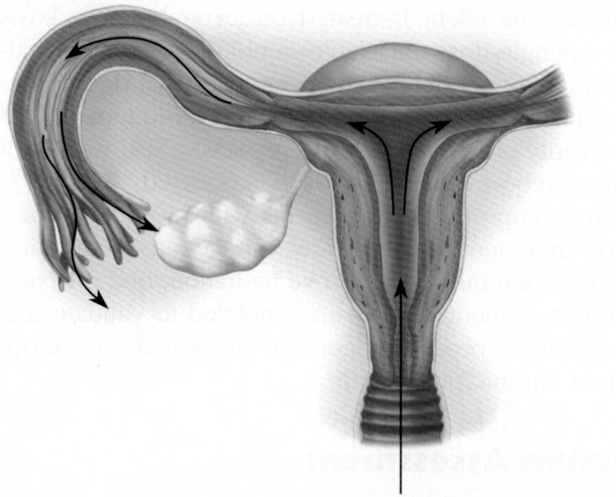

FIGURE 5.7 Pelvic inflammatory disease. Chlamydia or gonorrhea spreads up the vagina into the uterus and then to the fallopian tubes and ovaries.

HEALTHY PEOPLE 2020

STD-5 objective	Significance
Reduce the proportion of females who have ever required treatment for pelvic inflammatory disease (PID)	Educate women that abstinence is the only way to completely avoid contracting sexually transmitted infections
Reduce the proportion of childless females with fertility problems who have had a sexually transmitted disease or who have ever required treatment for PID.	Encourage women always to use condoms if participating in any sexual act Provide an open and confidential environment so women will report symptoms and seek treatment earlier

ectopic pregnancy, pelvic abscess, subfertility, recurrent or chronic episodes of the disease, chronic abdominal pain, pelvic adhesions, and depression (Gilbert, 2015). Because most PID cases are secondary to STIs, especially chlamydia, the most effective approach to control it is prevention. Because of the seriousness of the complications of PID, an accurate diagnosis is critical *Healthy People 2020*.

Therapeutic Management

Broad-spectrum antibiotic therapy is generally required to cover chlamydia, gonorrhea, and/or any anaerobic infection. A parenteral cephalosporin in a single injection with doxycycline 100 mg twice a day for 14 days is the current CDC recommendation (CDC, 2015a). PID in pregnancy is uncommon, but a combination of cefotaxime, azithromycin, and metronidazole for 14 days may be used. The client is treated on an ambulatory basis with a single-dose injectable antibiotic or is hospitalized and given antibiotics intravenously. The decision to hospitalize a woman is based on clinical judgment and the severity of her symptoms (e.g., severely ill with high fever, a tubo-ovarian abscess is suspected, woman is immunocompromised or presents with protracted vomiting). Treatment then includes intravenous antibiotics, increased oral fluids to improve hydration, bed rest, and pain management. Follow-up is needed to validate that the infectious process is gone to prevent the development of chronic pelvic pain.

Nursing Assessment

Nursing assessment of the woman with PID involves a complete health history and assessment of clinical manifestations, physical examination, and laboratory and diagnostic testing.

Health History and Clinical Manifestations

Explore the client's current and past medical health history for risk factors for PID, which may include:

- Adolescence or young adulthood
- Non-White female
- Having multiple sex partners
- Early onset of sexual activity
- History of PID or STI
- Sexual intercourse at an early age
- Alcohol or drug use
- Having intercourse with a partner who has untreated urethritis
- Recent insertion of an intrauterine contraceptive (IUC)
- Nulliparity
- Cigarette smoking
- Recent termination of pregnancy
- Lack of consistent condom use
- Lack of contraceptive use
- Douching
- Prostitution (Hay et al., 2015)

Assess the client for clinical manifestations of PID, keeping in mind that because of the wide variety of clinical manifestations of PID, clinical diagnosis can be challenging. To reduce the risk of missed diagnosis, the CDC has established criteria to establish the diagnosis of PID. Minimal criteria (all must be present) are lower abdominal tenderness, adnexal tenderness, and cervical motion tenderness. Additional supportive criteria that support a diagnosis of PID are:

- Abnormal cervical or vaginal mucopurulent discharge
- Oral temperature above 101°F
- Cervical motion tenderness
- Elevated erythrocyte sedimentation rate (inflammatory process)
- Elevated C-reactive protein level (inflammatory process)
- *N. gonorrhoeae* or *C. trachomatis* infection documented (causative bacterial organism)
- White blood cells on saline vaginal smear
- Prolonged or increased menstrual bleeding
- Dysmenorrhea
- Dysuria
- Painful sexual intercourse
- Nausea
- Vomiting (CDC, 2015n)

Physical Examination and Laboratory and Diagnostic Tests

Inspect the client for presence of fever (usually over 101°F) or vaginal discharge. Palpate the abdomen, noting tenderness over the uterus or ovaries. However, the only way to diagnose PID definitively is through an endometrial biopsy, transvaginal ultrasound, or laparoscopic examination.

Nursing Management

If the woman with PID is hospitalized, maintain hydration via intravenous fluids, if necessary and administer analgesics as needed for pain. Semi-Fowler's positioning facilitates pelvic drainage. A key element to treatment of PID is education to prevent recurrence. Depending on the clinical setting (hospital or community clinic) where the nurse encounters the woman diagnosed with PID, a risk assessment should be done to ascertain what interventions are appropriate to prevent a recurrence. To gain the woman's cooperation, explain the various diagnostic tests needed. Discuss the implications of PID and the risk factors for the infection; her sexual partner should be included if possible. Sexual counseling should include practicing safer sex, limiting the number of sexual partners, using barrier contraceptives consistently, avoiding vaginal douching, considering another contraceptive method if she has an intrauterine system (IUS) and has multiple sexual partners, and completing the course of antibiotics prescribed (Shepherd, 2015). Review the serious sequelae that may occur if the condition is not treated or if the woman does not comply with the treatment plan. Ask the woman to have her partner go for evaluation and treatment to prevent a repeat infection. Provide nonjudgmental support while stressing the importance of barrier contraceptive methods and follow-up care. Teaching Guidelines 5.4 gives further information related to PID prevention.

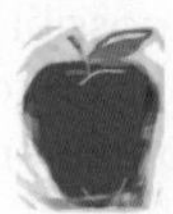

Teaching Guidelines 5.4

PREVENTING PELVIC INFLAMMATORY DISEASE

- Advise sexually active girls and women to insist their partners use condoms.
- Discourage routine vaginal douching, as this may lead to bacterial overgrowth.
- Encourage regular STI screening.
- Emphasize the importance of having each sexual partner receive antibiotic treatment.

VACCINE-PREVENTABLE STIS

Some STIs can be effectively prevented through preexposure vaccination. Vaccines are under development or are undergoing clinical trials for certain STIs, including HIV and HSV. However, the only vaccines currently available are for prevention of HAV, HBV, and HPV infection. Vaccination efforts focus largely on integrating the use of these available vaccines into STI prevention and treatment activities (CDC, 2014c).

Human Papillomavirus

HPV is the most common viral infection in the United States (CDC, 2015l). Genital warts or condylomata (Greek for "warts") are caused by HPV. Conservative estimates suggest that in the United States, approximately 80 million people have productive HPV infection, and 14 million Americans acquire it annually (CDC, 2015l). Clinical studies have confirmed that HPV is the cause of essentially all cases of cervical cancer, which is the fourth most common cancer in women in the United States, following lung, breast, and colorectal cancer (American Cancer Society [ACS], 2015). HPV-mediated oncogenesis is responsible for up to 95% of cervical squamous cell carcinomas and nearly all preinvasive cervical neoplasms (Gearhart et al., 2015). More than 30 types of HPV can infect the genital tract. HPV is most prevalent in young women between the ages of 20 and 24 years old, followed closely by the 15- to 19-year-old age group (Callahan, 2016).

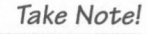

Take Note!

Most sexually active men and women will get HPV at some point in their lives. This means everyone is at risk (CDC, 2015l).

Nursing Assessment

Nursing assessment of the woman with HPV involves a complete health history and assessment of clinical manifestations, physical examination, and laboratory and diagnostic testing.

Health History and Clinical Manifestations

Assess the client's health history for risk factors for HPV, which include having multiple sex partners, age 15 to 25 years old, sex with a male who has had multiple sexual partners, and first intercourse at 16 years or younger (Dillner, 2015). Risk factors contributing to the development of cervical cancer include smoking, few or no screenings for cervical cancer, multiple sex partners, immunosuppressed state, nulliparity, long-term contraceptive use (more than 2 years), coinfection with another STI, pregnancy, nutritional deficiencies, and early onset of sexual activity (Coffey et al., 2015).

Assess the client for clinical manifestations of HPV. Most HPV infections are asymptomatic, unrecognized, or subclinical. Visible genital warts are usually caused by HPV types 6 or 11. In addition to the external genitalia, genital warts can occur on the cervix and in the vagina, urethra, anus, and mouth. Depending on the size and location, genital warts can be painful, friable, and pruritic, although most are typically asymptomatic (Fig. 5.8). The strains of HPV associated with genital warts are considered low risk for development of cervical cancer, but other HPV types (16, 18, 31, 33, 45, 52, and 58) have been strongly associated with cervical cancer (CDC, 2015l).

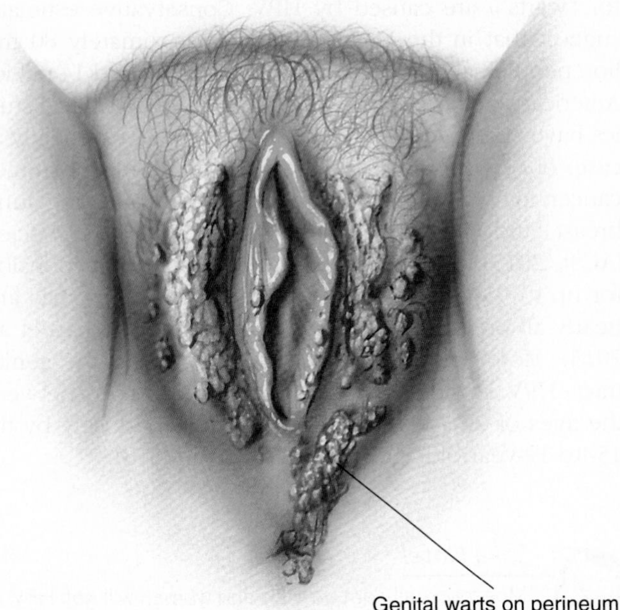

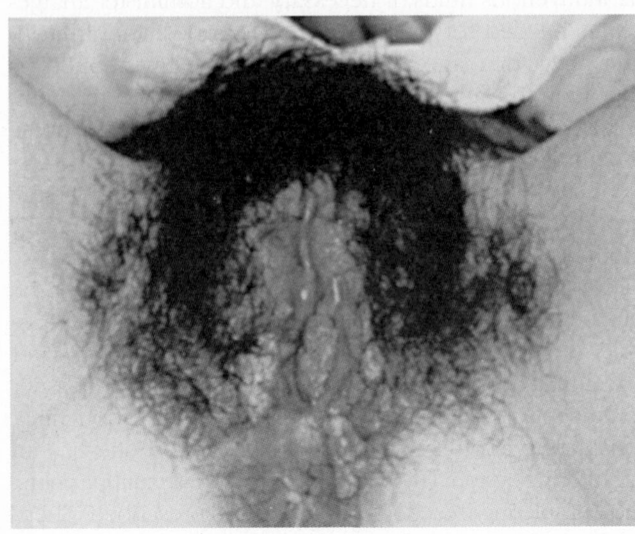

FIGURE 5.8 Genital warts. (Illustration provided by Anatomical Chart Co. Photograph from Sherwood L. Gorbach, John G. Bartlett, et al. *Infectious Diseases*. Philadelphia: Lippincott Williams & Wilkins, 2004.)

Physical Examination and Laboratory and Diagnostic Tests

Clinically, visible warts are diagnosed by inspection. The warts are fleshy papules with a warty, granular surface. Lesions can grow very large during pregnancy, affecting urination, defecation, mobility, and descent of the fetus (CDC, 2015l). Large lesions, which may resemble cauliflowers, exist in coalesced clusters and bleed easily.

Serial Pap smears are performed for low-risk women. These regular Pap smears will detect the cellular changes associated with HPV. The FDA has recently approved an HPV test as a follow-up for women who have an ambiguous Pap test. In addition, this HPV test may be a helpful addition to the Pap test for general screening of women aged 30 years and above. The HPV test is a diagnostic test that can determine the specific HPV strain, which is useful in discriminating between low-risk and high-risk HPV types. A specimen for testing can be obtained with a fluid-phase collection system such as Thin Prep. The HPV test can identify 13 of the high-risk types of HPV associated with the development of cervical cancer and can detect high-risk types of HPV even before there are any conclusive visible changes to the cervical cells. If the test is positive for the high-risk types of HPV, the woman should be referred for colposcopy.

Upon physical examination, it is determined that Sandy has genital warts. The nurse finds out that Sandy engaged in high-risk behavior with a stranger she "hooked up" with recently at college. She couldn't imagine that he would give her an STI because "he looked so clean-cut." She wonders how she could possibly have genital warts. What information should be given to Sandy about STIs in general? What specific information about HPV should be stressed?

Therapeutic Management

There is currently no medical treatment or cure for HPV. Instead, therapeutic management focuses heavily on prevention through the use of the HPV vaccine and education and on the treatment of lesions and warts caused by HPV. The FDA has approved three HPV vaccines to prevent cervical cancer: Cervarix, Gardasil, and Gardasil 9. The CDC's Advisory Committee on Immunization Practices (ACIP) has recommended the vaccine for routine administration to 11- and 12-year-old girls and boys. The ACIP also endorsed the use of a HPV vaccine for girls and boys as young as 9 years and recommended that women between the ages of 13 and 26 years receive the vaccination series, which consists of three injections over 6 months. All three are prophylactic HPV vaccines designed primarily for cervical cancer prevention. Cervarix is effective against HPV-16, 18, 31, 33, and 45, the five most common cancer-causing types, including most causes of adenocarcinoma for which we cannot screen adequately. Gardasil is effective against HPV-16, 18, and 31, three common squamous cell cancer-causing types.

In addition, Gardasil is effective against HPV-6 and 11, causes of genital warts and respiratory papillomatosis. The most important determinant of vaccine impact to reduce cervical cancer is its duration of efficacy. Cervarix is used only in females, whereas Gardasil 9 is used for both boys and girls. Gardasil 9 is effective against HPV types 6, 11, 16, 18, 31, 33, 45, 52, and 58. According to the FDA, the new vaccine (Gardasil 9) can potentially prevent about 90% of cervical, vulvar, vaginal, and anal cancers (Gearhart, Higgins, & Randall, 2015). Prophylactic HPV vaccines are safe, well tolerated, and highly efficacious in preventing persistent infections and cervical diseases associated with vaccine-HPV types among young females.

The vaccine is administered intramuscularly in three separate 0.5-mL doses. The first dose may be given to any individual 9 to 26 years old prior to infection with HPV. The second dose is administered 2 months after the first, and the third dose is given 6 months after the initial dose. The deltoid region of the upper arm or anterolateral area of the thigh may be used. The most common vaccine side effects include pain, fainting, redness, and swelling at the injection site; fatigue; headache; muscle and joint aches; and gastrointestinal distress. The vaccine is given in a series of three injections over a 6-month period (CDC, 2015l).

If the woman doesn't receive primary prevention with the vaccine, then secondary prevention would focus on education about the importance of receiving regular Pap smears and, for women over age 30 years, including an HPV test to determine whether the woman has a latent high-risk virus that could lead to precancerous cervical changes. Finally, treatment options for precancerous cervical lesions or genital warts caused by HPV are numerous and may include:

- Topical trichloroacetic acid 80% to 90%
- Liquid nitrogen cryotherapy
- Topical imiquimod 5% cream
- Topical podophyllin 10% to 25%
- Sinecatechins 15% ointment
- Laser carbon dioxide vaporization
- Client-applied podofilox 0.5% solution or gel
- Simple surgical excision
- Loop electrosurgical excisional procedure (LEEP)
- Intralesional interferon therapy (CDC, 2015a)

The goal of treating genital warts is to remove the warts and induce wart-free periods for the client. Treatment of genital warts should be guided by the preference of the client and available resources. No single treatment has been found to be ideal for all clients, and most treatment modalities appear to have comparable efficacy. Because genital warts can proliferate and become friable during pregnancy, they should be removed using a local agent. A cesarean birth is not indicated solely to prevent transmission of HPV infection to the newborn, unless the pelvic outlet is obstructed by warts (Gearhart et al., 2015).

Nursing Management

An HPV infection has many implications for the woman's health, but most women are unaware of HPV and its role in cervical cancer. The average age of sexual debut is in early adolescence; therefore, it is important to target this population for use of the HPV/cervical cancer vaccine.

Key nursing roles are teaching about prevention of HPV infection and client education and promotion of vaccines and screening tests in order to reduce the morbidity and mortality associated with cervical cancer caused by HPV infection. Teach all women that the only way to prevent HPV is to refrain from any genital contact with another person. Although the effect of condoms in preventing HPV infection is unknown, latex condom use has been associated with a lower rate of cervical cancer. Teach women about the link between HPV and cervical cancer. Explain that, in most cases, there are no signs or symptoms of infection with HPV. Strongly encourage all young women aged between 9 and 26 years to consider getting Gardasil 9, the vaccine against HPV. For all women, promote the importance of obtaining regular Pap smears and, for women over 30 years, suggest an HPV test to rule out the presence of a latent high-risk strain of HPV.

Education and counseling are important aspects of managing women with genital warts. Teach the woman that:

- Even after genital warts are removed, HPV still remains and viral shedding will continue.
- The likelihood of transmission to future partners and the duration of infectivity after treatment for genital warts are unknown.
- The recurrence of genital warts within the first few months after treatment is common and usually indicates recurrence rather than reinfection (CDC, 2015a).

Hepatitis A and B

Hepatitis is an acute, systemic, viral infection that can be transmitted sexually. The viruses associated with hepatitis or inflammation of the liver are hepatitis A, B, C, D, E, and G. Hepatitis A virus (HAV) is spread via the gastrointestinal tract. It can be acquired by drinking polluted water, by eating uncooked shellfish from sewage-contaminated waters or food handled by a hepatitis carrier with poor hygiene, and from oral/anal sexual contact. Approximately 33% of the United States population has serologic evidence of prior hepatitis A infection; the rate increases directly with age (Pyrsopoulos & Reddy, 2015). A person with hepatitis A can easily pass the disease to others within the same household.

Hepatitis B (HBV) is transmitted through saliva, blood serum, semen, menstrual blood, and vaginal secretions. The incubation period from the time of exposure to onset of symptoms is 6 weeks to 6 months (CDC, 2015h). In the early 2000s, transmission among heterosexual partners accounted for 40% of infections, and transmission among men who have sex with men accounted for 20% of infections. The World Health Organization (WHO) estimates that the prevalence of hepatitis B worldwide is 2 billion people, with about 240 million chronically infected with it. Worldwide, hepatitis B has the highest death rate of any STI except HIV (WHO, 2015b). Risk factors for infection include having multiple sex partners, engaging in unprotected receptive anal intercourse, and having a history of other STIs (CDC, 2015h). The most effective means to prevent the transmission of hepatitis A or B is pre-exposure immunization. Vaccines are available for the prevention of HAV and HBV, both of which can be transmitted sexually. Every person seeking treatment for an STI should be considered a candidate for hepatitis B vaccination, and some individuals (e.g., men who have sex with men, and injection-drug users) should be considered for hepatitis A vaccination (CDC, 2015h).

Therapeutic Management

Unlike other STIs, HBV and HAV are preventable through immunization. HAV is usually self-limiting and does not result in chronic infection. HBV can result in serious, permanent liver damage. Treatment is generally supportive. No specific treatment for acute HBV infection exists.

Nursing Assessment

Assess the client for clinical manifestations of hepatitis A and B. Hepatitis A produces flu-like symptoms with malaise, skin rashes, fatigue, anorexia, nausea, pruritus, fever, and upper right quadrant pain. Symptoms of hepatitis B are similar to those of hepatitis A, but with less fever and skin involvement. The diagnosis of hepatitis A cannot be made based on clinical manifestations alone and requires serologic testing. The presence of IgM antibody to HAV is diagnostic of acute HAV infection. Hepatitis B is detected by a blood test that looks for antibodies and proteins produced by the virus and is positively diagnosed by the presence of hepatitis B surface antibody (HBsAb) (Pyrsopoulos & Reddy, 2015).

Nursing Management

Nurses should encourage all women to be screened for hepatitis when they have their annual Pap smear, or sooner if high-risk behavior is identified. Nurses should also encourage women to undergo HBV screening at their first prenatal visit and repeat screening in the last trimester for women with high-risk behaviors (Lee & Lok, 2015). Nurses can also explain that hepatitis B vaccine is given to all infants after birth in most hospitals. The vaccination consists of a series of three injections given within 6 months. The vaccine has been shown to be safe and well tolerated by most recipients (CDC, 2015a). Hepatitis A vaccine is strongly encouraged for children between 12 and 23 months; persons 1 year of age and older traveling to countries with a high prevalence of hepatitis A, such as Central or South America, Mexico, Asia, Africa, and eastern Europe; men who have sex with men; persons who use street drugs; and persons with chronic liver disease (CDC, 2015g). For others, hepatitis A vaccine series (two doses 6 months apart) may be started whenever a person is at risk of infection.

Hepatitis C

Although HCV is not transmitted sexually, it deserves a brief mention here because injection-drug use by women places them at risk for it. Women at high risk include those with a history of injecting-drug use and those with a history of blood transfusion before 1992 (CDC, 2015i). The prevalence of HCV infection in pregnant women is approximately 1%. The majority of infected women are not aware they have HCV because they are not clinically ill. Perinatal transmission of HCV is relatively rare, except in women who are immunocompromised (HIV/AIDS) (Mattson & Smith, 2015).

ECTOPARASITIC INFECTIONS

Ectoparasites are a common cause of skin rash and pruritus throughout the world, affecting people of all ages, races, and socioeconomic groups. Overcrowding, delayed diagnosis and treatment, and poor public education contribute to the prevalence of ectoparasites in both industrial and nonindustrial nations. Approximately 300 million cases of ectoparasitic cases are reported worldwide each year (CDC, 2015d). These infections include infestations of scabies and pubic lice. Since these parasites are easily passed from one person to another during sexual intimacy, clients should be assessed for them when receiving care for other STIs. Scabies is an intensely pruritic dermatitis caused by a mite. The female mite burrows under the skin and deposits eggs, which hatch.

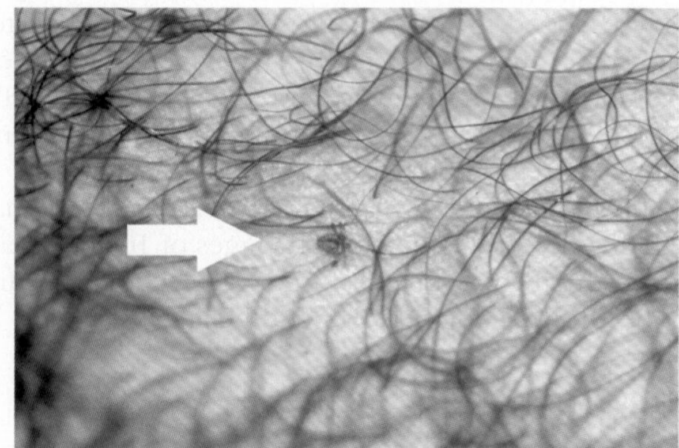

FIGURE 5.9 Pubic lice. A small brown living crab louse is seen at the base of hairs (*arrow*). (From Goodheart, H. (2009). *Goodheart's photoguide of common skin disorders*. Philadelphia, PA: Lippincott Williams & Wilkins.)

The lesions start as a small papule that reddens, erodes, and sometimes crusts. Diagnosis is based on history and appearance of burrows in the webs of the fingers and the genitalia (Guenther & Maguiness, 2015). Aggressive infestation can occur in immunodeficient, debilitated, or malnourished people, but healthy people do not usually suffer sequelae.

Clients with pediculosis pubis (pubic lice) usually seek treatment because of the pruritus, because of a rash brought on by skin irritation from scratching, or because they notice lice or nits in their pubic hair, axillary hair, abdominal and thigh hair, and sometimes in the eyebrows, eyelashes, and beards. Infestation is usually asymptomatic until after a week or so, when bites cause pruritus and secondary infections from scratching (Fig. 5.9). Diagnosis is based on history and the presence of nits (small, shiny, yellow, oval, dew-drop-like eggs) affixed to hair shafts or lice (a yellowish, oval, wingless insect) (Monsel & Chosidow, 2015).

Treatment is directed at the infested area, using permethrin 1% cream rinse and pyrethrin with piperonyl butoxide, which are FDA approved for treating head lice. Both are available as over-the-counter (OTC) preparations. Repeat treatment in 1 week is advised to eradicate eggs that may have hatched after treatment started (King et al., 2015). Bedding and clothing should be washed in hot water to decontaminate it. Sexual partners should be treated also, as well as family members who live in close contact with the infected person.

Nursing care of a woman infested with lice or scabies involves a three-tiered approach: eradicating the infestation with medication, removing nits, and preventing spread or recurrence by managing the environment. OTC products are safe for use and kill the active lice or mites. Nurses should provide education about these products (Teaching Guidelines 5.5). The nurse can follow these same guidelines to prevent the health care facility from becoming infested.

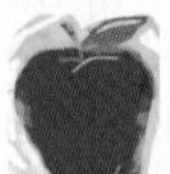

Teaching Guidelines 5.5

TREATING AND MINIMIZING THE SPREAD OF SCABIES AND PUBIC LICE

- Use the medication according to the manufacturer's instructions.
- Remove nits with a fine-toothed nit comb.
- Do not share any personal items with others or accept items from others.
- Treat objects, clothing, and bedding and wash them in hot water.
- Meticulously vacuum carpets to prevent a recurrence of infestation.

HUMAN IMMUNODEFICIENCY VIRUS (HIV)

An estimated 1 million people in the United States and 34 million globally currently live with HIV and new cases of HIV infection in the United States have remained stable at about 50,000 annually (National Institute of Allergy and Infectious Diseases, 2015). In terms of epidemiology, fatality rate, and its social, legal, ethical, and political aspects, HIV infection became a global public health crisis over 20 years ago and has generated more concern than any other infectious disease in modern medical history (Oyelowo & Johnson, 2016). To date, there is no cure for this fatal viral infection.

The HIV virus is transmitted by intimate sexual contact, by sharing needles for intravenous drug use, from mother to fetus during pregnancy, or by transfusion of infected blood or blood products. Men who have sex with men represent the largest proportion of new infections, followed by men and women infected through heterosexual sex (CDC, 2015k). Approximately one in four people living with HIV infection in the United States are women (CDC, 2015k). About 12,500 new cases of HIV infection among women in the United States occur each year (CDC, 2015k). HIV infection disproportionately affects African American and Hispanic women. Together they represent less than 25% of all US women, yet they account for more than 88% of HIV infection cases (CDC, 2015k).

Women are particularly vulnerable to heterosexual transmission of HIV due to substantial mucosal exposure to seminal fluids. This biologic fact amplifies the risk of HIV transmission when coupled with the high prevalence of nonconsensual sex, sex without condoms, and the unknown and/or high-risk behaviors of their partners (NIAID, 2015). Therefore, the face of HIV/AIDS is becoming the face of young women. That shift will ultimately exacerbate the incidence of HIV because women spread it not only through sex, but also through nursing and childbirth.

AIDS is a breakdown in the immune function caused by HIV, a retrovirus. The infected person develops opportunistic infections or malignancies that become fatal. Progression from HIV infection to AIDS varies within individuals. HIV affects CD4 cells in two ways: by depleting them and by impairing the remaining ones. This invasion of CD4 cells results in a gradual loss of immune function. If nothing is done to stop this invasion of CD4 cells, HIV can destroy as many as 1 billion CD4 cells daily (King et al., 2015).

Over 30 years (1981) have passed since HIV/AIDS began to affect our society. Since then, 1 million people have been infected by the virus, with AIDS being the fourth leading cause of death globally (CDC, 2015k). The morbidity and mortality of HIV continue to hold the attention of the medical community. While there has been a dramatic improvement in both morbidity and mortality with the use of antiretroviral therapy (ART), the incidence of HIV infection continues to be a public health challenge.

Take Note!

Once the HIV infection has progressed to AIDS, the survival period is usually less than 2 years in untreated clients (Bennett & Gilroy, 2015).

The fetal and neonatal effects of acquiring HIV through perinatal transmission can be devastating. If the HIV-infected infant goes untreated, progression to AIDS and eventual fatality will occur. An infected mother can transmit HIV infection to her newborn before or during birth and through breastfeeding. Current incidence of perinatal transmission is less than 1% if HIV+ mother is taking antiretroviral medication during pregnancy (CDC, 2015k).

HIV and Adolescents

As a typical function of development adolescents may view themselves as invincible, and thus delay seeking health care. They may be embarrassed or lack access to health care or may delay or refuse treatment if a diagnosis of HIV infection is made. Though the rates of HIV infection among adolescents have remained stable since 2006, the effects of HIV infection in this population continue to be of concern (CDC, 2015j). On average, the development of AIDS occurs about 11 years after infection, so most young adults with AIDS were infected during adolescence (Fairlie et al., 2015).

Most HIV-infected adolescents are exposed to the virus through heterosexual or homosexual contact. The majority of HIV-infected adolescent males are infected through sex with other males, while female teenagers are mostly exposed through heterosexual contact. Injected drug use accounts for a small percentage of HIV infection among male and female adolescents. Similar to HIV infection in women, African American and Hispanic adolescents represent a disproportionate percentage of HIV infection among teenagers (CDC, 2015j). More than 2 million adolescents between the ages of 10 and 19 are living with HIV, and many do not receive the care and support they need to stay in good health.

Clinical Manifestations

HIV infection undergoes three distinct phases—acute seroconversion, asymptomatic infection, and then progresses to AIDS. When a person is initially infected with HIV, he or she goes through an acute primary infection period for about 3 weeks. The HIV viral load drops rapidly because the host's immune system works well to fight this initial infection. The onset of the acute primary infection occurs 2 to 6 weeks after exposure. Symptoms include fever, pharyngitis, rash, and myalgia. Most people do not associate this flu-like condition with HIV infection. After initial exposure, there is a period of 3 to 12 months before seroconversion. The person is considered infectious during this time.

After the acute phase, the infected person becomes asymptomatic, but the HIV virus begins to replicate. Even though there are no symptoms, the immune system runs down. A normal person has a CD4 T-cell count of 450 to 1,200 cells per μL. When the CD4 T-cell count reaches 200 or less, the person has reached the stage of AIDS. The immune system begins a constant battle to fight this viral invasion, but over time it falls behind. A viral reservoir occurs in T cells that can store various stages of the virus. The onset and severity of the disease correlate directly with the viral load: the more HIV virus that is present, the worse the person will feel.

As profound immunosuppression begins to occur, an opportunistic infection will occur, qualifying the person for the diagnosis of AIDS. The diagnosis is finally confirmed when the CD4 count is below 200. As of now, AIDS will eventually develop in everyone who is HIV-positive.

World Health Organization (2015a) now recommends earlier initiation of ART for adults and adolescents, the delivery of more client-friendly antiretroviral (ARV) drugs, and prolonged use of ARVs to reduce the risk of mother-to-child transmission of HIV. ART should be started when the CD4 count reaches the 350 to 500 range. Also, WHO (2015a) recommends that HIV-positive mothers or their infants take ARVs while breastfeeding to prevent HIV transmission for up to 12 months after birth.

Diagnosis

HIV testing is regarded as the gateway to prevention and treatment. Several types of tests are approved to detect antigens, antibodies, or RNA. Screening for HIV infection is paramount, since infected individuals may remain asymptomatic for years while the infection progresses. Currently, there are two categories of screening methods: rapid HIV tests and confirmatory tests. The rapid tests allow for screening at the point of care and offer quick results. Five rapid HIV tests that are FDA approved are OraQuick Advance HIV tests (whole blood used); Uni-Gold Recombigen HIV test (whole blood used); Reveal G-3 Rapid HIV Antibody test (serum or plasma used); Multispot (serum or plasma used); and Clearview Stat-Pak (whole blood used). A positive result is followed up with one of two confirmatory tests: Western blot (WB) test or immunofluorescence assay (IFA) (Bennett & Gilroy, 2015).

Quick tests for HIV produce results in 10 to 20 minutes and also lower the health care worker's risk of occupational exposure by eliminating the need to draw blood. The CDC's Advancing HIV Prevention initiative, launched in 2003, has made increased testing a national priority. The initiative calls for testing to be incorporated into all routine medical care and to be delivered in more nontraditional settings.

Fewer than half of adults between the ages of 18 and 64 have ever had an HIV test, according to the CDC. The agency estimates that one fourth of the 1 million HIV-infected people in the United States do not know they are infected. This means they are not receiving treatment that can prolong their lives, and they may be unknowingly infecting others. In addition, even when people do get tested, one in three failed to return to the testing site to learn their results when there was a 2-week wait. The CDC hopes that the new "one-stop" approach to HIV testing changes that pattern. About 50,000 new HIV cases are reported each year in the United States, and that number has held steady for the past few years despite massive efforts in prevention education (CDC, 2015k).

People who are infected with HIV but not aware of it are not able to take advantage of the therapies that can keep them healthy and extend their lives, nor do they have the knowledge to protect their sex or drug-use partners from becoming infected. Knowing whether one is positive or negative for HIV confers great benefits in healthy decision making.

Rapid point of service HIV tests are becoming powerful screening tools in various health care settings because they offer the opportunity to not only screen for HIV, but also to educate the person regarding risk factors, and discuss their test results—all in one clinical visit. Most use a finger stick drop of blood or a swab of saliva taken from the mouth. Results are typically ready within 10 to 20 minutes. The CDC has specific protocols for confirmation of positive screening test results—confirmation tests include the WB test or IFA. Home HIV testing kits are available, accurate, and being used by many with the potential to increase testing, diagnosis, and ultimately reduce HIV prevalence (Dore, 2015).

If the confirmation test (WB or IFA) is positive, the person is infected with HIV and is capable of transmitting the virus to others. HIV antibody is detectable in at least 95% of people within 3 months after infection (CDC, 2015k).

Therapeutic Management

The goals of HIV drug therapy are to:

- Decrease the HIV viral load below the level of detection
- Restore the body's ability to fight off pathogens
- Improve the client's quality of life
- Reduce HIV morbidity and mortality (King et al., 2015)

Highly active antiretroviral therapy (HAART), which combines at least three ARV drugs, has dramatically improved the prognosis of HIV/AIDS. Treatment with HAART should begin for any person with an AIDS-defining illness or with a history of a CD4 count less than 350 cells/mm (WHO, 2016). The current HAART standard is a triple combination therapy, but some clients may be given a fourth or fifth agent.

Current therapy to prevent the transmission of HIV to the newborn includes a three-part regimen of having the mother take an oral ARV agent at 14 to 34 weeks of gestation; it is continued throughout pregnancy. During labor, an ARV agent is administered intravenously until delivery. An ARV syrup is administered to the infant within 12 hours after birth.

Dramatic new treatment advances with ARV medications have turned a disease that used to be a death sentence into a chronic, manageable one for individuals who live in countries where ART is available. Despite these advances in treatment, however, only a minority of HIV-positive people in the United States who take ARV medications are receiving the full benefits because they are not adhering to the prescribed regimen. Successful ART requires nearly perfect adherence to a complex medication regimen; less-than-perfect adherence leads to drug resistance (King et al., 2015).

Adherence is difficult because of the complexity of the regimen and the lifelong duration of treatment. A typical ARV regimen may consist of three or more medications taken twice daily. Adherence is made even more difficult because of the unpleasant side effects, such as nausea and diarrhea. Women in early pregnancy already experience these, and the ARV medication only exacerbates them.

Nursing Management

Nurses can play a major role in caring for the HIV-positive woman by helping her accept the possibility of a shortened life span, cope with others' reactions to a stigmatizing illness, and develop strategies to maintain her physical and emotional health. Educate the woman about changes she can make in her behavior to prevent spreading HIV to others, and refer her to appropriate community resources such as HIV medical care services, substance abuse, mental health services, and social services. See Nursing Care Plan 5.1: Overview for the Woman With HIV (at the end of the chapter).

Providing Education About Drug Therapy

The goal of ART is to suppress viral replication so that the viral load becomes undetectable by diagnostic tests. This is done to preserve immune function and delay disease progression but is a challenge because of the side effects of nausea and vomiting, diarrhea, altered taste, anorexia, flatulence, constipation, headaches, anemia, and fatigue. Although not everyone experiences all of the side effects, the majority do have some of them. Current research hasn't documented the long-term safety of exposure of the fetus to ARV agents during pregnancy, but collection of data is ongoing.

Help to reduce the development of drug resistance and thus treatment failure by identifying the barriers to adherence; identifying these barriers can help the woman to overcome them. Some of the common barriers exist because the woman:

- Does not understand the link between drug resistance and nonadherence
- Fears revealing her HIV status by being seen taking medication
- Hasn't adjusted emotionally to the HIV diagnosis
- Doesn't understand the dosing regimen or schedule
- Experiences unpleasant side effects frequently
- Feels anxious or depressed (Abdurakhmanov & Zandman-Goddard, 2015)

Educate the woman about the prescribed drug therapy and stress that it is very important to take the regimen as prescribed. Offer suggestions about how to cope with anorexia, nausea, and vomiting by:

- Separating the intake of food and fluids
- Eating dry crackers upon arising
- Eating six small meals daily
- Using high-protein supplements (Boost, Ensure) to provide quick and easy protein and calories
- Eating "comfort foods," which may appeal when other foods don't

Promoting Compliance

Remaining compliant with drug therapy is a huge challenge for many HIV-infected people. Compliance becomes difficult when the same pills that are supposed to thwart the disease are making the person sick. Nausea and diarrhea are just two of the possible side effects. It is often difficult to increase the client's quality of life when so much oral medication is required. The combination medication therapy is challenging for many people, and staying compliant over a period of years is extremely difficult. Stress the importance of taking the prescribed ARV drug therapies by explaining that they help prevent replication of the retroviruses and subsequent progression of the disease, as well as decreasing the risk of perinatal transmission of HIV. In addition, provide written materials describing diet, exercise, medications, and signs and symptoms of complications and opportunistic infections. Reinforce this information at each visit.

Preventing HIV Infection

The lack of information about HIV infection and AIDS causes great anxiety and fear of the unknown. It is vital to take a leadership role in educating the public about risky behaviors in the fight to control this disease. The core of HIV prevention is to abstain from sex until marriage, to be faithful, and to use condoms. This is all good advice for many women, but some simply do not have the economic and social power or choices or control over their lives to put that advice into practice. Recognize that fact, and address the factors that will give women more control over their lives by providing anticipatory guidance, giving ample opportunities to practice negotiation techniques and refusal skills in a safe environment, and encouraging the use of female condoms to protect against this deadly virus. Prevention is the key to reversing the current infection trends.

Providing Care During Pregnancy and Childbirth

Voluntary counseling and HIV testing should be offered to all pregnant women as early in the pregnancy as possible to identify HIV-infected women so that treatment can be initiated early. Once a pregnant woman is identified as being HIV-positive, she should be informed about the risk for perinatal infection. The risk of perinatal transmission of HIV from an infected mother to her newborn is about 25%. This risk falls to less than 1% if the mother receives ART during pregnancy (Adam, 2015). HIV can be spread to the infant through breastfeeding so that when acceptable alternative infant formulas are readily available, HIV-infected mothers should be counseled to avoid breastfeeding and use formula instead. WHO (2015a) recommendations indicate that transmission of HIV via breast milk is decreased when the mother is undergoing ART.

In addition, the woman needs instructions on ways to enhance her immune system by following these guidelines during pregnancy:

- Getting adequate sleep each night (7 to 9 hours)
- Avoiding infections (e.g., staying away from crowds, handwashing)

- Decreasing stress in her life
- Consuming adequate protein and vitamins
- Increasing her fluid intake to 2 L daily to stay hydrated
- Planning rest periods throughout the day to prevent fatigue

Despite the dramatic reduction in perinatal transmission, hundreds of infants will be born infected with HIV. The birth of each infected infant is a missed prevention opportunity. To minimize perinatal HIV transmission, identify HIV infection in women, preferably before pregnancy; provide information about disease prevention; and encourage HIV-infected women to follow the prescribed drug therapy.

Providing Appropriate Referrals

The HIV-infected woman may have difficulty coping with the normal activities of daily living because she has less energy and decreased physical endurance. She may be overwhelmed by the financial burdens of medical and drug therapies and the emotional responses to a life-threatening condition, as well as concern about her infant's future, if she is pregnant. A case management approach is needed to deal with the complexity of her needs during this time. Be an empathetic listener and make appropriate referrals for nutritional services, counseling, homemaker services, spiritual care, and local support groups. Many community-based organizations have developed programs to address the numerous issues regarding HIV/AIDS. The national AIDS hotline (1–800–342-AIDS) is a good resource. Table 5.4 provides a summary of perinatal effects of STIs during pregnancy.

PREVENTING SEXUALLY TRANSMITTED INFECTIONS

Education about safer sex practices—and the resulting increase in the use of condoms—can play a vital role in reducing STI rates all over the world. Clearly, knowledge and prevention are the best defenses against STIs. The prevention and control of STIs is based on the following concepts (CDC, 2014c).

1. Education and counseling of people at risk about safer sexual behavior
2. Identification of asymptomatic infected people and of symptomatic people unlikely to seek diagnosis and treatment
3. Effective diagnosis and treatment of infected people
4. Evaluation, treatment, and counseling of sex partners of people who are infected with an STI
5. Pre-exposure vaccination of people at risk for vaccine-preventable STIs

Nurses play an integral role in identifying and preventing STIs. They have a unique opportunity to educate the public about this serious public health issue by communicating the methods of transmission and symptoms associated with each condition, tracking the updated CDC treatment guidelines, and offering clients strategic preventive measures to reduce the spread of STIs.

It is not easy to discuss STI prevention when globally we are failing at it. Knowledge exists on how to prevent every single route of transmission, but the incidence continues to climb. Challenges to prevention of STIs include lack of resources and difficulty in changing the behaviors that contribute to their spread. Regardless of the challenging factors involved, nurses must continue to educate and meet the needs of all women to promote their sexual health. Successful treatment and prevention of STIs is impossible without education. Successful teaching approaches include giving clear, accurate messages that are age-appropriate and culturally sensitive.

Primary prevention strategies include education of all women, especially adolescents, regarding the risk of early sexual activity, the number of sexual partners, and STIs. Sexual abstinence is ideal but often not practiced; therefore, the use of barrier contraception (condoms) should be encouraged (see Teaching Guidelines 5.1).

Secondary prevention involves the need for annual pelvic examinations with Pap smears for all sexually active women, regardless of age. Many women with STIs are asymptomatic, so regular screening examinations are paramount for early detection. Understanding the relationship between poor socioeconomic conditions

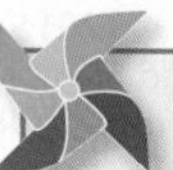

Consider This

I was thinking of my carefree college days, when the most important thing was having an active sorority life and meeting guys. I had been raised by very strict parents and was never allowed to date under their watch. Since I attended an out-of-state college, I figured that my parents' outdated advice and rules no longer applied. Abruptly, my thoughts of the past were interrupted by the HIV counselor asking about my feelings concerning my positive diagnosis. What was there to say at this point? I had a lot of fun but never dreamed it would haunt me for the rest of my life, which was going to be shortened considerably now. I only wish I could turn back the hands of time and listen to my parents' advice, which somehow doesn't seem so outdated now.

Thoughts: All of us have thought back on our lives to better times and wondered how our lives would have changed if we had made better choices or gone down another path. It is a pity that we have only one chance to make good, sound decisions at times. What would you have changed in your life if given a second chance? Can you still make a change for the better now?

TABLE 5.4 MATERNAL AND FETAL EFFECTS FROM STIS

STI	Maternal Effects	Fetal Effects
Candidiasis	Resistant to treatment during pregnancy Uncomfortable localized genital itching and discharge	Can acquire thrush in the mouth during birthing process if mother infected
Trichomoniasis	Has been implicated to cause PROM and preterm births	Risk of prematurity
Bacterial vaginosis	Increases risk for spontaneous abortion, PROM, chorioamnionitis, postpartum endometritis, and preterm labor	Risk of neonatal sepsis
Chlamydia	Postpartum endometritis, PROM, and preterm birth	Conjunctivitis, which can lead to blindness Low birth weight; and pneumonitis
Gonorrhea	Chorioamnionitis, preterm birth, PROM, fetal growth restriction, postpartum sepsis	Eye infection *gonococcal ophthalmia* which can cause blindness
Genital herpes	Spontaneous abortion, intrauterine infection, preterm labor, PROM, fetal growth restriction	Birth anomalies; transplacental infection
Syphilis	Spontaneous abortion, preterm birth, stillbirth	Congenital syphilis: multisystem organ failure, structural damage; mental retardation
Human papillomavirus (HPV)	May cause dystocia if large lesions	None known
Hepatitis B	May cause preterm birth; can be transmitted to fetus if active in last trimester	Can become chronic carrier of hepatitis B which may lead to liver cancer or cirrhosis
HIV	Fatigue, nausea, weight loss	Transmission can occur transplacentally, during childbirth or through breast milk

Sources: Callahan, T. L. (2016). *Tarascon OB/GYN pocketbook*. Burlington, MA: Jones & Bartlett Learning; King, T. L., Brucker, M. C., Kriebs, J. M., Fahey, J. O., Gegor, C. L., & Varney, H. (2015). *Varney's midwifery* (5th ed.), Burlington, MA: Jones & Bartlett Learning; Queenan, J. T., Spong, C. Y., & Lockwood, C. J. (2015). *Protocols for high-risk pregnancies: An evidence-based approach* (6th ed.). Somerset, NJ: John Wiley & Sons; and Silasi, M., Cardenas, I., Kwon, J. Y., Racicot, K., Aldo, P., & Mor, G. (2015). Viral infections during pregnancy. *American Journal of Reproductive Immunology, 73*(3), 199–213.

and poor patterns of sexual and reproductive self-care is significant in disease prevention and health promotion strategies.

Every successful form of prevention requires a change in behavior. The nursing role in teaching and rendering quality health care is invaluable evidence that the key to reducing the spread of STIs is through behavioral change. Nurses working in these specialty areas have a responsibility to educate themselves, their clients, their families, and the community about STIs, and to provide compassionate and supportive care to clients. Some strategies nurses can use to prevent the spread of STIs are detailed in Box 5.3.

Behavior Modification

Research validates that changing behaviors does result in a decrease in new STIs, but it must encompass all levels—governments, community organizations, schools, churches, parents, and individuals. Nurses can advocate for the development and implementation of educational initiatives to increase awareness of STIs (Alexander et al., 2015). Education must address ways to prevent becoming infected, ways to prevent transmitting infection, symptoms of STIs, and treatment. At this point in the STI epidemic, nurses do not have time to debate the relative merits of prevention versus treatment: both are underused and underfunded, and one leads to the other. But being serious about prevention and focusing on the strategies outlined above will bring about a positive change on everyone's part.

Contraception

The spread of STIs could be prevented by access to safe, efficient, appropriate, modern contraception for

BOX 5.3

SELECTED NURSING STRATEGIES TO PREVENT THE SPREAD OF STIS

- Provide basic information about STI transmission.
- Outline safer sexual behaviors for people at risk for STIs.
- Refer clients to appropriate community resources to reduce risk.
- Screen asymptomatic persons with STIs.
- Identify barriers to STI testing and remove them.
- Offer pre-exposure immunizations for vaccine-preventable STIs.
- Respond honestly about testing results and options available.
- Counsel and treat sexual partners of persons with STIs.
- Educate school administrators, parents, and teens about STIs.
- Support youth development activities to reduce sexual risk-taking.
- Promote the use of barrier methods (condoms, diaphragms) to prevent the spread of STIs.
- Assist clients to gain skills in negotiating safer sex.
- Discuss reducing the number of sexual partners to reduce risk.

everyone who wants it. Nurses can play an important role in helping women to identify their risk of STIs and to adopt preventive measures through the dual protection that contraceptives offer. Traditionally, family planning and STI services have been separate entities. Family planning services have addressed a woman's need for contraception without considering her or her partner's risk of STI; meanwhile, STI services have been heavily slanted toward men, ignoring the contraceptive needs of men and their partners.

Many women are at significant risk for unintended pregnancy and STIs, yet with this separation of services, there is limited evaluation of whether they need dual protection—that is, concurrent protection from STIs and unintended pregnancy. This lack of integration of services represents a missed opportunity to identify many at-risk women and to offer them counseling on dual protection (Zapata et al., 2015).

Nurses can expand their scopes in either setting by discussing dual protection by use of a male or female condom alone or by use of a condom along with a non-barrier contraceptive. Because barrier methods are not the most effective means of fertility control, they have not been typically recommended as a method alone for dual protection. Unfortunately, the most effective pregnancy prevention methods—sterilization, hormonal methods, and intrauterine devices—do not protect against STIs. Dual-method use protects against STIs and pregnancy.

NURSING CARE PLAN 5.1

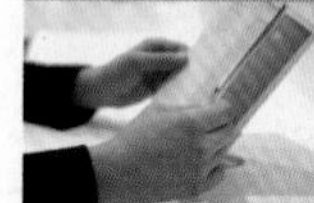

Overview of the Woman Who is HIV-Positive

Annie, a 28-year-old African American woman, is HIV-positive. She acquired HIV through unprotected sexual contact. She has been inconsistent in taking her antiretroviral medications and presents today stating she is tired and doesn't feel well.

NURSING DIAGNOSIS: Ineffective protection related to risk of infection secondary to inadequate immune system as manifested by client stating she has been inconsistent in taking her antiretroviral therapy medications.

Outcome Identification and Evaluation

Client will remain free of opportunistic infections as evidenced by temperature within acceptable parameters and absence of signs and symptoms of opportunistic infections.

Interventions: ***Minimizing the Risk of Opportunistic Infections***

- Assess CD4 count and viral loads *to determine disease progression* (CD4 counts 500/L and viral loads >10,000 copies/L = increased risk for opportunistic infections).
- Assess complete blood count *to identify presence of infection* (>10,000 cells/mm^3 may indicate infection).
- Assess oral cavity and mucous membranes for painful white patches in mouth *to evaluate for possible fungal infection*.
- Teach client to monitor for general signs and symptoms of infections, such as fever, weakness, and fatigue, *to ensure early identification*.

(continued)

NURSING CARE PLAN 5.1

Overview of the Woman Who is HIV-Positive (continued)

- Provide information explaining the importance of avoiding people with infections when possible *to minimize risk of exposure to infections.*
- Teach importance of keeping appointments so her CD4 count and viral load can be monitored *to alert the health care provider about her immune system status.*
- Instruct her to reduce her exposure to infections via:
  - Meticulous handwashing
  - Thorough cooking of meats, eggs, and vegetables
  - Wearing shoes at all times, especially when outdoors
- Encourage a balance of rest with activity throughout the day *to prevent overexertion.*
- Stress importance of maintaining prescribed antiretroviral drug therapies *to prevent disease progression and resistance.*
- If necessary, refer Annie to a nutritionist to help her understand what constitutes a well-balanced diet with supplements *to promote health and ward off infection.*

NURSING DIAGNOSIS: Knowledge deficit related to HIV infection and possible complications.

Outcome Identification and Evaluation

Client will demonstrate increased understanding of HIV infection as evidenced by verbalizing appropriate health care practices and adhering to measures to comply with therapy and reduce her risk of further exposure and reduce risk of disease progression.

Interventions: ***Providing Client Education***

- Assess her understanding of HIV and its treatment *to provide a baseline for teaching.*
- Establish trust and be honest with Annie; encourage her to talk about her fears and the impact of the disease *to provide an outlet for her concerns.* Encourage her to discuss reasons for her noncompliance.
- Provide a nonjudgmental, accessible, confidential, and culturally sensitive approach *to promote Annie's self-esteem and allow her to feel that she is a priority.*
- Explain measures, including safer sex practices and birth control options, to prevent disease transmission; determine her willingness to practice safer sex to protect others *to determine further teaching needs.*
- Discuss the signs and symptoms of disease progression and potential opportunistic infections *to promote early detection for prompt intervention.*
- Outline with the client the availability of community resources and make appropriate referrals as needed *to provide additional education and support.*
- Encourage Annie to keep scheduled appointments *to ensure follow-up and allow early detection of potential problems.*

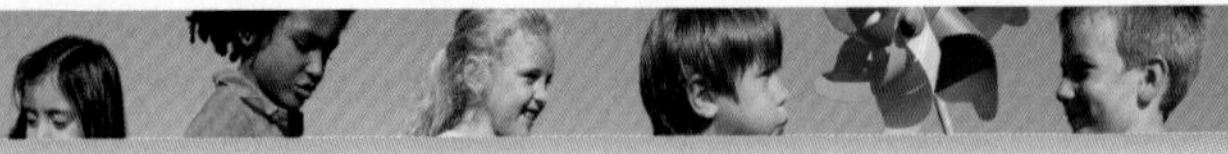

KEY CONCEPTS

- Avoiding risky sexual behaviors may preserve fertility and prevent chronic conditions later in life.
- An estimated 65 million people live with an incurable STI, and another 20 million are infected each year.
- The most reliable way to avoid transmission of STIs is to abstain from sexual intercourse (i.e., oral, vaginal, or anal sex) or to be in a long-term, mutually monogamous relationship with an uninfected partner.
- Barrier methods of contraception are recommended because they increase protection

from contact with urethral discharge, mucosal secretions, and lesions of the cervix or penis.

- The high rate of asymptomatic transmission of STIs calls for teaching high-risk women the nature of transmission and how to recognize infections.
- The CDC and ACOG recommend that all women be offered group B streptococcal screening by rectovaginal culture at 35 to 37 weeks of gestation, and that colonized women be treated with intravenous antibiotics at the time of labor or ruptured membranes.
- Nurses should practice good handwashing techniques and follow standard precautions to protect themselves and their clients from STIs.
- Nurses are in an important position to promote the sexual health of all women. Nurses should make their clients and the community aware of the perinatal implications and lifelong sequelae of STIs.

REFERENCES AND RECOMMENDED READINGS

Abdurakhmanov, A., & Zandman-Goddard, G. (2015). HIV spectrum and autoimmune diseases. In Y. Shoenfeld, N. Agmon-Levin, & N. Rose (Eds.), *Infection and autoimmunity* (2nd ed., pp. 371–392). St. Louis, MO: Elsevier.

Adam, S. (2015). HIV and pregnancy: review. *Obstetrics and Gynecology Forum* (Vol. 25(2), pp. 19–22). Sabinet Online.

Alexander, K. A., Jemmott, L. S., Teitelman, A. M., & D'Antonio, P. (2015). Addressing sexual health behavior during emerging adulthood: A critical review of the literature. *Journal of Clinical Nursing, 24*(1–2), 4–18.

Alexander, L. L., LaRosa, J. H., Bader, H., & Garfield, S. (2014). *New dimensions in women's health* (6th ed.). Sudbury, MA: Jones and Bartlett Publishers.

American Cancer Society. (2015). *HPV (human papilloma virus)*. Retrieved from http://www.cancer.org/cancer/cancercauses/othercarcinogens/infectiousagents/hpv/hpv-landing

Bennett, N. J., & Gilroy, S. A. (2015). *HIV disease*. Retrieved from http://emedicine.medscape.com/article/211316-overview

Brunham, R. C. (2015). A Chlamydia vaccine on the horizon. *Science, 348*(6241), 1322–1323.

Brunham, R. C., Gottlieb, S. L., & Paavonen, J. (2015). Pelvic inflammatory disease. *New England Journal of Medicine, 372*(21), 2039–2048.

Callahan, T. L. (2016). *Tarascon OB/GYN pocketbook*. Burlington, MA: Jones & Bartlett Learning.

Centers for Disease Control and Prevention. (2013). *Condom effectiveness*. Retrieved from http://www.cdc.gov/condomeffectiveness/docs/condomfactsheetinbrief.pdf

Centers for Disease Control and Prevention. (2014a). *Chlamydia – CDC fact sheet*. Retrieved from http://www.cdc.gov/std/chlamydia/stdfact-chlamydia.htm

Centers for Disease Control and Prevention. (2014b). *Reported STDs in the United States*. Retrieved from http://www.cdc.gov/nchhstp/ux-test-2015/newsroom/docs/factsheets/std-trends-508.pdf

Centers for Disease Control and Prevention. (2014c). *Sexually transmitted diseases*. Retrieved from http://www.cdc.gov/std/general/default.htm

Centers for Disease Control and Prevention. (2015a). *2015 Sexually transmitted diseases treatment guidelines*. Retrieved from http://www.cdc.gov/std/tg2015/

Centers for Disease Control and Prevention. (2015b). *Chlamydial infections*. Retrieved from http://www.cdc.gov/std/tg2015/chlamydia.htm

Centers for Disease Control and Prevention. (2015c). *Congenital syphilis*. Retrieved from http://www.cdc.gov/std/tg2015/congenital.htm

Centers for Disease Control and Prevention. (2015d). *Ectoparasitic infections*. Retrieved from http://www.cdc.gov/std/tg2015/ectoparasitic.htm

Centers for Disease Control and Prevention. (2015e). *Genital herpes*. Retrieved from http://www.cdc.gov/std/herpes/

Centers for Disease Control and Prevention. (2015f). *Gonorrhea*. Retrieved from http://www.cdc.gov/std/gonorrhea/default.htm

Centers for Disease Control and Prevention. (2015g). *Hepatitis A questions and answers for health professionals*. Retrieved from http://www.cdc.gov/hepatitis/hav/havfaq.htm#general

Centers for Disease Control and prevention. (2015h). *Hepatitis B FAQs for health professionals*. Retrieved from http://www.cdc.gov/hepatitis/hbv/hbvfaq.htm#overview

Centers for Disease Control and Prevention. (2015i). *Hepatitis C FAQs for health professionals*. Retrieved from http://www.cdc.gov/hepatitis/hcv/hcvfaq.htm#section1

Centers for Disease Control and Prevention. (2015j). *HIV among youth*. Retrieved from http://www.cdc.gov/hiv/group/age/youth/index.html

Centers for Disease Control and Prevention. (2015k). *HIV/AIDS*. Retrieved from http://www.cdc.gov/hiv/basics/index.html

Centers for Disease Control and Prevention. (2015l). *Human papillomavirus (HPV)*. Retrieved from http://www.cdc.gov/std/hpv/default.htm

Centers for Disease Control and Prevention. (2015m). *Minority health*. Retrieved from http://www.cdc.gov/minorityhealth/populations/REMP/aian.html

Centers for Disease Control and Prevention. (2015n). *Pelvic inflammatory disease (PID) – CDC fact sheet*. Retrieved from http://www.cdc.gov/std/pid/stdfact-pid-detailed.htm

Centers for Disease Control and Prevention. (2015o). *Sexual risk behaviors: HIV, STD, & teen pregnancy prevention*. Retrieved from http://www.cdc.gov/healthyyouth/sexualbehaviors/

Centers for Disease Control and Prevention. (2015p). *Syphilis*. Retrieved from http://www.cdc.gov/std/tg2015/syphilis.htm

Centers for Disease Control and Prevention [CDC] (2016). *Fungal Diseases: Candidiasis*. Retrieved from: http://www.cdc.gov/fungal/diseases/candidiasis/

Chen, M. Y., Klausner, J. D., Fairley, C. K., Guy, R., Wilson, D., & Donovan, B. (2015). Syphilis: A fresh look at an old foe. *Sexual Health, 12*(2), 93–95.

Coffey, K., Beral, V., Green, J., Reeves, G., & Barnes, I. (2015). Lifestyle and reproductive risk factors associated with anal cancer in women aged over 50 years. *British Journal of Cancer, 112*, 1568–1574. doi:10.1038/bjc.2015.89

Dillner, J. (2015). Prevention of human papillomavirus–Associated cancers. *Seminars in Oncology, 42*(2), 272–283.

Dore, M. (2015). Observations on home HIV testing. *AIDS, 29*(11), 1421–1422.

Euerle, B., Hogan, D. J., Weiss, E. L., Sachter, J. J., McCalmont, T., Sinert, R., et al. (2014). *Syphilis*. Retrieved from http://emedicine.medscape.com/article/229461-overview

Fairlie, L., Sipambo, N., Fick, C., & Moultrie, H. (2015). Focus on adolescents with HIV and AIDS. *South African Medical Journal, 104*(12), 897–904.

Gearhart, P. A., Higgins, R. V., Randall, T. C., & Buckley, R. M. (2015). *Human papillomavirus*. Retrieved from http://emedicine.medscape.com/article/219110-overview

Gilbert, L. (2015). Update on pelvic inflammatory disease. *Pathology-Journal of the RCPA, 47*, S49. doi: 10.1097/01.PAT.0000461451.11655.2 c

Guenther, L. C. C., & Maguiness, S. (2015). *Pediculosis and phthiriasis (lice infestation)*. Retrieved from: http://emedicine.medscape.com/article/225013-overview

Guttmacher Institute. (2014). *American teens' sexual and reproductive health*. Retrieved from http://www.guttmacher.org/pubs/FB-ATSRH.html

Hay, P. E., Kerry, S. R., Normansell, R., Horner, P. J., Reid, F., Kerry, S. M., et al. (2015). Which sexually active young female students are most at risk of pelvic inflammatory disease? A prospective study. *Sexually Transmitted Infections*, doi:10.1136/sextrans-2015–052063

Heller, D. S. (2015). Diseases of the fallopian tube. *OB-GYN pathology for the clinician* (pp. 135–145). New York, NY: Springer International Publishing.

King, T. L., Brucker, M. C., Kriebs, J. M., Fahey, J. O., Gegor, C. L., & Varney, H. (2015). *Varney's midwifery* (5th ed.). Burlington, MA: Jones & Bartlett Learning.

Lawrence, D., Cresswell, F., Whetham, J., & Fisher, M. (2015). Syphilis treatment in the presence of HIV: The debate goes on. *Current Opinion in Infectious Diseases, 28*(1), 44–52.

Lee, H., & Lok, A. S. F. (2015). Hepatitis B and pregnancy. UpToDate. Retrieved from http://www.uptodate.com/contents/hepatitis-b-and-pregnancy

March of Dimes. (2015). *Your top STD questions answered*. Retrieved from: http://newsmomsneed.marchofdimes.org/?tag=stis

Mattson, S., & Smith, J. E. (2015). *Core curriculum for maternal-newborn nursing* (5th ed.). St. Louis, MO: Saunders Elsevier.

Monsel, G., & Chosidow, O. (2015). 24. Scabies, lice, and myiasis. In S. David (Ed.): *Clinical Infectious Disease* (2nd ed., pp.162–166). Cambridge: Cambridge University Press.

Myers, J. L., Buhi, E. R., Marhefka, S., Daley, E., & Dedrick, R. (2015). Associations between individual and relationship characteristics and genital herpes disclosure. Journal of Health Psychology, doi: 10.1177/1359105315575039.

National Institute of Allergy and Infectious Diseases. (2015). *HIV/AIDS*. Retrieved from: http://www.niaid.nih.gov/topics/hivaids/Pages/Default.aspx

Oyelowo, T., & Johnson, J. L. (2016). *A guide to women's health* (2nd ed.). Burlington, MA: Jones & Bartlett Learning.

Petrova, D., & Garcia-Retamero, R. (2015). Effective evidence-based programs for preventing sexually-transmitted infections: A meta-analysis. *Current HIV Research, 13*(5), 432–438.

Public Health Agency of Canada. (2015). *Canadian guidelines on sexually transmitted infections*. Retrieved from http://www.phac-aspc.gc.ca/std-mts/sti-its/

Pyrsopoulos, N. T., & Reddy, K. R. (2015). *Hepatitis B. eMedicine*. Retrieved from http://emedicine.medscape.com/article/177632-overview

Queenan, J. T., Spong, C. Y. & Lockwood, C. J. (2015). *Protocols for high-risk pregnancies: An evidence-based approach* (6th ed.). Somerset, NJ: John Wiley & Sons.

Qureshi, S. (2015). Chlamydial genitourinary infections. eMedicine. Retrieved from http://emedicine.medscape.com/article/214823-overview.

Ross, C. E., Tao, G., Patton, M., & Hoover, K. W. (2015). Screening for human immunodeficiency virus and other sexually transmitted diseases among US women with prenatal care. *Obstetrics & Gynecology, 125*(5), 1211–1216.

Sangkomkamhang, U. S., Lumbiganon, P., Prasertcharoensuk, W., & Laopaiboon, M. (2015). Antenatal lower genital tract infection screening and treatment programs for preventing preterm delivery. *Cochrane Database of Systematic Reviews 2015, 2*: CD006178. doi: 10.1002/14651858.CD006178.pub3.

Selim, M. A., Parra, V., Sangueza, O. P., Requena, L., & Sangueza, M. A. (2015). Infectious diseases and infestations of the vulva. In Mai, P. H., & Selim, M. A., (Eds.) *Vulvar Pathology* (pp. 139–193). New York, NY: Springer.

Shepherd, S. M. (2015). Pelvic inflammatory disease. eMedicine. Retrieved from http://emedicine.medscape.com/article/256448-overview.

Silasi, M., Cardenas, I., Kwon, J. Y., Racicot, K., Aldo, P., & Mor, G. (2015). Viral infections during pregnancy. *American Journal of Reproductive Immunology, 73*(3), 199–213.

Smith, D. S., & Ramos, N. (2015). Trichomoniasis. eMedicine. Retrieved from http://emedicine.medscape.com/article/230617-overview.

Stamm, L. V. (2015). Syphilis: Antibiotic treatment and resistance. *Epidemiology and Infection, 143*(08), 1567–1574.

Thomas, J., Bates, C. M., & Mathew, T. (2015). P251 Treatment dilemma of chlamydia in pregnancy. *Sexually Transmitted Infections, 91*(Suppl 1), A98-A98.

U.S. Department of Health and Human Services. (2015). *Healthy People 2020*. Retrieved from http://www.healthypeople.gov/2020/topics-objectives.

U.S. Department of Health and Human Services Office of Adolescent Health. (2015). Sexually transmitted diseases. Retrieved from http://www.hhs.gov/ash/oah/adolescent-health-topics/reproductive-health/stds.html

World Health Organization. (2015a). *Breast is best, even for HIV-positive mothers.* Retrieved from: http://www.who.int/bulletin/volumes/88/1/10–030110/en/

World Health Organization. (2015b). *Hepatitis B.* Retrieved from http://www.who.int/mediacentre/factsheets/fs204/en/

World Health Organization (2016). *Antiretroviral therapy.* Retrieved from http://www.who.int/topics/antiretroviral_therapy/en/

Wong, B. (2015). Gonorrhea. eMedicine. Retrieved from http://emedicine.medscape.com/article/218059-overview.

Zapata, L. B., Tregear, S. J., Curtis, K. M., Tiller, M., Pazol, K., Mautone-Smith, N., et al. (2015). Impact of contraceptive counseling in clinical settings: A systematic review. *American Journal of Preventive Medicine, 49*(2), S31–S45.

CHAPTER WORKSHEET

MULTIPLE CHOICE QUESTIONS

1. Which of the following contraceptive methods offers protection against sexually transmitted infections (STIs)?
   a. Oral contraceptives
   b. Withdrawal
   c. Latex condom
   d. Intrauterine system

2. When teaching about HIV transmission, which of the following does the nurse explain that the virus cannot be transmitted by?
   a. Shaking hands
   b. Sharing drug needles
   c. Sexual intercourse
   d. Breastfeeding

3. A woman with HPV is likely to present with which nursing assessment finding?
   a. Profuse, pus-filled vaginal discharge
   b. Clusters of genital warts
   c. Single painless ulcer
   d. Multiple vesicles on genitalia

4. The nurse's discharge teaching plan for the woman with PID should reinforce which of the following potentially life-threatening complications?
   a. Involuntary infertility
   b. Chronic pelvic pain
   c. Depression
   d. Ectopic pregnancy

5. To confirm a finding of primary syphilis, the nurse would observe which of the following on the external genitalia?
   a. A highly variable skin rash
   b. A yellow-green vaginal discharge
   c. A nontender, indurated ulcer
   d. A localized gumma formation

6. A sexually active 19-year-old presents to the clinic with postcoital bleeding, dysuria, and a yellow discharge. Her cervix upon exam is red and friable. What might the nurse suspect?
   a. Cervical cancer
   b. A tampon injury
   c. Primary syphilis
   d. Chlamydia

   The correct response is "D" because these clinical manifestations are typical of a chlamydia infection (postcoital bleeding, dysuria, frequency, vaginal discharge, cervical tenderness with easily induced bleeding). Response "A" is incorrect because it would be rare to have cervical cancer at such a young age and the symptoms presented are not suggestive of this diagnosis. Response "B" is incorrect because the presenting symptoms are not suggestive of a cervical injury. Response "C" is incorrect because primary syphilis would present with a chancre lesion at the site where the bacteria entered the body, typically the vulva.

CRITICAL THINKING EXERCISE

1. Sally, age 17, comes to the teen clinic saying that she is in pain and has some "crud" between her legs. The nurse takes her into the examining room and questions her about her symptoms. Sally states she had numerous genital bumps that had been filled with fluid, then ruptured and turned into ulcers with crusts. In addition, she has pain on urination and overall body pain. Sally says she had unprotected sex with several men when she was drunk at a party a few weeks back, but she thought they were "clean."
   a. Which STI would the nurse suspect?
   b. The nurse should give immediate consideration to which of Sally's complaints?
   c. What should be the goal of the nurse in teaching Sally about STIs?

STUDY ACTIVITIES

1. Select a website at the end of the chapter to explore. Educate yourself about one specific STI thoroughly and share your expertise with your clinical group.

2. Contact your local health department and request current statistics regarding three STIs. Ask them to compare the current number of cases reported to last year's. Are they less or more? What may be some of the reasons for the change in the number of cases reported?

3. Request permission to attend a local STI clinic to shadow a nurse for a few hours. Describe the nurse's counseling role with clients and what specific information is emphasized to clients.

4. Two common STIs that appear together and commonly are treated together regardless of identification of the secondary one are ________________ and ________________.

5. Genital warts can be treated with which of the following? Select all that apply.
   a. Penicillin
   b. Podophyllin
   c. Imiquimod
   d. Cryotherapy
   e. Antiretroviral therapy
   f. Acyclovir

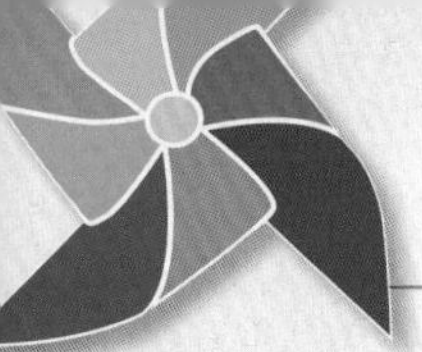

CHAPTER WORKSHEET

BRINGING IT ALL TOGETHER: A CASE STUDY

Charlotte, a 22 year old, has presented at the local clinic with concerns of having contracted a sexually transmitted infection (STI). During the nursing interview Charlotte identifies that she has been sexually active since the age of 15 and has had "at least 5 different sex partners". The health assessment confirms that Charlotte has been infected with pediculosis pubis (pubic lice) and treatment has been prescribed.

Go to thePoint to find questions to consider about this case.

6

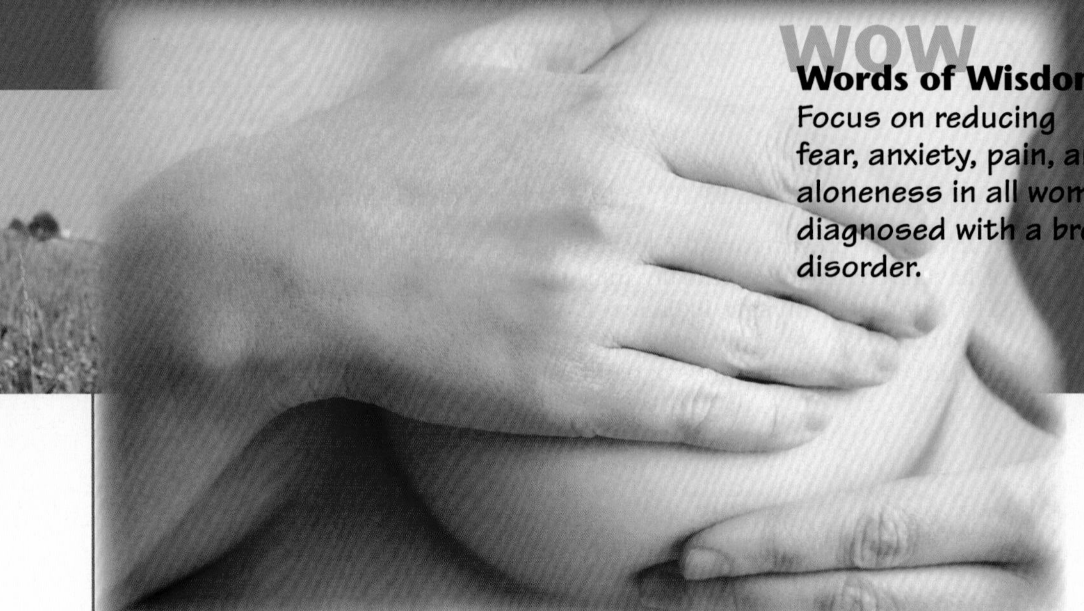

WOW
Words of Wisdom
Focus on reducing fear, anxiety, pain, and aloneness in all women diagnosed with a breast disorder.

Disorders of the Breasts

KEY TERMS
benign breast disorder
breast augmentation
breast cancer
breast-conserving surgery
breast implants
breast self-examination (BSE)
carcinoma
chemotherapy
duct ectasia
endocrine therapy
fibroadenomas
fibrocystic breast changes
mammography
mastitis
modified radical mastectomy
simple mastectomy

Learning Objectives

Upon completion of the chapter, you will be able to:

1. Identify the incidence, risk factors, screening methods, and treatment modalities for benign breast conditions.
2. Appraise reasons behind breast augmentation including the potential benefits and risks.
3. Outline preventive strategies for breast cancer through lifestyle changes and health screening.
4. Analyze the incidence, risk factors, treatment modalities, and nursing considerations related to breast cancer.
5. Develop an educational plan to teach BSE to a group of high-risk women.

***Nancy* hasn't been able to sleep well since she felt the lump in her left breast over a month ago, just after her 60th birthday. She knows she is at high risk because her mother died of breast cancer, but she can't bring herself to have it checked out.**

INTRODUCTION

The breasts are modified sweat glands, lying over the pectoralis major muscles of the chest wall. Physiologically, the breast is an organ specialized for milk formation to nourish their offspring. Each breast extends approximately from the second to the sixth rib. The female breasts are closely linked to womanhood in American culture. Women's breasts act as physical markers for transitions from one stage of life to another, and although the primary function of the breasts is lactation, they are perceived as a symbol of beauty and sexuality.

This chapter discusses assessments, screening procedures, and management of specific benign and malignant breast disorders. Nurses play a key role in helping women maintain breast health by providing education and screening. A good working knowledge of early detection techniques, diagnosis, and treatment options is essential.

BENIGN BREAST DISORDERS

A benign breast disorder is any noncancerous breast abnormality. Though not life-threatening, benign disorders can cause pain and discomfort, and they account for a large number of visits to primary care providers. Fully understanding benign breast disorders should enable the nurse to appropriately evaluate symptoms, determine which breast lesions require treatment, and identify women who are at increased risk for breast cancer.

Depending on the type of benign breast disorder, treatment might or might not be necessary. Although these disorders are benign, the emotional trauma women experience is phenomenal. Fear, anxiety, disbelief, helplessness, and depression are just a few of the reactions that a woman may have when she discovers a lump in her breast. Many women believe that all lumps are cancerous, but actually more than 80% of the lumps discovered are benign and need no treatment (Alexander et al., 2014). Patience, support, and education are essential components of nursing care.

The most commonly encountered benign breast disorders in women include fibrocystic changes of the breasts, **fibroadenomas**, and **mastitis**. Although these breast disorders are considered benign, fibrocystic changes of the breasts carry a cancer risk, with prolific masses and hyperplastic changes occurring within the breasts. Generally speaking, fibroadenomas and mastitis carry little cancer risk (Seetharam & Rodrigues, 2015). Table 6.1 summarizes benign breast conditions.

Fibrocystic Breast Changes

Fibrocystic breast changes, also known as *benign breast disease* (BBD), represent a variety of changes in the glandular and structural tissues of the breast. Because this condition affects 50% to 60% of all women at some point, it is more accurately defined as a "change" rather than a "disease." Fibrocystic changes are caused by an overgrowth of fibrous tissues in the connective tissues

TABLE 6.1 SUMMARY OF BENIGN BREAST DISORDERS

Breast Condition	Nipple Discharge	Site	Characteristics/ Age of Client	Tenderness	Diagnosis & Treatment
Fibrocystic breast changes	+ or –	Bilateral; upper outer quadrant	Round, smooth Several lesions Cyclic, palpable 30–50 yrs old	+	Aspiration and biopsy Limit caffeine; ibuprofen; supportive bra
Fibroadenomas	–	Unilateral; nipple area or upper outer quadrant	Round, firm, movable Palpable, rubbery Well delineated Single lesion 15–30 yrs old	–	Mammogram "Watchful waiting" Aspiration and biopsy Surgical excision
Mastitis	–	Unilateral; outer quadrant	Wedge shaped Warmth, redness Swelling Nipple cracked Breast engorged	+	Antibiotics Warm shower Supportive bra Breast-feeding Increase fluids

Adapted from Alexander, L. L., LaRosa, J. H., Bader, H., & Garfield, S. (2014). *New dimensions in women's health* (6th ed.). Sudbury, MA: Jones & Bartlett; American Cancer Society (ACS). (2015a). *Non-cancerous breast conditions.* Retrieved from http://www.cancer.org/Healthy/FindCancerEarly/WomensHealth/Non-CancerousBreastConditions/non-cancerous-breast-conditions-fibrocystic-changes; and Bope, E. T., & Kellerman, R. D. (2015). *Conn's current therapy 2015.* Philadelphia, PA: Saunders Elsevier.

supporting the breasts. This is frequently accompanied by the presence of fluid-filled cysts, which contribute to the lumpy feeling experienced by women. In contrast to malignant breast lesions, the cysts that develop move freely when palpated and symptoms decline after menopause when levels of estrogen and progesterone drop (Sabel, 2015). Fibrocystic changes do not increase the risk of breast cancer for most women except when the breast biopsy shows "atypia" or abnormal breast cells. The cause for concern for many women with fibrocystic changes is that breast examinations and **mammography** become more difficult to interpret with multiple cysts present, and early cancerous lesions may occasionally be overlooked (American Cancer Society [ACS], 2015a).

Fibrocystic breast changes are most common in women between the ages of 20 and 50. The condition is rare in postmenopausal women not taking hormone replacement therapy (HRT). According to the ACS (2015a), fibrocystic breast changes affect at least half of all women at some point in their lives and are the most common breast disorder today.

Therapeutic Management

Management of the symptoms of fibrocystic breast changes begins with self-care. For some women, diet and lifestyle changes help to reduce discomfort. Other options include wearing a supportive bra, taking over-the-counter pain relievers, and limiting salt consumption which can cause fluid retention (Files, Allen, & Pruthi, 2015). In severe cases drugs, including bromocriptine, tamoxifen, or danazol, can be used to reduce the influence of estrogen on breast tissue. However, several undesirable side effects, including masculinization, have been documented. Aspiration or surgical removal of breast lumps will reduce pain and swelling by removing the space-occupying mass.

Nursing Assessment

Nursing assessment consists of a health history, physical examination, and laboratory and diagnostic tests.

HEALTH HISTORY

Ask the woman about common clinical manifestations, which include lumpy, tender breasts, particularly during the week before menses. Changes in breast tissue produce pain by nerve irritation from edema in connective tissue and by fibrosis from nerve pinching. The pain is cyclic and frequently dissipates after the onset of menses. The pain is described as a dull, aching feeling of fullness. Masses or nodularities usually appear in both breasts and are often found in the upper outer quadrants. Some women also experience spontaneous clear to yellow nipple discharge when the breast is squeezed or manipulated.

PHYSICAL EXAMINATION

It is best to examine a woman's breast a week after menses, when swelling has subsided. The breast examination is performed using the Triple Touch Method in which the health care provider uses the pads of the middle three fingers and makes dime-sized overlapping circles to feel the breast tissue with three levels of pressure: light, medium, and firm (Jarvis, 2015). Observe the breasts for fibrosis, or thickening of the normal breast tissues, which occurs in the early stages. Cysts form in the later stages and feel like multiple, smooth, well-delineated tiny pebbles or bumpy oatmeal under the skin (Fig. 6.1). On physical examination of the breasts, a few characteristics might be helpful in differentiating a cyst from a cancerous lesion. Cancerous lesions typically are fixed and painless and may cause skin retraction (pulling). Cysts tend to be mobile and tender and do not cause skin retraction in the surrounding tissue.

LABORATORY AND DIAGNOSTIC TESTS

Mammography can be helpful in distinguishing fibrocystic changes from breast cancer. Ultrasound is a useful adjunct to mammography for breast evaluation because it helps to differentiate a cystic mass from a solid one (Dixon & Macaskill, 2015). Ultrasound produces images of the breasts by sending sound waves through a gel applied to the breasts. Fine-needle aspiration biopsy can also be done to differentiate a solid tumor, cyst, or malignancy. A fine-needle aspiration biopsy uses a thin needle guided by ultrasound to the mass. In a method called stereotactic needle biopsy, a computer maps the exact location of the mass using mammograms taken from two angles, and the map is used to guide the needle.

Nursing Management

A nurse caring for a woman with fibrocystic breast changes can teach her about the condition, provide tips for self-care (Teaching Guidelines 6.1), suggest lifestyle changes, and demonstrate how to perform monthly **breast self-examination (BSE)** after her menses to monitor the changes. Nursing Care Plan 6.1 (at the end of the chapter) presents a plan of care for a woman with fibrocystic breast changes.

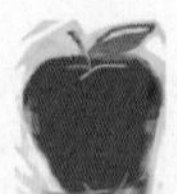

Teaching Guidelines 6.1

RELIEVING SYMPTOMS OF FIBROCYSTIC BREAST CHANGES

- Wear an extra-supportive bra to prevent undue strain on the ligaments of the breasts to reduce discomfort.
- Take oral contraceptives, as recommended by a health care practitioner, to stabilize the monthly hormonal levels.
- Eat a low-fat diet rich in fruits, vegetables, and grains to maintain a healthy nutritional lifestyle and ideal weight.

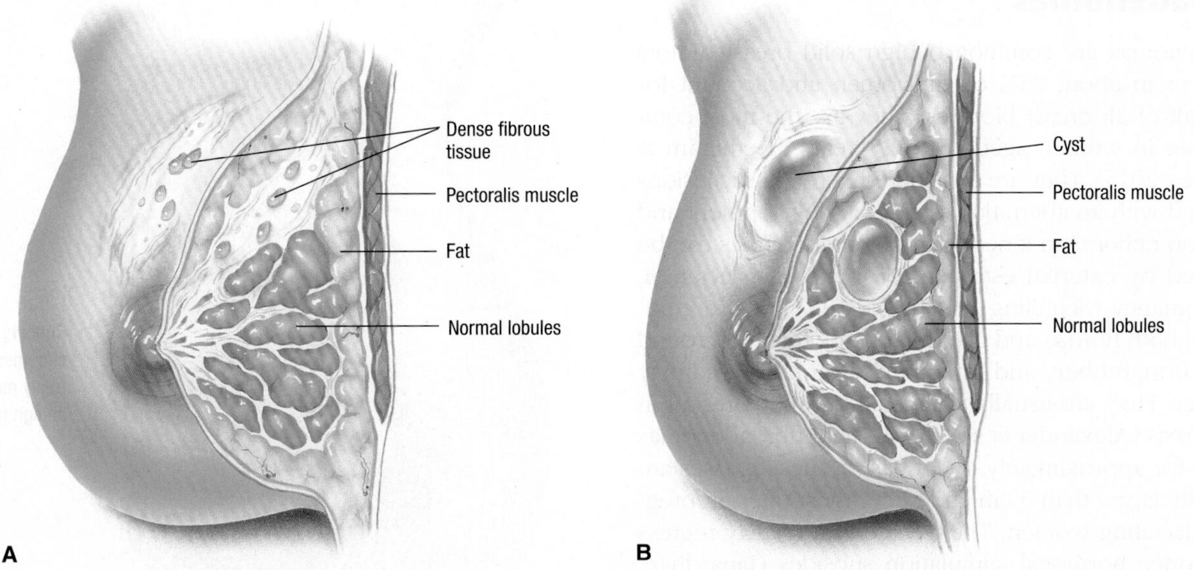

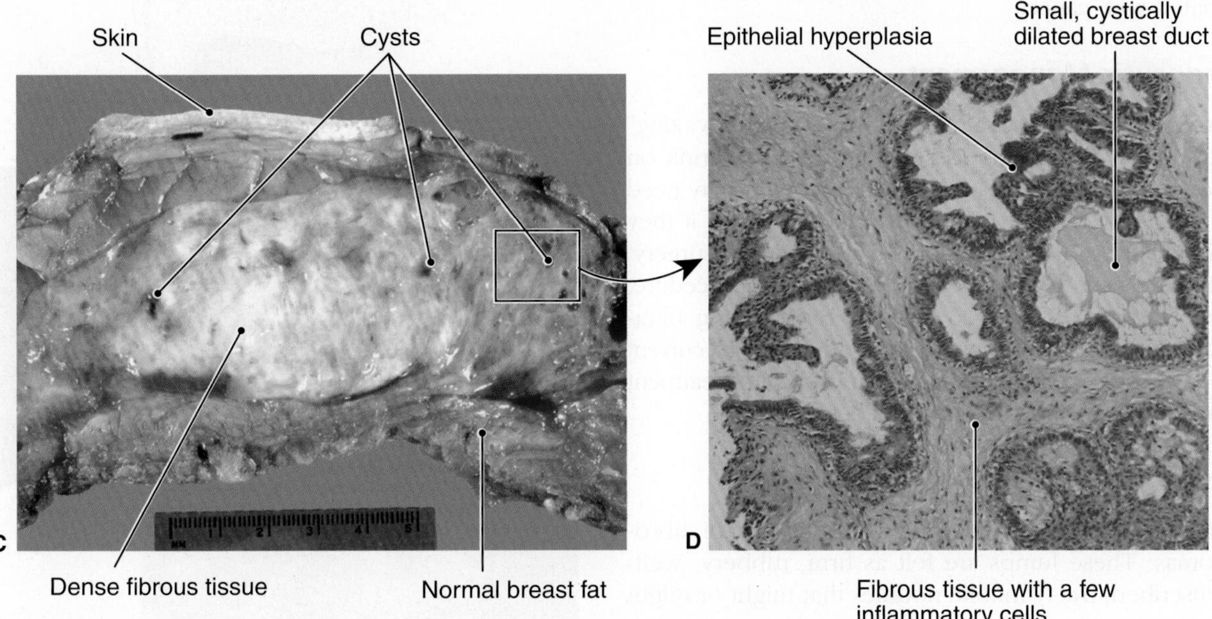

FIGURE 6.1 **A.** Fibrocystic breast changes. **B.** Breast cysts. **C.** This gross study shows that most of the abnormal tissue is fibrous. Cysts are relatively inconspicuous in this example. **D.** The microscopic study shows dense fibrous tissue containing dilated ducts lined by hyperplastic epithelium. (Images A & B are from The Anatomical Chart Company. (2006). *Atlas of pathophysiology*. Springhouse, PA: Springhouse Corporation. Images C & D courtesy of McConnell, T. H. (2014). *The nature of disease pathology for the health professions* (2nd ed.). Philadelphia, PA: Lippincott Williams & Wilkins.)

- Apply heat to the breasts to help reduce pain via vasodilation of vessels.
- Take diuretics, as recommended by a health care practitioner, to counteract fluid retention and swelling of the breasts.
- Reduce salt intake to reduce fluid retention and swelling in the breasts.
- Take over-the-counter medications, such as acetylsalicylic acid (Aspirin) or ibuprofen (Motrin, Advil, Nuprin), to reduce inflammation and discomfort.
- Use thiamine and vitamin E therapy. This has been found helpful for some women, but research has failed to demonstrate a direct benefit from either therapy.
- Take medications as prescribed (e.g., bromocriptine, tamoxifen, or danazol).
- Discuss the possibility of aspiration or surgical removal of breast lumps with a health care practitioner.
- Avoid caffeinated drinks (coffee, tea, soda) which tend to trigger breast discomfort.

Fibroadenomas

Fibroadenomas are common benign solid breast tumors that occur in about 25% of all women and account for up to half of all breast biopsies. They are the most common mass in women aged 15 to 25 years (Seetharam & Rodrigues, 2015). They are considered hyperplastic lesions associated with an aberration of normal development and involution rather than a neoplasm. Fibroadenomas can be stimulated by external estrogen, progesterone, lactation, and pregnancy (Schuiling & Likis, 2016). They are composed of both fibrous and glandular tissue that feels round or oval, firm, rubbery and smooth, and is mobile and may be tender. They are usually unilateral, but may present in both breasts (Alexander et al., 2014). Giant fibroadenomas account for approximately 4% of cases. These masses are frequently larger than 5 cm and occur most often in pregnant or lactating women. These large lesions may regress in size once hormonal stimulation subsides (Janardhan, Venkateshwar, & Rao, 2015). Fibroadenomas are rarely associated with cancer.

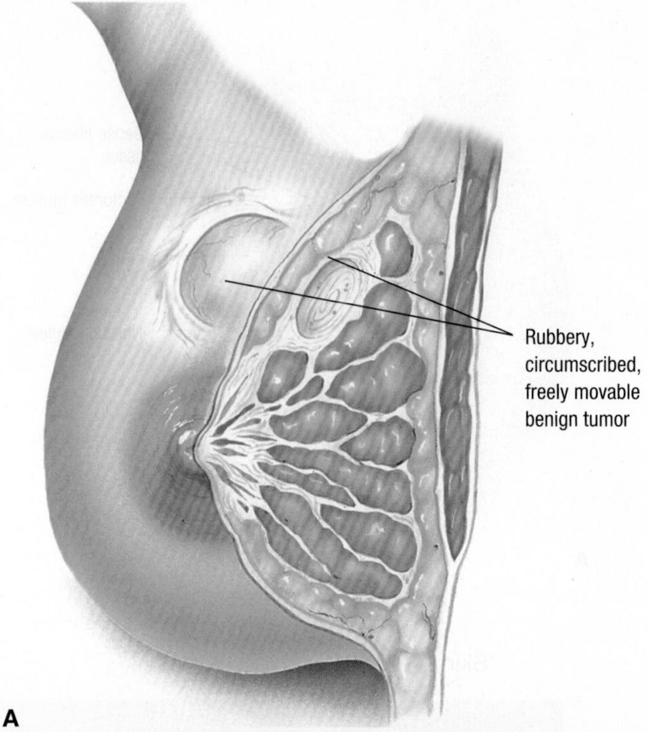

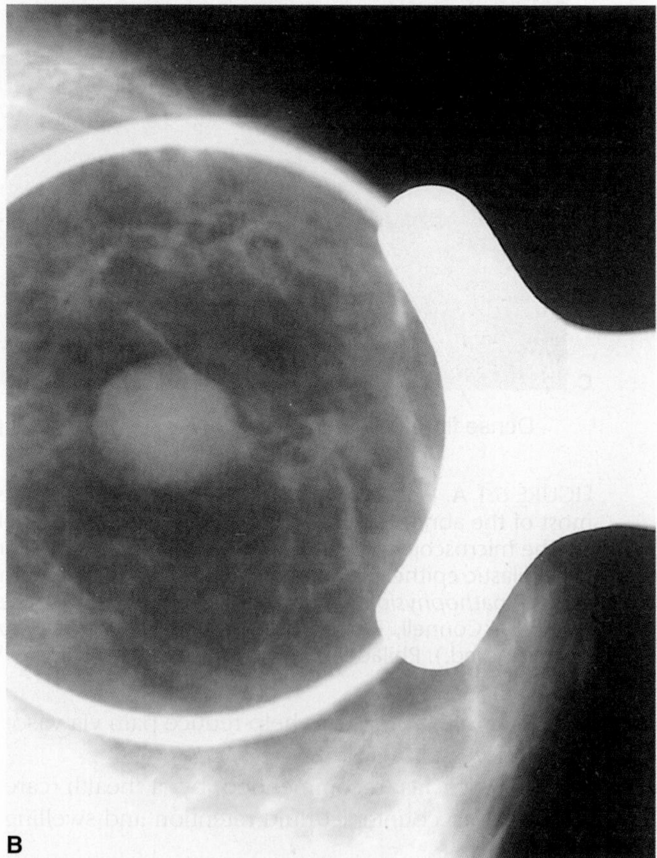

FIGURE 6.2 **A.** Fibroadenoma. (Asset provided by Anatomical Chart Co.) **B.** Spot compression view of a smoothly marinated mass proven to represent a fibroadenoma. Ultrasonography demonstrated a solid mass.

Therapeutic Management

Treatment may include a period of "watchful waiting" because many fibroadenomas stop growing or shrink on their own without any treatment. Other growths may need to be surgically removed if they do not regress or if they remain unchanged. Cryoablation, an alternative to surgery, can also be used to remove a tumor. In this procedure, extremely cold gas is piped into the tumor using ultrasound guidance. The tumor freezes and dies. The current trend is toward a more conservative approach to treatment after careful evaluation and continued monitoring.

Nursing Assessment

Ask the woman about clinical manifestations of fibroadenomas. These lumps are felt as firm, rubbery, well-circumscribed, freely mobile nodules that might or might not be tender when palpated.

Breast fibroadenomas are usually detected incidentally during clinical or self-examinations and are usually located in the upper outer quadrant of the breast; more than one may be present (Fig. 6.2). Several other breast lesions have similar characteristics, so every woman with a breast mass should be evaluated to exclude cancer. A clinical breast examination (CBE) by a health care provider is critical. In addition, diagnostic studies include imaging studies (mammography, ultrasound, or both) and some form of biopsy, most often a fine-needle aspiration, core needle biopsy, or stereotactic needle biopsy. The core needle biopsy removes a small cylinder of tissue from the breast mass, more than the fine-needle aspiration biopsy. If additional tissue needs to be evaluated, the advanced breast biopsy instrument (ABBI) is used. This instrument removes a larger cylinder of tissue for examination by using a rotating circular knife. The

ABBI procedure removes more tissue than any of the other methods except a surgical biopsy (ACS, 2015a).

Nursing Management

The nurse should urge the client to return for reevaluation in 6 months, perform monthly BSEs, and return annually for a CBE. Recent studies suggest that women with high breast density and proliferative BBD are at very high risk for future breast cancer. Women with low breast density are at low risk, regardless of their benign pathologic diagnosis (Slanetz, Freer, & Birdwell, 2015). This is all the more reason for women to have close monitoring over time.

Mastitis

Mastitis is an infection or inflammation of the connective tissue in the breast that occurs primarily in lactating or engorged women. The prevalence of it in breast-feeding women may be as high as 33% (Faguy, 2015). Mastitis is divided into lactational or nonlactational types. The usual causative organisms for lactational mastitis are *Staphylococcus aureus, Haemophilus influenzae,* and haemophilus and streptococcus species, the source of which is the baby's flora. Lactating mastitis typically occurs in the first 2 to 3 weeks of lactation, but can occur at any stage of lactation. One or more of the ducts drain poorly or become blocked, resulting in bacterial growth in the retained milk (Pluchinotta, 2015). The only evidence-based predisposing factor that may lead to mastitis is the development of milk stasis. However, other associated factors include damaged or cracked nipples, especially those colonized with *S. aureus;* irregular or missed feedings; failing to allow the infant to empty one breast completely before moving on to the next breast; poor latch and transfer of milk; illness of mother or infant; oversupply; a tight bra; blocked nipple pore or duct; being primiparous women; and maternal stress and fatigue (Miller & Kennedy, 2015).

Nonlactational mastitis can be caused by **duct ectasia**, which occurs when the milk ducts become congested with secretions and debris, resulting in periductal inflammation. It may be divided into central (periareolar) and peripheral breast lesions. Periareolar infections consist of active inflammation around nondilated subareolar breast ducts—a condition termed periductal mastitis. Peripheral nonlactating breast abscesses are less common than periareolar abscesses and are often associated with an underlying condition, such as diabetes, rheumatoid arthritis, steroid treatment, granulomatous lobular mastitis, and trauma (Faguy, 2015). Women with these types of abscesses present with greenish nipple discharge, nipple retraction, and noncyclical pain.

Therapeutic Management

Effective milk removal, pain medication, and antibiotic therapy have been the mainstays of treatment. Management of both types of mastitis involves the use of oral antibiotics (usually a penicillinase-resistant penicillin or cephalosporin), warm compresses to the inflamed area of the breast, continued breast-feeding, and acetaminophen (Tylenol) for pain and fever (King et al., 2015).

Nursing Assessment

Assess the client's health history for risk factors for mastitis, which include poor hand hygiene ductal abnormalities, nipple cracks and fissures, lowered maternal defenses due to fatigue, tight clothing, poor support of pendulous breasts, failure to empty the breasts properly while breast-feeding, or missing breast-feedings.

The diagnosis of mastitis is made clinically on the basis of a localized, unilateral area of erythema with associated fever. Assess the client for clinical manifestations of mastitis, which include flu-like symptoms of malaise, nausea, headache, leukocytosis, fever, fatigue, and chills. Physical examination of the breasts reveals increased warmth, swollen area of one breast, redness, tenderness, and swelling. The nipple is usually cracked or abraded and the breast is distended with milk (Fig. 6.3). In a lactating woman, severe engorgement can be differentiated from mastitis because engorgement is bilateral with general involvement of the whole breast. Ultrasound scans can be undertaken to differentiate between the types of mastitis or abscesses, but typically the diagnosis is made based on history and examination.

Nursing Management

Teach the woman about the etiology of mastitis and encourage her to continue to breast-feed, emphasizing that it is safe for her infant to do so. Stress to all breast-feeding mothers to check for medication safety before taking it. Drugs administered to mothers can accumulate in the bodies of their infants and can alter infant's bowel flora, causing diarrhea. Mothers should be

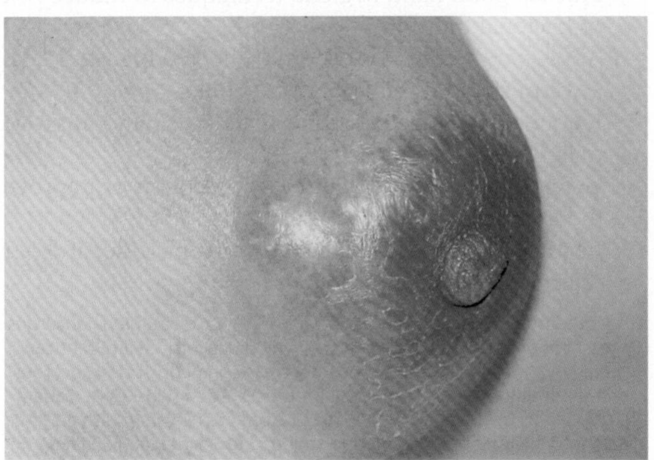

FIGURE 6.3 Mastitis. (From Sweet, R. L., & Gibbs, R. S. (2009). *Infectious diseases of the female genital tract.* Philadelphia, PA: Lippincott Williams & Wilkins.)

warned about this to reduce their anxiety. Once it has been declared safe to do so, the nurse should urge them to take the medication as prescribed until completed. Continued emptying of the breast or pumping improves the outcome, decreases the duration of symptoms, and decreases the incidence of breast abscess. Thus, continued breast-feeding is recommended in the presence of mastitis (King et al., 2015).

Although 80% of breast biopsy results prove to be benign, increased surveillance is necessary because of the risk of cancer development. The recommended follow-up schedule is imaging (mammography or ultrasound) and a CBE by a surgeon at 6, 12, and 24 months after a benign breast biopsy finding (Tharpe, Farley, & Jordan, 2016). Instructions for the woman with mastitis are detailed in Teaching Guidelines 6.2.

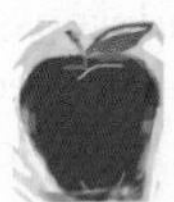

Teaching Guidelines 6.2

CARING FOR MASTITIS

- Take medications as prescribed to reduce inflammation and infection.
- Continue breast-feeding, as tolerated to keep the milk flowing.
- Begin feeding on most affected breast to allow it to be emptied first.
- Massage the breasts before and during breast-feeding to encourage milk extraction.
- Wear a supportive bra 24 hours a day to support the breasts for comfort.
- Increase fluid intake to stay hydrated.
- Gentle massage toward nipple several times daily.
- Vary the infants breast-feeding position—cradle, side-lying, football, & belly to belly.
- Make sure infant is positioned correctly on the nipple to prevent discomfort.
- Practice good hand hygiene techniques to reduce risk of bacterial transfer.
- Apply warm compresses to the affected breast or take a warm shower before breast-feeding.
- Frequently change positions while nursing to improve milk flow.
- Get adequate rest and nutrition to support or improve the immune system.
- Instruct to contact their health care provider if fever returns, chills, or worsening symptoms.

Adapted from American Cancer Society (ACS). (2015a). *Non-cancerous breast conditions.* Available at http://www.cancer.org/healthy/findcancerearly/womenshealth/non-cancerousbreastconditions/non-cancerous-breast-conditions-intro; King, T. L., Brucker, M. C., Kriebs, J. M., Fahey, J. O., Gegor, C. L., & Varney, H. (2015) *Varney's midwifery* (5th ed.). Berlington, MA: Jones & Bartlett Learning; and Tharpe, N. L., Farley, C. L., & Jordan, R. G. (2016). *Clinical practice guidelines for midwifery & women's health.* (4th ed.). Burlington, MA: Jones & Bartlett Learning.

MALIGNANT BREAST DISORDER

Breast cancer is a neoplastic disease in which normal body cells are transformed into malignant ones (National Cancer Institute [NCI], 2015a). It is the most common cancer in women and the second leading cause of cancer deaths (lung cancer is first) among American women. Breast cancer accounts for one of every three cancers diagnosed in the United States (ACS, 2015a). A new case is discovered every 2 minutes. It is estimated that one out of every eight women will develop the disease at some time during her life, and the mortality rate of those with breast cancer is 1 in 36 (NCI, 2015a).

Over 200,000 cases of invasive breast cancer are diagnosed in the United States each year (ACS, 2015a). Breast cancer can also affect men, but only 1% of all individuals diagnosed with breast cancer annually are men. About 2,000 men are diagnosed with breast cancer annually, with about a one in four mortality rate (Khan, Allerton, & Pettit, 2015). Because men are not routinely screened for breast cancer, the diagnosis is often delayed. The most common clinical manifestation of male breast cancer is a painless, firm, subareolar breast mass. Any suspicious breast mass in a male should undergo diagnostic biopsy. If a malignancy is diagnosed, typical treatment is mastectomy with assessment of the axillary nodes.

The cause of breast cancer, while not well understood, is thought to be a complex interaction between environmental, genetic, and hormonal factors. Breast cancer is a progressive rather than a systemic disease, meaning that most cancers grow from small size with low metastatic potential to larger size and greater metastatic potential. Tumor stage, size, and lymph node involvement are major predictors of metastatic potential (Arora et al., 2015).

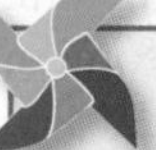

Consider This

It was pouring down rain and I was driving alone along dark wet streets to my 8 AM appointment for a breast ultrasound. I recently had my annual mammogram and the radiologist thought he saw something suspicious on my right breast. I was on my way to confirm or refute his suspicions, and I couldn't keep focused on the road ahead. For the past few days I had been a basket case, fearing the worst. I was playing in my mind, what I would do if...? What changes would I make in my life and how would I react when told? I have been through such personal turmoil since that doctor announced he wanted "more tests."

Thoughts: This woman is worrying and is emotionally devastated before she even has a conclusive diagnosis. Is this a typical reaction to a breast disorder? Why do women fear the worst? Many women use denial to mask their feelings and hope against hope the doctor made a mistake or misread their mammogram. How would you react if you or your sister, girlfriend, or mother were confronted with a breast disorder?

Pathophysiology

Cancer is not just one disease, but rather a group of diseases that result from unregulated cell growth. Without regulation, cells divide and grow uncontrollably until they eventually form a tumor. Extensive research has determined that all cancer is the result of changes in DNA or chromosome structure that cause the mutation of specific genes. Most genetic mutations that cause cancer are acquired sporadically, which means they occur by chance and are not necessarily due to inherited mutations (Shannon & Chittenden, 2015). Cancer development is thought to be clonal in nature, which means that each cell is derived from another cell. If one cell develops a mutation, any daughter cell derived from that cell will have that same mutation, and this process continues until a malignant tumor forms.

Breast cancer starts in the epithelial cells that line the mammary ducts within the breast. The growth rate depends on hormonal influences, mainly estrogen and progesterone. The two major categories of breast cancer are noninvasive and invasive. Noninvasive, or in situ, breast cancers are those that have not extended beyond their duct, lobule, or point of origin into the surrounding breast tissue. Conversely, invasive (infiltrating) breast cancers have extended into the surrounding breast tissue, with the potential to metastasize. Many researchers believe that most invasive cancers probably originate as noninvasive cancers (Cuzick & Thorat, 2015).

Breast cancer is considered to be a highly variable disease. While the process of metastasis is a complex and poorly understood phenomenon, there is evidence to suggest that new vascularization of the tumor plays an important role in the biologic aggressiveness of breast cancer (Toi et al., 2015). Breast cancer metastasizes widely and to almost all organs of the body, but primarily to the bone, lungs, lymph nodes, liver, and brain. The first sites of metastases are usually local or regional, involving the chest wall or axillary supraclavicular lymph nodes or bone (ACS, 2015a).

Invasive Ductal Carcinoma

By far the most common breast cancer is invasive ductal **carcinoma**, which represents 85% of all cases (ACS, 2015c). Carcinoma is a malignant tumor that occurs in epithelial tissue; it tends to infiltrate and give rise to metastases. The incidence of this cancer peaks in the sixth decade of life (>60 years old). It spreads rapidly to axillary and other lymph nodes, even while small. Infiltrating ductal carcinoma may take various histologic forms—well differentiated and slow growing, poorly differentiated and infiltrating, or highly malignant and undifferentiated with numerous metastases. This common type of breast cancer starts in the ducts, breaks through the duct wall, and invades the fatty breast tissue. This type of cancer accounts for 75% of all breast cancers (Stopeck, Chalasani, & Thompson, 2015).

Invasive Lobular Carcinoma

Invasive lobular carcinomas, which originate in the terminal lobular units of breast ducts, account for 10% of all cases of breast cancer. The peak incidence is in women aged 40 to 50 years old. It presents as an area of ill-defined thickening rather than a palpable mass. The tumor is frequently located in the upper outer quadrant of the breast, and by the time it is discovered the prognosis is usually poor (Selvi, 2015).

Other Invasive Carcinomas

Other invasive types of cancer include tubular carcinoma (29%), which is fairly uncommon and typically occurs in women aged 55 and older. Colloid carcinoma (2% to 4%) occurs in women 60 to 70 years of age and is characterized by the presence of large pools of mucus interspersed with small islands of tumor cells. Medullary carcinoma accounts for 5% to 7% of malignant breast tumors; it occurs frequently in younger women (<50 years of age) and grows into large tumor masses. Inflammatory breast cancer (<4%) often presents with skin edema, redness, and warmth and is associated with a poor prognosis. Paget disease (2% to 4%) originates in the nipple and typically occurs with invasive ductal carcinoma (Bope & Kellerman, 2015).

Staging of Breast Cancer

Breast cancers are classified into three stages based on:

1. Tumor size
2. Extent of lymph node involvement
3. Evidence of metastasis

The purposes of tumor staging are to determine the probability that the tumor has metastasized, to decide on an appropriate course of therapy, and to assess the client's prognosis. Table 6.2 gives details and characteristics of each stage (also Fig. 6.4). The overall 10-year survival rate for a woman with stage I breast cancer is 80% to 90%; for a woman with stage II, it is about 50%. The outlook is not as good for women with stage III or IV disease (Alexander et al., 2014).

There is no completely accurate way to know whether the cancer has micrometastasized to distant organs, but certain tests can help determine if the cancer has spread. A bone scan can be performed to assess the bones. Magnetic resonance imaging (MRI) can be used to detect metastases to the liver, abdominal cavity, lungs, or brain.

TABLE 6.2 STAGING OF BREAST CANCER

Stage	Characteristics
0	In situ, early type of breast cancer
I	Localized tumor <1 in in diameter
II	Tumor 1–2 in in diameter; spread to axillary lymph nodes
III	Tumor 2 in or larger; spread to other lymph nodes and tissues
IV	Cancer has metastasized to other body organs

Adapted from American Cancer Society (ACS). (2015h). *How is breast cancer staged?* Retrieved from http://www.cancer.org/Cancer/BreastCancer/DetailedGuide/breast-cancer-staging.

TABLE 6.3 ESTIMATED RISK OF BREAST CANCER AT SPECIFIC AGES

Ages 30–39	1 out of 233
Ages 40–49	1 out of 69
Ages 50–59	1 out of 42
Ages 60–69	1 out of 29

Adapted from American Cancer Society (ACS). (2015i) *How many women get breast cancer?* Retrieved from http://www.cancer.org/cancer/breastcancer/overviewguide/breast-cancer-overview-key-statistics

Risk Factors

An estimated 80% of women in whom breast cancer develops have no documented risk factors (Bope & Kellerman, 2015). Breast cancer is thought to develop in response to a number of related factors: aging; gender (99% of cases occur in women, delayed childbearing or never bearing children, genetic influences); BRCA1 and BRCA2 genetic mutations; history of receiving ionizing radiation; high breast density; postmenopausal obesity; family history of cancer; hormonal factors such as early menarche <12 years, late menopause >50 years, first term pregnancy >30 to 35 years of age; HRT with estrogen plus progestin; and ingestion of two drinks or more alcohol each day (ACS, 2015b). Other factors might contribute to breast cancer but have not been scientifically proven.

In 1970, the lifetime risk for developing breast cancer was 1 in 10; since then, the risk has gradually risen (NCI, 2015b). This slight increase in incidence might be explained in a variety of ways: better detection and screening tools are available, which have identified more cases; women are living to an older age, when their risk increases; and lifestyle changes in American women (having their first pregnancy at an older age, having fewer children, and using hormonal therapy to treat the symptoms of menopause) might have produced the higher numbers. Age is a significant risk factor. Because rates of breast cancer increase with age, estimates of risk at specific ages are more meaningful than estimates of lifetime risk. The estimated chances of a woman being diagnosed with breast cancer between the ages of 30 and 70 are detailed in Table 6.3.

Risk factors for breast cancer can be divided into those that cannot be changed (nonmodifiable risk factors) and those that can be changed (modifiable risk factors). Nonmodifiable risk factors (ACS, 2015b) are:

- Gender (female)
- Aging (>50 years old)
- Genetic mutations (BRCA1 and BRCA2 genes)
- Personal history of ovarian or colon cancer
- Increased breast density increases the risk three-to-fivefold
- Family history of breast cancer

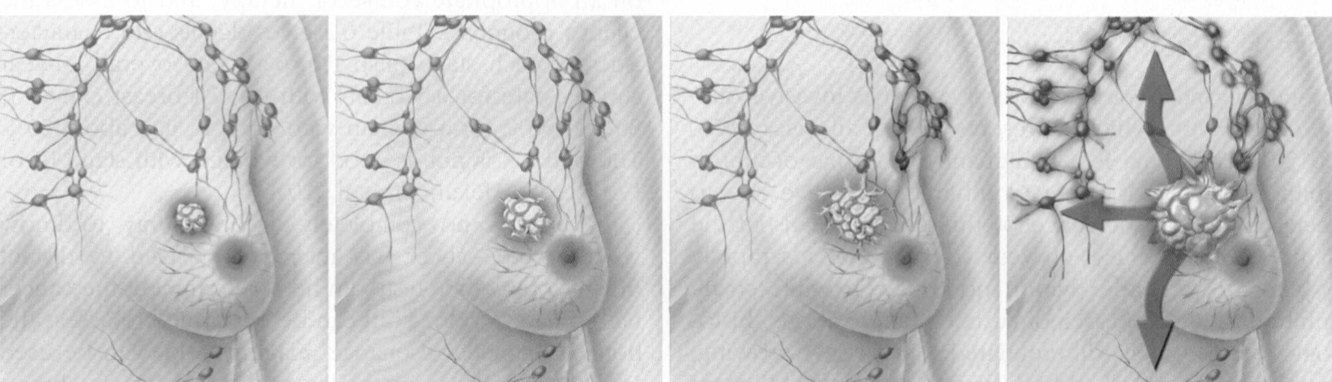

FIGURE 6.4 Stages I to IV of breast cancer.

- Personal history of breast cancer (three- to fourfold increase in risk for recurrence)
- Race/ethnicity (higher in White women, but African-American women are more likely to die of it)
- Previous abnormal breast biopsy (atypical hyperplasia)
- Exposure to chest radiation (radiation damages DNA)
- Previous breast radiation (12 times normal risk)
- Early menarche (<12 years old) or late onset of menopause (>55 years old), which represents increased estrogen exposure over the lifetime

Modifiable risk factors related to lifestyle choices (ACS, 2015b) include:

- Not having children at all or not having children until after age 30—this increases the risk of breast cancer by not reducing the number of menstrual cycles
- Postmenopausal use of estrogens and progestins—the Women's Health Initiative study (2002) reported increased risks with long-term (>5 years) use of HRT
- Failing to breast-feed for up to a year after pregnancy—increases the risk of breast cancer because it does not reduce the total number of lifetime menstrual cycles
- Alcohol consumption—boosts the level of estrogen in the bloodstream
- Smoking—exposure to carcinogenic agents found in cigarettes
- Obesity and consumption of high-fat diet—fat cells produce and store estrogen, so more fat cells create higher estrogen levels
- Sedentary lifestyle and lack of physical exercise—increases body fat, which houses estrogen

Breast cancer incidence rates are higher in non-Hispanic White women compared with African-American women for most age groups. However, African-American women have a higher incidence rate before 40 years of age and are more likely to die from breast cancer at every age (ACS, 2015b). Some of that gap is because of social factors such as poverty and restricted access to health care. Some studies have also found genetic differences in the type of breast cancer that develops in African American and White women. Little is known, however, about whether other risk factors have a different impact in women of different races. A new study's findings suggest that the risk factors are similar in both races (ACS, 2015b).

The presence of risk factors, especially several of them, calls for careful ongoing monitoring and evaluation to promote early detection. Even though risk factors are important considerations, many women with newly diagnosed breast cancer have no known risk factors. Although routine mammography and self-examination are prudent for high-risk women, these precautions may become lifesavers for early detection of cancerous lesions.

Consuming a low-fat diet with plenty of fruits, vegetables, legumes, and whole grains can provide all the vitamins and nutrients our bodies need and has been shown to significantly reduce the risk of developing many types of cancer. A plant-based diet can also reduce cancer recurrence: high-fiber, low-fat diets rich in fruits and vegetables, avoiding sugared beverages and calorie dense foods, and processed meats reduce breast cancer recurrence, according to Catsburg et al., (2015). They studied the effectiveness of a high-vegetable, low-fat diet, aimed at markedly raising circulating carotenoid concentrations from food sources, in reducing additional breast cancer events and early death in women with early-stage invasive breast cancer. It is a prescription for cancer prevention that has only positive side effects—lower cholesterol, weight loss, and a lower risk of heart disease. Adherence to a plant-based diet that limits red meat intake may be associated with reduced risk of breast cancer, particularly in postmenopausal women (Catsburg et al., 2015).

Screening for breast cancer begins with a routine history and physical examination. Nurses should take every opportunity to educate and emphasize the goal of breast cancer screening: early detection reduces mortality. Screening also includes a BSE, CBE, and mammography.

Diagnosis

Many studies can be performed to make an accurate diagnosis of a malignant breast lump. Diagnostic tests include:

- Diagnostic mammography or digital mammography
- Magnetic resonance mammography (MRM)
- Fine-needle aspiration
- Stereotactic needle-guided biopsy
- Sentinel lymph node biopsy
- Hormone receptor status
- Infrared thermal imaging
- DNA ploidy status
- Cell proliferative indices
- HER-2/neu genetic marker (Han et al., 2015)

Mammography

Mammography has become an accepted screening procedure that is sanctioned by most cancer organizations and is paid for annually by most health insurance agencies. Mammography serves a twofold purpose: to screen and to diagnose. Mammography involves taking x-ray pictures of a bare breast while it is compressed between two plastic plates. This procedure is a screening tool used to identify and characterize a breast mass and to detect an early malignancy. It remains the gold standard screening method for women at average risk

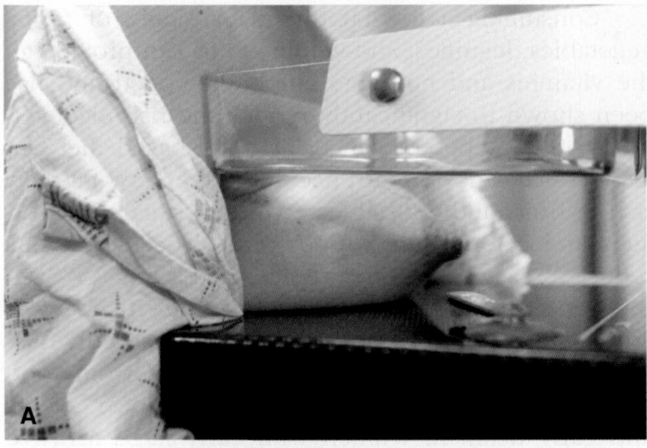

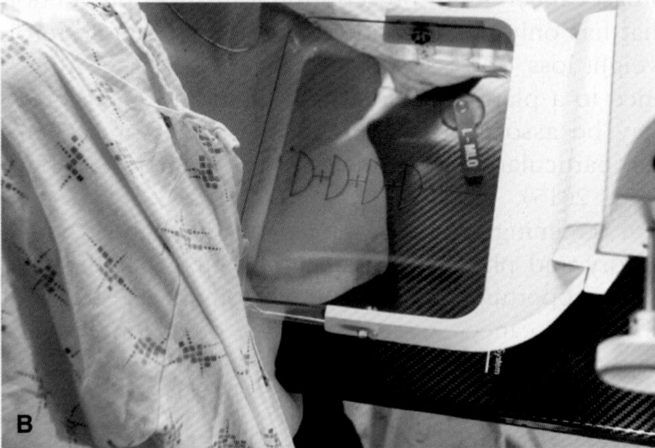

FIGURE 6.5 Mammography. **A.** A top-to-bottom view of the breast. **B.** A side view of the breast.

for breast cancer. It is relatively inexpensive, requires only a low dose of radiation, and reliably identifies malignant tumors, especially those that are too small to feel. It can also be used to investigate breast lumps and other symptoms. A screening mammogram typically consists of four views, two per breast (Fig. 6.5). It can detect lesions as small as 0.5 cm (the average size of a tumor detected by a woman practicing occasional BSE is approximately 2.5 cm) (Rifkin & Lazris, 2015).

A diagnostic mammogram is performed when a woman has suspicious clinical findings on a breast examination or an abnormality has been found on a screening mammogram. A diagnostic mammogram uses additional views of the affected breast as well as magnification views. Diagnostic mammography provides the radiologist with additional detail to render a more specific diagnosis. Currently, digital mammography is being used to diagnose breast lesions.

Most women find the 10-minute mammography procedure uncomfortable but not painful. Teaching Guidelines 6.3 offers tips for a client to follow before she undergoes this procedure.

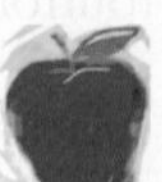

Teaching Guidelines 6.3

PREPARING FOR A SCREENING MAMMOGRAM

- Schedule the procedure just after menses, when breasts are less tender.
- Do not use deodorant or powder on the day of the procedure, because they can appear on the x-ray film as calcium spots.
- Acetaminophen (Tylenol) or acetylsalicylic acid (aspirin) can relieve any discomfort after the procedure.
- Remove all jewelry from around your neck, because the metal can cause distortions on the film image.
- Select a facility that is accredited by the American College of Radiology to ensure appropriate credentialed staff.

The U.S. Preventive Services Task Force (USPSTF) changed its recommendations for breast cancer screening in 2009, resulting in considerable controversy. The USPSTF now recommends biennial screening mammography for women aged 50 to 74 years. Previously, women 40 years and older were advised to start screening mammography. They stated that the decision to start regular, biennial screening mammography before the age of 50 years should be an individual one and take client context into account, including the client's values regarding specific benefits and harms. In addition, the USPSTF concluded that the current evidence is insufficient to assess the additional benefits and harms of screening mammography in women 75 years or older. Finally, the USPSTF recommended against teaching BSE because scientific evidence does not support this practice as a valid screening method for women since its sensitivity ranges from 12% to 41%, lower than that of the CBE done by a health care provider and mammography, and it is age dependent. The USPSTF is currently updating their breast cancer screening recommendation guidelines and may return to every 1 to 2 years for women age 40 or older for diagnostic mammograms (U.S. Preventive Services Task Force [USPSTF], 2015).

The American Cancer Society has different guidelines for women with no symptoms or family history of breast cancer than the USPSTF. They still recommend annual mammograms and CBEs for women starting at age 40 and do not recommend stopping them at any age. They also recommend a CBE about every 3 years for women in their 20s and 30s and every year for women >40. BSE is an option for women starting in their 20s (ACS, 2015d).

The American Congress of Obstetricians and Gynecologists (ACOG) recommends that mammography screening be offered annually to women beginning at age 40. Previous ACOG guidelines recommended mammograms every 1 to 2 years starting at age 40 and annually beginning at age 50. ACOG continues to recommend annual CBEs for women aged 40 and older, and every 1 to 3 years for women aged 20 to 39. Additionally, it encourages breast self-awareness for women ages 20 and older (American Congress of Obstetricians and Gynecologists [ACOG], 2015).

This conflicting information can be confusing to women trying to make decisions about breast cancer screening. Nurses can present the latest evidence-based research to help women make informed decisions based on their age, overall health status, and family history of cancer. (See Table 6.4 for a helpful outline.) There really isn't any clear direction given to women by the authoritative agencies; they in essence leave the decision up to the woman and her health care provider. The associated risk is delay in detecting a breast lesion early when it could be treated and her life saved.

Magnetic Resonance Mammography

MRM is a relatively new procedure that might allow for earlier detection because it can detect smaller lesions and provide finer detail. MRM is a highly accurate (>90% sensitivity for invasive carcinoma) but costly tool. Contrast infusion is used to evaluate the rate at which the dye initially enters the breast tissue. The basis of the high sensitivity of MRM is the tumor angiogenesis (vessel growth) that accompanies a majority of breast cancers, even early ones. Malignant lesions tend to exhibit increased enhancement within the first 2 minutes (Bhatti et al., 2015). Currently MRM is used as a complement to mammography and CBE because it is expensive, but recent research findings report that it is more accurate than mammography for size assessment of breast lesions (Poulos, 2015).

Fine-Needle Aspiration Biopsy or Core Biopsy

Fine-needle aspiration biopsy is done to identify a solid tumor, cyst, or malignancy. It is a simple office procedure that can be performed with or without anesthesia. A small (23- to 27-gauge) needle connected to a 10-mL or larger syringe is inserted into the breast mass and suction is applied to withdraw the contents. The aspirate is then sent to the cytology laboratory to be evaluated for abnormal cells.

A core needle biopsy is much like a fine-needle biopsy except that a larger needle is used to withdraw small cylinders or cores of tissue from the abnormal area of the breast. It takes longer than the fine-needle biopsy, but more tissue is sampled to be tested.

TABLE 6.4 SCREENING RECOMMENDATIONS FROM USPSTF, ACS, AND ACOG

The U.S. Preventive Services Task Force	In 2009, the USPSTF changed its recommendations for breast cancer screening for women with no symptoms or no family history of breast cancer. Previously they advised screening mammography for women ages 40 yrs and older. Updated recommendations include biennial screening mammography for women ages 50–74 yrs, and no breast self-examination (BSE) since scientific evidence does not support this practice as a valid screening method for women because its sensitivity ranges from 12–41%, which is lower than that of the clinical breast examination done by a health professional and mammography, and it is age dependent. The previous recommendations are now under review (2015). The USPSTF states that a woman's decision to start regular, biennial screening mammography before the age of 50 yrs should be an individual one and take client context into account, including the client's values regarding specific benefits and harms. The USPSTF also reports that current evidence is insufficient to assess the additional benefits and harmful aspects of screening mammography in women 75 yrs or older (USPSTF, 2015).
The American Cancer Society	Guidelines from the ACS differ from those of the USPSTF for women with no symptoms or no family history of breast cancer. The ACS still recommends annual mammograms and clinical breast examinations for women starting at age 40 and do not recommend stopping them at any age. They suggest that BSEs can be optional for women from age 20 onward (ACS, 2015d).
The American Congress of Obstetricians and Gynecologists	The ACOG recommends screening mammograms be offered annually to women beginning at age 40. Previous guidelines recommended a mammogram every 1–2 yrs starting at age 40 and annually beginning at age 50. Clinical breast examinations are still recommended every year, but BSEs are optional and not strongly recommended (ACOG, 2015).

Stereotactic Needle-Guided Biopsy

This diagnostic tool is used to target and identify mammographically detected nonpalpable lesions in the breast. This procedure is less expensive than an excisional biopsy. The procedure takes place in a specially equipped room and generally takes about an hour. Women are required to lie prone and must be able to remain still for approximately 20 minutes while the biopsy is taken. When proper placement of the breast mass is confirmed by digital mammograms, the breast is locally anesthetized and a spring-loaded biopsy gun is used to obtain two or three core biopsy tissue samples. After the procedure is finished, the biopsy area is cleaned and a sterile dressing is applied.

Sentinel Lymph Node Biopsy

The status of the axillary lymph nodes is an important prognostic indicator in early-stage breast cancer. The presence or absence of malignant cells in lymph nodes is highly significant: the more lymph nodes involved and the more aggressive the cancer, the more powerful **chemotherapy** will have to be, both in terms of the toxicity of drugs and the duration of treatment (Tsujimoto, 2015). With a sentinel lymph node biopsy, the clinician can determine whether breast cancer has spread to the axillary lymph nodes without having to do a traditional axillary lymph node dissection. Experience has shown that the lymph ducts of the breast typically drain to one lymph node first before draining through the rest of the lymph nodes under the arm. The first lymph node is called the sentinel lymph node.

This procedure can be performed under local anesthesia. A radioactive blue dye is injected 2 hours before the biopsy to identify the afferent sentinel lymph node. The surgeon usually removes one to three nodes and sends them to the pathologist to determine whether cancer cells are present. The sentinel lymph node biopsy is usually performed before a lumpectomy to make sure the cancer has not spread. Removing only the sentinel lymph node can allow women with breast cancer to avoid many of the side effects (lymphedema) associated with a traditional axillary lymph node dissection. This procedure is associated with less morbidity compared to the axillary lymph node dissection, which results in more accurate staging, better axillary tumor control and improved survival. It is considered a standard of care for initial evaluation of metastatic spread to the axillary lymph node chain (Chatterjee, Serniak, & Czerniecki, 2015).

Hormone Receptor Status

Normal breast epithelium has hormone receptors and responds specifically to the stimulatory effects of estrogen and progesterone. Most breast cancers retain estrogen receptors, and for those tumors estrogen will retain proliferative control over the malignant cells. It is therefore useful to know the hormone receptor status of the cancer to predict which women will respond to hormone manipulation. Hormone receptor status reveals whether the tumor is stimulated to grow by estrogen and progesterone. Postmenopausal women tend to be ER+; premenopausal women tend to be ER− (Kalinsky et al., 2015). To determine hormone receptor status, a sample of breast cancer tissue obtained during a biopsy or a tumor removed surgically during a lumpectomy or mastectomy is examined by a cytologist.

Therapeutic Management

Women diagnosed with breast cancer have many treatments available to them. Generally, treatments fall into two categories: local and systemic. Local treatments are surgery and radiation therapy. Effective systemic treatments include chemotherapy, hormonal therapy, and immunotherapy (Evidence-Based Practice 6.1).

Treatment plans are based on multiple factors, with the primary factors being whether the cancer is invasive or noninvasive, the tumor's size and grade, the number of cancerous axillary lymph nodes, the hormone receptor status, and the ability to obtain clear surgical margins (ACS, 2015e). A combination of surgical options and adjunctive therapy is often recommended.

Another consideration in making decisions about a treatment plan is genetic testing for BRCA1 and BRCA2 genetic mutations. This genetic testing became available in 1995 and can pinpoint women who have a significantly increased risk for breast, ovarian cancer and contralateral breast cancer: individuals with BRCA1 and BRCA2 mutations have a 75% lifetime risk of breast cancer and a 30% lifetime risk of ovarian cancer. Most cases of breast and ovarian cancer are sporadic in nature, but approximately 10% of breast and ovarian cancers are thought to result from genetic inheritance (Li et al., 2015). DNA (from a blood or saliva sample) is needed for mutation testing. The sample is sent to a laboratory for analysis. It usually takes about a month to get the results back. Testing positive for a BRCA1 or BRCA2 mutation can significantly alter health care decisions. In some cases, before genetic testing was available, lumpectomy with radiation or mastectomy was the treatment most often recommended. However, if the woman is found to have a BRCA1 mutation, she is most likely to be offered the option of bilateral prophylactic mastectomy and possible bilateral oophorectomy. A recent study found that current evidence does not support worse breast cancer survival of BRCA1/2 mutation carriers in the adjuvant setting; differences if any are likely to be small when compared to non-BRCA1/2 mutation carriers (van den Broek et al., 2015).

EVIDENCE-BASED PRACTICE 6.1 **COMBINATION (SEVERAL DRUGS AT A TIME) VERSES SEQUENTIAL CHEMOTHERAPY (SAME DRUG GIVEN ONE AFTER THE OTHER) FOR METASTATIC BREAST CANCER**

STUDY

Combination chemotherapy can cause greater tumor cell kill if the drug dose is not compromised, while sequential single agent chemotherapy may allow for greater dose intensity and treatment time, potentially meaning greater benefit from each single agent. In addition, sequentially using single agents might cause less toxicity and impairment of quality of life, but it is not known whether this might compromise survival time. The purpose of this study was to assess the effect of combination chemotherapy compared to the same drugs given sequentially in women with metastatic breast cancer.

Findings

Randomized controlled trials of combination chemotherapy compared to the same drugs used sequentially in women with metastatic breast cancer in the first-, second- or third-line setting were selected. Twelve trials reporting on nine treatment comparisons (2,317 patients randomized) were identified. The findings concluded that sequential single agent chemotherapy has a positive effect on progression-free survival, whereas combination chemotherapy has a higher response rate and a higher risk of febrile neutropenia in metastatic breast cancer. There was no difference in overall survival time between these treatment strategies, but when drugs were given one at a time, there was more time before the tumors grew back again. However, combination chemotherapy caused tumors to shrink more. Generally this study supports the recommendations by international guidelines to use sequential monotherapy unless there is rapid disease progression.

Nursing Implications

Although not entirely conclusive in its findings, nurses need to be aware of this study's findings to be able to counsel women when both therapies are being considered. This study suggests that accurate information about both therapies is needed for all women with metastatic breast cancer, for them to make an informed decision. Nurses need to remember that metastatic breast cancer is not currently curable, but can be effectively treated with chemotherapy. Average survival is about 2 years, but many women live much longer. The type of therapy chosen should take into consideration optimizing survival, minimizing side effects, and quality of life.

Adapted from Dear, R. F., McGeechan, K, Jenkins, M. C., Barratt, A., Tattersall, M. H. N, & Wilcken, N. (2015). Combination versus sequential single agent chemotherapy for metastatic breast cancer. *Cochrane Database of Systematic Reviews* 2013, 3:CD008792. doi: 10.1002/14651858.CD008792.pub2.

Discovery of mutations in the breast and ovarian cancer susceptibility genes BRCA1 and BRCA2 can have emotional consequences for both the tested individual and his or her relatives.

Severe psychological distress can occur as a result of genetic testing. Their distress relates to family cancer history, relationships, coping strategies, communication patterns, and mutation status (Wevers et al., 2015). Nurses might find it useful to explore these issues in order to prepare clients before BRCA1/BRCA2 testing and to support them through shifts in family dynamics after disclosure of results. Also, many women perceive their breasts as intrinsic to their femininity, self-esteem, and sexuality, and the risk of losing a breast can provoke extreme anxiety (Alexander et al., 2014). Nurses need to address the physical, emotional, and spiritual needs of the women they care for, as well as their families, since this mutation is inherited in an autosomal dominant fashion. Nurses should identify the woman's personal coping style which has an impact on her likelihood of experiencing distress after her diagnosis. Women who are emotionally expressive and/or have a "fighting spirit" usually experience lower levels of emotional distress. Based on Mendelian genetics, women with BRCA1 and BRCA2 mutations have a 5- to 20-fold increased risk of developing breast and ovarian cancer (Caple & Schub, 2015).

Surgical Options

Generally, the first treatment option for a woman diagnosed with breast cancer is surgery. A few women with tumors larger than 5 cm or inflammatory breast cancer may undergo neoadjuvant chemotherapy or radiotherapy to shrink the tumor before surgical removal is attempted (Debled et al., 2015). The surgical options depend on the type and extent of cancer. The choices are typically either **breast-conserving surgery** (lumpectomy with radiation) or mastectomy with or without reconstruction. The overall survival rate with lumpectomy and radiation is about the same as that with **modified radical mastectomy** (ACS, 2015f). Research has shown that the survival rates in women who have had mastectomies versus those who have undergone breast-conserving surgery followed by radiation are the same. However, lumpectomy may not be an option for some women, including those:

- Who have two or more cancer sites that cannot be removed through one incision
- Whose surgery will not result in a clean margin of tissue

- Who have active connective tissue conditions (lupus or scleroderma) that make body tissues especially sensitive to the side effects of radiation
- Who have had previous radiation to the affected breast
- Whose tumors are larger than 5 cm (2 in) (National Comprehensive Cancer Network [NCCN], 2015).

These decisions are made jointly between the woman and her surgeon. If mastectomy is chosen, because of either tumor characteristics or client preference, then discussion needs to include breast reconstruction and regional lymph node biopsy versus sentinel lymph node biopsy. The mastectomy techniques are a **simple mastectomy** with sentinel node biopsy or a radical mastectomy with regional node biopsy. Removal of numerous lymph nodes places the client at high risk for lymphedema.

BREAST-CONSERVING SURGERY

Breast-conserving surgery, the least invasive procedure, is the wide local excision (or lumpectomy) of the tumor along with a 1-cm margin of normal tissue. A lumpectomy is often used for early-stage localized tumors. The goal of breast-conserving surgery is to remove the suspicious mass along with tissue free of malignant cells to prevent recurrence. The results are less drastic and emotionally less scarring than having a mastectomy to the woman. Women undergoing breast-conserving therapy receive radiation after lumpectomy with the goal of eradicating residual microscopic cancer cells to limit locoregional recurrence. In women who do not require adjuvant chemotherapy, radiation therapy typically begins 2 to 4 weeks after surgery to allow healing of the lumpectomy incision site. Radiation is administered to the entire breast at daily doses over a period of several weeks (Corradini et al., 2015).

A sentinel lymph node biopsy may also be performed since the lymph nodes draining the breast are located primarily in the axilla. Theoretically, if breast cancer is to metastasize to other parts of the body, it will probably do so via the lymphatic system. If malignant cells are found in the nodes, more aggressive systemic treatment may be needed.

MASTECTOMY

A simple mastectomy is the removal of all breast tissue, the nipple, and the areola. The axillary nodes and pectoral muscles are spared. This procedure would be used for a large tumor or multiple tumors that have not metastasized to adjacent structures or the lymph system.

A modified radical mastectomy is another surgical option, conducive to breast reconstruction and results in greater mobility and less lymphedema (Alexander et al., 2014). This procedure involves removal of breast tissue, and a few positive axillary nodes. Breast-conserving surgeries do not increase the future risk of death from recurrent disease when compared with mastectomy (Schuiling & Likis, 2016).

In conjunction with the mastectomy, lymph node surgery (removal of underarm nodes) may need to be done to reduce the risk of distant metastasis and improve a woman's chance of long-term survival. For women with a positive sentinel node biopsy, 10 to 20 underarm lymph nodes may need to be removed. Complications associated with axillary lymph node surgery include nerve damage during surgery, causing temporary numbness down the upper aspect of the arm; seroma formation (fluid build-up) followed by wound infection; restrictions in arm mobility (some women need physiotherapy); and lymphedema (swelling related to the lymph glands). In many women lymphedema can be avoided by:

- Avoiding using the affected arm for drawing blood, inserting intravenous lines, or measuring blood pressure (can cause trauma and possible infection)
- Seeking medical care immediately if the affected arm swells
- Wearing gloves when engaging in activities such as gardening that might cause injury
- Wearing a well-fitted compression sleeve to promote drainage return

Women having mastectomies must decide whether to have further surgery to reconstruct the breast. If the woman decides to have reconstructive surgery, it ideally is performed immediately after the mastectomy. The woman must also determine whether she wants the surgeon to use saline implants or natural tissue from her abdomen (TRAM flap method) or back (LAT flap method).

If reconstructive surgery is desired, the ultimate decision regarding the method will be determined by the woman's anatomy (e.g., is there sufficient fat and muscle to permit natural reconstruction?) and her overall health status. Both procedures require a prolonged recovery period.

Some women opt for no reconstruction, and many of them choose to wear breast prostheses. Some prostheses are worn in the bra cup and others fit against the skin or into special pockets created into clothing.

Whether to have reconstructive surgery is an individual and very complex decision. Each woman must be presented with all of the options and then allowed to decide. The nurse can play an important role here by presenting the facts to the woman so that she can make an intelligent decision to meet her unique situation. Breast reconstruction surgery can help restore the look and feel of the breast after a mastectomy. Performed by a plastic surgeon, breast reconstruction can be done immediately after the mastectomy or at a later date. Breast reconstruction can be done with **breast implants** (filled with saline or silicone); natural tissue flaps (using skin

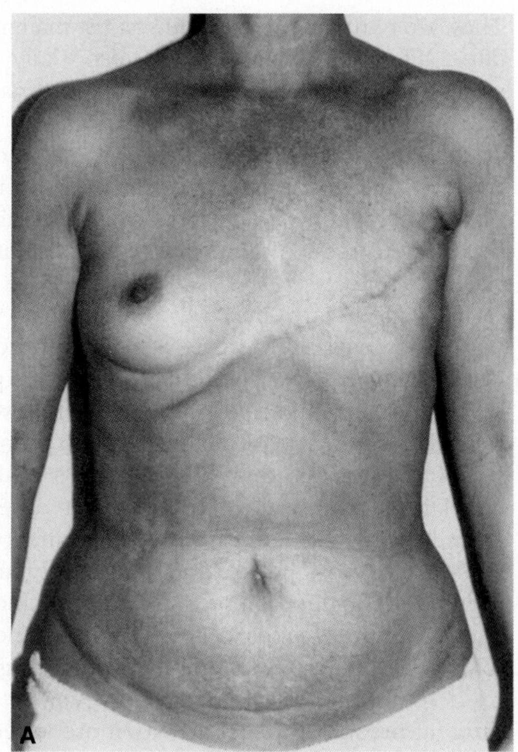

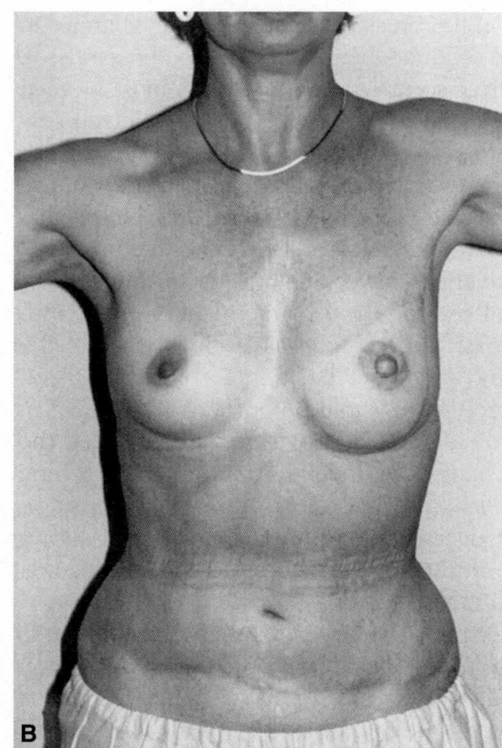

FIGURE 6.6 Before and after photos of postmastectomy and reconstruction.

fat and muscle from your own body); or a combination of both. Side effects or complications include risk of rupture, hardening of the tissues around the implant, infection, and pain. Nurses need to educate the woman about these potential problems and make sure they understand before consenting to breast reconstruction. See Figure 6.6 for examples of a postmastectomy (A) and reconstruction breast Augmentation (B).

BREAST AUGMENTATION

Breast augmentation is a common surgical procedure with women undergoing it with implants for a variety of reasons ranging from aesthetic to reconstructive surgery following a mastectomy. Saline-filled or silicone-filled implants are used in cosmetic enhancement and reconstructive surgeries. The exact anatomical placement of breast implants can vary, but the location typically is subglandular (over the pectoral muscle) or subpectoral (under the muscle). Breast implants are not lifetime devices, but most are guaranteed for approximately 10 years in case of rupture. Breast augmentation with implants is not without risks. Potential complications include capsular contracture, rippling, implant rupture, infection, or hematoma. Capsular contraction occurs when scar tissue forms, contracts, and hardens around the implant. Rippling most often occurs when wrinkles form in the implant or as a complication of contracture (Mugea, 2015).

Breast examination in women with reconstructive surgery is done exactly the same way as for natural breasts. Breasts with implants in place usually feel firmer than normal breast tissue on palpation due to the formation of a fibrotic band or capsule around the implant. If implants are used, press firmly inward at the edges of the implant to feel the ribs beneath.

Adjunctive Therapy

Adjunctive therapy is supportive or additional therapy that is recommended after surgery. Adjunctive therapies include local therapy such as radiation therapy and systemic therapies using chemotherapy, hormonal therapy, and immunotherapy.

RADIATION THERAPY

Radiation therapy (also called radiotherapy) uses high-energy rays to destroy cancer cells that might have been left behind in the breast, chest wall, or underarm area after a tumor has been removed surgically. Usually serial radiation doses are given 5 days a week to the tumor site for 6 to 8 weeks postoperatively. Each treatment takes only a few minutes, but the dose is cumulative. Women undergoing breast-conserving therapy receive radiation to the entire breast after lumpectomy with the goal of eradicating residual microscopic cancer cells to reduce the chance of recurrence (Chu et al., 2015).

Side Effects. Side effects of traditional radiation therapy include inflammation, local edema, anorexia, swelling, and heaviness in the breast; sunburn-like skin changes in the treated area; and fatigue. Changes to the breast tissue and skin usually resolve in about a year in most women (Lara et al., 2015). This type of therapy can be given several ways: external beam radiation, which delivers a carefully focused dose of radiation from a machine outside the body, or internal radiation, in which tiny pellets that contain radioactive material are placed into the tumor.

Several advances have taken place in the field of radiation oncology for the treatment of women with early-stage breast cancer that assist in reducing the side effects. The treatment position for external radiation has changed from supine to prone, with the arm on the affected side raised above the head, so that the treated breast hangs dependently through the opening of the treatment board. Treatment in the prone position improves dose distribution within the breast and allows for a decrease in the dose delivered to the heart, lung, chest wall, and other breast (NCCN, 2015).

High-dose brachytherapy is another advance that is an alternative to traditional radiation treatment. A balloon catheter is used to insert radioactive seeds into the breast after the tumor has been removed surgically. The seeds deliver a concentrated dose directly to the operative site; this is important because most cancer recurrences in the breast occur at or near the lumpectomy site (Chang et al., 2015). This allows a high dose of radiation to be delivered to a small target volume with a minimal dose to the surrounding normal tissue. This procedure takes 4 to 5 days as opposed to the 4 to 6 weeks that traditional radiation therapy takes; it also eliminates the need to delay radiation therapy to allow for wound healing. Brachytherapy is now used as a primary radiation treatment after breast-conserving surgery in selected women as an alternative to whole breast irradiation (Guinot et al., 2015). Side effects of brachytherapy include redness or discharge around catheters, fever, and infection. Daily cleansing of the catheter insertion site with a mild soap and application of an antibiotic ointment will minimize the risk of infection.

Intensity-modulated radiation therapy (IMRT) offers still another new approach to the delivery of treatment to reduce the dose within the target area while sparing surrounding normal structures. A computed tomography scan is used to create a three-dimensional model of the breast. Based on this model, a series of intensity-modulated beams is produced to the desired dose distribution to reduce radiation exposure to underlying structures. Acute toxicity is thus minimized (Muralidhar, Soubhagya, & Ahmed, 2015). Research is ongoing to evaluate the impact of all of these advances in radiation therapy.

CHEMOTHERAPY

Chemotherapy refers to the use of drugs that are toxic to all cells and interfere with a cell's ability to reproduce. They are particularly effective against malignant cells but affect all rapidly dividing cells, especially those of the skin, the hair follicles, the mouth, the gastrointestinal tract, and the bone marrow. Breast cancer is a systemic disease in which micrometastases are already present in other organs by the time the breast cancer is diagnosed. Chemotherapeutic agents perform a systemic "sweep" of the body to reduce the chances that distant tumors will start growing.

Chemotherapy may be indicated for women with tumors larger than 1 cm, positive lymph nodes, or cancer of an aggressive type. Chemotherapy is prescribed in cycles, with each period of treatment followed by a rest period. Treatment typically lasts 3 to 6 months, depending on the dose used and the woman's health status.

Different classes of drugs affect different aspects of cell division and are used in combinations or "cocktails." The most active and commonly used chemotherapeutic agents for breast cancer include alkylating agents, anthracyclines, antimetabolites, and vinca alkaloids. Fifty or more chemotherapeutic agents can be used to treat breast cancer; however, a combination drug approach appears to be more effective than a single drug treatment (ACS, 2015g). Refer to Evidence-Based Practice 6.1.

Side Effects. Side effects of chemotherapy depend on the agents used, the intensity of dosage, the dosage schedule, the type and extent of cancer, and the client's physical and emotional status. Nurses need to remain current in order to accommodate new treatments and the side effect profiles. This knowledge is vital to providing evidence-based care for breast cancer women receiving these treatments (Bourdeanu & Lui, 2015). However, typical side effects include nausea and vomiting, diarrhea or constipation, hair loss, weight loss, stomatitis, fatigue, and immunosuppression. The most serious is bone marrow suppression (myelosuppression). This causes an increased risk of infection, bleeding, and a reduced red blood cell count, which can lead to anemia. Treatment of the side effects can generally be addressed through appropriate support medications such as antinausea drugs. In addition, growth-stimulating factors, such as epoetin alfa (Procrit) and filgrastim (Neupogen), help keep blood counts from dropping too low. Counts that are too low would stop or delay the use of chemotherapy.

An aggressive systemic option, when other treatments have failed or when there is a strong possibility of relapse or metastatic disease, is high-dose chemotherapy with bone marrow and/or stem cell transplant. This therapy involves the withdrawal of bone marrow before the administration of toxic levels of chemotherapeutic agents. The marrow is frozen and then returned to the client after the high-dose chemotherapy is finished.

Clinical trials are still researching this experimental therapy (King et al., 2015).

HORMONAL THERAPY

One of estrogen's normal functions is to stimulate the growth and division of healthy cells in the breasts. However, in some women with breast cancer, this normal function contributes to the growth and division of cancer cells.

The objective of **endocrine therapy** is to block or counter the effect of estrogen. Estrogen plays a central role in the pathogenesis of cancer, and treatment with estrogen deprivation has proven to be effective. Approximately two thirds of women diagnosed with early-stage breast cancer have hormone-sensitive disease (estrogen receptor positive and/or progesterone receptor positive), and adjuvant hormone therapy plays an essential role in reducing the risk of recurrence and improving survival (Gradishar, 2015). Several different drug classes are used to interfere or block estrogen receptors. They include selective estrogen receptor modulators (SERMs), estrogen receptor downregulators, aromatase inhibitors, luteinizing hormone–releasing hormone, progestin, and biologic response modifiers (King et al., 2015). Current recommendations for most women with ER+ breast cancer are to take a hormone-like medication—known as a SERM antiestrogenic agent—daily for up to 5 years after initial treatment. Certain areas in the female body (breasts, uterus, ovaries, skin, vagina, and brain) contain specialized cells called hormone receptors that allow estrogen to enter the cell and stimulate it to divide. SERMs enter these same receptors and act like keys, turning off the signal for growth inside the cell (King et al., 2015). The best-known SERM is tamoxifen (Nolvadex, 20 mg daily for 5 years). Although it works well in preventing further spread of cancer, it is also associated with an increased incidence of endometrial cancer, pulmonary embolus, deep vein thrombosis, hot flashes, vaginal discharge and bleeding, stroke, and cataract formation (Jager et al., 2015).

Another SERM is the antiosteoporosis drug raloxifene (Evista), which has shown promising results. It has antiestrogen effects on the breast and uterus. In recent studies involving postmenopausal women at high risk for breast cancer, raloxifene worked as well as tamoxifen in preventing breast cancer, but with fewer serious adverse effects. Both drugs cut the cancer risk in half (Bevers, 2015). It was originally marketed solely for the prevention and treatment of osteoporosis but is now used as adjunctive breast cancer therapy.

Another class of endocrine agents, aromatase inhibitors, works by inhibiting the conversion of androgens to estrogens. Aromatase inhibitors include letrozole (Femara, 2.5 mg daily), exemestane (Aromasin, 25 mg daily), and anastrozole (Arimidex, 1 mg daily for 5 years), all of which are taken orally. These are usually given to women with advanced breast cancer. In recent clinical studies in postmenopausal women with breast cancer, third-generation aromatase inhibitors were shown to be superior to tamoxifen for the treatment of metastatic disease (Bevers, 2015).

Side Effects. The side effects associated with these endocrine therapies include hot flashes, bone pain, bone thinning, insomnia, weight gain, depression, fatigue, nausea, cough, dyspnea, and headache (Breast Cancer Organization, 2015). Women with hormone-sensitive cancers can live for long periods without any intervention other than hormonal manipulation, but quality-of-life issues need to be addressed in the balance between treatment and side effects.

IMMUNOTHERAPY

Immunotherapy, used as an adjunct to surgery, represents an attempt to stimulate the body's natural defenses to recognize and attack cancer cells. Trastuzumab (Herceptin, 2 to 4 mg/kg intravenous infusion) is the first monoclonal antibody approved for breast cancer (NCCN, 2015). Some tumors produce excessive amounts of HER-2/neu protein, which regulates cancer cell growth. Breast cancers that overexpress the HER-2/neu protein are associated with a more aggressive form of disease and a poorer prognosis. Trastuzumab blocks the effect of this protein to inhibit the growth of cancer cells. It can be used alone or in combination with other chemotherapy to treat clients with metastatic breast disease. Although immunotherapy has shown some promise against the fight against cancer, recent data suggests that greater success will be achieved by combining it with other therapies, such as radiation (Leavy, 2015).

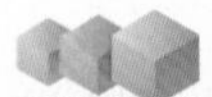

Concept Mastery Alert

Tamoxifen Versus Trastuzumab in Breast Cancer Treatment

Tamoxifen is a selective estrogen receptor modulator used to prevent further spread of breast cancer in women with ER-positive breast cancer. Trastuzumab is a monoclonal antibody used in the treatment of breast cancer and is considered immunotherapy.

Side Effects. Adverse effects of trastuzumab include cardiac toxicity, vascular thrombosis, hepatic failure, fever, chills, nausea, vomiting, and pain with first infusion (Skidmore-Roth, 2015).

NURSING PROCESS FOR THE CLIENT WITH BREAST CANCER

When a woman is diagnosed with breast cancer, she faces treatment that may alter her body shape, may make her feel unwell, and may not carry a certainty of cure. Nurses can support women from the time of diagnosis, through the treatments, and through follow-up after the surgical and adjunctive treatments have been completed. Allowing clients time to ask questions and to discuss any necessary preparations for treatment is critical. As our understanding of breast disorders keeps improving, treatments continue to change.

Although the goal of treatment remains improved survival, increasing emphasis is being focused on prevention. Breast cancer prevention measures focus on evaluating and reducing risk factors. Approaches for reducing breast cancer risk include lifestyle modifications (diet and physical exercise), chemoprevention (SERMs & AIs), and prophylactic surgery (bilateral salpingo-oophorectomy & bilateral prophylactic mastectomy) (Euhus & Diaz, 2015). Nurses can have an impact on early detection of breast disorders, treatment, and symptom management. Women with a cancer diagnosis often experience negative emotions and nurses' empathic response can help alleviate their distress (Alexander et al., 2014). A nurse who is involved in the woman's treatment plan from the beginning can effectively offer support throughout the whole experience.

Teamwork is important in breast screening and caring for women with breast disorders. Treatment is often fragmented between the hospital and community treatment centers, which can be emotionally traumatic for the woman and her family. The advances being made in the diagnosis and treatment of breast disorders mean that guidelines are constantly changing, requiring all health care providers to keep up to date. Informed nurses can provide support and information and, most importantly, continuity of care for the woman undergoing treatment for a breast problem.

The nurse plays a particularly important role in providing psychological support and self-care teaching to clients with breast cancer. Nurses can influence both physical and emotional recovery, which are both important aspects of care that help in improving the woman's quality of life and the ability to survive. The nurse's role should extend beyond helping clients; spreading the word in the community about screening and prevention is a big part in the ongoing fight against cancer. The community should see nurses as both educators and valued sources of credible information. This role will help improve clinical outcomes while achieving high levels of client satisfaction.

Despite the new guidelines issued by various governmental agencies regarding BSEs, a CBE done by a professional health care provider is essential for good breast health for all women. See Box 6.1 for additional information.

Remember Nancy from the chapter opener? Is her response typical of many women upon discovering a lump in their breast? Nancy confides her discovery of the lump and her worries to you. What advice would you give her?

Assessment

Early breast cancer has no symptoms. The earliest sign of breast cancer is often an abnormality seen on a screening mammogram before the woman or the health care provider feels it. A healthy, asymptomatic presentation is typical. However, symptoms may include a lump in the breast that is usually nontender, fixed, and hard with irregular borders. In the woman presenting with a breast disorder, take a thorough history of the problem and explore the woman's risk factors for breast cancer. Assess the woman for clinical manifestations of breast cancer, such as changes in breast appearance and contour, which become apparent with advancing breast cancer (ACS, 2015d). These changes include:

- Continued and persistent changes in the breast
- A lump or thickening in one breast
- Persistent nipple irritation
- Unusual breast swelling or asymmetry
- A lump or swelling in the axilla
- Changes in skin color or texture
- Nipple retraction, tenderness, or discharge

Complete a breast examination to validate the clinical manifestations and findings of the health history and risk factor assessment. The CBE involves both inspection and palpation (Box 6.1). Helpful characteristics in evaluating palpable breast masses are described in Table 6.5. If a lump can be palpated, the cancer has been there for quite some time.

Be cognizant of the impact that breast cancer has on a woman's emotional state, coping ability, and quality of life. Women may experience sadness, vulnerability, loss of control, alteration of body image and integrity, anger, the illness's impact on relationships, fear of mortality, the need to reprioritize her life, and guilt as a result of having breast cancer. However, despite potential negative outcomes, many women have a positive outlook for their future and adapt to treatment modalities with a good quality of life (Kleban & Glaser, 2015). Closely monitor clients for their psychosocial

BOX 6.1

CLINICAL BREAST EXAMINATION BY HEALTH CARE PROVIDER

If the woman is deemed high risk, the nurse would then teach the woman to perform a BSE to enhance breast awareness.

Purpose: To Assess Breasts For Abnormal Findings

1. Inspect the breast for size, symmetry, and skin texture and color. It is common for the left breast to be slightly larger than the right. Inspect the nipples and areola. Ask the client to sit at the edge of the examination table, with her arms resting at her sides.

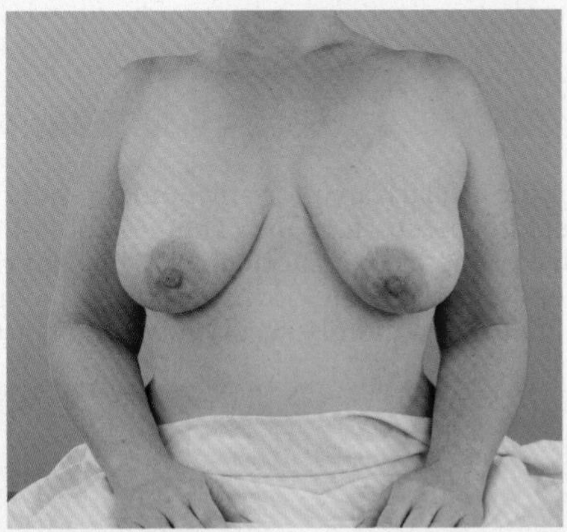

2. Inspect the breast for masses, retraction, dimpling, or ecchymosis.
   - The client places her hands on her hips.

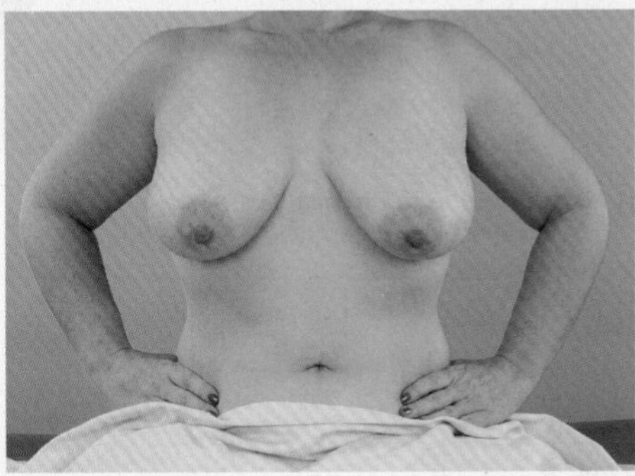

   - She then raises her arms over her head so the axillae can also be inspected.

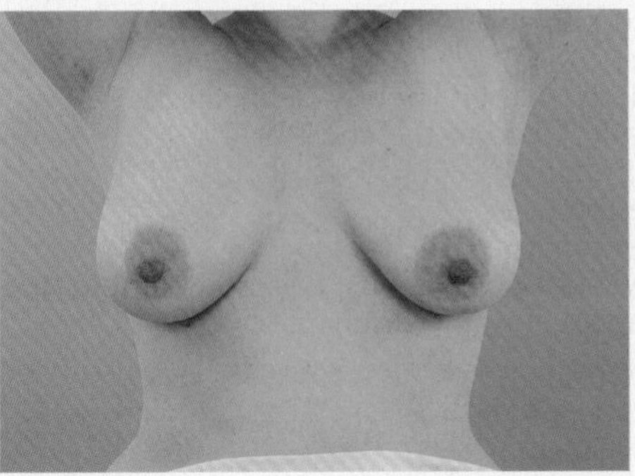

   - The client then stands, places her hands on her hips, and leans forward.

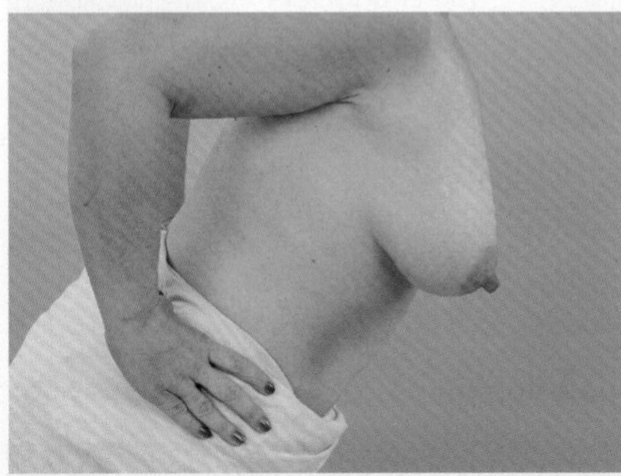

3. Palpate the breasts using the pads of your first three fingers and make a rotary motion on the breast. Assist the client into a supine position with her arms above her head. Place a pillow or towel under the client's head to help spread the breasts. Three patterns might be used to palpate the breasts:

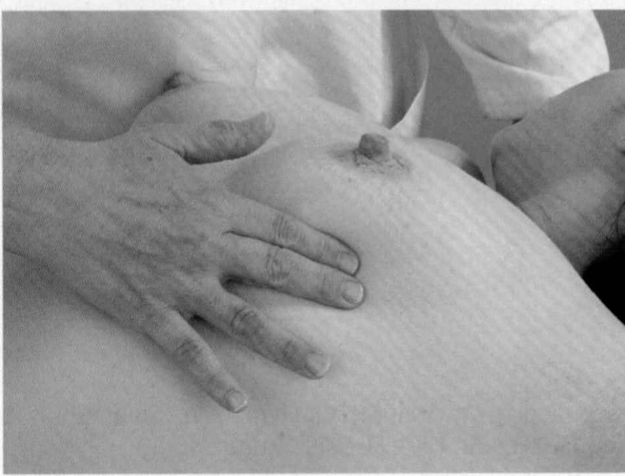

   - Spiral

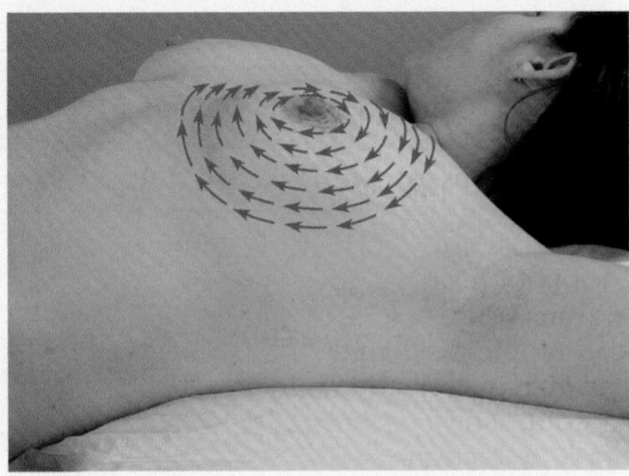

- Pie-shaped wedges

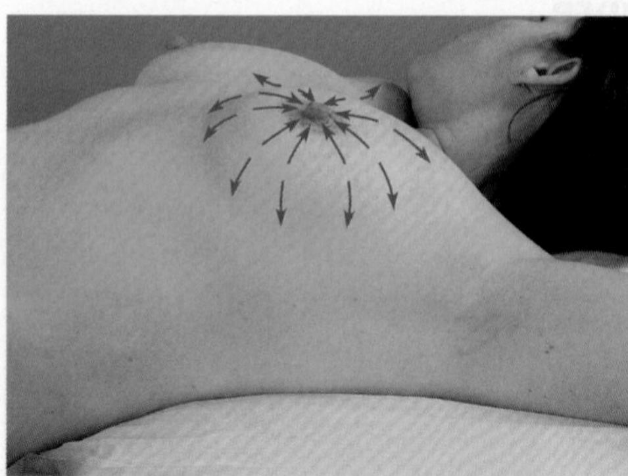

- Vertical strip

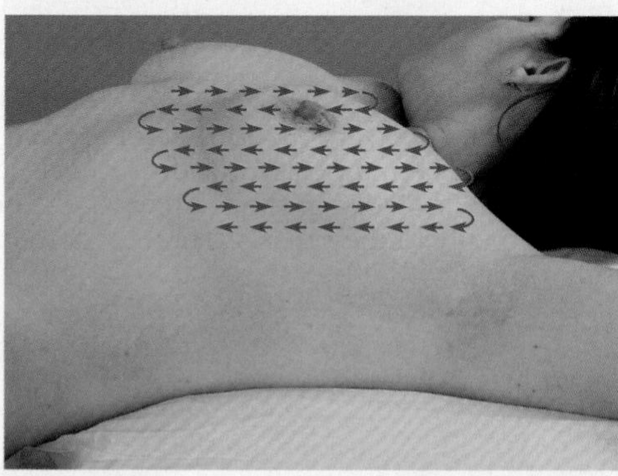

4. Compress the nipple gently between the thumb and index finger to evaluate for masses and squeeze to check for any discharge.

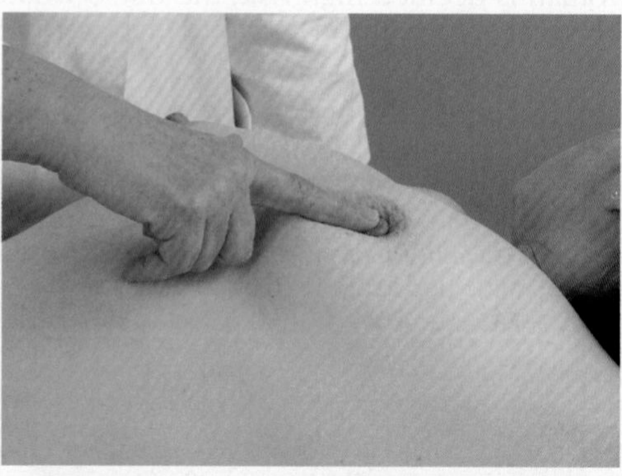

5. Palpate the axillary area for any tenderness or lymph node enlargement. Have the client sit up and move to the edge of the examination table. While supporting the client's arm, palpate downward from the armpit, palpating toward the ribs just below the breast.

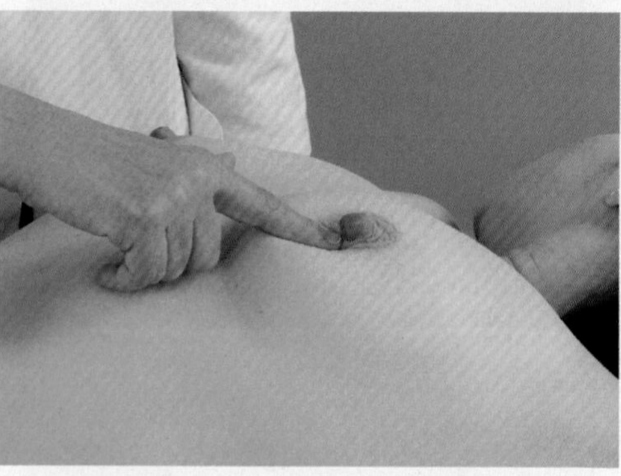

Adapted from Ball, J. W., Dains, J. E., Flynn, J. A., Soloman, B. S., & Stewart, R. W. (2015). *Seidel's guide to physical examination* (8th ed.). St. Louis, MO: Elsevier Saunders.

TABLE 6.5 CHARACTERISTICS OF BENIGN VERSUS MALIGNANT BREAST MASSES

Benign Breast Masses Are Described As	Malignant Breast Masses Are Described As
• Frequently painful • Firm, rubbery mass • Bilateral masses • Induced nipple discharge • Regular margins (clearly delineated) • No skin dimpling • No nipple retraction • Mobile, not affixed to the chest wall • No bloody discharge	• Hard to palpation • Painless • Irregularly shaped (poorly delineated) • Immobile, fixed to the chest wall • Skin dimpling • Nipple retraction • Unilateral mass • Bloody, serosanguineous, or serous nipple discharge • Spontaneous nipple discharge

adjustment to diagnosis and treatment and be able to identify those who need further psychological intervention. By giving practical advice, the nurse can help the woman adjust to her altered body image and to accept the changes in her life.

Because family members play a significant role in supporting women through breast cancer diagnosis and treatment, assess the emotional distress of both partners during the course of treatment and, if needed, make a referral for psychological counseling. By identifying interpersonal strains, negative psychosocial side effects of cancer treatment can be minimized.

Nursing Diagnosis

Appropriate nursing diagnoses for a woman with a diagnosis of breast cancer might include:

- Disturbed body image related to:
  - Loss of body part (breast)
  - Loss of femininity
  - Loss of hair due to chemotherapy
- Fear related to:
  - Diagnosis of cancer
  - Prognosis of disease
- Deficient knowledge related to:
  - Cancer treatment options
  - Reconstructive surgery decisions
  - Breast self-examination

Nursing Interventions

Offer information, support, and perioperative care to women diagnosed with breast cancer who are undergoing treatment. Implement health promotion and disease prevention strategies to minimize the risk for developing breast cancer and to promote optimal outcomes.

Remember Nancy, who discovered a breast lump? You offer to go with her to the doctor. After a full examination and several diagnostic tests, the results come back positive for breast cancer. What treatment options does Nancy have, and what factors need to be considered in selecting those options?

Providing Client Education

Help the woman and her partner to prioritize the voluminous amount of information given to them so that they can make informed decisions. Explain all treatment options in detail so the client and her family understand them. By preparing an individualized packet of information and reviewing it with the woman and her partner (if applicable), the nurse can help the woman understand her specific type of cancer, the diagnostic studies and treatment options she may choose, and the goals of treatment. For example, nurses play an important role in educating women about the use of endocrine therapies, observing women's experiences with treatment, and communicating those observations to their primary health care providers to make dosage adjustments, in addition to contributing to the knowledge base of endocrine therapy in the treatment of breast cancer.

Providing information is a central role of the nurse in caring for the woman with a diagnosis of breast cancer. This information can be given via telephone counseling, one-to-one contact, and pamphlets. Telephone counseling with women and their partners may be an effective method to improve symptom management and quality of life. Educate women on living with risk, maintaining quality of life, and participating in support groups (Strayer & Schub, 2014).

PROVIDING EMOTIONAL SUPPORT

The diagnosis of cancer affects all aspects of life for a woman and her family. The threatening nature of the disease and feelings of uncertainty about the future can lead to anxiety and stress. Address the woman's need for:

- Information about diagnosis and treatment
- Physical care while undergoing treatments
- Contact with supportive people
- Education about disease, options, and prevention measures
- Discussion and support by a caring, competent nurse

Reassure the client and her family that the diagnosis of breast cancer does not necessarily mean imminent death, a decrease in attractiveness, or diminished sexuality. Encourage the woman to express her fears and worries. Be available to listen and address the woman's concerns in an open manner to help her toward recovery. All aspects of care must include sensitivity to the client's personal efforts to cope and heal. Some women will become involved in organizations or charities that support cancer research; they may participate in breast cancer walks to raise awareness or become a *Reach to Recovery* volunteer to help others. Each woman copes in her own personal manner, and all of these efforts can be positive motivators for her own healing.

To help women cope with the diagnosis of breast cancer, the ACS launched *Reach to Recovery* more than 30 years ago. Specially trained breast cancer survivors give women and their families' opportunities to express their feelings, verbalize their fears, and get answers. Recovery volunteers can also, when appropriate, provide a temporary breast form and give information on types of permanent prostheses, as well as lists of where those items are available in the community. Most importantly, *Reach to Recovery* volunteers offer understanding, support, and hope through face-to-face visits or by telephone; they are proof that people can survive breast cancer and live productive lives. National contact information is 1-800-ACS-2345.

Providing Postoperative Care

For the woman who has had surgery to remove a malignant breast lump or an entire breast, excellent postoperative nursing care is crucial. Tell the woman what to expect in terms of symptoms and when they usually occur during treatment and after surgery. This allows women to anticipate these symptoms and proactively employ management strategies to improve their cancer experience. Postoperative care includes immediate postoperative care, pain management, care of the affected arm, wound care, mobility care, respiratory care, emotional care, referrals, and educational needs.

IMMEDIATE POSTOPERATIVE CARE

Assess the client's respiratory status by auscultating the lungs and observing the breathing pattern. Assess circulation; note vital signs, skin color, and skin temperature. Observe the client's neurologic status by evaluating the level of alertness and orientation. Monitor the wound for amount and color of drainage. Monitor the intravenous lines for patency, correct fluid, and rate. Assess the drainage tube for amount, color, and consistency of drainage.

PAIN MANAGEMENT

Provide analgesics as needed. Reassure the woman that her pain will be controlled. Teach the woman how to communicate her pain intensity on a scale of 0 to 10, with 10 being the worst pain imaginable. Assess the client's pain level frequently and anticipate pain before assisting the woman to ambulate.

AFFECTED ARM CARE

Elevate the affected arm on a pillow to promote lymph drainage. Make sure that no treatments are performed on the affected arm, including laboratory draws, intravenous lines, blood pressures, and so on. Place a sign above the bed to warn others not to touch the affected arm.

WOUND CARE

Observe the wound often and empty drainage reservoirs as needed. Tell the client to report any evidence of infection early, such as fever, chills, or any area of redness or inflammation along the incision line. Also tell the client to report any increase in drainage, foul odor, or separation at the incision site.

MOBILITY CARE

Perform active range-of-motion and arm exercises as ordered. Encourage self-care activities for successful rehabilitation. Perform dressing and drainage care; explain the care during the procedure.

RESPIRATORY CARE

Assist with turning, coughing, and deep breathing every 2 hours. Explain that this helps to expand collapsed alveoli in the lungs, promotes faster clearance of inhalation agents from the body, and prevents postoperative pneumonia and atelectasis.

EMOTIONAL CARE AND REFERRALS

Encourage the client to participate in her care. Assess her coping strategies preoperatively. Explain possible body image concerns after discharge. Promote the ACS web sites, which provide the latest cancer therapy news. Encourage the client to attend local support groups for breast cancer survivors, such as *Reach to Recovery*.

EDUCATIONAL NEEDS

Provide follow-up information about adjunctive therapy. Explain that radiation therapy may start within weeks postoperatively. Discuss chemotherapy, its side effects and cycles, home care during treatment, and future monitoring strategies. Explain hormonal therapy, including antiestrogens or aromatase inhibitors. Teach progressive arm exercises to minimize lymphedema. Explain that ongoing surveillance is needed to detect recurrence of cancer or a new primary site and that the client will typically see the health care provider every 6 months.

***Nancy* underwent a mastectomy with radiation and chemotherapy. What follow-up care is needed? How can the nurse assist Nancy to cope with her uncertain future? What community resources might help her?**

Implementing Health Promotion and Disease Prevention Strategies

In the past, most women assumed that there was little they could do to reduce their risk of developing breast cancer, but since the 1970s significant advances have been made in the diagnosis and treatment of breast cancer. Mortality rates have decreased since 1990, particularly in women <50 years old. The declining incidence of breast cancer and lower mortality rates have been attributed to early detection, improved treatment, and research (Sestak & Cuzick, 2015). However, research has found that the choices women make concerning breast cancer screening, diet, exercise, and other health practices have a profound impact on cancer risk. In the fight against cancer, nurses often assume a variety of roles, such as educator, counselor, advocate, and role model. Nurses can offer education about the following:

- Prevention
- Early detection
- Screening
- Dispelling myths and fears
- Self-examination techniques if needed
- Individual risk status and strategies for risk reduction

It is important to be knowledgeable about the most current evidence-based practices and cognizant of how the media presents this information. Offer prevention strategies within the context of a woman's life. Factors such as lifestyle choices, economic status, and multiple roles need to be taken into consideration when counseling women. Advocate for healthy lifestyles and making sound choices to prevent cancer. Nurses, like all health care providers, should offer guidance from a comprehensive perspective that acknowledges the unique needs of each individual. Nurses need to not only be proficient in the postoperative physical care of clients who undergo mastectomy but also demonstrate advanced skills related to the educational needs of clients and their families and to ensure care is delivered in a manner that is client-centered and individualized. Nurses require advanced skills to meet the social and psychological care needs of the woman and her family during this major life event (Fallowfield & Jenkins, 2015).

Breast cancer is a frightening experience for all women but is particularly burdensome on African American women, ranking second among the cause of cancer deaths in them. Although the incidence of breast cancer is highest in White women, African American women have a higher breast cancer mortality rate at every age and a lower survival rate than any other racial or ethnic group. Statistics indicate that the gap is widening (ACS, 2015e).

Like a black cloud hanging over their heads, with little regard for any victim, breast cancer stalks women everywhere they go. Many women are left with new health risks and lingering effects associated with treatment (e.g., limited mobility, memory problems, low social activity and support). Many have a close friend or relative who is battling the disease; many have watched their mothers and sisters die of this dreaded disease. Those with risk factors live with even greater anxiety and fear. No woman wants to hear those chilling words: "The biopsy is positive. You have breast cancer." Provide women with information about detection and risk factors, inform them about the new ACS screening guidelines, instruct them on BSE, and outline dietary changes that might reduce their risk of breast cancer.

Awareness is the first step toward a change in habits. Raising the level of awareness about breast cancer is of paramount importance, and nurses can play an important role in health promotion, disease prevention, and education.

Breast Cancer Screening

The three components of early detection are BSE, CBE, and mammography. The ACS (2015d) has issued breast cancer screening guidelines that, for the first time, offer specific guidance for the women and greater clarification of the role of breast examinations (Table 6.4). ACS screening guidelines are revised about every 5 years to include new scientific findings and developments.

Women are exposed to multiple sources of cancer prevention information, and much of it may not be sound. Discuss the benefits, risks, and potential limitations of BSE, CBE, and mammography with each woman and tailor the information to her specific risk factors (ACS, 2015b). Based on the new guidelines, make clinical judgments as to the appropriateness of recommending BSE, and reevaluate the need to teach the procedure to all women. The focus might instead be on encouraging regular mammograms (depending, of course, on the woman's individual risk factors).

Breast Self-Examination

BSE is a technique that enables a woman to detect any changes in her breasts. BSEs, once thought essential for early breast cancer detection, are now considered optional. Instead, breast awareness is stressed. Breast awareness refers to a woman being familiar with the normal consistency of both breasts and the underlying tissue. This emphasis is now on awareness of breast changes, not just discovery of cancer. Research has shown that BSE plays a small role in detecting breast cancer compared with self-awareness. However, doing BSE is one way for a woman to know how her breasts normally feel so that she can notice any changes that do occur (ACS, 2015d).

If appropriate, there are two steps to conducting a BSE: visual inspection and tactile palpation. The visual part should be done in three separate positions: with the arms up behind the head, with the arms down at the sides, and bending forward. Instruct the woman to look for:

- Changes in shape, size, contour, or symmetry
- Skin discoloration or dimpling, bumps/lumps
- Sores or scaly skin
- Discharge or puckering of the nipple

In the second part, the tactile examination, the health care provider feels the woman's breasts in one of three specific patterns: spiral, pie-shaped wedges, or a vertical strip (up and down). When using any of the three patterns, the woman should use a circular rubbing motion (in dime-sized circles) without lifting the fingers. The examiner checks not only the breasts but also between the breast and the axilla, the axilla itself, and the area above the breast up to the clavicle and across the shoulder. The pads of the three middle fingers on the right hand are used to assess the left breast; the pads of the three middle fingers on the left hand are used to assess the right breast. Instruct the woman to use three different degrees of pressure:

- Light (move the skin without moving the tissue underneath)
- Medium (midway into the tissue)
- Hard (down to the ribs)

Nutrition

Nutrition plays a critical role in health promotion and disease prevention. Cancer is considered to be a chronic disease that may be influenced at many stages by nutrition. These factors may affect prevention, progression, and treatment of the disease (Shrivastava, Shrivastava, & Ramasamy, 2015). Being overweight or obese is a risk factor for breast cancer in postmenopausal women. Excess body weight has been linked to an increased risk of postmenopausal breast cancer, and growing evidence also suggests that obesity is associated with poor prognosis in women diagnosed with early-stage breast cancer. Dozens of studies demonstrate that women who are overweight or obese at the time of breast cancer diagnosis are at increased risk of cancer recurrence and death compared with leaner women, and some evidence suggests that women who gain weight after breast cancer diagnosis may also be at increased risk of poor outcomes (Wright et al., 2015). *Healthy People 2020* identified being overweight or obese as one of the 10 leading health indicators and a major health concern (U.S. Department of Health and Human Services, 2010). Almost 65% of women over the age of 20 years are overweight; of these, 33.4% are obese (Carlson, 2015). A Mediterranean diet high in fruits, vegetables, and high-fiber carbohydrates and low in animal fats seems to offer protection against breast cancer as well as weight control. Women who followed these dietary guidelines decreased their risk of breast cancer. In addition, substantial evidence has shown that obesity, as measured by body mass index (BMI) is linked to breast cancer outcomes and greater mortality risks (Chan & Norat, 2015).

The Women's Health Initiative Dietary Modification Trial (Brasky et al., 2015) was designed to study a low-fat diet, a nutritional approach to prevention of chronic diseases. It found a marginally statistically significant reduction in breast cancer incidence among women in the low-fat dietary pattern group, and also disproved that "heart healthy eating" prevented future cardiac events in women.

The American Institute for Cancer Research, which conducts extensive research, made the following recommendations to reduce a woman's risk for developing breast cancer:

- Engaging in daily moderate exercise and weekly vigorous physical activity
- Consuming at least five servings of fruits and vegetables daily
- Not smoking or using any tobacco products
- Keeping a maximum BMI of 25 and limiting weight gain to no more than 11 lb since age 18
- Consuming seven or more daily portions of complex carbohydrates, such as whole grains and cereals
- Limiting intake of processed foods and refined sugar
- Limiting consumption of energy-dense foods and sugary drinks
- Avoiding use of dietary supplements which are unlikely to improve prognosis
- Restricting red meat intake to approximately 3 oz daily
- Limiting intake of fatty foods, particularly those of animal origin
- Restricting intake of salted foods and use of salt in cooking (Swisher et al., 2015).

The medical community is also starting to study the role of phytochemicals in health. The unique geographic variability of breast cancer around the world and the low rate of breast cancer in Asian countries compared with Western countries prompted this interest. This area of research appears hopeful for women seeking to prevent breast cancer as well as those recovering from it. Although the mechanism is not clear, certain foods demonstrate anticancer properties and boost the immune system. Phytochemical-rich foods include:

- Green tea and herbal teas
- Garlic
- Whole grains and legumes
- Onions and leeks
- Soybeans and soy products
- Tomato products (cooked tomatoes)
- Fruits (citrus, apricots, pumpkin, berries)
- Green leafy vegetables (spinach, collards, romaine)
- Colorful vegetables (carrots, squash, tomatoes)
- Cruciferous vegetables (broccoli, cabbage, cauliflower)
- Flax seeds (Bahadoran, Karimi, & Abedini, 2015).

Adopt a holistic approach when addressing the nutritional needs of women with breast cancer. Incorporate nutritional assessment into the general overall assessment of all women. Culturally sensitive nutritional assessment tools need to be developed and used to enhance this process. Providing examples of appropriate foods associated with the woman's current dietary habits, relating current health status to nutritional intake, and placing proposed modifications within a realistic personal framework may increase a woman's willingness to incorporate needed changes in her nutritional behavior. Be able to interpret research results and stay up to date on nutritional influences so that you can transmit this key information to the public.

NURSING CARE PLAN 6.1

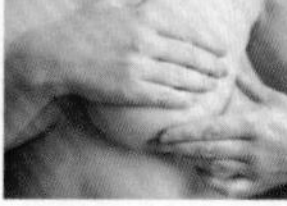

Overview of the Woman with Fibrocystic Breast Changes

Sheree Rollins is a 37-year-old woman who comes to the clinic for her routine checkup. During the examination, she says, "Sometimes my breasts feel so heavy and they ache a lot. I noticed a couple of lumpy areas in my breast last week just before I got my period. Is this normal? Now they feel like they're almost gone. Should I be worried?" Clinical breast examination reveals two small (pea-sized), mobile, slightly tender nodules in each breast bilaterally. No skin retraction noted. Previous mammogram revealed fibrocystic breast changes.

NURSING DIAGNOSIS: Pain related to changes in breast tissue

Outcome Identification and Evaluation

The client will demonstrate a decrease in breast pain as evidenced by a pain rating of 1 or 2 on a pain rating scale of 0 to 10 with statements made that her pain is lessened.

Interventions: *Relieving Pain*

- Ask client to rate her pain using a numeric pain rating scale to establish a baseline.
- Discuss with client any measures used to relieve pain to determine effectiveness of the measures.
- Encourage use of a supportive bra to aid in reducing discomfort.
- Instruct client in use of over-the-counter analgesics to promote pain relief.
- Advise the client to apply warm compresses or allow warm water from the shower to flow over her breasts to promote vasodilation and subsequent pain relief.
- Tell client to reduce her intake of salt to reduce risk of fluid retention and swelling leading to increased pain.

NURSING DIAGNOSIS: Deficient knowledge related to fibrocystic breast changes and appropriate care measures

Outcome Identification and Evaluation

The client will verbalize understanding of condition as evidenced by statements about the cause of breast changes and appropriate choices for lifestyle changes, and demonstration of self-care measures.

Interventions: *Providing Client Education*

- Assess client's knowledge of fibrocystic breast changes to establish a baseline for teaching.
- Explain the role of monthly hormonal level changes and describe the signs and symptoms to promote understanding of this condition.
- Teach the client how to perform breast self-examination after her menstrual period to monitor for changes.
- Encourage client to report any changes promptly to ensure early detection of problems.
- Suggest client speak with her primary care provider about the use of oral contraceptives to help stabilize monthly hormonal levels.
- Review lifestyle choices, such as eating a low-fat diet rich in fruits, vegetables, and grains, and adhering to screening recommendations to promote health.
- Discuss measures for pain relief to minimize discomfort associated with breast changes.

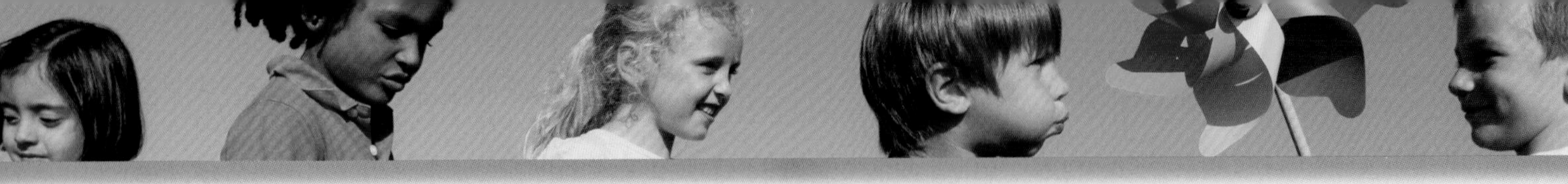

KEY CONCEPTS

- Many women believe that all lumps are cancerous, but actually more than 80% of the lumps discovered are benign and need no treatment (Alexander et al., 2014).
- The most commonly encountered benign breast disorders in women include fibrocystic breasts, fibroadenomas, and mastitis (Bope & Kellerman, 2015).
- Current research suggests that women with fibrocystic breast disease or other benign breast conditions are more likely to develop breast cancer later only if a breast biopsy shows "atypia" or abnormal breast cells (ACS, 2015a).
- Fibroadenomas are common benign solid breast tumors that can be stimulated by external estrogen, progesterone, lactation, and pregnancy.
- Mastitis is an infection of the connective tissue in the breast that occurs primarily in lactating or engorged women; it is divided into lactational or nonlactational types.
- Management of both types of mastitis involves the use of oral antibiotics (usually a penicillinase-resistant penicillin or cephalosporin) and acetaminophen (Tylenol) for pain and fever (Miller & Kennedy, 2015).
- Breast cancer is the most common cancer in women and the second leading cause of cancer deaths (lung cancer is first) among American women (ACS, 2015a).
- Breast cancer metastasizes widely and to almost all organs of the body, but primarily to the bone, lungs, lymph nodes, liver, and brain.
- The etiology of breast cancer is unknown, but the disease is thought to develop in response to a number of related factors: aging, delayed childbearing or never bearing children, high breast density, family history of cancer, late menopause, obesity, and hormonal factors.
- Breast cancer treatments fall into two categories: local and systemic. Local treatments are surgery and radiation therapy. Effective systemic treatments include chemotherapy, hormonal therapy, and immunotherapy.
- Women commonly perceive their breasts as intrinsic to their femininity, self-esteem, and sexuality, and the risk of losing a breast can provoke extreme anxiety.
- Nurses can influence both physical and emotional recovery, which are both important aspects of care that help in improving the woman's quality of life and the ability to survive.
- Providing up-to-date information and emotional support are central roles of the nurse in caring for the woman with a diagnosis of breast cancer.

REFERENCES AND RECOMMENDED READINGS

Alexander, L. L., LaRosa, J. H., Bader, H., & Garfield, S. (2014). *New dimensions in women's health* (6th ed.). Sudbury, MA: Jones & Bartlett.

American Cancer Society [ACS]. (2015a). *Breast cancer.* Retrieved from http://www.cancer.org/Cancer/BreastCancer/index

American Cancer Society [ACS]. (2015b). *Risk factors for breast cancer.* Available at: http://www.cancer.org/cancer/breast-cancer/detailedguide/breast-cancer-risk-factors

American Cancer Society [ACS]. (2015c). *Types of breast cancer.* Available at: http://www.cancer.org/cancer/breast-cancer/detailedguide/breast-cancer-breast-cancer-types

American Cancer Society [ACS]. (2015d). *Guidelines for the early detection of breast cancer.* Available at: http://www.cancer.org/healthy/findcancerearly/cancerscreeningguidelines/american-cancer-society-guidelines-for-the-early-detection-of-cancer

American Cancer Society [ACS]. (2015e). *Cancer facts & figures.* Available at: http://www.cancer.org/acs/groups/content/@epidemiologysurveilance/documents/document/acspc-036845.pdf

American Cancer Society [ACS]. (2015f). *How is breast cancer treated?* Available at: http://www.cancer.org/cancer/breastcancer/detailedguide/breast-cancer-treating-surgery

American Cancer Society [ACS]. (2015g). *Chemotherapy for breast cancer.* Available at: http://www.cancer.org/cancer/breastcancer/detailedguide/breast-cancer-treating-chemotherapy

American Cancer Society [ACS]. (2015h). *How is breast cancer staged?* Available at: http://www.cancer.org/cancer/breast-cancer/detailedguide/breast-cancer-staging

American Cancer Society [ACS]. (2015i). *How many women get breast cancer?* Retrieved from http://www.cancer.org/cancer/breastcancer/overviewguide/breast-cancer-overview-key-statistics.

American Congress of Obstetricians and Gynecologists [ACOG]. (2015). Annual mammograms now recommended for women beginning at age 40. Retrieved from http://www.acog.org/About%20ACOG/News%20Room/News%20Releases/2011/Annual%20Mammograms%20Now%20Recommended%20for%20Women%20Beginning%20at%20Age%2040.aspx

Arora, R., Schmitt, D., Karanam, B., Tan, M., Yates, C., & Dean-Colomb, W. (2015). Inhibition of the Warburg effect with a natural compound reveals a novel measurement for determining the metastatic potential of breast cancers. *Oncotarget, 6*(2), 662–678.

Bahadoran, Z., Karimi, Z., & Abedini, S. (2015). Healthy dietary patterns and the risk of breast cancer: A review of current data. *American Journal of Life Sciences, 3*(2–1), 1–5.

Ball, J. W., Dains, J. E., Flynn, J. A., Soloman, B. S., & Stewart, R. W. (2015). *Seidel's guide to physical examination* (8th ed.). St. Louis, MO: Elsevier Saunders.

Bevers, T. B. (2015). Breast cancer risk reduction therapy: The low-hanging fruit. *Journal of the National Comprehensive Cancer Network, 13*(4), 376–378.

Bhatti, L., Hoang, J. K., Dale, B. M., & Bashir, M. R. (2015). Advanced magnetic resonance techniques: 3 T. *Radiologic Clinics of North America, 53*(3), 441–455.

Bope, E. T., & Kellerman, R. D. (2015). *Conn's current therapy 2015.* Philadelphia, PA: Saunders Elsevier.

Bourdeanu, L., & Liu, E. A. (2015). Systemic treatment for breast cancer: Chemotherapy and biotherapy agents. In *Seminars in oncology nursing.* WB Saunders. doi:10.1016/j.soncn.2015.02.003

Brasky, T. M., Rodabough, R. J., Liu, J., Kurta, M. L., Wise, L. A., Orchard, T. S., et al. (2015). Long-chain -3 fatty acid intake and endometrial cancer risk in the Women's Health Initiative. *The American Journal of Clinical Nutrition, 101*(4), 824–834.

Breast Cancer Organization (2015). *Hormonal therapy side effects.* Available at: http://www.breastcancer.org/treatment/hormonal/comp_chart

Caple, C., & Schub, T. (2015). Breast cancer: Psychological adjustment. *CINAHL Information Systems.* (Online 4/17/15) Evidence-based Care Sheet. Retrieved from http://web.b.ebscohost.com.ezproxy.net.ucf.edu/ehost/pdfviewer/pdfviewer?sid=415529de-e3be-4ada-b09e-fde7fd22ec97%40sessionmgr111&vid=33&hid=118

Catsburg, C., Kim, R. S., Kirsh, V. A., Soskolne, C. L., Kreiger, N., & Rohan, T. E. (2015). Dietary patterns and breast cancer risk: A study in 2 cohorts. *The American Journal of Clinical Nutrition, 101*(4), 817–823.

Chan, D. S., & Norat, T. (2015). Obesity and breast cancer: Not only a risk factor of the disease. *Current Treatment Options in Oncology, 16*(5), 1–17.

Chang, Z., Craciunescu, O., Xu, X., Steffey, B., Meltsner, S., Cai, J., et al. (2015). Evaluating radiation-induced changes with diffusion weighted imaging in patients with gynecologic cancers treated with combined external beam radiation radiotherapy and high-dose-rate brachytherapy: Initial results. *Brachytherapy, 14,* S75-S76.

Chatterjee, A., Serniak, N., & Czerniecki, B. J. (2015). Sentinel lymph node biopsy in breast cancer: A work in progress. *The Cancer Journal, 21*(1), 7–10.

Carlson, R. H. (2015). Obesity and breast cancer: Research update. *Oncology Times, 37*(9), 33.

Chu, Q. D., Caldito, G., Miller, J. K., & Townsend, B. (2015). Postmastectomy radiation for N2/N3 breast cancer: Factors associated with low compliance rate. *Journal of the American College of Surgeons, 220*(4), 659–669.

Corradini, S., Niyazi, M., Niemoeller, O. M., Li, M., Roeder, F., Eckel, R., et al. (2015). Adjuvant radiotherapy after breast conserving surgery—A comparative effectiveness research study. *Radiotherapy & Oncology, 114*(1), 28–34. doi:10.1016/j.radonc.2014.08.027

Cuzick, J., & Thorat, M. (2015). PG 6.02 Preventing invasive breast cancer in women at high risk based on benign/in situ pathology. *The Breast, 24,* S11.

Dear, R. F., McGeechan, K, Jenkins, M. C., Barratt, A., Tattersall, M. H., & Wilcken, N. (2015). Combination versus sequential single agent chemotherapy for metastatic breast cancer. *Cochrane Database of Systematic Reviews,* 3:CD008792.

Debled, M., MacGrogan, G., Breton-Callu, C., Ferron, S., Hurtevent, G., Fournier, M., et al. (2015). Surgery following neoadjuvant chemotherapy for HER2-positive locally advanced breast cancer. Time to reconsider the standard attitude. *European Journal of Cancer, 51*(6), 697–704.

Dixon, J. M., & Macaskill, E. J. (2015). Management of benign breast disease. In *Breast disease* (pp. 51–77). New York, NY: Springer Publishers.

Euhus, D. M., & Diaz, J. (2015). Breast cancer prevention. *The Breast Journal, 21*(1), 76–81.

Faguy, K. (2015). Breast disorders in pregnant and lactating women. *Radiologic Technology, 86*(4), 419M–438M.

Fallowfield, L., & Jenkins, V. (2015). Psychosocial/Survivorship issues in breast cancer: Are we doing better? *Journal of the National Cancer Institute, 107*(1), 335.

Files, J. A., Allen, S. V., & Pruthi, S. (2015). Management of breast pain. In *Breast disease* (pp. 79–91). New York, NY: Springer Publishers.

Gradishar, W. J. (2015). Adjuvant therapy for breast cancer: Hormonal therapy. In *Breast disease* (pp. 353–362). New York, NY: Springer Publishers.

Guinot, J. L., Baixauli-Perez, C., Soler, P., Tortajada, M. I., Moreno, A., Santos, M. A., et al. (2015). High-dose-rate brachytherapy boost effect on local tumor control in young women with breast cancer. *International Journal of Radiation Oncology, Biology, Physics, 91*(1), 165–171.

Han, F., Shi, G., Liang, C., Wang, L., & Li, K. (2015). A simple and efficient method for breast cancer diagnosis based on infrared thermal imaging. *Cell Biochemistry and Biophysics, 71,* 491–498.

Jager, N. G. L., Linn, S. C., Schellens, J. H., & Beijnen, J. H. (2015). Tailored tamoxifen treatment for breast cancer patients: A perspective. *Clinical Breast Cancer, 15*(4), 241–244.

Janardhan, J., Venkateshwar, P., & Rao, K.S. (2015). Giant fibroadenoma of the breast: Conservative surgery. *International Archives of Integrated Medicine, 2*(4), 156–160.

Jarvis, C. (2015). *Physical examination & health assessment* (7th ed.). St. Louis, MO: Elsevier Health Sciences.

Kalinsky, K., Mayer, J. A., Xu, X., Pham, T., Wong, K. L., Villarin, E., et al. (2015). Correlation of hormone receptor status between circulating tumor cells, primary tumor, and metastasis in breast cancer patients. *Clinical and Translational Oncology, 17*(7):539–546.

Khan, M. H., Allerton, R., & Pettit, L. (2015). Hormone therapy for male breast cancer. *Clinical Breast Cancer, 15*(4), 245–250.

King, T.L., Brucker, M.C., Kriebs, J.M., Fahey, J.O., Gegor, C.L., & Varney, H. (2015) *Varney's midwifery* (5th ed.). Berlington, MA: Jones & Bartlett Learning.

Kleban, R., & Glaser, S. (2015). The many dimensions of breast cancer: Determining the scope of needed services. In *Handbook of oncology social work: Psychosocial care for people with cancer* (pp. 93–99). New York, NY: Oxford University press.

Lara, P. C., López-Peñalver, J. J., Farias, V. A., Ruiz-Ruiz, M. C., Oliver, F. J., & Ruiz de Almodóvar, J. M. (2015). Direct and bystander radiation effects: A biophysical model and clinical perspectives. *Cancer Letters, 356*(1), 5–16.

Leavy, O. (2015). Immunotherapy: A triple blow for cancer. *Nature Reviews Cancer, 15*, 258–259.

Li, J., Holm, J., Bergh, J., Eriksson, M., Darabi, H., Lindström, L. S., et al. (2015). Breast cancer genetic risk profile is differentially associated with interval and screen-detected breast cancers. *Annals of Oncology, 26*(3), 517–522.

Miller, A.C., & Kennedy, C. (2015). Breast abscess and masses. eMedicine. Available at: http://emedicine.medscape.com/article/781116-overview#a0104

Mills, S. (2013). Performing a clinical breast exam. *Nursing, 43*(9), 68.

Mugea, T. T. (2015). Complications of breast augmentation. In *Aesthetic surgery of the breast* (pp. 425–512). Berlin, Heidelberg; Springer.

Muralidhar, K. R., Soubhagya, B., & Ahmed, S. (2015). Intensity modulated radiotherapy versus volumetric modulated arc therapy in breast cancer: A comparative dosimetric analysis. *International Journal of Cancer Therapy and Oncology, 3*(2), 1–6.

National Cancer Institute [NCI]. (2015a). Breast cancer. Retrieved from http://www.cancer.gov/cancertopics/types/breast

National Cancer Institute [NCI]. (2015b). Probability of breast cancer in American women. Retrieved from http://www.cancer.gov/cancertopics/factsheet/detection/probability-breast-cancer

National Comprehensive Cancer Network [NCCN]. (2015). *Breast cancer treatment guidelines: NCCN patient guidelines.* Retrieved from http://www.nccn.org/patients/patient_gls/_english/_breast/5_treatment.asp

Pluchinotta, A. M. (2015). Inflammatory diseases of the breast. In *The outpatient breast clinic* (pp. 169–195). Springer International Publishing.

Poulos, A. (2015). Diagnostic breast imaging: Mammography, sonography, magnetic resonance imaging, and interventional procedures. *Journal of Medical Radiation Sciences, 62*(1), 86–87.

Rifkin, E., & Lazris, A. (2015). Breast cancer screening: Mammograms. In *Interpreting health benefits and risks* (pp. 33–41). Springer International Publishing.

Sabel, M.S. (2015). Overview of benign breast disease. UpToDate, Available from: http://www.uptodate.com/contents/overview-of-benign-breast-disease

Schuiling, K.D., & Likis, F.E. (2016). *Women's gynecological health* (3rd ed.). Burlington, MA: Jones & Bartlett Learning.

Seetharam, P., & Rodrigues, G. (2015). Benign breast disorders: An insight with a detailed literature review. *Webmed Central Breast, 6*(1) doi: 10.9754/journal.wmc.2015.004806

Selvi, R. (2015). Invasive lobular carcinoma. In *Breast diseases* (pp. 281–286). India: Springer Publishers.

Sestak, I., & Cuzick, J. (2015). Update on breast cancer risk prediction and prevention. *Current Opinion in Obstetrics and Gynecology, 27*(1), 92–97.

Shannon, K. M., & Chittenden, A. (2015). Breast cancer genetics and risk assessment. In *Breast cancer screening and diagnosis* (pp. 1–21). New York, NY: Springer Publishers.

Shrivastava, S. R., Shrivastava, P. S., & Ramasamy, J. (2015). Assessing the contribution of dietary factors in breast cancer. *Clinical Cancer Investigation Journal, 4*(1), 1–5.

Skidmore-Roth, L. (2015). *Mosby's 2015 nursing drug reference* (28th ed.). St. Louis, MO: Elsevier Health Science.

Slanetz, P. J., Freer, P. E., & Birdwell, R. L. (2015). Breast-density legislation—Practical considerations. *New England Journal of Medicine, 372*(7), 593–595.

Stopeck, A.T., Chalasani, P., & Thompson, P.A. (2015) Breast cancer. EMedicine. Available at: http://emedicine.medscape.com/article/1947145-overview

Strayer, D. A., & Schub, T. (2014). Breast cancer. Published by CINAHL Information Systems. Full Text, EBSCOhost

Swisher, A. K., Abraham, J., Bonner, D., Gilleland, D., Hobbs, G., Kurian, S., et al. (2015). Exercise and dietary advice intervention for survivors of triple-negative breast cancer: effects on body fat, physical function, quality of life, and adipokine profile. *Supportive Care in Cancer, 23*(10):2995–3003.

Tharpe, N.L., Farley, C.L., & Jordan, R.G. (2016). *Clinical practice guidelines for midwifery & women's health* (5th ed.). Burlington, MA: Jones & Bartlett Learning.

Toi, M., Winer, E.P., Benson, J.R., & Klimberg, S. (2015). *Personalized treatment of breast cancer.* Japan: Springer Publishers.

Tsujimoto, M. (2015). Recent advances in sentinel node biopsy in breast surgery. *Breast Cancer, 22*(3):211.

U.S. Department of Health and Human Services. (2015). Healthy people 2020. Retrieved from http://www.healthypeople.gov/2020/topicsobjectives2020/default.aspx

U.S. Preventive Services Task Force [USPSTF]. (2015). *Screening for breast cancer.* Available at: http://www.uspreventiveservicestaskforce.org/breastcancer.htm

van den Broek, A. J., Schmidt, M. K., van 't Veer, L. J., Tollenaar, R. M., & van Leeuwen, F. E. (2015). Worse breast cancer prognosis of BRCA1/BRCA2 mutation carriers: What's the evidence? A systematic review with meta-analysis. *Plos ONE, 10*(3), 1–29.

Wevers, M. R., Ausems, M. M., Verhoef, S., Bleiker, E. A., Hahn, D. E., Brouwer, T., et al. (2015). Does rapid genetic counseling and testing in newly diagnosed breast cancer patients cause additional psychosocial distress? Results from a randomized clinical trial. *Genetics in Medicine: Official Journal of the American College of Medical Genetics*. doi:10.1038/gim.2015.50.

Wright, C. E., Harvie, M., Howell, A., Evans, D. G., Hulbert-Williams, N., & Donnelly, L. S. (2015). Beliefs about weight and breast cancer: an interview study with high risk women following a 12 month weight loss intervention. *Hereditary Cancer in Clinical Practice, 13*(1), 1.

Writing Group for the Women's Health Initiative Investigators. (2002). Women's Health Initiative Study. *JAMA, 288*(3), 321–333.

CHAPTER WORKSHEET

MULTIPLE-CHOICE QUESTIONS

1. Breast self-examinations involve both touching of breast tissue and:
   a. Palpation of cervical lymph nodes
   b. Firm squeezing of both breast nipples
   c. Visualizing both breasts for any change
   d. A mammogram to evaluate breast tissue

2. Which of the following is the strongest risk factor for breast cancer?
   a. Advancing age and being female
   b. High number of children
   c. Genetic mutations in BRCA1 and BRCA2 genes
   d. Family history of colon cancer

3. A biopsy procedure that traces radioisotopes and blue dye from the tumor site through the lymphatic system into the axillary nodes is:
   a. Stereotactic biopsy
   b. Sentinel node biopsy
   c. Axillary dissection biopsy
   d. Advanced breast biopsy

4. The most serious potential adverse reaction from chemotherapy is:
   a. Thrombocytopenia
   b. Deep vein thrombosis
   c. Alopecia
   d. Myelosuppression

5. What suggestion would be helpful for the client experiencing painful fibrocystic breast changes?
   a. Increase her caffeine intake.
   b. Take a mild analgesic when needed.
   c. Reduce her intake of leafy vegetables.
   d. Wear a bra bigger than she needs.

6. A postoperative mastectomy client should be referred to which of the following organizations for assistance upon discharge from the hospital?
   a. National Organization for Women (NOW)
   b. Food and Drug Administration (FDA)
   c. March of Dimes Foundation (MDF)
   d. Reach to Recovery (RTR)

7. Breast cancer that is localized is referred to as:
   a. Primary
   b. In situ
   c. Metastasized
   d. Localized

8. A 25-year-old woman presents with an asymptomatic breast mass. Which of the following is true concerning her diagnosis and treatment?
   a. All breast masses should be considered premalignant
   b. The breast mass should be surgically removed immediately
   c. Ultrasound is typically used to determine the diagnosis
   d. Since it is asymptomatic, just reassurance is needed now

CRITICAL THINKING EXERCISES

1. Mrs. Gordon, 48, presents to the women's community clinic where you work as a nurse. She is very upset and crying. She tells you that she found lumps in her breast: "I know that it's cancer and I will die." When you ask her about her problem, she says she does not check her breasts monthly and hasn't had a mammogram for years because "they're too expensive." She also describes the intermittent pain she experiences.
   a. What specific questions would you ask this client to get a clearer picture?
   b. What education is needed for this client regarding breast health?
   c. What community referrals are needed to meet this client's future needs?

2. Ruth Davis, 51, stops in at the urgent care facility with an anxious look on her face. She tells the nurse practitioner that she has green discharge coming from her right breast and discomfort intermittently. She can't understand how this would happen since she hasn't previously had any nipple discharge or pain.
   a. What benign breast condition might the nurse practitioner suspect based on her description?
   b. What specific information should the nurse practitioner give Mrs. Davis about duct ectasia?
   c. The typical treatment of this benign breast condition would include what?

STUDY ACTIVITIES

1. Discuss with a group of women what their breasts symbolize to them and to society. Do they symbolize something different to each one?

2. When a woman experiences a breast disorder, what feelings might she be experiencing and how can a nurse help her sort them out?

3. Interview a woman who has fibrocystic breast changes and find out how she manages this condition.

4. An infection of the breast connective tissue that frequently occurs in the lactating woman is __________________.

CHAPTER WORKSHEET

BRINGING IT ALL TOGETHER: A CASE STUDY

A 67-year-old obese woman presented to her internist after a several year absence complaining of back pain that has persisted despite taking a nonsteroidal anti-inflammatory drug (NSAID) for several weeks. She also has recently noticed a 10-lb weight loss over the past 6 months and occasional right upper quadrant discomfort. She also states that she has been feeling tired over the last several months, but rationalized it as "old age" catching up with her.

ASSESSMENT

She has a family history of breast and colon cancer in her immediate family and both of her parents died from these (mother from breast cancer and father from colon cancer). Her aunt also had breast cancer, but is in remission now after treatment. She can't remember when the last time she had a pap smear or mammogram. She admits that she doesn't keep up with her health checkups, since she babysits for her grandchildren and has difficulty scheduling them. She confesses that her diet hasn't been what it should be, since her grandchildren prefer fast food and sodas for meals, rather than home-cooked ones. Thus, she gives into them and eats what they want.

1. Based on her chief complaint, what might be a reason for her current back pain?
2. What is concerning about her family health history that might have a bearing on her present symptoms?
3. How does her poor dietary intake and weight status impact her overall health status?

Breast cancer does metastasize to the bone and this could be the reason for her back pain that doesn't response to anti-inflammatory medications. Since she has first-degree relatives that had cancer, she is at high risk for it herself. Research in nutrition and obesity and its link to cancer suggests that high consumption of processed foods (fast foods) and low consumption of fruits and vegetables in addition to being obese places people at risk for cancer.

PLAN

1. What diagnostic tests might be ordered to determine her diagnosis?
2. What treatment modalities are available to her if metastatic cancer is found?
3. What health promotion instructions are needed for this client?
4. How can the nurse provide an open forum for this woman to discuss her feelings?

An MRI and a bone scan might be ordered to identify any "hot spots" or cancerous lesions on her bones as well as her liver, which are common areas cancer might have spread to. Depending on the extent of the metastasis, chemotherapy and radiation might be treatment modalities. Nutrition counseling and lifestyle changes to lose weight to promote better health are both health promotion areas that need to be addressed with this client. A thorough explanation of the treatments, their side effects and prognosis need to also be discussed to make sure she understands. Fear and anxiety are common feelings felt by anyone with a cancer diagnosis, so the nurse needs to be open and supportive to her and allow time for her to express her fears.

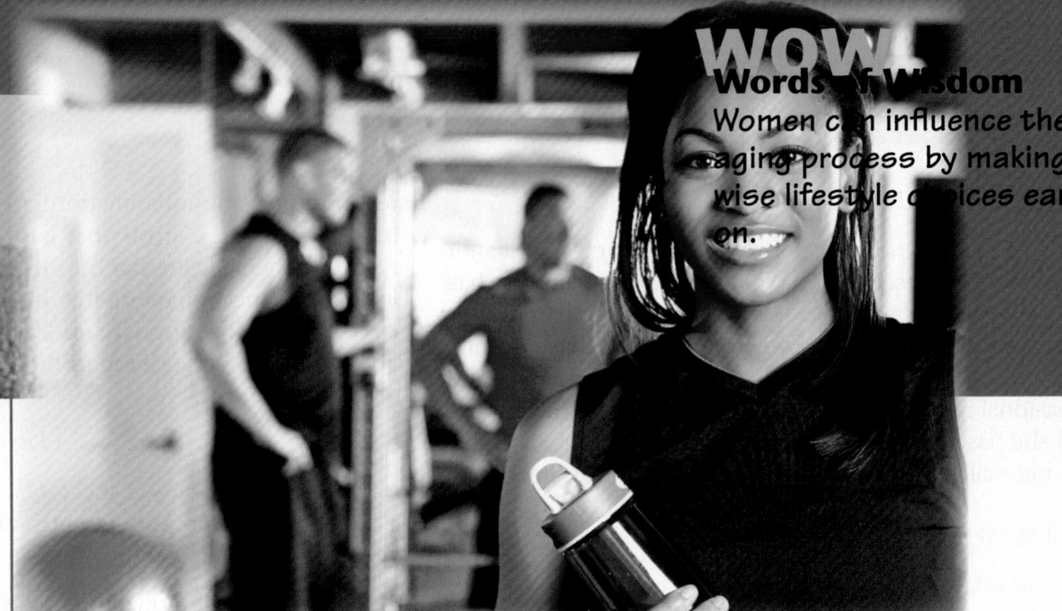
WOW
Words of Wisdom
Women can influence their aging process by making wise lifestyle choices early on.

7

Benign Disorders of the Female Reproductive Tract

KEY TERMS
cystocele
enterocele
ovarian cyst
pelvic floor muscle exercises (Kegel exercises)
pelvic organ prolapse (POP)
pessary
polycystic ovary syndrome (PCOS)
polyps
rectocele
urinary incontinence (UI)
uterine fibroids
uterine prolapse

Learning Objectives

Upon completion of the chapter, you will be able to:

1. Characterize the major pelvic relaxation disorders in terms of etiology, management, and nursing interventions.
2. Outline the nursing management needed for the most common benign reproductive disorders in women.
3. Evaluate urinary incontinence in terms of pathology, clinical manifestations, treatment options, and effect on quality of life.
4. Compare the various benign growths in terms of their symptoms and management.
5. Analyze the emotional impact of polycystic ovarian syndrome and the nurse's role as a counselor, educator, and advocate.

***Liz*, a 26-year-old, overweight woman, presented to the clinic with hirsutism and facial acne and told the nurse she was concerned about her irregular menstrual periods. She also said that recently the hair on top of her head seemed to be falling out. What diagnostic tests might the nurse anticipate with this client? How can the nurse prepare Liz for them?**

INTRODUCTION

The incidence of several benign pelvic disorders increases as women age. For instance, women may experience pelvic floor disorders related to pelvic relaxation or urinary incontinence (UI). These disorders generally develop after years of wear and tear on the muscles and tissues that support the pelvic floor—such as that which occurs with childbearing, chronic coughing, straining, surgery, or simply aging. In addition to pelvic floor disorders, woman may also experience various benign neoplasms of the reproductive tract, such as cervical polyps, uterine leiomyomas (fibroids), ovarian cysts, genital fistulas, and Bartholin cysts. This chapter provides an overview of various pelvic floor disorders and benign neoplasms, discussing the assessment, treatment, and prevention strategies for each. It also addresses female genital cutting in the context of it being a harmful practice that affects girls' and women's health.

PELVIC FLOOR DISORDERS

Pelvic floor disorders such as pelvic organ prolapse (POP) or genital prolapse and urinary and fecal incontinence are common in aging women. Researchers funded by the National Institutes of Health (NIH) (2015a) reported that more than one third of women in the United States have a pelvic floor disorder, and nearly one quarter of women in the United States have one or more pelvic floor disorders that cause symptoms. The study reported that the frequency of pelvic floor disorders increases with age, affecting more than 40% of women from 60 to 79 years of age, and about 50% of women 80 years and older. The NIH analysis is the first to document in a nationally representative sample the extent of pelvic floor disorders, a cluster of health problems that causes physical discomfort and limits activity.

Pelvic floor disorders cause significant physical and psychological morbidity and can diminish women's social interactions, emotional well-being, and overall quality of life. Because these disorders increase with age, the problem will grow worse as our population ages. The term "pelvic floor" refers to the group of muscles that form a sling or hammock across the pelvis. Together with their surrounding tissues, these muscles hold the pelvic organs (uterus, bladder, & bowel), in place so that they can function correctly. These disorders occur as a result of weakness of the connective tissue and muscular support of pelvic organs due to a number of factors: pregnancy, vaginal childbirth, obesity, lifting, chronic cough from smoking, straining at defecation secondary to constipation, radiation to the pelvis for cancer, and estrogen deficiency (American College of Obstetricians and Gynecologists [ACOG], 2015a). The female anatomy is susceptible to the development of pelvic floor disorders because of its vertical structures placement. The bony pelvis has an exaggerated lumbar spinal curve and downward tilt to it. The bladder rests on the symphysis and the posterior organs rest on the sacrum and coccyx. The pelvis holds the organs, but a woman's erect posture causes a funneling effect and constant downward pressure.

Pelvic Organ Prolapse

Pelvic organ prolapse (POP) (from the Latin *prolapsus,* "a slipping forth") refers to the abnormal descent or herniation of the pelvic organs from their original attachment sites or their normal position in the pelvis. POP occurs when structures of the pelvis shift and protrude into or outside of the vaginal canal. This disorder affects a woman's micturition, defecation, and sexual activity. The Egyptians were the first to describe prolapse of the genital organs. Hippocrates in 400 BC made reference to placing a pomegranate half into the vagina to treat organ prolapse. A disorder exclusive to women, POP rarely results in severe morbidity or mortality but can affect a woman's daily activities and quality of life (Brown, 2015). It is difficult to determine the incidence of POP, because the disorder is often asymptomatic and many women do not seek treatment. It has been estimated, however, that up to 75% of all women who have had a vaginal birth have POP (ACOG, 2015a). Each year, over 250,000 women undergo surgery to repair the prolapse at a cost of over $1 billion for hospitalization and physician or nurse practitioner fees alone (Maher & Haya, 2015). As the older adult population is expected to double in number by 2030, POP and its associated symptoms will become more prevalent (Mukwege, et al., 2015).

Obesity is associated with a high prevalence of pelvic floor disorders. Obesity can also aggravate symptoms of POP, fecal incontinence, sexual dysfunction, stress UI and increase the risk of endometrial polyps and symptomatic fibroids. Weight reduction enhances reproductive outcomes, diminishes symptoms of UI, improves sexual dysfunction, and reduces morbidity following gynecologic surgery. Sustained and substantial weight loss, however, is difficult to achieve for many women with their current lifestyle and dietary choices (Ramalingam & Monga, 2015).

The treatment and diagnosis of POP is challenging and problematic.

Types of Pelvic Organ Prolapse

The four most common types of pelvic or genital prolapse are cystocele, rectocele, enterocele, and uterine prolapse (Fig. 7.1):

- **Cystocele** occurs when the posterior bladder wall protrudes downward through the anterior vaginal wall.
- **Rectocele** occurs when the rectum sags and pushes against or into the posterior vaginal wall.

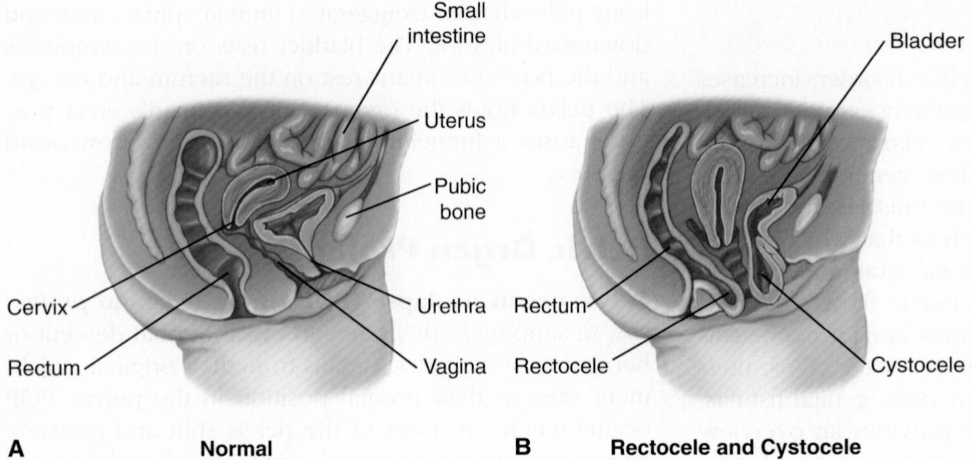

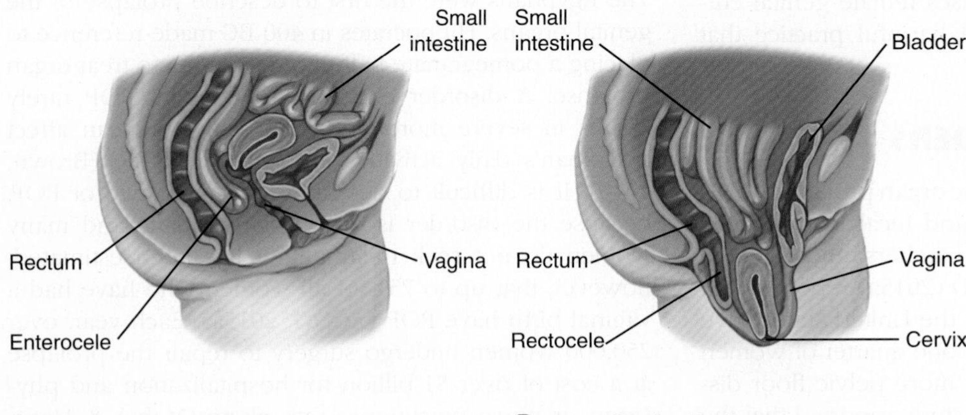

FIGURE 7.1 Types of pelvic prolapses. **A.** Normal. **B.** Rectocele and cystocele. **C.** Enterocele. **D.** Uterine prolapse.

- **Enterocele** occurs when the small intestine bulges through the posterior vaginal wall (especially common when straining).
- **Uterine prolapse** occurs when the uterus descends through the pelvic floor and into the vaginal canal. Multiparous women are at particular risk for uterine prolapse. The extent of uterine prolapse is classified in terms of stages:
  - *Stage 0:* No descent of pelvic structure during straining.
  - *Stage I:* The prolapsed descending organ is >1 cm above the hymenal ring.
  - *Stage II:* The prolapsed organ extends ~1 cm below the hymenal ring.
  - *Stage III:* The prolapsed organ extends 2 to 3 cm below the hymenal ring.
  - *Stage IV:* The vagina is completely everted or the prolapsed organ is >3 cm below the hymenal ring (Riss & Koch, 2015).

Etiology

Anatomic support of the pelvic organs is mainly provided by the levator ani muscle complex and the connective tissue attachments of the pelvic organ fascia. Dysfunction of one or both of these components can lead to loss of support and eventually POP. Weakened pelvic floor muscles also prevent complete closure of the urethra, resulting in urine leakage during physical stress. This problem is not limited to older women: UI has been documented in women of varying ages, including young (<25 years old) women (Walters, 2015).

Many risk factors for POP have been suggested, but the true cause is likely to be multifactorial. Causes might include:

- Constant downward gravity because of erect human posture
- Atrophy of supporting tissues with aging and decline of estrogen levels
- Weakening of pelvic support related to childbirth trauma
- Reproductive surgery, including hysterectomy
- Instrumental childbirth
- Multiparity
- Uncontrolled rapid birth
- Family history of POP
- Young age at first birth
- Connective tissue disorders
- Infant birth weight of more than 4,500 g

- Pelvic radiation
- Increased abdominal pressure secondary to:
  - Lifting of children or heavy objects
  - Straining due to chronic constipation
  - Respiratory problems or chronic coughing
- Obesity (Rodriguez-Mias et al., 2015)

Therapeutic Management

Treatment options for POP depend on the symptoms and their effect on the woman's quality of life. Important considerations when deciding on nonsurgical or surgical options include the severity of symptoms, the woman's preferences, the woman's health status, age, and suitability for surgery, and the presence of other pelvic conditions (urinary or fecal incontinence).

Conservative measures such as pelvic floor muscle exercises (PFMEs) or Kegel exercises supplemented by lifestyle interventions such as weight loss, avoidance of straining (reducing lifting heavy weights, treatment of chronic cough and constipation) are recommended as first-line management. PFME is aimed to increase the strength and endurance of the pelvic floor supports, prevent or delay worsening of prolapse and improve prolapse symptoms. PFME can help women delay or avert the need for surgery and pre- and postoperatively have been found to improve outcomes after surgery.

When surgery is being considered, the nature of the procedure and the likely outcome must be fully explained and discussed with the woman and her partner. Treatment options for POP include PFMEs, estrogen replacement therapy, dietary and lifestyle modifications, use of a pessary (a removable device placed into the vagina to support pelvic organs), and surgery (Evidence-Based Practice 7.1).

PELVIC FLOOR MUSCLE EXERCISES OR KEGEL EXERCISES

Pelvic floor muscle exercises strengthen the pelvic floor muscles to support the inner organs and prevent further prolapse. PFMEs are generally accepted as first-line treatment for stress and urge UI and they are also widely used for anal incontinence. Over the past 30 years a wealth of research has proven the benefits of PFMEs in treating both UI and POP (McClurg, Gerrard, & Hove, 2015). The purpose of pelvic floor exercises

EVIDENCE-BASED PRACTICE 7.1

PELVIC FLOOR MUSCLE TRAINING VERSES NO TREATMENT, OR INACTIVE CONTROL TREATMENTS, FOR URINARY INCONTINENCE IN WOMEN

STUDY

Involuntary leakage of urine (urinary incontinence) affects women of all ages, particularly older women who live in residential care such as nursing homes. Some women leak urine during exercise or when they cough or sneeze (stress urinary incontinence) and this may occur as a result of weakness of the pelvic floor muscles such as damage during childbirth. Other women leak urine before going to the toilet when there is a sudden and compelling need to pass urine (urgency urinary incontinence). This may be caused by involuntary contraction of the bladder muscle. Mixed urinary incontinence is the combination of both stress and urgency urinary incontinence. Pelvic floor muscle training is a supervised physical therapy treatment and it involves muscle-clenching exercises to strengthen the pelvic floor muscles. It is a common treatment used by women to stop urine leakage. Other treatments are also available which can either be used alone or in combination with pelvic floor muscle training (PFMT).

PFMT is a conservative treatment for urinary incontinence in women. This systematic review evaluated the effects of PFMT when compared to no treatment, placebo, or other inactive control treatments for urinary incontinence in women.

This study was done to compare the effects of PFMT to no treatment, placebo, or other inactive control treatments in the management of women with urinary incontinence.

Findings

Randomized or quasi-randomized trials were used. Twenty-one trials (1,281 women) met the eligibility criteria for inclusion, comprising women with stress urinary incontinence (SUI), urgency urinary incontinence (UUI), or mixed urinary incontinence (MUI), and they compared PFMT added to no treatment, placebo, or other inactive control treatments.

This systematic review found support for the widespread recommendation that PFMT be included in first-line conservative management programs for women with stress and any type of urinary incontinence. In women with stress incontinence, there was high-quality evidence that PFMT is associated with improvement or cure.

Nursing Implications

Overall, according to this study, there is sufficient evidence to support the widespread recommendation that PFMT should be included in a first-line conservative management program for women with stress, urge, or mixed urinary incontinence. Previous studies have validated that pelvic floor exercises do help in bringing tone to the muscles that control micturition. Nurses can continue to instruct women with urinary incontinence to perform PFMT daily to improve their urinary control and their quality of life.

Adapted from Dumoulin, C., Hay-Smith, E. J., Mac Habee-Sequin, G. M., & Mercier, J. (2015). Pelvic floor muscle training verses no treatment, or inactive control treatments, for urinary incontinence in women. *Neurourology & Urodynamics, 34*(4), 300–308.

is to increase the muscle volume, which will result in a stronger muscular contraction. PFMEs might limit the progression of mild prolapse and alleviate mild prolapse symptoms, including low back pain and pelvic pressure. They will not, however, help severe uterine prolapse.

HORMONE REPLACEMENT THERAPY

Hormone replacement therapy, or HRT (orally, transdermally, low-dose vaginal ring or vaginal cream) may improve the tone, natural thickness, and vascularity of the supporting tissue in perimenopausal and menopausal women by increasing blood perfusion and the elasticity of the vaginal wall. HRT has many benefits, as well as risks. It is essential that the benefits are weighed out against the risks before this therapy is initiated.

Take Note!

Before hormone therapy is considered, a thorough medical history must be taken to assess a woman's risk for complications (e.g., endometrial cancer, myocardial infarction, stroke, breast cancer, pulmonary emboli, and deep vein thrombosis). Because of these risks, estrogens, with or without progestins, should be given at the lowest effective dose and for the shortest duration consistent with the treatment goals and risks for the individual woman (ACOG, 2015a).

DIETARY AND LIFESTYLE MODIFICATIONS

Dietary and lifestyle modifications may help prevent pelvic relaxation and chronic problems later in life. Specific lifestyle changes would include avoiding constipation, bladder irritants, heavy lifting, high impact exercise, weight loss, and smoking cessation. Dietary habits can exacerbate the prolapse by causing constipation and consequently chronic straining. The stools of a constipated woman are hard and dry, and typically she must strain while bearing down to defecate. This straining to pass a hard stool increases intra-abdominal pressure, which over time causes the pelvic organs to prolapse. Dietary modifications can help to establish regular bowel movements without discomfort and eliminate flatus and bloating. A weight loss regimen might also need to be instituted if the woman is overweight.

PESSARIES

Vaginal **pessaries** are synthetic devices inserted in the vagina to provide support to the bladder and other pelvic organs as a corrective measure for UI and/or POP (Fig. 7.2). Today almost all pessaries are made of medical-grade silicone, which provides many advantages. Silicone pessaries are pliable and have a long shelf life; lack odor and secretion absorption; are biologically inert, nonallergenic, and noncarcinogenic; and they can be boiled or autoclaved for sterilization. Because most pessaries are made of silicone, pessary style and size are the main considerations when selecting a pessary (Colyar, 2015). Although many types and shapes are available, the most commonly used pessary is a firm ring that presses against the wall of the vagina and urethra to help decrease leakage and support a prolapsed vagina or uterus. Pessaries are a low-risk treatment option with the advantage of being cost effective and minimally invasive, and provide immediate relief of symptoms.

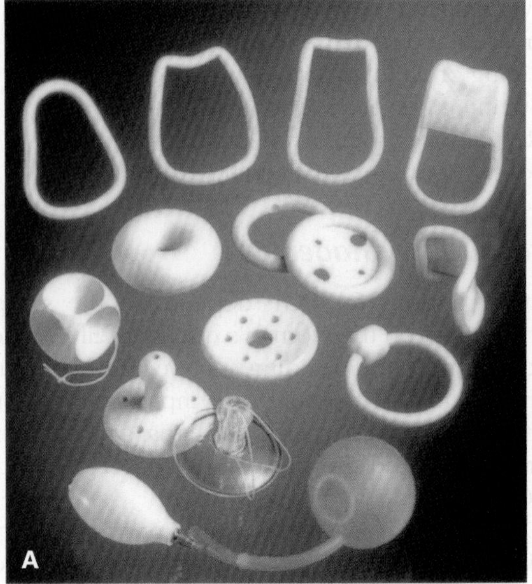

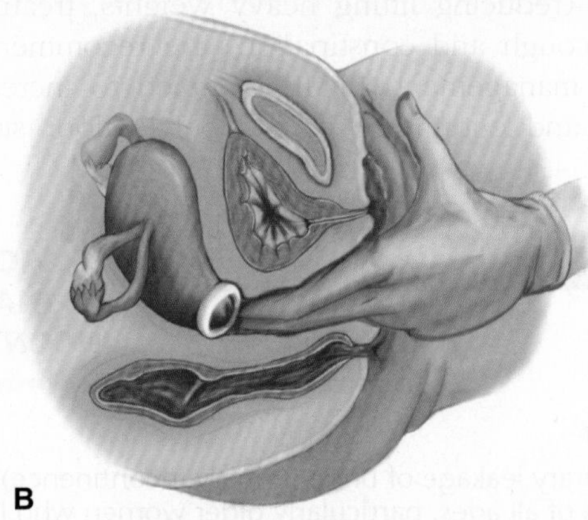

FIGURE 7.2 Examples of pessaries. A. Various shapes and sizes of pessaries available. B. Insertion of one type of pessary. A link to a web site for a picture of Colpexin Sphere is located on.

Indications for pessary use include uterine prolapse or cystocele, especially among elderly clients for whom surgery is contraindicated; younger women with prolapse who plan to have additional children; and women with marked prolapse who prefer to use a pessary rather than undergo surgery (Ralph & Tamussino, 2015). Many women use pessaries for only a short period of time and become free of symptoms. Long-term use can lead to pressure necrosis and the development of fistulas in some women; in this situation other methods of support should be explored. Pessaries are fitted by trial and error; the woman often needs to try several sizes or styles. The largest pessary that the woman can wear comfortably is generally the most effective. The woman should be instructed to report any discomfort or difficulty with urination or defecation while wearing the pessary and also to attend follow-up care appointments to check positioning.

Nurses need to be aware of the personal isolation and embarrassment and social and cultural implications that UI may cause as well as the subjective experiences of using a pessary. With appropriate support, vaginal pessaries can provide women with the freedom to lead active, engaged social lives.

SURGICAL INTERVENTIONS

Surgical interventions for pelvic or genital organ prolapse are designed to correct specific defects, with the goals being to restore normal anatomy and to preserve function. Approximately 260,000 stress incontinence surgical procedures are performed annually in the United States (Kirby, Tan-Kim, & Nager, 2015). Surgery is not an option for all women. Women who are at high risk of suffering recurrent prolapse after a surgical repair or who have morbid obesity, chronic obstructive pulmonary disease, or medical conditions in which general anesthesia would be risky are not good candidates for surgical repair (Alexander et al., 2015), and noninvasive treatment strategies should be discussed with them.

Surgical interventions might include anterior or posterior colporrhaphy (to repair a cystocele or rectocele) and vaginal hysterectomy (for uterine prolapse). This can be done laparoscopically whereby the uterus is removed through the vagina. An anterior and posterior colporrhaphy may be effective for a first-degree prolapse. This surgical procedure tightens the anterior and posterior vaginal wall, thus repairing a cystocele or rectocele. The pubocervical fascia (supportive tissue between the vagina and bladder) is folded and sutured to bring the bladder and urethra in proper position (Nilsson, 2015).

A vaginal hysterectomy is the treatment of choice for uterine prolapse because it removes the prolapsed organ that is bringing down the bladder and rectum with it. It can be combined with an anterior and posterior repair if a cystocele or rectocele is present.

Nursing Assessment

Nursing assessment for women with POP includes a thorough health history, a physical examination, and several laboratory and diagnostic tests.

HEALTH HISTORY AND CLINICAL MANIFESTATIONS

A history and general assessment of the client is important to exclude pathology and evaluate various factors that may influence choice and success of management. Evaluation of systems such as bowel, urinary and sexual function, coexistent morbidities, medical and surgical history, any physical or mental impairment, and lifestyle are noticeably very important, particularly in older women. The client's social circumstances and support systems, desire for treatment, and expectations will have implications on the management options.

The cause of prolapse is multifactorial, with vaginal childbirth, advancing age, heavy work, poor nutrition, vaginal surgery, and increasing body mass index being the most consistent risk factors (Rodriguez-Mias et al., 2015). Assessment of risk factors (chronic straining, hysterectomy, normal aging, and abnormalities of connective tissue) in the woman's history will assist the health care provider in the diagnosis and treatment of POP. The history should include questions about:

- The woman's obstetrical history (number of pregnancies, weight of newborns, pregnancy spacing)
- Chronic respiratory condition (chronic coughing)
- Menopausal status
- Weight history (loss or gain)
- Constipation (frequency and chronicity)
- Age
- Work history (e.g., physical labor or light office work)
- Nutritional assessment
- Family history (family member with POP)
- UI
- Previous pelvic surgeries

Assess for clinical manifestations of POP. POP is often asymptomatic, but when symptoms do occur, they are often related to the site and type of prolapse. Symptoms common to all types of prolapses are a feeling of dragging, a lump in the vagina, or something "coming down." Women with POP can present either with one symptom, such as vaginal bulging or pelvic pressure, or with several complaints, including many bladder, bowel, and pelvic symptoms. Symptoms associated with POP are summarized in Box 7.1.

Women present with varying degrees of uterine descent. Uterine prolapse is the most troubling type of pelvic relaxation because it is often associated with concomitant defects of the vagina in the anterior, posterior, and lateral compartments (Lazarou & Grigorescu, 2015).

PHYSICAL EXAMINATION

The pelvic examination performed by the health care provider includes an external genital inspection to visualize any obvious protrusion of the uterus, bladder, urethra, or vaginal wall occurring at the vaginal opening. Usually the woman is asked to perform the Valsalva maneuver (bearing down) while the examiner notes which organ prolapses first and the degree to which it occurs. Any urine leakage during the examination is important to note. The woman is asked to contract the pubococcygeal muscles (PFME); the health care provider inserts two fingers into

BOX 7.1

SYMPTOMS ASSOCIATED WITH PELVIC ORGAN PROLAPSE

- Urinary symptoms
  - Stress incontinence
  - Frequency (diurnal and nocturnal)
  - Urgency and urge incontinence
  - Hesitancy
  - Poor or prolonged stream
  - Feeling of incomplete emptying
- Bowel symptoms
  - Difficulty with defecation
  - Incontinence of flatus or liquid or solid stool
  - Urgency of defecation
  - Feeling of incomplete evacuation
  - Rectal protrusion or prolapse after defecation
- Sexual symptoms
  - Inability to have frequent intercourse
  - Dyspareunia
  - Lack of satisfaction or orgasm
  - Incontinence during sexual activity
- Other local symptoms
  - Pressure or heaviness in the vagina
  - Pain in the vagina or perineum
  - Low back pain after long periods of standing
  - Palpable bulge in the vaginal vault
  - Difficulty walking due to a protrusion from the vagina
  - Difficulty inserting or keeping a tampon in place
  - Vaginal-cervical mucosa hypertrophy, excoriation, ulceration, and bleeding
  - Abdominal pressure or pain

Adapted from American College of Obstetricians and Gynecologists [ACOG]. (2015a). Pelvic support problems. *ACOG Educational Pamphlet.* Retrieved from http://www.acog.org/~/media/For%20Patients/faq012.pdf?dmc=1&ts=20140128T1159591406; and Lazarou, G., & Grigorescu, B. A. (2015). Pelvic organ prolapse. *eMedicine.* Retrieved from http://emedicine.medscape.com/article/276259-overview

the vagina to assess the strength and symmetry of the contraction. Because pelvic or genital organ prolapse can cause urinary symptoms such as incontinence, bladder function should be assessed by determining postvoid residual with a catheter. If the woman has more than 100 mL of retained urine, she should be referred for further urodynamic evaluation and testing.

LABORATORY AND DIAGNOSTIC TESTS

Common laboratory tests that may be ordered to determine the cause of POP include a urinalysis to rule out a bacterial infection, urine culture to identify the specific organism if present, visualization of urine loss during the pelvic examination, and measurement of postvoid urine volume.

Nursing Management

Help the woman understand the nature of the condition, the treatment options, and the likely outcomes. Nursing considerations might include the following:

- Describe normal anatomy and causes of pelvic prolapse.
- Assess how this condition has affected the woman's life.
- Outline the options, with the advantages and disadvantages of each.
- Allow the client to make the decision that is right for her.
- Provide education.
- Schedule preoperative activities needed for surgery.
- Reassure the client that there is a solution for her symptoms.
- Provide community education about genital prolapse.

Nursing Care Plan 7.1 (at the end of the chapter) provides an overview of care for a woman with POP.

PROMOTE PREVENTION STRATEGIES

Limited data are available on ways to prevent POP, but a nurse needs first to understand its incidence, risk factors, prevalence, clinical implications, and treatment options to be an effective caretaker of the woman. The nurse's understanding will not only improve his or her ability to treat this growing client population, but will also help in developing preventive strategies to address a woman's suffering from this condition.

Approaches include lifestyle changes that reduce modifiable risk factors, such as losing weight, avoiding heavy lifting, and relieving constipation. Explore with the woman what factors in her lifestyle might be modified to reduce her risk of developing POP (primary prevention) or to improve her quality of life after receiving treatment (secondary prevention).

ENCOURAGE PELVIC FLOOR MUSCLE TRAINING

Encourage the woman to perform PFMEs daily (Teaching Guidelines 7.1). Discuss current research findings and educate the woman about estrogen therapy, allowing the woman to make her own decision on whether to use hormones. Controversy still exists regarding the benefits versus the risks of taking hormones, so the woman must weigh this option carefully (ACOG, 2015a).

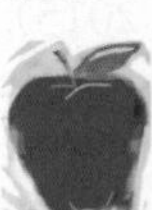

Teaching Guidelines 7.1

PERFORMING PELVIC FLOOR EXERCISES

- Squeeze the muscles in your rectum as if you are trying to prevent passing flatus.
- Stop and start urinary flow to help identify the pubococcygeus muscle.
- Tighten the pubococcygeus muscle for a count of three, and then relax it.
- Contract and relax the pubococcygeus muscle rapidly 10 times.
- Try to bring up the entire pelvic floor and bear down 10 times.
- Repeat pelvic floor muscle exercises at least five times daily.

ENCOURAGE DIETARY AND LIFESTYLE MODIFICATIONS

Instruct clients to increase dietary fiber and fluids to prevent constipation. A high-fiber diet with an increase in fluid intake alleviates constipation by increasing stool bulk and stimulating peristalsis. It is accomplished by replacing refined, low-fiber foods with high-fiber foods. The recommended daily intake of fiber for women is 25 g (Meyer, 2015). In addition to increasing the amount of fiber in her diet, also encourage the woman to drink eight 8-oz glasses of fluid daily and to engage in regular low-impact aerobic exercise, which promotes muscle tone and stimulates peristalsis.

Educate the client about other lifestyle changes that will assist with prolapse, such as:

- Achieve ideal weight to reduce intra-abdominal pressure and strain on pelvic organs, including pressure on the bladder.
- Wear a girdle or abdominal support to support the muscles surrounding the pelvic organs.
- Avoid lifting heavy objects to reduce the risk of increasing intra-abdominal pressure, which can push the pelvic organs downward.
- Avoid high-impact aerobics, jogging, or jumping repeatedly to minimize the risk of increasing intra-abdominal pressure, which places downward pressure on the organs.
- Give up smoking to minimize the risk for a chronic "smoker's cough," which increases intra-abdominal pressure and forces the pelvic organs downward.

PROVIDE TEACHING FOR PESSARY USE

Educate the woman about pessary use. Discuss complications as part of the instruction. Although the pessary is a safe device, it is still a foreign body in the vagina. Because of this, the most common side effects of the pessary are increased vaginal discharge, urinary tract infections, vaginitis, and odor. Odors can be reduced by douching with dilute vinegar or hydrogen peroxide. Postmenopausal women with thin vaginal mucosa are susceptible to vaginal ulceration with the use of a pessary. Advise the woman to use estrogen cream to make the vaginal mucosa more resistant to erosion and to strengthen the vaginal walls.

The woman must be capable of managing use of the pessary, either alone or with the help of a caretaker. The most common recommendations for pessary care include removing the pessary twice weekly and cleaning it with soap and water; using a lubricant for insertion; and having regular follow-up examinations every 6 to 12 months after an initial period of adjustment.

Besides cleaning, clients must properly reinsert the device into their vaginal cavity, and the woman must also be willing to participate in all aspects of care of the pessary for this treatment option to be successful. All women choosing this option must be instructed in the care of her pessary so she feels comfortable with all aspects of it before leaving the health care facility. Health care visits should allow adequate time for women to share their concerns, anxieties, and fears surrounding the transition to life with a pessary.

PROVIDE PERIOPERATIVE CARE

Prepare the woman for surgery by reinforcing the risks and benefits of surgery and describing the postoperative course. Explain that a Foley catheter will be in place for up to 1 week, and that she might not be able to urinate due to the swelling after the catheter has been removed. Provide home care instructions for the Foley catheter. She should cleanse the perineal area daily with mild soap and water, especially around where the catheter enters the urinary meatus. If the woman is provided with a leg bag to be worn during waking hours, instruct her to empty it frequently and keep it below the level of the bladder to prevent backflow. The same principles are applied to the primary Foley bag when emptying it.

During the recovery period, instruct the client to avoid for several weeks activities that cause an increase in abdominal pressure, such as straining, sneezing, and coughing. In addition, advise her to avoid lifting anything heavy or straining to push anything. Explain to the woman that stool softeners and gentle laxatives might be prescribed to prevent constipation and straining with bowel movements. Avoiding vaginal intercourse will be recommended until the operative area is healed in 6 weeks.

Urinary Incontinence

Urinary incontinence (UI) is defined by the International Continence Society (2015) as the involuntary loss of urine that represents a hygienic or social problem to the individual. This disorder affects over 15 million women in the United States (Walters, 2015), but is underreported. It has been estimated that 50% of all women experience UT at some time in their life, varying in severity from mild to severe (Files, Mayer, & Chutka, 2015). The psychosocial costs and morbidities are even more difficult to quantify. Embarrassment and depression are common. The affected individual may experience a decrease in social interactions, excursions out of the home, and sexual activity (Su, Sun, & Jiann, 2015). It is more common than diabetes and Alzheimer disease, both of which receive a great deal of press attention. Despite the considerable impact of incontinence on quality of life, many women are unlikely to bring up the subject of their lack of bladder control and very few women seek help or treatment for incontinence concerns. The following are several possible explanations for why clients do not talk about their bladder control issues. The client may:

- Feel that UI is inevitable and not amenable to treatment.
- Feel that UI is a "normal" part of aging.
- Believe that UI is part of being "female." Women tend to accept urinary symptoms such as UI more so than men.
- Feel embarrassment and try to deny that it is a real problem.
- Think that the only treatment option is surgical.
- The client may consider a UI a hygiene problem and not a medical condition.

Take Note!

Incontinence is preventable, treatable, and often curable. However, many women believe that loss of bladder function is a normal and expected part of aging.

Incontinence can have far-reaching effects. Some women experience anxiety, depression, social isolation, embarrassment, insomnia, fear, feelings of uncleanliness, worry, vulnerability, shame, limit her ability to travel far from home or have social engagements, and disruptions in their self-esteem and dignity. UI can cause the woman to stop working, traveling, socializing, and enjoying sexual relationships. In addition, incontinence can create a tremendous burden for caretakers and is a common reason for admission to a long-term care facility. Depression and high levels of stress are typical in these women (Kwak, Kwon, & Kim, 2015).

Women often try to cope with UI through lifestyle modifications such as wearing protective pads, avoiding certain activities, emptying the bladder frequently, and modifying diet/fluid intake. Women who experience UI are generally most distressed by the social implications and many go to great efforts to hide their symptoms. In some cultures, UI is abhorred to the point where women are shunned by their communities. A sense of control, normality, and self-esteem are central issues in living with UI. Generally with time and worsening of symptoms, women pursue medical evaluation and treatment (Waetjen et al., 2015).

The types of UI are defined based on their presenting symptoms and signs. The three most common types of incontinence are urgency UI (overactive bladder caused by detrusor muscle contractions), stress incontinence (inadequate urinary sphincter function), and mixed incontinence (involves both stress and urge incontinence) (King et al., 2015). Comparison Chart 7.1 details these types of UI.

Pathophysiology and Etiology

Urinary continence requires several factors, including effective functioning of the bladder, adequate pelvic floor muscles, neural control from the brain, and integrity of the neural connections that facilitate voluntary control. The bladder neck and proximal urethra function as a sphincter. During urination the sphincter relaxes and the bladder empties. The ability to control urination requires the integrated function of numerous components of the lower urinary tract, which must be structurally sound and functioning normally.

Incontinence can develop if the bladder muscles become overactive due to weakened sphincter muscles, if the bladder muscles become too weak to contract properly, or if signals from the nervous system to the urinary structures are interrupted. A major factor in women that contributes to urinary continence is the estrogen level, because this hormone helps maintain bladder sphincter tone. In perimenopausal or menopausal women, incontinence can be a problem as estrogen levels begin to decline and genitourinary changes occur. In simple terms, the bladder is the reservoir, the urethra is the seal, and the levator ani muscle is the gate that holds pressure against the outflow of urine by supporting the urethra and bladder from below. When any of these three structures is not functioning normally, incontinence occurs.

Contributing factors in UI include:

- Fluid intake, especially alcohol, carbonated drinks, and caffeinated beverages
- Constipation: alters the position of the pelvic organs and puts pressure on the bladder

COMPARISON CHART 7.1 URGE INCONTINENCE VERSUS STRESS INCONTINENCE

	Urge Incontinence	Stress Incontinence
Description	Precipitous loss of urine, preceded by a strong urge to void, with increased bladder pressure and detrusor contraction	Accidental leakage of urine that occurs with increased pressure on the bladder from coughing, sneezing, laughing, or physical exertion
Etiology	Causes might be neurologic, idiopathic, or infectious	Develops commonly in women in their 40s and 50s, usually as the result of weakened muscles and ligaments in the pelvis following childbirth
Signs and Symptoms	Urgency, frequency, nocturia, and a large amount of urine loss	Involuntary loss of a small amount of urine in response to physical activity that raises intra-abdominal pressure

- Habitual "preventive" emptying: may result in training the bladder to hold only small amounts of urine
- Menopause and depletion of estrogen
- Chronic disease such as stroke, multiple sclerosis, or diabetes
- Smoking: nicotine increases detrusor muscle contractions
- Advancing age: age-related anatomic changes provide less pelvic support
- Pregnancy and childbirth: damage to pelvic structures during childbirth
- Obesity: increases abdominal pressure (Schuiling & Likis, 2016).

Therapeutic Management

Treatment options depend on the type of UI. In general, the least invasive procedure with the fewest risks is the first choice for treatment. Surgery is used only if other methods have failed. There is a widespread belief that UI is an inevitable problem of getting older and that little or nothing can be done to relieve symptoms or reverse it. Nothing is further from the truth, and attitudes must change so that women will feel comfortable seeking help for this embarrassing condition.

For many women with urge incontinence, simple reassurance and lifestyle interventions might help. The promotion of a healthy weight can help to reduce incontinence related to obesity. However, if more than simple lifestyle measures are needed, effective treatments might include:

- Bladder training to establish normal voiding intervals (every 3 to 5 hours)
- Pelvic floor muscle exercises to strengthen the pelvic floor musculature
- Pessary ring to support pelvic structures that have weakened
- Pharmacotherapy to reduce the urge to void. Anticholinergic agents such as oxybutynin (Ditropan) or tolterodine (Detrol) or oxybutynin (Oxytrol) might be prescribed. The most common side effects of anticholinergic agents are dry mouth, blurred vision, constipation, nausea, dizziness, and headaches (King et al., 2015).

For women with stress incontinence, treatment is not always a cure, but it can minimize the impact of this condition on the woman's quality of life. Some treatment options for stress incontinence might include:

- Weight loss if needed
- Avoidance of constipation
- Smoking cessation
- PFMEs to strengthen the pelvic floor
- Pessaries
- Weighted vaginal cones to improve the tone of pelvic floor muscles
- Periurethral injection (injecting a bulking agent [collagen] to form a bulge that brings the urethral walls closer together to achieve a better closure)
- Medications such as duloxetine (Cymbalta, Yentreve) to increase urethral sphincter contractions during the storage phase of the urination cycle
- Estrogen replacement therapy to improve bladder sphincter tone
- Surgery to correct genital prolapse and improve urethral and bladder tone

Nursing Assessment

The assessment of the woman experiencing UI includes a history, physical examination, laboratory tests, and possibly urodynamic testing. The onset, frequency, severity, and pattern of incontinence should be determined, as well as any associated symptoms such as frequency, dysuria, urgency, and nocturia. Incontinence may be quantified by asking the woman if she wears a pad and how often the pad is changed. A review of the woman's current medications, including over-the-counter medications, should be included in the history.

A complete physical examination should be carried out by the health care provider; it should include a neurologic assessment and pelvic and rectal examinations. The presence of associated POP should be noted

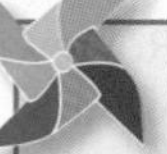

Consider This

Life can be complicated and embarrassing at times when we least expect it. I met a man in church who seemed interested in me, and he asked me out for coffee after Sunday services. I have been alone for 10 years and this prospect seemed exciting to me. We talked for hours over coffee and seemed to have a great deal in common, especially since both of us had lost our spouses to cancer. He asked me to go square dancing with him, since that was an activity we both had enjoyed in the past with our spouses. I hadn't been out or physically active for ages and didn't realize how my body had changed with age.

It was during the first dance that I noticed a wet sensation between my legs, which I was unable to control. I managed to continue on and pretend that all was fine, but then realized what many of my friends were talking about—stress incontinence. Not being able to control one's urine is very embarrassing and it complicates your life, but I made up my mind that it wasn't going to control me!

Thoughts: Gravity and childbirth take a toll on women's reproductive organs by pushing them downward. This woman is not going to let stress incontinence curtail her outside activity, which demonstrates a good attitude. What can be done about her embarrassing accidents? Were there any preventive strategies she could have used at an earlier age?

because it can contribute to the woman's voiding problems and may have an impact on diagnosis and treatment. A rectal examination is done to evaluate sphincter tone and perineal sensation. A "cough stress test" can be performed by asking the woman to cough with a full bladder and subsequently observing for leakage of urine from the urethra can also help in assessing the client's ability to control voiding.

A urinalysis is performed to look for hematuria, pyuria, glucosuria, or proteinuria. A urine culture is done if there is pyuria or bacteriuria. Postvoid residual should be measured either with pelvic ultrasound or directly with a catheter. If the residual exceeds the limit set, urodynamic testing is then used to diagnose the incontinence.

Nursing Management

Incontinence can be devastating and can cause psychosocial concerns and isolation. Nurses can encourage women with troublesome symptoms to seek help. Discuss the treatment options with the client, including benefits and potential outcomes, and encourage her to select the continence treatment best for her lifestyle. Provide education about good bladder habits and strategies to reduce the incidence or severity of incontinence (Teaching Guidelines 7.2). Provide support and encouragement to ensure adherence to the guidelines. Remember that aging can increase the risk of incontinence, but incontinence is not an inevitable part of aging. Review the anatomy and physiology of the urinary system and offer simple explanations to help the woman cope with urinary alterations. Therapeutic listening is important. Be aware of the courage it takes for a woman to disclose an embarrassing condition.

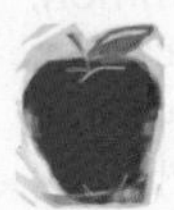

Teaching Guidelines 7.2

MANAGING URINARY INCONTINENCE

- Avoid drinking too much fluid (i.e., 1.5 L total daily limit), but do not decrease your intake of fluids.
- Reduce intake of fluids and foods that are bladder irritants and precipitate urgency, such as chocolate, caffeine, sodas, alcohol, artificial sweetener, hot spicy foods, orange juice, tomatoes, and watermelon.
- Increase fiber and fluids in your diet to reduce constipation.
- Control blood glucose levels to prevent polyuria.
- Treat chronic cough.
- Remove any barriers that delay you from reaching the toilet.
- Practice good perineal hygiene by using mild soap and water. Wipe from front to back to prevent urinary tract infections.
- Become aware of adverse drug effects.
- Take your medications as prescribed.
- Continue to do pelvic floor muscle exercises.

Adapted from Files, J. A., Mayer, A. P., & Chutka, D. S. (2015). Urinary incontinence: Not just a mid-laugh crisis. *Journal of Women's Health, 24*(1), 107–108; McClurg, D., Gerrard, J., & Hove, R. T. (2015). Reducing the incidence of incontinence. *British Journal of Midwifery, 23*(1), 17–20; and Vasavada, S. P., Carmel, M. E., & Rackley, R. (2015). Urinary incontinence. eMedicine. Retrieved from http://emedicine.medscape.com/article/452289-overview

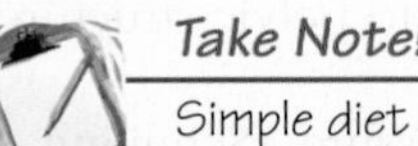

Take Note!

Simple diet and lifestyle alterations, combined with a proper pelvic floor muscle strengthening program, can often produce significant improvements for women of all ages.

BENIGN GROWTHS

The most common benign growths of the reproductive tract include cervical, endocervical, and endometrial polyps; uterine fibroids (leiomyomas); genital fistulas; Bartholin cysts; and ovarian cysts.

Polyps

Polyps are small, usually benign growths. The incidence of malignancy in cervical polyps is 1 in 1,000. Malignancy is more common in perimenopausal or postmenopausal women (Nelson, Papa, & Ritchie, 2015). The cause of polyp growth is not well understood, but they are frequently the result of infection. Polyps might be associated with chronic inflammation, an abnormal local response to increased levels of estrogen, or local congestion of the cervical vasculature (Stewart, 2016). Single or multiple polyps might occur. They are most common in multiparous women. Polyps can appear anywhere but are most common on the cervix and in the uterus (Fig. 7.3).

Cervical polyps often appear after menarche. They occur in 2% to 5% of women, and approximately 2% of these polyps have cancerous changes (Schuiling & Likis, 2016). Endocervical polyps are commonly found in multiparous women ages 40 to 60. Endocervical polyps are more common than cervical polyps, with a stalk of varied width and length. Endometrial polyps are benign tumors or localized overgrowths of the endometrium. Most endometrial polyps are solitary, and they rarely occur in women younger than 20 years of age. The incidence of these polyps rises steadily with increasing age, peaks in the fifth decade of life, and gradually declines after menopause. They are present in up to 25% of women being seen for abnormal bleeding (Lieng, 2015).

Therapeutic Management

Treatment of polyps usually consists of simple removal with small forceps done on an outpatient basis, removal during hysteroscopy, or dilation and curettage (D&C).

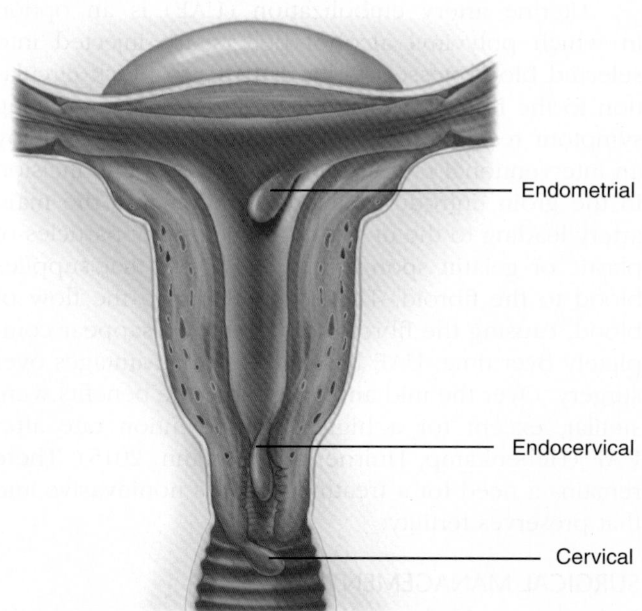

FIGURE 7.3 Cervical, endocervical, and endometrial polyps.

The polyp base can be removed by laser vaporization. Because many polyps are infected, an antibiotic may be ordered after removal as a preventive measure or to treat early signs of infection.

Although polyps are rarely cancerous, a specimen should be sent after surgery to a pathology laboratory to exclude malignancy. A cervical biopsy typically reveals mildly atypical cells and signs of infection. Polyps rarely return after they are removed. Regularly scheduled Pap smears are suggested for women with cervical polyps to detect any future abnormal growths that may be malignant.

Nursing Assessment

Nursing assessment for a woman with polyps includes assisting with the physical examination and preparing the collected specimen to be sent to the cytologist.

CLINICAL MANIFESTATIONS

Assess for clinical manifestations of polyps. Most endocervical polyps are cherry red, whereas most cervical polyps are grayish-white (Heller, 2015). Cervical and endocervical polyps are often asymptomatic, but they can produce mild symptoms such as abnormal vaginal bleeding (after intercourse or douching, between menses) or discharge. The most common clinical manifestation of endometrial polyps is metrorrhagia (irregular, acyclic uterine bleeding).

PHYSICAL EXAMINATION AND LABORATORY AND DIAGNOSTIC STUDIES

Typically, cervical polyps are diagnosed when the cervix is visualized through a speculum during the woman's annual gynecologic examination (Nelson et al., 2015). Endometrial polyps are not detected on physical examination, but rather with ultrasound or hysteroscopy (introduction of a small camera through the cervix to visualize the uterine cavity).

Nursing Management

Nursing management of polyps involves explaining the condition and the rationale for removal and giving follow-up care instructions. The nurse also assists the health care provider with the removal procedure.

Uterine Fibroids

Uterine fibroids, also known as myomasor leiomyomas, are benign tumors composed of smooth muscle and fibrous connective tissue in the uterus. Unlike cancerous tumors, fibroids usually grow slower responding to present estrogen levels and their cells do not break away and invade other parts of the body. Fibroids are classified according to their position in the uterus and on the uterine layer most involved (Fig. 7.4):

- *Subserosol fibroids:* lie underneath the outermost peritoneal layer of the uterus and grow outside the uterus. They are attached to the uterus by a stalk or peduncle.
- *Intramural fibroids:* grow within the wall of the uterus and are the most common type.

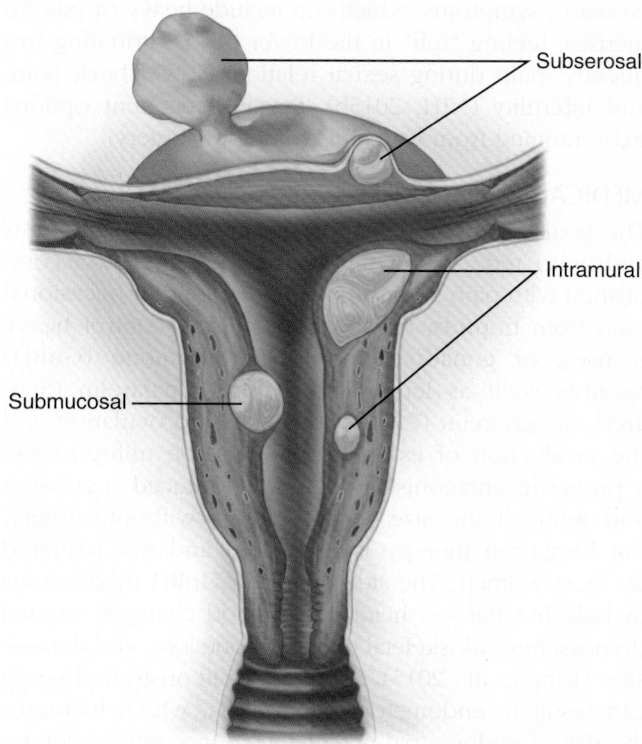

FIGURE 7.4 Submucosal, intramural, and subserosal fibroids.

- *Submucosal fibroids:* grow from immediately below the inner uterine surface (endometrium) into the uterine cavity (King et al., 2015).

Fibroids are estrogen-dependent and thus grow rapidly during the childbearing years, when estrogen is plentiful, but they shrink during menopause, when estrogen levels decline. It is believed that these benign tumors develop in up to 70% of all women over 30 years of age, but up to 50% are asymptomatic (Stewart, 2015). It is difficult to be precise because fibroids may cause no symptoms, and thus many women do not know they have them.

Fibroids are the most common indication for hysterectomy in the United States. The peak incidence occurs around age 45, and they are three times more prevalent in African American women than White women (Stewart, 2015).

Etiology

Although the cause of fibroids is unknown, several predisposing factors have been identified, including:

- Age (late reproductive years)
- Genetic predisposition
- African-American ethnicity
- Hypertension
- Nulliparity
- Obesity (Alexander et al., 2014).

Therapeutic Management

Treatment depends on the size of the fibroids and the woman's symptoms, which can include heavy or painful menses, feeling "full" in the lower pelvis, urinating frequently, pain during sexual relations, lower back pain, and infertility (NIH, 2015b). Several treatment options exist, ranging from watchful waiting to surgery.

MEDICAL MANAGEMENT

The goals of medical therapy are to reduce symptoms and/or to reduce the tumor size. This can be accomplished with pain medications to treat mild or occasional pain from fibroids; birth control pills to control heavy menses; or gonadotropin-releasing hormone (GnRH) agonists such as leuprolide (Lupron), nafarelin (Synarel), or goserelin (Zoladex), which stop ovulation and the production of estrogen, or low-dose mifepristone, a progestin antagonist. Both have produced regression and reduced the size of the tumors without surgery, but long-term therapy is expensive and not tolerated by most women. The side effects of GnRH medications include hot flashes, headaches, mood changes, vaginal dryness, musculoskeletal malaise, bone loss, and depression (King et al., 2015). Long-term mifepristone therapy can result in endometrial hyperplasia, which increases the risk of endometrial malignancy. Once either therapy is stopped, the fibroids typically recur.

Uterine artery embolization (UAE) is an option in which polyvinyl alcohol pellets are injected into selected blood vessels via a catheter to block circulation to the fibroid, causing it to shrink and producing symptom resolution. The procedure is carried out by an interventional radiologist who makes a tiny incision in the groin, introduces a fine catheter into the main artery leading to the uterus, and injects tiny particles of plastic or gelatin sponge into the artery that supplies blood to the fibroid. These particles stop the flow of blood, causing the fibroid to shrink or disappear completely over time. UAE has short-term advantages over surgery. Over the mid and long term, the benefits were similar, except for a higher reintervention rate after UAE (Hehenkamp, Huirne, & Brolmann, 2015). There remains a need for a treatment that is noninvasive and that preserves fertility.

SURGICAL MANAGEMENT

For women with large fibroids or severe menorrhagia, surgery is preferred over medical treatment. Surgical management might involve myomectomy, laser surgery, or hysterectomy.

Myomectomy. Myomectomy involves removing the fibroid alone. A myomectomy is performed via laparoscopy, through an abdominal incision or through a vaginal approach. The advantage is that only the fibroid is removed; fertility is not jeopardized because this procedure leaves the uterine muscle walls intact. Myomectomy relieves symptoms but does not affect the underlying process; thus, fibroids grow back and further treatment will be needed in the future.

Laser Surgery. Laser surgery (or electrocauterization) involves destroying small fibroids with lasers. Laser therapy can be done using a vaginal approach or laparoscopically. The laser treatment preserves the uterus, but the process may cause scarring and adhesions, thus impairing fertility (Shigetomi et al., 2015). Fibroids can return after this procedure. Controversy remains as to whether laser treatment weakens the uterine wall and thus may contribute to uterine rupture in the future.

Hysterectomy. A hysterectomy is the surgical removal of the uterus. It is the most effective treatment for symptomatic fibroids with no recurrence. After cesarean section, it is the second most frequently performed surgical procedure for women in the United States. Approximately 600,000 hysterectomies are performed annually in the United States (Centers for Disease Control and Prevention [CDC], 2015). The top three conditions associated with hysterectomies are fibroids, endometriosis, and uterine prolapse (CDC, 2015). A hysterectomy to remove fibroids eliminates both the symptoms and the risk of recurrence, but it also terminates the woman's ability to bear children. Three types of hysterectomy surgeries are available: vaginal hysterectomy, laparoscopically assisted vaginal hysterectomy, and abdominal hysterectomy.

In a vaginal hysterectomy, the uterus is removed through an incision in the posterior vagina. Advantages include a shorter hospital stay and recovery time and no abdominal scars. Disadvantages include a limited operating space and poor visualization of other pelvic organs.

In a laparoscopically assisted vaginal hysterectomy, the uterus is removed through a laparoscope, through which structures within the abdomen and pelvis are visualized. Small incisions are made in the abdominal wall to permit the laparoscope to enter the surgical site. Advantages include a better surgical field, less pain, lower cost, and a shorter recovery time. Disadvantages include potential injury to the bladder and the inability to remove enlarged uteruses and scar tissue.

In an abdominal hysterectomy, the uterus and other pelvic organs are removed through an incision in the abdomen. This procedure allows the surgeon to visualize all pelvic organs and is typically used when a malignancy is suspected or a very large uterus is present. Disadvantages include the need for general anesthesia, a longer hospital stay and recovery period, more pain, higher cost, and a visible scar on the abdomen.

Complications of hysterectomy vary based on route of surgery and technique. The most common complications include infection, venous thromboembolic, genitourinary and gastrointestinal injuries, and hemorrhage (Goldman et al., 2015). With astute nursing observations and assessments, these complications can be reduced or minimized. A summary of treatment options for uterine fibroids is presented in Table 7.1.

Nursing Assessment

Nursing assessment for the woman with uterine fibroids includes a thorough health history, physical examination, and laboratory and diagnostic studies.

HEALTH HISTORY AND CLINICAL MANIFESTATIONS

The history should include questions about the woman's menstrual cycle, including alterations in the menstrual pattern (e.g., pain or pressure, aggravating and alleviating factors), history of infertility, and any history of spontaneous abortion, which might indicate a space-occupying uterine lesion. Ask if any female relatives have had fibroids, because there is a familial predisposition. Assess for clinical manifestations of uterine fibroids. Symptoms of fibroids depend on their size and location and may include:

- Chronic pelvic pain
- Low back pain
- Iron-deficiency anemia secondary to bleeding
- Bloating
- Constipation
- Infertility (with large tumors)
- Dysmenorrhea
- Miscarriage
- Sciatica
- Dyspareunia
- Urinary frequency, urgency, incontinence
- Irregular vaginal bleeding (menorrhagia)
- Feeling of heaviness in the pelvic region

PHYSICAL EXAMINATION AND LABORATORY AND DIAGNOSTIC STUDIES

The bimanual examination performed by the health care provider typically shows an enlarged, irregular uterus. The uterus may be palpable abdominally if the fibroid

TABLE 7.1 SUMMARY OF TREATMENT OPTIONS FOR UTERINE FIBROIDS

Method	Advantages	Disadvantages
Hormones	Noninvasive Reduces size of fibroids Symptom improvement	Serious side effects with long-term use Fibroids regrow when meds stopped
Uterine artery embolization	Minimally invasive Dramatic decrease in symptoms Future fertility possible	Procedure frequently painful Requires radiation and contrast dye Permanently implanted material Possible negative fertility impact
Myomectomy	Performed as minor surgery Uterus is preserved	Requires general anesthesia New growth of fibroids occurs
Hysterectomy	Complete removal of fibroids Immediate symptom relief	Requires general anesthesia Major surgery with associated risks Fertility not preserved
Laser surgery	Can be done as an outpatient procedure to destroy small fibroids	Vaporization process can cause scarring and adhesions, affecting future fertility

is very large. Ultrasound may be used to confirm the diagnosis.

Nursing Management

The level of support that nurses can provide women with fibroids depends on the type of treatment offered and her choice of them. Nurses should be able to explain any current treatment options and the implications of a diagnosis of fibroids. Many women have not heard of fibroids previously and need reassurance that they are both common and benign. If medication is prescribed, it is essential to explain the possible side effects and why medication can only be taken for a limited duration. If surgery is selected, verbal and written information about it and the aftercare should be addressed (Box 7.2).

A woman undergoing a hysterectomy for the treatment of fibroids often needs special care and can benefit from presurgical and postsurgical support provided by nurses. Personalized nursing, tailored to the individual woman's needs, enhances the client's coping strategies and alleviates different adverse psychological sequelae following gynecologic surgery. Women must cope with a variety of psychological adjustment difficulties, related to the changes in self-image, self-esteem, loss of femininity or identity, and sexual dysfunction. The incidence of postsurgical problems can be reduced greatly with proper client-centered perioperative nursing care.

Genital Fistulas

Genital fistulas are an underestimated problem worldwide and have devastating consequences for women. Genital fistulas are abnormal openings between a genital tract organ and another organ, such as the urinary tract or the gastrointestinal tract. A fistula can result from a congenital anomaly, surgical complications, Bartholin gland abscesses, radiation, or malignancy, but the majority of fistulas that occur worldwide are related to obstetric trauma and female genital cutting (Spurlock, 2015). During normal labor, the bladder is displaced upward into the abdomen, and the anterior vaginal wall, the base of the bladder, and the urethra are compressed between the fetal head and the posterior pubis. When labor is obstructed or prolonged, this unrelieved compression

BOX 7.2

NURSING INTERVENTIONS FOR A WOMAN UNDERGOING A HYSTERECTOMY

Preoperative Care

- Instruct the client and her family about the procedure and aftercare.
- Provide interventions to reduce anxiety (due to perceived threats to the woman's self-concept and role functioning) and fear of alteration in body image, complications, and pain. Prepare the woman so she knows what to expect throughout her perioperative experience. Explain postoperative pain management procedures that will be used. Identify the high-risk woman early to reduce her stress.
- Teach turning, deep breathing, and coughing before surgery to prevent postoperative atelectasis and respiratory complications such as pneumonia.
- Encourage the woman to discuss her feelings. Some women equate their femaleness with their reproductive capability, and loss of the uterus could evoke grieving.
- Complete all preoperative orders in a timely manner to allow for rest.

Postoperative Care

- Provide comfort measures.
- Administer analgesics promptly or use a patient-controlled anesthesia (PCA) pump.
- Administer antiemetics to control nausea and vomiting per order.
- Change the client's linens and gown frequently to promote hygiene.
- Change the client's position frequently and use pillows for support to promote comfort and pain management.
- Assess the incision, the dressing, and vaginal bleeding and report if bleeding is excessive (soaking perineal pad within an hour).
- Monitor elimination and provide increased fluids and fiber to prevent constipation and straining.
- Encourage ambulation and active range-of-motion exercises when in bed to prevent thrombophlebitis and venous stasis.
- Monitor vital signs to detect early complications.
- Be comfortable discussing sexual concerns with the client.

Discharge Planning

- Advise the client to reduce her activity level to avoid fatigue, which might inhibit healing.
- Advise the client to rest when she is tired and to increase her activity level slowly.
- Educate the client on the need for pelvic rest (nothing in the vagina) for 6 weeks.
- Instruct the client to avoid heavy lifting or straining for about 6 weeks to prevent an increase in intra-abdominal pressure, which could weaken her sutures.
- Teach the client the signs and symptoms of infection.
- Advise the woman to take showers instead of tub baths to reduce the risk for infection.
- Encourage the client to eat a healthy diet with increased intake of fluids to prevent dehydration and fluid and electrolyte imbalance.
- Instruct the client to change her perineal pad frequently to prevent infection.
- Explain and schedule follow-up care appointments as needed.
- Provide information about community resources for support/help.

causes ischemia, which causes pressure necrosis and subsequent fistula formation.

Common types of fistulas include:

- *Vesicovaginal:* communication between the bladder and genital tract
- *Urethrovaginal:* communication between the urethra and the vagina
- *Rectovaginal:* communication between the rectum or sigmoid colon and the vagina

The direct consequences of this damage include UI and fecal incontinence if the rectum is involved. This tragic condition has plagued women since the beginning of history (Taylor & Rakinic, 2015). Another major cause of genital trauma leading to the development of genital fistulas is female genital cutting. This cultural practice, primarily carried out in Africa and Asia, is receiving worldwide attention as part of the international public health agenda to move toward reducing its incidence. Reasons for continuing this practice include rite of passage, preserving chastity, ensuring marriageability, religion, hygiene, improving fertility, and enhancing sexual pleasure for men (Nour, 2015). Because of migration, health care providers are increasingly confronted with the range of negative urogynecologic effects that result from this practice. Nurses need to have a deeper understanding of the history, cultural beliefs, medical complications, and methods of surgical reconstruction to provide culturally competent care to this unique group of women. This cultural practice will be addressed in detail in Chapter 9.

Therapeutic Management

Many small fistulas will heal without treatment, but large fistulas often require surgical repair; surgery may be postponed until the edema or inflammation in the surrounding tissues has dissipated. Surgical repair of fistulas is associated with a high success rate if it is done in a timely manner, but larger fistulas and those of long duration have a poorer prognosis (Jellison & Raz, 2015).

Nursing Assessment

The history should include questions about any changes in the woman's urinary and bowel patterns. Assess for common signs and symptoms of fistulas, which are related to the type of fistula. If the opening involves the rectum, feces and flatus will leak through the vagina. If it involves the bladder, urine will leak from the vagina. Depending on the location and size of the fistula, the woman may or may not experience discomfort. The health care provider can detect these abnormal openings through inspection and palpation during the pelvic examination. Diagnostic or laboratory tests are generally not ordered once this condition is found.

Nursing Management

Provide guidance and support. Offer information to help the woman learn about her condition and, with appropriate intervention, to improve her quality of life. Begin by making sure the woman understands her anatomy and why she is having such symptoms. Provide a thorough explanation of the treatment options so that she can make an informed decision. Be sensitive to the woman's feeling of shame and fear about her incontinence; these feelings may be why she delayed seeking treatment. Address all of the woman's needs, both physical and emotional.

Bartholin Cysts

A Bartholin cyst is a swollen, fluid-filled, sac-like structure that results when one of the ducts of the Bartholin gland becomes blocked. The cyst may become infected and an abscess may develop in the gland. The Bartholin glands are two mucus-secreting glandular structures with duct openings bilaterally at the base of the labia minora near the opening of the vagina that provide lubrication during sexual arousal. Normally these glands cannot be felt or seen unless they are infected. Bartholin cysts are the most common cystic growths in the vulva, affecting approximately 2% of women at some time in their life (Reif et al., 2015).

Therapeutic Management

Treatment can be conservative or surgical depending on the symptoms, the size of the cyst, and whether it is infected or not. Small asymptomatic cysts do not require treatment. Sitz baths along with analgesics are used to reduce discomfort. Antibiotics are prescribed if the gland is infected. The aim of treatment for a cyst or abscess is to create a fistulous tract from the dilated duct to the outside vulva by incision and drainage. However, cysts or abscesses tend to return if this option is used.

Other treatment options beyond incision and drainage include placement of a Word catheter or a small loop of plastic tubing secured in place to prevent closure and to allow drainage. The use of a carbon dioxide laser to remove the cyst is also possible. After the Word catheter is inserted, the balloon tip is inflated and it is left in place for 4 to 6 weeks. The follow-up of the plastic tubing for removal is in approximately 3 weeks. Both procedures are safe and effective alternatives to surgery (Prabhu & Gardella, 2015). Treatment for a pregnant woman with a Bartholin cyst depends on the severity of the symptoms and whether an infection is present. Surgery may be delayed until after the woman gives birth if there are no symptoms.

Nursing Assessment

Nursing assessment for the woman with a Bartholin cyst includes a thorough health history, physical examination, and laboratory and diagnostic tests.

HEALTH HISTORY

The history should include questions about the woman's sexual practices and protective measures used. Assess for common signs and symptoms of Bartholin cysts. The woman may be asymptomatic if the cyst is small (less than 5 cm) and not infected. If infection is present, symptoms include varying degrees of pain, especially when walking or sitting; unilateral edema; redness around the gland; and dyspareunia. Extensive inflammation may cause systemic symptoms. Abscess formation occurs when the cystic fluid becomes infected. An abscess usually develops rapidly over a 2- to 3-day period and may spontaneously rupture. A history of sudden relief of pain following profuse discharge is highly suggestive of spontaneous rupture (Schuiling & Likis, 2016).

PHYSICAL EXAMINATION AND LABORATORY AND DIAGNOSTIC STUDIES

The diagnosis of Bartholin cysts or abscesses is primarily made during a physical examination when a protruding tender labial mass is located. In women over the age of 40, there is an increased risk of malignancy, typically sarcomas which account for 2% of all invasive vulvar malignancies. They are characterized by rapid growth, high metastatic potential, frequent recurrences, aggressive behavior, and high mortality rate (Chokoeva et al., 2015). Cultures of the purulent abscess fluid and of the cervix should be obtained for *Neisseria gonorrhoeae* and *Chlamydia trachomatis* to rule out a sexually transmitted infection.

Nursing Management

Nurses must be aware of and knowledgeable about vulvar cysts and treatment options. The woman may be aware of a vulvar cyst secondary to the pain or may be unaware of it if it is asymptomatic. A Bartholin cyst may be an incidental finding during a routine pelvic examination. Explain the cause of the cyst and assist with cultures if needed. Provide reassurance and support.

Ovarian Cysts

An **ovarian cyst** is a fluid-filled sac that forms on the ovary (Fig. 7.5). These very common growths are benign 90% of the time and are asymptomatic in many women. The cysts are discovered incidentally during an ultrasound or routine pelvic examination. Ovarian cysts occur in 30% of women with regular menses, 50% of women with irregular menses, and 7% of postmenopausal women (Templeman, 2015). When the cysts grow large and exert pressure on surrounding structures, women often seek medical help.

Types of Ovarian Cysts

The most common benign ovarian cysts are follicular cysts, corpus luteum (lutein) cysts, theca lutein cysts, and polycystic ovarian syndrome (PCOS).

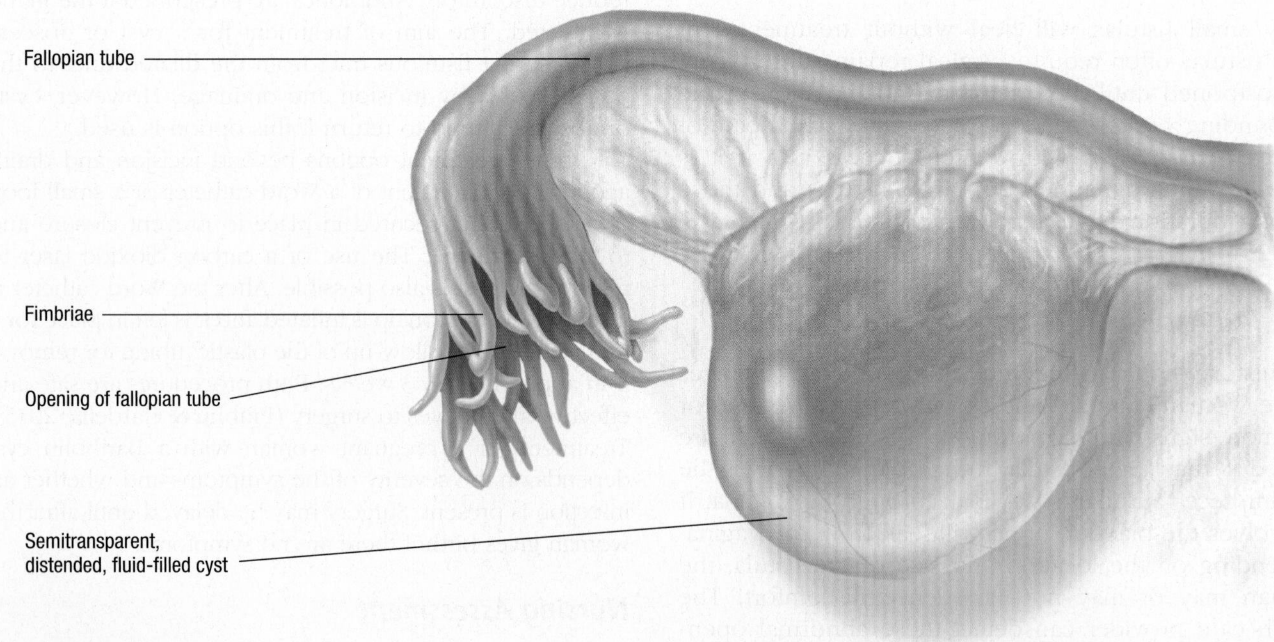

FIGURE 7.5 Ovarian cyst. (Asset provided by Anatomical Chart Co.)

FOLLICULAR CYSTS

Small follicular cysts are commonly found in the ovaries of prepubertal girls and women of reproductive age, and in most cases, they are of no clinical significance. They are usually self-limiting and resolve spontaneously. Follicular cysts are caused by the failure of the ovarian follicle to rupture at the time of ovulation. Follicular cysts seldom grow larger than 5 cm in diameter; most regress and require no treatment. They can occur at any age and are rare after menopause. They are detected by vaginal ultrasound.

CORPUS LUTEUM (LUTEIN) CYSTS

A corpus luteum cyst forms when the corpus luteum becomes cystic or hemorrhagic and fails to degenerate after 14 days. These cysts might cause pain and delay the next menstrual period. A pelvic ultrasound helps to make this diagnosis. Typically these cysts appear after ovulation and resolve without intervention.

THECA LUTEIN CYSTS

Prolonged abnormally high levels of human chorionic gonadotropin (hCG) stimulate the development of theca lutein cysts. Although rare, these cysts are associated with hydatidiform mole, choriocarcinoma, polycystic ovary syndrome, and Clomid therapy.

POLYCYSTIC OVARY SYNDROME

Polycystic ovary syndrome (PCOS) is the most common endocrine condition in women of reproductive age. It is a heterogeneous condition that involves the presence of multiple inactive follicle cysts within the ovary that interfere with ovarian function. It is a multifaceted disorder, and central to its pathogenesis are hyperandrogenemia and hyperinsulinemia, which are targets for treatment (King et al., 2015). It is associated with obesity, hyperinsulinemia, elevated luteinizing hormone levels (linked to ovulation), elevated androgen levels (virilization), hirsutism (male-pattern hair growth), obstructive sleep apnea, follicular atresia (ovarian growth failure), ovarian growth and cyst formation, anovulation (failure to ovulate), infertility, type 2 diabetes, sleep apnea, amenorrhea (absence of menstruation or irregular periods), metabolic syndrome, which is characterized by abdominal obesity (waist circumference > 35 in), dyslipidemia (triglyceride level > 150 mg/dL, high-density lipoprotein cholesterol level < 50 mg/dL), elevated blood pressure, a proinflammatory state characterized by an elevated C-reactive protein level, and a prothrombotic state characterized by elevated PAI-1 and fibrinogen levels. Recent studies also indicate that PCOS is associated with an increase in the risk of uterine fibroids, depression, adverse pregnancy outcomes, and neonatal complications. A recent meta-analysis found that women with PCOS demonstrated a significantly higher risk of developing gestational diabetes, gestational hypertension, preeclampsia, preterm birth, and had a higher cesarean section rate when compared to controls (Kyrou, Weickert, & Randeva, 2015). With an estimated prevalence of 5% to 10% of all females, PCOS is the most common cause of medically treatable infertility and is responsible for 70% of cases of anovulatory subfertility and up to 20% of couples' infertility cases (NIH, 2015c).

Take Note!

Careful attention should be given to this condition because affected women are at increased risk for long-term health problems such as cardiovascular disease, hypertension, dyslipidemia, type 2 diabetes (half of all women), infertility, and cancer (endometrial, breast, and ovarian) (Moran, Norman, & Teede, 2015).

Initially PCOS was called Stein–Leventhal syndrome after its researchers, but it is now recognized to be an anabolic syndrome. Unfortunately, less than two thirds of women are aware of their diagnosis or the concomitant high risk for developing type 2 diabetes mellitus and cardiovascular disease related to metabolic syndrome. Its etiology is not clearly understood, but studies suggest a genetic (autosomal-dominant) component. Women with PCOS have abnormalities in the metabolism of androgens and estrogen and in the control of androgen production. In addition, they have peripheral insulin resistance and hyperinsulinemia and obesity (Trikudanathan, 2015). All of these clinical manifestations must be addressed throughout the lifespan with an emphasis on prevention of cardiometabolic risks in the treatment plan.

Therapeutic Management

Treatment is centered on the clinical manifestations and should be initiated early to prevent/limit long-term complications such as metabolic syndrome, diabetes, endometrial carcinoma, and infertility (Ganie, Chakraborty, & Rehman, 2015). Oral contraceptives, antidiabetic agents, and statins are some of the common therapies used to address the symptoms of this complex hormonal condition. Weight loss and surgery may also be beneficial as nondrug options.

Treatment of ovarian cysts focuses on differentiating a benign cyst from a solid ovarian malignancy. Transvaginal ultrasound is useful in distinguishing fluid-filled cysts from solid masses. Laparoscopy may be needed to remove the cyst if it is large and pressing on surrounding structures. For smaller cysts, monitoring with repeat ultrasounds every 3 to 6 months might be in order (Lucidi, 2015). Oral contraceptives are often prescribed to suppress gonadotropin levels, which may help resolve the cysts. Pain medication is also prescribed if needed.

Medical management of PCOS is aimed at the treatment of metabolic derangements, anovulation, hirsutism, and menstrual irregularity. This includes both drug and nondrug therapy, along with lifestyle modifications. Goals of therapy focus on reducing the production and circulating levels of androgens, protecting the endometrium against the effects of unopposed estrogens, supporting lifestyle changes to achieve ideal body weight, lowering the risk of cardiovascular disease, avoiding the effects of hyperinsulinemia on the risk of cardiovascular disease and diabetes, and inducing ovulation to achieve pregnancy if desired (Evidence-Based Practice 7.2). Treatment modalities for PCOS are highlighted in Box 7.3.

Nursing Assessment

Nursing assessment for the woman with PCOS includes a thorough health history, physical examination, and laboratory and diagnostic tests.

HEALTH HISTORY

The history should include questions about the woman's symptoms, including onset, location, frequency, quality, intensity, and aggravating and alleviating factors of her discomfort. Note the last menstrual period and whether or not her cycles are regular. Ask about her overall

BOX 7.3

TREATMENT MODALITIES FOR PCOS

- Oral contraceptives to treat menstrual irregularities and acne
- Mechanical hair removal (shaving, waxing, plucking, or electrolysis) to treat hirsutism
- Glucophage (metformin), which improves insulin uptake by fat and muscle cells, to treat hyperinsulinemia; thiazolidinediones (Actos, Avandia) to decrease insulin resistance
- Ovulation induction agents (Clomid) to treat infertility
- Lifestyle changes (e.g., weight loss, exercise, balanced low-fat diet)
- Referral to support groups to help improve emotional state and build self-esteem

Adapted from King, T. L., Brucker, M. C., Kriebs, J. M., Fahey, J. O., Gegor, C. L., & Varney, H. (2015). *Varney's midwifery.* (5th ed.). Burlington, MA: Jones & Bartlett Learning; Kyrou, I., Weickert, M. O., & Randeva, H. S. (2015). Diagnosis and management of polycystic ovary syndrome (PCOS). In *Endocrinology and diabetes* (pp. 99–113). London, England: Springer Publishers; and Lucidi, R.S. (2015). Polycystic ovarian syndrome. *EMedicine.* Available at: http://emedicine.medscape.com/article/256806-overview

EVIDENCE-BASED PRACTICE 7.2

IT'S NOT JUST PHYSICAL: THE ADVERSE PSYCHOSOCIAL EFFECTS OF POLYCYSTIC OVARY SYNDROME IN ADOLESCENTS

STUDY

The prevalence of depression and other psychological disorders in women with PCOS is high and varies in numerous studies. In particular, women with PCOS have been found to be at an increased risk of social phobia and suicide attempts. The reasons for a higher prevalence of psychological disorders in women with PCOS are likely to be complex. Some investigators suggest that physical symptoms experienced by women with PCOS are the likely cause of psychological distress. However, evidence is inconsistent. While acne, hirsutism, and obesity have been linked to increased psychological distress in some studies, no link is demonstrated in others. It is likely that multiple factors contribute to the high prevalence of psychosocial disorders in women with PCOS.

This study sheds light on the fact that this gynecologic disorder of endocrine origin can be associated with a great number of psychological symptoms (e.g., depression, anxiety, body image dissatisfaction, eating and sexual disorders, and poor quality of life). The goal of the study was to address the prevalence of psychological disorders and determinants of well-being.

Findings

An overwhelming majority of scientific literature on PCOS has focused on the medical approach to analyze the disorder and only a few studies have investigated its predisposing psychological factors. The literature review revealed several psychological disorders that accompany this syndrome with limited attention given to them to help women cope. The symptoms typically associated with PCOS, including amenorrhea, oligomenorrhea, hirsutism, obesity, infertility, anovulation, and acne, can lead to symptoms of depression, withdrawal from society, emotional distress, embarrassment, lower self-esteem, anxiety, body image disturbances, eating disorders, marital and social maladjustment, and impaired sexual functioning.

Nursing Implications

PCOS is closely associated with psychological disorders with important implications that necessitate identification and treatment of the disorders. The high prevalence rate of these psychological disorders in this population suggests that initial evaluation of all women with PCOS should also include an assessment of their mental health. Psychological support by nurses should take on an important role in the management of the affected women with PCOS. This should not suggest that medical treatment of PCOS is not required, but a thorough cooperation between medical treatment and psychological support would improve the situation of PCOS-affected women. The physical and psychosocial aspects of management of PCOS go hand in hand. Meeting physical management goals (e.g., weight loss, reduction in hyperandrogenism manifestations) can lessen some of the distressing psychosocial effects, and enhance self-esteem.

Adapted from Lee, J. S. (2015). It's not just physical: The adverse psychosocial effects of polycystic ovary syndrome in adolescents. *Women's Healthcare, 3*(1), 20–28.

general health and any changes recently noticed, such as a change in abdominal girth without a concomitant weight gain. Assess for common signs and symptoms of ovarian cysts. Findings might include:

- Hirsutism (face and chin, upper lip, areola, lower abdomen, and perineum)
- Alopecia (frontal region and crown of head)
- Virilization (clitoral hypertrophy, deepening of voice, increased muscle mass, breast atrophy, male-pattern baldness)
- Menstrual irregularity and infertility (menorrhagia, anovulation)
- Polycystic ovaries (12 or more follicles on ovaries)
- Obesity (occurs in more than 50% of women with PCOS; occurs in abdominal region, with an increase in the waist–hip ratio)
- Insulin resistance (chronic hyperinsulinemia leads to type 2 diabetes)
- Metabolic syndrome (elevated cholesterol, triglycerides, low-density lipoprotein; risk of cardiovascular disease)
- Increased risk for endometrial cancer, ovarian cancer, breast cancer
- Psychological impact (depression, frustration, anxiety, eating disorders)
- Acne (face and shoulders) (Lucidi, 2015)

PHYSICAL EXAMINATION AND LABORATORY AND DIAGNOSTIC STUDIES

The physical examination includes inspection, auscultation, and palpation of the abdomen because large ovarian masses may cause visible changes in the abdomen. A complete pelvic examination is performed to assess the location, size, shape, texture, mobility, and tenderness of any palpable mass.

Diagnostic tests include a pregnancy test to rule out ectopic pregnancy. Gonorrhea and chlamydia testing is warranted if an ovarian abscess is suspected. An ultrasound may be ordered to differentiate between functional or simple ovarian cysts and a solid tumor. Additional tests may be performed depending on the findings.

Remember Liz, the client with irregular menses, facial hair, and acne? Her glucose level is elevated, multiple cysts were felt on her ovaries during the pelvic examination, and laboratory tests found elevated lipid and lipoprotein levels. What education should the nurse provide Liz regarding her PCOS diagnosis? What medications might be prescribed to address her abnormal laboratory values?

Nursing Management

Nursing care should include education about the condition, treatment options, diagnostic test arrangements, and referral for surgery if needed. Provide support and reassurance during the diagnostic period to allay anxiety in the client and her family. Reassure the woman that the majority of ovarian cysts are benign, but regardless stress the importance of follow-up care. Listen to the woman's concerns about her appearance, infertility, and facial hair growth. Offer suggestions to help the woman feel better about herself and her health.

Nurses can have a positive impact on women with PCOS through counseling and education. Provide support for women dealing with negative self-image secondary to the physical manifestations of PCOS. Through education, help the woman understand the syndrome and its associated risk factors to prevent long-term health problems. Encourage the woman to make positive lifestyle changes. Make community referrals to local support groups to help the woman build her coping skills.

***Liz* returns to the clinic a month later for reevaluation of her PCOS. She has been taking metformin to reduce her insulin resistance and has followed her exercise regimen and reduced her caloric intake to lose weight, but she still complains about her facial hair and acne. What interventions might be helpful to address this problem? What medication might also be prescribed to regularize her menses and relieve the hirsutism?**

NURSING CARE PLAN 7.1

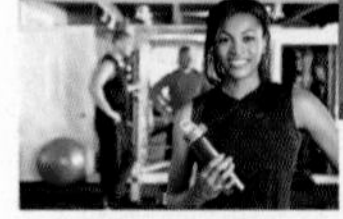

Overview of a Woman with Pelvic Organ Prolapse

Katherine, a 62-year-old multiparous woman, came to her gynecologist with complaints of a chronic dragging or heavy painful feeling in her pelvis, lower backache, constipation, and urine leakage. Her symptoms increase when she stands for long periods. She has not had menstrual cycles for at least a decade. She tells you, "I'm not taking any of those menopausal hormones." She also states she is very self-conscious and embarrassed about her urine leakage and restricts her outside activities.

(continued)

NURSING CARE PLAN 7.1

Overview of a Woman with Pelvic Organ Prolapse (continued)

NURSING DIAGNOSIS: Body image changes related to relaxation of pelvic support and elimination difficulties

Outcome Identification and Evaluation

The client will report an improved body image after management of pelvic organ prolapse and improved urinary control.

Interventions: *Providing Pain Management*

- Obtain a thorough history, including ongoing embarrassing experiences, methods of urine control used, what worked, what didn't, any changes in sexual practices related to this, and the effect of this condition on her activities of daily living *to provide a baseline and enable a systematic approach to address it.*
- Assess the frequency, severity, precipitating factors, and aggravating/alleviating factors *to identify characteristics of the client's abnormal urinary patterns to plan appropriate interventions.*
- Educate client about any medications prescribed (correct dosage, route, side effects, and precautions) *to increase the client's understanding of the therapy and promote compliance.*
- Assess problematic elimination patterns *to identify underlying factors from which to plan appropriate prevention strategies.*
- Encourage client to increase fluids and fiber in diet and increase physical activity daily *to promote peristalsis.*
- Assist client with establishing regular toileting patterns by setting aside time daily for bowel elimination *to promote regular bowel function and evacuation.*
- Urge client to avoid the routine use of laxatives *to reduce risk of compounding constipation.*

NURSING DIAGNOSIS: Deficient knowledge related to causes of structural disorders and treatment options

Outcome Identification and Evaluation

The client will demonstrate an understanding of current condition and treatments as evidenced by identifying treatment options, making health-promoting lifestyle choices, verbalizing appropriate health care practices, and adhering to treatment plan.

Interventions: *Providing Client Education*

- Assess client's understanding of pelvic organ prolapse and its treatment options *to provide a baseline for teaching.*
- Review information provided about surgical procedures and recommendations for healthy lifestyle, obtaining feedback frequently, *to validate client's understanding of instructions.*
- Discuss association between uterine, bladder, and rectal prolapse and symptoms *to help client understand the etiology of her symptoms and pain.*
- Have client verbalize and discuss information related to diagnosis, surgical procedure, preoperative routine, and postoperative regimen *to ensure adequate understanding and provide time for correcting or clarifying any misinformation or misconceptions.*
- Provide written material with pictures *to promote learning and help client visualize what has occurred to her body secondary to aging, weight gain, childbirth, and gravity.*
- Discuss pros and cons of hormone replacement therapy, osteoporosis prevention, and cardiovascular events common in postmenopausal women *to promote informed decision making by the client about available menopausal therapies.*
- Inform client about the availability of community resources and make appropriate referrals as needed *to provide additional education and support.*
- Document details of teaching and learning *to allow for continuity of care and further education, if needed.*

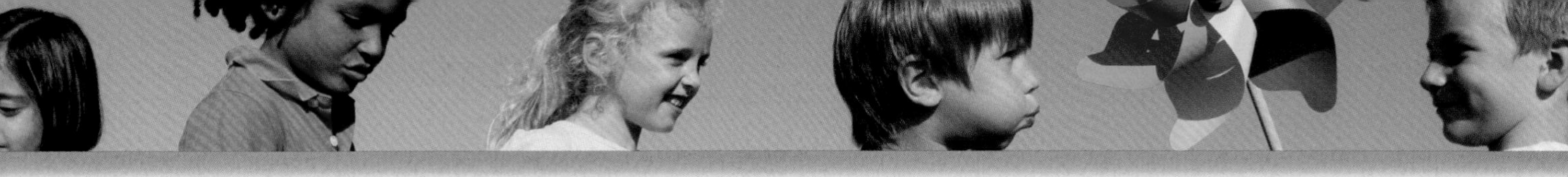

KEY CONCEPTS

- Pelvic floor disorders such as pelvic organ prolapse and urinary and fecal incontinence are prevalent conditions in aging women. They cause significant physical and psychological morbidity, with obvious detriment to women's social interactions, emotional well-being, and overall quality of life.
- The four most common types of genital prolapse are cystocele, rectocele, enterocele, and uterine prolapse.
- The purpose of pelvic floor muscle exercises is to increase the muscle volume, which will result in a stronger muscular contraction. These exercises might limit the progression of mild prolapse and alleviate mild prolapse symptoms, including low back pain and pelvic pressure.
- UI is the involuntary loss of urine sufficient enough to be a social or hygiene problem. It affects approximately 15 million women in the United States.
- The three most common types of incontinence are urge incontinence (overactive bladder caused by detrusor muscle contractions), stress incontinence (inadequate urinary sphincter function), and mixed incontinence (involves both stress and urge incontinence).
- The most common benign growths of the reproductive tract include cervical, endocervical, and endometrial polyps; uterine fibroids (leiomyomas); genital fistulas; Bartholin cysts; and ovarian cysts.
- PCOS involves the presence of multiple inactive follicle cysts within the ovary that interfere with ovarian function. Hyperandrogenism, insulin resistance, and chronic anovulation characterize PCOS. Careful attention should be given to this condition because women with it are at increased risk for long-term health problems such as cardiovascular disease, hypertension, dyslipidemia, infertility, type 2 diabetes, and cancer (endometrial, breast, and ovarian).

REFERENCES AND RECOMMENDED READINGS

Alexander, L. L., LaRosa, J. H., Bader, H., & Garfield, S. (2014). *New dimensions in women's health* (6th ed.). Sudbury, MA: Jones & Bartlett.

Alexander, L., Shakespeare, K., Barradell, V., & Orme, S. (2015). Management of urinary incontinence in frail elderly women. *Obstetrics, Gynecology & Reproductive Medicine, 25*(3), 75–82.

American College of Obstetricians and Gynecologists [ACOG]. (2015a). Pelvic support problems. ACOG Educational Pamphlet. Retrieved from http://www.acog.org/~/media/For%20Patients/faq012.pdf?dmc=1&ts=20140128T1159591406

Brown, D. N. (2015). Pelvic organ prolapse: A consequence of nature or nurture? *Menopause, 22*(5), 477–479.

Centers for Disease Control and Prevention [CDC]. (2015). Women's reproductive health: Hysterectomy. Retrieved from http://www.cdc.gov/reproductivehealth/WomensRH/Hysterectomy.htm

Chokoeva, A. A., Tchernev, G., Cardoso, J. C., Patterson, J. W., Dechev, I., Valkanov, S., et al. (2015). Vulvar sarcomas: Short guideline for histopathological recognition and clinical management. Part 1. *International Journal of Immunopathology and Pharmacology, 28*(2), 168–177.

Colyar, M.R. (2015). *Advanced practice nursing procedures* Philadelphia, PA: F.A. Davis Company.

Dumoulin, C., Hay-Smith, E.J., Mac Habee-Sequin, G. M., & Mercier, J. (2015). Pelvic floor muscle training verses no treatment, or inactive control treatments, for urinary incontinence in women. *Neurourology & Urodynamics, 34*(4), 300–308.

Files, J. A., Mayer, A. P., & Chutka, D. S. (2015). Urinary incontinence: Not just a mid-laugh crisis. *Journal of Women's Health, 24*(1), 107–108.

Ganie, M. A., Chakraborty, S., & Rehman, H. (2015). Treatment of polycystic ovary syndrome: Recent trial results. *Clinical Investigation, 5*(3), 337–350.

Goldman, N. A., Lynch, K., Jones, H., Rutledge, J., & Burke, W. M. (2015). Comparison of complications in patients undergoing robotic-assisted hysterectomy for large leiomyomas [107]. *Obstetrics & Gynecology, 125*, 40S.

Hehenkamp, W. J., Huirne, J. A., & Brölmann, H. A. (2015). Uterine artery embolization and new ablation techniques. In *Uterine myoma, myomectomy and minimally invasive treatments* (pp. 153–168). Springer International Publishing.

Heller, D. S. (2015). Diseases of the cervix. In *OB-GYN pathology for the clinician* (pp. 91–106). Springer International Publishing.

International Continence Society. (2015). Urinary incontinence. Retrieved from http://www.icsoffice.org/Home.aspx

Jellison, F. C., & Raz, S. (2015). Vaginal fistula repairs. In *Female pelvic surgery* (pp. 145–163). New York, NY: Springer Publishers.

King, T. L., Brucker, M. C., Kriebs, J. M., Fahey, J. O., Gegor, C. L., & Varney, H. (2015). *Varney's midwifery* (5th ed.). Burlington, MA: Jones & Bartlett Learning.

Kirby, A. C., Tan-Kim, J., & Nager, C. W. (2015). Dynamic maximum urethral closure pressures measured by high-resolution manometry increase markedly after sling surgery. *International Urogynecology Journal, 26*, 1–5.

Kwak, Y., Kwon, H., & Kim, Y. (2015). Health-related quality of life and mental health in older women with urinary incontinence. *Aging & Mental Health*, 1–8.

Kyrou, I., Weickert, M. O., & Randeva, H. S. (2015). Diagnosis and management of polycystic ovary syndrome (PCOS). In

Endocrinology and diabetes (pp. 99–113). London, England: Springer Publishers.

Lazarou, G., & Grigorescu, B. A. (2015). Pelvic organ prolapse. eMedicine. Retrieved from http://emedicine.medscape.com/article/276259-overview

Lee, J. S. (2015). It's not just physical: The adverse psychosocial effects of polycystic ovary syndrome in adolescents. *Women's Healthcare, 3*(1), 20–28.

Lieng, M. (2015). Endometrial polyps. In *Minimally invasive gynecological surgery* (pp. 61–73). Berlin, Heidelberg: Springer Publishers.

Lucidi, R. S. (2015). Polycystic ovarian syndrome. EMedicine. Available at: http://emedicine.medscape.com/article/256806-overview

Maher, C., & Haya, N. (2015). Changing trends in pelvic organ prolapse surgery. *Obstetrics, Gynecology & Reproductive Medicine, 25*(6), 147–151.

McClurg, D., Gerrard, J., & Hove, R. T. (2015). Reducing the incidence of incontinence. *British Journal of Midwifery, 23*(1), 17–20.

Meyer, D. (2015). Health benefits of prebiotic fibers. *Advances in Food and Nutrition Research, 74*, 47–91.

Moran, L. J., Norman, R. J., & Teede, H. J. (2015). Metabolic risk in PCOS: Phenotype and adiposity impact. *Trends in Endocrinology & Metabolism, 26*(3), 136–143.

Mukwege, A. A., El-Nashar, S. A., Rhodes, D., Dowdy, S. C., & Trabuco, E. C. (2015). Are demographic and clinical characteristics of women presenting with advanced pelvic organ prolapse different compared with women presenting in earlier stages?[374]. *Obstetrics & Gynecology, 125*, 116S–117S.

National Institutes of Health [NIH]. (2015a). *Pelvic floor disorders*. Retrieved from https://www.nichd.nih.gov/health/topics/pelvicfloor/Pages/default.aspx

National Institutes of Health [NIH]. (2015b). *Uterine fibroids*. Available at http://www.nichd.nih.gov/health/topics/uterine/conditioninfo/Pages/default.aspx

National Institutes of Health [NIH]. (2015c). *Polycystic ovarian syndrome*. Available at: http://www.nichd.nih.gov/health/topics/PCOS/Pages/default.aspx

Nelson, A. L., Papa, R. R., & Ritchie, J. J. (2015). Asymptomatic cervical polyps: Can we just let them be? *Women's Health, 11*(2), 121–126.

Nilsson, C. G. (2015). Creating a gold standard surgical procedure: the development and implementation of TVT. *International Urogynecology Journal*, 1–3. doi: 10.1007/s00192-014-2616-2.

Nour, N. M. (2015). Female genital cutting: Impact on women's health. *Seminars in Reproductive Medicine, 33*(1), 41–46.

Prabhu, A., & Gardella, C. (2015). Common vaginal and vulvar disorders. *Medical Clinics of North America, 99*(3), 553–574.

Ralph, G., & Tamussino, K. (2015). Conservative management of pelvic organ prolapse. In *Principles and practice of urogynecology* (pp. 115–122). India: Springer Publishers.

Ramalingam, K., & Monga, A. (2015). Obesity and pelvic floor dysfunction. *Best Practice & Research Clinical Obstetrics & Gynecology, 29*(4):541–547.

Reif, P., Ulrich, D., Bjelic-Radisic, V., Häusler, M., Schnedl-Lamprecht, E., & Tamussino, K. (2015). Management of Bartholin's cyst and abscess using the Word catheter–implementation, recurrence rates and costs. *European Journal of Obstetrics & Gynecology and Reproductive Biology, 190*, 81–84.

Riss, P., & Koch, M. (2015). Evaluation of pelvic organ prolapse. In *Principles and practice of urogynecology* (pp. 107–114). India: Springer Publishers.

Rodríguez-Mias, N. L., Martínez-Franco, E., Aguado, J., Sánchez, E., & Amat-Tardiu, L. (2015). Pelvic organ prolapse and stress urinary incontinence, do they share the same risk factors? *European Journal of Obstetrics & Gynecology and Reproductive Biology, 190*, 52–57.

Schuiling, K. D., & Likis, F. E. (2016). *Women's gynecologic health* (3rd ed.). Sudbury, MA: Jones & Bartlett.

Shigetomi, H., Oka, K., Seki, T., & Kobayashi, H. (2015). Design and preclinical validation of the composite-type optical fiberscope for minimally invasive procedure of intrauterine disease. *Journal of Minimally Invasive Gynecology, 190*, 52–57

Spurlock, J. (2015). Vesicovaginal fistula. eMedicine. Retrieved from http://emedicine.medscape.com/article/267943-overview#a0102

Stewart, E. A. (2015). Uterine fibroids. *New England Journal of Medicine, 372*(17), 1646–1655.

Stewart, E. A. (2016). Endometrial polyps. *UpToDate*, Retrieved from http://www.uptodate.com/contents/endometrial-polyps

Su, C. C., Sun, B. Y. C., & Jiann, B. P. (2015). Association of urinary incontinence and sexual function in women. *International Journal of Urology, 22*(1), 109–113.

Taylor, D., & Rakinic, J. (2015). Rectovaginal fistula. eMedicine. Retrieved from http://emedicine.medscape.com/article/193277-overview

Templeman, C. (2015). Ovarian cysts. *Journal of Pediatric and Adolescent Gynecology, 17*, 297–298.

Trikudanathan, S. (2015). Polycystic ovarian syndrome. *Medical Clinics of North America, 99*(1), 221–235.

Vasavada, S. P., Carmel, M. E., & Rackley, R. (2015). Urinary incontinence. eMedicine. Retrieved from http://emedicine.medscape.com/article/452289-overview

Waetjen, L. E., Xing, G., Johnson, W. O., Melnikow, J., Gold, E. B., & Study of Women's Health Across the Nation (SWAN). (2015). Factors associated with seeking treatment for urinary incontinence during the menopausal transition. *Obstetrics & Gynecology, 125*(5), 1071–1079.

Walters, M. (2015). Urinary incontinence in women comes and goes, and reasons remain elusive. *BJOG: An International Journal of Obstetrics & Gynecology, 122*, 824.

CHAPTER WORKSHEET

MULTIPLE-CHOICE QUESTIONS

1. When you are interviewing a client with uterine fibroids, what subjective data would you expect to find in her history?
   a. Cyclic migraine headaches
   b. Urinary tract infections
   c. Chronic pelvic pain
   d. Chronic constipation
2. Conservative treatment options available for women with pelvic organ prolapse are:
   a. Pessaries and PFM exercises
   b. External pelvic fixation devices
   c. Weight gain and yoga
   d. Firm panty-and-girdle garments
3. Which of the following dietary and lifestyle modifications might the nurse recommend to help prevent pelvic relaxation as women age?
   a. Eat a high-fiber diet to avoid constipation and straining.
   b. Avoid sitting for long periods; get up and walk around frequently.
   c. Limit the amount of exercise to prevent overdeveloping muscles.
   d. Space children a year apart to reduce wear and tear on the uterus.
4. Women with polycystic ovarian syndrome (PCOS) are at increased risk for developing which of the following long-term health problems?
   a. Osteoporosis
   b. Lupus
   c. Type 2 diabetes
   d. Migraine headaches
5. Side effects experienced by women taking gonadotropin-releasing hormone (GnRH) agonists for the treatment of fibroids closely resemble those of:
   a. Anorexia nervosa
   b. Osteoarthritis
   c. Depression
   d. Menopause
6. In securing a health history of a 65-year-old woman, which clinical manifestation described by the client would the nurse suspect is related to pelvic organ prolapse?
   a. Chronic abdominal pain
   b. Heavy feeling or dragging in vagina
   c. Uterine cramping and backache
   d. Weight gain and edema of ankles

CRITICAL THINKING EXERCISE

1. Faith, a 42-year-old multiparous woman, presents to the women's health clinic complaining of pelvic pain, menorrhagia, and vaginal discharge. She says she has been having these problems for several months. On examination, her uterus is enlarged and irregular in shape. Her blood studies reveal anemia.
   a. What condition might Faith have, based on her symptoms?
   b. What treatment options are available to address this condition?
   c. What educational interventions should the nurse discuss with Faith?

STUDY ACTIVITIES

1. Prepare an educational session to teach women how to do pelvic floor muscle exercises to prevent stress incontinence and pelvic floor relaxation.
2. In a small group, discuss the personal, social, and sexual issues that might affect a woman with pelvic organ prolapse. How might these issues affect her socialization? How might a support group help?
3. List the symptoms that a woman with uterine fibroids might have. Discuss how these symptoms might mimic a more frightening condition and why the woman might delay seeking treatment.
4. A bladder that herniates into the vagina is a ____________________.
5. A rectum that herniates into the vagina is a ____________________.

BRINGING IT ALL TOGETHER: A CASE STUDY

Elizabeth, a 52-year-old woman presented to the gynecologic clinic to discuss a "horrible personal problem" that was ruining her life. She appeared very distressed and only wanted to talk to the nurse in private about it. A few months ago when she was out walking her dog, she experienced a sudden rectal urgency that she thought was gas, but she expelled feces instead. Over the past few months, her fecal incontinence has increased in severity and frequency causing her extreme stress. To avoid embarrassment, she has had to cover and excuse herself from work situations and turn down social invitations. She now has to wear a protective pad and disposable pants.

CHAPTER **WORKSHEET**

ASSESSMENT

Elizabeth is otherwise healthy and takes no prescription medications presently. She has had five vaginal births with three episiotomies. She has a body mass index of 27, mild stress urinary incontinence, and a low-grade rectocele with slightly decreased anal sphincter tone. Her pelvic examination demonstrated pelvic organ prolapse. The digital rectal examination ruled out fecal impaction and any rectal mass. A detailed history of her incontinence episodes was also taken.

1. What risk factors are associated with fecal incontinence? Which does Elizabeth have?
2. Is her condition common in women of her age? If so, why?
3. What treatment options might help Elizabeth with her condition?

Risk factors for fecal incontinence include increasing age, anorectal procedures, obesity, urinary incontinence, vaginal births, pelvic organ prolapse, and female gender. Fecal incontinence is not a disease state, but rather is a symptom of an underlying pelvic disorder such as POP. It is a nonfatal condition, but can greatly reduce the individual's quality of life. Treatment options include nonoperative interventions such as bulking agents to improve stool consistency, pelvic floor muscle exercises, antidiarrheal agents, and surgery.

PLAN

1. What specific health promotion strategy can the nurse discuss to reduce her symptoms?
2. How can the nurse improve Elizabeth's coping strategies?
3. What dietary changes might be helpful for Elizabeth?
4. How can the nurse offer client-centered care to Elizabeth?

Since Elizabeth has a high BMI; a weight loss intervention would be helpful in reducing the intra-abdominal pressure on her pelvic organs. Obesity is a risk factor for this condition. The nurse can discuss ways to reduce her weight through diet and exercise. Coping strategies should include a discussion of continence products available, providing emotional and psychological support to her, the use of anal plugs, skin-care, odor control, bowel training, laundry advice and advice on preservation of dignity. Dietary changes might include starting a food and fluid diary to determine if there are food items increasing her stool frequency, advise her to modify one food at a time, and consuming foods that add bulk to her diet to increase formed stools. Management should be tailored to the needs of the individual. Information should be provided in a caring format in which Elizabeth can understand, so that she can participate in decisions about their treatment.

8

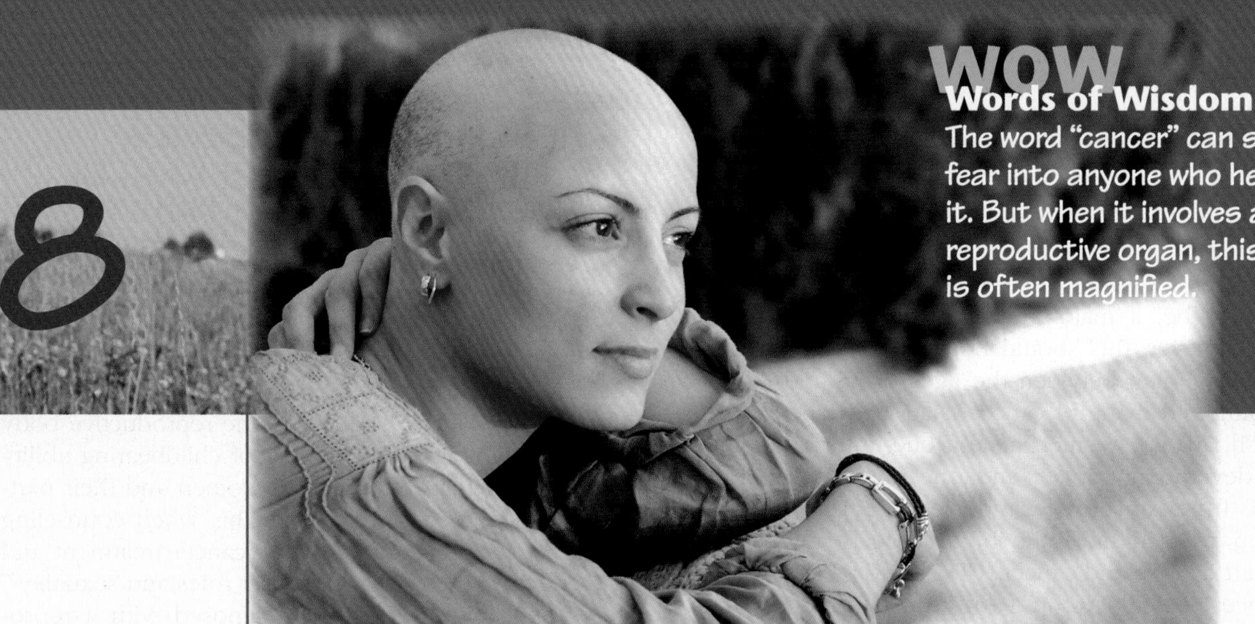
WOW
Words of Wisdom
The word "cancer" can strike fear into anyone who hears it. But when it involves a reproductive organ, this fear is often magnified.

Cancers of the Female Reproductive Tract

KEY TERMS

- cervical cancer
- cervical dysplasia
- colposcopy
- cone biopsy
- cryotherapy
- endometrial cancer
- human papillomavirus
- ovarian cancer
- Papanicolaou (Pap) test
- vaginal cancer
- vulvar cancer

Learning Objectives

Upon completion of the chapter, you will be able to:

1. Evaluate the major modifiable risk factors for reproductive tract cancers.
2. Analyze the screening methods and treatment modalities for cancers of the female reproductive tract.
3. Outline the nursing management needed for the most common malignant reproductive tract cancers in women.
4. Examine lifestyle changes and health screenings that can reduce the risk of or prevent reproductive tract cancers.
5. Assess at least three web site resources available for a woman diagnosed with cancer of the reproductive tract.
6. Appraise the psychological distress felt by women diagnosed with cancer, and outline information that can help them to cope.

Carmella **is an obese, 55-year-old woman who presents to her woman's health care provider with vaginal bleeding. She has been through menopause and wonders why she is having a period again. Her history includes infertility and hypertension. Three years ago she had a mastectomy for breast cancer, and she has been taking tamoxifen (Nolvadex) to prevent recurrent breast cancer since her surgery. What risk factors in Carmella's history might predispose her to a reproductive tract cancer? What additional information is needed to make a diagnosis?**

INTRODUCTION

Cancer is the second leading cause of death for women in the United States, surpassed only by cardiovascular disease (Centers for Disease Control and Prevention [CDC], 2015a). Cardiovascular disease is, and should continue to be, a major focus of efforts in women's health. However, this should not overshadow the fact that many women between the ages of 35 and 74 are developing and dying of cancer (National Cancer Institute [NCI], 2015a). Women have a one-in-three lifetime risk of developing cancer, and one out of every four deaths is from cancer (Alexander et al., 2014). African-American women have the highest death rates from both heart disease and cancer (CDC, 2015a). The American Cancer Society (ACS) (2016) estimated that in 2016 there will be 1,685,210 new cancer cases diagnosed and 595,690 cancer deaths in the United States. Scientific evidence suggested that about one-third of these cancer deaths expected to occur in 2015 were related to obesity, physical inactivity, and poor nutrition and thus could have been prevented. Certain cancers are related to infectious agents, such as hepatitis B virus (HBV), **human papillomavirus** (HPV), human immunodeficiency virus (HIV), and *Helicobacter pylori,* and can be prevented through behavioral changes, vaccines, or antibiotics (Herrington, Coates, & Duprex, 2015). In addition, many of the more than 2 million skin cancers that are diagnosed annually could be prevented by protecting the skin from the sun's rays and avoiding indoor tanning. Sunburns, especially if they occur repetitively in childhood, may lead to melanoma. Most melanomas are treated successfully if discovered early, but metastatic melanoma has no good treatment (Balk, 2015).

It has been estimated that in the United States half of all premature deaths, one-third of acute disabilities, and one-half of chronic disabilities are preventable, including some cancers (NCI, 2015b). Nurses need to focus their energies on screening, education, and early detection to reduce these numbers. Because cancer risk is strongly associated with lifestyle and behavior, screening programs are of particular importance for early detection. There is evidence that prevention and early detection have reduced cancer mortality rates and prevented reproductive cancers (CDC, 2015b).

This chapter begins with a nursing process overview of the care of women with reproductive cancer. It then describes selected cancers of the reproductive system: ovarian, endometrial, cervical, vaginal, and **vulvar cancer**. The chapter discusses the nurse's role through diagnosis, intervention, and follow-up care. Cancer management requires a multidisciplinary approach, including specialists in surgical, medical, and radiation oncology. The nurse can provide guidance and support to the client as she finds her way through the health care maze.

NURSING PROCESS OVERVIEW FOR THE WOMAN WITH CANCER OF THE REPRODUCTIVE TRACT

The word *cancer* is laden with fear and dread. These feelings may worsen when the cancer involves a woman's reproductive tract. The diagnosis of a reproductive tract cancer can have a profound impact on a woman's sexuality because it affects the very core of her identity as a female. The loss of the reproductive body part as well as the possible loss of childbearing ability can have a significant effect on women and their partners. Nurses need to remember this when counseling women and their partners about cancer treatment and side effects and changes in gender roles and sexuality.

When a woman is first diagnosed with a reproductive tract cancer, two primary needs arise: information and emotional support. When the diagnosis is made, the woman typically has many questions, such as "What is going to happen to me?" "How will this change my life?" and "Will I survive?" Nurses can play a major role in helping women find the answers to their questions and directing them to the resources they need. Two reliable sources of general cancer information are the NCI and the American Cancer Society. They can be reached via the Internet or by phone.

The nurse also plays a key role in offering emotional support, determining appropriate sources of support, and helping the woman use effective coping strategies. A recent research study found that social support from the woman's family, friends, and coworkers is one of the strongest predictors of how well she will cope (Garner et al., 2015). Implications for nurses working with women following a cancer diagnosis include assessing women's definitions and availability of support; respecting varied needs for informational support; providing a supportive clinical environment; educating clinicians, family, and friends regarding unsupportive responses within the cultural context; and validating women's control and balancing of support needs. Nurses are well positioned to provide women with anticipatory guidance from diagnosis to the end of treatment (Shirvani & Alhani, 2015). Women without a social support network may need a social work referral or may need to be guided toward support groups to receive the emotional support they need.

In addition, cancer clients have a strong need for hope. Strategies for inspiring hope may include active listening, touch, presence, and helping clients overcome communication barriers. Often it is not what nurses say or do but just their presence that counts.

Assessment

Assessment of a woman with cancer of the reproductive tract involves a thorough history and physical examination. In addition, various laboratory and diagnostic tests may be done to evaluate for malignancy.

Health History and Physical Examination

Interview the woman carefully to determine any current or past factors that might increase her risk of cancer, such as early menarche, late menopause, sexually transmitted infections (STIs), use of hormonal agents, or infertility. Find out if the woman has a family history of cancer. Be thorough in obtaining the woman's past medical history, especially her reproductive, obstetric, and gynecologic history. Ask about her lifestyle and behaviors, including risky behaviors such as engaging in unprotected sexual intercourse or sexual intercourse with multiple partners. Find out if she has had routine or recommended screening procedures.

Ask if the woman has had any symptoms, such as abnormal vaginal bleeding or discharge or vaginal discomfort. Often the symptoms of cancer are vague and nonspecific and the woman may attribute them to another problem, such as aging, stress, or improper diet.

Perform a complete physical examination, including a review of body systems and a pelvic examination. Observe for lesions or masses in the perineal area. Note any masses when palpating the abdomen or when performing the pelvic examination.

Laboratory and Diagnostic Testing

Some of the laboratory and diagnostic tests used to help diagnose cancer of the reproductive tract are discussed in Common Laboratory and Diagnostic Tests 8.1.

COMMON LABORATORY AND DIAGNOSTIC TESTS 8.1

Test	Explanation	Indications	Nursing Implications
Clinical breast examination	Assessment of the breast for abnormal findings; client may discover lump herself; high-risk history for breast cancer	Identifies palpable mass, skin change, inverted nipple, or unresolved rash	• Educate client to perform breast self-examination and report any abnormalities if high risk • Reinforce need for frequent clinical breast examinations if risk factors are present
Mammography	Screening modality for breast cancer or any distortion in breast tissue architecture	Detects calcifications, densities, and nonpalpable cancer lesions	Stress importance of annual mammograms for all women after the age of 40 or 50, depending on their risk history
Pap smear	Cervical cytology screening to diagnose cervical cancers	Aids in detecting abnormal cells of the cervix (from squamocolumnar junction of the cervix; most cervical cancers arise here)	Encourage all sexually active women to receive a pelvic examination, including a Pap smear if they have a high-risk profile, to promote early detection of cervical cancer
Transvaginal ultrasound	Screening for pelvic pathology to assist in diagnosing endometrial cancers	Allows measurement of endometrial thickness to determine if endometrial biopsy is needed for postmenopausal bleeding	• Review the risk factors for the development of endometrial cancer and reason for this screening test • Assist in preparing the client for this examination
CA-125	Nonspecific blood test used as a tumor marker	Elevation of marker suggests malignancy but is not specific to ovarian cancer	• Review risk factors for ovarian cancer and explain that a series of diagnostic tests may be performed (transvaginal ultrasound, CT scan, CA-125) to assist in the diagnosis and treatment plan • Elevated marker levels are not specific to ovarian cancer; they can be elevated in other types of cancer

Adapted from American Cancer Society [ACS]. (2015b). *American Cancer Society guidelines for the early detection of cancer.* Retrieved from http://www.cancer.org/Healthy/FindCancerEarly/CancerScreeningGuidelines/american-cancer-society-guidelines-for-the-early-detection-of-cancer; Centers for Disease Control and Prevention [CDC]. (2015b). Cancer prevention and control. Retrieved from http://www.cdc.gov/cancer/dcpc/prevention/other.htm; and National Cancer Institute [NCI]. (2015c). *General cancer prevention.* Retrieved from http://www.cancer.gov/cancertopics/prevention#General+Cancer+Prevention+Information

Nursing Diagnoses and Related Interventions

Upon completion of a thorough assessment, the nurse might identify several nursing diagnoses, including:

- Deficient knowledge
- Disturbed body image
- Anxiety
- Fear
- Pain

Nursing goals, interventions, and evaluation for the woman with reproductive cancer are based on the nursing diagnoses. Nursing Care Plan 8.1 (at the end of the chapter) may be used as a guide in planning nursing care for the woman with reproductive cancer. It should be individualized based on the woman's symptoms and needs.

Nurses have traditionally served as advocates in the health care arena and should continue to be on the forefront of health education and diagnosis, acting as leaders in the fight against cancer. Over half a million women in the United States will be diagnosed with cancer this year alone and more than half will die of it (Siegel, Miller, & Jemal, 2015). The public needs to know that not only are these deaths preventable, but many of the cancers themselves are preventable. Nurses need to work to improve the availability and quality of cancer-screening services, making them accessible to underserved and socioeconomically disadvantaged clients. Through a unified effort by health care providers, health policy experts, government agencies, health insurance companies, the media, educational institutions, and women themselves, along with consistency and continuity, nurses can offer quality care to all women with cancer.

Educating to Prevent Cancer

Globally, there are nearly 13 million new cases of cancer and 8 million deaths from cancer each year. The most important cause of cancer is tobacco, which causes 30% of cancer deaths. Dietary factors, including obesity, are estimated to cause around 25% of cancer deaths, and alcohol about 6% of cancer deaths. All of these factors associated with cancer are preventable (Key, 2015). Nurses need to provide clients with information to help prevent disease and enhance quality of life. Educate women about the importance of consistent and timely screenings to identify cancer early. Emphasize the importance of having an annual pelvic examination. Also stress the need for follow-up screenings as recommended. Provide clients with information if further diagnostic testing is required. Nurses also play a key role in promoting cancer awareness, prevention, and control. Advocate improving the availability of cancer-screening services and work to provide public education about risk factors for cancer.

Nurses can be instrumental in helping women to identify and change behaviors that put them at risk for various reproductive tract cancers (Teaching Guidelines 8.1). Do not limit your interventions to providing preventive education only: inform women about the consequences of doing nothing about their conditions and what the long-range outcomes might be without treatment. For example, stress the importance of visiting a health care provider if certain signs and symptoms appear:

- Blood in a bowel movement is considered abnormal
- Unusual vaginal discharge or chronic vulvar itching
- Persistent abdominal bloating or constipation
- Irregular vaginal bleeding
- Persistent low backache not related to standing
- Elevated or discolored vulvar lesions
- Bleeding after menopause
- Pain or bleeding after sexual intercourse

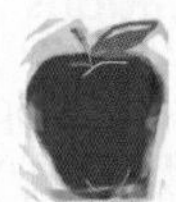

Teaching Guidelines 8.1

REDUCING YOUR RISK FOR CANCER

- Do not smoke; smoking is linked to lung cancer development.
- Drink alcohol only in moderation (no more than one drink daily).
- Be physically active daily.
- Eat a healthy diet.
- Stay current with immunizations.
- Use a condom with every sexual encounter.
- Reach and maintain a healthy weight.
- Take preventive medicines if needed.
- Get recommended screening tests:
- Body mass index (BMI) to identify obesity
- Mammogram every 1 to 2 years starting at age 40
- Pap smear every 1 to 3 years if sexually active, between the ages of 21 and 65
- Cholesterol checked annually starting at age 45
- Blood pressure checked at least every 2 years
- Diabetes test if hypertensive or hypercholesterolemia
- Check for STIs if sexually active

Adapted from Agency for Healthcare Research and Quality. (2014). *Cancer screening and treatment in women: Recent findings.* Retrieved from http://www.ahrq.gov/research/findings/factsheets/women/cancerwom/; American Cancer Society [ACS]. (2015b). *American Cancer Society guidelines for the early detection of cancer.* Retrieved from http://www.cancer.org/Healthy/FindCancerEarly/CancerScreeningGuidelines/american-cancer-society-guidelines-for-the-early-detection-of-cancer; Mayo Clinic. (2015). *Cancer prevention: 7 steps to reduce your risk.* Retrieved from http://www.mayoclinic.org/cancer-prevention/art-20044816; National Cancer Institute [NCI]. (2015c). *General cancer prevention.* Retrieved from http://www.cancer.gov/cancertopics/prevention#General+Cancer+Prevention+Information; World Health Organization. (2015). Cancer prevention and control. Retrieved from http://www.who.int/nmh/a5816/en/

Teaching the Client About Her Diagnosis

Provide information about tests that may be required to confirm or rule out the diagnosis. Review with the woman what she has been told about her diagnosis and her understanding of her condition. It is not unusual for the woman to hear the diagnosis and then become overwhelmed by the thought of cancer, blocking out whatever is said after that. Answer any questions she may have. Go slowly and repeat the information as necessary. Use written materials to explain and reinforce the teaching. Provide information about her condition and recommended therapies. For example, if a client is undergoing surgery, discuss postoperative issues such as incision care, pain, and activity level. Instruct the client on health maintenance activities after treatment, and inform her and her family about available support resources.

Providing Emotional Support

Once the diagnosis is made, provide the woman and her family with emotional support. Validate the client's feelings and provide realistic hope, using a nonjudgmental approach and therapeutic communication skills during all interactions. Nurses can be invaluable when assisting women who are coping with the uncertainty of their future by providing positive communication and support. Nurses need to focus on the physical, psychosocial, and economic concerns, from diagnosis through treatment and, if applicable, until the end of life, for all of the women for whom they care. Individualize the care based on the client's cultural traditions and beliefs, as explained in the following section.

ENSURING CULTURALLY COMPETENT CANCER CARE

Cultural diversity in America is increasing, and as diverse cultures interact, conflicts inevitably ensue. These conflicts can affect health care outcomes. Providing culturally competent cancer care can improve outcomes and decrease disparities in care. If nurses are to meet the needs of ethnically diverse populations, they must be culturally sensitive, appreciative of differing health beliefs and practices, and very flexible in the way they approach health care. It is we who must adapt, expand, and learn.

Nurses have the opportunity to learn about diverse cultures, religions, and faith traditions that support clients and families during their cancer journey and while facing a serious life-limiting illness. Nurses' care practices embrace all clients with whom they come in contact and, by having a better understanding of diverse groups, nurses can build trust in clients seeking oncology care needs that range from detection to diagnosis and treatment possibly through palliative care and end of life.

Be aware of the client's cultural background, religion, migration history, degree of acculturation, living conditions, educational level, and legal status, because each of these factors can affect the client's understanding of her diagnosis and the eventual outcome. A woman's reaction to a cancer diagnosis and her decisions about treatment are influenced by an individual's cultural values and how the community views cancer. A diagnosis of cancer carries deep physical, psychosocial, and cultural implications. Sensitive cross-cultural communication and cultural competence are vital for all nurses to deliver equal care to all cancer clients. Nurses need to understand the disparities and the influence of those disparities on health outcomes. Women with cancer reflect the demographic changes occurring in the United States and represent increasing differences in culture, religion, socioeconomic status, race, and lifestyle. Through embracing and learning from these differences, nurses become stronger care providers (Surbone, 2015).

In some cultures, sharing news of a serious illness like cancer is considered disrespectful and impolite. For example, some Europeans view such sharing as inhumane; the Asian culture views a cancer diagnosis as unnecessarily cruel. The Chinese, out of respect for aging family members, withhold discussions of serious illness to avoid causing unnecessary anxieties (Lofters, 2015). Integrate this knowledge in your care to ensure a culturally competent approach.

Take Note!

When a diagnosis of cancer is made, assessing an individual's strengths and weaknesses from a cultural perspective will help the nurse to provide culturally competent care.

As life becomes increasingly multilingual, multicultural, and multireligious, learning about clients' values and cultural beliefs becomes challenging. Be willing to learn about client preferences; doing so promotes caring and nurturing.

SUPPORTING THE PREGNANT WOMAN WITH CANCER

Pregnancy complicated by cancer is relatively rare, occurring in 1 out of every 1,000 pregnancies (Cancer.Net, 2015a). The incidence is increasing because women in Western societies are tending to delay childbearing to the third and fourth decade of life; this phenomenon is going to be encountered more often in the future by nurses. The most frequent malignancies diagnosed during pregnancy are breast cancer, **cervical cancer**, hematologic malignancies (lymphomas and acute leukemia), and melanoma. Breast cancer is the most common cancer diagnosed in pregnant women which affects approximately 1 in 3,000 pregnancies. Less common tumors during pregnancy include gastrointestinal, ovarian, urologic, and lung cancers (Amant et al., 2015).

Theoretically, changes in the mother's immune system during pregnancy can increase the risk of malignancy because cell-mediated immunity, which is suppressed in pregnant women, normally protects against cancerous tumors (Kim & Chu, 2015). Some research has hinted at an increased rate of progression and decreased survival times in women who develop breast and cervical cancer and then become pregnant, but this generally has not been validated by research studies. With the cooperation of multidisciplinary teams, treatment of cancer during pregnancy with normal fetal outcome is feasible (Andersson et al., 2015).

Ovarian cancer during pregnancy is rare because the disease typically occurs in older women. Because most pregnant women receive frequent medical care, including pelvic examinations, most ovarian cancers in pregnant women are found at early stages; this carries a good prognosis for both the mother and the newborn. The presence of ascites indicates advanced disease (de Haan, Verheecke, & Amant, 2015).

Endometrial cancer is the most common neoplasia of the female reproductive system, with the highest incidence among uterine malignancies. It is rarely associated with pregnancy. Adenocarcinoma associated with pregnancy is typically endometrioid, focal, well differentiated, and minimally invasive. Active treatment of endometrial cancer is incompatible with continuation of the pregnancy. Since routine screening for endometrial cancer is currently not recommended in the general population, few cases would be detected in the relatively young pregnant population (Cancer in Pregnancy, 2015a). Cervical cancer is more common in the pregnant population than other reproductive malignancies, and it can affect the woman's health status and the pregnancy. Approximately 30% of women diagnosed with cervical cancer are in their reproductive years, whereas 3% of cervical cancers are diagnosed during pregnancy (Cancer in Pregnancy, 2015b). Management of cervical cancer during pregnancy depends on the following factors:

- Stage of the disease (and the tumor size)
- Nodal status
- Histologic subtype of the tumor
- Term of the pregnancy
- Whether the client wishes to continue her pregnancy
- Woman's desire for future fertility

In women with early-stage disease and absence of nodal involvement who are diagnosed during the first two trimesters of pregnancy, there is an increasing tendency to preserve the pregnancy while awaiting fetal maturity. The birth (when the fetal maturity is attained) should be performed using a cesarean section (ACS, 2015c). Treatment decisions are influenced by the stage of the cancer, the histologic type, the stage of the pregnancy, and the client's wishes. Both maternal and fetal safety and well-being have to be taken into account. Termination of pregnancy is not indicated in all cases. Pregnancy preservation in tumors diagnosed during early gestation is feasible in carefully selected cases. Discussion with the client and her family is essential and treatment has to be individualized (ACS, 2015c).

Nurses caring for young clients with cervical cancer must be aware of the surgical fertility preservation options, which clients are candidates for these surgeries, and the options for future assisted reproductive technology. Nurses need to be able to coordinate care for these clients with gynecologic oncologists and reproductive endocrinologists in order to facilitate optimal outcomes.

Women diagnosed with any malignancy during pregnancy must confront the reality of the disease and its impact on their future fertility and live with the risk of recurrence. The prognosis for a pregnant woman with cancer is often the same as other women of the same age with the same type of cancer (Cancer.Net, 2015a). The wishes of the pregnant woman and her family are of paramount importance when making decisions about continuing the pregnancy and undergoing cancer treatment. Some women will decide to terminate the pregnancy for the sake of their own health; others will undergo treatment during the pregnancy to preserve the life of the unborn child. Regardless of the woman's decision, provide support, hope, and education during treatment, birth, and beyond.

OVARIAN CANCER

Ovarian cancer is malignant neoplastic growth of the ovary (Fig. 8.1). It is the ninth most common cancer among women and the fifth most common cause of cancer deaths for women in the United States. It accounts for more deaths than any other cancer of the reproductive system (ACS, 2015d). A woman's risk of getting invasive ovarian cancer in her lifetime is about 1 in 75. Her lifetime chance of dying from invasive ovarian cancer is about 1 in 100 (ACS, 2015d). This cancer mainly develops in older women. About half of the women who are diagnosed with ovarian cancer are 63 years or older. It is more common in White women than African-American women (ACS, 2015d).

The most important variable influencing the prognosis is the extent of the disease. Survival depends on the stage of the tumor, grade of differentiation, gross findings at surgery, amount of residual tumor after

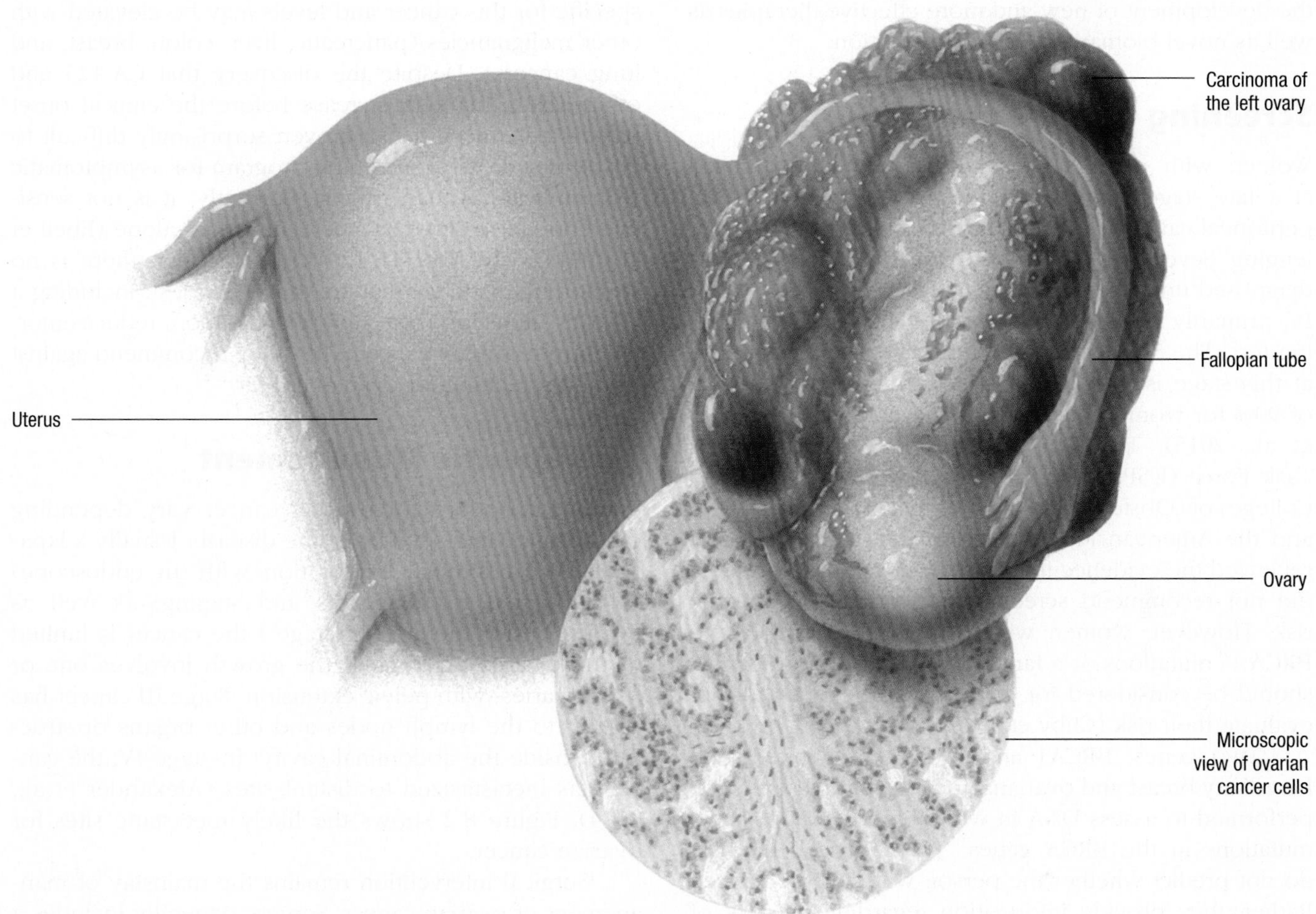

FIGURE 8.1 Ovarian cancer. (Asset provided by Anatomical Chart Co.)

surgery, and effectiveness of any adjunct treatment postoperatively. Many women with ovarian cancer will experience recurrence despite best efforts to eradicate the cancer through surgery, radiation, or chemotherapy to eliminate residual tumor cells. The likelihood of long-term survival in the event of recurrence is dismal (Matsumoto, Onada, & Yaegashi, 2015). The 5-year survival rates (the percentage of women who live at least 5 years after their diagnosis) are shown in Table 8.1 according to stage.

Pathophysiology

Ovarian cancer, the cause of which is unknown, can originate from different cell types. Most ovarian cancers are thought to originate in the ovarian epithelium. New insights now propose a pivotal role for the fallopian tube during ovarian cancer pathogenesis. Increasing evidence suggests that serous ovarian cancer originates from the fimbriated distal end of the fallopian tube, whereas the ovary gets only involved at a later stage. These represent 50% to 60% of all epithelial ovarian cancers. Based on this finding, a post-reproductive salpingectomy deserves consideration as a prophylactic intervention that may confer protection against an often deadly disease (Poole et al., 2015).

Tumors usually present as solid masses that have spread beyond the ovary and seeded into the peritoneum prior to diagnosis. Thorough understanding of the true pathogenesis of this cancer's origin could lead to

TABLE 8.1 FIVE-YEAR SURVIVAL RATES FOR OVARIAN CANCER

Stage	Five-Year Relative Survival Rates
I	80–94%
II	57–76%
III	34–45%
IV	18%

Adapted from American Cancer Society [ACS]. (2015o). *Survival rates for ovarian cancer by stage.* Retrieved from http://www.cancer.org/cancer/ovariancancer/detailedguide/ovarian-cancer-survival-rates

the development of new and more effective therapies as well as novel biomarkers in early detection.

Screening and Diagnosis

Women with ovarian cancer are typically diagnosed at a late stage, when the cancer has spread into the peritoneal cavity and complete surgical removal is challenging. Seventy-five percent of ovarian cancers are not diagnosed until the cancer has advanced to stage III or IV, primarily because there is still no adequate screening test. The 5-year survival time for women diagnosed at this stage is 30%, in contrast with a 5-year survival of 90% for women diagnosed at an early stage (Wright et al., 2015). The United States Preventive Services Task Force (USPSTF) (2015), along with the American College of Obstetricians and Gynecologists (ACOG), and the American Medical Association (AMA) recently reviewed the evidence for ovarian cancer screening and did not recommend screening for women at average risk. However, women with increased risk related to BRCA ½ mutations or a family history of ovarian cancer should be considered for genetic counseling to further evaluate their risk (Cliby et al., 2015).

Two genes, BRCA1 and BRCA2, are linked with hereditary breast and ovarian cancers. Blood tests can be performed to assess DNA in white blood cells to detect mutations in the BRCA genes. These genetic markers do not predict whether the person will develop cancer. Rather, they provide information regarding the risk of developing cancer: a woman who is BRCA positive may have up to an 80% chance of developing breast cancer and a 40% chance of developing ovarian cancer (Liede, Sun, & Narod, 2015).

To assist in screening, researchers have developed an ovarian cancer symptom index that includes pelvic and abdominal pain, urinary frequency and urgency, increased abdominal size (bloating), and difficulty eating (feeling full). But this symptom index is not much help in detecting the disease early, as these symptoms tend to go unrecognized, leading to delays in diagnosis. When the presentation of such symptoms triggers a medical evaluation for ovarian cancer, the disease is diagnosed in only 1 in 100 women. The NCI reports that the present symptom index has a "low positive predictive value," especially for early-stage disease discovery (NCI, 2015d).

Specific clinical guidelines for ovarian cancer screening have not been developed, so the disease is often not diagnosed until it has metastasized. The USPSTF recommends against routine screening for ovarian cancer with serum CA-125 or transvaginal ultrasound because earlier detection would have a small effect, at best, on mortality. CA-125 is a biologic tumor marker associated with ovarian cancer. Although levels are elevated in many women with ovarian cancer, CA-125 is not specific for this cancer and levels may be elevated with other malignancies (pancreatic, liver, colon, breast, and lung cancers). Despite the discovery that CA-125 and other serum markers increase before the clinical onset of ovarian cancer, it has proven surprisingly difficult to devise a successful screening program for asymptomatic women with ovarian cancer. Currently, it is not sensitive enough to serve as a screening tool alone (Ebell et al., 2015). The USPSTF (2015) reports that there is no supporting evidence that any screening test, including a CA-125, ultrasound, or pelvic examination, reduces mortality from ovarian cancer. Thus they recommend against routine screening for ovarian cancer.

Therapeutic Management

Treatment options for ovarian cancer vary depending on the stage and severity of the disease. Usually a laparoscopy (abdominal exploration with an endoscope) is performed for diagnosis and staging, as well as evaluation for therapy. In stage I the cancer is limited to the ovaries. In stage II the growth involves one or both ovaries, with pelvic extension. Stage III cancer has spread to the lymph nodes and other organs or structures inside the abdominal cavity. In stage IV, the cancer has metastasized to distant sites (Alexander et al., 2014). Figure 8.2 shows the likely metastatic sites for ovarian cancer.

Surgical intervention remains the mainstay of management of ovarian cancer. Surgery generally includes a total abdominal hysterectomy, bilateral salpingo-oophorectomy, peritoneal biopsies, omentectomy (excision of all or part of the omentum, which is a sheet of fat

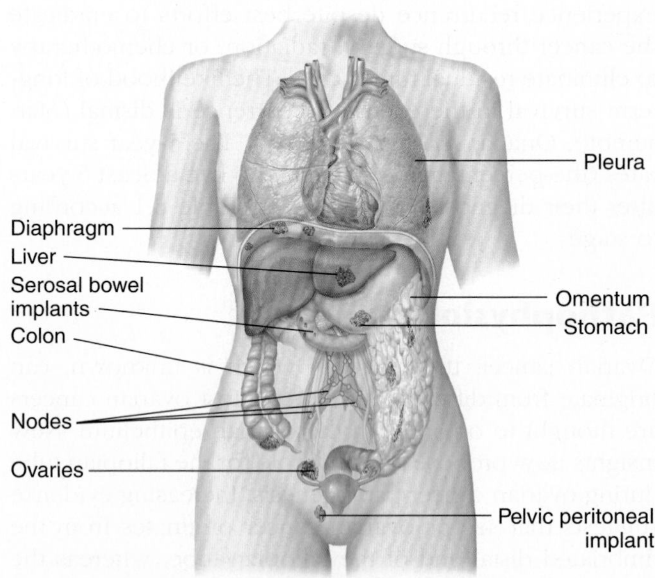

FIGURE 8.2 Common metastatic sites for ovarian cancer. (Asset provided by Anatomical Chart Co.)

covered by the peritoneum that protects the abdominal structures), and pelvic para-aortic lymph node sampling to evaluate cancer extension (Nick et al., 2015). Because most women are diagnosed with advanced-stage ovarian cancer, aggressive management involving debulking or cytoreductive surgery is commonly performed. This surgery involves resecting all visible tumors from the peritoneum, taking peritoneal biopsies, sampling lymph nodes, and removing all reproductive organs and the omentum. This aggressive surgery has been shown to improve long-term survival rates.

Additional therapy with radiation may be warranted. Chemotherapy is recommended for all stages of ovarian cancer. Intraperitoneal chemotherapy, combined with surgery, has produced encouraging results for overall survivals at acceptable morbidity and mortality rates. Despite all of these therapies, virtually the only agreement about treatment for advanced disease is that surgery and chemotherapy play a role, and that current treatment is effective in far too many women (Helm, 2015a).

Nursing Assessment

Ovarian cancers are considered the worst of all the gynecologic malignancies, primarily because they develop slowly and remain silent without symptoms until the cancer is far advanced. It has been described as the "overlooked disease" or "silent killer" because women and health care providers often ignore or rationalize early symptoms. For example, women may attribute gastrointestinal problems to stress and midlife changes. However, these vague complaints may precede more obvious symptoms by months. The most common early symptoms include abdominal bloating, early satiety, fatigue, vague abdominal pain, urinary frequency, diarrhea or constipation, malaise, and unexplained weight loss or gain. The later symptoms include anorexia, dyspepsia, ascites, a palpable abdominal mass, pelvic pain, and back pain (Goldstein et al., 2015).

Obtain a thorough history of the woman's symptoms, including their onset, duration, and frequency. Review the woman's history for risk factors such as:

- Nulliparity
- Early menarche (before 12 years old)
- Late menopause (after 55 years old)
- Increasing age (after menopause)
- High-fat diet
- Obesity
- Persistent ovulation over time
- First-degree relative with ovarian cancer
- Genetics (women of Ashkenazi Jewish decent)
- Use of perineal talcum powder or hygiene sprays
- Older than 30 years at first pregnancy
- Positive BRCA1 and BRCA2 mutations
- Personal history of breast, bladder, or colon cancer
- Hormone replacement therapy (HRT) for more than 10 years
- Infertility (CDC, 2015c)

Perform a complete physical examination. Inspect the abdomen, noting any distention or bloating. Palpate the abdomen. Be alert for a mass or pain on palpation. Anticipate further testing to confirm the diagnosis.

Nursing Management

The complexities of ovarian cancer make a multidisciplinary approach necessary for optimal management. With the subtle nature and high risk of recurrence and mortality of this condition, most women find it an emotionally exhausting and devastating experience. The presence of hope is essential for women at the time of the diagnosis; they want to believe in being cured and able to continue their life as usual with loved ones, friends, and relatives. Still, the newly received cancer diagnosis makes women oscillate between hope and hopelessness, between positive expectations of getting cured and frightening feelings of the disease taking command. Nurses are invaluable resources in inspiring clients to find hope in life when diagnosed with cancer. Nursing management needs to focus on measures to promote early detection, educate the woman about the disease and its treatments, and provide emotional support. Nurses should show a positive attitude that communicates understanding and reassurance.

Promoting Early Detection

Nurses need to ensure that women are aware of the risk factors for ovarian cancer. Urge women not to dismiss seemingly innocuous symptoms as "just a part of aging." Encourage women to describe such nonspecific complaints at health visits.

Assess the woman's family and personal history for risk factors and encourage genetic testing for women with affected family members. Outline screening guidelines for women with hereditary cancer syndrome and inform women at high risk about the appropriate screening strategies.

Urge women to have yearly bimanual pelvic examinations and a transvaginal ultrasound to allow identification of ovarian masses in their early stages. After menopause, a mass on an ovary is not a cyst: physiologic cysts can arise only from a follicle that has not ruptured or from the cystic degeneration of the corpus luteum. Ovarian cancer is not always silent, and may manifest with several vague gastrointestinal symptoms. Although screening the general population is not recommended, nurses need to know what factors place women at high risk and really listen to women's complaints to detect this type of cancer before it becomes advanced.

Take Note!

A small ovarian "cyst" found on ultrasound in an asymptomatic postmenopausal woman should arouse suspicion. Any mass or ovary palpated in a postmenopausal woman should be considered cancerous until proven otherwise (Helm, 2015b).

Educating the Client

Education is a major focus of nursing care. This teaching involves risk reduction and health promotion. Teach the woman about risk reduction strategies; for instance, pregnancy, use of oral contraceptives, and breast-feeding reduce the risk of ovarian cancer. Instruct women to avoid using talc and hygiene sprays on their genitals. Review the lifetime risks related to *BRCA1* and *BRCA2* genes and options available should the woman test positive for these genes. Help to promote community awareness of ovarian cancer by educating the public about risk-reducing behaviors. See research on reproductive cancer risk factor (Evidence-Based Practice 8.1).

Instruct the woman about the importance of healthy lifestyles. Stress the importance of maintaining a healthy weight to reduce risk. Encourage women to eat a low-fat diet. Factors associated with a reduced risk of ovarian cancer include the use of oral contraceptives for 3 years or longer, pregnancy and breast-feeding before the age of 30, bilateral tubal ligation, and removal of the ovaries (Memorial Sloan Kettering Cancer Center, 2015).

For the woman who is diagnosed with ovarian cancer, describe in simple terms the tests, treatment modalities, and follow-up needed. For example, if the woman will be having surgery, provide thorough teaching about what to expect before, during, and after surgery. Outline treatment options and the implications of choices. Assist the woman and her family to decipher the myriad of information related to staging, tests, and treatments. Teach the woman about additional treatment measures, such as radiation therapy or chemotherapy, including how to handle the common adverse effects of treatment.

Supporting the Client and Family

The diagnosis of ovarian cancer, like any cancer, can be overwhelming. In addition, the treatments and their effects can be highly stressful, both physically and emotionally. Provide one-to-one support for women facing treatment for ovarian cancer. Ovarian cancer involves the reproductive system, which has a direct impact on the woman's view of herself. Encourage open discussion of sexuality and the impact of cancer. Listen and support the woman and her family as they try to cope with this disease. By being aware of women's individual needs and different coping strategies, nurses can improve support to women in this vulnerable situation.

EVIDENCE-BASED PRACTICE 8.1

DOES OVARIAN STIMULATION FOR IVF INCREASE GYNECOLOGIC CANCER RISK? A SYSTEMATIC REVIEW AND META-ANALYSIS

STUDY

Drugs to stimulate ovulation have been widely used for various types of subfertility since the early 1960s, and their use has increased in recent years. The use of assisted reproductive techniques is increasing, but the possible link between fertility drugs and reproductive cancer remains controversial. Subfertile women are commonly exposed to these agents, which may be administered at high doses for long periods of time during treatment for subfertility. There is uncertainty about the safety of these drugs and the potential risk of causing cancers associated with their use. The objective of this study was to evaluate the risk of reproductive cancer in women previously treated with ovulation-stimulating drugs for infertility.

Findings

A systematic review and meta-analysis was conducted. Clinical trials that examined the association between ovarian stimulation for IVF and gynecologic cancers were included. Twelve cohort studies with 178,396 women exposed to IVF were included. The meat-analysis found no significant association between ovarian stimulation for IVF and increased ovarian, endometrial, cervical, and breast cancer risk. Ovarian stimulation for IVF, therefore, does not increase the gynecologic risk, whether hormone-dependent endometrial and breast cancer risk or non–hormone-dependent ovarian and cervical cancer. This study found no convincing evidence of an increased risk of reproductive cancer with fertility drug treatment.

Nursing Implications

Nurses can use the information from this study to reassure women that having experienced infertility and undergone in vitro fertilization treatments in the past are not increasing their risk of having reproductive cancer later in life. When women are trying to decide to undergo fertility treatment using drug therapy, it can be very anxiety producing for them as well as their partners. Knowing that in vitro fertilization treatment will not increase their risk of reproductive cancer as they age based on earlier exposure to ovulation-stimulating drug therapy can reduce their anxiety regarding their decision.

Adapted from Li, Y., Zhao, J., Zhang, Q., & Wang, Y. (2015). Does ovarian stimulation for IVF increase gynecological cancer risk? A systematic review and meta-analysis. *Reproductive BioMedicine Online, 31*(1), 20–29.

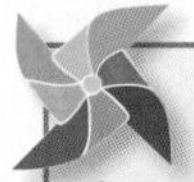

Consider This

I felt I was a lucky woman because I had been in remission from breast cancer for 12 years, and I had been given the gift of life to share with my beloved family. Recently I became ill with stomach problems: pain, indigestion, bloating, and nausea. My doctor treated me for gastric reflux disease, but the symptoms persisted. I then was referred to a gastroenterologist, a urologist, and then a gynecologist, who did an ultrasound, which was negative. I received reassurance from all three that there was nothing wrong with me. As time went by, I experienced more pain, more symptoms, and increased frustration. Six months after seeing all three specialists, a repeat ultrasound revealed I had ovarian cancer, and I needed surgery as soon as possible. I underwent a complete hysterectomy and my surgeon found I was in stage III. Since then, I have undergone chemotherapy and participated in a clinical cancer study that wasn't successful for me, and now I am facing the fact that I am going to die soon.

Thoughts: This woman has tried everything to save her life, but, alas, time has run out for her with advanced ovarian cancer. Women diagnosed with breast cancer are at a significant risk for developing ovarian cancer later in life. Of the string of doctors she saw, one has to ponder why none ordered more extensive testing, given her history of breast cancer. We are haunted with the question: If they had, would she be in stage III now? We will never know.

Encourage the use of appropriate coping strategies to allow for the best quality of life. Try to restore hope to women with ovarian cancer, and stress treatment compliance. Nurses should not forget about the family caregivers who need help with managing emotions about prognosis, balancing their own and the client's needs, work, and decision-making when there is uncertainty. If appropriate, encourage participation in clinical trials to offer hope for all women. Continue to offer support to the woman and her family members as they experience sadness and grief.

ENDOMETRIAL CANCER

Endometrial cancer (also known as uterine cancer) is malignant neoplastic growth of the uterine lining. It is the fourth most common gynecologic malignancy and accounts for 6% of all cancers in women in the United States or 1 in 37 women. The NCI (2015e) estimates that about 54,870 new cases will be diagnosed in women in 2015 and that approximately 10,170 of these women will die. Endometrial cancer is responsible for over 75,000 deaths annually among women worldwide (Siegel, Miller, & Jemal, 2015). It is uncommon before the age of 55, but as women age, their risk of endometrial cancer increases. Approximately 80% of these malignancies are carcinomas of the endometrium. Because endometrial cancer is usually diagnosed in the early stages, it has a better prognosis than cervical or ovarian cancer (ACS, 2015e).

The increasing incidence and prevalence of endometrial cancer can be explained by the increase in life expectancy, increased caloric intake, increased obesity rates, infertility, null parity (never bearing children), older age of first pregnancy, and long-term use of unopposed estrogens for HRT. Protection against endometrial cancer includes increased parity, daily physical activity, use of combined oral contraceptives, and increased age of women at last childbirth (Schmid et al., 2015).

Pathophysiology

Two mechanisms are believed to be involved in the development of endometrial cancer. A history of exposure to unopposed estrogen is the cause in approximately 80% of women. Those that are spontaneous and are unrelated to estrogen or endometrial hyperplasia represent the other 20% of endometrial cancers. There has been an increase in incidence over the past several decades associated with and increased use of estrogen replacement therapy (without progestin) and obesity (adipose fat converts androstenedione to estrone, thereby increasing circulating estrogen levels) (Temple, 2015).

Endometrial cancer may originate in a polyp or in a diffuse multifocal pattern. The pattern of spread partially depends on the degree of cellular differentiation. Well-differentiated tumors tend to limit their spread to the surface of the endometrium. Metastatic spread occurs in a characteristic pattern and most commonly involves the lungs, inguinal and supraclavicular nodes, liver, bones, brain, and vagina (NCI, 2015f). Early tumor growth is characterized by friable and spontaneous bleeding. Later tumor growth is characterized by myometrial invasion and growth toward the cervix (Fig. 8.3).

Adenocarcinoma of the endometrium is typically preceded by hyperplasia. Carcinoma in situ is found only on the endometrial surface. Type I carcinomas, the most common, begin as endometrial hyperplasia and progress to carcinomas. Giving estrogen preparations without progestin for HRT leads to an increased risk for endometrial cancer. Type I is generally found at an earlier stage and treatment results are more favorable.

Unlike type I endometrial carcinoma, type II carcinomas appear spontaneously, are associated with a poorly differentiated cell type, and have a poor prognosis. They account for less than 10% of all endometrial cancers but contribute to the majority of all endometrial deaths. This type is unrelated to estrogen or endometrial hyperplasia (ACS, 2015f).

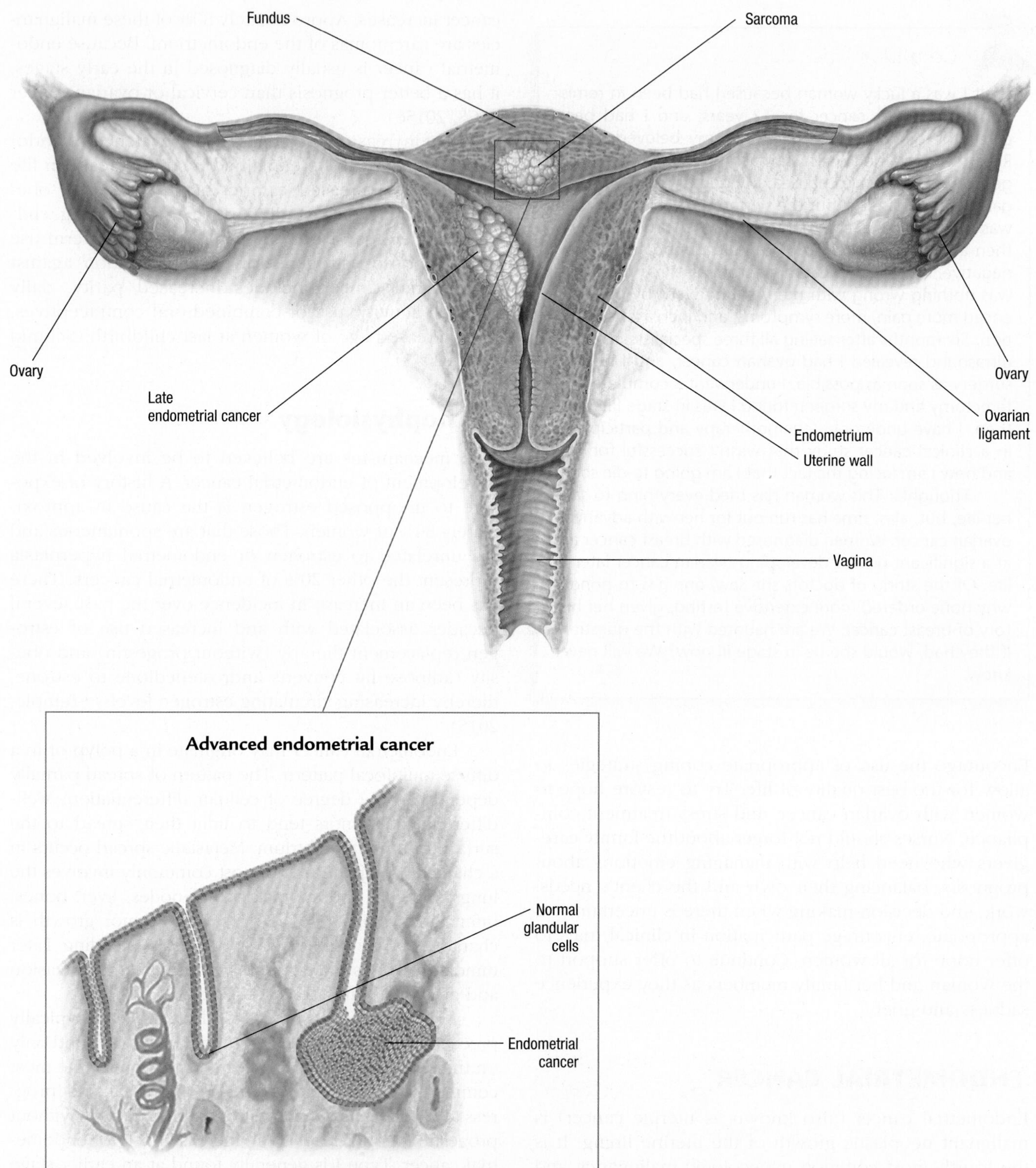

FIGURE 8.3 Progression of endometrial cancer. (Image 1 provided by Anatomical Chart Co.)

Remember Carmella, the woman with postmenopausal bleeding? In postmenopausal women, any bleeding is abnormal and warrants further assessment. What testing would the nurse anticipate as being ordered to confirm the diagnosis? What would be the nurse's role during this testing?

Screening and Diagnosis

There is no specific screening test currently available to detect endometrial cancer. Screening for endometrial cancer is not routinely done because it is not practical or cost effective. The ACS (2015f) recommends that women be informed about the risks and symptoms of endometrial cancer at the onset of menopause and strongly encouraged to report any unexpected bleeding or spotting to their health care provider. A pelvic examination is frequently normal in the early stages of the disease. Changes in the size, shape, or consistency of the uterus or its surrounding support structures may exist when the disease is more advanced.

During the past two decades, the role of ultrasound in the evaluation of postmenopausal bleeding has changed markedly, from little or no role to a major role today. In the intervening years, numerous studies have shown that ultrasound is at least as sensitive as endometrial biopsy for endometrial cancer and that ultrasound can reliably exclude cancer without the need for biopsy in some women with postmenopausal bleeding. The depth of myometrium is an important diagnostic factor. In particular, numerous studies have shown that women with an endometrial thickness of 4 mm or less have an extremely low likelihood of endometrial cancer and thus do not need to undergo endometrial biopsy. Ultrasound can also help in the selection of an appropriate biopsy technique. In a woman with postmenopausal bleeding and a thick endometrium, a sonohysterogram can determine whether the endometrium is diffusely thick or has focal areas of thickening. With diffuse thickening, an endometrial biopsy is appropriate. When one or more focal areas of thickening are present, hysteroscopic biopsy is likely to be the better choice. Typically, the noninvasive ultrasound is done first before an invasive endometrial biopsy is attempted (Dueholm et al., 2015).

Transvaginal ultrasound can be used to evaluate the endometrial cavity and measure the thickness of the endometrial lining. It can be used to detect endometrial hyperplasia. If the endometrium measures less than 4 mm, then the client is at low risk for malignancy. Large prospective studies have shown that an endometrial thickness of ≤4 mm on transvaginal ultrasound in postmenopausal women with bleeding has a low risk of malignancy. Thus, in postmenopausal clients with bleeding, biopsy is not indicted when endometrial thickness is ≤4 mm, thereby avoiding invasive diagnostics (Wong et al., 2015).

Endometrial biopsy is an office procedure that is also one of the first steps in the diagnosis of endometrial cancer in a woman with postmenopausal bleeding. The biopsy is obtained through the use of an endometrial suction catheter that is inserted through the cervix into the uterine cavity and a tissue sample is taken. The sensitivity and specificity of the biopsy procedure tend to be in the range of 95% for detection of endometrial cancer or other pathologies (King et al., 2015).

As indicated earlier, staging is the process of looking at all of the information the doctors have learned about the tumor to determine how much the cancer may have spread. The stage of an endometrial cancer is the most important factor in choosing a treatment plan. It can spread *locally* to other parts of the uterus or *regionally* to nearby lymph nodes. The regional lymph nodes are found in the pelvis and farther away along the aorta. Finally, the cancer can spread (*metastasize*) to distant lymph nodes or organs such as lung, liver, bone, brain, and others.

In stage I, the tumor is confined to the corpus uteri. In stage II, it has spread to the cervix, but not outside the uterus. In stage III, it has spread locally and regionally. In stage IV, it has invaded the bladder mucosa, bowel with distant metastases to the lungs, liver, and bone (International Federation of Gynecology & Obstetrics, 2015).

Therapeutic Management

Typically, the stage of the disease directs treatment. It usually involves surgery with adjunct therapy based on pathologic findings. Surgery most often involves removal of the uterus (hysterectomy) and the fallopian tubes and ovaries (salpingo-oophorectomy). Removal of the fallopian tubes and ovaries is recommended because tumor cells spread early to the ovaries, and any dormant cancer cells could be stimulated to grow by ovarian estrogen. In more advanced cancers, radiation and chemotherapy are used as adjuncts to surgery. Routine surveillance intervals for follow-up care are typically every 3 to 4 months for the first 2 years, since 85% of recurrences occur in the first 3 years after diagnosis (Brennan et al., 2015).

Nursing Assessment

Obtain a thorough history from the woman, ascertaining her primary complaint. Most commonly, the major initial symptom of endometrial cancer is abnormal and painless vaginal bleeding. Obtain a menstrual history and inquire if the woman is taking any hormones. Also ascertain if she has a personal or family history of breast, ovarian, or colon cancer. These key pieces of information will assist in identifying the woman at high risk for endometrial cancer.

Take Note!

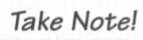

Any episode of bright-red bleeding that occurs after menopause should be investigated. Abnormal uterine bleeding is rarely the result of uterine malignancy in a young woman, but in the postmenopausal woman it should be regarded with suspicion.

Also review the woman's history for any risk factors, including:

- Nulliparity
- Obesity (more than 50 lb overweight)
- Liver disease
- Infertility
- Diabetes mellitus
- Hypertension
- History of pelvic radiation
- Polycystic ovary syndrome
- Early menarche (before 12 years old)
- High-fat diet
- Use of prolonged exogenous unopposed estrogen with an intact uterus
- Endometrial hyperplasia
- Family history of endometrial cancer
- Personal history of hereditary nonpolyposis colon cancer
- Personal history of breast, colon, or ovarian cancer
- History of uterine fibroids
- Late onset of menopause (after age 52 years)
- Tamoxifen use
- Chronic anovulation (Moses, 2015)

Assess the woman for additional manifestations, such as dyspareunia, low back pain, purulent genital discharge, dysuria, pelvic pain, weight loss, and a change in bladder and bowel habits. These may suggest advanced disease.

Perform a physical examination or assist with, as appropriate, a pelvic examination. Observe for vaginal discharge. Note any changes in the size, shape, or consistency of the uterus or surrounding structures or client reports of pain during examination. Anticipate the need for transvaginal ultrasound to identify endometrial hyperplasia (usually greater than 4 mm) and endometrial biopsy to identify malignant cells.

Nursing Management

Ensure that the woman understands all of the treatment options. Address any concerns the woman expresses, including questions about sexuality. Ensure that follow-up appointments are scheduled appropriately. Refer the client to a support group. Offer the woman and family explanations and emotional support throughout.

Educate the client about preventive measures or follow-up care if she has been treated for cancer. Education may be the most important tool currently available for the early detection of endometrial cancer. Many risk factors for endometrial cancer are modifiable or treatable, including obesity, hypertension, and diabetes. Educating women about risk factors and ways to decrease the risks is essential so that women can learn about their own risk and can become partners in the fight against the number-one gynecologic cancer (Teaching Guidelines 8.2).

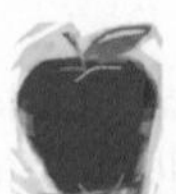

Teaching Guidelines 8.2

PREVENTIVE AND FOLLOW-UP MEASURES FOR ENDOMETRIAL CANCER

- Schedule regular pelvic examinations after the age of 21.
- Visit health care practitioner for early evaluation of any abnormal bleeding after menopause.
- Maintain a low-fat diet throughout life.
- Exercise daily.
- Manage weight to discourage hyperestrogenic states, which predispose to endometrial hyperplasia.
- Pregnancy serves as a protective factor by reducing estrogen.
- Ask your doctor about the use of combination estrogen and progestin pills.
- When combination oral contraceptives are taken to facilitate the regular shedding of the uterine lining, take risk reduction measures.
- Be aware of risk factors for endometrial cancer and make modifications as needed.
- Report any of the following symptoms immediately:
  - Bleeding or spotting after sexual intercourse
  - Bleeding that lasts longer than a week
  - Reappearance of bleeding after 6 months or more of no menses
- After cancer therapy, schedule follow-up appointments for the next few years.
- After cancer therapy, frequently communicate with your health care provider concerning your status.
- After surgery, maintain a healthy weight.

Carmella's **endometrial biopsy indicates endometrial adenocarcinoma. Her health care provider recommends surgery and adjuvant radiation therapy. How long will Carmella need to follow up after surgery? What lifestyle changes will the nurse need to stress with Carmella?**

CERVICAL CANCER

Cervical cancer is cancer of the uterine cervix. It is the third most common genital malignancy in women in the United States, after cancers of the endometrium and the ovary. The ACS (2015g) estimates that over 13,000 cases of invasive cervical cancer will be diagnosed in the United States in women in 2015 and that approximately 4,100 of these women will die. Some researchers estimate that noninvasive cervical cancer (carcinoma in situ) is about four times more common than invasive cervical cancer. The 5-year survival rate for all stages of cervical cancer is 72% (ACS, 2015g). Cervical cancer is five to eight times more common in women affected with HIV or AIDS than those who do not have this virus.

Hispanic women are most likely to get cervical cancer, followed by African Americans, Asians and Pacific Islanders, and Whites. Cervical cancer remains a disease of socioeconomic disparity. The high mortality rates of minorities are indicative of barriers to health care among those living in poverty. Hispanic women also have the highest rates of poverty, poor access to health care, and language and cultural barriers. Barriers to screening and prevention of cervical cancer include procrastination, fear of finding out that they have cancer, and embarrassment about having a **Papanicolaou (Pap) test**. In addition, most have little to no knowledge about HPV and its link with cancer (Strohl et al., 2015).

The incidence and mortality rates of cervical cancer have decreased noticeably in the past several decades, with most of the reduction attributed to the Pap test, which detects cervical cancer and some precancerous lesions. The Pap test (also known as a Pap smear) is a procedure used to obtain cells from the cervix for cytology screening. Cervical cancer is one of the most treatable cancers when detected at an early stage (ACS, 2015g). *Healthy People 2020* identifies several goals that address cervical cancer (Healthy People 2020 8.1; U.S. Department of Health & Human Services, 2015). Cervical cancer tends to occur in midlife. Most cases are found in women younger than age 50. It rarely develops in women younger than age 20. Many older women do not realize that the risk of developing cervical cancer is still present as they age. The probability of a woman in the United States developing cervical cancer is approximately 1 in 120, but this statistic is age dependent; the highest incidence is in women 40 to 49 years of age (Sawaya et al., 2015).

Pathophysiology

Cervical cancer starts with abnormal changes in the cellular lining or surface of the cervix. Typically, these changes occur in the squamous–columnar junction of the cervix. Here, cylindrical secretory epithelial cells (columnar) meet the protective flat epithelial cells (squamous) from the outer cervix and vagina in what is termed the transformation zone. The continuous replacement of columnar epithelial cells by squamous epithelial cells in this area makes these cells vulnerable to taking up foreign or abnormal genetic material (ACS, 2015h). Figure 8.4 shows the pathophysiology of cervical cancer.

HPV infection must be present for cervical cancer to occur. HPV infections occur in a high percentage of sexually active women, but a successful immune response results in viral control or clearance of HPV. Most people who have HPV are asymptomatic and, therefore, do not realize they have the virus. More than 90% of squamous cervical cancers contain HPV DNA, and the virus is now accepted as a major causative factor in the development of cervical cancer and its precursor, **cervical dysplasia** (disordered growth of abnormal cells). Since only a small proportion of HPV infections progress to cancer, other factors must be involved in the process of carcinogenesis.

HEALTHY PEOPLE 2020

Objectives	Nursing Significance
C-3 Reduce the female breast cancer death rate **C-4** Reduce the death rate from cancer of the uterine cervix	• Will help improve mortality rates and quality of life for women, and reduce health care costs related to treatment of malignancies.
C-10 Reduce invasive uterine cervical cancer **C-11** Reduce late-stage female breast cancer **C-15** Increase the proportion of women who receive a cervical cancer screening based on the most recent guidelines	• Will help to promote screening and early detection. The National Institutes of Health (2015) reported that half of the women diagnosed with invasive cervical cancer have never had a Pap smear and 10% have not had Pap smears during the past 5 years
C-17 Increase the proportion of women who receive a breast cancer screening based on the most recent guidelines	• Will raise awareness of cancer screening and prevention on a local and national level to improve and promote the health of all women.
C-18 Increase the proportion of women who were counseled about mammograms and Pap smear cancer screening consistent with current guidelines	• Will reduce the number of new cancer cases, as well as the illness, disability, and death caused by cancer.
C-20 Increase the proportion of persons who participate in behaviors that reduce their exposure to harmful ultraviolet (UV) irradiation and avoid sunburn	• Will reflect the importance of promoting evidence-based screening for cervical and breast cancer by lower mortality rates.

Note: *All cancer objectives project a 10% improvement from the baseline by 2020.*
Healthy People objectives based on data from http://www.healthypeople.gov

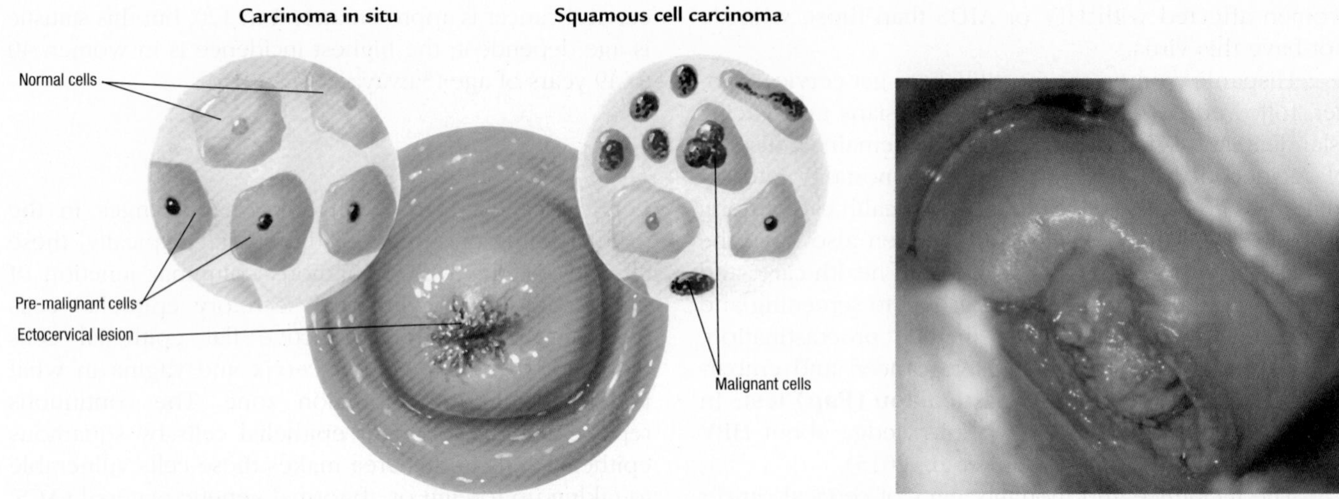

FIGURE 8.4 Cervical cancer. (Illustration is from The Anatomical Chart Company. [2009]. *Atlas of pathophysiology* [3rd ed.]. Philadelphia, PA: Lippincott Williams & Wilkins.)

Screening and Diagnosis

Screening for cervical cancer is very effective because the presence of a precursor lesion, cervical intraepithelial neoplasia, helps determine whether further tests are needed. Lesions start as *dysplasia* and progress in a predictable fashion over a long period, allowing ample opportunity for intervention at a precancerous stage. Progression from low-grade to high-grade dysplasia takes an average of 9 years, and progression from high-grade dysplasia to invasive cancer takes up to 2 years. Three main factors have been postulated to influence the progression of low-grade dysplasia to high grade. These include the type and duration of viral infection, with high-risk HPV type and persistent infection predicting a higher risk for progression; host conditions that compromise immunity, such as multiparity or poor nutritional status; and environmental factors such as smoking, oral contraceptive use, or vitamin deficiencies. In addition, various gynecologic factors, including age of menarche, age of first intercourse, and number of sexual partners, significantly increase the risk for cervical cancer (Broadman & Matthews, 2015).

Widespread use of the Pap test is credited with saving tens of thousands of women's lives and decreasing deaths from cervical cancer. Routine Pap smear testing for all sexually active women has been one of the primary screening methods for early detection of cervical irregularities related to HPV and is crucial for the prevention of cervical cancer.

Despite its outstanding record of success as a screening tool for cervical cancer (it detects approximately 90% of early cancer changes), the conventional Pap smear has a 20% false-negative rate. High-grade abnormalities missed by human screening are frequently detected by computerized instruments (NCI, 2015g). Thus, many technologies have been developed to improve the sensitivity and specificity of Pap testing, including:

- *Thin-Prep:* In this liquid-based technique, the cervical specimen is placed into a vial of preservative solution rather than on a glass slide.
- *Computer-assisted automated Pap test rescreening (Autopap):* An algorithm-based decision-making technology identifies slides that should be rescreened by cytopathologists by selecting samples that exceed a certain threshold for the likelihood of abnormal cells.
- *HPV-DNA typing (Hybrid Capture):* This system uses the association between certain types of HPV (16, 18, 31, 33, 35, 45, 51, 52, and 56) and the development of cervical cancer. This system can identify high-risk HPV types and improves detection and management.
- *Computer-assisted technology (Cytyc CDS-1000, AutoCyte, AcCell):* These computerized instruments can detect abnormal cells that are sometimes missed by technologists (CDC, 2015d).

The high rate of false-negative results may also be due to other factors, including errors in sampling the cervix, in preparing the slide, and in client preparation. Although cytology-based nationwide cervical screening has been helpful in identifying abnormal cervical cells, the sensitivity of cytology for the detection of high-grade precursor lesions is limited. Additionally, adenocarcinoma and its precursors are often missed by cytology. The current insight that infection with HPV is the causative agent of cervical cancer and its precursors has led to the development of molecular tests for the detection of HPV. Strong evidence now supports the use of HPV testing in the prevention of cervical cancer. It is evident that HPV can be detected in urine-based testing which might eventually become a helpful tool in cervical cancer screening and HPV surveillance efforts. Nurses need to keep up to date on the latest research developments as well as the strengths and weaknesses of various screening methods (Fontenot, 2015).

Although professional medical organizations disagree as to the recommended frequency of screening for cervical cancer, ACOG (2015) recommends that cervical cancer screening should begin at age 21 years (regardless of sexual history), since women younger than age 21 are at very low risk of cancer. In addition, ACOG advises Pap smears every 3 years for women between the ages of 21 and 29 years and every 3 years for women between ages 30 and 65 years old. An HPV co-test should be done every 5 years for this older age group. Cervical cancer screening can be stopped >65 years old with an adequate screening history. Women who have had a hysterectomy should stop screening. Women who have received the HPV vaccine should be screened according to the same guidelines as women who have not been vaccinated. In addition, women must have a clear understanding of the results of Pap smear testing and follow-up guidelines. High-risk women should continue to have annual Pap smears throughout their life (Table 8.2).

TABLE 8.2 PAP SMEAR GUIDELINES

First Pap	Cervical cancer screening should begin at age 21. Women under age 21 should not be tested.
Ages 21–30	Should have a Pap smear every 3 years. HPV testing should not be used in this age group unless it is needed after an abnormal Pap test result.
Ages 30–65	Should have a Pap smear plus an HPV test every 5 years. This is the preferred approach, but having a Pap smear alone every 3 years is also okay.
Age >65 years	Women who have had regular cervical testing with normal results should not be tested for cervical cancer. Women with a history of serious cervical precancer lesions should continue testing for at least 20 years after that diagnosis, even if it continues after age 65.
HPV vaccination	Women who have received the HPV vaccine should follow the screening recommendations for her age group.

Adapted from American Cancer Society [ACS]. (2015b). *American Cancer Society guidelines for the early detection of cancer.* Retrieved from http://www.cancer.org/healthy/findcancerearly/cancerscreeningguidelines/american-cancer-society-guidelines-for-the-early-detection-of-cancer

BOX 8.1

THE BETHESDA SYSTEM FOR CLASSIFYING PAP SMEARS

Specimen Type: Conventional Pap smear vs. liquid-based

Specimen Adequacy: Satisfactory or unsatisfactory for evaluation

General Categorization: (optional)
- Negative for intraepithelial lesion or malignancy
- Epithelial cell abnormality; see interpretation/result

Automated Review: If case was examined by automated device or not

Ancillary Testing: Provides a brief description of the test methods and report results so health care provider understands

Interpretation/Result:
- Negative for intraepithelial lesion or malignancy
- Organisms: *Trichomonas vaginalis;* fungus; bacterial vaginosis; herpes simplex
- Other non-neoplastic findings: Reactive cellular changes associated with inflammation, radiation, intrauterine devices, atrophy
- Other: Endometrial cells in a woman >40 years of age
- Epithelial cell abnormalities:
- *Squamous cell*
  - Atypical squamous cells
    - Of undetermined significance (ASC-US)
    - Cannot exclude HSIL (ASC-H)
  - Low-grade squamous intraepithelial lesion (LSIL)
    - Encompassing HPV/mild dysplasia/CIN-1
  - High-grade squamous intraepithelial lesion (HSIL)
  - Encompassing moderate and severe dysplasia CIS/CIN-2 and CIN-3
  - With features suspicious for invasion
  - Squamous cell carcinoma
- Glandular Cell: Atypical
  - Endocervical, endometrial, or glandular cells
    - Endocervical cells—favor neoplastic
    - Glandular cells—favor neoplastic
    - Endocervical adenocarcinoma in situ
  - Adenocarcinoma
    - Endocervical, endometrial, extrauterine
- Other malignant neoplasms (specify)

Educational Notes and Suggestions: (optional)

Adapted from American Society of Cytopathology (2015). *The Bethesda System for reporting cervical cytology: Definitions, criteria and explanatory notes.* Retrieved from http://www.cytopathology.org/the-bethesda-system-for-reporting-cervical-cytology-definitions-criteria-and-explanatory-notes-3rd-edition/; National Cancer Institute [NCI] (2015k). *Cervical cancer prevention.* Retrieved from http://www.cancer.gov/cancertopics/pdq/prevention/cervical/Patient/page3; Schuiling, K. D., & Likis, F. E. (2016). *Women's gynecologic health* (3rd ed.). Sudbury, MA: Jones & Bartlett.

Pap smear results are classified using the Bethesda System (Box 8.1), which provides a uniform diagnostic terminology that allows clear communication between the laboratory and the health care provider. The information provided by the laboratory is divided into three categories: specimen adequacy, general categorization of cytologic findings, and interpretation/result (ACS, 2015h).

Therapeutic Management

Treatment for abnormal Pap smears depends on the severity of the results and the health history of the woman. Therapeutic choices all involve destroying as many affected cells as possible. With the introduction of multimodality therapy for cervical cancer, many women will be long-term survivors in need of comprehensive surveillance care. Obesity and smoking are significant comorbidities that may complicate care in cervical cancer survivors. Nurses can focus their interventions at modifying these risk factors to increase the quality of life for cervical cancer survivors. Box 8.2 describes treatment options.

Using the Bethesda System, the following management guidelines for abnormal Pap results were developed by the NCI to provide direction to health care providers and clients:

- *ASC-US:* Repeat the Pap smear in 4 to 6 months or refer for **colposcopy**.
- *ASC-H:* Refer for colposcopy with HPV testing.
- *Atypical glandular cells (AGC) and adenocarcinoma in situ (AIS):* Immediate colposcopy; follow-up is based on the findings.

BOX 8.2

TREATMENT OPTIONS FOR CERVICAL CANCER

- **Cryotherapy**—destroys abnormal cervical tissue by freezing with liquid nitrogen, Freon, or nitrous oxide. Studies show a 90% cure rate (NCI, 2015g). Healing takes up to 6 weeks, and the client may experience a profuse, watery vaginal discharge for 3 to 4 weeks.
- **Cone biopsy or conization**—removes a cone-shaped section of cervical tissue. The base of the cone is formed by the ectocervix (outer part of the cervix) and the point or apex of the cone is from the endocervical canal. The transformation zone is contained within the cone sample. The cone biopsy is also a treatment and can be used to completely remove any precancers and very early cancers. Two methods are commonly used for cone biopsies:
- **LEEP (loop electrosurgical excision procedure) or LLETZ (large loop excision of the transformation zone)**—the abnormal cervical tissue is removed with a wire that is heated by an electrical current. For this procedure, a local anesthetic is used. It is performed in the health care provider's office in approximately 10 minutes. Mild cramping and bleeding may persist for several weeks after the procedure.
- **Cold knife cone biopsy**—a surgical scalpel or a laser is used instead of a heated wire to remove tissue. This procedure requires general anesthesia and is done in a hospital setting. After the procedure, cramping and bleeding may persist for a few weeks.
- **Laser therapy**—destroys diseased cervical tissue by using a focused beam of high-energy light to vaporize it (burn it off). After the procedure, the woman may experience a watery brown discharge for a few weeks. Very effective in destroying precancers and preventing them from developing into cancers.
- **Hysterectomy**—removes the uterus and cervix surgically.
- **Radiation therapy**—delivered by internal radium applications to the cervix or external radiation therapy that includes lymphatics of the pelvis.
- **Chemoradiation**—weekly cisplatin therapy concurrent with radiation. Investigation of this therapy is ongoing (ACS, 2015h).

Colposcopy is a microscopic examination of the lower genital tract using a magnifying instrument called a colposcope. Specific patterns of cells that correlate well with certain histologic findings can be visualized.

Nursing Assessment

Obtain a thorough history and physical examination of the woman. Investigate her history for risk factors such as:

- Early age at first intercourse (within 1 year of menarche)
- Lower socioeconomic status
- Promiscuous male partners
- Unprotected sexual intercourse
- Family history of cervical cancer (mother or sisters)
- Sexual intercourse with uncircumcised men
- Female offspring of mothers who took diethylstilbestrol (DES)
- Infections with genital herpes or chronic chlamydia
- Multiple sex partners
- Cigarette smoking
- Immunocompromised state
- HIV infection
- Oral contraceptive use
- Moderate dysplasia on Pap smear within past 5 years
- HPV infection (CDC, 2015e)

Question the woman about any signs and symptoms. Clinically, the first sign is abnormal vaginal bleeding, usually after sexual intercourse. Also be alert for reports of vaginal discomfort, malodorous discharge, and dysuria. In some cases the woman is asymptomatic, with detection occurring at an annual gynecologic examination and Pap test.

Perform a physical examination. Inspect the perineal area for vaginal discharge or genital warts. Perform or assist with a pelvic examination, including the collection of a Pap smear as indicated (Nursing Procedure 8.1).

Take Note!

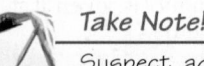

Suspect advanced cervical cancer in women with pelvic, back, or leg pain, weight loss, anorexia, weakness and fatigue, and fractures.

Prepare the woman for further diagnostic testing if indicated, such as a colposcopy. In a colposcopy, the woman is placed in the lithotomy position and her cervix is cleansed with acetic acid solution. Acetic acid makes abnormal cells appear white, which is referred to

NURSING PROCEDURE 8.1

Assisting with Collection of a Pap Smear

Purpose: To Obtain Cells from the Cervix for Cervical Cytology Screening

1. Explain procedure to the client (Fig. A).
2. Instruct client to empty her bladder.
3. Wash hands thoroughly.
4. Assemble equipment, maintaining sterility of equipment (Fig. B).

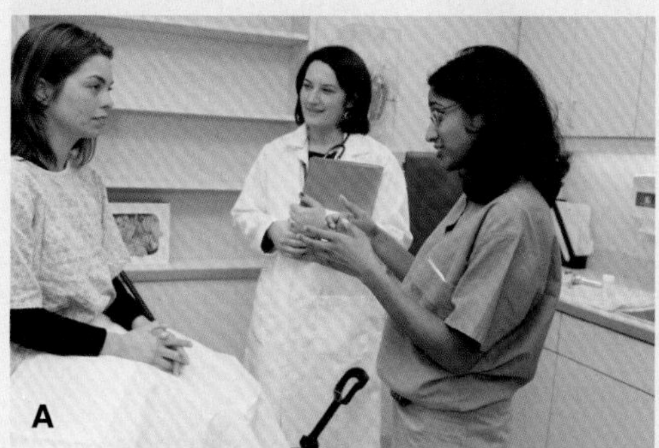
A

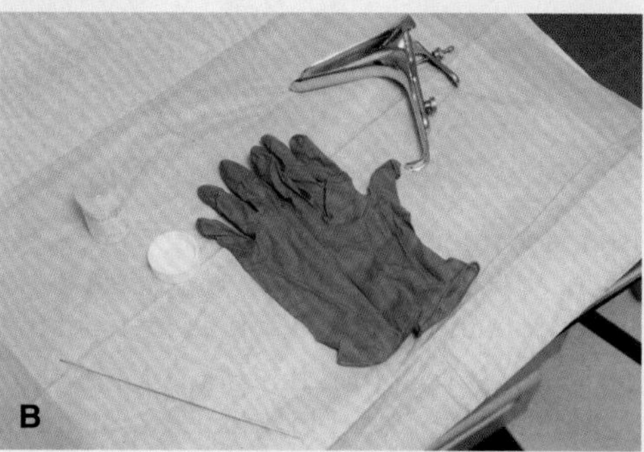
B

1. Position client on stirrups or foot pedals so that her knees fall outward.
2. Drape client with a sheet for privacy, covering the abdomen but leaving the perineal area exposed.
3. Open packages as needed.
4. Encourage client to relax.
5. Provide support to client as the practitioner obtains a sample by spreading the labia; inserting the speculum; inserting the cytobrush and swabbing the endocervix; and inserting the plastic spatula and swabbing the cervix (Figs. C–H).

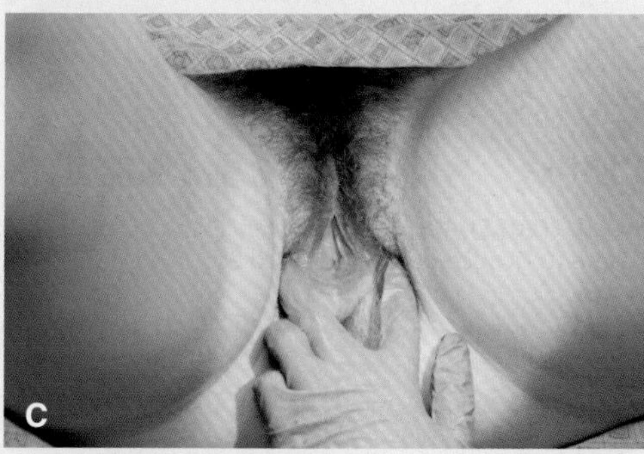
C

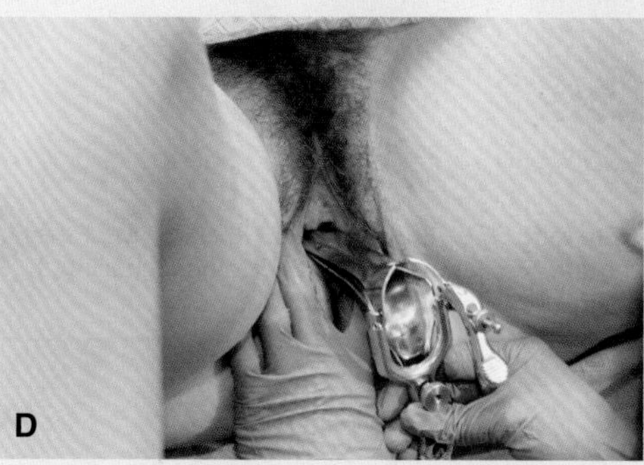
D

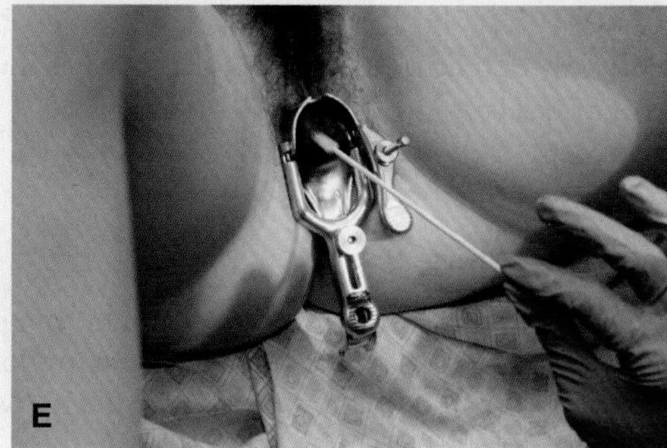
E

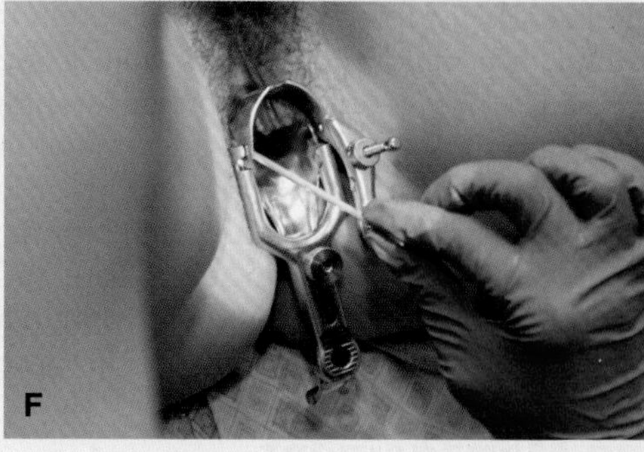
F

(continued)

NURSING PROCEDURE 8.1

Assisting with Collection of a Pap Smear (continued)

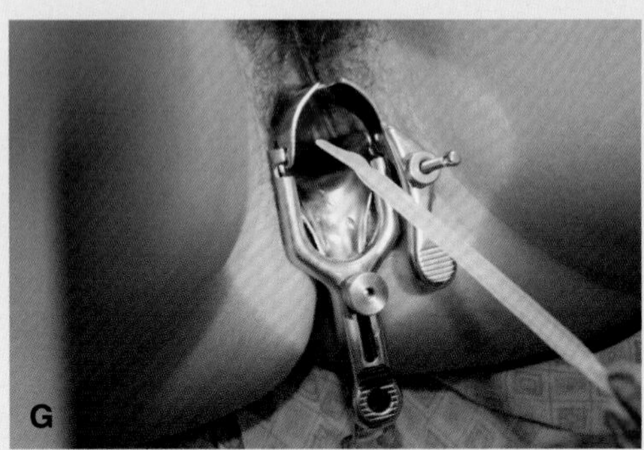

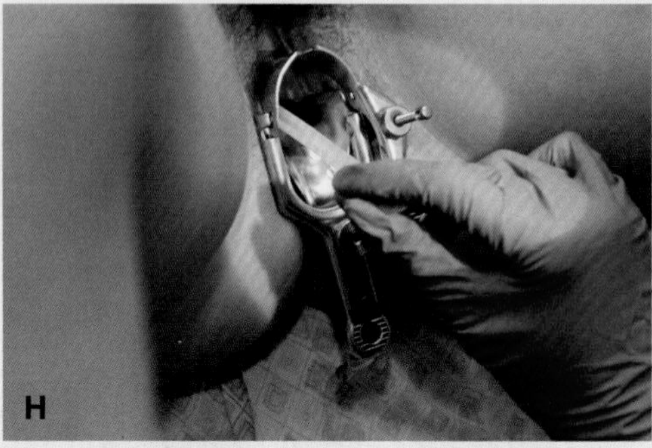

1. Transfer specimen to container (Fig. I) or slide. If a slide is used, spray the fixative on the slide holding the spray container about 12 in away from the slide.
2. Place sterile lubricant on the practitioner's fingertip when indicated for the bimanual examination.
3. Wash hands thoroughly.
4. Label specimen according to facility policy.
5. Rinse reusable instruments and dispose of waste appropriately (Fig. J).
6. Wash hands thoroughly.
7. Assist the client up after the examination is completed.

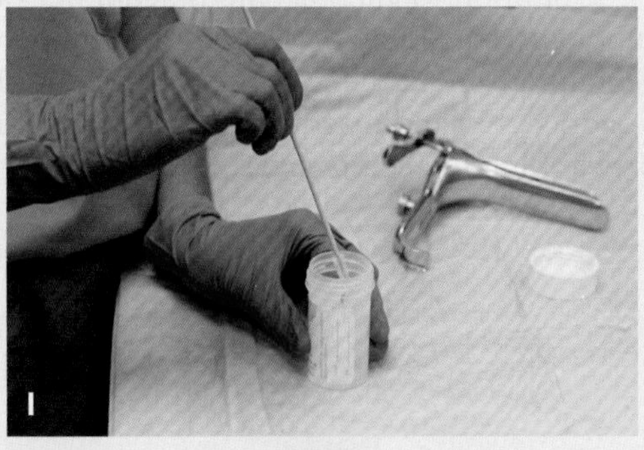

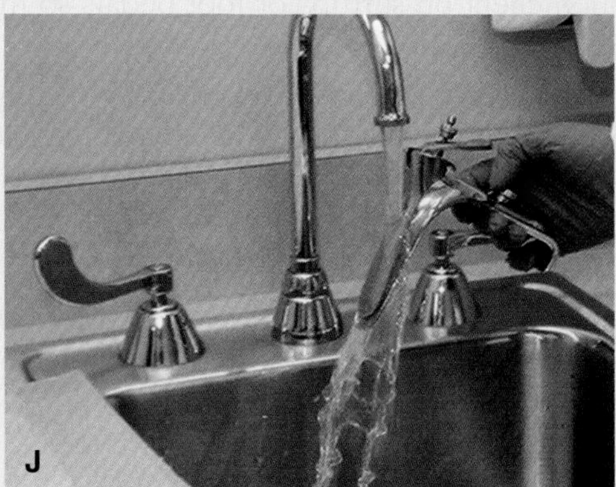

Adapted from King, T. L., Brucker, M. C., Kriebs, J. M., Fahey, J. O., Gegor, C. L., & Varney, H. (2015). *Varney's midwifery* (5th ed.). Burlington, MA: Jones & Bartlett Learning; Schuiling, K. D., & Likis, F. E. (2016). *Women's gynecologic health* (3rd ed.). Burlington, MA: Jones & Bartlett Learning.

as *acetowhite*. These white areas are then biopsied and sent to the pathologist for assessment. Although this test is not painful, has minor side effects (minor bleeding, cramping, and a risk of an infection developing after the biopsy), and can be performed safely in the clinic or office setting, women may be apprehensive or anxious about it because it is done to identify and confirm potential abnormal cell growth. Some health care providers request that the woman premedicate with a mild analgesic such as ibuprofen prior to undergoing the procedure.

Nursing Management

The nurse's role involves primary prevention by educating women about risk factors and ways to prevent cervical dysplasia. Cervical cancer rates have decreased in the United States because of the widespread use of Pap testing, which can detect precancerous lesions of the cervix before they develop into cancer.

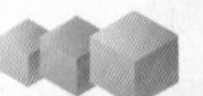
Concept Mastery Alert

Cervical Cancer Prevention

The key points to remember in cervical cancer prevention are smoking cessation, limiting alcohol consumption, and encouraging teens to refrain from early sexual activity.

Gardasil and Cervarix are vaccines approved by the United States Food and Drug Administration to protect girls and women from HPV and thus prevent cervical cancer. The vaccines prevent infection from four HPV types: HPV 6, 11, 16, and 18. These types are responsible for 70% of cervical cancers and 90% of genital warts (NCI, 2015h). Clinical trials indicate that the vaccine has high efficacy in preventing persistent HPV infection, cervical cancer precursor lesions, vaginal and vulvar cancer precursor lesions, and genital warts (NCI, 2015h). The vaccine is administered by intramuscular injection, and the recommended schedule is a three-dose series with the second and third doses administered 2 and 6 months after the first dose. The recommended age for vaccination of females is 9 to 26 years old (Castle & Schmeler, 2015). The vaccines protect against infection with these types of HPV for 6 to 8 years. It is not known if the protection lasts longer. The vaccines do not protect women who are already infected with HPV (NCI, 2015h). However, the vaccine is not a substitute for routine cervical cancer screening, and vaccinated women should have Pap smears as recommended.

Focus primary prevention education on the following:

- Identify high-risk behaviors in clients and teach them how to reduce such behaviors:
  - Take steps to prevent STIs.
  - Avoid early sexual activity.
  - Faithfully use barrier methods of contraception.
  - Avoid smoking and drinking.
  - Receive the HPV vaccine.
  - Instruct women on the importance of screening for cervical cancer by having annual Pap smears. Outline the proper preparation before having a Pap smear (Teaching Guidelines 8.3). Reinforce specific guidelines for screening.

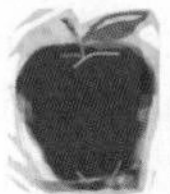

Teaching Guidelines 8.3

STRATEGIES TO OPTIMIZE PAP SMEAR RESULTS

- Schedule your Pap smear appointment about 2 weeks (10 to 18 days) after the first day of your last menses to increase the chance of getting the best sample of cervical cells without menses.
- Refrain from intercourse for 48 hours before the test because additional matter such as sperm can obscure the specimen.
- Do not douche within 48 hours before the test to prevent washing away cervical cells that might be abnormal.
- Do not use tampons, birth control foams, jellies, vaginal creams, or vaginal medications for 72 hours before the test, because they could cover up or obscure the cervical cell sample.
- Cancel your Pap appointment if vaginal bleeding occurs, because the presence of blood cells interferes with visual evaluation of the sample (Schuiling & Likis, 2016).

Nurses also can advocate for clients by making sure that the Pap smear is sent to an accredited laboratory for interpretation. Doing so reduces the risk of false-negative results. The identification and treatment of early precancerous lesions is critical to prevention of cervical cancer. Prevention measures should include educating women that the risk of infection can be reduced by delaying the onset of sexual activity, decreasing the number of sexual partners, using condoms consistently, and never start smoking.

Secondary prevention focuses on reducing or limiting the area of cervical dysplasia. Tertiary prevention focuses on minimizing disability or the spread of cervical cancer. Explain in detail all procedures that might be needed. Encourage the client who has undergone any cervical treatment to allow the pelvic area to rest for approximately 1 month. Discuss this rest period with the client and her partner to gain his cooperation. Outline alternatives to vaginal intercourse, such as cuddling, holding hands, and kissing. Remind the woman about any follow-up procedures that are needed and assist her with scheduling if necessary.

Tertiary prevention of cervical cancer involves the diagnosis and treatment of confirmed cases of cancer. Treatment is typically through surgery, radiotherapy, and frequently chemotherapy. Palliative care is provided to women when the disease has already reached an incurable stage. Knowing that the woman and her family have been told about her prognosis, the nurse is in a position to support them when the impact of the diagnosis is realized.

Throughout the process, provide emotional support to the woman and her family. During the decision-making process, the woman may be overwhelmed by the diagnosis and all the information being presented. Refer the woman and her family to appropriate community resources and support groups as indicated. It is crucial for all women to be given correct information regarding safe sexual practices, informed about the preventive role of the HPV vaccination, and become educated about the role of the Pap test as a secondary screening measure for cervical cancer. The emotional needs of the woman diagnosed with cancer can best be met by a warm, friendly personality, an attitude of empathy rather than sympathy, and skilled communication. Nurses across all settings are in a powerful position to be advocates for safe health care practices of women through education at personal, community, and national levels.

VAGINAL CANCER

Vaginal cancer is a rare malignant tissue growth arising in the vagina. Only about 1 of every 1,100 women will develop vaginal cancer in her lifetime. In 2015, the ACS

(2015i) estimate that more than 4,000 new cases will be diagnosed in women and that over 900 of those women will die from this cancer. The peak incidence of vaginal cancer occurs at 60 to 65 years of age. The prognosis of vaginal cancer depends largely on the stage of disease and the type of tumor. The overall 5-year survival rate for squamous cell carcinoma is about 42%; that for adenocarcinoma is about 78% (NCI, 2015i). Vaginal cancer can be effectively treated, and when found early it is often curable.

Pathophysiology

The etiology of vaginal cancer has not been identified. Malignant diseases of the vagina are either primary vaginal cancers or metastatic forms from adjacent or distant organs. About 80% of vaginal cancers are metastatic, primarily from the cervix and endometrium. These cancers invade the vagina directly. Cancers from distant sites that metastasize to the vagina through the blood or lymphatic system are typically from the colon, kidneys, skin (melanoma), or breast. Tumors in the vagina commonly occur on the posterior wall and spread to the cervix or vulva (NCI, 2015i).

Squamous cell carcinomas that begin in the epithelial lining of the vagina account for about 85% of vaginal cancers. This type of cancer usually occurs in women over the age of 50. The SCCs develop slowly over a period of years, commonly in the upper third of the vagina. They tend to spread early by directly invading the bladder and rectal walls. They also metastasize through blood and lymphatics. The remaining 15% are adenocarcinomas, which differ from SCC by an increase in pulmonary metastases and supraclavicular and pelvic node involvement (ACS, 2015j).

Therapeutic Management

Treatment of vaginal cancer depends on the type of cells involved and the stage of the disease. If the cancer is localized, radiation, laser surgery, or both may be used. If the cancer has spread, radical surgery might be needed, such as a hysterectomy, or removal of the upper vagina with dissection of the pelvic nodes in addition to radiation therapy.

Nursing Assessment

Begin the history and physical examination by reviewing for risk factors. Although direct risk factors for the initial development of vaginal cancer have not been identified, associated risk factors include advancing age (over 60 years old), previous pelvic radiation, exposure to DES in utero, vaginal trauma, history of genital warts (HPV infection), HIV infection, cervical cancer, chronic vaginal discharge, smoking, and low socioeconomic level (ACS, 2015k).

Question the woman about any symptoms. Most women with vaginal cancer are asymptomatic. Those with symptoms have painless vaginal bleeding (often after sexual intercourse), abnormal vaginal discharge, dyspareunia, dysuria, constipation, and pelvic pain (NCI, 2015i). During the physical examination, observe for any obvious vaginal discharge or genital warts or changes in the appearance of the vaginal mucosa. Anticipate colposcopy with biopsy of suspicious lesions to confirm the diagnosis.

Nursing Management

Nursing management for this cancer is similar to that for other reproductive cancers, with emphasis on sexuality counseling and referral to local support groups. Women undergoing radical surgery need intensive counseling about the nature of the surgery, risks, potential complications, changes in physical appearance and physiologic function, and sexuality alterations. Nurses should focus their care on client education, client pain and symptom management, communication with the woman and her family, and coordination of care across of all settings.

VULVAR CANCER

Vulvar cancer is an abnormal neoplastic growth on the external female genitalia including the clitoris, vaginal lips, and opening to the vagina (Fig. 8.5). Vulvar cancer accounts for approximately 5% of all female genital malignancies. In the United States, women have a 1 in 333 chance of developing vulvar cancer at some point in their lifetime. It is the fourth most common gynecologic cancer, after endometrial, ovarian, and cervical cancers (NCI, 2015j). The ACS (2015h) estimates that in 2015, over 5,000 cancers of the vulva will be diagnosed in the United States and over 1,000 women will die of this cancer. When detected early, it is highly curable. Typically, it can be advanced at diagnosis, though it is a visible cancer. Awareness is essential for early detection of this rare cancer.

Vulvar cancer is found most commonly in older women in their mid-60s to mid-70s, but the incidence in women younger than 35 years old has increased during the past few decades. The overall 5-year survival rate when lymph nodes are not involved is 90%, but it drops to 50% to 70% when the lymph nodes have been invaded (ACS, 2015m).

Pathophysiology

Vulvar cancer can be classified into two groups according to predisposing factors: the first type correlates

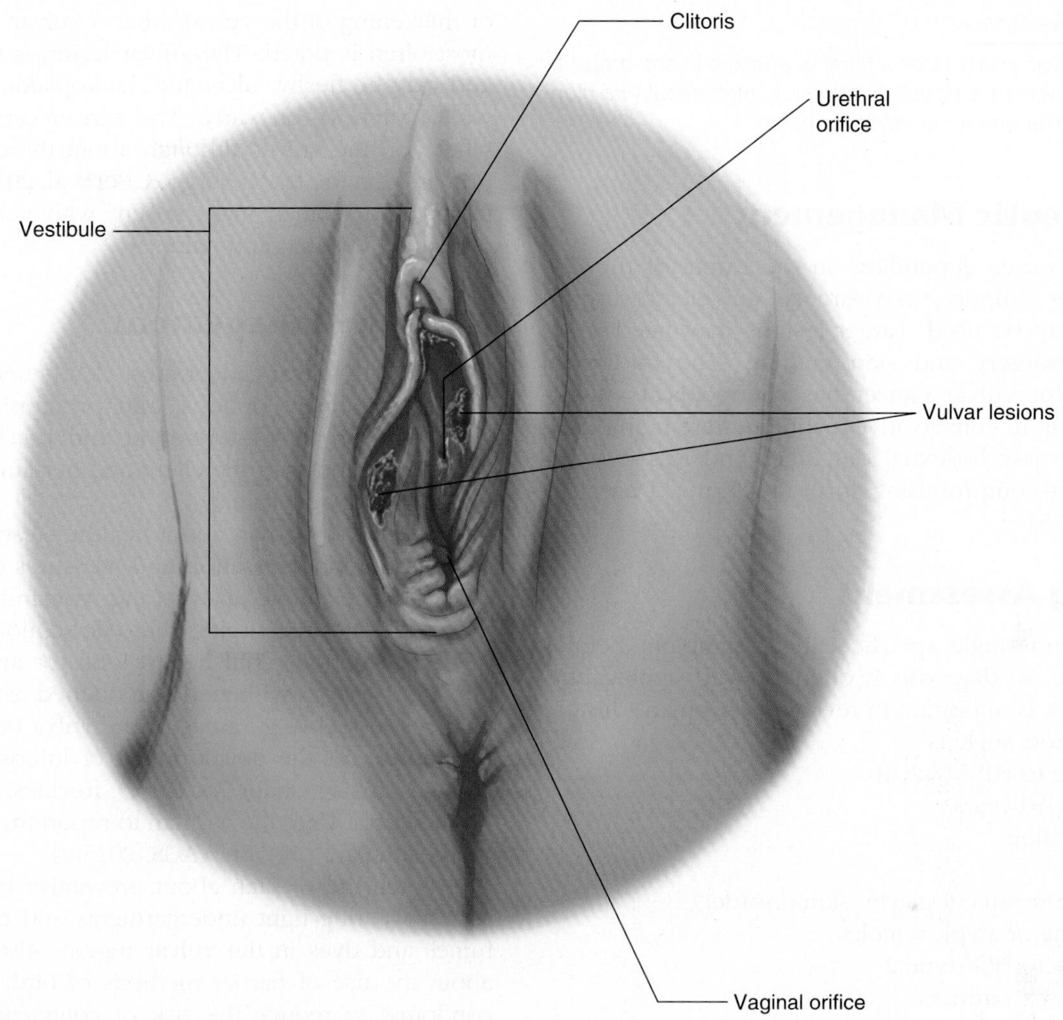

FIGURE 8.5 Vulvar cancer. (The Anatomical Chart Company. [2009]. *Atlas of pathophysiology* [3rd ed.]. Philadelphia, PA: Lippincott Williams & Wilkins.)

with a HPV infection and occurs mostly in younger women. The second group is not HPV associated and occurs in elderly women without cancerous disorders. Approximately 80% of vulvar tumors are squamous cell carcinomas. This type of cancer forms slowly over several years and is usually preceded by precancerous changes. These precancerous changes are termed vulvar intraepithelial neoplasia (VIN). The two major types of VIN are classic (undifferentiated) and simplex (differentiated). Classic VIN, the more common one, is associated with HPV infection (genital warts due to types 16, 18, 31, 33, 35, 45, and 54) and smoking (Alkatout et al., 2015). It typically occurs in women between 30 and 40 years. In contrast to classic VIN, simplex VIN usually occurs in postmenopausal women and is not associated with HPV but chronic irritation over time (Cancer.Net, 2015b).

Screening and Diagnosis

Annual vulvar examination is the most effective way to prevent vulvar cancer. Careful inspection of the vulva during routine annual gynecologic examinations remains the most productive diagnostic technique. Liberal use of biopsies of any suspicious vulvar lesion is usually necessary to make the diagnosis and to guide treatment. However, many women do not seek health care evaluation for months or years after noticing an abnormal lump or lesion. Leading presenting complaints of women with vulvar cancer include dyspareunia, long history of pruritus, ulcers on the "outside" genitalia, vulvar swelling, vulvar bleeding, and urinary problems (Alkatout et al., 2015). The diagnosis of vulvar cancer is made by a biopsy of the suspicious lesion, which is usually found on the labia majora.

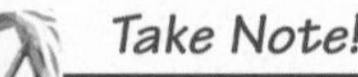

Take Note!

Vulvar pruritus or a lump is present in the majority of women with vulvar cancer. Lumps should be biopsied even if the woman is asymptomatic.

Therapeutic Management

Treatment varies depending on the extent of the disease. Laser surgery, cryosurgery, or electrosurgical incision may be used. Larger lesions may need more extensive surgery and skin grafting. The traditional treatment for vulvar cancer has been radical vulvectomy, but more conservative techniques are being used to improve psychosexual outcomes and less morbidity, without compromising survival (Forner, Dakhil, & Lampe, 2015).

Nursing Assessment

Typically, no single specific clinical symptom heralds this disease, so diagnosis is often delayed significantly. Therefore, it is important to review the woman's history for risk factors such as:

- Exposure to HPV type 16
- Age over 50 years
- HIV infection
- VIN
- Lichen sclerosus (a patchy skin disorder)
- Melanoma or atypical moles
- Exposure to HSV type 2
- Multiple sex partners
- Smoking
- Herpes simplex
- History of breast cancer
- Immune suppression
- Hypertension
- Diabetes mellitus
- Obesity (ACS, 2015n)

In most cases, the woman reports persistent vulvar itching, burning, and edema that do not improve with the use of creams or ointments. A history of condyloma, gonorrhea, and herpes simplex are some of the factors for greater risk for VIN. Diagnosis of vulvar carcinoma is often delayed. Women neglect to seek treatment for an average of 6 months from the onset of symptoms. In addition, a delay in diagnosis often occurs after the client presents to her physician or nurse practitioner. In many cases, a biopsy of the lesion is not performed until the problem fails to respond to numerous topical therapies. During the physical examination, observe for any masses or thickening of the vulvar area. A vulvar lump or mass most often is noted. The vulvar lesion is usually raised and may be fleshy, ulcerated, leukoplakic (looking like white patches), or warty. The cancer can appear anywhere on the vulva, although about three-fourths arise primarily on the labia (Vargo & Beriwal, 2015). Less commonly, the woman may present with vulvar bleeding, discharge, dysuria, and pain.

Nursing Management

Women with vulvar cancer must clearly understand their disease, treatment options, and prognosis. To accomplish this, provide information and establish effective communication with the client and her family. Act as an educator and advocate.

Teach the woman about healthy lifestyle behaviors, such as smoking cessation and measures to reduce risk factors. For example, instruct the woman how to examine her genital area, urging her to do so monthly between menstrual periods. Tell her to look for any changes in appearance (e.g., whitened or reddened patches of skin); changes in feel (e.g., areas of the vulva becoming itchy or painful); or the development of lumps, moles (e.g., changes in size, shape, or color), freckles, cuts, or sores on the vulva. Urge the woman to report these changes to the health care provider (ACS, 2015m).

Teach the woman about preventive measures such as not wearing tight undergarments and not using perfumes and dyes in the vulvar region. Also educate her about the use of barrier methods of birth control (e.g., condoms) to reduce the risk of contracting HIV, HSV, and HPV. Other prevention measures include delaying first sexual intercourse, avoiding sexual intercourse with multiple partners, not starting smoking or quitting if a smoker already, and getting the HPV vaccine available for all boys and girls and women between 9 and 26 years.

For the woman diagnosed with vulvar cancer, provide information and support. Discuss potential changes in sexuality if radical surgery is performed. Encourage her to communicate openly with her partner. Refer her to appropriate community resources and support groups. All nurses come in contact with women in their clinical practices who have the potential to become cancer clients, already have suspicious signs or symptoms of cancer, are already undergoing cancer treatment, or are terminal cancer clients. The nurse will be involved with all aspects of cancer, from diagnosis through palliative care. Each nurse has an obligation to keep informed of current developments in the cancer field to function effectively and be able to educate the woman and her family.

NURSING CARE PLAN 8.1

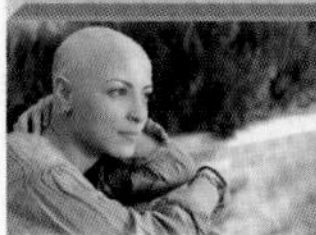

Overview of a Woman with a Reproductive Tract Cancer

Molly, a thin 28-year-old woman, comes to the free health clinic complaining of a thin, watery vaginal discharge and spotting after sex. Molly says she has had multiple sex partners since the age of 15 years. She had an abnormal Pap smear "a while back" but did not return to the clinic for follow-up. Cervical cancer is suspected.

NURSING DIAGNOSIS: Anxiety related to uncertainty of diagnosis, possible diagnosis of cancer, and eventual outcome as evidenced by client's report of signs and symptoms and statements of being worried and not knowing what she would do

Outcome Identification and Evaluation

The client will demonstrate measures to cope with anxiety *as evidenced by statements acknowledging anxiety, use of positive coping strategies, and verbalization that anxiety has decreased.*

Interventions: *Reducing Anxiety*

- Encourage client to express her feelings and concerns *to reduce her anxiety and to determine appropriate interventions.*
- Assess the meaning of the diagnosis to the client, clarify misconceptions, and provide reliable, realistic information *to enhance her understanding of her condition, subsequently reducing her anxiety.*
- Assess client's psychological status *to determine degree of emotional distress related to diagnosis and treatment options.*
- Identify and address verbalized concerns, providing information about what to expect *to decrease uncertainty about the unknown.*
- Assess the client's use of coping mechanisms in the past and their effectiveness *to foster use of positive strategies.*
- Teach client about early signs of anxiety and help her recognize them (e.g., fast heartbeat, sweating, or feeling flushed) *to minimize escalation of anxiety.*
- Provide positive reinforcement that the client's condition can be managed *to relieve her anxiety.*

NURSING DIAGNOSIS: Deficient knowledge related to diagnosis, prevention strategies, disease course, and treatment as evidenced by client's statements about hoping nothing bad is wrong, lack of follow-up for previous abnormal Pap test, and high-risk behaviors

Outcome Identification and Evaluation

The client will demonstrate an understanding of diagnosis, *as evidenced by making health-promoting lifestyle choices, verbalizing appropriate health care practices, describing condition once diagnosed, and adhering to measures to comply with therapy.*

Interventions: *Providing Client Teaching*

- Assess client's current knowledge about her diagnosis and proposed therapeutic regimen *to establish a baseline from which to develop a teaching plan.*
- Review contributing factors associated with development of reproductive tract cancer, including lifestyle behaviors, *to foster an understanding of the etiology of cervical cancer.*
- Review information about treatments and procedures and recommendations for healthy lifestyle, obtaining feedback frequently *to validate adequate understanding of instructions.*

(continued)

NURSING CARE PLAN 8.1

Overview of a Woman with a Reproductive Tract Cancer (continued)

- Discuss strategies, including using condoms and limiting the number of sexual partners, *to reduce the risk of transmission of STIs,* including HPV, which is associated with cervical cancer.
- Encourage client to obtain prompt treatment of any vaginal or cervical infections *to minimize the risk for cervical cancer.*
- Urge the client to have an annual Pap smear and/or HPV test *to allow screening and early detection.*
- Describe the treatment measures used *to provide client with knowledge of what may be necessary.*
- Provide written material with pictures *to allow for client review and to help her visualize what is occurring in her body.*
- Inform client about available community resources and make appropriate referrals as needed *to provide additional education and support.*
- Document details of teaching and learning *to allow for continuity of care and further education, if needed.*

NURSING DIAGNOSIS: Disturbed body image related to suspected reproductive tract cancer and impact on client's sexuality and sense of self as evidenced by statement of being worried about not being the same

Outcome Identification and Evaluation

The client will verbalize or demonstrate a positive self-esteem in relation to body image as evidenced by positive statements about self, sexuality, and participation in activities with others.

Interventions: *Promoting Healthy Body Image*

- Assess client's use of self-criticism *to determine client's current state of coping and adjustment.*
- Determine if the client's change in body image has contributed to social isolation *to provide a direction for care.*
- Provide opportunities for client to explore her feelings related to issues of sexuality, including past behaviors that may have placed her at risk, *to minimize feelings of guilt about her condition.*
- Acknowledge the client's feelings about possible changes in her body and sexuality and her illness *to foster trust and allow client to ventilate feelings and concerns.*
- Facilitate contact with other clients with the same type of cancer *to promote sharing of feelings and decrease feelings of isolation.*
- Initiate referrals for counseling and community support groups as necessary *to assist client in gaining a positive image of herself.*

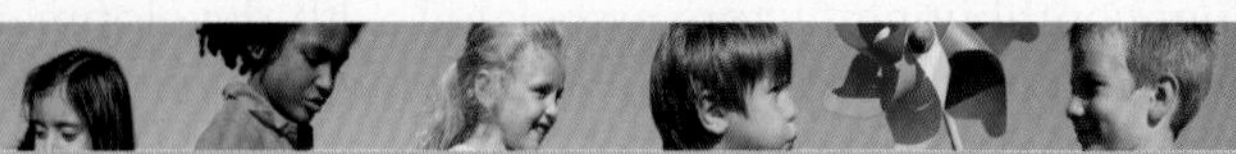

KEY CONCEPTS

- Women have a one-in-three lifetime risk of developing cancer, and one out of every four deaths is from cancer; thus, nurses must focus on screening and educating all women regardless of risk factors.
- The nurse plays a key role in offering emotional support, determining appropriate sources of support, and helping the woman use effective coping strategies when facing a diagnosis of cancer of the reproductive tract. Although reproductive

tract cancer is rare during pregnancy, the woman's vigilance and routine screenings should continue throughout.

- A woman's sexuality and culture are inextricably interwoven, and it is essential that nurses working with women of various cultures recognize this and remain sensitive to the vast changes that will take place when the diagnosis of cancer is made.
- Ovarian cancer is the eighth most common cancer among women and the fourth most common cause of cancer deaths for women in the United States, accounting for more deaths than any other cancer of the reproductive system.
- Ovarian cancer has been described as the "overlooked disease" or "silent killer" because women and health care practitioners often ignore or rationalize early symptoms. It is typically diagnosed in advanced stages.
- Unopposed endogenous and exogenous estrogens, obesity, nulliparity, menopause after the age of 52 years, and diabetes are the major etiologic risk factors associated with the development of endometrial cancer.
- The American Cancer Society recommends that women should be informed about risks and symptoms of endometrial cancer at the onset of menopause and strongly encouraged to report any unexpected bleeding or spotting to their health care providers.
- Malignant diseases of the vagina are either primary vaginal cancers or metastatic forms from adjacent or distant organs. Vaginal cancer tumors can be effectively treated and, when found early, are often curable.
- Cervical cancer incidence and mortality rates have decreased noticeably in the past several decades, with most of the reduction attributed to the Pap test, which detects cervical cancer and precancerous lesions.
- The nurse's role involves primary prevention of cervical cancer through education of women regarding risk factors and preventive vaccines to avoid cervical dysplasia.
- Diagnosis of about 80% of vaginal cancers is metastatic, primarily from the cervix and endometrium. These cancers invade the vagina directly. Vulvar cancer is often delayed significantly because there is no single specific clinical symptom that heralds it. The most common presentation is persistent vulvar itching that does not improve with the application of creams or ointments.

REFERENCES AND RECOMMENDED READINGS

Agency for Healthcare Research and Quality. (2014). *Cancer screening and treatment in women: Recent findings.* Retrieved from http://www.ahrq.gov/research/findings/factsheets/women/cancerwom/

Alexander, L. L., LaRosa, J. H., Bader, H., & Garfield, S. (2014). *New dimensions in women's health* (6th ed.). Sudbury, MA: Jones & Bartlett.

Alkatout, I., Schubert, M., Garbrecht, N., Weigel, M. T., Jonat, W., Mundhenke, C., et al. (2015). Vulvar cancer: Epidemiology, clinical presentation, and management options. *International Journal of Women's Health, 7,* 305–313.

Amant, F., Han, S. N., Gziri, M. M., Vandenbroucke, T., Verheecke, M., & Van Calsteren, K. (2015). Management of cancer in pregnancy. *Best Practice & Research Clinical Obstetrics & Gynecology, 29*(5), 741–753.

American Cancer Society [ACS]. (2015a). *Key statistics about lung cancer.* Retrieved from http://www.cancer.org/cancer/lungcancer-non-smallcell/detailedguide/non-small-cell-lung-cancer-key-statistics

American Cancer Society [ACS]. (2015b). *ACS guidelines for the early detection of cancer.* Retrieved from http://www.cancer.org/healthy/findcancerearly/cancerscreeningguidelines/american-cancer-society-guidelines-for-the-early-detection-of-cancer

American Cancer Society [ACS]. (2015c). *Cervical cancer and pregnancy.* Retrieved from http://www.cancer.org/cancer/cervicalcancer/overviewguide/cervical-cancer-overview-treating-pregnancy

American Cancer Society [ACS]. (2015d). *What are the key statistics about ovarian cancer?* Retrieved from http://www.cancer.org/cancer/ovariancancer/detailedguide/ovarian-cancer-key-statistics

American Cancer Society [ACS]. (2015e). *What are the key statistics about endometrial cancer?* Retrieved from http://www.cancer.org/cancer/endometrialcancer/detailedguide/endometrial-uterine-cancer-key-statistics

American Cancer Society [ACS]. (2015f). *Endometrial (uterine) cancer.* Retrieved from http://www.cancer.org/acs/groups/cid/documents/webcontent/003097-pdf.pdf

American Cancer Society [ACS]. (2015g). *What are the key statistics about cervical cancer?* Retrieved from http://www.cancer.org/cancer/cervicalcancer/detailedguide/cervical-cancer-key-statistics

American Cancer Society [ACS]. (2015h). *Cervical cancer.* Retrieved from http://www.cancer.org/acs/groups/cid/documents/webcontent/003094-pdf.pdf

American Cancer Society [ACS]. (2015i). *What are the key statistics about vaginal cancer?* Retrieved from http://www.cancer.org/cancer/vaginalcancer/detailedguide/vaginal-cancer-key-statistics

American Cancer Society [ACS]. (2015j). *Vaginal cancer.* Retrieved from http://www.cancer.org/cancer/vaginal-cancer/detailedguide/

American Cancer Society [ACS]. (2015k). *What are risk factors for vaginal cancer?* Retrieved from http://www.cancer.org/cancer/vaginalcancer/detailedguide/vaginal-cancer-risk-factors

American Cancer Society [ACS]. (2015l). *What are the key statistics about vulvar cancer?* Retrieved from http://www.

cancer.org/cancer/vulvarcancer/detailedguide/vulvar-cancer-key-statistics

American Cancer Society [ACS]. (2015m). *What is vulvar cancer?* Retrieved from http://www.cancer.org/cancer/vulvar-cancer/detailedguide/vulvar-cancer-what-is-vulvar-cancer

American Cancer Society [ACS]. (2015n). *What are the risk factors for vulvar cancer?* Retrieved from http://www.cancer.org/cancer/vulvarcancer/detailedguide/vulvar-cancer-risk-factors

American Cancer Society [ACS]. (2015o). *Survival rates for ovarian cancer by stage.* Retrieved from http://www.cancer.org/cancer/ovariancancer/detailedguide/ovarian-cancer-survival-rates

American cancer Society [ACS]. (2016). *Cancer facts & figures 2016.* Retrieved from http://www.cancer.org/research/cancerfactsstatistics/cancerfactsfigures2016/index

American College of Obstetricians and Gynecologists [ACOG]. (2015). *The ACOG cervical cancer screening guidelines: Key changes.* Retrieved from https://www.hpv16and18.com/hcp/cervical-cancer-screening-guidelines/acog-guidelines.html

American Society of Cytopathology. (2015). *The Bethesda System for reporting cervical cytology: Definitions, criteria and explanatory notes.* Retrieved from http://www.cytopathology.org/the-bethesda-system-for-reporting-cervical-cytology-definitions-criteria-and-explanatory-notes-3rd-edition/

Andersson, T. M., Johansson, A. L., Fredriksson, I., & Lambe, M. (2015). Cancer during pregnancy and the postpartum period: A population-based study. *Cancer, 121*(12), 2072–2077.

Balk, S. J. (2015). Pediatricians can play role in reducing skin cancer epidemic. *AAP News, 36*(1), 8–9.

Brennan, D. J., Hackethal, A., Mann, K. P., Mutz-Dehbalaie, I., Fiegl, H., Marth, C., et al. (2015). Serum HE4 detects recurrent endometrial cancer in patients undergoing routine clinical surveillance. *BMC Cancer, 15*(1), 33–36.

Broadman, C. H., & Matthews, K. J. (2015). *Cervical cancer. eMedicine.* Retrieved from http://emedicine.medscape.com/article/253513-overview

Cancer in Pregnancy. (2015a). *Endometrial cancer.* Retrieved from http://www.cancerinpregnancy.org/node/103

Cancer in Pregnancy. (2015b). *Cervical cancer.* Retrieved from http://www.cancerinpregnancy.org/node/52

Cancer.Net. (2015a). *Cancer during pregnancy.* Retrieved from http://www.cancer.net/coping/emotional-and-physical-matters/sexual-and-reproductive-health/cancer-during-pregnancy

Cancer.Net. (2015b). *Vulvar cancer.* Retrieved from http://www.cancer.net/cancer-types/vulvar-cancer/risk-factors-and-prevention

Castle, P. E., & Schmeler, K. M. (2015). HPV vaccination: For women of all ages? *The Lancet, 384*(9961), 2178–2180.

Centers for Disease Control and Prevention [CDC]. (2015a). *Cancer among women.* Retrieved from http://www.cdc.gov/cancer/dcpc/data/women.htm

Centers for Disease Control and Prevention [CDC]. (2015b). *Cancer prevention and control.* Retrieved from http://www.cdc.gov/cancer/dcpc/prevention/other.htm

Centers for Disease Control and Prevention [CDC]. (2015c). *Ovarian cancer risk factors.* Retrieved from http://www.cdc.gov/cancer/ovarian/basic_info/risk_factors.htm

Centers for Disease Control and Prevention [CDC]. (2015d). *Cervical cancer screening.* Retrieved from http://www.cdc.gov/cancer/cervical/basic_info/screening.htm

Centers for Disease Control and Prevention [CDC]. (2015e). *Cervical cancer risk factors.* Retrieved from http://www.cdc.gov/cancer/cervical/basic_info/risk_factors.htm

Cliby, W. A., Powell, M. A., Al-Hammadi, N., Chen, L., Miller, J. P., Roland, P. Y., et al. (2015). Ovarian cancer in the United States: Contemporary patterns of care associated with improved survival. *Gynecologic Oncology, 136*(1), 11–17.

de Haan, J., Verheecke, M., & Amant, F. (2015). Management of ovarian cysts and cancer in pregnancy. *Facts, Views & Vision in ObGyn, 7*(1), 25–31.

Dueholm, M., Marinovskij, E., Hansen, E. S., Møller, C., & Ørtoft, G. (2015). Diagnostic methods for fast-track identification of endometrial cancer in women with postmenopausal bleeding and endometrial thickness greater than 5 mm. *Menopause, 22*(6), 1.

Ebell, M. H., Culp, M., Lastinger, K., & Dasigi, T. (2015). A systematic review of the bimanual examination as a test for ovarian cancer. *American Journal of Preventive Medicine, 48*(3), 350–356.

Fontenot, H. B. (2015). Urine-Based HPV Testing as a method to screen for cervical cancer. *Nursing for Women's Health, 19*, 59–65.

Forner, D. M., Dakhil, R., & Lampe, B. (2015). Quality of life and sexual function after surgery in early stage vulvar cancer. *European Journal of Surgical Oncology (EJSO), 41*(1), 40–45.

Garner, M. J., McGregor, B. A., Murphy, K. M., Koenig, A. L., Dolan, E. D., & Albano, D. (2015). Optimism and depression: A new look at social support as a mediator among women at risk for breast cancer. *Psychooncology, 24*(12), 1708–1713.

Goldstein, C. L., Susman, E., Lockwood, S., Medlin, E. E., & Behbakht, K. (2015). Awareness of symptoms and risk factors of ovarian cancer in a population of women and healthcare providers. *Clinical Journal of Oncology Nursing, 19*(2), 206–212.

Helm, C. W. (2015a). Hyperthermic intraperitoneal chemotherapy for ovarian cancer: Is there a role? *Journal of Gynecologic Oncology, 26*(1), 1–2.

Helm, C. W. (2015b). *Ovarian cysts. eMedicine.* Retrieved from http://emedicine.medscape.com/article/255865-overview

Herrington, C., Coates, P., & Duprex, W. (2015). Viruses and disease: Emerging concepts for prevention, diagnosis and treatment. *Journal of Pathology, 235*, 149–152.

International Federation of Gynecology & Obstetrics. (2015). *Endometrial carcinoma staging.* Retrieved from http://www.figo.org/search/node/endometrial+cancer+staging

Key, T. (2015). Cancer prevention and treatment. In Bier, D. M., Mann, J., Alpers, D. H., Vorster, H. E., & Gibney, M. J. (Eds.), *Nutrition for the primary care provider* (pp. 111, 1234–129). Oxford, UK: Karger Publishers.

Kim, R. H., & Chu, Q. D. (2015). Breast cancer during pregnancy. In Chu, Q. D., Gibbs, J. F., & Zibari, G. B. (Eds.), *Surgical oncology: A practical and comprehensive approach* (pp. 163–168). New York, NY: Springer Publishers.

King, T. L, Brucker, M. C., Kriebs, J. M., Fahey, J. O., Gegor, C. L., & Varney, H. (2015). *Varney's midwifery* (5th ed.). Burlington, MA; Jones & Bartlett Learning.

Li, Y., Zhao, J., Zhang, Q., & Wang, Y. (2015). Does ovarian stimulation for IVF increase gynecological cancer risk? A systematic review and meta-analysis. *Reproductive BioMedicine Online, 31*(1), 20–29.

Liede, A., Sun, P., & Narod, S. (2015). Effect of breast cancer after ovarian cancer on mortality for BRCA mutation carriers. *JAMA Surgery, 150*(5), 490–491.

Lofters, A. K. (2015). Ethnicity and breast cancer stage at diagnosis: An issue of health equity. *Current Oncology, 22*(2), 80–81.

Matsumoto, K., Onda, T., & Yaegashi, N. (2015). Pharmacotherapy for recurrent ovarian cancer: Current status and future perspectives. *Japanese Journal of Clinical Oncology, 45*(5), 408–410.

Mayo Clinic. (2015). *Cancer prevention: 7 steps to reduce your risk.* Retrieved from http://www.mayoclinic.org/cancer-prevention/art-20044816

Memorial Sloan Kettering Cancer Center. (2015). *Ovarian cancer risk factors.* Retrieved from http://www.mskcc.org/cancer-care/adult/ovarian/risk-factors

Moses, S. (2015). *Endometrial cancer risk factors. Family practice notebook.* Retrieved from http://www.fpnotebook.com/Gyn/HemeOnc/EndmtrlCncrRskFctr.htm

National Cancer Institute [NCI]. (2015a). *SEER cancer statistics review.* Retrieved from http://seer.cancer.gov/csr/1975_2010/

National Cancer Institute [NCI]. (2015b). *The burden of cancer.* Retrieved from http://www.cancer.gov/cancertopics/pdq/prevention/overview/HealthProfessional

National Cancer Institute [NCI]. (2015c). *General cancer prevention.* Retrieved from http://www.cancer.gov/cancertopics/prevention#General+Cancer+Prevention+Information

National Cancer Institute [NCI]. (2015d). *General information about ovarian epithelial cancer.* Retrieved from: http://www.cancer.gov/cancertopics/pdq/treatment/ovarianepithelial/healthprofessional

National Cancer Institute [NCI]. (2015e). *Stat fact sheets: Endometrial cancer.* Retrieved from http://seer.cancer.gov/statfacts/html/corp.html

National Cancer Institute [NCI]. (2015f). *Endometrial cancer.* Retrieved from http://www.cancer.gov/cancertopics/types/endometrial

National Cancer Institute [NCI]. (2015g). *Screening and testing to detect cervical cancer.* Retrieved from http://www.cancer.gov/cancertopics/screening/cervical

National Cancer Institute [NCI]. (2015h). *Human papillomavirus (HPV) vaccines.* Retrieved from http://www.cancer.gov/cancertopics/factsheet/prevention/HPV-vaccine

National Cancer Institute [NCI]. (2015i). *General information about vaginal cancer.* Retrieved from http://www.cancer.gov/cancertopics/pdq/treatment/vaginal/Patient/page1

National Cancer Institute [NCI]. (2015j). *General information about vulvar cancer.* Retrieved from http://www.cancer.gov/cancertopics/pdq/treatment/vulvar/HealthProfessional/page1

National Cancer Institute [NCI]. (2015k). *Cervical cancer prevention.* Retrieved from http://www.cancer.gov/cancertopics/pdq/prevention/cervical/Patient/page3

National Institutes of Health [NIH]. (2015). *Cervical cancer.* Retrieved from http://report.nih.gov/nihfactsheets/viewfactsheet.aspx?csid=76

Nick, A. M., Coleman, R. L., Ramirez, P. T., & Sood, A. K. (2015). A framework for a personalized surgical approach to ovarian cancer. *Nature Reviews Clinical Oncology, 12*(4), 239–245.

Poole, E. M., Rice, M. S., Crum, C. P., & Tworoger, S. S. (2015). Salpingectomy as a potential ovarian cancer risk-reducing procedure. *Journal of the National Cancer Institute, 107*(2), dju490.

Sawaya, G. F., Kulasingam, S., Denberg, T., & Qaseem, A. (2015). Cervical cancer screening in average-risk women: Best practice advice from the clinical guidelines committee of the American College of Physicians. *Annals of Internal Medicine, 162*(12), 851–859.

Schmid, D., Behrens, G., Keimling, M., Jochem, C., Ricci, C., & Leitzmann, M. (2015). A systematic review and meta-analysis of physical activity and endometrial cancer risk. *European Journal of Epidemiology, 30*(5), 137–412.

Schuiling, K. D., & Likis, F. E. (2016). *Women's gynecologic health* (3rd ed.). Sudbury, MA: Jones & Bartlett.

Shirvani, H., & Alhani, F. (2015). Challenges nursing role on improving quality of life in women with breast cancer undergoing chemotherapy. *Journal of Clinical Nursing and Midwifery, 3*(4), 1–12.

Siegel, R. L., Miller, K. D., & Jemal, A. (2015). Cancer statistics, 2015. *CA: A Cancer Journal for Clinicians, 65*, 5–29.

Strohl, A. E., Mendoza, G., Ghant, M. S., Cameron, K. A., Simon, M. A., Schink, J. C., et al. (2015). Barriers to prevention: Knowledge of HPV, cervical cancer, and HPV vaccinations among African American women. *American Journal of Obstetrics and Gynecology, 212*(1), 65–70.

Surbone, A. (2015). A review of cultural attitudes about cancer. In Miller, K. D. & Simon, M. (Eds.), *Global perspectives on cancer: Incidence, care, and experience [2 volumes]* (pp. 19–37). Santa Barbara, CA: ABC-CLIO Publisher.

Temple, S. V. (2015). Cancers of the reproductive system. In Itano, J. K., Brant, J., Conde, F., & Saria, M. (Eds.), *Core curriculum for oncology nursing* (5th ed., 103–116). St. Louis, MO: Elsevier.

U.S. Department of Health and Human Services. (2015). *Healthy People 2020.* Retrieved from http://www.healthypeople.gov/2020/topicsobjectives2020.

U.S. Preventive Services Task Force [USPSTF]. (2015). *Screening for ovarian cancer. U.S. Preventive Services Task Force summary of recommendations.* Retrieved from http://www.ahrq.gov/clinic/pocketgd1011/gcp10s2.htm

Vargo, J. A., & Beriwal, S. (2015). Vulvar cancer. In Lee, N. Y., Riaz, N., & Lu, J. J. (Eds.), *Target volume delineation for conformal and intensity-modulated radiation therapy* (pp. 349–358). New York, NY: Springer Publishers.

Wong, A. S., Lao, T. T., Cheung, C. W., Yeung, S. W., Fan, H. L., Ng, P. S., et al. (2015). Reappraisal of endometrial thickness for the detection of endometrial cancer in postmenopausal bleeding: A retrospective cohort study. *BJOG, 123*(3), 439–446.

World Health Organization. (2015). *Cancer prevention and control.* Retrieved from http://www.who.int/nmh/a5816/en/

Wright, J. D., Chen, L., Tergas, A. I., Patankar, S., Burke, W. M., Hou, J. Y., et al. (2015). Trends in relative survival for ovarian cancer from 1975 to 2011. *Obstetrics & Gynecology, 125*(6), 1345–1352.

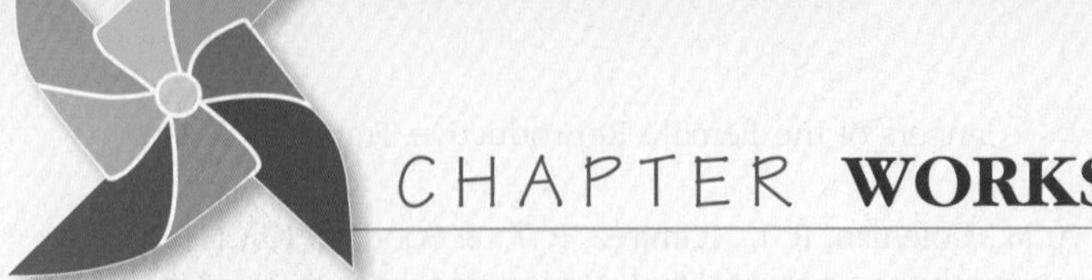

CHAPTER WORKSHEET

MULTIPLE-CHOICE QUESTIONS

1. When describing ovarian cancer to a local women's group, the nurse states that ovarian cancer often is not diagnosed early because:
   a. The disease progresses very slowly.
   b. The early stages produce very vague symptoms.
   c. The disease usually is diagnosed only at autopsy.
   d. Clients do not follow up on acute pelvic pain.
2. A postmenopausal woman reports that she has started spotting again. Which of the following would the nurse do?
   a. Instruct the client to keep a menstrual diary for the next few months.
   b. Tell her not to worry, since this a common but not serious event.
   c. Have her start warm-water douches to promote healing.
   d. Anticipate that the doctor will assess her endometrium thickness.
3. Which of the following would the nurse identify as the priority psychosocial need for a women diagnosed with reproductive cancer?
   a. Research findings
   b. Hand-holding
   c. Cheerfulness
   d. Offering of hope
4. When teaching a group of women about screening and early detection of cervical cancer, the nurse would include which of the following as most effective?
   a. Fecal occult blood test
   b. CA-125 blood test
   c. Pap smear and HPV test
   d. Sigmoidoscopy
5. After teaching a group of students about reproductive tract cancers, the nursing instructor determines that the teaching was successful when the students identify which of the following as the deadliest type of female reproductive cancer?
   a. Vulvar
   b. Ovarian
   c. Endometrial
   d. Cervical
6. The nurse is attempting to reassure her obese female client about the discovery of an ovarian cyst after her pelvic examination. Which of the following statements is true concerning ovarian cysts? They are:
   a. Frequently seen in polycystic kidney disease
   b. Always painful and need to be removed surgically
   c. A precursor to ovarian carcinoma
   d. Part of a syndrome that includes hypertension and diabetes
7. Which of the following is considered a risk factor for vulvar cancer?
   a. Vitamin B_{12} deficiency
   b. Epstein–Barr virus
   c. Human papillomavirus
   d. Adenovirus

CRITICAL THINKING EXERCISES

1. A 27-year-old sexually active White woman visits the Health Department family planning clinic and requests information about the various available methods of contraception. In taking her history, the nurse learns that she started having sex at age 15 and has had multiple sex partners since then. She smokes two packs of cigarettes daily. Because she has been unemployed for a few months, her health insurance policy has lapsed. She has never previously obtained any gynecologic care.
   a. Based on her history, which risk factors for cervical cancer are present?
   b. What recommendations would you make for her and why?
   c. What are this client's educational needs concerning health maintenance?
2. A 60-year-old nulliparous woman presents to the gynecologic oncology clinic after her health care provider palpated an adnexal mass on her right ovary. In taking her history, the nurse learns that she has experienced mild abdominal bloating and weight loss for the past several months but felt fine otherwise. She was diagnosed with breast cancer 15 years ago and was treated with a lumpectomy and radiation. She has occasionally used talcum powder in her perineal area over the past 20 years.

   A transvaginal ultrasound reveals a complex mass in the right adnexa. She undergoes a total abdominal hysterectomy and bilateral salpingo-oophorectomy and lymph node biopsy. Pathology confirms a diagnosis of stage III ovarian cancer with abdominal metastasis and positive lymph nodes.
   a. Is this client's profile typical for a woman with this diagnosis?
   b. What in her history might have increased her risk for ovarian cancer?
   c. What can the nurse do to increase awareness of this cancer for all women?

CHAPTER WORKSHEET

STUDY ACTIVITIES

1. During your surgical clinical rotation, interview a female client undergoing surgery for cancer of her reproductive organs. Ask her to recall the symptoms that brought her to the health care provider. Ask her what thoughts, feelings, and emotions went through her mind before and after her diagnosis. Finally, ask her how this experience will change her life in future.
2. Visit an oncology and radiology treatment center to find out about the various treatment modalities available for reproductive cancers. Contrast the various treatment methods and report your findings to your class.
3. Visit one of the web sites listed in the extensive list of web sites provided to explore a topic of interest concerning reproductive cancers. How correct and current is the content? What is its level? Share your assessment with your classmates.
4. Taking oral contraceptives provides protection against ____________________ cancer.
5. Two genes, *BRCA1* and *BRCA2,* are linked with hereditary ________________ and ________________ cancers.

BRINGING IT ALL TOGETHER: A CASE STUDY

Jill, a 38-year-old obese female with a history of infertility and irregular bleeding, returned to her OB/GYN doctor for a follow-up appointment. She had a D&C the week before to stop a profuse bleeding episode. She is informed by the doctor that her pathology report came back from the D&C showing endometrial adenocarcinoma. She is in shock over the diagnosis at her young age.

ASSESSMENT

The nurse took Jill's history, which included irregular menstrual cycles since her menarche. She has a BMI of 32. She takes medication to manage her diabetes and hypertension. She had been previously diagnosed with PCOS when she was a teenager. Her pelvic examination demonstrated an enlarged uterus. She had been to see her doctor several times because of her irregular bleeding, but she had been treated with medications until a D&C was done after months of unsuccessful drug therapy.

1. What risk factors for endometrial cancer does Jill have?
2. Is it unusual for a woman of Jill's age to have this diagnosis? Why or why not?
3. What treatment options might Jill need to consider after her diagnosis?

PLAN

Jill's histopathology at the time of surgery was reported as grade III adenocarcinoma with pelvic lymph node involvement. Jill underwent a total hysterectomy with bilateral salpingo-oophorectomy and went through three courses of chemotherapy also.

1. What health promotion instructions can the nurse impart to Jill when she returns for her postoperative office visit?
2. In what ways can the nurse assist Jill during this challenging time?
3. What is the "take-home" message learned from this case study?

9

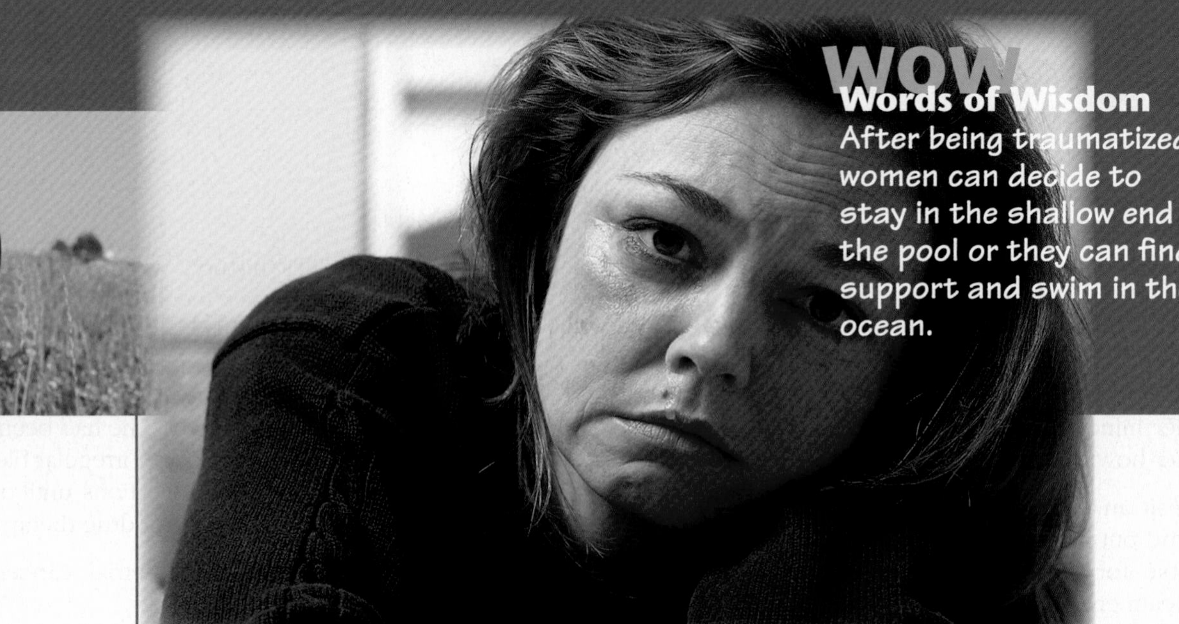
WOW
Words of Wisdom
After being traumatized, women can decide to stay in the shallow end of the pool or they can find support and swim in the ocean.

Violence and Abuse

KEY TERMS

acquaintance rape
battered women syndrome
cycle of violence
date rape
female genital cutting (FGC)
human trafficking
incest
intimate partner violence (IPV)
posttraumatic stress disorder (PTSD)
rape
sexual abuse
statutory rape

Learning Objectives

Upon completion of the chapter, you will be able to:

1. Examine the incidence of violence in women.
2. Characterize the cycle of violence and appropriate interventions.
3. Evaluate the various myths and facts about violence.
4. Analyze the dynamics of rape and sexual abuse.
5. Select the resources available to women experiencing abuse.
6. Outline the role of the nurse who cares for abused women.

***Dorothy* came to the prenatal clinic with a complaint of recurring headaches. She had been in twice this week already, but insisted she be seen today and started to cry. When the nurse called her into the examination room, Dorothy's cell phone rang. She hurried to answer it and told the person on the other end that she was at the store. When the nurse asked if she was afraid at home, Dorothy answered "at times." What cues did the nurse pick up on to ask that question? How frequent is this problem in women?**

INTRODUCTION

Imagine if you were subjected to assault, **rape**, sexual slavery, torture, verbal abuse, mutilation, even murder—all because of your gender. It is rarely acknowledged that violence against women and girls exists on the scale it does. Many of these females are brutalized from cradle to grave simply because of their gender. This abuse is the most pervasive human rights violation in the world today, and yet remains silent to many ears around the globe.

Gender-based violence is a major global public health and human rights problem and one that often goes unrecognized and unreported. It is a common source of physical, psychological, and emotional morbidity. It occurs in all countries, irrespective of social, economic, religious, or cultural group. It affects women across race, ethnicity, age, socioeconomic status, religion, sexual orientation, and geographic boundaries. No segments of society are immune from the vestiges of this problem. Due to the unequal power relations between men and women, women are violated either in the family, in the community, or in the country in which they live. The causes are multidimensional and are social, economic, cultural, political, and religious. Pregnancy is a time of unique vulnerability to **intimate partner violence (IPV)** victimization because of changes in women's physical, social, emotional, and economic needs during pregnancy. Although the true prevalence of violence during pregnancy is unclear, research suggests it is substantial and often continues into the postpartum period. Gender-based violence is one of the most rigorous challenges of women's health and well-being; it is a harrowing worldwide public health concern with serious consequences for individuals, families, and societies (Berthold, 2015).

Female-perpetrated violence against male partners receives little attention. Although women are victims of violence more frequently than men, the prevalence of violence among men nonetheless represents a significant public health concern. One out of every four men has experienced rape, physical violence, and/or stalking by an intimate partner in their lifetime. (National Coalition Against Domestic Violence, 2015).

Although women can be violent in relationships with men, and also in same-sex partnerships, the overwhelming burden of partner violence is borne by women at the hands of men. Nearly 4 in 10 women and 1 in 10 men in the United States have experienced rape, physical violence, and/or stalking by a partner with IPV-related impact (World Health Organization [WHO], 2015a).

Of all the strides American women have made in the past 100 years, obliterating violence against themselves is not one of them. Violence against women is a growing problem and in many countries is still accepted as part of normal behavior. According to the Federal Bureau of Investigation (FBI, 2015), up to half of all women in the United States will experience some form of physical violence during their lifetime. In North America 40% to 60% of murders of women are committed by intimate partners (FBI, 2015). Recently, the FBI has broadened its definition of rape. The new definition, as it appears on the FBI web site, is "Penetration, no matter how slight, of the vagina or anus with any body part or object, or oral penetration by a sex organ of another person, without the consent of the victim." This broader definition will have a dramatic impact on the way rape is tracked and reported nationwide (FBI 2015).

Federal funding for the problem is trickling down to local programs, but it is not reaching victims fast enough. For example, the United States has three times more shelters for animals than for battered women (Bouchet & Braswell, 2015). In many cases, a victim escapes her abuser only to be turned away from a local shelter because it is full. The number of abused women is staggering: one woman is being battered every 12 seconds in the United States (Centers for Disease Control & Prevention [CDC], 2015a).

Nurses play a major role in assessing women who have suffered some type of violence. Nurses have a central ethic of caring and an agenda of early intervention and health promotion for their clients to improve their health status and well-being. Often, after a woman is victimized, she will complain about physical ailments that will give her the opportunity to visit a health care setting. A visit to a health care agency is an ideal time for women to be assessed for violence. Because nurses are viewed as trustworthy and sensitive about very personal subjects, women often feel comfortable confiding in them and discussing these issues with them. As a professional nurse, the act of screening women seen in every health care setting is often the first step for a victim to start thinking about a better future. Remember, your words carry weight with your client who looks to you for help, support, and encouragement.

> ***Take Note!***
>
> *Nurses will come in contact with violence and sexual abuse no matter what health care setting they work in. Nurses must be ready to ask the right questions and to act on the answers, because such action could be lifesaving.*

This chapter addresses several types of gender-based violence: IPV, **female genital cutting (FGC)**, **human trafficking**, and **sexual abuse**. All of these types of violence against women have devastating and costly consequences for all of society.

INTIMATE PARTNER VIOLENCE

IPV is actual or threatened physical or sexual violence or psychological/emotional abuse. Research suggests that physical violence in intimate relationships is often

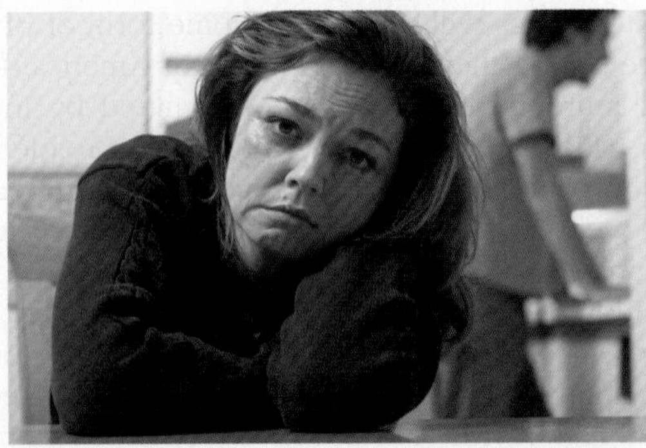

FIGURE 9.1 Intimate partner violence has significant physical, psychological, social, and economic consequences. An important role of the health care provider is to identify abusive or potentially abusive situations as soon as possible and provide support for the victim.

accompanied by psychological abuse and in one-third to over one-half of cases by sexual abuse (CDC, 2015b). Intimate partners include individuals who are currently in dating, cohabitating, or marital relationships, or those who have been in such relationships in the past. Some of the common terms used to describe IPV are domestic abuse, spouse abuse, domestic violence, gender-based violence, battering, and rape. IPV affects a distressingly high percentage of the population and has physical, psychological, social, and economic consequences (Fig. 9.1).

Because a nurse may be the first health care provider to assess and identify the signs of IPV, a nurse can have a profound impact on a woman's decision to seek help. Thus, it is important for nurses to be able to identify abuse and aid the victim. IPV can leave significant psychological scars, and a well-trained nurse can have a positive impact on the victim's mental and emotional health.

Incidence

Overall, lifetime, and 1-year estimates for sexual violence, stalking, and IPV are alarmingly high for adult Americans, with IPV alone affecting more than 12 million people each year. On average, 20 persons per minute are victims of rape, physical violence, or stalking by an intimate partner in the United States. Women are disproportionately affected. The estimated cost of violence in the United States exceeds $70 billion each year. Each year, IPV results in an estimated 2500 deaths and 3 million injuries among women (CDC, 2015c).

Women are at risk for violence at nearly every stage of their lives. Old, young, beautiful, unattractive, married, single—no woman is completely safe from the risk of IPV. Current or former husbands or lovers kill over half of the murdered women in the United States. IPV against women causes more serious injuries and deaths than automobile accidents, rapes, and muggings combined. IPV is expensive. The medical cost of IPV approaches $4.4 trillion each year globally to pay for medical and surgical care, counseling, child care, burden on the justice system, incarceration, attorney fees, and loss of work productivity (Lomborg, 2015).

IPV is pervasive and crosses all boundaries of sexual orientation, race, and class. The intimidation of another person through abusive acts and words is not a gender issue. Violence within these relationships may go unreported for fear of harassment or ridicule. The medical community's efforts to address IPV have often neglected members of the lesbian, gay, bisexual, and transgender (LGBT) population. Heterosexual women are primarily targeted for IPV screening and intervention despite the similar prevalence of IPV in LGBT individuals and its detrimental health effects (Cannon & Buttell, 2015). Perhaps because of the multiple barriers that confront LGBT abuse victims and the invisibility of the problem in the context of IPV services, the role of the nurse as their advocate is all the more critical.

Little is known about the national prevalence of IPV, sexual violence, and stalking among the LGBT community in the United States. Research documents that rates of IPV among LGBT individuals are equal to or greater than rates observed among heterosexual individuals. Risk factors are also similar to those documented among heterosexual individuals, in addition to help-seeking leaving, and recovery process (Edwards, Sylaska, & Neal, 2015). Current findings seem to also indicate some disparities in perceptions of what constitutes abuse among same and opposite sex couples (Russell & Chapleau, 2015). The *Violence against Women Act* has recently been renewed. It now includes coverage of same-sex partners—a big sign that attitudes are changing and improving for gays seeking shelters and help. As individuals and society come to realize same-sex partner violence as an existing problem, there is hope.

Background

Until the mid-1970 s, our society tended to legitimize a man's power and control over a woman. The United States legal and judicial systems considered intervention into family disputes wrong and a violation of the family's right to privacy. IPV was often tolerated and even socially acceptable. Fortunately, attitudes and laws have changed to protect women and punish abusers. There are 13 measurable violence prevention objectives displayed in the *Healthy People 2020* table that follows. In addition to the 13 objectives listed, there are 7 developmental objectives that focus on preventing sexual violence across the lifespan and preventing the different forms of partner violence including physical and sexual violence, emotional abuse, and stalking by a current or former partner.

HEALTHY PEOPLE *2020*

Violence Prevention Objectives	Baseline (Year)	Target (2020)
IVP-29 Reduce homicides per 100,000 population	6.1 (2007)	5.5
IVP-30 Reduce firearm-related deaths per 100,000 population	10.3 (2007)	9.3
IVP-31 Reduce nonfatal firearm-related injuries per 100,000 population	20.7 (2007)	18.6
IVP-32 Reduce nonfatal physical assault injuries per 100,000 population	512.5 (2008)	461.2
IVP-33 Reduce physical assaults per 1,000 population (12+ years)	21.2 (2008)	19.2
IVP-34 Reduce physical fighting among adolescents in grades 9–12	31.5 (2009)	28.4
IVP-35 Reduce bullying among adolescents in grades 9–12	19.9 (2009)	17.9
IVP-36 Reduce weapon carrying by adolescents on school property	5.6 (2009)	4.6
IVP-37Reduce child maltreatment deaths per 100,000 population	2.3 (2008)	2.1
IVP-38 Reduce nonfatal child maltreatment per 100,000 population	9.4 (2008)	8.5
IVP-41 Reduce nonfatal intentional self-harm injuries per 100,000 population	124.9 (2008)	112.4
IVP-42 Reduce children's exposure to violence <18 years old	58.8 (2008)	52.9
IVP-43 Increase the number of States that link data on violent deaths	16 states	50 states

Nursing Significance

- Will increase men and women's quality and years of healthy life
- Eliminate health disparities for survivors of violence
- Goal is to have improved adherence to screening for IPV by health care providers.
- Meeting these objectives will reflect the importance of early detection, intervention, and evaluation
- Eliminating LGBT health disparities and enhancing efforts to improve LGBT health are necessary to ensure that LGBT individuals can lead long, healthy lives

Healthy People objectives based on data from http://www.healthypeople.gov
Adapted from U.S. Department of Health and Human Services [(USDHHS]. (2015b). *Healthy People.gov.* Retrieved from www.healthypeople.gov/2020/default.aspx

Characteristics of Intimate Partner Violence

Although more research is needed in this area, studies have found certain risk factors for IPV in men. These risk factors can be divided into four different categories: individual factors, relationship factors, community factors, and societal factors. Specific risk factors within each category are listed in Table 9.1.

Generation-to-Generation Continuum of Violence

Violence is a learned behavior that, without intervention, is self-perpetuating. It is a cyclical health problem. The long-term effects of violence on victims and children can be profound. Children who witness one parent abuse another are more likely to become delinquents or batterers themselves because they see abuse as an integral part of a close relationship. Thus, an abusive relationship between father and mother can perpetuate future abusive relationships. Violence in childhood and adolescence is linked to the child's perception of the family as a hostile environment and of violence against women as a corrective measure, and insults, swearing, and humiliation by their partner as acceptable (Song et al., 2015). If one considers violence against children and spouses, the psychological consequences are huge, stemming from the paradox of the victim being abused by a member of the family with whom he or she expects to have a supportive, loving, and respectful relationship. Research has found that children who witness IPV are at risk for developing psychiatric disorders, **posttraumatic stress disorder (PTSD)**, developmental problems, school failure, violence against others, and low self-esteem (Cater et al., 2015).

TABLE 9.1 COMMON MYTHS AND FACTS ABOUT VIOLENCE

Myths	Facts
Battering of women occurs only in lower socioeconomic classes.	Violence occurs in all socioeconomic classes.
Substance abuse causes the violence.	Violence is a learned behavior and can be changed. The presence of drugs and alcohol can make a bad problem worse.
Men have the right to discipline their partners. Battering is not a crime	In the past, our patriarchal legal system afforded men the right to physically chastise their wives and children; we no longer live under that system. Women and children are no longer considered the property of men, and violence against them is a crime in every state.
Violence occurs to only a small percentage of women.	One in four women will be victims of violence.
Intimate partner violence (IPV) is typically a one time, isolated occurrence.	Battering is a pattern of coercion and control that one person exerts over another. It is repeated using a number of tactics, including intimidation, threats, physical injury, economic deprivation, isolation, and sexual abuse. The various forms of abuse utilized by batterers help to maintain power and control over their victims.
Women can easily choose to leave an abusive relationship.	Women stay in the abusive relationship because they feel they have no options.
Only men with mental health problems commit violence against women.	Abusers often seem normal and do not appear to suffer from personality disorders or other forms of mental illness.
Pregnant women are protected from abuse by their partners.	One in five women is physically abused during pregnancy. The effects of violence on infant outcomes can include preterm delivery, fetal distress, low birth weight, and child abuse.
Women provoke their partners to abuse them.	Women may be willing to blame themselves for someone else's bad behavior, but nobody deserves to be beaten.
Violent tendencies have gone on for generations and are accepted.	The police, justice system, and society are beginning to make IPV socially unacceptable.
IPV is only a heterosexual issue.	There is as much IPV in the lesbian/gay/bisexual/transgender (LGBT) population as in heterosexual relationships with the added psychological abuse of "outing" (when one partner threatens to disclose the others sexual preference in an effort to maintain power and control).

Adapted from Domestic Violence Organization. (2015a). *Common myths and why they are wrong.* Retrieved from http://www.domesticviolence.org/common-myths/; Tahoe Safe Alliance. (2015). *Myths about intimate partner violence in the LGBTQUA community.* Retrieved from http://tahoesafealliance.org/for-lgbqtia/lgbtqiamyths/; Medicine Net. (2015b). *Domestic violence.* Retrieved from http://www.medicinenet.com/domestic_violence/page4.htm#what_are_the_causes_or_risk_factors_for_intimate_partner_violence

Childhood maltreatment is a major health problem that is associated with a wide range of physical conditions and leads to high rates of psychiatric morbidity and social problems in adulthood. Consequences of violence extend far beyond the physical and mental suffering of victims and their families and have an impact on schools, neighborhoods, businesses, and the legal and health care systems. Women who were physically or sexually abused as children have an increased risk of victimization and fear of crime, poor general health, and in addition experience adverse mental health conditions such as depression, anxiety, and low self-esteem as adults (Barrios et al., 2015).

In many cases when a parent is abused, the children are abused as well. Approximately 1 in 8 children are abused annually in the United States. The lifetime economic cost to society due to childhood maltreatment is estimated to be $124 billion dollars (Jackson & Deye, 2015). Young children who live with family violence represent a disempowered group. Developmentally, young children have relatively limited verbal skills and emotional literacy. In addition, the environment becomes one of secrecy and intimidation, as well as reduced emotional availability from the child's main caretaker. Taken together, these factors severely restrict these young children's capacity and opportunity to make their voices and needs heard (Jackson & Deye, 2015). Exposure to violence has a negative impact on children's physical, emotional, and cognitive well-being. The cycle continues into another generation through learned responses and violent acting out. Although there are always exceptions, most children deprived of their basic physical, psychological, and spiritual needs do not develop healthy personalities. They grow up with feelings of fear, behavioral problems, substance abuse, relationship difficulties, inadequacy, anxiety, anger, hostility, guilt, and rage. They often lack coping skills, blame others, demonstrate poor impulse control, have early delinquent behavior, and generally struggle with authority (Huang et al., 2015). Unless this cycle is broken, more than half become abusers themselves (CDC, 2015e).

The Cycle of Violence

In an abusive relationship, the **cycle of violence** comprises three distinct phases: the tension-building phase, the acute battering phase, and the honeymoon phase (Lawrence, 2015). The cyclical behavior begins with a time of tension-building arguments, progresses to violence, and settles into a making-up or calm period. This cycle of violence increases in frequency and severity as it is repeated over and over again. The cycle can cover a long or short period of time. The honeymoon phase gradually shortens and eventually disappears altogether. Abuse in relationships typically becomes accelerated and thus more dangerous over time. The abuser no longer feels the need to apologize and indulge in a honeymoon phase as the woman becomes increasingly disempowered in the relationship.

PHASE 1: TENSION BUILDING

During the first—and usually the longest—phase of the cycle, tension escalates between the couple. Excessive drinking, jealousy, or other factors might lead to name-calling, hostility, and friction. The woman might sense that her partner is reacting to her more negatively, that he is on edge and reacts heatedly to any trivial frustration. A woman often will accept her partner's building anger as legitimately directed toward her. She internalizes what she perceives as her responsibility to keep the situation from exploding. In her mind, if she does her job well, he remains calm. But if she fails, the resulting violence is her fault.

PHASE 2: ACUTE BATTERING

The second phase of the cycle is the explosion of violence. The batterer loses control both physically and emotionally. This is when the victim may be assaulted or murdered. After a battering episode, most victims consider themselves lucky that the abuse was not worse, no matter how severe their injuries. They often deny the seriousness of their injuries and refuse to seek medical treatment.

PHASE 3: HONEYMOON

The third phase of the cycle is a period of calm, loving, contrite behavior on the part of the batterer. He may be genuinely sorry for the pain he caused his partner. He attempts to make up for his brutal behavior and believes he can control himself and never hurt the woman he loves. The victim wants to believe that her partner really can change. She feels responsible, at least in part, for causing the incident, and she feels responsible for her partner's well-being (Box 9.1).

Types of Abuse

Abusers may use whatever it takes to control a situation—from emotional abuse and humiliation to physical assault. Victims often tolerate emotional, physical, financial, and sexual abuse. Many remain in abusive relationships because they believe they deserve the abuse.

BOX 9.1

CYCLE OF VIOLENCE (FEMALE VICTIM AND MALE ABUSER)

- *Phase 1—Tension building:* Verbal or minor battery occurs. Almost any subject, such as housekeeping or money, may trigger the buildup of tension. There is a breakdown of communication. The victim attempts to calm the abuser. Victim feels like "walking on egg shells" around the abuser.
- *Phase 2—Acute battering:* Characterized by uncontrollable discharge of tension. Violence is rarely triggered by the victim's behavior: she is battered no matter what her response. The start of the battering episode is unpredictable and beyond the victim's control.
- *Phase 3—Reconciliation (honeymoon)/calm phase:* First, the abuser is ashamed of his behavior. The batterer tries to minimize the abuse and blame it on the partner. The batterer becomes loving, kind, and apologetic and expresses guilt. Then the abuser works on making the victim feel responsible. This loving behavior strengthens the bond between partners and will probably convince the victim, once again, that leaving the relationship is not necessary.

Adapted from Domestic Violence Organization. (2015b). *Cycle of violence*. Retrieved from http://www.domesticviolence.org/cycle-of-violence/; Domestic Violence Roundtable. (2015). *The cycle of domestic violence*. Retrieved from http://www.domesticviolenceroundtable.org/domestic-violence-cycle.html; National Stress Clinic. (2015). *Domestic abuse: Understanding and breaking the cycle of violence*. Retrieved from http://www.nationalstressclinic.com/domestic-abuse-understanding-and-breaking-the-cycle-of-violence/

Emotional Abuse

Emotional abuse includes:
- Promising, swearing, or threatening to hit the victim
- Forcing the victim to perform degrading or humiliating acts
- Threatening to harm children, pets, or close friends
- Humiliating the woman by name-calling and insults
- Threatening to leave her and the children
- Isolation from family and friends
- Destroying valued possessions
- Controlling the victim's every move

Physical Abuse

Physical abuse includes:
- Hitting or grabbing the victim so hard that it leaves marks
- Throwing things at the victim
- Slapping, spitting at, biting, burning, pushing, choking, or shoving the victim
- Kicking or punching the victim, or slamming her against things
- Attacking the victim with a knife, gun, rope, or electrical cord
- Controlling access to health care for injury

Financial Abuse

Financial abuse includes:
- Preventing the woman from getting a job
- Sabotaging a current job
- Controlling how all money is spent
- Failing to contribute financially

Sexual Abuse

Sexual abuse includes:
- Forcing the woman to have vaginal, oral, or anal intercourse against her will
- Biting the victim's breasts or genitals
- Shoving objects into the victim's vagina or anus
- Forcing the woman to do something sexual that she finds degrading or humiliating
- Forcing the victim to perform sexual acts on other people or animals

Myths and Facts About Intimate Partner Violence

Table 9.2 lists many of the myths about IPV. Health care providers should take steps to dispel these myths.

Abuse Profiles

Victims

Ironically, victims rarely describe themselves as abused. In **battered woman syndrome**, the woman has experienced deliberate and repeated physical or sexual assault by an intimate partner. She is terrified and feels trapped, helpless, and alone. She reacts to any expression of anger or threat by avoidance and withdrawal behavior. Some women believe that the abuse is caused by a personality flaw or inadequacy in themselves (e.g., inability to keep the man happy). These feelings of failure are reinforced and exploited by their partners. After being told repeatedly that they are "bad," some women begin to believe it. Many victims were abused as children and may have poor self-esteem, poor health, PTSD, depression, insomnia, low education achievement, or a history of suicide attempts, injury, or drug and alcohol abuse (Barrios et. al., 2015).

Abusers

Abusers come from all walks of life and often feel insecure, powerless, and helpless, feelings that are not in line with the macho image they would like to project. The abuser expresses his feelings of inadequacy through violence or aggression toward others (Lawson, 2015).

Violence typically occurs at home and is usually directed toward the man's intimate partner or the children who live there. Abusers refuse to share power and choose violence to control their victims. They often exhibit childlike aggression or antisocial behaviors. They may fail to accept responsibility or blame others for their own problems. They might also have a history of substance abuse problems, trouble with the justice system, few close relationships, being sensitive to criticism, having a tendency to hold grudges, involved in power struggles, emotionally disregulated, lacking in insight, prone to feeling misunderstood, mistreated, or victimized, mental illness, arrests, troubled relationships, obsessive jealousy, controlling behaviors, generally violent behavior, erratic employment history, and financial problems (Lawson, 2015).

Violence Against Pregnant Women

Many think of pregnancy as a time of celebration and planning for the unborn child's future, but in a troubled relationship it can be a time of escalating violence. The strongest predictor of abuse during pregnancy is prior abuse. Violence against pregnant women seems to be more prevalent than diseases routinely investigated during prenatal care, such as preeclampsia and diabetes (Lévesque & Chamberland, 2015). For women who have been abused before, beatings and violence during pregnancy are "business as usual" for them.

Women are at a higher risk for violence during pregnancy. Recent research findings indicate that having children does not protect women from IPV. On the contrary, the IPV appears to last longer if women have children, and this also seems to be the case even after the partnership has come to an end (Mauri et al., 2015). Pregnant women are vulnerable during this time, and abusers

TABLE 9.2 COMMON MYTHS AND FACTS ABOUT RAPE

Myths	Facts
Women who are raped get over it quickly.	It can take several years to recover emotionally and physically from rape.
Most rape victims tell someone about it.	The majority of women never tell anyone about it. In fact, almost two-thirds of victims never report it to the police.
Once the rape is over, a survivor can again feel safe in her life.	The victim feels vulnerable, betrayed, and insecure afterward.
If a woman does not want to be raped, it cannot happen.	A woman can be forced and overpowered by most men.
Women who feel guilty after having sex then say they were raped.	Few women falsely cry "rape." It is very traumatizing to be a victim.
Victims should report the violence to the police and judicial system.	Only 1% of rapists are arrested and convicted. Factoring unreported rapes together with the odds of being arrested and getting a felony conviction, only 6% of rapists will ever spend a day in jail. In other words: 15 of 16 rapists walk free.
Women blame themselves for the rape, believing they did something to provoke the rape.	Women should never blame themselves for being the victim of someone else's violence.
When it comes to sex, men can be provoked to "a point of no return."	Men are physically able to stop at any point during sexual activity. Rape is not an act of impulsive, uncontrolled passion; it is a premeditated act of violence.
Women who wear tight, short clothes are "asking for it."	No victim invites sexual assault, and what she wears is irrelevant.
Women have rape fantasies and want to be raped.	Reality and fantasy are different. Dreams have nothing to do with the brutal violation of rape.
Only attractive women are raped.	Anyone can be raped. Children, the elderly, and people with physical and mental disabilities are easy targets of rape because of their vulnerability.
Medication can help women forget about the rape.	Initially medication can help, but counseling is needed.

Adapted from Centers for Disease Control and Prevention [CDC]. (2015f). *Understanding sexual violence.* Retrieved from http://www.cdc.gov/violenceprevention/pdf/svfactsheet2013-a.pdf; Rape Crisis. (2015). *Common myths about rape.* Retrieved from http://www.rapecrisis.org.uk/commonmyths2.php; Women Against Violence Against Women [WAVAW]. (2015). *Rape myths.* Retrieved from http://www.wavaw.ca/mythbusting/rape-myths/; WELLWVU The Student's Center of Health. (2015). *Rape myths and facts.* Retrieved from https://well.wvu.edu/articles/rape_myths_and_facts

can take advantage of it. An estimated 325,000 pregnant women are abused by their partners each year (CDC, 2015a). Abuse during pregnancy poses special risks and dynamics. Various factors may lead to battering during pregnancy, including:

- Inability of the couple to cope with the stressors of pregnancy
- Young age at time of pregnancy
- Having less than a high school education for both partners
- Unemployment for either or both in partnership
- Violence in the family of origin
- Cohabitation and single marital status
- Sexual proprietariness on the part of the male partner
- Heavy drinking by partner
- Resentment toward the interference of the growing fetus and change in the woman's shape
- Doubts about paternity or the expectant mother's fidelity during pregnancy
- Perception that the baby will be a competitor
- Outside attention the pregnancy brings to the woman
- Unwanted pregnancy
- The woman's new interest in herself and her unborn baby
- Insecurity and jealousy about the pregnancy and the responsibilities it brings

- Financial burden related to expense of pregnancy and loss of income
- Stress of role transition from adult man to becoming the father of a child
- Physical and emotional changes of pregnancy that make the woman vulnerable
- Previous isolation from family and friends that limit the couple's support system

Abuse during pregnancy threatens the well-being of the mother and fetus. Physical violence may involve injuries to the head, face, neck, thorax, breasts, and abdomen. The mental health consequences are also significant. Several studies have confirmed the relationship between abuse and poor mental health, especially depression and PTSD; poor quality of life; increased distress, fearfulness, anxiousness, and stressfulness; and increased use of tobacco, alcohol, and/or illicit drugs (Lawson, 2015). For the pregnant woman, many of these conditions most often manifest during the postpartum period.

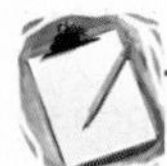

Take Note!

Frequently the fear of harm to her unborn child will motivate a woman to escape an abusive relationship.

Women assaulted during pregnancy are at risk for:

- Injuries to themselves and the fetus
- Depression
- Panic disorder
- Fetal and maternal deaths
- Chronic anxiety
- Miscarriage
- Stillbirth
- Poor nutrition
- Insomnia
- Placental abruption
- Uterine rupture
- Excessive weight gain or loss
- Smoking and substance abuse
- Delayed or no prenatal care
- Preterm labor
- Higher rate of surgical births
- Chorioamnionitis
- Vaginitis
- Sexually transmitted infections (STIs)
- Urinary tract infections
- Premature and low–birth-weight infants (Association of Women's Health, Obstetric and Neonatal Nurses [AWHONN], 2015).

Signs of abuse can emerge during pregnancy and may include poor attendance at prenatal visits, unrealistic fears, weight fluctuations, difficulty with pelvic examinations, and nonadherence to treatment. See Evidence-Based Practice 9.1 for an intervention utilized for pregnant women experiencing IPV.

Uncovering abuse in pregnant women requires a consistent and direct approach to every client by the nurse. Multiple assessments may enhance reporting by enabling the nurse to establish trust and rapport with the woman and identify changes in her behavior. Once abuse is discovered in a pregnant woman, interventions should include safety assessment, emotional support,

EVIDENCE-BASED PRACTICE 9.1

EFFECTIVENESS OF HOME VISITING IN REDUCING PARTNER VIOLENCE FOR FAMILIES EXPERIENCING ABUSE: A SYSTEMATIC REVIEW

STUDY

Intimate partner violence against women is a major, global societal problem with tremendous health consequences both for mother and child. Home-visiting interventions by nurses for families at risk of abuse seem promising in decreasing IVP. In this systematic review the effectiveness of home visiting was assessed as an intervention to reduce IPV experienced by mothers.

Findings

A systematic review was conducted of 1258 articles; 19 of them met the inclusion criteria and were examined in detail. Sixteen reported lower rates of physical assault with home visits by nurses and three studies showed no significant reduction of IPV. This systematic review found that home-visiting interventions that support abused women during their pregnancy and beyond to stop IPV seem to be effective in reducing the incidence of IPV. However, it is not known whether these results are effective long term.

Nursing Implications

By nurses making home visits, a trusting relationship can be established between the client and nurse. By addressing factors that may increase the risk of IPV in general, such as stress as well as other contributing factors, IPV can be reduced and the cycle of violence can be broken. A major benefit of home-visiting interventions is that they succeed in reaching high-risk young pregnant women, who are notoriously hard to reach for regular prenatal services during a vulnerable stage in their lives. Nurses can see the home environment and can detect risk factors and plan interventions to address them.

Adapted from Prosman, G. J., Wong, S. H. L. F., van der Wouden, J. C., & Lagro-Janssen, A. L. (2015). Effectiveness of home visiting in reducing partner violence for families experiencing abuse: A systematic review. *Family Practice*, (Online: 5/6/15) doi: 10.1093/fampra/cmu091 counseling, referral to community services, and ongoing prenatal care to avoid adverse health outcomes (Hewitt, 2015).

Violence Against Older Women

IPV affects women of all ages, but often the literature focuses on women in the childbearing years, ignoring the problems of aging women who experience abuse. Elder mistreatment (i.e., abuse and neglect) is defined as intentional actions that cause harm or create a serious risk of harm to a vulnerable elder by a caregiver or other person who stands in a trust relationship to the elder. All 50 states have laws requiring health care providers to report elder or vulnerable person abuse. Estimates suggest that 500,000 to 2 million cases of elder abuse and neglect occur annually in the United States. It is estimated that 1 in 10 older adults experience abuse, but only 1 in 5 to as little as 1 in 24 are reported. Research suggests that female elders are abused at a higher rate than males and that the older one is, the more likely one is to be abused. Elder abuse is expected to increase as the population ages (Wang et al., 2015). Types of abuse experienced by the older woman may include physical abuse, neglect, emotional abuse, sexual abuse, and financial/exploitation abuse (National Center on Elder Abuse, 2015).

Although an injury may bring the older woman into the health care system, the physical and emotional sequelae of IPV may be more subtle and may include depression, insomnia, chronic pain, difficulty trusting others, low self-esteem, thoughts of suicide, substance abuse, anger issues, atypical chest pain, or other kinds of somatic symptoms. Research suggests that older women usually have endured long-term abuse, have developed unhealthy strategies to cope (substance abuse, keeping the family together at all cost, and physical/mental health consequences), and shoulder blame from their adult children, yet have developed empowerment from within to be able to cope with the abuse (Policastro & Finn, 2015).

Accurate detection and assessment of abuse in older women are essential duties of all nurses. Nurses have frequent contact with older victims of abuse, providing them the opportunity to play a significant role in detecting, reporting, and intervening in such cases. As part of a thorough screening, nurses should determine what the client has done to attempt to resolve the abuse and the effectiveness of those strategies. Actions taken by the client, prior to revealing her abuse issue to the nurse, might have included passive acceptance, calling law enforcement, counseling, or other measures. In addition, taking time to establish rapport with older women builds a sense of trust, safety, and openness. Nurses must listen carefully and nonjudgmentally. Judging or criticizing the victim for her decisions might lead to the impression that she deserves the abuse or that she is to blame. Finally, nurses should attempt to stay current in their knowledge of referral resources to assist the older woman experiencing abuse. Some of these resources may be housing, transportation, medical services, employment, social services, and local support groups. A coordinated and comprehensive response to IPV is essential to reduce its sequelae.

Nursing Management of Intimate Partner Violence Victims

Nurses encounter thousands of abuse victims each year in their practice settings, but many victims slip through the cracks. As universal violence assessment has increased in recent years, nurses need to be aware of not only how to screen for violence, but how to respond in a way that is helpful, sincere, nonjudgmental, and legally adequate. This will require nurses to move beyond a description of violence toward a response that is action-oriented and evidence based, which includes safety planning and referrals. There are many things that nurses can do to help victims. Early recognition and intervention can significantly reduce the morbidity and mortality associated with IPV. To stop the cycle of violence, nurses need to know how to assess for and identify IPV and implement appropriate actions.

Assessment

Routine screening for IPV is the first way to detect abuse. The nurse should build rapport by listening, showing an interest in the concerns of the woman, and creating an atmosphere of openness. Communicating support through a nonjudgmental attitude and telling the woman that no one deserves to be abused are first steps toward establishing trust and rapport. Rather than overlooking abused women as "chronic complainers," astute nurses need to be vigilant for subtle clues of abuse. Learning how to assess for abuse is critical. Some basic assessment guidelines follow.

SCREEN FOR ABUSE DURING EVERY HEALTH CARE VISIT

Screening for violence takes only a few minutes and can have an enormously positive effect on the outcome for the abused woman. Any woman could be a victim; no single sign marks a woman as an abuse victim, but the following clues may be helpful:

- Injuries: bruises on their chest and abdomen, scars from blunt trauma, minor lacerations or weapon wounds on the face, head, and neck
- Injury sequelae: headaches, hearing loss from ruptured ear drums, joint pain, sinus infections, teeth marks, clumps of hair missing, dental trauma, pelvic pain, breast or genital injuries

- Reported history of injury that is not consistent with the actual presenting problem
- Mental health problems: depression, anxiety, substance abuse, eating disorders, suicidal ideation or suicide attempts, anger toward health care provider, PTSD
- Frequent tranquilizer or sedative use
- Delay in seeking medical attention and patterns of repeated injury
- Bruises to the upper arm, neck and face, abdomen, or breasts
- Comments about emotional or physical abuse of "a friend"
- STIs or pelvic inflammatory disease
- Appears nervous, ashamed, or evasive when asked questions
- Frequent health care visits for chronic, stress-related disorders such as chest pain, headaches, back or pelvic pain, insomnia, injuries, anxiety, and gastrointestinal disturbances
- Partner's behavior at the health care visit: appears overly solicitous or overprotective, is unwilling to leave her alone with the health care provider, answers questions for her, and attempts to control the situation (Ghandour, Campbell, & Lloyd, 2015).

***Dorothy*, who you met at the beginning of the chapter, has been frequenting the clinic with vague somatic complaints in recent weeks and admits she is sometimes afraid at home. She tells the nurse her partner doesn't want her to work, although he is only sporadically employed at low-paying jobs. What cues in her assessment might indicate abuse? What physical signs might the nurse observe?**

ISOLATE CLIENT IMMEDIATELY FROM FAMILY

If abuse is detected, immediately isolate the woman to provide privacy and to prevent potential retaliation from the abuser. Asking about abuse in front of the perpetrator may trigger an abusive episode during the interview or at home. Ways to ensure the woman's safety would be to take the victim to an area away from the abuser to ask questions. The assessment can take place anywhere that is private and away from the abuser, for example, x-ray area, ultrasound room, elevator, ladies' room, or laboratory.

If abuse is detected, the nurse can do the following to enhance the nurse–client relationship:

- Educate the woman about the connection between the violence and her symptoms.
- Help the woman acknowledge what has happened to her and begin to deal with the situation.
- Offer her referrals so she can get the help that will allow her to begin to heal.

***Dorothy* returns to the prenatal clinic a month later with anemia, inadequate weight gain, bruises on her face and neck, and second-trimester bleeding. This time she is accompanied by her partner, who stays close to Dorothy. What questions should the nurse ask to assess the situation? Where is the appropriate location to ask these questions? What legal responsibilities does the nurse have concerning her observations?**

ASK DIRECT OR INDIRECT QUESTIONS ABOUT ABUSE

Violence against women is often unseen, unknown, and hidden in families. Questions to screen for abuse should be routine and handled just like any other question. Many nurses feel uncomfortable asking questions of this nature, but broaching the subject is important even if the answer comes later. Opening up the possibility for women to express themselves about their experience of abuse to a nurse sends out a clear message that violence should never be tolerated and not kept hidden; it also conveys the message that nurses care about women's experiences and want to offer a best practice initial response. Just knowing that someone else knows about the abuse offers a victim some relief and may help her disclose it.

Ask difficult questions in an empathetic and nonthreatening manner and remain nonjudgmental in all responses and interactions. Choose the type of question that makes you most comfortable. Direct and indirect questions produce the same results. "Does your partner hit you?" or "Have you ever been or are you now in an abusive relationship?" are direct questions. If that approach feels uncomfortable, try indirect questions: "We see many women with injuries or complaints like yours and often they are being abused. Is that what is happening to you?" or "Many women in our community experience abuse from their partners. Is anything like that happening in your life?" With either approach, nurses need to maintain a nonjudgmental acceptance of whatever answers the woman offers. The SAVE Model is a screening protocol that nurses can use when assessing women for violence (Box 9.2).

ASSESS IMMEDIATE SAFETY

It is essential to assist the woman by assessing her safety and the safety of her children. To do this, speak to the woman alone and ask her:

- Does she feel safe going home after her meeting with you?
- Does she need an immediate place of safety for herself or her children?
- Does she have a plan of escape if she becomes at risk for her safety?
- Does she need to consider an alternative exit from this building?
- Who are the people she could contact for help or support?

BOX 9.2

SAVE MODEL

SCREEN all of your clients for violence by asking:
- Within the last year, have you been physically hurt by someone?
- Do you feel you are in control of your life?
- Within the last year, has anyone forced you to engage in sexual activities?
- Can you talk about your abuse with me now?
- In general, how would you describe your present relationship?

ASK direct questions in a nonjudgmental way:
- Begin by normalizing the topic to the woman.
- Make continuous eye contact with the woman.
- Stay calm; avoid emotional reactions to what she tells you.
- Never blame the woman, even if she blames herself.
- Do not dismiss or minimize what she tells you, even if she does.
- Wait for each answer patiently. Do not rush to the next question.
- Do not use formal, technical, or medical language.
- Avoid using leading questions; be direct and to the point.
- Use a nonthreatening, accepting approach.

VALIDATE the client by telling her:
- You believe her story.
- You do not blame her for what happened.
- It is brave of her to tell you this.
- Help is available for her.
- Talking with you is a hopeful sign and a first big step.

EVALUATE, educate, and refer this client by asking her:
- What type of violence was it?
- Is she now in any danger?
- How is she feeling now?
- Does she know that there are consequences to violence?
- Is she aware of community resources available to help her?

Adapted from U.S. Department of Health and Human Services [USDHHS]. (2015c). Screening for domestic violence in health care settings. *Office of the Assistant Secretary for Planning and Evaluation.* Retrieved from http://aspe.hhs.gov/hsp/13/dv/pb_screeningdomestic.cfm; Association of Women's Health, Obstetric and Neonatal Nurses [AWHONN]. (2015). Intimate partner violence. *Journal of Obstetric, Gynecologic, and Neonatal Nursing, 44*(3), 405–408.; Canadian Domestic Homicide Prevention Initiative. (2015). *Risk assessment, risk management and safety planning.* Retrieved from http://www.learningtoendabuse.ca/cdhpi/risk-assessment-risk-management-and-safety-planning

The Danger Assessment Tool (Box 9.3) helps women and health care providers assess the potential for homicidal behavior in an ongoing abusive relationship. It is based on research that showed several risk factors for abuse-related murders:

- Increased frequency or severity of abuse
- Presence of firearms
- Sexual abuse
- Substance abuse
- Precipitated by arguments and conflicts
- Generally violent behavior outside of the home
- Control issues (e.g., daily chores, friends, job, money)
- Physical abuse during pregnancy
- Suicide threats or attempts (victim or abuser)
- Child abuse (Sugg, 2015).

DOCUMENT AND REPORT YOUR FINDINGS

If the interview reveals a history of abuse, accurate documentation is critical because this evidence may support the woman's case in court. Documentation must include details about the frequency and severity of abuse; the location, extent, and outcome of injuries; and any treatments or interventions. When documenting, use direct quotes and be very specific: "He choked me." Describe any visible injuries, and use a body map (outline of a woman's body) to show where the injuries are. Obtain photos (with informed consent) or document her refusal if the woman declines photos. Pictures or diagrams can be worth a thousand words. Figure 9.2 shows a sample documentation form for IPV.

Laws in many states require health care providers to alert the police to any injuries that involve knives, firearms, or other deadly weapons or that present life-threatening emergencies. If assessment reveals suspicion or actual indication of abuse, nurses can explain to the woman that they are required by law to report it.

Nursing Diagnosis

When violence is suspected or validated, the nurse needs to formulate nursing diagnoses based on the completed assessment. Possible nursing diagnoses related to violence against women might include the following:

- Deficient knowledge related to understanding the cycle of violence and availability of resources
- Anxiety related to threat to self-concept, situational crisis of abuse
- Situational low self-esteem related to negative family interactions
- Powerlessness related to lifestyle of helplessness
- Compromised individual and family coping related to abusive patterns

Interventions

The response of nurses to battered women can have a profound effect on their willingness to open up or seek help. Some responses to assist successful communication in these circumstances could include:

- Listening—"I hear and understand what you are saying." Being listened to can be an empowering experience for a woman who has been abused.
- Communicating belief—"That must have been very frightening for you."

BOX 9.3

DANGER ASSESSMENT TOOL

Several risk factors have been associated with increased risk of homicides (murders) of women and men in violent relationships. No one can predict what will happen in your case, but we would like you to be aware of the danger of homicide in situations of abuse and for you to see how many of the risk factors apply to your situation. ("He" refers to your husband, partner, ex-husband, ex-partner, or whoever is currently physically hurting you.)

_____1. Has the physical violence increased in severity or frequency over the past year?
_____2. Does he own a gun?
_____3. Have you left him after living together during the past year?
_____4. Is he unemployed?
_____5. Has he ever used a weapon against you or threatened you with a lethal weapon?
_____6. Does he threaten to kill you?
_____7. Has he avoided being arrested for domestic violence?
_____8. Do you have a child that is not his?
_____9. Has he ever forced you to have sex when you did not wish to do so?
_____10. Does he ever try to choke you?
_____11. Does he use illegal drugs? By drugs, I mean "uppers" or amphetamines, "meth," speed, angel dust, cocaine, "crack," street drugs, or mixtures.
_____12. Is he an alcoholic or problem drinker?
_____13. Does he control most or all of your daily activities? For instance: does he tell you who you can be friends with, when you can see your family, how much money you can use, or when you can take the car?
_____14. Is he violently and constantly jealous of you? (For instance, does he say "If I can't have you, no one can.")
_____15. Have you ever been beaten by him while you were pregnant?
_____16. Has he ever threatened or tried to commit suicide?
_____17. Does he threaten to harm your children?
_____18. Do you believe he is capable of killing you?
_____19. Does he follow or spy on you, leave threatening notes or messages on answering machine, destroy your property, or call you when you don't want him to?
_____20. Have you ever threatened or tried to commit suicide?
_____ Total "Yes" Answers

Thank you. Please talk to your nurse, advocate, or counselor about what the Danger Assessment means in terms of your situation.

Source: March of Dimes Danger Assessment questionnaire. (From Campbell, J. (1986). Nursing assessment for risk of homicide with battered women. *Advances in Nursing Science, 8*(4), 36–51.)

- Validating the decision to disclose—"It must have been difficult for you to talk about this today."
- Emphasizing the unacceptability of this violence—"You don't deserve to be treated this way."

If abuse is identified, nurses can undertake interventions that can increase the woman's safety and improve her health. The goal of intervention is to enable the victim to gain control of her life. Provide sensitive, predictable care in an acceptable setting. Offer step-by-step explanations of procedures. Provide educational materials about violence. Allow the victim to actively participate in her care and have control over all health care decisions. Pace your nursing interventions and allow the woman to take the lead. Communicate support through a nonjudgmental attitude. Carefully document all of your assessment findings and nursing interventions.

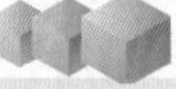
Concept Mastery Alert

Priorities in Intimate Partner Violence Interventions

Although it is certainly important that the woman in an abusive situation is safe, it is most important for a woman to regain a sense of control in her life. A lack of control is what prevents a woman from escaping an abusive situation.

A public health approach to violence prevention requires input from and coordination across sectors, including health, education, social services, justice, and policy. The goal of public health is to improve the health of the entire community or society. Depending on when in the cycle of violence the nurse encounters the abused woman, goals may fall into three groups:

Domestic Violence Screening/Documentation Form

DV Screen
☐ DV + (Positive)
☐ DV? (Suspected)

Date ________ Patient ID# ________
Patient Name ________
Provider Name ________
Patient Pregnant? ☐ Yes ☐ No

Assess Patient Safety

☐ Yes ☐ No Is abuser here now?
☐ Yes ☐ No Is patient afraid of their partner?
☐ Yes ☐ No Is patient afraid to go home?
☐ Yes ☐ No Has physical violence increased in severity?
☐ Yes ☐ No Has partner physically abused children?
☐ Yes ☐ No Have children witnessed violence in the home?
☐ Yes ☐ No Threats of homicide?
By whom? ________
☐ Yes ☐ No Threats of suicide?
By whom? ________
☐ Yes ☐ No Is there a gun in the home?
☐ Yes ☐ No Alcohol or substance abuse?
☐ Yes ☐ No Was safety plan discussed?

Referrals

☐ Hotline number given
☐ Legal referral made
☐ Shelter number given
☐ In-house referral made
Describe: ________
☐ Other referral made
Describe: ________

Reporting

☐ Law enforcement report made
☐ Child Protective Services report made
☐ Adult Protective Services report made

Photographs

☐ Yes ☐ No Consent to be photographed?
☐ Yes ☐ No Photographs taken?
Attach photographs and consent form

FIGURE 9.2 Intimate partner violence documentation form. (Reprinted from *Home Healthcare Nurse, 17*, Cassidy K, *How to assess and intervene in domestic violence situations,* 644–72, Copyright 1999, with permission from Lippincott Williams & Wilkins.)

- *Primary prevention:* aimed at breaking the abuse cycle through community educational initiatives by nurses, physicians and nurse practitioners, law enforcement, teachers, and clergy
- *Secondary prevention:* focuses on screening high-risk individuals and dealing with victims and abusers in early stages, with the goal of preventing progression of abuse
- *Tertiary prevention:* activities are geared toward helping severely abused women and children recover and become productive members of society and rehabilitating abusers to stop the cycle of violence. These activities are typically long term and expensive.

A modified tool developed by Holtz and Furniss (1993)—the ABCDES—provides a framework for providing sensitive nursing interventions to abused women (Box 9.4). Specific nursing interventions for the abused woman include educating her about community services, providing emotional support, and offering a safety plan.

BOX 9.4

THE ABCDES OF CARING FOR ABUSED WOMEN

- **A** is reassuring the woman that she is not alone. The isolation by her abuser keeps her from knowing that others are in the same situation and that health care providers can help her.
- **B** is expressing the belief that violence against women is not acceptable in any situation and that it is not her fault. Demonstrate by your actions and words that you believe her disclosure.
- **C** is confidentiality, since the woman might believe that if the abuse is reported, the abuser will retaliate. Interview her in private, without her partner or family members being present. Assure her that you will not release her information without her permission.
- **D** is documentation, which includes the following:
  1. A clear quoted statement about the abuse in the woman's own words.
  2. Accurate descriptions of injuries and the history of them.
  3. Information on the first, the worst, and the most recent abusive incident.
  4. Photos of the injuries (with the woman's consent).
- **E** is education about the cycle of violence and that it will escalate:
  1. Educate about abuse and its health effects.
  2. Help her to understand that she is not alone.
  3. Offer appropriate community support and referrals.
  4. Display posters and brochures to foster awareness of this public health problem.
- **S** is safety, the most important aspect of the intervention, to ensure that the woman has resources and a plan of action to carry out when she decides to leave.

Adapted from Centers for Disease Control & Prevention [CDC]. (2015a). *Understanding intimate partner violence: Fact sheet.* Retrieved from http://www.cdc.gov/violenceprevention/pub/ipv_factsheet.html; Human Rights Watch. (2015). *Abused and expelled.* Retrieved from http://www.hrw.org/sites/default/files/reports/morocco0214_ForUpload.pdf; Ghandour, R. M., Campbell, J. C., & Lloyd, J. (2015). Screening and counseling for intimate partner violence: A vision for the future. *Journal of Women's Health, 24*(1), 57–61.

EDUCATE THE WOMAN ABOUT COMMUNITY SERVICES

A wide range of support services are available to meet the needs of victims of violence. Nurses should be prepared to help the woman take advantage of these opportunities. Services will vary by community but might include psychological counseling, legal advice, social services, crisis services, support groups, hotlines, housing, vocational training, and other community-based referrals.

Give the woman information about shelters or services even if she initially rejects it. Give the woman the National Domestic Violence hotline number: (800) 799-7233. The Joint Commission on the Accreditation of Hospitals and Health care Organizations (JCAHO), American Medical Association (AMA), American College of Obstetrician Gynecologists (ACOG), and the United States Preventive Services Task Force (USPSTF) all recommend routine IVP screening, counseling, and referrals in all health care agencies (U.S. Department of Health and Human Services [USDHHS], 2015c).

PROVIDE EMOTIONAL SUPPORT

Providing reassurance and support to a victim of abuse is essential if the violence is to end. The physical, psychological, and emotional effects of IPV on women and their children can be severe and long lasting. Nurses in all clinical settings can help victims to feel a sense of personal power and provide them with a safe and supportive environment. Appropriate action can help victims to express their thoughts and feelings in constructive ways, manage stress, and move on with their lives. Appropriate interventions are:

- Strengthen the woman's sense of control over her life by:
  - Teach coping strategies to manage her stress
  - Assist with activities of daily living to improve her lifestyle
  - Allow her to make as many decisions as she can
  - Educate her about the symptoms of PTSD and their basis
- Encourage the woman to establish realistic goals for herself by:
  - Teaching problem-solving skills
  - Encouraging social activities to connect with other people
- Providing support and allow the woman to grieve for her losses by:
  - Listening to and clarifying her reactions to the traumatic event
  - Discussing shock, disbelief, anger, depression, and acceptance
- Explain to the woman that:
  - Abuse is never OK. She didn't ask for it and she doesn't deserve it
  - She is not alone and help is available

- Abuse is a crime and she is a victim
- Alcohol, drugs, money problems, depression, or jealousy does not cause violence, but these things can give the abuser an excuse for losing control and abusing her
- The actions of the abuser are not her fault
- Her history of abuse is believed
- Making a decision to leave an abusive relationship can be very hard and takes time

OFFER A SAFETY PLAN

The choice to leave must rest with the victim. Nurses cannot choose a life for the victim; they can only offer choices. Leaving is a process, not an event. Victims may try to leave their abusers as many as seven or eight times before succeeding. Frequently, the final attempt to leave may result in the death of the victim. Women planning to leave an abusive relationship should have a safety plan, if possible (Teaching Guidelines 9.1).

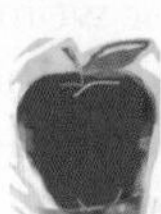

Teaching Guidelines 9.1

SAFETY PLAN FOR LEAVING AN ABUSIVE RELATIONSHIP

- When leaving an abusive relationship, take the following items:
  - Driver's license or photo ID
  - Social Security number or green card/work permit
  - Birth certificates for you and your children
  - Phone numbers for social services or women's shelter
  - The deed or lease to your home or apartment
  - Any court papers or orders
  - A change of clothing for you and your children
  - Pay stubs, checkbook, credit cards, and cash
  - Health insurance cards
  - If you need to leave a domestic violence situation immediately, turn to authorities for assistance in gathering this material
- Develop a "game plan" for leaving and rehearse it
- Don't use phone cards—they leave a trail to follow

Adapted from Burnett, L. B., & Adler, J. (2015). Domestic violence. *eMedicine.* Retrieved from http://emedicine.medscape.com/article/805546-overview; Murray, C. E., Horton, G. E., Johnson, C. H., Notestine, L., Garr, B., Pow, A. M., et al. (2015). Domestic violence service providers' perceptions of safety planning: A focus group study. *Journal of Family Violence, 30*(3), 381–392; Chang, J. C. (2015). Domestic violence: Epidemiology and risk factors. *Clinical Gynecology* (2nd ed., pp. 94–101), Cambridge, UK: Cambridge University Press.

Nurses need to remember that their role is that of a guide, not a savior. A woman will make the best decision she sees fit at that moment in time. A nurse may be her most effective resource in her stress-filled environment. Just allowing the woman to talk may be the most valuable intervention. The impact of the nurse's presence and support will stay with the woman, no matter what decision she makes.

SEXUAL VIOLENCE

Sexual violence is both a public health problem and a human rights violation. Sexual violence includes IPV, human trafficking, **incest**, FGC, forced prostitution, bondage, exploitation, neglect, infanticide, and sexual assault. It occurs worldwide and affects up to one-third of women over a lifetime (Bagwell-Gray et al., 2015). Once every 2 minutes, 30 times an hour, 1871 times a day, girls and women in America are raped. One in 5 women and 1 in 71 men will be sexually assaulted during their lifetime (Rape, Abuse, and Incest National Network [RAINN], 2015a). Rape has been reported against females from age 6 months to 93 years, but it still remains one of the most underreported violent crimes in the United States. Once every 2 minutes, a woman is sexually assaulted in the United States (RAINN, 2015a). The National Center for Prevention and Control of Sexual Assault estimates that two-thirds of sexual assaults will not be reported (CDC, 2015f). Over the course of their lives, women may experience more than one type of violence.

Sexual violence can have a variety of devastating short- and long-term effects. Women can experience psychological, physical, and cognitive symptoms that affect them daily. They can include chronic pelvic pain, headaches, backache, STIs, pregnancy, anxiety, denial, fear, withdrawal, sleep disturbances, guilt, nervousness, phobias, substance abuse, depression, sexual dysfunction, and PTSD. Many contemplate suicide (CDC, 2015f). A traumatic experience not only damages a woman's sense of safety in the world, but it can also reduce her self-esteem and her ability to continue her education, to earn money and be productive, to have children and, if she has children, to nurture and protect them. Overall, sexually assaulted women exhibit lower functioning as adults afterward (MacGregor et al., 2015).

Take Note!

Sexual violence has been called a "tragedy of youth." More than half of all rapes (54%) of women occur before age 18 (Medicine Net, 2015a).

Characteristics of Assailants

Assailants, like their victims, come from all walks of life and all ethnic backgrounds; there is no typical profile. More than half are under the age of 25, and the majority are married and leading "normal" sex lives. Why do men rape? No theory provides a satisfactory explanation. So few assailants are caught and convicted that a clear profile remains elusive. What is known is that many assailants have trouble dealing with the stresses of daily life. Such men become angry and experience feelings of powerlessness. They become jealous easily; do not view women as equals; frequently are hot tempered; have a need to be reassured of their manhood; and do not handle stress in their lives well. They commit a sexual assault as an expression of power and control (Kilmartin, 2015).

Sexual Abuse

Sexual abuse occurs when a woman is forced to have sexual contact of any kind (vaginal, oral, or anal) without her consent. Current estimates indicate that one of five girls is sexually abused, and the peak ages of such abuse are from 8 to 12 years of age. At every age in the life span, females are more likely to be sexually abused by father, brother, family member, neighbor, boyfriend, husband, partner, or ex-partner than by a stranger or anonymous assailant. Sexual abuse knows no economic or cultural barriers (de Jong et al., 2015). Marriage does not constitute a tacit agreement for a spouse to inflict one's demands on the other without permission.

Childhood sexual abuse is any type of sexual exploitation that involves a child younger than 18 years old. It might include disrobing, nudity, masturbation, fondling, digital penetration, forced performance of sexual acts on the perpetrator, and intercourse (Dutton, 2015). Childhood sexual abuse has a lifelong impact on its survivors. There is strong evidence that sexual assault in childhood or adolescence is a serious risk factor for mental illness (Brooker & Durmaz, 2015). Women who were sexually abused during childhood are at a heightened risk for repeat abuse. This is because the early abuse lowers their self-esteem and their ability to protect themselves and set firm boundaries. Childhood sexual abuse is a trauma that influences the way victims form relationships, deal with adversity, cope with daily problems, relate to their children and peers, protect their health, and live. See Evidence-Based Practice 9.2 for study regarding childhood sexual abuse. Studies have shown that the more victimization a woman experiences, the more likely it is she will be revictimized (Brenner & Ben-Amitay, 2015).

Interventions for sexually abused children or women should include referral for mental health counseling. Follow up for any medical problems (e.g., genitourinary complaints) should be arranged with the child's or woman's primary care physician or nurse practitioner. If the community has an abuse referral center, refer the victim there for follow-up care according to local protocol.

EVIDENCE-BASED PRACTICE 9.2 SIBLING SEXUAL ABUSE: AN EXPLORATORY STUDY OF LONG-TERM CONSEQUENCES FOR SELF-ESTEEM AND COUNSELING CONSIDERATIONS

Today, health care providers recognize childhood sexual abuse within the family as a significant and widespread problem with consequences lasting long into adulthood. Despite this progression, the research related to interfamilial incest conducted by researchers has focused primarily on father to daughter incest, largely ignoring the experience of sibling sexual assault, although it is more common than parental incest. Clearly, sibling incest is a pandemic problem that requires more attention from health care providers.

STUDY

This study addresses experiencing sibling sexual abuse as a child and how it inversely affects the level of self-esteem in adulthood. One hundred college students were used as the sample size; 67% were female and 33% were male with a diverse cultural representation. The age of the students ranged from 20 to 59 years old. A survey with two sections was used. The first section addressed recollection of the prevalence and severity of sibling abuse; the second section of the survey addressed self-esteem using the Rosenberg Self-Esteem Scale. Reliability and validity of this tool reflected a Cronbach alpha coefficient of 0.82.

Findings

This study supported the likelihood that sibling sexual abuse could be the most common form of child sexual abuse in the United States. In spite of the apparent prevalence of this, it is disturbing how little has been done to address the complexity surrounding this form of abuse. Both survivors and offenders of sibling sexual abuse experience the lasting impact of the abuse as they become adults in their social interactions, school, work, and family life. In addition to a low self-esteem, other mental health issues experienced include symptoms of PTSD, anxiety disorders, depression, eating disorders, angry outbursts, self-injury, somatic complaints, and suicidal ideation. Many engage in at-risk behaviors such as unprotected sex, self-medication with drugs and alcohol, and dating violence. Clearly, ignoring the problem of sibling sexual abuse has a negative effect on a sense of well-being as these children become adults.

Nursing Implications

One of the most important aspects is to establish trust with these clients and create a safe environment. An important role for nurses is in primary prevention of sibling sexual abuse through educating parents. When parents understand how to promote positive parent–child relationships and sibling interactions, the risk of abuse in the entire family tends to be reduced. Nurses can take a lead role through promotion of structured parent education programs within their communities and referrals to national networks such as Family Support America.

Adopted from Morrill, M. (2014). Sibling sexual abuse: An exploratory study of long term consequences for self-esteem and counseling considerations. *Journal of Family Violence. 29*(2), 205–213.

The medical consequences of sexual abuse require the prophylaxis and treatment of STIs, emergency contraception, and treatment of any injuries that resulted from the abuse. Victims with postassault bleeding require an emergent evaluation and may need emergency treatment by a gynecologist for repair of genital injury. The psychosocial aspects of sexual abuse must also be addressed because appropriate therapeutic follow-up is essential to the victim's future emotional well-being.

Incest

Incest is defined as sexual activity between persons so closely related that marriage between them is legally or culturally prohibited (Dorland, 2015). The exact incidence of child sexual victimization is unknown. Such sexual abuse is not only a crime but also a symptom of acute and irreversible family dysfunction. Childhood incest abuse involves any kind of sexual exploitation between a child and another person that violates the social taboos of family roles; children cannot yet understand these activities and cannot give informed consent. Adult women with a history of incest exhibit a clinical syndrome that includes low self-esteem, difficulty with intimate relationships, sexual dysfunction, flashbacks and nightmares, repeated victimization, as well as suicidality, depressive symptomatology, eating disorders, and substance abuse (Harkins, 2015). Survivors of incest are often tricked, coerced, or manipulated. All adults appear to be powerful to children. Perpetrators might threaten victims so that they are afraid to disclose the abuse or might tell them the abuse is their fault. Often these threats serve to silence victims.

Incestuous relationships in the home endanger not only the child's intellectual and moral development, but also the health of the child. Many children do not ask for help because they do not want to expose their "secret." For this reason, just the tip of the iceberg is statistically visible: serious injuries, internal damage, STIs, or pregnancy. Incest can have serious long-term effects on its victims, which may include eating disorders, sexual problems in adult life, difficulty in interpersonal relationships, anxiety, PTSD, intense guilt and shame, low self-esteem, depression, and self-destructive behavior (National Center for Victims of Crime [NCVC], 2015a).

Whether an incest victim endured an isolated incident of abuse or ongoing assaults over an extended period, recovery can be painful and difficult. The recovery process begins with admission of abuse and the recognition that help and services are needed. Resources for incest victims include books, self-help groups, workshops, therapy programs, and possibly legal remedies. In addition to listening to and believing incest victims, nurses need to search for ways to prevent future generations from enduring such abuse and from continuing the cycle of abuse in their own family and relationships. Nurses have the ability and the responsibility to function within an interdisciplinary system responsible for the assessment and ongoing treatment of incestuous families. Nurses can fulfill their roles as advocates for children, while at the same time adding necessary referrals to social services and legal authorities. Forming this partnership with the social service and judicial communities will help protect the child from future abuse and ensure the child a safe environment in which to grow and develop.

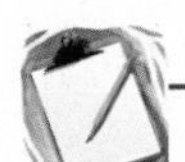

Take Note!

Childhood sexual abuse is a trauma that can affect every aspect of the victim's life.

Rape

Rape is an expression of violence, not a sexual act. Rape distorts one of the most intimate forms of human interaction. It is not an act of lust or an overzealous release of passion: it is a violent, aggressive assault on the victim's body and integrity. Those who rape do so for a number of reasons, but they basically involve the motives of anger, power, eroticized cruelty, and opportunistic mating (Keygnaert, Vettenburg, & Temmerman, 2015). Rape is a legal rather than a medical term. It denotes penile penetration of the vagina, mouth, or rectum of the female or male without consent. It may or may not include the use of a weapon. **Statutory rape** is sexual activity between an adult and a person under the age of 18 and is considered to have occurred even if the underage person was willing (RAINN, 2015b). Nine out of every 10 rape victims are female (Alexander et al., 2014). Enforcement of laws, education, and community empowerment are all needed to prevent rape.

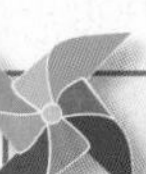

Consider This

At 53 years old, I stood and looked at myself in the mirror. The image staring back at me was one of a frightened, middle-aged, cowardly woman hiding her past. I had been sexually abused by my father for many years as a child and never told anyone. My mother knew of the abuse but felt helpless to make it stop. I married right out of high school to escape and felt I lived a "happy normal life" with my husband and three children. My children have left home and live away, and my husband recently died of a sudden heart attack. I am now experiencing dreams and thoughts about my past abuse and feeling afraid again.

Thoughts: This woman suppressed her abusive past for most of her life and now her painful experience has surfaced. What can be done to reach out to her at this point? Did her health care providers miss the "red flags" that are common to women with a history of childhood sexual abuse all those years?

Many people believe that rape usually occurs on a dark night when a stranger assaults a provocatively dressed, promiscuous woman. They believe that rapists are sex-starved people seeking sexual gratification. Rape myths are destructive beliefs about sexual aggression (i.e., its scope, causes, context, and consequences) that serve to deny, downplay, or justify sexually aggressive behavior that men commit against women. A rape victim's recovery is frequently complicated by the public's failure to believe the victim and restore justice (Klaus, Buczkowski, & Wiktorska, 2015). Rape myths serve to blame victims and exonerate perpetrators. Such myths and the facts are presented in Table 9.3.

Acquaintance Rape

In **acquaintance rape**, someone is forced to have sex by a person he or she knows. Rape by a coworker, a teacher, a husband's friend, or a boss is considered acquaintance rape. **Date rape**, an assault that occurs within a dating relationship or marriage without consent of one of the participants, is a form of acquaintance rape. Acquaintance and date rapes commonly occur on college campuses. One in four college women has been raped—that is, has been forced, physically or verbally, actively or implicitly, to engage in sexual activity (Wilson & Miller, 2015).

TABLE 9.3 FOUR PHASES OF RAPE RECOVERY

Phase	Survivor's Response
Acute phase (disorganization)	Shock, fear, disbelief, anger, shame, guilt, feelings of uncleanliness; insomnia, nightmares, and sobbing
Outward adjustment phase (denial)	Appears outwardly composed and returns to work or school; refuses to discuss the assault and denies need for counseling
Reorganization	Denial and suppression do not work, and the survivor attempts to make life adjustments by moving or changing jobs and uses emotional distancing to cope
Integration and recovery	Survivor begins to feel safe and starts to trust others. She may become an advocate for other rape victims

Adapted from National Center for Victims of Crime [NCVC]. (2015b). *The trauma of victimization.* Retrieved from http://victimsofcrime.org/help-for-crime-victims/get-help-bulletins-for-crime-victims/trauma-of-victimization#ptsd; Rape, Abuse, and Incest National Network [RAINN]. (2015d). *Recovery from sexual assault.* Retrieved from http://www.rainn.org/get-information/sexual-assault-recovery; The Advocacy Center. (2015). The path toward recovery for survivors of sexual violence. Retrieved from http://advocacycenter.syr.edu/students/path-of-recovery/

These forms of rape are physically and emotionally devastating for the victims. Research has indicated that the survivors of acquaintance rape report similar levels of depression, anxiety, complications in subsequent relationships, and difficulty attaining prerape levels of sexual satisfaction to those reported by survivors of stranger rape. Acquaintance rape remains a controversial topic because there is lack of agreement on the definition of consent. Despite the violation and reality of physical and emotional trauma, victims of acquaintance assault often do not identify their experience as sexual assault. Instead of focusing on the violation of the sexual assault, victims of acquaintance rape often blame themselves for the assault (RAINN, 2015c).

Although acquaintance rape and date rape do not always involve drugs, a rapist might use alcohol or other drugs to sedate his victim. In 1996 the federal government passed a law making it a felony to give an unsuspecting person a "date rape drug" with the intent of raping him or her. Even with penalties of large fines and up to 20 years in prison, the use of date rape drugs is growing (USDHHS, 2015a). Date rape drugs are also known as "club drugs" because they are often used at dance clubs, fraternity parties, and all-night raves. The most common is Rohypnol (also known as "roofies," "forget pills," "mind erasers," and the "drop drug"). It comes in the form of a liquid or pill that quickly dissolves in liquid with no odor, taste, or color. This drug is 10 times as strong as diazepam (Valium). The effects can be felt within 30 minutes and produces memory loss for up to 8 hours. Gamma hydroxybutyrate (GHB; called "liquid ecstasy" or "easy lay") produces euphoria, an out-of-body high, sleepiness, increased sex drive, and memory loss. GHB takes effect in about 15 minutes and can last 3 to 4 hours. It comes in a white powder or liquid and may cause unconsciousness, depression, and coma. The third date rape drug, ketamine (known as "Special K," "vitamin K," or "super acid"), acts on the central nervous system very quickly to separate perception and sensation. Combining ketamine with other drugs can be fatal. Date rape drugs can be very dangerous, and women can protect themselves against them in a variety of ways (Teaching Guidelines 9.2).

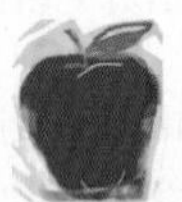

Teaching Guidelines 9.2

PROTECTING YOURSELF AGAINST DATE RAPE DRUGS

- Avoid parties where alcohol is being served.
- Never leave a drink of any kind unattended.
- Don't accept a drink from someone else.
- Accept drinks from a bartender or in a closed container only.
- If a drink is left unattended, pour it out, don't drink it
- Don't drink anything that tastes or smells strange
- Don't drink from a punch bowl or a keg.
- If you think someone drugged you, call 911.

TABLE 9.4 RISK FACTORS FOR INTIMATE PARTNER VIOLENCE IN MEN

Individual Factors	Relationship Factors	Community Factors	Societal Factors
Young age	Martial conflict	Weak sanctions against IPV	Traditional gender norms
Heavy drinking	Economic stress	Poverty	Social norms supportive of violence
Personality disorders	Dysfunctional family	Low social capital	
Depression	Marital instability		
Low academic achievement	Male dominance in family		
Witnessing violence as a child	Cohabitation		
Low income and/or unemployment	Having outside sexual partners		
Experiencing violence as a child			
Desire for power and control in all relationships			
Anger and hostility	Taking aggression out on others while growing up		

Adapted from Centers for Disease Control and Prevention [CDC]. (2015d) *Intimate partner violence: Risk and protective factors.* Retrieved from http://www.cdc.gov/violenceprevention/intimatepartnerviolence/riskprotectivefactors.html; The Christian Broadcasting Network [CBN]. (2015). *12 traits of an abuser.* Retrieved from http://www.cbn.com/family/marriage/petherbridge_abusertraits.aspx; Ghandour, R. M., Campbell, J.C., & Lloyd, J. (2015). Screening and counseling for intimate partner violence: A vision for the future. *Journal of Women's Health*, 24(1), 57–61.

Rape Recovery

Rape survivors take a long time to heal from their traumatic experience. Some women never heal and never get professional counseling, but most can cope. Rape is viewed as a situational crisis that the survivor is unprepared to handle because it is an unforeseen event. Survivors typically go through four phases of recovery following rape (Table 9.4).

A significant proportion of women who are raped also experience symptoms of PTSD. PTSD develops when an event outside the range of normal human experience occurs that produces marked distress in the person. Symptoms of PTSD are divided into three groups:

- **Intrusion** (re-experiencing the trauma, including nightmares, flashbacks, recurrent thoughts)
- **Avoidance** (avoiding trauma-related stimuli, social withdrawal, emotional numbing)
- **Hyperarousal** (increased emotional arousal, exaggerated startle response, irritability)

Not every traumatized female develops full-blown or even minor PTSD. Symptoms usually begin within 3 months of the incident, but occasionally may only emerge years later. They must last more than a month to be considered PTSD. The condition varies from person to person. Some women recover within months, while others have symptoms for much longer. In some people, the condition becomes chronic (Darnell et al., 2015; Friedman, 2015).

Nursing Management of Rape Victims

Health care providers, along with sexual assault nurse examiners (SANE), can make a difference in the lives of survivors by understanding the facts, the effects this violence can have on mental and physical health, where to find information for themselves and their clients, and how to properly care for a survivor. A SANE is a registered nurse specially trained to conduct sexual assault evidentiary exams for rape victims. In addition to the collection of forensic evidence, they also provide access to crisis intervention, STI testing, and emergency contraception (International Association of Forensic Nurses, 2015).

Research has found that rape survivors undergo a profound and complex trauma. Exposure therapy has been used to help victims confront their trauma-related memories, feelings, and stimuli that evoke fear and anxiety (Nacasch, Rachamim, & Foa, 2015). The survivor should be provided with a safe and comfortable environment for a forensic examination. Nursing care of the rape survivor should focus on providing supportive care, collecting and documenting evidence, assessing for STIs, preventing pregnancy, and assessing for PTSD. Once initial treatment and evidence collection have been completed, follow-up care should include counseling, medical treatment, and crisis intervention. There is mounting evidence that early intervention and immediate counseling speed a rape survivor's recovery. By early intervention, it means interventions implemented in the initials hours, days, or weeks after the traumatic event (Bryant, 2015). Nursing Care Plan 9.1 (at the end of the chapter) highlights a sample plan of care for a victim of rape.

Take Note!

Many rape survivors seek treatment in the hospital emergency department if no rape crisis center is available. Unfortunately, many emergency department doctors and nurses have little training in how to treat rape survivors or in collecting evidence. To make matters worse, if they have to wait for hours in public waiting rooms, survivors may leave the hospital, never to receive treatment or supply the evidence needed to arrest and convict their assailants.

PROVIDING SUPPORTIVE CARE

Establishing a therapeutic and trusting relationship will help the survivor describe her experience. Take the woman to a secure, isolated area away from family, friends, and other clients and staff so she can be open and honest when asked about the assault. Provide a change of clothes, access to a shower and toiletries, and a private waiting area for family and friends.

COLLECTING AND DOCUMENTING EVIDENCE

The victim should be instructed to bring all clothing, especially undergarments, worn at the time of the assault to the medical facility. The victim should not shower or bathe before presenting for care. Typically a specially trained nurse will collect the evidence from the victim.

ASSESSING FOR SEXUALLY TRANSMITTED INFECTIONS

As part of the assessment, a pelvic examination will be done to collect vaginal secretions to rule out any STIs. This examination is very emotionally stressful for most women and should be carried out very gently and sensitively.

PREVENTING PREGNANCY

An essential element in the care of rape survivors involves offering them pregnancy prevention. After unprotected intercourse, including rape, pregnancy can be prevented by using an emergency contraceptive pill, sometimes called postcoital contraception. Emergency contraceptive pills involve high doses of the same oral contraceptives that millions of women take every day. The emergency regimen consists of one dose taken within 72 to 120 hours of the unprotected intercourse. Emergency contraception works by preventing ovulation, fertilization, or implantation. It does not disrupt an established pregnancy and should not be confused with mifepristone (RU-486), a drug approved by the Food and Drug Administration for abortion in the first 49 days of gestation. Emergency contraception is most effective if it is taken within 12 hours of the rape; it becomes less effective with every 12 hours of delay thereafter.

ASSESSING FOR POSTTRAUMATIC STRESS DISORDER

Nurses can begin to assess the extent to which a survivor is suffering from PTSD by asking the following questions:

- To assess the presence of intrusive thoughts:
  - Do upsetting thoughts and nightmares of the trauma bother you?
  - Do you feel as though you are actually reliving the trauma?
  - Does it upset you to be exposed to anything that reminds you of that event?
- To assess the presence of avoidance reactions:
  - Do you find yourself trying to avoid thinking about the trauma?
  - Do you stay away from situations that remind you of the event?
  - Do you have trouble recalling exactly what happened?
  - Do you feel numb emotionally?
- To assess the presence of physical symptoms:
  - Are you having trouble sleeping?
  - Have you felt irritable or experienced outbursts of anger?
  - Do you have heart palpitations and sweating?
  - Do you have muscle aches and pains all over? (NCVC, 2015b).

With a growing body of knowledge about rape-related PTSD, help is available through most rape crisis and trauma centers. Support groups have been established where survivors can meet regularly to share experiences to help relieve the symptoms of PTSD. For some survivors, medication prescribed along with therapy is the best combination to relieve the pain. Just as in the treatment of any other illness, at the first opportunity, the woman should be encouraged to talk about the traumatic experience. This ventilating provides a chance to receive needed support and comfort, as well as an opportunity to begin making sense of the experience. To diminish symptoms of PTSD, survivors must work on two fronts: coming to terms with the past and alleviating stress in the present (Bryant, 2015).

In order to have a better understanding of the aftermath of criminal victimization such as sexual assault, nurses must begin to accept the reality that crime is random, senseless, and can happen to anyone regardless of the precautions that are taken to prevent it. Nurses must also understand that a victim's life is turned upside down when he or she becomes a victim of crime. In order to help victims to trust society again and regain a sense of balance and self-worth, nurses must educate all those who come in contact with victims and survivors to be sensitive to their needs.

Female Genital Cutting

FGC, also referred to as female genital mutilation (FGM) or female circumcision, is defined as a procedure involving any injury of the external female genitalia for cultural or nontherapeutic reasons. It confers severe health consequences for girls and women. The international community views this practice as a human rights violation (Gayle & Rymer, 2015). It is the surgical removal of a portion or portions of the genitalia of female infants, girls, and women, including the clitoris (type I), clitoris and labia minora (type II), and clitoris, labia minora, labia majora, and then suturing of the remaining tissue, known as fibulation, to leave only a small opening for urination, menstruation, intercourse, and childbirth (type III). There is a type IV, which encompasses all other mutilations of the female genital area such as pricking, piercing, cutting, cauterizing, and scraping of the vaginal tissue, incisions to the clitoris and vagina, and burning, scarring, or cauterizing of tissue with the aim of tightening or narrowing the vagina (Nour, 2015).

FGC is a worldwide practice that affects millions of women and girls. According to the World Health Organization (WHO) (2015b) and UNICEF, 140 million women are victims of FGC with about 130 million girls between infancy and age 15 undergoing FGC every year. Countries where this is practiced include 30 African countries and parts of the Middle East and Asia. Prevalence in countries such as Sudan and Egypt has been estimated as high as 99% (Johnsdotter, 2015). The exact origins of FGC are not known. Although FGC may be interwoven into the culture, it is not mandated by any religion. This practice predates both Islam and Christianity (Gruenbaum & Wirtz, 2015). In some cultures, it is associated with feminine beauty and often signifies a rite of passage from childhood to adulthood. Female cutting is performed to decrease a woman's sexual desires and to ensure her chastity until marriage and receipt of a dowry from the prospective groom (Farage et al., 2015). Ultimately, the reality of being ostracized by the community and the possibility of being ineligible to marry create enormous social pressure to have FGC carried out, pressure that outweighs the known physical and emotional damage of this practice (Nour, 2015).

Complications vary, depending on the type of cutting and the way it was performed. It is frequently performed without anesthesia under nonsterile conditions. Cutting tools can be anything from razors blades to knives to pieces of glass or tin can lids. Complications can include infertility, dysmenorrhea, dyspareunia, sexual dysfunction, infection, hemorrhage after the procedure, vaginal stenosis, chronic vaginitis, pelvic inflammatory disease, chronic urinary tract infections, incontinence, genital fistulas, recurrent abscesses, transmission of HIV and hepatitis during the procedure, severe pain and shock after the procedure, difficulty walking or using stairs due to severe scarring, urinary retention, inability to experience orgasm, and difficulty in giving birth. Long-term complications related to FGC include chronic pain, dyspareunia, and difficult childbirth. The most common long-term complication is the formation of inclusion clitoral dermoid cysts and labial fusion. These become large as a grapefruit and can lead to difficulty in walking, sitting and can cause psychological distress from the deformity. The psychological effects range from eating disorders, insomnia, depression, PTSD, and negative effects on the women's self-esteem and identity (Creighton, 2015).

As immigration to the United States increases, nurses are increasingly likely to encounter women affected by FGC and its complications. The psychological pressure and trauma of being torn between two cultures and feeling different may lie heavily on the women in a new setting where FGC is foreign and banned. Nurses need updated education regarding women with FGC so that appropriate care for this population can be provided for this very sensitive health care problem. Well-informed nurses are the best tool for providing culturally sensitive care to this population. Nurses are in a unique position to contact and educate women who have been cut or are at risk for mutilation. To advocate for these women, a thorough understanding of the practice of FGC, its cultural overtones, religious implications, and psychosocial effects is needed.

Take Note!

From a Western perspective, FGC is hard to comprehend. Because it is not talked about openly in communities that practice it, women who have undergone it accept it without question and assume it is done to all girls (Gruenbaum & Wirtz, 2015).

Background

Reasons for performing the ritual reflect the ideology and cultural values of each community that practices it. Some consider it a rite of passage into womanhood; others use it as a means of preserving virginity until marriage. In cultures where it is practiced, it is an important part of culturally defined gender identity. In any case, all the reasons are cultural and traditional and are not rooted in any religious texts (Research Action and Information Network for the Bodily Integrity of Women [RAINBO], 2015). Since FGC has no health benefits and often leaves women with lifelong physical and

BOX 9.5

FOUR MAJOR TYPES OF FEMALE GENITAL MUTILATION PROCEDURES

Type I: Excision of the prepuce with excision of part or the entire clitoris

Type II: Excision of the clitoris and part or all of the labia minora

Type III (Infibulation): Excision of all or part of the external genitalia and stitching/narrowing of the vaginal opening

Type IV: Pricking, piercing, or incision of the clitoris or labia

- Stretching of the clitoris and/or labia
- Cauterizing by burning the clitoris and surrounding tissues
- Scraping or cutting the vaginal orifice
- Introduction of a corrosive substance into the vagina
- Placing herbs into the vagina to narrow it

Adapted from World Health Organization [WHO]. (2015b). *Female genital mutilation.* Retrieved from http://www.who.int/mediacentre/factsheets/fs241/en/print.html; Nour, N. M. (2015). Female genital cutting: Impact on women's health. In *Seminars in Reproductive Medicine. 33*(1), 41–46; and Research Action and Information Network for the Bodily Integrity of Women [RAINBO]. (2015). *Caring for women with circumcision: Fact sheet for physicians.* Retrieved from http://www.rainbo.org/factsheet.html

emotional trauma, there is a human rights justification to end the practice. International pressure to end FGC has been mounting since 1997, when the WHO, UNICEF, and UNFPA issued a joint statement to call on governments to ban the practice (Borsand et al., 2015). Box 9.5 lists types of FGC procedures.

Nursing Management of Female Genital Cutting Client

Because of increasing migration, nurses throughout the world are increasingly exposed to women who have experienced these procedures and thus need to know about its impact on women's reproductive health. Helping women who have had an FGC procedure requires good communication skills and often an interpreter, since many may not speak English. As nurses, we are educated to provide comprehensive, culturally sensitive care regardless of our client's circumstances. Nurses must keep in mind that FGC is considered normal in many cultures and to not have it done would be unthinkable. Nurses have the opportunity to educate clients by providing accurate information and positive health care experiences. Make sure that you are comfortable with your own feelings about this practice before dealing with clients. Some guidelines are as follows:

- Let the client know you are concerned and interested and want to help.
- Speak clearly and slowly, using simple, accurate terms.
- Use the term or name for this practice that the recipient uses, not "FGC."
- Use pictures and diagrams to help the woman understand what you are saying.
- Be patient in allowing the client to answer questions.
- Include men in any education, as they are influential in this practice.
- Repeat back your understanding of the client's statements.
- Always look and talk directly to the client, not the interpreter.
- Place no judgment on the cultural practice.
- Maintain respect for older women who have experienced FGC.
- Encourage the client to express herself freely.
- Maintain strict confidentiality.
- Provide culturally attuned care to all women.

In short, FGC is a form of violence against women, and it is only through education and empowerment of women that real changes in this practice can be made. Because this practice often defines a woman and becomes a part of her identity, nurses must understand this to be able to assist women who have had this done to them. Only through intense education will the next generation of girls be saved from this practice.

Human Trafficking

The United Nations defines human trafficking as the recruitment, transportation, transfer, harboring or receipt of persons, by means of the threat or use of force, of abduction, of fraud, or deception to achieve the consent of a person having control over another person, for the purpose of exploitation (United Nations Office on Drugs and Crime [UNODC], 2015).

A girl who was just 14 years old was held captive in a tiny trailer room, where she was forced to have sex with as many as 30 men a day. On her nightstand was a teddy bear that reminded her of her childhood in Mexico from where she was abducted and forced into sexual slavery.

This scenario describes human trafficking, the enslavement of immigrants for profit in America. Within our borders, thousands of foreign nationals and US citizens, many of them children, are forced or coerced into sex work or various forms of labor every year (Weitzer, 2015). Human trafficking is both a global problem and a domestic problem. The United States is a major receiver of trafficked persons. Human trafficking is a modern form of slavery that affects nearly 1 million people worldwide and approximately 20,000 persons in the United States annually (U.S. Department of State, 2015). Women and children are the primary victims of human trafficking, many in the sex trade as described above and others through forced-labor domestic servitude.

Poverty and lack of economic opportunity make women and children potential victims of traffickers associated with international criminal organizations. They are vulnerable to false promises of job opportunities in other countries. Many of those who accept these offers from what appear to be legitimate sources find themselves in situations where their documents are destroyed, they or their families threatened with harm, or they are bonded by a debt that they have no chance of repaying

Trafficking persons is hugely profitable: one estimate places global profits at approximately $35 billion annually. Among illegal enterprises, trafficking is second only to drug dealing and is tied with the illegal arms industry in its ability to generate dollars (Aronowitz & Koning, 2015).

The United States is a profitable destination country for traffickers, and these profits contribute to the development of organized criminal enterprises worldwide. According to findings of the (Victims of Trafficking and Violence Protection Act of 2000):

- Victims are primarily women and children who lack education, employment, and economic opportunities in their own countries.
- Traffickers promise victims employment as nannies, maids, dancers, factory workers, sales clerks, or models in the United States.
- Traffickers transport the victims from their counties to unfamiliar destinations away from their support systems.
- Once they are here, traffickers coerce them, using rape, torture, starvation, imprisonment, threats, or physical force, into prostitution, pornography, the sex trade, forced labor, or involuntary servitude.

These victims are exposed to serious and numerous health risks such as rape; physical injury such as cigarette burns, fractures, bruises; torture; HIV/AIDS; STIs; cervical cancer; violence; hazardous work environments; poor nutrition; and drug and alcohol addiction (Greenbaum et al., 2015). Health care is one of the most pressing needs of these victims, but no comprehensive care is available to undocumented immigrants. Nurses and other health care providers who encounter victims of trafficking often do not realize it, and opportunities to intervene are lost. Although no one sign can demonstrate with certainty when someone is being trafficked, clinicians should be aware of several indicators. It is important to be alert for trafficking victims in any setting and to recognize cues (Box 9.6).

Nursing interventions in the case of trafficking victims would include the following:

- Building trust is the number-one priority
- Take the time to listen and develop rapport
- Screen in a private place to ensure confidentiality and safety
- Reassure the potential victim
- One-on-one interactions are ideal
- Specifically ask about the client's safety
- Offer reworded stories
- Stay calm and on an even keel
- Understand the risk these victims are taking by disclosing their plight
- ALWAYS document your suspicion in your notes, at the very least
- Call the human trafficking hotline for guidance: 1-866-US-TIPLINE

Human trafficking is a violation of human rights. Few crimes are more repugnant than the sex trafficking of helpless and innocent victims. Nurses are one of the few groups of professionals likely to interact with trafficked victims while they are still in captivity. They have the opportunity to screen, identify, intervene, and rescue

BOX 9.6

IDENTIFYING VICTIMS OF HUMAN TRAFFICKING

Look beneath the surface and ask yourself: Is this person

- A female or a child in poor health?
- Foreign-born and doesn't speak English?
- Lacking immigration documents?
- Giving an inconsistent explanation of injury?
- Reluctant to give any information about self, injury, home, or work?
- Fearful of authority Figure or "sponsor" if present? ("Sponsor" might not leave victim alone with health care provider.)
- Living with the employer?

Sample questions to ask the potential victim of human trafficking:

- Can you leave your job or situation if you wish?
- Can you come and go as you please?
- Have you been threatened if you try to leave?
- Has anyone threatened your family with harm if you leave?
- What are your working and living conditions?
- Do you have to ask permission to go to the bathroom, eat, or sleep?
- Is there a lock on your door so you cannot get out?
- What brought you to the United States? Are your plans the same now?
- Are you free to leave your current work or home situation?
- Who has your immigration papers? Why don't you have them?
- Are you paid for the work you do?
- Are there times you feel afraid?
- How can your situation be changed?

Adapted from United Nations Office on Drugs and Crime [UNODC]. (2015). *Human trafficking.* Retrieved from http://www.unodc.org/unodc/en/human-trafficking/what-is-human-trafficking.html; Sanchez, R., & Stark, S. (2014). The hard truth about human trafficking. *Nursing Management, 45*(1), 18–23; Weitzer, R. (2015). Human trafficking and contemporary slavery. *Annual Review of Sociology, 41*(1). Retrieved from http: //www.annualreviews.org/doi/abs/10.1146/annurev-soc-073014–112506

these victims. If you suspect a trafficking situation, notify local law enforcement and a regional social service organization that has experience in dealing with trafficking victims. It is imperative to reach out to these victims and stop the cycle of abuse by following through on your suspicions. Nurses can also reach out within their communities to bring about awareness through community education to human trafficking to uncover the hard truth about it to our nation's blind eyes.

SUMMARY

The causes of violence against women are complex. Previously, violence against women was largely invisible, natural, and trivial. Many laughed at the notion that intimate or community violence against women should be seen as a human rights violation. Raising awareness and developing evidence-based programs, practices and policies to prevent IPV and sexual assault are essential in stopping violent behavior before it starts. Many women will experience some type of violence in their lives, and it can have a debilitating effect on their health and future relationships. Nurses have the skills, professional experience, and perspective to be an important part of comprehensive violence prevention efforts in communities. Violence is a preventable public health problem if multiple sectors understand patterns of violence and implement prevention strategies to reduce it (Copelon, 2015).

Violence frequently leaves a "legacy of pain" to future generations. Nurses can empower women and encourage them to move forward and take control of their lives. When women live in peace and security, free from violence, they have an enormous potential to contribute to their own communities and to the national and global society. Nurses can play an important role in working toward the creation of a violence-free community, but they must first become informed. Nurses must insist that health care agencies that employ them accept this responsibility and work together to reach out to those being abused. The time is ripe for nurses to act and ensure serious inroads are made in improving the health and well-being of all women across the globe.

Violence against women is not normal, legal, or acceptable and it should never be tolerated or justified. It can and must be stopped by the entire world community. Early education and prevention provide the best hope for creating healthy futures and fostering a global society without violence.

NURSING CARE PLAN 9.1

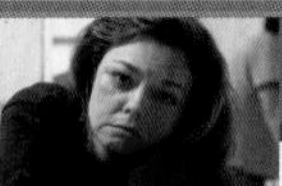

Overview of the Woman Who is a Victim of Rape

Lucia, a 20-year-old college junior, was admitted to the emergency room after police found her when a passerby called 911 to report an assault. She stated, "I was raped a few hours ago while I was walking home through the park." Assessment reveals the following: numerous cuts and bruises of varying sizes on her face, arms, and legs; lip swollen and cut; right eye swollen and bruised; jacket and shirt ripped and bloodied; hair matted with grass and debris; vital signs within acceptable parameters; client tearful, clutching her clothing, and trembling; perineal bruising and tearing.

NURSING DIAGNOSIS: Rape-trauma syndrome related to report of recent sexual assault

Outcome Identification and Evaluation

Client will demonstrate adequate coping skills related to effects of rape as evidenced by her ability to discuss the event, verbalize her feelings and fears, and exhibit appropriate actions to return to her precrisis level of functioning.

Interventions: ***Promoting Adequate Coping Skills***

- Stay with the client to promote feelings of safety.
- Explain the procedures to be completed based on facility's policy to help alleviate client's fear of the unknown.
- Assist with physical examination for specimen collection to obtain evidence for legal proceedings.
- Administer prophylactic medication as ordered to prevent pregnancy and STIs.
- Provide care to wounds as ordered to prevent infection.
- Assist client with hygiene measures as necessary to promote self-esteem.
- Allow client to describe the events as much as possible to encourage ventilation of feelings about the incident; engage in active listening and offer nonjudgmental support to facilitate coping and demonstrate understanding of the client's situation and feelings.

NURSING CARE PLAN 9.1

Overview of the Woman Who is a Victim of Rape (continued)

- Help the client identify positive coping skills and personal strengths used in the past to aid in effective decision making.
- Assist client in developing additional coping strategies and teach client relaxation techniques to help deal with the current crisis and anxiety.
- Contact the rape counselor in the facility to help the client deal with the crisis.
- Arrange for follow-up visit with rape counselor to provide continued care and to promote continuity of care.
- Encourage the client to contact a close friend, partner, or family member to accompany her home to provide support.
- Provide the client with the telephone number of a counseling service or community support groups to help her cope and obtain ongoing support.
- Provide written instructions related to follow-up appointments, care, and testing to ensure adequate understanding.

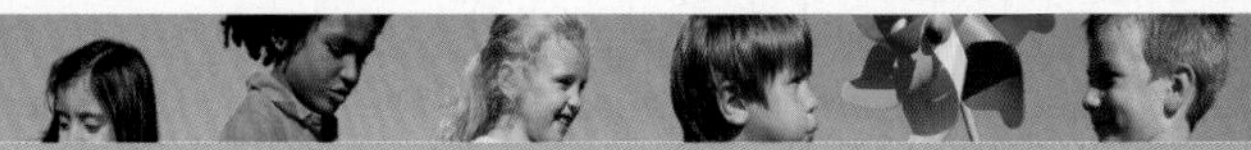

KEY CONCEPTS

- Violence against women is a major public health and social problem because it violates a woman's very being and causes numerous mental and physical health sequelae.
- Every woman has the potential to become a victim of violence.
- Several *Healthy People 2020* objectives focus on reducing the rate of physical assaults and the number of rapes and attempted rapes.
- Abuse may be mental, physical, or sexual in nature or a combination of all of these.
- The cycle of violence includes three phases: tension building, acute battering, and honeymoon.
- Many women experience PTSD after being sexually assaulted. PTSD can inhibit a survivor from adapting or coping in a healthy manner.
- Pregnancy can precipitate violence toward the woman or escalate it.
- FGC is practiced worldwide and nurses in the United States need to become knowledgeable about it and place no judgment on this cultural practice.
- Human trafficking is a violation against human rights, and nurses who suspect it should report it to stop the cycle of abuse against young children and women.
- The nurse's role in dealing with survivors of violence is to establish rapport; open up lines of communication; apply the nursing process to assess and screen all clients in all settings; and implement and intervene as appropriate.

REFERENCES AND RECOMMENDED READINGS

Alexander, L. L., LaRosa, J. H., Bader, H., & Garfield, S. (2014). *New dimensions in women's health* (6th ed.). Sudbury, MA: Jones & Bartlett.

Aronowitz, A. A., & Koning, A. (2015). Understanding human trafficking as a market system: Addressing the demand side of trafficking for sexual exploitation. *Revue International de droit Pénal, 85*(3), 669–696.

Association of Women's Health, Obstetric and Neonatal Nurses [AWHONN]. (2015). Intimate partner violence. *Journal of Obstetric, Gynecologic, and Neonatal Nursing, 44*(3), 405–408.

Bagwell-Gray, M. E., Messing, J. T., & Baldwin-White, A. (2015). Intimate partner sexual violence: A review of terms, definitions, and prevalence. *Trauma, Violence, & Abuse, 16*(3), 316–335.

Barrios, Y. V., Gelaye, B., Zhong, Q., Nicolaidis, C., Rondon, M. B., Garcia, P. J., et al. (2015). Association of childhood physical and sexual abuse with intimate partner violence, poor general health and depressive symptoms among pregnant women. *PLoS One, 10*(1), e0116609.

Berthold, S. M. (2015). Intimate partner violence and a rights-based approach to healing. In *Human rights-based approaches to clinical social work* (pp. 85–113). Springer International Publishing.

Borsand, M., Friedman, B., Mirzayan, N., & Borsand, A. (2015). Female genital cutting: An ancient practice embedded in an ever-evolving world. *American Journal of Cosmetic Surgery, 32*(1), 31–36.

Bouchet, S., & Braswell, K. (2015). *Beyond silence and violence.* Dunwoody, GA: Fathers Incorporated. www.fathersincorporated.com

Brenner, I., & Ben-Amitay, G. (2015). Sexual revictimization: The impact of attachment anxiety, accumulated trauma, and response to childhood sexual abuse disclosure. *Violence and Victims, 30*(1), 49–65.

Brooker, C., & Durmaz, E. (2015). Mental health, sexual violence and the work of Sexual Assault Referral centres

(SARCs) in England. *Journal of Forensic and Legal Medicine, 31*, 47–51.

Bryant, R. A. (2015). Early intervention after trauma. In *Evidence based treatments for trauma-related psychological disorders* (pp. 125–142). Springer International Publishing.

Burnett, L. B., & Adler, J. (2015). Domestic violence. eMedicine. Retrieved from http://emedicine.medscape.com/article/805546-overview

Canadian Domestic Homicide Prevention Initiative. (2015). *Risk assessment, risk management and safety planning*. Retrieved from http://www.learningtoendabuse.ca/cdhpi/risk-assessment-risk-management-and-safety-planning

Cannon, C., & Buttell, F. (2015). Illusion of inclusion: The failure of the gender paradigm to account for intimate partner violence in LGBT relationships. *Partner Abuse, 6*(1), 65–70.

Cater, Å. K., Miller, L. E., Howell, K. H., & Graham-Bermann, S. A. (2015). Childhood exposure to intimate partner violence and adult mental health problems: Relationships with gender and age of exposure. *Journal of Family Violence*, 1–12. doi: 10.1007/s10896–015–9703–0

Centers for Disease Control & Prevention [CDC]. (2015a). *Understanding intimate partner violence: Fact sheet*. Retrieved from http://www.cdc.gov/violenceprevention/pub/ipv_factsheet.html

Centers for Disease Control and Prevention [CDC]. (2015b). *Intimate partner violence: definitions*. Retrieved from http://www.cdc.gov/violenceprevention/intimatepartnerviolence/definitions.html

Centers for Disease Control & Prevention [CDC]. (2015c). *CDC grand rounds: A public health approach to prevention of intimate partner violence*. Retrieved from http://www.cdc.gov/violenceprevention/intimatepartnerviolence/definitions.html

Centers for Disease Control & Prevention [CDC]. (2015d). *Intimate partner violence: Risk and protective factors*. Retrieved from http://www.cdc.gov/violenceprevention/intimatepartnerviolence/riskprotectivefactors.html

Centers for Disease Control and Prevention [CDC]. (2015e). *Understanding child mistreatment*. Retrieved from http://www.cdc.gov/violenceprevention/pdf/cm-factsheet–2013.pdf

Centers for Disease Control and Prevention [CDC]. (2015f). *Understanding sexual violence*. Retrieved from http://www.cdc.gov/violenceprevention/pdf/svfactsheet2013-a.pdf

Chang, J. C. (2015). *Domestic violence: Epidemiology and risk factors. Clinical gynecology* (2nd ed., pp. 94–101), Cambridge, UK: Cambridge University Press.

Copelon, R. (2015). Violence against women: The potential and challenge of a human rights perspective. *Women's Health Journal, (2–3)*, 62–67.

Creighton, S. M. (2015). Female genital mutilation (FGM) and the lower urinary tract. *International Journal of Urological Nursing*. *9*(2), 69–73.

Darnell, D., Peterson, R., Berliner, L., et al. (2015). Factors associated with follow-up attendance among rape victims seen in acute medical care. *Psychiatry, 78*(1), 89–101.

de Jong, R., Alink, L., Bijleveld, C., Finkenauer, C., & Hendriks, J. (2015). Transition to adulthood of child sexual abuse victims. *Aggression and Violent Behavior*, 24, 175–187.

Domestic Violence Organization. (2015a). *Common myths and why they are wrong*. Retrieved from http://www.domesticviolence.org/common-myths/

Domestic Violence Organization. (2015b). *Cycle of violence*. Retrieved from http://www.domesticviolence.org/cycle-of-violence/

Domestic Violence Roundtable. (2015). *The cycle of domestic violence*. Retrieved from http://www.domesticviolenceroundtable.org/domestic-violence-cycle.html

Dorland, W. A. N. (2015). *Dorland's dictionary of medical acronyms & abbreviations* (7th ed.). Philadelphia, PA: Elsevier Health Sciences.

Dutton, M. A. (2015). Mindfulness-based stress reduction for underserved trauma populations. In *Mindfulness-oriented interventions for trauma: Integrating contemplative practices (Chapter 15)*. New York, NY: The Guilford Press.

Edwards, K. M., Sylaska, K. M., & Neal, A. M. (2015). Intimate partner violence among sexual minority populations: A critical review of the literature and agenda for future research. *Psychology of Violence, 5*(2), 112–121.

Farage, M. A., Miller, K. W., Tzeghai, G. E., Azuka, C. E., Sobel, J. D., & Ledger, W. J. (2015). Female genital cutting: Confronting cultural challenges and health complications across the lifespan. *Women's Health, 11*(1), 79–94.

Federal Bureau of Investigation [FBI]. (2015). *Intimate partner violence*. Retrieved from http://www.justice.gov/usao-cdca/victimwitness/domestic-violence-laws

Friedman, M. J. (2015). Overview of posttraumatic stress disorder (PTSD). In *Posttraumatic and acute stress disorders* (pp. 1–8). Springer International Publishing.

Gayle, C. M., & Rymer, J. M. (2015) Female genital mutilation. In *Clinical gynecology* (2nd ed., pp. 102–111), Cambridge, UK: Cambridge University Press.

Ghandour, R. M., Campbell, J. C., & Lloyd, J. (2015) Screening and counseling for intimate partner violence: A vision for the future. *Journal of Women's Health, 24*(1), 57–61.

Greenbaum, J., Crawford-Jakubiak, J. E., Christian, C. W., Flaherty, E. G., Leventhal, J. M., Lukefahr, J. L., et al. (2015). Child sex trafficking and commercial sexual exploitation: Health care needs of victims. *Pediatrics, 135*(3), 566–574.

Gruenbaum, E., & Wirtz, E. (2015). Female genital cutting debates. *The International Encyclopedia of Human Sexuality*. (Online 4/20/15), doi: 10.1002/9781118896877.wbiehs147

Harkins, G. (2015). Incest. *The International Encyclopedia of Human Sexuality*. 583–625. doi: 10.1002/9781118896877.wbiehs231

Hewitt, L. N. (2015). Intimate partner violence: The role of nurses in protection of patients. *Critical Care Nursing Clinics of North America, 27*(2), 271–275.

Holtz, H., & Furniss, K. K. (1993). The health care provider's role in domestic violence. *Trends in Health Care Law and Ethics, 15*, 519–522.

Huang, C. C., Vikse, J. H., Lu, S., & Yi, S. (2015). Children's exposure to intimate partner violence and early delinquency. *Journal of Family Violence, 30*(8), 1–13.

Human Rights Watch. (2015). *Abused and expelled*. Retrieved from http://www.hrw.org/sites/default/files/reports/morocco0214_ForUpload.pdf

International Association of Forensic Nurses. (2015). *Sexual assault nurse examiners*. Retrieved from http://www.forensicnurses.org/?page=aboutsane

Jackson, A. M., & Deye, K. (2015). Aspects of abuse: Consequences of childhood victimization. *Current Problems in Pediatric and Adolescent Health Care, 45*(3), 86–93.

Joint Commission. (2015). *The Joint Commission accreditation manual for hospitals.* Chicago, IL: Author.

Johnsdotter, S. (2015). Genital cutting, female. *The International Encyclopedia of Human Sexuality.* (Online 4/20/15), doi: 10.1002/9781118896877.wbiehs180

Keygnaert, I., Vettenburg, N., & Temmerman, M. (2015). Hidden violence is silent rape. *Culture, Health and Sexuality: An Introduction,* 189–206.

Kilmartin, C. (2015). Men's violence against women: An overview. In *Religion and Men's Violence against Women* (pp. 15–25). New York, NY: Springer Publishers.

Klaus, W., Buczkowski, K., & Wiktorska, P. (2015). Empowering the victims of crime: A real goal of the criminal justice system or no more than a pipe dream? In *Trust and Legitimacy in Criminal Justice* (pp. 65–91). Springer International Publishing.

Lawrence, D. (2015). Breaking the cycle of violence. *Nursing Standard (1987), 29,* 18–21.

Lawson, D. M. (2015). *Family violence: Explanations and evidence-based clinical practice.* Hoboken, NJ: John Wiley & Sons.

Lévesque, S., & Chamberland, C. (2015). Intimate partner violence among pregnant young women. A qualitative inquiry. *Journal of Interpersonal Violence,* doi: 10.1177/0886260515584349.

Lomborg, B. (2015) *Why domestic violence costs more than war. World Economic Forum.* Retrieved from https://agenda.weforum.org/2015/09/domestic-violence-cost-war-development-goals/

MacGregor, K. E., Villalta, L., Clarke, V., Viner, R. M., Kramer, T., & Khadr, S. N. (2015). G146 A systematic review of mental health outcomes in young people following sexual assault. *Archives of Disease in Childhood, 100*(Suppl 3), A63.

Mauri, E. M., Nespoli, A., Persico, G., & Zobbi, V. F. (2015). Domestic violence during pregnancy: Midwives' experiences. *Midwifery, 31*(5), 498–504.

Medicine Net. (2015a). *Sexual assault.* Retrieved from http://www.medicinenet.com/rape_sexual_assault/article.htm#rape_sexual_assault_facts

Medicine Net (2015b). *Domestic violence.* Retrieved from http://www.medicinenet.com/domestic_violence/page4.htm#what_are_the_causes_or_risk_factors_for_intimate_partner_violence

Morrill, M. (2014). Sibling sexual abuse: An exploratory study of long term consequences for self-esteem and counseling considerations. *Journal of Family Violence, 29*(2), 205–213.

Murray, C. E., Horton, G. E., Johnson, C. H., Notestine, L., Garr, B., Pow, A. M., et al. (2015). Domestic violence service providers' perceptions of safety planning: A focus group study. *Journal of Family Violence, 30*(3), 381–392.

Nacasch, N., Rachamim, L., & Foa, E. B. (2015). Prolonged exposure treatment. In *Future directions in post-traumatic stress disorder* (pp. 245–251). Philadelphia, PA: Springer Publishers.

National Center for Victims of Crime [NCVC]. (2015a). *Incest.* Retrieved from http://www.victimsofcrime.org/

National Center for Victims of Crime [NCVC]. (2015b). *The trauma of victimization.* Retrieved from http://victimsofcrime.org/help-for-crime-victims/get-help-bulletins-for-crime-victims/trauma-of-victimization#ptsd

National Center on Elder Abuse. (2015). *Statistics/data: Elder abuse: The size of the problem.* Retrieved from http://www.ncea.aoa.gov/Library/Data/

National Coalition Against Domestic Violence. (2015). *Fact sheet: National Statistics.* Retrieved from http://www.ncadv.org/learn/statistics

National Stress Clinic. (2015). *Domestic abuse: Understanding and breaking the cycle of violence.* Retrieved from http://www.nationalstressclinic.com/domestic-abuse-understanding-and-breaking-the-cycle-of-violence/

Nour, N. M. (2015). Female genital cutting: Impact on women's health. In *Seminars in reproductive medicine, 33*(1), 41–46.

Policastro, C., & Finn, M. A. (2015). Coercive control and physical violence in older adults analysis using data from the National Elder Mistreatment Study. *Journal of Interpersonal Violence,* (Online 5/14/15), doi: 10.1177/0886260515585545.

Prosman, G. J., Wong, S. H. L. F., van der Wouden, J. C., & Lagro-Janssen, A. L. (2015). Effectiveness of home visiting in reducing partner violence for families experiencing abuse: a systematic review. *Family Practice,* (Online: 5/6/15) doi: 10.1093/fampra/cmu091

Rape, Abuse, and Incest National Network [RAINN]. (2015a). *Statistics.* Retrieved from https://www.rainn.org/statistics

Rape, Abuse, and Incest National Network [RAINN]. (2015b). *Who are the victims?* Retrieved from http://rainn.org/get-information/statistics/sexual-assault-victims

Rape, Abuse, and Incest National Network [RAINN]. (2015c). *Acquaintance rape.* Retrieved from https://www.rainn.org/get-information/types-of-sexual-assault/acquaintance-rape

Rape, Abuse, and Incest National Network [RAINN]. (2015d). *Recovery from sexual assault.* Retrieved from http://www.rainn.org/get-information/sexual-assault-recovery

Research Action and Information Network for the Bodily Integrity of Women [RAINBO]. (2015). *Caring for women with circumcision: Fact sheet for physicians.* Retrieved from http://www.rainbo.org/factsheet.html

Russell, B., & Chapleau, K. (2015). When is it abuse? How assailant gender, sexual orientation, and protection orders influence perceptions of intimate partner abuse. *Partner Abuse, 6*(1), 47–64.

Sanchez, R., & Stark, S. (2014). The hard truth about human trafficking. *Nursing Management, 45*(1), 18–23.

Song, A., Wenzel, S. L., Kim, J. Y., & Nam, B. (2015). Experience of domestic violence during childhood, intimate partner violence, and the deterrent effect of awareness of legal consequences. *Journal of Interpersonal Violence,* doi: 10.1177/0886260515586359.

Sugg, N. (2015). Intimate partner violence: prevalence, health consequences, and intervention. *Medical Clinics of North America, 99*(3), 629–649.

TahoeSafe Alliance. (2015). *Myths about intimate partner violence in the LGBTQUA community.* Retrieved from http://tahoesafealliance.org/for-lgbqtia/lgbtqiamyths/

The Advocacy Center. (2015). *The path toward recovery for survivors of sexual violence.* Retrieved from http://www.theadvocacycenter.org/adv_violencewhatis.html

The Christian Broadcasting Network [CBN]. (2015). *12 traits of an abuser.* Available at: http://www.cbn.com/family/marriage/petherbridge_abusertraits.aspx

United Nations Office on Drugs and Crime [UNODC]. (2015). *Human trafficking*. Retrieved from http://www.unodc.org/unodc/en/human-trafficking/what-is-human-trafficking.html

U.S. Department of Health and Human Services [USDHHS]. (2015a). *Date rape drugs fact sheet. National Women's Health Information Center.* Retrieved from http://www.womenshealth.gov/publications/our-publications/fact-sheet/date-rape-drugs.html

U.S. Department of Health and Human Services [USDHHS]. (2015b). *Healthy People 2020*. Retrieved from http://www.healthypeople.gov/document/HTML/Volume2/15Injury.htm#_Toc490549392

U.S. Department of Health and Human Services [USDHHS]. (2015c). Screening for domestic violence in health care settings. *Office of the Assistant Secretary for Planning and Evaluation*. Retrieved from http://aspe.hhs.gov/hsp/13/dv/pb_screeningdomestic.cfm

U.S. Department of State. (2015). *What is modern slavery?* Retrieved from http://www.state.gov/j/tip/what/index.htm

Victims of Trafficking and Violence Protection Act of 2000. (2000).*Pub. Law No. 106–386 [H.R. 3244] (2000)*. Retrieved from http://ojp.gov/vawo/laws/vawo2000/stitle_a.htm

Wang, X. M., Brisbin, S., Loo, T., & Straus, S. (2015). Elder abuse: An approach to identification, assessment and intervention. *Canadian Medical Association Journal, 187*(8), 575–581.

Weitzer, R. (2015). Human trafficking and contemporary slavery. *Annual Review of Sociology, 41*(1), 223–242. Retrieved from http://www.annualreviews.org/doi/abs/10.1146/annurev-soc-073014–112506

WELLWVU The Student's Center of Health. (2015). *Rape myths and facts*. Retrieved from https://well.wvu.edu/articles/rape_myths_and_facts

Wilson, L. C., & Miller, K. E. (2015). Meta-analysis of the prevalence of unacknowledged rape. *Trauma, Violence, & Abuse,* (Online 3/17/15) doi: 10.1177/1524838015576391.

Women Against Violence Against Women [WAVAW]. (2015). *Rape myths*. Retrieved from http://www.wavaw.ca/myth-busting/rape-myths/

World Health Organization [WHO]. (2015a). *Violence against women fact sheet*. Retrieved from http://www.who.int/mediacentre/factsheets/fs239/en/

World Health Organization [WHO]. (2015b). *Female genital mutilation*. Retrieved from http://www.who.int/media centre/factsheets/fs241/en/print.html

CHAPTER WORKSHEET

MULTIPLE-CHOICE QUESTIONS

1. The primary goal of intervention in working with abused women is to:
   a. Set up an appointment with a mental health counselor for the victim
   b. Convince them to set up a safety plan to use when they leave
   c. Help them to develop courage and financial support to leave the abuser
   d. Empower them and improve their self-esteem to regain control of their lives

2. The first phase of the abuse cycle is characterized by:
   a. The woman provoking the abuser to bring about battering
   b. Tension building and verbal or minor battery
   c. A honeymoon period that lulls the victim into forgetting
   d. An acute episode of physical battering

3. Women recovering from abusive relationships need to learn ways to improve their:
   a. Educational level by getting a college degree
   b. Earning power so they can move to a better neighborhood
   c. Self-esteem and communication skills to increase assertiveness
   d. Relationship skills so they will be better prepared to deal with their partners

4. Which of the following statements might empower abuse victims to take action?
   a. "You deserve better than this."
   b. "Your children deserve to grow up in a two-parent family."
   c. "Try to figure out what you do to trigger his abuse and stop it."
   d. "Give your partner more time to come to his senses about this."

5. If a woman thinks she is being stalked when driving, a good safety measure is to:
   a. Drive to a local police or fire department
   b. Take short cuts through back streets to lose them
   c. Wave a handgun to intimidate them
   d. Roll down her window and confront them

6. Nurses play an important role in screening and assessment of any client abuse/violence. Which of the following statements is correct?
   a. Most clients are extremely reluctant to come forth with private matters.
   b. Any intimate partner violence questions should be asked in the presence of both partners.
   c. To invite disclosure, assure the woman that you won't document her statements.
   d. The best statement to make to the abused victim is: "You don't deserve this."

7. What should the nurse do if a victim of intimate partner violence chooses not to disclose information about her abusive relationship during your interview?
   a. Confront the victim with the physical evidence and telltale signs of abuse
   b. Contact family members to tell you about their abusive relationship
   c. Call the local police department to inquire about domestic disturbance calls
   d. Respect the client's right of self-determination and provide her with resources

CRITICAL THINKING EXERCISE

1. Mrs. Boggs has three children under the age of 5 and is 6 months pregnant with her fourth child. She has made repeated unscheduled visits to your clinic with vague somatic complaints regarding the children as well as herself, but has missed several scheduled prenatal appointments. On occasion she has worn sunglasses to cover bruises around her eyes. As a nurse you sense there is something else bothering her, but she doesn't seem to want to discuss it with you. She appears sad and the children cling to her.
   a. Outline your conversation when you broach the subject of abuse with Mrs. Boggs.
   b. What is your role as a nurse in caring for a family in which you suspect abuse is occurring?
   c. What ethical/legal considerations are important in planning care for this family?

STUDY ACTIVITIES

1. Visit the BellaOnline Domestic Violence web site for victims of violence. Discuss what you discovered on this site and your reactions to it.

2. Research the statistics about violence against women in your state. Are law enforcement and community interventions reducing the incidence of sexual assault and intimate partner violence?

3. Attend a dorm orientation at a local college to hear about measures in place to protect women's safety on campus. Find out the number of sexual assaults reported and what strategies the college uses to reduce this number.

4. Volunteer to spend a weekend evening at the local sheriff's department 911 hotline desk to observe the number and nature of calls received reporting domestic violence. Interview the dispatch operator about the frequency and trends of these calls.
5. Identify three community resources that could be useful to a victim of violence. Identify their sources of funding and the services they provide.

BRINGING IT ALL TOGETHER: A CASE STUDY

A 23-year-old pregnant female presents to the public health maternity clinic for the third time in a month with a myriad of vague complaints including insomnia, diffuse body aches and pains, poor appetite, fatigue, and constipation. This is her first pregnancy, and it was unplanned. Her recent OB examination and laboratory survey are within normal limits. Her past medical history is remarkable for anxiety and depression. According to the client, she does not drink or smoke. She does not work outside of the home.

ASSESSMENT

On physical examination the nurse notes a well-dressed, pleasant, but anxious young female. Her husband of a year usually accompanies her to the office visits, but is absent today. She tends to avoid eye contact with the nurse when asked questions about her symptoms. Her vital signs and fetal heart rate are all within the normal range. On further examination, the nurse notices several bruises on her upper arms and thighs. When questioned about these marks, the client looks away.

QUESTIONS

1. Based on her frequent visits and diversity of symptoms with no abnormal findings, what might the nurse suspect?
2. What makes this woman vulnerable to IPV?
3. If she is experiencing abuse, what are the health consequences of it?

PLAN

1. What is the next step for the nurse in managing this client?
2. What information does the nurse need to know prior to questioning this client?
3. What important resource for abused clients is vital to inform her about for help?
4. What message does the nurse need to convey to any abused client?

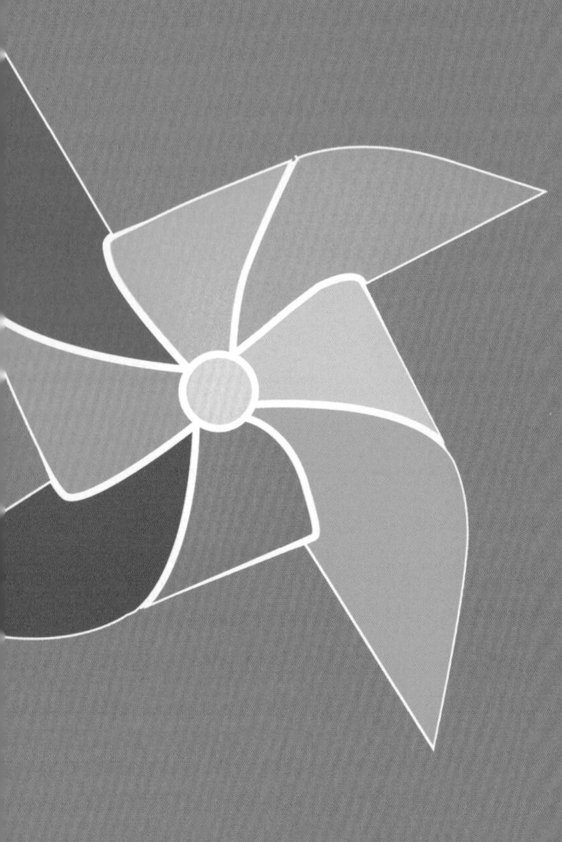

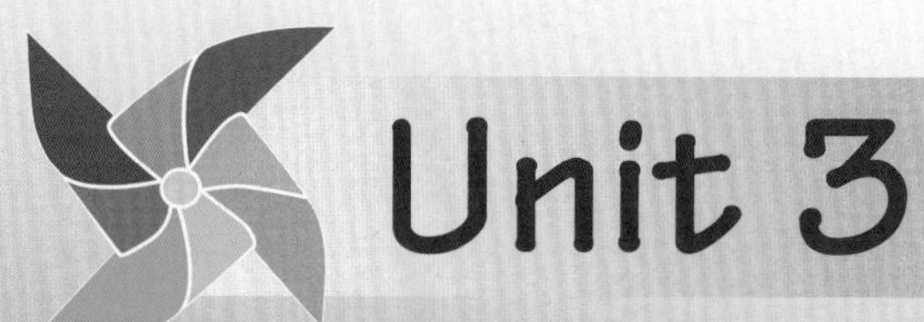

Pregnancy

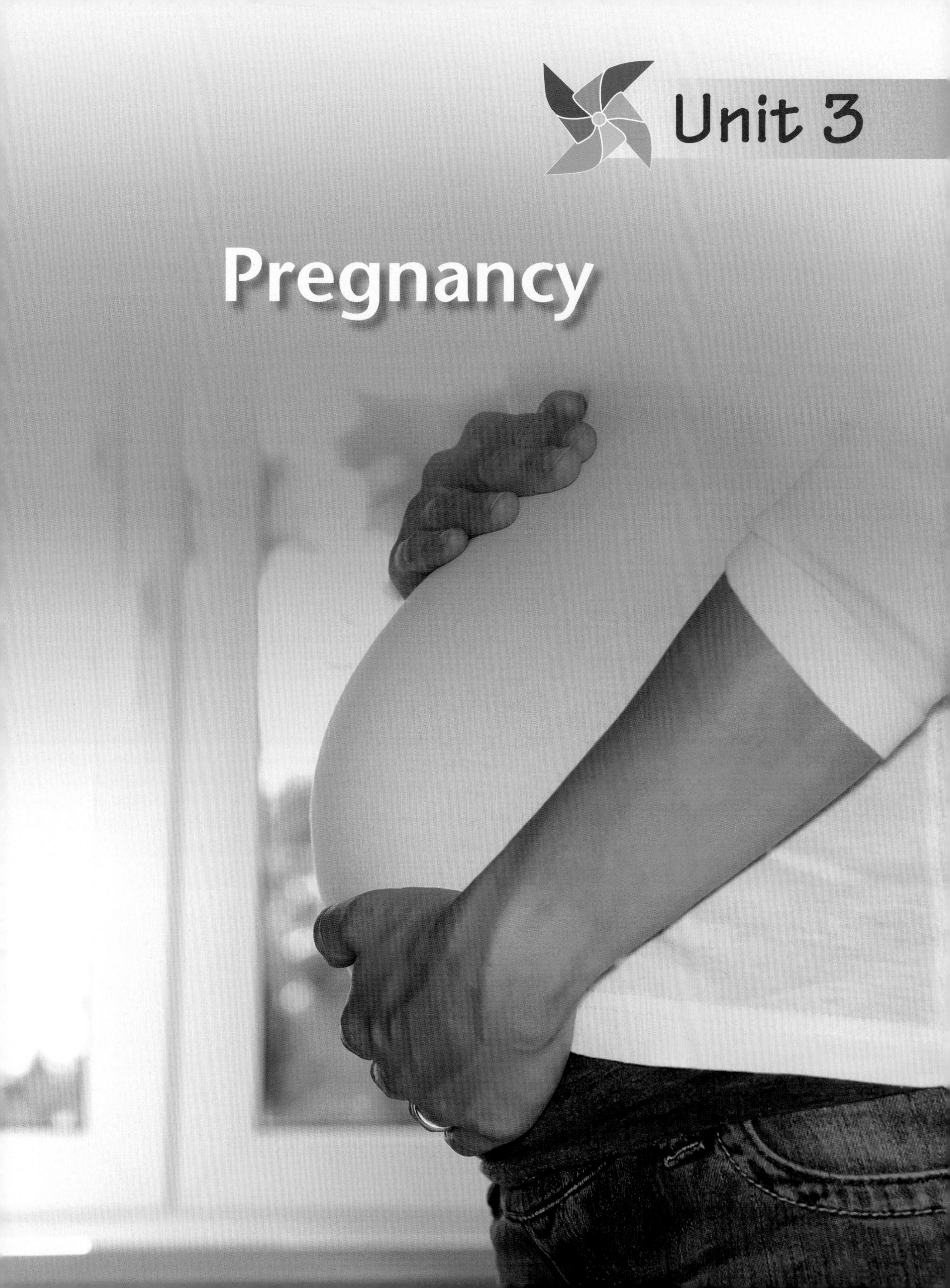

10

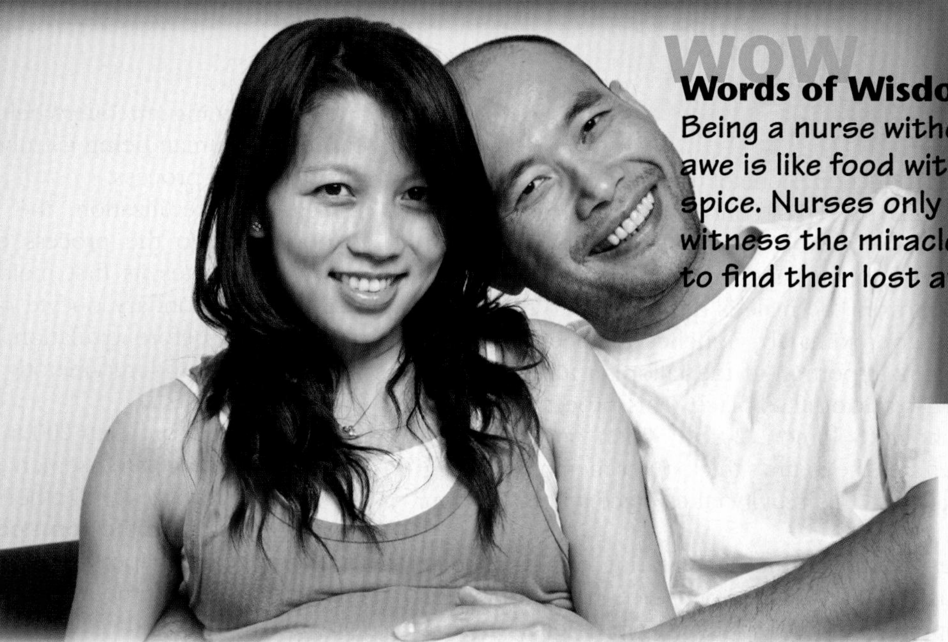

WOW

Words of Wisdom

Being a nurse without awe is like food without spice. Nurses only have to witness the miracle of life to find their lost awe.

Fetal Development and Genetics

KEY TERMS

- allele
- blastocyst
- embryonic stage
- fertilization
- fetal stage
- genes
- genetic counseling
- genetics
- genome
- genomics
- genotype
- heterozygous
- homozygous
- karyotype
- mosaicism
- monosomy
- morula
- mutation
- phenotype
- placenta
- preembryonic stage
- teratogen
- trisomy
- trophoblast
- umbilical cord
- zona pellucida
- zygote

Learning Objectives

Upon completion of the chapter, you will be able to:

1. Characterize the process of fertilization, implantation, and cell differentiation.
2. Examine the functions of the placenta, umbilical cord, and amniotic fluid.
3. Outline normal fetal development from conception through birth.
4. Compare the various inheritance patterns, including nontraditional patterns of inheritance.
5. Analyze examples of ethical and legal issues surrounding genetic testing.
6. Research the role of the nurse in genetic counseling and genetic-related activities.

Robert and Kate Shafer **have just received the good news that Kate's pregnancy test is positive. It had been a long and anxious 3 years of trying to start a family. Although both are elated about the prospect of becoming parents, they are concerned about the possibility of a genetic problem because Kate is 38 years old. What might be their first step in looking into their genetic concern? As a nurse, what might raise concerns for you?**

INTRODUCTION

Human reproduction is one of the most intimate spheres of an individual's life. For conception to occur, a healthy ovum from the woman is released from the ovary, passes into an open fallopian tube, and starts its journey downward. Sperm from the male is deposited into the vagina and swims approximately 7 inches to meet the ovum at the outermost portion of the fallopian tube, the area where **fertilization** takes place. This process occurs in about an hour (Solomon, 2015). When one spermatozoon penetrates the ovum's thick outer membrane, pregnancy begins. All this activity takes place within a 5-hour time span.

Nurses caring for the childbearing family need to have a basic understanding of conception and prenatal development so they can identify problems or variations and can initiate appropriate interventions should any problems occur. This chapter presents an overview of fetal development, beginning with conception. It also discusses hereditary influences on fetal development and the nurse's role in **genetic counseling**.

FETAL DEVELOPMENT

Fetal development during pregnancy is measured in number of weeks after fertilization. The duration of pregnancy is about 40 weeks from the time of fertilization. This equates to 9 calendar months or approximately 266 to 280 calendar days. The three stages of fetal development during pregnancy are:

1. **Preembryonic stage**: fertilization through the second week
2. **Embryonic stage**: end of the second week through the eighth week
3. **Fetal stage**: end of the eighth week until birth

Fetal circulation is a significant aspect of fetal development that spans all three stages.

Preembryonic Stage

The preembryonic stage begins with fertilization, also called *conception*. Fertilization is the union of ovum and sperm, which is the starting point of pregnancy. Fertilization typically occurs around 2 weeks after the last normal menstrual period in a 28-day cycle (Mader & Windelspecht, 2015). Fertilization requires a timely interaction between the release of the mature ovum at ovulation and the ejaculation of enough healthy, mobile sperm to survive the hostile vaginal environment through which they must travel to meet the ovum. All things considered, the act of conception is difficult at best. To say merely that it occurs when the sperm unites with the ovum is overly simple because this union requires an intricate interplay of hormonal preparation and overcoming an overwhelming number of natural barriers. A human being is truly an amazing outcome of this elaborate process.

Prior to fertilization, the ovum and the spermatozoon undergo the process of meiosis. The primary oocyte completes its first meiotic division before ovulation. The secondary oocyte begins its second meiotic division just before ovulation. Primary and secondary spermatocytes undergo meiotic division while still in the testes (Fig. 10.1).

Although more than 200 million sperm/mL are contained in the ejaculated semen, only one is able to enter the ovum to fertilize it. All others are blocked by the clear protein layer called the **zona pellucida**. The zona pellucida disappears in about 5 days. Once the sperm reaches the plasma membrane, the ovum resumes meiosis and forms a nucleus with half the number of chromosomes (23). When the nucleus from the ovum and the nucleus of the sperm make contact, they lose their respective nuclear membranes and combine their maternal and paternal chromosomes. Because each nucleus contains a haploid number of chromosomes (23), this union restores the diploid number (46). The resulting **zygote** begins the process of a new life. The genetic information from both ovum and sperm establishes the unique physical characteristics of the individual. Sex determination is also determined at fertilization and depends on whether the ovum is fertilized by a Y-bearing sperm or an X-bearing sperm. Approximately half of sperm carry the XX chromosome and the other half carries XY. An XX zygote will become a female and an XY zygote will become a male (Fig. 10.2). That is why it is scientifically correct to say that the sex of the infant is determined by the father and not by the mother.

Fertilization takes place in the outer third of the ampulla of the fallopian tube. When the ovum is fertilized by the sperm (now called a zygote), a great deal of activity immediately takes place. Mitosis, or *cleavage,* occurs as the zygote is slowly transported into the uterine cavity by tubal muscular movements (Fig. 10.3). After a series of four cleavages, the 16 cells appear as a solid ball of cells, or **morula**, meaning "little mulberry." The morula reaches the uterine cavity about 72 hours after fertilization. As fluid, which provides nutrients, from the uterine cavity enters the morula, the **blastocyst** is formed (Mader & Windelspecht, 2015).

With additional cell division, the morula divides into specialized cells that will later form fetal structures. Within the morula, an off-center, fluid-filled space appears, transforming it into a hollow ball of cells called a blastocyst (Fig. 10.4). The inner surface of the blastocyst will form the embryo and amnion. The outer layer of cells surrounding the blastocyst cavity is called a **trophoblast**. Eventually, the trophoblast develops into one of the embryonic membranes, the chorion, and helps to form the **placenta**.

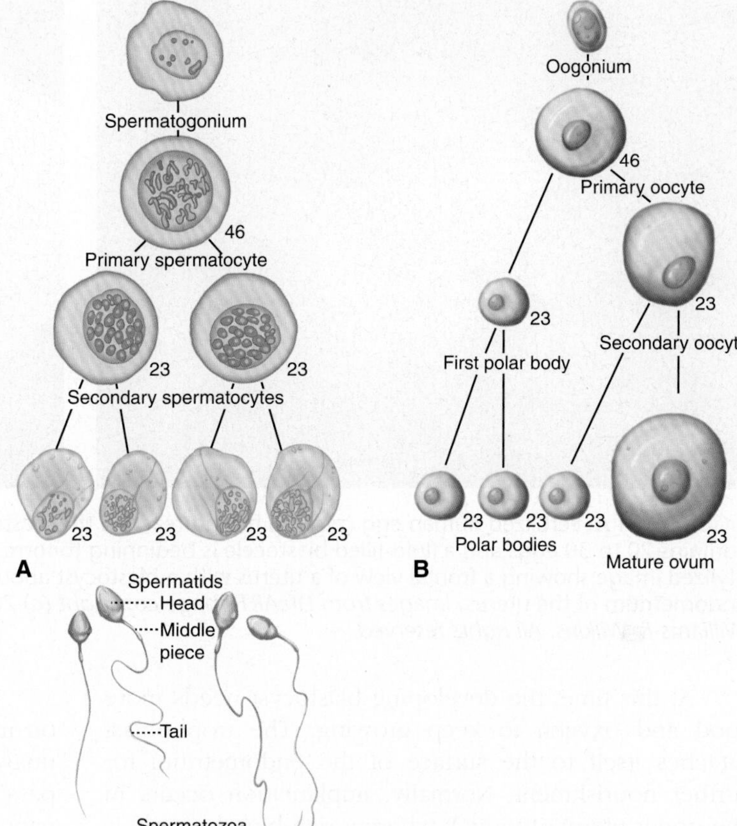

FIGURE 10.1 The formation of gametes by the process of meiosis is known as gametogenesis. **A.** Spermatogenesis. One spermatogonium gives rise to four spermatozoa. **B.** Oogenesis. From each oogonium, one mature ovum and three abortive cells are produced. The chromosomes are reduced to one-half the number characteristic for the general body cells of the species. In humans, the number in the body cells is 46, and that in the mature spermatozoon and secondary oocyte is 23.

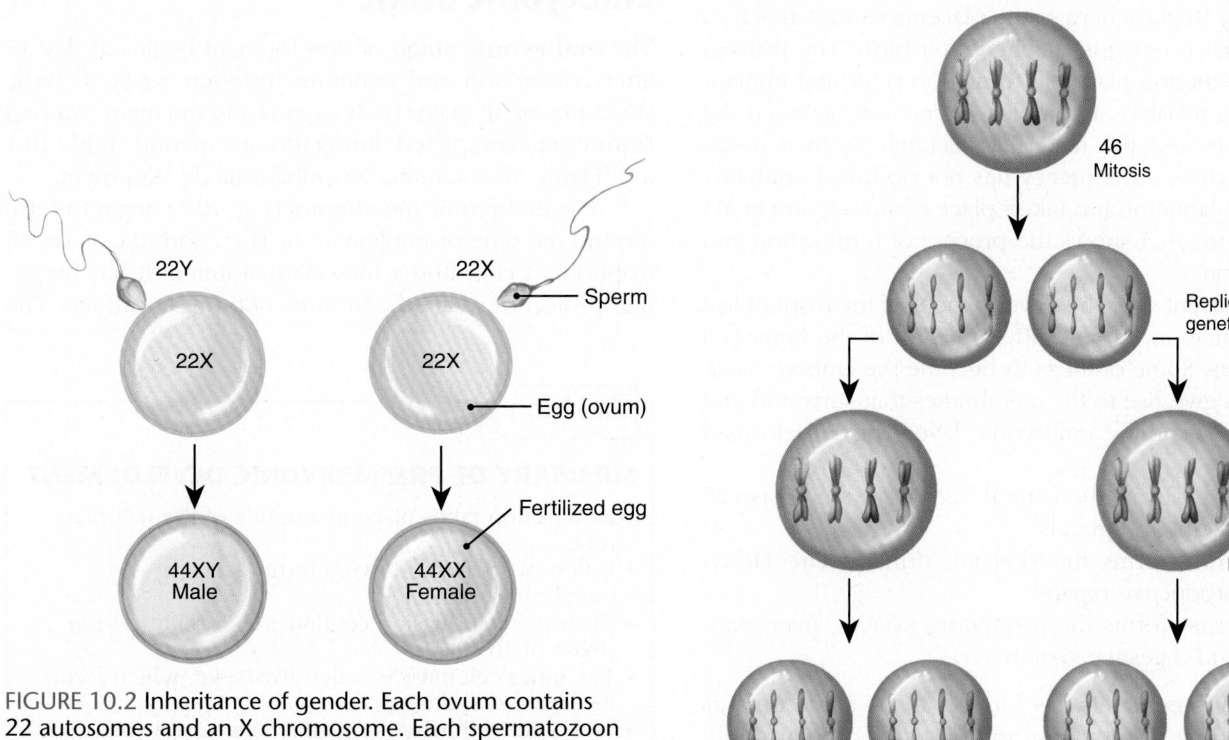

FIGURE 10.2 Inheritance of gender. Each ovum contains 22 autosomes and an X chromosome. Each spermatozoon (sperm) contains 22 autosomes and either an X chromosome or a Y chromosome. The gender of the zygote is determined at the time of fertilization by the combination of the sex chromosomes of the sperm (either X or Y) and the ovum (X).

FIGURE 10.3 Mitosis of the stoma cells.

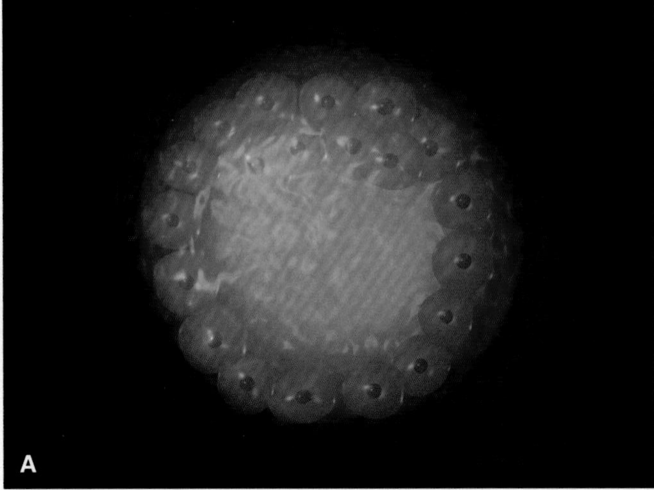

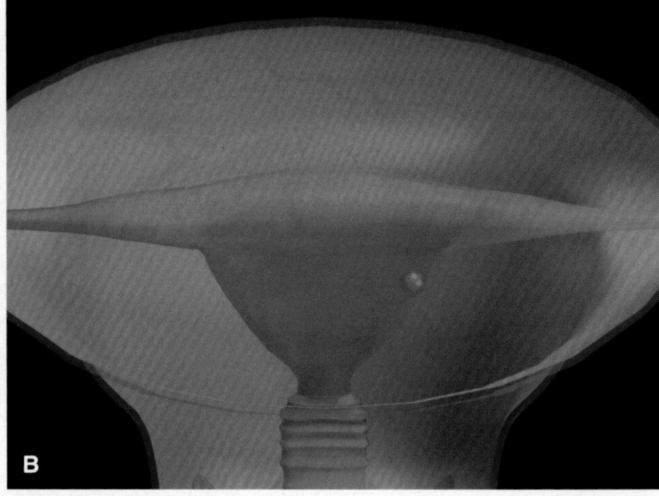

FIGURE 10.4 **A.** Fertilized human egg (zygote) having reached the blastocyst stage. Zygote contains 20 to 30 eggs and a fluid-filled blastocele is beginning to form. **B.** Implantation. Stylized image showing a frontal view of a uterus with a blastocyst about to implant into endometrium of the uterus. *Images from LifeART image copyright (c) 2011 Lippincott Williams & Wilkins. All rights reserved.*

At this time, the developing blastocyst needs more food and oxygen to keep growing. The trophoblast attaches itself to the surface of the endometrium for further nourishment. Normally, implantation occurs in the upper uterus (fundus), where a rich blood supply is available. This area also contains strong muscular fibers, which clamp down on blood vessels after the placenta separates from the inner wall of the uterus. Additionally, the lining is thickest here so the placenta cannot attach so strongly that it remains attached after birth. The process of attachment and placental formation is termed implantation. This involves a complex interaction between the trophoblasts and the maternal decidua. From a medical perspective, a pregnancy has not occurred until successful implantation has taken place (Cunningham et al., 2014). Figure 10.5 shows the process of fertilization and implantation.

Concurrent with the development of the trophoblast and implantation, further differentiation of the inner cell mass occurs. Some of the cells become the embryo itself, and others give rise to the membranes that surround and protect it. The three embryonic layers of cells formed are:

1. Ectoderm—forms the central nervous system, special senses, skin, and glands
2. Mesoderm—forms the skeletal, urinary, circulatory, and reproductive organs
3. Endoderm—forms the respiratory system, liver, pancreas, and digestive system

These three layers are formed at the same time as the embryonic membranes, and all tissues, organs, and organ systems develop from these three primary germ cell layers (Jones & Lopez, 2014). Box 10.1 summarizes preembryonic development.

Despite the intense and dramatic activities going on internally to create a human life, many women are unaware that pregnancy has begun. Several weeks will pass before even one of the presumptive signs of pregnancy—missing the first menstrual period—will take place.

Embryonic Stage

The **embryonic stage** of development begins at day 15 after conception and continues through week 8. Basic structures of all major body organs and the main external features are completed during this time period. Table 10.1 and Figure 10.6 summarize embryonic development.

The embryonic membranes (Fig. 10.7) begin to form around the time of implantation. The chorion consists of trophoblast cells and a mesodermal lining. It has finger-like projections called *chorionic villi* on its surface. The

BOX 10.1

SUMMARY OF PREEMBRYONIC DEVELOPMENT

- Fertilization takes place in ampulla of the fallopian tube.
- Union of sperm and ovum forms a *zygote* (46 chromosomes).
- Cleavage cell division continues to form a *morula* (mass of 16 cells).
- The inner cell mass is called *blastocyst,* which forms the embryo and amnion.
- The outer cell mass is called *trophoblast,* which forms the placenta and chorion.
- Implantation occurs 7 to 10 days after conception in the endometrium.

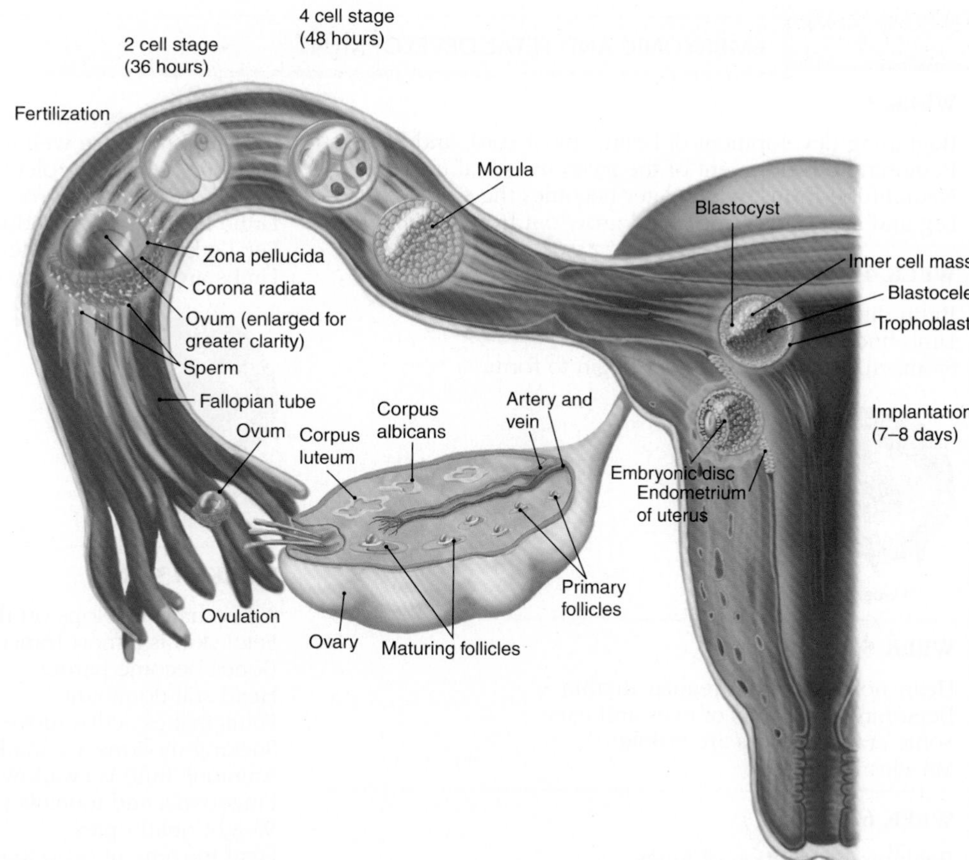

FIGURE 10.5 Fertilization and tubal transport of the zygote. From fertilization to implantation, the zygote travels through the fallopian tube, experiencing rapid mitotic division (cleavage). During the journey toward the uterus the zygote evolves through several stages, including morula and blastocyst.

amnion originates from the ectoderm germ layer during the early stages of embryonic development. It is a thin protective membrane that contains amniotic fluid. As the embryo grows, the amnion (inner layer) expands until it touches the chorion (outer layer). These two fetal membranes form the fluid-filled amniotic sac, or bag of waters, that protects the floating embryo (Cunningham et al., 2014).

Amniotic fluid surrounds the embryo and increases in volume as the pregnancy progresses, reaching approximately 1 L at term. Amniotic fluid is derived from two sources: fluid transported from the maternal blood across the amnion and fetal urine. Its volume changes constantly as the fetus swallows and voids. Sufficient amounts of amniotic fluid help maintain a constant body temperature for the fetus, permit

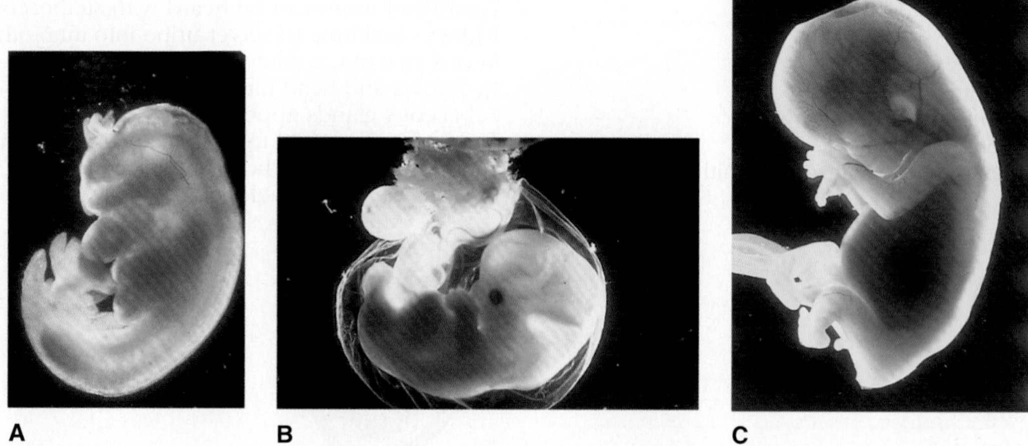

FIGURE 10.6 Embryonic development. **A.** 4-week embryo. **B.** 5-week embryo. **C.** 6-week embryo.

TABLE 10.1 EMBRYONIC AND FETAL DEVELOPMENT

WEEK 3

Beginning development of brain, spinal cord, and heart
Beginning development of the gastrointestinal tract
Neural tube forms, which later becomes the spinal cord
Leg and arm buds appear and grow out from body

WEEK 4

Brain differentiates
Limb buds grow and develop more
Stomach, pancreas, and liver begin to form

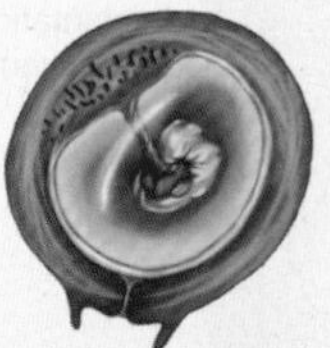

4 weeks

WEEK 5

Heart now beats at a regular rhythm
Beginning structures of eyes and ears
Some cranial nerves are visible
Muscles innervated

WEEK 6

Beginning formation of lungs
Fetal circulation established
Liver produces RBCs
Further development of the brain
Primitive skeleton forms
Central nervous system forms
Brain waves detectable

WEEK 7

Straightening of trunk
Nipples and hair follicles form
Elbows and toes visible
Arms and legs move
Diaphragm formed
Fetal heartbeat can be heard
Mouth with lips and early tooth buds

WEEK 8

Rotation of intestines
Facial features continue to develop
Heart development complete
Resembles a human being (Mattson & Smith, 2015).

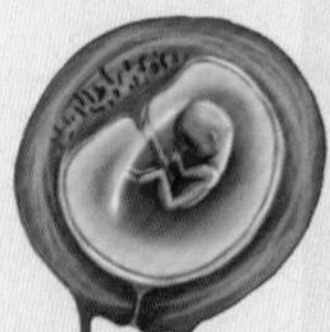

8 weeks

WEEKS 9–12

Sexual differentiation continues
Buds for all 20 temporary teeth laid down
Digestive system shows activity
Head comprises nearly half the fetus size
Face and neck are well formed
Urogenital tract completes development
Red blood cells are produced in the liver
Urine begins to be produced and excreted
Fetal gender can be determined by week 12
Limbs are long and thin; digits are well formed

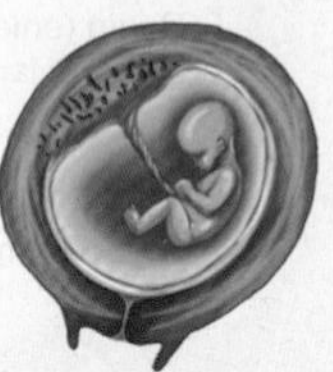

12 weeks

WEEKS 13–16

A fine hair develops on the head called lanugo
Fetal skin is almost transparent
Bones become harder
Head still dominant
Fetus makes active movement
Sucking motions are made with the mouth
Amniotic fluid is swallowed
Fingernails and toenails present
Weight quadruples
Fetal movement (also known as quickening) detected by mother

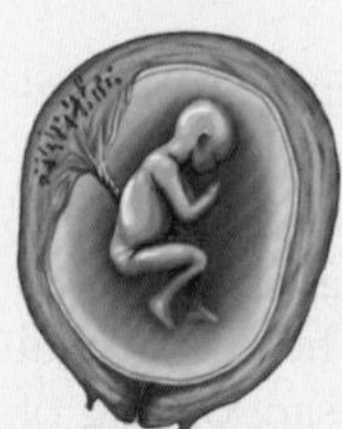

16 weeks

WEEKS 17–20

Rapid brain growth occurs
Fetal heart tones can be heard with stethoscope
Kidneys continue to secret urine into amniotic fluid
Vernix caseosa, a white greasy film, covers the fetus
Eyebrows and head hair appear
Sebaceous glands appear
Brown fat deposited to help maintain temperature
Nails are present on both fingers and toes
Muscles are well developed

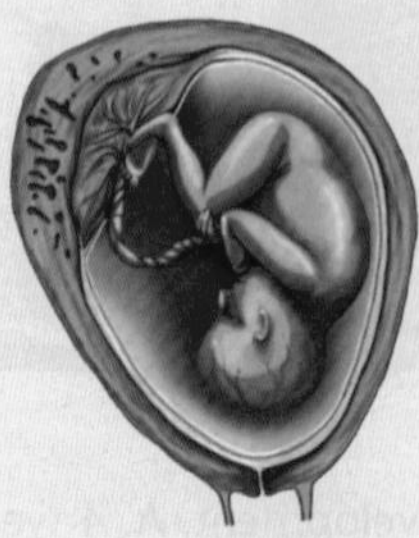

20 weeks

TABLE 10.1 EMBRYONIC AND FETAL DEVELOPMENT (continued)

WEEKS 21–24

Eyebrows and eyelashes are well formed
Fetus has a hand grasp and startle reflex
Alveoli forming in lungs
Body is lean but fairly well proportioned
Skin is translucent and red
Lungs begin to produce surfactant

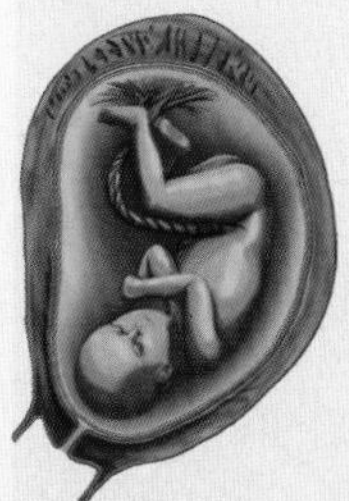

25 weeks

WEEKS 25–28

Fetus reaches a length of 15 inches
Rapid brain development
Eyelids open and close
Nervous system controls some functions
Fingerprints are set
Blood formation shifts from spleen to bone marrow
Fetus usually assumes head-down position

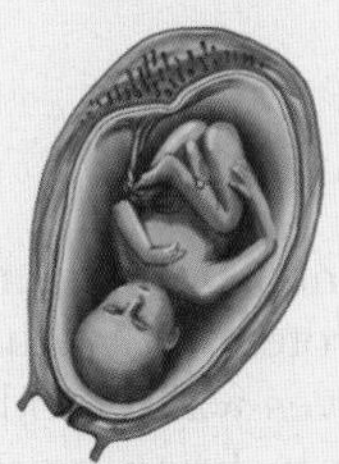

28 weeks

WEEKS 29–32

Rapid increase in amount of body fat
Increased central nervous system control over body functions
Rhythmic breathing movements occur
Lungs are not fully mature
Fetus stores iron, calcium, and phosphorus

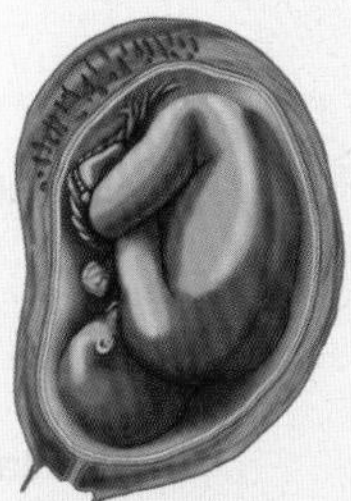

32 weeks

WEEKS 33–38

Testes are in scrotum of male fetus
Lanugo begins to disappear
Increase in body fat
Fingernails reach the ends of fingertips
Small breast buds are present on both sexes
Mother supplies fetus with antibodies against disease
Fetus is considered full term at 38 weeks
Fetus fills uterus (El-Mazny, 2014)

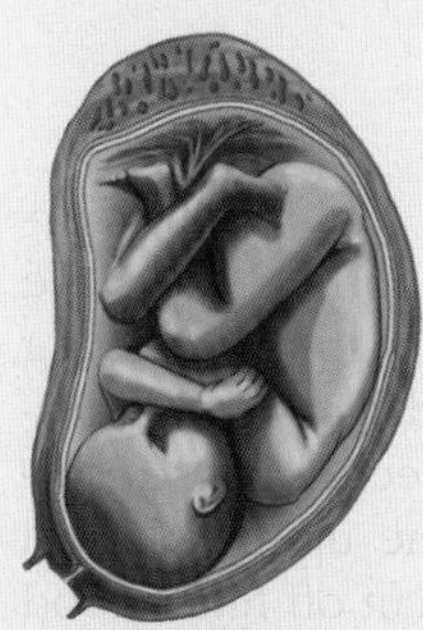

37 weeks

symmetric growth and development, cushion the fetus from trauma, allow the **umbilical cord** to be relatively free from compression, and promote fetal movement to enhance musculoskeletal development. Amniotic fluid is composed of 98% water and 2% organic matter. It is slightly alkaline and contains albumin, urea, bile pigments, renin, glucose, hormones, uric acid, creatinine, bilirubin, lecithin, sphingomyelin, epithelial cells, vernix, and fine hair called lanugo. The composition of amniotic fluid changes with gestation. Adequate amniotic fluid volume is necessary for proper fetal growth and development. (Magann & Ross, 2014).

The volume of amniotic fluid is important in determining fetal well-being. It gradually fluctuates throughout the pregnancy. Alterations in amniotic fluid volume can be associated with problems in the fetus. Too little amniotic fluid (<500 mL at term), termed *oligohydramnios,* is associated with uteroplacental insufficiency, fetal renal abnormalities, and a higher risk of surgical births and low birth weight infants. Too much amniotic fluid (>2000 mL at term), termed *polyhydramnios,* is associated with maternal diabetes, neural tube defects, chromosomal deviations, and malformations of the central nervous system and/or gastrointestinal tract that prevent normal swallowing of amniotic fluid by the fetus. Polyhydramnios may threaten premature rupture of membranes due to uterine overdistention (Moore, 2015).

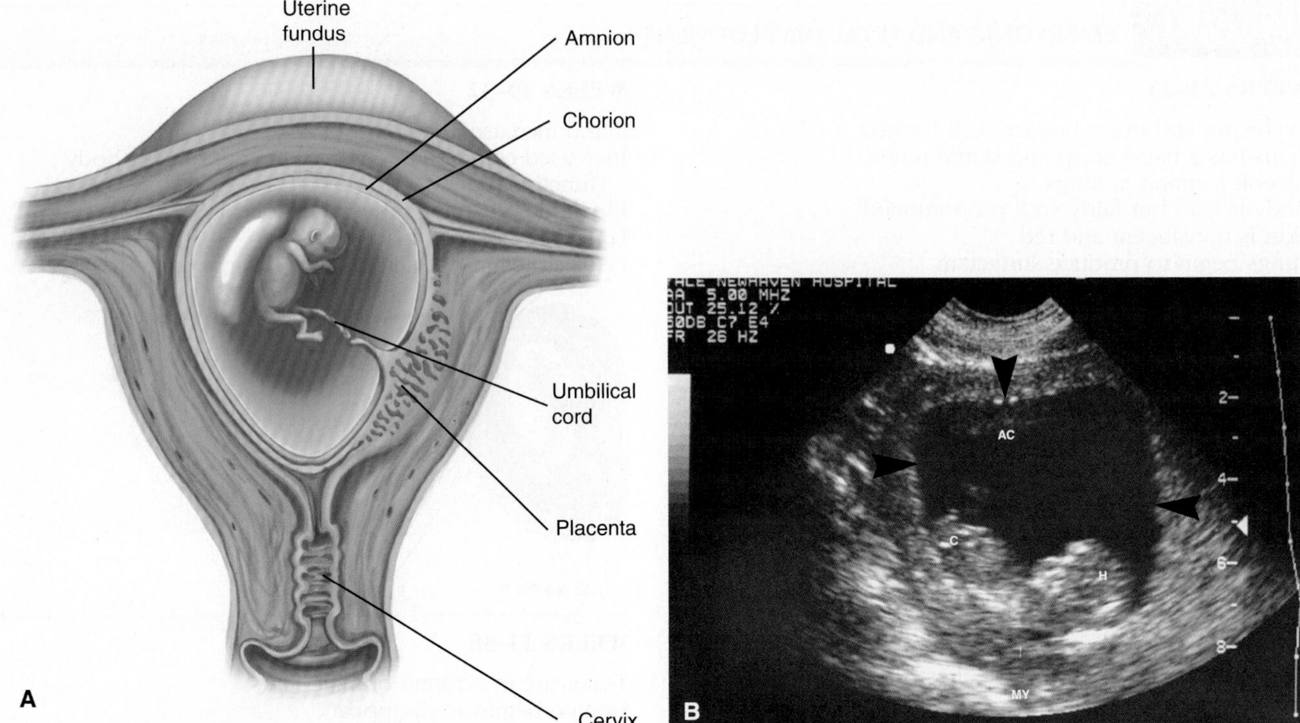

FIGURE 10.7 **A.** The embryo is floating in amniotic fluid, surrounded by the protective fetal membranes (amnion and chorion). **B.** Longitudinal sonogram of a pregnant uterus at 11 weeks showing the intrauterine gestational sac (black arrowheads) and the amniotic cavity (AC) filled with amniotic fluid; the fetus is seen in longitudinal section with the head (H) and coccyx (C) well displayed. The myometrium (MY) of the uterus can be identified. (*Figure B is courtesy of L Scoutt.*)

While the placenta is developing (end of the second week), the umbilical cord is also formed from the amnion. It is the lifeline from the mother to the growing embryo. It contains one large vein and two small arteries. Wharton's jelly (a specialized connective tissue) surrounds these three blood vessels in the umbilical cord to prevent compression, which would cut off fetal blood and nutrient supply. The cord reaches its maximum length by 30 weeks of gestation. Its length is determined by **genetics** and intrauterine space and fetal activity, which places tension on the cord. At term, the average umbilical cord is 22 inches long and about 1 inch wide (King et al., 2015).

The precursor cells of the placenta—the trophoblasts—first appear 4 days after **fertilization** as the outer layer of cells of the blastocyst. These early blastocyst trophoblasts differentiate into all the cells that form the placenta. When fully developed, the placenta serves as the interface between the mother and the developing fetus. As early as 3 days after conception, the trophoblasts make human chorionic gonadotropin (hCG), a hormone that ensures that the endometrium will be receptive to the implanting embryo. During the next few weeks the placenta begins to make hormones that control the basic physiology of the mother in such a way that the fetus is supplied with the nutrients and oxygen needed for growth. The placenta also protects the fetus from immune attack by the mother, removes waste products from the fetus, induces the mother to bring more food to the placenta and, near the time of childbirth, produces hormones that ready fetal organs for life outside the uterus. Placenta function depends on the maternal blood pressure supplying circulation. If there is an interference with blood flow to the placenta, it cannot carry out its functions to the embryo or fetus (Mattson & Smith, 2015).

Theoretically, at no time during pregnancy does the mother's blood mix with fetal blood because there is no direct contact between their bloods; layers of fetal tissue always separate the maternal blood and the fetal blood. These fetal tissues are called the *placental barrier*. Materials can be interchanged only through diffusion. The maternal uterine arteries deliver the nutrients to the placenta, which in turn provides nutrients to the developing fetus; the mother's uterine veins carry fetal waste products away. The structure of the placenta is usually completed by week 12.

The placenta is not only a transfer organ but a hormone factory as well. Placental hormones have profound effects on maternal metabolism, initially building up her energy reserves and then releasing these to support fetal growth in later pregnancy and lactation postnatally. Several hormones are produced that are necessary for normal pregnancy:

- hCG—preserves the corpus luteum and its progesterone production so that the endometrial lining of the uterus is maintained; this is the basis for pregnancy tests
- Human placental lactogen (hPL)—modulates fetal and maternal metabolism, participates in the development of maternal breasts for lactation, and decreases maternal insulin sensitivity to increase its availability for fetal nutrition
- Estrogen (estriol)—causes enlargement of a woman's breasts, uterus, and external genitalia; stimulates myometrial contractility
- Progesterone (progestin)—maintains the endometrium, decreases the contractility of the uterus, stimulates maternal metabolism and breast development, provides nourishment for the early conceptus
- Relaxin—acts synergistically with progesterone to maintain pregnancy, causes relaxation of the pelvic ligaments, softens the cervix in preparation for birth (Freemark, 2015).

The placenta acts as a pass-through between the mother and fetus, not a barrier. Almost everything the mother ingests (food, alcohol, drugs) passes through to the developing conceptus. This is why it is so important to advise pregnant women not to use unprescribed drugs, alcohol, and tobacco, because they can be harmful to the conceptus.

During the embryonic stage, the conceptus grows rapidly as all organs and structures are forming. During this critical period of differentiation the growing embryo is most susceptible to damage from external sources, including **teratogen**s (substances that cause birth defects, such as alcohol and drugs), infections (such as rubella or cytomegalovirus), radiation, and nutritional deficiencies.

Fetal Stage

The average pregnancy lasts 280 days from the first day of the last menstrual period. The fetal stage is the time from the end of the eighth week until birth. It is the longest period of prenatal development. During this stage, the conceptus is mature enough to be called a fetus. Although all major systems are present in their basic form, dramatic growth and refinement of all organ systems take place during the fetal period (see Table 10.1). Figure 10.8 depicts a 12- to 15-week-old fetus.

Fetal Circulation

Fetal circulation differs from adult circulation due to the presence of certain vessels and shunts. These shunts will close after birth and most of the vessels will be seen as remnants in the adult circulation. The function of these shunts is to direct oxygen-rich venous blood to the systemic circulation and to ensure that oxygen-depleted venous blood bypasses the underdeveloped pulmonary circulation. The lungs finish their development after birth. Prior to birth, the lungs function is taken over by the placenta during fetal life (Finnemore & Groves, 2015). The circulation through the fetus during uterine life differs from that of a child or an adult. In the extrauterine world, oxygenation occurs in the lungs and oxygenated blood returns via the pulmonary veins to the left side of the heart to be ejected by the left ventricle into the systemic circulation. In contrast, fetal circulation oxygenation occurs in the placenta, and the fetal lungs are nonfunctional as far as the transfer of oxygen and carbon dioxide is concerned. For oxygenated blood derived from the placenta to reach the fetus's systemic circulation, it has to travel through a series of shunts to accomplish this.

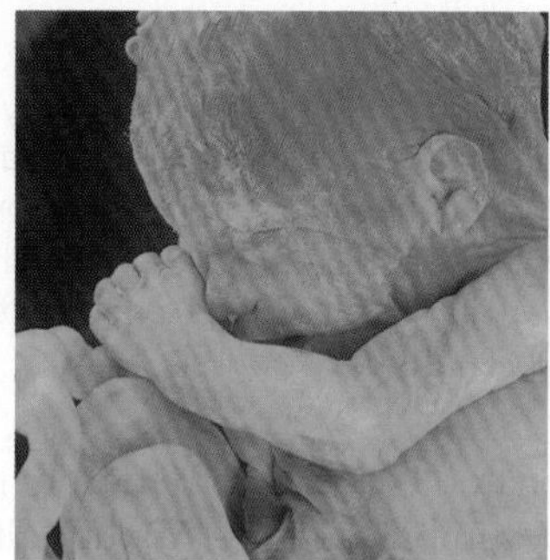

FIGURE 10.8 Fetal development: 12- to 15-week fetus.

Thus, fetal circulation involves the circulation of blood from the placenta to and through the fetus, and back to the placenta. A properly functioning fetal circulation system is essential to sustain the fetus. Before it develops, nutrients and oxygen diffuse through the extraembryonic coelom and the yolk sac from the placenta. As the embryo grows, its nutrient needs increase and the amount of tissue easily reached by diffusion increases. Thus, the circulation must develop quickly and accurately (Jones & Lopez, 2014).

The circulatory system of the fetus functions much differently from that of a newborn. The most significant difference is that oxygen is received from the placenta during fetal life and via the lungs after birth. In addition, the fetal liver does not perform the metabolic functions that it will after birth because the mother's body performs these functions. Three shunts also are present during fetal life:

1. Ductus venosus—connects the umbilical vein to the inferior vena cava
2. Ductus arteriosus—connects the main pulmonary artery to the aorta
3. Foramen ovale—anatomic opening between the right and left atrium

Take Note!

Fetal circulation functions to carry highly oxygenated blood to vital areas (e.g., heart, brain) while first shunting it away from less important ones (e.g., lungs, liver). The placenta essentially takes over the functions of the lungs and liver during fetal life. As a result, large volumes of oxygenated blood are not needed.

The oxygenated blood is carried from the placenta to the fetus via the umbilical vein. About half of this blood passes through the hepatic capillaries and the rest flows through the ductus venosus into the inferior vena cava. Blood from the vena cava is mostly deflected through the foramen ovale into the left atrium, then to the left ventricle, into the ascending aorta, and on to the head and upper body. This allows the fetal coronary circulation and the brain to receive the blood with the highest level of oxygenation.

Deoxygenated blood from the superior vena cava flows into the right atrium, the right ventricle, and then the pulmonary artery. Because of high pulmonary vascular resistance, only a small percentage (5% to 10%) of the blood in the pulmonary artery flows to the lungs; the majority is shunted through the patent ductus arteriosus and then to the descending aorta (American Heart Association, 2015). The fetal lungs are essentially nonfunctional because they are filled with fluid, making them resistant to incoming blood flow. They receive only enough blood for proper nourishment. Finally, two umbilical arteries carry the unoxygenated blood from the descending aorta back to the placenta.

At birth, a dramatic change in the fetal circulatory pattern occurs. The foramen ovale, ductus arteriosus, ductus venosus, and umbilical vessels are no longer needed. With the newborn's first breath, the lungs inflate, which leads to an increase in blood flow to the lungs from the right ventricle. This increase raises the pressure in the left atrium, causing a one-way flap on the left side of the foramen ovale, called the septum primum, to press against the opening, creating a functional separation between the two atria. Blood flow to the lungs increases because blood entering the right atrium can no longer bypass the right ventricle. As a result, the right ventricle pumps blood into the pulmonary artery and on to the lungs. Typically the foramen ovale is functionally closed within 1 to 2 hours after birth. It is physiologically closed by 1 month with deposits of fibrin to seal the shunt. Permanent closure occurs by the sixth month of life.

The ductus venosus, which links the inferior vena cava with the umbilical vein, usually closes with the clamping of the umbilical cord and inhibition of blood flow through the umbilical vein. This fetal structure closes by the end of the first week. The ductus arteriosus constricts partly in response to the higher arterial oxygen levels that occur after the first few breaths. This closure prevents blood from the aorta from entering the pulmonary artery. Functional closure of the ductus arteriosus in a term infant usually occurs within the first 72 hours after birth. Permanent closure occurs at 3 to 4 weeks of age. Frequently a functional or innocent murmur is auscultated by the nursery nurse when there are delayed fetal shunt closures, but they usually are not associated with a heart lesion (Lawford & Tulloh, 2015). All of these changes at birth leave the newborn with the typical adult pattern of circulation with right ventricle output equaling that of the left. Figure 10.9 shows fetal circulation. Go to thePoint for a web link to a video depicting fetal circulation.

GENETICS

Genetics is the study of heredity and its variation (Nussbaum, McInnes, & Willard, 2016). **Genomics**, a relatively new science, is the study of all genes and includes interactions among genes as well as interactions between genes and the environment. Genomics plays a role in complex conditions such as heart disease and diabetes. Another emerging area of research is that of pharmacogenomics, the study of genetic and genomic influences on pharmacodynamics and pharmacotherapeutics. It aims to use an individual's genetic information in order to treat diseases more efficiently and minimize adverse events (Meyer zu Schwabedissen, 2015). An individual's genetics influences wellness and health issues throughout that person's lifespan. The challenge for health care providers is to find the link between the client's genetic makeup and diseases (Brazeau, 2015).

According to the Centers for Disease Control and Prevention (CDC), birth defects occur in about 3% of all infants born in the United States, or 1 in every 33 infants. Every 5 minutes an infant is born with a birth defect in the United States with nearly 120,000 infants affected annually (Centers for Disease Control and Prevention, 2015). Traditionally, genetics has been associated with making decisions about childbearing and caring for children with genetic disorders. Recently, genetic and technologic advances are expanding our understanding of how genetic changes affect human diseases such as diabetes, cancer, Alzheimer's disease, and other multifactorial diseases that are prevalent in adults. Today's genetic technologies are not yet a crystal ball for seeing a child's future, but scientists are closer to routinely glimpsing at the genetic blueprints of a fetus just months after sperm meets egg (Kumar, Kingsley, & DiStefano, 2015). Newborn screening is perhaps the most widely used application of genetics in perinatal and neonatal care. Our ability to diagnose genetic conditions is more advanced than our ability to cure or treat the disorders. However, accurate diagnosis has led to improved treatment and outcomes for those affected with these disorders.

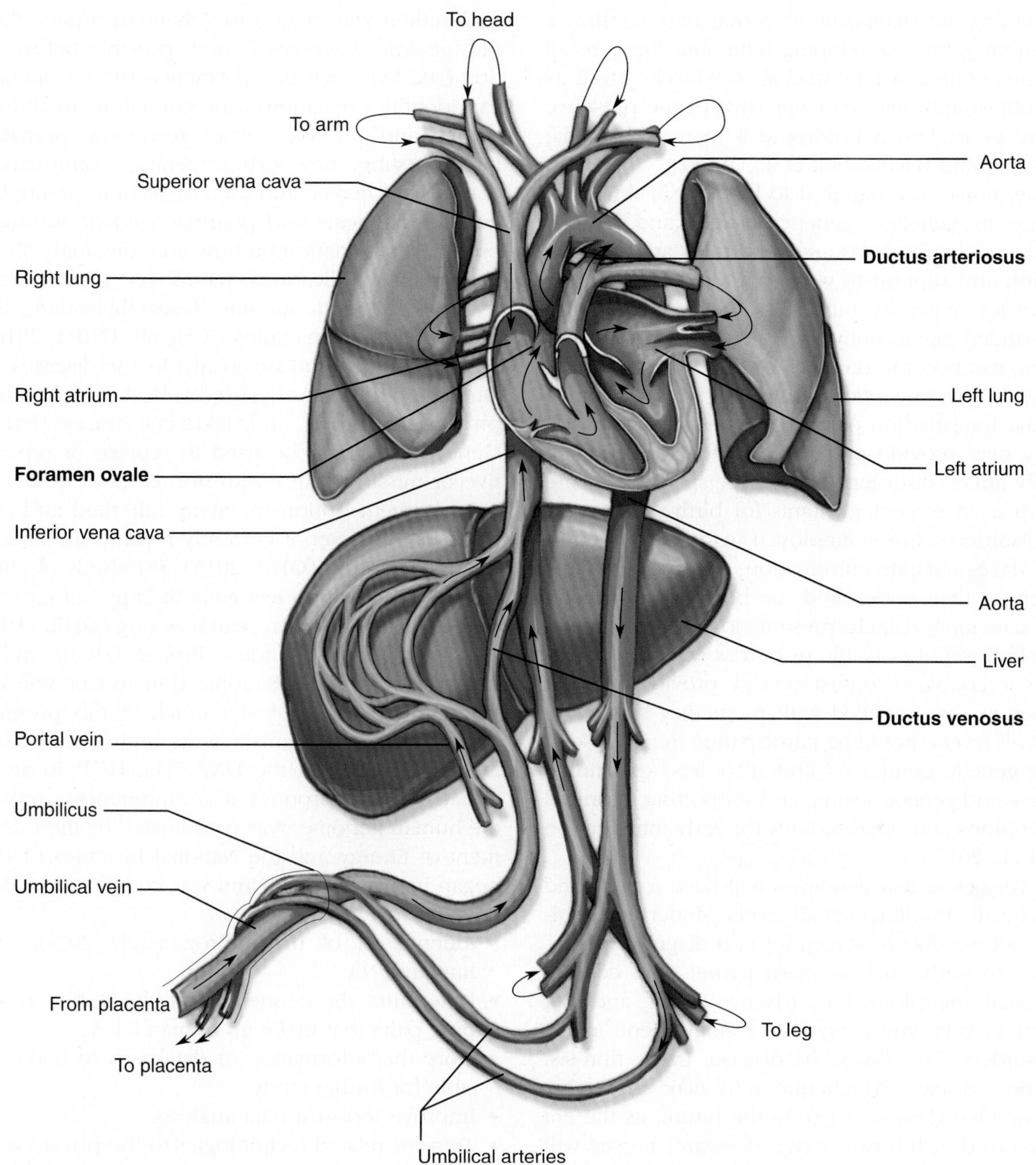

FIGURE 10.9 Fetal circulation. Arrows indicate the path of blood. The umbilical vein carries oxygen-rich blood from the placenta to the liver and through the ductus venosus. From there it is carried to the inferior vena cava to the right atrium of the heart. Some of the blood is shunted through the foramen ovale to the left side of the heart, where it is routed to the brain and upper extremities. The rest of the blood travels down to the right ventricle and through the pulmonary artery. A small portion of the blood travels to the nonfunctioning lungs, while the remaining blood is shunted through the ductus arteriosus into the aorta to supply the rest of the body.

Take Note!

Genetic science has the potential to revolutionize health care with regard to national screening programs, predisposition testing, detection of genetic disorders, and pharmacogenetics.

Genetics has been a part of perinatal care for decades. Rapid development and implementation of advanced genetics technology in prenatal settings includes the ability to screen for and diagnose a broader range of diseases and conditions of the fetus in early gestational ages. Ultrasounds and maternal serum screening have become routine elements of prenatal care. Preconception carrier screening for conditions such as Tay–Sachs disease has been in place among high-risk populations such as Ashkenazi Jews. Amniocentesis and chorionic villus sampling are diagnostic tests that may confirm a genetic anomaly in a developing fetus, but they are all invasive procedures. A fetal nuchal translucency test, as seen on ultrasound, may be suggestive of the presence of trisomy 21 or Down syndrome if increased nuchal thickness is found (Lichtenbelt et al., 2015).

Today, nurses are required to have basic skills and knowledge in genetics, genetic testing, and genetic counseling so they can assume new roles and provide information and support to women, children, and families. Roles for maternity nurses in genetic health care have expanded significantly as genetics education and counseling has become standard of care. Today, nurses may provide preconception counseling for women at risk for the transmission of a genetic disorder. In addition, they may provide prenatal care for women with genetically linked disorders that require specialized care or participate in screening infants for birth defects and genetic disorders. Nurses employed in prenatal settings need to have accurate information they can provide to women so they understand the benefits and limitations of screening. Timely presentation of information and identification of available resources will help nurses minimize a couple's confusion and provide support for women as they proceed with pregnancy screening. Nurses at all levels should be participating in risk assessment for genetic conditions and disorders, explaining genetic risk and genetic testing, and supporting informed health decisions and opportunities for early intervention (Seven et al., 2015).

It is very clear that genomics will have a profound effect on health and illness at all levels. Modern technology makes it possible to screen for and diagnose conditions prior to birth, such as open neural tube defects, chromosomal aneuploids (i.e., trisomy 13, 18, and 21), congenital defects, and a myriad of single gene inheritable disorders (i.e., Tay-Sachs disease, cystic fibrosis, Huntington's disease, Duchenne muscular dystrophy, and hemophilia) (Lewis, 2015). In the future, as the era of personalized health care moves forward, nurses will be responsible for ensuring that our practice includes the scientific principles, ethical standards, and professional accountability of genetics and genomics practice. Nurses are increasingly incorporating genetics into their practice as they gain the knowledge and skills necessary to do so. The strength of the nursing voice in genetics and genomic research will be the link to the bedside and the commitment to ensure that new knowledge is translated into competent, safe, effective evidence-based client care (Latendresse & Deneris, 2015).

Advances in Genetics

Recent advances in genetic knowledge and technology have affected all areas of health. These advances have increased the number of health interventions that can be undertaken with regard to genetic disorders. For example, genetic diagnosis is now possible before conception (see Evidence-Based Practice 10.1). Genetic testing can identify presymptomatic conditions in children and adults, and provide carrier screening, prenatal diagnostic testing, newborn screening, confirmation of a diagnosis, forensic and identity testing, preimplantation genetic diagnosis and pharmacogenetic testing, which provides information on how an individual will respond to certain medications based on genetic variability (National Human Genome Research Institute [NHGRI], 2015a; National Institutes of Health (NIH), 2016). Over 2,000 genetic tests are available for diseases such as Duchenne muscular dystrophy/Becker muscular dystrophy, cystic fibrosis, and sickle cell disease (NIH, 2013). Gene therapy can be used to replace or repair defective or missing genes with normal ones. It is a promising treatment option for many inherited and incurable diseases; however, it currently remains an experimental treatment option (GHR, 2015). Hundreds of clinical trials are underway to test gene therapy but currently it is only available in the research setting (GHR, 2015).

The Human Genome Project (HGP) and continued research by the National Human Genome Research Institute has helped foster much of this progress. The **genome** of an organism is its entire hereditary information encoded in the DNA. The HGP, in an international effort to produce a comprehensive sequence of the human genome, was coordinated by the U.S. Department of Energy and the National Institutes of Health. It began in October 1990 and was completed in May 2003. Its goals included:

- Identify all of the approximately 20,500 genes in human DNA.
- Determine the sequences of the 3 billion chemical base pairs that make up human DNA.
- Store this information in databases to make it accessible for further study.
- Improve tools for data analysis.
- Transfer related technologies to the private sector.
- Address the ethical, legal, and social implications of this discovery (U.S. Department of Energy Genome Programs, 2014).

The HGP has led to the discovery of the genetic basis for hundreds of disorders and has advanced our understanding of basic genetic processes at the molecular level. A link to additional information about the HGP is available at thePoint.

One goal of the HGP was to translate the findings into new and more effective strategies for the prevention, diagnosis, and treatment of genetic diseases and disorders.

Current and potential applications for the HGP to health care include rapid and more specific diagnosis of disease, with hundreds of genetic tests available in

EVIDENCE-BASED PRACTICE 10.1

THE EVIDENCE BASE REGARDING THE EXPERIENCES OF AND ATTITUDES TO PREIMPLANTATION GENETIC DIAGNOSIS IN PROSPECTIVE PARENTS

STUDY

Technology now allows scientists to know the sequence of people's genomes and to act on this knowledge. Preimplantation genetic diagnosis was developed for IVF couples with a family history of genetic disease. It involves obtaining cells from a developing embryo in culture, which is then subjected to genetic diagnostic analysis. The resulting information is used to guide which embryos are transferred into the uterus. Previous research has suggested that couples wishing to avoid having a child with an inherited genetic condition favor preimplantation genetic testing to prevent the need for pregnancy termination following a prenatal diagnosis of an affected fetus. The purpose of this study was to understand the experiences of couples who have used or considered this technique.

Findings

A systematic review was conducted using nine studies that met the inclusion criteria. Results of the studies were analyzed and synthesized with three main themes emerging: 1) motivating factors; 2) emotional labor; 3) choices and uncertainty. The review identified an emotional and difficult journey for couples pursing preimplantation genetic diagnosis. While this technique gave them hope to prevent transmission of a genetic disease, both the decision-making and uncertainty were challenging. Lack of information was a major barrier to accessing this reproductive option.

Nursing Implications

Based on the findings, more education is needed for nurses regarding various reproductive screening tests that are available for couples with a family history of a genetic disease or at risk for them. Being aware of the spectrum of genetic disorders and linking them with the appropriate genetic tests when counseling couples would assist them greatly. The nurse needs to know which genetic problems this option would help. They might include autosomal recessive diseases in which both parents are known carriers, such as cystic fibrosis, Tay–Sachs disease, or sickle cell disease; autosomal dominant diseases, such as Huntington's disease; genetic mutations with important consequences, such as BRCA gene (breast cancer); and X linked diseases, such as hemophilia. With greater understanding and current knowledge of the various options available for couples, nurses can improve communication and provide psychological support to couples.

Source: Cunningham, J., Goldsmith, L., & Skirton, H. (2015). The evidence base regarding the experiences of and attitudes to preimplantation genetic diagnosis in prospective parents. *Midwifery, 31*(2), 288–296.

research or clinical practice; earlier detection of genetic predisposition to disease; less emphasis on treating the symptoms of a disease and more emphasis on looking at the fundamental causes of the disease; new classes of drugs; avoiding environmental conditions that may trigger disease; and repair or replacement of defective genes through gene therapy (U.S. Department of Energy Genome Programs, 2015). This new genetic knowledge and technology, along with the commercialization of this knowledge, will change both professional and parental understanding of genetic disorders.

The potential benefits of these discoveries are vast, but so is the potential for misuse. These advances challenge all health care professionals to consider the many ethical, legal, and social ramifications of genetics in human lives. In the near future, risk profiling based on an individual's unique genetic makeup will be used to tailor prevention, treatment, and ongoing management of health conditions. This profiling will raise issues associated with privacy and confidentiality related to workplace discrimination and access to health insurance. Issues of autonomy are equally problematic as society considers how to address the injustices that will inevitably surface when disease risk can be determined years in advance of its occurrence. Nurses will play an important role in developing policies and providing direction and support in this arena, and to do so they will need a basic understanding of genetics, including inheritance and inheritance patterns. Visit thePoint for links to websites sharing additional information on the ethical, social, and legal issues surrounding human genetic research and advances.

Inheritance

The nucleus within the cell is the controlling factor in all cellular activities because it contains chromosomes, long continuous strands of deoxyribonucleic acid (DNA) that carry genetic information. Each chromosome is made up of genes. **Genes** are individual units of heredity of all traits and are organized into long segments of DNA that occupy a specific location on a chromosome and determine a particular characteristic in an organism.

DNA stores genetic information and encodes the instructions for synthesizing specific proteins needed to maintain life. DNA is double-stranded and takes the form of a double helix. The side pieces of the double helix are made up of a sugar, deoxyribose, and a phosphate, occurring in alternating groups. The cross connections or rungs of the ladder are attached to the sides and are

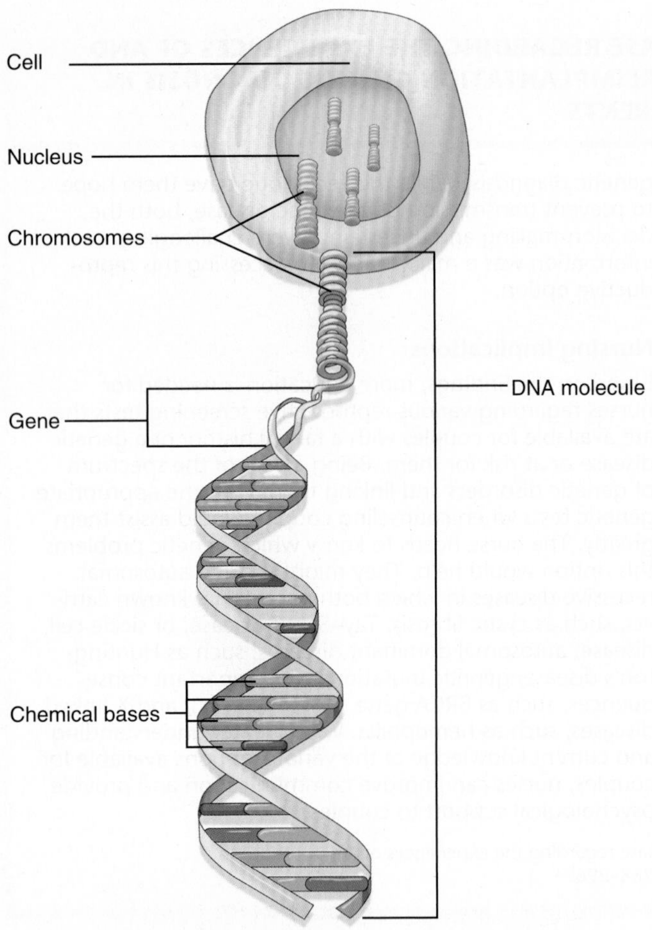

FIGURE 10.10 DNA is made up of four chemical bases. Tightly coiled strands of DNA are packaged in units called chromosomes, housed in the cell's nucleus. Working subunits of DNA are known as genes. (From the National Institutes of Health and National Cancer Institute. [1995]. Understanding gene testing [NIH Pub. No. 96–3905]. Washington, DC: U.S. Department of Human Services.)

made up of four nitrogenous bases: adenine, cytosine, thymine, and guanine. The sequence of the base pairs as they form each rung of the ladder is referred to as the genetic code (Fig. 10.10) (Travers & Muskhelishvili, 2015).

Each gene has a segment of DNA with a specific set of instructions for making proteins needed by body cells for proper functioning. Genes control the types of proteins made and the rate at which they are produced (Snustad, 2015). Any change in gene structure or location leads to a **mutation**, which may alter the type and amount of protein produced (Fig. 10.11). Genes never act in isolation; they always interact with other genes and the environment. They are arranged in a specific linear formation along a chromosome.

The **genotype**, the specific genetic makeup of an individual, usually in the form of DNA, is the internally coded inheritable information. It refers to the particular **allele**, which is one of two or more alternative versions of gene at a given position or locus on a chromosome that imparts the same characteristic of that gene. For instance, each human has a gene that controls height, but there are variations of these genes, which are alleles, in accordance with the specific height for which the gene codes. A gene that controls eye color may have an allele that can produce blue eyes or an allele that produces brown eyes. The genotype, together with environmental variation that influences the individual, determines the **phenotype**, or the observed, outward characteristics of an individual. A human inherits two genes, one from each parent. Therefore, one allele comes from the mother and one from the father. These alleles may be the same for the characteristic (**homozygous**) or different (**heterozygous**). For example, WW stands for homozygous dominant; ww stands for homozygous recessive. Heterozygous would be indicated as Ww. If the two

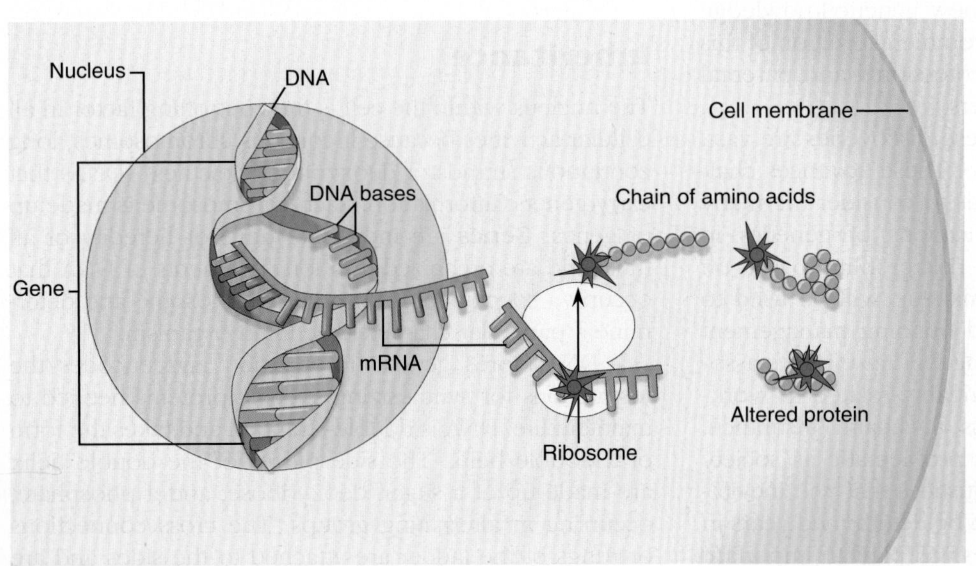

FIGURE 10.11 When a gene contains a mutation, the protein encoded by that gene will be abnormal. Some protein changes are insignificant, while others are disabling. (From the National Institutes of Health and National Cancer Institute. [1995]. *Understanding gene testing* [NIH Pub. No. 96–3905]. Washington, DC: U.S. Department of Human Services.)

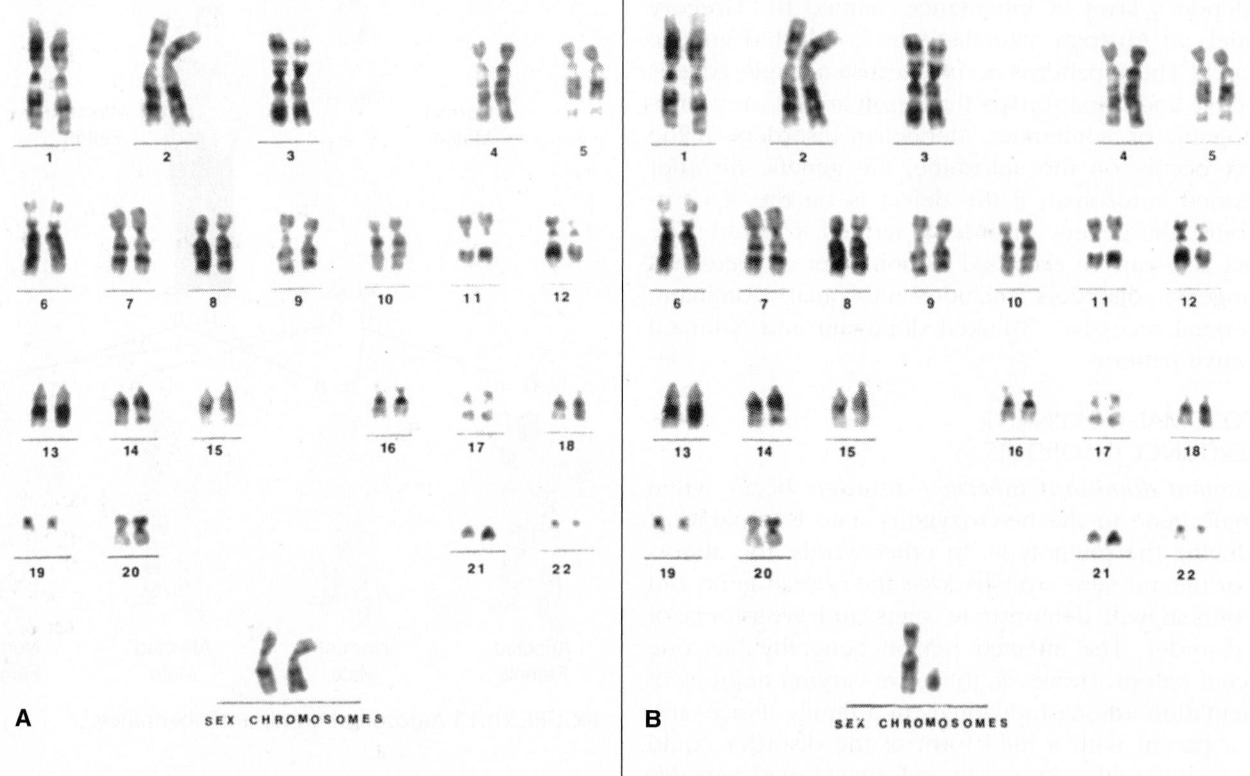

FIGURE 10.12 Karyotype pattern. **A.** Normal female karyotype. **B.** Normal male karyotype.

alleles differ, such as Ww, the dominant one will usually be expressed in the phenotype of the individual.

Human beings typically have 46 chromosomes. This includes 22 pairs of non-sex chromosomes or autosomes and 1 pair of sex chromosomes (two X chromosomes in females, and an X chromosome and a Y chromosome in males). Offspring receive one chromosome of each of the 23 pairs from each parent.

The pictorial analysis of the number, form, and size of an individual's chromosomes is termed the **karyotype**. This analysis commonly uses white blood cells and fetal cells in amniotic fluid. The chromosomes are numbered from the largest to the smallest, 1 to 22, and the sex chromosomes are designated by the letter X or Y. A female karyotype is designated as 46, XX and a male karyotype is designated as 46, XY. Figure 10.12 illustrates an example of a karyotyping pattern.

Regulation and expression of the thousands of human genes is very complex and is the result of many intricate interactions within each cell. Alterations in gene structure, function, transcription, translation, and protein synthesis can influence an individual's health (Jones & Lopez, 2014). Gene mutations are a permanent change in the sequence of DNA. Some mutations have no significant effect, whereas others can have a tremendous impact on the health of the individual. Several genetic disorders can result from these mutations, such as cystic fibrosis, sickle cell disease, phenylketonuria, or hemophilia.

Patterns of Inheritance for Genetic Disorders

Patterns of inheritance demonstrate how genetic abnormalities can be passed on to offspring. Although diagnosis of a genetic disorder is usually based on clinical signs and symptoms or on laboratory confirmation of an altered gene associated with the disorder, accurate diagnosis can be aided by the recognition of the pattern of inheritance within a family. In addition, nurses must understand the patterns of inheritance so they can teach and counsel families about the risks of genetic disorders occurring in future pregnancies. Some genetic disorders occur in multiple family members, while others may occur in only a single family member. A genetic disorder is caused by completely or partially altered genetic material, whereas a familial disorder is more common in relatives of the affected individual but may be caused by environmental influences and not genetic alterations. For a more detailed discussion of specific types of genetic disorders, see Chapter 49.

Mendelian or Monogenic Laws of Inheritance

Principles of inheritance of single-gene disorders are the same principles that govern the inheritance of other traits, such as eye and hair color. These are known as Mendel's laws of inheritance, named for Gregory Mendel, an Austrian naturalist who conducted genetic research. These patterns occur because a single gene is defective and the disorders that result are referred to as monogenic or, sometimes, Mendelian disorders. If the defect occurs on the autosome, the genetic disorder is termed autosomal; if the defect is on the X chromosome, the genetic disorder is termed X-linked. The defect also can be classified as dominant or recessive. Monogenic disorders include autosomal dominant, autosomal recessive, X-linked dominant and X-linked recessive patterns.

AUTOSOMAL DOMINANT INHERITANCE DISORDERS

Autosomal dominant inherited disorders occur when a single gene in the heterozygous state is capable of producing the phenotype. In other words, the abnormal or mutant gene overshadows the normal gene and the person will demonstrate signs and symptoms of the disorder. The affected person generally has one affected parent. However, there are varying degrees of presentation among individuals in a family. For example, a parent with a mild form of the disorder could have a child with a more severe form (termed *variable expression*). In some autosomal dominant disorders there may be no history of an affected family member. This can be due to the child representing a new mutation or the result of incomplete or reduced penetrance, which means that a person with the genetic mutation does not develop phenotypic features of the disorder. Incomplete or reduced penetrance may result from a combination of genetic, environmental, and lifestyle factors, age, and gender.

Offspring of an affected parent will have a 50% chance of inheriting two normal genes (disorder free) and a 50% chance of inheriting one normal and one abnormal gene (and, thus, the disorder) (Fig. 10.13) (NIH, 2013). Females and males are equally affected by autosomal dominant disorders and an affected male can pass the disorder on to his son (NIH, 2013). This male-to-male transmission is important in distinguishing autosomal dominant inheritance from X-linked inheritance. Common types of genetic disorders that follow the autosomal dominant pattern of inheritance include neurofibromatosis (genetic disorders affecting the development and growth of neural cells and tissues), Huntington's disease (a genetic disorder affecting the nervous system characterized by abnormal involuntary movements and progressive dementia), achondroplasia (a genetic disorder resulting in disordered growth and abnormal body proportion), and polycystic kidney disease (a genetic disorder involving the growth of multiple, bilateral, grapelike clusters of fluid-filled cysts in the kidneys that eventually compress and replace functioning renal tissue).

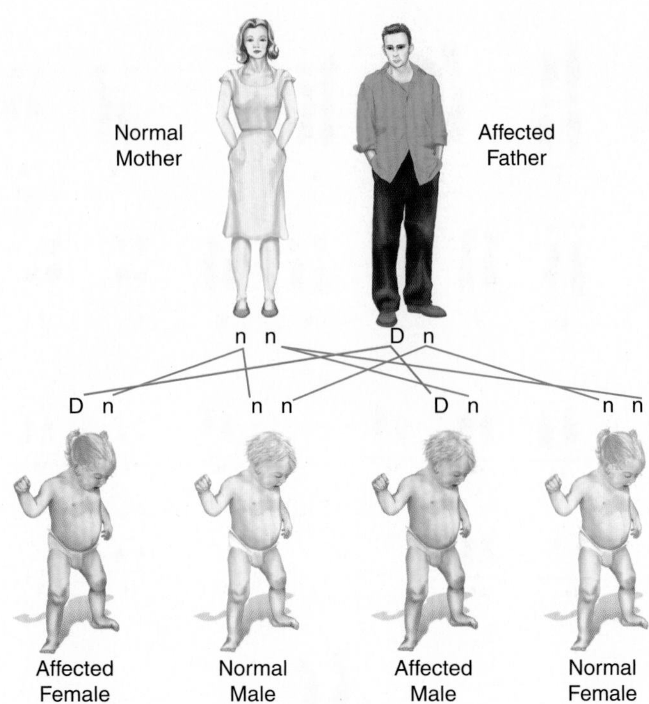

FIGURE 10.13 Autosomal dominant inheritance.

AUTOSOMAL RECESSIVE INHERITANCE DISORDERS

Autosomal recessive inherited disorders occur when two copies of the mutant or abnormal gene in the homozygous state are necessary to produce the phenotype. In other words, two abnormal genes are needed for the individual to demonstrate signs and symptoms of the disorder. Both parents of the affected person must be heterozygous carriers of the gene (clinically normal but carriers of the gene). Offspring of two carriers of the abnormal gene have a 25% chance of inheriting two normal genes; a 50% chance of inheriting one normal gene and one abnormal gene (carrier); and a 25% chance of inheriting two abnormal genes (and, thus, the disorder) (Fig. 10.14) (NIH, 2013). Affected people are usually present in only one generation of the family. Females and males are equally affected and a male can pass the disorder on to his son. The chance that any two parents will both be carriers of the mutant gene is increased if the couple has consanguinity (relationship by blood or common ancestry) (NIH, 2013). Common types of genetic disorders that follow the autosomal recessive inheritance pattern include cystic fibrosis (a genetic disorder involving generalized dysfunction of the exocrine glands), phenylketonuria (a disorder involving a deficiency in a liver enzyme that leads to the inability to process the essential amino acid phenylalanine), Tay–Sachs disease (a disorder due to insufficient activity of the enzyme hexosaminidase, which is necessary for the breakdown of certain fatty substances in the brain and nerve cells), and sickle cell disease (a genetic disorder in which the red blood cells

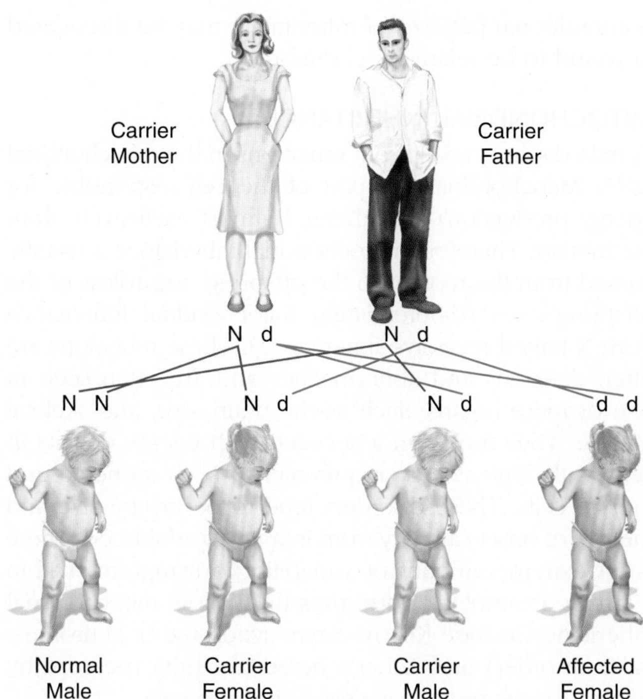

FIGURE 10.14 Autosomal recessive inheritance.

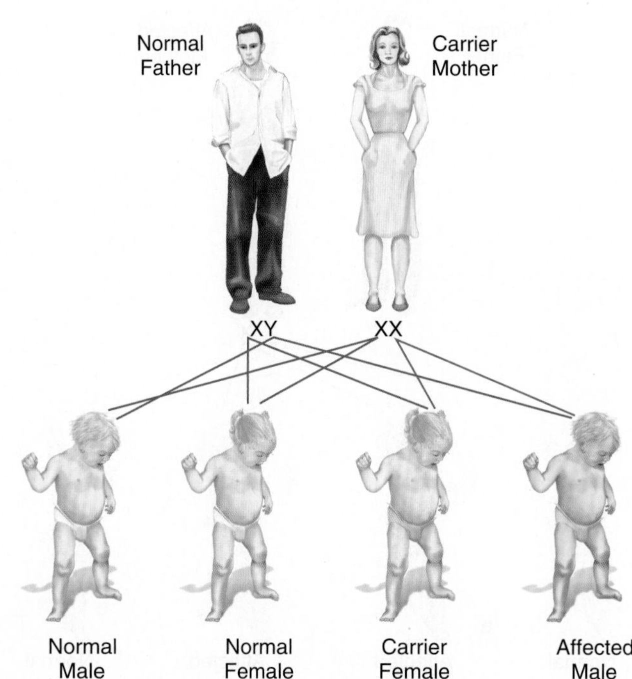

FIGURE 10.15 X-linked recessive inheritance.

carry an ineffective type of hemoglobin instead of the normal adult hemoglobin).

X-LINKED INHERITANCE DISORDERS

X-linked inherited disorders are those associated with altered genes present on the X chromosome. They differ from autosomal disorders. If a male inherits an X-linked altered gene, he will express the condition. This is because a male has only one X chromosome, therefore all the genes on his X chromosome will be expressed (the Y chromosome carries no normal allele to compensate for the altered gene). Because females inherit two X chromosomes, they can be either heterozygous or homozygous for any allele. Therefore, X-linked disorders in females are expressed similarly to autosomal disorders.

X-LINKED RECESSIVE INHERITANCE

Most X-linked disorders demonstrate a recessive pattern of inheritance (Snustad, 2015). There are more affected males than females because all the genes on a man's X chromosome will be expressed since a male has only one X chromosome (Snustad, 2015). On the other hand, a female will usually need two abnormal X chromosomes to exhibit the disease, and one normal and one abnormal X chromosome to be a carrier of the disease. There is no male-to-male transmission (since no X chromosome from the male is transmitted to male offspring), but any man who is affected with an X-linked recessive disorder will have carrier daughters. If a woman is a carrier, there is a 25% chance she will have an affected son, a 25% chance that her daughter will be a carrier, a 25% chance that she will have an unaffected son, and a 25% chance her daughter will be a noncarrier (Fig. 10.15) (Conley, 2014). Common types of genetic disorders that follow X-linked recessive inheritance patterns include hemophilia, color blindness, and Duchenne muscular dystrophy (NIH, 2013).

X-LINKED DOMINANT INHERITANCE

X-linked dominant inheritance occurs when a male has an abnormal X chromosome or a female has one abnormal X chromosome. All of the daughters and none of the sons of an affected male will inherit the condition, while both male and female offspring of an affected woman have a 50% chance of inheriting the condition (Fig. 10.16) (NIH, 2013). Males are more severely affected than females. Many X-linked dominant disorders have lethal results in males (Slavotinek & Ali, 2015). In females, even though the gene is dominant, having a second normal X gene offsets the effects of the dominant gene to some extent resulting in decreasing severity of the disorder. X-linked dominant disorders are rare; examples include hypophosphatemic (vitamin D–resistant) rickets and fragile X syndrome. Fragile X syndrome causes a range of developmental problems including learning disabilities and cognitive impairment (Van Esch, 2014). A characteristic of X-linked dominant inheritance is that fathers cannot pass X-linked traits to their sons (no male-to-male transmission) (GHR, 2015).

Multifactorial Inheritance Disorders

Many of the common congenital malformations, such as cleft lip, cleft palate, spina bifida, pyloric stenosis, clubfoot,

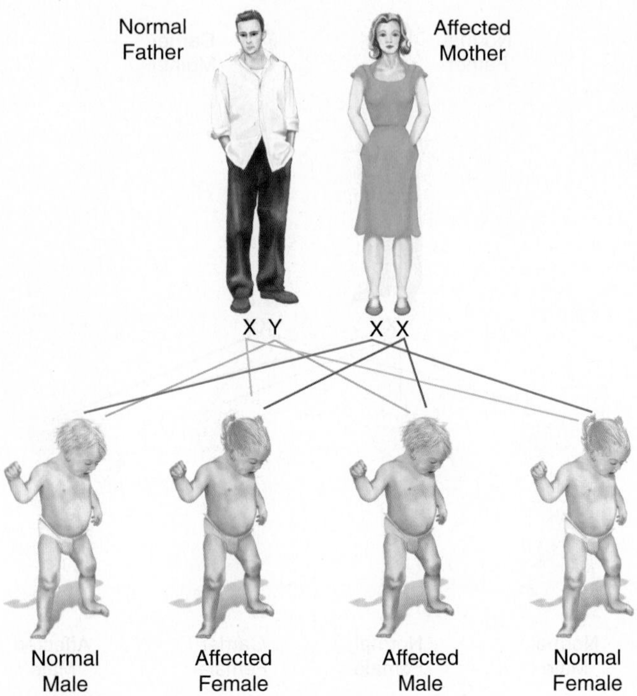

FIGURE 10.16 **X-linked dominant inheritance.**

congenital hip dysplasia, and cardiac defects, are attributed to multifactorial inheritance (Snustad, 2015). These conditions are thought to be caused by multiple gene and environmental factors. That is, a combination of genes from both parents, along with unknown environmental factors, produces the trait or condition. An individual may inherit a predisposition to a particular anomaly or disease. The anomalies or diseases vary in severity, and often a sex bias is present. For example, pyloric stenosis is seen more often in males, while congenital hip dysplasia is much more likely to occur in females. Multifactorial conditions tend to run in families, but the pattern of inheritance is not as predictable as with single-gene disorders. The chance of recurrence is also less than in single-gene disorders, but the degree of risk is related to the number of genes in common with the affected individual. The closer the degree of relationship, the more genes an individual has in common with the affected family member, resulting in a higher chance the individual's offspring will have a similar defect. In multifactorial inheritance the likelihood that both identical twins will be affected is not 100%, indicating that there are nongenetic factors involved.

Nontraditional Inheritance Patterns

Molecular studies have revealed that some genetic disorders are inherited in ways that do not follow the typical patterns of dominant, recessive, X-linked, or multifactorial inheritance. Examples of nontraditional inheritance patterns include mitochondrial inheritance and genomic imprinting. As the science of molecular genetics advances and more is learned about inheritance patterns, other nontraditional patterns of inheritance may be discovered or found to be relatively common.

MITOCHONDRIAL INHERITANCE

Certain diseases result from mutations in the mitochondrial DNA. Mitochondria (the part of the cell responsible for energy production) are inherited almost exclusively from the mother. Therefore, mitochondrial inheritance is usually passed from the mother to the offspring, regardless of the offspring's sex (differentiating mitochondrial inheritance from X-linked recessive inheritance). These mutations are often deletions and abnormalities and are often seen in one or more organs, such as the brain, eye, and skeletal muscle. They are often associated with energy deficits in cells with high energy requirements, such as nerve and muscle cells. These disorders tend to be progressive and the age of onset can vary from infancy to adulthood. There is an extreme amount of variability in symptoms within a family. Examples of disorders that follow mitochondrial inheritance include Kearns–Sayre syndrome (a neuromuscular disorder) and Leber's hereditary optic neuropathy (which causes progressive visual impairment).

GENOMIC IMPRINTING

Another nontraditional inheritance pattern results from a process called genomic imprinting. Genomic imprinting plays a critical role in fetal growth and development and placental functioning. It is a phenomenon by which the expression of a gene is determined by its parental origin. In genomic imprinting both the maternal and paternal alleles are present, but only one is expressed; the other is inactive. Genomic imprinting does not alter the genetic sequence itself, but affects the phenotype observed. In these cases, the altered genes in a certain region of the genome have very different expressions depending on whether they were inherited from the mother or the father. Several human syndromes are known to be associated with defects in gene imprinting. Disorders that result from a disruption of imprinting usually involve a growth phenotype and include varying degrees of developmental problems. Common examples include Prader–Willi syndrome (a condition resulting in severe hypotonia and hyperphagia, leading to obesity and intellectual disability), Angelman syndrome (a neurodevelopmental disorder associated with intellectual disability, jerky movements, and seizures), and Beckwith–Wiedemann syndrome (characterized by somatic overgrowth, congenital malformations, and a predisposition to embryonic neoplasia).

Chromosomal Abnormalities

In some cases of genetic disorders, the abnormality occurs due to problems with the chromosomes. Chromosomal abnormalities do not follow straightforward patterns of inheritance. Although some chromosomal disorders can be inherited, most others occur due to random events during the formation of reproductive cells or in early fetal development. Most chromosomal abnormalities occur due to an error in the egg or sperm. Therefore, the abnormality is present in every cell of the body. Some abnormalities can happen after fertilization, during mitotic cell division, and result in mosaicism. **Mosaicism** or the mosaic form is when the chromosomal abnormalities do not show up in every cell; only some cells or tissues carry the abnormality. In mosaic forms of the disorder the symptoms are usually less severe than if all the cells were abnormal.

Chromosomal abnormalities occur in about 1 in 150 live-born infants (March of Dimes, 2015). Congenital anomalies and intellectual disability are often associated with chromosomal abnormalities (Bacino & Lee, 2016). These abnormalities occur on autosomal or nonsex chromosomes as well as sex chromosomes and can result from abnormalities of either chromosome number or chromosome structure.

As mentioned, a karyotype is a pictorial analysis of chromosomes. It depicts a systematic arrangement of chromosomes of a single cell by pairs (see Fig. 10.12). Karyotyping is often used in prenatal testing to diagnose or predict genetic diseases.

Abnormalities of Chromosome Number

Chromosomal abnormalities of number often result due to nondisjunction (failure of separation of the chromosome pair during cell division, meiosis, or mitosis). Few chromosomal numerical abnormalities are compatible with full-term development and most result in spontaneous abortion (Snustad, 2015).

There are some numerical abnormalities that do support development to term because the chromosome on which the abnormality is present carries relatively few genes (such as chromosome 13, 18, 21, or X). Two common abnormalities of chromosome number are monosomy and trisomy. In **monosomy**, there is only one copy of a particular chromosome instead of the usual pair (an entire single chromosome is missing). In these cases, all fetuses spontaneously abort in early pregnancy. Survival is seen only in mosaic forms of these disorders. In **trisomy**, there are three of a particular chromosome instead of the usual two (an entire single chromosome is added). The most common trisomies include trisomy 21 (Down syndrome), trisomy 18, and trisomy 13. Figure 10.17 shows the karyotype of a child with Down syndrome. (See Chapter 49 for a detailed discussion of these disorders.) Trisomies may be present in every cell or may present in the mosaic form.

Abnormalities of Chromosome Structure

Abnormalities of chromosome structure usually occur when there is a breakage and loss of a portion of one or more chromosomes, and during the repair process the broken ends are rejoined incorrectly. Structural abnormalities usually lead to having too much or too little genetic material. Altered chromosome structure can take on several forms. Deletions occur when a portion of the chromosome is missing or deleted, resulting in a loss of that portion of the chromosome. Duplications are seen when a portion of the chromosome is duplicated and an extra chromosomal segment is present. Clinical findings vary depending on how much chromosomal material is involved. Inversions occur when a portion of the chromosome breaks off at two points and is turned upside down and reattached; therefore, the genetic material is inverted. With inversion, there is no loss or gain of chromosomal material and carriers are phenotypically normal, but they do have an increased risk for miscarriage and having chromosomally abnormal offspring (GHR, 2015). Ring chromosomes are seen when a portion of a chromosome has broken off in two places and formed a circle or ring. The most clinically significant structural abnormality is a translocation. This occurs when a portion of one chromosome is transferred to another chromosome and an abnormal rearrangement is present.

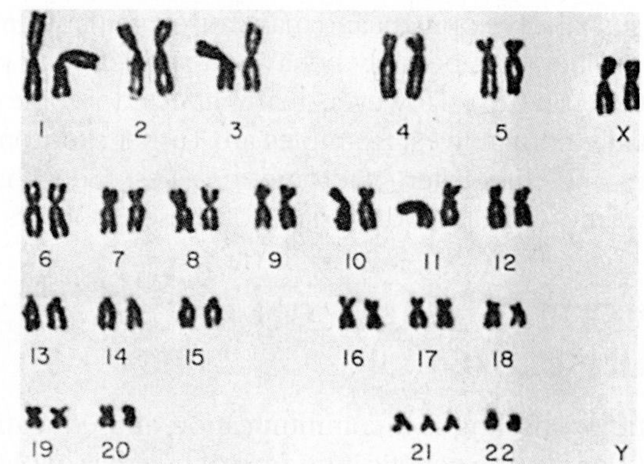

FIGURE 10.17 Karyotype of a child with Down syndrome.

Structural abnormalities can be balanced or unbalanced. Balanced abnormalities involve the rearrangement of genetic material with neither an overall gain nor loss. Individuals who inherit a balanced structural abnormality are usually phenotypically normal but are at a higher risk for miscarriages and having chromosomally abnormal offspring. Examples of structural rearrangements that can be balanced include inversions, translocation, and ring chromosomes. Unbalanced structural abnormalities are similar to numerical abnormalities because genetic material is either gained or lost. Unbalanced structural abnormalities can encompass several genes and result in severe clinical consequences.

Sex Chromosome Abnormalities

Chromosomal abnormalities can also involve sex chromosomes. These cases are usually less severe in their clinical effects than autosomal chromosomal abnormalities. Sex chromosome abnormalities are gender-specific and involve a missing or extra sex chromosome. They affect sexual development and may cause infertility, growth abnormalities, and possibly behavioral and learning problems (Chen, 2015). However, many affected people lead essentially normal lives. Examples are Turner syndrome in females and Klinefelter syndrome in males. (See Chapter 49 for a more detailed discussion of these disorders.)

GENETIC EVALUATION AND COUNSELING

Genetic counseling is a communication and educational process where the genetic influence of health is explained along with information regarding a specific genetic disorder, its transmission, inheritance, and options available in management and family planning (Nussbaum et al., 2016). There are a variety of reasons a person should be referred for genetic counseling (Box 10.2). In many cases, geneticists and genetic counselors provide information to families regarding genetic diseases. However, an experienced family physician, pediatrician, or nurse who has received special training in genetics may also provide the information. A genetic consultation involves evaluation of an individual or a family. Its purpose is to confirm, diagnose, or rule out genetic conditions; identify medical management issues; calculate and communicate genetic risks to a family; discuss ethical and legal issues; and assist in providing and arranging psychosocial support. Genetic counselors serve as educators and resource persons for other health care providers and the general public. Nurses have long been on the forefront of genetic counseling for their clients. The knowledge gained from the Human Genome Project is transforming the health care model, with implications for nurses in genetic counseling, practice and research (International Society of Nurses in Genetics [ISONG], 2014).

The ideal time for genetic counseling is before conception. Preconception counseling allows couples to identify and reduce potential pregnancy risks, plan for known risks, and establish early prenatal care. Unfortunately, many women delay seeking prenatal care until their second or third trimester, after the crucial time of organogenesis. Therefore, it is important that preconception counseling is offered to all women as they seek health care throughout their childbearing years, especially if they are contemplating pregnancy. This requires health care providers to take an active role. Consideration of genetics is rapidly becoming a part of routine health care, and all nurses need to be up to date and confident in their understanding of this topic.

BOX 10.2

THOSE WHO MAY BENEFIT FROM GENETIC COUNSELING

- Maternal age 35 years or older when the baby is born
- Paternal age 50 years or older
- Previous child, parents, or close relatives with an inherited disease, congenital anomalies, metabolic disorders, developmental disorders, or chromosomal abnormalities
- Consanguinity or incest
- Pregnancy screening abnormality, including alpha-fetoprotein, triple/quadruple screen, amniocentesis, or ultrasound
- Stillborn with congenital anomalies
- Two or more pregnancy losses
- Exposure to drugs, medications, radiation, chemicals, or infection
- Teratogen exposure or risk
- Concerns about genetic defects that occur frequently in their ethnic or racial group (e.g., those of African descent are most at risk for having a child with sickle cell anemia)
- Abnormal newborn screening
- Couples with a family history of X-linked disorders
- Carriers of autosomal recessive or dominant diseases
- Child born with one or more major malformations in a major organ system
- Child with abnormalities of growth
- Child with developmental delay, intellectual disability, blindness, or deafness

Adapted from March of Dimes. (2013). *Genetic counseling.* Retrieved from http://www.marchofdimes.org/pregnancy/genetic-counseling.aspx; National Human Genome Research Institute. (2015b). *Frequently asked questions about genetic counseling.* Retrieved from http://www.genome.gov/19016905; Lewis, R. (2015). *Human genetics: Concepts and applications* (11th ed.). New York: McGraw-Hill Companies, Incorporated.

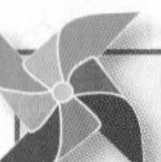

Consider This

As I waited for the genetic counselor to come into the room, my mind was filled with numerous fears and questions. What does an inconclusive amniocentesis really mean? What if this pregnancy produced an abnormal baby? How would I cope with a special child in my life? If only I had gone to the midwife sooner when I thought I was pregnant, but still in denial. Why did I wait so long to admit this pregnancy and get prenatal care? If only I had started to take my folic acid pills when prescribed. Why didn't I research my family's history to know of any hidden genetic conditions? What about my sister with a Down syndrome child? What must I have been thinking? I guess I could play the "what-if" game forever and never come up with answers. It was too late to do anything about this pregnancy because I was in my last trimester. I started to pray silently when the counselor opened the door....

Thoughts: This woman is reviewing the last several months, looking for answers to her greatest fears. Inconclusive screenings can introduce emotional torment for many women as they wait for validating results. Are these common thoughts and fears for many women facing potential genetic disorders? What supportive interventions might the nurse offer?

Preconception counseling plays a key role in preparing for a pregnancy. In couples with a history of recurrent early pregnancy loss, counseling is of particular importance because women are invariably more distressed and require reassurance to avoid future pregnancy losses. Several interventions ranging from genetic testing to lifestyle changes and medications may have a positive effect on the chances of a successful pregnancy. Early pregnancy monitoring and support increases the chance of a live birth and helps to predict potential future pregnancy complications. Recent research suggests that events that occur in the uterine decidua, even before a woman knows she is pregnant, may have a significant impact on fetal growth and the outcome of pregnancy. With this in mind, shifting future research and clinical practice to focus on the periconceptual period and the very early stages of pregnancy should offer significant benefits to the health of both the mother and her infant. The overall aim should be to effectively use every pregnancy as the health care opportunity of two lifetimes (Lopes, de Omena Bomfim, & Floria-Santos, 2015).

Preconception screening and counseling can raise serious ethical and moral issues for a couple. The results of prenatal genetic testing can lead to the decision to terminate a pregnancy, even if the results are not conclusive but indicate a strong possibility that the child will have an abnormality. The severity of the abnormality may not be known, and some may find the decision to terminate unethical. Another difficult situation that provides an example of the ethical and moral issues surrounding genetic screening and counseling involves disorders that affect only one gender of offspring. A mother may find she is a carrier of a gene for a disorder for which there is no prenatal screening test available. In these cases the couple may decide to terminate any pregnancy where the fetus is the affected sex, even though there is a 50% chance that the child will not inherit the disorder. In these situations, the choice is the couple's and information and support must be provided in a nondirective, nonjudgmental manner.

Genetic counseling is particularly important if a congenital anomaly or genetic disease has been diagnosed prenatally or when a child is born with a life-threatening congenital anomaly or genetic disease. In these cases families need information urgently so they can make immediate decisions. If a diagnosis with genetic implications is made later in life, if a couple with a family history of a genetic disorder or a previous child with a genetic disorder is planning a family, or if there is suspected teratogen exposure, urgency of information is not such an issue. In these situations, the family needs to take in all the information and explore their options. This may occur during several meetings over a longer period of time.

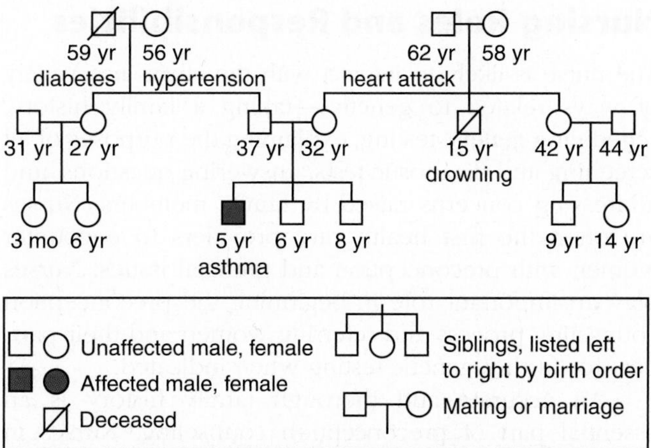

FIGURE 10.18 A pedigree is a diagram made using symbols that demonstrates the links between family members and focuses on medical and health information for each relative.

Genetic counseling involves extensive information gathering about birth history, past medical history, and current health status as well as a family history of congenital anomalies, mental retardation, genetic diseases, reproductive history, general health, and causes of death. A detailed family history is imperative and in most cases will include the development of a pedigree, which is like a family tree (Fig. 10.18). Information is ideally gathered on three generations, but if the family history is complicated, information from more distant relatives may be needed. Families receiving genetic counseling should be told that this information will be necessary so that they can discuss these sensitive issues with family members in advance. When necessary, medical records may be requested for family members, especially those who have a genetic disorder, to help ensure accuracy of the information. Sometimes the process of preparing a pedigree may reveal information that is not known by all family members, such as an adoption, a child conceived through in vitro fertilization, or a husband not being the father of a baby. Therefore, it is extremely important to take steps to maintain confidentiality. After careful analysis of the data obtained, referral to a genetic counselor when indicated is appropriate.

Medical genetic knowledge has increased dramatically over the past few decades. This has greatly expanded the role of the genetic counselor. It is possible not only to detect specific diseases with genetic mutations, but also to test for a genetic predisposition to various diseases or conditions and certain physical characteristics. This leads to complex ethical, moral, and social issues. Health care providers need to maintain privacy and confidentiality and administer care in a nondiscriminatory manner while maintaining sensitivity to cultural differences. It is essential to respect the individual's autonomy and present information in a nondirective manner.

Nursing Roles and Responsibilities

The nurse is likely to interact with the client in a variety of ways related to genetics—taking a family history, scheduling genetic testing, explaining the purposes of all screening and diagnostic tests, answering questions, and addressing concerns raised by family members. Nurses are often the first health care providers to encounter women with preconception and prenatal issues. Nurses play an important role in beginning the preconception counseling process and referring women and their partners for further genetic testing when indicated.

An accurate and thorough family history is an essential part of preconception counseling. Nurses in any practice setting can obtain a client's history during the initial encounter. The purpose is to gather client and family information that may provide clues as to whether the client has a genetic trait, inherited condition, or inherited predisposition (ISONG, 2014). At a basic level, all nurses should be able to take a family medical history to help identify those at risk for genetic conditions, and then initiate a referral when appropriate. (Box 10.3) presents examples of focused assessment questions that can be used. Based on the information gathered during the history, the nurse must decide whether a referral to a genetic specialist is necessary or whether further evaluation is needed. Families identified with genetic issues need unique clinical care including management of acute illnesses, screening for long-term complications, discussion of the etiology of the condition, connections to social supports, and clarification of the recurrence risks and prenatal testing and treatment options (ISONG, 2014). Prenatal testing to assess for genetic risks and defects might be used to identify genetic disorders. These tests are described in Common Laboratory and Diagnostic Tests 10.1.

BOX 10.3

FOCUSED HEALTH ASSESSMENT: GENETIC HISTORY

What was the cause and age of death for deceased family members?
Does any consanguinity exist between relatives?
Do any serious illnesses or chronic conditions exist? If so, what was the age of onset?
Do any female family members have a history of miscarriages, stillbirths, or diabetes?
Do any female members have a history of alcohol or drug use during pregnancy?
What were the ages of female members during childbearing, especially if older than 35?
Do any family members have mental retardation or developmental delays?
Do any family members have a known or suspected metabolic disorder such as PKU?
Do any family members have an affective disorder such as bipolar disorder?
Have any close relatives been diagnosed with any type of cancer?
What is your ethnic background (explore as related to certain disorders)?
Do any family members have a known or suspected chromosomal disorder?
Do any family members have a progressive neurologic disorder?

Sources: Edelman, C. L., Kudzma, E. C., & Mandle, C. L. (2014). *Health promotion throughout the lifespan* (8th ed.). St. Louis, MO: Mosby Elsevier; Nussbaum, R. L., McInnes, R. R., & Willard, H. F. (2016). *Thompson & Thompson genetics in medicine* (8th ed.), Philadelphia, PA: Elsevier; and Genetic Alliance. (n. d.). *Family health history.* Retrieved from http://www.geneticalliance.org/programs/genesinlife/fhh

Remember Robert and Kate Shafer? Based on the information gathered from their genetic history, they were referred to a genetic specialist. What prenatal tests might be ordered to assess their risk for genetic disorders? What would be the nurse's role related to genetic counseling?

Nurses working with families involved with genetic counseling typically have certain responsibilities. These include:

- Using interviewing and active listening skills to identify genetic concerns
- Knowing basic genetic terminology and inheritance patterns
- Explaining basic concepts of probability and disorder susceptibility
- Safeguarding the privacy and confidentiality of clients' genetic information
- Providing complete informed consent to facilitate decisions about genetic testing
- Discussing costs of genetic services and the benefits and risks of using health insurance to pay for genetic services, including potential risks of discrimination
- Recognizing and defining ethical, legal, and social issues
- Providing accurate information about the risks and benefits of genetic testing
- Providing culturally appropriate methods to convey genetic information
- Monitoring clients' emotional reactions after receiving genetic analysis
- Providing information on appropriate local support groups
- Knowing their own limitations and making appropriate referrals (Sermon & Viville, 2014)

Talking with families who have recently been diagnosed with a genetic disorder or who have had a child born with congenital anomalies is very difficult. Many times the nurse may be the one who has first

COMMON LABORATORY AND DIAGNOSTIC TESTS 10.1

PRENATAL TESTS TO ASSESS RISK FOR GENETIC DISORDERS

Test	Description	Indication	Timing
Alpha-fetoprotein	A sample of the woman's blood is drawn to evaluate plasma protein that is produced by the fetal liver, yolk sac, and GI tract, and crosses from the amniotic fluid into the maternal blood	Increased levels might indicate a neural tube defect, Turner syndrome, tetralogy of Fallot, multiple gestation, omphalocele gastroschisis, or hydrocephaly. Decreased levels might indicate Down syndrome or trisomy 18	Typically performed between 15 and 18 weeks' gestation
Amniocentesis	Amniotic fluid aspirated from the amniotic sac; safety concerns include infection, pregnancy loss, and fetal needle injuries	To perform chromosome analysis, alpha-fetoprotein, DNA markers, viral studies, karyotyping, and identify inborn errors of metabolism	Usually performed between 15 and 20 weeks' gestation to allow for adequate amniotic fluid volume to accumulate; results take 2–4 weeks
Chorionic villus sampling	Removal of small tissue specimen from the fetal portion of the placenta, which reflects the fetal genetic makeup; main complications include severe transverse limb defects and spontaneous pregnancy loss	To detect fetal karyotype, sickle cell anemia, phenylketonuria, Down syndrome, Duchenne muscular dystrophy, and numerous other genetic disorders	Typically performed between 10 and 12 weeks' gestation, with results available in less than 1 week
Percutaneous umbilical blood sampling	Insertion of a needle directly into a fetal umbilical vessel under ultrasound guidance; two potential complications: fetal hemorrhage and risk of infection	Used for prenatal diagnosis of inherited blood disorders such as hemophilia A, karyotyping, detection of fetal infection, determination of acid–base status, and assessment and treatment of isoimmunization	Generally performed after 16 weeks' gestation
Fetal nuchal translucency (FNT)	An intravaginal ultrasound that measures fluid collection in the subcutaneous space between the skin and the cervical spine of the fetus	To identify fetal anomalies; abnormal fluid collection can be associated with genetic disorders (trisomies 13, 18, and 21), Turner syndrome, cardiac deformities, and/or physical anomalies. When the FNT is greater than 2.5 mm, the measurement is considered abnormal	Performed between 10 and 14 weeks' gestation
Level II ultrasound/fetal scan	Use of high-frequency sound waves to visualize the fetus	Enables evaluation of structural changes to be identified early	Typically performed after 18 weeks' gestation
Triple and quad screening tests	Triple screening includes alpha-fetoprotein, estriol, and beta-hCG; quad screening includes alpha-fetoprotein, estriol, beat-hCG, and inhibin A	To identify risk for Down syndrome, neural tube defects, and other chromosomal disorders. Elevated hCG combined with lower-than-normal estriol and MSAFP levels indicate increased risk for Down syndrome or other trisomy condition.	Performed between 15 and 18 weeks' gestation
Preimplantation genetic diagnosis	Genetic testing of embryos produced through in vitro fertilization (IVF)	Identifies embryos carrying specific genetic alterations that can cause disease, and transfer those without genetic alterations into the woman's uterus to start a pregnancy; prevents inheritable genetic disease before implantation	Usually on day 3 after egg retrieval and 2 days after fertilization, a single blastomere is removed from the developing embryo to be evaluated
Cell-free fetal DNA (CffDNA)	A noninvasive prenatal test using maternal plasma which hold a mixture of maternal and fetal DNA after 4 weeks' gestation	Determines fetal sex in pregnancies at risk of sex-linked conditions; RhD genotyping in pregnancies at risk of hemolytic disease of the newborn and fetal chromosomal abnormalities such as Down syndrome.	A maternal blood sample is taken and next generation sequencing is used to analyze the cffDNA at approximately 10 weeks' gestation.

Sources: Latendresse, G., & Deneris, A. (2015). An update on current prenatal testing options: First trimester and noninvasive prenatal testing. *Journal of Midwifery & Women's Health*, 60(1), 24–36; Dayal, M. B. & Athanasiadia, I. (2013). *Preimplantation genetic diagnosis*. Retrieved from http://emedicine.medscape.com/article/273415-overview; Khalil, A., & Coates, A. (2015). Prenatal diagnosis of chromosomal abnormalities. In A. Bhide, S. Arulkumaran, K. R. Damania, & S. N. Daftary (Eds.), *Arias' practical guide to high-risk pregnancy and delivery: A South Asian perspective* (4th ed., pp. 1–13). New Delhi, India: Elsevier; Van Leeuwen, A. M., & Bladh, M. L. (2015). *Davis's comprehensive handbook of laboratory & diagnostic tests with nursing implications* (6th ed.). Philadelphia, PA: F. A. Davis Company..

contact with these parents and will be the one to provide follow-up care.

Genetic disorders are significant, life-changing, and possibly life-threatening situations. The information is highly technical and the field is undergoing significant technologic advances. Nurses need an understanding of who will benefit from genetic counseling and must be able to discuss the role of the genetic counselor with families. The nurse wants to ensure that families at risk are aware that genetic counseling is available before they attempt to have another baby.

Based on the results of their genetic tests, Robert and Kate are placed at moderate risk for having an infant with an autosomal recessive genetic disorder. The couple asks the nurse what all of this means. What information should the nurse provide about concepts of probability and disorder susceptibility for this couple? How can the nurse help this couple to make knowledgeable decisions concerning their reproductive future?

Nurses play an essential role in providing emotional support to the family through this challenging time. Genetics permeates all aspects of health care. Today, everyone is embracing quality and evidence-based care. Nurses who have an understanding of genetics and genomics will possess the foundation to provide quality, evidence-based care especially with follow-up counseling after the couple or family has been to the genetic specialist (Verklan & Walden, 2015).

Take Note!

Nurses need to be actively engaged with clients and their families and help them consider the facts, values, and context in which they are making decisions. Nurses need to be open and honest with families as they discuss these sensitive and emotionally laden choices.

The nurse is in an ideal position to help families review what has been discussed during the genetic counseling sessions and to answer any additional questions they might have. Referral to appropriate agencies, support groups, and resources, such as a social worker, a chaplain, or an ethicist, is another key role when caring for families with suspected or diagnosed genetic disorders. Couples need unique clinical care which includes screening for genetic disorders, discussion of the etiology of a potential condition, connections to social supports, and clarification of the recurrence risks and prenatal testing and treatment options. Nurses need to be involved in all aspects of this care.

KEY CONCEPTS

- Fertilization, which takes place in the outer third of the ampulla of the fallopian tube, leads to the formation of a zygote. The zygote undergoes cleavage, eventually implanting in the endometrium about 7 to 10 days after conception.
- Three embryonic layers of cells are formed and include the ectoderm, which forms the central nervous system, special senses, skin, and glands; the mesoderm, which forms the skeletal, urinary, circulatory, and reproductive systems; and the endoderm, which forms the respiratory system, liver, pancreas, and digestive system.
- Amniotic fluid surrounds the embryo and increases in volume as the pregnancy progresses, reaching approximately 1 L in volume by term.
- At no time during pregnancy is there any direct connection between the blood of the fetus and the blood of the mother, so there is no mixing of blood. A specialized connective tissue known as Wharton's jelly surrounds the three blood vessels in the umbilical cord to prevent compression, which would choke off the blood supply and nutrients to the growing life inside.
- The placenta protects the fetus from immune attack by the mother, removes waste products from the fetus, induces the mother to bring more food to the placenta and, near the time of birth, produces hormones that mature fetal organs in preparation for life outside the uterus.
- The purpose of fetal circulation is to carry highly oxygenated blood to vital areas (heart and brain) while first shunting it away from less vital ones (lungs and liver).
- Humans have 46 paired chromosomes that are found in all cells of the body, except the ovum and sperm cells, which have just 23 chromosomes. Each person has a unique genetic constitution, or genotype.
- Research from the Human Genome Project has provided a better understanding of the genetic contribution to disease.
- Genetic disorders can result from abnormalities in patterns of inheritance or chromosomal abnormalities involving chromosomal number or structure.
- Autosomal dominant inheritance occurs when a single gene in the heterozygous state is capable

of producing the phenotype. Autosomal recessive inheritance occurs when two copies of the mutant or abnormal gene in the homozygous state are necessary to produce the phenotype. X-linked inheritance disorders are those associated with altered genes present on the X chromosome. They can be dominant or recessive. Multifactorial inheritance is thought to be caused by multiple genetic and environmental factors.

- In some cases of genetic disorders, a chromosomal abnormality occurs. Chromosomal abnormalities do not follow straightforward patterns of inheritance. These abnormalities occur on autosomal as well as sex chromosomes and can result from changes in the number or structure of the chromosomes.
- Genetic counseling involves evaluation of an individual or a family. Its purpose is to confirm, diagnose, or rule out genetic conditions; identify medical management issues; calculate and communicate genetic risks to a family; discuss ethical and legal issues; and assist in providing and arranging psychosocial support.
- Legal, ethical, and social issues can arise related to genetic testing and may include the privacy and confidentiality of genetic information, who should have access to personal genetic information, psychological impact and stigmatization due to individual genetic differences, use of genetic information in reproductive decision making and reproductive rights, and whether testing should be performed if no cure is available.
- Preconception screening and counseling can raise serious ethical and moral issues for a couple. The results of prenatal genetic testing can lead to the decision to terminate a pregnancy.
- Nurses play an important role in beginning the preconception counseling process and referring women and their partners for further genetic information when indicated. Many times the nurse is the one who has first contact with these women and will be the one to provide follow-up care.
- Nurses need to have a solid understanding of who will benefit from genetic counseling and be able to discuss the role of the genetic counselor with families, ensuring that families at risk are aware that genetic counseling is available before they attempt to have another baby.
- Nurses play an essential role in providing emotional support and referrals to appropriate agencies, support groups, and resources when caring for families with suspected or diagnosed genetic disorders. Nurses can assist clients with their decision making by referring them to a social worker, chaplain, or ethicist.

REFERENCES AND RECOMMENDED READINGS

American Heart Association. (2015). *Fetal Circulation.* Retrieved from http://www.heart.org/HEARTORG/Conditions/CongenitalHeartDefects/SymptomsDiagnosisofCongenitalHeartDefects/Fetal-Circulation_UCM_315674_Article.jsp

Bacino, C. A., & Lee, B. (2016). Chapter 81: Cytogenetics. In R. M. Kleigman, B. F. Stanton, J. W. St. Geme III, & N. F. Schor (Eds.), *Nelson textbook of pediatrics* (20th ed., pp. 604–626). Philadelphia, PA: Elsevier.

Brazeau, G. (2015). Chapter 10: Pharmacogenomics/pharmacogenetics and interprofessional education and practice. In D. H. Lea, D. J. Cheek, D. Brazeau, & G. Brazeau (Eds.), *Mastering pharmacogenomics: A nurse's handbook for success* (pp. 191–204). Indianapolis, IN: Sigma Theta Tau International.

Burke, W., Tarini, B., Press, N., & Evans, J. (2011). Genetic screening. *Epidemiologic Reviews, 33,* 148–164.

Carcio, H. A., & Secor, M. C. (2010). *Advanced health assessment of women* (2nd ed.). New York, NY: Springer Publishing Company, Inc.

Centers for Disease Control and Prevention. (2015). *Birth defects.* Retrieved from http://www.cdc.gov/ncbddd/birthdefects/index.html

Chen, H. (2015). *Klinefelter syndrome.* Retrieved from http://emedicine.medscape.com/article/945649-overview

Conley, Y. P. (2014). Chapter 4: Genetics and health applications. In S. M. Nettina (Ed.), *Lippincott manual of nursing practice* (10th ed., pp. 33–44). Philadelphia, PA: Wolters Kluwer Health/Lippincott Williams & Wilkins.

Cunningham, J., Goldsmith, L., & Skirton, H. (2015). The evidence base regarding the experiences of and attitudes to preimplantation genetic diagnosis in prospective parents. *Midwifery, 31*(2), 288–296.

Cunningham, F. G., Leveno, K. J., Bloom, S. L., Spong, C. Y., Dashe, J. S., Hoffman, B. L., et al. (2014). *William's obstetrics* (24th ed.). New York, NY: McGraw Education.

Dayal, M. B., & Athanasiadia, I. (2013). *Preimplantation genetic diagnosis.* Retrieved from http://emedicine.medscape.com/article/273415-overview

Edelman, C. L., Kudzma, E. C., & Mandle, C. L. (2014). *Health promotion throughout the lifespan* (8th ed.). St. Louis, MO: Mosby Elsevier.

El-Mazny, A. (2014). *Human reproduction: Basic anatomy and physiology.* Charleston, SC: Amazon CreateSpace Publishers.

Finnemore, A., & Groves, A. (2015). Physiology of the fetal and transitional circulation. *Seminars in Fetal and Neonatal Medicine, 20*(4), 210–216.

Freemark, M. (2015). Placental hormones and the control of fetal growth. *International Journal of Pediatric Endocrinology, 2015* (Suppl 1), O13.

Genetic Alliance. (n. d.). *Family health history.* Retrieved from http://www.geneticalliance.org/programs/genesinlife/fhh

International Society of Nurses in Genetics. (2014). *What is a genetics nurse?* Retrieved from http://www.isong.org/ISONG_genetic_nurse.php

Jones, R. E., & Lopez, K. H. (2014). *Human reproductive biology* (4th ed.). Waltham, MA: Elsevier Health Sciences.

Khalil, A., & Coates, A. (2015). Prenatal diagnosis of chromosomal abnormalities. In A. Bhide, S. Arulkumaran, K. R.

Damania, & S. N. Daftary (Eds.), *Arias' practical guide to high-risk pregnancy and delivery: A South Asian perspective* (4th ed., pp. 1–13). New Delhi, India: Elsevier.

King, T. L., Brucker, M. C., Kriebs, J. M., Fahey, J. O., Gegor, C. L., & Varney, H. (2015). *Varney's midwifery*. (5th ed.). Burlington, MA: Jones & Bartlett Learning.

Kumar, S., Kingsley, C., & DiStefano, J. K. (2015). The Human Genome Project: Where are we now and where are we going? In R. Dugurala, L. Almasy, S. Williams-Blangero, S. F. D. Paul, & C. Kole (Eds.), *Genome mapping and genomics in human and non-human primates* (pp. 7–31). New York, NY: Springer-Verlag Berlin Heidelberg.

Latendresse, G., & Deneris, A. (2015). An update on current prenatal testing options: First trimester and noninvasive prenatal testing. *Journal of Midwifery & Women's Health, 60*(1), 24–36.

Lawford, A., & Tulloh, R. M. (2015). Cardiovascular adaptation to extra uterine life. *Pediatrics and Child Health, 25*(1), 1–6.

Lea, D., Skirton, H., Read, C. Y., & Williams, J. K. (2011). Implications for educating the next generation of nurses on genetics and genomics in the 21st century. *Journal of Nursing Scholarship, 43*(1), 3–12.

Lee, B. (2011). Chapter 72: Integration of genetics into pediatric practice. In R. M. Kliegman Lee, B, B. F. Stanton, J. W. St. Geme, N. F. Schor, & R. E. Behrman, (Eds.), (*Nelson's textbook of pediatrics* (19th ed., p. 376–380). Philadelphia, PA: Saunders.

Lewis, R. (2015). *Human genetics: Concepts and applications* (11th ed.). New York, NY: McGraw-Hill Companies, Incorporated.

Lichtenbelt, K. D., Diemel, B. D., Koster, M. P., Manten, G. T., Siljee, J., Schuring-Blom, G. H., et al. (2015). Detection of fetal chromosomal anomalies: Does nuchal translucency measurement have added value in the era of non-invasive prenatal testing? *Prenatal Diagnosis, 35*, 663–668.

Lopes, L. C., de Omena Bomfim, E., & Flória-Santos, M. (2015). Genomics-based health care: Implications for nursing. *International Journal of Nursing Didactics, 5*(02), 11–15.

Mader, S., & Windelspecht, M. (2015). *Human biology* (14th ed.). New York, NY: McGraw-Hill Higher Education.

Magann, E., & Ross, M. G. (2014). *Assessment of amniotic fluid volume*. Retrieved from http://www.uptodate.com/contents/assessment-of-amniotic-fluid-volume

March of Dimes. (2013). *Genetic counseling*. Retrieved from http://www.marchofdimes.org/pregnancy/genetic-counseling.aspx

March of Dimes. (2015). *Understanding basic biological processes*. Retrieved from http://www.marchofdimes.org/research/understanding-basic-biological-processes.aspx

Mattson, S., & Smith, J. E. (2015). *Core curriculum for maternal-newborn nursing*. (5th ed.). St. Louis, MO: Saunders Elsevier.

Meyer zu Schwabedissen, H. E. (2015). The role of pharmacogenomics in individualized medicine. In T. Fischer, M. Langanke, P. Marschall, & S. Michl (Eds.), *Individualized medicine: Ethical, economical, and historical perspectives* (pp. 93–112). New York, NY: Springer International Publishing.

Moore, T. R. (2015). Abnormal amniotic fluid. In J. T. Queenan, C. Y. Spong, & C. J. Lockwood (Eds.), *Protocols for high-risk pregnancies: An evidence-based approach* (6th ed., pp. 315–328). West Sussex, UK: Wiley Blackwell Publishers.

National Human Genome Research Institute. (2015a). *All about the Human Genome Project (HGP)*. Retrieved from http://www.genome.gov/10001772

National Human Genome Research Institute. (2015b). *Frequently asked questions about genetic counseling*. Retrieved from http://www.genome.gov/19016905

National Human Genome Research Institute. (2015c). *Frequently asked questions about genetic testing*. Retrieved from http://www.genome.gov/19516567

National Institutes of Health. (2013). *Genetic testing: How it is used for healthcare*. Retrieved from http://www.report.nih.gov/NIHfactsheets/ViewFactSheet.aspx?csid=43&key=G

National Institutes of Health. (2016). *Genetics home reference: Guide to understanding genetic conditions*. Retrieved from https://ghr.nlm.nih.gov/

Nussbaum, R. L., McInnes, R. R., & Willard, H. F. (2016). *Thompson & Thompson genetics in medicine* (8th ed.). Philadelphia, PA: Elsevier.

Scott, D. A. & Lee, B. (2011). Chapter 80: Patterns of Genetic Transmission. In R. M. Kliegman, B. F. Stanton, J. W. St. Geme, & N. F. Schor (Eds.), *Nelson's textbook of pediatrics* (20th ed., pp. 593–603). Philadelphia, PA: Elsevier.

Sermon, K., & Viville, S. (2014). *Textbook of human reproductive genetics*. New York, NY: Cambridge University Press.

Seven, M., Akyüz, A., Elbüken, B., Skirton, H., & Öztürk, H. (2015). Nurses' knowledge and educational needs regarding genetics. *Nurse Education Today, 35*(3), 444–449.

Slavotinek, A., & Ali, M. (2015). Recognizable syndromes in the newborn period. *Clinics in Perinatology, 42*(2), 263–280.

Snustad, D. P. (2015). *Principles of genetics* (7th ed.). New York, NY: Wiley Publishers.

Solomon, E. P. (2015). *Introduction to human anatomy and physiology* (4th ed.). Philadelphia, PA: Elsevier Health Sciences.

Travers, A. & Muskhelishvili, G. (2015). DNA structure and function. *FEBS Journal, 282*, 2279–2295.

U.S. Department of Energy Genome Programs. (2014). *Human Genome Project information archive*. Retrieved from http://www.ornl.gov/sci/techresources/Human_Genome/home.shtml

U.S. Department of Energy Genome Programs. (2015). *Human Genome Project information: Gene testing*. Retrieved from http://doegenomestolife.org/program/index.shtml

Van Esch, H. (2014). *Fragile X syndrome: Clinical features and diagnosis in children and adolescents*. Retrieved from http://www.uptodate.com/contents/fragile-x-syndrome-clinical-features-and-diagnosis-in-children-and-adolescents

Van Leeuwen, A. M., & Bladh, M. L. (2015). *Davis's comprehensive handbook of laboratory & diagnostic tests with nursing implications* (6th ed.). Philadelphia, PA: F. A. Davis Company.

Verklan, M. T., & Walden, M. (2015). *Core curriculum for neonatal intensive care nursing* (4th ed.). St. Louis, MO: Saunders Elsevier.

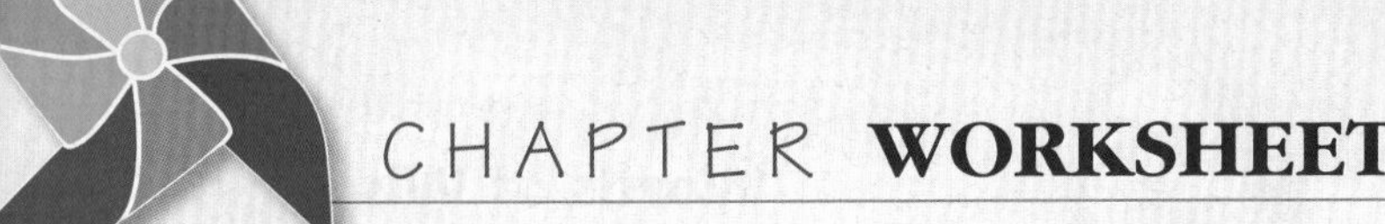

CHAPTER WORKSHEET

MULTIPLE-CHOICE QUESTIONS

1. After teaching a group of students about fertilization, the instructor determines that the teaching was successful when the group identifies which as the usual site of fertilization?
   a. Fundus of the uterus
   b. Endometrium of the uterus
   c. Distal portion of fallopian tube
   d. Follicular tissue of the ovary
2. A client comes to the clinic for pregnancy testing. The nurse explains that the test detects the presence of which hormone?
   a. Human placental lactogen (hPL)
   b. Human chorionic gonadotropin (hCG)
   c. Follicle stimulating hormone (FSH)
   d. Thyroid stimulating hormone (TSH)
3. The nurse is counseling a couple, one of whom is affected by an autosomal dominant disorder. They express concerns about the risk of transmitting the disorder. What is the best response by the nurse regarding the risk that their baby may have for the disease?
   a. "You have a one in four (25%) chance."
   b. "The risk is 12.5%, or a one in eight chance."
   c. "The chance is 100%."
   d. "Your risk is 50%, or a one in two chance."
4. What is the first step in determining a couple's risk for a genetic disorder?
   a. Observing the client and family over time
   b. Conducting extensive psychological testing
   c. Obtaining a thorough family health history
   d. Completing an extensive exclusionary list
5. A nurse is working in a women's health clinic. Which woman would genetic counseling be most appropriate for?
   a. Had her first miscarriage at 10 weeks
   b. Is 30 years old and planning to conceive
   c. Has a history with a close relative with Down syndrome
   d. Is 18 weeks pregnant with a normal triple screen result
6. Which of the following is an example of an autosomal dominant disorder?
   a. Phenylketonuria
   b. Tay–Sachs disease
   c. Polycystic kidney disease
   d. Cystic fibrosis
7. Which of the following is the major goal of genetic counseling?
   a. Diagnose and determine the role of heredity
   b. Reinforce previously presented test data
   c. Emphasize good communication skills
   d. Offer referral to community support groups

CRITICAL THINKING EXERCISE

1. Mr. and Mrs. Martin wish to start a family, but they can't agree on something important. Mr. Martin wants his wife to be tested for cystic fibrosis (CF) to see if she is a carrier. Mr. Martin had a brother with CF and watched his parents struggle with the hardship and the expense of caring for him for years, and he doesn't want to experience it in his own life. Mr. Martin has found out he is a CF carrier. Mrs. Martin doesn't want to have the test because she figures that once a baby is in their arms, they will be glad, no matter what.
   a. What information/education should this couple consider before deciding whether to have the test?
   b. How can you assist this couple in their decision-making process?
   c. What is your role in this situation if you don't agree with their decision?

STUDY ACTIVITIES

1. Obtain the video *Miracle of Life,* which shows conception and fetal development. What are your impressions? Is the title of this video realistic?
2. Select one of the websites listed in thePoint to explore the topic of genetics. Critique the information presented. Was it understandable to a layperson? What specifically did you learn? Share your findings with your classmates during a discussion group.
3. Draw your own family pedigree, identifying inheritance patterns. Share it with your family to validate its accuracy. What did you discover about your family's past health?
4. Select one of the various prenatal screening tests (alpha-fetoprotein, amniocentesis, chorionic villus sampling, or fetal nuchal translucency) and research it in depth. Role-play with another nursing student how you would explain its purpose, the procedure, and potential findings to an expectant couple at risk for a fetal abnormality.

BRINGING IT ALL TOGETHER: A CASE STUDY

Rebecca and Jon are a couple seeking genetic counseling. Rebecca, 43 years old, is 10 weeks pregnant with their first baby. The couple is concerned about the possibility of their child demonstrating trisomy 21 (Down syndrome).

Go to thePoint to find questions to consider about this case.

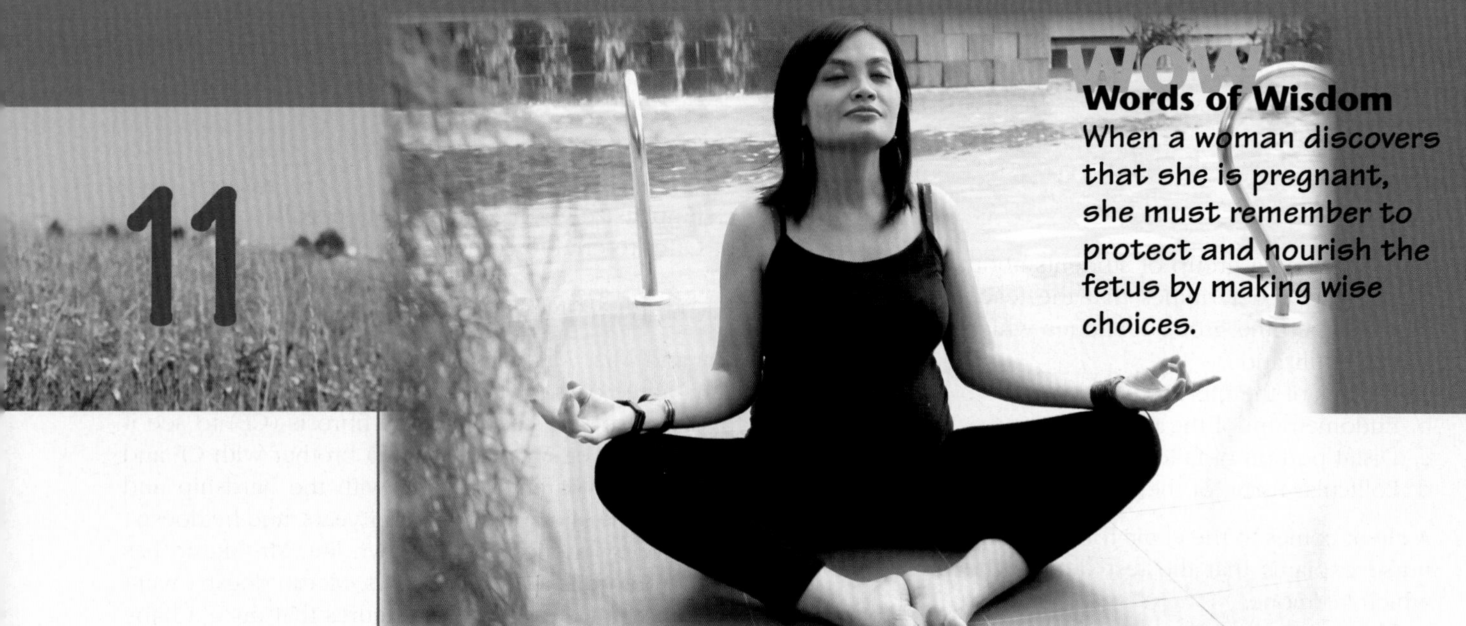
WOW
Words of Wisdom
When a woman discovers that she is pregnant, she must remember to protect and nourish the fetus by making wise choices.

11 Maternal Adaptation During Pregnancy

KEY TERMS

ballottement
Braxton Hicks contractions
Chadwick's sign
dietary reference intakes (DRIs)
Goodell's sign
Hegar's sign
linea nigra
physiologic anemia of pregnancy
pica
quickening
trimester

Learning Objectives

Upon completion of the chapter, you will be able to:

1. Differentiate between subjective (presumptive), objective (probable), and diagnostic (positive) signs of pregnancy.
2. Describe maternal physiologic changes that occur during pregnancy.
3. Summarize the nutritional needs of the pregnant woman and her fetus.
4. Characterize the emotional and psychological changes that occur during pregnancy.

***Marva*, age 17, appeared at the health department clinic complaining that she had a stomach virus and needed to be seen right away. When the nurse asked her additional questions about her illness, Marva reported that she had been sick to her stomach and "beat tired" for days. She had stopped eating to avoid any more nausea and vomiting.**

INTRODUCTION

Pregnancy is a normal life event that involves considerable physical and psychological adjustments for the mother. A pregnancy is divided into three trimesters of 13 weeks each (Edelman, Kudzma, & Mandle, 2014). Within each **trimester**, numerous adaptations take place that facilitate the growth of the fetus. The most obvious are physical changes to accommodate the growing fetus, but pregnant women also undergo psychological changes as they prepare for parenthood. A thorough understanding of these numerous changes and adaptations is essential for all nurses caring for women during pregnancy.

SIGNS AND SYMPTOMS OF PREGNANCY

Traditionally, signs and symptoms of pregnancy have been grouped into the following categories: presumptive, probable, and positive (Box 11.1). The only signs that can determine a pregnancy with 100% accuracy are positive signs.

What additional information is necessary to complete the assessment of Marva, the 17-year-old with nausea and vomiting? What diagnostic tests might be done to confirm the nurse's suspicion that she is pregnant?

Subjective (Presumptive) Signs

Presumptive signs are those signs that the mother can perceive. The most obvious presumptive sign of pregnancy is the absence of menstruation. Skipping a period is not a reliable sign of pregnancy by itself, but if it is accompanied by consistent nausea, fatigue, breast tenderness, and urinary frequency, pregnancy would seem very likely.

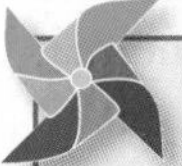

Consider This

Jim and I decided to start our family, so I stopped taking the pill 3 months ago. One morning when I got out of bed to take the dog out, I felt queasy and light-headed. I sure hoped I wasn't coming down with the flu. By the end of the week, I was feeling really tired and started taking naps in the afternoon. In addition, I seemed to be going to the bathroom frequently, despite not drinking much fluid. When my breasts started to tingle and ache, I decided to make an appointment with my doctor to see what "illness" I had contracted.

After listening to my list of physical complaints, the office nurse asked me if I might be pregnant. My eyes opened wide: I had somehow missed the link between my symptoms and pregnancy. I started to think about when my last period was, and it had been 2 months ago. The office ran a pregnancy test and much to my surprise it was positive!

Thoughts: Many women stop contraceptives in an attempt to achieve pregnancy but miss the early signs of pregnancy. This woman was experiencing several signs of early pregnancy—urinary frequency, fatigue, morning nausea, and breast tenderness. What advice can the nurse give this woman to ease these symptoms? What additional education related to her pregnancy would be appropriate at this time?

BOX 11.1

SIGNS AND SYMPTOMS OF PREGNANCY

Presumptive (Time of Occurrence)	Probable (Time of Occurrence)	Positive (Time of Occurrence)
Fatigue (12 wks)	Braxton Hicks contractions (16–28 wks)	Ultrasound verification of embryo or fetus (4–6 wks)
Breast tenderness (3–4 wks)	Positive pregnancy test (4–12 wks)	Fetal movement felt by experienced clinician (20 wks)
Nausea and vomiting (4–14 wks)	Abdominal enlargement (14 wks)	Auscultation of fetal heart tones via Doppler (10–12 wks)
Amenorrhea (4 wks)	Ballottement (16–28 wks)	
Urinary frequency (6–12 wks)	Goodell's sign (5 wks)	
Hyperpigmentation of the skin (16 wks)	Chadwick's sign (6–8 wks)	
Fetal movements (quickening; 16–20 wks)	Hegar's sign (6–12 wks)	
Uterine enlargement (7–12 wks)		
Breast enlargement (6 wks)		

Adapted from Bope, E. T., & Kellerman, R. D. (2015). *Conn's current therapy 2015*. Philadelphia, PA: Saunders Elsevier; Shields, A. D. (2015). Pregnancy diagnosis. *eMedicine*. Retrieved from http://emedicine.medscape.com/article/262591-overview; Jordan, R.G., Engstrom, J., Matrfell, J., & Farley, C. L. (2014). *Prenatal and postnatal care: A woman-centered approach*. Ames, IA: Wiley-Blackwell.

Presumptive changes are the least reliable indicators of pregnancy because any one of them can be caused by conditions other than pregnancy (Shields, 2015). For example, amenorrhea can be caused by early menopause, endocrine dysfunction, malnutrition, anemia, diabetes mellitus, long-distance running, cancer, or stress. Nausea and vomiting can be caused by gastrointestinal disorders, food poisoning, acute infections, or eating disorders. Fatigue could be caused by anemia, stress, or viral infections. Breast tenderness may result from chronic cystic mastitis, premenstrual changes, or the use of oral contraceptives. Urinary frequency could have a variety of causes other than pregnancy, such as infection, cystocele, structural disorders, pelvic tumors, or emotional tension (Tharpe, Farley, & Jordan, 2016).

Objective (Probable) Signs

Physical Signs

Probable signs of pregnancy are those that can be detected on physical examination by a health care provider. Common probable signs of pregnancy include softening of the lower uterine segment or isthmus (**Hegar's sign**), softening of the cervix (**Goodell's sign**), and a bluish-purple coloration of the vaginal mucosa and cervix (**Chadwick's sign**). Other probable signs include changes in the shape and size of the uterus, abdominal enlargement, Braxton Hicks contractions, and **ballottement** (the examiner pushes against the woman's cervix during a pelvic examination and feels a rebound from the floating fetus).

Pregnancy Tests

Along with these physical signs, pregnancy tests are also considered a probable sign of pregnancy. In-home pregnancy testing became available in the United States in late 1977. In-home testing appealed to the general public because of convenience, cost, and confidentiality. Several pregnancy tests are available (Table 11.1). The tests vary in sensitivity, specificity, and accuracy and are influenced by the length of gestation, specimen concentration, presence of blood, and the presence of some drugs. Human chorionic gonadotropin (hCG) is detectable in the serum of approximately 5% of clients 8 days after conception and in more than 98% of clients by day 11 (Shields, 2015). At least 25 different home pregnancy tests are currently marketed in the United States. Most of these tests claim "99% accuracy" according to a U.S. Food and Drug Administration (FDA) guideline or make other similar statements on the packaging or product insert. The 99% accuracy statement in reference to the FDA guideline is misleading in that it has no bearing on the ability of the home pregnancy test to detect early pregnancy (Shields, 2015). The limitations of these tests must be understood so that pregnancy detection is not delayed significantly. Early pregnancy detection allows for the commencement of prenatal care, potential medication changes, and lifestyle changes to promote a healthy pregnancy.

Human chorionic gonadotropin (hCG) is a glycoprotein and the earliest biochemical marker for pregnancy. Many pregnancy tests are based on the recognition of hCG or a beta subunit of hCG. hCG levels in normal pregnancy usually double every 48 to 72 hours until they peak approximately 60 to 70 days after fertilization. At this point, they decrease to a plateau at 100 to 130 days of pregnancy. The hCG doubling time has been used as a marker by clinicians to differentiate normal from abnormal gestations. Low levels are associated with an

TABLE 11.1 SELECTED PREGNANCY TESTS

Type	Specimen	Example	Remarks
Agglutination inhibition tests	Urine	Pregnosticon, Gravindex	If hCG is present in urine, agglutination does not occur, which is positive for pregnancy; reliable 14–21 days after conception; 95% accurate in diagnosing pregnancy
Immunoradiometric assay	Blood serum	Neocept, Pregnosis	Measures ability of blood sample to inhibit the binding of radiolabeled hCG to receptors; reliable 6–8 days after conception; 99% accurate in diagnosing pregnancy
Enzyme-linked immunosorbent assay (ELISA)	Blood serum or urine	Over-the-counter home/office pregnancy tests; precise	Uses an enzyme to bond with hCG in the urine if present; reliable 4 days after implantation; 99% accurate if hCG specific

Adapted from Jordan, R. G., Engstrom, J., Matrfell, J., & Farley, C. L. (2014). *Prenatal and postnatal care: A woman-centered approach*. Ames, IA: Wiley-Blackwell; King, T. L., Brucker, M. C., Kriebs, J. M., Fahey, J. O., Gegor, C. L., & Varney, H. (2015). *Varney's midwifery* (5th ed.). Burlington, MA: Jones & Bartlett Learning; Shields, A. D. (2015). Pregnancy diagnosis. *eMedicine.* Retrieved from http://emedicine.medscape.com/article/262591-overview

ectopic pregnancy and higher-than-normal levels may indicate a molar pregnancy or multiple-gestational pregnancies (Zinaman, Johnson, & Marriott, 2015).

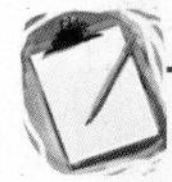

Take Note!

This elevation of hCG corresponds to the morning sickness period of approximately 6 to 12 weeks during early pregnancy.

Although probable signs suggest pregnancy and are more reliable than presumptive signs, they still are not 100% reliable in confirming a pregnancy. For example, uterine tumors, polyps, infection, and pelvic congestion can cause changes to uterine shape, size, and consistency. And although pregnancy tests are used to establish the diagnosis of pregnancy when the physical signs are still inconclusive, they are not completely reliable, because conditions other than pregnancy (e.g., ovarian cancer, choriocarcinoma, hydatidiform mole) can also elevate hCG levels.

Positive Signs

Usually within 2 weeks after a missed period, enough subjective symptoms are present so that a woman can be reasonably sure she is pregnant. However, an experienced health care provider can confirm her suspicions by identifying positive signs of pregnancy that can be directly attributed to the fetus. The positive signs of pregnancy confirm that a fetus is growing in the uterus. Visualizing the fetus by ultrasound, palpating for fetal movements, and hearing a fetal heartbeat are all signs that make the pregnancy a certainty.

If the pregnancy test is positive, the clinical visit should include an estimation of gestational age so that appropriate counseling can be provided. In addition, clients should receive information about the normal signs and symptoms of early pregnancy, and should be instructed to report any concerns to the health care provider for further evaluation. Once pregnancy has been confirmed, the health care provider will set up a schedule of prenatal visits to assess the woman and her fetus throughout the entire pregnancy. Assessment and education begins at the first visits and continues throughout the pregnancy (see Chapter 12).

Remember Marva, who thought she had a stomach virus? Her pregnancy test was positive. On questioning by the nurse, she acknowledged missing two menstrual periods and being sexually active with her boyfriend without using protection. What is the nurse's role at this point with Marva? What instructions might be given to her while she waits for her first prenatal visit?

PHYSIOLOGIC ADAPTATIONS DURING PREGNANCY

Every system of a woman's body changes during pregnancy to accommodate the needs of the growing fetus, and these changes occur with startling rapidity. The physical changes of pregnancy can be uncomfortable, although every woman reacts uniquely.

Reproductive System Adaptations

Significant changes occur throughout the woman's body during pregnancy to accommodate the growing human being within her. Many have a protective role for maternal homeostasis and are essential to meet the demands of both the mother and the fetus. Many adaptations are reversible after the woman gives birth, but some persist for life.

Uterus

The uterus grows at a steady, predictable rate during pregnancy. During the first few months of pregnancy, estrogen stimulates uterine growth, and the uterus undergoes a tremendous increase in size, weight, length, width, depth, volume, and overall capacity throughout pregnancy. The weight of the uterus increases from 70 g to about 1,100 to 1,200 g at term; its capacity increases from 10 to 5,000 mL or more at term (King et al., 2015). The uterine walls thin to 1.5 cm or less; the shape changes from pear shape to a solid globe in the first trimester, and then expands to become a hollow vessel.

Uterine growth occurs as a result of both hyperplasia and hypertrophy of the myometrial cells, which do not increase much in number but do increase in size. In early pregnancy, uterine growth is due to hyperplasia of uterine smooth muscle cells within the myometrium; however, the major component of myometrial growth occurs after mid-gestation due to smooth muscle cell hypertrophy caused by mechanical stretch of uterine tissue by the growing fetus (Osol & Moore, 2014). Blood vessels elongate, enlarge, dilate, and sprout new branches to support and nourish the growing muscle tissue, and the increase in uterine weight is accompanied by a large increase in uterine blood flow, which is necessary to perfuse the uterine muscle and accommodate the growing fetus. As pregnancy progresses, 80% to 90% of uterine blood flow goes to the placenta, with the remainder distributed between the endometrium and myometrium. During pregnancy, the diameter of the main uterine artery approximately doubles in size. This enlargement from a narrow to a larger-caliber vessel enhances the capacity of the uteroplacental vessels to accommodate the increased blood volume needed to supply the placenta (Osol & Moore, 2014).

Uterine contractility is enhanced as well. Spontaneous, irregular, and painless contractions, called **Braxton Hicks contractions**, begin during the first trimester. These contractions continue throughout pregnancy, becoming especially noticeable during the last month, when they function to thin out or efface the cervix before birth (see Chapter 12 for more information).

The lower portion of the uterus (the isthmus) does not undergo hypertrophy and becomes increasingly thinner as pregnancy progresses, thereby forming the lower uterine segment. Changes in the lower uterus occurring during the first 6 to 8 weeks of gestation produce some of the typical findings, including a positive Hegar's sign. This softening and compressibility of the lower uterine segment results in exaggerated uterine anteflexion during the early months of pregnancy, which adds to urinary frequency (Heffner & Schust, 2014).

The uterus remains in the pelvic cavity for the first 3 months of pregnancy, after which it progressively ascends into the abdomen (Fig. 11.1). As the uterus grows, it presses on the urinary bladder and causes the increased frequency of urination experienced during early pregnancy. In addition, the heavy gravid uterus in the last trimester can fall back against the inferior vena cava in the supine position, resulting in

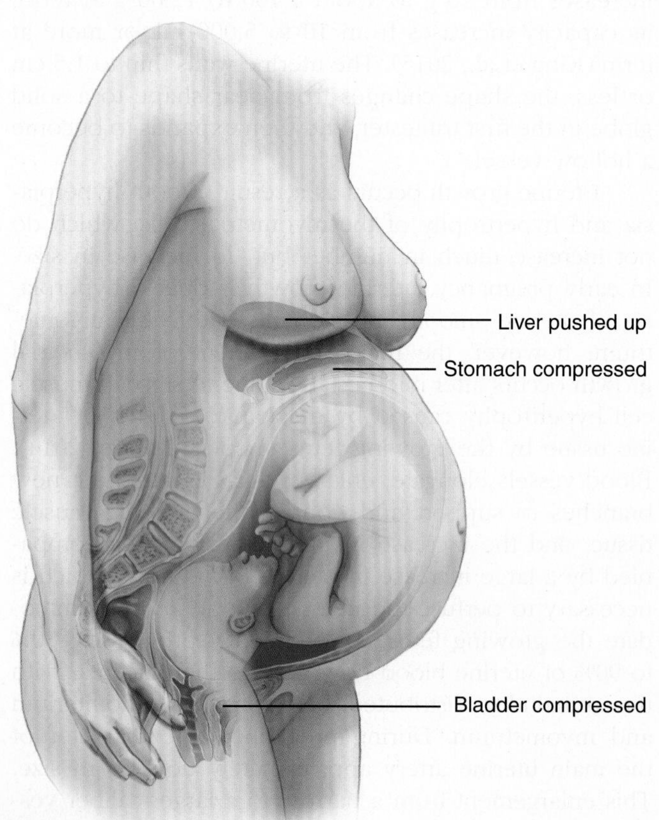

FIGURE 11.1 The growing uterus in the abdomen.

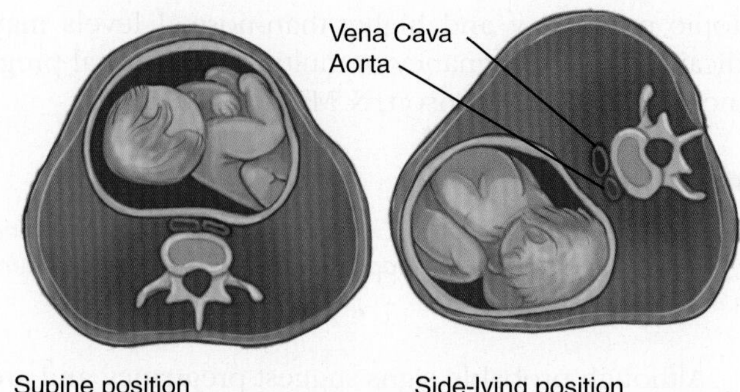

FIGURE 11.2 Supine hypotensive syndrome.

vena cava compression, which reduces venous return and decreases cardiac output and blood pressure, with increasing orthostatic stress. This occurs when the woman changes her position from recumbent to sitting to standing. This acute hemodynamic change, termed supine hypotensive syndrome, causes the woman to experience symptoms of weakness, light-headedness, nausea, dizziness, or syncope (Fig. 11.2). These changes are reversed when the woman is in the side-lying position, which displaces the uterus to the left and off the vena cava.

The uterus, which starts as a pear-shaped organ, becomes ovoid as length increases over width. By 20 weeks' gestation, the fundus, or top of the uterus, is at the level of the umbilicus and measures 20 cm. A monthly measurement of the height of the top of the uterus in centimeters, which corresponds to the number of gestational weeks, is commonly used to date the pregnancy.

> **Take Note!**
>
> Fundal height usually can be correlated with gestational weeks most accurately between 18 and 32 weeks. Obesity, hydramnios, and uterine fibroids interfere with the accuracy of this correlation.

The fundus reaches its highest level, at the xiphoid process, at approximately 36 weeks. Between 38 and 40 weeks, fundal height drops as the fetus begins to descend and engage into the pelvis. Because it pushes against the diaphragm, many women experience shortness of breath. By 40 weeks, the fetal head begins to descend and engage in the pelvis, which is termed *lightening*. For the woman who is pregnant for the first time, lightening usually occurs approximately 2 weeks before the onset of labor; for the woman who is experiencing her second or subsequent pregnancy, it usually occurs at the onset of labor. Although breathing becomes easier because of this descent, the pressure on the urinary bladder now increases and the woman now experiences urinary frequency again, as she did in the first trimester of pregnancy.

Cervix

Between weeks 6 and 8 of pregnancy, the cervix begins to soften (Goodell's sign) due to vasocongestion and the influence of estrogen. Along with the softening, the endocervical glands increase in size and number and produce more cervical mucus. Under the influence of progesterone, a thick mucus plug is formed that blocks the cervical os and protects the opening from bacterial invasion. At about the same time, increased vascularization of the cervix causes Chadwick's sign, a cyanosis or bluish purple discoloration Cervical ripening (softening, effacement, and increased distensibility) begins about 4 weeks before birth. The connective tissues of the cervix undergo biochemical modifications in preparation for labor that result in changes to its elasticity and strength. These changes are mediated through several factors, including inflammation, cervical stretch, pressure of the fetal presenting part, and release of hormones, including oxytocin, relaxin, nitric oxide, and prostaglandins (Myers et al., 2015).

Vagina

During pregnancy, vascularity increases because of the influences of estrogen, resulting in pelvic congestion and hypertrophy of the vagina in preparation for the distention needed for birth. The vaginal mucosa thickens, the connective tissue begins to loosen, the smooth muscle begins to hypertrophy, and the vaginal vault begins to lengthen (Bope & Kellerman, 2015). Vaginal secretions become more acidic, white, and thick. Most women experience an increase in a whitish vaginal discharge, called leukorrhea, during pregnancy. This is normal except when it is accompanied by itching and irritation, possibly suggesting *Candida albicans,* a monilial vaginitis, which is a very common occurrence in this glycogen-rich environment (King et al., 2015). Symptomatic vulvovaginal candidiasis affects 15% of pregnant women (Krapf, 2015). It is a benign fungal condition that is uncomfortable for the woman and can be transmitted from an infected mother to her newborn at birth. Neonates develop an oral infection known as thrush, which presents as white patches on the mucous membranes of their mouths. It is self-limiting and is treated with local antifungal agents.

Ovaries

The increased blood supply to the ovaries causes them to enlarge until approximately the 12th to 14th week of gestation. The ovaries are not palpable after that time because the uterus fills the pelvic cavity. Ovulation ceases during pregnancy because of the elevated levels of estrogen and progesterone, which block secretion of follicle-stimulating hormone (FSH) and luteinizing hormone (LH) from the anterior pituitary. The ovaries are very active in hormone production to support the pregnancy until about weeks 6 to 7, when the corpus luteum regresses and the placenta takes over the major production of progesterone.

Breasts

The breasts increase in fullness, become tender, and grow larger throughout pregnancy under the influence of estrogen and progesterone. The breasts become highly vascular, and veins become visible under the skin. The nipples become larger and more erect. Both the nipples and the areola become deeply pigmented, and tubercles of Montgomery (sebaceous glands) become prominent. These sebaceous glands keep the nipples lubricated for breast-feeding.

Changes that occur in the connective tissue of the breasts, along with the tremendous growth, lead to striae (stretch marks) in approximately half of all pregnant women (Jordan et al., 2014). Initially they appear as pink to purple lines on the skin, but they eventually fade to a silver color. Although they become less conspicuous in time, they never completely disappear.

Creamy, yellowish breast fluid called colostrum can be expressed by the third trimester. This fluid provides nourishment for the breast-feeding newborn during the first few days of life (see Chapters 15 and 16 for more information). Table 11.2 summarizes reproductive system adaptations.

General Body System Adaptations

In addition to changes in the reproductive system, the pregnant woman also experiences changes in virtually every other body system in response to the growing fetus.

Gastrointestinal System

The gastrointestinal system begins in the oral cavity and ends at the rectum. During pregnancy, the gums become hyperemic, swollen, and friable and tend to bleed easily. This change is influenced by estrogen and increased proliferation of blood vessels and circulation to the mouth. In addition, the saliva produced in the mouth becomes more acidic. Some women complain about excessive salivation, termed *ptyalism,* which may be caused by the decrease in unconscious swallowing by the woman when nauseated. Ptyalism typically resolves spontaneously, although in some women it endures throughout the pregnancy. Some women get temporary relief from gum chewing or sucking on hard candies (King et al., 2015). Dental plaque, calculus, and debris deposits increase during pregnancy and are all associated with gingivitis. An increased production of

TABLE 11.2 SUMMARY OF REPRODUCTIVE SYSTEM ADAPTATIONS

Reproductive Organ	Adaptations
Uterus	Size increases to 20 times that of nonpregnant size Capacity increases by 2,000 times to accommodate the developing fetus Weight increases from 2 oz to approximately 2 lb at term Uterine growth occurs as a result of both hyperplasia and hypertrophy of the myometrial cells Increased strength and elasticity allow uterus to contract and expel fetus during birth
Cervix	Increases in mass, water content, and vascularization Changes from a relatively rigid to a soft, distensible structure that allows the fetus to be expelled Under the influence of progesterone, a thick mucus plug is formed, which blocks the cervical os and protects the developing fetus from bacterial invasion
Vagina	Increased vascularity because of estrogen influences, resulting in pelvic congestion and hypertrophy Increased thickness of mucosa, along with an increase in vaginal secretions to prevent bacterial infections
Ovaries	Increased blood supply to the ovaries causes them to enlarge until approximately the 12th to 14th week of gestation. They actively produce hormones to support the pregnancy until weeks 6 to 7 when the placenta takes over the production of progesterone.
Breasts	Breast changes begin soon after conception; they increase in size and areolar pigmentation The tubercles of Montgomery enlarge and become more prominent, and the nipples become more erect The blood vessels become more prominent, and blood flow to the breast doubles

female hormones during pregnancy contributes to the development of gingivitis and periodontitis because vascular permeability and possible tissue edema are both increased. It is reported that as many as 50% to 70% of pregnant women will have some level of gingivitis during pregnancy as a result of hormonal changes that promote inflammation (Anil et al., 2015). Previous studies linked periodontal disease with preterm birth, preeclampsia, low–birth-weight risk, stillbirth, and early-onset neonatal sepsis, but more recent research findings indicated no reduction in preterm births with the treatment of periodontal disease during pregnancy (Trivedi, Lal, & Singhal, 2015).

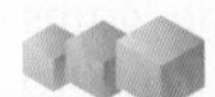

Concept Mastery Alert

Gum Fragility in Pregnancy

Bleeding of gums during pregnancy results from increased estrogen levels that cause blood vessel proliferation. This then leads to increased blood vessels in the gums and an increased chance of bleeding.

Smooth muscle relaxation and decreased peristalsis occur related to the influence of progesterone. Elevated progesterone levels cause smooth muscle relaxation, which results in delayed gastric emptying and decreased peristalsis. Transition time of food throughout the gastrointestinal tract may be so much slower that more water than normal is reabsorbed, leading to bloating and constipation. Constipation can also result from low-fiber food choices, reduced fluid intake, use of iron supplements, decreased activity level, and intestinal displacement secondary to a growing uterus. Constipation, increased venous pressure, and the pressure of the gravid uterus contribute to the formation of hemorrhoids.

The slowed gastric emptying combined with relaxation of the cardiac sphincter allows reflux, which causes heartburn. Acid indigestion or heartburn (pyrosis) seems to be a universal problem for pregnant women. It is caused by regurgitation of the stomach contents into the upper esophagus and may be associated with the generalized relaxation of the entire digestive system. Over-the-counter antacids will usually relieve the symptoms, but they should be taken with the health care provider's knowledge and only as directed.

The emptying time of the gallbladder is prolonged secondary to the smooth muscle relaxation from progesterone. Hypercholesterolemia can follow, increasing the risk of gallstone formation. Other risk factors for gallbladder disease include obesity, Hispanic ethnicity, and increasing maternal age (Heuman, Mihas, & Allen, 2015).

Nausea and vomiting, better known as morning sickness, plague about 80% of pregnant women. This condition is usually self-limiting, but the symptoms can be distressing and interfere with work, social activities, and interrupt sleep. Recently, the FDA approved doxylamine succinate 10 mg/pyridoxine hydrochloride 10 mg (Diclegis) as the first medication to specifically treat morning sickness in pregnancy (Pope, Maltepe, & Koren, 2015). Although it occurs most often in the morning, the nauseated feeling can last all day in some women. The highest incidence of morning sickness occurs between 6 and 12 weeks. The physiologic basis for morning sickness is still debatable. It has been linked to the high levels of hCG, high levels of circulating estrogens, prostaglandins, reduced stomach acidity, advancing maternal age, slowed peristalsis, genetic factors, and the lowered tone and motility of the digestive tract (King et al., 2015).

Cardiovascular System

Cardiovascular changes occur early during pregnancy to meet the demands of the enlarging uterus and the placenta for more blood and more oxygen. The changes include an increase in heart rate (25%); cardiac output increases by 30% to 50% and peaks at 25 to 30 weeks' gestation; reduced total peripheral resistance; increased blood volume; increased plasma volume which leads to physiologic anemia. Perhaps the most striking cardiac alteration occurring during pregnancy is the increase in blood volume.

BLOOD VOLUME

Blood volume increases by approximately 1,500 mL, or up to 50% above nonpregnant levels, by the 32nd week of gestation, and remains more or less constant thereafter (Foo et al., 2015). The increase is made up of 1,000 mL plasma plus 450 mL red blood cells. It begins at weeks 10 to 12, peaks at weeks 32 to 34, and decreases slightly by week 40.

Take Note!

The rise in blood volume correlates directly with fetal weight, supporting the concept of the placenta as an arteriovenous shunt in the maternal vascular compartment.

This increase in blood volume is needed to provide adequate hydration of fetal and maternal tissues, to supply blood flow to perfuse the enlarging uterus, and to provide a reserve to compensate for blood loss at birth and during postpartum. The maternal blood volume expansion occurs at a larger proportion than the increase in red blood cell mass, which results in physiologic anemia and hemodilution. Criteria of physiologic anemia include hemoglobin 10 g or less, red blood cells 3.5 million/mm^3, and normal morphology with central pallor (Sabina et al., 2015). This increase is also necessary to meet the increased metabolic needs of the mother and to meet the need for increased perfusion of other organs, especially the woman's kidneys, because she is excreting waste products for herself and the fetus.

CARDIAC OUTPUT AND HEART RATE

Cardiac output, the product of stroke volume and heart rate, is a measure of the functional capacity of the heart. It increases from 30% to 50% over the nonpregnant rate by the 32nd week of pregnancy and declines to about a 20% increase at 40 weeks' gestation. The increase in cardiac output is associated with an increase in venous return and greater right ventricular output, especially in the left lateral position (Bope & Kellerman, 2015). Heart rate increases by 10 to 15 bpm between 14 and 20 weeks of gestation, and this persists to term. There is slight hypertrophy or enlargement of the heart during pregnancy. This is probably to accommodate the increase in blood volume and cardiac output. The heart works harder and pumps more blood to supply the oxygen needs of the fetus as well as those of the mother. Both heart rate and venous return are increased in pregnancy, contributing to the increase in cardiac output seen throughout gestation. A woman with preexisting heart disease may become symptomatic and begin to decompensate during the time the blood volume peaks. Close monitoring is warranted during 28 to 35 weeks' gestation.

BLOOD PRESSURE

Blood pressure, especially the diastolic pressure, declines slightly during pregnancy as a result of peripheral vasodilation caused by progesterone. It usually reaches a low point at midpregnancy and thereafter increases to prepregnancy levels until term. During the first trimester, blood pressure typically remains at the prepregnancy level. During the second trimester, the blood pressure decreases 5 to 10 mmHg and thereafter returns to first-trimester levels (Gaillard & Jaddoe, 2015). Any significant rise in blood pressure during pregnancy should be investigated to rule out gestational hypertension. Gestational hypertension is a clinical diagnosis defined by the new onset of hypertension (systolic of 140 mmHg or higher and/or diastolic of 90 mmHg or higher) after 20 weeks' gestation.

BLOOD COMPONENTS

The number of red blood cells also increases throughout pregnancy to a level 25% to 33% higher than nonpregnant values, depending on the amount of iron available. This increase is necessary to transport the additional oxygen required during pregnancy. Although there is an increase in red blood cells, there is a greater increase in the plasma volume as a result of hormonal factors and sodium and water retention. Because the plasma increase exceeds the increase of red blood cell production, normal hemoglobin and hematocrit values decrease. This state of hemodilution is referred to as **physiologic anemia of pregnancy**. Changes in red blood cell volume are due to increased circulating erythropoietin and accelerated red blood cell production. The rise in erythropoietin in the last two trimesters is stimulated by progesterone, prolactin, and human placental lactogen (Jones & Lopez, 2014).

Iron requirements during pregnancy increase because of the demands of the growing fetus and the increase in maternal blood volume. The fetal tissues prevail over the mother's tissues with respect to use of iron stores. With the accelerated production of red blood cells, iron is necessary for hemoglobin formation, the oxygen-carrying component of red blood cells.

Take Note!

Many women enter pregnancy with insufficient iron stores and thus need supplementation to meet the extra demands of pregnancy.

Both fibrin and plasma fibrinogen levels increase, along with various blood-clotting factors. These factors make pregnancy a hypercoagulable state. These changes, coupled with venous stasis secondary to venous pooling, which occurs during late pregnancy after long periods of standing in the upright position with the pressure exerted by the uterus on the large pelvic veins, contribute to slowed venous return, pooling, and dependent edema. These factors also increase the woman's risk for venous thrombosis (DeLoughery, 2015).

Respiratory System

The growing uterus and the increased production of the hormone progesterone cause the lungs to function differently during pregnancy. Oxygen consumption reflects the uptick of maternal metabolism by increasing between 20% and 30% by the time full term is reached. During pregnancy, the amount of space available to house the lungs decreases as the uterus puts pressure on the diaphragm and causes it to shift upward by 4 cm above its usual position. The growing uterus does change the size and shape of the thoracic cavity, but diaphragmatic excursion increases, chest circumference increases by 2 to 3 inches, and the transverse diameter increases by an inch, allowing a larger tidal volume, as evidenced by deeper breathing (tidal volume, or the volume of air inhaled, increases by 30% to 40% (from 500 to 700 mL) as the pregnancy progresses. This increase results in maternal hyperventilation and hypocapnia. As a result of these changes, the woman's breathing becomes more diaphragmatic than abdominal. Concomitant with the increase in tidal volume is a 30% to 40% increase in maternal oxygen consumption due to the increased oxygen requirements of the developing fetus, placenta, and maternal organs.

Anatomic and physiologic changes of pregnancy predispose the mother to increased morbidity and mortality and increase the risks of a less than optimal outcome for the fetus. The frequency and significance of acute and chronic respiratory conditions in pregnant women have increased in recent years. Because of these various changes, pregnant women with asthma, pneumonia, or other respiratory pathology are more susceptible to early decompensation (Mehta et al., 2015).

A pregnant woman breathes faster and more deeply because she and the fetus need more oxygen. Oxygen consumption increases during pregnancy even as airway resistance and lung compliance remain unchanged. Changes in the structures of the respiratory system take place to prepare the body for the enlarging uterus and increased lung volume (Alexander et al., 2014). As muscles and cartilage in the thoracic region relax, the chest broadens, with a conversion from abdominal breathing to thoracic breathing. This leads to a 50% increase in air volume per minute. All of these structural alterations are temporary and revert back to their prepregnant state at the end of the pregnancy.

Increased vascularity of the respiratory tract is influenced by increased estrogen levels, leading to congestion. Rising levels of sex hormones and heightened sensitivity to allergens may influence the nasal mucosa, precipitating epistaxis (nosebleed) and rhinitis. This congestion gives rise to nasal and sinus stuffiness and changes in the tone and quality of the woman's voice (Jordan et al., 2014).

Renal/Urinary System

Hormonal changes during pregnancy allow for increased blood flow to the kidneys. The renal system must handle the effects of increased maternal intravascular and extracellular volume and metabolic waste products as well as excretion of fetal wastes. The predominant structural change in the renal system during pregnancy is dilation of the renal pelvis and uterus. Changes in renal structure occur as a result of the hormonal influences of estrogen and progesterone, pressure from an enlarging uterus, and an increase in maternal blood volume. Like the heart, the kidneys work harder throughout the pregnancy. Changes in kidney function occur to accommodate a heavier workload while maintaining a stable electrolyte balance and blood pressure. As more blood flows to the kidneys, the glomerular filtration rate (GFR) increases, leading to an increase in urine flow and volume, substances delivered to the kidneys, and filtration and excretion of urea, uric acid, creatinine, water and solutes (Cox & Reid, 2015).

Anatomically, the kidneys enlarge during pregnancy. Each kidney increases in length by approximately 1 to 1.5 cm and weight as a result of hormonal effects that cause increased tone and decreased motility of the smooth muscle. The renal pelvis becomes dilated. The ureters (especially the right ureter) elongate, widen, and become more curved above the pelvic rim as early as the 10th gestational week (Thadhani & Maynard, 2015). Progesterone is thought to cause both of these changes because of its relaxing influence on smooth muscle.

Blood flow to the kidneys increases by 50% to 80% as a result of the increase in cardiac output and relaxin, which causes a decrease in both efferent and afferent resistance. This in turn leads to an increase in the GFR by as much as 40% to 60% starting during the second trimester, resulting in hyperfiltration. This elevation continues until birth. This change has important clinical implications for medication use because renally excreted drugs may require higher doses and more frequent administration for therapeutic blood levels during pregnancy (Larson, 2015).

The activity of the kidneys normally increases when a person lies down and decreases on standing. This difference is amplified during pregnancy, which is one reason a pregnant woman feels the need to urinate frequently while trying to sleep. Late in the pregnancy, the increase in kidney activity is even greater when the woman lies on her side rather than her back. Lying on either side relieves the pressure that the enlarged uterus puts on the vena cava carrying blood from the legs. Subsequently, venous return to the heart increases, leading to increased cardiac output. Increased cardiac output results in increased renal perfusion and glomerular filtration. As a rule, all the physiologic changes maximize by the end of the second trimester and then start to return to the prepregnant level. However, changes in the anatomy take up to 3 months postpartum to subside (King et al., 2015).

Musculoskeletal System

Changes in the musculoskeletal system are progressive, resulting from the influence of hormones, fetal growth, and maternal weight gain. Pregnancy is characterized by changes in posture and gait. By the 10th to 12th week of pregnancy, the ligaments that hold the sacroiliac joints and the pubis symphysis in place begin to soften and stretch, and the articulations between the joints widen and become more movable (Bope & Kellerman, 2015). The relaxation of the joints peaks by the beginning of the third trimester. The purpose of these changes is to increase the size of the pelvic cavity and to make delivery easier.

The postural changes of pregnancy—an increased swayback and an upper spine extension to compensate for the enlarging abdomen—coupled with the loosening of the sacroiliac joints may result in lower back pain. The woman's center of gravity shifts forward, requiring a realignment of the spinal curvatures. Factors thought to contribute to these postural changes include the alteration to the center of gravity that come with pregnancy, the influence of the pregnancy-related hormone relaxin on the pelvic joints, and the increasing weight and position of the growing fetus.

An increase in the normal lumbosacral curve (lordosis) occurs and a compensatory curvature in the cervicodorsal area develops to assist her in maintaining her balance (Fig. 11.3). In addition, relaxation and increased mobility of joints occur because of the hormones progesterone and relaxin, which lead to the characteristic "waddle" gait that pregnant women demonstrate toward term. Increased weight gain can add to this discomfort by accentuating the lumbar and dorsal curves (Kouhkan et al., 2015).

Integumentary System

There are a variety of skin changes that are associated with pregnancy. Increased activity of the maternal

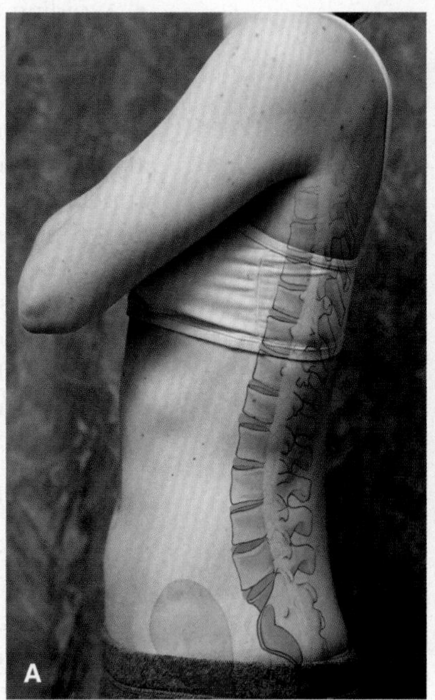

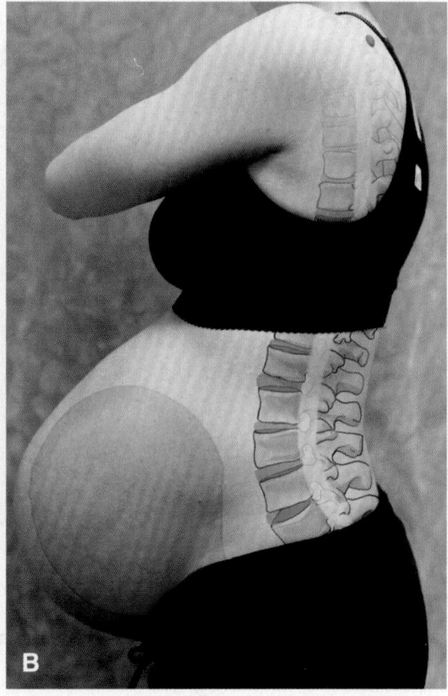

FIGURE 11.3 Postural changes during (**A**) the first trimester and (**B**) the third trimester.

adrenal and pituitary glands, along with a contribution for the developing fetal endocrine glands, increasing cortisone levels, accelerated metabolism, and enhanced production of progesterone and estrogenic hormones are responsible for most skin changes in pregnancy (Tyler, 2015). Up to 90% of pregnant women will show signs of hyperpigmentation during pregnancy, and it is typically generalized and mild. The skin of pregnant women undergoes hyperpigmentation primarily as a result of estrogen, progesterone, and melanocyte-stimulating hormone levels. These changes are mainly seen on the nipples, areola, umbilicus, perineum, and axilla. Although many integumentary changes disappear after giving birth, some only fade. Many pregnant women express concern about stretch marks, skin color changes, and hair loss. Unfortunately, little is known about how to avoid these changes.

Complexion changes are not unusual. The increased pigmentation that occurs on the breasts and genitalia also develops on the face to form the "mask of pregnancy," which is also called facial melasma. It occurs in up to 70% of pregnant women. There is a genetic predisposition toward melasma, which is exacerbated by the sun, and it tends to recur in subsequent pregnancies. This blotchy, brownish pigment covers the forehead and cheeks in dark-haired women. Most facial pigmentation fades as the hormones subside at the end of the pregnancy, but some may linger. The skin in the middle of the abdomen may develop a pigmented line called **linea nigra**, which extends from the umbilicus to the pubic area (Fig. 11.4).

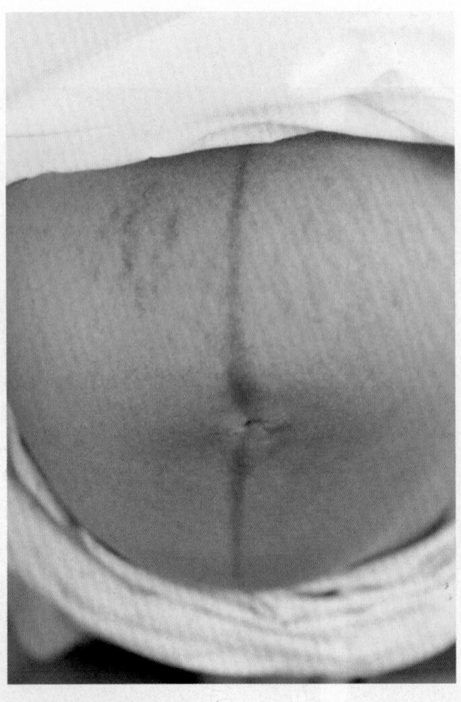

FIGURE 11.4 Linea nigra.

Striae gravidarum, or stretch marks, are irregular reddish streaks that appear on the abdomen, breasts, and buttocks in up to 90% of pregnant women. Striae are most prominent by 6 to 7 months. They result from genetics, reduced connective tissue strength resulting from the elevated adrenal steroid levels, and stretching of the structures secondary to growth (Tyler, 2015). They are more common in younger women, women with larger infants, and women with higher body mass indices. Nonwhites and women with a history of breast or thigh striae or a family history of striae gravidarum also are at higher risk. Several creams and lotions such as cocoa butter and olive oil have been touted as being able to prevent striae gravidarum, but research currently doesn't validate these claims. A study done by Tretti Clementoni and Lavagno (2015) did find that laser treatments did improve pigmentation, volume, and textural appearance of striae gravidarum in >50% of the women enrolled in the study.

Vascular-Related Skin Changes

Vascular changes during pregnancy manifested in the integumentary system include varicosities of the legs, vulva, and perineum. Varicose veins commonly are the result of distention, instability, and poor circulation secondary to prolonged standing or sitting and the heavy gravid uterus placing pressure on the pelvic veins, preventing complete venous return. Interventions to reduce the risk of developing varicosities include:

- Elevating both legs when sitting or lying down
- Avoiding prolonged standing or sitting; changing position frequently
- Resting in the left lateral position
- Walking daily for exercise
- Avoiding tight clothing or knee-high hosiery
- Wearing support hose if varicosities are a preexisting condition to pregnancy

Another skin manifestation, believed to be secondary to vascular changes and high estrogen levels, is the appearance of small blood vessels called vascular spiders. They may appear on the neck, thorax, face, and arms. They are especially obvious in White women and typically disappear after childbirth. Palmar erythema is a well-delineated pinkish area on the palmar surface of the hands. This integumentary change is also related to elevated estrogen levels (Trupin, 2015).

Hair and Nails

Some women also notice a decline in hair growth during pregnancy. The hair follicles normally undergo a growing and resting phase. The resting phase is followed by a loss of hair; the hairs are then replaced by new ones. During pregnancy, fewer hair follicles go into the resting phase. After delivery, the body catches up with subsequent hair loss for several months. Nails typically grow faster during pregnancy. Pregnant women may experience increased brittleness, distal separation of the nail bed, whitish discoloration, and transverse grooves on the nails, but most of these conditions resolve in the postpartum period (King et al., 2015).

Endocrine System

The endocrine system undergoes many changes during pregnancy because hormonal changes are essential in meeting the needs of the growing fetus. Hormonal changes play a major role in controlling the supplies of maternal glucose, amino acids, and lipids to the fetus. Although estrogen and progesterone are the main hormones involved in pregnancy changes, other endocrine glands and hormones also change during pregnancy.

THYROID GLAND

The thyroid gland enlarges slightly and becomes more active during pregnancy as a result of increased vascularity and hyperplasia. Increased gland activity results in an increase in thyroid hormone secretion starting during the first trimester; levels taper off within a few weeks after birth and return to normal limits. Maternal thyroid hormone is transferred to the fetus beginning soon after conception and is critical for fetal brain development, neurogenesis, and organizational processes prior to 20 weeks when fetal thyroid production is low. However, even after the fetal thyroid is producing increasing amounts of hormone, much of the thyroxin (T_4) needed for development continues to be provided by the mother. Low maternal thyroid levels with thyroid insufficiency, hypothyroidism, or low or inadequate iodine intake may compromise fetal neurologic development (Pearce, 2015). With an increase in the secretion of thyroid hormones, the basal metabolic rate (the amount of oxygen consumed by the body over a unit of time in milliliters per minute) progressively increases by 25%, along with heart rate and cardiac output (Medici et al., 2015).

PITUITARY GLAND

During pregnancy, major endocrine and metabolic alterations occur due to the physiologic hormonal secretion from the placenta. The pituitary gland adapts to these changes and all secretory axes are affected. During pregnancy, the pituitary gland enlarges; it returns to normal size after birth.

The anterior lobe of the pituitary is glandular tissue and produces multiple hormones. The release of these hormones is regulated by releasing and inhibiting hormones produced by the hypothalamus. Some of these anterior pituitary hormones induce other glands to secrete their hormones. The increase in blood levels of the hormones produced by the final target glands (e.g., the ovary or thyroid) inhibits the release of anterior pituitary hormones. Changes in levels of pituitary hormones are discussed in the following paragraphs.

FSH and LH secretion are inhibited during pregnancy, probably as a result of hCG produced by the placenta and corpus luteum, and the increased secretion of prolactin by the anterior pituitary gland. Levels remain decreased until after delivery.

Thyroid-stimulating hormone (TSH) is reduced during the first trimester but usually returns to normal for the remainder of the pregnancy. Decreased TSH is thought to be one of the factors, along with elevated hCG levels, associated with morning sickness, nausea, and vomiting during the first trimester.

Growth hormone (GH) is an anabolic hormone that promotes protein synthesis. It stimulates most body cells to grow in size and divide, facilitating the use of fats for fuel and conserving glucose. During pregnancy, there is a decrease in the number of GH-producing cells and a corresponding decrease in GH blood levels. The action of human placental lactogen (hPL) is thought to decrease the need for and use of GH. During pregnancy, prolactin is secreted in pulses and increases 10-fold to promote breast development and the lactation process. High levels of progesterone secreted by the placenta inhibit the direct influence of prolactin on the breast during pregnancy, thus suppressing lactation. At birth, as soon as the placenta is expelled and there is a drop in progesterone, lactogenesis can begin. Prolactin, released from the anterior pituitary gland in response to suckling by the newborn is the major hormonal signal responsible for stimulation in the breasts (Crowley, 2015).

Melanocyte-stimulating hormone (MSH), another anterior pituitary hormone, increases during pregnancy. For many years, its increase was thought to be responsible for many of the skin changes of pregnancy, particularly changes in skin pigmentation (e.g., darkening of the areola, melasma, and linea nigra). However, currently it is thought that the skin changes are due to estrogen (and possibly progesterone) as well as the increase in MSH.

The two hormones oxytocin and antidiuretic hormone (ADH) released by the posterior pituitary are actually synthesized in the hypothalamus. They migrate along nerve fibers to the posterior pituitary and are stored until stimulated to be released into the general circulation. Oxytocin is released by the posterior pituitary gland, and its production gradually increases as the fetus matures (Kim, Bennett, & Terzidou, 2015). Oxytocin is responsible for uterine contractions, both before and after delivery. The muscle layers of the uterus (myometrium) become more sensitive to oxytocin near term. Toward the end of a term pregnancy, levels of progesterone decline and contractions that were previously suppressed by progesterone begin to occur more frequently and with stronger intensity. This change in the hormonal levels is believed to be one of the initiators of labor.

Oxytocin is responsible for stimulating the uterine contractions that bring about delivery. Contractions lead to cervical thinning and dilation. They also exert pressure, helping the fetus to descend in the pelvis for eventual delivery. After delivery, oxytocin secretion continues, causing the myometrium to contract and helping to constrict the uterine blood vessels, decreasing the amount of vaginal bleeding after delivery. Oxytocin is also responsible for milk ejection during breast-feeding. Stimulation of the breasts through sucking or touching stimulates the secretion of oxytocin from the posterior pituitary gland. Oxytocin causes contraction of the myoepithelial cells in the lactating mammary gland.

Women experience cramping pain and discomfort following childbirth as the uterus contracts and returns to its prepregnant size. These after pains are caused by involuntary contractions and usually last for a few days after childbirth. They are more evident in women who have previously had a baby. Breastfeeding, signals the release of oxytocin, which stimulates the uterus to contract and increases the severity of after birth pains.

Vasopressin, also known as antidiuretic hormone (ADH) functions to inhibit or prevent the formation of urine via vasoconstriction, which results in increased blood pressure. Vasopressin also exhibits an antidiuretic effect and plays an important role in the regulation of water balance (Cheng, 2015).

PANCREAS

The pancreas is an exocrine organ, supplying digestive enzymes and buffers, and an endocrine organ. The endocrine pancreas consists of the islets of Langerhans, which are groups of cells scattered throughout, each containing four cell types. One of the cell types is the beta cell, which produces insulin. Insulin lowers blood glucose by increasing the rate of glucose uptake and utilization by most body cells. The growing fetus needs significant amounts of glucose, amino acids, and lipids. Even during early pregnancy the fetus makes demands on the maternal glucose stores. Ideally, hormonal changes of pregnancy help meet fetal needs without putting the mother's metabolism out of balance.

A woman's insulin secretion works on a supply versus demand mode. As the demand to meet the needs of pregnancy increases, more insulin is secreted. Maternal insulin does not cross the placenta, so the fetus must produce his or her own supply to maintain glucose control. (Box 11.2 gives information about pregnancy, glucose, and insulin.)

Maternal glucose metabolism during pregnancy differs from the nongravid state to allow the mother to meet her own and the growing fetus's energy needs. During the first half of pregnancy, much of the maternal glucose is diverted to the growing fetus, and thus the mother's glucose levels are low. Human placental lactogen and other hormonal antagonists increase during the second half of pregnancy. Therefore, the mother must produce more insulin to overcome the resistance by these hormones. Insulin resistance (the inability of insulin to increase glucose uptake and utilization) in pregnancy is consequent to the physiologic adaptation necessary to provide glucose to the growing fetus. Disturbance in the maternal metabolism can induce structural and functional adaptations during fetal development (Nas, Breyer, & Tuu, 2015).

If the mother has normal beta cells of the islets of Langerhans, there is usually no problem meeting the demands for extra insulin. However, if the woman has inadequate numbers of beta cells, she may be unable to produce enough insulin and will develop glucose intolerance during pregnancy. If the woman has glucose intolerance, she is not able to meet the increasing demands and her blood glucose level increases.

BOX 11.2

PREGNANCY, INSULIN, AND GLUCOSE

- During early pregnancy, maternal glucose levels decrease because of the heavy fetal demand for glucose. The fetus is also drawing amino acids and lipids from the mother, decreasing the mother's ability to synthesize glucose. Maternal glucose is diverted across the placenta to assist the growing embryo/fetus during early pregnancy, and thus levels decline in the mother. As a result, maternal glucose concentrations decline to a level that would be considered "hypoglycemic" in a nonpregnant woman.
- During early pregnancy there is also a decrease in maternal insulin production and insulin levels. The pancreas is responsible for the production of insulin, which facilitates entry of glucose into cells. Although glucose and other nutrients easily cross the placenta to the fetus, insulin does not. Therefore, the fetus must produce its own insulin to facilitate the entry of glucose into its own cells.
- After the first trimester, hPL from the placenta and steroids (cortisol) from the adrenal cortex act against insulin. hPL acts as an antagonist against maternal insulin, and thus more insulin must be secreted to counteract the increasing levels of hPL and cortisol during the last half of pregnancy.
- Prolactin, estrogen, and progesterone are also thought to oppose insulin. As a result, glucose is less likely to enter the mother's cells and is more likely to cross over the placenta to the fetus.

Adapted from Cunningham, F. G., Leveno, K. J., Bloom, S. L., Spong, C. Y., Dashe, J. S., Hoffman, B. L., et al. (2014). *William's Obstetrics* (24th ed.). New York, NY: McGraw Hill Education.

ADRENAL GLANDS

Pregnancy does not cause much change in the size of the adrenal glands themselves, but there are changes in some secretions and activity. One of the key changes is the marked increase in cortisol secretion, which regulates carbohydrate and protein metabolism and is helpful in times of stress. Although pregnancy is considered a normal condition, it is a time of stress for a woman's body. The rate of secretion of cortisol by maternal adrenals is not increased in pregnancy, but the rate of clearance is decreased. Cortisol increases in response to increased estrogen levels throughout pregnancy and returns to normal levels within 6 weeks postpartum (Banerjee & Williamson, 2015). During the stress of pregnancy, cortisol:

- Helps keep up the level of glucose in the plasma by breaking down noncarbohydrate sources, such as amino and fatty acids, to make glycogen. Glycogen, stored in the liver, is easily broken down to glucose when needed so that glucose is available in times of stress
- Breaks down proteins to repair tissues and manufacture enzymes
- Has anti-insulin, anti-inflammatory, and antiallergic actions
- Is needed to make the precursors of adrenaline, which the adrenal medulla produces and secretes (Jones & Lopez, 2014)

The amount of aldosterone, also secreted by the adrenal glands, is increased during pregnancy. It normally regulates absorption of sodium from the distal tubules of the kidney. During pregnancy, progesterone allows salt to be wasted (or lost) in the urine. Aldosterone is a key regulator of electrolyte and water homeostasis and plays a central role in blood pressure regulation. Hormonal changes during pregnancy, among them increased progesterone and aldosterone production, lead to the required plasma volume expansion of the maternal body as an accommodation mechanism for fetus growth. Aldosterone is produced in increased amounts by the adrenal glands as early as 15 weeks of pregnancy (Rossier, Baker, & Studer, 2015).

PROSTAGLANDIN SECRETION DURING PREGNANCY

Prostaglandins are not protein or steroid hormones; they are chemical mediators, or local hormones. Although hormones circulate in the blood to influence distant tissues, prostaglandins act locally on adjacent cells. The fetal membranes of the amniotic sac—the amnion and chorion—are both believed to be involved in the production of prostaglandins. Various maternal and fetal tissues, as well as the amniotic fluid itself, are considered to be sources of prostaglandins, but details about their composition and sources are limited. It is widely believed that prostaglandins play a part in softening the cervix and initiating and/or maintaining labor, but the exact mechanism is unclear. What is theorized is that when progesterone levels drop at term, an increased production of prostaglandins occurs, which facilitates uterine contractions and increases myometrial sensitivity to oxytocin that is needed for the labor process (King et al., 2015). Along with oxytocin, the influence of prostaglandins on the uterine myometrium predominates to promote uterine contractile activity.

PLACENTAL SECRETION

The placenta is an organ that serves to prevent the direct exchange between the blood of the fetus and the blood of the mother. The placenta is not only a transfer organ but a factory as well. It is capable of synthesizing enzymes and proteins, and manufactures fats and carbohydrates that serve as a source of stored energy. The placenta also functions as an endocrine gland, manufacturing and secreting hormones. The placenta has a feature possessed by no other endocrine organ—the ability to form protein and steroid hormones. Very early during pregnancy, the placenta begins to produce the following hormones:

- hCG
- hPL
- Relaxin
- Progesterone
- Estrogen

Table 11.3 summarizes the role of these hormones.

Immune System

The immune system is made up of organs and specialized cells whose primary purpose is to defend the body from foreign substances (antigens) that may cause tissue injury or disease. The mechanisms of innate and adaptive immunity work cooperatively to prevent, control, and eradicate foreign antigens in the body.

A general enhancement of innate immunity (inflammatory response and phagocytosis) and suppression of adaptive immunity (protective response to a specific foreign antigen) take place during pregnancy. These immunologic alterations help prevent the mother's immune system from rejecting the fetus (foreign body), increase her risk of developing certain infections such as urinary tract infections, and influence the course of chronic disorders such as autoimmune diseases. Some chronic conditions worsen (diabetes) while others seem to stabilize (asthma) during pregnancy, but this is individualized and not predictable. In general, immune function in pregnant women is similar to immune function in nonpregnant women. Table 11.4 summarizes the general body systems' adaptations to pregnancy.

Marva **returns for her first prenatal appointment and tells the nurse that her whole body is "out of sorts." She is overwhelmed and feels poorly. Outline the bodily changes Marva can expect each trimester to help her understand the adaptations taking place. What guidance can the nurse give Marva to help her understand the changes of pregnancy?**

TABLE 11.3 PLACENTAL HORMONES

Hormone	Description
Human chorionic gonadotropin (hCG)	• Responsible for maintaining the maternal corpus luteum, which secretes progesterone and estrogens, with synthesis occurring before implantation • Production by fetal trophoblast cells until the placenta is developed sufficiently to take over that function • Basis for early pregnancy tests because it appears in the maternal bloodstream soon after implantation • Production peaks at 8 weeks and then gradually declines
hPL (also known as human chorionic somatomammotropin [hCS])	• Preparation of mammary glands for lactation and involved in the process of making glucose available for fetal growth by altering maternal carbohydrate, fat, and protein metabolism • Antagonist of insulin because it decreases tissue sensitivity or alters the ability to use insulin • Increase in the amount of circulating free fatty acids for maternal metabolic needs and decrease in maternal metabolism of glucose to facilitate fetal growth
Relaxin	• Secretion by the placenta as well as the corpus luteum during pregnancy • Thought to act synergistically with progesterone to maintain pregnancy • Increase in flexibility of the pubic symphysis, permitting the pelvis to expand during delivery • Dilation of the cervix, making it easier for the fetus to enter the vaginal canal; thought to suppress the release of oxytocin by the hypothalamus, thus delaying the onset of labor contractions
Progesterone	• Often called the "hormone of pregnancy" because of the critical role it plays in supporting the endometrium of the uterus • Supports the endometrium to provide an environment conducive to fetal survival • Produced by the corpus luteum during the first few weeks of pregnancy and then by the placenta until term • Initially, causes thickening of the uterine lining in anticipation of implantation of the fertilized ovum. From then on, it maintains the endometrium, inhibits uterine contractility, and assists in the development of the breasts for lactation
Estrogen	• Promotes enlargement of the genitals, uterus, and breasts, and increases vascularity, causing vasodilatation • Relaxation of pelvic ligaments and joints • Associated with hyperpigmentation, vascular changes in the skin, increased activity of the salivary glands, and hyperemia of the gums and nasal mucous membranes • Aids in developing the ductal system of the breasts in preparation for lactation

Adapted from Cunningham, F. G., Leveno, K. J., Bloom, S. L., Spong, C. Y., Dashe, J. S., Hoffman, B. L., et al. (2014). *William's obstetrics* (24th ed.). New York, NY: McGraw Hill Education; Edelman, C. L., Kudzma, E. C., & Mandle, C. L. (2014). *Health promotion throughout the lifespan* (8th ed.). St. Louis, MO: Mosby Elsevier; Shields, A. D. (2015). Pregnancy diagnosis. *eMedicine*. Retrieved from http://emedicine.medscape.com/article/262591-overview

CHANGING NUTRITIONAL NEEDS OF PREGNANCY

Maternal body weight and diet quality, even prepregnancy, can affect the uterine environment, birth weight, and the infant's subsequent health into adulthood. Healthy eating during pregnancy enables optimal gestational weight gain and reduces complications, both of which are associated with positive birth outcomes. During pregnancy, maternal nutritional needs change to meet the demands of the pregnancy. Healthy eating can help ensure that adequate nutrients are available for both mother and fetus.

Nutritional intake during pregnancy has a direct effect on fetal well-being and birth outcome. Inadequate nutritional intake, for example, is associated with preterm birth, low birth weight, and congenital anomalies. Excessive nutritional intake is connected with fetal macrosomia (>4,000 g), leading to a difficult birth, neonatal hypoglycemia, and continued obesity in the mother and the potential for childhood obesity and the components of metabolic syndrome (Ojha et al., 2015).

Since the requirements for so many nutrients increase during pregnancy, pregnant women should take a vitamin and mineral supplement daily. Prenatal vitamins are prescribed routinely as a safeguard

TABLE 11.4 SUMMARY OF GENERAL BODY SYSTEM ADAPTATIONS

System	Adaptation
Gastrointestinal system	*Mouth and pharynx:* Gums become hyperemic, swollen, and friable and tend to bleed easily. Saliva production increases. *Esophagus:* Decreased lower esophageal sphincter pressure and tone, which increases the risk of developing heartburn. *Stomach:* Decreased tone and mobility with delayed gastric emptying time, which increases the risk of gastroesophageal reflux and vomiting; decreased gastric acidity and histamine output, which improves symptoms of peptic ulcer disease. *Intestines:* Decreased intestinal tone motility with increased transit time, which increases risk of constipation and flatulence. *Gallbladder:* Decreased tone and motility, which may increase risk of gallstone formation.
Cardiovascular system	*Blood volume:* Marked increase in plasma (50%) and RBCs (25–33%) compared to nonpregnant values; causes hemodilution, which is reflected in a lower hematocrit and hemoglobin. *Cardiac output and heart rate:* CO increases from 30–50% over the nonpregnant rate by the 32nd week of pregnancy. The increase in CO is associated with an increase in venous return and greater right ventricular output, especially in the left lateral position. Heart rate increases by 10–15 bpm between 14 and 20 weeks of gestation, and this increase will persist to term. *Blood pressure:* Diastolic pressure decreases typically 10–15 mmHg to reach its lowest point by mid-pregnancy; it then gradually returns to nonpregnant baseline values by term. *Blood components:* The number of RBCs increases throughout pregnancy to a level 25–33% higher than nonpregnant values. Both fibrin and plasma fibrinogen levels increase, along with various blood-clotting factors. These factors make pregnancy a hypercoagulable state.
Respiratory system	Enlargement of the uterus shifts the diaphragm up to 4 cm above its usual position. As muscles and cartilage in the thoracic region relax, the chest broadens, with conversion from abdominal breathing to thoracic breathing. This leads to a 50% increase in air volume per minute. Tidal volume, or the volume of air inhaled, increases gradually by 30–40% (from 500 to 700 mL) as the pregnancy progresses.
Renal/urinary system	The renal pelvis becomes dilated. The ureters (especially the right ureter) elongate, widen, and become more curved above the pelvic rim. Bladder tone decreases and bladder capacity doubles by term. GFR increases 40–60% during pregnancy. Blood flow to the kidneys increases by 50–80% as a result of the increase in cardiac output.
Musculoskeletal system	Distention of the abdomen with growth of the fetus tilts the pelvis forward, shifting the center of gravity. The woman compensates by developing an increased curvature (lordosis) of the spine. Relaxation and increased mobility of joints occur because of the hormones progesterone and relaxin, which lead to the characteristic "waddle gait" that pregnant women demonstrate toward term.
Integumentary system	Hyperpigmentation of the skin is the most common alteration during pregnancy. The most common areas include the areola, genital skin, axilla, inner aspects of the thighs, and linea nigra. Striae gravidarum, or stretch marks, are irregular reddish streaks that may appear on the abdomen, breasts, and buttocks in about half of pregnant women. The skin in the middle of the abdomen may develop a pigmented line called linea nigra, which extends from the umbilicus to the pubic area. Melasma ("mask of pregnancy") occurs in up to 70% of pregnant women. It is characterized by irregular, blotchy areas of pigmentation on the face, most commonly on the cheeks, chin, and nose.
Endocrine system	Controls the integrity and duration of gestation by maintaining the corpus luteum via hCG secretion; production of estrogen, progesterone, hPL, and other hormones and growth factors via the placenta; release of oxytocin (by the posterior pituitary gland), prolactin (by the anterior pituitary), and relaxin (by the ovary, uterus, and placenta).
Immune system	A general enhancement of innate immunity (inflammatory response and phagocytosis) and suppression of adaptive immunity (protective response to a specific foreign antigen) take place during pregnancy. These immunologic alterations help prevent the mother's immune system from rejecting the fetus (foreign body), increase her risk of developing certain infections, and influence the course of chronic disorders such as autoimmune diseases.

against a less-than-optimal diet. In particular, iron and folic acid need to be supplemented because their increased requirements during pregnancy are usually too great to be met through diet alone. With the exception of folic acid, there is little scientific evidence to support giving vitamin supplements to healthy pregnant women, but it seems to be a standard of care today. Prenatal vitamins are prescribed in the United States almost universally (Jordan et al., 2014). Iron and folic acid are needed to form new blood cells for the expanded maternal blood volume and to prevent anemia. Iron is essential for fetal growth and brain development and in the prevention of maternal anemia. An increase in folic acid is essential before pregnancy and in the early weeks of pregnancy to prevent neural tube defects in the fetus. For most pregnant women, supplements of 27 mg of ferrous iron and 400 to 800 mcg of folic acid per day are recommended by the **dietary reference intakes (DRIs)** (American College of Obstetricians and Gynecologists [ACOG], 2015a; Hankey, 2015; U.S. Preventive Services Task Force [USPSTF], 2015). Women with a previous history of a fetus with a neural tube defect are often prescribed a higher dose of folic acid.

There is an abundance of conflicting advice about nutrition during pregnancy and what is good or bad to eat. Overall, the following guidelines are helpful:

- Increase consumption of fruits and vegetables.
- Replace saturated fats with unsaturated ones.
- Make half the plate fruits and vegetables.
- Choose whole grains in place of refined grains.
- Choose foods with a lot of fiber to prevent constipation.
- Avoid hydrogenated or partially hydrogenated fats.
- Do not consume any alcoholic beverages.
- Use reduced-fat spreads and dairy products instead of full-fat ones.
- Eat at least two servings of fish weekly, with one of them being an oily fish.
- Consume at least 2 quarts of water daily (U.S. Department of Agriculture [USDA], 2015).

In the months before conception, food choices are key. The foods and vitamins consumed can ensure that the woman and her fetus will have the nutrients that are essential for the very start of pregnancy.

While most women recognize the importance of healthy eating during pregnancy, some find it challenging to achieve. Many women say they have little time and energy to devote to meal planning and preparation. Another barrier to healthy eating is conflicting messages from various sources, resulting in a lack of clear, reliable, and relevant information. Moreover, many women are eating less in an effort to control their weight, putting them at greater risk of inadequate nutrient intake.

Nutritional Requirements During Pregnancy

Pregnancy is one of the most nutritionally demanding periods of a woman's life. Gestation involves rapid cell division and organ development, and an adequate supply of nutrients is essential to support this tremendous fetal growth. Optimal maternal health via good nutritional practices during pregnancy reduces the risk of suboptimal fetal development.

Most women are usually motivated to eat properly during pregnancy for the sake of the fetus. The Food and Nutrition Board of the National Research Council has made recommendations for nutrient intakes for people living in the United States. The DRIs are more comprehensive than previous nutrient guidelines issued by the Board. They have replaced previous recommendations because they are not limited to preventing deficiency diseases. Rather, the DRIs incorporate current concepts about the role of nutrients and food components in reducing the risk of chronic disease, developmental disorders, and other related problems. The DRIs can be used to plan and assess diets for healthy people (Kruger & Butte, 2015).

These dietary recommendations also include information for women who are pregnant or lactating, because growing fetal and maternal tissues require increased quantities of essential dietary components. For example, the current DRIs suggest an increase in the pregnant woman's intake of protein from 60 to 80 g/day, iron from 18 to 27 g/day, and folic acid from 400 to 800 mcg/day, along with an increase of 300 calories/day over the recommended intake of 1,800 to 2,200 calories/day for nonpregnant women (Walsh & McAuliffe, 2015; Storck, 2015) (Table 11.5).

Gluten Free Diet During Pregnancy

In recent years, gluten free foods have become popular, fueling a growing market for the Food Industry. Pregnant women may be missing out on important nutrients if they adopt gluten-free diets as many are also joining the ever-expanding "G-free" bandwagon. Many people feel that these products are healthier than their conventional counterparts. But is it really a health-promotion diet or just another trend during pregnancy? Gluten may have gotten its bad rap because it is frequently found in many processed, unhealthy foods. Several gluten free foods contain more fat, including saturated, and sodium, but fewer minerals and vitamins than their equivalents with gluten (Pellegrini & Agostoni, 2015). Skipping processed foods altogether and focusing on fruits, vegetables, lean protein, and whole grains would provide a well-balanced healthy diet.

TABLE 11.5 DIETARY RECOMMENDATIONS FOR THE PREGNANT AND LACTATING WOMAN

Nutrient	Nonpregnant Women	Pregnant Woman	Lactating Woman
Calories	2,200	2,500	2,700
Protein	60 g	80 g	80 g
Water/fluids	6–8 glasses daily	8 glasses daily	8 glasses daily
Vitamin A	700 mcg	770 mcg	1,300 mcg
Vitamin C	75 mg	85 mg	120 mg
Vitamin D	5 mcg	5 mcg	5 mcg
Folate	400 mcg	600 mcg	500 mcg
Calcium	1,000 mg	1,000 mg	1,000 mg
Iodine			
Iron	18 mg	27 mg	9 mg

Adapted from American Pregnancy Association. (2015). *Pregnancy nutrition.* Retrieved from http://americanpregnancy.org/pregnancyhealth/pregnancynutrition.html; Ural, S. H. (2015). Prenatal nutrition. *eMedicine.* Retrieved from http://emedicine.medscape.com/article/259059-overview; Lutz, C.A., Mazur, E., & Litch, N. (2014). *Nutrition and diet therapy* (6th ed.). Philadelphia, PA: F. A. Davis.

Eating a gluten free diet can make it hard to get the recommended amount of folate, vitamin B, iron, calcium, fiber, and grain-servings that all pregnant women need. That is why, unless there is medical reason in which gluten must be eliminated from the diet due to celiac disease or a gluten allergy, there isn't a scientific reason to cut out wholesome, nutrient-dense grains from the diet (Neifeld, 2015).

USDA and MyPlate

For a pregnant woman to meet recommended DRIs, she should eat according to the U.S. Department of Agriculture (USDA) Food Guide *MyPlate* (Fig. 11.5). The USDA Food Guide *MyPlate* replaced the Food Guide Pyramid in 2011 as the government's primary food group symbol. *MyPlate* is an easy-to-understand visual cue to help consumers adopt healthy eating habits by encouraging them to build a healthy plate, consistent with the *Dietary Guidelines for Americans, 2015* (USDA & U.S. Department of Health and Human Services [USDHHS], 2015), which are the basis for federal nutrition policy (USDA & USDHHS, 2015). This new tool will serve as a basis for dietary instruction and it can be tailored to meet each woman's individual needs.

MyPlate provides guidance to help implement the dietary guidelines. The USDA has designed an interactive online diet-planning program called the Daily Food Plan for Moms that helps pregnant women personalize their dietary intake throughout their pregnancy. (Refer to thePoint for additional information about this food plan.) A summary of the new guidelines is as follows:

- Eat a variety of food from all food groups using portion control.
- Increase intake of vitamins, minerals, and dietary fiber.
- Lower intake of saturated fats, trans fats, and cholesterol.
- Consume adequate synthetic folic acid from supplements or from fortified foods.
- Increase intake of fruits, vegetables, and whole grains.
- Balance calorie intake with exercise to maintain ideal healthy weight (USDA, 2015).

An eating plan that follows *MyPlate* should provide sufficient nutrients for a healthy pregnancy. Except for iron, folic acid, and calcium, most of the nutrients a woman needs during pregnancy can be obtained by making healthy food choices. However, a vitamin and mineral supplement is generally prescribed.

Take Note!

Good food sources of folic acid include dark green vegetables, such as broccoli, romaine lettuce, and spinach; baked beans; black-eyed peas; citrus fruits; peanuts; and liver.

Food Concerns During Pregnancy

ARTIFICIAL SWEETENERS

Artificial sweeteners or intense sweeteners are sugar substitutes that are used as an alternative to table sugar.

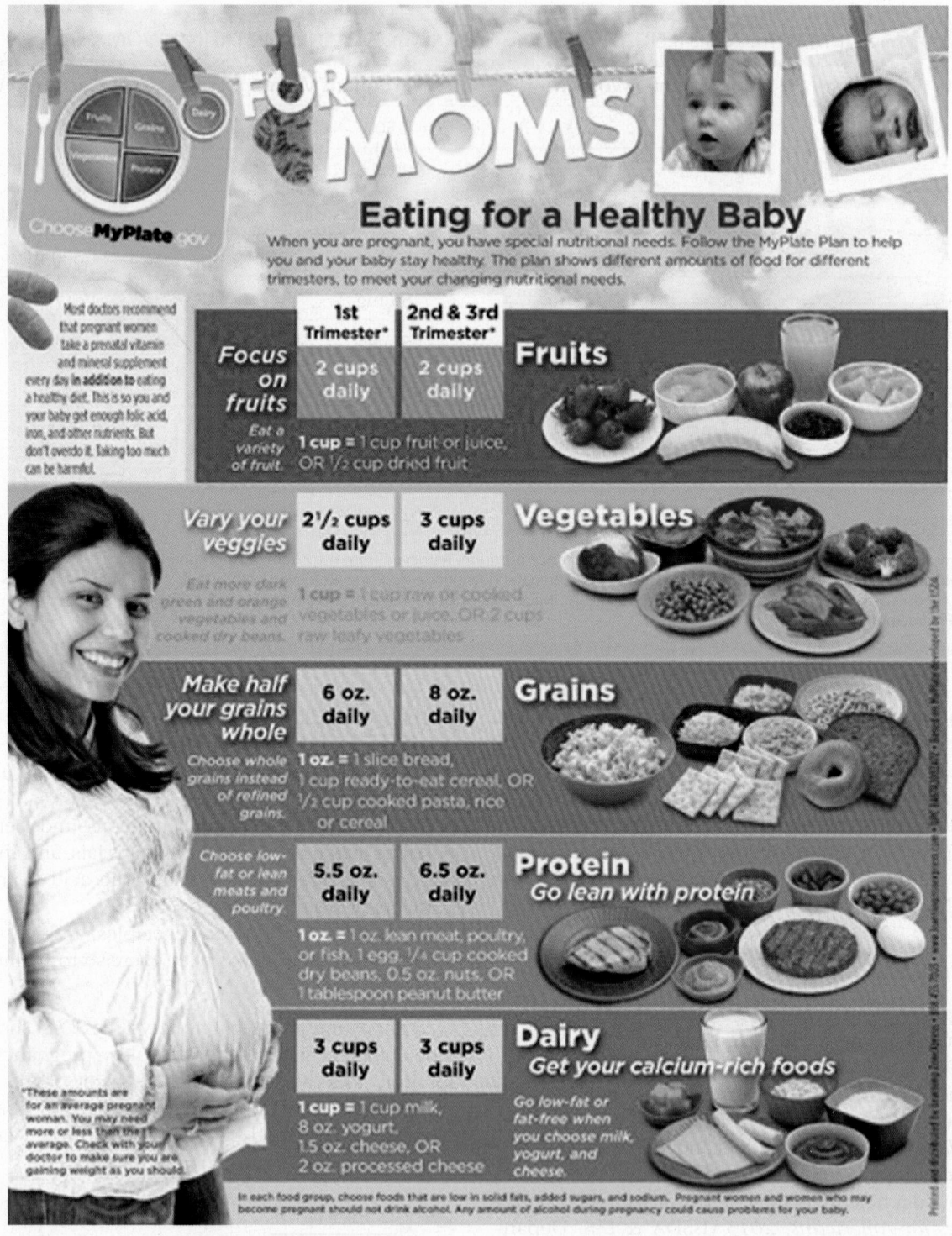

FIGURE 11.5 Food Guide *MyPlate* for pregnancy.

They are many times sweeter than natural sugar and contain no calories. Extensive scientific research has demonstrated the safety of the six low-calorie sweeteners currently approved for use in foods in the United States and Europe (stevia, acesulfame-K, aspartame, neotame, saccharin, and sucralose), if taken in acceptable quantities daily. But there is an ongoing debate over whether artificial sweeteners pose a health threat (Qurrat-ul-Ain & Khan, 2015).

The safety of artificial sweeteners consumed during pregnancy remains controversial also. Some health care providers advise their pregnant clients to avoid all nonnutritive sweeteners during pregnancy, while others suggest they can be used in moderation (Hankley,

2015). The debate continues on this matter until additional research can be completed.

FISH, SHELLFISH, AND LEVELS OF MERCURY

Fish and shellfish are an important part of a healthy diet because they contain high-quality protein, are low in saturated fat, and contain omega-3 fatty acids. However, nearly all fish and shellfish contain traces of mercury and some contain higher levels of mercury that may harm a developing fetus if ingested by pregnant women in large amounts. Human exposure to mercury occurs primarily through the consumption of fish contaminated through atmospheric mercury releases. The U.S. Environmental Protection Agency (EPA) and the United Nations Environment Program have identified coal-fired power plants as the source of 50% to 75% of the atmospheric mercury pollution in the United States and worldwide. Once airborne, rainfall transfers mercury particles into waterways where it is converted to the neurotoxic methylmercury form through a microbial process. Plankton absorbs the methylmercury and as the smaller fish eat the plankton and the larger predatory fish consume the smaller fish, the methylmercury bioaccumulates up the food chain to humans. Mercury exposure in pregnancy has been associated with both pregnancy complications and developmental problems in infants. Apart from the environmental exposure, mercury is likely to arise from predatory fish consumption. It would be prudent to advise all pregnant women to avoid these potential problems and minimize any risk.

All fish contain methylmercury regardless of the size or the geographic location of the waters from which the fish is caught, although size and type of fish as well as the geographic location of waters can influence lower or higher amounts of methylmercury. In addition, because methylmercury resides in the tissue of the fish, no method of cleaning or cooking will reduce the amount of mercury in a meal of contaminated fish (Nelson, 2015).

With this in mind, the FDA and the EPA are advising women who may become pregnant, pregnant women, and nursing mothers to do the following:

- Avoid consumption of fish with moderate-to-high mercury levels (e.g., for 6 to 12 months prior to conception and throughout pregnancy).
- Avoid eating shark, swordfish, king mackerel, orange roughy, ahi tuna, and tilefish because they are high in mercury levels.
- Eat up to 12 ounces (two average meals) weekly of low-mercury-level fish such as shrimp, canned light tuna, salmon, pollock, and catfish.
- Check local advisories about the safety of fish caught by family and friends in local lakes, rivers, and coastal areas (FDA, 2015).

LISTERIOSIS AND PREGNANCY

Another food issue concern for pregnant women is consumption of food contaminated with the gram-positive bacillus *Listeria*. *Listeria* is a type of bacteria found in soil, water, and sometimes on plants. *Listeria* is commonly found in processed and prepared foods and in raw or unpasteurized milk. Listeriosis is associated with high morbidity and mortality. Though *Listeria* is all around our environment, most *Listeria* infections in people result from eating contaminated foods. Listeriosis during pregnancy usually presents as an unremarkable febrile illness in the mother, but can be fatal for the fetus and newborn. Reliable laboratory testing for early diagnosis is lacking. Listeriosis can be passed to an unborn baby through the placenta even if the mother is not showing signs of illness. This can lead to preterm births, miscarriages, stillbirths, and high neonatal mortality rates (Allerberger & Huhulescu, 2015). The Food Safety and Inspection Service and the FDA (2015) the following advice for pregnant women:

- Do not eat hot dogs, luncheon meats, or deli meats unless they are reheated until steaming hot.
- Avoid getting fluid from hot dog packages on other foods, utensils, and food preparation surfaces, and wash hands after handling hot dogs, luncheon meats, and deli meats.
- Do not eat soft cheeses such as feta, Brie, Camembert, and blue-veined cheeses.
- It is safe to eat hard cheeses, semi-soft cheeses such as mozzarella, pasteurized processed cheese slices and spreads, cream cheese, and cottage cheese.
- Do not eat refrigerated pâté or meat spreads.
- It is safe to eat canned or shelf-stable pâté and meat spreads.
- Do not eat refrigerated smoked seafood unless it is an ingredient in a cooked dish such as a casserole. Examples of refrigerated smoked seafood include salmon, trout, whitefish, cod, tuna, and mackerel and are most often labeled as "nova-style," "lox," "kippered," "smoked," or "jerky." This fish is found in the refrigerated section or sold at deli counters of grocery stores and delicatessens.
- It is safe to eat canned fish such as salmon and tuna or shelf-stable smoked seafood.
- Do not drink raw (unpasteurized) milk or eat foods that contain unpasteurized milk.
- Use all refrigerated perishable items that are precooked or ready-to-eat as soon as possible.
- Use a refrigerator thermometer to make sure that the refrigerator always stays at 40°F (about 5 °C) or below.
- Do not eat salads made in the store such as ham salad, chicken salad, egg salad, tuna salad, or seafood salad.
- Clean your refrigerator regularly.

Maternal Weight Gain

The amount of weight that a woman gains during pregnancy is not as important as what she eats. A woman can lose extra weight after a pregnancy, but she can

TABLE 11.6 NORMAL DISTRIBUTION OF WEIGHT GAIN DURING PREGNANCY

Component	Weight (lb)
Infant birth weight	7.5
Blood volume increase	4
Uterus	2
Increase in breast tissue	2
Placenta	1.5
Maternal fluid volume	4
Maternal fat tissue	7
Amniotic fluid	2
Approximate total weight gain	30

Adapted from American College of Obstetricians and Gynecologists [ACOG]. (2015b). *Weight gain guidelines by ACOG for pregnancy.* Retrieved from http://www.womenshealthcaretopics.com/weight_gain_during_pregnancy.htm; Lutz, C.A., Mazur, E., & Litch, N. (2014). *Nutrition and diet therapy* (6th ed.). Philadelphia, PA: F. A. Davis.

BOX 11.3

BODY MASS INDEX

Body mass index (BMI) provides an accurate estimate of total body fat and is considered a good method to assess overweight and obesity in people. BMI is a weight-to-height ratio calculation that can be determined by dividing a woman's weight in kilograms by her height in meters squared. BMI can also be calculated by weight in pounds divided by the height in inches squared, multiplied by 704.5.

The Centers for Disease Control and Prevention (2015) categorizes BMI as follows:

- Underweight: <18.5
- Healthy weight: 18.5–24.9
- Overweight: 25–29.9
- Obese: 30 or higher

Use this example to calculate BMI:

Mary is 5 feet 5 inches tall and weighs 150 lb.

1. Convert weight into kilograms: 150 divided by 2.2 lb/kg = 68.18 kg.
2. Convert height into meters:
   a. 5 feet 5 inches = 65 inches ÷ 2.54 cm/in. = 165.1 cm
   b. 165.1 cm/100 cm = 1.65 m
3. Then square the height in meters: 1.65 × 1.65 = 2.72
4. Calculate BMI: 68.18 kg divided by 2.72 = 25.

Adapted from Centers for Disease Control and Prevention [CDC]. (2015). *BMI for adults: Body mass index calculator.* Retrieved from http://www.cdc.gov/nc cdphp/dnpa/bmi/calc-bmi.htm

never make up for a poor nutritional status during the pregnancy. Earlier guidelines recommended weight gain that would be optimal for the infant, but new guidelines take into account the well-being of the mother too (Table 11.6).

In 2009 Health and Medicine Division revised the recommendations regarding maternal gestational weight gain. The revisions took into account that presently American women (1) have more multiple pregnancies; (2) are becoming pregnant at an older age; (3) are exceeding the ideal weight gain during pregnancy; and (4) tend to be more overweight and obese when becoming pregnant. The new recommendations are based on the woman's pregnancy body mass index (BMI) as follows (Box 11.3):

- Underweight (BMI < 18.5) total weight gain range = 28 to 40 lb
- Normal weight (BMI = 18.5–24.9) total weight gain range = 25 to 35 lb
- Overweight (BMI = 25–29.9) total weight gain range = 15 to 25 lb
- Obese (BMI = 30 or higher) total weight gain range = 11 to 20 lb

A woman who is underweight before pregnancy or who has a low maternal weight gain pattern should be monitored carefully because she is at risk of giving birth to a low-birth-weight infant (<2,500 g or 5.5 lb). Frequently these women simply need advice on what to eat to add weight. Encourage the woman to eat snacks that are high in calories such as nuts, peanut butter, milkshakes, cheese, fruit, yogurt, and ice cream. Any woman who has a prepregnancy BMI of less than 18.5 is considered to be high risk and should be referred to a nutritionist (Sharma et al., 2015).

Conversely, women who start a pregnancy while overweight (BMI >25–29) run the risk of having a high-birth-weight infant, with resulting cephalopelvic disproportion and, potentially, a surgical birth. Two thirds of reproductive-age women in the United States are overweight or obese and at risk for numerous adverse pregnancy outcomes, in additional to a surgical birth. Some researchers have suggested that the uterine environment may influence the potential development of offspring obesity later in life. In a recent study, just a 10% weight loss before conception was associated with at least a 10% lower risk of preeclampsia, gestational diabetes, preterm birth, macrosomia, and stillbirth (Schummers et al., 2015). Dieting during pregnancy is never recommended, even for women who are obese. Severe restriction of caloric intake is associated with a decrease in birth weight. Because of the expansion of maternal blood volume and the development of fetal and placental tissues, some weight gain is essential for a healthy pregnancy. Women who gain more than the recommended weight during pregnancy and who fail to lose this weight 6 months after giving birth are at much higher risk of being obese nearly a decade later (ACOG, 2015a). Women who are overweight when beginning a pregnancy should gain no more than 15 to 25 lb during the pregnancy, depending on their nutritional status and degree of obesity (ACOG, 2015a).

The best way to assess whether a pregnant woman is consuming enough calories is to follow her pattern of weight gain. All pregnant women should aim for a steady rate of weight gain throughout pregnancy. If she is gaining in a steady, gradual manner, then she is taking in enough calories. However, consuming an adequate amount of calories does not guarantee that her nutrients are sufficient. It is critical to evaluate both the quantity and the quality of the foods eaten.

During the first trimester, for women whose prepregnancy weight is within the normal weight range, weight gain should be about 3.5 to 5 lb. For underweight women, weight gain should be at least 5 lb. For overweight women, weight gain should be about 2 lb. Much of the weight gained during the first trimester is caused by growth of the uterus and expansion of the blood volume.

During the second and third trimesters, the following pattern is recommended: for women whose prepregnancy weight is within the normal weight range, weight gain should be about 1 pound per week. For underweight women, weight gain should be slightly more than 1 pound per week. For overweight women, weight gain should be about two thirds of a pound per week (Hankley, 2015).

Nutrition Promotion

Through education, nurses can play an important role in ensuring adequate nutrition for pregnant women. During the initial prenatal visit, health care providers conduct a thorough assessment of a woman's typical dietary practices and address any conditions that may cause inadequate nutrition, such as nausea and vomiting or lack of access to adequate food. Assess and reinforce dietary information at every prenatal visit to promote good nutrition. A normal pregnancy and a well-balanced diet generally provide most of the recommended nutrients except iron and folate, both of which must be supplemented in the form of prenatal vitamins. See Teaching Guidelines 11.1.

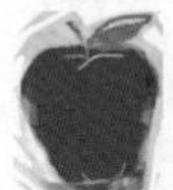

Teaching Guidelines 11.1

TEACHING TO PROMOTE OPTIMAL NUTRITION DURING PREGNANCY

- Follow the USDA Food Guide *MyPlate* and select a variety of foods from each group.
- Gain between 15 and 40 lb in a gradual and steady manner depending on prepregnancy weight as follows:
    - Underweight (BMI >18.5) total weight gain range = 28–40 lb
    - Normal weight (BMI = 18.5–24.0) total weight gain range = 25–35 lb
    - Overweight (BMI = 25–29) total weight gain range = 15–25 lb
    - Obese (BMI = 30 or higher) total weight gain range = 11–20 lb (Health and Medicine Division [HMD], 2009)
- Take your prenatal vitamin/mineral supplementation daily.
- Avoid weight-reduction diets during pregnancy.
- Do not skip meals; eat three meals with one or two snacks daily.
- Limit the intake of sodas and caffeine-rich drinks.
- Avoid the use of diuretics during pregnancy.
- Do not restrict the use of salt unless instructed to do so by your health care provider.
- Engage in reasonable physical activity daily.

Special Nutritional Considerations

Many factors play an important role in shaping a person's food habits, and these factors must be taken into account if nutritional counseling is to be realistic and appropriate. Nurses need to be aware of these factors to ensure individualized teaching and care.

Cultural Variations and Restrictions

Food is important to every cultural group. It is often part of celebrations and rituals. When working with women from various cultures, the nurse needs to adapt American nutritional guidelines to meet their nutritional needs within their cultural framework. Food choices and variations for different cultures might include the following:

- Bread, cereal, rice, and pasta group:
    - Bolillo
    - Couscous
    - Flaxseed
    - Hau juan
- Vegetable group:
    - Agave
    - Bok choy
    - Jicama
    - Okra
    - Water chestnuts
- Protein group:
    - Bean paste
    - Blood sausage
    - Legumes
    - Shellfish
- Fruit group:
    - Catalpa
    - Kumquats

- Plantain
- Yucca fruit
- Zapote
- Milk and dairy:
  - Buffalo milk
  - Buttermilk
  - Soybean milk (Academy of Nutrition and Dietetics [AND], 2015a)

Lactose Intolerance

The best source of calcium is milk and dairy products, but for women with lactose intolerance, adaptations are necessary. Women with lactose intolerance lack an enzyme (lactase) needed for the breakdown of lactose into its component simple sugars, glucose and galactose. Without adequate lactase, lactose passes through the small intestine undigested and causes abdominal discomfort, gas, and diarrhea. Lactose intolerance is especially common among women of African, Asian, and Middle Eastern descent (Szilagyi, 2015).

Additional or substitute sources of calcium may be necessary. These may include peanuts, almonds, sunflower seeds, broccoli, salmon, kale, and molasses (McIndoo, 2015). In addition, encourage the woman to drink lactose-free dairy products or calcium-enriched orange juice or soy milk (Evidence-Based Practice 11.1).

Vegetarians

Vegetarian diets are becoming increasing prevalent in the United States. People choose a vegetarian diet for various reasons including environmental, animal rights, philosophical, religious, and health beliefs (Dunlevy, 2015). Vegetarians choose not to eat meat, poultry, and fish. Their diets consist mostly of plant-based foods, such as legumes, vegetables, whole grains, nuts, and seeds. Vegetarians fall into groups defined by the types of foods they eat. Lacto-ovo-vegetarians omit red meat, fish, and poultry, but eat eggs, milk, and dairy products in addition to plant-based foods. Lacto-vegetarians consume milk and dairy products along with plant-based foods;

EVIDENCE-BASED PRACTICE 11.1 INTERVENTIONS FOR NAUSEA AND VOMITING IN EARLY PREGNANCY

Nausea, retching or dry heaving, and vomiting in early pregnancy are very common and can be very distressing for women. Many treatments are available to women with 'morning sickness,' including drugs and complementary and alternative therapies. Because of concerns that taking medications may adversely affect the development of the fetus, this review aimed to examine if these treatments have been found to be effective and safe.

STUDY

The purpose of this study was to assess the effectiveness and safety of all interventions for nausea and vomiting in early pregnancy, up to 20 weeks' gestation. Thirty-seven trials involving 5,049 women met the inclusion criteria. These trials covered many interventions, including acupressure, acustimulation, acupuncture, ginger, chamomile, lemon oil, mint oil, vitamin B6, and several antiemetic drugs.

Evidence regarding the effectiveness of P6 acupressure, auricular (ear) acupressure, and acustimulation of the P6 point was limited. Acupuncture (P6 or traditional) showed no significant benefit to women in pregnancy. The use of ginger products may be helpful to women, but the evidence of effectiveness was limited and not consistent, though two recent studies support ginger over placebo. There was only limited evidence from trials to support the use of pharmacological agents including vitamin B6, and anti-emetic drugs to relieve mild or moderate nausea and vomiting. There was little information on maternal and fetal adverse outcomes and on psychological, social, or economic outcomes. The methodological quality of the included studies was mixed.

Findings

This review found a lack of high-quality evidence to back up any advice on which interventions to use. Some of the studies showed a benefit in improving nausea and vomiting symptoms for women, but generally effects were inconsistent and limited. Studies were carried out in a way that meant they were at high risk of bias and, therefore, it was difficult to draw firm conclusions. Most studies had different ways of measuring the symptoms of nausea and vomiting and therefore, could not be looked at these findings together. Few studies reported maternal and fetal adverse outcomes and there was very little information on the effectiveness of treatments for improving women's quality of life.

Nursing Implications

Given the high prevalence of nausea and vomiting in early pregnancy, women and nurses caring for them need clear guidance about effective and safe interventions based on systematically reviewed evidence. Diclegis is the only FDA approved medicine for treatment of morning sickness presently, but causes drowsiness, so women should avoid engaging in activities requiring complete mental alertness, such as driving. There is a lack of high-quality evidence to support any particular intervention at this time. This is not the same as saying that the interventions studied are ineffective, but that there is insufficient strong evidence for any one intervention. Advice provided by nurses to pregnant clients experiencing morning sickness should remain general and individualized, based on the findings of this study.

Adapted from Matthews, A., Haas, D. M., O'Mathúna, D. P., Dowswell, T., & Doyle, M. (2014). Interventions for nausea and vomiting in early pregnancy. *Cochrane Database of Systematic Reviews* 2014, 3, CD007575.

they omit eggs, meat, fish, and poultry. Vegans eliminate all foods from animals, including milk, eggs, and cheese, and eat only plant-based foods (Foster & Samman, 2015).

The concern with any form of vegetarianism, especially during pregnancy, is that the diet may be inadequate in nutrients. Other risks of vegetarian eating patterns during pregnancy may include low gestational weight gain, iron-deficiency anemia, compromised protein utilization, and decreased mineral absorption (Piccoli et al., 2015). A diet can become so restrictive that a woman is not gaining weight or is consistently not eating enough from one or more of the food groups. Generally, the more restrictive the diet is, the greater the chance of nutrient deficiencies.

Well-balanced vegetarian diets that include dairy products provide adequate caloric and nutrient intake and do not require special supplementation; however, vegan diets do not include any meat, eggs, or dairy products. Pregnant vegetarians must pay special attention to their intake of protein, iron, calcium, and vitamin B_{12}. Suggestions include:

- *For protein:* substitute soy foods, beans, lentils, nuts, grains, and seeds.
- *For iron:* eat a variety of meat alternatives, along with vitamin C–rich foods.
- *For calcium:* substitute soy, calcium-fortified orange juice, and tofu.
- *For vitamin B_{12}:* eat fortified soy foods and a B_{12} supplement.

The AND (2015b) used an evidence-based review to show that well-planned vegetarian diets are appropriate for individuals during all stages of the life cycle, including pregnancy, lactation, infancy, childhood, and adolescence, and for athletes.

Pica

Pica is a term used to describe the intense craving for and eating of non-food items. Many women experience unusual food cravings during their pregnancy. Having cravings during pregnancy is perfectly normal. Sometimes, however, women crave substances that have no nutritional value and can even be dangerous to themselves and their fetus. Pica is the compulsive ingestion of nonfood substances. Pica is derived from the Latin term for magpie, a bird that is known to consume a variety of nonfood substances. Unlike the bird, however, pregnant women who develop a pica habit typically have one or two specific cravings.

The exact cause of pica is not known. Many theories have been advanced to explain it, but none has been proven scientifically. The incidence of pica is difficult to determine, since it is underreported. It is more common in the United States among African American women compared with other ethnicities, but the practice of pica is not limited to any one geographic area, race, creed, or culture. In the United States, pica is also common in women from rural areas and women with a family history of it. Common substances ingested include dirt, clay, and laundry starch. Other pica cravings are burnt matches, stones, charcoal, mothballs, ice, cornstarch, toothpaste, soap, sand, plaster, coffee grounds, paint chips, coffee grounds, baking soda, and cigarette ashes (Jyothi, 2015).

The three main substances consumed by women with pica are soil or clay (geophagia), ice (pagophagia), and laundry starch (amylophagia). Nutritional implications include:

- *Soil:* replaces nutritive sources and causes iron-deficiency anemia
- *Clay:* produces constipation; can contain toxic substances and cause parasitic infection
- *Ice:* can cause iron-deficiency anemia, tooth fractures, freezer burn injuries
- *Laundry starch:* replaces iron-rich foods, leads to iron deficiencies, and replaces protein metabolism, thus depriving the fetus of amino acids needed for proper development (American Pregnancy Association, 2015)

Clinical manifestations of anemia often precede the identification of pica because the health care provider rarely addresses the behavior and the woman does not usually volunteer such information (King et al., 2015). Secrecy surrounding this habit makes research and diagnosis difficult because some women fail to view their behavior as anything unusual, harmful, or worth reporting. Because of the clinical implications, pica should be discussed with all pregnant women as a preventive measure. The topic can be part of a general discussion of cravings, and the nurse should stress the harmful effects outlined above.

Suspect pica when the woman exhibits anemia although her dietary intake is appropriate. Ask about her usual dietary intake, and include questions about the ingestion of nonfood substances. Consider the potential negative outcomes for the pregnant woman and her fetus, and take appropriate action.

PSYCHOSOCIAL ADAPTATIONS DURING PREGNANCY

Pregnancy is a unique time in a woman's life. It is a time of dramatic alterations in her body and her appearance, as well as a time of change in her social status. All of these changes occur simultaneously. Concurrent with the physiologic changes within her body systems are psychosocial changes within the mother and family members as they face significant role and lifestyle changes.

Maternal Emotional Responses

Motherhood, perhaps more than any role in society, has acquired a special significance for women. Women are taught they should find fulfillment and satisfaction in the role of the "ever-bountiful, ever-giving, self-sacrificing mother." Pregnancy and transitioning to motherhood are critical experiences in a woman's life, stirring a whole range of powerful emotions (Einstein, 2015). With such high expectations, many pregnant women experience various emotions throughout their pregnancy. The woman's approach to these emotions is influenced by her emotional makeup, her sociologic and cultural background, her acceptance or rejection of the pregnancy, whether the pregnancy was planned, if the father is known, and her support network (Alexander et al., 2014).

Despite the wide-ranging emotions associated with the pregnancy, many women experience similar responses. These responses commonly include ambivalence, introversion, acceptance, mood swings, and changes in body image.

Ambivalence

The realization of a pregnancy can lead to fluctuating responses, possibly at the opposite ends of the spectrum. For example, regardless of whether the pregnancy was planned, the woman may feel proud and excited by the news, while at the same time fearful and anxious of the implications. The reactions are influenced by several factors, including the way the woman was raised, her current family situation, the quality of the relationship with the expectant father, and her hopes for the future. Some women express concern over the timing of the pregnancy, wishing that goals and life objectives had been met before becoming pregnant. Other women may question how a newborn or infant will affect their career or their relationships with friends and family. These feelings can cause conflict and confusion about the pregnancy.

Ambivalence, or having conflicting feelings at the same time, is a universal feeling and is considered normal when preparing for a lifestyle change and new role. Pregnant women commonly experience ambivalence during the first trimester. Usually ambivalence evolves into acceptance by the second trimester, when fetal movement is felt. The woman's personality, her ability to adapt to changing circumstances and the reactions of her partner will affect her adjustment to being pregnant and her acceptance of impending motherhood.

Introversion

Introversion, or focusing on oneself, is common during the early part of pregnancy. The woman may withdraw and become increasingly preoccupied with herself and her fetus. As a result, she may participate less with the outside world, and she may appear passive to her family and friends.

This introspective behavior is a normal psychological adaptation to motherhood for most women. Introversion seems to heighten during the first and third trimesters, when the woman's focus is on behaviors that will ensure a safe and health pregnancy outcome. Couples need to be aware of this behavior and should be informed about measures to maintain and support the focus on the family.

Acceptance

During the second trimester, the physical changes of the growing fetus, including an enlarging abdomen and fetal movement, bring reality and validity to the pregnancy. There are many tangible signs that someone separate from herself is present. The pregnant woman feels fetal movement and may hear the heartbeat. She may see the fetal image on an ultrasound screen and feel distinct parts, recognizing independent sleep and wake patterns. She becomes able to identify the fetus as a separate individual and accepts this.

Many women will verbalize positive feelings about the pregnancy and will conceptualize the fetus. The woman may accept her new body image and talk about the new life within. Generating a discussion about the woman's feelings and offering support and validation at prenatal visits are important.

Mood Swings

Emotional lability is characteristic throughout most pregnancies. One moment a woman can feel great joy, and within a short time she can feel shock and disbelief. Frequently, pregnant women will start to cry without any apparent cause. Some women feel as though they are riding an emotional "roller-coaster." These extremes in emotion can make it difficult for partners and family members to communicate with the pregnant woman without placing blame on themselves for their mood changes. Clear explanations about how common mood swings are during pregnancy are essential.

Change in Body Image

The way in which pregnancy affects a woman's body image varies greatly from person to person. Some women feel as if they have never been more beautiful, whereas others spend their pregnancy feeling overweight and uncomfortable. For some women pregnancy is a relief from worrying about weight, whereas for others it only exacerbates their fears of weight gain. Changes in body image are normal but can be very stressful for the pregnant woman. Offering a thorough explanation and initiating discussion of the expected bodily changes may help the family to cope with them.

Becoming a Mother

Reva Rubin (1984) identified maternal tasks that a woman must accomplish to incorporate the maternal role into her personality. Accomplishing these tasks helps the expectant mother to develop her self-concept as a mother and to form a mutually gratifying relationship with her infant. These tasks are listed in Box 11.4.

Pregnancy and Sexuality

Sexuality is an important part of health and well-being. Sexual behavior modifies as pregnancy progresses, influenced by biologic, psychological, and social factors. The way a pregnant woman feels and experiences her body during pregnancy can affect her sexuality. The woman's changing shape, emotional status, fetal activity, changes in breast size, pressure on the bladder, and other discomforts of pregnancy result in increased physical and emotional demands. These can produce stress on the sexual relationship between the pregnant woman and her partner. As the changes of pregnancy ensue, many partners become confused, anxious, and fearful of how the relationship may be affected.

The sexual desire of pregnant women may change throughout the pregnancy. During the first trimester, the woman may be less interested in sex because of fatigue, nausea, and fear of disturbing the early embryonic development. During the second trimester, her interest may increase because of the stability of the pregnancy. During the third trimester, her enlarging size may produce discomfort during sexual activity (Bope & Kellerman, 2015).

Potential complications of sex during pregnancy include preterm labor, pelvic inflammatory disease, antepartum hemorrhage in placenta previa, and venous air embolism. Generally, sexual relations are generally considered safe in pregnancy. Abstinence is usually only recommended for women who are at risk for preterm labor or for antepartum hemorrhage because of placenta previa (Boynton, 2015).

A woman's sexual health is intimately linked to her own self-image. Sexual positions to increase comfort as the pregnancy progresses as well as alternative noncoital modes of sexual expression, such as cuddling, caressing, and holding, should be discussed. Giving permission to talk about and then normalizing sexuality can help enhance the sexual experience during pregnancy and, ultimately, the couple's relationship. If avenues of communication are open regarding sexuality during pregnancy, any fears and myths the couple may have can be dispelled.

BOX 11.4

BECOMING A MOTHER

- **Ensuring safe passage throughout pregnancy and birth**
  - Primary focus of the woman's attention
  - First trimester: woman focuses on herself, not on the fetus
  - Second trimester: woman develops attachment of great value to her fetus
  - Third trimester: woman has concern for herself and her fetus as a unit
  - Participation in positive self-care activities related to diet, exercise, and overall well-being
- **Seeking acceptance of infant by others**
  - First trimester: acceptance of pregnancy by herself and others
  - Second trimester: family needs to relate to the fetus as member
  - Third trimester: unconditional acceptance without rejection
- **Seeking acceptance of self in maternal role to infant ("binding in")**
  - First trimester: mother accepts idea of pregnancy, but not of infant
  - Second trimester: with sensation of fetal movement (**quickening**), mother acknowledges fetus as a separate entity within her.
  - Third trimester: mother longs to hold infant and becomes tired of being pregnant.
- **Learning to give of oneself**
  - First trimester: identifies what must be given up to assume new role
  - Second trimester: identifies with infant, learns how to delay own desires
  - Third trimester: questions her ability to become a good mother to infant

Adapted from Rubin, R. (1984). *Maternal identity and the maternal experience*. New York, NY: Springer.

Pregnancy and the Partner

Nursing care related to childbirth has expanded from a narrow emphasis on the physical health needs of the mother and infant to a broader focus on family-related social and emotional needs. One prominent feature of this family-centered approach is the recent movement toward promoting the mother–infant bond. To achieve a truly family-centered practice, nursing must make a comparable commitment to understanding and meeting the needs of the partner in the emerging family. Recent studies suggest that the partner's potential contribution to the infant's overall development has been misperceived or devalued and that the partner's ability and willingness to assume a more active role in the infant's care may have been underestimated.

Reactions to pregnancy and to the psychological and physical changes by the woman's partner vary greatly. Some enjoy the role of being the nurturer, whereas others experience alienation and may seek comfort or companionship elsewhere. Some expectant fathers may view pregnancy as proof of their masculinity and assume the dominant role, whereas others see their role as minimal, leaving the pregnancy up to the woman entirely. Each expectant partner reacts uniquely.

Emotionally and psychologically, expectant partners may undergo fewer visible changes than women, but most of these changes remain unexpressed and unappreciated (Davies, 2015). Expectant partners also experience a multitude of adjustments and concerns. Physically, they may gain weight around the middle and experience nausea and other GI disturbances—a reaction termed *couvade syndrome* that is a sympathetic response to their partner's pregnancy. They also experience ambivalence during early pregnancy, with extremes of emotions (e.g., pride and joy versus an overwhelming sense of impending responsibility).

During the second trimester of pregnancy, partners go through acceptance of their role of breadwinner, caretaker, and support person. They come to accept the reality of the fetus when movement is felt, and they experience confusion when dealing with the woman's mood swings and introspection. During the third trimester, the expectant partner prepares for the reality of this new role and negotiates what the role will be during the labor and birthing process. Many express concern about being the primary support person during labor and birth and worry how they will react when faced with their loved one in pain. Expectant partners share many of the same anxieties as their pregnant partners. However, it is uncommon for them to reveal these anxieties to the pregnant partner or health care providers. Often, how the expectant partner responds during the third trimester depends on the state of the marriage or partnership. When the marriage or partnership is struggling, the impending increase in responsibility toward the end of pregnancy acts to drive the expectant partner further away. Often it manifests as working late, staying out late with friends, or beginning new or superficial relationships. In the stable marriage or partnership, the expectant partner who may have been struggling to find his or her place in the pregnancy now finds concrete tasks to do—for example, painting the nursery, assembling the car seat, or attending Lamaze classes.

Pregnancy and Siblings

A sibling's reaction to pregnancy is age dependent. Some children might express excitement and anticipation, whereas others might have negative reactions. A young toddler might regress in toilet training or ask to drink from a bottle again. An older school-aged child may ignore the new addition to the family and engage in outside activities to avoid the new member. The introduction of an infant into the family is often the beginning of sibling rivalry, which results from the child's fear of change in the security of the relationship with his or her parents (Jordan et al., 2014). Preparation of the siblings for the anticipated birth is imperative and must be designed according to the age and life experiences of the sibling at home. Constant reinforcement of love and caring will help to reduce the older child's fear of change and worry about being replaced by the new family member.

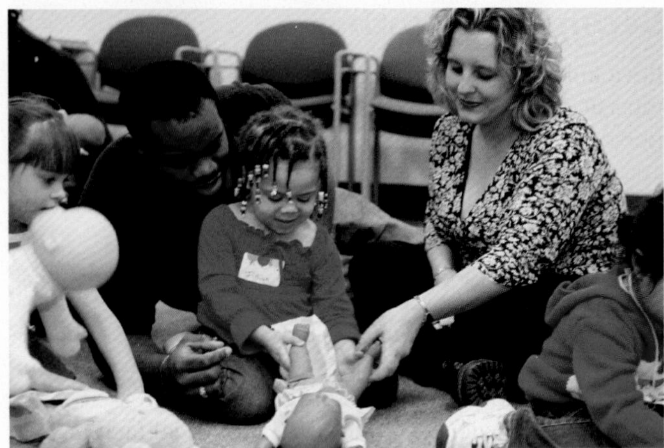

FIGURE 11.6 Parents preparing sibling for the birth of a new baby.

If possible, parents should include siblings in preparation for the birth of the new baby to help them feel as if they have an important role to play (Fig. 11.6). Parents must also continue to focus on the older sibling after the birth to reduce regressive or aggressive behavior toward the newborn.

Pregnancy is an extremely busy time, not only in terms of the bodily changes taking place, but tasks that must be done such as choosing a provider to care for them, preparing for the new family member in a matter of months, and making lifestyle modifications to promote the best possible pregnancy outcome. We will explore this more in Chapter 12.

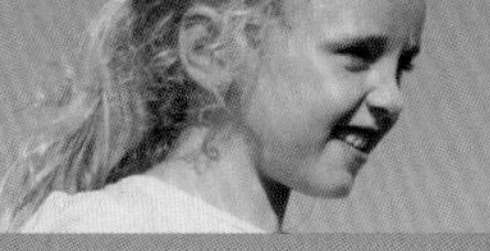
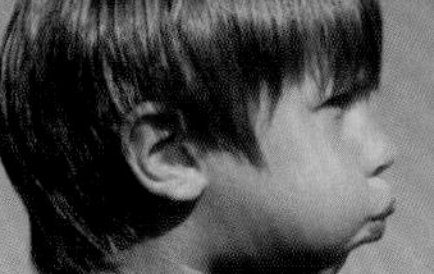
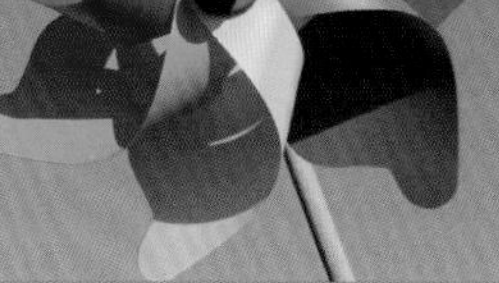
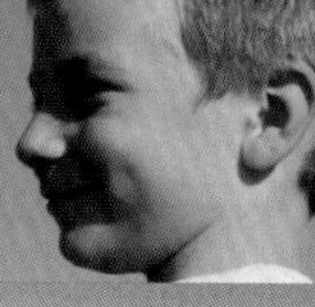

KEY CONCEPTS

- Pregnancy is a normal life event that involves considerable physical, psychosocial, emotional, and relationship adjustments.
- The signs and symptoms of pregnancy have been grouped into those that are subjective (presumptive) and experienced by the woman herself, those that are objective (probable) and observed by the health care provider, and those that are the positive, certain signs.
- Physiologically, almost every system of a woman's body changes during pregnancy with startling rapidity to accommodate the needs of the growing fetus. A majority of the changes are influenced by hormonal changes.
- The placenta is a unique kind of endocrine gland; it has a feature possessed by no other endocrine organ—the ability to form protein and steroid hormones.
- Occurring in conjunction with the physiologic changes in the woman's body systems are psychosocial changes occurring within the mother and family members as they face significant role and lifestyle changes.
- Commonly experienced emotional responses to pregnancy in the woman include ambivalence, introversion, acceptance, mood swings, and changes in body image.
- Reactions of expectant partners to pregnancy and to the physical and psychological changes in the woman vary greatly.
- A sibling's reaction to pregnancy is age dependent. The introduction of a new infant to the family is often the beginning of sibling rivalry, which results from the established child's fear of change in security of their relationships with their parents. Therefore, preparation of the siblings for the anticipated birth is imperative.

REFERENCES AND RECOMMENDED READINGS

Academy of Nutrition and Dietetics [AND]. (2015a). *Eat right, your way, every day with foods from all ethnic traditions.* Retrieved from http://www.eatright.org/Media/content.aspx?id=6442474621#.U3DyestOXL8

Academy of Nutrition and Dietetics [AND]. (2015b). *Vegetarian pregnancy.* Retrieved from http://www.eatright.org/Public/content.aspx?id=6442478249&terms=vegetarian%20and%20pregnancy

Alexander, L. L., LaRosa, J. H., Bader, H., & Garfield, S. (2014). *New dimensions in women's health* (6th ed). Sudbury, MA: Jones & Bartlett.

Allerberger, F., & Huhulescu, S. (2015). Pregnancy related listeriosis: Treatment and control. *Expert Review of Anti-infective Therapy, 13*(3), 395–403.

American College of Obstetricians and Gynecologists [ACOG]. (2015a). *Nutrition during pregnancy.* Retrieved from http://www.acog.org/ /media/For%20Patients/faq001.pdf?dmc=1&ts=20140510T1230032319

American College of Obstetricians and Gynecologists [ACOG]. (2015b). *Weight gain guidelines by ACOG for pregnancy.* Retrieved from http://www.womenshealthcaretopics.com/weight_gain_during_pregnancy.htm

American Pregnancy Association. (2015). *Pregnancy and pica: Non-food cravings.* Retrieved from http://www.american-pregnancy.org/pregnancyhealth/unusualcravingspica.html

Anil, S., Alrowis, R. M., Chalisserry, E. P., Chalissery, V. P., AlMoharib, H. S., & Al-Sulaimani, A. F. (2015). Chapter 28: Oral health and adverse pregnancy outcomes. In Virdi, M. (Ed.), *Emerging trends in oral health sciences and dentistry* (pp. 631–662). Retrieved from http://dx.doi.org/10.5772/59517

Banerjee, A., & Williamson, C. (2015). Chapter 5: Endocrine and metabolic emergencies in pregnancy. In Matfin, G. (Ed.), *Endocrine and metabolic medical emergencies.* Retrieved from http://dx.doi.org/10.1210/EME.9781936704811.ch5

Bope, E. T., & Kellerman, R. D. (2015). *Conn's current therapy 2015.* Philadelphia, PA: Elsevier.

Boynton, P. M. (2015). Pregnancy: relationships advice. In Whelehan, P., & Bolin, A. (Eds.), *The international encyclopedia of human sexuality* (pp. 861–1042). Retrieved from http://dx.doi.org/10.1002/9781118896877.wbiehs372

Centers for Disease Control and Prevention. (2015). *BMI for adults: Body mass index calculator.* Retrieved from http://www.cdc.gov/nc cdphp/dnpa/bmi/calc-bmi.htm

Cheng, H. M. (2015). Water balance. In *Physiology question-based learning* (pp. 127–135). New York, NY: Springer International Publishing.

Cox, S., & Reid, F. (2015). Urogynecological complications in pregnancy: an overview. *Obstetrics, Gynecology & Reproductive Medicine, 25*(5), 123–127.

Crowley, W. R. (2015). Neuroendocrine regulation of lactation and milk production. *Comprehensive Physiology, 5,* 255–291.

Cunningham, F. G., Leveno, K. J., Bloom, S. L., Spong, C. Y., Dashe, J. S., Hoffman, B. L., et al. (2014). *William's obstetrics* (24th ed.). New York, NY: McGraw Hill Education.

Davies, J. (2015). Fatherhood Institute: Supporting fathers to play their part. *Community Practitioner, 88*(1), 13–14.

DeLoughery, T. G. (2015). Bleeding and thrombosis: Women's issues. In *Hemostasis and thrombosis* (pp. 151–155). New York, NY: Springer International Publishing.

Dunlevy, F. (2015). Nutritional assessment during pregnancy. *Topics in Clinical Nutrition, 30*(1), 71–79.

Edelman, C. L., Kudzma, E. C., & Mandle, C. L. (2014). *Health promotion throughout the lifespan* (8th ed.). St. Louis, MO: Mosby Elsevier.

Einstein, A. (2015). *Thinking about emotions. Thinking about thinking: Cognition, science, and psychotherapy* (pp. 68–85). New York, NY: Routledge.

Foo, L., Tay, J., Lees, C. C., McEniery, C. M., & Wilkinson, I. B. (2015). Hypertension in pregnancy: Natural history and treatment options. *Current Hypertension Reports, 17*(5), 1–18.

Food Safety and Inspection Service and Food and Drug Administration [FDA]. (2013). *Listeriosis and pregnancy*. Retrieved from http://www.fsis.usda.gov/Factsheets/Protect_Your_Baby/index.asp

Foster, M., & Samman, S. (2015). Vegetarian diets across the lifecycle: Impact on zinc intake and status. *Advances in Food and Nutrition Research, 74*, 93–131.

Gaillard, R., & Jaddoe, V. W. (2015). Assessment of maternal blood pressure development during pregnancy. *Journal of Hypertension, 33*(1), 61–62.

Hankey, C. R. (2015). Chapter 1: Importance of good health and nutrition before and during pregnancy. In Stewart, L., & Thompson, J. (Eds.), *Early years nutrition and healthy weight* (pp. 1–13). Somerset, NJ: John Wiley & Sons.

Health and Medicine Division [HMD]. (2009). *Weight gain during pregnancy: Reexamining the guidelines*. Retrieved from http://www.iom.edu/Reports/2009/Weight-Gain-During-Pregnancy-Reexamining-the-Guidelines.aspx

Heffner, L. J., & Schust, D. J. (2014). *The reproductive system at a glance* (4th ed.). Somerset, NJ: Wiley Blackwell.

Heuman, D. M., Mihas, A. A., & Allen, J. (2015). Gallstones (cholelithiasis). *eMedicine*. Retrieved from http://emedicine.medscape.com/article/175667-overview

Jones, R. E., & Lopez, K. H. (2014). *Human reproductive biology* (4th ed.). Waltham, MA: Elsevier.

Jordan, R. G., Engstrom, J., Matrfell, J., & Farley, C. L. (2014). *Prenatal and postnatal care: A woman-centered approach*. Ames, IA: Wiley-Blackwell.

Jyothi, N. (2015). Case study on post pregnancy related complication of pica. *International Journal of Nursing Care, 3*(1), 42–45.

Kim, S. H., Bennett, P. R., & Terzidou, V. (2015). Diverse roles of oxytocin. *Inflammation and Cell Signaling, 2*(1), 10–14.

King, T. L., Brucker, M. C., Kriebs, J. M., Fahey, J. O., Gegor, C. L., & Varney, H. (2015). *Varney's midwifery* (5th ed.). Burlington, MA: Jones & Bartlett Learning.

Kouhkan, S., Rahimi, A., Ghasemi, M., Naimi, S. S., & Baghban, A. A. (2015). Postural changes during first pregnancy. *British Journal of Medicine and Medical Research, 7*(9), 744–753.

Krapf, J. M. (2015). Vulvovaginitis. *eMedicine*. Retrieved from http://emedicine.medscape.com/article/2188931-overview

Kruger, H. S., & Butte, N. F. (2015). Nutrition in pregnancy and lactation. In Bier, D. M., Mann, J., Alpers, D. H., Vorster, H. E., & Gibney, M. J. (Eds.), *Nutrition for the primary care provider* (pp. 64–70). Basel: Karger.

Larson, L. (2015). Renal disease in pregnancy. In Rosene-Montella, K. (Ed.), *Medical management of the pregnant patient* (pp. 261–272). New York, NY: Springer Publishers.

Lutz, C. A., Mazur, E., & Litch, N. (2014). *Nutrition and diet therapy* (6th ed.). Philadelphia, PA: F. A. Davis.

Matthews, A., Haas, D. M., O'Mathúna, D. P., Dowswell, T., & Doyle, M. (2014). Interventions for nausea and vomiting in early pregnancy. *Cochrane Database of Systematic Reviews 2014*, 3, CD007575.

McIndoo, H. (2015). The best plant-based milks. *Environmental Nutrition, 38*(1), 5–6.

Medici, M., Korevaar, T. I., Visser, W. E., Visser, T. J., & Peeters, R. P. (2015). Thyroid function in pregnancy: What is normal? *Clinical chemistry, 61*(5), 704–713.

Mehta, N., Chen, K., Hardy, E., & Powrie, R. (2015). Respiratory disease in pregnancy. *Best Practice & Research Clinical Obstetrics & Gynecology, 29*(5), 598–611.

Myers, K. M., Feltovich, H., Mazza, E., Vink, J., Bajka, M., Wapner, R. J., et al. (2015). The mechanical role of the cervix in pregnancy. *Journal of Biomechanics, 48*(9), 1511–1523.

Nas, K., Breyer, H., & Tuu, L. (2015). The role of tailored treatment on conception and pregnancy at patients with insulin resistance. *Endocrine Abstracts, 37*. doi: 10.1530/endoabs.37.EP189.

Neifeld, R. (2015) Gluten free for the gluten tolerant during pregnancy. *BabyMed*. Retrieved from http://www.babymed.com/food-and-nutrition/gluten-free-gluten-tolerant-during-pregnancy

Nelson, R. (2015). To eat fish or not to eat fish. *American Journal of Nursing, 115*(2), 18–19.

Ojha, S., Fainberg, H. P., Sebert, S., Budge, H., & Symonds, M. E. (2015). Maternal health and eating habits: Metabolic consequences and impact on child health. *Trends in Molecular Medicine, 21*(2), 126–133.

Osol, G., & Moore, L. G. (2014). Maternal uterine vascular remodeling during pregnancy. *Microcirculation, 21*(1), 38–47.

Pearce, E. N. (2015). Thyroid disorders during pregnancy and postpartum. *Best Practice & Research Clinical Obstetrics & Gynecology, 29*(5), 700–706.

Pellegrini, N., & Agostoni, C. (2015). Nutritional aspects of gluten-free products. *Journal of the Science of Food and Agriculture, 95*(12), 2380–2385.

Piccoli, G., Clari, R., Vigotti, F., Leone, F., Attini, R., Cabiddu, G., et al. (2015). Vegan-vegetarian diets in pregnancy: Danger or panacea? A systematic narrative review. *BJOG: An International Journal of Obstetrics & Gynecology, 122*(5), 623–633..

Pope, E., Maltepe, C., & Koren, G. (2015). Comparing pyridoxine and doxylamine succinate-pyridoxine HCl for nausea and vomiting of pregnancy: A matched, controlled cohort study. *Journal of Clinical Pharmacology, 55*(7), 809–814.

Qurrat-ul-Ain, & Khan, S. A. (2015). Artificial sweeteners: safe or unsafe? *JPMA. The Journal of the Pakistan Medical Association, 65*(2), 225–227.

Rossier, B. C., Baker, M. E., & Studer, R. A. (2015). Epithelial sodium transport and its control by aldosterone: The story of our internal environment revisited. *Physiological Reviews, 95*(1), 297–340.

Rubin, R. (1984). *Maternal identity and the maternal experience*. New York, NY: Springer.

Sabina, S., Iftequar, S., Zaheer, Z., Khan, M. M., & Khan, S. (2015). An overview of anemia in pregnancy. *Journal of Innovations in Pharmaceuticals and Biological Sciences, 2*(2), 144–151.

Samra-Latif, O. M. (2015). Vulvovaginitis. *eMedicine*. Retrieved from http://emedicine.medscape.com/article/2188931-overview#a0101

Schummers, L., Hutcheon, J. A., Bodnar, L. M., Lieberman, E., & Himes, K. P. (2015). Risk of adverse pregnancy outcomes by prepregnancy body mass index: A population-based study to inform prepregnancy weight loss counseling. *Obstetrics & Gynecology, 125*(1), 133–143.

Sharma, A. J., Vesco, K. K., Bulkley, J., Callaghan, W. M., Bruce, F. C., Staab, J., et al. (2015). Associations of gestational weight gain with preterm birth among underweight and normal weight women. *Maternal and Child Health Journal, 19*(9), 2066-2073.

Shields, A. D. (2015). Pregnancy diagnosis. *eMedicine.* Retrieved from http://emedicine.medscape.com/article/262591-overview

Storck, S. (2015). Eating right during pregnancy. *MedlinePlus.* Retrieved from http://www.nlm.nih.gov/medlineplus/ency/patientinstructions/000584.htm

Szilagyi, A. (2015). Adult lactose digestion status and effects on disease. *Canadian Journal of Gastroenterology & Hepatology, 29*(3), 149–156.

Thadhani, R. I., & Maynard, S. E. (2015). Renal and urinary physiology in normal pregnancy. *UpToDate.* Retrieved from http://www.uptodate.com/contents/renal-and-urinary-tract-physiology-in-normal-pregnancy

Tharpe, N. L., Farley, C. L., & Jordan, R. (2016). *Clinical practice guidelines for midwifery & women's health* (5th ed.). Sudbury, MA: Jones & Bartlett.

Tretti Clementoni, M., & Lavagno, R. (2015). A novel 1565 nm non-ablative fractional device for stretch marks: A preliminary report. *Journal of Cosmetic and Laser Therapy, 17*(3), 148–155.

Trivedi, S., Lal, N., & Singhal, R. (2015). Periodontal diseases and pregnancy. *Journal of Orofacial Sciences, 7*(1), 67–68.

Trupin, S. R. (2015). Common pregnancy complaints and questions. *eMedicine.* Retrieved from http://emedicine.medscape.com/article/259724-overview

Tyler, K. H. (2015). Physiological skin changes during pregnancy. *Clinical Obstetrics and Gynecology, 58*(1), 119–124.

U.S. Department of Agriculture [USDA]. (2015). *Health and nutrition information for pregnant and breastfeeding women.* Retrieved from http://www.choosemyplate.gov/pregnancy-breastfeeding/pregnancy-nutritional-needs.html

U.S. Department of Agriculture [USDA] & U.S. Department of Health and Human Services [USDHHS]. (2015). *Dietary guidelines for Americans, 2015* (8th ed.). Retrieved from http://www.health.gov/dietaryguidelines/2015.asp

U.S. Food and Drug Administration [FDA]. (2015). *What you need to know about mercury in fish and shellfish.* Retrieved from http://www.fda.gov/food/resourcesforyou/consumers/ucm110591.htm

U.S. Preventive Services Task Force [USPSTF]. (2015) *Folic acid for the prevention of neural tube defects: U.S. Preventive Services Task Force recommendation statement.* Retrieved from http://www.ahrq.gov/clinic/pocketgd1011/gcp10 s2.htm

Walsh, J. M., & McAuliffe, F. M. (2015). Impact of maternal nutrition on pregnancy outcome–Does it matter what pregnant women eat? *Best Practice & Research Clinical Obstetrics & Gynecology, 29*(1), 63–78.

Zinaman, M. J., Johnson, S., & Marriott, L. (2015). Analysis of human chorionic gonadotropin levels in normal and failing pregnancies [40]. *Obstetrics & Gynecology, 125*, 21S–22S.

CHAPTER WORKSHEET

MULTIPLE-CHOICE QUESTIONS

1. What factors would change during a pregnancy if the hormone progesterone were reduced or withdrawn?
   a. The woman's gums would become red and swollen and would bleed easily.
   b. The uterus would contract more and peristalsis would increase.
   c. Morning sickness would increase and would be prolonged.
   d. The secretion of prolactin by the pituitary gland would be inhibited.

2. Which of the following is a presumptive sign or symptom of pregnancy?
   a. Restlessness
   b. Elevated mood
   c. Urinary frequency
   d. Low backache

3. When obtaining a blood test for pregnancy, which hormone would the nurse expect the test to measure?
   a. Human chorionic gonadotropin (hCG)
   b. Human placental lactogen (hPL)
   c. Follicle-stimulating hormone (FSH)
   d. Luteinizing hormone (LH)

4. During pregnancy, which of the following should the expectant mother reduce or avoid?
   a. Raw meat or uncooked shellfish
   b. Fresh, washed fruits and vegetables
   c. Whole grains and cereals
   d. Protein and iron from meat sources

5. A feeling expressed by most women upon learning they are pregnant is:
   a. Acceptance
   b. Depression
   c. Jealousy
   d. Ambivalence

6. Reva Rubin identified four major tasks that the pregnant woman undertakes to form a mutually gratifying relationship with her infant. What is "binding in"?
   a. Ensuring safe passage through pregnancy, labor, and birth
   b. Seeking acceptance of this infant by others
   c. Seeking acceptance of self as mother to the infant
   d. Learning to give of oneself on behalf of the infant

7. A pregnant client close to term comes into the clinic for an exam. The woman complains about experiencing shortness of breath. The nurse knows that this complaint can be explained as the:
   a. Fetus is needing more oxygen now that his/her size is larger.
   b. Fundus of the uterus is high and pushing the diaphragm upwards.
   c. Woman is experiencing an allergic reaction because of high histamine levels.
   d. Oxygen partial pressure concentration is lower in the third trimester.

8. Which of the following fish should be limited in a pregnant woman's diet because of the high mercury content?
   a. Salmon
   b. Cod
   c. Shrimp
   d. Sword fish

CRITICAL THINKING EXERCISES

1. When interviewing a woman at her first prenatal visit, the nurse asks about her feelings. The woman replies, "I'm frightened and confused. I don't know whether I want to be pregnant or not. Being pregnant means changing our whole life, and now having somebody to care for all the time. I'm not sure I would be a good mother. Plus I'm a bit afraid of all the changes that would happen to my body. Is this normal? Am I okay?"
   a. How should the nurse answer this question?
   b. What specific information is needed to support the client during this pregnancy?

2. Sally, age 23, is 9 weeks pregnant. At her clinic visit she says, "I'm so tired I can barely make it home from work. Then once I'm home, I don't have the energy to make dinner." She says she is so sick in the morning that she is frequently late to work and spends much of the day in the bathroom. Sally's current lab work is within normal limits.
   a. What explanation can the nurse offer Sally about her discomforts?
   b. What interventions can the nurse offer to Sally?

3. Bringing a new infant into the family affects the siblings. What strategies can a nurse discuss when a mother asks how to deal with this?

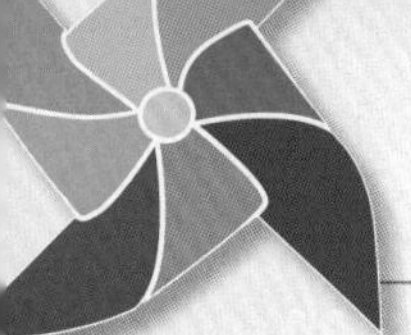

CHAPTER WORKSHEET

STUDY ACTIVITIES

1. Go to your local health department's maternity clinic and interview several women regarding their feelings and the bodily changes that have taken place since they became pregnant. Based on your findings, place them into appropriate trimesters of their pregnancy.
2. Search the Internet for information about the psychological changes that occur during pregnancy. Share information from the websites you found with your clinical group.
3. During pregnancy, the plasma volume increases by 50% but the RBC volume increases by only 25% to 33%. This disproportion is manifested as __________________.
4. When a pregnant woman in her third trimester lies on her back and experiences dizziness and light-headedness, the underlying cause of this is __________________.

BRINGING IT ALL TOGETHER: A CASE STUDY

A 22-year-old pregnant client presents to the maternity clinic with a 4-day history of loss of appetite, constipation, and abdominal pain. She is in the first trimester of her first pregnancy and came to this country recently from India. Her mother accompanies her and answers most of the questions for her daughter. After much questioning, the mother reveals that her daughter frequently eats dirt, which was common practice in her country.

Go to thePoint to find questions to consider about this case.

12

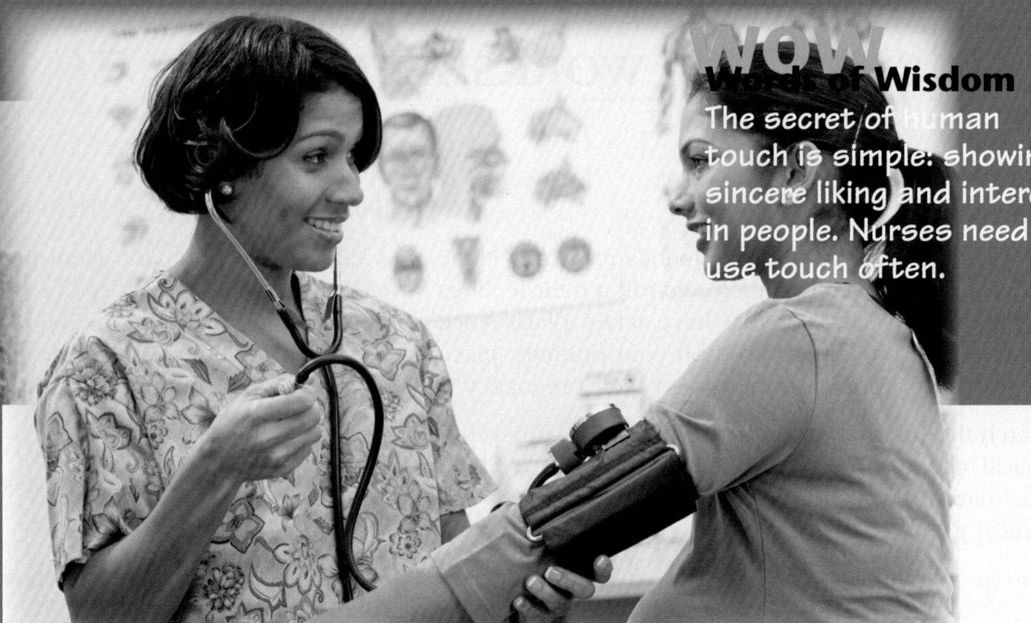
WOW
Words of Wisdom
The secret of human touch is simple: showing a sincere liking and interest in people. Nurses need to use touch often.

Nursing Management During Pregnancy

KEY TERMS

alpha-fetoprotein
amniocentesis
biophysical profile (BPP)
chorionic villus sampling (CVS)
gravida
high-risk pregnancy
linea nigra
natural childbirth
para
perinatal education
preconception care

Learning Objectives

Upon completion of the chapter, you will be able to:

1. Relate the information typically collected at the initial prenatal visit.
2. Determine an appropriate reproductive life plan based on a couple's risk profile.
3. Select the assessments completed at follow-up prenatal visits.
4. Evaluate the tests used to assess maternal and fetal well-being, including nursing management for each.
5. Outline appropriate nursing management to promote maternal self-care and to minimize the common discomforts of pregnancy.
6. Examine the key components of perinatal education.

***Linda and her husband, Rob*, are eager to start a family within the next year. They are stable in their careers and financially secure. They decide to investigate a new nurse-midwife practice associated with the local hospital, and they go for a preconception appointment. They leave their appointment overwhelmed with all the information they were given about having a healthy pregnancy.**

INTRODUCTION

Pregnancy is a time of many physiologic and psychological changes that can positively or negatively affect the woman, her fetus, and her family. Misconceptions, inadequate information, and unanswered questions about pregnancy, birth, and parenthood are common. The ultimate goal of any pregnancy is the birth of a healthy newborn, and nurses play a major role in helping the pregnant woman and her partner achieve this goal. Ongoing assessment and education are essential.

This chapter describes the nursing management required during pregnancy. It begins with a brief discussion of **preconception care** and then describes the assessment of the woman at the first prenatal visit and on follow-up visits. The chapter discusses tests commonly used to assess maternal and fetal well-being, including specific nursing management related to each test. The chapter also identifies important strategies to minimize the common discomforts of pregnancy and promote self-care. Finally, the chapter discusses **perinatal education**, including childbirth education, birthing options, health care provider options, preparation for breast-feeding or bottle-feeding, and final preparation for labor and birth.

PRECONCEPTION CARE

Ideally, couples thinking about having a child should schedule a visit with their health care provider for preconception counseling to ensure that they are in the best possible state of health before pregnancy. Preconception care is the promotion of the health and well-being of a woman and her partner before pregnancy. The goal of preconception care is to identify and modify biomedical, behavioral, and social risks to a woman's health or pregnancy outcome through prevention and management interventions (Centers for Disease Control and Prevention [CDC], 2015a).

Preconception care is advocated throughout the world as a tool for improving perinatal outcomes. Preconception care should occur any time a health care provider sees a woman of reproductive age. Primary care for all women of childbearing age by nurses should include a routine assessment of a woman's reproductive goals and planning. Women who could potentially become pregnant should be assessed for preconception risks and educated about the importance of maternal health in ensuring healthy pregnancies. Women may be motivated to address modified health risks by learning about the way their present health will affect a future pregnancy. For women not intending a pregnancy soon, preconception care should focus on contraception counseling (Callegari, Ma, & Schwartz, 2015). Personal and family history, physical examination, laboratory screening, reproductive plan, nutrition, supplements, weight, exercise, vaccinations, and injury prevention should be reviewed in all women. Encourage folic acid 400 to 800 mcg per day depending on risk profile, as well as proper diet and exercise. Women should receive the influenza vaccine if planning pregnancy during flu season; the rubella and varicella vaccines if there is no evidence of immunity to these viruses; and tetanus/diphtheria/pertussis if lacking adult vaccination. Offer specific interventions to reduce morbidity and mortality for both the woman who has been identified with chronic diseases or exposed to teratogens or illicit substances and her baby. Several interventions have been proven to effectively improve pregnancy outcome when provided as preconception care. Recent research suggests that events that occur in the uterine decidua, even before a woman knows she is pregnant, may have a significant impact on fetal growth and the outcome of pregnancy. In addition, an intact immune system optimizes placental development and function and is essential for fetal survival (Regal, Gilbert, & Burwick, 2015). New insights reveal that the early embryo is extremely sensitive to signals from gametes, trophoblastic tissue, and periconception maternal lifestyles. Also, environmental factors prior to and after conception have an enormous impact on the developing embryo and cause long-term health problems. There is a growing body of evidence that environmental factors during embryonic development can cause irreversible alteration in epigenetic markers and induce various adult diseases, such as cardiovascular, neurologic, and metabolic disorders later in life (Keytash, Jones, & Frances, 2015). With this in mind, shifting the focus on the periconception period and the very early stages of pregnancy should offer significant benefits to the health of both the mother and her infant. The overall aim should be to effectively use every pregnancy as the health care opportunity of two lifetimes (Steeggers-Theunissen & Steegers, 2015).

The CDC (2015b) formulated 10 guidelines for preconception care (Box 12.1).

Risk Factors for Adverse Pregnancy Outcomes

Preconception care is just as important as prenatal care to reduce adverse pregnancy outcomes such as maternal and infant mortality, preterm births, and low-birth-weight infants. Adverse pregnancy outcomes constitute a major public health challenge: 13% of infants are born premature; 8.3% are born with low birth weight; 1 in 33 live births have major birth defects; and 32% of women suffer pregnancy complications (CDC, 2015c). Risk factors for these adverse pregnancy outcomes are prevalent among women of reproductive age, as demonstrated by the following statistics:

- 10% of women smoke during pregnancy, contributing to fetal addiction to nicotine.

BOX 12.1

TEN GUIDELINES FOR PRECONCEPTION CARE

- **Recommendation 1.** Individual responsibility across the life span: Each woman, man, and couple should be encouraged to have a reproductive life plan.
- **Recommendation 2.** Consumer awareness: Increase public awareness of the importance of preconception health behaviors and preconception care services by using information and tools appropriate across various ages; literacy, including health literacy; and cultural/linguistic contexts.
- **Recommendation 3.** Preventive visits: As a part of primary care visits, provide risk assessment and educational and health promotion counseling to all women of childbearing age to reduce reproductive risks and improve pregnancy outcomes.
- **Recommendation 4.** Interventions for identified risks: Increase the proportion of women who receive interventions as follow-up to preconception risk screening, focusing on high-priority interventions (i.e., those with evidence of effectiveness and greatest potential impact).
- **Recommendation 5.** Interconception care: Use the interconception period to provide additional intensive interventions to women who have had a previous pregnancy that ended in an adverse outcome (i.e., infant death, fetal loss, birth defects, low birth weight, or preterm birth).
- **Recommendation 6.** Prepregnancy checkup: Offer, as a component of maternity care, one prepregnancy visit for couples and persons planning pregnancy.
- **Recommendation 7.** Health insurance coverage for women with low incomes: Increase public and private health insurance coverage for women with low incomes to improve access to preventive women's health and preconception and interconception care.
- **Recommendation 8.** Public health programs and strategies: Integrate components of preconception health into existing local public health and related programs, including emphasis on interconception interventions for women with previous adverse outcomes.
- **Recommendation 9.** Research: Increase the evidence base and promote the use of the evidence to improve preconception health.
- **Recommendation 10.** Monitoring improvements: Maximize public health surveillance and related research mechanisms to monitor preconception health.

Adapted from Centers for Disease Control and Prevention. (2015b). *Preconception care recommendations.* Retrieved from http://www.cdc.gov/preconception/hcp/recommendations.html

- 7.6% consume alcohol during pregnancy, leading to fetal alcohol spectrum disorder.
- 70% of women do not take folic acid supplements, increasing the risk of neural tube defects in the newborn. Taking folic acid reduces the incidence of neural tube defects by two thirds.
- 35% of women starting a pregnancy are obese, which may increase their risk of developing hypertension, diabetes, and thromboembolic disease and may increase the need for cesarean birth.
- 3% take prescription or over-the-counter drugs that are known teratogens (substances harmful to the developing fetus).
- 5% of women have pre-existing medical conditions that can negatively affect pregnancy if unmanaged (CDC, 2015d).

All of the preceding factors pose risks to pregnancy and could be addressed with early interventions if the woman seeks preconception health care. Specific recognized risk factors for adverse pregnancy outcomes that fall into one or more of these categories are listed in Box 12.2.

The period of greatest environmental sensitivity and consequent risk for the developing embryo is between days 17 and 56 after conception. The first prenatal visit, which is usually a month or later after a missed menstrual period, may occur too late to affect reproductive outcomes associated with abnormal organogenesis secondary to poor lifestyle choices. In some cases, such as with unplanned pregnancies, women may delay seeking health care because they deny that they are pregnant. Thus, commonly used prevention practices may begin too late to avert the morbidity and mortality associated with congenital anomalies and low birth weight. A more global preventative strategy is needed to reduce the high rates of pregnancy complications in all populations. Securing international level political priority for maternal and newborn care remains critical to accomplish the goal of better health for all families. All couples should take on the responsibility of developing their reproductive life plan and share it with their health care providers at office visits (Darmstadt, Shiffman, & Lawn, 2015).

What is the purpose of couples like Linda and Rob going for preconception counseling? What are the goals of preconception care for this couple? What psychologic support can be offered by the nurse to this couple at this stage?

Nursing Management

In the United States, rates of maternal mortality, unintended pregnancies, low birth weight and preterm infants continue to rise, making the need for preconception care a priority for all nurses. Traditionally, women have thought that preconception care is a single visit made before getting pregnant; however, the maximum benefits are obtained when the woman and her partner receive care throughout her reproductive years. The nurse's role is vital in identifying risk factors and encouraging healthier behaviors that potentially improve maternal and

BOX 12.2

RISK FACTORS FOR ADVERSE PREGNANCY OUTCOMES

- **Isotretinoins**. Use of isotretinoins (e.g., Accutane®) in pregnancy to treat acne can result in high risk of congenital malformations which may include craniofacial, cardiac, and central nervous systems injuries. It is contraindicated in pregnancy
- **Alcohol misuse.** No time during pregnancy is safe to drink alcohol, and harm can occur early, before a woman has realized that she is or might be pregnant. Fetal alcohol syndrome and other alcohol-related birth defects can be prevented if women cease intake of alcohol before conception.
- **Antiepileptic drugs.** Certain antiepileptic drugs are known teratogens (e.g., valproic acid). Recommendations suggest that before conception, women who are on a regimen of these drugs and who are contemplating pregnancy should be prescribed a lower dosage of these drugs.
- **Diabetes (preconception).** The threefold increase in the prevalence of birth defects among infants of women with type 1 and type 2 diabetes is substantially reduced through proper management of diabetes.
- **Folic acid deficiency.** Daily use of vitamin supplements containing folic acid (400 mcg) has been demonstrated to reduce the occurrence of neural tube defects by two thirds.
- **Hepatitis B.** Vaccination is recommended for men and women who are at risk for acquiring hepatitis B virus (HBV) infection. Preventing HBV infection in women of childbearing age prevents transmission of infection to infants and eliminates risk to the woman of HBV infection and sequelae, including hepatic failure, liver carcinoma, cirrhosis, and death.
- **HIV/AIDS.** If HIV infection is identified before conception, timely antiretroviral treatment can be administered, and women (or couples) can be given additional information that can help prevent mother-to-child transmission.
- **Rubella seronegativity.** Rubella vaccination provides protective seropositivity and prevents congenital rubella syndrome.
- **Obesity.** Adverse perinatal outcomes associated with maternal obesity include neural tube defects, preterm delivery, diabetes, cesarean section, and hypertensive and thromboembolic disease. Appropriate weight loss and nutritional intake before pregnancy reduce these risks.
- **STIs.** *Chlamydia trachomatis* and *Neisseria gonorrhoeae* have been strongly associated with ectopic pregnancy, infertility, and chronic pelvic pain. STIs during pregnancy might result in fetal death or substantial physical and developmental disabilities, including intellectual disability and blindness. Early screening and treatment prevents these adverse outcomes.
- **Smoking.** Preterm birth, low birth weight, and other adverse perinatal outcomes associated with maternal smoking in pregnancy can be prevented if women stop smoking before or during early pregnancy. Because only 20% of women successfully control tobacco dependency during pregnancy, cessation of smoking is recommended before pregnancy.

Adapted from Centers for Disease Control and Prevention [CDC]. (2015a). *Preconception care and health care.* Retrieved from http://www.cdc.gov/preconception/hcp/; March of Dimes. (2015a). *Pregnancy complications.* Retrieved from http://www.marchofdimes.com/pregnancy/pregnancy-complications.aspx; National Institutes of Health [NIH] (2015). *Health problems in pregnancy.* Retrieved from http://www.nlm.nih.gov/medlineplus/healthproblemsinpregnancy.html; and Senie, R. T. (2014). *Epidemiology of women's health.* Burlington, MA: Jones & Bartlett Learning.

perinatal outcomes. Preconception care involves obtaining a complete health history and physical examination of the woman and her partner. Key areas include:

- Immunization status of the woman
- Underlying medical conditions, such as cardiovascular and respiratory problems or genetic disorders
- Reproductive health data, such as pelvic examinations, use of contraceptives, and sexually transmitted infections (STIs)
- Sexuality and sexual practices, such as safer-sex practices and body image issues
- Nutrition history and present status
- Lifestyle practices, including occupation and recreational activities
- Psychosocial issues such as levels of stress and exposure to abuse and violence
- Medication and drug use, including use of tobacco, alcohol, over-the-counter and prescription medications, and illicit drugs
- Support system, including family, friends, and community

Figure 12.1 gives a sample preconception screening tool.

This information provides a foundation for planning health promotion activities and education. For example, to have a positive impact on the pregnancy:

- Ensure that the woman's immunizations are up to date.
- Create a reproductive life plan to address and outline their reproductive needs.
- Take a thorough history of both partners to identify any medical or genetic conditions that need treatment or a referral to specialists.
- Identify history of STIs and high-risk sexual practices so they can be modified.
- Complete a dietary history combined with nutritional counseling.
- Gather information regarding exercise and lifestyle practices to encourage daily exercise for well-being and weight maintenance.
- Stress the importance of taking folic acid to prevent neural tube defects.

PRECONCEPTION SCREENING AND COUNSELING CHECKLIST

NAME | BIRTHPLACE | AGE

DATE: / / ARE YOU PLANNING TO GET PREGNANT IN THE NEXT SIX MONTHS? ___ Y ___N

IF YOUR ANSWER TO A QUESTION IS YES, PUT A CHECK MARK ON THE LINE IN FRONT OF THE QUESTION. FILL IN OTHER INFORMATION THAT APPLIES TO YOU.

DIET AND EXERCISE

What do you consider a healthy weight for you?_________
___Do you eat three meals a day?
___Do you follow a special diet (vegetarian, diabetic, other)?
___Which do you drink (__ coffee __ tea __ cola __ milk __ water __ soda/pop other_________________________)?
___Do you eat raw or undercooked food (meat, other)?
___Do you take folic acid?
___Do you take other vitamins daily (__ multivitamin __ vitamin A __ other)?
___Do you take dietary supplements (__ black cohosh __ pennyroyal __ other)?
___Do you have current/past problems withh eating disorders?
___Do you exercise? Type/frequency:_________

Notes:

LIFESTYLE

___Do you smoke cigarettes or use other tobacco products?
How many cigarettes/packs a day?__________
___Are you exposed to second-hand smoke?
___Do you drink alcohol?
What kind?_________How often?_________How much?_________
___Do you use recreational drugs (cocaine, heroin, ecstasy, meth/ice, other?
List:
___Do you see a dentist regularly?
What kind of work do you do?__________
___Do you work or live near possible hazards (chemicals, x-ray or other radiation, lead)? List:__________________
___Do you use saunas or hot tubs?

Notes:

MEDICATION /DRUGS

___Are you taking prescribed drugs (Accutane, valproic acid, blood thinners)? List them__________
___Are you taking non-prescribed drugs?
List them:__________________
___Are you using birth control pills?
___Do you get injectable contraceptives or shots for birth control?
___Do you use any herbal remedies or alternative medicine?
List:__________________

NOTES:

MEDICAL/FAMILY HISTORY

Do you have or have you ever had:
___Epilepsy?
___Diabetes?
___Asthma?
___High blood pressure?
___Heart disease?
___Anemia?
___Kidney or bladder disorders?
___Thyroid disease?
___Chickenpox?
___Hepatitis C?
___Digestive problems?
___Depression or other mental health problem?
___Surgeries?
___Lupus?
___Scleroderma?
___Other conditions?

Have you ever been vaccinated for:
___Measles, mumps, rubella?
___Hepatitis B?
___Chickenpox?

NOTES:

WOMEN'S HEALTH

___Do you have any problems with your menstrual cycle?
___How many times have you been pregnant?
What was/ were the outcomes(s)?__________________
___Did you have difficulty getting pregnant last time?
___Have you been treated for infertility?
Have you had surgery on your uterus, cervix, ovaries, or tubes?
___Did you mother take the hormone DES during pregnancy?
Have you ever had HPV, genital warts or chlamydia?
___Have you ever been treated for a sexually transmitted infection (genital herpes, gonorrhea, syphilis, HIV/AIDS, other)? List:__________

NOTES:

GENETICS

Does your family have a history of Or Your partner's family
___Hemophilia? ___
___Other bleeding disorders? ___
___Tay-Sachs disease? ___
___Blood diseases (sickle cell, thalassemia, other)? ___
___Muscular dystrophy? ___
___Down syndrome/mental retardation? ___
___Cystic fibrosis? ___
___Birth defects (spine/heart/kidney)? ___

Your ethnic background is:__________________
Your partner's ethnic background is:__________________

NOTES:

HOME ENVIRONMENT

___Do you feel emotionally supported at home?
___Do you have help from relatives or friends if needed?
___Do you feel you have serious money/financial worries?
___Are you in a stable relationship?
___Do you feel safe at home?
___Does anyone threaten or physically hurt you?
___Do you have pets (cats, rodents, exotic animals)? List:__________
___Do have any contact with soil, cat litter, or sandboxes?

Baby preparation (if planning pregnancy):
___Do you have a place for a baby to sleep?
___Do you need any baby items?

NOTES:

OTHER

IS THERE ANYTHING ELSE YOU'D LIKE ME TO KNOW?

ARE THERE ANY QUESTIONS YOU'D LIKE TO ASK ME?

FIGURE 12.1 Sample preconception screening tool. (Used with permission. Copyright March of Dimes.)

- Urge the woman to achieve optimal weight before a pregnancy.
- Identify work environment and any needed changes to promote health.
- Address substance use issues, including smoking and drugs.
- Identify victims of violence and assist them to get help.
- Manage chronic conditions such as diabetes and asthma.
- Educate the couple about environmental hazards, including metals and herbs.
- Offer genetic counseling to identify carriers.
- Suggest the availability of support systems, if needed (Hurst & Linton, 2015; Templeton, 2015).

Nurses can act as advocates and educators, creating healthy, supportive communities for women and their partners in the childbearing phases of their lives. It is important to enter into a collaborative partnership with the woman and her partner, enabling them to examine their own health and its influence on the health of their future baby. Provide information to allow the woman and her partner to make an informed decision about having a baby, but keep in mind that this decision rests solely with the couple.

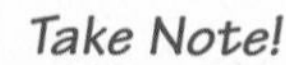

Take Note!

Because all women of reproductive age, from menarche to menopause, benefit from preventive care, preconception care should be an integral part of that continuum (Boggess & Berggren, 2015).

Linda and Rob **decide to change several aspects of their lifestyle and nutritional habits before conceiving a baby, based on advice from the nurse-midwife. They both want to lose weight, stop smoking, and increase their intake of fruits and vegetables. How will these lifestyle and dietary changes benefit Linda's future pregnancy? What other areas might need to be brought up to date to prepare for a future pregnancy?**

THE FIRST PRENATAL VISIT

Once a pregnancy is suspected and, in some cases, tentatively confirmed by a home pregnancy test, the woman should seek prenatal care to promote a healthy outcome. Although the most opportune window (preconception) for improving pregnancy outcomes may be missed, appropriate nursing management starting at conception and continuing throughout the pregnancy can have a positive impact on the health of pregnant women and their unborn children.

The assessment process begins at this initial prenatal visit and continues throughout the pregnancy. The initial visit is an ideal time to screen for factors that might place the woman and her fetus at risk for problems such as preterm delivery. The initial visit also is an optimal time to begin educating the client about changes that will affect her life.

Prenatal care can be delivered in one of two methods: individually or in a group format termed *centering*. The first method is the traditional model whereby a pregnant woman sees her health care provider at specified interims throughout her pregnancy and all visits occur on a one-to-one basis. The centering pregnancy model of group prenatal care involves groups of up to a dozen women in similar gestational ages meeting with their health care provider for 10 sessions of approximately 1.5 to 2 hours each. The centering group method has been theorized to produce better birth outcomes than traditional individually delivered prenatal care due to increased client–provider interaction, increased social support, and greater perceived empowerment (Tracy, 2014). See Evidence-Based Practice 12.1.

The International Association of Diabetes and Pregnancy Study Groups (IADPSG) recently issued recommendations on the diagnosis and classification of hyperglycemia in pregnancy. Specific recommendations for diagnosing hyperglycemic disorders in pregnancy include the following:

- At the *first prenatal visit,* measure fasting plasma glucose, HbA1c, or random plasma glucose of all women or all high-risk women based on her risk factors, weight status, and family history. Thresholds for diagnosis of overt diabetes during pregnancy are shown in Box 12.3.
- If glucose testing is not diagnostic of overt diabetes, the woman should be tested for gestational diabetes from 24 to 28 weeks of gestation with a 2-hour 75-g oral glucose tolerance test (American Diabetes Association [ADA], 2015).

Given our society's poor food choices, sedentary tendencies, obesity, increasing life stresses, and the increasing immigration of high-risk populations (Hispanic, African American, Southeast Asian, Arab, Afro-Caribbean, Mediterranean, and Native American), the incidence of gestational diabetes is growing. The American College of Obstetricians and Gynecologists (ACOG),

BOX 12.3

THRESHOLDS FOR DIAGNOSIS OF OVERT DIABETES DURING PREGNANCY

The thresholds for the diagnosis of overt diabetes during pregnancy are:

- Fasting plasma glucose: 126 mg/dL
- Hemoglobin A1c level: at least 6.5%
- Random plasma glucose: 200 mg/dL

EVIDENCE-BASED PRACTICE 12.1 **THE EFFECTS OF CENTERING PREGNANCY GROUP PRENATAL CARE ON GESTATIONAL AGE, BIRTH WEIGHT, AND FETAL DEMISE**

STUDY

Although rates of infant mortality in the United States have declined over the last several decades, rates of preterm births (<27 weeks' gestation) and low birth weight (<2,500 g) have increased. Access to quality prenatal care has demonstrated improvement of maternal and child outcomes, and may help reduce infant mortality, preterm birth, and low weight infants. The centering group prenatal care model has been theorized to produce better birth outcomes than traditional individually delivered prenatal care due to increased patient–provider interaction, increased social support, greater perceived empowerment, and increased exposure to useful skills and information about pregnancy, birthing, and childcare.

This study compared birth outcomes for women who received two different forms of prenatal care. The objective of this study was to examine the effects of centering prenatal care versus individually delivered prenatal care on gestational age, birth weight, and fetal demise. Samples of 6,155 women were divided into two groups—individual prenatal care and group prenatal care at five sites. The sample included women who received prenatal care at one of five sites that offered both individual and group prenatal care.

Findings

Results indicated that women in the centering pregnancy group prenatal care, compared with women in traditional individually delivered prenatal care, had significantly longer gestational ages (b = 0.35, 95% CI [0.29, 0.41]) and higher overall birth weights (b = 28.6, 95% CI [4.8, 52.3]). Results also indicated that group delivered prenatal care was associated with significantly and substantially lower odds of very low birth weight and fetal demise.

Nursing Implications

At present there is support to provide centering group prenatal care where possible according to guidelines. The results indicated largely beneficial effects of group prenatal care on women's birth outcomes. Health policy reforms aimed at reducing adverse birth outcomes may consider group prenatal care a promising alternative format for delivering prenatal care. Nurses should continue to encourage all women to obtain prenatal care (group or traditional) as part of their reproductive plan to enhance the outcomes of their pregnancy and all of their future children. Given the evidence of beneficial effects of centering group prenatal care and the cost implications of widespread implementation will be critical for informing state and local health policies aimed at improving maternal and perinatal health outcomes.

Adapted from Tanner-Smith, E., Steinka-Fry, K., & Lipsey, M. (2014). The effects of centering pregnancy group prenatal care on gestational age, birth weight, and fetal demise. *Maternal & Child Health Journal, 18*(4), 801–809.

the American Diabetes Association (ADA), and the World Health Organization have all recommended screening at the first prenatal visit for women who are over 25 years old, overweight, have polycystic ovary syndrome, history of gestational diabetes, and a positive family history of diabetes (Satyan et al., 2015). Global guidelines for screening, diagnosis, and classification have been established, and offer the potential to stop the cycle of diabetes and obesity caused by hyperglycemia in pregnancy. Normoglycemia is the goal in all aspects of pregnancy and offers the benefits of decreased short-term and long-term complications of diabetes.

Counseling and education of the pregnant woman and her partner are critical to ensure healthy outcomes for mother and her infant. Pregnant women and their partners frequently have questions, misinformation, or misconceptions about what to eat, weight gain, physical discomforts, drug and alcohol use, sexuality, and the birthing process. The nurse needs to allow time to answer questions and provide anticipatory guidance during the pregnancy and to make appropriate community referrals to meet the needs of these clients. To address these issues and foster the overall well-being of pregnant women and their fetuses, specific national health goals have been established (see *Healthy People 2020*).

Comprehensive Health History

During the initial visit, a comprehensive health history is obtained, including age, menstrual history, prior obstetric history, past medical and surgical history, psychological screening, family history, genetic screening, dietary habits, lifestyle and health practices, medication or drug use, and history of exposure to STIs (Moses, 2015a). Often, use of a prenatal history form (Fig. 12.2) is the best way to document the data collected (Evidence-Based Practice 12.2.)

The initial health history typically includes questions about three major areas: the reason for seeking care; the client's past medical, surgical, and personal history, including that of the family and her partner; and the client's reproductive history. During the history-taking process, the nurse and client establish the foundation of a trusting relationship and jointly develop a plan of

(text continues on page 404)

HEALTHY PEOPLE 2020

Objective	Nursing Significance
MICH-10 Increase the proportion of pregnant women who receive early and adequate prenatal care by 10% over *HP 2010* goal.	Will contribute to reduced rates of perinatal illness, disability, and death by helping to identify possible risk factors and implementing measures to lessen these factors that contribute to poor outcomes
MICH-12 (Developmental) Increase the proportion of pregnant women who attend a series of prepared childbirth classes.	Will contribute to a positive birthing experience because women will be prepared for what they will face; will also help in reducing pain and anxiety
MICH-13 (Developmental) Increase the proportion of mothers who achieve a recommended weight gain during their pregnancies.	Will reduce the risks associated with weight for better perinatal outcomes for mother and infant
MICH-16 Increase the proportion of women delivering a live birth who received preconception care services and practiced key recommended preconception health behaviors: • Took multivitamins/folic acid prior to pregnancy • Did not smoke prior to pregnancy • Did not drink alcohol prior to pregnancy • (Developmental) Used contraception to plan pregnancy	The risk of maternal and infant mortality and pregnancy-related complications can be reduced by increasing access to quality preconception care. This will enhance healthy birth outcomes and early identification and treatment of health.

Adapted from U.S. Department of Health and Human Services. (2010). *Healthy People 2020*. Retrieved from http://www.healthypeople.gov/2020/topicsobjectives2020/objectiveslist.aspx?topicId=26.

EVIDENCE-BASED PRACTICE 12.2 ANTENATAL DIETARY EDUCATION AND SUPPLEMENTATION TO INCREASE ENERGY AND PROTEIN INTAKE

STUDY

Gestational weight gain is positively associated with fetal growth, and observational studies of food supplementation in pregnancy have reported increases in gestational weight gain and fetal growth. During pregnancy, the fetus develops based on the nutrition of the mother. Inadequate intake during pregnancy can lead to malnutrition and poor outcomes for the fetus. The objective of this study was to assess the effects of education during pregnancy to increase energy and protein intake, or of actual energy and protein supplementation, on energy and protein intake, and the effect on maternal and infant health outcomes.

Findings

The review included 17 randomized controlled trials, involving 9,030 women. Four main findings included (1) providing nutritional advice resulted in an increase in the mother's protein intake with resulting fewer preterm births and low birth weights; (2) giving mothers balanced energy and protein supplements was associated with fewer infants dying during labor and infants had an increase in birth weights; (3) high protein supplementation showed no benefit for women and potential harm for the infant with more becoming small for gestational age at birth; and (4) isocaloric protein supplementations showed no benefit for higher birth weight in the infant and weekly gestational gain for the mothers.

Nursing Implications

This review provides encouraging evidence that prenatal nutritional education with the aim of increasing energy and protein intake in the maternal population appears to be effective in reducing the risk of preterm birth, low birth weight, increasing head circumference at birth, increasing birth weight among undernourished women, and increasing protein intake. There remains question about high protein supplementation being beneficial. Nurses can continue to provide good sound evidence-based nutritional education to their pregnant clients to bring about healthy outcomes.

Adapted from Ota, E., Hori, H., Mori, R., Tobe-Gai, R., & Farrar, D. (2015). Antenatal dietary education and supplementation to increase energy and protein intake. *Cochrane Database of Systematic Reviews, 6*, CD000032.

Health History Summary

Maternal/Newborn Record System

Page 1 of 2

Patient's name ______

ID. No. ______

Demographic data

Date of birth ______ Age ____ Language ☐ English ☐ ______ Interpreter ☐ None ☐ ______

Religion ☐ N/A ☐ ______ Race/ethnicity ______

Marital status S M SEP D W Name of baby's father ______

Education	Occupation	Full	Part	Self	Unemp	Work Tel No	Home Tel No
Patient		☐	☐	☐	☐		
Father of baby		☐	☐	☐	☐		

Allergy/sensitivity

☐ **None** ☐ **Latex**

☐ Other ______

Primary/referring physician

Menstrual history	Menarche yrs	Interval days	Length days	Abnormalities ☐ None

LMP ___/___/___ Certain ☐ Yes ☐ No Normal ☐ Yes ☐ No Positive pregnancy test ___/___/___ ☐ Blood ☐ Urine

EDD By dates ___/___/___ By ultrasound ___/___/___ Date of ultrasound ___/___/___

Pregnancy history	Gravida	Full term	Premature	Spontaneous Ab	Induced Ab	Ectopic	Multiple births	Live

No	Month/ year	Infant sex	Weight at birth	Wks gest	Hours in labor	Type of delivery	Anesthesia	Comments/complications
1								
2								
3								
4								
5								
6								
7								

Medical history

Check and detail positive findings below. Use reference numbers.

Obstetric (Patient)

1. Anemia ______ ☐
2. Fetal/neonatal death or anomaly ______ ☐
3. Gestational diabetes ______ ☐
4. Hemorrhage ______ ☐
5. Hyperemesis ______ ☐
6. Incompetent cervix ______ ☐
7. Intrauterine growth retardation ______ ☐
8. Isoimmunization ______ ☐
9. Polyhydramnios ______ ☐
10. Postpartum depression ______ ☐
11. Pregnancy-induced hypertension ______ ☐
12. Preterm labor or birth ______ ☐
13. PROM-chorioamnionitis ______ ☐
14. Rhogam given ______ ☐
15. RH neg ______ ☐

Gynecologic

16. Contraceptive use ______ ☐
17. Abnormal PAP ______ ☐
18. Fibroids ______ ☐
19. Gyn· surgery ______ ☐

Gynecologic (cont'd.) (Patient)

20. Infertility ______ ☐
21. In utero exposure to DES ______ ☐
22. Uterine/cervical anomaly ______ ☐

Sexally transmitted diseases

23. Chlamydia ______ ☐
24. Gonorrhea ______ ☐
25. Herpes (HSV) ______ ☐
26. Syphilis ______ ☐

Vaginal/genital infections

27. Trichomonas ______ ☐
28. Condylomata ______ ☐
29. Candidiasis ______ ☐

Other infections

30. Toxoplasmosis ______ ☐
31. Group B streptococcus ______ ☐
32. Rubella or immunization ______ ☐
33. Varicella or immunization ______ ☐
34. Cytomegalovirus (CMV) ______ ☐
35. AIDS (HIV) ______ ☐
36. Hepatitis (type ______) ______ ☐ or immunization (type ______)

FIGURE 12.2 Sample prenatal history form. (Used with permission. Copyright Briggs Corporation, 2001.)

Health History Summary
Maternal/newborn record system

Page 2 of 2

Patient's name ______

ID. No. ______

Check and detail positive findings below. Use reference numbers.

Cardiovascular	Patient	Family
37. Myocardial infarction	☐	☐
38. Heart disease	☐	☐
39. Rheumatic fever	☐	
40. Valve disease	☐	
41. Chronic hypertension	☐	☐
42. Disease of the aorta	☐	☐
43. Varicosities Thrombophlebitis	☐	☐
44. Previous pulmonary embolism	☐	
45. Blood disorders	☐	☐
46. Anemia/ hemoglobinopathy	☐	☐
47. Blood transfusions	☐	
48. Other	☐	
Pulmonary		
49. Asthma	☐	
50. Tuberculosis	☐	☐
51. Chronic obstructive pulmonary disease	☐	☐
Endocrine		
52. Diabetes	☐	☐
53. Thyroid dysfunction	☐	☐
54. Maternal PKU	☐	
55. Endocrinopathy	☐	☐
56. Gastrointestinal	☐	
57. Liver disease	☐	

Renal disease	Patient	Family
58. Cystitis	☐	
59. Pyelonephritis	☐	
60. Asymptomatic bacteriuria	☐	
61. Chronic renal disease	☐	☐
62. Autoimmune disease	☐	☐
63. Cancer	☐	☐
Neurologic disease		
64. Cerebrovascular accident	☐	☐
65. Seizure disorder	☐	☐
66. Migraine headaches	☐	☐
67. Degenerative disease	☐	☐
68. Other	☐	
Psychological/surgical		
69. Psychiatric disease Mental lillness	☐	☐
70. Physical abuse or neglect	☐	☐
71. Emotional abuse or neglect	☐	☐
72. Addiction	☐	
(drug, alcohol, nicotine)	☐	☐
73. Major accidents	☐	
74. Surgery	☐	
75. Anesthetic complications	☐	
76. Non-surgical hospitalization	☐	
77. Other	☐	
78. **No known disease/problems**	☐	

Genetic history	Patient	Father of baby	Family
79. Age 35 or older (female) 50 or older (male)	☐	☐	☐
80. Cerebral palsy	☐	☐	☐
81. Cleft lip/palate	☐	☐	☐
82. Congenital anomalies	☐	☐	☐
83. Congenital heart disease	☐	☐	☐
84. Consanguinity	☐	☐	☐
85. Cystic fibrosis	☐	☐	☐
86. Down's syndrome	☐	☐	☐
87. Hemophilia	☐	☐	☐
88. Huntington's chorea	☐	☐	☐
89. Mental retardation	☐	☐	☐
90. Muscular dystrophy	☐	☐	☐
91. Neural tube defect	☐	☐	☐
92. Sickle cell disease or trait	☐	☐	☐
93. Tay-sachs disease	☐	☐	☐
94. Test for fragile X	☐	☐	☐
95. Thalassemia A or B	☐	☐	☐
96. Other	☐	☐	☐
97. Other	☐	☐	☐
98. Other	☐	☐	☐

Historical risk status ☐ **No risk factors noted**

☐ **At risk (identify)**

Signature

FIGURE 12.2 *(continued)*

care for the pregnancy. They tailor this plan to the client's lifestyle as much as possible and focus primarily on education for overall wellness during the pregnancy. The ultimate goal for the first prenatal visit is to collect baseline data about the woman and her partner and to detect any risk factors that need to be addressed to facilitate a healthy pregnancy (King et al., 2015). See *Healthy People 2020.*

Reason for Seeking Care

The woman commonly comes for prenatal care based on the suspicion that she is pregnant. She may report that she has missed her menstrual period or has had a positive result on a home pregnancy test. Ask the woman for the date of her last normal menstrual period (LMP). Also ask about any presumptive or probable signs of pregnancy that she might be experiencing. Typically a urine or blood test to check for evidence of human chorionic gonadotropin (hCG) is done to confirm the pregnancy.

Past History

Ask about the woman's past medical and surgical history. This information is important because conditions that the woman experienced in the past (e.g., urinary tract infections) may recur or be exacerbated during pregnancy. Also, chronic illnesses, such as diabetes or heart disease, can increase the risk for complications during pregnancy for the woman and her fetus. Ask about any history of allergies to medications, foods, or environmental substances. Ask about any mental health problems, such as depression or anxiety. Gather similar information about the woman's family and her partner.

The woman's personal history also is important. Ask about her occupation, possible exposure to teratogens, exercise and activity level, recreational patterns (including the use of substances such as alcohol, tobacco, and drugs), use of alternative and complementary therapies, sleep patterns, nutritional habits, and general lifestyle. Each of these may have an impact on the outcome of the pregnancy. For example, if the woman smokes during pregnancy, nicotine in the cigarettes causes vasoconstriction in the mother, leading to reduced placental perfusion. As a result, the newborn may be small for gestational age. The newborn will also go through nicotine withdrawal soon after birth. In addition, no safe level of alcohol ingestion in pregnancy has been determined. Many fetuses exposed to heavy alcohol levels during pregnancy develop fetal alcohol syndrome, a collection of deformities and disabilities.

Reproductive History

The woman's reproductive history includes a menstrual, obstetric, and gynecologic history. Typically, this history begins with a description of the woman's menstrual cycle, including her age at menarche, number of days in her cycle, typical flow characteristics, and any discomfort experienced. The use of contraception also is important, including when the woman last used any contraception.

Establishing an accurate due date is one of the most important assessments for a pregnant woman, one that has both social and medical significance. For women and their families, this estimated due date (EDD) represents the long-awaited birthday of their child and is a time frame around which many economic and social activities are planned. This end point date provides guidance for the timing of specific maternal and fetal testing throughout pregnancy, gauges fetal growth parameters, and provides well-established timelines for specific interventions in the management of prenatal complications. In fact, critical decisions, such as preterm labor management, timing of postdate induction of labor, and identification of fetal growth restriction (FGR), are all based on the presumed gestational age of the fetus, which is calculated backward from the EDD (Bond, 2015).

Ask the woman the date of her LMP to determine the estimated or EDD. Several methods may be used to estimate the date of birth. Nagele rule can be used to establish the EDD (Box 12.4). Using this rule, subtract 3 months from the month of her LMP and then add 7 days to the first day of the LMP. Then correct the year by adding 1 to it where necessary. An alternative way is to add 7 days and then add 9 months = year where needed. This date has a margin of error of plus or minus 2 weeks. For instance, if a woman reports that her LMP was October 14, 2015, you would subtract 3 months (July) and add 7 days (21), then add 1 year (2016). The woman's EDD is July 21, 2016.

Because of the normal variations in women's menstrual cycles, differences in the normal length of gestation among ethnic groups, and errors in dating methods, there is no such thing as an exact due date. In general, a birth 2 weeks before or 2 weeks after the EDD is considered normal. Nagele rule is less accurate if the woman's menstrual cycles are irregular, if the woman conceives while breast-feeding or before her regular menstrual cycle is established after childbirth, if she is ovulating

BOX 12.4

NAGELE RULE FOR CALCULATING THE ESTIMATED DUE DATE (EDD)

1. Use the first day of the last normal menstrual period	10/14/15
2. Subtract 3 from the number of months	7/14/15
3. Add 7 to the number of days	7/21/15
4. Adjust the year by adding one year	7/21/16
5. Estimated due date (+ or – 2 weeks) = July 21st 2016	

although she is amenorrheic, or after she discontinues oral contraceptives (Schuiling & Likis, 2016).

A gestational or birth calculator or wheel can also be used to calculate the due date (Fig. 12.3). Some practitioners use ultrasound to more accurately determine the gestational age and date the pregnancy. Ultrasound is typically the most accurate method of dating a pregnancy.

Typically, an obstetric history provides information about the woman's past pregnancies, including any problems encountered during the pregnancy, labor, birth, and postpartum. Such information can provide clues to problems that might develop in the current pregnancy. Some common terms used to describe and document an obstetric history include gravid, **gravida**, gravida I (primigravida), gravida II (secundigravida), multigravida, and para (Table 12.1).

Other systems may be used to document a woman's obstetric history. These systems often break down the category of para more specifically (Box 12.5).

Information about the woman's gynecologic history is important. Ask about any reproductive tract surgeries the woman has undergone. For example, surgery on the uterus may affect its ability to contract effectively during labor. A history of tubal pregnancy increases

BOX 12.5

OBSTETRIC HISTORY TERMS: GTPAL OR TPAL

G = gravida, T = term births, P = preterm births, A = abortions, L = living children

- G—the current pregnancy to be included in count
- T—the number of term gestations delivering between 38 and 42 weeks
- P—the number of preterm pregnancies ending >20 weeks or viability but before completion of 37 weeks
- A—the number of pregnancies ending before 20 weeks or viability
- L—the number of children currently living

Consider this example:

Mary Johnson is pregnant for the fourth time. She had one abortion at 8 weeks' gestation.

She has a daughter who was born at 40 weeks' gestation and a son born at 34 weeks.

Mary's obstetric history would be documented as follows:

- Using the gravida/para method: gravida 4, para 2
- Using the TPAL method: 1112 (T = 1 [daughter born at 40 weeks]; P = 1 [son born at 34 weeks]; A = 1 [abortion at 8 weeks]; L = 2 [two living children])

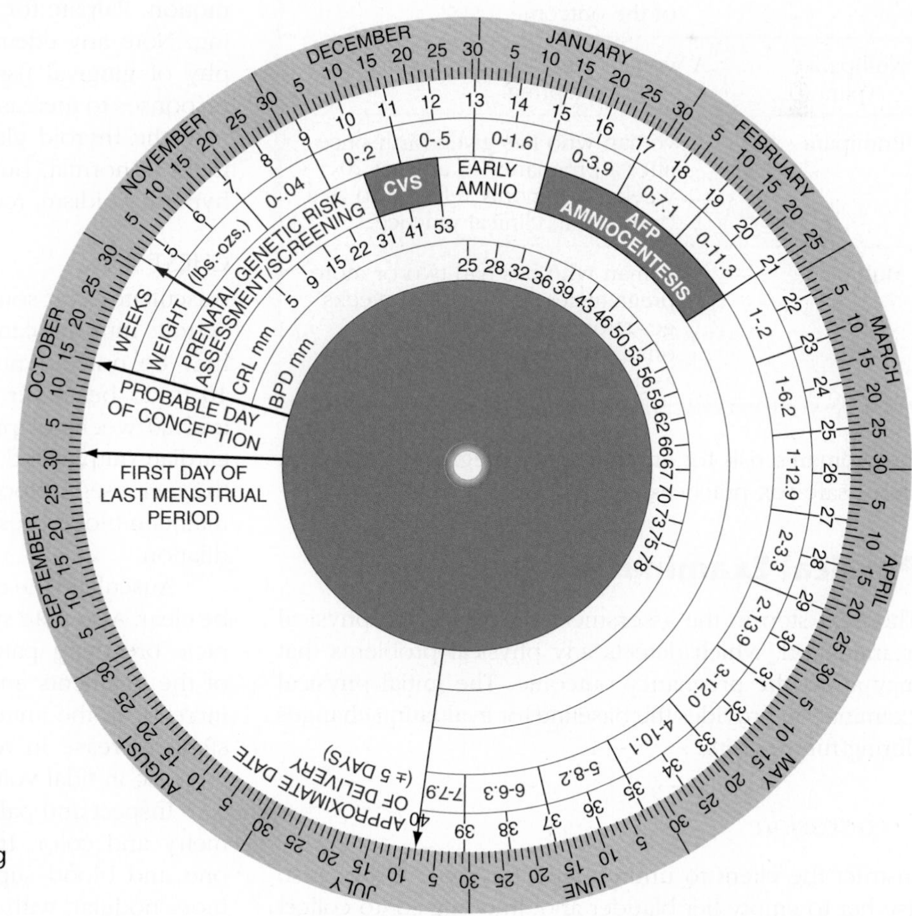

FIGURE 12.3 EDD using a birth wheel. The first day of the woman's last normal menstrual period was October 1. Using the birth wheel, her EDD would be approximately July 8 of the following year. (Used with permission. Copyright March of Dimes, 2015.)

TABLE 12.1 PREGNANCY TERMS

Term	Definition
Gravid	The state of being pregnant
Gravida/ Gravidity	The total number of times a woman has been pregnant, regardless of whether the pregnancy resulted in a termination or if multiple infants were born from a pregnancy.
Nulligravida	A woman who has never experienced pregnancy
Primigravida	A woman pregnant for the first time
Secundigravida	A woman pregnant for the second time
Multigravida	A woman pregnant for at least the third time
Para	The number of times a woman has given birth to a fetus of at least 20 gestational weeks (viable or not), counting multiple births as one birth event.
Parity	Refers to the number of pregnancies, not the number of fetuses, carried to the point of viability, regardless of the outcome
Nullipara (para 0)	A woman who has not produced a viable offspring.
Primipara	A woman who has given birth once after a pregnancy of at least 20 weeks, commonly referred to as a "'primip" in clinical practice.
Multipara	A woman who has had two or more pregnancies of at least 20 weeks' gestation resulting in viable offspring. Commonly referred to as a "multip."

the woman's risk for another tubal pregnancy. Also ask about safe-sex practices and any history of STIs.

Physical Examination

The next step in the assessment process is the physical examination, which detects any physical problems that may affect the pregnancy outcome. The initial physical examination provides the baseline for evaluating changes during future visits.

Preparation

Instruct the client to undress and put on a gown. Also ask her to empty her bladder and, in doing so, to collect a urine specimen. Typically this specimen is a clean-catch urine specimen that is sent to the laboratory for a urinalysis to detect a possible urinary tract infection.

Begin the physical examination by obtaining vital signs, including blood pressure, respiratory rate, temperature, and pulse. Also measure the client's height and weight. Abnormalities such as an elevated blood pressure may suggest pregestational hypertension, requiring further evaluation. Abnormalities in pulse rate and respiration require further investigation for possible cardiac or respiratory disease. If the woman weighs less than 100 lb or more than 200 lb or there has been a sudden weight gain, report these findings to the primary care provider; medical treatment or nutritional counseling may be necessary.

Head-to-Toe Assessment

A complete head-to-toe assessment is usually performed by the health care provider. Every body system is assessed. Some of the major areas are discussed here. Throughout the assessment, be sure to drape the client appropriately to ensure privacy and prevent chilling.

HEAD AND NECK

Assess the head and neck area for any previous injuries and sequelae. Evaluate for any limitations in range of motion. Palpate for any enlarged lymph nodes or swelling. Note any edema of the nasal mucosa or hypertrophy of gingival tissue in the mouth; these are typical responses to increased estrogen levels in pregnancy. Palpate the thyroid gland for enlargement. Slight enlargement is normal, but marked enlargement may indicate hyperthyroidism, requiring further investigation.

CHEST

Auscultate heart sounds, noting any abnormalities. A soft systolic murmur caused by the increase in blood volume may be noted. Anticipate an increase in heart rate by 10 to 15 beats per minute (bpm) (starting between 14 and 20 weeks of pregnancy) secondary to increases in cardiac output and blood volume. The body adapts to the increase in blood volume with peripheral dilation to maintain blood pressure. Progesterone causes peripheral dilation.

Auscultate the chest for breath sounds, which should be clear. Also note symmetry of chest movement and thoracic breathing patterns. Estrogen promotes relaxation of the ligaments and joints of the ribs, with a resulting increase in the anteroposterior chest diameter. Expect a slight increase in respiratory rate to accommodate the increase in tidal volume and oxygen consumption.

Inspect and palpate the breasts and nipples for symmetry and color. Increases in estrogen and progesterone and blood supply make the breasts feel full and more nodular, with increased sensitivity to touch. Blood vessels become more visible and there is an increase in breast size. Striae gravidarum (stretch marks) may be visible in women with large breasts. Darker pigmentation of the nipple and areola is present, along with enlargement of Montgomery glands. Colostrum (yellowish secretion that precedes mature breast milk) is excreted typically in the third trimester.

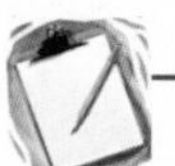

Take Note!

Use this opportunity to reinforce and teach breast self-examination if the woman has a high-risk history.

ABDOMEN

The appearance of the abdomen depends on the number of weeks of gestation. The abdomen enlarges progressively as the fetus grows. Inspect the abdomen for striae, scars, shape, and size. Inspection may reveal striae gravidarum (stretch marks) and **linea nigra**, a thin brownish black pigmented line running from the umbilicus to the symphysis pubis, depending on the duration of the pregnancy. Palpate the abdomen, which should be rounded and nontender. A decrease in muscle tone may be noted due to the influence of progesterone.

Typically, the height of the fundus is measured when the uterus arises out of the pelvis to evaluate fetal growth. At 12 weeks' gestation the fundus can be palpated at the symphysis pubis. At 16 weeks' gestation the fundus is midway between the symphysis and the umbilicus. At 20 weeks the fundus can be palpated at the umbilicus and measures approximately 20 cm from the symphysis pubis. By 36 weeks the fundus is just below the xiphoid process and measures approximately 36 cm. The uterus maintains a globular/ovoid shape throughout pregnancy (Bope & Kellerman, 2015).

EXTREMITIES

Inspect and palpate both legs for dependent edema, pulses, and varicose veins. If edema is present in early pregnancy, further evaluation may be needed to rule out gestational hypertension. During the third trimester, dependent edema is a normal finding. Ask the woman if she has any pain in her calf that increases when she ambulates. This might indicate a deep vein thrombosis (DVT). High levels of estrogen during pregnancy place women at higher risk for DVT.

Pelvic Examination

The pelvic examination provides information about the internal and external reproductive organs. In addition, it aids in assessing some of the presumptive and probable signs of pregnancy and allows for determination of pelvic adequacy. During the pelvic examination, remain in the examining room to assist the health care provider with any specimen collection, fixation, and labeling. Also provide comfort and emotional support for the woman, who might be anxious. Throughout the examination, explain what is happening and why, and answer any questions as necessary.

EXTERNAL GENITALIA

After the client is placed in the lithotomy position and draped appropriately, the external genitalia are inspected visually. They should be free from lesions, discharge, hematomas, varicosities, and inflammation upon inspection. A culture for STIs may be collected at this time.

INTERNAL GENITALIA

Next, the internal genitalia are examined via a speculum. The cervix should be smooth, long, thick, and closed. Because of increased pelvic congestion, the cervix will be softened (Goodell sign), the uterine isthmus will be softened (Hegar sign), and there will be a bluish coloration of the cervix and vaginal mucosa (Chadwick sign).

The uterus typically is pear shaped and mobile, with a smooth surface. It will undergo cell hypertrophy and hyperplasia so that it enlarges throughout the pregnancy to accommodate the growing fetus.

During the pelvic examination, a Papanicolaou (Pap) smear may be obtained. Additional cultures, such as for gonorrhea and chlamydia screening, also may be obtained. Ensure that all specimens obtained are labeled correctly and sent to the laboratory for evaluation. A rectal examination is done last to assess for lesions, masses, prolapse, or hemorrhoids.

Once the examination of the internal genitalia is completed and the speculum is removed, a bimanual examination is performed to estimate the size of the uterus to confirm dates and to palpate the ovaries. The ovaries should be small and nontender, without masses. At the conclusion of the bimanual examination, the health care provider reinserts the index finger into the vagina and the middle finger into the rectum to assess the strength and regularity of the posterior vaginal wall.

PELVIC SIZE, SHAPE, AND MEASUREMENTS

The size and shape of the women's pelvis can affect her ability to deliver vaginally. Pelvic shape is typically classified as one of four types: gynecoid, android, anthropoid, and platypelloid. Refer to Chapter 13 for an in-depth discussion of pelvic size and shape.

Taking internal pelvic measurements determines the actual diameters of the inlet and outlet through which the fetus will pass. This is extremely important if the woman has never given birth vaginally. Taking pelvic measurements is unnecessary for the woman who has given birth vaginally before (unless she has experienced some type of trauma to the area) because vaginal delivery demonstrates that the pelvis is adequate for the passage of the fetus.

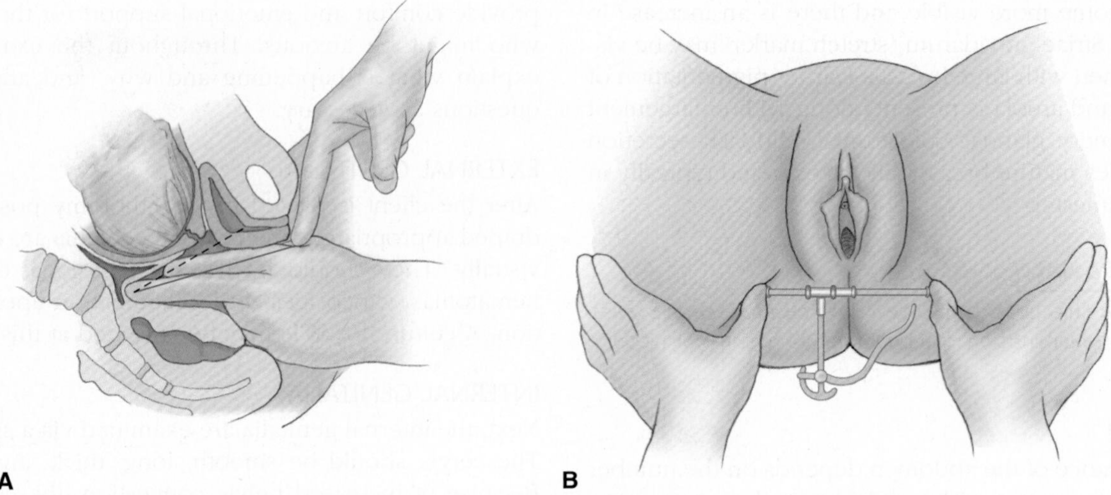

FIGURE 12.4 Pelvic measurements. **A.** Diagonal conjugate (*solid line*) and true conjugate (*dotted line*). **B.** Ischial tuberosity diameter.

Three measurements are assessed: diagonal conjugate, true conjugate, and ischial tuberosity (Fig. 12.4). The diagonal conjugate is the distance between the anterior surface of the sacral prominence and the anterior surface of the inferior margin of the symphysis pubis (Bope & Kellerman, 2015). This measurement, usually 12.5 cm or greater, represents the anteroposterior diameter of the pelvic inlet through which the fetal head passes first. The diagonal conjugate is the most useful measurement for estimating pelvic size because a misfit with the fetal head occurs if it is too small.

The true conjugate, also called the obstetric conjugate, is the measurement from the anterior surface of the sacral prominence to the posterior surface of the inferior margin of the symphysis pubis. This diameter cannot be measured directly; rather, it is estimated by subtracting 1 to 2 cm from the diagonal conjugate measurement. The average true conjugate diameter is at least 11.5 cm (Cunningham et al., 2014). This measurement is important because it is the smallest front-to-back diameter through which the fetal head must pass when moving through the pelvic inlet.

The ischial tuberosity diameter is the transverse diameter of the pelvic outlet. This measurement is made outside the pelvis at the lowest aspect of the ischial tuberosities. A diameter of 10.5 cm or more is considered adequate for passage of the fetal head (Tharpe, Farley, & Jordan, 2016).

Laboratory Tests

A series of tests is generally ordered during the initial visit so that baseline data can be obtained, allowing for early detection and prompt intervention if any problems occur. Tests that are generally conducted for all pregnant women include urinalysis and blood studies. The urine is analyzed for albumin, glucose, ketones, and bacteria casts. Blood studies usually include a complete blood count (hemoglobin, hematocrit, red and white blood cell counts, and platelets), blood typing and Rh factor, glucose screening for high-risk women, a rubella titer, hepatitis B surface antibody antigen, HIV, venereal disease research laboratory (VDRL) or rapid plasma reagin (RPR) tests, and cervical smears to detect STIs (Common Laboratory and Diagnostic Tests 12.1). In addition, most offices and clinics have ultrasound equipment available to validate an intrauterine pregnancy and assess early fetal growth.

The need for additional laboratory studies is determined by a woman's history, physical examination findings, current health status, and risk factors identified in the initial interview. Additional tests can be offered (e.g., screening for genetic diseases, blood lead screening, rubeola, and so on), but ultimately the woman and her partner make the decision about undergoing them. Educate the client and her partner about the tests, including the rationale. In addition, support the client and her partner in their decision-making process, regardless of whether you agree with the couple's decision. The couple's decisions about their health care are based on the ethical principle of autonomy, which allows an individual the right to make decisions about his or her own body.

Remember Linda and Rob, the couple who want to start a family? Ten months after the preconception appointment, Linda calls to make a first prenatal appointment. What key areas will be addressed at this first prenatal visit? What interventions might be suggested for Linda to implement in order to ensure a healthy newborn? What emotional support might be needed by Linda at this time in her first trimester of pregnancy?

COMMON LABORATORY AND DIAGNOSTIC TESTS 12.1

Test	Explanation
Complete blood cell count (CBC)	Evaluates hemoglobin (12–14 g) and hematocrit (42% ± 5) levels and red blood cell count (4.2–5.4 million/mm^3) to detect presence of anemia; identifies white blood cell level (5,000–10,000/mm^3), which if elevated may indicate an infection; determines platelet count (150,000–450,000 mL^3) to assess clotting ability
Blood typing	Determines woman's blood type and Rh status to rule out any blood incompatibility issues early; Rh-negative mother would likely receive RhoGAM (at 28 wks' gestation) and again within 72 hrs after childbirth, if she is Rh sensitive
Rubella titer	Detects antibodies for the virus that causes German measles; if titer is 1:8 or less, the woman is not immune; requires immunization after birth; and woman is advised to avoid people with undiagnosed rashes
Hepatitis B	Determines if mother has hepatitis B by detecting presence of hepatitis antibody surface antigen (HbsAg) in her blood
HIV testing	Detects HIV antibodies and if positive requires more specific testing, counseling, and treatment during pregnancy with antiretroviral medications to prevent transmission to fetus
STI screening: Venereal Disease Research Laboratory (VDRL) or rapid plasma reagin (RPR) serologic tests or by cervical smears, cultures, or visual identification of suspicious lesions	Detects STIs (such as syphilis, herpes, HPV, gonorrhea) so that treatment can be initiated early to prevent transmission to fetus
Cervical smears	Detects abnormalities such as cervical cancer (Pap test) or infections such as gonorrhea, chlamydia, or group B streptococcus so that treatment can be initiated if positive

Adapted from Fischbach, F., & Dunning, M. B. (2014). *A manual of laboratory and diagnostic tests* (9th ed.). Philadelphia, PA: Lippincott Williams & Wilkins; and Ferri, F. F. (2014). *Ferri's best test: A practical guide to laboratory medicine and diagnostic imaging* (3rd ed.). Philadelphia, PA: Elsevier Health Sciences.

FOLLOW-UP VISITS

Continuous prenatal care is important for a successful pregnancy outcome. The recommended follow-up visit schedule for a healthy pregnant woman is as follows:

- Every 4 weeks up to 28 weeks (7 months)
- Every 2 weeks from 29 to 36 weeks
- Every week from 37 weeks to birth

At each subsequent prenatal visit the following assessments are completed:

- Weight and blood pressure, which are compared with baseline values
- Urine testing for protein, glucose, ketones, and nitrites
- Fundal height measurement to assess fetal growth
- Assessment for quickening/fetal movement to determine fetal well-being
- Assessment of fetal heart rate (should be 110 to 160 bpm)

At each follow-up visit answer questions, provide anticipatory guidance and education, review nutritional guidelines, and evaluate the client for adherence to prenatal vitamin therapy. Throughout the pregnancy, encourage the woman's partner to participate if possible.

Follow-Up Visit Intervals and Assessments

Up to 28 weeks' gestation, follow-up visits involve assessment of the client's blood pressure and weight. The urine is tested for protein and glucose. Fundal height and fetal heart rate are assessed at every office visit.

The best procedure for screening and diagnosing gestational diabetes remains controversial. All strategies involve an oral glucose test, but there remains disagreement about how many grams of glucose (50, 75, or 100) the woman ingests and how long afterward, her blood sample is drawn. A recent *Cochrane Review* concluded that there was insufficient evidence to permit assessment of which is the best method to use to identify women who have gestational diabetes (Farrar et al., 2015). Screening for gestational diabetes is best done between 24 and 28 weeks' gestation, unless screening is warranted in the first trimester for high-risk reasons (obesity, >25 years old, family history of diabetes, history of gestational diabetes, or woman is of a certain ethnic group: Hispanic, Native Americans, Asian, or African American) (U.S. Preventive Services Task Force [USPSTF], 2015). Between weeks 24 and 28, a blood glucose level is obtained using an oral 50-g glucose load followed by a 1-hour plasma glucose determination. If the result is more than 130 (ADA) to 140 (ACOG) mg/dL, further testing, such as a 3-hour 100-g glucose tolerance test, is warranted to determine whether gestational diabetes is present (Farrar et al., 2015). Because insulin resistance increases as pregnancy advances, testing at this gestational point yields a higher rate of abnormal test results.

During this time, review the common discomforts of pregnancy, evaluate any client complaints, and answer questions. Reinforce the importance of good nutrition and use of prenatal vitamins, along with daily exercise.

Between 29 and 36 weeks' gestation, all the assessments of previous visits are completed, along with assessment for edema. Special attention is focused on the presence and location of edema during the last trimester. Pregnant women commonly experience dependent edema of the lower extremities from constriction of blood vessels secondary to the heavy gravid uterus. Periorbital edema around the eyes, edema of the hands, and pretibial edema (edema on the front, or shin part of the leg) are abnormal and could be signs of gestational hypertension. Inspecting and palpating both extremities, listening for complaints of tight rings on fingers, and observing for swelling around the eyes are important assessments. Abnormal findings in any of these areas need to be reported.

If the mother is Rh negative, her antibody titer is evaluated. RhoGAM is given if indicated. RhoGAM is used to prevent development of antibodies to Rh^+ red cells whenever fetal cells are known or suspected of entering the maternal circulation such as after a spontaneous abortion or **amniocentesis**. It is also recommended for prophylaxis at 28 weeks' gestation and following birth if the infant is Rh^+ (King et al., 2015). The client also is evaluated for risk of preterm labor. At each visit, ask if she is experiencing any common signs or symptoms of preterm labor (e.g., uterine contractions, dull backache, feeling of pressure in the pelvic area or thighs, increased vaginal discharge, menstrual-like cramps, vaginal bleeding). If the woman has had a previous preterm birth, she is at risk for another and close monitoring is warranted. An initial preterm labor evaluation if the woman reports signs and symptoms of preterm labor includes review of prenatal record for risk factors, evaluation of reported symptoms (uterine contractions, vital signs, fetal heart rate, pelvic examination for cervical dilation and effacement assessment, and status of fetal membranes), and a urine culture to diagnose asymptomatic bacteriuria (Jordan et al., 2014). If positive for preterm labor, the woman may be requested to rest and medications to stop contractions may be in order.

Counsel the woman about choosing a health care provider for the newborn, if she has not selected one yet. Along with completion of a breast assessment, the nurse should discuss and educate the client about the choice of breast-feeding versus bottle-feeding. The American Academy of Pediatrics does encourage all mothers to breast-feed their offspring, but the decision to do so is the woman's ultimately. The nurse can refer the client to *Nursing Mothers* and *La Leche League* web sites for further information to assist her in making that decision. Reinforce the importance of daily fetal movement monitoring as an indicator of fetal well-being. Reevaluate hemoglobin and hematocrit levels to assess for anemia.

Between 37 and 40 weeks' gestation, the same assessments are done as for the previous weeks. In addition, screening for group B streptococcus, gonorrhea, and chlamydia is done. Fetal presentation and position (via Leopold maneuvers) are assessed. Review the signs and symptoms of labor and forward a copy of the prenatal record to the hospital labor department for future reference. Review the client's desire for family planning after birth as well as her decision to breast-feed or bottle-feed. Remind the client that an infant car seat is required by law and must be used to drive the newborn home from the hospital or birthing center.

Fundal Height Measurement

Fundal height is the distance (in centimeters) measured with a tape measure from the top of the pubic bone to the top of the uterus (fundus) with the client lying on her back with her knees slightly flexed (Fig. 12.5). Measurement in this way is termed the McDonald method. Fundal height typically increases as the pregnancy progresses; it reflects fetal growth and provides a gross estimate of the duration of the pregnancy.

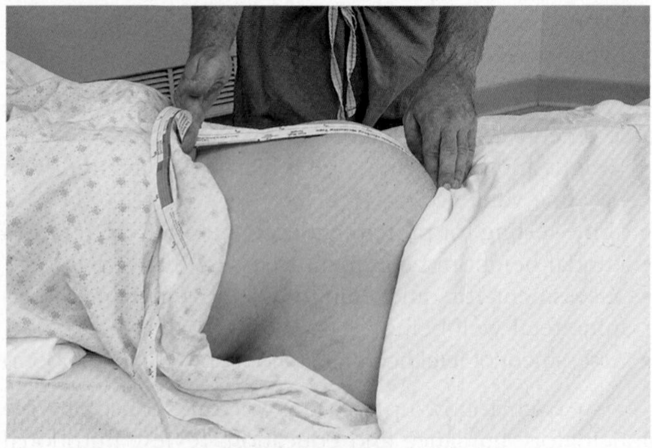

FIGURE 12.5 Fundal height measurement.

Between 12 and 14 weeks' gestation, the fundus can be palpated above the symphysis pubis. The fundus reaches the level of the umbilicus at approximately 20 weeks and measures 20 cm. Fundal measurement should approximately equal the number of weeks of gestation until week 36. For example, a fundal height of 24 cm suggests a fetus at 24 weeks' gestation. After 36 weeks, the fundal height then drops due to lightening and may no longer correspond with the week of gestation.

It is expected that the fundal height will increase progressively throughout the pregnancy, reflecting fetal growth. However, if the growth curve flattens or stays stable, it may indicate the presence of FGR. If the fundal height measurement is greater than 4 cm from the estimated gestational age, further evaluation is warranted if a multifetal gestation has not been diagnosed or hydramnios has not been ruled out (Weber & Kelley, 2014).

Fetal Movement Determination

Perception of fetal movement typically begins in the second trimester, and occurs earlier in multiparous women verses nulliparous women. The mother's first perception of fetal movement, termed "quickening," is commonly described as a gentle fluttering. This perceived fetal movement is most often related to trunk and limb motion and rollovers, or flips (Moses, 2015b). Maternal perception of fetal movement is an important screening method for fetal well-being, because decreased fetal movement is associated with a range of pregnancy pathologies and poor pregnancy outcomes. Decreased fetal movement may indicate asphyxia and FGR. If compromised, the fetus decreases its oxygen requirements by decreasing activity. Reduced fetal movement is thought to represent fetal compensation in a chronic hypoxic environment due to inadequacies in the placental supply of oxygen and nutrients (Fretts, 2014). A decrease in fetal movement may also be related to other factors as well, such as maternal use of central nervous system depressants, fetal sleep cycles, hydrocephalus, bilateral renal agenesis, stillbirth, placental dysfunction, and bilateral hip dislocation (Heazell, 2015).

Fetal movement counting is a method used by the mother to quantify her fetus's movement. However, the optimal number of movements and the ideal duration of counting them remain controversial. Many variations for determining fetal movement, also called fetal movement counts, have been developed, but the one most common method is described as follows. Determining fetal movement is a noninvasive method of screening and can be easily taught to all pregnant women. Any technique used requires client participation and cooperation.

Instruct the client about how to count fetal movements, the reasons for doing so, and the significance of decreased fetal movements. Urge the client to perform the counts in a relaxed environment and a comfortable position, such as semi-Fowler's or side-lying. Provide the client with detailed information concerning fetal movement counts and stress the need for consistency in monitoring (at approximately the same time each day) and the importance of informing the health care provider promptly of any reduced movements. Providing clients with "fetal kick count" charts to record movement helps promote adherence to your instructions. No values for fetal movement have been established that indicate fetal well-being, so the woman needs to be aware of a decrease in the number of movements when last assessed. The most common method used is "Count to 10," whereby a woman focuses her attention on her fetus's movement and records how long it takes to document 10 movements. If it takes longer than 2 hours, the woman should contact her health care provider for further evaluation. Fetal kick counting in current prenatal care appears to be underutilized and nurses need to educate women about this assessment in their pregnancy care.

Fetal Heart Rate Measurement

Fetal heart rate measurement is integral to fetal surveillance throughout the pregnancy. Auscultating the fetal heart rate with a handheld Doppler at each prenatal visit helps confirm that the intrauterine environment is still supportive to the growing fetus. The purpose of assessing fetal heart rate is to determine rate and rhythm. The normal fetal heart rate range is 110 to 160 bpm. Nursing Procedure 12.1 lists the steps in measuring fetal heart rate.

Teaching About the Danger Signs of Pregnancy

It is important to educate the client about danger signs during pregnancy that require further evaluation. Explain that she should contact her health care provider immediately if she experiences any of the following:

- *During the first trimester:* spotting or bleeding (miscarriage), painful urination (infection), severe persistent vomiting (hyperemesis gravidarum), fever >100°F (37.7°C; infection), and lower abdominal pain with dizziness and accompanied by shoulder pain (ruptured ectopic pregnancy)
- *During the second trimester:* regular uterine contractions (preterm labor); pain in calf, often increased with foot flexion (blood clot in deep vein); sudden gush or leakage of fluid from vagina (premature rupture of membranes); and absence of fetal movement for more than 12 hours (possible fetal distress or demise)
- *During the third trimester:* sudden weight gain; periorbital or facial edema, severe upper abdominal pain, or headache with visual changes (gestational hypertension and/or preeclampsia); and a decrease in fetal

NURSING PROCEDURE 12.1

Measuring Fetal Heart Rate

Purpose: To assess fetal well-being

1. Assist the woman onto the examining table and have her lie down.
2. Cover her with a sheet to ensure privacy, and then expose her abdomen.
3. Palpate the abdomen to determine the fetal lie, position, and presentation.
4. Locate the back of the fetus (the ideal position to hear the heart rate).
5. Apply lubricant gel to abdomen in the area where the back has been located.
6. Turn on the handheld Doppler device and place it on the spot over the fetal back.
7. Listen for the sound of the amplified heart rate, moving the device slightly from side to side as necessary to obtain the loudest sound. Assess the woman's pulse rate and compare it to the amplified sound. If the rates appear the same, reposition the Doppler device.
8. Once the fetal heart rate has been identified, count the number of beats in 1 minute and record the results.
9. Remove the Doppler device and wipe off any remaining gel from the woman's abdomen and the device.
10. Record the heart rate on the woman's medical record; normal range is 110 to 160 bpm.
11. Provide information to the woman regarding fetal well-being based on findings.

daily movement for more than 24 hours (possible demise). Any of the previous warning signs and symptoms can also be present in this last trimester (March of Dimes, 2015a).

Early Contractions

One of the warning signs that should be emphasized is early contractions, which can lead to preterm birth. The woman should not confuse these early preterm contractions with Braxton Hicks contractions, which are not true labor pains because they go away when walking around or resting. They often go away when the woman goes to sleep. Braxton Hicks contractions are usually felt in the abdomen versus in the lower back with true preterm labor contractions. Signs of preterm labor that a woman may experience include contractions every 10 minutes or more frequently, change in vaginal discharge, pelvic pressure, low, dull backache, pelvic cramps, and diarrhea (Nagtalon-Ramos, 2014).

All pregnant women need to be able to recognize early signs of contractions to prevent preterm labor, which is a major public health problem in the United States. Approximately 12% of all live births—or one out of nine infants—is born too soon. Our nation's rate of premature births has increased by 36% over the last 25 years. Worldwide, 15 million infants are born too soon each year (March of Dimes, 2015b). These preterm infants (born at less than 37 weeks' gestation) can suffer lifelong health consequences such as intellectual disability, chronic lung disease, cerebral palsy, seizure disorders, and blindness (March of Dimes, 2015c). Preterm labor can happen to any pregnant women at any time. In many cases it can be stopped with medications if it is recognized early, before significant cervical dilation has taken place. If the woman experiences menstrual-like cramps occurring every 10 minutes accompanied by a low, dull backache, she should stop what she is doing and lie down on her left side for 1 hour and drink two or three glasses of water. If the symptoms worsen or do not subside after 1 hour, she should contact her health care provider.

ASSESSMENT OF FETAL WELL-BEING

During the antepartum period, several tests are performed routinely to monitor fetal well-being and to detect possible problems. When a **high-risk pregnancy** is identified, additional antepartum testing can be initiated to promote positive maternal, fetal, and neonatal outcomes. High-risk pregnancies include those that are complicated by maternal or fetal conditions (coincidental with or unique to pregnancy) that jeopardize the health status of the mother and put the fetus at risk for uteroplacental insufficiency, hypoxia, and death (CDC, 2015d). However, additional antepartum fetal testing should take place only when the results obtained will guide future care, whether it is reassurance, more frequent testing, admission to the hospital, or the need for immediate delivery (Brown, 2015).

Ultrasonography

Since its introduction in the late 1950s, ultrasonography has become a very useful diagnostic tool in obstetrics. Real-time scanners can produce a continuous picture of the fetus on a monitor screen. A transducer that emits high-frequency sound waves is placed on the mother's abdomen and moved to visualize the fetus (Fig. 12.6).

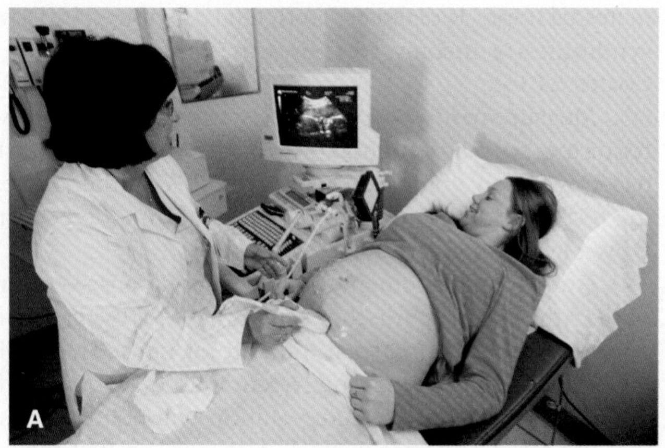

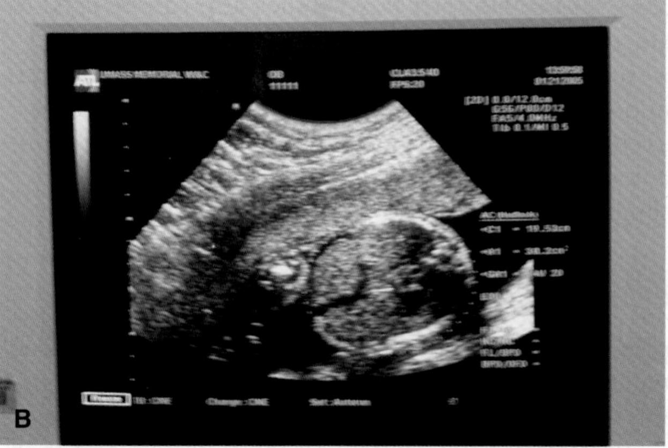

FIGURE 12.6 Ultrasound. **A.** Ultrasound device being applied to client's abdomen. **B.** View of monitor.

The fetal heartbeat and any malformations in the fetus can be assessed and measurements can be made accurately from the picture on the monitor screen.

Obstetric ultrasound is a standard component of prenatal care used to identify pregnancy complications and to establish an accurate gestational age in order to improve pregnancy outcomes. Because the ultrasound procedure is noninvasive, it is a safe, but not evidence-based practice for low-risk women, accurate, and cost-effective tool. It provides important information about fetal activity, growth, and gestational age; assesses fetal well-being; and determines the need for invasive intrauterine tests (Maeda, 2015).

There are no hard-and-fast rules as to the number of ultrasounds a woman should have during her pregnancy. A low-risk woman does not necessarily require any, but most practices do them as part of their prenatal care routine. A transvaginal ultrasound may be performed in the first trimester to confirm pregnancy, exclude ectopic (in which a fertilized egg implants somewhere other than the main cavity of the uterus) or molar (hydatidiform mole, a benign tumor that develops in the uterus) pregnancies, and confirm cardiac pulsation. A second abdominal scan may be performed at about 18 to 20 weeks to look for congenital malformations, exclude multifetal pregnancies, and verify dates and growth. A third abdominal scan may be done at around 34 weeks to evaluate fetal size, assess fetal growth, and verify placental position (Everett & Peebles, 2015). An ultrasound is used to confirm placental location during amniocentesis and to provide visualization during **chorionic villus sampling (CVS)**. An ultrasound is also ordered whenever an abnormality is suspected.

During the past several years, ultrasound technology has advanced significantly. Now available for expecting parents is 3D/4D ultrasound imaging. Unlike traditional 2D imaging, which takes a look at the developing fetus from one angle (thus creating the "flat" image), 3D imaging takes a view of the fetus from three different angles. Software then takes these three images and merges them to produce a three-dimensional image. Because the fourth dimension is time and movement, with 4D parents are able to watch the live movements of their fetus in 3D.

Nursing management during the ultrasound procedure focuses on educating the woman about the ultrasound test and reassuring her that she will not experience any sensation from the sound waves during the test. No special client preparation is needed before performing the ultrasound, although in early pregnancy the woman may need to have a full bladder. Inform her that she may experience some discomfort from the pressure on the full bladder during the scan, but it will last only a short time. Tell the client that the conducting gel used on the abdomen during the scan may feel cold initially.

Doppler Flow Studies

Comprehensive assessment of fetal well-being involves monitoring of fetal growth, placental function, central venous pressure, and cardiac function. Ultrasound evaluation of the fetus using 2D, color Doppler, and pulse-wave Doppler techniques forms the foundation of prenatal diagnosis of structural anomalies, rhythm abnormalities, and altered fetal circulation (Pruetz, Votava-Smith, & Miller, 2015). Doppler flow studies can be used to measure the velocity of blood flow via ultrasound. Doppler flow studies can detect fetal compromise in high-risk pregnancies. The test is noninvasive and has no contraindications. The color images produced help to identify abnormalities in diastolic flow within the umbilical vessels. The velocity of the fetal red blood cells can be determined by measuring the change in the frequency of the sound wave reflected off the cells. Thus, Doppler flow studies can detect the movement of red blood cells in vessels (Everett & Peebles, 2015). In pregnancies complicated by hypertension or FGRs diastolic blood flow may be absent or even reversed (Alfirevic, Stampalija, &

Medley, 2015). Doppler flow studies also can be used to evaluate the blood flow through other fetal blood vessels, such as the aorta and those in the brain. Research continues to determine the indications for Doppler flow studies to improve pregnancy outcomes. Nursing management of the woman undergoing Doppler flow studies is similar to that described for an ultrasound.

Alpha-Fetoprotein Analysis

Alpha-fetoprotein (AFP) is a glycoprotein produced initially by the yolk sac and fetal gut, and later predominantly by the fetal liver. In a fetus, the serum AFP level increases until approximately 14 to 15 weeks, and then falls progressively. In normal pregnancies, AFP from fetal serum enters the amniotic fluid (in microgram quantities) through fetal urination, fetal gastrointestinal secretions, and transudation across fetal membranes (amnion and placenta). About 30 years ago, elevated levels of maternal serum AFP (MSAFP) or amniotic fluid AFP were first linked to the occurrence of fetal neural tube defects. This biomarker screening test is now recommended for all pregnant women along with other prenatal screening test depending on risk profile (Alexander et al., 2014; American College of Obstetricians and Gynecologists, 2015b).

AFP is present in amniotic fluid in low concentrations between 10 and 14 weeks of gestation and can be detected in maternal serum beginning at approximately 12 to 14 weeks of gestation (Callahan, 2016). If a developmental defect is present, such as failure of the neural tube to close, more AFP escapes into amniotic fluid from the fetus. AFP then enters the maternal circulation by crossing the placenta, and the level in maternal serum can be measured. The optimal time for AFP screening is 16 to 18 weeks of gestation. Currently, ACOG recommends offering screening and diagnostic tests to all pregnant women, regardless of age or risk factors present (2015b). Correct information about gestational dating, maternal weight, race, number of fetuses, and insulin dependency is necessary to ensure the accuracy of this screening test. If incorrect maternal information is submitted or the blood specimen is not drawn during the appropriate time frame, false-positive results may occur, increasing the woman's anxiety. Subsequently, further testing might be ordered based on an inaccurate interpretation, resulting in additional financial and emotional costs to the woman.

A variety of situations can lead to elevation of MSAFP, including open neural tube defect, underestimation of gestational age, the presence of multiple fetuses, gastrointestinal defects, low birth weight, oligohydramnios, maternal age, diabetes, and decreased maternal weight (King et al., 2015). Lower-than-expected MSAFP levels are seen when fetal gestational age is overestimated or in cases of fetal death, hydatidiform mole, increased maternal weight, maternal type 1 diabetes, and fetal trisomy 21 (Down syndrome) or trisomy 18 (Edwards syndrome) (Khalil & Coates, 2015).

Measurement of MSAFP is minimally invasive, requiring only a venipuncture for a blood sample. AFP has now been combined with other biomarker screening tests to determine the risk of neural tube defects and Down syndrome.

Nursing management for AFP testing consists of preparing the woman for this screening test by gathering accurate information about the date of her LMP, weight, race, and gestational dating. Accurately determining the window of 16 to 18 weeks' gestation will help to ensure that the test results are correct. Also explain that the test involves obtaining a blood specimen.

Marker Screening Tests

Using maternal serum is an effective, noninvasive method for identifying fetal risk for aneuploidy (trisomies 13, 18, & 21) and neural tube defects. Prenatal screening for Down syndrome in the early second trimester with multiple maternal serum markers has been available for more than 15 years. Abnormalities in maternal serum marker levels and fetal measurements obtained during the first trimester screening can be markers for not only certain chromosomal disorders and anomalies in the fetus, but also for specific pregnancy complications. Pregnancy-associated plasma protein A (PAPP-A) is a key regulator of insulin-like growth factor essential for normal fetal development. In maternal blood, this protein increases with gestational age. It is routinely used for Down syndrome screening in the first trimester. A low maternal serum PAPP-A, at 11 to 13 weeks of gestation, is associated with stillbirth, infant death, preterm birth, preeclampsia, and chromosomal abnormalities (Kalousova, Muravska, & Zima, 2014; Patil, Panchanadikar, & Wagh, 2014). Multiple blood screening tests may be used to determine the risk of open neural tube defects and Down syndrome: the triple-marker screen (AFP, hCG, and unconjugated estriol) or the quad screen, which includes the triple screening tests with the addition of a fourth marker, inhibin A (glycoprotein secreted by the placenta). The quad screen is used to enhance the accuracy of screening for Down syndrome in women younger than 35 years of age. Low inhibin A levels indicate the possibility of Down syndrome (ACOG, 2015b). These biomarkers are merely screening tests and identify women who need further definitive procedures (i.e., ultrasound, amniocentesis, and genetic counseling) to make a diagnosis of neural tube defects (anencephaly, spina bifida, and encephalocele) or Down syndrome in the fetus. Most screening tests are performed between 15 to 22 weeks of gestation (16 to 18 weeks is ideal), except for the cffDNA test which can be performed around 9 to 10 weeks' gestation (Dempsey & Overton, 2015).

With these multiple screening tests, low MSAFP, unconjugated estriol levels, and a high hCG level suggest the possibility of Down syndrome. Elevated levels of MSAFP are associated with open neural tube defects, ventral wall defects, some renal abnormalities, multiple gestation, certain skin disorders, fetal demise, and placental abnormality. The multiple marker combination with the highest screening performance currently available is AFP, unconjugated estriol (uE3), hCG, and inhibin A, together with maternal age (the so-called quad marker test). With this combination, a detection rate of 80% at a 5% false-positive rate is achieved (Hixson et al., 2015).

A number of factors influence the interpretation of an MSAFP value. The most important is the accuracy of the gestational age determination. A variation of 2 weeks can be misleading and lead to a wrong interpretation. Maternal weight (>250 lb), ethnicity, maternal smoking habits, fetal gender, gravidity, para status, and women with insulin-dependent diabetes also may alter the levels of MSAFP and need to be taken into consideration when interpreting the results (Latendresse & Deneris, 2015). Recent research studies indicate prenatal testing with the use of cell free DNA (cfDNA) has significantly lower false positives and high positive predictive values for detection of trisomies than standard testing (Greeley, Kessler, & Vohra, 2015).

Nursing Management

Accurate test interpretation and risk determination are dependent on accurate pregnancy dating and reporting of relevant maternal characteristics. This is why it is so important for nurses, if an abnormal test result is reported, for them to confirm pregnancy dating and report any significant maternal factors relevant to test accuracy. In addition, nurses have a big role in providing education about the tests to the couples. Prenatal screening has become standard in prenatal care. However, for many couples it remains confusing, emotionally charged, and filled with uncertain risks. Offer a thorough explanation of the test, reinforcing the information given by the health care professional. Provide couples with a description of the risks and benefits of performing these screens, emphasizing that these tests are for screening purposes only. Remind the couple that a definitive diagnosis is not made without further tests such as an amniocentesis. Answer any questions about these prenatal screening tests and respect the couple's decision if they choose not to have them done. Many couples may choose not to know because they would not consider having an abortion regardless of the test results.

Nuchal Translucency Screening

Nuchal translucency screening (ultrasound) is also done in the first trimester between 11 and 14 weeks. This allows for early detection and diagnosis of some fetal chromosomal and structural abnormalities. Over the years, it has become clear that increased nuchal translucency is a marker for chromosomal abnormalities, and is also associated with a wide spectrum of structural anomalies, genetic syndromes, and high risk of abortion and fetal death (Rayburn, Jolley, & Simpson, 2015). Ultrasound is used to identify an increase in nuchal translucency, which is due to the subcutaneous accumulation of fluid behind the fetal neck. Increased nuchal translucency is associated with chromosomal abnormalities such as trisomy 21, 18, and 13. Infants with trisomies tend to have more collagen and elastic connective tissue, allowing for accumulation. In addition, diaphragmatic hernias, cardiac defects, and fetal skeletal and neurologic abnormalities have been associated with increased nuchal translucency measurements (Evans, Andriole, & Evans, 2015). See Chapter 10 for more information.

Amniocentesis

Amniocentesis involves a transabdominal puncture of the amniotic sac to obtain a sample of amniotic fluid for analysis. The fluid contains fetal cells that are examined to detect chromosomal abnormalities and several hereditary metabolic defects in the fetus before birth. In addition, amniocentesis is used to confirm a fetal abnormality when other screening tests detect a possible problem.

Amniocentesis is performed in the second trimester, usually between 15 and 18 weeks' gestation. At this age, the amount of fluid is adequate (approximately 150 mL), and the ratio of viable to nonviable cells is greatest (Hehir, Dalrymple, & Malone, 2015). More than 40 different chromosomal abnormalities, inborn errors of metabolism, and neural tube defects can be diagnosed with amniocentesis. It can replace a genetic probability with a diagnostic certainty, allowing the woman and her partner to make an informed decision about the option of therapeutic abortion.

Amniocentesis can be performed in any of the three trimesters of pregnancy. An early amniocentesis (performed between weeks 11 and 14) is done to detect genetic anomalies. However, early amniocentesis has been associated with a high risk of spontaneous miscarriage and postprocedural amniotic fluid leakage compared with transabdominal chorionic villus screening (King et al., 2015).

In the second trimester the procedure is performed between 15 and 20 weeks to detect chromosomal abnormalities, evaluate the fetal condition when the woman is sensitized to the Rh-positive blood, diagnose intrauterine infections, and investigate amniotic fluid AFP when the MSAFP level is elevated (March of Dimes, 2015d).

In the third trimester amniocentesis is most commonly indicated to determine fetal lung maturity after the 35th week of gestation via analysis of lecithin-to-

TABLE 12.2 AMNIOTIC FLUID ANALYSIS AND IMPLICATIONS

Test Component	Normal Findings	Fetal Implications of Abnormal Findings
Color	Clear with white flecks of vernix caseosa in a mature fetus	Blood of maternal origin is usually harmless. "Port wine" fluid may indicate abruptio placentae. Fetal blood may indicate damage to the fetal, placental, or umbilical cord vessels.
Bilirubin	Absent at term	High levels indicate hemolytic disease of the neonate in isoimmunized pregnancy.
Meconium	Absent (except in breech presentation)	Presence indicates fetal hypotension or distress.
Creatinine	More than 2 mg/dL in a mature fetus	Decrease may indicate immature fetus (less than 37 wks).
Lecithin-to-sphingomyelin ratio (L/S ratio)	More than 2 generally indicates fetal pulmonary maturity.	A ratio of less than 2 indicates pulmonary immaturity and subsequent respiratory distress syndrome.
Phosphatidylglycerol	Present	Absence indicates pulmonary immaturity.
Glucose	Less than 45 mg/dL	Excessive increases at term or near term indicate hypertrophied fetal pancreas and subsequent neonatal hypoglycemia.
Alpha-fetoprotein	Variable, depending on gestation age and laboratory technique; highest concentration (about 18.5 ng/mL) occurs at 13–14 wks	Inappropriate increases indicate neural tube defects such as spina bifida or anencephaly, impending fetal death, congenital nephrosis, or contamination of fetal blood.
Bacteria	Absent	Presence indicates chorioamnionitis.
Chromosomes	Normal karyotype	Abnormal karyotype may indicate fetal sex and chromosome disorders.
Acetylcholinesterase	Absent	Presence may indicate neural tube defects, exomphalos, or other serious malformations.

Adapted from Cunningham, F., Leveno, K., Bloom, S., Spong, K., Dashe, J. S., Hoffman, B.L., et al. (2014). *Williams obstetrics* (24th ed.). New York, NY: McGraw-Hill Education; March of Dimes. (2015d). *Aminocentesis.* Retrieved from http://www.marchofdimes.com/pregnancy/amniocentesis.aspx; and Springer, S. C. (2015). Prenatal diagnosis and fetal therapy. *eMedicine.* Retrieved from http://emedicine.medscape.com/article/936318-overview

sphingomyelin ratios and to evaluate the fetal condition with Rh isoimmunization. Table 12.2 lists amniotic fluid analysis findings and their implications.

Procedure

Amniocentesis is performed after an ultrasound examination identifies an adequate pocket of amniotic fluid free of fetal parts, the umbilical cord, or the placenta (Fig. 12.7). The health care provider inserts a long pudendal or spinal needle, a 22-gauge, 5-in needle, into the amniotic cavity and aspirates amniotic fluid, which is placed in an amber or foil-covered test tube to protect it from light. When the desired amount of fluid has been withdrawn, the needle is removed and slight pressure is applied to the site. If there is no evidence of bleeding, a sterile bandage is applied to the needle site. The specimens are then sent to the laboratory immediately for the cytologist to evaluate.

Examining a sample of fetal cells directly produces a definitive diagnosis rather than a "best guess" diagnosis based on indirect screening tests. It is an invaluable diagnostic tool, but the risks include lower abdominal discomfort and cramping that may last up to 48 hours after the procedure, spontaneous abortion (1 in 200), maternal or fetal infection, postamniocentesis chorioamnionitis that has an insidious onset, fetal–maternal hemorrhage, leakage of amniotic fluid in 2% to 3% of women after the procedure, and higher rates of fetal loss in earlier amniocentesis procedures (<15 weeks' gestation) versus later ones (Akolekar et al., 2015). Obtaining the test results may take up to 3 weeks. Women

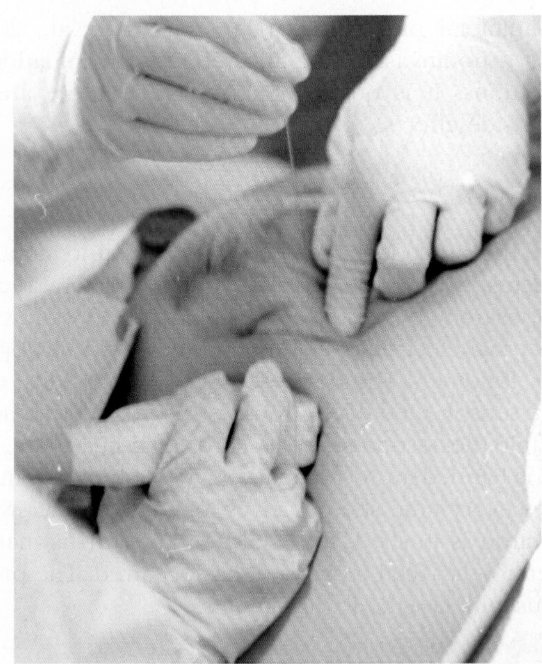

FIGURE 12.7 Technique for amniocentesis: Inserting needle.

today are choosing noninvasive prenatal testing rather than undergoing invasive testing such as amniocentesis or CVS despite those tests not being 100% correct. Women with reassuring noninvasive results and normal ultrasound findings seem satisfied over the risk of procedure-related pregnancy loss (Biswas & Choolani, 2015). The number of invasive procedures has declined since the availability of noninvasive prenatal testing, and it is predicted that they will replace the more invasive procedures in the future.

Nursing Management

When preparing the woman for an amniocentesis, explain the procedure and its potential complications, and encourage her to empty her bladder just before the procedure to avoid the risk of bladder puncture. Inform her that a 20-minute electronic fetal monitoring strip usually is obtained to evaluate fetal well-being and obtain a baseline to compare after the procedure is completed. Obtain and record maternal vital signs.

After the procedure, assist the woman to a position of comfort and administer RhoGAM intramuscularly if the woman is Rh negative to prevent potential sensitization to fetal blood. Assess maternal vital signs and fetal heart rate every 15 minutes for an hour after the procedure. Observe the puncture site for bleeding or drainage. Instruct the client to rest after returning home and remind her to report fever, leaking amniotic fluid, vaginal bleeding, or uterine contractions or any changes in fetal activity (increased or decreased) to the health care provider.

When the test results come back, be available to offer support, especially if a fetal abnormality is found. Also prepare the woman and her partner for the need for genetic counseling. Trained genetic counselors can provide accurate medical information and help couples to interpret the results of the amniocentesis so they can make the decisions that are right for them as a family.

Chorionic Villus Sampling

CVS is an invasive procedure involving an 18-gauge needle stick through the abdomen or passage of a suction catheter through the cervix under ultrasound guidance. This test is used to obtain a sample of the chorionic villi from the placenta for prenatal evaluation of chromosomal disorders such as Down syndrome or cystic fibrosis, enzyme deficiencies, and fetal gender determination and to identify sex-linked disorders such as hemophilia, sickle cell anemia, and Tay–Sachs disease (Greeley, Kessler, & Vohra, 2015). Chorionic villi are finger-like projections that cover the embryo and anchor it to the uterine lining before the placenta is developed. Because they are of embryonic origin, sampling provides information about the developing fetus. CVS can be used to detect numerous genetic disorders, with the exception of neural tube defects (Latendresse & Deneris, 2015).

There has been an impetus to develop earlier prenatal diagnostic procedures so that couples can make an early decision to terminate the pregnancy if an anomaly is confirmed. Early prenatal diagnosis by CVS has been proposed as an alternative to routine amniocentesis, which carries fewer risks if done later in the pregnancy. In addition, results of CVS testing are available sooner than those of amniocentesis, usually within 48 hours.

Procedure

CVS is generally performed 10 to 13 weeks after the LMP. Earlier, chorionic villi may not be sufficiently developed for adequate tissue sampling and the risk of limb defects is increased (Khalil & Coates, 2015). First, an ultrasound is done to confirm gestational age and viability. Then, under continuous ultrasound guidance, CVS is performed using either a transcervical or transabdominal approach. With the transcervical approach, the woman is placed in the lithotomy position and a sterile catheter is introduced through the cervix and inserted in the placenta, where a sample of chorionic villi is aspirated. This approach requires the client to have a full bladder to push the uterus and placenta into a position that is more accessible to the catheter. A full bladder also helps in better visualization of the structures. With the transabdominal approach, an 18-gauge spinal needle is inserted through the abdominal wall into the placental tissue and a sample of chorionic villi is aspirated. Regardless of the approach used, the sample is sent to the cytogenetics laboratory for analysis.

Potential complications of CVS include postprocedure vaginal bleeding and cramping (most common), hematomas, spontaneous abortion, limb abnormalities, rupture of membranes, infection, chorioamnionitis, and fetal–maternal hemorrhage (March of Dimes, 2015e). The pregnancy loss rate or procedure-related miscarriage rate is approximately 0.5% to 1.0%, which is the same rate for amniocentesis. In addition, women who are Rh negative should receive immune globulin (RhoGAM) to avoid isoimmunization (Jordan et al., 2014).

Nursing Management

Explain to the woman that the procedure will last about 15 minutes. An ultrasound will be done first to locate the embryo, and a baseline set of vital signs will be taken before starting. Make sure she is informed of the risks related to the procedure, including their incidence. If a transabdominal CVS procedure is planned, advise her to fill her bladder by drinking increased amounts of water. Inform her that a needle will be inserted through her abdominal wall and samples will be collected. Once the samples are collected, the needle will be withdrawn and the samples will be sent to the genetics laboratory for evaluation.

For transcervical CVS, inform the women that a speculum will be placed into the vagina under ultrasound guidance. Then the vagina is cleaned and a small catheter is inserted through the cervix. The samples obtained through the catheter are then sent to a laboratory.

After either procedure, assist the woman to a position of comfort and clean any excess lubricant or secretions from the area. Instruct her about signs to watch for and report, such as fever, cramping, and vaginal bleeding. Urge her not to engage in any strenuous activity for the next 48 hours. Assess the fetal heart rate for changes and administer RhoGAM to an unsensitized Rh-negative woman after the procedure.

Nonstress Test

The nonstress test (NST) is the most common method of prenatal testing used in practice today. The NST provides an indirect measurement of uteroplacental function. Unlike the fetal movement counting done by the mother alone, this procedure requires specialized equipment and trained personnel. The basis for the NST is that the normal fetus produces characteristic fetal heart rate patterns in response to fetal movements. In the healthy fetus there is an acceleration of the fetal heart rate with fetal movement. Currently, an NST is recommended twice weekly (after 28 weeks of gestation) for clients with diabetes and other high-risk conditions, such as IUGR, preeclampsia, postterm pregnancy, renal disease, and multifetal pregnancies (Cunningham et al., 2014). NST is a noninvasive test that requires no initiation of contractions. It is quick to perform and there are no known side effects.

Procedure

Before the procedure the client eats a meal to stimulate fetal activity. Then she is placed in the left lateral recumbent position to avoid supine hypotension syndrome. An external electronic fetal monitoring device is applied to her abdomen. The device consists of two belts, each with a sensor. One of the sensors records uterine activity, while the second sensor records fetal heart rate. The client is handed an "event marker" with a button that she pushes every time she perceives fetal movement. When the button is pushed, the fetal monitor strip is marked to identify that fetal movement has occurred. The procedure usually lasts 20 to 30 minutes.

Nursing Management

Prior to the NST, explain the testing procedure and have the woman empty her bladder. Position her in a semi-Fowler position and apply the two external monitor belts. Document the date and time the test is started, client information, the reason for the test, and the maternal vital signs. Obtain a baseline fetal monitor strip over 15 to 30 minutes.

During the test, observe for signs of fetal activity with a concurrent acceleration of the fetal heart rate. Interpret the NST as reactive or nonreactive. A reactive NST includes at least two fetal heart rate accelerations from the baseline of at least 15 bpm for at least 15 seconds within the 20-minute recording period. If the test does not meet these criteria after 40 minutes, it is considered nonreactive. A nonreactive NST is characterized by the absence of two fetal heart rate accelerations using the 15-by-15 criterion in a 20-minute time frame. A nonreactive test has been correlated with a higher incidence of fetal distress during labor, fetal mortality, and IUGR. Additional testing, such as a **biophysical profile (BPP)**, should be considered (King et al., 2015).

After the NST procedure, assist the woman off the table, provide her with fluids, and allow her to use the restroom. Typically the health care provider discusses the results with the woman at this time. Provide teaching about signs and symptoms to report. If serial NSTs are being done, schedule the next testing session.

Biophysical Profile

A BPP uses a real-time ultrasound and NST to allow assessment of various parameters of fetal well-being. A BPP includes ultrasound monitoring of fetal movements, fetal tone, and fetal breathing and ultrasound assessment of amniotic fluid volume with or without assessment of the fetal heart rate. A BPP is performed in an effort to identify infants who may be at risk of poor pregnancy outcome, so that additional assessments of well-being may be performed, or labor may be induced or a caesarean section performed to expedite birth. The primary objectives of the BPP are to reduce stillbirth and to detect hypoxia early enough to allow delivery in time to avoid permanent fetal damage resulting from fetal asphyxia. These parameters, together with the NST, constitute the BPP. Each parameter is controlled by a different structure in the fetal brain: fetal tone by the cortex; fetal movements by the cortex and motor nuclei; fetal breathing movements by the centers close to the fourth ventricle; and the NST by the posterior hypothalamus and medulla. The amniotic fluid is the result of fetal urine volume. Some facilities do not perform an NST unless other parameters of the profile are abnormal (King et al., 2015). The BPP is based on the concept that a fetus that experiences hypoxia loses certain behavioral parameters in the reverse order in which they were acquired during fetal development (normal order of development: tone at 8 weeks; movement at 9 weeks; breathing at 20 weeks; and fetal heart rate reactivity at 24 weeks).

Scoring and Interpretation

The BPP is a scored test with five components, each worth 2 points if present. A total score of 10 is possible if the NST is used. Thirty minutes are allotted for testing, although less than 10 minutes is usually needed. The following criteria must be met to obtain a score of 2; anything less is scored as 0 (Moses, 2015c):

- *Body movements:* three or more discrete limb or trunk movements
- *Fetal tone:* one or more instances of full extension and flexion of a limb or trunk
- *Fetal breathing:* one or more fetal breathing movements of more than 30 seconds
- *Amniotic fluid volume:* one or more pockets of fluid measuring 2 cm
- *NST:* normal NST = 2 points; abnormal NST = 0 points

Interpretation of the BPP score can be complicated, depending on several fetal and maternal variables. Because it is indicated as a result of a nonreassuring finding from previous fetal surveillance tests, this test can be used to quantify the interpretation, and intervention can be initiated if appropriate. A maximum score of 10 can be achieved and the test is complete once all of the variables have been observed. For the test to be judged abnormal and a score of zero awarded for the absence of fetal movement, fetal tone, or fetal breathing movements, a period of not less than 30 minutes must have elapsed. Because of the excellent sensitivity of fetal NST for fetal acidemia, it has been proposed that this acute marker alone may be used for fetal assessment in combination with the amniotic fluid volume assessment, a chronic marker. This combination, also known as the modified BPP, has been shown to have excellent false-negative rates that compare with that of the complete BPP. In addition, a recent study reported that BPP scores correlate fairly closely with the APGAR scores obtained after birth (Nisa et al., 2015).

One of the important factors is the amniotic fluid volume, taken in conjunction with the results of the NST. Amniotic fluid is largely composed of fetal urine. As placental function decreases, perfusion of fetal organs, such as kidneys, decreases, and this can lead to a reduction of amniotic fluid. If oligohydramnios or decreased amniotic fluid is present, the potential exists for antepartum or intrapartum fetal compromise (Lakshmi & Jyothsna, 2015).

Overall, a score of 8 to 10 is considered normal if the amniotic fluid volume is adequate. A score of 6 or below is suspicious, possibly indicating a compromised fetus; further investigation of fetal well-being is needed.

Because the BPP is an ultrasonographic assessment of fetal behavior, it requires more extensive equipment and more highly trained personnel than other testing modalities. The cost is much greater than with less sophisticated tests. It permits conservative therapy and prevents premature or unnecessary intervention. There are fewer false-positive results than with the NST alone (Callahan, 2016).

Nursing Management

Nursing management focuses primarily on offering the client support and answering her questions. Expect to complete the NST before scheduling the BPP, and explain why further testing might be needed. Tell the woman that the ultrasound will be done in the diagnostic imaging department.

NURSING MANAGEMENT FOR THE COMMON DISCOMFORTS OF PREGNANCY

Most women experience common discomforts during pregnancy and ask a nurse's advice about ways to minimize them. However, other women will not bring up their concerns unless asked. Therefore, the nurse needs to address the common discomforts that occur in each trimester at each prenatal visit and provide realistic measures to help the client deal with them (Teaching Guidelines 12.1). Nursing Care Plan 12.1 (at the end of the chapter) applies the nursing process to the care of a woman experiencing some discomforts of pregnancy.

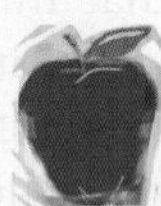

Teaching Guidelines 12.1

TEACHING TO MANAGE THE DISCOMFORTS OF PREGNANCY

Urinary Frequency or Incontinence

- Try pelvic floor exercises to increase control over leakage.
- Empty your bladder when you first feel a full sensation.
- Avoid caffeinated drinks, which stimulate voiding.
- Reduce your fluid intake after dinner to reduce nighttime urination.

Fatigue

- Attempt to get a full night's sleep, without interruptions.
- Eat a healthy balanced diet.
- Schedule a nap in the early afternoon daily.
- When you are feeling tired, rest.

Nausea and Vomiting

- Avoid an empty stomach at all times.
- Eat dry crackers/toast in bed before arising.
- Eat several small meals throughout the day.
- Avoid brushing teeth immediately after eating to avoid gag reflex.
- Acupressure wristbands can be worn daily.
- Drink fluids between meals rather than with meals.
- Avoid greasy, fried foods or ones with a strong odor, such as cabbage or Brussels sprouts.

Backache

- Avoid standing or sitting in one position for long periods.
- Apply heating pad (low setting) to the small of your back.
- Support your lower back with pillows when sitting.
- Use proper body mechanics for lifting anything.
- Avoid excessive bending, lifting, or walking without rest periods.
- Wear supportive low-heeled shoes; avoid high heels.
- Stand with your shoulders back to maintain correct posture.

Leg Cramps

- Elevate legs above heart level frequently throughout the day.
- If you get a cramp, straighten both legs and flex your feet toward your body.
- Ask your health care provider about taking additional calcium supplements, which may reduce leg spasms.

Varicosities

- Walk daily to improve circulation to extremities.
- Elevate both legs above heart level while resting.
- Avoid standing in one position for long periods of time.
- Don't wear constrictive stockings and socks.
- Don't cross the legs when sitting for long periods.
- Wear support stockings to promote better circulation.

Hemorrhoids

- Establish a regular time for daily bowel elimination.
- Avoid constipation and straining during defecation.
- Prevent straining by drinking plenty of fluids and eating fiber-rich foods and exercising daily.
- Use warm sitz baths and cool witch hazel compresses for comfort.

Constipation

- Increase your intake of foods high in fiber and drink at least eight 8-oz glasses of fluid daily.
- Ingest prunes or prune juice which are natural laxatives.
- Consume warm liquids (tea) on rising, to stimulate peristalsis.
- Exercise each day (brisk walking) to promote movement through the intestine.
- Reduce the amount of cheese consumed.

Heartburn/Indigestion

- Avoid spicy or greasy foods and eat small frequent meals.
- Sleep on several pillows so that your head is elevated 30 degrees.
- Stop smoking and avoid caffeinated drinks to reduce stimulation.
- Avoid lying down for at least 3 hours after meals.
- Try drinking sips of water to reduce burning sensation.
- Avoid foods that trigger symptoms—fried foods, citrus, soda, chocolate.
- Take antacids sparingly if burning sensation is severe.

Braxton Hicks Contractions

- Keep in mind that these contractions are a normal sensation. Try changing your position or engaging in mild exercise to help reduce the sensation.
- Drink more fluids if possible.

First-Trimester Discomforts

During the first 3 months of pregnancy, the woman's body is undergoing numerous changes. Some women experience many discomforts, but others have few. These discomforts are caused by the changes taking place within the body and they pass as the pregnancy progresses.

Urinary Frequency or Incontinence

Urinary frequency or incontinence is common in the first trimester because the growing uterus compresses the bladder. This also is a common complaint during the third trimester, especially when the fetal head settles into the pelvis. However, the discomfort tends to improve in the second trimester, when the uterus becomes an abdominal organ and moves away from the bladder region.

After infection and gestational diabetes have been ruled out as causative factors of increased urinary frequency, suggest that the woman decrease her fluid intake 2 to 3 hours before bedtime and limit her intake of caffeinated beverages. Increased voiding is normal, but encourage the client to report any pain or burning during urination. Also explain that increased urinary frequency may subside as she enters her second trimester, only to recur in the third trimester. Teach the client to perform pelvic floor muscle training exercises, formally termed Kegel exercises, to increase support of the uterus, bladder, small intestine, and rectum throughout the day to help strengthen perineal muscle tone, thereby enhancing urinary control and decreasing the possibility of incontinence.

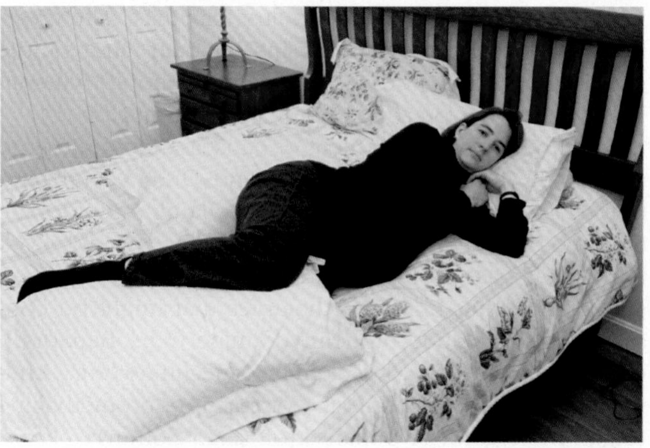

FIGURE 12.8 Using pillows for support in the side-lying position.

Fatigue

Fatigue plagues all pregnant women, primarily in the first and third trimesters (the highest energy levels typically occur during the second trimester), even if they get their normal amount of sleep at night. First-trimester fatigue most often is related to the many physical changes (e.g., increased oxygen consumption, increased levels of progesterone and relaxin, increased metabolic demands) and psychosocial changes (e.g., mood swings, multiple role demands) of pregnancy. Third-trimester fatigue can be caused by sleep disturbances from increased weight (many women cannot find a comfortable sleeping position due to the enlarging abdomen), physical discomforts such as heartburn, and insomnia due to mood swings, multiple role anxiety, and a decrease in exercise (Rigby, 2015).

Once anemia, infection, and blood dyscrasias have been ruled out as contributing to the client's fatigue, advise her to arrange work, child care, and other demands in her life to permit additional rest periods. Work with the client to devise a realistic schedule for rest. Using pillows for support in the left-side-lying position relieves pressure on major blood vessels that supply oxygen and nutrients to the fetus when resting (Fig. 12.8). Also recommend the use of relaxation techniques, providing instructions as necessary, and suggest she increase her daily exercise level.

Nausea and Vomiting

It is estimated that somewhere between 70% to 80% of pregnant women experience nausea and vomiting. In the United States, this translates to approximately 4 million women. It is found more often in Western countries and urban populations, and is rare among Africans, Native Americans, Eskimos, and most Asian populations (Callahan, 2016). The problem is generally time limited, with the onset about the fifth week after the LMP, a peak at 8 to 12 weeks, and resolution by 16 to 18 weeks. Despite popular use of the term *morning sickness,* nausea and vomiting of pregnancy persists throughout the day in the majority of affected women and has been found to be limited to the morning in less than 2% of women (Tyler & Nagtalon-Ramos, 2015). The physiologic changes that cause nausea and vomiting are unknown, but research suggests that unusually high levels of estrogen, progesterone, and hCG and a vitamin B_6 deficiency may be contributing factors. Symptoms generally last until the second trimester and are generally associated with a positive pregnancy outcome, in terms of lower rates of miscarriages, congenital malformations, and preterm births (Cunningham et al., 2014). In summary, the etiology of nausea and vomiting in pregnancy is physiologic, thus assessment of the condition focuses on severity, and the management is largely supportive.

Nausea and vomiting of pregnancy can take a physical and psychologic toll on the pregnant woman, and may have an adverse effect on her partner, family members, and even coworkers. The burden it places on the woman is usually minimized, as it is considered a normal part of pregnancy, thus it may not be worthy of evaluation, diagnosis, management, and emotional support. As a result, it may not be taken seriously because it is so common and time-limited; leading some women to feel frustrated and feel guilty that they are even complaining about their symptoms. Nurses need to pick up on this, address it and provide support for her.

The goal of treatment is to improve symptoms while minimizing risks to mother and fetus. Treatment management ranges from simple dietary modifications to drug therapy. To help alleviate nausea and vomiting, advise the woman to eat small, frequent meals that are bland and low in fat (five or six a day) to prevent her stomach from becoming completely empty. Other helpful suggestions include eating dry crackers, Cheerios, or cheese or drinking lemonade before getting out of bed in the morning and increasing her intake of foods high in vitamin B_6, such as meat, poultry, bananas, fish, green leafy vegetables, peanuts, raisins, walnuts, and whole grains, or making sure she is receiving enough vitamin B_6 by taking her prescribed prenatal vitamins.

Pharmacologic treatment of nausea and vomiting in pregnancy is limited. The Food and Drug Administration (FDA) recently approved doxylamine-pyridoxine therapy for use in pregnancy, which seems to work fairly well based on the current reviews (Slaughter et al., 2014). Other pharmacotherapies that might be considered may include diphenhydramine (e.g., Benadryl), dimenhydrinate (e.g., Dramamine), meclinine (e.g., Antivert), prochlorperazine (e.g., Compazine), promethazine (e.g., Phenergan), or ondansetron (e.g., Zofran).

Other helpful tips to deal with nausea and vomiting include:

- Get out of bed in the morning very slowly.
- Avoid sudden movements.
- Avoid triggers that stimulate or exacerbate nausea—strong food odors.
- Eat a high-protein snack before retiring at night to prevent an empty stomach.
- Take ginger (up to 1 g in divided doses daily; 250-mg capsules QID), which increases tone and peristalsis in the gastrointestinal tract.
- Open a window to remove odors of food being cooked.
- Eat more protein than carbohydrates and take in more liquids than solids.
- Limit intake of fluids or soups during meals (drink them between meals).
- Avoid fried foods and foods cooked with grease, oils, or fatty meats, because they tend to upset the stomach.
- Avoid highly seasoned foods such as those cooked with garlic, onions, peppers, and chili.
- Drink a small amount of caffeine-free carbonated beverage (ginger ale) if nauseated.
- Trying acupressure using a wristband has been FDA approved for nausea.
- Avoid wearing tight or restricting clothes, which might place increased pressure on the expanding abdomen.
- Avoid stress(Bope & Kellerman, 2015; Jordan et al., 2014; King et al., 2015).

Breast Tenderness

As a result of increased estrogen and progesterone levels, which cause the fat layer of breasts to thicken and the number of milk ducts and glands to increase during the first trimester, many women experience breast tenderness. Offering a thorough explanation to the woman about the reasons for the breast discomfort is important. Wearing a larger bra with good support can help alleviate this discomfort. Advise her to wear a supportive bra, even while sleeping. As her breasts increase in size, advise her to change her bra size to ensure adequate support.

Constipation

Constipation affects up to 38% of pregnancies (Verghese, Futaba, & Latthe, 2015). Increasing levels of progesterone during pregnancy lead to decreased contractility of the gastrointestinal tract, slowed movement of substances through the colon, and a resulting increase in water absorption. All of these factors lead to constipation. Lack of exercise or too little fiber or fluids in the diet can also promote constipation. In addition, the large bowel is mechanically compressed by the enlarging uterus, adding to this discomfort. The iron and calcium in prenatal vitamins can also contribute to constipation during the first and third trimesters.

Explain how pregnancy exacerbates the symptoms of constipation and offer the following suggestions:

- Eat fresh or dried fruit daily.
- Eat more raw fruits and vegetables, including their skins.
- Eat whole-grain cereals and breads such as raisin bran or bran flakes.
- Participate in physical activity every day.
- Engage in pelvis floor exercises, stretching exercises, and yoga daily.
- Eat meals at regular intervals.
- Establish a time of day to defecate, and elevate feet on a stool to avoid straining.
- Drink six to eight glasses of water daily.
- Decrease intake of refined carbohydrates.
- Drink warm fluids on arising to stimulate bowel motility.
- Decrease consumption of sugary sodas.
- Avoid eating large amounts of cheese.

If the suggestions above are ineffective, suggest that the woman use a bulk-forming laxative such as Metamucil®.

Nasal Stuffiness, Bleeding Gums, Epistaxis (Nosebleeds)

Increased levels of estrogen cause edema of the mucous membranes of the nasal and oral cavities. Advise the woman to drink extra water for hydration of the mucous membranes or to use a cool mist humidifier in her bedroom at night. If she needs to blow her nose to relieve nasal stuffiness, advise her to blow gently, one nostril at a time. Advise her to avoid the use of nasal decongestants and sprays.

If a nosebleed occurs, advise the woman to loosen the clothing around her neck, sit with her head tilted forward, pinch her nostrils with her thumb and forefinger for 10 to 15 minutes, and apply an ice pack to the bridge of her nose.

If the woman has bleeding gums, encourage her to practice good oral hygiene by using a soft toothbrush and flossing daily. Warm saline mouthwashes can relieve discomfort. If the gum problem persists, instruct her to see her dentist.

Cravings

Food craving refers to an intense desire to consume a specific food. Desires for certain foods and beverages are likely to begin during the first trimester but do not appear to reflect any physiologic need. Foods with a high sodium or sugar content often are the ones craved. At times, some women crave nonfood substances such as clay, cornstarch, laundry detergent, baking soda, soap, paint chips, dirt, ice, or wax. As explained in Chapter 11, this craving for nonfood substances, termed *pica,* may indicate a severe dietary deficiency of minerals or vitamins, or it may have cultural roots (Jyothi, 2015).

Leukorrhea

Increased vaginal discharge begins during the first trimester and continues throughout pregnancy. The physiologic changes behind leukorrhea arise from the high levels of estrogen, which cause increased vascularity and hypertrophy of cervical glands as well as vaginal cells (Cunningham et al., 2014). The result is progressively increasing vaginal secretions throughout pregnancy.

Advise the woman to keep the perineal area clean and dry, washing the area with mild soap and water during her daily shower. Also recommend that she avoid wearing pantyhose and other tight-fitting nylon clothes that prevent air from circulating to the genital area. Encourage the use of cotton underwear and suggest wearing a nightgown rather than pajamas to allow for increased airflow. Also instruct the woman to avoid douching and tampon use.

Second-Trimester Discomforts

A sense of well-being typically characterizes the second trimester for most women. By this time, the fatigue, nausea, and vomiting have subsided and the uncomfortable changes of the third trimester are a few months away. Not every woman experiences the same discomforts during this time, so nursing assessments and interventions must be individualized.

Backache

Musculoskeletal pain is a common occurrence in pregnancy and postpartum. Half of women report having back pain at some point during pregnancy. This can seriously impact the quality of life of women and have socioeconomic issues from loss days at work. The pain can be lumbar or sacroiliac. The pain may also be present only at night. Back pain is thought to be due to multiple factors, which include shifting of the center of gravity caused by the enlarging uterus, increased joint laxity due to an increase in relaxin, stretching of the ligaments (which are pain-sensitive structures), and pregnancy-related circulatory changes.

Treatment is heat and ice, acetaminophen, massage, proper posturing, good support shoes, and a good exercise program for strength and conditioning. Pregnant women may also relieve back pain by placing one foot on a stool when standing for long periods of time and placing a pillow between the legs when lying down (Plastaras & Appasamy, 2015). After exploring other reasons that might cause backache, such as uterine contractions, urinary tract infection, ulcers, or musculoskeletal back disorders, the following instructions may be helpful:

- Maintain correct posture, with head up and shoulders back.
- Wear low-heeled shoes with good arch support.
- When standing for long periods, place one foot on a stool or box.
- Use good body mechanics when lifting objects.
- When sitting, use foot supports and pillows behind the back.
- Try pelvic tilt or rocking exercises to strengthen the back (ACOG, 2015c).

The pelvic tilt or pelvic rock is used to alleviate pressure on the lower back during pregnancy by stretching the lower back muscles. It can be done sitting, standing, or on all fours. To do it on all fours, the hands are positioned directly under the shoulders and the knees under the hips. The back should be in a neutral position with the head and neck aligned with the straight back. The woman then presses up with the lower back and holds this position for a few seconds, then relaxes to a neutral position. This action of pressing upward is repeated frequently throughout the day to prevent a sore back (Rigby, 2015).

Leg Cramps

Many women experience leg cramps in pregnancy. They become more common as pregnancy progresses and are especially troublesome at night. They occur primarily in the second and third trimesters and could be related to the pressure of the gravid uterus on pelvic nerves and blood vessels. During pregnancy, up to 50% of women can be affected by leg cramps, and up to 25% can be affected by restless legs syndrome (King et al., 2015). Along with lack of exercise, diet can also be a contributing factor if the woman is not consuming enough of certain minerals, such as calcium and magnesium. The sudden stretching of leg muscles may also play a role in causing leg cramps (Kondhare & Khodgire, 2015).

Encourage the woman to gently stretch the muscle by dorsiflexing the foot up toward the body. Wrapping a warm, moist towel around the leg muscle can also help the muscle to relax. Advise the client to avoid stretching her legs, pointing her toes, and walking excessively. Stress the importance of wearing low-heeled shoes and support hose and arising slowly from a sitting position. If the leg cramps are due to deficiencies in minerals, the condition can be remedied by eating more foods rich in these nutrients. Also instruct the woman on calf-stretching exercises: have her stand 3 ft from the wall and lean toward it, resting her lower arms against it, while keeping her heels on the floor. This may help reduce cramping if it is done before going to bed.

Elevating the legs throughout the day will help relieve pressure and minimize strain. Wearing support hose and avoiding curling the toes may help to relieve leg discomfort. Also instruct the client to avoid standing in one spot for a prolonged period or crossing her legs. If she must stand for prolonged periods, suggest that she change her position at least every 2 hours by walking or sitting to reduce the risk of leg cramps. Encourage her to drink eight 8-oz glasses of fluid throughout the day to ensure adequate hydration. Taking daily walks can also help reduce leg cramping because ambulation improves circulation to the muscles.

Varicosities of the Vulva and Legs

Varicosities of the vulva and legs are associated with the increased venous stasis caused by the pressure of the gravid uterus on pelvic vessels and the vasodilation resulting from increased progesterone levels. Progesterone relaxes the vein walls, making it difficult for blood to return to the heart from the extremities; pooling can result. Genetic predisposition, inactivity, obesity, and poor muscle tone are also contributing factors.

Encourage the client to wear support hose and teach her how to apply them properly. Advise her to elevate her legs above her heart while lying on her back for 10 minutes before she gets out of bed in the morning, thus promoting venous return before she applies the hose. Instruct the client to avoid crossing her legs and avoid wearing knee-high stockings. They cause constriction of leg vessels and muscles and contribute to venous stasis. Also encourage the client to elevate both legs above the level of the heart for 5 to 10 minutes at least twice a day (Fig. 12.9); to wear low-heeled shoes; and to avoid long periods of standing or sitting, frequently changing her position. If the client has vulvar varicosities, suggest she apply ice packs to the area when she is lying down.

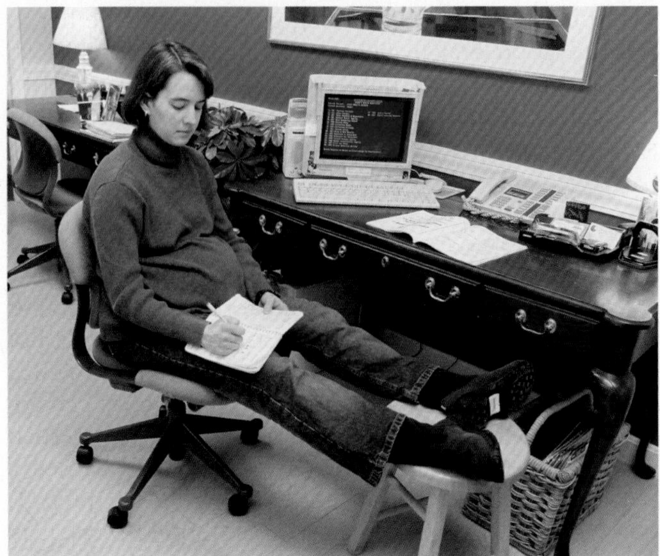

FIGURE 12.9 Woman elevating her legs while working.

Hemorrhoids

Hemorrhoids are varicosities of the rectum and may be external (outside the anal sphincter) or internal (above the sphincter) (ACOG, 2015d). They occur as a result of progesterone-induced vasodilation and from pressure of the enlarged uterus on the lower intestine and rectum. Hemorrhoids are more common in women with constipation, poor fluid intake or poor dietary habits, smokers, or those with a previous history of hemorrhoids (Zielinski, Searing, & Deibel, 2015).

Instruct the client in measures to prevent constipation, including increasing fiber intake and drinking at least 2 L of fluid per day. Recommend the use of topical anesthetics (e.g., Preparation H®, Anusol, witch hazel compresses such as Tucks®) to reduce pain, itching, and swelling, if permitted by the health care provider. Teach the client about local comfort measures such as warm sitz baths, witch hazel compresses, or cold compresses. To minimize her risk of straining while defecating, suggest that she elevate her feet on a stool. Also encourage her to avoid prolonged sitting or standing (ACOG, 2015d).

Flatulence With Bloating

Flatulence and gas pain are another result of decreased gastrointestinal motility. The physiologic changes that result in constipation (reduced gastrointestinal motility and dilation secondary to progesterone's influence) may also result in increased flatulence. As the enlarging uterus compresses the bowel, it delays the passage of food through the intestines, thus allowing more time for gas to be formed by bacteria in the colon. The woman usually reports increased passage of rectal gas, abdominal bloating, or belching. Instruct the woman to avoid gas-forming foods, such as beans, cabbage, and onions, as well as foods that have a high content of white sugar. Adding more fiber to the diet, increasing fluid intake, and increasing physical exercise are also helpful in reducing flatus. In addition, reducing the amount of swallowed air, if chewing gum, will reduce gas build-up. The knee-chest position may also help with discomfort from unexpelled gas. Reducing the intake of carbonated beverages and cheese and eating mints can also help reduce flatulence during pregnancy (Almansa, De Vault, & Houghton, 2015).

Third-Trimester Discomforts

As women enter their third trimester, many experience a return of the first-trimester discomforts of fatigue, urinary frequency, leukorrhea, and constipation. These discomforts are secondary to the ever-enlarging uterus compressing adjacent structures, increasing hormone levels, and the metabolic demands of the fetus. In addition to these discomforts, many women experience shortness of breath, heartburn and indigestion, swelling, and Braxton Hicks contractions.

Shortness of Breath and Dyspnea

Dyspnea is a common complaint in pregnant women. Physiologic and hemodynamic changes can result in a significant dyspnea in such cases. In some women, dyspnea in normal daily activities can be a sign of heart and lung disease and may be associated with poor perinatal and cardiac outcome in which early detection can prevent adverse events. The increasing growth of the uterus prevents complete lung expansion late in pregnancy. As the uterus enlarges upward in the second and third trimesters, the expansion of the diaphragm is limited. Dyspnea can occur when the woman lies on her back and the pressure of the gravid uterus against the vena cava reduces venous return to the heart (Tara et al., 2015).

Explain to the woman that dyspnea is normal and will improve when the fetus drops into the pelvis (lightening). Instruct her to adjust her body position to allow for maximum expansion of the chest and to avoid large meals, which increase abdominal pressure. Raising the head of the bed on blocks or placing pillows behind her back is helpful too. Under normal circumstances, resting with the head elevated while taking slow, deep breaths reduces shortness of breath symptoms. In addition, stress to her that lying on her left side will displace the uterus off the vena cava and improve her breathing. Having the woman periodically stand up and stretch her arms above her head and take a deep breath is helpful to relieve dyspnea. Also, advise the woman to avoid exercise that precipitates dyspnea, to rest after exercise, and to avoid overheating in warm climates. If she still smokes, encourage her to stop.

Heartburn and Indigestion

Heartburn and indigestion result when high progesterone levels cause relaxation of the cardiac sphincter, allowing food and digestive juices to flow backward from the stomach into the esophagus. Irritation of the esophageal lining occurs, causing the burning sensation known as heartburn. It occurs in up to 70% of women at some point during pregnancy, with an increased frequency seen in the third trimester (King et al., 2015). The pain may radiate to the neck and throat. It worsens when the woman lies down, bends over after eating, or wears tight clothes. Indigestion (vague abdominal discomfort after meals) results from eating too much or too fast; from eating when tense, tired, or emotionally upset; from eating food that is too fatty or spicy; and from eating heavy food or food that has been badly cooked or processed (Nagtalon-Ramos, 2014). In addition, the stomach is displaced upward and compressed by the large uterus in the third trimester, thus limiting the stomach's capacity to empty quickly. Food sits, causing heartburn and indigestion.

Review the client's usual dietary intake and suggest that she limit or avoid gas-producing or fatty foods and large meals. Instruct the woman to pay attention to the timing of the discomfort. Usually it is heartburn when the pain occurs 30 to 45 minutes after a meal. Encourage the client to maintain proper posture and remain in the sitting position for 1 to 3 hours after eating to prevent reflux of gastric acids into the esophagus by gravity. Urge the client to consume small, frequent meals, to eat slowly, chewing her food thoroughly to prevent excessive swallowing of air, which can lead to increased gastric pressure. Instruct the client to avoid foods that act as triggers such as caffeinated drinks, greasy, gas-forming foods, citrus, spiced foods, chocolate, coffee, alcohol, and spearmint or peppermint. These items stimulate the release of gastric digestive acids, which may cause reflux into the esophagus. Avoid late-night or large meals and gum chewing. Avoid lying down within 3 hours after eating. Finally, elevate the head of the bed by 10 to 30 degrees.

Dependent Edema

Swelling is the result of increased capillary permeability caused by elevated hormone levels and increased blood volume. Sodium and water are retained and thirst increases. Edema occurs most often in dependent areas such as the legs and feet throughout the day due to gravity; it improves after a night's sleep. Warm weather or prolonged standing or sitting may increase edema. Generalized edema, appearing in the face, hands, and feet, can signal preeclampsia if accompanied by dizziness, blurred vision, headaches, upper quadrant pain, or nausea (Rigby, 2015). This edema should be reported to the health care provider. Appropriate suggestions to minimize dependent edema include:

- Elevate your feet and legs above the level of the heart periodically throughout the day.
- Wear support hose when standing or sitting for long periods.
- Change position frequently throughout the day.
- Walk at a sensible pace to help contract leg muscles to promote venous return.
- When taking a long car ride, stop to walk around every 2 hours.
- When standing, rock from the ball of the foot to the toes to stimulate circulation.
- Lie on your left side to keep the gravid uterus off the vena cava to return blood to the heart.
- Avoid foods high in sodium, such as lunch meats, potato chips, and bacon.
- Avoid wearing knee-high stockings.
- Drink six to eight glasses of water daily to replace fluids lost through perspiration.
- Avoid high intake of sugar and fats, because they cause water retention.

Braxton Hicks Contractions

Braxton Hicks contractions are irregular, painless contractions that occur without cervical dilation. Typically they intensify in the third trimester in preparation for labor. In reality, they have been present since early in the pregnancy but may have gone unnoticed. They are thought to increase the tone of uterine muscles for labor purposes (Grant, Strevens, & Thornton, 2015).

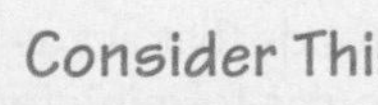

Consider This

One has to wonder sometimes why women go through what they do. During my first pregnancy I was sick for the first 2 months. I would experience waves of nausea from the moment I got out of bed until midmorning. Needless to say, I wasn't the happiest camper around. After the third month, my life seemed to settle down and I was beginning to think that being pregnant wasn't too bad after all. For the moment, I was fooled. Then, during my last 2 months, another wave of discomfort struck—heartburn and constipation—a double whammy! I now feared eating anything that might trigger acid indigestion and also might remain in my body too long. I literally had to become the "fiber queen" to combat these two challenges. Needless to say, my "suffering" was well worth our bright-eyed baby girl in the end.

Thoughts: Despite the various discomforts associated with pregnancy, most women wouldn't change their end result. Do most women experience these discomforts? What suggestions could be made to reduce them?

Reassure the client that these contractions are normal. Instruct the client in how to differentiate between Braxton Hicks and labor contractions. Explain that true labor contractions usually grow longer, stronger, and closer together and occur at regular intervals. Walking usually strengthens true labor contractions, whereas Braxton Hicks contractions tend to decrease in intensity and taper off. Advise the client to keep herself well hydrated and to rest in a left-side-lying position to help relieve the discomfort. Suggest that she use breathing techniques such as Lamaze techniques to ease the discomfort.

NURSING MANAGEMENT TO PROMOTE SELF-CARE

Pregnancy is considered a time of health, not illness. Health promotion and maintenance activities are essential to promoting an optimal outcome for the woman and her fetus. Pregnant women commonly have many questions about the changes occurring during pregnancy: how these changes affect their usual routine, such as working, traveling, exercising, or engaging in sexual activity; how the changes influence their typical self-care activities, such as bathing, perineal care, or dental care; and whether these changes are signs of a problem.

Take Note!

Women may have heard stories about or been told by others what to do and what not to do during pregnancy, leading to many misconceptions and much misinformation.

Nurses can play a major role in providing anticipatory guidance and teaching to foster the woman's responsibility for self-care, helping to clarify misconceptions and correct any misinformation. Educating the client to identify threats to safety posed by her lifestyle or environment and proposing ways to modify them to avoid a negative outcome are important. Counseling should also include healthy ways to prepare food, advice to avoid medications unless they are prescribed for her, and advice on identifying teratogens within her environment or at work and how to reduce her risk from exposure. The pregnant client can better care for herself and the fetus if her concerns are anticipated and identified by the nurse and are incorporated into teaching sessions at each prenatal visit.

Personal Hygiene

Hygiene is a necessity for the maintenance of good health. Cleansing the skin removes dirt, bacteria, sweat, dead skin cells, and body secretions. Counsel women to wash their hands and under their fingernails frequently throughout the day in order to lower the bacterial count on both. During pregnancy a woman's sebaceous (sweat) glands become more active under the influence of hormones, and sweating is more profuse. This increase may make it necessary to use a stronger deodorant and shower more frequently. The cervical and vaginal glands also produce more secretions during pregnancy. Frequent showering helps to keep the area dry and promotes better hygiene. Encourage the use of cotton underwear to allow greater air circulation. Taking a tub bath in early pregnancy is permitted, but closer to term, when the woman's center of gravity shifts, it is safer to shower to prevent the risk of slipping.

Hot Tubs and Saunas

Caution pregnant women to avoid using hot tubs, saunas, whirlpools, and tanning beds during pregnancy. The heat may cause fetal tachycardia as well as raise the maternal temperature. Exposure to bacteria in hot tubs that have not been cleaned sufficiently is another reason to avoid them during pregnancy.

Perineal Care

The glands in the cervical and vaginal areas become more active during pregnancy secondary to hormonal influences. This increase in activity will produce more vaginal secretions, especially in the last trimester. Advise pregnant women to shower frequently and wear all-cotton underwear to minimize the effects of these secretions. Caution pregnant women not to douche, because douching can increase the risk of infection, and not to wear panty liners, which block air circulation and promote moisture. Explain that they should also avoid perfumed soaps, lotions, perineal sprays, and harsh laundry detergents to help prevent irritation and potential infection.

Dental Care

Physiologic changes that occur in pregnant women can adversely affect oral health. Elevations in estrogen and progesterone enhance the inflammatory response and consequently alter gingival tissue. During pregnancy, the incidence of gingivitis and periodontitis increases (Anil et al., 2015). Pregnancy is a time when a woman can be very receptive to health messaging. Pregnancy is no longer a contraindication for dental treatment; it is also a time when nurses can help clients understand that good oral health is important to a healthy pregnancy and can decrease the risk of dental caries in their children. When women see oral health as a priority for themselves, they are more likely to place a high priority on their children's oral health.

Periodontal disease is a contributing factor to systemic conditions, such as heart disease, respiratory diseases, diabetes mellitus, adverse pregnancy outcomes (preterm births, low-birth-weight infants, and small-for-gestational-age infants), anemia, and stroke (Trivedi, Lal, & Singhal, 2015). Research has established that the elevated levels of estrogen and progesterone during pregnancy cause women to be more sensitive to the effects of bacterial dental plaque, which can cause gingivitis, an oral infection characterized by swollen and bleeding gums (ACOG, 2013). Brushing and flossing teeth twice daily will help reduce bacteria in the mouth. Advise the woman to visit her dentist early in the pregnancy to address any dental caries and have a thorough cleaning to prevent possible infection later in the pregnancy. Advise her to avoid exposure to x-rays by informing the hygienist of the pregnancy. If x-rays are necessary, the abdomen should be shielded with a lead apron.

Researchers have reported an association between prematurity and periodontitis, an oral infection that spreads beyond the gum tissues to invade the supporting structures of the teeth. Periodontitis is characterized by bleeding gums, loss of tooth attachment, loss of supporting bone, and bad breath due to pus formation. Unfortunately, because this infection is chronic and often painless, women frequently do not realize they have it and a preterm birth can result. During pregnancy, gingivitis occurs in 35% to 100% of women, depending upon the study (Trivedi, Lal, & Singhal, 2015). Nurses should assess all pregnant women's oral health status by taking an oral health history; checking their mouths for swollen or bleeding gums, untreated dental decay, mucosal lesions, and signs of infection; and document findings in the prenatal record.

Additional guidelines that the nurse should stress regarding maintaining dental health include:

- Seek professional dental care during the first trimester for assessment and care.
- Be reassured that oral health care is safe during pregnancy.
- Obtain treatment for dental pain and infection promptly during pregnancy.
- Brush twice daily for 2 minutes, especially before bed, with fluoridated toothpaste and rinse well. Use a soft-bristled toothbrush and be sure to brush at the gum line to remove food debris and plaque to keep gums healthy.
- Floss teeth daily with dental floss and rinse well afterward with plain water.
- Eat healthy foods, especially those high in vitamins A, C, and D and calcium.
- Avoid sugary snacks.
- Chew sugar-free gum for 10 minutes after a meal if brushing is not possible.
- After vomiting, rinse your mouth immediately with baking soda (¼ teaspoon) and warm water (1 cup) to neutralize the acid (National Maternal and Child Oral Health Resource Center, 2015).

Breast Care

Because the breasts enlarge significantly and become heavier throughout pregnancy, stress the need to wear a firm, supportive bra with wide straps to balance the weight of the breasts. Instruct the woman to anticipate buying a larger-sized bra about halfway through her pregnancy because of the increasing size of the breasts. Advise her to avoid using soap on the nipple area because it can be very drying. Encourage her to rinse the nipple area with plain water while bathing to keep it clean. The Montgomery glands (located in the areolar part of the nipple) secrete a lubricating substance that keeps the nipples moist and discourages growth of bacteria, so there is no need to use alcohol or other antiseptics on the nipples.

If the mother has chosen to breast-feed, nipple preparation is unnecessary unless her nipples are inverted and do not become erect when stimulated. Breast shells can be worn during the last 2 months to address this issue (Alexander et al., 2014).

Around week 16 of pregnancy, colostrum secretion begins, which the woman may notice as moisture in her bra. Advise the woman to place breast pads or a cotton cloth in her bra and change them frequently to prevent build-up, which may lead to excoriation.

Clothing

Many contemporary clothes are loose fitting and layered, so the woman may not need to buy an entirely new wardrobe to accommodate her pregnancy. Some pregnant women may continue to wear tight clothes. Point out that loose clothing will be more comfortable for the client and her expanding waistline.

Advise pregnant women to avoid wearing constricting clothes and girdles that compress the growing abdomen. Urge the woman to avoid knee-high hose, which might impede lower-extremity circulation and increase the risk of developing DVT. Low-heeled shoes will minimize pelvic tilt and possible backache. Wearing layered clothing that can be removed as the temperatures fluctuate may be more comfortable, especially toward term, when the woman may feel overheated.

Exercise

A physically inactive lifestyle is associated with an increase in chronic diseases such as cardiovascular disease, type 2 diabetes, osteoporosis, and cancer. The proportion of pregnant women who are overweight or obese is increasing globally, thus exercise is essential to reduce these risks and promote a healthy pregnancy. Exercise is well tolerated by a healthy woman during pregnancy. It promotes a feeling of well-being; improves circulation; helps reduce constipation, bloating, and swelling; may help prevent or treat gestational diabetes; promotes muscle tone, strength, and endurance; may improve the woman's ability to cope with labor; increases energy level; improves posture; helps sleep and promotes relaxation and rest; and relieves the lower back discomfort that often arises as the pregnancy progresses (Barakat, Lucia, & Ruiz, 2015). However, the duration and difficulty of exercise should be modified throughout pregnancy because of a decrease in performance efficiency with gestational age. Some women continue to push themselves to maintain their prior level of exercise, but most find that as their shape changes and their abdominal area enlarges, they must modify their exercise routines. Modification also helps to reduce the risk of injury caused by laxity of the joints and connective tissue due to the hormonal effects (Petrov Fieril, Glantz, & Fagevik Olsen, 2015).

Exercise during pregnancy is contraindicated in women with preterm labor, poor weight gain, anemia, facial and hand edema, pain, hypertension, threatened abortion, dizziness, shortness of breath, multiple gestation, decreased fetal activity, cardiac disease, and palpitations (Rigby, 2015).

Federal physical activity guidelines recommend at least 150 minutes of moderate-intensity exercise per week during pregnancy (Dietz, 2015) (Fig. 12.10). It is believed that pregnancy is a unique time for behavior modification and that healthy behaviors maintained or adopted during pregnancy may improve the woman's health for the rest of her life. The excess weight gained in pregnancy, which some women never lose, is a major public health problem (Truong et al., 2015). Exercise helps the woman avoid gaining excess weight during pregnancy.

Exercise during pregnancy helps return a woman's body to good health after the baby is born. The long-term benefits of exercise that begin in early pregnancy include improved posture, weight control, and improved muscle tone. Exercise also aids in the prevention of osteoporosis after menopause, reduces the risk of hypertension and diabetes, and assists in keeping the birth weight of the fetus within the normal range (Barakat, Lucia, & Ruiz, 2015). Teaching Guidelines 12.2 highlights recommendations for exercise during pregnancy.

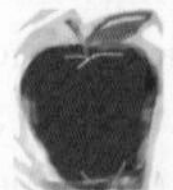

Teaching Guidelines 12.2

TEACHING TO PROMOTE EXERCISE DURING PREGNANCY

- Consume liquids before, during, and after exercising.
  - Ask your health care provider before you start a new exercise routine.
  - Avoid exercising in hot, humid weather or when you have a fever.
  - Stop exercising if you experience vaginal bleeding, dizziness, chest pain, headache, muscle

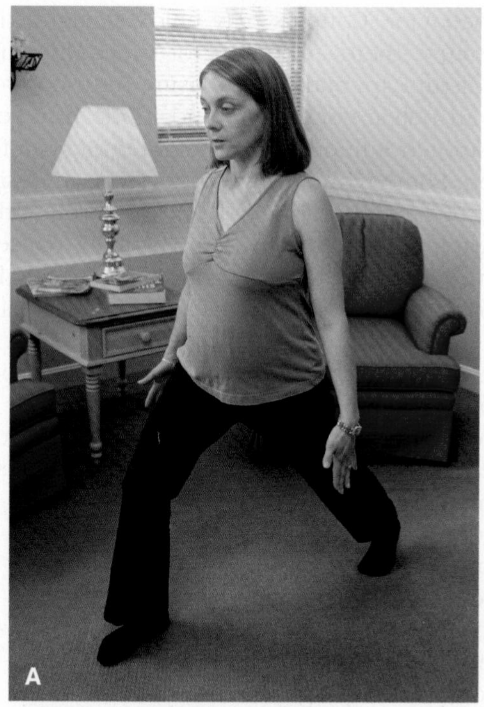

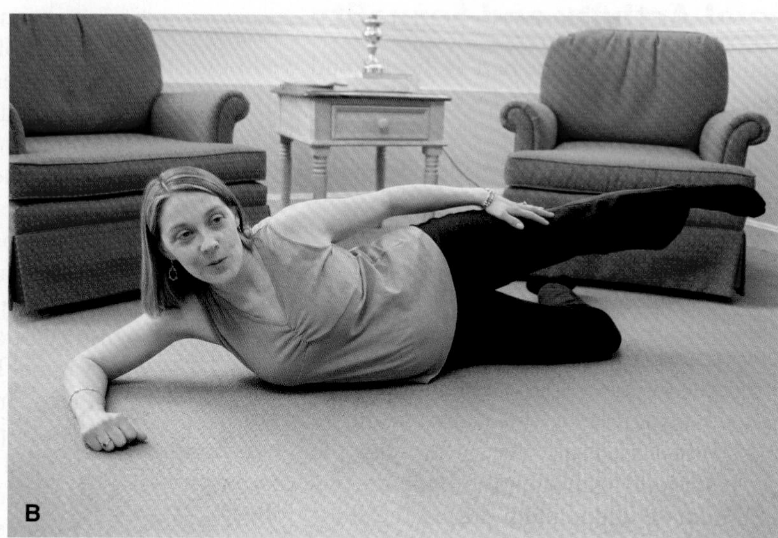

FIGURE 12.10 Exercising during pregnancy.

weakness, calf pain or swelling, uterine contractions, decreased fetal movement, or fluid leaking from the vagina.
- Exercise three or four times each week, not sporadically.
- Engage in brisk walking, swimming, biking, or low-impact aerobics; these are considered ideal activities.
- Avoid getting overheated during exercise.
- Wear comfortable exercise footwear that gives strong ankle and arch support.
- Contact sports should be avoided during pregnancy.
- Include relaxation and stretching before and after your exercise program.
- Reduce the intensity of workouts in late pregnancy.
- Avoid jerky, bouncy, or high-impact movements.
- Avoid lying flat (supine) after the fourth month because of hypotensive effect.
- Use pelvic tilt and pelvic rocking to relieve backache.
- Start with 5 to 10 minutes of stretching exercises.
- Rise slowly following an exercise session to avoid dizziness.
- Avoid activities such as skiing, surfing, scuba diving, and ice hockey.
- Never exercise to the point of exhaustion.

Adapted from Kader, M., & Naim-Shuchana, S. (2014). Physical activity and exercise during pregnancy. *European Journal of Physiotherapy, 16*(1), 2–9. doi:10.3109/21679169.2013.861509; American College of Obstetricians & Gynecologists [ACOG]. (2015e). *Exercise during pregnancy.* Retrieved from https://www.acog.org/Search?Keyword=exercise+guidelines; and American Pregnancy Association [APA]. (2014b). *Pregnancy exercise guidelines.* Retrieved from http://americanpregnancy.org/pregnancyhealth/exerciseguidelines.html

Sleep and Rest

Getting enough sleep helps a person feel better and promotes optimal performance levels during the day. The body releases its greatest concentration of growth hormone during sleep, helping the body to repair damaged tissue and grow. Also, with the increased metabolic demands during pregnancy, fatigue is a constant challenge to many pregnant women, especially during the first and third trimesters. The following tips can help promote adequate sleep:

- Stay on a regular schedule by going to bed and waking up at the same times.
- Eat regular meals at regular times to keep external body cues consistent.
- Take time to unwind and relax before bedtime.
- Establish a bedtime routine or pattern and follow it.
- Create a proper sleep environment by reducing the light and lowering the room temperature.
- Go to bed when you feel tired; if sleep does not occur, read a book until you are sleepy.
- Reduce caffeine intake later in the day.
- Limit fluid intake after dinner to minimize trips to the bathroom.
- Exercise daily to improve circulation and well-being.
- Use a modified Sims position to improve circulation in the lower extremities.
- Avoid lying on your back after the fourth month, which may compromise circulation to the uterus.
- Avoid sharply bending your knees, which promotes venous stasis below the knees.

- Keep anxieties and worries out of the bedroom. Set aside a specific area in the home or time of day for them.

Sexual Activity and Sexuality

Sexuality is an important part of health and well-being. Pregnancy is characterized by intense biologic, psychological, and social changes. These changes have direct and indirect, conscious and unconscious effects on a woman's sexuality. The woman experiences dramatic alterations in her physiology, her appearance, and her body, as well as her relationships. A woman's sexual responses during pregnancy vary widely. Common symptoms such as fatigue, nausea, vomiting, breast soreness, and urinary frequency may reduce her desire for sexual intimacy. However, many women report enhanced sexual desire due to increasing levels of estrogen. Usually sexual satisfaction does not change in pregnancy compared with the prepregnancy patterns despite a decline of sexual activity during the third trimester. A discussion of expected changes in sexuality should be routinely done in order to improve couples' perception of possible sexual modifications induced by pregnancy. It is clear that, despite some difficulties related to sexual activity during pregnancy, its need and importance are recognized for both participants.

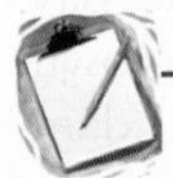

Take Note!

Fluctuations in sexual desire are normal and a highly individualized response throughout pregnancy.

The physical and emotional adjustments of pregnancy can cause changes in body image, fatigue, mood swings, and sexual activity. The woman's changing shape, emotional status, fetal activity, changes in breast size, pressure on the bladder, and other common discomforts of pregnancy result in increased physical and emotional demands. These can produce stress on the sexual relationship of the pregnant woman and her partner. However, most women adjust well to the alterations and experience a satisfying sexual relationship. Research indicates that sexual intercourse is safe in the absence of ruptured membranes, bleeding, or placenta previa, but pregnant women engage in sex less often as the pregnancy progresses (ACOG, 2015f).

Often pregnant women ask whether sexual intercourse is allowed during pregnancy or whether there are specific times when they should refrain from having sex. This is a good opportunity to educate clients about sexual behavior during pregnancy and also to ask about their expectations and individual experience related to sexuality and possible changes. It is also a good time for nurses to address the impact of the changes associated with pregnancy on sexual desire and behavior. Couples may enjoy sexual activity more because there is no fear of pregnancy and no need to disrupt spontaneity by using birth control. An increase in pelvic congestion and lubrication secondary to estrogen influence may heighten orgasm for many women. Some women have a decrease in desire because of a negative body image, fear of harming the fetus by engaging in intercourse, and fatigue, nausea, and vomiting (Boynton, 2015). Condom use can be recommended to decrease the release of prostaglandins in the semen that may stimulate contractions. A couple may need assistance to adjust to the various changes brought about by pregnancy.

Reassure the women and her partner that sexual activity is permissible during pregnancy unless there is a history of any of the following:

- Vaginal bleeding
- Placenta previa
- Risk of preterm labor
- Cervical insufficiency
- Premature rupture of membranes
- Presence of infection (Rigby, 2015)

Inform the couple that the fetus will not be injured by intercourse. Suggest that alternative positions may be more comfortable (e.g., woman on top, side-lying), especially during the later stages of pregnancy. Some of the physical changes in pregnancy, which can affect a couple's relationship, for example, halitosis which can result from dehydration, but can be alleviated through extra fluids and better oral hygiene. Women can have breast tenderness and skin changes that can cause them feel unattractive to their partner during pregnancy. In addition, they can be worried about increases in vaginal discharge and need to know what is normal and what can be a sign of infection. Nurses should make women feel comfortable talking about their fears, encouraging them to take pride in their changing bodies.

Many women feel a particular need for closeness during pregnancy, and the woman should communicate this need to her partner (Halford, Petch, & Creedy, 2015). Emphasize to the couple that closeness and cuddling need not culminate in intercourse, and that other forms of sexual expression, such as mutual masturbation, foot massage, holding hands, kissing, and hugging can be very satisfying (Halford, Petch, & Creedy, 2015).

Sex in pregnancy is normal. Research suggests that prepregnancy sexuality plays an important role in maintaining sexuality during pregnancy and postpartum (Yildiz, 2015). There are very few proven contraindications and risks to intercourse in low-risk pregnancies, and therefore these clients should be reassured. In pregnancies complicated by placenta previa or an increased risk of preterm labor, the evidence to support abstinence is lacking, but it is a reasonable benign recommendation given the theoretical catastrophic consequences (Yeniel & Petri, 2014).

Women will experience a myriad of symptoms, feelings, and physical sensations during their pregnancy. Having a satisfying sexual relationship during pregnancy is certainly possible, but it requires honest communication between partners to determine what works best for them and a good relationship with their health care provider to ensure safety (March of Dimes, 2015f).

Employment

Nearly three quarters of pregnant women in the United States will continue to work outside the home until the last month of pregnancy (Jordan et al., 2014). For the most part, women can continue working until giving birth if they have no complications during their pregnancy and the workplace does not present any special hazards (Zolotor & Carlough, 2014). Hazardous occupations include health care workers, daycare providers, laboratory technicians, chemists, painters, hairstylists, veterinary workers, and carpenters (Guidotti, 2014). Jobs requiring strenuous work such as heavy lifting, climbing, carrying heavy objects, and standing for prolonged periods place a pregnant woman at risk if modifications are not instituted.

Assess for environmental and occupational factors that place a pregnant women and her fetus at risk for injury. Interview the woman about her employment environment. Ask about possible exposure to teratogens (substances with the potential to alter the fetus permanently in form or function) and the physical demands of employment: Is she exposed to temperature extremes? Does she need to stand for prolonged periods in a fixed position? A description of the work environment is important in providing anticipatory guidance to the woman. Stress the importance of taking rest periods throughout the day, because constant physically intensive workloads increase the likelihood of low birth weight and preterm labor and birth (Cunningham et al., 2014).

Because of the numerous physiologic and psychosocial changes that women experience during their pregnancies, the employer may need to make special accommodations to reduce the pregnant woman's risk of hazardous exposures and heavy workloads. The employer may need to provide adequate coverage so that the woman can take rest breaks; remove the woman from any areas where she might be exposed to toxic substances; and avoid work assignments that require heavy lifting, hard physical labor, continuous standing, or constant moving. Some recommendations for working while pregnant are given in Teaching Guidelines 12.3.

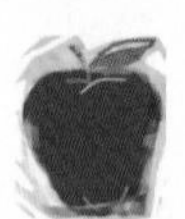

Teaching Guidelines 12.3

TEACHING FOR THE PREGNANT WORKING WOMAN

- Plan to take two 10- to 15-minute breaks within an 8-hour work day.
- Be sure there is a place available for you to rest, preferably in the side-lying position, with a restroom readily available.
- Avoid jobs that require strenuous workloads; if this is not possible, then request a modification of work duties (lighter tasks) to reduce your workload.
- Change your position from standing to sitting or vice versa at least every 2 hours.
- Ensure that you are allowed time off without penalty, if necessary, to ensure a healthy outcome for you and your fetus.
- Make sure the work environment is free of toxic substances.
- Ensure the work environment is smoke-free so passive smoking is not a concern.
- Minimize heavy lifting if associated with bending.

Travel

Pregnancy does not curtail a woman's ability to travel in a car or in a plane. However, women should follow a few safety guidelines to minimize risk to themselves and their fetuses. According to ACOG (2015g), pregnant women can travel safely throughout their pregnancy, although the second trimester is perhaps the best time to travel because there is the least chance of complications. Pregnant women considering international travel should evaluate the problems that could occur during the journey as well as the quality of medical care available at the destination.

A woman in the third trimester should be advised to defer overseas travel because of concerns about access to medical care in case of problems such as hypertension, phlebitis, or premature labor (CDC, 2015e). Pregnant women should be advised to consult with their health care providers before making any travel decisions.

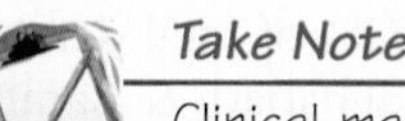

Take Note!

Clinical manifestations that indicate the need for immediate medical attention while traveling are vaginal bleeding, passing tissue or clots, abdominal pain or cramps, contractions, ruptured membranes, excessive leg swelling or pain, headaches, or visual problems (Leggat & Zuckerman, 2015).

Advise pregnant women to be aware of the potential for injuries and traumas related to traveling, and teach women ways to prevent these from occurring. Teaching Guidelines 12.4 offers tips for safe travel on planes and to foreign areas.

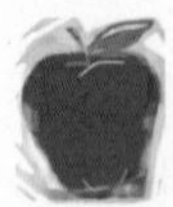

Teaching Guidelines 12.4

TEACHING TO PROMOTE SAFE TRAVEL ON PLANES AND IN FOREIGN COUNTRIES

- Bring along a copy of the prenatal record if your travel will be prolonged in case there is a medical emergency away from home.
- When traveling abroad, carry a foreign dictionary that includes words or phrases for the most common pregnancy emergencies.
- Travel with at least one companion at all times for personal safety.
- Check with your health care provider before receiving any immunizations necessary for foreign travel; some may be harmful to the fetus.
- When in a foreign country, avoid fresh fruit, vegetables, and local water.
- Avoid any milk that is not pasteurized.
- Eat only meat that is well cooked to avoid exposure to toxoplasmosis.
- Request an aisle seat and walk about the airplane every 2 hours.
- While sitting on long flights, practice calf-tensing exercises to improve circulation to the lower extremities.
- Be aware of typical problems encountered by pregnant travelers, such as fatigue, heartburn, indigestion, constipation, vaginal discharge, leg cramps, urinary frequency, and hemorrhoids.
- Always wear support hose while flying to prevent the development of blood clots.
- Drink plenty of water to keep well hydrated throughout the flight.
- Postpone travel if risks outweigh benefits.

Adapted from American College of Obstetricians and Gynecologists. (2015e). *Travel during pregnancy: FAQ 055.* Retrieved from http://www.acog.org/~/media/for%20patients/faq055.ashx; and Centers for Disease Control and Prevention [CDC]. (2015e). *Pregnant travelers.* Retrieved from http://wwwnc.cdc.gov/travel/yellowbook/2014/chapter-8-advising-travelers-with-specific-needs/pregnant-travelers

When traveling by car, the major risk is a car accident. Motor vehicle accidents account for more than 50% of all traumas during pregnancy and 82% of fetal deaths occurring during these accidents (Eshaghabadi & Barati, 2015). The impact and momentum can lead to traumatic separation of the placenta from the wall of the uterus. Shock and massive hemorrhage might result. Tips that nurses can offer to promote safety during ground travel include:

- Always wear a three-point seat belt, no matter how short the trip, to prevent ejection or serious injury from collision.
- Apply a nonpadded shoulder strap properly; it should cross between the breasts and over the upper abdomen, above the uterus (Fig. 12.11).

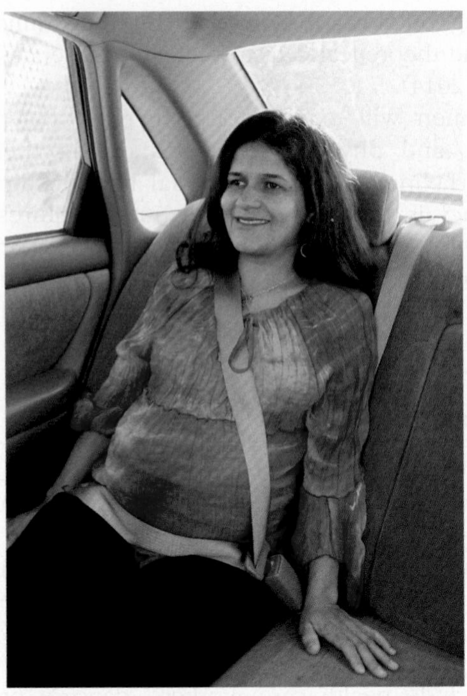

FIGURE 12.11 **Proper application of a seat belt during pregnancy.**

- If no seat belts are available (buses or vans), ride in the back seat of the vehicle.
- Use a lap belt that crosses over the pelvis below the uterus.
- Deactivate the airbag if possible. If you can't, move the seat as far back from the dashboard as possible to minimize impact on the abdomen.
- Never use a cellular phone while driving to prevent distraction.
- Avoid driving when very fatigued in the first and third trimesters.
- Avoid late-night driving, when visibility might be compromised.
- Direct a tilting steering wheel away from the abdomen (CDC, 2015e).

Immunizations and Medications

Vaccines are among the greatest public health achievements of the 21st century, credited with significant reduction of morbidity and mortality from many diseases caused by bacteria and viruses (Senie, 2014). Ideally, clients should receive all childhood immunizations before conception to protect the fetus from any risk of congenital anomalies. If the client comes for a preconception visit, discuss immunizations such as measles, mumps, and rubella (MMR), hepatitis B, and diphtheria/tetanus (every 10 years); administer them at this time if needed.

The risk to a developing fetus from vaccination of the mother during pregnancy is primarily theoretical. Routine immunizations are not usually indicated during pregnancy. However, no evidence exists of risk from vaccinating pregnant women with inactivated virus or bacterial vaccines or toxoids. A number of other vaccines have not been adequately studied, and thus theoretical risks of vaccination must be weighed against the risks of the disease to mother and fetus (CDC, 2015f).

Take Note!

Advise pregnant women to avoid live virus vaccines (MMR and varicella) and to avoid becoming pregnant within 1 month of having received one of these vaccines because of the theoretical risk of transmission to the fetus (CDC, 2015f).

CDC guidelines for vaccine administration are highlighted in Box 12.6.

Little is known about the effects of taking most medications during pregnancy. Less than 10% of medications approved by the FDA since 1980 have enough information to determine their risk for birth defects (CDC, 2015g). Based on this lack of evidence, it is best for pregnant women not to take any medications during their pregnancy. At the very least, encourage them to discuss with the health care provider their current medications and any herbal remedies they take so that they can learn about any potential risks should they continue to take them during pregnancy. Generally, if the woman is taking medicine for seizures, high blood pressure, asthma, or depression, the benefits of continuing the medicine during pregnancy outweigh the risks to the fetus. The safety profile of some medications may change according to the gestational age of the fetus. Embryogenesis is completed by the end of the first trimester, when all fetal organs are complete. Thus, to cause a malformation, fetal drug exposure must occur in the first 12 weeks of gestation (Gadot & Koren, 2015).

The FDA has developed a system of ranking drugs that appears on drug labels and package inserts. These risk categories are summarized in Box 12.7. Always advise women to check with the health care provider for guidance.

A common concern of many pregnant women involves the use of over-the-counter medications and herbal agents. Many women consider these products benign simply because they are available without a

BOX 12.6

CDC GUIDELINES FOR VACCINE ADMINISTRATION DURING PREGNANCY

Vaccines That Should be Considered if Otherwise Indicated

- Hepatitis B
- Influenza (inactivated) injection
- Tetanus/diphtheria (Tdap)
- Meningococcal
- Rabies

Vaccines Contraindicated During Pregnancy

- Influenza (live, attenuated vaccine) nasal spray
- Measles
- Mumps
- Rubella
- Varicella
- BCG (tuberculosis)
- Meningococcal
- Typhoid

Adapted from Centers for Disease Control and Prevention [CDC]. (2015f). *Vaccines for pregnant women.* Retrieved from http://www.cdc.gov/vaccines/adults/rec-vac/pregnant.html; and March of Dimes (2015h). *Vaccinations during pregnancy.* Retrieved from http://www.marchofdimes.com/pregnancy/vaccinations-during-pregnancy.aspx

BOX 12.7

FDA PREGNANCY RISK CLASSIFICATION OF DRUGS

- *Category A:* These drugs have been tested and found safe during pregnancy. Examples: folic acid, vitamin B_6, and thyroid medicine.
- *Category B:* These drugs have been used frequently during pregnancy and do not appear to cause major birth defects or other fetal problems. Examples: antibiotics, acetaminophen (Tylenol), aspartame (artificial sweetener), famotidine (Pepcid), prednisone (cortisone), insulin, and ibuprofen. (Ibuprofen should not be used after 36 weeks of pregnancy to avoid increased blood loss during parturition and to avoid premature closure of the ductus arterious in the fetus.)
- *Category C:* These drugs are more likely to cause problems and safety studies have not been completed. Examples: prochlorperazine (Compazine), fluconazole (Diflucan), ciprofloxacin (Cipro), and some antidepressants.
- *Category D:* These drugs have clear health risks for the fetus. Examples: alcohol, lithium (treats bipolar disorders), phenytoin (Dilantin); all chemotherapeutic agents used to treat cancer.
- *Category X:* These drugs have demonstrated positive evidence of fetal abnormalities and are contraindicated in women who are or may become pregnant. Examples: Accutane (treats cystic acne), androgens (treat endometriosis), Coumadin (prevents blood clots), antithyroid medications for overactive thyroid; radiation therapy (cancer treatment), Tegison or Soriatane (treats psoriasis), streptomycin (treats tuberculosis); thalidomide (treats insomnia), diethylstilbestrol (DES) (treats menstrual disorders), and organic mercury from contaminated food.

Adapted from King, T. L., Brucker, M. C., Kriebs, J. M., Fahey, J. O., Gegor, C. L., & Varney, H. (2015). *Varney's midwifery* (5th ed.). Burlington, MA: Jones & Bartlett Learning; and Rigby, F.B. (2015). Common pregnancy complaints and questions. *eMedicine.* Retrieved from http://emedicine.medscape.com/article/259724-overview

prescription (King et al., 2015). Although herbal medications are commonly thought of as "natural" alternatives to other medicines, they can be just as potent as some prescription medications. A major concern about herbal medicine is the lack of consistent potency in the active ingredients in any given batch of product, making it difficult to know the exact strength by reading the label. Also, many herbs contain chemicals that cross the placenta and may cause harm to the fetus.

Nurses are often asked about the safety of over-the-counter medicines and herbal agents. Unfortunately, many drugs have not been evaluated in controlled studies, and it is difficult to make general recommendations for these products. Therefore, encourage pregnant women to check with their health care provider before taking anything. Questions about the use of over-the-counter and herbal products are part of the initial prenatal interview.

NURSING MANAGEMENT TO PREPARE THE WOMAN AND HER PARTNER FOR LABOR, BIRTH, AND PARENTHOOD

Pregnancy and birth are unique to every woman. Women and families hold different expectations during childbearing based on their knowledge, experiences, belief systems, culture, and social and family backgrounds. These differences should be understood and respected by the nurse, and care to them adapted to meet the individual needs of the women and families. Knowing a woman's needs, values, cultural background, preferences, and expectations during childbirth helps nurses to provide high-quality care to them. Childbirth today is a very different experience from childbirth in previous generations. In the past, women were literally "put to sleep" with anesthetics, and they woke up with a baby. Most women never remembered the details and had a passive role in childbirth as the physician delivered the newborn. In the 1950s, consumers began to insist on taking a more active role in their health care, and couples desired to be together during the extraordinary event of childbirth. Beginning in the 1970s, the father or significant other support person remained with the mother throughout labor and birth. Fathers today want to be seen as individuals who are part of the laboring couple. If fathers are left out, they tend to feel helpless; this can result in a feeling of panic and can put their support for their partner at risk (Schytt & Bergstrom, 2014).

Health beliefs related to pregnancy and childbirth exist in various cultures globally. A woman's perception of her own status is critical to her decision-making process, because her personal behaviors can significantly alter her pregnancy-related risks. Pregnant women of diverse cultures hold a number of beliefs related to diet, behavior related to prenatal care, and the use of herbs during pregnancy and postnatally. Nurses need to be aware of these cultural beliefs so as to incorporate those into their practices, while those posing a health risk should be discouraged respectfully (M'soka, Mabuza, & Pretorius, 2015).

Childbirth education began because women demanded to become more involved in their birthing experience rather than simply turning control over to a health care provider. Nurses played a pivotal role in bringing about this change by providing information and supporting clients and their families, fostering a more active role in preparing for the upcoming birth.

Traditional childbirth education classes focused on developing and practicing techniques for use in managing pain and facilitating the progress of labor. Recently, the focus of this education has broadened: it now encompasses not only preparation for childbirth, but also preparation for breast-feeding, infant care, transition to new parenting roles, relationship skills, family health promotion, and sexuality (Varner, 2015). The term used to describe this broad range of topics is perinatal education. Subjects commonly addressed in perinatal education include:

- Anatomy and physiology of reproduction
- Fetal growth and development
- Prenatal maternal exercise
- Physiologic and emotional changes during pregnancy
- Sex during pregnancy
- Infant growth and development
- Nutrition and healthy eating habits during pregnancy
- Teratogens and their impact on the fetus
- Signs and symptoms of labor
- Preparation for labor and birth (for parents, siblings, and other family members)
- Options for birth
- Infant nutrition, including preparation for breast-feeding
- Infant care, including safety, CPR, and first aid
- Family planning (March of Dimes, 2015g)

Childbirth Education Classes

Childbirth education classes teach pregnant women and their support person about pregnancy, birth, and parenting. The classes are offered in local communities or online and are usually taught by certified childbirth educators. Most childbirth classes support the concept of **natural childbirth** (a birth without pain-relieving medications) so that the woman can be in control throughout the experience as much as possible. The classes differ in their approach to specific comfort techniques and breathing patterns. The three most common childbirth methods are the Lamaze (psychoprophylactic) method, the Bradley (partner-coached childbirth) method, and the Dick-Read (natural childbirth) method.

Lamaze Method

Lamaze is a psychoprophylactic ("mind prevention") method of preparing for labor and birth that promotes the use of specific breathing and relaxation techniques. Dr. Fernand Lamaze, a French obstetrician, popularized this method of childbirth preparation in the 1960s. Lamaze believed that conquering fear through knowledge and support was important. He also believed women needed to alter the perception of suffering during childbirth. This perception change would come about by learning conditioned reflexes that, instead of signaling pain, would signal the work of producing a child, and thus would carry the woman through labor awake, aware, and in control of her own body (Lamaze International, 2015). Lamaze felt strongly that all women have the right to deliver their babies with minimal or no medication while maintaining their dignity, minimizing their pain, maximizing their self-esteem, and enjoying the miracle of birth.

Lamaze classes include information on toning exercises, relaxation exercises and techniques, and breathing methods for labor. The breathing techniques are used in labor to enhance relaxation and to reduce the woman's perception of pain. The goal is for women to become aware of their own comfortable rate of breathing in order to maintain relaxation and adequate oxygenation of the fetus. The following breathing techniques are an effective attention-focusing strategy to reduce pain:

- *Paced breathing* involves breathing techniques used to decrease stress responses and therefore decrease pain. This type of breathing implies self-regulation by the woman. The woman starts off by taking a cleansing breath at the onset and end of each contraction. This cleansing breath symbolizes freeing her mind from worries and concerns. This breath enhances oxygenation and puts the woman in a relaxed state.
- *Slow-paced breathing* is associated with relaxation and should be half the normal breathing rate (six to nine breaths per minute). This type of breathing is the most relaxed pattern and is recommended throughout labor. Abdominal or chest breathing may be used. It is generally best to breathe in through the nose and breathe out either through the nose or mouth, whichever is more comfortable for the woman.
- *Modified-paced breathing* can be used for increased work or stress during labor to increase alertness or focus attention or when slow-paced breathing is no longer effective in keeping the woman relaxed. The woman's respiratory rate increases, but it does not exceed twice her normal rate. Modified-paced breathing is a quiet upper chest breath that is increased or decreased according to the intensity of the contraction. The inhalation and the exhalation are equal. This breathing technique should be practiced during pregnancy for optimal use during labor.
- *Patterned-paced breathing* is similar to modified-paced breathing but with a rhythmic pattern. It uses a variety of patterns, with an emphasis on the exhalation breath at regular intervals. Different patterns can be used, such as 4/1, 6/1, 4/1. A 4/1 rhythm is four upper chest breaths followed by an exhalation (a sighing out of air, like blowing out a candle). Random patterns can be chosen for use as long as the basic principles of rate and relaxation are met.

Couples practice these breathing patterns typically during the last few months of the pregnancy until they feel comfortable using them. Focal points (visual fixation on a designated object), effleurage (light abdominal massage by woman or partner), massage, and imagery (journey of the mind to a relaxing place) are also added to aid in relaxation. From the nurse's perspective, encourage the woman to breathe at a level of comfort that allows her to cope. Always remain quiet during the woman's periods of imagery and focal point visualization to avoid breaking her concentration.

Bradley (Partner-Coached) Method

The Bradley method uses various exercises and slow, controlled abdominal breathing to accomplish relaxation. Dr. Robert Bradley, a Denver-based obstetrician, advocated a completely unmedicated labor and birth experience. The Bradley method emphasizes the pleasurable sensations of childbirth, teaching women to concentrate on these sensations while "turning on" to their own bodies (Bradley Method, 2014). In 1965, Bradley wrote *Husband-Coached Childbirth,* which advocated the active participation of the husband as labor coach.

A woman is conditioned to work in harmony with her body using breath control and deep abdominopelvic breathing to promote general body relaxation during labor. This method stresses that childbirth is a joyful, natural process and emphasizes the partner's involvement during pregnancy, labor, birth, and the early newborn period. Thus, the training techniques are directed toward the coach, not the mother. The coach is educated in massage/comfort techniques to use on the mother throughout the labor and birth process.

Dick-Read Method

In 1944 Grantly Dick-Read, a British obstetrician, wrote *Childbirth Without Fear.* He believed that the attitude of a woman toward her birthing process had a considerable influence on the ease of her labor, and he believed that fear is the primary pain-producing agent in an otherwise normal labor. He felt that fear builds a state of tension, creating an antagonistic effect on the laboring muscles of the uterus, which results in pain. A private, undisturbed and dark environment, where women can feel safe can promote the release of oxytocin, the hormone responsible for uterine contractions and though to promote the release of the pain-relieving hormones endorphins. When this is not achieved, women can experience fear–tension–pain syndrome, impeding labor progress and causing increased levels of pain (Westbury, 2015). Dick-Read sought to interrupt the circular pattern of fear, tension, and pain during the labor and birthing process. He promoted the belief that the degree of fear could be diminished with increased understanding of the normal physiologic response to labor (Alexander et al., 2014).

Dick-Read believed that prenatal instruction was essential for pain relief and that emotional factors during labor interfered with the normal labor progression. The woman achieves relaxation and reduces pain by arming herself with the knowledge of normal childbirth and using abdominal breathing during contractions.

Nursing Management and Childbirth Education

Childbirth education is less about methods than about mastery. The overall aim of any of the methods is to promote an internal locus of control that will enable each woman to yield her body to the process of birth. As the woman gains success and tangible benefits from the exercises she is taught, she begins to reframe her beliefs and gains practical knowledge, and the impetus will be there for her to engage in the conscious use of the techniques (Fig. 12.12). Nurses play a key role in supporting and encouraging each couple's use of the techniques taught in childbirth education classes.

Every woman's labor is unique, and it is important for nurses not to generalize or stereotype women. The most effective support a nurse can offer a couple using prepared childbirth methods is encouragement and presence. These nursing measures must be adapted to each individual throughout the labor process. Offering encouraging phrases such as "great job" or "you can do it" helps to reinforce their efforts and at the same time empowers them to continue. Using eye-to-eye contact to engage the woman's total attention is important if she appears overwhelmed or appears to lose control during the transition phase of labor.

Nurses play a significant role in enhancing the couple's relationship by respecting the involvement of the partner and demonstrating concern for his needs throughout labor. Offering to stay with the woman to give him a break periodically allows him to meet his needs while at the same time still actively participating. Offer anticipatory guidance to the couple and assist during critical times in labor. Demonstrate many of the coping techniques to the partner and praise their successful use, which increases self-esteem. Focus on their strengths and the positive elements of the labor experience. Congratulating the couple for a job well done is paramount.

Throughout the labor experience, demonstrate personal warmth and project a friendly attitude. Frequently, a nurse's touch may help to prevent a crisis by reassuring the mother that she is doing fine.

Options for Birth Settings and Care Providers

From the moment a woman discovers she is pregnant, numerous decisions await her—where the infant will be born, what birth setting is best, and who will assist with the birth. The majority of women are well and healthy and can consider the full range of birth settings—hospital, birth center, or home setting—and care providers.

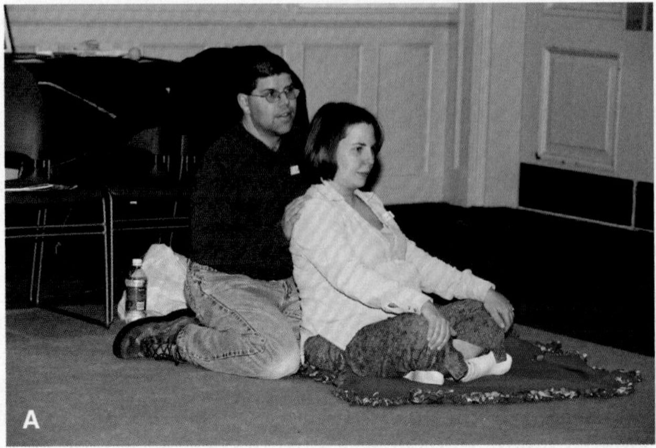

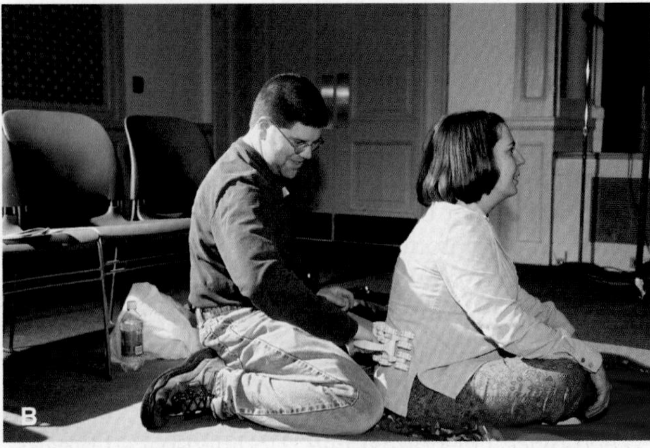

FIGURE 12.12 A couple practicing the techniques taught in a childbirth education class.

They should be given information about each to ensure the most informed decision.

Birth Settings

HOSPITALS

Hospitals are the most common site for birth in the United States. If the woman has a serious medical condition or is at high risk for developing one, she will probably need to plan to give birth in a hospital setting under the care of an obstetrician. Giving birth in a hospital is advantageous for several reasons. Hospitals are best equipped to diagnose and treat women and newborns with complications; trained personnel are available if necessary; and no transportation is needed if a complication should arise during labor or birth. Disadvantages include the high-tech atmosphere; strict policies and restrictions that might limit who can be with the woman; and the medical model of care.

Within the hospital setting, however, choices do exist regarding birth environments. The conventional delivery room resembles an operating room, where the health care professional delivers the newborn from the woman, who is positioned in stirrups. The woman is then transferred to the recovery area on a stretcher and then again to the postpartum unit. The birthing suite is the other option within the hospital setting. In the birthing suite, the woman and her partner remain in one place for labor, birth, and recovery. The birthing suite is a private room decorated to look as homelike as possible. For example, the bed converts to allow for various birthing positions, and there may be a rocking chair or an easy chair for the woman's partner. Despite the homey atmosphere, the room is still equipped with emergency resuscitative obstetric equipment and electronic fetal monitors in case they are needed quickly (Fig. 12.13A). Such settings provide a more personal childbirth experience in a less formal and intimidating atmosphere compared to the traditional delivery room.

FREESTANDING BIRTH CENTER

A freestanding birth center offers women a comfortable setting where they can receive maternity care with appropriate levels of intervention. A freestanding birth center (Fig. 12.13B) can be a good choice for a woman who wants more personalized care than in a hospital but does not feel comfortable with a home birth. In contrast to the institutional environment in hospitals, most freestanding birth centers have a homelike atmosphere, and many are, in fact, located in converted homes. Some are located on hospital property and are affiliated with them. Birth centers are designed to provide maternity care to women judged to be at low risk for obstetric complications. Women are allowed and encouraged to give birth in the position most comfortable for them. Care in birth centers is often provided by midwives and is more relaxed, with no routine intravenous lines, fetal monitoring, and restrictive protocols. A disadvantage of the birth center is the need to transport the woman to a hospital quickly if an emergency arises, because emergency equipment is not readily available. In a research study comparing homelike to conventional institutional settings, the author concluded that there appeared to be some benefits from homelike settings for childbirth, although increased support from caregivers may be more important (Alliman, Jolles, & Summers, 2015).

HOME BIRTHS

Rates of planned home births have been increasing since the 1970s, with 1 in 49 non-Hispanic White women giving birth outside the hospital setting now (Zielinski, Ackerson, & Low, 2015). Most women who choose a home birth believe that birth is a natural process that requires little medical intervention (Lewis, 2015). Research has shown that women believe that planned home births increase privacy, comfort, and convenience; are associated with reduced rates of medical interventions; and facilitate family involvement in a relaxed, peaceful atmosphere (Budin, 2015).

A

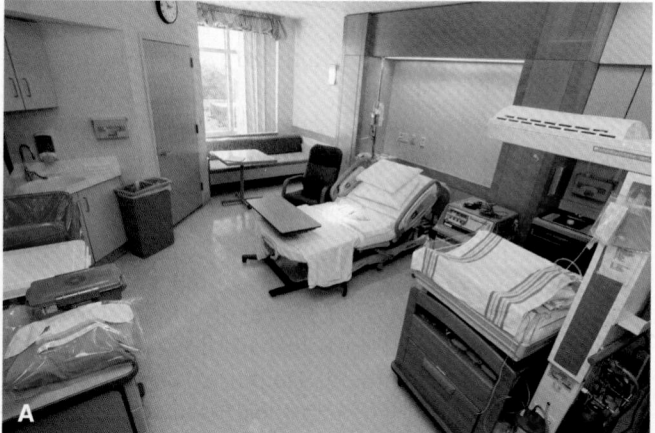

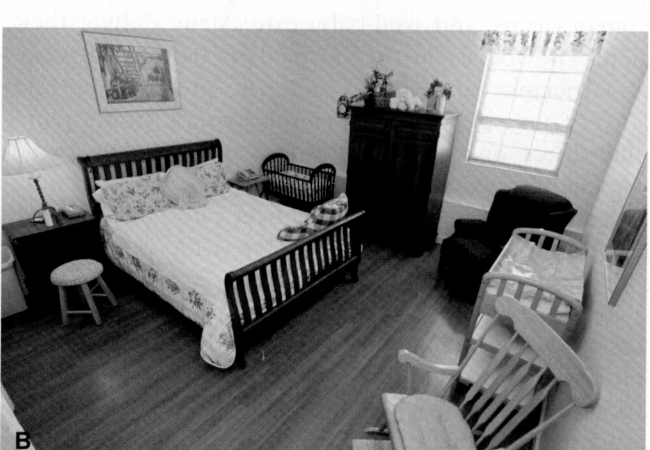

FIGURE 12.13 **A.** Birthing suite in hospital setting. **B.** Childbirth room in Birthing Center.

The safety of home births is an ongoing debate in the United States. The American College of Nurse Midwives (ACNM), the American Public Health Association (APHA), and World Health Organization (WHO) state that planned home births is safe, as long as the woman falls under certain criteria, such as a low-risk pregnancy, singleton fetus, cephalic fetus at term, and the absence of pre-existing conditions (Declercq & Stotland, 2015). Home births can be safe if there are qualified, experienced attendants and an emergency transfer system in place in case of serious complications. Many women choose the home setting out of a strong desire to control their child's birth and to give birth surrounded by family members. Most home birth caregivers are midwives who have provided continuous care to the woman throughout the pregnancy. Disadvantages include the need to transport the woman to the hospital during or after labor if a problem arises, and the limited pain management available in the home setting.

Care Providers

While most women in the United States still receive pregnancy care from an obstetrician, an increasing number are choosing a midwife for their care. The difference is a matter of degrees. Obstetricians must finish a 4-year residency in obstetrics and gynecology in addition to medical school. Certified nurse-midwives are registered nurses who have graduated from a nurse-midwifery education program accredited by the Accreditation Commission for Midwifery Education (ACME) and have passed a national certification examination to receive the professional designation of certified nurse-midwife. As of 2010, a graduate degree is required for entry into midwifery practice in the United States. Midwives usually care for low-risk women in a variety of settings. They are able to write prescriptions, provide prenatal care, childbirth care, postpartum care, newborn care, and well women's care throughout the life span. Family practice doctors also provide maternity, woman's care, and well-baby care. Many deliver their clients' newborns in the hospital or birthing centers. Obstetricians can handle high-risk pregnancies and delivery emergencies; can administer or order pain-relief drugs; and are assisted by a support staff in the hospital setting. Midwives work in hospitals, birthing centers, and home settings to deliver care. They believe in the normalcy of birth and tolerate wide variations of what is considered normal during labor, which leads to fewer interventions applied during the childbirth process. Midwives attend approximately 8% of total United States births (American College of Nurse-Midwives, 2015). Midwives do handle high risk and emergency births because many are not always predictable—they typically have an obstetrician as back up when they do occur to assist them.

In addition to the woman's primary health care provider, some women hire a doula to be with them during the childbearing process. *Doula* is a Greek word that means "woman's servant." A doula is a laywoman trained to provide women and their families with encouragement, emotional and physical support, and information through late pregnancy, labor, birth, and postpartum. Doulas provide the woman with continuous support throughout labor but do not perform any clinical procedures.

Preparation for Breast-Feeding or Bottle-Feeding

Pregnant women are faced with a decision about which method of feeding to choose. Educate the pregnant client about the advantages and disadvantages of each method, allowing the woman and her partner to make an informed decision about the best method for their situation. Providing the client and her partner with this information will increase the likelihood of a successful experience regardless of the method of feeding chosen. As part of health promotion/evidence-based interventions, nurses should be encouraging and educating all women on breast-feeding.

Breast-Feeding

Substantial scientific evidence exists documenting the health benefits of breast-feeding for newborns. Current evidence cited by the American Academy of Pediatrics (AAP) showed improved outcomes for breast-fed infants with regard to otitis media, lower respiratory infections, gastroenteritis, atopic dermatitis, childhood asthma, childhood obesity, type 1 and type 2 diabetes, childhood leukemia, sudden infant death syndrome, and cognitive development and for their mothers with regard to breast cancer, ovarian cancer, and type 2 diabetes. The AAP recommends that infants be breast-fed exclusively until the age 6 months, and continue to be breast-fed for a year and for as long as it is mutually desired (2012). In addition, a lack of breast-feeding has a negative impact on the health care system by increasing the number of client visits, hospital admissions, rate of obesity, and health care costs. Most researchers agree that the duration of breast-feeding is inversely associated with overweight risk. Breast-feeding is a cost-effective, natural, and effective prevention strategy for reducing childhood obesity. A recent study estimates that $13 billion a year would be saved and 1,000 deaths prevented each year if 90% of infants in the United States were exclusively breast-fed until 6 months (Office on Women's Health, 2014).

Human milk provides an ideal balance of nutrients for newborns (ACOG, 2015h). Breast-feeding is advantageous for the following reasons:

- Human milk is digestible and economical and requires no preparation.
- Bonding between mother and child is promoted.
- Cost is less than purchasing formula.
- Ovulation is suppressed (however, this is not a reliable birth control method).
- The risk of ovarian cancer and the incidence of premenopausal breast cancer are reduced for the woman.
- Extra calories are used, which promotes weight loss gradually without dieting.
- Oxytocin is released to promote more rapid uterine involution with less bleeding.
- Sucking helps to develop the muscles in the infant's jaw.
- Absorption of lactose and minerals in the newborn is improved.
- The immunologic properties of breast milk help prevent infections in the baby.
- The composition of breast milk adapts to meet the infant's changing needs.
- Constipation in the baby is not a problem with adequate intake.
- Food allergies are less likely to develop in the breast-fed baby.
- The incidence of otitis media and upper respiratory infections in the infant is reduced.
- Breast-fed babies are less likely to be overfed, thus reducing the risk of adult obesity.
- Breast-fed newborns are less prone to vomiting (American Academy of Family Physicians (2015); AAP (2015); ACOG (2015h); and Women, Infant & Children [WIC], 2015).

One could say that lactation and breast-feeding are so natural that they should just happen on their own accord, but this is not the case. Learning to breast-feed takes practice, requires support from the partner, and requires dedication and patience on the part of the mother; it may be necessary to work closely with a lactation consultant to be successful and comfortable when breast-feeding (Fig. 12.14 shows the different positions that may be used for breast-feeding). Nurses can encourage breast-feeding for all mothers except those who are HIV+, and are untreated, have active tuberculosis, use illicit drugs, or take prescribed cancer chemotherapeutic agents.

Breast-feeding also has some side effects. These include breast discomfort, sore nipples, mastitis, engorgement, milk stasis, vaginal dryness, and decreased libido (Alekseev, Vladimir, & Nadezhda, 2015). The most common cause of nipple pain is an improper latch and such discomfort is piercing, immediate and short lived, typically occurring as soon as the baby starts nursing and gradually subsiding during the feeding. Some mothers feel it is inconvenient or embarrassing, limits other activities, limits partner involvement, increases their dependency by being tied to the infant all the time, and restricts their use of alcohol or drugs. Nurses can help mothers to cope with their fear of dependency and feelings of obligation by emphasizing the positive aspects of breast-feeding and encouraging bonding experiences. Nurses can be instrumental in helping mothers prepare and continue to breast-feed after they return to work.

PREPARATION FOR BREAST-FEEDING

Nipple preparation is not necessary during the prenatal period unless the nipples are inverted and do not become erect when stimulated. Assess for this by placing the forefinger and thumb above and below the areola and compressing behind the nipple. If it flattens or inverts, advise the client to wear breast shields during the last 2 months of pregnancy. Breast shields exert a continuous pressure around the areola, pushing the nipple through a central opening in the inner shield (La Leche League International, 2016). The shields are worn inside the bra. Initially the shields are worn for 1 hour, and then the woman progressively increases the wearing time up to 8 hours daily. The client maintains this schedule until after childbirth, and then she wears the shield 24 hours a day until the infant latches on easily (La Leche League International, 2016). In addition, suggest that the woman wear a supportive nursing bra 24 hours a day.

Encourage the woman to request a certified lactation specialist (CLS) at the hospital, if giving birth there. Lactation specialists are health care providers who specialize in the clinical management of breast-feeding. Some run their own breast-feeding support groups as well. In addition, suggest that the woman attend a breast-feeding support group (e.g., La Leche League), provide her with sources of information about infant feeding, and suggest that she read a good reference book about lactation. All of these activities will help in her decision-making process and will be invaluable to her should she choose to breast-feed her newborn. Women returning to work can pump their breasts and store the milk in the freezer for future use.

Bottle-Feeding

Recent research indicates that infants who are fed formula within the first 6 months do have an increased incidence of otitis media, diabetes, asthma, atopic dermatitis, reflux, diarrhea, colic, constipation, and lower respiratory infections (Schram, 2014). It is important to inform mothers and their partners of this.

Bottle-feeding an infant is not just a matter of "open, pour, and feed." Parents need information on types of formulas, preparation and storage of formula, equipment, and feeding positions. It is recommended that normal full-term infants receive conventional cow's milk-based formula; the physician should direct this choice. If the infant has a reaction (diarrhea, vomiting, abdominal pain, excessive gas) to the first formula, another formula should be tried. Sometimes a soy-based formula is

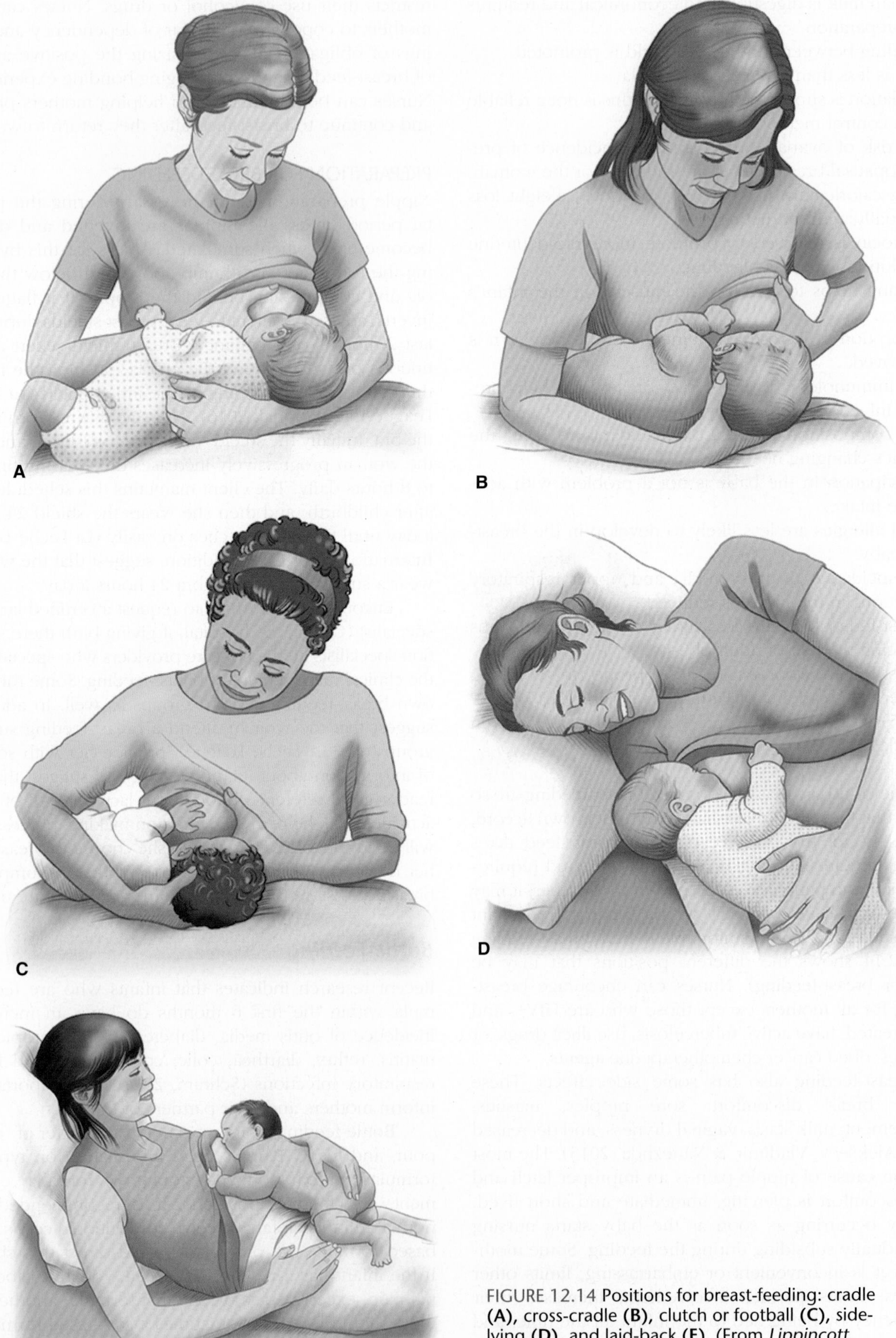

FIGURE 12.14 Positions for breast-feeding: cradle **(A)**, cross-cradle **(B)**, clutch or football **(C)**, side-lying **(D)**, and laid-back **(E)**. (From *Lippincott Procedures.*)

substituted. In terms of preparation of formula and its use, the following guidelines should be stressed:

- Obtain adequate equipment (six 4-oz bottles, eight 8-oz bottles, and nipples).
- Consistency is important. Stay with a nipple that is comfortable to the infant.
- Frequently assess nipples for any loose pieces of rubber at the opening.
- Correct formula preparation is critical to the health and development of the infant. Formula is available in three forms: ready-to-feed, concentrate, and powder.
- Read the formula label thoroughly before mixing.
- Correct formula dilution is important to avoid fluid imbalances. For ready-to-use formula, use as is without dilution. For concentrated formulas, dilute with equal parts of water. For powdered formulas, mix one scoop of powder with 2 oz of water.
- If the water supply is safe, sterilization is not necessary.
- Bottles and nipples should be washed in hot, sudsy water using a bottle brush.
- Formula should be served at room temperature.
- If the water supply is questionable, water should be boiled for 5 minutes before use.
- Formula should not be heated in a microwave oven, because it is heated unevenly.
- Formula can be prepared 24 hours ahead of time and stored in the refrigerator.

Teach the woman and other caretakers to feed the infant in a semi-upright position using the cradle hold in the arms. This position allows for face-to-face contact between the infant and caretaker. Advise the caretaker to hold the bottle so that the nipple is kept full of formula to prevent excessive air swallowing. Instruct the caretaker to feed the infant every 3 to 4 hours and adapt the feeding times to the infant's needs. Frequent burping of the infant (every ounce) helps prevent gas from building up in the stomach. Caution the caretaker not to prop the bottle; propping the bottle can cause choking.

Bottle-feeding should mirror breast-feeding as closely as possible. While nutrition is important, so are the emotional and interactive components of feeding. Encourage the caretaker to cuddle the infant closely and position the infant so that his or her head is in a comfortable position. Also encourage communication with the infant during feedings. Nurses should know the different types of formulas available to provide advice to mothers who have made the informed choice not to breast-feed or to stop breast-feeding.

Take Note!

Warn the caretaker about the danger of putting the infant to bed with a bottle. This can lead to "baby bottle tooth decay" (nursing caries) because sugars in the formula stay in contact with the infant's developing teeth for prolonged periods.

Final Preparation for Labor and Birth

The nurse has played a supportive/education role for the couple throughout the pregnancy and now needs to assist in preparing them for their "big event" by making sure they have made informed decisions and completed the following checklist:

- Attended childbirth preparation classes and practiced breathing techniques
- Selected a birth setting and made arrangements there
- Know what to expect during labor and birth
- Toured the birthing facility
- Packed a suitcase to take to the birthing facility when labor starts
- Made arrangements to have siblings and/or pets taken care of during labor
- Been instructed on signs and symptoms of labor and what to do
- Know what to do if membranes rupture prior to going into labor
- Know how to reach their health care provider when labor starts
- Communicated their needs and desires concerning pain management
- Discussed the possibility of a cesarean birth if complications occur
- Discussed possible names for the newborn
- Selected a feeding method (breast or bottle) with which they feel comfortable
- Made a decision regarding circumcision if they have a boy
- Purchased an infant safety car seat in which to bring their newborn home
- Decided on a pediatrician
- Have items needed to prepare for the newborn's homecoming:
  - Infant clothes in several sizes
  - Nursing bras
  - Infant crib with spaces between the slats that are 2 in or less apart
  - Diapers (cloth or disposable)
  - Feeding supplies (bottles and nipples if bottle-feeding)
  - Infant thermometer
- Selected a family planning method to use after the birth

At each prenatal visit the nurse has had the opportunity to discuss and reinforce the importance of being prepared for the birth of the child with the parents. It is now up to the parents to use the nurse's guidance and put it into action to be ready for the upcoming birth.

A recent national survey entitled *Listening to Mothers III: Pregnancy and Birth* revealed concerns about overuse of maternity care practices and women's readiness to make informed decisions. Key findings point to the need for quality improvement, consumer engagement, and shared decision making (Declercq, Sakala, Corry, Applebaum, & Herrlick, 2014). These findings present a challenge for all nurses caring for maternity clients to thoroughly explain all procedures, along with their rationales, and truly listen to what the woman desires to make her childbirth experience outcome a positive one for her.

All nurses have the responsibility to impart their knowledge to all women and their families—and that starts with teaching themselves first. The evidence is clear that women have better outcomes when nurses intervene only when needed in the childbirth process. Nurses need to personalize their care to every woman based on her needs, her desires, and her state of health. Nurses must focus on teaching women and their families to understand the value of birth and its long-lasting effects on the family. In addition, nurses must provide birth settings that are safe, whether in the hospital, birth center, or at home. This includes, but is not limited to, providing continuous support in labor, allowing women the freedom to move and assume positions of choice, offering nourishment of the woman's body and spirit, using nonpharmacologic pain relief modalities whenever possible, and ensuring seamless, collaborative teamwork. Continuous labor support is a nonpharmacologic, evidence-based strategy associated with reduced cesarean rates (Baum, Crawford, & Humphrey-Shelton, 2015).

NURSING CARE PLAN 12.1

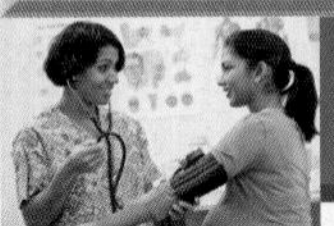

Overview of the Woman Experiencing Common Discomforts of Pregnancy

Alicia, a 32-year-old, G1 P0, at 10 weeks' gestation, comes to the clinic for a visit. During the interview she tells you, "I'm running to the bathroom to urinate it seems like all the time, and I'm so nauseous that I'm having trouble eating." She denies any burning or pain on urination. Vital signs are within acceptable limits.

NURSING DIAGNOSIS: Impaired urinary elimination related to frequency secondary to physiologic changes of pregnancy

Outcome Identification and Evaluation

The client will report a decrease in urinary complaints, as evidenced by a decrease in the number of times she uses the bathroom to void, reports that she feels her bladder is empty after voiding, and use of Kegel exercises.

Interventions: *Promoting Normal Urinary Elimination Patterns*

- Assess client's usual bladder elimination patterns to establish a baseline for comparison.
- Obtain a urine specimen for analysis to rule out infection or glucosuria.
- Review with client the physiologic basis for the increased frequency during pregnancy; inform client that frequency should abate during the second trimester and that it most likely will return during her third trimester. This will promote understanding of the problem.
- Encourage the client to empty her bladder when first feeling a sensation of fullness to minimize risk of urinary retention.
- Suggest client avoid caffeinated drinks, which can stimulate the need to void.
- Encourage client to drink adequate amounts of fluid throughout the day; however, have client reduce her fluid intake before bedtime to reduce nighttime urination.
- Urge client to keep perineal area clean and dry to prevent irritation and excoriation from any leakage.
- Instruct client in Kegel exercises to increase perineal muscle tone and control over leakage.
- Teach client about the signs and symptoms of urinary tract infection and urge her to report them should they occur to ensure early detection and prompt intervention.

NURSING DIAGNOSIS: Imbalanced nutrition, less than body requirements, related to nausea and vomiting

NURSING CARE PLAN 12.1

Overview of the Woman Experiencing Common Discomforts of Pregnancy (continued)

Outcome Identification and Evaluation

The client will ingest adequate amounts of nutrients for maternal and fetal well-being as evidenced by acceptable weight gain pattern and statements indicating an increase in food intake with a decrease in the number of episodes of nausea and vomiting.

Interventions: ***Promoting Adequate Nutrition***

1. Obtain weight and compare to baseline to determine effects of nausea and vomiting on nutritional intake.
2. Review client's typical dietary intake over 24 hours to determine nutritional intake and patterns so that suggestions can be individualized.
3. Encourage client to eat five or six small frequent meals throughout the day to prevent her stomach from becoming empty.
4. Suggest that she munch on dry crackers, toast, cereal, or cheese or drink a small amount of lemonade before arising to minimize nausea.
5. Encourage client to arise slowly from bed in the morning and avoid sudden movements to reduce stimulation of the vomiting center.
6. Advise client to drink fluids between meals rather than with meals to avoid overdistention of the abdomen and subsequent increase in abdominal pressure.
7. Encourage her to increase her intake of foods high in vitamin B_6 such as meat, poultry, bananas, fish, green leafy vegetables, peanuts, raisins, walnuts, and whole grains, as tolerated, to ensure adequate nutrient intake.
8. Advise the client to avoid greasy, fried, or highly spiced foods and to avoid strong odors, including foods such as cabbage, to minimize gastrointestinal upset.
9. Encourage the client to avoid wearing tight or restricting clothes to minimize pressure on the expanding abdomen.
10. Arrange for consultation with nutritionist as necessary to assist with diet planning.

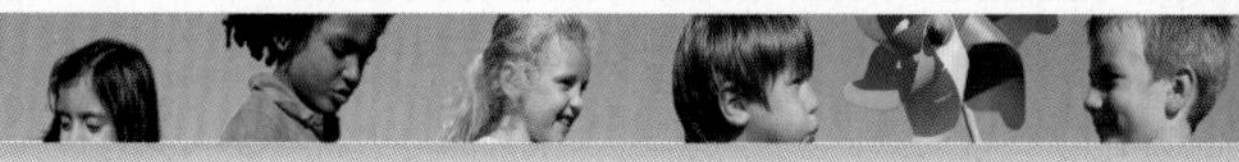

KEY CONCEPTS

- Preconception care is the promotion of the health and well-being of a woman and her partner before pregnancy. The goal of preconception care is to identify any areas such as health problems, lifestyle habits, or social concerns that might unfavorably affect pregnancy.
- A thorough history and physical examination are performed on the initial prenatal visit.
- A primary aspect of nursing management during the antepartum period is counseling and educating the pregnant women and her partner to promote healthy outcomes for all involved.
- Nagele rule can be used to establish the estimated date of birth. Using this rule, subtract 3 months from the month of their last LMP, add 7 days to the first day of the last normal menstrual period, then correct the year by adding 1 to it. This date is within plus or minus 2 weeks (margin of error).
- Pelvic shape is typically classified as one of four types: gynecoid, android, anthropoid, and platypelloid. The gynecoid type is the typical female pelvis and offers the best shape for a vaginal delivery.
- Continuous prenatal care is important for a successful outcome. The recommended schedule is every 4 weeks up to 28 weeks (7 months); every 2 weeks from 29 to 36 weeks; and every week from 37 weeks to birth.

- The height of the fundus is measured when the uterus arises out of the pelvis to evaluate fetal growth.
- The fundus reaches the level of the umbilicus at approximately 20 weeks and measures 20 cm. The fundal measurement should approximately equal the number of weeks of gestation until week 36.
- At each visit the woman is asked whether she is having any common signs or symptoms of preterm labor, which might include uterine contractions, dull backache, pressure in the pelvic area or thighs, increased vaginal discharge, menstrual-like cramps, and vaginal bleeding.
- Prenatal screening has become standard in prenatal care to detect neural tube defects and genetic abnormalities.
- The nurse should address matter of factly common discomforts that occur in each trimester at all prenatal visits and should provide realistic measures to help the client deal with them effectively.
- The pregnant client can better care for herself and the fetus if her concerns are anticipated by the nurse and incorporated into guidance sessions at each prenatal visit.
- Iron and folic acid need to be supplemented because their increased requirements during pregnancy are usually too great to be met through diet alone.
- Throughout pregnancy, a well-balanced diet is critical for a healthy baby.
- Perinatal education has broadened its focus to include preparation for pregnancy and family adaptation to the new parenting roles. Childbirth education began because of increasing pressure from consumers who wanted to become more involved in their birthing experience.
- Three common childbirth education methods are Lamaze (psychoprophylactic), Bradley (partner-coached childbirth), and Dick-Read (natural childbirth).
- The great majorities of women in the United States are well and healthy and can consider the full range of birth settings: hospital, birth center, or home setting.
- All pregnant women need to be able to recognize early signs of contractions to prevent preterm labor.

REFERENCES AND RECOMMENDED READINGS

Akolekar, R., Beta, J., Picciarelli, G., Ogilvie, C., & D'Antonio, F. (2015). Procedure-related risk of miscarriage following amniocentesis and chorionic villus sampling: A systematic review and meta-analysis. *Ultrasound in Obstetrics & Gynecology, 45*(1), 16–26.

Alekseev, N. P., Vladimir, I. I., & Nadezhda, T. E. (2015). Pathological postpartum breast engorgement: Prediction, prevention, and resolution. *Breastfeeding Medicine, 10*(4), 203–208.

Alexander, L. L., LaRosa, J. H., Bader, H., & Garfield, S. (2014). *New dimensions in women's health* (6th ed.). Sudbury, MA: Jones & Bartlett.

Alfirevic Z, Stampalija T, Medley N. (2015). Fetal and umbilical Doppler ultrasound in normal pregnancy. *Cochrane Database of Systematic Reviews, 4*, CD001450.

Alliman, J., Jolles, D., & Summers, L. (2015). The innovation imperative: Scaling freestanding birth centers, centering pregnancy, and midwifery-led maternity health homes. *Journal of Midwifery & Women's Health, 60*, 244–249.

Almansa, C., DeVault, K., & Houghton, L. A. (2015). *Gas and bloating. In Functional and motility disorders of the gastrointestinal tract* (pp. 113–123). New York, NY: Springer Publishers.

American Academy of Family Physicians. (2015). *Summary of recommendations for clinical preventive services.* Retrived from http://www.aafp.org/dam/AAFP/documents/patient_care/clinical_recommendations/cps-recommendations.pdf

American Academy of Pediatrics [AAP]. (2012). Breastfeeding and the use of human milk. *Pediatrics, 129*(3), 827–841.

American Academy of Pediatrics. (2015). *Breastfeeding.* Retrieved from https://www2.aap.org/breastfeeding/index.html

American College of Nurse-Midwives. (2015). *About midwives.* Retrieved from http://www.midwife.org/About-Midwives

American College of Obstetricians & Gynecologists [ACOG]. (2013). *Oral health care during pregnancy and through the lifespan.* Retrieved from http://www.acog.org/Resources-And-Publications/Committee-Opinions/Committee-on-Health-Care-for-Underserved-Women/Oral-Health-Care-During-Pregnancy-and-Through-the-Lifespan

American College of Obstetricians and Gynecologists [ACOG]. (2015a). *Routine tests in pregnancy FAQ 133.* Retrieved from http://www.acog.org/For_Patients/Search_FAQs?Topics=906bff1e-0656–4579-a7df-4a22f9bce483&pipe;fb741a4b-41f7–4b37–8307-f4844738b26f

American College of Obstetricians and Gynecologists [ACOG]. (2015b). *Screening tests for birth defects.* Retrieved from http://www.acog.org/~/media/For%20Patients/faq165.pdf?dmc=1&ts=20140517T0925037578

American College of Obstetricians and Gynecologists [ACOG]. (2015c). *Easing back pain during pregnancy.* Retrieved from http://www.acog.org/~/media/For%20Patients/faq115.pdf?dmc=1&ts=20140517T1536210126

American College of Obstetricians and Gynecologists [ACOG]. (2015d). *Problems of the digestive system.* Retrieved from http://www.acog.org/~/media/For%20Patients/faq120.pdf?dmc=1&ts=20140518T1321141397

American College of Obstetricians & Gynecologists [ACOG]. (2015e). *Exercise during pregnancy.* Retrieved from https://www.acog.org/Search?Keyword=exercise+guidelines

American College of Obstetricians & Gynecologists [ACOG]. (2015f). *Sexuality and sexual problems.* Retrieved from http://pause.acog.org/topics/sexuality-and-sexual-problems

American College of Obstetricians & Gynecologists [ACOG]. (2015g). *Travel during pregnancy.* Retrieved from http://www.acog.org/~/media/For%20Patients/faq055.pdf?dmc=1&ts=20140519T1526511729

American College of Obstetricians & Gynecologists [ACOG]. (2015h). *Breastfeeding your baby.* Retrieved from http://www.acog.org/~/media/For%20Patients/faq029.pdf?dmc=1&ts=20140520T0943394126

American Diabetes Association [ADA]. (2015). Classification and diagnosis of diabetes. *Diabetes Care, 38*(Suppl 1), S8–S16.

American Pregnancy Association [APA]. (2014a). *Maternal serum alpha-fetoprotein screening (MSAFP).* Retrieved from http://americanpregnancy.org/prenataltesting/afp.html

American Pregnancy Association [APA]. (2014b). *Pregnancy exercise guidelines.* Retrieved from http://americanpregnancy.org/pregnancyhealth/exerciseguidelines.html

Anil, S., Alrowis, R. M., Chalisserry, E. P., Chalissery, V. P., AlMoharib, H. S., & Al-Sulaimani, A. F. (2015). Oral health and adverse pregnancy outcomes. In *Emerging trends in oral health sciences and dentistry.* (pp. 631–662). http://dx.doi.org/10.5772/59517

Barakat, R., Lucía, A., & Ruiz, J. (2015). Exercise and pregnancy, In M. L. Mountjoy (Ed.), *Handbook of sports medicine and science: The female athlete.* Hoboken, NJ, USA: John Wiley & Sons, Inc.

Baum, A., Crawford, P., & Humphrey-Shelton, M. (2015). Clinical inquiry: Does the presence of a trained support person during labor decrease C-section rates? *The Journal of Family Practice, 64*(3), 192–193.

Biswas, A., & Choolani, M. (2015). Prenatal diagnosis of chromosomal abnormalities–shifting paradigm. *Annals of the Academy of Medicine, Singapore, 44*(2), 40–42.

Boggess, K. A., & Berggren, E. K. (2015). Preconception care has the potential for a high return on investment. *American Journal of Obstetrics & Gynecology, 212*(1), A1–A20.

Bond, S. (2015). American College of Obstetricians and Gynecologists releases committee opinion on estimation of due date. *Journal of Midwifery & Women's Health, 60*(2), 220–224.

Bope, E. T., & Kellerman, R. D. (2015). *Conn's current therapy 2015.* Philadelphia, PA: Saunders Elsevier.

Boynton, P. M. (2015). Pregnancy: Relationships advice. *The International Encyclopedia of Human Sexuality,* 861–1042.

Bradley Method. (2014). *Introduction to the Bradley method.* Retrieved from http://www.bradleybirth.com

Brown, H. L. (2015). ACOG guidelines at a glance: Antepartum fetal surveillance. Contemporary OB/GYN. Retrieved from http://contemporaryobgyn.modernmedicine.com/contemporary-obgyn/news/acog-guidelines-glance-antepartum-fetal-surveillance?page=full

Budin, W. C. (2015). Choosing wisely for birth. *The Journal of Perinatal Education, 24*(1), 3–5.

Callahan, T. L. (2016). *Tarascon Ob/Gyn Pocketbook.* Burlington, MA: Jones & Bartlett Learning.

Callegari, L. S., Ma, E. W., & Schwarz, E. B. (2015). Preconception care and reproductive planning in primary care. *Medical Clinics of North America, 99*(3), 663–682.

Centers for Disease Control and Prevention [CDC]. (2015a). *Preconception care and health care.* Retrieved from http://www.cdc.gov/preconception/hcp/

Centers for Disease Control and Prevention [CDC]. (2015b). *Preconception care recommendations.* Retrieved from http://www.cdc.gov/preconception/hcp/recommendations.html

Centers for Disease Control and Prevention [CDC]. (2015c). *Facts about birth defects.* Retrieved from http://www.cdc.gov/ncbddd/birthdefects/facts.html

Centers for Disease Control and Prevention [CDC]. (2015d). *Pregnancy complications.* Retrieved from http://www.cdc.gov/reproductivehealth/MaternalInfantHealth/PregComplications.htm#n5

Centers for Disease Control and Prevention [CDC]. (2015e). *Pregnant travelers.* Retrieved from http://wwwnc.cdc.gov/travel/yellowbook/2014/chapter-8-advising-travelers-with-specific-needs/pregnant-travelers

Centers for Disease Control and Prevention [CDC]. (2015f). *Vaccines for pregnant women.* Retrieved from http://www.cdc.gov/vaccines/adults/rec-vac/pregnant.html

Centers for Disease Control and Prevention [CDC]. (2015g). *Mediations and pregnancy.* Retrieved from http://www.cdc.gov/pregnancy/meds/

Cunningham, F., Leveno, K, Bloom, S., Spong, K., Dashe, J. S., Hoffman, B. L., et al. (2014). *Williams obstetrics* (24th ed.). New York, NY: McGraw-Hill Education.

Darmstadt, G. L., Shiffman, J., & Lawn, J. E. (2015). Advancing the newborn and stillbirth global agenda: Priorities for the next decade. *Archives of Disease in Childhood, 100*(Suppl 1), S13–S18.

Declercq, E. R., Sakala, C., Corry, M. P., Applebaum, S., & Herrlich, A. (2014). Major survey findings of listening to mothers (SM) III: New mothers speak out: Report of national surveys of women's childbearing experiences conducted October 2102 and January-April 2013. *Journal of Perinatal Education.* Winter, 23(1), 17–24. Doi: 10.1891/1058-1243.23.1.17

Declercq, E., & Stotland, N. E. (2015). *Planned home birth.* UpToDate. Retrieved from http://0-www.uptodate.com.ksclib.keene.edu/contents/planned-homebirth?source=search_result&search=planned+home+birth&selectedTitle=1~150

Dempsey, Á. C., & Overton, T. G. (2015). Advances in fetal therapy. *Obstetrics, Gynecology & Reproductive Medicine. 25*(7), 203–207.

Dietz, W. H. (2015). The response of the US Centers for Disease Control and Prevention to the obesity epidemic. *Annual Review of Public Health, 36,* 575–596.

Eshaghabadi, A., & Barati, P. (2015). P97: Motor vehicle accident during the pregnancy. *The Neuroscience Journal of Shefaye Khatam, 2*(4), 147–147.

Evans, M. I., Andriole, S., & Evans, S. M. (2015). Genetics: Update on prenatal screening and diagnosis. *Obstetrics and Gynecology Clinics of North America, 42*(2), 193–208.

Everett, T. R., & Peebles, D. M. (2015). Antenatal tests of fetal wellbeing. In *Seminars in fetal and neonatal medicine.* WB Saunders.

Farrar, D., Duley, L., Medley, N., & Lawlor D.A. (2015). Different strategies for diagnosing gestational diabetes to improve maternal and infant health. *Cochrane Database of Systematic Reviews* , *1*, CD007122.

Ferri, F.F. (2014). *Ferri's best test: A practical guide to laboratory medicine and diagnostic imaging* (3rd ed.). Philadelphia, PA: Elsevier Health Sciences.

Fischbach, F., & Dunning, M. B. (2014). *A manual of laboratory and diagnostic tests.* (9th ed.). Philadelphia, PA: Lippincott Williams & Wilkins.

Fretts, R.C. (2014). Evaluation of decreased fetal movements. UpToDate. Retrieved from http://www.uptodate.com/contents/evaluation-of-decreased-fetal-movements

Gadot, Y., & Koren, G. (2015). Medications in pregnancy: Can we treat the mother while protecting the unborn? In *Optimizing treatment for children in the developing world* (pp. 65–70). Springer International Publishing.

Grant, N., Strevens, H., & Thornton, J. (2015). Physiology of labor. In *Epidural labor analgesia* (pp. 1–10). Springer International Publishing.

Greeley, E. T., Kessler, K. A., & Vohra, N. (2015). Clinical applications of noninvasive prenatal testing. *Journal of Fetal Medicine, 2*(1):11–17.

Guidotti, T. L. (2014). Demystifying reproductive hazards in the workplace. *Archives of Environmental & Occupational Health, 69*(2), 125–126.

Halford, W. K., Petch, J., & Creedy, D. (2015). Caring and sexuality. In *Clinical guide to helping new parents* (pp. 131–150). New York, NY: Springer Publishers.

Heazell, A. (2015). A kick in the right direction-reduced fetal movements and stillbirth prevention. *BMC Pregnancy and Childbirth, 15*(Suppl 1), A7.

Hehir, M. P., Dalrymple, J., & Malone, F. D. (2015). Decision-support guide and use of prenatal genetic testing. *JAMA, 313*(2), 199–199.

Hixson, L., Goel, S., Schuber, P., Faltas, V., Lee, J., Narayakkadan, A., et al. (2015). An overview on prenatal screening for chromosomal aberrations. *Journal of Laboratory Automation, 20*(5),562–573.

Hurst, H. M., & Linton, D. M. (2015). Preconception care: Planning for the future. *The Journal for Nurse Practitioners, 11*(3), 335–340.

Jordan, R. G., Engstrom, J., Marfell, J., & Farley, C. L. (2014). *Prenatal and postnatal care: A women-centered approach.* Ames, Iowa: John Wiley & Sons.

Jyothi, M. N. (2015). A case report on pica: A rare pregnancy related complication. *Asian Journal of Nursing Education and Research, 5*(1), 137–139.

Kader, M., & Naim-Shuchana, S. (2014). Physical activity and exercise during pregnancy. *European Journal of Physiotherapy, 16*(1), 2–9.

Kalousová, M., Muravská, A., & Zima, T. (2014). Pregnancy-associated plasma protein A (PAPP-A) and preeclampsia. *Advances in Clinical Chemistry, 63*, 169–209.

Keytash, A., Jones, L., & Frances, A. (2015). Strong healthy behavioral change program for women. *Australian Nursing and Midwifery Journal, 22*(9), 45–46.

Khalil, A., & Coates, A. (2015). Prenatal diagnosis of chromosomal abnormalities. *Arias' practical guide to high-risk pPregnancy and delivery: A south asian perspective* (4th ed., pp. 1–13). Elsevier Health Sciences.

King, T. L., Brucker, M. C., Kriebs, J. M., Fahey, J. O., Gegor, C. L., & Varney, H. (2015). *Varney's midwifery* (5th ed.). Burlington, MA: Jones & Bartlett Learning.

Kondhare, M. M., & Khodgire, U. (2015). Benefits of exercises on selected physiological common complaints during pregnancy. *Journal of Physical Education Research, 1*, 13–26.

Lakshmi, G. R., & Jyothsna, D. (2015). Influence of amniotic fluid index on fetal outcome. *Journal of Evidence Based Medicine and Healthcare, 2*(10), 1455–1463.

La Leche League International. (2016). *Breastfeeding help.* Retrieved from http://www.llli.org/resources/assistance.html?m=0,0

Lamaze International. (2015). *Healthy birth practices.* Retrieved from http://www.lamaze.org

Latendresse, G., & Deneris, A. (2015). An update on current prenatal testing options: First trimester and noninvasive prenatal testing. *Journal of Midwifery & Women's Health, 60*(1), 24–36.

Leggat, P. A., & Zuckerman, J. N. (2015). Pre-travel health risk assessment. *Essential Travel Medicine,* (pp.23–34). West Sussex, UK: John Wiley & Sons.

Lewis, R. (2015). As home births increase, recent studies illuminate controversies and complexities. *JAMA, 313*(6), 553–555.

Maeda, K. (2015). Ultrasound diagnosis of the fetus in-utero. *Journal of Health Medical Informatics, 6*(174), 2.

March of Dimes. (2015a). *Pregnancy complications.* Retrieved from http://www.marchofdimes.com/pregnancy/pregnancy-complications.aspx

March of Dimes. (2015b). *The serious problem of premature birth.* Retrieved from http://www.marchofdimes.com/mission/prematurity-campaign.aspx

March of Dimes. (2015c). *Preterm labor.* Retrieved from http://www.marchofdimes.com/pregnancy/preterm-labor-and-birth.aspx

March of Dimes. (2015d). *Aminocentesis.* Retrieved from http://www.marchofdimes.com/pregnancy/amniocentesis.aspx

March of Dimes. (2015e). *Chorionic villus sampling.* Retrieved from http://www.marchofdimes.com/pregnancy/chorionic-villus-sampling.aspx

March of Dimes. (2015f). *Sex during pregnancy.* Retrieved from http://www.marchofdimes.com/pregnancy/physicalactivity_sex.html

March of Dimes. (2015g). *Childbirth education classes.* Retrieved from http://www.marchofdimes.com/pregnancy/childbirth-education-classes.aspx

March of Dimes. (2015h). *Vaccinations during pregnancy.* Retrieved from http://www.marchofdimes.com/pregnancy/vaccinations-during-pregnancy.aspx

Moses, S. (2015a). *Routine obstetric visit-Family Practice Notebook.* Retrieved from http://www.fpnotebook.com/ob/Exam/RtnObstrcVst.htm

Moses, S. (2015b). *Fetal movement count-Family Practice Notebook.* Retrieved from http://www.fpnotebook.com/ob/fetus/FtlMvmntCnt.htm

Moses, S. (2015c). *Biophysical profile- Family Practice Notebook.* Retrieved from http://www.fpnotebook.com/ob/fetus/BphysclPrfl.htm

M'soka, N. C., Mabuza, L. H., & Pretorius, D. (2015). Cultural and health beliefs of pregnant women in Zambia regarding pregnancy and child birth. *Curationis, 38*(1), 1–7.

Nagtalon-Ramos, J. (2014). *Best evidence-based practices in maternal-newborn care*. Philadelphia, PA: F. A. Davis Company.

National Institutes of Health. (2015). *Health problems in pregnancy.* Retrieved from http://www.nlm.nih.gov/medlineplus/healthproblemsinpregnancy.html

National Maternal and Child Health Resource Center. (2015). *Oral health care during pregnancy: A national consensus statement.* Retrieved from http://www.mchoralhealth.org/materials/consensus_statement.html

Nisa, M. U., Hamid, N., Nasreen, F., & Khanum, F. (2015). Corelation of biophysical profile with APGAR score. *Cell, 92.* doi: 321–9001662.

Office on Women's Health. (2014). Why breastfeeding is important. *Womenshealth.gov.* Retrieved from http://www.womenshealth.gov/breastfeeding/why-breastfeeding-is-important/

Ota E, Hori H, Mori R, Tobe-Gai R, & Farrar D. (2015). Antenatal dietary education and supplementation to increase energy and protein intake. *Cochrane Database of Systematic Reviews, 6*, CD000032.

Patil, M., Panchanadikar, T., & Wagh, G. (2014). Variation of PAPP-A level in the first trimester of pregnancy and its clinical outcome. *Journal of Obstetrics and Gynecology of India, 64*(2), 116–119.

Petrov Fieril, K., Glantz, A., & Fagevik Olsen, M. (2015). The efficacy of moderate to vigorous resistance exercise during pregnancy: A randomized controlled trial. *Acta Obstetricia et Gynecologica Scandinavica, 94*(1), 35–42.

Plastaras, C. T., & Appasamy, M. (2015). Interventional procedures for musculoskeletal pain in pregnancy and postpartum: Efficacy and safety. In *Musculoskeletal health in pregnancy and postpartum* (pp. 115–133). Springer International Publishing.

Pruetz, J. D., Votava-Smith, J., & Miller, D. A. (2015). Clinical relevance of fetal hemodynamic monitoring: Perinatal implications. In *Seminars in fetal and neonatal medicine.* WB Saunders. doi:10.1016/j.siny.2015.03.007

Rayburn, W. F., Jolley, J. A., Simpson, L. L. (2015). Advances in ultrasound imaging for congenital malformations during early gestation. *Birth Defects Research Part A: Clinical and Molecular Teratology, 103*,260–268. doi: 10.1002/bdra.23353

Regal, J. F., Gilbert, J. S., & Burwick, R. M. (2015). The complement system and adverse pregnancy outcomes. *Molecular Immunology, 67*(1), 56–70.

Rigby, F. B. (2015). Common pregnancy complaints and questions. *Emedicine.* Retrieved from http://emedicine.medscape.com/article/259724-overview

Satyan, M. T., Grothusen, J., Drummond, K., Kennedy, B., Weiner, C., & Lee, G. (2015). 200: A retrospective review of the impact of HAPO based screening guidelines for gestational diabetes. *American Journal of Obstetrics & Gynecology, 212*(1), S113–S114.

Schram, J. (2014). Food for thought. *World of Irish Nursing & Midwifery, 22*(3), 46–47.

Schuiling, K. D., & Likis, F. E. (2016). *Women's gynecologic health* (3rd ed.). Burlington, MA: Jones & Bartlett Learning.

Schytt, E., & Bergström, M. (2014). First-time fathers' expectations and experiences of childbirth in relation to age. *Midwifery, 30*(1), 82–88.

Senie, R.T. (2014). *Epidemiology of women's health.* Burlington, MA: Jones & Bartlett Learning.

Slaughter, S., Hearns-Stokes, R., van der Vlugt, T., & Joffe, H. (2014). FDA approval of doxylamine-pyridoxine therapy for use in pregnancy. *New England Journal of Medicine, 370*(12), 1081–1083.

Springer, S. C. (2015). Prenatal diagnosis and fetal therapy. *eMedicine.* Retrieved from http://emedicine.medscape.com/article/ 936318-overview#aw2aab6b5

Steegers-Theunissen, R. P., & Steegers, E. A. (2015). Embryonic health: New insights, health and personalized patient care. *Reproduction, Fertility and Development, 27*(4), 712–715.

Tara, F., Vakilian, F., Moosavi-Baigy, F., Salehi, M., & Moghiman, T. (2015). Prenatal and cardiovascular outcome in pregnant patients with dyspnea. *Research in Cardiovascular Medicine, 4*(2). doi: 10.5812/cardiovascmed.20950

Tanner-Smith, E., Steinka-Fry, K., & Lipsey, M. (2014). The effects of centering pregnancy group prenatal care on gestational age, birth weight, and fetal demise. *Maternal & Child Health Journal, 18*(4), 801–809.

Templeton, A. (2015). The public health importance of antenatal care. *Facts, Views & Vision in ObGyn, 7*(1), 5–6.

Tharpe, N. L., Farley, C. L., & Jordan, R. (2016). *Clinical practice guidelines for midwifery & women's health* (5th ed.). Sudbury, MA: Jones & Bartlett.

Tracy, M. (2014). Centering pregnancy: An alternative model of prenatal care. *The Citizen.* Retrieved from http://www.auburnhospital.org/news-events/articles/centering-pregnancy-an-alternate-model-of-prenatal-care

Trivedi, S., Lal, N., & Singhal, R. (2015). Periodontal diseases and pregnancy. *Journal of Orofacial Sciences, 7*(1), 67–68.

Truong, Y. N., Yee, L. M., Caughey, A. B., & Cheng, Y. W. (2015). Weight gain in pregnancy: Does the Health and Medicine Division have it right? *American Journal of Obstetrics and Gynecology, 212*(3), 362–370.

Tyler, S., & Nagtalon-Ramos, J. (2015). Managing nausea and vomiting of pregnancy. *NP Women's Healthcare, 3*(2), 7–13.

U.S. Department of Health and Human Services. (2010). *Healthy People 2020.* Retrieved from http://www.healthypeople.gov/2020/topicsobjectives2020/objectiveslist.aspx?topicId=26

U.S. Preventive Services Task Force [USPSTF]. (2015). *Screening for gestational diabetes mellitus.* Retrieved from http://www.uspreventiveservicestaskforce.org/uspstf/uspsgdm.htm

Varner, C. A. (2015). Comparison of the Bradley method and HypnoBirthing childbirth education classes. *The Journal of Perinatal Education, 24*(2), 128–136.

Verghese, T. S., Futaba, K., & Latthe, P. (2015). Constipation in pregnancy. *The Obstetrician & Gynecologist, 17*(2), 111–115.

Weber, J., & Kelley, J. H. (2014). *Health assessment in nursing* (5th ed.). Philadelphia, PA: Lippincott Williams & Wilkins.

Westbury, B. (2015). The power of environment. *The Practicing Midwife, 18*(6), 24–26.

Women, Infants and Children [WIC]. (2015). *Breastfeeding promotion and support in WIC.* Retrieved from http://www.fns.usda.gov/wic/breastfeeding-promotion-and-support-wic

Yeniel, A. A., & Petri, E. E. (2014). Pregnancy, childbirth, and sexual function: Perceptions and facts. *International Urogynecology Journal, 25*(1), 5–14.

Yildiz, H. (2015). The relation between prepregnancy sexuality and sexual function during pregnancy and the postpartum period: A prospective study. *Journal of Sex & Marital Therapy, 41*(1), 49–59.

Zielinski, R., Ackerson, K., & Low, L. K. (2015). Planned home birth: Benefits, risks, and opportunities. *International Journal of Women's Health, 7,* 361–377.

Zielinski, R., Searing, K., & Deibel, M. (2015). Gastrointestinal distress in pregnancy: Prevalence, assessment, and treatment of 5 common minor discomforts. *The Journal of Perinatal & Neonatal Nursing, 29*(1), 23–31.

Zolotor, A., & Carlough, M. (2014). Update on prenatal care. *American Family Physician, 89*(3), 199–208.

CHAPTER WORKSHEET

MULTIPLE-CHOICE QUESTIONS

1. Which of the following biophysical profile findings indicate poor oxygenation to the fetus?
   a. Two pockets of amniotic fluid
   b. Well-flexed arms and legs
   c. Nonreactive fetal heart rate
   d. Fetal breathing movements noted
2. The nurse teaches the pregnant client how to perform Kegel exercises as a way to accomplish which of the following?
   a. Prevent perineal lacerations
   b. Stimulate labor contractions
   c. Increase pelvic muscle tone
   d. Lose pregnancy weight quickly
3. During a clinic visit, a pregnant client at 30 weeks' gestation tells the nurse, "I've had some mild cramps that are pretty irregular. What does this mean?" The cramps are probably:
   a. The beginning of labor in the very early stages
   b. An ominous finding indicating that the client is about to have a miscarriage
   c. Related to over hydration of the woman
   d. Braxton Hicks contractions, which occur throughout pregnancy
4. The nurse is preparing her teaching plan for a woman who has just had her pregnancy confirmed. Which of the following should be included in it? Select all that apply.
   a. Prevent constipation by taking a daily laxative
   b. Balance your dietary intake by increasing your calories by 300 daily
   c. Continue your daily walking routine just as you did before this pregnancy
   d. Tetanus, measles, mumps, and rubella vaccines will be given to you now
   e. Avoid tub baths now that you are pregnant to prevent vaginal infections
   f. Sexual activity is permitted as long as your membranes are intact
   g. Increase your consumption of milk to meet your iron needs
5. A pregnant client's last normal menstrual period was on August 10. Using Nagele rule, the nurse calculates that her estimated due date (EDD) will be which of the following?
   a. June 23
   b. July 10
   c. July 30
   d. May 17
6. Which of the following is not true about breast-feeding?
   a. Breast-fed infants experience more obesity and allergies
   b. Breast milk is perfectly suited to the infant's nutritional needs
   c. Breast milk contains maternal antibodies to stimulate infant's immunity
   d. Breast-feeding enhances maternal bonding and attachment
7. Practicing good oral hygiene is important for all women throughout their pregnancy. As a nurse providing anticipatory guidance for pregnant women, what condition can result from periodontal disease if good dental care isn't practiced?
   a. Post-dates pregnancy
   b. Large for gestational age infant
   c. Advanced reproductive cancer
   d. Preterm or low-birth-weight infant
8. Anticipatory guidance regarding sexual activity during pregnancy includes which of the following? Select all that apply:
   a. Sexual activity is contraindicated throughout pregnancy
   b. Most women don't desire intimacy after the first trimester
   c. Sexual activity may continue up until the end of the second trimester
   d. Sexual intercourse is prohibited if a history of preterm labor exists
   e. Women's sexual desire may change throughout the pregnancy
   f. Couples can try a variety of positions of comfort during pregnancy
9. Which of the following would be considered risk factors for psychologic well-being in pregnancy? Select all that apply:
   a. Limited support system and network of friends and family
   b. Introverted personality at any point in the pregnancy
   c. Ambivalence any time during the pregnancy
   d. High levels of stress due to family discord
   e. History of previous high-risk pregnancy with complications
   f. Depression prior to pregnancy and on medication

CHAPTER WORKSHEET

CRITICAL THINKING EXERCISES

1. Mary Jones comes to the Women's Health Center, where you work as a nurse. She is in her first trimester of pregnancy and tells you her main complaints are nausea and fatigue, to the point that she wants to sleep most of the time and eats one meal daily. She appears pale and tired. Her mucous membranes are pale. She reports that she gets 8 to 9 hours of sleep each night but still can't seem to stay awake and alert at work. She tells you she knows that she is not eating as she should, but she isn't hungry. Her hemoglobin and hematocrit are low.
   a. What subjective and objective data do you have to make your assessment?
   b. What is your impression of this woman?
   c. What nursing interventions would be appropriate for this client?
   d. How will you evaluate the effectiveness of your interventions?
2. Monica, a 16-year-old African American high school student, is here for her first prenatal visit. Her last normal menstrual period was 2 months ago, and she states she has been "sick ever since." She is 5 ft, 6 in tall, and weighs 110 lb. In completing her dietary assessment, the nurse asks about her intake of milk and dairy products. Monica reports that she doesn't like "that stuff" and doesn't want to put on too much weight because it "might ruin my figure."
   a. In addition to the routine obstetric assessments, which additional ones might be warranted for this teenager?
   b. What dietary instruction should be provided to this teenager based on her history?
   c. What follow-up monitoring should be included in subsequent prenatal visits?
3. Maria, a 27-year-old Hispanic woman in her last trimester of pregnancy (34 weeks), complains to the clinic nurse that she is constipated and feels miserable most of the time. She reports that she has started taking laxatives, but they don't help much. When questioned about her dietary habits, she replies that she eats beans and rice and drinks tea with most meals. She says she has tried to limit her fluid intake so she doesn't have to go to the bathroom so much because she doesn't want to miss any of her daytime soap operas on television.
   a. What additional information would the nurse need to assess her complaint?
   b. What interventions would be appropriate for Maria?
   c. What adaptations will Maria need to make to alleviate her constipation?

STUDY ACTIVITIES

1. Visit a freestanding birth center and compare it to a traditional hospital setting in terms of restrictions, type of pain management available, and costs.
2. Arrange to shadow a nurse-midwife for a day to see her role in working with the childbearing family.
3. Visit the student resources on and select two of the supplied websites that correspond to this chapter. Note their target audience, the validity of information offered, and their appeal to expectant couples. Present your findings.
4. Request permission to attend a childbirth education class in your local area and help a woman without a partner practice the paced breathing exercises. Present the information you learned and think about how you can apply it while taking care of a woman during labor.
5. A laywoman with a specialized education and experience in assisting women during labor is a ________________.

BRINGING IT ALL TOGETHER: A CASE STUDY

A 19-year-old female came to the public health clinic. This was her first prenatal visit, although she was 8 months pregnant. Her explanation as to why she hadn't been there before was: "It was summer and everything had been going good until my back started hurting two days ago."

ASSESSMENT

Her vital signs were within normal range. Weight was 175 lb. On physical examination, the back area was normal without tenderness when palpated. Fundal height was 36 cm; fetal heart rate was 150 bpm; urinalysis was negative for blood, glucose, or leukocytes. The pelvic examination showed the cervix to be long, thick, and closed. Missed routine prenatal lab work was done since this was her first visit. When questioned further about when her back seemed to cause her the most discomfort, she stated that she was a waitress and when she finished her shift, she could barely walk home.

1. What additional information is needed to make a diagnosis?
2. Based on the assessment, what might be suspected as the cause of her back pain?
3. What lab work might be included in her routine prenatal assessment that was missed?

It would be important to know what her prepregnant weight was to compare it with her present weight. If she has gained a large amount of weight during this pregnancy, it might be a contributing factor to her low back pain. Low back pain can also be a symptom of early labor, but in her case, she hasn't noticed any contractions and no cervical changes have taken place based on the examination. Low back pain in the lumbosacral region generally occurs in the last trimester and increases in intensity as the pregnancy progresses secondary to the increasing weight of the enlarged uterus and relaxation of the sacroiliac ligaments. The normal lordosis of pregnancy strains the back muscles and causes pain. Routine lab work may include a complete blood count (CBC), blood type, Rh type, and antibody screen, Hepatitis B surface antigen, HIV screening test, syphilis screening test, diabetic screening, and urinalysis or dipstick for protein.

PLAN

1. What health teaching by the nurse is needed for this client?
2. What specific relief measures are helpful to address her concern?
3. What changes in her work environment might be suggested?
4. How can her lack of prenatal care be addressed by the nurse?

Since this is her first prenatal visit, she has not had the benefit of any health teaching throughout her pregnancy thus far. Since she is in her last trimester, focus should be on preparing her for labor and birth, making arrangements for her childbirth at a local hospital, and referring her to obtain Women/Infants/Children (WIC) and other community resources available. Specific relief measures for low back pain would include instructing her to rest in a side-lying position to take the weight off her back; use proper body mechanics for lifting, stooping rather than bending so that the legs, rather than the back bear the weight and strain; and wearing low-heeled shoes. Excessive standing for long periods of time can contribute to low back pain, so periodic rest periods may need to be instituted in her work environment to reduce her low back pain. Since this client is already in her 8th month of pregnancy, the nurse should encourage her to keep her weekly prenatal appointments without placing judgment on her previous behavior. Making judgments and placing blame are not therapeutic interventions that provide an accepting environment to any client. Stressing the importance of prenatal care to the health of her baby and herself are important.

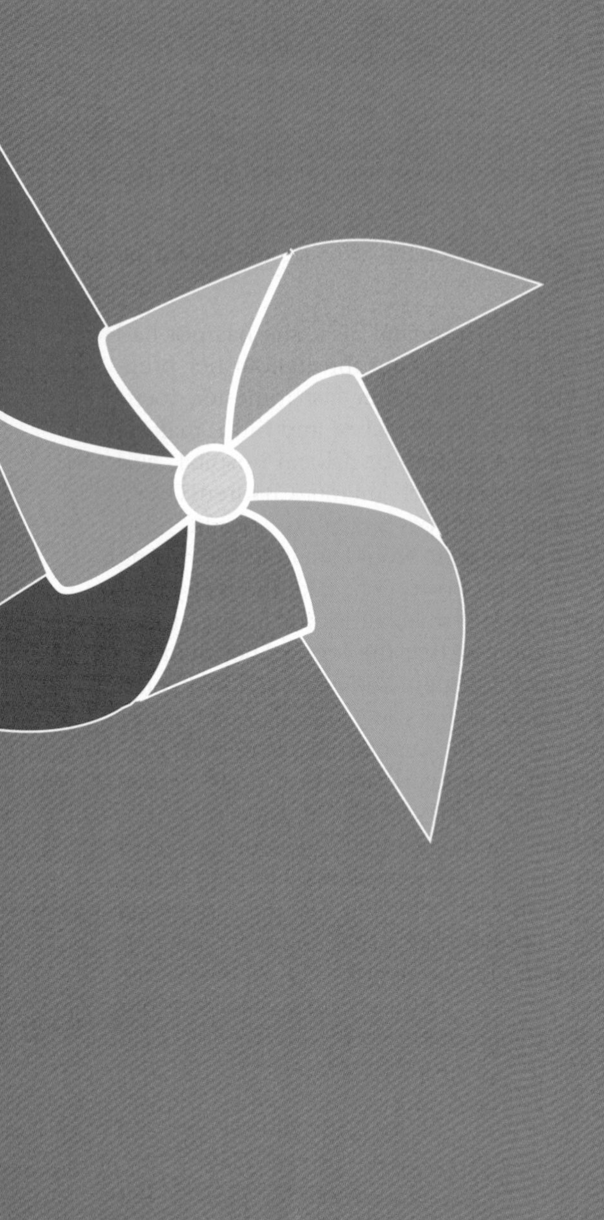

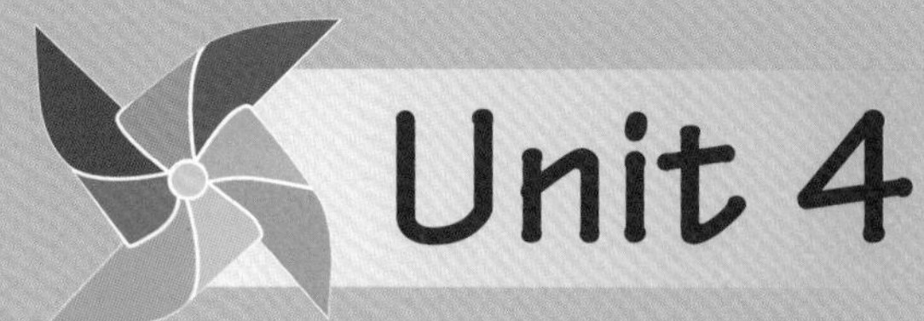

Labor and Birth

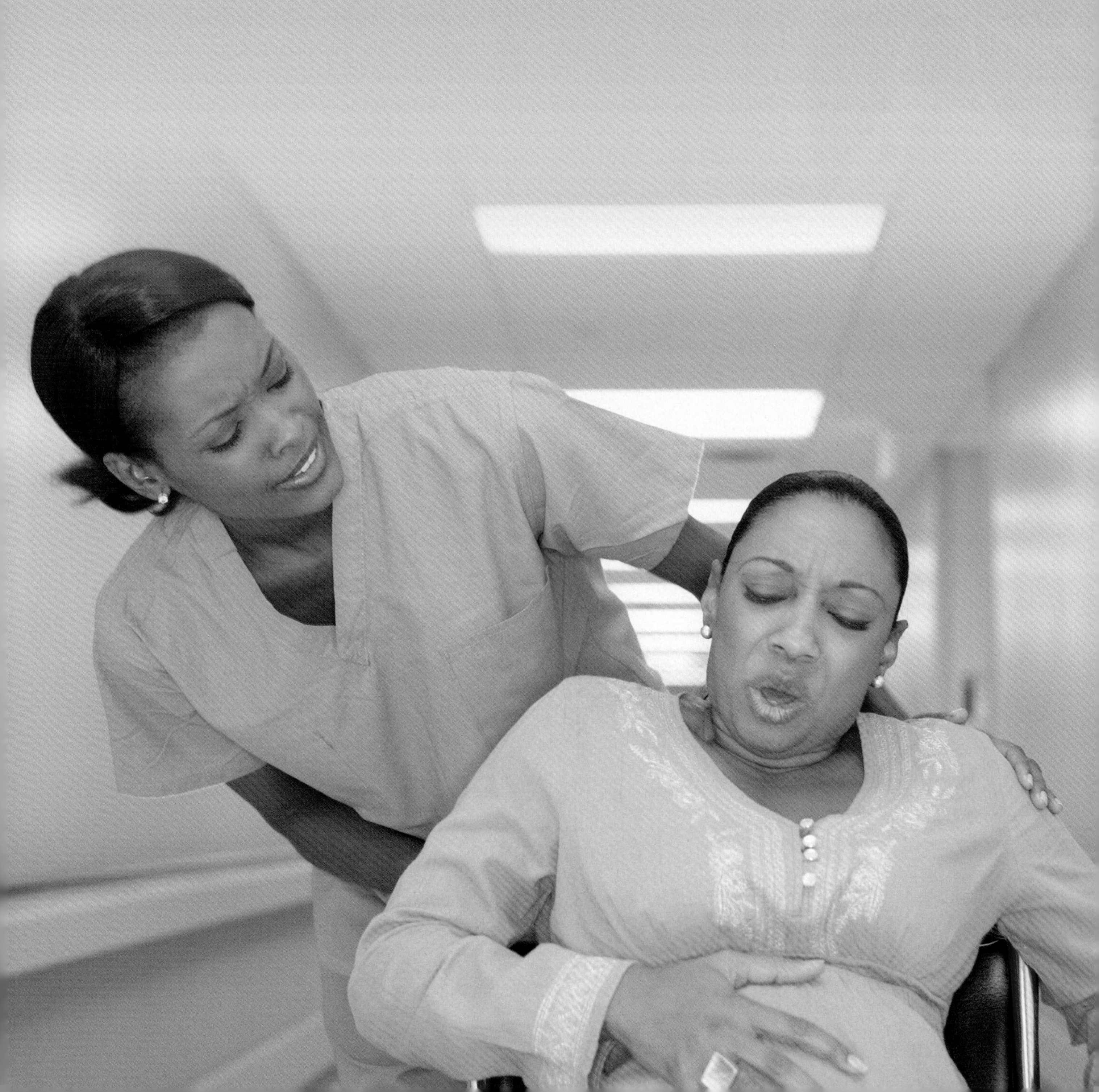

13

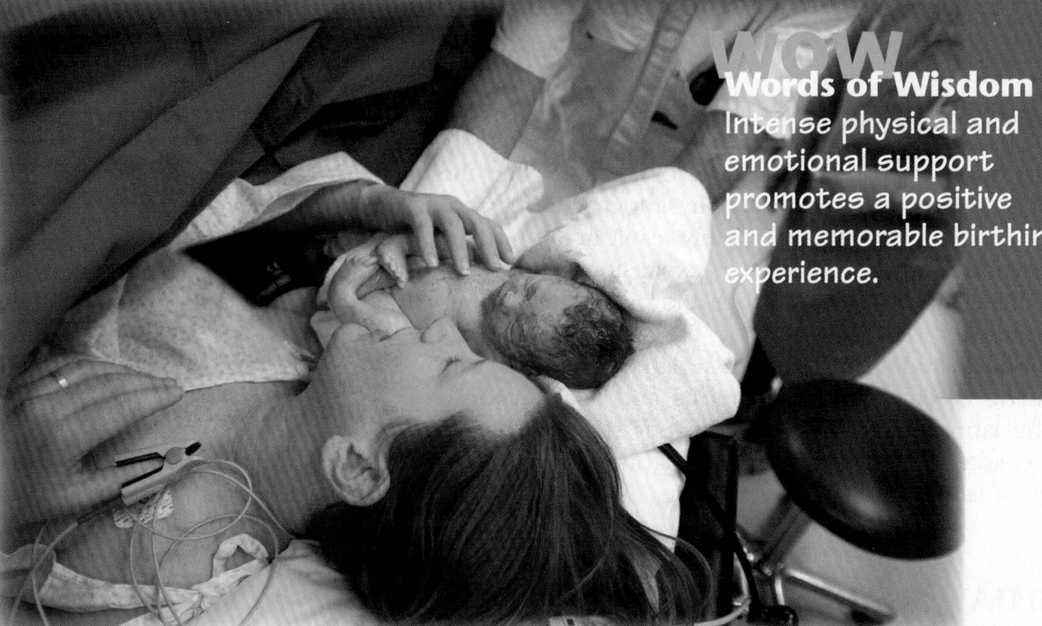

WOW

Words of Wisdom

Intense physical and emotional support promotes a positive and memorable birthing experience.

Labor and Birth Process

KEY TERMS

attitude
dilation
doula
duration
effacement
engagement
frequency
intensity
lie
lightening
molding
position
presentation
station

Learning Objectives

Upon completion of the chapter, you will be able to:

1. Relate premonitory signs of labor.
2. Compare and contrast true versus false labor.
3. Categorize the critical factors affecting labor and birth.
4. Analyze the cardinal movements of labor.
5. Evaluate the maternal and fetal responses to labor and birth.
6. Classify the stages of labor and the critical events in each stage.
7. Characterize the normal physiologic/psychological changes occurring during all four stages of labor.
8. Formulate the concept of pain as it relates to the woman in labor.

***Kathy and Chuck* have been eagerly awaiting the birth of their first child for what seems to them an eternity. When Kathy finally feels contractions in her abdomen, she and Chuck rush to the birthing center. After the OB nurse finishes a complete history and physical assessment, she informs Kathy and her husband that she must have experienced "false labor" and that they should return home until she starts true labor.**

INTRODUCTION

The process of labor and birth involves more than the birth of a newborn. Numerous physiologic and psychological events occur that ultimately result in the birth of a newborn and the creation or expansion of the family. This chapter describes labor and birth as a process. It addresses initiation of labor, the premonitory signs of labor, including true and false labor, critical factors affecting labor and birth, maternal and fetal response to the laboring process, and the four stages of labor. The chapter also identifies critical factors related to each stage of labor: the "10 P's of labor."

INITIATION OF LABOR

Labor is a physiologic event involving a sequential, integrated set of changes within the myometrium, decidua, and cervix that occurs gradually over a period of days to weeks in order to expel the fetus from the uterus. It is difficult to determine exactly why labor begins and what initiates it. Although several theories have been proposed to explain the onset and maintenance of labor, none of these has been proved scientifically. It is widely believed that labor is influenced by a cascade of events, including uterine stretch from the fetus and amniotic fluid volume, progesterone withdrawal to estrogen dominance, increased oxytocin sensitivity, and increased release of prostaglandins.

One theory suggests that labor is initiated by a change in the estrogen-to-progesterone ratio. During the last trimester of pregnancy, estrogen levels increase and progesterone levels decrease. This change leads to an increase in the number of myometrium gap junctions. Gap junctions are proteins that connect cell membranes and facilitate coordination of uterine contractions and myometrial stretching (Norwitz, 2015).

Although physiologic evidence for the role of oxytocin in the initiation of labor is inconclusive, the number of oxytocin receptors in the uterus increases at the end of pregnancy. This creates an increased sensitivity to oxytocin. Estrogen, the levels of which are also rising, increases myometrial sensitivity to oxytocin. With the increasing levels of oxytocin in the maternal blood in conjunction with increasing fetal cortisol levels that synthesize prostaglandins, uterine contractions are initiated. Oxytocin also aids in stimulating prostaglandin synthesis through receptors in the decidua. Prostaglandins lead to additional contractions, cervical softening, gap junction induction, and myometrial sensitization, thereby leading to a progressive cervical **dilation** (the opening or enlargement of the external cervical os). Uterine contractions have two main functions: to dilate the cervix and to push the fetus through the birth canal (Funai & Norwitz, 2015).

PREMONITORY SIGNS OF LABOR

Before the onset of labor, a pregnant woman's body undergoes several changes in preparation for the birth of the newborn. The changes that occur often lead to characteristic signs and symptoms that suggest that labor is near. These premonitory signs and symptoms can vary, and not every woman experiences every one of them.

Cervical Changes

Before labor begins, cervical softening and possible cervical dilation with descent of the presenting part into the pelvis occur. These changes can occur 1 month to 1 hour before actual labor begins.

As labor approaches, the cervix changes from an elongated structure to a shortened, thinned segment. Cervical collagen fibers undergo enzymatic rearrangement into smaller, more flexible fibers that facilitate water absorption, leading to a softer, more stretchable cervix. These changes occur secondary to the effects of prostaglandins and pressure from Braxton Hicks contractions. The ripening and softening of the cervix are essential for **effacement** and dilation, which reflect the enhanced collagen breakdown that was previously inhibited by progesterone (Grant, Strevens, & Thornton, 2015).

Lightening

Lightening occurs when the fetal presenting part begins to descend into the true pelvis. The uterus lowers and moves into a more anterior **position**. The shape of the abdomen changes as a result of the change in the uterus. With this descent, the woman usually notes that her breathing is much easier and that there is a decrease in gastric reflux. However, she may complain of increased pelvic pressure, leg cramping, dependent edema in the lower legs, and low back discomfort. She may notice an increase in vaginal discharge and more frequent urination. In primiparas, lightening can occur 2 weeks or more before labor begins; among multiparas it may not occur until labor starts (Cheng & Caughey, 2015a).

Increased Energy Level

Some women report a sudden increase in energy before labor. This is sometimes referred to as nesting, because many women will focus this energy toward childbirth preparation by cleaning, cooking, preparing the nursery, and spending extra time with other children in the household. The increased energy level usually occurs 24 to 48 hours before the onset of labor. It is thought to be the result of an increase in epinephrine release caused by a decrease in progesterone (Jordan, et al., 2014).

Bloody Show

At the onset of labor or before, the mucous plug that fills the cervical canal during pregnancy is expelled as a result of cervical softening and increased pressure of the presenting part. These ruptured cervical capillaries release a small amount of blood that mixes with mucus, resulting in the pink-tinged secretions known as bloody show.

Braxton Hicks Contractions

Braxton Hicks contractions, which the woman may have been experiencing throughout the pregnancy, may become stronger and more frequent. Braxton Hicks contractions are typically felt as a tightening or pulling sensation of the top of the uterus. They occur primarily in the abdomen and groin and gradually spread downward before relaxing. In contrast, true labor contractions are more commonly felt in the lower back. These contractions aid in moving the cervix from a posterior position to an anterior position. They also help in ripening and softening the cervix. However, the contractions are irregular and can be decreased by walking, voiding, eating, increasing fluid intake, or changing position.

Braxton Hicks contractions usually last about 30 seconds but can persist for as long as 2 minutes. As birth draws near and the uterus becomes more sensitive to oxytocin, the **frequency** and **intensity** of these contractions increase. However, if the contractions last longer than 30 seconds and occur more often than four to six times an hour, advise the woman to contact her health care provider so that she can be evaluated for possible preterm labor, especially if she is less than 38 weeks pregnant.

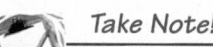

Take Note!

An infant born between 34 0/7 and 36 6/7 weeks of gestation is identified as "late preterm" and experiences many of the same health issues as other preterm birth infants (Horgan, 2015).

Spontaneous Rupture of Membranes

Rupture of membranes with loss of amniotic fluid prior to the onset of labor is termed prelabor rupture of membranes (PROM). It occurs in 8% to 10% of women with term pregnancies, the majority of whom will begin labor spontaneously within 24 hours (King, et al., 2015). The rupture of membranes can result in either a sudden gush or a steady leakage of amniotic fluid. Although much of the amniotic fluid is lost when the rupture occurs, a continuous supply is produced to ensure protection of the fetus until birth.

After the amniotic sac has ruptured, the barrier to infection is gone and an ascending infection is possible. In addition, there is a danger of cord prolapse if **engagement** has not occurred with the sudden release of fluid and pressure with rupture. Due to the possibility of these complications, advise women to notify their health care provider and go in for an evaluation.

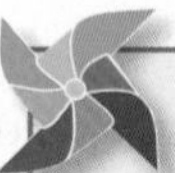

Consider This

I always pictured myself a dignified woman and behaved in ways to demonstrate that, for that was the way I was raised. My mother and grandmother always stressed that you should look good, dress well, and do nothing to embarrass yourself in public. I did a fairly good job of living up to their expectations until an incident occurred at the end of my first pregnancy. I recall I was overdue according to my dates and was miserable in the summer heat. I decided to go to the store for some ice cream. As I waddled down the grocery aisles, all of a sudden my water broke and came pouring down my legs all over the floor. Not wanting to make a spectacle of myself and remembering what my mother always said about being dignified at all times in public, I quickly reached up onto the grocery shelf and "accidentally" knocked off a large jar of pickles right where my puddle was. As I walked hurriedly away from that mess without my ice cream, I heard on the store loudspeaker, "Clean-up on aisle 13!"

Thoughts: We tend to live by what we are taught, and in this case, this woman needed to save face from her ruptured membranes. Many women experience ruptured membranes before the onset of labor, so it is not out of the ordinary for this to happen in public. What risks can occur when membranes do rupture? What action should this woman take now to minimize these risks? How will the nurse validate this woman's ruptured membranes?

TRUE VERSUS FALSE LABOR

False labor is a condition occurring during the latter weeks of some pregnancies in which irregular uterine contractions are felt, but the cervix is not affected. In contrast, true labor is characterized by contractions occurring at regular intervals that increase in frequency, **duration**, and intensity. True labor contractions bring about progressive cervical dilation and effacement. Table 13.1 summarizes the differences between true and false labor. False labor, prodromal labor, and Braxton Hicks contractions are all names for contractions that do not contribute in a measurable way toward the goal of birth. Distinguishing between true and false labor is an essential nursing assessment skill and one that develops with experience.

TABLE 13.1 DIFFERENCES BETWEEN TRUE AND FALSE LABOR

Parameters	True Labor	False Labor
Contraction timing	Regular, becoming closer together, usually 4–6 min apart, lasting 30–60 sec	Irregular, not occurring close together
Contraction strength	Become stronger with time, vaginal pressure is usually felt	Frequently weak, not getting stronger with time or alternating (a strong one followed by weaker ones)
Contraction discomfort	Starts in the back and radiates around toward the front of the abdomen	Usually felt in the front of the abdomen
Any change in activity	Contractions continue no matter what positional change is made	Contractions may stop or slow down with walking or making a position change
Stay or go?	Stay home until contractions are 5 min apart, last 45–60 sec, and are strong enough so that a conversation during one is not possible—then go to the hospital or birthing center.	Drink fluids and walk around to see if there is any change in the intensity of the contractions; if the contractions diminish in intensity after either or both—stay home.

Adapted from Curningham, F. G., Leveno, K. J., Bloom, S. L., Spong, C. Y., Dashe, J. S., Hoffman, B. L., Casey, B. M., & Sheffield, J. S. (2014). *Williams obstetrics* (24th ed.). New York, NY: McGraw-Hill Education; King, T. L., Brucker, M. C., Kriebs, J. M., Fahey, J. O., Gegor, C. L., & Varney, H. (2015). *Varney's midwifery* (5th ed.). Burlington, MA: Jones & Bartlett Learning; and Tharpe, N. L., Farley, C. L., & Jordan, R. (2016). *Clinical practice guidelines for midwifery & women's health*(4th ed.). Sudbury, MA: Jones & Bartlett.

Many women fear being sent home from the hospital with false labor. All women feel anxious when they feel contractions, but they should be informed that labor could be a long process, especially if it is their first pregnancy. Encourage the woman to think of false labor or prelabor signs as positive, because they are part of the entire labor continuum. With first pregnancies, the cervix can take up to 20 hours to dilate completely (Cunningham et al., 2014).

Remember Kathy and Chuck, the anxious couple who came to the hospital too early? Kathy felt sure she was in labor and is now confused. What explanations and anticipatory guidance should be offered to this couple? What term would describe her earlier contractions?

FACTORS AFFECTING THE LABOR PROCESS

Traditionally, the critical factors that affect the process of labor and birth are outlined as the "five P's":

1. **P**assageway (birth canal)
2. **P**assenger (fetus and placenta)
3. **P**owers (contractions)
4. **P**osition (maternal)
5. **P**sychological response

These critical factors are commonly accepted and discussed by health care providers. However, five additional "P's" can also affect the labor process:

1. **P**hilosophy (low tech, high touch)
2. **P**artners (support caregivers)
3. **P**atience (natural timing)
4. **P**atient (client) preparation (childbirth knowledge base)
5. **P**ain management (comfort measures)

These five additional P's are helpful in planning care for the laboring family. These client-focused factors are an attempt to foster labor that can be managed through the use of high touch, patience, support, knowledge, and pain management.

Passageway

The birth passageway is the route through which the fetus must travel to be born vaginally. Compared to other primates, childbirth is remarkably difficult in humans because the head of the neonate is large relative to the birth-relevant dimensions of the maternal pelvis. The passageway consists of the maternal pelvis and soft tissues. Of the two, however, the maternal bony pelvis is more important because it is relatively unyielding (except for the coccyx). Typically the pelvis is assessed and measured during the first trimester, often at the first visit to the health care provider, to identify any abnormalities that might hinder a successful vaginal birth. As the pregnancy progresses, the hormones relaxin and estrogen cause the connective tissues to become more relaxed and elastic and cause the joints to become more flexible to prepare the mother's pelvis for birth. Additionally, the soft tissues usually yield to the forces of labor.

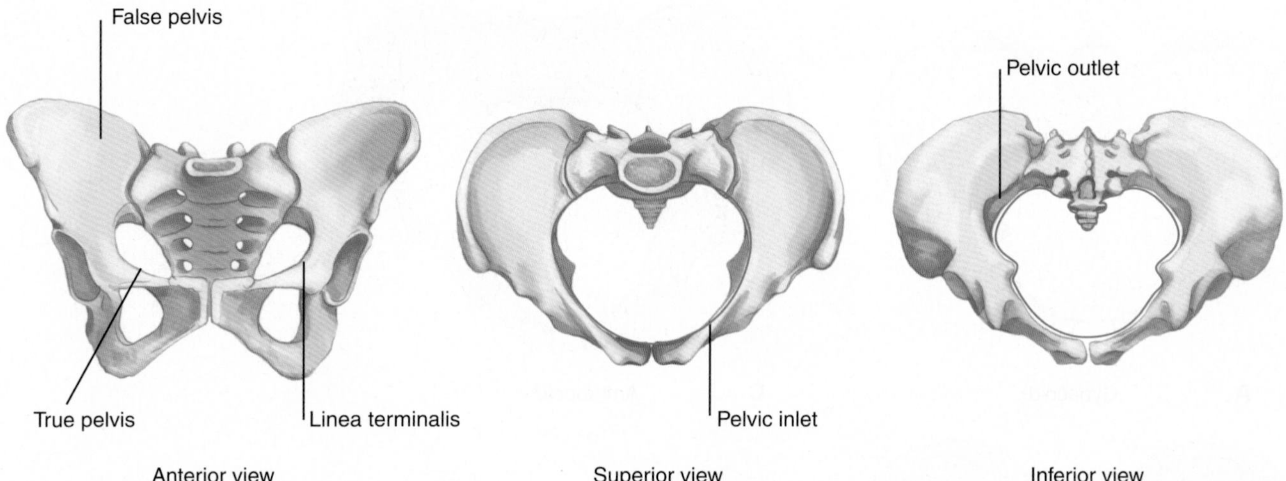

FIGURE 13.1 The bony pelvis.

Bony Pelvis

The maternal bony pelvis can be divided into the true and false portions. The false (or greater) pelvis is composed of the upper flared parts of the two iliac bones with their concavities and the wings of the base of the sacrum. The false pelvis is divided from the true pelvis by an imaginary line drawn from the sacral prominence at the back to the superior aspect of the symphysis pubis at the front of the pelvis. This imaginary line is called the linea terminalis. The false pelvis lies above this imaginary line; the true pelvis lies below it (Fig. 13.1). The true pelvis is the bony passageway through which the fetus must travel. It is made up of three planes: the inlet, the mid-pelvis (cavity), and the outlet.

PELVIC INLET

The pelvic inlet allows entrance to the true pelvis. It is bounded by the sacral prominence in the back, the ilium on the sides, and the superior aspect of the symphysis pubis in the front (Jones & Lopez, 2014). The pelvic inlet is wider in the transverse aspect (sideways) than it is from front to back.

MID-PELVIS

The mid-pelvis (cavity) occupies the space between the inlet and outlet. It is through this snug, curved space that the fetus must travel to reach the outside. As the fetus passes through this small area its chest is compressed, causing lung fluid and mucus to be expelled. This expulsion removes the space-occupying fluid so that air can enter the lungs with the newborn's first breath.

PELVIC OUTLET

The pelvic outlet is bound by the ischial tuberosities, the lower rim of the symphysis pubis, and the tip of the coccyx. In comparison with the pelvic inlet, the outlet is wider from front to back. For the fetus to pass through the pelvis, the outlet must be large enough. To ensure the adequacy of the pelvic outlet for vaginal birth, the following pelvic measurements are assessed:

- Diagonal conjugate of the inlet (distance between the anterior surface of the sacral prominence and the anterior surface of the inferior margin of the symphysis pubis)
- Transverse or ischial tuberosity diameter of the outlet (distance at the medial and lowest aspect of the ischial tuberosities, at the level of the anus; a known hand span or clenched-fist measurement is generally used to obtain this measurement)
- True or obstetric conjugate (distance estimated from the measurement of the diagonal conjugate; 1.5 cm is subtracted from the diagonal conjugate measurement)

For more information about pelvic measurements, see Chapter 12.

If the diagonal conjugate measures at least 11.5 cm and the true or obstetric conjugate measures 10 cm or more (1.5 cm less than the diagonal conjugate, or about 10 cm), then the pelvis is large enough for a vaginal birth of what would be considered a normal-size newborn.

Pelvic Shape

In addition to size, the shape of a woman's pelvis is a determining factor for a vaginal birth. Each plane of the pelvis has a shape, which is defined by the anterior-posterior and transverse diameters. The pelvis is divided into four main shapes: gynecoid, anthropoid, android, and platypelloid (Fig. 13.2).

GYNECOID PELVIS

The gynecoid pelvis is considered the true female pelvis, occurring in about 40% of all women; it is less common

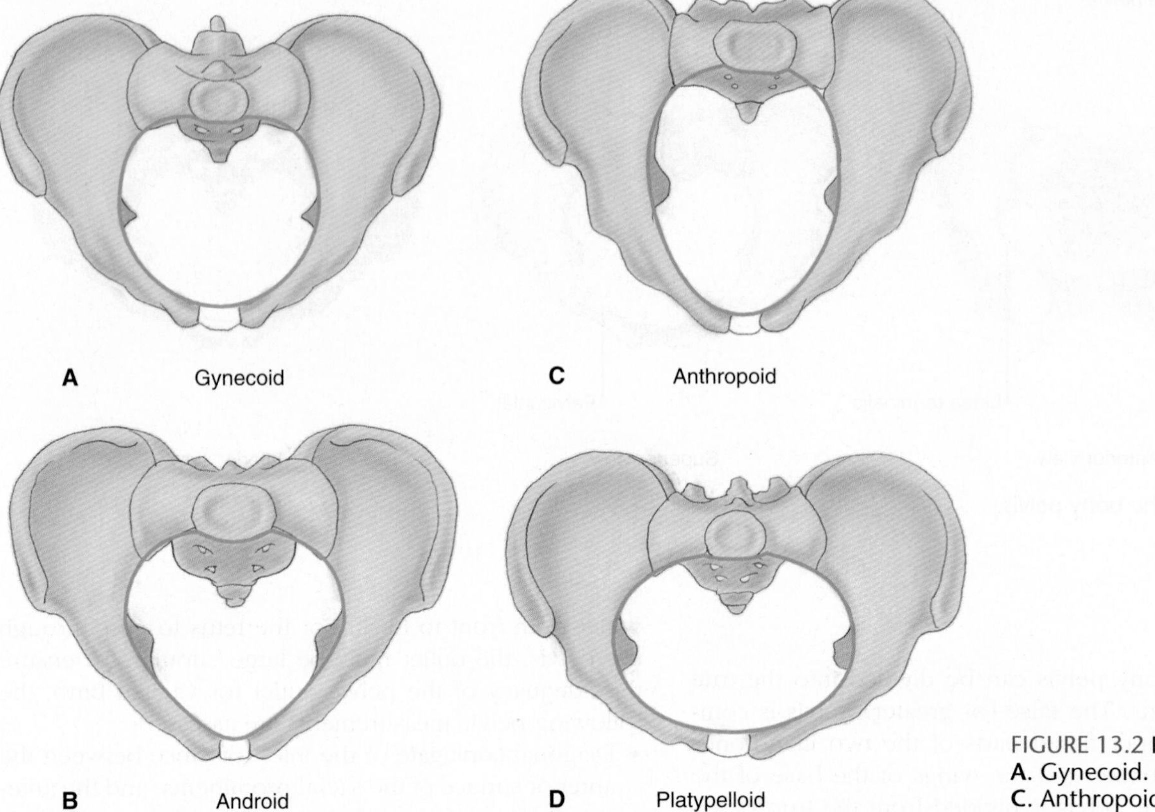

FIGURE 13.2 Pelvic shapes. **A**. Gynecoid. **B**. Android. **C**. Anthropoid. **D**. Platypelloid.

in men (Fischer & Mitteroecker, 2015). Vaginal birth is most favorable with this type of pelvis because the inlet is round and the outlet is roomy. This shape offers the optimal diameters in all three planes of the pelvis. This type of pelvis allows early and complete fetal internal rotation during labor.

ANTHROPOID PELVIS

The anthropoid pelvis is common in men and is most common in non-White women. It occurs in approximately 25% of women (Marani & Koch, 2014). The pelvic inlet is oval and the sacrum is long, producing a deep pelvis (wider front to back [anterior to posterior] than side to side [transverse]). Vaginal birth is more favorable with this pelvic shape compared with the android or platypelloid shape (Tharpe, Farley, & Jordan, 2016).

ANDROID PELVIS

The android pelvis is considered the male-shaped pelvis and is characterized by a funnel shape. It occurs in approximately 20% of women (Cunningham et al., 2014). The pelvic inlet is heart-shaped and the posterior segments are reduced in all pelvic planes. Descent of the fetal head into the pelvis is slow, and failure of the fetus to rotate is common. The prognosis for labor is poor, subsequently leading to cesarean birth.

PLATYPELLOID (FLAT) PELVIS

The platypelloid or flat pelvis is the least common type of pelvic structure among men and women, with an approximate incidence of 3% (King, et al., 2015). The pelvic cavity is shallow but widens at the pelvic outlet, making it difficult for the fetus to descend through the mid-pelvis. Labor prognosis is poor with arrest at the inlet occurring frequently. It is not favorable for a vaginal birth unless the fetal head can pass through the inlet. Women with this type of pelvis usually require cesarean birth.

An important principle is that most pelvises are not purely defined but occur in nature as mixed types. Many women have a combination of these four basic pelvis types, with no two pelves being exactly the same. Regardless of the shape, the newborn can be born vaginally if size and positioning remain compatible. The narrowest part of the fetus attempts to align itself with the narrowest pelvic dimension (e.g., biparietal to interspinous diameters, which means the fetus generally tends to rotate to the most ample portion of the pelvis).

Soft Tissues

The soft tissues of the passageway consist of the cervix, the pelvic floor muscles, and the vagina. Through effacement, the cervix effaces (thins) to allow the presenting fetal part to descend into the vagina.

Take Note!

The process of cervical effacement and dilation is similar to that of pulling a turtleneck sweater over your head.

The pelvic floor muscles help the fetus to rotate anteriorly as it passes through the birth canal. The soft tissues of the vagina expand to accommodate the fetus during birth.

Passenger

The fetus (with placenta) is the passenger. The fetal head (size and presence of **molding**), fetal **attitude** (degree of body flexion), fetal lie (relationship of body parts), fetal **presentation** (first body part), fetal position (relationship to maternal pelvis), fetal station, and fetal engagement are all important factors that have an impact on the ultimate outcome in the birthing process.

Fetal Head

The fetal head is the largest fetal structure, making it an important factor in relation to labor and birth. Considerable variation in the size and diameter of the fetal skull is often seen.

Compared with an adult's head, the fetal head is large in proportion to the rest of the body, usually about one quarter of the body surface area (Martin, Fanaroff, & Walsh, 2014). The bones that make up the face and cranial base are fused and essentially fixed. However, the five bones that make up the rest of the cranium (two frontal bones, two parietal bones, and the occipital bone) are not fused; rather, they are soft and pliable, with gaps between the plates of bone. These gaps, membranous spaces between the cranial bones, are called sutures, and the intersections of these sutures are called fontanelles. Sutures are important because they allow the cranial bones to overlap in order for the head to adjust in shape (elongate) when pressure is exerted on it by uterine contractions or the maternal bony pelvis. Some diameters shorten, whereas others lengthen as the head is molded during the labor and birthing process. This malleability of the fetal skull may decrease fetal skull dimensions by 0.5 to 1 cm (King, et al., 2015). After birth, the sutures close as the bones grow and the brain reaches its full growth.

The changed (elongated) shape of the fetal skull at birth as a result of overlapping of the cranial bones is known as molding. Along with molding, fluid can also collect in the scalp (caput succedaneum) or blood can collect beneath the scalp (cephalohematoma), further distorting the shape and appearance of the fetal head. Caput succedaneum can be described as edema of the scalp at the presenting part. This swelling crosses suture lines and disappears within 3 to 4 days. Cephalohematoma is a

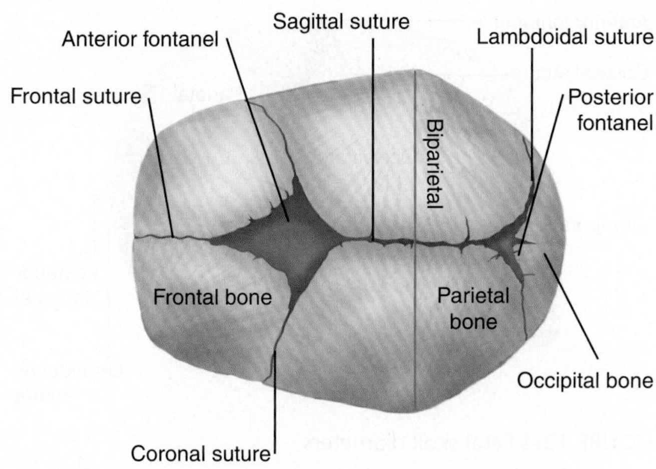

FIGURE 13.3 Fetal skull.

collection of blood between the periosteum and the bone that occurs several hours after birth. It does not cross suture lines and is generally reabsorbed over the next 6 to 8 weeks (Collins & Reed, 2014).

Take Note!

Parents may become concerned about the distortion of their newborn's head. However, reassurance that the oblong shape is only temporary is usually all that is needed to reduce their anxiety.

Sutures also play a role in helping to identify the position of the fetal head during a vaginal examination. Figure 13.3 shows a fetal skull. During a pelvic examination, palpation of these sutures by the examiner reveals the position of the fetal head and the degree of rotation that has occurred.

The anterior and posterior fontanelles are also useful in helping to identify the position of the fetal head. They allow for molding, and are important when evaluating the newborn. The anterior fontanelle is the famous "soft spot" of the newborn's head. It is a diamond-shaped space that measures from 1 to 4 cm. It remains open for 12 to 18 months after birth to allow for growth of the brain (Verklan & Walden, 2014). The posterior fontanelle corresponds to the anterior one but is located at the back of the fetal head; it is triangular. This one closes within 8 to 12 weeks after birth and measures, on average, 1 to 2 cm at its widest diameter (Weber & Kelley, 2014).

The diameter of the fetal skull is an important consideration during the labor and birth process. Fetal skull diameters are measured between the various landmarks of the skull. Diameters include occipitofrontal, occipitomental, suboccipitobregmatic, and biparietal (Fig. 13.4). The two most important diameters that can affect the birth process are the suboccipitobregmatic (approximately 9.5 cm at term) and the biparietal (approximately 9.25 cm at term) diameters. The suboccipitobregmatic diameter, measured from the base of the occiput to the

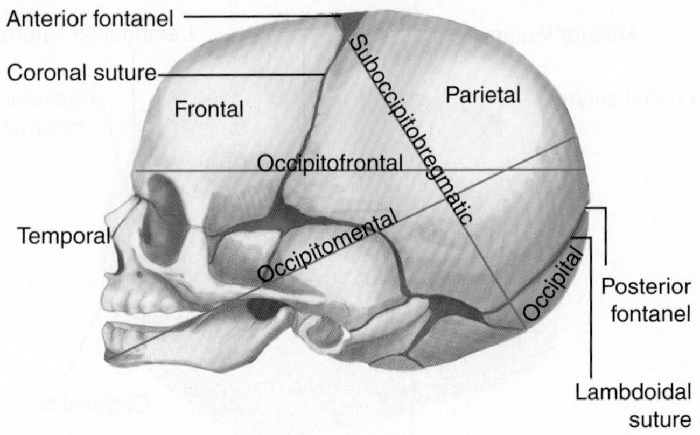

FIGURE 13.4 Fetal skull diameters.

center of the anterior fontanelle, identifies the smallest anteroposterior diameter of the fetal skull. The biparietal diameter measures the largest transverse diameter of the fetal skull: the distance between the two parietal bones. In a cephalic (head first) presentation, which occurs in 95% of all term births, if the fetus presents in a flexed position in which the chin is resting on the chest, the optimal or smallest fetal skull dimensions for a vaginal birth are demonstrated. If the fetal head is not fully flexed at birth, the anteroposterior diameter increases. This increase in dimension might prevent the fetal skull from entering the maternal pelvis.

Fetal Attitude

Fetal attitude is another important consideration related to the passenger. Fetal attitude refers to the posturing (flexion or extension) of the joints and the relationship of fetal parts to one another. The most common fetal attitude when labor begins is with all joints flexed—the fetal back is rounded, the chin is on the chest, the thighs are flexed on the abdomen, and the legs are flexed at the knees (Fig. 13.5). This normal fetal position is most favorable for vaginal birth, presenting the smallest fetal skull diameters to the pelvis.

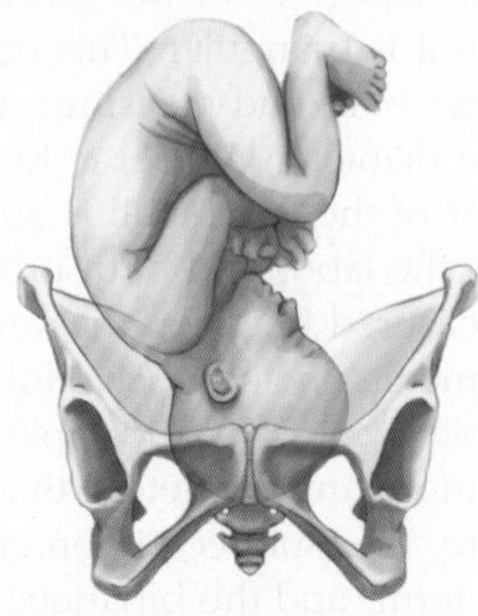

FIGURE 13.5 Fetal attitude: full flexion. Note that the smallest diameter presents to the pelvis.

When the fetus presents to the pelvis with abnormal attitudes (no flexion or extension), their nonflexed position can increase the diameter of the presenting part as it passes through the pelvis, increasing the difficulty of birth. An attitude of extension tends to present larger fetal skull diameters, which may make birth difficult.

Fetal Lie

Fetal **lie** refers to the relationship of the long axis (spine) of the fetus to the long axis (spine) of the mother. There are three possible lies: longitudinal (which is the most common), transverse (Fig. 13.6), and oblique.

A longitudinal lie occurs when the long axis of the fetus is parallel to that of the mother (fetal spine to maternal spine side-by-side). A transverse lie occurs when the long axis of the fetus is perpendicular to the long axis of the mother (fetal spine lies across the maternal abdomen and crosses her spine). In an oblique lie, the fetal long axis is at an angle to the bony inlet, and no palpable fetal part is presenting. This lie is usually transitory and occurs during fetal conversion between other lies. A fetus in a transverse or oblique lie position cannot be delivered vaginally (Cunningham, et al., 2014).

Fetal Presentation

Fetal presentation refers to the body part of the fetus that enters the pelvic inlet first (the "presenting part"). This is the fetal part that lies over the inlet of the pelvis or the cervical os. Knowing which fetal part is coming first

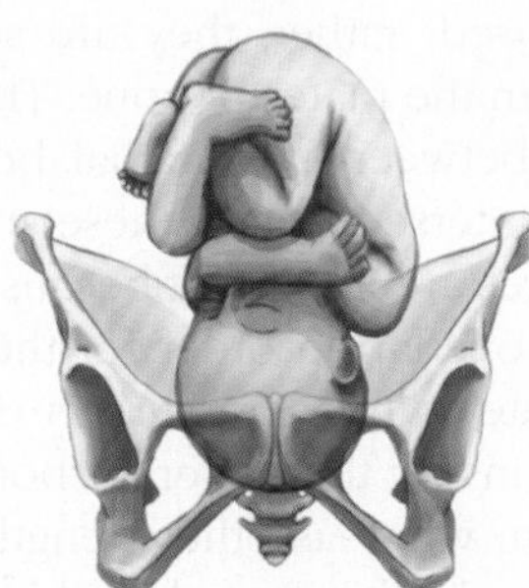

A. Longitudinal lie

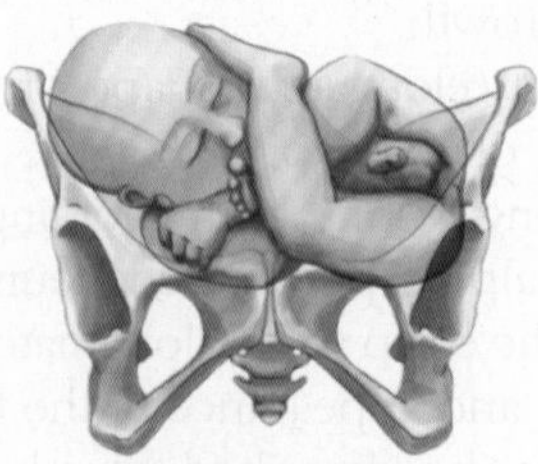

B. Transverse lie

FIGURE 13.6 Fetal lie.

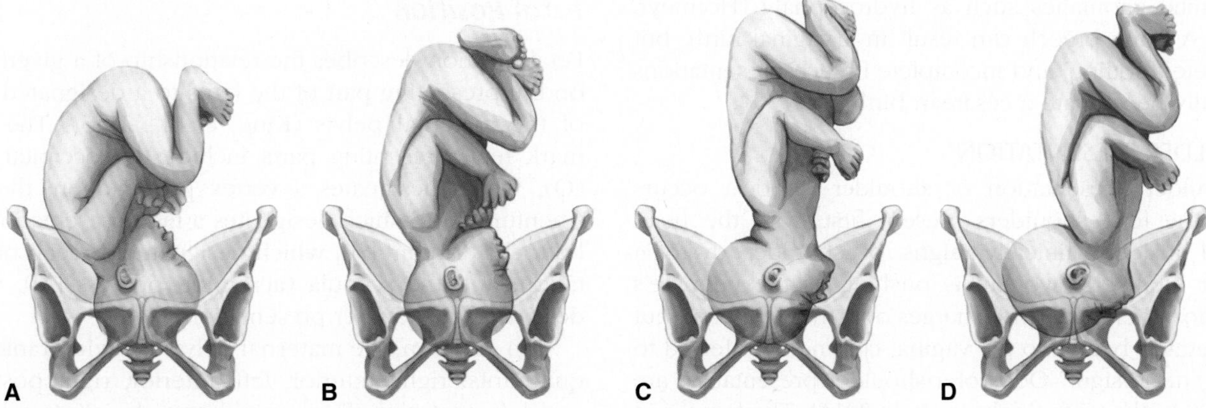

FIGURE 13.7 Fetal presentation: cephalic presentations. **A.** Vertex. **B.** Military. **C.** Brow. **D.** Face.

at birth is critical for planning and initiating appropriate interventions.

The three main fetal presentations are cephalic (head first), breech (pelvis first), and shoulder (scapula first). The majority of term newborns (95%) enter this world in a cephalic presentation; breech presentations account for 3% of term births, and shoulder presentations for approximately 2% (Tharpe et al., 2016).

In a cephalic presentation, the presenting part is usually the occipital portion of the fetal head (Fig. 13.7). This presentation is also referred to as a vertex presentation. Variations in a vertex presentation include the military, brow, and facial presentations.

BREECH PRESENTATION

By term, approximately 97% of infants actively turn to a cephalic presentation. It is determined by abdominal palpation (Hofmeyr, 2015). Breech presentation occurs when the fetal buttocks or feet enter the maternal pelvis first and the fetal skull enters last. This abnormal presentation poses several challenges at birth. Primarily, the largest part of the fetus (skull) is born last and may become "hung up" or stuck in the pelvis. In addition, the umbilical cord can become compressed between the fetal skull and the maternal pelvis after the fetal chest is born because the head is the last to exit. Moreover, unlike the hard fetal skull, the buttocks are soft and are not as effective as a cervical dilator during labor compared with a cephalic presentation. Finally, there is the possibility of trauma to the head as a result of the lack of opportunity for molding.

The types of breech presentations are determined by the positioning of the fetal legs (Fig. 13.8). In a frank breech (50% to 70%), the buttocks present first with both legs extended up toward the face. In a full or complete breech (5% to 10%), the fetus sits crossed-legged above the cervix. In a footling or incomplete breech (10% to 30%), one or both legs are presenting. Breech presentations are associated with prematurity, placenta previa, multiparity, uterine abnormalities (fibroids), and some

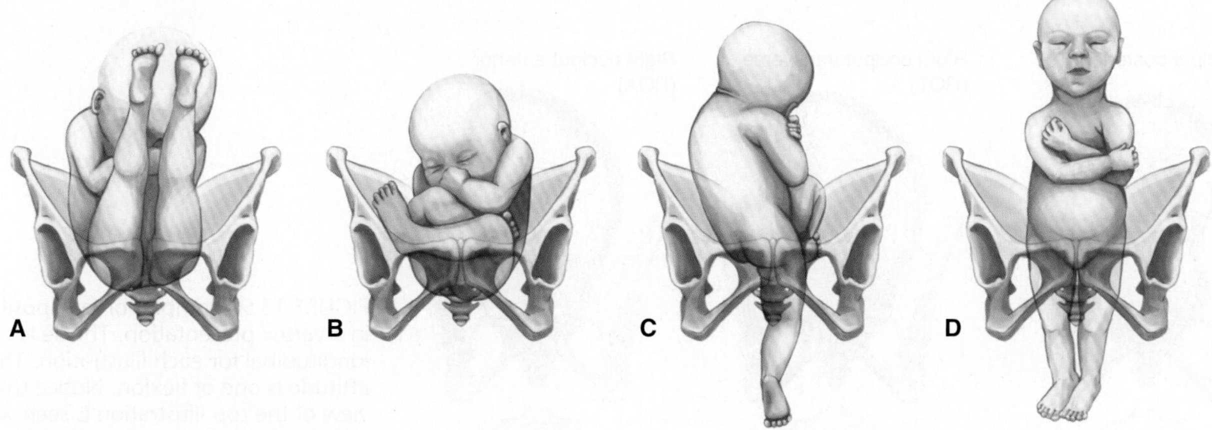

FIGURE 13.8 Breech presentations. **A.** Frank breech. **B.** Complete breech. **C.** Single footling breech. **D.** Double footling breech.

congenital anomalies such as hydrocephaly (Hofmeyr, 2015). A frank breech can result in a vaginal birth, but complete, footling, and incomplete breech presentations generally necessitate a cesarean birth.

SHOULDER PRESENTATION

A shoulder presentation or shoulder dystocia occurs when the fetal shoulders present first, with the head tucked inside. Clinically, signs of shoulder dystocia appear while the woman is pushing as the neonate's head slowly extends and emerges over the perineum, but then retracts back into the vagina, commonly referred to as the "turtle sign." Odds of a shoulder presentation are 1 in 300 births (Cunningham et al., 2014). The fetus is in a transverse lie with the shoulder as the presenting part. Conditions associated with shoulder dystocia include placenta previa, prematurity, high parity, premature rupture of membranes, multiple gestation, or fetal anomalies. A cesarean birth is usually necessary if identified before labor begins, but will be evaluated based on the length of gestation, the size of the fetus, the position of the placenta, and whether the membranes have ruptured (Sharshiner & Silver, 2015).

Fetal Position

Fetal position describes the relationship of a given point on the presenting part of the fetus to a designated point of the maternal pelvis (King, et al., 2015). The landmark fetal presenting parts include the occipital bone (O), which designates a vertex presentation; the chin (mentum [M]), which designates a face presentation; the buttocks (sacrum [S]), which designate a breech presentation; and the scapula (acromion process [A]), which designates a shoulder presentation.

In addition, the maternal pelvis is divided into four quadrants: right anterior, left anterior, right posterior, and left posterior. These quadrants designate whether the presenting part is directed toward the front, back, left, or right side of the pelvis. Fetal position is determined by identifying first the presenting part and then the maternal quadrant the presenting part is facing (Fig. 13.9). Position is indicated by a three-letter abbreviation as follows:

- The first letter defines whether the presenting part is tilted toward the left (L) or the right (R) side of the maternal pelvis.

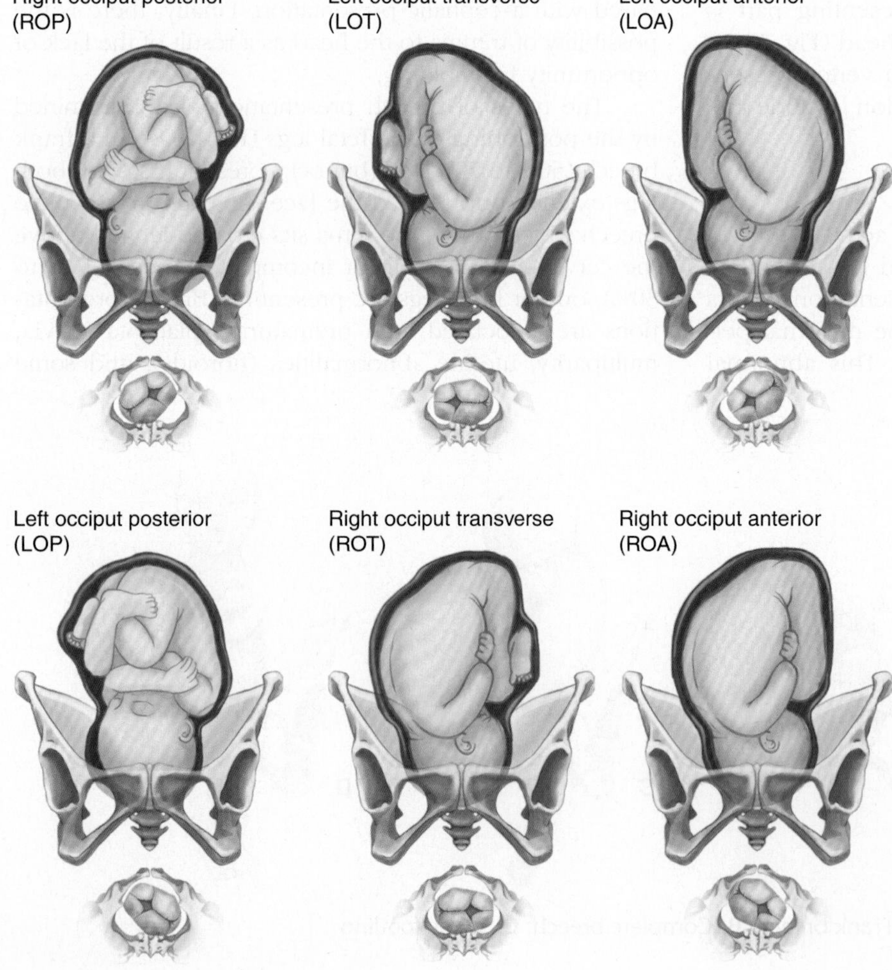

FIGURE 13.9 Examples of fetal positions in a vertex presentation. The lie is longitudinal for each illustration. The attitude is one of flexion. Notice that the view of the top illustration is seen when facing the pregnant woman. The bottom view is that seen with the woman in a dorsal recumbent position.

- The second letter represents the particular presenting part of the fetus: O for occiput, S for sacrum (buttocks), M for mentum (chin), A for acromion process, and D for dorsal (refers to the fetal back) when denoting the fetal position in shoulder presentations (Cheng & Caughey, 2015a).
- The third letter defines the location of the presenting part in relation to the anterior (A) portion of the maternal pelvis or the posterior (P) portion of the maternal pelvis. If the presenting part is directed to the side of the maternal pelvis, the fetal presentation is designated as transverse (T).

For example, if the occiput is facing the left anterior quadrant of the pelvis, then the position is termed left occiput anterior and is recorded as LOA.

Take Note!

LOA is the most common (and most favorable) fetal position for birthing today, followed by right occiput anterior (ROA). The positioning of the fetus allows the fetal head to contour to the diameters of the maternal pelvis. LOA and ROA are optimal positions for a vaginal birth.

An occiput posterior position may lead to a long and difficult birth, and other positions may or may not be compatible with vaginal birth.

Fetal Station

Fetal **station** refers to the relationship of the presenting part to the level of the maternal pelvic ischial spines. Fetal station is measured in centimeters and is referred to as a minus or plus, depending on its location above or below the ischial spines. Typically, the ischial spines are the narrowest part of the pelvis and are the natural measuring point for the birth progress.

Zero (0) station is designated when the presenting part is at the level of the maternal ischial spines. When the presenting part is above the ischial spines, the distance is recorded as minus stations. When the presenting part is below the ischial spines, the distance is recorded as plus stations. For instance, if the presenting part is above the ischial spines by 1 cm, it is documented as being a –1 station; if the presenting part is below the ischial spines by 1 cm, it is documented as being a +1 station.

An easy way to understand this concept is to think in terms of meeting the goal, which is the birth. If the fetus is descending downward (past the ischial spines) and moving toward meeting the goal of birth, then the station is positive and the centimeter numbers grow bigger from +1 to +4. If the fetus is not descending past the ischial spines, then the station is negative and the centimeter numbers grow bigger from –1 to –4. The farther away the presenting part from the outside, the larger the negative number (–4 cm). The closer the presenting part of the fetus is to the outside, the larger the positive number (+4 cm). Figure 13.10 shows stations of the presenting part.

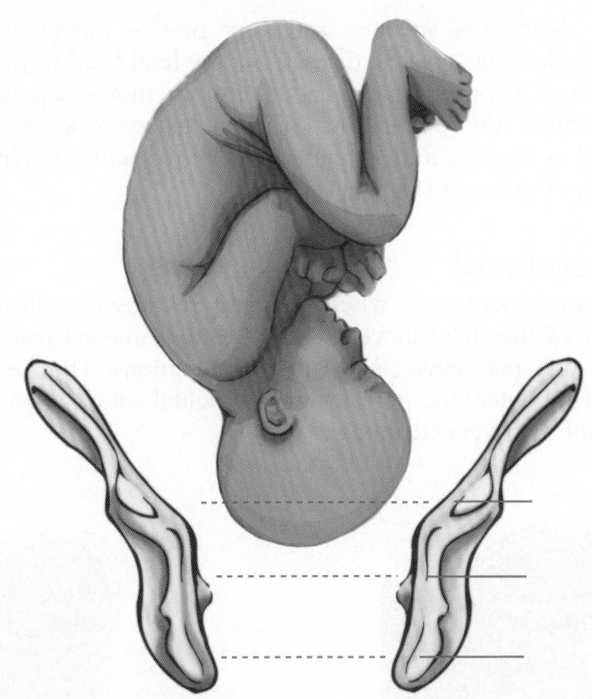

FIGURE 13.10 Fetal stations.

Fetal Engagement

Fetal engagement signifies the entrance of the largest diameter of the fetal presenting part (usually the fetal head) into the smallest diameter of the maternal pelvis (Alexander, et al., 2014). The fetus is said to be engaged in the pelvis when the presenting part reaches 0 station. Engagement is determined by pelvic examination.

The largest diameter of the fetal head is the biparietal diameter. It extends from one parietal prominence to the other. It is an important factor in the navigation through the maternal pelvis. Engagement typically occurs in primigravidas 2 weeks before term, whereas multiparas may experience engagement several weeks before the onset of labor or not until labor begins.

Take Note!

The term floating is used when engagement has not occurred, because the presenting part is freely movable above the pelvic inlet.

Cardinal Movements of Labor

The fetus goes through many positional changes as it travels through the passageway. These positional changes are known as the cardinal movements of labor. They are deliberate, specific, and very precise movements that allow the smallest diameter of the fetal head to pass through a corresponding diameter of the mother's pelvic structure. Although cardinal movements are conceptualized as separate and sequential, the movements are typically concurrent (Fig. 13.11).

ENGAGEMENT

Engagement occurs when the greatest transverse diameter of the head in vertex (biparietal diameter) passes through the pelvic inlet (usually 0 station). The head usually enters the pelvis with the sagittal suture aligned in the transverse diameter.

DESCENT

Descent is the downward movement of the fetal head until it is within the pelvic inlet. Descent occurs intermittently with contractions and is brought about by one or more of the following forces:

- Pressure of the amniotic fluid
- Direct pressure of the fundus on the fetus's buttocks or head (depending on which part is located in the top of the uterus)
- Contractions of the abdominal muscles (second stage)
- Extension and straightening of the fetal body

Descent occurs throughout labor, ending with birth. During this time, the mother experiences discomfort, but

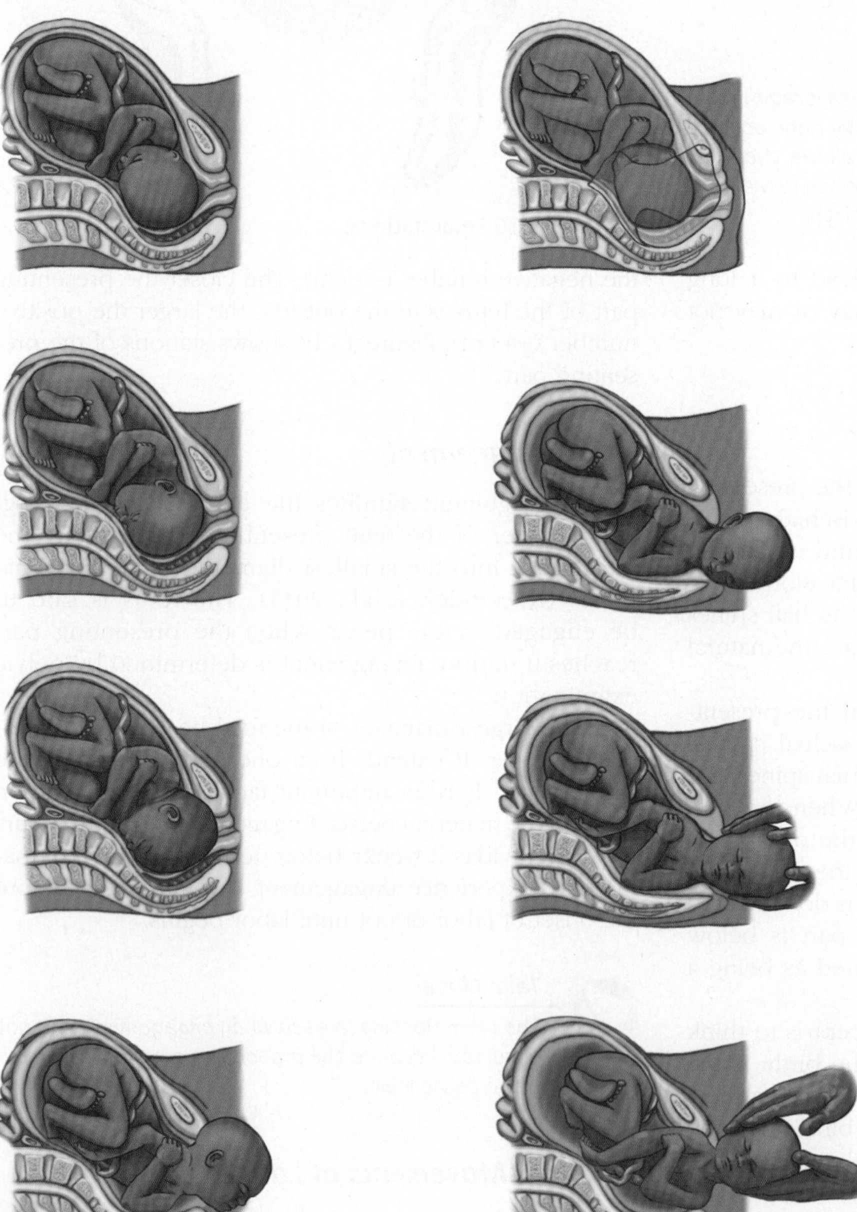

FIGURE 13.11 Cardinal movements of labor.

she is unable to isolate this particular fetal movement from her overall discomfort.

FLEXION

Flexion occurs as the vertex meets resistance from the cervix, the walls of the pelvis, or the pelvic floor. As a result, the chin is brought into contact with the fetal thorax and the presenting diameter is changed from occipitofrontal to suboccipitobregmatic (9.5 cm), which achieves the smallest fetal skull diameter presenting to the maternal pelvic dimensions.

INTERNAL ROTATION

After engagement, as the head descends, the lower portion of the head (usually the occiput) meets resistance from one side of the pelvic floor. As a result, the head rotates about 45 degrees anteriorly to the midline under the symphysis. This movement is known as *internal rotation*. Internal rotation brings the anteroposterior diameter of the head in line with the anteroposterior diameter of the pelvic outlet. It aligns the long axis of the fetal head with the long axis of the maternal pelvis. The widest portion of the maternal pelvis is the anteroposterior diameter, and thus the fetus must rotate to accommodate the pelvis.

EXTENSION

With further descent and full flexion of the head, the nucha (the base of the occiput) becomes impinged under the symphysis. Resistance from the pelvic floor causes the fetal head to extend so that it can pass under the pubic arch. *Extension* occurs after internal rotation is complete. The head emerges through extension under the symphysis pubis along with the shoulders. The anterior fontanel, brow, nose, mouth, and chin are born successively.

EXTERNAL ROTATION (RESTITUTION)

After the head is born and is free of resistance, it untwists, causing the occiput to move about 45 degrees back to its original left or right position (restitution). The sagittal suture has now resumed its normal right-angle relationship to the transverse (bisacromial) diameter of the shoulders (i.e., the head realigns with the position of the back in the birth canal). *External rotation* of the fetal head allows the shoulders to rotate internally to fit the maternal pelvis.

EXPULSION

Expulsion of the rest of the body occurs more smoothly after the birth of the head and the anterior and posterior shoulders (Cheng & Caughey, 2015a). See Figure 13.3 for an image of a fetal skull.

Powers

The primary stimulus powering labor is uterine contraction. Contractions cause complete dilation and effacement of the cervix during the first stage of labor. The secondary powers in labor involve the use of intra-abdominal pressure (voluntary muscle contractions) exerted by the woman as she pushes and bears down during the second stage of labor.

Uterine Contractions

Uterine contractions are involuntary and therefore cannot be controlled by the woman experiencing them, regardless of whether they are spontaneous or induced. Uterine contractions are rhythmic and intermittent, with a period of relaxation between contractions. This pause allows the woman and the uterine muscles to rest. In addition, this pause restores blood flow to the uterus and placenta, which is temporarily reduced during each uterine contraction.

Uterine contractions are responsible for thinning and dilating the cervix, then thrusting the presenting part toward the lower uterine segment. The cervical canal reduces in length from 2 cm to a paper-thin entity and is described in terms of percentages from 0% to 100%. In primigravidas, effacement typically starts before the onset of labor and usually begins before dilation; in multiparas, however, neither effacement nor dilation may start until labor ensues (Fig. 13.12). On clinical examination the following may be assessed:

- Cervical canal 2 cm in length would be described as 0% effaced.

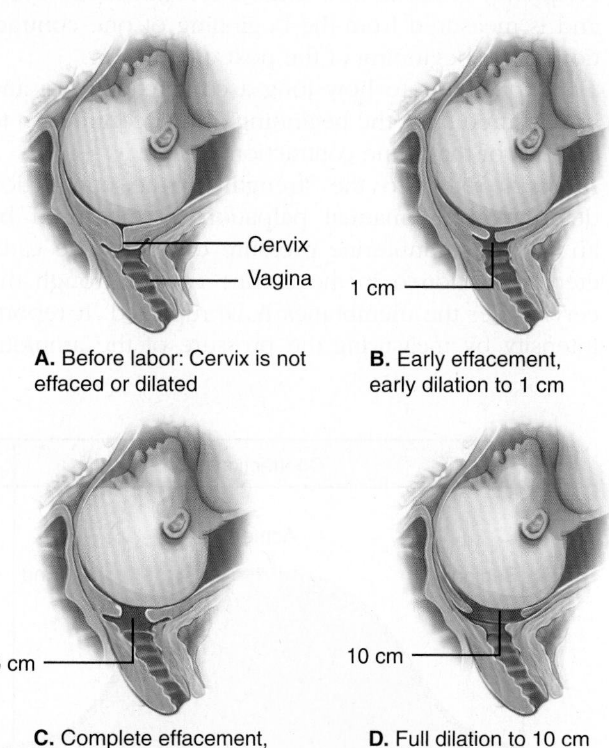

FIGURE 13.12 Cervical effacement and dilation. Cervical dilation is expressed in centimeters. **A.** Shows cervix not effaced or dilated. **B.** 50% effaced. **C.** 100% effaced. **D.** Fully dilated at 10 centimeters.

- Cervical canal 1 cm in length would be described as 50% effaced.
- Cervical canal 0 cm in length would be described as 100% effaced.

Dilation is dependent on the pressure of the presenting part and the contraction and retraction of the uterus. The diameter of the cervical os increases from less than 1 cm to approximately 10 cm to allow for birth. When the cervix is fully dilated, it is no longer palpable on vaginal examination. Descriptions may include the following:

- External cervical os closed: 0 cm dilated
- External cervical os half open: 5 cm dilated
- External cervical os fully open: 10 cm dilated

During early labor, uterine contractions are described as mild, they last about 30 seconds, and they occur about every 5 to 7 minutes. As labor progresses, contractions last longer (60 seconds), occur more frequently (2 to 3 minutes apart), and are described as being moderate to high in intensity. Each contraction has three phases: increment (buildup of the contraction), acme (peak or highest intensity), and decrement (descent or relaxation of the uterine muscle fibers; Fig. 13.13).

Uterine contractions are monitored and assessed according to three parameters: frequency, duration, and intensity.

1. *Frequency* refers to how often the contractions occur and is measured from the beginning of one contraction to the beginning of the next contraction.
2. *Duration* refers to how long a contraction lasts and is measured from the beginning of one contraction to the end of that same contraction.
3. *Intensity* refers to the strength of the contraction determined by manual palpation or measured by an internal intrauterine pressure catheter. The catheter is positioned in the uterine cavity through the cervix after the membranes have ruptured. It reports intensity by measuring the pressure of the amniotic fluid inside the uterus in millimeters of mercury. It is not recommended for routine use in low-risk laboring women due to the potential risk of infection and injury to the placenta or fetus. In a recent meta-analysis involving >2,000 laboring women, the researchers found an increase in surgical births and no advantages of using internal intrauterine pressure catheters over external monitoring during labor augmentation (Milton, Chelmow, & Ramus, 2015).

Intra-Abdominal Pressure

Increased intra-abdominal pressure (voluntary muscle contractions) compresses the uterus and adds to the power of the expulsion forces of the uterine contractions (Grant, Strevans, & Thornton, 2015). Coordination of these forces in unison promotes birth of the fetus and expulsion of the fetal membranes and placenta from the uterus. Interference with these forces (such as when a woman is highly sedated or extremely anxious) can compromise the effectiveness of these powers.

Position (Maternal)

Positioning for normal labor and birth has evolved. Until about 250 years ago, women were depicted in art and described in essays as sitting upright with flexed hips, squatting, or less commonly standing or kneeling during the childbirth process. These positions maintain flexion at the hip joint and somewhat straighten the pelvis (Nieuwenhuijze, et al., 2014). In the past 250 years, dorsal and dorsal lithotomy positions evolved for unclear reasons and have been ascribed to Western medicine. Childbirth medicalization has reduced laboring women's opportunity for a spontaneous position of choice to a recumbent one. Medical historians say the evolution was to facilitate forceps usage, to promote men's power over women, and for convenience after administration of anesthesia (Marani & Koch, 2014).

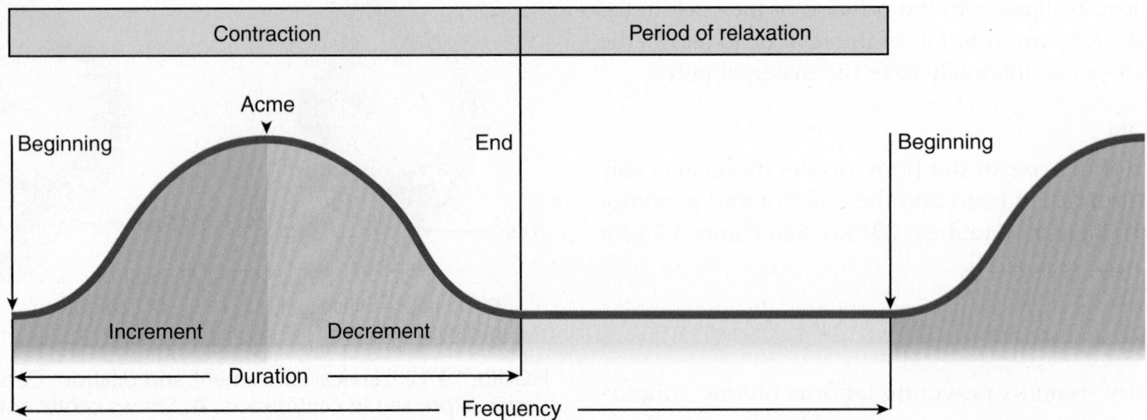

FIGURE 13.13 The three phases of a uterine contraction.

Maternal positioning during labor has only recently been the subject of well-controlled research. Scientific evidence has shown that nonmoving, back-lying positions during labor are not healthy (Gizzo, et al., 2014). However, despite this evidence to the contrary, many women continue to lie flat on their backs during labor. Some of the reasons why this practice continues include the beliefs that:

- laboring women need to conserve their energy and not tire themselves
- nurses cannot keep track of the whereabouts of ambulating women
- it is the preference of the health care provider
- the fetus can be monitored better in this position
- the supine position facilitates vaginal examinations and external belt adjustment
- a bed is "where one is supposed to be" in a hospital setting
- the position is more convenient for the delivering health care provider
- laboring women are "connected to things" that impede movement (Hanson & VandeVusse, 2014).

Although many labor and birthing facilities claim that all women are allowed to adopt any position of comfort during their laboring experience, many women spend their time on their backs during labor and birth. Women should be encouraged to assume any position of comfort for them. In a recent randomized, controlled study, the use of a peanut-shaped ball during labor decreased the length of labor and increased the rate of vaginal births. The peanut ball was associated with a significantly lower incidence of cesarean births. The peanut ball can be a potentially successful nursing intervention to help progress labor and support vaginal birth for women laboring under epidural analgesia (Tussey, et al., 2015).

Take Note!

If the only furniture provided is a bed, this is what the woman will use. Furnishing rooms with comfortable chairs, beanbags, and other birth props allows a woman to choose from a variety of positions and to be free to move during labor.

Changing positions and moving around during labor and birth offer several benefits. Maternal position can influence pelvic size and contours. Changing position and walking affect the pelvis joints, which may facilitate fetal descent and rotation. Squatting enlarges the pelvic inlet and outlet diameters, whereas a kneeling position removes pressure on the maternal vena cava and helps to rotate the fetus from a posterior position to an anterior one to facilitate birth (Budin, 2015). The use of any upright or lateral position, compared with supine or lithotomy positions, may:

- Reduce the length of the first stage of labor
- Reduce the duration of the second stage of labor
- Reduce the number of assisted deliveries (vacuum and forceps)
- Reduce episiotomies and perineal tears
- Contribute to fewer abnormal fetal heart rate patterns
- Increase comfort/reduce requests for pain medication
- Enhance a sense of control by the mother
- Alter the shape and size of the pelvis, which assists in descent
- Assist gravity to move the fetus downward (Cox & King, 2015).

Using the research available can bring better outcomes, heightened professionalism, and evidence-based practice to childbearing practices. The National Institute for Health and Care Excellence [NICE] guidelines recommend discouraging women from lying supine or semi-supine during labor and encourage them to adapt to any other position that they find comfortable since lying on their backs is associated with longer labors, increase in surgical births, increased pain, and a higher incidence of FHR abnormalities. The Cochrane collaboration supports the current NICE guidance of positions (Camorcia, 2015).

Psychological Response

Childbearing can be one of the most life-altering experiences for a woman. The experience of childbirth goes beyond the physiologic aspects: it influences a woman's self-confidence, self-esteem, and view of life, relationships, and children. Her state of mind (psyche) throughout the entire process is critical to bringing about a positive outcome for her and her family. Factors promoting a positive birth experience include:

- Clear information about procedures
- Support, not being alone
- Sense of mastery, self-confidence
- Trust in staff caring for her
- Positive reaction to the pregnancy
- Personal control over breathing
- Preparation for the childbirth experience.

Having a strong sense of self and meaningful support from others can often help women manage labor well. Feeling safe and secure typically promotes a sense of control and ability to withstand the challenges of the childbearing experience. Anxiety and fear, however, decrease a woman's ability to cope with the discomfort of labor. Maternal catecholamines secreted in response to anxiety and fear can inhibit uterine blood flow and placental perfusion. In contrast, relaxation can augment the natural process of labor (Leonard, 2015). Preparing mentally for childbirth is important so that the woman can work with, rather than against, the natural forces of labor.

Philosophy

Not everyone views childbirth in the same way. A philosophical continuum exists that extends from viewing labor as a disease process to a normal process. One philosophy assumes that women cannot manage the birth experience adequately and therefore need constant expert monitoring and management. The other philosophy assumes that women are capable, reasoning individuals who can actively participate in their birth experience.

The health care system in the United States today appears to be leaning toward the former philosophy, applying technological interventions to most mothers who enter the hospital system. Giving birth in a hospital in the 21st century for many women has become "intervention intensive"—designed to start, continue, and end labor through medical management rather than allowing the normal process of birth to unfold. Advances in medical care have improved the safety for women with high-risk pregnancies. However, the routine use of intravenous therapy, electronic fetal monitoring, augmentation, and epidural anesthesia has not necessarily improved birth outcomes for all women (Leonard, 2015). Perhaps a middle-of-the-road philosophy for intervening when circumstances dictate, along with weighing the risks and benefits before doing so, may be appropriate.

During the 1970s, family-centered maternity care was developed in response to the consumer reaction to the depersonalization of birth. The hope was to shift the philosophy from "technologization" to personalization to humanize childbirth. The term *family-centered birthing* is more appropriate today to denote the low-tech, high-touch approach requested by many childbearing women, who view childbirth as a normal process.

Certified nurse midwives (CNMs) are champions of family-centered birthing, and their participation in the childbirth process is associated with fewer unnecessary interventions when compared with obstetricians. CNMs subscribe to a normal birth process where the woman uses her own instincts and bodily signs during labor. In short, midwives empower women within the birthing environment (Casey, et al., 2015).

No matter what philosophy is held, it is ideal if everyone involved in the particular birth process—from the health care provider to the mother—shares the same philosophy toward the birth process.

Partners

Women desire support and attentive care during labor and birth. Caregivers can convey emotional support by offering their continued presence and words of encouragement. Throughout the world, few women are left to labor totally alone: emotional, physical, or spiritual support during labor is the norm for most cultures. According to the Childbirth Connection's ongoing *Listening to Mothers Initiative III* survey, almost all women (99%) reported having received some type of supportive care during labor (Edmonds, Cwiertniewicz, & Stoll, 2015). A caring partner can use massage, light touch, acupressure, handholding, stroking, and relaxation; can help the woman communicate her wishes to the staff; and can provide a continuous, reassuring presence, all of which bring some degree of comfort to the laboring woman (Capogna, 2015). Although the presence of the mother's significant other at the birth provides special emotional support, a partner can be anyone who is present to support the woman throughout the experience. For many women, the essential ingredients for a safe and satisfying birth include a sense of empowerment and success in coping with or transcending the experience, in addition to having solid, positive encouragement from a support companion.

Worldwide, women usually support other women in childbirth. ***Doula*** is a Greek word meaning woman servant or caregiver. It now commonly refers to a woman who offers emotional and practical support to a mother or couple before, during, and after childbirth. A doula believes in "mothering the mother," but clinical support remains the job of the midwife or medical staff (Ahlemeyer & Mahon, 2015). The continuous presence of a trained female support person reduces the need for medication for pain relief, the use of vacuum or forceps delivery, and the need for cesarean births. Continuous support was also associated with a slight reduction in the length of labor. The doula, who is an experienced labor companion, provides the woman and her partner with emotional and physical support and information throughout the entire labor and birth experience.

A recent study in the United States found that nursing care decreases the likelihood of negative evaluations of the childbirth experience, feelings of tenseness during labor, and finding labor worse than expected. Also reported were less perineal trauma, reduced difficulty in mothering, and reduced likelihood of early cessation of breast-feeding. Continuous support by nurses included reassurance, encouragement, praise, and explaination (Iravani, et al., 2015).

Given the many benefits of intrapartum support, laboring women should always have the option to receive partner support, whether from nurses, doulas, significant others, or family. Whoever the support partner is, he or she should provide the mother with continuous presence and hands-on comfort and encouragement. The overall objective of providing support for women during childbirth is to create a positive experience for her, while preserving her physical and psychologic health.

Patience

The birth process takes time. If more time were allowed for women to labor naturally without intervention, the cesarean birth rate would most likely be reduced. In one study, continuous support provided by midwives during labor reduced the duration of labor and the number of cesarean births; this model of support should be available to all women (Cox & King, 2015). The literature suggests that delaying interventions can give a woman enough time to progress in labor and reduce the need for surgical intervention (American College of Obstetricians and Gynecologists [ACOG], 2015) .

Healthy People 2020 has two goals related to cesarean births in the United States:

1. Reduce the rate of cesarean births among low-risk (full-term, singleton, vertex presentation) women having their first child to 23.9% of live births, from a baseline of 26.5%.
2. Reduce the rate of cesarean births among women who have had a prior cesarean birth to 81.7% of live births, from a baseline of 90.8% (U.S. Department of Health and Human Services, 2010).

We are a long way from achieving these goals—the current cesarean birth rate in the United States, at 32.7%, approximately one in three births, is the highest since these data first became available from birth certificates in 1989. Cesarean birth rate is associated with increased morbidity and mortality for both mother and infant as well as increased inpatient length of stay and health care costs (Centers for Disease Control and Prevention [CDC], 2014a).

It is difficult to predict how a labor will progress and therefore equally difficult to determine how long a woman's labor will last. There is no way to estimate the likely strength and frequency of uterine contractions, the extent to which the cervix will soften and dilate, and how much the fetal head will mold to fit the birth canal. We cannot know beforehand whether the complex fetal rotations needed for an efficient labor will take place properly. All of these factors are unknowns when a woman starts labor.

Induction of Labor

There is a trend in health care to attempt to manipulate the process of labor through medical means such as artificial rupture of membranes (amniotomy) and augmentation of labor with oxytocin (Kriebs, 2015). The labor induction rate has doubled in the United States since the 1990s (Moses, 2015).

Approximately one in four women are induced or have labor augmented with uterine-stimulating drugs or artificial rupture of membranes to accelerate her progress, and early term (in the 37th and 38th week) inductions have increased also. An amniotomy (artificial rupture of the fetal membranes) may be performed to augment or induce labor when the membranes have not ruptured spontaneously. Doing so allows the fetal head to have more direct contact with the cervix to dilate it. This procedure is performed with the fetal head at −2 station or lower, with the cervix dilated to at least 3 cm. Synthetic oxytocin (Pitocin) is also used to induce or augment labor by stimulating uterine contractions. It is administered piggybacked into the primary intravenous line with an infusion pump titrated to uterine activity.

Elective induction of labor is at an all-time high in the United States despite known associated risks. It can lead to birth of an infant too early, a long labor, exposure to a high-alert medication with its potential side effects, unnecessary cesarean birth, and maternal and neonatal morbidity. Elective induction has a cascade of related interventions, such as an intravenous line, continuous electronic fetal monitoring, confinement to bed, amniotomy, pharmacologic labor-stimulating agents, parental pain medications, and regional anesthesia, each with its own set of potential complications and risks. These risks apply to all women having the procedure; however, for nulliparous women before 41 weeks of gestation with an unfavorable cervix, the main risk is cesarean birth after unsuccessful labor induction with the potential for maternal and neonatal morbidity and increased health care costs. When cesarean occurs, subsequent births are likely to be via cesarean as well (Caughey, 2014). Compelling evidence indicates that elective induction of labor may increase the risk of cesarean birth, especially for nulliparous women (Le Ray, et al., 2015). Elective induction of labor in nulliparas is associated with increased rates of cesarean, postpartum hemorrhage, neonatal resuscitation, and longer hospitalizations without improvement in neonatal outcomes (Glavind & Uldbjerg, 2015). The belief is that many cesarean births could be avoided if women were allowed to labor longer and if the natural labor process were allowed to complete the job. The longer wait (using the intervention of patience) usually results in less intervention.

The ACOG attributes the dramatic increase in inductions in part to pressure from women, convenience for physicians, and liability concerns. Other reasons for the increase in inductions include the availability of better cervical ripening agents and a more relaxed attitude toward marginal indications for inductions. They recommend a cautious approach regarding elective induction until clinical trials can validate a more liberal use of labor inductions (ACOG, 2015). Current medical indications for inducing labor include:

- Spontaneous rupture of membranes and when labor does not start
- Large-size fetus not expected to navigate the maternal pelvis
- Fetal growth restriction (FGR) where external intervention is needed
- A pregnancy of more than 42 weeks' gestation
- Maternal hypertension, diabetes, or lung disease
- A uterine infection (March of Dimes, 2015).

When the laboring woman feels the urge to bear down, pushing begins. Most women respond extremely well to messages from their body without being directed by the nurse. A more natural, undirected approach allows the woman to wait and bear down when she feels the urge to push. Having patience and letting nature take its course will reduce the incidence of physiologic stress in the mother, resulting in less trauma to her perineal tissue.

Patient (Client) Preparation: Prenatal Education

Basic prenatal education can help women manage their labor process and feel in control of their birthing experience. The literature indicates that if a woman is prepared before the labor and birth experience, the labor is more likely to remain normal or natural (without the need for medical intervention) (Byrne, et al., 2014). An increasing body of evidence also indicates that the well-prepared woman, with good labor support, is less likely to need analgesia or anesthesia and is unlikely to require cesarean birth (Hoang, 2014).

Prenatal education teaches the woman about the childbirth experience and increases her sense of control. She is then able to work as an active participant during the labor and birth experience (Jordan, et al., 2014). The research also suggests that prenatal preparation may affect intrapartum and postpartum psychosocial outcomes (Budin, 2014). For example, prenatal education covering parenting communication classes had a significant effect on postpartum anxiety and postpartum adjustment. In a recent study of Hispanic women attending a community prenatal education program, they found that many women experienced anguish from unknowns during their pregnancy, leading to a yearning to learn and understand more, but with a desire to do so without sacrificing their cultural identity (Fitzgerald, Cronin, & Boccella, 2015). In another study involving Somali couples, most did not attend prenatal classes because their religion doesn't allow women and men to learn in the same room, and the men are not allowed to look at naked figures displayed in photos and videos (Wojnar, 2015). If the prenatal educational setting were more respectful of their beliefs, attendance would improve. These findings have important implications for nurses teaching prenatal classes to diverse cultures. Prenatal education should be viewed as an opportunity to strengthen families by providing anticipatory guidance and improving family members' life skills. In short, prenatal education helps to promote healthy families during the transition to parenthood and beyond (Woods & Chesser, 2015).

There is increasing evidence that women use herbs to induce labor and also during labor for pain relief. Desire to have control over their health has been cited as the strongest motive for women to use herbal medicine. A few of the herbs used include *Caulophyllum*, made from the herb blue cohosh to induce labor contractions; blue and black cohosh, raspberry leaves, castor oil and evening primrose oil used for cervical ripening and induction of labor; and *Chanlibao* to shorten the second stage of labor by strengthening the contractions (Ramasubramaniam, et al., 2015). The use of herbs during labor have been found to benefit some women by easing the labor process without side effects, but clinical trials are lacking to prove the safety and effectiveness of them.

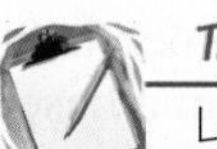

Take Note!

Learning about labor and birth allows women and couples to express their needs and preferences, enhance their confidence, and improve communication between themselves and the staff.

Pain Management

Labor and birth, although a normal physiologic process, can produce significant pain. Pain during labor is a nearly universal experience. Controlling the uterine discomfort without harm to the fetus or labor process is the major focus of pain management during childbirth. Pain is a subjective experience involving a complex interaction of physiologic, spiritual, psychosocial, cultural, and environmental influences (Van der Gucht & Lewis, 2015). Cultural values and learned behaviors influence perception and response to pain, as do anxiety and fear, both of which tend to heighten the sense of pain (Jones, 2015). The challenge for care providers is to find the right combination of pain/coping management methods to keep the discomfort manageable while minimizing the negative effect on the fetus, the normal physiology of labor, maternal–infant bonding, breast-feeding, and a woman's perception of the labor itself (King, et al., 2015). Chapter 14 presents a full discussion of pain management during labor and birth.

PHYSIOLOGIC RESPONSES TO LABOR

Labor is the process by which the birth canal is prepared to allow the fetus to pass from the uterine cavity to the outside world. During pregnancy, progesterone secreted from the placenta suppresses the spontaneous contractions of a typical uterus, keeping the fetus within the uterus. In addition, the cervix remains firm and noncompliant. At term, however, changes occur in the cervix that make it softer. In addition, uterine contractions become more frequent and regular, signaling the onset of labor.

The labor process involves a series of rhythmic, involuntary, usually quite uncomfortable uterine muscle contractions. The contractions bring about a shortening that causes effacement and dilation of the cervix and a bursting of the fetal membranes. Uterine contractions of an intensity of 30 mmHg or greater promote cervical dilation. Then, accompanied by both reflex and voluntary contractions of the abdominal muscles (pushing), the uterine contractions result in the birth of the baby (Grant, Strevens, & Thornton, 2015). During labor, the mother and fetus make several physiologic adaptations.

Maternal Responses

As the woman progresses through childbirth, numerous physiologic responses occur that assist her to adapt to the labor process. The labor process stresses several of the woman's body systems, which react through numerous compensatory mechanisms. Maternal physiologic responses include:

- Heart rate increases by 10 to 20 bpm.
- Cardiac output increases by 12% to 31% during the first stage of labor and by 50% during the second stage of labor.
- Blood pressure increases by up to 35 mmHg during uterine contractions in all labor stages.
- The white blood cell count increases to 25,000 to 30,000 cells/mm^3, perhaps as a result of tissue trauma.
- Respiratory rate increases and more oxygen is consumed related to the increase in metabolism.
- Gastric motility and food absorption decrease, which may increase the risk of nausea and vomiting during the transition stage of labor.
- Gastric emptying and gastric pH decrease, increasing the risk of vomiting with aspiration.
- Temperature rises slightly, possibly due to an increase in muscle activity.
- Muscular aches/cramps occur as a result of the stressed musculoskeletal system.
- Basal metabolic rate increases and blood glucose levels decrease because of the stress of labor (Cheng & Caughey, 2015a).

A woman's ability to adapt to the stress of labor is influenced by her psychological and physical state. Among the many factors that affect her coping ability are:

- Previous birth experiences and their outcomes (complications and previous birth outcomes)
- Current pregnancy experience (planned versus unplanned, discomforts experienced, age, risk status of pregnancy, chronic illness, weight gain)
- Cultural considerations (values and beliefs about health status)
- Support system (presence and support of a valued partner during labor)
- Childbirth preparation (attended childbirth classes and has practiced paced breathing techniques)
- Exercise during pregnancy (muscles toned; ability to assist with intra-abdominal pushing)
- Expectations of the birthing experience (viewed as a meaningful or stressful event)
- Anxiety level (excessive anxiety may interfere with labor progress)
- Fear of labor and loss of control (fear may enhance pain perception, augmenting fear)
- Fatigue and weariness (not up for the challenge/duration of labor) (King, et al., 2015).

Fetal Responses

Although the focus during labor may be on assessing the mother's adaptations, several physiologic adaptations occur in the fetus as well. The fetus is experiencing labor along with the mother. If the fetus is healthy, the stress of labor usually has no adverse effects. The nurse needs to be alert to any abnormalities in the fetus's adaptation to labor. Fetal responses to labor include:

- Periodic fetal heart rate accelerations and slight decelerations related to fetal movement, fundal pressure, and uterine contractions
- Decrease in circulation and perfusion to the fetus secondary to uterine contractions (a healthy fetus is able to compensate for this drop)
- Increase in arterial carbon dioxide pressure (PCO_2)
- Decrease in fetal breathing movements throughout labor
- Decrease in fetal oxygen pressure with a decrease in the partial pressure of oxygen (PO_2) (Verklan & Walden, 2014).

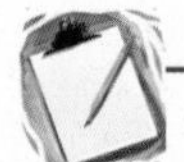

Take Note!

Respiratory changes during labor help to prepare the fetus for extrauterine respiration immediately after birth.

STAGES OF LABOR

Labor is typically divided into four stages: dilation, expulsive, placental, and restorative. Table 13.2 summarizes the major events of each stage.

The first stage is the longest: it begins with the first true contraction and ends with full dilation (opening) of the cervix. Because this stage lasts so long, it is divided into three phases, each corresponding to the progressive dilation of the cervix.

Stage two of labor, or the expulsive stage, begins when the cervix is completely dilated and ends with the birth of the newborn. The expulsive stage can last from minutes to hours. The contractions typically occur every 2 to 3 minutes, lasting 60 to 90 seconds, and are strong by palpation. The woman is usually intent on the work of pushing during this stage.

The third stage, or placental expulsion, starts after the newborn is born and ends with the separation and

TABLE 13.2 STAGES AND PHASES OF LABOR

	First Stage	Second Stage	Third Stage	Fourth Stage
Description	From 0 to 10 cm dilation; consists of three phases	From complete dilation (10 cm) to birth of the newborn; may last up to 3 hrs	Separation and delivery of the placenta; usually takes 5–10 min, but may take up to 30 min	1–4 hrs after the birth of the newborn; time of maternal physiologic adjustment
Phases	**Latent phase** (0–3 cm dilation) • Cervical dilation from 0 to 3 cm • Cervical effacement from 0% to 40% • Nullipara, lasts up to 9 hrs; multipara, lasts up to 5–6 hrs • Contraction frequency every 5–10 min • Contraction duration 30–45 sec • Contraction intensity mild to palpation **Active phase** (4–7 cm dilation) • Cervical dilation from 4 to 7 cm • Cervical effacement from 40% to 80% • Nullipara, lasts up to 6 hrs; multipara, lasts up to 4 hrs • Contraction frequency every 2–5 min • Contraction duration 45–60 sec • Contraction intensity moderate to palpation **Transition phase** (8–10 cm dilation) • Cervical dilation from 8 to 10 cm • Cervical effacement from 80% to 100% • Nullipara lasts up to 1 hr; multipara, lasts up to 30 min • Contraction frequency every 1–2 min • Contraction duration 60–90 sec • Contraction intensity strong by palpation	**Pelvic phase** (period of fetal descent) **Perineal phase** (period of active pushing) • Nullipara, lasts up to 1 hr; multipara, lasts up to 30 min • Contraction frequency every 2–3 min or less • Contraction duration 60–90 sec • Contraction intensity strong by palpation • Strong urge to push during the later perineal phase	**Placental separation:** detaching from uterine wall **Placental expulsion:** coming outside the vaginal opening	

Adapted from Cheng, Y. W., & Caughey, A. B. (2015a). Normal labor and delivery. *eMedicine*. Retrieved from http://emedicine.medscape.com/article/260036-overview; Cunningham, F. G., Leveno, K. J., Bloom, S. L., Spong, C. Y., Dashe, J. S., Hoffman, B. L., Casey, B. M., & Sheffield, J. S. (2014). *Williams obstetrics* (24th ed.). New York, NY: McGraw-Hill Education; and King, T. L., Brucker, M. C., Kriebs, J. M., Fahey, J. O., Gegor, C. L., & Varney, H. (2015). *Varney's midwifery* (5th ed.). Burlington, MA: Jones & Bartlett Learning.

birth of the placenta. Continued uterine contractions typically cause the placenta to be expelled within 5 to 30 minutes. If the newborn is stable, bonding of infant and mother takes place during this stage through touching, holding, and skin-to-skin contact.

The fourth stage, or the restorative stage or immediate postpartum period, lasts from 1 to 4 hours after birth. This period is when the mother's body begins to stabilize after the hard work of labor and the loss of the products of conception. The fourth stage is often not recognized as a true stage of labor, but it is a critical period for maternal physiologic transition as well as new family attachment. Close monitoring of both the mother and her newborn are done during this stage (Green, 2015).

First Stage

During the first stage of labor, the fundamental change underlying the process is progressive dilation of the cervix. Cervical dilation is gauged subjectively by vaginal examination and is expressed in centimeters. The first stage ends when the cervix is dilated to 10 cm in diameter and is large enough to permit the passage of a fetal head of average size. The fetal membranes, or bag of waters, usually rupture during the first stage, but they may have burst earlier or may even remain intact until birth. For the primigravida, the first stage of labor lasts about 12 hours. However, this time can vary widely; for the multiparous woman, it is usually only half that.

During the first stage of labor, women usually perceive the visceral pain of diffuse abdominal cramping and uterine contractions. Pain during the first stage of labor is primarily a result of the dilation of the cervix and lower uterine segment, and the distention (stretching) of these structures during contractions. The first stage is divided into three phases: latent or early phase, active phase, and transition phase.

Latent or Early Phase

The latent or early phase gives rise to the familiar signs and symptoms of labor. This phase begins with the start of regular contractions and ends when rapid cervical dilation begins. Cervical effacement occurs during this phase, and the cervix dilates from 0 to 3 cm.

Contractions usually occur every 5 to 10 minutes, last 30 to 45 seconds, and are described as mild by palpation by the nurse. Assessment of intensity is evaluated by pressing down on the fundus during a contraction to see if it can be dented with the nurse's fingers. The ability to indent the fundus at the peak of the contraction would typically indicate a mild contraction. Effacement of the cervix is from 0% to 40%. Most women are very talkative during this period, perceiving their contractions to be similar to menstrual cramps. Women may remain at home during this phase, contacting their health care provider about the onset of labor.

For the nulliparous woman, the latent phase typically lasts about 9 hours; in the multiparous woman, it lasts about 6 hours (Cheng & Caughey, 2015a). During this phase, women are apprehensive but excited about the start of their labor after their long gestational period.

Think back to the couple who were sent home from the hospital birthing center. Three days later Kathy awoke with a wet sensation and intense discomfort in her back, spreading around to her abdomen. She decided to go for a walk, but her contractions didn't diminish. Instead, her contractions continued to occur every few minutes and grew stronger in intensity. She and Chuck decided to go back to the hospital birthing center. Was there a difference in the location of Kathy's discomfort this time? What changes will the admission nurse find in Kathy if this is true labor?

Active Phase

The active phase of labor encompasses the time from an increase in the rate of cervical dilation (end of latent phase of labor) until completion of cervical dilation. Cervical dilation begins to occur more rapidly during the active phase. The cervix usually dilates from 4 to 7 cm, with 40% to 80% effacement taking place. This phase can last up to 6 hours for the nulliparous woman and 4.5 hours for the multiparous woman (Leap & Hunter, 2015). The fetus descends farther in the pelvis. Contractions become more frequent (every 2 to 5 minutes) and increase in duration (45 to 60 seconds). The woman's discomfort intensifies (moderate to strong by palpation). She becomes more intense and inwardly focused, absorbed in the serious work of her labor. She limits interactions with those in the room. If she and her partner have attended childbirth education classes, she will begin to use the relaxation and paced breathing techniques that they learned to cope with the contractions. The typical dilation rate for the nulliparous woman is 1.2 cm/hr; for the multiparous woman, it is 1.5 cm/hr (Cunningham et al., 2014).

Transition Phase

The transition phase is the last phase of the first stage of labor. During this phase, dilation slows, progressing from 8 to 10 cm, with effacement from 80% to 100%. The transition phase is the most difficult and, fortunately, the shortest phase for the woman, lasting approximately 1 hour in the first birth and perhaps 15 to 30 minutes in successive births (Tharpe et al., 2016). During transition, the contractions are stronger (hard by palpation), more painful, more frequent (every 1 to 2 minutes), and they last longer (60 to 90 seconds). The average rate of fetal descent is 1 cm/hr in nulliparous women and 2 cm/hr in multiparous women. Pressure on the rectum is great, and there is a strong desire to contract the abdominal muscles and push.

Other maternal symptoms during the transitional phase include nausea and vomiting, trembling extremities, backache, increased apprehension and irritability, restless movement, increased bloody show from the vagina, inability to relax, diaphoresis, feelings of loss of control, and being overwhelmed (the woman may say, "I can't take it anymore") (Cunningham et al., 2014).

In assessing Kathy, the nurse finds she is 4 cm dilated and 50% effaced with ruptured membranes. In what stage and phase of labor would this assessment finding place Kathy?

Second Stage

The second stage of labor begins with complete cervical dilation (10 cm) and effacement and ends with the birth of the newborn. Although the previous stage of labor primarily involved the thinning and opening of the cervix, this stage involves moving the fetus through the birth canal and out of the body. The cardinal movements of labor occur during the early phase of passive descent in the second stage of labor.

Contractions occur every 2 to 3 minutes, last 60 to 90 seconds, and are described as strong by palpation. The average length of the second stage of labor in a nullipara is approximately 1 hour and less than half that time for a multipara. During this expulsive stage, the mother usually feels more in control and less irritable and agitated. She is focused on the work of pushing. The maternal urge to push is generally felt when there is direct contact of the fetus to the pelvic floor. Stretch receptors in the wall of the vagina, rectum, and perineum communicate the pressure of the fetus descending in the birth canal that, along with increased abdominal pressure, causes the overwhelming urge to push described by laboring women (Camorcia, 2015).

Pushing

The second stage of labor has two phases (pelvic and perineal) related to the existence and quality of the maternal urge to push and to obstetric conditions related to fetal descent. The early phase of the second stage is called the pelvic phase, because it is during this phase that the fetal head is negotiating the pelvis, rotating, and advancing in descent. The later phase is called the perineal phase, because at this point the fetal head is lower in the pelvis and is distending the perineum. The occurrence of a strong urge to push characterizes the later phase of the second stage and has also been called the phase of active pushing (Cheng & Caughey, 2015b).

The later perineal phase occurs when the mother feels a tremendous urge to push as the fetal head is lowered and is distending the perineum. The perineum bulges and there is an increase in bloody show. The fetal head becomes apparent at the vaginal opening but disappears between contractions. When the top of the head no longer regresses between contractions, it is said to have crowned. The fetus rotates as it maneuvers out. Evidence now shows that labor actually progresses slower than we thought in the past. Many women might need a little more time to labor and give birth vaginally instead of moving to a surgical birth (ACOG, 2014b). The second stage commonly lasts up to 3 hours in a first labor and up to an hour in subsequent ones (Fig. 13.14).

SPONTANEOUS PUSHING VERSUS DIRECTED PUSHING

There are two ways of conducting the second stage of labor: *spontaneous pushing* (following the mother's spontaneous urge) and *directed pushing* (pushing directed by the caregiver). Spontaneous pushing represents a natural way of managing the second stage of labor. However, lately, and as a result of epidural analgesia, health care providers frequently resort to directed pushing without taking into account the negative repercussions it has on the woman and her fetus.

Evidence is mounting that the management of the second stage, particularly pushing, is a modifiable risk factor in long-term perinatal outcomes (ACOG, 2015). Research supports spontaneous physiologic approaches to second stage labor care; however, many women in hospital settings continue to receive direction from nurses to use prolonged Valsalva (holding breath) bearing-down efforts as soon as the cervix is completely dilated. Traditionally, women have been taught to hold their breath to the count of 10, inhale again, push again, and repeat the process several times during a contraction. This sustained, strenuous style of pushing, that is, Valsalva bearing-down and supine maternal positions, is linked to hemodynamic changes in the mother and interferes with oxygen exchange between the mother and the fetus. In addition, it is associated with pelvic floor damage: the longer the push, the more damage to the pelvic floor.

In clinical practice, health care providers sometimes resist delaying the onset of pushing after the second stage of labor has begun because of a belief that it will increase labor time. Delaying maternal bearing-down efforts during the second stage until the woman feels the urge to push (laboring down) allows for optimal use of maternal energy, has no detrimental maternal effects, and results in improved fetal oxygenation (Osborne & Hanson, 2014). Research shows that delaying pushing for up to 90 minutes after complete cervical dilation resulted in a significant decrease in the time mothers spend pushing without a significant increase in total time in second stage of labor (King, et al., 2015). Because research does not support a policy of directed pushing, and some evidence suggests it may be harmful, the practice of directed pushing should be abandoned (Brodric, 2014). The newest protocol from the Association of Women's Health, Obstetric and Neonatal Nurses (AWHONN, 2014) recommends an open-glottis method in which air is released during pushing to prevent the buildup of intrathoracic pressure. Doing so also supports mother's involuntary bearing-down efforts (Holvey, 2014). The adoption of a physiologic, woman-directed approach to bearing down is advocated (King, et al. 2015).

Behaviors demonstrated by laboring women during this time include pushing at the onset of the urge to bear down; using their own pattern and technique of bearing down in response to sensations they experience; using open-glottis bearing down with contractions; pushing with variations in strength and duration; pushing down with progressive intensity; and using multiple positions to increase progress and comfort. This approach is in stark contrast to management by arbitrary time limits

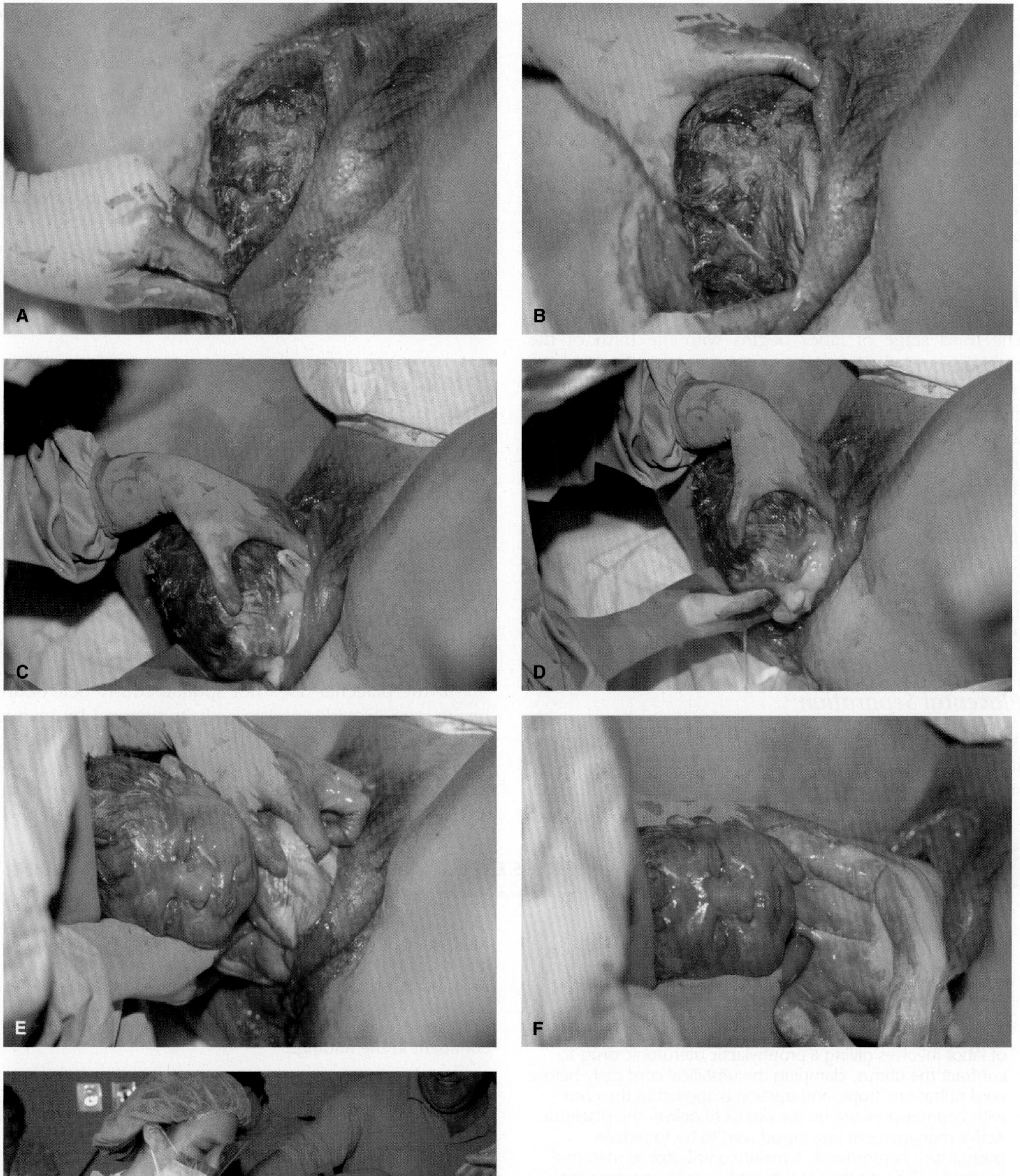

FIGURE 13.14 Birth sequence from crowning through birth of the newborn. **A.** Early crowning of the fetal head. Notice the bulging of the perineum. **B.** Late crowning. Notice that the fetal head is appearing face down. This is the normal OA position. **C.** As the head extends, you can see that the occiput is to the mother's right side—ROA position. **D.** The cardinal movement of extension. **E.** The shoulders are born. Notice how the head has turned to line up with the shoulders—the cardinal movement of external rotation. **F.** The body easily follows the shoulders. **G.** The newborn is held for the first time. (© B. Proud.)

and the directed bearing-down efforts seen in practice today. Labor nurses need to develop an evidence-based approach that acknowledges and reinforces women's innate ability to birth and refrain from trying to direct women's pushing behaviors (Reed, 2015).

Laboring down (promotion of passive descent) is an alternative strategy for second-stage management in women with epidurals. Using this approach, the fetus descends and is born without coached maternal pushing.

Third Stage

The third stage of labor begins with the birth of the newborn and ends with the separation and birth of the placenta. It consists of two phases: placental separation and placental expulsion. Worldwide, approximately 800 women die each day from preventable causes related to childbirth. The single most common cause is severe bleeding, which can kill a woman within hours if care is delayed. Prompt and effective management is paramount to saving the lives of these women and prevention measures can be initiated in the third stage of labor. Controversy continues about active verses expectant management of the third stage of labor. See Evidence-Based Practice 13.1.

Placental Separation

After the infant is born, the uterus continues to contract strongly and can now retract, decreasing markedly in size. These contractions cause the placenta to pull away from the uterine wall. The following signs of separation indicate that the placenta is ready to deliver:

- The uterus rises upward.
- The umbilical cord lengthens.
- A sudden trickle of blood is released from the vaginal opening.
- The uterus changes its shape to globular.

Spontaneous birth of the placenta occurs in one of two ways: the fetal side (shiny gray side) presenting first (called Schultz's mechanism or more commonly called "shiny Schultz's") or the maternal side (red raw side) presenting first (termed Duncan's mechanism or "dirty Duncan").

Placental Expulsion

After separation of the placenta from the uterine wall, continued uterine contractions cause the placenta to be expelled within 2 to 30 minutes unless there is gentle external traction to assist. After the placenta is expelled, the uterus is massaged briefly by the attending physician, nurse practitioner, or midwife until it is firm so that uterine blood vessels constrict, minimizing the possibility of hemorrhage. Normal blood loss is approximately 500 mL for a vaginal birth and 1,000 mL for a cesarean birth. Blood loss of over 1,000 mL is considered severe (Pavord & Maybury, 2015).

If the placenta does not spontaneously deliver, the health care provider assists with its removal by manual extraction. On expulsion, the placenta is inspected for its intactness by the health care provider and the nurse to make sure all sections are present. If any piece is still

EVIDENCE-BASED PRACTICE 13.1 **ACTIVE VERSUS EXPECTANT MANAGEMENT FOR WOMEN IN LABOR**

STUDY

Once birth has taken place, the uterus continues to contract, causing the placenta to separate from the wall of the uterus. The mother then delivers the placenta without outside intervention. This is termed expectant management of the third stage of labor. Active management of the third stage of labor involves giving a prophylactic uterotonic drug to contract the uterus, clamping the umbilical cord early before cord pulsations stops, and traction is applied to the cord with counter-pressure on the uterus to deliver the placenta. Active management was introduced to try to reduce postpartum hemorrhage, a major contributor to maternal mortality. The objective of this study was to compare the effectiveness of active verses expectant management of the third stage of labor.

Findings

Seven studies involving 8,247 women were analyzed. Because of the clinical heterogeneity of the sample, random-effects were used in the analysis. Active management showed a significant decrease in primary blood loss greater than 500 mL and subsequent anemia. However it reduced the newborn's birthweight and increased the mother's blood pressure. Overall, the quality of the evidence was low and more data is needed to be confident in the findings.

Nursing Implications

Although there was lack of high-quality evidence in this review, active management of the third stage of labor reduced the risk of hemorrhage after childbirth, but adverse effects were identified. Women should be provided information on the benefits and harms of both methods to support informed choice. Given the concerns about early cord clamping and the potential adverse effects of uterotonic drugs, it is important to look at the individual components of third-stage management and work toward modifications to bring about the best outcomes.

Adapted from Begley, C. M., Gyte, G. M. L., Devane, D., McGuire, W., & Weeks, A. (2015). Active versus expectant management for women in the third stage of labor. *Cochrane Database of Systematic Reviews* 2015, 3:CD007412.

attached to the uterine wall, it places the woman at risk for postpartum hemorrhage because it becomes a space-occupying object that interferes with the ability of the uterus to contract fully and effectively.

Fourth Stage

The fourth stage begins with completion of the expulsion of the placenta and membranes and ends with the initial physiologic adjustment and stabilization of the mother (1 to 4 hours after birth). This stage initiates the postpartum period. The mother usually feels a sense of peace and excitement, is wide awake, and is very talkative initially. The attachment process begins with her inspecting her newborn and desiring to cuddle and breast-feed him or her. The mother's fundus should be firm and well contracted. Typically it is located at the midline between the umbilicus and the symphysis, but it then slowly rises to the level of the umbilicus during the first hour after birth (Jordan, et al., 2014). If the uterus becomes boggy, it is massaged to keep it firm. The lochia (vaginal discharge) is red, mixed with small clots, and of moderate flow. If the woman has had an episiotomy during the second stage of labor, it should be intact, with the edges approximated and clean and no redness or edema present.

The focus during this stage is to monitor the mother closely to prevent hemorrhage, bladder distention, and venous thrombosis. Usually the mother is thirsty and hungry during this time and may request food and drink. Her bladder is hypotonic and thus she has limited sensation to acknowledge a full bladder or to void. Vital signs, the amount and consistency of the vaginal discharge (lochia), and the uterine fundus are usually monitored every 15 minutes for at least 1 hour. The woman will be feeling cramp-like discomfort during this time due to the contracting uterus.

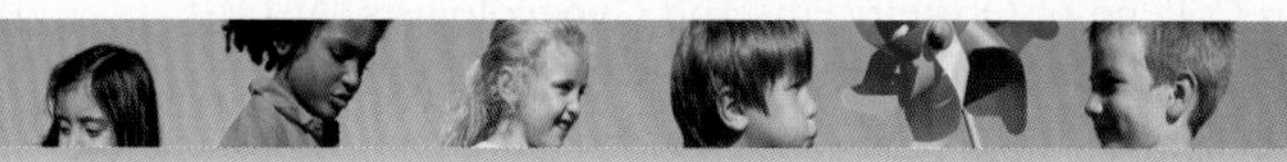

KEY CONCEPTS

- Labor is a complex, multifaceted interaction between the mother and fetus. Thus, it is difficult to determine exactly why labor begins and what initiates it.
- Before the onset of labor, a pregnant woman's body undergoes several changes in preparation for the birth of the newborn, often leading to characteristic signs and symptoms that suggest that labor is near. These changes include cervical changes, lightening, increased energy level, bloody show, Braxton Hicks contractions, and spontaneous rupture of membranes.
- False labor is a condition seen during the latter weeks of some pregnancies in which irregular uterine contractions are felt, but the cervix is not affected.
- The critical factors in labor and birth are designated as the 10 P's: passageway (birth canal), passenger (fetus and placenta), powers (contractions), position (maternal), psychological response, philosophy (low tech, high touch), partners (support caregivers), patience (natural timing), patient (client) preparation (childbirth knowledge base), and pain management (comfort measures).
- The size and shape of a woman's pelvis are determining factors for a vaginal birth. The female pelvis is classified according to four main shapes: gynecoid, anthropoid, android, and platypelloid.
- The labor process is comprised of a series of rhythmic, involuntary, usually quite uncomfortable uterine muscle contractions that bring about a shortening (effacement) and opening (dilation) of the cervix, and a bursting of the fetal membranes. Important parameters of uterine contractions are frequency, duration, and intensity.
- The diameters of the fetal skull vary considerably, with some diameters shortening and others lengthening as the head is molded during the labor and birth process.
- Pain during labor is a nearly universal experience for childbearing women. Having a strong sense of self and meaningful support from others can often help women manage labor well and reduce their sensation of pain.
- Preparing mentally for childbirth is important for women to enable them to work with the natural forces of labor and not against them.
- As the woman experiences and progresses through childbirth, numerous physiologic responses occur that assist her adaptation to the laboring process.
- Labor is typically divided into four stages that are unequal in length.
- During the first stage, the fundamental change underlying the process is progressive dilation of the cervix. It is further divided into three phases: latent phase, active phase, and transition.

- The second stage of labor is from complete cervical dilation (10 cm) and effacement through the birth of the infant.
- The third stage is that of separation and birth of the placenta. It consists of two phases: placental separation and placental expulsion.
- The fourth stage begins after the birth of the placenta and membranes and ends with the initial physiologic adjustment and stabilization of the mother (1 to 4 hours).

REFERENCES AND RECOMMENDED READING

Ahlemeyer, J., & Mahon, S. (2015). Doulas for childbearing women. *MCN: The American Journal of Maternal/Child Nursing, 40*(2), 122–127.

Alexander, L. L., LaRosa, J. H., Bader, H., & Garfield, S. (2014). *New dimensions in women's health* (6th ed.). Sudbury, MA: Jones & Bartlett.

American College of Obstetricians and Gynecologists [ACOG]. (2014a). *Labor induction: FAQ 154.* Retrieved from http://www.acog.org/For_Patients/Search_FAQs

American College of Obstetricians & Gynecologists [ACOG]. (2014b). *Nation's OB/GYNs take aim at preventing cesareans: New guidelines recommends allowing women to labor longer to help avoid cesarean.* Retrieved from http://www.acog.org/About_ACOG/News_Room/News_Releases/2014/Nations_Ob-Gyns_Take_Aim_at_Preventing_Cesareans

American College of Obstetricians and Gynecologists [ACOG] (2015) Practice Bulletin 107 reaffirmed: Induction of labor. *Obstetrics & Gynecology*, 113:386–397.

Association of Women's Health, Obstetric and Neonatal Nurses [AWHONN]. (2014). *Nursing care and management of the* 2nd *stage of labor* (2nd ed.). Retrieved from https://www.awhonn.org/awhonn/content.do?name=08_Store/08_labormanagement.htm

Begley, C. M., Gyte, G. M., Devane, D., McGuire, W., & Weeks, A. (2015). Active versus expectant management for women in the third stage of labor. *Cochrane Database of Systematic Reviews*, 3, CD007412. doi: 10.1002/14651858.CD007412.pub4.

Brodric, A. (2014). Too afraid to push: Dealing with fear of childbirth. *Practicing Midwife, 17*(3), 15–17.

Budin, W. C. (2014). What to Teach? *Journal of Perinatal Education, 23*(2), 59–61.

Budin, W. C. (2015). Choosing wisely for birth. *The Journal of Perinatal Education, 24*(1), 3–5.

Byrne, J., Hauck, Y., Fisher, C., Bayes, S., & Schutze, R. (2014). Effectiveness of a mindfulness-based childbirth education pilot study on maternal self-efficacy and fear of childbirth. *Journal of Midwifery & Women's Health, 59*(2), 192–197.

Camorcia, M. (2015). Chapter 9: The second and third stage of labor. In Capogna, G. (Ed.), *Epidural labor analgesia* (pp. 103–119). New York, NY: Springer International Publishing.

Capogna, G. (2015). Chapter 24: Humanization of childbirth and epidural analgesia. In Capogna, G. (Ed.), *Epidural labor analgesia* (pp. 315–323). New York, NY: Springer International Publishing.

Casey, M., Fealy, G., Kennedy, C., Hegarty, J., Prizeman, G., McNamara, M., et al. (2015) Nurses', midwives' and key stakeholders' experiences and perceptions of a scope of nursing and midwifery practice framework. *Journal of Advanced Nursing, 71*(6), 1227–1237.

Caughey, A. (2014). Induction of labor: Does it increase the risk of cesarean delivery? *BJOG: An International Journal of Obstetrics & Gynecology, 121*(6), 658–661.

Centers for Disease Control and Prevention [CDC]. (2014a). Primary cesarean delivery rates, by state: Results from the revised birth certificate, 2006–2012. *National vital statistics reports, 63*(1), Hyattsville, MD: National Center for Health Statistics.

Cheng, Y. W., & Caughey, A. B. (2015a). Normal labor and delivery. *eMedicine.* Retrieved from http://emedicine.medscape.com/article/260036-overview

Cheng, Y. W., & Caughey, A. B. (2015b). Second stage of labor. *Clinical Obstetrics and Gynecology, 58*(2), 227–240.

Collins, K. A., & Reed, R. C. (2014). Chapter 6: Birth trauma. In Collins, K. A., & Byard, R. W. (Eds.), *Forensic pathology of infancy and childhood* (pp. 139–168). New York, NY: Springer International Publishing.

Cox, K. J., & King, T. L. (2015). Preventing primary cesarean births: Midwifery care. *Clinical Obstetrics and Gynecology, 58*(2), 282–293.

Cunningham, F. G., Leveno, K. J., Bloom, S. L., Spong, C. Y., Dashe, J. S., Hoffman, B. L., et al. (2014). *Williams obstetrics* (24th ed.). New York, NY: McGraw-Hill Education.

Edmonds, J. K., Cwiertniewicz, T., & Stoll, K. (2015). Childbirth education prior to pregnancy? Survey findings of childbirth preferences and attitudes among young women. *The Journal of Perinatal Education, 24*(2), 93–101.

Fischer, B., & Mitteroecker, P. (2015). Covariation between human pelvis shape, stature, and head size alleviates the obstetric dilemma. *Proceedings of the National Academy of Sciences, 112*(18), 5655–5660.

Fitzgerald, E. M., Cronin, S. N., & Boccella, S. H. (2015). Anguish, yearning, and identity: Toward a better understanding of the pregnant Hispanic woman's prenatal care experience. *Journal of Transcultural Nursing*, pii: 1043659615578718. (Online 4/2/15), doi: 10.1177/1043659615578718.

Funai, E. F., & Norwitz, E. R. (2015). Mechanism of normal labor and delivery. *UpToDate.* Retrieved from http://www.uptodate.com/contents/mechanism-of-normal-labor-and-delivery

Gizzo, S., Di Gangi, S., Noventa, M., Bacile, V., Zambon, A., & Nardelli, G. B. (2014). Women's choice of positions during labor: Return to the past or a modern way to give birth? *BioMed Research International*, 2014. Retrieved from http://dx.doi.org/10.1155/2014/638093

Glavind, J., & Uldbjerg, N. (2015). Elective cesarean delivery at 38 and 39 weeks: Neonatal and maternal risks. *Current Opinion in Obstetrics and Gynecology, 27*(2), 121–127.

Grant, N., Strevens, H., & Thornton, J. (2015). Chapter 1: Physiology of labor. In Capogna, G. (Ed.), *Epidural labor analgesia* (pp. 1–10). New York, NY: Springer International Publishing.

Green, C. J. (2015). *Maternal newborn nursing care plans.* (3rd ed.), Burlington, MA: Jones & Bartlett Learning.

Hanson, L., & VandeVusse, L. (2014). Supporting labor progress toward physiologic birth. *Journal of Perinatal & Neonatal Nursing*, *28*(2), 101–107.

Hoang, S. (2014). Pregnancy and anxiety. *International Journal of Childbirth Education*, *29*(1), 67–70.

Hofmeyr, G. J. (2015). Breech delivery. *Protocols for high-risk pregnancies: An evidence-based approach* (6th ed., pp. 423–427). West Sussex, UK: John Wiley & Sons.

Holvey, N. (2014). Supporting women in the second stage of labor. *British Journal of Midwifery*, *22*(3), 182–186.

Horgan, M. J. (2015). Management of the late preterm infant: Not quite ready for prime time. *Pediatric Clinics of North America*, *62*(2), 439–451.

Iravani, M., Zarean, E., Janghorbani, M., & Bahrami, M. (2015). Women's needs and expectations during normal labor and delivery. *Journal of Education and Health Promotion*, *4*, 6.

Jones, L. V. (2015). Non-pharmacological approaches for pain relief during labor can improve maternal satisfaction with childbirth and reduce obstetric interventions. *Evidence Based Nursing*, 18(3), 70.

Jones, R. E., & Lopez, K. H. (2014). *Human reproductive biology* (4th ed.). Waltham, MA: Elsevier Health Sciences.

Jordan, R. G., Engstrom, J., Marfell, J., & Farley, C. L. (2014). *Prenatal and postnatal care: A women-centered approach*. Ames, IA: John Wiley & Sons.

King, T. L., Brucker, M. C., Kriebs, J. M., Fahey, J. O., Gegor, C. L., & Varney, H. (2015). *Varney's midwifery* (5th ed.). Burlington, MA: Jones & Bartlett Learning.

Kriebs, J. M. (2015). Patient safety during induction of labor. *The Journal of Perinatal & Neonatal Nursing*, *29*(2), 130–137.

Leap, N., & Hunter, B. (2015). *Supporting women for labor and birth: A companion*. Florence, KY: Routledge.

Leonard, P. (2015). Childbirth education: A handbook for nurses. *Nursing spectrum*. Retrieved from http://ce.nurse.com/60057/Childbirth-Education-A-Handbook-for-Nurses

Le Ray, C., Blondel, B., Prunet, C., Khireddine, I., Deneux-Tharaux, C., & Goffinet, F. (2015). Stabilizing the caesarean rate: Which target population? British Journal of Obstetrics and Gynaecology, *122*, 690–699.

March of Dimes. (2015). *Inducing labor: Medical reasons*. Retrieved from http://www.marchofdimes.org/videos/inducing-labor-medical-reasons.aspx

Marani, E., & Koch, W. (2014). *The pelvis: Structure, gender and society*. Philadelphia, PA: Springer Healthcare.

Martin, R. J., Fanaroff, A. A., & Walsh, M. C. (2014). *Neonatal-perinatal medicine* (10th ed.). St. Louis, MO: Elsevier Health Sciences.

Moses, S. (2015). Labor induction. *Family practice notebook*, Retrieved from http://www.fpnotebook.com/ob/ld/LbrIndctn.htm

Nieuwenhuijze, M., Low, L., Korstjens, I., & Lagro-Janssen, T. (2014). The role of maternity care providers in promoting shared decision making regarding birthing positions during the second stage of labor. *Journal of Midwifery & Women's Health*, 59(3), 277–285.

Milton, S. K., Chelmow, D., & Ramus, R. M. (2015). Maternal and fetal outcomes with internal compared with external tocometry: A meta-analysis [218]. *Obstetrics & Gynecology*, *125*, 71S.

Norwitz, E. R. (2015). Physiology of parturition. *UpToDate*. Retrieved from http://www.uptodate.com/contents/physiology-of-parturition

Osborne, K., & Hanson, L. (2014). Labor down or bear down: A strategy to translate second-stage labor evidence to perinatal practice. *Journal of Perinatal & Neonatal Nursing*, *28*(2), 117–126.

Pavord, S., & Maybury, H. (2015). How I treat postpartum hemorrhage. *Blood*, *125*(18), 2759–2770.

Ramasubramaniam, S., Renganathan, L., Vijayalakshmi, G., & Mallo-Banatao, M. V. (2015). Use of herbal preparations among parturient women: Is there enough evidence - A review of literature. *International Journal of Herbal Medicine*, *2*(5), 20–26.

Reed, R. (2015). Supporting women's instinctive pushing behavior during birth. *The Practicing Midwife*, *18*(6), 13–15.

Sharshiner, R., & Silver, R. M. (2015). Management of fetal malpresentation. *Clinical Obstetrics and Gynecology*, *58*(2), 246–255.

Tharpe, N. L., Farley, C. L., & Jordan, R. (2016). *Clinical practice guidelines for midwifery & women's health* (5th ed.). Sudbury, MA: Jones & Bartlett.

Tussey, C. M., Botsios, E., Gerkin, R. D., Kelly, L. A., Gamez, J., & Mensik, J. (2015). Reducing length of labor and cesarean surgery rate using a peanut ball for women laboring with an epidural. *The Journal of Perinatal Education*, *24*(1), 16–24.

U.S. Department of Health and Human Services (2010). *Healthy People 2020*. Retrieved from http://www.healthypeople.gov/2020/topicsobjectives2020

Van der Gucht, N., & Lewis, K. (2015). Women's experiences of coping with pain during childbirth: A critical review of qualitative research. *Midwifery*, *31*(3), 349–358.

Verklan, T., & Walden, M. (2014). *Core curriculum for neonatal intensive care nursing* (4th ed.). St. Louis, MO: Saunders Elsevier.

Weber, J., & Kelley, J. (2014). *Health assessment in nursing* (5th ed.). Philadelphia, PA: Lippincott Williams & Wilkins.

Wojnar, D. M. (2015). Perinatal experiences of Somali couples in the United States. *JOGNN: Journal of Obstetric, Gynecologic & Neonatal Nursing*, *44*(3), 358–369.

Woods, N. K., & Chesser, A. (2015). Becoming a mom: Improving birth outcomes through a community collaborative prenatal education model. *Journal of Family Medicine & Disease Prevention*, *1*(002), 1–4.

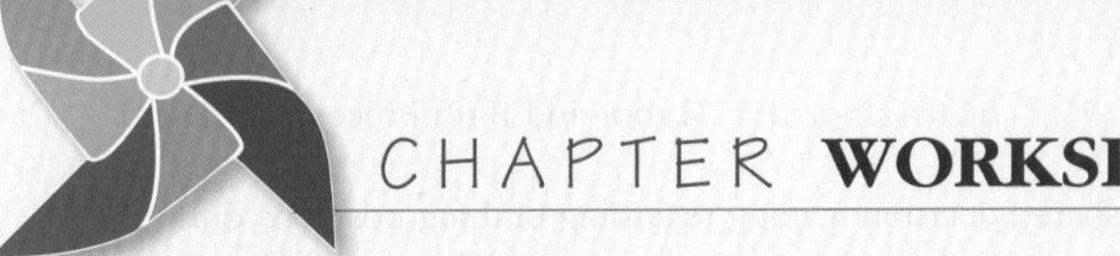

CHAPTER WORKSHEET

MULTIPLE-CHOICE QUESTIONS

1. When determining the frequency of contractions, the nurse would measure which of the following?
   a. Start of one contraction to the start of the next contraction
   b. Beginning of one contraction to the end of the same contraction
   c. Peak of one contraction to the peak of the next contraction
   d. End of one contraction to the beginning of the next contraction
2. Which fetal lie is most conducive to a spontaneous vaginal birth?
   a. Transverse
   b. Longitudinal
   c. Perpendicular
   d. Oblique
3. Which of the following observations would suggest that placental separation is occurring?
   a. Uterus stops contracting altogether.
   b. Umbilical cord pulsations stop.
   c. Uterine shape changes to globular.
   d. Maternal blood pressure drops.
4. As the nurse is explaining the difference between true versus false labor to her childbirth class, she states that the major difference between them is:
   a. Discomfort level is greater with false labor.
   b. Progressive cervical changes occur in true labor.
   c. There is a feeling of nausea with false labor.
   d. There is more fetal movement with true labor.
5. The shortest but most intense phase of labor is the:
   a. Latent phase
   b. Active phase
   c. Transition phase
   d. Placental expulsion phase
6. A laboring woman is admitted to the labor and birth suite at 6 cm dilation. She would be in which phase of the first stage of labor?
   a. Latent
   b. Active
   c. Transition
   d. Early
7. Which assessment would indicate that a woman is in true labor?
   a. Membranes are ruptured and fluid is clear.
   b. Presenting part is engaged and not floating.
   c. Cervix is 4 cm dilated, 90% effaced.
   d. Contractions last 30 seconds, every 5 to 10 minutes.
8. Interventions that are underutilized in promoting a normal birth. Select all that apply.
   a. Oral nutrition and fluids in labor
   b. Open glottis pushing in the second stage of labor
   c. Skin-to-skin contact after birth for infant bonding
   d. Routine artificial rupture of membranes (amniotomy)
   e. Labor induction with Pitocin given intravenously
   f. Routine episiotomy to shorten labor length
9. Physiologic preparation for labor would be demonstrated by:
   a. Decrease in Braxton Hicks contractions felt by mother
   b. Weight gain and increase in appetite by mother
   c. Lightening, whereby the fetus drops into true pelvis
   d. Fetal heart rate accelerations and increased movements

CRITICAL THINKING EXERCISES

1. Cindy, a 20-year-old primipara, calls the birthing center where you work as a nurse and reports that she thinks she is in labor because she feels labor pains. Her due date is this week. The midwives have been giving her prenatal care throughout this pregnancy.
   a. What additional information do you need to respond appropriately?
   b. What suggestions/recommendations would you make to her?
   c. What instructions need to be given to guide her decision making?
   d. What other premonitory signs of labor might the nurse ask about?
   e. What manifestations would be found if Cindy is experiencing true labor?
2. You are assigned to lead a community education class for women in their third trimester of pregnancy to prepare them for their upcoming birth. Prepare an outline of topics that should be addressed.

STUDY ACTIVITIES

1. During clinical post-conference, share with the other nursing students how the critical forces of labor influenced the length of labor and the birthing process for a laboring woman assigned to you.
2. The cardinal movements of labor include which of the following? Select all that apply.
   a. Extension and rotation
   b. Descent and engagement
   c. Presentation and position
   d. Attitude and lie
   e. Flexion and expulsion

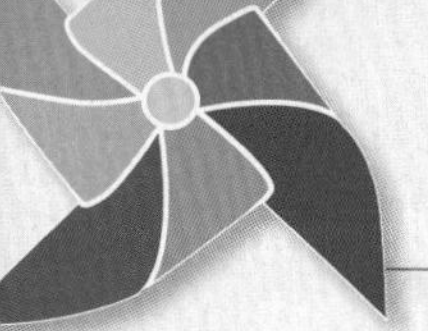

CHAPTER WORKSHEET

3. Interview a woman on the mother–baby unit who has given birth within the past few hours. Ask her to describe her experience and examine psychological factors that may have influenced her laboring process.

4. On the following illustration, identify the parameters of uterine contractions by marking an "X" where the nurse would measure the duration of the contraction.

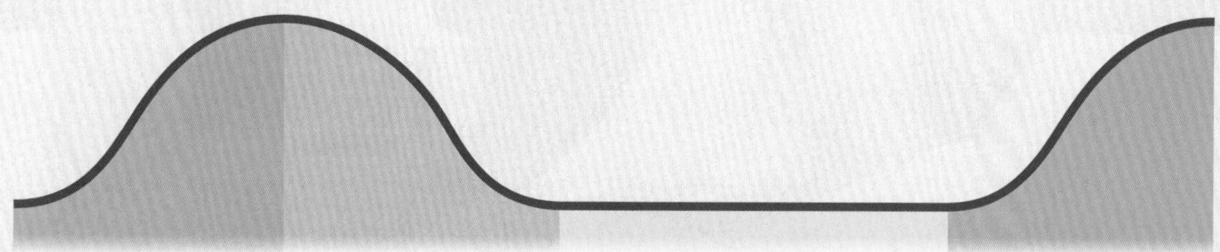

BRINGING IT ALL TOGETHER: A CASE STUDY

Moritza is a 20-year-old pregnant female who comes to the prenatal clinic with her boyfriend for her prenatal visit at 39 weeks' gestation. This is her first pregnancy and she has missed several of her previous prenatal office visits. Her pregnancy has been uneventful thus far, but she is concerned today about impending labor and how she will know when to go to the hospital. She feels unprepared for labor and admits she is very afraid of the pain since many of her friends and family members have shared their 'horror' stories about their experiences. She admits she is scared about having an IV in her arm at the hospital. She wants a normal physiologic childbirth.

Go to thePoint **to find questions to consider about this case.**

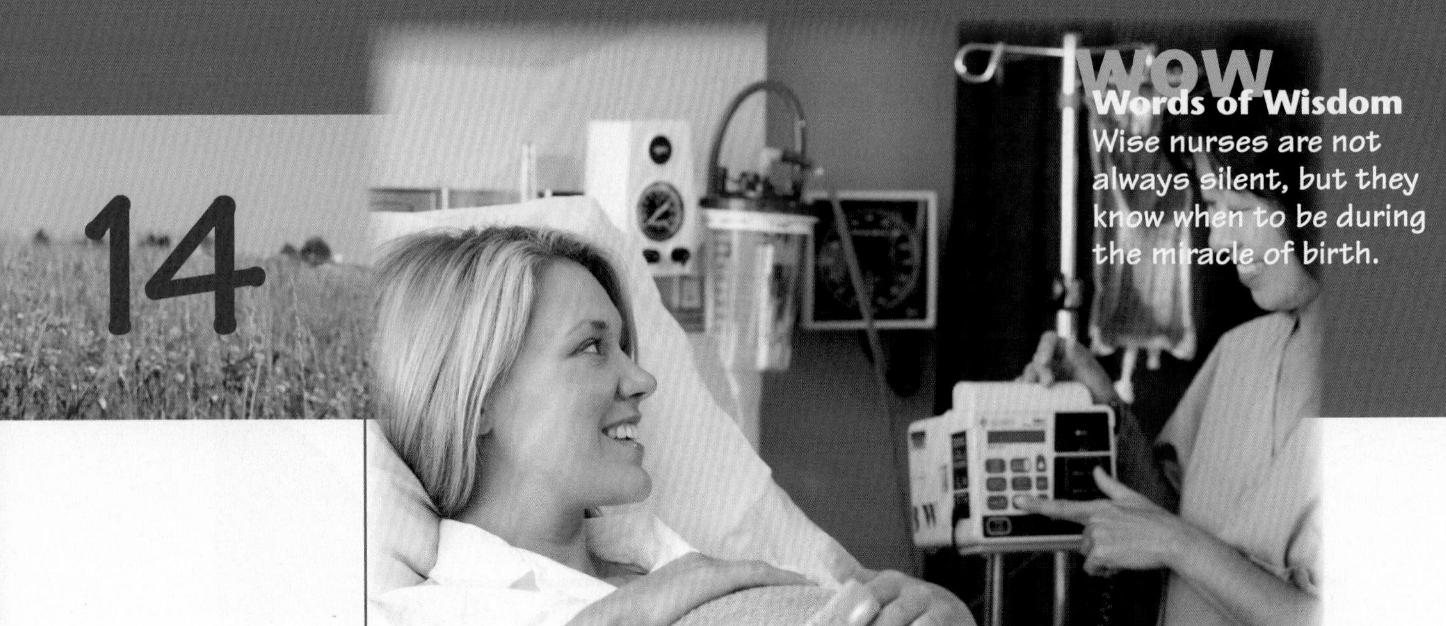

Nursing Management During Labor and Birth

KEY TERMS

accelerations
artifact
baseline fetal heart rate
baseline variability
crowning
deceleration
electronic fetal monitoring (EFM)
episiotomy
Leopold maneuvers
neuraxial analgesia/anesthesia
periodic baseline changes

Learning Objectives

1. Examine the measures used to evaluate maternal status during labor and birth.
2. Differentiate the advantages and disadvantages of external and internal fetal monitoring, including the appropriate use for each.
3. Choose appropriate nursing interventions to address nonreassuring fetal heart rate patterns.
4. Outline the nurse's role in fetal assessment.
5. Appraise the various comfort promotion and pain relief strategies used during labor and birth.
6. Summarize the assessment data collected on admission to the perinatal unit.
7. Relate the ongoing assessments involved in each stage of labor and birth.
8. Analyze the nurse's role throughout the labor and birth process.

Sheila **was admitted in active labor to the labor and birth unit. She has progressed to the transition phase (dilated 8 cm) and is becoming increasingly more uncomfortable. She is using a patterned-paced breathing pattern now, but is thrashing around in the hospital bed.**

INTRODUCTION

The laboring and birthing process is a life-changing event for many women. Nurses need to be respectful, available, encouraging, supportive, and professional in dealing with all women. Nursing management for labor and birth involves assessment, comfort measures, emotional support, information and instruction, advocacy, and support for the partner. Providing the highest quality in maternity care is dependent on nurses valuing the childbirth experience and recognizing it as a life-changing experience for women and their families; caring nurse practice encompasses technical skills and caring behaviors; giving care that protects, promotes, and supports physiologic childbirth; providing optimal, evidence-based care; and recognizing health disparity and cultural diversity in all women cared for to improve their childbirth experience across time, settings, and disciplines. One of the components for evidence-based care and woman-centered care is women's preferences to guide their own care during the birthing process. In a recent study, women's needs and expectations during labor and birth were assessed. Seven themes emerged—physiologic needs (nutrition, room environment, hygiene, comfort, and privacy); psychologic needs (empathy and advocacy, constant emotional support and encouragement); informational needs (about labor process and hospital policies); communication needs (health care provider and familiar attendant); esteem needs (sense of value, confidence, involvement in decisions); security needs (calming fears); and medical needs (pain relief and prevention of unnecessary interventions during labor and birth) (Iravani et al., 2015). It is important that nurses identify the expectations and needs of women in their care, so as to empower them to fully participate in their childbirth experience.

The health of mothers and their infants is of critical importance, both as a reflection of the current health status of a large segment of our population and as a predictor of the health of the next generation. The United States Department of Health and Human Services [USDHHS] (2010) addresses maternal health in two objectives: reducing maternal deaths and reducing maternal illness and complications due to pregnancy (complications during hospitalized labor and delivery). In addition, two more objectives address increasing the proportion of pregnant women who receive early and adequate prenatal care. A goal in development seeks to increase the proportion of pregnant women who attend a series of prepared childbirth classes. (See Chapter 12 for more information on these objectives.)

This chapter provides information about nursing management during labor and birth. First, the essentials for in-depth assessment of maternal and fetal status during labor and birth are discussed. This is followed by a thorough description of the major methods of promoting comfort and providing pain management during the labor and birth process. The chapter concludes by putting all the information together with a discussion of the nursing care specific to each stage of labor, including the necessary data to be obtained with the admission assessment, methods to evaluate labor progress during the first stage of labor, and key nursing measures that focus on maternal and fetal assessments and pain relief for all stages of labor.

MATERNAL ASSESSMENT DURING LABOR AND BIRTH

During labor and birth, various techniques are used to assess maternal status. These techniques provide an ongoing source of data to determine the woman's response and her progress in labor:

- Assess maternal vital signs, including temperature, blood pressure, pulse, respiration, and pain, which are primary components of the physical examination and ongoing assessment.
- Also review the prenatal record to identify risk factors that may contribute to a decrease in uteroplacental circulation during labor.
- If there is no vaginal bleeding on admission, a vaginal examination is performed to assess cervical dilation, after which it is monitored periodically as necessary to identify progress.
- Evaluate maternal pain and the effectiveness of pain management strategies at regular intervals during labor and birth.

Vaginal Examination

The World Health Organization [WHO] recommends digital vaginal examinations at intervals of 4 hours for routine assessment and identification of a delay in active labor (2014). Although not all nurses perform vaginal examinations on laboring women in all practice settings, most nurses working in community hospitals do so because physicians are not routinely present in labor and birth suites. Since most newborns in the United States are born in community hospitals, nurses are performing vaginal examinations along with midwives and physicians (American Hospital Association, 2015).

Take Note!

A vaginal examination is an assessment skill that takes time and experience to develop; only by doing it frequently in clinical practice can the practitioner's skill level improve.

The purpose of performing a vaginal examination is to assess the amount of cervical dilation, the percentage of cervical effacement, and the fetal membrane status and to gather information on presentation, position,

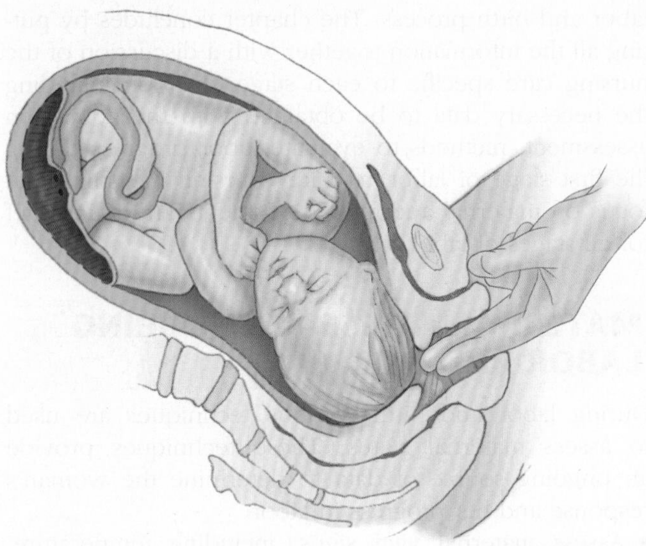

FIGURE 14.1 Vaginal examination to determine cervical dilation and effacement.

station, degree of fetal head flexion, and presence of fetal skull swelling or molding (Fig. 14.1). Prepare the woman by informing her about the procedure, what information will be obtained from it, how she can assist with the procedure, how it will be performed, and who will be performing it.

The woman is typically on her back during the vaginal examination. The vaginal examination is performed gently, with concern for the woman's comfort. If it is the initial vaginal examination to check for membrane status, water is used as a lubricant.

After donning sterile gloves, the examiner inserts his or her index and middle fingers into the vaginal introitus. Next, the cervix is palpated to assess dilation, effacement, and position (e.g., posterior or anterior). If the cervix is open to any degree, the presenting fetal part, fetal position, station, and presence of molding can be assessed. In addition, the membranes can be evaluated and described as intact, bulging, or ruptured.

At the conclusion of the vaginal examination, the findings are discussed with the woman and her partner to bring them up to date about labor progress. In addition, the findings are documented either electronically or in writing and reported to the primary health care provider in charge of the case.

Cervical Dilation and Effacement

The amount of cervical dilation (opening) and the degree of cervical effacement (thinning) are key areas assessed during the vaginal examination as the cervix is palpated with the gloved index finger. Although this finding is somewhat subjective, experienced examiners typically come up with similar findings. The width of the cervical opening determines dilation, and the length of the cervix assesses effacement. Effacement and dilation are used to assess cervical changes as follows:

- Effacement:
  - 0%: cervical canal is 2 cm long
  - 50%: cervical canal is 1 cm long
  - 100%: cervical canal is obliterated
- Dilation:
  - 0 cm: external cervical os is closed
  - 5 cm: external cervical os is halfway dilated
  - 10 cm: external os is fully dilated and ready for birth passage

The information yielded by this examination serves as a basis for determining which stage of labor the woman is in and what her ongoing care should be.

Fetal Descent and Presenting Part

In addition to cervical dilation and effacement findings, the vaginal examination can also determine fetal descent (station) and presenting part. During the vaginal examination, the gloved index finger is used to palpate the fetal skull (if vertex presentation) through the opened cervix or the buttocks in the case of a breech presentation. Station is assessed in relation to the maternal ischial spines and the presenting fetal part. These spines are not sharp protrusions but rather blunted prominences at the midpelvis. The ischial spines serve as landmarks and have been designated as zero station. If the presenting part is palpated higher than the maternal ischial spines, a negative number is assigned; if the presenting fetal part is felt below the maternal ischial spines, a plus number is assigned, denoting how many centimeters below zero station (see Chapter 13 for a more detailed discussion).

Progressive fetal descent (–5 to +4) is the expected norm during labor—moving downward from the negative stations to zero station to the positive stations in a timely manner. If progressive fetal descent does not occur, a disproportion between the maternal pelvis and the fetus might exist and needs to be investigated.

Rupture of Membranes

The integrity of the membranes can be determined during the vaginal examination. Typically, if intact, the membranes will be felt as a soft bulge that is more prominent during a contraction. If the membranes have ruptured, the woman may have reported a sudden gush of fluid. Membrane rupture also may occur as a slow trickle of fluid. When membranes rupture, the priority focus should be on assessing fetal heart rate (FHR) first to identify a **deceleration**, which might indicate cord compression secondary to cord prolapse. If the membranes are ruptured when the woman comes to the hospital, the health care provider should ascertain when it occurred. Prolonged ruptured membranes increase the risk of infection as a result of ascending vaginal pathologic organisms for both mother and fetus. Signs of intrauterine infection to be alert for include maternal fever, fetal and maternal tachycardia, foul odor of vaginal discharge, and an increase in white blood cell count.

To confirm that membranes have ruptured, a sample of fluid is taken from the vagina via a nitrazine yellow dye swab to determine the fluid's pH. Vaginal fluid is acidic, whereas amniotic fluid is alkaline and turns a nitrazine swab blue. Sometimes, however, false-positive results can occur, especially in women experiencing a large amount of bloody show, because blood is alkaline. The membranes are most likely intact if the nitrazine swab remains yellow to olive green, with pH between 5 and 6. The membranes are probably ruptured if the nitrazine swab turns a blue-green to deep blue, with pH ranging from 6.5 to 7.5 (Tharpe, Farley, & Jordan, 2016).

If the nitrazine test is inconclusive, an additional test, called the *fern test*, can be used to confirm rupture of membranes. With this test, a sample of vaginal fluid is obtained, applied to a microscope slide, and allowed to dry. Using a microscope, the slide is examined for a characteristic fern pattern that indicates the presence of amniotic fluid.

Assessing Uterine Contractions

The primary power of labor is uterine contractions, which are involuntary. Uterine contractions increase intrauterine pressure, causing tension on the cervix. This tension leads to cervical dilation and thinning, which in turn eventually forces the fetus through the birth canal. Normal uterine contractions have a contraction (systole) and a relaxation (diastole) phase. The contraction resembles a wave, moving downward to the cervix and upward to the fundus of the uterus. Each contraction starts with a building up (increment), gradually reaching an acme (peak intensity), and then a letting down (decrement). Each contraction is followed by an interval of rest, which ends when the next contraction begins. At the acme (peak) of the contraction, the entire uterus is contracting, with the greatest intensity in the fundal area. The relaxation phase follows and occurs simultaneously throughout the uterus.

Uterine contractions during labor are monitored by palpation and by electronic monitoring. Assessment of the contractions includes frequency, duration, intensity, and uterine resting tone (see Chapter 13 for a more detailed discussion). Uterine contractions with intensity of 30 mm Hg or greater initiate cervical dilation. During active labor, the intensity usually reaches 50 to 80 mm Hg. Resting tone is normally between 5 and 10 mm Hg in early labor and between 12 and 18 mm Hg in active labor (Hiersch et al., 2015).

To palpate the fundus for contraction intensity, place the pads of your fingers on the fundus and describe

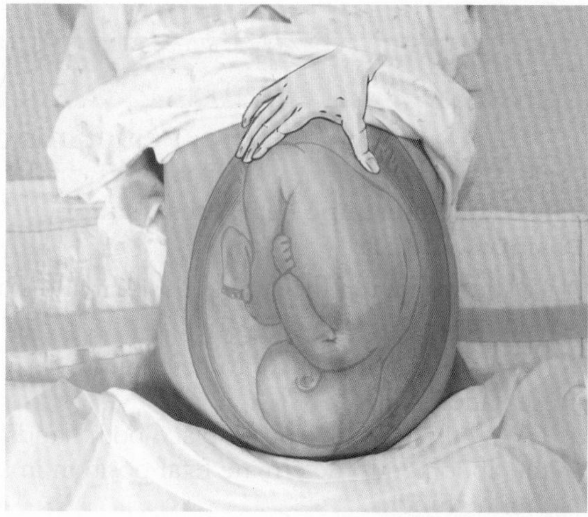

FIGURE 14.2 Nurse palpating the woman's fundus during a contraction.

how it feels: like the tip of the nose (mild), like the chin (moderate), or like the forehead (strong). Palpation of intensity is a subjective judgment of the indentability of the uterine wall; a descriptive term is assigned (mild, moderate, or strong) (Fig. 14.2).

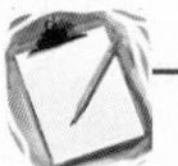

Take Note!

Frequent clinical experience is needed to gain accuracy in assessing the intensity of uterine contractions.

The second method used to assess the intensity of uterine contractions is electronic monitoring, either external or internal. Both methods provide a reasonable measurement of the intensity of uterine contractions. Although the external fetal monitor is sometimes used to estimate the intensity of uterine contractions, it is not as accurate an assessment tool.

Performing Leopold Maneuvers

Leopold maneuvers are a method for determining the presentation, position, and lie of the fetus through the use of four specific steps. This method involves inspection and palpation of the maternal abdomen as a screening assessment for malpresentation. A longitudinal lie is expected, and the presentation can be cephalic, breech, or shoulder. Each maneuver answers a question:

- *Maneuver 1*: What fetal part (head or buttocks) is located in the fundus (top of the uterus)?
- *Maneuver 2*: On which maternal side is the fetal back located? (Fetal heart tones are best auscultated through the back of the fetus.)
- *Maneuver 3*: What is the presenting part?
- *Maneuver 4*: Is the fetal head flexed and engaged in the pelvis?

Leopold maneuvers are described in Nursing Procedure 14.1. Also see Chapter 12.

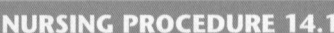

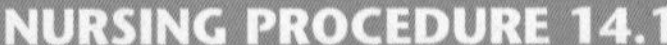

NURSING PROCEDURE 14.1

Performing Leopold Maneuvers

Purpose: To Determine Fetal Presentation, Position, and Lie

1. Place the woman in the supine position and stand beside her.
2. Perform the first maneuver to determine presentation.
   a. Facing the woman's head, place both hands on the abdomen to determine fetal position in the uterine fundus.
   b. Feel for the buttocks, which will feel soft and irregular (indicates vertex presentation); feel for the head, which will feel hard, smooth, and round (indicates a breech presentation).

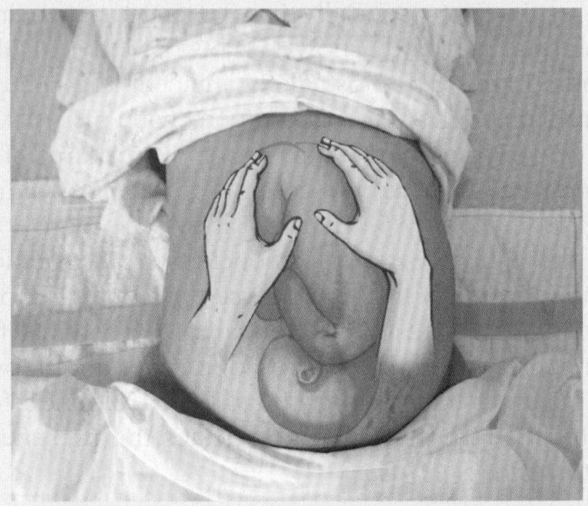

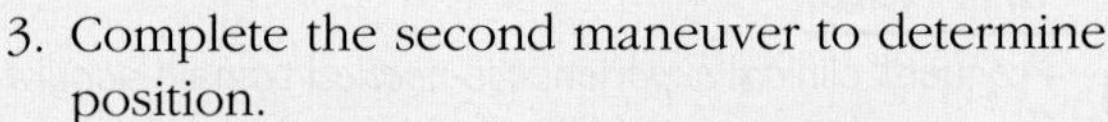

3. Complete the second maneuver to determine position.
   a. While still facing the woman, move hands down the lateral sides of the abdomen to palpate on which side the back is located (feels hard and smooth).
   b. Continue to palpate to determine on which side the limbs are located (irregular nodules with kicking and movement).

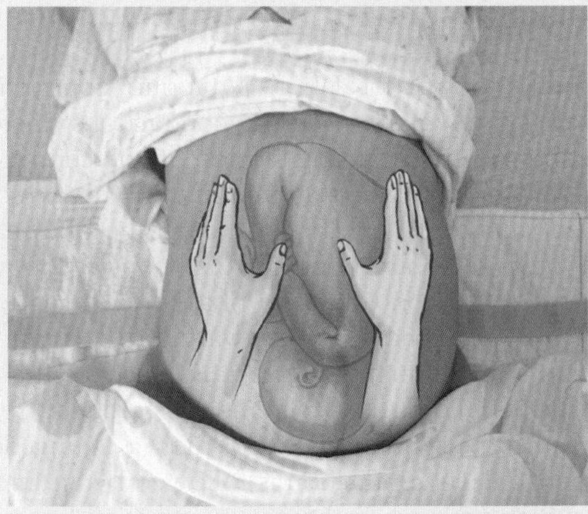

4. Perform the third maneuver to confirm presentation.
   a. Move hands down the sides of the abdomen to grasp the lower uterine segment and palpate the area just above the symphysis pubis.
   b. Place thumb and fingers of one hand apart and grasp the presenting part by bringing fingers together.
   c. Feel for the presenting part. If the presenting part is the head, it will be round, firm, and ballottable; if it is the buttocks, it will feel soft and irregular.

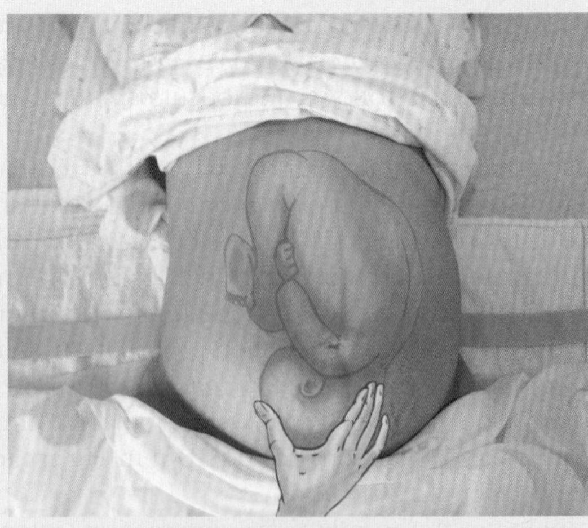

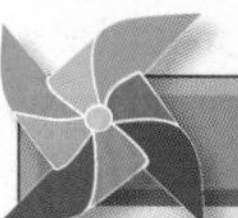

NURSING PROCEDURE 14.1

Performing Leopold Maneuvers (continued)

5. Perform the fourth maneuver to determine attitude.
   a. Turn to face the client's feet and use the tips of the first three fingers of each hand to palpate the abdomen.
   b. Move fingers toward each other while applying downward pressure in the direction of the symphysis pubis. If you palpate a hard area on the side opposite the fetal back, the fetus is in flexion, because you have palpated the chin. If the hard area is on the same side as the back, the fetus is in extension, because the area palpated is the occiput.

Also, note how your hands move. If the hands move together easily, the fetal head is not descended into the woman's pelvic inlet. If the hands do not move together and stop because of resistance, the fetal head is engaged into the woman's pelvic inlet (Walker & Sabrosa, 2014).

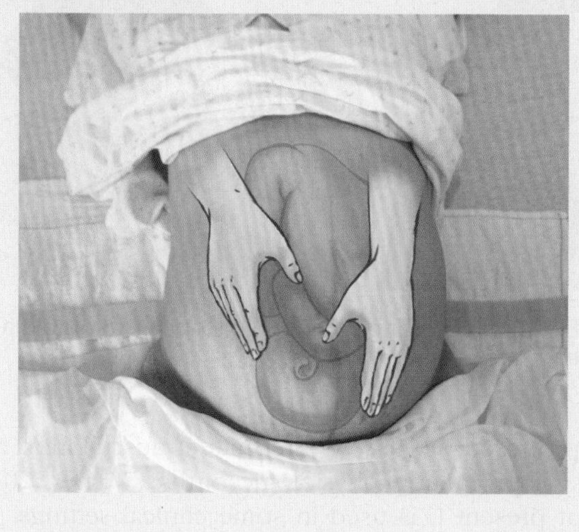

FETAL ASSESSMENT DURING LABOR AND BIRTH

A fetal assessment identifies well-being or signs that indicate compromise. The character of the amniotic fluid is assessed, but the fetal assessment focuses primarily on determining the FHR pattern. Umbilical cord blood analysis and fetal scalp stimulation are additional assessments performed as necessary in the case of questionable FHR patterns.

Analysis of Amniotic Fluid

Amniotic fluid should be clear when the membranes rupture. Rupturing of membranes is either spontaneous or artificial by means of an amniotomy, during which a disposable plastic hook (an amnihook) is used to perforate the amniotic sac. Cloudy or foul-smelling amniotic fluid indicates infection. Green fluid may indicate that the fetus has passed meconium secondary to transient hypoxia, prolonged pregnancy, cord compression, intrauterine growth restriction (IUGR), maternal hypertension, diabetes, or chorioamnionitis; however, it is considered a normal occurrence if the fetus is in a breech presentation. If it is determined that meconium-stained amniotic fluid is due to fetal hypoxia, the maternity and pediatric teams work together to prevent meconium aspiration syndrome. This would necessitate suctioning after the head is born before the infant takes a breath and perhaps direct tracheal suctioning after birth if the Apgar score is low. In some cases an amnioinfusion (introduction of warmed, sterile normal saline or Ringer lactate solution into the uterus) is used to dilute moderate to heavy meconium released in utero to assist in preventing meconium aspiration syndrome.

Analysis of the FHR

Analysis of the FHR is one of the primary evaluation tools used to determine fetal oxygen status indirectly. FHR assessment can be done intermittently using a fetoscope (a modified stethoscope attached to a headpiece) or a Doppler (ultrasound) device, or continuously with an electronic fetal monitor applied externally or internally. The object of FHR monitoring is to reduce the mortality/morbidity by ensuring that all fetal hypoxic insults are identified in time to allow removal or alteration of the reason for it, or to enable a safe birth of the fetus before irreversible asphyxia damage occurs (Hastings, 2015).

Intermittent FHR Monitoring

Intermittent FHR monitoring involves auscultation via a fetoscope or a handheld Doppler device that uses ultrasound waves that bounce off the fetal heart, producing echoes or clicks that reflect the rate of the fetal heart (Fig. 14.3). Traditionally, a fetoscope was used to assess FHR, but the handheld Doppler device has been found to have a greater sensitivity than the fetoscope. Intermittent auscultation of the FHR is an acceptable option for low-risk laboring women, yet it is underutilized in the hospital setting. Recently several professional organizations

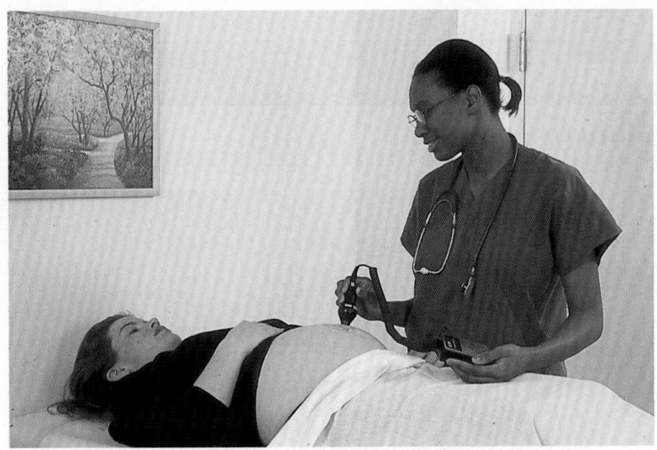

FIGURE 14.3 Nurse using a handheld Doppler to obtain a fetal heart rate.

have proposed the use of intermittent auscultation as a means of promoting physiologic births (Wisner, 2015); thus, at present it is used in some clinical settings. See Evidence-Based Practice 14.1 for more information.

Take Note!

Doppler devices to detect FHRs are relatively low in cost and are used in hospitals and in home births and birthing centers routinely. Many nurses use them in their work settings.

Intermittent FHR monitoring allows the woman to be mobile in the first stage of labor. She is free to move around and change position at will since she is not attached to a stationary electronic fetal monitor. However, intermittent monitoring does not provide a continuous FHR recording and does not document how the fetus responds to the stress of labor (unless listening is done during the contraction). The best way to assess fetal well-being would be to start listening to the FHR at the end of the contraction (not after one) so that late decelerations could be detected. However, the pressure of the device during a contraction is uncomfortable and can distract the woman from using her paced-breathing patterns.

Intermittent FHR auscultation can be used to detect FHR baseline and rhythm and changes from baseline. However, it cannot detect variability and types of decelerations, as **electronic fetal monitoring (EFM)** can (Wisner, 2015). During intermittent auscultation to establish a baseline, the FHR is assessed for a full minute after a contraction. From then on, unless there is a problem, listening for 30 seconds and multiplying the value by two is sufficient. If the woman experiences a change in condition during labor, auscultation assessments should be more frequent. Changes in condition include ruptured membranes or the onset of bleeding. In addition, more frequent assessments occur after periods of ambulation, a vaginal examination, administration of pain medications, or other clinically important events (King et al., 2015).

The FHR is heard most clearly at the fetal back. In a cephalic presentation, the FHR is best heard in the lower quadrant of the maternal abdomen. In a breech presentation, it is heard at or above the level of the maternal umbilicus (Fig. 14.4). As labor progresses, the FHR location will change accordingly as the fetus descends into the maternal pelvis for the birthing

EVIDENCE-BASED PRACTICE 14.1 INTRAPARTUM FETAL MONITORING

STUDY

Electronic fetal monitoring is a widely utilized means of assessing fetal status during labor and has been a central component of intrapartum care. Currently, electronic fetal monitoring (EFM) is the most common method used to evaluate the fetus during labor without substantial evidence to suggest a benefit. Clinicians spend valuable time and energy trying to characterize and distinguish between different types of FHR decelerations even though most of them have been shown to have little association with fetal acidosis. The purpose of this review was to determine if continuous electronic fetal monitoring versus intermittent auscultation improved perinatal outcomes.

Findings

A Cochrane review of 13 trials, which included over 37,000 women, found that continuous EFM provided no significant improvement in perinatal death rate (risk rate 0.86; confidence interval 0.59–1.23) or cerebral palsy rate (risk rate 1.75; confidence interval 0.84–3.63) as compared with intermittent auscultation; however, there was a significant increase in cesarean births (risk rate 1.63; confidence interval 1.29–2.07) and operative vaginal births (risk rate 1.15; confidence interval 1.01–1.33).

Nursing Implications

Despite the lack of scientific evidence to support routinely using continuous electronic fetal monitoring to reduce adverse perinatal outcomes, its use is almost universal in the hospital setting and very likely has contributed to the rise in cesarean birth rates. Nurses are uniquely positioned to influence the monitoring method used in labor by offering intermittent auscultation to low-risk women, and requesting orders from the health care providers that include it as an option. The high-touch nature of intermittent auscultation may help nurses reconnect to their clients and to the essence of nursing practice.

Adapted from Cahill, A. G., & Spain, J. (2015). Intrapartum fetal monitoring. *Clinical Obstetrics and Gynecology, 58*(2), 263–268.

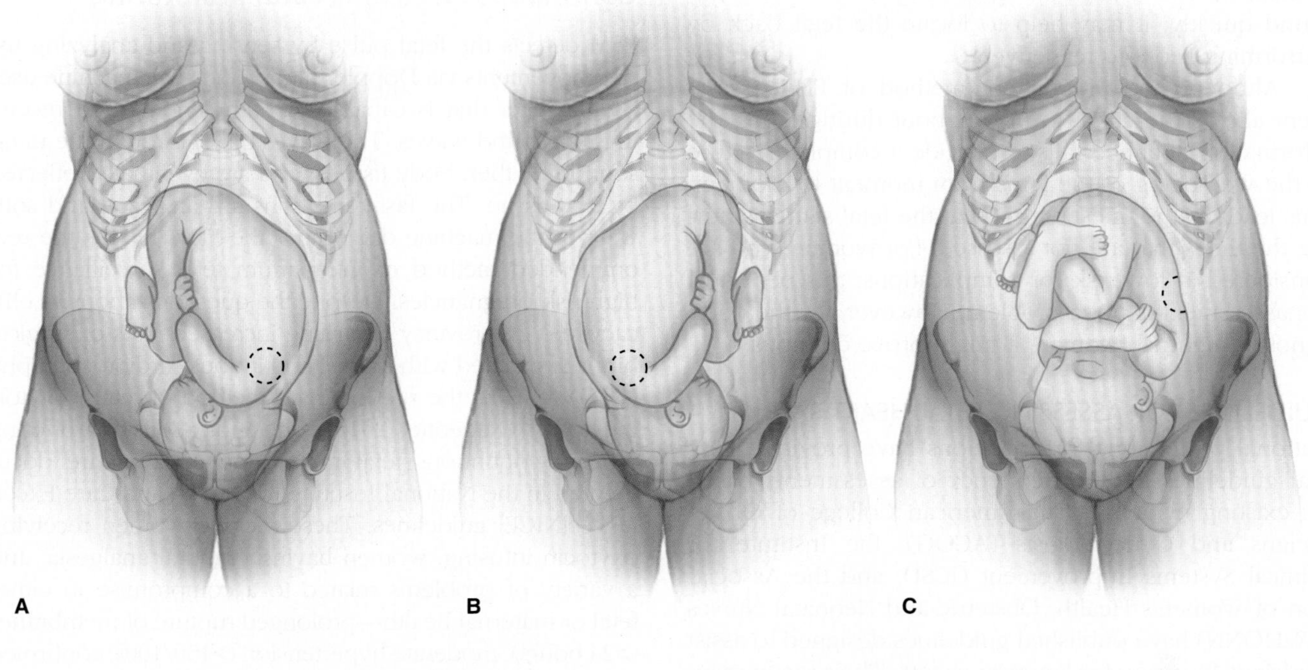

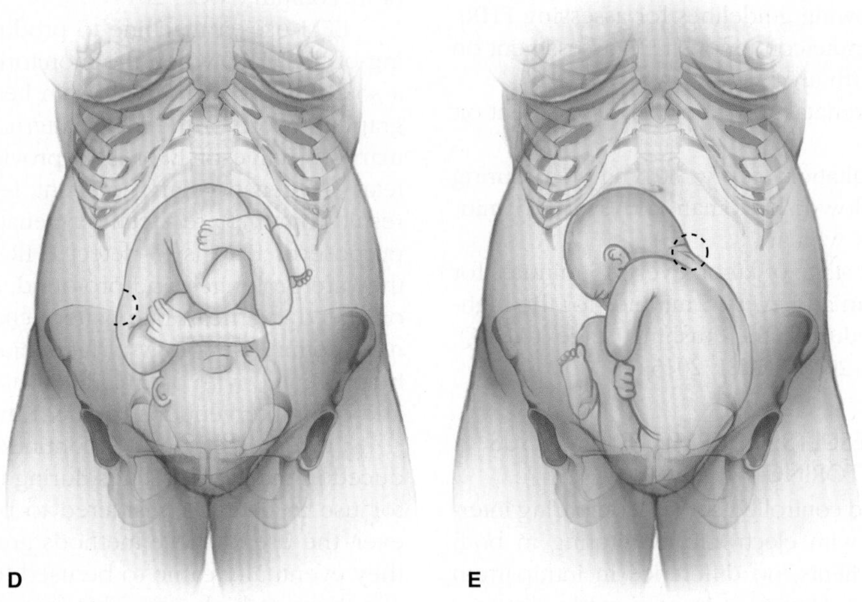

FIGURE 14.4 Locations for auscultating fetal heart rate based on fetal position. **A.** Left occiput anterior (LOA). **B.** Right occiput anterior (ROA). **C.** Left occiput posterior (LOP). **D.** Right occiput posterior (ROP). **E.** Left sacral anterior (LSA).

process. To ensure that the maternal heart rate is not confused with the FHR, palpate the client's radial pulse simultaneously while the FHR is being auscultated through the abdomen.

For low-risk women, the FHR and contraction characteristics should be assessed every 15 to 30 minutes in active labor and every 5 to 15 minutes while pushing, as well as before and after any digital vaginal examinations, membrane rupture, medication administered, and ambulation to the restroom (Freeman, 2015).

Nursing Procedure 12.1 in Chapter 12 lists detailed steps for using a Doppler device to assess FHR. In brief, a small amount of water-soluble gel is applied to the woman's abdomen or ultrasound device before auscultation with the Doppler device to promote sound wave transmission. Usually the FHR is best heard in the woman's lower abdominal quadrants; if the FHR is not found quickly, it may help to locate the fetal back by performing Leopold maneuvers.

Although the intermittent method of FHR assessment allows the client to move about during labor, the information obtained fails to provide a complete picture of the well-being of the fetus from moment to moment. This leads to the question of what the fetal status is during the times that are not assessed. For women who are considered at low risk for complications, this period of nonassessment is not a problem. However, for the undiagnosed high-risk woman, it might prove ominous.

GUIDELINES FOR ASSESSING FETAL HEART RATE

National professional organizations have provided general guidelines for the frequency of assessments based on existing evidence. The American College of Obstetricians and Gynecologists (ACOG), the Institute for Clinical Systems Improvement (ICSI), and the Association of Women's Health, Obstetric and Neonatal Nurses (AWHONN) have published guidelines designed to assist clinicians in caring for laboring clients. Their recommendations are supported by large controlled studies. They recommend the following guidelines for assessing FHR:

- Initial 10- to 20-minute continuous FHR assessment on entry into labor/birth area
- Completion of a prenatal and labor risk assessment on all clients
- Intermittent auscultation every 30 minutes during active labor for a low-risk woman and every 15 minutes for a high-risk woman
- During the second stage of labor, every 15 minutes for the low-risk woman and every 5 minutes for the high-risk woman and during the pushing stage (AHRQ, 2014); (AWHONN, 2015); (ICSI, 2015a).

EVIDENCE-BASED RESULTS: INTERMITTENT VERSUS ELECTRONIC MONITORING

In several randomized controlled studies comparing intermittent auscultation with electronic monitoring in both low- and high-risk clients, no difference in intrapartum fetal death was found. However, in each study a nurse–client ratio of 1:1 was consistently maintained during labor (ICSI, 2015a). This suggests that adequate staffing is essential with intermittent FHR monitoring to ensure optimal outcomes for the mother and fetus. There is insufficient evidence to indicate specific situations where continuous electronic FHR monitoring might result in better outcomes when compared to intermittent assessment. However, in pregnancies involving an increased risk of perinatal death, cerebral palsy, or neonatal encephalopathy and when oxytocin is used for induction or augmentation, it is recommended that continuous EFM be used rather than intermittent fetal auscultation (Society of Obstetricians and Gynecologists of Canada, 2015).

Continuous Electronic Fetal Monitoring

EFM detects the fetal pulse by sensing and analyzing tissue movements via Doppler ultrasound. The machine uses a transducer that is capable of both sending and receiving ultrasound waves. The waves travel through the ultrasound gel, then body tissues, and are eventually reflected by any tissue. The fast reflections are analyzed and software in the machine determines the FHR. EFM is the recommended method of intrapartum fetal surveillance for high-risk pregnancies. Despite the questions about its efficacy and controversy regarding increased rates of surgical births associated with its use, continuous cardiotocography (CTG) remains the predominant method of fetal monitoring today (Nageotte, 2015). The indications for offering women continuous fetal monitoring in labor are documented in the National Institute for Health and Care Excellence [NICE] guidelines. These include women receiving oxytocin infusing; women having epidural analgesia; and a variety of problems related to a compromise in either fetal or maternal health—prolonged rupture of membranes (>24 hours), moderate hypertension (>150/100), confirmed delay in the first or second stage of labor; and the presence of meconium (NICE, 2014).

EFM uses a machine to produce a continuous tracing of the FHR. When the monitoring device is in place, a sound is produced with each heartbeat. In addition, a graphic record of the FHR pattern is produced. The primary objective of EFM is to provide information about fetal oxygenation and prevent fetal injury that could result from impaired fetal oxygenation during labor. The purpose of EFM is to detect FHR changes early before they are prolonged and profound. Fetal hypoxia is demonstrated in a heart rate pattern change and is by far the most common etiology of fetal injury and death that can be prevented with optimal fetal surveillance during labor and early interventions (Cox & King, 2015).

Current methods of continuous EFM were introduced in the United States during the 1970s, specifically for use in clients considered to be at high risk. However, the use of these methods gradually increased and they eventually came to be used for women other than just those at high risk. This increased use has become controversial because it is suspected of being associated with the steadily increasing rates of cesarean births with no decrease in the rate of cerebral palsy (Omo-Aghoja, 2015). Many studies suggest that when compared with standardized intermittent auscultation, the use of intrapartum continuous EFM seems to increase the number of preterm and surgical births but has no significant effect on reducing the incidence of intrapartum death or long-term neurologic injury. When a woman is admitted to the labor unit, a fetal monitor is applied and the FHR is monitored continuously. An impetus for this is the litigious nature of current society, but the benefits have not been proven scientifically. EFM has been given excessive importance in legal cases. Before assigning fault on events at birth, a better understanding of developmental neurobiology and limitations of the present biomarkers is warranted (Freeman, 2015). To date, continuous EFM is not evidence based for determining fetal health status.

With EFM, there is a continuous record of the FHR: no gaps exist, as they do with intermittent auscultation. The concept of hearing and evaluating every beat of the fetus's heart to allow for early intervention seems logical. On the downside, however, using continuous monitoring can limit maternal movement and encourages the woman to lie in the supine position, which reduces placental perfusion. Despite the criticisms, EFM remains an accurate method for determining fetal health status by providing a moment-to-moment printout of FHR status.

Various groups within the medical community have criticized the use of continuous fetal monitoring for all pregnant clients, whether high risk or low risk. Concerns about the efficiency and safety of routine EFM in labor have led expert panels in the United States to recommend that such monitoring be limited to high-risk pregnancies. However, its use in low-risk pregnancies continues globally (Maso et al., 2015; Prior & Kumar, 2015). This remains an important research issue.

Continuous EFM can be performed externally (indirectly), with the equipment attached to the maternal abdominal wall, or internally (directly), with the equipment attached to the fetus. Both methods provide a continuous printout of the FHR, but they differ in their specificity. The efficacy of EFM depends on the accurate interpretation of the tracings, not necessarily which method (external vs. internal) is used.

CONTINUOUS EXTERNAL MONITORING

In external or indirect monitoring, two ultrasound transducers, each of which is attached to a belt, are applied around the woman's abdomen. They are similar to the handheld Doppler device. One transducer is called a tocotransducer, a pressure-sensitive device that is applied against the uterine fundus. It detects changes in uterine pressure and converts the pressure registered into an electronic signal that is recorded on graph paper (Farine, 2015). The tocotransducer is placed over the uterine fundus in the area of greatest contractility to monitor uterine contractions. The other ultrasound transducer records the baseline FHR, long-term variability, **accelerations**, and decelerations. It is positioned on the maternal abdomen in the midline between the umbilicus and the symphysis pubis. The diaphragm of the ultrasound transducer is moved to either side of the abdomen to obtain a stronger sound and is then attached to the second elastic belt. This transducer converts the fetal heart movements into beeping sounds and records them on graph paper (Fig. 14.5).

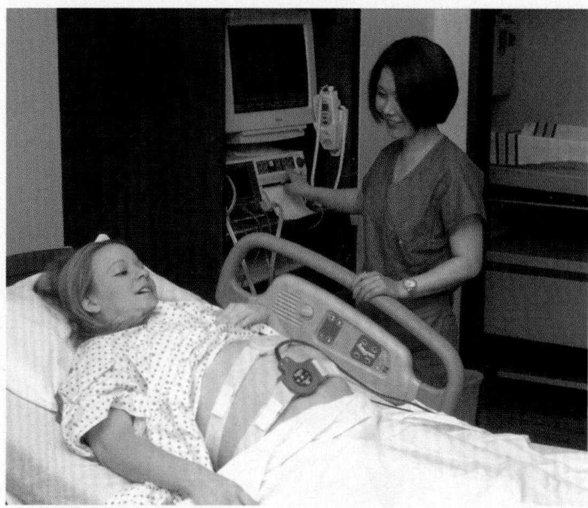

FIGURE 14.5 Continuous external electronic fetal monitoring device applied to the woman in labor.

Good continuous data are provided on the FHR. External monitoring can be used while the membranes are still intact and the cervix is not yet dilated, but also can be used with ruptured membranes and a dilating cervix. It is noninvasive and can detect relative changes in abdominal pressure between uterine resting tone and contractions. External monitoring also measures the approximate duration and frequency of contractions, providing a permanent record of FHR (Casanova, 2015).

However, external monitoring can restrict the mother's movements. It also cannot detect short-term variability. Signal disruptions can occur due to maternal obesity, fetal malpresentation, and fetal movement as well as by **artifact**. The term *artifact* is used to describe irregular variations or absence of the FHR on the fetal monitor record that result from mechanical limitations of the monitor or electrical interference. For instance, the monitor may pick up transmissions from citizen's band (CB) radios used by truck drivers on nearby roads and translate them into a signal. Additionally, gaps in the monitor strip can occur periodically without explanation.

CONTINUOUS INTERNAL MONITORING

Continuous internal monitoring is usually indicated for women or fetuses considered to be at high risk. Possible conditions might include multiple gestation, decreased fetal movement, abnormal FHR on auscultation, IUGR, maternal fever, preeclampsia, dysfunctional labor, preterm birth, or medical conditions such as diabetes or hypertension. It involves the placement of a spiral electrode into the fetal presenting part, usually the head, to assess FHR, and a pressure transducer placed internally within the uterus to record uterine contractions (Fig. 14.6). The fetal spiral electrode is considered the most accurate method of detecting fetal heart characteristics and patterns because it involves receiving a signal directly from the fetus (Nageotte, 2015). Specially trained labor and

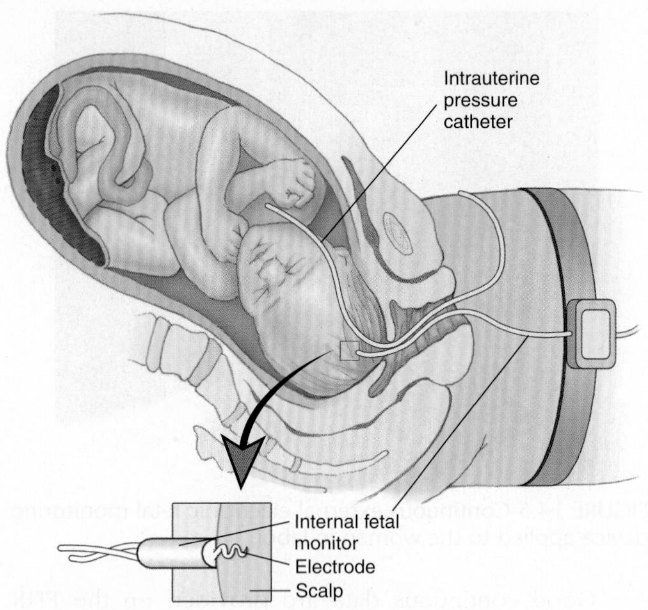

FIGURE 14.6 Continuous internal electronic fetal monitoring.

birth nurses are permitted to place the spiral electrode on the fetal head when the membranes rupture to assess the FHR in some health care facilities, but they do not place the intrauterine pressure catheter in the uterus. Internal monitoring does not have to include both an intrauterine pressure catheter and a scalp electrode. A fetal scalp electrode can be used to monitor the fetal heartbeat without monitoring the maternal intrauterine pressure.

Both the FHR and the duration and interval of uterine contractions are recorded on the graph paper. This method permits evaluation of baseline heart rate and changes in rate and pattern.

Four specific criteria must be met for this type of monitoring to be used:

- Ruptured membranes
- Cervical dilation of at least 2 cm
- Presenting fetal part low enough to allow placement of the scalp electrode
- Skilled practitioner available to insert spiral electrode (ICSI, 2015b).

Compared with external monitoring, continuous internal monitoring can accurately detect both short-term (moment-to-moment) changes and variability (fluctuations within the baseline) and FHR dysrhythmias. In addition, maternal position changes and movement do not interfere with the quality of the tracing.

Determining FHR Patterns

Due to the rising costs of litigations related to birth asphyxia of the newborn and increasing complexity of obstetric populations, it has become absolutely mandatory that all nurses responsible for the care of women in labor are trained adequately in interpretation and documentation of CTG tracings, as well as the guidelines for interventions based on the assessment of the tracing and overall clinical situation. Assessment parameters of the FHR include baseline FHR and variability, presence of accelerations, periodic or episodic decelerations, and changes or trends of FHR patterns over time. The nurse must be able to interpret the various parameters to determine if the FHR pattern is a *category I*, which is strongly predictive of normal fetal acid–base status at the time of observation and needs no intervention; a *category II*, which is not predictive of abnormal fetal acid–base status and but does require evaluation and continued monitoring; or a *category III*, which is predictive of abnormal fetal acid–base status at the time of observation and requires prompt evaluation and interventions such as giving maternal oxygen, changing maternal position, discontinuing labor augmentation medication, and/or treating maternal hypotension (Freeman, 2015). Table 14.1 summarizes these categories.

BASELINE FHR

Baseline FHR refers to the average FHR that occurs during a 10-minute segment that excludes periodic or episodic rate changes, such as tachycardia or bradycardia. It is assessed when the woman has no contractions and the fetus is not experiencing episodic FHR changes. The normal baseline FHR ranges between 110 and 160 beats per minute (bpm) (National Institute of Child Health and Human Development [NICHD], 2015). The normal baseline FHR can be obtained by auscultation, ultrasound, or Doppler, or by a continuous internal direct fetal electrode.

Fetal bradycardia occurs when the FHR is below 110 bpm and lasts 10 minutes or longer (Maso et al., 2015). It can be the initial response of a healthy fetus to asphyxia. Causes of fetal bradycardia might include fetal hypoxia, prolonged maternal hypoglycemia, fetal acidosis, administration of analgesic drugs to the mother, hypothermia, anesthetic agents (epidural), maternal hypotension, fetal hypothermia, prolonged umbilical cord compression, and fetal congenital heart block (Nageotte, 2015). Bradycardia may be benign if it is an isolated event, but it is considered an ominous sign when accompanied by a decrease in baseline variability and late decelerations.

Fetal tachycardia is a baseline FHR greater than 160 bpm that lasts for 10 minutes or longer (NICHD, 2015). It can represent an early compensatory response to asphyxia. Other causes of fetal tachycardia include fetal hypoxia, maternal fever, maternal dehydration, amnionitis, drugs (e.g., cocaine, amphetamines, nicotine), maternal hyperthyroidism, maternal anxiety, fetal anemia, prematurity, fetal infection, chronic hypoxemia, congenital anomalies, fetal heart failure, and fetal arrhythmias. Fetal tachycardia is considered an ominous sign if it is accompanied by a decrease in variability and late decelerations (Yuan, 2015).

TABLE 14.1 INTERPRETING FHR PATTERNS

Category I: normal	*Predictive of normal fetal acid–base status and do not require intervention* • Baseline rate (110–160 bpm) • Baseline variability moderate • Present or absent accelerations • Present or absent early decelerations • No late or variable decelerations Can be monitored with intermittent auscultation during labor
Category II: indeterminate	*Not predictive of abnormal fetal acid–base status, but require evaluation and continued surveillance* • Fetal tachycardia (>160 bpm) present • Bradycardia (<110 bpm) not accompanied by absent baseline variability • Absent baseline variability not accompanied by recurrent decelerations • Minimal or marked variability • Recurrent late decelerations with moderate baseline variability • Recurrent variable decelerations accompanied by minimal or moderate baseline variability, overshoots, or shoulders • Prolonged decelerations >2 min but <10 min
Category III: abnormal	*Predictive of abnormal fetus acid–base status and require intervention* • Fetal bradycardia (<110 bpm) • Recurrent late decelerations • Recurrent variable decelerations—declining or absent • Sinusoidal pattern (smooth, undulating baseline)

Adapted from Association of Women's Health, Obstetric and Neonatal Nurses [AWHONN]. (2015). *Fetal heart monitoring: Principles and practices.* Washington, D.C.: AWHONN; Cibils, L. A. (2014). *Electronic fetal-maternal monitoring: Antepartum/intrapartum* (2nd ed.). New York, NY: Springer Publishers; Hersh, S., Megregian, M., & Emeis, C. (2014). Intermittent auscultation of the fetal heart rate during labor: An opportunity for shared decision making. *Journal of Midwifery & Women's Health,* 59, 344–349. doi: 10.1111/jmwh.12178; and Martin, R. J., Fanaroff, A. A., & Walsh, M. C. (2014). *Neonatal-perinatal medicine* (10th ed.). Philadelphia, PA: Elsevier Health Sciences.

BASELINE VARIABILITY

Baseline variability is defined as irregular fluctuations in the baseline FHR, which is measured as the amplitude of the peak to trough in bpm (Sholapurkar, 2015). It represents the interplay between the parasympathetic and sympathetic nervous systems. The constant interplay (push-and-pull effect) on the FHR from the parasympathetic and sympathetic systems produces a moment-to-moment change in the FHR. Because variability is in essence the combined result of autonomic nervous system branch function, its presence implies that the both branches are working and receiving adequate oxygen (Timmins & Clark, 2015). Thus, variability is one of the most important characteristics of the FHR. Variability is described in four categories as follows:

- fluctuation range undetectable
- fluctuation range observed at <5 bpm
- fluctuation range from 6 to 25 bpm
- fluctuation range >25 bpm

Absent or minimal variability typically is caused by fetal acidemia secondary to uteroplacental insufficiency, cord compression, a preterm fetus, maternal hypotension, uterine hyperstimulation, abruptio placenta, or a fetal dysrhythmia. Interventions to improve uteroplacental blood flow and perfusion through the umbilical cord include lateral positioning of the mother, increasing the IV fluid rate to improve maternal circulation, administering oxygen at 8 to 10 L/min by mask, considering internal fetal monitoring, documenting findings, and reporting to the health care provider. Preparation for a surgical birth may be necessary if no changes occur after attempting the interventions.

Moderate viability indicates that the autonomic and central nervous systems (CNSs) of the fetus are well developed and well oxygenated. It is considered a good sign of fetal well-being and correlates with the absence of significant metabolic acidosis (Fig. 14.7).

Marked variability occurs when there are more than 25 beats of fluctuation in the FHR baseline. Causes of this include cord prolapse or compression, maternal hypotension, uterine hyperstimulation, and abruptio placenta. Interventions include determining the cause if possible, lateral positioning, increasing intravenous fluid rate, administering oxygen at 8 to 10 L/min by mask, discontinuing oxytocin infusion, observing for changes in tracing, considering internal fetal monitoring, communicating an abnormal pattern to the health care provider, and preparing for a surgical birth if no change in pattern is noted (Freeman, 2015).

FHR variability is an important clinical indicator that is predictive of fetal acid–base balance and cerebral tissue perfusion. It is influenced by fetal oxygenation status, cardiac output, and drug effects (King et al., 2015). As the CNS is desensitized by hypoxia and acidosis, FHR decreases until a smooth baseline pattern appears. Loss of variability may be associated with a poor outcome.

> **Take Note!**
>
> External electronic fetal monitoring cannot assess variability accurately. Therefore, if external monitoring shows a baseline that is smoothing out, use of an internal spiral electrode should be considered to gain a more accurate picture of the fetal health status.

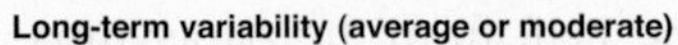

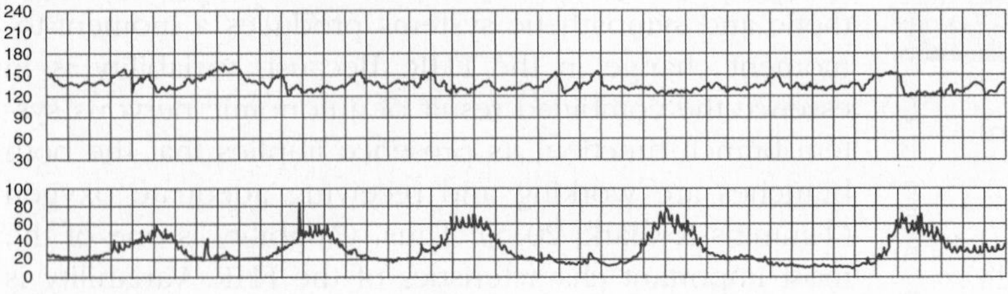

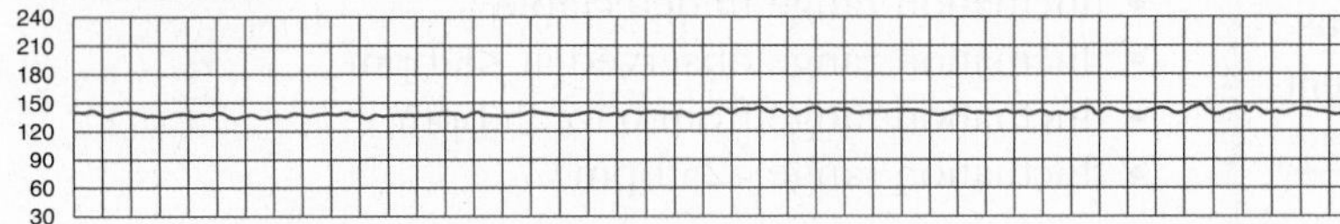

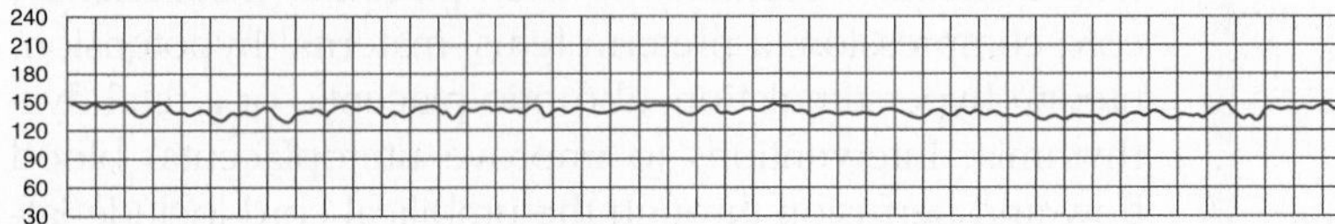

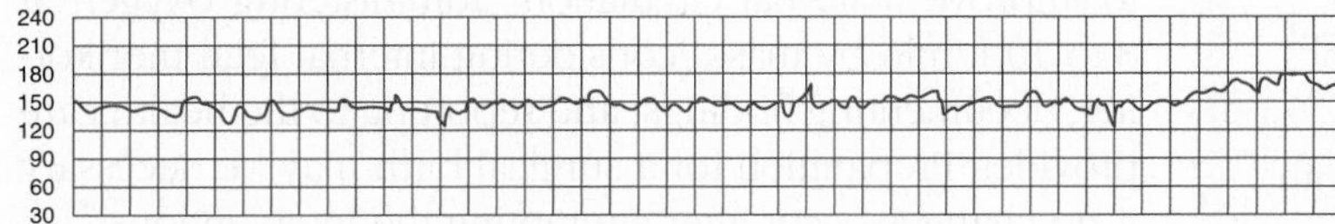

FIGURE 14.7 Examples of fetal monitoring strips. **A.** Long-term variability (average or moderate); **B.** minimal variability **C.** moderate variability **D.** marked variability.

PERIODIC BASELINE CHANGES

Periodic baseline changes are temporary, recurrent changes made in response to a stimulus such as a contraction. The FHR can demonstrate patterns of acceleration or deceleration in response to most stimuli. Fetal accelerations are transitory abrupt increases in the FHR above the baseline that last <30 seconds from onset to peak. They are associated with sympathetic nervous stimulation. They are visually apparent, with elevations of FHR of more than 15 bpm above the baseline, and their duration is >15 seconds, but less than 2 minutes (NICHD, 2015). They are generally considered reassuring and require no intervention. Accelerations denote fetal movement and fetal well-being and are the basis for nonstress testing.

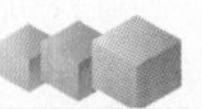

Concept Mastery Alert

Responding to Fetal Heart Rate Distress During Labor

During possible fetal distress that involves lack of variability, late decelerations, and fetal tachycardia, simply changing the woman's position is inadequate. The nurse should notify the health care provider immediately regarding the situation.

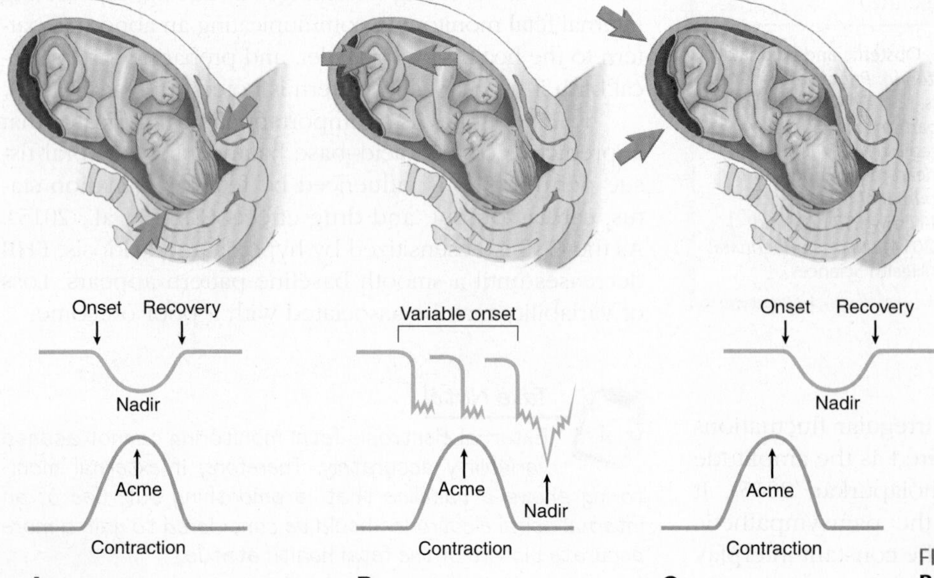

FIGURE 14.8 Decelerations. **A.** Early. **B.** Variable. **C.** Late.

A deceleration is a transient fall in FHR caused by stimulation of the parasympathetic nervous system. Decelerations are described by their shape and association to a uterine contraction. They are classified as early, late, and variable only (Fig. 14.8).

Early decelerations are visually apparent, usually symmetrical, and characterized by a gradual decrease in the FHR in which the nadir (lowest point) occurs at the peak of the contraction. They rarely decrease more than 30 to 40 bpm below the baseline. Typically, the onset, nadir, and recovery of the deceleration occur at the same time as the onset, peak, and recovery of the contraction. They are most often seen during the active stage of any normal labor, during pushing, **crowning**, or vacuum extraction. They are thought to be a result of fetal head compression that results in a reflex vagal response with a resultant slowing of the FHR during uterine contractions. Early decelerations are not indicative of fetal distress and do not require intervention.

Late decelerations are visually apparent, usually symmetrical, transitory decreases in FHR that occur after the peak of the contraction. The FHR does not return to baseline levels until well after the contraction has ended. Delayed timing of the deceleration occurs, with the nadir of the uterine contraction. Late decelerations are associated with uteroplacental insufficiency, which occurs when blood flow within the intervillous space is decreased to the extent that fetal hypoxia or myocardial depression exists (Martin, Fanaroff, & Walsh, 2014). Conditions that may decrease uteroplacental perfusion with resultant decelerations include maternal hypotension, gestational hypertension, placental aging secondary to diabetes and postmaturity, hyperstimulation via oxytocin infusion, maternal smoking, anemia, and cardiac disease. They imply some degree of fetal hypoxia. Recurrent or intermittent late decelerations are always category II (indeterminate) or category III (abnormal) regardless of depth of deceleration. Acute episodes with moderate variability are more likely to be correctable, whereas chronic episodes with loss of variability are less likely to be correctable (Sholapurkar, 2015). Box 14.1 highlights interventions for category III decelerations.

Variable decelerations present as visually apparent abrupt decreases in FHR below baseline and have an unpredictable shape on the FHR baseline, possibly demonstrating no consistent relationship to uterine contractions. The shape of variable decelerations may be U, V, or W, or they may not resemble other patterns (Cahill & Spain, 2015). Variable decelerations usually occur abruptly with quick deceleration. They are the most common deceleration pattern found in the laboring woman and are usually transient and correctable (Ugwumadu, 2015). Variable decelerations are associated with cord compression. However, they are classified either as category II or III depending on the accompanying change in baseline variability (ICSI, 2015a). The pattern of variable deceleration consistently related to the contractions with a slow return to FHR baseline warrants further monitoring and evaluation.

BOX 14.1

INTERVENTIONS FOR CATEGORY III PATTERNS

- Notify the health care provider about the pattern and obtain further orders, making sure to document all interventions and their effects on the FHR pattern.
- Discontinue oxytocin or other uterotonic agent as dictated by the facility's protocol, if it is being administered.
- Turn the client on her left or right lateral, knee-chest, or hands and knees to increase placental perfusion or relieve cord compression.
- Administer oxygen via nonrebreather face mask to increase fetal oxygenation.
- Increase the intravenous fluid rate to improve intravascular volume and correct maternal hypotension.
- Assess the client for any underlying contributing causes.
- Provide reassurance that interventions are to effect pattern change.
- Modify pushing in the second stage of labor to improve fetal oxygenation.
- Document any and all interventions and any changes in FHR patterns.
- Prepare for an expeditious surgical birth if the pattern is not corrected in 30 minutes.

Adapted from American College of Obstetricians and Gynecologists [ACOG]. (2014). Safe prevention of the primary cesarean delivery. Obstetric Care Consensus 1. *Obstetrics & Gynecology, 123,* 693–711; Freeman, R. K. (2015) Intrapartum fetal heart rate monitoring. In J. T. Queenan, C. Y. Spong and C. J. Lockwood (Eds.), Protocols for high-risk pregnancies: An evidence-based approach. Chichester, UK: John Wiley & Sons, Ltd; and Cahill, A. G., & Spain, J. (2015). Intrapartum fetal monitoring. *Clinical Obstetrics and Gynecology, 58*(2), 263–268.

Prolonged decelerations are abrupt FHR declines of at least 15 bpm that last longer than 2 minutes, but less than 10 minutes (NICHD, 2015). The rate usually drops to less than 90 bpm. Many factors are associated with this pattern, including prolonged cord compression, abruptio placenta, cord prolapse, supine maternal position, vaginal examination, fetal blood sampling, maternal seizures, regional anesthesia, or uterine rupture (ACOG & Society for Maternal Fetal Medicine [SMFM], 2014). Prolonged decelerations can be remedied by identifying the underlying cause and correcting it.

A *sinusoidal pattern* is described as having a visually apparent smooth, sinewave-like undulating pattern in the FHR baseline with a cycle frequency of 3 to 5 bpm that persists for >20 minutes. It is attributed to a derangement of CNS control of FHR and occurs when a severe degree of hypoxia secondary to fetal anemia and hypovolemia is present. It is always considered a category III pattern, and to correct it a fetal intrauterine transfusion would be needed (Nageotte, 2015).

Combinations of FHR patterns obtained by EFM during labor are not infrequent. Category II and III patterns are more significant if they are mixed, persist for long periods, or have frequent prolonged late decelerations, absent or minimal variability, bradycardia or tachycardia, and prolonged variable decelerations lower than 60 bpm. The likelihood of fetal compromise is increased if category II and III patterns are associated with decreased baseline variability or abnormal contraction patterns (ICSI, 2015a).

Other Fetal Assessment Methods

In situations suggesting the possibility of fetal compromise, such as category II or category III FHR patterns, further ancillary testing such as umbilical cord blood analysis and fetal scalp stimulation may be used to validate the FHR findings and assist in planning interventions.

Take Note!

In recent years, the use of fetal scalp sampling has decreased, being replaced by techniques that yield similar information. It has been shown to have a poor positive predictive value for intrapartum hypoxia and recent systematic reviews have reported no evidence of benefit in reducing cesarean section rates (Chandraharan, 2014).

Umbilical Cord Blood Analysis

Neonatal and childhood mortality and morbidity, including cerebral palsy, are often attributed to fetal acidosis, as defined by a low cord pH at birth. Umbilical cord blood acid–base analysis drawn at birth provides an objective method of evaluating a newborn's condition, identifying the presence of intrapartum hypoxia and acidemia. This test is considered a good indicator of fetal oxygenation and acid–base condition at birth (Martin et al., 2014). The normal mean pH value range is 7.2 to 7.3. The pH values are useful for planning interventions for the newborn born with low 5-minute Apgar scores, severe FGR, category II and III patterns during labor, umbilical cord prolapse, uterine rupture, maternal fever, placental abruption, meconium-stained amniotic fluid, and postterm births (Gujral & Nayar, 2015). The interventions needed for the compromised newborn might include providing an optimal extrauterine environment, fluids, oxygen, medications, and other treatments.

Fetal Scalp Stimulation

An indirect method used to evaluate fetal oxygenation and acid–base balance to identify fetal hypoxia is fetal scalp stimulation or vibroacoustic stimulation. If the fetus does not have adequate oxygen reserves, carbon dioxide builds up, leading to acidemia and hypoxemia. These metabolic states are reflected in abnormal FHR patterns as well as fetal inactivity. Fetal stimulation is performed to promote fetal movement with the hope that FHR accelerations will accompany the movement.

Fetal movement can be stimulated with a vibroacoustic stimulator (artificial larynx) applied to the woman's lower abdomen and turned on for 3 to 5 seconds to produce sound and vibration or by placing a gloved finger on the fetal scalp and applying firm pressure. A well-oxygenated fetus will respond when stimulated (tactile or by noise) by moving in conjunction with an acceleration of 15 bpm above the baseline heart rate that lasts at least 15 seconds. This FHR acceleration reflects a pH of more than 7 and a fetus with an intact CNS. Fetal scalp stimulation is not done if the fetus is preterm, or if the woman has an intrauterine infection, a diagnosis of placenta previa (which could lead to hemorrhage), or a fever (which increases the risk of an ascending infection) (King et al., 2015). If no acceleratory response by the fetus is exhibited with either scalp stimulation or vibroacoustic stimulation, further evaluation of the fetus is warranted.

Nurses play an essential role in the evaluation of maternal and fetal status during labor, continued surveillance, initiation of corrective measures when indicated, and reevaluation. A vital attribute of nursing surveillance is that it is a systematic process for assessment, intervention, and evaluation.

PROMOTING COMFORT AND PROVIDING PAIN MANAGEMENT DURING LABOR

Pain during labor is a universal experience, although the intensity of the pain may vary. Labor pain is unique to every woman based on various contributing physiologic, emotional, social, and cultural factors. Although labor and childbirth are viewed as natural processes, both can produce significant pain and discomfort. The physical causes of pain during labor include cervical stretching, hypoxia of the uterine muscle due to a decrease in perfusion during contractions, pressure on the urethra, bladder, and rectum, and distention of the muscles of the pelvic floor (Leonard, 2015).

Pain during labor is a physiologic phenomenon. The etiology of pain during the first stage of labor is associated with ischemia of the uterus during contractions. In the second stage, pain is caused by the stretching of the vagina and perineum and compression of the pelvic structures. A woman's pain perception can be influenced by her previous experiences with pain, fatigue, pain anticipation, genetics, positive or negative support system, health care provider's presence and encouragement, labor and birth environment, cultural expectations, and level of emotional stress and anxiety. Pain perception during labor changes in intensity and nature as labor progresses, and this is associated with behavioral changes in the laboring woman (Liu, Fernando, & Mon, 2015).

The techniques used to manage the pain of labor vary according to geography and culture. For example, some Appalachian women believe that placing a hatchet or knife under the bed of a laboring woman may help "cut the pain of childbirth," and a woman from this background may wish to do so in the hospital setting (Bowers, 2015). Asian, Latino, and Orthodox Jewish women may request that their own mothers, not their husbands, attend their births; husbands do not actively participate in the birthing process. Cherokee, Hmong, and Japanese women will often remain quiet during labor and birth and not complain of pain because outwardly expressing pain is not appropriate in their cultures. Never interpret their quietness as freedom from pain. The concept of pain and pain expression during labor has different meanings for women of different cultures. Several points for the nurse to consider when caring for diverse cultural clients include using a qualified interpreter to communicate about pain as needed, offer and support culturally acceptable forms of pain relief, and assess for pain frequently (Wojnar & Narruhn, 2016).

Immigrating to a new country is a stressful process of readjustment and change. Effective verbal communication and understanding nonverbal social cues is invaluable when providing care to diverse cultures. Culturally diverse childbearing families present to the labor and birth suites with the same needs and desires of all families. Give them the same respect and sense of welcome shown to all families. Make sure they have a high-quality birth experience: uphold their religious, ethnic, and cultural values and integrate them into care.

Today, women have many safe nonpharmacologic and pharmacologic choices for the management of pain during labor and birth, which may be used separately or in combination with one another. Pharmacologic approaches are directed at eliminating the physical sensation of labor pain, whereas nonpharmacologic approaches are largely directed at prevention of suffering.

Nurses are in an ideal position to provide childbearing women with balanced, clear, concise information about effective nonpharmacologic and pharmacologic measures to relieve pain. Pain management standards issued by the Joint Commission mandate that pain be assessed in all clients admitted to a health care facility. Attention to the pain that occurs during labor and childbirth should be a priority of care for all nurses (Jones et al., 2015). A pain assessment tool named the *Coping with Labor Algorithm* uses the FOCUS format "Plan, Do, Check, and Act" cycle in laboring women. This tool provides a mechanism for pain documentation and links it to nursing care interventions (Roberts et al., 2010). Thus, it is important for nurses to be knowledgeable about the most recent scientific research on labor pain relief modalities, to make sure that accurate and unbiased information about effective pain relief measures is available to laboring women, to be sure that the woman determines what is an acceptable labor pain level for her, and to allow the woman the choice of pain relief method.

Nonpharmacologic Measures

Nonpharmacologic measures may include continuous labor support, hydrotherapy, hypnosis, ambulation and maternal position changes, transcutaneous electrical nerve stimulation (TENS), acupuncture and acupressure, attention focusing and imagery, therapeutic touch and massage, breathing techniques, and effleurage. Most of these methods are based on the *gate control theory of pain*, which proposes that local physical stimulation can interfere with pain stimuli by closing a hypothetical gate in the spinal cord, thus blocking pain signals from reaching the brain (McGeary, Swanholm, & Gatchel, 2015). It has long been a standard of care for labor nurses to first provide or encourage a variety of nonpharmacologic measures before moving to the pharmacologic interventions.

Nonpharmacologic measures are usually simple, safe, and inexpensive to use. Many of these measures are taught in childbirth classes, and women should be encouraged to try a variety of methods prior to the real labor. Many of the measures need to be practiced for best results and coordinated with the partner/coach. The nurse provides support and encouragement for the woman and her partner using nonpharmacologic methods. Although women cannot consciously direct the labor contractions, they can control how they respond to them, thereby enhancing their feelings of control. See Evidence-Based Practice 14.2 for more information.

Continuous Labor Support

Continuous labor support involves offering a sustained presence to the laboring woman by providing emotional support, comfort measures, advocacy, information and advice, and support for the partner. It is a nonpharmacologic, evidence-based strategy associated with reduced cesarean rates (Jackson & Gregory, 2015). A woman's family, a midwife, a nurse, a doula, or anyone else close to the woman can provide this continuous presence. A support person can assist the woman to ambulate, reposition herself, and use breathing techniques. A support person can also aid with the use of acupressure, massage, music therapy, or therapeutic touch. During the natural course of childbirth, a laboring woman's functional ability is limited secondary to pain, and she often has trouble making decisions. The support person can help make them based on his or her knowledge of the woman's birth plan and personal wishes.

Research has validated the value of continuous labor support versus intermittent support in terms of fewer operative deliveries, cesarean births, and requests for pain

EVIDENCE-BASED PRACTICE 14.2 EFFECTIVENESS OF AROMATHERAPY AND BIOFEEDBACK IN PROMOTION OF LABOR OUTCOME DURING CHILDBIRTH AMONG PRIMIGRAVIDAS

STUDY

Labor pain is described as the most severe form of pain that every woman may experience during their lifetime. When considering labor analgesia, one is faced with a number of choices each with different advantages and disadvantages depending on the woman's expectations and preferences. Many women would like to avoid taking medications or invasive methods for pain management because of the potential negative impact on their fetus during labor. Severe pain triggers a stress response which may lead to harmful effects on both mother and fetus. The purpose of this study was to evaluate the effect of aromatherapy (essential oils from plants are massaged in the skin and inhaled) and biofeedback (mother was asked to experience both the fetal heart sound and variation in contractions and consciously regulate them) in promotion of labor outcome during childbirth.

Findings

Six hundred nulliparous women were selected randomly and assigned to an aromatherapy group ($n = 200$), a biofeedback group ($n = 200$), or a control group ($n = 200$). The researchers rated pain by using a visual pain analog scale during their labors. Sixty nine percent of cases in the aromatherapy group expressed it was helpful, provided pain relief and emotional well-being during their labors. Biofeedback was also effective in reducing pain and duration of labor during childbirth compared with the control group.

Nursing Implications

The results of this study indicated that the use of aromatherapy and biofeedback, as nonpharmacologic methods were both effective methods of reducing pain perception and duration of labor among women during labor. As a nonpharmacologic nursing intervention, these are easy to administer, cost-effective, harmless, and appealing to the mother without any apparent maternal or neonatal adverse effects.

Adopted from Janula, R., & Mahipal, S. (2015). Effectiveness of aromatherapy and biofeedback in promotion of labor outcome during childbirth among primigravidas. *Health Science Journal, 9*(1), 1–5.

medication. Continuous labor support has shown to have beneficial effects on the mother and the newborn primarily due to the reduction in anxiety during the laboring experience. Most women expressed greater satisfaction with their childbirth experience (Iravani et al., 2015).

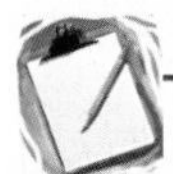

Take Note!

The human presence is of immeasurable value to make the laboring woman feel secure.

Hydrotherapy

Hydrotherapy is a nonpharmacologic measure that may involve showering or soaking in a regular tub or whirlpool bath. When showering is the selected method of hydrotherapy, the woman stands or sits in a shower chair in a warm shower and allows the water to gently glide over her abdomen and back. If a tub or whirlpool is chosen, the woman immerses herself in warm water for relaxation and relief of discomfort. When the woman enters the warm water, the warmth and buoyancy help to release muscle tension and can impart a sense of well-being (Taghavi, Barband, & Khaki, 2015). Warm water provides soothing stimulation of nerves in the skin, promoting vasodilation, reversal of sympathetic nervous response, and a reduction in catecholamines (Dalal, 2015). Contractions are usually less painful in warm water because the warmth and buoyancy of the water have a relaxing effect. Recent research findings reported that women who used hydrotherapy had significantly reduced surgical birth rates, a shorter second stage of labor, reduced analgesic requirements, and a lower incidence of perineal trauma (Taghavi et al., 2015). The research concluded that hydrotherapy during labor significantly aids the labor process, minimizes the use of analgesic medications, offers fast- and short-acting pain and anxiety relief, and should be considered as a safe and effective birthing aid (Taghavi et al., 2015).

A wide range of hydrotherapy options are available, from ordinary bathtubs to whirlpool baths and showers, combined with low lighting and music. Many hospitals provide showers and whirlpool baths for laboring women for pain relief. However, hydrotherapy is more commonly practiced in birthing centers managed by midwives. The recommendation for initiating hydrotherapy is that the woman be in active labor (more than 5 cm dilated) to prevent the slowing of labor contractions secondary to muscular relaxation. The woman's membranes can be intact or ruptured. Women are encouraged to stay in the bath or shower as long as they feel they are comfortable. The water temperature should not exceed body temperature.

Hydrotherapy is an effective pain management option for many women. Women who are experiencing a healthy pregnancy can be offered this option. The potential risks associated with hydrotherapy include hyperthermia, hypothermia, changes in maternal heart rate, fetal tachycardia, and unplanned underwater birth. The benefits include reducing pain, relieving anxiety, and promoting a sense of control during labor (Nutter, 2016).

Ambulation and Position Changes

Ambulation and position changes during labor are another extremely useful comfort measure. Historically, women adopted a variety of positions during labor, rarely using the recumbent position until during the first half of the twentieth century. The medical profession has favored recumbent positions during labor, but without evidence to demonstrate their appropriateness. A recent Cochrane database systematic review reported there is evidence that walking and upright positions in the first stage of labor reduce the length of labor and do not seem to be associated with increased intervention or negative effects on mothers' and babies' well-being. In an upright posture, gravity directs the weight of the fetus and amniotic fluid downward, successively dilating the cervix and the birth canal. Uterine contractions have been shown to be better spaced, stronger and more efficient in dilating the cervix when the mother is in an upright position than when she is supine (Cox & King, 2015). Women should be encouraged to take up whatever position they find most comfortable in the first stage of labor (Cheng & Caughey, 2015a).

Changing position frequently (every 30 minutes or so) – sitting, walking, kneeling, standing, lying down, getting on hands and knees, and using a birthing ball – helps relieve pain (Fig. 14.9). Position changes also

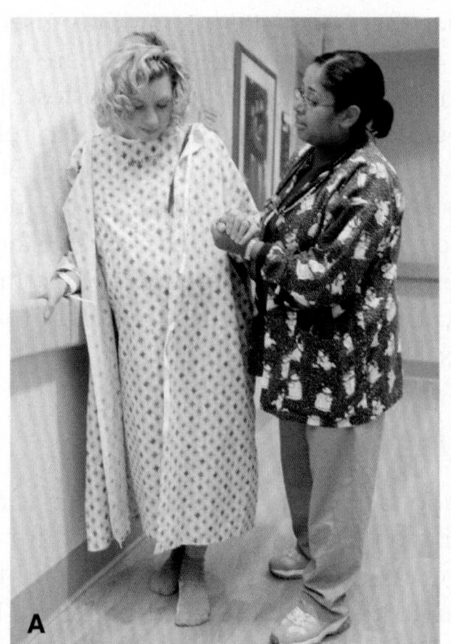

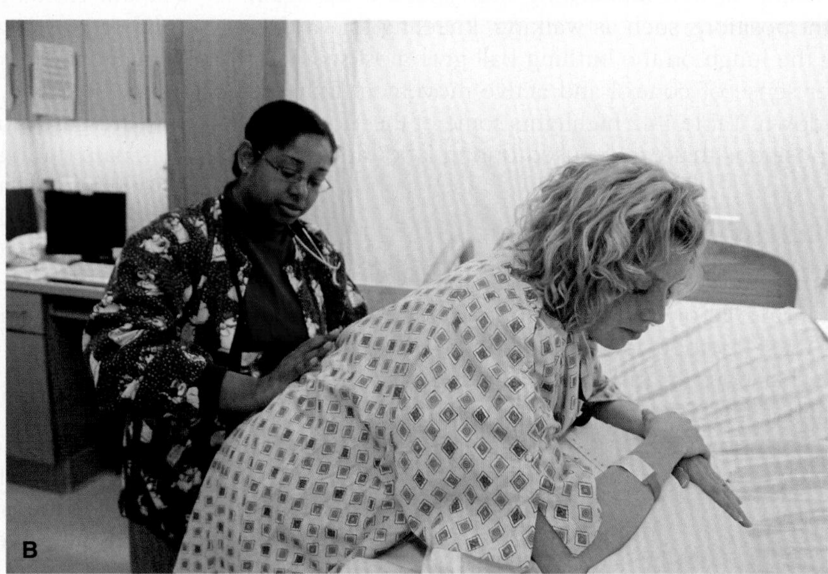

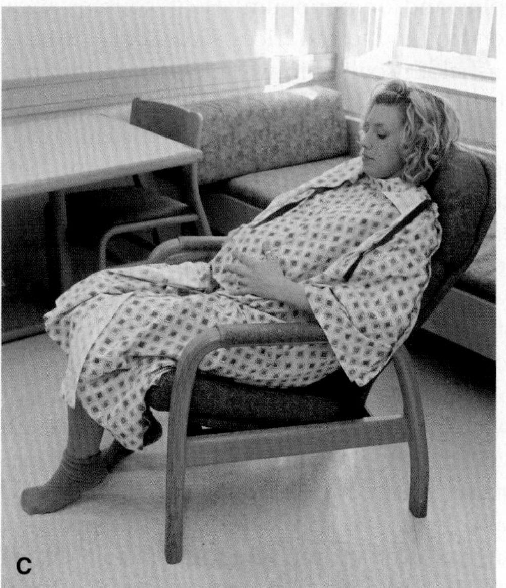

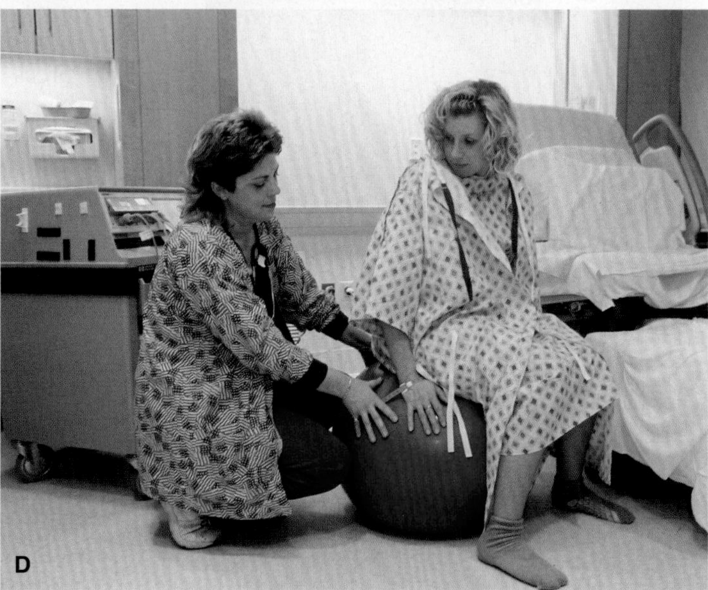

FIGURE 14.9 Various positions for use during labor. **A.** Ambulation. **B.** Leaning forward. **C.** Sitting in a chair. **D.** Using a birthing ball.

may help to speed labor by adding the benefits of gravity and changing the shape of the pelvis. Research has found that the position that the woman assumes and the frequency of position changes have a profound effect on uterine activity and efficiency. Allowing the woman to obtain a position of comfort frequently facilitates a favorable fetal rotation by altering the alignment of the presenting part with the pelvis. As the mother continues to change position based on comfort, the optimal presentation is afforded (King et al., 2015). Supine positions should be avoided, since they may interfere with labor progress and can cause compression of the vena cava and decrease blood return to the heart.

Swaying from side to side, rocking, or other rhythmic movements may also be comforting. If labor is progressing slowly, ambulating may speed it up again. Upright positions such as walking, kneeling forward, or doing the lunge on the birthing ball give most women a greater sense of control and active movement than just lying down. Table 14.2 highlights some of the more common positions that can be used during labor and birth.

Acupuncture and Acupressure

Acupuncture and acupressure can be used to relieve pain during labor. Although controlled research studies of these methods are limited, there is adequate evidence that both are useful in relieving pain associated with labor and birth. However, both methods require a trained, certified clinician, and such a person is not available in many birth facilities (Halpern & Garg, 2015).

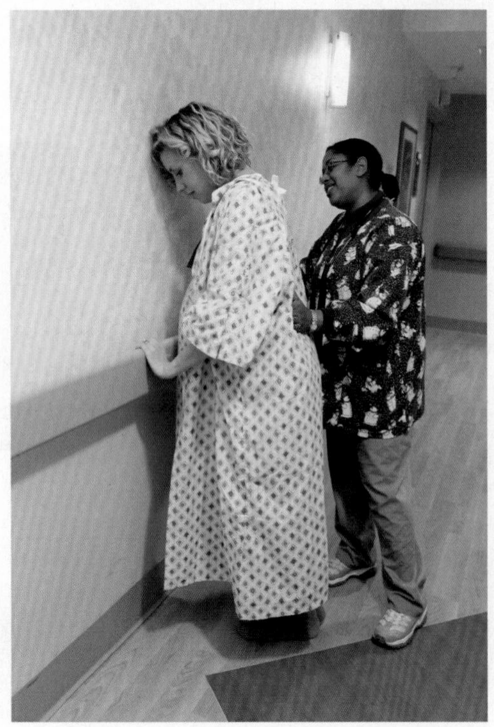

FIGURE 14.10 Nurse massaging the client's back during a contraction while she ambulates during labor.

Acupuncture involves stimulating key trigger points with needles. This form of Chinese medicine has been practiced for approximately 3,000 years. Classical Chinese teaching holds that throughout the body there are meridians or channels of energy (*qi*) that when in balance regulate body functions. Pain reflects an imbalance or obstruction of the flow of energy. The purpose of acupuncture is to restore thus diminishing pain (Adams et al., 2015). Stimulating the trigger points causes the release of endorphins, reducing the perception of pain.

Acupressure involves the application of a firm finger or massage used in acupuncture to reduce the pain sensation. The amount of pressure is important. The intensity of the pressure is determined by the needs of the woman. Holding and squeezing the hand of a woman in labor may trigger the point most commonly used for both techniques. Some acupressure points are found along the spine, neck, shoulder, toes, and soles of the feet. Pressure along the side of the spine can help relieve back pain during labor (Mollart, Adam, & Foureur, 2015). A Cochrane collaboration review found that acupuncture may indeed reduce labor pain, increasing satisfaction with pain management and reduced use of pharmacologic management. However, there is a need for further research (Simkin & Klein, 2015).

Application of Heat and Cold

Superficial applications of heat and/or cold, in various forms, are popular with laboring women. They are easy to use, inexpensive, require no prior practice, and have minimal negative side effects when used properly. Heat is typically applied to the woman's back, lower abdomen, groin, and/or perineum. Heat sources include a hot water bottle, heated rice-filled sock, warm compress (washcloth soaked in warm water and wrung out), electric heating pad, warm blanket, and warm bath or shower. In addition to being used for pain relief, heat is used to relieve chills or trembling, decrease joint stiffness, reduce muscle spasm, and increase connective tissue extensibility (Liu et al., 2015).

Cold therapy, or cryotherapy, is usually applied on the woman's back, chest, and/or face during labor. Forms of cold include a bag or surgical glove filled with ice, a frozen gel pack, camper's "ice," a hollow, plastic rolling pin or bottle filled with ice, a washcloth dipped in cold water, soda cans chilled in ice, and even a frozen bag of vegetables. "Instant" cold packs, often available in hospitals, usually are not cold enough to effectively relieve labor pain. Women who feel cold usually need to feel warm before they can comfortably tolerate using a cold pack. Chilled soda cans and rolling pins filled with ice give the added benefit of mechanical pressure when rolled on the low back. Cold has the additional effects of

TABLE 14.2 COMMON POSITIONS FOR USE DURING LABOR AND BIRTH

Position	Advantages
Standing	• Takes advantage of gravity during and between contractions • Makes contractions feel less painful and be more productive • Helps fetus line up with angle of maternal pelvis • Helps to increase urge to push in second stage of labor
Walking	• Has the same advantages as standing • Causes changes in the pelvic joints, helping the fetus move through the birth canal
Standing and leaning forward on partner, bed, birthing ball	• Has the same advantages as standing • Is a good position for a backrub • May feel more restful than standing • Can be used with electronic fetal monitor
Slow dancing (standing with woman's arms around partner's neck, head resting on his chest or shoulder, with his hands rubbing woman's lower back, sway to music and breathe in rhythm if it helps)	• Has the same advantages as walking • Back pressure helps relieve back pain • Rhythm and music help woman relax and provide comfort
The lunge (standing facing a straight chair with one foot on the seat with knee and foot to the side; bending raised knee and hip, and lunging sideways repeatedly during a contraction, holding each lunge for 5 seconds; partner holds chair and helps with balance)	• Widens one side of the pelvis (the side toward lunge) • Encourages rotation of baby • Can also be done in a kneeling position
Sitting upright	• Helps promote rest • Has more gravity advantage than lying down • Can be used with electronic fetal monitor
Semi-sitting (setting the head of the bed at a 45-degree angle with pillows used for support)	• Has the same advantages as sitting upright • Is an easy position if on a bed
Sitting on toilet or commode	• Has the same advantages as sitting upright • May help relax the perineum for effective bearing down
Rocking in a chair	• Has the same advantages as sitting upright • May help speed labor (rocking movement)
Sitting, leaning forward with support	• Has the same advantages as sitting upright • Is a good position for a backrub
On all fours, on hands and knees	• Helps relieve backache • Assists rotation of baby in posterior position • Allows for pelvic rocking and body movement • Relieves pressure on hemorrhoids • Allows for vaginal examinations • Is sometimes preferred as a pushing position by women with back labor
Kneeling, leaning forward with support on a chair seat, the raised head of the bed, or on a birthing ball	• Has the same advantages as all-fours position • Puts less strain on wrists and hands
Side-lying	• Is a very good position for resting and convenient for many kinds of medical interventions • Helps lower elevated blood pressure • May promote progress of labor when alternated with walking • Is useful to slow a very rapid second stage • Avoids vena cava syndrome • May offer increased control of pushing efforts • Takes pressure off hemorhoids • Facilitates relaxation between contractions

(continued)

TABLE 14.2 COMMON POSITIONS FOR USE DURING LABOR AND BIRTH (continued)

Position	Advantages
Squatting	• May relieve backache • Takes advantage of gravity • Requires less bearing-down effort • Widens pelvic outlet by approximately 28% • Pressure is evenly distributed to the perineum, reducing the need for episiotomy • May help fetus turn and move down in a difficult birth • Helps if the woman feels no urge to push • Allows freedom to shift weight for comfort • Offers an advantage when pushing, since upper trunk presses on the top of the uterus
Supported squat (leaning back against partner, who supports woman under the arms and takes the entire woman's weight; standing up between contractions)	• Requires great strength in partner • Lengthens trunk, allowing more room for fetus to maneuver into position • Lets gravity help
Dangle (partner sitting high on bed or counter with feet supported on chairs or footrests and thighs spread; woman leaning back between partner's legs, placing flexed arms over partner's thighs; partner gripping sides with his thighs; woman lowering herself and allowing partner to support her full weight; standing up between contractions)	• Has the same advantages of a supported squat • Requires less physical strength from the partner

Adapted from Gizzo, S., Di Gangi, S., Noventa, M., Bacile, V., Zambon, A., & Nardelli, B. (2014). Women's choice of positions during labor: Return to the past or a modern way to give birth? A cohort study in Italy. *BioMed Research International*, ID 638093, http://dx.doi.org/10.1155/2014/638093; Hanson, L., & VandeVusse, L. (2014). Supporting labor progress toward physiologic birth. *Journal of Perinatal & Neonatal Nursing*, 28(2), 101–107; and Magowan, B., Owen, P., & Thomson, A. (2014). *Clinical obstetrics & gynecology* (3rd ed.). St. Louis, MO: Saunders Elsevier.

relieving muscle spasms and reducing inflammation and edema (Tharpe et al., 2016).

To date, no randomized controlled studies have evaluated the use of heat and cold, so further study is needed to determine if either approach is efficacious. With appropriate safety precautions, heat and cold offer comfort and relief, and their use should be dictated by the desires and responses of the laboring woman.

Attention Focusing and Imagery

Attention focusing and imagery use many of the senses and the mind to focus on stimuli. The woman can focus on tactile stimuli such as touch, massage, or stroking. She may focus on auditory stimuli such as music, humming, or verbal encouragement. Visual stimuli might be any object in the room, or the woman can imagine the beach, a mountaintop, a happy memory, or even the contractions of the uterine muscle pulling the cervix open and the fetus pressing downward to open the cervix. Some women focus on a particular mental activity such as a song, a chant, counting backward, or a Bible verse. Breathing, relaxation, positive thinking, and positive visualization work well for mothers in labor. The use of these techniques keeps the sensory input perceived during the contraction from reaching the pain center in the cortex of the brain (Capogna, 2015a).

Effleurage and Massage

Effleurage is a light, stroking, superficial touch of the abdomen, in rhythm with breathing during contractions. It is used as a relaxation and distraction technique from discomfort. External fetal monitor belts may interfere with the ability to accomplish this.

Effleurage and massage use the sense of touch to promote relaxation and pain relief. Massage works as a form of pain relief by increasing the production of endorphins in the body. Endorphins reduce the transmission of signals between nerve cells and thus lower the perception of pain. Because touch receptors go to the brain faster than pain receptors, massage – anywhere on the body – can block the pain message to the brain. In addition, light touch has been found to release endorphins and induce a relaxed state. In addition, touching and massage distract the woman from discomfort. Massage involves manipulation of the body's soft tissues. It is commonly used to help relax tense muscles and to soothe and calm the individual. Massage may help to relieve pain by assisting with relaxation, inhibiting sensory transmission in the pain pathways, or improving blood flow and oxygenation of tissues (Neetu & Panchal, 2015).

Breathing Techniques

Conscious use of breath by the woman has the power to profoundly influence her labor and how she engages with it. The first action anyone takes in any situation is a breath. The breath affects the lungs, immediately cueing the nervous system. The nervous system responds by sending messages, which impact our entire psychophysiologic system. Messages sent from the nervous system affect us physically, emotionally, and mentally. If we alter how we breathe, we alter the constellation of messages and reactions in our entire mind–body experience (Cheng & Caughey, 2015a).

Breathing techniques are effective in producing relaxation and pain relief through the use of distraction. If the woman is concentrating on slow-paced rhythmic breathing, she is not likely to fully focus on contraction pain. Breathing techniques are often taught in childbirth education classes (see Chapter 12 for additional information).

Controlled breathing helps reduce the pain experienced by using stimulus–response conditioning. The woman selects a focal point within her environment to stare at during the first sign of a contraction. This focus creates a visual stimulus that goes directly to her brain. The woman takes a deep cleansing breath, which is followed by rhythmic breathing. Verbal commands from her partner supply an ongoing auditory stimulus to her brain. Benefits of practicing patterned breathing include breathing:

- becomes an automatic response to pain.
- increases relaxation and can be used to deal with life's everyday stresses.
- is calming during labor.
- provides a sense of well-being and a measure of control.
- brings purpose to each contraction, making them more productive.
- provides more oxygen for the mother and fetus (American Pregnancy Association, 2015).

Many couples learn patterned-paced breathing during their childbirth education classes. Three levels may be taught, each beginning and ending with a cleansing breath or sigh after each contraction. In the first pattern, also known as slow-paced breathing, the woman inhales slowly through her nose and exhales through pursed lips. The breathing rate is typically 6 to 9 bpm. In the second pattern, the woman inhales and exhales through her mouth at a rate of four breaths every 5 seconds. The rate can be accelerated to two breaths per second to assist her to relax. The third pattern, is similar to the second pattern except that the breathing is punctuated every few breaths by a forceful exhalation through pursed lips. All breaths are kept equal and rhythmic and can increase as contractions increase in intensity (Lindholm & Hildingsson, 2015).

Many childbirth educators do not recommend specific breathing techniques or try to teach parents to breathe the "right" way during labor and birth. Couples are encouraged to find breathing styles that enhance their relaxation and use them. There are numerous benefits to controlled and rhythmic breathing in childbirth (outlined previously), and many women choose these techniques to manage their discomfort during labor.

Pharmacologic Measures

With varying degrees of success, generations of women have sought ways to relieve the pain of childbirth. Pharmacologic pain relief during labor includes systemic analgesia and regional or local anesthesia. Women have seen dramatic changes in pharmacologic pain management options over the years. Methods have evolved from biting down on a stick to control their pain, experiencing "twilight sleep" during their labors and not remembering what happened, to a more complex pharmacologic approach such as epidural/intrathecal analgesia. Systemic analgesia and regional analgesia/anesthesia have become less common, while newer **neuraxial analgesia/anesthesia** techniques involving minimal motor blockade have become more popular. Neuraxial analgesia/anesthesia is the administration of analgesic (opioids) or anesthetic (capable of producing a loss of sensation in an area of the body) agents, either continuously or intermittently, into the epidural or intrathecal space to relieve pain. Low-dose and ultra-low-dose epidural analgesia, spinal analgesia, and combined spinal–epidural (CSE) analgesia have replaced the traditional epidural for labor. Neuraxial analgesia does not interfere with the progress or outcome of labor. There is no need to withhold neuraxial analgesia until the active stage of labor (Grant et al., 2015). This shift in pain management techniques allows a woman to be an active participant in labor.

Take Note!

Regardless of which approach is used during labor, the woman has the right to choose the methods of pain control that will best suit her and meet her needs.

Systemic Analgesia

Systemic analgesia involves the use of one or more drugs administered orally, intramuscularly, or intravenously; they become distributed throughout the body via the circulatory system. Depending on which administration method is used, the therapeutic effect of pain relief can occur within minutes and last for several hours. The most important complication associated with the use of this class of drugs is respiratory depression. Therefore, women given these drugs require careful monitoring. Opioids given close to the time of birth can cause CNS depression in the newborn, necessitating the administration of naloxone (Narcan) to reverse the depressant effects of the opioids.

Several drug categories may be used for systemic analgesia:

- *Opioids*, such as butorphanol (Stadol), nalbuphine (Nubain), meperidine (Demerol), morphine, or fentanyl (Sublimaze)
- *Ataractics*, such as hydroxyzine (Vistaril), promethazine (Phenergan), or prochlorperazine (Compazine)
- *Benzodiazepines*, such as diazepam (Valium) or midazolam (Versed)

Drug Guide 14.1 highlights some of the major drugs used for systemic analgesia.

Systemic analgesics are typically administered parenterally, usually through an existing intravenous line. Nearly all medications given during labor cross the placenta and have a depressant effect on the fetus; therefore, it is important for the woman to receive the least amount of systemic medication that relieves her discomfort so that it does not cause any harm to the fetus (Cheng & Caughey, 2015a). Historically opioids have been administered by nurses, but in the past decade there has been increasing use of client-controlled intravenous analgesia (patient-controlled analgesia). With this system, the woman is given a button connected to a computerized pump on the intravenous line. When the woman desires analgesia, she presses the button and the pump delivers a preset amount of medication. This system provides the woman with a sense of control over her own pain management and active participation in the childbirth process.

OPIOIDS

Opioids are morphine-like medications that are most effective for the relief of moderate to severe pain. Opioids typically are administered intravenously. All opioids are lipophilic and cross the placental barrier, but do not affect labor progress in the active phase. Opioids are associated with newborn respiratory depression, decreased alertness, inhibited sucking, and a delay in effective feeding (King et al., 2015).

Opioids decrease the transmission of pain impulses by binding to receptor site pathways that transmit the pain signals to the brain. The effect is increased tolerance to pain and respiratory depression related to a decrease in sensitivity to carbon dioxide (Skidmore-Roth, 2015). All opioids are considered good analgesics. However, respiratory depression can occur in the mother and fetus depending on the dose given. They may also cause a decrease in FHR variability identified on the fetal monitor strip. This FHR pattern change is usually transient. Other systemic side effects include nausea, vomiting, pruritus, delayed gastric emptying, drowsiness, hypoventilation, and newborn depression. To reduce the incidence of newborn depression, birth should occur within 1 hour or after 4 hours of administration to prevent the fetus from receiving the peak concentration (Cheng & Caughey, 2015a).

A recent study reported that parenteral opioids provide some relief from pain in labor, but are associated with neonatal respiratory distress. Maternal satisfaction with opioid analgesia appeared moderate at best (Kerr, Taylor, & Evans, 2015)

Opioid antagonists such as naloxone (Narcan) are given to reverse the effects of the CNS depression, including respiratory depression, caused by opioids. Opioid antagonists also are used to reverse the side effects of neuraxial opioids, such as pruritus, urinary retention, nausea, and vomiting, without significantly decreasing analgesia (Skidmore-Roth, 2015). Consult a current drug guide for more specifics on these drug categories.

ANTIEMETICS

The antiemetic group of medications is used in combination with an opioid to decrease nausea and vomiting and lessen anxiety. These adjunct drugs potentiate the effectiveness of the opioid so that a lesser dose can be given. They may also be used to increase sedation. Promethazine (Phenergan) can be given intravenously, but hydroxyzine (Vistaril) must be given by mouth or by intramuscular injection into a large muscle mass. Neither drug affects the progress of labor, but either may cause a decrease in FHR variability and possible newborn depression (Skidmore-Roth, 2015). Prochlorperazine (Compazine) is typically given intravenously or intramuscularly with morphine sulfate for sleep during a prolonged latent phase. It counteracts the nausea associated with opioids (King et al., 2015).

BENZODIAZEPINES

Benzodiazepines are used for minor tranquilizing and sedative effects. Diazepam (Valium) also is given intravenously to stop seizures resulting from eclampsia. It can be administered to calm a woman who is out of control, thereby enabling her to relax enough so that she can participate effectively during her labor process rather than fighting against it. Lorazepam (Ativan) can also be used for its tranquilizing effect, but increased sedation is experienced with this medication (Skidmore-Roth, 2015). Midazolam (Versed), also given intravenously, produces good amnesia but no analgesia. It is most commonly used as an adjunct for anesthesia. Diazepam and midazolam cause CNS depression for both the woman and the newborn.

DRUG GUIDE 14.1 COMMON AGENTS USED FOR SYSTEMIC ANALGESIA

Type	Drug	Comments
Opioids	Morphine 2–5 mg IV	May be given IV or epidurally Rapidly crosses the placenta, causes a decrease in FHR variability Can cause maternal and neonatal CNS depression Decreases uterine contractions
	Meperidine (Demerol) 25–75 mg IV	May be given IV, intrathecally, or epidurally with maximal fetal uptake 2–3 hr after administration Can cause CNS depression Decreases fetal variability
	Butorphanol (Stadol) 1–2 mg IV	Is given IV
	q2–4h	Is rapidly transferred across the placenta Causes neonatal respiratory depression
	Nalbuphine (Nubain) 10–20 mg IV	Is given IV Causes less maternal nausea and vomiting Causes decreased FHR variability, fetal bradycardia, and respiratory depression
	Fentanyl (Sublimaze) 50–100 mcg IV	Is given IV or epidurally Can cause maternal hypotension, maternal and fetal respiratory depression Rapidly crosses placenta
Antiemetics	Hydroxyzine (Vistaril) 50–100 mg IM	Does not relieve pain but reduces anxiety and potentiates opioid analgesic effects; cannot be given IV Is used to decrease nausea and vomiting
	Promethazine (Phenergan) 25–50 mg IV or IM	Is used for antiemetic effect when combined with opioids Causes sedation and reduces apprehension May contribute to maternal hypotension and neonatal depression
	Prochlorperazine (Compazine) 5–10 mg IV or IM	Frequently given with morphine sulfate for sleep during prolonged latent phase; counteracts the nausea that opioids can produce
Benzodiazepines	Diazepam (Valium) 2–5 mg IV	Is given to enhance pain relief of opioid and cause sedation May be used to stop eclamptic seizures Decreases nausea and vomiting Can cause newborn depression; therefore, lowest possible dose should be used
	Midazolam (Versed) 1–5 mg IV	Is not used for analgesic but amnesia effect Is used as adjunct for anesthesia Is excreted in breast milk

IV, intravenous.
Adapted from Cheng, Y., & Caughey, A. B. (2015a). *Normal labor and delivery*. Retrieved from http://emedicine.medscape.com/article/260036-overview#aw2aab6b2; King, T.L., Brucker, M. C., Kriebs, J. M., Fahey, J. O., Gegor, C. L., & Varney, H. (2015). *Varney's midwifery* (5th ed.). Burlington, MA: Jones & Bartlett Learning; and Skidmore-Roth, L. (2015). *Mosby's 2015 nursing drug reference* (28th ed.). St. Louis, MO: Mosby Elsevier.

Inhaled Analgesics

Nitrous oxide is known by most people as "laughing gas." For labor pain, half nitrous oxide gas (50%) is mixed with half oxygen (50%) and breathed through a mask or mouthpiece. This has been recently introduced in the United States, but has been in widespread use in Europe and Canada for many years. Women have generally reported satisfaction with the use of nitrous oxide for pain relief in labor. An additional factor that may contribute to the decreased perception of pain is maternal control—it is self-administered. Self-administration is not only empowering for women, but it also acts as a safety mechanism because it is almost impossible to overdose when it is self-administered (Halpern & Garg, 2015). Potential side effects of N2O/O2 include nausea and vomiting, dizziness, and dysphoria, although these are rare. No FHR abnormalities have been attributed to its use (Badve & Vallejo, 2015).

Regional Analgesia/Anesthesia

Regional analgesia/anesthesia provides pain relief without loss of consciousness. It involves the use of local anesthetic agents, with or without added opioids, to bring about pain relief or numbness through the drug's effects on the spinal cord and nerve roots. Obstetric regional analgesia generally refers to a partial or complete loss of pain sensation below the T8 to T10 level of the spinal cord (Stocks & Griffiths, 2015).

The routes for regional pain relief include epidural block, CSE, local infiltration, pudendal block, and intrathecal (spinal) analgesia/anesthesia. Local and pudendal routes are used during birth for episiotomies (surgical incision into the perineum to facilitate birth); epidural and intrathecal routes are used for pain relief during active labor and birth. The major advantage of regional pain management techniques is that the woman can participate in the birthing process and still have good pain control.

EPIDURAL ANALGESIA

Women requesting epidural analgesia in labor will do so when they feel they need pain relief, and for some it might be quite early in their labor. Epidural analgesia for labor and birth involves the injection of a local anesthetic agent (e.g., lidocaine or bupivacaine) and an opioid analgesic agent (e.g., morphine or fentanyl) into the lumbar epidural space. A small catheter is then passed through the epidural needle to provide continuous access to the epidural space for maintenance of analgesia throughout labor and birth (Fig. 14.11). Epidural analgesia does increase the duration of the second stage of labor and may increase the rate of instrument-assisted vaginal deliveries as well as that of oxytocin administration (Camorcia, 2015). Approximately 60% of laboring women in the United States receive an epidural for pain relief during labor, but one in eight women who have an epidural during labor still need to use other methods of pain relief. In urban areas, many hospitals approach 90% use of epidurals (Capogna, 2015b).

An epidural involves the injection of a drug into the epidural space, which is located outside the dura mater between the dura and the spinal canal. The epidural space is typically entered through the third and fourth lumbar vertebrae with a needle, and a catheter is threaded into the epidural space. An epidural can be used for both vaginal and cesarean births. It has evolved from a regional block producing total loss of sensation to analgesia with minimal blockade. The effectiveness of epidural analgesia depends on the technique and medications used. Theoretically, epidural local anesthetics could block all labor pain if used in large volumes and high concentrations. However, pain relief is balanced against other goals such as walking during the first stage of labor, pushing effectively in the second stage, and minimizing maternal and fetal side effects.

An epidural is contraindicated for women with a previous history of spinal surgery or spinal abnormalities, coagulation defects, cardiac disease, obesity, infections,

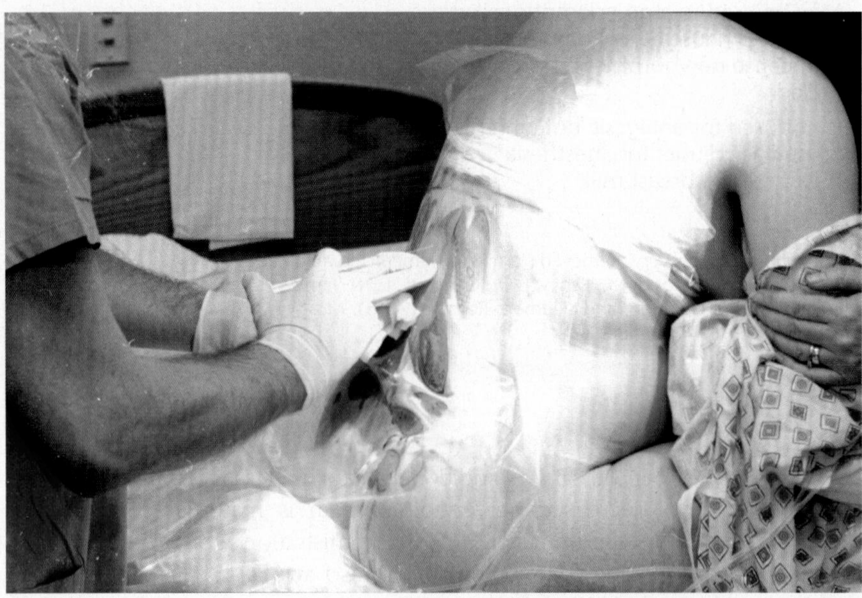

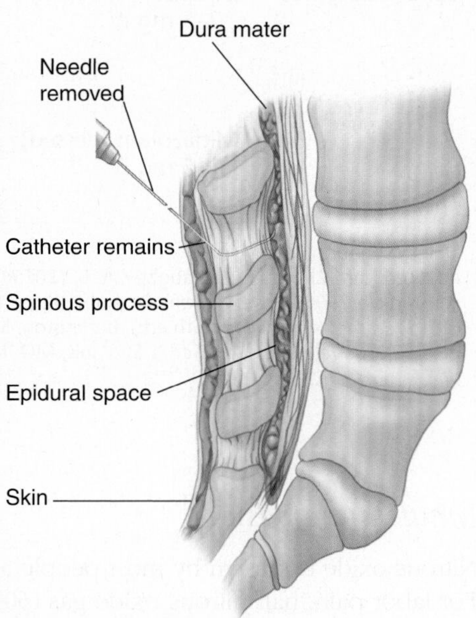

FIGURE 14.11 Epidural catheter insertion. **A.** A needle is inserted into the epidural space. **B.** A catheter is threaded into the epidural space; the needle is then removed. The catheter allows medication to be administered intermittently or continuously to relieve pain during labor and childbirth.

and hypovolemia. It also is contraindicated for the woman who is receiving anticoagulation therapy.

Complications include nausea and vomiting, hypotension, fever, pruritus, intravascular injection, maternal fever, allergic reaction, and respiratory depression. Effects on the fetus during labor include fetal distress secondary to maternal hypotension (Ibrahim et al., 2015). Ensuring that the woman avoids a supine position after an epidural catheter has been placed will help to minimize hypotension.

The addition of opioids, such as fentanyl or morphine, to the local anesthetic helps decrease the amount of motor block obtained. Continuous infusion pumps can be used to administer the epidural analgesia, allowing the woman to be in control and administer a bolus dose on demand (Patkar et al., 2015).

COMBINED SPINAL–EPIDURAL ANALGESIA

Another epidural technique is CSE analgesia. This technique involves inserting the epidural needle into the epidural space and subsequently inserting a small-gauge spinal needle through the epidural needle into the subarachnoid space. An opioid, without a local anesthetic, is injected into this space. The spinal needle is then removed and an epidural catheter is inserted for later use.

CSE is advantageous because of its rapid onset of pain relief (within 3 to 5 minutes) that can last up to 3 hours. It also allows the woman's motor function to remain active. Her ability to bear down during the second stage of labor is preserved because the pushing reflex is not lost, and her motor power remains intact. The CSE technique provides greater flexibility and reliability for labor than either spinal or epidural analgesia alone (Stocks & Griffiths, 2015). When compared with traditional epidural or spinal analgesia, which often keeps the woman lying in bed, CSE allows her to ambulate ("walking epidural"). A recent Cochrane review contrasting the CSE analgesia approach with traditional and low-dose epidural analgesia in labor identified that CSE analgesia was associated with a greater incidence of pruritus, but a lower incidence of urinary retention and need for rescue analgesia, than epidural alone. In addition, CSE analgesia had a faster onset of pain relief, and there were no differences in labor outcomes (Heesen et al., 2015). Ambulating during labor provides several benefits: it may help control pain better, shorten the first stage of labor, increase the intensity of the contractions, and decrease the possibility of an operative vaginal or cesarean birth.

Although women can walk with CSE, they often choose not to because of sedation and fatigue. Often health care providers do not encourage or assist women to ambulate for fear of injury. Nurses need to evaluate for ambulation safety that includes no postural hypotension and normal leg strength by demonstrating a partial knee bend while standing; they also need to assist with ambulation at all times (Capogna, 2015b). Currently, anesthesiologists are performing walking epidurals using continuous infusion techniques as well as CSE and client-controlled epidural analgesia (Grant et al., 2015).

Complications include maternal hypotension, intravascular injection, accidental intrathecal blockade, postdural puncture headache, inadequate or failed block, maternal fever, and pruritus. Hypotension and associated FHR changes are managed with maternal positioning (semi-Fowler position), intravenous hydration, and supplemental oxygen (Ibrahim et al., 2015).

PATIENT-CONTROLLED EPIDURAL ANALGESIA

Patient-controlled epidural analgesia (PCEA) involves the use of an indwelling epidural catheter with an infusion of medication and a programmed pump that allows the woman to control the dosing. This method allows

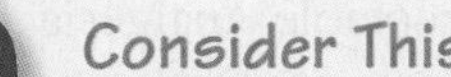

Consider This

When I was expecting my first child, I was determined to put my best foot forward and do everything right. I was an experienced OB nurse, and in my mind doing everything right was expected behavior. I was already 2 weeks past my calculated due date and I was becoming increasingly worried. That particular day I went to work with a backache but felt no contractions.

I managed to finish my shift but felt completely wiped out. As I walked to my car outside the hospital, my water broke and I felt the warm fluid run down my legs. I went back inside to be admitted for this much-awaited event.

Although I had helped thousands of women go through their childbirth experience, I was now the one in the bed and not standing alongside it. My husband and I had practiced our breathing techniques to cope with the discomfort of labor, but this "discomfort" in my mind was more than I could tolerate. So despite my best intentions of doing everything right, within an hour I begged for a painkiller to ease the pain. While the medication took the edge off my pain, I still felt every contraction and truly now appreciate the meaning of the word "labor." Although I wanted to use natural childbirth without any medication, I know that I was a full participant in my son's birthing experience, and that is what "doing everything right" was for me!

Thoughts: Doing what is right varies for each individual, and as nurses we need to support whatever that is. Having a positive outcome from the childbirth experience is the goal; the means it takes to achieve it is less important. How can nurses support women in making their personal choices to achieve a healthy outcome? Are any women "failures" if they ask for pain medication to tolerate labor? How can nurses help women overcome this stigma of being a "wimp"?

the woman to have a sense of control over her pain and reach her own individually acceptable analgesia level. When compared with traditional epidural analgesia, PCEA provides equivalent analgesia with lower anesthetic use, lower rates of supplementation, and higher client satisfaction (Van De Velde, 2015).

With PCEA, the woman uses a handheld device connected to an analgesic agent that is attached to an epidural catheter. When she pushes the button, a bolus dose of agent is administered via the catheter to reduce her pain. This method allows her to manage her pain at will without having to ask a staff member to provide pain relief. Evidence supports the use of PCEA which appears to result in greater maternal satisfaction and lower overall medication use (Sng et al., 2015).

LOCAL INFILTRATION

Local infiltration involves the injection of a local anesthetic, such as lidocaine, into the superficial perineal nerves to numb the perineal area. This technique is done by the physician or midwife just before performing an **episiotomy** or before suturing a laceration. Local infiltration does not alter the pain of uterine contractions, but it does numb the immediate area of the episiotomy or laceration. Local infiltration does not cause side effects for the woman or her newborn.

PUDENDAL NERVE BLOCK

A pudendal nerve block refers to the injection of a local anesthetic agent (e.g., bupivacaine, ropivacaine) into the pudendal nerves near each ischial spine. It provides pain relief in the lower vagina, vulva, and perineum (Fig. 14.12).

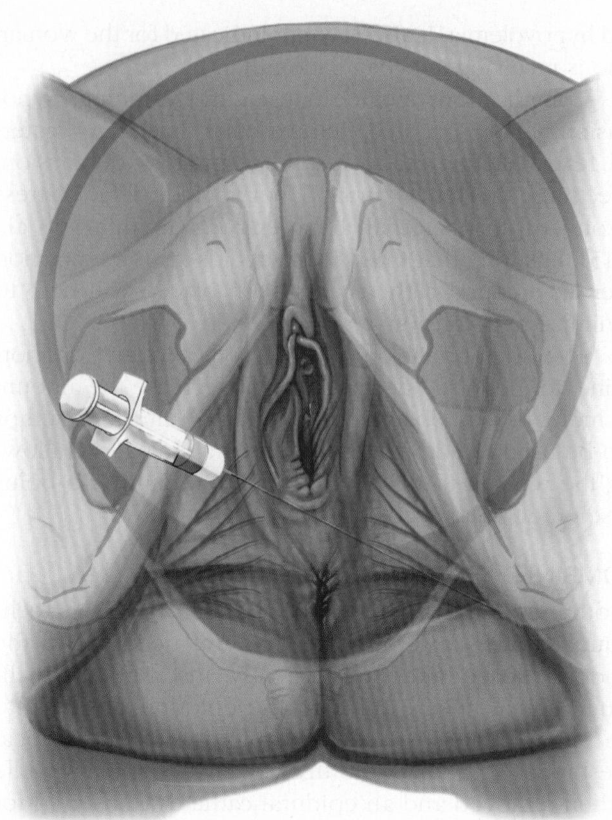

FIGURE 14.12 Pudendal nerve block.

A pudendal block is used for the second stage of labor, an episiotomy, or an operative vaginal birth with outlet forceps or vacuum extractor. It must be administered about 15 minutes before it would be needed to ensure its full effect. A transvaginal approach is generally used to inject an anesthetic agent at or near the pudendal nerve branch. Neither maternal nor fetal complications are common.

SPINAL (INTRATHECAL) ANALGESIA/ANESTHESIA

The spinal (intrathecal) pain management technique involves injection of an anesthetic "caine" agent, with or without opioids, into the subarachnoid space to provide pain relief during labor or cesarean birth. The subarachnoid space is a fluid-filled area located between the dura mater and the spinal cord. Spinal anesthesia is frequently used for elective and emergent cesarean births. The contraindications are similar to those for an epidural block. Adverse reactions for the woman include hypotension and spinal headache.

The subarachnoid injection of opioids alone, a technique termed intrathecal narcotics, has been gaining popularity since it was introduced in the 1980s. A narcotic is injected into the subarachnoid space, providing rapid pain relief while still maintaining motor function and sensation (Sng, Kwok, & Sia, 2015). An intrathecal narcotic is given during the active phase (more than 5 cm of dilation) of labor. Compared with epidural blocks, intrathecal narcotics are easy to administer, require a smaller volume of medication, produce excellent muscular relaxation, provide rapid-onset pain relief, are less likely to cause newborn respiratory depression, and do not cause motor blockade (Badve & Vallejo, 2015). Although pain relief is rapid with this technique, it is limited by the narcotic's duration of action, which may be only a few hours and not last through the labor. Additional pain measures may be needed to sustain pain management.

General Anesthesia

General anesthesia is typically reserved for emergency cesarean births when there is not enough time to provide spinal or epidural anesthesia or if the woman has a contraindication to the use of regional anesthesia. It can be started quickly and causes a rapid loss of consciousness. General anesthesia can be administered by intravenous injection, inhalation of anesthetic agents, or both. Commonly, thiopental, a short-acting barbiturate, or propofol is given intravenously to produce unconsciousness. This is followed by administration of a muscle relaxant. After the woman is intubated, nitrous oxide and oxygen are administered. A volatile halogenated agent may also be administered to produce amnesia (Cheng & Caughey, 2015a).

All anesthetic agents cross the placenta and affect the fetus. The primary complication with general anesthesia is fetal depression, along with uterine relaxation and potential maternal vomiting and aspiration. General anesthesia complications are usually due to maternal aspiration or the inability to intubate the woman. The incidence of these complications has decreased greatly as a result of improved techniques (Hawkins, 2015).

Although the anesthesiologist or nurse anesthetist administers the various general anesthesia agents, the nurse needs to be knowledgeable about the pharmacologic aspects of the drugs used and must be aware of airway management. Ensure that the woman is not taking anything by mouth (NPO) and has a patent intravenous line. In addition, administer a nonparticulate (clear) oral antacid (e.g., Bicitra or sodium citrate) or a proton pump inhibitor (Protonix) as ordered to reduce gastric acidity. Assist with placement of a wedge under the woman's right hip to displace the gravid uterus and prevent vena cava compression in the supine position. Once the newborn has been removed from the uterus, assist the perinatal team in providing supportive care.

NURSING CARE DURING LABOR AND BIRTH

Childbirth, a physiologic process that is fundamental to all human existence, is one of the most significant cultural, psychological, spiritual, and behavioral events in a woman's life. Although the act of giving birth is a universal phenomenon, it is a unique experience for each woman. Continuous evaluation and appropriate intervention for women during labor are essential to promoting a positive outcome for the family.

The nurse's role in childbirth is to ensure a safe environment for the mother and her newborn. Nurses begin evaluating the mother and fetus during the admission procedures at the health care agency and continue to do so throughout labor. It is critical to provide anticipatory guidance and explain each procedure (fetal monitoring, intravenous therapy, medications given, and expected reactions) and what will happen next. This will prepare the woman for the upcoming physical and emotional challenges, thereby helping to reduce her anxiety. Acknowledging members of her support system (family or partner) helps allay their fears and concerns, thereby assisting them in carrying out their supportive role. Knowing how and when to evaluate a woman during the various stages of labor is essential for all labor and birth nurses to ensure a positive maternal experience and a healthy newborn.

A major focus of care for the woman during labor and birth is assisting her with maintaining control over her pain, emotions, and actions while being an active participant. Nurses can help and support women to be actively involved in their childbirth experience by allowing time for discussion, offering companionship, listening to worries and concerns, paying attention to the woman's emotional needs, and offering information to help her understand what is happening in each stage of labor.

Nursing Management During the First Stage of Labor

Depending on how far advanced the woman's labor is when she arrives at the facility; the nurse will determine assessment parameters of maternal–fetal status and plan care accordingly. The nurse will provide high-touch, low-tech supportive nursing care during the first stage of labor when admitting the woman and orienting her to the labor and birth suite. The nurse is usually the primary gatekeeper of observations, interventions, treatments, and often the management of labor in the inpatient perinatal setting. Nursing care during this stage will include taking an admission history (reviewing the prenatal record); checking the results of routine laboratory tests and any special tests such as chorionic villi sampling, amniocentesis, genetic studies, and biophysical profile done during pregnancy; asking the woman about her childbirth preparation (birth plan, classes taken, coping skills); and completing a physical assessment of the woman to establish baseline values for future comparison.

Key nursing interventions include:

- Identifying the estimated date of birth from the client and the prenatal chart
- Validating the client's prenatal history to determine fetal risk status
- Determining fundal height to validate dates and fetal growth
- Performing Leopold maneuvers to determine fetal position, lie, and presentation
- Checking FHR
- Performing a vaginal examination (as appropriate) to evaluate effacement and dilation progress
- Instructing the client and her partner about monitoring techniques and equipment
- Assessing fetal response and FHR to contractions and recovery time
- Interpreting fetal monitoring strips
- Checking FHR baseline for accelerations, variability, and decelerations
- Repositioning the client to obtain an optimal FHR pattern
- Recognizing FHR problems and initiating corrective measures
- Checking amniotic fluid for meconium staining, odor, and amount

- Comforting client throughout testing period and labor
- Documenting times of notification for team members if problems arise
- Knowing appropriate interventions when abnormal FHR patterns present
- Supporting the client's decisions regarding intervention or avoidance of intervention
- Assessing the client's support system and coping status frequently

In addition to these interventions to promote optimal outcomes for the mother and fetus, the nurse must document care accurately and in a timely fashion. Accurate and timely documentation helps to decrease professional liability exposure, minimize the risk of preventable injuries to women and infants during labor and birth, and preserve families (Simpson, 2015). Guidelines for recording care include documenting:

- All care rendered, to prove that standards were met
- Conversations with all providers, including notification times
- Nursing interventions before and after notifying provider
- Use of the chain of command and response at each level
- All flow sheets and forms, to validate care given
- All education given to client and response to it
- Facts, not personal opinions
- Detailed descriptions of any adverse outcome
- Initial nursing assessment, all encounters, and discharge plan
- All telephone conversations (Callahan, 2016).

This standard of documentation is needed to prevent or defend against litigation, which is prevalent in the childbirth arena.

Assessing the Woman Upon Admission

The nurse usually first comes in contact with the woman either by phone or in person. The nurse should ascertain whether the woman is in true or false labor and whether she should be admitted or sent home. Upon admission to the labor and birth suite, the highest priorities include assessing FHR, assessing cervical dilation/effacement, and determining whether membranes have ruptured or are intact. These assessment data will guide the critical thinking in planning care for the client.

If the initial contact is by phone, establish a therapeutic relationship with the woman. Speaking in a calm caring tone facilitates this. Nurses providing a telephone triage service need to have sufficient clinical experience and have clear lines of responsibility to enable sound decision making. When completing a phone assessment, include questions about the following:

- Estimated date of birth, to determine if term or preterm
- Fetal movement (frequency in the past few days)
- Other premonitory signs of labor experienced
- Parity, gravida, and previous childbirth experiences
- Time from start of labor to birth in previous labors
- Characteristics of contractions, including frequency, duration, and intensity
- Appearance of any vaginal bloody show
- Membrane status (ruptured or intact)
- Presence of supportive adult in household or if she is alone

When speaking with the woman over the telephone, review the signs and symptoms that denote true versus false labor, and suggest various positions she can assume to provide comfort and increase placental perfusion. Also suggest walking, massage, and taking a warm shower to promote relaxation. Outline what foods and fluids are appropriate for oral intake in early labor. Throughout the phone call, listen to the woman's concerns and answer any questions clearly.

Reducing the risk of liability exposure and avoiding preventable injuries to mothers and fetuses during labor and birth can be accomplished by adhering to two basic tenets of clinical practice: (1) use applicable evidence and/or published standards and guidelines as the foundation of care, and (2) whenever a clinical choice is presented, choose client safety (Miller, 2014). With these two tenets in mind, advise the woman on the phone to contact her health care provider for further instructions or to come to the facility to be evaluated, since ruling out true labor and possible maternal–fetal complications cannot be done accurately over the phone. Additional nursing responsibilities associated with a phone assessment include:

- Consulting the woman's prenatal record for parity status, estimated date of birth, and untoward events
- Calling the health care provider to inform him or her of the woman's status
- Preparing for admission to the perinatal unit to ensure adequate staff assignment
- Notifying the admissions office of a pending admission

If the nurse's first encounter with the woman is in person, an assessment is completed to determine whether she should be admitted to the perinatal unit or sent home until her labor advances. Recent research findings suggest that women admitted before active labor are approximately twice as likely to be augmented with oxytocin and give birth via cesarean when compared with women admitted in active labor (Neal et al., 2014). Nurses need to make careful assessment of labor progression *prior* to labor admission to decrease early admissions and to improve labor safety and birth outcomes.

Entering a facility is often an intimidating and stressful event for women since it is an unfamiliar environment. Giving birth for the first time is a pivotal event in the lives of most women. Therefore, demonstrate respect when addressing the client; listen carefully and express interest and concern. Nurses must value and respect women and promote their self-worth and sense of control by allowing them to participate in making decisions. Allowing them a fair amount of autonomy in their childbirth decisions, supporting their personal worth, knowing them holistically, and using caring communication will increase client satisfaction (Ivory, 2014).

An admission assessment includes maternal health history, physical assessment, fetal assessment, laboratory studies, and assessment of psychological status. Usually the facility has a form that can be used throughout labor and birth to document assessment findings (Fig. 14.13).

MATERNAL HEALTH HISTORY AND CULTURAL ASSESSMENT

A maternal health history should include typical biographical data such as the woman's name and age and the name of the delivering health care provider. Other information that is collected includes reason for admission, such as labor, cesarean birth, or observation for a complication; the prenatal record data, including the estimated date of birth, a history of the current pregnancy, and the results of any laboratory and diagnostic tests, such as blood type, Rh status, and group B streptococcal status; past pregnancy and obstetric history; past health history and family history; prenatal education; list of medications; risk factors such as diabetes, hypertension, and use of tobacco, alcohol, or illicit drugs; pain management plan; history of potential domestic violence; history of previous preterm births; allergies; time of last food ingestion; method chosen for infant feeding; name of birth attendant (MD or midwife)(s) and pediatrician.

Ascertaining this information is important so that an individualized plan of care can be developed for the woman. If, for example, the woman's due date is still 2 months away, it is important to establish this information so interventions can be initiated to arrest the labor immediately or notify the intensive perinatal team to be available. In addition, if the woman has diabetes, it is critical to monitor her glucose levels during labor, to prepare for a surgical birth if dystocia of labor occurs, and to alert the newborn nursery of potential hypoglycemia in the newborn after birth. By collecting important information about each woman they care for, nurses can help improve the outcomes for all concerned.

Be sure to observe the woman's emotions, support system, verbal interaction, cultural background and language spoken, body language and posture, perceptual acuity, and energy level. This psychosocial information provides cues about the woman's emotional state, culture, and communication systems. For example, if the woman arrives at the labor and birth suite extremely anxious, alone, and unable to communicate in English, how can the nurse meet her needs and plan her care appropriately? It is only by assessing each woman physically and psychosocially that the nurse can make astute decisions regarding proper care. In this case, an interpreter would be needed to assist in the communication process between the staff and the woman to initiate proper care.

It is important to acknowledge and try to understand the cultural differences in women with cultural backgrounds different from that of the nurse. Attitudes toward childbirth are heavily influenced by the culture in which the woman has been raised. As a result, within every society, specific attitudes and values shape the woman's childbearing behaviors. Be aware of what these are. When carrying out a cultural assessment during the admission process, ask questions (Box 14.2) to help plan culturally competent care during labor and birth.

BOX 14.2

QUESTIONS FOR PROVIDING CULTURALLY COMPETENT CARE DURING LABOR AND BIRTH

- Where were you born? How long have you lived in the United States?
- What languages do you speak and read?
- Who are your major support people?
- What are your religious practices?
- How do you view childbearing?
- Are there any special precautions or restrictions that are important?
- Is birth considered a private or a social experience?
- How would you like to manage your labor discomfort?
- Who will provide your labor support?

Adapted from Bowers, P. (2015). Cultural perspectives in childbearing. *Nursing spectrum*. Retrieved from http://ce.nurse.com/ce263-60/cultural-perspectives-in-childbearing; and Anderson, L. (2014). Cultural competence in the nursing practice. *Nursetogether*. Retrieved from http://www.nursetogether.com/cultural-competence-in-the-nursing-practice

PHYSICAL EXAMINATION

The physical examination typically includes a generalized assessment of the woman's body systems, including hydration status, vital signs, auscultation of heart and lung sounds, and measurement of height and weight. The physical examination also includes the following assessments:

1. Pain level and coping behaviors demonstrated
2. Uterine activity, including contraction frequency, duration, and intensity
3. Fetal status, including heart rate, position, and station
4. Cervical dilation and degree of effacement
5. Status of membranes (intact or ruptured)
6. Assess vital signs: temperature, pulse, respirations, & blood pressure
7. Perform Leopold maneuvers to determine fetal lie
8. Fundal height measurement
9. Ability to ambulate safely

These assessment parameters form a baseline against which the nurse can compare all future values

ADMISSION ASSESSMENT OBSTETRICS

▲ PATIENT IDENTIFICATION ▲

ADMISSION DATA

Date | Time | Via ☐ Ambulatory ☐ Wheelchair ☐ Stretcher

Grav. | Term | Pre-term | Ab. | Living | EDC | LMP | GA

Prev. adm. date ________ Reason ________
Obstetrician ________ Pediatrician ________
Ht.______ Wt. ______ Wt. gain ______
Allergies (meds/food) ☐ None ________ ☐ Hx latex sensitivity
BP ______ T ______ P ______ R ______
FHR ______ Vag exam ______

Reason for Admission

☐ Labor / SROM ☐ Induction ________
☐ Primary C/S ________ ☐ Repeat C/S
☐ Observation ________
☐ OB / Medical complication ________

Onset of labor: ☐ Not in labor
Date ______ Time ______
Membranes: ☐ Intact
☐ Ruptured / Date ______ Time ______
☐ Clear ☐ Meconium ☐ Bloody ☐ Foul
Vaginal bleeding: ☐ None
☐ Normal show ☐ ________

Current Pregnancy Labs ☐ NPC

☐ POL ☐ PPROM ☐ Cerclage
☐ PIH ☐ Chr. HTN ☐ Other ________
☐ Diabetes ________ Diet ________
☐ Insulin ________
☐ Amniocentesis ________ Results ________

Bld type / RH____Date Rhogam____
Antibody screen ☐ Neg ☐ Pos
Rubella ☐ Non-immune ☐ Immune
Diabetic screen ☐ Normal ☐ Abnormal
Recent exposure to chick pox ☐
Current meds:________

	Pos	Neg	Tested
Hepatitis B	☐	☐	☐ No
HIV	☐	☐	☐ No
Group B strep	☐	☐	☐ No
GC	☐	☐	☐ No
Chlamydia	☐	☐	☐ No
RPR	☐	☐	☐ No

Previous OB History

☐ POL ☐ Multiple gestation
☐ Prev C/S type ________ Reason ________
☐ PIH ☐ Chronic HTN ☐ Diabetes
☐ Stillbirth/demise ☐ Neodeath ☐ Anomalies
☐ Precipitous labor (<3 H) ☐ Macrosomia
☐ PP Hemorrhage
☐ Hx Transfusion reaction ☐ Yes ☐ No
☐ Other ________

Latest risk assessment ☐ None
1. ________ 3. ________
2. ________ 4. ________

Date ________
Signature ________ Time ________

NEUROLOGICAL

☐ WNL
Variance: ☐ HA
☐ Scotoma / visual changes
Reflexes ☐ < 2 + ☐ > 2 +
☐ Clonus___ bts
☐ Numbness ☐ Tingling
☐ Hx Seizures
☐ ________

RESPIRATORY

☐ WNL
Variance: ☐ Hx Asthma ☐ URI
Respirations: ☐ < 12 ☐ > 24
Effort: ☐ SOB
☐ Shallow ☐ Labored
Auscultation:
☐ Diminished ☐ Crackles
☐ Wheezes ☐ Rhonchi

	No	Yes
Cough for greater than 2 weeks?	☐	☐
Is the cough productive?	☐	☐
Blood in the sputum?	☐	☐
Experiencing any fever or night sweats?	☐	☐
Ever had TB in the past?	☐	☐
Recent exposure to TB?	☐	☐
Weight loss in last 3 weeks?	☐	☐

If the patient answers yes to any three of the above questions implement policy and procedure # 5725-0704.

GASTROINTESTINAL

☐ WNL
Variance: ☐ Heartburn
☐ Epigastric pain Nausea
☐ Vomiting ☐ Diarrhea
☐ Constipation ☐ Pain
☐ Wt. Gain < 2lbs / month**
☐ Recent change in appetite of < 50% of usual intake for > 5 days
☐ ________

INTEGUMENTARY

☐ WNL
Variance: ☐ Rash ☐ Lacerations
☐ Abrasion ☐ Swelling
☐ Uticaria ☐ Bruising
☐ Diaphoretic/hot
☐ Clammy/cold
☐ Scars
☐ ________

FETAL ASSESSMENT

☐ WNL
Variance:
☐ NRFS
FHR ☐ < 110 ☐ > 160
LTV ☐ Absent ☐ Minimal
☐ Increased
STV Absent
Decelerations:________
☐ Decreased fetal movement
☐ IUGR
☐ ________

CARDIOVASCULAR

☐ WNL
Variance:
☐ MVP
Heart rate: ☐ < 60 ☐ > 100
B/P: Systolic: ☐ < 90 ☐ > 140
Diastolic: ☐ < 50 ☐ > 90
☐ Edema ________
☐ Chest pain / palpitations
☐ ________

MUSCULOSKELETAL

☐ WNL
Variance:
☐ Numbness ☐ Tingling
☐ Paralysis ☐ Deformity
☐ Scoliosis
☐ ________

GENITOURINARY

☐ WNL
Variance: ☐ Albumin
Output: ☐ < 30 cc/Hr.
☐ UTI ☐ Rx ☐ Frequency
☐ Dysuria ☐ Hematuria
☐ CVA Tenderness
☐ Hx STD ________
☐ Vag. discharge ________
☐ Rash ☐ Blisters
☐ Warts ☐ Lesions
☐ ________

EARS, NOSE, THROAT, AND EYES

☐ WNL
Variance:
☐ Sore throat ☐ Eyeglasses
☐ Runny nose ☐ Contact lenses
☐ Nasal congestion
☐ ________

PSYCHOSOCIAL

☐ WNL
Variance: ☐ Hx depression
☐ Yes ☐ No
☐ Emotional behavioral care
Affect: ☐ Flat ☐ Anxious
☐ Uncooperative ☐ Combative
Living will ☐ Yes ☐ No
☐ On chart
Healthcare surrogate ☐ Yes ☐ No
☐ On chart
Are you being hurt, hit, frightened by anyone at home or in your life? ☐ Yes ☐ No
Religious preference ________

Tobacco use ☐ Denies ☐ Yes Amt ________
Alcohol use ☐ Denies ☐ Yes Amt ________
Drug use ☐ Denies ☐ Yes Amt type ________
Primary language ☐ English ☐ Spanish ☐ ________

PAIN ASSESSMENT

1. Do you have any ongoing pain problems? ☐ No ☐ Yes
2. Do you have any pain now? ☐ No ☐ Yes
3. If any of the above questions are answered yes, the patient has a positive pain screening.
4. *Patient to be given pain management education material. Complete pain / symptom assessment on flowsheet.*
5. *Please proceed to complete pain assessment.*

FIGURE 14.13 Sample documentation form used for admission to the perinatal unit. (Used with permission. Briggs Corporation, 2001.)

throughout labor. The findings should be similar to those of the woman's prepregnancy and pregnancy findings, with the exception of her pulse rate, which might be elevated secondary to her anxious state with beginning labor.

LABORATORY STUDIES

On admission, laboratory studies typically are done to establish a baseline. Although the exact tests may vary among facilities, they usually include a urinalysis via clean-catch urine specimen and complete blood count. Blood typing and Rh factor analysis may be necessary if the results of these are unknown or unavailable. In addition, if the following test results are not included in the maternal prenatal history, it may be necessary to perform them at this time. They include syphilis screening, hepatitis B (HbsAg) screening, group B streptococcus (GBS), human immune deficiency virus (HIV) testing (if woman gives consent), and possible drug screening if the history is positive.

GBS is a gram-positive organism that colonizes in the female genital tract and rectum and is present in 10% to 30% of all healthy women (King et al., 2015). These women are asymptomatic carriers but can cause GBS disease of the newborn through vertical transmission during labor and horizontal transmission after birth. The mortality rate of infected newborns varies according to time of onset (early or late). Risk factors for GBS include maternal intrapartum fever, prolonged ruptured membranes (>12 to 18 hours), previous birth of an infected newborn, and GBS bacteriuria in the present pregnancy.

The Centers for Disease Control and Prevention (CDC), ACOG, and the American Academy of Pediatrics have guidelines that advised universal screening of pregnant women at 35 to 37 weeks' gestation for GBS and intrapartum antibiotic therapy for GBS carriers. These new guidelines reaffirmed the major prevention strategy—universal antenatal GBS screening and intrapartum antibiotic prophylaxis for culture-positive and high-risk women. Also included are new recommendations for laboratory methods for identification of GBS colonization during pregnancy, algorithms for screening and intrapartum prophylaxis for women with preterm labor and premature rupture of membranes, updated prophylaxis recommendations for women with a penicillin allergy, and a revised algorithm for the care of newborn infants (CDC, 2014). Maternal infections associated with GBS include acute chorioamnionitis, endometritis, and urinary tract infection. Neonatal clinical manifestations include pneumonia and sepsis. Identified GBS carriers receive intravenous antibiotic prophylaxis (penicillin G or ampicillin) at the onset of labor or ruptured membranes.

The ACOG, CDC, AWHONN, and the United States Preventive Services Task Force all recommend that all pregnant women be offered a screening test for HIV antibodies on their first prenatal visit, again during the third trimester if engaging in high-risk behaviors, and on admission to the labor and birth area. The CDC estimates that 50,000 individuals contract HIV in the United States each year, and 250,000 individuals have undiagnosed HIV infections (CDC, 2015).

If her HIV status is not documented, the woman being admitted to the labor and birth suite should have rapid HIV testing done. To reduce perinatal transmission, women who are HIV-positive are given zidovudine (2 mg/kg intravenously over an hour, and then a maintenance infusion of 1 mg/kg/hr until birth) or a single 200-mg oral dose of nevirapine at the onset of labor; the newborn is given zidovudine orally (2 mg/kg body weight every 6 hours) and should be continued for 6 weeks (Verklan & Walden, 2014). To further reduce the risk of perinatal transmission, ACOG and the United States Public Health Service recommend that women who are infected with HIV and have plasma viral loads of more than 1,000 copies/mL be counseled regarding the benefits of elective cesarean birth. In the absence of any medical intervention, the rate of vertical transmission of HIV to the fetus can range from 15% to 45% (Ashimi et al., 2015).

Additional interventions to reduce the transmission risk would include avoiding use of a scalp electrode for fetal monitoring or doing a scalp blood sampling for fetal pH, delaying amniotomy, encouraging formula feeding after birth, and avoiding invasive procedures such as forceps or vacuum-assisted devices. The nurse stresses the importance of all interventions and the goal to reduce transmission of HIV to the newborn.

Continuing Assessment During the First Stage of Labor

After the admission assessment is complete and the woman and her support person have been orientated to the room, equipment, and procedures, assessment continues for changes that would indicate that labor is progressing as expected. Assess the woman's knowledge, experience, and expectations of labor. Typically, blood pressure, pulse, and respirations are assessed every hour during the latent phase of labor unless the clinical situation dictates that vital signs be taken more frequently. During the active and transition phases, they are assessed every 30 minutes. The temperature is taken every 4 hours throughout the first stage of labor and every 2 hours after membranes have ruptured to detect an elevation indicating an ascending infection.

Vaginal examinations are performed periodically to track labor progress. This assessment information is shared with the woman to reinforce that she is making progress toward the goal of birth. Uterine contractions are monitored for frequency, duration, and intensity every 30 to 60 minutes during the latent phase, every 15 to 30 minutes during the active phase, and every 15 minutes during transition. Note the changes in the character of the contractions as labor progresses, and inform the woman of her progress. Continually determine the woman's level of pain and her ability to cope and use relaxation techniques effectively.

When the fetal membranes rupture, spontaneously or artificially, assess the FHR and check the amniotic fluid for color, odor, and amount. Assess the FHR intermittently or continuously via electronic monitoring. During the latent phase of labor, assess the FHR every 30 to 60 minutes; in the active phase, assess FHR at least every 15 to 30 minutes. Also, be sure to assess the FHR before ambulation, before any procedure, and before administering analgesia or anesthesia to the mother. Table 14.3 summarizes assessments for the first stage of labor.

Remember Sheila from the chapter-opening scenario? What is the nurse's role with Sheila in active labor? What additional comfort measures can the labor nurse offer Sheila?

Nursing Interventions

Nursing interventions during the admission process should include:

- Asking about the client's expectations of the birthing process
- Providing information about labor, birth, pain management options, and relaxation techniques
- Presenting information about fetal monitoring equipment and the procedures needed
- Monitoring FHR and identifying patterns that need further intervention
- Monitoring the mother's vital signs to obtain a baseline for later comparison
- Reassuring the client that her labor progress will be monitored closely and nursing care will focus on ensuring fetal and maternal well-being throughout

As the woman progresses through the first stage of labor, nursing interventions include:

- Encouraging the woman's partner to participate
- Keeping the woman and her partner up to date on the progress of the labor
- Orienting the woman and her partner to the labor and birth unit and explaining all of the birthing procedures

TABLE 14.3 SUMMARY OF ASSESSMENTS DURING THE FIRST STAGE OF LABOR

Assessments[a]	Latent Phase (0–3 cm)	Active Phase (4–7 cm)	Transition (8–10 cm)
Vital signs (BP, pulse, respirations)	Every 30–60 min	Every 30 min	Every 15–30 min
Temperature	Every 4 hr; more frequently if membranes are ruptured	Every 4 hr; more frequently if membranes are ruptured	Every 4 hr; more frequently if membranes are ruptured
Contractions (frequency, duration, intensity)	Every 30–60 min by palpation or continuously if EFM	Every 15–30 min by palpation or continuously if EFM	Every 15 min by palpation or continuously if EFM
Fetal heart rate	Every hour by Doppler or continuously by EFM	Every 30 min by Doppler or continuously by EFM	Every 15–30 min by Doppler or continuously by EFM
Vaginal examination	Initially on admission to determine phase and as needed based on maternal cues to document labor progression	As needed to monitor labor progression	As needed to monitor labor progression
Behavior/psychosocial	With every client encounter: talkative, excited, anxious	With every client encounter: self-absorbed in labor; intense and quiet now	With every client encounter: discouraged, irritable, feels out of control, declining coping ability

[a]The frequency of assessments is dictated by the health status of the woman and fetus and can be altered if either one of their conditions changes.
EFM, electronic fetal monitoring.
Adapted from King, T.L., Brucker, M.C., Kriebs, J. M., Fahey, J. O., Gegor, C. L., & Varney, H. (2015). *Varney's midwifery* (5th ed.). Burlington, MA: Jones & Bartlett Learning; and Green, C. J. (2016). *Maternal newborn nursing care plans* (3rd ed.). Burlington, MA: Jones & Bartlett Learning.

- Providing clear fluids (e.g., ice chips) as needed or requested
- Maintaining the woman's parenteral fluid intake at the prescribed rate if she has an IV
- Initiating or encouraging comfort measures, such as backrubs, cool cloths to the forehead, frequent position changes, ambulation, showers, slow dancing, leaning over a birth ball, side-lying, or counterpressure on lower back (Teaching Guidelines 14.1)

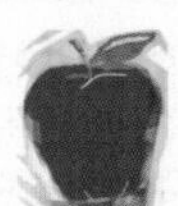

Teaching Guidelines 14.1

POSITIONING DURING THE FIRST STAGE OF LABOR

- Walking with support from the partner (adds the force of gravity to contractions to promote fetal descent)
- Slow-dancing position with the partner holding the woman (adds the force of gravity to contractions and promotes support from and active participation of your partner)
- Side lying with pillows between the knees for comfort (offers a restful position and improves oxygen flow to the uterus)
- Semi-sitting in bed or on a couch leaning against the partner (reduces back pain because fetus falls forward, away from the sacrum)
- Sitting in a chair with one foot on the floor and one on the chair (changes pelvic shape)
- Leaning forward by straddling a chair, a table, or a bed or kneeling over a birth ball (reduces back pain, adds the force of gravity to promote descent; possible pain relief if partner can apply sacral pressure)
- Encourage any position of comfort the woman choses to labor in and give birth.
- Sitting in a rocking chair or on a birth ball and shifting weight back and forth (provides comfort because rocking motion is soothing; uses the force of gravity to help fetal descent)
- Lunge by rocking weight back and forth with foot up on chair during contraction (uses force of gravity by being upright; enhances rotation of fetus through rocking)
- Open knee-chest position (helps to relieve back discomfort) (Gizzo et al., 2014; Tharpe et al., 2016).

- Encouraging the partner's involvement with breathing techniques
- Assisting the woman and her partner to focus on breathing techniques
- Informing the woman that the discomfort will be intermittent and of limited duration; urging her to rest between contractions to preserve her strength; and encouraging her to use distracting activities to lessen the focus on contractions
- Changing bed linens and gown as needed
- Keeping the perineal area clean and dry
- Supporting the woman's decisions about pain management
- Monitoring maternal vital signs frequently and reporting any abnormal values
- Ensuring that the woman takes deep cleansing breaths before and after each contraction to enhance gas exchange and oxygen to the fetus
- Educating the woman and her partner about the need for rest and helping them plan strategies to conserve strength
- Monitoring FHR for baseline, accelerations, variability, and decelerations
- Checking on bladder status and encouraging voiding at least every 2 hours to make room for birth
- Repositioning the woman as needed to obtain optimal heart rate pattern
- Communicating requests from the woman to appropriate personnel
- Respecting the woman's sense of privacy by covering her when appropriate
- Offering human presence by being present with the woman, not leaving her alone for long periods
- Being patient with the natural labor pattern to allow time for change
- Encouraging maternal movement throughout labor to increase the woman's level of comfort
- Dimming the lights in the room when pushing and request softened voices be used to maintain a calm and centered ambiance
- Reporting any deviations from normal to the health care professional so that interventions can be initiated early to be effective (Lucas et al., 2015; Green, 2016; and Nagtalon-Ramos, 2014).

See Nursing Care Plan 14.1 (at the end of the chapter).

Nursing Management During the Second Stage of Labor

Management of the second stage of labor often follows tradition-based routines rather than evidence-based practices. Current evidence for management of the second stage of labor supports the practices of delayed pushing, spontaneous (nondirected) pushing, and maternal choice positions (Cox & King, 2015). To be able to help women through the second stage of labor requires the nurse to have a comprehensive understanding of physiology and be aware of the latest evidence-based research and apply it to practice (Green, 2016).

Nursing care during the second stage of labor focuses on supporting the woman and her partner in making active decisions about her care and labor management, implementing strategies to prolong the early passive phase of fetal descent, supporting involuntary bearing-down efforts, providing instruction and assistance, and using maternal positions that can enhance descent and reduce pain (King et al., 2015). Women in the past gave birth unaided by following their bodies signals to birth their babies, so the role of the nurse should be to support the woman in her choice of pushing method and to encourage confidence in her maternal instinct of when and how to push.

In the absence of any complications, nurses should not be controlling this stage of labor, but empowering women to achieve a satisfying experience. The primary rationale for directing women to push is to shorten the second stage of labor. Common practice in many labor units is still to coach women to use closed glottis pushing with every contraction, starting at 10 cm of dilation, a practice that is not supported by research. Research suggests that directed pushing during the second stage may be accompanied by a significant decline in fetal pH and may cause maternal muscle and nerve damage if done too early (Reed, 2015). Shortening the phase of active pushing and lengthening the early phase of passive descent can be achieved by encouraging the woman not to push until she has a strong desire to do so and until the descent and rotation of the fetal head are well advanced. Effective pushing can be achieved by assisting the woman to assume a more upright or squatting position. Supporting spontaneous pushing and encouraging women to choose their own method of pushing should be accepted as best clinical practice (Cheng & Caughey, 2015b).

Perineal lacerations or tears can occur during the second stage when the fetal head emerges through the vaginal introitus. The extent of the laceration is defined by depth: a first-degree laceration extends through the skin; a second-degree laceration extends through the muscles of the perineal body; a third-degree laceration continues through the anal sphincter muscle; and a fourth-degree laceration also involves the anterior rectal wall. Special attention needs to be paid to third- and fourth-degree lacerations to prevent fecal incontinence. Risks for third- or fourth-degree lacerations included nulliparity, being Asian or Pacific Islander, increased birth weight of newborn, operative vaginal birth, episiotomy, and longer second stage of labor. Increasing body mass index was associated with fewer lacerations (Sides et al., 2015). The primary care provider should repair any lacerations during the third stage of labor.

An episiotomy is an incision made in the perineum to enlarge the vaginal outlet and theoretically to shorten the second stage of labor. Alternative measures such as warm compresses and continual massage with oil have been successful in stretching the perineal area to prevent cutting it. Certified nurse midwives can cut and repair episiotomies, but they frequently use alternative measures if possible.

Take Note!

Restrictive use of episiotomy has been recommended by ACOG given the risks of the procedure and unclear benefits of routine use (Friedman et al., 2015).

The midline episiotomy has been the most commonly used one in the United States because it can be easily repaired and causes the least amount of pain. The application of warmed compresses and/or intrapartum perineal massage is associated with a decrease in trauma to the perineal area and reduced the need for an episiotomy (Green, 2016). Routine episiotomy has declined since liberal usage has been discouraged by ACOG, except to avoid several maternal lacerations or to expedite difficult births. Anal sphincter laceration rates with spontaneous vaginal delivery have decreased, likely reflecting the decreased usage of episiotomy. The decline in operative vaginal delivery corresponds with a sharp increase in cesarean births, which may indicate that health care providers are favoring cesarean births for difficult births (Faisal-Cury et al., 2015). Figure 14.14 shows episiotomy locations.

Continuous Assessment During the Second Stage of Labor

Assessment is continuous during the second stage of labor. Hospital policies dictate the specific type and timing of assessments, as well as the way in which they are documented. Assessment involves identifying the signs typical of the second stage of labor, including:

- Increase in apprehension or irritability
- Spontaneous rupture of membranes
- Sudden appearance of sweat on upper lip
- Increase in blood-tinged show
- Low grunting sounds from the woman
- Complaints of rectal and perineal pressure
- Beginning of involuntary bearing-down efforts

Other ongoing assessments include the contraction frequency, duration, and intensity; maternal vital signs every 5 to 15 minutes; fetal response to labor as indicated by FHR monitor strips; amniotic fluid for color, odor, and amount when membranes are ruptured; and the copying status of the woman and her partner (Table 14.4).

Assessment also focuses on determining the progress of labor. Associated signs include bulging of the perineum, labial separation, advancing and retreating of the newborn's head during and between bearing-down efforts, and crowning (fetal head is visible at vaginal opening; Fig. 14.15).

A vaginal examination is completed to determine if it is appropriate for the woman to push. Pushing is appropriate if the cervix has fully dilated to 10 cm and the woman feels the urge to do so.

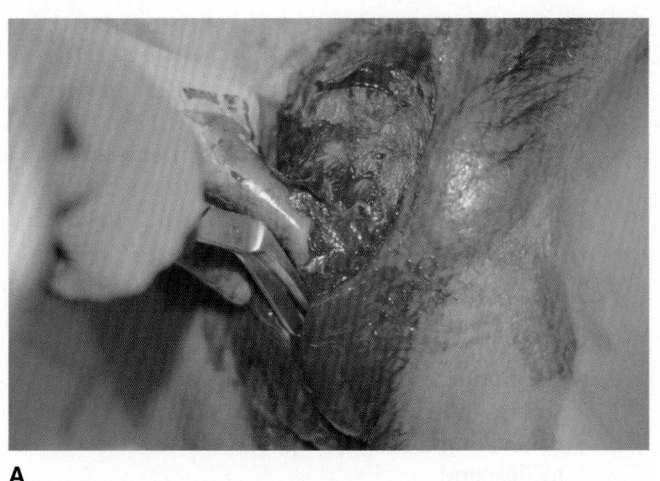

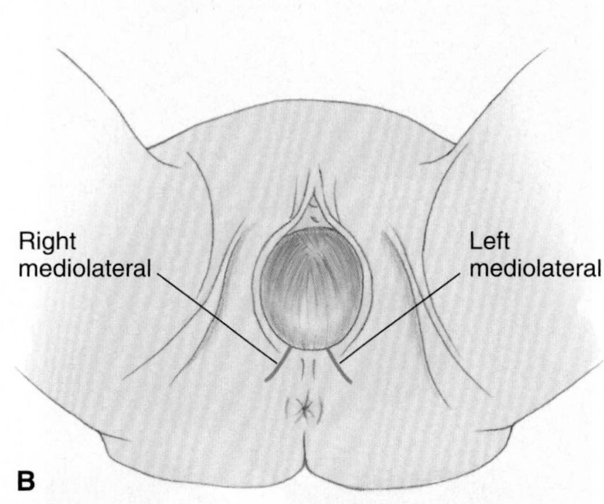

A B

FIGURE 14.14 **Location of an episiotomy. A. Midline episiotomy. B. Right and left mediolateral episiotomies.**

Nursing Interventions

Nursing interventions during this stage focus on motivating the woman, assisting with positioning and encouraging her to put all her efforts to pushing this newborn to the outside world, and giving her feedback on her progress. If the woman is pushing without progress, suggest that she keep her eyes open during the contractions and look toward where the newborn is coming out. Changing positions frequently will also help in making progress. Positioning a mirror so the woman can visualize the birthing process and how successful her pushing efforts are can help motivate her.

TABLE 14.4 SUMMARY OF ASSESSMENTS DURING THE SECOND, THIRD, AND FOURTH STAGES OF LABOR

Assessments[a]	Second Stage of Labor (Birth of Neonate)	Third Stage of Labor (Placenta Expulsion)	Fourth Stage of Labor (Recovery)
Vital signs (BP, pulse, respirations)	Every 5–15 min	Every 15 min	Every 15 min
Fetal heart rate	Every 5–15 min by Doppler or continuously by EFM	Apgar scoring at 1 and 5 min	Newborn—complete head-to-toe assessment; vital signs every 15 min until stable
Contractions/uterus	Palpate every one	Observe for placental separation	Palpating for firmness and position every 15 min for first hour
Bearing down/ pushing	Assist with every effort	None	None
Vaginal discharge	Observe for signs of descent—bulging of perineum, crowning	Assess bleeding after expulsion	Assess every 15 min with fundus firmness
Behavior/ psychosocial	Observe every 15 min: cooperative, focus is on work of pushing newborn out	Observe every 15 min: often feelings of relief after hearing newborn crying; calmer	Observe every 15 min: usually excited, talkative, awake; needs to hold newborn, be close, and inspect body

[a]The frequency of assessments is dictated by the health status of the woman and fetus and can be altered if either one of their conditions changes.

EFM, electronic fetal monitoring.

Adapted from Holvey, N. (2014). Supporting women in the second stage of labor. *British Journal of Midwifery, 22*(3), 182–186; American Hospital Association. (2015). *RNs role in labor and delivery*. Retrieved from http://www.aha.org/search?q=RNs+role+in+labor+and+delivery&start-date; and Wenner, L. (2015). It's the little things. *Nursing for Women's Health, 19*(2), 203–204.

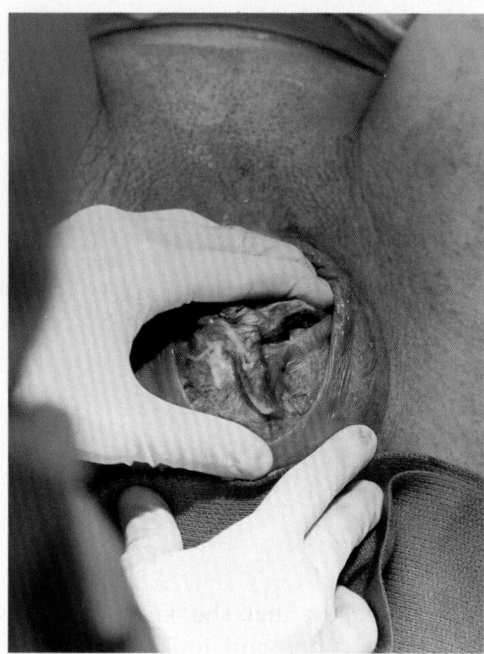

FIGURE 14.15 Crowning.

During the second stage of labor, an ideal position would be one that opens the pelvic outlet as wide as possible, provides a smooth pathway for the fetus to descend through the birth canal, takes advantage of gravity to assist the fetus to descend, and gives the mother a sense of being safe and in control of the labor process (Capogna, 2015a). Some suggestions for positions in the second stage include:

- Lithotomy with feet up in stirrups: most convenient position for caregivers, although EBP findings do not support this position physiologically
- Semi-sitting with pillows underneath knees, arms, and back
- Lateral/side-lying with curved back and upper leg supported by partner
- Sitting on birthing stool: opens pelvis, enhances the pull of gravity, and helps with pushing
- Squatting/supported squatting: gives the woman a sense of control
- Kneeling with hands on bed and knees comfortably apart

Other important nursing interventions during the second stage include:

- Providing continuous comfort measures such as mouth care, encouraging position changes, changing bed linen and underpads, and providing a quiet, focused environment
- Instructing the woman on the following bearing-down positions and techniques:
  - Pushing only when she feels an urge to do so
  - Delaying pushing for up to 90 minutes after complete dilation
  - Using abdominal muscles when bearing down
  - Using short pushes of 6 to 7 seconds
  - Focusing attention on the perineal area to visualize the newborn
  - Relaxing and conserving energy between contractions
  - Pushing several times with each contraction
  - Pushing with an open glottis and slight exhalation (Petrocnik & Marshall, 2015)
- Continuing to monitor contraction and FHR patterns to identify problems
- Providing brief, explicit directions throughout this stage
- Continuing to provide psychosocial support by reassuring and coaching
- Facilitating the upright position to encourage the fetus to descend
- Continuing to assess blood pressure, pulse, respirations, uterine contractions, bearing-down efforts, FHR, and coping status of the client and her partner
- Providing pain management if needed
- Providing a continuous nursing presence
- Offering praise for the client's efforts
- Preparing for and assisting with delivery by:
  - Notifying the health care provider of the estimated time frame for birth
  - Preparing the delivery bed and positioning client
  - Preparing the perineal area according to the facility's protocol
  - Offering a mirror and adjusting it so the woman can watch the birth
  - Explaining all procedures and equipment to the client and her partner
  - Setting up delivery instruments needed while maintaining sterility
  - Using standard precautions during the birthing process to avoid body fluid splashes
  - Recording the time of birth, time of placenta, and type of birth
  - Receiving newborn and transporting him or her to a warming environment, or covering the newborn with a warmed blanket on the woman's abdomen
  - Providing initial care and assessment of the newborn (see the Birth section that follows)

***Sheila* is completely dilated now and experiencing the urge to push. How can the nurse help Sheila with her pushing efforts? What additional interventions can the labor nurse offer Sheila now? In addition to encouraging Sheila to rest between pushing and offering praise for her efforts, what is the nurse's role during the birthing process?**

BIRTH

The second stage of labor ends with the birth of the newborn. The maternal position for birth varies from the standard lithotomy position to side-lying to squatting to standing or kneeling, depending on the birthing location, the woman's preference, and standard protocols. Once the woman is positioned for birth, cleanse the vulva and perineal areas. The primary health care provider then takes charge after donning protective eyewear, masks, gowns, and gloves and performing hand hygiene.

Once the fetal head has emerged, the primary care provider explores the fetal neck to see if the umbilical cord is wrapped around it. If it is, the cord is slipped over the head to facilitate delivery. As soon as the head emerges, the health care provider suctions the newborn's mouth first (because the newborn is an obligate nose breather) and then the nares with a bulb syringe to prevent aspiration of mucus, amniotic fluid, or meconium (Fig. 14.16). The umbilical cord is double-clamped and cut between the clamps by the birth attendant or the woman's partner if desired. With the first cries of the newborn, the second stage of labor ends. For care of the woman undergoing a surgical birth, the reader is referred to Chapter 21.

In addition to encouraging Sheila to rest between pushing and offering praise for her efforts, what is the nurse's role during the birthing process?

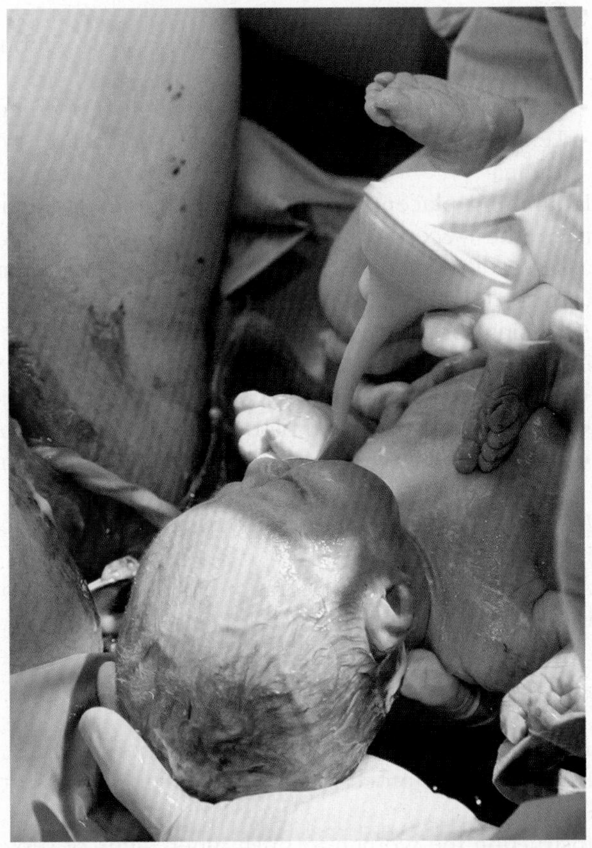

FIGURE 14.16 Suctioning the newborn immediately after birth.

IMMEDIATE CARE OF THE NEWBORN

Once birth takes place, the newborn is placed under a radiant warmer, dried, assessed, wrapped in warmed blankets, and placed on the woman's abdomen for warmth and closeness. In some health care facilities, the newborn is placed on the woman's abdomen immediately after birth and covered with a warmed blanket without being dried or assessed. In either scenario, the stability of the newborn dictates the location of aftercare. The nurse can also assist the mother with breast-feeding her newborn for the first time.

Assessment of the newborn begins at the moment of birth and continues until the newborn is discharged. Drying the newborn and providing warmth to prevent heat loss by evaporation is essential to help support thermoregulation and provide stimulation. Placing the newborn under a radiant heat source and putting on a stockinette/knitted cap will further reduce heat loss after drying.

Assess the newborn by assigning an Apgar score at 1 and 5 minutes. The Apgar score assesses five parameters – (1) heart rate (absent, slow, or fast), (2) respiratory effort (absent, weak cry, or good strong yell), (3) muscle tone (limp, or lively and active), (4) response to irritation stimulus, and (5) color – that evaluate a newborn's cardiorespiratory adaptation after birth. The parameters are arranged from the most important (heart rate) to the least important (color). The newborn is assigned a score of 0 to 2 in each of the five parameters. The purpose of the Apgar assessment is to evaluate the physiologic status of the newborn; see Chapter 18 for additional information on Apgar scoring.

Secure two identification bands on the newborn's wrist and ankle that match the band on the mother's wrist to ensure the newborn's identity. This identification process is completed in the birthing suite before anyone leaves the room. Some health care agencies also take an early photo of the newborn for identification in the event of abduction (National Center for Missing and Exploited Children [NCMEC], 2015).

Other types of newborn security systems can also be used to prevent abduction. Some systems have sensors that are attached to the newborn's identification bracelet or cord clamp. An alarm is set off if the bracelet or clamp activates receivers near exits. Others have an alarm that is activated when the sensor is removed from the newborn (Fig. 14.17). Even with the use of electronic sensors, the parents, nursing staff, and security personnel are responsible for prevention strategies and ensuring the safety and protection of all newborns (NCMEC, 2015). Nurses can help in preventing newborn abduction by educating parents about abduction risks, using identically numbered bands on the baby and parents, by instructing couples to keep their newborn in their direct line of vision within their hospital room at all times, taking color photographs of the infant, wearing color photograph ID badges themselves, discouraging parents/families from publishing

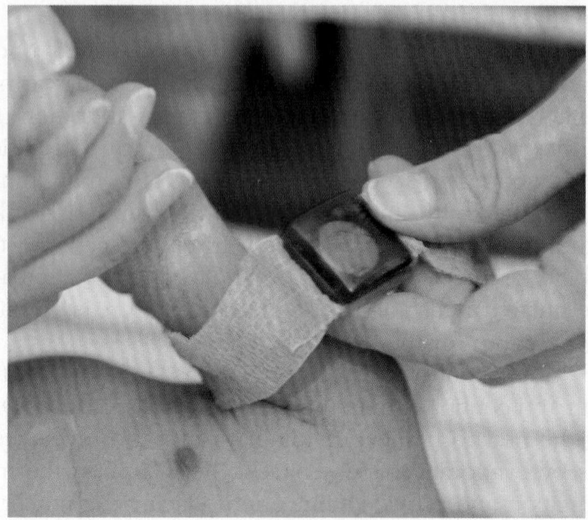

FIGURE 14.17 An example of a security sensor applied to a newborn's arm.

birth notices in the public media with mother's name and address, controlling access to nursery/postpartum unit with locked doors, and utilizing infant security tags or abduction alarm systems (NCMEC, 2015).

Sheila gave birth to a healthy 7-lb, 7-oz baby girl. She is eager to hold and nurse her newborn. What is the initial care of the newborn? How can the nurse meet the needs of both the newborn and Sheila, who is exhausted but eager to bond with her newborn?

Nursing Management During the Third Stage of Labor

During the third stage of labor, strong uterine contractions continue at regular intervals under the continuing influence of oxytocin. The uterine muscle fibers shorten, or retract, with each contraction, leading to a gradual decrease in the size of the uterus, which helps shear the placenta away from its attachment site. The third stage is complete when the placenta is delivered. Nursing care during the third stage of labor primarily focuses on immediate newborn care and assessment and observing for signs of placental separation, being available to assist with the delivery of the placenta, recording the time of expulsion and inspecting it for intactness. The nurse should also be assessing by palpating the uterus before and after placental expulsion.

Three hormones play important roles in the third stage. During this stage the woman experiences peak levels of oxytocin and endorphins, while the high adrenaline levels that occurred during the second stage of labor to aid with pushing begin falling. The hormone oxytocin causes uterine contractions and helps the woman to enact instinctive mothering behaviors such as holding the newborn close to her body and cuddling the baby.

Skin-to-skin contact immediately after birth and the newborn's first attempt at breast-feeding further augment maternal oxytocin levels, strengthening the uterine contractions that will help the placenta to separate and the uterus to contract to prevent hemorrhage. Endorphins, the body's natural opiates, produce an altered state of consciousness and aid in blocking out pain. In addition, the drop in adrenaline level from the second stage, which had kept the mother and baby alert at first contact, causes most women to shiver and feel cold shortly after giving birth.

Take Note!

A crucial role for nurses during this time is to protect the natural hormonal process by ensuring unhurried and uninterrupted contact between mother and newborn after birth, providing warmed blankets to prevent shivering, and allowing skin-to-skin contact with initial breast-feeding.

Continuing Assessment During the Third Stage of Labor

Assessment during the third stage of labor includes:

- Monitoring placental separation by looking for the following signs:
  - Firmly contracting uterus
  - Change in uterine shape from discoid to globular ovoid
  - Sudden gush of dark blood from vaginal opening
  - Lengthening of umbilical cord protruding from vagina
- Examining placenta and fetal membranes for intactness the second time (the health care provider assesses the placenta for intactness the first time) (Fig. 14.18)
- Assessing for any perineal trauma, such as the following, before allowing the birth attendant to leave:
  - Firm fundus with bright-red blood trickling: laceration
  - Boggy fundus with red blood flowing: uterine atony
  - Boggy fundus with dark blood and clots: retained placenta
- Inspecting the perineum for condition of episiotomy, if performed
- Assessing for perineal lacerations and ensuring repair by birth attendant

Nursing Interventions

Interventions during the third stage of labor include:

- Describing the process of placental separation to the couple
- Instructing the woman to push when signs of separation are apparent

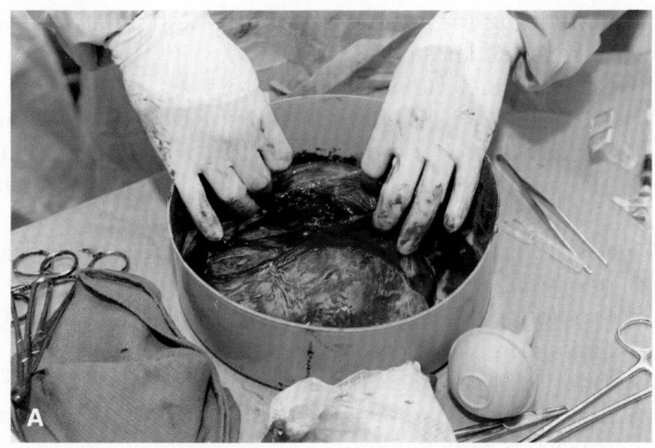

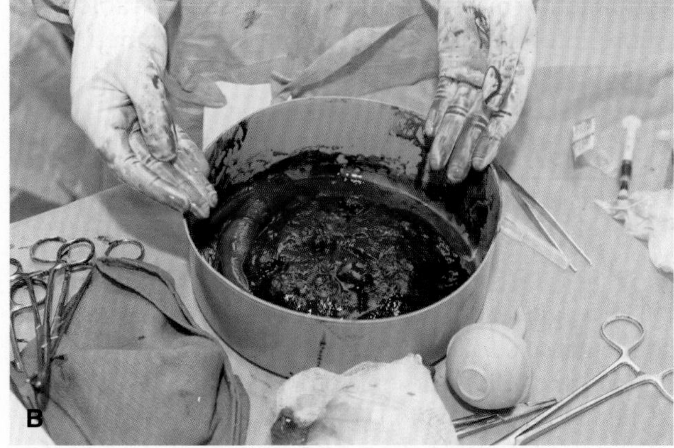

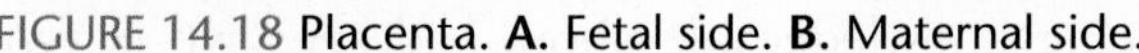

FIGURE 14.18 Placenta. **A.** Fetal side. **B.** Maternal side.

- Administering an oxytocic agent if ordered and indicated after placental expulsion
- Providing support and information about episiotomy and/or laceration if applicable
- Cleaning and assisting client into a comfortable position after birth, making sure to lift both legs out of stirrups (if used) simultaneously to prevent strain
- Assess the woman's knowledge of breast-feeding to determine educational needs
- Instruct her about latching on, positioning, infant sucking, and swallowing
- Repositioning the birthing bed to serve as a recovery bed if applicable
- Assisting with transfer to the recovery area if applicable
- Providing warmth by replacing warmed blankets over the woman
- Applying an ice pack to the perineal area to provide comfort to episiotomy if indicated
- Explaining what assessments will be carried out over the next hour and offering positive reinforcement for actions
- Ascertaining any needs
- Monitoring maternal physical status by assessing:
  - Vaginal bleeding: amount, consistency, and color
  - Vital signs: blood pressure, pulse, and respirations taken every 15 minutes
  - Uterine fundus, which should be firm, in the midline, and at the level of the umbilicus
- Recording all birthing statistics and securing primary caregiver's signature
- Documenting birthing event in the birth book (official record of the facility that outlines every birth event), detailing any deviations

Nursing Management During the Fourth Stage of Labor

The fourth stage of labor begins after the placenta is expelled and lasts up to 4 hours after birth, during which time recovery takes place. This recovery period may take place in the same room where the woman gave birth, in a separate recovery area, or in her postpartum room. During this stage, the woman's body is beginning to undergo the many physiologic and psychological changes that occur after birth. The focus of nursing management during the fourth stage of labor involves frequent close observation for hemorrhage, provision of comfort measures, and promotion of family attachment.

Assessment

Assessments during the fourth stage center on the woman's vital signs, status of the uterine fundus and perineal area, comfort level, lochia amount, and bladder status. During the first hour after birth, vital signs are taken every 15 minutes, then every 30 minutes for the next hour if needed. The woman's blood pressure should remain stable and within normal range after giving birth. A decrease may indicate uterine hemorrhage; an elevation might suggest preeclampsia.

The pulse usually is typically slower (60 to 70 bpm) than during labor. This may be associated with a decrease in blood volume following placental separation. An elevated pulse rate may be an early sign of blood loss. The blood pressure usually returns to its prepregnancy level and therefore is not a reliable early indicator of shock. Fever is indicative of dehydration (less than 100.4°F or 38°C) or infection (above 101°F), which may involve the genitourinary tract. Respiratory rate is usually between 16 and 24 breaths per minute and regular. Respirations should be unlabored unless there is an underlying preexisting respiratory condition.

Assess fundal height, position, and firmness every 15 minutes during the first hour following birth. The fundus needs to remain firm to prevent excessive postpartum bleeding. The fundus should be firm (feels like the size and consistency of a grapefruit), located in the midline and below the umbilicus. If it is not firm (boggy), gently massage it until it is firm (see Table 22.2 for more information). Once firmness is obtained, stop massaging.

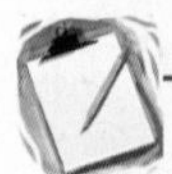

Take Note!

If the fundus is displaced to the right of the midline, suspect a full bladder as the cause.

The vagina and perineal areas are quite stretched and edematous following a vaginal birth. Assess the perineum, including the episiotomy if present, for possible hematoma formation. Suspect a hematoma if the woman reports excruciating pain or cannot void or if a mass is noted in the perineal area. Also assess for hemorrhoids, which can cause discomfort.

Assess the woman's comfort level frequently to determine the need for analgesia. Ask the woman to rate her pain on a scale of 1 to 10; it should be less than 3. If it is higher, further evaluation is needed to make sure there aren't any deviations contributing to her discomfort.

Assess vaginal discharge (lochia) every 15 minutes for the first hour and every 30 minutes for the next hour. Palpate the fundus at the same time to ascertain its firmness and help to estimate the amount of vaginal discharge. In addition, palpate the bladder for fullness, since many women receiving an epidural block experience limited sensation in the bladder region. Voiding should produce large amounts of urine (diuresis) each time. Palpating the woman's bladder after each voiding helps in assessing it and ensuring complete emptying. A full bladder will displace the uterus to either side of the midline and potentiate uterine hemorrhage secondary to bogginess.

Nursing Interventions

Nursing interventions during the fourth stage might include:

- Providing support and information to the woman regarding episiotomy repair and related pain relief and self-care measures
- Applying an ice pack to the perineum to promote comfort and reduce swelling
- Assisting with hygiene and perineal care; teaching the woman how to use the perineal bottle after each pad change and voiding; helping the woman into a new gown
- Monitoring for return of sensation and ability to void (if regional anesthesia was used)
- Encouraging the woman to void by ambulating to the bathroom, listening to running water, or pouring warm water over the perineal area with the peribottle
- Monitoring vital signs and fundal and lochia status every 15 minutes and documenting them
- Assessing for postpartum hemorrhage and urinary retention via uterine palpation
- Promoting comfort by offering analgesia for afterpains and warm blankets to reduce chilling
- Offering fluids and nourishment if desired
- Encouraging parent–infant attachment by providing privacy for the family
- Being knowledgeable about and sensitive to typical cultural practices after birth
- Assisting and encouraging the mother to nurse, if she chooses, during the recovery period to promote uterine firmness (the release of oxytocin from the posterior pituitary gland stimulates uterine contractions)
- Teaching the woman how to assess her fundus for firmness periodically and to massage it if it is boggy
- Describing the lochia flow and normal parameters to observe for postpartum
- Teaching safety techniques to prevent newborn abduction
- Demonstrating the use of the portable sitz bath as a comfort measure for her perineum if she had a laceration or an episiotomy repair
- Explaining comfort/hygiene measures and when to use them
- Assisting with ambulation when getting out of bed for the first time
- Providing information about the routine on the mother–baby unit or nursery for her stay
- Observing for signs of early parent–infant attachment: fingertip touch to palm touch to enfolding of the infant (Leonard, 2015; Green, 2016).

The nurse's role in labor and birth is a privileged one, supporting women at one of their most vulnerable times—childbirth. The nurse's focus during this time should be on supporting, protecting, advocating, and empowering women. The nurse should also provide informational support, which would allow the woman to realize her aspirations and goals by making decisions through informed choice. Nurses make a long-term difference in the lives of childbearing women with small things they do for their clients that make a big difference to them.

NURSING CARE PLAN 14.1

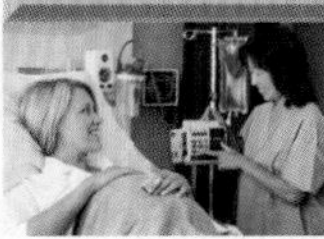

Overview of a Woman in the Active Phase of the First Stage of Labor

Candice, a 23-year-old gravida 1, para 0 (G1, P0), is admitted to the labor and birth suite at 39 weeks' gestation having contractions of moderate intensity every 5 to 6 minutes. A vaginal examination reveals that her cervix is 80% effaced and 5 cm dilated. The presenting part (vertex) is at 0 station and her membranes ruptured spontaneously 4 hours ago at home. She is admitted and an intravenous line is started for hydration and vascular access. An external fetal monitor is applied. FHR is 140 bpm and regular. Her partner is present at her bedside. Candice is now in the active phase of the first stage of labor, and her assessment findings are as follows: cervix dilated 7 cm, 80% effaced; moderate to strong contractions occurring regularly, every 3 to 5 minutes, lasting 45 to 60 seconds; at 0 station on pelvic examination; FHR auscultated loudest below umbilicus at 140 bpm; vaginal show—pink or bloody vaginal mucus; currently apprehensive, inwardly focused, with increased dependency; voicing concern about ability to cope with pain; limited ability to follow directions.

NURSING DIAGNOSIS: Anxiety related to labor and birth process and fear of the unknown related to client's first experience

Outcome Identification and Evaluation

The client will remain calm and in control as evidenced by ability to make decisions and use positive coping strategies.

Interventions: *Promoting Positive Coping Strategies*

- Provide instruction regarding the labor process to allay anxiety.
- Orient the woman to the physical environment and equipment as necessary to keep her informed of events.
- Encourage verbalization of feelings and concerns to reduce anxiety.
- Listen attentively to woman and partner to demonstrate interest and concern.
- Inform woman and partner of standard procedures/processes to ensure adequate understanding of events and procedures.
- Frequently update woman of progress and labor status to provide positive reinforcement for actions.
- Reinforce relaxation techniques and provide instruction if needed to aid in coping.
- Encourage participation of the partner in the coaching role; role-model to facilitate partner participation in labor process to provide support and encouragement to the client.
- Provide a presence and remain with the client as much as possible to provide comfort and support.

NURSING DIAGNOSIS: Acute pain related to uterine contractions and stretching of the cervix and birth canal

Outcome Identification and Evaluation

The client will maintain a tolerable level of pain and discomfort as evidenced by statements of pain relief, pain rating of 2 or less on pain rating scale, and absence of adverse effects in client and fetus from analgesia or anesthesia.

Interventions: *Providing Pain Relief*

- Monitor vital signs, observe for signs of pain, and have client rate pain on a scale of 0 to 10 to provide baseline for comparison.
- Encourage client to void every 1 to 2 hours to decrease pressure from a full bladder.
- Assist woman to change positions frequently to increase comfort and promote labor progress.
- Encourage use of distraction to reduce focus on contraction pain.

(continued)

NURSING CARE PLAN 14.1

Overview of a Woman in the Active Phase of the First Stage of Labor (continued)

- Suggest pelvic rocking, massage, or back counter pressure to reduce pain.
- Assist with use of relaxation and breathing techniques to promote relaxation.
- Use touch appropriately (backrub) when desired by the woman to promote comfort.
- Integrate use of nonpharmacologic measures for pain relief, such as warm water, birthing ball, or other techniques to facilitate pain relief.
- Administer pharmacologic agents as ordered when requested to control pain.
- Provide reassurance and encouragement between contractions to foster self-esteem and continued participation in labor process.

NURSING DIAGNOSIS: Risk of infection related to multiple vaginal examinations following rupture of membranes and tissue trauma

Outcome Identification and Evaluation

The client will remain free of infection as evidenced by the absence of signs and symptoms of infection, vital signs and FHR within acceptable parameters, lab test results within normal limits, and clear amniotic fluid without odor.

Interventions: *Preventing Infection*

- Monitor vital signs (every 2 hours after rupture of membranes [ROM]) and FHR frequently as per protocol to allow for early detection of problems; report fetal tachycardia (early sign of maternal infection) to ensure prompt treatment.
- Provide frequent perineal care and pad changes to maintain good perineal hygiene.
- Change linens and woman's gown as needed to maintain cleanliness.
- Ensure that vaginal examinations are performed only when needed to prevent introducing pathogens into the vaginal vault.
- Monitor lab test results such as white blood cell count to assess for elevations indicating infection.
- Use aseptic technique for all invasive procedures to prevent infection transmission.
- Carry out good handwashing techniques before and after procedures and use standard precautions as appropriate to minimize risk of infection transmission.
- Document amniotic fluid characteristics – color, odor – to establish baseline for comparison.

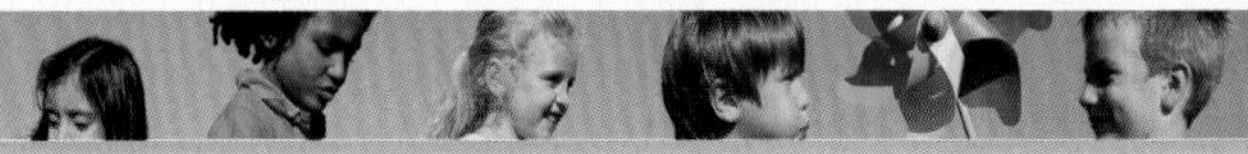

KEY CONCEPTS

- A nurse provides physical and emotional support during the labor and birth process to assist a woman to achieve her goals.
- When a woman is admitted to the labor and birth area, the admitting nurse must assess and evaluate the risk status of the pregnancy and initiate appropriate interventions to provide optimal care for the client.
- Completing an admission assessment includes taking a maternal health history; performing a physical assessment on the woman and fetus, including her emotional and psychosocial status; and obtaining the necessary laboratory studies.
- The nurse's role in fetal assessment for labor and birth includes determining fetal well-being and interpreting signs and symptoms of possible compromise. Determining the fetal heart rate (FHR) pattern and assessing amniotic fluid characteristics are key.
- FHR can be assessed intermittently or continuously. Although the intermittent method allows the client to move about during labor, the information obtained intermittently does not provide a complete picture of fetal well-being from moment to moment.
- Assessment parameters of the FHR are classified as baseline rate, baseline variability, and periodic changes in the rate (accelerations and decelerations).

- The nurse monitoring the laboring client needs to be knowledgeable about which category the FHR pattern is in so that appropriate interventions can be instituted.
- For a category III FHR pattern, the nurse should notify the health care provider about the pattern and obtain further orders, making sure to document all interventions and their effects on the FHR pattern.
- In addition to interpreting assessment findings and initiating appropriate inventions for the laboring client, accurate and timely documentation must be carried out continuously.
- Today's women have many safe nonpharmacologic and pharmacologic choices for the management of pain during childbirth. They may be used individually or in combination to complement one another.
- Nursing management for the woman during labor and birth includes comfort measures, emotional support, information and instruction, advocacy, and support for the partner.
- Nursing care during the first stage of labor includes taking an admission history (reviewing the prenatal record), checking the results of routine laboratory work and special tests done during pregnancy, asking the woman about her childbirth preparation (birth plan, classes taken, coping skills), and completing a physical assessment of the woman to establish baseline values for future comparison.
- Nursing care during the second stage of labor focuses on supporting the woman and her partner in making decisions about her care and labor management, implementing strategies to prolong the early passive phase of fetal descent, supporting involuntary bearing-down efforts, providing support and assistance, and encouraging the use of maternal positions that can enhance descent and reduce the pain.
- Nursing care during the third stage of labor primarily focuses on immediate newborn care and assessment and being available to assist with the delivery of the placenta and inspecting it for intactness.
- The focus of nursing management during the fourth stage of labor involves frequently observing the mother for hemorrhage, providing comfort measures, and promoting family attachment.

REFERENCES AND RECOMMENDED READINGS

Adams, J., Frawley, J., Steel, A., Broom, A., & Sibbritt, D. (2015). Use of pharmacological and non-pharmacological labor pain management techniques and their relationship to maternal and infant birth outcomes: Examination of a nationally representative sample of 1835 pregnant women. *Midwifery, 31*(4), 458–463.

Agency for Healthcare Research and Quality [AHRQ]. (2014). *Intrapartum fetal heart rate monitoring: Nomenclature, and general management principles*. Retrieved from http://www.guideline.gov/content.aspx?id=14885

American College of Obstetricians and Gynecologists [ACOG], & Society for Maternal Fetal Medicine [SMFM]. (2014). Safe prevention of the primary cesarean delivery. Obstetric Care Consensus 1. *Obstetrics & Gynecology, 123*, 693–711.

American Hospital Association. (2015). *RNs role in labor and delivery*. Retrieved from http://www.aha.org/search?q=RNs+role+in+labor+and+delivery&start-date

American Pregnancy Association. (2015). *Patterned breathing during labor*. Retrieved from http://www.americanpregnancy.org/labornbirth/patternedbreathing.htm

Anderson, L. (2014). Cultural competence in the nursing practice. *Nursetogether*. Retrieved from http://www.nursetogether.com/cultural-competence-in-the-nursing-practice

Ashimi, O., Hoff, E., Sibai, B., & Hardwicke, R. (2015). 212: Should the current DHHS recommendations for use of antiretroviral drugs in maternal HIV-1 RNA undergo a review? An urban academic experience. *American Journal of Obstetrics & Gynecology, 212*(1), S119–S120.

Association of Women's Health, Obstetric and Neonatal Nurses [AWHONN]. (2015). *Fetal heart monitoring: Principles and practices* (5th ed.). Washington, DC: AWHONN.

Badve, M., & Vallejo, M. C. (2015). Obstetric anesthesia. In *Basic clinical anesthesia* (pp. 501–527). New York, NY: Springer Publishers.

Bowers, P. (2015). Cultural perspectives in childbearing. *Nursing spectrum*. Retrieved from http://ce.nurse.com/ce263-60/cultural-perspectives-in-childbearing

Cahill, A. G., & Spain, J. (2015). Intrapartum fetal monitoring. *Clinical Obstetrics and Gynecology, 58*(2), 263–268.

Callahan, T. L. (2016). *Tarascon's OB/GYN pocketbook*. Burlington, MA: Jones & Bartlett Learning.

Camorcia, M. (2015). The second and third stage of labor. In *Epidural labor analgesia* (pp. 103–119). Switzerland: Springer International Publishing.

Capogna, G. (2015a). Humanization of childbirth and epidural analgesia. In *Epidural labor analgesia* (pp. 315–323). Switzerland: Springer International Publishing.

Capogna, G. (2015b). Maintenance of labor analgesia. In *Epidural labor analgesia* (pp. 89–101). Switzerland: Springer International Publishing.

Casanova, R. (2015). *Shelf-life obstetrics and gynecology*. Philadelphia, PA: Lippincott Williams & Wilkins.

Centers for Disease Control and Prevention [CDC]. (2014). *Group B strep (GBS) guidelines*. Retrieved from http://www.cdc.gov/groupbstrep/guidelines/new-differences.html

Centers for Disease Control and Prevention [CDC]. (2015). *HIV/AIDS testing*. Retrieved from http://www.cdc.gov/hiv/basics/testing.html

Chandraharan, E. (2014). Fetal scalp sampling during labor: Is it a useful diagnostic test or a historical test that no longer has a place in modern obstetrics? *An International Journal of Obstetrics & Gynaecology, 121*, 1056–1062.

Cheng, Y., & Caughey, A. B. (2015a). Normal labor and delivery. *eMedicine*. Retrieved from http://emedicine.medscape.com/article/260036-overview#aw2aab6b2

Cheng, Y. W., & Caughey, A. B. (2015b). Second stage of labor. *Clinical Obstetrics and Gynecology, 58*(2), 227–240.

Cibils, L. A. (2014). *Electronic fetal-maternal monitoring: Antepartum/intrapartum* (2nd ed.). New York, NY: Springer Publishers.

Cox, K. J., & King, T. L. (2015). Preventing primary cesarean births: Midwifery care. *Clinical Obstetrics and Gynecology, 58*(2), 282–293.

Dalal, S. M. (2015). Newer aspects in labor analgesia. *Research Chronicle in Health Sciences*, 1(2), 130–138.

Faisal-Cury, A., Menezes, P. R., Quayle, J., Matijasevich, A., & Diniz, S. G. (2015). The relationship between mode of delivery and sexual health outcomes after childbirth. *The Journal of Sexual Medicine, 12*(5), 1212–1220.

Farine, D. (Ed.). (2015). *New technologies for managing labor.* Boston, MA: Walter de GruyterGmbH & Co KG.

Freeman, R. K. (2015) Intrapartum fetal heart rate monitoring. In J. T. Queenan, C. Y. Spong and C. J. Lockwood (Eds.), Protocols for high-risk pregnancies: An evidence-based approach. Chichester, UK: John Wiley & Sons, Ltd. doi: 10.1002/9781119001256.ch50

Friedman, A. M., Ananth, C. V., Prendergast, E., D'Alton, M. E., & Wright, J. D. (2015). Variation in and factors associated with use of episiotomy. *Journal of the American Medical Association, 313*(2), 197–199.

Gizzo, S., Di Gangi, S., Noventa, M., Bacile, V., Zambon, A., & Nardelli, B. (2014). Women's choice of positions during labor: Return to the past or a modern way to give birth? A cohort study in Italy. *BioMed Research International,2014*, 638093, http://dx.doi.org/10.1155/2014/638093

Grant E. N., Tao W., Craig M., McIntire D., & Leveno K. (2015). Neuraxial analgesia effects on labor progression: Facts, fallacies, uncertainties and the future. *British Journal of Obstetrics and Gynaecology, 122*(3), 288–293.

Green, C. J. (2016). *Maternal newborn nursing care plans* (3rd ed.). Burlington, MA: Jones & Bartlett Learning.

Gujral, K., & Nayar, S. (2015). Current trends in management of fetal growth restriction. *Journal of Fetal Medicine, 1*(3), 125–129.

Halpern, S. H., & Garg, R. (2015). Evidence-based medicine and labor analgesia. In *Epidural labor analgesia* (pp. 285–295). Switzerland: Springer International Publishing.

Hanson, L., & VandeVusse, L. (2014). Supporting labor progress toward physiologic birth. *Journal of Perinatal & Neonatal Nursing, 28*(2), 101–107.

Hastings, C. (2015). The role of fetal monitoring in intrapartum care. *British Journal of Healthcare Management,* [serial online], *21*(4), 166–170.

Hawkins, J. L. (2015). Excess in moderation: General anesthesia for cesarean delivery. *Anesthesia & Analgesia, 120*(6), 1175–1177.

Heesen, M., Van de Velde, M., Klöhr, S., Lehberger, J., Rossaint, R., & Straube, S. (2015). Meta-analysis of the success of block following combined spinal-epidural vs epidural analgesia during labor. *Survey of Anesthesiology, 59*(3), 131–133.

Hersh, S., Megregian, M., & Emeis, C. (2014). Intermittent auscultation of the fetal heart rate during labor: An opportunity for shared decision making. *Journal of Midwifery & Women's Health, 59*(3), 344–349.

Hiersch, L., Rosen, H., Salzer, L., Aviram, A., Ben-Haroush, A., & Yogev, Y. (2015). Does artificial rupturing of membranes in the active phase of labor enhance myometrial electrical activity? *The Journal of Maternal-Fetal & Neonatal Medicine, 28*(5), 515–518.

Holvey, N. (2014). Supporting women in the second stage of labor. *British Journal of Midwifery, 22*(3), 182–186.

Ibrahim, S. E. H., Fridman, M., Korst, L. M., & Gregory, K. D. (2015). Anesthesia complications as a childbirth patient safety indicator. *Survey of Anesthesiology, 59*(3), 127–129.

Institute for Clinical Systems Improvement [ICSI]. (2015a). *Fetal monitoring*. Retrieved from http://link.springer.com/chapter/10.1007/978-1-4614-8557-5_42#page-1

Institute for Clinical Systems Improvement [ICSI]. (2015b). *Health care guideline: Management of labor.* Retrieved from https://www.icsi.org/_asset/br063k/LaborMgmt.pdf

Iravani, M., Zarean, E., Janghorbani, M., & Bahrami, M. (2015). Women's needs and expectations during normal labor and delivery. *Journal of Education and Health Promotion, 4,* 6.

Ivory, C. H. (2014). Standardizing the words nurses use to document elements of perinatal failure to rescue. *JOGNN: Journal of Obstetric, Gynecologic & Neonatal Nursing, 43*(1), 13–24.

Jackson, S., & Gregory, K. D. (2015). Management of the first stage of labor: Potential strategies to lower the cesarean delivery rate. *Clinical Obstetrics and Gynecology, 58*(2), 217–226.

Janula, R., & Mahipal, S. (2015). Effectiveness of aromatherapy and biofeedback in promotion of labor outcome during childbirth among primigravidas. *Health Science Journal, 9*(1), 1–5.

Jones, L. E., Whitburn, L. Y., Davey, M. A., & Small, R. (2015). Assessment of pain associated with childbirth: Women's perspectives, preferences and solutions. *Midwifery, 31*(7), 708–712.

Kerr, D., Taylor, D., & Evans, B. (2015). Patient-controlled intranasal fentanyl analgesia: A pilot study to assess practicality and tolerability during childbirth. *International Journal of Obstetric Anesthesia, 24*(2), 117–123.

King, T. L., Brucker, M. C., Kriebs, J. M., Fahey, J. O., Gegor, C. L., & Varney, H. (2015). *Varney's midwifery* (5th ed.). Burlington, MA: Jones & Bartlett Learning.

Leonard, P. (2015). Childbirth education: A handbook for nurses. *Nursing spectrum*. Retrieved from http://ce.nurse.com/60057/childbirth-education-a-handbook-for-nurses

Lindholm, A., & Hildingsson, I. (2015). Women's preferences and received pain relief in childbirth—a prospective longitudinal study in a northern region of Sweden. *Sexual & Reproductive Healthcare, 6*(2), 74–81.

Liu, Y. M., Fernando, R., & Mon, W. Y. (2015). Labor pain. In *Epidural labor analgesia* (pp. 21–37). Switzerland: Springer International Publishing.

Lucas, M. T. B., da Rocha, M. J. F., de Medonça Costa, K. M., de Oliveira, G. G., & Melo, J. O. (2015). Nursing care during labor in a model maternity unit: Cross-sectional study. *Online Brazilian Journal of Nursing, 14*(1), 32–40.

Magowan, B., Owen, P., & Thomson, A. (2014). *Clinical obstetrics & gynecology* (3rd ed.). St. Louis, MO: Saunders Elsevier.

Martin, R. J., Fanaroff, A. A., & Walsh, M. C. (2014). *Neonatal-perinatal medicine* (10th ed.). Philadelphia, PA: Elsevier Health Sciences.

Maso, G., Piccoli, M., De Seta, F., Parolin, S., Banco, R., Camacho, M. L., et al. (2015). Intrapartum fetal heart rate monitoring interpretation in labor: A critical appraisal. *Minerva Ginecologica, 67*(1), 65–79.

McGeary, C. A., Swanholm, E., & Gatchel, R. J. (2015). Pain management. *The Encyclopedia of Clinical Psychology*, 1–6. DOI: 10.1002/9781118625392.wbecp144

Miller, L. A. (2014). Ask an expert: Frequently asked questions on nursing liability issues. *Journal of Perinatal & Neonatal Nursing, 28*(1), 9–11.

Mollart, L. J., Adam, J., & Foureur, M. (2015). Impact of acupressure on onset of labor and labor duration: A systematic review. *Women and Birth*, *28*(3), 199–206.

Nageotte, M. P. (2015). Fetal heart rate monitoring. *Seminars in Fetal and Neonatal Medicine*, *20*(3), 144–148.

Nagtalon-Ramos, J. (2014). *Best evidence-based practices in maternal-newborn nursing care*. Philadelphia, PA: F. A. Davis Company.

National Center for Missing and Exploited Children [NCMEC]. (2015). *Infant abductions*. Retrieved from http://www.missingkids.com/InfantAbduction

National Institute for Health and care Excellence [NICE]. (2014). *Intrapartum care: Care of healthy women and their babies during childbirth*. CG190. London, UK: NICE.

National Institute of Child Health and Human Development [NICHD]. (2015). NICHD terminology for fetal heart rate characteristics. Retrieved from http://www.nichd.nih.gov/search.cfm?search_string=electronic+fetal+monitoring

Neal, J. L., Lamp, J. M., Buck, J. S., Lowe, N. K., Gillespie, S. L., & Ryan, S. L. (2014). Outcomes of nulliparous women with spontaneous labor onset admitted to hospitals in preactive versus active labor. *Journal of Midwifery & Women's Health*, *59*(1), 28–34.

Neetu, P. S., & Panchal, R. (2015). A study to assess the effectiveness of abdominal effleurage on labor pain intensity and labor outcomes among nullipara mothers during first stage of labor in selected Hospitals of District Ambala, Haryana. *International Journal of Science & Research*, *4*(1), 1585–1590.

Nutter, E. (2016). Decreasing vulnerability in childbirth: Waterbirth in military treatment facilities. *Caring for the vulnerable* (4th ed., pp. 253–262). Burlington, MA: Jones & Bartlett Learning.

Omo-Aghoja, L. (2015). Maternal and fetal acid-base chemistry: A major determinant of perinatal outcome. *Annals of Medical and Health Sciences Research*, *4*(1), 8–17.

Patkar, C. S., Vora, K., Patel, H., Shah, V., Modi, M. P., & Parikh, G. (2015). A comparison of continuous infusion and intermittent bolus administration of 0.1% ropivacaine with 0.0002% fentanyl for epidural labor analgesia. *Journal of Anesthesiology, Clinical Pharmacology*, *31*(2), 234–238.

Petrocnik, P., & Marshall, J. E. (2015). Hands-poised technique: The future technique for perineal management of second stage of labor? A modified systematic literature review. *Midwifery*, *31*(2), 274–279.

Prior, T., & Kumar, S. (2015). Expert review—identification of intra-partum fetal compromise. *European Journal of Obstetrics & Gynecology and Reproductive Biology*, *190*, 1–6.

Reed, R. (2015). Supporting women's instinctive pushing behaviour during birth. *The Practicing Midwife*, *18*(6), 13–15.

Roberts, L., Gulliver, B., Fisher, J., & Cloyes, K. G. (2010). The coping with labor algorithm: An alternate pain assessment tool for the laboring woman. *Journal of Midwifery & Women's Health*, *55*, 107–116.

Sholapurkar, M. S. L. (2015). Intrapartum fetal monitoring: Overview, controversies and pitfalls. *The Health Foundation*, 1–8.

Sholapurkar, S. (2014). Algorithm for management of category II fetal heart rate tracings: A standardization of right sort? *American Journal of Obstetrics and Gynecology*, *210*(2), 175.

Sides, C., Rios, A. R., Lam, M. C., Ward, A. R., Stoltzfus, J., & Lucente, V. R. (2015). Above all, do no harm: Modifiable risk factors for high-risk perineal lacerations [139]. *Obstetrics & Gynecology*, *125*, 49S.

Simkin, P., & Klein, M.C. (2015). Nonpharmacologic approaches to management of labor pain. *UpToDate*. Retrieved from http://www.uptodate.com/contents/nonpharmacological-approaches-to-management-of-labor-pain

Simpson, K. R. (2015). Electronic health records. *MCN: The American Journal of Maternal/Child Nursing*, *40*(1), 68.

Skidmore-Roth, L. (2015). *Mosby's 2015 nursing drug reference* (28th ed.). St. Louis, MO: Mosby Elsevier.

Sng, B. L., Kwok, S. C., & Sia, A. T. (2015). Modern neuraxial labor analgesia. *Current Opinion in Anesthesiology*, *28*(3), 285–289.

Sng, B. L., Zhang, Q., Leong, W. L., Ocampo, C., Assam, P. N., & Sia, A. T. (2015). Incidence and characteristics of breakthrough pain in parturients using computer-integrated patient-controlled epidural analgesia. *Journal of Clinical Anesthesia*, *27*(4), 277–284.

Society of Obstetricians and Gynecologists of Canada. (2015). Fetal health surveillance in labor (SOGC Clinical Practice Guidelines). *Journal of Obstetrics and Gynecology in Canada*. Retrieved from http://www.sogc.org

Stocks, G. M., & Griffiths, S. K. (2015). Initiation of labor analgesia: Epidural, CSE. In *Epidural labor analgesia* (pp. 73–88). Switzerland: Springer International Publishing.

Taghavi, S., Barband, S., & Khaki, A. (2015). Effect of hydrotherapy on pain of labor process. *BALTICA*, *28*(1), 116–121.

Tharpe, N. L., Farley, C. L., & Jordan, R. (2016). *Clinical practice guidelines for midwifery & women's health* (5th ed.). Sudbury, MA: Jones and Bartlett.

Timmins, A. E., & Clark, S. L. (2015). How to approach intrapartum category II tracings. *Obstetrics and Gynecology Clinics of North America*, *42*(2), 363–375.

U.S. Department of Health and Human Services. (2010). *Healthy people 2020*. Retrieved from http://www.healthypeople.gov/2020/topicsobjectives2020

Ugwumadu, A. (2015). Author's reply re: Are we (mis)guided by current guidelines on intrapartum fetal heart rate monitoring? Case for a more physiological approach to interpretation. *BJOG: An International Journal of Obstetrics & Gynecology*, *122*, 589.

Van de Velde, M. (2015). Patient-controlled intravenous analgesia remifentanil for labor analgesia: Time to stop, think and reconsider. *Current Opinion in Anesthesiology*, *28*(3), 237–239.

Verklan, T., & Walden, M. (2014). *Core curriculum for neonatal intensive care nursing* (4th ed.). St. Louis, MO: Saunders Elsevier.

Walker, S., & Sabrosa, R. (2014). Assessment of fetal presentation: Exploring a woman-centered approach. *British Journal of Midwifery*, *22*(4), 240–244.

Wenner, L. (2015). It's the little things. *Nursing for Women's Health*, *19*(2), 203–204.

Wisner, K. (2015). Intermittent auscultation in low-risk labor. *MCN: The American Journal of Maternal/Child Nursing*, *40*(1), 58.

Wojnar, D. M., & Narruhn, R. A. (2016). *Transcultural aspects of perinatal health care of Somali women. Caring for the vulnerable* (4th ed., pp. 287–302). Burlington, MA: Jones & Bartlett Learning.

World Health Organization [WHO]. (2014). *WHO recommendations for augmentation of labor*. Retrieved from http://apps.who.int/iris/bitstream/10665/112825/1/9789241507363_eng.pdf

Yuan, S. M. (2015). Fetal cardiac interventions. *Pediatrics & Neonatology*, *56*(2), 81–87.

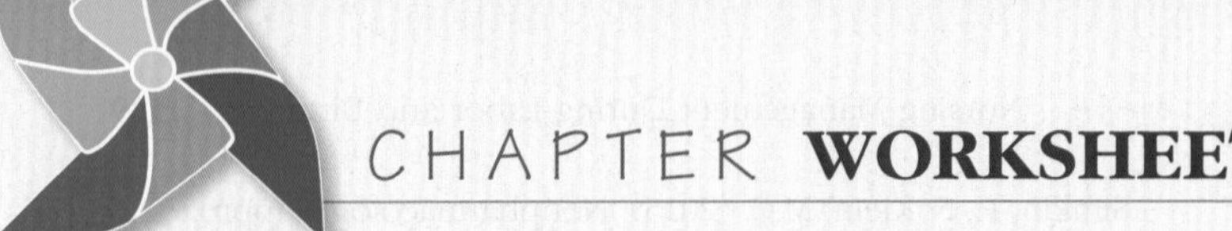

CHAPTER WORKSHEET

MULTIPLE-CHOICE QUESTIONS

1. When a client in labor is fully dilated, which instruction would be most effective to assist her in encouraging effective pushing?
   a. Hold your breath and push through entire contraction.
   b. Use chest-breathing with the contraction.
   c. Pant and blow during each contraction.
   d. Wait until you feel the urge to push.
2. During the fourth stage of labor, the nurse assesses the woman at frequent intervals after giving childbirth. What assessment data would cause the nurse the most concern?
   a. Moderate amount of dark red lochia drainage on peripad
   b. Uterine fundus palpated to the right of the umbilicus
   c. An oral temperature reading of 100.6°F
   d. Perineal area bruised and edematous beneath her ice pack
3. When managing a client's pain during labor, nurses should:
   a. Make sure the agents given do not prolong labor
   b. Know that all pain relief measures are similar
   c. Support the client's decisions and requests
   d. Not recommend nonpharmacologic methods
4. When caring for a client during the active phase of labor without continuous electronic fetal monitoring, the nurse would intermittently assess FHR every:
   a. 15 to 30 minutes
   b. 5 to 10 minutes
   c. 45 to 60 minutes
   d. 60 to 75 minutes
5. The nurse notes the presence of transient fetal accelerations on the fetal monitoring strip. Which intervention would be most appropriate?
   a. Reposition the client on the left side.
   b. Begin 100% oxygen via face mask.
   c. Document this as indicating a normal pattern.
   d. Call the health care provider immediately.
6. By the end of the second stage of labor, the nurse would expect which of the following events? The
   a. cervix is fully dilated and effaced
   b. placenta is detached and expelled
   c. fetus is born and on mother's chest
   d. woman to request pain medication
7. Which of the following practices would not be included in a physiologic birth?
   a. Early induction of labor <39 weeks' gestation
   b. Freedom of movement for the laboring woman
   c. Continuous presence and support throughout labor
   d. Encouraging spontaneous pushing when urge felt

CRITICAL THINKING EXERCISES

1. A 20-year-old primigravida at term, comes to the birthing center in active labor (dilation 5 cm and 80% effaced, –1 station) with ruptured membranes. She states she wants an "all-natural" birth without medication. Her partner is with her and appears anxious but supportive. On the admission assessment, this client's prenatal history is unremarkable; vital signs are within normal limits; FHR via Doppler ranges between 140 and 144 bpm and is regular.
   a. Based on your assessment data and the woman's request not to have medication, what nonpharmacologic interventions could you offer her?
   b. What positions might be suggested to facilitate fetal descent?
2. Several hours later, the client complains of nausea and turns to her partner and angrily tells him to not touch her and to go away.
   a. What assessment needs to be done to determine what is happening?
   b. What explanation can you offer this client's partner regarding her change in behavior?

STUDY ACTIVITIES

1. Share experiences within a post clinical conference group regarding the pain management interventions of the clients to which you were assigned. Compare and evaluate the effectiveness of different methods used, maternal behavior observed, and neonatal outcome in terms of Apgar scores.
2. On the fetal heart monitor, the nurse notices an elevation of the fetal baseline with the onset of contractions. This elevation would describe ____________.
3. Compare and contrast a local birthing center to a community hospital's birthing suite in terms of the pain management techniques and fetal monitoring used.
4. Select a childbirth website for expectant parents and critique the information provided in terms of its educational level and amount of advertising.

CHAPTER WORKSHEET

BRINGING IT ALL TOGETHER: A CASE STUDY

A 30-year-old woman at term presents to the emergency room with abdominal pain. This is her first pregnancy and she is accompanied by her partner and her very anxious sister. She is 40 weeks and 6 days based on her last ultrasound. All pregnancy blood tests have been normal. Earlier in the day she had a mucus-like dark red discharge followed by the onset of irregular period-type cramps. Two hours ago she felt a gush of clear fluid from her vagina and since then she has felt miserable. She took two Tylenol at home for the pain, but she is now in distress and came to the hospital for assessment.

Go to thePoint **to find questions to consider about this case.**

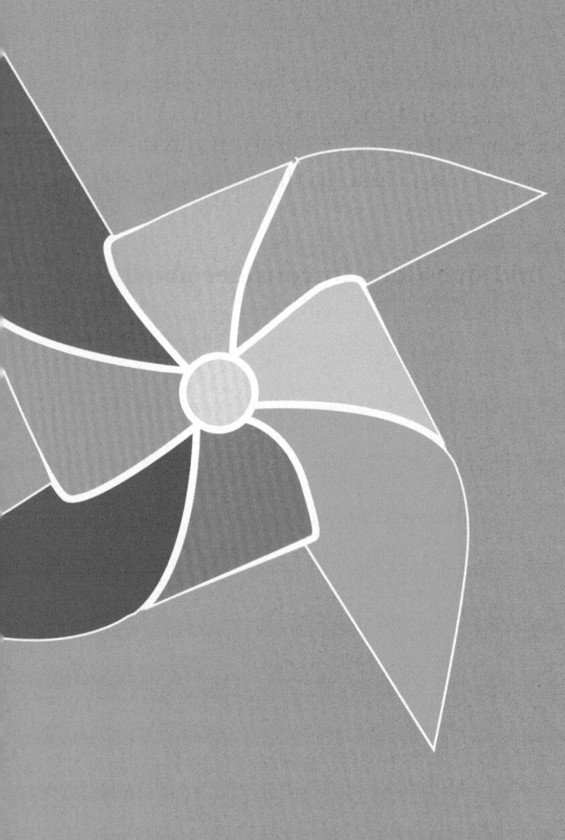

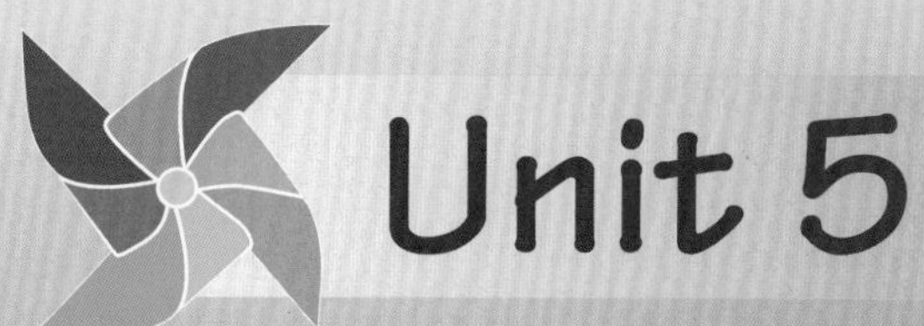

Postpartum Period

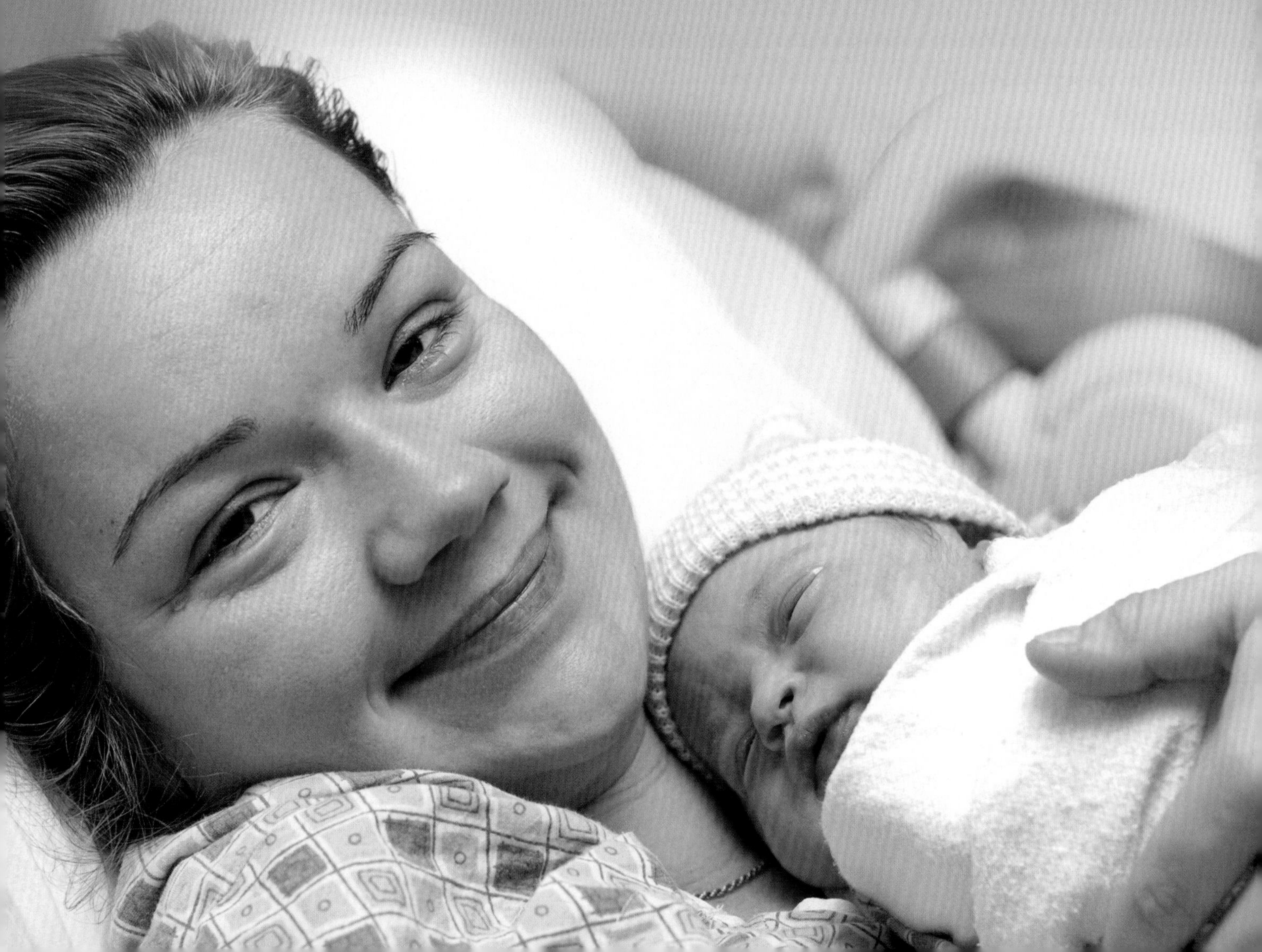

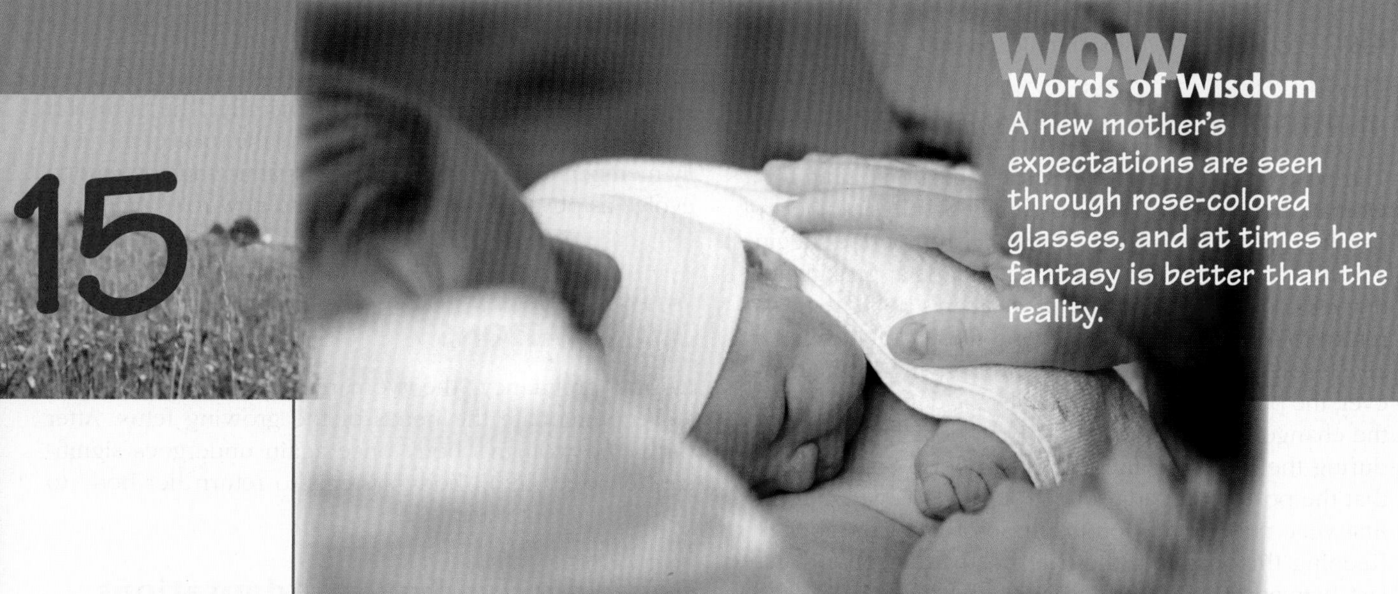

15

Postpartum Adaptations

KEY TERMS
attachment
engorgement
engrossment
involution
lactation
letting-go phase
lochia
puerperium
taking-hold phase
taking-in phase
uterine atony

Learning Objectives

Upon completion of the chapter, you will be able to:

1. Examine the systemic physiologic changes occurring in the woman after childbirth.
2. Determine the psychological changes that occur in women in the postpartum period.
3. Relate effective maternal self-care measures to be implemented in the postpartum period.
4. Integrate dimensions of postpartum care for the multicultural family.
5. Plan postpartum nursing care with interventions to foster maternal/infant bonding.
6. Assess the phases of maternal role adjustment and accompanying behaviors.
7. Analyze the psychological adaptations occurring in the mother's partner after childbirth.

Betsy **had been home only 3 days when she called the OB unit where she had given birth and asked to speak to the lactation consultant. She reported pain in both breasts. Her nipples were tender due to frequent breast-feeding and she described her breasts as heavy, hard, and swollen.**

INTRODUCTION

The postpartum period is a critical transitional time for a woman, her newborn, and her family on physiologic and psychological levels. The **puerperium** period begins after the delivery of the placenta and lasts approximately 6 weeks. During this period the woman's body begins to return to its prepregnant state, and these changes generally resolve by the sixth week after giving birth. However, the postpartum period can also be defined to include the changes in all aspects of the mother's life that occur during the first year after a child is born. Some believe that the postpartum adjustment period lasts well into the first year, making the fourth phase of labor the longest. Keeping this in mind, the true postpartum period may last between 9 and 12 months as the mother works to lose the weight she gained while pregnant, adjusts psychologically to the changes in her life, and takes on the new role of mother.

Nurses caring for childbearing families should consider all aspects of culture, including communication, space, and family roles. Communication encompasses an understanding of not only a person's language, and loudness of speech, but also the meaning of touch and gestures. The concept of personal space and the dimensions of comfort zones differ from culture to culture. Touching, placing clients in proximity to others, and taking away personal possessions can reduce a client's personal security and heighten her anxiety. Nurses must be sensitive to how people respond when being touched and should refrain from touching if the client's response indicates that it is unwelcome. Cultural norms also have an impact on family roles, expectations, and behaviors associated with a member's position in the family. For example, culture may influence whether a man actively participates in the pregnancy and childbirth. Maternity health care professionals in the United States expect men to be involved, but this role expectation may conflict with that of many of the diverse groups now living in the United States. Mexican Americans, Arab Americans, Asian Americans, and Orthodox Jewish Americans, for example, usually view the birthing experience as a woman's affair (Purnell, 2014).

Our major role as nurses is to provide safe and evidence-based care to promote optimal birth outcomes for all women, regardless of their cultural background. Nurses need to remember that there is more than one way to provide this care. Nurses are important cultural brokers as they welcome women and their families into our obstetrical units, where nurses share with those families one of the most intimate experiences of their lives (Bowers & Ceballos, 2015).

This chapter describes the major physiologic and psychological changes that occur in a woman after childbirth. Various systemic adaptations take place throughout the woman's body. In addition, the mother and the family adjust to the new addition psychologically. The birth of a child changes the family structure and the roles of the family members. The adaptations are dynamic and continue to evolve as physical changes occur and new roles emerge.

MATERNAL PHYSIOLOGIC ADAPTATIONS

During pregnancy, the woman's entire body changes to accommodate the needs of the growing fetus. After birth, the woman's body once again undergoes significant changes in all body systems to return her body to its prepregnant state.

Reproductive System Adaptations

The reproductive system goes through tremendous adaptations to return to the prepregnancy state. All organs and tissues of the reproductive system are involved. The female reproductive system is unique in its capacity to remodel itself throughout the woman's reproductive life. The events after birth, with the shedding of the placenta and subsequent uterine **involution**, involve substantial tissue destruction and subsequent repair and remodeling. For example, the woman's menstrual cycle, interrupted during pregnancy, will begin to return several weeks after childbirth, if the woman is not breast-feeding. Ovulation can return any time, thus breast-feeding should not be considered as a safe contraceptive and other methods should be used to prevent pregnancy. The uterus, which has undergone tremendous expansion during pregnancy to accommodate progressive fetal growth, will return to its prepregnant size over several weeks. The mother's breasts have grown to prepare for **lactation** and do not return to their prepregnant size as the uterus does.

Uterine Involution

The uterus returns to its normal size through a gradual process of involution, which involves retrogressive changes that return it to its nonpregnant size and condition. Involution involves three retrogressive processes:

1. Contraction of muscle fibers to reduce those previously stretched during pregnancy
2. Catabolism, which shrinks enlarged, individual myometrial cells
3. Regeneration of uterine epithelium from the lower layer of the decidua after the upper layers have been sloughed off and shed during lochial discharge (Mattson & Smith, 2015).

The uterus, which weighs approximately 1,000 g (2.2 lb) soon after birth, undergoes physiologic involution as it returns to its nonpregnant state. Approximately 1 week after birth, the uterus shrinks in size by 50% and weighs about 500 g (1 lb); at the end of 6 weeks,

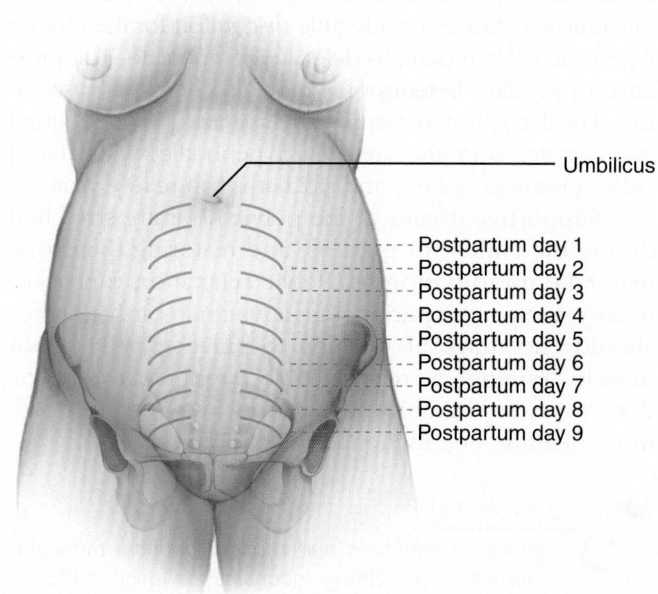

FIGURE 15.1 Uterine involution.

it weighs approximately 60 g (2 oz), about the weight before the pregnancy (Jordan et al., 2014) (Fig. 15.1). During the first few days after birth, the uterus typically descends from the level of the umbilicus at a rate of 1 cm (1 fingerbreadth) per day. By 3 days, the fundus lies 2 to 3 fingerbreadths below the umbilicus (or slightly higher in multiparous women). By the end of 10 days, the fundus usually cannot be palpated because it has descended into the true pelvis.

If these retrogressive changes do not occur as a result of retained placental fragments or infection, then subinvolution of the uterus typically results (delayed or absent involution). Subinvolution is generally responsive to early diagnosis and treatment. Factors that facilitate uterine involution include complete expulsion of amniotic membranes and placenta at birth, a complication-free labor and birth process, breast-feeding, and early ambulation. Factors that inhibit involution include a prolonged labor and difficult birth, incomplete expulsion of amniotic membranes and placenta, uterine infection, over-distention of uterine muscles (such as by multiple gestation, hydramnios, or a large singleton fetus), a full bladder (which displaces the uterus and interferes with contractions), anesthesia (which relaxes uterine muscles), and close childbirth spacing (frequent and repeated distention decreases tone and causes muscular relaxation).

LOCHIA

Lochia is the vaginal discharge that occurs after birth and continues for approximately four to eight weeks. It results from involution, during which the superficial layer of the decidua basalis becomes necrotic and is sloughed off. Immediately after childbirth, lochia is bright red and consists mainly of blood, fibrinous products, decidual cells, and red and white blood cells. The lochia from the uterus is alkaline but becomes acidic as it passes through the vagina. It is roughly equal to the amount occurring during a heavy menstrual period. The average amount of lochial discharge is 240 to 270 mL (8 to 9 oz) (Bope & Kellerman, 2015).

Women who have had cesarean births tend to have less flow because the uterine debris is removed manually along with delivery of the placenta. Lochia is present in most women for at least 3 weeks after childbirth, but it persists in some women for as long as 6 weeks.

Lochia passes through three stages:

- *Lochia rubra* is a deep-red mixture of mucus, tissue debris, and blood that occurs for the first 3 to 4 days after birth. As uterine bleeding subsides, it becomes paler and more serous.
- *Lochia serosa* is the second stage. It is pinkish brown and is expelled 3 to 10 days postpartum. Lochia serosa primarily contains leukocytes, decidual tissue, red blood cells, and serous fluid.
- *Lochia alba* is the final stage. The discharge is creamy white or light brown and consists of leukocytes, decidual tissue, and reduced fluid content. It occurs from days 10 to 14 but can last 3 to 6 weeks postpartum in some women and still be considered normal.

Lochia at any stage should have a fleshy smell; an offensive odor usually indicates an infection, such as endometritis.

Take Note!

A danger sign is the reappearance of bright-red blood after lochia rubra has stopped. Reevaluation by a health care provider is essential if this occurs.

AFTERPAINS

Part of the involution process involves uterine contractions. Subsequently, many women are frequently bothered by painful uterine contractions termed *afterpains*. All women experience afterpains, but they are more acute in multiparous and breast-feeding women secondary to repeated stretching of the uterine muscles from multiple pregnancies or stimulation during breast-feeding with oxytocin released from the pituitary gland. Primiparous women typically experience mild afterpains because their uterus is able to maintain a contracted state. Breast-feeding and administration of exogenous oxytocin both cause powerful and painful uterine contractions. Afterpains usually respond to oral analgesics.

Take Note!

Afterpains are usually stronger during breast-feeding because oxytocin released by the sucking reflex strengthens the contractions. Mild analgesics can reduce this discomfort.

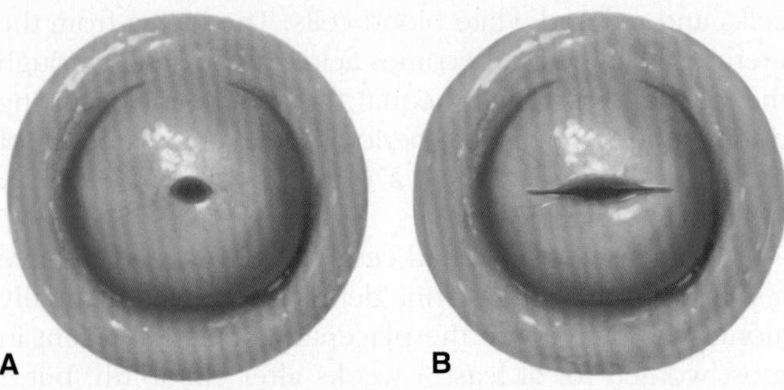

FIGURE 15.2 Appearance of the cervical os, (**A**) before the first pregnancy, and (**B**) after pregnancy.

Cervix

The cervix typically returns to its prepregnant state by week 6 of the postpartum period. The cervix gradually closes but never regains its prepregnant appearance. Immediately after childbirth, the cervix is shapeless and edematous and is easily distensible for several days. The internal cervical os gradually closes and returns to normal by 2 weeks, whereas the external os widens and never appears the same after childbirth. The external cervical os is no longer shaped like a circle, but instead appears as a jagged slit-like opening, often described as a "fish mouth" (Fig. 15.2).

Vagina

Shortly after birth, the vaginal mucosa is edematous and thin, with few rugae. As ovarian function returns and estrogen production resumes, the mucosa thickens and rugae return in approximately 3 weeks. The vagina gapes at the opening and is generally lax. The vagina returns to its approximate prepregnant size by 6 to 8 weeks postpartum but will always remain a bit larger than it had been before pregnancy.

Normal mucus production and thickening of the vaginal mucosa usually return with ovulation. The vagina gradually decreases in size and regains tone over several weeks. By 3 to 4 weeks, the edema and vascularity have decreased. The vaginal epithelium is generally restored by 6 to 8 weeks postpartum (Mattson & Smith, 2015). Localized dryness and coital discomfort (dyspareunia) usually plague most women until menstruation returns. Water-soluble lubricants can reduce discomfort during intercourse.

Perineum

The perineum is often edematous and bruised for the first day or two after birth. If the birth involved an episiotomy or laceration, complete healing may take as long as 4 to 6 months in the absence of complications at the site, such as hematoma or infection. The muscle tone may or may not return to normal, depending on the extent of injury to muscle, nerve, and connecting tissues (Spiliolpoulos & Mastrogiannis, 2014). Perineal lacerations may extend into the anus and cause considerable discomfort for the mother when she is attempting to defecate or ambulate. The presence of swollen hemorrhoids may also heighten discomfort. Local comfort measures such as ice packs, pouring warm water over the area via a peribottle, witch hazel pads, anesthetic sprays, and sitz baths can relieve pain.

Supportive tissues of the pelvic floor are stretched during the childbirth process, and restoring their tone may take up to 6 months. Pelvic relaxation can occur in any woman experiencing a vaginal birth. Nurses should encourage all women to practice pelvic floor muscle training exercises (PFMT) to improve pelvic floor tone, strengthen the perineal muscles, and promote healing. See Evidence-Based Practice 15.1.

Take Note!

Failure to maintain and restore perineal muscular tone leads to urinary incontinence later in life for many women.

Cardiovascular System Adaptations

The cardiovascular system undergoes dramatic changes after birth. During pregnancy, the heart is displaced slightly upward and to the left. This reverses as the uterus undergoes involution. Cardiac output remains high for the first few days postpartum and then gradually declines to nonpregnant values within 3 months of birth.

Blood volume, which increases substantially during pregnancy, drops rapidly after birth and returns to normal within 4 weeks postpartum. The decrease in both cardiac output and blood volume reflects the birth-related blood loss (an average of 500 mL with a vaginal birth and 1,000 mL with a cesarean birth). The cardiac output deceases to prelabor values 24 to 72 hours postpartum, rapidly falls over the next 2 weeks and usually returns to nonpregnant levels within 6 to 8 weeks postpartum. Blood plasma volume is further reduced through diuresis, which occurs during the early postpartum period (Cheng & Caughey, 2015). Despite the decrease in blood volume, the hematocrit level remains relatively stable and may even increase, reflecting the predominant loss of plasma. Thus, an acute decrease in hematocrit is not an expected finding and may indicate hemorrhage.

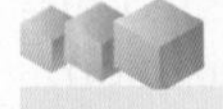
Concept Mastery Alert

Prioritizing Postpartum Vital Signs

It is not uncommon for women to have a temperature elevation up to 100.4°F in the first 24 hours postpartum. There may also be a slight decrease in blood pressure. The nurse should be most concerned about a blood pressure elevation because preeclampsia may occur during the early postpartum period.

EVIDENCE-BASED PRACTICE 15.1

PELVIC FLOOR MUSCLE TRAINING VERSUS NO TREATMENT, OR INACTIVE CONTROL TREATMENTS, FOR URINARY INCONTINENCE IN WOMEN

Stress incontinence is the involuntary leakage of urine with a physical activity that increases intra-abdominal pressure such as coughing or sneezing. This incontinence can occur after childbirth secondary to perineal trauma. Pelvic floor muscle training (PFMT) is the most common intervention for women that experience stress urinary incontinence. The objective of this study was to determine the effects of PFMT for women with urinary incontinence when compared with no treatment, placebo, or other inactive control treatments.

STUDY

Randomized or quasi-randomized trials in women experiencing stress incontinence were reviewed. Twenty-one trials involving 1,281 women met the inclusion criteria. Women with stress urinary incontinence who were in the PFMT groups were 8 times more likely than the controls to report that they were cured (46/82 [56.1%] vs. 5/83 [6.0%], RR 8.38, 95% CI 3.68 to 19.07) and 17 times more likely to report cure or improvement (32/58 [55%] vs. 2/63 [3.2%], RR 17.33, 95% CI 4.31 to 69.64). In trials in women with any type of urinary incontinence, PFMT groups were also more likely to report cure, or more cure and improvement, than the women in the control groups, although the effect size was reduced. Women with stress urinary incontinence were also more satisfied with the active treatment, while women in the control groups were more likely to seek further treatment. Women treated with PFMT leaked urine less often, lost smaller amounts on the short office-based pad test, and emptied their bladders less often during the day.

Findings

The review of trials found that PFMT (muscle-clenching exercises) helps women cure and improve stress urinary incontinence in particular, and all types of incontinence.

Nursing Implications

The review provides support for the widespread recommendation that PFMT be included in first-line conservative management programs for women with stress and any type of urinary incontinence. Long-term effectiveness of PFMT needs to be further researched. The take-away message for nurses working with postpartum women should be to instruct them how to perform PFMT exercises at home to assist in restoring pelvic floor strength and tone. In addition to PFMT exercises, the promotion of healthy weight can also help prevent or reduce incontinence as a woman ages.

Adapted from Dumoulin C., Hay-Smith, E. J. C, & Mac Habée-Séguin, G. (2014). Pelvic floor muscle training versus no treatment, or inactive control treatments, for urinary incontinence in women. *Cochrane Database of Systematic Reviews, 5,* CD005654.

Pulse and Blood Pressure

The increase in cardiac output and stroke volume during pregnancy begins to diminish after birth once the placenta has been delivered. This decrease in cardiac output is reflected in bradycardia (40 to 60 bpm) for up to the first 2 weeks postpartum. This slowing of the heart rate is related to the increased blood that flows back to the heart and to the central circulation after it is no longer perfusing the placenta. This increase in central circulation brings about an increased stroke volume and allows a slower heart rate to provide ample maternal circulation. Gradually, cardiac output returns to prepregnant levels by 3 months after childbirth (Mahendru et al., 2014).

Tachycardia (heart rate above 100 bpm) in the postpartum woman warrants further investigation. It may indicate hypovolemia, dehydration, or hemorrhage. However, because of the increased blood volume during pregnancy, a considerable loss of blood may be well tolerated and not cause a compensatory cardiovascular response such as tachycardia. In most instances of postpartum hemorrhage, blood pressure and cardiac output remain increased because of the compensatory increase in heart rate. Thus, a decrease in blood pressure and cardiac output are not expected changes during the postpartum period. Early identification is essential to ensure prompt intervention.

Blood pressure falls mostly in the first 2 days and then increases 3 to 7 days after childbirth, and returns to prepregnancy levels by 6 weeks (Parpaglioni, 2015). A significant increase accompanied by headache might indicate preeclampsia and requires further investigation. Decreased blood pressure may suggest an infection or a uterine hemorrhage.

Coagulation

Normal physiologic changes of pregnancy, including alterations in hemostasis that favor coagulation, reduced fibrinolysis, and pooling and stasis of blood in the lower limbs, place women at risk for blood clots. These changes, which usually return to prepregnant levels 3 weeks postpartum, are important for minimizing blood loss at childbirth. Smoking, obesity, immobility, and postpartum factors such as infection, bleeding, and emergency surgery (including emergency cesarean section) also increase the risk of coagulation disorders (Creasy et al., 2014).

Clotting factors that increased during pregnancy tend to remain elevated during the early postpartum period. Giving birth stimulates this hypercoagulability state further. As a result, these coagulation factors remain elevated for 2 to 3 weeks postpartum (King et al., 2015). This hypercoagulable state, combined with vessel damage during birth and immobility, places the woman at risk for thromboembolism (blood clots) in the lower extremities and the lungs.

Blood Cellular Components

Red blood cell production ceases early in the puerperium, causing mean hemoglobin and hematocrit levels to decrease slightly in the first 24 hours. During the next 2 weeks, both levels rise slowly. The white blood count, which increases in labor, remains elevated for first 4 to 6 days after birth but then falls to 6,000 to 10,000/mm^3. This white blood cell elevation can complicate a diagnosis of infection in the immediate postpartum period.

Urinary System Adaptations

Pregnancy and birth can have profound effects on the urinary system. During pregnancy, the glomerular filtration rate and renal plasma flow increase significantly. Both usually return to normal by 6 weeks after birth. There is a gradual return of bladder tone and normal size and function of the bladder, ureters, and renal pelvis, all of which were dilated during pregnancy.

Many women have difficulty feeling the sensation to void after giving birth if they received an anesthetic block during labor (which inhibits neural functioning of the bladder) or if they received oxytocin to induce or augment their labor (antidiuretic effect). These women will be at risk for incomplete emptying, bladder distention, difficulty voiding, and urinary retention. In addition, urination may be impeded by:

- Perineal lacerations
- Generalized swelling and bruising of the perineum and tissues surrounding the urinary meatus
- Hematomas
- Decreased bladder tone as a result of regional anesthesia
- Diminished sensation of bladder pressure as a result of swelling, poor bladder tone, and numbing effects of regional anesthesia used during labor (Bope & Kellerman, 2015).

Difficulty voiding can lead to urinary retention, bladder distention, and ultimately urinary tract infection. Urinary retention and bladder distention can cause displacement of the uterus from the midline to the right and can inhibit the uterus from contracting properly, which increases the risk of postpartum hemorrhage. Urinary retention is a major cause of **uterine atony**, which allows excessive bleeding. Frequent voiding of small amounts (less than 150 mL) suggests urinary retention with overflow, and catheterization may be necessary to empty the bladder to restore tone.

Postpartum diuresis occurs as a result of several mechanisms: the large amounts of intravenous fluids given during labor, a decreasing antidiuretic effect of oxytocin as its level declines, the buildup and retention of extra fluids during pregnancy, and a decreasing production of aldosterone—the hormone that decreases sodium retention and increases urine production (Evans & De Franco, 2014). All of these factors contribute to rapid filling of the bladder within 12 hours of birth. Diuresis begins within 12 hours after childbirth and continues throughout the first week postpartum. Normal function returns within a month after birth (Cunningham et al., 2014).

Consider This

Have you ever felt like a real idiot by not being able to complete a simple task in life? I had a beautiful baby boy after only 6 hours of labor. My epidural worked well and I actually felt very little discomfort throughout my labor. Because it was in the middle of the night when they brought me to my postpartum room, I felt a few hours of sleep would be all I needed to be back to normal. During an assessment early the next morning, the nurse found my uterus had shifted to the right from my midline, and I was instructed to empty my bladder. I didn't understand why the nurse was concerned about where my uterus was located and, besides, I didn't feel any sensation of a full bladder. But I did get up anyway and tried to comply. Despite all the nurse's tricks of running the faucet for sound effects, in addition to having warm water poured over my thighs via the peribottle, I was unable to urinate. How could I not accomplish one of life's simplest tasks?

Thoughts: Women who receive regional anesthesia frequently experience reduced sensation to their perineal area and do not feel a full bladder. The nursing assessment revealed a displaced uterus secondary to a full bladder. What additional "tricks" can be used to assist this woman to void? What explanation should be offered to her regarding why she is having difficulty urinating?

Gastrointestinal System Adaptations

The gastrointestinal system quickly returns to normal after birth because the gravid uterus is no longer filling the abdominal cavity and producing pressure on the abdominal organs. Progesterone levels, which caused relaxation of smooth muscle during pregnancy and diminished bowel tone, also are declining.

Regardless of the type of delivery, most women experience decreased bowel tone and sluggish bowels for several days after birth. Decreased peristalsis occurs in response to analgesics, surgery, diminished intra-abdominal pressure, low-fiber diet, insufficient fluid intake, and diminished muscle tone. In addition, women with an episiotomy, perineal laceration, or hemorrhoids may fear pain or damage to the perineum with their first bowel movement and may attempt to delay it. Subsequently, constipation is a common problem during the postpartum period. A stool softener can be prescribed for this reason.

Most women are hungry and thirsty after childbirth, commonly related to nothing-by-mouth (NPO) restrictions and the energy expended during labor. Their appetite returns to normal immediately after giving birth.

Take Note!

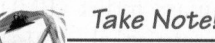

Anticipate the woman's need to replenish her body with food and fluids, and provide both soon after she gives birth.

Musculoskeletal System Adaptations

The effects of pregnancy on the muscles and joints vary widely. Musculoskeletal changes associated with pregnancy, such as increased ligament laxity, weight gain, change in the center of gravity, and carpal tunnel syndrome, revert back during the postpartum period. During pregnancy, the hormones relaxin, estrogen, and progesterone relax the joints. After birth, levels of these hormones decline, resulting in a return of all joints to their prepregnant state, with the exception of the woman's feet. Parous women will note a permanent increase in their shoe size (Jordan et al., 2014).

Women commonly experience fatigue and activity intolerance and have a distorted body image for weeks after birth secondary to declining relaxin and progesterone levels, which cause hip and joint pain that interferes with ambulation and exercise. Good body mechanics and correct positioning are important during this time to prevent low back pain and injury to the joints. Within 6 to 8 weeks after delivery, joints are completely stabilized and return to normal.

During pregnancy, stretching of the abdominal wall muscles occurs to accommodate the enlarging uterus. This stretching leads to a loss in muscle tone and possibly separation of the longitudinal muscles (rectus abdominis muscles) of the abdomen. Separation of the rectus abdominis muscles, called diastasis recti, is more common in women who have poor abdominal muscle tone before pregnancy. After birth, muscle tone is diminished and the abdominal muscles are soft and flabby. Specific exercises are necessary to help the woman regain muscle tone. Fortunately, diastasis responds well to exercise, and abdominal muscle tone can be improved. (See Chapter 16 for more information about exercises to improve muscle tone.)

Take Note!

If rectus muscle tone is not regained through exercise, support may not be adequate during future pregnancies.

Integumentary System Adaptations

Another system that experiences lasting effects of pregnancy is the integumentary system. As estrogen and progesterone levels decrease, the darkened pigmentation on the abdomen (linea nigra), face (melasma), and nipples gradually fades. Some women experience hair loss during pregnancy and the postpartum periods. Approximately 90% of hairs are growing at any one time, with the other 10% entering a resting phase. Because of the high estrogen levels present during pregnancy, an increased number of hairs go into the resting phase, which is part of the normal hair loss cycle. The most common period for hair loss is within 3 months after birth, when estrogen returns to normal levels and more hairs are allowed to fall out. This hair loss is temporary, and regrowth generally returns to normal levels in 4 to 6 months in two thirds of women and by 15 months in the remainder, although hair may be less abundant than before pregnancy (King et al., 2015).

Striae gravidarum (stretch marks) that developed during pregnancy on the breasts, abdomen, and hips gradually fade to silvery lines. However, these lines do not disappear completely. Although many products on the market claim to make stretch marks disappear, their effectiveness is highly questionable.

The profuse diaphoresis (sweating) that is common during the early postpartum period is one of the most noticeable adaptations in the integumentary system. Many women will wake up drenched with perspiration during the puerperium. This postpartum diaphoresis is a mechanism to reduce the amount of fluids retained during pregnancy and restore prepregnant body fluid levels. It can be profuse at times. It is common, especially at night during the first week after birth. Reassure the client that this is normal and encourage her to change her gown to prevent chilling.

Respiratory System Adaptations

Respirations usually remain within the normal adult range of 16 to 24 breaths per minute. As the abdominal organs resume their nonpregnant position, the diaphragm returns to its usual position. Anatomic changes in the thoracic cavity and rib cage caused by increasing uterine growth resolve quickly. As a result, discomforts such as shortness of breath and rib aches are relieved. Tidal volume, minute volume, vital capacity, and functional residual capacity return to prepregnant values, typically within 1 to 3 weeks of birth (Mattson & Smith, 2015).

Endocrine System Adaptations

The endocrine system rapidly undergoes several changes after birth. Levels of circulating estrogen and progesterone drop quickly with delivery of the placenta. Decreased estrogen levels are associated with breast **engorgement** and with the diuresis of excess extracellular fluid accumulated during pregnancy (Creasy et al., 2014). Estrogen is at its lowest level a week after birth. For the woman who is not breast-feeding, estrogen levels begin to increase by 2 weeks after birth. For the breast-feeding woman, estrogen levels remain low until breast-feeding frequency decreases.

Other placental hormones (human chorionic gonadotropin [hCG], human placental lactogen [hPL], progesterone) decline rapidly after birth. The hCG levels are nonexistent at the end of the first postpartum week, and hPL is undetectable within 1 day after birth (Mattson & Smith, 2016). Progesterone levels are undetectable by 3 days after childbirth, and production is reestablished with the first menses. Prolactin is a hormone secreted by the anterior pituitary gland involved with lactation and reproduction. Prolactin levels decline within 2 weeks for the woman who is not breast-feeding, but remain elevated for the lactating woman (Jin et al., 2015).

Weight Loss After Childbirth

For all women of reproductive age, excessive weight gain and postpartum weight retention can increase their risk of obesity. Breast-feeding has been shown to have many health benefits for both mother and infant; however, its role in postpartum weight loss is unclear. More research studies are needed to reliably assess the impact of breast-feeding on postpartum weight management (Neville et al., 2014).

The rate and amount of weight loss in the postpartum period seem to be determined by the same factors that determine weight loss at any point in a woman's life, including existing weight/body mass index (BMI), diet, age, and activity level (Nascimento et al., 2014). Thus, there is benefit from overall lifestyle interventions on weight loss in postpartum women which include exercise plus dietary changes to achieve their weight reduction goals. See Evidence-Based Practice 15.2.

Think back to Betsy, the woman experiencing painful changes in her breasts. What is Betsy describing to the lactation consultant? Why has the condition of her breasts changed compared with when she was in the hospital?

EVIDENCE-BASED PRACTICE 15.2 REDUCING POSTPARTUM WEIGHT RETENTION AND IMPROVING BREAST-FEEDING OUTCOMES IN OVERWEIGHT WOMEN: A PILOT RANDOMIZED CONTROLLED TRIAL

Women naturally gain weight during pregnancy and many gradually lose it afterward. Some women, though, find it difficult to lose the pregnancy-related weight during the postpartum period and there is concern that this may be a health risk. The retention of weight gained during pregnancy may contribute to obesity. Obesity in the general population increases the risk of diabetes, heart disease, and high blood pressure. It is suggested that women who return to their prepregnancy weight by about 6 months after childbirth have a lower risk of being overweight 10 years later. Weight gain is also associated with lower rates of breast-feeding initiation and duration. The purpose of this randomized study was to help women reduce their postpartum weight retention and improve breast-feeding outcomes.

STUDY

Thirty-six women with a BMI of >25 were recruited, stratified by BMI and randomized to one of three groups with follow-up to 6 months postpartum. Women received a dietary intervention with or without breast-feeding support from a lactation consultant. All participants initiated breast-feeding, but the group that had lactation support had a longer duration of breast-feeding than the group without the lactation support. In addition, the women with longer breast-feeding duration also lost the most weight during the 6-month period.

Findings

The study provided evidence to support the feasibility of providing overweight and obese women with targeted dietary advice and breast-feeding support to improve weight and breast-feeding outcomes.

Nursing Implications

Based on the findings of this study, nurses can recommend to their postpartum mothers desiring to lose their pregnancy weight should be encouraged to breast-feed and sustain it for at least six months to lose their pregnancy weight gained. Research findings associate breast-feeding with postpartum weight loss due to the increase in women's metabolic rates which burn calories. This information should be reported to postpartum mothers desiring to lose weight and breast-feed. Overall, if gained weight through the pregnancy isn't lost, their risk of cardiovascular diseases, diabetes, hypertension, and cancer will be increased as they age. The weight loss will help prevent these conditions or at the very least reduce their risks.

Adapted from Martin, J., MacDonald-Wicks, L., Hure, A., Smith, R., & Collins, C. E. (2015). Reducing postpartum weight retention and improving breastfeeding outcomes in overweight women: A pilot randomized controlled trial. *Nutrients, 7*(3), 1464–1479.

Global Health of Childbearing Women

Globalization has changed our society in numerous ways, yet the health of women is remaining stagnant or growing worse in many parts of the world. Many women in developing counties are denied their fundamental right to enjoy a complete state of health as defined by the World Health Organization (Boyd-Judson & James, 2014). More than half a million women die each year from complications during and after childbirth (bleeding and infections), the vast majority of them in Africa and Asia (Webber & Chirangi, 2014).

Women throughout the world continue to face enormous obstacles in attempting to access obstetric care. Skilled attendance at childbirth is critical for decreasing maternal and neonatal mortality, yet many women in developing countries give birth outside health facilities, without skilled help. Nurses throughout the world can help advocate for cost-effective, evidence-based interventions to prevent and battle complications from childbirth to save women's lives. The challenge is to guarantee that every pregnant woman who needs care gets it. Nurses can make a difference outside their own country's borders by advocating for all international women through their governmental political systems and encouraging those governments to offer help and save lives.

Lactation

Lactation is the secretion of milk by the breasts. It is thought to be brought about by the interaction of progesterone, estrogen, prolactin, and oxytocin. Breast milk typically appears within 4 to 5 days after childbirth.

BREAST-FEEDING

Breast-feeding is a dynamic process, which requires coupling between periodic motions of the infant's jaws, undulation of the tongue, and breast milk ejection reflex. All mechanisms must be coordinated to be successful. All major health organizations recommend breast-feeding. The American Academy of Pediatrics recommends exclusive breast-feeding for 6 months, followed by the introduction of appropriate complementary foods and continued breast-feeding to 1 year and beyond (AAP, 2015). This recommendation is considered to be the standard of care today. Nurses have an important role in promoting, supporting and protecting breast-feeding. Proper positioning, latching-on, sucking, and swallowing are the foundation for successful breast-feeding. Although breast-feeding is recommended by international and national organizations, the nurse must respect and support all mothers in either infant feeding method chosen.

During pregnancy, the breasts increase in size and functional ability in preparation for breast-feeding. Estrogen stimulates growth of the milk collection (ductal) system, whereas progesterone stimulates growth of the milk production system. Within the first month of gestation, the ducts of the mammary glands grow branches, forming more lobules and alveoli. These structural changes make the breasts larger, more tender, and heavy. Each breast gains nearly 1 pound in weight by term, the glandular cells fill with secretions, blood vessels increase in number, and the amounts of connective tissue and fat cells increase (Engel et al., 2015).

Prolactin from the anterior pituitary gland, secreted in increasing levels throughout pregnancy, triggers the synthesis and secretion of milk after the woman gives birth. During pregnancy, prolactin, estrogen, and progesterone cause synthesis and secretion of *colostrum*, which contains protein and carbohydrate but no milk fat. It is only after birth takes place, when the high levels of estrogen and progesterone are abruptly withdrawn, that prolactin is able to stimulate the glandular cells to secrete milk instead of colostrum. This takes place within 4 to 5 days after giving birth.

Oxytocin acts so that milk can be ejected from the alveoli to the nipple. Therefore, sucking by the newborn will release milk. A decrease in the quality of stimulation causes a decrease in prolactin surges and thus a decrease in milk production. Prolactin levels increase in response to nipple stimulation during feedings. Prolactin and oxytocin result in milk production if stimulated by sucking (Stuebe et al., 2015) (Fig. 15.3). If the stimulus (sucking) is not present, as with a woman who is not breast-feeding, breast engorgement and milk production will subside within days postpartum.

Skin-to-skin contact during the first hour following birth is the gold standard to initiate breast-feeding, if the mother decides this is the method of feeding for her newborn. Researchers realized that a newborn's instinct was to seek nourishment after birth. They move on their mother's abdomen up to her breast instinctively. Researchers termed this movement the *breast crawl* that helps initiate breast-feeding immediately after childbirth. This instinct arises when a newborn, left undisturbed and skin-to-skin on the mother's trunk following birth, moves toward her/his mother's breast for the purpose of locating and self-attaching for the first feeding. From there, the newborn uses leg and arm movements to propel her/himself toward the breast. Upon reaching the sternum, the newborn will bounce her/his head up and down and side to side. As the newborn approaches the nipple, her/his mouth opens and, after several attempts, latch-on and suckling take place. Newborns have senses and skills that enable early initiation of feeding at the breast. Nurses can help facilitate the breast crawl as a continuation of the birthing process. Nurses have a responsibility to promote the health of their childbearing families and provide evidence-based care. Encouraging use of the breast crawl can be the first step in health promotion for every newborn (Zanardo & Straface, 2015).

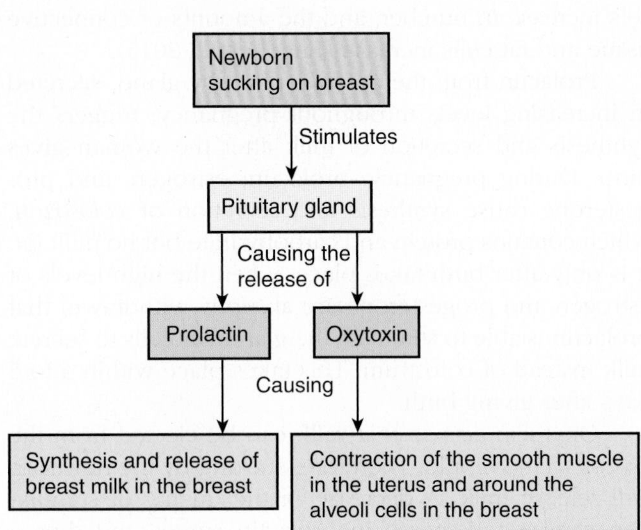

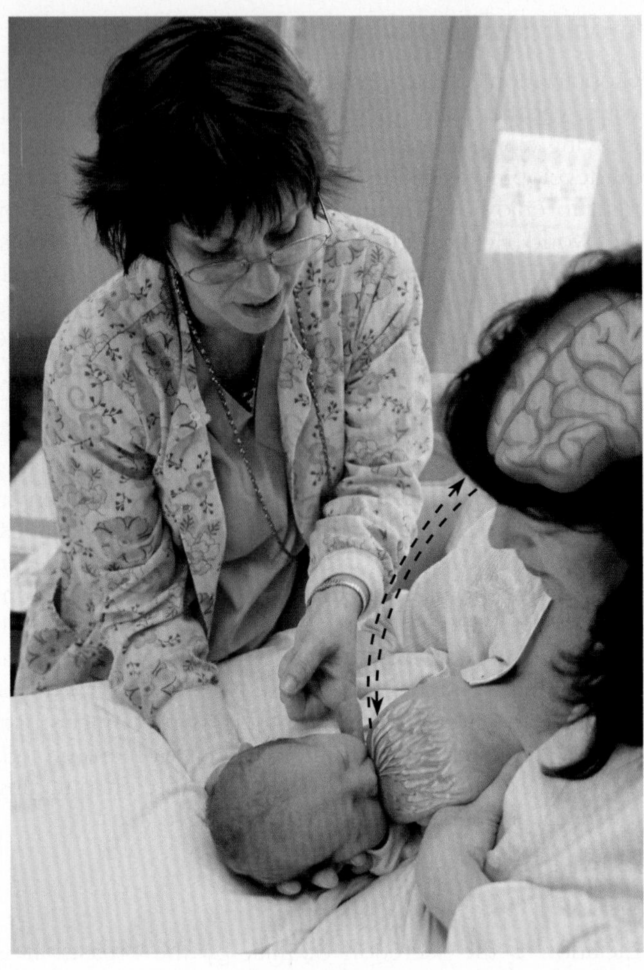

FIGURE 15.3 Physiology of lactation.

Breast milk production can be summarized as follows:

- Prolactin levels increase at term with a decrease in estrogen and progesterone levels.
- Estrogen and progesterone levels decrease after the placenta is delivered.
- Prolactin is released from the anterior pituitary gland and initiates milk production.
- Oxytocin is released from the posterior pituitary gland to promote milk let-down.
- Infant sucking at each feeding provides continuous stimulus for prolactin and oxytocin release (Wambach & Riordan, 2014).

Typically, during the first 2 days after birth, the breasts are soft and nontender. The woman also may report a tingling sensation in both breasts, which is the "let-down reflex" that occurs immediately before or during breast-feeding. After this time, breast changes depend on whether the mother is breast-feeding or taking measures to prevent lactation.

Engorgement is a postnatal physiologic painful condition in which distension and swelling of the breast tissue occurs as a result of an increase in blood and lymph supply as a precursor to lactation (Fig. 15.4). Breast engorgement usually peaks in 3 to 5 days postpartum and usually subsides within the following 24 to 36 hours (Alekseev, Vladimir, & Nadezhda, 2015). Engorgement can occur from infrequent feeding or ineffective emptying of the breasts and typically lasts about 24 hours. Breasts increase in vascularity and swell in response to prolactin 2 to 4 days after birth. If engorged, the breasts will be hard and tender to touch. They are temporarily full, tender, and very uncomfortable until the milk supply is ready. Frequent emptying of the breasts helps to minimize discomfort and resolve engorgement. Standing in a warm shower or applying warm compresses immediately before feedings will help to soften the breasts and nipples in order to allow the newborn to latch on more easily.

Treatments to reduce the pain of breast engorgement include heat or cold applications, cabbage leaf compresses, breast massage and milk expression, ultrasound, breast pumping, and anti-inflammatory agents (King et al., 2015). A nonprescription anti-inflammatory medication can also be taken for the breast discomfort and swelling resulting from engorgement. These measures will also enhance the let-down reflex. Between

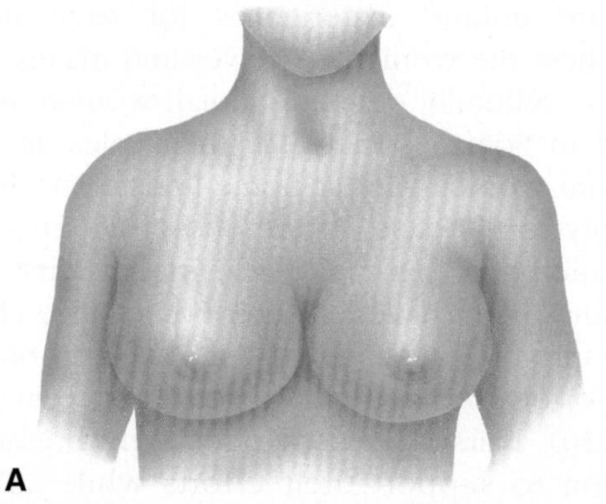

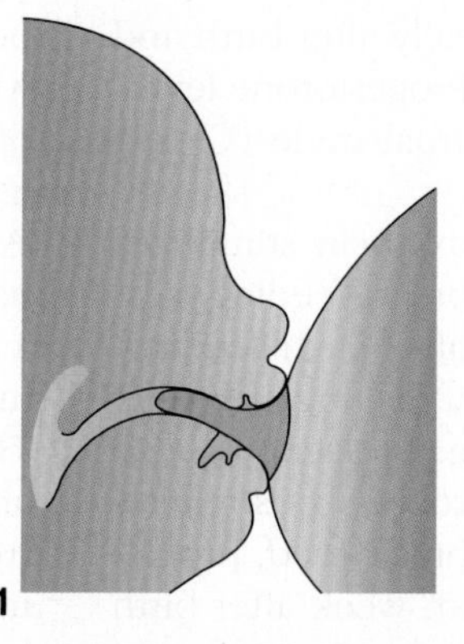

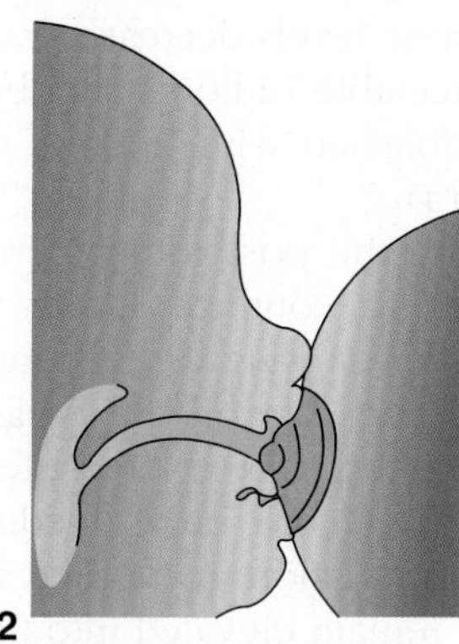

FIGURE 15.4 **A.** Image of engorged breasts. Note swelling and inflammation of both breasts. **B.** Breast engorgement can disrupt breast-feeding: (1) When sucking at a normal breast, the infant's lips compress the areola and fit neatly against the sides of the nipple. The infant also has adequate room to breathe. (2) When a breast is engorged, however, the infant has difficulty grasping the nipple and breathing ability is compromised. (From Pillitteri, A. [2014]. Maternal and Child Nursing (7th ed.). Philadelphia, PA: Lippincott Williams & Wilkins.)

feedings, applying cold compresses to the breasts helps to reduce swelling. To maintain milk supply, the breasts need to be stimulated by a nursing infant, a breast pump, or manual expression of the milk (Fig. 15.5).

Remember Betsy, with the breast discomfort? The lactation consultant explained that she was experiencing normal breast engorgement and offered several suggestions to help her. What relief measures might she have suggested? What reassurance can be given to Betsy at this time?

SUPPRESSING LACTATION

Various pharmacologic and nonpharmacologic interventions have been used to suppress lactation after childbirth and relieve associated symptoms. Despite the large volume of literature on the subject, there is currently no universal guideline on the most appropriate approach for suppressing lactation in postpartum women (Cunningham et al., 2014). It is estimated that more than 30% of women in the United States do not breast-feed their infants, and a larger proportion discontinues breast-feeding within 2 weeks of childbirth (Senie, 2014). Although physiologic cessation of lactation eventually occurs in the absence of physical stimulus such as infant suckling, a large number of women experience moderate to severe milk leakage and discomfort before lactation ceases.

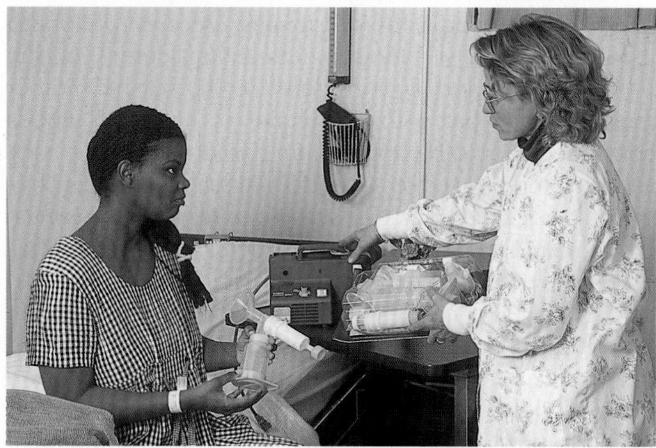

FIGURE 15.5 Nurse instructs the new breast-feeding mother about use of a breast pump. (Copyright B. Proud.)

Up to two thirds of non–breast-feeding women experience moderate to severe engorgement and breast pain when no treatment is applied (Spencer, 2015). If a woman does not desire to breast-feed, some relief measures include wearing a tight, supportive bra 24 hours daily, applying ice to her breasts for approximately 15 to 20 minutes every other hour, avoiding sexual stimulation, and not stimulating the breasts by squeezing or manually expressing milk from the nipples. In addition, avoiding exposing the breasts to warmth (e.g., a hot shower) will help relieve breast engorgement. In women who are not breast-feeding, engorgement typically subsides within 2 to 3 days with application of these measures.

Ovulation and Return of Menstruation

Changing hormone levels constantly interact with one another to produce bodily changes. Four major hormones are influential during the postpartum period: estrogen, progesterone, prolactin, and oxytocin. Estrogen plays a major role during pregnancy, but levels drop profoundly at birth and reach their lowest level a week into the postpartum period. Progesterone quiets the uterus to prevent a preterm birth during pregnancy, and its increasing levels during pregnancy prevent lactation from starting before birth takes place. As with estrogen, progesterone levels decrease dramatically after birth and are undetectable 72 hours after birth. Progesterone levels are reestablished with the first menstrual cycle (Creasy et al., 2014).

During the postpartum period, oxytocin stimulates the uterus to contract during the breast-feeding session and for as long as 20 minutes after each feeding. Oxytocin also acts on the breast by eliciting the milk let-down reflex during breast-feeding. Prolactin is also associated with the breast-feeding process by stimulating milk production. In women who breast-feed, prolactin levels remain elevated into the sixth week after birth (Bope & Kellerman, 2015). The levels of prolactin fluctuate in proportion to nipple stimulation. Prolactin levels decrease in nonlactating women, reaching prepregnant levels by the third postpartum week. High levels of prolactin have been found to delay ovulation by inhibiting ovarian response to follicle-stimulating hormone (Bernard et al., 2015).

The timing of first menses and ovulation after birth differs between women who are breast-feeding and women who are not breast-feeding. For nonlactating women, menstruation may resume as early as 7 to 9 weeks after giving birth, but the majority take up to 3 months, with the first cycle being anovulatory (Barrett et al., 2014). The return of menses in the lactating woman depends on breast-feeding frequency and duration. It can return any time after childbirth, depending on whether the woman is exclusively breast-feeding or supplementing with formula.

Take Note!

Ovulation may occur before menstruation. Therefore, breast-feeding is not a totally reliable method of contraception unless the mother exclusively breast-feeds, has had no menstrual period since giving birth, and whose infant is younger than 6 months old (Alexander et al., 2014).

***Betsy* tries several of the measures the lactation consultant suggested to relieve her breast discomfort, but is still having heaviness and pain. She feels discouraged and tells the nurse she is thinking of reducing her breast-feeding and using formula to feed her newborn. Is that a good choice? Why or why not? What interventions will help Betsy get through this difficult time?**

CULTURAL CONSIDERATIONS FOR THE POSTPARTUM PERIOD

Cultures vary in their postpartum beliefs, practices, and customs. Nurses practice in an increasingly multicultural society. Therefore, they must be open, respectful, nonjudgmental, and willing to learn about ethnically diverse populations. Although childbirth and the postpartum period are unique experiences for each individual woman, how the woman perceives and makes meaning of them is culturally defined. Somali women are highly regarded in Somali society for their roles as mothers. Postpartum women stay at home and refrain from sexual activity for 40 days. At the end of 40 days, there is a celebration and this typically marks the first time the mother and infant have left their home since childbirth. The majority of Somalian and Arab women breast-feed and do so for extended periods of time (Wojnar & Narruhn, 2016). Nurses need to offer early breast-feeding instruction to support their efforts while still in the hospital setting before discharge.

Balance of Hot and Cold

Two areas that are significantly different from Western culture involve beliefs about the balance of hot and cold and confinement after childbirth. Vietnamese women view the postpartum period as a cold state (duong) and protect themselves through warmth. Cultural practices include warm water for hygiene and stimulation of lactation, consuming warm foods, and staying indoors. In the United States, childbearing and recovery are viewed as healthy states and mothers receive little formal support for both their recovery and infant care. In China, childbearing and postpartum are viewed as states which disturb the normal health balance between yin and yang. In order to restore balance in health, postpartum women engage in practices for a month related to the maternal role, physical activity, maintenance of body warmth, and certain food consumption that will restore their balance. Recent research findings in a small sample of Chinese women found that postpartum confinement negatively correlated with aerobic endurance and positively correlated with depression. These findings may challenge the assumption that practices of confinement are healthy for Chinese women's recovery after childbirth (Liu, Maloni, & Petrini, 2014).

For many cultures, good health requires the balancing of hot and cold substances. Because childbirth involves the loss of blood, which is considered hot, the postpartum period is considered cold, so the mother must balance that with the intake of hot food. Foods consumed should be hot in nature, and cold foods, such as fruits and vegetables, avoided. Western practices frequently use cold packs or sitz baths to reduce perineal swelling and discomfort. These practices are not acceptable to women of many cultures and can be viewed as harmful. Hot–cold beliefs are common among Latin American, African, and Asian people (Purnell, 2014).

To reduce infant and mother vulnerability and potential illness, women may practice a month-long confinement period after childbirth. During this confinement period, new mothers rest and recuperate. The postpartum period is a time to avoid cold—both in temperature and foods. Women are kept warm, stay inside to prevent becoming chilled, bathe infrequently, and avoid exercise (Rice & Manderson, 2014).

Postpartum Cultural Beliefs

With increasing multiculturalism in the United States, understanding various cultures' views of the postnatal period as it relates to their recovery and well-being after childbirth is important for all nurses. Postpartum nurses need to understand these diverse cultural beliefs and provide creative strategies for encouraging hygiene (sponge baths, perineal care), exercise, and balanced nutrition, while remaining respectful of the cultural significance of these practices. The best approach is to ask each woman to describe what cultural practices are important to her and plan accordingly.

PSYCHOLOGICAL ADAPTATIONS

The process of becoming a mother (BAM) requires extensive psychological, social, and physical work. Women experience heightened vulnerability and face tremendous challenges as they make this transition. Nurses have a remarkable opportunity to help women learn, gain confidence, and experience growth as they assume the mother identity.

The transition to parenthood, while an exciting time to celebrate the life of their child, causes parents to face new challenges such as physical exhaustion, role overload, and less time for themselves and their partners (Velotti, Castellano, & Zavattini, 2015). Mothers' and fathers' experiences of pregnancy are necessarily different, and this difference continues after childbirth as they both adjust to their new parenting roles. Many couples struggle to adapt to parenthood. Parenting involves caring for infants physically and emotionally to foster the growth and development of responsible, caring adults. A substantial body of research finds no biologically based differences between mothers and fathers in sensitivity to infants, capacity to provide care, or acquisition of parenting skills. Within 15 minutes of holding a newborn, men experience raised levels of oxytocin, cortisol, and prolactin. The increased levels of these nurturing hormones are the same in men and women exposed to infants (Davies, 2015). Other members of the newborn's family, such as siblings and grandparents, also experience changes related to the birth of the newborn (see Chapter 16). Early parent–infant contact after birth improves **attachment** behaviors.

Parental Attachment Behaviors

The postpartum period is a unique time distinguished by the inseparable relationship parents have with their newborn. To enable an attachment to be built, closeness of this family unit is essential. Attachment is the formation of a relationship between a parent and his or her newborn through a process of physical and emotional interactions. Attachment between a woman and her newborn has lifelong implications (King et al., 2015). Maternal attachment has the potential to affect both child development and parenting. The bond between a parent and their newborn is one of strength, power, and potential. Attachment begins before birth, during the prenatal period where acceptance and nurturing of the growing fetus takes place. It continues after giving birth as parents learn to recognize their newborn's cues, adapt to their newborn's behaviors and responses, and meet their newborn's needs.

Several factors take place during the early postpartum period that can have a large influence on the attachment/bonding that occurs during this time. Oxytocin plays an essential role in the chemistry aspect of bonding, and its effects can be enhanced by skin-to-skin contact, breast-feeding, eye contact, social vocalizations, maternal and milk odors, which are soothing for the newborn, and newborn message during the first postpartum hour (Hutcheson & Cheeseman, 2015; Buckley, 2015). Early and sustained contact between newborns and their parents is vital for initiating their relationship.

Nurses play a crucial role in assisting the attachment process by promoting early parent–newborn interactions. In addition, nurses can facilitate skin-to-skin contact (kangaroo care) by placing the infant onto the bare chests of mothers and fathers to enhance parent–newborn attachment. This activity will enable them to get close to their newborn and experience an intense feeling of connectedness and evoke feelings of being nurturing parents. Encouraging breast-feeding is another way to foster attachment between mothers and their newborns. Finally, nurses can encourage nurturing activities and contact such as touching, talking, singing, comforting, changing diapers, feeding—in short, participating in routine newborn care.

The process of attachment is complex and is influenced by many factors including environmental circumstances, the newborn's health status, and the quality of nursing care (Buckley, 2015). Nurses need to minimize parent–newborn separation by promoting parent–newborn interactions through kangaroo care, breast-feeding, and participation in their newborn care. Nurses who provide positive psychosocial support and clear communication to parents will help support the attachment process within family units.

Maternal Psychological Adaptations

Childbirth is supposed to be the most joyous period in a woman's life and involves the almost spiritual experience of giving birth and being able to give life to another being. For many, this can be a life-changing event and through the centuries has been anticipated with excitement and joy and has even been referred to as a blessing. In reality, childbirth and child rearing are very stressful, financially challenging, and emotionally demanding.

Mood Disorders

Many people consider childbirth a time of happiness and well-being, but it is common for women to experience changes in their mood during this time. This may include being fatigued, irritable, or worried, and frequently these mood symptoms become severe enough to need medical intervention. In the postpartum period, mood disorders can be divided into three distinct entities in ascending order of severity: maternal (baby) blues, postpartum depression, and psychosis. These disorders, however, have not been clearly demarcated and it is a matter of much debate whether they are discrete disorders or a single disorder that ranges along a continuum of severity (Finley & Brizendine, 2015).

Up to 85% of new mothers suffer from the short-lived postpartum mood disorder termed "baby blues" or maternal blues, which are characterized by mild depressive symptoms, anxiety, irritability, mood swings, loss of appetite, trouble with sleeping, tearfulness (often for no discernible reason), increased sensitivity, and fatigue (Flynn, 2015). The "blues" typically peak on postpartum days 4 and 5, may last hours to days, and usually resolve by day 10. Although these symptoms may be distressing, they do not reflect psychopathology, and they typically do not affect the mother's ability to function and care for her child. For additional information, see Chapter 22.

Phases of Maternal Adaptation to Parenthood

Parenthood is a highly anticipated and positive event for most women. Society has constructed many ideal images of motherhood, giving standards for women to live up to, and frequently setting them up for disappointment. Most women are able to experience this mismatch between their ideal and actual self and adapt with minimal discrepancy (Adams, 2015). The woman experiences a variety of responses as she adjusts to a new family member and to postpartum discomforts, changes in her body image, and the reality of change in her life. In the early 1960s, Reva Rubin identified three phases that a mother goes through to adjust to her new maternal role. Rubin's maternal role framework can be used to monitor the client's progress as she "tries on" her new role as a mother. The absence of these processes or inability to progress through the phases satisfactorily may impede the appropriate development of the maternal role (Rubin, 1984). Although Rubin's maternal role development theories are of value, some of her observations regarding the length of each phase may not be completely relevant for the contemporary woman of the 21st century. Today, many women know their infant's gender, have "seen" their fetus in utero through four-dimensional ultrasound, and have a working knowledge of childbirth and child care. They are less passive than in years past and progress through the phases of attaining the maternal role at a much faster pace than Rubin would have imagined. Still, Rubin's framework is timeless for assessing and monitoring expected role behaviors when planning care and appropriate interventions.

TAKING-IN PHASE

The **taking-in phase** is the time immediately after birth when the client needs sleep, depends on others to meet her needs, and relives the events surrounding the birth process. This phase is characterized by dependent behavior. During the first 24 to 48 hours after giving birth, mothers often assume a very passive role in meeting their own basic needs for food, fluids, and rest, allowing the nurse to make decisions for them concerning activities and care. They spend time recounting their labor experience to anyone who will listen. Such actions help the mother integrate the birth experience into reality—that is, the pregnancy is over and the newborn is now a unique individual, separate from herself. When interacting with the newborn, new mothers spend time claiming the newborn and touching him or her, commonly identifying specific features in the newborn, such as "he has my nose" or "his fingers are long like his father's" (Fig. 15.6).

Take Note!

The taking-in phase typically lasts 1 to 2 days and may be the only phase observed by nurses in the hospital setting because of the shortened postpartum stays that are the norm today.

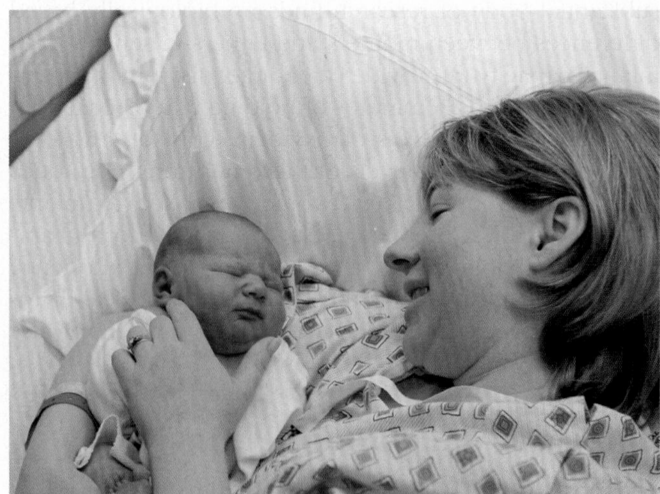

FIGURE 15.6 Mother bonding with newborn during the taking-in phase.

TAKING-HOLD PHASE

The **taking-hold phase**, the second phase of maternal adaptation, is characterized by dependent and independent maternal behavior. This phase typically starts on the second to third day postpartum and may last several weeks.

As the client regains control over her bodily functions during the next few days, she will be taking hold and becoming preoccupied with the present. She will be particularly concerned about her health, the infant's condition, and her ability to care for her or him. She demonstrates increased autonomy and mastery of her own body's functioning, and a desire to take charge with support and help from others. She will show independence by caring for herself and learning to care for her newborn, but she still requires assurance that she is doing well as a mother. She expresses a strong interest in caring for the infant by herself.

LETTING-GO PHASE

In the **letting-go phase**, the third phase of maternal adaptation, the woman reestablishes relationships with other people. She adapts to parenthood through her new role as a mother. She assumes the responsibility and care of the newborn with a bit more confidence now (Edelman, Kudzma, & Mandle, 2014). The focus of this phase is to move forward by assuming the parental role and to separate herself from the symbiotic relationship that she and her newborn had during pregnancy. She establishes a lifestyle that includes the infant. The mother relinquishes the fantasy infant and accepts the real one.

Nurses have recognized the importance of the process of becoming a mother (BAM) to maternal–infant nursing since Rubin's report on maternal role attainment (MRA). Mothers' perceptions of their competence or confidence, or both, in mothering and their expressions of love for their infants include age, relationship with the father, socioeconomic status, birth experience, experienced stress, available support, personality traits, self-concept, child-rearing attitudes, role strain, health status, preparation during pregnancy, relationships with own mother, depression, and anxiety. Infant variables identified as influencing MRA/BAM include appearance, responsiveness, temperament, and health status (DiPietro et al., 2015). More current research has led to renaming the four stages a woman progresses through in establishing a maternal identity in BAM:

1. Commitment, attachment to the unborn baby, and preparation for delivery and motherhood during pregnancy
2. Acquaintance/attachment to the infant, learning to care for the infant, and physical restoration during the first 2 to 6 weeks following birth
3. Moving toward a new normal
4. Achievement of a maternal identity through redefining self to incorporate motherhood (around 4 months). The mother feels self-confident and competent in her mothering and expresses love for and pleasure interacting with her infant (Mercer & Walker, 2006)

The woman's work in the first stage is to make a commitment to the pregnancy and to the safe birth and care of her unborn child. This commitment is associated with a positive adaptation to motherhood. During the second stage while the mother is placing the infant in her family context and learning how to care for her infant, her attachment and attitude toward her infant, and her self-confidence or sense of competence in mothering, or both, consistently indicate an interdependence of these two variables. The nursing care provided during the first two stages is especially important in assisting mothers as they begin to mother. Follow-up by nurses is needed as mothers move toward a new normal and recognize that a transformation of self in BAM. Nurses can continue to reinforce their new mothering capabilities (Mercer, 2006).

To foster maternal role attainment, three specific interventions for nurses were identified in a review of the literature (Ferrarello & Hatfield, 2014). First, instructions about infant care and the infant's capabilities are more effective if they are specifically focused on that particular mother's infant. Second, mothers prefer live classes rather than videotapes so they can ask questions. In short, interactive nurse–client relationships are associated with positive maternal growth. Third, identifying barriers that reduce skin-to-skin periods of mother-to-infant during the postpartum hospital stay and intervening to reduce them have implications for both maternal role development and breast-feeding success, if she has chosen this method. Providing times for skin-to-skin mother and infant contact has a positive impact on the long-term health of both. Nurses who interact with clients long term during pregnancy, childbirth, and during well child care help build maternal competence. Pregnancy, birth, and becoming a mother collectively represent a critical period of physical and emotional upheaval in a woman's life. The need for a holistic care approach that supports the emotional and physical health of the dyad is imperative (Spiteri et al., 2014).

Transition to motherhood theories (Rubin and Mercer) describe women in a prescribed role—that of being a mother and indeed a predetermined type of mother. In that sense transition to motherhood theory is baby-centered. New theories needs to be developed that are woman-centered and which conceptualize the woman as an embodied self who is powerful in her own life.

Partner Psychological Adaptations

For partners, whether they are husbands, significant others, boyfriends, same-sex life partners, or just friends, becoming a parent or just sharing the childbirth experience can be a perplexing time as well as a time of great change. This transition is influenced by many factors, including participation in childbirth, relationships with significant others, competence in child care, the family role organization, the individual's cultural background, and the method of infant feeding.

The transition from being merely a partner to being a parent can propel many partners to reorganize their lifestyles. During the postpartum period, partners frequently find themselves struggling to balance personal and work needs with the new demands of parent status and their new self-image. The complexities of the transitional process involved in forging a parenthood identity can be viewed at three different levels: readjustment to a new self-image, formation of a triadic family relationship, and adaptation to redefining themselves and their relationship with their partner: the "more united tag team" (Halford, Petch, & Creedy, 2015).

Nurses can play a key role in supporting a partner's transition to parenthood by keeping partners informed about birth and postpartum routines, reporting on their newborn's health status, and reviewing infant development. They can also contribute by creating participative space for new partners during the postpartum period. This can be achieved, for example, by helping partners take on their new role by supporting and promoting their degree of involvement in the process. They can also be encouraged to actively participate in caring for, and maintaining contact with, their newborns.

Take Note!

Most research findings stress the importance of early contact between the partner or significant other and the newborn, as well as participation in infant care activities, to foster the relationship (Nolan, 2015).

Infants have a powerful effect on their parents and others, who become intensely involved with them (Fig. 15.7). The father's or significant other's developing bond with the newborn—a time of intense absorption, preoccupation, and interest—is called *engrossment.*

Engrossment

Engrossment is characterized by seven behaviors:

1. Visual awareness of the newborn—the partner perceives the newborn as attractive, pretty, or beautiful.
2. Tactile awareness of the newborn—the partner has a desire to touch or hold the newborn and considers this activity to be pleasurable.
3. Perception of the newborn as perfect—the partner does not "see" any imperfections.
4. Strong attraction to the newborn—the partner focuses all attention on the newborn when they are in the room.

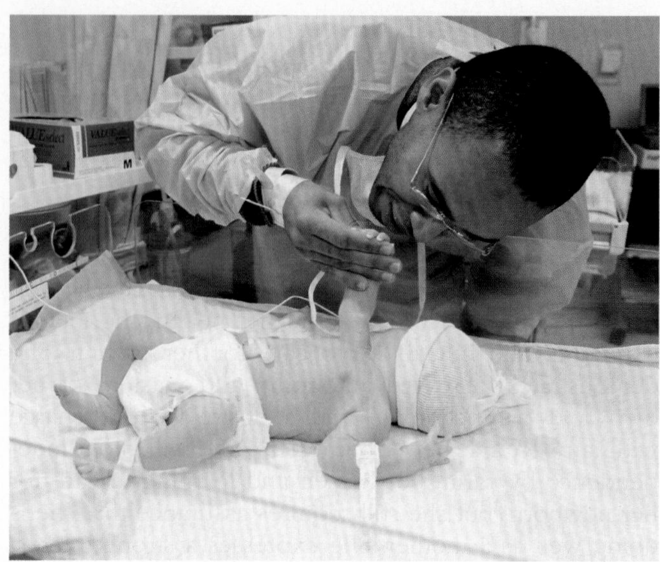

FIGURE 15.7 Engrossment of the father and his newborn.

5. Awareness of distinct features of the newborn—the partner can distinguish his/her newborn from others in the nursery.
6. Extreme elation—the partner feels a "high" after the birth of his/her child.
7. Increased sense of self-esteem—the partner feels proud, "bigger," more mature, and older after the birth of his/her child (Sears & Sears, 2015).

Frequently, partners are portrayed as well-meaning but bumbling when caring for newborns. However, they have their own unique way of relating to their newborns and can become as nurturing as mothers. A partner's nurturing responses may be less automatic and slower to unfold than a mother's, but they are capable of a strong bonding attachment to their newborns (Sears & Sears, 2015). Encouraging partners to express their feelings by seeing, touching, and holding their son or daughter and by cuddling, talking to, and feeding him or her will help to cement this new relationship. Reinforcement of this engrossing behavior helps partners to make a positive attachment during this critical period.

Three-Stage Role Development Process

Similar to mothers, partners also go through a predictable three-stage process during the first 3 weeks as they too "try on" their roles as parents. The three stages are expectations, reality, and transition to mastery (Sears & Sears, 2015).

STAGE 1: EXPECTATIONS

New partners pass through stage 1 (expectations) with preconceptions about what home life will be like with a newborn. Many partners may be unaware of the dramatic changes that can occur when this newborn comes home to live with them. For some, it is an eye-opening experience.

STAGE 2: REALITY

Stage 2 (reality) occurs when partners realize that their expectations in stage 1 are not realistic. Their feelings change from elation to sadness, ambivalence, jealousy, and frustration. Many wish to be more involved in the newborn's care and yet do not feel prepared to do so. Some find parenting fun but at the same time do not feel fully prepared to take on that role.

Partner's stress, irritability, and frustration in the days, weeks, and months after the birth of their child can turn into depression, just like new maternal experience. Unfortunately, partners rarely discuss their feelings or ask for help, especially during a time when they are supposed to be the "strong one" for the new mother. Depression in partners can cause marital conflicts, reckless or violent behavior, withdrawn parental interactions with the newborn, poor job performance, and substance abuse. In addition, paternal depression following childbirth can have a detrimental effect on a couple's relationship, on the parent–child relationship, and on their children's future development (Sethna et al., 2015).

Risk factors for partner postpartum depression include previous history of depression, financial problems, a poor relationship with his/her partner, and an unplanned pregnancy. Symptoms of depression appear 1 to 3 weeks after birth and can include feelings of being very stressed and anxious, being discouraged or fatigued, resentment toward the infant and the attention he or she is getting, and headaches. Partners experiencing these symptoms should understand that it is not a sign of weakness and professional help can be helpful for them.

STAGE 3: TRANSITION TO MASTERY

In stage 3 (transition to mastery), the partner makes a conscious decision to take control and be at the center of his/her newborn's life regardless of his/her preparedness. This adjustment period is similar to that of the mother's letting-go phase, when she incorporates the newest member into the family.

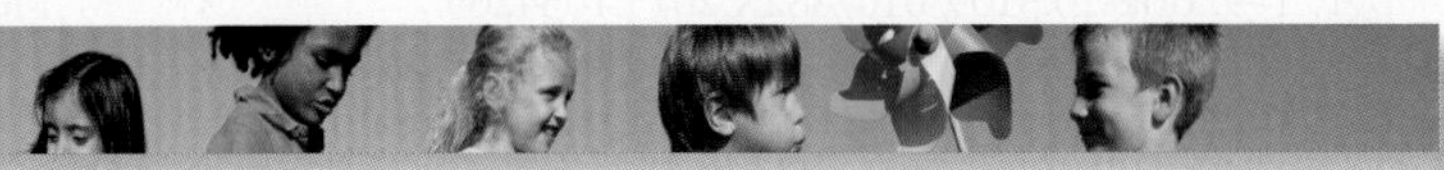

KEY CONCEPTS

- The puerperium period refers to the first 6 weeks after delivery. During this period, the mother experiences many physiologic and psychological adaptations to return her to the prepregnant state.
- Involution involves three processes: contraction of muscle fibers to reduce stretched ones, catabolism (which reduces enlarged, individual cells), and regeneration of uterine epithelium from the lower layer of the decidua after the upper layers have been sloughed off and shed in lochia.
- Lochia passes through three stages—lochia rubra, lochia serosa, and lochia alba—during the postpartum period.
- Maternal blood plasma volume decreases rapidly after birth and returns to normal within 4 weeks postpartum.
- Reva Rubin (1984) identified three phases the mother goes through to adjust to her new maternal role: the taking-in, taking-hold, and letting-go phases.
- The transition to fatherhood is influenced by many factors, including participation in childbirth, relationships with significant others, competence in child care, the family role organization, the father's cultural background, and the method of infant feeding.
- Like mothers, partners go through a predictable three-stage process during the first 3 weeks as they too "try on" their roles as partners. The three stages include expectations, reality, and transition to mastery.

REFERENCES AND RECOMMENDED READING

Adams, M. (2015). Motherhood: A discrepancy theory. *Research and Theory for Nursing Practice, 29*(2), 143–157.

Alekseev, N. P., Vladimir, I. I., & Nadezhda, T. E. (2015). Pathological postpartum breast engorgement: Prediction, prevention, and resolution. *Breastfeeding Medicine, 10*(4), 203–208.

Alexander, L. L., LaRosa, J. H., Bader, H., & Garfield, S. (2014). *New dimensions in women's health* (6th ed.). Sudbury, MA: Jones & Bartlett.

American Academy of Pediatrics [AAP]. (2015). *Caring for your baby and young child: Birth to age 5* (6th ed.). Elk Grove Village, IL: AAP.

Barrett, E. S., Parlett, L. E., Windham, G. C., & Swan, S. H. (2014). Differences in ovarian hormones in relation to parity and time since last birth. *Fertility & Sterility, 101*(6), 1773–1780.

Bernard, V., Young, J., Chanson, P., & Binart, N. (2015). New insights in prolactin: pathological implications. *Nature Reviews Endocrinology, 11*(5), 265–275.

Bope, E., & Kellerman, R. (2015). *Conn's current therapy 2015*. Philadelphia, PA: Saunders Elsevier.

Bowers, P., & Ceballos, K. (2015). Cultural perspectives in childbearing. Nurse.com. Retrieved from http://ce.nurse.com/course/ce263-60/cultural-perspectives-in-childbearing

Boyd-Judson, L., & James, P. (2014). *Women's global health: Norms and state policies*. Plymouth, UK: Lexington Books.

Buckley, S. (2015). *Hormonal physiology of childbearing: Evidence and implications for women, babies and maternity care*. Washington, DC: Childbirth Connection, National Partnership for Women & Families.

Cheng, Y. W., & Caughey, A. B. (2015). Normal labor and delivery. *eMedicine*. Retrieved from http://emedicine.medscape.com/article/260036-overview

Creasy, R. K., Resnik, R., Iams, J. D., Lockwood, C. J., Moore, T. R., & Greene, M. F. (2014). *Creasy & Resnik's maternal-fetal medicine: Principles and practice* (7th ed.). Philadelphia, PA: Elsevier Saunders.

Cunningham, F. G., Leveno, K. J., Bloom, S. L., Spong, C., Dashe, J. S., Hoffman, B. L., et al. (2014). *Williams obstetrics* (24th ed.). New York, NY: McGraw-Hill Publishers.

Davies, J. (2015). Fatherhood Institute: Supporting fathers to play their part. *Community Practitioner, 88*(1), 13–14.

DiPietro, J. A., Goldshore, M. A., Kivlighan, K. T., Pater, H. A., & Costigan, K. A. (2015). The ups and downs of early mothering. *Journal of Psychosomatic Obstetrics & Gynecology*, 1–9. doi: 10.3109/0167482X.2015.1034269.

Dumoulin, C., Hay-Smith, E. J., & Mac Habée-Séguin, G. (2014). Pelvic floor muscle training versus no treatment, or inactive control treatments, for urinary incontinence in women. *Cochrane Database of Systematic Reviews*, 5, CD005654. doi: 10.1002/14651858.CD005654.pub3.

Edelman, C. L., Kudzma, E. C., & Mandle, C. L. (2014). *Health promotion throughout the lifespan* (8th ed.). St. Louis, MO: Mosby Elsevier.

Engel, S., Kon, S. K., Mawson, E. H., & Folley, S. J. (2015). Discussion of some recent developments in knowledge of the physiology of the breast. *Proceedings of the Royal Society of Medicine, 40*, 899–906.

Evans, A. T., & De Franco, E. (2014). *Manual of obstetrics* (8th ed.). Philadelphia, PA: Lippincott Williams & Wilkins.

Ferrarello, D., & Hatfield, L. (2014). Barriers to skin-to-skin care during the postpartum stay. *MCN. The American Journal of Maternal Child Nursing, 39*(1), 56–61.

Finley, P. R., & Brizendine, L. (2015). Enhancing our understanding of perinatal depression. *CNS Spectrums, 20*(1), 9–10.

Flynn, R. (2015). Mood disorders during and after pregnancy. *South African Journal of Diabetes, 8*(2), 27–33.

Halford, W. K., Petch, J., & Creedy, D. (2015). *Clinical guide to helping new parents: The couple CARE for parents program*. New York, NY: Springer Publishers.

Halford, W. K., Petch, J., & Creedy, D. (2015). Taking baby home. In *Clinical guide to helping new parents* (pp. 87–109). New York, NY: Springer Publishers.

Hutcheson, J. L., & Cheeseman, S. E. (2015). An innovative strategy to improve family–infant bonding. *Neonatal Network, 34*(3), 189–191.

Jin, B., Yu, H., Jin, M., Du, X., & Yang, S. (2015). Measurement of prolactin and estradiol to estimate menses return of breastfeeding mothers. *Reproduction and Contraception, 14*(2), 111–117.

Jordan, R. G., Engstrom, J., Marfell, J., & Farley, C. L. (2014). *Prenatal & postnatal care: A women-centered approach*. Ames, IA: John Wiley & Sons.

King, T. L., Brucker, M. C., Kriebs, J. M., Fahey, J. O., Gegor, C. L., & Varney, H. (2015) *Varney's midwifery* (5th ed.). Burlington, MA: Jones & Bartlett Learning.

Liu, Y., Maloni, J. A., & Petrini, M. A. (2014). Effect of postpartum practices of doing the month on Chinese women's physical and psychological health. *Biological Research for Nursing, 16*(1), 55–63.

Mahendru, A., Everett, T., Wilkinson, I., Lees, C., & McEniery, C. (2014). A longitudinal study of maternal cardiovascular function from preconception to the postpartum period. *Journal of Hypertension, 32*(4), 849–856.

Martin, J., MacDonald-Wicks, L., Hure, A., Smith, R., & Collins, C. E. (2015). Reducing postpartum weight retention and improving breastfeeding outcomes in overweight women: A pilot randomized controlled trial. *Nutrients, 7*(3), 1464–1479.

Mattson, S., & Smith, J. (2016). *Core curriculum for maternal–newborn nursing*. (5th ed.). St. Louis, MO: Elsevier Saunders.

Mercer, R. (2006). Nursing support of the process of becoming a mother. *Journal of Obstetric, Gynecologic & Neonatal Nursing, 35*(5), 649–651.

Mercer, R., & Walker, L. (2006). A review of nursing interventions to foster becoming a mother. *Journal of Obstetric, Gynecologic & Neonatal Nursing, 35*(5), 568–582.

Nascimento, S., Pudwell, J., Surita, F., Adamo, K., & Smith, G. (2014). The effect of physical exercise strategies on weight loss in postpartum women: A systematic review and meta-analysis. *International Journal of Obesity, 38*(5), 626–635.

Neville, C., McKinley, M., Holmes, V., Spence, D., & Woodside, J. (2014). The relationship between breastfeeding and postpartum weight change—A systematic review and critical evaluation. *International Journal of Obesity, 38*(4), 577–590.

Nolan, M. (2015). Why it is important to involve new fathers in the care of their child: Mary Nolan explores research into the often-neglected role of men and suggests how primary care nurses can develop services to increase their involvement. *Primary Health Care, 25*(3), 18–23.

Norwitz, E. R., & Schorge, J. O. (2015). *Obstetrics & gynecology at a glance* (5th ed.). Oxford, UK: Wiley-Blackwell.

Parpaglioni, R. (2015). Anatomo-physiological changes during labor and after delivery. In *Epidural labor analgesia* (pp. 11–20). New York, NY: Springer International Publishing.

Purnell, L. D. (2014). *Guide to culturally competent health care* (3rd ed.). Philadelphia, PA: F. A. Davis.

Rice, P. L., & Manderson, L. (2014). *Maternity and reproductive health in Asian societies*. Abingdon, Oxon: Routledge.

Rubin, R. (1984). *Maternal identity and the maternal experience*. New York, NY: Springer.

Sears, R. W., & Sears, J. M. (2015). Father–newborn bonding. *Ask Dr. Sears*. Retrieved from http://www.askdrsears.com/topics/pregnancy-childbirth/tenth-month-post-partum/bonding-with-your-newborn/father-newborn-bonding

Senie, R. T. (2014). *Epidemiology of women's health*. Burlington, MA: Jones & Bartlett Learning.

Sethna, V., Murray, L., Netsi, E., Psychogiou, L., & Ramchandani, P. G. (2015). Paternal depression in the postnatal period and early father–infant interactions. *Parenting, 15*(1), 1–8.

Spencer, B. (2015). Medications and breastfeeding for mothers with chronic illness. *Journal of Obstetric, Gynecologic, & Neonatal Nursing, 44*(4), 543–552.

Spiliopoulos, M., & Mastrogiannis, D. (2014). Normal and abnormal puerperium. *eMedicine*. Retrieved from http://emedicine.medscape.com/article/260187-overview#a1

Spiteri, G., Borg Xuereb, R., Carrick-Sen, D., Kaner, E., & Martin, C. R. (2014). Preparation for parenthood: A concept analysis. *Journal of Reproductive & Infant Psychology, 32*(2), 148–165. doi: 10.1080/02646838.2013.869578.

Stuebe, A. M., Meltzer-Brody, S., Pearson, B., Pedersen, C., & Grewen, K. (2015). Maternal neuroendocrine serum levels in exclusively breastfeeding mothers. *Breastfeeding Medicine, 10*(4), 197–202.

Wambach, K., & Riordan, J. (2014). *Breastfeeding and human lactation*. (5th ed.). Burlington, MA: Jones and Bartlett Learning.

Webber, G. C., & Chirangi, B. (2014). Women's health in women's hands: A pilot study assessing the feasibility of providing women with medications to reduce postpartum hemorrhage and sepsis in rural Tanzania. *Health Care for Women International, 35*(7-9), 758–770.

Wojnar, D. M., & Narruhn, R. A. (2015). Chapter 18: Transcultural aspects of perinatal health care of Somali women. In De Chesnay, M., & Anderson, B. A. (Eds.), *Caring for the Vulnerable* (4th ed., pp. 287–302). Burlington, MA: Jones & Bartlett Learning.

Zanardo, V., & Straface, G. (2015). The higher temperature in the areola supports the natural progression of the birth to breastfeeding continuum. *PloS One, 10*(3), e0118774.

CHAPTER WORKSHEET

MULTIPLE-CHOICE QUESTIONS

1. Postpartum breast engorgement occurs 48 to 72 hours after giving birth. What physiologic change influences breast engorgement?
   a. An increase in blood and lymph supply to the breasts
   b. An increase in estrogen and progesterone levels
   c. Colostrum production increases dramatically.
   d. Fluid retention in the breasts due to the intravenous fluids given during labor

2. In the taking-in maternal role phase described by Rubin (1984), the nurse would expect the woman's behavior to be characterized as which of the following?
   a. Gaining self-confidence
   b. Adjusting to her new relationships
   c. Being passive and dependent
   d. Resuming control over her life

3. The nurse is explaining to a postpartum woman 48 hours after her giving childbirth that the afterpains she is experiencing can be the result of which of the following?
   a. Abdominal cramping is a sign of endometriosis.
   b. A small infant weighing less than 8 pounds
   c. Pregnancies that were too closely spaced
   d. Contractions of the uterus after birth

4. The nurse would expect a postpartum woman to demonstrate lochia in which sequence?
   a. Rubra, alba, serosa
   b. Rubra, serosa, alba
   c. Serosa, alba, rubra
   d. Alba, rubra, serosa

5. The nurse is assessing Ms. Smith, who gave birth to her first child 5 days ago. What findings by the nurse would be expected?
   a. Cream-colored lochia; uterus above the umbilicus
   b. Bright-red lochia with clots; uterus 2 fingerbreadths below umbilicus
   c. Light pink or brown lochia; uterus 4 to 5 fingerbreadths below umbilicus
   d. Yellow, mucousy lochia; uterus at the level of the umbilicus

6. Prioritize the postpartum mother's needs 4 hours after giving birth by placing a number 1, 2, 3, or 4 in the blank before each need.
   a. ________ Learn how to hold and cuddle the infant.
   b. ________Watch a baby bath demonstration given by the nurse.
   c. ________ Sleep and rest without being disturbed for a few hours.
   d. ________ Interaction time (first 30 minutes) with the infant to facilitate bonding

7. Immediately after childbirth in the recovery area, the nurse observes the mother's partner's fascination and interest in the new son. This behavior is often termed:
   a. Attachment
   b. Engrossment
   c. Bonding
   d. Temperament

8. After the nurse provides instructions to a postpartum woman about postpartum blues, which statement would indicate understanding of it? I will
   a. "Need to take medication daily to treat the anxiety and sadness."
   b. "Call the OB support line only if I start to hear voices."
   c. "Contact my doctor if I become dizzy and fell nauseated."
   d. "Feel like laughing 1 minute and crying the next minute."

CRITICAL THINKING EXERCISES

1. A new nurse assigned to the postpartum mother–baby unit makes a comment to the oncoming shift that, a 25-year-old primipara patient, seems lazy and shows no initiative in taking care of herself or her baby. The nurse reported that this new mother talks excessively about her labor and birth experience and seems preoccupied with herself and her needs, not her newborn's care. She wonders if something is wrong with this mother because she seems so self-centered and has to be directed to do everything.
   a. Is there something "wrong" with this mother's behavior? Why or why not?
   b. What maternal role phase is being described by the new nurse?
   c. What role can the nurse play to support the mother through this phase?

CHAPTER WORKSHEET

2. Mrs. Lenhart, a primipara, gave birth to a healthy baby boy yesterday. Her partner seemed elated at the birth, calling their friends and family on his cell phone minutes after the birth. He passed out cigars and praised his wife for her efforts. Today, when the nurse walked into their room, her partner seemed very anxious around his new son and called for the nurse whenever the baby cried or needed a diaper change. He seemed standoffish when asked to hold his son, and he spent time talking to other fathers in the waiting room, leaving his wife alone in the room.
   a. Would you consider Mr. Lenhart's paternal behavior to be normal at this time?
   b. What might Mr. Lenhart be feeling at this time?
   c. How can the nurse help this new father adjust to his new role?

STUDY ACTIVITIES

1. Find an Internet resource that discusses general postpartum care for new mothers who might have questions after discharge. Evaluate the web site's information as to how credible, accurate, and current the information is.
2. Prepare a teaching plan for new mothers, outlining the various physiologic changes that will take place after discharge.
3. The term that describes the return of the uterus to its prepregnant state is ____________.
4. A deviated fundus to the right side of the abdomen would indicate a ____________.

BRINGING IT ALL TOGETHER: A CASE STUDY

A 29-year-old married Latina mother of four children lived with her migrant husband and his parents in a small rural border town. She had given birth to her fourth child 7 weeks ago. She now had four children in the past 4 years. Her pregnancy, labor, and birth had been uneventful, and an untrained neighbor woman helped conduct the home birth. Because pregnancy was viewed as a normal occurrence that did not require any medical attention, she did not receive any prenatal care for any of her four pregnancies. For the first month after birth, she felt normal, but then began to exhibit bizarre behaviors. She became isolated from her family, stopped speaking to them, and ceased to care for her newborn or other children. Her family wondered about her isolation, but seemed indifferent to her condition, as they were all busy with their own lives. One day when all of her family members and her children had gone to work in the fields, she ended her life.

Go to thePoint to find questions to consider about this case.

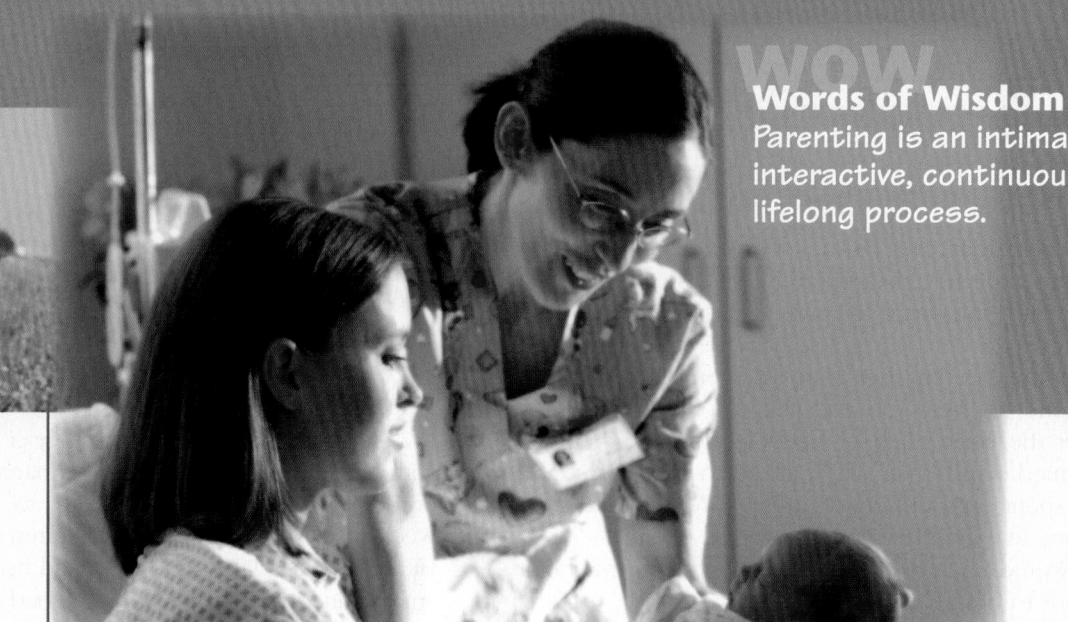

16

WOW

Words of Wisdom

Parenting is an intimate, interactive, continuous, lifelong process.

Nursing Management During the Postpartum Period

KEY TERMS

attachment

bonding

en face position

pelvic floor exercises

peribottle

postpartum blues

sitz bath

Learning Objectives

Upon completion of the chapter, you will be able to:

1. Characterize the normal physiologic and psychological adaptations to the postpartum period.
2. Determine the parameters that need to be assessed during the postpartum period.
3. Compare and contrast bonding to the attachment process.
4. Select behaviors that enhance or inhibit the attachment process.
5. Outline nursing management for the woman and her family during the postpartum period.
6. Examine the role of the nurse in promoting successful breast-feeding.
7. Plan areas of health education needed for discharge planning, home care, and follow-up.

A 24-year-old Muslim primipara has just been admitted to the postpartum unit. Her husband sits at the bedside but doesn't seem to give her any physical or emotional support after her lengthy labor and difficult birth.

INTRODUCTION

The postpartum period is a time of major adjustments and adaptations not just for the mother, but for all members of the family. It is during this time that parenting starts and a relationship with the newborn begins. A positive, loving relationship between parents and their newborn promotes the emotional well-being of all. This relationship endures and has profound effects on the child's growth and development.

Take Note!

Parenting is a skill that is often learned by trial and error, with varying degrees of success. Successful parenting, a continuous and complex interactive process, requires the parents to learn new skills and to integrate the new member into the family.

Once the infant is born, each system in the mother's body takes several weeks to return to its nonpregnant state. The physiologic changes in women during the postpartum period are dramatic. Nurses should be aware of these changes and should be able to make observations and assessments to validate normal occurrences and detect any deviations.

This chapter describes the nursing management of the woman and her family during the postpartum period. (See Chapter 21 for a detailed discussion of the postpartum care of the woman undergoing a surgical birth.) Nursing management during the postpartum period focuses on assessing the woman's ability to adapt to the physiologic and psychological changes occurring at this time (see Chapter 15 for a detailed discussion of these adaptations). The chapter outlines physical assessment parameters for new mothers and newborns. It also focuses on **bonding** and **attachment** behaviors; nurses need to be aware of these behaviors so they can perform appropriate interventions. Family members are also assessed to determine how well they are making the transition to this new stage.

Based on assessment findings, the nurse plans and implements care to address the family's needs. Steps to address physiologic needs such as comfort, self-care, nutrition, and contraception are described. Ways to help the woman and her family adapt to the birth of the newborn are also discussed (Fig. 16.1). Because of today's shortened lengths of stay, the nurse may be able to focus only on priority needs and may need to arrange for follow-up in the home to ensure that all the family's needs are met.

SOCIAL SUPPORT AND CULTURAL CONSIDERATIONS

In addition to physical assessment and care of the woman in the postpartum period, strong social support is vital to help her integrate the baby into the family. A key to providing effective postpartum care is to understand the woman in her social and cultural context so that all care provided is culturally competent and sensitive. In today's mobile society, extended families may live far away and may be unable to help care for the new family. As a result, many new parents turn to health care providers for information as well as physical and emotional support during this adjustment period. Nurses can be an invaluable resource by serving as mentors, teaching about self-care measures and baby care basics, and providing emotional support. Nurses can "mother" the new mother by offering physical care, emotional support, information, and practical help. The nurse's support and care through this critical time can increase the new parents' confidence, giving them a sense of accomplishment in their parenting skills. One important intervention during the postpartum period is promotion of breast-feeding. *Healthy People 2020* includes breast-feeding as a goal for maternal, infant, and child health (U.S. Department of Health and Human Resources [USDHHS], 2010).

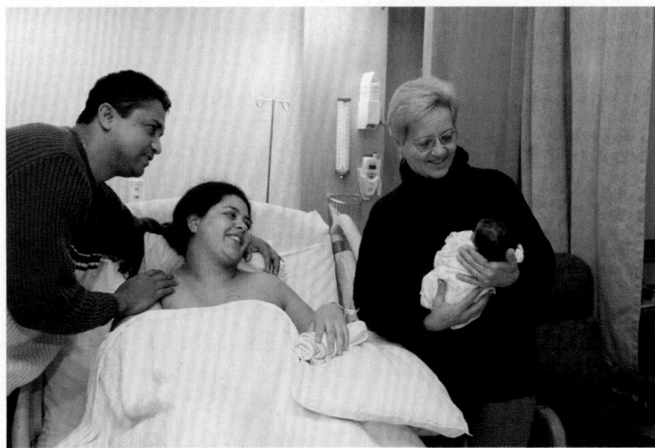

FIGURE 16.1 Parents and grandmother interacting with the newborn.

As in all nursing care, nurses should provide culturally competent care during the postpartum period. The nurse should engage in ongoing cultural self-assessment and overcome any stereotypes that perpetuate prejudice or discrimination against any cultural group (Bowers & Ceballos, 2015). Providing culturally competent nursing care during the postpartum period requires time, open-mindedness, and patience. The global migration of diverse populations presents nurses with the challenge of providing care to unprecedented numbers of clients and their families with health care beliefs and practices that differ from their own. Sensitivity cannot be assumed; it needs to be nurtured and developed. The skill set needed by nurses to provide culturally competent care to postpartum clients and their families includes understanding their beliefs, experiences, and family environment; facilitating their language through appropriate use of interpreters so that the information provided can be understood; and compassionately respecting clients and their human rights. The Chinese culture values

HEALTHY PEOPLE 2020

Objective	Nursing Significance
Increase the proportion of mothers who breast-feed their babies.	• Will provide infants with the most complete form of nutrition, improving their health, growth and development, and immunity
Increase the number of mothers who breast-feed ever from a baseline of 74% to 81.9%.	• Will improve maternal health via breast-feeding's beneficial effects
Increase the number of mothers who breast-feed at 6 months from a baseline of 43.5% to 60.6%.	• Will increase the rate of breast-feeding, particularly among low-income and certain racial and ethnic populations who are less likely to begin breast-feeding in the hospital or to sustain it through the infant's first year
Increase the number of mothers who breast-feed at 1 year from a baseline of 22.7% to 34.1%.	
Increase the number of mothers who breast-feed exclusively through 3 months from a baseline of 33.6% to 46.2%.	
Increase the number of mothers who breast-feed exclusively through 6 months from a baseline of 14.1% to 25.5%.	

Healthy People objectives based on data from http://www.healthypeople.gov.

traditions and the involvement of elders in the extended family. Some Chinese women living in the United States practice transnational parenting, a process of sending their American-born child to China to be raised by the extended family there. This obviously has implications for breast-feeding success among these mothers (Lee & Brann, 2015). To promote positive outcomes, the nurse should be sensitive to the woman's and family's culture, religion, and ethnic influences (see "Providing Optimal Cultural Care" in the Nursing Interventions section).

Remember the couple introduced at the beginning of the chapter? When the postpartum nurse comes to examine Raina, her husband quickly leaves the room and returns a short time later after the examination is complete. How do you interpret his behavior toward his wife? What might you communicate to this couple?

NURSING ASSESSMENT IN THE POSTPARTUM PERIOD

Many adaptations and adjustments must be made to accommodate the new family member. The nurse's focus is on assistance for families to maximize their adjustment, surveillance for maladaptation, and education, consultation, collaboration as needed. Comprehensive nursing assessment begins within an hour after the woman gives birth and continues through discharge.

Take Note!

Nurses need a firm grasp of normal findings to be able to recognize abnormal findings and intervene appropriately.

This postpartum assessment includes vital signs and physical and psychosocial assessments. It also includes assessing the parents and other family members, such as siblings and grandparents, for attachment and bonding with the newborn. Although the exact protocol may vary among facilities, postpartum assessment typically is performed as follows:

- During the first hour: every 15 minutes
- During the second hour: every 30 minutes
- During the first 24 hours: every 4 hours
- After 24 hours: every 8 hours (Jordan et al., 2014; Mattson & Smith, 2016).

During each assessment, keep in mind risk factors that may lead to complications, such as infection or hemorrhage, during the recovery period (Box 16.1). Early identification is critical to ensure prompt intervention.

The postpartum period is a time of transition for women. The end of the pregnancy and childbirth initiates physiologic changes as many body systems return to their nonpregnant state. Nurses need to be aware of the normal physiologic and psychological changes that take place in clients' bodies and minds in order to provide comprehensive care during the postpartum period. In addition to client and family teaching, one of the most significant responsibilities of the postpartum nurse is to recognize potential complications after childbirth.

As with any assessment, always review the woman's medical record for information about her pregnancy, labor, and birth. Note any pre-existing conditions, any complications that occurred during pregnancy, labor, birth, and immediately afterward, and any treatments provided.

Postpartum assessment of the mother typically includes vital signs, pain level, epidural site inspection for infection, and a systematic head-to-toe review of body systems. The acronym **BUBBLE-EE** – **b**reasts, **u**terus, **bl**adder, **b**owels, **l**ochia, **e**pisiotomy/perineum/epidural site, **e**xtremities, and **e**motional status – can be used as a guide for this head-to-toe review (Cunningham et al., 2014).

BOX 16.1

FACTORS INCREASING A WOMAN'S RISK FOR POSTPARTUM COMPLICATIONS

Risk Factors for Postpartum Infection

- Operative procedure (forceps, cesarean birth, vacuum extraction)
- History of diabetes, including gestational-onset diabetes
- Prolonged labor (more than 24 hours)
- Use of indwelling urinary catheter
- Anemia (hemoglobin < 10.5 mg/dL)
- Multiple vaginal examinations during labor
- Prolonged rupture of membranes (>24 hours)
- Manual extraction of placenta
- Compromised immune system (HIV positive)

Risk Factors for Postpartum Hemorrhage

- Precipitous labor (less than 3 hours)
- Uterine atony
- Placenta previa or abruptio placenta
- Labor induction or augmentation
- Operative procedures (vacuum extraction, forceps, cesarean birth)
- Retained placental fragments
- Prolonged third stage of labor (more than 30 minutes)
- Multiparity, more than three births closely spaced
- Uterine overdistention (large infant, twins, hydramnios)

While assessing the woman and her family during the postpartum period, be alert for danger signs (Box 16.2). Notify the primary health care provider immediately if any are noted.

Vital Signs Assessment

Obtain vital signs and compare them with the previous values, noting and reporting any deviations. Vital sign changes can be an early indicator of complications.

BOX 16.2

POSTPARTUM DANGER SIGNS

- Fever more than 100.4°F (38°C)
- Foul-smelling lochia or an unexpected change in color or amount
- Large blood clots, or bleeding that saturates a peripad in an hour
- Severe headaches or blurred vision
- Visual changes, such as blurred vision or spots, or headaches
- Calf pain with dorsiflexion of the foot
- Swelling, redness, or discharge at the episiotomy, epidural, or abdominal sites
- Dysuria, burning, or incomplete emptying of the bladder
- Shortness of breath or difficulty breathing without exertion
- Depression or extreme mood swings

Temperature

Use a consistent measurement technique (oral, axillary, or tympanic) to get the most accurate readings. Typically, the new mother's temperature during the first 24 hours postpartum is within the normal range or a low-grade elevation. Some women experience a slight fever, up to 100.4°F (38°C), during the first 24 hours. This elevation may be the result of dehydration because of fluid loss during labor. Temperature should be normal after 24 hours with replacement of fluids lost during labor and birth (Green, 2016).

A temperature above 100.4°F (38°C) at any time or an abnormal temperature after the first 24 hours may indicate infection and must be reported. Abnormal temperature readings warrant continued monitoring until an infection can be ruled out through cultures or blood studies. An elevated temperature can identify maternal sepsis, which results in significant maternal morbidity and mortality worldwide. To improve the outcome, it is essential that nurses be vigilant in obtaining accurate values and monitoring their client's temperature.

Pulse

Pulse rates of 60 to 80 beats per minute (bpm) at rest are normal during the first week after birth. This pulse rate is called puerperal bradycardia. During pregnancy, the heavy gravid uterus causes a decreased flow of venous blood to the heart. After giving birth, there is an increase in intravascular volume. The cardiac output is most likely caused by an increased stroke volume from the venous return now. The elevated stroke volume leads to a decreased heart rate (Creasy et al., 2014). Tachycardia in the postpartum woman can suggest anxiety, excitement, fatigue, pain, excessive blood loss or delayed hemorrhage, infection, or underlying cardiac problems. Any pulse rate higher than 100 bpm warrants further investigation to rule out complications.

Respirations

Respiratory rates in the postpartum woman should be within the normal range of 12 to 20 bpm at rest. Pulmonary function typically returns to the prepregnant state after childbirth when the diaphragm descends and the organs revert to their normal positions. Any change in respiratory rate out of the normal range might indicate pulmonary edema, atelectasis, a side effect of epidural anesthesia, or pulmonary embolism and must be reported. Lungs should be clear on auscultation.

Blood Pressure

Assess the woman's blood pressure and compare it with her usual range. Report any deviation from this range. Immediately after childbirth, the blood pressure should remain the same as during labor. An increase in blood pressure could indicate gestational hypertension, whereas a decrease could indicate shock or orthostatic hypotension or dehydration, a side effect of epidural anesthesia. Blood pressure readings should not be higher than 140/90 mm Hg or lower than 85/60 mmHg (King et al., 2015). Blood pressure also may vary based on the woman's position, so assess blood pressure with the woman in the same position every time. Be alert for orthostatic hypotension, which can occur when the woman moves rapidly from a lying or sitting position to a standing one.

Pain

Pain, the fifth vital sign, is assessed along with the other four parameters. Question the woman about the type of pain and its location and severity. Have the woman rate the pain using a numeric scale from 0 to 10 points. Nursing care should focus on providing comfort measures to ease pain which might include perineal care, clean gown, mouth care, providing warm blankets, ensuring adequate fluid intake to facilitate healing, reposition frequently, and encouraging rest between assessments (Nagtalon-Ramos, 2014).

Many postpartum orders will have the nurse premedicate the woman routinely for afterbirth pains rather than wait for her to experience them first. The goal of pain management is to have the woman's pain scale rating maintained between 0 and 2 points at all times, especially after breast-feeding. This can be accomplished by assessing the woman's pain level frequently and preventing pain by administering analgesics. If the woman has severe pain in the perineal region despite use of physical comfort measures, check for a hematoma by inspecting and palpating the area. If one is found, notify the health care provider immediately.

Physical Examination

Physical examination of the postpartum woman focuses on assessing the breasts, uterus, bladder, bowels, lochia, episiotomy/perineum and epidural site and extremities.

Breasts

Inspect the breasts for size, contour, asymmetry, engorgement, or erythema. Check the nipples for cracks, redness, fissures, or bleeding, and note whether they are erect, flat, or inverted. Flat or inverted nipples can make breast-feeding challenging for both mother and infant. Cracked, blistered, fissured, bruised, or bleeding nipples in the breast-feeding woman are generally indications that the baby is improperly positioned on the breast. Palpate the breasts lightly to ascertain if they are soft, filling, or engorged, and document your findings. For women who are not breast-feeding, use a gentle, light touch to avoid breast stimulation, which would exacerbate engorgement.

Lactogenesis (the onset of milk secretion) is initially triggered by the delivery of the placenta, which results in falling levels of estrogen and progesterone, with the continued presence of prolactin. If the mother is not breast-feeding, the prolactin levels fall and return to normal levels within 2 to 3 weeks. As milk is starting to come in, the breasts become firmer; this is charted as "filling." Engorged breasts are hard, tender, and taut. Ask the woman if she is having any nipple discomfort. Palpate the breasts for any nodules, masses, or areas of warmth, which may indicate a plugged duct that may progress to mastitis if not treated promptly. Any discharge from the nipple should be described and documented if it is not colostrum (creamy yellow) or foremilk (bluish white). Over the first week, the breast milk matures and contains all necessary nutrients in the neonatal period. The breast milk continues to change throughout the period of breast-feeding to meet the changing demands of the growing infant.

Uterus

Assess the fundus (top portion of the uterus) to determine the degree of uterine involution. If possible, have the woman empty her bladder before assessing the fundus and auscultate her bowel sounds prior to uterine palpation. If the client has had a cesarean birth and has a patient-controlled anesthesia (PCA) pump, instruct her to self-medicate prior to fundal assessment to decrease her discomfort.

Using a two-handed approach with the woman in the supine position with her knees flexed slightly and the bed in a flat position or as low as possible, palpate the abdomen gently, feeling for the top of the uterus while the other hand is placed on the lower segment of the uterus to stabilize it (Fig. 16.2).

The fundus should be midline and should feel firm. A boggy or relaxed uterus is a sign of uterine atony (loss of muscle tone in the uterus). This can be the result of bladder distention, which displaces the uterus upward and to the right, or retained placental fragments. Either situation predisposes the woman to hemorrhage.

Once the fundus is located, place your index finger on the fundus and count the number of fingerbreadths between the fundus and the umbilicus (1 fingerbreadth is approximately equal to 1 cm). One to 2 hours after birth, the fundus typically is between the umbilicus and the symphysis pubis. Approximately 6 to 12 hours after birth, the fundus usually is at the level of the umbilicus. If the fundal height is above the umbilicus, which would be an abnormal finding, investigate this immediately to prevent excessive bleeding. Frequently the woman's bladder is full, thus displacing the uterus up and to either

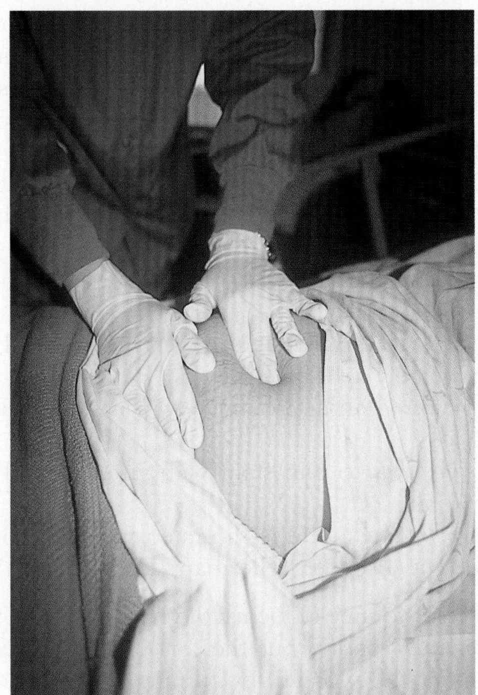

FIGURE 16.2 Palpating the fundus.

side of the midline. Ask the woman to empty her bladder and reassess the uterus again.

Normally, the fundus progresses downward at a rate of 1 fingerbreadth (or 1 cm) per day after childbirth and should be nonpalpable by 10 to 14 days postpartum. By day 14, the uterus has descended below the rim of the symphysis pubis and is no longer palpable (Cunningham et al., 2014). On the first postpartum day, the top of the fundus is located 1 cm below the umbilicus and is recorded as u/1. Similarly, on the second postpartum day, the fundus would be 2 cm below the umbilicus and should be recorded as u/2, and so on. Health care agencies differ according to how fundal heights are charted, so follow their protocols for this. If the fundus is not firm, gently massage the uterus using a circular motion until it becomes firm.

Bladder

Considerable diuresis – as much as 3,000 mL/day – begins within 12 hours after childbirth and continues for several days. A single voiding may be 500 mL or more. By 21 days postpartum, the diuresis is usually complete (Jordan et al., 2014). However, many postpartum women do not sense the need to void even if their bladder is full. In this situation the bladder can become distended and displace the uterus upward and to the side, which prevents the uterine muscles from contracting properly and can lead to excessive bleeding. Urinary retention as a result of decreased bladder tone and emptying can lead to urinary tract infections. It is imperative that nurses monitor clients for signs of urinary tract infections, including fever, urinary frequency and/or urgency, difficult or painful urination, and tenderness over the costovertebral angle (Wilson et al., 2015). Women who received regional anesthesia during labor are at risk for urinary tract infections due to continuous urinary catheterization to prevent urinary retention during labor, which is thought to delay fetal descent. They also experience difficulty voiding and loss of sensation and must wait until it returns to feel a full bladder which might be several hours after childbirth.

Assess for voiding problems by asking the woman the following questions:

- Have you (voided, urinated, gone to the bathroom) yet?
- Have you noticed any burning or discomfort with urination?
- Do you have any difficulty passing your urine?
- Do you feel that your bladder is empty when you finish urinating?
- Do you have any signs of infection such as urgency, frequency, or pain?
- Are you able to control the flow of urine by squeezing your muscles?
- Have you noticed any leakage of urine when you cough, laugh, or sneeze?

Assess the bladder for distention and adequate emptying after efforts to void. Palpate the area over the symphysis pubis. If empty, the bladder is not palpable. Palpation of a rounded mass suggests bladder distention. Also percuss the area: a full bladder is dull to percussion. If the bladder is full, lochia drainage will be more than normal because the uterus cannot contract to suppress the bleeding.

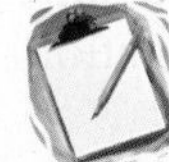

Take Note!

Note the location and condition of the fundus; a full bladder tends to displace the uterus up and to the right.

After the woman voids, palpate and percuss the area again to determine adequate emptying of the bladder. If the bladder remains distended, the woman may be retaining urine in her bladder, and measures to initiate voiding should be instituted. Be alert for signs of infection, including infrequent or insufficient voiding (less than 200 mL), discomfort, burning, urgency, or foul-smelling urine (Mattson & Smith, 2016). Document all urine output.

Bowels

Spontaneous bowel movements may not occur for 1 to 3 days after giving birth because of a decrease in muscle tone in the intestines as a result of elevated progesterone levels. Normal patterns of bowel elimination usually return within a week after birth (Verghese, Futaba, & Latthe, 2015). Often women are hesitant to have a bowel movement due to pain in the perineal area resulting from an episiotomy, lacerations, or hemorrhoids. Some are fearful that they may "rip their stitches" should they strain. Nurses should reassure their clients that stool softeners and/or laxatives to treat constipation have been prescribed for them to reduce discomfort.

Inspect the woman's abdomen for distention, auscultate for bowel sounds in all four quadrants prior to palpating the uterine fundus, and palpate for tenderness. The abdomen typically is soft, nontender, and nondistended. Bowel sounds are present in all four quadrants. Ask the woman if she has had a bowel movement or has passed gas since giving birth, because constipation is a common problem during the postpartum period and many women do not offer this information unless asked about it. Normal assessment findings are active bowel sounds, passing gas, and a nondistended abdomen.

Lochia

Assess lochia in terms of amount, color, odor, and change with activity and time. To assess how much a woman is bleeding, ask her how many perineal pads she has used in the past 1 to 2 hours and how much drainage was on each pad. For example, did she saturate the pad completely, or was only half of the pad covered with drainage? Ask about the color of the drainage, odor, and the presence of any clots. Lochia has a definite musky scent, with an odor similar to that of menstrual flow without any large clots (fist size). Foul-smelling lochia suggests an infection, and large clots suggest poor uterine involution, necessitating additional intervention.

To determine the amount of lochia, observe the amount of lochia saturation on the perineal pad and relate it to time (Fig. 16.3). Also, take into consideration the specific type of peripad used, because some are more absorbent than others. Lochia flow will increase when the woman gets out of bed (lochia pools in the vagina and the uterus while she is lying down) and when she breast-feeds (oxytocin release causes uterine contractions). A woman who saturates a perineal pad within 30 to 60 minutes is bleeding much more than one who saturates a pad in 2 hours.

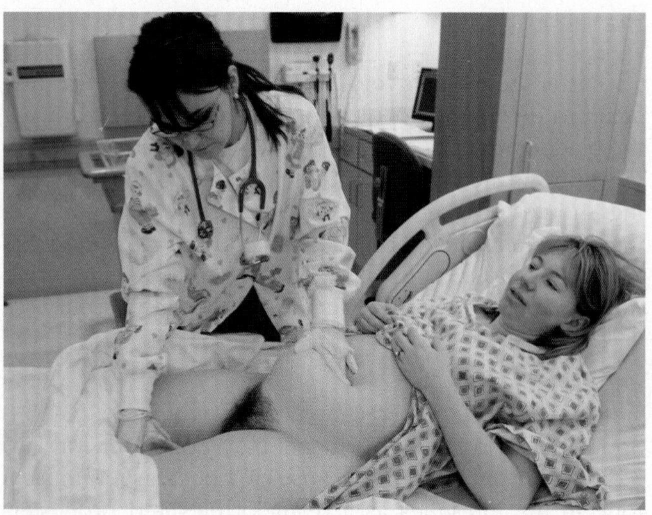

FIGURE 16.3 Assessing lochia.

Typically, the amount of lochia is described as follows:

- *Scant:* a 1- to 2-in lochia stain on the perineal pad or approximately a 10-mL loss
- *Light or small:* an approximately 4-in stain or a 10- to 25-mL loss
- *Moderate:* a 4- to 6-in stain with an estimated loss of 25 to 50 mL
- *Large or heavy:* a pad is saturated within 1 hour after changing it (Bope & Kellerman, 2015).

The total volume of lochial discharge varies in women based on their parity, but the amount decreases daily. Check under the woman, by turning her over to either side, to make sure additional blood is not hidden and not being absorbed on her perineal pad. This also a good time to assess for the presence and condition of hemorrhoids since the nurse is visually inspecting the perineum.

Report any abnormal findings, such as heavy, bright-red lochia with large tissue fragments or a foul odor. If excessive bleeding occurs, the first step would be to massage the boggy fundus until it is firm to reduce the flow of blood. Document all findings.

Women who had a cesarean birth will have less lochia discharge than those who had a vaginal birth, but stages and color changes remain the same. Although the woman's abdomen will be tender after surgery, the nurse must palpate the fundus and assess the lochia to make sure they are within the normal range and that there is no excessive bleeding.

Anticipatory guidance to give the woman at discharge should include information about lochia and the expected changes. Urge the woman to notify her health care provider if lochia rubra returns after the serosa and alba transitions have taken place. This is abnormal and may indicate subinvolution or that the woman is too active and needs to rest more. Lochia is an excellent medium for bacterial growth. Explain to the woman that frequent changing of perineal pads, continued use of her **peribottle** for rinsing her perineal area, and hand hygiene before and after pad changes are important infection control measures.

Episiotomy/Perineum and Epidural Site

If the woman has an episiotomy, which is not routinely done currently, to assess the episiotomy and perineal area, position the woman on her side with her top leg

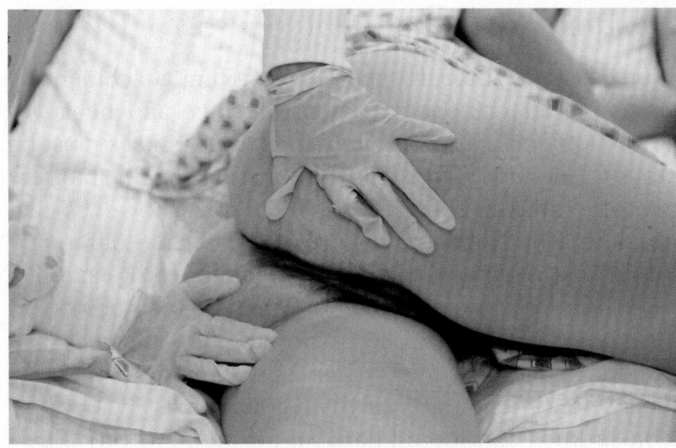

FIGURE 16.4 Inspecting the perineum.

flexed upward at the knee and drawn up toward her waist. If necessary, use a penlight to provide adequate lighting during the assessment. Wearing gloves and standing at the woman's side with her back to you, gently lift the upper buttock to expose the perineum and anus (Fig. 16.4). Inspect the episiotomy for irritation, ecchymosis, tenderness, or hematomas. Assess for hemorrhoids and their condition.

During the early postpartum period, the perineal tissue surrounding the episiotomy is typically edematous and slightly bruised. The normal episiotomy site should not have redness, discharge, or edema. The majority of healing takes place within the first 2 weeks, but it may take 4 to 6 months for the episiotomy to heal completely (King et al., 2015).

Lacerations to the perineal area sustained during the birthing process that were identified and repaired also need to be assessed to determine their healing status. Lacerations are classified based on their severity and tissue involvement:

- *First-degree laceration:* involves only skin and superficial structures above muscle
- *Second-degree laceration:* extends through perineal muscles
- *Third-degree laceration:* extends through the anal sphincter muscle
- *Fourth-degree laceration:* continues through anterior rectal wall

Assess the episiotomy and any lacerations at least every 8 hours to detect hematomas or signs of infection. Large areas of swollen, bluish skin with complaints of severe pain in the perineal area indicate pelvic or vulvar hematomas. Redness, swelling, increasing discomfort, or purulent drainage may indicate infection. Both findings need to be reported immediately.

A white line running the length of the episiotomy is a sign of infection, as well as swelling or discharge. Severe, intractable pain, perineal discoloration, and ecchymosis indicate a perineal hematoma, a potentially dangerous condition. Report any unusual findings. Ice can be applied to relieve discomfort and reduce edema; **sitz bath**s also can promote comfort and perineal healing (see "Promoting Comfort" in the Nursing Interventions section).

If the woman has had an epidural during her labor, assessment of the epidural wound site is important as well as checking for any side effects of the medication injected such as itching, nausea and vomiting, or urinary retention. Visual inspection of the epidural site and an accurate documentation of intake and output are essential.

Extremities

Pregnancy is associated with an increased risk of venous thromboembolism (VTE), which includes pulmonary embolism and deep vein thrombosis. During pregnancy, the state of hypercoagulability protects the mother against excessive blood loss during childbirth and placental separation. However, this hypercoagulable state can increase the risk of thromboembolic disorders during pregnancy and postpartum. Three factors predispose women to thromboembolic disorders during pregnancy: stasis (compression of the large veins because of the gravid uterus), altered coagulation (state of pregnancy), and localized vascular damage (may occur during the birthing process). All of these factors increase the risk of clot formation and having it travel to the lungs.

While inspecting the woman's extremities, also determine the degree of sensory and motor function return (recovery from anesthesia) by asking the woman if she feels sensation at various areas the nurse touches and also by observing her ambulation stability.

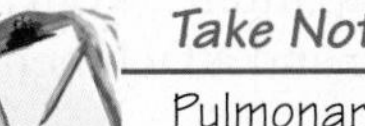

Take Note!

Pulmonary embolism occurs in up to 3 per 1,000 births and is a major cause of maternal mortality (Kim et al., 2015).

Pulmonary emboli typically result from dislodged deep vein thrombi in the lower extremities. Risk factors associated with thromboembolic conditions include:

- Anemia
- Diabetes mellitus
- Cigarette smoking
- Obesity
- Preeclampsia
- Hypertension
- Severe varicose veins
- Pregnancy
- Multiple pregnancies
- Cardiovascular disease
- Sickle cell disease
- Postpartum hemorrhage
- Oral contraceptive use

- Cesarean birth
- Severe infection
- Previous thromboembolic disease
- Multiparity
- Bed rest or immobility for 4 days or more
- Advanced maternal age > 35 years (Kline & Kabrhel, 2015).

Because of the subtle presentation of thromboembolic disorders, the physical examination may not be enough to detect them. An accurate diagnosis of pulmonary embolism is needed because it requires (1) prolonged therapy (≤9 months of heparin during pregnancy), (2) prophylaxis during future pregnancies, and (3) avoidance of oral contraceptive pills. The woman may report lower extremity tightness or aching when ambulating that is relieved with rest and elevation of the leg. Edema in the affected leg (typically the left), along with warmth and tenderness, and a low-grade fever may also be noted. A duplex ultrasound (two-dimensional ultrasound and Doppler ultrasound that compresses the vein to assess for changes in venous flow) in conjunction with the physical findings frequently is needed for a conclusive diagnosis (Sucker & Zotz, 2015).

Women with an increased risk for this condition during the postpartum period should wear antiembolism stockings or use sequential compression devices to reduce the risk of venous stasis by preventing blood from pooling in the calves of the legs. Encouraging the client to ambulate after childbirth reduces the incidence of thrombophlebitis.

Psychosocial Assessment

Psychosocial assessment of the postpartum woman focuses on emotional status and bonding and attachment.

Emotional Status

Assess the woman's emotional status by observing how she interacts with her family, her level of independence, energy levels, eye contact with her infant (within a cultural context), posture and comfort level while holding the newborn, and sleep and rest patterns. Be alert for mood swings, irritability, or crying episodes.

Remember Raina and her "quiet" husband, the Muslim couple? The postpartum nurse informs Raina that her doctor, Nancy Schultz, has been called away for emergency surgery and won't be available the rest of the day. The nurse explains that Dr. Robert Nappo will be making rounds for her. Raina and her husband become upset. Why? Is culturally competent care being provided to this couple?

Bonding and Attachment

Nurses can be instrumental in promoting attachment by assessing attachment behaviors (positive and negative) and intervening appropriately if needed. Nurses must be able to identify any family discord that might interfere with the attachment process. Remember, however, that mothers from different cultures may behave differently from what is expected in your own culture. For example, Native American mothers tend to handle their newborns less often and use cradle boards to carry them. Native American mothers and many Asian American mothers delay breast-feeding until their milk comes in, because colostrum is considered harmful for the newborn (Bowers & Ceballos, 2015) Do not assume that different behavior is wrong.

Meeting the newborn for the first time after birth can be an exhilarating experience for parents. Although the mother has spent many hours dreaming of her unborn and how he or she will look, it is not until after birth that they meet face to face. They both need to get to know one another and to develop feelings for one another.

Bonding is the close emotional attraction to a newborn by the parents that develops during the first 30 to 60 minutes after birth. It is unidirectional, from parent to infant. It is thought that optimal bonding of the parents to a newborn requires a period of close contact within the first few minutes to a few hours after birth. Bonding is really a continuation of the relationship that began during pregnancy (Sears & Sears, 2015a). It is affected by a multitude of factors, including the parent's socioeconomic status, family history, role models, support systems, cultural factors, and birth experiences. The mother initiates bonding when she caresses her infant and exhibits certain behaviors typical of a mother tending her child. The infant's responses to this, such as body and eye movements, are a necessary part of the process. During this initial period, the infant is in a quiet, alert state, looking directly at the holder.

Take Note!

The length of time necessary for bonding depends on the health of the infant and mother, as well as the circumstances surrounding the labor and birth (Tester-Jones et al., 2015).

Attachment is the development of strong affection between an infant and a significant other (mother, father, sibling, and caretaker). This attachment is reciprocal; both the significant other and the newborn exhibit attachment behaviors. The attachment relationship formed between the infant and primary caregiver influences the child's view of the world and future relationships (Sette, Coppola, & Cassibba, 2015). This tie between two people is psychological rather than biologic, and it does not occur overnight. The process of attachment follows a progressive or developmental course that changes over time. Attachment is an individualized and multifactorial process that differs based on the health of the infant, the mother, environmental circumstances, and the quality of care the infant receives. The newborn responds to the significant other by cooing, grasping, smiling, and crying. Nurses can assess for attachment behaviors by observing the interaction between the newborn and the person holding him or her (Mattson & Smith, 2016). It occurs through mutually satisfying experiences. Maternal attachment begins during pregnancy as the result of fetal movement and maternal fantasies about the infant and continues through the birth and postpartum periods. Attachment behaviors include seeking, physical caretaking behaviors, emotional attentiveness to infant's needs, staying close to, touching, kissing, cuddling, choosing the ***en face*** (face-to-face) **position** while holding or feeding the newborn, expressing pride in the newborn and exchanging gratifying experiences with the infant (McComish, 2015). In a high-risk pregnancy, the attachment process may be complicated by premature birth (lack of time to develop a relationship with the unborn baby) and by parental stress due to the fetal and/or maternal vulnerability.

Bonding is a vital component of the attachment process and is necessary in establishing parent–infant attachment and a healthy, loving relationship. During this early period of acquaintance, mothers touch their infants in a very characteristic manner. Mothers visually and physically "explore" their infants, initially using their fingertips on the infant's face and extremities and progressing to massaging and stroking the infant with their fingers. This is followed by palm contact on the trunk. Eventually, mothers draw their infant toward them and hold the infant (Fig. 16.5).

Generally, research on attachment has found that the process is similar for partners as for mothers, but the pace may be different. Like mothers, partners manifest attachment behaviors during pregnancy. Indeed, Baltes, Featherman, & Lerner (2014) found that the best predictors of early postnatal attachment for fathers or significant others were those who viewed the paternal caregiving role as important and also had greater marital quality. Higher levels of paternal sensitivity were associated with better infant–father attachment. Becoming a father or significant partner requires the person to build on the experiences he/she has had throughout childhood and adolescence. Fathers or significant other partners develop an emotional tie with their infants in a variety of ways. They seek and maintain closeness with the infant and can recognize characteristics of the infant. Another study further described paternal attachment as a permanent, cyclical concept characterized by changes in response to the child's developmental stage. When children have a secure, supportive, and sensitive relationship with their fathers or mother's significant other, they are generally better adjusted than those that have a nonsupportive relationship (Lickenbrock & Braungart-Rieker, 2015).

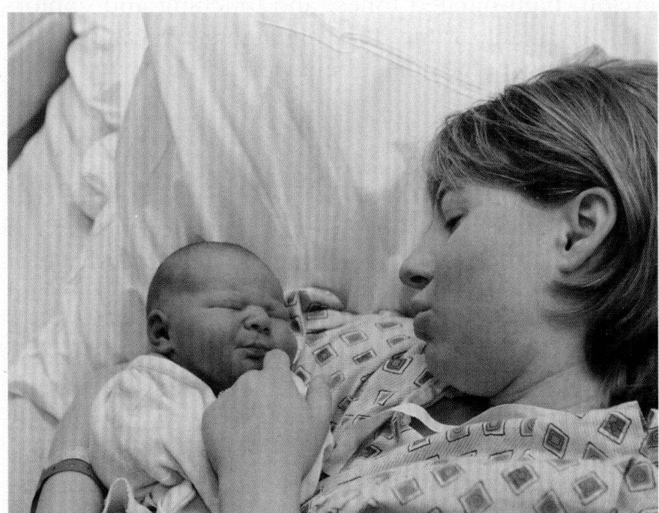

FIGURE 16.5 *En face* position.

Attachment is a process; it does not occur instantaneously, even though many parents believe in a romanticized version of attachment, which happens right after birth. A delay in the attachment process can occur if a mother's physical and emotional states are adversely affected by exhaustion, pain, and the absence of a support system; if she has an infant in NICU and is separated from it; or had a traumatic birth experience, anesthesia, or an unwanted outcome, such as an ill infant (Lee et al., 2014).

Take Note!

Touch is a basic instinctual interaction between a parent and his or her infant and has a vital role in the infant's early development. Parents provide a variety of tactile stimulation while addressing their infant's daily care routines (Hugill, 2015).

The developmental task for the infant is learning to differentiate between trust and mistrust. If the mother or caretaker is consistently responsive to the infant's care, meeting the baby's physical and psychological needs, the infant will likely learn to trust the caretaker, view the world as a safe place, and grow up to be secure, self-reliant, trusting, cooperative, and helpful. However, if the infant's needs are not met, the child is more likely to face developmental delays, neglect, and child abuse (Klebanov & Travis, 2015).

"Becoming" a parent may take 4 to 6 months. The transition to parenthood, according to Mercer (2006), involves four stages:

1. Commitment, attachment, and preparation for an infant during pregnancy
2. Acquaintance with and increasing attachment to the infant, learning how to care for the infant, and physical restoration during the first weeks after birth

3. Moving toward a new normal routine in the first 4 months after birth
4. Achievement of a parenthood role around 4 months

The stages overlap, and the timing of each is affected by variables such as the environment, family dynamics, and the partners (Mercer, 2006).

FACTORS AFFECTING ATTACHMENT

Attachment behaviors are influenced by three major factors:

1. Parents' background (includes the care that the parents received when growing up, cultural practices, relationship within the family, experience with previous pregnancies and planning and course of events during pregnancy, postpartum depression)
2. Infant (includes the infant's temperament and health at birth)
3. Care practices (the behaviors of physicians, nurse practitioners, midwives, nurses, and hospital personnel, care and support during labor, first day of life in separation of mother and infant, and rules of the hospital or birthing center) (Lewis & Rudolph, 2014).

Attachment occurs more readily with the infant whose temperament, health, appearance, and gender fit the parent's expectations. If the infant does not meet these expectations, attachment can be delayed (Lickenbrock & Braungart-Rieker, 2015).

Factors associated with the health care facility or birthing unit can also hinder attachment. These include:

- Separation of infant and parents immediately after birth and for long periods during the day
- Policies that discourage unwrapping and exploring the infant
- Intensive care environment, restrictive visiting policies
- Staff indifference or lack of support for parent's caretaking attempts and abilities

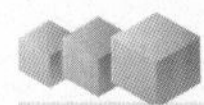

Concept Mastery Alert

Grief After Delivery of a Child with Special Needs

It is important for the mother to visit the child in the special care nursery, but the priority is to assist the mother in dealing with the grief that accompanies giving birth to a child with special needs. The mother must first mourn the loss of the "perfect child."

CRITICAL ATTRIBUTES OF ATTACHMENT

The terms *bonding* and *attachment* are often used interchangeably, even though they involve different time frames and interactions. Attachment stages include proximity, reciprocity, and commitment.

Proximity refers to the physical and psychological experience of the parents being close to their infant. This attribute has three dimensions:

1. *Contact:* The sensory experiences of touching, holding, and gazing at the infant are part of proximity-seeking behavior.
2. *Emotional state:* The emotional state emerges from the affective experience of the new parents toward their infant and their parental role.
3. *Individualization:* Parents are aware of the need to differentiate the infant's needs from themselves and to recognize and respond to them appropriately, making the attachment process also, in some way, one of detachment.

Reciprocity is the process by which the infant's abilities and behaviors elicit parental response. Reciprocity is described by two dimensions: complementary behavior and sensitivity. Complementary behavior involves taking turns and stopping when the other is not interested or becomes tired. An infant can coo and stare at the parent to elicit a similar parental response to complement his or her behavior. Parents who are sensitive and responsive to their infant's cues will promote their development and growth. Parents who become skilled at recognizing the ways their infant communicates will respond appropriately by smiling, vocalizing, touching, and kissing.

Commitment refers to the enduring nature of the relationship. The components of this are twofold: centrality and parent role exploration. In centrality, parents place the infant at the center of their lives. They acknowledge and accept their responsibility to promote the infant's safety, growth, and development. Parent role exploration is the parents' ability to find their own way and integrate the parental identity into themselves (Sears & Sears, 2015b).

POSITIVE AND NEGATIVE ATTACHMENT BEHAVIORS

Positive bonding behaviors include maintaining close physical contact, making eye-to-eye contact, speaking in soft, high-pitched tones, and touching and exploring the infant. Table 16.1 highlights typical positive and negative attachment behaviors.

NURSING INTERVENTIONS

In terms of postpartum hospital stays today, "less is more." If the woman had a vaginal delivery, she may be discharged within 48 hours or sooner. If she had a cesarean birth, she may remain hospitalized for up to 72 hours. This shortened stay leaves little time for nurses to prepare the woman and her family for the many changes that will occur when she returns home. Research shows that mothers feel unprepared, uninformed, and unsupported during the postpartum period as they struggle with physical and emotional issues, infant caregiving, breast-feeding concerns, and lifestyle

TABLE 16.1 POSITIVE AND NEGATIVE ATTACHMENT BEHAVIORS

	Positive Behaviors	Negative Behaviors
Infant	Smiles; is alert; demonstrates strong grasp reflex to hold parent's finger; sucks well, feeds easily; enjoys being held close; makes eye-to-eye contact; follows parent's face; appears facially appealing; is consolable when crying	Feeds poorly, regurgitates often; cries for long periods, colicky and inconsolable; shows flat affect, rarely smiles even when prompted; resists holding and closeness; sleeps with eyes closed most of time; stiffens body when held; is unresponsive to parents; doesn't pay attention to parents' faces
Parent	Makes direct eye contact; assumes *en face* position when holding infant; claims infant as family member, pointing out common features; expresses pride in infant; assigns meaning to infant's actions; smiles and gazes at infant; touches infant, progressing from fingertips to holding; names infant; requests to be close to infant as much as allowed; speaks positively about infant	Expresses disappointment or displeasure in infant; fails to "explore" infant visually or physically; fails to claim infant as part of family; avoids caring for infant; finds excuses not to hold infant close; has negative self-concept; appears uninterested in having infant in room; frequently asks to have infant taken back to nursery to be cared for; assigns negative attributes to infant and calls infant inappropriate, negative names (e.g., frog, monkey, tadpole)

Adapted from Bope, E., & Kellerman, R. (2015). *Conn's current therapy 2015*. Philadelphia, PA: Saunders Elsevier; Park, S., Kim, S., & Kang, K. (2014). Integrative review of nursing intervention studies on mother-infant interactions. *Child Health Nursing Research*, 20(2), 75–86; and Barnes, D. L. (2014). *Women's reproductive mental health across the lifespan*. New York, NY: Springer Publishers.

adjustments (Walker, Murphey, & Nichols, 2015). Nurses need to focus on pain and discomfort, immunizations, nutrition, activity and exercise, infant care, lactation instruction, discharge teaching, sexuality and contraception, and follow-up with the limited time they have with their clients (see Nursing Care Plan 16.1, at the end of the chapter). Planning home visits to reinforce postpartum instructions may enhance maternal-infant wellness. (See Evidence-Based Practice 16.1.)

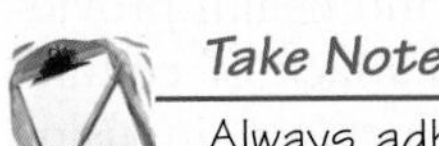

Always adhere to standard precautions when providing direct care to reduce the risk of disease transmission.

EVIDENCE-BASED PRACTICE 16.1 ENHANCING NEONATAL WELLNESS WITH HOME VISITATION

STUDY

According to the AAP, there is sufficient evidence that breast-feeding provides the best nutrition for newborns and should be continued for the first 6 months followed by continued breast-feeding during the first year or more, as solid foods are introduced. The purpose of this study was to measure the effectiveness of home visits by RNs on neonatal wellness as measured by the continuance of breast-feeding at 6 months, reduce readmissions for newborn jaundice and identify any maternal or newborn health issues. The home visits were made on days three and seven after discharge from the hospital. A complete physical assessment on both mother and infant was performed at each home visit.

Findings

The study used a longitudinal, mixed method, within-subject design involving 1,705 participants. Quantitative data were compared to regional and national benchmarks. Qualitative data from study participant interviews were analyzed to identify common themes. The data indicated the home visits did help mothers to continue to breast-feed longer when compared to the regional and national statistics and the home visits also effectively identified newborn jaundice with a reduction in the average length of stay for infants readmitted in comparison to benchmarks.

Nursing Implications

The study's results reinforce the need for extended breast-feeding support beyond the hospital setting discharge for new mothers to continue to breast-feed longer. New mothers need to have access to community-based interventions after discharge to reinforce their postpartum education. Nurses can be instrumental in making referrals for home visitations to promote the safe transition from the hospital to the home.

Adapted from Parker, C., Warmuskerken, G., & Sinclair, L. (2015). Enhancing neonatal wellness with home visitation. *Nursing for Women's Health, 19*(1), 36–45.

Providing Optimal Cultural Care

As the face of America is becoming more diverse, nurses must be prepared to care for childbearing families from various cultures. In many cultures, women and their families are cared for and nurtured by their community for weeks and even months after the birth of a new family member. Overall, the culturally competent care for all childbearing families include understanding of traditional folk beliefs; involvement and support by family members; respect; presence of a significant other; breast-feeding and eating healthy; observing the principles of hot and cold; avoidance of sexual intercourse postnatally; encouragement; empowerment; their spiritual dimensions as important; avoidance of evil spirits; and the hope that nurses will anticipate the needs of the mother and infant (McFarland & Wehbe-Alamah, 2015). Box 16.3 highlights some of the major cultural variants during the postpartum period.

Nurses need to remember that childbearing practices and beliefs vary from culture to culture. To provide appropriate nursing care, the nurse should determine the client's preferences before intervening. Cultural practices may include dietary restrictions, certain clothes, taboos, activities for maintaining mental health, and the use of silence, prayer, or meditation. Restoring health may involve taking folk medicines or conferring with a tribal healer. A language barrier might interfere with communication between the woman and health providers, followed by health care provider's lack of cultural sensitivity, leading to a woman's reluctance in using health services (Santiago & Figueiredo, 2015). Providing culturally diverse care within our global community is challenging for all nurses, because they must remember that one's culture cannot be easily summarized in a reference book, but must be viewed through one's own life experiences.

The Muslim woman and her husband are upset at the thought of having a male doctor care for her because Muslim women are very modest and prefer having a same-sex care provider. What should the nurse do in this situation?

Promoting Comfort

The postpartum woman may have discomfort and pain from a variety of sources, such as an episiotomy, perineal lacerations, backache as a result of the epidural, pain from a full bladder, an edematous perineum, inflamed hemorrhoids, engorged breasts, afterbirth pains secondary to uterine contractions in breast-feeding and multiparous mothers, and sore nipples if breast-feeding. Relieving the underlying problem is the first step in pain management. Most practices traditionally employed for postpartum discomforts are not evidence based, so both nonpharmacologic and pharmacologic measures are often used in tandem (King et al., 2015).

Applications of Cold and Heat

COLD

Commonly, an ice pack is the first measure used after a vaginal birth to relieve perineal discomfort from edema, an episiotomy, or a laceration. An ice pack seems to minimize edema, reduce inflammation, decrease capillary permeability, and reduce nerve conduction to the site. It is applied during the fourth stage of labor and can be used for the first 24 hours to reduce perineal edema and to prevent hematoma formation, thus reducing pain and promoting healing. Ice packs are wrapped in a disposable covering or clean washcloth and are applied to the perineal area. Usually the ice pack is applied intermittently for 20 minutes and removed for 10 minutes. Many commercially prepared ice packs are available, but a surgical glove filled with crushed ice and covered can also be used if the mother is not allergic to latex. Ensure that the ice pack is changed frequently to promote good hygiene and to allow for periodic assessments.

HEAT

The **peribottle** is a plastic squeeze bottle filled with warm tap water that is sprayed over the perineal area after each voiding and before applying a new perineal pad. Usually the peribottle is introduced to the woman when she is assisted to the bathroom to freshen up and void for the first time—in most instances, once vital signs are stable after the first hour. Provide the woman with instructions on how and when to use the peribottle. Reinforce this practice each time she changes her pad, voids, or defecates, making sure that she understands to direct the flow of water from front to back. The woman can take the peribottle home and use it over the next several weeks until her lochia discharge stops. The peribottle can be used by women who had either vaginal or cesarean births to provide comfort and hygiene to the perineal area.

After the first 24 hours, a **sitz bath** with room temperature water may be prescribed and substituted for the ice pack to reduce local swelling and promote comfort for an episiotomy, perineal trauma, or inflamed hemorrhoids. The change from cold to room temperature therapy enhances vascular circulation and healing. When compared with an infrared light to promote healing and reduce perineal pain, sitz baths were significantly more effective in promoting episiotomy wound healing (Sukhwinder et al., 2014). Before using a sitz bath, the woman should cleanse the perineum with a peribottle or take a shower using mild soap.

Most health care agencies use plastic disposable sitz baths that women can take home. The plastic sitz bath consists of a basin that fits on the commode; a

BOX 16.3

CULTURAL INFLUENCES DURING THE POSTPARTUM PERIOD

African American

- Mother may share care of the infant with extended family members.
- Experiences of older women within the family influence infant care.
- Mothers may protect their newborns from strangers for several weeks.
- Mothers may not bathe their newborns for the first week. Oils are applied to skin and hair to prevent dryness and cradle cap.
- Silver dollars may be taped over the infant's umbilicus in an attempt to flatten the slightly protruding umbilical stump.
- Sleeping with parents is a common practice.

Amish

- Women consider childbearing their primary role in society.
- They generally oppose birth control.
- Pregnancy and childbirth are considered a private matter; they may conceal it from public knowledge.
- Women typically do not respond favorably when hurried to complete a self-care task. Nurses need to take cues from women indicating their readiness to complete morning self-care activities.

Appalachian

- Infant colic is treated by passing the newborn through a leather horse's collar or administering weak catnip tea.
- An *asafetida* bag (a gum resin with a strong odor) is tied around the infant's neck to ward off disease.
- Women may avoid eye contact with nurses and health care providers.
- Women typically avoid asking questions even though they do not understand directions.
- The grandmother may rear the infant for the mother.

Filipino American

- Grandparents often assist in the care of their grandchildren.
- Breast-feeding is encouraged, and some mothers breast-feed their children for up to 2 years.
- Women have difficulty discussing birth control and sexual matters.
- Strong religious beliefs prevail and bedside prayer is common.
- Families are very close-knit and numerous visitors can be expected at the hospital after childbirth.

Japanese American

- Cleanliness and protection from cold are essential components of newborn care. Nurses should bathe the infant daily.
- Newborns routinely are not taken outside the home because it is believed that they should not be exposed to outside or cold air. Infants should be kept in a quiet, clean, warm place for the first month of life.
- Breast-feeding is the primary method of feeding.
- Many women stay in their parents' home for 1 to 2 months after birth.
- Bathing the infant can be the center of family activity at home.

Mexican American

- The newborn's grandmother lives with the mother for several weeks after birth to help with housekeeping and child care.
- Most women will breast-feed for more than 1 year. The infant is carried in a *rebozo* (shawl) that allows easy access for breast-feeding.
- Women may avoid eye contact and may not feel comfortable being touched by a stranger. Nurses need to respect this feeling.
- Some women may bring religious icons to the hospital and may want to display them in their room.

Muslim

- Modesty is a primary concern; nurses need to protect the client's modesty.
- Muslims are not permitted to eat pork; check all food items before serving.
- Muslims prefer a same-sex health care provider; male–female touching is prohibited except in an emergency situation.
- A Muslim woman stays in the house for 40 days after birth, being cared for by the female members of her family.
- Most women will breast-feed, but religious events call for periods of fasting, which may increase the risk of dehydration or malnutrition.
- Women are exempt from obligatory five-times-daily prayers as long as lochia is present.
- Extended family is likely to be present throughout much of the woman's hospital stay. They will need an empty room to perform their prayers without having to leave the hospital.

Native American

- Women are secretive about pregnancies and do not reveal them early.
- Touching is not a typical female behavior and eye contact is brief.
- They resent being hurried and need time for sitting and talking.
- Most mothers breast-feed and practice birth control.

Adapted from Bowers, P., & Caballos, K. (2015). *Cultural perspectives in childbearing.* Retrieved from http://ce.nurse.com/ce263-60/Cultural-Perspectives-in-Childbearing;

Dayer-Berenson, L. (2014). *Cultural competencies of nurses: Impact on health and illness* (2nd ed.). Burlington, MA: Jones & Bartlett Learning; and Andrews, M. M., & Boyle, J. S. (2012). *Transcultural concepts in nursing care* (6th ed.). Philadelphia, PA: Wolters Kluwer Health.

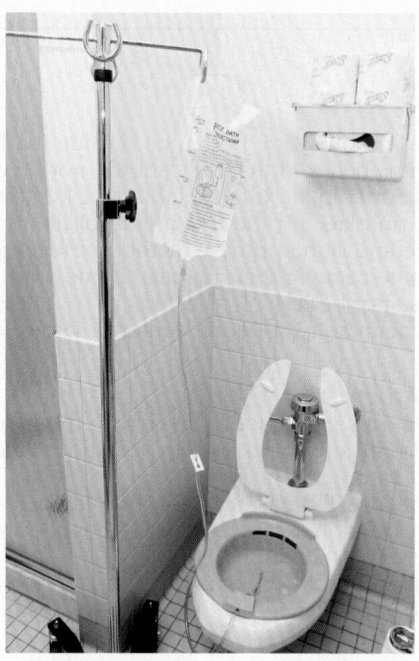

FIGURE 16.6 Sitz bath setup.

bag filled with warm water is hung on a hook and connected via a tube onto the front of the basin (Fig. 16.6). Teaching Guidelines 16.1 highlights the steps in using a sitz bath.

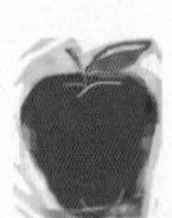

Teaching Guidelines 16.1
USING A SITZ BATH

1. Close clamp on tubing before filling bag with water to prevent leakage.
2. Fill sitz bath basin and plastic bag with room-temperature water (comfortable to touch).
3. Place the filled basin on the toilet with the seat raised and the overflow opening facing toward the back of the toilet.
4. Hang the filled plastic bag on a hook close to the toilet or an IV pole.
5. Attach the tubing to the opening on the basin.
6. Sit on the basin positioned on the toilet seat and release the clamp to allow warm water to irrigate the perineum.
7. Remain sitting on the basin for approximately 15 to 20 minutes.
8. Stand up and pat the perineum area dry. Apply a clean peripad.
9. Tip the basin to remove any remaining water and flush the toilet.
10. Wash the basin with warm water and soap and dry it in the sink.
11. Store basin and tubing in a clean, dry area until the next use.
12. Wash hands with soap and water.

Advise the woman to use the sitz bath several times daily to provide hygiene and comfort to the perineal area. Encourage her to continue this measure after discharge. Some facilities have hygienic sitz baths called Suri-Gators in the bathroom that spray an antiseptic, water, or both onto the perineum. The woman sits on the toilet with legs apart so that the nozzle spray reaches her perineal area.

Keep in mind that tremendous hemodynamic changes are taking place within the mother during this early postpartum period, and her safety must be a priority. Fatigue, blood loss, the effects of medications, and lack of food may cause her to feel weak when she stands up. Assisting the woman to the bathroom to instruct her on how to use the peribottle and sitz bath is necessary to ensure her safety. Many women become light-headed or dizzy when they get out of bed and need direct physical assistance. Staying in the woman's room, ensuring that the emergency call light is readily available, and being available if needed during this early period will ensure safety and prevent accidents and falls.

Recent reviews of the use of postpartum local cooling and warming interventions for perineal pain found limited evidence supporting their effectiveness. Additional studies are needed in the area of perineal pain and healing in order to develop evidence-based interventions in the future (Mooventhan & Nivethitha, 2014).

Topical Preparations

Several treatments may be applied topically for temporary relief of perineal pain and discomfort. One such treatment is a local anesthetic spray such as benzocaine topical. These agents numb the perineal area and are used after cleansing the area with water via the peribottle and/or a sitz bath.

Postpartum women are predisposed to hemorrhoid development due to pressure during vaginal birth, constipation, relaxation of the smooth muscles in vein walls, and impaired blood return, all related to increased pressure from the heavy gravid uterus. Nonpharmacologic measures to reduce hemorrhoid discomfort include ice packs, ice sitz baths, and application of cool witch hazel pads, such as Tucks®. The pads are placed at the rectal area, between the hemorrhoids and the perineal pad. These pads cool the area, help relieve swelling, and minimize itching. Pharmacologic methods used to reduce hemorrhoid pain include local anesthetics (dibucaine) or steroids (hydrocortisone acetate). Prevention or correction of constipation, encouraging the use of the side-lying position, proper toileting habits, assuming positions that minimize putting pressure on the hemorrhoids, and not straining during defecation will be helpful in reducing discomfort (King et al., 2015).

Nipple pain is difficult to treat, although a wide variety of topical creams, ointments, and gels are available to do so. This group includes beeswax, glycerin-based products, petrolatum, lanolin, and hydrogel products. Many women find these products comforting. Beeswax, glycerin-based products, and petrolatum all need to be removed before breast-feeding. These products should be avoided in order to limit infant exposure because the process of removal may increase nipple irritation. Applying expressed breast milk to nipples and allowing it to dry has been suggested to reduce nipple pain. Usually the pain is due to incorrect latch-on and/or removal of the nursing infant from the breast. Early assistance with breast-feeding to ensure correct positioning can help prevent nipple trauma.

Analgesics

Analgesics such as acetaminophen and oral nonsteroidal anti-inflammatory drugs (NSAIDs) such as ibuprofen or naproxen are prescribed to relieve mild postpartum discomfort. For moderate to severe pain, a narcotic analgesic such as codeine or oxycodone in conjunction with aspirin or acetaminophen may be prescribed. Instruct the woman about adverse effects of any medication prescribed. Common adverse effects of oral analgesics include dizziness, light-headedness, nausea and vomiting, constipation, and sedation (Skidmore-Roth, 2015).

Also inform the woman that the drugs are secreted in breast milk. Nearly all medications that the mother takes are passed into her breast milk; however, the mild analgesics (e.g., acetaminophen or ibuprofen) are considered relatively safe for breast-feeding mothers (King et al., 2015). Administering a mild analgesic approximately an hour before breast-feeding will usually relieve afterpains and/or perineal discomfort.

Assisting With Elimination

The bladder is edematous, hypotonic, and congested immediately postpartum. Consequently, bladder distention, incomplete emptying, and inability to void are common. A full bladder interferes with uterine contraction and may lead to hemorrhage, because it will displace the uterus out of the midline. Encourage the woman to void. Often, assisting her to assume the normal voiding position on the commode facilitates this. If the woman has difficulty voiding, pouring warm water over the perineal area, hearing the sound of running tap water, blowing bubbles through a straw, taking a warm shower, drinking fluids, providing her with privacy, or placing her hand in a basin of warm water may stimulate voiding. If these actions do not stimulate urination within 4 to 6 hours after giving birth, catheterization may be needed. Palpate the bladder for distention and ask the woman if she is voiding in small amounts (less than 100 mL) frequently (retention with overflow). If catheterization is necessary, use sterile technique to reduce the risk of infection.

Decreased bowel motility during labor, high iron content in prenatal vitamins, postpartum fluid loss, and the adverse effects of pain medications and/or anesthesia may predispose the postpartum woman to constipation. In addition, the woman may fear that bowel movements will cause pain or injury, especially if she had an episiotomy or a laceration that was repaired with sutures.

Usually a stool softener, such as docusate, with or without a laxative might be helpful if the client has difficulty with bowel elimination. Other measures, such as ambulating and increasing fluid and fiber intake, may also help. Nutritional instruction might include increasing fruits and vegetables in the diet; drinking plenty of fluids (8 to 12 cups daily) to keep the stool soft; drinking small amounts of prune juice and/or hot liquids to stimulate peristalsis; eating high-fiber foods such as bran cereals, whole grains, dried fruits, fresh fruits, and raw vegetables; and walking daily.

Promoting Activity, Rest, and Exercise

The postpartum period is an ideal time for nurses to promote the importance of physical fitness, help women incorporate exercise into their lifestyle, and encourage them to overcome barriers to exercise. The lifestyle changes that occur postpartum may affect a woman's health for decades. Early ambulation is encouraged to reduce the risk of thromboembolism and to improve strengthening.

Many changes occur postpartum, and caring for a newborn alters the woman's eating and sleeping habits, work schedules, and time allocation. Postpartum fatigue is common during the early days after childbirth, and it may continue for weeks or months. Having adequate sleep is critical for new mothers because shorter sleep time, a high percentage of sleep disturbances, and greater fatigue are associated with depressive symptoms in postpartum women (Bhati & Richards, 2015). Working partners with newborns experience fatigue during early parenthood and are unable to recover due to interrupted and poor sleep patterns. This sleep deficit can compromise their work safety (Parfitt & Ayers, 2014). For women, it affects the mother's relationships with significant others and her ability to fulfill household and child care responsibilities. Be sure that the mother recognizes her need for rest and sleep and is realistic about her expectations. Some suggestions include the following:

- Nap when the infant is sleeping, because getting uninterrupted sleep at night is difficult.
- Reduce participation in outside activities and limit the number of visitors.
- Determine the infant's sleep–wake cycles and attempt to increase wakeful periods during the day so the baby sleeps for longer periods at night.

- Eat a balanced diet to promote healing and to increase energy levels.
- Share household tasks to conserve your energy.
- Ask the father or other family members to provide infant care during the night periodically so that mothers can get an uninterrupted night of sleep, if they are not breast-feeding.
- Review your family's daily routine and see if you can "cluster" activities to conserve energy and promote rest.

The demands of parenthood may reduce or prevent exercise in even the most committed person. A targeted exercise program and proper body mechanics can help new mothers deal with the physical challenges of motherhood. Emphasize the benefits of a regular exercise program, which include:

- Helps the woman to lose pregnancy weight
- Reduces the risk of obesity later in life
- Increases overall postpartum well-being
- Increases energy level so the woman can cope with her new responsibilities
- Speeds the return to prepregnant size and shape
- Reduces risk of postpartum depression
- Reduces risk of constipation
- Reduces mental fatigue
- Provides an outlet for stress (Covan, 2015).

Overweight and obesity are epidemic in the United States. Obesity is a risk factor for numerous conditions, including diabetes, hypertension, high cholesterol, stroke, heart disease, cancer, and arthritis. More than one third of American women are overweight (American College of Obstetricians & Gynecologists [ACOG], 2014). Although the average gestational weight gain is small (approximately 25 to 35 lb), excess weight gain and failure to lose weight after pregnancy are important predictors of long-term obesity. The postpartum period is a vulnerable time for excessive weight retention, particularly for the increasing number of women who are overweight at the start of their pregnancy and subsequently find it difficult to lose the additional weight gained during pregnancy. Breast-feeding and exercise may help to control weight in the long term (Neville et al., 2014).

Take Note!

Women who are unable to return to a healthy weight by 6 months postpartum increase their risk factors for the development of chronic diseases including metabolic syndrome, obesity, and cardiovascular disease (Brekke et al., 2014). Encourage women to lose their pregnancy weight by 6 months postpartum, and refer those who don't to community weight-loss programs.

The postpartum woman may face some obstacles to exercising, including physical changes (ligament laxity), competing demands (newborn care), lack of information about weight retention (inactivity equates to weight gain), and stress incontinence (leaking of urine during activity).

A healthy woman with an uncomplicated vaginal birth can resume exercise in the immediate postpartum period. Advise the woman to start slowly and increase the level of exercise over a period of several weeks as tolerated. Infant strollers/carriers may be an option for some women, allowing them to walk with their newborns for exercise. Jogging strollers can be used later when the infant is 6 to 12 months old and can hold his or her head up. Also, exercise videos and home exercise equipment allow mothers to work out while the newborn naps.

Exercising after giving birth promotes feelings of well-being and restores muscle tone lost during pregnancy. Routine exercise should be resumed gradually, beginning with **pelvic floor exercises** on the first postpartum day and, by the second week, progressing to abdominal, buttock, and thigh-toning exercises. Most postpartum women fail to meet national guidelines for physical activity which may elevate their risk for morbidity and contribute to the intergenerational impact of obesity on their offspring (Downs, Evenson, & Chasan-Taber, 2014). Walking is an excellent form of early exercise as long as the woman avoids jarring and bouncing movements, because joints do not stabilize until 6 to 8 weeks postpartum. Exercising too much too soon can cause the woman to bleed more and her lochia may return to bright red. If this occurs, instruct the woman to stop exercising and rest lying down until the bleeding slows. This increase in bleeding should be a warning to the woman that she is over doing it and needs to slow down her exercise routine.

Recommended exercises for the first few weeks postpartum include abdominal breathing, head lifts, modified sit-ups, double knee roll, and pelvic tilt (Teaching Guidelines 16.2). The number of exercises and their duration is gradually increased as the woman gains strength.

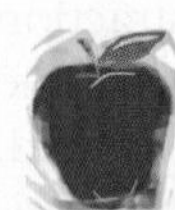

Teaching Guidelines 16.2
POSTPARTUM EXERCISES

Abdominal Breathing

1. While lying on a flat surface (floor or bed), take a deep breath through your nose and expand your abdominal muscles (they will rise up from your midsection).
2. Slowly exhale and tighten your abdominal muscles for 3 to 5 seconds.
3. Repeat this several times.

Head Lift

1. Lie on a flat surface with knees flexed and feet flat on the surface.
2. Lift your head off the flat surface, tuck it onto your chest, and hold for 3 to 5 seconds.

3. Relax your head and return to the starting position.
4. Repeat this several times.

Modified Sit-Ups

1. Lie on a flat surface and raise your head and shoulders 6 to 8 in so that your outstretched hands reach your knees.
2. Keep your waist on the flat surface.
3. Slowly return to the starting position.
4. Repeat, increasing in frequency as your comfort level allows.

Double Knee Roll

1. Lie on a flat surface with your knees bent.
2. While keeping your shoulders flat, slowly roll your knees to your right side to touch the flat surface (floor or bed).
3. Roll your knees back over your body to the left side until they touch the opposite side of the flat surface.
4. Return to the starting position on your back and rest.
5. Repeat this exercise several times.

Pelvic Tilt

1. Lie on your back on a flat surface with your knees bent and your arms at your side.
2. Slowly contract your abdominal muscles while lifting your pelvis up toward the ceiling.
3. Hold for 3 to 5 seconds and slowly return to your starting position.
4. Repeat several times.

Remember that cultures have different attitudes toward exercise. Some cultures (e.g., Haitian, Arab American, Chinese, and Mexican) expect new mothers to observe a specific period of bed rest or activity restriction; thus, it would be inappropriate to recommend active exercise during the early postpartum period (Bowers & Ceballos, 2015).

Preventing Stress Incontinence

Fifty percent of all parous women develop some degree of pelvic prolapse in their lifetime that is associated with stress incontinence. Stress incontinence causes reduced quality of life and withdrawal from fitness and exercise activities typically. Research suggests that having a vaginal delivery results in direct pelvic muscle trauma and disruption of fascial supports, and also causes damage to the levator ani muscle and pudendal nerve injury. Offering pelvic floor muscle exercise instruction to all women during their first pregnancy and again after having a vaginal birth is recommended by the National Institute for Health and Care Excellence (NICE) guidelines. Nurses can offer them as a first-line intervention in the prevention of urinary incontinence postpartum (Hall & Woodward, 2015). The more vaginal deliveries a woman has had, the more likely she is to have stress incontinence. Stress incontinence can occur with any activity that causes an increase in intra-abdominal pressure. Postpartum women might consider low-impact activities such as walking, biking, swimming, or low-impact aerobics so they can resume physical activity while strengthening the pelvic floor.

Suggestions to prevent stress incontinence are:

- Start a regular program of pelvic floor muscle exercises after childbirth.
- Lose weight if necessary; obesity is associated with stress incontinence.
- Avoid smoking; limit intake of alcohol and caffeinated beverages, which irritate the bladder.
- Adjust fluid intake to produce a 24-hourly urine output of 1,000 to 2,000 mL.
- Use either an intravaginal or intraurethral device that puts pressure onto the urethra so that urine will not leak when bladder pressure rises (Laliberte, 2015).

Pelvic floor exercises (Kegel exercises) help to strengthen the pelvic floor muscles if done properly and regularly (Ciaghi, Bianco, & Guarese, 2015). These pelvic floor strengthening exercises were originally developed by Dr. Arnold Kegel in the 1940s as a method of controlling incontinence in women after childbirth. The principle behind these exercises is that strengthening the muscles of the pelvic floor improves urethral sphincter function.

While providing postpartum care, instruct women on primary prevention of stress incontinence by discussing the value and purpose of pelvic floor muscle exercises. Approach the subject sensitively, avoiding the term *incontinent*. The terms *leakage*, *loss of urine*, or *bladder control issues* are more acceptable to most women.

Take Note!

When properly performed, pelvic floor exercises have been effective in preventing or improving urinary continence (Jones & Hawkes, 2015).

Women can perform pelvic floor exercises, doing ten 5-second contractions, whenever they change diapers, talk on the phone, or watch TV. Teach the woman to perform pelvic floor exercises properly; help her to identify the correct muscles by trying to stop and start the flow of urine when sitting on the toilet (Teaching Guidelines 16.3). Pelvic floor exercises can be done without anyone knowing.

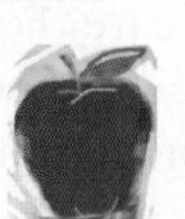

Teaching Guidelines 16.3

PERFORMING PELVIC FLOOR MUSCLE EXERCISES

1. Identify the correct pelvic floor muscles by contracting them to stop the flow of urine while sitting on the toilet.
2. Repeat this contraction several times to become familiar with it.

3. Start the exercises by emptying the bladder.
4. Tighten the pelvic floor muscles and hold for 10 seconds.
5. Relax the muscle completely for 10 seconds.
6. Perform 10 exercises at least three times daily. Progressively increase the number that you perform.
7. Perform the exercises in different positions, such as standing, lying, and sitting.
8. Keep breathing during the exercises.
9. Don't contract your abdominal, thigh, leg, or buttocks muscles during these exercises.
10. Relax while doing pelvic floor exercises and concentrate on isolating the right muscles.
11. Attempt to tighten your pelvic muscles before sneezing, jumping, or laughing.
12. Remember that you can perform these exercises anywhere without anyone noticing.

Assisting With Self-Care Measures

Demonstrate and discuss with the woman ways to prevent infection during the postpartum period. Because she may experience lochia drainage for as long as a month after childbirth, describe practices to promote well-being and healing. These measures include:

- Frequently change perineal pads, applying and removing them from front to back to prevent spreading contamination from the rectal area to the genital area.
- Avoid using tampons after giving birth to decrease the risk of infection.
- Shower once or twice daily using a mild soap. Avoid using soap on nipples.
- Use a sitz bath after every bowel movement to cleanse the rectal area and relieve enlarged hemorrhoids.
- Use the peribottle filled with warm water after urinating and before applying a new perineal pad.
- Avoid tub baths for 4 to 6 weeks, until joints and balance are restored, to prevent falls.
- Wash your hands before changing perineal pads, after disposing of soiled pads, and after voiding (Mattson & Smith, 2016).

To reduce the risk of infection at the episiotomy site, reinforce proper perineal care with the client, showing her how to rinse her perineum with the peribottle after she voids or defecates. Stress the importance of always patting gently from front to back and washing her hands thoroughly before and after perineal care. For hemorrhoids, have the client apply witch hazel-soaked pads (Tucks®), ice packs to relieve swelling, or hemorrhoidal cream or ointment if ordered.

Ensuring Safety

One of the safety concerns during the postpartum period is orthostatic hypotension. When the woman rapidly moves from a lying or sitting position to a standing one, her blood pressure can suddenly drop, causing her pulse rate to increase. She may become dizzy and faint. Be aware of this problem and initiate the following safeguards:

- Check blood pressure first before ambulating the client.
- Elevate the head of the bed for a few minutes before ambulating the client.
- Have the client sit on the side of the bed for a few moments before getting up.
- Help the client to stand up, and stay with her.
- Ambulate alongside the client and provide support if needed.
- Frequently ask the client how her head feels.
- Stay close by to assist if she feels light-headed.

Additional topics to address orthostatic hypotension that may concern infant safety include instructing the woman to place the newborn back in the crib on his or her back if she is feeling sleepy to prevent a fall. If the woman falls asleep while holding the infant, she might drop him or her. Also, instruct mothers to keep the door to their room closed when their infant is in their room with them. They should check the identification of anyone who enters their room or who wants to take the infant out of the room. This will prevent infant abduction.

Counseling About Sexuality and Contraception

Pregnancy and childbirth are special periods in a woman's life that involve significant physical, hormonal, psychological, social, and cultural changes that may influence her own sexuality as well as the health of a couple's sexual relationship. This is often a time period filled with excitement, changes, and challenges. Mothers often face changes in their own sexuality in their adjustment to motherhood. Sexuality is an important part of every woman's life. Women want to get back to "normal" as soon as possible after giving birth, but a couple's sexual relationship cannot be isolated from the psychological and psychosocial adjustments that both partners are going through.

Childbirth is a significant life transition that has a measurable impact on postpartum women's sexual function. There are physical (perineal pain), psychological (depression), and contextual factors (motherhood) that contribute to the change in many women's sex lives after experiencing childbirth. Postpartum women may hesitate to resume sexual relations for a number of reasons. Many postpartum women have fatigue, weakness, loss of sexual desire, perception of decreased attractiveness, change in body appearance, vaginal bleeding, perineal discomfort, hemorrhoids, sore breasts, decreased vaginal lubrication resulting from low estrogen levels, and dyspareunia. Fatigue, the physical demands made by the infant, and the stress of new roles and responsibilities may stress the emotional reserves of couples. New parents may not get much privacy or rest, both of which are necessary for sexual pleasure (Whittock, 2015).

Men may feel they now have a secondary role within the family, and they may not understand their partner's daily routine. The delicate nature of postpartum sexuality makes it difficult for couples to discuss. These issues, combined with the woman's increased investment in the mothering role, can strain the couple's sexual relationship.

Although couples are reluctant to ask, they often want to know when they can safely resume sexual intercourse after childbirth. Typically, sexual intercourse can be resumed once bright-red bleeding has stopped and the perineum is healed from an episiotomy or lacerations. This is usually by the third to the sixth week postpartum. However, there is no set, prescribed time at which to resume sexual intercourse after childbirth. There is no scientific basis for the traditional recommendation to delay sexual activity until the 6-week postpartum check-up. Each couple must set their own time frame when they feel it is appropriate to resume sexual intercourse. Despite fears and myths about sexual activity during pregnancy, maintaining a couple's sexual interactions throughout pregnancy and the postpartum period can promote sexual health and well-being and a greater depth of intimacy.

Postpartum sexual health and sexual problems are common, which receive little attention from health care providers during the postpartum period, need to be addressed (Halford, Petch, & Creedy, 2015). When counseling the couple about sexuality, determine what knowledge and concerns the couple have about their sexual relationship. Inform the couple that fluctuations in sexual interest are normal. Reassure the breast-feeding mother that she may notice a let-down reflex during orgasm and find her breasts are very sensitive when touched by her partner. Also inform the couple about how to prevent discomfort. Precoital vaginal lubrication may be impaired during the postpartum period, especially in women who are breast-feeding. Use of water-based gel lubricants (K-Y® jelly, Astroglide) can help. Pelvic floor exercises, in addition to preventing stress incontinence, can also enhance sensation.

Initiation of contraception during the postpartum period is important to prevent unintended pregnancy and short birth intervals, which can lead to negative health outcomes for mother and infant. Contraceptive options should be included in the discussions with the couple so that they can make an informed decision before resuming sexual activity. Many couples are overwhelmed with the amount of new information given to them during their brief hospitalization, so many are not ready for a lengthy discussion about contraceptives. Presenting a brief overview of the options, along with literature, may be appropriate. It may be suitable to ask them to think about contraceptive needs and preferences and advise them to use a barrier method (condom with spermicidal gel or foam) until they choose another form of contraception. This advice is especially important if the follow-up appointment will not occur for 4 to 6 weeks after childbirth, because many couples will resume sexual activity before this time. Some postpartum women ovulate before their menstrual period returns and thus need contraceptive protection to prevent another pregnancy.

Recently, the CDC assessed evidence regarding the safety of estrogen-containing contraceptive methods use during the postpartum period. They recommend that postpartum women not use combined hormonal contraceptives during the first 21 days after childbirth because of the high risk for VTE during this period. During days 21 to 42 postpartum, women without risk factors for VTE generally can initiate estrogen-containing contraceptives, but women with risk factors for VTE (e.g., previous VTE or recent cesarean delivery) generally should not use these methods. After 42 days postpartum, no restrictions on the use of combined hormonal contraceptives based on postpartum status apply (Centers for Disease Control & Prevention [CDC], 2015a).

Open and effective communication is necessary for effective contraceptive counseling so that information is clearly understood. Provide clear, consistent information appropriate to the woman and her partner's language, culture, and educational level. This will help the couple select the best contraceptive method. Research supports that postpartum education about contraception leads to more contraception use and fewer unplanned pregnancies and that both short-term and multiple-contact interventions had effects. The use of contraceptives was highest when contraceptive counseling was provided prenatally and again in the postpartum period (Zapata et al., 2015).

Promoting Maternal Nutrition

The postpartum period can be a stressful one for myriad reasons, such as fatigue, the physical stress of pregnancy and birth, and the nonstop work required to take care of the newborn and to meet the needs of other family members. As a result, the new mother may ignore her own nutrition needs. Whether she is breast-feeding or bottle-feeding, encourage the new mother to take good care of herself and eat a healthy diet so that the nutrients lost during pregnancy can be replaced and she can return to a healthy weight. In general, nutrition recommendations for the postpartum woman include the following:

- Eat a wide variety of foods with high nutrient density.
- Eat meals that require little or no preparation.
- Avoid high-fat fast foods.

- Drink plenty of fluids daily—at least 2,500 mL (approximately 84 oz).
- Avoid fad weight-reduction diets and harmful substances such as alcohol, tobacco, and drugs.
- Avoid excessive intake of fat, salt, sugar, and caffeine.
- Eat the recommended daily servings from each food group (Box 16.4).

Nutrition for the Breast-Feeding Mother

The breast-feeding mother's nutritional needs are higher than they were during pregnancy. The mother's diet and nutritional status influence the quantity and quality of breast milk. Recently, the American Academy of Pediatrics [AAP] (2014a)recommended that breast-feeding women consume foods that contain iodine, an element that is crucial to healthy brain development and may be lacking in their present diets. Iodine is necessary to produce thyroid hormone, which in turn helps brain development. To meet the needs for breast milk production, the woman's nutritional needs increase as follows:

- *Calories:* + 500 cal/day for the first and second 6 months of lactation
- *Protein:* + 20 g/day, adding an extra 2 cups of skim milk
- *Calcium:* + 400 mg daily—consumption of four or more servings of milk
- *Iodine:* 290 mcg daily—dairy products, seafood, and iodized salt

BOX 16.4

NUTRITIONAL RECOMMENDATIONS FOR NUTRITION DURING THE POSTPARTUM PERIOD

Recommendations for the Lactating Woman From the Food Guide *MyPlate*

- Fruits: 4 servings
- Vegetables: 4 servings
- Milk: 4 to 5 servings
- Bread, cereal, pasta: 12 or more servings
- Meat, poultry, fish, eggs: 7 servings
- Fats, oils, and sweets: 5 servings (Dudek, 2014).

General Dietary Guidelines for Americans from the Food Guide on *MyPlate* (for the Nonlactating Woman)

- Fruits: Make half of your plate fruits and vegetables.
- Vegetables: Eat red, orange, and dark-green vegetables.
- Milk: Switch to skim milk or 1%.
- Breads, grains, and cereals should be whole grains.
- Meat, poultry, fish, eggs: Eat seafood twice a week and beans, which are high in fiber.
- Eat the right amount of calories for you; enjoy your food, but eat less.
- Be physically active your way in activities that you enjoy.
- Fats, oils, and sweets: Cut back on these.
- Use food labels to help you make better choices (U. S. Department of Agriculture [USDA] & USDHHS, 2014).

- *Fluid:* + 2 to 3 quarts of fluids daily (milk, juice, or water); no sodas

Some foods eaten by the breast-feeding mother may affect the flavor of the breast milk or cause gastrointestinal problems for the infant. Not all infants are affected by the same foods. It is suggested that the mother identify the food item that may be causing a problem for the infant and reduce or eliminate her intake of it.

Nutritional needs for breast-feeding mothers are based on the nutritional content of breast milk and the energy expended to produce it. If intake of calories exceeds the energy expended, weight gain occurs. The highest incidence of obesity in women occurs during the childbearing years. Women need to be made aware that weight gained during their reproductive years will have a negative impact on their health as they age. Nurses can assist women in their postpartum weight management program by assessing their readiness to change to lose their pregnancy weight gain; assessing their breast-feeding status, dietary intake, and activity levels; and assessing them for stress and depressive symptoms, which might hinder their weight loss (Green, 2016).

Take Note!

During a woman's brief stay in a health care facility, she may demonstrate a healthy appetite and eat well. Nutritional problems usually start at home when the mother needs to make her own food selections and prepare her own meals. This is a crucial area to address during follow-up.

Supporting the Woman's Choice of Infant Feeding Method

The AAP, WHO, ANA, IOA, USDHHS, ADA, & USPSTF have all released position statements in support of breast-feeding and nurses, should be encouraging it as part of evidence-based practice (Edelman, Kudzma, & Mandle, 2014). Although there is considerable evidence that breast-feeding has numerous health benefits for both mother and infant, many mothers choose to feed their infants formula for the first year of life. Nurses must be able to deliver sound, evidence-based information to help the new mother choose the best way to feed her infant and must support her in her decision. Research findings indicate that parents do listen to nurse's instruction on feeding practices (Stagg & Ustianov, 2015). Many factors affect a woman's choice of feeding method, such as culture, employment demands, support from significant others and family, and knowledge base. Although breast-feeding is encouraged, be sure that couples have the information they need to make an informed decision. Whether a couple chooses to breast-feed or bottle-feed the newborn, support and respect their choice.

Women Who Should Not Breast-Feed

Certain women should not breast-feed. Drugs such as antithyroid drugs, antineoplastic drugs, alcohol, herpes infection on the breasts, or street drugs (methamphetamines, cocaine, PCP, marijuana) enter the breast milk and would harm the infant, so women taking these substances should not breast-feed. To prevent HIV transmission to the newborn, women who are HIV positive should not breast-feed. Other contraindications to breast-feeding include a newborn with an inborn error of metabolism such as galactosemia or phenylketonuria (PKU), active tuberculosis, or a mother with a serious mental health disorder that would prevent her from remembering to feed the infant consistently (Denne, 2015).

Providing Assistance With Breast-Feeding and Bottle-Feeding

First-time mothers often have many questions about feeding, and even women who have had experience with feeding may have questions. Regardless of whether the postpartum woman is breast-feeding or bottle-feeding her newborn, she can benefit from instruction.

PROVIDING ASSISTANCE WITH BREAST-FEEDING

The AAP (2014b) recommends breast-feeding for all full-term newborns. Exclusive breast-feeding is sufficient to support optimal growth and development for approximately the first 6 months of life. Breast-feeding should be continued for at least the first year of life and beyond for as long as mutually desired by mother and child. Educating a mother about breast-feeding will increase the likelihood of a successful breast-feeding experience.

At birth, all newborns should be quickly dried, assessed, and, if stable, placed immediately in uninterrupted skin-to-skin contact (kangaroo care) with their mother. This is good practice whether the mother is going to breast-feed or bottle-feed her infant. Numerous benefits of kangaroo care have been reported related to physiologic (thermoregulation, cardiorespiratory stability), behavioral (sleep, breast-feeding duration, and degree of exclusivity), domains, as an effective therapy to relieve procedural pain, and improve neurodevelopment. In addition, kangaroo care provides the newborn with optimal physiologic stability, warmth, and opportunities for the first feed (Campbell-Yeo et al., 2015).

The benefits of breast-feeding for infants are clear (see Chapter 18). To promote breast-feeding, the Baby-Friendly Hospital Initiative, an international program of the World Health Organization (WHO) and the United Nations International Children's Emergency Fund (UNICEF), was started in 1991. This global health promotion initiative was put forth to improve maternal-infant health by improving rates of exclusive breast-feeding. As part of this program, the hospital or birth center should take the following 10 steps to provide "an optimal environment for the promotion, protection, and support of breast-feeding":

1. Have a written breast-feeding policy that is communicated to all staff.
2. Educate all staff to implement this written policy.
3. Inform all women about the benefits and management of breast-feeding.
4. Show all mothers how to initiate breast-feeding within 30 minutes of birth.
5. Give no food or drink other than breast milk to all newborns.
6. Demonstrate to all mothers how to initiate and maintain breast-feeding.
7. Encourage breast-feeding on demand.
8. Allow no pacifiers to be given to breast-feeding infants.
9. Establish breast-feeding support groups and refer mothers to them.
10. Practice rooming-in 24 hours daily (CDC, 2015a; Cleminson et al., 2015; WHO, 2014a).

The nurse is responsible for protecting, promoting, and supporting breast-feeding when appropriate. For the woman who chooses to breast-feed her infant, the nurse or lactation consultant will need to spend time instructing her about how to do so successfully. Many women have the impression that breast-feeding is simple. Although it is a natural process, women may experience some difficulty in breast-feeding their newborns. Nurses can assist mothers in smoothing out this transition. Assist and provide one-to-one instruction to breast-feeding mothers, especially first-time breast-feeding mothers, to ensure correct technique. Suggestions are highlighted in Teaching Guidelines 16.4. (See Evidence-Based Practice 16.2.)

> ***Take Note!***
>
> *Some newborns "latch on and catch on" right away, and others take more time and patience. Inform new mothers about this to reduce their frustration and uncertainty about their ability to breast-feed.*

Tell mothers that they need to believe in themselves and their ability to accomplish this task. They should not panic if breast-feeding does not go smoothly at first; it takes time and practice. Additional suggestions to help mothers relax and feel more comfortable breast-feeding, especially when they return home, include the following:

- Select a quiet corner or room where you won't be disturbed.
- Use a rocking chair to soothe both you and your infant.
- Take long, slow deep breaths to relax before nursing.
- Drink while breast-feeding to replenish body fluids.
- Listen to soothing music while breast-feeding.
- Cuddle and caress the infant while feeding.
- Set out extra cloth diapers within reach to use as burping cloths.

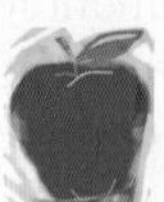

Teaching Guidelines 16.4

BREAST-FEEDING SUGGESTIONS

1. Explain that breast-feeding is a learned skill for both parties.
2. Offer a thorough explanation about the procedure.
3. Instruct the mother to wash her hands before starting.
4. Inform her that her afterpains will increase during breast-feeding.
5. Make sure the mother is comfortable (pain-free) and not hungry.
6. Tell the mother to start the feeding with an awake and alert infant showing hunger signs.
7. Assist the mother to position herself correctly for comfort.
8. Urge the mother to relax to encourage the let-down reflex.
9. Guide the mother's hand to form a "C" to access the breast with thumb on top and other four fingers under the breast.
10. Have the mother lightly tickle the infant's upper lip with her nipple to stimulate the infant to open the mouth wide.
11. Aid her in helping the infant to latch on by bringing the infant rapidly to the breast with a wide-open mouth.
12. Show her how to check that the newborn's mouth position is correct, and tell her to listen for a sucking noise.
13. Demonstrate correct removal from the breast, using her finger to break the suction.
14. Instruct the mother on how to burp the infant before changing from one breast to another.
15. Show her different positions, such as cradle and football holds and side-lying positions (see Chapter 18).
16. Reinforce and praise the mother for her efforts.
17. Allow ample time to answer questions and address concerns.
18. Refer the mother to support groups and community resources.

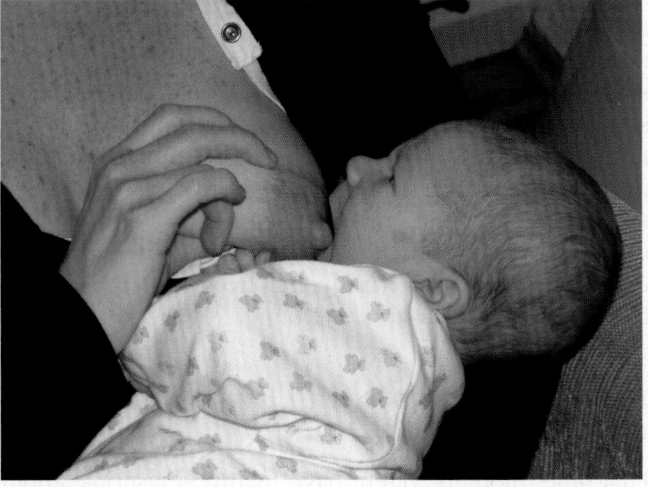

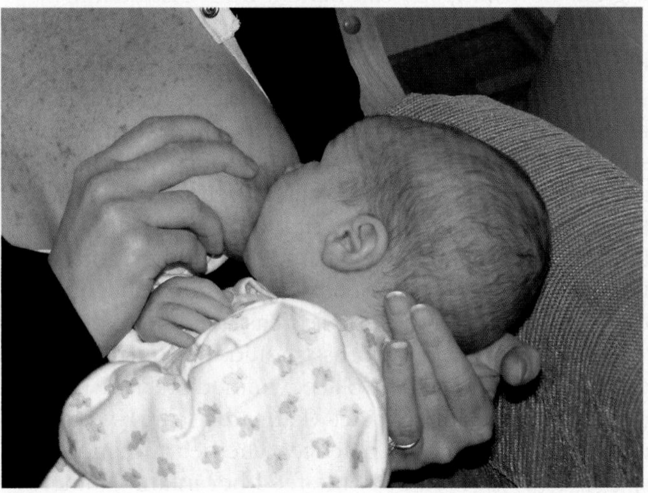

- Allow sufficient time to enjoy each other in an unhurried atmosphere.
- Involve other family members in all aspects of the infant's care from the start.
- Contact a local La Leche or Nursing Mother's group for continued guidance/support.

Because obesity in America is increasing in all walks of life, it is important for nurses to be knowledgeable about how it impacts breast-feeding and ways to support the obese mother. Research shows that mothers who are obese (BMI > 30) are less likely to initiate lactation, have difficulties with latching on, have delayed lactogenesis, experience mechanical challenges, and are prone to early cessation of breast-feeding (Shannon, Chao, & Ramos, 2015). Obesity rates are highest among African American women, who have the lowest rate of breast-feeding initiation and shortest duration when compared with Hispanic and White women. Women who are overweight and obese have lowered prolactin responses to infant sucking, thus milk production may be inhibited. Lactation plays a significant role in preventing future obesity in both the mother and the infant (Masho, Cha, & Morris, 2015).

Nurses can assist in managing obesity-related lactation challenges by keeping the mother and newborn together to facilitate early and frequent sucking to trigger prolactin and oxytocin production, which will help negate the obesity-related blunting of the prolactin response. Suggesting a sandwich technique to insert the mother's breast into the newborn's mouth to elicit sucking

EVIDENCE-BASED PRACTICE 16.2 NURSES IMPROVING THE HEALTH OF MOTHERS AND INFANTS BY DANCING THE 10 STEPS TO SUCCESSFUL BREAST-FEEDING

STUDY

The Baby Friendly Hospital Initiative has gained momentum in the United States in recent years. The principles of it are evidence-based and that promoting breast-feeding improves health outcomes and neurocognitive development in infants. The purpose of this study was to implement the Ten Steps to Successful Breast-feeding and see if the rates and duration of breast-feeding improved. The implementation strategies included assessment of current practices, identification of barriers and opportunities, and strategies to support changes in 89 hospitals that participated. The initiative was to increase the number of Baby Friendly designated hospitals over a 2-year process-improvement time frame.

Findings

Results included heightened professional environment of competence, enhanced delivery of client-centered care, improved health of mothers and infants, increased client satisfaction, and achievement of benchmarks. The implementation of the Ten Steps to Successful Breast-feeding resulted in improved rates of breast-feeding in all 89 hospitals.

Nursing Implications

This study demonstrated the positive effect of a nurse-led initiative that improved the continuum of care for mothers and infants from the prenatal period through post discharge community care. Nurses can be instrumental by applying principles of evidence-based practices and bring forth change within their health care agencies to improve the outcomes for mothers and their infants.

Adapted from Allen, M., & Schafer, D. J. (2015). Nurses improving the health of mothers and infants by dancing the 10 steps to successful breastfeeding. *Journal of Obstetric, Gynecologic, & Neonatal Nursing, 44,* S52.

might be helpful for the mother with large breasts. In the sandwich technique, the mother is taught to grasp her breast by making a "C" with her thumb and index finger. The thumb stabilizes the top of the breast while the remaining four fingers support her breast from below. Massage or pumping the breast may soften and extend the nipple for easier infant latch-on. In short, nurses can make a difference by observing lactation, assessing infant hydration and satisfaction, and reassuring the mother about her breast-feeding capacity.

PROVIDING ASSISTANCE WITH BOTTLE-FEEDING

If the mother or couple has chosen to bottle-feed their newborn, the nurse should respect and support their decision. Discuss with the parents what type of formula they will use. Commercial formulas are classified as cow's milk-based (Enfamil, Similac), soy protein-based (Isomil, Prosobee, Nursoy), or specialized or therapeutic formulas for infants with protein allergies (Nutramigen, Pregestimil, Alimentum). Commercial formulas can also be purchased in various forms: powdered (must be mixed with water), condensed liquid (must be diluted with equal amounts of water), ready to use (poured directly into bottles), and prepackaged (ready to use in disposable bottles).

Breast milk is a dynamic fluid with compositional changes occurring throughout the period of lactation that reflects the growth rate and developmental needs of the infant. Infant formula, in contrast, has a static composition, intended to meet the nutritional requirements of infants from birth to 12 months of age (Lonnerdal & Hernell, 2015). Nurses need to bring this information to the attention of mothers who choose to formula feed their infants that changes may be needed in different stages of growth to meet the nutritional needs of their infant.

Newborns need about 108 cal/kg or approximately 650 cal/day (Dudek, 2014). Therefore, explain to parents that a newborn will need 2 to 4 oz to feel satisfied at each feeding. Until about age 4 months, most bottle-fed infants need six feedings a day. After this time, the number of feedings declines to accommodate other foods in the diet, such as fruits, cereals, and vegetables (Dudek, 2014). For more information on newborn nutrition and bottle-feeding, see Chapter 18.

When teaching the mother about bottle-feeding, provide the following guidelines:

- Wash hands with soap and water and dry using a clean or disposable cloth.
- Make sure all bottles, nipples, and other utensils are clean.
- Make feeding a relaxing time, a time to provide both food and comfort to your newborn.
- Use the feeding period to promote bonding by smiling, singing, making eye contact, and talking to the infant.
- Powdered formula mixes more easily and the lumps dissolve faster if you use room-temperature water.
- Store any formula prepared in advance in the refrigerator to keep bacteria from growing.
- Do not microwave formula; the microwave won't heat it evenly, causing hot spots.
- Always hold the newborn when feeding. Never prop the bottle.

- Use a comfortable position when feeding the newborn. Place the newborn in your dominant arm, which is supported by a pillow. Or have the newborn in a semi-upright position supported in the crook of your arm. (This position reduces choking and the flow of milk into the middle ear.)
- Tilt the bottle so that the nipple and the neck of the bottle are always filled with formula. This prevents the infant from taking in too much air.
- Stimulate the sucking reflex by touching the nipple to the infant's lips.
- Refrigerate any powdered formula that has been combined with tap water.
- Discard any formula not taken; do not keep it for future feedings.
- Burp the infant frequently, and place the baby on his or her back for sleeping.
- Use only iron-fortified infant formula for the first year (Moses, 2014).

Teaching About Breast Care

Regardless of whether or not the mother is breast-feeding her newborn, urge her to wear a very supportive, snug bra 24 hours a day to support enlarged breasts and promote comfort. A woman who is breast-feeding should wear a supportive bra throughout the lactation period. A woman who is not nursing should wear it until engorgement ceases, and then should wear a less restrictive one. The bra should fit snugly while still allowing the mother to breathe without restriction. All new mothers should use plain water to clean their breasts, especially the nipple area; soap is drying and should be avoided.

Assessing the Breasts

Instruct the mother how to examine her breasts daily. Daily assessment includes the milk supply (breasts will feel full as they are filling), the condition of the nipples (red, bruised, fissured, or bleeding), and the success of breast-feeding. The fullness of the breasts may progress to engorgement in the breast-feeding mother if feedings are delayed or breast-feeding is ineffective. Palpating both breasts will help identify whether the breasts are soft, filling, or engorged. A similar assessment of the breasts should be completed on the nonlactating mother to identify any problems, such as engorgement or mastitis.

Alleviating Breast Engorgement

Breast engorgement usually occurs during the first week postpartum. It is a common response of the breasts to the sudden change in hormones and the presence of an increased amount of milk. Reassure the woman that this condition is temporary and usually resolves within 72 hours.

ALLEVIATING BREAST ENGORGEMENT IN THE BREAST-FEEDING WOMAN

If the mother is breast-feeding, encourage frequent feedings, at least every 2 to 3 hours, using manual expression just before feeding to soften the breast so the newborn can latch on more effectively. Advise the mother to allow the newborn to feed on the first breast until it softens before switching to the other side. See Chapter 18 for more information on alleviating breast engorgement and other common breast-feeding concerns.

ALLEVIATING BREAST ENGORGEMENT AND SUPPRESSING LACTATION IN THE BOTTLE-FEEDING WOMAN

If the woman is bottle-feeding, explain that breast engorgement is a self-limiting phenomenon that disappears as increasing estrogen levels suppress milk formation (i.e., lactation suppression). Encourage the woman to use ice packs, to wear a snug, supportive bra 24 hours a day, and to take mild analgesics such as acetaminophen. Encourage her to avoid any stimulation to the breasts that might foster milk production, such as warm showers or pumping or massaging the breasts. Medication is no longer given to hasten lactation suppression because these agents had limited effectiveness and adverse side effects. Teaching Guidelines 16.5 provides tips on lactation suppression.

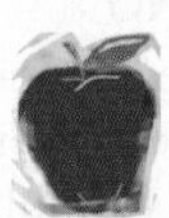

Teaching Guidelines 16.5

SUPPRESSING LACTATION

1. Wear a supportive, snugly fitting bra 24 hours daily, but not one that binds the breasts too tightly or interferes with your breathing.
2. Suppression may take 5 to 7 days to accomplish.
3. Take mild analgesics to reduce breast discomfort.
4. Let shower water flow over your back rather than your breasts.
5. Avoid any breast stimulation in the form of sucking or massage.
6. Drink to quench your thirst. Restricting your fluid intake will not dry up your milk.
7. Reduce your salt intake to decrease fluid retention.
8. Use ice packs or cool compresses (e.g., cool cabbage leaves) inside the bra to decrease local pain and swelling; change them every 30 minutes (King et al., 2015).

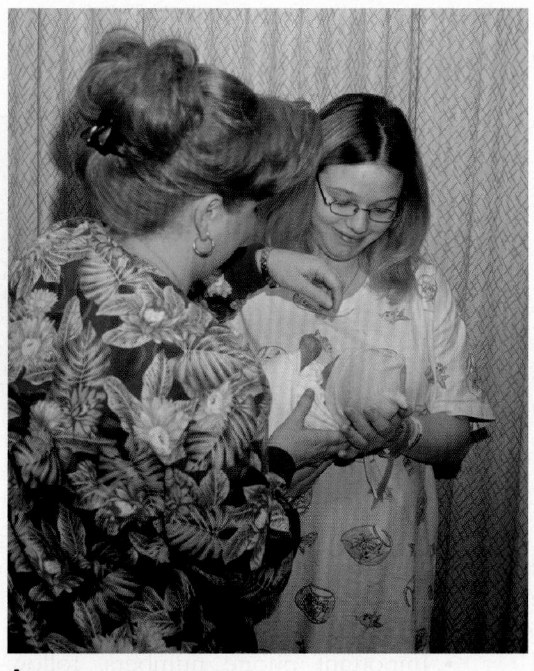

A

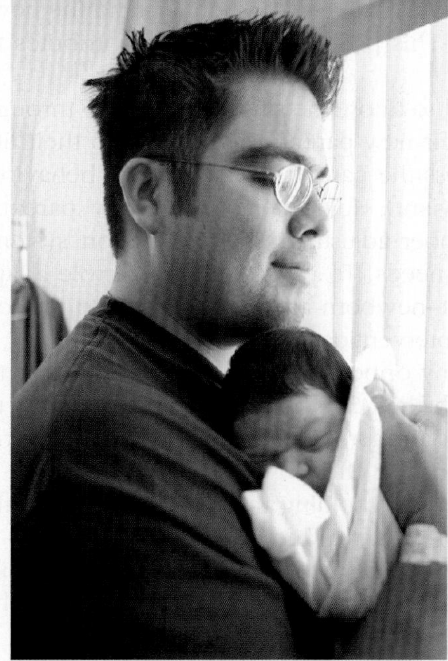

B

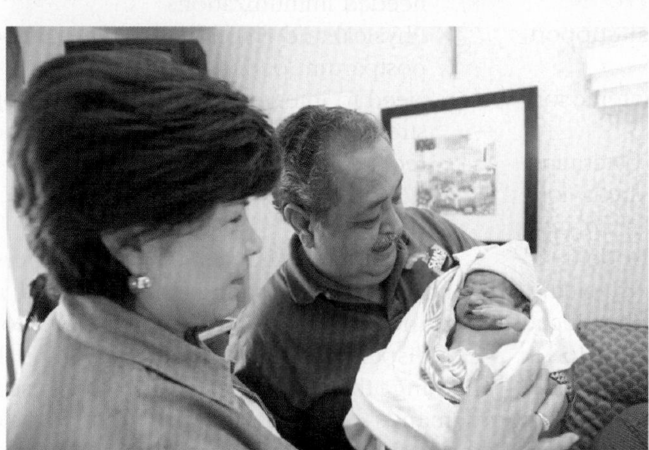

C

FIGURE 16.7 Examples of family members carrying out roles to promote adjustment and well-being. **A.** An aunt admiring the newest member of the family. **B.** A father holding his newborn closely on his chest. **C.** Grandparents welcoming the newest little one to the family circle.

Promoting Family Adjustment and Well-Being

The postpartum period involves extraordinary physiologic, psychological, and sociocultural changes in the life of a woman and her family. Adapting to the role of a parent is not an easy process. The postpartum period is a "getting-to-know-you" time when parents begin to integrate the newborn into their lives as they reconcile the fantasy child with the real one. This can be a very challenging period for families. Nurses play a major role in assisting families to adapt to the changes, promoting a smooth transition into parenthood. Appropriate and timely interventions can help parents adjust to the role changes and promote attachment to the newborn (Fig. 16.7).

For couples who already have children, the addition of a new member may bring role conflict and challenges. The nurse should provide anticipatory guidance about siblings' responses to the new baby, increased emotional tension, child development, and meeting the multiple needs of the expanding family. Although the multiparous woman has had experience with newborns, do not assume that her knowledge is current and accurate, especially if some time has elapsed since her previous child was born. Reinforcing information is important for all families.

Promoting Parental Roles

Parents' roles develop and grow when they interact with their newborn (see Chapter 15 for information on maternal and paternal adaptation). The pleasure they derive from this interaction stimulates and reinforces this behavior. With repeated, continued contact with the newborn, parents learn to recognize cues and understand the newborn's behavior. This positive interaction contributes to family harmony.

Nurses need to know the stages parents go through as they make their new parenting roles fit into their life experience. Assess the parents for attachment behaviors (normal and deviant), adjustment to the new parental role, family member adjustment, social support system, and educational needs. To promote parental role adaptation and parent–newborn attachment, provide the following nursing interventions:

- Provide as many opportunities as possible for parents to interact with their newborn. Encourage parents to explore, hold, and provide care for their newborn. Praise them for their efforts.
- Model behaviors by holding the newborn close, calling the newborn's name, and speaking positively.
- Speak directly to the newborn in a calm voice, while pointing out the newborn's positive features to the parents.
- Evaluate the family's strengths and weaknesses and readiness for parenting.
- Assess for risk factors such as lack of social support and the presence of stressors.
- Observe the effect of culture on the family interaction to determine healthy family dynamics.
- Monitor parental attachment behaviors to determine whether alterations require referral. Positive behaviors include holding the newborn closely or in an *en face* position, talking to or admiring the newborn, or demonstrating closeness. Negative behaviors include avoiding contact with the newborn, calling it names, or showing a lack of interest in caring for the newborn (see Table 16.1).
- Monitor the parents' coping behaviors to determine alterations that need intervention. Positive coping behaviors include positive conversations between the partners, both parents wanting to be involved with newborn care, and lack of arguments between the parents. Negative behaviors include not visiting, limited conversations or periods of silence, and heated arguments or conflict.
- Identify the support systems available to the new family and encourage them to ask for help. Ask direct questions about home or community support. Make referrals to community resources to meet the family's needs.
- Arrange for community home visits in high-risk families to provide positive reinforcement of parenting skills and nurturing behaviors with the newborn.
- Provide anticipatory guidance about the following before discharge to reduce the new parents' frustration:
  - Newborn sleep–wake cycles (they may be reversed)
  - Variations in newborn appearance and developmental milestones (growth spurts)
  - How to interpret crying cues (hunger, wet, discomfort) and what to do about them
  - Sensory enrichment/stimulation (colorful mobile)
  - Signs and symptoms of illness and how to assess for fever
  - Important phone numbers, follow-up care, and needed immunizations
  - Physical and emotional changes associated with the postpartum period
  - Need to integrate siblings into care of the newborn; stress that sibling rivalry is normal and offer ways to reduce it
  - Ways to make time together for the couple.

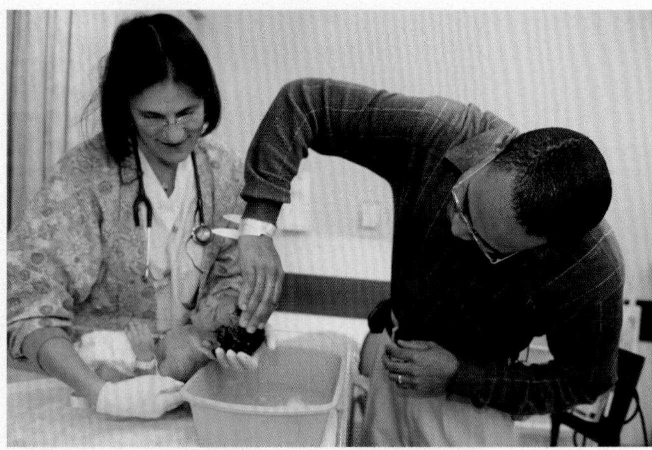

FIGURE 16.8 **Father participating in newborn care.**

In addition, nurses can help fathers to feel more competent in assuming their parental role by teaching and providing information (Fig. 16.8). Education can dispel any unrealistic expectations they may have, helping them to cope more successfully with the demands of fatherhood and thereby fostering a nurturing family relationship.

Explaining Sibling Roles

It can be overwhelming to a young child to have another family member introduced into his or her small, stable world. Although most parents try to prepare siblings for the arrival of their new little brother or sister, many young children experience stress. They may view the new infant as competition, or fear that they will be replaced in the parents' affection. All siblings need extra attention from their parents and reassurance that they are loved and important. Many parents need reassurance that sibling rivalry is normal. Suggest the following to help parents minimize sibling rivalry:

- Expect and tolerate some regression (thumb sucking, bedwetting).
- Explain childbirth in an appropriate way for the child's age.
- Encourage discussion about the new infant during relaxed family times.

- Encourage the sibling(s) to participate in decisions, such as the baby's name and toys to buy.
- Take the sibling on a tour of the maternity suite.
- Buy a T-shirt that says "I'm the [big brother or big sister]."
- Spend "special time" with the child.
- Read with the child. Some suggested titles include *Things to Do With a New Baby* (Ormerod, 1984); *Betsy's Baby Brother* (Wolde, 1975); *The Berenstain Bears' New Baby* (Berenstain, 1974); and *Mommy's Lap* (Horowitz & Sorensen, 1993).
- Plan time for each child throughout the day.
- Role-play safe handling of a newborn, using a doll. Give the preschooler or school-age child a doll to care for.
- Encourage older children to verbalize emotions about the newborn.
- Purchase a gift that the child can give to the newborn.
- Purchase a gift that can be given to the child by the newborn.
- Arrange for the child to come to the hospital to see the newborn (Fig. 16.9).
- Move the sibling from his or her crib to a youth bed months in advance of the birth of the newborn.
- Show the older sibling photos of the baby growing in mommy's belly. Let them pat the baby beneath the bulge, talk to baby, and feel the baby kick.
- Make the older sibling feel important by giving them a title "mommy's helper."
- Encourage grandparents to pay attention to the older child when visiting.
- Tell the older sibling that their friends come and go, but siblings are forever.
- Encourage "Do unto others as you would have them do unto you" (Sears & Sears, 2015c).

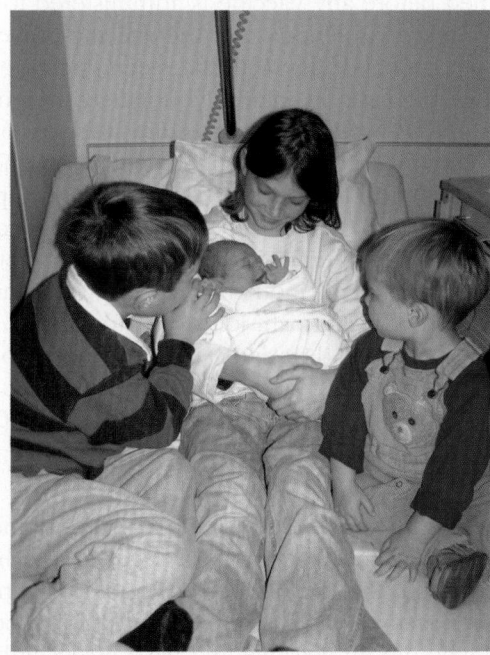

FIGURE 16.9 Sibling visitation.

Consider This

Katie and Molly have been excited about having a new baby sister ever since they were told about their mother's pregnancy. The 6-year-old twins are eagerly looking out the front window, waiting for their parents to bring their new sister, Jessica, home. The girls are big enough to help their mother care for their new sibling, and for the past few months they have been fixing up the new nursery and selecting baby clothes. They practiced diapering their dolls – their mother was specific about not using any powder or lotion on Jessica's bottom – and holding them correctly to feed them bottles. Finally, their mother arrives home from the hospital with Jessica in her arms!

The girls notice that their mother is very protective of Jessica and watches them carefully when they care for her. They fight over the opportunity to hold her or feed her. What is special to both of them is the time they spend alone with their parents. Although a new family member has been added, the twins still feel special and loved by their parents.

Thoughts: Bringing a new baby into an established family can cause conflict and jealousy. What preparation did the older siblings have before Jessica arrived? Why is it important for parents to spend time with each sibling separately?

Discussing Grandparents' Role

Grandparents can be a source of support and comfort to the postpartum family if effective communication skills are used and roles are defined. The grandparents' role and involvement will depend on how close they live to the family, their willingness to become involved, and cultural expectations of their role. Just as parents and siblings go through developmental changes, so too do grandparents. These changes can have a positive or negative effect on the relationship.

Newborn care, feeding, and child-rearing practices have changed since the grandparents raised the parents. New parents may lack parenting skills but nonetheless want their parents' support without criticism. A grandparent's "take-charge approach" may not be welcome by new parents who are testing their own parenting roles, and family conflict may ensue. However, many grandparents respect their adult children's wishes for autonomy and remain "resource people" for them when requested.

Take Note!

Grandparents' involvement can enrich the lives of the entire family if accepted in the right context and dose by the family.

Nurses can assist in the grandparents' role transition by assessing their communication skills, role expectations, and support skills during the prenatal period. Find out whether the grandparents are included in the couple's social support network and whether their support is wanted or helpful. If they are, and it is, then encourage the grandparents to learn about the parenting, feeding, and child-rearing skills their children have learned in childbirth classes. This information is commonly found in "grandparenting" classes, which introduce new parenting concepts and bring the grandparents up to date on today's childbirth practices.

Teaching About Postpartum Blues

The postpartum period is typically a happy yet stressful time, because the birth of an infant is accompanied by enormous physical, social, and emotional changes. The postpartum woman may report feelings of emotional lability, such as crying 1 minute and laughing the next. (See Chapter 15 for **Postpartum Blues** discussion.) Although postpartum blues is usually benign and self-limited, these mood changes can be frightening to the woman. It is prudent to ask two questions—about having pleasure and interest in things, or feeling predominately down, depressed, or hopeless. Once postpartum blues are determined to be the likely cause of her mood symptoms, the nurse can offer anticipatory guidance that these mood swings are commonly experienced and usually resolve spontaneously within a week and offer reassurance. Women should also be counseled to seek further evaluation if these moods do not resolve within 2 weeks, as postpartum depression may be developing (King et al., 2015).

Take Note!

Postpartum blues have been regarded as brief, benign, and without clinical significance, but several studies have proposed a link between blues and subsequent depression in the 6 months following childbirth (Cristescu et al., 2015).

Postpartum blues require no formal treatment other than support and reassurance because they do not usually interfere with the woman's ability to function and care for her infant. Nurses can ease a mother's distress by encouraging her to vent her feelings and by demonstrating patience and understanding with her and her family. Suggest that getting outside help with housework and infant care might help her to feel less overwhelmed until the blues ease. Provide telephone numbers she can call when she feels down during the day. Making women aware of this disorder while they are pregnant will increase their knowledge about this mood disturbance, which may lessen their embarrassment and increase their willingness to ask for and accept help if it does occur.

The postpartum woman also is at risk for postpartum depression and postpartum psychosis; these conditions are discussed in Chapter 22.

Preparing for Discharge

The WHO recommends that the length of stay in the health care facility should be individualized for each mother and baby, but should be at least 24 hours after birth (2014b). A shortened hospital stay may be indicated if the following criteria are met:

- Mother is afebrile and vital signs are within normal range.
- Lochia is appropriate amount and color for stage of recovery.
- Hemoglobin and hematocrit values are within normal range.
- Uterine fundus is firm; urinary output is adequate.
- ABO blood groups and RhD status are known and, if indicated, anti-D immunoglobulin has been administered.
- Surgical wounds are healing and no signs of infection are present.
- Mother is able to ambulate without difficulty.
- Food and fluids are taken without difficulty.
- Self-care and infant care are understood and demonstrated.
- Family or other support system is available to care for both.
- Mother is aware of possible complications (WHO, 2014b)

Providing Immunizations

Prior to discharge, check the immunity status for rubella for all mothers and give a subcutaneous injection of rubella vaccine if they are not serologically immune (titer less than 1:8). Be sure that the client signs a consent form to receive the vaccine. The rubella vaccine should not be given to any woman who is immune compromised, and the immune status of her close contacts needs to be determined before any vaccine is administered to her to prevent a more virulent case of the vaccine-preventable illness or potential death. With the recent increase in the number of pertussis in infants younger than 3 months of age, the CDC is also recommending vaccination with (Tdap) (combination of diphtheria, pertussis, and tetanus vaccines) for the mother during her postpartum stay (CDC, 2015b). Nursing mothers can be vaccinated because the live, attenuated rubella virus is not communicable. Inform all mothers receiving immunization about adverse effects (rash, joint symptoms, and a low-grade fever 5 to 21 days later) and the need to avoid pregnancy for at least 28 days after being vaccinated because of the risk of teratogenic effects (CDC, 2015b).

Rh Status

If the client is Rh-negative, check the Rh status of the newborn. Verify that the woman is Rh-negative and has not been sensitized, that her indirect Coombs test (antibody screen) is negative, and that the newborn is Rh-positive. Mothers who are Rh-negative and have given birth to an infant who is Rh-positive should receive an injection of

Rh immunoglobulin within 72 hours after birth to prevent a sensitization reaction in the Rh-negative woman who received Rh-positive blood cells during the birthing process. Administering RhoGAM prevents initial isoimmunization in Rh-negative mothers by destroying fetal erythrocytes in the maternal system before maternal antibodies can develop and maternal memory cells become sensitized. This is a classic passive immunization technique. The usual protocol for the Rh-negative woman is to receive two doses of Rh immunoglobulin (RhoGAM), one at 28 weeks' gestation and the second dose within 72 hours after childbirth. The standard dose of Rho(D) immune globulin (RhoGAM) is 300 mcg given intramuscularly, which prevents the development of antibodies for an exposure of up to 15 mL of fetal red blood cells (King et al., 2015). A signed consent form is needed after a thorough explanation is provided about the procedure, including its purpose, possible adverse effects, and effect on future pregnancies.

RhoGam contains actual Rh antibodies produced by people who have become sensitized. It is therefore, a blood product. Each dose contains enough anti-D to suppress the immune response of 15 mL of Rh-positive red blood cells (Jordan et al., 2014). Jehovah's Witnesses and others who belong to religions prohibiting the use of blood products should consult their conscience and possibly ecclesiastical leaders about the use of RhoGam. Nurses need to respect whatever their decision is.

BOX 16.5

CHALLENGES FACING FAMILIES AFTER DISCHARGE

- Lack of role models for breast-feeding and infant care
- Lack of support from the new mother's own mother if she did not breast-feed
- Increased mobility of society, which means that extended family may live far away and cannot help care for the newborn and support the new family
- Feelings of isolation and limited community ties for women who work full time
- Shortened hospital stays: parents may be overwhelmed by all the information they are given in the brief hospital stay
- Prenatal classes usually focus on the birth itself rather than on skills needed to care for themselves and the newborn during the postpartum period
- Limited access to education and support systems for families from diverse cultures

Adapted from Bope, E., & Kellerman, R. (2015). *Conn's current therapy 2015*. Philadelphia, PA: Saunders Elsevier; and Bang, K., Huh, B., & Kwon, M. (2014). The effect of a postpartum nursing intervention program for immigrant mothers. *Child Health Nursing Research, 20*(1), 11–19.

Ensuring Follow-Up Care

New mothers and their families need to be attended to over an extended period of time by nurses knowledgeable about mother care, infant feeding (breast-feeding and bottle-feeding), infant care, and nutrition. Although continuous nursing care stops on discharge from the hospital or birthing center, extended episodic nursing care needs to be provided at home. Some of the challenges faced by families after discharge are described in Box 16.5.

Many new mothers are reluctant to "cut the cord" after their brief stay in the health care facility and need expanded community services. Women who are discharged too early from the hospital run the risk of uterine subinvolution, discomfort at an episiotomy or cesarean site, infection, fatigue, and maladjustment to their new role. Postpartum nursing care should include a range of family-focused care, including telephone calls, outpatient clinics, and home visits. Typically, public health nurses, community and home health nurses, and the health care provider's office staff will provide postpartum care after hospital discharge.

PROVIDING TELEPHONE FOLLOW-UP

Telephone follow-up typically occurs during the first week after discharge to check on how things are going at home. Calls can be made by perinatal nurses within the agency as part of follow-up care or by the local health department nurses. One disadvantage of a phone call assessment is that the nurse cannot see the client and thus must rely on the mother or the family's observations. The experienced nurse needs to be able to recognize distress and give appropriate advice and referral information if needed.

PROVIDING OUTPATIENT FOLLOW-UP

For mothers with established health care providers such as private pediatricians and obstetricians, visits to the office are arranged soon after discharge. For the woman with an uncomplicated vaginal birth, an office visit is usually scheduled for 4 to 6 weeks after childbirth. A woman who had a cesarean birth frequently is seen within 2 weeks after hospital discharge. Hospital discharge orders will specify when these visits should be made. Newborn examinations and further diagnostic laboratory studies are scheduled within the first week.

Take Note!

The hospital stay of the mother and her healthy term newborn should be long enough to allow identification of early problems and to ensure that the family is able and prepared to care for the infant at home (WHO, 2014b).

Outpatient clinics are available in many communities. If family members run into a problem, the local clinic is available to provide assessment and treatment. Clinic visits can replace or supplement home visits. Although these clinics are open during daytime hours only and the staff members are unfamiliar with the family, they can be a valuable resource for the new family with a problem or concern.

(text continues on page 589)

Maternal Assessment

Maternal/Newborn Record System

Page 1 of 2

PATIENT IDENTIFICATION

Record No. ______

Name ______

Home address ______ STREET

CITY STATE ZIP

Date MO / DAY / YR Time begin: ______ Date of delivery MO / DAY / YR

Time end: ______

Medication allergy ☐ None Identify ______

Significant health history ☐ None Identify ______

PHYSICAL

TEMP.	PULSE	RESP.	BP /

Breasts ☐ Nursing ☐ Non-nursing

Color ☐ Normal ☐ Reddened

Condition ☐ Soft ☐ Firm ☐ Engorged ☐ Blocked ducts

Secretion ☐ Colostrum ☐ Milk ☐ Other ______

Support bra ☐ No ☐ Yes, fit ☐ Appropriate ☐ Inappropriate

Nipples (If nursing) ☐ Erect ☐ Flat ☐ Inverted

Condition ☐ Intact ☐ Bruised ☐ Blistered ☐ Fissured ☐ Bleeding ☐ Scabbed

Care ☐ Water only ☐ Soap ☐ Air dry ☐ Topical agent (type/frequency) ______ ☐ Other ______

Self-exam ☐ Accurate ☐ Inaccurate/instructed

Abdomen

Diastasis recti ☐ Absent ☐ Present ______ cm ☐ Exercise taught

Incision ☐ None

Type ☐ Transverse ☐ Vertical ☐ Umbilical

Closure ☐ Staples ☐ Sutures ☐ Steri-strips

Condition ☐ Approximated ☐ Open ______ cm ☐ Redness ______ ☐ Swelling ______ ☐ Discharge ______ ☐ Other ______

Reproductive Tract

Uterus ☐ Firm ☐ Firm with massage ☐ Boggy

Height ______ ☐ Midline ☐ Displaced L R

☐ Non tender ☐ Tender ☐ With touch ☐ Constant

Lochia ☐ Rubra ☐ Serosa ☐ Alba ☐ Clots (describe) ______ ☐ Fleshy odor ☐ Foul odor

Pads Type ______ Number/day ______

Saturation % 0 25 50 75 100

Perineum ☐ Intact ☐ Laceration ☐ Episiotomy Type ______ Extension ______

Condition ☐ Redness ______ ☐ Edema ______ ☐ Ecchymosis ______ ☐ Discharge ______ ☐ Approximation ______

Care ☐ Front-to-back cleansing ☐ Peri-bottle ☐ Soap/water ☐ Ice ☐ Sitz bath ☐ Warm ☐ Cool ☐ Topical agent (type/frequency) ______ ☐ Other ______

Elimination

Urinary tract

Voiding pattern ☐ Normal ☐ Incontinence ☐ Bladder distention ☐ Catheter (type) ______

Signs of infection ☐ None/reviewed ☐ Urgency ☐ Frequency ☐ Dysuria ☐ CVA tenderness L R

Gastrointestinal tract

Bowel pattern ☐ Normal ☐ No BM ☐ Constipation ☐ Diarrhea ☐ Meds/treatments (type, frequency, effect) ______

Hemorrhoids ☐ No ☐ Yes (describe) ______ ☐ Meds/treatments (type, frequency, effect) ______

Lower Extremities

Edema ☐ None ☐ Pedal ☐ Ankle ☐ Pretibial ☐ Thigh ☐ Pitting (describe) ______

Signs of thrombophlebitis ☐ None

	L	R		L	R
Homan's sign	☐	☐	Redness	☐	☐
Pain	☐	☐	Warmth	☐	☐
Swelling	☐	☐			

Pain	No	Yes Managed	Yes Problematic
Abdominal incision	☐	☐	☐
Back	☐	☐	☐
Breasts	☐	☐	☐
Headache	☐	☐	☐
Hemorrhoid	☐	☐	☐
Nipple	☐	☐	☐
Perineum	☐	☐	☐
Uterine cramping	☐	☐	☐
Other ______	☐	☐	☐

Analgesic ☐ No ☐ Yes (type/dose/frequency) ______

Reportable danger signs ☐ Aware ☐ Unaware/instructed

TESTS ☐ None ☐ Urinalysis ☐ CBC ☐ ______

IDENTIFIED NEEDS

Signature ______

A

FIGURE 16.10 Sample postpartum home visit assessment form. A. Maternal assessment. B. Newborn assessment. (Used with permission: Copyright Briggs Corporation. Professional Nurse Associates.)

Maternal Assessment

Maternal/Newborn Record System

Page 2 of 2

PATIENT IDENTIFICATION

Record No. ________

Name ________

Home address ________ STREET

CITY STATE ZIP

ACTIVITIES OF DAILY LIVING - 24 HOUR HISTORY

Date MO / DAY / YR

Nutrition

Appetite ☐ Good ☐ Fair ☐ Poor

Usual pattern ☐ Yes ☐ No ________

Special diet ☐ No ☐ Yes ________

Food intolerance/allergy ☐ No ☐ Yes ________

Vitamin/mineral supplement ☐ No ☐ Yes ________

Fluid intake (type/amount) ________

BREAKFAST	LUNCH	DINNER	SNACKS

General Hygiene ☐ Adequate ☐ Inadequate (describe)

Sleep/Activity

Amount of Activity

Night, uninterrupted ________ hrs

Naps ☐ No ☐ Yes ________ hrs

Fatigue ☐ None ☐ Minimal ☐ Moderate ☐ Exhausted

Activities

Limitations ☐ None Identify ________

☐ Self-care ☐ Infant care

	Appropriate	Inappropriate/instructed
Stair climbing	☐	☐
Lifting	☐	☐
Household tasks	☐	☐
Outside home	☐	☐

Other ________

Exercise

☐ None

	Accurate	Inaccurate/instructed
Kegel	☐	☐
Postpartum	☐	☐

Other ________

PSYCHOLOGICAL

Review of Labor and Birth

Missing pieces ☐ No ☐ Yes

Unmet expectations ☐ No ☐ Yes

Unresolved feelings ☐ No ☐ Yes

Pertinent data ________

Postpartum Timetable (Key on reverse side)

☐ Taking in ☐ Taking hold ☐ Letting go

Emotional Status ☐ Happy ☐ Ambivalent ☐ Anxious ☐ Sad ☐ Other ________

Postpartum-depression (Key on reverse side)

☐ 0 ☐ 1 ☐ 2 ☐ 3 ☐ 4

☐ Signs/Symptoms Reviewed

General Comments (body image, role changes, concerns) ________

SEXUALITY

	Aware	Unaware/ instructed
Relationship with partner		
Adjustment	☐	☐
Expressions of affection	☐	☐
Resuming Intercourse		
Timing (lack of lochia, comfort)	☐	☐
Vaginal dryness	☐	☐
Milk ejection (if lactating)	☐	☐
Position variation	☐	☐
Libidinal changes	☐	☐
Return of Menses	☐	☐

Contraceptive Method

☐ None ☐ Undecided/aware of options

☐ Natural family planning

☐ Cervical cap

☐ Condom

☐ Diaphragm

☐ Hormones ☐ Pill ☐ Injection ☐ Implant

☐ IUD

☐ Spermicide

☐ Sterilization ☐ Female ☐ Male

☐ Other ________

Accurate use ☐ Yes ☐ No/instructed

IDENTIFIED NEEDS ________

Signature ________

FIGURE 16.10 *(continued)*

Maternal Assessment

Maternal/Newborn Record System

PATIENT IDENTIFICATION

Record No. ____________

Name ____________

Home address ____________ STREET

CITY STATE ZIP

Date MO / DAY / YR Time begin: ________ Date of Birth MO / DAY / YR

Time end: ________

Significant history ☐ None Identify ____________

PHYSICAL

Temp ________ Pulse (rate/rhythm) ________ Resp ________

Weight ________ Birth weight ________ % Change ________

Length ________ Head ________ Chest ________

HEAD/NECK

	Level	Bulging	Depressed
1. Fontanels			
Anterior	☐	☐	☐
Posterior	☐	☐	☐

Sutures ☐ Open ☐ Closed ☐ Overriding

2. Variations ☐ Molding ☐ Caput ☐ Cephalhematoma

	NORMAL	ABNORMAL	DETAIL VARIATIONS/ ABNORMAL FINDINGS
3. Face (symmetry)	☐	☐	
4. Eyes (symmetry, conjunctiva, sciera, eyelids, PERL)	☐	☐	
5. Ears (shape, position, auditory response)	☐	☐	
6. Nose (patency)	☐	☐	
7. Mouth (lip, mucous membranes, tongue, palate)	☐	☐	
8. Neck (ROM, symmetry)	☐	☐	
Chest			
9. Appearance (shape, breasts, nipples)	☐	☐	
10. Breath sounds	☐	☐	
11. Clavicles	☐	☐	
Cardiovascular			
12. Heart sounds	☐	☐	
13. Brachial/femoral pulses (compare strength, equality)	☐	☐	
Abdomen			
14. Appearance (shape, size)	☐	☐	
15. Cord (condition)	☐	☐	
16. Liver (less than or equal to 3 cm ↓ ®costal margin)	☐	☐	
Genitalia			
17. Female (labia, introitus, discharge	☐	☐	
18. Male (meatus, scrotum, testes)	☐	☐	
19. Circumcision ☐ No ☐ Yes	☐	☐	
Musculoskeletal			
20. Muscle tone	☐	☐	
21. Extremities (symmetry, digits, ROM)	☐	☐	
22. Hips (symmetry, ROM)	☐	☐	
23. Spine (alignment, integrity)	☐	☐	
Neurologic			
24. Reflexes (presence, symmetry)			
Moro	☐	☐	
Grasp	☐	☐	
Babinski	☐	☐	
25. Cry (presence, quality)	☐	☐	

PHYSICAL (CONT'D)

Skin

Turgor ☐ Good ☐ Poor

Condition ☐ Smooth ☐ Dry, cracked ☐ Peeling

Color ☐ Pink ☐ Ruddy ☐ Cyanotic ☐ Pale

☐ Jaundice (note levels)

- ☐ Head (3 mg/dl)
- ☐ Head and upper chest (6 mg/dl)
- ☐ Head and entire chest (9 mg/dl)
- ☐ Head, chest and abdomen to umbilicus (12 mg/dl)
- ☐ Head, chest and entire abdomen (15 mg/dl)
- ☐ Head, chest, abdomen, legs and feet (18 mg/dl)

Variations (Rashes, lesions, birthmarks). ____________

NUTRITION

Feeding

Reflexes ☐ Root ☐ Suck ☐ Swallow

Hunger cues identified ☐ Yes ☐ No/instructed

BREAST	FORMULA
Frequency ___ times in ___ hours	Type ________
Time per breast ___ min ___ min	Amount ________ oz.
Positioning ☐ Correct	Frequency ________
☐ Incorrect ________	Preparation ☐ Correct
Latch ☐ Correct	☐ Incorrect ________
☐ Incorrect ________	________
Appropriate audible swallows	☐ Correct
☐ Yes ☐ No ________	☐ ________

Satiation demonstrated ☐ Yes

☐ No (describe) ________

Regurgitation ☐ No ☐ Yes (describe) ________

Pacifier use ☐ No ☐ Yes (type/pattern) ________

Stool (number/day, color, consistency) ________

Urine (number/day, color) ________

BEHAVIOR

Sleep/Activity Pattern (24 hours)

Sleep (16–20 hrs) ☐ Yes ☐ No (describe) ________

Awake-alert (2–3 hrs) ☐ Yes ☐ No (describe) ________

Awake-crying (2–4 hrs) ☐ Yes ☐ No (describe) ________

Consolability (Key on reverse) ☐ 0 ☐ 1 ☐ 2 ☐ 3 ☐ 4

TESTS ☐ None Time

☐ Metabolic screen kit no. ________ ________

☐ Bilirubin ________

☐ Hematocrit ________

☐ ________ ________

☐ ________ ________

INENTIFIED NEEDS ________

Signature ________

B

FIGURE 16.10 *(continued)*

PROVIDING HOME VISIT FOLLOW-UP

Home visits are usually made within the first week after discharge to assess the mother and newborn. During the home visit, the nurse assesses for and manages common physical and psychosocial problems. In addition, the home nurse can help the new parents adjust to the change in their lives. The postpartum home visit usually includes the following:

- *Maternal assessment:* general well-being, vital signs, breast health and care, abdominal and musculoskeletal status, voiding status, fundus and lochia status, psychological and coping status, family relationships, proper feeding technique, environmental safety check, newborn care knowledge, and health teaching needed (Fig. 16.10 shows sample assessment forms.)
- *Infant assessment:* physical examination, general appearance, vital signs, home safety check, child development status, any education needed to improve parents' skills

The home care nurse must be prepared to support and educate the woman and her family in the following areas:

- Breast-feeding or bottle-feeding technique and procedures
- Appropriate parenting behavior and problem solving
- Maternal/newborn physical, psychosocial, and culture–environmental needs
- Emotional needs of the new family
- Warning signs of problems and how to prevent or eliminate them
- Sexuality issues, including contraceptive use
- Immunization needs for both mother and infant
- Family dynamics for smooth transition
- Links to health care providers and community resources

NURSING CARE PLAN 16.1

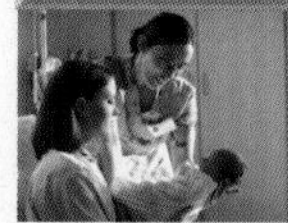

Overview of the Postpartum Woman

A 26-year-old G2P2, is a client on the mother–baby unit after giving birth to a term 8-lb, 12-oz baby boy yesterday. The night nurse reports that she has an episiotomy, complains of a pain rating of 7 points on a scale of 1 to 10, is having difficulty breast-feeding, and had heavy lochia most of the night. The nurse also reports that the client seems focused on her own needs and not on those of her infant. Assessment this morning reveals the following:

B: **Breasts** are soft with colostrum leaking; nipples cracked
U: **Uterus** is 1 fingerbreadth below the umbilicus; deviated to right
B: **Bladder** is palpable; client states she hasn't been up to void yet
B: **Bowels** have not moved; bowel sounds present; passing flatus
L: **Lochia** is moderate; peripad soaked from night accumulation
E: **Episiotomy** site intact; swollen, bruised; hemorrhoids present
E: **Extremities**; no edema over tibia, no warmth or tenderness in calf
E: **Emotional status** is "distressed" as a result of discomfort and fatigue

NURSING DIAGNOSIS: Impaired tissue integrity related to episiotomy

Outcome Identification and Evaluation

The client will remain free of infection, without any signs and symptoms of infection, and exhibit evidence of progressive healing as demonstrated by clean, dry, decreased/absent edema, and an intact episiotomy site.

Interventions: ***Promoting Tissue Integrity***

- Monitor episiotomy site for redness, edema, warmth, or discharge *to identify infection.*
- Assess vital signs at least every 4 hours *to identify changes suggesting infection.*
- Apply ice pack to episiotomy site *to reduce swelling.*
- Instruct client on use of sitz bath *to promote healing, hygiene, and comfort.*
- Encourage frequent perineal care and peripad changes *to prevent infection.*
- Recommend ambulation *to improve circulation and promote healing.*
- Instruct client on positioning *to relieve pressure on perineal area.*
- Demonstrate use of anesthetic sprays *to numb perineal area.*

(continued)

NURSING CARE PLAN 16.1

Overview of the Postpartum Woman (continued)

NURSING DIAGNOSIS: Pain related to episiotomy, sore nipples, and hemorrhoids

Outcome Identification and Evaluation

The client will experience a decrease in pain as evidenced by reporting that her pain has diminished to a tolerable level and rating it as 2 points or less.

Interventions: ***Providing Pain Relief***

- Thoroughly inspect perineum to rule out hematoma as cause of pain.
- Administer analgesic medication as ordered as needed to promote comfort.
- Carry out comfort measures to episiotomy as outlined earlier to reduce pain.
- Explain discomforts and reassure the client that they are time limited to assist in coping with pain.
- Apply Tucks® to swollen hemorrhoids to induce shrinkage and reduce pain.
- Suggest frequent use of sitz bath to reduce hemorrhoid pain.
- Administer stool softener and laxative to prevent straining with first bowel movement.
- Observe positioning and latching-on technique while breast-feeding. Offer suggestions based on observations to correct positioning/latching on to minimize trauma to the breast.
- Suggest air-drying of nipples after breast-feeding and use of plain water to prevent nipple cracking.
- Teach relaxation techniques when breast-feeding to reduce anxiety and discomfort.

NURSING DIAGNOSIS: Risk for ineffective coping related to mood alteration and pain

Outcome Identification and Evaluation

The client will cope with mood alterations, as evidenced by positive statements about newborn and participation in newborn care.

Interventions: ***Promoting Effective Coping***

- Provide a supportive, nurturing environment and encourage the mother to vent her feelings and frustrations *to relieve anxiety.*
- Provide opportunities for the mother to rest and sleep *to combat fatigue.*
- Encourage the mother to eat a well-balanced diet *to increase her energy level.*
- Provide reassurance and explanations that mood alterations are common after birth secondary to waning hormones after pregnancy *to increase the mother's knowledge.*
- Allow the mother relief from newborn care *to afford opportunity for self-care.*
- Discuss with partner expected behavior from mother and how additional support and help are needed during this stressful time *to promote partner's participation in care.*
- Make appropriate community referrals for mother–infant support *to ensure continuity of care.*
- Encourage frequent skin-to-skin contact and closeness between mother and infant *to facilitate bonding and attachment behaviors.*
- Encourage client to participate in infant care and provide instructions as needed *to foster a sense of independence and self-esteem.*
- Offer praise and reinforcement of positive mother–infant interactions *to enhance self-confidence in care.*

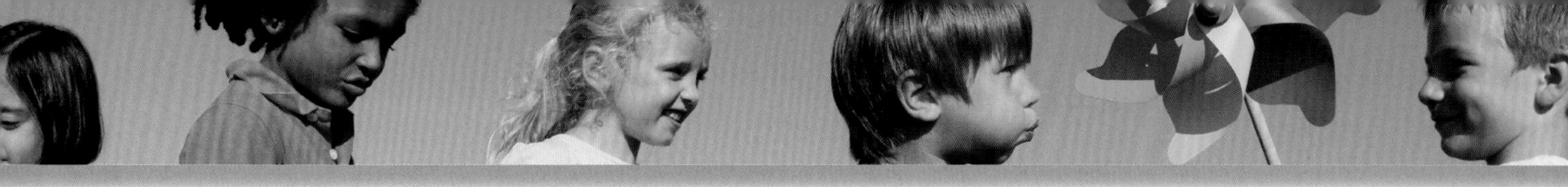

KEY CONCEPTS

- The transitional adjustment period between birth and parenthood includes education about baby care basics, the role of the new family, emotional support, breast-feeding or bottle-feeding support, and maternal mentoring.
- Sensitivity to how childbearing practices and beliefs vary for multicultural families and how best to provide appropriate nursing care to meet their needs are important during the postpartum period.
- A thorough postpartum assessment is key to preventing complications as is frequent hand hygiene by the nurse, especially between handling mothers and infants.
- The postpartum assessment that uses the acronym BUBBLE-EE (breasts, uterus, bowel, bladder, lochia, episiotomy/perineum/epidural site, extremities, and emotions) is a helpful guide in performing a systematic head-to-toe postpartum assessment.
- Lochia is assessed according to its amount, color, and change with activity and time. It proceeds from lochia rubra to serosa to alba.
- Because of shortened agency stays, nurses must use this brief time with the client to address areas of comfort, elimination, activity, rest and exercise, self-care, sexuality and contraception, nutrition, family adaptation, discharge, and follow-up.
- The AAP advocates breast-feeding for all full-term newborns, maintaining that, ideally, breast milk should be the sole nutrient for the first 6 months and continued with foods until 12 months of life or longer.
- Successful parenting is a continuous and complex interactive process that requires the acquisition of new skills and the integration of the new member into the existing family unit.
- Bonding is a vital component of the attachment process and is necessary in establishing parent–infant attachment and a healthy, loving relationship; attachment behaviors include seeking and maintaining proximity to, and exchanging gratifying experiences with, the infant.
- Nurses can be instrumental in facilitating attachment by first understanding attachment behaviors (positive and negative) of newborns and parents, and intervening appropriately to promote and enhance attachment.
- New mothers and their families need to be attended to over an extended period of time by nurses knowledgeable about mother care, newborn feeding (breast-feeding and bottle-feeding), newborn care, and nutrition.

REFERENCES AND RECOMMENDED READINGS

Allen, M., & Schafer, D. J. (2015). Nurses improving the health of mothers and infants by dancing the 10 steps to successful breastfeeding. *Journal of Obstetric, Gynecologic, & Neonatal Nursing, 44*, S52.

American Academy of Pediatrics [AAP]. (2014a). Iodine deficiency: Pregnant and breastfeeding women need supplementation. *AAP News*. Retrieved from http://aapnews.aappublications.org/content/35/6/11.1.extract

American Academy of Pediatrics [AAP]. (2014b). *Ten steps to support parent's choice to breastfeed their baby*. Retrieved from http://www2.aap.org/breastfeeding/files/pdf/tenstepsposter.pdf

American College of Obstetricians & Gynecologists [ACOG]. (2014). Challenges for overweight and obese women. *Obstetrics & Gynecology, 1234*(3), 726–730.

Andrews, M. M., & Boyle, J. S. (2012). *Transcultural concepts in nursing care* (6th ed.). Philadelphia, PA: Wolters Kluwer Health.

Baltes, P. B., Featherman, D. L., & Lerner, R. M. (2014). *Life-span development and behavior* (10th ed.). New York, NY: Psychology Press.

Bang, K., Huh, B., & Kwon, M. (2014). The effect of a postpartum nursing intervention program for immigrant mothers. *Child Health Nursing Research, 20*(1), 11–19.

Barnes, D. L. (2014). *Women's reproductive mental health across the lifespan*. New York, NY: Springer Publishers.

Bhati, S., & Richards, K. (2015). A systematic review of the relationship between postpartum sleep disturbance and postpartum depression. *JOGNN: Journal of Obstetric, Gynecologic & Neonatal Nursing, 44*(3), 350–357.

Bope, E., & Kellerman, R. (2015). *Conn's current therapy 2015*. Philadelphia, PA: Saunders Elsevier.

Bowers, P., & Ceballos, K. (2015). Cultural perspectives in childbearing. Retrieved from http://ce.nurse.com/ce263-60/Cultural-Perspectives-in-Childbearing

Brekke, H. K., Bertz, F., Rasmussen, K. M., Bosaeus, I., Ellegård, L., & Winkvist, A. (2014). Diet and exercise interventions among overweight and obese lactating women: Randomized trial of effects on cardiovascular risk factors. *Plos ONE, 9*(2), 1–8.

Campbell-Yeo, M. L., Disher, T. C., Benoit, B. L., & Johnston, C. C. (2015). Understanding kangaroo care and its benefits to preterm infants. *Pediatric Health, Medicine & Therapeutics, 6*, 15–33.

Centers for Disease Control and Prevention [CDC]. (2015a). Reproductive health. Retrieved from http://www.cdc.gov/reproductivehealth/unintendedpregnancy/usmec.htm

Centers for Disease Control and Prevention [CDC]. (2015b). Tdap for pregnant women: Information for providers. Retrieved from http://www.cdc.gov/vaccines/vpd-vac/pertussis/tdap-pregnancy-hcp.htm

Ciaghi, F., Bianco, A. D., & Guarese, O. (2015). Prevalence of pelvic floor disorders during the postpartum period. A prospective study and a proposal of a multidisciplinary prevention strategy. *Scienza Riabilitativa, 17*(1), 5–15.

Cleminson, J., Oddie, S., Renfrew, M. J., & McGuire, W. (2015). Being baby friendly: Evidence-based breastfeeding support. *Archives of Disease in Childhood-Fetal and Neonatal Edition, 100*(2), 173–178.

Covan, E. K. (2015). Benefits of exercise for body, mind, and spirit. *Health Care for Women International, 36*(3), 255.

Creasy, R. K., Resnik, R., Iams, J. D., Lockwood, C. J., Moore, T. R., & Greene, M. F. (2014). *Creasy & Resnik's maternal-fetal medicine: Principles and practice* (7th ed.). Philadelphia, PA: Elsevier Saunders.

Cristescu, T., Behrman, S., Jones, S. V., Chouliaras, L., & Ebmeier, K. P. (2015). Be vigilant for perinatal mental health problems. *The Practitioner, 259*(1780), 19–23.

Cunningham, F. G., Leveno, K. J., Bloom, S. L., Spong, C., Dashe, J. S., Hoffman, B. L., et al. (2014). *Williams' obstetrics* (24th ed.). New York, NY: McGraw-Hill Publishers.

Dayer-Berenson, L. (2014). *Cultural competencies of nurses: Impact on health and illness* (2nd ed.). Berlington, MA: Jones & Bartlett Learning.

Denne, S. C. (2015). Neonatal nutrition. *Pediatric Clinics of North America, 62*(2), 427–438.

Downs, D. S., Evenson, K. R., & Chasan-Taber, L. (2014). Obesity and physical activity during pregnancy and postpartum: Evidence, guidelines, and recommendations. In *Obesity during pregnancy in clinical practice* (pp. 183–227). London, England: Springer.

Dudek, S. G. (2014). *Nutrition essentials for nursing practice* (7th ed.). Philadelphia, PA: Lippincott Williams & Wilkins.

Edelman, C. L., Kudzma, E. C., & Mandle, C. L. (2014). *Health promotion throughout the lifespan* (8th ed.). St. Louis, MO: Elsevier Mosby.

Green, C. J. (2016). *Maternal-newborn nursing care plans* (3rd ed.). Burlington, MA: Jones & Bartlett Learning.

Halford, W. K., Petch, J., & Creedy, D. (2015). Caring and sexuality. In *Clinical guide to helping new parents* (pp. 131–150). New York, NY: Springer Publishers.

Hall, B., & Woodward, S. (2015). Pelvic floor muscle training for urinary incontinence postpartum. *British Journal of Nursing, 24*(11), 576–579.

Hugill, K. (2015). The senses of touch and olfaction in early mother-infant interaction. *British Journal of Midwifery, 23*(4), 238–243.

Jones, C., & Hawkes, R. (2015). Managing pregnancy-related pelvic floor dysfunction. *Primary Health Care, 25*(1), 24–28.

Jordan, R. G., Engstrom, J., Marfell, J., & Farley, C. L. (2014). *Prenatal & postnatal care: A women-centered approach*. Ames, IA: John Wiley & Sons.

Kim, Y. K., Kim, K. B., Kim, C. H., & Ha, H. (2015). Pulmonary embolism and uterine venous plexus thrombosis in the postpartum period. *Korean Journal of Legal Medicine, 39*(2), 41–44.

King, T. L., Brucker, M. C., Kriebs, J. M., Fahey, J. O., Gegor, C. L., & Varney, H. (2015). *Varney's midwifery* (5th ed.). Burlington, MA: Jones & Bartlett Learning.

Klebanov, M. S., & Travis, A. D. (2015). *The critical role of parenting in human development*. New York, NY: Routledge, Taylor & Francis Group.

Kline, J. A., & Kabrhel, C. (2015). Emergency evaluation for pulmonary embolism, Part 1: Clinical factors that increase risk. *The Journal of Emergency Medicine, 49*(1), 104–117.

Laliberte, R. (2015). Leaky bladder. *Prevention, 67*(7), 52–54.

Lee, A., & Brann, L. (2015). Influence of cultural beliefs on infant feeding, postpartum and childcare practices among Chinese-American mothers in New York City. *Journal of Community Health, 40*(3), 476–483.

Lee, L. A., Carter, M., Stevenson, S. B., & Harrison, H. (2014). Improving family-centered care practices in the NICU. *Neonatal Network, 33*(3), 125–132.

Lewis, M., & Rudolph, K. D. (2014). *Handbook of developmental psychopathology* (3rd ed.). New York, NY: Springer Publishers.

Lickenbrock, D. M., & Braungart-Rieker, J. M. (2015). Examining antecedents of infant attachment security with mothers and fathers: An ecological systems perspective. *Infant Behavior & Development, 39*, 173–187.

Lönnerdal, B., & Hernell, O. (2015). An opinion on" staging" of infant formula-A developmental perspective on infant feeding. *Journal of Pediatric Gastroenterology and Nutrition*, 62(1), 9–21.

Masho, S. W., Cha, S., & Morris, M. R. (2015). Prepregnancy obesity and breastfeeding non-initiation in the United States: An examination of racial and ethnic differences. *Breastfeeding Medicine, 10*(5), 253–262.

Mattson, S., & Smith, J. E. (2016). *Core curriculum for maternal-newborn nursing* (5th ed.). St. Louis, MO: Saunders Elsevier.

McComish, J. F. (2015). Infant mental health and attachment. *Journal of Child & Adolescent Psychiatric Nursing, 28*(2), 63–64.

McFarland, M. R., & Wehbe-Alamah, H. B. (2015). *Leininger's cultural care and diversity and universality: A worldwide nursing theory* (3rd ed.). Burlington, MA: Jones & Bartlett Learning.

Mercer, R. T. (2006). Nursing support of the process of becoming a mother. *Journal of Obstetric, Gynecologic, and Neonatal Nursing, 35*(5), 649–651.

Mooventhan, A., & Nivethitha, L. (2014). Scientific evidence-based effects of hydrotherapy on various systems of the body. *North American Journal of Medical Sciences, 6*(5), 199–209.

Moses, S. (2014). Formula feeding. *Family Practice Notebook*. Retrieved from http://www.fpnotebook.com/pharm/NICU/FrmlFdng.htm

Nagtalon-Ramos, J. (2014). *Best evidence-based practices in maternal-newborn nursing care*. Philadelphia, PA: F. A. Davis Company.

Neville, C., McKinley, M., Holmes, V., Spence, D., & Woodside, J. (2014). The effectiveness of weight management interventions in breastfeeding women-a systematic review and critical evaluation. *Birth, 41*(3), 223–236.

Parfitt, Y., & Ayers, S. (2014). Transition to parenthood and mental health in first-time parents. *Infant Mental Health Journal, 35*, 263–273.

Park, S., Kim, S., & Kang, K. (2014). Integrative review of nursing intervention studies on mother-infant interactions. *Child Health Nursing Research, 20*(2), 75–86.

Parker, C., Warmuskerken, G., & Sinclair, L. (2015). Enhancing neonatal wellness with home visitation. *Nursing for Women's Health, 19*(1), 36–45.

Purnell, L. D. (2014). *Guide to culturally competent health care* (3rd ed.). Philadelphia, PA: F. A. Davis.

Santiago, M., & Figueiredo, M. (2015). Immigrant women's perspective on prenatal and postpartum care: Systematic review. *Journal of Immigrant & Minority Health, 17*(1), 276–284.

Sears, R. W., & Sears, J. M. (2015a). Bonding – What it means. Retrieved from http://www.askdrsears.com/topics/pregnancy-childbirth/tenth-month-post-partum/bonding-with-your-newborn/bonding-what-it-means

Sears, R. W., & Sears, J. M. (2015b). Attachment parenting. Retrieved from http://www.askdrsears.com/topics/parenting/attachment-parenting

Sears, R. W., & Sears, J. M. (2015c). Introducing a new baby: 11 smooth-entry tips. Retrieved from http://www.askdrsears.com/topics/parenting/discipline-behavior/bothersome-behaviors/sibling-rivalry/introducing-new-baby-11

Sette, G., Coppola, G., & Cassibba, R. (2015). The transmission of attachment across generations: The state of art and new theoretical perspectives. *Scandinavian Journal of Psychology, 56*(3), 315–326.

Shannon, C., Chao, M., & Ramos, D. E. (2015). A gap analysis of effective interventions for postpartum weight loss in obese new mothers. *Obstetrics & Gynecology, 125*, 56–59.

Skidmore-Roth, L. (2015). *Mosby's 2015 nursing drug reference* (28th ed.). St. Louis, MO: Mosby Elsevier.

Stagg, J., & Ustianov, J. (2015). Improving and sustaining breastfeeding practices through a statewide learning collaborative. *Journal of Obstetric, Gynecologic, & Neonatal Nursing, 44*, S55.

Sucker, C., & Zotz, R. B. (2015). Prophylaxis and treatment of venous thrombosis and pulmonary embolism in pregnancy. *Reviews in Vascular Medicine, 3*(2), 24–30.

Sukhwinder, K., Poonam, S., Sulakshna, C., & Jodibala, H. (2014). Comparison of infrared light therapy vs sitz bath on episiotomy in terms of wound healing and intensity of pain among postnatal mothers. *International Journal of Nursing Care, 2*(1), 37–41.

Tester-Jones, M., O'Mahen, H., Watkins, E., & Karl, A. (2015). The impact of maternal characteristics, infant temperament and contextual factors on maternal responsiveness to infant. *Infant Behavior & Development, 40*, 1–11.

U.S. Department of Agriculture [USDA] & U.S. Department of Health and Human Services [USDHHS]. (2014). Choose MyPlate. Center for Nutrition Policy and Promotion. Retrieved from http://www.DietaryGuidelines.gov

U.S. Department of Health and Human Resources [USDHHS]. (2010). Healthy people 2020. Retrieved from http://www.healthypeople.gov/2020/topicsobjectives2020

Verghese, T. S., Futaba, K., & Latthe, P. (2015). Constipation in pregnancy. *The Obstetrician & Gynecologist, 17*(2), 111–115.

Walker, L. O., Murphey, C. L., & Nichols, F. (2015). The broken thread of health promotion and disease prevention for women during the postpartum period. *Journal of Perinatal Education, 24*(2), 81–92.

Whittock, J. (2015). Promoting sexual health: Sex after childbirth. *MIDIRS Midwifery Digest, 25*(1), 77–80.

Wilson, B. L., Passante, T., Rauschenbach, D., Yang, R., & Wong, B. (2015). Bladder management with epidural anesthesia: A randomized controlled trial. *MCN. The American Journal of Maternal Child Nursing, 40*(4), 234–242.

World Health Organization [WHO]. (2014a). Implementation of the baby-friendly hospital initiative. Retrieved from http://www.who.int/elena/bbc/implementation_bfhi/en/

World Health Organization [WHO]. (2014b). WHO recommendations on postnatal care of the mother and newborn. Retrieved from http://apps.who.int/iris/bitstream/10665/97603/1/9789241506649_eng.pdf

Zapata, L. B., Murtaza, S., Whiteman, M. K., Jamieson, D. J., Robbins, C. L., Marchbanks, P. A., et al. (2015). Contraceptive counseling and postpartum contraceptive use. *American Journal of Obstetrics and Gynecology, 212*(2), 171–179.

CHAPTER WORKSHEET

MULTIPLE-CHOICE QUESTIONS

1. When assessing a postpartum woman, which of the following would lead the nurse to suspect postpartum blues?
   a. Panic attacks and suicidal thoughts
   b. Anger toward self and infant
   c. Periodic crying and insomnia
   d. Obsessive thoughts and hallucinations

2. Which of these activities would best help the postpartum nurse to provide culturally sensitive care for the childbearing family?
   a. Taking a transcultural course
   b. Caring for only families of his or her cultural origin
   c. Teaching Western beliefs to culturally diverse families
   d. Educating himself or herself about diverse cultural practices

3. Which of the following suggestions would be most appropriate to include in the teaching plan for a postpartum woman who needs to lose weight?
   a. Increase fluid intake and acid-producing foods in her diet.
   b. Avoid empty-calorie foods, breast-feed, increase exercise.
   c. Start a high-protein, low carbohydrate diet and restrict fluids.
   d. Eat no snacks or carbohydrates after dinner.

4. After teaching a group of breast-feeding women about nutritional needs, the nurse determines that the teaching was successful when the women state that they need to increase their intake of which nutrients?
   a. Carbohydrates and fiber
   b. Fats and vitamins
   c. Calories and protein
   d. Iron-rich foods and minerals

5. Which of the following would lead the nurse to suspect that a postpartum woman was developing a complication?
   a. Fatigue and irritability
   b. Perineal discomfort and pink discharge
   c. Pulse rate of 60 bpm
   d. Swollen, tender, hot area on breast

6. Which of the following would the nurse assess as indicating positive bonding between the parents and their newborn?
   a. Holding the infant close to the body
   b. Having visitors hold the infant
   c. Buying expensive infant clothes
   d. Requesting that the nurses care for the infant

7. Which activity would the nurse include in the teaching plan for parents with a newborn and an older child to reduce sibling rivalry when the newborn is brought home?
   a. Punishing the older child for bedwetting behavior
   b. Sending the sibling to the grandparents' house
   c. Planning a daily "special time" for the older sibling
   d. Allowing the sibling to share a room with the infant

8. The major purpose of the first postpartum homecare visit is to:
   a. Identify complications that require interventions
   b. Obtain a blood specimen for PKU testing
   c. Complete the official birth certificate
   d. Support the new parents in their parenting roles

9. The nurse is instructing the postpartum client who plans to bottle-feed her newborn about measures to prevent breast engorgement when she is discharged. Which of the following measures should the nurse include in the teaching plan?
   a. Decreasing her fluid intake for the first week at home
   b. Wearing a tight-fitting supportive bra 24 hours daily
   c. Take a diuretic to release the extra fluid in the breasts
   d. Manually express the milk that is accumulating

10. A new mother was brought to the postpartum unit who gave birth 12 hours ago. Because this is her first child, which of the following goals by the nurse is most appropriate?
    a. Early discharge for the mother and newborn
    b. Rapid transition into her role of being a parent/caretaker
    c. Minimal need for expression of her feelings now
    d. Effective education of both parents before discharge

CHAPTER WORKSHEET

CRITICAL THINKING EXERCISES

1. As a nurse working on a postpartum unit, you enter the room of, a 22-year-old primipara, and find her chatting on the phone while her newborn is crying loudly in the bassinette, which has been pushed into the bathroom. You pick up and comfort the newborn. While holding the baby, you ask the client if she was aware her newborn was crying. She replies, "That's about all that monkey does since she was born!" You hand the newborn to her and she places the newborn on the bed away from her and continues her phone conversation.
   a. What is your nursing assessment of this encounter?
   b. What nursing interventions would be appropriate?
   c. What specific discharge interventions may be needed?
2. A 34-year-old single primipara, left the hospital after a 36-hour stay with her newborn son. She lives alone in a one-bedroom walk-up apartment. As the postpartum home health nurse visiting her 2 days later, you find the following:
   - Tearful client pacing the floor holding her crying son
   - Home cluttered and in disarray
   - Fundus firm and displaced to right of midline
   - Moderate lochia rubra; episiotomy site clean, dry, and intact
   - Vital signs within normal range; pain rating less than 3 points on scale of 1 to 10
   - Breasts engorged slightly; supportive bra on
   - Newborn assessment within normal limits
   - Distended bladder upon palpation; reporting urinary frequency

   a. Which of these assessment findings warrants further investigation?
   b. What interventions are appropriate at this time, and why?
   c. What health teaching is needed before you leave this home?
3. The nurse walks into the room of a 24-year-old primigravida. She asks the nurse to hand her the bottle sitting on the bedside table, stating, "I'm going to finish it off because my baby only ate half of it 3 hours ago when I fed him."
   a. What response by the nurse would be appropriate at this time?
   b. What action should the nurse take?
   c. What health teaching is needed for this new mother prior to discharge?

STUDY ACTIVITIES

1. Identify two questions that a nurse would ask a postpartum woman to assess for postpartum blues.
2. Find a website that offers advice to new parents about breast-feeding. Critique the site, the author's credentials, and the accuracy of the content.
3. Outline instructions you would give to a new mother on how to use her peribottle.
4. Breast tissue swelling secondary to vascular congestion after childbirth and preceding lactation describes ____________________.
5. Listen to the postpartum story of one of your assigned clients and share it with your peers in class or as part of online discussion.

BRINGING IT ALL TOGETHER: A CASE STUDY

A 26-year-old African-American woman gave birth to a healthy term neonate yesterday and is preparing for discharge. The mother is illiterate and lives in a poor agricultural area of town not far from the hospital. This is her fourth infant in 5 years. The postpartum nurse comes into the room and observes that this mother has wrapped a piece of unclean cloth tightly around the infant's abdomen with a quarter which covers the cord stump. The take-home infant outfit is not clean and not appropriate for the weather conditions outside. The mother is waiting for a ride home from a friend. The postpartum nurse is here to provide her with discharge instructions.

Go to thePoint to find questions to consider about this case.

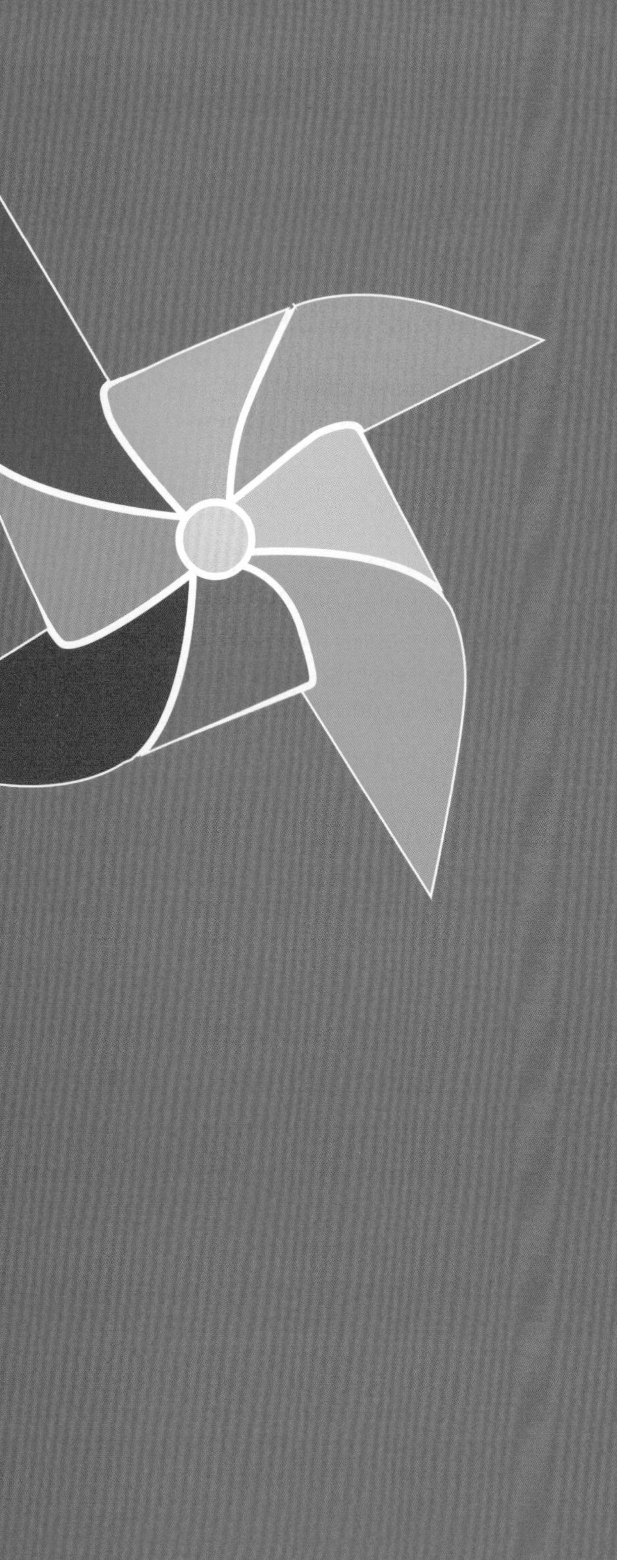

The Newborn

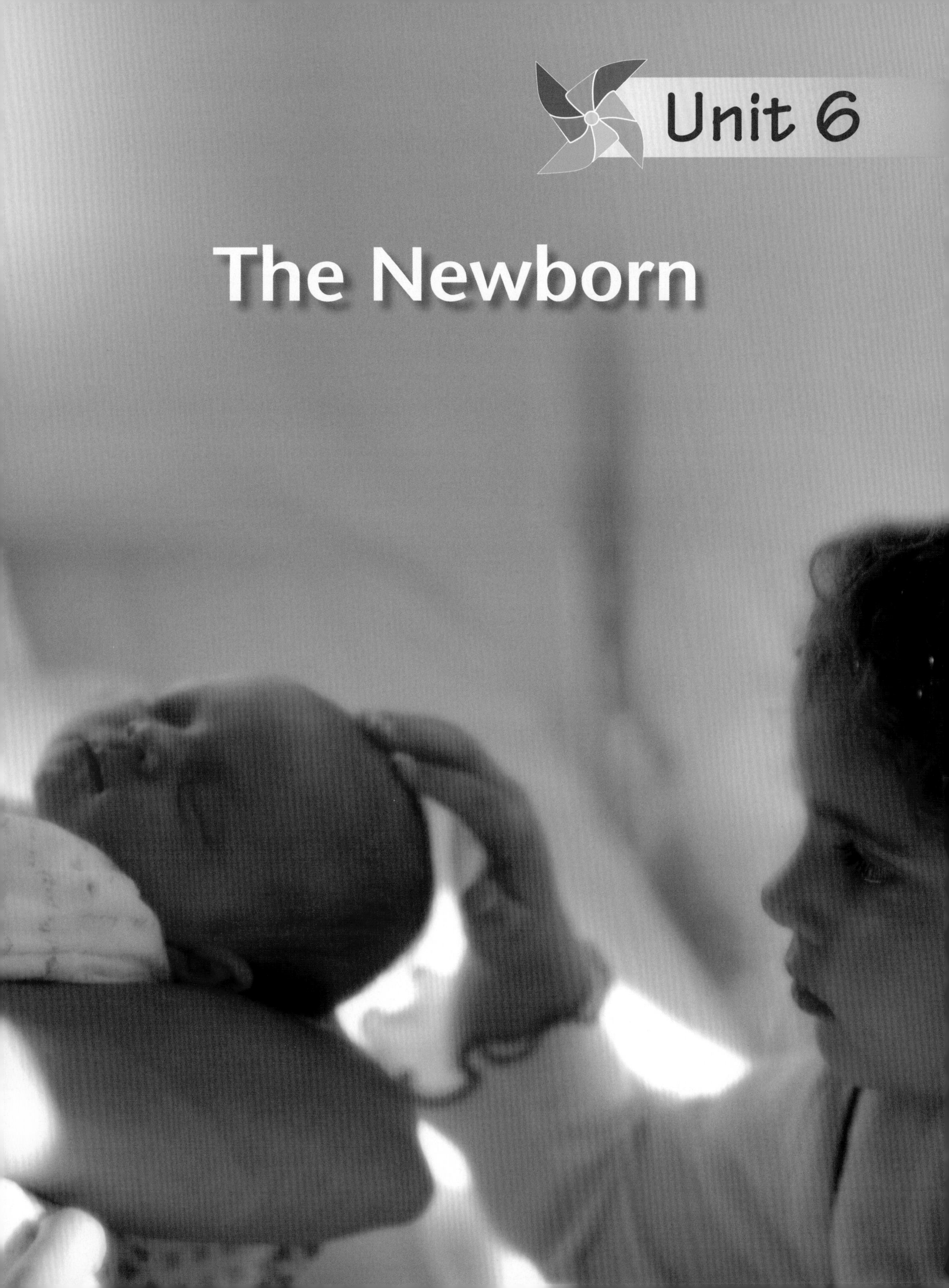

17

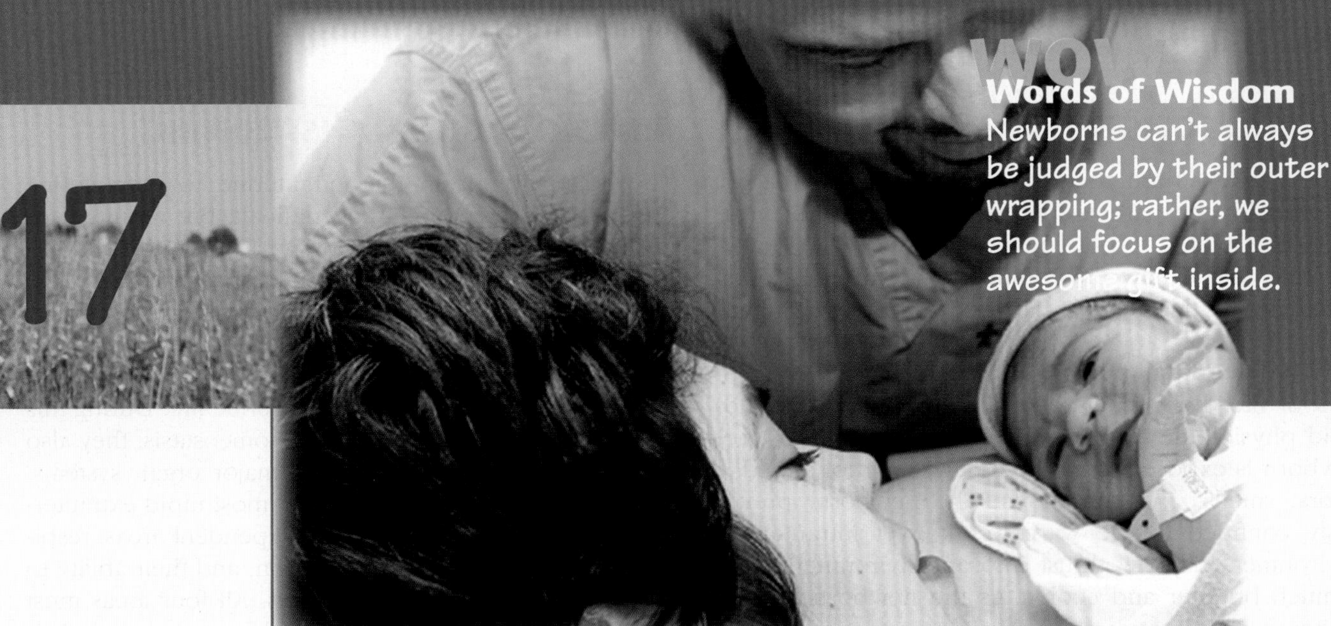
WOW
Words of Wisdom
Newborns can't always be judged by their outer wrapping; rather, we should focus on the awesome gift inside.

Newborn Transitioning

KEY TERMS

cold stress
jaundice
meconium
neonatal period
neurobehavioral response
neutral thermal environment
periodic breathing
reflex
surfactant
thermoregulation

Learning Objectives

Upon completion of the chapter, you will be able to:

1. Examine the major physiologic changes that occur as the newborn transitions to extrauterine life.
2. Determine the primary challenges faced by the newborn during the transition to extrauterine life.
3. Interpret the factors that influence the initiation of newborn respirations.
4. Compare and contrast the cardiovascular changes that take place from fetal circulation to extrauterine circulation after birth.
5. Relate three characteristics that predispose newborns to heat loss after birth.
6. Distinguish three primary immunoglobulins that help strengthen the newborn's immunologic system.
7. Differentiate the three behavioral patterns that newborns progress through after birth.
8. Assess the five typical behavioral responses triggered by external stimuli of the newborn.

The Healthy Start home care nurse reviewed the client's file in her car before she got out: 18-year-old primipara, 1 week postpartum with a term newborn girl weighing 7 lb. The new mother, Maria, greeted the nurse at the door and let her inside the house. After performing a postpartum assessment on Maria and an assessment of her newborn daughter, the nurse asked Maria if she had any questions or concerns. Maria's eyes welled up with tears: she is worried that her daughter can't see.

INTRODUCTION

When a child is born, the exhaustion and stress of labor are over for the parents, but now the newborn must begin the work of physiologically and behaviorally adapting to the new environment. The first 24 hours of life can be the most precarious (Swanson & Sinkin, 2015).

The **neonatal period** is defined as the first 28 days of life. It is a period of the most dramatic and rapid physiologic changes in humans. After birth, the newborn is exposed to a whole new world of sounds, colors, smells, and sensations. The newborn, previously confined to the warm, dark, wet intrauterine environment, is now thrust into an environment that is much brighter and cooler. As the newborn adapts to life after birth, numerous physiologic changes occur (Table 17.1).

Awareness of the adaptations that are occurring forms the foundation for providing support to the newborn during this crucial time. Physiologic and behavioral changes occur quickly during this transition period. Being aware of any deviations from the norm is crucial to ensure early identification and prompt intervention.

This chapter describes the physiologic changes of the newborn's major body systems. It also discusses the behavioral adaptations, including behavioral patterns and the newborn's behavioral responses, which occur during this transition period.

PHYSIOLOGIC TRANSITIONING

The adaptation from the intrauterine to extrauterine environment is complex and difficult, but required for all humans. Maternal medical and fetal conditions can have a profound effect on the successful transition. The mechanics of birth require a change in the newborn for survival outside the uterus. Immediately at birth, respiratory gas exchange, along with circulatory modifications, must occur to sustain extrauterine life. During this time, as newborns strive to attain homeostasis, they also experience complex changes in major organ systems. The newborn's most dramatic and most rapid extrauterine transitions occur in four interdependent areas: respiratory, circulatory, thermoregulation, and their ability to stabilize their blood glucose levels. All four areas must all make successful transitions for the newborn to adapt to extrauterine life. Although the transition usually takes place within the first 6 to 10 hours of life, many adaptations take weeks to attain full maturity.

Cardiovascular System Adaptations

During fetal life, the heart relies on certain unique structures that assist it in providing adequate perfusion of vital body parts. The umbilical vein carries oxygenated blood from the placenta to the fetus. The ductus venosus allows the majority of the umbilical vein blood to bypass the liver and merge with blood moving through the vena

TABLE 17.1 ANATOMIC AND PHYSIOLOGIC COMPARISON OF THE FETUS AND NEWBORN

Topic of Comparison	Fetus	Newborn
Respiratory system	Fluid-filled, high-pressure system causes blood to be shunted from the lungs through the ductus arteriosus to the rest of the body.	Air-filled, low-pressure system encourages blood flow through the lungs for gas exchange; increased oxygen content of blood in the lungs contributes to the closing of the ductus arteriosus (becomes a ligament).
Site of gas exchange	Placenta	Lungs
Circulation through the heart	Pressures in the right atrium are greater than in the left, encouraging blood flow through the foramen ovale.	Pressures in the left atrium are greater than in the right, causing the foramen ovale to close.
Hepatic portal circulation	Ductus venosus bypasses; maternal liver performs filtering functions.	Ductus venosus closes (becomes a ligament); hepatic portal circulation begins.
Thermoregulation	Body temperature is maintained by maternal body temperature and the warmth of the intrauterine environment.	Body temperature is maintained through a flexed posture and brown fat.

Adapted from Sharma, A., Ford, S., & Calvert, J. (2014). Adaptation for life: A review of neonatal physiology. *Anesthesia & Intensive Care Medicine, 15*(3), 89–95; Stave, U. (2014). *Perinatal physiology*. New York, NY: Springer Publishers; and King, T. L., Brucker, M. C., Kriebs, J. M., Fahey, J. O., Gegor, C. L., & Varney, H. (2015). *Varney's midwifery* (5th ed.). Burlington, MA: Jones & Bartlett Learning.

cava, bringing it to the heart sooner. The foramen ovale allows more than half the blood entering the right atrium to cross immediately to the left atrium, bypassing the pulmonary circulation. The ductus arteriosus connects the pulmonary artery to the aorta, which allows bypassing of the pulmonary circuit. Only a small portion of blood passes through the pulmonary circuit for the main purpose of perfusion of the structure, rather than for oxygenation. The fetus depends on the placenta to provide oxygen and nutrients and to remove waste products.

At birth, the circulatory system must switch from fetal to newborn circulation and from placental to pulmonary gas exchange. Successful transition from fetal to postnatal circulation requires increased pulmonary blood flow, removal of the placenta, and closure of the intracardiac (foramen ovale) and extracardiac shunts (ductus venosus and ductus arteriosus). These changes are needed to equalize the right ventricular output with that of the left (Steinhorn, 2015). The physical forces of the contractions of labor and birth, mild asphyxia, increased intracranial pressure as a result of cord compression and uterine contractions, and the cold stress experienced immediately after birth lead to an increased release of catecholamines that is critical for the changes involved in the transition to extrauterine life. The increased levels of epinephrine and norepinephrine stimulate increased cardiac output and contractility, surfactant release, and promotion of pulmonary fluid clearance (Sharma, Ford, & Calvert, 2014).

Fetal to Neonatal Circulation Changes

Changes in circulation occur immediately at birth as the fetus separates from the placenta (Fig. 17.1). When the umbilical cord is clamped, the first breath is taken and the lungs begin to function. As a result, systemic vascular resistance increases and blood return to the heart via the inferior vena cava decreases. Concurrently with these changes, there is a rapid decrease in pulmonary vascular resistance and an increase in pulmonary blood flow (Cuneo, 2014). The foramen ovale functionally closes with a decrease in pulmonary vascular resistance, which leads to a decrease in right-sided heart pressures. An increase in systemic pressure, after clamping of the cord, leads to an increase in left-sided heart pressures. The ductus arteriosus, ductus venosus, and umbilical vessels that were vital during fetal life are no longer needed. Over a period of months these fetal vessels form nonfunctional ligaments.

Before birth, the foramen ovale allowed most of the oxygenated blood entering the right atrium from the inferior vena cava to pass into the left atrium of the heart. With the newborn's first breath, air pushes into the lungs, triggering an increase in pulmonary blood flow and pulmonary venous return to the left side of the heart. As a result, the pressure in the left atrium becomes higher than in the right atrium. The increased left atrial pressure causes the foramen ovale to close, thus allowing the output from the right ventricle to flow entirely to the lungs. With closure of this fetal shunt, oxygenated blood is now separated from nonoxygenated blood. The subsequent increase in tissue oxygenation further promotes the increase in systemic blood pressure and continuing blood flow to the lungs. The foramen ovale normally closes functionally at birth when left atrial pressure increases and right atrial pressure decreases. Permanent anatomic closure, though, really occurs throughout the next several weeks.

During fetal life, the ductus arteriosus, located between the aorta and the pulmonary artery, protected the lungs against circulatory overload by shunting blood (right to left) into the descending aorta, bypassing the pulmonary circulation. Its patency during fetal life is promoted by continual production of prostaglandin E2 (PGE2) by the ductus arteriosus (van Vonderen et al., 2014). The ductus arteriosus becomes functionally closed within the first few hours after birth. Oxygen is the most important factor in controlling its closure. Closure depends on the high oxygen content of the aortic blood that results from aeration of the lungs at birth. At birth, pulmonary vascular resistance decreases, allowing pulmonary blood flow to increase and oxygen exchange to occur in the lungs. It occurs secondary to an increase in PO_2 coincident with the first breath and umbilical cord occlusion when it is clamped.

The ductus venosus shunted blood from the left umbilical vein to the inferior vena cava during intrauterine life. It closes within a few days after birth, because this shunting is no longer needed as a result of activation of the liver. The activated liver now takes over the functions of the placenta (which was expelled at birth). The ductus venosus becomes a ligament in extrauterine life.

The two umbilical arteries and one umbilical vein begin to constrict at birth, because with placental expulsion, blood flow ceases. In addition, peripheral circulation increases. Thus, the vessels are no longer needed and they too become ligaments. Successful transition and closure of the three fetal shunts creates a neonatal circulation where deoxygenated blood returns to the heart through the inferior and superior vena cava. It enters the right atrium to the right ventricle and travels through the pulmonary artery to the pulmonary vascular bed. Oxygenated blood returns through pulmonary veins to the left atrium, the left ventricle, and through the aorta to the systemic circulation (Stave, 2014). Box 17.1 provides a summary of fetal to neonatal circulation.

Heart Rate

During the first few minutes after birth, the newborn's heart rate is approximately 110 to 160 bpm. Thereafter, it begins to decrease to an average of 120 to 130 bpm

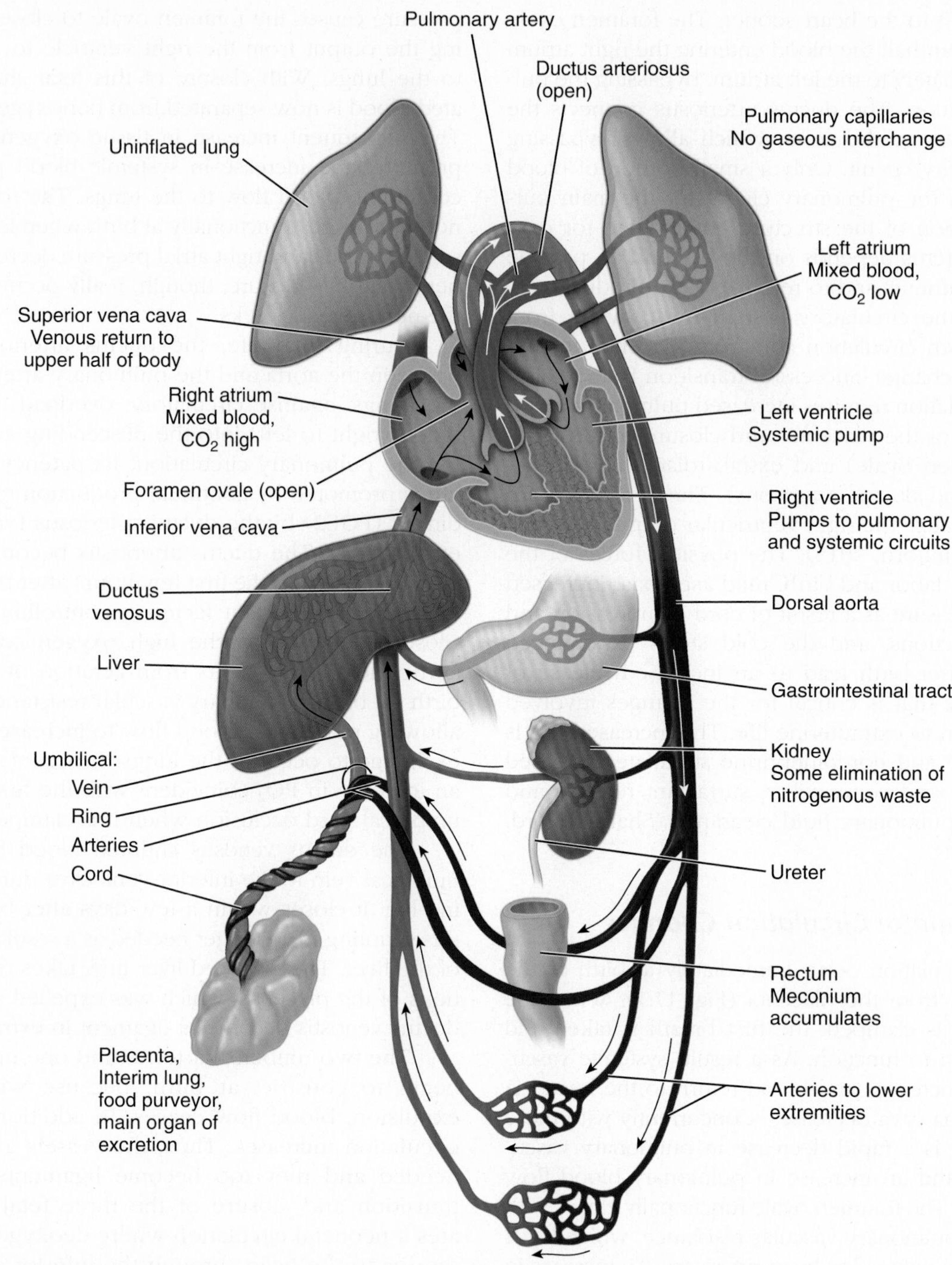

FIGURE 17.1 Cardiovascular adaptations of the newborn. Note the changes in oxygenation between (A) prenatal circulation and (B) postnatal (pulmonary) circulation.

(Creasy et al., 2014). The newborn is highly dependent on heart rate for maintenance of cardiac output and blood pressure. Although the blood pressure is not taken routinely in the healthy term newborn, it is usually highest after birth and reaches a plateau within a week after birth. Cardiac defects may be identified in the newborn nursery by conducting a thorough and systematic physical assessment, including inspection, palpation, auscultation, and measurement of blood pressure and oxygen saturations. The ability of the nurse to identify irregular findings during physical assessment aids rapid identification and treatment.

Take Note!

Transient functional cardiac murmurs may be heard during the neonatal period as a result of the changing dynamics of the cardiovascular system at birth (Fillipps & Bucciarelli, 2015).

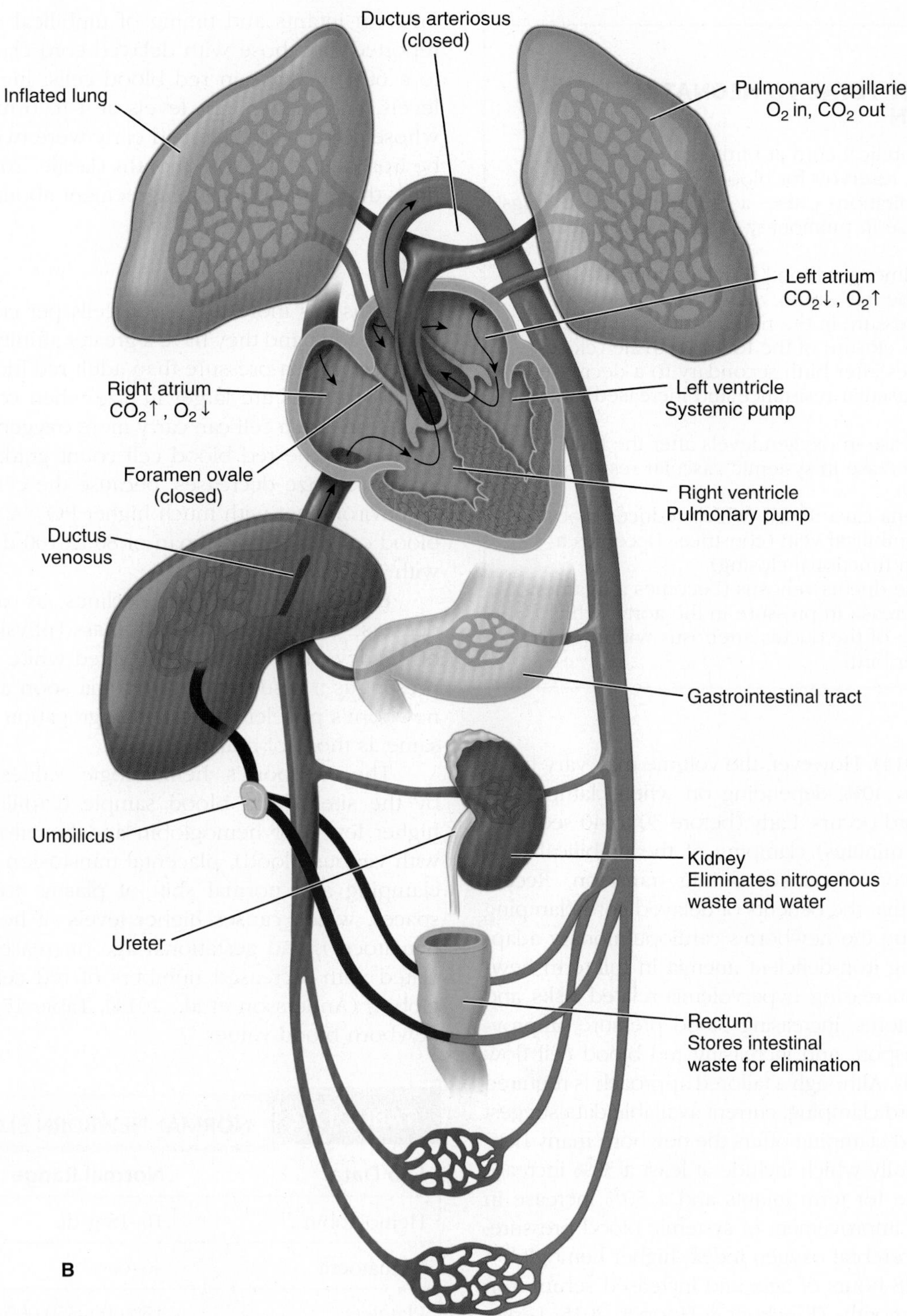

FIGURE 17.1 *(continued)*

The fluctuations in both the heart rate and blood pressure tend to follow the changes in the newborn's behavioral state. An increase in activity, such as wakefulness, movement, or crying, corresponds to an increase in heart rate and blood pressure. In contrast, the compromised newborn demonstrates markedly less physiologic variability overall. Tachycardia may be found with volume depletion, cardiorespiratory disease, drug withdrawal, and hyperthyroidism. Bradycardia is often associated with apnea and is often seen with hypoxia.

Blood Volume

The blood volume of the newborn depends on the amount of blood transferred from the placenta at birth. It is usually estimated to be 80 to 85 mL/kg of body weight in the term

BOX 17.1

SUMMARY OF FETAL TO NEONATAL CIRCULATION

- Clamping umbilical cord at birth eliminates the placenta as a reservoir for blood.
- Onset of respirations causes a rise in PO_2 in the lungs and a decrease in pulmonary vascular resistance, *which...*
- Increases pulmonary blood flow and increases pressure in the left atrium, *which...*
- Decreases pressure in the right atrium of the heart, which causes closure of the foramen ovale (closes within minutes after birth secondary to a decreased pulmonary vascular resistance and increased left heart pressure).
- With an increase in oxygen levels after the first breath, an increase in systemic vascular resistance occurs, *which...*
- Decreases vena cava return, which reduces blood flow in the umbilical vein (constricts, becomes a ligament with functional closing).
- Closure of the ductus venosus (becomes a ligament) causes an increase in pressure in the aorta, which forces closure of the ductus arteriosus within 10 to 15 hours after birth.

infant (Stave, 2014). However, the volume may vary by as much as 25% to 40%, depending on when clamping of the umbilical cord occurs. Early (before 30 to 40 seconds) or late (after 3 minutes) clamping of the umbilical cord changes circulatory dynamics during transition. Recent studies indicate that the benefits of delayed cord clamping include improving the newborn's cardiopulmonary adaptation, preventing iron-deficient anemia in full-term newborns without increasing hypervolemia-related risks and increased iron stores, increasing blood pressure, improving oxygen transport, and increasing red blood cell flow (McAdams, 2014). Although a tailored approach is required in the case of cord clamping, current available data suggest that delayed cord clamping offers the newborn many benefits physiologically which include at least a 30% increase in blood volume for term infants and a 50% increase in preterm infants; improvement of systemic blood pressure; increase in the cerebral oxygen index; higher hemoglobin levels at 24 to 48 hours of age; and increased serum iron levels at 4 to 6 months (Kluckow & Hooper, 2015; Leslie, 2015). Cord blood has also been described as "nature's first stem cell transplant" because it possesses regenerative properties and can grow into different types of cells in the body (van Vonderen et al., 2014).

Professional organizations AAP (2013) and ACOG (2014) have released opinions that support delayed cord clamping for preterm infants, but endorse further research on this procedure for term infants. WHO (2014) released a report recommending delayed cord clamping for "all births" as a best practice. A recent Cochrane review on term infants and timing of umbilical cord clamping reported that those with delayed cord clamping had up to a 60% increase in red blood cells, high hemoglobin levels, and higher iron levels at 4 to 6 months. Infants whose cords were clamped early were twice as likely to be iron deficit at 3 to 6 months (Leslie, 2015). So, at this time, there is no uniform agreement about this practice.

Blood Components

The fetus has more red blood cells per cubic millimeter than an adult and they have a greater affinity for oxygen at a lower oxygen pressure than adult red blood cells. Fetal red blood cells are larger in size when compared to an adult, thus each cell can carry more oxygen (Stave, 2014). After birth, the red blood cell count gradually increases as the cell size decreases, because the cells now live in an environment with much higher PO_2. A newborn's red blood cells have a life span of 80 to 100 days, compared with 120 days in adults.

Hemoglobin initially declines as a result of a decrease in neonatal red cell mass (physiologic anemia of infancy). Leukocytosis (elevated white blood cells) is present as a result of birth trauma soon after birth. The newborn's platelet count and aggregation ability are the same as those of adults.

The newborn's hematologic values are affected by the site of the blood sample (capillary blood has higher levels of hemoglobin and hematocrit compared with venous blood), placental transfusion (delayed cord clamping and normal shift of plasma to extravascular spaces, which causes higher levels of hemoglobin and hematocrit), and gestational age (increased age is associated with increased numbers of red cells and hemoglobin) (Andersson et al., 2014). Table 17.2 lists normal newborn blood values.

TABLE 17.2 NORMAL NEWBORN BLOOD VALUES

Lab Data	Normal Range
Hemoglobin	16–18 g/dL
Hematocrit	46–68%
Platelets	150,000–350,000/μL
Red blood cells	4.5–7.0 (1,000,000/μL)
White blood cells	10–30,000/mm^3

Adapted from Fischbach, F., & Dunning, M. B. (2014). *Manual of laboratory and diagnostic tests* (9th ed.). Philadelphia, PA: Lippincott Williams & Wilkins; Verklan, T., & Walden, M. (2014). *Core curriculum for neonatal intensive care nursing* (4th ed.). St. Louis, MO: Saunders Elsevier; and Davidson, M.R. (2014) *Fast facts for the neonatal nurse: A nursing orientation and care guide in a nutshell.* New York, NY: Springer.

Respiratory System Adaptations

The newborn's transition from fetal to neonatal life includes aeration of the lungs, establishment of pulmonary gas exchange, and changing the fetal circulation into the adult type. Lung aeration leads to the establishment of functional residual capacity, allowing pulmonary gas exchange to start. The first breath of life is a gasp that generates an increase in transpulmonary pressure and results in diaphragmatic descent. Hypercapnia, hypoxia, and acidosis resulting from normal labor become stimuli for initiating respirations. Inspiration of air and expansion of the lungs allow for an increase in tidal volume (amount of air brought into the lungs). **Surfactant** is a surface tension–reducing lipoprotein found in the newborn's lungs that prevents alveolar collapse at the end of expiration and loss of lung volume. It lines the alveoli to enhance aeration of gas-free lungs, thus reducing surface tension and lowering the pressure required to open the alveoli. Normal lung function depends on surfactant, which permits a decrease in surface tension at end expiration (to prevent atelectasis) and an increase in surface tension during lung expansion (to facilitate elastic recoil on inspiration). Surfactant provides the lung stability needed for gas exchange. The newborn's first breath, in conjunction with surfactant, overcomes the surface forces to permit aeration of the lungs. The chest wall of the newborn is floppy because of the high cartilage content and poorly developed musculature. Thus, accessory muscles to help in breathing are ineffective.

One of the most crucial adaptations that the newborn makes at birth is adjusting from a fluid-filled intrauterine environment to a gaseous extrauterine environment. During fetal life, the lungs are expanded with an ultrafiltrate of the amniotic fluid. During and after birth, this fluid must be removed and replaced with air. Passage through the birth canal allows intermittent compression of the thorax, which helps eliminate the fluid in the lungs. Pulmonary capillaries and the lymphatics remove the remaining fluid.

If fluid is removed too slowly or incompletely (e.g., with decreased thoracic squeezing during birth or diminished respiratory effort), transient tachypnea (respiratory rate above 60 breaths per minute) of the newborn occurs. Examples of situations involving decreased thoracic compression and diminished respiratory effort include cesarean birth and sedation in newborns. Research findings support the need for thoracic compression because the absence of the neonate's exposure to labor contractions, which may occur with cesarean births or heavy sedation during the labor process or general anesthesia administered during the surgical birth, is associated with an increased risk of transient tachypnea at term, with oxygen supplementation being needed for a longer duration (Hooper, Polglase, & Roehr, 2015).

Take Note!

A neonate born by cesarean section does not have the same benefit of the birth canal squeeze as does the newborn born by vaginal delivery. Closely observe the respirations of the newborn after cesarean delivery.

Lungs

Before the newborn's lungs can maintain respiratory function, the following events must occur:

- Initiation of respiratory movement
- Expansion of the lungs
- Establishment of functional residual capacity (ability to retain some air in the lungs on expiration)
- Increased pulmonary blood flow
- Redistribution of cardiac output (Bope & Kellerman, 2015)

Initial breathing is probably the result of a reflex triggered by pressure changes, noise, light, temperature changes, touching, compression of the fetal chest during the birthing process, and high carbon dioxide and low oxygen concentrations of the newborn's blood. Central chemoreceptors stimulated by hypoxia and hypercapnia further increase the respiratory drive. Many theories address the initiation of respiration in the newborn, but most are based on speculation from observations rather than on empirical research (Sharma et al., 2014). Research continues to search for answers to these questions.

Respirations

After respirations are established in the newborn, they are shallow and irregular, ranging from 30 to 60 breaths per minute, with short periods of apnea (less than 15 seconds). The newborn's respiratory rate varies according to his or her activity; the more active the newborn, the higher the respiratory rate, on average. Signs of respiratory distress to observe for include cyanosis, tachypnea, expiratory grunting, sternal retractions, and nasal flaring. Respirations should not be labored, and the chest movements should be symmetric. In some cases, **periodic breathing** may occur, which is the cessation of breathing that lasts 5 to 10 seconds without changes in color or heart rate (Davidson, 2014). Periodic breathing may be observed in newborns within the first few days of life and requires close monitoring.

Take Note!

Apneic periods lasting more than 15 seconds with cyanosis and heart rate changes require further evaluation (Mattson & Smith, 2015).

Body Temperature Regulation

Newborns are dependent on their environment for the maintenance of body temperature, much more so immediately after birth than later in life. One of the most important elements in a newborn's survival is obtaining a stable body temperature to promote an optimal transition to extrauterine life. On average, a newborn's temperature ranges from 97.9° to 99.7°F (36.6° to 37.6°C). Since newborns lose heat easily after birth, having skin-to-skin contact with their mothers is recommended as the initial method for maintaining newborn body temperature. Skin-to-skin contact should be the first line of treatment for hypothermia and as a measure to reduce discomfort from painful procedures. See Evidence-Based Practice 17.1.

Thermoregulation is the process of maintaining the balance between heat loss and heat production in order to maintain its core internal temperature. It is a critical physiologic function that is closely related to the transition and survival of the newborn. An appropriate thermal environment is essential for maintaining a normal body temperature. Compared with adults, newborns tolerate a narrower range of environmental temperatures and are extremely vulnerable to both under heating and overheating. Nurses play a key role in providing an appropriate environment to help newborns maintain thermal stability (Fig. 17.2).

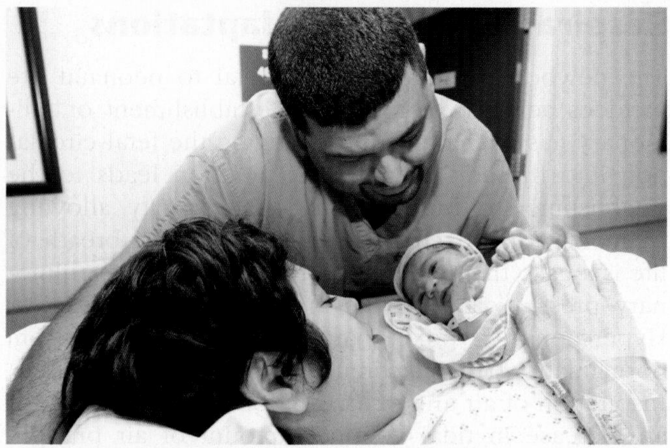

FIGURE 17.2 Father and mother looking at their newborn after birth. Note the newborn's hat and warm blanket to preserve body heat.

Heat Loss

Newborns have several characteristics that predispose them to heat loss:

- Thin skin with blood vessels close to the surface
- Lack of shivering ability to produce heat until 3 months old
- Limited stores of metabolic substrates (glucose, glycogen, fat)

EVIDENCE-BASED PRACTICE 17.1

EFFECT OF EARLY MATERNAL/NEWBORN SKIN-TO-SKIN CONTACT AFTER BIRTH ON THE DURATION OF THIRD STAGE OF LABOR AND INITIATION OF BREAST-FEEDING

STUDY

The holding of a newborn with vertical skin-to-skin contact typically in an upright position with the swaddled newborn on the chest of the mother, is commonly referred to as kangaroo care. It has been recommended that this skin-to-skin contact is a feasible, natural, and cost-effective intervention for breast-feeding initiation, and thermoregulation. The aim of this study was to determine the effect of early maternal-newborn skin-to-skin contact after birth on the duration of the third stage of labor and initiation of breast-feeding.

Findings

A nonrandomized controlled clinical trial was conducted using a sample of 100 laboring women. The project included a study group (50) who had skin-to-skin contact and a control group (50) who received routine hospital care. Tools used to collect data included a structured interview, assessment of mothers during the third stage of labor, and an outcome assessment of first breast-feeding. The results revealed that success in first time breast-feeding during, complete separation of the placenta, and immediate contraction of the uterus was higher in the study group compared to the control group. There were statistically significant differences between the study and control groups in third stage of labor duration (9 minutes shorter), complete placental separation, and immediate contraction of the uterus or excessive bleeding. The study concluded that mothers who practice early mother/newborn skin-to-skin contact immediately after giving birth experienced a shorter third stage duration and early successful initiation of breast-feeding.

Nursing Implications

Based on these findings, it would make sense to incorporate early skin-to-skin contact immediate postbirth and delay routine infant care until the success of the first breast-feeding process for the benefits it provides to both mother and newborn. Nurses need to apply evidence-based research into their care since this application would improve maternal and child health outcomes.

Adapted from Essa, R. M., & Ismail, N. I. A. A. (2015). Effect of early maternal/newborn skin-to-skin contact after birth on the duration of third stage of labor and initiation of breastfeeding. *Journal of Nursing Education and Practice*, *5*(4), 98–107.

- Limited use of voluntary muscle activity or movement to produce heat
- Large body surface area relative to body weight
- Lack of subcutaneous fat, which provides insulation
- Little ability to conserve heat by changing posture (fetal position)
- No ability to adjust their own clothing or blankets to achieve warmth
- Inability to communicate that they are too cold or too warm

Every newborn struggles to maintain body temperature from the moment of birth, when the newborn's wet body is exposed to the much cooler environment of the birthing room. The amniotic fluid covering the newborn cools as it evaporates rapidly in the low humidity and air-conditioning of the room. The newborn's temperature may decrease 3° to 5°F (−16.1° to −15°C) within minutes after leaving the warmth of the mother's uterus (99.6°F [37.5°C]). The skin of newborns adjusts quickly to the challenging environmental conditions of extrauterine life. However, certain functions, for example, microcirculation, continue to develop even beyond the neonatal period (McCall et al., 2014).

The transfer of heat depends on the temperature of the environment, air speed, and water vapor pressure or humidity. Heat exchange between the environment and the newborn involves the same mechanisms as those with any physical object and its environment. Heat can be lost by four mechanisms including conduction (3%), convection (34%), evaporation (24%), and radiation (39%) (Sharma et al., 2014). Prevention of heat loss is a key nursing intervention (Fig. 17.3).

Consider This

When I look down at my little miracle of life in my arms, I can't help but beam with pride at this great accomplishment. She seems so vulnerable and defenseless, and yet is equipped with everything she needs to survive at birth. When the nurse brought my daughter in for the first time after birth, I wanted to see and feel every part of her. Much to my dismay, she was wrapped up like a mummy in a blanket and she had a pink knit cap on her head. I asked the nurse why all the babies had to look like they were bound for the North Pole with all these layers on. Wasn't the nurse aware it was summertime and probably at least 85°F (29.4°C) outside?

The nurse explained that newborns lose body heat easily and need to be kept warm until their temperature stabilizes. Even though I wanted to get up close and personal with my baby, I decided to keep the pink polar bear outfit on her.

Thoughts: Newborns may be born with "everything they need to survive" on the outside, but they still experience temperature instability and lose heat through radiation, evaporation, convection, and conduction. Because the newborn's head is the largest body part, a great deal of heat can be lost if a cap is not kept on the head. What guidance can be given to this mother before discharge to stabilize her daughter's temperature while at home? What simple examples can be used to demonstrate your point?

CONDUCTION

Conduction involves the transfer of heat from one object to another when the two objects are in direct contact with each other. Conduction refers to heat fluctuation between the newborn's body surface when in contact with other solid surfaces, such as a cold mattress, scale, or circumcision restraining board. Heat loss by conduction can also occur when touching a newborn with cold hands or when the newborn has direct contact with a colder object such as a metal scale. Using a warmed cloth diaper or blanket to cover any cold surface touching a newborn directly helps to prevent heat loss through conduction. Placing the newborn skin-to-skin with the mother also helps prevent heat loss through conduction.

CONVECTION

Convection involves the flow of heat from the body surface to cooler surrounding air or to air circulating over a body surface. An example of convection-related heat loss would be a cool breeze that flows over the newborn. To prevent heat loss by this mechanism, keep the newborn out of direct cool drafts (open doors, windows, fans, air conditioners) in the environment, work inside an isolette as much as possible and minimize opening portholes that allow cold air to flow inside, and warm any oxygen or humidified air that comes in contact with the newborn. Using clothing and blankets in isolettes is an effective means of reducing the newborn's exposed surface area and providing external insulation. Also, transporting the newborn to the nursery in a warmed isolette, rather than carrying him or her, helps to maintain warmth and reduce exposure to the cool air.

EVAPORATION

Evaporation involves the loss of heat when a liquid is converted to a vapor. Evaporative loss may be insensible (such as from skin and respiration) or sensible (such as from sweating). Insensible loss occurs, but the individual is not aware of it. Sensible loss is objective and can be noticed. It depends on air speed and the absolute humidity of the air. For example, when the baby is born, the body is covered with amniotic fluid. The fluid evaporates into the air, leading to heat loss. Heat loss via evaporation also occurs when bathing a newborn. Drying newborns immediately after birth with warmed blankets and placing a cap on their head will help to prevent heat loss through evaporation. In addition, drying the newborn after bathing will help prevent heat loss through

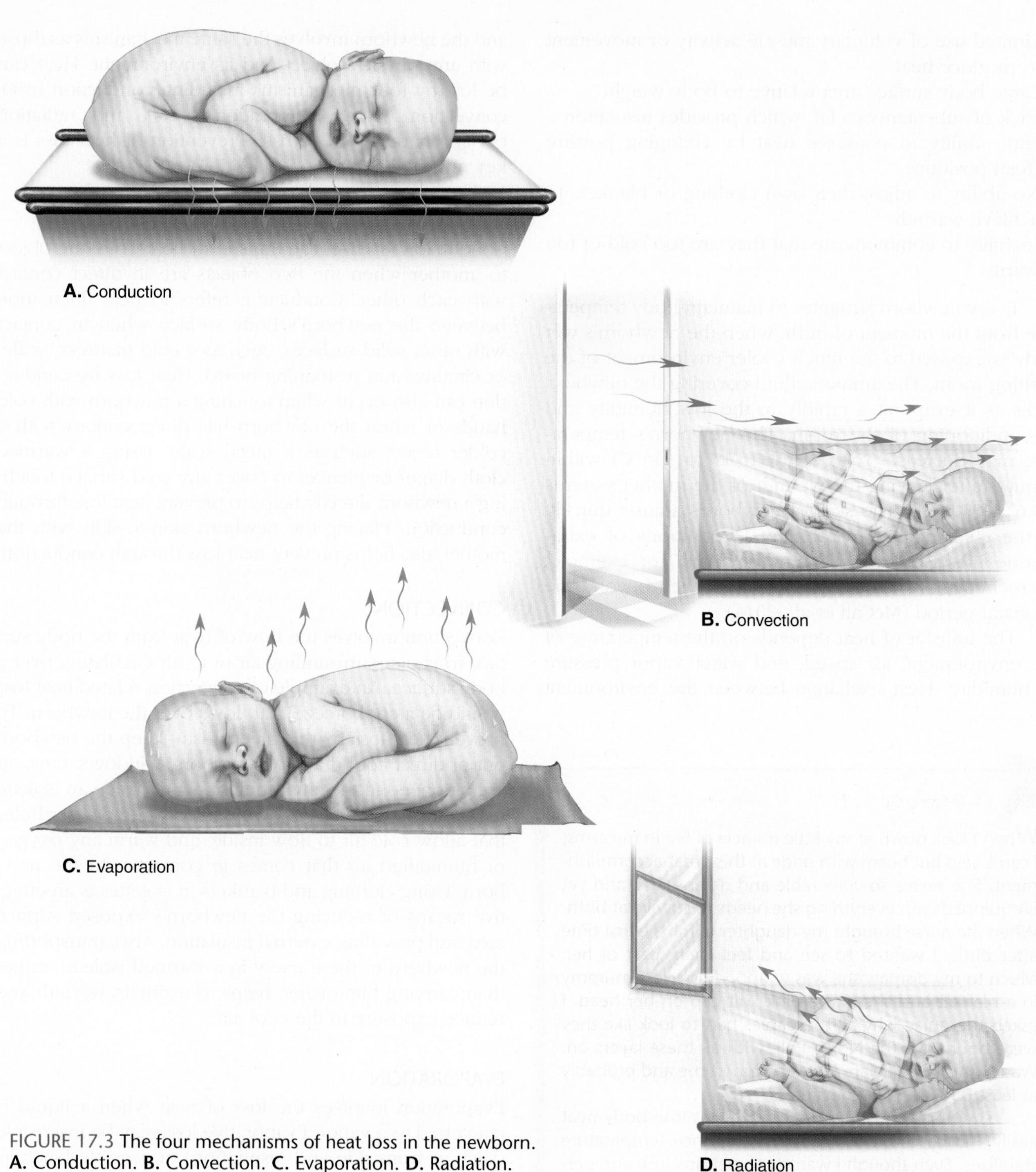

FIGURE 17.3 The four mechanisms of heat loss in the newborn. A. Conduction. B. Convection. C. Evaporation. D. Radiation.

evaporation. Promptly changing wet linens, clothes, or diapers will also reduce heat loss and prevent chilling.

RADIATION

Radiation involves the loss of body heat to cooler, solid surfaces that are in proximity but not in direct contact with the newborn. The amount of heat loss depends on the size of the cold surface area, the surface temperature of the newborn's body, and the temperature of the receiving surface area. For example, when a newborn is placed in a single-wall isolette next to a cold window, heat loss from radiation occurs. Newborns will become cold even though they are in a heated isolette. To reduce heat loss by radiation, keep cribs and isolettes away from outside walls, cold windows, and air conditioners. Also, using radiant warmers for transporting newborns and when performing procedures that may expose the newborn to the cooler environment will help reduce heat loss.

A warmed transporter is an enclosed isolette on wheels. A radiant warmer is an open bed with a radiant heat source above. This type of environment allows health care providers to reach the newborn to carry out procedures and treatments.

Overheating

The newborn is also prone to overheating. Limited insulation and limited sweating ability can predispose any newborn to overheating. Control of body temperature is achieved via a complex negative feedback system that creates a balance between heat production, heat gain, and heat loss. The primary heat regulator is located in the hypothalamus and the central nervous system. The immaturity of the newborn's central nervous system makes it difficult to create and maintain this balance. Therefore, the newborn can become overheated easily. For example, an isolette that is too warm or one that is left too close to a sunny window may lead to hyperthermia. Although heat production can substantially increase in response to a cool environment, basal metabolic rate and the resultant heat produced cannot be reduced. Overheating increases fluid loss, the respiratory rate, and the metabolic rate considerably.

Thermoregulation

Humans have the ability to regulate their body temperature within a narrow range. Newborns have a decreased ability to regulate their body temperature, producing heat through nonshivering thermogenesis. Thermoregulation, the balance between heat loss and heat production, is related to the newborn's rate of metabolism and oxygen consumption. The newborn attempts to conserve heat and increase heat production by increasing the metabolic rate, increasing muscular activity through movement, increasing peripheral vasoconstriction, and assuming a fetal position to hold in heat and minimize exposed body surface area.

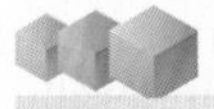
Concept Mastery Alert

Effects of Cold Stress in the Newborn's Brown Fat Metabolism

The newborn first experiences an increase in norepinephrine in response to a cold environment. This then influences the triglycerides to stimulate brown fat metabolism.

An environment in which body temperature is maintained without an increase in metabolic rate or oxygen use is called a **neutral thermal environment**. Within a neutral thermal environment, the rates of oxygen consumption and metabolism are minimal, and internal body temperature is maintained because of thermal balance. A neutral thermal environment promotes growth and stability, conserves energy for basic bodily functions, and minimizes heat (energy) and water loss (Knobel, 2014). Because newborns have difficulty maintaining their body heat through shivering or other mechanisms, they need a higher environmental temperature to maintain a neutral thermal environment. If the environmental temperature decreases, the newborn responds by consuming more oxygen. The respiratory rate increases (tachypnea) in response to the increased need for oxygen. As a result, the newborn's metabolic rate increases.

As noted earlier, the newborn's primary method of heat production is through nonshivering thermogenesis. This is a process in which brown fat (adipose tissue) is oxidized in response to cold exposure. Brown fat is a special kind of highly vascular fat found only in newborns. Brown adipose tissue is a unique tissue that is able to convert chemical energy directly into heat when activated by the sympathetic nervous system. It is produced during the third trimester; ordinarily disappears by 3 to 5 weeks after birth and is vital for thermogenesis. The brown coloring is derived from the fat's rich supply of blood vessels and nerve endings. These fat deposits, which are capable of intense metabolic activity – and thus can generate a great deal of heat – are found between the scapulae, axillae, at the nape of the neck, in the mediastinum, and in areas surrounding the kidneys and adrenal glands. Brown fat makes up about 6% of term body weight in the full-term newborn (Betz & Enerback, 2015). When the newborn experiences a cold environment, norepinephrine is released. This in turn stimulates brown fat metabolism by breaking down triglycerides. Cardiac output increases, increasing blood flow through the brown fat tissue. Subsequently, this blood becomes warmed as a result of the increased metabolic activity of the brown fat (Fig. 17.4).

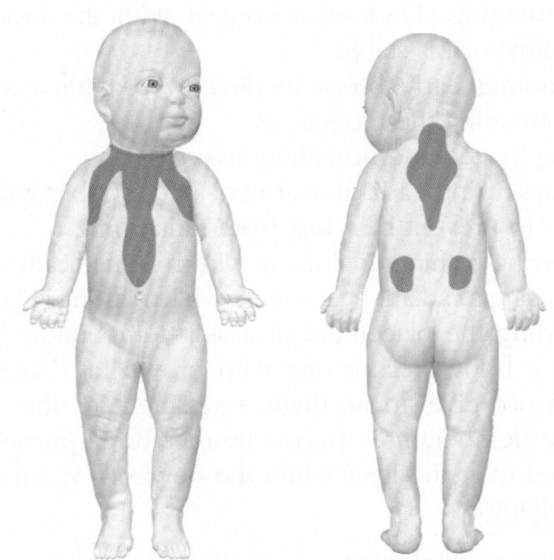

FIGURE 17.4 Areas of brown fat in a newborn.

Newborns can experience heat loss through all four mechanisms, ultimately resulting in cold stress. **Cold stress** is excessive heat loss that requires a newborn to use compensatory mechanisms (such as nonshivering thermogenesis and tachypnea) to maintain core body temperature (Davidson, 2014). The consequences of cold stress can be quite severe. As the body temperature decreases, the newborn becomes less active, lethargic, hypotonic, and weaker. All newborns are at risk for cold stress, particularly within the first 12 hours of life. However, preterm newborns are at the greatest risk for cold stress and experience more profound effects than full-term newborns because they have fewer fat stores, poorer vasomotor responses, and less insulation to cope with a hypothermic event.

Cold stress in the newborn can lead to the following problems if not reversed: depleted brown fat stores, increased oxygen needs, respiratory distress, increased glucose consumption leading to hypoglycemia, metabolic acidosis, jaundice, hypoxia, and decreased surfactant production (Mattson & Smith, 2015).

Take Note!

Nurses must be aware of the thermoregulatory needs of the newborn and must ensure that these needs are met to provide the newborn with the best start possible. Maintenance of temperature stability should be focused on preventative measures.

To minimize the effects of cold stress and maintain an neutral thermal environment, the following interventions are helpful:

- Prewarming blankets and hats to reduce heat loss through conduction
- Keeping the infant transporter (warmed isolette) fully charged and heated at all times
- Drying the newborn completely after birth to prevent heat loss from evaporation
- Encouraging skin-to-skin contact with the mother if the newborn is stable
- Promoting early breast-feeding to provide fuels for nonshivering thermogenesis
- Using heated and humidified oxygen
- Always using radiant warmers and double-wall isolettes to prevent heat loss from radiation
- Deferring bathing until the newborn is medically stable, and using a radiant heat source while bathing (Fig. 17.5)
- Avoiding the placement of a skin temperature probe over a bony area or one with brown fat, because it does not give an accurate assessment of the whole body temperature (most temperature probes are placed over the liver when the newborn is supine or side-lying)

The preceding interventions allow the newborn to minimize his or her metabolic rate and oxygen consumption, thereby conserving vital energy stores required for optimum growth.

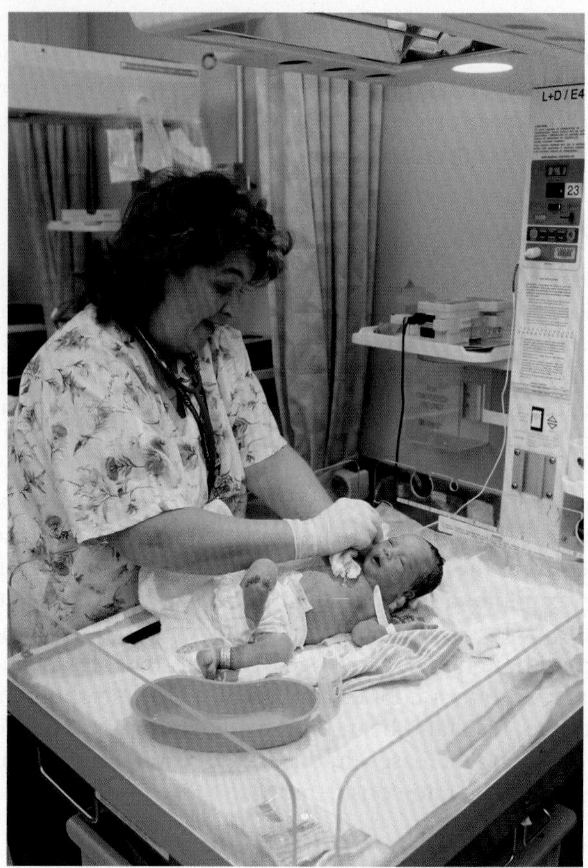

FIGURE 17.5 Bathing a newborn under a radiant warmer to prevent heat loss.

Hepatic System Function

The liver has an essential role in the synthesis, degradation, and regulation of pathways involved in the metabolism of carbohydrates, proteins, lipids, trace elements, and vitamins. At birth, the newborn's liver slowly assumes the functions that the placenta handled during fetal life. Most enzymatic pathways are present in the newborn, but are inactive at birth and generally become fully active at 3 months of age. These functions include blood coagulation, and also iron storage, carbohydrate metabolism, and conjugation of bilirubin, as discussed next. Glycogen reserves provide energy and may become depleted if the metabolic needs of the newborn increase, such as during cold or respiratory stress.

Iron Storage

As red blood cells are destroyed after birth, their iron is released and stored by the liver until new red cells need to be produced. Newborn iron stores are determined by total body hemoglobin content and length of gestation.

If the mother's iron intake was adequate during pregnancy, sufficient iron has been stored in the newborn's liver for use during the first 6 months of age.

Carbohydrate Metabolism

Glucose is an essential fuel for brain metabolism. When the placenta is lost at birth, the maternal glucose supply is cut off. Initially, the newborn's serum glucose levels decline. Newborns must learn to regulate their blood glucose concentration and adjust to an intermittent feeding schedule. Usually, a term newborn's blood glucose level is 70% to 80% of the maternal blood glucose level at birth. Hypoglycemia is one of the most frequent problems encountered, and maintaining glucose homeostasis is one of the important physiologic events during the fetal-to-newborn transition. During the first 24 to 48 hours of life, as normal neonates transition from intrauterine to extrauterine life, their plasma glucose levels are usually lower than later in life (Thornton et al., 2015).

Glucose is the main source of energy for the first several hours after birth. With the newborn's increased energy needs after birth, the liver releases glucose from glycogen stores for the first 24 hours. Initiating early breast- or bottle-feedings helps to stabilize the newborn's blood glucose levels. No evidence supports universal invasive routine measurement of glucose in healthy term newborns. Selective screening of at-risk newborns is more appropriate (Adamkin, 2015).

Bilirubin Conjugation

The liver is also responsible for the conjugation of bilirubin—a yellow to orange bile pigment produced by the breakdown of red blood cells. In utero, elimination of bilirubin in the blood is handled by the placenta and the mother's liver. However, once the cord is cut, the newborn must now assume this function.

Bilirubin normally circulates in plasma, is taken up by liver cells, and is changed to a water-soluble pigment that is excreted in the bile. This conjugated form of bilirubin is excreted from liver cells as a constituent of bile.

The principal source of bilirubin in the newborn is the hemolysis of erythrocytes. This is a normal occurrence after birth, when fewer red blood cells are needed to maintain extrauterine life. When red blood cells die after approximately 80 days of life, the heme in their hemoglobin is converted to bilirubin. Bilirubin is released in an unconjugated form called indirect bilirubin, which is fat soluble. Enzymes, proteins, and different cells in the reticuloendothelial system and liver process the unconjugated bilirubin into conjugated bilirubin or direct bilirubin. This form is water soluble and now enters the gastrointestinal system via the bile and is eventually excreted through feces. The kidneys also excrete a small amount.

Newborns produce bilirubin at a rate of approximately 6 to 8 mg/kg/day. This is more than twice the production rate in adults, primarily because of relative polycythemia and increased red blood cell turnover. Bilirubin production typically declines to the adult level within 10 to 14 days after birth (Bhutani et al., 2015). In addition, the metabolic pathways of the liver are relatively immature and thus cannot conjugate bilirubin as quickly as needed.

Failure of the liver cells to break down and excrete bilirubin can cause an increased amount of bilirubin in the bloodstream, leading to jaundice (Sharma et al., 2014). Bilirubin is toxic to the body and must be excreted. Blood tests ordered to determine bilirubin levels measure bilirubin in the serum. Total bilirubin is a combination of indirect (unconjugated) and direct (conjugated) bilirubin. When unconjugated bilirubin pigment is deposited in the skin and mucous membranes as a result of increased bilirubin levels, **jaundice**, also known as icterus, develops, with a yellowing of the skin, sclera, and mucous membranes. Visible jaundice as a result of increased blood bilirubin levels occurs in more than half of all healthy newborns. Even in healthy term newborns, extremely elevated blood levels of bilirubin during the first week of life can cause bilirubin encephalopathy, a permanent and devastating form of brain damage (Wong & Bhutani, 2015).

Common risk factors for the development of jaundice include fetal–maternal blood group incompatibility, prematurity, asphyxia at birth, an insufficient intake of milk during breast-feeding, drugs (such as diazepam [Valium], oxytocin [Pitocin], sulfisoxazole/erythromycin [Pediazole], and chloramphenicol [Chloromycetin]), maternal gestational diabetes, infrequent feedings, male gender, trauma during birth resulting in cephalhematoma, cutaneous bruising from birth trauma, polycythemia, previous sibling with hyperbilirubinemia, intrauterine infections such as TORCH (toxoplasmosis, other viruses, rubella, cytomegalovirus, herpes simplex viruses), and ethnicity such as Asian or Native American (Moses, 2015).

The causes of newborn jaundice can be classified into three groups based on the mechanism of accumulation:

1. Bilirubin overproduction, such as from blood incompatibility (Rh or ABO), drugs, trauma at birth, polycythemia, delayed cord clamping, and breast milk jaundice
2. Decreased bilirubin conjugation, as seen in physiologic jaundice, hypothyroidism, and breast-feeding
3. Impaired bilirubin excretion, as seen in biliary obstruction (biliary atresia, gallstones, neoplasm), sepsis, hepatitis, chromosomal abnormality (Turner syndrome, trisomies 18 and 21), and drugs (aspirin, acetaminophen, sulfa, alcohol, steroids, antibiotics) (Nagtalon-Ramos, 2014).

Jaundice in the newborn is discussed in more detail in Chapter 24.

Gastrointestinal System Adaptations

The full-term newborn has the capacity to swallow, digest, metabolize, and absorb food taken in soon after birth. At birth, the pH of the stomach contents is mildly acidic, reflecting the pH of the amniotic fluid. The once-sterile gut changes rapidly, depending on what feeding is received. Bowel sounds are normally heard shortly after birth, but may be hypoactive on the first day.

Mucosal Barrier Protection

Humans start their development in a sterile intrauterine environment, but from the very moment of birth all epithelial surfaces in direct contact with the environment (skin, respiratory, gastrointestinal and urogenital tract) are colonized by microorganisms. An important adaptation of the gastrointestinal system is the development of a mucosal barrier to prevent the penetration of harmful substances (bacteria, toxins, and antigens) present within the intestinal lumen. At birth, the newborn must be prepared to deal with bacterial colonization of the gut. Colonization is dependent on oral intake. Nutrition, be it breast milk or formula, plays a major role in early colonization patterns in the neonatal gut. It usually occurs within 24 hours of age and is required for the production of vitamin K (Gritz & Bhandari, 2015). After birth, environmental, oral, and cutaneous microbes from the mother will be mechanically transferred to the newborn by several processes including suckling, kissing, and caressing. Thus, the proximity of the birth canal and the anus, as well as parental expression of neonatal care, is effective methods of ensuring transmission of microbes from one generation to the next. If harmful substances are allowed to penetrate the mucosal epithelial barrier under pathologic conditions, they can cause inflammatory and allergic reactions (Nylund et al., 2014).

Take Note!

Human breast milk provides a passive mechanism to protect the newborn against the dangers of a deficient intestinal defense system. It contains antibodies, viable leukocytes, and many other substances that can interfere with bacterial colonization and prevent harmful penetration.

Stomach and Digestion

The newborn must rapidly adapt from receiving all nutrient and energy requirements via the placenta to obtaining them orally after birth. The physiologic capacity of the newborn stomach is considerably less than its anatomic capacity. There is a rapid gain in physiologic capacity during the first 4 days of life. After the first 4 days, the anatomic and physiologic capacities more closely approximate each other. Researchers have found that for the first 24 hours after birth, the newborn's small stomach does not stretch to hold more, as it will within a day or two later (Batchelor, 2014). This explains the experience of countless hospital nurses who have learned the hard way that when newborns are fed an ounce or two by bottle during the first day of life, most of it tends to come right back up. The walls of the newborn stomach stay firm, expelling extra milk rather than stretching to hold it.

For bottle-fed newborns, small, frequent feedings set up a healthy eating pattern right from the start (breast-fed newborns self-regulate how much they consume). Experts now advise adults that it is healthier to eat smaller amounts more often and the same is true for babies and children. Coaxing an infant to take more milk leads to overfeeding. If feeling overfull at feedings becomes the norm for a young infant, this may lead to unhealthy eating habits that contribute to childhood and adult obesity later. Early-onset obesity is a precursor to a lifelong weight struggle and numerous comorbidities (Redsell et al., 2015; Reilly & Hughes, 2015).

The cardiac sphincter and nervous control of the stomach is immature, which may lead to uncoordinated peristaltic activity and frequent regurgitation. Immaturity of the pharyngoesophageal sphincter and absence of lower esophageal peristaltic waves also contribute to the reflux of gastric contents. Avoiding overfeeding and stimulating frequent burping may minimize regurgitation. Most digestive enzymes are available at birth, allowing newborns to digest simple carbohydrates and protein. However, they have limited ability to digest complex carbohydrates and fats, because amylase and lipase levels are low at birth. As a result, newborns excrete a fair amount of lipids, resulting in fatty stools.

Adequate digestion and absorption are essential for newborn growth and development. Normally, term newborns lose 5% to 10% of their birth weight as a result of insufficient caloric intake within the first week after birth, shifting of intracellular water to extracellular space, and insensible water loss. To gain weight, the term newborn requires an intake of 108 kcal/kg/day from birth to 6 months of age. Understanding the role and importance of nutrition in early postnatal life on growth and development is vital, but how it links to later health has the potential of health benefits for all future generations (Robinson, 2015).

Bowel Elimination

The frequency, consistency, and type of stool passed by newborns vary widely. The evolution of a stool pattern begins with a newborn's first stool, which is meconium. **Meconium** is composed of amniotic fluid, shed mucosal cells, intestinal secretions, and blood. It is greenish black, has a tarry consistency, and is usually passed within 12 to 24 hours of birth. The first meconium stool passed is semisterile, but this changes rapidly with ingestion of bacteria through feedings. After feedings are initiated, a transitional stool develops, which is greenish brown to yellowish brown, thinner in consistency, and seedy in appearance. If breast-fed, the stools will resemble light mustard with seed-like particles. If formula-fed, the stools will be tan or yellow in color and firmer. The frequency of bowel movements varies widely from one infant to another.

Take Note!

Newborns that are fed early pass stools sooner, which helps to reduce bilirubin buildup (Mattson & Smith, 2015).

The last development in the stool pattern is the milk stool. Its characteristics differ in breast-fed and formula-fed newborns. The stools of the breast-fed newborn are yellow-gold, loose, and stringy to pasty in consistency, and typically sour-smelling. The stools of the formula-fed newborn vary depending on the type of formula ingested. They may be yellow, yellow-green, or greenish and loose, pasty, or formed in consistency, and they have an unpleasant odor.

Renal System Changes

A full complement of one million nephrons is present by 34 weeks' gestation. The glomeruli and nephrons are functionally immature at birth, resulting in a reduced glomerular filtration rate (GFR) and limited concentrating ability. A limited ability to concentrate urine and the reduced GFR make the newborn susceptible to both dehydration and fluid overload (Sharma et al., 2014). Frequently the newborn's kidneys are described as immature, but they are able to carry out their usual responsibilities and can handle the challenge of excretion and maintaining acid–base balance. Only when the newborn is faced with unexpected imbalances of water, electrolytes, or a disruption of acid–base status secondary to a preterm birth or illness does it lack the ability to handle the body's fluid homeostasis. A newborn infant's body mass is 75% water, the highest proportion of body water at any stage of a person's life. The majority of term newborns void immediately after birth, indicating adequate renal function. Although the newborn's kidneys can produce urine, they are limited in their ability to concentrate it until about 3 months of age, when the kidneys mature more. Until that time, a newborn voids frequently and the urine has a low specific gravity (1.001 to 1.020). About six to eight voidings daily is average for most newborns; this indicates adequate fluid intake (Harshman & Brophy, 2014).

The renal cortex is relatively underdeveloped at birth and does not reach maturity until 12 to 18 months of age. The GFR is the amount of fluid filtered each minute by all the glomeruli of both kidneys and is one index of kidney function. At birth, the newborn's GFR is approximately 30% of normal adult values, reaching approximately 50% of normal adult values by the tenth day of life and full adult values by the first year of life (Chishti, 2014). The low GFR and the limited excretion and conservation capability of the kidney affect the newborn's ability to excrete salt, water loads, and drugs.

Take Note!

The possibility of fluid overload is increased in newborns; keep this in mind when administering intravenous therapy to a newborn.

Immune System Adaptations

Essential to the newborn's survival is the ability to respond effectively to hostile environmental forces. The newborn's immune system begins working early in gestation, but many of the responses do not function adequately during the early neonatal period. The newborn is protected from certain infections, in part because of maternal antibodies circulating in their system until about 6 months of age. Immunoglobulin G (IgG) crosses the placenta to the fetus while in utero. Newborns who are breast-fed receive antibodies from the breast milk which includes IgE, IgA, IgM, and IgG (Nagtalon-Ramos, 2014). The risk of acquiring an infection is great because a newborn's immune system is immature and not able to respond for long periods of time to fight infections. The intrauterine environment usually protects the fetus from harmful microorganisms and the need for defensive immunologic responses. With exposure to a wide variety of microorganisms at birth, the newborn must develop a balance between its host defenses and the hostile environmental organisms to ensure a safe transition to the outside world. Healthy infants begin to produce their own antibodies, starting at 2 to 3 months of age.

Responses of the immune system serve three purposes: defense (protection from invading organisms), homeostasis (elimination of worn-out host cells), and surveillance (recognition and removal of enemy cells). The newborn's immune system response involves recognition of the pathogen or other foreign material, followed by activation of mechanisms to react against and eliminate it. All immune responses primarily involve leukocytes (white blood cells).

The immune system's responses can be divided into two categories: natural and acquired immunity. These mechanisms are interrelated and interdependent; both are required for immunocompetency.

Natural Immunity

Natural immunity includes responses or mechanisms that do not require previous exposure to the microorganism or antigen to operate efficiently. Physical barriers (such as intact skin and mucous membranes), chemical barriers (such as gastric acids and digestive enzymes), and resident nonpathologic organisms make up the newborn's natural immune system. Natural immunity involves the most basic host defense responses: ingestion and killing of microorganisms by phagocytic cells.

Acquired Immunity

Acquired immunity involves two primary processes: (1) the development of circulating antibodies or immunoglobulins capable of targeting specific invading agents (antigens) for destruction and (2) formation of activated lymphocytes designed to destroy foreign invaders. Acquired immunity is absent until after the first invasion by a foreign organism or toxin.

Immunologic ability depends heavily on immunoglobulins such as IgG, IgM, and IgA. The newborn depends largely on these three immunoglobulins for defense against microorganisms associated with illness. Newborns remain very susceptible to infections for months.

IgG is the major immunoglobulin and the most abundant, making up about 80% of all circulating antibodies (Martin, Fanaroff & Walsh, 2014). It is found in serum and interstitial fluid. It is the only class able to cross the placenta, with active placental transfer beginning at approximately 20 to 22 weeks' gestation. IgG produces antibodies against bacteria, bacterial toxins, and viral agents.

IgA is the second most abundant immunoglobulin in the serum. IgA does not cross the placenta, and maximum levels are reached during childhood. This immunoglobulin is believed to protect mucous membranes from viruses and bacteria. IgA is predominantly found in the gastrointestinal and respiratory tracts, tears, saliva, colostrum, and breast milk.

Take Note!

A major source of IgA is human breast milk, so breast-feeding is believed to have significant immunologic advantages over formula feeding (Walker, 2014).

IgM is found in blood and lymph fluid and is the first immunoglobulin to respond to infection. It does not cross the placenta, and levels are generally low at birth unless a congenital intrauterine infection is present. IgM offers a major source of protection from blood-borne infections. The predominant antibodies formed during neonatal or intrauterine infection are of this class.

Integumentary System Adaptations

The newborn skin is critical to its transition from intrauterine to extrauterine environments and to the journey to self-sufficiency. The newborn's skin is a large organ, making up approximately 13% of body weight in contrast to 3% of body weight in an adult. It is sensitive, fragile, with a neutral pH on the surface, lower lipid content and higher water content when compared with adults. Because of these characteristics, newborn skin is vulnerable to injury and infections (Visscher et al., 2015). The most important function of the skin is to provide a protective barrier between the body and the environment. It limits the loss of water, prevents absorption of harmful agents, protects thermoregulation and fat storage, and protects against physical trauma. The epidermal barrier begins to develop during midgestation and is fully formed by about 32 weeks' gestation. Although the neonatal epidermis is similar to the adult epidermis in thickness and lipid composition, skin development is not complete at birth (King et al., 2015). Although the basic structure is the same as that of an adult, the less mature the newborn, the less mature the skin functions. Fewer fibrils connect the dermis and epidermis in the newborn compared with the adult. Also in a newborn, the risk of injury producing a break in the skin from the use of tapes and monitors and from handling is greater than for an adult. Improper handling of the newborn during daily skin care practices, such as bathing, can cause damage, prevent healing, and interfere with the normal maturation process.

Newborns vary greatly in appearance. Many of the variations are temporary and reflect the physiologic adaptations that the newborn is experiencing. Skin coloring varies, depending on the newborn's age, race or ethnic group, temperature, and whether he or she is crying. Skin color changes with both the environment and health status. At birth, the newborn's skin is dark red to purple. As the newborn begins to breathe air his or her skin color changes to red. This redness normally begins to fade the first day.

Neurologic System Adaptations

The nervous system is immature and continues to develop to achieve a full complement of cortical and brainstem cells by 1 year of age. The brain increases its size threefold during the first year of life. The nervous system consists of the brain, spinal cord, 12 cranial nerves, and a variety of spinal nerves that come from the spinal cord. Neurologic development follows cephalocaudal (head-to-toe) and proximal–distal (center-to-outside) patterns. Myelin develops early on in sensory impulse transmitters. Thus, the newborn has an acute sense of hearing, smell, and taste. The newborn's sensory capabilities include the following:

- *Hearing*—well developed at birth, responds to noise by turning to sound
- *Taste*—ability to distinguish between sweet and sour by 72 hours old
- *Smell*—ability to distinguish between mother's breast milk and breast milk from others
- *Touch*—sensitivity to pain, responds to tactile stimuli
- *Vision*—is incomplete at birth. Maturation is dependent on nutrition and visual stimulation. Newborns have ability to focus only on close objects (8 to 10 in away) with a visual acuity of 20/140; they can track objects in midline or beyond (90 in). This is the least mature sense at birth. The ability to fix, follow, and be alert is indicative of an intact CNS (King et al., 2015).

Remember Maria, the new mother who is worried that her daughter can't see? What might the new mother notice about her daughter's behavior? What might be the new mother's expectations?

Congenital Reflexes

Successful adaptations demonstrated by the respiratory, circulatory, thermoregulatory, and musculoskeletal systems indirectly indicate the central nervous system's successful transition from fetal to extrauterine life, because the central nervous system plays a major role in all these adaptations. In the newborn, congenital reflexes are the hallmarks of maturity of the central nervous system, viability, and adaptation to extrauterine life.

The presence and strength of a reflex is an important indication of neurologic development and function. A **reflex** is an involuntary muscular response to a sensory stimulus. It is built into the nervous system and does not need the intervention of conscious thought to take effect. The physical assessment of the neurologic system of the newborn includes evaluating the major reflexes (gag, Babinski, Moro, and Galant) and minor ones (finger grasp, toe grasp, rooting, sucking, head righting, stepping, and tonic neck).

To assess each reflex, the nurse progresses methodically, taking care to document each finding (Weber & Kelly, 2014). Many neonatal reflexes disappear with maturation, although some remain throughout adulthood. The arcs of these reflexes end at different levels of the spine and brain stem, reflecting the function of the cranial nerves and motor systems. The ways newborns blink, move their limbs, focus on a caretaker's face, turn toward sound, suck, swallow, and respond to the environment are all indications of their neurologic abilities. Congenital defects within the central nervous system are frequently not overt but may be revealed in abnormalities in tone, posture, or behavior (Davidson, 2014). Damage to the nervous system (birth trauma, perinatal hypoxia) during the birthing process can cause delays in the normal growth, development, and functioning of the newborn. Early identification may help to identify the cause and to start early intervention to decrease long-term complications or permanent sequelae.

Newborn reflexes are assessed to evaluate neurologic function and development. Absent or abnormal reflexes in a newborn, persistence of a reflex past the age when it is normally lost, or redevelopment of an infantile reflex in an older child or adult may indicate neurologic pathology. (See Chapter 18 for a description of newborn reflex assessment.)

The Healthy Start nurse explained to Maria that all newborns are born with some degree of myopia (inability to see distances) and that 20/20 vision is not generally achieved until 2 years of age. What developmental information should the nurse discuss with Maria?

BEHAVIORAL ADAPTATIONS

In addition to adapting physiologically, the newborn also adapts behaviorally. All newborns progress through a specific pattern of events after birth, regardless of their gestational age or the type of birth they experienced.

Behavioral Patterns

The newborn usually demonstrates a predictable pattern of behavior during the first several hours after birth, characterized by two periods of reactivity separated by a sleep phase. Behavioral adaptation is a defined progression of events triggered by stimuli from the extrauterine environment after birth.

First Period of Reactivity

The first period of reactivity begins at birth and may last from 30 minutes up to 2 hours. The newborn is alert and moving and may appear hungry. This period is characterized by myoclonic movements of the eyes, spontaneous Moro reflexes, sucking motions, chewing, rooting, and fine tremors of the extremities. Muscle tone and motor activity are increased (Healy & Fallon, 2014). Respiration and heart rate are elevated but gradually begin to slow as the next period begins.

This period of alertness allows parents to interact with their newborn and to enjoy close contact with their new baby (Fig. 17.6). The appearance of sucking and rooting behaviors provides a good opportunity for initiating breast-feeding. Many newborns latch on the nipple and suck well at this first experience.

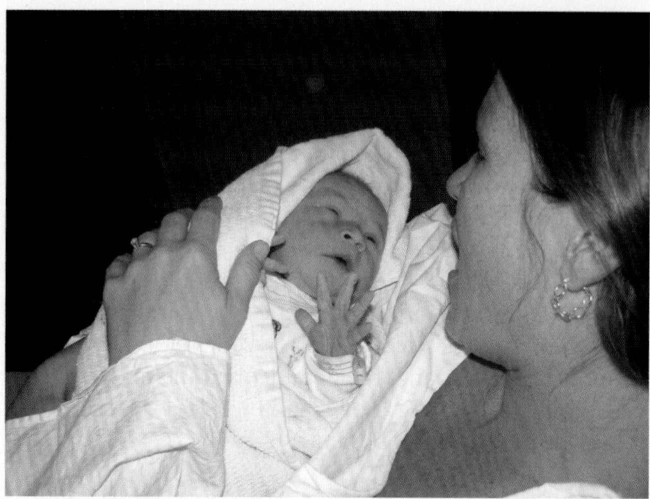

FIGURE 17.6 The first period of reactivity is an optimal time for interaction.

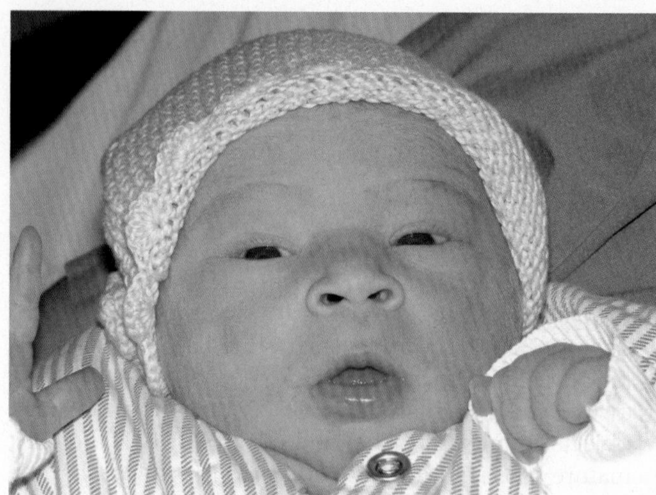

FIGURE 17.7 Newborn during the second period of reactivity. Note the newborn's wide-eyed interest.

Period of Decreased Responsiveness

At 30 to 120 minutes of age, the newborn enters the second stage of transition—that of the *sleep period* or a decrease in activity. This phase is referred to as a period of decreased responsiveness. Movements are less jerky and less frequent. Heart and respiratory rates decline as the newborn enters the sleep phase. The muscles become relaxed, and responsiveness to outside stimuli diminishes. During this phase, it is difficult to arouse or interact with the newborn. No interest in sucking is shown. This quiet time can be used for both mother and newborn to remain close and rest together after labor and the birthing experience.

Second Period of Reactivity

The second period of reactivity begins as the newborn awakens and shows an interest in environmental stimuli. This period lasts 2 to 8 hours in the normal newborn (Davidson, 2014). Heart and respiratory rates increase. Peristalsis also increases. Thus, it is not uncommon for the newborn to pass meconium or void during this period. In addition, motor activity and muscle tone increase in conjunction with an increase in muscular coordination (Fig. 17.7).

Interaction between the mother and the newborn during this second period of reactivity is encouraged if the mother has rested and desires it. This period also provides a good opportunity for the parents to examine their newborn and ask questions.

Take Note!

Teaching about feeding, positioning for feeding, and diaper-changing techniques can be reinforced during this time.

Behavioral Responses

Newborn development is a reflection of the dynamic relationship between endowment and environment. Newborns demonstrate several predictable responses when interacting with their environment. How they react to the world around them is termed as **neurobehavioral response**. It comprises predictable periods that are probably triggered by external stimuli. Expected newborn behaviors include orientation, habituation, motor maturity, self-quieting ability, and social behaviors. Any deviation in behavioral responses requires further assessment, because it may indicate a complex neurobehavioral problem.

Orientation

The response of newborns to stimuli is called *orientation*. They become more alert when they sense a new stimulus in their environment. Orientation reflects newborns' response to auditory and visual stimuli, demonstrated by their movement of head and eyes to focus on that stimulus. Newborns prefer the human face and bright shiny objects. As the face or object comes into their line of vision, newborns respond by staring at the object intently. Newborns use this sensory capacity to become familiar with people and objects in their surroundings.

Remember Maria, who was concerned about her newborn daughter's vision? She told the nurse that her daughter did not show any interest in her pastel-colored homemade mobile she had hung across the room from her crib. What suggestions can the nurse make to Maria regarding the placement of the mobile and the types and colors of objects used to promote orientation in her newborn daughter?

Habituation

Habituation is the newborn's ability to process and respond to visual and auditory stimuli. It is a measure of how well and appropriately an infant responds to the environment. Habituation is the ability to block out external stimuli after the newborn has become accustomed to the activity. During the first 24 hours after birth, newborns should increase their ability to habituate to environmental stimuli and sleep. Habituation provides a useful indicator of their neurobehavioral intactness.

Motor Maturity

Motor maturity depends on gestational age and involves evaluation of posture, tone, coordination, and movements. These activities enable newborns to control and coordinate movement. When stimulated, newborns with good motor organization demonstrate movements that are rhythmic and spontaneous. Bringing the hand up to the mouth is an example of good motor organization. As newborns adapt to their new environment, smoother movements should be observed. Such motor behavior is a good indicator of the newborn's ability to respond and adapt accordingly; it indicates that the central nervous system is processing stimuli appropriately.

Self-Quieting Ability

Self-quieting ability (also called self-soothing) refers to newborns' ability to quiet and comfort themselves. Newborns vary in their ability to console themselves or to be consoled. "Consolability" is how newborns are able to change from the crying state to an active alert, quiet alert, drowsy, or sleep state. They console themselves by hand-to-mouth movements and sucking, alerting to external stimuli and motor activity (Karp, 2014). Recent research outlines five things (the five "**S**'s") that parents can do to calm a fussy infant:

1. **S**waddling tightly;
2. **S**ide/stomach position on the lap of the caretaker;
3. **S**hushing loudly or continuous white noise;
4. **S**winging using any rhythmic movement; and
5. **S**ucking (Karp, 2014).

Assisting parents to identify consoling behaviors to quiet their newborn if the newborn is not able to self-quiet is important.

Social Behaviors

Newborns begin extrauterine life able to engage in it with their sensory capabilities and communicate with their environment through a complex repertoire of behaviors. Social behaviors include cuddling and snuggling into the arms of the parent when the newborn is held. Usually newborns are very sensitive to being touched, cuddled, and held. Cuddliness is very important to parents, because they frequently gauge their ability to care for their newborn by the newborn's acceptance or positive response to their actions. This can be assessed by the degree to which the newborn nestles into the contours of the holder's arms. Most newborns cuddle, but some will resist. Assisting parents to assume comforting behaviors (e.g., by cooing while holding their newborn) and praising them for their efforts can help foster cuddling behaviors.

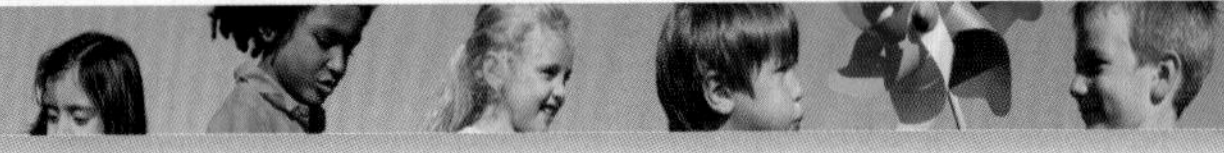

KEY CONCEPTS

- The neonatal period is defined as the first 28 days of life. As the newborn adapts to life after birth, numerous physiologic changes occur.
- At birth, the cardiopulmonary system must switch from fetal to neonatal circulation and from placental to pulmonary gas exchange.
- One of the most crucial adaptations that the newborn makes at birth is the adjustment of a fluid medium exchange from the placenta to the lungs and that of a gaseous environment.
- Neonatal red blood cells have a life span of 80 to 100 days in comparison with the adult red blood cell life span of 120 days. This difference in red blood cell life span causes several adjustment problems.
- Thermoregulation is the maintenance of balance between heat loss and heat production. It is a critical physiologic function that is closely related to the transition and survival of the newborn.
- The newborn's primary method of heat production is through nonshivering thermogenesis, a process in which brown fat (adipose tissue) is oxidized in response to cold exposure. Brown fat is a special kind of highly vascular fat found only in newborns.
- Heat loss in the newborn is the result of four mechanisms: conduction, convection, evaporation, and radiation.
- Responses of the immune system serve three purposes: defense (protection from invading organisms), homeostasis (elimination of worn-out host

cells), and surveillance (recognition and removal of enemy cells).

- In the newborn, congenital reflexes are the hallmarks of maturity of the CNS, viability, and adaptation to extrauterine life.
- The newborn usually demonstrates a predictable pattern of behavior during the first several hours after birth, characterized by two periods of reactivity separated by a sleep phase.

REFERENCES AND RECOMMENDED READING

Adamkin, D. H. (2015). Metabolic screening and postnatal glucose homeostasis in the newborn. *Pediatric Clinics of North America, 62*(2), 385–409.

American Academy of Pediatrics [AAP]. (2013). Statement of endorsement: Timing of umbilical cord clamping after birth. *Pediatrics, 131*(4), e1323.

American College of Obstetricians & Gynecologists [ACOG]. (2014). Committee opinion no. 543: Timing of umbilical cord clamping after birth. *Obstetrics & Gynecology, 120*(6), 1522–1526.

Andersson, O., Domellöf, M., Andersson, D., & Hellström-Westas, L. (2014). Effect of delayed vs early umbilical cord clamping on iron status and neurodevelopment at age 12 months: A randomized clinical trial. *JAMA Pediatrics, 168*(6), 547–554.

Batchelor, H. (2014). Pediatric development: Gastrointestinal. In *Pediatric formulations* (pp. 43–54). New York, NY: Springer.

Betz, M. J., & Enerbäck, S. (2015). Human brown adipose tissue: What we have learned so far. *Diabetes, 64*(7), 2352–2360.

Bhutani, V. K., Wong, R. J., Vreman, H. J., & Stevenson, D. K. (2015). Bilirubin production and hour-specific bilirubin levels. *Journal of Perinatology, 35*(9), 735–738.

Bope, E. T., & Kellerman, R. D. (2015). *Conn's current therapy 2015.* Philadelphia, PA: Elsevier.

Chishti, A. S. (2014). Assessment of renal function. In *Kidney and urinary tract diseases in the newborn* (pp. 117–126). Berlin, Heidelberg, Germany: Springer.

Creasy, R. K., Resnik, R., Iams, J. D., Lockwood, C. J., Moore, T. R., & Greene, M. F. (2014). *Creasy & Resnik's maternal-fetal medicine: Principles and practice* (7th ed.). St. Louis, MO: Elsevier.

Cuneo, B. (2014). Transition from fetal to neonatal circulation. *Pediatric and Congenital Cardiology, Cardiac Surgery and Intensive Care,* 179–199.

Davidson, M. R. (2014). *Fast facts for the neonatal nurse: A nursing orientation and care guide in a nutshell.* New York, NY: Springer.

Essa, R. M., & Ismail, N. I. A. A. (2015). Effect of early maternal/newborn skin-to-skin contact after birth on the duration of third stage of labor and initiation of breastfeeding. *Journal of Nursing Education and Practice, 5*(4), 98–107.

Fillipps, D. J., & Bucciarelli, R. L. (2015). Cardiac evaluation of the newborn. *Pediatric Clinics of North America, 62*(2), 471–489.

Fischbach, F., & Dunning, M. B. (2014). *Manual of laboratory and diagnostic tests* (9th ed.). Philadelphia, PA: Lippincott Williams & Wilkins.

Gritz, E. C., & Bhandari, V. (2015). The human neonatal gut microbiome: a brief review. *Frontiers in Pediatrics, 3,* 17–26.

Harshman, L. A., & Brophy, P. D. (2014). Development of renal function in the fetus and newborn. In *Kidney and urinary tract diseases in the newborn* (pp. 59–76). Berlin, Heidelberg, Germany: Springer.

Healy, P., & Fallon, A. (2014). Developments in neonatal care and nursing responses. *British Journal of Nursing, 23*(1), 21–24.

Hooper, S. B., Polglase, G. R., & Roehr, C. C. (2015). Cardiopulmonary changes with aeration of the newborn lung. *Pediatric Respiratory Reviews, 16*(3), 147–150.

Karp, H. (2014). *The happiest baby on the block.* New York, NY: Bantam Dell.

King, T. L., Brucker, M. C., Kriebs, J. M., Fahey, J. O., Gegor, C. L., & Varney, H. (2015). *Varney's midwifery* (5th ed.). Burlington, MA: Jones & Bartlett Learning.

Kluckow, M., & Hooper, S. B. (2015). Using physiology to guide time to cord clamping. *Seminars in Fetal and Neonatal Medicine, 20*(4), 225–231.

Knobel, R. B. (2014). Fetal and neonatal thermal physiology. *Newborn and Infant Nursing Reviews, 14*(2), 45–49.

Leslie, M. S. (2015). Perspectives on implementing delayed cord clamping. *Nursing for Women's Health, 19*(2), 164–176.

Martin, R. J., Fanaroff, A. A., & Walsh, M. C. (2014). *Neonatal-perinatal medicine* (10th ed.). Philadelphia, PA: Elsevier.

Mattson, S., & Smith, J. (2015). *Core curriculum for maternal-newborn nursing* (5th ed.). Philadelphia, PA: Elsevier.

McAdams, R. M. (2014). Time to implement delayed cord clamping. *Obstetrics & Gynecology, 123*(3), 549–552.

McCall, E., Alderdice, F., Halliday, H., Johnston, L., & Vohra, S. (2014). Challenges of minimizing heat loss at birth: A narrative overview of evidence-based thermal care interventions. *Newborn and Infant Nursing Reviews, 14*(2), 56–63.

Moses, S. (2015). Jaundice in newborns. *Family Practice Notebook.* Retrieved from http://www.fpnotebook.com/NICU/GI/JndcInNwbrns.htm.

Nagtalon-Ramos, J. (2014). *Maternal-newborn nursing care: Best evidence-based practices.* Philadelphia, PA: F.A. Davis Company.

Nylund, L., Satokari, R., Salminen, S., & de Vos, W. M. (2014). Intestinal microbiota during early life–impact on health and disease. *Proceedings of the Nutrition Society,* 1–13.

Redsell, S. A., Edmonds, B., Swift, J. A., Siriwardena, A. N., Weng, S., Nathan, D., et al. (2015). Systematic review of randomized controlled trials of interventions that aim to reduce the risk, either directly or indirectly, of overweight and obesity in infancy and early childhood. *Maternal & Child Nutrition.* doi: 10.1111/mcn.12184.

Reilly, J. J., & Hughes, A. R. (2015). Early life risk factors for childhood obesity. *Early Years Nutrition and Healthy Weight,* 40–45.

Robinson, S. M. (2015). Infant nutrition and lifelong health: Current perspectives and future challenges. *Journal of Developmental Origins of Health and Disease,* 6(5), 384–389.

Sharma, A., Ford, S., & Calvert, J. (2014). Adaptation for life: A review of neonatal physiology. *Anesthesia & Intensive Care Medicine, 15*(3), 89–95.

Stave, U. (2014). *Perinatal physiology*. New York, NY: Springer.

Steinhorn, R. H. (2015). Persistent pulmonary hypertension of the newborn. *PanVascular Medicine*, 4135–4155. doi: 10.1007/978-3-642-37078-6_157.

Swanson, J. R., & Sinkin, R. A. (2015). Transition from fetus to newborn. *Pediatric Clinics of North America, 62*(2), 329–343.

Thornton, P. S., Stanley, C. A., De Leon, D. D., Harris, D., Haymond, M. W., Hussain, K., et al. (2015). Recommendations from the Pediatric Endocrine Society for evaluation and management of persistent hypoglycemia in neonates, infants, and children. *The Journal of Pediatrics, 167*(2), 238–245.

van Vonderen, J. J., Roest, A. A., Siew, M. L., Walther, F. J., Hooper, S. B., & te Pas, A. B. (2014). Measuring physiological changes during the transition to life after birth. *Neonatology, 105*(3), 230–242.

Verklan, T., & Walden, M. (2014). *Core curriculum for neonatal intensive care nursing*. (4th ed.). St. Louis, MO: Elsevier.

Visscher, M. O., Adam, R., Brink, S., & Odio, M. (2015). Newborn infant skin: Physiology, development, and care. *Clinics in Dermatology, 33*(3), 271–280.

Walker, M. (2014). *Breastfeeding management for the clinician: Using the evidence* (3rd ed.). Burlington, MA: Jones & Bartlett Learning.

Weber, J., & Kelley, J. (2014). *Health assessment in nursing* (5th ed.). Philadelphia, PA: Lippincott Williams & Wilkins.

Wong, R. J., & Bhutani, V. K. (2015). Clinical manifestations of unconjugated hyperbilirubinemia in term and late preterm infants. *UpToDate*. Retrieved from http://www.uptodate.com/contents/clinical-manifestations-of-unconjugated-hyperbilirubinemia-in-term-and-late-preterm-infants

World Health Organization [WHO]. (2014). *Delayed clamping of the umbilical cord to reduce infant anemia* (Doc. No. WHO/RHR/14.19 ed.). Geneva, Switzerland: Author.

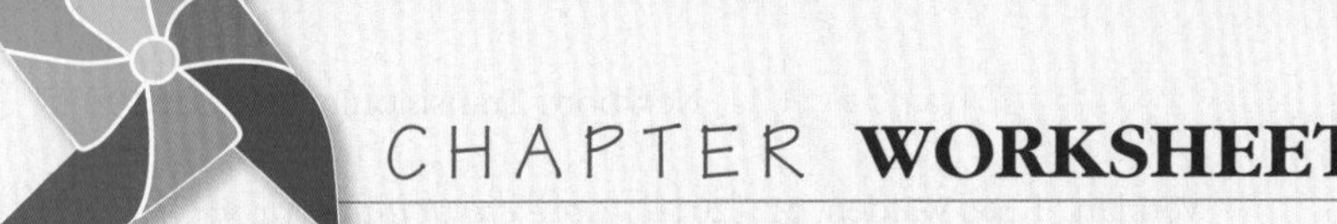

CHAPTER WORKSHEET

MULTIPLE-CHOICE QUESTIONS

1. When assessing the term newborn, the following are observed: newborn is alert, heart and respiratory rates have stabilized, and meconium has been passed. The nurse determines that the newborn is exhibiting behaviors indicating:
   a. Initial period of reactivity
   b. Second period of reactivity
   c. Decreased responsiveness period
   d. Sleep period for newborns
2. A nurse observes a 3-day-old term newborn that is starting to appear mildly jaundiced. What might explain this condition?
   a. Physiologic jaundice secondary to breast-feeding
   b. Hemolytic disease of the newborn due to blood incompatibility
   c. Exposing the newborn to high levels of oxygen
   d. Overfeeding the newborn with too much glucose water
3. After teaching a group of nursing students about thermoregulation and appropriate measures to prevent heat loss by evaporation, which of the following student behaviors would indicate successful teaching?
   a. Transporting the newborn in an isolette
   b. Maintaining a warm room temperature
   c. Placing the newborn on a warmed surface
   d. Drying the newborn immediately after birth
4. After birth, the nurse would expect which fetal structure to close as a result of increases in the pressure gradients on the left side of the heart?
   a. Foramen ovale
   b. Ductus arteriosus
   c. Ductus venosus
   d. Umbilical vein
5. Which of the following newborns could be described as breathing normally?
   a. Newborn A is breathing deeply, with a regular rhythm, at a rate of 20 bpm.
   b. Newborn B is breathing diaphragmatically with sternal retractions, at a rate of 70 bpm.
   c. Newborn C is breathing shallowly, with 40-second periods of apnea and cyanosis.
   d. Newborn D is breathing shallowly, at a rate of 36 bpm, with short periods of apnea.
6. When assessing a term newborn (6 hours old), the nurse auscultates bowel sounds and documents recent passing of meconium. These findings would indicate:
   a. Abnormal gastrointestinal newborn transition and needs to be reported
   b. An intestinal anomaly that needs immediate surgery
   c. A patent anus with no bowel obstruction and normal peristalsis
   d. A malabsorption syndrome resulting in fatty stools
7. A nursing student questions the nursery nurse why they don't bathe the newborn immediately upon admission to the nursery observation area after birth. The nurse states that this would increase the risk of:
   a. Jaundice
   b. Infection
   c. Hypothermia
   d. Anemia
8. Because the newborn's red blood cells break down much sooner than those of an adult, what might result?
   a. Anemia
   b. Bruising
   c. Apnea
   d. Jaundice
9. The nurse performs a physical examination on a newborn 2 hours after birth. Which of the following findings indicate a need for a pediatric consultation? Select all that apply:
   a. Respiratory rate of 50 breaths per minute
   b. Intermittent episodes of apnea, lasting <10 seconds each
   c. Absent Moro reflex when startled
   d. Preauricular skin tag noted on left ear
   e. White raised bumps noted on nose and face
   f. Yellow blanching of the skin when pressure applied to the nose

CRITICAL THINKING EXERCISES

1. As the nurse manager, you have been orienting a new nurse in the nursery for the past few weeks. Although she has been demonstrating adequacy with most procedures, today you observe her bathing several newborns without covering them, weighing them on the scale without a cover, leaving the storage door open with the transporter nearby, and leaving the newborns' head covers and blankets off after showing them to family members through the nursery observation window.
   a. What is your impression of this behavior?
   b. What principles concerning thermoregulation need to be reinforced?
   c. How will you evaluate whether your instructions have been effective?

CHAPTER WORKSHEET

2. The most important adaptations for the newborn to make after birth are to establish respirations, make cardiovascular adjustments, and establish thermoregulation. Nursing care focuses on monitoring and supporting adjustments to extrauterine adaptation. Write appropriate nursing interventions to help achieve the following newborn adaptations:
   a. Respiratory adaptation
   b. Safety, including prevention of infection
   c. Thermoregulation

STUDY ACTIVITIES

1. While in the nursery clinical setting, identify the period of behavioral reactivity (first, inactivity, or second period) for two newborns born at different times. Share your findings during the post conference for that clinical day.
2. Dramatic changes occur in the cardiovascular system at birth. When the umbilical cord is clamped and the placenta is separated, there is a resultant increase in systemic blood pressure and changes to the three major fetal shunts (ductus venosus, foramen ovale, and ductus arteriosus) occur. Outline what happens to cause their functional closures during this period of transition.
3. Find two web sites about the transition to extrauterine life that can be shared with other nursing students as well as nursery nurses. Critique the information presented in terms of how accurate and current it is.
4. The most common mechanism of heat loss in the newborn is ________________.
5. The newborn creates heat in three ways—shivering, muscle activity and through thermogenesis by the metabolism of brown adipose tissue. Which is the most effective?

BRINGING IT ALL TOGETHER: A CASE STUDY

An 18-year-old woman gave birth to her first infant 3 days ago, but she doesn't smile when the *Healthy Start* nurse greets her at a home visit. The nurse questions her about what has happened since she was discharged from the hospital 2 days ago. She tells the nurse that her breasts are swollen, hot, and very painful when touched. She states she knows that breast-feeding is best for her child, but she is not sure she wants to continue to breast-feed because of the pain. Her infant is lying on the bare kitchen table in only a diaper crying.

Go to thePoint to find questions to consider about this case.

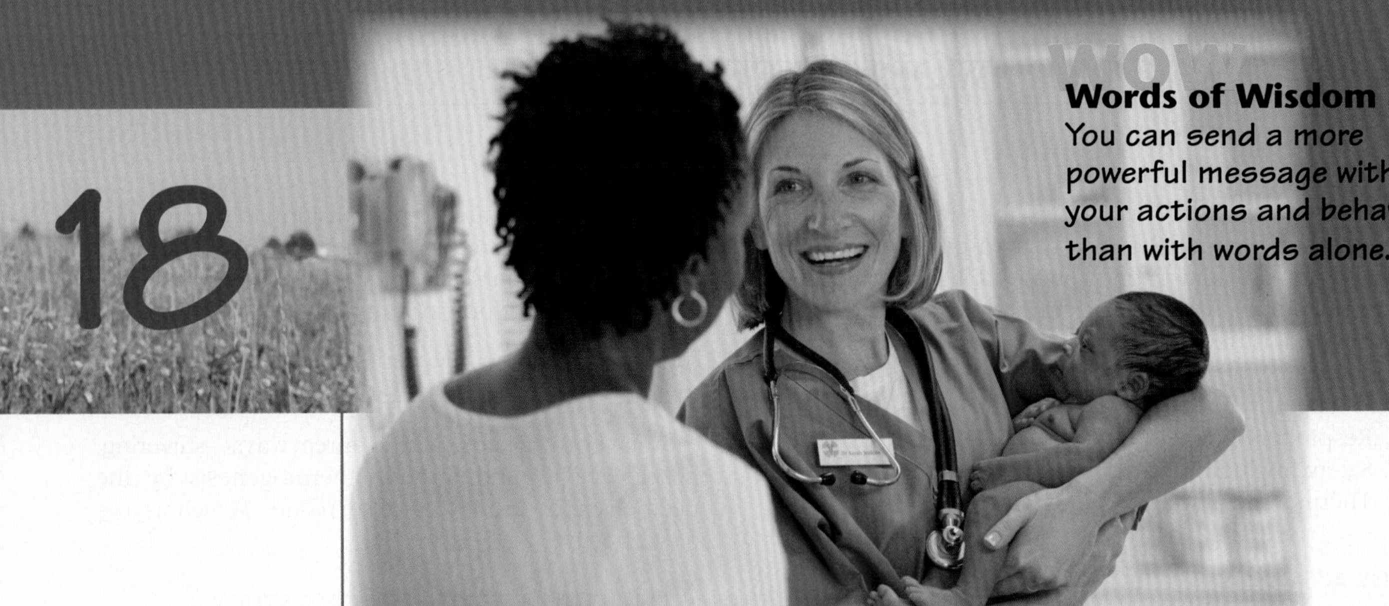
18
Words of Wisdom
You can send a more powerful message with your actions and behavior than with words alone.

Nursing Management of the Newborn

KEY TERMS

acrocyanosis
Apgar score
caput succedaneum
cephalhematoma
circumcision
Epstein pearls
erythema toxicum
gestational age
harlequin sign
immunizations
infant abduction
milia
molding
Mongolian spots
nevus flammeus
nevus vasculosus
ophthalmia neonatorum
phototherapy
pseudo-menstruation
stork bites
vernix caseosa

Learning Objectives

Upon completion of the chapter, you will be able to:

1. Perform the assessments needed during the immediate newborn period.
2. Employ interventions that meet the immediate needs of the term newborn.
3. Demonstrate the components of a typical physical examination of a newborn.
4. Distinguish common variations that can be noted during a newborn's physical examination.
5. Characterize common concerns in the newborn and appropriate interventions.
6. Compare the importance of the newborn screening tests.
7. Plan for common interventions that are appropriate during the early newborn period.
8. Analyze the nurse's role in meeting the newborn's nutritional needs.
9. Outline discharge planning content and education needed for the family with a newborn.

***Kelly*, a 16-year-old first-time mother, calls the hospital maternity unit 3 days after being discharged home. She tells the nurse that her newborn son "looks yellow, like a canary" and "isn't nursing well." She wonders what is wrong.**

INTRODUCTION

Immediately after the birth of a newborn, all mother and father/support persons/significant others are faced with the task of learning and understanding as much as possible about caring for this new family member, even if the parents already have other children. In their new or expanded role as parents, they will face many demands and challenges. For most, this is a wonderful, exciting time filled with many discoveries and much information.

Mother and father/support persons or significant others learn as they watch the nurse interacting with their newborn. Nurses play a major role in teaching the newborn's caretakers about normal newborn characteristics and about ways to foster optimal growth and development. This role is even more important today because of limited hospital stays.

The newborn has come from a dark, small, enclosed space in the mother's uterus into the bright, cold extrauterine environment. Nurses can easily forget that they are caring for a small human being who is experiencing his or her first taste of human interaction outside the uterus. The newborn period is an extremely important one, and two national health goals have been developed to address this critical period (see the *Healthy People 2020* feature; U.S. Department of Health and Human Services [USDHHS], 2010).

It is also easy to overlook the intensity with which mother and father/support persons/significant others and visitors observe the actions of nurses as they care for the new family member. Nurses need to serve as a model for giving nurturing care to newborns. This chapter provides information about assessment and interventions in the period immediately following the birth of a newborn and during the early newborn period.

NURSING MANAGEMENT DURING THE IMMEDIATE NEWBORN PERIOD

The period of transition from intrauterine to extrauterine life occurs during the first several hours after birth. During this time, the newborn is undergoing numerous adaptations, many of which are occurring simultaneously (see Chapter 17 for more information on the newborn's adaptation). The neonate's temperature, respiration, and car-

HEALTHY PEOPLE 2020

Objective	Nursing Significance
• Increase the proportion of mothers who breast-feed their babies during the early postpartum period from a baseline of 74% to 81.9%. • Increase the proportion of mothers who breast-feed at 6 months from a baseline of 43.5% to 60.6%. • Increase the proportion of mothers who breast-feed at 1 year from a baseline of 22.7% to 34.1%.	• Will emphasize the importance of breast milk as the most complete form of nutrition for infants. • Will help to promote infant health, growth, immunity, and development throughout the newborn and infant periods.
• Ensure appropriate newborn bloodspot screening and follow-up testing. • Increase the number of states and the District of Columbia that verify through linkage with vital records that all newborns are screened shortly after birth for conditions mandated by their state-sponsored screening program. • Increase the proportion of screen-positive children who receive follow-up testing within the recommended time period. • (Developmental) Increase the proportion of children with a diagnosed condition identified through newborn screening who have an annual assessment of services needed and received. • Increase the proportion of newborns who are screened for hearing loss by no later than age 1 month, have audiologic evaluation by age 3 months, and are enrolled in appropriate intervention service no later than age 6 months.	• Will help to foster early detection and prompt treatment for conditions, thereby lessening the incidence of illness, disability, and death associated with these conditions and their overall effects on the newborn, infant, and family.

Healthy People objectives based on data from http://www.healthypeople.gov.

diovascular dynamics stabilize during this period. Close observation of the newborn's status is essential. Careful examination of the newborn at birth allows for detection of anomalies, birth injuries, and disorders that can compromise adaptation to extrauterine life. Problems that occur during this critical time can have a lifelong impact.

Assessment

The initial newborn assessment is completed in the birthing area to determine whether the newborn is stable enough to stay with the parents or whether resuscitation or other immediate interventions are necessary. Recently, an easy, rapid newborn assessment tool, the RAPP, has been developed to enhance the nurse's ability to quickly and accurately assess the newborn's physiologic condition. The RAPP assessment (**r**espiratory **a**ctivity, **p**erfusion, and **p**osition) provides a method to swiftly evaluate the newborn's condition so that decisions can be made regarding newborn stability (Ludington-Hoe & Morgan, 2014). A second assessment may be performed within the first 2 to 4 hours, when the newborn is admitted to the nursery or the labor and birth room. A third assessment is usually completed before discharge, according to the hospital policy. The purpose of these assessments is to determine the newborn's overall health status, to provide information to the mother and father/support persons/ significant others about their newborn, and to identify apparent physical abnormalities (Davidson, 2014).

During the initial newborn assessment, look for signs that might indicate a problem, including:

- Nasal flaring
- Chest retractions
- Grunting on exhalation
- Labored breathing
- Generalized cyanosis
- Abnormal breath sounds: rhonchi, crackles (rales), wheezing, and stridor
- Abnormal respiratory rates (tachypnea, more than 60 breaths/min; bradypnea, less than 25 breaths/min)
- Flaccid body posture
- Pallor
- Apneic episodes
- Abnormal heart rates (tachycardia, more than 160 bpm; bradycardia, less than 100 bpm)
- Abnormal newborn size: small or large for **gestational age**

If any of these findings is noted, medical intervention may be necessary.

Apgar Scoring

The **Apgar score**, introduced in 1952 by Dr. Virginia Apgar, is used worldwide to evaluate a newborn's physical condition at 1 minute and 5 minutes after birth. An additional Apgar assessment is done at 10 minutes if the 5-minute score is less than 7 points. The heart rate was found to be the most important diagnostic and prognostic of the five signs (Apgar, 2015). It can be used as a rapid method for assessing the survival of a neonate. Assessment of the newborn at 1 minute provides data about the newborn's initial adaptation to extrauterine life. Assessment at 5 minutes provides a clearer indication of the newborn's overall central nervous system status.

Five parameters are assessed with Apgar scoring. A quick way to remember the parameters of Apgar scoring is as follows:

- **A** = appearance (color)
- **P** = pulse (heart rate)
- **G** = grimace (reflex irritability)
- **A** = activity (muscle tone)
- **R** = respiratory (respiratory effort)

Each parameter is assigned a score ranging from 0 to 2 points. A score of 0 points indicates an absent or poor response; a score of 2 points indicates a normal response (Table 18.1). A normal newborn's score should be 8 to 10 points. The higher the score indicates the better condition of the newborn. If the Apgar score is 8 points or higher, no intervention is needed other than supporting normal respiratory efforts and maintaining thermoregulation. Scores of 4 to 7 points signify moderate difficulty and scores of 0 to 3 points represent severe distress in adjusting to extrauterine life. The Apgar score is influenced by the presence of infection, newborn maturity, mother's age, congenital anomalies, physiologic immaturity, maternal sedation via medications, labor management, and neuromuscular disorders (Rudiger & Konstantelos, 2015).

When the newborn experiences physiologic depression, the Apgar score characteristics disappear in a predictable manner: first the pink coloration is lost, next the respiratory effort, and then the tone, followed by reflex irritability and finally heart rate (Apgar, 2015).

Take Note!

Although Apgar scoring is done at 1 and 5 minutes, it also can be used as a guide during the immediate newborn period to evaluate the newborn's status for any changes because it focuses on critical parameters that must be assessed throughout the early transition period.

Length and Weight

Parents are eager to know their newborn's length and weight. These measurements are taken soon after birth. A disposable tape measure or a built-in measurement board located on the side of some scales can be used. Length is measured from the head of the newborn to the heel with the newborn unclothed (Fig. 18.1). Because of the flexed position of the newborn after birth, place the newborn in a supine position and extend the leg completely when measuring the length. The expected length range of

TABLE 18.1 APGAR SCORING FOR NEWBORNS

Parameter (Assessment Technique)	0 Point	1 Point	2 Points
Heart rate (auscultation of apical heart rate for 1 full minute)	Absent	Slow (<100 bpm)	>100 bpm
Respiratory effort (observation of the volume and vigor of the newborn's cry; auscultation of depth and rate of respirations)	Apneic	Slow, irregular, shallow	Regular respirations (usually 30–60 breaths/min), strong, good cry
Muscle tone (observation of extent of flexion in the newborn's extremities and newborn's resistance when the extremities are pulled away from the body)	Limp, flaccid	Some flexion, limited resistance to extension	Tight flexion, good resistance to extension with quick return to flexed position after extension
Reflex irritability (flicking of the soles of the feet or suctioning of the nose with a bulb syringe)	No response	Grimace or frown when irritated	Sneeze, cough, or vigorous cry
Skin color (inspection of trunk and extremities with the appropriate color for ethnicity appearing within minutes after birth)	Cyanotic or pale	Appropriate body color; blue extremities (acrocyanosis)	Completely appropriate color (pink on both trunk and extremities)

Data from Cunningham, F. G., Leveno, K. J., Bloom, S. L., Spong, C. Y., Dashe, J. S., Hoffman, B. L., et al. (2014). *William's obstetrics* (24th ed.). New York, NY: McGraw-Hill Medical; and Marcdante, K. J., & Kliegman, R. M. (2014). *Nelson essentials of pediatrics* (7th ed.). Philadelphia, PA: Elsevier Science Health.

a full-term newborn is usually 44 to 55 cm (17 to 22 in). **Molding** can affect measurement (Weber & Kelley, 2014).

Most often, newborns are weighed using a digital scale that reads the weight in grams. Typically, the term newborn weighs 2,500 to 4,000 g (5 lb, 8 oz to 8 lb, 14 oz; Fig. 18.2). Birth weights less than 10% or more than 90% on a growth chart are outside the normal range and need further investigation. Weights taken at later times are compared with previous weights and are documented with regard to gain or loss on a nursing flow sheet. Newborns can lose up to 10% of their initial birth weight by 3 to 4 days of age secondary to loss of meconium, extracellular fluid, and limited food intake. This weight loss is usually regained by the 10th day of life (Fonseca et al., 2014).

Newborns can be classified by their birth weight regardless of their gestational age (American Academy of Pediatrics [AAP], 2015a) as follows:

- Low birth weight: >2,500 g (>5.5 lb)
- Very low birth weight: >1,500 g (>3.5 lb)
- Extremely low birth weight: >1,000 g (>2.5 lb)

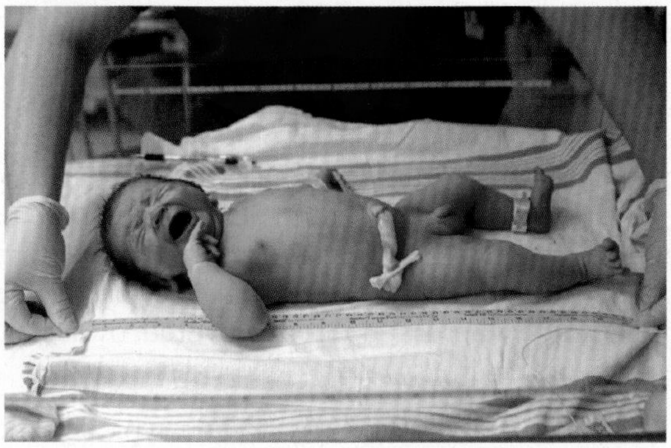

FIGURE 18.1 Measuring a newborn's length.

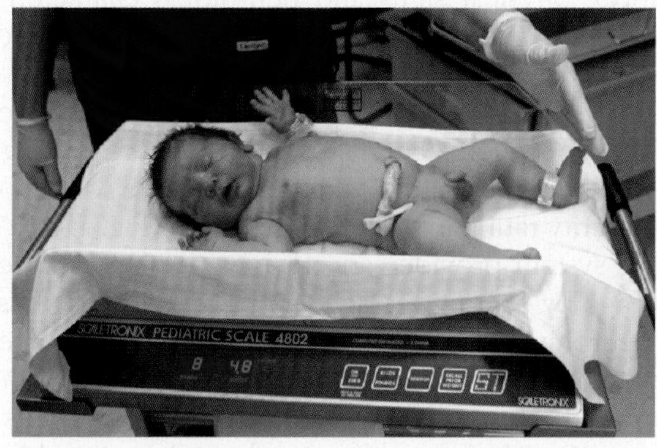

FIGURE 18.2 Weighing the newborn. Note how the nurse guards the newborn with her hand to prevent falling.

Vital Signs

Heart rate and respiratory rate are assessed immediately after birth with Apgar scoring. Heart rate, obtained by taking an apical pulse for 1 full minute, typically is 110 to 160 bpm. Newborns' respirations are assessed when they are quiet or sleeping. Place a stethoscope on the right side of the chest and count the breaths for 1 full minute to identify any irregularities. The newborn respiratory rate is 30 to 60 breaths/min with symmetric chest movement. Heart and respiratory rates are usually assessed every 30 minutes until stable for 2 hours after birth. Once stable, the heart rate and respiratory rates are checked every 8 hours. These assessment time frames may vary per hospital protocols, so nurses should follow the facility's procedures (Nagtalon-Ramos, 2014).

Vital signs are assessed at birth, within 1 to 4 hours after birth according to hospital policy. Vital signs are used for identifying a variety of complications and for ensuring well-being of the newborn. In some health care agencies, temperatures are taken immediately after the Apgar score has been taken to allow for identification of hypothermia, which then requires a glucose check, but nurses need to follow their hospital protocols on this assessment timing. In term newborns, the normal axillary temperature range should be maintained at 97.7° to 99.5°F (36.5° to 37.5°C).Rectal temperatures are no longer taken because of the risk of perforation (AAP, 2015b). The thermometer or temperature probe is held in the midaxillary space according to manufacturer's directions and hospital protocol. Blood pressure is not usually assessed as part of a normal newborn examination unless there is a clinical indication or low Apgar scores. If assessed, an oscillometer (Dinamap) is used. The typical range is 50 to 75 mm Hg (systolic) and 30 to 45 mm Hg (diastolic). Crying, moving, and late clamping of the umbilical cord will increase systolic pressure (Weber & Kelley, 2014). Typical values for newborn vital signs are provided in Table 18.2.

TABLE 18.2 NEWBORN VITAL SIGNS

Newborn Vital Signs	Ranges of Values
Temperature	97.7°–99.5°F (36.5°–37.5°C)
Heart rate (pulse) to 180 during crying	110–160 bpm; can increase
Respirations	30–60 breaths/min at rest; will increase with crying
Blood pressure	50–75 mm Hg systolic, 30–45 mm Hg diastolic

Data from Moses, S. (2015). Pediatric vital signs. *Family practice notebook*. Retrieved from http://www.fpnotebook.com/cv/exam/pdtrcvtlsgns.htm; and Kliegman, R. M., Behrman, R. E., Jenson, H. B., & Stanton, B. F. (2014). *Nelson's textbook of pediatrics* (20th ed.). St. Louis, MO: Saunders Elsevier.

Gestational Age Assessment

To determine a newborn's gestational age (the stage of maturity), physical signs and neurologic characteristics are assessed. Typically, gestational age is determined by using a tool such as the Ballard gestational age assessment or Ballard scale. It determines a newborn's gestational age between 20 and 44 weeks. A score is assigned to the various parameters, and the total score corresponds to a maturity rating in weeks of gestation (Fig. 18.3). This scoring system provides an objective estimate of gestational age by scoring the specific parameters of physical and neuromuscular maturity. Points are given for each assessment parameter, with a low score of −1 point or −2 points for extreme immaturity to 4 or 5 points for postmaturity. The scores from each section are added to correspond to a specific gestational age in weeks.

The physical maturity section of the examination is done during the first 2 hours after birth. The physical maturity assessment section of the Ballard examination evaluates physical characteristics that appear different at different stages depending on a newborn's gestational maturity. Newborns that are physically mature have higher scores than those who are not. The areas assessed on the physical maturity examination include:

- *Skin texture*—typically ranges from sticky and transparent to smooth, with varying degrees of peeling and cracking, to parchment-like or leathery with significant cracking and wrinkling
- *Lanugo*—soft downy hair on the newborn's body, which is absent in preterm newborns, appears with maturity, and then disappears again with postmaturity
- *Plantar creases*—creases on the soles of the feet, which range from absent to covering the entire foot, depending on maturity (the greater the number of creases, the greater the newborn's maturity)
- *Breast tissue*—the thickness and size of breast tissue and areola (the darkened ring around each nipple), which range from being imperceptible to full and budding
- *Eyes and ears*—eyelids can be fused or open and ear cartilage and stiffness determine the degree of maturity (the greater the amount of ear cartilage with stiffness, the greater the newborn's maturity)
- *Genitals*—in males, evidence of testicular descent and appearance of scrotum (which can range from smooth to covered with rugae) determine maturity; in females, appearance and size of clitoris and labia determine maturity (a prominent clitoris with flat labia suggests prematurity, whereas a clitoris covered by labia suggests greater maturity)

The neuromuscular maturity section typically is completed within 24 hours after birth. Six activities or maneuvers

NEUROMUSCULAR MATURITY

NEUROMUSCULAR MATURITY SIGN	SCORE −1	0	1	2	3	4	5	RECORD SCORE HERE
POSTURE								
SQUARE WINDOW (Wrist)	>90°	90°	60°	45°	30°	0°		
ARM RECOIL		180°	140°–180°	110°–140°	90°–110°	<90°		
POPLITEAL ANGLE	180°	160°	140°	120°	100°	90°	<90°	
SCARF SIGN								
HEEL TO EAR								
							TOTAL NEUROMUSCULAR MATURITY SCORE	

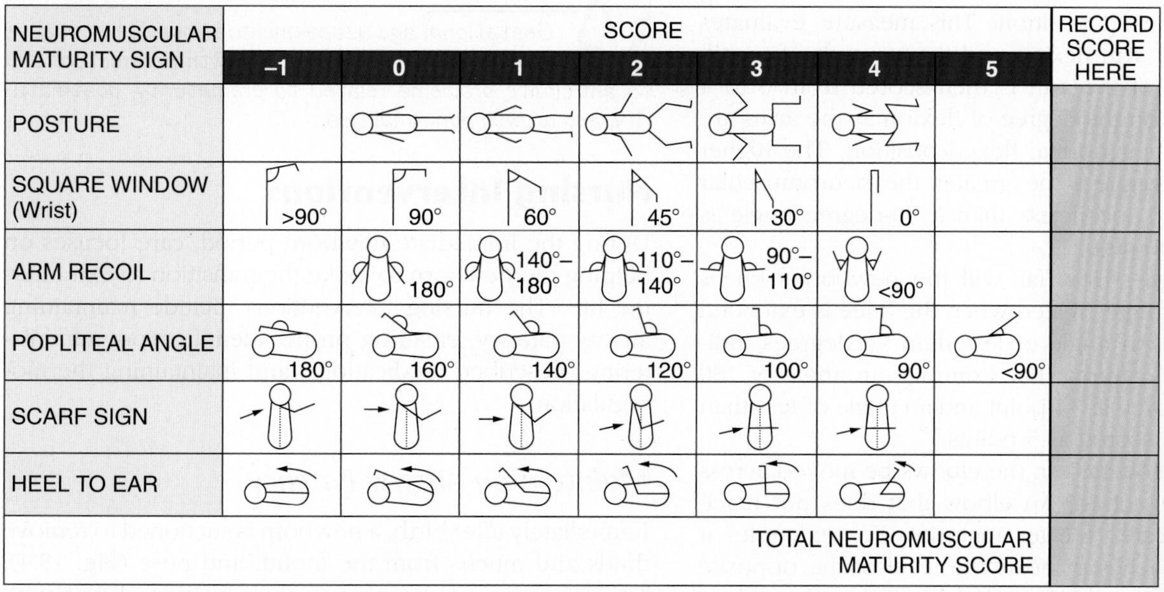

SCORE

Neuromuscular ____
Physical ____
Total ____

MATURITY RATING

Score	Weeks
−10	20
−5	22
0	24
5	26
10	28
15	30
20	32
25	34
30	36
35	38
40	40
45	42
50	44

PHYSICAL MATURITY

PHYSICAL MATURITY SIGN	SCORE −1	0	1	2	3	4	5	RECORD SCORE HERE
SKIN	sticky, friable, transparent	gelatinous, red, translucent	smooth, pink, visible veins	superficial peeling and/or rash, few veins	cracking pale areas, rare veins	parchment, deep cracking, no vessels	leathery, cracked, wrinkled	
LANUGO	none	sparse	abundant	thinning	bald areas	mostly bald		
PLANTAR SURFACE	heel-toe 40–50 mm: −1 <40 mm: −2	>50 mm no crease	faint red marks	anterior transverse crease only	creases ant. 2/3	creases over entire sole		
BREAST	impercep-tible	barely perceptible	flat areola no bud	stippled areola 1–2 mm bud	raised areola 3–4 mm bud	full areola 5–10 mm bud		
EYE-EAR	lids fused loosely: −1 tightly: −2	lids open pinna flat stays folded	sl. curved pinna; soft; slow recoil	well-curved pinna; soft but ready recoil	formed and firm instant recoil	thick cartilage, ear stiff		
GENITALS (Male)	scrotum flat, smooth	scrotum empty, faint rugae	testes in upper canal, rare rugae	testes descending, few rugae	testes down, good rugae	testes pendulous, deep rugae		
GENITALS (Female)	clitoris prominent and labia flat	prominent clitoris and small labia minora	prominent clitoris and enlarging minora	majora and minora equally prominent	majora large, minora small	majora cover clitoris and minora		
							TOTAL PHYSICAL MATURITY SCORE	

FIGURE 18.3 Gestational age assessment tool. The New Ballard Score (2014). (Adapted from http://www.ballardscore.com.)

that the newborn performs with various body parts are evaluated to determine the newborn's degree of maturity:

1. *Posture*—How does the newborn hold his or her extremities in relation to the trunk? The greater the degree of flexion, the greater the maturity. For example, extension of arms and legs is scored as 0 points and full flexion of arms and legs is scored as 4 points.
2. *Square window*—How far can the newborn's hands be flexed toward the wrist? The angle is measured and scored from more than 90 degrees to 0 degrees to determine the maturity rating. As the angle decreases, the newborn's maturity increases. For example, an angle of more than 90 degrees is scored as −1 point and an angle of 0 degrees is scored as 4 points.

3. *Arm recoil*—How far do the newborn's arms "spring back" to a flexed position? This measure evaluates the degree of arm flexion and the strength of recoil. The reaction of the arm is then scored from 0 to 4 points based on the degree of flexion as the arms are returned to their normal flexed position. The higher the points assigned, the greater the neuromuscular maturity (e.g., recoil less than a 90-degree angle is scored as 4 points).
4. *Popliteal angle*—How far will the newborn's knees extend? The angle created when the knee is extended is measured. An angle of less than 90 degrees indicates greater maturity. For example, an angle of 180 degrees is scored as –1 point and an angle of less than 90 degrees is scored as 5 points.
5. *Scarf sign*—How far can the elbows be moved across the newborn's chest? An elbow that does not reach midline indicates greater maturity. For example, if the elbow reaches or nears the level of the opposite shoulder, this is scored as –1 point; if the elbow does not cross the proximate axillary line, it is scored as 4 points.
6. *Heel to ear*—How close can the newborn's feet be moved to the ears? This maneuver assesses hip flexibility: the lesser the flexibility, the greater the newborn's maturity. The heel-to-ear assessment is scored in the same manner as the scarf sign.

After the scoring is completed, the 12 scores are totaled and then compared with standardized values to determine the appropriate gestational age in weeks. Scores range from very low in preterm newborns to very high for mature and postmature newborns.

Typically newborns are also classified according to gestational age as:

- *Preterm or premature*—born prior to 37 completed weeks' gestation, regardless of birth weight
- *Term*—born between 38 and 42 weeks' gestation
- *Postterm or postdates*—born after completion of week 42 of gestation
- *Postmature*—born after 42 weeks and demonstrating signs of placental aging

Using the information about gestational age and then considering birth weight, newborns can also be classified as follows:

- *Small for gestational age (SGA)*—weight less than the 10th percentile on standard growth charts (usually >5.5 lb)
- *Appropriate for gestational age (AGA)*—weight between 10th and 90th percentiles
- *Large for gestational age (LGA)*—weight more than the 90th percentile on standard growth charts (usually >9 lb)

Chapter 23 describes these variations in birth weight and gestational age in greater detail.

Take Note!

Gestational age assessment is important because it allows the nurse to plot growth parameters and to anticipate problems related to prematurity, postmaturity, and growth abnormalities.

Nursing Interventions

During the immediate newborn period, care focuses on helping the newborn to make the transition to extrauterine life. The nursing interventions include maintaining airway patency, ensuring proper identification, administering prescribed medications, and maintaining thermoregulation.

Maintaining Airway Patency

Immediately after birth, a newborn is suctioned to remove fluids and mucus from the mouth and nose (Fig. 18.4). Typically, the newborn's mouth is suctioned first with a bulb syringe to remove debris and then the nose is suctioned. Suctioning in this manner helps to prevent aspiration of fluid into the lungs by an unexpected gasp. Recent studies, along with recommendations from leading maternal health experts and the WHO, support using a towel to wipe secretions from the mouth and nose of newborns for stable newborns. Routine suctioning of the mouth and airways is not required. Despite evidence showing that the use of routine suctioning shows no benefit and may produce harm, the practice remains commonplace (Bond, 2015; Saugstad, 2015).

When suctioning a newborn with a bulb syringe, compress the bulb before placing it into the oral or nasal cavity. Release bulb compression slowly, making sure the tip is placed away from the mucous membranes to draw up the excess secretions. Remove the bulb syringe

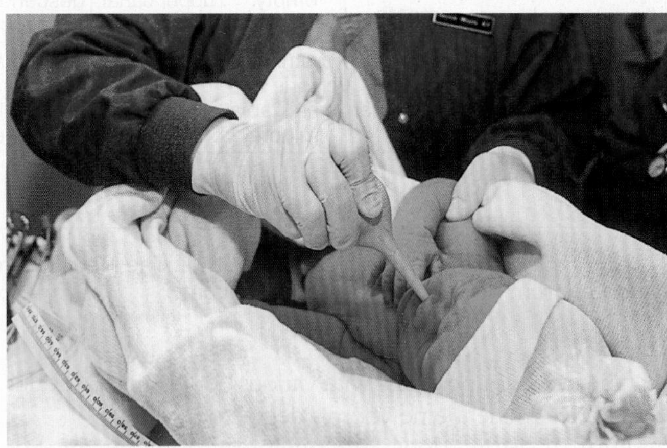

FIGURE 18.4 A newborn is suctioned by means of a bulb syringe to remove mucus from the mouth and nose. The head-down-and-to-the-side position facilitates drainage. Care is given with the infant under a radiant heat source. (Copyright Caroline Brown, RNC, MS, DEd.)

from the mouth or nose, and then, while holding the bulb syringe tip over an emesis basin lined with paper towel or tissue, compress the bulb to expel the secretions. Repeat the procedure several times until all secretions are removed or use a towel to wipe away secretions per hospital policy.

Take Note!

Always keep a bulb syringe near the newborn in case he or she develops sudden choking or a blockage in the nose. It may be lifesaving.

Ensuring Proper Identification

Infant abduction continues to be a threat in hospitals and health care organizations across the country. The abduction by nonfamily members of newborns from health care facilities has clearly become a subject of concern for parents, maternal-child care nurses, health care security and risk management administrators, law enforcement officials, and the National Center for Missing & Exploited Children (NCMEC). Staff ID badges, training, video surveillance, access control, and tagging systems can help prevent a newborn from being abducted from the hospital. Proactive security measures must become everyone's responsibility to ensure the safety of all newborns and their families in all hospital settings.

Before the newborn and family leave the birthing area, be sure that agency policy about identification has been followed. Typically, the mother, the newborn, and the father or any significant other or support person of the mother's choosing receive identification (ID) bracelets. The newborn commonly receives two ID bracelets, one on a wrist and one on an ankle. The mother receives a matching one, usually on her wrist. The ID bands usually state name, gender, date and time of birth, and identification number. The same identification number is on the bracelets of all family members.

These ID bracelets provide for the safety of the newborn and must be secured before the mother and newborn leave the birthing area. The ID bracelets are checked by all nurses to validate that the correct newborn is brought to the right mother if they are separated for any period of time (Fig. 18.5). They also serve as the official newborn identification and should be checked before initiating any procedure on that newborn and on discharge from the unit (NCMEC, 2015). Taking the newborn's picture within 2 hours after birth with a color camera or color video/digital image also helps prevent mix-ups and abduction. Many facilities use electronic devices that sound an alarm if a newborn is taken beyond a certain point on the unit or removed from the area.

Newborns' footprints may also be taken, using a form that includes the mother's fingerprint, name, date, and time of the birth. Some states require footprints of

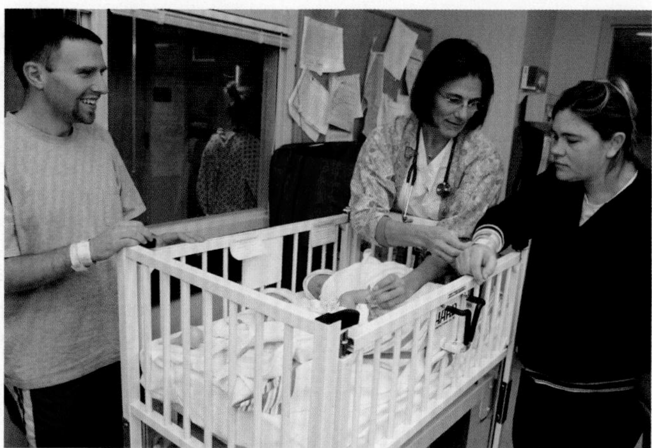

FIGURE 18.5 The nurse checks the newborn's identification band against the mother's.

the newborn, although many studies point out that birthing room staff does not take consistently legible footprints suitable for identification purposes (Goyal, Nagar, & Kumar, 2014). Many states have stopped requiring newborn footprints, and thus other means of identification are needed, such as collecting cord blood at the time of birth for DNA testing, facial biometric recognition, and live scans to capture digital forensic-quality prints that are suitable for identification purposes (Otsuka, 2014).

Prevention of infant abductions has been successful through a combination of increased security measures in hospitals, including video cameras and alarm devices, and education of staff and parents about precautions to take while in the hospital. It is critical not to allow anyone without identification to take an infant for any reason and to keep the infant within sight of the parent or nursery staff at all times. These measures should be largely invisible and create a sense of security rather than increasing parental fears about abduction.

Although infant abduction rates are rare, the safety and security of mothers and infants should remain a high priority for nurses. By being aware of physical security of maternity units, educating expectant parents on the methods used by potential abductors, and working with community resources, these tragic incidents can be prevented.

Administering Prescribed Medications

During the immediate newborn period, two medications are commonly ordered: vitamin K and eye prophylaxis with either erythromycin or tetracycline ophthalmic ointment (Drug Guide 18.1).

VITAMIN K

Prophylactic treatment of newborns with intramuscular vitamin K has been the standard of care for decades in the United States. Vitamin K, a fat-soluble vitamin, promotes blood clotting by increasing the synthesis of

DRUG GUIDE 18.1 DRUGS FOR THE NEWBORN

Drug	Action/Indication	Nursing Implications
Phytonadione (vitamin K [Aqua-MEPHYTON, Konakion, Mephyton])	Provides the newborn with vitamin K (necessary for production of adequate clotting factors II, VII, IX, and X by the liver) during the first week of birth until newborn can manufacture it Prevents vitamin K deficiency bleeding (VKDB) of the newborn	Administer within 1–2 hr after birth. Give as an IM injection at a 90-degree angle into the outer middle third of the vastus lateralis muscle. Use a 25-gauge, 5/8-in needle for injection. Hold the leg firmly and inject medication slowly. Adhere to standard precautions. Assess for bleeding at injection site after administration.
Erythromycin ophthalmic ointment 0.5% or tetracycline ophthalmic ointment 1%	Provides bactericidal and bacteriostatic actions to prevent *Neisseria gonorrhea* and *Chlamydia trachomatis* conjunctivitis Prevents ophthalmia neonatorum	Be alert for chemical conjunctivitis for 1–2 days. Wear gloves, and open eyes by placing thumb and finger above and below the eye. Gently squeeze the tube or ampoule to apply medication into the conjunctival sac from the inner canthus to the outer canthus of each eye. Do not touch the tip to the eye. Close the eye to make sure the medication permeates. Wipe off excess ointment after 1 min.

Adapted from King, T. L., Brucker, M. C., Kriebs, J. M., Fahey, J. O., Gegor, C. L., & Varney, H. (2015). *Varney's midwifery* (5th ed.). Burlington, MA: Jones & Bartlett Learning; and Skidmore-Roth, L. (2015). *Mosby's 2015 nursing drug reference* (28th ed.). St. Louis, MO: Elsevier Health Sciences.

prothrombin by the liver. A deficiency of this vitamin delays clotting and might lead to hemorrhage. Newborns are at risk for vitamin K deficiency and subsequent bleeding unless supplemented at birth. Vitamin K deficiency is an acquired coagulopathy in newborn infants because of an accumulation of inactive vitamin K coagulation factors, which leads to an increased bleeding tendency. Supplementation of vitamin K at birth has been recommended in the United States since 1961 and successfully reduces the risk of bleeding in newborns (Bellini, 2015).

Generally, the bacteria of the intestine produce vitamin K in adequate quantities. However, the newborn's bowel is sterile, so vitamin K is not produced in the intestine until after microorganisms have been introduced, such as with the first feeding. Usually it takes about a week for the newborn to produce enough vitamin K to prevent vitamin K deficiency bleeding. An oral vitamin K preparation is also being given to newborns outside the United States, but at least three doses are needed over a 1-month period (Abrams & Savelli, 2014).

The efficacy of vitamin K in preventing early vitamin K deficiency bleeding is firmly established and has been the standard of care since the AAP recommended it in the early 1960s. The AAP (2015c) recommends that vitamin K be administered to all newborns soon after birth in a single intramuscular dose of 0.5 to 1 mg (Fig. 18.6). The AAP also suggests that additional research is needed to validate the efficacy and safety of oral forms of vitamin

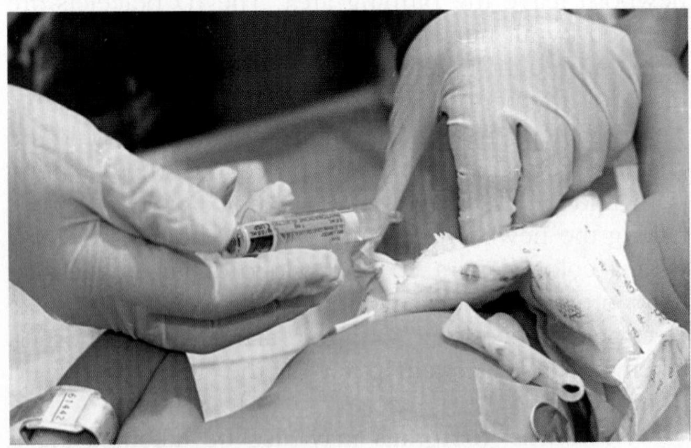

FIGURE 18.6 The nurse administers vitamin K IM to the newborn.

K, which have been used in many parts of the world, but currently are not recommended in the United States.

EYE PROPHYLAXIS

All newborns in the United States, whether delivered vaginally or by cesarean birth, must receive an installation of a prophylactic agent in their eyes within an hour or two of birth. This is mandated in all 50 states to prevent **ophthalmia neonatorum**, which can cause neonatal blindness (Centers for Disease Control and Prevention [CDC], 2015a). Ophthalmia neonatorum is a hyperacute purulent conjunctivitis occurring during the first 10 days of life. It is usually contracted during birth when the baby comes in contact with vaginal discharge of the mother infected with gonorrhea and chlamydia (CDC, 2015a). Most often both eyelids become swollen and red with purulent discharge.

Prophylactic agents that are currently recommended (and in most states legally required) include erythromycin 0.5% ophthalmic ointment or tetracycline 1% ophthalmic ointment in a single application. Silver nitrate solution was formerly used but has little efficacy in preventing chlamydial eye disease (Moore & MacDonald, 2015).

Regardless of which agent is used, instillation should be done as soon as possible after birth (Fig. 18.7). If instillation is delayed to allow visualization and bonding, the nursery staff should make sure the agent is administered when the newborn reaches the nursery for observation and assessment.

Inform all parents about the eye treatment, including why it is recommended, what problems may arise if the treatment is not given, and possible adverse effects of the treatment.

Take Note!

Ophthalmia neonatorum is a severe form of conjunctivitis caused by chlamydia and/or gonococcal infections that is potentially a blinding condition in newborns.

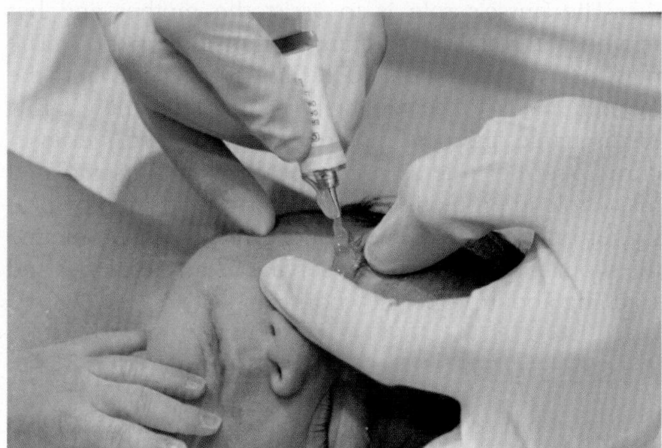

FIGURE 18.7 The nurse administers eye prophylaxis.

Maintaining Thermoregulation

Newborns have trouble regulating their temperature; especially during the first few hours after birth (see Chapter 17 for a complete discussion). Therefore, maintaining body temperature is crucial.

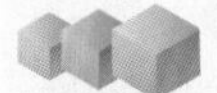

Concept Mastery Alert

Use of a Radiant Heater in Preventing Newborn Heat Loss

A 1-day-old infant should have adequate thermoregulation to remain out of the radiant heater. The best way to prevent heat loss is to ensure that the infant does not come in contact with cold surfaces.

Assess body temperature frequently during the immediate newborn period. The baby's temperature should be taken every 30 minutes for the first 2 hours or until the temperature has stabilized, and then every 8 hours until discharge or follow hospital protocols (King et al., 2015). Commonly a thermistor probe (automatic sensor) is attached to the newborn to record body temperature on a monitoring device. The probe is taped to the newborn's abdomen, usually in the right upper quadrant, which allows for position changes without having to readjust the probe. The other end of the thermistor probe is inserted into the radiant heat control panel. Temperature parameters are set on an alarm system connected to the heat panel that will sound if the newborn's temperature falls out of the set range. Check the probe connection periodically to make sure that it remains secure. Remember the potential for heat loss in newborns, and perform all nursing interventions in a way that minimizes heat loss and prevents hypothermia.

Axillary temperatures can also be used to assess the newborn's body temperature. Place thermometer under the newborn's axilla and place the arm over the chest to keep the thermometer in place and provide comfort to the newborn.

Nursing interventions to help maintain body temperature include:

- Dry the newborn immediately after birth to prevent heat loss through evaporation.
- Wrap the baby in warmed blankets to reduce heat loss via convection.
- Skin-to-skin contact with mother as soon as stabilized.
- Use a warmed cover on the scale to weigh the unclothed newborn.
- Warm stethoscopes and hands before examining the baby or providing care.
- Avoid placing newborns in drafts or near air vents to prevent heat loss through convection.
- Delay the initial bath until the baby's temperature has stabilized to prevent heat loss through evaporation.

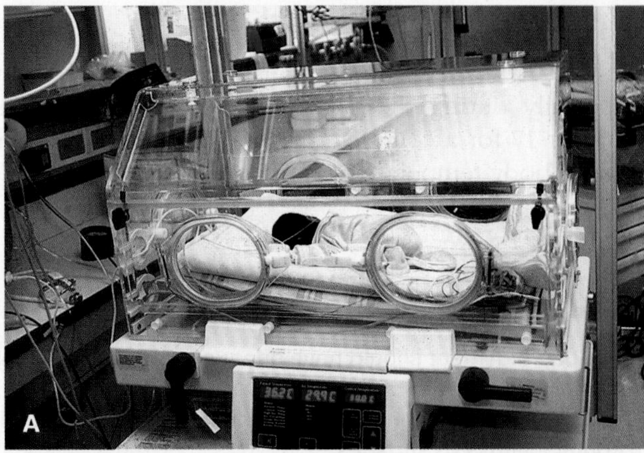

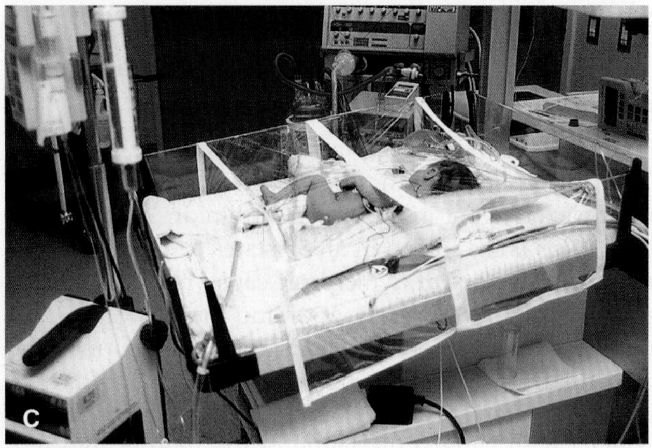

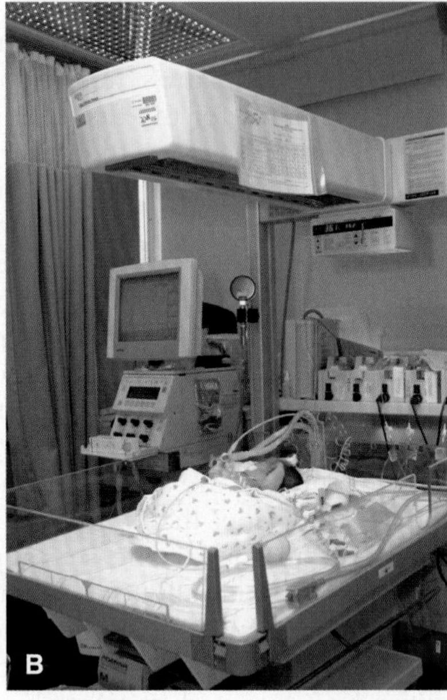

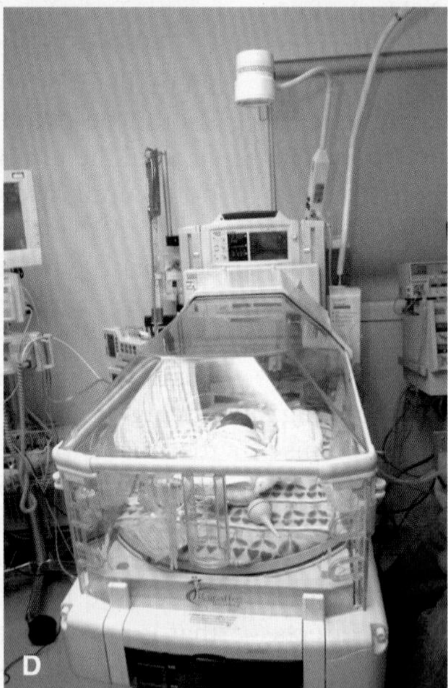

FIGURE 18.8 Maintaining thermoregulation. **A.** Isolette. **B.** Radiant warmer. **C.** Plastic wrap. **D.** Combination unit: radiant warmer and isolette.

- Avoid placing cribs near cold outer walls to prevent heat loss through radiation.
- Put a cap on the newborn's head after it is thoroughly dried after birth.
- Place the newborn under a temperature-controlled radiant warmer (Fig. 18.8).

NURSING MANAGEMENT DURING THE EARLY NEWBORN PERIOD

The early newborn period is a time of great adjustment for both the mother and the newborn, both of whom are adapting to many physiologic and psychological changes. In the past, mothers and newborns remained in the health care facility while these dramatic changes were taking place, with nurses and doctors readily available. However, today shorter hospital stays are the norm, and new mothers can easily be overwhelmed by having to go through all of these changes in such a short time: the woman gives birth, experiences marked physiologic and psychological changes, and must adapt to her newborn and learn the skills needed to care for herself and the baby, all within 24 to 48 hours.

The nurse's role is to assist the mother and her newborn through this dramatic transition period. The newborn needs continued health assessment, and the mother needs to be taught to care for the new baby. At discharge, the new mother may panic and feel insecure about her role as primary caretaker. Nurses play a major role in promoting the newborn's transition by providing ongoing assessment and care and in promoting the woman's confidence by serving as a role model and teaching about proper newborn care.

Assessment

The newborn requires ongoing assessment after leaving the birthing area to ensure that his or her transition to extrauterine life is progressing without problems. The nurse uses the data gathered during the initial assessment as a baseline for comparison.

Perinatal History

Pertinent maternal and fetal data are vital to formulate a plan of care for the mother and her newborn. Historical information is obtained from the medical record and from interviewing the mother. Review the maternal history because it provides pertinent information, such as the presence of certain risk factors that could affect the newborn. Keep in mind that a comprehensive maternal history may not be available, especially if the mother has had limited or no prenatal care. Historical information usually includes the following:

- Mother's name, medical record number, blood type, serology result, rubella and hepatitis status, and history of substance abuse
- Other maternal tests that are relevant to the newborn and care, such as human immunodeficiency virus (HIV) and group B streptococcus status
- Intrapartum maternal antibiotic therapy (type, dose, and duration)
- Maternal illness that can affect the pregnancy, evidence of chorioamnionitis, maternal use of medications such as steroids
- Prenatal care, including timing of first visit and subsequent visits
- Risk for blood group incompatibility, including Rh status and blood type
- Fetal distress or any nonreassuring fetal heart rate patterns during labor
- Known inherited conditions such as sickle cell anemia and phenylketonuria (PKU)
- Birth weights of previous live-born children, along with identification of any newborn problems
- Social history, including tobacco, alcohol, and recreational drug use
- History of depression or domestic violence
- Cultural factors, including primary language and educational level
- Pregnancy complications associated with abnormal fetal growth, fetal anomalies, or abnormal results from tests of fetal well-being
- Information on the progress of labor, birth, labor complications, duration of ruptured membranes, and presence of meconium in the amniotic fluid
- Medications given during labor, at birth, and immediately after birth
- Time and method of delivery, including presentation and the use of forceps or a vacuum extractor
- Status of the newborn at birth, including Apgar scores at 1 and 5 minutes, the need for suctioning, weight, gestational age, vital signs, and umbilical cord status
- Medications administered to the newborn
- Postbirth maternal information, including placental findings, positive cultures, and presence of fever

Newborn Physical Examination

The initial newborn physical examination, which may demonstrate subtle differences related to the newborn's age, is carried out within the first 24 hours after birth. For example, a newborn who is 30 minutes old has not yet completed the normal transition from intrauterine to extrauterine life, and thus variability may exist in vital signs and in respiratory, neurologic, gastrointestinal, skin, and cardiovascular systems. Therefore, a comprehensive examination should be delayed until after the newborn has completed the transition.

The physical examination should not be initiated if the newborn is crying or appears to be upset. Instead, it is best to postpone the assessment until the newborn is calm. In a quiet newborn, begin the examination with the least invasive and noxious elements of the examination (auscultation of heart and lungs). Then examine the areas most likely to irritate the newborn (e.g., examining the hips and eliciting the Moro reflex). A general visual assessment provides an enormous amount of information about the well-being of a newborn. Initial observation gives an impression of a healthy (stable) versus an ill newborn and a term versus a preterm newborn.

A typical physical examination of a newborn includes a general survey of skin color, posture, state of alertness, head size, overall behavioral state, respiratory status, gender, and any obvious congenital anomalies. Check the overall appearance for anything unusual. Then complete the examination in a systematic fashion.

Remember Kelly, who called the home health nurse and said her newborn son "looks like a canary"? What additional information is needed about the baby? What might be causing his yellow color?

ANTHROPOMETRIC MEASUREMENTS

Shortly after birth, after the gender of the child is revealed, most women and their partners/significant others want to know the vital statistics of their newborn – length and weight – to report to their family and friends. Additional measurements, including head and chest circumference, are also taken and recorded. Abdominal measurements are not routinely obtained unless there is a suspicion of pathology that causes abdominal distention. The newborn's progress from that point on will be validated based on these early measurements. These measurements will be compared with future serial measurements to determine growth patterns, which are plotted on growth charts to evaluate normalcy. Therefore, accuracy is paramount.

Length. The average length of most newborns is 50 cm (20 in), but it can range from 44 to 55 cm (17 to 22 in). Measure length with the unclothed newborn lying on a warmed blanket placed on a flat surface with the knees held in an extended position. Then run a tape measure down the length of the newborn – from the head to the soles of the feet – and record this measurement in the newborn's record (Fig. 18.1).

Weight. At birth the average newborn weighs 3,400 g (7.5 lb), but normal birth weights can range from 2,500 to 4,000 g (5 lb, 8 oz to 8 lb, 13 oz). Newborns are weighed immediately after birth and then daily. Newborns usually lose up to 6% of their birth weight within the first few days of life, but regain it in approximately 10 days.

Newborns are weighed on admission to the nursery or are taken to a digital scale to be weighed and returned to the mother's room. First, balance the scale if it is not balanced. Place a warmed protective cloth or paper as a barrier on the scale to prevent heat loss by conduction; recalibrate the scale to zero after applying the barrier. Next, place the unclothed newborn in the center of the scale. Keep a hand above the newborn for safety (Fig. 18.2).

Weight is affected by racial origin, genetics, maternal age, size of the parents, maternal nutrition, maternal weight prenatally, and placental perfusion (Tawia & McGuire, 2014). Weight should be correlated with gestational age. A newborn who weighs more than normal might be LGA or an infant of a diabetic mother; a newborn who weighs less than normal might be SGA, preterm, or have a genetic syndrome. It is important to identify the cause for the deviation in size and to monitor the newborn for complications common to that etiology.

Head Circumference. The average newborn head circumference is 32 to 38 cm (13 to 15 in). Measure the circumference at the head's widest diameter (the occipitofrontal circumference). Wrap a flexible or paper measuring tape snugly around the newborn's head and record the measurement (Fig. 18.9A).

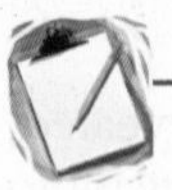

Take Note!

Head circumference may need to be remeasured at a later time if the shape of the head is altered from birth.

The head circumference should be approximately one fourth of the newborn's length or about half the infant's body length plus 10 cm. Expected head circumference for a term infant is between 32 and 37 cm (12.5 to 14.5 in) (Nagtalon-Ramos, 2014). A small head might indicate microcephaly caused by rubella, toxoplasmosis, or SGA status; an enlarged head might indicate hydrocephalus or increased intracranial pressure. Both need to be documented and reported for further investigation.

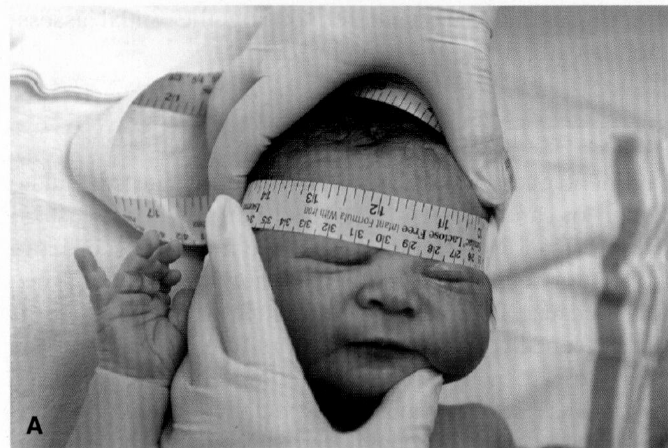

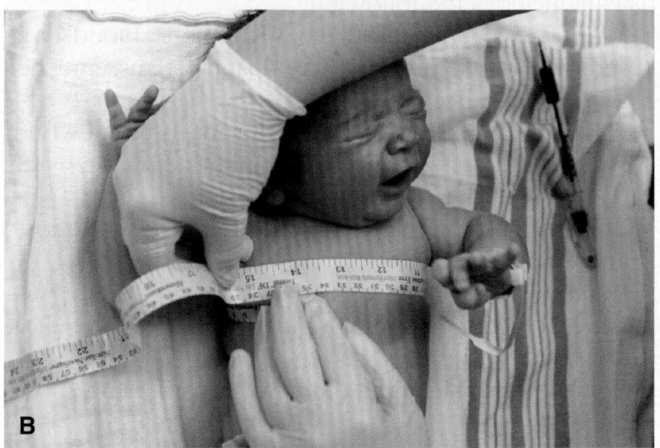

FIGURE 18.9 **A.** Measuring head circumference. **B.** Measuring chest circumference.

Chest Circumference. The average chest circumference is 30 to 36 cm (12 to 14 in). It is generally equal to or about 2 to 3 cm less than the head circumference (Weber & Kelley, 2014). Place a flexible or paper tape measure around the unclothed newborn's chest just below the nipple line without pulling it taut (Fig. 18.9B).

Take Note!

The head and chest circumferences are usually equal by about 1 year of age.

VITAL SIGNS

In the newborn, temperature, pulse, and respirations are monitored frequently and compared with baseline data obtained immediately after birth. Generally, vital signs (excluding blood pressure) are taken:

- On admission to the nursery or in the labor and birth room after the woman/parents are allowed to hold and bond with the newborn

- Once every 30 minutes until the newborn has been stable for 2 hours
- Then once every 4 to 8 hours until discharge (Davidson, 2014)

Blood pressure is not routinely assessed in a normal newborn unless the baby's clinical condition warrants it. This schedule can change depending on the baby's health status.

Obtain a newborn's temperature by placing an electronic temperature probe in the midaxillary area or by monitoring the electronic thermistor probe that has been taped to the abdominal skin (applied when the newborn was placed under a radiant heat source). Monitor the newborn's temperature frequently per hospital protocol for changes until it stabilizes. If the temperature is higher, adjust the environment, such as removing some clothing or blankets. If the temperature is lower, check the radiant warmer setting or add a warmed blanket. Report any abnormalities to the primary health care provider if simple adjustments to the environment do not change the baby's temperature.

Obtain an apical pulse by placing the stethoscope over the fourth intercostal space on the chest. Listen for a full minute, noting rate, rhythm, and abnormal sounds such as murmurs. In the typical newborn, the heart rate is 120 to 160 bpm, with wide fluctuations with activity and sleep. Sinus arrhythmia is a normal finding. Murmurs detected during the newborn period do not necessarily indicate congenital heart disease, but they need to be evaluated further if they persist. Also palpate the apical, femoral, and brachial pulses for presence and equality (Fig. 18.10). Report any abnormalities to the primary health care provider for evaluation.

Assess respirations by observing the rise and fall of the chest for 1 full minute. Respirations should be symmetric, slightly irregular, shallow, and unlabored at a rate of 30 to 60 breaths/min. The newborn's respirations are predominantly diaphragmatic, but they are synchronous with abdominal movements. Also auscultate breath sounds. Note any abnormalities, such as tachypnea, bradypnea, grunting, gasping, periods of apnea lasting longer than 20 seconds, asymmetry or decreased chest expansion, abnormal breath sounds (rhonchi, crackles), or sternal retractions. Some variations might exist early after birth, but if the abnormal pattern persists, notify the primary health care provider.

SKIN

The newborn's skin is similar in structure to the adult's, but many of the functions are not fully developed. Observe the overall appearance of the skin, including color, texture, turgor, and integrity. The newborn's skin should be smooth and flexible, and the color should be consistent with genetic background.

Skin Condition and Color. Check skin turgor by pinching a small area of skin over the chest or abdomen and note how quickly it returns to its original position. In a well-hydrated newborn, the skin should return to its normal position immediately. Skin that remains "tented" after being pinched may indicate dehydration. A small amount of lanugo (fine downy hair) may be observed

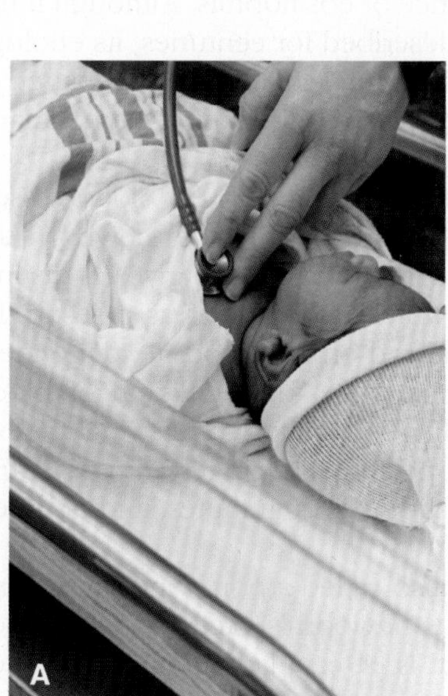

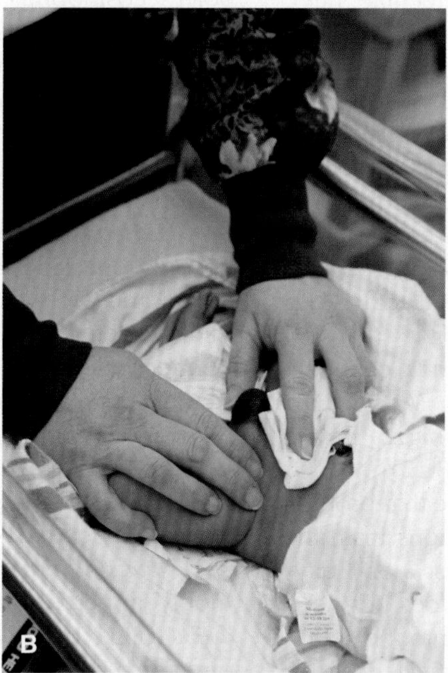

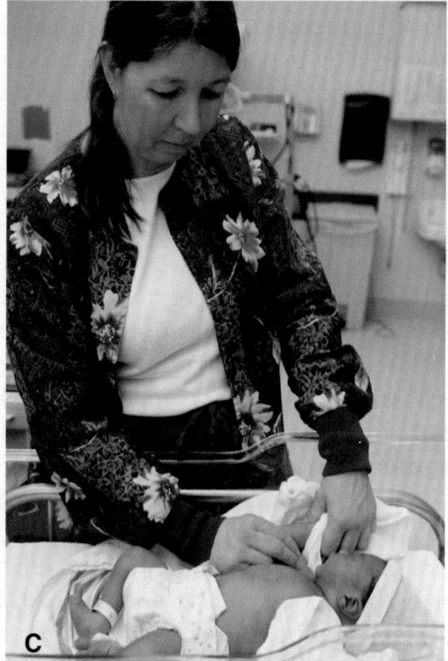

FIGURE 18.10 Assessing the newborn's vital signs. **A.** Assessing the apical pulse. **B.** Palpating the femoral pulse. **C.** Palpating the brachial pulse.

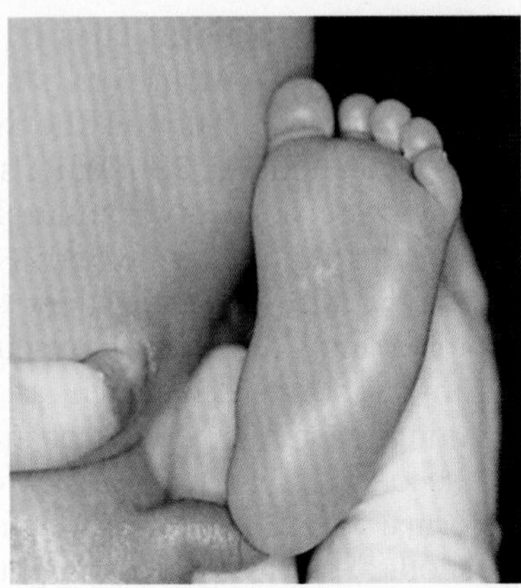

FIGURE 18.11 Acrocyanosis. This commonly appears on the feet and hands of babies shortly after birth. This infant is a 32-week newborn. (From Fletcher M. (1998). *Physical diagnosis in neonatology*. Philadelphia, PA: Lippincott-Raven Publishers.)

over the shoulders and on the sides of the face and upper back. There may be some cracking and peeling of the skin. The skin should be warm to the touch and intact.

The newborn's skin often appears blotchy or mottled, especially in the extremities. Persistent cyanosis of fingers, hands, toes, and feet with mottled blue or red discoloration and coldness is called **acrocyanosis** (Fig. 18.11). It may be seen in newborns during the first few weeks of life in response to exposure to cold. Acrocyanosis is normal and intermittent. Any change in color of the newborn skin needs further investigation.

Newborn Skin Variations. While assessing the skin, make note of any rashes, ecchymoses or petechiae, nevi, or dark pigmentation. Skin lesions can be congenital or transient; they may be a result of infection or may result from the mode of birth. If any are present, observe the anatomic location, arrangement, type, and color. Bruising may result from the use of devices such as a vacuum extractor during delivery. Petechiae may be the result of pressure on the skin during the birth process. Forceps marks may be observed over the cheeks and ears. A small puncture mark may be seen if internal fetal scalp electrode monitoring was used during labor.

Common skin variations include **vernix caseosa**, **stork bites** or salmon patches, **milia**, **Mongolian spots**, **erythema toxicum**, **harlequin sign**, **nevus flammeus**, and **nevus vasculosus** (Fig. 18.12).

Vernix caseosa is a thick white substance that protects the skin of the fetus. It is formed by secretions from the fetus's oil glands and is found during the first 2 or 3 days after birth in body creases and the hair. It does not need to be removed because it will be absorbed into the skin.

Stork bites or salmon patches are superficial vascular areas found on the nape of the neck, on the eyelids, and between the eyes and upper lip (Fig. 18.12A). The name comes from the marks on the back of the neck where, as myth goes, a stork may have picked up the baby. They are caused by a concentration of immature blood vessels and are most visible when the newborn is crying. They are considered a normal variant, and most fade and disappear completely within the first year.

Milia are multiple pearly-white or pale yellow unopened sebaceous glands frequently found on a newborn's nose. They may also appear on the chin and forehead (Fig. 18.12B). They form from oil glands and disappear on their own within 2 to 4 weeks. When they occur in a newborn's mouth and gums, they are termed **Epstein pearls**. They occur in approximately 80% of newborns. As most lesions break spontaneously within the first few weeks of life, no therapy is indicated (El-Radhi, 2015).

Mongolian spots are benign blue or purple splotches that appear solitary on the lower back and buttocks of newborns, but may occur as multiple over the legs and shoulders (Fig. 18.12C). They tend to occur in African American, Asian, Hispanic, and Indian newborns but can occur in dark-skinned newborns of all races. The spots are caused by a concentration of pigmented cells and usually disappear spontaneously within the first 4 years of life. They should not be confused with bruises caused by trauma (Silverberg, 2015).

Erythema toxicum (newborn rash) is a benign, idiopathic, generalized, transient rash that occurs in up to 70% of all newborns during the first week of life. It consists of small papules or pustules on the skin resembling flea bites. It is often mistaken for staphylococcal pustules. The rash is common on the face, chest, and back (Fig. 18.12D). One of the chief characteristics of this rash is its lack of pattern. It is caused by the newborn's eosinophils reacting to the environment as the immune system matures. Histologically, erythema toxicum shows an abundance of eosinophils. Although it has been recognized and described for centuries, its etiology and pathogenesis remain unclear (Gloster, Gebauer, & Mistur, 2016a). It does not require any treatment and disappears in a few days.

Harlequin sign refers to the dilation of blood vessels on only one side of the body, giving the newborn the appearance of wearing a clown suit. It gives a distinct midline demarcation, which is described as pale on the nondependent side and red on the opposite, dependent side. It results from immature autoregulation of blood flow and is commonly seen in low-birth-weight newborns when there is a positional change (Lomax, 2015). It is transient, lasting as long as 20 minutes, and no intervention is needed.

Nevus flammeus, also called a port-wine stain, commonly appears on the newborn's face or other body areas (Fig. 18.12E). It is a capillary angioma located directly below the dermis. It is flat with sharp demarcations and is purple-red. This skin lesion is made up of mature capillaries that are congested and dilated. It

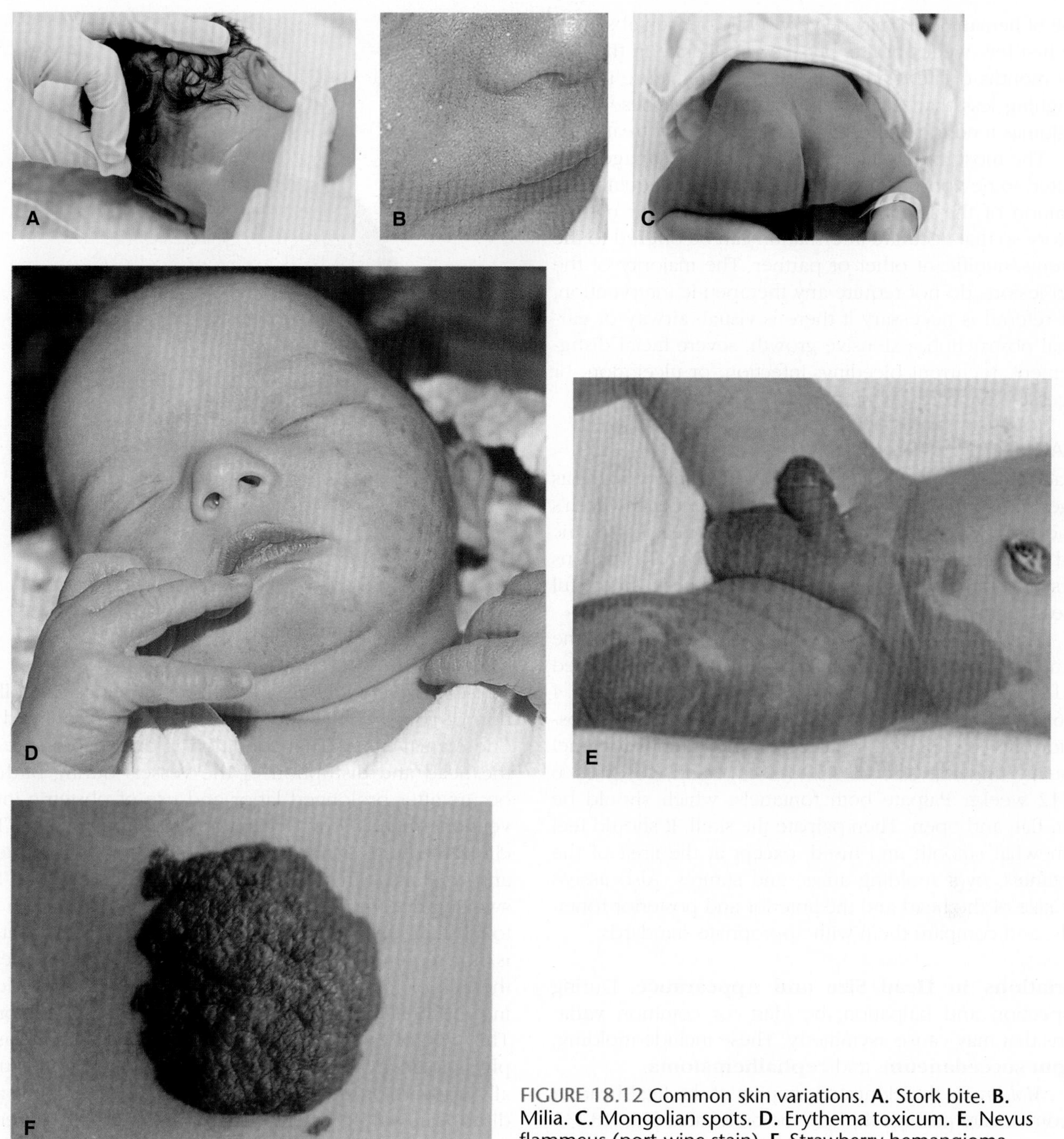

FIGURE 18.12 Common skin variations. **A.** Stork bite. **B.** Milia. **C.** Mongolian spots. **D.** Erythema toxicum. **E.** Nevus flammeus (port-wine stain). **F.** Strawberry hemangioma.

ranges in size from a few millimeters to large, occasionally involving as much as half the body surface. Although it does not grow in area or size, it is permanent and will not fade. Although they may occur anywhere on the body, the majority are located in the head and neck areas. Port-wine stains may be associated with structural malformations, bony or muscular overgrowth, and certain cancers. Recent studies have noted an association between port-wine birthmarks and childhood cancer, so newborns with these lesions should be monitored with periodic eye examinations, neurologic imaging, and extremity measurements. Lasers and intense pulsed light have been used to remove larger lesions with some success. The optimal timing of treatment is before 1 year of age (Giese & Richter, 2015).

Nevus vasculosus, also called a strawberry mark or strawberry hemangioma, is a benign capillary hemangioma in the dermal and subdermal layers. It is raised, rough, dark red, and sharply demarcated (Fig. 18.12F). It is commonly found in the head region within a few weeks after birth and can increase in size or number. They are commonly found in about 10% of children. This type of hemangioma may be very subtle or even absent in the first few weeks of life, but they proliferate in the first few months of life. Commonly seen in premature infants weighing less than 1,500 g (El-Radhi, 2015), these hemangiomas tend to resolve by age 3 without any treatment.

The most important aspects of nursing management related to newborn skin variations include adequate recognition of the lesions and knowledge of their natural history so that accurate information can be offered to the parents/significant other or partner. The majority of the skin lesions do not require any therapeutic intervention, but referral is necessary if there is visual, airway or ear-canal obstruction, extensive growth, severe facial disfigurement, recurrent bleeding, infection, or ulceration, or excessive concern by the parents.

HEAD

Head size varies with age, gender, and ethnicity and has a general correlation with body size. Inspect a newborn's head from all angles. The head should appear symmetric and round. As many as 90% of the congenital malformations present at birth are visible on the head and neck, so careful assessment is very important (Pfister & Ramel, 2014).

The newborn has two fontanels at the juncture of the cranial bones. The anterior fontanel is diamond shaped and closes by 18 to 24 months. Typically it measures 4 to 6 cm at the largest diameter (bone to bone). The posterior one is triangular, smaller than the anterior fontanel (usually fingertip size or 0.5 to 1 cm), and closes by 6 to 12 weeks. Palpate both fontanels, which should be soft, flat, and open. Then palpate the skull. It should feel somewhat smooth and fused, except at the area of the fontanels, over molding areas, and sutures. Also assess the size of the head and the anterior and posterior fontanels, and compare them with appropriate standards.

Variations in Head Size and Appearance. During inspection and palpation, be alert for common variations that may cause asymmetry. These include molding, **caput succedaneum**, and **cephalhematoma**.

Molding is the elongated shaping of the fetal head to accommodate passage through the birth canal (Fig. 18.13). It occurs with a vaginal birth from a vertex position in which elongation of the fetal head occurs with prominence of the occiput and overriding sagittal suture line. It typically resolves within a week after birth without intervention.

Caput succedaneum describes localized edema on the scalp that occurs from the pressure of the birth process. It is commonly observed after prolonged labor. Clinically, it appears as a poorly demarcated soft tissue swelling that crosses suture lines. Pitting edema and overlying petechiae and ecchymosis are noted (Fig. 18.14A). The swelling will gradually dissipate in about 3 days without any treatment. Newborns who were delivered via vacuum extraction usually have a caput in the area where the cup was used.

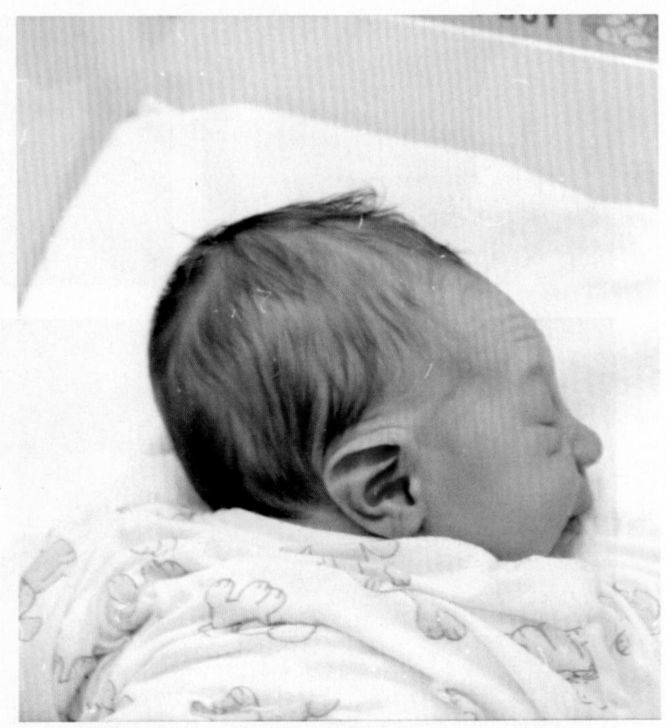

FIGURE 18.13 Molding in a newborn's head.

*Cephalhematoma*is a localized subperiosteal collection of blood of the skull which is always confined by one cranial bone. This condition is due to pressure on the head and disruption of the vessels during birth. It occurs after prolonged labor and use of obstetric interventions such as low forceps or vacuum extraction. The clinical features include a well-demarcated, often fluctuant swelling with no overlying skin discoloration. The swelling does not cross suture lines and is firmer to the touch than an edematous area (Fig. 18.14B). Aspiration is not required for resolution and is likely to increase the risk of infection. Hyperbilirubinemia occurs following the breakdown of the RBCs within the hematoma. This type of hyperbilirubinemia occurs later than classic physiologic hyperbilirubinemia. Cephalhematoma usually appears on the second or third day after birth and disappears within weeks or months. Large cephalhematomas can lead to increased bilirubin levels and subsequent jaundice (Lomax, 2015).

Common Abnormalities in Head or Fontanel Size. Common abnormalities in head or fontanel size that may indicate a problem include:

- *Microcephaly*—a head circumference more than 2 standard deviations below average or less than 10% of normal parameters for gestational age, caused by failure of brain development. There is a reduced production of neurons leading to a reduction of brain volume and as a consequence of that a reduced skull size. Microcephaly is common, affecting more than 25,000 infants in the United States each year. Children

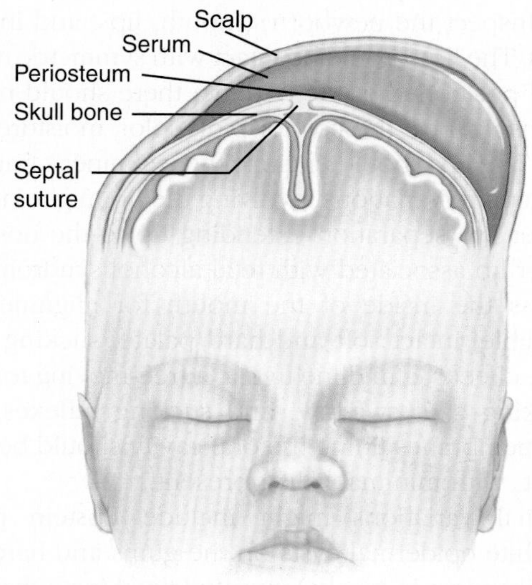

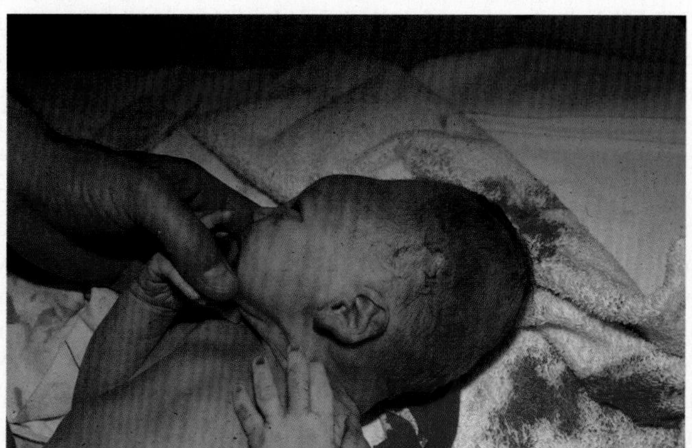

Scalp
Periosteum
Skull bone
B1

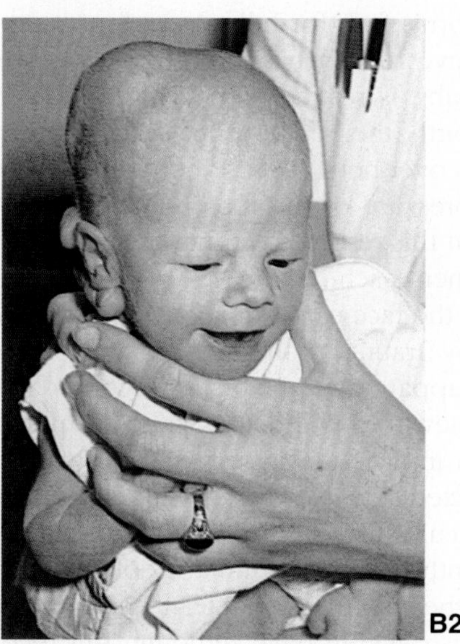

FIGURE 18.14 **A1 and A2.** Caput succedaneum involves the collection of serous fluid and often crosses the suture line. **B1 and B2.** Cephalhematoma involves the collection of blood and does not cross the suture line. (**A1**, **B1**, and **B2**, photos from O'Doherty N. *Atlas of the newborn.* Philadelphia: J B Lippincott, 1979:136, and 1979:117, 143, with permission. A2, photo from Chung, E. K., Atkinson-McEvoy, L. R., Boom, J. A., & Matz, P. S. (2010). *Visual diagnosis and treatment in pediatrics* (2nd ed.). LWW, Courtesy of the late Peter Sol, MD.)

with severe microcephaly, defined as more than 3 standard deviations below the mean for age and sex, are more likely to have imaging abnormalities and more severe developmental impairments than those with milder microcephaly. About 40% of children with microcephaly also have epilepsy, 20% have cerebral palsy, 50% have intellectual disability, and 20% to 50% have ophthalmologic and hearing disorders (Boom, 2015a). It can be familial, with autosomal dominant or recessive inheritance, and it may be associated with infections (cytomegalovirus), rubella, toxoplasmosis, and syndromes such as trisomy 13, 18, or 21 and fetal alcohol syndrome. Genetic counseling and clinical management through carrier detection/prenatal diagnosis in families can help reduce the incidence of these disorders (Alcantara & O'Driscoll, 2014).

- *Macrocephaly*—a head circumference more than 90% of normal, typically related to hydrocephalus (Boom, 2015b). It is often familial (with autosomal dominant inheritance) and can be either an isolated anomaly or a manifestation of other anomalies, including hydrocephalus and skeletal disorders (achondroplasia).
- *Large fontanels*—more than 6 cm in the anterior diameter bone to bone or more than a 1-cm diameter in the posterior fontanel; possibly associated with malnutrition, hydrocephaly, congenital hypothyroidism, trisomies 13, 18, and 21, and various bone disorders such as osteogenesis imperfecta.
- *Small or closed fontanels*—smaller-than-normal anterior and posterior diameters or fontanels that are closed at birth. Craniosynostosis and abnormal brain development are associated with a small fontanel or early fontanel closure associated with microcephaly (Sheth, Ranalli, & Aldana, 2014).

FACE

Observe the newborn's face for fullness and symmetry. The face should have full cheeks and should be symmetric when the baby is resting and crying. If forceps were used during birth, the newborn may have bruising and reddened areas over both cheeks and parietal bones secondary to the pressure of the forceps blades. Reassure the parents that this resolves without treatment, and point out improvement each day.

Problems with the face can also involve facial nerve paralysis caused by trauma from the use of forceps. Paralysis is usually apparent on the first or second day of life. Typically, the newborn will demonstrate asymmetry of the face with an inability to close the eye and move the lips on the affected side. Newborns with facial nerve paralysis have difficulty making a seal around the nipple, and consequently milk or formula drools from the paralyzed side of the mouth. Most facial nerve palsies resolve spontaneously within days, although full recovery may require weeks to months. Attempt to determine the cause from the newborn's history.

Nose. Inspect the nose for size, symmetry, position, and lesions. The newborn's nose is small and narrow. The nose should have a midline placement, patent nares, and an intact septum. The nostrils should be of equal size and should be patent. A slight mucous discharge may be present, but there should be no actual drainage. The newborn is a preferential nose breather and will use sneezing to clear the nose if needed. The newborn can smell after the nasal passages are cleared of amniotic fluid and mucus (Clark-Gambelunghe & Clark, 2015).

Mouth. Inspect the newborn's mouth, lips, and interior structures. The lips should be intact with symmetric movement and positioned in the midline; there should not be any lesions. Inspect the lips for pink color, moisture, and cracking. The lips should encircle the examiner's finger to form a vacuum. Variations involving the lip might include cleft upper lip (separation extending up to the nose) or thin upper lip associated with fetal alcohol syndrome.

Assess the inside of the mouth for alignment of the mandible, intact soft and hard palate, sucking pads inside the cheeks, a midline uvula, a free-moving tongue, and working gag, swallow, and sucking reflexes. The mucous membranes lining the oral cavity should be pink and moist, with minimal saliva present.

Normal variations might include Epstein pearls (small, white epidermal cysts on the gums and hard palate that disappear in weeks), erupted natal teeth that may need to be removed to prevent aspiration (Fig. 18.15), and thrush (white plaque inside the mouth caused by exposure to *Candida albicans* during birth), which cannot be wiped away with a cotton-tipped applicator.

Eyes. Inspect the external eye structures, including the eyelids, lashes, conjunctiva, sclera, iris, and pupils, for position, color, size, and movement. There may be marked edema of the eyelids and subconjunctival hemorrhages due to pressure during birth. The eyes should be clear and symmetrically placed. Test the blink reflex by bringing an object close to the eye; the newborn should respond quickly by blinking. Also test the newborn's pupillary reflex: pupils should be equal, round, and reactive to light bilaterally. Assess the newborn's gaze: he or she should be able to track objects to the midline. Movement may be uncoordinated during the first few weeks of life. Many newborns have transient strabismus (deviation or wandering of eyes independently) and searching nystagmus (involuntary repetitive eye movement), which is caused by immature muscular control. These are normal for the first 3 to 6 months of age.

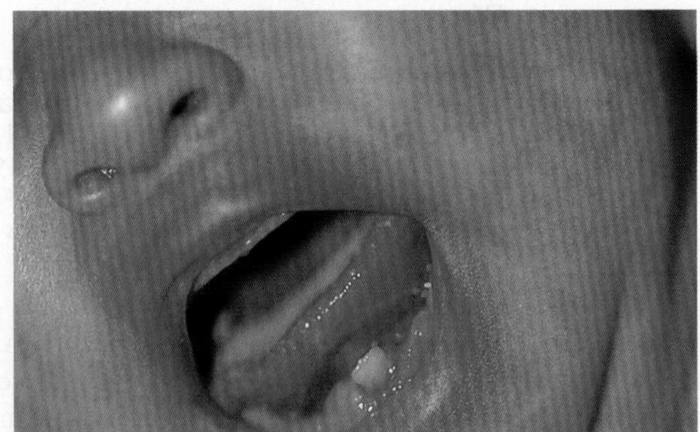

FIGURE 18.15 A natal tooth in a 16-day-old neonate. Natal teeth can be present at birth and are usually considered benign. No treatment is needed if they don't interfere with feeding.

Examine the internal eye structures. A red reflex (luminous red appearance seen on the retina) should be seen bilaterally on retinoscopy. The red reflex normally shows no dullness or irregularities.

Chemical conjunctivitis commonly occurs within 24 hours of instillation of eye prophylaxis after birth. There is lid edema with sterile discharge from both eyes. Usually it resolves within 48 hours without treatment.

Ears. Inspect the ears for size, shape, skin condition, placement, amount of cartilage, and patency of the auditory canal. The ears should be soft and pliable and should recoil quickly and easily when folded and released. Ears should be aligned with the outer canthi of the eyes. Low-set ears and abnormally shaped ears are characteristic of many syndromes and genetic abnormalities, such as trisomy 13 or 18, and internal organ abnormalities involving the renal system. Findings of sinuses or preauricular skin tags should prompt further evaluation for possible renal abnormalities since both systems develop at the same time.

An otoscopic examination is not typically done because the newborn's ear canals are filled with amniotic fluid and vernix caseosa, which would make visualization of the tympanic membrane difficult.

Newborn hearing screening is required by law in most states (discussed later in the chapter). Hearing loss is the most common birth defect in the United States: 1 in 1,000 newborns are profoundly deaf and 3 in 1,000 have some degree of hearing impairment (March of Dimes, 2015a). Delays in identification and intervention may affect the child's cognitive, verbal, behavioral, and emotional development. Screening at birth has reduced the age at which newborns with hearing loss are identified and has improved early intervention rates dramatically. Available treatments include cochlear implantation, hearing augmentation, and follow-up by an audiologist, otolaryngologist, pediatrician, geneticist, and deaf education specialist (Nikolopoulos, 2015). Prior to universal newborn screening, children were usually older than 2 years before significant congenital hearing loss was detected; by this time it had already affected their speech and language skills (CDC, 2015b).

Causes of hearing loss can be conductive, sensorineural, or central. Risk factors for congenital hearing loss include cytomegalovirus infection and preterm birth necessitating a stay in the neonatal intensive care unit.

To assess for hearing ability generally, observe the newborn's response to noises and conversations. The newborn typically turns toward these noises and startles with loud ones.

NECK

Inspect the newborn's neck for movement and ability to support the head. The newborn's neck will appear almost nonexistent because it is so short. Creases are usually noted. The neck should move freely in all directions and should be capable of holding the head in a midline position. The newborn should have enough head control to be able to hold it up briefly without support. Report any deviations such as restricted neck movement or absence of head control.

Also inspect the clavicles (collar bone), which should be straight and intact. The clavicles are the bones mostly commonly broken in infants, especially large ones experiencing difficult births, in operative vaginal births, abnormal fetal positions, and in maternal obesity. In most cases, the fractured clavicle is asymptomatic, but edema, crepitus, and decreased or absent movement and pain or tenderness on movement of the arm on the affected side may be noted. Major risk factors for clavicle fractures are typically vacuum births and large newborn birth weights (Ahn et al., 2015). If the newborn with clavicular fracture is in pain, the affected arm should be immobilized, with the arm abducted more than 60 degrees and the elbow flexed more than 90 degrees. In addition to immobilization, treatment involves minimizing pain overall.

CHEST

Inspect the newborn's chest for size, shape, and symmetry. The newborn's chest should be round, symmetric, and 2 to 3 cm smaller than the head circumference. The xiphoid process may be prominent at birth, but it usually becomes less apparent when adipose tissue accumulates. Nipples may be engorged and may secrete a white discharge. This discharge, which occurs in both boys and girls, is a result of exposure to high levels of maternal estrogen while in utero. This enlargement and milky discharge usually dissipates within a few weeks. Some newborns may have extra nipples, called supernumerary nipples. They are typically small, raised, pigmented areas vertical to the main nipple line, 5 to 6 cm below the normal nipple. Supernumerary nipples may be unilateral or bilateral, and they may include an areola, nipple, or both. They tend to be familial and do not contain glandular tissue. Supernumerary nipples are generally thought to be benign. Some studies have suggested an association with renal or urogenital anomalies, whereas other studies have failed to show this association. There is insufficient evidence to recommend imaging studies or removal in the absence of other clinical concerns or physical findings (Gloster, Gebauer, & Mistur, 2016b). Reassure parents that these extra small nipples are harmless.

The newborn chest is usually barrel shaped, with equal anteroposterior and lateral diameters, and symmetric. Auscultate the lungs bilaterally for equal breath sounds. Normal breath sounds should be heard, with little difference between inspiration and expiration. Fine crackles can be heard on inspiration soon after birth as a result of amniotic fluid being cleared from the lungs. Diminished breath sounds might indicate atelectasis or pneumonia (Weber & Kelley, 2014).

Listen to the heart when the newborn is quiet or sleeping. S1 and S2 heart sounds are accentuated at birth. The point of maximal impulse is a lateral to midclavicular line located at the fourth intercostal space. A displaced point of maximal impulse may indicate tension pneumothorax or cardiomegaly. Murmurs are common during the first few hours as the foramen ovale is closing. Although cardiac murmurs in the neonatal period do not necessarily indicate heart disease, they should be evaluated if they persist (Fillipps & Bucciarelli, 2015).

ABDOMEN

Inspect the abdomen for shape and movement. Typically the newborn's abdomen is protuberant but not distended. This contour is a result of the immaturity of the abdominal muscles. Abdominal movements are synchronous with respirations because newborns are, at times, abdominal breathers.

Auscultate bowel sounds in all four quadrants and then palpate the abdomen for consistency, masses, and tenderness. Perform auscultation and palpation systematically in a clockwise fashion until all four quadrants have been assessed. Palpate gently to feel the liver, the kidneys, and any masses. The liver is normally palpable 1 to 3 cm below the costal margin in the midclavicular line. The kidneys are 1 to 2 cm above and to both sides of the umbilicus. Normal findings would include bowel sounds in all four quadrants and no masses or tenderness on palpation. Absent or hyperactive bowel sounds might indicate an intestinal obstruction. Abdominal distention might indicate ascites, obstruction, infection, masses, or an enlarged abdominal organ. The newborn may also show signs of abdominal tenderness (Springer & Glasser, 2015). Imaging is a mainstay to diagnosis abdominal pathology and should be readily performed in a newborn with abdominal distention to determine the underlying etiology.

Inspect the umbilical cord area for the correct amount of blood vessels (two arteries and one vein). The umbilical vein is larger than the two umbilical arteries. Evidence of only a single umbilical artery is associated with renal and gastrointestinal anomalies. Also inspect the umbilical area for signs of bleeding, infection, inflammation, redness, swelling, purulent drainage or bleeding, erythema around the umbilicus, granuloma, or abnormal communication with the intra-abdominal organs. Umbilical infections can occur because of an embryologic remnant or poor hygiene. Traditionally, gram-positive organisms, such as *Staphylococcus aureus* and *Streptococcus pyogens,* were most commonly identified, but gram-negative and polymicrobial infections are seen today. An umbilical cord infection (omphalitis) can spread to adjacent tissue, causing peritonitis, hepatic vein thrombosis, and hepatic abscess. Immediate evaluation and referral is needed (Lomax, 2015).

GENITALIA

Male. Inspect the penis and scrotum in the male. In the circumcised male newborn, the glans should be smooth, with the meatus centered at the tip of the penis. It will appear reddened until it heals. For the uncircumcised male, the foreskin should cover the glans. Check the position of the urinary meatus: it should be in the midline at the glans tip. If it is on the ventral surface of the penis, the condition is termed hypospadias; if it is on the dorsal surface of the penis, it is termed epispadias. In either case, **circumcision** should be avoided until further evaluation.

Inspect the scrotum for size, symmetry, color, presence of rugae, and location of testes. The scrotum usually appears relatively large with well-formed rugae and that should cover the scrotal sac. There should not be bulging, edema, or discoloration (Fig. 18.16A).

Palpate the scrotum for evidence of the testes, which should be in the scrotal sac. The testes should feel firm and smooth and should be of equal size on both sides of the scrotal sac in the term newborn. Undescended testes (cryptorchidism) might be palpated in the inguinal canal in preterm infants; they can be unilateral or bilateral. If the testes are not palpable within the scrotal sac, further investigation is needed.

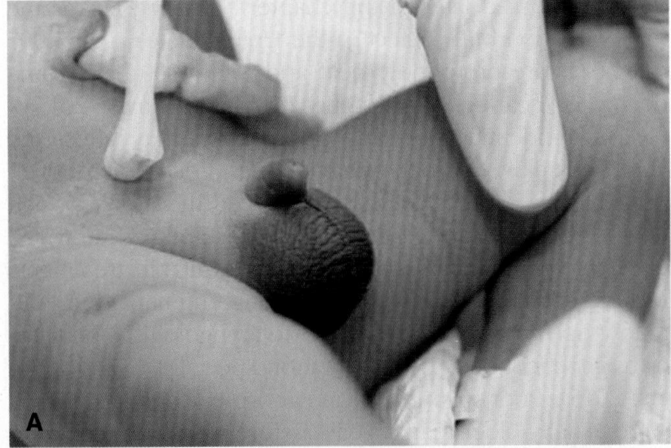

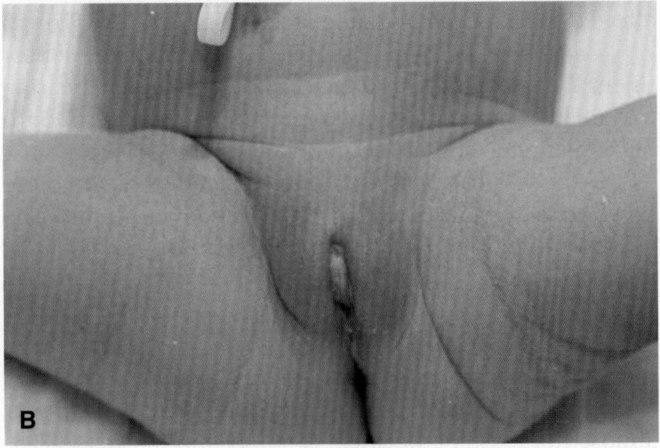

FIGURE 18.16 Newborn genitalia. **A.** Male genitalia. Note the darkened color of the scrotum. **B.** Female genitalia.

Female. In the female newborn, inspect the external genitalia. The urethral meatus is located below the clitoris in the midline (Mutter & Prat, 2014). In contrast to the male genitalia, the female genitalia will be engorged: the labia majora and minora may both be edematous. The labia majora is large and covers the labia minora. The clitoris is large and the hymen is thick. These findings are due to the maternal hormones estrogen and progesterone (Fig. 18.16B). A vaginal discharge composed of mucus mixed with blood may also be present during the first few weeks of life. This discharge, called **pseudomenstruation**, requires no treatment. Explain this phenomenon to the parents.

Variations in female newborns may include a labial bulge, which might indicate an inguinal hernia, ambiguous genitalia, a rectovaginal fistula with feces present in the vagina, and an imperforate hymen.

Male and Female. Inspect the anus in both male and female newborns for position and patency. Passage of meconium indicates patency. If meconium is not passed, a lubricated rectal thermometer can be inserted or a digital examination can be performed to determine patency. Abnormal findings would include anal fissures or fistulas and no meconium passed within 24 hours after birth.

EXTREMITIES AND BACK

Upper Extremities. Inspect the newborn's upper extremities for appearance and movement. Inspect the hands for shape, number, and position of fingers and presence of palmar creases. The newborn's arms and hands should be symmetric and should move through range of motion without hesitation. Observe for spontaneous movement of the extremities. Each hand should have five digits. Note any extra digits (polydactyly) or fusing of two or more digits (syndactyly). Most newborns have three palmar creases on the hand. A single palmar crease, called a simian line, is frequently associated with Down syndrome.

A brachial plexus injury can occur during a difficult birth involving shoulder dystocia. Erb palsy is an injury resulting from damage to the upper plexus, and palsies associated with the lower brachial plexus are termed Klumpke palsies. Factors associated with obstetric brachial plexus paralysis include large birth weight, breech delivery, labor anomalies, operative vaginal birth, and shoulder dystocia. Obstetric brachial plexus paralysis results from excessive lateral traction on the head away from the shoulder. This force on the brachial plexus can cause varying degrees of injury to the nerves. The affected arm hangs limp alongside the body, and the affected shoulder and arm are adducted, extended, and internally rotated with a pronated wrist. The Moro reflex is absent on the affected side in brachial palsy. Complete recovery may take 6 months or longer. Current research studies support endogenous labor forces as the etiology of this injury. Despite training in the management of shoulder dystocia and a rising institutional cesarean section rate, the incidence of brachial plexus injuries has remained unchanged compared with 10 years earlier (Tung & Moore, 2015).

Lower Extremities. Assess the lower extremities in the same manner. They should be of equal length, with symmetric skinfolds. Inspect the feet for clubfoot (a turning-inward position), which is secondary to intrauterine positioning. This may be positional or structural. Perform the Ortolani and Barlow maneuvers to identify congenital hip dislocation, commonly termed developmental dysplasia of the hip (DDH). Nursing Procedure 18.1 highlights the steps for performing these maneuvers. Table 18.3 summarizes the newborn assessment.

NEUROLOGIC STATUS

Assess the newborn's state of alertness, posture, muscle tone, and reflexes.

Newborn Alertness, Posture, and Muscle Tone. The newborn should be alert and not persistently lethargic. The normal posture is hips abducted and partially flexed, with knees flexed. Arms are adducted and flexed at the elbow. Fists are often clenched, with fingers covering the thumb.

To assess for muscle tone, support the newborn with one hand under the chest. Observe how the neck muscles hold the head. The neck extensors should be able to hold the head in line briefly. There should be only slight head lag when pulling the newborn from a supine position to a sitting one.

Newborn Reflexes. Assess the newborn's reflexes to evaluate neurologic function and development. Absent or abnormal reflexes in a newborn, persistence of a reflex past the age when the reflex is normally lost, or return of an infantile reflex in an older child or adult may indicate neurologic pathology (Table 18.4). Reflexes commonly assessed in the newborn include sucking, Moro, stepping, tonic neck, rooting, Babinski, palmar grasp, and plantar grasp reflexes. Spinal reflexes tested include truncal incurvation (Galant reflex) and anocutaneous reflex (anal wink).

The *sucking reflex* is elicited by gently stimulating the newborn's lips by touching them. The newborn will typically open the mouth and begin a sucking motion. Placing a gloved finger in the newborn's mouth will also elicit a sucking motion (Fig. 18.17A).

The *Moro reflex*, also called the embrace reflex, occurs when the neonate is startled. To elicit this reflex, place the newborn on his or her back. Support the upper body weight of the supine newborn by the arms, using a lifting motion, without lifting the newborn off the surface. Then release the arms suddenly. The newborn will

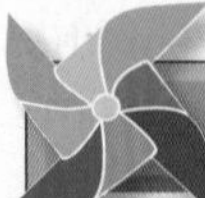

NURSING PROCEDURE 18.1

Performing Ortolani and Barlow Maneuvers

Purpose: To Detect Congenital Developmental Dysplasia of the Hip

Ortolani Maneuver

1. Place the newborn in the supine position and flex the hips and knees to 90 degrees at the hip.
2. Grasp the inner aspect of the thighs and abduct the hips (usually to approximately 180 degrees) while applying upward pressure.

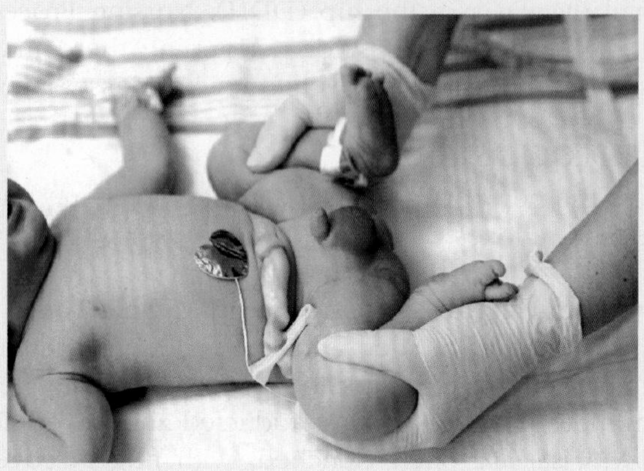

3. Listen for any sounds during the maneuver. There should be no "cluck" or "click" heard when the legs are abducted. Such a sound indicates the femoral head hitting the acetabulum as the head reenters the area. This suggests developmental hip dysplasia.

Barlow Maneuver

1. With the newborn still lying supine and grasping the inner aspect of the thighs (as just mentioned), adduct the thighs while applying outward and downward pressure to the thighs.

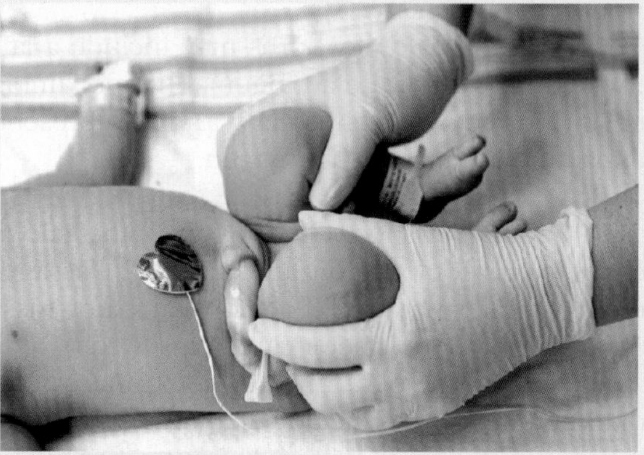

2. Feel for the femoral head slipping out of the acetabulum; also listen for a click.

Adapted from Tamai, J., & McCarthy, J. J. (2015). Developmental dysplasia of the hip. *eMedicine*. Retrieved from http://emedicine.medscape.com/article/1248135-overview; and Weber, J., & Kelley, J. (2014). *Health assessment in nursing* (5th ed.). Philadelphia, PA: Lippincott Williams & Wilkins.

throw the arms outward and flex the knees; the arms then return to the chest. The fingers also spread to form a C. The newborn initially appears startled and then relaxes to a normal resting position (Fig. 18.17B).

Assess the *stepping reflex* by holding the newborn upright and inclined forward with the soles of the feet touching a flat surface. The baby should make a stepping motion or walking, alternating flexion and extension with the soles of the feet (Fig. 18.17C).

The *tonic neck reflex* resembles the stance of a fencer and is often called the fencing reflex. Test this reflex by having the newborn lie on the back. Turn the baby's head to one side. The arm toward which the baby is facing should extend straight away from the body with the hand partially open, whereas the arm on the side away from the face is flexed and the fist is clenched tightly. Reversing the direction to which the face is turned reverses the position (Fig. 18.17D).

Elicit the *rooting reflex* by stroking the newborn's cheek. The newborn should turn toward the side that was stroked and should begin to make sucking movements (Fig. 18.17E).

The *Babinski reflex* should be present at birth and disappears at approximately 1 year of age. It is elicited by stroking the lateral sole of the newborn's foot from the heel toward and across the ball of the foot. The toes should fan out. A diminished response indicates a neurologic problem and needs follow-up (Fig. 18.17F).

The newborn exhibits two grasp reflexes: *palmar grasp and plantar grasp*. Elicit the palmar grasp reflex by placing a finger on the newborn's open palm. The baby's hand will close around the finger. Attempting to remove the finger causes the grip to tighten. Newborns have strong grasps and can almost be lifted from a flat surface if both hands are used. The grasp should

TABLE 18.3 NEWBORN ASSESSMENT SUMMARY

Assessment	Usual Findings	Variations and Common Problems
Anthropometric measurements	Head circumference: 33–37 cm (13–14 in) Chest circumference: 30–33 cm (12–13 in) Weight: 2,500–4,000 g (5.5–8.5 lb) Length: 45–55 cm (17–21 in)	SGA, LGA, preterm, postterm
Vital signs	Temperature: 97°–99°F (36.5°–37.5°C) Apical pulse: 110–160 bpm Respirations: 30–60 breaths/min	
Skin	Normal: smooth, flexible, good skin turgor, well hydrated; warm	Jaundice, acrocyanosis, milia, Mongolian spots, stork bites
Head	Normal: varies with age, gender, ethnicity	Microcephaly, macrocephaly, enlarged fontanels
Face	Normal: full cheeks, facial features symmetric	Facial nerve paralysis, nevus flammeus, nevus vasculosus
Nose	Normal: small, placement in the midline and narrow, ability to smell	Malformation or blockage
Mouth	Normal: aligned in midline, symmetric, intact soft and hard palate	Epstein pearls, erupted precocious teeth, thrush
Neck	Normal: short, creased, moves freely, baby holds head in midline	Restricted movement, clavicular fractures
Eyes	Normal: clear and symmetrically placed on face; online with ears	Chemical conjunctivitis, subconjunctival hemorrhages
Ears	Normal: soft and pliable with quick recoil when folded and released	Low-set ears, hearing loss
Chest	Normal: round, symmetric, smaller than head	Nipple engorgement, whitish discharge
Abdomen	Normal: protuberant contour, soft, three vessels in umbilical cord	Distended, only two vessels in umbilical cord
Genitals	Normal male: smooth glans, meatus centered at tip of penis Normal female: swollen female genitals as a result of maternal estrogen	Edematous scrotum in males, vaginal discharge in females
Extremities and spine	Normal: extremities symmetric with free movement	Congenital hip dislocation; tuft or dimple on spine

Data from Davidson, M. R. (2014). *Fast facts for the neonatal nurse: A nursing orientation and care guide in a nutshell.* New York, NY: Springer Publishing Company; and Weber, J., & Kelley, J. (2014). *Health assessment in nursing* (5th ed.). Philadelphia, PA: Wolters Kluwer.

be equal bilaterally (Fig. 18.17G). The plantar grasp is similar to the palmar grasp. Place a finger just below the newborn's toes. The toes typically curl over the finger (Fig. 18.17H).

Blinking, sneezing, gagging, and *coughing* are all protective reflexes and are elicited when an object or light is brought close to the eye (blinking), something irritating is swallowed or a bulb syringe is used for suctioning (gagging and coughing), or an irritant is brought close to the nose (sneezing).

The *truncal incurvation reflex (Galant reflex)* is present at birth and disappears in a few days to 4 weeks (Fig. 18.18). With the newborn in a prone position or held in ventral suspension, apply firm pressure and run a finger down either side of the spine. This stroking will cause the pelvis to flex toward the stimulated side. This

TABLE 18.4 NEWBORN REFLEXES: APPEARANCE AND DISAPPEARANCE

Reflex	Appearance	Disappearance
Blinking	Newborn	Persists into adulthood
Moro	Newborn	3–6 mo
Grasp	Newborn	3–4 mo
Stepping	Birth	1–2 mo
Tonic neck	Newborn	3–4 mo
Sneeze	Newborn	Persists into adulthood
Rooting	Birth	4–6 mo
Gag reflex	Newborn	Persists into adulthood
Cough reflex	Newborn	Persists into adulthood
Babinski sign	Newborn	12 mo

indicates T2–S1 innervation. Lack of response indicates a neurologic or spinal cord problem.

The *anocutaneous reflex (anal wink)* is elicited by stimulating the perianal skin close to the anus. The external sphincter will constrict (wink) immediately with stimulation. This indicates S4–S5 innervations (Marcdante & Kliegman, 2014).

Nursing Interventions

Developing confidence in caring for their newborn is challenging for most parents/significant others/partners. It takes time and patience and a great deal of instruction provided by the nurse. "Showing and telling" parents about their newborn and all the procedures (e.g., feeding, bathing, changing, handling) involved in daily care are key nursing interventions.

Providing General Newborn Care

Generally, newborn care involves bathing and hygiene, elimination and diaper area care, cord care, circumcision care, environmental safety measures, and prevention of infection. Nurses should teach these skills to parents and should serve as role models for appropriate and consistent interaction with newborns. Demonstrating respect for the newborn and family helps foster a positive atmosphere to promote the newborn's growth and development.

BATHING AND HYGIENE

Immediately after birth, drying the newborn and removing blood may minimize the risk of infection caused by hepatitis B, herpes virus, and HIV, but the specific benefits of this practice remain unclear. Until the newborn has been thoroughly bathed, standard precautions should be used when handling the newborn. Nurses need to follow their hospital policies regarding the timing and procedures for newborn bathing and hygiene.

Newborns are bathed primarily for aesthetic reasons, and bathing is postponed until thermal and cardiorespiratory stability is ensured. Traditional reasons why nurses

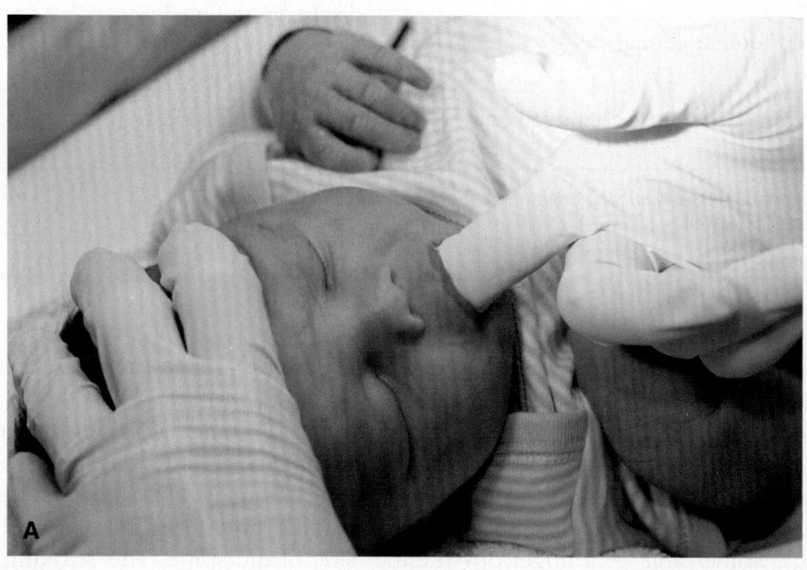

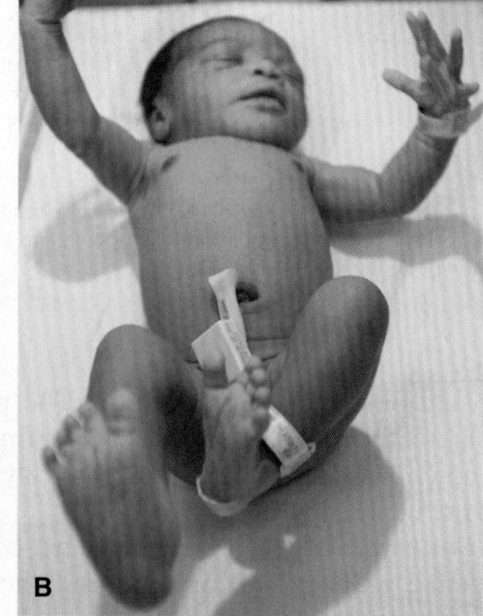

FIGURE 18.17 Newborn reflexes. **A.** Sucking reflex. **B.** Moro reflex.

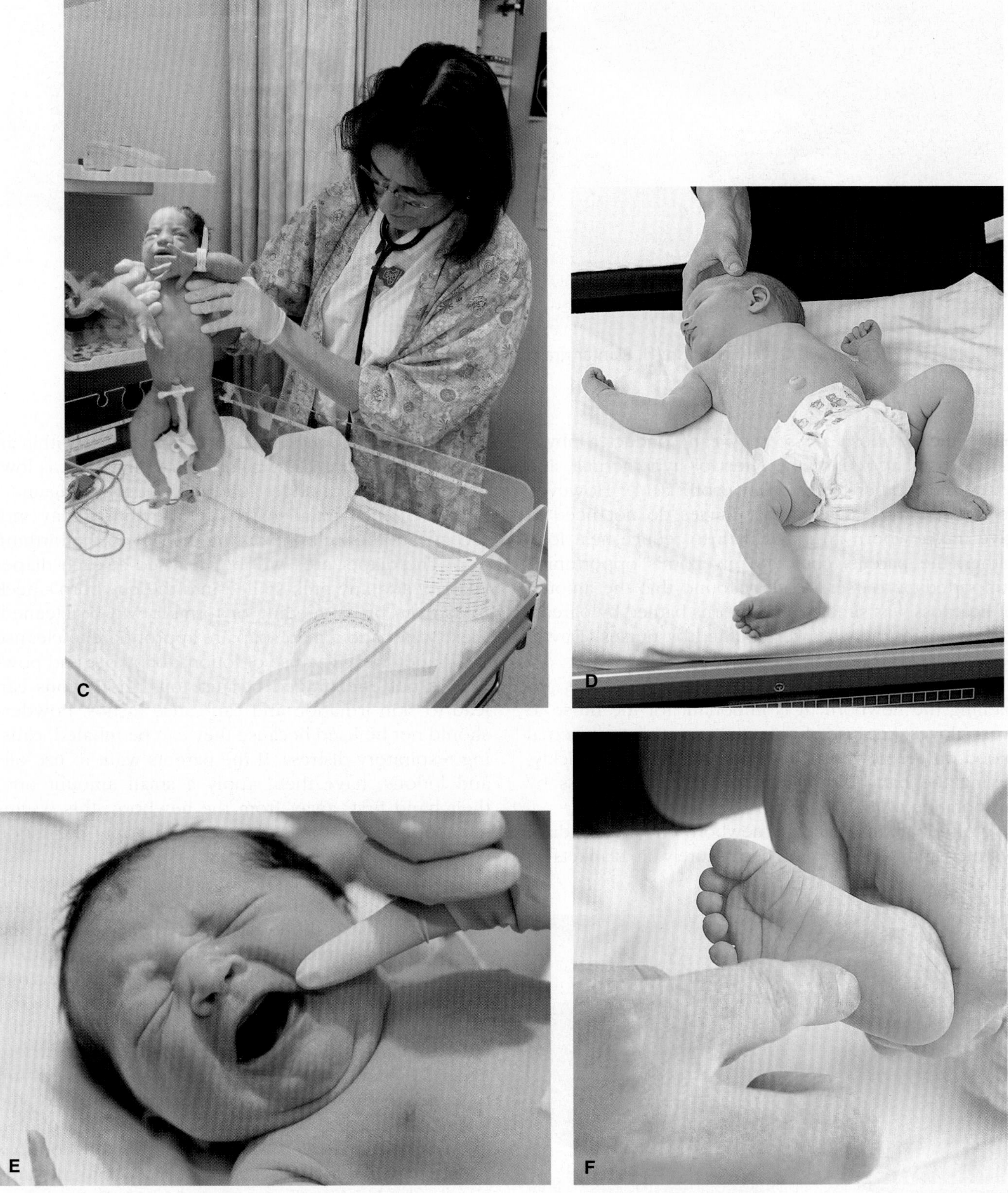

FIGURE 18.17 *(continued)* **C.** Stepping reflex. **D.** Tonic neck reflex. **E.** Rooting reflex. **F.** Babinski reflex. *(continued)*

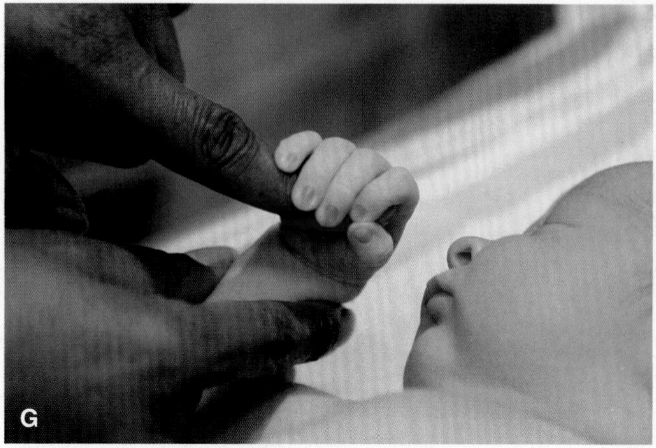

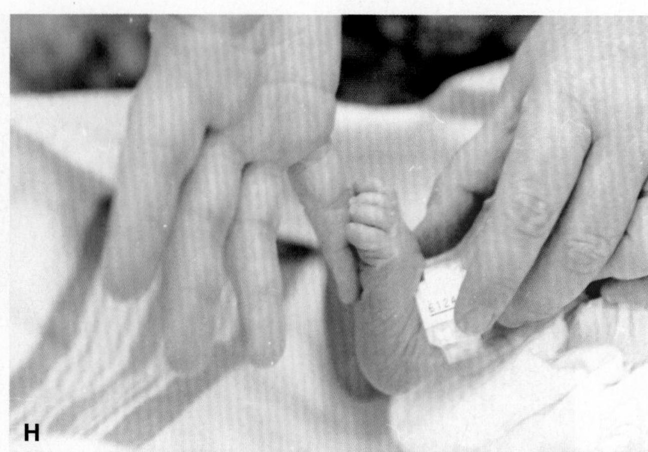

FIGURE 18.17 *(continued)* **G.** Palmar grasp. **H.** Plantar grasp.

bathe the newborn are so they can conduct a physical assessment, reduce the effect of hypothermia, and allow the mother to rest (Davidson, 2014). However, recent research suggests that nurses do not need to give the newborn an initial bath to reduce heat loss; rather, the parents could be given this opportunity, supported by nurses. A study found that the amount of heat loss was similar in newborns bathed by parents versus newborns who were bathed by nurses (Davidson, 2014).

Nursing Procedure 18.2 explains the steps for bathing the newborn. It is important for the nurse to wear gloves, because of potential exposure to maternal blood on the newborn, and perform the bath quickly, drying the baby thoroughly to prevent heat loss by evaporation.

After bathing, place the newborn under the radiant warmer and wrap him or her securely in blankets to prevent chilling. Check the baby's temperature within an hour to make sure it is within normal limits. If it is low, place the newborn under a radiant heat source again.

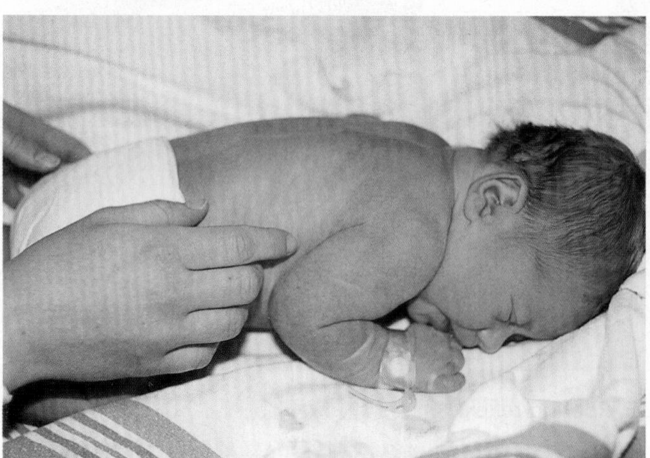

FIGURE 18.18 Trunk incurvation reflex. When the paravertebral area is stroked, the newborn flexes his or her trunk toward the direction of the stimulation. (Copyright Caroline Brown, RNC, MS, DEd.)

After the initial bath, the newborn may not receive another full one during the stay in the birthing unit. The diaper area will be cleansed at each diaper change, and any milk spilled into the newborn's neck folds from breast-feeding or formula will be cleaned. Clear water and a mild soap are appropriate to cleanse the diaper area. The use of lotions, baby oil, and powders is not encouraged because oils and lotions can lead to skin irritation and can cause rashes. Powders should not be used because they can be inhaled, causing respiratory distress. If the parents want to use oils and lotions, have them apply a small amount onto their hand first, away from the newborn; this warms the lotion. Then the parents should apply the lotion or oil sparingly.

Encourage the parents to gather all items needed before starting the bath: a soft, clean washcloth; two cotton balls to clean the eyes; mild, unscented soap and shampoo; towels or blankets; a tub or basin with warm water; a clean diaper; and a change of clothes. Instruct parents that a bath two or three times weekly is sufficient for the first year; more frequent bathing may dry the skin. Parents should not fully immerse the newborn into water until the umbilical cord area is healed—up to 2 weeks after birth. Encourage parents to give the infant a sponge bath until the umbilical cord falls off and the navel area is healed completely. If the newborn has been circumcised, advise parents to wait until that area has also healed (usually 1 to 2 weeks). Until then, clean the penis with mild soap and water and apply a small amount of petroleum jelly to the tip to prevent the diaper from adhering to the penis. Instruct parents to apply the diaper loosely and place the newly circumcised male infant on his side or back to prevent pressure and irritation on the penis.

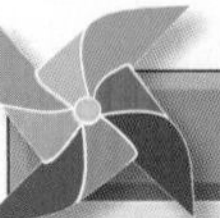

NURSING PROCEDURE 18.2

Bathing the Newborn

It is important that the nurse wear gloves, because of potential exposure to maternal blood on the newborn, and performs the bath quickly, drying the baby thoroughly to prevent heat loss by evaporation. Keep the newborn covered to prevent heat loss during the bathing procedure.

1. Begin the newborn bath starting from the cleanest area (the eyes) and proceeding to the most soiled area (the diaper area) to prevent cross-contamination. Use plain warm water on the face and eyes, adding a mild soap (e.g., Dove) to cleanse the remainder of the body. Wash, rinse, and dry each area before proceeding to the next one.

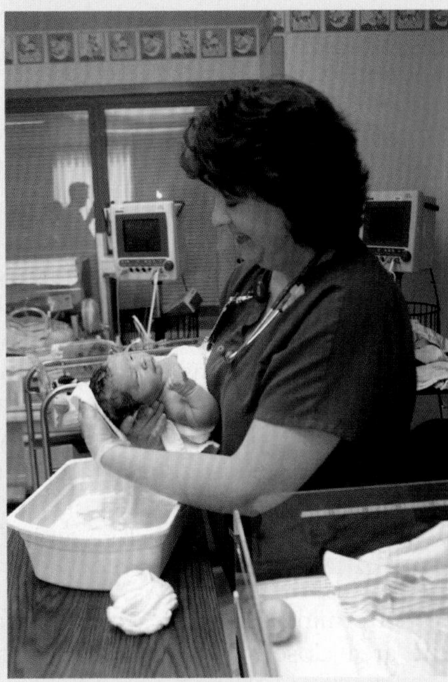

2. Wash the hair using running water so that the scalp can be thoroughly rinsed. A mild shampoo or soap can be used. Wash both fontanel areas. Frequently parents avoid these "soft spots" because they fear that they will "hurt the baby's brain" if they rub too hard. Reassure parents that there is a strong membrane providing protection. Urge the parents to clean and rinse these areas well. If the anterior fontanel is not rinsed well after shampooing, cradle cap (dry flakes on the scalp) can develop. Avoid getting water in ears to prevent infection.

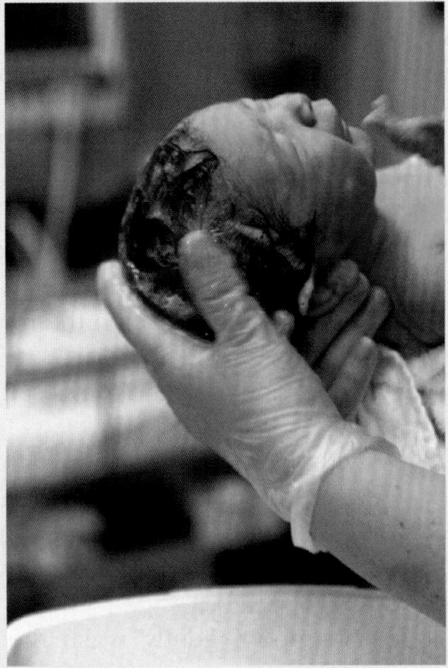

3. Make sure to cleanse all body creases, especially the neck folds to remove any milk that may have dripped into these areas.

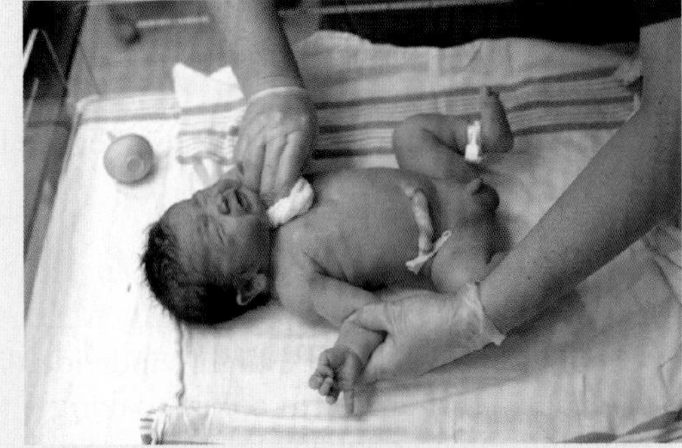

4. Continue downward washing the trunk and extremities ending up with the diaper area last.

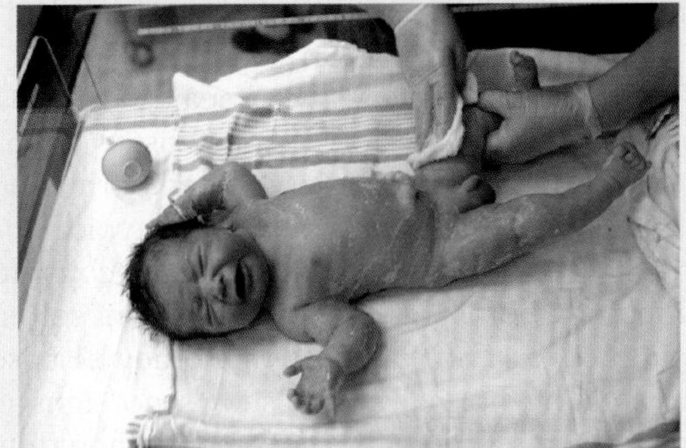

Other guidelines for bathing newborns are given in Teaching Guidelines 18.1.

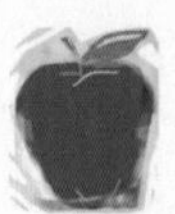

Teaching Guidelines 18.1
BATHING A NEWBORN

- Select a warm room with a flat surface at a comfortable working height.
- Before the bath, gather all supplies needed so they will be within reach.
- Never leave the newborn alone or unattended at any time during the bath.
- Undress the newborn down to shirt and diaper.
- Always support the newborn's head and neck when moving or positioning him or her.
- Place a blanket or towel underneath the newborn for warmth and comfort.
- In this order, progressing from the cleanest to the dirtiest areas:
  - Wipe eyes with plain water, using either cotton balls or a washcloth. Wipe from the inner corner of the eyes to the outer with separate wipes.
  - Wash the rest of the face, including ears, with plain water.
  - Using baby shampoo, gently wash the hair and rinse with water.
  - Pay special attention to body creases, and dry thoroughly.
  - Wash extremities, trunk, and back. Wash, rinse, dry, cover.
  - Wash diaper area last, using soap and water, and dry; observe for rash.
- Put on a clean diaper and clean clothes after the bath.

ELIMINATION AND DIAPER AREA CARE

Newborn elimination patterns are highly individualized. Usually the urine is light amber in color. Soaking 6 to 12 diapers a day indicates adequate hydration. Stools can change in color, texture, and frequency without signaling a problem. Meconium is passed for the first 48 hours after birth; the stools appear thick, tarry, sticky, and dark green. Transitional stools (thin, brown to green, less sticky than meconium) typically appear by day 3 after initiation of feeding. The stool characteristics after transitional stool depend on whether the newborn is breastfed or bottle-fed. Breast-fed newborns typically pass mustard-colored, soft stool with a seedy consistency; formula-fed newborns pass yellow to brown, soft stools with a pasty consistency. As long as the newborn seems content, is eating normally, and shows no signs of illness, minor changes in bowel movements should not be a concern.

The newborn needs to be checked frequently to see whether a diaper change is needed, especially after feeding. Adhere to standard precautions when providing diaper area care. Instruct parents to keep the top edge of the diaper folded down below the umbilical cord area to prevent irritation and to allow air to help dry the cord. For a male infant, point the penis down to prevent urine from wetting the top of the diaper where the umbilicus is located.

Meconium can be difficult to remove from the skin. Use plain water or special cleansing wipes if necessary to clean the area. Teach parents how to clean the diaper area properly and how to prevent skin irritation. Encourage them to avoid products such as powder and fragranced items, which could irritate the newborn's skin.

Discuss the pros and cons of using cloth diapers versus disposable diapers so that the parents can make informed decisions. Regardless of the type of diapers used, up to 10 diapers a day, or about 70 a week, will be needed.

Additional information about diapering might include:

- Before diapering, make sure all supplies are within reach, including clean diaper, cleaning agent or wipes, and ointment.
- Lay the newborn on a changing table and remove the dirty diaper.
- Use water and mild soap or wipes to gently wipe the genital area clean; wipe from front to back for girls to avoid urinary tract infections.
- Wash your hands thoroughly before and after changing diapers.

While performing diaper area care, parents should observe the area closely for irritation or rash. Tips for preventing or healing a diaper rash include:

- Change diapers frequently, especially after bowel movements.
- Apply a "barrier" cream, such as A&D ointment or Desitin, after cleaning with mild soap and water.
- Use dye- and fragrance-free detergents to wash cloth diapers.
- Avoid the use of plastic pants, because they tend to hold in moisture.
- Expose the newborn's bottom to air several times a day.
- Place the newborn's buttocks in warm water after he or she has had a diaper on all night.

Take Note!

Advise parents that a rash that persists for more than 3 days may be fungal in origin and may require additional treatment. Encourage the parents to notify the health care provider.

CORD CARE

The umbilical cord begins drying within hours after birth and is shriveled and blackened by the second or third day. Within 7 to 10 days, it sloughs off and the umbilicus heals. During this transition, frequent assessments of the area are necessary to detect any bleeding or signs of infection. Cord bleeding is abnormal and may occur if the cord clamp is loosened. Any cord drainage is also abnormal and is generally caused by infection, which requires immediate treatment.

To protect the cord area during each diaper change, apply the appropriate agent (e.g., triple dye, alcohol, or an antimicrobial agent), according to facility policy, to the cord stump to prevent any ascending infections. Single-use agents for cleaning are recommended to prevent cross-contamination with other newborns. Expect to remove the cord clamp approximately 24 hours after birth by using a cord-cutting clamp. However, if the cord is still moist, keep the clamp in place and ensure a referral to home health care so that the home care nurse can remove it after discharge. Always adhere to agency policies regarding cord care; changes in policy may be necessary based on new research findings.

Many parents avoid contact with the cord site to make sure they don't "bother" it. Teach them how to care for the cord site when they go home to prevent complications (Teaching Guidelines 18.2).

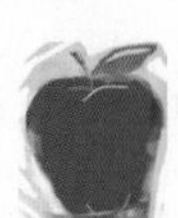

Teaching Guidelines 18.2
UMBILICAL CORD CARE

- Observe for bleeding, redness, drainage, or foul odor from the cord stump and report it to your newborn's primary care provider immediately.
- Avoid tub baths until the cord has fallen off and the area has healed.
- Expose the cord stump to the air as much as possible throughout the day.
- Fold diapers below the level of the cord to prevent contamination of the site and to promote air-drying of the cord.
- Observe the cord stump, which will change color from yellow to brown to black. This is normal.
- Never pull the cord or attempt to loosen it; it will fall off naturally.

CIRCUMCISION AND CARE OF THE PENIS

Circumcision is one of the oldest and most common surgical procedures performed worldwide, but remains controversial. It is performed for medical, religious, cultural, and social reasons. Circumcision is the surgical removal of all or part of the foreskin (prepuce) of the penis (Freedman & Hurwitz, 2015). This has been traditionally done for hygiene and medical reasons and is the oldest known religious rite. In the Jewish faith, circumcision is a ritual that is performed by a *mohel* (ordained circumciser) on the eighth day after birth if possible. The circumcision is followed by a *bris* (the Jewish religious ceremony), typically in the home, during which the newborn is named and symbolically enters the Jewish religious community.

Most other circumcisions are performed in the hospital before the newborn is discharged as this is convenient for parents or taken to the doctor's outpatient office after discharge, is practical, and has a demonstrated record of safety. There are three commonly used methods of circumcision: the Gomco clamp, the Hollister Plastibell device, and the Mogen clamp. During the circumcision procedure, part of the foreskin is removed by clamping and cutting with a scalpel (Gomco or Mogen clamp) or by using a Plastibell. The Plastibell is fitted over the glans, and the excess foreskin is pulled over the plastic ring. A suture is tied around the rim to apply pressure to the blood vessels, creating hemostasis. The excess foreskin is cut away. The plastic rim remains in place until healing occurs. The plastic ring typically loosens and falls off in approximately 1 week. Petroleum jelly should be applied to the circumcised area after the procedure is done with the Gomco or Mogen clamp (Sinkey et al., 2015) (Fig. 18.19).

The debate over routine newborn circumcision continues in the United States. For many years, the purported benefits and harms of circumcision have been debated in the medical literature and society at large, with no clear consensus to date. Despite the controversy, circumcision is the most common surgical procedure performed on newborns, and almost two thirds (61%) of American male newborns are circumcised (CDC, 2015c).

Policy Statement by American Academy of Pediatrics. A policy statement by the AAP indicates that newborn circumcision has potential disadvantages and risks as well as medical benefits and advantages. Risks to the newborn include infection, hemorrhage, skin dehiscence, adhesions, urethral fistula, and pain. Benefits to the newborn include the following:

- Urinary tract infections are slightly less common in circumcised boys. However, rates are low in both circumcised and uncircumcised boys and are easily treated without long-term sequelae.
- Sexually transmitted infections are less common in circumcised males, but the risk is believed to be related more to behavioral factors than to circumcision status. However, circumcised males have a 50% lower risk of acquiring HIV infection, herpes simplex virus, human papillomavirus (HPV), genital ulcer disease, bacterial vaginosis, and trichomoniasis (Tobian, Kacker, & Quinn, 2014).

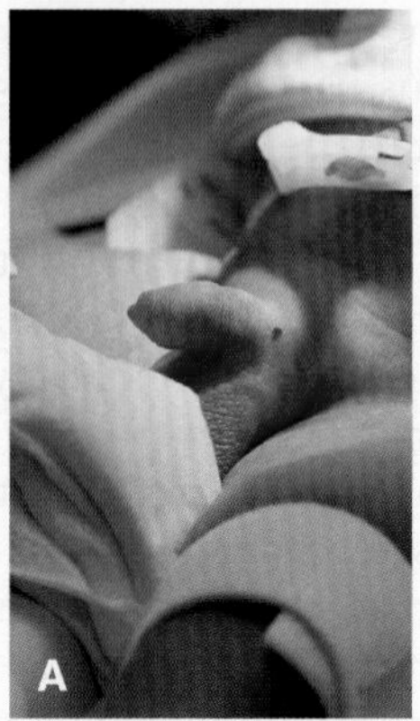

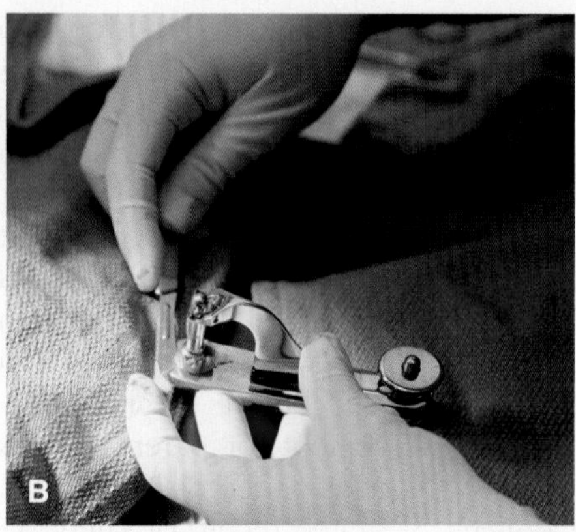

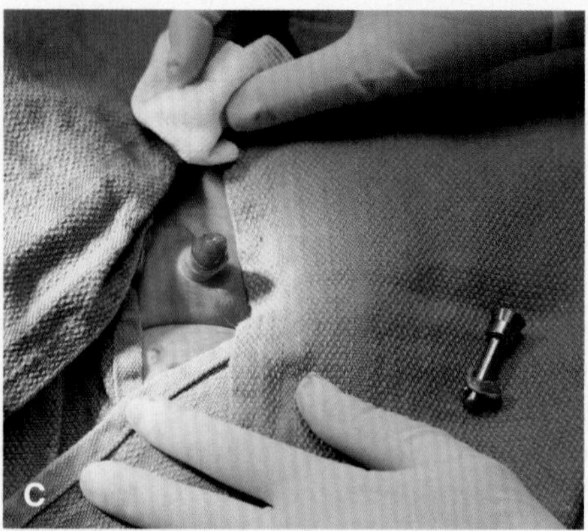

FIGURE 18.19 Circumcision. **A.** Before the procedure. **B.** Clamp applied and foreskin removed. **C.** Appearance after circumcision.

- There appears to be a slightly lower rate of penile cancer in circumcised males. However, penile cancer is rare and risk factors such as genital warts, infection with HPV, multiple sex partners, and cigarette smoking seem to play a much larger role in causing penile cancer than circumcision status (Marcdante & Kliegman, 2014).

The new AAP recommendations state that if parents decide to circumcise their newborn, pain relief must be provided. Research has found that newborns circumcised without analgesia experience pain and stress, indicated by changes in heart rate, blood pressure, oxygen saturation, and cortisol levels (Morrison et al., 2014). Analgesic methods may include EMLA® cream (a topical mixture of local anesthetics, lidocaine and prilocaine), a dorsal penile nerve block with buffered lidocaine, acetaminophen, skin-to-skin contact, a sucrose pacifier, and swaddling (Cunningham et al., 2014).

The AAP (2015e) recommends that parents be given accurate and unbiased information about the risks and benefits of circumcision. As with other newborn procedures, research continues. Nurses must keep informed about current medical research to allow parents to make informed decisions. The absence of compelling medical evidence in favor of or against newborn circumcision makes informed consent of parents of paramount importance. The circumcision discussion involves cultural, religious, medical, and emotional considerations. Nurses may have difficulty remaining unbiased and unemotional as they present the facts to parents. Circumcision is a very personal decision for parents, and the nurse's major responsibility is to inform the parents of the risks and benefits of the procedure and to address concerns so that the parents can reach a fully informed decision.

Take Note!

The decision to circumcise the male newborn is often a social one, with the strongest factor being whether the newborn's father is himself circumcised (Mielke, 2014).

Preoperative circumcision preparation should include confirmation of the following:

- Infant is at least 12 hours old or older
- Infant has received standard vitamin K prophylaxis
- Infant has voided normally at least once since birth
- Infant has not eaten for at least an hour prior to the procedure
- Written parental consent has been obtained
- Correct identification of the infant brought to procedure room

Immediately after circumcision, the tip of the penis is usually covered with petroleum jelly–coated gauze to keep the wound from sticking to the diaper. Continued care of this site includes:

- Assess for bleeding every 30 minutes for at least 2 hours.
- Document the first voiding to evaluate for urinary obstruction or edema.
- Squeeze soapy water over the area daily and then rinse with warm water. Pat dry.
- Apply a small amount of petroleum jelly with every diaper change if the Plastibell was used; clean with mild soap and water if other techniques were used.
- Fasten the diaper loosely over the penis and avoiding placing the newborn on his abdomen to prevent friction.

If a Plastibell has been used, it will fall off by itself in about a week. Inform parents of this and advise them not to pull it off sooner. Also instruct the parents to check daily for any foul-smelling drainage, bleeding, or unusual swelling.

If the newborn is uncircumcised, wash the penis with mild soap and water after each diaper change and do not force the foreskin back; it will retract normally over time.

SAFETY

Newborns are completely dependent on those around them to ensure their safety. Their safety must be ensured while in the health care facility and after they are discharged. Parental education is key, especially as the newborn grows and develops and begins to respond to and explore his or her surroundings (Teaching Guidelines 18.3).

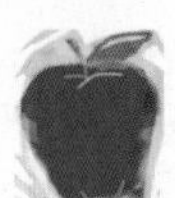

Teaching Guidelines 18.3

GENERAL NEWBORN SAFETY

- Have emergency telephone numbers readily available, such as those for emergency medical assistance and the poison control center.
- Keep small or sharp objects out of reach to prevent them from being aspirated.
- Put safety plugs in wall sockets within the child's reach to prevent electrocution.
- Do not leave the infant alone in any room without a portable intercom on.
- Always supervise the newborn in the tub: a newborn can drown in 2 in of water.
- Make sure the crib or changing table is sturdy, without any loose hardware, and is painted with lead-free paint.
- Avoid placing the crib or changing table near blinds or curtain cords.
- Provide a smoke-free environment for all infants.
- Place all infants on their backs to sleep to prevent sudden infant death syndrome.
- To prevent falls, do not leave the newborn alone on any elevated surface.
- Use sun shields on strollers and hats to avoid overexposing the newborn to the sun.
- To prevent infection, thoroughly wash your hands before preparing formula.
- Thoroughly investigate any infant care facility before using it.

Adapted from Centers for Disease Control and Prevention [CDC]. (2015d). *Infants and toddlers – Safety in the home and community.* Retrieved from http://www.cdc.gov/parents/infants/safety.html

Environmental Safety. People who enter a health care facility for treatment expect to be safe there until they return home, but ensuring a safe environment can be a daunting challenge to a health care facility.

Consider this scenario: A woman dressed in nurse's clothing entered the hospital room of a new mother soon after she had given birth. This "nurse" told the mother she needed to take her newborn to the nursery to have him weighed. Sometime later, a staff nurse making her routine rounds realized something was wrong when she saw that the newborn's bassinet in the mother's room was empty and the mother was sound asleep in her bed. The staff nurse called security immediately because she suspected that a newborn abduction had taken place.

This is a typical abduction scenario that is repeated many times throughout the United States each year. In infant abduction, someone who is not a family member takes a child less than 1-year old (NCMEC, 2015). Infant abductions are traumatic for the parents, the community, and the health care facility. The facility may also face huge financial liability if a lawsuit is filed by the parents.

Abductions typically occur during the day and are usually carried out by women who are not criminally sophisticated. Many of these women experienced a pregnancy loss in the past; they are often emotionally immature and compulsive, with low self-esteem. Most female abductors can play the role of a hospital employee convincingly. Infants usually are abducted when taken for testing, during return to the nursery, when left unattended in the nursery, or while a mother was napping or showering (Joint Commission, 2015).

Health care agencies are challenged to prevent infant abduction by instituting sound security practices and systems (Joint Commission, 2015). Such measures include the following:

- All newborns must be transported in cribs and not carried.
- Nurses must respond immediately to any security alarm that sounds on the unit.
- Newborns must never be unattended at any time, especially in hallways.
- All staff must wear appropriate identification at all times.
- Encourage mothers to keep their baby/bassinet on their far side, away from the door.
- Personnel should be wary of visitors who do not seem to be visiting a specific mother.
- The electronic security system should be checked to make sure it works.
- Footprint the newborn, take a color photograph, and record the newborn's physical examination within 2 hours of birth.
- Discontinue publication of birth notices in local newspapers.
- Develop and implement a proactive infant abduction prevention plan.
- Ensure the proper functioning and placement of any electronic sensors used on newborns.
- Parents should be taught what infant abduction is; why infant security is important; the schedule of nursery, feeding, and visiting hours; rules about visitor access; the facility's security policies and procedures; what parents can do to protect their infant in the hospital; which staff members are allowed to handle the newborn; and what a proper ID looks like.

Educating staff, educating mothers, and access control are the three key steps to preventing abductions from any health care facility. Providing a safe and secure environment is a shared responsibility of the facility, staff, and parents. Preventing abductions requires everyone to learn and follow the rules and policies.

Car Safety. Every state requires the use of car seats for infants and children, because motor vehicle accidents are still the leading cause of unintentional injury and death in children under age 5. National Highway Traffic Safety Administration statistics show that nearly one half of deaths and injuries in infants occurred because they were not properly restrained. Child safety seats, when installed and used properly, can prevent injuries and save lives (AAP, 2015f).

Despite evidence that the use of car seats can reduce the morbidity and mortality of motor vehicle crashes, parents who lack knowledge about them may underuse or misuse them (Hodges & Smith, 2014). Make sure that both parents understand the importance of safely transporting their newborn in a federally approved safety car seat every time the infant rides in a car. Do not release any newborn unless the parents have a car seat in place for their newborn's ride home (Fig. 18.20). If they cannot afford one, many community organizations will provide one for them. According to the AAP's policy statement on child passenger safety (2015f), no one car seat is considered to be the "safest" or the "best," but rather consistent and proper use is the key to preventing injuries and deaths. Instruct parents in the following:

- Select a car seat that is appropriate for the child's size and weight.
- Caution caregivers against the placement of car seats on elevated or soft surfaces outside the car to prevent falling.
- Use the car seat correctly, every time the child is in the car.
- Use rear-facing car safety seats for most infants up to 2 years of age or until they reach the highest weight or height allowed by the manufacturer of their CSS.
- Make sure the harness (most seats have a three- to five-point harness) is in the slots at or below the shoulders.

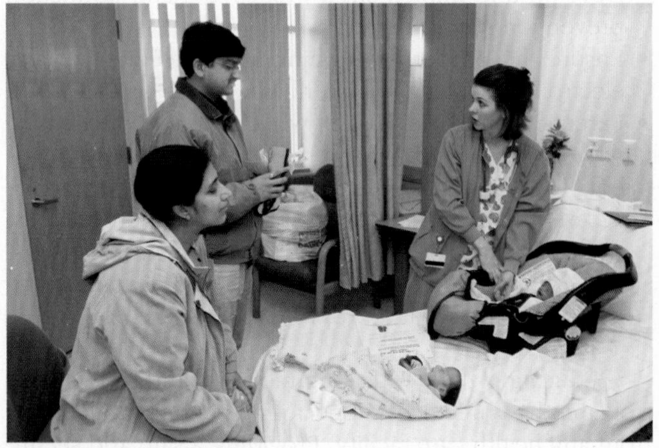

FIGURE 18.20 Newborn in a properly secured car seat.

INFECTION PREVENTION

The nurse plays a major role in preventing infection in the newborn environment. Ways to control infection are as follows:

- Minimize exposure of newborns to organisms.
- Wash your hands before and after providing care, and insist that all personnel wash their hands before handling any newborn.
- Do not allow ill staff or visitors to visit or handle newborns.
- Avoid sharing any infant supplies with another infant.
- Monitor the umbilical cord stump and circumcision site for signs of infection.
- Provide eye prophylaxis by instilling prescribed medication soon after birth.
- Educate parents about appropriate home measures that will prevent infections, such as practicing good hand hygiene before and after diaper changes, keeping the newborn well hydrated, avoiding taking the infant into crowds (which may expose him or her to colds and flu viruses), observing for early signs of infection (fever, vomiting, loss of appetite, lethargy, labored breathing, green watery stools, drainage from umbilical cord site or eyes), and keeping pediatrician appointments for routine **immunizations**.

Promoting Sleep

Although many parents feel their newborns need them every minute of the day, babies actually need to sleep much of the day initially. Usually newborns sleep up to 15 hours daily. They sleep for 2 to 4 hours at a time but do not sleep through the night because their stomach capacity is too small to go long periods without nourishment.

Take Note!

All newborns develop their own sleep patterns and cycles, but it may take several months before the newborn sleeps through the night. Frequently, newborns have their day and night hours reversed and tend to sleep more during the daytime and less during the night.

Parents should place the newborn on his or her back to sleep. To prevent suffocation, all fluffy bedding, quilts, sheepskins, stuffed animals, and pillows should be removed from the crib. Parents should be informed that the practice of "co-sleeping" (sharing a bed) is not safe. For example, infants who sleep in adult beds are up to 40 times more likely to suffocate than those who sleep in cribs (AAP, 2015g). Suffocation can occur when the infant gets entangled in bedding or caught under pillows, or slips between the bed and the wall or the headboard and mattress. The parent may accidentally roll against or on top of the baby. The safest place for a newborn to sleep is in a crib, without any movable objects close by. Benefits versus risks of co-bedding, bed sharing, or co-sleeping include:

- *Benefits*—Promotes breast-feeding practices; increases bonding time between infant and mother; promotes skin-to-skin contact; and increases maternal vigilance over infant.
- *Risks*—Increases risk for SIDS for infants younger than 4 months; risk of death if parent rolls over the infant; interrupts infant sleeping patterns; risk of asphyxia due to entrapment or airway obstruction; and unsafe design of adult beds for infants (Gaydos et al., 2014).

Teach parents to avoid other unsafe conditions, such as placing the newborn in the prone position, using a crib that does not meet federal safety guidelines, allowing window cords to hang loose and in proximity to the crib, placing blankets and pillows in the crib (can potentially smother infant), exposure to tobacco smoke, alcohol, and illicit drugs or setting the room temperature too high (can cause overheating) (CDC, 2015d). Recommendations for safe infant sleeping practices are an important aspect of education for new parents. It is important for nurses to assess families' cultural beliefs and their prior practices to fully understand how to make recommendations in a culturally sensitive manner.

The *Safe to Sleep Campaign* (NICHD, 2014) recommends the following to reduce the risk of SIDS:

- Always place baby on his or her back to sleep for all sleep times, including naps
- Room share—keep baby's sleep area in the same room next to where you sleep
- Use a firm sleep surface, free from soft objects, toys, blankets, and crib bumpers

Enhancing Bonding

Encourage and enhance parent–newborn interaction by involving both parents with the baby and demonstrating appropriate nurturing behaviors:

- Say "hello" and introduce yourself to the newborn.
- Ask the parents' permission to care for and hold their newborn. This helps parents to realize that they are responsible for their child and reminds nurses of their role.
- Show parents the power of a soothing voice to calm the newborn (Fig. 18.21).
- Provide care to the newborn in the least stressful way.
- Demonstrate ways to gently wake up the newborn for better feeding.
- Tell parents what you are doing, why you are doing it, and how they can duplicate what you are doing at home.
- Offer the opportunity for parents to perform care while you observe them. Support their efforts to soothe the newborn throughout the care process.

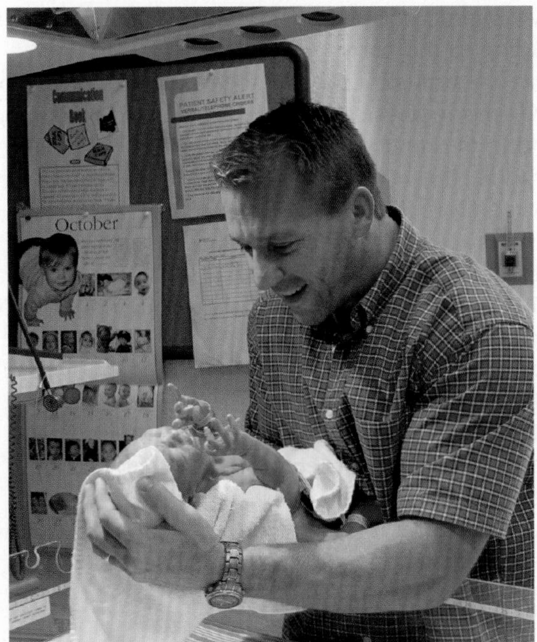

FIGURE 18.21 The father uses a soothing voice to calm the newborn.

- Help parents to interpret the communication cues the newborn uses.
- Point out the efforts the newborn is making to connect with the parents (e.g., alerting to the familiar voice, following the parents while they are speaking, quieting when held securely).

One of the most pleasurable aspects of newborn care is being close to them. Bonding begins soon after birth when parents cradle their newborn and gently stroke him or her with their fingers. Provide parents with opportunities for "skin-to-skin" contact with the newborn, holding the baby against their own skin when feeding or cradling. Many newborns respond very positively to gentle massage. If necessary, recommend books and videos that cover the subject.

For newborns, crying is their only way to communicate that something is wrong. Try to find out the reason why: Is the diaper wet? Is the room too hot or too cold? Is the baby uncomfortable (e.g., diaper rash or tight clothing)? Suggest the following ways in which parents can soothe an upset newborn:

- Try feeding or burping to relieve air or stomach gas.
- Lightly rub the newborn's back and speak softly to him or her.
- Gently sway side to side, or rock back and forth in a rocking chair.
- Talk with the newborn while making eye contact.
- Take the newborn for a walk in a stroller or carriage to get fresh air.
- Change the baby's position from back to side or vice versa.

- Try singing, reciting poetry and nursery rhymes, or reading to the baby.
- Turn on a musical mobile above the newborn's head.
- Give more physical contact by walking, rocking, or patting the newborn.
- Swaddle the newborn to provide a sense of security and comfort. To do this:
  - Spread out a receiving blanket, with one corner folded slightly.
  - Lay the newborn face up with head at the folded corner.
  - Wrap the left corner over the baby's body and tuck it beneath the baby.
  - Bring the bottom corner over the baby's feet.
  - Wrap the right corner around the baby, leaving only the head exposed.
  - Arms can be released from the blanket to allow for self-comforting.

Assisting With Screening Tests

Newborn screening has been among the most successful public health programs of the 21st century. Approximately 4 million infants are screened annually in the United States (Adamkin, 2015). Screening newborns for problems is important because some potentially life-threatening metabolic diseases may not be obvious at birth. Newborn screening tests that are required in most states before discharge are used to check for certain genetic and inborn errors of metabolism and hearing. Early identification and initiation of treatment can prevent significant complications and can minimize the negative effects of untreated disease.

GENETIC AND INBORN ERRORS OF METABOLISM SCREENING

Although each state mandates which conditions must be tested, the most common screening tests are for PKU, hypothyroidism, galactosemia, and sickle cell disease (Table 18.5).

The trend toward early discharge of newborns can affect the timing of screening and the accuracy of some test results. For example, the newborn needs to ingest enough breast milk or formula to elevate phenylalanine levels for the screening test to identify PKU accurately, so newborn screening for PKU testing should not be performed before 24 hours of age.

Screening tests for genetic and inborn errors of metabolism require a few drops of blood taken from the newborn's heel (Fig. 18.22). These tests are usually performed shortly before discharge. Newborns that are discharged before 24 hours of age need to have repeat tests done within a week in an outpatient facility.

Be aware of which conditions your state regularly screens for at birth to ensure that the parents are taught about the tests and the importance of early treatment. Also be familiar with the optimal time frame for screening and conditions that could affect the results. Ensure that a satisfactory specimen has been obtained at the appropriate time and that circumstances that could cause false results have been minimized. Send out specimens and completed forms within 24 hours of collection to the appropriate laboratory (Nagtalon-Ramos, 2014).

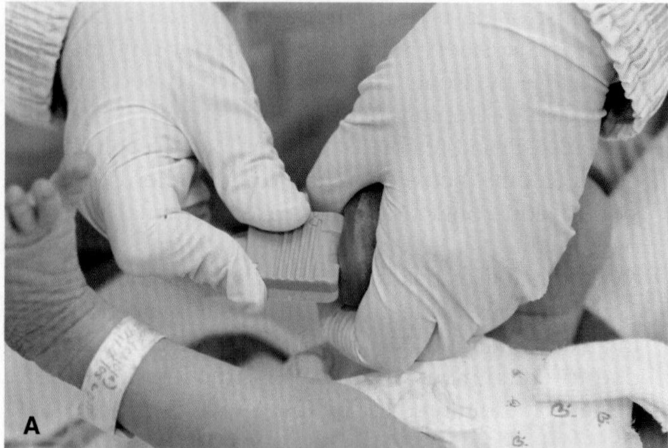

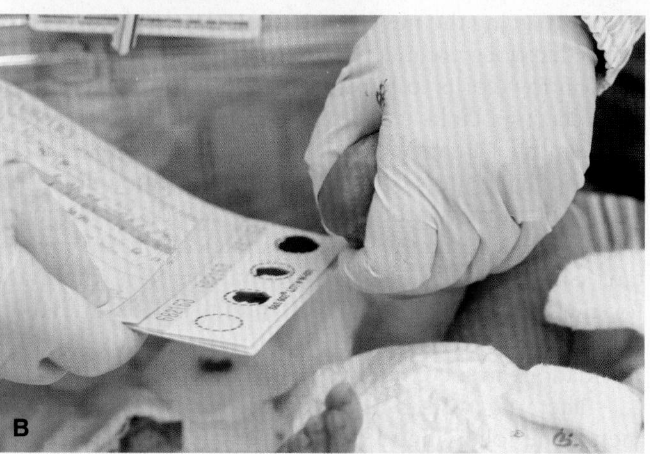

FIGURE 18.22 **Screening for PKU. A. Performing a heel stick. B. Applying the blood specimen to the card for screening.**

HEARING SCREENING

Hearing loss is the most common birth disorder in the United States: approximately 3 to 5 newborns out of every 1,000 live births have some degree of hearing loss. Unlike a physical deformity, hearing loss is not clinically detectable at birth and thus remains difficult to assess (CDC, 2015b). Factors associated with an increased risk of hearing loss include:

- Family history of hereditary childhood sensory hearing loss
- Congenital infections such as cytomegalovirus, rubella, toxoplasmosis, or herpes
- Craniofacial anomalies involving the pinna or ear canal
- Low birth weight (less than 1,500 g)

TABLE 18.5 SELECTED CONDITIONS SCREENED FOR IN THE NEWBORN

Condition	Description	Clinical Picture/Effect If Not Treated	Treatment	Timing of Screening
PKU	Autosomal recessive inherited deficiency in one of the enzymes necessary for the metabolism of phenylalanine to tyrosine—essential amino acids found in most foods	Irritability, vomiting of protein feedings, and a musty odor to the skin or body secretions of the newborn; if not treated, mental and motor retardation, seizures, microcephaly, and poor growth and development	Lifetime diet of foods low in phenylalanine (low protein) and monitoring of blood levels; special newborn formulas available: Phenex and Lofenalac	Universally screened for in the United States; testing is done 24–48 hrs after protein feeding (PKU)
Congenital hypothyroidism	Deficiency of thyroid hormone necessary for normal brain growth, calorie metabolism, and development; may result from maternal hypothyroidism	Increased risk in newborns with birth weight <2,000 g or >4,500 g, and those of Hispanic and Asian ethnic groups; feeding problems, growth and breathing problems; if not treated, irreversible brain damage and intellectual disability before age one	Lifelong thyroid replacement therapy	Testing (measures thyroxin [T_4] and TSH) is done between days 4 and 6 of life
Galactosemia	Absence of the enzyme needed for the conversion of the milk sugar galactose to glucose	Poor weight gain, vomiting, jaundice, mood changes, loss of eyesight, seizures, and intellectual disability; if untreated, galactose buildup causing permanent damage to the brain, eyes, and liver, and eventually death	Eliminate milk from diet; substitute soy milk	First test done on discharge from the hospital with a follow-up test within 1 mo
Sickle cell anemia	Recessively inherited abnormality in hemoglobin structure, most commonly found in African American newborns	Anemia developing shortly after birth; increased risk for infection, growth restriction, vasoocclusive crisis	Maintenance of hydration and hemodilution, rest, electrolyte replacement, pain management, blood replacement, and antibiotics	Bloodspot obtained at same time of other newborn screening tests or prior to 3 mo of age

Adapted from Bhattacharya, K., Wotton, T., & Wiley, V. (2014). The evolution of blood-spot newborn screening. *Translational Pediatrics, 3*(2), 63–70; Boyle, C. A., Bocchini, J. A., & Kelly, J. (2014). Reflections on 50 years of newborn screening. *Pediatrics, 133*(6), 961–963; and Greene, C. L., & Matern, D. (2014). Newborn screening for inborn errors of metabolism. In *Physician's guide to the diagnosis, treatment, and follow-up of inherited metabolic diseases* (pp. 719–735). Berlin Heidelberg, Germany: Springer Publishers.

- Postnatal infections such as bacterial meningitis
- Head trauma
- Hyperbilirubinemia requiring an exchange transfusion
- Exposure to ototoxic drugs, especially aminoglycosides
- Perinatal asphyxia (Nikolopoulos, 2015)

Delays in identification and intervention may affect the child's language development, academic performance, and cognitive development. Detection before 3 months greatly improves outcomes. Because of this, auditory screening programs for all newborns are recommended by the AAP (2015d) and are mandated by law in over 30 states. Screening only infants with risk factors is not enough, because as many as 50% of infants born with hearing loss have no known risk factors (CDC, 2015b). Early identification and intervention can prevent severe psychosocial, educational, and language development delays.

The current goals of *Healthy People 2020* (USDHHS, 2010) are to screen all infants by 1 month of age, confirm hearing loss with an audiologic examination by 3 months of age, and treat with comprehensive early intervention services before 6 months of age (see the *Healthy People 2020* feature earlier in this chapter and Box 18.1 for screening methods). All newborns should be screened prior to discharge to ensure that any newborn with a hearing loss is not missed. Those with suspected hearing loss should be referred for follow-up assessment. In addition, nurses should ensure that testing is accurate to facilitate early diagnosis and intervention services and to optimize the newborn's developmental potential. The implementation of newborn hearing screenings has lowered the mean age of hearing loss identification and many deaf children are now diagnosed in the early age of months old.

BOX 18.1

NEWBORN HEARING SCREENING METHODS

Newborn hearing screening is the standard of care in hospitals nationwide. The primary purpose of newborn hearing screening is to identify newborns who are likely to have a hearing loss and who require further evaluation. A newborn's hearing can be screened in one of two ways: otoacoustic emission (OAE) or automated auditory brain stem response (ABR).

In OAE, an earphone is placed in the infant's ear canal and the sounds produced by the newborn's inner ear are measured in response to certain tones or clicks presented through the earphone. Preset parameters in the equipment decide whether the OAEs are sufficient for the newborn to pass or whether a referral is necessary for further evaluation.

In ABR, an earphone is placed in the ear canal or an earmuff is placed over the newborn's ear, and a soft, rapid tapping noise is presented. Electrodes placed around the newborn's head, neck, and shoulders record neural activity from the infant's brain stem in response to the tapping noises. The ABR tests how well the ear and the nerves leading to the brain work. Like OAEs, automated ABR screening is sensitive to more than mild degrees of hearing loss, but a "pass" does not guarantee normal hearing.

Adapted from Mersch, J., Kibby, J. E., & Bredenkamp, J. K. (2014). Newborn infant hearing screening. *MedicineNet.com.* Retrieved from http://www.medicinenet.com/newborn_infant_hearing_screening/article.htm; American Speech-Language-Hearing Association [ASHA]. (2014). *Newborn infant hearing screening.* Retrieved from http://www.asha.org/Practice-Portal/Professional-Issues/Newborn-Infant-Hearing-Screening/; and American Academy of Pediatrics [AAP]. (2015d). *Purpose of newborn hearing screening.* Retrieved from http://www.healthychildren.org/English/ages-stages/baby/Pages/Purpose-of-Newborn-Hearing-Screening.aspx

Common Concerns

During the newborn period of transition, certain conditions can develop that require intervention. These conditions, although not typically life-threatening, can be a source of anxiety for the parents. Common concerns include transient tachypnea of the newborn, physiologic jaundice, and hypoglycemia.

TRANSIENT TACHYPNEA OF THE NEWBORN

Transient tachypnea of the newborn appears soon after birth. It occurs when the fetal liquid in the lungs is removed slowly or incompletely. This can be due to the lack of thoracic squeezing that occurs during a cesarean birth or diminished respiratory effort if the mother received central nervous system depressant medication. Prolonged labor, macrosomia of the fetus, and maternal asthma also have been associated with this condition. A vaginal birth appears to be protective against transient tachypnea of the newborn (Cunningham et al., 2014).

Transient tachypnea is accompanied by retractions, expiratory grunting, or cyanosis and is relieved by low-dose oxygen therapy. Mild or moderate respiratory distress typically is present at birth or within 6 hours of birth. Transient tachypnea of the newborn is generally a self-limited disorder without significant morbidity. Transient tachypnea of the newborn resolves over a 24-hour to 72-hour period.

Nursing interventions include providing supportive care: giving oxygen, ensuring warmth, observing respiratory status frequently, and allowing time for the pulmonary capillaries and the lymphatics to remove the remaining fluid. The clinical course is relatively benign, but any newborn respiratory issue can be very frightening to the parents. Provide a thorough explanation and reassure them that the condition will resolve over time.

PHYSIOLOGIC JAUNDICE

Physiologic jaundice is very common in newborns, with the majority demonstrating yellowish skin, mucous membranes, and sclera within the first 3 days of life. In any given year, approximately 65% of the newborns in the United States will experience clinical jaundice (King et al., 2015). Jaundice is the visible manifestation of hyperbilirubinemia. It typically results from the deposition of unconjugated bilirubin pigment in the skin and mucous membranes.

Physiologic jaundice can be best understood as an imbalance between the production and elimination of bilirubin, with a multitude of factors and conditions affecting each of these processes. When an imbalance results because of an increase in circulating bilirubin (or the bilirubin load) to significantly high levels, it may go on to cause acute neurologic sequelae (acute bilirubin encephalopathy). In most infants, an increase in bilirubin production (e.g., due to hemolysis) is the primary cause of physiologic jaundice, and thus reducing bilirubin production is a rational approach for its management.

Factors that contribute to the development of physiologic jaundice in the newborn include an increased bilirubin load because of relative polycythemia, a shortened erythrocyte life span (80 days compared with the adult 120 days), and immature hepatic uptake and conjugation processes (Chu, 2014). Normally the liver removes bilirubin from the blood and changes it into a form that can be excreted. As the red blood cell breakdown continues at a fast pace, the newborn's liver cannot keep up with bilirubin removal. Thus, bilirubin accumulates in the blood, causing a yellowish discoloration on the skin.

AAP Guidelines for Prevention and Management of Hyperbilirubinemia in Newborns. The AAP has recently released guidelines for the prevention and management of hyperbilirubinemia in newborns:

- Promote and support successful breast-feeding practices to make sure the newborn is well hydrated and stooling frequently to promote elimination of bilirubin.
- Advise mothers to nurse their infants at least 8 to 12 times per day for the first several days.
- Avoid routine supplementation of nondehydrated breast-fed infants with water or dextrose water because that will not lower bilirubin levels.
- Ensure that all infants are routinely monitored for the development of jaundice and that nurseries have established protocols for the assessment of jaundice. Jaundice should be assessed whenever the infant's vital signs are measured but no less than every 8 to 12 hours.
- Before discharge, complete a systematic assessment for the risk of severe hyperbilirubinemia.
- Provide early and focused follow-up based on the risk assessment.
- When indicated, treat newborns with **phototherapy** or exchange transfusion to prevent acute bilirubin encephalopathy (AAP, 2015h)

In newborn infants, jaundice can be detected by blanching the skin with digital pressure on the bridge of the nose, sternum, or forehead, revealing the underlying color of the skin and subcutaneous tissue. If jaundice is present, the blanched area will appear yellow before the capillary refill. The assessment of jaundice must be performed in a well-lit room or, preferably, in daylight at a window. Jaundice is usually seen first in the face and progresses caudally to the trunk and extremities (AAP, 2015h).

Measures that parents can take to reduce the risk of jaundice include exposing the newborn to natural sunlight for short periods of time throughout the day to help oxidize the bilirubin deposits on the skin, providing breast-feeding on demand to promote elimination of bilirubin through urine and stooling, and avoiding glucose water supplementation, which hinders elimination.

If or when the levels of unconjugated serum bilirubin increase and do not return to normal levels with increased hydration, phototherapy is used. The serum level of bilirubin at which phototherapy is initiated is a matter of clinical judgment by the physician, but it is often begun when bilirubin levels reach 12 to 15 mg/dL in the first 48 hours of life in a term newborn (Davidson, 2014). Phototherapy involves exposing the newborn to ultraviolet light, which converts unconjugated bilirubin into products that can be excreted through feces and urine. Phototherapy is the most common treatment for hyperbilirubinemia and has virtually eliminated the need for exchange transfusions in newborns now.

Take Note!

Exposure of newborns to sunlight represents the first documented use of phototherapy in the medical literature. Sister J. Ward, a charge nurse in Essex, England, recognized in 1956 that when jaundiced newborns were exposed to the sun they became less yellow. This observation changed the entire treatment of jaundice in newborns (Maisels, 2015).

Phototherapy reduces bilirubin levels in the blood by breaking down unconjugated bilirubin into colorless compounds. These compounds can then be excreted in the bile. Phototherapy aims to curtail the increase in bilirubin blood levels; thereby preventing kernicterus, a condition in which unconjugated bilirubin enters the brain. If not treated, kernicterus can lead to brain damage and death.

During the past several decades, phototherapy has generally been administered with either banks of fluorescent lights or spotlights. Factors that determine the dosage of phototherapy include spectrum of light emitted, irradiance of light source, design of light unit, surface area of newborn exposed to the light, and distance of the newborn from the light source (McDermott, 2015). For phototherapy to be effective, the rays must penetrate as much of the skin as possible. Thus, the newborn must be naked and turned frequently to ensure maximum exposure of the skin. Several side effects of standard phototherapy have been identified: frequent loose stools, increased insensible water loss, transient rash, and potential retinal damage if the newborn's eyes are not covered sufficiently.

Recently, fiberoptic pads (Biliblanket or Bilivest) have been developed that can be wrapped around the newborn or on which the newborn can lie. The light is delivered from a tungsten–halogen bulb through a fiberoptic cable and is emitted from the sides and ends of the fibers inside a plastic pad (Plavskii, Tret'yakova, & Mostovnikova, 2014). These products work on the premise that phototherapy can be improved by delivering higher-intensity therapeutic light to decrease bilirubin levels. The pads do not produce appreciable heat like the banks of lights or spotlights do, so insensible water loss is not increased. Eye patches also are not needed; thus, parents can feed and hold their newborns continuously to promote bonding.

When caring for newborns receiving phototherapy for jaundice, nurses must do the following:

- Closely monitor body temperature and fluid and electrolyte balance.
- Document frequency, character, and consistency of stools.
- Monitor hydration status (weight, specific gravity of urine and urine output).
- Turn frequently to increase the infant's skin exposure to phototherapy.
- Observe skin integrity (as a result of exposure to diarrhea and phototherapy lights).
- Provide eye protection to prevent corneal injury related to phototherapy exposure.
- Encourage parents to participate in their newborn's care to prevent parent–infant separation.

See Chapter 24 for a more detailed discussion of hyperbilirubinemia.

The home health nurse made a postpartum visit to Kelly to assess the situation. Kelly's son was slightly jaundiced when the home health nurse pressed gently over his sternum, but Kelly said he was nursing better compared with the previous 2 days. What home suggestions can the nurse make to Kelly to reduce the jaundice? What specific education about physiologic jaundice is needed?

HYPOGLYCEMIA

During the first 24 to 48 hours of life, as normal newborns transition from intrauterine to extrauterine life, their plasma glucose levels are typically lower than later in life. Hypoglycemia affects as many as 40% of all full-term newborns. It is defined as a blood glucose level of less than 30 mg/dL or a plasma concentration of less than 40 mg/dL in the first 72 hours of life (Thornton et al., 2015). From a physiologic perspective, a newborn may be said to be hypoglycemic when glucose supply is inadequate to meet demand. In newborns, blood glucose levels fall to a low point during the first few hours of life because the source of maternal glucose is removed when the placenta is expelled. This period of transition is usually smooth, but certain newborns are at greater risk for hypoglycemia: infants of mothers who have diabetes, preterm newborns, and newborns with intrauterine growth restriction (IUGR), inadequate caloric intake, sepsis, asphyxia, hypothermia, polycythemia, glycogen storage disorders, and endocrine deficiencies (Adamkin, 2015).

Most newborns experience transient hypoglycemia and are asymptomatic. The symptoms, when present, are nonspecific and include jitteriness, lethargy, cyanosis, apnea, seizures, high-pitched or weak cry, hypothermia, and poor feeding. If hypoglycemia is prolonged or is left untreated, serious, long-term adverse neurologic sequelae such as learning disabilities and intellectual disabilities can occur (Stanley et al., 2015).

Treatment of hypoglycemia in the newborn includes administration of a rapid-acting source of glucose such as a sugar/water mixture or early formula-feeding. In acute, severe cases, intravenous administration of glucose may be required. Continuous monitoring of glucose levels is not only prudent but mandatory in high-risk newborns. Although there is no specific means of preventing hypoglycemia in newborns, it is wise and cautious to monitor for symptoms and intervene as soon as symptoms are noted. Subsequently, early diagnosis and appropriate intervention are essential for all newborns.

Nursing care of the hypoglycemic newborn includes monitoring for signs of hypoglycemia or identifying high-risk newborns prone to this disorder based on their perinatal history, physical examination, body measurements, and gestational age. Glucose screening should be performed only on at-risk infants and those with clinical symptoms compatible with hypoglycemia (National Guideline Clearinghouse, 2015).

Prevent hypoglycemia in newborns at risk by initiating early feedings with breast milk or formula. If hypoglycemia persists despite feeding, notify the primary health care provider for orders such as intravenous therapy with dextrose solutions. Anticipate hypoglycemia in certain high-risk newborns and begin assessments immediately on nursery admission.

Promoting Nutrition

Several physiologic changes dictate the type and method of feeding throughout the newborn's first year. Some of these changes include the following:

- Stomach capacity is limited at birth. The emptying time is short (2 to 3 hours) and peristalsis is rapid.

Therefore, small, frequent feedings are needed at first, with amounts progressively increasing with maturity.
- The immune system is immature at birth, so the baby is at a high risk for food allergies during the first 4 to 6 months of life. Introducing solid foods prior to this time increases the risk of developing food allergies.
- Pancreatic enzymes and bile to assist in digestion of fat and starch are in limited supply until about 3 to 6 months of age. Infants cannot digest cereal prior to this time.
- The kidneys are immature and unable to concentrate urine until about 4 to 6 weeks of age. Excess protein and mineral intake can place a strain on kidney function and can lead to dehydration. Infants need to consume more water per unit of body weight than adults do as a result of their high body weight from water.
- Immature muscular control at birth changes over time to assist in the feeding process by improving head and neck control, hand–eye coordination, swallowing, and ability to sit, grasp, and chew. At about 4 to 6 months, inborn reflexes disappear, head control develops, and the infant can sit to be fed, making spoon-feeding possible (Dudek, 2014).

NEWBORN NUTRITIONAL NEEDS

As newborns grow, their energy and nutrient requirements change to meet their body's changing needs. During infancy, energy, protein, vitamin, and mineral requirements per pound of body weight are higher than at any other time of life. These high levels are needed to fuel the rapid growth and development during this stage of life. Generally, an infant's birth weight doubles in the first 4 to 6 months of life and triples within the first year (Walker, 2014).

A newborn's caloric needs range from 110 to 120 cal/kg body weight. Breast milk and formulas contain approximately 20 cal/oz, so the caloric needs of young infants can be met if several feedings are given throughout the day. Most term infants need a basic formula if the mother chooses not to breast-feed. These formulas are modeled after breast milk, which contains 20 cal/oz. There is no evidence to recommend one brand over the other since all of them are nutritionally interchangeable. All formulas are classified based on three parameters: caloric density, carbohydrate source, and protein composition (Table 18.6).

Fluid requirements for the newborn and infant range from 100 to 150 mL/kg daily. This requirement can be met through breast- or bottle-feeding. Additional water supplementation is not necessary. Adequate carbohydrates, fats, protein, and vitamins are achieved through consumption of breast milk or formula. The AAP (2015i) recommends that bottle-fed infants be given iron supplementation, because iron levels are low in all types of formula milk. This can be achieved by giving iron-fortified formula from birth. The breast-fed infant draws on iron reserves for the first 6 months and then needs iron-rich foods or supplementation added at 6 months of age. The AAP (2015i) also has recommended that all infants (breast- and bottle-fed) receive a daily supplement of 400 IU of vitamin D starting within the first few days of life to prevent rickets and vitamin D deficiency. It is also recommended that fluoride supplementation be given to infants not receiving fluoridated water after the age of 6 months (AAP, 2015i). Recently the AAP recommended that all pregnant and lactating women use iodized salt and take a supplement of 150 mcg of iodine daily. An iodine deficiency can affect fetal and early childhood neurocognitive development (AAP, 2015j).

SUPPORTING THE CHOICE OF FEEDING METHOD

The benefits of breast-feeding are significant and well documented. Numerous health-related professional organizations promote breast-feeding because of the health benefits for both the mother and infant. Nurses should encourage and advocate breast-feeding for their clients and provide support for the family throughout their breast-feeding experiences. Parents typically decide about the method of feeding well before the infant is born. Prenatal and childbirth classes present information about breast-feeding versus bottle-feeding and allow the parents to make up their minds about which method is best for them. Various factors can influence their decision, including socioeconomic status, culture, sexual objectification, fear of a negative community reaction, personal inconvenience, dietary restrictions, lack of social support, lack of self-efficacy, high frequency of violence, employment, level of education, lack of access to breast pumps, lack of time, free formula provided by government programs, range of care interventions provided during pregnancy, childbirth, and the early postpartum period, and especially partner support (Dunn et al., 2015). Nurses can provide evidence-based information to assist the couple in making their decision. Regardless of which method is chosen, the nurse needs to respect and support the couple's decision.

FEEDING THE NEWBORN

The newborn can be fed at any time during the transition period if assessments are normal and a desire is demonstrated. Before the newborn can be fed, determine his or her ability to suck and swallow. Clear any mucus in the nares or mouth with a bulb syringe before initiating feeding. Auscultate bowel sounds, check for abdominal distention, and inspect the anus for patency. If these parameters are within normal limits, newborn feeding may be started. Most newborns are on demand feeding schedules and are allowed to feed when they awaken. When they go home, mothers are encouraged to feed their newborns every 2 to 4 hours during the day and only when the newborn awakens during the night for the first few days after birth.

TABLE 18.6 COMPARISON OF BREAST MILK WITH SELECTED FORMULA COMPOSITION

Type	Brand Names	Calories/ Ounce	Carbohydrate Source	Protein Source	Indications
Breast milk	None	20	Lactose	Human milk	Preferred for all infants
Term formula	Enfamil; Similac; Carnation Good Start	20	Lactose	Cow's milk	Appropriate for all term infants
Term formula with DHA and ARA	Enfamil Lipil; Good Start DHA & ARA; Similac Advance	20	Lactose	Cow's milk	Marketed to promote good vision and brain development; to make them more like breast milk
Preterm formula	Enfamil 24 Premature; Preemie SMA 24	24	Lactose	Cow's milk	Usually given to preterm infants <34 wks' gestation
Soy formula	Enfamil Prosobee; Good Start Soy	20	Corn based	Soy	For infants with galactosemia
Hypoallergenic formula	Similac Alimentum; Enfamil Nutramigen; Enfamil Pregestimil	20	Corn or sucrose	Extensively hydrolyzed	For infants with a milk protein allergy
Nonallergenic formula	Neocate; Nutramigen AA	20	Corn or sucrose	Amino acids	For infants with a milk protein allergy
Antireflux formula	Enfamil AR; Similac Sensitive RS	20	Lactose thickened with rice starch	Cow's milk	For infants with gastric reflux disorder

Adapted from Lönnerdal, B. (2014). Infant formula and infant nutrition: Bioactive proteins of human milk and implications for composition of infant formulas. *The American Journal of Clinical Nutrition*, 99(3), 712S–717S; Kent, G. (2014). Regulating fatty acids in infant formula: Critical assessment of US policies and practices. *International Breastfeeding Journal*, 9(1), 2–10; and Abrams, S. A., & Schanler, R. J. (2014). Data do not support claims that 'supplement formulas' are better than standard formulas for breastfed infants. *AAP News*, 35(6), 26–27.

Parents often have many questions about feeding. Generally, newborns should be fed on demand whenever they seem hungry. Most newborns will give clues about their hunger status by crying, placing their fingers or fist in their mouth, rooting around, and sucking.

Newborns differ in their feeding needs and preferences, but most breast-fed ones need to be fed every 2 to 3 hours, nursing for 10 to 20 minutes on each breast. The length of feedings is up to the mother and newborn. Encourage the mother to respond to cues from her infant and not feed according to a standard or preset schedule.

Formula-fed newborns usually feed every 3 to 4 hours, finishing a bottle in 30 minutes or less. Daily formula intake for an infant should be 1.5 to 2 oz/lb of body weight, but growth is a better measure of health than the amount of formula consumed (Schlenker & Gilbert, 2015). If the newborn seems satisfied, wets 6 to 10 diapers daily, produces several stools a day, sleeps well, and is gaining weight regularly, then he or she is probably receiving sufficient breast milk or formula.

Newborns swallow air during feedings, which causes discomfort and fussiness. Parents can prevent this by burping them frequently throughout the feeding. Tips about burping include:

- Hold the newborn upright with his or her head on the parent's shoulder (Fig. 18.23A).
- Support the head and neck while the parent gently pats or rubs the newborn's back (Fig. 18.23B).
- Have the newborn sit on the parent's lap, while supporting the baby's chest and head. Gently rub the newborn's back with the other hand.
- Lay the newborn on the parent's lap with the baby's back facing up.
- Support the newborn's head in the crook of the parent's arm and gently pat or rub the back.

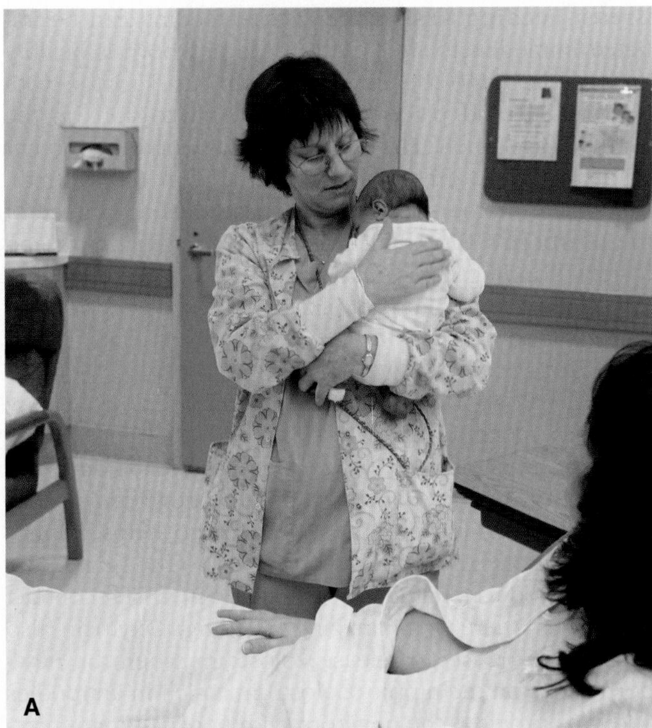

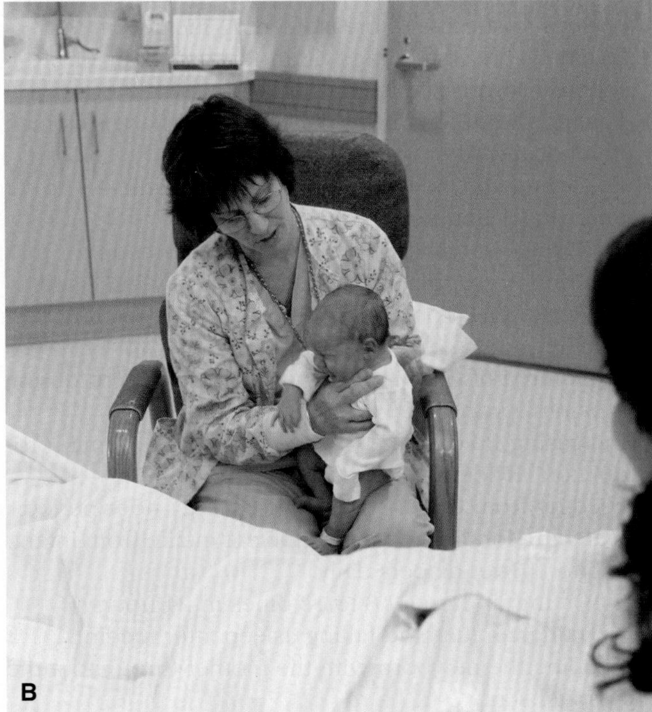

FIGURE 18.23 The nurse demonstrates (**A**) holding the newborn upright over the shoulder and (**B**) sitting the newborn upright, supporting the neck and chin.

Take Note!

It is the upright position, not the strength of the patting or rubbing that allows the newborn to release air accumulated in the stomach.

Stress to parents that feeding time is more than an opportunity to get nutrients into their newborn; it is also a time for closeness and sharing. Feedings are as much for the baby's emotional pleasure as his or her physical well-being. Encourage parents to maintain eye contact with the newborn during the feeding, hold him or her comfortably close to them, and talk softly during the feeding to promote closeness and security.

BREAST-FEEDING

There is consensus in the medical community that breast-feeding is optimal for all newborns. The AAP and the American Dietetic Association recommend breast-feeding exclusively for the first 6 months of life, continuing it in conjunction with other food at least until the newborn's first birthday. An estimated 75% of American mothers attempt to breast-feed, but just 13% are able to exclusively by 6 months (Busch, Logan, & Wilkinson, 2014). Box 18.2 highlights the advantages of breast-feeding for the mother and newborn. In addition, breast-feeding is associated with lower incidence of necrotizing enterocolitis and diarrhea during the early period of life and with lower incidence of inflammatory bowel diseases, type 2 diabetes, and obesity later in life (Martin, Fanaroff, & Welsh, 2014). Mothers should continue to breast-feed during mild illnesses such as colds or the flu. However, in the United States mothers with HIV are advised not to breast-feed.

The composition of breast milk changes over time from colostrum, to transitional milk, and finally to mature milk. Colostrum is a thick, yellowish substance secreted during the first few days after birth. It is high in protein, minerals, and fat-soluble vitamins. It is rich in immunoglobulins (IgA), which help protect the newborn's gastrointestinal tract against infections. It is a natural laxative that helps rid the intestinal tract of meconium quickly (Gephart & Weller, 2014).

Transitional milk occurs between colostrum and mature milk and contains all the nutrients in colostrum, but it is thinner and less yellow than colostrum. This transitional milk is replaced by true or mature milk around day 10 after birth. Mature milk appears bluish and is not as thick as colostrum. It provides 20 cal/oz and contains:

- *Protein*—Although the content is lower than formula, it is ideal to support growth and development for the newborn. The majority of the protein is whey, which is easy to digest.
- *Fat*—Approximately 58% of total calories are fat, but they are easy to digest. Essential fatty acid content is high, as is the level of cholesterol, which helps develop enzyme systems capable of handling cholesterol later in life.
- *Carbohydrate*—Approximately 35% to 40% of total calories are in the form of lactose, which stimulates the growth of natural defense bacteria in the gastrointestinal system and promotes calcium absorption.

BOX 18.2

ADVANTAGES OF BREAST-FEEDING

Advantages for the Newborn

- Contributes to the development of a strong immune system
- Stimulates growth of positive bacteria in digestive tract
- Reduces incidence of stomach upset, diarrhea, and colic
- Begins the immunization process at birth by providing passive immunity
- Promotes optimal mother–infant bonding
- Reduces risk of newborn constipation
- Promotes greater developmental gains in preterm infants
- Provides easily tolerated and digestible formula that is sterile, at proper temperature, and readily available with no artificial colorings, flavorings, or preservatives
- Is less likely to result in overfeeding, leading to obesity
- Promotes better tooth and jaw development as a result of sucking hard
- Provides protection against food allergies
- Lowers health care costs due to fewer illnesses
- Is associated with avoidance of type 1 diabetes and heart disease

Advantages for the Mother

- Can facilitate postpartum weight loss by burning extra calories
- Stimulates uterine contractions to control bleeding
- Lowers risk for ovarian and endometrial cancers
- Facilitates bonding with newborn infant
- Lowers risk of type 2 diabetes
- Breastmilk is free verses formula costs
- Reduces risk of postpartum depression
- Promotes uterine involution as a result of release of oxytocin
- Lowers risk of breast cancer and osteoporosis
- Affords some protection against conception, although it is not a reliable contraceptive method

Data from Schlenker, E., & Gilbert, J. A. (2015). *William's essentials of nutrition and diet therapy* (11th ed.). St. Louis, MO: Mosby Elsevier; Christopher, G. C., & Krell, J. K. (2014). Changing the breastfeeding conversation and our culture. *Breastfeeding Medicine, 9*(2), 53–55; and Walker, M. (2014). *Breastfeeding management for the clinician: Using the evidence* (3rd ed.). Burlington, MA: Jones & Bartlett Learning.

- *Water*—Water, the major nutrient in breast milk, makes up 85% to 95% of the total volume. Total milk volume varies with the age of the infant and demand.
- *Minerals*—Breast milk contains calcium, phosphorus, chlorine, potassium, and sodium, with trace amounts of iron, copper, and manganese. Iron absorption is about 50%, compared with about 4% for iron-fortified formulas.
- *Vitamins*—All vitamins are present in breast milk; vitamin D is the lowest in amount. Vitamin D supplementation is recommended by the AAP now.
- *Enzymes*—Lipase and amylase are found in breast milk to assist with digestion (Dudek, 2014).

Breast-Feeding Assistance. Breast-feeding can be initiated immediately after birth. If the newborn is healthy and stable, wipe the newborn from head to toe with a dry cloth and place him or her skin-to-skin on the mother's abdomen. Then cover the newborn and mother with another warmed blanket to hold in the warmth. Immediate mother–newborn contact takes advantage of the newborn's natural alertness after a vaginal birth and fosters bonding. This immediate contact also reduces maternal bleeding and stabilizes the newborn's temperature, blood glucose level, and respiratory rate (Khan et al., 2014).

Left alone on the mother's abdomen, a healthy newborn scoots upward, pushing with the feet, pulling with the arms, and bobbing the head until finding and latching on to the mother's nipple. A newborn's sense of smell is highly developed, which also helps in finding the nipple. As the newborn moves to the nipple, the mother produces high levels of oxytocin, which contract the uterus, thereby minimizing bleeding. Oxytocin also causes the breasts to release colostrum when the newborn sucks on the nipple. Colostrum is rich in antibodies and thus provides the newborn with her "first immunization" against infection.

Keys to successful breast-feeding include:

- Initiating breast-feeding within the first hour of life if the newborn is stable
- Placing the newborn on the mother's chest/abdomen immediately after birth
- Following the newborn's feeding schedule—8 to 12 times in 24 hours
- Providing unrestricted periods of breast-feeding
- Offering no supplement unless medically indicated
- Having a lactation consultant observe a feeding session
- Avoiding artificial nipples and pacifiers except during a painful procedure
- Increasing fluid intake to encourage greater milk production (Evidence-Based Practice Box 18.1)
- Feeding from both breasts over each 24-hour period
- Watching for indicators of sufficient intake from infant:
  - 6 to 10 wet diapers daily
  - Waking up hungry 8 to 12 times in 24 hours
  - Acting content and falling asleep after feeding
- Keeping the newborn with the mother throughout the hospital stay
- The nurse or lactation consultant should be available to guide and support the breast-feeding mother while on the postpartum unit

Help position the newborn so that latching-on is effective and is not painful for the mother. Placing pillows or a folded blanket under the mother's head may help, or rolling her to one side and tucking the newborn next to her. Assess both the mother and newborn during this initial session to determine needs for assistance

EVIDENCE-BASED PRACTICE 18.1 **PRIMARY CARE SETTING: A COMMUNITY PILOT PROJECT APPLYING THE TRI-CORE BREAST-FEEDING MODEL: BEYOND THE BASICS**

STUDY

Ongoing evidence-based practice findings strongly indicate that the lifelong health and economic benefits of breast-feeding contributes greatly to the health status of the infant, the mother, family, and society at large. Promotional lactation interventions are needed in the community to initiate and foster breast-feeding efforts beyond the hospital after discharge. The purpose of this study was to develop a primary care breast-feeding support program, bridging the gap from hospital discharge into primary care to improve breast-feeding rates. The study incorporated the three core interventions of the Tri-Core Model—(1) improving lactation support; (2) enhancing maternal and staff lactation education; and (3) fostering maternal confidence in their ability to breast-feed.

Findings

The study population ($N = 50$) included middle to low-income families that had recently given birth to a healthy full-term infant who desired to breast-feed within the early postpartum period. Outcomes were measured by the assessment of breast-feeding rates, durations, and reported maternal self-efficacy levels at 1-month, and a 2-month visit. Ongoing office support was provided with lactation visits and phone calls. Findings indicated significant gains in all three areas especially in overall breast-feeding rates when compared to previous rates, especially in rates of exclusive breast-feeding.

Nursing Implications

Based on the results of this study, nurses should remain instrumental in promoting successful breast-feeding practices by initiating breast-feeding as soon as possible after birth, assisting the mother to find a comfortable position for breast-feeding, assessing the infant's latch on to the mother's breast, and reassuring her that the infant is getting adequate amount of breast milk. In addition, utilizing multiprofessional community resources to encourage and support continued breast-feeding efforts is essential. Community referrals are important to help support the novice breast-feeding mother to reinforce breast-feeding instruction once she is discharged from the hospital. Nurses involved in improving breast-feeding rates benefit all ages and its greatest impact will be improving short- and long-term health care outcomes for all families.

Adapted from Busch, D., Nassar, L., & Silbert-Flagg, J. (2015). The necessity of breastfeeding–promoting breastfeeding in the primary care setting: A community pilot project applying the Tri-Core Breastfeeding Model: Beyond the basics. *Journal of Pregnancy & Child Health, 2*(3), 2–7. doi:10.4172/2376-127X.1000158

and education. One tool used frequently in this assessment is the LATCH scoring tool (Abbas & Hasan, 2015). The LATCH scoring tool is a breast-feeding charting system that provides a systematic method for gathering information about individual breast-feeding sessions. The system assigns a numerical score of 0, 1, or 2 to five key components of breast-feeding. Each letter of the acronym LATCH denotes an area of assessment. "L" is for how well the infant latches onto the breast. "A" is for the amount of audible swallowing noted. "T" is for the mother's nipple type. "C" is for the mother's level of comfort. "H" is for the amount of help the mother needs to hold her infant to the breast. The system is visually represented in the same form as the Apgar scoring grid, and the numbers are handled in the same way. With the LATCH system, the nurse can assess maternal and infant variables, define areas of needed intervention, and determine priorities in providing client care and teaching (Table 18.7). The higher the score, the less nursing intervention is needed by the mother and baby.

Breast-Feeding Positioning. The mother and infant must be in comfortable positions to ensure breast-feeding success. The four most common positions for breast-feeding are the football, cradle, across-the-lap, and side-lying holds. Each mother, on experimentation, can decide which positions feel most comfortable for her (Fig. 18.24).

- In the football hold, the mother holds the infant's back and shoulders in her palm and tucks the infant under her arm. Remind the mother to keep the infant's ear, shoulder, and hip in a straight line. The mother supports the breast with her hand and brings it to the infant's lips to latch on. She continues to support the breast until the infant begins to nurse. This position allows the mother to see the infant's mouth as she guides her infant to the nipple. This is a good choice for mothers who have had a cesarean birth because it avoids pressure on the incision.
- The cradling position is the one most commonly used. The mother holds the baby in the crook of her arm, with the infant facing the mother. The mother supports the breast with her opposite hand.
- In the across-the-lap position, the mother places a pillow across her lap, with the infant facing the mother. The mother supports the infant's back and shoulders with her palm and supports her breast from underneath. After the infant is in position, the infant is pulled forward to latch on.
- In the side-lying position, the mother lies on her side with a pillow supporting her back and another pillow supporting the newborn in the front. To start, the

TABLE 18.7 THE LATCH SCORING TOOL

Parameters	0 Point	1 Point	2 Points
L: latch	Sleepy infant, no sustained latch achieved	Must hold nipple in infant's mouth to sustain latch and suck; must stimulate infant to continue to suck	Grasps nipple; tongue down; rhythmic sucking
A: audible swallowing	None	A few observed with stimulation	Spontaneous and intermittent both <24-hr old and afterward
T: type of nipple	Inverted (drawn inward into breast tissue)	Flat (not protruding)	Everted or protruding out after stimulation
C: comfort of nipple	Engorged, cracked bleeding; severe discomfort	Filling; reddened, small blisters or bruises; mild to moderate discomfort	Soft, nontender
H: hold (positioning)	Nurse must hold infant to breast	Minimal assistance; help with positioning, then mother takes over	No assistance needed by nurse

Adapted from Walker, M. (2014). *Breastfeeding management for the clinician: Using the evidence* (3rd ed.). Burlington, MA: Jones & Bartlett Learning; Altuntas, N., Turkyilmaz, C., Yildiz, H., Kulali, F., Hirfanoglu, I., Onal, E., et al. (2014). Validity and reliability of the infant breastfeeding assessment tool, the mother baby assessment tool, and the LATCH scoring system. *Breastfeeding Medicine*, 9(4), 191–195; and Giordano, J. (2014). Cultivating better outcomes for mothers and newborns through integrated best practice models. In *Association of Women's Health, Obstetric and Neonatal Nurses (June 14–18, 2014)*. AWHONN.

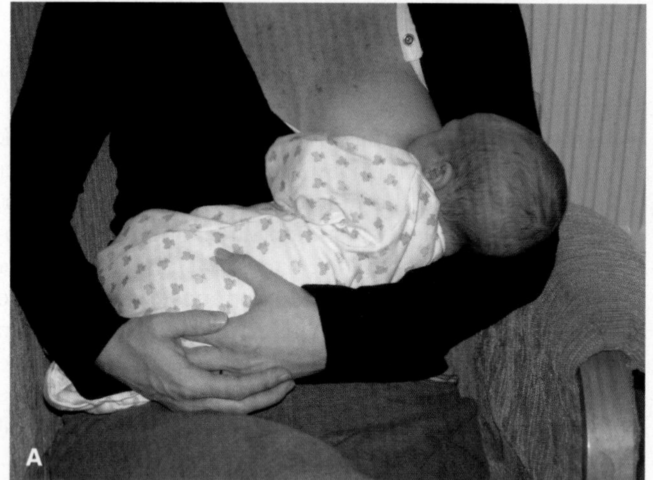

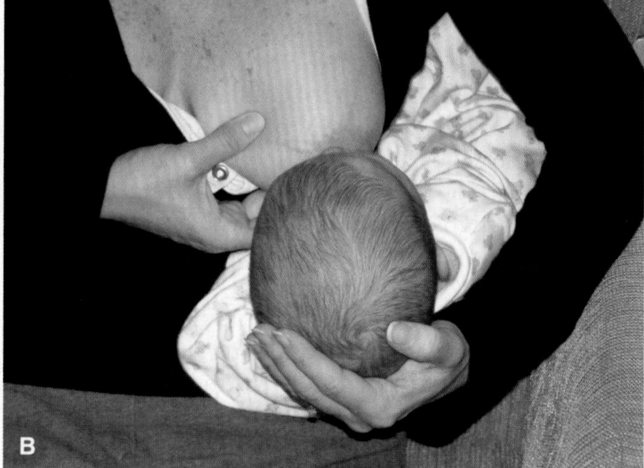

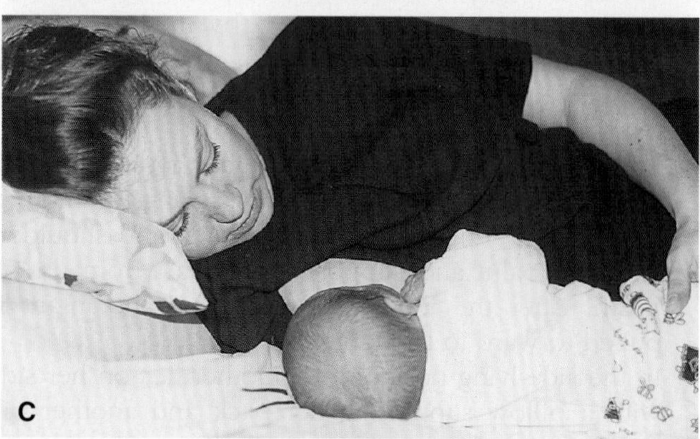

FIGURE 18.24 Breast-feeding positions. Cradling position (**A**) football hold position (**B**) and side-lying position (**C**).

mother props herself up on an elbow and supports the newborn with that arm, while holding her breast with the opposite hand. Once nursing is started, the mother lies down in a comfortable position.

To promote latching-on, instruct the mother to make a C or a V with her fingers. In the C hold, the mother places her thumb well above the areola and the other four fingers below the areola and under the breast. In the V hold, the mother places her index finger above the areola and her other three fingers below the areola and under the breast. Either method can be used as long as the mother's hand is well away from the nipple so the infant can latch on.

Breast-Feeding Education. Breast-feeding is not an innate skill in human mothers. Almost all women have the potential to breast-feed successfully, but many fail because of inadequate knowledge. Nursing Care Plan 18.1 (at the end of the chapter) gives typical nursing diagnoses, outcomes, and interventions. For many mothers and newborns, breast-feeding goes smoothly from the start, but for others it is a struggle. Nurses can help throughout the experience by not being judgmental and by demonstrating techniques and offering encouragement and praise for success. Correct positioning will enhance good attachment and will ensure effective milk transfer. Nurses should emphasize that the key to successful breast-feeding is correct positioning and latching-on.

Teaching by nurses has been shown to have a significant effect on both the ability to breast-feed successfully and the duration of lactation (Dudek, 2014). During the first few breast-feeding sessions, mothers want to know how often they should be nursing, whether breast-feeding is going well, if the newborn is getting enough nourishment, and what problems may ensue and how to cope with them. Education for the breast-feeding mother is highlighted in Teaching Guidelines 18.4.

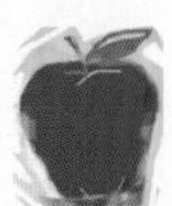

Teaching Guidelines 18.4
BREAST-FEEDING

- Set aside a quiet place where you can be relaxed and won't be disturbed. Relaxation promotes milk let-down.
- Sit in a comfortable chair or rocking chair or lie on a bed. Try to make each feeding calm, quiet, and leisurely. Avoid distractions.
- Listen to soothing music and sip a nutritious drink during feedings.
- Initially, nurse the newborn every few hours to stimulate milk production. Remember that the supply of milk is equal to the demand—the more sucking, the more milk.
- Watch for signals from the infant to indicate that he or she is hungry, such as:
  - Nuzzling against the mother's breasts
  - Demonstrating the rooting reflex by making sucking motions
  - Placing fist or hands in mouth to suck on
  - Crying and squirming
  - Smacking the lips
- Stimulate the rooting reflex by touching the newborn's cheek to initiate sucking.
- Look for signs indicating that the newborn has latched on correctly: wide-open mouth with the nipple and much of the areola in the mouth, lips rolled outward, and tongue over lower gum, visible jaw movement drawing milk out, rhythmic sucking with an audible swallowing (soft "ka" or "ah" sound indicates the infant is swallowing milk).
- Hold the newborn closely, facing the breast, with the newborn's ear, shoulder, and hip in direct alignment.
- Nurse the infant on demand, not on a rigid schedule. Feed every 2 to 3 hours within a 24-hour period for a total of 8 to 12 feedings.
- Alternate the breast you offer first; identify with a safety pin on bra.
- Vary your position for each feeding to empty breasts and reduce soreness.
- Look for signs that the newborn is getting enough milk:
  - At least six wet diapers and two to five loose yellow stools daily
  - Steady weight gain after the first week of age
  - Pale-yellow urine, not deep yellow or orange
  - Sleeping well, yet looks alert and healthy when awake
- Wake up the newborn if he or she has nursed less than 5 minutes by unwrapping him or her.
- Before removing the baby from the breast, break the infant's suction by inserting a finger.
- Burp the infant to release air when changing breasts and at the end of the breast-feeding session.
- Avoid supplemental formula feedings unless indicated for a medical reason. Do not take drugs or medications unless approved by the health care provider.
- Avoid drinking alcohol or caffeinated drinks because they pass through milk.
- Do not smoke while breast-feeding; it increases the risk of sudden infant death syndrome.
- Always wash your hands before expressing or handling milk to store.
- Wear nursing bras and clothes that are easy to undo.

Adapted from Dyson, L., McCormick, F. M., & Renfrew, M. J. (2014). Interventions for promoting the initiation of breastfeeding. *Sao Paula Medical Journal, 132*(1), 68–72; La LecheLeague. (2015a). *Lactation support and health care providers*. Retrieved from http://www.llli.org/resources/providers.html?m=0,2; and Walker, M. (2014). *Breastfeeding management for the clinician: Using the evidence* (3rd ed.). Sudbury, MA: Jones & Bartlett.

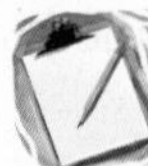

Take Note!

Remember that the supply of milk is equal to the demand—the more sucking, the more milk.

Remember Kelly, who was concerned about jaundice in her newborn son? At her son's 2-week well-baby checkup at the clinic, his bilirubin level came back within normal limits. Kelly still felt he was not getting enough to eat and stated that she might switch to formula-feeding her son. What information can the nurse present to promote and reinforce breast-feeding? Should the nurse make a referral to the lactation consultant?

Breast Milk Storage and Expression. If the breast-feeding mother becomes separated from the newborn for any reason (e.g., work, travel, illness), she needs instruction on how to express and store milk safely. Expressing milk can be done manually (hand compression of breast) or by using a breast pump. Manual or handheld pumps are inexpensive and can be used by mothers who occasionally need an extra bottle if they are going out (Fig. 18.25A). Electric breast pumps are used for mothers who experience a lengthy separation from their infants and need to pump their breasts regularly, for example, while at the work place (Fig. 18.25B).

To ensure the safety of expressed breast milk, instruct the mother in the following:

- Wash your hands before expressing milk or handling breast milk.
- Find a quiet, clean place to express milk if returned to workplace
- Use clean containers to store expressed milk.
- Use sealed and chilled milk within 24 hours.
- Discard any milk that has been refrigerated more than 24 hours.
- Use any frozen expressed milk within 3 months.
- Do not use microwave ovens to warm chilled milk.
- Discard any used milk; never refreeze it.
- Store milk in quantities to be used for each feeding (2 to 4 oz).
- Thaw milk in warm water before using (La Leche League, 2015b).

Common Breast-Feeding Concerns. Breast-feeding women may experience problems such as cracked nipples, engorgement (the painful overfilling of the breasts with milk), or mastitis (inflammation of the breast). Breast-feeding should not be painful for the mother. If she has sore, cracked nipples, the first step is to find the cause. Incorrect positioning or latching-on, removing the infant from the breast without first breaking the suction, or wearing a bra that is too tight can cause cracked or sore nipples. Cracked nipples can increase the risk of mastitis because a break in the skin may allow *S. aureus* or other organisms to enter the body.

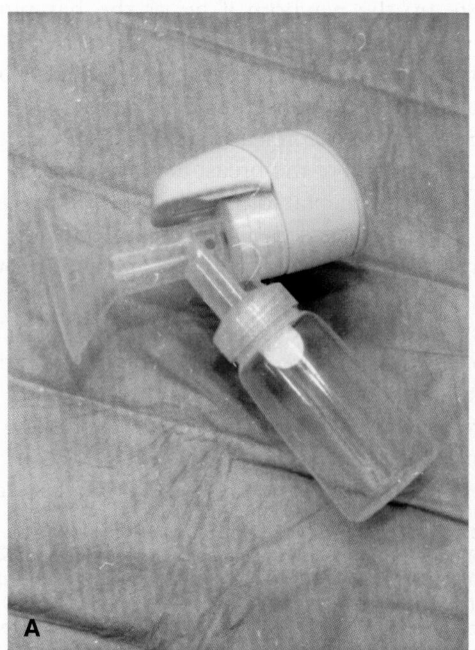

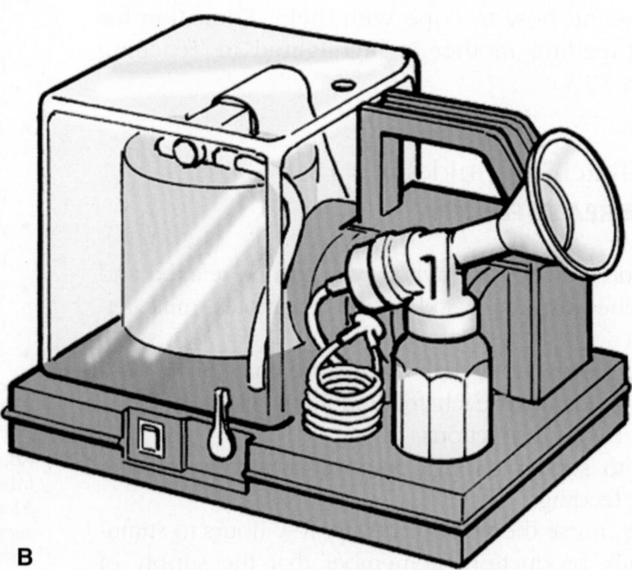

FIGURE 18.25 **A.** Handheld breast pump. **B.** Electric breast pump. (Part B from Lippincott's Nursing Procedures and Skills, 2007.)

Sore nipples usually are caused by improper infant attachment, which traumatizes the tissue. The nurse should review techniques for proper positioning and latching-on. It is important to get this correct from the first feed to assist in the prevention of incorrect attachment and associated nipple trauma. Recommend the following to the mother:

- Use only warm water, not soap, to clean the nipples to prevent dryness.
- Express some milk before feeding to stimulate the milk ejection reflex.
- Avoid using breast pads with plastic liners, and change pads when they are wet.
- Wear a comfortable bra that is not too tight.
- Apply a few drops of breast milk to the nipples after feeding.
- Take systemic anti-inflammatory such as ibuprofen for discomfort.
- Rotate positions when feeding the infant to promote complete breast emptying.
- Leave the nursing bra flaps down after feeding to allow nipples to air-dry.
- Inspect the nipples daily for redness or cracks (Walker, 2014).

To ease nipple pain and trauma, reinforce appropriate latching-on techniques and remind the woman about the need to break the suction at the breast before removing the newborn from the breast. Additional measures may include applying cold compresses over the area and massaging breast milk onto the nipple after feeding.

Engorgement may occur as the milk comes in around day 3 or 4 after birth of the newborn. Explain to the mother that engorgement, though uncomfortable, is self-limited and will resolve as the newborn continues to nurse. The mother should continue to nurse during engorgement to avoid a plugged milk duct, which could lead to mastitis. Provide the following tips for relieving engorgement:

- Take warm to hot showers to encourage milk release.
- Express some milk manually before breast-feeding.
- Wear a supportive nursing bra 24 hours a day to provide support.
- Feed the newborn in a variety of positions—sitting up and then lying down.
- Massage the breasts from under the axillary area down toward the nipple.
- Increase the frequency of feedings.
- Apply warm compresses to the breasts prior to nursing.
- Stay relaxed while breast-feeding.
- Use a breast pump if nursing or manual expression is not effective.
- Remember that this condition is temporary and resolves quickly.

Mastitis, or inflammation of the breast, causes flu-like symptoms, chills, fever, and malaise. These symptoms may occur before the development of soreness, aching, swelling, and redness in the breast (usually the upper outer quadrant). This condition usually occurs in just one breast when a milk duct becomes blocked, causing inflammation, or through a cracked or damaged nipple, allowing bacteria to infect a portion of the breast. Treatment consists of rest, warm compresses, antibiotics, breast support, and continued breast-feeding (the infection will not pass into the breast milk). Explain to the mother that it is important to keep the milk flowing in the infected breast, whether it is through nursing or manual expression or with a breast pump.

FORMULA-FEEDING

Despite the general acknowledgment that breast-feeding is the most desirable means of feeding infants, many mothers choose formula-feeding and need education about this procedure. Formula-fed infants grow more rapidly than breast-fed infants not only in weight but also in length.

Formula-feeding requires more than just opening, pouring, and feeding. Parents need information about the types of formula available, preparation and storage of formula, equipment, feeding positions, and the amount to feed their newborn. The mother also needs to know how to prevent lactation (see Chapter 16 for more information).

Commercially prepared formulas are regulated by the Food and Drug Administration (FDA), which sets minimum and maximum levels of nutrients. Formulas are manufactured by numerous manufacturers in the United States. Normal full-term infants usually receive conventional cow's milk–based formula, but the health care provider makes this decision. If the infant shows signs of a reaction or lactose intolerance, a switch to another formula type is recommended.

The general recommendation is for all infants to receive iron-fortified formula until the age of 1 year. The latest generation of infant formulas includes some fortification with docosahexaenoic acid (DHA) and arachidonic acid (ARA), two natural components of breast milk. Many feel the FDA does not adequately regulate the use of fatty acid additives (DHA and ARA) to infant formula before they are marketed, and there is no systematic assessment after marketing is underway. Researchers are calling for more FDA regulation over additives in infant formulas (Kent, 2014). Commercial formulas come in three forms: powder, concentrate, and easy to feed or ready to use. All are similar in terms of nutritional content but differ in expense. Powdered formula is the least expensive, with concentrated formula the next most expensive. Both must be mixed with water before using. Ready-to-feed formula is the most expensive; it can be opened and poured into a bottle and fed directly to the infant.

Parents need information about the equipment needed for formula-feeding. Basic supplies are four to six 4-oz bottles, eight to ten 8-oz bottles, eight to ten nipple units, a bottle brush, and a nipple brush. A key area of instruction is assessing for flow of formula through the nipple and checking for any nipple damage. When the bottle is filled and turned upside down, the flow from the nipple should be approximately one drop per second. If the parents are using bottles with disposable bags, instruct them to make sure they have a tight-fitting nipple to prevent leaks. Frequent observation of the flow rate from the nipple and the condition of the nipple will prevent choking and aspiration associated with too fast a rate of delivery. Ask the parents to fill a bottle with formula and then turn it upside down and observe the rate at which the formula drips from the bottle. If it is too fast (more than one drop/sec), then the nipple should be replaced.

Correct formula preparation is critical to the newborn's health and development. Mistakes in dilution may result if the parents do not understand how to prepare the formula or make measurement errors. The safety of the water supply should be considered. If well water is used, parents should sterilize the water by boiling it or should use bottled water. Many health care providers still recommend that all water used in formula preparation be brought to a rolling boil for 1 to 2 minutes and then cooled to room temperature before use.

Opened cans of readymade or concentrated formula should be covered and refrigerated after being prepared for the day (24 hours). Instruct parents to discard any unused portions after 48 hours.

Take Note!

Any formula left in the bottle after feeding should also be discarded, because the infant's saliva has been mixed with it.

To warm refrigerated formula, advise the parents to place the bottle in a pan of hot water or an electric bottle warmer and test the temperature by letting a few drops fall on the inside of the wrist. If it is comfortably warm to the mother, it is the correct temperature.

Formula-Feeding Assistance. The process of feeding a newborn formula from a bottle should mirror breast-feeding as closely as possible. Although nutrition is important, so are the emotional and interactive components of feeding. Encourage parents to cuddle their newborn closely and position him or her so that the head is in a comfortable position, not too far back or turned, which makes swallowing difficult (Fig. 18.26). Also urge parents to communicate with their newborn during the feedings by talking and singing to him or her.

Although it may seem that bottle-feeding is not a difficult task, many new parents find it awkward. At first glance, holding an infant and a bottle appears simple enough, but both the position of the baby and the angle of the bottle must be correct.

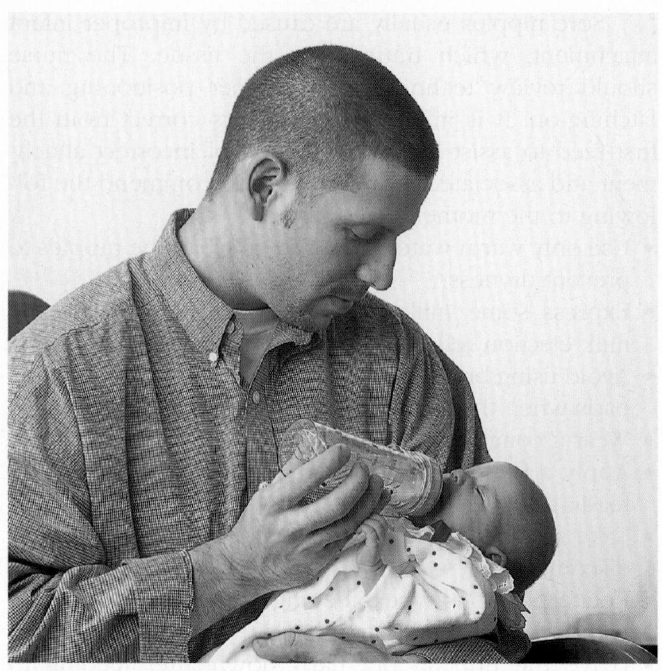

FIGURE 18.26 Father holding his newborn securely while feeding.

Formula-Feeding Positions. Advise mothers to feed their newborns in a relaxed and quiet setting to create a sense of calm for themselves and the baby. Make sure that comfort is a priority for both mother and newborn. The mother can sit in a comfortable chair, using a pillow to support the arm in which she is holding the baby. The mother can cradle the newborn in a semi-upright position, supporting the newborn's head in the crook of her arm. Holding the newborn close during feeding provides stimulation and helps prevent choking. Holding the newborn's head raised slightly will help prevent formula from washing backward into the eustachian tubes in the ears, which can lead to an ear infection.

Formula-Feeding Education. Parents require teaching about the correct preparation and storage of formula as well as the techniques for feeding. See Teaching Guidelines 18.5.

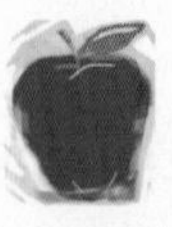

Teaching Guidelines 18.5
FORMULA-FEEDING

- Wash your hands with soap and water before preparing formula.
- Mix the formula and water amounts exactly as the label specifies.
- Always hold the newborn and bottle during feedings; never prop the bottle.
- Never freeze formula or warm it in the microwave.

- Place refrigerated formula in a pan of hot water for a few minutes to warm.
- Test the temperature of the formula by shaking a few drops on the wrist.
- Hold the bottle like a pencil, keeping it tipped to prevent air from entering. Position the bottle so that the nipple remains filled with milk.
- Burp the infant after every few ounces to allow air swallowed to escape.
- Move the nipple around in the infant's mouth to stimulate sucking.
- Always keep a bulb syringe close by to use if choking occurs.
- Avoid putting the infant to bed with a bottle to prevent "baby bottle tooth decay."
- Feed the newborn approximately every 3 to 4 hours.
- Use an iron-fortified formula for the first year.
- Prepare enough formula for the next 24 hours.
- Check nipples regularly and discard any that are sticky, cracked, or leaking.
- Store unmixed, open liquid formula in the refrigerator for up to 48 hours.
- Throw away any formula left in the bottle after each feeding.

Proper positioning makes bottle-feeding easier and more enjoyable for both mother and newborn. As in breast-feeding, frequent burping is key. Advise the parents to hold the bottle so that formula fills the nipple, thus allowing less air to enter. Infants get fussy when they swallow air during feedings and need to be relieved of it every 2 to 3 oz.

Emphasize to parents that an electrolyte imbalance can occur in infants who are fed formula that has been incorrectly mixed. Mixing the formula with too *little* water (i.e., too thickly), can cause hypernatremia because the high concentration of sodium is too much for the baby's immature kidneys to handle. As a result, sodium is excreted along with water, leading to dehydration. Mixing the formula with too *much* water in an effort to save money can lead to failure to thrive, diminished nutrition, fluoride overdose, and lack of weight gain (Monahan, 2014).

WEANING AND INTRODUCTION OF SOLID FOODS

Weaning. Eventually, breast-feeding or formula-feeding comes to an end. Weaning involves the transition from breast to bottle, from breast or bottle to cup, or from liquids to solids. Weaning from breast-feeding to cup has several advantages over weaning to a bottle because it eliminates the step of weaning first to a bottle and then to a cup. Another advantage is that the bottle does not become a security object for the infant.

Weaning can be done because the mother is returning to work and cannot keep breast-feeding, or because the infant is losing interest in breast-feeding and showing signs of independence. There is no "right" time to wean; it depends on the desires of the mother and infant. Weaning represents a significant change in the way the mother and infant interact, and each mother must decide for herself when she and her infant are ready to take that step. Either one can start the weaning process, but usually it occurs between 6 months and 1 year of age.

To begin weaning from the breast, instruct mothers to substitute breast-feeding with a cup or bottle. Often the midday feeding is the easiest feeding to replace. A trainer cup with two handles and a snap-on lid with a spout is appropriate and minimizes spilling. Because weaning is a gradual process, it may take months. Instruct parents to proceed slowly and let the infant's willingness and interest guide them.

Weaning from the bottle to the cup also needs to be timed appropriately for mother and infant. Typically, the night bottle is the last to be given up, with cup drinking substituted throughout the day. Slowly diluting the formula with water over a week can help in this process; the final result is an all-water bottle. To prevent the baby from sucking on the bottle during the night, remove it from the crib after the infant falls asleep.

Introduction of Solid Foods. When infants double their birth weight and weigh at least 13 lb, it is time to consider introducing solid foods. Readiness cues include:

- Consumption of 32 oz of formula or breast milk daily (estimated)
- Ability to sit up with minimal support and turn head away to indicate fullness
- Reduction of protrusion reflex so cereal can be propelled to back of throat
- Demonstration of interest in food others around them are eating
- Ability to open mouth automatically when food approaches it

When introducing solid foods, certain principles apply:

- New foods should be introduced one at a time and a week apart so that if a problem develops, the responsible item can be identified.
- Infants should be allowed to set the pace regarding how much they wish to eat.
- New foods should not be introduced more frequently than every 3 to 5 days.
- Fruits are added after cereals; then vegetables and meats are introduced; eggs are introduced last.
- A relaxed, unhurried, calm atmosphere for meals is important.
- A variety of foods are provided to ensure a balanced diet.
- Infants should never be force-fed (Schlenker & Gilbert, 2015).

Nurses can promote good feeding practices by actively listening to new mothers, helping them clarify their feelings, and discussing solutions. A warm, sincere manner and tone of voice will put an anxious mother at ease. Giving accurate information, making suggestions, and presenting options will enable the mother to decide what is best for her and her infant. Nurses should be sensitive to the individual, family, and economic and cultural differences among mothers before offering suggestions for feeding practices that may not be appropriate.

Preparing for Discharge

Preparing the parents for discharge is an essential task for the nurse. Because of today's shorter hospital stays, the nurse must identify the major teaching topics that need to be covered. Nurses should assess the parents' baseline knowledge and learning needs and plan how to meet them. Using the following principles fosters a learner-centered approach:

- Make the environment conducive to learning. Encourage the parents to feel comfortable during this stressful time by using support and praise.
- Allow the parents to provide input about the content and the process of learning. What do they want and need to learn?
- Build the parents' self-esteem by confirming that their responses to the entire birthing process and aftercare are legitimate, and others have felt the same way.
- Ensure that what the parents learn is relevant to their day-to-day home situation.
- Encourage responsibility by reinforcing that their emotional and physical responses are within the normal range.
- Respect cultural beliefs and practices that are important to the family by taking into account their heritage and health beliefs regarding newborn care. Examples include placing a bellyband over the newborn's navel (Hispanics and African Americans), delaying naming the newborn (Asian Americans and Haitians), and delaying breast-feeding (Native Americans; they regard colostrum as "bad") (Bowers, 2015).

While in the hospital, women have ready access to support and hands-on instruction regarding feeding and newborn care. When the new mother is discharged, this close supervision and support by nurses should not end abruptly. Providing the new parents with the phone number of the mother–baby unit will help them through this stressful transitional period. Giving the new family information and offering backup support via the telephone will increase parenting success. (See Evidence-Based Practice 18.1.)

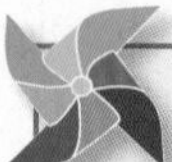

Consider This

I have always prided myself on being very organized and in control in most situations, but survival at home after childbirth wasn't one of them. I left the hospital 24 hours after giving birth to my son because my doctor said I could. The postpartum nurse encouraged me to stay longer, but wanting to be in control and sleeping in my own bed again won out. I thought my baby would be sleeping while I sent out birth announcements to my friends and family—wrong! What happened instead was my son didn't sleep as I imagined and my nipples became sore after breast-feeding every few hours. I was weary and tired and wanted to sleep, but I couldn't. Somehow I thought I would be getting a full night's sleep because I was up throughout the day, but that was a fantasy too. At 2 o'clock in the morning when you are up feeding your baby, you feel you are the only one in the world up at that time and feel very much alone. My feelings of being organized and in control all the time have changed dramatically since I left the hospital. I have learned to yield to the important needs of my son and derive satisfaction from being able to bring comfort to him and to let go of my control.

Thoughts: It is interesting to see how a newborn changed this woman's need to organize and control her environment. What "tips of survival" could the nurse offer this woman to help in her transition to home with her newborn? How can friends and family help when women arrive home from the hospital with their newborns?

ENSURING FOLLOW-UP CARE

Most newborns are scheduled for their first health follow-up appointment within 2 to 4 days after discharge so they can have additional laboratory work done as part of the newborn screening series, especially if they were discharged within 48 hours. After this first visit, the typical schedule of health care visits is as follows: 2 to 4 weeks of age; 2, 4, and 6 months of age for checkups and vaccines; 9 months of age for a checkup; 12 months for a checkup and tuberculosis testing; 15 and 18 months for checkups and vaccines; and 2 years of age for a checkup. These appointments provide an opportunity for parents to ask questions and receive anticipatory guidance as their newborn grows and develops.

In addition to encouraging parents to keep follow-up appointments, advise parents to call their health care provider if they notice signs of illness in their newborn. They should know which over-the-counter medicines should be kept on hand. Review the following warning signs of illness with parents:

- Temperature of 101°F (38.3°C) or higher
- Forceful, persistent vomiting, not just spitting up
- Refusal to take feedings
- Two or more green, watery diarrheal stools
- Infrequent wet diapers and change in bowel movements from normal pattern
- Lethargy or excessive sleepiness
- Inconsolable crying and extreme fussiness
- Abdominal distention
- Difficult or labored breathing

PROVIDING IMMUNIZATION INFORMATION

In the last century, vaccinations have been the most effective medical intervention to reduce mortality and morbidity caused by communicable diseases. It is believed that vaccines save at least two to three million lives annually worldwide (Delany, Rappuoli, & De Gregorio, 2014). Parents also need instructions about immunizations for their newborn. Immunization is the process of rendering an individual immune or of becoming immune to certain communicable diseases (Verklan & Walden, 2015). The purpose of the immune system is to identify unknown (nonself) substances in the body and develop a defense against these invaders. Disease prevention by immunization is a public health priority and is one of the leading health indicators as part of *Healthy People 2020*. Despite many advances in vaccine delivery, the goal of universal immunization has not been reached (Davidson, 2014). Nurses can help to meet this national goal by educating new parents about the importance of disease prevention through immunizations.

Immunity can be provided either passively or actively. Passive immunity is protection transferred via already formed antibodies from one person to another. Passive immunity includes transplacental passage of antibodies from a mother to her newborn, immunity passed through breast milk, and immunity from immunoglobulins. Passive immunity provides limited protection and decreases over a period of weeks or months (Chu & Englund, 2014). Active immunity is protection produced by an individual's own immune system. It can be obtained by having the actual disease or by receiving a vaccine that produces an immunologic response by that person's body. Active immunity may be lifelong either way. (See Chapter 17.)

Young infants and children are susceptible to various illnesses because their immune systems are not yet mature. Many of these illnesses can be prevented by following the recommended schedule of childhood immunizations. Figure 18.27 shows the *2015 Childhood Immunization Schedule*. Refer to *The Point* website for

Figure 1. Recommended immunization schedule for persons aged 0 through 18 years – United States, 2015.
(FOR THOSE WHO FALL BEHIND OR START LATE, SEE THE CATCH-UP SCHEDULE [FIGURE 2]).
These recommendations must be read with the footnotes that follow. For those who fall behind or start late, provide catch-up vaccination at the earliest opportunity as indicated by the green bars in Figure 1. To determine minimum intervals between doses, see the catch-up schedule (Figure 2). School entry and adolescent vaccine age groups are shaded.

Vaccine	Birth	1 mo	2 mos	4 mos	6 mos	9 mos	12 mos	15 mos	18 mos	19–23 mos	2-3 yrs	4-6 yrs	7-10 yrs	11-12 yrs	13–15 yrs	16–18 yrs
Hepatitis B[1] (HepB)	1st dose	←2nd dose→			←3rd dose→											
Rotavirus[2] (RV) RV1 (2-dose series); RV5 (3-dose series)			1st dose	2nd dose	See footnote 2											
Diphtheria, tetanus, & acellular pertussis[3] (DTaP: <7 yrs)			1st dose	2nd dose	3rd dose			←4th dose→				5th dose				
Tetanus, diphtheria, & acellular pertussis[4] (Tdap: ≥7 yrs)														(Tdap)		
Haemophilus influenzae type b[5] (Hib)			1st dose	2nd dose	See footnote 5		←3rd or 4th dose, See footnote 5→									
Pneumococcal conjugate[6] (PCV13)			1st dose	2nd dose	3rd dose		←4th dose→									
Pneumococcal polysaccharide[6] (PPSV23)																
Inactivated poliovirus[7] (IPV: <18 yrs)			1st dose	2nd dose	←3rd dose→							4th dose				
Influenza[8] (IIV; LAIV) 2 doses for some: See footnote 8					Annual vaccination (IIV only) 1 or 2 doses						Annual vaccination (LAIV or IIV) 1 or 2 doses		Annual vaccination (LAIV or IIV) 1 dose only			
Measles, mumps, rubella[9] (MMR)					See footnote 9		←1st dose→					2nd dose				
Varicella[10] (VAR)							←1st dose→					2nd dose				
Hepatitis A[11] (HepA)							←2-dose series, See footnote 11→									
Human papillomavirus[12] (HPV2: females only; HPV4: males and females)														(3-dose series)		
Meningococcal[13] (Hib-MenCY ≥ 6 weeks; MenACWY-D ≥9 mos; MenACWY-CRM ≥ 2 mos)			See footnote 13											1st dose		Booster

Range of recommended ages for all children | Range of recommended ages for catch-up immunization | Range of recommended ages for certain high-risk groups | Range of recommended ages during which catch-up is encouraged and for certain high-risk groups | Not routinely recommended

This schedule includes recommendations in effect as of January 1, 2015. Any dose not administered at the recommended age should be administered at a subsequent visit, when indicated and feasible. The use of a combination vaccine generally is preferred over separate injections of its equivalent component vaccines. Vaccination providers should consult the relevant Advisory Committee on Immunization Practices (ACIP) statement for detailed recommendations, available online at http://www.cdc.gov/vaccines/hcp/acip-recs/index.html. Clinically significant adverse events that follow vaccination should be reported to the Vaccine Adverse Event Reporting System (VAERS) online (http://www.vaers.hhs.gov) or by telephone (800-822-7967). Suspected cases of vaccine-preventable diseases should be reported to the state or local health department. Additional information, including precautions and contraindications for vaccination, is available from CDC online (http://www.cdc.gov/vaccines/recs/vac-admin/contraindications.htm) or by telephone (800-CDC-INFO [800-232-4636]).

This schedule is approved by the Advisory Committee on Immunization Practices (http//www.cdc.gov/vaccines/acip), the American Academy of Pediatrics (http://www.aap.org), the American Academy of Family Physicians (http://www.aafp.org), and the American College of Obstetricians and Gynecologists (http://www.acog.org).

NOTE: The above recommendations must be read along with the footnotes of this schedule.

FIGURE 18.27 Recommended childhood immunization schedule. *(continued)*

FIGURE 2. Catch-up immunization schedule for persons aged 4 months through 18 years who start late or who are more than 1 month behind —United States, 2015.
The figure below provides catch-up schedules and minimum intervals between doses for children whose vaccinations have been delayed. A vaccine series does not need to be restarted, regardless of the time that has elapsed between doses. Use the section appropriate for the child's age. Always use this table in conjunction with Figure 1 and the footnotes that follow.

Children age 4 months through 6 years					
Vaccine	Minimum Age for Dose 1	Minimum Interval Between Doses			
		Dose 1 to Dose 2	Dose 2 to Dose 3	Dose 3 to Dose 4	Dose 4 to Dose 5
Hepatitis B[1]	Birth	4 weeks	8 weeks *and* at least 16 weeks after first dose. Minimum age for the final dose is 24 weeks.		
Rotavirus[2]	6 weeks	4 weeks	4 weeks[2]		
Diphtheria, tetanus, and acellular pertussis[3]	6 weeks	4 weeks	4 weeks	6 months	6 months[3]
Haemophilus influenzae type b[5]	6 weeks	4 weeks if first dose was administered before the 1st birthday. 8 weeks (as final dose) if first dose was administered at age 12 through 14 months. No further doses needed if first dose was administered at age 15 months or older.	4 weeks[5] if current age is younger than 12 months **and** first dose was administered at younger than age 7 months, **and** at least 1 previous dose was PRP-T (ActHib, Pentacel) or unknown. 8 weeks *and* age 12 through 59 months (as final dose)[5] • if current age is younger than 12 months **and** first dose was administered at age 7 through 11 months; OR • if current age is 12 through 59 months **and** first dose was administered before the 1st birthday, **and** second dose administered at younger than 15 months; OR • if both doses were PRP-OMP (PedvaxHIB; Comvax) **and** were administered before the 1st birthday. No further doses needed if previous dose was administered at age 15 months or older.	8 weeks (as final dose) This dose only necessary for children age 12 through 59 months who received 3 doses before the 1st birthday.	
Pneumococcal[6]	6 weeks	4 weeks if first dose administered before the 1st birthday. 8 weeks (as final dose for healthy children) if first dose was administered at the 1st birthday or after. No further doses needed for healthy children if first dose administered at age 24 months or older.	4 weeks if current age is younger than 12 months and previous dose given at <7months old. 8 weeks (as final dose for healthy children) if previous dose given between 7-11 months (wait until at least 12 months old); OR if current age is 12 months or older and at least 1 dose was given before age 12 months. No further doses needed for healthy children if previous dose administered at age 24 months or older.	8 weeks (as final dose) This dose only necessary for children aged 12 through 59 months who received 3 doses before age 12 months or for children at high risk who received 3 doses at any age.	
Inactivated poliovirus[7]	6 weeks	4 weeks[7]	4 weeks[7]	6 months[7] (minimum age 4 years for final dose).	
Meningococcal[13]	6 weeks	8 weeks[13]	See footnote 13	See footnote 13	
Measles, mumps, rubella[9]	12 months	4 weeks			
Varicella[10]	12 months	3 months			
Hepatitis A[11]	12 months	6 months			
Children and adolescents age 7 through 18 years					
Tetanus, diphtheria; tetanus, diphtheria, and acellular pertussis[4]	7 years[4]	4 weeks	4 weeks if first dose of DTaP/DT was administered before the 1st birthday. 6 months (as final dose) if first dose of DTaP/DT was administered at or after the 1st birthday.	6 months if first dose of DTaP/DT was administered before the 1st birthday.	
Human papillomavirus[12]	9 years	Routine dosing intervals are recommended.[12]			
Hepatitis A[11]	Not applicable (N/A)	6 months			
Hepatitis B[1]	N/A	4 weeks	8 weeks **and** at least 16 weeks after first dose.		
Inactivated poliovirus[7]	N/A	4 weeks	4 weeks[7]	6 months[7]	
Meningococcal[13]	N/A	8 weeks[13]			
Measles, mumps, rubella[9]	N/A	4 weeks			
Varicella[10]	N/A	3 months if younger than age 13 years. 4 weeks if age 13 years or older.			

NOTE: The above recommendations must be read along with the footnotes of this schedule.

FIGURE 18.27 *(continued)*

information about how to view the latest CDC immunization schedule. The schedule for immunizations should be reviewed with parents, stressing the importance of continued follow-up health care to preserve their infant's health.

The newborn's first immunization (hepatitis B) is received in the hospital soon after birth. The first dose can also be given by age 2 months if the mother is HbsAg negative. If the mother is HbsAg positive, then the newborn should receive hepatitis B vaccine and hepatitis B immunoglobulin within 12 hours of birth (Cunningham et al., 2014).

Education for the parents should include the risks and benefits for each vaccine and possible adverse effects. Federal law requires a consent form to be signed before administering a vaccine. Parents have the right to refuse immunizations based on their religious beliefs and can sign a waiver noting their decision. When consent has been received, the nurse administering the vaccine must document the date and time it was given, name and manufacturer, lot number and expiration date of the vaccine given, site and route of administration, and the name and title of the nurse who administered the vaccine. Despite overwhelming evidence of vaccine safety, suspicion and misconception continues in small groups of hesitant or resistant parents/partners/significant others, often leading to outbreaks of vaccine-preventable infections. On the front lines of vaccinations, nurses can improve vaccination rates by developing trust with parents/partners/significant others and arming them with information based on sound evidence.

NURSING CARE PLAN 18.1

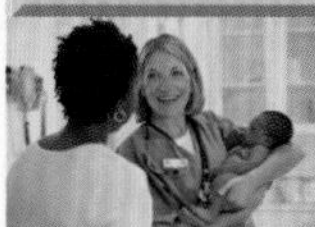

Overview of the Mother and Newborn Having Difficulty With Breast-Feeding

Baby boy James, weight 7 lb, 4 oz, was born a few hours ago. His mother is a 19-year-old gravida 1, para 1. His Apgar scores were 9 points at both 1 and 5 minutes. Labor and birth were unremarkable, and James was admitted to the nursery for assessment. After stabilization, James was brought to his mother, who had said she wished to breast-feed. The postpartum nurse assisted the new mother with positioning and latching-on and left the room for a few minutes. On returning, the mother was upset, James was crying, and she stated she wanted a bottle of formula to feed him since she didn't have milk and her nipples hurt.

Assessment reveals a young, inexperienced mother placed in an uncomfortable situation with limited knowledge of breast-feeding. Anxiety from the mother transferred to James, resulting in crying. The mother, apprehensive about breast-feeding, needs additional help.

NURSING DIAGNOSIS: Ineffective breast-feeding related to pain and limited skill

Outcome Identification and Evaluation

The mother will demonstrate understanding of breast-feeding skills as evidenced by use of correct positioning and technique, and verbalization of appropriate information related to breast-feeding.

Interventions: ***Providing Education***

- Instruct mother on proper positioning for breast-feeding; suggest use of football hold, side-lying position, modified cradle, and across-the-lap position *to ensure comfort and to promote ease in breast-feeding.*
- Review breast anatomy and milk letdown reflex *to enhance mother's understanding of lactation.*
- Observe newborn's ability to suck and latch on to the nipple *to assess whether newborn has adequate ability.*
- Monitor sucking and newborn swallowing for several minutes *to ensure adequate latching on and to assess intake.*
- Reinforce nipple care with water and exposure to air *to maintain nipple integrity.*

NURSING DIAGNOSIS: Anxiety related to breast-feeding ability and irritable, crying newborn

Outcome Identification and Evaluation

The mother will verbalize increased comfort with breast-feeding as evidenced by positive statements related to breast-feeding and verbalization of desire to continue to breast-feed newborn.

Interventions: ***Reducing Anxiety***

- Ensure that the environment is calm and soothing without distractions *to promote maternal and newborn relaxation.*
- Show mother correct latching-on technique *to promote breast-feeding.*
- Assist in calming newborn by holding and talking *to ensure that the newborn is relaxed prior to latching on.*
- Reassure mother she can be successful at breast-feeding *to enhance her self-esteem and confidence.*
- Encourage frequent trials and attempts *to enhance confidence.*
- Encourage the mother to verbalize her anxiety/fears *to reduce anxiety.*

(continued)

NURSING CARE PLAN 18.1

Overview of the Mother and Newborn Having Difficulty With Breast-Feeding (continued)

NURSING DIAGNOSIS: Pain related to breast-feeding and incorrect latching-on technique

Outcome Identification and Evaluation

The mother will experience a decrease in pain during breast-feeding as evidenced by statements of less nipple pain.

Interventions: ***Reducing Pain***

- Suggest several alternate positions for breast-feeding *to increase comfort.*
- Demonstrate how to break suction before removing infant from breast *to minimize trauma to nipple.*
- Inspect nipple area *to promote early identification of trauma.*
- Reinforce correct latching-on technique *to prevent nipple trauma.*
- Administer pain medication if indicated *to relieve pain.*
- Instruct about nipple care between feedings *to maintain nipple integrity.*

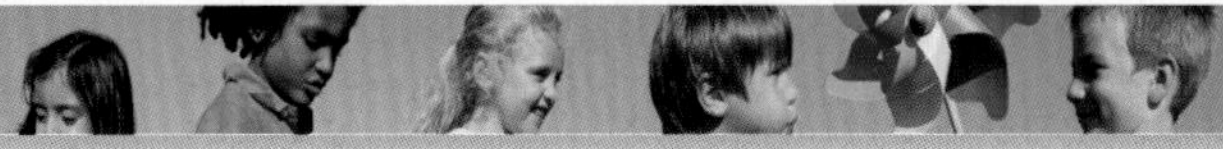

KEY CONCEPTS

- The period of transition from intrauterine to extrauterine life occurs during the first several hours after birth. It is a time of stabilization for the newborn's temperature, respiration, and cardiovascular dynamics.
- The newborn's bowel is sterile at birth. It usually takes about a week for the newborn to produce vitamin K in sufficient quantities to prevent VKDB.
- It is recommended that all newborns in the United States receive an installation of a prophylactic agent (erythromycin or tetracycline ophthalmic ointment) in their eyes within an hour or two of being born.
- Nursing measures to maintain newborns' body temperature include drying them immediately after birth to prevent heat loss through evaporation, wrapping them in prewarmed blankets, putting a hat on their head, and placing them under a temperature-controlled radiant warmer.
- The specific components of a typical newborn examination include a general survey of skin color, posture, state of alertness, head size, overall behavioral state, respiratory status, gender, and any obvious congenital anomalies.
- Gestational age assessment is pertinent because it allows the nurse to plot growth parameters and to anticipate potential problems related to prematurity/postmaturity and growth abnormalities such as SGA/LGA.
- After the newborn has passed the transitional period and stabilized, the nurse needs to complete ongoing assessments, vital signs, weight and measurements, cord care, hygiene measures, newborn screening tests, and various other tasks until the newborn is discharged home from the birthing unit.
- Important topics about which to educate parents include environmental safety, newborn characteristics, feeding and bathing, circumcision and cord care, sleep and elimination patterns of newborns, safe infant car seats, holding/positioning, and follow-up care.
- Newborn screening tests consist of hearing and certain genetic and inborn errors of metabolism tests required in most states for newborns before discharge from the birth facility.
- The AAP and the American Dietetic Association recommend breast-feeding exclusively for the first 6 months of life and that it continue along with other food at least until the first birthday.
- Parents who choose not to breast-feed need to know what types of formula are available, preparation and storage of formula, equipment, feeding positions, and how much to feed their infant.

- Common problems associated with the newborn include transient tachypnea, physiologic jaundice, and hypoglycemia.
- Transient tachypnea of the newborn appears soon after birth; is accompanied by retractions, expiratory grunting, or cyanosis; and is relieved by low-dose oxygen.
- Physiologic jaundice is a very common condition in newborns, with the majority demonstrating yellowish skin, mucous membranes, and sclera within the first 3 days of life. Newborns undergoing phototherapy in the treatment of jaundice require close monitoring of their body temperature and fluid and electrolyte balance; observation of skin integrity; eye protection; and parental participation in their care.
- The newborn with hypoglycemia requires close monitoring for signs and symptoms of hypoglycemia if present. In addition, newborns at high risk need to be identified based on their perinatal history, physical examination, body measurements, and gestational age.
- The schedule for immunizations should be reviewed with parents, stressing the importance of continual follow-up health care to preserve their infant's health.

REFERENCES AND RECOMMENDED READINGS

Abbas, I. M., & Hasan, R. T. (2015). Assessment of LATCH tool regarding initiation of breastfeeding among women after childbirth. *Assessment*, *5*(05), 38–44.

Abrams, S., & Savelli, S. L. (2014). Be prepared to address parents' concerns about vitamin K injection. *AAP News*, *35*(5), 1--1.

Abrams, S. A., & Schanler, R. J. (2014). Data do not support claims that 'supplement formulas' are better than standard formulas for breastfed infants. *AAP News*, *35*(6), 26–27.

Adamkin, D. H. (2015). Metabolic screening and postnatal glucose homeostasis in the newborn. *Pediatric Clinics of North America*, *62*(2), 385–409.

Ahn, E. S., Jung, M. S., Lee, Y. K., Ko, S. Y., Shin, S. M., & Hahn, M. H. (2015). Neonatal clavicular fracture: Recent 10 year study. *Pediatrics International*, *57*(1), 60–63.

Alcantara, D., & O'Driscoll, M. (2014). Congenital microcephaly. *In American Journal of Medical Genetics Part C: Seminars in Medical Genetics*, *166C*, 124–139.

Altuntas, N., Turkyilmaz, C., Yildiz, H., Kulali, F., Hirfanoglu, I., Onal, E., et al. (2014). Validity and reliability of the infant breastfeeding assessment tool, the mother baby assessment tool, and the LATCH scoring system. *Breastfeeding Medicine*, *9*(4), 191–195.

American Academy of Pediatrics [AAP]. (2015a). A recommendation for the definition of "late preterm" and the birth weight-gestational age classification system. Retrieved from http://www.aap.org/en-us/search/pages/results.aspx?k=newbornbirthweightclassification&s=ClinicalSupport

American Academy of Pediatrics [AAP]. (2015b). *Pediatric clinical practice guidelines & policies: A compendium of evidence-based research for pediatric practice* (14th ed.). American Academy of Pediatrics.

American Academy of Pediatrics [AAP]. (2015c). *Where we stand: Administration of vitamin K*. Retrieved from http://www.healthychildren.org/English/ages-stages/prenatal/delivery-beyond/Pages/Where-We-Stand-Administration-of-Vitamin-K.aspx

American Academy of Pediatrics [AAP]. (2015d). *Purpose of newborn hearing screening*. Retrieved from http://www.healthychildren.org/English/ages-stages/baby/Pages/Purpose-of-Newborn-Hearing-Screening.aspx

American Academy of Pediatrics [AAP]. (2015e). *Circumcision*. Retrieved from http://www.healthychildren.org/English/ages-stages/prenatal/decisions-to-make/Pages/Circumcision.aspx

American Academy of Pediatrics [AAP]. (2015f). *Car seats: Information for families for 2014*. Retrieved from http://www.healthychildren.org/English/safety-prevention/on-the-go/Pages/Car-Safety-Seats-Information-for-Families.aspx

American Academy of Pediatrics [AAP]. (2015g). *Co-sleeping*. Retrieved from http://www.aap.org/en-us/search/pages/results.aspx?k=co-sleeping

American Academy of Pediatrics [AAP]. (2015h). *Jaundice*. Retrieved from http://www.healthychildren.org/English/ages-stages/baby/Pages/Jaundice.aspx

American Academy of Pediatrics [AAP]. (2015i). *Vitamins and iron supplements*. Retrieved from http://www.healthychildren.org/English/ages-stages/baby/feeding-nutrition/Pages/Vitamin-Iron-Supplements.aspx

American Academy of Pediatrics [AAP]. (2015j). Iodine deficiency: Pregnant, breastfeeding women need supplementation, AAP says. *AAP News*, *35*(6). Retrieved from http://aapnews.aappublications.org/content/35/6/11.1.extract

American Speech-Language-Hearing Association [ASHA]. (2014). *Newborn infant hearing screening*. Retrieved from http://www.asha.org/Practice-Portal/Professional-Issues/Newborn-Infant-Hearing-Screening/

Apgar, V. (2015). A proposal for a new method of evaluation of the newborn infant. *Anesthesia & Analgesia*, *120*(5), 1056–1059.

Bellini, S. (2015). What parents need to know about vitamin K administration at birth. *Nursing for Women's Health*, *19*, 261–265.

Bhattacharya, K., Wotton, T., & Wiley, V. (2014). The evolution of blood-spot newborn screening. *Translational Pediatrics*, *3*(2), 63–70.

Bond, S. (2015). Rethinking old practices: Evidence supports wiping, not suctioning, newborn secretions at birth. *Journal of Midwifery & Women's Health*, *60*(2), 220–224.

Boom, J. A. (2015a). Microcephaly in infants and children: Etiology and evaluation. *UpToDate*. Retrieved from http://www.uptodate.com/contents/microcephaly-in-infants-and-children-etiology-and-evaluation

Boom, J. A. (2015b). Macrocephaly in infants and children: Etiology and evaluation. *UpToDate*. Retrieved from http://www.uptodate.com/contents/macrocephaly-in-infants-and-children-etiology-and-evaluation

Boyle, C.A., Bocchini, J.A., & Kelly, J. (2014). Reflections on 50 years of newborn screening. *Pediatrics*, *133*(6), 961–963.

Bowers, P. (2015). Cultural perspectives of childbearing. *Nursing Spectrum*. Retrieved from http://ce.nurse.com/ce263-60/CoursePage

Busch, D., Nassar, L., & Silbert-Flagg, J. (2015). The necessity of breastfeeding–promoting breastfeeding in the primary care setting: A community pilot project applying the Tri-Core Breastfeeding Model: Beyond the basics. *Journal of Pregnancy & Child Health, 2*(3), 2–7.

Busch, D. W., Logan, K., & Wilkinson, A. (2014). Clinical practice breastfeeding recommendations for primary care: Applying a tri-core breastfeeding conceptual model. *Journal of Pediatric Health Care, 28*(6), 486–496.

Centers for Disease Control and Prevention [CDC]. (2015a). *Conjunctivitis in newborns.* Retrieved from http://www.cdc.gov/conjunctivitis/newborns.html

Centers for Disease Control and Prevention [CDC]. (2015b). *Hearing loss in children: Recommendations and guidelines.* Retrieved from http://www.cdc.gov/ncbddd/hearingloss/recommendations.html

Centers for Disease Control and Prevention [CDC]. (2015c). *Trends in circumcision for male newborns in U.S. Hospitals.* Retrieved from http://www.cdc.gov/nchs/data/hestat/circumcision_2013/circumcision_2013.htm

Centers for Disease Control and Prevention [CDC]. (2015d). *Infants and toddlers – Safety in the home and community.* Retrieved from http://www.cdc.gov/parents/infants/safety.html

Christopher, G. C., & Krell, J. K. (2014). Changing the breastfeeding conversation and our culture. *Breastfeeding Medicine, 9*(2), 53–55.

Chu, J. (2014). Approach to jaundice in infancy. *Mount Sinai Expert Guides: Hepatology*, 374–381. doi: 10.1002/9781118748626.ch36

Chu, H. Y., & Englund, J. A. (2014). Maternal immunization. *Clinical Infectious Diseases*, ciu327. (Online June 16, 2014). doi: 10.1093/cid/ciu327

Clark-Gambelunghe, M. B., & Clark, D. A. (2015). Sensory development. *Pediatric Clinics of North America, 62*(2), 367–384.

Cunningham, F. G., Leveno, K. J., Bloom, S. L., Spong, C. Y., Dashe, J. S., Hoffman, B. L., et al. (2014). *William's obstetrics* (24th ed.). New York, NY: McGraw-Hill Medical.

Davidson, M. R. (2014). *Fast facts for the neonatal nurse: A nursing orientation and care guide in a nutshell.* New York, NY: Springer Publishing Company.

Delany, I., Rappuoli, R., & De Gregorio, E. (2014). Vaccines for the 21st century. *EMBO Molecular Medicine, 6*(6), 708–720.

Dudek, S. G. (2014). *Nutrition essentials for nursing practice* (7th ed.). Philadelphia, PA: Lippincott Williams & Wilkins.

Dunn, R. L., Kalich, K. A., Henning, M. J., & Fedrizzi, R. (2015). Engaging field-based professionals in a qualitative assessment of barriers and positive contributors to breastfeeding using the social ecological model. *Maternal and Child Health Journal, 19*(1), 6–16.

Dyson, L., McCormick, F. M., & Renfrew, M. J. (2014). Interventions for promoting the initiation of breastfeeding. *Sao Paulo Medical Journal, 132*(1), 68–72.

El-Radhi, A. S. (2015). Management of common neonatal problems. *British Journal of Nursing, 24*(5), 258–266.

Fillipps, D. J., & Bucciarelli, R. L. (2015). Cardiac evaluation of the newborn. *Pediatric Clinics of North America, 62*(2), 471–489.

Fonseca, M. J., Severo, M., Barros, H., & Santos, A. C. (2014). Determinants of weight changes during the first 96 hours of life in full term newborns. *Birth, 41*(2), 160–168.

Freedman, A. L., & Hurwitz, R. S. (2015). Complications of newborn circumcision: Prevention, diagnosis and treatment. In P. P. Godbole, M. A. Koyle, & D. T. Wilcox (Eds.), *Pediatric Urology: Surgical Complications and Management* (2nd ed.). Hoboken, NJ: John Wiley & Sons. doi: 10.1002/9781118473382.ch25

Gaydos, L. M., Blake, S. C., Gazmararian, J. A., Woodruff, W., Thompson, W. W., & Dalmida, S. G. (2014). Revisiting safe sleep recommendations for African-American Infants: Why current counseling is insufficient. *Maternal and Child Health Journal, 19*(3), 496–503.

Gephart, S. M., & Weller, M. (2014). Colostrum as oral immune therapy to promote neonatal health. *Advances in Neonatal Care, 14*(1), 44–51.

Giese, R. A., & Richter, G. T. (2015). Capillary malformations. *Head and neck vascular anomalies: A practical casebased approach* (pp. 127–128), San Diego, CA: Plural Publishing.

Giordano, J. (2014). Cultivating better outcomes for mothers and newborns through integrated best practice models. In *Association of Women's Health, Obstetric and Neonatal Nurses (June 14–18, 2014)*. AWHONN.

Gloster, H. M. Jr, Gebauer, L. E., & Mistur, R. L. (2016a). Erythema toxicum neonatorum. In *Absolute dermatology review* (pp. 87–89). Springer International Publishing.

Gloster, H. M. Jr, Gebauer, L. E., & Mistur, R. L. (2016b). Supernumerary nipples. In *Absolute dermatology review* (pp. 355–356). Springer International Publishing.

Goyal, D., Nagar, S., & Kumar, B. (2014). An enhanced approach for face recognition of newborns using HMM and SVD coefficients. *International Journal of Computer Applications, 88*(14), 17–23.

Greene, C. L., & Matern, D. (2014). Newborn screening for inborn errors of metabolism. In *Physician's guide to the diagnosis, treatment, and follow-up of inherited metabolic diseases* (pp. 719–735). Berlin Heidelberg, Germany: Springer Publishers.

Hodges, N. L., & Smith, G. A. (2014). Car safety. *Pediatrics in Review, 35*(4), 155–161.

Joint Commission. (2015). Infant abductions: Preventing future occurrences. Retrieved from http://www.jointcommission.org/SentinelEvents/SentinelEventAlert/sea_9.htm

Kent, G. (2014). Regulating fatty acids in infant formula: Critical assessment of US policies and practices. *International Breastfeeding Journal, 9*(1), 2–10.

Khan, J., Vesel, L., Bahl, R., & Martines, J. C. (2014). Timing of breastfeeding initiation and exclusivity of breastfeeding during the first month of life: Effects on neonatal mortality and morbidity—A systematic review and meta-analysis. *Maternal and Child Health Journal*, 1–12. (Online June 4, 2014). doi: 10.1007/s10995-014-1526-8

King, T. L., Brucker, M. C., Kriebs, J. M., Fahey, J. O., Gegor, C. L., & Varney, H. (2015). *Varney's midwifery* (5th ed.). Burlington, MA: Jones & Bartlett Learning.

Kliegman, R. M., Behrman, R. E., Jenson, H. B., & Stanton, B. F. (2014). *Nelson's textbook of pediatrics* (20th ed.). St. Louis, MO: Elsevier.

La LecheLeague. (2015a). *Lactation support and health care providers.* Retrieved from http://www.llli.org/resources/providers.html?m=0,2

La LecheLeague. (2015b). *Expressing and storing milk.* Retrieved from http://www.llli.org/nb/nbjulaug07p168.html

Lomax, A. (2015). *Examination of the newborn: An evidence-based guide* (2nd ed.). West Sussex, UK: John Wiley & Sons.

Lönnerdal, B. (2014). Infant formula and infant nutrition: Bioactive proteins of human milk and implications for composition of infant formulas. *The American Journal of Clinical Nutrition, 99*(3), 712S–717S.

Ludington-Hoe, S. M., & Morgan, K. (2014). Infant assessment and reduction of sudden unexpected postnatal collapse risk during skin-to-skin contact. *Newborn and Infant Nursing Reviews, 14*(1), 28–33.

Maisels, M. J. (2015). Sister Jean Ward, phototherapy, and jaundice: A unique human and photochemical interaction. *Journal of Perinatology.* doi:10.1038/jp.2015.56

Marcdante, K. J., & Kliegman, R. M. (2014). *Nelson essentials of pediatrics* (7th ed.). Philadelphia, PA: Elsevier.

March of Dimes. (2015a). *Hearing loss.* Retrieved from http://www.marchofdimes.com/baby/hearing-impairment.aspx

Martin, R. J., Fanaroff, A. A., & Walsh, M. C. (2014). *Fanaroff & Martin's neonatal-perinatal medicine* (10th ed.). Philadelphia, PA: Elsevier.

McDermott, J. L. (2015). G586 (P) Phototherapy management in jaundiced babies: Jaundice management tool. *Archives of Disease in Childhood, 100*(Suppl 3), A268--A269.

Mersch, J., Kibby, J. E., & Bredenkamp, J. K. (2014). Newborn infant hearing screening. *MedicineNet.com.* Retrieved from http://www.medicinenet.com/newborn_infant_hearing_screening/article.htm

Mielke, R. T. (2014). Counseling parents who are considering newborn male circumcision. *Journal of Midwifery & Women's Health, 59*(2), 225.

Monahan, E. (2014). What are the dangers of diluted baby formula? *Livestrong.* Retrieved from http://www.livestrong.com/article/97662-dangers-diluted-baby-formula/

Moore, D. L., & MacDonald, N. E. (2015). Preventing ophthalmia neonatorum. *Pediatrics & Child Health, 20*(2), 93–96.

Morrison, K., Herbst, K., Corbett, S., & Herndon, C. D. (2014). Pain management practice patterns for common pediatric urology procedures. *Urology, 83*(1), 206–210.

Moses, S. (2015). Pediatric vital signs. *Family Practice Notebook.* Retrieved from http://www.fpnotebook.com/cv/exam/pdtrcvtlsgns.htm

Mutter, G. L., & Prat, J. (2014). *Pathology of the female reproductive tract.* Philadelphia, PA: Elsevier Health Sciences.

Nagtalon-Ramos, J. (2014). *Maternal-newborn nursing care: Best evidence-based practices.* Philadelphia, PA: F.A. Davis Company.

National Center for Missing & Exploited Children [NCMEC]. (2015). *Infant abductions.* Retrieved from http://www.missingkids.com/InfantAbduction

National Guideline Clearinghouse. (2015). *Guidelines for glucose monitoring and treatment of hypoglycemia in neonates.* Retrieved from http://www.guideline.gov/content.aspx?id=11218&search=glucose+monitoring+of+hypoglycemia+in+neonates

National Institute of Child Health and Human Development [NICHD]. (2014). *Safe to sleep public education campaign.* Retrieved from http://www.nichd.nih.gov/sts/news/downloadable/Pages/infographic_horizontal.aspx

Nikolopoulos, T. P. (2015). Neonatal hearing screening: What we have achieved and what needs to be improved. *International Journal of Pediatric Otorhinolaryngology, 79*(5), 635–637.

Otsuka, Y. (2014). Face recognition in infants: A review of behavioral and near-infrared spectroscopic studies. *Japanese Psychological Research, 56,* 76–90.

Pfister, K. M., & Ramel, S. E. (2014). Linear growth and neurodevelopmental outcomes. *Clinics in Perinatology, 41*(2), 309–321.

Plavskii, V. Y., Tret'yakova, A. I., & Mostovnikova, G. R. (2014). Phototherapeutic systems for the treatment of hyperbilirubinemia of newborns. *Journal of Optical Technology, 81*(6), 341–348.

Rüdiger, M., & Konstantelos, D. (2015). Apgar score and risk of cause-specific infant mortality. *The Lancet, 385*(9967), 505–506.

Saugstad, O. D. (2015). Delivery room management of term and preterm newly born infants. *Neonatology, 107*(4), 365–371.

Schlenker, E., & Gilbert, J. A. (2015). *William's essentials of nutrition and diet therapy* (11th ed.). St. Louis, MO: Elsevier.

Sheth, R. D., Ranalli, N., & Aldana, P. (2014). Pediatric craniosynostosis. *eMedicine.* Retrieved from http://emedicine.medscape.com/article/1175957-overview

Silverberg, N. B. (2015). Normal color variations in children of color. In *Pediatric skin of color* (pp. 63–68). New York, NY: Springer.

Sinkey, R. G., Eschenbacher, M. A., Walsh, P. M., Doerger, R. G., Lambers, D. S., Sibai, B. M., et al. (2015). The GoMo study: A randomized clinical trial assessing neonatal pain with Gomco vs. Mogen clamp circumcision. *American Journal of Obstetrics and Gynecology, 212*(5), 664-e1.

Skidmore-Roth, L. (2015). *Mosby's 2015 nursing drug reference* (28th ed.). St. Louis, MO: Elsevier.

Springer, S. C., & Glasser, J. G. (2015). Bowel obstruction in the newborn. *eMedicine.* Retrieved from http://emedicine.medscape.com/article/980360-overview

Stanley, C. A., Rozance, P. J., Thornton, P. S., De Leon, D. D., Harris, D., Haymond, M. W., et al. (2015). Re-evaluating "transitional neonatal hypoglycemia": Mechanism and implications for management. *The Journal of Pediatrics, 166*(6), 1520–1525.

Tamai, J., & McCarthy, J. J. (2015). Developmental dysplasia of the hip. *eMedicine.* Retrieved from http://emedicine.medscape.com/article/1248135-overview

Tawia, S., & McGuire, L. (2014). Early weight loss and weight gain in healthy, full-term, exclusively-breastfed infants. *Breastfeeding Review, 22*(1), 31–42.

Thornton, P. S., Stanley, C. A., De Leon, D. D., Harris, D., Haymond, M. W., Hussain, K., et al. (2015). Recommendations from the Pediatric Endocrine Society for evaluation and management of persistent hypoglycemia in neonates, infants, and children. *The Journal of Pediatrics, 167*(2), 238--245.

Tobian, A. A., Kacker, S., & Quinn, T. C. (2014). Male circumcision: A globally relevant but under-utilized method for the prevention of HIV and other sexually transmitted infections. *Annual Review of Medicine, 65,* 293–306.

Tung, T. H., & Moore, A. M. (2015). 14 brachial plexus injuries. *Nerve surgery* (pp. 391–479). New York, NY: Thieme-Medical Publishers.

U.S. Department of Health and Human Services [USDHHS]. (2010). *Healthy people 2020.* Retrieved from http://www.healthypeople.gov/2020/topicsobjectives2020

Verklan, M.T., & Walden, M. (2015). *Core curriculum for neonatal intensive care nursing* (5th ed.). St. Louis, MO: Elsevier.

Walker, M. (2014). *Breastfeeding management for the clinician: Using the evidence* (3rd ed.). Burlington, MA: Jones & Bartlett Learning.

Weber, J., & Kelley, J. (2014). *Health assessment in nursing* (5th ed.). Philadelphia, PA: Lippincott Williams & Wilkins.

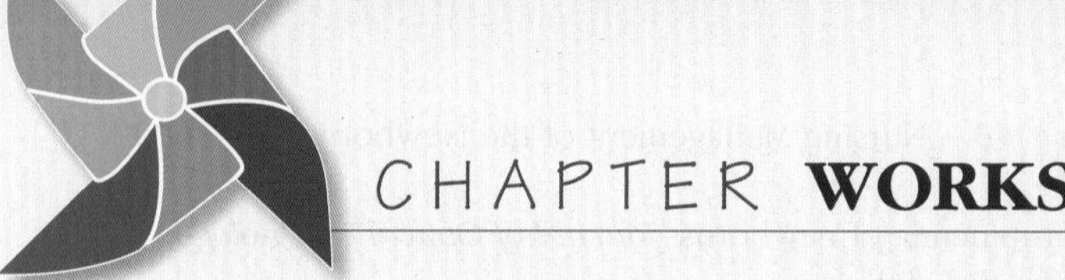

CHAPTER WORKSHEET

MULTIPLE-CHOICE QUESTIONS

1. At birth, a newborn's assessment reveals the following: heart rate of 140 bpm, loud crying, some flexion of extremities, crying when bulb syringe is introduced into the nares, and a pink body with blue extremities. The nurse would document the newborn's Apgar score as:
   a. 5 points
   b. 6 points
   c. 7 points
   d. 8 points
2. The nurse is explaining phototherapy to the parents of a newborn. The nurse would include which of the following as the purpose?
   a. Increase surfactant levels
   b. Stabilize the newborn's temperature
   c. Destroy Rh-negative antibodies
   d. Oxidize bilirubin on the skin
3. The nurse administers a single dose of vitamin K intramuscularly to a newborn after birth to promote:
   a. Conjugation of bilirubin
   b. Blood clotting
   c. Foreman ovale closure
   d. Digestion of complex proteins
4. A prophylactic agent is instilled in both eyes of all newborns to prevent which of the following conditions?
   a. Gonorrhea and chlamydia
   b. Thrush and enterobacter
   c. *Staphylococcus* and syphilis
   d. Hepatitis B and herpes
5. The AAP recommends that all newborns be placed on their backs to sleep to reduce the risk of:
   a. Respiratory distress syndrome
   b. Bottle mouth syndrome
   c. Sudden infant death syndrome
   d. GI regurgitation syndrome
6. Which one of the following immunizations is most commonly received by newborns before hospital discharge?
   a. Pneumococcus
   b. Varicella
   c. Hepatitis A
   d. Hepatitis B
7. Which condition would be missed if a newborn were screened before he had tolerated protein feedings for at least 48 hours?
   a. Hypothyroidism
   b. Cystic fibrosis
   c. Phenylketonuria
   d. Sickle cell disease
8. Which of the following findings in a newborn would the nurse document as abnormal when assessing the newborn head?
   a. Two soft spots palpated between the cranial bones
   b. A spongy area of edema outlined on the head
   c. Head circumference 32 cm, chest 34 cm
   d. Asymmetry of the head with overriding bones
9. Which of the following findings in a newborn would be considered normal?
   a. Passage of meconium within the first 24 hours
   b. Respiratory rate of 80 breaths per minute
   c. Yellow skin tones at 10 hours after birth
   d. Bleeding from the umbilicus area

CRITICAL THINKING EXERCISE

1. An African-American mother who delivered her first baby and is on the mother–baby unit, calls the nursery nurse into her room and expresses concern about how her daughter looks. The mother tells the nurse that her baby's head looks like a "banana" and is mushy to the touch, and she has "white spots" all over her nose. In addition, there appear to be "big bluish bruises" all over her baby's buttocks. She wants to know what is wrong with her baby and whether these problems will go away.
   a. How should the nurse respond to this mother's questions?
   b. What additional newborn instruction might be appropriate at this time?
   c. What reassurance can be given to this new mother regarding her daughter's appearance?

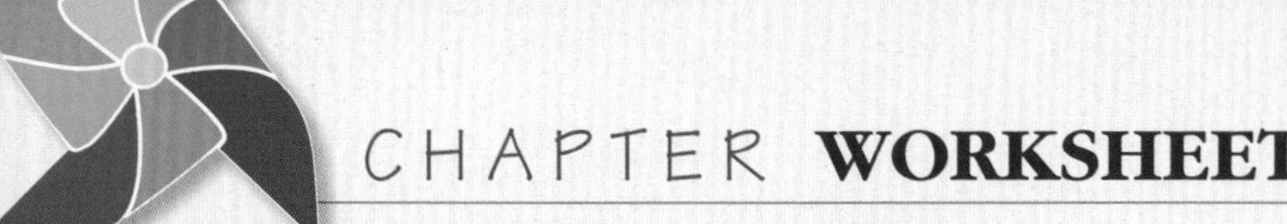

CHAPTER WORKSHEET

2. At approximately 12:30 AM on a Friday, a woman enters a hospital through a busy emergency department. She is wearing a white uniform and a lab coat with a stethoscope around her neck. She identifies herself as a new nurse coming back to check on something she had left on the unit on an earlier shift. She enters a postpartum client's room containing the mother's newborn, pushes the open crib down a hallway, and escapes through an exit. The security cameras aren't working. The infant isn't discovered missing until the 2 AM check by the nurse.
   a. What impact does an infant abduction have on the family and the hospital?
   b. What security measure was the weak link in the chain of security?
   c. What can hospitals do to prevent infant abduction?

STUDY ACTIVITIES

1. Obtain a set of vital signs (temperature, pulse, respiration) of a newborn on admission to the nursery. Repeat this procedure and compare changes in the values several hours later. Discuss what changes in the vital signs you would expect during this transitional period.

   The discussion of newborn changes noticed will vary from student to student, depending on the interview information obtained from the new mother.

2. Interview a new mother on the postpartum unit on her second day about the changes she has noticed in her newborn's appearance and behavior within the past 24 hours. Discuss your interview findings at postconference. This discussion will vary depending on questions asked during the bath demonstration as well as each individual mother's response to it.

3. Demonstrate a newborn bath to a new mother in her room, using the principle of bathing from the cleanest to the dirtiest body part. Discuss the questions asked by the mother and her reaction to the demonstration in post conference.

4. Go to the La Leche League website (refer to The Point website). Review the information it provides on breast-feeding. How helpful would it be to a new mother?

5. Debate the risks and benefits of neonatal circumcision within your nursing group at postconference. Did either side present a stronger position? What is your opinion, and why?

BRINGING IT ALL TOGETHER: A CASE STUDY

Two days after having a difficult birth to her first child at 37 weeks' gestation, 25-year-old Molly and her partner take their son home from the hospital. That evening while she is breast-feeding him, Molly notices that the whites of her son's eyes seem slightly yellow, a condition that worsens noticeably by the next day. Molly calls the *Healthy Start* Home Health nurse and requests a visit to evaluate her newborn.

Go to thePoint to find questions to consider about this case.

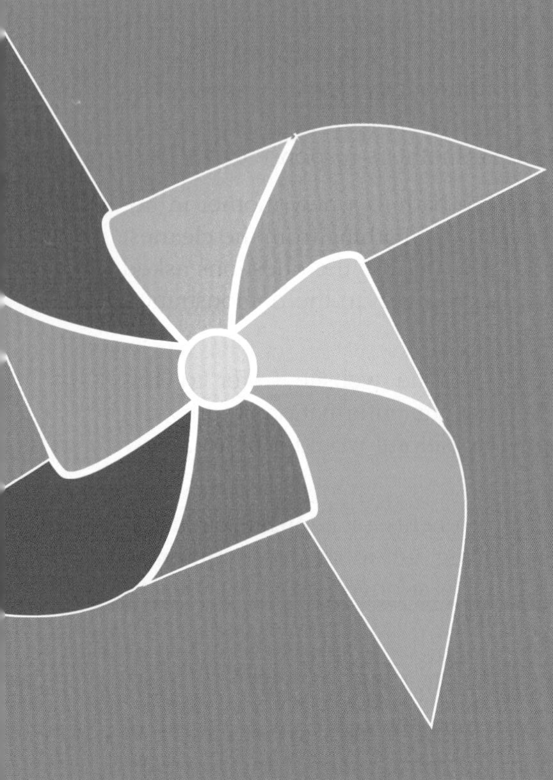

Childbearing at Risk

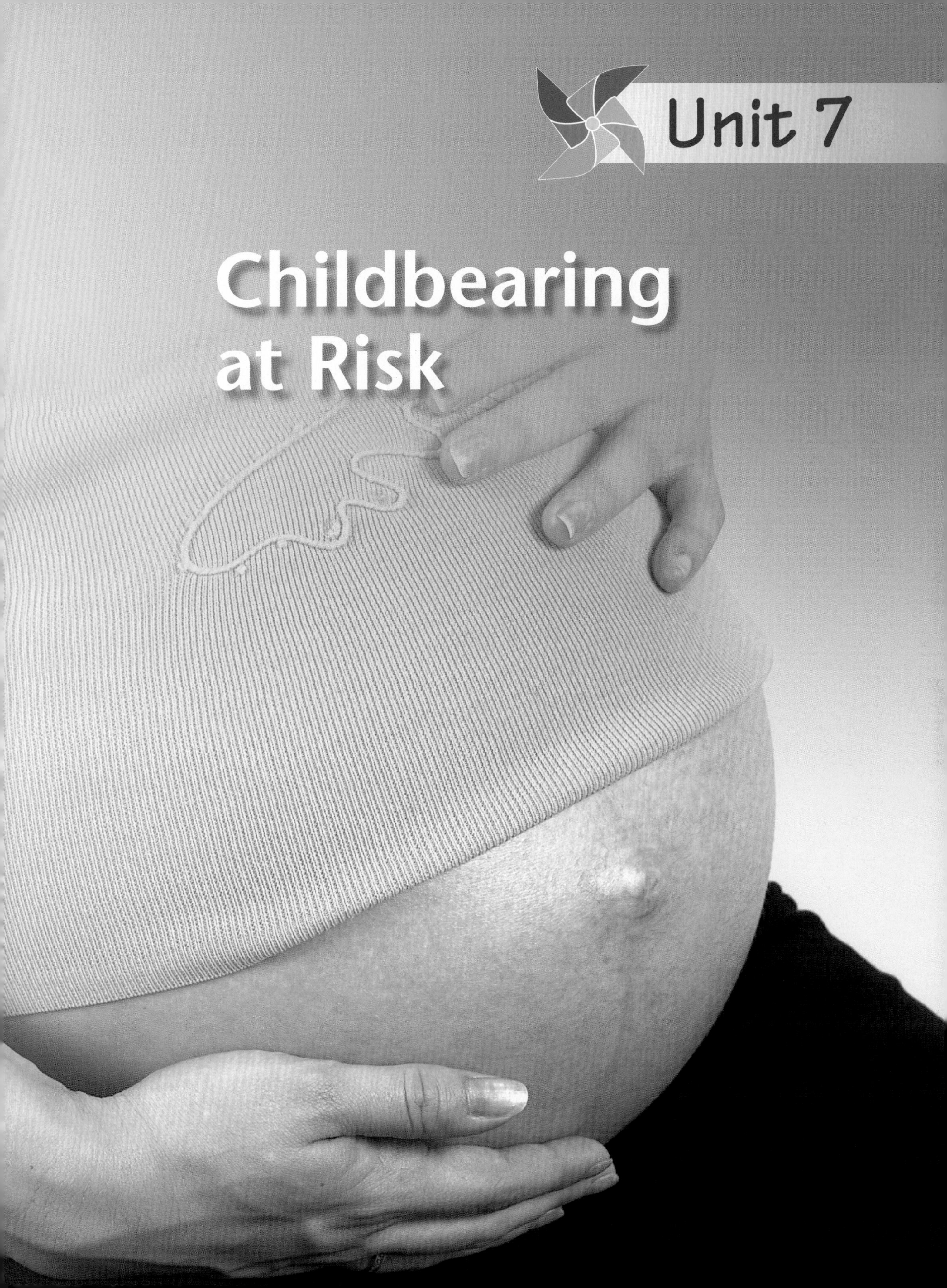

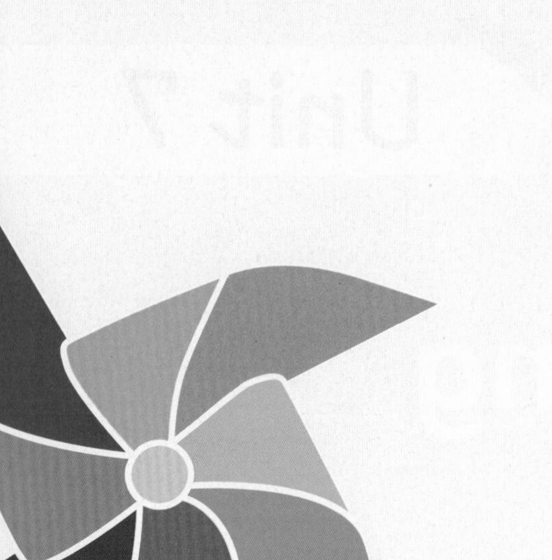

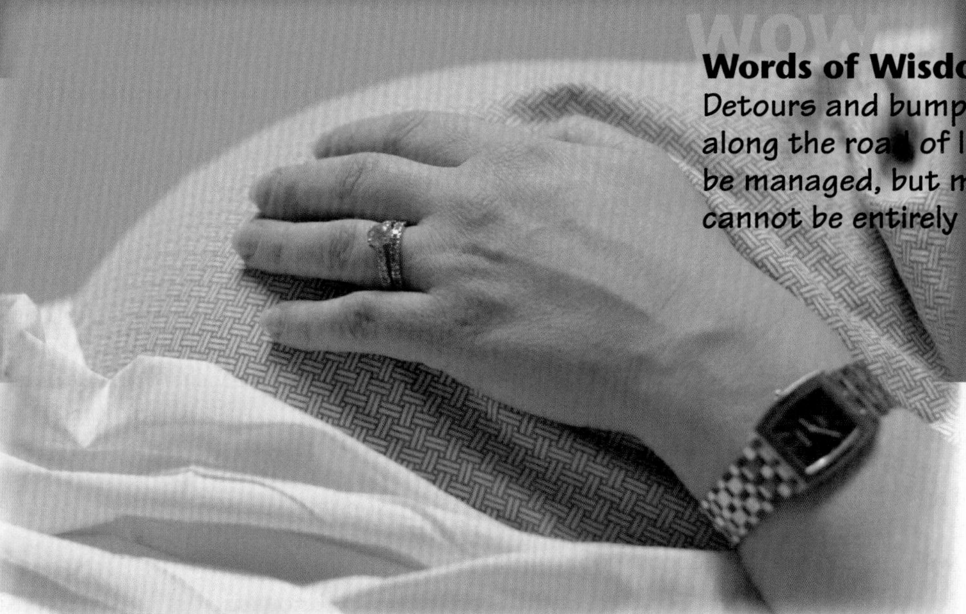
WOW
Words of Wisdom
Detours and bumps along the road of life can be managed, but many cannot be entirely cured.

19

Nursing Management of Pregnancy at Risk: Pregnancy-Related Complications

KEY TERMS

abortion
abruptio placentae
eclampsia
ectopic pregnancy
gestational hypertension
gestational trophoblastic disease (GTD)
high-risk pregnancy
polyhydramnios
hyperemesis gravidarum
multiple gestation
oligohydramnios
placenta accreta
placenta previa
preeclampsia
premature rupture of membranes (PROM)
preterm premature rupture of membranes (PPROM)

Learning Objectives

Upon completion of the chapter, you will be able to:

1. Compare and contrast a normal pregnancy to a high risk one. Determine the common factors that might place a pregnancy at high risk.
2. Detect the causes of vaginal bleeding during early and late pregnancy.
3. Outline nursing assessment and management for the pregnant woman experiencing vaginal bleeding.
4. Develop a plan of care for the woman experiencing preeclampsia, eclampsia, and HELLP syndrome.
5. Examine the pathophysiology of hydramnios and subsequent management.
6. Evaluate factors in a woman's prenatal history that place her at risk for premature rupture of membranes (PROM).
7. Formulate a teaching plan for maintaining the health of pregnant women experiencing a high-risk pregnancy.

***Helen*, a 35-year-old G5 P4, presented to the labor and birth suite with severe abdominal pain. She reports that the pain began suddenly about an hour ago while she was resting. She has had two prior cesarean births and thus far has had an uneventful past 32 weeks. Helen appears distressed and is moaning. What additional assessments do you need to do to care for Helen? What might be your immediate nursing action?**

INTRODUCTION

Most people view pregnancy as a natural process with a positive outcome—the birth of a healthy newborn. Unfortunately, conditions can occur that may result in negative outcomes for the fetus, mother, or both. A **high-risk pregnancy** is one in which a condition exists that jeopardizes the health of the mother, her fetus, or both. The condition may result from the pregnancy, or it may be a condition that was present before the woman became pregnant.

Approximately one in four pregnant women is considered to be at high risk or diagnosed with complications (Nagtalon-Ramos, 2014). Women who are considered to be at high risk have a higher morbidity and mortality compared with mothers in the general population. The risk status of a woman and her fetus can change during the pregnancy, with a number of problems occurring during labor, birth, or afterward, even in women without any known previous antepartal risk. Examples of high-risk conditions include gestational diabetes and **ectopic pregnancy**. Many obstetric complications and conditions are life-threatening emergencies with high morbidity and mortality rates. It is essential that these be identified early to ensure the best possible outcome for the mother and infant. These conditions are specifically addressed in *Healthy People 2020* (U.S. Department of Health and Human Services, 2010). Early identification of the woman at risk is essential to ensure that appropriate interventions are instituted promptly, increasing the opportunity to change the course of events and provide a positive outcome.

The term *risk* may mean different things to different groups. For example, health care providers may focus on the disease processes and treatments to prevent complications. Nurses may focus on nursing care and on the psychosocial impact on the woman and her family. Insurance companies may concentrate on the economic issues related to the high-risk status. The woman's attention may be focused on her own needs and those of her family. Together, working as a collaborative team, the ultimate goal of care is to ensure the best possible outcome for the woman, her fetus, and her family.

Risk assessment begins at the first antepartal visit and continues with each subsequent visit because factors may be identified in later visits that were not apparent during earlier visits. For example, as the nurse and client develop a trusting relationship, previously unidentified or unsuspected factors (such as drug abuse or intimate partner violence) may be revealed. Through education and support, the nurse can encourage the client to inform her health care provider of these concerns, and necessary interventions or referrals can be made.

Various factors must be considered when determining a woman's risk for adverse pregnancy outcomes, and a comprehensive approach to high-risk pregnancy is needed. For example, prenatal stress and distress have been shown to have significant consequences for the mother, child, and family. Pregnancy-specific stress such as depression, anxiety, and perceived stress may increase the risk for adverse birth outcomes and is associated with preterm births (Staneva et al., 2015). Risks are grouped into broad categories based on threats to health and pregnancy outcome. Current categories of risk are biophysical, psychosocial, sociodemographic, and environmental (Cunningham et al., 2014) (Box 19.1).

This chapter describes the major conditions directly related to pregnancy that can complicate a pregnancy, possibly affecting maternal and fetal outcomes. These include bleeding during pregnancy (spontaneous **abortion**, ectopic pregnancy, **gestational trophoblastic disease (GTD)**, cervical insufficiency, **placenta previa**, **abruptio placentae**, and **placenta accreta**), hyperemesis gravidarum, **gestational hypertension**, HELLP syndrome, gestational diabetes, blood incompatibility, amniotic fluid imbalances (**polyhydramnios** and **oligohydramnios**), multiple gestation, and **premature rupture of membranes (PROM)**. Chapter 20 addresses pre-existing conditions that can complicate a woman's pregnancy as well as populations that are considered to be at high risk.

HEALTHY PEOPLE 2020

Objective	Nursing Significance
MICH-6 Reduce maternal illness and complications due to pregnancy (complications during hospitalized labor and delivery).	Will reduce perinatal morbidity and mortality and optimize pregnancy outcomes.
MICH-9 Reduce preterm births.	Will help to preserve the health and well-being of the growing fetus if the pregnancy goes to term.

Healthy People objectives based on data from http://www.healthypeople.gov.

BLEEDING DURING PREGNANCY

Bleeding at any time during pregnancy is potentially life-threatening. Every minute of every day, a woman dies in pregnancy or childbirth. The biggest killer is obstetric hemorrhage, the successful treatment of which is a challenge for both the developed and developing worlds. The presence of an attendant at every birth and access to emergency obstetric care are strategic to reducing maternal morbidity and mortality (World Health Organization [WHO], 2015). Management of obstetric hemorrhage involves early recognition, assessment, and resuscitation.

BOX 19.1

FACTORS PLACING A WOMAN AT RISK DURING PREGNANCY

Biophysical Factors

- Genetic conditions
- Chromosomal abnormalities
- Multiple pregnancy
- Defective genes
- Inherited disorders
- ABO incompatibility
- Large fetal size
- Medical and obstetric conditions
- Preterm labor and birth
- Cardiovascular disease
- Chronic hypertension
- Cervical insufficiency
- Placental abnormalities
- Infection
- Diabetes
- Maternal collagen diseases
- Thyroid disease
- Asthma
- Postterm pregnancy
- Hemoglobinopathies
- Nutritional status
- Inadequate dietary intake
- Food fads
- Excessive food intake
- Under- or overweight status
- Hematocrit value less than 33%
- Eating disorder

Psychosocial Factors

- Smoking
- Caffeine
- Alcohol and substance abuse
- Maternal obesity
- Inadequate support system
- Situational crisis
- History of violence
- Emotional distress
- Unsafe cultural practices

Sociodemographic Factors

- Poverty status
- Lack of prenatal care
- Age younger than 15 years or older than 35 years
- Parity—all first pregnancies and more than five pregnancies
- Marital status—increased risk for unmarried women
- Accessibility to health care
- Ethnicity—increased risk in non-White women

Environmental Factors

- Infections
- Radiation
- Pesticides
- Illicit drugs
- Industrial pollutants
- Second-hand cigarette smoke
- Personal stress

Adapted from Martin, R. J., Fanaroff, A. A., & Walsh, M. C. (2014). *Fanaroff & Martin's neonatal-perinatal medicine* (10th ed.). Philadelphia, PA: Elsevier Health Sciences; Foley, M., Strong, T. M., & Garite, T. (2014). *Obstetric intensive care manual* (4th ed.). New York, NY: McGraw-Hill Publishers; & Cunningham, F. G., Leveno, K. J., Bloom, S. L., Spong, C. Y., Dashe, J. S., Hoffman, B. L., et al. (2014). *Williams' obstetrics* (24th ed.). New York, NY: McGraw-Hill Education.

Various methods are available to try to stop the bleeding, ranging from pharmacologic methods to aid uterine contraction (e.g., oxytocin, ergometrine, and prostaglandins) to surgical methods to stem the bleeding (e.g., balloon tamponade, compression sutures, or arterial ligation). Bleeding can occur early or late in the pregnancy and may result from numerous conditions. Bleeding is experienced by approximately 20% of women during the first trimester of pregnancy (Knez, Day, & Jurkovic, 2014). Conditions commonly associated with early bleeding (first half of pregnancy) include spontaneous abortion, uterine fibroids, ectopic pregnancy, GTD, and cervical insufficiency. Conditions associated with late bleeding include placenta previa, abruptio placentae, and placenta accreta, which usually occur after the 20th week of gestation.

Spontaneous Abortion

Abortion is considered not only a major reproductive health matter, but also a health risk factor for women's well-being. Spontaneous abortion is the most common complication of early pregnancy (Tulandi & Al-Fozan, 2015). An abortion is the loss of an early pregnancy, usually before week 20 of gestation. Abortion can be spontaneous or induced. A spontaneous abortion refers to the loss of a fetus resulting from natural causes, that is, not elective or therapeutically induced by a procedure. A stillbirth is the loss of a fetus after the 20th week of development, whereas a miscarriage refers to a loss before the 20th week. Nonmedical people often use the term *miscarriage* to denote an abortion that has occurred spontaneously. A miscarriage can occur during early pregnancy, and many women who miscarry may not even be aware that they are pregnant. About 80% of spontaneous abortions occur within the first trimester. The terms *stillbirth* and *miscarriage* can sometimes be confusing. Both refer to the loss of an early pregnancy; however, stillbirth occurs later in pregnancy. Some stillbirths can occur right up to the time of labor and delivery. Stillbirths are much less common than miscarriages, occurring in only 1 out of every 160 pregnancies (March of Dimes, 2015a).

The overall rate for spontaneous abortion in the United States is reported to be 15% to 20% of recognized pregnancies in the United States. However, with the development of highly sensitive assays for human chorionic gonadotropin (hCG) levels that detect pregnancies prior to the expected next menses, the incidence of pregnancy loss increases significantly—to about 60% to 70% (King et al., 2015). The frequency of spontaneous abortion increases further with maternal age.

Pathophysiology

The causes of spontaneous abortion are varied and often unknown. The most common cause for first-trimester abortions is fetal genetic abnormalities, usually unrelated to the mother. Chromosomal abnormalities are more likely causes in the first trimester and maternal disease is more likely in the second trimester. Those occurring during the second trimester are more likely related to maternal conditions, such as cervical insufficiency, congenital or acquired anomaly of the uterine cavity (uterine septum or fibroids), hypothyroidism, diabetes mellitus, chronic nephritis, use of crack cocaine, inherited and acquired thrombophilias, lupus, polycystic ovary syndrome, severe hypertension, and acute infection such as rubella virus, cytomegalovirus, herpes simplex virus, bacterial vaginosis, and toxoplasmosis (Jones & Lopez, 2014).

Women experiencing a first-trimester abortion at home without a dilation and curettage (D&C) to resolve it require frequent monitoring of hCG levels to validate that all the conceptus tissues have been expelled. Women going through a second-trimester abortion are admitted to the hospital to have an augmented labor and delivery. Nursing care would focus on care of the laboring women with tremendous attention paid to providing emotional support to the woman and her family.

Nursing Assessment

When a pregnant woman calls and reports vaginal bleeding, she must be seen as soon as possible by a health care professional to ascertain the etiology. Varying degrees of vaginal bleeding, low back pain, abdominal cramping, and passage of products of conception tissue may be reported. Ask the woman about the color of the vaginal bleeding (bright red is significant) and the amount—for example, question her about the frequency with which she is changing her peripads (saturation of one peripad hourly is significant) and the passage of any clots or tissue. Instruct her to save any tissue or clots passed and bring them with her to the health care facility. Also, obtain a description of any other signs and symptoms the woman may be experiencing, along with a description of their severity and duration. It is important to remain calm and listen to the woman's description.

When the woman arrives at the health care facility, assess her vital signs and observe the amount, color, and characteristics of the bleeding. Ask her to rate her current pain level, using an appropriate pain assessment tool. Also, evaluate the amount and intensity of the woman's abdominal cramping or contractions, and assess the woman's level of understanding about what is happening to her. A thorough assessment helps in determining the type of spontaneous abortion, such as threatened abortion, inevitable abortion, incomplete abortion, complete abortion, missed abortion, and habitual abortion, that the woman may be experiencing (Table 19.1).

Nursing Management

Nursing management of the woman with a spontaneous abortion focuses on providing continued monitoring and psychological support, for the family is experiencing acute loss and grief. An important component of this support is reassuring the woman that spontaneous abortions usually result from an abnormality and that her actions did not cause the abortion.

PROVIDING CONTINUED MONITORING

Continued monitoring and ongoing assessments are essential for the woman experiencing a spontaneous abortion. Monitor the amount of vaginal bleeding through pad counts and observe for passage of products of conception tissue. Assess the woman's pain and provide appropriate pain management to address the cramping discomfort.

Assist in preparing the woman for procedures and treatments such as surgery to evacuate the uterus or medications such as misoprostol or PGE2. If the woman is Rh negative and not sensitized, expect to administer RhoGAM within 72 hours after the abortion is complete. Drug Guide 19.1 gives more information about these medications.

PROVIDING SUPPORT

A woman's emotional reaction may vary depending on her desire for this pregnancy and her available support network. Provide both physical and emotional support. In addition, prepare the woman and her family for the assessment process and answer their questions.

Explaining some of the causes of spontaneous abortions can help the woman to understand what is happening and may allay her fears and guilt that she did something to cause the pregnancy loss. Most women experience an acute sense of loss and go through a grieving process with a spontaneous abortion. Providing sensitive listening, counseling, and anticipatory guidance to the woman and her family will allow them to verbalize their feelings and ask questions about future pregnancies.

The grieving period may last as long as 2 years after a pregnancy loss, with each person grieving in his or her own way. Encourage friends and family to be supportive but give the couple space and time to work through their loss. Referral to a community support group for parents who have experienced a miscarriage can be very helpful during this grief process.

TABLE 19.1 CATEGORIES OF ABORTION

Category	Assessment Findings	Diagnosis	Therapeutic Management
Threatened abortion	Vaginal bleeding (often slight) early in a pregnancy No cervical dilation or change in cervical consistency Mild abdominal cramping Closed cervical os No passage of fetal tissue	Vaginal ultrasound to confirm if sac is empty Declining maternal serum hCG and progesterone levels to provide additional information about viability of pregnancy	Conservative supportive treatment Possible reduction in activity in conjunction with nutritious diet and adequate hydration
Inevitable abortion	Vaginal bleeding (greater than that associated with threatened abortion) Rupture of membranes Cervical dilation Strong abdominal cramping Possible passage of products of conception	Ultrasound and hCG levels to indicate pregnancy loss	Vacuum curettage if products of conception are not passed, to reduce risk of excessive bleeding and infection Prostaglandin analogs such as misoprostol to empty uterus of retained tissue (only used if fragments are not completely passed)
Incomplete abortion (passage of some of the products of conception)	Intense abdominal cramping Heavy vaginal bleeding Cervical dilation	Ultrasound confirmation that products of conception still in uterus	Client stabilization Evacuation of uterus via D&C or prostaglandin analog
Complete abortion (passage of all products of conception)	History of vaginal bleeding and abdominal pain Passage of tissue with subsequent decrease in pain and significant decrease in vaginal bleeding	Ultrasound demonstrating an empty uterus	No medical or surgical intervention necessary Follow-up appointment to discuss family planning
Missed abortion (nonviable embryo retained in utero for at least 6 wks)	Absent uterine contractions Irregular spotting Possible progression to inevitable abortion	Ultrasound to identify products of conception in uterus	Evacuation of uterus (if inevitable abortion does not occur): suction curettage during first trimester, dilation and evacuation during second trimester Induction of labor with intravaginal PGE2 suppository to empty uterus without surgical intervention
Habitual abortion	History of three or more consecutive spontaneous abortions Not carrying the pregnancy to viability or term	Validation via client's history	Identification and treatment of underlying cause (possible causes such as genetic or chromosomal abnormalities, reproductive tract abnormalities, chronic diseases, or immunologic problems) Cervical cerclage in second trimester if incompetent cervix is the cause

Ectopic Pregnancy

An ectopic pregnancy is any pregnancy in which the fertilized ovum implants outside the uterine cavity. The term *ectopic* is derived from the Greek word *ektopos,* meaning "out of place," and refers to the implantation of a fertilized egg in a location outside of the uterine cavity, including the fallopian tubes, cervix, ovary, and the abdominal cavity. This abnormally implanted embryo grows and draws its blood supply from the site of abnormal implantation. As the embryo enlarges, it creates

DRUG GUIDE 19.1 MEDICATIONS RELATED TO ABORTIONS

Medication	Action/Indications	Nursing Implications
Misoprostol (Cytotec)	Stimulates uterine contractions to terminate a pregnancy; to evacuate the uterus after abortion to ensure passage of all the products of conception	• Monitor for side effects such as diarrhea, abdominal pain, nausea, vomiting, dyspepsia. • Assess vaginal bleeding and report any increased bleeding, pain, or fever. • Monitor for signs and symptoms of shock, such as tachycardia, hypotension, and anxiety.
Mifepristone (RU-486)	Acts as progesterone antagonist, allowing prostaglandins to stimulate uterine contractions; causes the endometrium to slough; may be followed by administration of misoprostol within 48 hrs	• Monitor for headache, vomiting, diarrhea, and heavy bleeding. • Anticipate administration of antiemetic prior to use to reduce nausea and vomiting. • Encourage client to use acetaminophen to reduce discomfort from cramping.
PGE2, dinoprostone (Cervidil, Prepidil Gel, Prostin E2)	Stimulates uterine contractions, causing expulsion of uterine contents; to expel uterine contents in fetal death or missed abortion during second trimester, or to efface and dilate the cervix in pregnancy at term	• Bring gel to room temperature before administering. • Avoid contact with skin. • Use sterile technique to administer. • Keep client supine for 30 min after administering. • Document time of insertion and dosing intervals. • Remove insert with retrieval system after 12 hrs or at the onset of labor. • Explain purpose and expected response to client.
Rh(D) immunoglobulin (Gamulin, HydroRho-D, RhoGAM, MICRhoGAM)	Suppresses immune response of nonsensitized Rh-negative clients who are exposed to Rh-positive blood; to prevent isoimmunization in Rh-negative women exposed to Rh-positive blood after abortions, miscarriages, and pregnancies	• Administer intramuscularly in deltoid area. • Give only MICRhoGAM for abortions and miscarriages <12 wks unless fetus or father is Rh negative (unless client is Rh positive, Rh antibodies are present). • Educate woman that she will need this after subsequent deliveries if newborns are Rh positive; also check lab study results prior to administering the drug.

Adapted from King, T. L., Brucker, M. C., Kriebs, J. M., Fahey, J. O., Grgor, C. L., & Varney, H. (2015). *Varney's midwifery* (5th ed.). Burlington, MA: Jones & Bartlett Learning; and Skidmore-Roth, L. (2015). *Mosby's 2015 nursing drug reference* (28th ed.). Philadelphia, PA: Elsevier.

the potential for organ rupture because only the uterine cavity is designed to expand and accommodate fetal development. Ectopic pregnancy can lead to massive hemorrhage, infertility, or death.

Ectopic pregnancies occur in 1 in every 50 pregnancies in the United States or roughly 2% of all pregnancies are diagnosed as ectopic; this rate has increased dramatically during the past 30 years (March of Dimes, 2015b). It is a major health concern for women of reproductive age and is the primary cause of death during the first trimester of pregnancy in the United States (Szypulski, 2015). The discovery of ectopic pregnancies prior to rupture has increased dramatically in the past few decades as a result of improved diagnostic techniques such as the development of sensitive and specific radioimmunoassays for hCG, high-resolution ultrasonography, and the widespread availability of laparoscopy (Desai et al., 2014).

With an ectopic pregnancy, rupture and hemorrhage may occur due to the growth of the embryo. A ruptured ectopic pregnancy is a medical emergency; therefore, prediction of any tubal rupture before its occurrence is extremely important. It is a potentially life-threatening condition and involves pregnancy loss. Even in the United States, women can and do still die from ectopic pregnancy, although early diagnosis has helped prevent that.

Pathophysiology

Normally, the fertilized ovum implants in the uterus. In ectopic pregnancy the journey along the fallopian tube is arrested or altered in some way. With an ectopic pregnancy, the ovum implants outside the uterus. The most common site for implantation is the fallopian tubes, but some ova may implant in the ovary, the intestine, the

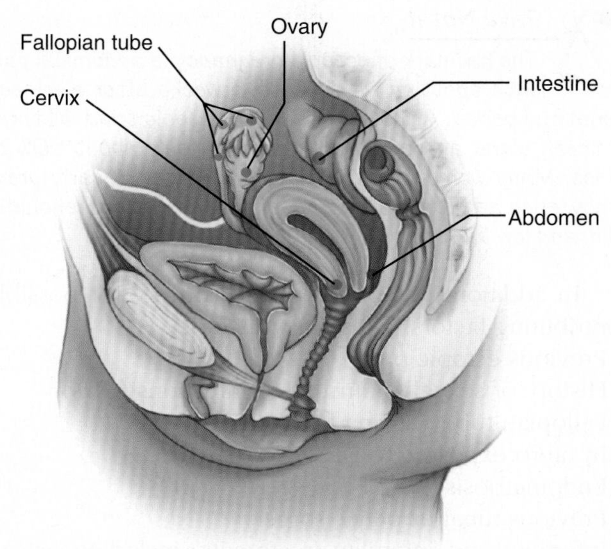

FIGURE 19.1 Possible sites for implantation with an ectopic pregnancy.

cervix, or the abdominal cavity (Fig. 19.1) (Sepilian & Wood, 2015). None of these anatomic sites can accommodate placental attachment or a growing embryo.

Risk Factors

Ectopic pregnancies usually result from conditions that obstruct or slow the passage of the fertilized ovum through the fallopian tube to the uterus. This may be a physical blockage in the tube, or failure of the tubal epithelium to move the zygote (the cell formed after the egg is fertilized) down the tube into the uterus. In the general population, most cases are the result of tubal scarring secondary to pelvic inflammatory disease (PID). Organisms such as *Neisseria gonorrhea* and *Chlamydia trachomatis* preferentially attack the fallopian tubes, producing silent infections. A recent study reported a two-fold increased risk for ectopic pregnancy in women with a history of a chlamydia infection, secondary to tubal damage (Randall & LaMontagne, 2015). Other associated risk factors for ectopic pregnancy include previous tubal surgery, infertility, PID, previous pregnancy loss (induced or spontaneous), use of an intrauterine contraceptive system, previous ectopic pregnancy, uterine fibroids, sterilization, smoking (which alters tubal motility), history of multiple sexual partners, use of progestin-only oral contraceptives, douching, and exposure to diethylstilbestrol (DES) (Ardehali & Casikar, 2015).

Therapeutic Management

The diagnosis of ectopic pregnancy can be challenging because many women are asymptomatic before tubal rupture. The classic clinical triad of ectopic pregnancy includes abdominal pain, amenorrhea, and vaginal bleeding. Unfortunately, only about half of women present with all three symptoms.

Diagnostic procedures used for a suspected ectopic pregnancy include a urine pregnancy test to confirm the pregnancy, beta-hCG concentrations to exclude a false-negative urine test, and a transvaginal ultrasound to visualize the misplaced pregnancy (Bourne, 2015).

Historically, the treatment of ectopic pregnancy was limited to surgery. The therapeutic management of ectopic pregnancy depends on whether the tube is intact or has ruptured, creating a medical emergency. In the event of a surgical intervention, preservation of the affected fallopian tube is attempted (King et al., 2015).

MEDICAL INTERVENTION

With early diagnosis, most women with ectopic pregnancy could be treated with methotrexate. The overall success rate of medical treatment in properly selected women is nearly 90% To be eligible for medical therapy, the client must be hemodynamically stable, with no signs of active bleeding in the peritoneal cavity, low beta-hCG levels (<5,000 mIU/mL) and the mass (which must measure less than 4 cm as determined by ultrasound) must be unruptured. Contraindications to medical treatment include an unstable client, severe persistent abdominal pain, renal or liver disease, immunodeficiency, active pulmonary disease, peptic ulcer, suspected intrauterine pregnancy, and poor client compliance (Tulandi, 2015). The potential advantages include avoidance of surgery, the preservation of tubal patency and function, and a lower cost.

The medical approach today for an unruptured tubal pregnancy most often consists of a single-dose IM injection of methotrexate (Rheumatrex; Trexall) with outpatient follow-up. Medical management with methotrexate, though not approved by the Food and Drug Administration for this purpose, has been endorsed by the American College of Obstetricians and Gynecologists. Prostaglandins, misoprostol, and actinomycin have also been used in the medical (nonsurgical) management of ectopic pregnancy, with a reported success rate of approximately 90%. Methotrexate is a folic acid antagonist that inhibits cell division in the developing embryo. It typically has been used as a chemotherapeutic agent in the treatment of leukemia, lymphomas, and carcinomas. It has been shown to produce results similar to that for surgical therapy in terms of high success rate, low complication rate, and good reproductive potential (Dalia et al., 2015). Adverse effects associated with methotrexate include nausea, vomiting, stomatitis, diarrhea, gastric upset, increased abdominal pain, and dizziness. Methotrexate for an ectopic pregnancy is ordered based on the client's body surface area. The administration of methotrexate should be limited to people who have had education and training in the handling and administration of hazardous drugs. In some facilities internal policies require that only nurses who have completed a chemotherapy certification and/or hazardous drug competency program can administer this product (Cohen et al., 2015).

Prior to receiving the single-dose intramuscular injection to treat unruptured pregnancies, the woman needs to be counseled on the risks, benefits, adverse effects, and the possibility of failure of medical therapy, which would result in tubal rupture, necessitating surgery (Tulandi, 2015). The woman is then instructed to return weekly for follow-up laboratory studies for the next several weeks until beta-hCG titers decrease. Beta-hCG level changes between days 0 and 4 after methotrexate therapy have clinical significance and predictive value. A decreasing beta-hCG level is highly predictive of treatment success (Agarwal & Odejinmi, 2014).

SURGICAL INTERVENTION

Surgical management for the unruptured fallopian tube might involve a linear salpingostomy to preserve the tube—an important consideration for the woman wanting to preserve her future fertility. It may also be considered when medical treatment is considered unsuitable.

With a ruptured ectopic pregnancy, surgery is necessary as a result of possible uncontrolled hemorrhage. A laparotomy with a removal of the tube (salpingectomy) may be necessary. With earlier diagnosis and medical management, the focus has changed from preventing maternal death to facilitating rapid recovery and preserving fertility.

Regardless of the treatment approach (medical or surgical), the woman's beta-hCG level is monitored until it is undetectable to ensure that any residual trophoblastic tissue that forms the placenta is gone. Also, all Rh-negative unsensitized clients are given Rh immunoglobulin to prevent isoimmunization in future pregnancies.

Nursing Assessment

Nursing assessment focuses on determining the existence of an ectopic pregnancy and whether or not it has ruptured. A woman with a suspected ectopic pregnancy may have to undergo several diagnostic tests, some of which are invasive. Consider how she might feel during all of these tests, anticipate her questions, and offer her thorough explanations and reassurances.

HEALTH HISTORY AND PHYSICAL EXAMINATION

Assess the client thoroughly for signs and symptoms that may suggest an ectopic pregnancy. The onset of signs and symptoms varies, but they usually begin at about the seventh or eighth week of gestation. A missed menstrual period, adnexal fullness, and tenderness may indicate an unruptured tubal pregnancy. As the tube stretches, the pain increases. Pain may be unilateral, bilateral, or diffuse over the abdomen.

Take Note!

The hallmark of ectopic pregnancy is abdominal pain with spotting within 6 to 8 weeks after a missed menstrual period. Although this is the classic triad, all three of these signs and symptoms occur in only about 50% of cases. Many women have symptoms typical of early pregnancy, such as breast tenderness, nausea, fatigue, shoulder pain, and low back pain.

In addition, review the client's history for possible contributing factors. These may include:

- Previous ectopic pregnancy
- History of sexually transmitted infections (STIs)
- Fallopian tube scarring from PID
- In utero exposure to DES
- Endometriosis
- Previous tubal or pelvic surgery
- Infertility and infertility treatments, including use of fertility drugs
- Uterine abnormalities such as fibroids
- Presence of intrauterine contraception
- Use of progestin-only mini-pill (slows ovum transport)
- Postpartum or postabortion infection
- Altered estrogen and progesterone levels (interferes with tubal motility)
- Increasing age (older than 35 years)
- Cigarette smoking (Ardehali & Casikar, 2015).

If rupture or hemorrhage occurs before treatment begins, symptoms may worsen and include severe, sharp, and sudden pain in the lower abdomen as the tube tears open and the embryo is expelled into the pelvic cavity; feelings of faintness; referred pain to the shoulder area, indicating bleeding into the abdomen, caused by phrenic nerve irritation; hypotension; marked abdominal tenderness with distention; and hypovolemic shock (Cunningham et al., 2014).

LABORATORY AND DIAGNOSTIC TESTING

The use of transvaginal ultrasound to visualize the misplaced pregnancy and low levels of serum beta-hCG assist in diagnosing an ectopic pregnancy. The ultrasound determines whether the pregnancy is intrauterine, assesses the size of the uterus, and provides evidence of fetal viability. The visualization of an adnexal mass and the absence of an intrauterine gestational sac are diagnostic of ectopic pregnancy (Kao et al., 2014). In a normal intrauterine pregnancy, beta-hCG levels typically double every 2 to 4 days until peak values are reached 60 to 90 days after conception. Concentrations of hCG decrease after 10 to 11 weeks and reach a plateau at low levels by 100 to 130 days (Ko & Cheung, 2014). Therefore, low beta-hCG levels are suggestive of an ectopic pregnancy or impending abortion. Additional tests may be done to rule out other conditions such as spontaneous abortion, ruptured ovarian cyst, appendicitis, and salpingitis.

Nursing Management

Nursing management for the woman with an ectopic pregnancy focuses on preparing the woman for treatment, providing support, and providing education about preventive measures.

PREPARING THE WOMAN FOR TREATMENT

Administer analgesics as ordered to promote comfort and relieve discomfort from abdominal pain. Although the intensity of the pain can vary, women often report a great deal of pain. If the woman is treated medically, explain the medication that will be used and what she can expect. Also review signs and symptoms of possible adverse effects. If treatment will occur on an outpatient basis, outline the signs and symptoms of ectopic rupture (severe, sharp, stabbing, unilateral abdominal pain; vertigo/fainting; hypotension; and increased pulse) and advise the woman to seek medical help immediately if they occur.

If surgery is needed, close assessment and monitoring of the client's vital signs, bleeding (peritoneal or vaginal), and pain status are critical to identify hypovolemic shock, which may occur with tubal rupture. Prepare the client physiologically and psychologically for surgery or any procedure. Provide a clear explanation of the expected outcome. Astute vigilance and early referral will help reduce short- and long-term morbidity.

PROVIDING EMOTIONAL SUPPORT

The woman with an ectopic pregnancy requires support throughout diagnosis, treatment, and aftercare. A woman's psychological reaction to an ectopic pregnancy is unpredictable. However, it is important to recognize she has experienced a pregnancy loss in addition to undergoing treatment for a potentially life-threatening condition. The woman may find it difficult to comprehend what has happened to her because events occur so quickly. In the woman's mind, she had just started a pregnancy and now it has ended abruptly. Bleeding during any pregnancy is traumatic because of the uncertainty of the outcome. Help her to make this experience more "real" by encouraging her and her family to express their feelings and concerns openly, and by validating that this is a loss of pregnancy and that it is okay to grieve over the loss. Although the woman may have physically recovered following an ectopic pregnancy, she may still experience significant emotional distress for a long time.

Provide emotional support, spiritual care, and information about community support groups (such as *Resolve through Sharing*) as the client grieves for the loss of her unborn child and comes to terms with the medical complications of the situation. Acknowledge the client's pregnancy and allow her to discuss her feelings about what the pregnancy means. Also, stress the need for follow-up blood testing for several weeks to monitor hCG titers until they return to zero, indicating resolution of the ectopic pregnancy. Ask about her feelings and concerns about her future fertility, and provide teaching about the need to use contraceptives for at least three menstrual cycles to allow her reproductive tract to heal and the tissue to be repaired. Include the woman's partner in this discussion to make sure both parties understand what has happened, what intervention is needed, and what the future holds regarding childbearing.

EDUCATING THE CLIENT

Preventing ectopic pregnancies through screening and client education is essential. Many can be prevented by avoiding conditions that might cause scarring of the fallopian tubes. In addition, a contributing factor to the development of ectopic pregnancy is a previous ectopic pregnancy. Therefore, educating the woman is crucial. Prevention education may include the following:

- Reduce risk factors such as sexual intercourse with multiple partners or intercourse without a condom.
- Avoid contracting STIs that lead to PID.
- Obtain early diagnosis and adequate treatment of STIs.
- If an intrauterine contraceptive system is chosen, descriptions of the signs of PID should be included to reduce the risk of repeat ascending infections, which can be responsible for tubal scarring.
- Avoid smoking during childbearing years since a correlation and increase in risk exists.
- Use condoms to decrease the risk of infections that cause tubal scarring.
- Seek prenatal care early to confirm the location of pregnancy.

Gestational Trophoblastic Disease

GTD comprises a spectrum of neoplastic disorders that originate in the placenta. There is abnormal hyperproliferation of trophoblastic cells that normally would develop into the placenta during pregnancy. GTDs encompass hydatidiform mole (complete and partial), invasive mole, gestational choriocarcinoma, placental-site trophoblastic tumor, and epithelioid trophoblastic tumor (Nguyen & Slim, 2014). Gestational tissue is present, but the pregnancy is not viable. The incidence is hard to determine due to uncommon diagnosis and inaccuracy of documentation of pregnancy loss, but it is thought to occur in about 1 in 1,000 pregnancies in the United States; in Asian countries, the rate is 1 of every 120 pregnancies (American Cancer Society [ACS], 2015). The two most common types of GTD are hydatidiform mole (partial or complete) and choriocarcinoma.

Pathophysiology

The pathogenesis is unique because the maternal tumor arises from gestational rather than maternal tissue. Hydatidiform mole is a benign neoplasm of the chorion in

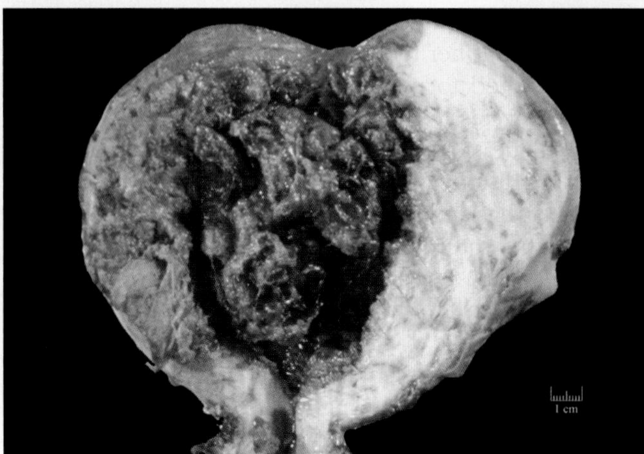

FIGURE 19.2 Complete hydatidiform mole as seen in a cutaway of a uterus. The chorionic villi degenerate and become filled with a viscid fluid, forming transparent vesicles. (From Reichert. (2011). *Diagnostic Gynecologic and Obstetric Pathology*, Courtesy of Dr. Enrique Higa. Philadelphia: LWW.)

which the chorionic villi degenerate and become transparent vesicles containing clear, viscid fluid. Hydatidiform mole is classified as complete or partial, distinguished by differences in clinical presentation, pathology, genetics, and epidemiology (Strohl & Lurain, 2014). The complete mole contains no fetal tissue and develops from an "empty egg," which is fertilized by a normal sperm (the paternal chromosomes replicate, resulting in 46 all-paternal chromosomes) (Fig. 19.2). The embryo is not viable and dies. No circulation is established, and no embryonic tissue is found. The complete mole is associated with the development of choriocarcinoma. Surgery can totally remove most complete moles, but as many as one in five women will have some persistent molar tissue and require further treatment (ACS, 2015). Most women with a classic complete mole present with vaginal bleeding, anemia, excessively enlarged uterus, **preeclampsia**, and hyperemesis.

The partial mole has a triploid karyotype (69 chromosomes), because two sperm have provided a double contribution by fertilizing the ovum. Women with a partial mole usually present with the clinical features of a missed or incomplete abortion, including vaginal bleeding and a small or normal size for date uterus (Dickson & Mullany, 2015).

The exact cause of molar pregnancy is unknown, but researchers are looking into a genetic basis. Other theories include an ovular defect, stress, or a nutritional deficiency (carotene). Although the etiology remains uncertain, at some point in the pregnancy trophoblastic cells that normally would form the placenta proliferate and the chorionic villi become edematous. The latter changes become the grape-like clusters that characterize the molar pregnancy (King et al., 2015). Studies have revealed some remarkable features about molar pregnancies, including:

- Ability to invade into the wall of the uterus
- Tendency to recur in subsequent pregnancies
- Possible development into choriocarcinoma, a virulent cancer with metastasis to other organs
- Influence of nutritional factors, such as protein deficiency
- Tendency to affect older women more often than younger women

Having a molar pregnancy (partial or complete) results in the loss of the pregnancy and the possibility of developing choriocarcinoma, a chorionic malignancy from the trophoblastic tissue. Typically asymptomatic, the first symptoms of choriocarcinoma in 80% of cases are shortness of breath, indicative of metastasis to the lungs. Choriocarcinoma affects women of all ages and can occur during pregnancy, after childbirth, or even years remote from the antecedent pregnancy. The most frequent sites of metastases are the lungs, lower genital tract, brain, and liver. Choriocarcinoma is highly responsive to chemotherapy, with an overall remission rate greater than 90% (Hensley & Shviraga, 2014). Partial moles rarely transform into choriocarcinoma.

Therapeutic Management

Treatment consists of immediate evacuation of the uterine contents as soon as the diagnosis is made and long-term follow-up of the client to detect any remaining trophoblastic tissue that might become malignant. D&C is used to empty the uterus. The tissue obtained is sent to the laboratory for analysis to evaluate for choriocarcinoma. Serial levels of hCG are used to detect residual trophoblastic tissue for 1 year. If any tissue remains, hCG levels will not regress. In 80% of women with a benign hydatidiform mole, serum hCG titers steadily drop to normal within 8 to 12 weeks after evacuation of the molar pregnancy. In the other 20% of women with a malignant hydatidiform mole, serum hCG levels begin to rise (Berkowitz, Goldstein, & Horowitz, 2014).

As a result of the increased risk for cancer, the client is advised to receive extensive follow-up therapy for the next 12 months. The follow-up protocol may include:

- Baseline hCG level, chest x-ray, and pelvic ultrasound
- Quantitative hCG levels every week until undetectable for 3 consecutive weeks; then serial hCG levels monthly for 1 year
- Chest x-ray every 6 months to detect pulmonary metastasis
- Regular pelvic examinations to assess uterine and ovarian regression
- Systemic assessments for symptoms indicative of lung, brain, liver, or vaginal metastasis
- Strong recommendation to avoid pregnancy for 1 year because the pregnancy can interfere with the monitoring of hCG levels

- Use of a reliable contraceptive for at least 1 year (Cunningham et al., 2014)

Nursing Assessment

The nurse plays a crucial role in identifying and bringing this condition to the attention of the health care provider based on sound knowledge of the typical clinical manifestations and through astute antepartal assessments.

Clinical manifestations of GTD are very similar to those of spontaneous abortion at about 12 weeks of pregnancy. Assess the woman for potential clinical manifestations at each antepartal visit. Be alert for the following:

- Report of early signs of pregnancy, such as amenorrhea, breast tenderness, fatigue
- Brownish vaginal bleeding/spotting
- Anemia
- Inability to detect a fetal heart rate after 10 to 12 weeks' gestation
- Fetal parts not evident with palpation
- Bilateral ovarian enlargement caused by cysts and elevated levels of hCG
- Persistent, often severe, nausea and vomiting (due to high hCG levels)
- Fluid retention and swelling
- Uterine size larger than expected for pregnancy dates
- Extremely high hCG levels present; no single value considered diagnostic
- Early development of preeclampsia (usually not present until after 24 weeks)
- Absence of fetal heart rate or fetal activity
- Expulsion of grape-like vesicles (possible in some women)

The diagnosis is made by very high hCG levels and the characteristic appearance of the vesicular molar pattern in the uterus via transvaginal ultrasound.

Nursing Management

Nursing management of the woman with GTD focuses on preparing her for a D&C, providing emotional support to deal with the loss and potential risks, and educating her about the risk that cancer may develop after a molar pregnancy and the strict adherence needed with the follow-up program. The woman must understand the need for the continued follow-up care regimen to improve her chances of future pregnancies and to ensure her continued quality of life.

PREPARING THE CLIENT

Upon diagnosis, the client will need an immediate evacuation of the uterus. Perform preoperative care, preparing the client physically and psychologically for the procedure.

PROVIDING EMOTIONAL SUPPORT

To aid the client and her family in coping with the loss of the pregnancy and the possibility of a cancer diagnosis, use the following interventions:

- Listen to their concerns and fears.
- Allow them time to grieve for the pregnancy loss.
- Acknowledge their loss and sad feelings (say you are sorry for their loss).
- Encourage them to express their grief; allow them to cry.
- Provide them with as much factual information as possible to help them make sense of what is happening.
- Enlist support from additional family and friends as appropriate and with the client's permission.

EDUCATING THE CLIENT

After GTD is diagnosed, teach the client about the condition and appropriate interventions that may be necessary to save her life. Explain each phase of treatment accurately and provide support for the woman and her family as they go through the grieving process.

As with any facet of health care, be aware of the latest research and new therapies. Inform the client about her follow-up care, which will probably involve close clinical

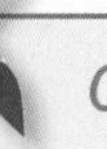

Consider This

We had lived across the dorm hall from each other during nursing school but really didn't get to know each other except for a casual hello in passing. When we graduated, Rose went to work in the emergency room and I worked in OB. We saw each other occasionally in the employee cafeteria, but a quick hello was all that we usually exchanged. I heard she married one of the paramedics who worked in the ER and was soon pregnant. I finally got to say more than hello when she was admitted to the OB unit bleeding during her fourth month of pregnancy. Gestational trophoblastic disease was discovered instead of a normal pregnancy. I remember holding her in my arms as she wept. She was told she had a complete molar pregnancy after surgery, and she would need extensive follow-up for the next year. I lost track of her that summer as my life became busier. Around Thanksgiving time, I heard she had died from choriocarcinoma. I attended her funeral, finally, to get the time to say a final hello and good-bye, but this time with sadness and tears.

Thoughts: Rose was only 26 years old when she succumbed to this very virulent cancer. I think back and realize I missed knowing this brave young woman and wished that I had taken the time to say more than hello. Could her outcome have been different? Why wasn't it recognized earlier? Did she not follow up after her diagnosis? I can only speculate regarding the whom, what, and where. She lived a short but purposeful life, and hopefully continued research will change other women's outcomes in the future.

surveillance for approximately 1 year, and reinforce its importance in monitoring the client's condition. Tell the client that serial serum beta-hCG levels are used to detect residual trophoblastic tissue. Continued high or increasing hCG titers are abnormal and need further evaluation.

Inform the client about the possible use of chemotherapy, such as methotrexate, which may be started prophylactically. Strongly urge the client to use a reliable contraceptive to prevent pregnancy for 1 year, because a pregnancy would interfere with tracking the serial beta-hCG levels used to identify a potential malignancy. Stress the need for the client to cooperate and adhere to the plan of therapy throughout this yearlong follow-up period.

Cervical Insufficiency

Cervical insufficiency, also called premature dilation of the cervix, describes a weak, structurally defective cervix that spontaneously dilates in the absence of uterine contractions in the second trimester, or early third trimester, resulting in the loss of the pregnancy. Since this typically occurs in the fourth or fifth month of gestation before the point of fetal viability, the fetus dies unless the dilation can be arrested. The incidence of cervical insufficiency is less than 1% in the obstetrical population (Agency for Healthcare Research and Quality [AHRQ], 2015).

Pathophysiology

The exact mechanism contributing to cervical insufficiency is not known. The cervix may have less elastin, less collagen, and greater amounts of smooth muscle than the normal cervix, and thus results in loss of sphincter tone (Magowan, Owen, & Thomson, 2014). Several theories have been proposed that focus on damage to the cervix as a key component of hormonal factors, such as increased amounts of relaxin. When the pressure of the expanding uterine contents becomes greater than the ability of the cervical sphincter to remain closed, the cervix suddenly relaxes, allowing effacement and dilation to proceed. The cervical dilation is typically rapid, relatively painless, and accompanied by minimal bleeding (Norwitz & Conroy, 2015).

Cervical insufficiency is likely to be the clinical end point of many pathologic processes, such as congenital cervical hypoplasia, in utero DES exposure that caused cervical hypoplasia, or trauma to the cervix (conization, amputation, obstetric laceration, or forced cervical dilation [may occur during elective pregnancy termination]). Other conditions such as previous precipitous birth, a prolonged second stage of labor, increased amounts of relaxin and progesterone, or increased uterine volume (multiple gestation, hydramnios) are associated with cervical insufficiency (Berghella, 2014). However, the exact etiology of cervical insufficiency is not known.

Cervical length also has been associated with cervical insufficiency and, subsequently, preterm birth. Recent studies have examined the association between a short cervical length and the risk of preterm birth. Some have demonstrated a continuum of risk between a shorter cervix on ultrasound and a higher risk of preterm birth, leading to the hypothetical argument that women with a short cervix on ultrasound might benefit from cervical cerclage (the sewing closed of the cervix). The American Congress of Obstetricians and Gynecologists (ACOG) does not recommend cerclage placement for women with a short cervix who do not have a history of preterm birth, as it has not been shown to be beneficial in this population (2014a).

Therapeutic Management

Cervical insufficiency may be treated in a variety of ways: bed rest; pelvic rest; avoidance of heavy lifting; progesterone supplementation in women at risk for preterm birth; placement of a cervical pessary (a round, silicone device at the mouth of the cervix) or surgically, via a cervical cerclage procedure in the second trimester. Cerclage was devised more than 50 years ago based on the hypothesis that for some women, weakness or malfunction of the cervix has a causative role in the pathway to preterm birth. It can either be performed transvaginally or transabdominally. Cervical cerclage involves using a heavy purse-string suture to secure and reinforce the internal os of the cervix (Fig. 19.3).

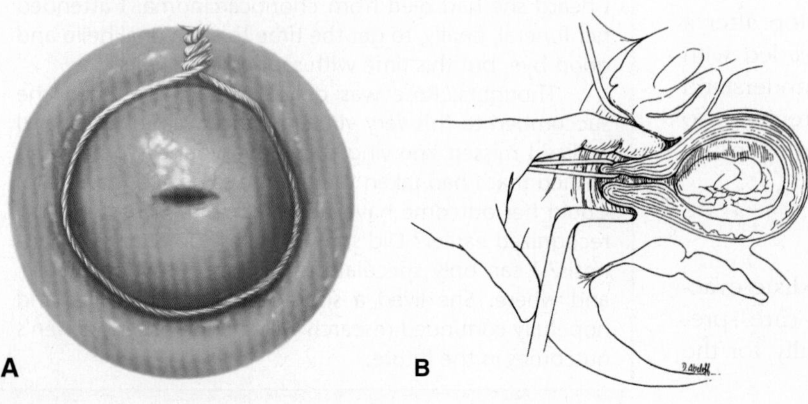

FIGURE 19.3 **A.** Cervical cerclage. **B.** Suturing the cervix for cervical insufficiency.

According to the American College of Obstetricians and Gynecologists (ACOG) (2014a), if a short cervix is identified at or after 20 weeks and no infection (chorioamnionitis) is present, the decision to proceed with cerclage should be made with caution. ACOG recommends the following indications for cervical cerclage: history of second-trimester pregnancy loss with painless dilatation; prior cerclage placement for cervical insufficiency; history of spontaneous preterm birth prior to 34 weeks' gestation; and painless cervical dilatation on physical examination in the second trimester (2014a). Complications associated with cerclage placement are suture displacement, rupture of membranes, and chorioamnionitis, and their incidence varies widely in relation to the timing and indications for the cerclage (Abu Hashim, Al-Inany, & Kilani, 2014). The optimal timing for cerclage removal is unclear, but ACOG (2014a) supports cerclage placement up to 28 weeks' gestation. A recent meta-analysis of randomized controlled trials concluded that either vaginal progesterone or cerclage are equally efficacious in the prevention of preterm birth in women with a short cervix in the mid trimester, singleton gestation, and previous preterm birth (Jena et al., 2015).

Nursing Assessment

RISK FACTORS

Nursing assessment focuses on obtaining a thorough history to determine any risk factors that might have a bearing on this pregnancy: previous cervical trauma, preterm labor, fetal loss in the second trimester, or previous surgeries or procedures involving the cervix. History may reveal a previous loss of pregnancy around 20 weeks.

Also be alert for complaints of vaginal discharge or pelvic pressure. Commonly with cervical insufficiency the woman will report a pink-tinged vaginal discharge or an increase in low pelvic pressure, cramping to vaginal bleeding, and loss of amniotic fluid. Cervical dilation also occurs. If this continues, rupture of the membranes, release of amniotic fluid, and uterine contractions occur, subsequently resulting in delivery of the fetus, often before it is viable.

Take Note!

The diagnosis of cervical insufficiency remains difficult in many circumstances. The cornerstone of diagnosis is a history of a pregnancy loss during the second or early third trimester associated with painless cervical dilation without evidence of uterine activity.

DIAGNOSTIC TESTS

Transvaginal Ultrasound. Transvaginal ultrasound typically is done between 16 and 24 weeks' gestation to determine cervical length, evaluate for shortening, and attempt to predict an early preterm birth. Cervical shortening occurs from the internal os outward and can be viewed on ultrasound as funneling. The amount of funneling can be determined by dividing funnel length by cervical length. The most common time at which a short cervix or funneling develops is 16 to 24 weeks, so ultrasound screening should be performed during this interval (Herrera & Lewis, 2014). A cervical length of less than 25 mm is abnormal between 16 and 24 weeks and may increase the risk of preterm labor. Among clients with a short cervix, provide education concerning the signs and symptoms of preterm labor, especially as the pregnancy approaches potential viability. Prenatal visits/contacts may be scheduled at more frequent intervals to increase client interaction with the care provider, especially between 20 and 34 weeks' gestation, which may decrease the rate of extremely early preterm births.

Expect the woman (particularly a woman with pelvic pressure, backache, or increased mucoid discharge) to undergo serial transvaginal ultrasound evaluations every few days to avoid missing rapid changes in cervical dilation or until the trend in cervical length can be characterized (Cunningham et al., 2014).

Home Uterine Activity Monitoring. For a woman at risk for preterm birth, home uterine activity monitoring can be used to screen for prelabor uterine contractility so that escalating contractility can be identified, allowing earlier intervention to prevent preterm birth. The home uterine activity monitor consists of a pressure sensor attached to a belt that is held against the abdomen and a recording/storage device that is carried on a belt or hung from the shoulder. Uterine activity is typically recorded by the woman for 1 hour twice daily, while she is performing routine activities. The stored data are transmitted via telephone to a perinatal nurse, and a receiving device prints out the data. The woman is contacted if there are any problems.

Although in theory identifying early contractions to initiate interventions to arrest the labor sounds reasonable, a recent Cochrane Review study found that uterine activity monitoring in asymptomatic high-risk women is inadequate for predicting preterm birth. There was no impact on maternal or perinatal outcomes or prediction of preterm births (Urquhart et al., 2015). This practice continues even though numerous randomized trials have found no relationship between monitoring and actual reduction of preterm labor. In more recent research findings, cervical length is predictive of preterm birth in all populations studied. A cervical length of less than 25 mm warrants intervention to improve the health outcomes of pregnant women and their infants (Boots et al., 2014).

Nursing Management

Nursing management focuses on monitoring the woman very closely for signs of preterm labor: backache, increase

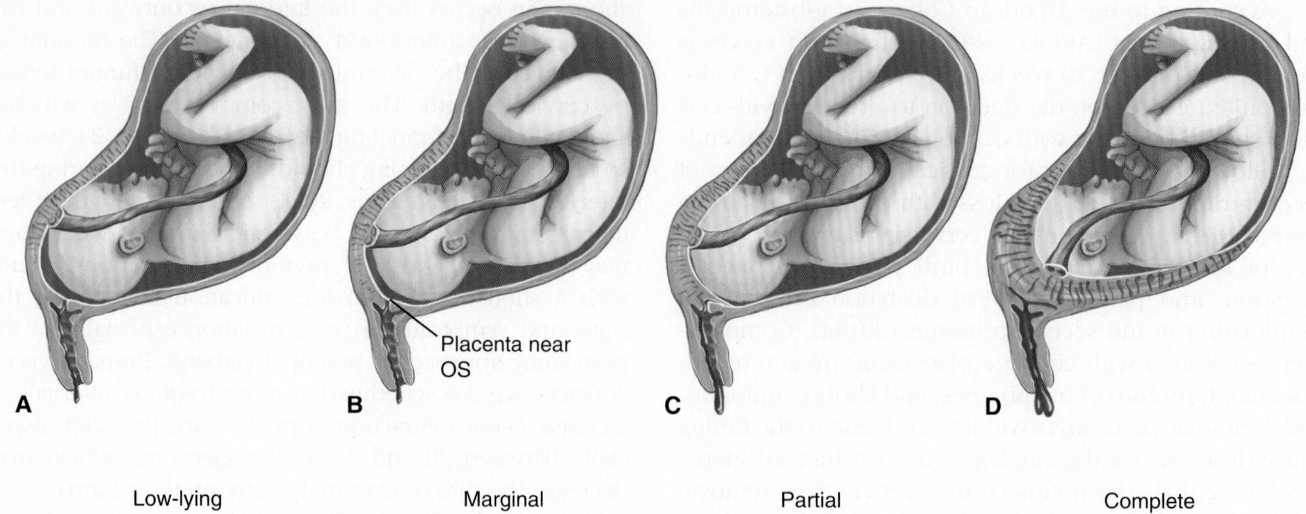

FIGURE 19.4 Classification of placenta previa. **A.** Low-lying. **B.** Marginal. **C.** Partial. **D.** Complete.

in vaginal discharge, rupture of membranes, and uterine contractions. Provide emotional support and education to allay the couple's anxiety about the well-being of their fetus. Provide preoperative care and teaching as indicated if the woman will be undergoing cerclage. Teach the client and her family about the signs and symptoms of preterm labor and the need to report any changes immediately. Also reinforce the need for activity restrictions (if appropriate) and continued regular follow-up. Continuing surveillance throughout the pregnancy is important to promote a positive outcome for the family. The nurse can play a pivotal role in identifying preterm labor through risk assessment, physical examination, and client advocacy.

Placenta Previa

Placenta previa is a bleeding condition that occurs during the last two trimesters of pregnancy. In placenta previa (literally, "afterbirth first"), the placenta implants over the cervical os. It may cause serious morbidity and mortality to the fetus and mother. The risk of placenta previa in a first pregnancy is 1 in 400, but it rises to 1 in 160 after one cesarean section; 1 in 60 after two; 1 in 30 after three; and 1 in 10 after four cesarean sections and is associated with potentially serious consequences from hemorrhage, abruption (separation) of the placenta, or emergency cesarean birth (Joy & Temming, 2015). With the rising incidence of cesarean section operations combined with increasing maternal age and more infertility treatments, the number of cases of placenta previa is increasing dramatically. The cesarean section rate must be reduced to decrease maternal morbidity and mortality. Comprehensive risk assessment, combined with advances in ultrasound, can provide earlier detection of this impaired placental implantation (Wiedaseck & Monchek, 2014).

Pathophysiology

The exact cause of placenta previa is unknown. It is initiated by implantation of the embryo in the lower uterus, perhaps due to uterine endometrial scarring or damage in the upper segment, which may incite placental growth in the unscarred lower uterine segment. Uteroplacental underperfusion may also be present, which may increase the surface area required for placental attachment and may cause the placenta to encroach on the lower uterine segment. With placental attachment and growth, the cervical os may become covered by the developing placenta. Placental vascularization is defective, allowing the placenta to attach directly to the myometrium (accreta), deeply attach to the myometrium (increta), or infiltrate the myometrium (percreta).

Placenta previa is generally classified according to the degree of coverage or proximity to the internal os, as follows (Fig. 19.4):

- Total placenta previa: the internal cervical os is completely covered by the placenta
- Partial placenta previa: the internal os is partially covered by the placenta
- Marginal placenta previa: the placenta is at the margin or edge of the internal os
- Low-lying placenta previa: the placenta is implanted in the lower uterine segment and is near the internal os but does not reach it

Therapeutic Management

Therapeutic management depends on the extent of bleeding, the amount of placenta over the cervical os, whether the fetus is developed enough to survive outside the uterus, the position of the fetus, the mother's parity, and the presence or absence of labor (Cunningham et al.,

2014). With the increase in the rate of previous cesarean sections, the frequency of placenta previa has increased. Most women continue to present in emergency departments, therefore the associated morbidity due to hemorrhage remains high. Efforts should be made to avoid primary cesarean section where possible. In addition, prenatal care and timely diagnosis of placenta previa on ultrasound can decrease the associated morbidity.

If the mother and fetus are both stable, therapeutic management may involve expectant ("wait-and-see" or watchful waiting) care. This care can be carried out at home or on an antepartal unit in the health care facility. If there is no active bleeding and the client has ready access to reliable transportation, can maintain bed rest at home, and can comprehend instructions, expectant care at home is appropriate. However, if the client requires continuous care and monitoring and cannot meet the home care requirements, the antepartal unit is the best environment.

Nursing Assessment

Nursing assessment involves a thorough history, including possible risk factors, and physical examination. Evaluate the client closely for these risk factors:

- Advancing maternal age (more than 35 years)
- Previous cesarean birth
- Multiparity
- Uterine insult or injury
- Cocaine use
- Prior placenta previa
- Infertility treatment
- Multiple gestations
- Previous induced surgical abortion
- Smoking
- Previous myomectomy to remove fibroids
- Short interval between pregnancies
- Hypertension or diabetes (Archibong & Ahmed, 2015).

HEALTH HISTORY AND PHYSICAL EXAMINATION

Ask the client if she has any problems associated with bleeding, now or in the recent past. The classical clinical presentation is painless, bright-red vaginal bleeding occurring during the second or third trimester. The initial bleeding usually is not profuse and it ceases spontaneously, only to recur again. The first episode of bleeding occurs (on average) at 27 to 32 weeks' gestation. The bleeding is thought to arise secondary to the thinning of the lower uterine segment in preparation for the onset of labor. When the bleeding occurs at the implantation site in the lower uterus, the uterus cannot contract adequately and stop the flow of blood from the open vessels. Typically with normal placental implantation in the upper uterus, minor disruptive placental attachment is not a problem, because there is a larger volume of myometrial tissue able to contract and constrict bleeding vessels.

Assess the client for uterine contractions, which may or may not occur with the bleeding. Palpate the uterus; typically it is soft and nontender on examination. Auscultate the fetal heart rate; it commonly is within normal parameters. Fetal distress is usually absent but may occur when cord problems arise, such as umbilical cord prolapse or cord compression, or when the client has experienced blood loss to the extent that maternal shock or placental abruption has occurred (King et al., 2015).

LABORATORY AND DIAGNOSTIC TESTING

To validate the position of the placenta, a transvaginal ultrasound is done. In addition, magnetic resonance imaging (MRI) may be ordered when preparing for delivery because it allows identification of placenta accreta (placenta abnormally adherent to the myometrium), increta (placenta accreta with penetration of the myometrium), or percreta (placenta accreta with invasion of the myometrium to the peritoneal covering, causing rupture of the uterus) in addition to placenta previa. These placental abnormalities, although rare, carry a very high morbidity and mortality rate, possibly necessitating a hysterectomy at delivery.

Nursing Management

Whether the care setting is in the client's home or in the health care facility, the nurse focuses on monitoring the maternal-fetal status, including assessing for signs and symptoms of vaginal bleeding and fetal distress and providing support and education to the client and her family, including providing information about the diagnostic studies and procedures that are performed. For the majority of women, a cesarean birth will be planned. Nursing Care Plan 19.1 (at the end of the Chapter) discusses the nursing process for the woman with placenta previa.

MONITORING MATERNAL-FETAL STATUS

Assess the degree of vaginal bleeding; inspect the perineal area for blood that may be pooled underneath the woman. Estimate and document the amount of bleeding. Perform a peripad count on an ongoing basis, making sure to report any changes in amount or frequency to the health care provider. If the woman is experiencing active bleeding, prepare for blood typing and cross-matching in the event a blood transfusion is needed.

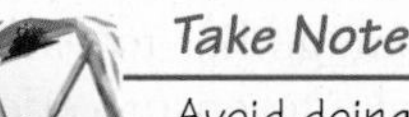
Take Note!

Avoid doing vaginal examinations in the woman with placenta previa because they may disrupt the placenta and cause hemorrhage.

Monitor maternal vital signs and uterine contractility frequently for changes. Have the client rate her level of pain using an appropriate pain rating scale. Assess fetal heart rates via Doppler or electronic monitoring to detect fetal distress. Monitor the woman's cardiopulmonary status, reporting any difficulties in respirations, changes in skin color, or complaints of difficulty breathing. Have oxygen equipment readily available should fetal or maternal distress develop. Encourage the client to lie on her side to enhance placental perfusion.

If the woman has an intravenous (IV) line inserted, inspect the IV site frequently. Alternately, anticipate the insertion of an intermittent IV access device such as a saline lock, which can be used if quick access is needed for fluid restoration and infusion of blood products. Obtain laboratory tests as ordered, including complete blood count (CBC), coagulation studies, and Rh status if appropriate.

Administer pharmacologic agents as necessary. Give Rh immunoglobulin if the client is Rh negative at 28 weeks' gestation. Monitor tocolytic (anticontraction) medication if prevention of preterm labor is needed.

PROVIDING SUPPORT AND EDUCATION

Determine the woman's level of understanding about placenta previa and the associated procedures and treatment plan. Doing so is important to prevent confusion and gain her cooperation. Provide information about the condition and make sure that all information related is consistent with information from the primary care provider. Explain all assessments and treatment measures as needed.

Act as a client advocate in obtaining information for the family. Teach the woman how to perform and record daily fetal movement. This action serves two purposes: (1) It provides valuable information about the fetus and (2) it is an activity in which the client can participate, thereby fostering some feeling of control over the situation.

If the woman will require prolonged hospitalization or home bed rest, assess the physical and emotional impact that this may have on her. Evaluate her coping mechanisms to help determine how well she will be able to adjust and adhere to the treatment plan. Allow the client to verbalize her feelings and fears, and provide emotional support. Also, provide opportunities for distraction – educational videos, arts and crafts, computer games, reading books – and evaluate the client's response.

In addition to the emotional impact of prolonged bed rest, thoroughly assess the woman's skin to prevent skin breakdown and to help alleviate her discomfort secondary to limited physical activity. Instruct the woman in appropriate skin care measures. Encourage her to eat a balanced diet with adequate fluid intake to ensure adequate nutrition and hydration and prevent complications associated with urinary and bowel elimination secondary to bed rest.

Teach the client and family about any signs and symptoms that should be reported immediately. In addition, prepare the woman for the possibility of a cesarean birth. The woman must notify her health care provider about any bleeding episodes or backaches (may indicate preterm labor contractions) and must adhere to the prescribed bed rest regimen. To ensure adherence to the plan and a positive outcome, the client needs to be aware of and understand the rationales for the ongoing observations.

Abruptio Placentae

Abruptio placentae is the premature separation of a normally implanted placenta after the 20th week of gestation prior to birth, which leads to hemorrhage. It is a significant cause of third-trimester bleeding, with a high mortality rate. It occurs in about 1% of all pregnancies throughout the world, or approximately 1 in 100 pregnancies. There is a 10 to 20 times greater risk of reoccurrence in a subsequent pregnancy. It typically peaks between 24 and 26 weeks' gestation.

Maternal risks include obstetric hemorrhage, need for blood transfusions, emergency hysterectomy, disseminated intravascular coagulopathy, and renal failure. Maternal death is rare, but seven times higher than the overall maternal mortality rate. Perinatal consequences include low birth weight, preterm delivery, asphyxia, stillbirth, and perinatal death. In developed countries, approximately 10% of all preterm births and 10% to 20% of all perinatal deaths are caused by placental abruption (Mukherjee et al., 2014). The overall fetal mortality rate for placental abruption is up to 50%, depending on the extent of the abruption. Maternal mortality is approximately 6% in abruptio placentae and is related to cesarean birth and/or hemorrhage/coagulopathy (Jaju, Kulkarni, & Mundada, 2014).

Pathophysiology

The etiology of this condition is unknown; however, it has been proposed that abruption starts with degenerative changes in the small maternal blood vessels, resulting in blood clotting, degeneration of the decidua (uterine lining), and possible rupture of a vessel. Bleeding from the blood vessel forms a blood clot between the placenta and the uterine wall. The continued bleeding causes increased pressure behind the placenta and results in separation from the uterine wall (Moses, 2015a). Fetal blood supply is compromised and fetal distress develops in proportion to the degree of placental separation. This is caused by the insult of the abruption itself and by issues related to prematurity when early birth is required to alleviate maternal or fetal distress.

Abruptio placentae is classified according to the extent of separation and the amount of blood loss from the maternal circulation. Classifications include:

- *Mild (grade 1):* minimal bleeding (less than 500 mL), marginal separation (10% to 20%), tender uterus, no coagulopathy, no signs of shock, no fetal distress

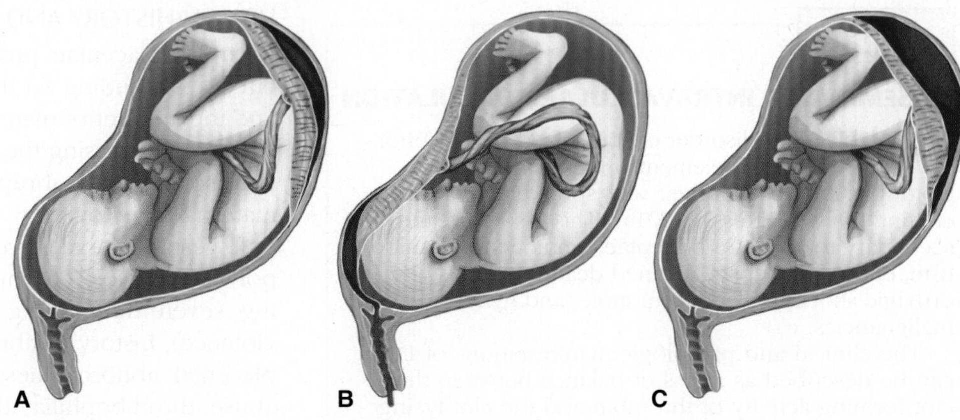

FIGURE 19.5 Classifications of abruptio placentae. **A.** Partial abruption with concealed hemorrhage. **B.** Partial abruption with apparent hemorrhage. **C.** Complete abruption with concealed hemorrhage.

- *Moderate (grade 2):* moderate bleeding (1,000 to 1,500 mL), moderate separation (20% to 50%), continuous abdominal pain, mild shock, normal maternal blood pressure, maternal tachycardia
- *Severe (grade 3):* absent to moderate bleeding (more than 1,500 mL), severe separation (more than 50%), profound shock, dark vaginal bleeding, agonizing abdominal pain, decreased maternal blood pressure, significant maternal tachycardia, and development of DIC (Atkinson et al., 2015).

Abruptio placentae also may be classified as partial or complete, depending on the degree of separation. Alternately, it can be classified as concealed or apparent, by the type of bleeding (Fig. 19.5).

Remember Helen, the pregnant woman with severe abdominal pain? Electronic fetal monitoring revealed uterine hypertonicity with absent fetal heart sounds. Palpation of her abdomen revealed rigidity and extreme tenderness in all four quadrants. Her vital signs were as follows: temperature, afebrile; pulse, 94; respirations, 22; blood pressure, 130/90 mm Hg. What might you suspect as the cause of Helen's abdominal pain? What course of action would you anticipate for Helen?

Therapeutic Management

Treatment of abruptio placentae is designed to assess, control, and restore the amount of blood lost; provide a positive outcome for both mother and newborn; and prevent coagulation disorders, such as DIC (Box 19.2). Emergency measures include starting two large-bore IV lines with normal saline or lactated Ringer solution to combat hypovolemia, obtaining blood specimens for evaluating hemodynamic status values and for typing and cross-matching, and frequently monitoring fetal and maternal well-being. After the severity of abruption is determined and appropriate blood and fluid replacement is given, cesarean birth is done immediately if fetal distress is evident. If the fetus is not in distress close monitoring continues, with delivery planned at the earliest signs of fetal distress. Because of the possibility of fetal blood loss through the placenta, a neonatal intensive care team should be available during the birth process to assess and treat the newborn immediately for shock, blood loss, and hypoxia.

If the woman develops DIC, treatment focuses on determining the underlying cause of DIC and correcting it. Replacement therapy of the coagulation factors is achieved by transfusion of fresh-frozen plasma along with cryoprecipitate to maintain the circulating volume and provide oxygen to the cells of the body. Anticoagulant therapy (low-molecular-weight heparin), packed red cells, platelet concentrates, antithrombin concentrates, and nonclotting protein-containing volume expanders, such as plasma protein fraction or albumin, are also used to combat this serious condition. The use of blood products must be dictated by the clinical picture and not simply to normalize laboratory test results (Holt, 2015). Prompt identification and early intervention are essential for a woman with acute DIC associated with abruptio placentae to treat DIC and possibly save her life.

Nursing Assessment

Abruptio placentae is a medical emergency. The nurse plays a critical role in assessing the pregnant woman presenting with abdominal pain and/or experiencing vaginal bleeding, especially in a concealed hemorrhage, in which the extent of bleeding is not recognized. Rapid assessment is essential to ensure prompt, effective interventions to prevent maternal and fetal morbidity and mortality. Comparison Chart 19.1 compares placenta previa with abruptio placentae.

BOX 19.2

DISSEMINATED INTRAVASCULAR COAGULATION

DIC is a bleeding disorder characterized by an abnormal reduction in the elements involved in blood clotting resulting from their widespread intravascular clotting (Davis & Kessler, 2014). This disorder can occur secondary to abruptio placentae, amniotic fluid embolism, endotoxin sepsis, retained dead fetus, posthemorrhagic shock, hydatidiform mole, and gynecologic malignancies.

The clinical and pathologic manifestations of DIC can be described as a loss of balance between the clot-forming activity of thrombin and the clot-lysing activity of plasmin. Therefore, too much thrombin tips the balance toward the prothrombic state and the client develops clots. Alternately, too much clot lysis (fibrinolysis) results from plasmin formation and the client hemorrhages. Small clots form throughout the body, and eventually the blood-clotting factors are used up, rendering them unavailable to form clots at sites of tissue injury. Clot-dissolving mechanisms are also increased, which results in bleeding (possibly severe).

DIC is usually associated with high mortality and morbidity rates. No single laboratory test is sensitive or specific enough to diagnose DIC definitively, but it can be diagnosed by using a combination of multiple clinical and laboratory tests that reflect the pathophysiology of the syndrome.

Laboratory studies that assist in the diagnosis include:

- Decreased fibrinogen and platelets
- Prolonged PT and aPTT
- Positive D-dimer tests and fibrin (split) degradation products (objective evidence of the simultaneous formation of thrombin and plasmin) (Martina, 2010)

Adapted from Davis, S. J., & Kessler, C. M. (2014). Disseminated intravascular coagulation: Diagnosis and management. In *Hemostasis and thrombosis: Practical guidelines in clinical management* (pp. 151–168). Hoboken, NJ: Wiley Blackwell; and Kobayashi, T. (2014). Obstetrical disseminated intravascular coagulation score. *Journal of Obstetrics and Gynecology Research, 40*(6), 1500–1506.

HEALTH HISTORY AND PHYSICAL EXAMINATION

Abruptio placentae produces a wide range of clinical effects, depending on the extent of placental separation and the amount of maternal blood loss. Begin the health history by assessing the woman for risk factors that may predispose her to abruptio placentae, such as advanced maternal age (over 35 years old), poor nutrition, multiple gestation, excessive intrauterine pressure caused by polyhydramnios, chronic hypertension, cigarette smoking, severe trauma (e.g., auto accident, intimate partner violence), history of abruption in a previous pregnancy, placental abnormalities, cocaine or methamphetamine abuse, thrombophilia, alcohol ingestion, and multiparity (Deering, 2015). In addition, be alert for other notable risk factors, such as male fetal gender, chorioamnionitis, prolonged premature ruptured membranes (more than 24 hours), oligohydramnios, preeclampsia, and low socioeconomic status (Nagtalon-Ramos, 2014).

Assess the woman for bleeding. As the placenta separates from the uterus, hemorrhage ensues. It can be apparent, appearing as vaginal bleeding, or it can be concealed. Vaginal bleeding is present in 80% of women diagnosed with abruptio placentae and may be significant enough to jeopardize both maternal and fetal health within a short time frame. The remaining 20% of abruptions are associated with a concealed hemorrhage and the absence of vaginal bleeding. Monitor the woman's level of consciousness, noting any signs or symptoms that may suggest shock.

Take Note!

Vital signs can be within normal range, even with significant blood loss, because a pregnant woman can lose up to 40% of her total blood volume without showing signs of shock (Schultz & McConachie, 2015).

Assess the woman for complaints of pain, including the type, onset, and location. Ask if she has had

COMPARISON CHART 19.1 PLACENTA PREVIA VERSUS ABRUPTIO PLACENTAE

Manifestation	Placenta Previa	Abruptio Placentae
Onset	Insidious	Sudden
Type of bleeding	Always visible; slight, then more profuse	Can be concealed or visible
Blood description	Bright red	Dark
Discomfort/pain	None (painless)	Constant; uterine tenderness on palpation
Uterine tone	Soft and relaxed	Firm to rigid
Fetal heart rate	Usually in normal range	Fetal distress or absent
Fetal presentation	May be breech or transverse lie; engagement is absent	No relationship

any contractions. Palpate the abdomen, noting any contractions, uterine tenderness, tenseness, or rigidity. Ask if she has noticed any changes in fetal movement and activity. Decreased fetal movement may be the presenting complaint, resulting from fetal jeopardy or fetal death (Cunningham et al., 2014). Assess fetal heart rate and continue to monitor it electronically.

Take Note!

Classic manifestations of abruptio placentae include painful, dark-red vaginal bleeding (port-wine color) because the bleeding comes from the clot that was formed behind the placenta; "knife-like" abdominal pain; uterine tenderness; contractions; and decreased fetal movement. Rapid assessment is essential to ensure prompt, effective interventions to prevent maternal and fetal morbidity and mortality.

LABORATORY AND DIAGNOSTIC TESTING

Laboratory and diagnostic tests may be helpful in diagnosing the condition and guiding management. These studies may include:

- *CBC*—determines the current hemodynamic status; however, it is not reliable for estimating acute blood loss
- *Fibrinogen levels*—typically are increased in pregnancy (hyperfibrinogenemia); thus, a moderate dip in fibrinogen levels might suggest DIC and, if profuse bleeding occurs, the clotting cascade might be compromised
- *Prothrombin time (PT)/activated partial thromboplastin time (aPTT)*—determines the client's coagulation status, especially if surgery is planned
- *Type and cross-match*—determines blood type if a transfusion is needed
- *Nonstress test*—demonstrates findings of fetal jeopardy manifested by late decelerations or bradycardia
- *Biophysical profile*—aids in evaluating clients with chronic abruption; a low score (less than 6 points) suggests possible fetal compromise (Creasy et al., 2014).

Ultrasound is not useful for making a definitive diagnosis because the clot is sonographically visible in less than 50% of the cases. A CT scan is a more reliable method for evaluation of placental abruption (Hosein, Abdel-Kariem, & Shriki, 2014).

Nursing Management

Nursing management of the woman with abruptio placentae warrants immediate care to provide the best outcome for both mother and fetus.

ENSURING ADEQUATE TISSUE PERFUSION

When the woman arrives at the facility, place her on strict bed rest and in a left lateral position to prevent pressure on the vena cava. This position provides uninterrupted perfusion to the fetus. Expect to administer oxygen therapy via nasal cannula to ensure adequate tissue perfusion. Monitor oxygen saturation levels via pulse oximetry to evaluate the effectiveness of interventions.

Obtain maternal vital signs frequently, as often as every 15 minutes as indicated, depending on the woman's status and amount of blood loss. Observe for changes in vital signs suggesting hypovolemic shock and report them immediately. Also expect to insert an indwelling urinary (Foley) catheter to assess hourly urine output and initiate an IV infusion for fluid replacement using a large-bore catheter.

Assess fundal height for changes. An increase in size would indicate bleeding. Monitor the amount and characteristics of any vaginal bleeding as frequently as every 15 to 30 minutes. Be alert for signs and symptoms of DIC, such as bleeding gums, tachycardia, oozing from the IV insertion site, and petechiae, and administer blood products as ordered if DIC occurs.

Institute continuous electronic fetal monitoring. Assess uterine contractions and report any increased uterine tenseness or rigidity. Also observe the tracing for tetanic uterine contractions or changes in fetal heart rate patterns suggesting that the fetus has been compromised.

PROVIDING SUPPORT AND EDUCATION

A woman diagnosed with abruptio placentae may be filled with a sense of heightened anxiety and apprehension for her own health as well as for the health of her fetus. Communicate empathy and understanding of the client's experience, and provide emotional support throughout this frightening time. Remain with the woman and her partner, acknowledge their emotions and fears, and address their spiritual and cultural needs. Answer their questions about the status of their fetus openly and honestly, being sure to explain indicators of fetal well-being. Provide information about the various diagnostic tests, treatments, and procedures that may be done, including the possible need for a cesarean birth. Depending on the client's status, extent of bleeding, and length of gestation, the fetus may not survive. If the fetus does survive, he or she most likely will require neonatal intensive care. Assist the client and family to deal with the loss or with the birth of a newborn in the neonatal intensive care unit.

Although abruptio placentae is not a preventable condition, client education is important to help reduce the risk for a recurrence of this condition. Encourage the woman to avoid drinking, smoking, or using drugs during pregnancy. Urge her to seek early and continuous prenatal care and to receive prompt health care if any signs and symptoms occur in future pregnancies.

Think back to Helen, the pregnant woman described at the beginning of the chapter. She was diagnosed with abruptio placentae and was prepared for an emergency cesarean birth. On exploration, there was almost a 75% abruption, with approximately 800 mL of concealed blood

between the uterus and the placenta. In addition, she lost an additional 500 mL during surgery. What in Helen's history may have placed her at increased risk for abruption? What assessments and interventions would be essential during her postpartum recovery secondary to her large blood loss? What psychosocial interventions would be necessary due to her fetal loss?

Placenta Accreta

Placenta accreta is a potentially life-threatening obstetrical hemorrhagic condition that requires a multidisciplinary approach to management. The incidence of placenta accreta has increased and seems to parallel the increasing cesarean birth rate or intrauterine procedures. Placenta accreta is a condition in which the placenta attaches itself too deeply into the wall of the uterus but does not penetrate the uterine muscle. It is further subcategorized as *placenta increta*, when the placenta invades the myometrium, and *placenta percreta*, when it has extended through the myometrium and uterine serosa and adjacent tissue. A common risk of placenta accreta during the birthing process is the possibility of hemorrhaging during manual attempts to detach the placenta. According to the March of Dimes (2015c), 1 in 530 births results in this condition. The specific cause of placenta accreta is unknown, but it can be related to placenta previa, advanced maternal age, smoking, and previous cesarean births. According to the literature, a cesarean birth increases the possibility of a future placenta accreta; the more cesarean births that are done, the greater the incidence.

According to ACOG (2014b), postpartum hemorrhage is a complication associated with placenta accreta. Ninety percent of accretas have postpartum hemorrhage, and 50% of these will result in a hysterectomy (ACOG, 2014b). Women at highest risk of emergency hysterectomy are those who are multiparous, had a cesarean birth in either a previous or the present pregnancy, or had abnormal placentation. The essential management issues are early detection and immediate and appropriate intervention. If a placenta accreta diagnosis is made, the client should be counseled that a cesarean section and possible hysterectomy may be necessary interventions (Creasy et al., 2014).

Placenta accreta is typically diagnosed after birth when the placenta fails to normally separate from the uterine wall. A prenatal screening diagnosis via ultrasound and MRI would decrease maternal and fetal morbidities and mortalities. A profuse hemorrhage may result because the uterus cannot contract to close off the open blood vessels. Management will depend on the severity of the bleeding and frequently necessitates a prompt hysterectomy (Humphrey, 2015). Nurses need to be prepared to assist in this emergency situation as dictated by the health care provider.

HYPEREMESIS GRAVIDARUM

Hyperemesis gravidarum is a severe form of nausea and vomiting of pregnancy associated with significant costs and psychosocial impacts. At least 70% to 85% of women experience nausea and vomiting during their pregnancy (Castillo & Phillippi, 2015). The term *morning sickness* is often used to describe this condition when symptoms are relatively mild. Studies have shown that nausea and vomiting of pregnancy is associated with improved fetal outcomes, such as lower rates of miscarriage (Ayyavoo et al., 2014). Such symptoms usually disappear after the first trimester. This mild form mostly affects the quality of life of the woman and her family, whereas the severe form – **hyperemesis gravidarum** – results in dehydration, weight loss, electrolyte imbalance, and the need for hospitalization (Taylor, 2014).

Unlike morning sickness, hyperemesis gravidarum is a complication of pregnancy characterized by persistent, uncontrollable nausea and vomiting that begins in the first trimester and causes dehydration, ketosis, and weight loss of more than 5% of prepregnancy body weight. Risk factors for hyperemesis include previous pregnancy complicated by hyperemesis, molar pregnancies, history of helicobacter pylori infection, **multiple gestation**, prepregnancy history of genitourinary disorders, clinical hyperthyroid disorders, and prepregnancy psychiatric diagnosis (King et al., 2015).

Hyperemesis (uncontrollable vomiting) is estimated to occur in approximately 2% of pregnant women. The prevalence increases in molar pregnancies and multiple gestations. The peak incidence is at 8 to 12 weeks of pregnancy, and symptoms usually resolve by week 20 (Maltepe et al, 2015).

Take Note!

Every pregnant woman needs to be instructed to report any episodes of severe nausea and vomiting or episodes that extend beyond the first trimester.

Pathophysiology

Although the exact cause of nausea and vomiting is unknown, its effects – decreased placental blood flow, decreased maternal blood flow, and acidosis – can threaten the health of the mother and fetus. Dehydration can also lead to preterm labor (Festin, 2014). Numerous theories abound, but few studies have produced scientific evidence to identify the etiology of this condition. It is likely that multiple factors contribute to it.

Elevated levels of hCG are present in all pregnant women during early pregnancy, usually declining after 12 weeks. This corresponds to the usual duration of morning sickness. In hyperemesis gravidarum, the hCG levels are often higher and extend beyond the first trimester. Symptoms exacerbate the disease. Decreased fluid intake and prolonged vomiting cause dehydration; dehydration increases the serum concentration of hCG, which in turn exacerbates the nausea and vomiting—a vicious cycle. A few other theories that have been proposed to explain its etiology include:

- *Endocrine theory*—high levels of hCG and estrogen during pregnancy
- *Metabolic theory*—vitamin B_6 deficiency
- *Genetic factors* that may predispose the woman to this condition
- *Psychological theory*—psychological stress increases the symptoms

Therapeutic Management

Hyperemesis gravidarum is a diagnosis of exclusion. Careful consideration of other conditions must be assessed when a client experiences nausea and vomiting for the first time after 9 weeks' gestation.

Conservative management in the home is the first line of treatment for the woman with hyperemesis gravidarum. This usually focuses on dietary and lifestyle changes. If conservative management fails to alleviate the client's symptoms and nausea and vomiting continue, hospitalization is necessary to reverse the effects of severe nausea and vomiting.

On admission to the hospital, blood tests are ordered to assess the severity of the client's dehydration, electrolyte imbalance, ketosis, and malnutrition. Parenteral fluids and drugs are ordered to rehydrate the woman and reduce the symptoms. The first choice for fluid replacement is generally normal saline, which aids in preventing hyponatremia, with vitamins (pyridoxine [B_6]) and electrolytes added. Oral food and fluids are withheld for the first 24 to 36 hours to allow the gastrointestinal tract to rest. Antiemetics may be administered rectally or intravenously to control the nausea and vomiting initially because the woman is considered NPO (not able to ingest anything by mouth). Once her condition stabilizes and she is allowed oral intake, medications may be administered orally.

If the client does not improve after several days of bed rest, "gut rest," IV fluids, and antiemetics, total parenteral nutrition or feeding through a percutaneous endoscopic gastrostomy tube is instituted to prevent malnutrition. Administering antiemetics intravenously or intramuscularly is typically the second pillar of treatment for hyperemesis gravidarum. Finding a drug that works for any given client is largely a matter of trial and error. If one drug is ineffective, another class of drugs with a different mechanism of action may help. Promethazine (Phenergan) and prochlorperazine (Compazine) are among the older preparations usually tried first. If they fail to relieve symptoms, newer drugs such as ondansetron (Zofran) may be tried. Most drugs are given intravenously or intramuscularly. There is no evidence that any antiemetic class is superior to another with respect to effectiveness (King et al., 2015) (Drug Guide 19.2).

Few women receive complete relief of symptoms from any one therapy. Complementary and alternative

DRUG GUIDE 19.2 MEDICATIONS USED FOR HYPEREMESIS GRAVIDARUM

Medication	Action/Indications	Nursing Implications
Promethazine (Phenergan)	Diminishes vestibular stimulation and acts on the chemoreceptor trigger zone (CTZ) Symptomatic relief of nausea and vomiting, and motion sickness	Be alert for urinary retention, dizziness, hypotension, and involuntary movements. Institute safety measures to prevent injury secondary to sedative effects. Offer hard candy and frequent rinsing of mouth for dryness.
Prochlorperazine (Compazine)	Acts centrally to inhibit dopamine receptors in the CTZ and peripherally to block vagus nerve stimulation in the gastrointestinal tract Controls severe nausea and vomiting	Be alert for abnormal movements and for neuroleptic malignant syndrome such as seizures, hyper/hypotension, tachycardia, and dyspnea. Assess mental status, intake/output. Caution client not to drive as a result of drowsiness or dizziness. Advise to change position slowly to minimize effects of orthostatic hypotension.
Ondansetron (Zofran)	Blocks serotonin release, which stimulates the vagal afferent nerves, thus stimulating the vomiting reflex	Monitor for possible side effects such as diarrhea, constipation, abdominal pain, headache, dizziness, drowsiness, and fatigue. Monitor liver function studies as ordered.

Adapted from King, T. L., Brucker, M. C., Kriebs, J. M., Fahey, J. O., Grgor, C. L., & Varney, H. (2015). *Varney's midwifery* (5th ed.). Burlington, MA: Jones & Bartlett Learning; and Ogunyemi, D. A., Fong, A., & Herrero, T. C. (2015). Hyperemesis gravidarum. *eMedicine*. Retrieved from http://emedicine.medscape.com/article/254751-overview

medicine therapies appeal to many women as supplements to traditional ones. Some popular therapies include acupressure, massage, therapeutic touch, ginger, and the wearing of Sea-Bands to prevent nausea and vomiting. Recent research has reported a positive effect of using acupressure (provided by Sea-Bands) over the *nei guan* acupoint on the wrist to control nausea and vomiting associated with pregnancy (Matthews et al., 2014).

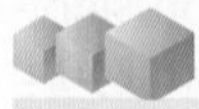
Concept Mastery Alert

Priority Interventions in Hyperemesis Gravidarum

Hyperemesis gravidarum is nausea and vomiting in early pregnancy that prevents the woman from ingesting adequate nutrition. IV fluids may be required for rehydration, but the priority is to stop all intake of food and fluid for a period of time until vomiting has stopped.

Nursing Assessment

Nursing assessment of the woman with hyperemesis gravidarum requires a thorough history and physical examination to identify signs and symptoms associated with this disorder. The client is extremely uncomfortable. She may experience many hours of lost work productivity and sleep, and hyperemesis may damage family relationships. If hyperemesis progresses untreated, it may cause neurologic disturbances, renal damage, dehydration, ketosis, alkalosis from loss of hydrochloric acid, hypokalemia, retinal hemorrhage, or death (Peled et al., 2014). Laboratory and diagnostic tests aid in determining the severity of the disorder.

Health History and Physical Examination

Begin the history by asking the client about the onset, duration, and course of her nausea and vomiting. Ask her about any medications or treatments she used and how effective they were in relieving her nausea and vomiting. Obtain a diet history from the client, including a dietary recall for the past week. Note the client's knowledge of nutrition and need for appropriate nutritional intake. Be alert for patterns that may contribute to or trigger her distress. Also ask about any complaints of ptyalism (excessive salivation), anorexia, indigestion, and abdominal pain or distention. Ask if she has noticed any blood or mucus in her stool.

Review the client's history for possible risk factors, such as young age, nausea and vomiting with previous pregnancy, history of intolerance of oral contraceptives, nulliparity, trophoblastic disease, multiple gestation, emotional or psychological stress, gastroesophageal reflux disease, primigravida status, obesity, hyperthyroidism, and *Helicobacter pylori* seropositivity (Ogunyemi, Fong, & Herrero, 2015). Weigh the client and compare this weight with her weight before she began experiencing symptoms and to her prepregnancy weight to estimate the degree of loss. With hyperemesis, weight loss usually exceeds 5% of body mass.

Inspect the mucous membranes for dryness and check skin turgor for evidence of fluid loss and dehydration. Assess blood pressure for changes, such as hypotension, that may suggest a fluid volume deficit. Also note any complaints of weakness, fatigue, activity intolerance, dizziness, or sleep disturbances.

Assess the client's perception of the situation. Note any evidence of depression, anxiety, irritability, mood changes, and decreased ability to concentrate, which can add to her emotional distress. Much of the psychological distress is self-limiting in this condition and probably in the causal pathway (Tan et al., 2014). Determine the woman's support systems that are available for help.

Laboratory and Diagnostic Testing

The results of laboratory and diagnostic tests may provide clues to the severity or etiology of the disorder. These may include:

- *Liver enzymes*—to rule out hepatitis, pancreatitis, and cholestasis; elevations of aspartate aminotransferase (AST) and alanine aminotransferase (ALT) are usually present
- *CBC*—elevated levels of red blood cells and hematocrit, indicating dehydration
- *Urine ketones*—positive when the body breaks down fat to provide energy in the absence of adequate intake
- *TSH and T4* to rule out thyroid disease
- *Blood urea nitrogen*—increased in the presence of salt and water depletion
- *Urine specific gravity*—greater than 1.025, possibly indicating concentrated urine linked to inadequate fluid intake or excessive fluid loss; ketonuria
- *Serum electrolytes*—decreased levels of potassium, sodium, and chloride resulting from excessive vomiting and loss of hydrochloric acid in stomach
- *Ultrasound*—evaluation for molar pregnancy or multiple gestation (Cunningham et al., 2014).

Nursing Management

Nursing management for the client with hyperemesis gravidarum focuses on promoting comfort by controlling the client's nausea and vomiting and promoting adequate nutrition. In addition, the nurse plays a major role in supporting and educating the client and her family.

Promoting Comfort and Nutrition

During the initial period, expect to withhold all oral food and fluids, maintaining NPO status to allow the gastrointestinal tract to rest. In addition, administer prescribed antiemetics to relieve the nausea and vomiting and IV fluids to replace fluid losses. Monitor the rate of infusion to prevent overload and assess the IV insertion site to prevent infiltration or infection. Also administer electrolyte replacement therapy as ordered to correct any imbalances, and periodically check serum electrolyte levels to evaluate the effectiveness of therapy.

Provide physical comfort measures such as hygiene measures and oral care. Pay special attention to the environment, making sure to keep the area free of pungent odors. As the client's nausea and vomiting subside, gradually introduce oral fluids and foods in small amounts. Monitor intake and output and assess the client's tolerance to the increase in intake.

Providing Support and Education

Women with hyperemesis gravidarum commonly are fatigued physically and emotionally. Many are exhausted, frustrated, and anxious. Offer reassurance that all interventions are directed toward promoting positive pregnancy outcomes for both the woman and her fetus. Providing information about the expected plan of care may help to alleviate the client's anxiety. Listen to her concerns and feelings, answering all questions honestly. Educate the woman and her family about the condition and its treatment options (Teaching Guidelines 19.1). Teach the client about therapeutic lifestyle changes, such as avoiding stressors and fatigue that may trigger nausea and vomiting. Offer ongoing support and encouragement and promote active participation in care decisions, thereby empowering the client and her family. Attempting to provide the client with a sense of control may help her overcome the feeling that she has lost control. If necessary, refer the client to a spiritual advisor or counseling. Also suggest possible local or national support groups that the client may contact for additional information. Arrange for possible home care follow-up for the client and reinforce discharge instructions to promote understanding. Timely counseling, balanced nutrition, pharmacotherapy, and emotional support are associated with favorable outcomes for the woman with this condition. Collaborate with community resources to ensure continuity of care.

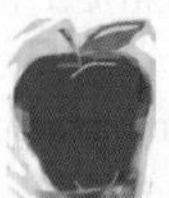

Teaching Guidelines 19.1

TEACHING TO MINIMIZE NAUSEA AND VOMITING

- Avoid noxious stimuli – such as strong flavors, perfumes, or strong odors such as frying bacon – that might trigger nausea and vomiting.
- Avoid tight waistbands to minimize pressure on abdomen.
- Eat small, frequent meals throughout the day—six small meals.
- Separate fluids from solids by consuming fluids in between meals.
- Avoid lying down or reclining for at least 2 hours after eating.
- Use high-protein supplement drinks.
- Avoid foods high in fat.
- Increase your intake of carbonated beverages.
- Increase your exposure to fresh air to improve symptoms.
- Eat when you are hungry, regardless of normal mealtimes.
- Drink herbal teas containing peppermint or ginger.
- Avoid fatigue and learn how to manage stress in life.
- Schedule daily rest periods to avoid becoming overtired.
- Eat foods that settle the stomach, such as dry crackers, toast, or soda.

HYPERTENSIVE DISORDERS OF PREGNANCY

Hypertension remains the most commonly encountered medical condition in pregnant women, complicating up to 15% of all pregnancies. It results in frequent hospital admissions, maternal morbidity and mortality, and preterm births with concomitant neonatal morbidity and mortality. Hypertensive disorders of pregnancy comprise a spectrum of severity ranging from a mild elevation of blood pressure to severe preeclampsia and hemolysis. Recent data show that hypertensive disorders of pregnancy are associated with long-term cardiovascular risks in women (Miller & Carpenter, 2015).

Hypertensive disorders of pregnancy include chronic hypertension, gestational hypertension, preeclampsia, **eclampsia**, and chronic hypertension with superimposed preeclampsia. Preeclampsia complicates about 3% to 5% of pregnancies. All hypertensive disorders, which affect up to 15% of pregnancies, are on the rise. Hypertensive disorders are associated with higher rates of maternal, fetal, and infant mortality and with severe morbidity, especially in cases of severe preeclampsia, eclampsia, and HELLP syndrome (ACOG, 2014c).

ACOG (2010c) and the National High Blood Pressure Education Program Working Group on High Blood Pressure in Pregnancy (2002) have identified a classification system for hypertensive disorders. Hypertension may be a pre-existing condition (chronic hypertension) or it may present for the first time during pregnancy (gestational hypertension). Both chronic hypertension and preeclampsia can be subclassified as either mild or severe. For chronic hypertension, subclassification is dependent on systolic and diastolic values. For preeclampsia, subclassification is dependent on the severity of end organ involvement (Foley, Strong, & Garite, 2014). Regardless of its onset or subclassification, hypertension jeopardizes the well-being of the mother as well as the fetus.

The classification of hypertensive disorders in pregnancy currently consists of five categories:

1. *Chronic hypertension*: hypertension that exists prior to pregnancy or that develops before 20 weeks' gestation.
2. *Gestational hypertension*: blood pressure elevation (140/90 mm Hg) identified after 20 weeks' gestation without proteinuria. Blood pressure returns to normal by 12 weeks' postpartum.
3. *Preeclampsia*: most common hypertensive disorder of pregnancy, which develops with proteinuria after 20 weeks' gestation. It is a multisystem disease process, which is classified as mild or severe, depending on the severity of the organ dysfunction.
4. *Eclampsia*: Onset of seizure activity in a woman with preeclampsia.
5. *Chronic hypertension with superimposed preeclampsia*: occurs in approximately 20% of pregnant women with increased maternal and fetal morbidity rates (King et al., 2015).

Population-based data indicate that approximately 1% of pregnancies are complicated by chronic hypertension, 5% to 6% by gestational hypertension (without proteinuria), and 3% to 5% by preeclampsia (Carson & Gibson, 2015). Worldwide, 50,000 to 60,000 women die from preeclampsia each year, corresponding to 12% of all maternal deaths (Clausen & Bergholt, 2014).

Chronic Hypertension

Chronic hypertension is defined as blood pressure exceeding 140/90 mm Hg before pregnancy or before 20 weeks' gestation. When hypertension is first identified during a woman's pregnancy and she is less than 20 weeks' gestation, blood pressure elevations usually represent chronic hypertension. Chronic hypertension occurs in about 20% of women of childbearing age, with the prevalence varying according to age, race, and body mass index (BMI). As our nation's obesity rate rises, more women will start pregnancies with elevated blood pressures. About 25% of women with chronic hypertension develop preeclampsia during pregnancy (Clausen & Bergholt, 2014). Women with chronic hypertension in pregnancy should be monitored for the development of worsening hypertension and/or the development of superimposed preeclampsia.

Women with mild chronic hypertension often do not require antihypertensive therapy during most of pregnancy. Pharmacologic treatment of mild hypertension does not reduce the likelihood of developing preeclampsia later in gestation and increases the likelihood of intrauterine growth restriction. If maternal blood pressure exceeds 160/100 mm Hg, however, drug treatment is recommended (Magee et al., 2015). Nurses can play a large role in educating their hypertensive clients to help them understand potential complications and how simple changes in their lifestyles might be helpful in influencing the pregnancy outcome positively.

Gestational Hypertension

The gestational hypertension category is used in women with nonproteinuric hypertension of pregnancy, in which the pathophysiologic disturbances of the preeclampsia syndrome do not develop before giving birth. Gestational hypertension is a temporary diagnosis for hypertensive pregnant women who do not meet the criteria for preeclampsia (both hypertension and possibly proteinuria) or chronic hypertension (hypertension first detected before the 20th week of pregnancy).

Gestational hypertension is characterized by hypertension (>140/90) without proteinuria after 20 weeks' gestation resolving by 12 weeks' postpartum (Magowan et al., 2014). Previously, gestational hypertension was known as pregnancy-induced hypertension or toxemia of pregnancy, but these terms are no longer used. Gestational hypertension is defined as systolic blood pressure >140 mm Hg and/or diastolic >90 mm Hg on at least two occasions at least 4 to 6 hours apart after the 20th week of gestation, in women known to be normotensive prior to this time and prior to pregnancy (King et al., 2015). Gestational hypertension can be differentiated from chronic hypertension, which appears before the 20th week of gestation; or hypertension before the current pregnancy, which continues after the woman gives birth.

A recent study found that progesterone supplementation during the first trimester significantly reduced the incidence of gestational hypertension and fetal distress in primigravida women. This supplementation might be a future therapy with addition studies to validate it (Zainul et al., 2014).

Preeclampsia and Eclampsia

Normal physiologic adaptations to pregnancy are altered in the woman who develops preeclampsia. Preeclampsia can be described as a multisystem, vasopressive disorder that targets the cardiovascular, hepatic, renal, and central nervous systems. Preeclampsia can be classified as mild or severe with a potential progression to eclampsia. Each is associated with specific criteria. Comparison Chart 19.2 highlights these classifications.

Pathophysiology

Preeclampsia remains an enigma. The condition can be devastating to both the mother and fetus, yet the etiology still remains a mystery to medical science despite decades of research. Many theories exist, but none has truly explained the widespread pathologic changes that result in pulmonary edema, oliguria, seizures, thrombocytopenia,

COMPARISON CHART 19.2 PREECLAMPSIA VERSUS ECLAMPSIA

	Mild Preeclampsia	Severe Preeclampsia	Eclampsia
Blood pressure	>140/90 mm Hg after 20 weeks' gestation	>160/110 mm Hg	>160/110 mm Hg
Proteinuria	300 mg/24 hr or greater than 1+ protein on a random dipstick urine sample	>500 mg/24 hr; greater than 3+ on random dipstick urine sample	Marked proteinuria
Seizures/coma	No	No	Yes
Hyperreflexia	No	Yes	Yes
Other signs and symptoms	Mild facial or hand edema Weight gain	Headache Oliguria Blurred vision, scotomata (blind spots) Pulmonary edema Thrombocytopenia (platelet count <100,000 platelets/mm^3) Cerebral disturbances Epigastric or RUQ pain HELLP	Severe headache Generalized edema RUQ or epigastric pain Visual disturbances Cerebral hemorrhage Renal failure HELLP

and abnormal liver enzymes (Cunningham et al., 2014). Despite the results of several research studies, the use of aspirin or supplementation with calcium, magnesium, zinc, or antioxidant therapy (vitamin C and E), salt restriction, diuretic therapy, or fish oils has not proved to prevent this destructive condition.

Preeclampsia is a two-stage event; the underlying mechanisms involved are vasospasm and hypoperfusion. In the first stage, the key feature is widespread vasospasm. In addition, endothelial injury occurs, leading to platelet adherence, fibrin deposition, and the presence of schistocytes (fragment of an erythrocyte). The second stage of preeclampsia is the woman's response to abnormal placentation, when symptoms appear, that is, hypertension, proteinuria, and edema due to hypoperfusion.

The first stage of generalized vasospasm results in elevation of blood pressure and reduced blood flow to the brain, liver, kidneys, placenta, and lungs. Decreased liver perfusion leads to impaired liver function and subcapsular hemorrhage. This is demonstrated by epigastric pain and elevated liver enzymes in the maternal serum. Decreased brain perfusion leads to small cerebral hemorrhages and symptoms of arterial vasospasm such as headaches, visual disturbances, blurred vision, and hyperactive deep tendon reflexes (DTRs). A thromboxane/prostacyclin imbalance leads to increased thromboxane (potent vasoconstrictor and stimulator of platelet aggregation) and decreased prostacyclin (potent vasodilator and inhibitor of platelet aggregation), which contribute to the hypertensive state. Decreased kidney perfusion reduces the glomerular filtration rate, resulting in decreased urine output and increased serum levels of sodium, BUN, uric acid, and creatinine, further increasing extracellular fluid and edema. Increased capillary permeability in the kidneys allows albumin to escape, which reduces plasma colloid osmotic pressure and moves more fluid into extracellular spaces; this leads to pulmonary edema and generalized edema. Poor placental perfusion resulting from prolonged vasoconstriction helps to contribute to intrauterine growth restriction, premature separation of the placenta (abruptio placentae), persistent fetal hypoxia, and acidosis. In addition, hemoconcentration (resulting from decreased intravascular volume) causes increased blood viscosity and elevated hematocrit (ACOG, 2014c).

Therapeutic Management

Management of the woman with preeclampsia varies depending on the severity of her condition and its effects on the fetus. Typically the woman is managed conservatively if she is experiencing mild symptoms. However, if the condition progresses, management becomes more aggressive. The "cure" for preeclampsia/eclampsia is always delivery of the placenta. The resolution following expulsion of the placenta supports theories related to the placental influence on the disease (Dekker, 2014). According to recent studies, prevention of preeclampsia should be considered with daily low-dose aspirin from 12 weeks' gestation and onward to women identified at high risk for it. While women with chronic hypertension or a personal history of preeclampsia should receive aspirin during pregnancy, further research should be ongoing to predict preeclampsia in low-risk women (Bujold, 2015).

MANAGEMENT FOR MILD PREECLAMPSIA

Conservative strategies for mild preeclampsia are used if the woman exhibits no signs of renal or hepatic dysfunction or coagulopathy. A woman with mild elevations in blood pressure may be placed on bed rest at home. She is encouraged to rest as much as possible in the lateral recumbent position to improve uteroplacental blood flow, reduce her blood pressure, and promote diuresis. In addition, antepartal visits and diagnostic testing – such as CBC, clotting studies, liver enzymes, and platelet levels – increase in frequency. The woman will be asked to monitor her blood pressure daily (every 4 to 6 hours while awake) and report any increased readings; she will also measure the amount of protein found in urine using a dipstick and will weigh herself for any weight gain. She also should take daily fetal movement counts, and if there is any decrease in movement, she needs to be evaluated by her health care provider that day. A balanced, nutritional diet with no sodium restriction is advised. In addition, she is encouraged to drink six to eight 8-oz glasses of water daily. If home management fails to reduce the blood pressure, admission to the hospital is warranted and the treatment strategy is individualized based on the severity of the condition and the gestational age at the time of diagnosis.

During the hospitalization, the woman with mild preeclampsia is monitored closely for signs and symptoms of severe preeclampsia or impending eclampsia (e.g., persistent headache, hyperreflexia). Blood pressure measurements are frequently recorded along with daily weights to detect excessive weight gain resulting from edema. Fetal surveillance is instituted in the form of daily fetal movement counts, nonstress testing, and serial ultrasounds to evaluate fetal growth and amniotic fluid volume to confirm fetal well-being. Expectant management (watchful waiting) usually continues until the pregnancy reaches term, fetal lung maturity is documented, or complications develop that warrant immediate birth. Women with mild preeclampsia are at greatest risk for postpartum hypertension (King et al., 2015).

Prevention of disease progression is the focus of treatment during labor. Blood pressure is monitored frequently and a quiet environment is important to minimize the risk of stimulation and to promote rest. IV magnesium sulfate is infused to prevent any seizure activity, along with antihypertensives if blood pressure values begin to rise. Calcium gluconate is kept at the bedside in case the magnesium level becomes toxic. Continued close monitoring of neurologic status is warranted to detect any signs or symptoms of hypoxemia, impending seizure activity, or increased intracranial pressure. An indwelling urinary (Foley) catheter usually is inserted to allow for accurate measurement of urine output.

MANAGEMENT FOR SEVERE PREECLAMPSIA

Severe preeclampsia may develop suddenly and bring with it high blood pressure of more than 160/110 mm Hg, proteinuria of more than 5 g in 24 hours, oliguria of less than 400 mL in 24 hours, cerebral and visual symptoms, and rapid weight gain. This clinical picture signals severe preeclampsia, and immediate hospitalization is needed.

Treatment is highly individualized and based on disease severity and fetal age. Birth of the infant is the only cure, because preeclampsia depends on the presence of trophoblastic tissue. Therefore, the exact age of the fetus is assessed to determine viability.

Severe preeclampsia is treated aggressively because hypertension poses a serious threat to mother and fetus. The goal of care is to stabilize the mother–fetus dyad and prepare for birth. Therapy focuses on controlling hypertension, preventing seizures, preventing long-term morbidity, and preventing maternal, fetal, or newborn death (Foo et al., 2015). Intense maternal and fetal surveillance starts when the mother enters the hospital and continues throughout her stay.

The woman in labor with severe preeclampsia typically receives oxytocin to stimulate uterine contractions and magnesium sulfate to prevent seizure activity. Oxytocin and magnesium sulfate can be given simultaneously via infusion pumps to ensure both are administered at the prescribed rate. Magnesium sulfate is given intravenously via an infusion pump. A loading dose of 4 to 6 g is given over 5 minutes. Then, a maintenance dose of 2 g/hr is given.

The client is evaluated closely for magnesium toxicity. If at all possible, a vaginal delivery is preferable to a cesarean birth for better maternal outcomes and less risk associated with a surgical birth. PGE2 gel may be used to ripen the cervix. A cesarean birth may be performed if the client is seriously ill. A pediatrician/neonatologist or neonatal nurse practitioner should be available in the birthing room to care for the newborn. A newborn whose mother received high doses of magnesium sulfate needs to be monitored for respiratory depression, hypocalcemia, and hypotonia. Decreased fetal heart rate variability may occur but, in general, magnesium sulfate does not pose a risk to the fetus. The newborn may exhibit respiratory depression, loss of reflexes, muscle weakness, and neurologic depression (Martin, Fanaroff, & Walsh, 2014).

MANAGEMENT OF ECLAMPSIA

In the woman who develops an eclamptic seizure, the convulsive activity begins with facial twitching, followed by generalized muscle rigidity. The woman's face initially may become distorted, with protrusion of the eyes, and foaming at the mouth may occur. Respirations cease for the duration of the seizure, resulting from muscle spasms, thus compromising fetal oxygenation. Seizure complications can include tongue biting, head trauma, broken bones, and aspiration. Coma usually follows the seizure activity, with respiration resuming. Eclamptic seizures are life-threatening emergencies and require immediate treatment to decrease maternal morbidity and mortality.

As with any seizure, the initial management is to clear the airway and administer adequate oxygen. Positioning the woman on her left side and protecting her from injury during the seizure are key. Suction equipment must be readily available to remove secretions from her mouth after the seizure is over. IV fluids are administered after the seizure at a rate to replace urine output and additional insensible losses. Fetal heart rate is monitored closely. Magnesium sulfate is administered intravenously to prevent further seizures. Serum magnesium levels, respiratory rate, reflexes, and urine output in women receiving magnesium sulfate are closely monitored to avoid magnesium toxicity and prevent cardiac arrest. Calcium gluconate (1 g intravenously) is typically ordered to counteract magnesium toxicity. Hypertension is controlled with antihypertensive medications. After the woman's seizures are controlled, her stability is assessed. If she is found stable, birth via induction or cesarean birth is performed (Amorim et al., 2015). If the woman's condition remains stable, she will be transferred to the postpartum unit for care. If she becomes unstable after giving birth, she may be transferred to the critical care unit for closer observation.

Nursing Assessment

Preventing complications related to preeclampsia requires the use of assessment, advocacy, and counseling skills. Assessment begins with the accurate measurement of the client's blood pressure at each encounter. In addition, nurses need to assess for subjective complaints that may indicate progression of the disease—visual changes, severe headaches, unusual bleeding or bruising, or epigastric pain (Nagtalon-Ramos, 2014). The significant signs of preeclampsia – proteinuria and hypertension – occur without the woman's awareness. Unfortunately, by the time symptoms are noticed, gestational hypertension can be severe.

Take Note!

The absolute blood pressure (value that validates elevation) of 140/90 mm Hg should be obtained on two occasions 4 to 6 hours apart to be diagnostic of preeclampsia. Proteinuria is defined as 300 mg or more of urinary protein per 24 hours or more than 1+ protein by chemical reagent strip or dipstick of at least two random urine samples collected at least 4 to 6 hours apart with no evidence of urinary tract infection (ACOG, 2014c).

HEALTH HISTORY AND PHYSICAL EXAMINATION

Take a thorough history during the first antepartal visit to identify whether the woman is at risk for preeclampsia. Risk factors include:

- Primigravida status
- Chromosomal abnormalities
- Structural congenital anomalies
- Multiple gestation
- History of preeclampsia in a previous pregnancy
- Excessive placental tissue, as is seen in women with GTD
- Chronic stress
- Use of ovulation drugs
- Family history of preeclampsia (mother or sister)
- Lower socioeconomic status
- History of diabetes, hypertension, or renal disease
- Poor nutrition
- Lower socioeconomic status
- African-American ethnicity
- Age extremes (younger than 20 or older than 35)
- Obesity (Ross, 2015).

In addition, complete a nutritional assessment that includes the woman's usual intake of protein, calcium, daily calories, and fluids.

Women at risk for preeclampsia require more frequent prenatal visits throughout their pregnancy, and they require teaching about problems so that they can report them promptly.

Blood pressure must be measured carefully and consistently. Obtain all measurements with the woman in the same position (blood pressure is highest in the sitting position and lowest in the side-lying position) and by using the same technique (automated vs. manual). This standardization in position and technique will yield the most accurate readings (Norwitz, 2015).

Obtain the client's weight (noting gain since last visit), and assess for amount and location of edema. Asking questions such as "Do your rings still fit on your fingers?" or "Is your face puffy when you get up in the morning?" will help to determine whether fluid retention is present or if the woman's status has changed since her last visit.

Take Note!

Although edema is not a cardinal sign of preeclampsia, weight should be monitored frequently to identify sudden gains in a short time span. Current research relies less on the classic triad of symptoms (hypertension, proteinuria, and edema or weight gain) and more on decreased organ perfusion, endothelial dysfunction (capillary leaking and proteinuria), and elevated blood pressure as key indicators (Carson & Gibson, 2015).

If edema is present, assess the distribution, degree, and pitting. Document your findings and identify whether the edema is dependent or pitting. Dependent edema is present on the lower half of the body if the client is ambulatory, where hydrostatic pressure is greatest. It is usually observed in the feet and ankles or in the sacral area if the client is on bed rest. Pitting edema is edema that leaves a small depression or pit after finger pressure is applied to a swollen area (Carson & Gibson, 2014). Record the depth of pitting demonstrated when pressure is applied. Although subjective, the following is used to record relative degrees:

- 1+ pitting edema = 2-mm depression into skin; disappears rapidly
- 2+ pitting edema = 4-mm skin depression; disappears in 10 to 15 seconds
- 3+ pitting edema = 6-mm depression into skin; lasts more than 1 minute
- 4+ pitting edema = 8-mm depression into skin; lasts 2 to 3 minutes

At every antepartal visit, assess the fetal heart rate with a Doppler device. Also check a clean-catch urine specimen for protein using a dipstick.

LABORATORY AND DIAGNOSTIC TESTING

Various laboratory tests may be performed to evaluate the woman's status. Typically these include a CBC, serum electrolytes, BUN, creatinine, and hepatic enzyme levels. Urine specimens are checked for protein; if levels are 1 to 2+ or greater, a 24-hour urine collection is completed.

Nursing Management

Nursing management of the woman with preeclampsia focuses on close monitoring of blood pressure and ongoing assessment for evidence of disease progression. Throughout the client's pregnancy, fetal surveillance is essential.

INTERVENING FOR PREECLAMPSIA

The woman with mild preeclampsia requires frequent monitoring to detect changes because preeclampsia can progress rapidly. Instruct all women in the signs and symptoms of preeclampsia and urge them to contact their health care professional for immediate evaluation should any occur.

Typically, women with mild preeclampsia can be managed at home if they have a good understanding of the disease process, blood pressure and vital signs are stable, there are no abnormal laboratory test results, and if good fetal movement is demonstrated (Teaching Guidelines 19.2). The home care nurse makes frequent visits and follow-up phone calls to assess the woman's condition, to assist with scheduling periodic evaluations of the fetus (such as nonstress tests), and to evaluate any changes that might suggest a worsening of the woman's condition.

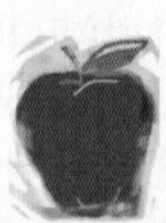

Teaching Guidelines 19.2

TEACHING FOR THE WOMAN WITH MILD PREECLAMPSIA

- Rest in a quiet environment to prevent cerebral disturbances.
- Drink 8 to 10 glasses of water daily.
- Consume a balanced, high-protein diet including high-fiber foods.
- Obtain intermittent bed rest to improve circulation to the heart and uterus.
- Limit your physical activity to promote urination and subsequent decrease in blood pressure.
- Enlist the aid of your family so that you can obtain appropriate rest time.
- Perform self-monitoring as instructed, including:
  - Taking your own blood pressure twice daily
  - Checking and recording weight daily
  - Performing urine dipstick twice daily
  - Recording the number of fetal kicks daily
- Contact the home health nurse if any of the following occurs:
  - Increase in blood pressure
  - Protein present in urine
  - Gain of more than 1 pound in 1 week
  - Burning or frequency when urinating
  - Decrease in fetal activity or movement
  - Headache (forehead or posterior neck region)
  - Dizziness or visual disturbances
  - Increase in swelling in hands, feet, legs, and face
  - Stomach pain, excessive heartburn, or epigastric pain
  - Decreased or infrequent urination
  - Contractions or low back pain
  - Easy or excessive bruising
  - Sudden onset of abdominal pain
  - Nausea and vomiting

Early detection and management of mild preeclampsia is associated with the greatest success in reducing progression of this condition. As long as the client carries out the guidelines of care as outlined by the health care provider and remains stable, home care can continue to maintain the pregnancy until the fetus is mature. If disease progression occurs, hospitalization is required.

INTERVENING FOR SEVERE PREECLAMPSIA

The woman with severe preeclampsia requires hospitalization. Maintain the client on complete bed rest in the left lateral lying position. Ensure that the room is dark and quiet to reduce stimulation. Give sedatives as ordered to encourage quiet bed rest. The client is at risk for seizures if the condition progresses. Therefore, institute and maintain seizure precautions, such as padding the side rails and having oxygen, suction equipment, and call light readily available to protect the client from injury.

Take Note!

Preeclampsia increases the risk of placental abruption, preterm birth, intrauterine growth restriction, and fetal distress during childbirth. Always be prepared if you see symptoms of preeclampsia!

Closely monitor the client's blood pressure. Administer antihypertensives as ordered to reduce blood pressure (Drug Guide 19.3). Assess the client's vision and level of consciousness. Report any changes and any complaints of headache or visual disturbances. Offer a high-protein diet with 8 to 10 glasses of water daily. Monitor the client's intake and output every hour and administer fluid and electrolyte replacements as ordered. Assess the woman for signs and symptoms of pulmonary edema, such as crackles and wheezing heard on auscultation, dyspnea, decreased oxygen saturation levels, cough, neck vein distention, anxiety, and restlessness.

DRUG GUIDE 19.3 MEDICATIONS USED WITH PREECLAMPSIA AND ECLAMPSIA

Medication	Action/Indications	Nursing Implications
Magnesium sulfate	Blockage of neuromuscular transmission, vasodilation Prevention and treatment of eclamptic seizures	Loading dose of 4–6 g by IV in 100 mL of fluid administered over 15–20 minutes, followed by a maintenance dose of 2 g as a continuous intravenous infusion. Monitor serum magnesium levels closely. Assess DTRs and check for ankle clonus. Have calcium gluconate readily available in case of toxicity. Monitor for signs and symptoms of toxicity, such as flushing, sweating, hypotension, and cardiac and central nervous system depression.
Hydralazine hydrochloride (Apresoline)	Vascular smooth muscle relaxant, thus improving perfusion to renal, uterine, and cerebral areas Reduction in blood pressure	Administer 5–10 mg by slow intravenous bolus every 20 min as needed. Use parenteral form immediately after opening ampule. Withdraw drug slowly to prevent possible rebound hypertension. Monitor for adverse effects such as palpitations, headache, tachycardia, anorexia, nausea, vomiting, and diarrhea.
Labetalol hydrochloride (Normodyne)	Alpha-1 and beta blocker Reduction in blood pressure	Be aware that drug lowers blood pressure without decreasing maternal heart rate or cardiac output. Administer IV dose of 20–40 mg every 15 min as needed and then administer intravenous infusion of 2 mg/min until desired blood pressure value achieved. Monitor for possible adverse effects such as gastric pain, flatulence, constipation, dizziness, vertigo, and fatigue.
Nifedipine (Procardia)	Calcium channel blocker/dilation of coronary arteries, arterioles, and peripheral arterioles Reduction in blood pressure, stoppage of preterm labor	Administer 10–20 mg orally for three doses and then every 4–8 hr. Monitor for possible adverse effects such as dizziness, peripheral edema, angina, diarrhea, nasal congestions, cough.
Sodium nitroprusside	Rapid vasodilation (arterial and venous) Severe hypertension requiring rapid reduction in blood pressure	Administer via continuous IV infusion with dose titrated according to blood pressure levels. Wrap intravenous infusion solution in foil or opaque material to protect from light. Monitor for possible adverse effects, such as apprehension, restlessness, retrosternal pressure, palpitations, diaphoresis, and abdominal pain.
Furosemide (Lasix)	Diuretic action, inhibiting the reabsorption of sodium and chloride from the ascending loop of Henle Pulmonary edema (used only if condition is present)	Administer via slow IV bolus at a dose of 10–40 mg over 1–2 min. Monitor urine output hourly. Assess for possible adverse effects such as dizziness, vertigo, orthostatic hypotension, anorexia, vomiting, electrolyte imbalances, muscle cramps, and muscle spasms.

Adapted from King, T. L., Brucker, M. C., Kriebs, J. M., Fahey, J. O., Grgor, C. L., & Varney, H. (2015). *Varney's midwifery* (5th ed.). Burlington, MA: Jones & Bartlett Learning; and Skidmore-Roth, L. (2015). *Mosby's 2015 nursing drug reference* (28th ed.). Philadelphia, PA: Elsevier Health Science.

The treatment of acute pulmonary edema is symptomatic and includes the administration of vasodilating agents and of diuretics. The development of acute pulmonary edema in women with hypertension during pregnancy is associated with high levels of IV fluid administration (Pauli & Repke, 2015).

To achieve a safe outcome for the fetus, prepare the woman for possible testing to evaluate fetal status as preeclampsia progresses. Testing may include the nonstress test, serial ultrasounds to track fetal growth, amniocentesis to determine fetal lung maturity, Doppler velocimetry to screen for fetal compromise, and biophysical profile to evaluate ongoing fetal well-being (Mattson & Smith, 2016).

Other laboratory tests may be performed to monitor the disease process and to determine if it is progressing into HELLP syndrome. These include liver enzymes such as lactic dehydrogenase (LDH), ALT, and AST; chemistry panel, such as creatinine, BUN, uric acid, and glucose; CBC, including platelet count; coagulation studies, such as PT, PTT, fibrinogen, and bleeding time; and a 24-hour urine collection for protein and creatinine clearance.

Administer parenteral magnesium sulfate as ordered to prevent seizures. Assess DTRs to evaluate the effectiveness of therapy. Clients with preeclampsia commonly present with hyperreflexia. Severe preeclampsia causes changes in the cortex, which disrupts the equilibrium of impulses between the cerebral cortex and the spinal cord. Brisk reflexes (hyperreflexia) are the result of an irritable cortex and indicate central nervous system (CNS) involvement (Marik, 2015). Diminished or absent reflexes occur when the client develops magnesium toxicity. Because magnesium is a potent neuromuscular blockade, the afferent and efferent nerve pathways do not relay messages properly and hyporeflexia develops. Common sites used to assess DTRs are biceps reflex, triceps reflex, patellar reflex, Achilles reflex, and plantar reflex. Nursing Procedure 19.1 highlights the steps for assessing the patellar reflex.

The National Institute of Neurological Disorders and Stroke, a division of the National Institutes of Health, published a scale in the early 1990s that, although subjective, is used widely today. It grades reflexes from 0 to 4+. Grades 2+ and 3+ are considered normal, whereas grades 0 and 4 may indicate pathology (Table 19.2). Because these are subjective assessments, to improve communication of reflex results, condensed descriptor categories such as absent, average, brisk, or clonus should be used rather than numeric codes (Magowan et al., 2014).

Clonus is the presence of rhythmic involuntary contractions, most often at the foot or ankle. Sustained clonus confirms CNS involvement. Nursing Procedure 19.2 highlights the steps when testing for ankle clonus.

With magnesium sulfate administration, the client is at risk for magnesium toxicity. Closely assess the client for signs of toxicity, which include a respiratory rate of less than 12 breaths per minute, absence of DTRs, and a decrease in urinary output (<30 mL/hr). Also monitor serum magnesium levels. Although exact levels may vary among agencies, serum magnesium levels ranging from 4 to 7 mEq/L are considered therapeutic, whereas levels more than 8 mEq/dL are generally considered toxic. As levels increase, the woman is at risk for severe problems:

- 10 mEq/L: possible loss of DTRs
- 15 mEq/L: possible respiratory depression
- 25 mEq/L: possible cardiac arrest (Skidmore-Roth, 2015).

NURSING PROCEDURE 19.1

Assessing the Patellar Reflex

Purpose: To Evaluate for Nervous System Irritability Related to Preeclampsia

1. Place the woman in the supine position (or sitting upright with the legs dangling freely over the side of the bed or examination table).
2. If lying supine, have the woman flex her knee slightly.
3. Place a hand under the knee to support the leg and locate the patellar tendon. It should be midline just below the knee cap.
4. Using a reflex hammer or the side of your hand, strike the area of the patellar tendon firmly and quickly.
5. Note the movement of the leg and foot. A patellar reflex occurs when the leg and foot move (documented as 2+).
6. Repeat the procedure on the opposite leg.

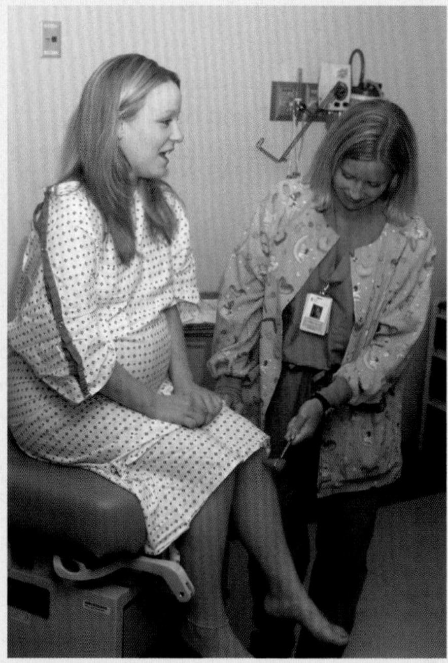

TABLE 19.2 GRADING DEEP TENDON REFLEXES

Description of Finding	Grade
Reflex absent, none elicited	0
Hypoactive response, sluggish	1
Reflex in lower half of normal range	2
Reflex in upper half of normal range	3
Hyperactive, brisk, clonus present	4

Adapted from King, T. L., Brucker, M. C., Kriebs, J. M., Fahey, J. O., Grgor, C. L., & Varney, H. (2015). *Varney's midwifery* (5th ed.). Burlington, MA: Jones & Bartlett Learning; & Nagtalon-Ramos, J. (2014). *Maternal-newborn nursing care: Best evidence-based practices.* Philadelphia, PA: F. A. Davis Company.

If signs and symptoms of magnesium toxicity develop, expect to administer calcium gluconate as the antidote.

Throughout the client's stay, closely monitor her for signs and symptoms of labor. Perform continuous electronic fetal monitoring to assess fetal well-being. Note trends in baseline rate and presence or absence of accelerations or decelerations. Also observe for signs of fetal distress and report them immediately. Administer glucocorticoid treatment as ordered to enhance fetal lung maturity and prepare for labor induction if the mother's condition warrants.

Keep the client and family informed of the woman's condition and educate them about the course of treatment. Provide emotional support for the client and family. Severe preeclampsia is very frightening for the client and her family, and most expectant mothers are very anxious about their own health as well as that of the fetus. To allay anxiety, use light touch to comfort and reassure her that the necessary actions are being taken. Actively listening to her concerns and fears and communicating them to the health care provider are important to keep open the lines of communication. Offering praise for small accomplishments can provide positive reinforcement for effective behaviors.

INTERVENING FOR ECLAMPSIA

The onset of seizure activity identifies eclampsia. Typically, eclamptic seizures are generalized and start with facial twitching. The body then becomes rigid, in a state of tonic muscular contraction. The clonic phase of the seizure involves alternating contraction and relaxation of all body muscles. Respirations stop during seizure

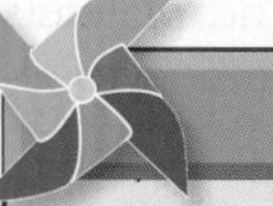

NURSING PROCEDURE 19.2

Testing for Ankle Clonus

Purpose: To Evaluate for Nervous System Irritability Related to Preeclampsia

1. Place the woman in the supine position.
2. Have the client slightly bend her knee and place a hand under the knee to support it.
3. Dorsiflex the foot briskly and then quickly release it.
4. Watch for the foot to rebound smoothly against your hand. If the movement is smooth without any rapid contractions of the ankle or calf muscle, then clonus is not present; if the movement is jerky and rapid, clonus is present.
5. Repeat on the opposite side.

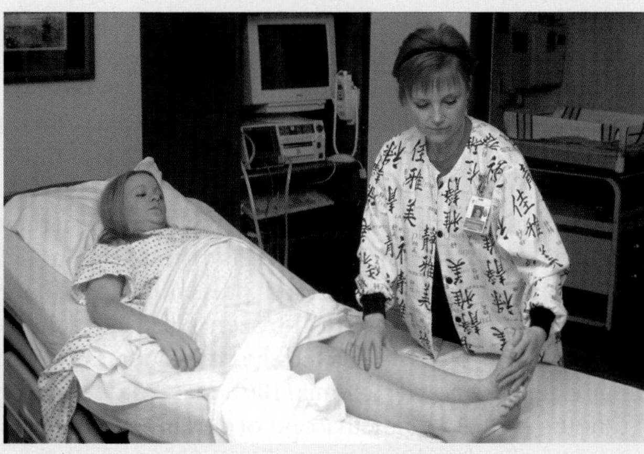

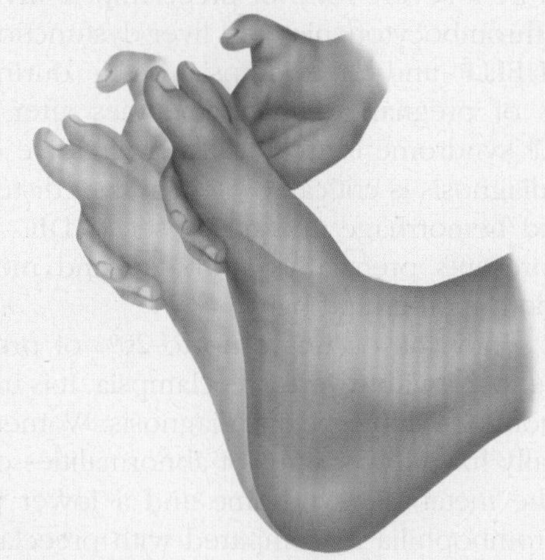

activity and resume shortly after it ends. Client safety is the primary concern during eclamptic seizures. If possible, turn the client to her side and remain with her. Make sure that the side rails are up and padded. Dim the lights and keep the room quiet.

Document the time and sequence of events as soon as possible. After the seizure activity has ceased, suction the nasopharynx as necessary and administer oxygen. Continue the magnesium sulfate infusion to prevent further seizures. Ensure continuous electronic fetal monitoring, evaluating fetal status for changes. Also assess the client for uterine contractions. After the client is stabilized, prepare her for the birthing process as soon as possible to reduce the risk of perinatal mortality.

PROVIDING FOLLOW-UP CARE

After delivery of the newborn, continue to monitor the client for signs and symptoms of preeclampsia/eclampsia for at least 48 hours. Expect to continue to administer magnesium sulfate infusion for 24 hours to prevent seizure activity, and monitor serum magnesium levels for toxicity.

Assess vital signs at least every 4 hours, along with routine postpartum assessments: fundus, lochia, breasts, bladder, bowels, and the woman's emotional state. Monitor urine output closely. Diuresis is a positive sign that, along with a decrease in proteinuria, signals resolution of the disease.

HELLP SYNDROME

HELLP syndrome is an acronym for hemolysis, elevated liver enzymes, and low platelet count. It is a variant of the preeclampsia/eclampsia syndrome that occurs in 10% to 20% of clients whose conditions are labeled as severe. Women with HELLP syndrome are at increased risk for complications such as cerebral hemorrhage, retinal detachment, hematoma/liver rupture, acute renal failure, disseminated intravascular coagulation (DIC), placental abruption and maternal death (Vigil-De Gracia, 2015). It is a life-threatening obstetric complication considered by many to be a severe form of preeclampsia involving hemolysis, thrombocytopenia, and liver dysfunction.

Both HELLP and preeclampsia occur during the later stages of pregnancy, and sometimes after childbirth. HELLP syndrome is a clinically progressive condition. Early diagnosis is critical to prevent liver distention, rupture, and hemorrhage and the onset of DIC. If the condition presents prenatally, morbidity and mortality can affect both mother and baby.

HELLP syndrome occurs in up to 20% of pregnant women diagnosed with severe preeclampsia. It is unique, as it is a laboratory-value specific diagnosis. Women with HELLP usually have fewer signs of abnormalities consistent with the metabolic syndrome and a lower prevalence of thrombophilia as compared with preeclampsia women without HELLP (Sibai, 2015). Although it has been reported as early as 17 weeks' gestation, most of the time it is diagnosed between 22 and 36 weeks' gestation (Cunningham et al., 2014). It can present prior to the presence of an elevated blood pressure. HELLP syndrome leads to an increased maternal risk for developing liver hematoma or rupture, stroke, cardiac arrest, seizure, pulmonary edema, DIC, subendocardial hemorrhage, adult respiratory distress syndrome, renal damage, sepsis, hypoxic encephalopathy, and maternal or fetal death (Moses, 2015b). The recognition of HELLP syndrome and an aggressive multidisciplinary approach and prompt transfer of these women to obstetric centers with expertise in this field are required for the improvement of maternal-fetal prognosis.

Pathophysiology

The hemolysis that occurs is termed microangiopathic hemolytic anemia. This cascade of events is thought to happen when red blood cells become fragmented as they pass through small, damaged blood vessels. Elevated liver enzymes are the result of reduced blood flow to the liver secondary to obstruction from fibrin deposits. At the same time, endothelial damage and fibrin deposition in the liver may lead to liver impairment and can result in hemorrhagic necrosis, indicated by right upper quadrant tenderness, nausea, and vomiting. Hyperbilirubinemia and jaundice result from liver impairment. Low platelets result from vascular damage, the result of vasospasm, and platelets aggregate at sites of damage, resulting in thrombocytopenia in multiple sites (Khan & Meirowitz, 2015).

Therapeutic Management

The treatment for HELLP syndrome is based on the severity of the disease, the gestational age of the fetus, and the condition of the mother and fetus. The mainstay of treatment is lowering of high blood pressure with rapid-acting antihypertensive agents, prevention of convulsions or further seizures with magnesium sulfate, and use of steroids for fetal lung maturity if necessary, followed by the birth of the infant and placenta (Foley et al., 2014). The client should be admitted or transferred to a tertiary center with a neonatal intensive care unit. Additional treatment includes correction of the coagulopathies that accompany HELLP syndrome. After this syndrome is diagnosed and the woman's condition is stable, birth of the infant is indicated.

Magnesium sulfate is used prophylactically to prevent seizures. Antihypertensives such as hydralazine or labetalol are given to control blood pressure. Blood component therapy – such as fresh-frozen plasma, packed red blood cells, or platelets – is transfused to address the microangiopathic hemolytic anemia. Birth may be delayed up to 96 hours so that betamethasone or dexamethasone can be given to stimulate lung maturation in the preterm fetus.

Nursing Assessment

Nursing assessment of the woman with HELLP is similar to that for the woman with severe preeclampsia. Be alert for complaints of nausea (with or without vomiting), malaise, epigastric or right upper quadrant pain, and demonstrable edema. Perform systematic assessments frequently, as indicated by the woman's condition and response to therapy.

A diagnosis of HELLP syndrome is made based on laboratory test results, including:

- Low hematocrit that is not explained by any blood loss
- Elevated LDH (liver impairment)
- Elevated AST (liver impairment)
- Elevated ALT (liver impairment)
- Elevated BUN
- Elevated bilirubin level
- Elevated uric acid and creatinine levels (renal involvement)
- Low platelet count (less than 100,000 cells/mm^3)

Nursing Management

Nursing management of the woman diagnosed with HELLP syndrome is the same as that for the woman with severe preeclampsia. If possible, the woman with HELLP syndrome should be transferred to a tertiary care center once she has been assessed and stabilized. Closely monitor the client for changes and provide ongoing support throughout this experience.

GESTATIONAL DIABETES

Gestational diabetes is a condition involving glucose intolerance that occurs during pregnancy. It is discussed in greater detail in Chapter 20.

BLOOD INCOMPATIBILITY

Blood incompatibility most commonly involves one of two issues: blood type or the Rh factor. *Blood type incompatibility*, also known as ABO incompatibility, arises when a mother with blood type O becomes pregnant with a fetus with a different blood type (type A, B, or AB). The mother's serum contains naturally occurring anti-A and anti-B, which can cross the placenta and hemolyze fetal red blood cells. It is usually less severe than Rh incompatibility. One reason is that fetal red blood cells express less of the ABO blood group antigens compared with adult levels. In addition, in contrast to the Rh antigens, the ABO blood group antigens are expressed by a variety of fetal (and adult) tissues, reducing the chances of anti-A and anti-B binding their target antigens on the fetal red blood cells. ABO incompatibility rarely causes significant hemolysis, and prenatal treatment is not warranted.

Rh isoimmunization occurs when a pregnant woman's immune system creates antibodies against fetal Rh blood factors. Although the mother will exhibit no symptoms of Rh incompatibility, Rh antibodies adversely affect fetal health. Rh antibodies can cause fetal heart problems, breathing difficulties, jaundice, and a form of anemia known as hemolytic disease of the newborn. Rh sensitization occurs in approximately 1 in 1,000 births to Rh-negative women (March of Dimes, 2015d). Today Rh isoimmunization in pregnant women and hemolytic disease of the newborn are rarely seen, primarily because women who are Rh negative are given anti-D immune globulin prophylaxis (RhoGAM) in the third trimester of pregnancy and after childbirth if the newborn is Rh positive.

Pathophysiology

ABO Incompatibility

Hemolysis associated with ABO incompatibility is limited to type O mothers with fetuses who have type A or B blood. In mothers with type A and B blood, naturally occurring antibodies are of the IgM class, which do not cross the placenta, whereas in type O mothers, the antibodies are predominantly IgG in nature. Because A and B antigens are widely expressed in a variety of tissues besides red blood cells, only a small portion of the antibodies crossing the placenta is available to bind to fetal red cells. In addition, fetal red cells appear to have less surface expression of A or B antigen, resulting in few reactive sites—hence the low incidence of significant hemolysis in affected neonates.

With ABO incompatibility, usually the mother is blood type O, with anti-A and anti-B antibodies in her serum; the infant is blood type A, B, or AB. The incompatibility arises as a result of the interaction of antibodies present in maternal serum and the antigen sites on the fetal red cells.

Rh Incompatibility

Rh incompatibility is a condition that develops when a woman with Rh-negative blood type is exposed to Rh-positive blood cells and subsequently develops circulating titers of Rh antibodies. Individuals with Rh-positive blood type have the D antigen present on their red cells, whereas individuals with an Rh-negative blood type do not. The presence or absence of the Rh antigen on the RBC membrane is genetically controlled.

In the United States, about 15% of the White population, 5% to 8% of the African American and Hispanic populations, and 1% to 2% of the Asian and Native American populations are Rh negative. The vast majority (85%) of individuals is considered Rh positive (March of Dimes, 2015d).

Rh incompatibility most commonly arises with exposure of an Rh-negative mother to Rh-positive fetal blood during pregnancy or birth, during which time erythrocytes from the fetal circulation leak into the maternal circulation.

Isoimmunization can also occur during an amniocentesis, ectopic pregnancy, placenta previa, placenta abruption, in utero fetal death, spontaneous abortion, or abdominal/ pelvic trauma. After a significant exposure, alloimmunization or sensitization occurs. As a result, maternal antibodies are produced against the foreign Rh antigen.

Theoretically, fetal blood and maternal blood do not mix during pregnancy. In reality, however, small placental accidents (transplacental bleeds secondary to minor separation), abortions, ectopic pregnancy, abdominal trauma, trophoblastic disease, amniocentesis, placenta previa, and abruptio placentae allow fetal blood to enter the maternal circulation and initiate the production of antibodies to destroy Rh-positive blood. The amount of fetal blood necessary to produce Rh incompatibility varies. In one study, less than 1 mL of Rh-positive blood was shown to result in sensitization of women who are Rh negative (Salem & Singer, 2015).

Once sensitized, it takes approximately a month for Rh antibodies in the maternal circulation to cross over into the fetal circulation. In 90% of cases, sensitization occurs during delivery (Cunningham et al., 2014). Thus, most first-born infants with Rh-positive blood type are not affected because the short period from first exposure of Rh-positive fetal erythrocytes to the birth of the infant is insufficient to produce a significant maternal IgG antibody response.

The risk and severity of alloimmune response increase with each subsequent pregnancy involving a fetus with Rh-positive blood. A second pregnancy with an Rh-positive fetus often produces a mildly anemic infant, whereas succeeding pregnancies produce infants with more serious hemolytic anemia.

Nursing Assessment

At the first prenatal visit, determine the woman's blood type and Rh status. Also obtain a thorough health history, noting any reports of previous events involving hemorrhage to delineate the risk for prior sensitization. When the client's history reveals an Rh-negative mother who may be pregnant with an Rh-positive fetus, prepare the client for an antibody screen (indirect Coombs test) to determine whether she has developed isoimmunity to the Rh antigen. This test detects unexpected circulating antibodies in a woman's serum that could be harmful to the fetus (Davidson, 2014).

Nursing Management

If the indirect Coombs test is negative (meaning no antibodies are present), then the woman is a candidate for RhoGAM. If the test is positive, RhoGAM is of no value because isoimmunization has occurred. In this case, the fetus is carefully monitored for hemolytic disease.

The incidence of isoimmunization has declined dramatically as a result of prenatal and postnatal RhoGAM administration after any event in which blood transfer may occur. The standard dose is 300 mcg, which is effective for 15 mL of fetal blood cells. Rh immunoglobulin helps to destroy any fetal cells in the maternal circulation before sensitization occurs, thus inhibiting maternal antibody production. This provides temporary passive immunity, thereby preventing maternal sensitization.

The current recommendation is for every Rh-negative nonimmunized woman to receive RhoGAM at some point between 28 and 32 weeks' gestation and again within 72 hours after giving birth. Other indications for RhoGAM include:

- Ectopic pregnancy
- Chorionic villus sampling
- Amniocentesis
- Prenatal hemorrhage
- Molar pregnancy
- Maternal trauma
- Percutaneous umbilical sampling
- Therapeutic or spontaneous abortion
- Fetal death
- Fetal surgery (King et al., 2015).

Despite the availability of RhoGAM and laboratory tests to identify women and newborns at risk, isoimmunization remains a serious clinical reality that continues to contribute to perinatal and neonatal mortality. Nurses, as client advocates, are in a unique position to make sure test results are brought to the health care provider's attention so appropriate interventions can be initiated. In addition, nurses must stay abreast of current literature and research regarding isoimmunization and its management. Stress to all women that early prenatal care can help identify and prevent this condition. Because Rh incompatibility is preventable with the use of RhoGAM, prevention remains the best treatment. Nurses can make a tremendous impact to ensure positive outcomes for the greatest possible number of pregnancies through education.

AMNIOTIC FLUID IMBALANCES

Amniotic fluid develops from several maternal and fetal structures, including the amnion, chorion, maternal blood, fetal lungs, gastrointestinal tract, kidneys, and skin. Any alteration in one or more of the various sources will alter the amount of amniotic fluid. Polyhydramnios and oligohydramnios are two imbalances associated with amniotic fluid.

Polyhydramnios

Polyhydramnios, also called hydramnios, is a condition in which there is too much amniotic fluid (more than 2,000 mL) surrounding the fetus between 32 and 36 weeks. It occurs in approximately 2% of all pregnancies and is associated with fetal anomalies of development such as upper gastrointestinal obstruction or atresias, neural tube defects, and anterior abdominal wall defects, together with impaired swallowing in fetuses with chromosomal anomalies, such as trisomy 13 and 18 (Carter & Boyd, 2015). Approximately 18% of all women with diabetes will develop polyhydramnios during their pregnancy. There is an increase in cesarean births for fetal labor intolerance, low 5-minute Apgar scores, increased neonatal birth weight, congenital anomalies, and newborn intensive care unit admissions for women with too much amniotic fluid at term (Moore, 2015). Overall, it is associated with poorer fetal outcomes because of the increased incidence of preterm births, fetal malpresentation, and cord prolapse.

There are several causes of polyhydramnios. Generally, too much fluid is being produced, there is a problem with the fluid being taken up, or both. It can be associated with maternal disease and fetal anomalies, but it can also be idiopathic (of unknown cause) in nature.

Therapeutic Management

Treatment may include close monitoring and frequent follow-up visits with the health care provider if the polyhydramnios is mild to moderate. In severe cases in which the woman is in pain and experiencing shortness of breath, an amniocentesis or artificial rupture of the membranes is done to reduce the fluid and the pressure. Removal of fluid by amniocentesis is only transiently effective. A noninvasive treatment may involve the use of a prostaglandin synthesis inhibitor (indomethacin) to decrease amniotic fluid volume by decreasing fetal urinary output, but this may cause premature closure of the fetal ductus arteriosus (King et al., 2015).

Nursing Assessment

Begin the assessment with a thorough history, being alert to risk factors such as maternal diabetes or multiple gestations. Review the maternal history for information about possible fetal anomalies including fetal esophageal or intestinal atresia, neural tube defects, chromosomal deviations, fetal hydrops, CNS or cardiovascular anomalies, and hydrocephaly.

Determine the gestational age of the fetus and measure the woman's fundal height. With polyhydramnios, there is a discrepancy between fundal height and gestational age, or a rapid growth of the uterus is noted. Assess the woman for complaints of discomfort in her abdomen, such as being severely stretched and tight. Also note any reports of uterine contractions, which may result from overstretching of the uterus. Assess for shortness of breath resulting from pressure on her diaphragm and inspect her lower extremities for edema, which results from increased pressure on the vena cava. Palpate the abdomen and obtain fetal heart rate. Often the fetal parts and heart rate are difficult to obtain because of the excess fluid present.

Prepare the woman for possible diagnostic testing to evaluate for the presence of possible fetal anomalies. An ultrasound usually is done to measure the pockets of amniotic fluid to estimate the total volume. In some cases, ultrasound also is helpful in finding the etiology of polyhydramnios, such as multiple pregnancy or a fetal structural anomaly.

Nursing Management

Nursing management of the woman with polyhydramnios focuses on ongoing assessment and monitoring for symptoms of abdominal pain, dyspnea, uterine contractions, and edema of the lower extremities. Explain to the woman and her family that this condition can cause her uterus to become overdistended and may lead to preterm labor and preterm rupture of membranes. Outline the signs and symptoms of both conditions and instruct the woman to contact her health care provider if they occur. If a therapeutic amniocentesis is performed, assist the health care provider and monitor maternal and fetal status throughout for any changes.

Oligohydramnios

Oligohydramnios is a decreased amount of amniotic fluid (less than 500 mL) between 32 and 36 weeks' gestation. It occurs in approximately 4% of all pregnancies. Oligohydramnios may result from any condition that prevents the fetus from making urine or blocks it from going into the amniotic sac. Oligohydramnios occurs in about 4 out of every 100 pregnancies. It is most common in the last trimester of pregnancy, but it can develop at any time in the pregnancy. About one out of eight women whose pregnancies last 2 weeks past the due date develops oligohydramnios. This happens as amniotic fluid levels naturally decline. This condition puts the fetus at an increased risk of perinatal morbidity and mortality (March of Dimes, 2015e). Reduction in amniotic fluid reduces the ability of the fetus to move freely without risk of cord compression, which increases the risk for fetal death and intrapartal hypoxia.

Therapeutic Management

The woman with oligohydramnios can be managed on an outpatient basis with serial ultrasounds and fetal surveillance through nonstress testing and biophysical profiles. As long as fetal well-being is demonstrated with frequent testing, no intervention is necessary. If fetal well-being is compromised, however, birth is planned along with amnioinfusion (the transvaginal infusion of crystalloid fluid to compensate for the lost amniotic fluid). The fluid is introduced into the uterus through an intrauterine pressure catheter. The infusion is administered in a controlled fashion to prevent overdistention of the uterus. Amnioinfusion is thought to improve abnormal fetal heart rate patterns, decrease cesarean births, and possibly minimize the risk of neonatal meconium aspiration syndrome, but more studies need to be done to validate this (Carter & Boyd, 2015).

Nursing Assessment

Review the maternal history for factors associated with oligohydramnios, including:

- Uteroplacental insufficiency
- PROM prior to labor onset
- Hypertension of pregnancy
- Maternal diabetes
- Intrauterine growth restriction
- Postterm pregnancy
- Fetal renal agenesis
- Polycystic kidneys
- Urinary tract obstructions

Assess the client for complaints of fluid leaking from the vagina. Leaking of amniotic fluid from the vagina occurs with rupture of the amniotic sac. Leaking in conjunction with a uterus that is small for expected dates of gestation also suggests oligohydramnios. Unfortunately, the woman may not present with any symptoms. Typically, the reduced volume of amniotic fluid is identified on ultrasound.

Nursing Management

Nursing management of the woman with oligohydramnios involves continuous monitoring of fetal well-being during nonstress testing or during labor and birth by identifying category II and III patterns on the fetal monitor. Variable decelerations indicating cord compression are common. Changing the woman's position might be therapeutic in altering this fetal heart rate pattern. After the birth, evaluate the newborn for signs of postmaturity, congenital anomalies, and respiratory difficulty.

Assist with amnioinfusion as indicated and continue to assess the woman's vital signs and contraction status and the fetal heart rate throughout the procedure. Provide comfort measures such as changing the bed linens and the woman's bed clothes frequently because of the constant leakage of fluid from the vagina. Also provide frequent perineal care during the infusion.

MULTIPLE GESTATION

Multiple gestation is defined as a pregnancy with two or more fetuses. This includes twins, triplets, and higher-order multiples such as quadruplets. In the past two decades, the number of multiple gestations in the United States has jumped dramatically because of the widespread use of fertility drugs, older age of women having babies, and the development of assisted reproductive technologies to treat infertility. About one third of live births from assisted reproductive technology result in more than one infant, and twins represent 85% of those multiple-birth children (De Sutter, 2015).

In the United States, the overall prevalence of twins is approximately 12 per 1,000, and two thirds are dizygotic (derived from two separate ova, March of Dimes, 2015f). The increasing number of multiple gestations is a concern because women who are expecting more than one infant are at high risk for preterm labor, polyhydramnios, hyperemesis gravidarum, anemia, preeclampsia, and antepartum hemorrhage. Fetal/newborn risks or complications include prematurity, respiratory distress syndrome, birth asphyxia/perinatal depression, congenital anomalies (CNS, cardiovascular, and gastrointestinal defects), twin-to-twin transfusion syndrome (transfusion of blood from one twin [i.e., donor] to the other twin [i.e., recipient]), intrauterine growth restriction, and becoming conjoined twins (Martin et al., 2014).

The two types of twins are monozygotic and dizygotic (Fig. 19.6). Monozygotic twins develop when a single,

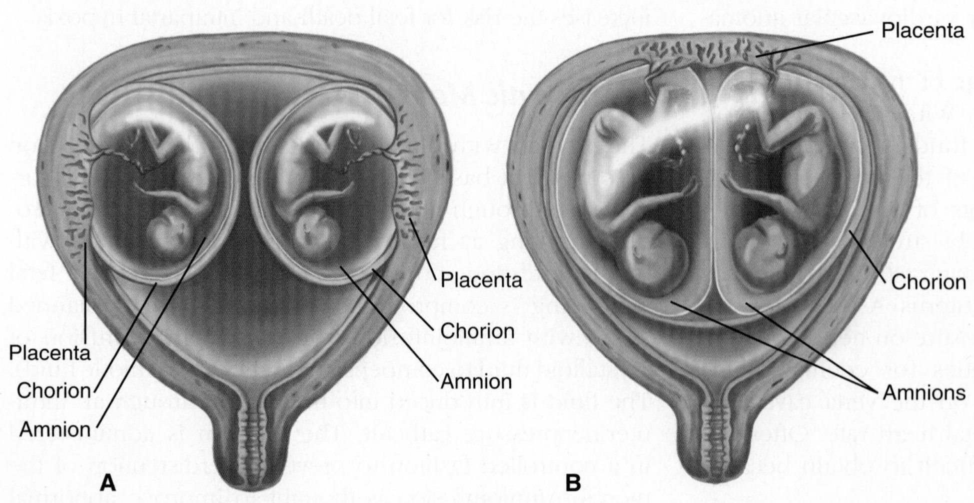

FIGURE 19.6 Multiple gestation with twins. **A.** Dizygotic twins, where each fetus has its own placenta, amnion, and chorion. **B.** Monozygotic twins, where the fetuses share one placenta, two amnions, and one chorion.

fertilized ovum splits during the first 2 weeks after conception. Monozygotic twins also are called identical twins. Two sperm fertilizing two ova produce dizygotic twins, which are called fraternal twins. Separate amnions, chorions, and placentas are formed in dizygotic twins. Triplets can be monozygotic, dizygotic, or trizygotic.

Therapeutic Management

When a multiple gestation is confirmed, the woman is followed with serial ultrasounds to assess fetal growth patterns and development. Biophysical profiles along with nonstress tests are ordered to determine fetal well-being. Many women are hospitalized in late pregnancy to prevent preterm labor and receive closer surveillance. During the intrapartum period the woman is closely monitored, with a perinatal team available to assist after birth. Operative delivery is frequently needed due to fetal malpresentation.

Nursing Assessment

Obtain a health history and perform a physical examination. Be alert for complaints of fatigue and severe nausea and vomiting. Assess the woman's abdomen and fundal height. Typically with a multiple gestation the uterus is larger than expected based on the estimated date of birth. Laboratory test results may reveal anemia. Prepare the woman for ultrasound, which typically confirms the diagnosis of a multiple gestation.

Nursing Management

During the prenatal period, provide education and support for the woman regarding nutrition, increased rest periods, and close observation for pregnancy complications such as anemia, excessive weight gain, proteinuria, edema, vaginal bleeding, and hypertension. Instruct the woman to be alert for and report immediately any signs and symptoms of preterm labor: contractions, uterine cramping, low back ache, increase in vaginal discharge, loss of mucous plug, pelvic pain, and pressure.

With the onset of labor, expect to monitor fetal heart rates continuously. Prepare the woman for an ultrasound to assess the presentation of each fetus to determine the best delivery approach. Ensure that extra nursing staff and the perinatal team are available for any birth or newborn complications.

After the babies are born, closely assess the woman for hemorrhage by frequently assessing uterine involution. Palpate the uterine fundus and monitor the amount and characteristics of lochia.

Throughout the entire pregnancy, birth, and hospital stay, inform and support the woman and her family. Encourage them to ask questions and verbalize any fears and concerns.

PREMATURE RUPTURE OF MEMBRANES

Premature rupture of membranes (**PROM**) is the rupture of the bag of waters before the onset of true labor. There are a number of associated conditions and complications, such as infection, prolapsed cord, abruptio placentae, and preterm labor. High-risk factors associated with preterm PROM include low socioeconomic status, multiple gestation, low BMI, tobacco use, history of preterm labor, placenta previa, abruptio placentae, urinary tract infection, vaginal bleeding at any time in pregnancy, cerclage, and amniocentesis (Jazayeri, 2015).

If prolonged (greater than 24 hours), the woman's risk for infection (chorioamnionitis, endometritis, sepsis, and neonatal infections) increases and continues to increase the longer the time since the bag of waters ruptured. The time interval from rupture of membranes to the onset of regular contractions is termed the latent period.

Women with PROM present with leakage of fluid, vaginal discharge, vaginal bleeding, and pelvic pressure, but they are not having contractions. PROM is diagnosed by speculum vaginal examination of the cervix and vaginal cavity. Pooling of fluid in the vagina or leakage of fluid from the cervix, ferning of the dried fluid under microscopic examination, and alkalinity of the fluid as determined by nitrazine paper (ph indicator) confirm the diagnosis.

The terminology of PROM can be confusing. PROM is rupture of the membranes prior to the onset of labor and is used appropriately when referring to a woman who is beyond 37 weeks' gestation, has presented with spontaneous rupture of the membranes, and is not in labor. A related term is **preterm premature rupture of membranes (PPROM)**, which is defined as rupture of membranes prior to the onset of labor in a woman who is *less* than 37 weeks' gestation. Perinatal risks associated with PPROM may stem from immaturity, including respiratory distress syndrome, intraventricular hemorrhage, patent ductus arteriosus, and necrotizing enterocolitis. Eighty-five percent of neonatal morbidity and mortality is a result of prematurity. PPROM is associated with 30% to 40% of preterm deliveries and is the leading identifiable cause of preterm delivery. PPROM complicates 3% of all pregnancies and occurs in approximately 150,000 pregnancies yearly in the United States (Jazayeri, 2015).

The exact cause of PROM is not known, but may be associated with vaginal bleeding, placental abruption, microbial invasion of the amniotic cavity, and defective placentation. In many cases, PROM occurs spontaneously. Increasing evidence associates abnormalities in vaginal flora during pregnancy with preterm labor and birth with potential neonatal sequelae due to prematurity and poor perinatal outcome (Gilbert, 2014). A recent study found that women with previous PPROM are at increased risk for recurrence, and a short interval between pregnancies is associated with increased risk (Gibbins et al., 2014).

Therapeutic Management

Treatment of PROM typically depends on the gestational age. Under no circumstances is an unsterile digital cervical examination done until the woman enters active labor, to minimize infection exposure. If the fetal lungs are mature, induction of labor is initiated. PROM is not a lone indicator for surgical birth. If the fetal lungs are immature, expectant management is carried out with adequate hydration, reduced physical activity, pelvic rest, and close observation for possible infection, such as with frequent monitoring of vital signs and laboratory test results (e.g., the white blood cell count). Corticosteroids may be given to enhance fetal lung maturity if lungs are immature, although this remains controversial. Recent studies have shown clear benefits of antibiotics to decrease neonatal morbidity associated with PPROM (Mattson & Smith, 2016).

Nursing Assessment

Nursing assessment focuses on obtaining a complete health history and performing a physical examination to determine maternal and fetal status. An accurate assessment of the gestational age and knowledge of the maternal, fetal, and neonatal risks are essential to appropriate evaluation, counseling, and management of women with PROM and PPROM. Nurses need to be aware that the risk of infection increases with the duration of PPROM.

Health History and Physical Examination

Review the maternal history for risk factors such as infection, increased uterine size (polyhydramnios, macrosomia, multiple gestation), uterine and fetal anomalies, lower socioeconomic status, STIs, cervical insufficiency, vaginal bleeding, and cigarette smoking during pregnancy. Ask about any history or current symptoms of urinary tract infection (frequency, urgency, dysuria, or flank pain) or pelvic or vaginal infection (pain or vaginal discharge).

Assess for signs and symptoms of labor, such as cramping, pelvic pressure, or back pain. Also assess her vital signs, noting any signs indicative of infection such as fever and elevated white blood cell count (more than 18,000 cells/mm^3) (Nagtalon-Ramos, 2014).

Institute continuous electronic fetal heart rate monitoring to evaluate fetal well-being. Conduct a vaginal examination to ascertain the cervical status in PROM. If PPROM exists, a sterile speculum examination (where the examiner inspects the cervix but does not palpate it) is done rather than a digital cervical examination because it may diminish latency (period of time from rupture of membranes to birth) and increase newborn morbidity (Cunningham et al., 2014).

Observe the characteristics of the amniotic fluid. Note any evidence of meconium, or a foul odor. When meconium is present in the amniotic fluid, it typically indicates fetal distress related to hypoxia. Meconium stains the fluid yellow to greenish brown, depending on the amount present. A foul odor of amniotic fluid indicates infection. Also observe the amount of fluid. A decreased amount of amniotic fluid reduces the cushioning effect, thereby making cord compression a possibility. Some research shows that restoring the volume of lost amniotic fluid will help to reduce the risk of infection and reduce cord compression. See Evidence-Based Practice 19.1. Key assessments are summarized in Box 19.3.

Laboratory and Diagnostic Testing

To diagnose PROM or PPROM, several procedures may be used: the Nitrazine test, fern test, or ultrasound. After the insertion of a sterile speculum, a sample of the fluid in the vaginal area is obtained. With a Nitrazine test, the pH of the fluid is tested; amniotic fluid is more basic (7.0) than normal vaginal secretions (4.5). Nitrazine paper turns blue in the presence of amniotic fluid. However, false-positive results can occur if blood, urine, semen, or antiseptic chemicals are also present; all will increase the pH.

For the fern test, a sample of vaginal fluid is placed on a slide to be viewed directly under a microscope. Amniotic fluid will develop a fern-like pattern when it dries because of sodium chloride crystallization. If both of these tests are inconclusive, a transvaginal ultrasound can also be used to determine whether membranes have ruptured by demonstrating a decreased amount of amniotic fluid (oligohydramnios) in the uterus (Jazayeri, 2015).

Other laboratory and diagnostic tests that may be used include:

- Urinalysis and urine culture for UTI or asymptomatic bacteriuria
- Cervical test or culture for chlamydia or gonorrhea
- Vaginal culture for bacterial vaginosis and trichomoniasis
- Vaginal introital/rectal culture for group B streptococcus

Nursing Management

Nursing management for the woman with PROM or PPROM focuses on preventing infection and identifying uterine contractions. The risk for infection is great because of the break in the amniotic fluid membrane and its proximity to vaginal bacteria. Therefore, monitor maternal vital signs closely. Be alert for a temperature

EVIDENCE-BASED PRACTICE 19.1

A LOW-DOSE ASPIRIN FOR PREVENTING PREECLAMPSIA AND ITS COMPLICATIONS: A META-ANALYSIS

STUDY

Preeclampsia is a major cause of perinatal mortality and morbidity worldwide. The etiology of it remains unclear, but it is thought that the condition arises because of abnormal trophoblastic invasion of uterine vessels or endothelial cell activation and dysfunction. Low-dose aspirin is thought to prevent preeclampsia in high-risk pregnancy, but it is not universally used because of safety concerns. The World Health Organization [WHO] and the US Preventive Services Task Force [USPSTF] both recommend using low-dose aspirin in women at high risk for preeclampsia. A systematic review and meta-analysis were analyzed using 29 studies involving 21,403 women.

Findings

The meta-analysis showed that low-dose aspirin significantly reduced the incidence of preeclampsia. Risk of preeclampsia was reduced when initiated before 16 weeks' gestation. Prophylactic low-dose aspirin, especially initiated before 16 weeks' gestation, is effective at preventing preeclampsia, preterm birth, and fetal growth restriction in high-risk pregnancies.

Nursing Implications

Based on the study's results, nurses can be involved in prenatal assessments of the high-risk mother to identify them early so that prophylactic low-dose aspirin can be prescribed if deemed appropriate by the health care provider. The nurse can provide instruction and rationales for the use and timing of this therapy to the clients. Two major professional health organizations have recommended this therapy to prevent preeclampsia, so nurses can view this therapy as an evidence-based intervention to promote better outcomes for mothers and their infants.

Adapted from Xu, T. T., Zhou, F., Deng, C. Y., Huang, G. Q., Li, J. K., & Wang, X. D. (2015). Low dose aspirin for preventing preeclampsia and its complications: A meta analysis. *The Journal of Clinical Hypertension, 17*(7), 567–573.

BOX 19.3

KEY ASSESSMENTS WITH PREMATURE RUPTURE OF MEMBRANES

For the woman with PROM, the following assessments are essential:

- Determining the date, time, and duration of membrane rupture by client interview
- Ascertaining gestational age of the fetus based on date of mother's last menstrual period, fundal height, and ultrasound dating
- Questioning the woman about possible history of or recent UTI or vaginal infection that might have contributed to PROM
- Assessing for any associated labor symptoms, such as back pain or pelvic pressure
- Assisting with or performing diagnostic tests to validate leakage of fluid, such as Nitrazine test, "ferning" on slide, and ultrasound. Contamination of Nitrazine tape with lubricant or insufficient fluid will render the assessment unreliable.
- Continually assessing for signs of infection including:
  - Elevation of maternal temperature and pulse rate
  - Abdominal/uterine tenderness
  - Fetal tachycardia more than 160 bpm
  - Elevated white blood cell count and C-reactive protein
  - Cloudy, foul-smelling amniotic fluid

Adapted from Nagtalon-Ramos, J. (2014). *Maternal-newborn nursing care: Best evidence-based practices.* Philadelphia, PA: F. A. Davis Company; Cunningham, F. G., Leveno, K. J., Bloom, S. L., Spong, C. Y., Dashe, J. S., Hoffman, B. L., et al. (2014). *Williams' obstetrics* (24th ed.). New York, NY: McGraw-Hill Education; and Magowan, B. A., Owen, P., & Thomson, A. (2014). *Clinical obstetrics & gynecology* (3rd ed.). St. Louis, MO: Saunders Elsevier.

elevation or an increase in pulse, which could indicate infection. Also monitor the fetal heart rate continuously, reporting any fetal tachycardia (which could indicate a maternal infection) or variable decelerations (suggesting cord compression). If variable decelerations are present, anticipate amnioinfusion based on agency policy. Evaluate the results of laboratory tests such as a CBC. An elevation in white blood cells would suggest infection. Administer antibiotics if ordered.

Encourage the woman and her partner to verbalize their feelings and concerns. Educate them about the purpose of the protective membranes and the implications of early rupture. Keep them informed about planned interventions, including potential complications and required therapy. As appropriate, prepare the woman for induction or augmentation of labor as appropriate if she is near term.

If labor does not start within 48 hours, the woman with PPROM may be discharged home on expectant management, which may include:

- Antibiotics if cervicovaginal cultures are positive
- Activity restrictions
- Education about signs and symptoms of infection and when to call with problems or concerns (Teaching Guidelines 19.3)
- Frequent fetal testing for well-being
- Ultrasound every 3 to 4 weeks to assess amniotic fluid levels
- Possible corticosteroid treatment depending on gestational age
- Daily kick counts to assess fetal well-being

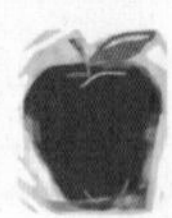

Teaching Guidelines 19.3

TEACHING FOR THE WOMAN WITH PPROM

- Monitor your baby's activity by performing fetal kick counts daily.
- Check your temperature daily and report any temperature increases to your health care provider.
- Watch for signs related to the beginning of labor. Report any tightening of the abdomen or contractions.
- Avoid any touching or manipulating of your breasts, which could stimulate labor.
- Do not insert anything into your vagina or vaginal area—no tampons, avoid vaginal intercourse
- Do not swim in pools or in the ocean or sit in a hot tub or Jacuzzi.
- Take showers for daily hygiene needs; avoid sitting in a tub bath.
- Maintain any specific activity restrictions as recommended.
- Wash your hands thoroughly after using the bathroom and make sure to wipe from front to back each time.
- Keep your perineal area clean and dry.
- Take your antibiotics as directed if your health care provider has prescribed them.
- Call your health care provider with changes in your condition, including fever, uterine tenderness, feeling like your heart is racing, and foul-smelling vaginal discharge.

NURSING CARE PLAN 19.1

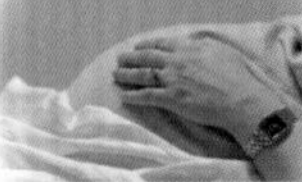

Overview of the Woman with Placenta Previa

A 39-year-old G5, P4, multigravida client at 32 weeks' gestation, was admitted to the labor and birth suite with sudden vaginal bleeding. She had no further active bleeding and did not complain of any abdominal discomfort or tenderness. She did complain of occasional "tightening" in her stomach. Her abdomen palpated soft. Fetal heart rates were in the 140s with accelerations with movement. She was placed on bed rest with bathroom privileges. Ultrasound identified a low-lying placenta with a viable, normal-growth fetus. She was diagnosed with placenta previa and admitted for observation and surveillance of fetal well-being. Her history revealed two previous cesarean births, smoking half a pack of cigarettes per day, and endometritis infection after birth of her last newborn. Additional assessment findings included painless, bright-red vaginal bleeding with initial bleeding ceasing spontaneously; irregular, mild, and sporadic uterine contractions; fetal heart rate and maternal vital signs within normal range; fetus in transverse lie; anxiety related to the outcome of pregnancy; and expression of feelings of helplessness.

NURSING DIAGNOSIS: Risk for injury (fetal and maternal) related to threat to uteroplacental perfusion and hemorrhage

Outcome Identification and Evaluation

The client will maintain adequate tissue perfusion as evidenced by stable vital signs, decreased blood loss, few or no uterine contractions, normal fetal heart rate patterns and variability, and positive fetal movement.

NURSING CARE PLAN 19.1

Overview of the Woman with Placenta Previa (continued)

Interventions: ***Maintaining Adequate Tissue Perfusion***

- Establish intravenous access to allow for administration of fluids, blood, and medications as necessary.
- Obtain type and cross-match for at least 2 units blood products to ensure availability should bleeding continue.
- Obtain specimens as ordered for blood studies, such as CBC and clotting studies, to establish a baseline and use for future comparison.
- Monitor output to evaluate adequacy of renal perfusion.
- Administer intravenous fluid replacement therapy as ordered to maintain blood pressure and blood volume.
- Palpate for abdominal tenderness and rigidity to determine bleeding and evidence of uterine contractions.
- Institute bed rest to reduce oxygen demands.
- Assess for rupture of membranes to evaluate for possible onset of labor.
- Avoid vaginal examinations to prevent further bleeding episodes.
- Complete an Rh titer to identify need for RhoGAM.
- Avoid nipple stimulation to prevent uterine contractions.
- Continuously monitor for contractions or PROM to allow for prompt intervention.
- Administer tocolytic agents as ordered to stall preterm labor.
- Monitor vital signs frequently to identify possible hypovolemia and infection.
- Assess frequently for active vaginal bleeding to minimize risk of hemorrhage.
- Continuously monitor fetal heart rate with electronic fetal monitor to evaluate fetal status.
- Assist with fetal surveillance tests as ordered to aid in determining fetal well-being.
- Observe for abnormal fetal heart rate patterns, such as loss of variability, decelerations, tachycardia, to identify fetal distress.
- Position client in side-lying position with wedge for support to maximize placental perfusion.
- Assess fetal movement to evaluate for possible fetal hypoxia.
- Teach woman to monitor fetal movement to evaluate well-being.
- Administer oxygen as ordered to increase oxygenation to mother and fetus.

NURSING DIAGNOSIS: Anxiety related to threat to self and fetus, unknown future

Outcome Identification and Evaluation

The client will experience a decrease in anxiety as evidenced by verbal reports of less anxiety, use of effective coping measures, and calm demeanor.

Interventions: ***Minimizing Anxiety***

- Provide factual information about diagnosis and treatment, and explain interventions and the rationale behind them *to provide client with understanding of her condition.*
- Answer questions about health status honestly *to establish a trusting relationship.*
- Speak calmly to client and family members *to minimize environmental stress.*
- Encourage the use of past effective techniques for coping *to promote relaxation and feelings of control.*
- Acknowledge and facilitate the woman's spiritual needs *to promote effective coping.*
- Involve the woman and family in the decision-making process *to foster self-confidence and control over situation.*
- Maintain a presence during stressful periods *to allay anxiety.*
- Use the sense of touch if appropriate *to convey caring and concern.*
- Encourage talking as a means *to release tension.*

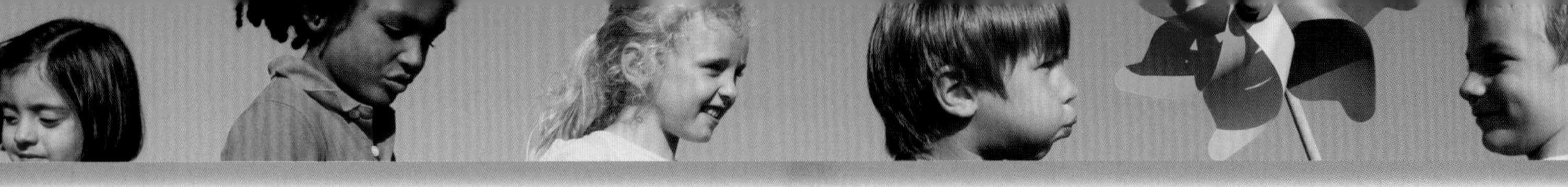

KEY CONCEPTS

- Identifying risk factors early on and throughout the pregnancy is important to ensure the best outcome for every pregnancy. Risk assessment should start with the first prenatal visit and continue with subsequent visits.
- The three most common causes of hemorrhage early in pregnancy (first half of pregnancy) are spontaneous abortion, ectopic pregnancy, and GTD.
- Ectopic pregnancies occur in about 1 in 50 pregnancies and have increased dramatically during the past few decades.
- Having a molar pregnancy results in the loss of the pregnancy and the possibility of developing choriocarcinoma, a chronic malignancy from the trophoblastic tissue.
- The classic clinical picture presentation for placenta previa is painless, bright-red vaginal bleeding occurring during the third trimester.
- Treatment of abruptio placentae is designed to assess, control, and restore the amount of blood lost; to provide a positive outcome for both mother and infant; and to prevent coagulation disorders.
- DIC can be described in simplest terms as a loss of balance between the clot-forming activity of thrombin and the clot-lysing activity of plasmin.
- Hyperemesis gravidarum is a complication of pregnancy characterized by persistent, uncontrollable nausea and vomiting before the 20th week of gestation.
- Gestational hypertension is the leading cause of maternal death in the United States and the most common complication reported during pregnancy.
- HELLP is an acronym for hemolysis, elevated liver enzymes, and low platelets.
- Rh incompatibility is a condition that develops when a woman of Rh-negative blood type is exposed to Rh-positive fetal blood cells and subsequently develops circulating titers of Rh antibodies.
- Polyhydramnios occurs in approximately 3% to 4% of all pregnancies and is associated with fetal anomalies of development.
- Nursing care related to the woman with oligohydramnios involves continuous monitoring of fetal well-being during nonstress testing or during labor and birth by identifying category II and III patterns on the fetal monitor.
- The increasing number of multiple gestations is a concern because women who are expecting more than one infant are at high risk for preterm labor, hydramnios, hyperemesis gravidarum, anemia, preeclampsia, and antepartum hemorrhage.
- Nursing care related to PROM centers on infection prevention and identification of preterm labor contractions.
- Monitoring maternal vital signs for changes and the fetal hearth rate once PPROM occurs is essential to increasing the changes of a good outcome.
- It is essential that nurses educate all pregnant women how to detect the early signs of PROM and what action is needed if it happens.

REFERENCES AND RECOMMENDED READINGS

Abu Hashim, H., Al-Inany, H., & Kilani, Z. (2014). A review of the contemporary evidence on rescue cervical cerclage. *International Journal of Gynecology & Obstetrics, 124*(3), 198–203.

Agarwal, N., & Odejinmi, F. (2014). Early abdominal ectopic pregnancy: Challenges, update and review of current management. *Obstetrician & Gynecologist, 16*(3), 193–198.

Agency for Healthcare Research and Quality [AHRQ]. (2015). *Cerclage for the management of cervical insufficiency.* Retrieved from http://www.guideline.gov/content.aspx?id=47771

American Cancer Society [ACS]. (2015). *Gestational trophoblastic disease.* Retrieved from http://www.cancer.org/cancer/gestationaltrophoblasticdisease/detailedguide/gestational-trophoblastic-disease-key-statistics

American College of Obstetricians and Gynecologists [ACOG]. (2014a). Practice bulletin no. 142: Cerclage for the management of cervical insufficiency. *Obstetrics & Gynecology, 123*(2), 372–379.

American College of Obstetricians and Gynecologists [ACOG]. (2014b). *Placenta accreta.* Retrieved from http://www.acog.org/Resources-And-Publications/Committee-Opinions/Committee-on-Obstetric-Practice/Placenta-Accreta

American College of Obstetricians and Gynecologists [ACOG]. (2014c). ACOG task force on hypertension in pregnancy—A step forward in management. *Contemporary OB/GYN.* Retrieved from http://contemporaryobgyn.modernmedicine.com/contemporary-obgyn/news/acog-task-force-hypertension-pregnancy-step-forward-management?page=full

Amorim, M. M., Katz, L., Barros, A. S., Almeida, T. S., Souza, A. S. R., & Faúndes, A. (2015). Maternal outcomes according to mode of delivery in women with severe preeclampsia: A cohort study. *The Journal of Maternal-Fetal & Neonatal Medicine, 28*(6), 654–660.

Ananth, C. V., & Kinzler, W. L. (2015). *Placental abruption: Clinical features and diagnosis.* UpToDate. Retrieved from http://www.uptodate.com/contents/placental-abruption-clinical-features-and-diagnosis

Archibong, E. I., & Ahmed, E. S. (2015). Risk factors maternal and neonatal outcome in major placenta previa: A prospective study. *Annals of Saudi Medicine, 21*(3--4), 245–247.

Ardehali, A., & Casikar, I. (2015). Identification of risk factors of ectopic pregnancy. In *Ectopic pregnancy* (pp. 1–10). Springer International Publishing.

Atkinson, A. L., Santolaya-Forgas, J., Blitzer, D. N., Santolaya, J. L., Matta, P., Canterino, J., et al. (2015). Risk factors for perinatal mortality in patients admitted to the hospital with the diagnosis of placental abruption. *The Journal of Maternal-Fetal & Neonatal Medicine, 28*(5), 594–597.

Ayyavoo, A., Derraik, J. B., Hofman, P. L., & Cutfield, W. S. (2014). Hyperemesis gravidarum and long-term health of the offspring. *American Journal of Obstetrics & Gynecology, 210*(6), 521–525.

Berghella, V. (2014). Cervical insufficiency. *UpToDate.* Retrieved from http://www.uptodate.com/contents/cervical-insufficiency

Berkowitz, R. S., Goldstein, D. P., & Horowitz, N. S. (2014). Management options of gestational trophoblastic disease. *Current Obstetrics and Gynecology Reports, 3*(1), 76–83.

Boots, A. B., Sanchez-Ramos, L., Bowers, D. M., Kaunitz, A. M., Zamora, J., & Schlattmann, P. (2014). The short-term prediction of preterm birth: A systematic review and diagnostic metaanalysis. *American Journal of Obstetrics and Gynecology, 210*(1), 54. e1–e54.

Bourne, T. (2015). A missed opportunity for excellence: The NICE guideline on the diagnosis and initial management of ectopic pregnancy and miscarriage. *Journal of Family Planning and Reproductive Health Care, 41*(1), 13–19.

Bujold, E. (2015). Low-dose aspirin reduces morbidity and mortality in pregnant women at high-risk for preeclampsia. *Evidence Based Nursing, 18*(3), 71.

Carson, M. P., & Gibson, P. S. (2015). Hypertension and pregnancy. *eMedicine.* Retrieved from http://emedicine.medscape.com/article/261435-overview

Carter, B. S., & Boyd, R. L. (2015). Polyhydramnios and oligohydramnios. *eMedicine.* Retrieved from: http://reference.medscape.com/article/975821-overview

Castillo, M. J., & Phillippi, J. C. (2015). Hyperemesis gravidarum: A holistic overview and approach to clinical assessment and management. *The Journal of Perinatal & Neonatal Nursing, 29*(1), 12–22.

Clausen, T. D., & Bergholt, T. (2014). Chronic hypertension during pregnancy. *BMJ: British Medical Journal, 348*, g2655. [CE: Please check the page range.]

Cohen, A., Zakar, L., Gil, Y., Amer-Alshiek, J., Bibi, G., Almog, B., et al. (2015). Methotrexate success rates in progressing ectopic pregnancies: A reappraisal. *Obstetrical & Gynecological Survey, 70*(2), 88–89.

Creasy, R. K., Resnik, R., Iams, J. D., Lockwood, C. J., Moore, T. R., & Greene, M.F. (2014). *Creasy and Resnik's maternal-fetal medicine: Principles and practice* (7th ed.). Philadelphia, PA: Elsevier.

Cunningham, F. G., Leveno, K. J., Bloom, S. L., Spong, C. Y., Dashe, J. S., Hoffman, B.L., et al. (2014). *Williams' obstetrics* (24th ed.). New York, NY: McGraw-Hill Education.

Dalia, S., Price, S., Forsyth, P., Sokol, L., & Jaglal, M. (2015). What is the optimal dose of high dose methotrexate in the initial treatment of primary Central Nervous System lymphoma? *Leukemia & Lymphoma, 56*(2), 500--502.[CE: As per pubmed the reference has been updated. The year also changed from 2014 to 2015. Pls check is this correct or not.]

Davidson, M. R. (2014). *Fast facts for the neonatal nurse: A nursing orientation & care guide in a nutshell.* New York, NY: Springer Publishing Company.

Davis, S. J., & Kessler, C. M. (2014). Disseminated intravascular coagulation: Diagnosis and management. In *Hemostasis and thrombosis: Practical guidelines in clinical management* (pp. 151–168). Hoboken, NJ: Wiley Blackwell.

Deering, S. H. (2015). Abruptio placenta. *eMedicine.* Retrieved from http://emedicine.medscape.com/article/252810-overview

Dekker, G. A. (2014). Management of preeclampsia. *Pregnancy hypertension: An International Journal of Women's Cardiovascular Health, 4*(3), 246–247.

Desai, D., Lu, J., Wyness, S. P., Greene, D. N., Olson, K. N., Wiley, C. L., et al. (2014). Human chorionic gonadotropin discriminatory zone in ectopic pregnancy: Does assay harmonization matter? *Fertility and Sterility, 101*(6), 1671–1674.

De Sutter, P. (2015). The challenge of multiple pregnancies. In *Reducing risk in fertility treatment* (pp. 1–17). London, England: Springer Publishers.

Dickson, E. L., & Mullany, S. A. (2015). Gestational trophoblastic disease. In *Gynecologic oncology* (pp. 175–201). New York: Springer.

Festin, M. (2014). Nausea and vomiting in early pregnancy. *BMJ Clinical Evidence, 2014*, pii: 1405. Available from: MEDLINE, Ipswich, MA.

Foley, M., Strong, T.M., & Garite, T. (2014). *Obstetric intensive care manual* (4th ed.). New York, NY: McGraw-Hill Publishers.

Foo, L., Tay, J., Lees, C. C., McEniery, C. M., & Wilkinson, I. B. (2015). Hypertension in pregnancy: Natural history and treatment options. *Current Hypertension Reports, 17*(5), 1–18.

Gibbins, K., Esplin, M. S., Varner, M., Eller, A., & Manuck, T. (2014). 835: Subsequent pregnancy outcomes among women with a history of preterm premature rupture of membranes (PPROM)< 24.0 weeks gestation. *American Journal of Obstetrics & Gynecology, 210*(1), S405--S406.

Gilbert, R. (2014). Immediate delivery for group B streptococci-colonized women with preterm premature rupture of membranes. Don't forget the antibiotics. *BJOG: An International Journal of Obstetrics & Gynecology.* doi: 10.1111/1471-0528.12940

Hensley, J., & Shviraga, B. (2014). Metastatic choriocarcinoma in a term pregnancy: A case study. *MCN: The American Journal of Maternal Child Nursing, 39*(1), 8–15.

Herrera, K., & Lewis, D. (2014). Cervical insufficiency and cerclage. *Postgraduate Obstetrics & Gynecology, 34*(3), 1–5.

Holt, J. L. (2015). Multidisciplinary care of a woman experiencing obstetric hemorrhage. *Journal of Obstetric, Gynecologic, & Neonatal Nursing, 44*, S85–S86.

Hosein, H., Abdel-Kariem, R., & Shriki, J. E. (2014). Placental abruption imaging. *eMedicine.* Retrieved from http://emedicine.medscape.com/article/402314-overview

Humphrey, J. (2015). Primary cesarean delivery results in emergency hysterectomy due to placenta accreta: A case study. *AANA Journal, 83*(1), 28–34.

Infante, F., Menakaya, U., & Condous, G. (2014). Medical treatment of ectopic pregnancy. *Fertility and Sterility,*

101(3), e16–e22. doi: http://dx.doi.org/10.1016/j.fertnstert.2013.12.013

Jaju, K. G., Kulkarni, A. P. & Mundada, S. K. (2014). Study of perinatal outcome in relation to abruptio placentae. *International Journal of Recent Trends in Science and Technology, 11*(3), 355–358.

Jazayeri, A. (2015). Premature rupture of membranes. *eMedicine*. Retrieved from http://emedicine.medscape.com/article/261137-overview

Jena, S. K., Samal, S., Behera, B. K., & Allms, B. (2015). Cervical cerclage in modern obstetrics: A review. *Health, 3*(1), 9–14.

Jones, R. E., & Lopez, K. H. (2014). *Human reproductive biology* (4th ed.). Waltham, MA: Academic Press/Elsevier.

Joy, S., & Temming, L. (2015). Placenta previa. *eMedicine*. Retrieved from http://emedicine.medscape.com/article/262063-overview

Kao, L., Scheinfeld, M., Chernyak, V., Rozenblit, A., Oh, S., & Dym, R. (2014). Beyond ultrasound: CT and MRI of ectopic pregnancy. *American Journal of Roentgenology, 202*(4), 904–911.

Khan, H., & Meirowitz, N. B. (2015). HELLP syndrome. *eMedicine*. Retrieved from http://emedicine.medscape.com/article/1394126-overview

King, T. L., Brucker, M. C., Kriebs, J. M., Fahey, J. O., Grgor, C. L., & Varney, H. (2015). *Varney's midwifery* (5th ed.). Burlington, MA: Jones & Bartlett Learning.

Knez, J., Day, A., & Jurkovic, D. (2014). Ultrasound imaging in the management of bleeding and pain in early pregnancy. *Best Practice & Research Clinical Obstetrics & Gynecology, 28*(5), 621–636.

Ko, J., & Cheung, V. (2014). Time to revisit the human chorionic gonadotropin discriminatory level in the management of pregnancy of unknown location. *Journal of Ultrasound in Medicine, 33*(3), 465–471.

Kobayashi, T. (2014). Obstetrical disseminated intravascular coagulation score. *Journal of Obstetrics and Gynecology Research, 40*(6), 1500–1506.

Magee, L. A., Pels, A., Helewa, M., Rey, E., von Dadelszen, P., Audibert, F., et al. (2015). The hypertensive disorders of pregnancy (29.3). *Best Practice & Research Clinical Obstetrics & Gynecology, 29*(5):643–657.

Magowan, B.A., Owen, P., & Thomson, A. (2014). *Clinical obstetrics & gynecology* (3rd ed.). St. Louis, MO: Saunders Elsevier.

Maltepe, C., Popa, M. V., Bertucci, C., Farine, D., Koren, G., & Nulman, I. (2015). The effects of counseling and predictors of pregnancy outcomes in women with hyperemesis gravidarum [316]. *Obstetrics & Gynecology, 125*, 101S.

March of Dimes. (2015a). *Pregnancy loss*. Retrieved from http://www.marchofdimes.com/loss/stillbirth.aspx

March of Dimes. (2015b). *Ectopic pregnancy*. Retrieved from http://www.marchofdimes.com/loss/ectopic-pregnancy.aspx

March of Dimes. (2015c). *Placenta accreta, increta, and percreta*. Retrieved from http://www.marchofdimes.com/pregnancy/placental-accreta-increta-and-percreta.aspx

March of Dimes. (2015d). *Rh disease*. Retrieved from http://www.marchofdimes.com/baby/rh-disease.aspx

March of Dimes. (2015e). *Oligohydramnios*. Retrieved from http://www.marchofdimes.com/pregnancy/oligohydramnios.aspx

March of Dimes. (2015f). *Multiples: Twins, triplets and beyond*. Retrieved from http://www.marchofdimes.com/pregnancy/multiples-twins-triplets-and-beyond.aspx

Marik, P. E. (2015). Pregnancy related disorders. In *Evidence-based critical care* (pp. 759–772). Springer International Publishing.

Martin, R. J., Fanaroff, A. A., & Walsh, M. C. (2014). *Fanaroff & Martin's neonatal-perinatal medicine* (10th ed.). Philadelphia, PA: Elsevier Health Sciences.

Matthews, A., Haas, D. M., O'Mathúna, D. P., Dowswell, T., & Doyle, M. (2014). Interventions for nausea and vomiting in early pregnancy. *Cochrane Database of Systematic Reviews*, 3, CD007575.

Mattson, S., & Smith, J. E. (2016). *Core curriculum for maternal-newborn nursing* (5th ed.). St. Louis, MO: Saunders Elsevier.

Miller, M. A., & Carpenter, M. (2015). Hypertensive disorders of pregnancy. In *Medical management of the pregnant patient* (pp. 177–193). New York, NY: Springer Publishers.

Moore, T. R. (2015). Abnormal amniotic fluid. *Protocols for high-risk pregnancies: An evidence-based approach* (pp. 315–328). West Sussex, UK: John Wiley & Sons.

Moses, S. (2015a). Placental abruption. *Family Practice Notebook*. Retrieved from http://www.fpnotebook.com/ob/Bleed/PlcntlAbrptn.htm

Moses, S. (2015b). HELLP syndrome. *Family Practice Notebook*. Retrieved from http://www.fpnotebook.com/heme-onc/OB/HlpSyndrm.htm

Mukherjee, S., Bawa, A. K., Sharma, S., Nandanwar, Y. S., & Gadam, M. (2014). Retrospective study of risk factors and maternal and fetal outcome in patients with abruptio placentae. *Journal of Natural Science, Biology and Medicine, 5*(2), 425–428.

Nagtalon-Ramos, J. (2014). *Maternal-newborn nursing care: Best evidence-based practices*. Philadelphia, PA: F. A. Davis Company.

National High Blood Pressure Education Program Working Group on High Blood Pressure in Pregnancy. (2002). Working Group in High Blood Pressure in Pregnancy report. *American Journal of Obstetrics and Gynecology, 183*, S1–S22.

Nguyen, N., & Slim, R. (2014). Genetics and epigenetics of recurrent hydatidiform moles: Basic science and genetic counselling. *Current Obstetrics and Gynecology Reports, 3*, 55–64.

Norwitz, E. R. (2015). Eclampsia. *UpToDate*, Retrieved from http://www.uptodate.com/contents/eclampsia

Norwitz, E. R., & Conroy, K. E. (2015). Cervical insufficiency. *eMedicine*. Retrieved from http://emedicine.medscape.com/article/1979914-overview

Ogunyemi, D. A., Fong, A., & Herrero, T. C. (2015). Hyperemesis gravidarum. *eMedicine*. Retrieved from http://emedicine.medscape.com/article/254751-overview

Pauli, J. M., & Repke, J. T. (2015). Preeclampsia: Short-term and long-term implications. *Obstetrics and Gynecology Clinics of North America, 42*(2), 299–313.

Peled, Y., Melamed, N., Hiersch, L., Pardo, J., Wiznitzer, A., & Yogev, Y. (2014). The impact of total parenteral nutrition support on pregnancy outcome in women with hyperemesis gravidarum. *Journal of Maternal-Fetal & Neonatal Medicine, 27*(11), 1146–1150.

Randall, S., & LaMontagne, D. S. (2015). Screening for chlamydia: Seize the day. *Journal of Family Planning and Reproductive Health Care, 31*(2), 98–100.

Ross, M. G. (2015). Eclampsia. *eMedicine.* Retrieved from http://emedicine.medscape.com/article/253960-overview

Salem, L., & Singer, K. R. (2015). Rh incompatibility. *eMedicine.* Retrieved from http://emedicine.medscape.com/article/797150-overview

Schultz, W., & McConachie, I. (2015). Vital signs after hemorrhage–caution is appropriate. *Trends in Anesthesia and Critical Care.* doi: http://dx.doi.org/10.1016/j.tacc.2015.04.001

Sepilian, V., & Wood, E. (2015). Ectopic pregnancy. *eMedicine.* Retrieved from http://emedicine.medscape.com/article/2041923-overview

Sibai, B. M. (2015). HELLP syndrome. *UpToDate.* Retrieved from http://www.uptodate.com/contents/hellp-syndrome

Skidmore-Roth, L. (2015). *Mosby's 2015 nursing drug reference* (28th ed.). Philadelphia, PA: Elsevier Health Science.

Staneva, A., Bogossian, F., Pritchard, M., & Wittkowski, A. (2015). The effects of maternal depression, anxiety, and perceived stress during pregnancy on preterm birth: A systematic review. *Women and Birth. 28*(3), 179–193.

Strohl, A. E., & Lurain, J. R. (2014). Clinical epidemiology of gestational trophoblastic disease. *Current Obstetrics and Gynecology Reports, 3*(1), 40–43.

Szypulski, H. (2015). Practice guideline to prevent ectopic pregnancy rupture. *International Journal of Childbirth Education, 30*(1), 59–62.

Tan, P., Zaidi, S., Azmi, N., Omar, S., & Khong, S. (2014). Depression, anxiety, stress and hyperemesis gravidarum: Temporal and case controlled correlates. *Plos ONE, 9*(3), 1–7.

Taylor, T. (2014). Treatment of nausea and vomiting in pregnancy. *Australian Prescriber, 37*(2), 42–45.

Tulandi, T. (2015). Medical treatment of ectopic pregnancy. In *Ectopic pregnancy* (pp. 49–53). Springer International Publishing.

Tulandi, T., & Al-Fozan, H. M. (2015). Spontaneous abortion: Risk factors, etiology, clinical manifestations, and diagnostic evaluation. *UpToDate.* Retrieved from http://www.uptodate.com/contents/spontaneous-abortion-risk-factors-etiology-clinical-manifestations-and-diagnostic-evaluation

Urquhart C., Currell R., Harlow F., & Callow L. (2015). Home uterine monitoring for detecting preterm labor. *Cochrane Database of Systematic Reviews*, 1, CD006172.

U.S. Department of Health and Human Services. (2010). *Healthy People 2020.* Retrieved from http://www.healthypeople.gov/2020/topicsobjectives2020/

Verklan, T., & Walden, M. (2014). *Core curriculum for neonatal intensive care nursing* (4th ed.). St. Louis, MO: Saunders Elsevier.

Vigil-De Gracia, P. (2015). HELLP syndrome. *Ginecología Y Obstetricia De México, 83*(1), 48–57.

Wiedaseck, S., & Monchek, R. (2014). Placental and cord insertion pathologies: Screening, diagnosis, and management. *Journal of Midwifery & Women's Health, 59*(3), 328–335.

World Health Organization [WHO]. (2015). *Skilled birth attendants.* Retrieved from http://www.who.int/reproductivehealth/topics/mdgs/skilled_birth_attendant/en/

Xu, T. T., Zhou, F., Deng, C. Y., Huang, G. Q., Li, J. K., & Wang, X. D. (2015). Low dose aspirin for preventing preeclampsia and its complications: A meta analysis. *The Journal of Clinical Hypertension, 17*(7), 567–573.

Zainul Rashid, M. R., Lim, J., Nawawi, N. M., Luqman, M., Zolkeplai, M., Rangkuty, H., et al. (2014). A pilot study to determine whether progestogen supplementation using dydrogesterone during the first trimester will reduce the incidence of gestational hypertension in primigravidae. *Gynecological Endocrinology, 30*(3), 217–220.

CHAPTER **WORKSHEET**

MULTIPLE-CHOICE QUESTIONS

1. Which of the following women should receive RhoGAM postpartum?
   a. Nonsensitized Rh-negative mother with a Rh-negative newborn
   b. Nonsensitized Rh-negative mother with a Rh-positive newborn
   c. Sensitized Rh-negative mother with a Rh-positive newborn
   d. Sensitized Rh-negative mother with a Rh-negative newborn

2. A woman is suspected of having abruptio placentae. Which of the following would the nurse expect to assess as a classic symptom?
   a. Painless, bright-red bleeding
   b. "Knife-like" abdominal pain
   c. Excessive nausea and vomiting
   d. Hypertension and headache

3. RhoGAM is given to Rh-negative women to prevent maternal sensitization. In addition to pregnancy, Rh-negative women would also receive this medication after which of the following?
   a. Therapeutic or spontaneous abortion
   b. Head injury from a car accident
   c. Blood transfusion after a hemorrhage
   d. Unsuccessful artificial insemination procedure

4. After teaching a woman about hyperemesis gravidarum and how it differs from the typical nausea and vomiting of pregnancy, which statement by the woman indicates that the teaching was successful?
   a. "I can expect the nausea to last through my second trimester."
   b. "I should drink fluids with my meals instead of in between them."
   c. "I need to avoid strong odors, perfumes, or flavors."
   d. "I should lie down after I eat for about 2 hours."

5. A pregnant woman, approximately 12 weeks' gestation, comes to the emergency department after calling her health care provider's office and reporting moderate vaginal bleeding. Assessment reveals cervical dilation and moderately strong abdominal cramps. She reports that she has passed some tissue with the bleeding. The nurse interprets these findings to suggest which of the following?
   a. Threatened abortion
   b. Inevitable abortion
   c. Incomplete abortion
   d. Missed abortion

6. When administering magnesium sulfate to a client with preeclampsia, the nurse explains to her that this drug is given to:
   a. Reduce blood pressure
   b. Increase the progress of labor
   c. Prevent seizures
   d. Lower blood glucose levels

7. A woman is being discharged after receiving treatment for a hydatidiform molar pregnancy. The nurse should include which of the following in her discharge teaching?
   a. Do not become pregnant for at least a year; use contraceptives to prevent it
   b. Have the client's blood pressure checked weekly in the clinic
   c. RhoGAM must be given within the next month to her at the clinic
   d. An amniocentesis can detect a recurrence of this disorder in the future

CRITICAL THINKING EXERCISES

1. A 16-year-old primigravida, presents to the maternity clinic complaining of continual nausea and vomiting for the past 3 days. She states she is approximately 15 weeks pregnant and has been unable to hold anything down or take any fluids in without throwing up for the past 3 days. She reports she is dizzy and weak. On examination, Suzanne appears pale and anxious. Her mucous membranes are dry, skin turgor is poor, and her lips are dry and cracked.
   a. What is your impression of this condition?
   b. What risk factors does Suzanne have?
   c. What intervention is appropriate for this woman?

2. An obese 39-year-old primigravida of African-American descent who is diagnosed with gestational hypertension presents to the prenatal clinic. Her history reveals that her sister developed preeclampsia during her pregnancy. When describing her diet to the nurse, this client mentions that she tends to eat a lot of fast food.
   a. What risk factors does this client have that increase her risk for gestational hypertension?
   b. When assessing this client, what assessment findings would lead the nurse to suspect that this client has developed severe preeclampsia?

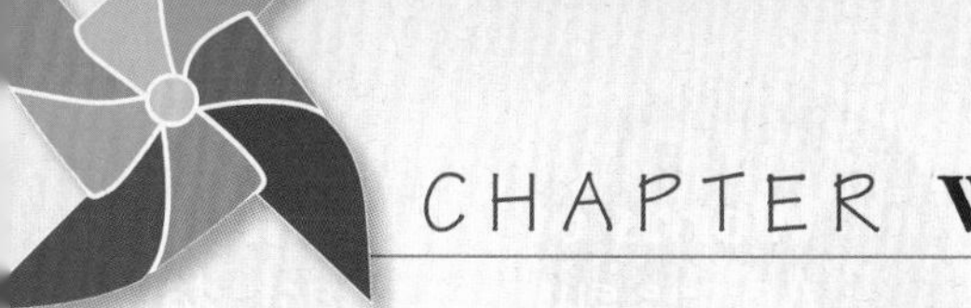

CHAPTER WORKSHEET

STUDY ACTIVITIES

1. Ask a community health maternity nurse how the signs and symptoms of gestational hypertension (including preeclampsia and eclampsia) are taught, and how effective efforts have been to reduce the incidence in the area.
2. Find a website designed to help parents who have suffered a pregnancy loss secondary to a spontaneous abortion. What is its audience level? Is the information up to date?
3. A pregnancy in which the blastocyst implants outside the uterus is an ________________ pregnancy.
4. The most serious complication of hydatidiform mole is the development of ________________ afterward.
5. Discuss various activities a woman with a multiple gestation could engage in to help pass the time when ordered to be on bed rest at home for 2 months.

BRINGING IT ALL TOGETHER: A CASE STUDY

A 21-year-old women presented to the local Public Health maternity clinic with a chief complaint of intermittent vaginal bleeding, abdominal cramping, and nausea. She stated her last menstrual period was 8 weeks ago and she had done a home pregnancy test prior to her coming here, which was positive. She was taking no medications and had no known drug allergies. She did admit she was a half-pack a day smoker, but had been trying to quit.

Go to thePoint to find questions to consider about this case.

20

WOW
Words of Wisdom
As the sun sets each day, nurses should make sure they have done something for others, and should try to be understanding even under the most difficult of conditions.

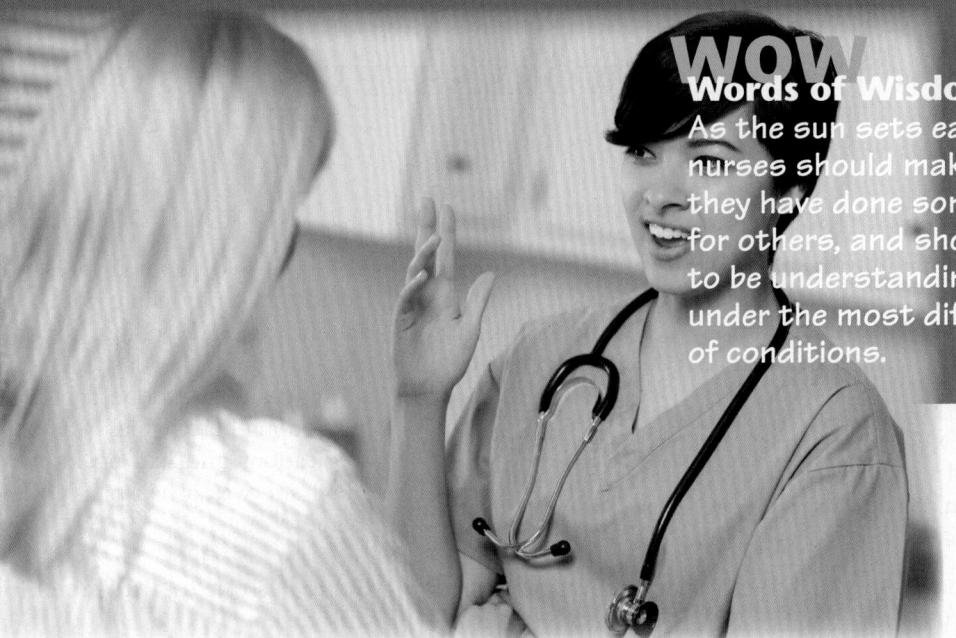

KEY TERMS
acquired immunodeficiency syndrome (AIDS)
adolescence
anemia
fetal alcohol spectrum disorder (FASD)
gestational diabetes mellitus
glycosylated hemoglobin (HbA1C) level
human immunodeficiency virus (HIV)
impaired fasting glucose
impaired glucose tolerance
multiple sclerosis (MS)
neonatal abstinence syndrome (NAS)
perinatal drug abuse
pica
pregestational diabetes
rheumatoid arthritis (RA)
systemic lupus erythematosus (SLE)
teratogen
type 1 diabetes
type 2 diabetes

Nursing Management of the Pregnancy at Risk: Selected Health Conditions and Vulnerable Populations

Learning Objectives

Upon completion of the chapter, you will be able to:

1. Select at least two conditions present before pregnancy that can have a negative effect on a pregnancy.
2. Examine how a condition present before pregnancy can affect the woman physiologically and psychologically when she becomes pregnant.
3. Evaluate the nursing assessment and management for a pregnant woman with diabetes from that of a pregnant woman without diabetes.
4. Explore how congenital and acquired heart conditions can affect a woman's pregnancy.
5. Design the nursing assessment and management of a pregnant woman with cardiovascular disorders and respiratory conditions.
6. Differentiate among the types of anemia affecting pregnant women in terms of prevention and management.
7. Relate the nursing care needed for the pregnant woman with an autoimmune disorder.
8. Compare the most common infections that can jeopardize a pregnancy, and propose possible preventive strategies.
9. Develop a plan of care for the pregnant woman who is HIV positive.
10. Outline the nurse's role in the prevention and management of adolescent pregnancy.
11. Determine the impact of pregnancy on a woman over the age of 35.
12. Analyze the effects of substance abuse during pregnancy.

***Rose*, a thin 16-year-old appearing very pregnant, came into the clinic wheezing and having difficulty catching her breath. She had missed several previous prenatal visits but arrived at the clinic today in distress. Rose has a history of asthma since she was 5 years old. How might Rose's current condition affect her pregnancy? Is this picture typical of the pregnant woman with asthma?**

INTRODUCTION

Pregnancy and childbirth are exciting yet complex facets within the continuum of women's health. Pregnancy is a special time in most women's lives, but the 9-month waiting period can be very anxiety-producing if it is complicated by a medical condition which might complicate the pregnancy and jeopardize the fetal outcome. Ideally the pregnant woman is free of any conditions that can affect a pregnancy, but in reality many women enter pregnancy with a multitude of health-related or psychosocial issues that can have a negative impact on the outcome. Currently, because of the obesity epidemic in the nation and women postponing their pregnancies until later in their lives, nurses will increasingly see more women with medical conditions that affect their pregnancies.

Many pregnant women express the wish "I hope my baby is born healthy." Nurses can play a major role in helping this become a reality by educating women before they become pregnant. Conditions such as diabetes, cardiac and respiratory disorders, **anemia**, autoimmune disorders, and specific infections frequently can be controlled through close prenatal management so that their impact on pregnancy is minimized. Nurses can provide pregnancy prevention strategies when counseling teenagers. Meeting the developmental needs of pregnant adolescents is a challenge. Finally, lifestyle choices can place many women at risk during pregnancy, and nurses need to remain nonjudgmental when working with these special populations. Lifestyle choices such as use of alcohol, nicotine, and illicit substances during pregnancy are addressed in a *Healthy People 2020* goal.

Chapter 19 described pregnancy-related conditions that place the woman at risk. This chapter addresses common conditions that can have a negative impact on the pregnancy and special populations at risk, outlining appropriate nursing assessment and management for each condition or situation. The unique skills of nurses, in conjunction with the other members of the health care team, can increase the potential for a positive outcome in many high-risk pregnancies.

HEALTHY PEOPLE 2020

Objective	Nursing Significance
• Increase abstinence from alcohol, cigarettes, and illicit drugs among pregnant women • Increase in reported abstinence in the past month from substances by pregnant women • Alcohol from a baseline of 89.4% to 98.3% • Binge drinking from a baseline of 95% to 100% • Cigarette smoking from a baseline of 89.6% to 98.6% • Illicit drugs from a baseline of 94.9% to 100%	Will help to focus attention on measures for reducing substance exposure and use, thereby minimizing the effects of these substances on the fetus and newborn

Healthy People objectives based on data from http://www.healthypeople.gov.

DIABETES MELLITUS

Diabetes mellitus is a chronic disease characterized by a relative lack of insulin or absence of the hormone that is necessary for glucose metabolism. The chronic hyperglycemia of diabetes is associated with long-term damage, dysfunction, and failure of the eyes, kidneys, nerves, heart, and blood vessels. The prevalence of diabetes in the United States is increasing at an alarming rate, already reaching epidemic proportions. Contributing factors to these increasing rates are more sedentary lifestyles, dietary changes, continued immigration by high-risk populations, and the growing epidemic of childhood and adolescent obesity. Currently, an estimated 20% of people over the age of 20 have undiagnosed prediabetes. This group of people is the pool from which childbearing women are drawn. Current estimates project that by 2025, one in three adults in the United States will have diabetes mellitus (Knox, Delaney, & Winterstein, 2014). The Institute for Alternative Futures (2015) estimates that the number of Americans living with diabetes (diagnosed and undiagnosed) will increase 64% by 2025. The resulting medical and societal cost of diabetes will be approximately $515 billion.

Diabetes commonly is classified based on disease etiology (American Diabetes Association [ADA], 2015a). These groups include:

- **Type 1 diabetes:** absolute insulin deficiency (due to an autoimmune process); usually appears before the age of 30 years; approximately 5% of those diagnosed have type 1 diabetes.
- **Type 2 diabetes:** insulin resistance or deficiency (related to obesity, sedentary lifestyle); diagnosed primarily in adults older than 30 years of age but now being seen in children; the most common type of diabetes. It is more common in African Americans, Latinos, Native Americans, and Asian Americans/Pacific Islanders, as well as older adults.
- **Impaired fasting glucose and impaired glucose tolerance:** characterized by hyperglycemia at a level lower than what qualifies as a diagnosis of diabetes (fasting blood glucose level between 100 and 125 mg/dL; blood glucose level between 140 and 199 mg/dL after a 2-hour glucose tolerance test, respectively);

symptoms of diabetes are absent; newborns are at risk for being large for gestational age (LGA).

- **Gestational diabetes mellitus:** glucose intolerance with its onset during pregnancy usually around the 24th week or first detected in pregnancy. The prevalence of gestational diabetes has been increasing in the United States and is as high as up to 10% in the United States.

During pregnancy, diabetes typically is categorized into two groups: **pregestational diabetes** (alteration in carbohydrate metabolism identified before conception), which includes women with type 1 or type 2 disease and gestational diabetes, which develops during pregnancy.

The International Association of Diabetes and Pregnancy Study Group has issued recommendations for diagnosing and classifying hyperglycemia in pregnancy (see Table 20.1).

Gestational diabetes is associated with either neonatal complications such as macrosomia, hypoglycemia, and birth trauma or maternal complications such as preeclampsia and cesarean birth. All women of childbearing age with diabetes should be counseled about the importance of strict glycemic control prior to conception. Observational studies show an increased risk of anencephaly, microcephaly, and congenital heart disease, which increases directly with elevations in A1C (Lapolla & Dalfra, 2015).

Before the discovery of insulin in 1922, most women with diabetes were infertile or experienced spontaneous abortion (March of Dimes, 2015a). During the past several decades, great strides have been made in improving the outcomes of pregnancy in women with diabetes, but this chronic metabolic disorder remains a high-risk condition during pregnancy. A favorable outcome requires commitment on the woman's part to adhere to frequent prenatal visits, dietary restrictions, self-monitoring of blood glucose levels, frequent laboratory tests, intensive fetal surveillance, and perhaps hospitalization.

Pathophysiology

Diabetes is a complex and progressive disease that has major societal and economic impact. It is a multifactorial disease, the pathophysiology of which involves not only the pancreas but also the liver, skeletal muscle, adipose tissue, gastrointestinal tract, brain, and kidney. Reduced sensitivity to insulin in the liver, muscle, and adipose tissue, and a progressive decline in pancreatic beta-cell function, leads to impaired insulin secretion, eventually resulting in hyperglycemia, the hallmark of diabetes (Cornell, 2015). Current understanding of the pathophysiology of gestational diabetes includes two key components. These are the existence of pancreatic beta-cell dysfunction prior to pregnancy and the unmasking of this problem by the development of insulin resistance during pregnancy, which requires enhanced insulin production to maintain normal blood glucose ranges.

Normal pregnancy is characterized by increasing peripheral resistance to insulin and a compensatory increase in insulin secretion. Therefore, pregnancy might be viewed as a stress test for the glucose homeostasis mechanisms. That is, women who have some degree of chronic insulin resistance and compensatory increased insulin production resulting in beta-cell dysfunction before pregnancy may be unable to mount a sufficiently robust beta-cell response to pregnancy-mediated insulin resistance. Pregnancy is accompanied by insulin resistance, mediated by placental secretion of diabetogenic hormones. These and other metabolic changes that occur during pregnancy ensure that the fetus has an ample supply of nutrients.

TABLE 20.1 RECOMMENDATIONS FOR DIAGNOSING AND CLASSIFYING HYPERGLYCEMIA IN PREGNANCY

When	Diagnosis	Test	Cutoff for Diagnosis
First prenatal visit	Overt (pregestational) diabetes or high-risk history—physical inactivity, first-degree relative with diabetes, hypertension, high-risk race/ethnicity, obesity, polycystic ovarian syndrome, hypercholesterolemia, previous large infant >9 lb; and smoker.	Fasting HbA1C Random	126 mg/dL <7% 200 mg/dL
24–28 weeks	Gestational diabetes	Fasting 75 g OGTT—1 hr 75 g OGTT—2 hrs	92 mg/dL 180 mg/dL 153 mg/dL

OGTT, oral glucose tolerance test.

Adapted from International Association of Diabetes and Pregnancy Study Group. (2012). Screening for gestational diabetes mellitus. *Diabetes Care, 35*(2). Retrieved from http://care.diabetesjournals.org/content/early/2012/01/23/dc11-1643;ACOG (2014a). ACOG guidelines at a glance: Gestational diabetes mellitus. *Contemporary OB/GYN*. Retrieved from http://contemporaryobgyn.modernmedicine.com/contemporary-obgyn/news/acog-guidelines-glance-gestational-diabetes-mellitus?page=full; and Roglie, G., & Colagiuri, S. (2014). Gestational diabetes mellitus: Squaring the circle. *Diabetes Care, 37*(6), 143–144.

With diabetes, there is a deficiency of or resistance to insulin. This alteration interferes with the body's ability to obtain essential nutrients for fuel and storage. If a pregnant woman has pregestational diabetes or develops gestational diabetes, the profound metabolic alterations that occur during pregnancy and that are necessary to support the growth and development of the fetus are greatly affected.

Maternal metabolism is directed toward supplying adequate nutrition for the fetus. In pregnancy, placental hormones cause insulin resistance at a level that tends to parallel the growth of the fetoplacental unit. As the placenta grows, more placental hormones are secreted. Human placental lactogen (hPL) and growth hormone (somatotropin) increase in direct correlation with the growth of placental tissue, rising throughout the last 20 weeks of pregnancy and causing insulin resistance. Subsequently, insulin secretion increases to overcome the resistance of these two hormones. In the pregnant woman without diabetes, the pancreas can respond to the demands for increased insulin production to maintain normal glucose levels throughout the pregnancy (Toledano, Hadar, & Hod, 2015). However, the woman with glucose intolerance or diabetes during pregnancy cannot cope with changes in metabolism resulting from insufficient insulin to meet the needs during gestation.

Over the course of pregnancy, insulin resistance does change. It peaks in the last trimester to provide more nutrients to the fetus. The insulin resistance typically results in postprandial hyperglycemia, although some women also have an elevated fasting blood glucose level (Aktas et al., 2014). With this increased demand on the pancreas in late pregnancy, women with diabetes or glucose intolerance cannot accommodate the increased insulin demand; glucose levels rise as a result of insulin deficiency, leading to hyperglycemia. Subsequently, the mother and her fetus can experience major problems, as shown in Table 20.2.

Screening

Currently, there are inconsistent standards around the world for how women are tested for gestational diabetes, as well cutoff values to diagnose it. The American College of Obstetricians and Gynecologists (ACOG) and ADA currently recommend a risk analysis of all pregnant women at their first prenatal visit and additional

TABLE 20.2 DIABETES AND PREGNANCY: EFFECTS ON THE MOTHER AND FETUS

Effects on the Mother	Effects on the Fetus/Neonate
• Hydramnios due to fetal diuresis caused by hyperglycemia • Gestational hypertension of unknown etiology • Ketoacidosis due to uncontrolled hyperglycemia • Preterm labor secondary to premature membrane rupture • Stillbirth in pregnancies complicated by ketoacidosis and poor glucose control • Hypoglycemia as glucose is diverted to the fetus (occurring in first trimester) • Urinary tract infections resulting from excess glucose in the urine (glucosuria), which promotes bacterial growth • Chronic monilial vaginitis due to glucosuria, which promotes growth of yeast • Difficult labor, cesarean birth, postpartum hemorrhage secondary to an overdistended uterus to accommodate a macrosomic infant	• Cord prolapse secondary to polyhydramnios and abnormal fetal presentation • Congenital anomaly due to hyperglycemia in the first trimester (cardiac problems, neural tube defects, skeletal deformities, and genitourinary problems) • Macrosomia resulting from hyperinsulinemia stimulated by fetal hyperglycemia • Birth trauma due to increased size of fetus, which complicates the birthing process (shoulder dystocia) • Preterm birth secondary to polyhydramnios and an aging placenta, which places the fetus in jeopardy if the pregnancy continues • Fetal asphyxia secondary to fetal hyperglycemia and hyperinsulinemia • Intrauterine growth restriction secondary to maternal vascular impairment and decreased placental perfusion, which restricts growth • Perinatal death due to poor placental perfusion and hypoxia • Respiratory distress syndrome resulting from poor surfactant production secondary to hyperinsulinemia inhibits the production of phospholipids that make up the surfactant • Polycythemia due to excessive red blood cell (RBC) production in response to hypoxia • Hyperbilirubinemia due to excessive RBC breakdown from hypoxia and an immature liver unable to break down bilirubin • Neonatal hypoglycemia resulting from ongoing hyperinsulinemia after the placenta is removed • Subsequent childhood obesity and carbohydrate intolerance

Adapted from Cunningham, F. G., Leveno, K. J., Bloom, S.L., Spong, C., & Dashe, J. (2014). *Williams' obstetrics* (24th ed.). New York, NY: McGraw-Hill Professional Publishing; Moore, T. R. (2015). Diabetes mellitus and pregnancy. *eMedicine.* Retrieved from http://emedicine.medscape.com/article/127547 and March of Dimes. (2015a). *Gestational diabetes.* Retrieved from http://www.marchofdimes.com/pregnancy/gestational-diabetes.aspx.

screening of all high-risk pregnant women again at 24 to 28 weeks, or earlier if risk factors are present. If the initial screening risk assessment is low, additional screening may not be necessary. Pregnant women who fulfill all of the following criteria need not be screened at their first prenatal visit:

- No history of glucose intolerance
- Less than 25 years old
- Normal body weight
- No family history (first-degree relative) of diabetes
- No history of poor obstetric outcome
- Not from an ethnic/racial group with a high prevalence of diabetes (ADA, 2015b)

If the initial risk assessment is high, rescreening should take place between 24 and 28 weeks. A woman with abnormal early results may have had diabetes before the pregnancy, and her fetus is at great risk for congenital anomalies. An elevated glycosylated hemoglobin supports the likelihood of gestational diabetes. Combining the use of HbA1c and plasma glucose measurements for the diagnosis of diabetes offers the benefits of each test and reduces the risk of systematic bias inherent in HbA1c testing alone (Petry, 2014).

There is little consensus regarding the appropriate screening method. Typically, screening is based on a 75-g 1-hour glucose challenge test, usually performed between week 24 and 28 of gestation (McIntyre, Dyer, & Metzger, 2015). A 75-g oral glucose load is given, without regard to the timing or content of the last meal. Blood glucose is measured 1 hour later; a level above 140 mg/dL is abnormal. If the result is abnormal, a 3-hour glucose tolerance test is done. Normal values are:

- Fasting blood glucose level: less than 92 mg/dL
- At 1 hour: less than 180 mg/dL
- At 2 hours: less than 153 mg/dL
- At 3 hours: less than 140 mg/dL

A diagnosis of gestational diabetes can be made only after an abnormal result is obtained on the glucose tolerance test. One or more abnormal values confirm a diagnosis of gestational diabetes (Farrar et al., 2015). A newer, more controlled screening (HbA1C) has been adopted by the ADA and ACOG because of mounting evidence that diagnosing and treating even mild gestational diabetes reduces morbidity for both the mother and infant (ADA, 2015c).If adopted universally, the new guidelines are expected to have immediate, widespread clinical implications.

Therapeutic Management

Care for the Woman With Pregestational Diabetes

Pregestational diabetes is a significant public health problem that increases the risk for structural birth defects affecting both maternal and neonatal pregnancy outcomes. Women who have pregestational diabetes (the alteration in carbohydrate metabolism is identified before conception) need comprehensive prenatal care. Achieving good metabolic control during the period prior to conception is essential to reducing congenital malformations that can occur in pregnancies complicated by diabetes. The primary goals of care are to maintain glycemic control and minimize the risks of the disease on the fetus. Key aspects of treatment include nutritional management, exercise, insulin regimens, and close maternal and fetal surveillance (Fig. 20.1).

Preconception counseling is essential for the woman with pregestational diabetes to ensure that her disease state is stable. The problem is that as many as half of all pregnancies in the United States are unplanned. Thus, women with chronic medical conditions such as diabetes might not have the opportunity to take steps to

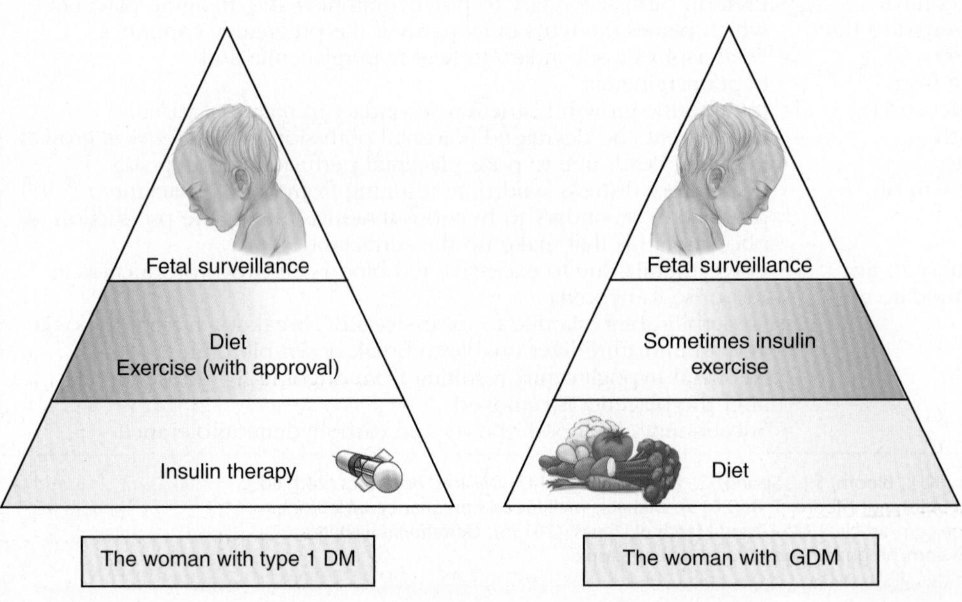

FIGURE 20.1 Treatment overview for diabetes in pregnancy. For women with pregestational type 1 DM, the foundation of glycemic management is insulin therapy along with dietary management, exercise, and fetal surveillance. For the woman who develops gestational diabetes, dietary modification is generally the foundation of treatment. Some women may require insulin along with dietary modifications, whereas others will not require insulin therapy at all. Exercise and fetal surveillance are also important facets of care.

optimize management of their diabetes before becoming pregnant. When preconception care is possible, women with pregestational diabetes should be taught how to improve their metabolic control prior to conception to reduce the risk of birth defects. Nurses caring for women of reproductive age can contribute to preconception care by helping to counsel someone who is prediabetic to avoid progression to diabetes and its attendant risks during pregnancy. The goals of preconception care are to:

- Integrate the woman into the management of her diabetes
- Achieve the lowest glycosylated hemoglobin A1C test results without excessive hypoglycemia
- Ensure effective contraception until stable glycemia is achieved
- Identify and evaluate long-term diabetic complications such as retinopathy, nephropathy, neuropathy, cardiovascular disease (CVD), and hypertension (Gabbay-Benziv et al., 2015).

Excellent control of blood glucose, as evidenced by normal fasting blood glucose levels and **glycosylated hemoglobin (HbA1C) levels** (a measurement of the average glucose levels during the past 100 to 120 days), is crucial to achieve the best pregnancy outcome. A glycosylated hemoglobin level of less than 7% indicates good control; a value of more than 8% indicates poor control and warrants intervention. A pregestational diabetic pregnant woman has up to a nine-fold increase in birth defects, compared with the rate seen in nondiabetic pregnancies, if she does not have glycemic control (Mitanchez et al., 2015).

Preconception counseling is also important in helping to reduce the risk of congenital malformation. The most common malformations associated with diabetes occur in the renal, cardiac, skeletal, and central nervous systems. Since these defects occur by the eighth week of gestation, preconception counseling is critical. The rate of congenital anomalies in women with pregestational diabetes can be reduced if excellent glycemic control is achieved at the time of conception (Simeone et al., 2015). This information needs to be stressed with all women with diabetes who are contemplating a pregnancy. In addition, the woman with pregestational diabetes needs to be evaluated for complications of diabetes. This evaluation should be part of baseline screening and continuing assessment during pregnancy.

Care During Pregnancy for the Woman With Gestational Diabetes

Lifestyle modification, nutritional changes, and encouragement of physical activities form the primary mode of therapy for diabetes during pregnancy. Therapeutic management for the woman with **gestational diabetes mellitus** (defined as glucose intolerance with its onset during pregnancy or first detected during pregnancy) focuses on tight glucose control. The ADA (2015b) recommends maintaining a fasting blood glucose level below 92 mg/dL, with 1-hour postprandial levels below 180 mg/dL and 2-hour postprandial levels below 153 mg/dL. In comparison, for pregnant women without diabetes, near-normal glucose values include a fasting value of 60 to 90 mg/dL, a 1-hour postprandial value of 100 to 120 mg/dL, and a 2-hour postprandial value of 60 to 120 mg/dL. Such tight control has been advocated because it is associated with a reduction in macrosomia. In addition, maternal prepregnancy weight and weight gain during pregnancy appear to be significant and independent risk factors for macrosomia in women with gestational diabetes also (Grandy et al., 2015).

Nutritional management focuses on maintaining balanced glucose levels and providing enough energy and nutrients for the pregnant woman, while avoiding ketosis, and minimizing the risk of hypoglycemia in women treated with insulin. Nutrition therapy is the cornerstone of therapy for women with gestational diabetes. Women should receive ethically appropriate nutritional advice on how to change their dietary habits from a dietitian. The diet counseling must be in keeping with their present cultural dietary patterns and not radically different to become adopted and followed. If rice is a staple of a Chinese client's diet, then it must be incorporated into the diet counseling plan and not eliminated (He et al., 2015). A low-glycemic index diet is considered safe and has positive effects on the glycemic control and pregnancy outcomes for both healthy women, those with **type 2 diabetes** and gestational diabetes. A moderately low carbohydrate diet with a carbohydrate content of 40% of the calories results in good glycemic control for most (Roskjær et al., 2014). Eating for two during pregnancy for a woman who has diabetes means eating not volume for two, but rather quality and timing to support both the mother and fetus. Women who receive dietary instruction and follow it have been shown to have a better pregnancy outcome than those who do not receive dietary advice (Ma et al., 2015).

PHARMACOLOGIC THERAPY FOR GESTATIONAL DIABETES

For the woman with gestational diabetes, nutritional management and exercise may be all that is necessary. Pharmacologic therapy is considered if nutrition and exercise fail to maintain target glucose levels. Blood glucose levels in the woman can be controlled by nutritional therapy and exercise, but in uncontrolled cases, where target glycemic levels cannot be reached, insulin is also required. Insulin, which does not cross the placenta, historically has been the medication of choice for treating hyperglycemia in pregnancy. Insulin is calculated based on the woman's weight. Combining intermediate and short-acting insulin yields the best result for most women. Two insulin doses are given daily with two thirds of the total insulin in the morning to cover energy needs of the active day and one third at night.

Oral Medications for Management of Gestational Diabetes. Women tend to manage oral medications better than insulin, so the standard of care may be moving toward the oral route (King et al., 2015). Recent studies have examined the use of oral hypoglycemic medications in pregnancy with much success. Several studies have used glyburide (DiaBeta) with promising results. Many health care providers are using glyburide and metformin as an alternative to insulin therapy because they do not cross the placenta and therefore do not cause fetal/neonatal hypoglycemia. Some oral hypoglycemic medications are considered safe and may be used if nutrition and exercise are not adequate alone. Maternal and newborn outcomes are similar to those seen in women who are treated with insulin. Oral hypoglycemic agents, however, must be further investigated to determine their safety with confidence and provide better treatment options for diabetes in pregnancy. Currently, there is a growing acceptance of glyburide (glibenclamide) use as a primary therapy for gestational diabetes. Glyburide and metformin (Glucophage) have also been found to be safe, effective, and economical for the treatment of gestational diabetes, although neither drug has been approved by the FDA for use in pregnancy. Insulin, however, still has an important role to play in gestational diabetes (Buschur, Brown, & Wyckoff, 2015). Gestational diabetes offers a window of opportunity, which needs to be seized, for prevention of diabetes in future life (Nagtalon-Ramos, 2014).

The ADA (2015c) recommends that women diagnosed with gestational diabetes by a 3-hour glucose tolerance test receive nutritional counseling from a registered dietitian. The ADA also recommends insulin therapy or oral diabetic medications if diet is unsuccessful in achieving a fasting glucose level below 92 mg/dL, a 1-hour postprandial level below 180 mg/dL, or a 2-hour postprandial level below 153 mg/dL (ADA, 2015c).

The ACOG (2014a) recommends the use of diet or insulin or oral diabetic medications to achieve a 1-hour postprandial blood glucose level of 130 mg/dL. Randomized studies show that glyburide and insulin are equally effective in achieving glycemic control. Glycemic control—regardless of whether it involves diet, insulin, or oral agents—leads to fewer cases of shoulder dystocia, hyperbilirubinemia requiring phototherapy, nerve palsy, bone fracture, LGA status, and fetal macrosomia (ACOG, 2014a).

Exercise is another important component of comprehensive prenatal care for the pregnant woman with glucose intolerance. Regular exercise helps maintain glucose control by increasing the uptake of glucose into the cells and decreasing central obesity, hypertension, and dyslipidemia, which will ultimately decrease the woman's insulin requirements (Jordan et al., 2014). Regular physical activity has been proven to result in marked benefits for mother and fetus. Maternal benefits include improved cardiovascular function, limited pregnancy weight gain, decreased musculoskeletal discomfort, reduced incidence of muscle cramps and lower limb edema, mood stability, and reduction of gestational diabetes mellitus and gestational hypertension. Fetal benefits include decreased fat mass, improved stress tolerance, and advanced neurobehavioral maturation. Research also suggests the role of physical activity in prevention of gestational diabetes (Bain et al., 2015).

Insulin for Management of Gestational Diabetes. Insulin remains the medication of choice for glycemic control if oral medications, diet, or exercise fail to yield results in pregnant and lactating women with any type of diabetes (Moore, 2015). Generally, insulin doses are reduced in the first trimester to prevent hypoglycemia resulting from increased insulin sensitivity as well as from nausea and vomiting. Newer short-acting insulins such as lispro (Humalog) and aspart (NovoLog), which do not cross the placenta, may help reduce postprandial hyperglycemia, episodes of hypoglycemia between meals. Target fasting glucose values of 60 to 90 mg/dL and 1-hour postprandial values less than 120 mg/dL are necessary to provide good glycemic control and good pregnancy outcomes (Moore, 2015). Changes in diet and activity level add to the need for changes in insulin dosages throughout pregnancy.

Insulin regimens vary, and controversy remains over the best strategy for insulin delivery in pregnancy. Many health care providers use a split-dose therapy (two thirds of the daily dose in the morning and the remaining one third in the evening). Others advocate the use of an insulin pump to deliver a continuous subcutaneous insulin infusion. Regardless of which protocol is used, frequent blood glucose measurements are necessary, and the insulin dosage is adjusted on the basis of daily glucose levels. Insulin therapy or oral hypoglycemic agents, in addition to diet and exercise, are main elements of achieving glycemic control. See Evidence-Based Practice 20.1.

Close maternal and fetal surveillance is also essential. Frequent laboratory tests are done during pregnancy to monitor the woman's status and glucose control. Fetal surveillance via diagnostic testing aids in evaluating fetal well-being and assisting in determining the best time for birth.

Care During and After Labor for the Woman With Gestational Diabetes

For the laboring woman with diabetes, intravenous saline or lactated Ringer's is given and blood glucose levels are monitored every 1 to 2 hours. Glucose levels are maintained below 110 mg/dL throughout labor to reduce the

EVIDENCE-BASED PRACTICE 20.1

PREVENTION OF GESTATIONAL DIABETES IN PREGNANT WOMEN WITH RISK FACTORS FOR GESTATIONAL DIABETES: A SYSTEMATIC REVIEW AND META-ANALYSIS OF RANDOMIZED TRIALS

STUDY

Gestational diabetes mellitus (GDM) is defined as the diabetes diagnosed during pregnancy that is not clearly overt diabetes. According to this definition, glycemic levels meeting the thresholds of overt diabetes are considered to have pre-existing diabetes and the rest are given diagnosis of GDM. The objective of the systematic review was to identify any intervention that could be used for primary prevention of gestational diabetes in women with risk factors for it.

A systematic review and meta-analysis was conducted by including randomized controlled trials comparing any form of therapeutic intervention in comparison to usual antenatal care. A literature search was conducted using electronic databases together with a hand search of relevant journals and conference proceedings.

Findings

A total of 2,422 women from 14 randomized trials were included which compared diet, exercise, lifestyle changes, and metformin with standard care in women with risk factors for gestational diabetes. Dietary intervention was associated with statistically significant lower incidence of gestational diabetes and gestational hypertension compared to standard of care. There was no statistically significant difference in the incidence of gestational diabetes with exercise, lifestyle changes, or metformin used compared to standard care.

Nursing Implications

Based on these findings, nurses can encourage healthy dietary changes as a primary prevention strategy to prevent gestational diabetes for high-risk women, since this intervention was shown to be a statistically significant intervention over standard care. Instructing them on health dietary habits either preconceptually or at the first prenatal visit may help prevent gestational diabetes and turn the tide for better pregnancy outcomes for both the mother and infant.

Adapted from Madhuvrata, P., Govinden, G., Bustani, R., Song, S., & Farrell, T. A. (2015). Prevention of gestational diabetes in pregnant women with risk factors for gestational diabetes: A systematic review and meta-analysis of randomized trials. *Obstetric Medicine: The Medicine of Pregnancy, 8*(2), 68–85.

likelihood of neonatal hypoglycemia. If necessary, an infusion of regular insulin may be given to maintain this level (King et al., 2015). If the woman was receiving insulin during her pregnancy, adjustments in dosage may be necessary after birth since glucose diversion across the placenta to supply the growing fetus is no longer present and insulin resistance is now removed. Frequently, the woman with gestational diabetes can remain controlled through diet and weight management; the woman with type 1 diabetes usually returns to prepregnant levels of insulin administration (Kim, 2014).

After giving birth, the overt glycemic abnormalities of gestational diabetes usually resolve. This phenomenon suggests that the diabetes is transient and that the consequences of gestational diabetes end with the birth of the infant. However, for the woman, childbirth is not the end of the story. The diagnosis of gestational diabetes heralds future health risks. Knowledge of this "failed" stress test conveys new information about her future risk for type 2 diabetes, which warrants further screening and prevention efforts during the postpartum period and beyond.

Nursing Assessment

Nursing assessment begins at the first prenatal visit. A thorough history and physical examination in conjunction with specific laboratory and diagnostic testing aids in developing an individualized plan of care for the woman with diabetes.

Health History and Physical Examination

For the woman with pregestational diabetes, obtain a thorough history of the preexisting diabetic condition. Ask about her duration of disease, management of glucose levels (insulin injections, insulin pump, or oral hypoglycemic agents), dietary adjustments, presence of vascular complications and current vascular status, current insulin regimen, and technique used for glucose testing. Review any information that she may have received as part of her preconception counseling and measures that were implemented during this time.

Be knowledgeable about the woman's nutritional requirements and assess the adequacy and pattern of her dietary intake. Assess her blood glucose self-monitoring in terms of technique, frequency, and her ability to adjust the insulin dose based on the changing patterns. Ask about the frequency of episodes of hypoglycemia or hyperglycemia to ascertain the woman's ability to recognize and treat them. Continue to assess her for signs and symptoms of hypo- and hyperglycemia.

During antepartum visits, assess the client's knowledge about her disease, including the signs and symptoms of hypoglycemia, hyperglycemia, and diabetic ketoacidosis, insulin administration techniques, and the impact of pregnancy on her chronic condition. If possible, have the woman demonstrate her technique for blood glucose monitoring and insulin administration for correctness. It is essential that the nurse keeps in mind that there is a

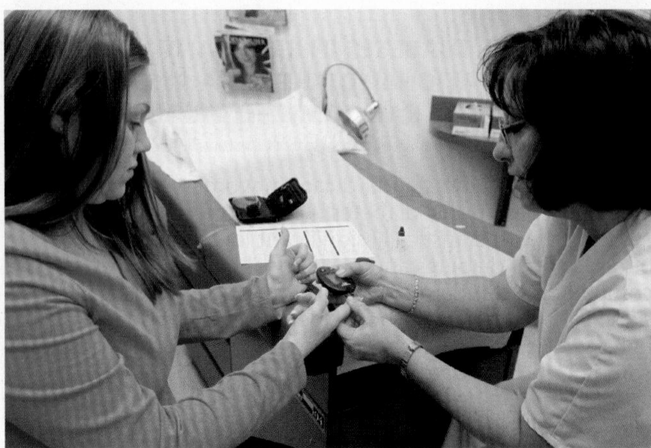

FIGURE 20.2 The nurse is demonstrating the technique for self-blood glucose monitoring with a pregnant client who has diabetes.

huge learning curve for women with diabetes concerning the need for dietary changes, frequency of blood glucose monitoring, exercise, and insulin or oral medication administration. Suddenly, the woman is expected to make rapid changes in her life, which can be overwhelming. The nurse can help facilitate these changes by exercising patience and understanding and reinforcing all verbal instructions with written material. Frequent encouragement is also needed to assist the woman in her lifestyle changes. Although the client may have had diabetes for some time, do not assume that she has a firm knowledge base about her disease process or management of it (Fig. 20.2).

Assess the woman's risk for gestational diabetes at the first prenatal visit. The clinical presentation of diabetes mellitus in pregnancy may be quite varied, but the classical triad of the symptoms of polydipsia, polyphagia, and polyuria may not be reported by most women during pregnancy. Instead, the women may present with previous history of medical complications of diabetes (chronic hypertension/chronic renal disease) and obesity. All of these conditions can influence pregnancy outcome. The ADA (2015a) recommends assessing all women for risk factors and then determining the need for additional testing in the high-risk group only. Factors that place a woman at high risk include:

- Previous infant with congenital anomaly (skeletal, renal, central nervous system, cardiac)
- History of gestational diabetes or polyhydramnios in a previous pregnancy
- Family history of diabetes
- Medications: corticosteroids or antipsychotics
- Age 35 years or older
- Polycystic ovarian syndrome
- Multiple pregnancy (twins, triplets)
- Previous infant weighing more than 9 lb (4,000 g)
- Previous unexplained fetal demise or neonatal death
- Maternal obesity (body mass index [BMI] >30)
- Hypertension before pregnancy or in early pregnancy
- Hispanic, Native American, Pacific Islander, or African American ethnicity
- Recurrent monilia infections that do not respond to treatment
- Signs and symptoms of glucose intolerance (polyuria, polyphagia, polydipsia, fatigue)
- Presence of glycosuria or proteinuria (Gupta, 2015).

Women with clinical characteristics consistent with a high risk for gestational diabetes should undergo glucose testing as soon as feasible.

Provide a close ongoing assessment throughout the antepartum period. Women with gestational diabetes mellitus are at increased risk for preeclampsia and glucose control-related complications such as hypoglycemia, hyperglycemia, and ketoacidosis. Gestational diabetes of any severity increases the risk of fetal macrosomia, as noted earlier. It is also associated with an increased frequency of maternal hypertensive disorders and operative births. This may be the result of fetal growth disorders (ADA, 2015a).Even though gestational diabetes is diagnosed during pregnancy, the woman may have had glucose intolerance before the pregnancy. Therefore, monitor the woman closely for signs and symptoms of possible complications.

Also assess the woman's psychosocial adaptation to her condition. This assessment is critical to gain her cooperation for a change in regimen or the addition of a new regimen throughout pregnancy. Identify her support systems and note any financial constraints, because she will need intense monitoring and frequent fetal surveillance.

Laboratory and Diagnostic Testing

The results of laboratory and diagnostic tests provide valuable information about maternal and fetal well-being. Women with pregestational diabetes and those discovered to have gestational diabetes require ongoing maternal and fetal surveillance to promote the best outcome.

SURVEILLANCE

Maternal surveillance may include the following:

- Urine check for protein (may indicate the need for further evaluation for preeclampsia) and for nitrates and leukocyte esterase (may indicate a urinary tract infection)
- Urine check for ketones (may indicate the need for evaluation of eating habits)
- Kidney function evaluation every trimester for creatinine clearance and protein levels
- Eye examination in the first trimester to evaluate the retina for vascular changes
- HbA1c every 4 to 6 weeks to monitor glucose trends (Jordan et al., 2014).

Fetal surveillance may include ultrasound to provide information about fetal growth, activity, and amniotic fluid volume and to validate gestational age. Alpha-fetoprotein levels may be obtained to detect congenital anomalies such as an open neural tube or ventral wall defects of omphalocele or gastroschisis, and a fetal echocardiogram may be necessary to rule out cardiac anomalies. A biophysical profile helps to monitor fetal well-being and uteroplacental profusion, and nonstress tests are commonly performed weekly after 28 weeks' gestation to evaluate fetal well-being. As the pregnancy progresses, an amniocentesis may be done to determine the lecithin/sphingomyelin (L/S) ratio and the presence of phosphatidyl glycerol (PG) to evaluate whether the fetal lung is mature enough for birth (Moore, 2015).

Nursing Management

The ideal outcome of every pregnancy is a healthy newborn and mother. Nurses can be pivotal in realizing this positive outcome for women with pregestational or gestational diabetes by implementing measures to minimize risks and complications. Since the woman with diabetes is considered to be at high risk, antepartum visits occur more frequently (every 2 weeks up to 28 weeks and then twice a week until birth), providing the nurse with numerous opportunities for ongoing assessment, education, and counseling (Nursing Care Plan 20.1, at the end of the chapter).

Promoting Optimal Glucose Control

At each visit, review the mother's blood glucose levels, including any laboratory tests and self-monitoring results. Reinforce the woman the need to perform blood glucose monitoring (usually four times a day: before meals and at bedtime) and to keep a record of the results. If appropriate, obtain a fingerstick blood glucose level to evaluate the accuracy of self-monitoring results. Also assess the woman's techniques for monitoring blood glucose levels and for administering insulin if ordered, and offer support and guidance. If the woman is receiving insulin therapy, assist with any changes needed if glucose levels are not controlled. Obtain a urine specimen and check for glucose, protein, and ketones. Ask the woman if she has had any episodes of hypoglycemia and what she did to alleviate them. Discuss dietary measures related to blood glucose control (Fig. 20.3). In addition, recommend the following:

- Avoid weight loss and dieting during pregnancy.
- Ensure that food intake is adequate to prevent ketone formation and promote weight gain.
- Eat three meals a day plus three snacks to promote glycemic control:
  - 40% of calories from good-quality complex carbohydrates.
  - 35% of calories from protein sources.

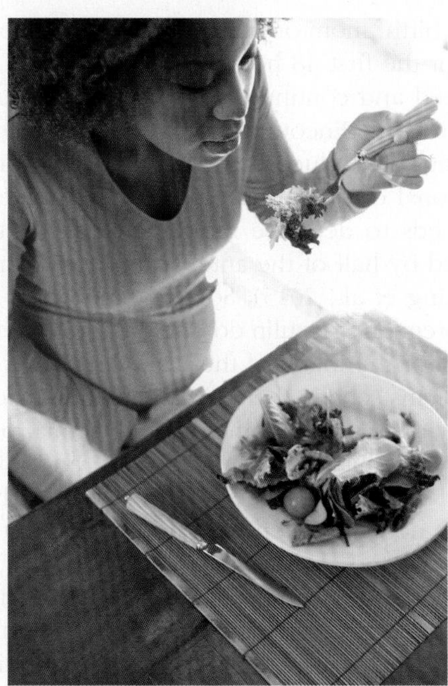

FIGURE 20.3 The pregnant client with diabetes eating a nutritious meal to ensure adequate glucose control.

  - 25% of calories from unsaturated fats.
  - Small frequent feedings throughout the day are recommended.
  - Bedtime snacks are recommended for all women.
  - Include protein and fat at each meal (National Diabetes Information Clearing House, 2015).

Take Note!

Nutrient requirements and recommendations for weight gain for the pregnant woman with diabetes are the same as those for the pregnant nondiabetic woman.

If necessary, arrange for consultation with a dietitian or nutritionist to individualize the dietary plan. Also encourage the women to participate in an exercise program that includes at least three sessions lasting at least 30 minutes daily. Exercise may lessen the need for insulin or dosage adjustments.

When caring for the laboring woman with pregestational or gestational diabetes, adjust the intravenous flow rate and the rate of supplemental regular insulin based on the blood glucose levels as ordered. Monitor blood glucose levels every 1 to 2 hours or more frequently if necessary. Keep a syringe with 50% dextrose solution at the bedside to treat profound hypoglycemia. Monitor fetal heart rate patterns throughout labor to detect category II and III patterns. Assess maternal vital signs every hour, in addition to assessing the woman's urinary output with an indwelling catheter. If a cesarean birth is scheduled, monitor the woman's blood glucose levels hourly and administer short-acting insulin or glucose based on the blood glucose levels as ordered.

After birth, monitor blood glucose levels every 2 to 4 hours for the first 48 hours to determine the woman's insulin need and continue intravenous fluid administration as ordered. Encourage breast-feeding to assist in maintaining good glucose control. For the woman with pregestational diabetes and type 1 or 2 diabetes, expect insulin needs to decrease rapidly after birth: they may be reduced by half of the antepartum dose as meals are started (King et al., 2015). Some women may return to their prepregnancy insulin dosage. In addition, the nurse must monitor the infant of the diabetic mother for common problems seen in them, which include macrosomia, respiratory distress syndrome, hypoglycemia, polycythemia, hypocalcemia, hyperbilirubinemia, and a variety of congenital anomalies (Green, 2016). Frequently, admission to the neonatal intensive care unit (NICU) for close observational and glucose control is needed.

The therapy plan after childbirth is individualized. If recommended dietary modifications are carried out along with weight loss, the woman with gestational diabetes may return to her normal glucose levels. This is also true for the woman with pregestational diabetes, except that she will return to her prepregnancy insulin administration levels. This provides the nurse with a wonderful opportunity to reinforce healthy lifestyle interventions on the postpartum unit. Nurses can also become involved with community-based education to continue to offer their expertise.

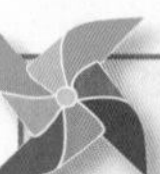

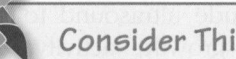

Consider This

Scott and I had been busy all day setting up the new crib in our nursery, and we finally sat down to rest. I was due any day, and we had been putting this off until we had a long weekend to complete the task. I was excited to think about all the frilly pinks that decorated her room. I was sure that my new daughter would love it as much as I loved her already. A few days later I barely noticed any fetal movement, but I thought that she must be as tired as I was by this point.

That night I went into labor and kept looking at the worried faces of the nurses and the midwife in attendance. I had been diagnosed with gestational diabetes a few months ago and had tried to follow the instructions regarding diet and exercise, but old habits are hard to change when you are 38 years old. I was finally told after a short time in the labor unit that they couldn't pick up a fetal heartbeat and an ultrasound was to be done—still no heartbeat was detected. Scott and I were finally told that our daughter was a stillborn. All I could think about was that she would never get to see all the pink colors in the nursery.

Preventing Complications

Assess the woman closely for signs and symptoms of complications at each visit. Anticipate possible complications and plan appropriate interventions or referrals. Check the woman's blood pressure for changes and evaluate for proteinuria when obtaining a urine specimen. These might suggest the development of preeclampsia. Measure the fundal height and review gestational age. Note any discrepancies between the fundal height and gestational age or a sudden increase in uterine growth. These may suggest polyhydramnios.

Encourage the woman to perform daily fetal movement counts to monitor fetal well-being. Tell her specifically when she should notify her health care provider. Also prepare the woman for the need for frequent laboratory and diagnostic testing to evaluate fetal status. Assist with serial ultrasounds to monitor fetal growth and with nonstress tests and biophysical profiles to assess fetal well-being.

Providing Client Education and Counseling

The pregnant woman with diabetes requires counseling and education about the need for strict glucose monitoring, diet and exercise, and signs and symptoms of complications. Encourage the client and her family to make any lifestyle changes needed to optimize the pregnancy outcome. Providing dietary education, weight control measures, and lifestyle advice that extends beyond pregnancy may lower the risk that the woman will have gestational diabetes in subsequent pregnancies as well as type 2 diabetes (Hashemi-Beni et al., 2015). At each visit, stress the importance of performing blood glucose screening and documenting the results. With proper instruction, the client and her family will be able to cope with all the changes in her body during pregnancy (Teaching Guidelines 20.1).

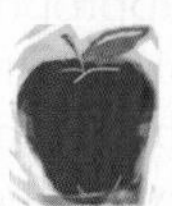

Teaching Guidelines 20.1

TEACHING FOR THE PREGNANT WOMAN WITH DIABETES

- Be sure to keep your appointments for frequent prenatal visits and tests for fetal well-being.
- Perform blood glucose self-monitoring as directed, usually before each meal and at bedtime. Keep a record of your results and call your health care provider with any levels outside the established range. Bring your results to each prenatal visit.
- Perform daily "fetal kick counts." Document them and report any decrease in activity.
- Drink eight to ten 8-ounce glasses of water each day to prevent bladder infections and maintain hydration.
- Wear proper, well-fitted footwear when walking to prevent injury.
- Engage in a regular exercise program such as walking to aid in glucose control, but avoid exercising in temperature extremes.

- Consider breast-feeding your infant to lower your blood glucose levels.
- If you are taking insulin:
  - Administer the correct dose of insulin at the correct time every day.
  - Eat breakfast within 30 minutes after injecting regular insulin to prevent a reaction.
  - Plan meals, as well as snacks, at a fixed time to prevent extremes in glucose levels.
- Avoid simple sugars (cake, candy, cookies), which raise blood glucose levels.
- Know the signs and symptoms of hypoglycemia and treatment needed:
  - Sweating, tremors, cold, clammy skin, headache
  - Feeling hungry, blurred vision, disorientation, irritability
  - Treatment: Drink 8 ounces of milk and eat two crackers or take two glucose tablets
- Carry "glucose boosters" (such as Life Savers) to treat hypoglycemia.
- Know the signs and symptoms of hyperglycemia and treatment needed:
  - Dry mouth, frequent urination, excessive thirst, rapid breathing
  - Feeling tired, flushed, hot skin, headache, drowsiness
  - Treatment: Notify health care provider, because hospitalization may be needed
- Wear a diabetic identification bracelet at all times.
- Wash your hands frequently to prevent infections.
- Report any signs and symptoms of illness, infection, and dehydration to your health care provider, because these can affect blood glucose control.

Review discussions about the timing of birth and the rationale. Counsel the client about the possibility of cesarean birth for an LGA infant, or inform the woman who will be giving birth vaginally about the possible need for augmentation with oxytocin (Pitocin).

Take Note!

In the woman with well-controlled diabetes, birth is typically not induced before term unless complications arise, such as preeclampsia or fetal compromise. An early delivery date might be set for the woman with poorly controlled diabetes or a large-sized fetus who is having complications.

Instruct the client about the benefits of breast-feeding related to blood glucose control. Breast-feeding helps to normalize blood glucose levels. Therefore, encourage the woman to breast-feed her newborn. Also teach the woman receiving insulin for her diabetes that her insulin needs after birth will drastically decrease. Inform her that she will need a repeat glucose challenge test at a postpartum visit (ADA, 2015d).

For the woman with gestational diabetes, the focus is on lifestyle education. Women with gestational diabetes have a greater than 50% increased risk of developing type 2 diabetes (ADA, 2015d). Inform the woman that screening most likely will be done at the postpartum follow-up appointment in 6 weeks. Women with normal results at that visit typically are screened every 3 years thereafter (ADA, 2015d). Teach her how to maintain an optimal weight to reduce her risk of developing diabetes. If necessary, refer the woman to a dietitian to help outline a balanced nutritious diet.

CARDIOVASCULAR DISORDERS

Despite an increase in awareness of a wide range of health concerns, the myth still exists that CVD is a man's disease and women do not need to be concerned about it. Every minute, an American woman dies of CVD and more than one in three women is living with a cardiovascular disorder, including nearly half of all African American women and 34% of White women (American Heart Association [AHA], 2015). CVD is the leading cause of death for men and women in the United States and is more deadly than all forms of cancer. It kills nearly 500,000 women each year. Despite the prominent reduction in cardiovascular mortality among men, the rate has not declined for women. Cardiovascular disease has killed more women than men since 1984 (AHA, 2015). In addition to being the number-one killer of women, at the time of diagnosis, women have both a poorer overall prognosis and a higher risk of death than men diagnosed with heart disease. Women represent 53% of deaths from CVD than the next three causes of death combined, including all forms of cancer (Worel & Hayman, 2015). In both men and women, risk factors such as hypertension, high blood cholesterol level, smoking, lack of physical activity, and obesity increase the probability of developing CVD. Menopause, gestational diabetes, oral contraceptive use, and bilateral oophorectomy in premenopausal women also affect the risk of CVD in women (Chomistek, Chiuve, & Eliassen, 2015).

More women die of heart disease, stroke, and other CVDs than men; yet many women do not realize they are at risk. These diseases kill more women each year than the next three causes of death combined, including all types of cancer (AHA, 2015). Approximately 3% of pregnant women have cardiac disease, which is responsible for 10% to 25% of maternal deaths (Cunningham et al., 2014). The prevalence of cardiac disease is increasing as a result of lifestyle patterns, including cigarette smoking, diabetes, and stress. As women are delaying childbearing, the incidence of cardiac disease in pregnancy will continue to increase. The cardiovascular adaptations during pregnancy are well tolerated by the normal heart, but may unveil undiagnosed underlying heart disease, or tip the hemodynamic balance and lead to decompensation in those with existing heart disease (Harvey, Coffman, & Miller, 2015).

Rheumatic heart disease used to represent the majority of cardiac conditions during pregnancy, but congenital heart disease now constitutes nearly half of all cases of heart disease encountered during pregnancy. Classic symptoms of heart disease mimic common symptoms of late pregnancy, such as palpitations, shortness of breath with exertion, and occasional chest pain. Few women with heart disease die during pregnancy, but they are at risk for other complications, such as heart failure, arrhythmias, and stroke. Their offspring are also at risk for complications, such as premature birth, low birth weight for gestational age, respiratory distress syndrome, intraventricular hemorrhage, and death (Gilstrap & Wood, 2014).

Congenital and Acquired Heart Disease

Congenital heart disease often involves structural defects that are present at birth but may not be discovered at that time (Table 20.3). Until recently, women with congenital heart disease did not live long enough to bear children. Today, due to new surgical techniques to correct these defects, many of these women can complete a successful pregnancy at relatively low risk when appropriate counseling and optimal care are provided. Increasing numbers of women with complex congenital heart disease are reaching childbearing age. Complications such as growth restriction, preterm and premature birth, and fetal and neonatal mortality are more common among children of women with congenital heart disease. The risk of complications is determined by the severity of the cardiac lesion, the presence of cyanosis, the maternal functional class, and the use of anticoagulation therapy (Choreño-Machain, Barrios, & Reta, 2015).

Women with certain congenital conditions should avoid pregnancy. These include uncorrected tetralogy of Fallot or transposition of the great arteries, and Eisenmenger's syndrome, a defect with both cyanosis and pulmonary hypertension (Brickner, 2014).

Acquired heart diseases are conditions affecting the heart and its associated blood vessels that develop during a person's lifetime, in contrast with congenital heart diseases, which are present at birth. Acquired heart diseases include coronary artery disease, coronary heart disease, rheumatic heart disease, diseases of the pulmonary vessels and the aorta, diseases of the tissues of the heart, and diseases of the heart valves. The incidence of rheumatic heart disease has declined dramatically in the past several decades because of prompt identification of streptococcal throat infections and treatment with antibiotics. When the heart is involved, valvular lesions, such as mitral stenosis, prolapse, or aortic stenosis, are common (see Table 20.3).

Many women are postponing childbearing until their 30s and 40s. With advancing maternal age, underlying medical conditions such as hypertension, diabetes, and hypercholesterolemia contributing to ischemic heart disease become more common and increase the incidence of acquired heart disease complicating pregnancy. Coronary artery disease and myocardial infarction may result.

A woman's ability to function during the pregnancy is often more important than the actual diagnosis of the cardiac condition. The following is a functional classification system developed by the Criteria Committee of the New York Heart Association (1994) based on past and present disability and physical signs. It provides a simple way of classifying the extent of heart failure by placing people in one of four categories based on how much they are limited during physical activity, normal breathing, and varying degrees of shortness of breath and/or chest pain:

- *Class I:* asymptomatic with no limitation of physical activity; no objective evidence of cardiac disease. Ordinary physical activity does not cause undue fatigue, palpitation, dyspnea, or chest pain.
- *Class II:* symptomatic (dyspnea, chest pain) with increased activity resulting in slight limitation of physical activity. They are comfortable at rest. Ordinary physical activity results in fatigue, palpitation, dyspnea, or anginal pain. Minimal CVD present.
- *Class III:* symptomatic (fatigue, palpitations) with normal activity resulting in marked limitation of physical activity. They are comfortable at rest. Less than ordinary activity causes fatigue, palpitation, dyspnea, or anginal pain. Moderately severe CVD present.
- *Class IV:* symptomatic at rest or with any physical activity resulting in inability to carry on any physical activity without discomfort. Symptoms of heart failure or the anginal syndrome may be present even at rest. If any physical activity is undertaken, discomfort is increased. Severe CVD present.

The classification may change as the pregnancy progresses and the woman's body must cope with the increasing stress on the cardiovascular system resulting from the numerous physiologic changes taking place. Typically, a woman with class I or II cardiac disease can go through a pregnancy without major complications. A woman with class III disease usually has to maintain bed rest during pregnancy. A woman with class IV disease typically should be advised to avoid pregnancy (Grewal, Silversides, & Coleman, 2014). Women with cardiac disease may benefit from preconception counseling so that they know the risks before deciding to become pregnant.

Maternal mortality varies directly with the functional class at pregnancy onset. The ACOG has adopted a three-tiered classification according to the risk of death during pregnancy (Box 20.1).

TABLE 20.3 SELECTED HEART CONDITIONS AFFECTING PREGNANCY

Condition	Description	Management
Congenital		
Tetralogy of Fallot	Congenital defect involving four structural anomalies: obstruction to pulmonary flow; ventricular septal defect (abnormal opening between the right and left ventricles); dextroposition of the aorta (aortic opening overriding the septum and receiving blood from both ventricles); and right ventricular hypertrophy (increase in volume of the myocardium of the right ventricle)	Hospitalization and bed rest possible after the 20th week with hemodynamic monitoring via a pulmonary artery catheter to monitor volume status Oxygen therapy may be necessary during labor and birth.
Atrial septal defect (ASD)	Congenital heart defect involving a communication or opening between the atria with left-to-right shunting due to greater left-sided pressure. Arrhythmias present in some women.	Treatment with atrioventricular nodal blocking agents, and at times with electrical cardioversion.
Ventricular septal defect (VSD)	Congenital heart defect involving an opening in the ventricular septum, permitting blood flow from the left to the right ventricle. Complications include arrhythmias, heart failure, and pulmonary hypertension.	Rest with limited activity if symptomatic.
Patent ductus arteriosus	Abnormal persistence of an open lumen in the ductus arteriosus between the aorta and the pulmonary artery after birth; results in increased pulmonary blood flow and redistribution of flow to other organs.	Surgical ligation of the open ductus during infancy; subsequent problems minimal after surgical correction
Acquired		
Mitral valve prolapse	Very common in the general population, occurring most often in younger women. Leaflets of the mitral valve prolapse into the left atrium during ventricular contraction. The most common cause of mitral valve regurgitation if present during pregnancy. Usually improvements in mitral valve function due to increased blood volume and decreased systemic vascular resistance of pregnancy; most women are able to tolerate pregnancy well.	Most women are asymptomatic; diagnosis is made incidentally. Occasional palpations, chest pain, or arrhythmias in some women, possibly requiring beta blockers Usually no special precautions are necessary during pregnancy.
Mitral valve stenosis	Most common chronic rheumatic valvular lesion in pregnancy. Causes obstruction of blood flow from the atria to the ventricle, thereby decreasing ventricular filling and causing a fixed cardiac output. Resultant pulmonary edema, pulmonary hypertension, and right ventricular failure. Most pregnant women with this condition can be managed medically.	General symptomatic improvement with medical management involving diuretics, beta blockers, and anticoagulant therapy. Activity restriction, reduction in sodium, and potentially bed rest if condition is severe
Aortic stenosis	Narrowing of the opening of the aortic valve, leading to an obstruction to left ventricular ejection. Women with mild disease can tolerate hypervolemia of pregnancy; with progressive narrowing of the opening, cardiac output becomes fixed. Diagnosis can be confirmed with echocardiography. Most women can be managed with medical therapy, bed rest, and close monitoring.	Diagnosis confirmed with echocardiography Pharmacologic treatment with beta blockers and/or antiarrhythmic agents to reduce risk of heart failure and/or dysrhythmias Bed rest/limited activity and close monitoring

(continued)

TABLE 20.3 SELECTED HEART CONDITIONS AFFECTING PREGNANCY (continued)

Condition	Description	Management
Peripartum cardiomyopathy	Rare congestive cardiomyopathy that may arise during pregnancy. Multiparity, age, multiple fetuses, hypertension, an infectious agent, autoimmune disease, or cocaine use may contribute to its presence. Development of heart failure in the last month of pregnancy or within 5 months of giving birth without any preexisting heart disease or any identifiable cause.	Preload reduction with diuretic therapy Afterload reduction with vasodilators Improvement in contractility with inotropic agents Nonpharmacologic approaches include salt restriction and daily exercise such as walking or biking. The question of whether another pregnancy should be attempted is controversial due to the high risk of repeat complications.
Myocardial infarction (MI)	Rare during pregnancy but incidence is expected to increase as older women are becoming pregnant and the risk factors for coronary artery disease become more prevalent. Factors contributing to MI include family history, stress, smoking, age, obesity, multiple fetuses, hypercholesterolemia, and cocaine use. Increased plasma volume and cardiac output during pregnancy increase the cardiac workload as well as the myocardial oxygen demands; imbalance in supply and demand may contribute to myocardial ischemia.	Usual treatment modalities for any acute MI along with consideration for the fetus Anticoagulant therapy, rest, and lifestyle changes to preserve the health of both parties

Adapted from Brickner, M. E. (2014). Cardiovascular management in pregnancy congenital heart disease. *Circulation, 130*(3), 273–282; Gilstrap, L. G., & Wood, M. J. (2014). Cardiovascular disease in women and pregnancy. In *MGH cardiology board review* (pp. 205–223). London: Springer Publishers; Jordan, R. G., Engstrom, J. L., Marfell, J. A., & Farley, C. L. (2014). *Prenatal and postnatal care: A woman-centered approach.* Ames, IO: John Wiley & Sons, Inc. and Mohamad, T. N., Fakhri, H. A., Bernal, J. M., Thatai, D., & Peterson, E. (2015). Cardiovascular disease and pregnancy. *eMedicine.* Retrieved from http://emedicine.medscape.com/article/162004-overview.

Pathophysiology

Numerous hemodynamic changes occur in all pregnant women. These normal physiologic changes can overstress the woman's cardiovascular system, increasing her risk for problems. Increased cardiac workload and greater myocardial oxygen demand during pregnancy place the woman's cardiovascular system at high risk for morbidity and mortality.

Pregnancy causes cardiac output to rise as early as the first trimester, reaching peak values at 20 to 24 weeks, and continues to increase until it plateaus between 28 and 34 weeks' gestation. This rise in cardiac output is due to a 30% to 50% increase in blood volume (stroke

BOX 20.1

CLASSIFICATION OF MATERNAL MORTALITY RISK

Group I (minimal risk) has a mortality rate of 1% and comprises women with:

- Patent ductus arteriosus
- Tetralogy of Fallot, corrected
- Atrial septal defect
- Ventricular septal defect
- Mitral stenosis, class I and II

Group II (moderate risk) has a mortality rate of 5% to 15% and comprises women with:

- Tetralogy of Fallot, uncorrected
- Mitral stenosis with atrial fibrillation
- Aortic stenosis, class III and IV
- Aortic coarctation without valvular involvement
- Artificial valve replacement

Group III (major risk) has a 25% to 50% mortality rate and comprises women with:

- Pulmonary hypertension
- Complicated aortic coarctation
- Previous myocardial infarction

Adapted from American Heart Association [AHA]. (2015). *Women and heart disease.* Retrieved from https://www.goredforwomen.org/about-heart-disease/facts_about_heart_disease_in_women-sub-category/statistics-at-a-glance/;Alonso-Gonzalez, R., & Swan, L. (2014). Treating cardiac disease in pregnancy. *Women's Health, 10*(1), 79–90; and Mohamad, T. N., Fakhri, H. A., Bernal, J. M., Thatai, D., & Peterson, E. (2015). Cardiovascular disease and pregnancy. *eMedicine.* Retrieved from http://emedicine.medscape.com/article/162004-overview.

volume) and a 30% increase in heart rate. A normal resting heart rate for any pregnant woman can be on average 20 beats per minute above her normal values.

Take Note!

Uterine blood flow increases by at least 1 liter per minute, requiring the body to produce more blood during pregnancy. This results in a 25% increase in red blood cells, a 50% expansion of plasma volume during pregnancy, and an overall hemodilution. In addition, the increase in total red blood cellular volume includes an increase in clotting factors and platelets, defining the hypercoagulable state of pregnancy (Swan, 2014). These changes start as early as the second month of gestation.

Similarly, cardiac output increases steadily during pregnancy by 30% to 50% over prepregnancy levels. Stroke volume increases 20% to 30% from prepregnant levels, and the maternal heart rate increases by 10 to 20 beats per minute (bpm). The increase is due to both the expansion in blood volume and the augmentation of stroke volume and heart rate. Other hemodynamic changes associated with pregnancy include a decrease in both the systemic vascular resistance and pulmonary vascular resistance, thereby lowering the systolic and diastolic blood pressure. In addition, the hypercoagulability associated with pregnancy might increase the risk of arterial thrombosis and embolization. These normal physiologic changes are important for a successful adaptation to pregnancy but create unique physiologic challenges for the woman with cardiac disease (Comparison Chart 20.1).

Therapeutic Management

Ideally, a woman with a history of congenital or acquired heart disease should consult her health care provider and undergo a risk assessment before becoming pregnant. This risk assessment must consider the woman's functional capacity, exercise tolerance, degree of cyanosis, medication needs, and history of arrhythmias. Data needed for risk assessment can be acquired from a thorough cardiovascular history and examination, a 12-lead electrocardiogram (ECG), and evaluation of oxygen saturation levels by pulse oximetry. The impact of heart disease on a woman's childbearing potential needs to be clearly explained, and providing information on how pregnancy may affect her and the fetus is important. This allows women to make an informed choice about whether they wish to accept the risks associated with pregnancy. When possible, any surgical procedures, such as valve replacement, should be done before pregnancy to improve fetal and maternal outcomes (Sliwa et al., 2015).

If the woman presents for care after she has become pregnant, prenatal counseling focuses on the impact of the hemodynamic changes of pregnancy, the signs and symptoms of cardiac compromise, and dietary and lifestyle changes needed. More frequent prenatal visits (every 2 weeks until the last month and then weekly) are usually needed to ensure the health and safety of the mother and fetus.

Nursing Assessment

Frequent and thorough assessments are crucial during the antepartum period to ensure early detection of and prompt intervention for problems. Assess the woman's vital signs, noting any changes. Auscultate the apical heart rate and heart sounds, being especially alert for abnormalities, including irregularities in rhythm or murmurs. Check the client's weight and compare with baseline and weights obtained on previous visits. Report any weight gain outside recommended parameters. Inspect the extremities for edema and note any pitting.

COMPARISON CHART 20.1 **CARDIOVASCULAR CHANGES: PREPREGNANCY VS. PREGNANCY**

Measurement	Prepregnancy	Pregnancy
Heart rate	72 (±10 bpm)	+10%–20%
Cardiac output	4.3 (±0.9 L/min)	+30%–50%
Blood volume	5 L	+20%–50%
Stroke volume	73.3 (±9 mL)	+30%
Systemic vascular resistance	1,530 (±520 dyne/cm/sec)	−20%
Oxygen consumption	250 mL/min	+20%–30%

Adapted from American Heart Association [AHA]. (2015). *Women and heart disease.* Retrieved from https://www.goredforwomen.org/about-heart-disease/facts_about_heart_disease_in_women-sub-category/statistics-at-a-glance/;Mohamad, T. N., Fakhri, H. A., Bernal, J. M., Thatai, D., & Peterson, E. (2015). Cardiovascular disease and pregnancy. *eMedicine.* Retrieved from http://emedicine.medscape.com/article/162004-overview; and King, T. L., Brucker, M. C., Kriebs, J. M., Fahey, J. O., Gegor, C. L., & Varney, H. (2015). *Varney's midwifery* (5th ed.). Burlington, MA: Jones & Bartlett Learning.

Question the woman about fetal activity, and ask if she has noticed any changes. Report any changes such as a decrease in fetal movements. Ask the woman about any symptoms of preterm labor, such as low back pain, uterine contractions, and increased pelvic pressure and vaginal discharge, and report them immediately. Assess the fetal heart rate and review serial ultrasound results to monitor fetal growth.

Assess the client's lifestyle and her ability to cope with the changes of pregnancy and its effect on her cardiac status and ability to function. Evaluate the client's understanding of her condition and what restrictions and lifestyle changes may be needed to provide the best outcome for her and her fetus. A healthy infant and mother at the end of pregnancy is the ultimate goal. As the client's pregnancy advances, expect her functional class to be revised based on her level of disability. Suggest realistic modifications.

The nurse plays a major role in recognizing the signs and symptoms of cardiac decompensation. Decompensation refers to the heart's inability to maintain adequate circulation. As a result, tissue perfusion in the mother and fetus is impaired. Common complaints of normal pregnancy, such as dyspnea, fatigue, palpitations, orthpnea, and pedal edema, mimic symptoms of worsening cardiac disease and create challenges when trying to evaluate pregnant women with cardiac disease. The pregnant woman is most vulnerable for this complication from 28 to 32 weeks of gestation and in the first 48 hours postpartum (Gandhi & Martin, 2015). Assess the woman for the following signs and symptoms:

- Shortness of breath on exertion, dyspnea
- Cyanosis of lips and nail beds
- Swelling of face, hands, and feet
- Jugular vein engorgement
- Rapid respirations
- Abnormal heartbeats, reports of heart racing or palpitations
- Chest pain with effort or emotion
- Syncope with exertion
- Increasing fatigue
- Moist, frequent cough

Take Note!

Assessing the pregnant woman with heart disease for cardiac decompensation is vital because the mother's hemodynamic status determines the health of the fetus.

Nursing Management

Nursing management of the pregnant woman with heart disease focuses on assisting with measures to stabilize the mother's hemodynamic status, because a decrease in maternal blood pressure or volume will cause blood to be shunted away from the uterus, thus reducing placental perfusion. Pregnant women with cardiac disease also need assistance in reducing risks that would lead to complications or further cardiac compromise; therefore, education and counseling are critical. Collaboration between the cardiologist, obstetrician, perinatologist, and nurse is needed to promote the best possible outcome.

Drug therapy may be indicated for the pregnant woman with a cardiac disorder. Possible drugs include diuretics, such as Lasix, to prevent heart failure; digitalis to increase contractility and decrease heart rates; antiarrhythmic agents (lidocaine); beta blockers (labetalol); calcium channel blockers (nifedipine) to treat hypertension; and anticoagulants (low-molecular-weight heparin). Warfarin (Coumadin) is not recommended because it crosses the placenta and may have teratogenic effects. It has been associated with spontaneous abortion, multiple birth defects, fetal growth restriction, and stillbirth (Lichtin & Philipson, 2014). The FDA's risk categories are as follows:

The FDA has changed their drug risk categories as of 6/30/15. They are no longer using categories A, B, C, D, and X. The new rule requires removal of the previous letter pregnancy categories. The package inserts will now include three separate categories that provide information in a narrative format. The goal of the new labeling is to provide information about the drug to the consumer. They now use specific subheadings under each of the three categories: Pregnancy; lactation; and females and males of reproductive potential. For specific changes under each category, please access the following FDA web site: http://www.fda.gov/Drugs/DevelopmentApprovalProcess/DevelopmentResources/Labeling/ucm425415.htm.

Encourage the woman to continue taking her cardiac medications as prescribed. Review the indications, actions, and potential side effects of the medications. Reinforce the importance of frequent antepartum visits and close medical supervision throughout the pregnancy.

Discuss the need to conserve energy. Help the client to prioritize household chores and child care to allow rest periods. Encourage the client to rest in the side-lying position, which enhances placental perfusion.

Encourage the client to eat nutritious foods and consume a high-fiber diet to prevent straining and constipation. Discuss limiting sodium intake if indicated to reduce fluid retention. Contact a dietitian to assist the woman in planning nutritionally appropriate meals.

Assist the woman in preparing for diagnostic tests to evaluate fetal well-being. Describe the tests that may be done, such as ECG and echocardiogram, and explain the need for serial nonstress testing, usually beginning at approximately 32 weeks' gestation. Instruct the woman in how to monitor fetal activity and movements. Urge her to do this daily and report any changes in activity immediately.

Although the morbidity and mortality rates of pregnant women with cardiac disease have decreased greatly, hemodynamic changes during pregnancy (increased heart rate, stroke volume, cardiac output and blood volume) have a profound effect, which may increase cardiac work and might exceed the functional capacity of the diseased heart. These changes may result in pulmonary hypertension, pulmonary edema, heart failure, or maternal death (Alonso-Gonzalez & Swan, 2014). Explain the signs and symptoms of these complications and review the sign and symptoms of cardiac decompensation, encouraging the woman to notify her health care provider if any occur.

Provide support and encouragement throughout the antepartum period. Assess the support systems available to the client and her family, and encourage her to use them. If necessary, assist with referrals to community services for additional support.

During labor, anticipate the need for invasive hemodynamic monitoring, and make sure the woman has been prepared for this beforehand. Monitor her fluid volume carefully to prevent overload. Anticipate the use of epidural anesthesia if a vaginal birth is planned. After birth, assess the client for fluid overload as peripheral fluids mobilize. This fluid shift from the periphery to the central circulation taxes the heart, and signs of heart failure such as cough, progressive dyspnea, edema, palpitations, and crackles in the lung bases may ensue before postpartum diuresis begins. Because hemodynamics do not return to baseline for several days after childbirth, women at intermediate or high risk require monitoring for at least 48 hours postpartum (Cunningham et al., 2014).

Pregnancy offers a unique window through which women at risk of future CVD may be identified. Nurses have the opportunity to implement health monitoring, lifestyle modifications, and other needed interventions to reduce the burden of future CVD in all of their pregnant clients. Dispelling the myths surrounding CVD in women versus men (it is a man's disease only) would be huge in promoting awareness.

Hypertension in Pregnancy

The ACOG has recently published revised guidelines for management of hypertension in pregnancy. They have outlined four categories to describe hypertension in pregnancy: preeclampsia–eclampsia, chronic hypertension, chronic hypertension with superimposed preeclampsia, and gestational hypertension. "Mild" is no longer used to categorize the severity of preeclampsia. The woman has it or not, with or without severe features (thrombocytopenia, renal insufficiency, impaired liver function, pulmonary edema, visual or cerebral changes). Proteinuria is no longer required to diagnose preeclampsia now. The ACOG recommends women with preeclampsia without severe features should give birth at 37 0/7 weeks; and women with preeclampsia with severe features give birth at 34 0/7 weeks (ACOG, 2013).

Chronic Hypertension

Entering pregnancy with chronic hypertension is increasingly common. It is an important risk factor for pregnancy complications, including for the fetus or newborn, poor fetal growth, preterm birth, low birth weight, admission to the NICU and death, and for the mother, superimposed preeclampsia/eclampsia, acute renal failure, pulmonary edema, surgical birth, placental abruption, stoke, postpartum cardiomyopathy, and mortality (Solomon & Greene, 2015). Chronic hypertension exists when the woman has high blood pressure before pregnancy or before the 20th week of gestation, or when hypertension persists for more than 12 weeks postpartum. The *Eighth Report of the Joint National Committee on Prevention, Detection, Evaluation, and Treatment of High Blood Pressure* (Joint National Committee [JNC 8], 2014) previously classified blood pressure that remained unchanged as follows:

- *Normal:* systolic less than 120 mm Hg, diastolic less than 80 mm Hg
- *Prehypertension*: systolic 120 to 139 mm Hg, diastolic 80 to 89 mm Hg
- *Mild hypertension:* systolic 140 to 159 mm Hg, diastolic 90 to 99 mm Hg
- *Severe hypertension*: systolic 160 mm Hg or higher, diastolic 100 mm Hg or higher (James et al., 2014).

Chronic hypertension occurs in up to 22% of women of childbearing age, with the prevalence varying according to age, race, and BMI. It complicates at least 5% of pregnancies, with one in four women developing preeclampsia during pregnancy (Sibai, 2015). Chronic hypertension is typically seen in older, obese women with glucose intolerance. The most common complication is preeclampsia, which is seen in approximately 25% of women who enter the pregnancy with hypertension. Worldwide, about 60,000 women die from preeclampsia each year, corresponding to 12% of all maternal deaths (Raio, Bolla, & Baumann, 2015). (See Chapter 19 for more information about preeclampsia.)

Therapeutic Management

Preconception counseling is important in fostering positive outcomes. Typically, it involves lifestyle changes such as diet, exercise, weight loss, and smoking cessation. Treatment for women with chronic hypertension focuses on maintaining normal blood pressure, preventing superimposed preeclampsia/eclampsia, and ensuring normal fetal development.

Once the woman is pregnant, antihypertensive agents are typically reserved for severe hypertension >160 mm Hg systolic and >100 mm Hg diastolic. Methyldopa (Aldomet) is commonly prescribed because of its safety record during pregnancy. This slow-acting antihypertensive agent helps to improve uterine perfusion. Other antihypertensive agents that can be used include labetalol (Trandate), atenolol (Tenormin), and nifedipine (Procardia) (Foo et al., 2015).

The U.S. Preventive Services Task Force (USPTF) (2015) recommends daily low-dose aspirin (81 mg/day) after 12 weeks of pregnancy in women with chronic hypertension and other risk factors who are at high risk for preeclampsia to reduce its occurrence.

Lifestyle changes are needed and should continue throughout gestation. The woman with chronic hypertension will be seen more frequently (every 2 weeks until 28 weeks and then weekly until birth) to monitor her blood pressure and to assess for any signs of preeclampsia. At approximately 24 weeks' gestation, the woman will be instructed to document fetal movement. At this same time, serial ultrasounds will be ordered to monitor fetal growth and amniotic fluid volume. Additional tests will be included if the client's status changes.

Nursing Assessment

Nursing assessment of the woman with chronic hypertension involves a thorough history and physical examination. Review the woman's history closely for risk factors. The pathogenesis of hypertension is multifactorial and includes many modifiable risk factors such as smoking, obesity, caffeine intake, excessive alcohol intake, excessive salt intake, and use of nonsteroidal anti-inflammatory drugs (NSAIDs). Also be alert for nonmodifiable risk factors such as increasing age and African American race (Miller & Carpenter, 2015). Ask if the woman has received any preconception counseling and what measures have been used to prevent or control hypertension.

Assess the woman's vital signs, in particular her blood pressure. Evaluate her blood pressure in all three positions (sitting, lying, and standing) and note any major differences in the readings. Assess her for orthostatic hypertension when she changes her position from sitting to standing. Document your findings.

Ask the woman if she monitors her blood pressure at home; if so, inquire about the typical readings. Ask the woman if she uses any medications for blood pressure control, including the drug, dosage, and frequency of administration, as well as any side effects. Ask the woman about lifestyle modifications that she has used to address any modifiable risk factors, and their effectiveness.

Hypertension during pregnancy decreases uteroplacental perfusion. Therefore, fetal well-being must be assessed and closely monitored. Anticipate serial ultrasounds to assess fetal growth and amniotic fluid volume. Question the woman about fetal movement and evaluate her report of daily "kick counts." Assess fetal heart rate at every visit.

Nursing Management

Preconception counseling is the ideal time to discuss lifestyle changes to prevent or control hypertension. One area to cover during this visit would be the Dietary Approaches to Stop Hypertension (DASH) diet, which contains an adequate intake of potassium, magnesium, and calcium. Sodium is usually limited to 2.4 g. Suggest aerobic exercise as tolerated. Encourage smoking cessation and avoidance of alcohol. If the woman is overweight, encourage her to lose weight before becoming pregnant, not during the pregnancy (Killion, 2015). Stressing the positive benefits of a healthy lifestyle might help motivate the woman to make the necessary modifications and change unhealthy habits.

Assist the woman in scheduling appointments for antepartum visits every 2 weeks until 28 weeks' gestation and then weekly. Prepare the woman for frequent fetal assessments. Explaining the rationale for the need to monitor fetal growth is important to gain the woman's cooperation. Carefully monitor the woman for signs and symptoms of abruptio placenta (abdominal pain, rigid abdomen, vaginal bleeding), as well as superimposed preeclampsia (elevation in blood pressure, weight gain, edema, proteinuria). Alerting the woman to these risks can mean early identification and prompt intervention.

Stress the importance of daily periods of rest (1 hour) in the left lateral recumbent position to maximize placental perfusion. Encourage women with chronic hypertension to use home blood pressure monitoring devices. Urge the woman to report any elevations. As necessary, instruct the woman and her family how to take and record a daily blood pressure, and reinforce the need for her to take her medications as prescribed to control her blood pressure and to ensure the well-being of her unborn child. Praising her for her efforts at each prenatal visit may motivate her to continue the regimen throughout her pregnancy.

The close monitoring of the woman with chronic hypertension continues during labor and birth and during the postpartum period to prevent or identify the onset of preeclampsia. Accurate and frequent blood pressure readings and careful administration of antihypertensive medications, if prescribed, are essential components of care. Stressing the need for continued medical supervision after childbirth is vital to motivate the woman to maintain or initiate lifestyle changes and dietary habits and stay compliant with her medication regimen.

RESPIRATORY CONDITIONS

During pregnancy, the respiratory system is affected by hormonal changes, mechanical changes, and prior respiratory conditions. These changes can cause a woman with a history of compromised respiration to decompensate during pregnancy. Although upper respiratory infections are typically self-limiting, chronic respiratory conditions, such as asthma or tuberculosis (TB), can have a negative effect on the growing fetus when alterations in oxygenation occur in the mother. The outcome of pregnancy in a woman with a respiratory condition depends on the severity of the oxygen alteration as well as the degree and duration of hypoxia on the fetus.

Asthma

Worldwide, the prevalence of asthma among pregnant women is on the rise; pregnancy leads to a worsening of asthma for many women (Nagtalon-Ramos, 2014). Asthma affects approximately up to 13% of pregnancies globally, ranging between 200,000 and 376,000 women annually in the United States. It affects over 20 million Americans and is one of the most common and potentially serious medical conditions to complicate pregnancy (Jordan et al., 2014). Maternal asthma is associated with an increased risk of infant death, preeclampsia, intrauterine growth restriction (IUGR), preterm birth, and low birth weight. These risks are linked to the severity of asthma: more severe asthma increases the risk (National Asthma Education and Prevention Program [NAEPP], 2015).

Remember Rose, the pregnant teenager with asthma in acute distress described at the beginning of the chapter. What therapies might be offered to control her symptoms? Should she be treated differently than someone who is not pregnant? Why or why not?

Pathophysiology

Asthma is an allergic-type inflammatory response of the respiratory tract to various stimuli such as allergens (pollen and animal dander), irritants (cigarette smoke and chemicals), stress, infections (colds or flu), and physical exertion. It is also known as reactive airway disease because the bronchioles constrict in response to these stimuli. Asthma is characterized by paroxysmal or persistent symptoms of bronchoconstriction including breathlessness, wheezing, chest tightness, cough, and sputum production. In addition to bronchoconstriction, inflammation of the airways produces thick mucus that further limits the movement of air and makes breathing difficult.

The normal physiologic changes of pregnancy affect the respiratory system. Although the respiratory rate does not change, hyperventilation increases at term by 48% due to high progesterone levels. Diaphragmatic elevation and a decrease in functional lung residual capacity occur late in pregnancy, which may reduce the woman's ability to inspire deeply to take in more oxygen. Oxygen consumption and the metabolic rate both increase, placing additional stress on the woman's respiratory system (American Academy of Allergy, Asthma, & Immunology [AAAAI], 2015).

Both the woman and her fetus are at risk if asthma is not well managed during pregnancy. When a pregnant woman has trouble breathing, her fetus also has trouble getting the oxygen it needs for adequate growth and development. Severe persistent asthma has been linked to the development of maternal hypertension, low birth weight, preterm birth, preeclampsia, placenta previa, uterine hemorrhage, and oligohydramnios. Women whose asthma is poorly controlled during pregnancy are at increased risk of preterm birth, low birth weight, and stillbirth (Vanders & Murphy, 2015).

The severity of the condition improves in one third of pregnant women, remains unchanged in one third, and worsens in one third (Cunningham et al., 2014). However, the effect of pregnancy on asthma is unpredictable. The greatest increase in asthma attacks usually occurs between 24 and 36 weeks' gestation; flare-ups are rare during the last 4 weeks of pregnancy and during labor (AAAAI, 2015).

Therapeutic Management

Asthma should be treated as aggressively in pregnant women as in nonpregnant women because the benefits of averting an asthma attack outweigh the risks of medications. The ultimate goal of asthma therapy is to prevent hypoxic episodes to preserve continuous fetal oxygenation; improved maternal and perinatal outcomes are achieved with optimal control of asthma. One third of women with asthma develop worsening of control during pregnancy; therefore, close monitoring and reevaluation are essential. Four important aspects of asthma treatment ensure optimal control: close monitoring, education of clients, avoidance of asthma triggers, and pharmacologic therapy.

Many women with asthma have positive skin tests to allergens, the most common being animal dander, dust mites, cockroach antigens, pollens, and molds. There are nonimmune triggers as well, including strong odors, tobacco smoke, air pollutants, and drugs such as aspirin and beta blockers. For exercise-triggered asthma, the use of a bronchodilator 5 to 60 minutes before exercise may reduce symptoms. Avoidance of these allergens and triggers can significantly reduce the need for medication and the occurrence of exacerbations during and after pregnancy. All women should be strongly encouraged to stop smoking, but especially those with asthma because they are at increased risk for worsening chronic and acute asthma sequelae.

Allergy injections may benefit those with allergies and asthma, called allergic asthma. Also called immunotherapy, allergy shots do not "cure" asthma in the manner in which an injection of, say, antibiotics might cure an infection. Instead, allergy shots work a bit more like a vaccine. Allergy injections for asthma actually contain a very small amount of an allergen (substance causing allergy). Over time, the dosage is increased. Exposure to progressive amounts of the allergen is likely to help the body develop a tolerance to it. If the allergen buildup is effective, the allergic reaction will become much less severe. Allergy injections can reduce the symptoms of allergies and prevent the development of asthma.

Medical therapy includes a stepwise approach in an attempt to use the least amount of medication necessary to control a woman's asthma and keep her severity in the mild range. Goals of therapy include having normal or near-normal pulmonary function and minimal or no chronic symptoms, exacerbations, or limitations on activities. The final goal is to minimize the adverse effects of treatment. Inhaled corticosteroids are preferred for the management of all levels of persistent asthma in pregnancy. Corticosteroids are the most effective treatment for the airway inflammation of asthma and reduce the hyperresponsiveness of airways to allergens and triggers.

NAEPP (2015) recommends three specific drugs to be used during pregnancy to control asthma:

- Budesonide (inhaled corticosteroid)
- Albuterol (short-acting beta$_2$ agonist)
- Salmeterol (long-acting beta$_2$ agonist)

Oral corticosteroids are not recommended for the long-term treatment of asthma during pregnancy, but they can be used to treat severe asthma attacks during pregnancy (AAAAI, 2015). In addition, two prostaglandins (hemabate and misoprostol [Cytotec]) used for treating postpartum hemorrhage and cervical ripening are contraindicated for clients with asthma due to the risk of bronchial spasm and bronchoconstriction (King et al., 2015).

Nursing Assessment

Obtain a thorough history of the disease, including the woman's usual therapy and control measures. Question the woman about asthma triggers and strategies used to reduce exposure to them (Box 20.2). Review the client's medication therapy regimen.

Auscultate the lungs and assess respiratory and heart rates. Include the rate, rhythm, and depth of respirations; skin color; blood pressure and pulse rate; and signs of fatigue. Clients with an acute asthma attack often present with wheezing, chest tightness, tachypnea, nonproductive coughing, shortness of breath, and dyspnea. Lung auscultation findings might include diffuse wheezes and rhonchi, bronchovesicular sounds, and a more prominent expiratory phase of respiration compared to the inspiratory phase (Kelly, Massoumi, & Lazarus, 2015). If the pregnancy is far enough along, the fetal heart rate is measured and routine prenatal assessments (weight, blood pressure, fundal height, urine for protein) are completed.

Laboratory studies usually include a complete blood count with differential (to assess the degree of nonspecific inflammation and identify anemia) and pulmonary function tests (to assess the severity of an attack and to provide a baseline to evaluate the client's response to treatment).

BOX 20.2

COMMON ASTHMA TRIGGERS

- Smoke and chemical irritants
- Air pollution
- Dust mites
- Animal dander
- Seasonal changes with pollen, molds, and spores
- Upper respiratory infections
- Esophageal reflux
- Medications, such as aspirin and nonsteroidal anti-inflammatory drugs (NSAIDs)
- Exercise
- Cold air
- Emotional stress

Adapted from American Academy of Allergy, Asthma & Immunology [AAAAI]. (2015). *Asthma and pregnancy.* Retrieved from http://www.aaaai.org/conditions-and-treatments/library/asthma-library/asthma-and-pregnancy.aspx;March of Dimes. (2015l). *Asthma during pregnancy.* Retrieved from http://www.marchofdimes.org/pregnancy/asthma-during-pregnancy.aspx; and Cunningham, F. G., Leveno, K. J., Bloom, S. L., Spong, C., & Dashe, J. (2014). *Williams' obstetrics* (24th ed.). New York, NY: McGraw-Hill Professional Publishing.

Nursing Management

Nursing management focuses on client education about the condition and the skills necessary to manage it: self-monitoring, correct use of inhalers, identifying and limiting exposure to asthma triggers, and following a long-term plan for managing asthma and for promptly handling signs and symptoms of worsening asthma. Client education fosters adherence to the treatment regimen, thereby promoting an optimal environment for fetal growth and development.

Client education should begin at the first prenatal visit. The importance of optimal asthma control and the risks of poor control for the woman and her fetus should be discussed early in pregnancy. Clients should be taught signs and symptoms, which should be of concern, as well as who to contact in emergent situations. Women should be observed using their inhalers and correct use reinforced. Frank discussion about the importance of continuing asthma medications and the possible severe consequences for the woman and her fetus with discontinuation is vital.

Ensure that the woman understands drug actions and interactions, the uses and potential abuses of asthma medications, and the signs and symptoms that require medical evaluation. Reviewing potential perinatal complications with the woman is helpful in motivating her to adhere to the prescribed regimen. At each antepartum visit, reassess the efficacy of the treatment plan to determine whether adjustments are needed.

Taking control of asthma in pregnancy is the responsibility of the client along with her health care team. Providing the client with the knowledge and tools to monitor her condition, control triggers and her environment (Teaching Guidelines 20.2), and use medications to prevent acute exacerbations assist the client in taking control. Facilitating a partnership with the woman will improve perinatal outcomes.

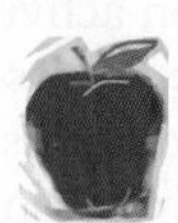

Teaching Guidelines 20.2

TEACHING TO CONTROL ASTHMA LINKED TO ENVIRONMENTAL TRIGGERS

- Remove any carpeting in the house, especially the bedroom, to reduce dust mites.
- Use allergen-proof encasing on the mattress, box spring, and pillows.
- Wash all bedding in hot water.
- Remove dust collectors in house, such as stuffed animals, books, knickknacks.
- Avoid pets in the house to reduce exposure to pet dander.
- Keep humidity <50% to reduce dust mites
- Use a high-efficiency particulate air-filtering system in the bedroom.
- Do not smoke, and avoid places where you can be exposed to passive cigarette smoke from others.
- Dust and vacuum frequently using vacuum with a high-efficiency HEPA air filter
- Avoid use of wood stove heaters within the house
- Stay indoors and use air conditioning when the pollen or mold count is high or air quality is poor.
- Wear a covering over your nose and mouth when going outside in the cold weather.
- Avoid exposure to persons with colds, flu, or viruses.

When teaching the pregnant woman with asthma, cover the following topics:

- Signs and symptoms of asthma progression and exacerbation
- Importance and safety of medication to the fetus and to herself
- Warning signs that indicate the need to contact the health care provider
- Potential harm to the fetus and to herself by undertreatment or delay in seeking help
- Prevention and avoidance of known triggers
- Home use of metered-dose inhalers
- Adverse effects of medications

Nurses should instruct and strongly urge women to remain on asthma medications during pregnancy because one third of clients have worsening of their asthma, including those women with mild asthma. There are proven negative effects from exacerbations and poor control on pregnancy outcome, whereas there are clear benefits of good control. Client education about the importance of good asthma control is essential for improving pregnancy outcomes.

During labor, monitor the client's oxygenation saturation by pulse oximetry and provide pain management through epidural analgesia to reduce stress, which may trigger an acute attack. Continuously monitor the fetus for distress during labor and assess fetal heart rate patterns for hypoxia. Assess the newborn for signs and symptoms of hypoxia.

***Rose*, the pregnant teenager described earlier, is concerned about passing her asthma on to her baby. What should the nurse discuss with her? What questions should the nurse ask to help in identifying triggers in Rose's environment to prevent future asthma attacks?**

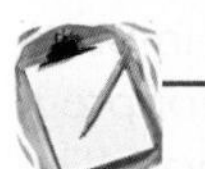

Take Note!

Successful asthma management can reduce adverse perinatal outcomes: preeclampsia, preterm birth, and low birth weight.

Tuberculosis

TB is known as the great masquerader, and manifestation of the disease can be vague and widespread. It is a disease that has been around for years but never seems to go away completely. TB is curable and preventable. Globally, TB is second only to HIV/AIDS as a cause of illness and death in adults, accounting for over 9 million cases of active disease and 2 million deaths each year. Someone in the world is newly infected with TB every second. Overall, one third of the world's population is currently infected with TB (World Health Organization [WHO], 2015b).

Although it is not prevalent in the United States, a resurgence was noted starting in the mid-1980s secondary to the AIDS epidemic and immigration. Left undiagnosed and untreated, each person with active TB will infect on average between 10 and 15 people each year (WHO, 2015b). The link between poverty and TB is strong. With the large numbers of immigrants coming to the United States, all nurses must be skilled in screening for and managing this condition.

In many cultures, the social consequences associated with the diagnosis of TB fall most heavily on women. Difficulties finding a marriage partner and divorce or abandonment among those already married are significant consequences for women from Pakistan, Vietnam, and India. Fear of social consequences can translate into delayed or absent health-seeking behavior. In pregnancy, TB that is treated early and adequately has outcomes equivalent to those in nonpregnant women. By contrast, studies have reported an increase in obstetrical mortality with increased incidence of spontaneous abortion, preterm labor, and preeclampsia in cases where TB was diagnosed late (Bates et al., 2015).

A person becomes infected by inhaling the infectious organism *Mycobacterium tuberculosis*, which is carried on droplet nuclei and spread by airborne transmission. The lung is the major site of involvement, but the lymph glands, meninges, bones, joints, and kidneys can become infected. Women can remain asymptomatic for long periods of time as the organism lies dormant. Pregnant women with untreated TB are more likely to have an underweight infant, an infant with a low Apgar score, and perinatal death (Mehta et al., 2015).

The newborn is at risk of postnatally acquired TB if the mother still has active TB at the time of birth. Therefore, prenatal diagnosis and effective treatment of the mother are essential.

Therapeutic Management

The WHO recommends that the treatment of TB in pregnant women should be the same as that in nonpregnant women and the rest of the general population. The only exception is that streptomycin should be avoided in pregnancy because it is ototoxic to the fetus.

Medications are the cornerstone of treatment to prevent infection from progressing. The FDA developed pregnancy categories that rank the risk of teratogenic effects of drugs to be used in drug labeling (see the list earlier in the chapter in the discussion of heart disease). The safety of the first-line drugs for the management of active TB in pregnancy has been established, and therapy improves both maternal and neonatal outcomes.

Pregnant women should start treatment as soon as TB is suspected. The preferred initial treatment regimen is INH, rifampin, and ethambutol daily for two months, followed by INH and rifampin daily, or twice weekly for 7 months. Women taking INH should also be taking pyridoxine (vitamin B_6) supplementation (CDC, 2015b).

Nursing Assessment

Review the woman's history for risk factors such as immunocompromised status, recent immigration status, homelessness or overcrowded living conditions, and injectable drug use. Women emigrating from developing countries such as Latin America, Asia, the Indian subcontinent, Eastern Europe, Russia, China, Mexico, Haiti, and Africa with high rates of TB also are at risk.

At antepartum visits, be alert for clinical manifestations of TB, including fatigue, fever or night sweats, nonproductive cough, weakness, slow weight loss, anemia, hemoptysis, fatigue, and anorexia (Herchline & Amorosa, 2015). If TB is suspected or the woman is at risk for developing TB, anticipate screening with purified protein derivative (PPD) administered by intradermal injection. If the client has been exposed to TB, a reddened induration will appear within 72 hours. If the test is positive, anticipate a follow-up chest x-ray with lead shielding over the abdomen, as well as sputum cultures to confirm the diagnosis.

Nursing Management

Adherence to the multidrug therapy is critical to protect the woman and her fetus from progression of TB. Provide education about the disease process, the mode of transmission, prevention, potential complications, and the importance of adhering to the treatment regimen.

Stressing the importance of health promotion activities throughout the pregnancy is important. Some suggestions might include avoiding crowded living conditions, avoiding sick people, maintaining adequate hydration, eating a nutritious, well-balanced diet, keeping all prenatal appointments to evaluate fetal growth and well-being, and getting plenty of fresh air outside. Determining the woman's understanding of her condition and treatment plan is important for adherence. A language interpreter may be needed to validate and reinforce her understanding if she does not speak English.

Breast-feeding is not contraindicated during the time the mother is on the medication regimen and should in fact be encouraged. If the mother is untreated for TB at the time of childbirth, they should not breastfeed or be in direct contact with their newborn until at least two weeks after starting anti-tuberculin medications. Untreated mothers can be encouraged to pump their milk to feed their newborns until they can breastfeed directly (AAP, 2015). Nurses should consult their hospital policies regarding mothers with TBfor guidance. Management of the newborn of a mother with TB involves preventing transmission by teaching the parents not to cough, sneeze, or talk directly into the newborn's face. Nurses need to stay current about new therapies and screening techniques to treat this centuries-old disease.

HEMATOLOGIC CONDITIONS

Anemia, a reduction in red blood cell volume, is measured by hematocrit (Hct) or a decrease in the concentration of hemoglobin (Hgb) in the peripheral blood. This results in reduced capacity of the blood to carry oxygen to the vital organs of the mother and fetus. Anemia is a sign of an underlying problem but does not indicate its origin.

Iron-Deficiency Anemia

Iron deficiency is the most common pathologic cause of anemia in pregnancy. Increased risk during pregnancy is due to increased maternal iron needs and demands from the growing fetus, increased erythrocyte mass; and, in the third trimester, expanded maternal blood volume (Cantor et al., 2015). Anemia affects one fourth of the world's population, and iron deficiency is the predominate cause. Iron-deficiency anemia mainly reflects poor nutrition, principally attributed to poor economic status worldwide. A recent study supports that and found that iron-deficiency anemia is strongly associated with low socioeconomic status, which affects women's knowledge and health-seeking behaviors. The study concludes that empowering women in terms of education and economic status is the key factor in combating anemia in pregnancy to prevent the vicious cycle of associated problems (Friedman et al., 2015).

Iron-deficiency anemia accounts for 75% to 95% of the cases of anemia in pregnant women (affecting one in four pregnancies), and is usually related to an iron-deficient diet, gastrointestinal issues affecting absorption, or a short pregnancy interval (Jimenez, Kulnigg-Dabsch, & Gasche, 2015). A woman who is pregnant often has insufficient iron stores to meet the demands of pregnancy.

The clinical consequences of iron-deficiency anemia include preterm delivery, perinatal mortality, and postpartum depression. Fetal and neonatal consequences include low birth weight and poor mental and psychomotor performance (Subramaniam & Girish, 2015). With significant maternal iron depletion, the fetus will attempt to store iron, but at a cost to the mother. Anemia at term increases the perinatal risk for both the mother and newborn. The risks of hemorrhage (impaired platelet function) and infection during and after birth also are increased. Clinical symptoms of iron-deficiency anemia include fatigue, diminished quality of life, impaired cognitive function, increased risk for thromboembolic events, headache, restless legs syndrome, and **pica** (consuming nonfood substances) eating behaviors (Camaschella, 2015).

Therapeutic Management

The goals of treatment for iron-deficiency anemia in pregnancy are to eliminate symptoms, correct the deficiency, and replenish iron stores. The Centers for Disease Control and Prevention (CDC), Health and Medicine Division (HMD), and the ACOG recommend routine iron supplementation for all pregnant women starting at a low dose of 30 mg/day beginning at the first prenatal visit (Moses, 2015). Attempting to meet maternal iron requirements solely through diet in the face of diminished iron stores is difficult.

Nursing Assessment

Review the mother's history for factors that may contribute to the development of iron-deficiency anemia, including poor nutrition, hemolysis, pica, multiple gestation, limited intervals between pregnancies, and blood loss. Assess the woman's dietary intake as well as the quantity and timing of ingestion of substances that interfere with iron absorption, such as tea, coffee, chocolate, and high-fiber foods. Ask the woman if she has fatigue, weakness, malaise, anorexia, or increased susceptibility to infection, such as frequent colds. Inspect the skin and mucous membranes, noting any pallor. Obtain vital signs and report any tachycardia.

Prepare the woman for laboratory testing. Laboratory tests usually reveal low Hgb (<11 g/dL), low Hct (<35%), low serum iron (<30 mcg/dL), microcytic and hypochromic cells, and low serum ferritin (<100 mg/dL).

> *Take Note!*
>
> *Hemoglobin and hematocrit decrease normally during pregnancy in response to an increase in blood plasma in comparison to red blood cells. This hemodilution can lead to physiologic anemia of pregnancy, which does not indicate a decrease in oxygen-carrying capacity or true anemia.*

Nursing Management

Nursing management of the woman with iron-deficiency anemia focuses on encouraging adherence to drug therapy and providing dietary instruction about the intake of iron-rich foods. Although iron constitutes a minimal percentage of the body's total weight, it has several major roles: it assists in the transport of oxygen and carbon dioxide throughout the body, aids in the production of red blood cells, and plays a role in the body's immune response.

Stress the importance of taking the prenatal vitamin and iron supplement consistently. Encourage the woman to take the iron supplement with vitamin C-containing fluids such as orange juice, which will promote absorption, rather than milk, which can inhibit iron absorption. Taking iron on an empty stomach improves its absorption, but many women cannot tolerate the gastrointestinal discomfort it causes. In such cases, advise the woman to take it with meals. Instruct the woman about adverse effects, which are predominantly gastrointestinal and include gastric discomfort, nausea, vomiting, anorexia, diarrhea, metallic taste, and constipation. Suggest that the woman take the iron supplement with meals and increase her intake of fiber and fluids to help overcome the most common side effects.

Provide dietary counseling. Recommend foods high in iron, such as dried fruits, whole grains, green leafy vegetables, meats, peanut butter, and iron-fortified cereals (Dudek, 2014). Anticipate the need for a referral to a dietitian. Teaching Guidelines 20.3 highlights instructions for the pregnant woman with iron-deficiency anemia.

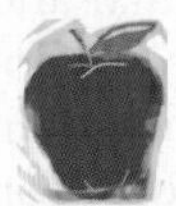

Teaching Guidelines 20.3

TEACHING FOR THE WOMAN WITH IRON-DEFICIENCY ANEMIA

- Take your prenatal vitamin daily; if you miss a dose, take it as soon as you remember.
- For best absorption, take iron supplements between meals.
- Awareness of the side effects of iron supplementation
- Avoid taking iron supplements with coffee, tea, chocolate, and high-fiber foods.
- Eat foods rich in iron, such as:
  - Meats, green leafy vegetables, legumes, dried fruits, whole grains
  - Peanut butter, bean dip, whole-wheat fortified breads and cereals

- For best iron absorption from foods, consume the food along with a food high in vitamin C.
- Increase your exercise, fluids, and high-fiber foods to reduce constipation.
- Plan frequent rest periods during the day.

Thalassemia

Thalassemia is a group of hereditary anemic disorders in which synthesis of one or both chains of hemoglobin molecules (alpha and beta) is defective. Inheritance is autosomal recessive. A low Hgb and a microcytic, hypochromic anemia results. The prevalence and severity of thalassemia depend on the woman's racial background: persons of Mediterranean, Asian, Italian, or Greek heritage and African Americans are most frequently affected. Beta-thalassemia is the most common form found in the United States (March of Dimes, 2015b).

Thalassemia occurs in two forms: alpha-thalassemia and beta-thalassemia. Alpha-thalassemia (minor), the heterozygous form, results from the inheritance of one abnormal gene from either parent, placing the offspring in a carrier trait state. These women have little or no hematologic disease and are clinically asymptomatic (silent carrier state). Beta-thalassemia (major) is the form involving inheritance of the gene from both parents. Beta-thalassemia major can be very severe. Genetic counseling might be necessary when decisions about childbearing are being made.

Thalassemia minor has little effect on pregnancy, although the woman will have mild, persistent anemia. This anemia does not respond to iron therapy, and iron supplements should not be prescribed. Several recent studies suggest that pregnancy appears safe for a woman with well-treated beta-thalassemia major who does not have heart disease (Rigby, 2015).

Management of thalassemia during pregnancy depends on the severity of the disease. Apart from the routine prenatal visit schedule, thalassemic pregnant women need additional care which includes regular and periodic evaluation of cardiac function by a cardiologist to prevent fluid overload; and frequent hemoglobin and ferritin levels should be monitored to avoid iron overload. Identification and screening are important to plan care. The woman's ethnic background, medical history, and blood studies are analyzed. If the woman is determined to be a carrier, screening of the father of the child is indicated. Knowledge of the carrier state of each parent provides the genetic counselor with knowledge about the risk that the fetus will be a carrier or will have the disease (Karimi, Cohan, & Parand, 2015). Mild anemia may be present, and instructions to rest and avoid infections are helpful. Nurses should provide supportive care and expectant management throughout the pregnancy.

Sickle Cell Anemia

Sickle cell anemia is an autosomal recessive inherited condition that results from a defective hemoglobin molecule (hemoglobin S). It is found most commonly in African Americans, Southeast Asians, and Middle Eastern populations. Sickle cell disease affects millions of people across the globe. In the United States, approximately 90,000 to 100,000 people have the disease, and 2 million have the sickle cell trait. Sickle cell disease occurs once in every 500 African American births, and once in 36,000 Hispanic American births. One in 12 African Americans has the sickle cell trait (CDC, 2015c).

Women with sickle cell disease can have more adverse maternal outcomes such as preeclampsia, eclampsia, preterm labor, placental abruption, intrauterine growth restriction, low birth weight, and maternal mortalities (Costa, Viana, & Aguiar, 2015). The gene offers protection against malaria, but can be a cause of chronic pain and early death. Life expectancy is shortened as a consequence of renal damage, cardiac damage, and infection (March of Dimes, 2015c). People with only one gene for the trait (heterozygous) will have sickle cell trait without obvious symptoms of the disease and with little effect on the pregnancy.

Pathophysiology

In the human body, the hemoglobin molecule serves as the oxygen-carrying component of the red blood cells. Most people have several types of circulating hemoglobin (HbA and HbA2) that make up the majority of their circulatory system. In sickle cell disease, the abnormal hemoglobin S (HbS) replaces HbA and HbA2. This abnormal hemoglobin (HbS) becomes "sickle" shaped as a result of any stress or trauma such as infection, fever, acidosis, dehydration, physical exertion, excessive cold exposure, or hypoxia. The sickle shape of the hemoglobin causes clumping together, which blocks the microvasculature. Significant anemia usually results.

Sickle cell anemia during pregnancy is associated with more severe anemia and frequent vaso-occlusive crises, with increased maternal and perinatal morbidity and mortality. In pregnant women with sickle cell anemia, complications can occur at any time during gestation, labor and birth, or postpartum. This is believed to be secondary to hormonal modifications, hypercoagulable state, and increased susceptibility to infection. Microvascular sickling in the placental circulation is associated with miscarriages, placental abruption, preeclampsia, preterm labor, intrauterine growth restriction, fetal distress, and low birth weight (Vichinsky, 2016).

Therapeutic Management

Ideally, women with hemoglobinopathies are screened before conception and are made aware of the risks of sickle cell anemia to themselves and to the fetus. A blood hemoglobin electrophoresis (lab study used for both DNA and RNA analysis) is done for all women from high-risk ancestry at their first prenatal visit to determine the types and percentages of hemoglobin present. This information should help them in making reproductive decisions.

Treatment depends on the health status of the woman. The effect of sickle cell disease on pregnancy depends on which manifestations the woman is experiencing. For example, sickle cell anemia combined with the increased blood volume in pregnancy increases the risks for heart failure, should fluid overload occur in therapy for the anemia (Cunningham et al., 2014).

Early and continuous prenatal care is needed to safeguard the fetus/infant from potential complications during the antepartum, intrapartum, and postpartum periods. Toward this end, prenatal visits for the first and second trimester should be scheduled more frequently. During pregnancy, only supportive therapy is used: blood transfusions for severe anemia, analgesics for pain, and antibiotics for infection.

Nursing Assessment

Assess the woman for signs and symptoms of sickle cell anemia. Ask the woman if she has anorexia, dyspnea, or malaise. Inspect the color of the skin and mucous membranes, noting any pallor. Be alert for indicators of sickle cell crisis, including severe abdominal pain, muscle spasms, leg pains, joint pain, fever, stiff neck, nausea and vomiting, and seizures (Jordan et al., 2014).

Nursing Management

Clients require emotional support, education, and follow-up care to deal with this chronic condition, which can have a great impact on the woman and her family. Monitor vital signs, fetal heart rate, weight gain, and fetal growth. Assess hydration status at each visit and urge the client to drink 8 to 10 glasses of fluid daily to prevent dehydration. Teach the client about the need to avoid infections (including meticulous hand hygiene), cigarette smoking, alcohol consumption, and temperature extremes.

Assist the woman in scheduling frequent fetal well-being assessments, such as biophysical profiles, nonstress tests, and contraction stress tests, and monitor laboratory test results for changes. Throughout the antepartum period, be alert for early signs and symptoms of crisis.

During labor, encourage rest and provide pain management. Oxygen supplementation is typically used throughout labor, along with intravenous fluids to maintain hydration. The fetal heart rate is monitored closely. After giving birth, the woman is fitted with antiembolism stockings to prevent blood clot formation. Before discharge from the facility after birth of the newborn, discuss family planning options.

The ability to predict the clinical course of sickle cell anemia during pregnancy is difficult. Outcomes have improved for pregnant women with the disease, and currently the majority can achieve a successful live birth. However, pregnancy is associated with an increased incidence of morbidity and mortality. Optimal management during pregnancy should be directed at preventing pain crises, chronic organ damage, and early mortality using a multidisciplinary team approach and prompt, effective, and safe relief of acute pain episodes. Although these measures do not remove the risk of maternal and fetal complications, they are thought to minimize them, promoting a successful pregnancy outcome. As part of the obstetric health care team, the nurse provides nursing interventions for the labor and postpartum client aimed at pain management, maternal/fetal safety, and client education. The overall objective is a healthy outcome for the childbearing family. The nurse has a vital role in making this happen.

AUTOIMMUNE DISORDERS

Autoimmune disorders are a group of more than 80 distinct diseases that emerge when the immune system launches an immune response against its own cells and tissues. Two distinct types of autoimmune disease occur:

1. Localized disorders target specific organs such as the thyroid gland in Hashimoto's thyroiditis and Graves' disease.
2. Systemic disorders affect multiple organs. For example, in **systemic lupus erythematosus** (SLE), the immune system can target the lungs, hearts, joints, kidneys, brain, and red blood cells.

Autoimmune disorders may cause mild insidious symptoms that come and go or debilitating conditions with high mortality.

Women suffer from autoimmune disease more than men. According to the CDC (2015d), autoimmune diseases affect approximately 8% of the population, 78% of whom are women. Autoimmune diseases are the third most common category of disease in the United States after cancer and heart disease; they affect approximately 5% to 8% of the population or 14 to 22 million people (CDC, 2015d). Previously, the general advice to women with autoimmune diseases, especially SLE, **multiple sclerosis (MS)**, or rheumatoid syndromes, was to avoid pregnancy because there was a high risk of maternal and fetal morbidity and mortality. However, it is now clear that these risks can be reduced in general by avoiding pregnancy when the diseases are active and continuing appropriate medication to reduce the chances of disease flare during pregnancy.

Systemic Lupus Erythematosus

Lupus disease, also known as SLE, is diagnosed based on laboratory values, symptoms, and signs; SLE is a chronic, relapsing autoimmune disease of the connective tissues that can affect various organs, such as the skin, joints, kidneys, and serosal membranes. Lupus disease is of unknown etiology, but it is thought to be a failure of the regulatory mechanisms of the autoimmune system. It is usually managed with anti-inflammatory and anti-rheumatic medications. Several triggers that cause the disease to activate include estrogen; cigarette smoking; infections, especially Epstein–Barr virus; physical or psychological stress; exposure to ultraviolet light; and pregnancy. Lupus symptoms may include swollen joints, extreme fatigue, oral ulcers, skin rashes, and sensitivity to sunlight (Mohindra & Marwah, 2015). Lupus is a complex disorder characterized by periods of relative inactivity and periods of disease exacerbation (flare-ups). To be diagnosed with SLE, a woman must have at least four out of eleven positive American College of Rheumatology Criteria which include red rash on face, photosensitivity, oral ulcers, arthritis, serositis, renal disease, seizures, fatigue, weight changes, anemia, and a positive anti-nuclear antibody test (Wasserman & Clowse, 2014).

The overall incidence of lupus in the United States is 150 per 100,000 people. The peak onset occurs between ages 15 and 45 with over 80% of the cases being diagnosed in women who are in their childbearing years. SLE is more common among those of African American, Afro-Caribbean, Asian, Native American, and Hispanic descent (Schur & Hahn, 2015).

Pathophysiology

The autoimmune responses in SLE prevent the body from recognizing "self" from "nonself," thus allowing antibodies to be formed that attack the body's own cells and proteins. This activity causes suppression of the body's normal immunity and damage to the body tissue. The autoimmune response may initially involve one organ or several. The most common organs/organ systems involved are the cardiovascular, integumentary, musculoskeletal, nervous systems, kidneys, and lungs. In pregnancy, inflammation of the connective tissue of the deciduas can result in placental implantation problems and poor functioning (Bartels & Muller, 2015).

Women with SLE are at increased risk for adverse pregnancy outcomes and cardiovascular disease. A pregnancy with lupus is prone to complications, including flares of disease activity during pregnancy or in the postpartum period, preeclampsia, pregnancy loss, miscarriage, stillbirth, fetal growth restriction, and preterm birth. Active lupus nephritis poses the greatest risk. The recognition of a lupus flare during pregnancy may be difficult because the signs and symptoms may mimic those of normal pregnancy (Singh & Chowdhary, 2015).

Therapeutic Management

The focus of therapy is to control disease flare-ups, suppress symptoms, and prevent organ damage. Treatment decisions are based on severity of the condition and organ involvement. Treatment of SLE in pregnancy is generally limited to NSAIDs (e.g., ibuprofen [Advil]), prednisone (Deltasone), and an antimalarial agent, hydroxychloroquine (Plaquenil). During pregnancy in the woman with SLE, the goal is to keep drug therapy to a minimum (King et al., 2015).

Nursing Assessment

The time at which the nurse comes in contact with the woman in her childbearing life cycle will determine the focus of the assessment. If the woman is considering pregnancy, it is recommended that she postpone conception until the disease has been stable or in remission for 6 months. Active disease at time of conception and history of renal disease increase the likelihood of a poor pregnancy outcome (Cunningham et al., 2014). In particular, if pregnancy is planned during periods of inactive or stable disease, the result often is giving birth to healthy full-term babies without increased risks of pregnancy complications. Nonetheless, pregnancies in most autoimmune diseases are still classified as high risk because of the potential for major complications. Preconception counseling should include the medical and obstetric risks of spontaneous abortion, stillbirth, fetal death, fetal growth restriction, preeclampsia, preterm labor, and neonatal death and the need for more frequent visits for monitoring her condition (Hadar, Ashwal, & Hod, 2014).

If the woman is already pregnant when the nurse encounters her, the nurse needs to assess for the following:

- Duration and presence of SLE signs and symptoms (fatigue, fever, malaise, polyarthritis, skin rashes, and multiorgan involvement)
- Evidence of anemia, thrombocytopenia, and thrombophilias
- Underlying renal disease (check the urine for protein and specific gravity)
- Signs of flare-ups
- Abnormalities in laboratory tests
- Signs of infection (check at each prenatal visit especially urinary tract infections and upper respiratory infections, since prednisone can mask signs of infection and lower resistance)
- Fetal well-being and growth (check using ultrasound, fundal height measurements, nonstress tests, and biophysical profiles)

Nursing Management

The nurse should discuss with the woman the importance of having good control over her SLE condition throughout the pregnancy. Discussions should focus on the effects of SLE during the pregnancy and possible risk for exacerbations. Emphasize the importance of frequent prenatal visits to detect early preeclampsia, preterm labor, or infections. Instruction should cover the implications and potential side effects of all drug therapies prescribed. Teach energy conservation techniques to prevent fatigue, signs and symptoms to report (extreme fatigue, edema, confusion, abdominal pain, weight loss, leg pain, anorexia), and the need for frequent and close monitoring for fetal well-being.

After childbirth, a discussion on birth control and the effects of the various methods on the disease is essential. Referral to self-help groups and local and national SLE organizations is important for further education of the woman and her family.

SLE can greatly complicate a pregnancy if close supervision is not maintained. The keys to a successful outcome for the mother and her infant include an accurate assessment of the disease and of the various systems involved, and vigilance during the pregnancy for disease progression, effects on the fetus, and development of complications. Nursing care should be directed at early detection of problematic signs and symptoms, education of the mother and family, careful evaluation of the fetal status, and providing support to assist the mother in strengthening her coping strategies.

Multiple Sclerosis

MS is a chronic inflammatory, demyelinating autoimmune disorder of the central nervous system. The Multiple Sclerosis Association of America [MSAA] (2015) estimates that approximately 400,000 people in the United States have MS. It is more commonly seen in women than in men, and the mean age of onset is 30 years. Globally, approximately 2.5 million are affected. There is no cure for the disease, and the disease usually becomes a chronic condition (2015).

In the early, inflammatory course of MS, autoreactive T cells cross the blood–brain barrier, attacking myelin proteins and leading to inflammation and demyelination. As the inflammatory process continues, repeated injury causes progressive neurodegeneration to the myelin membrane. The pathologic hallmark of MS can be described as multicentric, multiphasic central nervous system inflammation with resultant demyelination (Armon et al., 2015).

Uncomplicated MS does not have adverse effects on fertility, labor, or birth. Rates of spontaneous abortion, congenital anomalies, and fetal mortality are no higher among women with MS when compared with women in the general population (Vukusic & Marignier, 2015). There is no indication that women with MS require different care or management during the labor and birth process. Pregnant women with MS tend to have fewer relapses during gestation with a subsequent increase in disease activity in the first 3 months postpartum. Breastfeeding does not seem to have an influence on severity or frequency of exacerbations or the health of mothers, and has been shown to decrease MS relapse rates during the first six months postpartum (Walker, 2014). Breastfeeding should be encouraged as long as the woman is not being treated with disease-modifying agents.

The clinical presentation of MS can be similar to common pregnancy-related symptoms, especially fatigue, weakness, constipation, urinary frequency, balance problems, back pain, and visual changes. The similarity of the symptoms makes it difficult to attribute any symptoms that may develop during an established pregnancy to the disease process. These symptoms should be assessed carefully to assess MS exacerbations (Novotna & Ehler, 2014).

The focus of therapy for MS is to prevent clinical relapse and postpone neurodegeneration and the subsequent disability. Current medications include anti-inflammatories, immunosuppressants, immunomodulators/biologic agents, and a variety of complementary and alternative therapies such as vitamin/mineral supplementation, homeopathy, botanical products, and antioxidants. The complementary or alternative therapies have not been proven to reduce relapse rates or disease progression, but many MS sufferers turn to them (King et al., 2015). Most medications used in MS treatment during pregnancy are not FDA approved, but many have been used 'off label' and have not shown to have any adverse effects.

Nursing care is similar to that outlined previously under SLE. The need for support at this life-changing time is crucial. Continuity of care, access to information tailored to their needs, when requested by the woman or her family, and having a point of contact are all important aspects of nursing care.

Rheumatoid Arthritis

Rheumatoid arthritis (RA) is characterized by joint inflammation and progressive disability and is one of the most common chronic autoimmune disorders. It predominates in women, commonly affecting women of childbearing age and may complicate pregnancy. RA primarily affects synovial joints and tissues of the hands and feet, but any joint can be involved. Over time, bone and cartilage are damaged by the chronic inflammation process, resulting in joint deformity and loss of function. Progression of the disease and ensuing disability is unpredictable.

RA affects approximately 1.3 million adults in the United States. It is present in nearly all geographic areas and affects all ethnic groups. The disease typically presents between 30 and 50 years of age and affects twice as many women as men (American College of Rheumatology, 2015). The course of RA during pregnancy is usually benign. In about three fourths of pregnancies, the symptoms of the disease lessen. In these cases, most women experience relief in the first trimester that continues throughout the pregnancy. For many women with RA, pregnancy can provide a reprieve from long-term joint pain and inflammation, but others will not experience remission and will continue to need medication. RA does not adversely affect pregnancy outcome. With occasional exceptions, RA returns after the third to fourth month postpartum (Strangfeld et al., 2015).

Individuals with RA typically present with pain, swelling, and tenderness in joints; decreased mobility; and stiffness after periods of inactivity. Treatment of RA focuses on reducing joint inflammation, managing pain, and preventing joint destruction. The categories of medications used to accomplish this are NSAIDs, glucocorticoids, hydroxychloroquine, methotrexate, immunomodulators/biologic agents and complementary alternative therapies such as physical therapy, exercise, acupuncture, and joint splinting for pain relief. During pregnancy, medications are limited to hydroxychloroquine, glucocorticoids, and NSAIDs. Methotrexate is contraindicated during pregnancy (Brucker & King, 2017). Careful preconception counseling and risk assessment is important in women with RA. Antibody status and all medications need to be reviewed before pregnancy. Maintaining low disease activity before and during pregnancy is essential for optimal outcomes.

Nursing care should address the teratogenicity (the ability to cause birth defects) and adverse effects of some of the medications used to treat RA. Women with RA must be monitored closely following childbirth because most are likely to have arthritis flare-ups during the postpartum period. The general nursing care is similar to that outlined for the low-risk pregnant woman. Nurses caring for women with any disability (physical or cognitive) in general need to provide level-appropriate education on all reproductive health issues and improved access to health care. The woman's specific disability, her resources, and her approach to pregnancy and childbirth all help shape her experience. The nurse can play a role in making her experience a positive, memorable time in her life. Care for the woman with a disability should be well planned and coordinated by ensuring all documentation of the woman's needs and concerns is readily available to all personnel involved in her care. All members of the health care team should be involved in the plan of care and kept up to date of any changes. It is essential that the nurse facilitate care to ensure continuity of care throughout the woman's pregnancy and childbirth experience (Ostensen, 2014).

INFECTIONS

A wide variety of infections can affect the progression of pregnancy, possibly having a negative impact on the outcome. The effect of the infection depends on the timing and severity of the infection and the body systems involved. Common viral infections include cytomegalovirus, rubella, herpes simplex, hepatitis B, varicella, parvovirus B19, and several sexually transmitted infections (STIs; Table 20.4). Toxoplasmosis and group B streptococcus are common nonviral infections. Only the most common infections will be discussed here.

Cytomegalovirus

Human cytomegalovirus (CMV) infects greater than 50% of the human population. Humans are the only known hosts of CMV, which is transmitted via body fluids. Worldwide, the birth prevalence is estimated at seven per 1,000 births with the highest rates seen in developing countries. It is typically asymptomatic in most individuals. CMV is the most common congenital and perinatal viral infection in the world (Fig. 20.4). CMV is the leading cause of congenital infection, with morbidity and mortality at birth and sequelae. Each year approximately 1% to 7% of pregnant women acquire a primary CMV infection (Kovacs & Briggs, 2015). Of these, about 30% to 40% transmit the infection to their fetuses. The risk of serious fetal injury is greatest when maternal infection develops in the first trimester or early in the second trimester. Between 10% and 15% of congenitally infected infants are acutely symptomatic at birth and most of the survivors have serious long-term complications (March of Dimes, 2015d). It is a leading cause of hearing loss and intellectual disability in the United States. As a result of its substantial disease burden, congenital CMV is associated with an estimated $1 billion to $2 billion in direct economic costs each year. However, there has been limited progress in developing interventions to prevent or treat CMV infection (Bialas, Swamy, & Permar, 2015). Pregnant women acquire active disease primarily from sexual contact, blood transfusions, kissing, and contact with children in daycare centers. It can also be spread through vertical transmission from mother to child in utero (causing congenital CMV), during birth, or through breast-feeding. The virus can be found in virtually all body fluids. Prevalence rates in women in the United States range from 50% to 85% (CDC, 2015e). In the United States, approximately 1 in 60 people undergo seroconversion each year. Although prevalent in the United States population, CMV is not easily transmitted from host to recipient. The incidence of primary CMV infection in pregnant women in the United States ranges from 1% to 4% (CDC, 2015e). CMV infection during pregnancy may result in abortion, stillbirth, low birth weight, IUGR, microcephaly, deafness, blindness, intellectual disability,

TABLE 20.4 SEXUALLY TRANSMITTED INFECTIONS AFFECTING PREGNANCY

Infection/Organism	Effect on Pregnancy and Fetus/Newborn	Implications
Syphilis (*Treponema pallidum*)	Maternal infection increases the risk of premature labor and birth. Newborn may be born with congenital syphilis—jaundice, rhinitis, anemia, IUGR, and CNS involvement.	All pregnant women should be screened for this STI and treated with benzathine penicillin G 2.4 million units IM to prevent placental transmission.
Gonorrhea (*Neisseria gonorrhoeae*)	Majority of women are asymptomatic. It causes ophthalmia neonatorum in the newborn from birth through infected birth canal.	All pregnant women should be screened at first prenatal visit, with repeat screening in the third trimester. All newborns receive mandatory eye prophylaxis with tetracycline or erythromycin within the first hour of life. Mother is treated with ceftriaxone (Rocephin) 125 mg IM in single dose before going home.
Chlamydia (*Chlamydia trachomatis*)	Majority of women are asymptomatic. Infection is associated with infertility and ectopic pregnancy, spontaneous abortions, preterm labor, premature rupture of membranes, low birth weight, stillbirth, and neonatal mortality. Infection is transmitted to newborn through vaginal birth. Neonate may develop conjunctivitis or pneumonia.	All pregnant women should be screened at first prenatal visit and treated with erythromycin.
Human papillomavirus (HPV)	Infection causes warts in the anogenital area, known as condylomata acuminata. These warts may grow large enough to block a vaginal birth. Fetal exposure to HPV during birth is associated with laryngeal papillomas.	Warts are treated with trichloroacetic acid, liquid nitrogen, or laser therapy under colposcopy. Two HPV vaccines have been FDA approved (Gardasil and Cervarix) against the viral types most likely to cause cervical cancer (types 16 and 18) and genital warts (types 6 and 11) has been licensed in the United States for girls and women 9 to 26 years old. The vaccines are 95% to 100% effective. The vaccines are now recommended for young boys also.
Trichomonas (*Trichomonas vaginalis*)	Infection produces itching and burning, dysuria, strawberry patches on cervix, and vaginal discharge. Infection is associated with premature rupture of membranes and preterm birth.	Treatment is with a single 2-g dose of metronidazole (Flagyl).

Adapted from King, T. L., Brucker, M. C., Kriebs, J. M., Fahey, J. O., Gegor, C. L., & Varney, H. (2015). *Varney's midwifery* (5th ed.). Burlington, MA: Jones & Bartlett Learning; Kumar, B., & Gupta, S. (2014). *Sexually transmitted infections* (2nd ed.). Philadelphia, PA: Elsevier Health Sciences; and Centers for Disease Control and Prevention [CDC]. (2015r). *Sexually transmitted diseases*. Retrieved from http://www.cdc.gov/std/.

jaundice, or congenital or neonatal infection. The first or primary infection, if it occurs during pregnancy, is the most dangerous to the fetus: the fetus has a 30% to 40% chance of being infected.

There are three time periods during which mother-to-child transmission can occur: in utero, during birth, and after birth. However, permanent disability only occurs in association with in utero infection. Such disability can result from maternal infection during any point in the pregnancy, but more severe disabilities are usually associated with maternal infection during the first trimester.

Most women are asymptomatic and do not know that they have been exposed to CMV. Symptoms of CMV

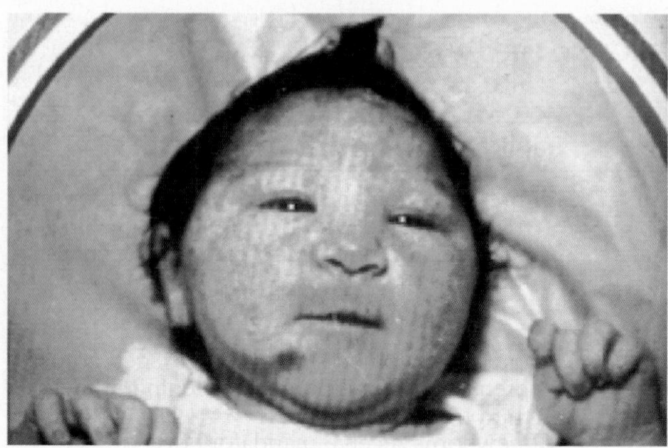

FIGURE 20.4 Clinical appearance of infant with congenital CMV with stigmata of disease, including petechial rash, microcephaly, jaundice, and abnormal posture of upper extremities secondary to CNS damage.

in the fetus and newborn, known as CMV inclusion disease, include hepatomegaly, thrombocytopenia, IUGR, jaundice, microcephaly, hearing loss, chorioretinitis, and intellectual disability. Newborns that are asymptomatic at birth may go on to develop late neurodevelopmental sequelae, with sensorineural hearing loss being the most common condition (Silasi et al., 2015). Prenatal screening for CMV infection is not routinely performed. Unfortunately, a preventive vaccine remains elusive. Since there is no therapy to prevent or treat CMV infections, nurses are responsible for educating and supporting childbearing-age women at risk for CMV infection. Stressing the importance of good hand hygiene and the use of sound hygiene practices can help to reduce transmission of the virus. A few specific hygiene guidelines for pregnant women include the following:

- Wash hands frequently with soap and water and wear gloves, especially after diaper changes, feeding, wiping nose or drool, and handling children's toys.
- Do not share cups, plates, utensils, food, or toothbrushes.
- Do not share towels or washcloths.
- Do not put a child's pacifier in your mouth.
- Clean toys, countertops, and other surfaces that come in contact with children's urine or saliva.
- Practice safe sex, including limiting sexual partners and use condoms consistently

Rubella

Rubella, commonly called German measles, is spread by droplets or through direct contact with a contaminated object. The risk of a pregnant woman transmitting this virus through the placenta to her fetus increases with earlier exposure to the virus. When infection occurs within the first month after conception, 50% of fetuses show signs of infection; in the second month following conception, 25% of fetuses will be infected; and in the third month, 10% of fetuses will be affected. Congenital rubella can manifest with a diverse range of symptoms in the newborn, including congenital cataracts, glaucoma, cardiac defects, microcephaly, as well as hearing and intellectual disabilities (Jyoti, Shirke, & Matalia, 2015).

Preconception care has been defined as a set of interventions designed to identify and modify risks to a woman's health or pregnancy outcome through prevention and management. This care should be provided any time any health care provider sees a reproductive age woman. Personal and family history, physical exam, laboratory screening, reproductive plan, nutrition, supplements, weight, exercise, vaccinations, and injury prevention should be reviewed in all women. Folic acid 400 mcg per day, as well as proper diet and exercise, should be encouraged. Women should receive the influenza vaccine if planning pregnancy during flu season; the rubella and varicella vaccines if there is no evidence of immunity to these viruses; and tetanus/diphtheria/pertussis if lacking adult vaccination (Lambert et al., 2015).

Education for primary prevention is key. Ideally, all women have been vaccinated and have adequate immunity against rubella. However, all women are still screened at their first prenatal visit to determine their status. A rubella antibody titer of 1:8 or greater proves evidence of immunity. Women who are not immune should be vaccinated during the immediate postpartum period so they will be immune before becoming pregnant again (Agent, 2015). Nurses need to check the rubella immune status of all new mothers and should make sure all mothers with a titer of less than 1:8 are immunized prior to discharge after birth of the newborn.

Herpes Simplex Virus

Genital herpes is an STI caused by the herpes simplex virus (HSV) type 1 or type 2. Both types can cause genital infections, although in recent years HSV-1 has become the predominant cause of genital herpes. Approximately 45 million people are infected with genital herpes in the United States, and 1.5 million new cases are diagnosed annually, including 1,500 newborns. Untreated neonatal HSV infection is associated with a mortality rate of 60%, and survivors experience considerable disability (Ural, 2015). Despite strategies designed to prevent perinatal transmission, the number of cases of newborn HSV infection continues to rise, mirroring the rising prevalence of genital herpes infection in women of childbearing age (Fig. 20.5) (James & Kimberlin, 2015).

HSV is a DNA virus with two subtypes: HSV-1 and HSV-2. HSV-1 infections were traditionally associated with oral lesions (fever blisters), whereas HSV-2 infections occurred in the genital region. Currently, either

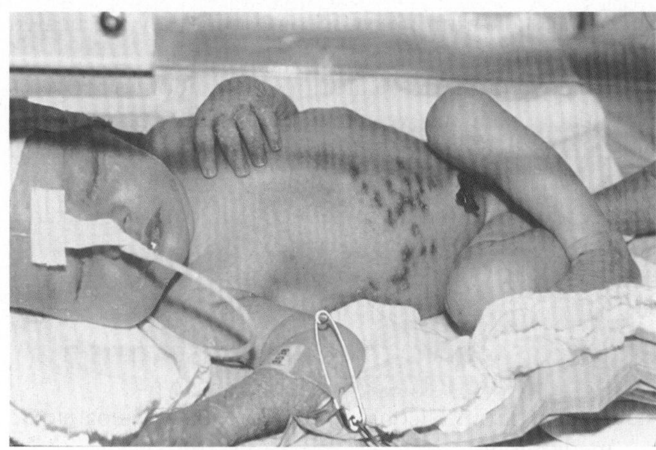

FIGURE 20.5 Newborn with disseminated herpes simplex virus infection. Note the healing ulcerations on the abdomen of the infant. (From Sweet, R. L., Gibbs, R. S. (2009). *Infectious diseases of the female genital tract* (5th ed.). Philadelphia, PA: Lippincott Williams & Wilkins.)

type can be found in either location, but HSV-1 is predominately causing genital herpes now (Ural, 2015).

Infection occurs by direct contact of the skin or mucous membranes with an active lesion through such activities as kissing, sexual (vaginal, oral, anal) contact, or routine skin-to-skin contact. HSV is associated with infections of the genital tract that when acquired during pregnancy can result in severe systemic symptoms in the mother and significant morbidity and mortality in the newborn. In addition, it may cause spontaneous abortion, birth anomalies, IUGR, or preterm labor. A 60% mortality rate may occur if the neonatal exposure is with an active primary infection (Silasi et al., 2015). Once the virus enters the body, it never leaves.

Infants born to mothers with a primary HSV infection have a 30% to 50% risk of acquiring the infection via perinatal transmission near or during birth. Recurrent genital HSV infections carry a 1% to 3% risk of neonatal infection if the recurrence occurs around the time of vaginal birth (March of Dimes, 2015e). About one in four pregnant women is infected with genital herpes, although most do not know it. Fortunately, only a small number pass the infection on to their newborns (March of Dimes, 2015e).

The greatest risk of transmission is when the mother develops a primary infection near term and it is not recognized. Most neonatal infections are acquired at or around the time of birth through either ascending infection after ruptured membranes or contact with the virus at the time of birth. The method and timing of birth in a woman with genital herpes are controversial. The CDC (2015f) recommends that in the absence of active lesions, a vaginal birth is acceptable, but if the woman has active herpetic lesions near or at term, a cesarean birth might be planned. All invasive procedures that might cause a break in the infant's skin should be avoided, such as artificial rupture of membranes, fetal scalp electrode, or forceps and vacuum extraction (Jordan et al., 2014).

Management for the woman with genital herpes during pregnancy involves caring for her as well as reducing the risk of newborn herpes. Some health care providers start the mother on prophylactic antiviral medications to prevent an active HSV outbreak at time of childbirth. No therapy can eradicate HSV, and this chronic infection is noted for its frequent asymptomatic viral shedding. Because the majority of newborn herpes cases result from perinatal transmission of the virus during vaginal birth, and because transmission can result in severe neurologic impairment or death, treatment of the mother with an antiviral agent such as acyclovir (Zovirax) must be started as soon as the culture comes back positive. Since the introduction of acyclovir, newer second-generation antivirals have been introduced (e.g., valacyclovir [Valtrex] and famciclovir [Famvir]) and are available (King et al., 2015). Use of condoms and antiviral medications assist in preventing transmission. Evidence does not support routine HSV serologic screening among asymptomatic pregnant women currently (Workowski & Bolan, 2015), so nurses need to remain knowledgeable about current practice to provide accurate and sensitive care to all women. Despite the surge in vaccine research, there is unfortunately no readily available or preventative or therapeutic vaccine for HSV to date.

Hepatitis B Virus

Hepatitis B is one of the most prevalent chronic diseases in the world. It is a serious global public health problem in Asia, Africa, Southern Europe, and Latin America, especially. Hepatitis B virus (HBV) has infected approximately 2 billion people worldwide, of whom more than 350 million are chronically infected. Life-threatening liver disease (cirrhosis, liver failure, and hepatocellular carcinoma) occurs in as many as 40% of people with hepatitis B. HBV infection causes about 5,000 deaths annually in the United States (Contag & Arrabal, 2015). HBV can be transmitted through contaminated blood, illicit drug use, and sexual contact. The virus is 100 times more infectious than HIV and, unlike HIV, it can live outside the body in dried blood for more than a week (Salman et al., 2015).

Sexual transmission accounts for most adult HBV infections in the United States. Acutely infected women develop hepatitis with anorexia, nausea, vomiting, fever, abdominal pain, and jaundice. In women with acute hepatitis B, vertical transmission occurs in approximately 10% of newborns when infection occurs in the first trimester and in 80% to 90% of newborns when acute infection occurs in the third trimester. Without intervention, 40% of infants born to women who are positive for hepatitis B will have chronic hepatitis B by 6 months of age (CDC, 2015g). In addition, hepatitis B infection during pregnancy is associated with an increased risk of preterm birth, fetal distress during labor, meconium peritonitis, low birth weight, and neonatal death. Newborns infected with HBV are likely to become chronic carriers of the virus, becoming reservoirs for continued infection in the population (CDC, 2015g). The fetus is at particular risk during birth because of the possible contact with contaminated blood at this time.

The CDC (2015g) recommends that all pregnant women should be tested for hepatitis B surface antigen (HBsAg) regardless of previous HBV vaccine or screening. Infants born to HBsAg-positive mothers should receive single-antigen HBV vaccine and hepatitis B immunoglobulin (HBIG) within 12 hours of birth. Completion of the vaccine schedule is recommended by HBV vaccination at 1 and 6 months (CDC, 2015g). There is a growing body of literature supporting the safety and efficacy of antiviral therapies administered in the third trimester of pregnancy to the reduce the vertical transmission of the HBV from the mother to the fetus, but to date there has not been any formal recommendations (Lamberth et al., 2015).

Nursing Assessment

Review the woman's history for factors placing her at high risk:

- History of STIs
- Household contacts with HBV-infected persons
- Employment as a health care provider
- Abuse of intravenous drugs
- Prostitution
- Foreign born
- Multiple sexual partners
- Chinese, Southeast Asian, or African heritage
- Sexual partners who are HBV infected (CDC, 2015g)

At the first prenatal visit, all pregnant women should be screened for HbsAg via blood studies, even if they were previously vaccinated or tested. Expect to repeat this screening later in pregnancy for women in high-risk groups (Park & Pan, 2014).

Nursing Management

If a woman tests positive for HBV, expect to administer HBIG (Hep-B-Gammagee). The newborn will also receive HBV vaccine (Recombivax-HB, Engerix-B) within 12 hours of birth. The second and third doses of the vaccine are given at 1 and 6 months of age (CDC, 2015g). The CDC recommends routine vaccination of all newborns.

Women who are HbsAg negative may be vaccinated safely during pregnancy. No current research supports the use of surgical births to reduce vertical transmission of HBV. Breast-feeding by mothers with chronic HBV infection does not increase the risk of viral transmission to their newborns, nor is it a contraindication to breast-feeding, unless the woman is taking antiviral medication and has bleeding nipples. Women with bleeding nipples should abstain from breast-feeding until they are healed (Jhaveri, 2015).

Client education related to prevention of HBV is essential. Teach the woman about safer sex practices, good hand hygiene techniques, and the use of standard precautions (Teaching Guidelines 20.4). Protection can be afforded with the highly effective hepatitis B vaccine.

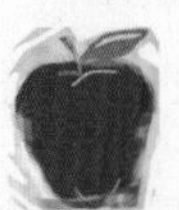

Teaching Guidelines 20.4

TEACHING TO PREVENT HEPATITIS B VIRUS PROGRESSION

- Abstain from alcohol and potentially hepatotoxic medications.
- Avoid intravenous drug exposure or sharing of needles.
- Encourage all household contacts and sexual partners to be vaccinated.
- Receive immediate treatment for any STI.
- Know that your newborn will receive hepatitis B vaccine soon after birth.
- Use good hand hygiene techniques at all times.
- Avoid contact with blood or body fluids.
- Use barrier methods such as condoms during sexual intercourse.
- Avoid sharing any personal items, such as razors, toothbrushes, or eating utensils.
- Inform all health care providers of your HBV status

Permanent remission of the disease even with treatment rarely occurs. Therefore, therapy is directed at long-term suppression of viral replication and prevention of end-stage liver disease. Urge the woman to consume a high-protein diet and avoid fatigue. A healthy lifestyle can help delay disease progression. Initiate an open discussion about the modes of transmission and use of condoms to prevent spread.

Varicella Zoster Virus

Varicella zoster virus (VZV) is one of the eight herpes family viruses. It is the virus that causes both varicella (chickenpox) and herpes zoster (shingles). Primary VZV leads to varicella (chicken pox) and establishes latency in dorsal root ganglia. Reactivation of VZV causes herpes zoster, commonly called shingles. Herpes zoster can occur once immune response against the virus wanes, usually with advancing age.

Pregnant women are at risk for developing varicella when they come in close contact with children who have active infection. Varicella occurs year round, but there is a higher incidence during winter and spring months. Maternal varicella can be transmitted to the fetus through the placenta, leading to congenital varicella syndrome, if the mother is infected during the first half of pregnancy, via an ascending infection during birth, or by direct contact with infectious lesions, leading to infection after birth. Varicella occurs in approximately 1/1,000 pregnancies (Charlier et al., 2014).

Congenital varicella syndrome can occur in newborns of mothers infected during early pregnancy. The vertical transmission rate is estimated to be between 2% and 10%. It is characterized by low birth weight, skin lesions in a dermatomal distribution, spontaneous abortion, chorioretinitis, cataracts, fetal growth restriction, delayed milestones, cutaneous scarring, limb hypoplasia, microcephaly, ocular abnormalities, intellectual disability, and early death (Swamy & Heine, 2015).

Preconception counseling is important for preventing this condition. A major component of counseling involves determining the woman's varicella immunity. Vaccination is the cornerstone of prevention. The vaccine is administered if needed. Varicella vaccine is a live attenuated viral vaccine. It should be administered to all adolescents and adults 13 years of age and older who do not have evidence of varicella immunity (King et al., 2015). Provide education to women who work in occupations that increase the risk of exposure to the virus, such as daycare workers, teachers of young children, and staff caring for children in institutional settings.

Varicella during pregnancy can be associated with severe illnesses for both the mother and her newborn. If contracted in the first half of pregnancy, some pregnant women are at risk for developing varicella pneumonia, which may put them at risk of life-threatening ventilatory compromise and death. Risk of varicella pneumonia appears to increase during pregnancy (Zhang, Patenaude, & Abenhaim, 2014). If the mother develops varicella rashes close to her due date, generalized neonatal varicella leading to death in about 20% of cases can be expected (Jordan et al., 2014).

Parvovirus B19

Parvovirus B19 infection occurs worldwide with most infected persons asymptomatic. The incidence of acute B19 infection in pregnancy is about 3%. Approximately 30% to 50% of pregnant women are not immune, and vertical transmission is common following maternal infection in pregnancy. Fetal infection may be associated with a normal outcome, but fetal death may also occur without ultrasound evidence of infectious sequelae (Desai & Brustman, 2014). Parvovirus B19 is a common, self-limiting, benign childhood virus that causes erythema infectiosum, also known as Fifth disease (referring to its fifth place in a list of common childhood infections). Approximately 65% of women of reproductive age have developed immunity to parvovirus B19. Infection with parvovirus B19 affects 1 in 400 pregnant women, but the majority has no adverse pregnancy outcome; those that do may experience spontaneous abortion and severe fetal anemia. There is no treatment for the pregnant woman with parvovirus B19 infection (Malee, 2015).

Pathophysiology

The infection is spread transplacentally, by the oropharyngeal route in casual contact, and through infected blood. Infection of the fetus occurs through transplacental passage of the virus. Acute infection in pregnancy can cause B19 infection in the fetus, leading to nonimmune fetal hydrops (a serious abnormal accumulation of fluid in 2 or more fetal compartments, including ascites, pleural effusion, pericardial effusion, and skin edema), secondary to severe anemia or fetal loss, depending on the gestational age at the time of infection. The risk to the fetus is greatest when the woman is exposed and infected within the first 20 weeks of gestation. In addition to hydrops, other fetal effects of parvovirus include spontaneous abortion, congenital anomalies (central nervous system, craniofacial, and eye), and long-term effects such as hepatic insufficiency, myocarditis, and learning disabilities (Edwards, 2014). Fetal infection with B19V is also associated with intrauterine fetal death, nonimmune hydrops fetalis, thrombocytopenia, myocarditis, and neurologic manifestations. Fetal infection can also remain clinically unrecognized (Suliman & Seopela, 2015).

Therapeutic Management

Generally, a diagnosis of parvovirus is based on clinical symptoms and serologic antibody testing for parvovirus immunoglobulin G (IgG) and parvovirus immunoglobulin M (IgM). Parvovirus B19 infection is followed by lifelong immunity, which is shown by positive serum B19 IgG. Pregnant women who have been exposed to or who develop symptoms of parvovirus B19 require assessment to determine whether they are susceptible to infection (nonimmune). If the woman is immune, she can be reassured that she will not develop infection and that the virus will not adversely affect her pregnancy. If she is nonimmune, then referral to a perinatologist is recommended and counseling regarding the risks of fetal transmission, fetal loss, and hydrops is necessary. Knowledge of how best to manage this infection during pregnancy lags behind our understanding of the potential adverse consequences.

Intrauterine B19 infection is a cause of fetal anemia, hydrops, and demise, and perhaps also of congenital anomalies. The best strategy for surveillance of the infected pregnant woman is serial ultrasounds for detection of hydropic changes and fetal anemia, and treatment for severe fetal anemia. Serial ultrasounds are advocated because the rates of fetal death and complications peak 4 to 6 weeks after exposure, but they can occur as late as 3 months following onset of symptoms. The infected newborn is assessed for any anomaly and followed for up to 6 years to identify any sequelae (Smith, 2015).

Nursing Assessment

Review the mother's history for any risk factors. Schoolteachers, daycare workers, and women living with school-aged children are at the highest risk for being seropositive for parvovirus B19, especially if a recent outbreak has occurred in those settings. Also assess the woman for specific signs and symptoms. The characteristic rash starts on the face with a "slapped-cheeks" appearance and is followed by a generalized maculopapular rash. Fever, arthralgia, and generalized malaise are usually present in the mother. Prepare the mother for antibody testing.

Nursing Management

Prevention is the best strategy. Stress the need for hand hygiene after handling children; cleaning toys and surfaces that children have been in contact with; and avoiding the sharing of food and drinks. Screening for parvovirus B19 during early pregnancy may help in early diagnosis, but the cost-effectiveness of a national screening program has not been accepted to date. The nurse can provide information regarding risk factors and potential complications if exposed and support the parent's decision.

Group B Streptococcus

Group B streptococcus (GBS) is a naturally occurring bacterium found in approximately 50% of healthy adults. Women who test positive for the GBS bacteria are considered carriers. Carrier status is transient and does not indicate illness. Approximately 25% of pregnant women carry GBS in the rectum or vagina, thus introducing the risk of colonization of the fetus during birth. GBS affects about 1 in every 2,000 newborns in the United States (March of Dimes, 2015f). Approximately 1 out of every 100 to 200 newborns born to mothers who carry GBS will develop signs and symptoms of GBS disease. Although GBS is rarely serious in adults, it can be life threatening to newborns. GBS is the most common cause of sepsis and meningitis in newborns and is a frequent cause of newborn pneumonia (Puopolo, Madoff, & Baker, 2015). Newborns with early-onset (within a week after birth) GBS infections may have pneumonia or sepsis, whereas late-onset (after the first week) infections often manifest with meningitis (CDC, 2015i).

Genital tract colonization poses the most serious threat to the newborn because of exposure during birth and to the mother because of ascending infection after the membranes rupture. GBS colonization in the mother is thought to cause chorioamnionitis, endometritis, and postpartum wound infection.

Therapeutic Management

Antibiotic therapy usually is effective in treating women with GBS infections of the urinary tract or uterus, or chorioamnionitis without any sequelae. According to the CDC guidelines, all pregnant women should be screened for GBS at 35 to 37 weeks' gestation and treated (2015i). Vaginal and rectal specimens are cultured for the presence of the bacterium. Both pregnant women and women during labor who have positive cultures are treated with a penicillin-based anti-infective agent.

Penicillin G is the treatment of choice for GBS infection because of its narrow spectrum. Alternative antibiotics can be prescribed for clients with a penicillin allergy. The drug is usually administered intravenously at least 4 hours before birth so that it can reach adequate levels in the serum and amniotic fluid to reduce the risk of newborn colonization. Close monitoring is required during the administration of intravenous antibiotics because severe allergic reactions can occur rapidly.

Nursing Assessment

Review the woman's prenatal history, and ask about any previous infection. Determine if the woman's membranes have ruptured and the time of rupture. Rupture of amniotic membranes more than 18 hours increases the risk for infection. Monitor the mother's vital signs, reporting any maternal fever greater than 100.4°F (38°C). Assess the woman for other risk factors for perinatal transmission of GBS, including previous colonization with GBS, low socioeconomic status, African American race, age less than 20 years, positive colonization at 35 to 37 weeks' gestation, GBS in urine sample, previous birth of GBS-positive newborn, preterm birth, and use of invasive obstetric procedures (March of Dimes, 2015f). Document this information to help prevent vertical transmission to the newborn.

Many women with GBS infection are asymptomatic, but they may have urinary tract infections, uterine infections, and chorioamnionitis.

Nursing Management

Nurses play major roles as educators and advocates for all women and newborns to reduce the incidence of GBS infections. Ensure that pregnant women between 35 and 37 weeks' gestation are screened for GBS infection during a prenatal visit. Record the results and notify the birth attendant if the woman has tested positive for GBS. During labor, be prepared to administer intravenous antibiotics to all women who are GBS positive.

Toxoplasmosis

Toxoplasmosis is a relatively widespread parasitic infection caused by a one-celled organism, *Toxoplasma gondii*. It is found all over the world, and can affect any warm-blooded animal, including humans, although the primary host is the cat. When a pregnant woman is exposed to this protozoan, the infection can pose serious risks to her fetus through transplacental transfer from the mother to the fetus. Between 1 in 1,000 and 8,000 newborns are born infected with toxoplasmosis in the United States (Hokelek, 2015). Cats are the definitive hosts of this parasite and shed it in their feces. It is transferred by hand to mouth after touching cat feces while changing the cat litter box or through gardening in contaminated soil. Consuming undercooked infected meat, such as pork, lamb, or venison drinking contaminated water, and eating unwashed fruits and vegetables can also transmit this organism.

A pregnant woman that contracts toxoplasmosis for the first time has an approximately 40% chance of passing the infection to her fetus. Toxoplasmosis acquired during pregnancy means high risk of damage for the fetus (March of Dimes, 2015g). Although the woman typically remains asymptomatic, transmission to her fetus can occur throughout pregnancy. A fetus that contracts congenital toxoplasmosis typically has a low birth weight, enlarged liver and spleen, chorioretinitis, jaundice, IUGR, hydrocephalus, microcephaly, neurologic damage, and anemia. Severity varies with gestational age; usually, the earlier the infection, the more severe the effects (Silasi et al., 2015).

Treatment of the woman during pregnancy to reduce the risk of congenital infection is a combination of pyrimethamine and sulfadiazine. Treatment with sulfonamides during pregnancy has been shown to reduce the risk of congenital infection.

Although there is much to learn about the best approach to the identification and treatment of toxoplasmosis, it is known that early treatment leads to the best neurodevelopmental outcomes in infants. Prevention is the key to managing this infection. Nurses play a key role in educating the woman about measures to prevent toxoplasmosis (Teaching Guidelines 20.5).

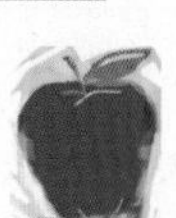

Teaching Guidelines 20.5

TEACHING TO PREVENT TOXOPLASMOSIS

- Avoid eating raw or undercooked meat, especially lamb or pork. Cook all meat to an internal temperature of 160°F (71°C) throughout.
- Clean cutting boards, work surfaces, and utensils with hot soapy water after contact with raw meat or unwashed fruits and vegetables.
- Peel or thoroughly wash all raw fruits and vegetables before eating them.
- Wash hands thoroughly with warm water and soap after handling raw meat.
- Avoid feeding the cat raw or undercooked meats.
- Avoid emptying or cleaning the cat's litter box. Have someone else do it daily.
- Keep outdoor sandboxes covered to prevent cat feces contamination
- Keep the cat indoors to prevent it from hunting and eating birds or rodents.
- Avoid uncooked eggs and unpasteurized milk.
- Wear gardening gloves when in contact with outdoor soil.
- Avoid contact with children's sandboxes, because cats can use them as litter boxes.

Women Who Are HIV Positive

The **human immunodeficiency virus (HIV)** is a chronic infection caused by the retrovirus HIV, which infects T cells that causes immunodeficiency. Once the CD4-positive cell count falls below a certain level, HIV infection causes increased susceptibility to infections, cancers, and neurologic damage (Hardy, Esposti, & Nee, 2015). HIV is transmitted by blood and body fluids. The number of people contracting HIV infection annually is estimated at nearly 50 million, including approximately 20 million women of childbearing age and 2.5 million children, most of whom acquired HIV from mother-to-child transmission. According to the most recent incidence estimates, more than one million people in the United States are living with HIV infection, and almost 1 in 6 are unaware of their infection (CDC, 2015j).

Despite the revolutionary strides that have been made in treatment and detection and recent clinical advances and cautious optimism associated with combination therapies and vaccines, the number of individuals who are HIV positive continues to climb worldwide. Intensive efforts notwithstanding, no real "cure" can be seen on the horizon. To achieve a durable end to the HIV pandemic, a vaccine remains essential in the fight against this virus (Fauci, Folkers, & Marston, 2014). Also, despite dramatic reductions in perinatal transmission of HIV in the United States, barriers to prevention still exist and perinatal HIV infections continue.

Historically, HIV/AIDS was associated with the male homosexual community and intravenous drug users, but currently the prevalence of HIV/AIDS is now increasing more rapidly among women than men. Women account for one in four people living with HIV in the United States, and are the fastest-growing segment of persons becoming infected with HIV; transmission in women occurs most frequently from sexual contact (84%) and from intravenous drug use (15%) (CDC, 2015k). Most women, a large number of whom are mothers, have acquired the disease through heterosexual contact. The risk of acquiring HIV through heterosexual contact is greater for women due to exposure to the higher viral concentration in semen. In addition, sexual intercourse may cause breaks in the vaginal lining, increasing the chances that the virus will enter the woman's body.

Fifty percent of all HIV/AIDS cases worldwide occur in women. AIDS is the third leading cause of death among all US women aged 25 to 44 years and the leading cause of death among African American women in this age group. At some point in their lifetimes, an estimated 1 in 32 African American women will be diagnosed with HIV infection (CDC, 2015k).

Pathophysiology

The three recognized modes of HIV transmission are unprotected sexual intercourse with an infected partner, contact with infected blood or blood products, and perinatal transmission.

Take Note!

HIV is not transmitted by doorknobs, faucets, toilets, dirty dishes, mosquitoes, wet towels, coughing or sneezing, shaking hands, or being hugged or by any other indirect method.

The virus attacks the T4 cells, decreases the CD4 cell count, and disables the immune system. The HIV condition can progress to a severe immunosuppressed state termed **acquired immunodeficiency syndrome (AIDS)**. AIDS is a progressive, debilitating disease that suppresses cellular immunity, predisposing the infected person to opportunistic infections and malignancies. The CDC defines AIDS as an HIV-infected person with a specific opportunistic infection or a CD4 count of less than 200. Eventually, death occurs. The time from infection with HIV to development of AIDS is a median of 11 years but varies depending on whether the client is taking current antiretroviral therapy (ART) (Maartens, Celum, & Lewin, 2014). Research indicates that pregnancy does not accelerate the progression of HIV to AIDS or death (Calvert & Ronsmans, 2015).

Once infected with HIV, the woman develops antibodies that can be detected with the enzyme-linked immunosorbent assay (ELISA) and confirmed with the Western blot test. Antibodies develop within 6 to 12 weeks after exposure, although this latent period is much longer in some women. Table 20.5 highlights the four stages of HIV infection according to the CDC (2015l).

Impact of HIV on Pregnancy

When a woman who is infected with HIV becomes pregnant, the risks to herself, her fetus, and the newborn are great. The risks are compounded by problems such as drug abuse, lack of access to prenatal care, poverty, poor nutrition, and high-risk behaviors such as unsafe sex practices and multiple sex partners, which can predispose the woman to additional STIs such as herpes, syphilis, or human papillomavirus (HPV). Additional risk factors to assess for include women who exchange sex for money or drugs or have sex partners who do; a woman whose past or present sex partners were HIV infected; and women who had a blood transfusion between 1978 and 1985. Early identification of maternal HIV seropositivity allows early antiretroviral treatment to prevent mother-to-child transmission, allows a provider to avoid obstetric practices that may increase the risk of transmission, and allows an opportunity to counsel the mother against breast-feeding (also known to increase the risk of transmission) (U.S. Preventive Services Task Force [USPSTF], 2014). Subsequently, pregnant women

TABLE 20.5 STAGES OF HIV INFECTION OUTLINED BY THE CDC

Stages	Description	Clinical Picture
I	Acute infection	Early stage with pervasive viral production Flu-like symptoms 2–4 weeks after exposure Signs and symptoms: weight loss, low-grade fever, fatigue, sore throat, night sweats, and myalgia. Ability to spread HIV is highest during this stage because large amounts of HIV are being produced in the body and the CD4 count drops.
II	Asymptomatic infection or clinical latency	Viral replication continues within lymphatics, but slows down Usually free of symptoms; lymphadenopathy
III	Persistent generalized lymphadenopathy	Possibly remaining in this stage for years; AIDS develops in most within 7–10 yr Opportunistic infections occur
IV	End-stage disease (AIDS)	Severe immune deficiency; very vulnerable to infections High viral load and low CD4 counts Signs and symptoms: bacterial, viral, or fungal opportunistic infections, fever, wasting syndrome, fatigue, neoplasms, and cognitive changes

Adapted from Centers of Disease Control and Prevention [CDC]. (2015s). *About HIV/AIDS*. Retrieved from http://www.cdc.gov/hiv/basics/whatishiv.html.

who are HIV positive are at risk for preterm delivery, fetal growth restriction, premature rupture of membranes, intrapartal or postpartum hemorrhage, postpartum infection, poor wound healing, and genitourinary tract infections (CDC, 2015m).

Perinatal transmission of HIV (from the mother to the fetus or child) also can occur. However, such cases have decreased in the past several years in the United States, primarily due to the use of antiretroviral therapy in pregnant women infected with HIV. This has not been the case in poor countries without similar resources. The Joint United Nations programs on HIV/AIDS (UNAIDS) estimates that over 2,000 new infections due to mother-to-child transmission occur daily. This number is expected to increase rapidly as the prevalence rises in Southeast Asia (Rakhmanina & van den Anker, 2014). Perinatal transmission rates are as high as 35% when there is no intervention (ART) and below 1% when antiretroviral treatment and appropriate care are available. African American and Hispanic women make up 82% of HIV/AIDS cases among women, and according to CDC data (2015j), the majority of prenatally infected children were African American or Hispanic. Lack of timely HIV testing during pregnancy is a major contributor to this outcome. Interventions are needed that will address knowledge barriers to HIV testing among African American and Hispanic women. Research has found that women who have information about methods to prevent perinatal HIV transmission and the importance of testing for the baby's or mother's health are more likely to be HIV tested. Media campaigns addressing the benefits of HIV testing may be a significant intervention. Media campaigns are not only successful in promoting HIV testing but, in populations with high HIV prevalence, they also are cost-effective (International AIDS Society, 2015).

With perinatal transmission, approximately half of children manifest AIDS within the first year of life, and about 80% have clinical symptoms of the disease within 3 to 5 years (Rivera & Frye, 2014). Breast-feeding is a major contributing factor for mother-to-child transmission, and the infected mother must be informed about this (March of Dimes, 2015i). The U.S. Public Health Service recommends that women who are HIV positive should avoid breast-feeding to prevent HIV transmission to the newborn. Given the devastating effects of HIV infection on children, preventing its transmission is critical (NIH, 2014).

In addition to perinatal transmission, the fetus and newborn also are at risk for prematurity, IUGR, low birth weight, and infection. Prompt treatment with antiretroviral medications for the infant with an HIV infection may slow the progression of the disease.

Therapeutic Management

Women who are seropositive for HIV require counseling about the risk of perinatal transmission and the potential for obstetric complications. The risk of perinatal transmission directly correlates with the viral load (Drake et al., 2014). A discussion of the options on continuing the pregnancy, medication therapy, risks, perinatal outcomes, and treatment is warranted. Women who elect to continue with the pregnancy should be treated with ART regardless of their CD4 count or viral load. Interventions to reduce HIV transmission include antiretroviral therapy to the mother and the newborn, consideration of elective cesarean section in women with elevated plasma viral load, and the avoidance of breastfeeding. With these interventions, the risk of HIV transmission is now less than 1% (Giles, 2015).

Drug therapy is the mainstay of treatment for pregnant women infected with HIV. The standard treatment is oral antiretroviral drugs given twice daily until giving birth, intravenous administration during labor, and oral zidovudine (AZT) for the newborn within 6 to 12 hours of birth (Vogler, 2014). The goal of therapy is to reduce the viral load as much as possible, which reduces the risk of transmission to the fetus.

Decisions about the birthing method to be used are made on an individual basis based on several factors involving the woman's health. Some reports suggest that cesarean birth may reduce the risk of HIV infection (King et al., 2015). Efforts to reduce instrumentation, such as avoiding the use of an episiotomy, fetal scalp electrodes, and fetal scalp sampling, will reduce the newborn's exposure to body fluids.

With appropriate therapies, the prognosis for pregnant women with HIV infection has improved significantly. In addition, the newborns of women with HIV infection who have received treatment usually do not become infected. Unfortunately, therapy is complicated and medications are expensive. Moreover, the medications are associated with numerous adverse effects and possible toxic reactions. These therapies offer a dual purpose: reduce the likelihood of mother-to-infant transmission and provide optimal suppression of the viral load in the mother. The core goal of all medical therapy is to bring the client's viral load to an undetectable level, thus minimizing the risk of transmission to the fetus and newborn.

Nursing Assessment

Nursing assessment begins with a thorough history and physical examination. In addition, the woman is offered screening for HIV antibodies. Screening and effective intervention for women who are HIV positive are essential components of prenatal services, which also include education, counseling, testing, treatment, and continued care.

HEALTH HISTORY AND PHYSICAL EXAMINATION

Review the woman's history for risk factors, such as unsafe sex practices, multiple sex partners, and injectable drug use. Also have the woman complete a risk assessment survey. In addition, question the woman about any flu-like symptoms such as a low-grade fever, fatigue, sore throat, night sweats, diarrhea, cough, skin lesions, or muscle pain. Numerous factors influence perinatal transmission. Factors that increase risk of perinatal transmission include high maternal viral load; maternal immune depletion (low CD4 T cell counts); maternal genital tract infections; nutritional deficiencies; drug abuse; cigarette smoking; unprotected sexual intercourse; other opportunistic and coexisting infections (TB, malaria); prolonged ruptured membranes; and breast-feeding. Nurses need to take a thorough history to identify risk factors present.

Perform a complete physical examination. Obtain the woman's weight and determine if she has lost weight recently. Assess for signs and symptoms of STIs, such as vulvovaginal candidiasis, bacterial vaginosis, HSV, chancroid, CMV, or chlamydia because of the increased risk for STIs.

Take Note!

Women who request an HIV test despite reporting no individual risk factors should be considered at risk, since many are not likely to disclose their high-risk behaviors.

LABORATORY AND DIAGNOSTIC TESTING

The USPSTF (2014) recommends that all pregnant women be offered HIV antibody testing, regardless of their risk of infection, and that testing be done during the initial prenatal evaluation. Testing is essential because treatments are available that can reduce the likelihood of perinatal transmission and maintain the health of the woman.

Take Note!

Screening only women who are identified as high risk based on their histories is inadequate due to the prolonged latency period that can exist after exposure. Also, research indicating that treatment with antiretroviral agents could reduce vertical transmission from the infected mother to the newborn has dramatically increased the importance of HIV antibody screening in pregnancy.

Offer all women who are pregnant or planning a pregnancy HIV testing using ELISA. Prepare the woman with a reactive screening test for an additional test, such as the Western blot or an immunofluorescence assay. The Western blot is the confirmatory diagnostic test. A positive antibody test confirmed by a supplemental test indicates that the woman has been infected with HIV and can pass it on to others. HIV antibodies are detectable in at least 95% of women within 3 months after infection (Rayment, Asboe, & Sullivan, 2014).

In addition to the usual screening tests done in normal pregnancy, additional testing for STIs may be necessary. Women infected with HIV have high rates of STIs, especially HPV, vulvovaginal candidiasis, bacterial vaginosis, syphilis, HSV, chancroid, CMV, gonorrhea, chlamydia, and hepatitis B (March of Dimes, 2015i).

Nursing Management

Women infected with HIV should have comprehensive prenatal care, which starts with pretest and post-test counseling. In pretest counseling, the client completes a risk assessment survey and the nurse explains the meaning of positive versus negative test results, obtains informed consent for HIV testing, and educates the woman on how to prevent HIV infection by changing lifestyle behaviors if needed. Post-test counseling includes informing the client of the test results, reviewing the meaning of the results again, and reinforcing safer sex guidelines. All pretest and post-test counseling should be documented in the client's chart.

EDUCATING THE CLIENT

Pregnant clients are dealing with many issues at their first prenatal visit. The confirmation of pregnancy may be accompanied by feelings of joy, anxiety, depression, or other emotions. Simultaneously, the client is given many pamphlets and receives advice and counseling about many important health issues (e.g., nutrition, prenatal development, appointment schedules). This health teaching may be done while the woman feels excited, tired, and anxious. To expect women to understand detailed explanations of a complex disease entity (HIV/AIDS) too may be unrealistic. Determine the client's readiness for this discussion. Identify the client's individual needs for teaching, emotional support, and physical care. Nurses need to approach education and counseling of HIV-positive pregnant women in a caring, sensitive manner. Address the following information:

- Infection control issues at home
- Safer sex precautions
- Stages of the HIV disease process and treatment for each stage
- Symptoms of opportunistic infections
- Preventive drug therapies for her unborn infant
- Avoidance of breast-feeding
- Referrals to community support, counseling, and financial aid
- Client's support system and potential caretaker
- Importance of continual prenatal care
- Need for a well-balanced diet
- Measures to reduce exposure to infections

Be knowledgeable about HIV infection and how HIV is transmitted and share this knowledge with all women. Nurses also can work to influence legislators, public health officials, and the entire health establishment toward policies to address the HIV epidemic. Research toward treatment and cure is tremendously important, but the major key to prevention of the spread of the virus is education. Nurses play a major role in this education.

SUPPORTING THE CLIENT

Be aware of the psychosocial sequelae of HIV/AIDS. A diagnosis of HIV can put a woman into an emotional tailspin, during which she is worried about her own health and that of her unborn infant. She may experience grief, fear, or anxiety about the future of her children. Along with the medications that are so important to her health maintenance, address the woman's mental health needs, family dynamics, capacity to work, and social concerns and provide appropriate support and guidance.

A stigma against both mothers and newborns who are HIV-exposed or infected persists as a challenge on many maternity care units. As nurses work to address this preventable disease, they should do so in a respectful conscientious manner. Beyond basic nursing care, nurses should strive to provide respectful care for all mothers and their newborns together. To accomplish this, be aware of your personal beliefs and attitudes toward women who are HIV positive or have AIDS. Incorporate this awareness in your actions as you help the woman face the reality of the diagnosis and treatment options. Empathy, understanding, caring, and assistance are key to helping the client and her family.

PREPARING FOR LABOR, BIRTH, AND AFTERWARD

Current evidence suggests that cesarean birth performed before the onset of labor and before the rupture of membranes significantly reduces the rate of perinatal transmission. The ACOG recommends that HIV-positive women be offered elective cesarean birth to reduce the rate of transmission beyond that which may be achieved through ART. They further suggest that operative births be performed at 38 weeks' gestation and that amniocentesis be avoided to prevent contamination of the amniotic fluid with maternal blood. Decisions concerning the method of delivery should be based on the woman's viral load, the duration of ruptured membranes, the progress of labor, and other pertinent clinical factors (USPSTF, 2014).

Prepare the woman physically and emotionally for the possibility of cesarean birth and assist as necessary. Ensure that she understands the rationale for the surgical birth.

After the birth of the newborn, the motivation for taking antiretroviral medications may be lower, thus affecting the woman's adherence to therapy. Encourage the woman to continue therapy for her own sake as well as that of the newborn. Nurses can make a difference in helping women to adhere to their complex drug regimens.

Reinforce family planning methods during this time, incorporating a realistic view of her disease status. It is clear that hormonal contraceptives are not protective against HIV infection and that dual protection with condoms should be the goal for women using hormonal contraception (U.S. Agency for International Development [USAID] 2014). Advise the woman that breast-feeding is not recommended. Instruct the woman who is HIV positive in self-care measures, including the proper method for disposing of perineal pads to reduce the risk of exposing others to infected body fluids. Finally, teach her the signs and symptoms of infection in newborns and infants, encouraging her to report any to the health care provider.

The evolution of HIV infection into a chronic disease has implications across all clinical care settings. Every nurse should be knowledgeable about the prevention, testing, treatment, and chronicity of the disease in order to provide high-quality care to people with or at risk for HIV. Breakthroughs in the prevention of HIV important to public health include male circumcision, antiretrovirals to prevent mother-to-child transmission, ART in HIV+ people to prevent transmission, and antiretrovirals for pre-exposure prophylaxis. Nurses, therefore, need to have an understanding of the changing epidemiology of the disease, the most recent testing recommendations, developments in screening technology, the implications of aging with HIV infection, and the nursing implications of this ongoing epidemic.

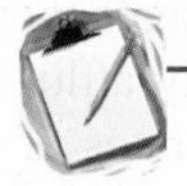

Take Note!

When providing direct care, **ALWAYS** follow standard precautions.

VULNERABLE POPULATIONS

Every year there are an estimated 208 million pregnancies worldwide, with about 6.6 million of them in the United States (Alan Guttmacher Institute, 2015b). Each pregnancy runs the risk of an adverse outcome for the mother and the baby, but risks are dramatically increased for certain vulnerable populations: adolescents, women over the age of 35, women who are obese, and women who engage in substance abuse. Although risks cannot be totally eliminated once pregnancy has begun, they can be reduced through appropriate and timely interventions.

Every woman's experience with pregnancy is unique and personal. The circumstances each one faces and what pregnancy means to her involve emotions and experiences that belong solely to her. Many women in these special population groups go through this experience in confusion and isolation, feeling desperately in need of help but not knowing where to go. Although all pregnant women experience these emotions to a certain extent, they are heightened in women who have numerous psychosocial issues. Pregnancy is a stressful time. Pregnant women face wide-ranging changes in their lives, relationships, and bodies as they move toward parenthood. These changes can be challenging for a woman without any additional stresses but are even more so in the face of age extremes, illness, or substance abuse.

Skilled nursing interventions are essential to promote the best outcome for the client and her baby. Timely support and appropriate interventions during the perinatal period can have long-standing implications for the mother and her newborn, ultimately with the goal of stability and integration of the family as a unit.

Pregnant Adolescent

Adolescence lasts from the onset of puberty to the cessation of physical growth, roughly from 11 to 19 years of age. Adolescents vacillate between being children and being adults. They need to adjust to the physiologic changes their bodies are undergoing and establish a sexual identity during this time. They search for personal identity and desire freedom and independence of thought and action. However, they continue to have a strong dependence on their parents (Crockett & Crouter, 2014).

Adolescent pregnancy has emerged as one of the most significant social problems facing our society. The latest estimates show that approximately one million teens become pregnant each year in the United States (Alan Guttmacher Institute, 2015a; CDC, 2015a). Among these approximately half will give birth, slightly over one third will opt for abortions, and the remaining 14% will have miscarriages or stillbirths. Despite being an advanced and relatively affluent nation, teens in the United States have higher rates of pregnancy and childbearing than any other industrialized country (Sedgh et al., 2015). It is estimated that 11% of births worldwide are to adolescents 15 to 19 years old (Ganchimeg et al., 2014). In addition, about half of all teen pregnancies occur within 6 months of first having sexual intercourse. About one in four teen mothers under age 18 have a second baby within 2 years after the birth of their first baby. Most of these girls are unmarried, and many are not ready for the emotional, psychological, and financial responsibilities of parenthood. Teens are least likely of all maternal age groups to get early and regular prenatal care (March of Dimes, 2015j). Adolescent pregnancy is further complicated by the adolescent's lack of financial resources: the income of teen mothers is half that of women who have given birth in their 20s (March of Dimes, 2015j).

Although the incidence of teenage pregnancy has steadily declined since the early 1990s, it continues to be higher in the United States than in any other industrialized country (Alan Guttmacher Institute, 2015a). Even this reduced incidence represents what is considered an unacceptably high level of pregnancy in an age group that is most likely to suffer the social consequences of early pregnancy. Although teen birth rates in the United States have declined, they remain high, especially among African American and Hispanic teens and in southern states. The highest rate of unintended teenage pregnancies occurs in Hispanics and African Americans.

Currently, fewer high school students are having sexual intercourse, and more sexually active students are using some method of contraception. However, many teens who have had sexual intercourse have not spoken with their parents about sex, and use of contraceptives remains rare (CDC, 2015a). Subsequently, adolescent pregnancy is considered a major health problem and is addressed in *Healthy People 2020* (see *Healthy People 2020*).

Impact of Pregnancy in Adolescence

The impact of adolescent pregnancy is evident in maternal and perinatal morbidity and mortality. Nonetheless, in addition to the age involved in precocious pregnancy, it also reflects previous conditions such as malnutrition, communicable diseases, and deficiencies in the health care given to pregnant adolescents. The most important impact lies in the psychosocial area: it contributes to a loss of self-esteem, societal discrimination, a destruction of life projects, and the maintenance of the circle of poverty (WHO, 2015a).

Adolescents are a unique group with special needs related to their stage of development. Adolescent pregnancy can be an emotionally charged situation, laden with ethical dilemmas and decisions. Topics such as abstinence, safer sex, abortion, and the decision to have a child are sensitive issues.

A nurse's moral convictions may influence the care that he or she provides to pregnant adolescents depending on his or her beliefs. Nurses need to examine their own beliefs about teen sexuality to identify personal assumptions. Putting aside one's moral convictions may be difficult, but it is necessary when working with pregnant adolescents. To be effective, health care providers must be able to communicate with adolescents in a manner they can understand and respect them as individuals.

The idea of it taking "a village to raise a child," as suggested by former First Lady Hillary Clinton in 1996, is perhaps even more valid than previously thought regarding teen pregnancy. The evidence suggests that it's not enough to teach teens to "just say no," nor is it enough to give them information about contraceptive methods; teens need to be connected to their parents, their peers, and their community (Whitworth & Cockerill, 2014). Nurses should feel that there is always hope and the chance of positive outcomes; nurses see that every day, often in the faces of their youngest clients. Nurses have to believe in that and work toward "*connecting*" with their teen clients. Nurses are on the front line of health care, and are often the first to interact and build rapport with teenagers. Teens who engage in risky sexual behavior may seek out nurses first. Nurse's scope of practice includes providing education and a source of comfort and support to all ages. It is therefore imperative for all nurses to be able to provide age-appropriate information about sexual health. In

HEALTHY PEOPLE 2020

Objective	Nursing Significance
FP-8 Reduce pregnancy rates among adolescent females by 10 percent by 2020. **FP-9** Increase the proportion of adolescents ages 17 years and under who have never had sexual intercourse by 10 percent by 2020. **FP-10** Increase the proportion of sexually active persons ages 15 to 19 years who use condoms to both effectively prevent pregnancy and provide barrier protection against disease by 10 percent by 2020. **FP-11** Increase the proportion of sexually active persons ages 15 to 19 years who use condoms and hormonal or intrauterine contraception to both effectively prevent pregnancy and provide barrier protection against disease by 10 percent by 2020. **FP-12** Increase the proportion of adolescents who received formal instruction on reproductive health topics before they were 18 years old by 10 percent by 2020. **FP-13** Increase the proportion of adolescents who talked to a parent or guardian about reproductive health topics before they were 18 years old by 10 percent by 2020.	Will help to foster a continued decline in adolescent pregnancy rates by focusing on interventions related to pregnancy prevention, including safe sex practices and teaching about the complications associated with adolescent pregnancy.
HIV-8 Reduce the number of perinatally acquired HIV and AIDS cases by 10 percent by 2020.	Education for the pregnant mothers about the need and rationale for antiretroviral drug therapy to prevent vertical transmission of HIV to their fetus will help reduce this incidence.
MICH-11 Increase abstinence from alcohol, cigarettes, and illicit drugs among pregnant women by 10 percent by 2020. **MICH-25** Reduce the occurrence of fetal alcohol syndrome (FAS) by 10 percent by 2020.	Education and support offered to pregnant women regarding the hazards of alcohol, cigarettes, and illicit drugs will reduce the abuse of these substances to enhance the perinatal outcomes.
NWS-22 Reduce iron deficiency among pregnant females.	Providing nutritional instruction on iron-rich foods will help reduce the incidence of iron deficiency anemia during pregnancy.

Healthy People objectives based on data from http://www.healthypeople.gov.

providing this care, the quality of life and outcome of both the mother and her infant can be improved.

Developmental Issues

An adolescent must accomplish certain developmental tasks to advance to the next stage of maturity. These developmental tasks include:

- Seeking economic and social stability
- Adjusting to sexually maturing bodies and feelings
- Developing a personal value system
- Building meaningful relationships with others (Fig. 20.6)
- Becoming comfortable with their changing bodies
- Working to become independent from their parents
- Learning to verbalize conceptually (CDC, 2015n)

Adolescents have special needs when working to accomplish their developmental tasks and making a smooth transition to young adulthood. One of the biggest areas of need is sexual health. Adolescents commonly lack the information, skills, and services necessary to make informed choices related to their sexual and reproductive health. Developmentally, adolescents are trying to figure out who they are and how they fit into society. As adolescents mature, their parents become less influential and peers become more influential. Peer pressure can lead adolescents to participate in sexual activity, as can the typical adolescent's belief that "it won't happen to me" (Box 20.3). As a result, unplanned pregnancies occur. Work on the developmental tasks of **adolescence**, especially identity, can be interrupted as the adolescent

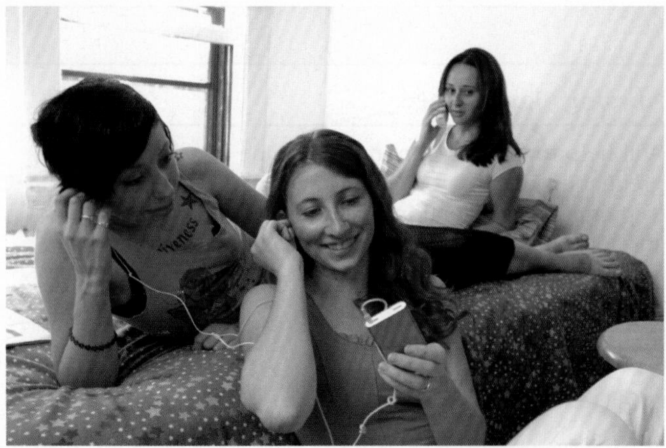

FIGURE 20.6 Adolescent girls sharing time together.

attempts to integrate the tasks of pregnancy, bonding, and preparing to care for another with the tasks of developing self-identity and independence. A pregnant adolescent must try to meet her own needs along with those of her fetus. The process of learning how to separate from the parents while learning how to bond and attach to a newborn brings conflict and stress. A pregnancy can exacerbate an adolescent's feeling of loss of control and helplessness (American Academy of Pediatrics, 2014).

Health and Social Issues

Adolescent pregnancy has a negative impact in terms of both health and social consequences. For example, 7 out of 10 adolescents will drop out of school. More than 75% will receive public assistance within 5 years of having their first child. In addition, children of adolescent mothers are at greater risk of preterm birth, low birth weight, child abuse, neglect, poverty, and death. The younger the adolescent is at the time of the first pregnancy, the more likely it is that she will have another pregnancy during her teens (March of Dimes, 2015j). Adolescent pregnancy also places them at high risk for obstetric complications such as preterm labor and births, low–birth-weight infants, STIs, poor maternal weight gain, preeclampsia, iron-deficiency anemia, poor eating habits, and inadequate nutrition and postpartum depression (Rajoriya & Kalra, 2015).

BOX 20.3

POSSIBLE FACTORS CONTRIBUTING TO ADOLESCENT PREGNANCY

- Early menarche
- Peer pressure to become sexually active
- Sexual or other abuse as a child
- Lack of accurate contraceptive information
- Fear of telling parents about sexual activity
- Feelings of invulnerability
- Poverty (85% of births occur in poor families)
- Culture or ethnicity (high incidence in Hispanic and African American girls)
- Unprotected sex
- Low self-esteem and inability to negotiate
- Lack of appropriate role models
- Strong need for someone to love
- Drug use, truancy from school, or other behavioral problems
- Wish to escape a bad home situation
- Early dating without supervision

Adapted from Alan Guttmacher Institute.(2015a). *Facts on American teens' sexual and reproductive health.* Retrieved from http://www.guttmacher.org/pubs/FB-ATSRH.html; Ross, S., Baird, A. S., & Porter, C. C. (2014). Teenage pregnancy: Strategies for prevention. *Obstetrics, Gynecology, & Reproductive Medicine, 24*(9), 266–273.; and March of Dimes. (2015j). *Teenage pregnancy.* Retrieved from http://www.marchofdimes.com/professionals/14332_1159.asp.

The psychosocial risks associated with early childbearing often have an even greater impact on mothers, families, and society than the obstetric or medical risks (Northridge & Coupey, 2015). Pregnant adolescents experience higher rates of domestic violence and substance abuse. Those experiencing abuse are more likely to abuse substances, receive inadequate prenatal care, and have lower pregnancy weight compared with those who are not (Smith et al., 2016). Moreover, substance abuse (cigarettes, alcohol, or illicit drugs) can contribute to low birth weight, fetal growth restriction, preterm births, newborn addiction, and sepsis (March of Dimes, 2015j).

Although early childbearing (12 to 19 years of age) occurs in all socioeconomic groups, it is more prevalent among poor women and those from minority backgrounds, who face more obstetric and newborn risks than their more affluent counterparts (March of Dimes, 2015j). Poverty often contributes to delayed prenatal care and medical complications related to poor nutrition, such as anemia.

The financial burden of adolescent pregnancy is high and costs taxpayers an estimated $11 billion annually in the United States (Alan Guttmacher Institute, 2015b). Much of the expense stems from Medicaid, food stamps, state health department maternity clinics, the federal Aid to Families with Dependent Children program, and direct payments to health care providers. However, this amount does not address the costs to society in terms of the loss of human resources and the far-reaching intergenerational effects of adolescent parenting. For some adolescents, pregnancy may be seen as a hopeless situation: a grim story of poverty and lost dreams, of being trapped in a life that was never wanted. Health-related behaviors, such as smoking, diet, sexual behavior, and help-seeking behaviors, which are developed during adolescence often, endure into later life (Fedorowicz et al., 2014). The consequences associated with an adolescent's less-than-optimal health status at this age due to pregnancy can ultimately affect her long-term health and that of her children. However, some adolescents can create a happy, stable life for themselves and their children by facing their challenges and working hard to beat the odds.

Recall Rose, the pregnant teenager with asthma. What issues would be important for the nurse to discuss with her related to her pregnancy, her asthma, and her age?

Nursing Assessment

Assessment of the pregnant adolescent is the same as that for any pregnant woman. However, when dealing with pregnant teens, the nurse also needs to ask:

- How does the girl see herself in the future?
- Are realistic role models available to her?
- How much does she know about child development?
- What financial resources are available to her?
- Does she work? Does she go to school?
- What emotional support is available to her?
- Can she resolve conflicts and manage anger?
- What does she know about health and nutrition for herself and her child?
- Will she need help dealing with the challenges of the new parenting role?
- Does she need information about community resources?

Having an honest regard for adolescents requires getting to know them and being able to appreciate the important aspects of their life. Doing so forms a basis for the nurse's clinical judgment and promotes care that takes into account the concerns and practical circumstances of the teen and her family. Skillful practice includes knowing how and when to advise a teen and when to listen and refrain from giving advice. Giving advice can be misinterpreted as "preaching," and the adolescent will probably ignore the information. The nurse must be perceptive, flexible, and sensitive and must work to establish a therapeutic relationship.

Nursing Management

For adolescents, as for all women, pregnancy can be a physically, emotionally, and socially stressful time. The pregnancy is often both the result of and cause of social problems and stressors that can be overwhelming to them. Nurses must support adolescents during the transition from childhood into adulthood, which is complicated by their emergence into motherhood. Assist the adolescent in identifying family and friends who want to be involved and provide support throughout the pregnancy.

Help the adolescent identify the options for this pregnancy, such as abortion, self-parenting of the child, temporary foster care for the baby or herself, or placement of the child for adoption. Explore with the adolescent if the pregnancy was planned or unintended. Becoming aware of why she decided to have a child is necessary to help with the development of the adolescent and her ability to parent. Identify barriers to seeking prenatal care, such as lack of transportation, too many problems at home, financial concerns, the long wait for an appointment, and lack of sensitivity on the part of the health care system. Encourage the girl to set goals and work toward them. Assist her in returning to school and furthering her education. As appropriate, initiate a referral for career or job counseling.

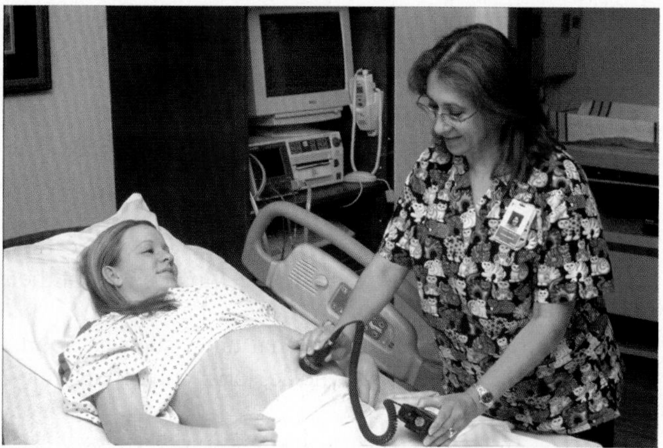

FIGURE 20.7 A pregnant adolescent receiving care during labor.

Stress that the girl's physical well-being is important for both herself and her developing fetus, which depends on her for its own health-related needs. Assist with arrangements for care, including stress management and self-care. Having a healthy newborn eases the transition to motherhood somewhat, rather than having to deal with the added stress of caring for an unhealthy baby (Rajoriya & Kalra, 2015). Monitor weight gain, sleep and rest patterns, and nutritional status to promote positive outcomes for both the mother and child. Stress the importance of attending prenatal education classes. Provide appropriate teaching based on the adolescent's developmental level and emphasize the importance of continued prenatal and follow-up care. Monitor maternal and fetal well-being throughout pregnancy and labor (Fig. 20.7).

Nurses can also play a major role in preventing adolescent pregnancies, perhaps by volunteering to talk to teen groups. Teaching Guidelines 20.6 highlights the key areas for teaching adolescents about pregnancy prevention.

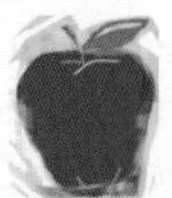

Teaching Guidelines 20.6

TOPICS FOR TEACHING ADOLESCENTS TO PREVENT PREGNANCY

- High-risk behaviors that lead to pregnancy
- Involvement in programs such as Free Teens, Teen Advisors, or Postponing Sexual Involvement
- Planning and goal setting to visualize their futures in terms of career, college, travel, and education
- Choice of abstinence or taking a step back to become a "second-time virgin"

- Discussions about sexuality with a wiser adult—someone they respect can help put things in perspective
- Protection against STIs and pregnancy if they choose to remain sexually active
- Critical observation and review of peers and friends to make sure they are creating the right atmosphere for friendship
- Empowerment to make choices that will shape their life for years to come, including getting control of their own lives now
- Appropriate use of recreational time, such as sports, drama, volunteer work, music, jobs, church activities, and school clubs

Adapted from Yoost, J. L., Hertweck, S. P., & Barnett, S. N. (2014). The effect of an educational approach to pregnancy prevention among high-risk early and late adolescents. *Journal of Adolescent Health, 55*(2), 222–227; Koh, H. (2014). The teen pregnancy prevention program: An evidence-based public health program model. *Journal of Adolescent Health, 54*(3), S1–S2; March of Dimes. (2015j). *Teenage pregnancy.* Retrieved from http://www.marchofdimes.com/professionals/14332_1159.asp.

Tackling the many issues surrounding adolescent pregnancy is difficult. Making connections with clients is crucial regardless of how complex their situation is. The future challenges nurses to find solutions to teenage pregnancies. Nurses must take proactive positions while working with adolescents, parents, schools, and communities to reduce the problems associated with early childbearing.

Nurses who provide care to adolescents have an opportunity to discuss future pregnancies and to use health care visits to teach about preconception health. Teaching adolescents who both express a desire for pregnancy and those who do not express such a desire is an important part of comprehensive nursing care. Teens require a thorough teaching about health care risks such as smoking cessation, body weight control, interpersonal violence, and the need for folic acid. Adolescents should be prime recipients of preconception education at every health care visit.

Teen childbearing is associated with adverse consequences for mothers and their children and imposes high public sector costs. Prevention of teen pregnancy requires evidence-based sex education, support for parents in talking with their children about pregnancy prevention and other aspects of sexual and reproductive health, and ready access to effective and affordable contraception for teens who are sexually active (CDC, 2015o).

The Advanced Maternal Age Woman

It is estimated that by the year 2025 about 25% of mothers will begin their childbearing period at an "advanced age."Advanced age is a risk factor for female infertility, pregnancy loss, fetal anomalies, stillbirth, and obstetric complications (Sauer, 2015). A few decades ago, a woman having a baby after the age of 35probably was giving birth to the last of several children, but today she may be having her first. With advances in technology and the tendency of women to seek career advancement prior to childbearing, the dramatic increase in women having first pregnancies after the age of 35 will likely continue.

Impact of Pregnancy on the Advanced Maternal Age Woman

Whether childbearing is delayed by choice or by chance, women starting a family at age 35 or older are not doing so without risk. Women in this age group may already have chronic health conditions that can put the pregnancy at risk. In addition, numerous studies have shown that increasing maternal age is a risk factor for infertility and spontaneous abortions, gestational diabetes, chronic hypertension, postpartum hemorrhage, preeclampsia, preterm labor and birth, multiple pregnancy, genetic disorders and chromosomal abnormalities, placenta previa, fetal growth restriction, low Apgar scores, and surgical births (Schimmel et al., 2015). However, even though increased age implies increased complications, most women today who become pregnant after age 34 have healthy pregnancies and healthy newborns. Today, one in five women in the United States has her first child after age 34 (March of Dimes, 2015m).

Nursing Assessment

Nursing assessment of the pregnant woman over age 34 is the same as that for any pregnant woman. For a woman of this age, a preconception visit is important to identify chronic health problems that might affect the pregnancy and also to address lifestyle issues that may take time to modify. Encourage the advanced maternal aged woman to plan for the pregnancy by seeing her health care provider before getting pregnant to discuss preexisting medical conditions, medications, and lifestyle choices. Assess the woman for risk factors such as cigarette smoking, poor nutrition, overweight or underweight, alcohol use, or illicit drug use.

A preconception visit also provides the opportunity to educate the woman about risk factors and provide information on how to modify her lifestyle habits to improve the pregnancy outcome. Assist the woman with lifestyle changes so that she can begin pregnancy in an optimal state of health. For example, if the woman is overweight, educate her about weight loss so that she can start the pregnancy at a healthy weight. If the woman smokes, encourage smoking cessation to reduce the effects of nicotine on herself and her fetus.

Prepare the woman for laboratory and diagnostic testing to establish a baseline for future comparisons. The risk of having a baby with Down syndrome increases with age, especially over age 34. Amniocentesis is routinely offered to all older women to allow the early detection of numerous chromosomal abnormalities, including Down syndrome. Additionally, a quadruple blood test screen (alpha fetoprotein [AFP], human chorionic gonadotropin [hCG], unconjugated estriol [UE], and inhibin A [placental hormone]) drawn between 15 and 20 weeks of pregnancy can be helpful in screening for Down syndrome and neural tube defects.

Nursing Management

During routine prenatal visits, the nurse can play a key role in promoting a healthy pregnancy. Consider social, genetic, and environmental factors that are unique to the advanced maternal aged pregnant women and prepare to address these factors when providing care. In a study by Mills and Lavender (2014), compared with the younger women, older women had statistically similar rates of gestational hypertension, gestational diabetes, preterm premature rupture of membranes/preterm labor, and abnormal placentation. Cesarean birth was higher in older women versus younger ones. Neonatal outcomes of gestational age and birth weight were excellent and similar between groups. Despite the increased risks, there are potential psychological and social advantages to delaying childbirth, and absolute numbers of complications are small.

Assess the woman's knowledge about risk factors and measures to reduce them. Educate her about measures to promote a positive outcome. Encourage her to get early and regular prenatal care. Advise her to eat a variety of nutritious foods, especially fortified cereals, enriched grain products, and fresh fruits and vegetables, and drink at least six to eight glasses of water daily and to take the prescribed vitamin containing 400 mcg of folic acid daily. Also stress the need for her to avoid alcohol intake during pregnancy, avoid exposure to secondhand smoke, and take no drugs unless they are prescribed. Provide continued surveillance of the mother and fetus throughout the pregnancy.

The Obese Pregnant Woman

Obese pregnant women are a particularly vulnerable group because their disability (obesity) is highly visible. In the United States, nearly 36% of adults are obese, including one out of three women (CDC, 2015p). Excess weight and obesity have gained attention as serious health care threats globally. Obesity during pregnancy is defined as a BMI of 30 kg/m^2 or more calculated using the height and weight measured at the first prenatal visit. Compared to normal weight women, overweight and obese women tend to gain excessive weight in pregnancy and are at high risk for maternal and birth outcomes. Excessive gestational weight gain is strongly associated with postpartum weight retention which increases the risk of additional weight gains in subsequent pregnancies (Chang et al., 2015). Obesity contributes to social, psychological, and economic problems throughout a woman's lifetime. Negative attitudes and discrimination by society can have negative consequences for the woman's quality of life. The number of women who are overweight or obese during pregnancy has also increased. During pregnancy, excess weight increases both obstetric and neonatal risks, including:

- Gestational diabetes
- Hypertension
- Thromboembolism
- Preeclampsia
- Preterm labor and birth
- Congenital anomalies
- Childhood and adolescent obesity
- Fetal macrosomia (birth weight >4,000 grams)
- Difficulty fighting postpartum infections
- Depression
- Tendency to remain overweight/obesity between pregnancies
- Prolongation of pregnancy/increased likelihood of post-term infant
- Increased risk of stillbirth
- Higher rate of cesarean births
- Increased risk of maternal mortality
- High risk for postpartum hemorrhage (ACOG, 2014b)

Negative or judgmental attitudes toward overweight or obese individuals can be encountered within the health care community and its providers, including nurses. Nurses can find it difficult to discuss weight issues during prenatal visits with obese women (Knight-Agarwal et al., 2014). Preconception assessment and counseling are needed for obese women, which should include specific information about maternal and fetal risks of obesity in pregnancy, as well as encouragement to undertake a weight-reduction program, including diet, exercise, and behavior modification, to achieve a healthy weight prior to conception.

Obese pregnant women require individualized nursing care. Extra time may be needed to promote healthful practices, which should include dealing with issues of weight, diet, and exercise. Specialist dietary interventions and evidence-based guidelines for working with childbearing women must be seen as a public health priority by all nurses. This care must be done with honesty and respect for all of the woman's needs. There is an opportunity for health promotion aimed at disseminating information about the risks of obesity in pregnancy to overweight and obese women of childbearing age.

The Pregnant Woman and Substance Abuse

Substance abuse in pregnancy is a significant public health crisis causing increased morbidity in two individuals, the mother and the fetus. The epidemic of substance abuse continues to pose a significant challenge to all nations. Although there is a tendency to simply associate drug abuse with poverty, the problem affects every social stratum, gender, and race; and pregnant women are no exception. **Perinatal drug abuse** is the use of alcohol and other drugs by pregnant women. The incidence of substance abuse during pregnancy is highly variable because most pregnant women are reluctant to reveal the extent of their use. The National Institute on Drug Abuse (NIDA) (2015a) estimates that 7% or more of the women in the United States have used illicit drugs while pregnant. These include cocaine, marijuana, heroin, and psychotherapeutic drugs that were not prescribed by a health care provider. More than 20% used alcohol and 19% smoked cigarettes during their pregnancy (2015a).

Impact of Substance Abuse on Pregnancy

Substance use can be viewed along a continuum between social recreational drug use and addiction. Substance abuse is very prevalent remains and continues to remain undetected and underdiagnosed in many pregnant women. Substance abuse rarely starts during pregnancy. More often, women enter pregnancy already abusing or dependent on drugs.

Prenatal education and counseling is essential to successfully impacting this high-risk population. The positive overall impact of adequate prenatal care on birth outcomes is well documented. For pregnant substance users, the receipt of adequate prenatal care is especially critical. Several studies have reported that increasing the adequacy of prenatal care utilization in pregnant substance users reduces risks for prematurity, low birth weight, and perinatal mortality. However, many pregnant women who are substance users do not seek prenatal care for fear of being reported to Child Protective Services (SAMHSA, 2015).

The use of drugs, legal or not, increases the risk of medical complications in the mother and poor birth outcomes in the newborn. The placenta acts as an active transport mechanism, not as a barrier, and substances pass from a mother to her fetus through the placenta. Thus, along with the mother, the fetus experiences substance use, abuse, and addiction. Additionally, fetal vulnerability to drugs is much greater because the fetus has not developed the enzymatic system needed to metabolize drugs (Doulatram, Raj, & Govindaraj, 2015).

EFFECTS OF ADDICTION

Addiction is a multifaceted process that is affected by environmental, psychological, family, and physical factors. Women who use drugs, alcohol, or tobacco come from all socioeconomic backgrounds, cultures, and lifestyles. Factors associated with substance abuse during a pregnancy may include low self-esteem, inadequate support systems, low self-expectations, high levels of anxiety, socioeconomic barriers, involvement in abusive relationships, chaotic familial and social systems, and a history of psychiatric illness or depression. Women often become substance abusers to relieve their anxieties, previous physical, sexual, and emotional traumas in their life, depression, and feelings of worthlessness (Slater, 2015).

Societal attitudes regarding women and substance abuse may prohibit them from admitting the problem and seeking treatment. Society sanctions women for failing to live up to expectations of how a pregnant woman "should" behave, thereby possibly driving them further away from the treatment they so desperately need. For many reasons, pregnant women who abuse substances feel unwelcome in prenatal clinics or medical settings. Often they seek prenatal care late or not at all. They may fear being shamed or reported to legal or child protection authorities. A nonjudgmental atmosphere and unbiased teaching to all pregnant women regardless of their lifestyle is crucial. A caring, concerned manner is critical to help these women feel safe and respond honestly to assessment questions.

Pregnancy can be a motivator for some who want to try treatment. The goal of therapy is to help the client deal with pregnancy by developing a trusting relationship. Providing a full spectrum of medical, social, and emotional care is needed.

EFFECTS OF COMMONLY ABUSED SUBSTANCES

Substance abuse in pregnancy has increased during the past three decades in the United States, resulting in approximately 250,000 infants being born yearly with prenatal exposure to illicit substances (CDC, 2015q). Routine screening and education of women of childbearing age remain the most important ways to reduce addiction in pregnancy.

Substance abuse during pregnancy, particularly in the first trimester, has a negative effect on the health of the mother and the growth and development of the fetus. The fetus experiences the same systemic effects as the mother, but often more severely. The fetus cannot metabolize drugs as efficiently as the expectant mother and will experience the effects long after the drugs have left the women's system. Substance abuse during pregnancy is associated with preterm labor, abortion, IUGR, abruptio placenta, depressed Apgar scores, third trimester bleeding, meconium staining at birth, fetal demise, low birth weight, neurobehavioral abnormalities, and long-term childhood developmental consequences (WHO, 2015c). Table 20.6 summarizes the effects of selected drugs during pregnancy. *Healthy People 2020* also addresses the goals for perinatal substance abuse.

TABLE 20.6 EFFECTS OF SELECTED DRUGS ON PREGNANCY

Substance	Effect on Pregnancy
Alcohol	Spontaneous abortion, inadequate weight gain, IUGR, fetal alcohol spectrum disorder, the leading cause of intellectual disability
Caffeine	Vasoconstriction and mild diuresis in mother; fetal stimulation, but teratogenic effects not documented via research
Nicotine	Vasoconstriction, reduced uteroplacental blood flow, decreased birth weight, abortion, prematurity, abruptio placentae, fetal demise
Cocaine	Vasoconstriction, gestational hypertension, abruptio placentae, abortion, "snow baby syndrome," CNS defects, IUGR
Marijuana	Anemia, inadequate weight gain, "amotivational syndrome," hyperactive startle reflex, newborn tremors, prematurity, IUGR
Opiates and Narcotics	Maternal and fetal withdrawal, abruptio placentae, preterm labor, premature rupture of membranes, perinatal asphyxia, newborn sepsis and death, intellectual impairment, malnutrition
Sedatives	CNS depression, newborn withdrawal, maternal seizures in labor, newborn abstinence syndrome, delayed lung maturity

Adapted from Centers for Disease Control and Prevention [CDC]. (2015q). *Illegal drug use.* Retrieved from http://www.cdc.gov/nchs/fastats/drug-use-illegal.htm; March of Dimes. (2015k). *Smoking, alcohol, and drugs and pregnancy.*Retrieved from http://www.marchofdimes.org/pregnancy/illicit-drug-use-during-pregnancy.aspx; and McKeever, A. E., Spaeth-Brayton, S., & Sheerin, S. (2014). The role of nurses in comprehensive care management of pregnant women with drug addiction. *Nursing for Women's Health, 18*(4), 284–293.

Alcohol. Alcohol abuse is a major public health issue in the United States. Alcohol is a **teratogen**, a substance known to be toxic to human development. The true rate of prenatal alcohol consumption is unknown. It is recognized that **fetal alcohol spectrum disorder (FASD)** is entirely preventable through alcohol abstinence, but worldwide approximately 30% of pregnant women consume alcohol during pregnancy (Vall, Salat-Batlle, & Garcia-Algar, 2015). Theoretically, no mother would give a glass of wine, beer, or hard liquor to her newborn, but when she drinks, her embryo or fetus is exposed to the same blood alcohol concentration as she is.

The teratogenic effects of heavy maternal drinking have been recognized since 1973, when fetal alcohol syndrome was first described. Fetal alcohol syndrome is now a classification under the broader term of FASD; this disorder includes the full range of birth defects, such as structural anomalies and behavioral and neurocognitive disabilities caused by prenatal exposure to alcohol (Vaux & Chambers, 2015). FASD affects 1 in 100 infants each year, more than autism, Down syndrome, cerebral palsy, cystic fibrosis, spina bifida, and sudden infant death syndrome (SIDS) combined (National Organization on Fetal Alcohol Syndrome [NOFAS], 2015). Each year in the United States, up to 50,000 infants are born with FASD. It is the leading cause of nongenetic intellectual disability in the United States, possibly exceeding even Down syndrome, which is currently approaching 1 in 500 live births. Alcohol consumption during pregnancy results in brain, craniofacial, and heart defects, neurotoxicity, and immune systems dysfunction.

Characteristics of FASD include craniofacial dysmorphia (thin upper lip, small head circumference, and small eyes), IUGR, microcephaly, and congenital anomalies such as limb abnormalities and cardiac defects. Long-term sequelae include postnatal growth restriction, attention deficits, delayed reaction time, and poor scholastic performance (NOFAS, 2015). The complex neurobehavioral problems typically manifest themselves insidiously. Children with prenatal alcohol exposure struggle with cognitive, academic, social, emotional, and behavioral challenges. These challenges reduce the child's ability to learn and function successfully in many structured environments (Mohammadzadeh & Farhat, 2014). Common cognitive and behavioral problems are listed in Box 20.4, and Figure 20.8 illustrates the characteristic facial features. See Chapter 24 for a more detailed discussion of the newborn with FASD.

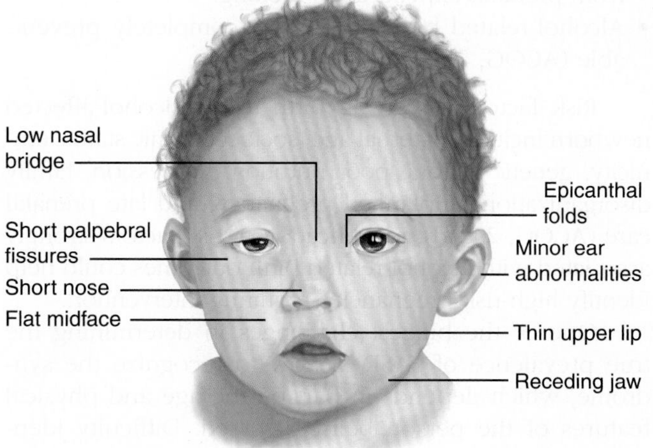

FIGURE 20.8 Typical facial characteristics of a newborn with FASD.

BOX 20.4

COMMON COGNITIVE AND BEHAVIORAL PROBLEMS ASSOCIATED WITH FASD AND ATTENTION DEFICIT/HYPERACTIVITY DISORDER

- Inability to foresee consequences
- Inability to learn from previous experience
- Lack of organization
- Intellectual disability or low IQ
- Difficulty in school, especially with math
- Learning difficulties
- Poor abstract thinking
- Poor reasoning and judgment skills
- Poor memory
- Poor impulse control
- Speech and language delays
- Poor judgment

Adapted from Centers for Disease Control and Prevention [CDC]. (2015h). *Fetal alcohol spectrum disorders.* Retrieved from http://www.cdc.gov/ncbddd/fasd/alcohol-use.html.

The preferred action taken to prevent alcohol consumption during pregnancy is abstinence. However, the detection, diagnosis, and treatment of FASD remain major public health needs in this country and throughout the world. Not every woman who drinks during pregnancy will give birth to an affected child. Based on the best research available, the following is known about alcohol consumption during pregnancy:

- Intake increases the risk of alcohol-related birth defects, including growth deficiencies, facial abnormalities, central nervous system impairment, behavioral disorders, and intellectual development.
- No amount of alcohol consumption is considered safe during pregnancy.
- Damage to the fetus can occur at any stage of pregnancy, even before a woman knows she is pregnant.
- Cognitive defects and behavioral problems resulting from prenatal exposure are lifelong.
- Alcohol-related birth defects are completely preventable (ACOG, 2014c).

Risk factors for giving birth to an alcohol-affected newborn include maternal age, socioeconomic status, ethnicity, genetic factors, poor nutrition, depression, family disorganization, unplanned pregnancy, and late prenatal care (ACOG, 2014d). Identification of risk factors strongly associated with alcohol-related birth outcomes could help identify high-risk pregnancies requiring intervention.

One of the biggest challenges in determining the true prevalence of FASD is how to recognize the syndrome, which depends in part on the age and physical features of the person being assessed. Difficulty identifying alcohol abuse results from the client's denial of alcohol use, unwillingness to report alcohol consumption, underreporting, and limited ability to recollect the frequency, quantity, and type of alcohol consumed. This makes it difficult to identify women who are drinking during pregnancy, institute preventive measures, or refer them for treatment.

Women who drink excessively while pregnant are at high risk for giving birth to children with birth defects. To prevent these defects, women should stop drinking during all phases of a pregnancy. Unfortunately, many women continue to drink during their pregnancy despite warnings from professionals.

Currently, it is not known whether there is a minimal amount of alcohol safe to drink during pregnancy; an occasional glass of wine might be harmless or might not be. Therefore, eliminating alcohol consumption during pregnancy is the ultimate goal to prevent FASD. Most women know they should not drink during pregnancy, but the window of vulnerability—i.e., the time lag between conception and the discovery of pregnancy—may put substantial numbers of children at risk. Additionally, traditional alcohol-screening questionnaires, such as the Michigan Alcoholism Screening Test (MAST) and the CAGE Questionnaire, are not sensitive enough to detect low levels of alcohol consumption among women.

Several challenges remain in preventing birth defects due to alcohol consumption:

- Ways to improve clinical recognition of high-risk women who drink alcohol
- Ways to intervene more effectively to modify drinking behaviors
- In utero approaches to prevent or minimize fetal injury
- Strategies to address the neurodevelopmental problems of children affected by maternal alcohol ingestion

Sedatives. Sedatives relax the central nervous system and are used medically for inducing relaxation and sleep, relieving tension, and treating seizures. Sedatives easily cross the placenta and can cause birth defects and behavioral problems. Infants born to mothers who abuse sedatives during pregnancy may be physically dependent on the drugs themselves and are more prone to respiratory problems, feeding difficulties, disturbed sleep, sweating, irritability, and fever (Alexander et al., 2014).

Nicotine. Cigarette smoking during pregnancy is the biggest preventable cause of death and illness in women and infants and is associated with numerous obstetric, fetal, and developmental complications, as well as an increased risk of adverse health consequences in the adult offspring. Nicotine replacement therapy has been developed as a pharmacotherapy for smoking cessation and is considered to be a safer alternative for women to smoking during pregnancy. The safety of nicotine replacement therapy (transdermal patches and bupropion) use during pregnancy has been evaluated in a limited number of short-term human trials, but there is currently no information on the long-term effects of developmental nicotine exposure in humans (Dhalwani et al., 2015).

Nicotine is found in cigarettes, and is another substance that is harmful to the pregnant women and her fetus. Nicotine, which causes vasoconstriction, transfers across the placenta and reduces blood flow to the fetus, contributing to fetal hypoxia. When compared with alcohol, marijuana, and other illicit drug use, tobacco use is less likely to decline as the pregnancy progresses (Velez & Jansson, 2015). Smoking is associated with adverse pregnancy outcomes. However, these adverse outcomes can be avoided if the woman stops smoking before becoming pregnant.

Smoking increases the risk of spontaneous abortion, tubal ectopic pregnancy, preterm labor and birth, fetal growth restriction, stillbirth, premature rupture of membranes, low fetal iron stores, maternal hypertension, placenta previa, and abruptio placentae. The perinatal death rate among infants of smoking mothers is 20% to 35% higher than that of nonsmoking mothers (Varner et al., 2014). Perinatal and childhood risks associated with mothers smoking during their pregnancies include increased risk of cleft lip and palate, clubfoot, asthma, middle ear infections, SIDS, reduced head circumference, altered brainstem development, and cerebral palsy (Cunningham et al., 2014).

Smoking has also been considered an important risk factor for low birth weight, SIDS, and cognitive deficits, especially in language, reading, and vocabulary, as well as poorer performances on tests of reasoning and memory. Researchers have also reported behavior problems, such as increased activity, inattention, impulsivity, opposition, and aggression (Skoglund et al., 2014). Women who smoke during the pregnancy often continue to smoke after giving birth, and thus the infant will be exposed to nicotine after birth. This environmental or passive exposure affects the child's development and increases the risk of childhood respiratory disorders.

Caffeine. Caffeine is a widely used and accepted pharmacologically active substance. The socially sanctioned nature of caffeinated beverages promotes caffeine's popularity and at the same time obscures the fact that as a drug it can definitely be abused. The effect of caffeine intake during pregnancy on fetal growth and development is still unclear. A recent study found that caffeine intake of no more than 300 mg/day during pregnancy does not affect pregnancy duration and the condition of the newborn (Procter & Campbell, 2014). Caffeine, a stimulant of the central nervous system, is present in varying amounts in common products such as coffee, tea, colas, and chocolate. It is also in cold remedies and analgesics. Birth defects have not been linked to caffeine consumption, but maternal coffee consumption decreases iron absorption and may increase the risk of anemia during pregnancy.

Moderate caffeine consumption (less than 300 mg/day) does not appear to be a major contributing factor in miscarriage or preterm birth. The relationship of caffeine to growth restriction remains undetermined. A final conclusion cannot be made at this time as to whether there is a correlation between high caffeine intake and miscarriage, due to lack of sufficient studies (Calhoun & Lewis, 2016).

Energy drinks represent a new class of caffeinated beverages that are marketed to improve energy, athletic performance, concentration, endurance, and weight loss, although the claims have not been supported by rigorous scientific evidence (Higgins, Yarlagadda, & Yang, 2015). All energy drinks surpass the FDA official soft drink concentration of caffeine limit, typically 2 to 4 times the amount seen in one serving of soda or tea. Adverse effects of energy drinks can occur in healthy people; however, pregnant women would be considered in an at-risk group and should avoid excessive caffeine intake which has been linked to adverse reproductive outcomes, such as low birth weight. Consumption of energy drinks is associated with increased demand of the heart causing hypertension, tachycardia, dysrhythmias, coronary artery spasm, and sudden cardiac death (James, 2015). Given the rise in emergency room visits for complications of energy drink consumption, nurses should advise their pregnant clients to refrain from drinking them.

Marijuana. Marijuana is the most commonly used illicit drug in America, with over 90 million people having tried it at least once. Its estimated prevalence in pregnant women is about 10% to 15%. It is often called pot, reefer, herb, widow, hash, grass, weed, Mary Jane, or MJ (NIDA, 2015c). Marijuana is a preparation of the leaves and flowering tops of *Cannabis sativa*, the hemp plant, which contains a number of pharmacologically active agents. Tetrahydrocannabinol (THC) is the most active ingredient of marijuana. With heavy smoking, THC narrows the bronchi and bronchioles and produces inflammation of the mucous membranes. Smoking marijuana causes tachycardia and a reduction in blood pressure, resulting in orthostatic hypotension. Although the federal government considers marijuana a schedule I substance (having no medicinal uses and high risk for abuse), a few states have legalized it for adult recreational use, and many states have passed laws allowing its use as a treatment for medical conditions (pain, nausea and vomiting, HIV/AIDS, cancer).

The effects of marijuana smoking on pregnancy are not yet fully understood because there are very few studies on its long-term effects on child development. One can speculate that the effects of marijuana on the immature nervous system may be subtle and not detected until more complex functions are required, usually in a formal educational setting. There is some evidence that marijuana increases the risk of spontaneous abortion and preterm delivery (Desai, Mark, & Terplan, 2014). Although marijuana is not considered teratogenic, many newborns display altered responses to visual stimuli, increased tremulousness, and a high-pitched cry, which might indicate insults against the central nervous system (Volkow et al., 2014). A strong correlation exists between the use of marijuana and the use of alcohol and cigarettes.

Opiates and Narcotics. Opiates and narcotics include opium, heroin (known as horse, junk, smack, downtown), morphine, codeine, hydromorphone (Dilaudid; little D), oxycodone (Percodan, perkies), meperidine (Demerol, demise), and methadone (meth, dollies). Opiates can be inhaled, injected, snorted, ingested, or used subcutaneously. These drugs are central nervous system depressants that soothe and lull. They may be used medically for pain, but all have a high potential for abuse. Most cause an intense addiction in both the mother and newborn.

Narcotic dependence is particularly problematic in pregnant women. It leads to medical, nutritional, and social neglect by the woman due to the long-term risks of physical dependence, malnutrition, compromised immunity, hepatitis, and fatal overdose (Alexander et al., 2014). Taking opiates or narcotics during pregnancy places the woman at increased risk for preterm labor, fetal growth restriction, abruptio placenta, perinatal mortality, preterm rupture of membranes, and preeclampsia (Prasad, 2014).

Heroin is the most common illicitly used opioid. It is derived from the seeds of the poppy plant and can be sniffed, smoked, or injected. It crosses the placenta via simple diffusion within 1 hour of maternal consumption (ACOG, 2014e). Use of heroin during pregnancy is believed to affect the developing brain of the fetus and may cause behavioral abnormalities in childhood. Risks of perinatal opiate exposure are not limited to the fetus. Maternal opiate overdose deaths have increased dramatically, which translates to 18 women dying per day, and for every woman who dies, 30 are being treated in emergency departments for abuse (Alexander et al., 2014).

The most common harmful effect of heroin and other narcotics on newborns is withdrawal, or **neonatal abstinence syndrome** (see Chapter 24). This collection of symptoms may include irritability, hypertonicity, jitteriness, fever, excessive and often high-pitched cry, vomiting, diarrhea, feeding disturbances, respiratory distress, disturbed sleeping, excessive sneezing and yawning, nasal stuffiness, diaphoresis, fever, poor sucking, tremors, and seizures (Slater, 2015).

Withdrawal from opiates during pregnancy is extremely dangerous for the fetus, so a prescribed oral methadone maintenance program combined with psychotherapy is recommended for the pregnant woman. This closely supervised treatment program reduces withdrawal symptoms in the newborn, reduces drug cravings, and blocks the euphoric effects of narcotic drugs in order to reduce illicit drug use. Management of opioid addiction in pregnancy includes maintenance therapy with methadone or buprenorphine in addition to traditional prenatal care and psychosocial treatment of substance abuse, such as self-help, 12-step groups, individual and group substance abuse counseling, and psychotherapy. Maintenance therapy drugs provide a steady state of opiate levels, thus reducing the risk of withdrawal to the fetus and exposure to HIV and other STIs because the mother is no longer injecting drugs. However, maintenance therapy drugs have the same withdrawal consequences for women and newborns as heroin does (McKeever, Spaeth-Brayton, & Sheerin, 2014).

Methamphetamines. Methamphetamine use is now more common than cocaine use in pregnancy, and its use by women of childbearing age is increasing in the United States. This highly addictive stimulant is commonly known as speed, meth, or chalk. In its smoked form, it is often referred to as ice, crystal, crank, and glass. Smoking or injecting the drug quickly delivers it to the brain for an immediate, intense euphoria. Because the pleasure also fades quickly, users often take repeated doses, in a "binge and crash" pattern. It is a white, odorless, bitter-tasting powder that was developed from its parent drug, amphetamine, and was used originally in nasal decongestants and bronchial inhalers. The maternal effects include increased energy and alertness, an intense rush, decreased appetite, tachycardia, and tachypnea. Chronic use can lead to psychosis, including paranoia, hallucinations, memory loss, and aggressive or violent behavior. Signs of methamphetamine use include track marks from intravenous injection, malnutrition, severe dental decay (meth mouth), and skin abscesses from skin picking (ACOG, 2014f). Few studies have been done on the effects of methamphetamine abuse during pregnancy, but the few done indicate an increased risk for preterm births, low birth weight, placental abruption, fetal growth restriction, and congenital anomalies (NIDA, 2015d). These findings are hard to interpret, however, due to small sample size and polydrug use of the participants.

Cocaine. Cocaine use is second only to marijuana use in women who abuse drugs during pregnancy. The incidence of cocaine exposure in utero is approximately 1 to 10 per 1,000 live births (Brandt et al., 2014). There is evidence that cocaine affects infant development both directly, via in utero exposure, and indirectly, via alterations in maternal care after birth.

Cocaine is a psychoactive drug derived from the leaves of the coca plant, which grows in the Andes Mountains of Peru, Ecuador, and Bolivia. The freebase form, called "crack" because of the cracking or popping noise made in its preparation, is less expensive, easily made, and smokable. Cocaine is a powerful vasoconstrictor. When sniffed into the mucous membranes of the nose, it produces an intense "rush" that some have compared to an orgasmic experience. Smoked crack is absorbed rapidly by the pulmonary vasculature and reaches the brain's circulation in 6 to 8 seconds (NIDA, 2015b).

Cocaine use produces vasoconstriction, dilates pupils, increases body temperature, tachycardia, and hypertension in both the mother and fetus (Kahn, Mikhael, & Vadivelu, 2015). Uteroplacental insufficiency may result from reduced blood flow and placental perfusion. Chronic use can result in low birth weight, the most common effect of cocaine use in pregnancy (NIDA, 2015b).

Studies suggest that perinatal cocaine use increases the risk of preterm labor, abortion, abruptio placentae, fetal growth restriction, intrauterine fetal distress and demise, seizures, withdrawal, and cerebral infarcts. Cocaine may increase the risk of uterine rupture and congenital anomalies (NIDA, 2015b). Fetal anomalies associated with cocaine use in early pregnancy involve neurologic problems such as neural tube defects and microcephaly; cardiovascular anomalies such as congenital heart defects; genitourinary conditions such as prune belly syndrome, hydronephrosis, and ambiguous genitalia; and gastrointestinal system problems such as necrotizing enterocolitis (Connery, 2014). Some infants exposed to cocaine in utero show increased irritability and are difficult to calm and soothe to sleep.

Nonmedical Use of Prescription Drugs. In addition to alcohol and illicit drug use, a new worldwide trend has emerged and may soon exceed illicit drug use; that is, the nonmedical use of prescription drugs found in many home medicine cabinets. Prescription drug abuse has reached epidemic levels in the United States. Estimates of prescription drug abuse rates during pregnancy range from 5% to 20%. Common drugs of choice include analgesics, stimulants, sedatives, and tranquilizers. A frequent belief among abusers is that prescribed medications are less dangerous than street drugs and using a friend's medication is safe. Unfortunately, unintentional poisoning deaths occur frequently. In addition, the development of a counterfeit market has developed utilizing the Internet, thereby creating a global counterfeit drug market (McHugh, Nielsen, & Weiss, 2015).

Early detection through a comprehensive evaluation is essential to improve overall treatment outcomes. New research supports screening all pregnant women for substance abuse. A major role of the nurse is to focus on prevention by educating all women about the dangers associated with misuse of prescription medications. Community education is vital to manage risks to prevent problems from developing.

Nursing Assessment

Complete a thorough history and physical examination to evaluate a client for substance use and abuse. Substance abuse screening in pregnancy is done to detect the use of any substance known or suspected to exert a deleterious effect on the client or her fetus. Routinely ask about substance abuse with all women of childbearing age, inform them of the risks involved, and advise them against continuing. Screening questionnaires are helpful in identifying potential users, may reduce the stigma of asking clients about substance abuse, and may result in a more accurate and consistent evaluation. The questions in Box 20.5 may be helpful in assessing a client who is at risk for substance abuse during pregnancy. Using "accepting" terminology may encourage the woman to give honest answers without fear of reproach.

A woman who claims to have taken no drugs while pregnant may be unaware that substances such as hair dye, diet cola, paint, or over-the-counter medications for colds or headaches are still considered drugs. Thus, it is very difficult to get a true picture of the real use of drugs by pregnant women.

Many drugs are considered to have a teratogenic effect on growing fetuses. A teratogen is any environmental substance that can cause physical defects in the

BOX 20.5

SAMPLE QUESTIONS FOR ASSESSING SUBSTANCE USE

- Have you ever used recreational drugs? If so, when and what?
- Have you ever taken a prescription drug other than as intended?
- What are your feelings about drug use during pregnancy?
- How often do you smoke cigarettes? How many per day?
- How often do you drink alcohol?
- Have you ever felt guilty about drinking or drug use?

If the assessment reveals substance use, obtain additional information by using the RAFFT questionnaire, which is a sensitive screening instrument for identifying substance abuse (Weekes & Lee, 2014):

R: Do you drink or take drugs to **R**elax, improve your self-image, or fit in?
A: Do you ever drink or take drugs while **A**lone?
F: Do you have any close **F**riends who drink or take drugs?
F: Does a close **F**amily member have a problem with alcohol or drugs?
T: Have you ever gotten in **T**rouble from drinking or taking drugs?

developing embryo and fetus. Pregnant women with substance abuse commonly present with polysubstance abuse, which is likely to be more damaging than the use of any single substance. Thus, it is inherently difficult to ascribe a specific perinatal effect to any one substance (McKeever, Spaeth-Brayton, & Sheerin, 2014).

A urine toxicology screen may also be helpful in determining drug use, although a urine screen identifies only recent or heavy use of drugs. The length of time a drug is present in urine is as follows:

- Cocaine: 24 to 48 hours in an adult, 72 to 96 hours in an infant
- Heroin: 24 hours in an adult, 24 to 48 hours in an infant
- Marijuana: 1 week to 1 month in an adult, up to a month or longer in an infant
- Methadone: up to 10 days in an infant (Wang, 2015).

Nursing Management

If the woman's drug screen is positive, use this as an opportunity to discuss prenatal exposure to substances that may be harmful. The discussion may lead the nurse to refer the client for a diagnostic assessment or identify an intervention such as counseling that may be helpful. Being nonjudgmental is a key to success; a client is more apt to trust and reveal patterns of abuse if the nurse does not judge her and her lifestyle choices.

A positive drug screen in a newborn warrants an investigation by the state protection agency. In the interim, institute measures to reduce stress and stimuli to promote the newborn's comfort (see Chapter 24 for a more in-depth discussion).

Be proactive, supportive, and accepting when caring for the client. Assure women with substance abuse problems that sharing information of a confidential nature with health care providers will not render them liable to criminal prosecution. Provide counseling and education, emphasizing the following:

- Effects of substance exposure on the fetus
- Interventions to improve mother–child attachment and improve parenting
- Psychosocial support if treatment is needed to reduce substance abuse
- Referral to outreach programs to improve access to treatment facilities
- Hazardous legal substances to avoid during pregnancy
- Follow-up of children born to substance-dependent mothers
- Dietary counseling to improve the pregnancy outcome for both mother and child
- Drug screening to identify all drugs a client is using
- More frequent prenatal visits to monitor fetal well-being
- Maternal and fetal benefits of remaining drug free
- Cultural sensitivity
- Coping skills, support systems, and vocational assistance

There is nothing categorically different about addiction in pregnancy compared with addiction in general. Pregnant women who use drugs are women who use drugs, get pregnant, and cannot stop using drugs. The fact that they are condemned in society leads to their further marginalization, which does nothing to improve their lives or the lives of their children.

Substance abuse is a complex problem that requires sensitivity to each woman's unique situation and contributing factors. Be sure to address individual psychological and sociocultural factors to help the woman regain control of her life. Nurses must be aware of these women's unique needs and the related legal and ethical ramifications surrounding pregnancy. Treatment must combine different approaches and provide ongoing support for women learning to live drug free. Developing personal strengths, such as communication skills, assertiveness, and self-confidence, will help the woman to resist drug use. Encourage the use of appropriate coping skills. Enhancing self-esteem also helps provide a foundation to avoid drugs. Through therapeutic communication, nursing interventions, clinical assessment, and building trusting relationships, nurses can have a significant impact in managing clients with substance abuse.

NURSING CARE PLAN 20.1

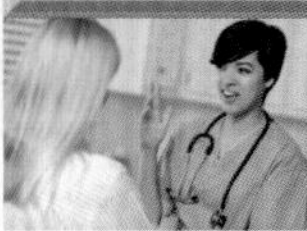

Overview of the Pregnant Woman with Type 1 Diabetes

Donna, a 30-year-old woman with type 1 diabetes, presents to the maternity clinic for preconception care. She has had diabetes for 8 years and takes insulin twice daily by injection. She does blood glucose self-monitoring four times daily. She reports that her disease is fairly well controlled, but "I'm worried about how my diabetes will affect a pregnancy and my baby. Will I need to make changes in my routine? Will my baby be normal?" She reports that she recently had a foot infection and needed to go to the emergency department because it led to an episode of ketoacidosis. She states that her last glycosylated hemoglobin A1c test results were abnormal.

NURSING DIAGNOSIS: Ineffective health maintenance: related to deficient knowledge regarding care in diabetic condition in pregnancy as evidenced by questions about effect on pregnancy, possible changes in regimen, and pregnancy outcome

Outcome Identification and Evaluation

The client will demonstrate increased knowledge of type 1 diabetes and effects on pregnancy as evidenced by proper techniques for blood glucose monitoring and insulin administration, ability to modify insulin doses and dietary intake to achieve control, and verbalization of need for glycemic control prior to pregnancy, with blood glucose levels remaining within normal range.

Interventions: *Providing Client Teaching*

- Assess client's knowledge of diabetes and pregnancy *to establish a baseline from which to develop an individualized teaching plan.*
- Review the underlying problems associated with diabetes and how pregnancy affects glucose control *to provide client with a firm knowledge base for decision-making.*
- Review signs and symptoms of hypoglycemia and hyperglycemia and prevention and management measures *to ensure client can deal with them should they occur.*
- Provide written materials describing diabetes and care needed for control *to provide opportunity for client's review and promote retention of learning.*
- Observe client administering insulin and self-glucose testing for technique and offer suggestions for improvement if needed *to ensure adequate self-care ability.*
- Discuss proper foot care to prevent future infections.
- Teach home treatment for symptomatic hypoglycemia to minimize risk to client and fetus.
- Outline acute and chronic diabetic complications to reinforce the importance of glucose control.
- Discuss use of contraceptives until blood glucose levels can be optimized before conception occurs *to promote the best possible health status before conception.*
- Explain the rationale for good glucose control and the importance of achieving excellent glycemic control before pregnancy to promote a positive pregnancy outcome.
- Review self-care practices (blood glucose monitoring and frequency of testing; insulin administration; adjustment of insulin dosages based on blood glucose levels) to foster independence in self-care and feelings of control over the situation.
- Refer client for dietary counseling to ensure optimal diet for glycemic control.
- Outline obstetric management and fetal surveillance needed for pregnancy to provide client with information on what to expect.
- Discuss strategies for maintaining optimal glycemic control during pregnancy to minimize risks to client and fetus.

(continued)

NURSING CARE PLAN 20.1

Overview of the Pregnant Woman with Type 1 Diabetes (continued)

NURSING DIAGNOSIS: Anxiety related to threat to self and fetus as evidenced by questions about her condition's effect on the baby and baby being normal

Outcome Identification and Evaluation

The client will openly express her feelings related to her diabetes and pregnancy as evidenced by statements of feeling better about her preexisting condition and pregnancy outlook, and statements of understanding related to future childbearing by linking good glucose control with positive outcomes for both herself and offspring.

Interventions: ***Minimizing Anxiety***

- Review the need for a physical examination to evaluate for any effects of diabetes on the client's health status.
- Explain the rationale for assessing client's blood pressure, vision, and peripheral pulses at each visit to provide information related to possible effects of diabetes on health status.
- Identify any alterations in present diabetic condition that need intervention to aid in minimizing risks that may increase client's anxiety level.
- Review potential effects of diabetes on pregnancy to promote client understanding of risks and ways to control or minimize them.
- Encourage active participation in decision-making and planning pregnancy to promote feelings of control over the situation and foster self-confidence.
- Discuss feelings about future childbearing and managing pregnancy to help reduce anxiety related to uncertainties.
- Encourage client to ask questions or voice concerns to help decrease anxiety related to the unknown.
- Emphasize the use of frequent and continued surveillance of client and fetal status during pregnancy to reduce the risk of complications and aid in alleviating anxieties related to the unknown.
- Provide positive reinforcement for healthy behaviors and actions to foster continued use and enhancement of self-esteem.

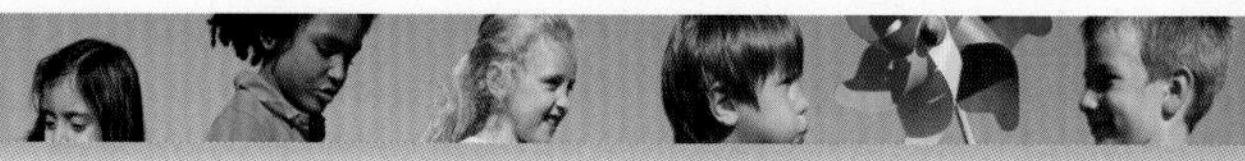

KEY CONCEPTS

- Preconception counseling for the woman with diabetes is helpful in promoting blood glucose control to prevent congenital anomalies.
- The classification system for diabetes is based on disease etiology and not pharmacology management; the classification includes type 1 diabetes, type 2 diabetes, gestational diabetes, and impaired fasting glucose and impaired glucose tolerance.
- A functional classification for heart disease during pregnancy is based on past and present disability: class I, asymptomatic with no limitation of physical activity; class II, symptomatic (dyspnea, chest pain) with increased activity; class III, symptomatic (fatigue, palpitation) with normal activity; and class IV, symptomatic at rest or with any physical activity.
- Chronic hypertension exists when the woman has a blood pressure of 140/90 mm Hg or higher before pregnancy or before the 20th week of gestation or when hypertension persists for more than 12 weeks' postpartum.
- Successful management of asthma in pregnancy involves elimination of environmental triggers, drug therapy, and client education.

- Ideally, women with hematologic conditions are screened before conception and are made aware of the risks to themselves and to a pregnancy.
- A wide variety of infections, such as cytomegalovirus, rubella, herpes simplex, hepatitis B, varicella, parvovirus B19, and many sexually transmitted infections can affect a pregnancy, having a negative impact on its outcome.
- The prevalence of HIV/AIDS is increasing more rapidly among women than men: half of all the HIV/AIDS cases worldwide now occur in women. There are only three recognized modes of HIV transmission: unprotected sexual intercourse with an infected partner, contact with infected blood or blood products, and perinatal transmission. Breastfeeding is a major contributing factor in mother-to-child transmission of HIV.
- Cases of perinatal AIDS have decreased in the past several years in the United States, primarily because of the use of zidovudine (ZDV) therapy in pregnant women with HIV. The U.S. Preventive Services Task Force recommends that all pregnant women should be offered HIV antibody testing regardless of their risk of infection, and that testing should be done during the initial prenatal evaluation.
- The younger an adolescent is at the time of her first pregnancy, the more likely it is that she will have another pregnancy during her teens. About 1 million teenagers between the ages of 15 and 19 become pregnant each year; about half give birth and keep their infants.
- The nurse's role in caring for the pregnant adolescent is to assist her in identifying the options for this pregnancy, including abortion, self-parenting of the child, temporary foster care for the baby or herself, or placement for adoption.
- Pregnant women with substance abuse problems commonly abuse several substances, making it difficult to ascribe a specific perinatal effect to any one substance. Societal attitudes regarding pregnant women and substance abuse may prohibit them from admitting the problem and seeking treatment.
- Substance abuse during pregnancy is associated with preterm labor, abortion, low birth weight, central nervous system and fetal anomalies, and long-term childhood developmental consequences.
- Fetal alcohol spectrum disorder is a lifelong yet completely preventable set of physical, mental, and neurobehavioral birth defects; it is the leading cause of intellectual disability in the United States.
- Nursing management for the woman with substance abuse focuses on screening and preventing substance abuse to reduce the high incidence of obstetric and medical complications as well as the morbidity and mortality among passively addicted newborns.

REFERENCES AND RECOMMENDED READINGS

Agent, O. E. (2015). 19 Classic viral exanthems. In D. Schlossberg (Ed.), *Clinical infectious disease* (2nd ed., Chapter 19). Cambridge, MA: Cambridge University Press.

Aktas, G., Alcelik, A., Ozlu, T., Tosun, M., Tekce, B. K., Savli, H., et al. (2014). Association between omentin levels and insulin resistance in pregnancy. *Experimental and Clinical Endocrinology & Diabetes, 122*(03), 163–166.

Alan Guttmacher Institute. (2015a). *Facts on American teens' sexual and reproductive health*. Retrieved from http://www.guttmacher.org/pubs/FB-ATSRH.html

Alan Guttmacher Institute. (2015b). *Pregnancy fact sheets*. Retrieved from http://www.guttmacher.org/in-the-know/pregnancy.html

Alexander, L. L., LaRosa, J. H., Bader, H., & Garfield, S. (2014). *New dimensions in women's health* (6th ed.). Sudbury, MA: Jones & Bartlett.

Alonso-Gonzalez, R., & Swan, L. (2014). Treating cardiac disease in pregnancy. *Women's Health, 10*(1), 79–90.

American Academy of Allergy, Asthma & Immunology [AAAAI]. (2015). *Asthma and pregnancy*. Retrieved from http://www.aaaai.org/conditions-and-treatments/library/asthma-library/asthma-and-pregnancy.aspx

American Academy of Pediatrics. (2014). Adolescent pregnancy: Current trends and issues. *AAP News, 35*(5), 19–25.

American Academy of Pediatrics [AAP]. (2015). *Serious illnesses and breastfeeding*. Retrieved from https://healthychildren.org/English/ages-stages/baby/breastfeeding/Pages/Serious-Illnesses-and-Breastfeeding.aspx

American College of Obstetricians & Gynecologists [ACOG]. (2013). Executive summary: Hypertension in pregnancy. *Obstetrics & Gynecology, 122*, 1122–1131.

American College of Obstetricians & Gynecologists [ACOG]. (2014a). ACOG guidelines at a glance: Gestational diabetes mellitus. *Contemporary OB/GYN*. Retrieved from http://contemporaryobgyn.modernmedicine.com/contemporary-obgyn/news/acog-guidelines-glance-gestational-diabetes-mellitus?page=full

American College of Obstetricians & Gynecologists [ACOG]. (2014b). Obesity in pregnancy. *Obstetrics & Gynecology, 121*, 213–217.

American College of Obstetricians & Gynecologists [ACOG]. (2014c). *Fetal alcohol spectrum disorders prevention handbook*. Retrieved from http://www.acog.org/About-ACOG/ACOG-Districts/District-II/Fetal-Alcohol-Spectrum-Disorders-Prevention-Handbook

American College of Obstetricians & Gynecologists [ACOG]. (2014d). *Tobacco, alcohol, drugs, and pregnancy*. Retrieved from http://www.acog.org/Patients/FAQs/Tobacco-Alcohol-Drugs-and-Pregnancy

American College of Obstetricians & Gynecologists [ACOG]. (2014e). *Opioid abuse, dependence, and addiction in pregnancy*. Retrieved from http://www.acog.org/Resources-And-Publications/Committee-Opinions/Committee-on-Health-Care-for-Underserved-Women/Opioid-Abuse-Dependence-and-Addiction-in-Pregnancy

American College of Obstetricians & Gynecologists [ACOG]. (2014f). *Methamphetamine abuse in women of reproductive age*. Retrieved from http://www.acog.org/Resources-And-Publications/Committee-Opinions/Committee-on-Health-Care-for-Underserved-Women/Methamphetamine-Abuse-in-Women-of-Reproductive-Age

American College of Rheumatology. (2015). *Prevalence statistics*. Retrieved from http://www.rheumatology.org/Research/Prevalence_Statistics/

American Diabetes Association [ADA]. (2015a). *Diabetes basics*. Retrieved from http://www.diabetes.org/diabetes-basics/

American Diabetes Association [ADA]. (2015b). *What is gestational diabetes?* Retrieved from http://www.diabetes.org/diabetes-basics/gestational/what-is-gestational-diabetes.html

American Diabetes Association [ADA]. (2015c). *How to treat gestational diabetes*. Retrieved from http://www.diabetes.org/diabetes-basics/gestational/how-to-treat-gestational.html

American Diabetes Association [ADA]. (2015d). Living with diabetes: After delivery. Retrieved from http://www.diabetes.org/living-with-diabetes/

American Heart Association [AHA]. (2015). *Women and heart disease*. Retrieved from https://www.goredforwomen.org/about-heart-disease/facts_about_heart_disease_in_women-sub-category/statistics-at-a-glance/

Anderson, B., & Cu-Uvin, S. (2015). HIV and pregnancy (beyond the basics). *UpToDate*. Retrieved from http://www.uptodate.com/contents/hiv-and-pregnancy-beyond-the-basics

Armon, C., Baquis, G. D., Howard, G. F., & Krupa, M. J. (2015). Neurologic disease and pregnancy. *eMedicine*. Retrieved from http://emedicine.medscape.com/article/1149405-overview#a7

Bain, E., Crane, M., Tieu, J., Han, S., Crowther, C. A., & Middleton, P. (2015). Diet and exercise interventions for preventing gestational diabetes mellitus. *Cochrane Database of Systematic Reviews 2015*, Issue 4. Art. No.: CD010443.

Bartels, C. M., & Muller, D. (2015). Systemic lupus erythematosus. *eMedicine*. Retrieved from http://emedicine.medscape.com/article/332244-overview

Bates, M., Ahmed, Y., Kapata, N., Maeurer, M., Mwaba, P., & Zumla, A. (2015). Perspectives on tuberculosis in pregnancy. *International Journal of Infectious Diseases*, *32*, 124–127.

Bialas, K. M., Swamy, G. K., & Permar, S. R. (2015). Perinatal cytomegalovirus and varicella zoster virus infections: Epidemiology, prevention, and treatment. *Clinics in Perinatology*, *42*(1), 61–75.

Brandt, L., Leifheit, A. K., Finnegan, L. P., & Fischer, G. (2014). Management of substance abuse in pregnancy: Maternal and neonatal aspects. In M. Galbally, M. Snellen, & A. Lewis (Eds.), *Psychopharmacology and pregnancy* (pp. 169–195). Berlin: Springer Publishers.

Brickner, M. E. (2014). Cardiovascular management in pregnancy congenital heart disease. *Circulation*, *130*(3), 273–282.

Brucker, M. C., & King, T. L. (2017). *Pharmacology for women's health* (2nd ed.). Burlington, MA: Jones & Bartlett Learning.

Buschur, E., Brown, F., & Wyckoff, J. (2015). Using oral agents to manage gestational diabetes: What have we learned? *Current Diabetes Reports*, *15*(2), 1–8.

Calvert, C., & Ronsmans, C. (2015). Pregnancy and HIV disease progression: A systematic review and meta-analysis. *Tropical Medicine & International Health*, *20*, 122–145.

Camaschella, C. (2015). Iron-deficiency anemia. *New England Journal of Medicine*, *372*(19), 1832–1843.

Cantor, A. G., Bougatsos, C., Dana, T., Blazina, I., & McDonagh, M. (2015). Routine iron supplementation and screening for iron deficiency anemia in pregnancy: A systematic review for the US Preventive Services Task Force. *Annals of Internal Medicine*, *162*(8), 566–576.

Cennimo, D. J., & Dieudonne, A. (2015). Parvovirus B19 infection. *eMedicine*. Retrieved from http://emedicine.medscape.com/article/961063-overview

Centers for Disease Control and Prevention [CDC]. (2015a). *Teen pregnancy in the United States*. Retrieved from http://www.cdc.gov/teenpregnancy/aboutteenpreg.htm

Centers for Disease Control and Prevention [CDC]. (2015b). *Tuberculosis and pregnancy*. Retrieved from http://www.cdc.gov/tb/publications/factsheets/specpop/pregnancy.htm

Centers for Disease Control and Prevention [CDC]. (2015c). *Fact sheet: Sickle cell disease*. Retrieved from http://www.cdc.gov/ncbddd/sicklecell/documents/scd-factsheet_what-is-scd.pdf

Centers for Disease Control and Prevention [CDC]. (2015d). *Women and autoimmune diseases*. Retrieved from http://wwwnc.cdc.gov/eid/article/10/11/14-0367_article

Centers for Disease Control and Prevention [CDC]. (2015e). *Cytomegalovirus and pregnant women*. Retrieved from http://www.cdc.gov/cmv/risk/preg-women.html

Centers for Disease Control and Prevention [CDC]. (2015f). *Genital herpes – CDC fact sheet*. Retrieved from http://www.cdc.gov/std/herpes/stdfact-herpes.htm

Centers for Disease Control and Prevention [CDC]. (2015g). *Hepatitis B information for health professionals: Perinatal transmission*. Retrieved from http://www.cdc.gov/hepatitis/HBV/PerinatalXmtn.htm

Centers for Disease Control and Prevention [CDC]. (2015h). *Fetal alcohol spectrum disorders*. Retrieved from http://www.cdc.gov/ncbddd/fasd/alcohol-use.html

Centers for Disease Control and Prevention [CDC]. (2015i). *Group B strep (GBS)*. Retrieved from http://www.cdc.gov/groupbstrep/about/fast-facts.html

Centers for Disease Control and prevention [CDC]. (2015j). *HIV in the United States: At a glance*. Retrieved from http://www.cdc.gov/hiv/statistics/basics/ataglance.html

Centers for Disease Control and Prevention [CDC]. (2015k). *HIV among women*. Retrieved from http://www.cdc.gov/hiv/risk/gender/women/facts/index.html

Centers for Disease Control and Prevention [CDC]. (2015l). *HIV transmission*. Retrieved from http://www.cdc.gov/hiv/basics/transmission.html

Centers for Disease Control and Prevention [CDC]. (2015m). *HIV among pregnant women, infants, and children*. Retrieved from http://www.cdc.gov/hiv/risk/gender/pregnantwomen/facts/

Centers for Disease Control and Prevention [CDC]. (2015n). *Child development: Teenagers (15–17 years old)*. Retrieved from http://www.cdc.gov/ncbddd/childdevelopment/positiveparenting/adolescence2.html

Centers for Disease Control and Prevention [CDC]. (2015o). *Health care providers and teen pregnancy prevention*. Retrieved from http://www.cdc.gov/teenpregnancy/health-careproviders.htm

Centers for Disease Control and Prevention [CDC]. (2015p). *Pregnancy complications: Obesity*. Retrieved from http://www.cdc.gov/reproductivehealth/maternalinfanthealth/pregcomplications.htm#n5

Centers for Disease Control and Prevention [CDC]. (2015q). *Illegal drug use*. Retrieved from http://www.cdc.gov/nchs/fastats/drug-use-illegal.htm

Centers for Disease Control and Prevention [CDC] (2015r). *Sexually transmitted diseases*. Retrieved from http://www.cdc.gov/std/

Centers of Disease Control and Prevention [CDC]. (2015s). *About HIV/AIDS*. Retrieved from http://www.cdc.gov/hiv/basics/whatishiv.html

Chang, M. W., Brown, R., Nitzke, S., Smith, B., & Eghtedary, K. (2015). Stress, sleep, depression and dietary intakes among low-income overweight and obese pregnant women. *Maternal and Child Health Journal*, *19*(5), 1047–1059.

Charlier, C., Le Mercier, D., Salomon, L. J., Ville, Y., Kermorvant-Duchemin, E., Frange, P., et al. (2014). Varicella-zoster virus and pregnancy. *Presse Medicale*, *43*(6), 665–675.

Cherry A. L., & Dillon, M. E. (Eds.). (2014). Adolescent pregnancy and mental health. *International handbook of adolescent pregnancy* (pp. 79–102). New York, NY: Springer Publishers.

Chomistek, A. K., Chiuve, S. E., & Eliassen, A. H. (2015). Healthy lifestyle in young women greatly reduces CHD and development of CVD risk factors. *Journal of American College of Cardiology*, *65*(1), 43–51.

Choreño-Machain, T. C., Barrios, J., & Reta, E. B. (2015). Congenital and acquired heart disease in pregnancy. *Journal of the American College of Cardiology*, *65*(10_S). doi:10.1016/S0735-1097(15)60548-4.

Connery, H. S. (2014). *Substance abuse during pregnancy, an issue of Obstetrics and Gynecology Clinics*, *41*(2). Philadelphia, PA: Elsevier Health Sciences.

Contag, S. A., & Arrabal, P. P. (2015). Hepatitis in pregnancy. *eMedicine*. Retrieved from http://emedicine.medscape.com/article/1562368-overview#a1

Cornell, S. (2015). Continual evolution of type 2 diabetes: An update on pathophysiology and emerging treatment options. *Therapeutics and Clinical Risk Management*, *11*, 621–632.

Costa, V. M., Viana, M. B., & Aguiar, R. A. (2015). Pregnancy in patients with sickle cell disease: Maternal and perinatal outcomes. *The Journal of Maternal-Fetal & Neonatal Medicine*, *28*(6), 685–689.

Crockett, L. J., & Crouter, A. C. (Eds.). (2014). *Pathways through adolescence: Individual development in relation to social contexts*. New York, NY: Psychology Press.

Cunningham, F. G., Leveno, K. J., Bloom, S.L., Spong, C., & Dashe, J. (2014). *Williams' obstetrics* (24th ed.). New York, NY: McGraw-Hill Professional Publishing.

Desai, A., Mark, K., & Terplan, M. (2014). Marijuana use and pregnancy: Prevalence, associated behaviors, and birth outcomes. *Obstetrics and Gynecology*, *123*, 46S.

Desai, K. N., & Brustman, L. E. (2014). Parvovirus in pregnancy. *Postgraduate Obstetrics & Gynecology*, *34*(8), 1–5.

Dhalwani, N. N., Szatkowski, L., Coleman, T., Fiaschi, L., & Tata, L. J. (2015). Nicotine replacement therapy in pregnancy and major congenital anomalies in offspring. *Pediatrics*, *135*(5), 859–867.

Doulatram, G., Raj, T. D., & Govindaraj, R. (2015). Pregnancy and substance abuse. In A. D. Kaye, N. Vadivelu, & R. D. Urman (Eds.), *Substance abuse* (pp. 453–494). New York, NY: Springer Publishers.

Drake, A. L., Wagner, A., Richardson, B., & John-Stewart, G. (2014). Incident HIV during pregnancy and postpartum and risk of mother-to-child HIV transmission: A systematic review and meta-analysis. *PLoS Medicine*, *11*(2), e1001608.

Dudek, S. G. (2014). *Nutrition essentials for nursing practice* (7th ed.). Philadelphia, PA: Lippincott Williams & Wilkins.

Edwards, M. S. (2014). Adverse fetal outcomes: Expanding the role of infection. *Journal of American Medical Association*, *311*(11), 1115–1116.

Farrar, D., Duley, L., Medley, N., & Lawlor, D. A. (2015). Different strategies for diagnosing gestational diabetes to improve maternal and infant health. *Cochrane Database of Systematic Reviews*, 1, CD007122.

Fauci, A. S., Folkers, G. K., & Marston, H. D. (2014). Ending the global HIV/AIDS pandemic: The critical role of an HIV vaccine. *Clinical Infectious Diseases*, *59*(Suppl. 2), S80–S84.

Fedorowicz, A. R., Hellerstedt, W. L., Schreiner, P. J., & Bolland, J. M. (2014). Associations of adolescent hopelessness and self-worth with pregnancy attempts and pregnancy desire. *American Journal of Public Health*, *104*(8), e133–e140.

Foo, L., Tay, J., Lees, C. C., McEniery, C. M., & Wilkinson, I. B. (2015). Hypertension in pregnancy: Natural history and treatment options. *Current Hypertension Reports*, *17*(5), 1–18.

Friedman, A. J., Shander, A., Martin, S. R., Calabrese, R. K., Ashton, M. E., Lew, I., et al. (2015). Iron deficiency anemia in women: A practical guide to detection, diagnosis, and treatment. *Obstetrical & Gynecological Survey*, *70*(5), 342–353.

Gabbay-Benziv, R., Reece, E. A., Wang, F., & Yang, P. (2015). Birth defects in pregestational diabetes: Defect range, glycemic threshold and pathogenesis. *World Journal of Diabetes*, *6*(3), 481–488.

Ganchimeg, T., Ota, E., Morisaki, N., Laopaiboon, M., Lumbiganon, P., Zhang, J., et al. (2014). Pregnancy and childbirth outcomes among adolescent mothers: A World Health Organization multicountry study. *BJOG: An International Journal of Obstetrics & Gynecology*, *121*(s1), 40–48.

Gandhi, M., & Martin, S. R. (2015). Cardiac disease in pregnancy. *Obstetrics and Gynecology Clinics of North America*, *42*(2), 315–333.

Giles, M. L. (2015). HIV in pregnancy—Diagnosis, management and follow up of the neonate. *Pathology*, *47*, S49.

Calhoun, B. C., & Lewis, T. (2016). *Tobacco cessation and substance abuse treatment in women's healthcare: A clinical guide*. Switzerland: Springer International Publishing.

Gilstrap, L. G., & Wood, M. J. (2014). Cardiovascular disease in women and pregnancy. In *MGH cardiology board review* (pp. 205–223). London: Springer Publishers.

Grandy, M., Purnell, J. Q., Thornburg, K. L., & Marshall, N. E. (2015). Gestational weight gain and maternal diet composition [272]. *Obstetrics & Gynecology*, *125*, 87S–88S.

Green, C. J. (2016). *Maternal newborn nursing care plans* (3rd ed.). Burlington, MA: Jones & Bartlett Learning.

Grewal, J., Silversides, C. K., & Colman, J. M. (2014). Pregnancy in women with heart disease: Risk assessment and management of heart failure. *Heart Failure Clinics, 10*(1), 117–129.

Gupta, Y. (2015). Updated guidelines on screening for gestational diabetes. *International Journal of Women's Health, 7*, 539–550.

Hadar, E., Ashwal, E., & Hod, M. (2014). The preconceptional period as an opportunity for prediction and prevention of non-communicable disease. *Best Practice & Research Clinical Obstetrics & Gynecology, 29*(1), 54–62.

Hamdan, A. H. (2015). Neonatal abstinence syndrome. *eMedicine.* Retrieved from http://emedicine.medscape.com/article/978763-overview

Hardy, E. J., DegliEsposti, S., & Nee, J. (2015). Viral infection in pregnancy: HIV and viral hepatitis. In *Medical management of the pregnant patient* (pp. 197–216). New York, NY: Springer Publishers.

Harvey, R. E., Coffman, K. E., & Miller, V. M. (2015). Women-specific factors to consider in risk, diagnosis and treatment of cardiovascular disease. *Women's Health, 11*(2), 239–257.

Hashemi-Beni, M., Rahimi-Madiseh, M., Khosravi, A., Malekpur-Thehrani, A., Alijani, Z., & Ayazi, Z. (2015). Educational needs assessment of gestational diabetes in pregnant women for safe delivery and healthy baby birth. *Journal of Clinical Nursing and Midwifery, 4*(1), 59–67.

He, J. R., Yuan, M. Y., Chen, N. N., Lu, J. H., Hu, C. Y., Mai, W. B., et al. (2015). Maternal dietary patterns and gestational diabetes mellitus: A large prospective cohort study in China. *British Journal of Nutrition, 113*(08), 1292–1300.

Herchline, T. E. & Amorosa, J. K. (2015). Tuberculosis. *eMedicine.* Retrived from http://emedicine.medscape.com/article/230802-overview

Higgins, J. P., Yarlagadda, S., & Yang, B. (2015). Cardiovascular complications of energy drinks. *Beverages, 1*(2), 104–126.

Hilfiker-Kleiner, D., & Arany, Z. (2014). Focus on pregnancy-mediated heart and vascular disease. *Cardiovascular Research, 101*(4), 543–544.

Hokelek, M. (2015). Toxoplasmosis. *eMedicine.* Retrieved from http://emedicine.medscape.com/article/229969-overview

Institute for Alternative Futures. (2015). *Diabetes 2015 – U.S., state, and metropolitan trends.* Retrieved from http://altfutures.org/diabetes2025/

International AIDS Society. (2015). *Mass media campaigns effective for condom use and HIV knowledge.* Retrieved from http://www.iasociety.org/Default.aspx?pageId=5&elementId=15969

James, J. E. (2015). Review: Higher caffeine intake during pregnancy increases risk of low birth weight. *Evidence Based Nursing, 18*(4), 111.

James, P. A., Oparil, S., Carter, B. L., Cushman, W. C., Dennison-Himmelfarb, C., Handler, J., et al. (2014). 2014 evidence-based guideline for the management of high blood pressure in adults: Report from the panel members appointed to the Eighth Joint National Committee (JNC 8). *Journal of American Medical Association, 311*(5), 507–520.

James, S. H., & Kimberlin, D. W. (2015). Neonatal herpes simplex virus infection: Epidemiology and treatment. *Clinics in Perinatology, 42*(1), 47–59.

Jhaveri, R. (2015). Prevention of hepatitis B virus vertical transmission: Time for the next step. *Pediatrics, 135*(5), e1286–e1287.

Jimenez, K., Kulnigg-Dabsch, S., & Gasche, C. (2015). Management of iron deficiency anemia. *Gastroenterology & Hepatology, 11*(4), 241–250.

Joint National Committee. (2014). *Eighth report of the Joint National Committee on prevention, detection, evaluation, and treatment of high blood pressure* (NIH Publication No. 035233). Washington, DC: National Institutes of Health.

Jordan, R. G., Engstrom, J. L., Marfell, J. A., & Farley, C. L. (2014). *Prenatal and postnatal care: A woman-centered approach.* Ames, IO: John Wiley & Sons, Inc.

Jyoti, M., Shirke, S., & Matalia, H. (2015). Congenital rubella syndrome: Global issue. *Journal of Cataract & Refractive Surgery, 41*(5), 1127–1134.

Kahn, E., Mikhael, H., & Vadivelu, N. (2015). Cocaine abuse. In *Substance abuse* (pp. 143–154). New York, NY: Springer Publishers.

Karimi, M., Cohan, N., & Parand, S. (2015). Thalassemia and women's health. *Women's Health Bulletin, 2*(3), E29440.

Kelly, W., Massoumi, A., & Lazarus, A. (2015). Asthma in pregnancy: Physiology, diagnosis, and management. *Postgraduate Medicine, 127*(4), 349–358.

Killion, M. (2015). New hypertension in pregnancy guidelines. *MCN: The American Journal of Maternal/Child Nursing, 40*(2), 128.

Kim, C. (2014). Maternal outcomes and follow-up after gestational diabetes mellitus. *Diabetic Medicine, 31*(3), 292–301.

King, T. L., Brucker, M. C., Kriebs, J. M., Fahey, J. O., Gegor, C. L., & Varney, H. (2015). *Varney's midwifery* (5th ed.), Burlington, MA: Jones & Bartlett Learning.

Knight-Agarwal, C. R., Kaur, M., Williams, L. T., Davey, R., & Davis, D. (2014). The views and attitudes of health professionals providing antenatal care to women with a high BMI: A qualitative research study. *Women and Birth, 27*(2), 138–144.

Knox, C. A., Delaney, J. A., & Winterstein, A. G. (2014). Anti-diabetic drug utilization of pregnant diabetic women in us managed care. *BMC Pregnancy and Childbirth, 14*(1), 28–34.

Koh, H. (2014). The teen pregnancy prevention program: An evidence-based public health program model. *Journal of Adolescent Health, 54*(3), S1–S2.

Kovacs, G., & Briggs, P. (Eds.). (2015). Infections during pregnancy—Varicella, herpes, cytomegalovirus, toxoplasma, listeria, Group B Streptococcus. *Lectures in obstetrics, gynecology and women's health* (pp. 133–137). Springer International Publishing.

Kumar, B., & Gupta, S. (2014). *Sexually transmitted infections* (2nd ed.). Philadelphia, PA: Elsevier Health Sciences.

Lambert, N., Strebel, P., Orenstein, W., Icenogle, J., & Poland, G. A. (2015). Rubella. *The Lancet, 385*(9984), 2297–2230.

Lamberth, J. R., Reddy, S. C., Pan, J. J., & Dasher, K. J. (2015). Chronic hepatitis B infection in pregnancy. *World Journal of Hepatology, 7*(9), 1233–1237.

Lapolla, A., & Dalfrà, M. G. (2015). Pregnancy and diabetes. In D. Bruttomesso, & G. Grassi (Eds.), *Frontiers in diabetes (Vol. 24*, pp. 11–22). Karger Medical & Scientific Publishers.

Lichtin, A., & Philipson, E. H. (2014). Pregnancy. In *The coagulation consult* (pp. 249–269). New York, NY: Springer Publishers.

Ma, W. J., Huang, Z. H., Huang, B. X., Qi, B. H., Zhang, Y. J., Xiao, B. X., et al. (2015). Intensive low-glycemic-load dietary intervention for the management of glycemia and serum lipids among women with gestational diabetes: A randomized control trial. *Public Health Nutrition, 18*(08), 1506–1513.

Maartens, G., Celum, C., & Lewin, S. R. (2014). HIV infection: Epidemiology, pathogeneses, treatment, and prevention. *The Lancet, 384*(9939), 258–271.

Madhuvrata, P., Govinden, G., Bustani, R., Song, S., & Farrell, T. A. (2015). Prevention of gestational diabetes in pregnant women with risk factors for gestational diabetes: A systematic review and meta-analysis of randomized trials. *Obstetric Medicine: The Medicine of Pregnancy, 8*(2), 68–85.

Malee, M. P. (2015). Protocol 30: Parvovirus B19 infection. In J. T. Queenan, C. Y. Spong, & C. J. Lockwood (Eds.), *Protocols for high-risk pregnancies: An evidence-based approach* (pp. 245–250). Chichester, UK: John Wiley & Sons.

March of Dimes. (2015a). *Gestational diabetes.* Retrieved from http://www.marchofdimes.com/pregnancy/gestational-diabetes.aspx

March of Dimes. (2015b). *Thalassemia.* Retrieved from http://www.marchofdimes.com/baby/thalassemia.aspx

March of Dimes. (2015c). *Sickle cell disease and pregnancy.* Retrieved from http://www.marchofdimes.com/pregnancy/sickle-cell-disease-and-pregnancy.aspx

March of Dimes. (2015d). *Cytomegalovirus and pregnancy.* Retrieved from http://www.marchofdimes.com/pregnancy/cytomegalovirus-and-pregnancy.aspx

March of Dimes. (2015e). *Genital herpes.* Retrieved from http://www.marchofdimes.com/pregnancy/genital-herpes.aspx

March of Dimes. (2015f). *Group B strep infection.* Retrieved from http://www.marchofdimes.com/pregnancy/group-b-strep-infection.aspx

March of Dimes. (2015g). *Toxoplasmosis.* Retrieved from http://www.marchofdimes.com/pregnancy/toxoplasmosis.aspx

March of Dimes. (2015h). *Keeping breastfeeding safe.* Retrieved from http://www.marchofdimes.org/baby/keeping-breastfeeding-safe.aspx

March of Dimes. (2015i). *Pregnancy complications: Sexually transmitted diseases.* Retrieved from http://www.marchofdimes.org/sexually-transmitted-diseases.aspx

March of Dimes. (2015j). *Teenage pregnancy.* Retrieved from http://www.marchofdimes.org/materials/teenage-pregnancy.pdf

March of Dimes. (2015k). *Smoking, alcohol, and drugs and pregnancy.* Retrieved from http://www.marchofdimes.org/pregnancy/illicit-drug-use-during-pregnancy.aspx

March of Dimes. (2015l). *Asthma during pregnancy.* Retrieved from http://www.marchofdimes.org/pregnancy/asthma-during-pregnancy.aspx

March of Dimes. (2015m). *A mommy after 35.* Retrieved from http://www.marchofdimes.org/pregnancy/a-mommy-after-35.aspx?gclid = CKqBr5zEwMACFWoR7AoddGQASQ

McHugh, R. K., Nielsen, S., & Weiss, R. D. (2015). Prescription drug abuse: From epidemiology to public policy. *Journal of Substance Abuse Treatment, 48*(1), 1–7.

McIntyre, H. D., Dyer, A. R., & Metzger, B. E. (2015). Odds, risks and appropriate diagnosis of gestational diabetes. *The Medical Journal of Australia, 202*(6), 309–311.

McKeever, A. E., Spaeth-Brayton, S., & Sheerin, S. (2014). The role of nurses in comprehensive care management of pregnant women with drug addiction. *Nursing for Women's Health, 18*(4), 284–293.

Mehta, N., Chen, K., Hardy, E., & Powrie, R. (2015). Respiratory disease in pregnancy. *Best Practice & Research Clinical Obstetrics & Gynecology, 29*(5), 598–611.

Miller, M. A., & Carpenter, M. (2015). Hypertensive disorders of pregnancy. In K. R. Montella (Ed.), *Medical management of the pregnant patient* (pp. 177–193). New York, NY: Springer Publishers.

Mills, T. A., & Lavender, T. (2014). Advanced maternal age. *Obstetrics, Gynecology & Reproductive Medicine, 24*(3), 85–90.

Mitanchez, D., Yzydorczyk, C., Siddeek, B., Boubred, F., Benahmed, M., & Simeoni, U. (2015). The offspring of the diabetic mother – short-and long-term implications. *Best Practice & Research Clinical Obstetrics & Gynecology, 29*(2), 256–269.

Mohamad, T. N., Fakhri, H. A., Bernal, J. M., Thatai, D., & Peterson, E. (2014). Cardiovascular disease and pregnancy. *eMedicine.* Retrieved from http://emedicine.medscape.com/article/162004-overview

Mohammadzadeh, A., & Farhat, A. (2014). Fetal alcohol syndrome. *Asia Pacific Journal of Medical Toxicology, 3,* 10.

Mohindra, R., & Marwah, S. (2015). Systemic lupus erythematosus in pregnancy-intricate, but wieldy. *International Journal of Reproduction, Contraception, Obstetrics and Gynecology, 4*(2), 295–300.

Moore, T. R. (2015). Diabetes mellitus and pregnancy. *eMedicine.* Retrieved from http://emedicine.medscape.com/article/127547-overview

Moses, S. (2015). Anemia in pregnancy. *Family practice notebook.* Retrieved from http://www.fpnotebook.com/heme-onc/OB/AnmInPrgncy.htm

Multiple Sclerosis Association of America [MSAA]. (2015). *MS Overview.* Retrieved from http://mymsaa.org/about-ms/overview/

Nagtalon-Ramos, J. (2014). *Best evidence-based practices: Maternal-newborn nursing care.* Philadelphia, PA: F.A. Davis Company.

National Asthma Education and Prevention Program [NAEPP]. (2015). *Guidelines for the diagnosis and management of asthma.* Retrieved from http://www.nhlbi.nih.gov/health-pro/guidelines/current/asthma-guidelines/index.htm

National Diabetes Information Clearing House. (2015). *What is gestational diabetes?* Retrieved from http://www.diabetes.niddk.nih.gov/dm/pubs/pregnancy

National Institute on Drug Abuse [NIDA]. (2015a). *What are the unique needs of pregnant women with substance abuse disorders?* Retrieved from http://www.drugabuse.gov/publications/principles-drug-addiction-treatment-research-based-guide-second-edition/frequently-asked-questions/what-are-unique-needs-pregnant-women

National Institute on Drug Abuse [NIDA]. (2015b). *Drug facts: Cocaine.* Retrieved from http://www.drugabuse.gov/publications/drugfacts/cocaine

National Institute on Drug Abuse [NIDA]. (2015c). *Drug facts: Marijuana.* Retrieved from http://www.drugabuse.gov/publications/drugfacts/marijuana

National Institute on Drug Abuse [NIDA]. (2015d). *Drug facts: Methamphetamine.* Retrieved from http://www.drugabuse.gov/publications/drugfacts/methamphetamine

National Institutes of Health [NIH]. (2014). Recommendations for use of antiretroviral drugs in pregnant HIV-infected women for maternal health and interventions to reduce perinatal transmission in the United States. *United Public Health Service*. Retrieved from http://aidsinfo.nih.gov/contentfiles/lvguidelines/PerinatalGL.pdf

National Organization on Fetal Alcohol Syndrome [NOFAS]. (2015). *What is fetal alcohol syndrome?* Retrieved from http://www.nofas.org/main/what_is_FAS.htm.

New York Heart Association, Criteria Committee. (1994). *Nomenclature and criteria for diagnosis of diseases of the heart and great vessels* (9th ed., pp. 253–256). Boston, MA: Little, Brown.

Northridge, J. L., & Coupey, S. M. (2015). Realizing reproductive health equity for adolescents and young adults. *American Journal of Public Health, 105*(7), 1284.

Novotna, A., & Ehler, E. (2014). Multiple sclerosis and pregnancy. *Clinical Neurophysiology, 125*(5), e27.

Østensen, M. (2014). Contraception and pregnancy counseling in rheumatoid arthritis. *Current Opinion in Rheumatology, 26*(3), 302–307.

Park, J. S., & Pan, C. (2014). Current recommendations of managing HBV infection in preconception or pregnancy. *Frontiers of Medicine, 8*(2), 158–165.

Petry, C. J. (2014). *Gestational diabetes: Origins, complications, and treatment*. Boca Raton, FL: CRC Press Taylor & Francis Group.

Prasad, M. (2014). When opiate abuse complicates pregnancy. *Contemporary OB/GYN* (Online, February 1, 2014).

Procter, S. B., & Campbell, C. G. (2014). Position of the Academy of Nutrition and Dietetics: Nutrition and lifestyle for a healthy pregnancy outcome. *Journal of the Academy of Nutrition and Dietetics, 114*(7), 1099–1103.

Puopolo, K. M., Madoff, L. C., & Baker, C. J. (2015). Group B streptococcal infection in pregnant women. *UpToDate*. Retrieved from http://www.uptodate.com/contents/group-b-streptococcal-infection-in-pregnant-women

Raio, L., Bolla, D., & Baumann, M. (2015). Hypertension in pregnancy. *Current Opinion in Cardiology, 30*(4), 411–415.

Rajoriya, M., & Kalra, R. (2015). Challenges of motherhood in adolescent girls. *International Journal of Reproduction, Contraception, Obstetrics and Gynecology, 4*(3), 696–700.

Rakhmanina, N. Y., & van den Anker, J. N. (2014). Pharmacologic prevention of perinatal HIV infection. *Early Human Development, 90*(1), S13–S15.

Rayment, M., Asboe, D., & Sullivan, A. K. (2014). HIV testing and management of newly diagnosed HIV. *British Medical Journal, 349*, g4275.

Rigby, F. B. (2015). Anemias in pregnancy. *eMedicine*. Retrieved from http://emedicine.medscape.com/article/261586-overview

Rivera, D. M., & Frye, R. E. (2014). Pediatric HIV infection. *eMedicine*. Retrieved from http://emedicine.medscape.com/article/965086-overview

Roglie, G., & Colagiuri, S. (2014). Gestational diabetes mellitus: Squaring the circle. *Diabetes Care, 37*(6), 143–144.

Roskjær, A. B., Andersen, J. R., Ronneby, H., Damm, P., & Mathiesen, E. R. (2014). Dietary advices on carbohydrate intake for pregnant women with type 1 diabetes. *The Journal of Maternal-Fetal & Neonatal Medicine, 28*(2), 229–233; 1–15.

Ross, S., Baird, A. S., & Porter, C. C. (2014). Teenage pregnancy: Strategies for prevention. *Obstetrics, Gynecology and Reproductive Medicine, 24*(9), 266–273.

Salman, K., Priti, S., Molly, M., Kumar, V. S., & Zeenat, S. (2015). Hepatitis B virus infection in pregnant women and transmission to newborns. *Asian Pacific Journal of Tropical Disease, 5*(6), 421–429.

Sauer, M. V. (2015). Reproduction at an advanced maternal age and maternal health. *Fertility and Sterility, 103*(5), 1136–1143.

Schimmel, M. S., Bromiker, R., Hammerman, C., Chertman, L., Ioscovich, A., Granovsky-Grisaru, S., et al. (2015). The effects of maternal age and parity on maternal and neonatal outcome. *Archives of Gynecology and Obstetrics, 291*(4), 793–798.

Schur, P. H., & Hahn, B. H. (2015). Epidemiology and pathogenesis of systemic lupus erythematosus. *UpToDate*. Retrieved from http://www.uptodate.com/contents/epidemiology-and-pathogenesis-of-systemic-lupus-erythematosus

Sedgh, G., Finer, L. B., Bankole, A., Eilers, M. A., & Singh, S. (2015). Adolescent pregnancy, birth, and abortion rates across countries: Levels and recent trends. *Journal of Adolescent Health, 56*(2), 223–230.

Seely, E. W., & Ecker, J. (2014). Chronic hypertension in pregnancy. *Circulation, 129*(11), 1254–1261.

Sibai, B. M. (2015). Protocol 25: Chronic hypertension. In J. T. Queenan., C. Y. Spong, & C. J. Lockwood (Eds.), *Protocols for high-risk pregnancies: An evidence-based approach*. Chichester, UK: John Wiley & Sons, Ltd.

Silasi, M., Cardenas, I., Kwon, J. Y., Racicot, K., Aldo, P., & Mor, G. (2015). Viral infections during pregnancy. *American Journal of Reproductive Immunology, 73*(3), 199–213.

Simeone, R. M., Devine, O. J., Marcinkevage, J. A., Gilboa, S. M., Razzaghi, H., Bardenheier, B. H., et al. (2015). Diabetes and congenital heart defects: A systematic review, meta-analysis, and modeling project. *American Journal of Preventive Medicine, 48*(2), 195–204.

Singh, A. G., & Chowdhary, V. R. (2015). Pregnancy-related issues in women with systemic lupus erythematosus. *International Journal of Rheumatic Diseases, 18*, 172–181.

Skoglund, C., Chen, Q., D Onofrio, B. M., Lichtenstein, P., & Larsson, H. (2014). Familial confounding of the association between maternal smoking during pregnancy and ADHD in offspring. *Journal of Child Psychology and Psychiatry, 55*, 61–68.

Slater, L. (2015). Substance use in pregnancy. *The Practicing Midwife, 18*(1), 10–13.

Sliwa, K., Johnson, M. R., Zilla, P., & Roos-Hesselink, J. W. (2015). Management of valvular disease in pregnancy: A global perspective. *European Heart Journal, 36*(18), 1078–1089.

Smith, B. (2015). *Neonatal-perinatal infections: An update. Clinics in Perinatology, 42*(1), 77–104. Philadelphia, PA: Elsevier Health Sciences.

Smith, M. V., Gotman, N., & Yonkers, K. A. (2016). Early childhood adversity and pregnancy outcomes. *Maternal and Child Health Journal, 20*(4), 790–798.

Solomon, C. G., & Greene, M. F. (2015). Control of hypertension in pregnancy—If some is good, Is more worse? *The New England Journal of Medicine, 372*(5), 475–476.

Strangfeld, A., Pattloch, D., Spilka, M., Manger, B., Krummel-Lorenz, B., Gräßler, A., et al. (2015). Pregnancies in patients with rheumatoid arthritis: Treatment decisions, course of the disease, and pregnancy outcomes. *Annals of the Rheumatic Diseases, 74*(Suppl. 2), 70–71.

Subramaniam, G., & Girish, M. (2015). Iron deficiency anemia in children. *The Indian Journal of Pediatrics, 82*(6), 558–564.

Substance Abuse and Mental Health Services Administration [SAMHSA]. (2015). *Pregnant women, new mothers, and substance abuse.* Retrieved from http://www.samhsa.gov/samhsaNewsLetter/Volume_17_Number_3/PregnancySubstanceAbuse.aspx

Suliman, S., & Seopela, L. (2015). Congenital and neonatal infections: Review. *Obstetrics and Gynecology Forum, 25*(2), 27–32.

Swamy, G. K., & Heine, R. (2015). Vaccinations for pregnant women. *Obstetrics & Gynecology, 125*(1), 212–226.

Swan, L. (2014). Congenital heart disease in pregnancy. *Best Practice & Research Clinical Obstetrics & Gynecology, 28*(4), 495–506.

Toledano, Y., Hadar, E., & Hod, M. (2015). Diabetes in pregnancy. In R. A. DeFronzo, E. Ferrannini, P. Zimmet., & K. G. M. M. Alberti (Eds.), *International textbook of diabetes mellitus* (4th ed.). Chichester, UK: John Wiley & Sons.

Ural, S. H. (2015). Genital herpes in pregnancy. *eMedicine.* Retrieved from http://emedicine.medscape.com/article/274874-overview

U.S. Agency for International Development [USAID]. (2014). *Contraceptives for clients with STIs, HIV, and AIDS.* Retrieved from https://www.fphandbook.org/contraceptives-clients-stis-hiv-and-aids

U.S. Department of Health and Human Services. (2010). *Healthy people 2020.* Retrieved from http://www.healthypeople.gov/2020/topicsobjectives2020

U.S. Preventive Services Task Force [USPSTF]. (2014). *Screening for HIV.* Retrieved from http://www.uspreventiveservicestaskforce.org/uspstf13/hiv/hivfinalrs.htm#summary

U.S. Preventive Services Task Force [USPTF]. (2015). *Low-dose aspirin use for the prevention of morbidity and mortality from preeclampsia: Preventive medication.* Retrieved from http://www.uspreventiveservicestaskforce.org/Page/Topic/recommendation-summary/low-dose-aspirin-use-for-the-prevention-of-morbidity-and-mortality-from-preeclampsia-preventive-medication

Vall, O., Salat-Batlle, J., & Garcia-Algar, O. (2015). Alcohol consumption during pregnancy and adverse neurodevelopmental outcomes. *Journal of Epidemiology and Community Health, 69*(10), 927–929.

Vanders, R. L., & Murphy, V. E. (2015). Maternal complications and the management of asthma in pregnancy. *Women's Health, 11*(2), 183–191.

Varner, M. W., Silver, R. M., Hogue, C. J. R., Willinger, M., Parker, C. B., Thorsten, V. R., et al. (2014). Association between stillbirth and illicit drug use and smoking during pregnancy. *Obstetrics & Gynecology, 123*(1), 113–125.

Vaux, K. K., & Chambers, C. (2015). Fetal alcohol syndrome. *eMedicine.* Retrieved from http://emedicine.medscape.com/article/974016-overview

Vichinsky, M. L., & Jansson, L. M. (2016). Perinatal addictions: Intrauterine exposures. In *Textbook of addiction treatment: International perspectives* (pp. 2333–2363). Springer Publishers.

Vinchinski, E. P. (2015).Pregnancy in women with sickle cell disease. *UpToDate.* Retrieved from http://www.uptodate.com/contents/pregnancy-in-women-with-sickle-cell-disease

Vogler, M. A. (2014). HIV and pregnancy. *Current Treatment Options in Infectious Diseases, 6*(2), 183–195.

Volkow, N. D., Baler, R. D., Compton, W. M., & Weiss, S. R. (2014). Adverse health effects of marijuana use. *New England Journal of Medicine, 370*(23), 2219–2227.

Vukusic, S., & Marignier, R. (2015). Multiple sclerosis and pregnancy in the 'treatment era'. *Nature Reviews Neurology, 11*, 280–289.

Walker, M. (2014). *Breastfeeding management for the clinician: Using the evidence* (3rd ed.). Burlington, MA: Jones & Bartlett Learning.

Wang, M. (2015). Perinatal drug abuse and neonatal withdrawal. *eMedicine.* Retrieved from http://emedicine.medscape.com/article/978492-overview

Wasserman, S., & Clowse, M. E. (2014). Systemic lupus erthematosus. In L. R. Sammaritano, & B. L. Bermas (Eds.), *Contraception and pregnancy in patients with rheumatic disease* (pp. 79–97). New York, NY: Springer Publishers.

Weber, J. R., & Kelley, J. H. (2014). *Health assessment in nursing* (5th ed.). Philadelphia, PA: Lippincott Williams & Wilkins.

Weekes, A. J., & Lee, D. S. (2014). Pediatric cocaine abuse clinical presentation. *eMedicine.* Retrieved from http://emedicine.medscape.com/article/917385-clinical

Whitworth, M., & Cockerill, R. (2014). Antenatal management of teenage pregnancy. *Obstetrics, Gynecology & Reproductive Medicine, 24*(1), 23–28.

Worel, J. N., & Hayman, L. L. (2015). Cardiovascular disease prevention in women: Reducing the major threat to women's health. *Journal of Cardiovascular Nursing, 30*(1), 5–7.

Workowski, K. A., & Bolan, G. A. (2015). Sexually transmitted diseases treatment guidelines, 2015. *MMWR. Recommendations and Reports: Morbidity and Mortality Weekly Report. Recommendations and Reports/Centers for Disease Control, 64*(RR-03), 1–137.

World Health Organization [WHO]. (2015a). *Health for the world's adolescents: A second chance in the second decade.* Geneva, Switzerland: Department of Maternal, Newborn, Child and Adolescent Health, WHO

World Health Organization [WHO]. (2015b). *Tuberculosis: Key facts.* Retrieved from http://www.who.int/mediacentre/factsheets/fs104/en/

World Health Organization [WHO]. (2015c). *Guidelines for the identification and management of substance abuse use disorders in pregnancy.* Retrieved from http://www.cdc.gov/nchs/fastats/drug-use-illegal.htm

Worley, J. (2014). Identification and management of prescription drug abuse in pregnancy. *The Journal of Perinatal & Neonatal Nursing, 28*(3), 196–203.

Yoost, J. L., Hertweck, S. P., & Barnett, S. N. (2014). The effect of an educational approach to pregnancy prevention among high-risk early and late adolescents. *Journal of Adolescent Health, 55*(2), 222–227.

Zhang, H. J., Patenaude, V., & Abenhaim, H. (2014). Maternal outcomes in pregnancies affected by varicella zoster virus infections. *Obstetrics & Gynecology, 123*, 86S–87S.

CHAPTER WORKSHEET

MULTIPLE CHOICE QUESTIONS

1. Which of the following would the nurse include when teaching a pregnant woman about the pathophysiologic mechanisms associated with gestational diabetes?
   a. Pregnancy fosters the development of carbohydrate cravings.
   b. There is progressive resistance to the effects of insulin.
   c. Hypoinsulinemia develops early in the first trimester.
   d. Glucose levels decrease to accommodate fetal growth.
2. When providing prenatal education to a pregnant woman with asthma, which of the following would be important for the nurse to do?
   a. Explain that she should avoid steroids during her pregnancy.
   b. Demonstrate how to assess her blood glucose levels.
   c. Teach correct administration of subcutaneous bronchodilators.
   d. Ensure she seeks treatment for any acute exacerbation.
3. Which of the following conditions would most likely cause a pregnant woman with type 1 diabetes the greatest difficulty during her pregnancy?
   a. Placenta previa
   b. Hyperemesis gravidarum
   c. Abruptio placentae
   d. Rh incompatibility
4. Women who drink alcohol during pregnancy:
   a. Often produce more alcohol dehydrogenase
   b. Usually become intoxicated faster than before
   c. Can give birth to an infant with fetal alcohol spectrum disorder
   d. Gain fewer pounds throughout the gestation
5. When explaining to a pregnant woman about HIV infection and transmission, which of the following would the nurse include?
   a. It primarily occurs when there is a large viral load in the blood.
   b. HIV is most commonly transmitted via sexual contact.
   c. It affects the majority of infants of mothers with HIV infection.
   d. Nurses are most frequently affected due to needlesticks.
6. Women who are obese have a greater risk of developing which of the following during pregnancy?
   a. Type 1 diabetes
   b. Hypotension
   c. Low birth weight infant
   d. Gestational hypertension
7. Maintenance on methadone or buprenorphine is the most common medical treatment for which of the following drug addictions?
   a. Alcohol
   b. Nicotine
   c. Opiates
   d. Marijuana

CRITICAL THINKING EXERCISES

1. A client at 26 weeks' gestation came to the clinic to follow up on her previous 1-hour glucose screening. Her results had come back outside the accepted screening range, and a 3-hour glucose tolerance test (GTT) had been ordered. It resulted in three abnormal values, confirming a diagnosis of gestational diabetes. As the nurse in the prenatal clinic you are seeing her for the first time.
   a. What additional information will you need to provide care for her?
   b. What education will she need to address this new diagnosis?
   c. How will you evaluate the effectiveness of your interventions?
2. A 14-year-old girl comes to the public health clinic with her mother. The mother tells you that her daughter has been "out messing around and has gotten herself pregnant." The girl is crying quietly in the corner and avoids eye contact with you. The mother reports that her daughter "must be following in my footsteps" because she became pregnant when she was only 15 years old. The client's mother goes back out into the waiting room and leaves the client with you.
   a. What is your first approach with the client to gain her trust?
   b. List the client's educational needs during this pregnancy.
   c. What prevention strategies are needed to prevent a second pregnancy?

3. A 27-year-old G3P2 is admitted to the labor and birth suite because of preterm rupture of membranes at an estimated 35 weeks' gestation. She has received no prenatal care and reports this was an unplanned pregnancy. Linda appears distracted and very thin. She reports that her two previous children have been in foster care since birth because the child welfare authorities "didn't think I was an adequate mother." She denies any recent use of alcohol or drugs, but you smell alcohol on her breath. She has a spontaneous vaginal birth a few hours later, producing a 4-lb baby boy with Apgar scores of 8 at 1 minute and 9 at 5 minutes.
   a. What aspects of this woman's history may lead the nurse to suspect that this infant may be at risk for fetal alcohol spectrum disorder?
   b. What additional screening or laboratory tests might validate your suspicion?
   c. What physical and neurodevelopmental deficits might present later in life if the infant has fetal alcohol spectrum disorder?
4. Outline a discussion you might have with an HIV-positive pregnant woman who doesn't see the need to take antiretroviral agents to prevent perinatal transmission.
5. The nurse is preparing a teaching session about breast-feeding for a group of pregnant women who have various infections listed below. The nurse would include women with which of the following conditions? Select all that apply.
   a. Hepatitis B
   b. Parvovirus B19
   c. Herpesvirus type 2
   d. HIV-positive status
   e. Cytomegalovirus
   f. Varicella-zoster virus

STUDY ACTIVITIES

1. In the maternity clinic or hospital setting, interview a pregnant woman with a preexisting medical condition (e.g., diabetes, asthma, sickle cell anemia) and find out how this condition affects her life and this pregnancy, especially her lifestyle choices.
2. You have a close friend who has a problem with alcohol but denies it. She now admits to you that she thinks she is pregnant because she missed her period. What specific information and advice should you give her concerning alcohol use during pregnancy?
3. Should marijuana be legalized in the United States? What impact might your view (pro or con) have on pregnant women and their offspring?

BRINGING IT ALL TOGETHER: A CASE STUDY

Linda is an 18-year-old, very thin client who has been abusing alcohol since the age of twelve. She lived in foster care for much of her life and is recently on her own with a part-time job. She reports she had experienced both emotional and sexual abuse during her childhood. At 16, she was introduced to crack cocaine. So many of her friends and relatives were using, that it was impossible for her to see any other lifestyle or want to seek help for her addiction. She states she wanted to start a new life and get clean when she found out she was pregnant, but admitted she ended up partying and using drugs for the past four months of this pregnancy. She presents today for her first prenatal visit. She claims that she is ready to commit to a positive change.

Go to thePoint to find questions to consider about this case.

21

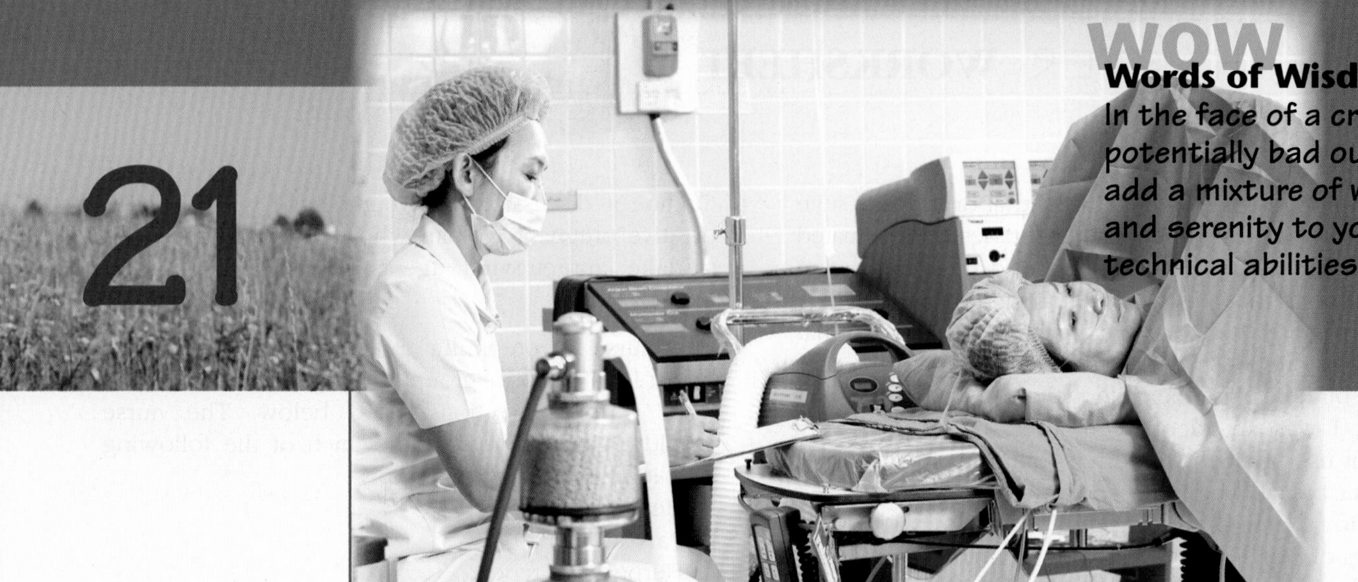

WOW

Words of Wisdom

In the face of a crisis or a potentially bad outcome, add a mixture of warmth and serenity to your technical abilities.

Nursing Management of Labor and Birth at Risk

KEY TERMS

amnioinfusion
arrest disorders
cesarean birth
dystocia
forceps
hypertonic uterine dysfunction
hypotonic uterine dysfunction
labor induction
macrosomia
multiple gestation
precipitate labor
preterm labor
postterm pregnancy
protracted disorders
shoulder dystocia
tocolytic
umbilical cord prolapse
vacuum extractor
vaginal birth after cesarean (VBAC)

Learning Objectives

Upon completion of the chapter, you will be able to:

1. Propose at least five risk factors associated with dystocia.
2. Differentiate the four major abnormalities or problems associated with dysfunctional labor patterns, giving examples of each problem.
3. Examine the nursing management for the woman with dysfunctional labor experiencing a problem with the powers, passenger, passageway, or psyche.
4. Devise a plan of care for the woman experiencing preterm labor.
5. Relate the nursing assessment and management of the woman experiencing a prolonged pregnancy.
6. Assess four obstetric emergencies that can complicate labor and birth, including appropriate management for each.
7. Compare and contrast the nursing management for the woman undergoing labor induction or augmentation, forceps- and vacuum-assisted birth.
8. Summarize the plan of care for a woman who is to undergo a cesarean birth.
9. Evaluate the key areas to be addressed when caring for a woman that undergoes a vaginal birth after cesarean (VBAC).

***Jennifer*, a 29-year-old G1P0, is at 41 weeks' gestation. Her health care provider has recommended that she come in for induction. She is very anxious about doing this since she has heard "horror stories" about the "hard painful contractions" that can result. What can the nurse do to calm her fears?**

INTRODUCTION

Most women describe pregnancy as an exciting time in their lives, but the development of an unexpected problem can suddenly change this description dramatically. Consider the woman who has had a problem-free pregnancy and then suddenly develops a condition during labor, changing a routine situation into a possible crisis. Many complications occur with little or no warning and present challenges for the perinatal health care team as well as the family. The nurse plays a major role in identifying the problem quickly and coordinating immediate intervention, ultimately achieving a positive outcome.

National health goals address maternal and newborn outcomes involving complications of labor and birth and **cesarean birth** (U.S. Department of Health and Human Services, 2010). These goals are highlighted in *Healthy People 2020*.

This chapter will address several conditions occurring during labor and birth that may increase the risk of an adverse outcome for the mother and fetus. It also describes birth-related procedures that may be necessary for the woman who develops a condition that increases her risk or that may be needed to reduce the woman's risk for developing a condition, thus promoting optimal maternal and fetal outcomes. Nursing management of the woman and her family focuses on professional support and compassionate care.

DYSTOCIA

Dystocia, defined as abnormal or difficult labor, can be influenced by a vast number of maternal and fetal factors. Dystocia is said to exist when the progress of labor deviates from normal; it is characterized by a slow and abnormal progression of labor. It occurs in approximately 8% to 11% of all labors and is the leading indicator for primary cesarean birth in the United States (Joy, Lyon, & Scott, 2015). It is of concern because of its fatiguing factor for both mother and fetus and frequently requires medical or surgical interventions, which increases risk.

To characterize a labor as abnormal, a basic understanding of normal labor is essential. Normal labor starts with regular uterine contractions that are strong enough to result in cervical effacement and dilation. Early in labor, uterine contractions are irregular and cervical effacement and dilation occurs gradually. When cervical dilation reaches 5 to 6 cm and uterine contractions become more powerful, the active phase of labor begins. It is usually during the active phase that dystocia becomes apparent. Because dystocia cannot be predicted or diagnosed with certainty, the term "failure to progress" is often used. This term includes lack of progressive cervical dilation, lack of descent of the fetal head, or both. An adequate trial of labor is needed to declare with confidence that dystocia or "failure to progress" exists.

Early identification of and prompt interventions for dystocia are essential to minimize risk to the woman and fetus. According to the American College of Obstetricians and Gynecologists (ACOG) (2014a) factors associated with an increased risk for dystocia include epidural analgesia, excessive analgesia, multiple pregnancy, hydramnios, maternal exhaustion, ineffective maternal pushing technique, occiput posterior position, longer first stage of labor, nulliparity, short maternal stature (less than 5 ft tall), fetal birth weight (more than 8.8 lb), **shoulder dystocia**, abnormal fetal presentation or position (breech), fetal anomalies (hydrocephalus), maternal age older than 34 years, high caffeine intake, overweight, gestational age more than 41 weeks, chorioamnionitis, ineffective uterine contractions, and high fetal station at complete cervical dilation.

One in three women who gives birth in the United States today does so by a cesarean birth. The most common indications for primary cesarean births include, in order of frequency, labor dystocia, abnormal fetal heart rate (FHR) tracing, fetal malpresentation, **multiple gestation**, and suspected **macrosomia**. It is time to revisit the definition of labor dystocia because recent studies show that contemporary labor progresses at a rate substantially slower than what was historically taught. Labors today are often longer which may in part be due to higher body mass index (BMI), higher rates of **labor induction**, and the significant increase in the use of epidural anesthesia (ACOG, 2014a).

Admitting women too early to the hospital while still in the early latent phase of labor may increase the diagnosis of dystocia and increase the risk of augmentation of labor and epidural analgesia. These two interventions may cascade into a surgical birth. Adequate

HEALTHY PEOPLE 2020

Objective	Nursing Significance
MICH-9 Reduce preterm births	• Will help to focus attention on the need for close antepartum surveillance and identification of risk factors for preterm labor/births and provide appropriate interventions to reduce it.
MICH-7 Reduce cesarean births among low-risk (full-term, singleton, vertex presentation) women	• Will help to reduce the number of surgical births with accompanying risk factors and costs by appropriate labor management, continual labor support, and practice patterns, while helping to ensure positive maternal and newborn outcomes.

Healthy People objectives based on data from http://www.healthypeople.gov.

hydration, rest, emotional and physical support, and, if needed, pharmacologic sedation can be encouraged as alternatives to early hospital admission. Patience should be the critical factor here.

Dystocia can result from problems or abnormalities involving the expulsive forces (known as the "powers"); presentation, position, and fetal development (the "passenger"); the maternal bony pelvis or birth canal (the "passageway"); and maternal stress (the "psyche"). Table 21.1 summarizes the diagnosis, therapeutic management, and nursing management of the common problems associated with dystocia.

Problems with the Powers

When the expulsive forces of the uterus become dysfunctional, the uterus may either never fully relax (hypertonic contractions), placing the fetus in jeopardy, or relax too much (hypotonic contractions), causing ineffective contractions. Still another dysfunction can occur when the uterus contracts so frequently and with such intensity that a very rapid birth will take place (**precipitate labor**).

Hypertonic uterine dysfunction occurs when the uterus never fully relaxes between contractions. Subsequently, contractions are ineffectual, erratic, and poorly coordinated because they involve only a portion of the uterus and because more than one uterine pacemaker is sending signals for contraction. Women in this situation experience a prolonged latent phase, stay at 2 to 3 cm, and do not dilate as they should. Placental perfusion becomes compromised, thereby reducing oxygen to the fetus. These hypertonic contractions exhaust the mother, who is experiencing frequent, intense, and painful contractions with little progression. This dysfunctional pattern occurs in early labor and affects nulliparous women more than multiparous women (Hinshaw & Kenyon, 2015).

Hypotonic uterine dysfunction occurs during active labor (dilation more than 5 to 6 cm) when contractions become poor in quality and lack sufficient intensity to dilate and efface the cervix. Factors associated with this abnormal labor pattern include overstretching of the uterus, a large fetus, multiple fetuses, hydramnios, multiple parity, bowel or bladder distention preventing descent, and excessive use of analgesia. Clinical manifestations of hypotonic uterine dysfunction include weak contractions that become milder, a uterine fundus that can be easily indented with fingertip pressure at the peak of each contraction, and contractions that become more infrequent and briefer (King et al., 2015). The major risk with this complication is hemorrhage after giving birth because the uterus cannot contract effectively to compress blood vessels.

Labor refers to uterine contractions resulting in progressive dilation and effacement of the cervix, and accompanied by descent and expulsion of the fetus. *Abnormal labor*, *dystocia*, and *failure to progress* are imprecise terms that have been used to describe a difficult labor pattern that deviates from that observed in the majority of women who have spontaneous vaginal deliveries. A better classification is to characterize labor abnormalities as protraction disorders (i.e., slower than normal progress) or **arrest disorders** (i.e., complete cessation of progress).

The term **protracted disorders** refers to a series of events including protracted active phase dilation (slower than normal rate of cervical dilation) and protracted descent (delayed descent of the fetal head in the active phase). A laboring woman with a slower than normal rate of cervical dilation is said to have a protraction labor pattern disorder. A slow progress may be the result of cephalopelvic disproportion. Most women, however, benefit greatly from adequate hydration and some nutrition, emotional reassurance, and position changes—these women may go on and give birth vaginally.

Precipitate labor is labor that is completed in less than 3 hours from the start of contractions to birth. Not only can labor be too slow, but it can be abnormally rapid. The prevailing opinion has been that too rapid a labor can result in maternal injury and place the fetus at risk for traumatic or asphyxia insults (Suzuki, 2015). Women experiencing precipitate labor typically have soft perineal tissues that stretch readily, permitting the fetus to pass through the pelvis quickly, or abnormally strong uterine contractions. Maternal complications are rare if the maternal pelvis is adequate and the soft tissues yield to a fast fetal descent. However, if the fetus delivers too fast, it does not allow the cervix to dilate and efface, which leads to cervical lacerations and the potential for uterine rupture. Potential fetal complications may include head trauma, such as intracranial hemorrhage or nerve damage, and hypoxia due to the rapid progression of labor (Cunningham et al., 2014).

Precipitate labor is an anxiety-producing situation and frequently very painful with little rest between contractions. Continuous monitoring, frequent updates on her labor progress, pain management, and reassurance about her condition can assist in reducing the mother's anxious state of mind. Management includes readiness of the health care team for this rapid birth.

Problems with the Passenger

Any presentation other than occiput anterior (head down and anterior facing) or a slight variation of the fetal position or size increases the probability of dystocia. These variations can affect the contractions or fetal descent through the maternal pelvis. Common problems involving the fetus include occiput posterior position, breech presentation, multifetal pregnancy, excessive size (macrosomia) as it relates to cephalopelvic disproportion, and structural anomalies.

(text continues on page 805)

TABLE 21.1 DIAGNOSIS AND MANAGEMENT OF COMMON PROBLEMS ASSOCIATED WITH DYSTOCIA

	Description	Diagnosis	Therapeutic Management	Nursing Management
Problems with the Powers				
Hypertonic uterine dysfunction	Occurring in the latent phase of the first stage of labor (cervical dilation of <4 cm); uncoordinated. Force of contraction typically in the midsection of uterus at the junction of the active upper and passive lower segments of the uterus rather than in the fundus. Loss of downward pressure to push the presenting part against the cervix. Woman commonly becomes discouraged due to lack of progress; also has increased pain secondary to uterine anoxia.	Characteristic hypertonicity of the contractions and the lack of labor progress	Therapeutic rest with the use of sedatives to promote relaxation and stop the abnormal activity of the uterus. Identification and intervention of any contributing factors. Ruling out abruptio placentae (also associated with high resting tone and persistent pain). Onset of a normal labor pattern occurs in many women after a 4- to 6-hr rest period.	Institute bed rest and sedation to promote relaxation and reduce pain. Assist with measures to rule out fetopelvic disproportion and fetal malpresentation. Evaluate fetal tolerance to labor pattern, such as monitoring of FHR patterns. Assess for signs of maternal infection. Promote adequate hydration through IV therapy. Provide pain management via epidural or IV analgesics. Assist with amniotomy to augment labor. Explain to woman and family about dysfunctional pattern. Plan for operative birth if normal labor pattern is not achieved.
Hypotonic uterine dysfunction	Often termed secondary uterine inertia because the labor begins normally and then the frequency and intensity of contractions decrease. Possible contributing factors: overdistended uterus with multifetal pregnancy or large single fetus, too much pain medicine given too early in labor, fetal malposition, and regional anesthesia	Evaluation of the woman's labor to confirm that she is having hypotonic active labor rather than a long latent phase. Evaluation of maternal pelvis and fetal presentation and position to ensure that they are not contributing to the prolonged labor without noticeable progress.	Identification of possible cause of inefficient uterine action (a malpositioned fetus, a too small maternal pelvis, overdistention of the uterus with fluid or a macrosomic fetus). Rupture of amniotic sac (amniotomy) if all causes ruled out. Possible augmentation with oxytocin (Pitocin) to stimulate effective uterine contractions. Cesarean birth if amniotomy and augmentation ineffective.	Administer oxytocin as ordered once fetopelvic disproportion is ruled out. Assist with amniotomy if membranes are intact. Provide continuous electronic fetal monitoring. Monitor vital signs, contractions, and cervix continually. Assess for signs of maternal and fetal infection. Explain to woman and family about dysfunctional pattern. Plan for surgical birth if normal labor pattern is not achieved or fetal distress occurs.
Precipitate labor	Abrupt onset of higher-intensity contractions occurring in a shorter period of time instead of the more gradual increase in frequency, duration, and intensity that typifies most spontaneous labors	Identification based on the rapidity of progress through the stages of labor	Vaginal delivery if maternal pelvis is adequate	Closely monitor woman with previous history. Anticipate use of scheduled induction to control labor rate. Administer pharmacologic agents, such as tocolytics, to slow labor. Stay in constant attendance to monitor progress.

(continued)

TABLE 21.1 DIAGNOSIS AND MANAGEMENT OF COMMON PROBLEMS ASSOCIATED WITH DYSTOCIA (continued)

	Description	Diagnosis	Therapeutic Management	Nursing Management
Problems with the Passenger				
Persistent occiput posterior position	Engagement of fetal head in the left or right occipitotransverse position with the occiput rotating posteriorly rather than into the more favorable occiput anterior position (fetus born facing upward instead of the normal downward position) Labor usually much longer and more uncomfortable (causing increased back pain during labor) if fetus remains in this position. Possible extensive caput succedaneum and molding from the sustained occiput posterior position.	Leopold maneuvers and vaginal examination to determine position of fetal head in conjunction with the mother's complaints of severe back pain (back of fetal head pressing on mother's sacrum and coccyx).	Labor to proceed, preparing the woman for a long labor (spontaneous resolution possible). Comfort measures and maternal positioning to help promote fetal head rotation.	Assess for complaints of intense back pain in first stage of labor. Anticipate possible use of forceps to rotate to anterior position at birth or manual rotation to anterior position at end of second stage. Assess for prolonged second stage of labor with arrest of descent (common with this malposition). Encourage maternal position changes to promote fetal head rotation: hands and knees and rocking pelvis back and forth; side-lying position; side lunges during contractions; sitting, kneeling, or standing while leaning forward; squatting position to give birth and enlarge pelvic outlet. Prepare for possible cesarean birth if rotation is not achieved. Administer agents as ordered for pain relief (effective pain relief crucial to help the woman to tolerate the back discomfort). Apply low back counter pressure during contractions to ease the discomfort. Use other helpful measures to attempt to rotate the fetal head, including lateral abdominal stroking in the direction that the fetal head should rotate; assisting the client into a hands-and-knees position (all fours); and squatting, pelvic rocking, stair climbing, assuming a side-lying position toward the side that the fetus should rotate, and side lunges. Provide measures to reduce anxiety. Continuously reinforce the woman's progress. Teach woman about measures to facilitate fetal head rotation.

Face and brow presentation	Face presentation with complete extension of the fetal head. Brow presentation: fetal head between full extension and full flexion so that the largest fetal skull diameter presents to the pelvis.	Diagnosis only once labor is well established via vaginal examination; palpation of facial features as the presenting part rather than the fetal head	Vaginal birth possible with face presentation with an adequate maternal pelvis and fetal head rotation; cesarean birth if head rotates backward. Cesarean birth for brow presentation unless head flexes.	Assist with evaluating for fetopelvic disproportion. Anticipate cesarean birth if vertex position is not achieved. Explain fetal malposition to the woman and her partner. Provide close observation for any signs of fetal hypoxia, as evidenced by late decelerations on the fetal monitor.
Breech presentation	Fetal buttocks, or breech, presenting first rather than the head. 1. Frank breech: buttock as the presenting part, with hips flexed and legs and knees extended upward 2. Complete breech (or full breech): buttock as presenting part, with hips flexed and knees flexed in a "cannonball" position 3. Footling or incomplete breech: One or two feet as the presenting part, with one or both hips extended	Vaginal examination to determine breech presentation. Ideally, ultrasound to confirm a clinically suspected presentation and to identify any fetal anomalies.	The optimal method of birth is controversial: cesarean birth by some providers unless the fetus is small and the mother has a large pelvis; vaginal birth by others with each occurrence treated individually and labor monitored very closely. Regardless of the birth method selected, the risk for trauma is high. Breech vaginal births are not recommended by ACOG and come with a higher risk to the mother and infant than a planned surgical birth. Vaginal delivery: fetus allowed to spontaneously deliver up to the umbilicus; then maneuvers to assist in the delivery of the remainder of the body, arms, and head; fetal membranes left intact as long as possible to act as a dilating wedge and to prevent cord prolapse; anesthesiologist and pediatrician present. Cesarean birth; use of external cephalic version to reduce the chance of breech presentation at birth; attempted after the 35th week of gestation but before the start of labor (some fetuses spontaneously turn to a cephalic presentation on their own) toward term, and some will return to the breech presentation if external cephalic version is attempted too early; variable success rates, with risk for fractured bones, ruptured viscera, abruptio placentae, fetomaternal hemorrhage, and umbilical cord entanglement. Tocolytic drugs to relax the uterus, as well as other methods, to facilitate external cephalic version at term. Individual evaluation of each woman for all factors before any interventions is initiated.	Assess for associated conditions such as placenta previa, hydramnios, fetal anomalies, and multifetal pregnancy. Arrange for ultrasound to confirm fetal presentation. Assist with external cephalic version possible after 36 weeks and administer tocolytics to assist with external cephalic version. Anticipate trial labor for 4–6 hrs to evaluate progress if version is unsuccessful. Plan for cesarean birth if no progress is seen or fetal distress occurs. After external cephalic version, administer RhoGAM to the Rh-negative woman to prevent a sensitization reaction if trauma has occurred and the potential for mixing of blood exists.

(continued)

TABLE 21.1 DIAGNOSIS AND MANAGEMENT OF COMMON PROBLEMS ASSOCIATED WITH DYSTOCIA (continued)

	Description	Diagnosis	Therapeutic Management	Nursing Management
Shoulder dystocia	Delivery of fetal head with neck not appearing; retraction of chin against the perineum; shoulders remaining wedged behind the mother's pubic bone, causing a difficult birth with potential for injury to both mother and baby. If shoulders still above the brim at this stage, no advancement. Newborn's chest trapped within the vaginal vault; chest unable to expand with respiration (although nose and mouth are outside). Risk of umbilical cord compression between the fetal body and the maternal pelvis.	Emergency, often unexpected complication. Diagnosis made when newborn's head delivers without delivery of neck and remaining body structures. Anticipate cesarean birth if no success in dislodging shoulders. Primary risk factors, including suspected infant macrosomia (weight > 4,500 g), maternal diabetes mellitus, excessive maternal weight gain, abnormal maternal pelvic anatomy, maternal obesity, postdated pregnancy, short stature, a history of previous shoulder dystocia, and use of epidural analgesia	If anticipated, preparatory tasks instituted: alerting of key personnel; education of woman and family regarding steps to be taken in the event of a difficult birth; emptying of woman's bladder to allow additional room for possible maneuvers needed for the birth. McRoberts maneuver. Suprapubic pressure (not fundal) (Fig. 21.1). Combination of maneuvers effective in more than 50% of cases of shoulder dystocia Newborn resuscitation team readily available.	Intervene immediately due to cord compression. Perform McRoberts maneuver and application of suprapubic pressure. Assist with positioning the woman in squatting position, hands-and-knees position, or lateral recumbent position for birth to free shoulder. Clear room of unnecessary clutter to make room for additional personnel and equipment. After the birth, assess newborn for crepitus, deformity, Erb palsy, or bruising, which might suggest neurologic damage or a fracture.
Multiple pregnancy	More than one fetus, leading to uterine overdistention and possibly resulting in hypotonic contractions and abnormal presentations of the fetuses.	Nearly all multiples are now diagnosed early by ultrasound. Most women go into labor before 37 wks.	Admission to facility with specialized care unit if woman goes into labor. Spontaneous progression of labor if woman has no complicating factors and first fetus is in longitudinal lie. Separate monitoring of each FHR during labor and birth.	Assess for hypotonic labor pattern due to overdistention. Evaluate for fetal presentation, maternal pelvic size, and gestational age to determine mode of delivery. Ensure presence of neonatal team for birth of multiples.

	Fetal hypoxia during labor is a significant threat due to placenta providing oxygen and nutrients to more than one fetus.		After birth of first fetus, clamping of cord and lie of the second twin assessed. Possible external cephalic version necessary to assist in providing a longitudinal lie. Second and subsequent fetuses at greater risk for birth-related complications, such as umbilical cord prolapse, malpresentation, and abruptio placentae. Cesarean birth if risk factors high.	Anticipate need for cesarean birth, which is common in multifetal pregnancy.
Excessive fetal size and abnormalities	Macrosomia leading to fetopelvic disproportion (fetus unable to fit through the maternal pelvis to be born vaginally). Reduced contraction strength due to overdistention by large fetus leading to a prolonged labor and the potential for birth injury and trauma. Fetal abnormalities possibly interfering with fetal descent, leading to prolonged labor and difficult birth.	A diagnosis of fetal macrosomia can be confirmed by measuring the birth weight after birth. Suspicion of macrosomia based on the findings of an ultrasound examination before onset of labor (if suspected due to conditions such as maternal diabetes or obesity, estimation of fetal weight via ultrasound). Leopold maneuvers to estimate fetal weight and position on admission to labor and birth unit.	Scheduled cesarean birth if diagnosis is made before the onset of labor to reduce the risk of injury to both the newborn and the mother. If identified by Leopold maneuvers, possible trial of labor to evaluate progress; however, providers usually opt to proceed with a cesarean birth in a primigravida with a macrosomic fetus.	Anticipate need for vacuum and forceps-assisted births (common). Plan for cesarean birth if maternal parameters are inadequate to give birth to large fetus.
Problems with the Passageway	Contraction of one or more of the three planes of the pelvis. Poorer prognosis for vaginal birth in women with android and platypelloid types of pelvis. Contracted pelvis involving reduction in one or more of the pelvic diameters interfering with progress of labor: inlet, midpelvis, and outlet contracture.	Shortest A-P diameter <10 cm or greatest transverse diameter <12 cm. (Approximation of A-P diameter via measurement of diagonal conjugate, which in the contracted pelvis is <11.5 cm.) X-ray pelvimetry to determine the smallest A-P diameter through which the fetal head must pass.	Focus on allowing natural forces of labor contractions to push the largest diameter (biparietal) of the fetal head beyond the obstruction or narrow passage. Possible forceps and vacuum extraction to assist navigation through this passageway.	Assess for poor contractions, slow dilation, prolonged labor. Evaluate bowel and bladder status to reduce soft tissue obstruction and allow increased pelvic space. Anticipate trial of labor; if no labor progression after an adequate trial, plan for cesarean birth.

(continued)

TABLE 21.1 DIAGNOSIS AND MANAGEMENT OF COMMON PROBLEMS ASSOCIATED WITH DYSTOCIA (continued)

	Description	Diagnosis	Therapeutic Management	Nursing Management
	Obstruction in the birth canal, such as placenta previa that partially or completely obstructs the internal os of the cervix, fibroids in the lower uterine segment, a full bladder or rectum, an edematous cervix caused by premature bearing-down efforts, and human papillomavirus (HPV) warts.	Interischial tuberous diameter of <8 cm possibly compromising outlet contracture (outlet and midpelvic contractures frequently occur together).		
Problems with the Psyche	Release of stress-related hormones (catecholamines, cortisol, epinephrine, beta-endorphin), which act on smooth muscle (uterus) and reduce uterine contractility. Excessive release of catecholamines and other stress-related hormones not therapeutic. Release also results in decreased uteroplacental perfusion and increased risk for poor newborn adjustment.	Ruling out of other possible causes of dystocia	Treatment dependent on woman's responses such as anxiety, fear, anger, frustration, or denial (highly variable due to woman's understanding of the condition itself, past experiences, previous coping mechanisms, and the amount of family and nursing support received). Appropriate medical or surgical interventions depending on the underlying condition.	Provide comfortable environment—dim lighting, music. Encourage partner to participate. Provide pain management to reduce anxiety and stress. Ensure continuous presence of staff to allay anxiety. Provide frequent updates concerning fetal status and progress. Provide ongoing encouragement to minimize the woman's stress and help her to cope with labor and to promote a positive, timely outcome. Assist in relaxation and comfort measures to help her body work more effectively with the forces of labor. Engage the woman in conversation about her emotional well-being; offer anticipatory guidance and reassurance to increase her self-esteem and ability to cope, decrease frustration, and encourage cooperation.

Adapted from American Academy of Pediatrics. (2015). *Delivery by cesarean section.* Retrieved from https://www.healthychildren.org/English/ages-stages/prenatal/delivery-beyond/Pages/Delivery-by-Cesarean-Section.aspx; Caughey, A. B., & Butler, J. R. (2015). Postterm pregnancy. *eMedicine.* Retrieved from http://emedicine.medscape.com/article/261369-overview; Cunningham, F. G., Leveno, K. J., Bloom, S. L., Spong, C. Y., Dashe, J., Hoffman, B. L., et al. (2014). *Williams' obstetrics* (24th ed.). New York, NY: McGraw-Hill; Fischer, R. (2015). Breech presentation. *eMedicine.* Retrieved from http://emedicine.medscape.com/article/262159-overview; Joy, S., Lyon, D., & Scott, P. L. (2015). Abnormal labor. *eMedicine.* Retrieved from http://emedicine.medscape.com/article/273053-overview; and King, T. L., Brucker, M. C., Kriebs, J. M., Fahey, J. O., Gegor, C. L., & Varney, H. (2015). *Varney's midwifery* (5th ed.). Burlington, MA: Jones & Bartlett Learning.

Persistent occiput posterior is the most common malposition, occurring in about 15% of laboring women. The reasons for this malposition are often unclear. This position presents slightly larger diameters to the maternal pelvis, thus slowing fetal descent. A fetal head that is poorly flexed may be responsible. In addition, poor uterine contractions may not push the fetal head down into the pelvic floor to the extent that the fetal occiput sinks into it rather than being pushed to rotate in an anterior direction.

Face and brow presentations are rare and are associated with fetal abnormalities (anencephaly), pelvic contractures, high parity, placenta previa, hydramnios, low birth weight, or a large fetus (World Health Organization [WHO], 2014a).

By 35 to 36 weeks' gestation, the majority of fetuses will spontaneously settle into the vertex presentation (head down, toward the birth canal). In about 3% to 4% of cases, however, the fetus will remain in a breech presentation with the buttocks or feet presenting. There is less risk to the fetus and mother when the head is down at the time of birth. This presentation frequently is associated with multifetal or multiple pregnancies, grand multiparity (more than five births), pregnancy over age 35 (advanced maternal age), placenta previa, hydramnios, preterm births, uterine malformations or fibroids, a scarred uterus, a female infant, and fetal anomalies such as hydrocephaly (Sharshiner & Silver, 2015). In a persistent breech presentation, an increased frequency of prolapsed cord, placenta previa, low birth weight from preterm birth, fetal or uterine anomalies, and perinatal morbidity and mortality from a difficult birth may occur (Cunningham et al., 2014). A breech presentation may be an indicator for subtle fetal abnormalities, as apparently healthy breech infants have on average poorer long-term neurodevelopmental scores than cephalic infants (Hofmeyr, 2015). Perinatal mortality is increased two- to fourfold with a breech presentation, regardless of the mode of delivery.

External cephalic version refers to a procedure in which the fetus is rotated from the breech to the cephalic presentation by manipulation through the mother's abdominal wall at or near term. Several national organizations (ACOG, WHO, AFP), recommend that this maneuver be offered to women between 36 and 38 weeks' gestation. It is performed only in a hospital setting under direct ultrasound guidance and continuous fetal monitoring. External cephalic version is successful in approximately 50% of cases. Women with a breech presentation today are often advised to have a surgical birth with no attempt to rotate the fetal position (Hofmeyr, Kulier, & West, 2015).

Shoulder dystocia is defined as the obstruction of fetal descent and birth by the axis of the fetal shoulders after the fetal head has been delivered. The incidence of shoulder dystocia is increasing due to increasing birth weight, with reports of it in up to 2% of vaginal births. It is an obstetric emergency that requires a coordinated team response, as there is no reliable way to predict it, and thus decrease the rate at which adverse outcomes occur (Gherman, 2015). It is one of the most anxiety-provoking emergencies encountered in labor. Failure of the shoulders to deliver spontaneously places both the woman and the fetus at risk for injury. Postpartum hemorrhage, secondary to uterine atony, vaginal lacerations, anal tears, and uterine rupture are major complications to the mother. Transient Erb or Duchenne brachial plexus palsies and clavicular or humeral fractures are the most common fetal injuries encountered with shoulder dystocia. The occurrence of neonatal brachial plexus palsy in the United States is 1.5 per 1,000 live births, with about one third suffering permanent upper extremity functional insufficiencies (Mehlman, 2015). Newborns experiencing shoulder dystocia typically have greater shoulder-to-head and chest-to-head disproportions compared with those delivered without dystocia (Cunningham et al., 2014). Prompt recognition and appropriate management, such as with McRoberts maneuver or suprapubic pressure, can reduce the severity of injuries to the mother and newborn (Fig. 21.1).

Take Note!

Prompt recognition and appropriate management of shoulder dystocia can reduce the severity of injuries to the mother and infant. Immediately assess the infant for signs of trauma such as a fractured clavicle, Erb palsy, or neonatal asphyxia. Assess the mother for excessive vaginal bleeding and blood in the urine from bladder trauma.

Multiple or multifetal gestation refers to twins, triplets, or more infants within a single pregnancy (Box 21.1). The incidence is increasing, primarily as a result of infertility treatment (both ovarian stimulation and in vitro fertilization) and an increased number of women giving birth at older ages. The incidence of twins, triples, and higher-order multiple gestations have now reached approximately 3% of all pregnancies (March of Dimes, 2015a). The incidence of twins is approximately 1 in 30 conceptions, with about two thirds of them due to the fertilization of two ova (dizygotic or fraternal) and about one third occurring from the splitting of one fertilized ovum (monozygotic or identical twins). One in approximately 8,100 pregnancies results in triplets (March of Dimes, 2015a). The most common maternal complication is postpartum hemorrhage resulting from uterine atony. Compared with singletons (one fetus), the risk of perinatal morbidity and mortality is markedly increased in multiple gestations. Based on recent level 1 evidence from a randomized controlled study, it was found that there was no difference in newborn outcomes between a planned surgical birth versus a planned vaginal birth for twins between 32 to 39 weeks' gestation. As long as

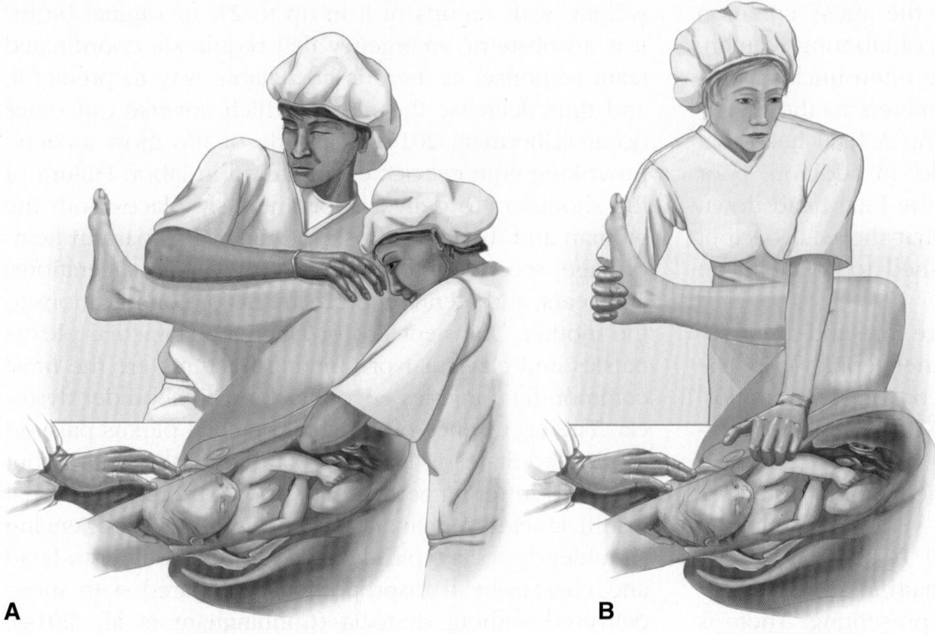

FIGURE 21.1 Maneuvers to relieve shoulder dystocia. **A.** McRoberts maneuver. The mother's thighs are flexed and abducted as much as possible to straighten the pelvic curve. **B.** Suprapubic pressure. Light pressure is applied just above the pubic bone, pushing the fetal anterior shoulder downward to displace it from above the mother's symphysis pubis. The newborn's head is depressed toward the mother's anus while light suprapubic pressure is applied.

BOX 21.1

MULTIPLE PREGNANCY

As the name implies, a multiple pregnancy or a multifetal pregnancy involves more than one fetus. These fetuses can result from fertilization of a single ovum or multiple ova. Monozygotic (identical) twins develop from one single ovum that divides into equal halves during early cleavage phase. Monozygotic twins are genetically identical; always the same gender, and look very similar in appearance. The number of amnions and chorions depends on the timing of division (cleavage). One fertilized ovum splitting into two separate individuals is termed *natural clones*. This type of twinning occurs in approximately 1 of 250 live births (March of Dimes, 2015a).

Twin pregnancies that are multiple-ova conceptions (dizygotic twins) result from two ova fertilized by two sperm. They are referred to as fraternal twins. Genetically, dizygotic twins are as alike (or unlike) as any other pair or siblings. There are separate amnions and chorions although the chorions and placentas may be fused. The incidence of dizygotic twinning is approximately 1 in 500 Asians, 1 in 125 Whites, and as high as 1 in 20 in African populations (March of Dimes, 2015a). Fraternal twins account for two thirds of all twins and there is a tendency to repeat within families. Currently the incidence of fraternal twins is increasing secondary to advancing maternal age when pregnancy occurs and an increase in use of fertility drugs and procedures being done.

Multiple births other than twins can be of the identical type, the fraternal type, or combinations of the two. Triplets can occur from the division of one zygote into two, with one dividing again, producing identical triplets, or they can come from two zygotes, one dividing into a set of identical twins, and the second zygote developing as a single fraternal sibling, or from three separate zygotes. Triplets are said to occur once in 7,000 births and quadruplets once in 660,000 births (March of Dimes, 2015a). In recent years, fertility drugs used to induce ovulation have resulted in a greater frequency of quadruplets, quintuplets, sextuplets, and even octuplets.

the presenting twin is vertex, a vaginal birth should be considered (Bibbo & Robinson, 2015).

Excessive fetal size and abnormalities can also contribute to labor and birth dysfunctions. Macrosomia, in which a newborn weighs 4,000 to 4,500 g (8.81 to 9.92 lb) or more at birth, complicates approximately 10% of all pregnancies. It is the result of a change in body composition in the neonate with an increase in both percentage of fat and fat mass. Macrosomia is associated with later life obesity, diabetes, and cardiovascular disease (Jazayeri, 2015). Fetal abnormalities may include hydrocephalus, ascites, or a large mass on the neck or head. Complications associated with dystocia related to excessive fetal size and anomalies include an increased risk for postpartum hemorrhage, shoulder dystocia, low Apgar scores, dysfunctional labor, fetopelvic disproportion, soft tissue laceration during vaginal birth, fetal injuries or fractures, and perinatal asphyxia (Hobbins, 2015).

Problems with the Passageway

Problems with the passageway (pelvis and birth canal) are related to a contraction of one or more of the three planes of the maternal pelvis: inlet, midpelvis, and outlet. The female pelvis can be classified into four types based on the shape of the pelvic inlet, which is bounded anteriorly by the posterior border of the symphysis pubis, posteriorly by the sacral promontory, and laterally by the linea terminalis. The four basic types are gynecoid, anthropoid, android, and platypelloid (see Chapter 12 for additional information). Contraction of the midpelvis is more common than inlet contraction and typically causes an arrest of fetal descent. Obstructions in the maternal birth canal, such as swelling of the soft maternal tissue and cervix, termed soft tissue dystocia, also can hamper fetal descent and impede labor progression outside the maternal bony pelvis.

Problems with the Psyche

Many women experience an array of emotions during labor, which may include fear, anxiety, helplessness, isolation, and weariness. These emotions can lead to psychological stress, which indirectly can cause dystocia. Hormones released in response to anxiety can cause dystocia. Intense anxiety stimulates the sympathetic nervous system, which releases catecholamines that can lead to myometrial dysfunction. Norepinephrine and epinephrine then lead to uncoordinated or increased uterine activity (Cheng & Caughey, 2015).

Nursing Assessment

Begin the assessment by reviewing the client's history to look for risk factors for dystocia which may include maternal short stature, obesity, hydramnios, uterine abnormalities, fetal malpresentation, cephalopelvic disproportion, over stimulation with oxytocin, maternal exhaustion, ineffective pushing, excessive size fetus, poor maternal positioning in labor, and maternal anxiety and fear (Green, 2016). Include in the assessment the mother's frame of mind to identify fear, anxiety, stress, lack of support, and pain, which can interfere with uterine contractions and impede labor progress. Helping the woman to relax will promote normal labor progress.

Assess the woman's vital signs. Note any elevation in temperature (might suggest an infection) or changes in heart rate or blood pressure (might signal hypovolemia). Evaluate the uterine contractions for frequency and intensity. Question the woman about any changes in her contraction pattern, such as a decrease or increase in frequency or intensity, and report these. Assess FHR and pattern, reporting any abnormal patterns immediately.

Assess fetal position via *Leopold maneuvers* (see Chapter 14 for more information) to identify any deviations in presentation or position, and report any deviations. Assist with or perform a vaginal examination to determine cervical dilation, effacement, and engagement of the fetal presenting part. Evaluate for evidence of membrane rupture. Report any malodorous fluid.

Nursing Management

Nursing management of the woman with dystocia, regardless of the etiology, requires patience. The nurse should provide physical and emotional support to the client and her family. The final outcome of any labor depends on the size and shape of the maternal pelvis, the quality of the uterine contractions, and the size, presentation, and position of the fetus. Thus, dystocia is diagnosed after labor has progressed for a time, not at the beginning of labor.

PROMOTING THE PROGRESS OF LABOR

The nurse plays a major role in determining the progress of labor. Continue to assess the woman, frequently monitoring cervical dilation and effacement, uterine contractions, and fetal descent, and document that all assessed parameters are progressing. Evaluate progress in active labor by using the simple rule of 1 cm per hour for cervical dilation. When the woman's membranes rupture, if they have not already ruptured, observe for visible cord prolapse.

Take Note!

If a dysfunctional labor occurs, contractions will slow or fail to advance in frequency, duration, or intensity; the cervix will fail to respond to uterine contractions by dilating and effacing; and the fetus will fail to descend.

Throughout labor, assess the woman's fluid balance status. Check skin turgor and mucous membranes. Monitor intake and output. Also monitor the client's bladder for distention at least every 2 hours and encourage her to empty her bladder often. In addition, monitor her bowel status. A full bladder or rectum can impede descent.

Continue to monitor fetal well-being. If the fetus is in the breech position, be especially observant for visible cord prolapse and note any variable decelerations in heart rate. If either occurs, report it immediately.

Be prepared to administer a labor stimulant such as oxytocin (Pitocin) if ordered to treat hypotonic labor contractions. Anticipate the need to assist with manipulations if shoulder dystocia is diagnosed. Prepare the woman and her family for the possibility of a cesarean birth if labor does not progress.

PROVIDING PHYSICAL AND EMOTIONAL COMFORT

Employ physical comfort measures to promote relaxation and reduce stress. Offer blankets for warmth and a backrub, if the client wishes, to reduce muscle tension. Provide an environment conducive to rest so the woman can conserve her energy. Lower the lights and reduce external noise by closing the hallway door. Offer a warm shower to promote relaxation (if not contraindicated). Use pillows to support the woman in a comfortable position, changing her position every 30 minutes to reduce tension and to enhance uterine activity and efficiency. Offer her fluids/food as appropriate to moisten her mouth and replenish her energy (Fig. 21.2).

Assist with providing counter pressure along with backrubs if the fetus is in the occiput posterior position. Encourage the woman to assume different positions to promote fetal rotation. Upright positions are helpful in facilitating fetal rotation and descent. Also encourage the woman to visualize the descent and birth of the fetus.

Assess the woman's level of pain and degree of distress. Administer analgesics as ordered or according to the facility's protocol. Evaluate the mother's level of fatigue throughout labor, such as verbal expressions of

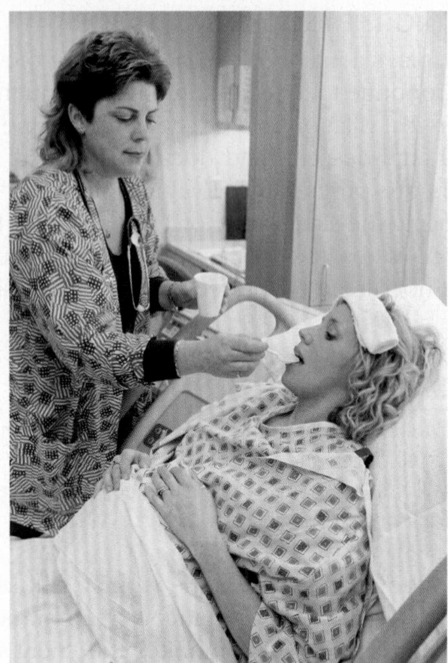

FIGURE 21.2 The nurse applies a cool, moist washcloth to the client's forehead and offers her ice chips to combat thirst and provide comfort to the woman experiencing dystocia.

feeling exhausted, inability to cope in early labor, or inability to rest or calm down between contractions. Praise the woman and her partner for their efforts. Provide empathetic listening to increase the client's coping ability, and remain with the client to demonstrate caring.

PROMOTING EMPOWERMENT

Educate the client and family about dysfunctional labor and its causes and therapies. Explain therapeutic interventions that may be needed to assist with the labor process. Encourage the client and her partner to participate in decision making about interventions.

Assist the woman and partner in expressing their fears and anxieties. Provide encouragement to help them to maintain control. Support the client and her partner in their coping efforts. Keep the woman and her partner informed of progress and advocate for them.

ALTERNATIVE/NONTRADITIONAL FAMILIES

There is a growing awareness of nontraditional families in the world. If one considers family forms cross-nationally, a variety of configurations exists. This awareness requires nurses to shift away from heterosexist thinking in caring for the childbearing family. Nurses must be adequately educated about lesbian-gay-bisexual-transgender-queer (LGBTQ) health issues to be empathetic and conscious of the needs of this population. With increasing numbers of LGBTQ couples getting married, and availability of alternative methods of conception, these couples are coming in contact with nurses through the birthing process. LGBTQ couples may face making complex childbearing decisions, navigating a health care system designed for heterosexual couples and confronting barriers such as insurance issues, nonaccepting negative attitudes by health care workers and uncertain legal rights (Holley & Pasch, 2015).

LGBTQ individuals are not a homogenous group and they are shaped by a range of factors including race, sexual orientation, ethnicity, socioeconomic status, and age. This community has been previously marginalized in society. Nurses caring for LGBTQ clients need to allow them to have their own identity, values, and beliefs. Every client should be treated with the kindness, with an individualized approach and be an advocate for their needs. Nurses need to consider the following when they are caring for the childbearing LGBTQ family by using appropriate language/identification and cultural representation by asking how they wish to be identified; and by personalizing their care that includes all intersecting aspects of their identity (Westwood et al., 2015).

PRETERM LABOR

Preterm labor is defined as the occurrence of regular uterine contractions accompanied by cervical effacement and dilation before the end of the 37th week of gestation. If not halted, it leads to preterm birth. Preterm births remain one of the biggest contributors to perinatal morbidity and mortality in the world. According to the March of Dimes (2015b), about 12% of births (one in eight infants) in the United States are premature.

Preterm birth is one of the most common obstetric complications, and its sequelae have a profound effect on the survival and health of the newborn. The rate of preterm births in the United States has increased 35% in the past 20 years. Preterm births account for 75% of neurodevelopmental disorders and other serious morbidities, as well as behavioral and social problems. They account for 85% of all perinatal morbidity and mortality. In addition, up to $30 billion is spent on maternal and infant care related to prematurity annually (March of Dimes, 2015b). Infants born prematurely also are at risk for serious sequelae such as respiratory distress syndrome, infections, congenital heart defects, thermoregulation problems that can lead to acidosis and weight loss, intraventricular hemorrhage, jaundice, hypoglycemia, feeding difficulties resulting from diminished stomach capacity and an underdeveloped suck reflex, and neurologic disorders related to hypoxia and trauma at birth. Many will face the prospect of numerous lifelong disabilities, such as cerebral palsy, intellectual impairment, vision defects, and hearing loss. A recent study's findings indicated that a single course of corticosteroids prenatally improved most neonate's neurodevelopmental outcomes if given before 34 weeks' gestation (Sotiriadis et al., 2015). Although great strides have been made in neonatal intensive care, prematurity remains the leading cause of death within the first month of life and is the second leading cause of all infant deaths (March of Dimes, 2015b). The exact cause of preterm labor is not known. Currently, prevention is the goal.

Therapeutic Management

Predicting the risk of preterm labor is valuable only if there is an available intervention that is likely to improve the situation. According to ACOG, many factors must be considered before selecting an intervention. Many factors influence the decision to intervene when women present with symptoms of preterm labor, including the probability of progressive labor, gestational age, and the risks of treatment. ACOG (2014b) recommends the following as guidelines:

- There are no clear first-line **tocolytic** drugs (drugs that promote uterine relaxation by interfering with uterine contractions) to manage preterm labor, and the results of research on their efficacy are mixed. Clinical circumstances and the health care provider's preference should dictate treatment.
- Antibiotics do not appear to prolong gestation and should be reserved for group B streptococcal prophylaxis in women in whom birth is imminent.
- Tocolytic drugs may prolong pregnancy for 2 to 7 days; during this time, steroids can be given to improve fetal lung maturity and the woman can be transported to a tertiary care center.
- A single course of corticosteroids is recommended for all pregnant women between 24 and 34 weeks of gestation who are at risk of preterm birth within 7 days. Prenatal corticosteroids significantly reduce the incidence and severity of neonatal respiratory distress syndrome.

With these recommendations, health care providers continue to prescribe pharmacologic treatment for preterm labor at home and in the hospital setting. This treatment often includes oral or intravenous tocolytics and varying degrees of activity restriction (Fig. 21.3). Antibiotics may also be prescribed to treat presumed or confirmed infections. Steroids may be given to enhance fetal lung maturity between 24 and 34 weeks' gestation.

Tocolytic Therapy

The decision to stop preterm labor is individualized based on risk factors, extent of cervical dilation, membrane status, fetal gestational age, and presence or absence of infection. Tocolytic therapy is most likely ordered if preterm labor occurs before the 34th week of gestation in an attempt to delay birth and thereby to reduce the severity of respiratory distress syndrome and other complications associated with prematurity. Tocolytic therapy does not typically prevent preterm birth, but it may delay it. It is contraindicated for abruptio placentae, acute fetal distress or death, eclampsia or severe preeclampsia, active vaginal bleeding, dilation of more than 6 cm, chorioamnionitis, and maternal hemodynamic instability (Locatelli, Consonni, & Ghidini, 2015).

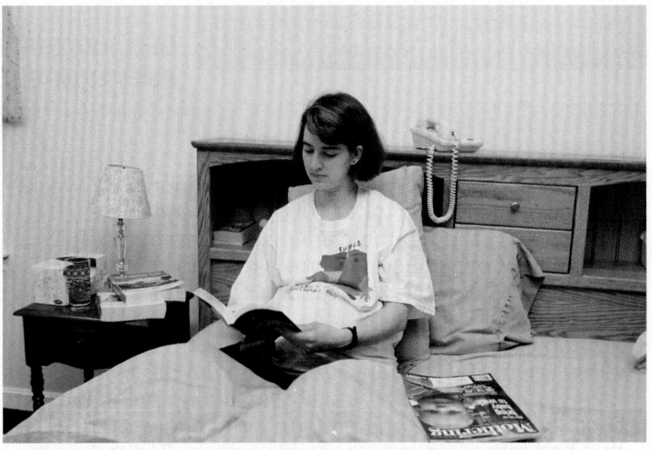

FIGURE 21.3 The mother with preterm labor resting in bed at home.

Medications commonly used for tocolysis include magnesium sulfate (which reduces the muscle's ability to contract), indomethacin (Indocin, a prostaglandin synthetase inhibitor), atosiban (Tractocile, Antocin, an oxytocin receptor antagonist), and nifedipine (Procardia, a calcium channel blocker). (Evidence-Based Practice box 21.1). These drugs are used "off label," which means that they are effective for this purpose but have not been officially tested and developed for this purpose by the U.S. Food and Drug administration (FDA) (Haas et al., 2014). In a recent Cochrane review study, calcium channel blockers were found to be better in preventing preterm labor when compared to beta-mimetics (Flenady et al., 2014). All of these medications have serious side effects, and the woman needs close supervision when they are being administered (Drug Guide 21.1).

Corticosteroids

Corticosteroids given to the mother in preterm labor can help prevent or reduce the frequency and severity of respiratory distress syndrome in premature infants delivered between 24 and 34 weeks' gestation. The beneficial effects of corticosteroids on fetal lung maturation have been reported within 48 hours of initial administration. A recent Cochrane review found that corticosteroids repeatedly administered to the woman in preterm labor provided short-term benefits to the preterm infant of less respiratory distress and fewer serious health problems in the first few weeks after birth. They supported the use of repeat dose(s) of

EVIDENCE-BASED PRACTICE 21.1 BED REST IN SINGLETON PREGNANCIES FOR PREVENTING PRETERM BIRTH

STUDY

Preterm birth, defined a birth occurring prior to 37 weeks of gestation occurs in up to 10% of all pregnancies worldwide. Although there are many different therapies available for preventing preterm birth, very few are proven to be effective and recommended for clinical use. One therapy, bed rest, has been traditionally been recommended for preventing preterm birth as a first step in treatment. This therapy is based on the observation that hard work and hard physical activity during pregnancy could be associated with preterm birth, and with the idea that bed rest could reduce uterine activity. Bed rest does have adverse effects such as increasing the incidence of venous thrombosis, muscle atrophy, and cardiovascular deconditioning. The purpose of this study was to evaluate the effect of bed rest in the hospital or at home for preventing preterm birth.

Findings

Randomized, cluster-randomized and quasi-randomized control studies were sought. Two studies met the inclusion criteria with 1,266 women participating. There was no evidence found to support or refute the use of bed rest at home or in the hospital to prevent preterm birth. Due to the potential adverse effects that bed rest can have on women, it is suggested that health care providers discuss this intervention thoroughly with their clients. Additional research is needed.

Nursing Implications

Although the study did not reveal results that were statistically significant, nurses need to be aware of the potential benefits and limitations associated with bed rest employed to delay a preterm birth so that they can provide women and their families with the most appropriate information about options to prolonged pregnancy. Potential benefits and harms should be discussed with women facing an increased risk of preterm birth. Nurses can integrate information from this study in their teaching about the risks associated with preterm labor and births. They can also use this information to help answer couple's questions about interventions currently used and their effectiveness as well as provide anticipatory guidance about the procedure. Doing so fosters empowerment of the woman and her family, promoting optimal informed decision making.

Adapted from Sosa, C. G., Althabe, F., Belizan, J. M., & Bergel, E. (2015). Bed rest in singleton pregnancies for preventing preterm birth. *Cochrane Database of Systematic Reviews*, (3), doi:10.1002/14651858.CD003581.pub3

DRUG GUIDE 21.1 MEDICATIONS USED WITH PRETERM LABOR

Drug	Action/Indication	Nursing Implications
Magnesium sulfate	Relaxes uterine muscles to stop irritability and contractions, to arrest uterine contractions for preterm labor (off-label use). Has been used in seizure prophylaxis and treatment of seizures in preeclamptic and eclamptic clients for almost 100 yrs	Administer IV with a loading dose of 4–6 g over 15–30 min initially, and then maintain infusion at 1–4 g/hr. Assess vital signs and deep tendon reflexes (DTRs) hourly; report any hypotension or depressed or absent DTRs. Monitor level of consciousness; report any headache, blurred vision, dizziness, or altered level of consciousness. Perform continuous electronic fetal monitoring; report any decreased FHR variability, hypotonia, or respiratory depression. Monitor intake and output hourly; report any decrease in output (<30 mL/hr). Assess respiratory rate; report respiratory rate <12 breaths/min; auscultate lung sounds for evidence of pulmonary edema. Monitor for common maternal side effects, including flushing, nausea and vomiting, dry mouth, lethargy, blurred vision, and headache. Assess for nausea, vomiting, transient hypotension, lethargy. Assess for signs and symptoms of magnesium toxicity, such as decreased level of consciousness, depressed respirations and DTRs, slurred speech, weakness, and respiratory and/or cardiac arrest. Have calcium gluconate readily available at the bedside to reverse magnesium toxicity.

DRUG GUIDE 21.1 MEDICATIONS USED WITH PRETERM LABOR (continued)

Drug	Action/Indication	Nursing Implications
Indomethacin (Indocin)	Inhibits prostaglandins, which stimulate contractions; inhibits uterine activity to arrest preterm labor	Continuously assess vital signs, uterine activity, and FHR. Administer oral form with food to reduce GI irritation. Do not give to women with peptic ulcer disease. Schedule ultrasound to assess amniotic fluid volume and function of ductus arteriosus before initiating therapy; monitor for signs of maternal hemorrhage. Be alert for maternal adverse effects such as nausea and vomiting, heartburn, rash, prolonged bleeding time, oligohydramnios, and hypertension. Monitor for neonatal adverse effects, including constriction of ductus arteriosus, premature ductus closure, necrotizing enterocolitis, oligohydramnios, and pulmonary hypertension. Contraindicated in >32 weeks' gestations, fetal growth restriction, history of asthma, urticaria, or allergic type reactions to aspirin or NSAIDs.
Nifedipine (Procardia)	Blocks calcium movement into muscle cells, inhibits uterine activity to arrest preterm labor	Use caution if giving this drug with magnesium sulfate because of increased risk for hypotension. Monitor blood pressure hourly if giving with magnesium sulfate; report a pulse rate >110 bpm. Monitor for fetal effects such as decreased uteroplacental blood flow manifested by fetal bradycardia, which can lead to fetal hypoxia. Monitor for adverse effects, such as flushing of the skin, headache, transient tachycardia, palpitations, postural hypertension, peripheral edema, and transient fetal tachycardia. Contraindicated in women with cardiovascular disease or hemodynamic instability.
Betamethasone (Celestone)	Promotes fetal lung maturity by stimulating surfactant production; prevents or reduces risk of respiratory distress syndrome and intraventricular hemorrhage in the preterm neonate less than 34 wks' gestation	Administer two doses intramuscularly 24 hr apart. Monitor for maternal infection or pulmonary edema. Educate parents about potential benefits of drug to preterm infant. Assess maternal lung sounds and monitor for signs of infection.

Adapted from Chandrasekaran, S., & Srinivas, S. K. (2014). Antenatal corticosteroid administration: Understanding its use as an obstetric quality metric. *American Journal of Obstetrics and Gynecology, 210*(2), 143–150; Jørgensen, J. S., Weile, L. K. K., & Lamont, R. F. (2014). Preterm labor: Current tocolytic options for the treatment of preterm labor. *Expert Opinion on Pharmacotherapy, 15*(5), 585–588; and King, T. L., Brucker, M. C., Kriebs, J. M., Fahey, J. O., Gegor, C. L., & Varney, H. (2015). *Varney's midwifery* (5th ed.). Burlington, MA: Jones & Bartlett Learning.

prenatal corticosteroids for women still at risk of preterm birth 7 days or more after an initial course. These benefits were associated with a small reduction in size at birth. The current available evidence reassuringly shows no significant harm in early childhood, although no benefit. Further research is needed on the long-term benefits and risks for the woman and baby. Individual client data meta-analysis may clarify how to maximize benefit and minimize harm (Cabbad et al., 2015). These drugs require at least 24 hours to become effective, so timely administration is crucial.

Nursing Assessment

The preterm birth rate cannot be reduced until there are ways to predict the risk for preterm birth. Because the etiology is often multifactorial, an individualized approach is needed.

Health History and Physical Examination

The signs of preterm labor are subtle and may be overlooked by the client as well as the health care provider. Obtain a thorough health history and be alert for risk factors associated with preterm labor and birth (Box 21.2).

Frequently, women are unaware that uterine contractions, effacement, and dilation are occurring, thus making early intervention ineffective in arresting preterm labor and preventing the birth of a premature newborn. Ask the woman about any complaints, being alert for the subtle symptoms of preterm labor, which may include:

- Change or increase in vaginal discharge with mucus, water, or blood in it
- Pelvic pressure (pushing-down sensation)
- Low, dull backache
- Menstrual-like cramps
- Urinary tract infection symptoms
- Feeling of pelvic pressure or fullness
- Gastrointestinal upset: nausea, vomiting, and diarrhea
- General sense of discomfort or unease
- Heaviness or aching in the thighs
- Uterine contractions, with or without pain
- More than six contractions per hour
- Intestinal cramping, with or without diarrhea (Jordan et al., 2014).

Assess the pattern of the contractions: the contractions must be persistent, such that four contractions occur every 20 minutes or eight contractions occur in 1 hour. Evaluate cervical dilation and effacement: cervical effacement is 80% or greater and cervical dilation is greater than 1 cm (ACOG, 2014b). On examination, engagement of the fetal presenting part will be noted.

BOX 21.2

RISK FACTORS ASSOCIATED WITH PRETERM LABOR AND BIRTH

- African-American race (double the risk)
- Maternal age extremes (<16 years and >40 years old)
- Low socioeconomic status
- Alcohol or other drug use, especially cocaine
- Poor maternal nutrition
- Maternal periodontal disease
- Cigarette smoking
- Low level of education
- History of prior preterm birth (triples the risk)
- Uterine abnormalities, such as fibroids
- Low pregnancy weight for height
- Pre-existing diabetes or hypertension
- Multiple pregnancy
- Premature rupture of membranes
- Late or no prenatal care
- Short cervical length
- Sexually transmitted infections: gonorrhea, *Chlamydia*, trichomoniasis
- Bacterial vaginosis (50% increased risk)
- Chorioamnionitis
- Hydramnios
- Gestational hypertension
- Cervical insufficiency
- Short interpregnancy interval (<1 year between births)
- Placental problems, such as placenta previa and abruption placenta
- Maternal anemia
- Urinary tract infection
- Domestic violence
- Stress, acute and chronic

Adapted from March of Dimes. (2015b). Preterm labor and birth: A serious pregnancy complication. Retrieved from http://www.marchofdimes.com/pregnancy/preterm_indepth.html

Laboratory and Diagnostic Testing

Commonly used diagnostic testing for preterm labor risk assessment includes a complete blood count to detect infection, which may be a contributing factor to preterm labor; urinalysis to detect bacteria and nitrites, which are indicative of a urinary tract infection; and an amniotic fluid analysis to determine fetal lung maturity and the presence of subclinical chorioamnionitis.

Other tests that may be used for preterm labor prediction include fetal fibronectin testing and cervical length evaluation by transvaginal ultrasound. Fetal fibronectin and cervical length examinations have a high negative predictive value and are thus better at predicting which pregnant women are unlikely to have a preterm birth as opposed to predicting those who will (van Baaren et al., 2015).

FETAL FIBRONECTIN

Fetal fibronectin, a glycoprotein produced by the chorion, is found at the junction of the chorion and decidua (fetal membranes and uterus). It acts as biologic glue, attaching the fetal sac to the uterine lining. It normally is present in cervicovaginal secretions up to 22 weeks of pregnancy and again at the end of the last trimester (1 to 3 weeks before labor). It usually cannot be detected between 24 and 34 weeks of pregnancy (5½ to 8½ months) unless there has been a disruption between the chorion and deciduas. It is present in cervicovaginal fluid prior to delivery, regardless of gestational age.

The test is a useful marker for impending membrane rupture within 7 to 14 days if the level increases to greater than 0.05 mcg/mL. The accuracy of fetal fibronectin is decreased in the presence of lubricants, blood, recent intercourse, or cervical manipulation within the previous 24 hours. Conversely, a negative fetal fibronectin test is a strong predictor that preterm labor in the next 2 weeks is unlikely (Abbott et al., 2015).

A sterile applicator is used to collect a cervicovaginal sample during an examination by speculum. The result is either positive (fetal fibronectin is present) or negative (fetal fibronectin is not present). Interpretation of fetal fibronectin results must always be viewed in conjunction with the clinical findings; it is not used as a lone indicator for predicting preterm labor. The primary importance of cervicovaginal fetal fibronectin lies in the high negative predictive values of the test for reducing preterm birth risk. Fibronectin testing can be a useful tool in the triaging of women symptomatic for preterm labor.

CERVICAL LENGTH MEASUREMENT

Transvaginal ultrasound of the cervix has been used as a tool to predict preterm labor in high-risk pregnancies and to differentiate between true and false preterm labor. Three parameters are evaluated during the transvaginal ultrasound: cervical length and width, funnel width and length, and percentage of funneling. Measurement of the closed portion of the cervix visualized during the transvaginal ultrasound is the single most reliable parameter for prediction of preterm delivery in high-risk women (van Baaren et al., 2014).

Cervical length varies during pregnancy and can be measured fairly reliably after 16 weeks' gestation using an ultrasound probe inserted in the vagina. A cervical length of 3 cm or more indicates that delivery within 14 days is unlikely. Women with a short cervical length of 2.5 cm during the mid trimester have a substantially greater risk of preterm birth prior to 35 weeks' gestation. As with fetal fibronectin testing, negative results can be reassuring and prevent unnecessary interventions (Souka et al., 2015).

Nursing Management

Nurses play a key role in reducing preterm labor and births to improve pregnancy outcomes for both mothers and their infants. Early detection of preterm labor is currently the best strategy to improve outcomes. Because of the numerous factors associated with preterm labor, it is challenging to identify and address all of them, especially when women experiencing contractions are frequently falsely reassured and not assessed thoroughly to determine the cause. This delay impedes initiation of interventions to reduce infant death and morbidity.

Preterm birth prevention programs for women at high risk have used self-monitoring of symptoms and patterns, weekly cervical examinations, clinical markers, telephone monitoring, home visiting, alone or in combination, with disappointing results. Preterm labor is currently thought to be a chronic, long-term multifactorial process with a genetic component. A recent study found a multiple pregnancy, prior preterm birth, low socioeconomic status, maternal medical disorders, and maternal infections were statistically significant risk factors for predicting spontaneous preterm labor (Patel, Pitre, & Bhooker, 2015). Despite technologic and pharmacologic advances in the identification and treatment of preterm labor, the incidence remains high and is growing in the United States.

Supportive nursing care is needed for the woman in preterm labor whether the contractions are stopped with tocolytic therapy or not. Nursing tasks include monitoring vital signs, measuring intake and output, encouraging bed rest on the woman's left side to enhance placental perfusion, monitoring the FHR via an external monitor continuously, limiting vaginal examinations to prevent an ascending infection, and monitoring the mother and fetus closely for any adverse effects from the tocolytic agents. Offering the couple ongoing explanations will help prepare them for the birth.

Administering Tocolytic Therapy

Tocolysis is the use of drugs to inhibit uterine contractions. The primary goals of tocolytic therapy are to arrest labor and delay birth long enough to initiate prophylactic corticosteroid therapy when indicated for stimulation of fetal lung maturity and to arrange for maternal-fetal transport to a perinatal tertiary care hospital. A firm diagnosis of preterm labor is necessary before treatment is considered. Diagnosis requires the presence of both uterine contractions and cervical change (or an initial cervical examination of more than 2 cm and/or more than 80% effacement in a nulliparous client). A cause for preterm labor should always be sought.

Absolute contraindications to administering tocolytic agents to stop labor include intrauterine infection, active hemorrhage, fetal distress, fetus before viability, fetal abnormality incompatible with life, fetal growth restriction, severe preeclampsia, heart disease, prolonged premature rupture of the membranes (PPROM), and intrauterine demise (Callahan, 2016). Bed rest and hydration are commonly recommended, but without proven efficacy.

Prevention of preterm labor remains an elusive goal. Presently, women at high risk for preterm labor are offered progesterone therapy at the start of their second trimester. Although progesterone therapy is recommended by ACOG, it has not been FDA approved for this purpose and has mixed results (Iams, 2015).

Magnesium sulfate may be ordered. This agent acts as a physiologic calcium antagonist and a general inhibitor of neurotransmission. Expect to administer it intravenously. Monitor the woman for nausea, vomiting, headache, weakness, hypotension, and cardiopulmonary arrest. Frequent monitoring of maternal respiratory effort and deep tendon reflexes is essential for early recognition of overdose. Because magnesium is exclusively excreted by the kidneys, adequate renal function is essential for safe administration. Assess the fetus for decreased FHR variability, drowsiness, and hypotonia. Magnesium has a wide margin of safety, but is not any more effective in delaying preterm birth as any other tocolytic agent. However, if administered prenatally, it is effective in helping women who develop preeclampsia and helping to protect fetal brains (Nakazawa et al., 2015).

Calcium channel blockers promote uterine relaxation by decreasing the influx of calcium ions into myometrium cells to inhibit contractions. Although calcium channel blockers may be prescribed to manage preterm labor, available literature provides little evidence that they have better efficacy in treating preterm labor than any other tocolytic agent. The perfect tocolytic drug that is 100% efficacious and 100% safe does not exist yet (van den Bosch, Ruys, & Roos-Hesselink, 2015). Administer calcium channel blockers (nifedipine) orally or sublingually every 4 to 8 hours as ordered. Monitor the woman for hypotension, reflex tachycardia, headache, nausea, and facial flushing.

Prostaglandin synthetase inhibitor (indomethacin [Indocin]) reduces prostaglandin synthesis from decidual macrophages. It readily crosses the placenta and can cause oligohydramnios due to a decrease in fetal renal blood flow if used for more than 48 hours. During treatment, urine output, maternal temperature, and amniotic fluid index (AFI) should be evaluated periodically. The initial recommended dose is 50 to 100 mg orally or per rectum followed by 25 to 50 mg every 6 hours for 8 doses. Indomethacin therapy is not recommended for gestations of 32 weeks or greater (Ross, 2015).

Educating the Client

Ensure that every pregnant woman receives basic education about preterm labor, including information about harmful lifestyles, the signs of genitourinary infections and preterm labor, and the appropriate response to these symptoms. Teach the client how to palpate for and time uterine contractions. Provide written materials to support this education at a level and in a language appropriate for the client. Also educate clients about the importance of prenatal care, risk reduction, and recognizing the signs and symptoms of preterm labor. Teaching Guidelines 21.1 highlights important instructions related to preventing preterm labor.

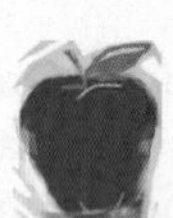

Teaching Guidelines 21.1

TEACHING TO PREVENT PRETERM LABOR

- Avoid traveling for long distances in cars, trains, planes, or buses.
- Avoid lifting heavy objects, such as laundry, groceries, or a young child.
- Avoid performing hard, physical work, such as yard work, moving of furniture, or construction.
- Mild to moderate levels of exercise are permitted such as walking daily.
- Achieve an appropriate prepregnancy weight.
- Achieve adequate iron stores through balanced nutrition.
- Wait at least 18 months between pregnancies.
- Visit a dentist in early pregnancy to evaluate and treat periodontal disease.
- Enroll in a smoking cessation program if you are unable to quit on your own.
- Curtail sexual activity until after 37 weeks if experiencing preterm labor symptoms.
- Consume a well-balanced nutritional diet to gain appropriate weight.
- Avoid the use of substances such as marijuana, cocaine, and heroin.
- Identify factors and areas of stress in your life, and use stress management techniques to reduce them.
- If you are experiencing intimate partner violence, seek resources to modify the situation.

Recognize the signs and symptoms of preterm labor and notify your birth attendant if any occur:

- Uterine contractions, cramping, or low back pain
- Feeling of pelvic pressure or fullness
- Increase in vaginal discharge
- Nausea, vomiting, and diarrhea
- Leaking of fluid from vagina

If you are experiencing any of these signs or symptoms, do the following:

- Stop what you are doing and rest for 1 hour.
- Empty your bladder.
- Lie down on your side.
- Drink two to three glasses of water.
- Feel your abdomen and make note of the hardness of the contraction. Call your health care provider and describe the contraction as:
  - Mild if it feels like the tip of the nose
  - Moderate if it feels like the tip of the chin
  - Strong if it feels like your forehead

Adapted from Jordan, R. G., Engstrom, J. L., Marfell, J. A., & Farley, C. L. (2014). *Prenatal and postnatal care: A woman-centered approach.* Ames, Iowa: John Wiley & Sons, Inc.; and Ross, M. G. (2015). Preterm labor. *eMedicine.* Retrieved from http://emedicine.medscape.com/article/260998-overview#aw2aab6b7

Explaining to the couple what is happening in terms of labor progress, the treatment regimen, and the status of the fetus is important to reduce the anxiety associated with the risk of giving birth to a preterm infant. Educate them about the importance of promotion of fetal lung maturity with corticosteroids. Include supportive family members in all education. Allow time for the woman and her family to express their concerns about the possible outcome for the infant and the possible side effects of the tocolytic therapy. Encourage them to vent any feelings, fears, and anger they may experience. Provide the woman and her family with an honest appraisal of the situation and plan of treatment throughout her care.

Providing Psychological Support

Preterm labor and birth present multifactorial challenges for everyone involved. If the woman's activities are restricted, additional stresses may be placed on the family, contributing to the crisis. Assess the stress levels of the client and family, and make appropriate referrals. Emphasize the need for more frequent supervision and office visits, and encourage clients to talk to their health care provider for reassurance.

Every case of spontaneous preterm labor is unique. Care must take into account the clinical circumstances, and the full and informed consent of the woman and her partner is needed. Half of all women who ultimately give birth prematurely have no identifiable risk factors. Nurses should be sensitive to any complaint and should provide appropriate assessment, information, and follow-up. Sensitivity to the subtle differences between normal pregnancy sensations and the prodromal symptoms of preterm labor is a key factor in ensuring timely care. Offer validation and clarification of the woman's symptoms.

If tocolytic therapy is not successful in stopping uterine contractions, support the couple through this stressful period to prepare them for the birth. Keep them informed of all progress and changes; for example, continuously monitor maternal and fetal vital signs, especially the maternal temperature to detect signs of early infection. Offer one-on-one contact and be available throughout this difficult and anxiety-producing period.

POSTTERM PREGNANCY

A term pregnancy usually lasts 38 to 42 weeks. A postterm or prolonged pregnancy is one that continues past the end of the 42nd week of gestation, or 294 days from the first day of the last menstrual period. A postterm or prolonged pregnancy is defined as a pregnancy that extends to 42 0/7 weeks and beyond. Within the United States, about 7% of singleton pregnancies extend beyond 41 weeks (Walker & Gan, 2015). Incorrect dates account for the majority of these cases: many women have irregular menses and thus cannot identify the date of their last menstrual period accurately.

Recall Jennifer described at the beginning of the chapter, who was at 41 weeks' gestation. What information would be most important to determine on admission to the facility? What interventions might the nurse anticipate when she arrives?

The exact etiology of a postterm or prolonged pregnancy is unknown because the mechanism for the initiation of labor is not completely understood. Theories suggest there may be a deficiency of estrogen and continued secretion of progesterone that prohibits the uterus from contracting, but no evidence has validated this. A woman who has one prolonged pregnancy is at greater risk for another in subsequent pregnancies.

Postterm pregnancies may adversely affect both the mother and fetus or newborn. Maternal risk is related to the large size of the fetus at birth, which increases the chances that a cesarean birth will be needed. Other issues might include dystocia, birth trauma, postpartum hemorrhage, and infection. Mechanical or artificial interventions such as **forceps** or vacuum-assisted birth and labor induction with oxytocin may be necessary. In addition, maternal exhaustion and feelings of despair over this prolonged gestation can add to the woman's anxiety level and reduce her coping ability. Women often blame themselves for prolonging the pregnancy, and a woman's negative feelings about herself can bring about strained relationships with the people closest to her.

Fetal risks associated with a **postterm pregnancy** include macrosomia, shoulder dystocia, brachial plexus injuries, low Apgar scores, postmaturity syndrome (loss of subcutaneous fat and muscle and meconium staining), and cephalopelvic disproportion. All of these conditions predispose this fetus to birth trauma or a surgical birth. The perinatal mortality rate at more than 42 weeks of gestation is twice that at term and increases sixfold and higher at 43 weeks of gestation and beyond. Uteroplacental insufficiency, meconium aspiration, and intrauterine infection contribute to the increased rate of perinatal deaths (Callahan, 2016). As the placenta ages, its perfusion decreases and it becomes less efficient at delivering oxygen and nutrients to the fetus. Amniotic fluid volume also begins to decline after 38 weeks of gestation, possibly leading to oligohydramnios, subsequently resulting in fetal hypoxia and an increased risk of cord compression because the cushioning effect offered by adequate fluid is no longer present. Hypoxia and oligohydramnios predispose the fetus to aspiration of meconium, which is released by the fetus in response to a hypoxic insult (Caughey & Butler, 2015). All of these issues can compromise fetal well-being and lead to fetal distress.

Nursing Assessment

Obtain a thorough history to determine the estimated date of birth. Many women are unsure of the date of their last menstrual period, so the date given may be unreliable. Despite numerous methods used to date pregnancies, many are still misdated. Accurate gestational dating via ultrasound is essential.

When expectant management is chosen versus labor induction for the postterm pregnancy, the nurse should anticipate that assessments for a postterm pregnancy will typically include daily fetal movement counts done by the woman, nonstress tests with amniotic fluid assessments as part of the biophysical profile done twice weekly, and weekly cervical examinations to evaluate for ripening. Induction can be deferred until 42 weeks if the fetal surveillance is reassuring. In addition, assess the following:

- Client's understanding of the various fetal well-being tests
- Client's stress and anxiety concerning her lateness
- Client's coping ability and support network

Nursing Management

Once the dates have been established and postterm status is confirmed, monitoring fetal well-being becomes critical. When determining the plan of care for a woman with a prolonged pregnancy, the first decision is whether to deliver the baby or wait. If the decision is to wait, then fetal surveillance is key. If the decision is to have the woman give birth, labor induction is initiated. Both decisions remain controversial, and there is no clear answer about which option is more appropriate. Therefore, the plan must be individualized.

Think back to Jennifer, who is scheduled for labor induction. What ongoing nursing assessments would be important when providing care for her?

Providing Support

The intense surveillance is time-consuming and intrusive, adding to the anxiety and worry already being experienced by the woman about her overdue status. Be alert to the woman's anxiety and allow her to discuss her feelings. Provide reassurance about the expected time range for birth and the well-being of the fetus based on the assessment tests. Validating the woman's stressful state due to the postterm pregnancy provides an opportunity for her to verbalize her feelings openly.

Educating the Woman and Her Partner

Teach the woman and her partner about the testing required and the reasons for each test. Also describe the methods that may be used for cervical ripening if indicated. Explain about the possibility of induction if the woman's labor is not spontaneous or if a dysfunctional labor pattern occurs. Also prepare the woman for the possibility of a surgical delivery if fetal distress occurs.

Providing Care During the Intrapartum Period

During the intrapartum period, continuously assess and monitor FHR to identify potential fetal distress early (e.g., late or variable decelerations) so that interventions can be initiated. Also monitor the woman's hydration status to ensure maximal placental perfusion. When the membranes rupture, assess amniotic fluid characteristics (color, amount, and odor) to identify previous fetal hypoxia and prepare for prevention of meconium aspiration. Report meconium-stained amniotic fluid immediately when the woman's membranes rupture. Anticipate the need for **amnioinfusion** to minimize the risk of meconium aspiration by diluting the meconium in the amniotic fluid expelled by the hypoxic fetus. In addition, monitor the woman's labor pattern closely because dysfunctional patterns are common (Soni, Vaishnav, & Gohil, 2015). Encourage the woman to verbalize her feelings and concerns, and answer all her questions. Provide support, presence, information, and encouragement throughout this time.

WOMEN REQUIRING LABOR INDUCTION AND AUGMENTATION

Ideally, all pregnancies go to term, with labor beginning spontaneously. However, many women need help to initiate or sustain the labor process. **Labor induction** involves the stimulation of uterine contractions by medical or surgical means before the onset of spontaneous labor. The labor induction rate is at an all-time high in the United States. The widespread use of artificial induction of labor for convenience has contributed to the recent increase in the number of cesarean births. Evidence is compelling that elective induction of labor significantly increases the risk of cesarean birth, instrumented delivery, use of epidural analgesia, and neonatal intensive care unit admission, especially for nulliparous women (Caughey, 2014a).

Labor induction is not an isolated event: it brings about a cascade of other interventions that may or may not produce a favorable outcome. Labor induction also involves intravenous therapy, bed rest, continuous electronic fetal monitoring, significant discomfort from stimulating uterine contractions, epidural analgesia/anesthesia, and a prolonged stay on the labor and birth unit (Vogel et al., 2014). Labor augmentation (stimulating the uterus, typically with oxytocin) enhances ineffective contractions after labor has begun. Continuous electronic FHR monitoring is necessary.

The World Health Organization [WHO] (2014b) has put forth recommendations regarding labor induction which includes:

- Labor induction should be performed only for a clear medical indication
- Women being induced should not be left unattended
- Labor induction should only be performed after CPD has been ruled out
- Labor induction should be applied to women with abnormal fetal presentations
- Close monitoring is needed of the FHR and uterine contraction pattern

There are multiple medical and obstetric reasons for inducing labor, the most common being prolonged gestation. Other indications for inductions include PPROM, gestational hypertension, cardiac disease, renal disease, chorioamnionitis, dystocia, intrauterine fetal demise (IUFD), isoimmunization, and diabetes (Jordan et al., 2014). Contraindications to labor induction include complete placenta previa, abruptio placentae, transverse fetal lie, prolapsed umbilical cord, a prior classic uterine incision that entered the uterine cavity, pelvic structure abnormality, previous myomectomy, vaginal bleeding with unknown cause, invasive cervical cancer, active genital herpes infection, and abnormal FHR patterns (Cunningham et al., 2014). In general, labor induction is indicated when the benefits of birth outweigh the risks to the mother or fetus for continuing the pregnancy. However, the balance between risk and benefit remains controversial.

Take Note!

Before labor induction is started, fetal maturity (dating, ultrasound, amniotic fluid studies) and cervical readiness (vaginal examination, Bishop scoring; Table 21.2) must be assessed. Both need to be favorable for a successful induction.

Therapeutic Management

The decision to induce labor is based on a thorough evaluation of maternal and fetal status. Typically, this includes an ultrasound to evaluate fetal size, position, and gestational age and to locate the placenta; engaged presenting fetal part; pelvimetry to rule out fetopelvic disproportion; a nonstress test to evaluate fetal well-being; a phosphatidylglycerol (PG) level to assess fetal lung maturity; confirmation of category I FHR pattern; complete blood count and urinalysis to rule out infection; and a vaginal examination to evaluate the cervix for inducibility (Kriebs, 2015). Accurate dating of the pregnancy also is essential before cervical ripening and induction are initiated to prevent a preterm birth.

Cervical Ripening

Cervical ripening is a process by which the cervix softens via the breakdown of collagen fibrils. It is the first step in the process of cervical effacement and dilation so that, on average, the cervix is approximately 50% effaced and 2 cm dilated at the onset of labor, although wide differences do exist. There has been increasing awareness that if the cervix is unfavorable or unripe, a successful vaginal birth is unlikely. Cervical ripeness is an important variable when labor induction is being considered. A ripe cervix is shortened, centered (anterior), softened, and partially dilated. An unripe cervix is long, closed, posterior, and firm. Cervical ripening usually begins prior to the onset of labor contractions and is necessary for cervical dilation and the passage of the fetus.

Various scoring systems to assess cervical ripeness have been introduced, but the Bishop score is most commonly used today. The Bishop score helps identify women who would be most likely to achieve a successful induction (Table 21.2). The duration of labor is inversely correlated with the Bishop score: a score over 8 indicates a successful vaginal birth. Bishop scores of less than 6 usually indicate that a cervical ripening method should be used prior to induction (Goldberg, 2015). Medical induction of labor has two components: cervical ripening and induction of contractions. When induction of labor is indicated, cervical readiness for labor is evaluated by pelvic examination and determination of a Bishop score is documented.

COMPLEMENTARY AND ALTERNATIVE MEDICINE METHODS

Nonpharmacologic methods for cervical ripening are less frequently used today, but nurses need to be aware of them and question clients about their use. Methods may include herbal agents such as evening primrose oil, black haw, black and blue cohosh, and red raspberry leaves. In addition, castor oil, hot baths, and enemas are used for cervical ripening and labor induction. The risks and benefits of these agents are unknown. None have

TABLE 21.2 BISHOP SCORING SYSTEM

Score	Dilation (cm)	Effacement (%)	Station	Cervical Consistency	Position of Cervix
0	Closed	0–30	−3	Firm	Posterior
1	1–2	40–50	−2	Medium	Midposition
2	3–4	60–70	−1 or 0	Soft	Anterior
3	5–6	80	+1 or +2	Very soft	Anterior

Modified from International Childbirth Education Association [ICEA]. (2014). *ICEA position paper: Induction.* Retrieved from http://www.icea.org/sites/default/files/Induction%20PP-FINAL.pdf

been evaluated scientifically, and thus, none can be recommended regarding their efficacy or safety.

Another nonpharmacologic method suggested for labor induction is sexual intercourse along with breast stimulation. This promotes the release of oxytocin, which stimulates uterine contractions. In addition, human semen is a biologic source of prostaglandins used for cervical ripening. According to a Cochrane review, sexual intercourse with breast stimulation would appear beneficial, but safety issues have not been fully evaluated, nor can this activity be standardized. It appears to shorten the latent phase of labor (King et al., 2015). Therefore, its use as a method for labor induction is not validated by research.

MECHANICAL METHODS

Mechanical methods are used to open the cervix and stimulate the progression of labor. All share a similar mechanism of action: application of local pressure stimulates the release of prostaglandins to ripen the cervix. Potential advantages of mechanical methods, compared with pharmacologic methods, may include simplicity or preservation of the cervical tissue or structure, lower cost, and fewer side effects. The risks associated with these methods include infection, bleeding, membrane rupture, and placental disruption (Sciscione, 2014). For example, an indwelling (Foley) catheter (e.g., 26 French) can be inserted into the endocervical canal to ripen and dilate the cervix. The catheter is placed in the uterus, and the balloon is filled. Direct pressure is then applied to the lower segment of the uterus and the cervix. This direct pressure causes stress in the lower uterine segment and probably the local production of prostaglandins. The risks, benefits, and expected side effects should be explained to the woman prior to the insertion of the balloon catheter (Fuks et al., 2015).

Hygroscopic dilators absorb endocervical and local tissue fluids; as they enlarge, they expand the endocervix and provide controlled mechanical pressure. The products available include natural osmotic dilators (laminaria, a type of dried seaweed) and synthetic dilators containing magnesium sulfate (Lamicel, Dilapan). Hygroscopic dilators are advantageous because they can be inserted on an outpatient basis and no fetal monitoring is needed. As many dilators are inserted in the cervix as will fit, and they expand over 12 to 24 hours as they absorb water. Absorption of water leads to expansion of the dilators and opening of the cervix. They are a reliable alternative when prostaglandins are contraindicated or unavailable (Goldberg, 2015).

Recently there has been a reduction in the use of hygroscopic and osmotic dilators for the induction of labor in favor of pharmacologic agents. The increased risk of maternal and fetal infections with hygroscopic and osmotic dilators when compared with that associated with the use of other pharmacologic agents and the ease of pharmacologic administration may be reasons for the decline. Placement of dilators also requires additional training and may be associated with rupture of membranes, vaginal bleeding, and client discomfort or pain (Drunecky et al., 2015).

Recent systematic review of randomized trials that compared cervical ripening with mechanical methods versus alternative pharmacologic agents or placebo demonstrated that maternal infection was increased in clients who underwent cervical ripening with mechanical methods. Thus, mechanical methods for cervical ripening have fallen into disfavor and are used infrequently today when compared with pharmacologic or surgical methods for induction (McCarthy & Kenny, 2014).

SURGICAL METHODS

Surgical methods used to ripen the cervix and induce labor include stripping of the membranes and performing an amniotomy. Stripping of the membranes is accomplished by inserting a finger through the internal cervical os and moving it in a circular direction. This motion causes the membranes to detach. Manual separation of the amniotic membranes from the cervix is thought to induce cervical ripening and the onset of labor (Afzal, Asif, & Miraj, 2015). However, there is no strong evidence at this time that membrane stripping significantly shortens the duration of pregnancy.

An amniotomy involves inserting a cervical hook (Amniohook) through the cervical os to deliberately rupture the membranes. This promotes pressure of the presenting part on the cervix and stimulates an increase in the activity of prostaglandins locally. Risks associated with these procedures include **umbilical cord prolapse** or compression, maternal or neonatal infection, FHR deceleration, bleeding, and client discomfort (King et al., 2015).

When either of these techniques is used, amniotic fluid characteristics (such as whether it is clear or bloody, or meconium is present) and the FHR pattern must be monitored closely.

PHARMACOLOGIC METHODS

The use of pharmacologic agents has revolutionized cervical ripening. The use of prostaglandins to attain cervical ripening has been found to be highly effective in producing cervical changes independent of uterine contractions (Grobman, 2015). In some cases, women will go into labor and require no additional stimulants for induction. Induction of labor with prostaglandins offers the advantage of promoting both cervical ripening and uterine contractility. A drawback of prostaglandins is their ability to induce excessive uterine contractions, which can increase maternal and perinatal morbidity (Callahan, 2016). Prostaglandin analogs commonly used for cervical ripening include dinoprostone gel (Prepidil), dinoprostone inserts (Cervidil), and misoprostol (Cytotec). Misoprostol (Cytotec), a synthetic

PGE1 analog, is a gastric cytoprotective agent used in the treatment and prevention of peptic ulcers. It can be administered intravaginally or orally to ripen the cervix or induce labor. It is available in 100-mcg or 200-mcg tablets, but doses of 25 to 50 mcg are typically used. It is important to note that only dinoprostone is approved by the FDA for use as a cervical ripening agent, although ACOG acknowledges the apparent safety and effectiveness of misoprostol for this purpose (King et al., 2015). A major adverse effect of the obstetric use of Cytotec is hyperstimulation of the uterus, which may progress to uterine tetany with marked impairment of uteroplacental blood flow, uterine rupture (requiring surgical repair, hysterectomy, and/or salpingooophorectomy), or amniotic fluid embolism (AFE) (Ahmed et al., 2015; Drug Guide 21.2). Furthermore, it is contraindicated for women with prior uterine scars and therefore should not be used for cervical ripening in women attempting a **vaginal birth after cesarean (VBAC)**.

Oxytocin

Oxytocin is a potent endogenous uterotonic agent used for both artificial induction and augmentation of labor. It is produced naturally by the posterior pituitary gland and stimulates contractions of the uterus. For women with low Bishop scores, cervical ripening is typically initiated before oxytocin is used. Once the cervix is ripe, oxytocin is the most popular pharmacologic agent used for inducing or augmenting labor.

DRUG GUIDE 21.2 DRUGS USED FOR CERVICAL RIPENING AND LABOR INDUCTION

Drug	Action/Indication	Nursing Implications
Dinoprostone (Cervidil insert; Prepidil gel)	Directly softens and dilates the cervix/to ripen cervix and induce labor FDA approved for cervical ripening	Provide emotional support. Administer pain medications as needed. Frequently assess degree of effacement and dilation. Monitor uterine contractions for frequency, duration, and strength. Assess maternal vital signs and FHR pattern frequently. Monitor woman for possible adverse effects such as headache, nausea and vomiting, and diarrhea.
Misoprostol (Cytotec)	Ripens cervix/to induce labor	Instruct client about purpose and possible adverse effects of medication. Ensure informed consent is signed per hospital policy. Assess vital signs and FHR patterns frequently. Monitor client's reaction to drug. Initiate oxytocin for labor induction at least 4 hours after last dose was administered. Monitor for possible adverse effects such as nausea and vomiting, diarrhea, uterine hyperstimulation, and category II FHR patterns.
Oxytocin (Pitocin)	Acts on uterine myofibrils to contract/to initiate or reinforce labor	Administer as an IV infusion via pump, increasing dose based on protocol until adequate labor progress is achieved. Assess baseline vital signs and FHR and then frequently after initiating oxytocin infusion. Determine frequency, duration, and strength of contractions frequently. Notify health care provider of any uterine hypertonicity or abnormal FHR patterns. Maintain careful I&O, being alert for water intoxication. Keep client informed of labor progress. Monitor for possible adverse effects such as hyperstimulation of the uterus, impaired uterine blood flow leading to fetal hypoxia, rapid labor leading to cervical lacerations or uterine rupture, water intoxication (if oxytocin is given in electrolyte-free solution or at a rate exceeding 20 mU/min), and hypotension.

Adapted from Goldberg, A. E. (2015). Cervical ripening. *eMedicine*. Retrieved from http://emedicine.medscape.com/article/263311-overview#aw2aab6b7; King, T. L., Brucker, M. C., Kriebs, J. M., Fahey, J. O., Gegor, C. L., & Varney, H. (2015). *Varney's midwifery* (5th ed.). Burlington, MA: Jones & Bartlett Learning; and Goetzl, L. (2014). Methods of cervical ripening and labor induction: Pharmacologic. *Clinical Obstetrics and Gynecology, 57*(2), 377–390.

Frequently, a woman with an unfavorable cervix is admitted the evening before induction to ripen her cervix with one of the prostaglandin agents. Then induction begins with oxytocin the next morning if she has not already gone into labor. Doing so markedly enhances the success of induction.

Response to oxytocin varies widely: some women are very sensitive to even small amounts. The most common adverse effect of oxytocin is uterine hyperstimulation, leading to fetal compromise and impaired oxygenation (King et al., 2015). The response of the uterus to the drug is closely monitored throughout labor so that the oxytocin infusion can be titrated appropriately. In addition, oxytocin has an antidiuretic effect, resulting in decreased urine flow that may lead to water intoxication. Symptoms to watch for include headache and vomiting.

Oxytocin is administered via an intravenous infusion pump piggybacked into the main intravenous line at the port most proximal to the insertion site. Typically, 10 units of oxytocin is added to 1 L of isotonic solution. The dose is titrated according to protocol to achieve stable contractions every 2 to 3 minutes lasting 40 to 60 seconds. Recent studies suggest that a more conservative oxytocin protocol with lower doses reduces the number of neonatal intensive care unit admissions and lower cesarean sections (Lewis et al., 2014; Manjula et al., 2015).

The uterus should relax between contractions. If the resting uterine tone remains above 20 mm Hg, uteroplacental insufficiency and fetal hypoxia can result. This underscores the importance of continuous FHR monitoring. Unfortunately, neither the optimal oxytocin administration regimen nor the maximum oxytocin dose has been established or agreed upon through research or expert opinion. Nurses assisting with labor inductions need to become familiar with their hospital protocols concerning dosage, infusion rates, and frequency of change.

Oxytocin has many advantages: it is potent and easy to titrate, it has a short half-life (1 to 5 minutes), and it is generally well tolerated. Induction using oxytocin has side effects (water intoxication, hypotension, and uterine hypertonicity), but because the drug does not cross the placental barrier, no direct fetal problems have been observed (Arrowsmith & Wray, 2014) (Fig. 21.4).

Remember Jennifer, the young woman described at the beginning of the chapter? After her cervix is ripened, an oxytocin infusion is started and her progress is slow. What encouragement can the nurse offer? After a few hours, her contractions begin to increase in intensity and frequency. What typical pain management measures can the nurse implement, and how would the nurse evaluate the effectiveness of these measures?

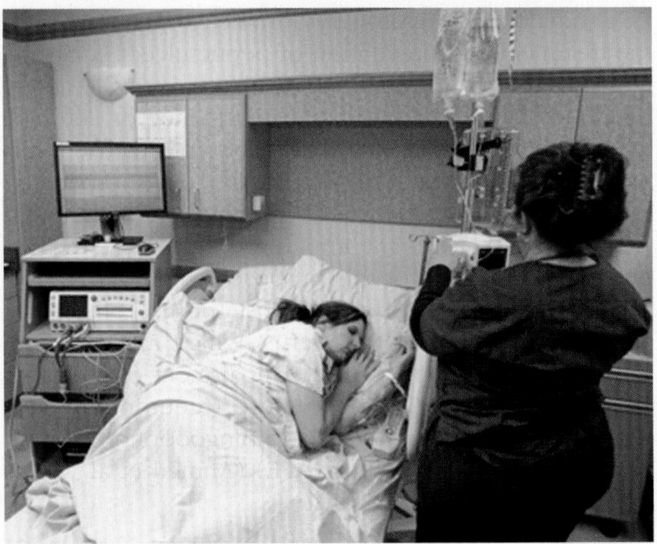

FIGURE 21.4 The nurse monitors an intravenous infusion of oxytocin being administered to a woman in labor who is being induced. (From Lippincott Professional Development, September 2014.)

Nursing Assessment

Nursing assessment of the woman who is undergoing labor induction or augmentation involves a thorough history and physical examination. Review the woman's history for relative indications for induction or augmentation, such as diabetes, hypertension, postterm status, dysfunctional labor pattern, prolonged ruptured membranes, and maternal or fetal infection, and for contraindications such as placenta previa, overdistended uterus, active genital herpes, fetopelvic disproportion, fetal malposition, or severe fetal distress.

Assist with determining the gestational age of the fetus to prevent a preterm birth. Assess fetal well-being to validate the client's and fetus's ability to withstand labor contractions. Evaluate the woman's cervical status, including cervical dilation and effacement, and station via vaginal examination as appropriate before cervical ripening or induction is started. Determine the Bishop score to determine the probable success of induction.

Take Note!

Nurses working with women in labor play an important role acting as the eyes and ears for the birth attendant because they remain at the client's bedside throughout the entire experience. Close, frequent assessment and follow-up interventions are essential to ensure the safety of the mother and her unborn child during cervical ripening and labor induction or augmentation.

Nursing Management

Explain to the woman and her partner about the induction or augmentation procedure clearly, using simple terms (Teaching Guidelines 21.2). Ensure that an informed consent has been signed after the client and her partner have received complete information about the procedure, including its advantages, disadvantages, and potential risks. Ensure that the Bishop score has been determined before proceeding. Nursing Care Plan 21.1 (at the end of the chapter) presents an overview of the nursing care for a woman undergoing labor induction.

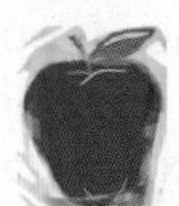

Teaching Guidelines 21.2

TEACHING IN PREPARATION FOR LABOR INDUCTION

- Your health care provider may recommend that you have your labor induced. This may be necessary for a variety of reasons, such as elevated blood pressure, a medical condition, prolonged pregnancy over 41 weeks, or problems with fetal heart rate patterns or fetal growth.
- Your health care provider may use one or more methods to induce labor, such as stripping the membranes, breaking the amniotic sac to release the fluid, administering medication close to or in the cervix to soften it, or administering a medication called oxytocin (Pitocin) to stimulate contractions.
- Labor induction is associated with some risks and disadvantages, such as overactivity of the uterus; nausea, vomiting, or diarrhea; and changes in fetal heart rate.
- Prior to inducing your labor, your health care provider may perform a procedure to ripen your cervix to help ensure a successful induction.
- Medication may be placed around your cervix the day before you are scheduled to be induced.
- During the induction, your contractions may feel stronger than normal. However, the length of your labor may be reduced with induction.
- Medications for pain relief and comfort measures will be readily available.
- Health care staff will be present throughout labor.

Administering Oxytocin

If not already done, prepare the oxytocin infusion by diluting 10 units of oxytocin in 1,000 mL of lactated Ringer solution or ordered isotonic solution. Use an infusion pump on a secondary line connected to the primary infusion. Start the oxytocin infusion in mU/min or milliliters per hour as ordered. Each hospital has its own standards/protocols for oxytocin infusion and dilution. The nurse needs to follow that procedure when administering this medication. Maintain the rate once the desired contraction frequency has been reached. To ensure adequate maternal and fetal surveillance during induction or augmentation, the nurse-to-client ratio should not exceed 1:2 (Mattson & Smith, 2016).

During induction or augmentation, monitoring of the maternal and fetal status is essential. Apply an external electronic fetal monitor or assist with placement of an internal device. Obtain the mother's vital signs and the FHR every 15 minutes during the first stage. Evaluate the contractions (frequency, duration, and intensity) and resting tone, and adjust the oxytocin infusion rate accordingly. Monitor the FHR, including baseline rate, baseline variability, and decelerations, to determine whether the oxytocin rate needs adjustment. Discontinue the oxytocin and notify the birth attendant if uterine hyperstimulation or a category II or III FHR pattern occurs. Perform or assist with periodic vaginal examinations to determine cervical dilation and fetal descent: cervical dilation of 1 cm/hr typically indicates satisfactory progress. Continue to monitor the FHR continuously and document it every 15 minutes during the active phase of labor and every 5 minutes during the second stage. Assist with pushing efforts during the second stage. Measure and record intake and output to prevent excess fluid volume. Encourage the client to empty her bladder every 2 hours to prevent soft tissue obstruction.

Providing Pain Relief and Support

Assess the woman's level of pain. Ask her frequently to rate her pain and provide pain management as needed. Offer position changes and other nonpharmacologic measures. Note her reaction to any medication given, and document its effect. Monitor her need for comfort measures as contractions increase.

Throughout induction and augmentation, frequently reassure the woman and her partner about the fetal status and labor progress. Provide them with frequent updates on the condition of the woman and the fetus. Assess the woman's ability to cope with stronger contractions, and follow protocols of the hospital about how frequent pain assessments are performed for each phase and stage of labor (Nagtalon-Ramos, 2014). Provide support and encouragement as indicated.

After a very long day, Jennifer gives birth to a healthy baby boy with Apgar scores of 9 at 1 minute and 10 at 5 minutes. When transferring her to the postpartum unit, what information is essential to include for the accepting nurse? What specific nursing information should be given to the nursery nurse regarding the laboring experience? With such a lengthy labor, what assessments might the postpartum nurse need to focus on for the first few hours after birth?

VAGINAL BIRTH AFTER CESAREAN

VBAC describes a woman who gives birth vaginally after having at least one previous cesarean birth. Despite evidence that some women who have had a cesarean birth are candidates for vaginal birth, most women who have had a cesarean birth once undergo another for subsequent pregnancies.

A multidisciplinary guideline group representing family medicine, epidemiology, obstetrics, and midwifery developed recommendations based on high-quality systematic evidence-based, peer-reviewed research, that individual assessment of risks and benefits be discussed with the pregnant woman with a history of one or more prior cesarean births who are deciding between a planned VBAC or a repeat cesarean birth. A planned VBAC is an appropriate option for most women with a history of prior cesarean birth (King et al., 2015).

Contraindications to VBAC include a prior classic uterine incision, prior transfundal uterine surgery (myomectomy), uterine scar other than low-transverse cesarean scar, contracted pelvis, and inadequate staff or facility if an emergency cesarean birth in the event of uterine rupture is required (Caughey, 2014b). Most women go through a trial of labor to see how they progress, but this must be performed in an environment capable of handling the emergency of uterine rupture. The use of cervical ripening agents increases the risk of uterine rupture and thus is contraindicated in VBAC clients. The woman considering induction of labor after a previous cesarean birth needs to be informed of the risks versus benefits with an induction than with spontaneous labor (Scott, 2015).

Women are the primary decision makers about the choice of birth method, but they need education about VBAC during their prenatal course. Management is similar for any women experiencing labor, but certain areas require special focus:

- *Consent:* Fully informed consent is essential for the woman who wants to have a trial of labor after cesarean birth. The client must be advised about the risks as well as the benefits. She must understand the ramifications of uterine rupture, even though the risk is small.
- *Documentation:* Record keeping is an important component of safe client care. If and when an emergency occurs, it is imperative to take care of the client, but also to keep track of the plan of care, interventions and their timing, and the client's response. Events and activities can be written right on the fetal monitoring tracing to correlate with the change in fetal status.
- *Surveillance:* A distressed fetal monitor tracing in a woman undergoing a trial of labor after a cesarean birth should alert the nurse to the possibility of uterine rupture. Terminal bradycardia must be considered an emergency situation, and the nurse should prepare the team for an emergency delivery.
- *Readiness for emergency:* According to ACOG (2010) criteria for a safe trial of labor for a woman who has had a previous cesarean birth, the physician or nurse practitioner, anesthesia provider, and operating room team must be immediately available. Anything less would place the women and fetus at risk.

Women and their health care providers are advised to consider VBAC in the context of potential risk, available resources, and the health care system. The ACOG (2010) guidelines state that VBACs are safe and appropriate for most women, but emphasize the need for thorough counseling, shared decision making, and client autonomy. Nurses must act as advocates, giving input on the appropriate selection of women who wish to undergo VBAC. Nurses also need to become experts at reading fetal monitoring tracings to identify fetal distress and set in motion an emergency birth. Including all of these nursing strategies will make VBAC safer for all.

INTRAUTERINE FETAL DEMISE

Pregnancy and childbirth are associated with hopes, expectations, joy, and happiness for the future. When an unborn life suddenly ends with fetal loss, the family members are profoundly affected. IUFD is fetal death that occurs after 20 weeks' gestation but before birth. The cause of IUFD is often unknown. The sudden loss of an expected child is tragic and the family's grief can be very intense: it can last for years and can cause extreme psychological stress and emotional problems (Sousou & Smart, 2015). The family's anticipation of a joyous birth is supplanted by despair, confusion, and loss. To women and their families who have gone through this harrowing experience, culturally appropriate and sensitive care is crucial. Particularly for the mother, fetal death in the last trimester of pregnancy, when she feels very close to the fetus due to its frequent movement in the uterus, must be similar to losing a part of her body.

Fetal demise can be due to an extensive range of risk factors and possible causes, such as postterm pregnancy, renal disease, substance abuse, infection, hypertension, advanced maternal age, multiple gestation, Rh disease, uterine rupture, diabetes, congenital anomalies, obesity, smoking, cord accident, abruption, blunt trauma, premature rupture of membranes, or hemorrhage—or it may go unexplained (Hugin & Sultani, 2015). Trauma in pregnancy remains one of the major contributors to maternal and fetal morbidity and mortality. Potential complications include maternal injury or death, shock, internal hemorrhage, IUFD, direct fetal injury, abruptio placentae, and uterine rupture. The leading causes of obstetric trauma are motor vehicle accidents, falls, assaults, and gunshots, and ensuing injuries are classified as blunt abdominal trauma, pelvic fractures, or penetrating trauma. In view of the significant impact of trauma on the pregnant woman and her fetus, preventive strategies are paramount (Kilpatrick, 2014).

Early pregnancy loss may be through a spontaneous abortion (miscarriage), an induced abortion (therapeutic abortion), or a ruptured ectopic pregnancy. A wide spectrum of feelings may be expressed, from relief to sadness and despair. A fetal death can occur at any gestational age, and typically there is little or no warning other than reduced fetal movement. The effects of childbearing loss may affect women and their families for a lifetime. The need to reflect, share, and regain strength is universal for all families dealing with loss. Grief, the typical response to the loss of a valued object, is not an intellectual response. Rather, it is personally experienced as a deep emotion of sadness and sorrow. Feelings such as helplessness, disbelief, unreality, and powerlessness are common. Emotional recovery from the pain of perinatal loss occurs with time, but it varies with each couple.

The moment that fetal death is diagnosed can frequently be described very clearly and in detail by most women. In many cases, the death was sudden, and women have no chance to prepare for the impending grief. Once IUFD is confirmed, most women choose to immediately undergo induction of labor. Approximately 90% of women will go into spontaneous labor within 2 weeks of fetal death (Green, 2016). With the death of a fetus or neonate, a couple's dreams and hopes for their expected child suddenly dissolve. To women who have experienced a sudden fetal death, the following processes may take place: experiencing a quiet birth without the infant, eclipsed by emptiness, anger, anxiety, loneliness, and sorrow; living without their infant, making it very difficult to see others with young infants; and experiencing differences with their partner over the loss (Callister, 2014). The process of grieving a death is not completed within a specific time frame, and for some, it is never complete. In general, the grief accompanying the loss of a fetus proceeds in the following order:

1. Accepting the reality of the loss
2. Getting over suffering from the loss
3. Adapting to the new environment without the deceased
4. Emotionally relocating the deceased and getting on with life (Grunebaum & Chervenak, 2014).

The period following a fetal death is extremely difficult for the family. For many women, emotional healing takes much longer than physical healing. The feelings of loss can be intense. The grief response in some women may be so great that their relationships become strained, and healing can become hampered unless appropriate interventions and support are provided.

Fetal death also affects the health care staff. Despite the trauma that the loss of a fetus causes, some staff members avoid dealing with the bereaved family, never talking about or acknowledging their grief. This seems to imply that not discussing the problem will allow the grief to dissolve and vanish. As a result, the family's needs go unrecognized. Failing to keep the lines of communication open with a bereaved client and her family closes off some of the channels to recovery and healing that may be desperately needed. Subsequently, the bereaved family members may feel isolated.

Nursing Assessment

A woman experiencing an IUFD is likely to seek care when she notices that the fetus is not moving or when she experiences contractions, loss of fluid, or vaginal bleeding. History and physical examination frequently are of limited value in the diagnosis of fetal death, since many times the only history tends to be recent absence of fetal movement and no fetal heart beat heard. An inability to obtain fetal heart sounds on examination suggests fetal demise, but an ultrasound is necessary to confirm the absence of fetal cardiac activity. Once fetal demise is confirmed, induction of labor or expectant management is offered to the woman.

Nursing Management

IUFD is associated with posttraumatic stress disorder (PTSD) and anxiety in a subsequent pregnancy (Robinson, 2014). The nurse can play a major role in assisting the grieving family. Nurses who can deal honestly with their own feelings regarding loss will be better able to help others cope with theirs. By working with couples who have suffered a significant loss, the nurse can grow personally and professionally and gain a deeper perspective about life. With skillful intervention, the bereaved family may be better prepared to resolve their grief and move forward.

To assist families in the grieving process, include the following measures:

- Provide accurate, understandable information to the family.
- Acknowledge that the woman's feeling of loss are legitimate.
- Reassure mother that there was likely nothing that she could have done to prevent it.
- Be knowledgeable about the grief process and comfortable in sharing another's grief.
- Utilize active listening to provide needed encouragement to the family members to open up to their feelings.
- Create a warm, receptive, accepting, and caring environment conducive to dialogue.
- Dispel guilt by saying that nothing the woman did caused the fetal death.
- Acknowledge their grief by saying that their feeling sad is appropriate.
- Recognize that each family member may express their grief differently.
- Provide reassurance about successful future pregnancies.
- Encourage discussion of the loss and venting of feelings of grief and guilt.

- Provide the family with baby mementos and pictures to validate the reality of death.
- Allow unlimited time with the stillborn infant after birth to validate the death; provide time for the family members to be together and grieve; offer the family the opportunity to see, touch, and hold the infant.
- Use appropriate touch, such as holding a hand or touching a shoulder.
- Inform the chaplain or the religious leader of the family's denomination about the death and request his or her presence.
- Assist the parents with the funeral arrangements or disposition of the body.
- Provide the parents with brochures offering advice about how to talk to other siblings about the loss.
- Refer the family to the support group SHARE Pregnancy and Infant Loss Support, Inc., which is designed for those who have lost an infant through abortion, miscarriage, fetal death, stillbirth, or other tragic circumstances.
- Make community referrals to promote a continuum of care after discharge.

Openness to talking with couples about their loss and grief is the basis for support provided by nurses, which can have a positive influence on the long-term adjustment of couples and families coping with perinatal loss. A sensitive nurse who is comfortable talking about loss and is able to assist couples in navigating the process of grief provides a starting point for preparation for future pregnancy. Couples need to talk about their loss, its meaning, and the emotions that accompany it while the nurse listens. Nurses play a significant role in linking women and men to appropriate professional support. As couples move through their grief and begin to consider another pregnancy, sensitive nursing care may mediate the understandable anxiety and concern that accompany this process. Nurses are a vital part of the interdisciplinary health care team caring for families with IUFD, who continue to require timely and sensitive care throughout the grieving process.

WOMEN EXPERIENCING AN OBSTETRIC EMERGENCY

Obstetric emergencies are challenging to all labor and birth personnel because of the increased risk of adverse outcomes for the mother and fetus. Quick clinical judgment and good critical decision making will increase the odds of a positive outcome for both mother and fetus. This section discusses a few of these emergencies: umbilical cord prolapse, placenta previa, placental abruption, uterine rupture, and AFE.

Umbilical Cord Prolapse

Umbilical cord prolapse is a rare obstetrical emergency that occurs when the cord precedes the fetus out. An umbilical cord prolapse is the protrusion of the umbilical cord alongside (occult) or ahead of the presenting part of the fetus (Fig. 21.5). This condition occurs in 1 out of every 300 births and requires prompt recognition and intervention for a positive outcome (March of Dimes, 2015c). Cord prolapse occurs in 3% of deliveries when the fetus is in the vertex position and in 3.7% of deliveries when the fetus is in the breech position. The risk is increased further when the presenting part does not fill the lower uterine segment, as is the case with incomplete breech presentations (5% to 10%), premature infants, and multiparous women (Bush, Eddleman, & Belogolovkin, 2015). With a 50% perinatal mortality rate, it is one of the most catastrophic events in the intrapartum period (Beall & Ross, 2014).

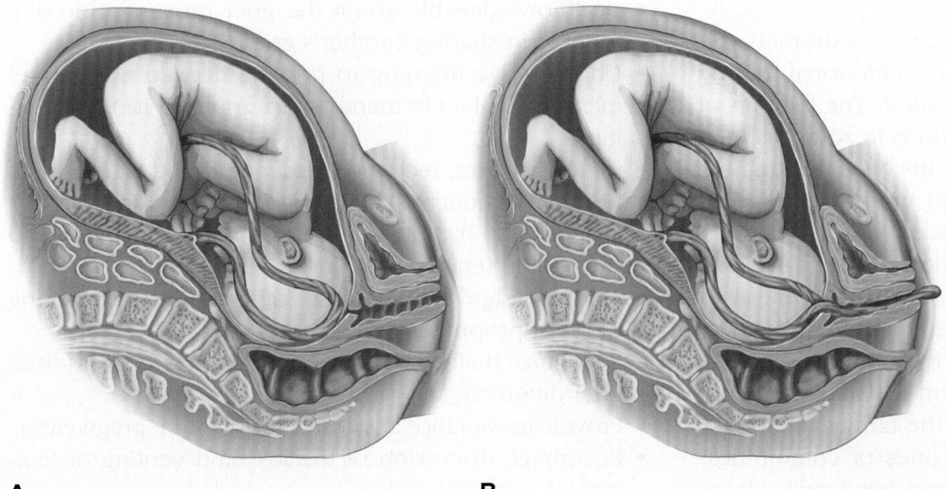

FIGURE 21.5 Prolapsed cord. **A.** Prolapse within the uterus. **B.** Prolapse with the cord visible at the vulva.

Pathophysiology

Prolapse usually leads to total or partial occlusion of the cord. Since this is the fetus's only lifeline, fetal perfusion deteriorates rapidly. Complete occlusion renders the fetus helpless and oxygen deprived. The fetus will die if the cord compression is not relieved.

Nursing Assessment

Prevention is the key to managing cord prolapse by identifying clients at risk for this condition. Carefully assess each client to help predict her risk status. Be aware that cord prolapse is more common in pregnancies involving malpresentation, growth restriction, prematurity, ruptured membranes with a fetus at a high station, hydramnios, grandmultiparity, and multiple gestation (Cunningham et al., 2014). Continuously assess the client and fetus to detect changes and to evaluate the effectiveness of any interventions performed.

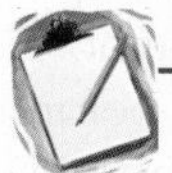

Take Note!

When the presenting part does not fully occupy the pelvic inlet, prolapse is more likely to occur.

Nursing Management

Prompt recognition of a prolapsed cord is essential to reduce the risk of fetal hypoxia resulting from prolonged cord compression. Often the first sign of cord prolapse is a sudden fetal bradycardia or recurrent variable decelerations that become progressively more severe. Call for help immediately and do not leave the woman. Inform the woman of what is happening and what options may be discussed by her health care provider. When membranes are artificially ruptured, assist with verifying that the presenting part is well applied to the cervix and engaged into the pelvis. If pressure or compression of the cord occurs, assist with measures to relieve the compression. Typically, the examiner places a sterile gloved hand into the vagina and holds the presenting part off the umbilical cord until delivery. Changing the woman's position to a modified Sims, Trendelenburg, or knee-chest position also helps relieve cord pressure. Do not attempt to replace the cord in the uterus. Monitor FHR, maintain bed rest, and administer oxygen if ordered. Provide emotional support and explanations as to what is going on to allay the woman's fears and anxiety. If the mother's cervix is not fully dilated, prepare the woman for an emergency cesarean birth to save the fetus's life if that is the intervention planned for by her health care provider.

Placenta Previa

Placenta previa is placental implantation in the lower uterine segment over or near the internal os of the cervix, typically during the second or third trimester of pregnancy. With uterine segment formation and cervical dilation, placental implantation over or near the cervical os, instead of along the uterine wall, inevitably results in spontaneous placental separation—and subsequent hemorrhage. This position can create a barrier for the fetus from the uterus during the birthing process. As the cervix begins to thin and dilate (open up) in preparation for labor, blood vessels that connect the placenta to the uterus may tear and cause bleeding. It is the most common cause of bleeding in the second half of pregnancy and should be suspected in any woman beyond 24 weeks' gestation presenting with vaginal bleeding; ultrasonography (e.g., transvaginal) is used to diagnose it. During labor and birth, bleeding can be severe, which can place the mother and fetus at risk. Reported incidence is approximately 1 in 200 births (March of Dimes, 2015d).

There is a direct relationship between the number of previous cesarean births and the risk of placenta previa, probably due to uterine scarring. The degree of occlusion of the internal cervical os may depend on the degree of cervical dilation, so what may appear to be a low-lying or marginal placenta previa prior to the onset of labor can progress to become more serious as the cervix effaces and opens up (King et al., 2015).

The incidence of maternal mortality is less than 1%, but common morbidities include septicemia, renal failure, hemorrhage and hypovolemic shock, invasive placenta (accrete, increta, and percreta), and postpartum anemia. Risk factors for placenta previa include previous cesarean section, advanced maternal age >34, multiparity, multiple gestation, prior placenta previa, and cigarette smoking. The risk for perinatal mortality is less than 10%, but common neonatal morbidities include stillbirth, prematurity, malpresentation, fetal growth restriction, and fetal anemia (Joy & Finneran, 2015).

Maternal signs and symptoms of placenta previa include sudden, painless bleeding (that may be heavy enough to be considered hemorrhaging), anemia, pallor, hypoxia, low blood pressure, tachycardia, soft and nontender uterus, and rapid, weak pulse. Bleeding may be episodic, with spontaneous initiation and cessation; in some cases, it is asymptomatic because there is intrauterine bleeding only without external signs.

Management of placenta previa varies by type and gestational age, and frequent medical surveillance may be sufficient in marginal cases; prompt treatment with bed rest, close monitoring, and control/replacement of blood loss greatly reduces risk for maternal and fetal complications and death. Vaginal delivery is possible when bleeding is minimal, placenta previa is marginal, or labor is rapid. Pregnancy termination, early birth by cesarean section, or a hysterectomy may be necessary in order to control severe bleeding, especially for clients with complete placenta previa. The overall maternal prognosis is good if hemorrhage is controlled and sepsis or other complications are prevented. Fetal prognosis is directly related to the amount of blood loss. The United States perinatal mortality rate associated with placental previa is 2% to 3%, and the maternal mortality rate is 0.03%. Risk for placenta previa recurrence in subsequent pregnancies is 4% to 8% (Lal & Hibbard, 2015).

Nursing management within the acute care setting includes the following: monitor maternal vital signs, intake and output, vaginal bleeding, and physiologic status for signs of hemorrhage, shock, or infection; closely monitor fetal heart tones for distress (e.g., bradycardia, tachycardia, baseline changes); and treat fetal distress, as ordered. Administer prescribed intravenous fluids, packed red blood cells platelets, and frozen plasma for transfusion, if ordered; Rho(D) immune globulin, if the client is Rh negative; intravenous-augmented oxytocin (Pitocin) to induce labor, if needed; and in cases of preterm labor, tocolytics (e.g., magnesium sulfate) to inhibit uterine contractions and corticosteroids (e.g., betamethasone) to enhance fetal lung maturity. Follow facility pre- and postsurgical protocols if woman becomes a surgical candidate (e.g., for cesarean section); reinforce pre- and postsurgical education and ensure completion of facility's informed consent documents; closely monitor postsurgically for bleeding, infection, and other complications; assess client's anxiety level and coping ability; and provide emotional support and reassurance.

Frequently there is expectant management for the woman after her first placenta previa bleed if it isn't severe and fetus well-being is validated. After she is assessed, she is released to go home. It is common for women to experience an initial bleeding episode, which then subsides. These women are monitored at home and instructed to report any additional bleeding episodes and come in to be evaluated (King et al., 2015).

Placental Abruption

Placental abruption refers to premature separation of a normally implanted placenta from the maternal myometrium. Placental abruption occurs in about 1% of all pregnancies throughout the world and is associated with significant perinatal mortality and morbidity (March of Dimes, 2015e). Risk factors include preeclampsia, gestational hypertension, seizure activity, advanced maternal age >34, uterine rupture, trauma, smoking, cocaine use, coagulation defects, chorioamnionitis, premature rupture of membranes, hydramnios, uterine trauma, external cephalic version for breech presentation, previous history of abruption, domestic violence, and placental pathology. These conditions may force blood into the underlayer of the placenta and cause it to detach (Deering, 2015).

Management of placental abruption depends on the gestational age, the extent of the hemorrhage, and maternal-fetal oxygenation perfusion/reserve status (see Chapter 19 for additional information on abruptio placentae). Treatment is based on the circumstances. Typically once the diagnosis is established, the focus is on maintaining the cardiovascular status of the mother and developing a plan to deliver the fetus quickly. A cesarean birth may take place quickly if the fetus is still alive with only a partial abruption. A vaginal birth may take place if there is fetal demise secondary to a complete abruption.

Uterine Rupture

Uterine rupture in pregnancy is a rare and often catastrophic complication with a high incidence of fetal and maternal morbidity. Uterine rupture is a catastrophic tearing of the uterus at the site of a previous scar into the abdominal cavity. Its onset is often marked only by sudden fetal bradycardia, and treatment requires rapid surgery for good outcomes. From the time of diagnosis to delivery, only 10 to 30 minutes are available before clinically significant fetal morbidity occurs. Fetal morbidity occurs secondary to catastrophic hemorrhage, fetal anoxia, or both.

Nursing Assessment

Review the mother's history for risk conditions such as uterine scars, prior cesarean births, prior rupture, trauma, prior invasive molar pregnancy, history of placenta percreta or increta, congenital uterine anomalies, multiparity, previous uterine myomectomy, malpresentation, labor induction with excessive uterine stimulation, and crack cocaine use (Nahum & Pham, 2015). Reviewing a client's history for risk factors might prove to be lifesaving for both mother and fetus.

Generally, the first and most reliable symptom of uterine rupture is sudden fetal distress. Other signs may include acute and continuous abdominal pain with or without an epidural, vaginal bleeding, hematuria, irregular abdominal wall contour, loss of station in the fetal presenting part, and hypovolemic shock in the woman, fetus, or both (Scott, 2015).

Timely management of uterine rupture depends on prompt detection. Because many women desire a trial of labor after a previous cesarean birth, the nurse must be familiar with the signs and symptoms of uterine rupture. It is difficult to prevent uterine rupture or to predict which women will experience rupture, so constant preparedness is necessary. Screening all women with previous uterine surgical scars is important, and continuous electronic fetal monitoring should be used during labor because this may provide the only indication of an impending rupture.

Nursing Management

Because the presenting signs may be nonspecific, the initial management will be the same as that for any other cause of acute fetal distress. Urgent delivery by cesarean birth is usually indicated. Monitor maternal vital signs and observe for hypotension and tachycardia, which might indicate hypovolemic shock. Assist in preparing for an emergency cesarean birth by alerting the operating room staff, anesthesia provider, and neonatal team. Insert an indwelling urinary (Foley) catheter if one is not in place already. Inform the woman of the seriousness of this event and remind her that the health care staff will be working quickly to ensure her health and that of her fetus. Remain calm and provide reassurance that everything is being done to ensure a safe outcome for both.

The life-threatening nature of uterine rupture is underscored by the fact that the maternal circulatory system delivers approximately 500 mL of blood to the term uterus every minute (Cunningham et al., 2014). Maternal death is a real possibility without rapid intervention. Newborn outcome after rupture depends largely on the speed with which surgical rescue is carried out. As in any case of acute obstetric emergency, preparation and timely mobilization of all necessary personnel is essential to optimizing outcome.

> **Take Note!**
> When excessive bleeding occurs during the childbirth process and it persists or signs such as bruising or petechiae appear, disseminated intravascular coagulation (DIC) should be suspected.

Amniotic Fluid Embolism

AFE is an unforeseeable, life-threatening complication of childbirth. AFE remains an enigmatic, but devastating obstetric condition associated with significant maternal and newborn morbidity and mortality. It is a rare and often fatal event characterized by the sudden onset of hypotension, hypoxia, and coagulopathy. Amniotic fluid containing particles of debris (e.g., hair, skin, vernix, or meconium) enters the maternal circulation and obstructs the pulmonary vessels, causing respiratory distress and circulatory collapse (Sadera & Vasudevan, 2015). Prediction and diagnosis of the event are nearly impossible. However, timely recognition and response is critical in saving a woman's life. Although estimates vary, AFE, also referred to as anaphylactoid syndrome of pregnancy, occurs in 1 in 15,000 births, with a reported mortality rate reaching 60% despite technologic advances in critical care life support (Moore, 2015).

Pathophysiology

The pathophysiology appears to involve an abnormal maternal response to fetal tissue exposure associated with breaches of the maternal-fetal physiologic barrier during the postpartum period. Normally, amniotic fluid does not enter the maternal circulation because it is contained within the uterus, sealed off by the amniotic sac. An embolus occurs when the barrier between the maternal circulation and the amniotic fluid is broken and amniotic fluid enters the maternal venous system via the endocervical veins, the placental site (if the placenta is separated), or a site of uterine trauma. This condition has a high mortality rate: as many as 50% of women die within the first hour after the onset of symptoms, and about 85% of survivors have permanent hypoxia-induced neurologic damage (Sadera & Vasudevan, 2015).

Although medical science has supplied many answers to questions about this condition, health care providers remain largely unable to predict or prevent an AFE or to decrease its mortality rate.

Nursing Assessment

Predisposing factors associated with AFE include placental abruption, uterine over distention, fetal demise, uterine trauma, oxytocin-stimulated labor, amnioinfusion, multiparity, advanced maternal age, and ruptured membranes. However, many women present without any of the risk factors.

Nurses must stay a step ahead and be prepared at all times in this obstetric emergency. A team response is essential because every person will be needed. No test can diagnose an AFE. Therefore, the nurse's assessment skills are critical. Immediate recognition and diagnosis of this condition are essential to improve maternal and fetal outcomes. Until recently, the diagnosis could be made only after an autopsy of the mother revealed squamous cells, lanugo hair, or other fetal and amniotic material in the pulmonary arterial vasculature (Baldisseri, 2014).

The clinical appearance is varied, but most women report difficulty breathing. Other symptoms include hypotension, cyanosis, hypoxemia, uterine atony, seizures, tachycardia, coagulation failure, disseminated intravascular coagulation (DIC), pulmonary edema, seizures, uterine atony with subsequent hemorrhage, adult respiratory distress syndrome, and cardiac arrest (Viswanathan, Venkateswaran, & Daniel, 2014).

> **Take Note!**
> Amniotic fluid embolism should be suspected in any pregnant women with an acute onset of dyspnea, hypotension, and DIC. By knowing how to intervene, the nurse can promote a better chance of survival for both the mother and her newborn. Most women are transferred to the intensive care unit.

Nursing Management

Upon recognizing the signs and symptoms of this life-threatening diagnosis, institute supportive measures: oxygenation (resuscitation and 100% oxygen), circulation (intravenous fluids, inotropic agents to maintain cardiac output and blood pressure), control of hemorrhage and coagulopathy (oxytocic agents to control uterine atony and bleeding), seizure precautions, and administration of steroids to control the inflammatory response. Monitor vital signs, pulse oximetry, skin color, and temperature and observe for clinical signs of coagulopathy (vaginal bleeding, bleeding from intravenous site, bleeding from gums) (Moses, 2015).

Care is largely supportive and aimed at maintaining oxygenation and hemodynamic function and correcting coagulopathy. There is no specific therapy that is lifesaving once this condition starts. Adequate oxygenation is necessary, with endotracheal intubation and mechanical ventilation for most women. Vasopressors are used to maintain hemodynamic stability. Management of DIC may involve replacement with packed red blood cells or fresh-frozen plasma as necessary. Oxytocin infusions and prostaglandin analogs can be used to address uterine atony.

Explain to the client and family what is happening and what therapies are being instituted. The woman is usually transferred to a critical care unit for intensive observation and care. Assist the family to express their feelings and provide support as needed. Inform and reassure the woman and family as much as possible during this crisis.

WOMEN REQUIRING BIRTH-RELATED PROCEDURES

Many women can give birth without the need for any operative obstetric interventions. Most do not anticipate the need for any medical intervention. However, in some situations interventions are necessary to safeguard the health of the mother and fetus. The most common birth-related procedures are amnioinfusion, forceps-assisted or vacuum-assisted birth, cesarean birth, episiotomy (see Chapter 14), and vaginal birth following a previous cesarean birth (see section earlier in this chapter). Nurses play a major role in helping couples to cope with any unanticipated procedures by offering thorough explanations of the procedure, its anticipated benefits and risks, and any other options available.

Amnioinfusion

Amnioinfusion is a technique in which a volume of warmed, sterile, normal saline or Ringer lactate solution is introduced into the uterus transcervically through an intrauterine pressure catheter to increase the volume of fluid when oligohydramnios is present. It is a procedure used during labor. It is used to change the relationship of the uterus, placenta, cord, and fetus to improve placental and fetal oxygenation. Instilling an isotonic glucose-free solution into the uterus helps to cushion the umbilical cord to prevent compression or dilute thick meconium. Studies support the use of this procedure a safe and effective in resolving FHR decelerations (Hofmeyr, Eke, & Lawrie, 2014).

This procedure is commonly indicated for severe variable decelerations due to cord compression, oligohydramnios due to placental insufficiency, postmaturity or rupture of membranes, preterm labor with premature rupture of membranes, and thick meconium fluid. However, it does not prevent meconium aspiration syndrome (Hofmeyr, Xu, & Eke, 2014). Contraindications to amnioinfusion include vaginal bleeding of unknown origin, umbilical cord prolapse, amnionitis, uterine hypertonicity, and severe fetal distress (Fong et al., 2014).

There is no standard protocol for amnioinfusion; nurses should follow their own institution protocols. After obtaining informed consent, a vaginal examination is performed to evaluate for cord prolapse, establish dilation, and confirm presentation. Next, 250 to 500 mL of warmed normal saline or lactated Ringer solution is administered using an infusion pump over 20 to 30 minutes. Overdistention of the uterus is a risk, so the amount of fluid infused must be monitored closely. Amnioinfusion should reach therapeutic result or increase the amniotic fluid volume in approximately 30 minutes (Mattson & Smith, 2016).

When caring for the woman who is receiving an amnioinfusion, include the following:

- Explain the need for the procedure, what it involves, and how it may solve the problem.
- Inform the mother that she will need to remain on bed rest during the procedure.
- Assess the mother's vital signs and associated discomfort level.
- Maintain intake and output records.
- Assess the duration and intensity of uterine contractions frequently to identify overdistention or increased uterine tone.
- Assess for fluid leakage by evaluating the chuck or pad under the woman to determine that it is not being retained in the uterus, which could lead to increased uterine pressure.
- Monitor the FHR pattern to determine whether the amnioinfusion is improving the fetal status.
- Prepare the mother for a possible cesarean birth if the FHR does not improve after the amnioinfusion.

Forceps- or Vacuum-Assisted Birth

Forceps or a **vacuum extractor** may be used to apply traction to the fetal head or to provide a method of

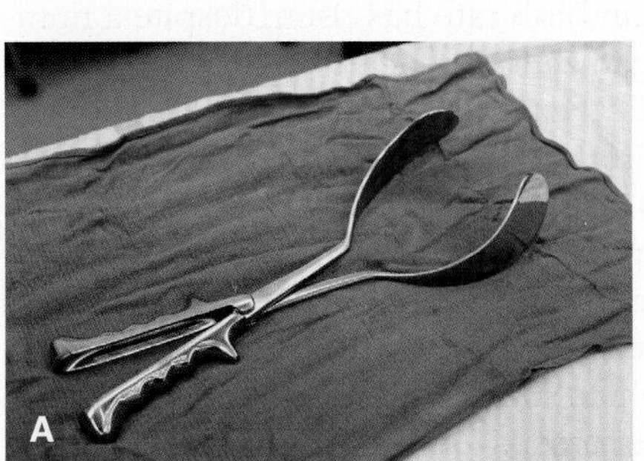
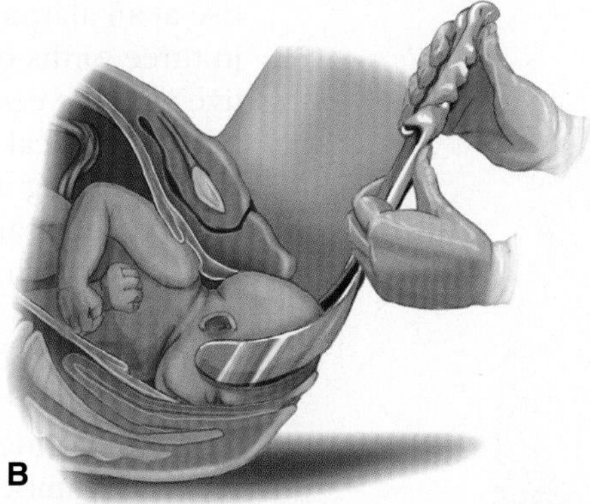
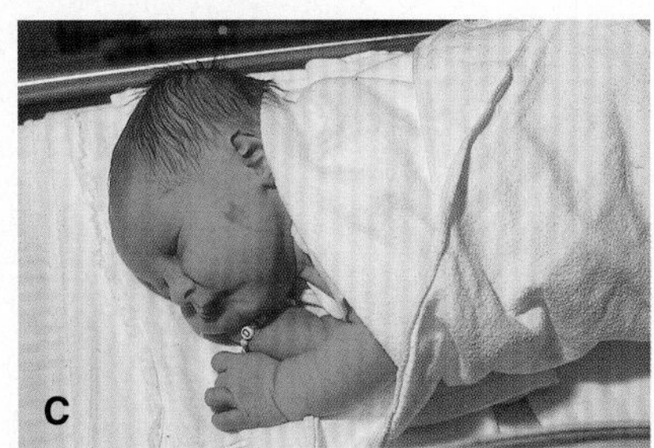

FIGURE 21.6 Forceps delivery (uncommon). **A.** Example of forceps. **B.** Forceps being applied to the fetus. **C.** Forceps marks are commonly found in newborns delivered by forceps. Such marks are transient and disappear in a day or two.

rotating the fetal head during birth. Forceps are stainless-steel instruments, similar to tongs, with rounded edges that fit around the fetus's head. Some forceps have open blades and some have solid blades. Outlet forceps are used when the fetal head is crowning and low forceps are used when the fetal head is at a +2 station or lower but not yet crowning. The forceps are applied to the sides of the fetal head. The type of forceps used is determined by the birth attendant. All forceps have a locking mechanism that prevents the blades from compressing the fetal skull. Use of forceps has declined in popularity recently because many obstetricians are not trained to use them in their residency since they are rarely used in obstetrical practice today (Fig. 21.6).

A vacuum extractor is a cup-shaped instrument attached to a suction pump used for extraction of the fetal head (Fig. 21.7). The suction cup is placed against the occiput of the fetal head. The pump is used to create negative pressure (suction) of approximately 50 to 60 mm Hg. The birth attendant then applies traction until the fetal head emerges from the vagina.

The indications for the use of either method are similar and include a prolonged second stage of labor, a distressed FHR pattern, failure of the presenting part to fully rotate and descend in the pelvis, limited sensation and inability to push effectively due to the effects of regional anesthesia, presumed fetal jeopardy or fetal distress, maternal heart disease, acute pulmonary edema, intrapartum infection, maternal fatigue, or infection. There is a clear trend to choose vacuum extraction over forceps to assist delivery, but the evidence supporting that trend is unconvincing. Recent literature confirms some advantages for forceps (e.g., a lower failure rate) and some disadvantages for vacuum extraction (e.g., increased neonatal injury), depending on the clinical circumstances (O'Grady & St. Andre, 2015).

The use of forceps or a vacuum extractor poses the risk of tissue trauma to the mother and the newborn. Maternal trauma may include lacerations of the cervix, vagina, or perineum; hematoma; extension of the episiotomy incision into the anus; hemorrhage; and infection. Potential newborn trauma includes ecchymoses, facial

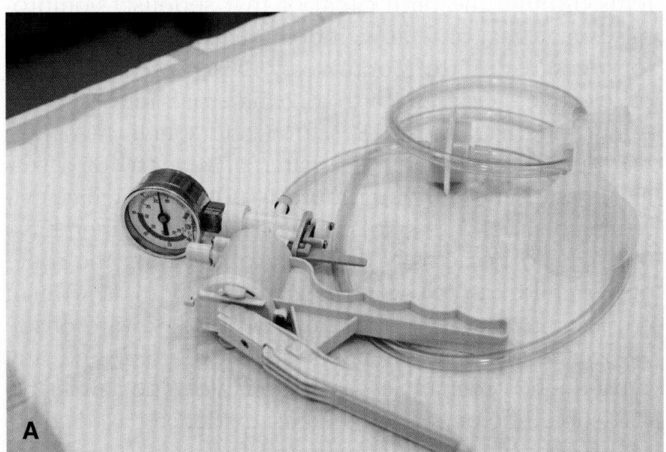
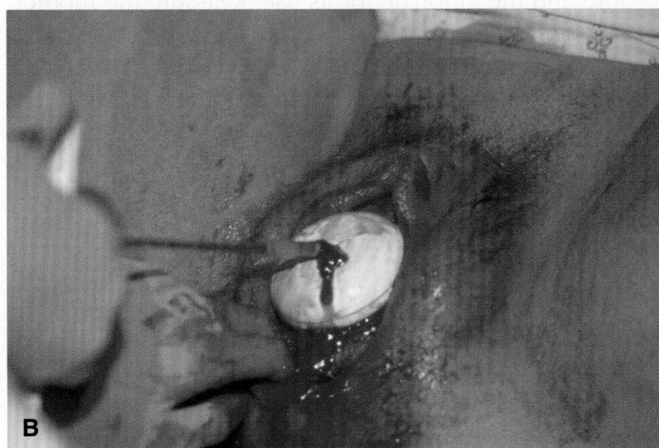

FIGURE 21.7 Vacuum extractor for delivery. **A.** Example of a vacuum extractor. **B.** Vacuum extractor applied to the fetal head to assist in delivery.

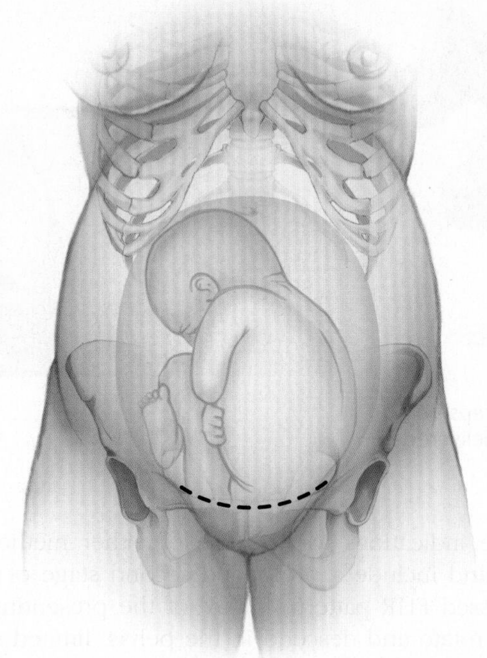

FIGURE 21.8 Low transverse incision for cesarean birth.

and scalp lacerations, facial nerve injury, cephalhematoma, and caput succedaneum (Cunningham et al., 2014). For forceps or a vacuum extractor to be applied, the following criteria need to be met: membranes ruptured, cervix completely dilated, fetus vertex and engaged, and an adequate maternal pelvis size.

Prevention is key to reducing the use of these techniques. Preventive measures include frequently changing the client's position, encouraging ambulation if permitted, frequently reminding the client to empty her bladder to allow maximum space for birth, and providing adequate hydration throughout labor. Additional measures include assessing maternal vital signs, the contraction pattern, the fetal status, and the maternal response to the procedure. Provide a thorough explanation of the procedure and the rationale for its use. Reassure the mother that any marks or swelling on the newborn's head or face will disappear without treatment within 2 to 3 days. Alert the postpartum nursing staff about the use of the technique so that they can observe for any bleeding or infection related to genital lacerations.

Cesarean Birth

A cesarean birth is the surgical birth of the fetus through an incision in the abdomen and uterine wall and is the most commonly performed surgery in the United States (Green, 2016). A classic (vertical) or low transverse (horizontal) incision may be used; however, the low transverse incision is more common today (Fig. 21.8).

High cesarean birth rates are an international concern. The cesarean birth rate in the United States is on the rise at an alarming rate. Today approximately 33% or one in three births occurs this way. This is the 14th consecutive year the cesarean birth rate has risen, despite a number of medical organizations, including the WHO and ACOG, urging medical care providers to work on lowering the cesarean birth rate (Centers for Disease Control and Prevention, 2015). Cesarean births may result from maternal, fetal, or placental factors that interfere with a vaginal birth. Several factors may explain this increased incidence of cesarean deliveries: the use of electronic fetal monitoring, which identifies fetal distress early; the reduced number of forceps-assisted births; older maternal age and reduced parity; increasing maternal obesity, with more nulliparous women having infants; convenience to the client and doctor; and an increase in malpractice suits. The leading indications for cesarean births are previous cesarean birth, breech presentation, dystocia, and fetal distress. Once a woman has experienced a primary cesarean birth, she has a 90% chance of having another one in a subsequent pregnancy (Joy & Contag, 2015).

Cesarean birth is a major surgical procedure with increased risks compared with a vaginal birth. The client is at risk for complications such as infection, hemorrhage, aspiration, pulmonary embolism, urinary tract trauma, thrombophlebitis, paralytic ileus, and atelectasis. Fetal injury and transient tachypnea of the newborn also may occur (Cunningham et al., 2014).

Spinal, epidural, or general anesthesia is used for cesarean births. Epidural anesthesia is most commonly used because it is associated with less risk and most women wish to be awake and aware of the birth experience.

Nursing Assessment

Review the woman's history for indications associated with cesarean birth and complete a physical examination. Any condition that prevents the safe passage of the fetus through the birth canal or that seriously compromises maternal or fetal well-being may be an indication for a cesarean birth. Controversy exists over the option of elective cesarean birth on maternal request. The Agency for Healthcare Research and Quality (AHRQ) has published a report on maternal request for a surgical birth, and although there is not high-quality evidence to support this, it is recognized that women have the right to be actively involved in choosing the route of her childbirth (Norwitz, 2015). The pregnant woman requesting a surgical birth must be made aware of the associated risks and benefits for the current and any subsequent pregnancies is reasonable. The clinician's role should be to provide the best evidence-based counseling possible to the woman and to respect her autonomy and decision-making capabilities when considering route of birth.

Examples of specific indications include active genital herpes, fetal macrosomia, fetopelvic disproportion, prolapsed umbilical cord, placental abnormality (placenta previa or abruptio placentae), previous classic uterine incision or scar, gestational hypertension, diabetes, positive human immunodeficiency virus (HIV) status, and dystocia. Fetal indications include malpresentation (nonvertex presentation), congenital anomalies (fetal neural tube defects, hydrocephalus, abdominal wall defects), and fetal distress (Joy & Contag, 2015).

Nursing Management

Once the decision has been made to proceed with a cesarean birth, assess the woman's knowledge of the procedure and necessary preparation. Assist with obtaining diagnostic tests as ordered. These tests are usually ordered to ensure the well-being of both parties and may include a complete blood count; urinalysis to rule out infection; blood type and cross-match so that blood is available for transfusion if needed; an ultrasound to determine fetal position and placental location; and an amniocentesis to determine fetal lung maturity if needed.

Although the nurse's role in a cesarean birth can be very technical and skill oriented at times, the focus must remain on the woman, not the equipment surrounding the bed. Care should be centered on the family, not the surgery. Provide education and minimize separation of the mother, father, and newborn. Remember that the client is anxious and concerned about her welfare as well as that of her child. Use touch, eye contact, therapeutic communication, and genuine caring to provide couples with a positive birth experience, regardless of the type of delivery.

PROVIDING PREOPERATIVE CARE

Client preparation varies depending on whether the cesarean birth is planned or unplanned. The major difference is the time allotted for preparation and teaching. In an unplanned cesarean birth, institute measures quickly to ensure the best outcomes for the mother and fetus. Ensure that the woman has signed an informed consent, and allow for discussion of fears and expectations. Provide essential teaching and explanations to reduce the woman's fears and anxieties.

Ascertain the client's and family's understanding of the surgical procedure. Reinforce the reasons for surgery given by the surgeon. Outline the procedure and expectations of the surgical experience. Ensure that all diagnostic tests ordered have been completed, and evaluate the results. Explain to the woman and her family about what to expect postoperatively. Reassure the woman that pain management will be provided throughout the procedure and afterward. Encourage the woman to report any pain. Ask the woman about the time she last had anything to eat or drink. Document the time and what was consumed. Throughout the preparations, assess maternal and fetal status frequently.

Provide preoperative teaching to reduce the risk of postoperative complications. Demonstrate the use of the incentive spirometer and deep-breathing and leg exercises. Instruct the woman on how to splint her incision.

Complete the preoperative procedures, which may include:

- Preparing the surgical site as ordered
- Starting an intravenous infusion for fluid replacement therapy as ordered
- Inserting an indwelling (Foley) catheter and informing the client about how long it will remain in place (usually 24 hours)
- Administering any preoperative medications as ordered; documenting the time administered and the client's reaction

Maintain a calm, confident manner in all interactions with the client and family. Help transport the client and her partner to the operative area.

PROVIDING POSTOPERATIVE CARE

Postoperative care for the mother who has had a cesarean delivery is similar to that for one who has had a vaginal birth, with a few additional measures. Assess vital signs and lochia flow every 15 minutes for the first hour, then every 30 minutes for the next hour, and then every 4 hours if stable. Assist with perineal care and instruct the client in the same. Inspect the abdominal dressing and document description, including any evidence of drainage. Assess uterine tone to determine fundal firmness. Check the patency of the intravenous line, making sure the infusion is flowing at the correct rate. Inspect the infusion site frequently for redness.

Assess the woman's level of consciousness if sedative drugs were administered. Institute safety precautions until the woman is fully alert and responsive. If a regional anesthetic was used, monitor for the return of sensation to the legs.

Assess for evidence of abdominal distention and auscultate bowel sounds. Assist with early ambulation to prevent respiratory and cardiovascular problems and to promote peristalsis. Monitor intake and output at least every 4 hours initially and then every 8 hours as indicated.

Encourage the woman to cough, perform deep-breathing exercises, and use the incentive spirometer every 2 hours. Enhance comfort and general well-being. Administer analgesics as ordered and provide comfort measures, such as splinting the incision and pillows for positioning. Assist the client to move in bed and turn side to side to improve circulation. Also encourage the woman to ambulate to promote venous return from the extremities. Prevent/minimize postoperative complications.

Encourage early touching and holding of the newborn to promote bonding. Promote family unity and bonding. Assist with breast-feeding initiation and offer continued support. Suggest alternate positioning techniques to reduce incisional discomfort while breast-feeding. (See Chapter 18 for breast-feeding positions.)

Review with the couple their perception of the surgical birth experience. Allow them to verbalize their feelings and assist them in positive coping measures. Promote a positive emotional response to the birth experience and parenting role. Prior to discharge, teach the woman about the need for adequate rest, activity restrictions such as lifting, and signs and symptoms of infection. Provide information about postpartum care at home upon discharge.

NURSING CARE PLAN 21.1

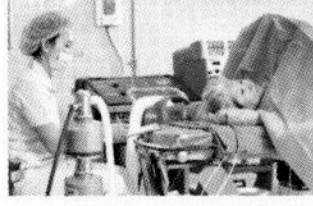

Overview of the Women Undergoing Labor Induction

Rose, a 29-year-old primipara, is admitted to the labor and birth suite at 40 weeks' gestation for induction of labor. Assessment reveals that her cervix is ripe and 80% effaced, and dilated to 2 cm. Rose says, "I'm a bit nervous about being induced. I've never been through labor before and I'm afraid that I'll have a lot of pain from the medicine used to start the contractions." She consents to being induced but wants reassurance that this procedure won't harm the baby. Upon examination, the fetus is engaged and in a cephalic presentation, with the vertex as the presenting part. Her partner is at her side. Induction is initiated with oxytocin. Rose reports that contractions have started and are beginning to get stronger.

NURSING DIAGNOSIS: Anxiety related to induction of labor and associated medical interventions needed as evidenced by statements about being nervous, not having gone through labor before, fear of pain and potential harm to fetus

Outcome Identification and Evaluation

The client will experience decrease in anxiety as evidenced by ability to verbalize understanding of procedures involved and use of positive coping skills to reduce anxious state.

Interventions: *Minimizing Anxiety*

- Provide a clear explanation of the labor induction process *to provide client and partner with a knowledge base.*
- Maintain continuous physical presence *to provide physical and emotional support and demonstrate concern for maternal and fetal well-being.*
- Explain each procedure before carrying it out and answer questions *to promote understanding of procedure and rationale for use and decrease fear of the unknown.*
- Review with client measures used in the past to deal with stressful situations *to determine effectiveness;* encourage use of past effective coping strategies *to aid in controlling anxiety.*
- Instruct client's partner in helpful measures to assist client in coping and encourage their use *to foster joint participation in the process and feelings of being in control and to provide support to the client.*
- Offer frequent reassurance of fetal status and labor progress *to help alleviate client's concerns and foster continued participation in the labor process.*

NURSING DIAGNOSIS: Risk for injury (maternal or fetal) related to induction procedure risk factors: hypertonic uterine contractions, potential preterm birth as evidenced by client's concerns about fetal well-being and possible adverse effects of oxytocin administration

Outcome Identification and Evaluation

The client will remain free of complications associated with induction as evidenced by progression of labor as expected, delivery of healthy newborn, and absence of signs and symptoms of maternal and fetal adverse effects.

NURSING CARE PLAN 21.1

Overview of the Women Undergoing Labor Induction (continued)

Interventions: ***Promoting Maternal and Fetal Safety***

- Follow agency's protocol for medication use and infusion rate *to ensure accurate, safe drug administration.*
- Set up oxytocin IV infusion to piggyback into the primary IV infusion line *to allow for prompt discontinuation should adverse effects occur.*
- Use an infusion pump *to deliver accurate dose as ordered.*
- Gradually increase oxytocin dose in increments based on assessment findings and protocol *to promote effective uterine contractions.*
- Maintain oxytocin rate once desired frequency of contractions has been reached *to ensure continued progress in labor.*
- Accurately monitor contractions for frequency, duration, and intensity and resting tone *to prevent development of hypertonic contractions.*
- Maintain a nurse-to-client ratio of 1:2 *to ensure maternal and fetal safety.*
- Monitor FHR via electronic fetal monitoring during induction and continuously observe the FHR response to titrated medication rate *to ensure fetal well-being and identify adverse effects immediately.*
- Obtain maternal vital signs every 1 to 2 hours or as indicated by agency's protocol, reporting any deviations, *to promote maternal well-being and allow for prompt detection of problems.*
- Communicate with birth attendant frequently concerning progress *to ensure continuity of care.*
- Discontinue oxytocin infusion if tetanic contractions (>90 seconds), uterine hyperstimulation (<2 minutes apart), elevated uterine resting tone, or a distressed FHR pattern occurs *to minimize risk of drug's adverse effects.*
- Provide client with frequent reassurance of maternal and fetal status *to minimize anxiety.*

NURSING DIAGNOSIS: Pain related to uterine contractions as evidenced by client's statements about contractions increasing in intensity and expected effect of oxytocin administration

Outcome Identification and Evaluation

The client will report a decrease in pain as evidenced by statements of increased comfort and pain rating of 3 or less on numeric pain rating scale.

Interventions: ***Promoting Maternal and Fetal Safety***

- Explain to the client that she will experience discomfort sooner than with naturally occurring labor *to promote client's awareness of events and prepare client for the experience.*
- Frequently assess client's pain using a pain rating scale *to quantify client's level of pain and evaluate effectiveness of pain relief measures.*
- Provide comfort measures, such as hygiene, backrubs, music, and distraction, and encourage the use of breathing and relaxation techniques *to help promote relaxation.*
- Provide support for her partner *to aid in alleviating stress and concerns.*
- Employ nonpharmacologic methods, such as position changes, birthing ball, hydrotherapy, visual imagery, and effleurage, *to help in managing pain and foster feelings of control over situation.*
- Administer pharmacologic agents such as analgesia or anesthesia as appropriate and as ordered *to control pain.*
- Continuously reassess client's pain level *to evaluate effectiveness of pain management techniques used.*

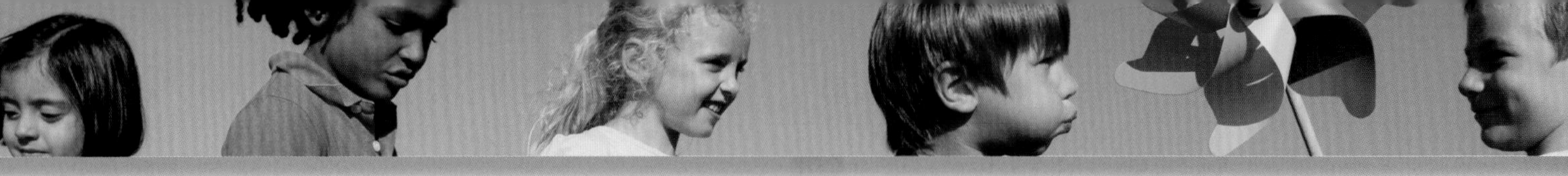

KEY CONCEPTS

- Risk factors for dystocia include epidural analgesia, occiput posterior position, longer first stage of labor, nulliparity, short maternal stature (<5 ft tall), high birth weight, maternal age older than 35 years, gestational age more than 41 weeks, chorioamnionitis, pelvic contractions, macrosomia, and high station at complete cervical dilation.
- Dystocia may result from problems in the powers, passenger, passageway, or psyche.
- Problems involving the powers that lead to dystocia include hypertonic uterine dysfunction, hypotonic uterine dysfunction, and precipitate labor.
- Management of hypertonic labor pattern involves therapeutic rest with the use of sedatives to promote relaxation and stop the abnormal activity of the uterus.
- Any presentation other than occiput or a slight variation of the fetal position or size increases the probability of dystocia.
- Multiple pregnancy may result in dysfunctional labor due to uterine overdistention, which may lead to hypotonic dystocia and abnormal presentations of the fetuses.
- During labor, evaluation of fetal descent, cervical effacement and dilation, and characteristics of uterine contractions are paramount to determine progress or lack thereof.
- Antepartum assessment for a postterm pregnancy typically includes daily fetal movement counts done by the woman, nonstress tests done twice weekly, amniotic fluid assessments as part of the biophysical profile, and weekly cervical examinations to check for ripening for induction.
- Once the cervix is ripe, oxytocin is the most popular pharmacologic agent used for inducing or augmenting labor.
- Generally, the first and most reliable symptom of uterine rupture is fetal distress.
- Amniotic fluid embolism is a rare but often fatal event characterized by the sudden onset of hypotension, hypoxia, and coagulopathy.
- Cesarean births have steadily risen in the United States; today, approximately one in three births occurs this way. Cesarean birth is a major surgical procedure and has increased risks over vaginal birth.

REFERENCES AND RECOMMENDED READINGS

Abbott, D. S., Hezelgrave, N. L., Seed, P. T., Norman, J. E., David, A. L., Bennett, P. R., et al. (2015). Quantitative fetal fibronectin to predict preterm birth in asymptomatic women at high risk. *Obstetrics & Gynecology, 125*(5), 1168–1176.

Afzal, M., Asif, U., & Miraj, B. (2015). Induction of labor: Efficacy of sweeping of membranes at term in previous one C-section. *Professional Medical Journal, 22*(4), 385–389.

Ahmed, Z. D., Garba, I., Nafi'ah, T., & Yakasai, I. A. (2015). Misoprostol: An effective agent for cervical ripening and labor induction: A 2-year review in a tertiary center. *Open Journal of Obstetrics and Gynecology, 5*(05), 274–279.

American Academy of Pediatrics. (2015). *Delivery by cesarean section*. Retrieved from http://www.healthychildren.org/English/ages-stages/prenatal/delivery-beyond/pages/Delivery-by-Cesarean-Section.aspx

American Academy of Pediatrics[AAP] & American College of Obstetricians and Gynecologists [ACOG]. (2010). *Guidelines for perinatal care* (6th ed.). Washington, DC: Author.

American College of Obstetricians and Gynecologists [ACOG]. (2010). ACOG practice bulletin no. 115: Vaginal birth after previous cesarean delivery. *Obstetrics and Gynecology, 116*, 450–463.

American College of Obstetricians & Gynecologists [ACOG]. (2014a). Safe prevention of primary cesarean delivery. *American Journal of Obstetrics & Gynecology, 123*, 693–711.

American College of Obstetricians & Gynecologists [ACOG]. (2014b). *Preterm labor practice guidelines*. Retrieved from http://www.acog.org/Womens-Health/Preterm-Premature-Labor-and-BirthAmerican

Arrowsmith, S., & Wray, S. (2014). Oxytocin: Its mechanism of action and receptor signaling in the myometrium. *Journal of Neuroendocrinology, 26*, 356–369.

Baldisseri, M. R. (2014). Amniotic fluid embolism syndrome. *UpToDate*. Retrieved from http://www.uptodate.com/contents/amniotic-fluid-embolism-syndrome

Beall, M. H., & Ross, M. G. (2014). Umbilical cord complications. *eMedicine*. Retrieved from http://emedicine.medscape.com/article/262470-overview

Bibbo, C., & Robinson, J. N. (2015). Management of twins: Vaginal or cesarean delivery? *Clinical Obstetrics & Gynecology, 58*(2), 294–308.

Bush, M., Eddleman, K., & Belogovkin, V. (2015). Umbilical cord prolapse. *UpToDate*. Retrieved from: http://www.uptodate.com/contents/umbilical-cord-prolapse

Cabbad, M. F., De Los Heros, D., Baltajian, K. Z., & Robertazzi, R. R. (2015). Corticosteroid use in the face of threatened preterm labor [165]. *Obstetrics & Gynecology, 125*, 56S.

Callahan, T. L. (2016). *Tarascon Ob/Gyn Pocketbook*. Burlington, MA: Jones & Bartlett Publishers.

Callister, L. C. (2014). Global perspectives on perinatal loss. *MCN: The American Journal of Maternal/Child Nursing, 39*(3), 207.

Caughey, A. (2014a). Induction of labor: Does it increase the risk of cesarean delivery? *BJOG, 121*, 658–661.

Caughey, A. B. (2014b). Vaginal birth after cesarean delivery. *eMedicine*. Retrieved from http://emedicine.medscape.com/article/272187-overview

Caughey, A. B., & Butler, J. R. (2015). Postterm pregnancy. *eMedicine*. Retrieved from http://emedicine.medscape.com/article/261369-overview

Centers for Disease Control and Prevention [CDC]. (2015). Primary cesarean delivery rates, by State. *National Vital Statistics Reports, 63*(1). Retrieved from http://www.cdc.gov/nchs/data/nvsr/nvsr63/nvsr63_01.pdf

Chandrasekaran, S., & Srinivas, S. K. (2014). Antenatal corticosteroid administration: Understanding its use as an obstetric quality metric. *American Journal of Obstetrics and Gynecology, 210*(2), 143–150.

Cheng, Y., & Caughey, A. B. (2015). Normal labor and delivery. *eMedicine*. Retrieved from http://emedicine.medscape.com/article/260036-overview

Cunningham, F. G., Leveno, K. J., Bloom, S. L., Spong, C.Y., Dashe, J.S., Hoffman, B.L., et al. (2014). *Williams' obstetrics* (24th ed.). New York, NY: McGraw-Hill.

Deering, S. H. (2015). Abruptio placenta. *eMedicine*. Retrieved from http://emedicine.medscape.com/article/252810-overview

Drunecký, T., Reidingerová, M., Plisová, M., Dudi , M., Gdovinová, D., & Stoy, V. (2015). Experimental comparison of properties of natural and synthetic osmotic dilators. *Archives of Gynecology and Obstetrics, 292*, 349–354.

Fischer, R. (2015). Breech presentation. *eMedicine*. Retrieved from http://emedicine.medscape.com/article/262159-overview

Flenady, V., Wojcieszek, A. M., Papatsonis, D. N. M., Stock, O. M., Murray, L., Jardine, L. A., et al. (2014). Calcium channel blockers for inhibiting preterm labor and birth. *Cochrane Database of Systematic Reviews, 6*, CD002255.

Fong, A., Chau, C., Pan, D., & Ogunyemi, D. (2014). Amniotic fluid embolism: Antepartum, intrapartum and demographic factors. *The Journal of Maternal-Fetal & Neonatal Medicine*, (Online June 30, 2014), 1–6.

Fuks, A. M., Robinson, J. V., Rothschild, T. J., Akinnawonu, K. F., & Salafia, C. (2015). Mechanical labor induction using the Foley catheter balloon compared with the cook cervical balloon [96]. *Obstetrics & Gynecology, 125*, 37S.

Gherman, R. (2015). Shoulder dystocia. In *Protocols for high-risk pregnancies: An evidence-based approach* (6th ed.). Hoboken, NJ: John Wiley & Sons.

Goetzl, L. (2014). Methods of cervical ripening and labor induction: Pharmacologic. *Clinical Obstetrics and Gynecology, 57*(2), 377–390.

Goldberg, A. E. (2015). Cervical ripening. *eMedicine*. Retrieved from http://emedicine.medscape.com/article/263311-overview

Green, C. J. (2016). *Maternal newborn nursing care plans* (3rd ed.). Burlington, MA: Jones & Bartlett Learning.

Grobman, W. (2015). Is it time for outpatient cervical ripening with prostaglandins? *BJOG: An International Journal of Obstetrics & Gynecology, 122*, 105.

Grunebaum, A., & Chervenak, F.A. (2014). Counseling parents after fetal demise and stillbirth. *UpToDate*. Retrieved from http://www.uptodate.com/contents/counseling-parents-after-fetal-demise-and-stillbirth

Haas, D. M., Benjamin, T., Sawyer, R., & Quinney, S. K. (2014). Short-term tocolytics for preterm delivery–current perspectives. *International Journal of Women's Health, 6*, 343–349.

Hinshaw, K., & Kenyon, S. (2015). Abnormal labor. In *Arias' practical guide to high-risk pregnancy & delivery* (4th ed.). New Delhi, India: Elsevier.

Hobbins, J. C. (2015). Macrosomia. *OB/GYN Clinical Alert, 32*(2), 13–16.

Hofmeyr, G. J. (2015). Protocol 51: Breech delivery. In J. T. Queenan, C. Y. Spong, & C. J. Lockwood (Eds.), *Protocols for high-risk pregnancies: An evidence-based approach*. Chichester, UK: John Wiley & Sons.

Hofmeyr, G. J., Eke, A. C., & Lawrie, T. A. (2014). Amnioinfusion for third trimester preterm premature rupture of membranes. *Cochrane Database of Systematic Reviews, 3*, CD000942.

Hofmeyr G. J., Kulier, R., & West, H. M. (2015). External cephalic version for breech presentation at term. *Cochrane Database of Systematic Reviews, 4*, CD000083.

Hofmeyr, G. J., Xu, H., & Eke, A. C. (2014). Amnioinfusion for meconium-stained liquor in labor. *Cochrane Database of Systematic Reviews, 1*, CD000014.

Holley, S. R., & Pasch, L. A. (2015). Counseling lesbian, gay, bisexual, and transgender patients. *Fertility counseling* (pp. 180–194). Cambridge, UK: Cambridge University Press.

Hugin, M. P., & Sultani, S. L. (2015). Evaluation of fetal death. *eMedicine*. Retrieved from http://emedicine.medscape.com/article/259165-overview

Iams, J. D. (2015). Clinical practice: Prevention of preterm parturition. *Obstetric Anesthesia Digest, 35*(1), 34–36.

International Childbirth Education Association [ICEA]. (2014). *ICEA position paper: Induction*. Retrieved from http://www.icea.org/sites/default/files/Induction%20PP-FINAL.pdf

Jazayeri, A. (2015). Macrosomia. *eMedicine*. [Online] Available: http://emedicine.medscape.com/article/262679-overview

Jordan, R. G., Engstrom, J. L., Marfell, J. A., & Farley, C. L. (2014). *Prenatal and postnatal care: A woman-centered approach*. Ames, Iowa: John Wiley & Sons, Inc.

Jørgensen, J. S., Weile, L. K. K., & Lamont, R. F. (2014). Preterm labor: Current tocolytic options for the treatment of preterm labor. *Expert Opinion on Pharmacotherapy, 15*(5), 585–588.

Joy, S., & Contag, S. A. (2015). Cesarean delivery. *eMedicine*. Retrieved from http://emedicine.medscape.com/article/263424-overview

Joy, S., & Finneran, M. M. (2015). Placenta previa. *eMedicine*. Retrieved from http://emedicine.medscape.com/article/262063-overview

Joy, S., Lyon, D., & Scott, P. L. (2015). Abnormal labor. *eMedicine*. Retrieved from http://emedicine.medscape.com/article/273053-overview

Kilpatrick, S. J. (2014). Trauma in pregnancy. *UpToDate*. Retrieved from http://www.uptodate.com/contents/trauma-in-pregnancy

King, T. L., Brucker, M. C., Kriebs, J. M., Fahey, J. O., Gegor, C. L., & Varney, H. (2015). *Varney's midwifery* (5th ed.). Burlington, MA: Jones & Bartlett Learning.

King, V. J., Fontaine, P. L., Atwood, L. A., Powers, E., Leeman, L., Ecker, J. L., et al. (2015). Clinical practice guideline executive summary: Labor after cesarean/planned vaginal birth after cesarean. *The Annals of Family Medicine, 13*(1), 80–81.

Kriebs, J. M. (2015). Patient safety during induction of labor. *The Journal of Perinatal & Neonatal Nursing*, *29*(2), 130–137.

Lal, A. K., & Hibbard, J. U. (2015). Placenta previa: An outcome-based cohort study in a contemporary obstetric population. *Archives of Gynecology and Obstetrics*, 299–305.

Lewis, L., Pan, H., Heine, R., Brown, H., Brancazio, L., & Grotegut, C. (2014). Labor and pregnancy outcomes after adoption of a more conservative oxytocin labor protocol. *Obstetrics & Gynecology*, *123*, 166S.

Locatelli, A., Consonni, S., & Ghidini, A. (2015). Preterm labor: Approach to decreasing complications of prematurity. *Obstetrics and Gynecology Clinics of North America*, *42*(2), 255–274.

Manjula, B. G., Bagga, R., Kalra, J., & Dutta, S. (2015). Labor induction with an intermediate-dose oxytocin regimen has advantages over a high-dose regimen. *Journal of Obstetrics & Gynecology*, *35*(4), 362–367.

March of Dimes. (2015a). Multiples: Twins, triplets and beyond. Retrieved from http://www.marchofdimes.com/professionals/14332_4545.asp

March of Dimes. (2015b). Preterm labor and birth: A serious pregnancy complication. Retrieved from http://www.marchofdimes.com/pregnancy/preterm_indepth.html

March of Dimes. (2015c). *Umbilical cord abnormalities*. Retrieved from http://www.marchofdimes.com/professionals/681_4546.asp.

March of Dimes. (2015d). *Placenta previa*. Retrieved from http://www.marchofdimes.org/pregnancy/placenta-previa.aspx

March of Dimes. (2015e). *Placental abruption*. Retrieved from http://www.marchofdimes.org/pregnancy/placental-abruption.aspx

Mattson, S., & Smith, J. E. (2016). *Core curriculum for maternal-newborn nursing* (5th ed.). Philadelphia, PA: Elsevier Health Sciences.

McCarthy, F. P., & Kenny, L. C. (2014). Induction of labor. *Obstetrics, Gynecology & Reproductive Medicine*, *24*(1), 9–15.

Mehlman, C. T. (2015). Neonatal brachial plexus palsy. *The pediatric upper extremity* (pp. 589–605). New York, NY: Springer Publishers.

Moore, L. E. (2015). Amniotic fluid embolism. *eMedicine*. Retrieved from http://emedicine.medscape.com/article/253068-overview#a5

Moses, S. (2015). Amniotic fluid embolism. *Family Practice Notebook*. Retrieved from: http://www.fpnotebook.com/Lung/OB/AmntcFldEmblsm.htm

Nagtalon-Ramos, J. (2014). *Best evidence-based practices-maternal-newborn nursing care*. Philadelphia, PA: F.A. Davis Company.

Nahum, G. G., & Pham, K. Q. (2015). Uterine rupture in pregnancy. *eMedicine*. Retrieved from http://emedicine.medscape.com/article/275854-overview

Nakazawa, H., Uchida, A., Minamitani, T., Makishi, A., Takamatsu, Y., Kiyoshi, K., et al. (2015). Factors affecting maternal serum magnesium levels during long-term magnesium sulfate tocolysis in singleton and twin pregnancy. *Journal of Obstetrics & Gynecology Research*. *41*(8), 1178–1184.

Norwitz, E. R. (2015). Cesarean delivery on maternal request. *UpToDate*. Retrieved from http://www.uptodate.com/contents/cesarean-delivery-on-maternal-request

O'Grady, J. P., & St. Andre, C. (2015). Vacuum extraction. *eMedicine*. Retrieved from http://emedicine.medscape.com/article/271175-overview#aw2aab6b4

Patel, P. K., Pitre, D. S., & Bhooker, S. P. (2015). Predictive value of various risk factors for preterm labor. *Community Medicine*, *6*(1), 121–125.

Robinson, G. E. (2014). Pregnancy loss. *Best Practice & Research Clinical Obstetrics & Gynecology*, *28*(1), 169–178.

Ross, M. G. (2015). Preterm labor. *eMedicine*. Retrieved from http://emedicine.medscape.com/article/260998-overview#aw2aab6b7

Sadera, G., & Vasudevan, B. (2015). Amniotic fluid embolism. *Journal of Obstetric Anesthesia and Critical Care*, *5*(1), 3–8.

Sciscione, A. C. (2014). Methods of cervical ripening and labor induction: Mechanical. *Clinical Obstetrics and Gynecology*, *57*(2), 369–376.

Scott, J. R. (2015). Vaginal birth after cesarean. *Protocols for high-risk pregnancies: An evidence-based approach* (6th ed., pp. 428–432). Hoboken, NJ: John Wiley & Sons.

Sharshiner, R., & Silver, R. M. (2015). Management of fetal malpresentation. *Clinical Obstetrics and Gynecology*, *58*(2), 246–255.

Soni, A., Vaishnav, G. D., & Gohil, J. (2015). Meconium and its significance and obstetric outcome. *Medicine Science International Medical Journal*, *4*(1), 1861–1868.

Sosa, C. G., Althabe, F., Belizan, J.M., & Bergel, E. (2015). Bed rest in singleton pregnancies for preventing preterm birth. *Cochrane Database of Systematic Reviews*, (3).

Sotiriadis, A., Tsiami, A., Papatheodorou, S., Baschat, A. A., Sarafidis, K., & Makrydimas, G. (2015). Neurodevelopmental outcome after a single course of antenatal steroids in children born preterm: A systematic review and meta-analysis. *Obstetrics & Gynecology*, *125*(6), 1385–1396.

Souka, A. P., Papastefanou, I., Papadopoulos, G., Chrelias, C., & Kassanos, D. (2015). Cervical length in late second and third trimester: A mixture model for predicting delivery. *Ultrasound in Obstetrics & Gynecology*, 308–312..

Sousou, J. & Smart, C. (2015). Care of the childbearing family with intrauterine fetal demise. *Nursing for Women's Health*, *19*, 236–247.

Suzuki, S. (2015). Clinical significance of precipitous labor. *Journal of Clinical Medicine Research*, *7*(3), 150–153.

U.S. Department of Health and Human Services. (2010). *Healthy People 2020*. Retrieved from http://www.healthypeople.gov/2020/topicsobjectives2020/default.aspx

van Baaren, G. J., Bruijn, M. M., Vis, J. Y., Wilms, F. F., Oudijk, M. A., Kwee, A., et al. (2015). Risk factors for preterm delivery: Do they add to fetal fibronectin testing and cervical length measurement in the prediction of preterm delivery in symptomatic women? *European Journal of Obstetrics & Gynecology and Reproductive Biology*. doi:10.1016/j.ejogrb.2015.05.004

van Baaren, G. J., Vis, J. Y., Wilms, F. F., Oudijk, M. A., Kwee, A., Porath, M. M., et al. (2014). Predictive value of cervical length measurement and fibronectin testing in threatened preterm labor. *Obstetrics & Gynecology*, *123*(6), 1185–1192.

van den Bosch, A. E., Ruys, T. P., & Roos-Hesselink, J. W. (2015). Use and impact of cardiac medication during pregnancy. *Future Cardiology*, *11*(1), 89–100.

Viswanathan, M., Venkateswaran, V. K., & Daniel, S. (2014). Amniotic fluid embolism: A comprehensive review.

International Journal of Reproduction, Contraception, Obstetrics and Gynecology, 3(2), 304–309.

Vogel, J. P., Gulmezoglu, A. M. M., Hofmeyr, G. J., & Temmerman, M. (2014). Global perspectives on elective induction of labor. *Clinical Obstetrics and Gynecology, 57*(2), 331–342.

Walker, N., & Gan, J. H. (2015). Prolonged pregnancy. *Obstetrics, Gynecology & Reproductive Medicine, 25*(3), 83–87.

Westwood, S., King, A., Almack, K., Suen, Y. T., & Bailey, L. (2015). Good practice in health and social care provision for LGBT older people in the UK. In *Lesbian, gay, bisexual and trans health inequalities: International perspectives in social work* (pp. 145–158). Chicago, IL: Policy Press.

World Health Organization [WHO]. (2014a). *Managing complications in pregnancy and childbirth: A guide for midwives and doctors.* Retrieved from http://www.who.int/maternal_child_adolescent/documents/9241545879/en/

World Health Organization [WHO]. (2014b). *WHO recommendations for augmentation of labor.* Retrieved from http://apps.who.int/iris/bitstream/10665/112825/1/9789241507363_eng.pdf

CHAPTER WORKSHEET

MULTIPLE-CHOICE QUESTIONS

1. When reviewing the medical record of a client, the nurse notes that the woman has a condition in which the fetus cannot physically pass through the maternal pelvis. The nurse interprets this as:
   a. Cervical insufficiency
   b. Contracted pelvis
   c. Maternal disproportion
   d. Fetopelvic disproportion
2. The nurse would anticipate a cesarean birth for a client who has which active infection present at the onset of labor?
   a. Hepatitis
   b. Herpes simplex virus
   c. Toxoplasmosis
   d. Human papillomavirus
3. After a vaginal examination, the nurse determines that the client's fetus is in an occiput posterior position. The nurse would anticipate that the client will have:
   a. Intense back pain
   b. Frequent leg cramps
   c. Nausea and vomiting
   d. A precipitous birth
4. When assessing the following women, which would the nurse identify as being at the greatest risk for preterm labor?
   a. Woman who had twins in a previous pregnancy
   b. Client living in a large city close to the subway
   c. Woman working full time as a computer programmer
   d. Client with a history of a previous preterm birth
5. The rationale for using a prostaglandin gel for a client prior to the induction of labor is to:
   a. Stimulate uterine contractions
   b. Numb cervical pain receptors
   c. Prevent cervical lacerations
   d. Soften and efface the cervix
6. A client who was in active labor and whose cervix had dilated to 4 cm experiences a weakening in the intensity and frequency of her contractions and exhibits no further progress in labor. The nurse interprets this as a sign of:
   a. Hypertonic labor
   b. Precipitate labor
   c. Hypotonic labor
   d. Dysfunctional labor
7. The nurse is developing a plan of care for a woman experiencing dystocia. Which of the following nursing interventions would be the nurse's high priority?
   a. Changing the woman's position frequently
   b. Providing comfort measures to the woman
   c. Monitoring the fetal heart rate patterns
   d. Keeping the couple informed of the labor progress
8. The nurse is caring for a woman experiencing hypertonic uterine dystocia. The woman's contractions are erratic in their frequency, duration, and of high intensity. The priority nursing intervention would be to:
   a. Encourage ambulation every 30 minutes
   b. Provide pain relief measures
   c. Monitor the Pitocin infusion rate closely
   d. Prepare the woman for an amniotomy

CRITICAL THINKING EXERCISES

1. A 26-year-old multipara, is admitted to the labor and birth suite in active labor. After a few hours, the nurse notices a change in her contraction pattern—poor contraction intensity and no progression of cervical dilatation beyond 5 cm. The client keeps asking about her labor progress and appears anxious about "how long this labor is taking."
   a. Based on the nurse's findings, what might you suspect is going on?
   b. How can the nurse address the client's anxiety?
   c. What are the appropriate interventions to change this labor pattern?
2. The woman activates her call light and states, "I feel increased wetness down below."
   a. What might be occurring?
   b. How will the nurse confirm the suspicions?
   c. What interventions are appropriate for this finding?

STUDY ACTIVITIES

1. Visit the SHARE Pregnancy and Infant Loss Support, Inc., website at the Point and assess its helpfulness to parents.
2. Outline the fetal and maternal risks associated with a prolonged pregnancy.
3. An abnormal or difficult labor describes ____________.

BRINGING IT ALL TOGETHER: A CASE STUDY

Tegan is a nulliparous woman who is now at 41 3/7 weeks' gestation with a male fetus. She presents for a routine prenatal visit. Fetal well-being is reassuring at this point with FHR 144, active fetal movement, no complaints voiced except for fatigue and a mild backache when she stands for long periods of time. She expresses concerned that she has not yet gone into labor.

Go to thePoint to find questions to consider about this case.

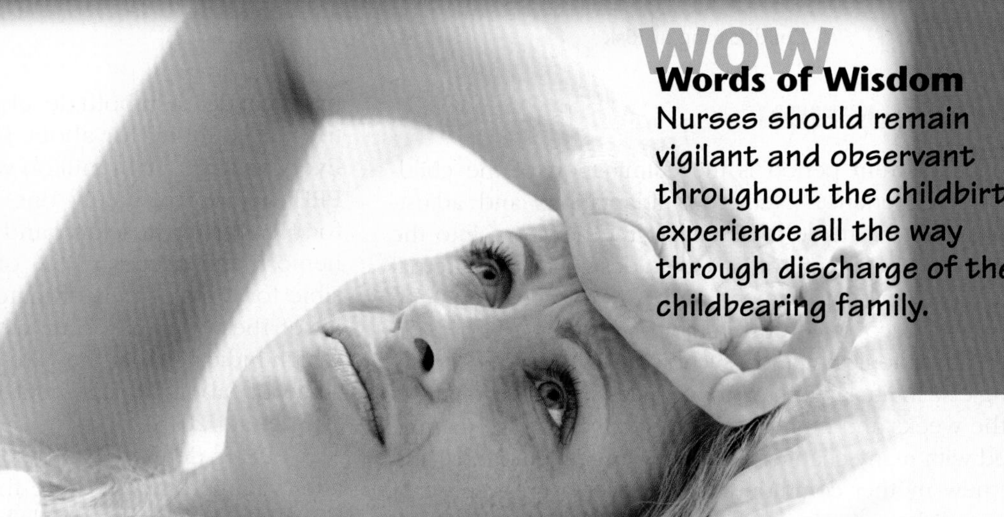

22

WOW

Words of Wisdom

Nurses should remain vigilant and observant throughout the childbirth experience all the way through discharge of the childbearing family.

Nursing Management of the Postpartum Woman at Risk

KEY TERMS

mastitis

metritis

postpartum depression (PPD)

postpartum hemorrhage (PPH)

subinvolution

uterine atony

uterine inversion

venous thromboembolism

Learning Objectives

Upon completion of the chapter, you will be able to:

1. Examine the major conditions that place the postpartum woman at risk.
2. Analyze the risk factors, assessment, preventive measures, and nursing management of common postpartum complications.
3. Differentiate the causes of postpartum hemorrhage based on the underlying pathophysiologic mechanisms.
4. Outline the nurse's role in assessing and managing the care of a woman with a thromboembolic condition.
5. Characterize the nursing management of a woman who develops a postpartum infection.
6. Compare and contrast at least two affective disorders that can occur in women after birth, describing specific therapeutic management for each.

Joan **gave birth about an hour ago to her fifth baby boy, who weighed 10 pounds, and she is resting in bed when the nurse comes in to assess her. She tells the nurse that she feels like there is "something really wet" between her legs. She also feels a bit light-headed. What would the nurse suspect is happening? What findings would support the nurse's suspicion? What should the nurse do first?**

INTRODUCTION

The postpartum period is the culmination of the childbearing experience. Numerous adaptations and adjustments must be made to assimilate the newborn into the established family unit. It is a time designed for maternal recovery, family attachment, and new role development. Typically, recovery from childbirth progresses normally both physiologically and psychologically. Just like everything else in life, a woman's body faces significant changes in the weeks and months following childbirth. It is a time filled with many changes and wide-ranging emotions, and the new mother commonly experiences a great sense of accomplishment. However, the woman can experience deviations from the norm, developing a postpartum condition that places her at risk. These high-risk conditions or complications can become life threatening. *Healthy People 2020* addresses these risks in two national health goals that were retained from the 2010 document.

This chapter addresses the nursing management of the most common conditions that place the postpartum woman at risk: hemorrhage, thromboembolic disease, infections, and postpartum affective disorders.

POSTPARTUM HEMORRHAGE

Postpartum hemorrhage (PPH) is a potentially life-threatening complication that can occur after both vaginal and cesarean births. It is the leading cause of maternal death in both developed and developing countries, accounting for about 35% of all maternal deaths. Every year about 14 million women globally suffer from PPH or approximately one in twenty births (Agency for Healthcare Research and Quality [AHRQ], 2015). A hemorrhage occurs in 5% of all births and is responsible for a major part of maternal mortality. The majority of these deaths occur within 4 hours of childbirth, which indicates that they are a consequence of the third stage of labor management (Crowe & Faulkner, 2014; Ekin et al., 2015).

PPH is defined as a blood loss greater than 500 mL after vaginal birth or more than 1,000 mL after a cesarean birth. However, this definition is arbitrary, because estimates of blood loss at birth are subjective and generally inaccurate. Moreover, average blood loss from birth frequently exceeds 500 or 1,000 mL, and symptoms of hemorrhage or shock from blood loss may be hidden by normal plasma volume increases that occur during pregnancy. Morbidity from PPH can be severe, with sequelae including organ failure, shock, edema, thrombosis, acute respiratory distress, sepsis, anemia, intensive care admissions, and prolonged hospitalization (AHRQ, 2015). A major obstetric hemorrhage is defined as a blood loss of more than 1,500 mL to 2,500 mL or bleeding that requires more than 5 units of transfused blood (Pavord & Maybury, 2015). Hemorrhage is the most common reason postpartum women are admitted to intensive care units and it is the most preventable cause of maternal death. Timely, accurate identification and initiation of appropriate interventions would improve outcomes (Clapp, 2015). Blood loss that occurs within 24 hours of birth is termed *primary (immediate or early) postpartum hemorrhage;* blood loss that occurs 24 hours to 12 weeks after birth is termed *delayed (late) postpartum hemorrhage.* A more objective definition of PPH would be any amount of bleeding that places the mother in hemodynamic jeopardy.

HEALTHY PEOPLE 2020

Objective	Nursing Significance
BDBS-15 Increase the proportion of women with von Willebrand disease (vWD) who are timely and accurately diagnosed by 10% by 2020.	• Will help foster the need for early identification of problems and prompt intervention to reduce the potential negative outcomes of pregnancy and birth.
MHMD-4 Reduce the proportion of persons who experience major depressive episodes by 10% by 2020.	• Will help to contribute to lower rates of rehospitalization, morbidity, and mortality by focusing on thorough assessments in the postpartum period. • Will help to minimize the devastating effects of complications during the postpartum period and the woman's ability to care for her newborn.

Healthy People objectives based on data from http://www.healthypeople.gov

Pathophysiology

Excessive bleeding can occur at any time between the separation of the placenta and its expulsion or removal. The most common cause of PPH is **uterine atony**, failure of the uterus to contract and retract after birth. The uterus must remain contracted after birth to control bleeding from the placental site. Uterine atony is responsible for 80% of primary or immediate PPH, while obstetric lacerations, **uterine inversion**, and rupture compromise about 20% of all primary or early PPHs (Kamel & Mastrogiannis, 2015). Any factor that causes the uterus to relax after birth will cause bleeding—even a full bladder that displaces the uterus.

During the third stage of labor the muscles of the uterus contract downward, causing constriction of the blood vessels that pass through the uterine wall to the placental surface and stopping the flow of blood. This action also causes the placenta to separate from the uterine wall. The absence of uterine contractions may result in excessive blood loss. Uterotonic medications promote uterine contractions to prevent atony and speed delivery of the placenta.

Over the course of pregnancy, maternal blood volume increases as much as 50% (from 4 to 6 L). The plasma volume increases twice as much in comparison to the total red blood cell volume. As a result, hemoglobin and hematocrit fall. The increase in blood volume meets the perfusion demands of the low-resistance uteroplacental unit and provides a reserve for the blood loss that occurs at delivery (Cunningham et al., 2014). Given this increase, the typical signs of hemorrhage (e.g., falling blood pressure, increasing pulse rate, and decreasing urinary output) do not appear until as much as 1,800 to 2,100 mL of blood has been lost. Current evidence on postpartum volume replacement suggests packed red blood cells, fresh frozen plasma, platelets, and recombinant factor VIIa be used for volume replacement (Nagtalon-Ramos, 2014). Clinical manifestations of shock resulting from blood loss are seen in Table 22.1.

In addition, accurate determination of actual blood loss is difficult because of blood pooling inside the uterus, on peripads, mattresses, and the floor. Because no universal clinical standard exists, nurses must remain vigilant, assessing for risk factors and checking clients carefully before the birth attendant leaves the birthing area.

Other causes of PPH include lacerations of the genital tract, episiotomy, retained placental fragments, uterine inversion, coagulation disorders, large for gestational age newborn, failure to progress during the second stage of labor, placenta accreta, induction or augmentation of labor with oxytocin, surgical birth, and hematomas of the vulva, vagina, or subperitoneal areas (Moses, 2015). A helpful way to remember the causes of postpartum hemorrhage is by using the 4 Ts:

1. **T***one*: uterine atony, distended bladder
2. **T***issue*: retained placenta and clots; uterine subinvolution
3. **T***rauma*: lacerations, hematoma, inversion, rupture
4. **T***hrombin*: coagulopathy (preexisting or acquired)

TABLE 22.1 CLINICAL MANIFESTATIONS OF SHOCK DUE TO BLOOD LOSS

Degree of Shock	Blood Loss	Signs and Symptoms
Mild	20%	Diaphoresis Increased capillary refilling Cool extremities Maternal anxiety
Moderate	20–40%	Tachycardia Postural hypotension Oliguria
Severe	>40%	Hypotension Agitation/confusion Hemodynamic instability

Adapted from Kolecki, P., & Menckhoff, C. R. (2015). Hypovolemic shock. *eMedicine.* Retrieved from http://emedicine.medscape.com/article/760145-overview; Belfort, M. A. (2015). Overview of postpartum hemorrhage. *UpToDate.* Retrieved from http://www.uptodate.com/contents/overview-of-postpartum-hemorrhage; and Cunningham, F. G., Leveno, K. J., Bloom, S. L., Spong, C., Dashe, J. S., Hoffman, B. L. et al. (2014). *Williams obstetrics* (24th ed.). New York, NY: McGraw-Hill.

Tone

Altered uterine muscle tone most commonly results from overdistention of the uterus. Overdistention can be caused by multiple gestation, fetal macrosomia, hydramnios, fetal abnormality, placenta previa, precipitous birth, or retained placental fragments. Other causes might include prolonged or rapid, forceful labor, especially if stimulated by oxytocin; bacterial toxins (e.g., chorioamnionitis, endomyometritis, septicemia); use of anesthesia, especially halothane; and magnesium sulfate used in the treatment of preeclampsia (Jordan et al., 2014). Overdistention of the uterus is a major risk factor for uterine atony, the most common cause of early postpartum hemorrhage, which can lead to hypovolemic shock. A distended bladder can also displace the uterus from the midline to either side, which impedes its ability to contract to reduce bleeding.

Tissue

Uterine contraction and retraction lead to detachment and expulsion of the placenta after birth. Classic signs of placental separation include a small gush of blood with lengthening of the umbilical cord and a slight rise of the uterus in the pelvis. Complete detachment and expulsion of the placenta permit continued contraction and optimal occlusion of blood vessels. Failure of complete placental separation and expulsion leads to retained fragments, which occupy space and prevent the uterus from contracting fully to clamp down on blood vessels; this can lead to hemorrhage. Clots can also occupy space, which inhibits uterine contractions.

After the placenta has been expelled, a thorough inspection is necessary to confirm its intactness; tears or fragments left inside may indicate an accessory lobe or placenta accreta (an uncommon condition in which the chorionic villi adhere to the myometrium, causing the placenta to adhere abnormally to the uterus and not separate and deliver spontaneously). Profuse hemorrhage results because the uterus cannot contract fully.

SUBINVOLUTION OF THE UTERUS

Subinvolution refers to incomplete involution of the uterus or failure to return to its normal size and condition after birth. Typically, subinvolution occurs when the myometrial fibers of the uterus do not contract effectively and causes relaxation. Complications of subinvolution include hemorrhage, pelvic peritonitis, salpingitis, and abscess formation (King et al., 2015). Causes of subinvolution include retained placental fragments, distended bladder, excessive maternal activity prohibiting proper recovery, uterine myoma, and infection. All of these conditions contribute to delayed postpartum bleeding. The clinical picture includes a postpartum fundal height that is higher than expected, with a boggy uterus; the lochia fails to change colors from red to serosa to alba within a few weeks. This condition is usually identified at the woman's postpartum examination 4 to 6 weeks after birth with a bimanual vaginal examination or ultrasound. Treatment is directed toward stimulating the uterus to expel fragments with a uterine stimulant, and antibiotics are given to prevent infection.

Trauma

Damage to the genital tract may occur spontaneously or through the manipulations used during birth. Lacerations and hematomas resulting from birth trauma can cause significant blood loss. Hematomas can present as pain or as a change in vital signs disproportionate to the amount of blood loss. Most often, hematoma formation is associated with episiotomy, instrumental birth, or nulliparity. Many hematomas can be prevented with gentle, controlled birth, and appropriate inspection and repair of lacerations or episiotomy (Jordan et al., 2014). Uterine inversion happens when the top of the uterus collapses into the inner cavity due to excessive fundal pressure or pulling on the umbilical cord when the placenta is still firmly attached to the fundus after the infant has been born. Treatment for uterine inversion includes giving uterine relaxants and immediate manual replacement by the health care provider. Additionally, uterine rupture can occur and cause damage to the genital tract and is more common in women with previous cesarean incisions or those who have undergone any procedure resulting in disruption of the uterine wall, including myomectomy, perforation of the uterus during a dilation and curettage (D&C), biopsy, or intrauterine system (IUS) insertion. Classically, its signs and symptoms combine pain, fetal heart rate abnormalities, and vaginal bleeding. Uterine rupture is a catastrophic complication that requires a rapid diagnosis and intervention, but initial clinical manifestations may be nonspecific (Nahum & Pham, 2015).

Trauma can also occur after prolonged or vigorous labor, especially if the uterus has been stimulated with oxytocin or prostaglandins. Trauma can also occur after extrauterine or intrauterine manipulation of the fetus.

Cervical lacerations commonly occur during a forceps delivery or in mothers who have not been able to resist bearing down before the cervix is fully dilated. Vaginal sidewall lacerations are associated with operative vaginal births but may occur spontaneously, especially if the fetal hand presents with the head. Lacerations can arise during manipulations to resolve shoulder dystocia. Lacerations should always be suspected in the face of a contracted uterus with bright-red blood continuing to trickle out of the vagina.

Thrombin

Thrombosis (formation of a blood clot) helps to prevent PPH immediately after birth by providing hemostasis. Fibrin deposits and clots in supplying vessels play a significant role in the hours and days after birth. Disorders that interfere with the clot formation can lead to postpartum hemorrhage. Medication used to prevent hemorrhage by stimulating uterine contractions may delay the appearance of coagulation disorders. Coagulopathies should be suspected when postpartum bleeding persists without any identifiable cause (AHRQ, 2015).

Disorders of coagulation are relatively uncommon as a sole cause of PPH. Coagulation disturbances should be suspected in women with a family history of such abnormalities and women with a history of menorrhagia. Clinical circumstances may also suggest coagulation defect as a cause of PPH. Diagnosis of a coagulation disorder often requires a high index of suspicion and should not be overlooked in the evaluation of obstetric hemorrhage (Yiadom & Carusi, 2015).

Ideally, the client's coagulation status is determined during pregnancy. However, if she received no prenatal care, coagulation studies should be ordered immediately to determine her status. Abnormal results typically include decreased platelet and fibrinogen levels; increased prothrombin time, partial thromboplastin time, and fibrin degradation products; and a prolonged bleeding time (Cunningham et al., 2014). Selected conditions associated with coagulopathies in the postpartum client include idiopathic thrombocytopenic purpura, von Willebrand disease, and disseminated intravascular coagulation (DIC).

IDIOPATHIC THROMBOCYTOPENIA PURPURA

Idiopathic thrombocytopenia purpura (ITP) is an autoimmune disorder of increased platelet destruction caused by autoantibodies, which can increase a woman's risk of hemorrhaging. There is a decrease in the number of circulating platelets in the absence of toxic exposure or a disease associated with a low platelet count. It is most common in young women during childbearing age and may be associated with maternal and fetal complications.

The incidence of ITP in adults is approximately 66 cases per 1,000,000 per year (Silverman, 2015). Glucocorticoids and immune globulin are the mainstays of medical therapy (Kessler & Sandler, 2015).

VON WILLEBRAND DISEASE

von Willebrand disease (vWD) is a congenital bleeding disorder that is inherited as an autosomal dominant trait. It is characterized by a prolonged bleeding time, a deficiency of von Willebrand factor, and impairment of platelet adhesion (CDC, 2015a). It is the most common hereditary bleeding disorder, affecting approximately 1% of the general population (National Hemophilia Foundation, 2015). Although vWD is thought to affect men and women equally, it is diagnosed more frequently in women because of menorrhagia, and it is more common among white women than African American women (ACOG, 2014a). Most cases remain undiagnosed due to lack of awareness, difficulty in diagnosis, a tendency to attribute bleeding to other causes, and variable symptoms.

The most common symptoms of vWD include bleeding gums, easy bruising, menorrhagia, blood in urine and stools, nosebleeds and hematomas. Prolonged bleeding from trivial wounds, oral cavity bleeding, and excessive menstrual bleeding are common. Gastrointestinal bleeding is rare. During pregnancy, the von Willebrand factor level increases in most women; thus, labor and birth usually proceed normally. However, all women should be monitored for excessive bleeding, particularly during the first week postpartum (Pollak, 2015).

DISSEMINATED INTRAVASCULAR COAGULATION

DIC is a life-threatening, acquired coagulopathy in which the clotting system is abnormally activated, resulting in widespread clot formation in the small vessels throughout the body, which leads to the depletion of platelets and coagulation factors. This is why DIC is also known as consumption coagulopathy.

DIC is not itself a specific illness; rather it is always a secondary diagnosis that occurs as a complication of abruptio placentae, amniotic fluid embolism, intrauterine fetal death with prolonged retention of the fetus, acute fatty liver of pregnancy, severe preeclampsia, HELLP syndrome (hemolysis, i.e., the breakdown of red blood cells, elevated liver enzymes, and low platelet count), septicemia, and postpartum hemorrhage. Clinical features include petechiae, ecchymoses, bleeding gums, fever, hypotension, acidosis, hematomas, tachycardia, proteinuria, uncontrolled bleeding during birth, and acute renal failure (Levi & Schmaier, 2015).Treatment goals are to maintain tissue perfusion through aggressive administration of fluid therapy, oxygen, heparin, and blood products. The most important treatment concept in DIC is that it is a secondary manifestation of an underlying disorder. The most important therapeutic maneuver is treating the initiating disorder. After treating the underlining cause, DIC will disappear, and the coagulation status will then become normalize. Without this, supportive measures ultimately fail (Erez, Mastrolia, & Thachil, 2015).

Therapeutic Management

Prompt diagnosis and understanding of the underlying triggers of this complication is essential for a favorable outcome. Team work and prompt treatment are essential for the successful management of women with DIC. Therapeutic management focuses on the underlying cause of the hemorrhage. For example, uterine massage is used to treat uterine atony. If retained placental fragments are the cause, the fragments are usually manually separated and removed and a uterine stimulant is given to promote the uterus to expel fragments. Antibiotics are administered to prevent infection. Lacerations are sutured or repaired. Glucocorticoids and intravenous immunoglobulin, intravenous anti-RhoD, and platelet transfusions may be given for ITP. Perinatal management of ITP should also include maintenance of maternal platelet count and regular monitoring of fetal growth along with prediction and prevention of fetal passive immune thrombocytopenia (Silverman, 2015).

The mainstays of therapy for vWD are desmopressin and plasma concentrates that contain von Willebrand factor. Delayed postpartum hemorrhage may occur, despite adequate prophylaxis. Frequent monitoring and continued prophylaxis and/or treatment are recommended for at least 2 weeks after childbirth (Pollak, 2015).

Nursing Assessment

Most women will not have identifiable risk factors. Nonetheless, primary prevention of a PPH begins with an assessment of identifiable risk factors. Pregnancy and childbirth involve significant health risks, even for women with no preexisting health problems. In the United States, where most births occur in hospitals and where resources are likely to be available as compared with developing countries, PPH still continues to be among the top causes of maternal deaths. Retrospective studies of these events suggest that some cases are preventable. As with many other sources of perinatal harm, delays in recognition, diagnosis, and treatment, problems with hierarchy and communication, and lack of knowledge, policies, and protocols were often cited as contributing factors (Shields et al., 2015).

The period after the birth and the first hours postpartum are crucial times for the prevention, assessment, and management of bleeding. Compared with other maternal risks such as infection, bleeding can rapidly become life threatening, and nurses, along with other health care providers, need to identify this condition quickly and intervene appropriately.

TABLE 22.2 FACTORS PLACING A WOMAN AT RISK FOR POSTPARTUM HEMORRHAGE

Clinical Risk Factors	Associated Clinical Conditions
***Tone* (abnormalities of uterine contractions)**	
Overdistention of uterus	Polyhydramnios Multifetal gestation Macrosomia
Uterine muscle exhaustion	Rapid labor Prolonged labor Oxytocin use
Uterine infection	Maternal fever Prolonged rupture of membranes
***Tissue* (retained in uterus)**	
Products of conception	Incomplete placenta at birth
Retained blood clots	Atonic uterus
***Trauma* (of the genital tract)**	
Lacerations anywhere	Precipitate birth or operative birth
Laceration extensions	Malposition of fetus Previous uterine surgery
Uterine inversion	Forceful pulling when placenta isn't separated yet; traction on the cord when uterus isn't contracted
***Thrombin* (coagulation abnormalities)**	
Preexisting conditions	Hereditary inheritance Hemophilia von Willebrand disease History of previous PPH Acquired in pregnancy Idiopathic thrombocytopenia purpura Bruising, elevated blood pressure Disseminated intravascular coagulation

Adapted from Centers for Disease Control and Prevention [CDC]. (2015a). *Facts about von Willebrand Disease*. Retrieved from http://www.cdc.gov/ncbddd/vwd/facts.html; King, T. L., Brucker, M. C., Kriebs, J. M., Fahey, J. O., Gegor, C. L., & Varney, H. (2015). *Varney's midwifery* (5th ed.). Burlington, MA: Jones & Bartlett Learning; and Mattson, S., & Smith, J. E. (2015). *Core curriculum for maternal-newborn nursing* (5th ed.). St. Louis, MO: Saunders Elsevier.

Begin by reviewing the mother's history, including labor and birth history, for risk factors associated with PPH (Table 22.2). The incidence of PPH has been rising, though the mortality has come down, suggesting improvement in the management of this condition. Although specific risk factors have been identified, PPH is often unanticipated and still occurs in approximately 5% of all births and increasing (Ekin et al., 2015).

Since the most common cause of immediate severe PPH is uterine atony (failure of the uterus to contract properly after birth), assess uterine tone after birth by palpating the fundus for firmness and location. A soft, boggy fundus indicates uterine atony.

Take Note!

A soft, boggy uterus that deviates from the midline suggests that a full bladder is interfering with uterine involution. If the uterus is not in correct position (midline), it will not be able to contract to control bleeding.

Assess the amount of bleeding. Visual estimation is the most frequently practiced method of determining blood loss during childbirth in the United States, and the results are usually included in the documentation of events pertaining to the birth. This method is used despite repeated studies showing its inaccuracy and underestimation. Weighing or counting peripads or using a Signaling a Postpartum Hemorrhage Emergency [SAPHE] mat would provide a more accurate estimate of blood loss. The mat was constructed so that each square on the mat would absorb up to 50 mL of blood. Blood loss is then calculated by multiplying the number of blood-saturated squares by 50 mL (Wilcox et al., 2015). In any method used, nurses should consult their hospital protocols and follow them. If bleeding continues even though there are no lacerations, suspect retained placental fragments. The uterus remains large with painless, dark-red bleeding mixed with clots. This cause of hemorrhage can be prevented by carefully inspecting the placenta for intactness.

If trauma is suspected, attempt to identify the source and document it. Typically, the uterus will be firm with a steady stream or trickle of unclotted bright-red blood noted in the perineum. Most deaths from PPH are not due to gross bleeding, but rather to inadequate management of slow, steady blood loss (Clapp, 2015).

Assess for hematoma which may require surgical treatment. The uterus would be firm, with bright-red bleeding. Observe for a localized bluish bulging area just under the skin surface in the perineal area (Fig. 22.1). Often the woman will report severe perineal or pelvic pain and will have difficulty voiding. In addition, she may exhibit hypotension, tachycardia, and anemia. Frequently, the health care provider will incise the skin bulge to evacuate the hematoma of trapped blood. A pressure dressing is applied to this area to prevent further bleeding (Green, 2016).

Inspect the skin and mucous membranes for gingival bleeding or petechiae and ecchymoses. Check venipuncture sites for oozing or prolonged bleeding. These findings might suggest a coagulopathy as a cause of PPH.

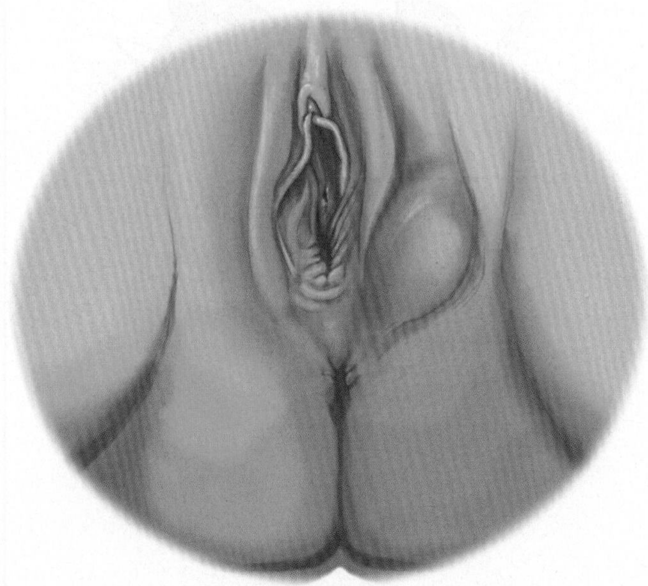

FIGURE 22.1 Perineal hematoma. Note the bulging swollen mass.

Also assess the amount of lochia, which would be much greater than usual. Urinary output would be diminished, with signs of acute renal failure. Vital signs would show an increased pulse rate and a decreased level of consciousness. However, signs of shock do not appear until hemorrhage is far advanced due to the increased fluid and blood volume of pregnancy.

Nursing Management

When excessive bleeding is encountered, initial management steps are aimed at improving uterine tone with immediate fundal massage, intravenous fluid resuscitation, and administration of uterotonic medications. If these methods fail to control bleeding, additional resources are mobilized and more aggressive interventions such as bimanual compression, internal uterine packing, and/or balloon tamponade techniques are employed by the health care provider. Other potential causes of bleeding should be thoroughly explored, and laboratory tests such as a complete blood count, type and cross-match, and coagulations studies should be obtained immediately. Transfusion of blood products should be instituted without hesitation once estimates of bleeding reach 1,500 mL (Nagtalon-Ramos, 2014).

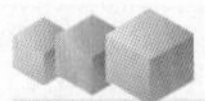

Concept Mastery Alert

Priority Intervention for Uterine Atony

Before initiating fundal massage, the nurse must first place a hand over the symphysis pubis to anchor the uterus and prevent possible uterine inversion.

Clearly, in all cases of unexpected hemorrhage, the interventions discussed as follows must be performed without delay. Postpartum hemorrhage is best managed by using a stepwise progressive approach. Manual message and pharmacologic therapies are first-line treatments. If the bleeding continues, second-line interventions might include the use of intrauterine balloon (or gauze) tamponade and uterine compression sutures. If these second-line therapies still don't stop the bleeding, women may need to undergo radiologic embolization, pelvic devascularization, or hysterectomy. Peripartum hysterectomy remains the last-resort lifesaving measure and carries with it a higher mortality rate compared with nonobstetric hysterectomy. It is a most demanding obstetric surgery performed under very trying circumstances of life-threatening hemorrhage (Van de Velde, Diez, & Varon, 2015). Moreover, high-volume transfusions are often required, and there are significant postsurgical morbidity risks such as renal failure, hepatic failure, respiratory distress syndrome, coagulopathies, septicemia, tissue hypoxia, and pituitary necrosis (Sheehan syndrome) (Rong, Yuna, & Yan, 2014). Postpartum hemorrhage outcomes can be improved by thorough preparation, anticipating the risks of PPH, and coordinating consultants for interventional procedures if warranted.

PPH is a serious complication of pregnancy that is often unanticipated. Even with prompt aggressive management, postpartum bleeding can quickly evolve into a life-threatening event. Perinatal nurses are often the first to observe significant postpartum bleeding and their prompt initial response and continued assessments are pivotal in the anticipation and coordination of necessary interventions. Multidisciplinary team support is critical because obstetric caregivers need a full array of medical and surgical strategies to manage intractable bleeding. Because all postpartum women are at risk for hemorrhage, nurses need to possess the knowledge and skills to practice active management of the third stage of labor to prevent hemorrhage and to recognize, assess, and respond rapidly to excessive blood loss in their clients.

Massage the Uterus

Massage the uterus if uterine atony is noted. The uterine muscles are sensitive to touch; massage stimulates the muscle fibers to contract. Massage the boggy uterus to stimulate contractions and expression of any accumulated blood clots while supporting the lower uterine segment. As blood pools in the vagina, stasis of blood causes clots to form. These clots need to be expelled as pressure is placed on the fundus. Note, however, that overly forceful massage can tire the uterine muscles, resulting in further uterine atony and increased pain. See Nursing Procedure 22.1 for the steps in massaging the fundus.

Administer a Uterotonic Drug

Administer an uterotonic drug if repeated fundal massage and expression of clots fail, medication is probably needed to cause the uterus to contract in order to control bleeding from the placental site. The injection of a uterotonic drug immediately after birth is an important intervention used to prevent PPH. Oxytocin (Pitocin); a synthetic analog of prostaglandin E1, misoprostol (Cytotec) or dinoprostone (Prostin E2); methylergonovine maleate (Methergine); and a derivative of prostaglandin (PGF2), carboprost (Hemabate), are drugs used to manage postpartum hemorrhage (Drug Guide 22.1). However, misoprostol is not approved by the U.S. Food

NURSING PROCEDURE 22.1

Massaging the Fundus

Purpose: To Promote Uterine Contraction

1. After explaining the procedure to the woman, place one gloved hand on the area above the symphysis pubis (this helps to support the lower uterine segment).
2. Place the other gloved hand (usually the dominant hand) on the fundus.
3. With the hand on the fundus, gently massage the fundus in a circular manner. Be careful not to over massage the fundus, which could lead to muscle fatigue and uterine relaxation.
4. Assess for uterine firmness (uterine tissue responds quickly to touch).
5. If firm, apply gentle yet firm pressure in a downward motion toward the vagina to express any clots that may have accumulated.
6. Do not attempt to express clots until the fundus is firm because the application of firm pressure on an uncontracted uterus could cause uterine inversion, leading to massive hemorrhage.
7. Assist the woman with perineal care and applying a new perineal pad.
8. Remove gloves and wash hands.

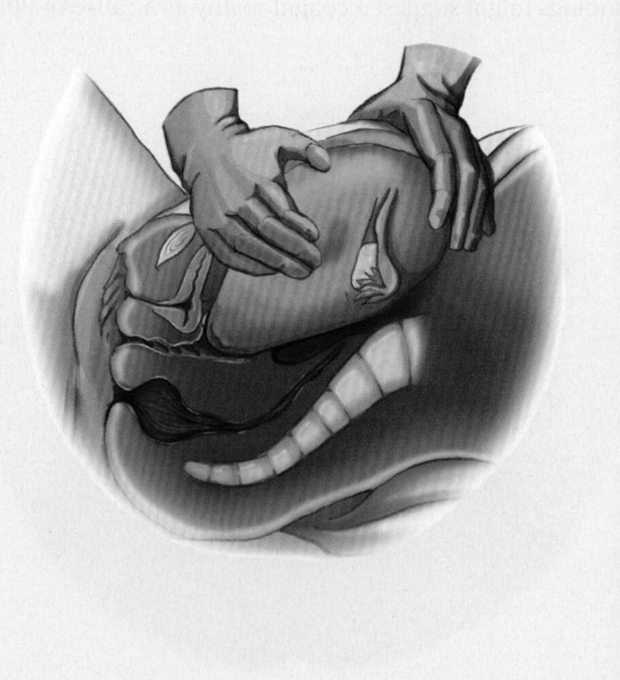

DRUG GUIDE 22.1 DRUGS USED TO CONTROL POSTPARTUM HEMORRHAGE

Drug	Action/Indication	Nursing Implications
Oxytocin (Pitocin) First-line therapy	Stimulates the uterus to contract/ to contract the uterus to control bleeding from the placental site 20–40 units in a liter IV Or 10 units IM	Assess fundus for evidence of contraction and compare amount of bleeding every 15 min or according to orders. Monitor vital signs every 15 min. Monitor uterine tone to prevent hyperstimulation. Reassure client about the need for uterine contraction and administer analgesics for comfort. Offer explanation to client and family about what is happening and the purpose of the medication. Provide nonpharmacologic comfort measures to assist with pain management. Set up the IV infusion to be piggybacked into a primary IV line. This ensures that the medication can be discontinued readily if hyperstimulation or adverse effects occur while maintaining the IV site and primary infusion.
Misoprostol (Cytotec)	Stimulates the uterus to contract/ to reduce bleeding; a prostaglandin analog 800 mcg per rectum, one dose (range, 400–1,000 mcg)	Contraindications: never give undiluted as a bolus injection IV. As above. Not FDA approved for this indication, but a very effective drug therapy for acute postpartum hemorrhage. Contraindications: allergy, active CVD, pulmonary or hepatic disease; use with caution in women with asthma.
Dinoprostone (Prostin E2)	20 mg vaginal or rectal suppository May be repeated every two hours.	Monitor blood pressure frequently since hypotension is a frequent side effect along with vomiting and diarrhea, nausea, temperature elevation.
Methylergonovine maleate (Methergine)	Stimulates the uterus/ to prevent and treat postpartum hemorrhage due to atony or subinvolution. 0.2 mg IM injection May be repeated in 5 min Thereafter every 2–4 hr	Assess baseline bleeding, uterine tone, and vital signs every 15 min or according to protocol. Offer explanation to client and family about what is happening and the purpose of the medication. Monitor for possible adverse effects, such as hypertension, seizures, uterine cramping, nausea, vomiting, and palpitations. Report any complaints of chest pain promptly. Contraindications: Hypertension
Prostaglandin (PGF2), Carboprost, (Hemabate)	Stimulates uterine contractions/ to treat postpartum hemorrhage due to uterine atony when not controlled by other methods. 0.25 mg IM injection May be repeated every 15–90 min up to 8 doses. Stimulates uterine contractions to reduce bleeding when not controlled by the first-line therapy of oxytocin.	Assess vital signs, uterine contractions, client's comfort level, and bleeding status as per protocol. Offer explanation to client and family about what is happening and the purpose of the medication. Monitor for possible adverse effects, such as fever, chills, headache, nausea, vomiting, diarrhea, flushing, and bronchospasm. Contraindications: asthma or active cardiovascular disease Same as above Contraindications: active cardiac, pulmonary, renal, or hepatic disease

Adapted from Callahan, T. L. (2016). *Tarascon's OB/GYN pocketbook*. Burlington, MA: Jones & Bartlett Learning; Bohlmann, M., & Rath, W. (2014). Medical prevention and treatment of postpartum hemorrhage: A comparison of different guidelines. *Archives of Gynecology & Obstetrics, 289*(3), 555–567. doi:10.1007/s00404-013-3016-4; and Skidmore-Roth, L. (2015). *Mosby's 2015 nursing drug reference* (28th ed.). St. Louis, MO: Mosby Elsevier.

and Drug Administration (FDA) for this purpose. The choice of which uterotonic drug to use for management of bleeding depends on the judgment of the health care provider, the availability of drugs, and the risks and benefits of the drug.

All nurses need to be aware of the contraindications of administering each of the medications used to control postpartum hemorrhage as follows:

- *Pitocin*—never give undiluted as a bolus injection intravenously
- *Cytotec*—allergy, active cardiovascular disease, pulmonary or hepatic disease
- *Prostin E2*—active cardiac, pulmonary, renal, or hepatic disease
- *Methergine*—if the woman is hypertensive, do not administer.
- *Hemabate*—contraindicated with asthma due to risk of bronchial spasm

Remember Joan, the woman described at the beginning of the chapter? The nurse assesses her and finds that her uterus is boggy. What would the nurse do next? What additional nursing measures might be used if Joan's fundus remains boggy? When should the health care provider be notified?

Maintain the Primary Intravenous Infusion

Maintain the primary intravenous infusion and be prepared to start a second infusion at another site if blood transfusions are necessary. Draw blood for type and cross-match and send it to the laboratory. Administer oxytocics as ordered, correlating and titrating the infusion rate to assessment findings of uterine firmness and lochia. Assess for visible vaginal bleeding, and count or weigh perineal pads.

Take Note!

Postpartum hemorrhage outcomes can be improved by thorough preparation, anticipating the risks factors of PPH in every woman admitted, and coordinating consultants for interventional procedures if warranted.

Check Vital Signs

Check vital signs every 15 to 30 minutes, depending on the acuity of the mother's health status. Monitor her complete blood count to identify any deficit or assess the adequacy of replacement. Assess the woman's level of consciousness to determine changes that may result from inadequate cerebral perfusion.

A Foley catheter is typically in place to keep the bladder empty to avoid displacement of her uterus. A fundus above the umbilicus and deviated laterally indicates a full bladder and interferes with uterine contractions to slow the bleeding.

Prepare the Woman for Removal of Retained Placental Fragments

Prepare the woman for removal of retained placental fragments. These fragments usually are manually separated and removed by the health care provider. Be sure that the health care provider remains long enough after birth to assess the bleeding status of the woman and determine the etiology. Assist the health care provider with suturing any lacerations immediately to control hemorrhage and repair the tissue.

Nurses should anticipate and prepare the woman for transfer to the operating room for surgical intervention if tamponade techniques fail to achieve hemostasis. The blood bank should be notified that additional transfusions may be required and the woman's condition closely monitored for signs of hypovolemic shock.

Continually Assess the Woman for Signs and Symptoms of Hemorrhagic Shock

Continually assess the woman for signs and symptoms of hemorrhagic shock, a condition in which inadequate perfusion of organs results in insufficient availability of oxygen to satisfy the metabolic needs of the tissues (Green, 2016). Hemorrhagic shock is the most common form of shock encountered in obstetric practice. Subsequently, a catabolic state develops, leading to inflammation, endothelial dysfunction, and disruption of normal metabolic processes in vital organs. Once these events become established, the process of shock is often irreversible, even if volume and red blood cell deficits are corrected. The main goals of treatment of hemorrhagic shock include fluid resuscitation, correction of the imbalance between oxygen delivery and consumption, and treating DIC (Tánczos, Németh, & Molnár, 2015).

A postpartum hemorrhage is a traumatic experience because medical complications are unexpected during what is anticipated as a joyful time. Assess the anxiety level of the woman; the woman going into hypovolemic shock is highly anxious and may lose consciousness. The woman's significant others experience a high level of anxiety as well and need a great deal of support.

Monitor the woman's blood pressure, pulse, capillary refill, mental status, and urinary output. These assessments allow estimation of the severity of blood loss and help direct treatment. If the woman develops hemorrhagic shock, interventions focus on controlling the source of blood loss; restoring adequate oxygen-carrying capacity; and maintaining adequate tissue perfusion. Successful treatment depends on efficient collaboration among all health care team members to meet the woman's specific needs.

For the woman with ITP, expect to administer glucocorticoids, intravenous immunoglobulin, intravenous anti-RhoD, and platelet transfusions. Prepare the woman for a splenectomy if the bleeding tissues do not respond to medical management. Be alert for women with abnormal bleeding tendencies, ensuring that they receive proper diagnosis and treatment. Teach them how to prevent severe hemorrhage by learning how to feel for and massage their fundus when boggy, assisting the nurse to keep track of the number of and amount of bleeding on perineal pads, and avoiding any medications with antiplatelet activity such as aspirin, antihistamines, or nonsteroidal anti-inflammatory drugs (NSAIDs).

Institute Emergency Measures If DIC Develops

If the woman develops DIC, institute emergency measures to control bleeding and impending shock and prepare to transfer her to the intensive care unit. Identification of the underlying condition and elimination of the causative factor are essential to correct the coagulation problem. Be ready to replace fluid volume, administer blood component therapy, and optimize the mother's oxygenation and perfusion status to ensure adequate cardiac output and end-organ perfusion. Continually reassess the woman's coagulation status via laboratory studies.

Monitor vital signs closely, being alert for changes that signal an increase in bleeding or impending shock. Observe for early signs of ecchymosis, including spontaneous bleeding from gums or nose, petechiae, excessive bleeding from the cesarean incision site or intravenous site, hematuria, and blood in the stool. Late signs include progressive changes in vital signs, skin color, and reduction of urinary output. Collectively, these findings correlate with decreased blood volume, decreased organ and peripheral tissue perfusion, and clots in the microcirculation (Levi & Schmaier, 2015).

Take Note!

Always remember the five causes of postpartum hemorrhage and the appropriate intervention for each: (1) uterine atony—massage and oxytocics; (2) retained placental tissue—evacuation and oxytocics; (3) lacerations or hematoma—surgical repair; (4) thrombin (bleeding disorders)—blood products; and (5) uterine inversion caused by too much cord traction—gentle replacement of uterus and oxytocics.

Institute measures to avoid tissue trauma or injury, such as giving injections and drawing blood. Also provide emotional support to the client and her family throughout this critical time by being readily available and providing explanations and reassurance.

Preventing Postpartum Hemorrhage

Avoid an episiotomy unless an emergency birth is necessary and the perineum is a limiting factor. It is important to have the continuous intrapartum presence of an experienced labor and birth nurse. Provide active management of the third stage of labor, including administration of a uterotonic medication after birth of anterior shoulder, controlled and gentle cord traction to deliver the placenta, and uterine massage after the placenta is out. Authors of a Cochrane review concluded that active management of the third stage of labor is associated with reduced blood loss, reduced risk of PPH, and a reduced prolonged third stage of labor (Mousa et al., 2014).

Frequent staff education and PPH drills will help keep skills up to date. Nurses must identify and correct anemia and screen for coagulopathies before labor and birth. After birth, it is important to inspect the placenta (once it is delivered) for completeness. Assess the woman for lower genital tract lacerations immediately after birth and reevaluate the woman's vital signs and vaginal flow after childbirth. Finally, it is important to be aware of the mother's beliefs about blood transfusions. Recently a workgroup representing all major women's health professional organizations developed an obstetric hemorrhage safety bundle for practice to improve PPH outcomes. Some of their selected readiness action domains include:

- Having a hemorrhage cart with supplies and instruction cards on every OB unit
- Having immediate access to medications used to treat a massive hemorrhage
- Establishing a response team within the hospital that can be called
- Developing emergency-release transfusion protocols in the blood bank
- Educating all staff on protocols and holding unit-based drills frequently

(Main et al., 2015).

In summary, careful monitoring of the mother's vital signs, laboratory tests (in particular, coagulation testing), and immediate diagnosis of the cause of PPH are important key factors to reduce maternal morbidity and mortality. Nurses must always be prepared to identify signs and symptoms of PPH, recognize maternal compromise and, deal with hemorrhage promptly. By identifying hemorrhage promptly and providing swift interventions, maternal mortality and morbidity can be reduced.

An intravenous oxytocin infusion is started for Joan. What assessments will need to be done frequently to make sure Joan is not losing too much blood? What discharge instructions need to be reinforced with Joan?

VENOUS THROMBOEMBOLIC CONDITIONS

Venous thromboembolism is one of the leading causes of maternal mortality and morbidity with an annual incidence of one per 1,000 pregnancies, a ten times higher risk than the nonpregnant population (Testa et al., 2015). A thrombosis (blood clot within a blood vessel) can cause an inflammation of the blood vessel lining (thrombophlebitis), which in turn can lead to a thromboembolism (obstruction of a blood vessel by a blood clot carried by the circulation from the site of origin). Thrombi can involve the superficial or deep veins in the legs or pelvis. Superficial venous thrombosis usually involves the saphenous venous system and is confined to the lower leg. Superficial thrombophlebitis may be caused by the use of the lithotomy position during birth. Deep venous thrombosis (DVT) can involve deep veins from the foot to the calf, to the thighs, or pelvis. In both locations, thrombi can dislodge and migrate to the lungs, causing a pulmonary embolism (PE).

DVT is a common condition that can have serious complications. Deep venous thrombi have a high probability of propagating and leading to pulmonary emboli, which may cause chest pain, breathlessness, and sudden death. Thus, an accurate and timely diagnosis of DVT is imperative. Although DVT is often clinically silent, it may present with a number of signs, including calf pain, edema, and venous distention.

The three most common venous thromboembolic conditions occurring during the postpartum period are superficial venous thrombosis, DVT, and PE. Although venous thromboembolic disorders occur in less than 1% of all postpartum women, pulmonary embolus can be fatal if a clot obstructs the lung circulation; thus, early identification and treatment are paramount. Risk for postpartum venous thromboembolism is highest during the first three weeks after childbirth. Women with obstetric complications are at highest risk for this, and this risk remains elevated throughout the first twelve weeks postpartum (Tepper et al., 2014).

Pathophysiology

Thrombus (blood clot) formation typically results from venous stasis, injury to the innermost layer of the blood vessel, and hypercoagulation. Venous stasis and hypercoagulation are both common in the postpartum period.

If a clot dislodges and travels to the pulmonary circulation, PE can occur. PE is a potentially fatal condition that occurs when the pulmonary artery is blocked by a blood clot that has traveled from another vein into the lungs, causing an obstruction and infarction. When the clot is large enough to block one or more of the pulmonary vessels that supply the lungs, it can result in sudden death. Approximately 600,000 PEs occur yearly in the United States, resulting in 60,000 to 100,000 deaths (CDC, 2015b). Only 25% of all clients with PE are actually diagnosed, indicating that thousands of PEs go undetected. Many deaths due to PE are unrecognized and the diagnosis is often made at autopsy. PE is the leading cause of pregnancy-related death in the United States, occurring in 2 out of 100,000 live births. It most commonly occurs up to 3 weeks postpartum and following a surgical birth (Conti et al., 2014). A national review of severe obstetric complications found a significant increase in the rate of PE associated with the increasing rate of cesarean births. Adequate treatment of thrombotic events in pregnancy is important to prevent progression of thrombosis to the development of pulmonary embolism (Sucker & Zotz, 2015).

Nursing Assessment

Assess the woman closely for risk factors and signs and symptoms of thrombophlebitis. Look for risk factors in the woman's history such as use of oral contraceptives before the pregnancy; smoking; employment that necessitates prolonged standing; history of thrombosis, thrombophlebitis, or endometritis; or evidence of current varicosities. Also look for other factors that can increase a woman's risk, such as prolonged bed rest, diabetes, obesity, cesarean birth, progesterone-induced distensibility of the veins of the lower legs during pregnancy, severe anemia, varicose veins, advanced maternal age (older than 34 years), and multiparity. The likelihood of thrombophlebitis is increased through most of pregnancy and for approximately 12 weeks after childbirth. This is partly due to increased platelet stickiness and partly due to reduced fibrinolytic activity (Guimicheva, Czuprynska, & Arya, 2015).

Ask the woman if she has pain or tenderness in the lower extremities. Suspect superficial venous thrombosis in a woman with varicose veins who reports tenderness and discomfort over the site of the thrombosis, most commonly in the calf area. The area appears reddened along the vein and is warm to the touch. The woman will report increased pain in the affected leg when she ambulates and bears weight.

Manifestations of DVT are often absent and diffuse. If present, they are caused by an inflammatory process and obstruction of venous return. Calf swelling, erythema, warmth, tenderness, and pedal edema may be noted. A positive Homans' sign (pain in the upper calf upon dorsiflexion) is not a definitive diagnostic sign as it is insensitive and nonspecific and is no longer recommended as an indicator of DVT. That is because calf pain can also be caused by a strained muscle, contusion, clients with herniated intervertebral discs, calf muscle spasm, neurogenic leg pain, ruptured Baker's cyst, and cellulitis (Heffline & Schmidt, 2014).

Be alert for signs and symptoms of pulmonary embolism, including unexplained sudden onset of shortness of breath and severe chest pain. The woman may be apprehensive and diaphoretic. Additional manifestations may include tachypnea, tachycardia, hypotension, syncope, distention of the jugular vein, decreased oxygen saturation (shown by pulse oximetry), cardiac arrhythmias, hemoptysis, and a sudden change in mental status as a result of hypoxemia (Quellette, Harrington, & Kamangar, 2015). Prepare the woman for a lung scan to confirm the diagnosis.

Nursing Management

Nursing management focuses on preventing thrombotic conditions, promoting adequate circulation if thrombosis occurs, and educating the client about preventive measures, anticoagulant therapy, and danger signs.

Preventing Thrombotic Conditions

Prevention of thrombotic conditions is an essential aspect of nursing management and can be achieved with the routine use of simple measures:

- Developing public awareness about risk factors, symptoms, and preventive measures
- Preventing venous stasis by encouraging activity that causes leg muscles to contract and promotes venous return (leg exercises and walking)
- Dorsi/plantar flexion of feet with prolonged sitting to promote venous return
- Using intermittent sequential compression devices to produce passive leg muscle contractions until the woman is ambulatory
- Elevating the woman's legs above her heart level to promote venous return
- Stopping smoking to reduce or prevent vascular vasoconstriction
- Applying compression stockings and removing them daily for inspection of legs
- Using postoperative deep-breathing exercises to improve venous return by relieving the negative thoracic pressure on leg veins
- Reducing hypercoagulability with the use of aspirin or anticoagulation therapy
- Preventing venous pooling by avoiding pillows under knees, not crossing legs for long periods, and not leaving legs up in stirrups for long periods
- Padding stirrups to reduce pressure against the popliteal angle
- Avoiding sitting or standing in one position for prolonged periods
- Avoiding trauma to legs to prevent injury to the vein wall
- Increasing fluid intake to prevent dehydration
- Avoiding the use of oral contraceptives

In women at risk, early ambulation is the easiest and most cost-effective method. Use of compression stockings decreases distal calf vein thrombosis by decreasing venous stasis and augmenting venous return (Wells, Forgie, & Rodger, 2014). Women who are at a high risk for thromboembolic disease based on risk factors or a previous history of DVT or PE may be placed on prophylactic anticoagulation therapy during pregnancy. A low-molecular-weight heparin such as enoxaparin (Lovenox) can be given or rivaroxaban (Xarelto), apixaban (Eliquis), or dabigatran etexilate (Pradaxa) can be given (Middeldorp, 2015). It is typically discontinued during labor and birth and then restarted during the postpartum period.

Promoting Adequate Circulation

The mainstay of venous thromboembolic conditions is anticoagulation, while interventions such as thrombolysis and inferior vena cava filters are reserved for limited circumstances. For the woman with superficial venous thrombosis, administer NSAIDs for analgesia, provide for rest and elevation of the affected leg, apply warm compresses to the affected area to promote healing, and use antiembolism stockings to promote circulation to the extremities.

Implement bed rest or limited ambulation if ordered and elevation of the affected extremity for the woman with DVT. These actions help to reduce interstitial swelling and promote venous return from that leg. Apply antiembolism stockings to both extremities as ordered. Fit the stockings correctly to avoid excess pressure and constriction and urge the woman to wear them at all times. Sequential compression devices can also be used for women with varicose veins, a history of thrombophlebitis, or a surgical birth.

Anticoagulant therapy using a continuous intravenous infusion of low-molecular-weight heparin along with vitamin K antagonists usually is initiated to prolong the clotting time and prevent extension of the thrombosis. Monitor the woman's coagulation studies closely; these might include activated partial thromboplastin time (aPTT), whole-blood partial thromboplastin time, and platelet levels. A therapeutic aPTT value typically ranges from 35 to 45 seconds, depending on which standard values are used (Pagana, Pagana & Pagana, 2014). Also apply warm moist compresses to the affected leg and administer analgesics as ordered to decrease the discomfort.

After several days of intravenous low-molecular-weight heparin therapy, expect to begin oral anticoagulant therapy as ordered. In most cases, the woman will continue to take this medication for several months after discharge.

For the woman who develops a pulmonary embolism, institute emergency measures immediately. The objectives of treatment are to prevent growth or multiplication of thrombi in the lower extremities, prevent more thrombi from traveling to the pulmonary vascular system, and provide cardiopulmonary support if needed. Administer oxygen via mask or cannula as ordered and initiate intravenous low-molecular-weight heparin therapy titrated according to the results of the coagulation studies. Maintain the client on bed rest, and administer analgesics as ordered for pain relief. Be prepared to assist with administering thrombolytic agents, such as alteplase (tPA), which might be used to dissolve pulmonary emboli and the source of the thrombus in the pelvis or deep leg veins, thus reducing the potential for a recurrence.

Educating the Client

Provide teaching about the use of anticoagulant therapy and danger signs that should be reported (Teaching Guidelines 22.1). Provide anticipatory guidance, support, and education about associated signs of complications and risks.

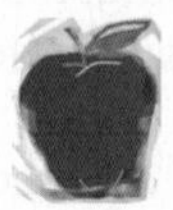

Teaching Guidelines 22.1

TEACHING TO PREVENT BLEEDING RELATED TO ANTICOAGULANT THERAPY

- Watch for possible signs of bleeding and notify your health care provider if any occur:
  - Nosebleeds
  - Bleeding from the gums or mouth
  - Black tarry stools
  - Brown "coffee grounds" vomitus
  - Red to brown speckled mucus from a cough
  - Oozing at incision, episiotomy site, cut, or scrape
  - Pink, red, or brown-tinged urine
  - Bruises, "black and blue marks"
  - Increased lochia discharge (from present level)
- Practice measures to reduce your risk of bleeding:
  - Brush your teeth gently using a soft toothbrush.
  - Use an electric razor for shaving.
  - Avoid activities that could lead to injury, scrapes, bruising, or cuts.
  - Do not use any over-the-counter products containing aspirin or aspirin-like derivatives.
  - Avoid consuming alcohol.
  - Inform other health care providers about the use of anticoagulants, especially dentists.
- Be sure to comply with follow-up laboratory testing as scheduled.
- If you accidentally cut or scrape yourself, apply firm direct pressure to the site for 5 to 10 minutes. Do the same after receiving any injections or having blood specimens drawn.
- Wear an identification bracelet or band that indicates that you are taking an anticoagulant.
- Elimination of modifiable risk factors for DVT (smoking, use of oral contraceptives, a sedentary lifestyle, and obesity)
- Importance of using compression stockings
- Avoidance of constrictive clothing and prolonged standing or sitting in a motionless, leg-dependent position
- Danger signs and symptoms (sudden onset of chest pain, dyspnea, and tachypnea) to report to the health care provider

POSTPARTUM INFECTION

Infection during the postpartum period is a common cause of maternal morbidity and mortality. Overall, postpartum infection is estimated to occur in up to 8% of all births and accounts for 15% of global maternal mortality. There is a higher occurrence in cesarean births than in vaginal births (Mattson, & Smith, 2016). Postpartum infection is defined as a fever of 100.4° F (38° C) or higher after the first 24 hours after childbirth, occurring on at least 2 of the first 10 days after birth, exclusive of the first 24 hours (Dalton & Castillo, 2014).

Risk factors include surgical birth, prolonged rupture of membranes, long labor with multiple vaginal examinations, inadequate hand hygiene, internal fetal monitoring, uterine manipulation, chorioamnionitis, instrumental birth, obesity, untreated infection prior to birth, retained placental fragments, obesity, gestational diabetes, extremes of client age, low socioeconomic status, and anemia during pregnancy (Jordan et al., 2014).

Infections can easily enter the female genital tract externally and ascend through the internal genital structures. Postpartum women possess an increased risk for infection due to tissue trauma during birth, vulnerability from placenta separation site, and the incision from cesarean section. In addition, the normal physiologic changes of childbirth increase the risk of infection by decreasing the vaginal acidity due to the presence of amniotic fluid, blood, and lochia, all of which are alkaline. An alkaline environment encourages the growth of bacteria.

Postpartum infections usually arise from organisms that constitute the normal vaginal flora, typically a mix of aerobic and anaerobic species. Generally, they are polymicrobial and involve the following microorganisms: *Staphylococcus aureus, Escherichia coli, Klebsiella, Gardnerella vaginalis,* gonococci, coliform bacteria, group A or B hemolytic streptococci, *Chlamydia trachomatis,* and the anaerobes that are common to bacterial vaginosis. Prevention can be achieved by screening and treating vaginal colonization during pregnancy (Callahan, 2016). Common postpartum infections include **metritis**, surgical site infections, urinary tract infections, and **mastitis**.

Metritis

Although usually referred to clinically as endometritis, postpartum uterine infections typically involve more than just the endometrial lining. **Metritis** is an infectious condition that involves the endometrium, decidua, and adjacent myometrium of the uterus. Extension of metritis can result in parametritis, which involves the broad ligament and possibly the ovaries and fallopian tubes, or septic pelvic thrombophlebitis, which results when the infection spreads along venous routes into the pelvis. It occurs within the first two days postpartum or as late as two to six weeks postpartum (King et al., 2015).

The uterine cavity is sterile until rupture of the amniotic sac. As a consequence of labor, birth, and associated manipulations, anaerobic and aerobic bacteria can contaminate the uterus. In most cases, the bacteria responsible for pelvic infections are those that normally reside in the bowel, vagina, perineum, and cervix, such as *E. coli, Klebsiella pneumoniae,* or *G. vaginalis.*

The risk of metritis increases dramatically after a cesarean birth; it complicates from 10% to 20% of cesarean births. This is typically an extension of chorioamnionitis that was present before birth (indeed, that may have been why the cesarean birth was performed). In addition, trauma to the tissues and a break in the skin (incision) provide entrances for bacteria to enter the body and multiply.

ACOG (2014b) recommends use of one dose of prophylactic antibiotic therapy administered one hour before any cesarean section and this has become standard practice in the United States today. Once rupture of the amniotic membranes occurs during labor and birth, the uterus becomes more susceptible to colonization and infection, especially if it is a prolonged labor. Any area traumatized during childbirth is susceptible to infection.

Surgical Site Infections

Any break in the skin or mucous membranes provides a portal for bacteria. In the postpartum woman, sites of wound infection include cesarean surgical incisions, the episiotomy site in the perineum, and genital tract lacerations (Fig. 22.2). Wound infections are usually not identified until the woman has been discharged from the hospital because symptoms may not show up until 24 to 48 hours after birth.

Urinary Tract Infections

Urinary tract infections are most commonly caused by bacteria often found in bowel flora, including *E. coli, Klebsiella, Proteus,* and *Enterobacter* species. Invasive manipulation of the urethra (e.g., urinary catheterization), frequent vaginal examinations, and genital trauma increase the likelihood of a urinary tract infection. It is the most common cause of a fever in the postpartum woman.

Mastitis

Mastitis is defined as inflammation of the mammary gland. A common problem that may occur within the first 2 days to 2 weeks postpartum. An estimated 5% of breast-feeding women develop lactational mastitis (Spiliopoulos & Mastrogiannis, 2015). Risk factors associated with mastitis include stasis of milk due to infrequent, inconsistent breastfeeding, and nipple trauma. As well as causing significant discomfort, it is a frequent reason for women to stop breast-feeding. It can result from any event that creates milk stasis: insufficient drainage of the breast, rapid weaning, oversupply of milk, pressure on the breast from a poorly fitting bra, a blocked duct, missed feedings, and breakdown of the nipple via fissures, cracks, or blisters (Nagtalon-Ramos, 2014). The most common infecting

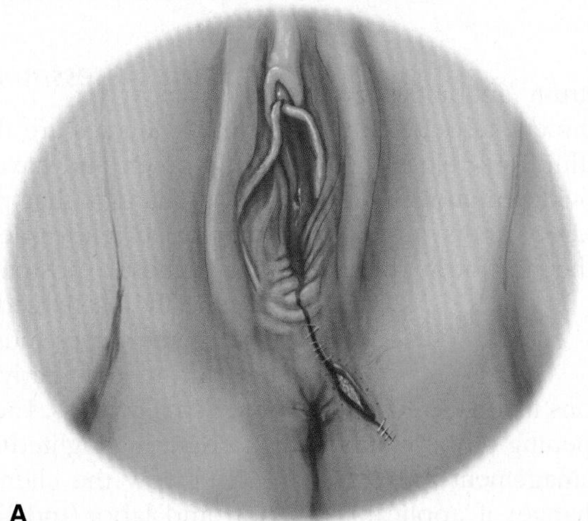

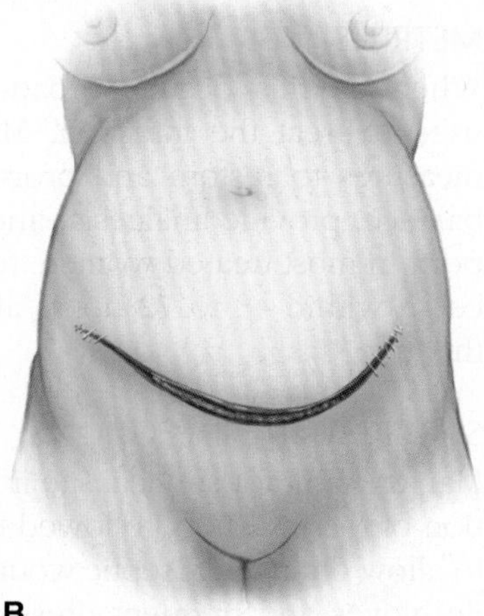

FIGURE 22.2 Postpartum wound infections. **A.** Infected episiotomy site. **B.** Infected cesarean birth incision.

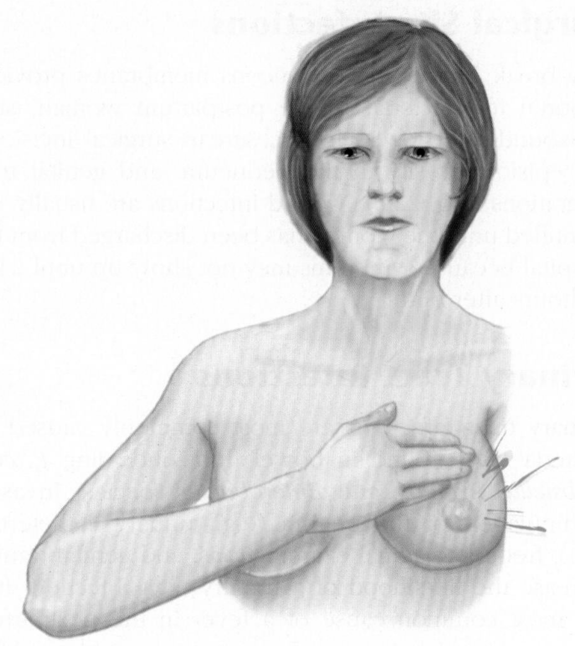

FIGURE 22.3 With mastitis, an area on one breast is tender, hot, red, and painful.

organism is *S. aureus,* which comes from the breast-feeding infant's mouth or throat. *Staphylococcus albus*, *E. coli*, and streptococci are also causative agents, but found less frequently. Infection can be transmitted from the lactiferous ducts to a secreting lobule, from a nipple fissure to periductal lymphatics, or by circulation (Amir, 2014) (Fig. 22.3). A breast abscess may develop if mastitis is not treated adequately. Flu-like symptoms are often the first symptoms experienced by the mother. Breasts are red, tender, and hot to the touch. The upper, outer quadrant of the breast is the most common site for mastitis to occur because most of the breast tissue is located there with both the right and left breasts being equally affected. Effective milk removal, pain medication, and antibiotic therapy have been the mainstays of treatment.

Therapeutic Management

METRITIS

When metritis occurs, broad-spectrum antibiotics are used to treat the infection. Management also includes measures to restore and promote fluid and electrolyte balance, provide analgesia, and provide emotional support. In most treated women, fever drops and symptoms cease within 48 to 72 hours after the start of antibiotic therapy.

SURGICAL SITE INFECTIONS

Management for surgical site infections involves recognition of the infection, followed by opening of the wound to allow drainage. Aseptic wound management with sterile gloves and frequent dressing changes if applicable, good hand hygiene, frequent perineal pad changes, hydration, and ambulation to prevent venous stasis and improve circulation are initiated to prevent development of a more serious infection or spread of the infection to adjacent structures. Parenteral antibiotics are the mainstay of treatment. Analgesics are also important, because women often experience discomfort at the wound site.

URINARY TRACT INFECTIONS

Urinary tract infections are common during the postpartum period and could be prevented by timely removal of urinary catheters used during labor or surgical births. Risk factors include catheterization, epidural anesthesia, and vaginal procedures. If the woman develops a urinary tract infection, fluids are used to treat dehydration. General nutrition measures include acidifying the urine by taking large doses of vitamin C or a regular intake of cranberry juice. Cranberry juice contains a substance with biologic activity that inhibits the growth of *E. coli* in the urinary tract (Wong & Rosh, 2015). Antibiotics may also be ordered if appropriate.

MASTITIS

Treatment of mastitis focuses on two areas: emptying the breasts and controlling the infection. Frequent breast emptying helps both infectious and noninfectious mastitis. The breast can be emptied either by the infant sucking or by manual expression. Increasing the frequency of nursing is advised. Lactation need not be suppressed. Control of infection is achieved with antibiotics. In addition, ice or warm packs and analgesics may be needed. In addition to antibiotics, management of lactational breast infections includes symptomatic treatment, assessment of the infant's attachment to the breast, and reassurance, emotional support, education, and support for ongoing breast-feeding.

Take Note!

Regardless of the etiology of mastitis, the focus is on reversing milk stasis, maintaining milk supply, and continuing breast-feeding, along with providing maternal comfort and preventing recurrence.

Nursing Assessment

Perinatal nurses are the primary caregivers for postpartum women and have a unique opportunity to identify subtle changes that place women at risk for infection. Nurses play a key role in identifying signs and symptoms that suggest a postpartum infection. Today women are commonly discharged 24 to 48 hours after giving birth. Therefore, nurses must assess new mothers for risk factors and identify early, subtle signs and symptoms of an infectious process. Factors that place a woman at risk for a PPI are highlighted in Box 22.1.

Review the client's history and physical examination and labor and birth record for factors that might

BOX 22.1

FACTORS PLACING A WOMAN AT RISK FOR POSTPARTUM INFECTION

- Prolonged (>18–24 hours) premature rupture of membranes (removes the barrier of amniotic fluid so bacteria can ascend)
- Cesarean birth (allows bacterial entry due to break in protective skin barrier)
- Urinary catheterization (could allow entry of bacteria into bladder due to break in aseptic technique)
- Regional anesthesia that decreases perception of need to void (causes urinary stasis and increases risk of urinary tract infection)
- Staff attending to woman are ill (promotes droplet infection from personnel)
- Compromised health status, such as anemia, obesity, smoking, drug abuse (reduces the body's immune system and decreases ability to fight infection)
- Preexisting colonization of lower genital tract with bacterial vaginosis, *Chlamydia trachomatis,* group B streptococci, *S. aureus,* and *E. coli* (allows microbes to ascend)
- Retained placental fragments (provides medium for bacterial growth)
- Manual removal of a retained placenta (causes trauma to the lining of the uterus and thus opens up sites for bacterial invasion)
- Insertion of fetal scalp electrode or intrauterine pressure catheters for internal fetal monitoring during labor (provides entry into uterine cavity)
- Instrument-assisted childbirth, such as forceps or vacuum extraction (increases risk of trauma to genital tract, which provides bacteria access to grow)
- Trauma to the genital tract, such as episiotomy or lacerations (provides a portal of entry for bacteria)
- Prolonged labor with frequent vaginal examinations to check progress (allows time for bacteria to multiply and increases potential exposure to microorganisms or trauma)
- Poor nutritional status (reduces body's ability to repair tissue)
- Gestational diabetes (decreases body's healing ability and provides higher glucose levels on skin and in urine, which encourages bacterial growth)
- Break in aseptic technique during surgery or birthing process (allows entry of bacteria)

Adapted from Salam, R. A., Mansoor, T., Mallick, D., Lassi, Z. S., Das, J. K., & Bhutta, Z. A. (2014). Essential childbirth and postnatal interventions for improved maternal and neonatal health. *Reproductive Health, 11*(Suppl 1), S3-20; Jordan, R. G., Engstrom, J. L., Marfell, J. A., & Farley, C. L. (2014). *Prenatal and postnatal care: A woman-centered approach.* Ames, Iowa: Wiley Blackwell; and Wong, A. W., & Rosh, A. J. (2015). Postpartum infections. *eMedicine.* Retrieved from http://emedicine.medscape.com/article/796892-overview

increase her risk for developing an infection. Then complete the assessment (using the "BUBBLE-EE" parameters discussed in Chapter 16), paying particular attention to areas such as the abdomen and fundus, breasts, urinary tract, episiotomy, lacerations, or incisions and being alert for signs and symptoms of infection (Table 22.3).

TABLE 22.3 SIGNS AND SYMPTOMS OF POSTPARTUM INFECTIONS

Postpartum Infection	Signs and Symptoms
Metritis	Lower abdominal tenderness or pain on one or both sides Temperature elevation (>38° C) Foul-smelling lochia Anorexia Nausea Fatigue and lethargy Leukocytosis and elevated sedimentation rate
Wound infection	Weeping serosanguineous or purulent drainage Separation of or unapproximated wound edges Edema Erythema Tenderness Discomfort at the site Maternal fever Elevated white blood cell count
Urinary tract infection	Urgency Frequency Dysuria Flank pain Low-grade fever Urinary retention Hematuria Urine positive for nitrates Cloudy urine with strong odor
Mastitis	Flu-like symptoms, including malaise, fever, and chills Tender, hot, red, painful area on one breast Inflammation of breast area Breast tenderness Cracking of skin around nipple or areola Breast distention with milk

Adapted from Dalton, E., & Castillo, E. (2014). Postpartum infections: A review for the non-OB/GYN. *Obstetric Medicine: The Medicine of Pregnancy,* (Online 2/27/14), 1753495X14522784. doi: 10.1177/1753495X14522784; Nagtalon-Ramos, J. (2014). *Maternal-newborn nursing care: Best evidence-based practices.* Philadelphia, PA: F.A. Davis Company; and Spiliopoulos, M., & Mastrogiannis, D. (2015). Normal and abnormal puerperium. *eMedicine.* Retrieved from http://emedicine.medscape.com/article/260187-overview#a1

Take Note!

A PPI is commonly associated with an elevated temperature, as mentioned previously. Other generalized signs and symptoms may include chills, foul-smelling vaginal discharge, headache, malaise, restlessness, anxiety, and tachycardia. In addition, the woman may have specific signs and symptoms based on the type and location of the infection.

The acronym REEDA is frequently used for assessing a woman's perineum status. It is derived from five components that have been identified to be associated with the healing process of the perineum. These include:

1. Redness—area may also feel warm to touch.
2. Edema—may indicate infection or a hematoma.
3. Ecchymosis—may indicate vaginal trauma.
4. Discharge—should follow the expected lochia pattern.
5. Approximation of skin edges—should be well aligned without gaps.

Each category is assessed and a number assigned (0 to 3 points) for a total REEDA score ranging from 0 to 15. The higher scores indicate increased tissue trauma (Kaur et al., 2015). See Figure 22.4 for the REEDA method for assessing perineum healing.

Monitor the woman's vital signs, especially her temperature. Changes may also signal an infection.

Nursing Management

Nursing management focuses on preventing postpartum infections. Use the following guidelines to reduce the incidence of postpartum infections:

- Maintain aseptic technique when performing invasive procedures such as urinary catheterization, when changing dressings, and during all surgical procedures.
- Use good hand hygiene technique before and after each client care activity.
- Reinforce measures for maintaining good perineal hygiene.
- Practice standard precautions whenever in contact with blood, body fluids, excretions.
- Use adequate lighting and turn the client to the side to assess the episiotomy site.
- Use extreme caution when handling sharp instruments, specimens, and waste disposal
- Screen all visitors for any signs of active infections to reduce the client's risk of exposure.
- Review the client's history for preexisting infections or chronic conditions.
- Monitor vital signs and laboratory results for any abnormal values.
- Monitor the frequency of vaginal examinations and length of labor.
- Assess frequently for early signs of infection, especially fever and the appearance of lochia.
- Inspect wounds frequently for inflammation and drainage.
- Encourage rest, adequate hydration, and healthy eating habits.
- Reinforce preventive measures during any interaction with the client.

If the woman develops an infection, review treatment measures, such as antibiotic therapy if ordered, and any special care measures, such as dressing changes, that might be needed (Nursing Care Plan 22.1, at the end of the chapter).

Postpartum women should be offered advice on the signs and symptoms of life-threatening conditions, including sepsis. Information should include the importance of good hand and perineal hygiene and of the need to seek immediate medical care if feeling unwell. Client teaching is a priority due to today's short lengths of stay after childbirth. Some infections may not manifest until after discharge. Review the signs and symptoms of infection, emphasizing the danger signs that need to be reported to the health care provider. Most importantly, stress proper hand hygiene, especially after perineal care and before and after breast-feeding. Also reinforce measures to promote breast-feeding, including proper breast care (see Chapter 16). Teaching Guidelines 22.2 highlights the major teaching points for a woman with a postpartum infection.

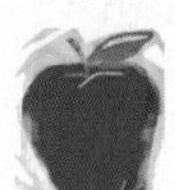

Teaching Guidelines 22.2

TEACHING FOR THE WOMAN WITH A POSTPARTUM INFECTION

- Continue your antibiotic therapy as prescribed.
- Take the medication exactly as ordered and continue with the medication until it is finished.
- Do not stop taking the medication even when you are feeling better.
- Check your temperature every day and call your health care provider if it is above 100.4° F (38° C).
- Watch for other signs and symptoms of infection, such as chills, increased abdominal pain, change in the color or odor of your lochia, or increased redness, warmth, swelling, or drainage from a wound site such as your cesarean incision or episiotomy. Report any of these to your health care provider immediately.
- Practice good infection prevention:
- Always wash your hands thoroughly before and after eating, using the bathroom, touching your perineal area, or providing care for your newborn.
- Wipe from front to back after using the bathroom.
- Remove your perineal pad using a front-to-back motion. Fold the pad in half so that the inner sides of the pad that were touching your body are against each other. Wrap in toilet tissue or place in a plastic bag and discard.
- Wash your hands before applying a new pad.
- Apply a new perineal pad using a front-to-back motion. Handle the pad by the edges (top and bottom or sides) and avoid touching the inner aspect of the pad that will be against your body.
- When performing perineal care with a peribottle, angle the spray of water so that it flows from front to back.
- Drink plenty of fluids each day and eat a variety of foods that are high in vitamins, iron, and protein.
- Be sure to get adequate rest at night and periodically throughout the day.

REEDA Method for Assessing Perineum Healing

- **R**edness
  - none = 0 points
  - Redness within .25 cm of incision bilaterally = 1
  - Redness within .50 cm of incision bilaterally = 2
  - Redness reaching beyond .5 cm of incision bilaterally = 3
- **E**dema – the more swelling present, the high the score
  - None = 0 points
  - < 1 cm from incision = 1 point
  - 1 to 2 cm from incision = 2 points
  - > 2 cm from incision = 3 points
- **E**cchymosis – the more bruising observed, the higher the score
  - None = 0 points
  - 1-2 cm from incision = 1 point
  - .25 cm-1 cm bilaterally or .5-2 cm unilaterally = 2 points
  - > 1 cm bilaterally or 2 cm unilaterally = 3 points
- **D**ischarge – range would be from none present to profuse
  - None = 0 points
  - Serum discharge present = 1 point
  - Serosanguineous discharge present = 2 points
  - Bloody, purulent discharge present = 3 points
- **A**pproximation of skin edges
  - Closed, skin edges approximated well = 0 points
  - Skin separated 3 cm or less = 1 point
  - Skin and subcutaneous fat separated = 2 points
  - Skin, subcutaneous fat and facial separation = 3 points

FIGURE 22.4 REEDA method for assessing perineum healing. (Adapted from Davidson, N. [1974]. REEDA: Evaluating postpartum healing. *Journal of Nurse Midwifery, 19*[2], 6–8; and Nikpour, M., Shirvani, M. A., Azadbakht, M., Zanjani, R., & Mousavi, E. [2014]. The effect of honey gel on abdominal wound healing in cesarean section: A triple blind randomized clinical trial. *Oman Medical Journal, 29*[4], 255–259.)

POSTPARTUM AFFECTIVE DISORDERS

The postpartum period involves extraordinary physiologic, psychological, and sociocultural changes in the life of a woman and her family. It is an exhilarating time for most women, but for others it may not be what they had expected. Women have varied reactions to their childbearing experiences, exhibiting a wide range of emotions. Typically, the delivery of a newborn is associated with positive feelings such as happiness, joy, and gratitude for the birth of a healthy infant. However, women may also feel weepy, overwhelmed, or unsure of what is happening to them. They may experience fear about loss of control; they may feel scared, alone, or guilty, or as if they have somehow failed. During the postpartum period, up to 85% of women experience some type of mood disorder (Joy, Mattingly, & Templeton, 2015).

Postpartum affective disorders have been documented for years, but only recently have they received medical attention. Plummeting levels of estrogen and progesterone immediately after birth can contribute to postpartum mood disorders. Reproductive hormones influence every biologic system and many women are particularly sensitive to the effects of perinatal changes in hormone levels after childbirth. It is believed that the greater the change in these hormone levels between pregnancy and postpartum, the greater the chance for developing a mood disorder (Schiller, Meltzer-Brody, & Rubinow, 2015).

Many types of affective disorders occur in the postpartum period. Although their description and classification may be controversial, the disorders are commonly classified on the basis of their severity as postpartum or baby blues, postpartum depression, and postpartum psychosis.

Postpartum Blues

Many postpartum women (approximately 80%) experience the "blues" (Callahan, 2016). The woman experiences rapid cycling mood symptoms during the first postpartum week typically. The woman exhibits mild depressive symptoms of anxiety, irritability, mood swings, tearfulness, increased sensitivity, despondency, feelings of being overwhelmed, difficulty thinking clearly, and fatigue (Pop et al., 2015). Emotional lability is the most prominent symptom of the maternity blues. The "blues" typically peak on postpartum days 4 and 5 and usually resolve by postpartum day 10. Biologic, psychological, and social factors have been hypothesized as relevant to blues causation, but no studies have validated this. Although the woman's symptoms may be distressing, they do not reflect psychopathology and usually do not affect the mother's ability to function and care for her infant.

Baby blues are usually self-limiting and require no formal treatment other than reassurance and validation of the woman's experience, as well as assistance in caring for herself and the newborn. However, follow-up of women with postpartum blues is important because up to 20% go on to develop postpartum depression (Alexander et al., 2014).

Postpartum Depression

Depression is more prevalent in women than in men, which may be related to biologic, hormonal, and psychosocial factors. **Postpartum depression (PPD)** is a form of clinical depression that can affect women, and less frequently men, after childbirth. It affects as many as 20% of all mothers in the United States, and as many as 60% of adolescent mothers (ACOG, 2014c; CDC,2015c; Joy et al., 2015). Unlike the postpartum blues, women with postpartum depression feel worse over time, and changes in mood and behavior do not go away on their own. Postpartum depression may persist for a minimum of six months if untreated. Different from the baby blues, the symptoms of PPD last longer, are more severe, and require treatment. Some signs and symptoms of PPD include feeling the following:

- Restless
- Worthless
- Guilty
- Hopeless
- Moody
- Sad
- Overwhelmed
- Loss of enjoyment
- Low energy level
- Loss of libido

The new mother may also:

- Cry a lot.
- Exhibit a lack of energy and motivation.
- Be unable to make decisions or focus.
- Lose her memory.
- Experience a lack of pleasure.
- Have changes in sleep or weight.
- Show a lack of concern for herself.
- Withdraw from friends and family.
- Have pains in her body that do not subside.
- Feel negatively toward her baby.
- Have appetite disturbances.
- Have feelings of isolation from others.
- Lack interest in her baby.
- Worry about hurting the baby.
- Act detached toward others and infant.
- Have recurrent thoughts of suicide and death (Bobo & Yawn, 2014).

Postpartum depression affects not only the woman but also the entire family. Identifying depression early can substantially improve the client and family outcomes. PPD usually has a gradual onset and becomes evident within the first 6 weeks postpartum.

The cause of PPD is not known, but research suggests that it is multifactorial. According to ACOG (2014c), "postpartum depression is likely to result from body, mind, and lifestyle factors combined." The levels of estrogen, progesterone, serotonin, and thyroid hormone decrease sharply and return to normal during the immediate postpartum period, which can trigger depression and can change a woman's mood and behavior. Other aspects that can lead to PPD include:

- Unresolved feelings about the pregnancy
- Fatigue after delivery from lack of sleep or broken sleep
- Feelings of being less attractive
- Inadequate assistance from partner
- Lack of social support network
- History of sexual or physical abuse
- Unemployment or financial insecurity
- Doubts about the ability to be a good mother
- Stress from changes in work and home routines
- Loss of freedom and old identity (Finley & Brizendine, 2015).

PPD may lend itself to prophylactic intervention because its onset is predictable, the risk period for illness is well defined, and women at high risk potentially could be identified using a screening tool. This is not the case for all women, however (see Evidence-Based Practice 22.1). Prophylaxis starts with a prenatal risk assessment and education. Based on the woman's history of prior depression, prophylactic antidepressant therapy may be needed during the third trimester or immediately after giving birth. Management mirrors that of any major depression: a combination of antidepressant medication, antianxiety medication, adequate sleep and rest, and psychotherapy in an outpatient or inpatient setting (Callahan, 2016). Marital counseling may be necessary if marital problems are contributing to the woman's depressive symptoms.

The significant other's or partner's emotional health should not be overlooked during the woman's pregnancy and throughout the first postpartum year. PPD, once expected only in new mothers, occurs in new significant others or partners as well. Up to 50% of significant others or partners whose partners suffer from PPD also have depressive symptoms, and little is known about the impact of maternal PPD on them. Depressive symptoms are likely to decrease their ability to provide maternal support. Significant other's or partner's PPD can be difficult to identify. New partners or significant others may seem more angry and anxious than sad, yet depression is present. When left untreated, partner's PPD limits the significant other's or partner's capacity to provide emotional support to their partners and children. The highest rates of depression among fathers have been reported between 3 and 6 months postpartum. Factors

EVIDENCE-BASED PRACTICE 22.1 A SYSTEMATIC REVIEW OF THE RELATIONSHIP OF BETWEEN POSTPARTUM SLEEP DISTURBANCE AND POSTPARTUM DEPRESSION

STUDY

Sleep is closely associated with psychological well-being. Insufficient sleep leads to adverse medical and psychological consequences and a poorer quality of life. Despite commonly held beliefs of joy and happiness after childbirth, women are vulnerable to mood disorders during the postpartum period. Nighttime feedings and frequent nocturnal awakenings contribute to sleep maternal mood disturbances. Poor and fragmented sleep patterns are associated with a poor quality of life, a decrease in attentiveness and general well-being. More importantly, it may be a risk factor for postpartum depression. Postpartum depression has been linked with a series of psychosocial sequelae for mothers and their newborns. The purpose of this review was to analyze the relationship between postpartum sleep disturbance and postpartum depression.

Findings

A systematic review was conducted on thirteen observational studies which included 3,793 women. The findings from all thirteen studies revealed a consistent strong relationship between sleep disturbance and postpartum depression. Short sleep duration and insomnia are related to a range of impaired functional outcomes that may negatively impact the daily life of postpartum women and their newborns.

Nursing Implications

Based on this evidence, nurses can counsel postpartum women about the importance of getting adequate sleep when they are discharged and the link between sleep disturbances and postpartum depression. Nurses can suggest several interventions to assist the new mother in obtaining adequate sleep such as bathing the newborn at night before bedtime, asking for help from family to assist in nighttime diaper changes, and taking naps throughout the day when the newborn sleeps. These simple helpful interventions may be a valuable prevention measure to assist in increasing the mother's wellness and reduce the risk of postpartum depression.

Adapted from Bhati, S., & Richards, K. (2015). A systematic review of the relationship between postpartum sleep disturbance and postpartum depression. *Journal of Obstetric, Gynecologic, & Neonatal Nursing, 44*(3), 350–357.

that increase the risk of paternal PPD include a personal history of depression and/or anxiety, a low level of marital satisfaction, excessive financial stressors, a lack of significant other or partner's parental leave, and the feeling that there is a great discrepancy between one's expectations of parenthood and its realities (Feeley et al., 2015).

Assessing partner's PPD is not easy. Nevertheless, it is important for all nurses who have contact with new partners to remain open to the notion that new partners are predisposed to PPD, particularly if their partner is afflicted. Delving deeper into understanding behaviors of withdrawing, indecisiveness, cynicism, avoiding, drinking, using drugs, fighting, partner violence, extramarital affairs, and feelings of heightened irritation will reveal important insights. Asking new partners candidly if they are feeling depressed, anxious, or angry can open the door to further exploration of these emotions (Weissman, 2014).

Although partner depression is only now beginning to be defined and measured, sufficient evidence exists to warrant nurses' attention and concern. Nurses may be most able to help a new partner devastated by PPD when they plant seeds of awareness that the disorder exists, that they are not alone, and that help is available.

Despite the negative outcomes associated with PPD, rates of diagnosis and treatment are low mainly because of lack of recognition by the health care provider. In addition, PPD is the most misinterpreted, frequently dismissed, and most undiagnosed postpartum complication. Early recognition of PPD can eliminate the length of time that women and men have to suffer with this debilitating condition and can decrease the potentially harmful effects on the infants involved.

Screening for symptoms of PPD in both men and women is an important preliminary step to diagnosis and treatment, but the effectiveness of depression screening is dependent on the reliability and validity of the screening instruments in the population. Both the Edinburgh Postnatal Depression Scale (EPDS) and the Postpartum Depression Predictor Scale (PDSS) have been used to screen mothers for PPD, but it is not clear which instrument best predicts a diagnosis of postpartum depression (Thombs et al., 2014).

The EPDS is a self-report, quick, and easy screening tool for PPD that consists of 10 questions with four possible responses. The couple fill out the tool according to their symptoms during the past 7 days, with each response given a score of 0 to 3 points, creating a maximum score of 30. Using a cutoff score of 9 or 10, the sensitivity is 86%; the specificity, 78%; and positive predictive value, 73% (Zhao et al., 2015).

The PDSS is a self-report, 35-item Likert-type response scale divided into seven conceptual domains:

1. Anxiety/insecurity
2. Sleep/eating disturbance
3. Emotional liability
4. Loss of self-esteem
5. Guilt/shame
6. Cognitive impairment
7. Suicidal thoughts

The scores range from 35 to 175. The scale has five symptoms for each domain, and the woman is asked to identify her degree of disagreement or agreement on the basis of her feelings over the past 2 weeks. The sensitivity of the PDSS is 91%; the specificity is 72% for detecting PPD. The PDSS takes 5 to 10 minutes to administer and is used during the postpartum period (King et al., 2015).

Early identification, screening, prevention, and treatment of PPD are crucial for improving overall outcomes for the mother and infant, as well as for decreasing mortality and morbidity. This is why it is crucial for nurses to understand and know about the risk factors, signs and symptoms, prevention, and use and interpretation of screening tools and to make appropriate referrals for treatment. Mass screening for PPD using a validated screening tool has been proven to improve the rates of detection and treatment of PPD and should be implemented in obstetricians' and pediatricians' offices and in primary care settings. The Edinburgh tool is shown in Figure 22.5.

Postpartum Psychosis

At the severe end of the continuum of postpartum emotional disorders is postpartum psychosis, which occurs in 1 in 1,000 live births (Doyle, Carballedo, & O'Keane, 2015). Postpartum psychosis, an emergency psychiatric condition, can result in a significant increased risk for suicide and infanticide. Symptoms of postpartum psychosis, such as mood lability, delusional beliefs, hallucinations, and disorganized thinking, can be frightening for the women who are affected and for their families. It generally surfaces within 3 months of giving birth and is manifested by sleep disturbances, fatigue, depression, and hypomania. The mother will be tearful, confused, and preoccupied with feelings of guilt and worthlessness. Early symptoms resemble those of depression, but they may escalate to delirium, hallucinations, extreme disorganization of thought, anger toward herself and her infant, bizarre behavior, delusions, disorientation, depersonalization, delirium-like appearance, manifestations of mania, and thoughts of hurting herself and the infant. The mother frequently loses touch with reality and experiences a severe regressive breakdown, associated with a high risk of suicide or infanticide (del Corral Serrano, 2015). Women with postpartum psychosis should not be left alone with their infants. Most women with postpartum psychosis are hospitalized for up to several months. Psychotropic drugs are almost always part of treatment, along with individual psychotherapy and support group therapy.

Edinburgh Postnatal Depression Scale

Name: ______________________ Address: ______________________

Your Date of Birth: ______________________ ______________________

Baby's Date of Birth: ______________________ Phone: ______________________

As you are pregnant or have recently had a baby, we would like to know how you are feeling. Please check the answer that comes closest to how you have felt **IN THE PAST 7 DAYS**, not just how you feel today.

Here is an example, already completed.

I have felt happy:
- ☐ Yes, all the time
- ☒ Yes, most of the time
- ☐ No, not very often
- ☐ No, not at all

This would mean: "I have felt happy most of the time" during the past week. Please complete the other questions in the same way.

In the past 7 days:

1. I have been able to laugh and see the funny side of things
   - ☐ As much as I always could
   - ☐ Not quite so much now
   - ☐ Definitely not so much now
   - ☐ Not at all

2. I have looked forward with enjoyment to things
   - ☐ As much as I ever did
   - ☐ Rather less than I used to
   - ☐ Definitely less than I used to
   - ☐ Hardly at all

*3. I have blamed myself unnecessarily when things went wrong
   - ☐ Yes, most of the time
   - ☐ Yes, some of the time
   - ☐ Not very often
   - ☐ No, never

4. I have been anxious or worried for no good reason
   - ☐ No, not at all
   - ☐ Hardly ever
   - ☐ Yes, sometimes
   - ☐ Yes, very often

*5 I have felt scared or panicky for no very good reason
   - ☐ Yes, quite a lot
   - ☐ Yes, sometimes
   - ☐ No, not much
   - ☐ No, not at all

*6. Things have been getting on top of me
   - ☐ Yes, most of the time I haven't been able to cope at all
   - ☐ Yes, sometimes I haven't been coping as well as usual
   - ☐ No, most of the time I have copied quite well
   - ☐ No, I have been coping as well as ever

*7 I have been so unhappy that I have had difficulty sleeping
   - ☐ Yes, most of the time
   - ☐ Yes, sometimes
   - ☐ Not very often
   - ☐ No, not at all

*8 I have felt sad or miserable
   - ☐ Yes, most of the time
   - ☐ Yes, quite often
   - ☐ Not very often
   - ☐ No, not at all

*9 I have been so unhappy that I have been crying
   - ☐ Yes, most of the time
   - ☐ Yes, quite often
   - ☐ Only occasionally
   - ☐ No, never

*10 The thought of harming myself has occurred to me
   - ☐ Yes, quite often
   - ☐ Sometimes
   - ☐ Hardly ever
   - ☐ Never

Administered/Reviewed by ______________________ Date ______________________

FIGURE 22.5 Adapted Edinburgh Postnatal Depression Scale (EPDS). (From Cox, J. L., Holden, J. M., & Sagovsky, R. [1987]. Detection of postnatal depression: Development of the 10-item Edinburgh Postnatal Depression Scale. *British Journal of Psychiatry, 150*, 782–786.)

Take Note!

The greatest hazard of postpartum psychosis is suicide. Infanticide and child abuse are also risks if the woman is left alone with her infant. Early recognition and prompt treatment of this disorder are imperative.

Nursing Assessment

Postpartum affective disorders are often overlooked and go unrecognized despite the large percentage of women who experience them. The postpartum period is a time of increased vulnerability, but few women receive education about the possibility of depression after birth. In addition, many women may feel ashamed of having negative emotions at a time when they "should" be happy; thus, they do not seek professional help. Nurses can play a major role in providing guidance about postpartum affective disorders, detecting manifestations, and assisting women to obtain appropriate care.

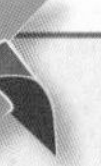

Consider This

Even though I was an assertive practicing attorney in my thirties, my first pregnancy was filled with nagging feelings of doubt about this upcoming event in my life. Throughout my pregnancy I was so busy with trial work that I never had time to really evaluate my feelings. I was always reading about the bodily changes that were taking place, and on one level I was feeling excited, but on another level I was emotionally drained. Shortly after the birth of my daughter, those suppressed nagging feelings of doubt surfaced big time and practically immobilized me. I felt exhausted all the time and was only too glad to have someone else care for my daughter. I didn't breast-feed because I thought it would tie me down too much. Although at the time I thought this "low mood" was normal for all new mothers, I have since found out it was postpartum depression. How could any woman be depressed about this wondrous event?

Thoughts: Now that postpartum depression has been "taken out of the closet" and recognized as a real emotional disorder, it can be treated. This woman showed tendencies during her pregnancy but was able to suppress the feelings and go forward. Her description of her depression is very typical of many women who suffer in silence, hoping to get over these feelings in time. What can nurses do to promote awareness of this disorder? Can it be prevented?

Begin the assessment by reviewing the history to identify general risk factors that could predispose a woman to depression:

- Poor coping skills
- First pregnancy
- Low self-esteem
- Numerous life stressors
- History of abuse
- Mood swings and emotional stress
- Previous psychological problems or a family history of psychiatric disorders
- Substance abuse
- Limited or lack of social support network

Also review the history for specific pregnancy and birth factors that may increase the woman's risk for depression. These may include a history of PPD, evidence of depression during the pregnancy, prenatal anxiety, a difficult or complicated pregnancy, traumatic birth experience, or birth of a high-risk or special-needs infant (Callahan, 2016).

Be alert for physical findings. Assess the woman's activity level, including her level of fatigue. Ask about her sleeping habits, noting any problems with insomnia. When interacting with the woman, observe for verbal and nonverbal indicators of anxiety as well as her ability to concentrate during the interaction. Difficulty concentrating and anxious behaviors suggest a problem. Also assess her nutritional intake: weight loss due to poor food intake may be seen. Assessment can identify women with a high-risk profile for depression, and the nurse can educate them and make referrals for individual or family counseling if needed. Some common assessment findings associated with PPD are listed in Box 22.2.

Nursing Management

Nurses need to educate themselves about this disorder to facilitate early recognition of signs and symptoms of it, which, in turn, would make early treatment possible, thus supporting recovery. Furthermore, greater knowledge could contribute to providing more effective and compassionate care to these women. Nursing management focuses on assisting any postpartum woman to cope with the changes of this period. Encourage the client to verbalize what she is going through and emphasize the importance of keeping her expectations realistic. Assist the woman in structuring her day to regain a sense of control over the situation. Encourage her to seek help if necessary, using available support systems. Also reinforce the need for good nutrition and adequate exercise and sleep (Bobo & Yawn, 2014).

The nurse can play an important role in assisting women and their partners with postpartum adjustment. Providing facts about the enormous changes that occur during the postpartum period is critical. This information would include changes in the woman's body. Review the signs and symptoms of all three affective disorders. This information is typically included as part of prenatal visits and childbirth education classes. Know the risk factors associated with these disorders and review the history of clients and their families. Use specific, nonthreatening questions to aid in early detection, such as, "Have you felt down, depressed, or hopeless lately?" and, "Have you felt little interest or pleasure in doing things recently?"

Discuss factors that may increase a woman's vulnerability to stress during the postpartum period, such

BOX 22.2

COMMON ASSESSMENT FINDINGS ASSOCIATED WITH POSTPARTUM DEPRESSION

- Loss of pleasure or interest in life
- Low mood, especially in the morning; sadness, tearfulness
- Exhaustion that is not relieved by sleep
- Feelings of guilt
- Weight loss
- Low energy
- Irritability
- Poor personal hygiene
- Constipation
- Being preoccupied and unfocused
- Indecisiveness
- Diminished concentration
- Anxiety
- Despair
- Compulsive thoughts
- Loss of libido
- Loss of confidence
- Sleep difficulties (insomnia)
- Loss of appetite
- Bleak and pessimistic view of the future
- Not responding to infant's cries or cues for attention
- Social isolation, not answering the door or the phone
- Feelings of failure as a mother

Adapted from American College of Obstetrics and Gynecology [ACOG]. (2014c). *Postpartum depression.* Retrieved from http://www.acog.org/Patients/FAQs/Postpartum-Depression#blues; Centers for Disease Control and Prevention [CDC]. (2015c). *Depression among women of reproductive age.* Retrieved from http://www.cdc.gov/reproductivehealth/depression/; and Joy, S., Mattingly, P. J., & Templeton, H. B. (2015). Postpartum depression: An overview of postpartum mood disorders. *eMedicine.* Retrieved from http://emedicine.medscape.com/article/271662-overview

as sleep deprivation and unrealistic expectations, so couples can understand and respond to those problems if they occur. Stress that many women need help after childbirth and that help is available from many sources, including people they already know. Assisting women to learn how to ask for help is important so they can gain the support they need. Also provide educational materials about postpartum emotional disorders. Have available referral sources for psychotherapy and support groups appropriate for women experiencing postpartum adjustment difficulties. See Evidence-Based Practice Study 22.1.

NURSING CARE PLAN 22.1

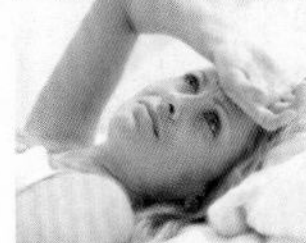

Overview of the Woman with a Postpartum Complication

Jennifer, a 16-year-old G1P1, gave birth to a boy 3 days ago. It was a cesarean birth due to cephalopelvic disproportion following 25 hours of labor with ruptured membranes. Her temperature is 102.6° F (39.2° C). She is complaining of chills and malaise and says, "My incision really hurts." Jennifer rates her pain as 7 to 8 out of 10. The incision site is red, swollen, and very warm to the touch. A 5-cm area of purulent drainage is noted on the dressing; a 3-cm area of the incision is slightly opened, with the wound edges separated. Jennifer's lochia is scant and dark red, with a strong odor. She asks the nurse to take her baby back to the nursery because she doesn't feel well enough to care for him.

NURSING DIAGNOSIS: Ineffective thermoregulation related to bacterial invasion as evidenced by fever, complaints of chills and malaise, and statement of not feeling well

Outcome Identification and Evaluation

The client will exhibit a return to normothermia as evidenced by a body temperature being maintained below 99° F (37.2° C), reports of a decrease in chills and malaise, and statements of feeling better.

Interventions: ***Promoting Fever Reduction***

- Assess vital signs every 2 to 4 hours and record results *to monitor progress of infection.*
- Administer antipyretics as ordered *to reduce temperature and help combat infection.*
- Encourage fluid intake *to promote fluid balance.*
- Document intake and output *to assess hydration status.*
- Offer cool bed bath or shower *to reduce temperature.*
- Place cool cloth on forehead and/or back of neck *to provide comfort.*
- Change bed linen and gown when damp from diaphoresis *to provide comfort and hygiene.*

(continued)

NURSING CARE PLAN 22.1

Overview of the Woman with a Postpartum Complication (continued)

NURSING DIAGNOSIS: Impaired skin integrity related to wound infection as evidenced by purulent drainage, redness, swelling, and separation of wound edges

Outcome Identification and Evaluation

The client will experience a resolution of wound infection as evidenced by a reduction in redness, swelling, and drainage from wound; absence of purulent drainage; and beginning signs and symptoms of wound healing.

Interventions: ***Promoting Wound Healing***

- Administer antibiotic therapy as ordered *to treat infection.*
- Perform frequent dressing changes and wound care as ordered *to promote wound healing;* monitor dressing for drainage, including amount, color, and characteristics, *to evaluate for resolution of infection.*
- Use aseptic technique *to prevent spread of infection.*
- Encourage fluid intake *to maintain fluid balance;* encourage adequate dietary intake, including protein, *to promote healing.*

NURSING DIAGNOSIS: Acute pain related to infectious process

Outcome Identification and Evaluation

The client will report a decrease in pain as evidenced by pain rating of 0 or 1 on pain scale, verbalization of relief with pain management, and statements of feeling better and ability to rest comfortably.

Interventions: ***Relieving Pain***

- Place client in semi-Fowler's position *to facilitate drainage and relieve pressure.*
- Assess pain level on pain scale of 0 to 10 *to quantify pain level*; reassess pain level after intervening *to determine effectiveness of intervention.*
- Assess fundus gently *to ensure appropriate involution.*
- Administer analgesics as needed and on time as ordered *to maintain pain relief.*
- Provide for rest periods *to allow for healing.*
- Assist with positioning in bed with pillows *to promote comfort.*
- Offer nonpharmacologic pain measures such as a backrub *to ease aches and discomfort if desired and enhance effectiveness of analgesics.*

NURSING DIAGNOSIS: Risk for impaired parent–infant attachment related to effects of postpartum infection as evidenced by mother's request to take baby back to the nursery

Outcome Identification and Evaluation

The client will begin to bond with newborn appropriately with each exposure as evidenced by desire to spend time with newborn, expression of positive feelings toward newborn when holding him, increasing participation in care of newborn as client's condition improves, and statements about help and support at home to care for self and newborn.

Interventions: ***Promoting Mother–Newborn Interaction***

- Promote adequate rest and sleep *to ensure adequate energy for interaction and wound healing.*
- Bring newborn to mother after she is rested and has had an analgesic *to allow mother to focus her energies on the child.*

NURSING CARE PLAN 22.1

Overview of the Woman with a Postpartum Complication (continued)

- Progressively allow the client to care for her infant or comfort him as her energy level and pain level improve *to promote self-confidence in caring for the newborn.*
- Offer praise and positive reinforcement for caretaking tasks; stress positive attributes of newborn to mother while caring for him *to facilitate bonding and attachment.*
- Contact family members to participate in care of the newborn *to allow mother to rest and recover from infection.*
- Encourage mother to care for herself first and then the newborn *to ensure adequate energy for newborn's care.*
- Arrange for assistance and support after discharge from hospital *to provide necessary backup.*
- Refer to community health nurse for follow-up care of mother and newborn at home *to foster continued development of maternal–infant relationship.*

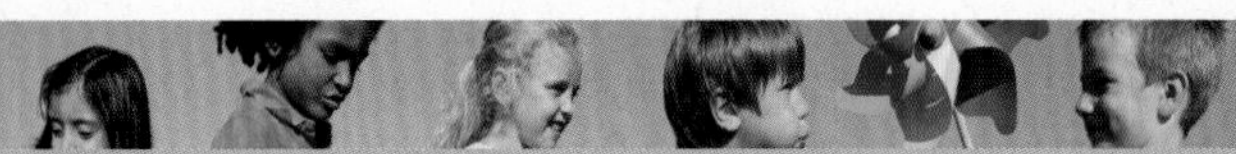

KEY CONCEPTS

- Postpartum hemorrhage is a potentially life-threatening complication of both vaginal and cesarean births. It is the leading cause of maternal mortality in the United States.
- A good way to remember the causes of postpartum hemorrhage is the "5 T's": tone, tissue, trauma, thrombin, and traction.
- Uterine atony is the most common cause of early postpartum hemorrhage, which can lead to hypovolemic shock.
- Oxytocin (Pitocin), misoprostol (Cytotec), dinoprostone (Prostin E2), methylergonovine maleate (Methergine), and prostaglandin PGF2α (carboprost [Hemabate]) are commonly used drugs used to manage postpartum hemorrhage.
- Failure of the placenta to separate completely and be expelled interferes with the ability of the uterus to contract fully, thereby leading to hemorrhage.
- Causes of subinvolution include retained placental fragments, distended bladder, uterine myoma, and infection.
- Lacerations should always be suspected when the uterus is contracted and bright-red blood continues to trickle out of the vagina.
- Conditions that cause coagulopathies may include idiopathic thrombocytopenic purpura (ITP), von Willebrand disease (vWD), and disseminated intravascular coagulation (DIC).
- Pulmonary embolism is a potentially fatal condition that occurs when the pulmonary artery is obstructed by a blood clot that has traveled from another vein into the lungs, causing obstruction and infarction.
- The major causes of a thrombus formation (blood clot) are venous stasis and hypercoagulation, both of which are common in the postpartum period.
- Postpartum infection is defined as a fever of 100.4° F (38° C) or higher after the first 24 hours after childbirth, occurring on at least 2 of the first 10 days exclusive of the first 24 hours.
- Common postpartum infections include metritis, wound infections, urinary tract infections, and mastitis.
- Postpartum emotional disorders are commonly classified on the basis of their severity: "baby blues," postpartum depression, and postpartum psychosis.
- Management of postpartum depression mirrors the treatment of any major depression: a combination of antidepressant medication, antianxiety medication, and psychotherapy in an outpatient or inpatient setting.

REFERENCES AND RECOMMENDED READING

Agency for Healthcare Research and Quality [AHRQ]. (2015). *Evidence-based practice: Management of postpartum hemorrhage.* Retrieved from http://www.effectivehealthcare.ahrq.gov/ehc/products/552/2078/hemorrhage-postpartum-report-150427.pdf

Alexander, L. L., LaRosa, J. H., Bader, H., & Garfield, S. (2014). *New dimensions in women's health* (6th ed.). Sudbury, MA: Jones & Bartlett.

American College of Obstetrics and Gynecologists [ACOG]. (2014a). *Von Willebrand Disease in women*. Retrieved from http://www.acog.org/Resources-And-Publications/Committee-Opinions/Committee-on-Adolescent-Health-Care/Von-Willebrand-Disease-in-Women

American College of Obstetrics and Gynecologists [ACOG]. (2014b). *Use of prophylactic antibiotics in labor and delivery*. Retrieved from http://www.guideline.gov/content.aspx?id=34024

American College of Obstetrics and Gynecology [ACOG]. (2014c). *Postpartum depression*. Retrieved from http://www.acog.org/Patients/FAQs/Postpartum-Depression#blues

Amir, L. H. (2014). The Academy of Breastfeeding Medicine Protocol Committee: Mastitis. *Breastfeeding Medicine. 9*(5): 239–243. doi:10.1089/bfm.2014.9984.

Anand, B., & Gujral, K. (2014). Monitoring of high-risk areas: Maternity wards. In Wattal, C., & Khardori, N. (Eds.), *Hospital infection prevention* (pp. 133–136). New Delhi, India: Springer Publishers.

Belfort, M.A. (2015). Overview of postpartum hemorrhage. *UpToDate*. Retrieved from http://www.uptodate.com/contents/overview-of-postpartum-hemorrhage

Bhati, S., & Richards, K. (2015). A systematic review of the relationship between postpartum sleep disturbance and postpartum depression. *Journal of Obstetric, Gynecologic, & Neonatal Nursing, 44*(3), 350–357.

Bobo, W. V., & Yawn, B. P. (2014). Concise review for physicians and other clinicians: Postpartum depression. *Mayo Clinic Proceedings. 89*(6), 835–844.

Bohlmann, M., & Rath, W. (2014). Medical prevention and treatment of postpartum hemorrhage: A comparison of different guidelines. *Archives of Gynecology & Obstetrics, 289*(3), 555–567. doi: 10.1007/s00404-013-3016-4.

Callahan, T. L. (2016). *Tarascon's OB/GYN pocketbook*. Burlington, MA: Jones & Bartlett Learning.

Centers for Disease Control and Prevention [CDC]. (2015a). *Facts about von Willebrand Disease*. Retrieved from http://www.cdc.gov/ncbddd/vwd/facts.html

Centers for Disease Control and Prevention [CDC]. (2015b). *Deep vein thrombosis (DVT)/Pulmonary embolism (PE)--Blood clot forming in a vein*. Retrieved from http://www.cdc.gov/ncbddd/dvt/data.html

Centers for Disease Control and Prevention [CDC] (2015c) *Depression among women of reproductive age*. Retrieved from http://www.cdc.gov/reproductivehealth/depression/

Clapp, J. C. (2015). A multidisciplinary team approach to management of postpartum hemorrhage. *Journal of Obstetric, Gynecologic, & Neonatal Nursing, 44*, S22. doi: 10.1111/1552-6909.12693.

Conti, E., Zezza, L., Ralli, E., Comito, C., Sada, L., Passerini, J. et al. (2014). Pulmonary embolism in pregnancy. *Journal of Thrombosis and Thrombolysis, 37*(3), 251–270.

Cox, J. L., Holden, J. M., & Sagovsky, R. (1987). Detection of postnatal depression: Development of the 10-item Edinburgh Postnatal Depression Scale. *British Journal of Psychiatry, 150*, 782–786.

Cox, J., Holden, J., & Henshaw, C. (2014). *Perinatal mental health: The Edinburgh Postnatal Depression Scale (EPDS) manual* (2nd ed.). London, England: RCPsychPublications.

Crowe, S. D., & Faulkner, B. (2014). Lean management system application in creation of a postpartum hemorrhage prevention bundle on postpartum units. *Obstetrics and Gynecology, 123*, 45S.

Cunningham, F. G., Leveno, K. J., Bloom, S. L., Spong, C., Dashe, J. S., Hoffman, B.L. et al. (2014). *Williams obstetrics* (24th ed.). New York, NY: McGraw-Hill.

Dalton, E., & Castillo, E. (2014). Postpartum infections: A review for the non-OB/GYN. *Obstetric Medicine: The Medicine of Pregnancy*, (Online 2/27/14), 1753495X14522784. doi: 10.1177/1753495X14522784.

del Corral Serrano, J. (2015). Puerperal psychosis. In Sáenz-Herrero, M. (Ed.), *Psychopathology in Women* (pp. 497–510). New York, NY: Springer International Publishing.

Doyle, M., Carballedo, A., & O'Keane, V. (2015). Perinatal depression and psychosis: an update. *Advances in Psychiatric Treatment, 21*(1), 5–14.

Ekin, A., Gezer, C., Solmaz, U., Taner, C. E., Dogan, A., & Ozeren, M. (2015). Predictors of severity in primary postpartum hemorrhage. *Archives of Gynecology and Obstetrics*, 1–8. doi: 10.1007/s00404-015-3771-5.

Erez, O., Mastrolia, S. A., & Thachil, J. (2015). Disseminated intravascular coagulation in pregnancy: Insights in pathophysiology, diagnosis and management. *American Journal of Obstetrics and Gynecology*. doi: http://dx.doi.org/10.1016/j.ajog.2015.03.054

Feeley, N., Bell, L., Hayton, B., Zelkowitz, P., & Carrier, M. E. (2015). Care for postpartum depression: What do women and their partners prefer? *Perspectives in Psychiatric Care*. doi: 10.1111/ppc.12107.

Finley, P. R., & Brizendine, L. (2015). Enhancing our understanding of perinatal depression. *CNS Spectrums, 20*(1), 9–10.

Green, C. J. (2016). *Maternal newborn nursing care plans* (3rd ed.). Burlington, MA: Jones & Bartlett Learning.

Guimicheva, B., Czuprynska, J. and Arya, R. (2015). The prevention of pregnancy-related venous thromboembolism. *British Journal of Hematology, 168*(2), 163–174. doi: 10.1111/bjh.13159.

Heffline, M., & Schmidt, M. K. (2014). Chapter 19: Superficial thrombophlebitis and deep vein thrombosis. In Christensen, C. R., & Lewis, P. A. (Eds.), *Core curriculum for vascular nursing* (pp. 370–399). Philadelphia, PA: WoltersKluwer.

Jordan, R. G., Engstrom, J. L., Marfell, J. A., & Farley, C. L. (2014). *Prenatal and postnatal care: A woman-centered approach*. Ames, Iowa: Wiley Blackwell.

Joy, S., Mattingly, P. J., & Templeton, H. B. (2015). Postpartum depression: An overview of postpartum mood disorders. *eMedicine*. Retrieved from http://emedicine.medscape.com/article/271662-overview

Kamel, I., & Mastrogiannis, D. S. (2015). The critically ill obstetric patient. Part 1: Epidemiology and pathophysiology. *Postgraduate Obstetrics & Gynecology, 35*(11), 1–7. doi: 10.1097/01.PGO.0000465723.98835.1e.

Kaur, P., Sagar, N., Deol, R., & Kaur, J. (2015). Effectiveness of infra-red therapy upon level of episiotomy pain and wound healing among postnatal mothers. *International Journal of Nursing Education, 7*(2), 184–187.

Kessler, C.M., & Sandler, S.G. (2015). Immune thrombocytopenic purpura. *eMedicine*. Retrieved from http://emedicine.medscape.com/article/202158-overview

King, T. L., Brucker, M. C., Kriebs, J. M., Fahey, J. O., Gegor, C. L., & Varney, H. (2015). *Varney's midwifery* (5th ed.). Burlington, MA: Jones & Bartlett Learning.

Kolecki, P., & Menckhoff, C. R. (2015). Hypovolemic shock. *eMedicine*. Retrieved from http://emedicine.medscape.com/article/760145-overview

Levi, M. M., & Schmaier, A. H. (2015). Disseminated intravascular coagulation. *eMedicine*. Retrieved from http://emedicine.medscape.com/article/199627-overview

Main, E. K., Goffman, D., Scavone, B. M., Low, L. K., Bingham, D., Fontaine, P. L. et al. (2015). National partnership for maternal safety: Consensus bundle on obstetric hemorrhage. *Journal of Obstetric, Gynecologic, & Neonatal Nursing*. doi: 10.1111/1552-6909.12723.

Mattson, S., & Smith, J. E. (2015). *Core curriculum for maternal-newborn nursing* (5th ed.). St. Louis, MO: Saunders Elsevier.

Middeldorp, S. (2015). New studies of low-molecular-weight heparin in pregnancy. *Thrombosis Research, 135*, S26-S29.

Moses, S. (2015). Postpartum hemorrhage. *Family Practice Notebook*. Retrieved from http://www.fpnotebook.com/ob/Bleed/PstprtmHmrhg.htm

Mousa, H. A., Blum, J., Abou El Senoun, G., Shakur, H., Alfirevic, Z. (2014). Treatment for primary postpartum hemorrhage. *Cochrane Database of Systematic Reviews*, (2). Art. No.: CD003249. doi: 10.1002/14651858.CD003249.pub3.

Nagtalon-Ramos, J. (2014). *Maternal-newborn nursing care: Best evidence-based practices*. Philadelphia, PA: F.A. Davis Company.

Nahum, G. G., & Pham, K. Q. (2015). Uterine rupture in pregnancy. *eMedicine*. Retrieved from http://reference.medscape.com/article/275854-overview

National Hemophilia Foundation. (2015). *Von Willebrand Disease*. Retrieved from https://www.hemophilia.org/Bleeding-Disorders/Types-of-Bleeding-Disorders/Von-Willebrand-Disease

Nikpour, M., Shirvani, M. A., Azadbakht, M., Zanjani, R., & Mousavi, E. (2014). The effect of honey gel on abdominal wound healing in cesarean section: A triple blind randomized clinical trial. *Oman Medical Journal, 29*(4), 255–259.

Pagana, K. D., Pagana, T. J., & Pagana, T. N. (2014). *Mosby's diagnostic and laboratory test reference* (12th ed.). St. Louis, MO: Mosby Elsevier.

Pavord, S., & Maybury, H. (2015). How I treat postpartum hemorrhage. *Blood, 125*(18), 2759–2770.

Pollak, E. S. (2015). von Willebrand disease. *eMedicine*. Retrieved from http://emedicine.medscape.com/article/206996-overview

Pop, V. J., Truijens, S. E., Spek, V., Wijnen, H. A., van Son, M. J., & Bergink, V. (2015). A new concept of maternity blues: Is there a subgroup of women with rapid cycling mood symptoms? *Journal of Affective Disorders, 177*, 74–79.

Quellette, D. R., Harrington, A., & Kamangar, N. (2015). Pulmonary embolism. *eMedicine*. Retrieved from http://emedicine.medscape.com/article/300901-overview

Rong, J., Yuna, G., & Yan, C. (2014). Risk factors associated with emergency peripartum hysterectomy. *Chinese Medical Journal, 127*(5), 900–904.

Salam, R. A., Mansoor, T., Mallick, D., Lassi, Z. S., Das, J. K., & Bhutta, Z. A. (2014). Essential childbirth and postnatal interventions for improved maternal and neonatal health. *Reproductive Health, 11*(Suppl 1), S3-20.

Schiller, C. E., Meltzer-Brody, S., & Rubinow, D. R. (2015). The role of reproductive hormones in postpartum depression. *CNS Spectrums, 20*(1), 48–59.

Shields, L. E., Wiesner, S., Fulton, J., & Pelletreau, B. (2015). Comprehensive maternal hemorrhage protocols reduce the use of blood products and improve patient safety. *American Journal of Obstetrics and Gynecology, 212*(3), 272–280.

Silverman, M. A. (2015). Idiopathic thrombocytopenic purpura. *eMedicine*. Retrieved from http://emedicine.medscape.com/article/779545-overview

Skidmore-Roth, L. (2015). *Mosby's 2015 nursing drug reference* (28th ed.). St. Louis, MO: Mosby Elsevier.

Spiliopoulos, M., & Mastrogiannis, D. (2015). Normal and abnormal puerperium. *eMedicine*. Retrieved from http://emedicine.medscape.com/article/260187-overview#a1

Sucker, C., & Zotz, R. B. (2015). Prophylaxis and treatment of venous thrombosis and pulmonary embolism in pregnancy. *Reviews in Vascular Medicine, 3*(2), 24–30. doi:10.1016/j.rvm.2015.05.003.

Tánczos, K., Németh, M., & Molnár, Z. (2015). What's new in hemorrhagic shock? *Intensive Care Medicine, 41*(4), 712–714.

Tepper, N. K., Boulet, S. L., Whiteman, M. K., Monsour, M., Marchbanks, P. A., Hooper, W. C. et al. (2014). Postpartum venous thromboembolism: Incidence and risk factors. *Obstetrics & Gynecology, 123*(5), 987–996.

Testa, S., Passamonti, S. M., Paoletti, O., Bucciarelli, P., Ronca, E., Riccardi, A. et al. (2015). The "Pregnancy Health-care Program" for the prevention of venous thromboembolism in pregnancy. *Internal and Emergency Medicine, 10*(2), 129–134.

Thombs, B. D., Arthurs, E., Coronado-Montoya, S., Roseman, M., Delisle, V. C., Leavens, A. et al. (2014). Depression screening and patient outcomes in pregnancy or postpartum: A systematic review. *Journal of Psychosomatic Research, 76*(6), 433–446.

U.S. Department of Health and Human Services. (2010). *Healthy people 2020*. Retrieved from http://www.healthypeople.gov/2020/topicsobjectives2020

Van de Velde, M., Diez, C., & Varon, A. J. (2015). Obstetric hemorrhage. *Current Opinion in Anesthesiology, 28*(2), 186–190.

Weissman, M. M. (2014). Treatment of depression: Men and women are different? *American Journal of Psychiatry, 171*(4), 384–387.

Wells, P. S., Forgie, M. A., & Rodger, M. A. (2014). Treatment of venous thromboembolism. *JAMA, 311*(7), 717–728.

Wilcox, L. L., Ramprasad, C., Gutierrez, A., Oden, M., Richards-Kortum, R., & Gandhi, M. (2015). Accuracy in estimation of blood loss using the SAPHE (Signaling a Postpartum Hemorrhage Emergency) Mat [51]. *Obstetrics & Gynecology, 125*, 25S. doi: 10.1097/AOG.0000000000000753.

Wong, A. W., & Rosh, A. J. (2015). Postpartum infections. *eMedicine*. Retrieved from http://emedicine.medscape.com/article/796892-overview

World Health Organization. (2010). *WHO recommendations for the prevention of postpartum hemorrhage*. Retrieved from http://www.who.int/making_pregnancy_safer/publications

World Health Organization [WHO]. (2014). *Postpartum hemorrhage*. Retrieved from http://www.who.int/medicines/areas/priority_medicines/Ch6_16PPH.pdf?ua=1

Yiadom, M. Y., & Carusi, D. (2015). Postpartum hemorrhage in emergency medicine. *eMedicine*. Retrieved from http://emedicine.medscape.com/article/796785-overview

Zhao, Y., Kane, I., Wang, J., Shen, B., Luo, J., & Shi, S. (2015). Combined use of the postpartum depression screening scale (PDSS) and Edinburgh postnatal depression scale (EPDS) to identify antenatal depression among Chinese pregnant women with obstetric complications. *Psychiatry Research, 226*(1), 113–119.

CHAPTER WORKSHEET

MULTIPLE-CHOICE QUESTIONS

1. A postpartum mother appears very pale and states she is bleeding heavily. The nurse should first:
   a. Call the client's health care provider immediately.
   b. Immediately set up an intravenous infusion of magnesium sulfate.
   c. Assess the fundus and ask her about her voiding status.
   d. Reassure the mother that this is a normal finding after childbirth.

2. A postpartum woman reports hearing voices and says, "The voices are telling me to do bad things to my baby." The clinic nurse interprets these findings as suggesting postpartum
   a. psychosis.
   b. anxiety disorder.
   c. depression.
   d. blues.

3. When implementing the plan of care for a multigravida postpartum woman who gave birth just a few hours ago, the nurse vigilantly monitors the client for which complication?
   a. Deep venous thrombosis
   b. Postpartum psychosis
   c. Uterine infection
   d. Postpartum hemorrhage

4. Which of the following would the nurse expect to include in the plan of care for a woman with mastitis who is receiving antibiotic therapy?
   a. Stop breast-feeding and apply lanolin.
   b. Administer analgesics and bind both breasts.
   c. Apply warm or cold compresses and administer analgesics.
   d. Remove the nursing bra and expose the breast to fresh air.

5. While assessing a postpartum multiparous woman, the nurse detects a boggy uterus midline 2 cm above the umbilicus. Which intervention would be the priority?
   a. Assessing vital signs immediately
   b. Measuring her next urinary output
   c. Massaging her fundus
   d. Notifying the woman's obstetrician

6. Methergine has been ordered for a postpartum woman because of excessive bleeding. The nurse should question this order if which of the following is present?
   a. Mild abdominal cramping
   b. Tender inflamed breasts
   c. Pulse rate of 68 beats per minute
   d. Blood pressure of 158/96 mmHg

7. Which of the following findings would lead the nurse to suspect that a woman is developing a postpartum complication?
   a. Moderate lochia rubra for the first 24 hours
   b. Clear lung sounds upon auscultation
   c. Temperature of 100 degrees F
   d. Chest pain experienced when ambulating

8. Which of the following factors in a postpartum woman's history would lead the nurse to monitor the woman closely for an infection?
   a. Hemoglobin of 12 mg/dL
   b. Manually extracted placenta
   c. Labor of 10 hours length
   d. Multiparity of 5 pregnancies

CRITICAL THINKING EXERCISES

1. Mrs. Griffin had a 22-hour labor before a cesarean birth. Her membranes ruptured 20 hours before she came to the hospital. Her fetus showed signs of fetal distress, so internal electronic fetal monitoring was used. Her most recent test results indicate she is anemic.
   a. What postpartum complication is this new mother at highest risk for? Why?
   b. What assessments need to be done to detect this complication?
   c. What nursing measures will the nurse use to prevent this complication?

2. Tammy, a 32-year-old G9P9, had a spontaneous vaginal birth 2 hours ago. Tammy has been having a baby each year for the past 9 years. Her lochia has been heavy, with some clots. She hasn't been up to void since she had epidural anesthesia and has decreased sensation to her legs.
   a. What factors place Tammy at risk for postpartum hemorrhage?
   b. What assessments are needed before planning interventions?
   c. What nursing actions are needed to prevent a postpartum hemorrhage?

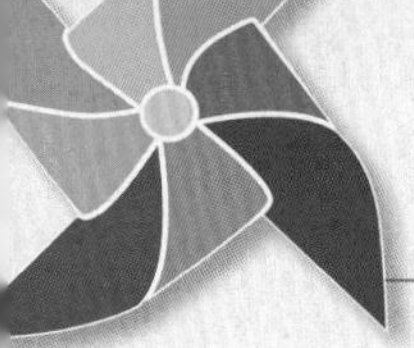

CHAPTER **WORKSHEET**

3. Lucy, a 25-year-old G2P2, gave birth 2 days ago and is expected to be discharged today. She had severe postpartum depression 2 years ago with her first child. Lucy has not been out of bed for the past 24 hours, is not eating, and provides no care for herself or her newborn. Lucy states she already has a boy at home and not having a girl this time is disappointing.
   a. What factors/behaviors place Lucy at risk for an affective disorder?
   b. Which interventions might be appropriate at this time?
   c. What education does the family need prior to discharge?

STUDY ACTIVITIES

1. Compare and contrast postpartum blues, postpartum depression, and postpartum psychosis in terms of their features and medical management.
2. Visit and select a website from the Student Resources for Chapter 22. Critique the website regarding its helpfulness to parents, the correctness of the information, and when it was last updated.
3. Interview a woman who has given birth and ask if she had any complications and what was most helpful to her during the experience.
4. The number one cause of postpartum hemorrhage is ___________________.
5. When giving report to the nurse who will be caring for a woman and her newborn in the postpartum period, what information should the labor nurse convey?

BRINGING IT ALL TOGETHER: A CASE STUDY

Sheila is an 18-year-old G1P1 Hispanic who had her first child two days ago via primary cesarean section. Her pregnancy was uneventful, but she didn't attend prenatal clinic very often. She presented to the hospital in labor at 39 weeks' gestation with ruptured membranes. The client reported that her membranes had been ruptured for a "couple of days," but she wasn't really sure. Upon admission, she was dilated 2 cm/40% effacement. She labored for about 7 hours when the health care provider came in to check her. She was only 5 cm/completely effaced at that time. The health care provider inserted an internal fetal monitor with a scalp electrode and also an intrauterine pressure catheter because she was obese and the nurse was having difficulty in picking up the FHR tracing. She had no progress for the next four hours and the fetus was noted to develop tachycardia with a baseline heart rate of 170 bpm. A primary cesarean section was performed and she was given perioperative antibiotic prophylaxis at the time of surgery. Infant was LGA and Apgar scores were 9/9 at one minute and five minutes, respectively.

Go to thePoint **to find questions to consider about this case.**

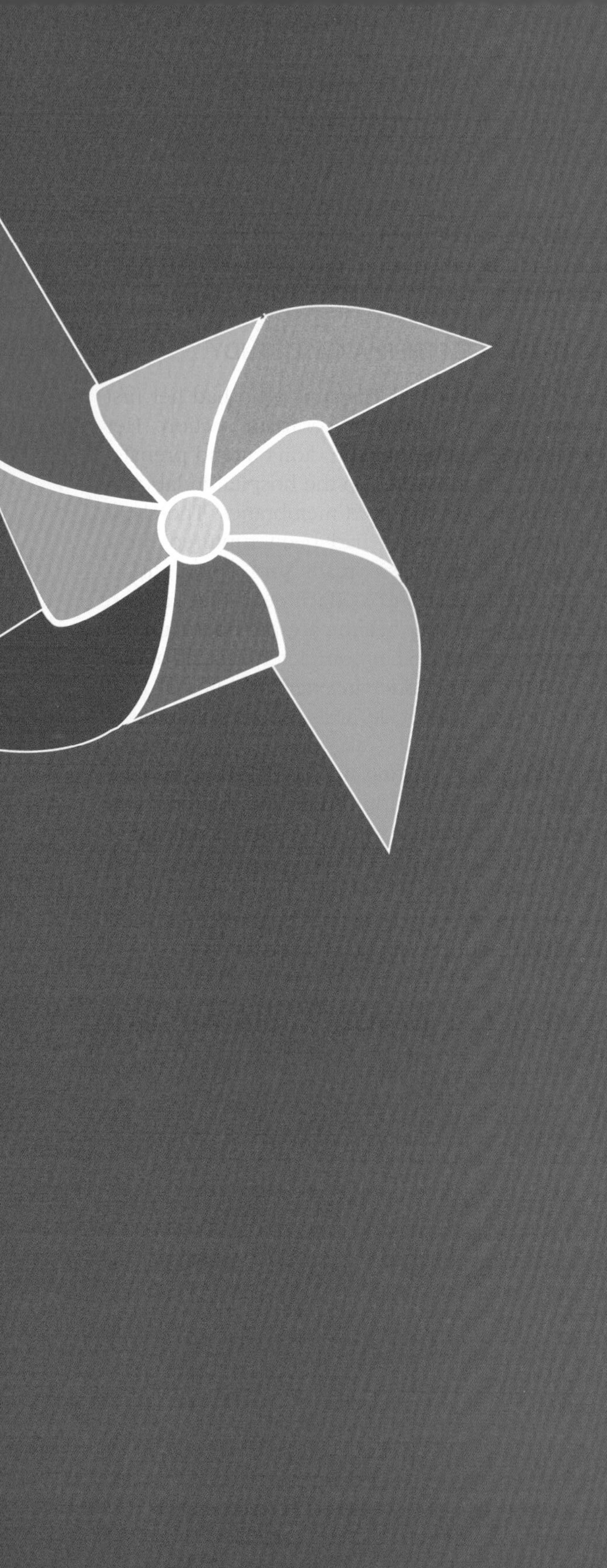

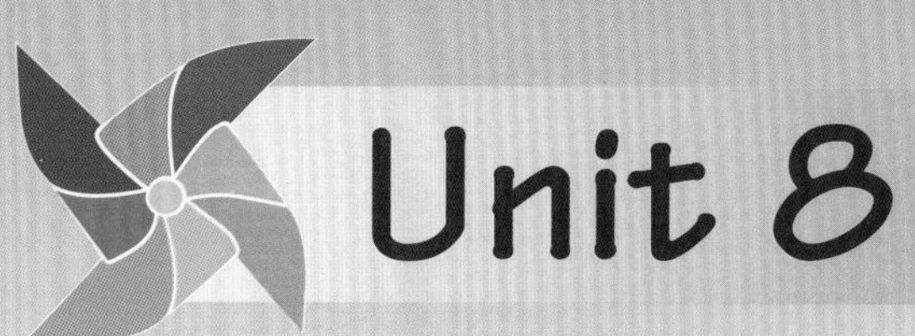

The Newborn at Risk

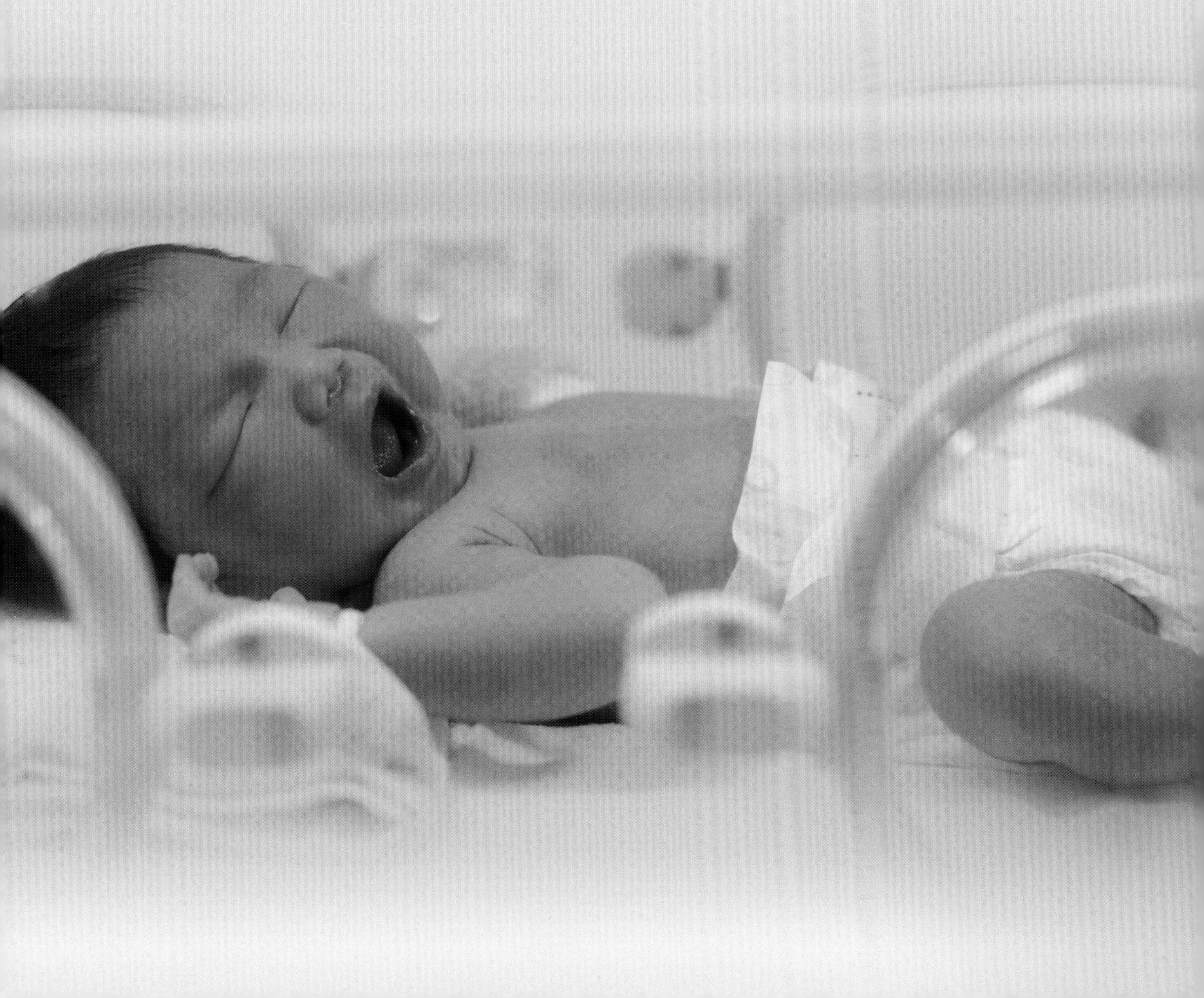

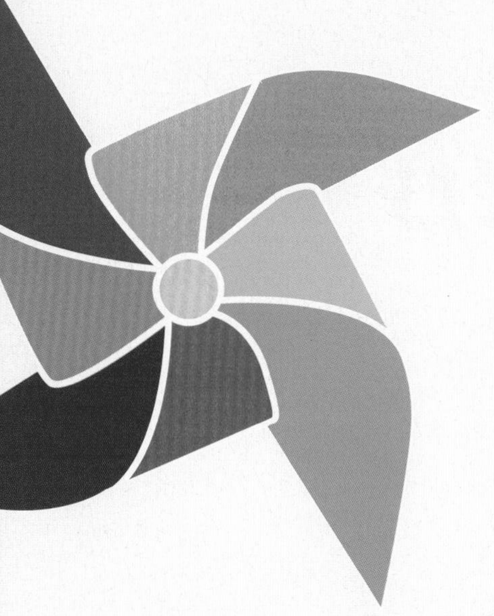

23

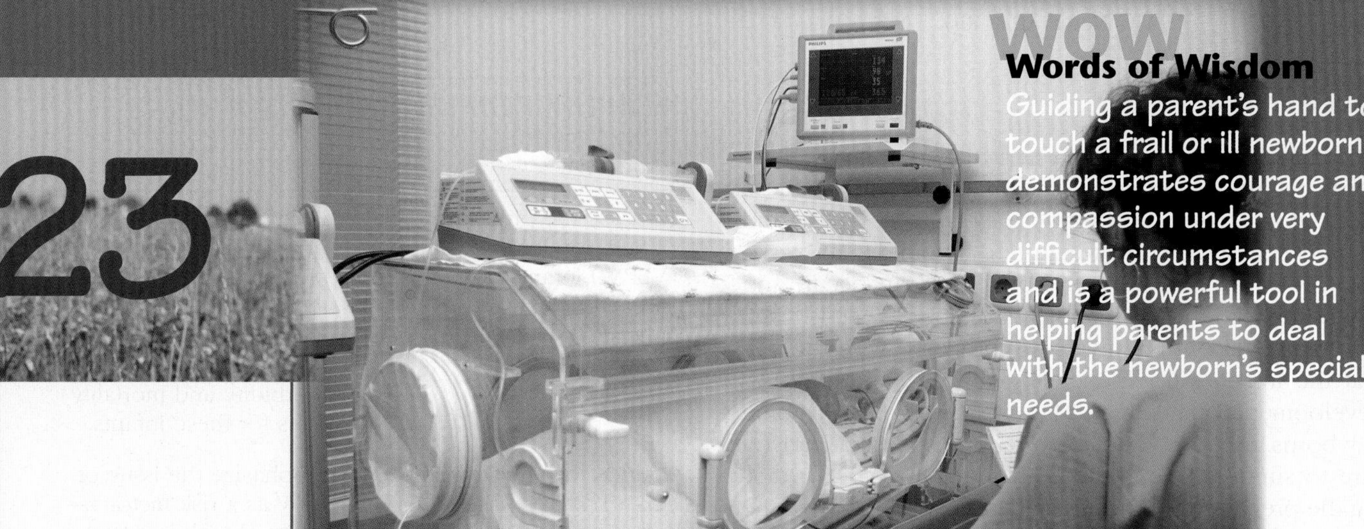

Words of Wisdom

Guiding a parent's hand to touch a frail or ill newborn demonstrates courage and compassion under very difficult circumstances and is a powerful tool in helping parents to deal with the newborn's special needs.

Nursing Care of the Newborn with Special Needs

KEY TERMS

appropriate for gestational age (AGA)
extremely low birthweight
fetal growth restriction (FGR)
large for gestational age (LGA)
late preterm newborn (near term)
low birthweight (LBW)
postterm newborn
preterm newborn
small for gestational age (SGA)
full term newborn
very low birthweight

Learning Objectives

Upon completion of the chapter, you will be able to:

1. Evaluate factors that assist in identifying a newborn at risk due to variations in birth weight and gestational age.
2. Select contributing factors and common complications associated with dysmature infants and their management.
3. Compare and contrast nursing assessment findings and nursing management of a small-for-gestational-age newborn and a large-for-gestational-age newborn; a postterm and a preterm newborn.
4. Analyze nursing assessment and management of newborn conditions associated with variations in birthweight and gestational ages.
5. Outline the nurse's role in helping parents experiencing perinatal grief or loss.
6. Integrate knowledge of the risks associated with late preterm births into nursing interventions, discharge planning, and parent education.

Anna **and her husband were stunned when she went into labor at 7 months' gestation. They couldn't understand what would cause her to give birth early, but it happened. When they approached the NICU, Anna took a deep breath and looked down at her tiny baby with tubes coming from everywhere. What feelings might they be experiencing at this moment?**

INTRODUCTION

All families look forward to the birth of a healthy newborn, but some pregnancy outcomes don't meet these expectations. Most newborns are born between 38 and 42 weeks' gestation and weigh 6 to 8 pounds, but variations in birthweight or gestational age can occur, and newborns with these variations have special needs. Gestational age at birth is inversely correlated with the risk that the infant will experience physical, neurologic, or developmental challenges (March of Dimes, 2013). Some newborns are born very ill and require special advanced care to survive. Unexpected difficulties may occur during the pregnancy or during childbirth which change the whole course of events for the families. *Healthy People 2020* includes the rate of preterm births and infant deaths as leading health indicators (U.S. Department of Health and Human Services [USDHHS], 2016). While reducing preterm births and low birthweight remain important objectives, the fact remains that 9.6% of infants are born prematurely and 8% are of low birthweight (National Center for Health Statistics, 2016).

When a woman gives birth to a newborn with problems involving immaturity or birthweight, especially one who is considered high risk, she may go through a grieving process in which she mourns the loss of the healthy full-term newborn she had expected. Through this process she learns to come to terms with the experience she now faces.

The key to identifying a newborn with special needs related to birthweight or gestational age variation is an awareness of the factors that could place a newborn at risk. These factors are similar to those that would suggest a high-risk pregnancy and include:

- Maternal nutrition (malnutrition or overweight)
- Substandard living conditions or low socioeconomic status
- Maternal age of less than 20 or more than 35 years old
- Substance abuse
- Lack of prenatal care
- Smoking or exposure to passive smoke
- Periodontal disease
- Multiple gestation
- Iron deficiency anemia
- Maternal obesity
- Extreme maternal stress
- Abuse and violence
- History of mental health disorders
- Placental complications (placenta previa or abruptio placentae)
- History of previous preterm birth
- Maternal disease (e.g., hypertension, diabetes, HIV)
- Maternal infection (e.g., urinary tract infection, chorioamnionitis)
- Exposure to occupational hazards, working long hours, or very physical labor (Simpson, 2015).

HEALTHY PEOPLE 2020

Objective	Nursing Significance
Increase the proportion of very low birthweight (VLBW) infants born at level III hospitals or subspecialty perinatal centers.	• Promote the delivery of high-risk infants in settings that have the technological capacity to care for them, ultimately reducing the morbidity and mortality rates for these infants.
Reduce **low birthweight (LBW)** from a baseline of 8.2% to a target of 7.8%; reduce very low birthweight (VLBW) from a baseline of 1.5% to 1.4%	• Emphasize the issue of LBW as a risk factor associated with newborn death. Promote measures to reduce this risk factor and contribute to significant reductions in infant mortality.
Reduce the total number of preterm births from a baseline of 12.7% to 11.4%.	• Emphasize the role of preterm birth as the leading cause of newborn deaths unrelated to birth defects.
Reduce the number of late preterm births or live births at 34 to 36 weeks' gestation from a baseline of 9% to 8.1% Reduce the number of live births at 32 to 33 weeks of gestation from a baseline of 1.6% to 1.4%. Reduce the number of very preterm or live births at less than 32 weeks' gestation from a baseline of 2% to 1.8%.	• Promote an overall reduction in infant illness, disability, and death.

USDHHS (2016).

The development of new technologies and regionalized care centers for the care of newborns with special needs has resulted in significant improvements in neonatal morbidity and mortality. Being able to anticipate the birth of a newborn at risk allows the birth to take place at a health care facility equipped with the resources to meet the mother's and newborn's needs. Nurses need to have a sound knowledge base to identify the newborn with special needs and to provide coordinated care.

This chapter discusses the nursing management of newborns with special needs related to variations in birthweight and gestational age. It also describes selected associated conditions affecting these newborns. Due to the frailty of these newborns, the care of the family experiencing perinatal loss and the role of the nurse in helping the family cope also are addressed.

BIRTHWEIGHT VARIATIONS

Fetal growth is influenced by maternal nutrition, genetics, placental function, environment, and a multitude of other factors. Assigning size to a newborn is a way to measure and monitor the growth and development of the newborn at birth. Newborns can be classified according to their birthweight and weeks of gestation. Knowing the group into which a newborn fits is important.

Appropriate for gestational age (AGA) describes a newborn with a weight that falls within the 10th to 90th percentile for that particular gestational age. This describes approximately 80% of all newborns (Mattson & Smith, 2015). Infants who are AGA have lower morbidity and mortality than other groups.

Small for gestational age (SGA) describes newborns that typically weigh less than 2,500 g (5 lb 8 oz) at term due to less growth than expected in utero. A newborn is also classified as SGA if his or her birthweight is at or below the 10th percentile as correlated with the number of weeks of gestation (Mandy, 2015a).

Large for gestational age (LGA) describes newborns whose birthweight is above the 90th percentile on a growth chart and who weigh more than 4,000 g (8 lb 13 oz) at term due to accelerated overgrowth for length of gestation (Mandy, 2015b).

The following terms describe other newborns with marginal weights at birth and of any gestational age:

- Low birthweight: less than 2,500 g (5.5 lb) (Fig. 23.1)
- **Very low birthweight**: less than 1,500 g (3 lb 5 oz)
- **Extremely low birthweight**: less than 1,000 g (2 lb 3 oz) (Cleary-Goldman & Robinson, 2015).

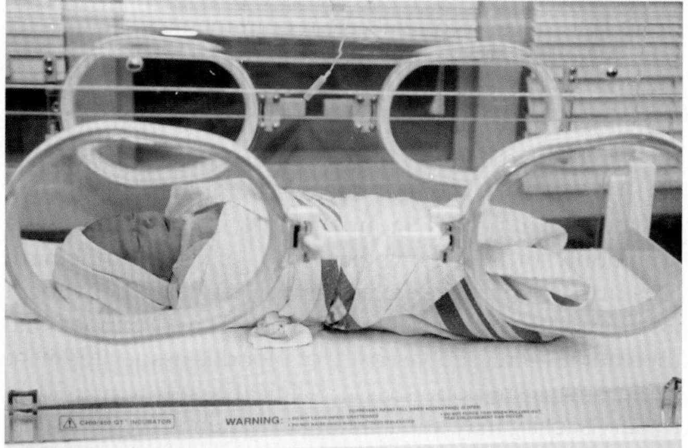

FIGURE 23.1 A low birthweight newborn in an isolette.

Small-for-Gestational-Age Newborns

Newborns are considered SGA when their weight falls below the 10th percentile for length, weight, or head circumference on a growth chart for gestational age. These infants can be preterm, term, or postterm. Some SGA newborns are constitutionally small; they are statistically small but otherwise healthy.

In some SGA newborns, the rate of growth does not meet the expected growth pattern. These infants are considered to have **fetal growth restriction (FGR)**. FGR is the pathologic counterpart of SGA. Newborns with FGR are considered at risk, having increased morbidity and mortality rates as compared to those of AGA newborns. FGR can result from aneuploidy, congenital malformations, infections, or uteroplacental insufficiency (Resnik, 2015). The fetus is thought to have an inherent growth potential that, under normal circumstances, yields a healthy newborn of appropriate size. The maternal–placental–fetal units act in harmony to meet the needs of the fetus during gestation. However, growth potential in the fetus can be limited, and this is analogous to failure to thrive in the infant. The causes of both can be intrinsic or environmental. Factors that can contribute to the birth of an SGA newborn are highlighted in (Box 23.1). FGR is usually categorized as symmetric or asymmetric. Symmetric FGR refers to fetuses with equally poor growth rates of the brain, the abdomen, and the long bones and is thought to result from an early global insult. All parameters of growth are affected. Asymmetric FGR refers to infants whose brain growth is spared compared to their abdomen and internal organs (Cunningham et al., 2014). Fetal growth is dependent on genetic, placental, and maternal factors. Cognitive and motor development during infancy forms the basis for children's subsequent development. Newborns that experience nutritional deficiencies in utero and are born with FGR are at risk for lifelong developmental deficits, and emotional and behavioral disorders (Verklan & Walden, 2015).

Nursing Assessment

Assessment of the SGA infant begins by reviewing the maternal history to identify risk factors such as smoking, drug abuse, alcohol consumption, preeclampsia, anemia, intrauterine viral infection, chronic maternal illness, hypertension, multiple gestation, or genetic disorders. This information allows the nurse to anticipate a possible problem and to be prepared to intervene quickly should one occur. At birth, perform a thorough physical examination, closely observing the newborn for typical characteristics, including:

- Head disproportionately large compared with rest of body (asymmetric)

BOX 23.1

FACTORS CONTRIBUTING TO THE BIRTH OF SGA NEWBORNS

- Maternal causes
  - Chronic hypertension
  - Diabetes mellitus with vascular disease
  - Autoimmune diseases
  - Living at a high altitude (hypoxia)
  - Smoking or exposure to passive smoke
  - Periodontal disease of the mouth
  - Maternal age of 20 or 35 years old
  - Failure to seek any prenatal care
  - Substandard living conditions
  - Low socioeconomic status
  - Abuse and violence
  - Substance abuse (heroin, cocaine, methamphetamines)
  - Hemoglobinopathies (sickle cell anemia)
  - Preeclampsia
  - Exposure to occupational hazards
  - Chronic renal disease
  - Maternal nutrition (malnutrition or obesity)
  - Extreme maternal stress
  - TORCH group infections
- Placental factors
  - Abnormal cord insertion
  - Chronic abruption
  - Decreased surface area, infarction
  - Decreased placental weight
  - Placenta previa
  - Placental insufficiency
- Fetal factors
  - Trisomy 13, 18, and 21
  - Turner's syndrome
  - Chronic fetal infection (cytomegalovirus [CMV], rubella, syphilis, toxoplasmosis)
  - Congenital anomalies (heart, diaphragmatic hernia, tracheoesophageal fistula)
  - Radiation exposure
  - Multiple fetal gestation

Adapted from Cunningham, F. G., Leveno, K. J., Bloom, S. L., Spong, C. Y., Dashe, J. S., Hoffman, B. L., Casey, B. M., & Sheffield, J. S. (2014). *Williams obstetrics* (24th ed.). New York, NY: McGraw-Hill; and Mandy, G. T. (2015a). Small for gestational age infant. *UpToDate.* Retrieved from http://www.uptodate.com/contents/small-for-gestational-age-infant

- Wasted appearance of extremities
- Reduced subcutaneous fat stores
- Jittery secondary to hypoglycemia
- Decreased amount of breast tissue
- Scaphoid abdomen (sunken appearance)
- Temperature instability
- Wide skull sutures secondary to inadequate bone growth
- Poor muscle tone over buttocks and cheeks
- Loose and dry skin that appears oversized
- Thin umbilical cord

Also assess the SGA newborn for any congenital malformations, neurologic insults, or indications of infection. SGA newborns commonly face problems after birth because of the decrease in placental function during gestation. Table 23.1 highlights some of the common problems associated with SGA newborns and others experiencing a variation in birthweight or gestational age. Anticipate the need for and provide resuscitation as indicated by the newborn's condition.

Nursing Management

Interventions for the SGA infant may include obtaining weight, length, and head circumference, comparing them with standards, and documenting the findings on a standardized growth chart. Perform frequent serial blood glucose measurements as ordered and monitor vital signs, being particularly alert for changes in respiratory status that might indicate respiratory distress. Institute measures to maintain a neutral thermal environment to prevent cold stress and acidosis.

Metabolic needs are increased for catch-up growth. Initiate early and frequent oral feedings unless contraindicated. At birth the newborn's glucose level is about 70% of the mother's serum glucose. Neonatal hypoglycemia is a major cause of brain injury since the brain needs glucose continuously as a primary source of energy (Verklan & Walden, 2015). A newborn stressed at birth uses up available glucose stores quickly with resulting hypoglycemia, a plasma glucose concentration at or below 40 mg/dL (Nagtalon-Ramos, 2014). With the loss of the placenta at birth, the newborn now must assume control of glucose homeostasis through intermittent oral feedings. If oral feedings are not accepted, an intravenous infusion with 10% dextrose in water may be needed to maintain the glucose level above 40 mg/dL. Monitor feeding tolerance, sucking, and swallowing ability. Weigh the newborn daily and ensure that he or she has adequate rest periods to decrease metabolic requirements.

Polycythemia is not uncommon and is a potentially serious disorder of newborns. It is defined as a venous hematocrit above 65% and hemoglobin of more than 20 grams. The hematocrit in a newborn peaks between 6 and 12 hours of age and decreases gradually after that. Polycythemia occurs in up to 12% of neonates, very commonly in SGA newborns 6 to 12 hours after birth (Lessaris, 2015). The relationship between hematocrit and viscosity is almost linear until 65% and exponential thereafter. Increased viscosity of blood is associated with symptoms of hypoperfusion. Clinical features related to hyperviscosity may affect all organ systems. Hyperviscosity of blood results in increased resistance to blood flow

(text continues on page 880)

TABLE 23.1 COMMON PROBLEMS ASSOCIATED WITH NEWBORNS EXPERIENCING A VARIATION IN BIRTHWEIGHT OR GESTATIONAL AGE

Problem	Occurrence	Etiology/Pathophysiology	Assessment Findings	Nursing Implications
Perinatal asphyxia	SGA newborns (common)	Poor tolerance to stress of labor, frequently leading to acidosis and hypoxia Living in hypoxic environment prior to birth due to placental insufficiency, leaving little to no oxygen reserves available to withstand stress of labor: – Uterine contractions increase hypoxic stress – Possible depletion of glycogen stores due to chronic hypoxic state, leading to fetal distress – Impaired uteroplacental circulation due to maternal and uterine conditions predisposing to perinatal depression Compromised newborn at birth experiencing difficulty adjusting to extrauterine environment	Fetal distress (bradycardia, decelerations) during labor Low Apgar scores Potential meconium passage into amniotic fluid	Anticipate possible problem; assess for maternal risk factors Initiate resuscitation measures immediately at birth
	Postterm newborns	Placental deprivation or oligohydramnios, leading to cord compression and subsequent reduction in perfusion to fetus		
	Preterm newborns (common)	Surfactant deficiency Unstable chest wall Immaturity of respiratory control centers in the CNS Small respiratory passages, increasing risk for obstruction Inability to clear mucus from airways		
Difficulty with thermoregulation	SGA newborns (common)	Less muscle mass, less brown fat, less heat-preserving subcutaneous fat, and limited ability to control skin capillaries	Temperature <36.4° C; temperature instability; skin cool to touch; cyanosis of hands and feet Bradypnea (<25 bpm) and tachypnea (>60 breaths/min) Tremors, irritability Wheezing, crackles, retractions Restlessness, lethargy Hypotonia Weak or high-pitched cry Seizures Poor feeding Grunting Acidosis	Maintain a neutral thermal environment to promote stabilization of newborn's temperature Assess skin temperature and respiration characteristics Monitor arterial blood gases and blood glucose levels Eliminate sources of heat loss: – Dry newborn thoroughly – Wrap in warmed blanket with stockinette cap on head – Use radiant heat source
	Postterm newborns	Associated with depleted glycogen stores, poor subcutaneous fat stores, and disturbances in CNS thermoregulation due to hypoxia Increased risk for acidosis and hypoglycemia secondary to metabolic stress Loss of subcutaneous fat second to placental insufficiency Use of stored nutrients for nutrition due to lost ability of placenta to nourish fetus Subsequent wasting of subcutaneous fat, muscle, or both		

(continued)

TABLE 23.1 COMMON PROBLEMS ASSOCIATED WITH NEWBORNS EXPERIENCING A VARIATION IN BIRTHWEIGHT OR GESTATIONAL AGE (continued)

Problem	Occurrence	Etiology/Pathophysiology	Assessment Findings	Nursing Implications
		Loss of natural insulation (subcutaneous fat) important in temperature regulation		
	Preterm newborns (common)	Immaturity of CNS (temperature-regulating center) interferes with ability to regulate body temperature Inadequate amounts of subcutaneous fat Lack of muscle tone and flexion to conserve heat		
	Late preterm infant (common)	Inadequate brown fat to generate heat Limited muscle mass activity, reducing ability to produce own heat Inability to shiver to generate heat		
Hypoglycemia	SGA newborns (common)	Increased metabolic rate and lack of adequate glycogen stores to meet newborn's metabolic needs	Often subtle Lethargy, tachycardia Respiratory distress Jitteriness Drowsiness Poor feeding, feeble sucking Hypothermia, temperature instability Diaphoresis Weak cry Seizures Hypotonia Blood glucose levels <40 mg/dL for term newborns, <20 mg/dL for preterm newborns	Monitor blood glucose levels, initially on arrival to nursery and hourly thereafter Maintain fluid and electrolyte balance Watch for subtle changes. Initiate early oral feedings if possible; if not, administer IV infusion with 10% dextrose in water
	LGA newborns (common)	Commonly associated with infants of diabetic mothers Abrupt cessation of high-glucose maternal blood supply with birth and continued insulin production by the newborn Limited ability to release glucagons and catecholamines, which normally stimulate glucagon breakdown and glucose release		
	Postterm newborns	Hypoxia secondary to depleted glycogen reserves Placental insufficiency secondary to placental aging contributing to chronic fetal nutritional deficiency further depleting glycogen stores		
	Preterm newborns	Immature sucking and swallowing leading to insufficient intake Perinatal hypoxia		
	Late preterm infants	Increased energy expenditure Decreased subcutaneous and brown fat with little to no glycogen stores		

Polycythemia	SGA newborns	Chronic mild hypoxia secondary to placental insufficiency Stimulation of erythropoietin release, leading to increased RBC production	Venous hematocrit >65% Plethora (ruddy appearance) Weak sucking reflex Tachypnea Jaundice Lethargy Jitteriness Hypotonia Irritability Feeding difficulties Difficulty in arousing Seizures	Ensure adequate hydration (orally or IV) Monitor hematocrit levels (goal is ~60%) Administer partial exchange transfusion, albumin, or normal saline IV to reduce RBC volume and increase fluid volume (controversial)
	LGA newborns	Secondary to fetal hypoxia, trauma with bleeding, increased erythropoietin production, or delayed cord clamping		
	Postterm newborns	Intrauterine hypoxia triggers increased RBC cell production to compensate for lower oxygen levels.		
Meconium aspiration	SGA newborns	Release of meconium into amniotic fluid prior to birth Inhalation of meconium-containing amniotic fluid by the newborn, leading to aspiration	Green amniotic fluid with rupture of membranes during labor Green staining of the umbilical cord or fingernails Difficulty initiating respirations	Initiate resuscitation measures as necessary Suction airways and support ventilation (see Chapter 24 for more information)
	Postterm newborns	Commonly associated with chronic intrauterine hypoxia Struggling by fetus making respiratory efforts and bearing down with abdominal muscles, leading to expulsion of meconium into amniotic fluid Normal sucking and swallowing by fetus leads to meconium filling airways		
Hyperbilirubinemia	LGA newborns (common)	Associated with polycythemia and RBC breakdown Inability to tolerate feedings in the first few days of life, leading to increased enterohepatic circulation of bilirubin	Elevated serum bilirubin levels Jaundice Tea-colored urine Clay-colored stools	Ensure adequate hydration Institute early feedings if possible Administer phototherapy (see Chapter 24 for more information)
	Preterm newborns	Excessive bruising secondary to birth trauma, leading to higher-than-normal bilirubin levels		
	Late preterm infants	Increased breakdown of RBCs and immature liver function to handle excess load		
Birth trauma	LGA newborns	Large size requiring use of operative birth procedure	Obvious deformities Bruising Edema Asymmetrical movement	Perform complete physical and neurologic assessment of the newborn. Note symmetry of structure and function Assist parents in understanding situation (see Chapter 24 for more information)

Adapted from Fanaroff, A. A., & Fanaroff, J. M. (2014). *Klaus and Fanaroff's care of the high-risk neonate* (6th ed.). Philadelphia, PA: Elsevier Health Sciences; Green, C. J. (2016). *Maternal newborn nursing care plans* (3rd ed.). Burlington, MA: Jones and Bartlett Learning; Lessaris, K. J. (2015). *Polycythemia of the newborn.* Retrieved from http://emedicine.medscape.com/article/976319-overview; and Verklan, M. T., & Walden, M. (2015). *Core curriculum for neonatal intensive care nursing* (5th ed.). St. Louis, MO: Saunders.

and decreased oxygen delivery. In the newborn, hyperviscosity can cause abnormalities of central nervous system function, hypoglycemia, decreased renal function, cardiorespiratory distress, and coagulation disorders. Hyperviscosity has been reported to be associated with long-term motor and cognitive neurodevelopmental disorders (Fanaroff & Fanaroff, 2014). Newborns born SGA, infants of diabetic mothers (IDM), and multiple births are at risk for polycythemia. They should therefore undergo screening at 2, 12, and 24 hours of age (Watchko, 2015).

Observe for clinical signs of polycythemia (respiratory distress, cyanosis, jitteriness, jaundice, ruddy skin color, and lethargy) and monitor blood results. Asymptomatic newborns with a hematocrit between 65% and 70% may simply be supported with fluids, close observation, and a repeat hematocrit level in 12 hours (Mahajan, Une, & Bansal, 2015). If the newborn is symptomatic, a partial exchange transfusion with replacement of removed red blood cell volume with volume expanders may be used, but this treatment is considered controversial and not validated by current evidence-based practice research.

Provide anticipatory guidance to parents about any treatments and procedures that are being done. Emphasize the need for close follow-up and careful monitoring of the infant's growth in length, weight, and head circumference and feeding patterns throughout the first year of life to confirm any "catch-up" growth taking place.

Large-for-Gestational-Age Newborns

A newborn whose weight is above the 90th percentile on growth charts or two standard deviations above the mean weight for gestational age is defined as LGA. LGA is also termed macrosomia. The infant's weight is over 4,000 g (>9 lb). LGA infants may be preterm, term, or postterm. Up to 10% of all infants are designated as LGA at birth. This large size can place both the mother and the newborn at risk for adverse outcomes (Jazayeri, 2015).

Because of the newborn's large size, vaginal birth may be difficult and occasionally results in birth injury. In addition, shoulder dystocia, clavicular fractures, and facial palsies are common. The incidence of cesarean births is very high with LGA newborns to avoid arrested labor and birth trauma.

> **Take Note!**
>
> Maternal diabetes is commonly associated with LGA newborns. However, due to poor placental perfusion, the newborn may experience fetal growth restriction and be SGA (Potter & Kicklighter, 2016).

Nursing Assessment

Assessment of the LGA newborn begins with a review of the maternal history, which can provide clues as to whether the woman has an increased risk of giving birth to a LGA newborn. Maternal factors that increase the chance of bearing an LGA newborn include diabetes mellitus or glucose intolerance, multiparity, prior history of a macrosomic infant, postterm gestation, maternal obesity, paternal height, gestational weight gain, male fetus, and genetics (Jazayeri, 2015).

At birth, assess the newborn for common characteristics. The typical LGA newborn has a large body and appears plump and full-faced. The increase in body size is proportional. However, the head circumference and body length are in the upper limits of intrauterine growth. These newborns have poor motor skills and have difficulty in regulating behavioral states. LGA newborns are more difficult to arouse to a quiet alert state (Mandy, 2015b).

Thoroughly assess the LGA newborn at birth to identify traumatic birth injuries such as fractured clavicles, brachial palsy, facial paralysis, phrenic nerve palsy, skull fractures, or hematomas. Perform a neurologic examination to identify any nerve palsies, looking for abnormalities such as immobility of the upper arm. Observe and document any injuries discovered to allow for early intervention and improved outcomes.

LGA infants are at risk for hypoglycemia related to early depletion of glycogen stores in their liver. Obtain frequent blood glucose levels as ordered to evaluate for hypoglycemia. The clinical signs are often subtle and include lethargy, apathy, drowsiness, irritability, tachypnea, weak cry, temperature instability, jitteriness, seizures, apnea, bradycardia, cyanosis or pallor, feeble suck and poor feeding, hypotonia, and coma. Other disorders, including septicemia, severe respiratory distress, and congenital heart disease, may present with similar findings. In addition, be alert for other common problems, such as polycythemia and hyperbilirubinemia (see Table 23.1).

Nursing Management

Hypoglycemia in a neonate is defined as blood glucose value below 40 mg/dL. It is commonly associated with a variety of neonatal conditions like prematurity, FGR, and maternal diabetes. It may be asymptomatic in some newborns. Essential nursing care activities include early identification of women at risk for diabetes, prevention of hypoglycemia, maintenance of fluid and electrolyte balance, and parental education and support. Screening for hypoglycemia in high-risk LGA infants is essential. Supervised breast-feeding or formula feeding may be initial treatment options in asymptomatic hypoglycemia. However, symptomatic hypoglycemia should always be treated with a continuous infusion of parenteral dextrose. LGA infants needing dextrose infusion rates above 12 mg/kg/min should be investigated for a definite cause of hypoglycemia. Hypoglycemia has been linked to poor neurodevelopmental outcome, and hence aggressive screening and treatment is recommended (Mattson & Smith, 2015).

Assist in stabilizing the LGA newborn. Monitor blood glucose levels within 30 minutes of birth and repeat the screening every hour. Recheck levels before feedings and also immediately in any infant suspected of having or showing clinical signs of hypoglycemia, regardless of age (Green, 2016). To help prevent hypoglycemia, initiate feedings, which can be formula or breast milk, with intravenous glucose supplementation as needed. Monitor and record intake and output and obtain daily weights to aid in evaluating nutritional intake.

Observe for signs of polycythemia and hyperbilirubinemia and report any immediately to the health care provider so that early interventions can be taken to prevent poor long-term neurologic development outcomes. Polycythemia and hyperviscosity are associated with fine and gross motor delays, speech delays, and neurologic sequelae (Mandy, 2015b). Increasing fluid volume aids in decreasing blood viscosity. Partial exchange transfusion with plasma or normal saline may be used to lower hematocrit and decrease blood viscosity, but this treatment remains controversial (Lessaris, 2015). Hydration, early feedings, and phototherapy are used to treat hyperbilirubinemia (see Chapter 24 for more information about hyperbilirubinemia). Provide parental guidance about the treatments and procedures being done and about the need for follow-up care for any abnormalities identified.

GESTATIONAL AGE VARIATIONS

The mean duration of pregnancy, calculated from the first day of the last normal menstrual period, is approximately 280 days, or 40 weeks. Gestational age is typically measured in weeks: a newborn born before completion of 37 weeks is classified as a **preterm newborn** and one born after completion of 42 weeks is classified as a **postterm newborn** (Cunningham et al., 2014). An infant born from the first day of the 38th week through 42 weeks is classified as a term newborn. A recent additional classification is that of the **late preterm newborn (near term)**—one that is born between 34 0/7 and 36 6/7 weeks of gestation. Late preterm births account for 72% of preterm births (Horgan, 2015).

- Preterm infant—born before 37 completed weeks of gestation
- Late preterm infant (near term)—34 0/7 to 36 6/7 weeks
- Full term infant—38 through 41 completed weeks of gestation
- Postterm infant—42 weeks or more

Precise knowledge of a newborn's gestational age is imperative for effective postnatal management. Determination of gestational age by the nurse assists in planning appropriate care for the newborn and provides important information regarding potential problems that need interventions. See Chapter 18 for more information on assessing gestational age.

> ***Take Note!***
>
> Although preterm and postterm newborns may appear to be at opposite ends of the gestational age spectrum and are very different in size and appearance, both are at high risk and need special care.

Postterm Newborn

A pregnancy that extends beyond 42 weeks' gestation (294 days) produces a postterm newborn. Other terms used to describe this late birth is a postmature infant. Postterm newborns may be LGA, SGA, or dysmature (newborn weighs less than established normal parameters for estimated gestational age [fetal growth restricted]), depending on placental function. A postmature infant's appearance typically shows the effects of progressive placental insufficiency.

The reason why some pregnancies last longer than others is not completely understood. What is known is that women who experience one postterm pregnancy are at increased risk in subsequent pregnancies. The incidence of prolonged pregnancy, beyond 42 weeks, is approximately 10% (Green, 2016).

The ability of the placenta to provide adequate oxygen and nutrients to the fetus after 42 weeks' gestation is thought to be compromised, leading to perinatal mortality and morbidity. After 42 weeks, the placenta begins aging. Deposits of fibrin and calcium, along with hemorrhagic infarcts, occur and the placental blood vessels begin to degenerate. All of these changes affect diffusion of oxygen to the fetus. As the placenta loses its ability to nourish the fetus, the fetus uses stored nutrients to stay alive, and wasting occurs. This wasted appearance at birth is secondary to the loss of muscle mass and subcutaneous fat. A recent study found that mortality in post-term infants was strongly related to FGR, not necessarily gestational age (Morken, Klungsoyr, & Skjaerven, 2014).

Nursing Assessment

Important nursing care activities include assessing neonate complications related to placental insufficiency, assessing for birth trauma, maintaining body temperature, and offering emotional support to the mother/partner. A thorough assessment of the postterm newborn upon admission to the nursery provides a baseline from which to identify changes in clinical status. Review the maternal history for any risk factors associated with postterm birth. Also be aware of the common physical characteristics and be able to identify any deviation from the expected. Postterm newborns typically exhibit the following characteristics:

- Dry, cracked, peeling, wrinkled skin
- Vernix caseosa and lanugo are absent.
- Long, thin extremities
- Creases that cover the entire soles of the feet
- Wide-eyed, alert expression
- Abundant hair on scalp
- Thin umbilical cord
- Long fingernails
- Limited vernix and lanugo
- Meconium-stained skin and fingernails (Mattson & Smith, 2015).

Assess the newborn's gestational age and complete a physical examination to identify any abnormalities. Review the medical record to determine the color of the amniotic fluid when membranes ruptured and observe for a meconium-stained umbilical cord and fingernails to assess for possible meconium aspiration. Careful suctioning at the time of birth and afterwards, if the condition dictates it, reduces the incidence of meconium aspiration (Verklan & Walden, 2015). Also be alert for other typical complications associated with a postterm newborn, such as perinatal asphyxia (caused by placental aging or oligohydramnios [decreased amniotic fluid]), hypoglycemia (caused by acute episodes of hypoxia related to cord compression which exhausts carbohydrate reserves), hypothermia (caused by loss of subcutaneous fat), and polycythemia (caused by an increased production of red blood cells to compensate for a reduced oxygen environment), and be prepared to initiate early interventions (see Table 23.1).

Nursing Management

The birth of a postterm newborn may create stress for the mother and her family. In most situations, birth of a newborn requiring special care was not anticipated. Postterm newborns are susceptible to several birth challenges secondary to placental dysfunction that place them at risk for asphyxia, hypoglycemia, and respiratory distress. The nurse must be vigilant for complications when managing these newborns.

The postterm newborn is at high risk for perinatal asphyxia, which is usually attributed to placental deprivation or oligohydramnios that leads to cord compression, thereby reducing perfusion to the fetus. Anticipating the need for newborn resuscitation is a priority. The newborn resuscitation team needs to be available in the birthing suite for immediate backup. The newborn may require transport to the neonatal intensive care unit (NICU) for continuous assessment, monitoring, and treatment, depending on his or her status after resuscitation.

Monitor and maintain the postterm newborn's blood glucose levels once stabilized. Intravenous dextrose 10% and/or early initiation of feedings will help stabilize the blood glucose levels to prevent central nervous system sequelae.

Also monitor the postterm newborn's skin temperature; respiration characteristics; results of blood studies, such as arterial blood gases (ABGs) and serum bilirubin levels; and neurologic status. Institute measures to prevent or reduce the risk of hypothermia by eliminating sources of heat loss: thoroughly dry the newborn at birth, wrap him or her in a warmed blanket, and place a stockinet cap on the newborn's head. Providing environmental warmth via a radiant heat source will help stabilize the newborn's temperature.

Closely assess all postterm newborns for polycythemia which contributes to hyperbilirubinemia due to red blood cell destruction. Providing adequate hydration helps to reduce the viscosity of the newborn's blood to prevent thrombosis. Be alert to the early, often subtle signs to promote early identification and prompt treatment to prevent any neurodevelopmental delays (Green, 2016).

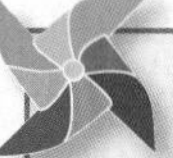

Consider This

I had been waiting for this baby since I can remember and now I was told to wait even longer. I was into my third week past my due date and was just told that if I didn't go into labor on my own, the doctor would induce me on Monday. As I walked out of his office into the hot summer sun, I thought about all the comments that would await me at the office: "You're not still pregnant, are you?" "Weren't you due last month?" "You look as big as a house." "Are you sure you aren't expecting triplets?" I started to get into my car when I felt warm fluid slide down my legs. Although I was embarrassed at my wetness, I was thrilled I wouldn't have to go back to the office and drove myself to the hospital. Within hours my wait was finally over with the birth of my son, a postterm infant with peeling skin and a thick head of hair. He was certainly worth the wait!

Thoughts: Although most due dates are within plus or minus 2 weeks, we can't "go to the bank with it" because so many factors influence the start of labor. This woman was anxious about her overdue status, but nature prevailed. The old adage, "When the fruit is ripe, it will fall," doesn't always bring a good outcome: many women need a little push to bring a healthy newborn forth. What happens when the fetus stays inside the uterus too long? What other features are typical of postterm infants?

Preterm Newborn

A preterm newborn is one who is born before the completion of 37 weeks of gestation. There has been an improved survival rate of preterm infants due to advancing technology and improved evidence-based perinatal care. Although the national birth rate has been declining since the 1990s, the preterm birth rate has been climbing rapidly. Approximately one in nine infants or nearly half a million infants are born before the 37th week of gestation (March of Dimes, 2016). Prematurity is now the leading cause of death worldwide within the first month of life and the second leading cause of all infant deaths.

The etiology of half of all preterm births is unknown (Cunningham et al., 2014). Preterm births take an enormous financial toll, estimated to be in the billions of dollars. They also take an emotional toll on those involved.

Changes in perinatal care practices, including regional care, have reduced newborn mortality rates. Transporting high-risk pregnant women to a tertiary center for birth rather than transferring the neonate after birth is associated with a reduction in neonatal mortality and morbidity (Kaneko et al., 2015). Despite increasing survival rates, preterm infants continue to be at high risk for neurodevelopmental disorders such as cerebral palsy or mental retardation, intraventricular hemorrhage, congenital anomalies, neurosensory impairment, behavioral problems, and chronic lung disease (Back, 2015). Making sure that all pregnant women receive quality prenatal care throughout pregnancy is a major method for preventing preterm births.

Preterm newborns face a myriad of possible complications as a result of their fragile health status or the procedures and treatments used. Some of the more common complications in preterm newborns include respiratory distress syndrome, periventricular-intraventricular hemorrhage, bronchopulmonary dysplasia, retinopathy of prematurity, hyperbilirubinemia, anemia, necrotizing enterocolitis, hypoglycemia, infection or septicemia, delayed growth and development, and mental or motor delays (Green, 2016). Several of these complications are described in Chapter 24.

Effects of Prematurity on Body Systems

Since the preterm newborn did not remain in utero long enough, every body system may be immature, affecting the newborn's transition from intrauterine to extrauterine life and placing him or her at risk for complications. Without full development, organ systems are not capable of functioning at the level needed to maintain extrauterine homeostasis (Carlo, 2015).

Recall Anna, who was described at the beginning of the chapter; she gave birth to a newborn at 7 months' gestation. What problems would you anticipate that her newborn might have?

RESPIRATORY SYSTEM

The respiratory system is one of the last body systems to mature. Therefore, the preterm newborn is at great risk for respiratory complications. A few of the problems that affect the preterm newborn's breathing ability and adjustment to extrauterine life include:

- Surfactant deficiency, leading to the development of respiratory distress syndrome
- Unstable chest wall, leading to atelectasis
- Immature respiratory control centers, leading to apnea
- Smaller respiratory passages, leading to an increased risk for obstruction
- Inability to clear fluid from passages, leading to transient tachypnea (Gardner et al., 2016).

CARDIOVASCULAR SYSTEM

The preterm newborn has great difficulty in making the transition from intrauterine to extrauterine life in terms of changing from a fetal to a newborn circulation pattern. Higher oxygen levels in the circulation once air breathing begins spur this transition. If the oxygen levels remain low secondary to perinatal asphyxia, the fetal pattern of circulation may persist, causing blood flow to bypass the lungs. Another problem affecting the cardiovascular system is the increased incidence of congenital anomalies associated with continued fetal circulation—patent ductus arteriosus and an open foramen ovale. In addition, impaired regulation of blood pressure in preterm newborns may cause fluctuations throughout the circulatory system. One of special note is cerebral blood flow, which may predispose the fragile blood vessels in the brain to rupture, causing intracranial hemorrhage (Fanaroff & Fanaroff, 2014).

GASTROINTESTINAL SYSTEM

Preterm newborns usually lack the neuromuscular coordination required to maintain the suck, swallowing, and breathing regimen necessary for sufficient calorie and fluid intake to support growth. Perinatal hypoxia causes shunting of blood from the gut to more important organs such as the heart and brain. Subsequently, ischemia and damage to the intestinal wall can occur. This combination of shunting, ischemia, damage to the intestinal wall, and poor sucking ability places the preterm infant at risk for malnutrition and weight loss.

In addition, preterm newborns have a small stomach capacity, weak abdominal muscles, compromised metabolic function, limited ability to digest proteins and absorb nutrients, and weak or absent suck and gag reflexes. All of these limitations place the preterm newborn at risk for nutritional deficiency and subsequent growth and development delays.

The preterm infant's ability to coordinate sucking, swallowing, and breathing is challenged. As a result, preterm infants often require enteral or intravenous feeding. Enteral tube feeding will help to conserve energy even in an infant who is able to suck. The exact nutritional needs of preterm infants depend on their gestational age, postnatal age, weight, route of nutritional intake, growth rate, activity, and thermal environment. Preterm infants that are ill or experiencing stressful situations have higher energy requirements. Preterm infants take time to establish enteral intakes, and parenteral nutrition is typically an integral component of care, but safe amounts of macronutrients, and the optimal amino acid and lipid composition remains an uncertainty (Brennan, Murphy, & Kiely, 2015).

Currently, minimal enteral feeding is used to prepare the preterm newborn's gut to overcome the many feeding difficulties associated with gastrointestinal immaturity. It involves the introduction of small amounts, usually 0.5 to 1 mL/kg/h, of enteral feeding to induce surges in gut hormones that enhance maturation of the intestine. This minute amount of breast milk or formula given via gavage (tube) feeding prepares the gut to absorb future introduction of nutrients. It builds mucosal bulk, stimulates development of enzymes, enhances pancreatic function, stimulates maturation of gastrointestinal hormones, reduces gastrointestinal distention and malabsorption, and enhances transition to oral feedings (Gardner et al., 2016).

RENAL SYSTEM

The renal system of the preterm newborn is immature, reducing the baby's ability to concentrate urine and slowing the glomerular filtration rate. As a result, the risk for fluid retention, with subsequent fluid and electrolyte disturbances, increases. In addition, preterm newborns have limited ability to clear drugs from their systems, thereby increasing the risk of drug toxicity. Close monitoring of the preterm newborn's acid–base and electrolyte balance is critical to identify metabolic inconsistencies. Prescribed medications require strict evaluation to prevent overwhelming the preterm baby's immature renal system (Mattson & Smith, 2015).

IMMUNE SYSTEM

The preterm newborn's immune system is very immature, increasing his or her susceptibility to infections. A deficiency of IgG may occur because transplacental transfer does not occur until after 34 weeks' gestation. This protection is lacking if the baby was born before this time. In addition, preterm newborns have an impaired ability to manufacture antibodies to fight infection if they were exposed to pathogens during the birth process. Moreover, the preterm newborn's thin skin and fragile blood vessels provide a limited protective barrier, adding to the increased risk for infection. Thus, anticipating and preventing infections is the goal; preventing infections has a better outcome than treating them (Gardner et al., 2016).

CENTRAL NERVOUS SYSTEM

The preterm newborn is susceptible to injury and insult to the central nervous system (CNS), increasing the potential for long-term disability into adulthood. Like all newborns, preterm newborns have difficulty in temperature regulation and maintaining stability. However, their risk for heat loss is compounded by inadequate amounts of insulating subcutaneous fat; lack of muscle tone and flexion to conserve heat; inadequate brown fat to generate heat; limited muscle mass activity, reducing the possibility of producing their own heat; inability to shiver to generate heat; and an immature temperature-regulating center in the brain (Kenner & Lott, 2014). It is crucial to prevent cold stress, which would increase the newborn's metabolic and oxygen needs. The goal is to create a neutral thermal environment in which oxygen consumption is minimal, but body temperature is maintained (Fanaroff & Fanaroff, 2014).

In addition, the preterm newborn is especially susceptible to hypoglycemia due to immature glucose control mechanisms, decreased glucose stores, and a reduced availability of alternative fuels such as ketone bodies.

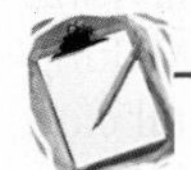

Take Note!

Glucose is needed by the brain and central nervous system to maintain and support numerous body system functions.

Nursing Assessment

Preterm newborns are at high risk for numerous problems and require special care. When preterm labor develops and cannot be stopped by medical interventions, plans are necessary for appropriate management of the mother and the preterm newborn, such as transporting them to a regional center with facilities to care for preterm newborns or notifying the facility's NICU. Depending on the degree of prematurity, the preterm newborn may be kept in the NICU for months.

A thorough assessment of the preterm newborn upon admission to the nursery provides a baseline from which to identify changes in clinical status. Be aware of the common physical characteristics and be able to identify any deviation from the expected (Fig. 23.2). Common physical characteristics of preterm infants may include:

- Birthweight of less than 5.5 lb
- Scrawny appearance
- Head disproportionately larger than chest circumference
- Poor muscle tone and flexion
- Fontanels wide and soft with overriding sutures
- Minimal subcutaneous fat
- Undescended testes in males
- Plentiful lanugo (soft, downy hair), especially over the face and back

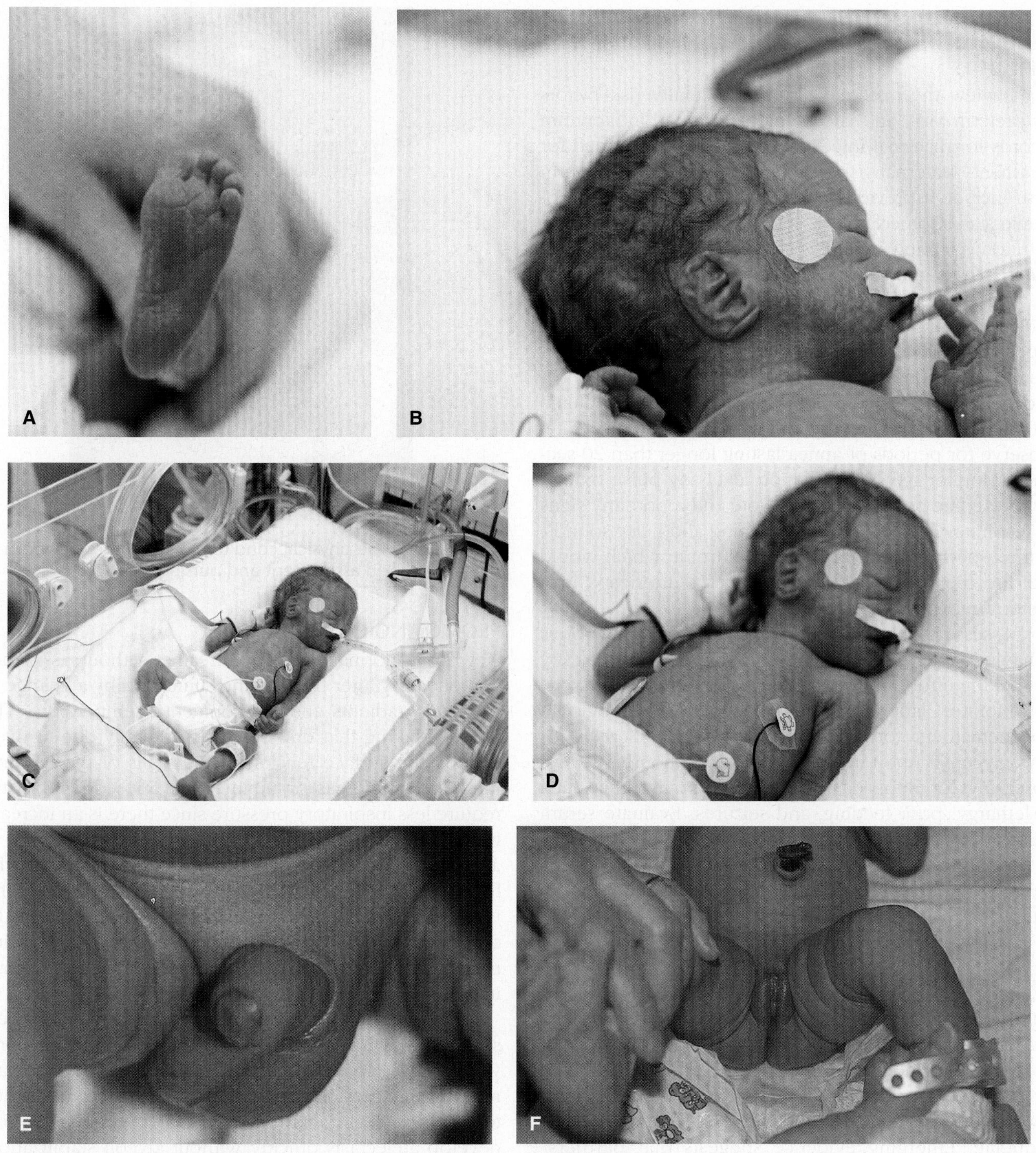

FIGURE 23.2 Characteristics of a preterm newborn. **A.** Few plantar creases. **B.** Soft, pliable ear cartilage, matted hair, and fused eyelids. **C.** Lax posture with poor muscle tone. **D.** Breast and nipple area barely visible. **E.** Male genitalia with minimal rugae on scrotum. **F.** Female genitalia with prominent labia and clitoris.

- Poorly formed ear pinna, with soft, pliable cartilage
- Fused eyelids
- Prominent clitoris and labia minora in females
- Soft and spongy skull bones, especially along suture lines
- Matted scalp hair, woolly in appearance
- Absent to a few creases in the soles and palms
- Minimal scrotal rugae in male infants
- Thin, transparent skin with visible veins
- Breast and nipples not clearly delineated
- Abundant vernix caseosa (Mattson & Smith, 2015).

Be alert for evidence that might suggest that the pre-term newborn is developing a complication (see Table 23.1).

Review the maternal history to identify risk factors for preterm birth and check antepartum and intrapartum records for maternal infections to anticipate the need for treatment. Maternal risk factors associated with preterm birth include a previous preterm delivery, low socioeconomic status, preeclampsia, hypertension, poor maternal nutrition, smoking, multiple gestation, infection, advanced maternal age, and substance abuse.

Assess the newborn's gestational age and assess for FGR if appropriate. Inspect the newborn's skin closely, especially skin color. Assess vital signs, including temperature via skin probe to identify hypothermia or fever, and heart rate for tachycardia or bradycardia. Evaluate the newborn's respiratory effort and respiratory rate. Observe for periods of apnea lasting longer than 20 seconds. Monitor oxygen saturation levels by pulse oximetry to validate perfusion status. Note and report any signs of respiratory distress. Auscultate lung and heart sounds, being especially alert for possible murmur, which would indicate the presence of patent ductus arteriosus in a preterm newborn.

Assess neurologic status by observing the newborn's behavior. Note any restlessness, hypotonia, or weak cry or sucking effort and report unusual findings.

Monitor laboratory studies such as hemoglobin and hematocrit for signs of polycythemia. Screen for hypoglycemia upon admission and then hourly, always observing for nonspecific signs of hypoglycemia such as lethargy, poor feeding, and seizures. Evaluate serum bilirubin concentrations.

Finally, assess the mother and family members. Identify family strengths and coping mechanisms to establish a basis for intervention.

Nursing Management

The birth of a preterm newborn creates a crisis for the mother and family. Multiple studies have found that hospitalization for preterm newborns is often followed by negative mental health/behavioral outcomes, anxiety and depressive disorders, and long-term neurologic sequelae. Emerging evidence suggests that partners/significant others experience high rates of psychological stress in the first few months after a preterm birth (Feinberg et al., 2015). Premature labor and birth are accompanied by feelings of helplessness, isolation, and loss of control (Gardner et al., 2016). Preterm newborns present with immaturity of all organ systems, abundant physiologic challenges, and significant morbidity and mortality globally (Verklan & Walden, 2015). The nurse must be vigilant for complications when managing preterm newborns (Fig. 23.3) (Nursing Care Plan 23.1, at the end of the chapter).

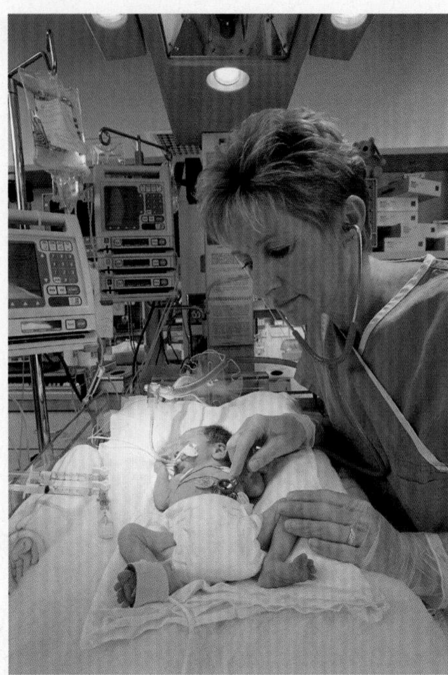

FIGURE 23.3 **The physical condition of a preterm newborn demands skilled assessment and nursing care.**

PROMOTING OXYGENATION

Newborns normally start to breathe without assistance and often cry after birth, being stimulated by a change in pressure gradients and environmental temperature. The work of taking that first breath is primarily due to overcoming the surface tension of the walls of the terminal lung units at the gas–tissue interface. Subsequent breaths require less inspiratory pressure since there is an increase in functional capacity and air retained. By 1 minute of age, most newborns are breathing well. A newborn who fails to establish adequate, sustained respiration after birth is said to have **asphyxia** (perinatal acidosis), which is the deprivation of oxygen during the birth process, resulting in fetal hypoxia that can lead to organ damage and brain injury (Herrera-Marschitz et al., 2015).

The preterm infant lacks surfactant, which lowers surface tension in the alveoli and stabilizes them to prevent their collapse. Even if preterm newborns can initiate respirations, they have a limited ability to retain air due to insufficient surfactant. Therefore, preterm newborns develop atelectasis quickly without alveoli stabilization. The inability to initiate and establish respirations leads to hypoxemia and ultimately hypoxia (decreased oxygen), acidosis (decreased pH), and hypercarbia (increased carbon dioxide). This change in the newborn's biochemical environment may inhibit the transition to extrauterine circulation, thus allowing fetal circulation patterns to persist (Boxwell, 2010).

Failure to initiate extrauterine breathing or failure to breathe well after birth leads to hypoxia (too little oxygen in the cells of the body). As a result, the heart rate falls, cyanosis develops, temperature decreases, blood pressure decreases, and respirations are altered (apnea, tachypnea, retractions, grunting, and nasal flaring) and the newborn becomes hypotonic and unresponsive. Although this can happen with any newborn, the risk is higher in preterm newborns.

Resuscitating the Newborn. Approximately 10% of newborns require some assistance to begin breathing at birth. The aim of neonatal resuscitation is to prevent neonatal death and adverse long-term neurodevelopmental sequelae associated with perinatal asphyxia (Yousaf, Hayat, & Afzal, 2015). Anticipation, adequate preparation, accurate evaluation, and prompt initiation of support are critical for successful newborn resuscitation. Have all basic equipment immediately available and in working order. Ensure that the equipment is evaluated daily, and document its condition and any needed repairs. Box 23.2 lists the equipment needed for basic newborn resuscitation.

Determine the need for resuscitation by performing a rapid assessment using the following questions:

- What is the newborn's heart rate?
- What is the gestational age of this newborn? Was the amniotic fluid clear of meconium?
- Is the newborn breathing or crying now?
- Does the newborn have good muscle tone?

If the answers are "yes" to all questions, then routine care is initiated: provide warmth, clear the airway, dry the newborn, and assess color. If the answer to any of these questions is "no," the newborn should receive one or more of the following actions, according to this sequence:

1. Stabilization—Dry the newborn thoroughly with a warm towel; provide warmth by placing him or her under a radiant heater to prevent rapid heat loss through evaporation; position the head in a neutral position to open the airway; clear the airway with a bulb syringe or suction catheter; stimulate breathing. At times, handling and rubbing the newborn with a dry towel may be all that is needed to stimulate respirations.
2. Assess for breathing—bag the newborn if not breathing.
3. Place pulse oximeter on the newborn's right hand to determine oxygen saturation.
4. Ventilation if needed
5. Assess heart rate.
6. Chest compressions if needed
7. Administration of epinephrine and/or volume expansion (Vali, Matthew, & Lakshminrusimha, 2015).

BOX 23.2

BASIC EQUIPMENT FOR NEWBORN RESUSCITATION

- A wall vacuum suction apparatus
- Infant-size stethoscopes
- Pulse oximeter
- Epinephrine
- Volume expander
- Intravenous fluids
- A wall source or tank source of 100% oxygen with a flow meter
- A neonatal self-inflating ventilation bag with correct-sized face masks
- A selection of endotracheal tubes (2.5, 3.0, or 3.5 mm) with introducers
- A laryngoscope with a small, straight blade and spare batteries and bulbs
- Ampules of naloxone (Narcan) with syringes and needles
- A wall clock to document timing of activities and events
- A supply of disposable gloves in a variety of sizes for staff to use

The decision to progress from one set of actions to the next and the need for further resuscitative efforts is determined by the assessment of respirations, heart rate, and color (American Academy of Pediatrics [AAP] & American Heart Association [AHA], 2014). Nurses need to remember that preterm infants have immature lungs that may be more difficult to ventilate and are also more vulnerable to injury by positive-pressure ventilation. They also have immature blood vessels in the brain that are prone to hemorrhage; thin skin and a large surface area, which contribute to rapid heat loss; increased susceptibility to infection; and increased risk of hypovolemic shock related to small blood volume. Anticipation, adequate preparation, accurate evaluation, and prompt initiation of support are critical for successful neonatal resuscitation.

When performing newborn resuscitation, use the mnemonic "ABCDs" (airway, breathing, circulation, and drugs) to remember the sequence of steps (Box 23.3).

Resuscitation measures are continued until the newborn has a pulse above 100 bpm, a good healthy cry or good breathing efforts, and a pink tongue. This last sign indicates a good oxygen supply to the brain. Effective ventilation is the key to successful resuscitation (Jaques & Kennea, 2015). Throughout the resuscitation period, keep the parents informed of what is happening to their newborn and what is being done and why. Provide support through this initial crisis. Once the newborn is stabilized, encourage bonding by having them stroke, touch, and when appropriate hold the newborn.

Administering Oxygen. Oxygen administration is a common therapy in the neonatal intensive care unit, though the normal oxygen concentration for a preterm infant remains unknown. Use of large concentrations of oxygen and sustained oxygen saturations higher than 95% while on supplemental oxygen have been associated with the development of retinopathy of prematurity (ROP) and further respiratory complications in the preterm newborn (Paul, 2015). For these reasons, oxygen

BOX 23.3

ABCDS OF NEWBORN RESUSCITATION

- **A**irway
  - Place infant's head in "sniffing" position.
  - Suction mouth, then nose.
  - Suction trachea if meconium-stained and newborn is NOT vigorous (strong respiratory effort, good muscle tone, and heart rate >100 bpm).
- **B**reathing
  - Use positive-pressure ventilation (PPV) for apnea, grasping, or pulse <100 bpm.
  - Ventilate at rate of 40 to 60 breaths/minute.
  - Listen for raising heart rate, audible breath sounds.
  - Look for slight chest movement with each breath.
  - Use carbon dioxide detector after intubation.
- **C**irculation
  - Start compressions if heart rate is <60 after 30 seconds of effective PPV.
  - Give 3 compressions: 1 breath every 2 seconds.
  - Compress one third of the anterior-posterior diameter of the chest.
- **D**rugs
  - Give epinephrine if heart rate is <60 after 30 seconds of compressions and ventilation.
  - *Caution:* Epinephrine dosage is different for endotracheal and IV routes!
- **E**pinephrine: 1:10,000 concentration
  - 0.1 to 0.3 mL/kg IV
  - 0.3 to 1 ml/kg via endotracheal tube

Adapted from AAP & AHA, 2014.

should be used judiciously to prevent the development of further complications. A guiding principle for oxygen therapy is it should be targeted to levels appropriate to the condition, gestational age, and postnatal age of the newborn. Current common practice is to maintain oxygen saturation levels in the high 80s to mid-90s, though a wide variation in practice may still occur. Room air is an emerging standard of care when initiating positive pressure ventilation during resuscitation (Ramji, Saugstad, & Jain, 2015). Refer to Chapter 39 for a more in-depth discussion of ROP.

Respiratory distress in preterm infants is commonly caused by a deficiency of surfactant, retained fluid in the lungs (wet lung syndrome), meconium aspiration, pneumonia, hypothermia, or anemia. The principles of care are the same regardless of the cause of respiratory distress.

- First, keep the newborn warm, preferably in a warmed isolette or with an overhead radiant warmer, to conserve the baby's energy and prevent cold stress.
- Handle the newborn as little as possible, because stimulation often increases the oxygen requirement.
- Provide energy through calories via intravenous dextrose or gavage or continuous tube feedings to prevent hypoglycemia.
- Treat cyanosis with an oxygen hood or blow-by oxygen placed near the newborn's face if respiratory distress is mild and short-term therapy is needed.
- Record the following important observations every hour or more frequently if indicated and document any deterioration in respiratory status:
  - Respiratory rate, quality of respirations, and respiratory effort
  - Airway patency, including removal of secretions per facility policy
  - Skin color, including any changes to duskiness, blueness, or pallor
  - Lung sounds on auscultation to differentiate breath sounds in upper and lower fields
  - Equipment required for oxygen delivery, such as:
    - Blow-by oxygen delivered via mask or tube for short-term therapy
    - Oxygen hood (oxygen is delivered via a plastic hood placed over the newborn's head)
    - Nasal cannula (oxygen is delivered directly through the nares) (Fig. 23.4A)
    - Continuous positive airway pressure (CPAP), which prevents collapse of unstable alveoli and delivers high levels of inspired oxygen into the lungs
    - Mechanical ventilation, which delivers consistent assisted ventilation and oxygen therapy, reducing the work of breathing for the fatigued infant (Fig. 23.4B)
- Correct placement of endotracheal tube (if present)
- Oxygen saturation levels via pulse oximetry
- Heart rate, including any changes
- Monitor the infant's respiratory status, clinically as well as by oxygen saturation, arterial blood gases, and chest x-ray.
- Oxygen saturation levels via pulse oximetry to evaluate need for therapy modifications based on hemoglobin
- Suction as needed to remove secretions to maintain a patent airway and enhance oxygenation
- Decrease stimulation; cluster all care to allow for rest.
- Maintain a neutral thermal environment.
- Administration of medication, such as exogenous surfactant
- Offer emotional support and progress reports on infant's condition to family.

If the newborn shows worsening cyanosis or if oxygen saturation levels fall below 87%, prepare to give additional oxygen as ordered. Evaluate arterial blood gas results periodically as ordered. Document any deterioration or changes in respiratory status. Administer exogenous surfactant as ordered. Throughout care, maintain strict asepsis and meticulous hand hygiene in order to reduce the risk of infection (Verklan & Walden, 2015).

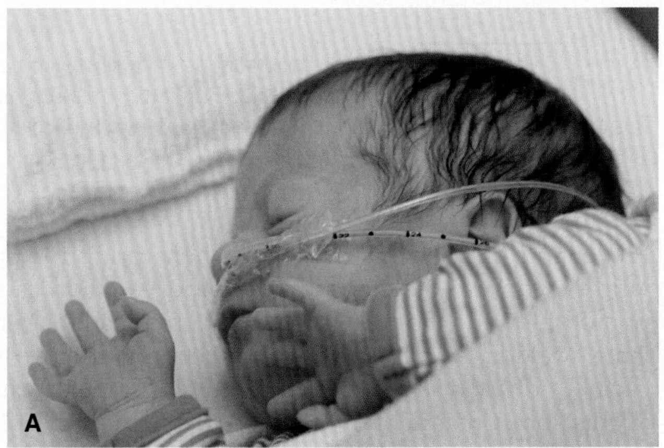

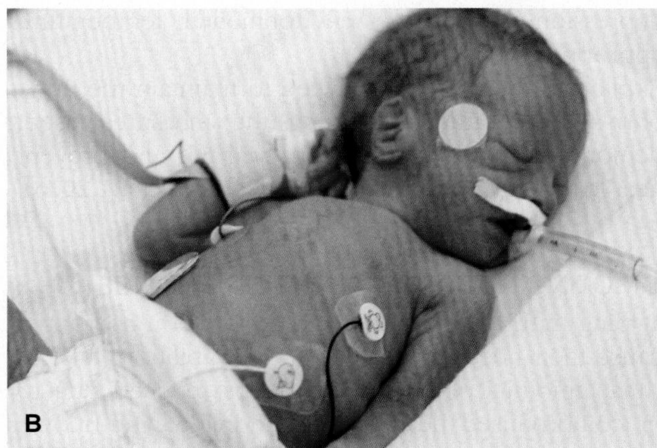

FIGURE 23.4 **A.** A preterm newborn receiving oxygen therapy via a nasal cannula. The newborn also has an enteral feeding tube inserted for nutrition. **B.** A preterm newborn receiving mechanical ventilation.

MAINTAINING THERMAL REGULATION

Providing an optimal thermal environment is important. When a newborn becomes chilled, it attempts to conserve body heat by vasoconstriction and thermogenesis by metabolizing brown adipose tissue and increasing oxygen consumption. This increase in energy expenditure reduces the neonate's ability to gain weight. Immediately after birth, dry the newborn with a warmed towel and then place him or her in a second warm, dry towel before performing the assessment. This drying prevents rapid heat loss secondary to evaporation. Newborns that are active, breathing well, and crying are stable and can be placed on their mother's chest ("kangaroo care") to promote warmth and prevent hypothermia. Preterm newborns that are not considered stable may be placed under a radiant warmer or in a warmed isolette after they are dried with a warmed towel.

Typically newborns use nonshivering thermogenesis for heat production by metabolizing their own brown adipose tissue. However, the preterm newborn has an inadequate supply of brown fat because he or she left the uterus early before the supply was adequate. The preterm newborn also has decreased muscle tone and thus cannot assume the flexed fetal position, which reduces the amount of skin exposed to a cooler environment. In addition, preterm newborns have large body surface areas compared to their weight. This allows an increased transfer of heat from their bodies to the environment.

Typically, a preterm newborn that is having problems with thermal regulation is cool to cold to the touch. The hands, feet, and tongue may appear cyanotic. Respirations are shallow or slow, or signs of respiratory distress are present. The newborn is lethargic and hypotonic, feeds poorly, and has a feeble cry. Blood glucose levels are probably low, leading to hypoglycemia, due to the energy expended to keep warm.

When promoting thermal regulation for the preterm newborn:

- Remember the four mechanisms for heat transfer and ways to prevent loss:
  - Convection: heat loss through air currents (avoid drafts near the newborn)
  - Conduction: heat loss through direct contact (warm everything the newborn comes in contact with, such as blankets, mattress, stethoscope)
  - Radiation: heat loss without direct contact (keep isolettes away from cold sources and provide insulation to prevent heat transfer)
  - Evaporation: heat loss by conversion of liquid into vapor (keep the newborn dry and delay the first bath until the baby's temperature is stable)
- Frequently assess the temperature of the isolette or radiant warmer, adjusting the temperature as necessary to prevent hypo- or hyperthermia.
- Utilize plastic wraps and bags, skin-to-skin contact, or transwarmer mattresses if available to keep infants warmer and decrease the incidence of hypothermia.
- Assess the newborn's temperature every hour until stable.
- Observe for clinical signs of cold stress, such as respiratory distress, central cyanosis, hypoglycemia, lethargy, weak cry, abdominal distention, apnea, bradycardia, and acidosis.
- Remember the complications of hypothermia and frequently assess the newborn for signs:
  - Metabolic acidosis secondary to anaerobic metabolism used for heat production, which results in the production of lactic acid
  - Hypoglycemia due to depleted glycogen stores
  - Pulmonary hypertension secondary to pulmonary vasoconstriction
- Monitor the newborn for signs of hyperthermia such as tachycardia, tachypnea, apnea, warm to touch, flushed skin, lethargy, weak or absent cry, and CNS

depression; adjust the environmental temperature appropriately.
- Explain to the parents the need to maintain the newborn's temperature, including the measures used; demonstrate ways to safeguard warmth and prevent heat loss (Mattson & Smith, 2015; Gardner et al., 2016).

PROMOTING NUTRITION AND FLUID BALANCE

Providing nutrition is challenging for preterm newborns because their needs are great but their ability to take in optimal amounts of energy/calories is reduced due to their compromised health status. Individual nutritional needs are highly variable.

Depending on their gestational age, preterm newborns receive nutrition orally, enterally, or parenterally via infusion. Several different methods can be used to provide nutrition: parenteral feedings administered through a percutaneous central venous catheter for long-term venous access with delivery of total parenteral nutrition (TPN); or enteral feedings, which can include oral feedings (formula or breast milk), continuous nasogastric tube feedings, or intermittent gavage tube feedings. Gavage feedings are commonly used for compromised newborns to allow them to rest during the feeding process. Many have a weak suck and become fatigued and thus cannot consume enough calories to meet their needs.

Most newborns born after 34 weeks' gestation without significant complications can feed orally. Those born before 34 weeks' gestation typically start with parenteral nutrition within the first 24 hours of life. Then enteral nutrition is introduced and advanced based on the degree of maturity and clinical condition. Ultimately, enteral nutrition methods replace parenteral nutrition.

To promote nutrition and fluid balance in the preterm newborn:

- Measure daily weight and plot it on a growth curve.
- Monitor intake; calculate fluid and caloric intake daily.
- Assess fluid status by monitoring weight; urinary output; urine specific gravity; laboratory test results such as serum electrolyte levels, blood urea nitrogen, creatinine, and hematocrit; skin turgor; and fontanels (Gardner et al., 2016). Be alert for signs of dehydration, such as a decrease in urinary output, sunken fontanels, temperature elevation, lethargy, and tachypnea.
- Continually assess for enteral feeding intolerance; measure abdominal girth, auscultate bowel sounds, and measure gastric residuals before the next tube feeding.
- Encourage and support breast-feeding by facilitating maternal breast pumping.
- Encourage nuzzling at the breast in conjunction with kangaroo care if the newborn is stable.

> *Take Note!*
>
> When assessing the fluid status of a preterm newborn, palpate the fontanels. Sunken fontanels suggest dehydration; bulging fontanels suggest overhydration.

PREVENTING INFECTION

Prevention of infection is critical when caring for preterm newborns. Infections are the most common cause of morbidity and mortality in the NICU population (Verklan & Walden, 2015). Sources of infection in a newborn can be divided into three categories: transplacental acquisition (intrauterine infection); perinatal acquisition during childbirth (intrapartum infection); and hospital acquisition in neonatal period (postnatal infection) from the mother, hospital environment, or staff (Gardner et al., 2016). Nursing assessment and early identification of infectious problems are imperative to improve outcomes.

Preterm newborns are at risk for infection because their early birth deprived them of maternal antibodies needed for passive protection. They are also susceptible to infection because of their limited ability to produce their own antibodies, asphyxia at birth, and thin, friable skin that is easily traumatized, providing an entry portal for microorganisms.

Early detection is crucial. The clinical manifestations can be nonspecific and subtle: apnea, diminished activity, poor feeding, temperature instability, respiratory distress, seizures, tachycardia, hypotonia, irritability, pallor, jaundice, and hypoglycemia. Report any of these to the primary care provider immediately so that treatment can be instituted.

Include the following interventions when caring for a preterm or postterm newborn to prevent infection:

- Assess for risk factors in maternal history that place the newborn at increased risk.
- Monitor for changes in vital signs such as temperature instability, tachycardia, or tachypnea.
- Assess oxygen saturation levels and initiate oxygen therapy as ordered if oxygen saturation levels fall below acceptable parameters.
- Assess feeding tolerance, typically an early sign of infection.
- Monitor laboratory test results for changes.
- Avoid using tape on the newborn's skin to prevent tearing.
- Use equipment that can be thrown away after use.
- Adhere to standard precautions; use clean gloves to handle dirty diapers and dispose of them properly.
- Use sterile gloves when assisting with any invasive procedure; attempt to minimize the use of invasive procedures.
- Remove all jewelry on your hands prior to washing hands; wash hands upon entering the nursery and in between caring for newborns.

- Administer antibiotics as ordered and monitor for therapeutic and adverse effects.
- Avoid coming to work when ill, and screen all visitors for contagious infections.

Remember Anna, who was in a state of shock when she entered the NICU to see her preterm baby for the first time? How could the nurse have prepared her for this event? What information needs to be given at the isolette to reduce her anxiety and fear now?

PROVIDING APPROPRIATE STIMULATION

Newborn stimulation involves a series of activities to encourage normal development. Research on developmental interventions shows that when preterm newborns, in particular, receive sensorimotor interventions such as rocking, nonnutritive sucking with a pacifier, skin-to-skin contact with parents, containment (swaddling and surrounded by blanket rolls), music, nonnutritive sucking, breast-feeding, massage, holding, or sleeping on waterbeds, they gain weight faster, progress in feeding abilities more quickly, and show improved interactive behavior compared to preterm newborns who were not stimulated (Verklan & Walden, 2015). Conversely, overstimulation may have negative effects by reducing oxygenation and causing stress. The NICU environment lends itself to persistent and unpredictable sounds that are in stark contrast to the protective sounds inside the mother. A newborn reacts to stress by flaying the hands or bringing an arm up to cover the face. When overstimulated, such as by noise, lights, excessive handling, alarms, and procedures, and stressed, heart and respiratory rates decrease and periods of apnea or bradycardia may follow (Gardner et al., 2016).

Appropriate developmental stimulation that would not overtax the compromised newborn might include kangaroo (skin-to-skin) holding, rocking, soft singing or music, cuddling, gentle stroking of the infant's skin, colorful mobiles, gentle massage, waterbed mattresses, and nonnutritive sucking opportunities (Fig. 23.5) or providing sucrose if tolerated.

The NICU environment can be altered to provide periods of calm and rest for the newborn by dimming the lights, lowering the volume and tone of conversations, closing doors gently, setting the telephone ringer to the lowest volume possible, clustering nursing activities, and covering the isolette with a blanket to act as a light shield to promote rest at night (Verklan & Walden, 2015).

Encourage parents to hold and interact with their newborn. Doing so helps to acquaint the parents with their newborn, promotes self-confidence, and fosters parent–newborn attachment (Fig. 23.6).

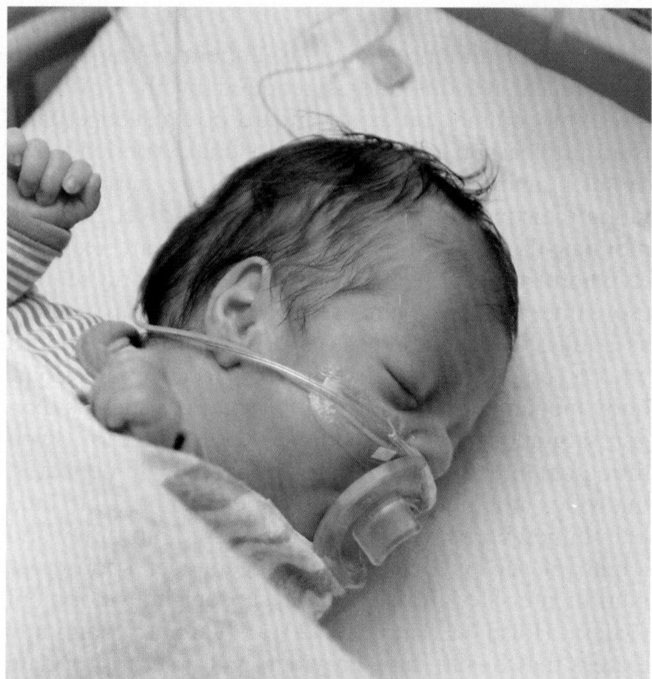

FIGURE 23.5 A preterm newborn receiving nonnutritive sucking.

Think back to Anna, the woman who gave birth to a preterm newborn at 7 months' gestation. Anna will be discharged but her newborn will be staying in the NICU for a while. What interventions would be appropriate to facilitate bonding despite their separation? What support can be provided specifically to her family?

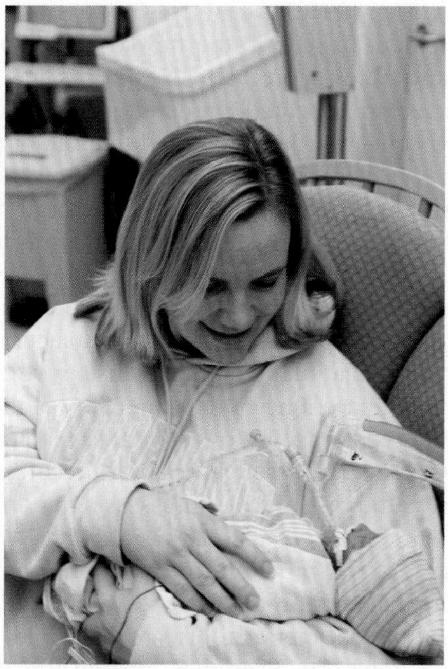

FIGURE 23.6 A mother bonding with her preterm newborn.

MANAGING PAIN

Pain control and prevention is imperative for ethical and clinical reasons and is required by the AAP and the Joint Commission as a standard of excellence. Pain is an unpleasant sensory and emotional experience felt by all humans. Unlike adults, infants are incapable of rating their pain on a scale of 0 to 10, and yet from the moment they take their first breath, they are exposed to painful procedures. Newborns feel pain and require the same level of pain assessment and management as adults. Common indicators of pain in the newborn who is unable to vocalize include facial expressions, body movements, and physiologic changes such as oxygen saturation (Harrison, Bueno, & Reszel, 2015). Even though pain may not be expressed verbally in neonates, this does not negate their experiencing it. Untreated pain in newborns may result in increased morbidity and length of stay in the NICU, exaggerated responses to pain in later life, and altered psychosocial development (Valeri, Holsti, & Linhares, 2015). Parents commonly expect that health care providers will use appropriate measures to prevent pain in their newborns, but there are gaps in knowledge about the most effective way to accomplish this.

Recent research findings suggested that infants be given an appropriate-sized pacifier for comfort during painful procedures. Administration of oral sucrose with and without nonnutritive sucking and warmth is also frequently used as a nonpharmacologic intervention for procedural pain relief in neonates. The recommended sucrose concentration is a 24% solution (Gray et al., 2015). Nurses need to be informed about the effectiveness of nonnutritive sucking, its analgesic mechanisms, and how to use and incorporate it into practice (Green, 2016).

Assessment of pain in the newborn remains a contentious and vexing problem. Newborns in the NICU are subjected to repeated procedures that cause them pain. Newborns, whether preterm, full term, or postterm, do experience pain, but the pain is difficult to validate with consistent behaviors. Considering that ill newborns undergo multiple noxious stimuli from invasive procedures, such as lumbar punctures, heel sticks, venipuncture, line insertions, chest tube placement, specimen collections, endotracheal intubation and suctioning, and mechanical ventilation, common sense would suggest that newborns experience pain from many of these activities and interventions. Historically, pain management in infants was not addressed formally but current guidelines address the nurse's role in assessing and managing neonatal pain (Yamada et al., 2015). Refer to Box 23.4 for an overview of the principles of newborn pain prevention and management that all nurses should utilize.

Several psychometric tools are available to assess pain in the newborn. Examples include the Premature Infant Pain Profile (PIPP), which assesses heart rate and oxygen saturation; the CRIES tool (cry, requires oxygen, increased vital signs, expression, and sleeplessness); and the Neonatal Infant Pain Scale (NIPS), which evaluates respiratory patterns. Most are based on facial expressions, crying patterns, change in vital signs, and body movements (Gardner et al., 2016). See Chapter 36 for a more in-depth discussion of pain assessment and management.

Nurses play a key role in assessing a newborn's pain level. Assess the newborn frequently. Pain is considered the "fifth vital sign" and should be assessed as frequently as the other four vital signs. Differentiate pain from agitation by observing for changes in vital signs, behavior, facial expression, and body movement. Suspect pain if the newborn exhibits the following:

- Sudden high-pitched cry
- Facial grimace with furrowing of brow and quivering chin
- Increased muscle tone
- Oxygen desaturation
- Increase in heart rate

BOX 23.4

NEWBORN PAIN PREVENTION AND MANAGEMENT GUIDELINES

- Newborn pain frequently goes unrecognized and undertreated.
- Pain assessment is an essential activity prior to pain management.
- Newborns experience pain, and analgesics should be given.
- A procedure considered painful for an adult should also be considered painful for a newborn.
- Developmental maturity and health status must be considered when assessing for pain in newborns.
- Newborns may be more sensitive to pain than adults.
- Pain behavior is frequently mistaken for irritability and agitation.
- Newborns are more susceptible to the long-term effects of pain.
- Adequate pain management may reduce complications and mortality.
- Nonpharmacologic measures can prevent, reduce, or eliminate newborn pain.
- Sedation does not provide pain relief and may mask pain responses.
- A newborn's response to both pharmacologic and nonpharmacologic pain therapy should be assessed within 30 minutes of administration or intervention.
- Health care professionals are responsible for pain assessment and treatment.
- Written guidelines are needed on each newborn unit.

Adapted from Kenner, C., & Lott, J. W. (2014). *Comprehensive neonatal care: An interdisciplinary approach* (5th ed.). St. Louis, MO: Saunders; Harrison, D., Bueno, M., & Reszel, J. (2015). Prevention and management of pain and stress in the neonate. *Research & Reports in Neonatology, 5*, 9–16; and Verklan, M. T., & Walden, M. (2015). *Core curriculum for neonatal intensive care nursing* (5th ed.). St. Louis, MO: Saunders.

- Body posturing, such as squirming, kicking, arching
- Limb withdrawal and thrashing movements
- Increased blood pressure, pulse, and respirations
- Fussiness and irritability (Verklan & Walden, 2015).

The goals of pain management are to minimize the amount, duration, and severity of pain and to assist the newborn in coping. It is essential that pain-related stress in preterm infants is accurately identified and appropriately managed, and that pain management strategies are evaluated for protective or adverse effects in the long term. Effective pain management strategies for newborns include preventing, limiting, or avoiding noxious stimuli; using nonpharmacologic techniques to reduce pain; and administering pharmacologic agents when appropriate. Box 23.5 lists some of the more commonly used nonpharmacologic pain management techniques for the preterm newborn.

Nonpharmacologic pain management strategies include nonnutritive sucking, breast-feeding, radiant heat to promote warmth, skin-to-skin contact, and sweetened solutions. Pharmacologic strategies include narcotic analgesics, but they are limited. Morphine and fentanyl, usually administered intravenously, are the most commonly used opioids for moderate to severe pain. Acetaminophen is effective for mild pain. Benzodiazepines are used as sedatives during painful procedures and can be combined with opioids for more effectiveness. Local or topical anesthetics (e.g., EMLA cream) also may be used before procedures such as venipuncture, lumbar puncture, and intravenous catheter insertion (Mattson & Smith, 2015).

Be vigilant in assessing for adverse effects (respiratory depression or hypotension) when administering pharmacologic agents for pain management, especially in preterm newborns with neurologic impairment. These negative effects are usually dose and route related, so be knowledgeable about the pharmacokinetics and therapeutic dosing of any drug administered.

BOX 23.5

NONPHARMACOLOGIC TECHNIQUES TO REDUCE PAIN IN THE PRETERM NEWBORN

- Gentle handling, rocking, caressing, cuddling, and massaging
- Rest periods before and after painful procedures
- Kangaroo care (skin-to-skin contact) during procedure
- Breast-feeding, if able, to reduce pain from minor procedures
- Use of a facilitated tuck (holding arms and legs in a flexed position)
- Application of topical anesthetics prior to venipuncture or lumbar puncture
- Swaddling and positioning to establish physical boundaries
- Nonnutritive sucking (pacifier dipped in sucrose) prior to procedure
- Minimal use of tape, with gentle removal to avoid skin tears
- Warm blankets for wrapping to facilitate relaxation
- Reduction of environmental stimuli by removing or turning down noxious stimuli such as noise from alarms, beepers, loud conversations, and bright lights
- Distraction, such as with colored objects or mobiles

Adapted from Adapted from Sabic, D., Blattner, C., & Metts, M. (2015). Newborn and infant pain control. *Clinical Pediatrics, 54*(7), 613–614; Nagtalon-Ramos, J. (2014) *Maternal-newborn nursing care: Best evidence-based practices.* Philadelphia, PA: F. A. Davis Company; and Verklan, M. T., & Walden, M. (2015). *Core curriculum for neonatal intensive care nursing* (5th ed.). St. Louis, MO: Saunders.

PROMOTING GROWTH AND DEVELOPMENT

In the late 1990s, researchers evaluated the NICU environment in terms of light and sound levels, caregiving activities, and handling of newborns. As a result of this research, many environmental modifications were made to reduce the stress and overstimulation of the NICU, and the concept of developmentally supportive care was introduced. Developmentally supportive care is defined as care of a newborn or infant to support positive growth and development. Developmental care focuses on what newborns or infants can do at that stage of development; it uses therapeutic interventions only to the point that they are beneficial; and it provides for the development of the newborn–family unit (White-Traut, 2015).

Family-centered developmental care is an essential element of neonatal intensive care. It is of particular importance when the infant is vulnerable and at greater risk for poor outcomes complicated by a family unit that is easily challenged by the unique needs of the infant, yet all newborns and their families deserve this philosophy of caregiving. Family-centered developmental care must continue to be tested through research to determine which interventions work, what does not work, and which interventions need further refinement (White & Wilson, 2015).

Developmental care is a philosophy of care that requires rethinking the relationships between newborns, families, and health care providers. It includes a variety of activities designed to manage the environment and individualize the care of the preterm or high-risk ill newborn based on behavioral observations (see Evidence-Based Practice 23.1).

Developmental care includes these strategies:

- Clustering care to promote rest and conserve the infant's energy
- Flexed positioning to simulate in utero positioning
- Environmental management to reduce noise and visual stimulation
- Kangaroo care to promote skin-to-skin sensation
- Placement of twins in the same isolette or open crib to reduce stress

EVIDENCE-BASED PRACTICE 23.1

EFFECT OF DEVELOPMENTAL CARE FOR THE VERY PREMATURE INFANTS ON NEURODEVELOPMENTAL OUTCOME AT 2 YEARS OF AGE

STUDY

Developmental care is a model for delivering individualized care to high-risk newborns within a family context that includes a developmentally supportive environment, flexible caregiving to meet the newborn's needs, parental involvement, and collaboration and communication with all individuals involved in the care. This study was done to determine the effect of developmental care on neurodevelopmental outcome in formerly preterm infants at the age of two years.

Findings

A prospective phase-lag study was performed which included 261 preterm infants divided into two groups. There were 124 placed in the conventional group and 137 placed in the developmental care group. It was found that the children in the developmental group showed less psychomotor delay than those in the control group. Not smoking in pregnancy and higher gestational age were also significant predictors for a better psychomotor outcome at two years of age. The data implicated that developmental care may result in an improved two-year psychomotor outcome in formerly preterm infants.

Nursing Implications

Based on the results of this study, nurses can feel confident in integrating the principles of developmental care into their practice to facilitate a positive impact on the infant's later neurodevelopmental outcome. Principles to incorporate into their nursing care would include clustering care to allow for rest periods, minimizing external stimuli (lights, noise, handling), respecting sleep states of the infant, utilizing comforting measures for painful procedures (swaddling, warmth, pacifiers, skin-to-skin), and engaging parents in their infant's care.

Source: Kiechl-Kohlendorfer, U., Merkle, U., Deufert, D., Neubauer, V., Peglow, U. P., & Griesmaier, E. (2015). Effect of developmental care for very premature infants on neurodevelopmental outcome at 2 years of age. *Infant Behavior & Development, 39*, 166–172.

- Activities to promote self-regulation and state regulation:
  - Surrounding the newborn with nesting rolls/devices
  - Swaddling with a blanket to maintain the flexed position
  - Providing sheepskin or a waterbed to simulate the uterine environment
  - Providing nonnutritive sucking (calms the infant)
  - Providing objects to grasp (comforts the newborn)
- Promotion of parent–infant bonding by making parents feel welcome in the NICU
- Open, honest communication with parents and staff
- Collaboration with the parents in planning the infant's care (Verklan & Walden, 2015; Gardner et al., 2016).

Developmental care can be fostered by clustering the lights in one area so that no lights are shining directly on newborns, installing visual alarm systems and limiting overhead pages to minimize noise, and monitoring continuous and peak noise levels. Nurses can play an active role by serving on committees that address these issues. In addition, nurses can provide direct developmentally supportive care. Doing so involves careful planning of nursing activities to provide the ideal environment for the newborn's development. For example:

- Dim the lights and cover isolettes at night to simulate nighttime.
- Support early extubation from mechanical ventilation.
- Encourage early and consistent feedings with breast milk.
- Administer prescribed antibiotics judiciously.
- Position the newborn as if he or she was still in utero (a nesting fetal position).
- Promote kangaroo care by encouraging parents to hold the newborn against the chest for extended periods each day.
- Coordinate care to respect sleep and awake states.

Throughout the newborn's stay, work with the parents, developing a collaborative partnership so they feel comfortable caring for their newborn. Be prepared to make referrals to community support groups to enhance coping (Hall et al., 2015).

PROMOTING PARENTAL COPING

Generally, pregnancy and the birth of a newborn are exciting times, but when the newborn has serious, perhaps life-threatening problems, the exciting experience suddenly changes to one of anxiety, fear, guilt, loss, and grief.

Parents are typically unprepared for the birth of a preterm newborn and commonly experience an array of emotions, including disappointment, fear for the survival of the newborn, and anxiety due to the separation from their newborn immediately after birth. Gaining insight into the experience of parents of premature infants can help nurses ensure services more effectively meet the needs of these families

(Discenza, 2015). Early interruptions in the bonding process and concern about the newborn's survival can create extreme anxiety and interfere with attachment (Mattson & Smith, 2015).

Nursing interventions aimed at reducing parental anxiety include:

- Reviewing with the parents the events that have occurred since birth
- Providing individualized support to parents while in NICU
- Providing simple relaxation and calming techniques (visual imagery, breathing)
- Exploring their perception of the newborn's condition and offering explanations
- Encouraging parental involvement with their newborn in NICU
- Validating their anxiety and behaviors as normal reactions to stress and trauma
- Providing a physical presence and support during emotional outbursts
- Providing anticipatory guidance about taking their infants home
- Exploring the coping strategies they used successfully in the past and encouraging their use now
- Encouraging frequent visits to the NICU
- Addressing their reactions to the NICU environment and explaining all equipment used
- Identifying family and community resources available to them (Rossman, Greene, & Meier, 2015; Cano Gimenez & Sanchez-Luna, 2015)

Preparing for Discharge

Discharge planning typically begins with evidence that recovery of the newborn is certain. However, the exact date of discharge may not be predictable. The goal of the discharge plan is to make a successful transition to home care. Essential elements for discharge are a physiologically stable infant, a family who can provide the necessary care with appropriate support services in place in the community, and a pediatrician or primary care physician or nurse practitioner available for ongoing care (Krowchuk, 2015; Verklan & Walden, 2015).

The care of each high-risk newborn after discharge requires careful coordination to provide ongoing multidisciplinary support for the family. The discharge planning team typically includes the parents, primary care physician, neonatologists, neonatal nurses, and a social worker. Other professionals, such as surgical specialists and pediatric subspecialists, occupational, physical, speech, and respiratory therapists, nutritionists, home health care nurses, and a case manager, may be included as needed (Fanaroff & Fanaroff, 2014; Verklan & Walden, 2015). Critical components of discharge planning are summarized in Box 23.6.

BOX 23.6

CRITICAL COMPONENTS OF DISCHARGE PLANNING

- Parental education—involvement and support in newborn care during NICU stay will ensure their readiness to care for the infant at home.
- Evaluation of unresolved medical problems—review of the active problem list and determination of what home care and follow-up is needed.
- Implementation of primary care—completion of newborn screening tests, immunizations, examinations such as funduscopic exam for ROP, and hematologic status evaluation
- Development of home care plan, including assessment of:
    - Equipment and supplies needed for care
    - In-home caregiver's preparation and ability to care for infant
    - Adequacy of the physical facilities in the home
    - An emergency care and transport plan if needed
    - Financial resources for home care costs
    - Family needs and coping skills
    - Community resources, including how they can be accessed

Nurses involved in the discharge process are instrumental in bridging the gap between the hospital and home. When planning for discharge of the high-risk infant, the nurse should:

- Assess the physical status of the mother and the newborn.
- Discuss the early signs of complications and what to do if they occur.
- Reinforce instructions for infant care and safety.
- Stress the importance of proper car seat use.
- Provide instructions for medication administration.
- Reinforce instructions for equipment operation, maintenance, and troubleshooting.
- Teach infant cardiopulmonary resuscitation and emergency care.
- Demonstrate techniques for special care procedures such as dressings, ostomy care, artificial airway maintenance, chest physiotherapy, suctioning, and infant stimulation.
- Provide breast-feeding support or instruction on gavage feedings.
- Assist with defining roles in the adjustment period at home.
- Assess the parents' emotional stability and coping status.
- Provide support and reassurance to the family.
- Report abnormal findings to the health care team for intervention.
- Follow up with parents to ensure that they have connected with appropriate support systems in the community (Krowchuk, 2015; Verklan & Walden, 2015).

Take Note!

Infants born prematurely between 34 0/7 and 36 6/7 weeks are at higher risk for morbidity and mortality than those born before 28 weeks or after 37 weeks due to their physiologic and metabolic immunity (Boyle et al., 2015).

LATE PRETERM NEWBORN ("NEAR TERM")

The late preterm is a newborn that is born between 34 weeks and 36 6/7 weeks of gestation. Previously, infants born during this time frame were called "near term" or "slightly premature," which was a misnomer because the infants have special care needs. Some of the most common complications for late preterm infants are cold stress, respiratory distress, hypoglycemia, sepsis, cognitive delays, hyperbilirubinemia, and feeding difficulties (Horgan, 2015). In recent years, the subject of late preterm birth has received much attention, since this population of preterm newborns represents more than 70% of all preterm births in the United States and has increased by 30% in the past 20 years (CDC, 2016). With the sharp rise in the number of cesarean births performed, the incidence of late preterm newborns will also rise. Perinatal nurses need to understand the risks of late preterm births and the unique needs of this population in order to facilitate timely assessment and intervention to improve outcomes. Some of the challenges facing the late preterm newborn include:

- Respiratory distress (related to pulmonary immaturity, lack of adequate surfactant, retained lung fluid, cesarean section)
- Thermoregulation issues (less brown and white, limited ability to flex the trunk and extremities to decrease exposed surface area)
- Hypoglycemia related to the first two challenges (respiratory distress and cold stress)
- Apnea (related to poor respiratory control and immaturity)
- Jaundice and hyperbilirubinemia (related to immature bilirubin conjugation and excretion)
- Feeding challenges related to immature suck and swallowing reflexes
- Sepsis because maternal antibodies are not fully transferred prior to the 37th week
- Neurodevelopmental delay (related to brain and central nervous system immaturity) (Gardner et al., 2016; Verklan & Walden, 2015).

These challenges are similar to those facing the preterm newborn and require similar management. Late preterm newborns have more clinical problems, longer lengths of stay, higher costs when compared with full-term newborns, and increased mortalities (Kenner & Lott, 2014). Anticipatory guidance for parents of late preterm infants should include recommending an infant cardiopulmonary resuscitation course, educating about sudden infant death syndrome prevention protocol (Back to Sleep), and advising the parents to avoid public places and limit visitors for the first few weeks after being discharged from the hospital. Consistent follow-up medical care, weekly weight checks, and up-to-date immunizations can help late preterm infants avoid complications (Baker, 2015). Nurses and parents must be aware of the risks associated with late preterm births to optimize care and outcomes for this group of newborns. For information related to discharge teaching for the family of the late preterm infant, refer to Teaching Guidelines 23.1.

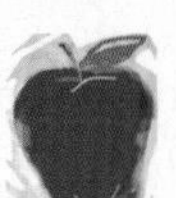

Teaching Guidelines 23.1

DISCHARGING THE LATE PRETERM INFANT

When discharge planning for the late preterm infant, validate parents' understanding of:

- Dressing the infant appropriately in order to maintain appropriate temperature
- Practicing good handwashing and limiting contact with ill persons
- Maintaining adequate nutritional and fluid intake to promote growth and development; breast-feeding is preferred
- Avoiding secondhand smoke exposure
- Practicing safe sleep practices: avoid soft mattresses or blankets, place infant supine to sleep
- Keeping appointments for health maintenance visits (check-ups) as scheduled
- Notifying the pediatrician or nurse practitioner immediately if the infant:
  - Has difficulty breathing or turns blue (call for emergency services in this case)
  - Has a temperature below 97° F (36.1° C) or above 100.4° F (38° C)
  - Displays a yellow color to the skin (jaundice)
  - Feeds poorly
  - Vomits
  - Fails to void for 12 hours, or to pass a bowel movement in 24 hours
  - Acts lethargic, irritable or "just not right"

Adapted from Baker, B. (2015). Evidence-based practice to improve outcomes for late preterm infants. *Journal of Obstetric, Gynecologic, & Neonatal Nursing, 44*, 127–134. doi: 10.1111/1552-6909.12533.

Dealing With Perinatal Loss

It is estimated that over 7 million perinatal losses occur globally each year. More than 1 million occur within the United States annually (Callister, 2014). Perinatal loss, defined as any pregnancy loss and/or neonatal death up to 1 month of age, continues to be a common occurrence even though major advances have taken place in perinatal health care. The prevalence of perinatal death reflects a very real possibility that all nurses will meet and care for a woman who has experienced the death of a baby (Rondinelli et al., 2015).

Perinatal loss is a profound experience for the family. It engenders a unique kind of mourning since the infant is so much a part of the parents' identity. Instead of celebrating a new life as they expected, parents are mourning the loss of dreams and hopes and the loss of an extension of themselves. NICU nurses face a difficult situation when caring for newborns who may not survive. Newborn death is incomprehensible to most parents/partners/significant others. They are commonly offered time to see their infant, memory items, and support. This can make the grieving process more difficult because of the denial the parents commonly experience: what is happening "can't be real." Deciding whether to see, touch, or hold the dying newborn is extremely difficult for many parents. Nurses play a major role in assisting parents/partners/significant others to make their dying newborn "real" to them by providing them with as many memories as possible and encouraging them to see, hold, touch, dress, and take care of the infant and take photographs. These actions help to validate the partners'/significant others'/parents' sense of loss, relive the experience, and attach significance to the meaning of loss. A lock of hair, a name card, or an identification bracelet may serve as important mementos that can ease the grieving process. The memories created by these interventions can be useful allies in the grieving process and in resolving grief (Mattson & Smith, 2015; Verklan & Walden, 2015).

A nurse's willingness to sit quietly and observe, to remain open and nonjudgmental, and to explore what might be helpful are useful strategies to bridge cultural differences. Statements such as, "Help me understand how your family cares for someone who is dying," or, "What would be important for me to know about how best to care for your baby's body?" convey a nurse's willingness to learn what is most important to each family. Parents' answers may help guide nurses in providing culturally appropriate care for diverse populations. Nurses who are attentive to learning what is most important to parents, and subsequently work to incorporate such interventions into their care, foster relationships between parents and their infant (Steen, 2015).

Parent–newborn interaction is vital to the normal processes of attachment and bonding. The detachment process involved in a newborn's death is equally important for parents. Nurses can aid in this process by helping parents to see their newborn through the maze of equipment, explaining the various procedures and equipment, encouraging them to express their feelings about the newborn's status, and providing time for them to be with their dying newborn (Gardner et al., 2016; Steen, 2015).

A common reaction by many people when learning that a newborn is not going to survive is one of avoidance. Nurses are no exception. It is difficult to initiate a conversation about such a sensitive issue without knowing how the parents are going to react and cope with the impending loss. One way to begin a conversation with the parents is to convey concern and acknowledge their loss. Active listening can give parents a safe place to begin the healing process. The relationship that the nurse establishes with the parents is a unique one, providing an opportunity for both the nurse and the parents to share their feelings.

Be aware of personal feelings about loss and how these feelings are part of one's own life and personal belief system. Actively listen to the parents when they are talking about their experiences. Communicate empathy (understanding and feeling what another person is feeling), respect their feelings, and respond to them in helpful and supportive ways (Cunningham et al., 2014). Table 23.2 highlights appropriate interventions for a family experiencing a perinatal loss before and after a newborn dies.

In a time of crisis or loss, people are often more sensitive to other people's reactions. For example, the parents may be extremely aware of the nurse's facial expressions, choice of words, and tone of voice. Talking quickly, in a businesslike fashion, or ignoring the loss may inhibit parents from discussing their pain or how they are coping with it. Parents may need to vent their frustrations and anger, and the nurse may become the target. Validate their feelings and attempt to reframe or refocus the anger toward the real issue of loss. An example would be to say, "I understand your frustration and anger about this situation. You have experienced a tremendous loss and it must be difficult not to have an explanation for it at this time." Doing so helps to defuse the anger while allowing them to express their feelings.

The death of an infant will more than likely be one of the toughest moments in a family's life. Giving families some sense of control in an otherwise hopeless situation can provide some comfort. Some ideas to provide them a sense of control include:

- Ask the family who they wish to have present as the infant dies.
- Give the family a choice of rooms in which they can say good-bye to their infant.
- Provide privacy for the family during this time period by placing a sign on the door.
- Provide ideas for making or selecting memorial items for a memory box.
- The family should never be left to handle their emotions alone unless they request it.
- Respect a family's wishes if they refuse to be with their infant during the dying process or afterward. Everyone grieves differently.

When assisting bereaved parents, start where the parents are in the grief process to avoid imposing your own agenda on them. You may feel uncomfortable at not being able to change the situation or take the pain away. The nurse's role is to provide immediate emotional

TABLE 23.2 ASSISTING PARENTS TO COPE WITH PERINATAL LOSS

Before the newborn's death	Respect variations in the family's spiritual needs and readiness. Assess cultural beliefs and practices that may bring comfort; respect culturally appropriate requests for truth telling and informed refusal. Initiate spiritual comfort by calling the hospital clergy if appropriate; offer to pray with the family if appropriate. Encourage the parents to take photographs, make memory boxes, and record their thoughts in a journal. Explore with family members how they dealt with previous losses. Discuss techniques to reduce stress, such as meditation and relaxation. Recommend that family members maintain a healthy diet and get adequate rest and exercise to preserve their health. Participate in early and repeated care conferencing to reduce family stress. Allow family to be present at both medical rounds and resuscitation; provide explanations of all procedures, treatments, and findings; answer questions honestly and as completely as possible. Provide opportunities for the family to hold the newborn if they so choose. Assess the family's support network. Provide suggestions as to how friends can be helpful to the family.
After the newborn's death	Help the family to accept the reality of death by using the word "died." Acknowledge their grief and the fact that their newborn has died. Help the family to work through their grief by validating and listening. Provide the family with realistic information about the causes of death. Offer condolences to the family in a sincere manner. Encourage the father to cry and grieve with his partner. Provide opportunities for the family to hold the newborn if they desire.
At the time of the release of the newborn's body	Reassure the family that their feelings and grieving responses are normal. Encourage the parents to have a funeral or memorial service to bring closure. Suggest that the parents plant a tree or flowers to remember the infant. Address attachment issues concerning subsequent pregnancies. Provide information about local support groups. Provide anticipatory guidance regarding the grieving process. Present information about any impact on future childbearing, and refer the parents to appropriate specialists or genetic resources.

Adapted from Gardner, S. L., Carter, B. S., Enzman-Hines, M., & Hernandez, J. A. (2016). *Merenstein & Gardner's handbook of neonatal intensive care* (8th ed.). St. Louis, MO: Mosby Elsevier; Steen, S. E. (2015). Perinatal death: Bereavement interventions used by US and Spanish nurses and midwives. *International Journal of Palliative Nursing, 21*(2), 79–86; and Fanaroff, A. A., & Fanaroff, J. M. (2014). *Klaus and Fanaroff's care of the high-risk neonate* (6th ed.). Philadelphia, PA: Elsevier Health Sciences.

support and facilitate the grieving process. Supporting and strengthening the family bond in the face of perinatal loss is essential.

Comforting the family after the infant's death is vital to give them a sense of closure and start the healing process. Some things the nurse can do to help the family during this time include:

- Sending the family a card from the nursing staff, signed by all who worked with their infant, within a week of leaving the hospital
- Attending the funeral to allow for a public good-bye and to support others in their time of loss
- Providing the family with a memory box, which might contain an outfit worn by their infant, a blanket used to cover their infant, a lock of hair, a card with hand and foot prints, and a photo with someone holding their infant
- Remembering their infant at various anniversaries by sending a card or calling the family to see how they are doing provides families much-needed comfort.
- Donating to a charity in memory of the infant, such as to March of Dimes
- Providing the family with resources that might help them. Information might include listings of local or online support groups as well as grief websites such as Share.org.

Being present during this traumatic event for families is tough. Serving infants and their families by bearing witness to their pain and grief is a special privilege. Being present for the family with compassion, comfort, support, and resources during their time of loss is truly an honorable gesture. Nurses are remembered years later for their kindness and guidance of the family members through this adverse event with dignity (Discenza, 2015).

NURSING CARE PLAN 23.1

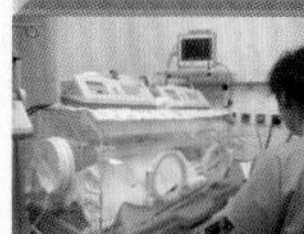

Overview of the Care of a Preterm Newborn

Alice, an 18-year-old, felt she had done everything right during her first pregnancy and certainly didn't anticipate giving birth to a preterm newborn at 32 weeks' gestation. When Mary Kaye was born, she had respiratory distress and hypoglycemia and couldn't stabilize her temperature. Assessment revealed the following: newborn described as scrawny in appearance; skin thin and transparent with prominent veins over abdomen; hypotonia with lax, extended positioning; weak sucking reflex when nipple offered; respiratory distress with tachypnea (70 breaths/min), nasal flaring, and sternal retractions; low blood glucose level suggested by lethargy, tachycardia, jitteriness; axillary temperature of 36° C (96.8° F) despite warmed blanket; weight 2,146 g (4.73 lb); length 45 cm (17.72 inches).

NURSING DIAGNOSIS: Ineffective breathing pattern related to immature respiratory system and respiratory distress as evidenced by tachypnea, nasal flaring, sternal retractions, and/or oxygen saturation <87%

Outcome Identification and Evaluation

Newborn's respiratory status returns to adequate level of functioning as evidenced by rate remaining within 30 to 60 breaths/min, maintenance of acceptable oxygen saturation levels, and minimal to absent signs of respiratory distress.

Interventions: *Promoting Optimal Breathing Pattern*

- Assess gestational age and risk factors for respiratory distress *to allow early detection.*
- Anticipate need for bag and mask setup and wall suction *to allow for prompt intervention should respiratory status continue to worsen.*
- Assess respiratory effort (rate, character, effort) *to identify changes.*
- Assess heart rate for tachycardia and auscultate heart sounds *to determine worsening of condition.*
- Observe for cues (grunting, shallow respirations, tachypnea, apnea, tachycardia, central cyanosis, hypotonia, increased effort) *to identify need for additional oxygen.*
- Maintain slight head elevation *to prevent upper airway obstruction.*
- Assess skin color *to evaluate tissue perfusion.*
- Monitor oxygen saturation level via pulse oximetry *to provide objective indication of perfusion status.*
- Provide supplemental oxygen as indicated and ordered *to ensure adequate tissue oxygenation.*
- Assist with any ordered diagnostic tests, such as chest x-ray and arterial blood gases, *to determine effectiveness of treatments.*
- Cluster nursing activities *to reduce oxygen consumption.*
- Maintain a neutral thermal environment *to reduce oxygen consumption.*
- Monitor hydration status *to prevent fluid volume deficit or overload.*
- Explain all events and procedures to the parents *to help alleviate anxiety and promote understanding of the newborn's condition.*

NURSING DIAGNOSIS: Ineffective thermoregulation related to lack of fat stores and hypotonia as evidenced by extended positioning, low axillary temperature despite warmed blanket/radiant heat source/isolette, respiratory distress, and lethargy

Outcome Identification and Evaluation

Newborn will demonstrate ability to regulate temperature as evidenced by temperature remaining in normal range (36.5° to 37.5° C) and absent signs of cold stress.

Interventions: *Promoting Thermoregulation*

- Assess the axillary temperature every hour or use a thermistor probe *to monitor for changes.*
- Review maternal history *to identify risk factors contributing to problem.*

(continued)

NURSING CARE PLAN 23.1

Overview of the Care of a Preterm Newborn (continued)

- Monitor vital signs, including heart rate and respiratory rate, every hour *to identify deviations.*
- Check radiant heat source or isolette *to ensure maintenance of appropriate temperature of the environment.*
- Assess environment for sources of heat loss or gain through evaporation, conduction, convection, or radiation *to minimize risk of heat loss.*
- Avoid bathing and exposing newborn *to prevent cold stress.*
- Warm all blankets and equipment that come in contact with newborn; place warmed cap on the newborn's head and keep it on *to minimize heat loss.*
- Encourage kangaroo care (mother or father holds preterm infant underneath clothing skin-to-skin and upright between breasts) *to provide warmth.*
- Educate parents on how to maintain a neutral thermal environment, including importance of keeping the newborn warm with a cap and double-wrapping with blankets and changing them frequently to keep dry *to promote newborn's adjustment.*
- Demonstrate ways to safeguard warmth and prevent heat loss.

NURSING DIAGNOSIS: Risk for imbalanced nutrition: less than body requirements to meet metabolic needs related to poor sucking and lack of glycogen stores necessary to meet the newborn's increased metabolic demands

Outcome Identification and Evaluation

Newborn will demonstrate adequate nutritional intake to progressively gain weight toward desired goal, remaining free of signs of hypoglycemia as evidenced by blood glucose levels being maintained above 45 mg/dL, enhanced sucking ability, and appropriate weight gain.

Interventions: ***Promoting Optimal Nutrition***

- Identify newborn at risk based on behavioral characteristics, body measurements, and gestational age *to establish a baseline and allow for early detection.*
- Assess blood glucose levels as ordered *to determine status and establish a baseline for interventions.*
- Obtain blood glucose measurements upon admission to nursery and every 1 to 2 hours as indicated *to evaluate for changes.*
- Observe behavior for signs of low blood glucose *to allow early identification.*
- Initiate early oral feedings or gavage feedings *to maintain blood glucose levels.*
- If oral or gavage feedings aren't tolerated, initiate an IV glucose infusion *to aid in stabilizing blood glucose levels.*
- Assess skin for pallor and sweating *to identify signs of hypoglycemia.*
- Assess neurologic status for tremors, seizures, jitteriness, and lethargy *to identify further drops in blood glucose levels.*
- Monitor weight daily for changes *to determine effectiveness of feedings.*
- Maintain temperature using warmed blankets, radiant warmer, or warmed isolette *to prevent heat loss and possible cold stress and reduce energy demands.*
- Monitor temperature *to prevent cold stress resulting in decreased blood glucose levels.*
- Offer opportunities for nonnutritive sucking on premature-size pacifier *to satisfy sucking needs.*
- Monitor for tolerance of oral feedings, including intake and output, *to determine effectiveness.*
- Administer IV dextrose if newborn is symptomatic *to raise blood glucose levels quickly.*
- Decrease energy requirements, including clustering care activities and providing rest periods, *to conserve glucose and glycogen stores.*
- Inform parents about procedures and treatments, including rationale for frequent blood glucose levels, *to help reduce their anxiety.*

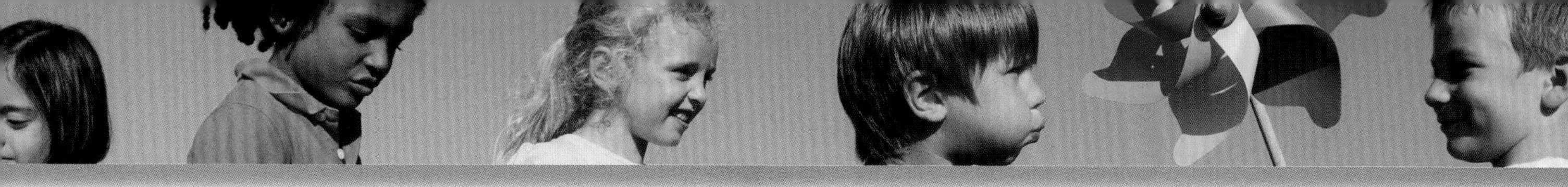

KEY CONCEPTS

- Variations in birthweight and gestational age can place a newborn at risk for problems that require special care.
- Variations in birthweight include the following categories: small for gestational age, appropriate for gestational age, and large for gestational age. Newborns who are small or large for gestational age have special needs.
- The small-for-gestational-age newborn faces problems related to a decrease in placental function in utero; these problems may include perinatal asphyxia, hypothermia, hypoglycemia, polycythemia, and meconium aspiration.
- Risk factors for the birth of a large-for-gestational-age infant include maternal diabetes mellitus or glucose intolerance, multiparity, prior history of a macrosomic infant, postdates gestation, maternal obesity, male fetus, and genetics. Large-for-gestational-age newborns face problems such as birth trauma due to cephalopelvic disproportion, hypoglycemia, and jaundice secondary to hyperbilirubinemia.
- Variations in gestational age include postterm and preterm newborns. Postterm newborns may be large or small for gestational age or dysmature, depending on placental function.
- The postterm newborn may develop complications after birth, including fetal hypoxia, hypoglycemia, hypothermia, polycythemia, and meconium aspiration.
- Preterm birth is the leading cause of death within the first month of life and the second leading cause of all infant deaths.
- The preterm newborn is at risk for complications because his or her organ systems are immature, thereby impeding the transition from intrauterine life to extrauterine life.
- Newborns can experience pain, but their pain is difficult to validate with consistent behaviors.
- Newborns with gestational age variations, primarily preterm newborns, benefit from developmental care, which includes a variety of activities designed to manage the environment and individualize the care based on behavioral observations.
- Nurses play a key role in assisting the parents and family of a newborn with special needs to cope with this crisis situation, including dealing with the possibility that the newborn may not survive. Nurses working with parents experiencing a perinatal loss can help by actively listening, understanding the parents' experiences, and communicating empathy.
- The goal of discharge planning is to make a successful transition to home care.

REFERENCES AND RECOMMENDED READINGS

Als, H. (2009). Newborn individualized developmental care and assessment program (NIDCAP): New frontier for neonatal and perinatal medicine. *Journal of Neonatal-Perinatal Medicine, 2*, 135–147.

American Academy of Pediatrics [AAP] and American Heart Association [AHA]. (2014). *Documentation of neonatal resuscitation. 23*(1), Retrieved from http://www2.aap.org/nrp/docs/IU/2014_SpringSummer_iu.pdf

Back, S. A. (2015). Brain injury in the preterm infant: New horizons for pathogenesis and prevention. *Pediatric Neurology, 53*(3), 185–192.

Baker, B. (2015). Evidence-based practice to improve outcomes for late preterm infants. *Journal of Obstetric, Gynecologic, & Neonatal Nursing, 44*, 127–134.

Boxwell, G. (ed.). (2010). *Neonatal intensive care nursing* (2nd ed.). New York: Routledge.

Boyle, E. M., Johnson, S., Manktelow, B., Seaton, S. E., Draper, E. S., Smith, L. K., et al. (2015). Neonatal outcomes and delivery of care for infants born late preterm or moderately preterm: A prospective population-based study. *Archives of Disease in Childhood: Fetal and Neonatal Edition, 100*(6), F479–F485.

Brennan, A. M., Murphy, B. P., & Kiely, M. (2015). Nutritional management and assessment of preterm infants: The Baby-Grow Longitudinal Nutrition and Growth study. *Topics in Clinical Nutrition, 30*(1), 80–93.

Callister, L. C. (2014). Global perspectives on perinatal loss. *MCN: The American Journal of Maternal/Child Nursing, 39*(3), 207–210.

Cano Giménez, E., & Sánchez-Luna, M. (2015). Providing parents with individualized support in a neonatal intensive care unit reduced stress, anxiety and depression. *Acta Paediatrica, 104*(7), e300–e305.

Carlo, W. A. (2015). Prematurity and intrauterine growth restriction. In R. M. Kliegman, B. R. Stanton, J. W. St. Geme, N. F. Schor, & R. E. Behrman (eds.), *Nelson textbook of pediatrics* (20th ed.). Philadelphia: Saunders.

Centers for Disease Control and Prevention [CDC]. (2016). *Birthweight and gestation.* Retrieved from http://www.cdc.gov/nchs/fastats/birthweight.htm

Cleary-Goldman, J., & Robinson, J. N. (2015). Delivery of the preterm low birth weight singleton fetus. *UpToDate.* Retrieved from http://www.uptodate.com/contents/delivery-of-the-preterm-low-birth-weight-singleton-fetus

Cunningham, F. G., Leveno, K. J., Bloom, S. L., Spong, C. Y., Dashe, J. S., Hoffman, B. L., et al. (2014). *Williams obstetrics* (24th ed.). New York, NY: McGraw-Hill.

Discenza, D. (2015). NICU helping hands: Supporting families through the whole journey. *Neonatal Network, 34*(1), 52–54. doi:10.1891/0730-0832.34.1.52.

Fanaroff, A. A., & Fanaroff, J. M. (2014). *Klaus and Fanaroff's care of the high-risk neonate* (6th ed.). Philadelphia, PA: Elsevier Health Sciences.

Feinberg, M. E., Roettger, M. E., Jones, D. E., Paul, I. M., & Kan, M. L. (2015). Effects of a psychosocial couple-based prevention program on adverse birth outcomes. *Maternal and Child Health Journal, 19*(1), 102–111.

Gardner, S. L., Carter, B. S., Enzman-Hines, M., & Hernandez, J. A. (2016). *Merenstein & Gardner's handbook of neonatal intensive care* (8th ed.). St. Louis, MO: Mosby Elsevier.

Gray, L., Garza, E., Zageris, D., Heilman, K. J., & Porges, S. W. (2015). Sucrose and warmth for analgesia in healthy newborns: An RCT. *Pediatrics, 135*(3), e607--e614.

Green, C. J. (2016). *Maternal newborn nursing care plans* (3rd ed.). Burlington, MA: Jones and Bartlett Learning.

Hall, S., Hynan, M., Phillips, R., Press, J., Kenner, C., & Ryan, D. J. (2015). Development of program standards for psychosocial support of parents of infants admitted to a neonatal intensive care unit: A national interdisciplinary consensus model. *Newborn & Infant Nursing Reviews, 15*(1), 24–27. doi:10.1053/j.nainr.2015.01.007.

Harrison, D., Bueno, M., & Reszel, J. (2015). Prevention and management of pain and stress in the neonate. *Research & Reports in Neonatology, 5*. 9–16.

Herrera-Marschitz, M., Neira-Peña, T., Leyton, L., Gebicke-Haerter, P., Rojas-Mancilla, E., Morales, P., et al. (2015). Short-and long-term consequences of perinatal asphyxia: Looking for neuroprotective strategies. In M. Antonelli (ed.), *Perinatal Programming of Neurodevelopment* (pp. 169–198). New York, NY: Springer Publishers.

Horgan, M. J. (2015). Management of the late preterm infant: Not quite ready for prime time. *Pediatric Clinics of North America, 62*(2), 439–451.

Jaques, S. C., & Kennea, N. (2015). Resuscitation of the newborn. *Obstetrics, Gynecology & Reproductive Medicine, 25*(3), 61–67.

Jazayeri, A. (2015). Macrosomia. *eMedicine*. Retrieved from http://emedicine.medscape.com/article/262679-overview

Kaneko, M., Yamashita, R., Kai, K., Yamada, N., Sameshima, H., & Ikenoue, T. (2015). Perinatal morbidity and mortality for extremely low birthweight infants: A population-based study of regionalized maternal and neonatal transport. *Journal of Obstetrics and Gynecology Research, 41*(7), 1056–1066.

Kelly, M. M. (2010). *Prematurity*. In P. J. Allen, J. A. Vessey, & N. A. Schapiro (eds.), *Primary care of the child with a chronic condition* (5th ed.). St. Louis: Mosby.

Kenner, C., & Lott, J. W. (2014). *Comprehensive neonatal care: An interdisciplinary approach* (5th ed.). St. Louis: Saunders.

Kiechl-Kohlendorfer, U., Merkle, U., Deufert, D., Neubauer, V., Peglow, U. P., & Griesmaier, E. (2015). Effect of developmental care for very premature infants on neurodevelopmental outcome at 2 years of age. *Infant Behavior & Development, 39*, 166–172.

Kliegman, R. M., Stanton, B., St. Geme, J., Schor, N., & Behrman, R. E. (eds.). (2015). *Nelson textbook of pediatrics* (20th ed.). St. Louis, MO: Saunders Elsevier.

Krowchuk, H. (2015). Toward evidence-based practice: Paternal and maternal concerns for their very low-birth-weight infants transitioning from the NICU to home. *MCN: The American Journal of Maternal Child Nursing, 40*(2), 134.

Lessaris, K. J. (2015). *Polycythemia of the newborn*. Retrieved from http://emedicine.medscape.com/article/976319-overview

Mahajan, R. C., Une, L., & Bansal, S. (2015). Study of clinical features and in newborn with polycythemia: Antenatal and natal factors. *MedPulse—International Medical Journal, 2*(2), 66–71.

Mandy, G. T. (2015a). Small for gestational age infant. *UpToDate*. Retrieved from http://www.uptodate.com/contents/small-for-gestational-age-infant

Mandy, G. T., (2015b). Large for gestational age newborn. *UpToDate*. Retrieved from http://www.uptodate.com/contents/large-for-gestational-age-newborn

March of Dimes. (2013). *Premature babies*. Retrieved from http://www.marchofdimes.org/baby/premature-babies.aspx

March of Dimes. (2014). *Low birthweight*. Retrieved from http://www.marchofdimes.org/complications/low-birth-weight.aspx

March of Dimes. (2015). *PeriStats*. Retrieved from http://www.marchofdimes.org/peristats/Peristats.aspx

March of Dimes. (2016). *Premature birth report cards 2015*, from http://www.marchofdimes.org/mission/prematurity-reportcard.aspx

Mattson, S., & Smith, J. E. (2015). *Core curriculum for maternal–newborn nursing* (5th ed.). St. Louis, MO: Saunders Elsevier.

Moore, T. R. (2014). Diabetes mellitus and pregnancy. *eMedicine*. Retrieved from http://emedicine.medscape.com/article/127547-overview

Morken, N. H., Klungsøyr, K., & Skjaerven, R. (2014). Perinatal mortality by gestational week and size at birth in singleton pregnancies at and beyond term: A nationwide population-based cohort study. *BMC Pregnancy and Childbirth, 14*(1), 172–175. doi:10.1186/1471-2393-14-172.

Nagtalon-Ramos, J. (2014). *Maternal-newborn nursing care: Best evidence-based practices*. Philadelphia, PA: F.A. Davis Company.

National Center for Health Statistics. (2016). *Birthweight and gestation*. Retrieved from http://www.cdc.gov/nchs/fastats/birthweight.htm

Neonatal eHandbook. (2014a). *Diabetic mother - infant care*. Retrieved from http://www.health.vic.gov.au/neonatalhandbook/conditions/diabetic-mother-infant-care.htm

Neonatal eHandbook. (2014b). *Polycythemia in neonates*. Retrieved from http://www.health.vic.gov.au/neonatalhandbook/conditions/polycythaemia.htm

Neonatal eHandbook. (2014c). *Nutrition*. Retrieved from http://www.health.vic.gov.au/neonatalhandbook/nutrition/index.htm

Paul, M. (2015). Oxygen administration to preterm neonates in the delivery room: Minimizing oxidative stress. *Advances in Neonatal Care, 15*(2), 94–103.

Potter, C. F., & Kicklighter, S. D. (2016) Infant of a diabetic mother. *eMedicine*. Retrieved from http://emedicine.medscape.com/article/974230-overview

Ramji, S., Saugstad, O. D., & Jain, A. (2015). Current concepts of oxygen therapy in neonates. *The Indian Journal of Pediatrics, 82*(1), 46–52.

Resnik, R. (2015). Fetal growth restriction: Evaluation and management. *UpToDate*. Retrieved from http://www.uptodate.com/contents/fetal-growth-restriction-evaluation-and-management

Rondinelli, J., Long, K., Seelinger, C., Crawford, C. L., & Valdez, R. (2015). Factors related to nurse comfort when caring for families experiencing perinatal loss. *Journal for Nurses in Professional Development, 31*(3), 158–163.

Rossman, B., Greene, M. M., & Meier, P. P. (2015). The role of peer support in the development of maternal identity for 'NICU moms'. *JOGNN: Journal of Obstetric, Gynecologic & Neonatal Nursing, 44*(1), 3–16.

Sabic, D., Blattner, C., & Metts, M. (2015). Newborn and infant pain control. *Clinical Pediatrics, 54*(7), 613–614

Simpson, L. (2015). *Best Practices in high-risk pregnancy: An issue of obstetrics and gynecology clinics, 42*(2). Philadelphia, PA: Elsevier Health Sciences.

Steen, S. E. (2015). Perinatal death: Bereavement interventions used by US and Spanish nurses and midwives. *International Journal of Palliative Nursing, 21*(2), 79–86.

U.S. Department of Health and Human Services. (2016). *Healthy People 2020*. Retrieved from http://www.healthypeople.gov/

Valeri, B. O., Holsti, L., & Linhares, M. B. (2015). Neonatal pain and developmental outcomes in children born preterm: A systematic review. *The Clinical Journal of Pain, 31*(4), 355–362.

Vali, P., Mathew, B., & Lakshminrusimha, S. (2015). Neonatal resuscitation: Evolving strategies. *Maternal Health, Neonatology and Perinatology, 1*(1), 4–23.

Verklan, M. T., & Walden, M. (2015). *Core curriculum for neonatal intensive care nursing* (5th ed.). St. Louis, MO: Saunders.

Watchko, J. F. (2015). Common hematologic problems in the newborn nursery. *Pediatric Clinics of North America, 62*(2), 509–524.

White, C., & Wilson, V. (2015). A longitudinal study of aspects of a hospital's family-centred nursing: Changing practice through data translation. *Journal of Advanced Nursing, 71*(1), 100–114. doi:10.1111/jan.12478.

White-Traut, R. (2015). Nurse management of the NICU environment is critical to optimal infant development. *Journal of Obstetric, Gynecologic, & Neonatal Nursing, 44*(2), 169–170.

Yamada, J., Stevens, B., Sidani, S., & Watt-Watson, J. (2015). Test of a process evaluation checklist to improve neonatal pain practices. *Western Journal of Nursing Research, 37*(5), 581–598.

Yousaf, U. F., Hayat, S., & Afzal, N. (2015). Resuscitation of newborn in high risk deliveries. *Journal of Ayub Medical College Abbottabad, 27*(2), 343–345.

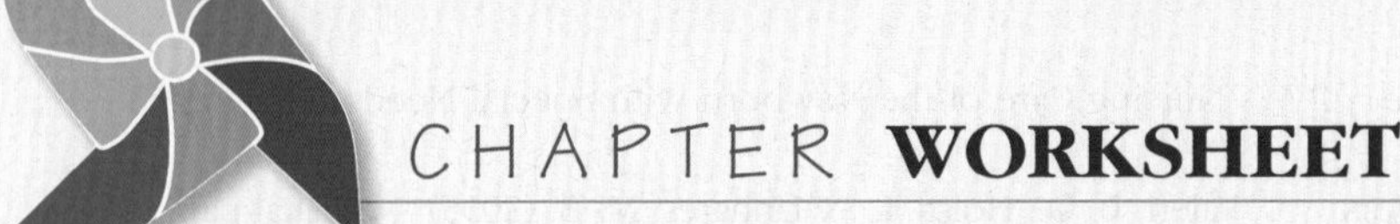

CHAPTER WORKSHEET

MULTIPLE-CHOICE QUESTIONS

1. The nurse documents that a newborn is postterm based on the understanding that he was born after:
   a. 38 weeks' gestation
   b. 40 weeks' gestation
   c. 42 weeks' gestation
   d. 44 weeks' gestation

2. SGA and LGA newborns have an excessive number of red blood cells related to:
   a. Hypoxia
   b. Hypoglycemia
   c. Hypocalcemia
   d. Hypothermia

3. Because subcutaneous and brown fat stores were used for survival in utero, the nurse would assess an SGA newborn for which of the following?
   a. Hyperbilirubinemia
   b. Hypothermia
   c. Polycythemia
   d. Hypoglycemia

4. In assessing a preterm newborn, which of the following findings would be of greatest concern?
   a. Milia over the bridge of the nose
   b. Thin transparent skin
   c. Poor muscle tone
   d. Heart murmur

5. In dealing with parents experiencing a perinatal loss, which of the following nursing interventions would be most appropriate?
   a. Sheltering the parents from the bad news
   b. Making all the decisions regarding care
   c. Encouraging them to participate in the newborn's care
   d. Leaving them by themselves to allow time to grieve

6. The nurse is providing care to several newborns with variations in gestational age and birthweight. When developing the plan of care for these newborns, the nurse focuses on energy conservation to promote growth and development. Which measures would the nurse include in the nursing plans of care? Select all that apply.
   a. Keeping the handling of the newborn to a minimum
   b. Maintaining a neutral thermal environment
   c. Decreasing environmental stimuli
   d. Initiating early oral feedings
   e. Using thermal warmers in all cribs

7. Which of the following concepts would the nurse incorporate into the plan of care when assessing pain in a newborn with special needs?
   a. Newborns experience pain primarily with surgical procedures.
   b. Preterm newborns in the NICU are at least risk for pain.
   c. Pain assessment needs to be comprehensive and frequent.
   d. A newborn's facial expression is the primary indicator of pain.

8. Evidence-based practice refers to the use of which of the following to validate your practice?
   a. Research findings
   b. Written guidelines
   c. Traditional practices
   d. Institutional policies

CRITICAL THINKING EXERCISES

1. After fetal distress was noted on the monitor, a postterm newborn was delivered via a difficult vacuum extraction. The newborn had low Apgar scores and had to be resuscitated before being transferred to the nursery. Once admitted, the nurse observed the following behaviors: jitteriness, tremors, hypotonia, lethargy, and rapid respirations.
   a. What might these behaviors indicate?
   b. For what other conditions might this newborn be at high risk?
   c. What intervention is needed to address this newborn's condition?

2. A preterm newborn was born at 35 weeks following an abruptio placenta due to a car accident. He was transported to the NICU at a nearby regional medical center. After being stabilized, he was placed in an isolette close to the door and placed on a cardiac monitor. A short time later, the nurse notices that he is cool to the touch and lethargic, has a weak cry, and has an axillary temperature of 36° C.
   a. What might have contributed to this newborn's hypothermic condition?
   b. What transfer mechanism may have been a factor?
   c. What intervention would be appropriate for the nurse to initiate?

CHAPTER WORKSHEET

3. A term SGA newborn weighing 4 pounds was brought to the nursery for admission a short time after birth. The labor and birth nurse reports the mother was a heavy smoker and a cocaine addict and experienced physical abuse throughout her pregnancy. After stabilizing the newborn and correcting the hypoglycemia with oral feedings, the nurse observes the following: acrocyanosis, ruddy color, poor circulation to the extremities, tachypnea, and irritability.
   a. What complication might this SGA newborn be manifesting?
   b. What factors may have contributed to this complication?
   c. What would be an appropriate intervention to manage this condition?

STUDY ACTIVITIES

1. At a community health department maternity clinic, secure permission to interview the parents of a special needs child. Ask about their feelings throughout the experience. How are they managing and coping now?
2. Visit the March of Dimes website and review this group's national campaign to reduce the incidence of prematurity. Are their strategies workable or not? Explain your reasoning.
3. A common metabolic disorder present in both SGA and LGA newborns after birth is ________________.
4. A 10-pound LGA newborn is brought to the nursery after a difficult vaginal birth. The nursery nurse should focus on detecting birth injuries such as ________________.

BRINGING IT ALL TOGETHER: A CASE STUDY

Taylor was born at 29 weeks. Her premature birth has resulted in an increased risk both for respiratory distress and for hypothermia. Her parents, Susan and Harvey, are interested and involved in Taylor's condition and care but are understandably anxious regarding their first child's health status. She is being cared for by nurses in the neonatal intensive care unit (NICU) of the university-affiliated medical center where she was born.

Go to thePoint to find questions to consider about this case.

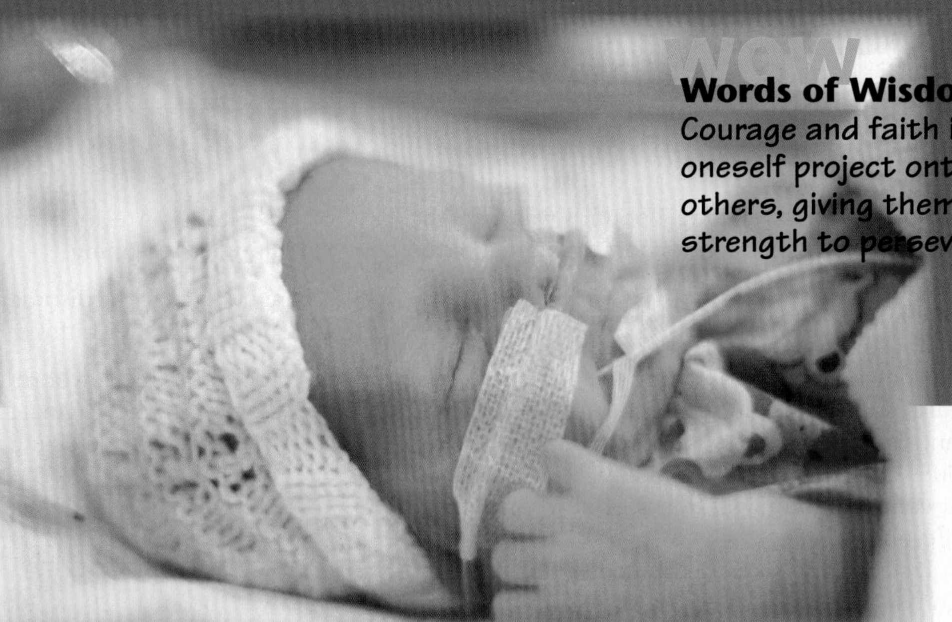

Words of Wisdom
Courage and faith in oneself project onto others, giving them the strength to persevere.

24

Nursing Management of the Newborn at Risk: Acquired and Congenital Newborn Conditions

KEY TERMS

alcohol-related birth defects
anencephaly
asphyxia
acute bilirubin encephalopathy
chronic bilirubin encephalopathy
fetal alcohol spectrum disorder (FASD)
gastroschisis
hyperbilirubinemia
infant of a diabetic mother (IDM)
kernicterus
meconium aspiration syndrome (MAS)
neonatal abstinence syndrome (NAS)
neonatal sepsis
neural tube defect (NTD)
omphalocele
respiratory distress syndrome (RDS)

Learning Objectives

After completion of the chapter, you will be able to:

1. Describe the most common acquired conditions affecting the newborn.
2. Characterize the nursing management of a newborn experiencing respiratory distress syndrome.
3. Outline the birthing room preparation and procedures necessary to prevent meconium aspiration syndrome in the newborn at birth.
4. Differentiate risk factors for the development of necrotizing enterocolitis.
5. Analyze the impact of maternal diabetes on the newborn and the care needed.
6. Evaluate the assessment and intervention for a newborn experiencing substance withdrawal after birth.
7. Develop assessment and nursing management for newborns sustaining trauma and birth injuries.
8. Outline the assessment, interventions, prevention, and management of hyperbilirubinemia in newborns.
9. Summarize the interventions appropriate for a newborn with neonatal sepsis.
10. Research four gastrointestinal system congenital anomalies that can occur in a newborn.
11. Formulate a plan of care for a newborn with an acquired or congenital condition.
12. Relate the importance of parental participation in care of the newborn with a congenital or acquired condition, including the nurse's role in facilitating parental involvement.

***Kelly*, a 27-year-old G2P1, comes to the labor and birth area in active labor. She tells you she is overdue and relieved to finally be giving birth. Her membranes rupture on admission, revealing meconium-stained fluid. What additional nursing assessments need to be carried out now? What risk factors need to be considered when developing Kelly's plan of care?**

INTRODUCTION

Advances in prenatal and neonatal medical and nursing care throughout the industrialized world have led to a marked increase in the number of newborns who have survived a high-risk pregnancy but experience acquired or congenital conditions. These newborns are considered one of our most vulnerable at-risk populations—that is, they are susceptible to morbidity and mortality because of the acquired or congenital disorder. One of the leading health indicators as identified by *Health People 2020* refers to decreasing the number of infant deaths. Acquired and congenital conditions account for a significant percentage of infant deaths. See *Healthy People 2020*.

During the past several decades technologic and pharmacologic advances, genomic discoveries, and standardized policies and procedures have significantly improved survival rates for at-risk newborns. However, the risk of morbidity remains an important sequela. For example, some of these newborns are at risk for continuing health problems that require long-term technologic support. Other newborns remain at risk for physical and developmental problems into the school years and beyond. Although challenges exist in application of these advances to improve the newborn's health, the high-risk newborn will increasingly benefit from them in the future. Providing the complex care needed to maintain the child's health and well-being will have a tremendous emotional and economic impact on the family. Nurses are challenged to provide support to mothers and their families when neonatal well-being is threatened.

Acquired disorders typically occur at or soon after birth. They may result from problems or conditions experienced by the woman during her pregnancy or at birth, such as diabetes, maternal infection, or substance abuse, or conditions associated with labor and birth, such as prolonged rupture of membranes or fetal distress. However, there may be no identifiable cause for the disorder.

Congenital disorders can be defined as structural or functional or metabolic abnormalities at birth. According to the World Health Organization (WHO) (2015), an estimated 1 in 33 infants or over three million fetuses and infants globally are born each year with major congenital disorders (2015). They are found in approximately 3% of all newborns (WHO, 2015). The most common serious defects are congenital heart defects, **neural tube defects**, and Down syndrome (WHO, 2015). Congenital disorders, which often involve a problem with inheritance, include structural anomalies (commonly referred to as birth defects), chromosomal disorders, and inborn errors of metabolism. Most congenital disorders have a complex etiology, involving many interacting genes, gene products, and social and environmental factors during organogenesis (the origin and development of organs). Some alterations can be prevented or compensated for with pharmacologic, nutritional, or other types of interventions, while others cannot be changed. Only through a better understanding of the complex interplay of genetic, environmental, social, and cultural factors can these devastating and life-changing outcomes be prevented (March of Dimes, 2016b).

The field of genomics and genetic medicine has witnessed an explosion of new knowledge, much of it learned from the Human Genome Project. Advances in understanding of the genetic basis of development and function, as well as the interaction of genes and the

HEALTHY PEOPLE 2020

Objective	Nursing Significance
Reduce the rate of fetal and infant deaths	• Foster early and consistent prenatal care.
Decrease the number of all infant deaths (within 1 year) from a baseline of 6.7/1,000 live births to 3.0/1,000 live births.	• Include education to place infants on their backs for naps and sleep to prevent sudden infant death syndrome (SIDS).
Decrease the number of neonatal deaths (within the first 28 days of life) from a baseline of 4.5 to 4.1 deaths/1,000 live births.	• Avoid exposing newborns to cigarette smoke.
Decrease the number of postneonatal deaths from a baseline of 2.2 to 2.0 deaths/1,000 live births.	• Ensure that infants with birth defects receive health care needed in order to thrive.
Reduce the number of deaths related to all birth defects from a baseline of 1.4 to 1.3 deaths/1,000 live births.	

Adapted from U.S. Department of Health and Human Services [USDHHS]. (2016). *Healthy People 2020*. Retrieved from http://healthypeople.gov/2020/default.aspx

environment, continue to foster new insights into human health. This chapter addresses selected acquired and congenital newborn conditions. In addition, it describes the nurse's role in assessment and management, emphasizing parental education and support. Nurses play a key role in helping the parents cope with the stress of having an ill newborn.

ACQUIRED DISORDERS

Acquired disorders are not passed genetically or caused by hereditary or developmental factors; they are obtained after birth by a reaction to environmental influences outside of the body. Examples of acquired disorders include perinatal **asphyxia**, **respiratory distress syndrome (RDS)**, **meconium aspiration syndrome (MAS)**, persistent pulmonary hypertension of the newborn (PPHN), intraventricular hemorrhage, necrotizing enterocolitis (NEC), retinopathy of prematurity, birth trauma, **hyperbilirubinemia**, and newborn infections.

Perinatal Asphyxia

At birth, the newborn's lungs are filled with fluid. This fluid must be cleared and replaced with air for successful respiration to begin after birth. As the newborn makes the transition to life outside the fluid-filled intrauterine environment, dramatic changes must occur to facilitate newborn respirations. Newborns normally start to breathe with routine warming, drying, airway suctioning, and mild stimulation. Most newborns make this transition such that by 1 minute of age, they are breathing well on their own. A newborn who fails to establish adequate, sustained respiration after birth is said to have asphyxia. Perinatal asphyxia, more appropriately known as hypoxic-ischemic encephalopathy, is characterized by clinical and laboratory evidence of acute or subacute brain injury due to systemic hypoxemia or reduced cerebral blood flow (Zanelli, Kaufman, & Stanley, 2015). Physiologically, asphyxia can be defined as impairment in gas exchange resulting in a decrease in blood oxygen levels (hypoxemia) and an excess of carbon dioxide or hypercapnia that leads to acidosis. It occurs when pulmonary oxygenation is delayed or interrupted.

Asphyxia is the most common clinical insult in the perinatal period. As many as 10% of United States' newborns require some degree of active resuscitation to stimulate breathing with 1.5% requiring extensive resuscitation (Cunningham et al., 2014). More than a million newborns who survive asphyxia at birth develop long-term problems such as cerebral palsy, intellectual disability, speech disorders, hearing and/or visual impairment, and learning disabilities (Zanelli et al., 2015).

Pathophysiology

Asphyxia occurs when oxygen delivery is insufficient to meet metabolic demands, resulting in hypoxia, hypercarbia, and metabolic acidosis. Any condition that reduces oxygen delivery to the fetus can result in asphyxia. These conditions may include maternal hypoxia, such as from cardiac or respiratory disease, anemia, or postural hypotension; maternal vascular disease that leads to placental insufficiency, such as diabetes or hypertension; cord problems such as compression or prolapse; and postterm pregnancies, which may trigger meconium release into the amniotic fluid.

Initially, the newborn uses compensatory mechanisms including tachycardia and vasoconstriction to help bring oxygen to the vital organs for a time. However, without intervention, these mechanisms fail, leading to hypotension, bradycardia, and eventually cardiopulmonary arrest.

With failure to breathe well after birth, the newborn will develop hypoxia (too little oxygen in the cells of the body). As a result, the heart rate falls, cyanosis develops, and the newborn becomes hypotonic and unresponsive. Newborn resuscitation is needed to help initiate breathing in newborns that fail to breathe spontaneously at birth.

Nursing Assessment

The key to successful treatment of newborn asphyxia is early identification and recognition of newborns that may be at risk. Review the perinatal history for risk factors, including:

- Trauma: injury to the central or peripheral nervous system secondary to a long or difficult labor, a precipitous birth, multiple gestation, abnormal presentation, cephalopelvic disproportion, shoulder dystocia, or extraction by forceps or vacuum
- Intrauterine asphyxia: for example, fetal hypoxia secondary to maternal hypoxia, diabetes, hypertension, anemia, cord compression, or meconium aspiration
- Sepsis: acquired bacterial or viral organisms from infected amniotic fluid, maternal infection, or direct contact while passing through the birth canal
- Malformation: congenital anomalies including facial or upper airway deformities, renal anomalies, pulmonary hypoplasia, neuromuscular disorders, esophageal atresia, or neural tube defects
- Hypovolemic shock: secondary to abruptio placentae, placenta previa, or cord rupture resulting in blood loss to the fetus
- Medication: drugs given to mother during labor that can affect the fetus by causing placental hypoperfusion and hypotension; use of hypnotics, analgesics, anesthetics, narcotics, oxytocin, and street drugs during pregnancy (Adcock & Stark, 2014).

At birth, assess the newborn immediately. Observe the infant's color, noting any pallor or cyanosis. Assess the work of breathing. Be alert for apnea, tachypnea, gasping respirations, grunting, nasal flaring, or retractions. Evaluate heart rate and note bradycardia. Assess the newborn's temperature, noting hypothermia. Determine the Apgar score at 1 and 5 minutes; if less than 7 at 5 minutes, repeat the assessment at 10 minutes of age. If the initial assessment is poor, begin resuscitation measures until the Apgar score is above 7.

Laboratory or diagnostic testing may be used to identify etiologies for the newborn's asphyxia. For example, a chest x-ray may identify structural abnormalities that might interfere with respiration. A blood culture may identify an infectious process. A blood toxicology screen may detect any maternal drugs in the newborn (Verklan & Walden, 2015).

Methods of testing to identify the fetus at risk for developing perinatal asphyxia continue to be developed and refined. The perinatal nurse needs to be knowledgeable of each test's purpose, capabilities, limitations, and clinical issues. Appropriate nursing interventions based on this knowledge facilitate the testing process and promote the goal of improved perinatal outcome.

Nursing Management

Management of the newborn experiencing asphyxia includes immediate resuscitation. Ensure that the equipment needed for resuscitation is readily available and in working order. Essential equipment includes a wall suction apparatus, an oxygen source, a newborn ventilation bag, endotracheal tubes (2 to 3 mm), infant warmer, surgical blue towels, a laryngoscope, and ampules of naloxone (Narcan) with syringes and needles for administration. Effective ventilation is essential to successful newborn resuscitation. Ventilation is frequently initiated with a manual resuscitation bag and face-mask followed by endotracheal intubation if respiratory depression continues (see Chapter 23 for a more detailed discussion of resuscitation).

Dry the newborn quickly with a warm towel and then place him or her under a radiant heater to prevent rapid heat loss through evaporation. Handling and rubbing the newborn with a dry towel may be all that is needed to stimulate the onset of breathing. If the newborn fails to respond to stimulation, then active resuscitation is needed.

The procedure for newborn resuscitation is easily remembered by the "ABCDs"—airway, breathing, circulation, and drugs (see Chapter 23, Box 23.3). Continue resuscitation until the newborn has a pulse above 100 bpm, a good healthy cry, or good breathing efforts and a pink tongue. This last sign indicates a good oxygen supply to the brain (Jaques & Kennea, 2015).

Take Note!

According to the American Heart Association and American Academy of Pediatrics Emergency Care Guidelines for Neonatal Resuscitation, resuscitation efforts may be stopped if the newborn exhibits no detectable heart rate after 10 minutes of continuous and adequate resuscitation (AHA & AAP, 2014).

Provide continued observation and assessment of the newborn that has been successfully resuscitated. Monitor the newborn's vital signs and oxygen saturation levels closely for changes. Maintain a neutral thermal environment to prevent hypothermia, which would increase the newborn's metabolic and oxygen demands. Check the blood glucose level and observe for signs of hypoglycemia; if this develops, it can further stress the newborn.

The need for resuscitative measures can be extremely upsetting for the parents/partners/significant others. Explain to them the initial resuscitation activities being performed and offer ongoing explanations about any procedures being done, equipment being used, or medications given. Provide presence and support to them throughout the procedure and give frequent updates about procedures being used on their newborn.

Therapeutic hypothermia is a promising neuroprotective intervention for newborns with moderate to severe perinatal encephalopathy after perinatal asphyxia and has currently been incorporated in many neonatal intensive care units (NICUs). However, some infants with encephalopathy will benefit from hypothermia therapy though some will still develop significant adverse outcomes. Cooling the whole body to 33.5°C for 3 days has significant effects on normal physiology as well as pathologic processes. Some of these effects are desirable and neuroprotective, whereas others are not. To enhance the outcome, specific diagnostic predictors are needed to identify newborns likely to benefit from hypothermia treatment (Groenendaal, 2015). This treatment decision must be made a collaborative one with the parents' full understanding of the risks involved. Nurses are in a unique position to detect parent anxiety and to maintain therapeutic communication that may help support them through this crisis.

Provide physical and emotional support to the parents through the initial crisis and throughout the newborn's stay. When the newborn is stable, allow parents to spend time with their newborn to promote bonding (Fig. 24.1). Point out the newborn's positive attributes (color, activity, healthy cry) and give frequent updates on his or her status. Role-model techniques for holding, interacting with, and caring for the newborn will assist to decrease the parents' anxiety.

Nurses need to remember developmental care practices for infants with perinatal asphyxia. A team

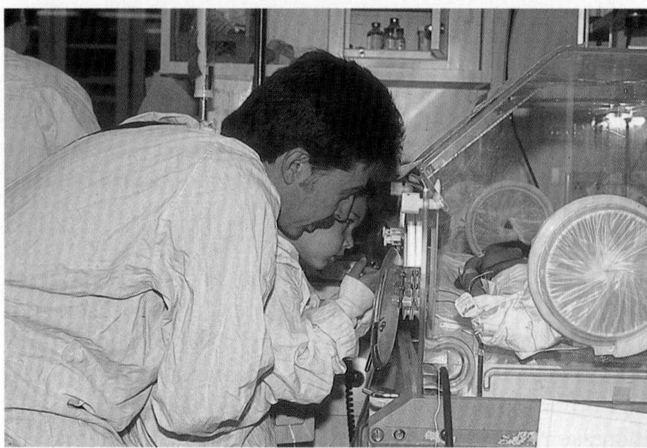

FIGURE 24.1 A father and sibling interacting with his newborn once the newborn's condition has stabilized.

approach incorporating developmental goals and intervention strategies into the nursing care of these infants is essential for optimal developmental outcome. Therapeutic management must always be appropriate for the infant's health status and gestational age. An understanding of the scientific basis for intervention and the therapeutic management techniques for newborns that are sick, recuperating, or convalescing will help the nurse to promote optimal development when caring for the asphyxiated infant (Smith et al., 2015).

Remember Kelly, the young woman described at the beginning of the chapter? Her son is intubated and tracheal suctioning is performed. Positive-pressure ventilation is also started with a self-inflating bag and 50% oxygen. Ventilation is continued for 1 minute and then gradually discontinued. The heart rate is now 120 bpm, and spontaneous respirations are noted. When free-flow oxygen is administered, the newborn begins to cry and turn pink. What continued care is needed in the special care nursery? What explanation should be offered to Kelly regarding her son?

Transient Tachypnea of the Newborn

Transient tachypnea of the newborn (TTN) is a self-limiting condition involving a mild degree of respiratory distress that requires minimal intervention, and resolves over 24 to 72 hours. It is described as the retention of lung fluid or transient pulmonary edema. It usually occurs within a few hours of birth and resolves by 72 hours of age. TTN occurs in approximately 1% to 2% of all live births and incidence is higher in males than females (Swanson & Sinkin, 2015).

Lower gestational age, cesarean birth, and male sex are independent risk factors for TTN. Performing elective cesarean sections no earlier than 39 weeks' gestation may decrease the risk of TTN. Labor before a cesarean section is not sufficient to decrease the frequency of TTN, even after 37 weeks of gestation, whereas vaginal birth appears to be protective against it (Pramanik, Rangaswamy, & Gates, 2015).

Pathophysiology

Most newborns make the transition from fetal to newborn life without incident. During fetal life, the lungs are filled with a serous fluid because the placenta, not the lungs, is used for nutrient and gas exchange. During and after birth, this fluid must be removed and replaced with air. An infant born by cesarean birth is at risk of having excessive pulmonary fluid as a result of not having experienced all the stages of labor. Passage through the birth canal during a vaginal birth compresses the thorax, which helps remove the majority of this fluid. Pulmonary circulation and the lymphatic drainage remove the remaining fluid shortly after birth. TTN occurs when the liquid in the lung is removed slowly or incompletely.

Nursing Assessment

Astutely observe the newborn with respiratory distress because TTN is a diagnosis of exclusion. Initially it might be difficult to distinguish this condition from RDS or group B streptococcal pneumonia, since the clinical picture is similar. However, the symptoms of transient tachypnea rarely last more than 72 hours and if they do, further investigation is warranted (Kim, Yang, & Kim, 2015).

HEALTH HISTORY AND PHYSICAL EXAMINATION

Review the perinatal history for risk factors related to TTN such as absence of labor, cesarean birth, precipitous delivery, prolonged labor, fetal macrosomia, infants born early, male gender, or maternal asthma and maternal smoking. Those factors are associated with a higher risk of TTN (Nagtalon-Ramos, 2014).

Closely assess the newborn for signs of TTN. Within the first few hours of birth, observe for tachypnea, expiratory grunting, retractions, labored breathing, nasal flaring, and mild cyanosis. Mild to moderate respiratory distress is present by 6 hours of age; with respiratory rates as high as 100 to 140 breaths per minute. Also inspect the newborn's chest for hyperextension or a barrel shape. Auscultate breath sounds, which may be slightly diminished secondary to reduced air entry (Fanaroff & Fanaroff, 2014).

LABORATORY AND DIAGNOSTIC TESTING

To aid in the diagnosis, a chest x-ray may be done. It usually reveals mild symmetric lung overaeration and prominent perihilar interstitial markings and streaking. These findings correlate with lymphatic engorgement of retained fetal fluid. In addition, an arterial blood gas (ABG) assessment is important to ascertain the degree of gas exchange and acid–base balance. It typically demonstrates mild hypoxemia, mildly elevated CO_2, and a normal pH (Martin, 2015).

Nursing Management

Management of TTN is supportive. As the retained lung fluid is absorbed by the infant's lymphatic system, the pulmonary status improves. Nursing management focuses on providing adequate oxygenation and determining whether the newborn's respiratory manifestations appear to be resolving or persisting. Provide supportive care while the retained lung fluid is reabsorbed. Administer intravenous (IV) fluids and/or gavage feedings until the respiratory rate decreases enough to allow safe oral feeding. Provide supplemental oxygen via a nasal cannula or oxygen hood to maintain adequate oxygen saturation. Maintain a neutral thermal environment with minimal stimulation to minimize oxygen demand.

Provide ongoing assessment of the newborn's respiratory status. As TTN resolves, the newborn's respiratory rate declines to 60 breaths per minute or less, the oxygen requirement decreases, and the chest x-ray shows resolution of the perihilar streaking. Provide reassurance and progress reports to the parents to help them cope with this crisis.

Respiratory Distress Syndrome

Despite improved survival rates and advances in perinatal care, many high-risk newborns are at risk for respiratory problems, particularly RDS, a breathing disorder resulting from lung immaturity and lack of alveolar surfactant, which keeps the air sacs in the lungs from collapsing and allows them to inflate easily. Without surfactant, the alveoli collapse at the end of expiration. Since the link between RDS and surfactant deficiency was discovered more than 30 years ago, tremendous strides have been made in understanding the pathophysiology and treatment of this disorder. The introduction of prenatal steroids to accelerate lung maturity and the development of synthetic surfactant can be credited with the dramatic improvements in the outcome of newborns with RDS (Pramanik & Rosenkrantz, 2015).

RDS affects an estimated 20,000 to 30,000 infants born alive in the United States annually. The incidence declines with degree of maturity at birth. It occurs in 50% of preterm newborns born at 26 to 28 weeks' gestation, and in 30% of those born at 30 to 31 weeks (Pramanik & Rosenkrantz, 2015). Intensive respiratory care, usually with mechanical ventilation, is necessary.

Pathophysiology

Lung immaturity and surfactant deficiency contribute to the development of RDS. Surfactant is a complex mixture of phospholipids and proteins that adheres to the alveolar surface of the lungs. Anatomically, the immature lung cannot support oxygenation and ventilation, because the alveolar sacs are insufficiently developed, causing a deficient surface area for gas exchange. Physiologically, the amount of surfactant is insufficient to prevent collapse of unstable alveoli. Surfactant forms a coating over the inner surface of the alveoli, reducing the surface tension and preventing alveolar collapse at the end of expiration. In the affected newborn, surfactant is deficient or lacking, and this deficit results in stiff lungs and alveoli that tend to collapse, leading to diffuse atelectasis. The work of breathing is increased because increased pressure similar to that required to initiate the first breath is needed to inflate the lungs with each successive breath. Hypoxemia and acidemia result, leading to vasoconstriction of the pulmonary vasculature. Right-to-left shunting occurs and alveolar capillary circulation is limited, further inhibiting surfactant production. As the disease progresses, fluid and fibrin leak from the pulmonary capillaries, causing hyaline membranes to form in the bronchioles, alveolar ducts, and alveoli. Hyaline membranes produce a glassy appearance in the lung membranes that can be seen on x-rays. These membranes further decrease gas exchange. These factors decrease the total surface area of the gas exchange membrane. The end result is hypoxemia, academia, and a worsening respiratory distress. A vicious cycle is created, compounding the problem (Cunningham et al., 2014).

Nursing Assessment

Nursing assessment focuses on keen observation to identify the signs and symptoms of respiratory distress. In addition, assessment aids in differentiating RDS from other respiratory conditions, such as TTN or group B streptococcal pneumonia.

HISTORY AND PHYSICAL EXAMINATION

Review the history for risk factors associated with RDS. The most common risk factor for the development of RDS is premature birth. Additional risk factors particularly in the term infant include cesarean birth in the absence of preceding labor (related to the lack of thoracic squeezing), male gender, previous birth of an infant with RDS, perinatal asphyxia, cold stress, and maternal diabetes, which produces high levels of insulin which inhibit surfactant production (Rubarth & Quinn, 2015).

Take Note!

Prolonged rupture of membranes, gestational or chronic maternal hypertension, maternal narcotic addiction, and use of prenatal corticosteroids reduce the newborn's risk for RDS because of the physiologic stress imposed on the fetus. Chronic stress experienced by the fetus in utero accelerates the production of surfactant before 35 weeks' gestation and thus reduces the incidence of RDS at birth (Pramanik, & Rosenkrantz, 2015).

The newborn with RDS usually demonstrates signs at birth or within a few hours of birth. Observe the infant for expiratory grunting, shallow breathing, nasal flaring, chest wall retractions (Fig. 24.2), seesaw respirations, and generalized cyanosis. Auscultate the heart and lungs, noting tachycardia (rates above 150 to 180), fine inspiratory crackles, and tachypnea (rates above 60 breaths per minute).

The Silverman–Anderson Index is an assessment scoring system that can be used to evaluate five parameters of work of breathing as it assigns a numerical score for each parameter. Each category is scored as "0" for normal, "1" for moderate impairment, or "2" for severe impairment. Parameters assessed are retractions of the upper chest, lower chest, and xiphoid; nasal flaring; and expiratory grunt. Normally functioning infants should have a cumulative score of 0, whereas critically ill and severely depressed infants will have scores closer to 10 (Fig. 24.3).

LABORATORY AND DIAGNOSTIC TESTING

The diagnosis of RDS is based on the clinical picture, a lung ultrasound, or x-ray findings and arterial blood gases that show hypoxemia and acidosis. A chest x-ray reveals hypoaeration, underexpansion, and a "ground glass" pattern (Pramanik et al., 2015).

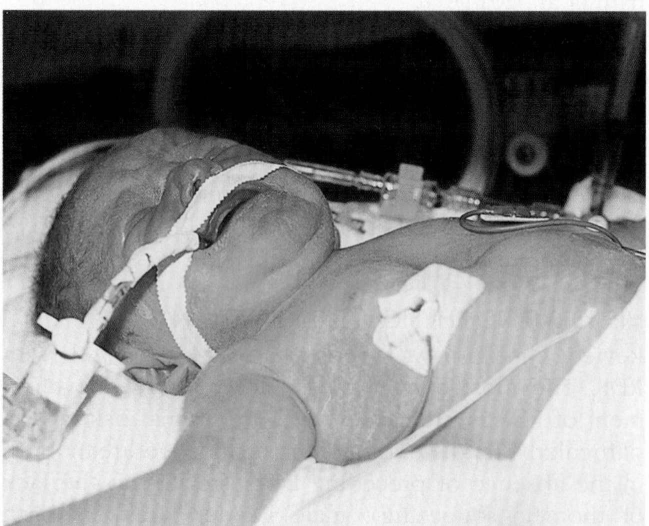

FIGURE 24.2 Sternal retractions are a sign of respiratory distress requiring immediate intervention, such as mechanical ventilation and other monitoring devices. (Copyright Caroline Brown, RNC, MS, DEd.)

Nursing Management

If untreated, RDS will worsen. In many infants respiratory symptoms decline after 72 hours, paralleling the production of surfactant in the alveoli (Gardner et al., 2016). The newborn needs supportive care until surfactant is produced. Effective therapies for established RDS include conventional mechanical ventilation, continuous positive airway pressure (CPAP), or positive end-expiratory pressure (PEEP) to prevent volume loss during expiration, and surfactant therapy. The use of exogenous surfactant replacement therapy to stabilize the newborn's lungs until postnatal surfactant synthesis matures has become a standard of care, but not necessarily evidence based. Knowledge of the surfactant proteins and lipids produced by the epithelial II cells were critical in the development of surfactant-replacement preparations used to treat RDS. This preparation has dramatically improved morbidity and mortality in preterm infants (Blennow & Bohlin, 2015; Whitsett, Wert, & Weaver, 2015).

Despite recent advances in the perinatal management of neonatal RDS, controversies still exist. Strong evidence exists for the role of a single course of prenatal steroids in RDS prevention, but the potential benefit and long-term safety of repeated courses are unclear. A Cochrane review concluded that the incidence of RDS was reduced in infants born before 48 hours and between 1 and 7 days of treatment of mothers with prenatal corticosteroids, but not those born <24 hours of administration (Gaur et al., 2015). Many practices involved in preterm neonatal stabilization at birth are not evidence based, including oxygen administration and positive-pressure lung inflation, and they may at times be harmful. Surfactant replacement therapy is crucial in the management of RDS, but the best preparation, optimal dose and timing of administration at different gestations has not been scientifically established. Respiratory support in the form of mechanical ventilation may also be lifesaving, but can cause lung injury, and protocols should be directed at avoiding mechanical ventilation where possible by using nasal CPAP or nasal ventilation. For newborns with RDS to have best outcomes, it is essential that they have optimal supportive care, including maintenance of a normal body temperature, proper fluid management, good nutritional support, and support of the circulation to maintain adequate tissue perfusion (Gardner et al., 2016).

As recommended, care of the newborn with RDS is primarily supportive and requires a multidisciplinary approach to obtain the best outcomes. Therapy focuses on improving oxygenation and maintaining optimal lung volumes. Expect to transfer the newborn to the NICU soon after birth. Apply the basic principles of

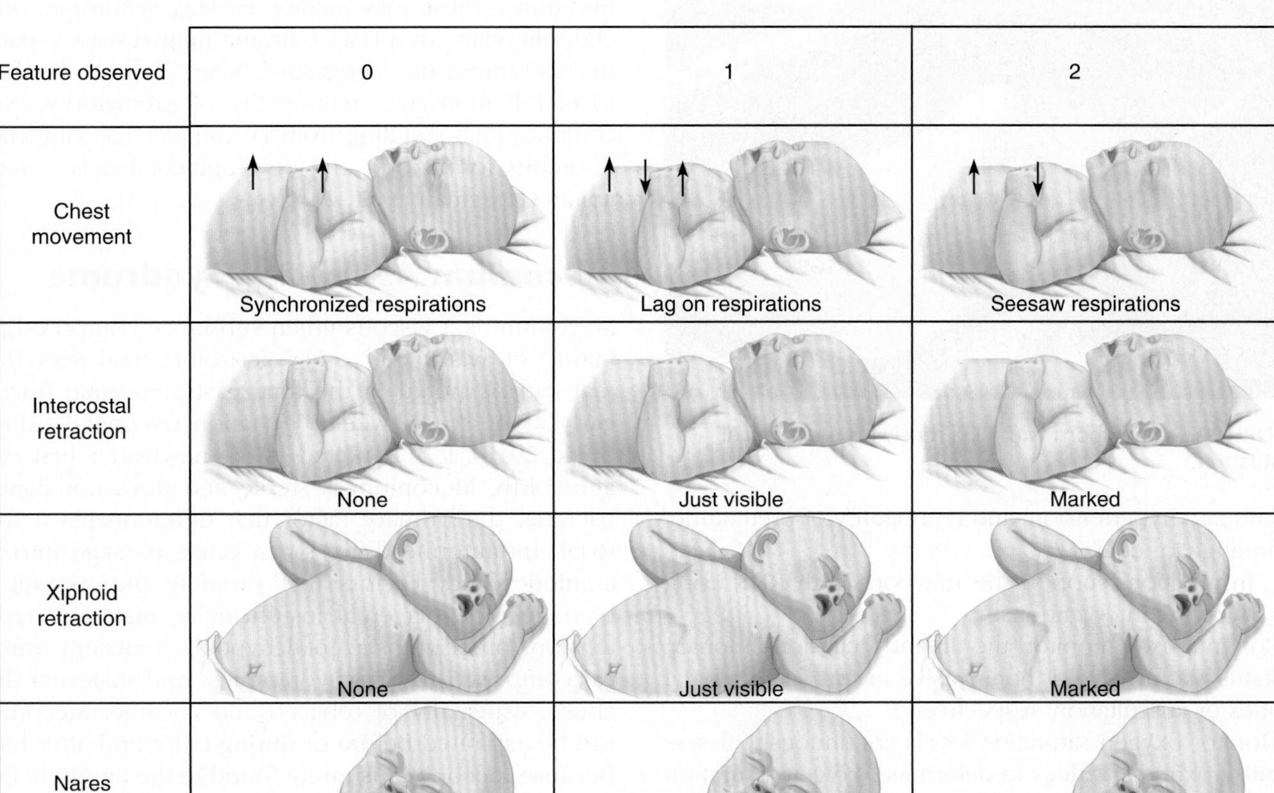

Score
Feature observed
0
1
2
Chest movement
Synchronized respirations
Lag on respirations
Seesaw respirations
Intercostal retraction
None
Just visible
Marked
Xiphoid retraction
None
Just visible
Marked
Nares dilation
None
Minimal
Marked
Expiratory grunt
None
Audible by stethoscope
Audible by unaided ear

FIGURE 24.3 Assessing the degree of respiratory distress. (Used with permission from Silverman, W. A., & Anderson, D. H. (1956). A controlled clinical trial of effects of water mist on obstructive respiratory signs, death rate, and necroscopy findings among premature infants. *Pediatrics, 17*(4), 1–9.)

newborn care, such as thermoregulation, cardiovascular and nutritional support, normal glucose level maintenance, and infection prevention, to achieve the therapeutic goals of reducing mortality and minimizing lung trauma.

Anticipate the administration of surfactant replacement therapy, prophylactically or as a rescue approach. With prophylactic administration, surfactant is given within minutes after birth, thus providing replacement surfactant before severe RDS develops. Rescue treatment is indicated for newborns with established RDS who require mechanical ventilation and supplemental oxygen. The earlier the surfactant is administered, the better the effect on gas exchange. Following surfactant administration, the newborn must be closely monitored, and preparation for reduced need for oxygen and ventilation should be anticipated (Mattson & Smith, 2015).

Administer the prescribed oxygen concentration via nasal cannula. Anticipate the need for ventilator therapy, which has greatly improved in the past several years, with significant advances in conventional and high-frequency ventilation therapies (Fig. 24.4). Recent studies show no difference in outcomes for newborns who received early treatment with high-frequency oscillatory ventilation compared with those receiving conventional mechanical ventilation. They are both equally effective (Jaecklin, Jarreau, & Kavanagh, 2015). Although mechanical ventilation has increased survival rates, it is also a contributing factor to bronchopulmonary dysplasia,

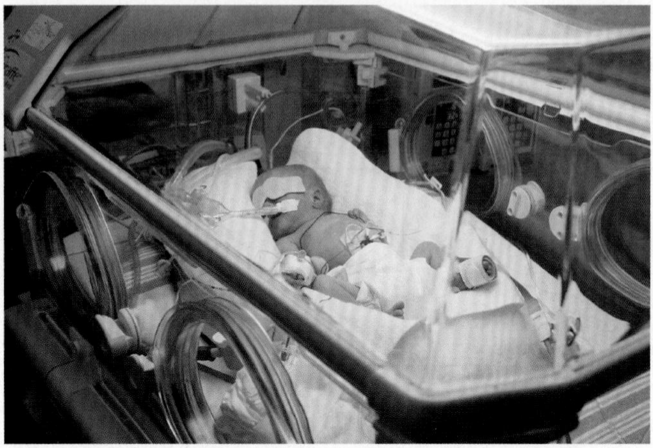

FIGURE 24.4 A newborn with RDS receiving mechanical ventilation.

pulmonary hypertension, and retinopathy of prematurity (Cunningham et al., 2014).

In addition, support the newborn with RDS using the following interventions:

- Continuously monitor the infant's cardiopulmonary status via invasive or noninvasive means (e.g., arterial lines or auscultation, respectively).
- Monitor oxygen saturation levels continuously; assess pulse oximeter values to determine oxygen saturation levels.
- Closely monitor vital signs, acid–base status, and arterial blood gases.
- Administer broad-spectrum antibiotics if blood cultures are positive.
- Administer sodium bicarbonate or acetate as ordered to correct metabolic acidosis.
- Provide fluids and vasopressor agents as needed to prevent or treat hypotension.
- Test blood glucose levels and administer dextrose as ordered for prevention or treatment of hypoglycemia.
- Cluster caretaking activities to avoid overtaxing and compromising the newborn.
- Place the newborn in the prone position to optimize respiratory status and reduce stress.
- Perform gentle suctioning to remove secretions and maintain a patent airway.
- Assess level of consciousness to identify intraventricular hemorrhage.
- Monitor x-ray studies to detect atelectasis or air leak.
- Maintain a neutral thermal environment to reduce metabolic and oxygen needs.
- Provide sufficient calories via gavage and IV feedings.
- Maintain adequate hydration and assess for signs of fluid overload.
- Provide information to the parents about treatment modalities; give thorough but simple explanations about the rationales for interventions.
- Encourage the parents to participate in care (Mattson & Smith, 2015; Verklan & Walken, 2015).

Provide ongoing assessment and be alert for complications. These may include air leak syndrome, bronchopulmonary dysplasia (chronic lung disease), patent ductus arteriosus, congestive heart failure, intraventricular hemorrhage, retinopathy of prematurity, NEC, complications resulting from IV catheter use (infection, thrombus formation), and developmental delay or disability (Kliegman et al., 2015).

Meconium Aspiration Syndrome

Meconium is a viscous green substance composed primarily of water and other gastrointestinal secretions that can be noted in the fetal gastrointestinal tract as early as 10 to 16 weeks' gestation (Neonatal eHandbook, 2015). It is expelled as the newborn's first stool after birth. Meconium is sterile and does not contain bacteria, the primary factor that differentiates it from stool. Intrauterine distress can cause passage into the amniotic fluid. Factors that promote the passage in utero include placental insufficiency, maternal hypertension, preeclampsia, fetal hypoxia, transient umbilical compression, oligohydramnios, and maternal drug abuse, especially of tobacco and cocaine. Meconium can be aspirated before or during labor and after birth. Because meconium is rarely found in the amniotic fluid prior to 34 weeks' gestation, it mainly impacts infants born at term and postterm (Haakonsen Lindenskov et al., 2015). It is usually expelled as the newborn's first stool after birth.

MAS occurs when the newborn inhales particulate meconium mixed with amniotic fluid into the lungs while still in utero or on taking the first breath after birth. It is a common cause of newborn respiratory distress and can lead to severe illness. Meconium staining of the amniotic fluid, with the possibility of aspiration, occurs in approximately 10% to 16% of births after 34 weeks' gestation (Garcia-Prats, 2015). Aspiration induces airway obstruction, surfactant dysfunction, hypoxia, and chemical pneumonitis with inflammation of pulmonary tissues. Only 5% of infants with meconium-stained amniotic fluid actually progress to MAS (Clark & Clark, 2014). Severe MAS can lead to persistent pulmonary hypertension and death. The use of surfactant and inhaled nitric oxide has led to the decreased mortality and the need for extracorporeal membrane oxygenation (ECMO).

Pathophysiology

The pathophysiology of MAS is complex, and the timing of the insult resulting in aspiration remains controversial. Meconium may be passed in utero secondary to hypoxic stress. Hypoxia induces the fetus to gasp or attempt to breathe. The fetus may bear down and pass meconium into the amniotic fluid or he or she may experience a vagal reflex that causes relaxation of the anal sphincter, allowing meconium to be passed into the amniotic fluid. The fetus then sucks or swallows this amniotic fluid in utero, or the infant may aspirate meconium with the first breath after birth as air rushes into the lungs.

Although the etiology is not well understood, the effects of meconium can be harmful to the fetus. Meconium alters the amniotic fluid by reducing antibacterial activity and subsequently increasing the risk of perinatal bacterial infection. Additionally, meconium is very irritating because it contains enzymes from the fetal pancreas.

When aspirated into the lungs, meconium blocks the bronchioles, causing an inflammatory reaction as well as a decrease in surfactant production. Gas exchange is impaired and atelectasis occurs. A ball-valve effect occurs when air is inspired into the alveoli but cannot be fully expired secondary to reduced airway diameter. Significant respiratory distress is followed by persistent pulmonary hypertension, right-to-left shunting of blood, and patent ductus arteriosus. Conventional mechanical ventilation, ECMO, nitric oxide, high-frequency ventilation, or liquid ventilation may be necessary (Clark & Clark, 2014).

Nursing Assessment

Review prenatal and birth records to identify newborns that may be at high risk for meconium aspiration. Predisposing factors for MAS include postterm pregnancy; breech presentation, forceps, or vacuum extraction births; nulliparity; ethnicity (Pacific Islander, Indigenous Australian, African-American); intrapartum fever; low Apgar score; prolonged or difficult labor associated with fetal distress in a term or postterm newborn; maternal drug abuse, especially of tobacco and cocaine; maternal infection/chorioamnionitis; maternal hypertension or diabetes; oligohydramnios; fetal growth restriction; prolapsed cord; or acute or chronic placental insufficiency (Choi et al., 2015).

Assess the amniotic fluid for meconium staining when the maternal membranes rupture. Green-stained amniotic fluid suggests the presence of meconium in the amniotic fluid and should be reported immediately. After birth, note any yellowish-green staining of the umbilical cord and nails and skin. This staining indicates that meconium has been present for some time.

Consider Kelly, the 27-year-old woman who gave birth to a son who required resuscitation. What findings would lead the nurse to suspect that her son aspirated meconium? What risk factors in Kelly's history would support the diagnosis of meconium aspiration syndrome?

Take Note!

Standard prevention and treatment for meconium aspiration syndrome previously included suctioning the mouth and nares upon head delivery before body delivery. However, recent evidence suggests that aspiration occurs in utero, not at delivery; therefore, the infant's birth should not be impeded for suctioning. After full delivery, the infant should be handed to a neonatal team for evaluation and treatment. Although infants previously have been given intubation and airway suctioning, routine tracheal suction is recommended only for depressed infants (e.g., nonvigorous with depressed tone and respirations and/or heart rate <100 bpm) and those with respiratory symptoms. Use of orogastric suctioning to prevent MAS is not supported by evidence from current studies. Guidelines suggest not stimulating infants born with meconium staining with vigorous sucking, to avoid aspiration (Gardner et al., 2016).

Observe the newborn for a barrel-shaped chest with an increased anterior-posterior (AP) chest diameter (similar to that found in a client with chronic obstructive pulmonary disease), prolonged tachypnea, progression from mild to severe respiratory distress, intercostal retractions, end-expiratory grunting, and cyanosis (Clark & Clark, 2014). Auscultate the lungs, noting coarse crackles and rhonchi.

Chest x-rays show patchy, fluffy infiltrates unevenly distributed throughout the lungs and marked hyperaeration mixed with areas of atelectasis. ABG analysis will indicate metabolic acidosis with a low blood pH, decreased PaO_2, and increased $PaCO_2$ (Gardner et al., 2016). Direct visualization of the vocal cords for meconium staining using an appropriate size laryngoscope is needed to confirm the presence of meconium below the larynx.

Nursing Management

Nursing management focuses on ensuring adequate tissue perfusion and minimizing oxygen demand and energy expenditure. Caring for the newborn with meconium aspiration begins in the birthing unit when the birth attendant identifies meconium-stained amniotic fluid with membrane rupture during labor. Upon delivery of the newborn's head, before the newborn takes the first breath, the nasal cavity and then the posterior pharynx are gently wiped to decrease the potential for aspiration. If the newborn is significantly depressed at birth, secondary clearing of the lower airways by direct tracheal suctioning may be necessary. Repeated suctioning and stimulation are limited to prevent overstimulation and further depression. In pregnancies complicated by meconium-stained amniotic fluid, suctioning of the hypopharynx before the birth of the infant's shoulders and postnatal suction of vigorous infants have been used in an effort to clear the airway and decrease the incidence and the severity of MAS. Based on the results of two large randomized controlled studies, international guidelines from scientific societies for intrapartum and postpartum management of pregnancies with meconium-stained amniotic fluid have radically changed. Intrapartum suction and postnatal intubation and suction of vigorous infants are no longer recommended (Hudson, 2015). Usually the newborn is transferred to the NICU for close monitoring.

Maintain a neutral thermal environment, including placing the newborn under a radiant warmer or in a warmed isolette, to prevent hypothermia. In addition, minimize handling to reduce energy expenditure and oxygen consumption that could lead to further hypoxemia and acidosis.

Administer oxygen therapy as ordered via nasal cannula or with positive-pressure ventilation. Monitor oxygen saturation levels via pulse oximetry to evaluate the newborn's response to treatment and to detect changes. Increased pulmonary pressures associated with meconium aspiration may cause blood to be shunted away from the lungs. The newborn may exhibit uneven pulmonary ventilation, with hyperinflation in some areas and atelectasis in others. This leads to poor perfusion and subsequent hypoxemia, which in turn may increase pulmonary vasoconstriction, resulting in a worsening of hypoxemia and acidosis.

Expect to administer hyperoxygenation to dilate the pulmonary vasculature and close the ductus arteriosus or nitric oxide inhalation to decrease pulmonary vascular resistance, or to use high-frequency oscillatory ventilation to increase the chance of air trapping (Clark & Clark, 2014). In addition, administer vasopressors and pulmonary vasodilators as prescribed and administer surfactant as ordered to counteract inactivation by meconium. Monitor ABG results for changes and assist with measures to correct acid–base imbalances to facilitate perfusion of tissues and prevent pulmonary hypertension (Cunningham et al., 2014). If these measures are ineffective, be prepared to assist with the use of ECMO, a modified type of heart–lung machine.

In addition, perform the following interventions:

- Cluster newborn care to minimize oxygen demand.
- Maintain an optimal thermal environment to minimize oxygen consumption.
- Prevent and treat any complications such as hypotension, metabolic acidosis, or anemia.
- Incorporate developmental care practices when applicable.
- Pay special attention to systemic blood volume and blood pressure to reduce right-to-left shunting through the patent ductus.
- Administer broad-spectrum antibiotics to treat bacterial pneumonia.
- Administer sedation to reduce agitation and oxygen consumption.
- Continuously monitor the newborn's condition (cardiac and respiratory status, oximetry).
- Provide continuous reassurance and support to the parents throughout the experience (Gardner et al., 2016; Verklan & Walden, 2015).

Persistent Pulmonary Hypertension of the Newborn

PPHN, previously referred to as persistent fetal circulation, is a cardiopulmonary disorder characterized by marked pulmonary hypertension that causes right-to-left extrapulmonary shunting of blood and hypoxemia. It occurs when the newborn's circulatory system does not have normal transition after birth. PPHN can occur idiopathically or as a complication of perinatal asphyxia, MAS, maternal smoking, maternal obesity, hypocalcemia, maternal asthma, pneumonia, congenital heart defects, metabolic disorders such as hypoglycemia, hypothermia, hypovolemia, hyperviscosity, acute hypoxia with delayed resuscitation, sepsis, and RDS. It occurs in 2 to 6 newborns per 1,000 live births of term, near-term, or postterm infants. Current research findings link increased risk of developing PPHN to exposure to selective serotonin reuptake inhibitors (SSRIs) (antidepressants) in late pregnancy (Huybrechts, 2015). Treatment of depression with antidepressants is complicated by the mother's needs. Careful consideration must be given to the risks, benefits, and alternatives of utero medication exposure, and this should be discussed with the woman.

Pathophysiology

Normally, pulmonary artery pressure decreases when the newborn takes the first breath. However, interference with this ability to breathe allows pulmonary pressures to remain increased. Hypoxemia and acidosis also occur, leading to vasoconstriction of the pulmonary artery. These events cause an elevation in pulmonary vascular resistance. Normally, the decrease in pulmonary artery pressure and pulmonary vascular resistance with breathing leads to the closure of the ductus arteriosus and foramen ovale. However, with PPHN pulmonary vascular resistance is elevated to the point that venous blood is diverted to some degree through fetal shunts (i.e., the ductus arteriosus and foramen ovale) into the systemic circulation, bypasses the lungs, and results in systemic arterial hypoxemia.

Nursing Assessment

Assess the newborn's status closely. A newborn with persistent pulmonary hypertension demonstrates tachypnea within 12 hours after birth. Observe for marked cyanosis, grunting, respiratory distress with tachypnea, and retractions. Auscultate the heart, noting a systolic ejection harsh sound (tricuspid insufficiency murmur), and measure blood pressure for hypotension resulting from both heart failure and persistent hypoxemia (Kenner & Lott, 2014). Measure oxygen saturation via pulse oximetry and report low values. Prepare the newborn for an echocardiogram, which will reveal right-to-left shunting of blood that confirms the diagnosis.

Nursing Management

Nursing management focuses on ensuring adequate tissue profusion and minimizing oxygen demand and energy expenditure. When caring for the newborn with persistent pulmonary hypertension, pay meticulous attention to detail, with continuous monitoring of the newborn's oxygenation and perfusion status and blood pressure. The goals of therapy include improving alveolar oxygenation, inducing metabolic alkalosis by administering sodium bicarbonate, correcting hypovolemia and hypotension with the administration of volume replacement and vasopressors, and anticipating use of ECMO when support has failed to maintain acceptable oxygenation (Kim et al., 2015).

Provide immediate resuscitation after birth and administer oxygen therapy as ordered. Early and effective resuscitation and correction of acidosis and hypoxia are helpful in preventing persistent pulmonary hypertension. Monitor arterial blood gases frequently to evaluate the effectiveness of oxygen therapy. Provide respiratory support, which frequently necessitates the use of mechanical ventilation. Administer prescribed medications, monitor cardiopulmonary status, cluster care to reduce stimulation, and provide ongoing support and education to the parents.

Take Note!

Almost any procedure, such as suctioning, weighing, changing diapers, or positioning, can precipitate severe hypoxemia due to the instability of the pulmonary vasculature. Therefore, minimize the newborn's exposure to stimulation as much as possible.

Periventricular-Intraventricular Hemorrhage

Periventricular-intraventricular hemorrhage (PVH-IVH) is defined as bleeding that usually originates in the subependymal germinal matrix region of the brain, often extending into the ventricular system (Annibale, 2014). IVH occurs in up to 50% of infants with birthweight less than 1,500 g and/or born at less than 35 weeks' gestation. It is uncommon in term neonates but may occur with birth trauma or asphyxia (Annibale, 2014). Complications resulting from IVH include hydrocephalus, seizure disorder, periventricular leukomalacia (an ischemic injury resulting from inadequate perfusion of the white matter adjacent to the ventricles), cerebral palsy, learning disabilities, vision or hearing deficits, and cognitive impairment (Adcock, 2015).

Pathophysiology

The pathogenesis of PVH-IVH is attributed to the intrinsic weakness of germinal vasculature and to the fluctuation in the cerebral blood flow. Genetics appear to play a role in this condition (Szpecht et al., 2015). The preterm newborn is at greatest risk for IVH because cerebral vascular development is immature, making it more vulnerable to injury. The earlier the newborn is, the greater the likelihood for brain damage. While all areas of the brain can be injured, the periventricular area is the most vulnerable (Gardner et al., 2016).

Each ventricular area contains a rich network of capillaries that are very thin, fragile, and easily ruptured. The causes of rupture vary and include fluctuations in systemic and cerebral blood flow, increases in cerebral blood flow from hypertension, IV infusions, seizure activity, increases in cerebral venous pressure due to vaginal delivery, hypoxia, and respiratory distress. With a preterm birth, the fetus is suddenly transported from a well-controlled uterine environment into a highly stimulating one. This tremendous physiologic stress and shock may contribute to the rupture of periventricular capillaries and subsequent hemorrhage. Most hemorrhages occur in the first 72 hours after birth (Annibale, 2014).

Nursing Assessment

The signs of intraventricular hemorrhage vary significantly and some infants may display no clinical signs. Approximately 50% of PVH-IVH occurs by 24 hours of age, and 90% by 72 hours of age (Noori & Seri, 2015). Assess for risk factors such as:

- Preterm birth
- Low birth weight
- Acidosis
- Asphyxia
- Unstable blood pressure
- Seizures
- Acute blood loss or hypovolemia
- Respiratory distress with mechanical ventilation, intubation, apnea, hypoxia, or suctioning
- Use of hyperosmolar solutions or rapid volume expansion

Evaluate the newborn for an unexplained drop in hematocrit, pallor, and poor perfusion as evidenced by respiratory distress and oxygen desaturation. Note seizures, lethargy or other changes in level of consciousness, bulging fontanel, weak sucking, metabolic acidosis, high-pitched cry, or hypotonia. Palpate the anterior fontanel for tenseness. Assess vital signs, noting bradycardia and hypotension. Evaluate laboratory data for changes indicating metabolic acidosis or glucose instability. Frequently a bleed can progress rapidly and result in shock and death. Prepare the newborn for cranial ultrasonography, the diagnostic tool of choice to detect hemorrhage (Verklan & Walden, 2015).

Nursing Management

Prevention of preterm birth is essential in preventing IVH. Identify risk factors that can lead to hemorrhage, and focus care on interventions to decrease the risk of hemorrhage. For example, institute measures to prevent perinatal asphyxia and birth trauma and provide developmental care in the NICU. If a preterm birth is expected, having the mother deliver at a tertiary care facility with an NICU would be most appropriate.

Care of the newborn with IVH is primarily supportive. Correct anemia, acidosis, and hypotension with fluids and medications. Administer fluids slowly to prevent fluctuations in blood pressure. Avoid rapid volume expansion to minimize changes in cerebral blood flow. Keep the newborn in a flexed, contained position with the head elevated to prevent or minimize fluctuations in intracranial pressure. Continuously monitor the newborn for signs of hemorrhage, such as changes in the level of consciousness, bulging fontanel, seizures, apnea, and reduced activity level. Also, measuring head circumference daily to assess for expansion in size is essential in identifying complications early.

Minimize handling of the newborn by clustering nursing care, and limit stimulation in the newborn's environment to reduce stress. Also reduce the newborn's exposure to noxious stimuli to avoid a fluctuation in blood pressure and energy expenditure. Provide adequate oxygenation to promote tissue perfusion but controlled ventilation to decrease the risk of pneumothorax. Developmental care principles include avoiding lifting the lower extremities above the midline with diaper changes, giving rapid fluid boluses, and high oxygen and ventilation, as these can increase the chance of more cranial hemorrhage (Green, 2016).

Support for the parents to cope with the diagnosis and potential long-term sequelae is essential. The long-term neurodevelopmental outcome is determined by the severity of the bleed. Provide education and emotional support for the parents throughout the newborn's stay. Discuss expectations for short-term and long-term care needs with the parents and assist them in obtaining the necessary support from appropriate community resources (Gardner et al., 2016).

Necrotizing Enterocolitis

NEC is an inflammatory disease of the bowel which can cause ischemic and necrotic injury in the gastrointestinal tract. It is the most common and most serious acquired gastrointestinal disorder among hospitalized preterm neonates and is associated with significant acute and chronic morbidity and mortality. NEC occurs in approximately 10% of infants who weigh less than 1,500 g, with mortality rates up to 50% (Johnson et al., 2015). Attempts to improve gastrointestinal function and reduce the risk of NEC include enteral antibiotics, judicious administration of parenteral fluids, human milk feedings, antenatal corticosteroids, enteral probiotics (*Lactobacillus acidophilus*), and slow continuous drip feedings (Springer & Annibale, 2016a).

Pathophysiology

The pathophysiology of NEC is not clearly understood and is thought to be multifactorial in nature. Current research points to three major pathologic mechanisms that lead to NEC: bowel hypoxic-ischemia events, perinatal stressors, an immature intestinal barrier, abnormal bacterial colonization, and formula feeding. The intestine of a preterm infant is characterized underdeveloped immune defenses and compromised mucosal barrier function. As a result, the immune intestine is susceptible to bacterial colonization by opportunistic pathogens, which follows oral feeding, which in turn incites an inflammatory response (Lim, Golden, & Ford, 2015).

During perinatal or postnatal stress, oxygen is shunted away from the gut to more important organs such as the heart and brain. Ischemia and intestinal wall damage occur, allowing bacteria to invade. High-solute feedings allow bacteria to flourish. Mucosal or transmucosal necrosis of part of the intestine occurs. Although any region of the bowel can be affected, the distal ileum and proximal colon are the regions most commonly involved. NEC usually occurs between 3 and 12 days of life, but it can occur weeks later in some newborns (Springer & Annibale, 2016). See for links to websites that provide additional information.

Nursing Assessment

NEC can be devastating, and astute assessment is crucial. Assessing the newborn for the development of NEC includes the health history and physical examination as well as laboratory and diagnostic testing. The onset of NEC is heralded by the development of feeding intolerance, abdominal distention, and bloody stools in a preterm infant receiving enteral feedings. As the disease worsens, the infant develops signs and symptoms of septic shock (respiratory distress, temperature instability, lethargy, hypotension, and oliguria). Nurses need to be suspicious of this condition in caring for this preterm infant.

HEALTH HISTORY AND PHYSICAL EXAMINATION

Assess the newborn's history for risk factors associated with NEC. In addition to preterm birth, prenatal and postnatal predisposing risk factors are highlighted in Box 24.1.

BOX 24.1

PREDISPOSING FACTORS FOR THE DEVELOPMENT OF NECROTIZING ENTEROCOLITIS

Prenatal Factors

- Preterm labor
- Prolonged rupture of membranes
- Preeclampsia
- Maternal sepsis
- Amnionitis
- Uterine hypoxia

Postnatal Factors

- Respiratory distress syndrome
- Patent ductus arteriosus
- Congenital heart disease
- Exchange transfusion
- Low birthweight
- Low Apgar scores
- Umbilical catheterization
- Hypothermia
- Gastrointestinal infection
- Hypoglycemia
- Asphyxia

Also observe the newborn for common signs and symptoms, which may include:

- Cardiorespiratory baseline changes
- Feeding intolerance
- Abdominal distention and tenderness
- Bloody or hemoccult-positive stools
- Diarrhea
- Respiratory distress
- Metabolic acidosis
- Temperature instability
- Decreased or absent bowel sounds
- Signs of sepsis
- Lethargy
- Apnea
- Shock (Fox, Thacker, & Hendricks-Munoz, 2015).

Always keep the possibility of NEC in mind when dealing with preterm newborns, especially when enteral feedings are being administered. Note respiratory distress, cyanosis, lethargy, decreased activity level, temperature instability, feeding intolerance, diarrhea, bile-stained emesis, or grossly bloody stools. Assess blood pressure, noting hypotension. Evaluate the neonate's abdomen for distention, tenderness, and visible loops of bowel. Measure the abdominal circumference, noting an increase. Determine residual gastric volume prior to feeding; when it is elevated, be suspicious for NEC (Verklan & Walden, 2015).

LABORATORY AND DIAGNOSTIC TESTING

Common laboratory and diagnostic tests ordered for assessment of NEC include:

- Kidney, ureter, and bladder (KUB) of the abdomen x-ray: confirms the presence of pneumatosis intestinalis (air in the bowel wall) and persistently dilated loops of bowel
- An abdominal x-ray to demonstrate dilated bowel loops, abnormal gas patterns, air bubbles that occur from bacteria, and thickened bowel walls
- Blood values: may demonstrate metabolic acidosis, increased white blood cells, thrombocytopenia, neutropenia, electrolyte imbalance, or disseminated intravascular coagulation (DIC) (Springer & Annibale, 2016)

Nursing Management

Nursing management of the newborn with NEC focuses on maintaining fluid and nutritional status, providing supportive care, and teaching the family about the condition and prognosis. Therapeutic management initially consists of bowel rest and antibiotic therapy. Serial kidney, ureter, and bladder x-rays and C-reactive protein levels are used to assess the resolution or progression of NEC. If medical treatment fails to stabilize the newborn or if free air is present on a left lateral decubitus film (where the infant is lying down on the left side), surgical intervention will be necessary to resect the portion of necrotic bowel while preserving as much of the intestinal length as possible. Surgery for NEC usually requires the placement of a proximal enterostomy until the anastomosis site is ready for reconnection. After surgery, post-op supportive care includes fluids, TPN, antibiotics, and bowel rest for 10 to 14 days.

MAINTAINING FLUID AND NUTRITIONAL STATUS

If NEC is suspected, immediately stop enteral feedings until a diagnosis is made. Administer IV fluids initially to restore proper fluid balance. If ordered, administer total parenteral nutrition (TPN) to keep the newborn supported nutritionally. Give prescribed IV antibiotics to prevent sepsis from the necrotic bowel (if surgery is required, antibiotics may be needed for an extended period of time). Institute gastric decompression as ordered with an orogastric tube attached to low intermittent suction. Carefully monitor intake and output. Restart enteral feedings once the disease has resolved (normal abdominal examination and KUB negative for pneumatosis) or as determined postoperatively by the surgeon.

PROVIDING SUPPORTIVE CARE

Manage pain by administering analgesics as ordered. Infection control is important, with an emphasis on careful handwashing. In addition, implement these interventions in an ongoing manner:

- Check stools for evidence of blood and report any positive findings.
- Measure the abdominal girth.
- Monitor blood pressure for hypotension.
- Palpate the abdomen for tenderness and rigidity.

- Auscultate for normal bowel sounds in all four quadrants.
- Monitor blood gases and oxygen saturation.
- Observe the abdomen for redness or shininess, which indicates peritonitis.
- Offer emotional support for parents/partners/significant others.

EDUCATING THE FAMILY

The diagnosis of NEC may cause significant family anxiety. Listen to the family's worries and fears. Answer their questions honestly. Inform the family that medically treated NEC is usually limited to a short period and resolves within 48 hours of stopping oral feedings, but surgically treated NEC can be a much lengthier process. The amount of bowel that has necrosed, as determined during the bowel resection, significantly increases the likelihood of long-term medical problems. Short bowel syndrome may result from a large resection (short bowel syndrome is discussed in Chapter 42). Reassure the family that although some infants have more involved cases of NEC, the improved parenteral nutrition formulations have improved the outcomes for these infants. Provide education about ostomy care if surgery is required (refer to Chapter 42 for a discussion of ostomy care). Promote interaction with their newborn. Nursing actions of active engagement with parents and the sick infant (providing NICU orientation and physical care), providing cautious guidance (offering information and instruction on infant care), and their subtle presence (overseeing parent's interaction with their infant) all contribute to fostering a positive, trusting relationship with parents (Nagtalon-Ramos, 2014; Verklan & Walden, 2015).

Infants of Diabetic Mothers

An **infant of a diabetic mother (IDM)** is one born to a woman with pregestational or gestational diabetes (see Chapter 20 for additional information). The newborn of a diabetic woman is at high risk for numerous health-related complications, especially hypoglycemia. Gestational diabetes mellitus (GDM) from all causes of diabetes is the most common medical complication of pregnancy and is increasing in incidence, particularly as type 2 diabetes continues to increase worldwide. Despite advances in perinatal care, IDMs remain at risk for a multitude of physiologic, metabolic, and congenital complications such as preterm birth, macrosomia, asphyxia, respiratory distress, hypoglycemia, hypocalcemia, hyperbilirubinemia, polycythemia and hyperviscosity, hypertrophic cardiomyopathy, and congenital anomalies, particularly of the central nervous system. Overt type 1 diabetes around conception produces marked risk of neural tube defects, cardiac defects, and caudal regression syndrome; later in gestation, severe and unstable type 1 maternal diabetes carries a higher risk of intrauterine growth restriction, asphyxia, and fetal death. IDMs born to mothers with type 2 diabetes are more commonly obese (macrosomic) with milder conditions of the common problems found in IDMs. IDMs from all causes of GDM also are predisposed to later-life risk of obesity, diabetes, and cardiovascular disease (Mattson & Smith, 2015).

Impact of Diabetes on the Newborn

For more than a century, it has been known that diabetes during pregnancy can have severe adverse effects on fetal and newborn outcomes. Infants of diabetic mothers have increased morbidity and mortality in the perinatal period. The incidence of major congenital anomalies is much greater for these newborns than for other newborns (Potter & Kicklighter, 2016). Poor glycemic control in the first trimester, during organogenesis, is thought to be a major reason for congenital malformations. The most common types of malformations in infants of diabetic mothers involve the cardiovascular, skeletal, central nervous, gastrointestinal, and genitourinary systems. Cardiac anomalies are the most common (Gardner et al., 2016).

Infants of diabetic mothers can be large for gestational age (LGA) or small for gestational age (SGA), depending on the vascular impact of this chronic systemic disease on the mother prior to and during the pregnancy. Fetal macrosomia occurs in 25% to 42% of diabetic pregnancies because of hyperinsulinemia (Gardner et al., 2016). LGA infants (>90th percentile on growth chart) are longer and weigh more than 4,000 g with the majority of the excess weight composed of fat. They also have increased organ weights (organomegaly) and excessive fat deposits on their shoulders and trunk, contributing to the increased overall body weight and predisposing them to shoulder dystocia, brachial plexus injury, fracture, neonatal depression, or cesarean birth. These oversized newborns frequently require cesarean births for cephalopelvic disproportion and dysfunctional labor patterns. They are frequently hypoglycemic in the first few hours after birth (Korkmazer, Solak, & Tokgoz, 2015).

SGA infants (<10th percentile on growth chart) of diabetic mothers usually suffer from intrauterine malnutrition and have few glucose reserves to tolerate the rigors of labor and birth. Uteroplacental circulation is often impaired, leading to poor growth patterns and hypoxemia.

Despite their increased or decreased size and weight, they may be remarkably frail, showing behaviors similar to those of a preterm newborn. Thus, birthweight may not be a reliable criterion of maturity. Newborns of women with diabetes but without vascular complications often tend to be LGA, whereas those of women with diabetes and vascular disease are usually SGA (Green, 2016).

Pathophysiology

The large size of the IDM arises secondary to exposure to high levels of maternal glucose crossing the placenta into the fetal circulation. Maternal hyperglycemia acts as a fuel to stimulate increased production of fetal insulin, which in turn promotes somatic growth within the fetus. The fetus responds to these high levels by producing more insulin, which acts as a growth factor in the fetus (Kliegman et al., 2015). How the fetus will be affected and the problems that the newborn experiences depend on the severity, duration, and control of the diabetes in the mother during the pregnancy. Table 24.1 summarizes the common problems that may occur in infants of diabetic mothers.

Nursing Assessment

Assessment begins in the prenatal period by identifying women with diabetes and taking measures to control maternal glucose levels (see Chapter 20 for information on management of the pregnant woman with diabetes).

TABLE 24.1 COMMON PROBLEMS OF INFANTS OF DIABETIC MOTHERS

Condition	Description	Effects
Macrosomia	Newborn with an excessive birthweight; arbitrarily defined as a birthweight >4,000 g (8 lb 8 oz) to 4,500 g (9 lb 9 oz) or >90% for gestational age Complication in 10% of all pregnancies in the United States	• Increased risk for shoulder dystocia, traumatic birth injury, birth asphyxia • Risks for newborn hypoglycemia and hypomagnesemia, polycythemia, and electrolyte disturbances • Increased maternal risk for surgical birth, postpartum hemorrhage and infection, and birth canal lacerations • Increased risk of developing type 2 diabetes later in life for both • Higher weight and accumulation of fat in childhood and a higher rate of obesity in adults
Respiratory distress syndrome (RDS)	Cortisol-induced stimulation of lecithin/sphingomyelin (phospholipids) necessary for lung maturation is antagonized due to the high insulin environment within the fetus due to mother's hyperglycemia Less mature lung development than expected for gestational age Decrease in the phospholipid phosphatidylglycerol (PG), which stabilizes surfactant, compounding risk	• Most commonly, breathing normally at birth but developing labored, grunting respiration with cough and a hoarse complaining cry within a few hours with chest retractions and varying degrees of cyanosis • IDMs with vascular disease seldom develop RDS because the chronic stress of poor intrauterine perfusion leads to increased production of steroids, which accelerates lung maturation
Hypoglycemia	Glucose is the major source of energy for organ function Typical characteristics: • Poor feedings • Jitteriness • Lethargy • High-pitched or weak cry • Apnea • Cyanosis and seizures Some newborns are asymptomatic	Low blood glucose levels are problematic during early postbirth period due to abrupt cessation of high-glucose maternal blood supply and the continuation of insulin production by the newborn Limited ability to release glucagon and catecholamines, which normally stimulate glucagon breakdown and glucose release Prolonged and untreated hypoglycemia leads to serious, long-term adverse neurologic sequelae such as learning disabilities and mental retardation
Hypocalcemia and hypomagnesemia	Hypocalcemia (drop in calcium levels) is manifested by tremors, hypotonia, apnea, high-pitched cry, and seizures due to abrupt cessation of maternal transfer of calcium to the fetus, primarily in the third trimester and experiencing birth asphyxia Associated hypomagnesemia is directly related to the maternal level before birth About half of IDMs affected	Newborn is at risk for a prolonged delay in parathyroid hormone production and cardiac dysrhythmias

(continued)

TABLE 24.1 COMMON PROBLEMS OF INFANTS OF DIABETIC MOTHERS (continued)

Condition	Description	Effects
Polycythemia	Venous hematocrit of >65% in the newborn Increased oxygen consumption by IDM secondary to fetal hyperglycemia and hyperinsulinemia Increased fetal erythropoiesis secondary to intrauterine hypoxia due to placental insufficiency from maternal diabetes Hypoxic stimulation of increased red blood cell (RBC) production as compensatory mechanism	Increased viscosity, resulting in poor blood flow predisposing newborn to decreased tissue oxygenation and development of microthrombi
Hyperbilirubinemia	Usually seen within the first few days after birth, manifested by a yellow appearance of the sclera and skin Excessive red cell hemolysis necessary to break down increased RBCs in circulation due to polycythemia Resultant elevated bilirubin levels Excessive bruising secondary to birth trauma of macrosomic infants, further adding to high bilirubin levels	If untreated, high levels of unconjugated bilirubin may lead to kernicterus (neurologic syndrome that results in irreversible damage) with long-term sequelae that include cerebral palsy, sensorineural hearing loss, and mental retardation
Congenital anomalies	Occur in up to 10% of infants of diabetic mothers, accounting for 30–50% of perinatal deaths Incidence is greatest among small-for gestational-age newborns Overall, infants of diabetic mothers have 3 times the usual incidence of congenital anomalies compared to newborns from the nondiabetic general population	Most common anomalies: • Coarctation of the aorta • Atrial and ventricular septal defects • Transposition of the great vessels • Sacral agenesis • Hip and joint malformations • Anencephaly • Spina bifida • Caudal dysplasia • Hydrocephalus

Adapted from Green, C. J. (2016). *Maternal newborn nursing care plans* (3rd ed.). Burlington, MA: Jones and Bartlett Learning; Gardner, S. L., Carter, B. S., Enzman-Hines, M., & Hernandez, J. A. (2016). *Merenstein & Gardner's handbook of neonatal intensive care* (8th ed.). St. Louis, MO: Mosby Elsevier; and Verklan, M. T., & Walden, M. (2015). *Core curriculum for neonatal intensive care nursing* (5th ed.). St. Louis, MO: Saunders.

PHYSICAL EXAMINATION

At birth, inspect the newborn for the following characteristic features. See also Figure 24.5.

- Full rosy cheeks with a ruddy skin color
- Short neck (some describe "no-neck" appearance)
- Buffalo hump over the nape of the neck
- Massive shoulders with a full intrascapular area
- Distended upper abdomen due to organ overgrowth
- Excessive subcutaneous fat tissue, producing fat extremities

Be alert for hypoglycemia, which may occur immediately after birth or within an hour. Assess blood glucose levels, which should remain above 40 mg/dL. Closely assess the newborn for signs of hypoglycemia, including listlessness, hypotonia, apathy, poor feeding, apneic episodes with a drop in oxygen saturation, cyanosis, temperature instability, pallor and sweating, tremors, irritability, and seizures.

Assess the newborn for signs of birth trauma involving the head (tense, bulging fontanels, cephalhematoma, skull fractures, and facial nerve paralysis), shoulders and extremities (posturing, paralysis), and skin (bruising). Inspect the newborn for compromised oxygenation by examining the skin for cyanosis, pallor, mottling, and sluggish capillary refill. Take the newborn's temperature frequently and provide a neutral thermal environment to prevent cold stress, which would increase the glucose utilization and contribute to the hypoglycemic state.

LABORATORY AND DIAGNOSTIC TESTING

Determine baseline serum calcium, magnesium, and bilirubin levels and monitor them frequently for changes (Table 24.2). Hypocalcemia is typically manifested in the first 2 to 3 days of life as a result of birth injury or a prolonged delay in parathyroid hormone production. Hypomagnesemia parallels calcium levels and is suspected

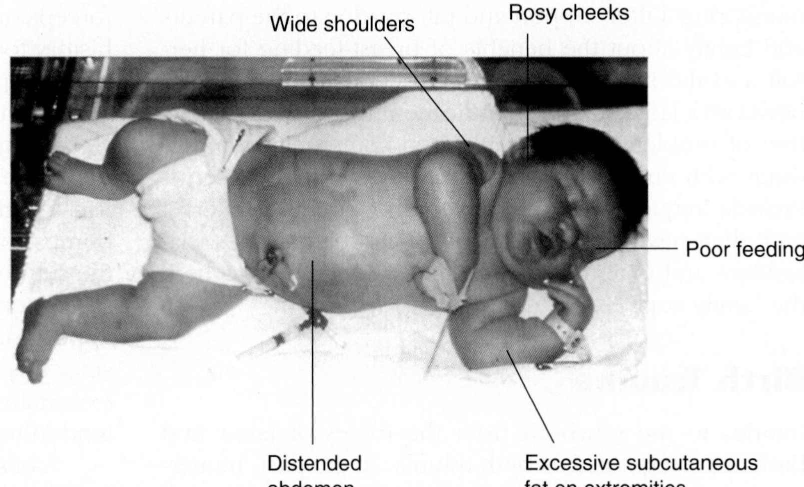

FIGURE 24.5 Characteristics of an infant of a diabetic mother. A macrosomic infant of a diabetic mother (IDM) has head circumference and length that are at the 90th percentile; the IDM's body weight greatly exceeds the 90th percentile. The IDM has considerable fat deposition in the shoulder and intrascapular area. (McDonald, M. G., Seshia, M. M. K. (2016). *Avery's neonatology: Pathophysiology & management of the newborn* (7th ed.). Philadelphia, PA: Wolters Kluwer.)

only when hypocalcemia does not respond to calcium replacement therapy. Red blood cell breakdown leads to increased hematocrit and polycythemia. In addition, hyperbilirubinemia may be caused by slightly decreased extracellular fluid volume, hepatic immaturity, and birth trauma forming enclosed hemorrhages. It can appear within the first 24 hours of life (pathologic) or after 24 hours of life (physiologic).

Nursing Management

The focus of care for these infants is early detection and initiation of therapy to address potential problems (Nursing Care Plan 24.1, at the end of the chapter). Perform a head-to-toe physical assessment to identify congenital anomalies. Institute measures to correct hypoglycemia, hypocalcemia, hypomagnesemia, dehydration, and jaundice. Provide oxygenation and ventilatory support as necessary. The focus of care includes correcting hypoglycemia and hypocalcemia, providing phototherapy for jaundice, administering fluid therapy, and maintaining oxygen and ventilation if needed.

TABLE 24.2 CRITICAL LABORATORY VALUES FOR INFANTS OF DIABETIC MOTHERS

Hypoglycemia	<40 mg/dL
Hypocalcemia	<7 mg/dL
Hypomagnesemia	<1.5 mg/dL
Hyperbilirubinemia	>12 mg/dL (term infant)
Polycythemia	>65% (venous hematocrit)

Adapted from Fanaroff, A. A., & Fanaroff, J. M. (2014). *Klaus and Fanaroff's care of the high-risk neonate* (6th ed.). Philadelphia, PA: Elsevier Health Sciences; Kenner, C., & Lott, J. W. (2014). *Comprehensive neonatal nursing care* (5th ed.). New York, NY: Springer Publishers; and Malcolm, W. (2015). *Beyond the NICU: Comprehensive care of the high risk infant.* New York, NY: McGraw Hill Education.

PREVENTING HYPOGLYCEMIA

Prevent hypoglycemia by providing early oral feedings with breast milk of formula at frequent intervals (every 2 to 3 hours). Feedings help to control glucose levels, reduce hematocrit, and promote bilirubin excretion. Maintain a neutral thermal environment to avoid cold stress, which may stimulate the metabolic rate, thereby increasing the demand for glucose. Provide rest periods to decrease energy demand and expenditure.

Monitor blood glucose levels via heel stick every hour for the first 4 hours of life and then every 3 to 4 hours until stable. Document the results. Report unstable glucose values if oral feedings do not maintain and stabilize the newborn's blood glucose levels. If glucose levels are not stabilized, initiate IV glucose infusions as ordered and monitor that the infusions are flowing at the prescribed rate.

MAINTAINING FLUID AND ELECTROLYTE BALANCE

Monitor serum calcium levels for changes indicating the need for supplementation, such as with oral or IV calcium gluconate. Assess the newborn for signs of hypocalcemia, such as tremors, jitteriness, twitching, seizures, and high-pitched cry.

Also administer fluid therapy as ordered to maintain adequate hydration. Monitor serum bilirubin levels and institute phototherapy if the newborn is over 24 hours old.

PROVIDING PARENTAL SUPPORT

Good communication between the nurse and the family is essential. It should be supported by evidence-based, written information tailored to meet the woman's individual needs. Assist the parents and family in understanding the newborn's condition and need for frequent monitoring. Offer support and information to the parents and family about the benefits of breast-feeding for herself and the infant. They may erroneously interpret the newborn's large size as an indication that the newborn is free of problems. Encourage open communication and listen with empathy to the family's fears and concerns. Provide frequent opportunities for the parents to interact with their newborn. Make appropriate referrals to social services and community resources as necessary to help the family cope.

Birth Trauma

Injuries to the newborn from the forces of labor and birth are categorized as birth trauma. In the past, numerous injuries were associated with difficult births requiring external or internal version or mid or high forceps deliveries. Today, however, cesarean births have contributed to the decline in birth trauma. Damage occurs to the tissues and organs of the newborn caused by mechanical forces during childbirth often accompanied by impaired blood circulation and organ functioning. The most frequent and significant birth injuries are to the skull, brain, and spinal cord (Malcolm, 2015).

Significant birth trauma accounts for fewer than 3% of neonatal deaths and stillbirths in the United States (Loroia, 2015). They estimate that birth trauma in the United States occurs in approximately 29 per 1,000 births with the three most frequently diagnosed birth trauma conditions being injuries to the scalp, injuries to the skeleton, and fracture of the clavicle (Gardner et al. 2016). Improved prenatal diagnosis and monitoring during labor have helped to reduce the incidence of birth injuries today.

Pathophysiology

The process of birth is a blend of compression, contractions, torques, and traction. When fetal size, presentation, or neurologic immunity complicates this process, the forces of labor and birth may lead to tissue damage, edema, hemorrhages, or fractures in the newborn. For example, birth trauma may result from the pressure of birth, especially in a prolonged or abrupt labor, abnormal or difficult presentation, cephalopelvic disproportion, or mechanical forces, such as forceps or vacuum used during delivery. Table 24.3 summarizes the most common types of birth trauma.

Nursing Assessment

Recognition of trauma and birth injuries is imperative so that early treatment can be initiated. Review the labor and birth history for risk factors, such as a prolonged or abrupt labor, abnormal or difficult presentation, cephalopelvic disproportion, or mechanical forces, such as forceps or vacuum used during delivery. Also review the history for multiple fetus deliveries, large-for-date infants, extreme prematurity, large fetal head, or newborns with congenital anomalies.

Complete a careful physical and neurologic assessment of every newborn admitted to the nursery to establish whether injuries exist. Inspect the head for lumps, bumps, or bruises. Note if swelling or bruising crosses the suture line. Assess the eyes and face for facial paralysis, observing for asymmetry of the face with crying or appearance of the mouth being drawn to the unaffected side. Ensure that the newborn spontaneously moves all extremities. Note any absence of or decrease in deep tendon reflexes or abnormal positioning of extremities.

Assess and document symmetry of structure and function. Be prepared to assist with scheduling diagnostic studies to confirm trauma or injuries, which will be important in determining treatment modalities.

Nursing Management

Nursing management is primarily supportive and focuses on assessing for resolution of the trauma or any associated complications along with providing support and education to the parents. Provide the parents with explanations and reassurance that these injuries usually resolve with minimal or no treatment. Parents are alarmed when their newborn is unable to move an extremity or demonstrates asymmetric facial movements. Provide parents with a realistic picture of the situation to gain their understanding and trust. Be readily available to answer questions and teach them how to care for the newborn, including any modifications that might be necessary. Allow parents adequate time to understand the implications of the birth trauma or injury and what treatment modalities are needed, if any. Provide them with information about the length of time until the injury will resolve and when and if they need to seek further medical attention for the condition. Spending time with the parents and providing them with support, information, and teaching are important to allow them to make decisions and care for their newborn. Anticipate the need for community referral for ongoing follow-up and care, if necessary.

Newborns of Substance-Abusing Mothers

It is generally assumed that all pregnant women want to provide a healthy environment for their unborn child and know how to avoid harm. However, women who use tobacco, alcohol, or illicit substances during pregnancy place themselves and their newborns at risk for numerous complications. Perinatal substance abuse is a persistent and significant public health issue particularly affecting children, with high rates of reported abuse,

TABLE 24.3 COMMON TYPES OF BIRTH TRAUMA

Type	Description	Findings	Treatment
Fractures	Most often occur during breech births or shoulder dystocia in newborns with macrosomia Midclavicular fractures are the most common type of fracture, secondary to shoulder dystocia Long bone fractures of the humerus or femur, usually midshaft, also can occur	Midclavicular fractures: The newborn is irritable and does not move the arm on the affected side either spontaneously or when the Moro reflex is elicited Femoral or humeral long bone fractures: The newborn shows loss of spontaneous leg or arm motion, respectively; usually swelling and pain accompany the limited movement X-rays confirm the fracture	Midclavicular fractures typically heal rapidly and uneventfully; arm motion may be limited by pinning the newborn's sleeve to the shirt Femoral and humeral shaft fractures are treated with splinting. Healing and complete recovery are expected within 2–4 wks without incident Explanation to the parents and reassurance are needed
Brachial plexus injury	Primarily in large babies, babies with shoulder dystocia, or breech delivery Results from stretching, hemorrhage within a nerve, or tearing of the nerve or the roots associated with cervical cord injury Associated traumatic injuries include fracture of the clavicle or humerus or subluxations of the shoulder or cervical spine Erb palsy is an upper brachial plexus injury Klumpke palsy is an injury to the lower brachial plexus (lower brachial injuries are less common)	In Erb palsy, the involved extremity usually presents adducted, prone, and internally rotated; shoulder movement is absent; Moro, bicep, and radial reflexes are absent, but the grasp reflex is usually present Klumpke palsy is manifested by weakness in the hand and wrist; grasp reflex is absent	Erb palsy usually involves immobilization of the upper arm across the upper abdomen/chest to protect the shoulder from excessive motion for the first week; then gentle passive range-of-motion exercises are performed daily to prevent contractures. There is usually no associated sensory loss, and this condition usually improves rapidly Treatment for Klumpke palsy involves placing the hand in a neutral position and using passive range-of-motion exercises In some cases deficits may persist, requiring continuing observation
Cranial nerve trauma	Most common is facial nerve palsy Frequently attributed to pressure resulting from forceps May also result from pressure on the nerve in utero, related to fetal positioning such as the head lying against the shoulder	Physical findings include asymmetry of the face when crying; mouth may be drawn toward the unaffected side; wrinkles are deeper on the unaffected side The paralyzed side may be smooth, with a swollen appearance. Eye is persistently open on the affected side	Most infants begin to recover in the first week, but full resolution may take up to several months; parents need reassurance about this In most cases, treatment is not necessary, only observation If the eye is affected and unable to close, protection with patches and synthetic tears may be necessary Parents need instruction about how to feed the newborn, since he or she cannot close the lips around the nipple without having milk seep out

(continued)

TABLE 24.3 COMMON TYPES OF BIRTH TRAUMA (continued)

Type	Description	Findings	Treatment
Head trauma	Mild trauma can cause soft tissue injuries such as cephalohematoma and caput succedaneum; greater trauma can cause depressed skull fractures **Cephalohematoma** (subperiosteal collection of blood secondary to the rupture of blood vessels between the skull and periosteum) occurs in 2.5% of all births and typically appears within hours after birth **Caput succedaneum** (soft tissue swelling) is caused by edema of the head against the dilating cervix during the birth process Subarachnoid hemorrhage (one of the most common types of intracranial trauma) may be due to hypoxia/ischemia, variations in blood pressure, and the pressure exerted on the head during labor. Bleeding is of venous origin, and underlying contusions also may occur Subdural hemorrhage (hematomas) occurs less often today because of improved obstetric techniques. Typically, tears of the major veins or venous sinuses overlying the cerebral hemispheres or cerebellum (most common in newborns of a primipara and large newborns, or after an instrumented birth) are the cause. Increased pressure on the blood vessels inside the skull leads to tears Depressed skull fractures (rare) may result from the pressure of a forceps delivery; can also occur during spontaneous or cesarean births and may be associated with other head trauma causing subdural bleeding, subarachnoid hemorrhage, or brain trauma	In cephalohematoma, suture lines delineate its extent; usually located on one side, over the parietal bone In caput succedaneum, swelling is not limited by suture lines: it extends across the midline and is associated with head molding. It does not usually cause complications other than a misshapen head. Swelling is maximal at birth and then rapidly decreases in size In subarachnoid hemorrhage, some RBCs may appear in the CSF of full-term newborns. Newborns may present with apnea, seizures, lethargy, or abnormal findings on a neurologic examination Subdural hemorrhage can be asymptomatic, or the neonate can exhibit seizures, enlarging head size, decreased level of consciousness, or abnormal findings on a neurologic examination, with hypotonia, a poor Moro reflex, or extensive retinal hemorrhages Depressed skull fractures can be observed and palpated as depressions. Confirmation by x-ray is necessary	Cephalohematoma resolves gradually over 2–3 wks without treatment Caput succedaneum usually resolves over the first few days without treatment Subarachnoid hemorrhage requires minimal handling to reduce stress Subdural hematoma requires aspiration; can be life-threatening if it is in an inaccessible location and cannot be aspirated Depressed skull fractures typically require a neurosurgical consultation

Adapted from Cunningham, F. G., Leveno, K. J., Bloom, S. L., Spong, C.Y., Dashe, J. S., Hoffman, B. L., et al. (2014). *Williams obstetrics* (24th ed.). New York, NY: McGraw-Hill; Gardner, S. L., Carter, B. S., Enzman-Hines, M., & Hernandez, J. A. (2016). *Merenstein & Gardner's handbook of neonatal intensive care* (8th ed.). St. Louis, MO: Mosby Elsevier; and Loroia, N. (2015). Birth trauma. *eMedicine.* Retrieved from http://emedicine.medscape.com/article/980112-overview

neglect, and foster care placement. Substance use during pregnancy exposes the fetus to the possibility of fetal growth restriction, prematurity, neurobehavioral and neurophysiologic dysfunction, birth defects, infections, and long-term developmental sequelae (Wang, 2014). Infants of mothers who abuse substances are more likely to suffer substantiated harm, enter foster care, and have more negative child protection outcomes. The effects of fetal alcohol syndrome (FAS) and spectrum disorders are well documented in the literature; studies attest to developmental delays, intellectual disabilities, attention disorders, and psychopathologies during the child's lifetime (Wang, 2014).

The full extent of the effects of prenatal drug exposure on a child is not known. However, studies show that various drugs of abuse may result in premature birth, miscarriage, low birthweight, and a variety of behavioral and cognitive problems.

It is difficult to establish the true prevalence of substance use in pregnant women; many women deny taking any nonprescribed substance because of the associated social stigma and legal implications. The National Institute on Drug Abuse (NIDA) suggests that over 15% of women use alcohol or illicit drugs thus exposing their fetuses to their effects (NIDA, 2015). Drug exposure may go unrecognized in these newborns, and they may be discharged from the newborn nursery at risk for medical and social problems, including abuse and neglect.

Tobacco, alcohol, and marijuana are the substances most commonly abused during pregnancy. Other drugs may include opioids such as morphine, codeine, methadone, meperidine, and heroin; CNS stimulants such as amphetamines and cocaine; CNS depressants such as barbiturates, diazepam (Valium), and sedative-hypnotics; and hallucinogens such as LSD, inhalants, glue, paint thinner, nail polish remover, and nitrous oxide (NIDA, 2015). Table 24.4 highlights commonly used substances and their effects on the fetus and newborn.

Substance abuse during pregnancy is the subject of much controversy. The type of substance used and the timing of drug ingestion during pregnancy usually determines the type and severity of damage to the fetus. Frequently, the woman uses more than one substance, which compounds the problem. Nurses must be knowledgeable about the issues of substance abuse and must be alert for opportunities to identify, prevent, manage, and educate women and families about this key public health issue.

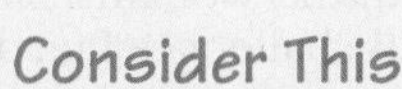

Consider This

I admit, I had led a reckless life since I was a teen. I rebelled against my mother's authority and started smoking and doing drugs just to "check out" of my painful world. It was one big blast after another with a high and then a low. I never considered the consequences of my behavior then and never thought it would hurt anyone until I learned I was about 4 months' pregnant. I convinced myself that if I cut back, everything would be fine.

Now, as I stand here in the NICU watching my tiny son struggle for air and tremble all over, I am not so convinced that I didn't hurt anyone except myself. As I witness my son fight against MY nicotine and drug addiction, my heart is heavy with guilt. I wonder how I could have thought that my troubles wouldn't become another's plight sooner or later. What must I have been thinking to isolate my addiction and not consider the impact that it would have on my mother and my son?

Thoughts: This woman honestly regrets what her addiction has done to her son as she stands watching him go through withdrawal. Her lifestyle choices do affect others, despite her previous denial. One problem with addiction is the difficulty in getting help after deciding to finally quit. There aren't enough rehab centers to deal with the large numbers needing their services and it can be difficult to get into one. What can be offered to pregnant women who abuse substances? How can nurses increase community awareness about the impact of this problem, especially during pregnancy?

Fetal Alcohol Spectrum Disorders (FASDs)

Alcohol abuse during pregnancy is currently among the fastest-growing health care challenges in the United States. Years ago, alcohol was not commonly recognized as a teratogen, an agent that can disrupt the development of a fetus. Today, it is known that prenatal alcohol exposure induces a variety of adverse effects on physical, neurologic, and behavioral development. Alcohol now is recognized as the leading preventable cause of birth defects and developmental disorders in the United States Substance Abuse & Mental Health Services Administration [SAMHSA] (2015). The adverse effects of alcohol consumption have been recognized for centuries, but the associated pattern of fetal anomalies was not labeled until the early 1970s. The distinctive pattern identified three specific findings: growth restriction (prenatal and postnatal), craniofacial structural anomalies, and CNS dysfunction. These distinctive findings were called FAS, characterized by physical and mental disorders that appear at birth and remain problematic throughout the child's life. However, there are also circumstances in which the effects of prenatal alcohol exposure are apparent, but the newborn does not meet the entire criteria specific to FAS. Other disorders included in the grouping **fetal alcohol spectrum disorders (FASDs)** are alcohol-related neurodevelopmental disorder (ARND) and

(text continues on page 930)

TABLE 24.4 COMMON TYPES OF ABUSED SUBSTANCES

Substance	Description	Effects on Fetus and Newborn	Nursing Implications
Alcohol	Consumption is pervasive and widely accepted, with use, abuse, and addiction affecting all levels of society It is a common misconception that a substance sold to the public without restriction is safe	Fetal alcohol syndrome (one of the most common known causes of mental retardation) Fetal alcohol spectrum disorders Alcohol-related birth defects	Provide education that decreasing or eliminating alcohol consumption during pregnancy is the only way to prevent fetal alcohol syndrome and fetal alcohol effects Assist pregnant woman in finding a treatment program if possible Inform all women who are pregnant or planning to become pregnant about the detrimental effects of alcohol during pregnancy Educate women using a nonjudgmental, culturally connected approach Warn women that there is no safe time to drink or amount of alcohol they can consume
Tobacco/nicotine	Nicotine is an addictive substance. It causes epinephrine release from the adrenal cortex, leading to initial stimulation followed by depression and fatigue, causing the user to seek more nicotine Increased numbers of women are smoking (at least 11% smoke during pregnancy) Over 2,500 chemicals are found in cigarette smoke, including nicotine, tar, carbon monoxide, and cyanide. It is unknown which are harmful, but nicotine and carbon monoxide are believed to play a role in causing adverse pregnancy outcomes	Impaired oxygenation of mother and fetus due to nicotine crossing placenta and carbon monoxide combining with hemoglobin Increased risk for low birthweight (risk almost doubled), small for gestational age, and preterm birth Increased risk for sudden infant death syndrome (SIDS) and chronic respiratory illness	Provide support for smoking cessation Individualize counseling based on factors associated with the woman's smoking and challenges faced (why woman smokes, stressors in life, and social support network) Suggest options such as group smoking cessation programs, relaxation techniques, individual counseling, hypnosis, and partner-support counseling
Marijuana	Most widely used illicit psychoactive substance in Western world and most commonly used illicit drug in the United States Derived from *Cannabis sativa* plant	Not shown to have teratogenic effects on fetus; no consistent types of malformations identified Fetal growth restriction (FGR) is common due to delivery of carbon monoxide to fetus Increased risk for small for gestational age Altered responses to visual stimuli, sleep-pattern abnormalities, photophobia, lack of motor control, hyperirritability, increased tremulousness, and high-pitched cry noted in infants of mothers who smoked marijuana Research related to long-term effects is continuing	Provide teaching to women about healthy behaviors Provide support for cessation of marijuana use

TABLE 24.4 COMMON TYPES OF ABUSED SUBSTANCES (continued)

Substance	Description	Effects on Fetus and Newborn	Nursing Implications
Methamphetamines	Addictive stimulant; use releases high levels of dopamine, which stimulates brain cells, enhancing mood and body movement High potential for abuse and addiction; can be inhaled, injected, smoked, or taken orally Many street names, such as speed, meth, ice, and chalk Primary effects include accelerated heart and respiratory rate, elevated blood pressure, papillary dilation; secondary effects include loss of appetite Used medically as treatment for obesity and narcolepsy in adults and hyperactivity in children	Little research on use during pregnancy because its use is less common than cocaine or narcotics Fetal effects similar to cocaine (suggesting vasoconstriction as possible underlying mechanism) Possible maternal malnutrition, leading to problems with fetal growth and development Increased risk for preterm birth and low-birthweight newborns Infants may have withdrawal symptoms, including dysphoria, agitation, jitteriness, poor weight gain, abnormal sleep patterns, poor feeding, frantic fist sucking, high-pitched cry, respiratory distress soon after birth, frequent infections, and significant lassitude Long-term effects not known	Provide teaching to women about healthy behaviors Provide support for cessation of methamphetamine use Monitor the woman for weight changes; emphasize the need for adequate nutritional intake to support fetal growth and development
Cocaine	Strong CNS stimulant that interferes with reabsorption of dopamine Physical effects: vasoconstriction; pupillary dilation; increased temperature, heart rate, and blood pressure Taken orally, sublingually, intranasally, intravenously, and via inhalation Estimated that 30–40% of cocaine addicts are female Maternal cocaine use during pregnancy is a significant health problem Increased potential for use of multiple drugs if mother using cocaine	Preterm birth and lower birthweight Unclear impact on later development Speculation that cocaine interferes with infant's cognitive development, leading to learning and memory difficulties later in life Associated congenital anomalies: GU, cardiac, and CNS defects, and prune belly syndrome Other typical newborn characteristics: smaller head circumference, piercing cry, limb defects, ambiguous genitalia, poor feeding, poor visual and auditory responses, poor sleep patterns, decreased impulse control, stiff, hyperextended positioning, irritability and hypersensitivity, inability to respond to caretaker. Elevated vital signs secondary to stimulating effect.	Educate the woman about the effects of cocaine use on the fetus and newborn Assess for use of other substances Provide teaching to women about healthy behaviors Provide support and guidance for cessation of cocaine and other substance use

(continued)

TABLE 24.4 COMMON TYPES OF ABUSED SUBSTANCES (continued)

Substance	Description	Effects on Fetus and Newborn	Nursing Implications
Heroin	Illegal, highly addictive opiate derived from morphine that can be sniffed, smoked, or injected Possible consequences include HIV infection, tuberculosis, crime, violence, and family disruption Severe physical addiction; CNS depressant producing mental dullness and drowsiness	Newborns of heroin-addicted mothers are born dependent on heroin Increased risk for transmission of hepatitis B and C and HIV to newborns when mothers share needles Significantly increased rates of stillbirth, fetal growth restriction, preterm birth, and newborn mortality (3–7 times greater) Small-for-gestational-age newborns, meconium aspiration, high incidence of SIDS, and delayed effects from subacute withdrawal (restlessness, continual crying, agitation, sneezing, vomiting, fever, diarrhea, seizures, irritability, and poor socialization [possibly persisting for 4–6 mo]); Intrauterine death or preterm birth is possible with abrupt cessation of heroin use	Educate the woman about the effects of heroin use on the fetus and newborn Assess for use of other substances Provide teaching to women about healthy behaviors Warn the woman not to abruptly stop heroin use. Encourage her to enroll in a methadone maintenance program
Methadone	Synthetic opiate narcotic used primarily as maintenance therapy for heroin addiction	Improvement in many of the detrimental fetal effects associated with heroin use Withdrawal symptoms are common in newborns. Possible low birthweight due to symmetric fetal growth restriction Increased severity and longer period of withdrawal (due to methadone's longer half-life) Seizures (commonly severe) do not usually occur until 2–3 wks of age, when the newborn is at home. Increased rate of SIDS (3–4 times higher)	Methadone maintenance programs are the standard of care for women with narcotic addiction Inform the woman about the benefits and risks of methadone use versus heroin use. Advantages include improved fetal and newborn growth, reduced risk of fetal death, and reduced risk of HIV infections Advise the woman that she will need to return consistently to receive the prescribed methadone dose Reinforce the need for continued prenatal care Inform the woman that she can breast-feed her newborn while receiving methadone Teach mother and caregivers about signs and symptoms of methadone withdrawal

alcohol-related birth defects (ARBD). Children with ARND primarily display intellectual disabilities related to behavior and learning while children with ARBD may have birth defects of the heart, kidneys, and/or bones. The problems associated with any of the FASDs are lifelong and are entirely preventable by avoiding alcohol consumption during pregnancy (Centers for Disease Control and Prevention [CDC], 2015). Box 24.2 summarizes the manifestations of FAS.

In the United States, about 40,000 babies are born each year with FASDs (March of Dimes, 2016). Current estimates indicate that approximately 1 in 8 women

BOX 24.2

CLINICAL PICTURE OF FETAL ALCOHOL SYNDROME

- Microcephaly (head circumference <10th percentile)[a]
- Small palpebral (eyelid) fissures[a]
- Abnormally small eyes
- Fetal growth restriction
- Maxillary hypoplasia (flattened or absent)
- Epicanthal folds (folds of skin of the upper eyelid over the eye)
- Thin upper lip[a]
- Missing vertical groove in median portion of upper lip[a]
- Short upturned nose
- Short birth length and low birthweight
- Joint and limb defects
- Small-for-gestational age
- Altered palmar crease pattern
- Prenatal or postnatal growth ≤10th percentile[a]
- Congenital cardiac defects (septal defects)
- Delayed fine and gross motor development
- Poor eye–hand coordination
- Clinically significant brain abnormalities[a]
- Mental retardation
- Narrow forehead
- Performance substantially below expected level in cognitive or developmental functioning, executive or motor functioning, and attention or hyperactivity; social or language skills[a]
- Inadequate sucking reflex and poor appetite

[a]Diagnosis of fetal alcohol syndrome requires the presence of three findings:

1. Documentation of all three facial abnormalities
2. Documentation of growth deficits (height, weight, or both <10th percentile)
3. Documentation of CNS abnormalities (structural, neurologic, or functional)

Adapted from Centers for Disease Control and Prevention. (2015). *Fetal alcohol spectrum disorders (FASDs)*. Retrieved from http://www.cdc.gov/ncbddd/fasd/facts.html; and Substance Abuse & Mental Health Services Administration [SAMHSA] (2015). *Fetal alcohol spectrum disorders.* Retrieved from http://fasdcenter.samhsa.gov/

HEALTHY PEOPLE 2020

Objective	Nursing Significance
Reduce the occurrence of fetal alcohol syndrome (FAS)	Counsel girls and women to avoid alcohol use during pregnancy. Participate in programs for at-risk groups, including adolescents, about the effects of substance abuse, especially alcohol, during pregnancy

Adapted from U.S. Department of Health and Human Services [USDHHS]. (2016). *Healthy People 2020.* Retrieved from http://healthypeople.gov/2020/default.aspx

drinks during pregnancy (CDC, 2015) while 1 in 30 admit to binge drinking. Heavy drinking and binge drinking place the fetus at highest risk (March of Dimes, 2016).

Decreasing or eliminating alcohol consumption during pregnancy is the only way to prevent FAS and fetal alcohol effects. Unfortunately, few treatment programs address the needs of pregnant women; so many newborns are exposed to alcohol in utero.

Neonatal Abstinence Syndrome

Neonatal abstinence syndrome (NAS) compromises a constellation of drug-withdrawal symptoms that result from chronic intrauterine exposure to a variety of substances, including opioids, barbiturates, SSRIs, alcohol, benzodiazepines, caffeine, and nicotine. Newborns of women who abuse tobacco, illicit substances, caffeine, and alcohol can exhibit withdrawal behavior. Withdrawal symptoms occur in 60% of all newborns exposed to drugs (March of Dimes, 2015a). Drug dependency acquired in utero is manifested by a constellation of neurologic and physical behaviors and is known as NAS. Although often treated as a single entity, NAS is not a single pathologic condition.

The manifestations of withdrawal are a function of the drug's half-life, the specific drug or combination of drugs used, dosage, route of administration, timing of drug exposure, and length of drug exposure (Hamdan, 2016). Typical newborn behaviors include CNS hypersensitivity, autonomic dysfunction, respiratory distress, temperature instability, hypoglycemia, tremors, seizures, abnormal cry patterns, feeding difficulties, and gastrointestinal disturbances (Gardner et al., 2016). NAS has both medical and developmental consequences for the newborn.

Nursing Assessment

A comprehensive prenatal medical and drug history, especially with respect to polydrug use, is vital. Fear of referral to child welfare agencies or the legal system has prompted women to conceal their drug abuse history. Frequently, the first inkling of drug use appears in the newborn when symptoms of withdrawal begin within 72 hours after birth. Typically the infant has been discharged by this time, unless the nurse has a high degree of suspicion that would prompt toxicology testing earlier. Several assessment tools can be used to assess a drug-exposed newborn. Figure 24.6 shows an example. Regardless of the tool used for assessment, address these key areas:

- Maternal history to identify risk behaviors for substance abuse:
    - Previous unexplained fetal demise
    - Lack of prenatal care
    - Incarceration

CENTRAL NERVOUS SYSTEM DISTURBANCES													
SIGNS AND SYMPTOMS	SCORE	AM							PM				
Excessive high-pitched cry	2												
Continuous high-pitched cry	3												
Sleeps <1 hour after feeding	3												
Sleeps <2 hours after feeding	2												
Sleeps <3 hours after feeding	1												
Hyperactive Moro reflex	2												
Markedly hyperactive Moro reflex	3												
Mild tremors disturbed	1												
Moderate–severe tremors disturbed	2												
Mild tremors undisturbed	1												
Moderate–severe tremors undisturbed	4												
Increased muscle tone	2												
Excoloration (specify area)	1												
Myoclonic jerks	3												
Generalized convulsions	5												
METABOLIC / VASOMOTOR/RESPIRATORY DISTURBANCES													
Sweating													
Fever <101 (99–100.8°F/37.2–38.2°C)	1												
Fever >101 (38.2°C and higher)	2												
Frequent yawning (>3–4 times/interval)	1												
Mottling	1												
Nasal stuffiness	1												
Sneezing (>3–4 times/interval)	1												
Nasal flaring	2												
Respiratory rate >60 / min	1												
Respiratory rate >60 / min, with retractions	2												
GASTROINTESTINAL DISTURBANCES													
Excessive sucking	1												
Poor feeding	2												
Regurgitation	2												
Projectile vomiting	3												
Loose stools	2												
Watery stools	3												
TOTAL SCORE													

FIGURE 24.6 Neonatal abstinence scoring system. (From Cloherty, J. P., Eichenwald, E. C., Hansen, A. R., & Stark, A. R. (2012). *Manual of neonatal care* (7th ed.). Philadelphia, PA: Lippincott Williams & Wilkins.)

BOX 24.3

WITHDRAWAL ACRONYM

Assess the newborn for signs of neonatal abstinence syndrome using the acronym WITHDRAWAL to focus the assessment:

W= **W**akefulness: sleep duration less than 3 hours after feeding
I = **I**rritability
T = **T**emperature variation, tachycardia, tremors
H = **H**yperactivity, high-pitched persistent cry, hyperreflexia, hypertonus
D = **D**iarrhea, diaphoresis, disorganized suck
R = **R**espiratory distress, rub marks, rhinorrhea
A = **A**pneic attacks, autonomic dysfunction
W= **W**eight loss or failure to gain weight
A = **A**lkalosis (respiratory)
L = **L**acrimation (Hamdan, 2016).

- Prostitution
- Cigarette smoking
- Fetal growth restriction
- Preterm birth
- History of STIs and/or HIV and/or HCV
- Mental health disorders
- History of intimate partner violence
- History of missed prenatal appointments
- Severe mood swings
- Precipitous labor
- Poor nutritional status
- Abruptio placentae
- Hypertensive episodes
- History of drug abuse

- Laboratory test results (toxicology) to identify substances in mother and newborn
- Signs of NAS (Use the WITHDRAWAL acronym; see Box 24.3.)
- Evidence of seizure activity and need for protective environment

The newborn's behavior often prompts the health care provider or nurse to suspect intrauterine drug exposure. The newborn physical examination may also reveal low birthweight for gestational age or drug or ARBD and dysfunction. Assess the newborn for signs of NAS (Box 24.4).

Take Note!

Cocaine-exposed newborns are typically fussy, irritable, and inconsolable at times. Cocaine-exposed infants demonstrate poor coordination of sucking and swallowing, making feeding time frustrating for the newborn and caregiver alike.

BOX 24.4

MANIFESTATIONS OF NEONATAL ABSTINENCE SYNDROME

CNS Dysfunction

- Tremors
- Generalized seizures
- Hyperactive reflexes
- Restlessness
- Hypertonic muscle tone, constant movement
- Shrill, high-pitched cry
- Disturbed sleep patterns

Metabolic, Vasomotor, and Respiratory Disturbances

- Fever
- Frequent yawning
- Mottling of the skin
- Sweating
- Frequent sneezing
- Nasal flaring
- Tachypnea >60 bpm
- Apnea

Gastrointestinal Dysfunction

- Poor feeding
- Frantic sucking or rooting
- Loose or watery stools
- Regurgitation or projectile vomiting

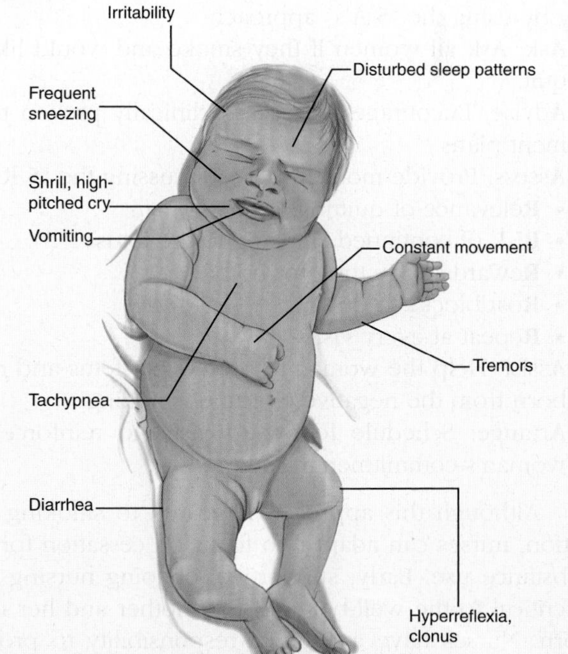

Adapted from Hamdan, A. H. (2016). Neonatal abstinence syndrome. *eMedicine.* Retrieved from http://emedicine.medscape.com/article/978763-overview; and Artigas, V. (2015). Management of neonatal abstinence syndrome in the newborn nursery. *Nursing for Women's Health, 18*(6), 509–514.

Assist with obtaining diagnostic studies to identify the severity of withdrawal. Toxicology screening of the newborn's blood, urine, and meconium identifies the substances to which the newborn has been exposed. Urine drug screening identifies only recent substance exposure, whereas meconium samples may reveal exposure from the second trimester to the present (Hamdan, 2016). Take care to avoid contamination of meconium with urine, as this may affect the accuracy of the sample.

Nursing Management

The needs of the substance-exposed newborn are multiple, complex, and costly, both to the health care system and to society. Substance abuse takes place among people of all colors, sizes, shapes, incomes, types, and conditions. Most pregnant women are unaware of the adverse impact their substance abuse can have on the newborn. Pregnant women dependent on opioids are maintained on methadone as the current standard of care, which provides multiple benefits including improved prenatal care, reduced fetal mortality, and improved fetal growth (Jansson, 2015).

Nurses are in a unique position to help because they interact with high-risk mothers and newborns in many settings, including the community, health care facilities, and family agencies. It is the responsibility of all nurses to identify, educate, counsel, and refer pregnant women with substance-abusing problems. For example, nurses can be instrumental in increasing the number of pregnant women who make a serious attempt to quit smoking by using the "5 A's" approach:

- **A**sk: Ask all women if they smoke and would like to quit.
- **A**dvise: Encourage the use of clinically proven treatment plans.
- **A**ssess: Provide motivation by discussing the "5 Rs":
  - **R**elevance of quitting to the woman
  - **R**isk of continued smoking to the fetus
  - **R**ewards of quitting for both
  - **R**oadblocks to quitting
  - **R**epeat at every visit
- **A**ssist: Help the woman to protect her fetus and newborn from the negative effects of smoking.
- **A**rrange: Schedule follow-up visits to reinforce the woman's commitment to quit.

Although this approach is geared to smoking cessation, nurses can adapt it to focus on cessation for any substance use. Early, supportive, ongoing nursing care is critical to the well-being of the mother and her newborn. Nurses have an ethical responsibility to provide evidence-based and nonjudgmental care to this highly vulnerable population.

Caring for a substance-exposed newborn remains a major challenge to health care providers. The major goals include providing comfort to the newborn by relieving symptoms, improving feeding and weight gain, preventing seizures, promoting mother–newborn interactions, and reducing the incidence of newborn mortality and abnormal development (Mattson & Smith, 2015).

PROMOTING COMFORT

Supportive interventions to promote comfort include swaddling, low lighting, gentle handling, quiet environment with minimal stimulation, use of soft voices, pacifiers to promote "self-soothing," frequent small feedings, vertical rocking during infant disorganization periods, and rooming-in and positioning (Artigas, 2015). Keep environmental stimuli to a minimum. For example, decrease stimuli by dimming the lights in the nursery, and swaddle the newborn tightly to decrease irritability behaviors. Other techniques such as gentle rocking, using a flexed position, and offering a pacifier can help manage CNS irritability. A pacifier also helps satisfy the newborn's need for nonnutritive sucking. Swaddling, pacifiers, low lighting, oscillating cribs, and avoidance of abrupt changes in the infant's environment can be helpful. Use a calm, gentle approach when handling the newborn and plan activities to avoid overstimulating the newborn, allowing time for rest periods.

MEETING NUTRITIONAL NEEDS

Newborns suffering from NAS have impaired feeding behaviors, such as excessive sucking, poor feeding, regurgitation, and diarrhea, which may cause weight loss. To improve weight gain, they are supplemented with high-calorie formula. When feeding the newborn, use small amounts and position the newborn upright to prevent aspiration and to facilitate rhythmic sucking and swallowing. Frequent small feedings are preferable and should provide 150 to 250 kcal/kg per 24 hours for proper growth of the infant undergoing significant withdrawal (Gardner et al., 2016).

Breast-feeding is encouraged unless the mother is still using drugs. Monitor the newborn's weight daily to evaluate the success of food intake. Assess hydration; check skin turgor and fontanels. Assess the frequency and characteristics of bowel movements and monitor the newborn's fluid and electrolyte and acid–base status.

PREVENTING COMPLICATIONS

Pharmacologic treatment is warranted if conservative measures, such as swaddling and decreased environmental stimulation, are not adequate. The AAP recommends that for newborns with confirmed drug exposure, drug therapy is indicated if the newborn has seizures, diarrhea, and vomiting resulting in excessive weight loss and dehydration, poor feeding, inability to sleep, and fever unrelated to infection (Jones & Fielder, 2015). Common medications used in the management of newborn withdrawal include an opioid (morphine or methadone) and phenobarbital as a second drug if the opiate does not adequately control symptoms (Artigas, 2015). Administer the prescribed medications and document the newborn's behavioral responses.

The newborn is at risk for skin breakdown. Weight loss, diarrhea, dehydration, and irritability can contribute to this risk. Provide meticulous skin care and protect the newborn's elbows and knees against friction and abrasions.

PROMOTING PARENT–NEWBORN INTERACTION

For a mother who abuses substances, the birth of a drug-exposed newborn is both a crisis and an opportunity. The mother may feel guilty about the newborn's condition. Many of these newborns are unresponsive and have disorganized sleeping and feeding patterns. When awake, they can be easily overstimulated and irritated. Such characteristics make parent–newborn interactions difficult and frustrating, leading to possible detachment and avoidance. Nursing support, which includes a description of symptoms and their management, is vital if maternal–infant attachment is to occur and potential neglect or abuse is avoided (Gardner et al., 2016). Instruct the mother or caretaker how to care for the newborn, including what to do after the newborn goes home (see Teaching Guidelines 24.1).

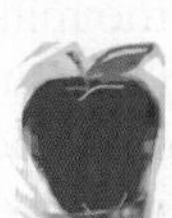

Teaching Guidelines 24.1

CARING FOR YOUR NEWBORN AT HOME

- Position your newborn with the head elevated to prevent choking.
- To aid your newborn's sucking and swallowing during feeding, position the chin downward and support it with your hand.
- Place your newborn on his or her back to sleep or nap, never on the stomach.
- Keep a bulb syringe close by to suction your newborn's mouth in case of choking.
- Cluster newborn care (bathing, feeding, dressing) to prevent overstimulation.
- If your newborn is fussy or crying, try these measures to help calm him or her:
    - Wrap your newborn snugly in a blanket and gently rock in rocking chair.
    - Take the baby for a ride in the car (using a newborn car seat).
    - Play soothing music and "dance" with the newborn.
    - Use a wind-up swing with music.
- To help your newborn get to sleep, try these measures:
    - Schedule a bath with a gentle massage prior to bedtime.
    - Change diaper and clothes to make the baby comfortable.
    - Feed the baby just prior to bedtime.
    - If the newborn cries when put in crib and all needs are met, allow him or her to cry.
    - Use a rocking chair to feed and sing a soft lullaby.
- Call your primary care provider if you observe withdrawal behaviors such as:
    - Slight tremors (shaking) of hands and legs
    - Stiff posture when held in your arms
    - Irritability and frequent fussiness
    - High-pitched cry, excessive sucking motions
    - Erratic sleep pattern
    - Frequent yawning, nasal stuffiness, sweating
    - Prolonged time needed to feed
    - Frequent vomiting after feeding

On the other hand, the newborn may be a powerful motivator for the mother to undergo treatment and seek recovery. Refer the mother to community agencies to address addiction and the infant's developmental needs (Mattson & Smith, 2015). The nurse can play a pivotal role in assisting her to abstain from drug use and to promote effective parenting skills.

Hyperbilirubinemia

Hyperbilirubinemia is a total serum bilirubin level above 5 mg/dL resulting from unconjugated bilirubin being deposited in the skin and mucous membranes (Hansen, 2016). Hyperbilirubinemia is exhibited as jaundice (yellowing of the body tissues and fluids). Newborn jaundice is one of the most common reasons for hospital readmission. It occurs in 60% to 80% of term newborns in the first week of life and in virtually all preterm newborns (Fanaroff & Fanaroff, 2014).

Pathophysiology

Bilirubin has two forms—unconjugated or indirect, which is fat-soluble and toxic to body tissues, and conjugated or direct, which is water-soluble and nontoxic. Elevated serum bilirubin levels are manifested as jaundice in the newborn. Typically the total serum bilirubin level rises over the first 3 to 5 days and then declines.

Newborn jaundice results from an imbalance in the rate of bilirubin production and bilirubin elimination. This imbalance determines the pattern and degree of newborn hyperbilirubinemia (Hansen, 2016).

During the newborn period, a rapid transition from the intrauterine to the extrauterine pattern of bilirubin physiology occurs. Fetal unconjugated bilirubin is normally cleared by the placenta and the mother's liver in utero, so total bilirubin at birth is low. After the umbilical cord is cut, the newborn must conjugate bilirubin (convert a lipid-soluble pigment into a water-soluble pigment) in the liver on his or her own. The rate and amount of bilirubin conjugation depend on the rate of red blood cell breakdown, the bilirubin load, the maturity of the liver, and the number of albumin-binding sites. Bilirubin levels rise in newborns by three main mechanisms: increased production (accelerated RBC breakdown), decreased removal (transient liver enzyme insufficiency), and increased reabsorption (delay in bowel excretion) (Gardner et al., 2016). Bilirubin production increases after birth mainly because of a shortened red blood cell lifespan (70 days in the newborn vs. 90 days in the adult) combined with an increased red blood cell mass. Therefore, the amount of bilirubin the newborn must deal with is large compared to that of an adult.

PHYSIOLOGIC JAUNDICE

Physiologic jaundice is an unconjugated hyperbilirubinemia that occurs after the first postnatal day and can last up to 1 week. Total serum bilirubin concentrations peak in the first 3 to 5 postnatal days and decline to adult values over the next several weeks.

It occurs in 60% of term infants and up to 80% of preterm infants (Blackburn, 2012). Serum bilirubin levels reach up to 10 mg/dL and then decline rapidly over the first week after birth (Cunningham et al., 2014). Most newborns have been discharged by the time this jaundice peaks (at about 72 hours).

Physiologic jaundice may result from an increased bilirubin load because of relative polycythemia, a shortened red blood cell lifespan, immature hepatic uptake and conjugation process, and increased enterohepatic circulation (Hansen, 2016). Newborns with delayed passage of meconium are more likely to develop physiologic jaundice because meconium contains high levels of bilirubin (Kenner & Lott, 2014).

Physiologic jaundice differs between breast-fed and bottle-fed newborns in relation to the onset of symptoms. Breast-fed newborns typically have peak bilirubin levels on the fourth day of life; levels for bottle-fed newborns usually peak on the third day of life. The rate of bilirubin decline is less rapid in breast-fed newborns compared to bottle-fed newborns because bottle-fed newborns tend to have more frequent bowel movements. Jaundice associated with breast-feeding presents in two distinct patterns: early-onset breast-feeding jaundice and late-onset breast milk jaundice.

Early-Onset Breast-Feeding Jaundice. Early-onset breast-feeding jaundice is probably associated with ineffective breast-feeding practices because of relative caloric deprivation in the first few days of life. Decreased volume and frequency of feedings may result in mild dehydration and the delayed passage of meconium. This delayed defecation allows enterohepatic circulation reuptake of bilirubin and an increase in the serum level of unconjugated bilirubin. To prevent this, strategies to promote early effective breast-feeding are important. The AAP guidelines recommend early and frequent breast-feeding without supplemental water or dextrose-water because they do not prevent hyperbilirubinemia and may lead to hyponatremia (Deshpande, 2015). Early frequent feedings can provide the newborn with adequate calories and fluid volume (via colostrum) to stimulate peristalsis and passage of meconium to eliminate bilirubin. Successful breast-feeding decreases the risk of hyperbilirubinemia. Infants need to be fed at least 8 to 12 times in the first few days after birth to help improve the mother's milk supply. The best way to judge successful breast-feeding is to monitor infant urine output, stool output, and weight. Newborns should have four to six wet diapers and three to four yellow, seedy stools per day by the fourth day after birth. Breast-feeding–associated jaundice is usually preventable through appropriate breast-feeding practices.

Late-Onset Breast-Feeding Jaundice. Late-onset breast-feeding jaundice occurs later in the newborn period, with the bilirubin level usually peaking in the first 6 to 14 days of life. It typically occurs between the fourth and seventh days of life, when mature milk begins to replace colostrum. Total serum bilirubin levels may reach as high as 12 mg/dL, but the level is not considered pathologic (Lauwers & Swisher, 2016). The specific cause of late-onset breast milk jaundice is not entirely understood, but it may be related to a change in the milk composition resulting in enhanced enterohepatic circulation. Additional research is needed to determine the cause. Interrupting breast-feeding is not recommended unless bilirubin levels reach dangerous levels; if this occurs, breast-feeding is stopped for only 1 or 2 days. Most cases require no interruption in breast-feeding. Frequent and effective breast-feeding soon after childbirth is associated with reducing the incidence and intensity of breast-feeding jaundice.

PATHOLOGIC JAUNDICE

Pathologic jaundice is manifested within the first 24 hours of life when total bilirubin levels increase by more than 5 mg/dL/day and the total serum bilirubin level is higher than 17 mg/dL in a full-term infant. This condition requires intervention (Ives, 2015). Conditions that alter the production, transport, uptake, metabolism, excretion, or reabsorption of bilirubin can cause pathologic jaundice in the newborn. A few conditions that contribute to red blood cell breakdown and thus higher bilirubin levels include polycythemia, blood incompatibilities, and systemic acidosis. These altered conditions can lead to high levels of unconjugated bilirubin, possibly reaching toxic levels and resulting in a severe condition called ***kernicterus*** or bilirubin encephalopathy. It can be acute or chronic.

Hyperbilirubinemia is a great concern because of the potential for brain injury. The spectrum of bilirubin-induced neurologic dysfunction ranges from **acute bilirubin encephalopathy** to the devastating and irreversible **chronic bilirubin encephalopathy** or kernicterus.

Acute bilirubin encephalopathy describes the effects of hyperbilirubinemia in the first weeks of life. Clinical signs include lethargy, poor feeding, high-pitched cry, poor tone, a poor Moro reflex with incomplete flexion of the extremities, and a high-pitched cry. As symptoms of acute bilirubin encephalopathy worsen, the newborn progresses to apnea, seizures, coma, and death (Gardner et al., 2016).

Chronic bilirubin encephalopathy or kernicterus is characterized by four clinical manifestations: movement disorder (athetosis, dystonia, spasticity, hypotonia), auditory dysfunction (deafness), oculomotor impairment, and dental enamel hypoplasia of deciduous teeth (Springer & Annibale, 2014). Unconjugated bilirubin enters the brain and acts as a neurotoxin causing long-term neurologic sequelae. Cases of kernicterus should not be occurring today, but delays in diagnosing pathologic causes of prolonged jaundice are still being missed or overlooked (Ives, 2015).

The most common condition associated with pathologic jaundice is hemolytic disease of the newborn secondary to incompatibility of blood groups of the mother and the newborn. The most frequent conditions are Rh factor and ABO incompatibilities.

Take Note!

Significant jaundice in the newborn less than 24 hours of age should be immediately reported to the physician, as it may indicate a pathologic process.

Nursing Assessment

Neonatal jaundice first becomes visible in the face and forehead. Identification is aided by pressure on the skin, since blanching reveals the underlying color. Jaundice then gradually becomes visible on the trunk and extremities. This cephalocaudal progression is well described. Jaundice disappears in the opposite direction. Nurses play an important role in early detection and identification of jaundice in the newborn. Keen observation skills are essential.

HEALTH HISTORY AND PHYSICAL EXAMINATION

Review the medical record for factors that might predispose the newborn to hyperbilirubinemia, such as:

- Polycythemia
- Significant bruising or cephalhematoma, which increases bilirubin production
- Infections such as TORCH (toxoplasmosis, hepatitis B, rubella, cytomegalovirus [CMV], herpes simplex virus)
- Use of drugs during labor and birth such as diazepam (Valium) or oxytocin (Pitocin)
- Prematurity
- Gestational age of 34 to 36 weeks
- Hemolysis due to ABO incompatibility or Rh isoimmunization
- Macrosomic IDM
- Delayed cord clamping, which increases the erythrocyte volume
- Decreased albumin binding sites to transport unconjugated bilirubin to the liver because of acidosis
- Delayed meconium passage, which increases the amount of bilirubin that returns to the unconjugated state and can be absorbed by the intestinal mucosa
- Siblings who had significant jaundice
- Inadequate breast-feeding leading to dehydration, decreased caloric intake, weight loss, and delayed passage of meconium
- Ethnicity, such as Asian American, Mediterranean, or Native American
- Male gender (Gardner et al., 2016; NICE, 2014)

Perform a complete physical examination. Assess the skin, mucous membranes, sclerae, and bodily fluids (tears, urine) for a yellow color. Detect jaundice by observing the infant in a well-lit room and blanching the skin with digital pressure over a bony prominence. Typically, jaundice begins on the head and gradually progresses to the abdomen and extremities. Also inspect for pallor (anemia), excessive bruising (bleeding), and dehydration (sluggish circulation), which may contribute to the development of jaundice and the risk for kernicterus.

Assess the newborn for Rh incompatibility. Be alert for clinical manifestations such as ascites, anemia, congestive heart failure, edema, pallor, jaundice, hepatosplenomegaly, polyhydramnios, thick placenta, and dilation of the umbilical vein (Salem & Singer, 2014).

Hydropic newborns appear pale, edematous, and limp at birth and typically require resuscitation. The newborn with immune hydrops exhibits severe generalized edema, organ hypertrophy and enlargement, and effusion of fluid into body cavities.

LABORATORY AND DIAGNOSTIC TESTING

Determine maternal and fetal blood types, checking for incompatibilities (Comparison Chart 24.1). Assess laboratory values for bilirubin (both unconjugated and conjugated). Bilirubin levels establish the diagnosis of hyperbilirubinemia. The newborn with Rh incompatibility demonstrates a rapidly rising unconjugated bilirubin level at birth or in the first 24 hours. Also expect to obtain alkaline phosphatase, liver enzymes, and prothrombin time and partial thromboplastin time, as well as the following:

- Direct Coombs test—to identify hemolytic disease of the newborn; positive results indicate that the newborn's red blood cells have been coated with antibodies and thus are sensitized

COMPARISON CHART 24.1 RH VERSUS ABO INCOMPATIBILITY

Clinical Picture	Rh Incompatibility	ABO Incompatibility
First-born	Rare	Common
Later pregnancies	More severe	No increase in severity
Jaundice	Moderate to severe	Mild
Hydrops fetalis	Frequent	Rare
Anemia	Frequently severe	Rare
Ascites	Frequent	Rare
Hepatosplenomegaly	Frequent	Common

- Hemoglobin concentration—for evidence of anemia
- Blood type—to determine Rh status and any incompatibility of the newborn
- Total serum protein—to detect reduced binding capacity of albumin
- Reticulocyte count—to identify an elevated level indicating increased hemolysis

Assist with obtaining blood specimens. Use cord blood for hemoglobin concentration measurements; use a heel stick for direct Coombs testing and bilirubin levels. Prepare the parents and newborn for radiologic evaluation if necessary to determine abnormalities that may be causing the jaundice.

Nursing Management

Nursing management of a newborn with hyperbilirubinemia requires a comprehensive approach. As members of the health care team, nurses share in the responsibility for early detection and identification, family education, management, and follow-up of the mother and newborn. Documentation of the timing of onset of jaundice is essential to differentiate between physiologic (>24 hours) and pathologic jaundice (<24 hours). Nurses can improve care by offering their presence and support and by following the AAP guidelines for preventing hyperbilirubinemia:

- Promote and support successful breast-feeding.
- Assess for risk factors that may increase bilirubin levels.
- Establish nursery protocols for identifying jaundice, including when a serum bilirubin can be ordered by a nurse.
- Measure total serum bilirubin on jaundiced infants in the first 24 hours.
- Interpret all bilirubin levels according to the infant's age in hours.
- Visual estimation of jaundice is inaccurate and shouldn't be used instead of labs.
- Infants <38 weeks, particularly if breast-fed, should be considered high risk.
- Perform risk assessment on all newborns prior to discharge.
- Jaundiced newborns should be treated, if indicated, with phototherapy.
- Provide parents with written and oral information about jaundice at discharge.
- Follow-up care and referrals should be based on time of discharge and risk.
- Empower parents to make appropriate decisions once home (Green, 2016; Mattson, & Smith, 2015).

REDUCING BILIRUIN LEVELS

Encourage early initiation of feedings to prevent hypoglycemia and provide protein to maintain the albumin levels to transport bilirubin to the liver. Ensure newborn feedings (breast milk or formula) every 2 to 3 hours to promote prompt emptying of bilirubin from the bowel. Encourage the mother to breast-feed (8 to 12 feedings per day) to prevent inadequate intake and thus dehydration. Supplement breast milk with formula to supply protein if bilirubin levels continue to increase with breast-feeding only. Monitor serum bilirubin levels frequently to reduce the risk of severe hyperbilirubinemia.

Phototherapy. For the newborn with jaundice, regardless of its etiology, phototherapy is used to convert unconjugated bilirubin to the less toxic water-soluble form that can be excreted. Phototherapy, via special lights placed above the newborn or a fiberoptic blanket placed under the newborn and wrapped around him or her, involves blue wavelengths of light to alter unconjugated bilirubin in the skin. For the newborn receiving phototherapy, place the newborn under the lights or on the fiberoptic blanket, exposing as much skin as possible. Cover the newborn's genitals and shield the eyes to protect these areas from becoming irritated or burned when using direct lights. Assess the intensity of the light

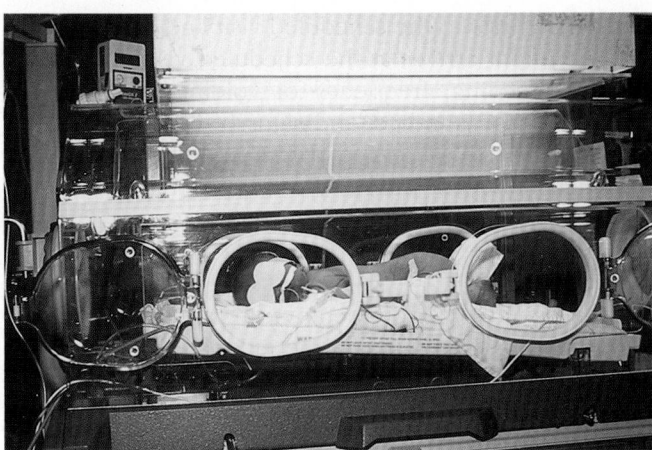

FIGURE 24.7 A newborn receiving phototherapy.

source to prevent burns and excoriation (Fig. 24.7). Turn the newborn every 2 hours to maximize the area of exposure, removing the newborn from the lights only for feedings. Maintain a neutral thermal environment to decrease energy expenditure, and assess the newborn's neurologic status frequently. Research is finding that intermittent versus continuous phototherapy is as efficacious to lower bilirubin levels (Evidence-Based Practice 24.1).

Assess the newborn's temperature every 3 to 4 hours as indicated. Monitor fluid intake and output closely and assess daily weights for gains or losses. Check skin turgor for evidence of dehydration.

With feedings, remove the newborn from the lights and remove the eye shields to allow interaction with the newborn. Encourage breast- or bottle-feedings every 2 to 3 hours. Follow agency policy about removing the eye shields periodically to assess the eyes for discharge or corneal irritation secondary to eye shield pressure. Typically, the eyes are assessed and eye shields removed once a shift.

Monitor stool for consistency and frequency. Unconjugated bilirubin excreted in the feces will produce a greenish appearance, and typically stools are loose. Lack of frequent green stools is a cause for concern.

Provide meticulous skin care. Assess skin surfaces frequently for dryness and irritation secondary to the dehydrating effects of phototherapy and irritation from highly acidic stool to prevent excoriation and skin breakdown (Green, 2016). Nursing responsibilities include ensuring effective irradiance delivery, maximizing skin exposure, providing eye protection and eye care, careful attention to thermoregulation, monitoring the newborn's skin turgor, maintaining adequate hydration, promoting elimination, and supporting parent–infant interaction (Nagtalon-Ramos, 2014).

A summary of the nursing care for the newborn undergoing phototherapy is as follows:

- Support parents, encouraging them to interact with their infant.

EVIDENCE-BASED PRACTICE 24.1

INTERMITTENT VERSUS CONTINUOUS PHOTOTHERAPY FOR THE TREATMENT OF NEONATAL NONHEMOLYTIC MODERATE HYPERBILIRUBINEMIA IN INFANTS MORE THAN 34 WEEKS OF GESTATION: A RANDOMIZED CONTROL TRIAL

STUDY

Neonatal hyperbilirubinemia is frequent reason for late preterm and full-term infants admitted to the NICU. Currently, phototherapy is the most effective therapy for management of neonatal hyperbilirubinemia. Phototherapy acts by three mechanisms to reduce the bilirubin level which include photooxidation, and photo and structural isomerization. The photochemical reaction requires a short period of time and the remaining time, the role of phototherapy is only minimal. With this process in mind, the purpose of this study was to compare intermittent phototherapy with 12 hours on and then 12 hours off with continuous phototherapy.

Findings

In this randomized control study, 75 healthy neonates >34 weeks' gestation were randomized either into intermittent or continuous phototherapy groups. The rate of fall of bilirubin was examined in each group. It was found that the rate of bilirubin fall was greater in the intermediate phototherapy group when compared to the continuous phototherapy group. This study concluded that intermittent phototherapy with 12-hour on and 12-hour off cycles is as efficacious as continuous phototherapy to reduce hyperbilirubinemia in neonates.

Nursing Implications

Nurses can begin the conversation within their clinical settings to bring about change in phototherapy protocols based on this study's findings. Although the sample size was small, it can be duplicated in larger clinical settings to demonstrate the effectiveness of intermittent phototherapy. This phototherapy protocol change could save costs and decrease the anxiety of parents/partners/significant others. Nurses can be instrumental in bringing evidence-based changes by serving on hospital policy and procedure committees.

Adapted from Sachdeva, M., Murki, S., Oleti, T. P., & Kandraju, H. (2015). Intermittent versus continuous phototherapy for the treatment of neonatal non-hemolytic moderate hyperbilirubinemia in infants more than 34 weeks of gestational age: A randomized controlled trial. *European Journal of Pediatrics, 174*(2),177–181.

- Support breast-feeding with one-on-one instruction and patience.
- Place infants on their back to expose as much naked skin as possible.
- Provide eye care/protection every time the infant is exposed to the light.
- Check temperature and environment around infant to prevent overheating.
- Take daily weights to make sure the infant isn't becoming dehydrated.

Exchange Transfusion. If the total serum bilirubin level remains elevated after intensive phototherapy, an exchange transfusion with albumin administered before the transfusion, the quickest method for lowering serum bilirubin levels, may be necessary (Hansen, 2016). In the presence of hemolytic disease, severe anemia, or a rapid rise in the total serum bilirubin level, an exchange transfusion is recommended. An exchange transfusion removes the newborn's blood and replaces it with nonhemolyzed red blood cells from a donor. During the transfusion, monitor the newborn's cardiovascular status continuously because serious complications can arise, such as acid–base imbalances, infection, hypovolemia, and fluid and electrolyte imbalances. Exchange transfusion is used only as a second-line therapy after phototherapy has failed to yield results. Intensive nursing care is needed.

Assist the physician or health care practitioner with an exchange transfusion if necessary. Monitor the newborn's status closely for changes, especially in vital signs and heart rate and rhythm, before, during, and after the procedure.

PROVIDING PARENT TEACHING AND SUPPORT

Nurses can help the parents to understand the diagnostic tests and treatment modalities by offering individualized teaching. Nurses are the ones who give discharge instructions to the family. Explore with the family their understanding of jaundice and treatment modalities to reduce anxiety and gain their cooperation in monitoring the infant. Teach the parents about jaundice and its potential risk using written and verbal material. Also show the parents how to identify newborn behaviors that might indicate rising bilirubin levels. Emphasize the need to seek treatment from their pediatrician should any of the following occur:

- Lethargy, sleepiness, poor muscle tone, floppiness
- Poor sucking, lack of interest in feeding
- High-pitched cry

Teach the parents how to assess their newborn for signs of jaundice because physiologic jaundice may not occur until after the newborn is discharged. After discharge is planned, parent education plays an important role in hyperbilirubinemia prevention, ensuring that the health care provider is contacted if concerning signs arise prior to the scheduled visit and also ensuring that the infant arrives at the scheduled visit. Frequency of breast-feeding, frequency of voiding and stooling, progression of jaundice, and signs of illness can all be monitored by the engaged parent and shared with the provider. Reinforce the need for appropriate follow-up with the primary care provider within 48 to 72 hours after discharge to assess jaundice status (Verklan & Walden, 2015).

The need for phototherapy can be anxiety-producing for the parents. Explain the rationale for the procedure and demonstrate techniques that the parents can use to interact with their newborn. Additional education about phototherapy may be necessary when home phototherapy is used (Teaching Guidelines 24.2).

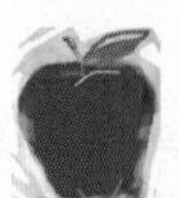

Teaching Guidelines 24.2

CARING FOR YOUR NEWBORN RECEIVING HOME PHOTOTHERAPY

- Inspect your newborn's skin, eyes, and mucous membranes for a yellow color.
- Remember that a home health nurse will come to visit and help set up the light system.
- Keep the lights about 12 to 30 in above your newborn.
- Cover your newborn's eyes with patches or cotton balls and gauze to protect them.
- Keep the newborn undressed except for the diaper area; fold the diaper down below the newborn's navel in the front and as far as possible in the back to expose as much skin area as possible.
- Turn your newborn every 2 hours so that all areas of the body are exposed.
- Remove the newborn from the lights only for feeding.
- Remove the eye patches during feedings so that you can interact with your newborn.
- Record your newborn's temperature, weight, and fluid intake daily.
- Document the frequency, color, and consistency of all stools; the stools should be loose and green as the bilirubin is broken down.
- Keep the skin clean and dry to prevent irritation.
- Feed your newborn frequently, including supplemental glucose water if allowed to provide added fluid, protein, and calories.
- Rock, cuddle, or hold the newborn to promote bonding when out of the lights.
- Contact your pediatrician or home health care agency with any questions or changes, including refusing feedings, fewer than five wet diapers in one day, vomiting of complete amounts of feeding, or elevated temperature.
- Keep appointments for follow-up laboratory testing to monitor bilirubin levels.

NEONATAL SEPSIS

Neonatal sepsis is defined as a clinical syndrome of bacteremia with systemic signs and symptoms of infection in the first month of life (Molyneux & Gest, 2015). Newborns have increased susceptibility to infections because their immune systems are immature and slow to react, and they have a poorly developed skin barrier. The antibodies that newborns received from their mother during pregnancy and from breast milk help protect them from invading organisms. However, these need time to reach optimal levels.

Bacterial infections of the newborn remain a major cause of illness and death in the neonatal period. The mortality rate from newborn sepsis may be as high as 50% if untreated. Infection is a major cause of death during the first month of life, contributing to 13% to 15% of all neonatal deaths (Anderson-Berry, Bellig, & Ohning, 2015).

Pathophysiology

When a pathologic organism overcomes the newborn's defenses, infection and sepsis result. Neonatal sepsis is the presence of bacterial, fungal, or viral microorganisms or their toxins in blood or other tissues. Infections that have an onset within the first month of life are termed *newborn infections*. Exposure to a pathogenic organism, whether a virus, fungus, or bacteria, occurs, and it enters the newborn's body and begins to multiply.

Newborn infections are usually grouped into three classes according to their time of onset: congenital infection, acquired in utero (intrauterine infections) by vertical transmission with onset before birth; early-onset infections, acquired by vertical transmission in the perinatal period, either shortly before or during birth; and late-onset infections, acquired by horizontal transmission in the nursery. About 85% of neonatal infections have their onset in the first 2 days of life and usually are pneumonia and meningitis (Deleon, Shattuck, & Jain, 2015). Comparison Chart 24.2 compares the three classes of newborn infections.

Early-onset neonatal infections (<72 hours) are associated with acquisition of microorganisms from the mother. Transplacental infection or an ascending infection from the cervix may be caused by organisms that colonize in the mother's genitourinary tract, with acquisition of the microbe by passage through a colonized birth canal at delivery. The microorganisms most commonly associated with early-onset infection include group B *Streptococcus* (GBS), *Escherichia coli,* coagulase-negative *Staphylococcus, Haemophilus influenzae,* and *Listeria monocytogenes.*

Late-onset infections (>72 hours), acquired in the postpartum period, are primarily through horizontal transmission from family members or caregivers or through environmental exposures. Infections such as human immunodeficiency virus (HIV) and CMV can be acquired through breast-feeding (discussed in more detail in Chapter 20) or by direct contact with family members or health care providers. These types of contacts and exposures are especially important in infants, primarily preterm, with prolonged hospital stays, where they are more likely to be exposed to multidrug-resistant hospital-associated organisms potentially from contact with caregivers or contaminated equipment. Organisms that cause late-onset sepsis include *Staphylococcus aureus, E. coli, Klebsiella, Pseudomonas, Enterobacter, Candida,* and *Anaerobes* (Mukhopadhyay & Puopolo, 2015). Comparison Chart 24.2 compares the three classes of newborn infections.

Nursing Assessment

Diagnosis of neonatal infections is challenging. Most infants will have some risk factors and the presenting symptoms are many and nonspecific, including poor feeding, breathing difficulty, apneas and bradycardia, gastrointestinal problems, increased oxygen requirement or ventilator support needs, lethargy or hypotension, decreased or elevated temperature, unusual skin rash or color change, persistent crying, or irritability. Adding to the challenge of correctly identifying the infection, the list of conditions to consider in the differential diagnosis is extensive, including metabolic and congenital abnormalities (Bengtsson, van Houten, & Oster, 2015).

Nursing assessment focuses on early identification of a newborn at risk for infection to allow for prompt treatment, thus reducing mortality and morbidity. Be aware of the myriad risk factors associated with newborn sepsis. Among the factors that contribute to the newborn's overall vulnerability to infection are poor skin integrity, invasive procedures, exposure to numerous caregivers, and an environment conducive to bacterial colonization (Green, 2016).

Few newborn infections are easy to recognize because manifestations usually are nonspecific. Early symptoms can be vague because of the newborn's inability to mount an inflammatory response. Often, the observation is that the newborn does not "look right." Assess the newborn for common nonspecific signs of infection, including:

- Temperature instability
- Hypotension
- Tachycardia
- Pallor or duskiness
- Hypotonia
- Cyanosis
- Poor weight gain
- Irritability
- Seizures
- Rash
- Petechiae
- Jaundice

COMPARISON CHART 24.2

INTRAUTERINE VERSUS EARLY-ONSET VERSUS LATE-ONSET NEWBORN INFECTIONS

	Intrauterine (Congenital)	Early-Onset Infections	Late-Onset Infections
Risk factors	• Immature immune system IgM, IgA, and T lymphocytes • Decreased gastric acid, which is needed to reduce organisms	• Prolonged rupture of membranes • Urinary tract infections • Preterm labor • Prolonged or difficult labor • Maternal fever • Colonization with group B streptococci • Maternal infections	• Low birthweight • Prematurity • Meconium staining • Need for resuscitation • Birth asphyxia • Improper handwashing
Common causative organisms	• Cytomegalovirus • Rubella • Toxoplasmosis • Syphilis	• *Escherichia coli* • Group B streptococci • *Klebsiella pneumoniae* • *Listeria monocytogenes* • Other enteric gram-negative bacilli	• *Candida albicans* • Coagulase-negative staphylococci • *Staphylococcus aureus* • *E. coli* • Enterobacter • Klebsiella • Serratia • Pseudomonas • Group B streptococci
Mechanism of infection	• Organism crossing placenta into fetal circulatory system; organism residing in amniotic fluid • Ascent of organism via the vagina, ultimately infecting membranes and causing rupture and leading to respiratory and gastrointestinal tract infections	• Most occur during birthing process when newborn comes into contact with infected birth canal (newborn cannot defend against host organisms) • Newborn susceptibility to infection by exogenous organisms possibly due to inadequacy of physical barriers (thin, friable skin with little subcutaneous tissue) • Lack of gastric acidity, possibly resulting in easy colonization by environmental organisms • Aspiration of microorganisms during birth with development of pneumonia	More common in newborns undergoing invasive procedures such as endotracheal intubation or catheter insertion; break in skin or mucosal protection barrier

Adapted from Anderson-Berry, A. L., Bellig, L. L., & Ohning, B. L. (2015). *Neonatal sepsis.* Retrieved from http://emedicine.medscape.com/article/978352-overview; Molyneux, E., & Gest, A. (2015). Neonatal sepsis: An old issue needing new answers. *The Lancet Infectious Diseases, 15*(5), 503–505; and Gardner, S. L., Carter, B. S., Enzman-Hines, M., & Hernandez, J. A. (2016). *Merenstein & Gardner's handbook of neonatal intensive care* (8th ed.). St. Louis, MO: Mosby Elsevier.

- Grunting
- Nasal flaring
- Apnea
- Lethargy
- Hypoglycemia
- Poor feeding (lack of interest in feeding)
- Abdominal distention (Gardner et al., 2016)

Since infection can be confused with other newborn conditions, laboratory and radiographic tests are needed to confirm the presence of infection. Be prepared to coordinate the timing of the various tests and assist as necessary.

Evaluate the complete blood count with a differential to identify anemia, leukocytosis, or leukopenia. Elevated C-reactive protein levels may indicate inflammation. As ordered, obtain x-rays of the chest and abdomen, which may reveal infectious processes located there. Blood, cerebrospinal fluid, and urine cultures are indicated to identify the location and type of infection present. Positive cultures confirm that the newborn has an infection. Initially, treatment is with ampicillin plus either gentamicin or cefotaxime, then narrowed down to organism-specific drugs as soon as the cultures identify the specific organism. This practice of empirically treating at-risk neonates leads to potentially harmful exposure for many uninfected infants, but in the absence of accurate rapid diagnostic tests, it is prudent to be safe (Oliver et al., 2015).

Nursing Management

To enhance the newborn's chance of survival, early recognition and diagnosis are essential. Often the diagnosis of sepsis is based on a suspicious clinical picture. Antibiotic therapy is usually started before the laboratory results identify the infecting pathogen. Along with antibiotic therapy, circulatory, respiratory, nutritional, and developmental support is important. Antibiotic therapy is continued for 7 to 21 days if cultures are positive, or it is discontinued within 72 hours if cultures are negative. With the use of antibiotics along with early recognition and supportive care, mortality and morbidity rates have been reduced greatly.

Nurses possess the education and assessment tools to decrease the incidence of and reduce the impact of infections on women (see Chapter 20 for additional information) and their newborns. Implement measures for prevention and early recognition, including:

- Formulate a sepsis prevention plan that includes education of all members of the health care team on identification and treatment of sepsis.
- Maintain medical and surgical asepsis for all providing care.
- Screen all newborns daily for signs of sepsis.
- Monitor sepsis cases and outcomes to reinforce continued quality-improvement measures or to modify current practices.
- Outline and carry out measures to prevent hospital-acquired infections, such as:
    - Thorough handwashing hygiene for all staff
    - Monitor and support nutritional status
    - Frequent oral care and inspections of mucous membranes
    - Proper positioning and turning to prevent skin breakdown
    - Use of strict aseptic technique for all wound care
    - Frequent monitoring of invasive catheter sites for signs of infection.
- Identify newborns at risk for sepsis by reviewing risk factors.
- Monitor vital sign changes and observe for subtle signs of infection.
- Monitor for signs of organ system dysfunction:
    - Cardiovascular compromise—tachycardia and hypotension
    - Respiratory compromise—respiratory distress and tachypnea
    - Renal compromise—oliguria or anuria
    - Systemic compromise—abnormal blood values
- Provide comprehensive sepsis treatment:
    - Circulatory support with fluids and vasopressors
    - Supplemental oxygen and mechanical ventilation
    - Obtaining culture samples as requested
    - Antibiotic administration as ordered, observing for side effects
    - Promote newborn comfort and pain management measures.
    - Assess the family's educational needs and providing instructions as necessary.

Perinatal infections continue to be a public health problem, with severe consequences for those affected. By promoting a better understanding of newborn infections and appropriate use of therapies, nurses can lower the mortality rates associated with severe sepsis, especially with appropriate timing of interventions. The potential for nursing interventions to identify, prevent, and minimize the risk for sepsis is significant. Primary disease prevention must be a major focus for nurses. Family education plays a key role in the prevention of perinatal infections, in addition to following accepted practices in immunization.

CONGENITAL CONDITIONS

The human and economic toll of birth defects is significant and tragic. Each year an estimated 8 million children – 6% of the total births globally – are born with a serious birth defect. Approximately 120,000 infants are born with a birth defect in the United States (March of Dimes, 2016b). Congenital conditions can arise from many etiologies, including single-gene disorders, chromosome aberrations, exposure to teratogens, and many sporadic conditions of unknown cause. Congenital conditions may be inherited or sporadic, isolated or multiple, apparent or hidden, gross or microscopic. They cause nearly half of all deaths in term newborns and cause long-term sequelae for many. The incidence varies according to the type of defect. When a serious anomaly is identified prenatally, the parents can decide whether or not to continue the pregnancy. When an anomaly is identified at or after birth, parents need to be informed promptly and given a realistic appraisal of the severity of the condition, the prognosis, and treatment options so that they can participate in all decisions pertaining to their child.

Congenital conditions can affect virtually any body system. This chapter describes common congenital conditions identified at or after birth. Some of these conditions warrant immediate treatment soon after birth. Other conditions, although identified in the newborn period, are long term with ongoing effects into childhood.

Ultimately, surveillance and research activities are translated into concrete strategies to prevent birth defects. In 1992, with solid evidence from epidemiologic research studies, the United States Public Health Service recommended that all women of childbearing age consume 400 micrograms (400 mcg or 0.4 mg) of folic acid daily to reduce the risk (up to 70%) of having a pregnancy affected by a neural tube defect such as spina bifida and **anencephaly**. All women between 15 and 45 years of age should consume folic acid daily because half of the United States' pregnancies are unplanned and birth defects occur very early in pregnancy (3 to 4 weeks after conception), before most women know they are pregnant. This has spurred prevention activities at local and national levels to promote the folic acid message (CDC, 2016).

Becoming a parent for most people implies a transition to something new and unknown in life. If the infant is born with a congenital defect, it is a very traumatic and challenging period for this overwhelmed family. In order to provide the best management for the infant and the family, guidelines based on scientific findings and recommendations should be followed. Nurses need to actively involve the parents/partners/significant others in the decision-making process, treatment options, and care of their infant in order to increase attachment and bonding.

Esophageal Atresia and Tracheoesophageal Fistula

Esophageal atresia and tracheoesophageal fistula are gastrointestinal anomalies in which the esophagus and trachea do not separate normally during embryonic development. Esophageal atresia refers to a congenitally interrupted esophagus where the proximal and distal ends do not communicate; the upper esophageal segment ends in a blind pouch and the lower segment ends a variable distance above the diaphragm (Fig. 24.8).

Tracheoesophageal fistula is an abnormal communication between the trachea and esophagus. When associated with esophageal atresia, the fistula most commonly occurs between the distal esophageal segment and the trachea. The incidence of esophageal atresia is 1 per 3,000 to 4,500 live births. The etiology has been attributed to genetic factors, infections, and teratogens, but in most cases, no cause is identifiable (Tewfik, Karsan, & Laberge, 2015).

Pathophysiology

Several types of esophageal atresia exist, but the most common anomaly is a fistula between the distal esophagus and the trachea, which occurs in 90% of newborns with an esophageal defect. Esophageal atresia and tracheoesophageal fistula are thought to be the result of incomplete separation of the lung bed from the foregut during early fetal development. A large percentage of these newborns have other congenital anomalies involving the vertebra, kidneys, heart, and musculoskeletal and gastrointestinal systems (Kliegman et al., 2015); most have several anomalies.

Nursing Assessment

Review the maternal history for polyhydramnios. Often this is the first sign of esophageal atresia because the fetus cannot swallow and absorb amniotic fluid in utero, leading to accumulation. Soon after birth, the newborn may exhibit copious, frothy bubbles of mucus in the mouth and nose, accompanied by drooling. Abdominal distention develops as air builds up in the stomach. In esophageal atresia, a gastric tube cannot be inserted beyond a certain point because the esophagus ends in a blind pouch. The newborn may have rattling respirations, excessive salivation, and drooling, and "the three Cs" (coughing, choking, and cyanosis) if feeding is attempted. The presence of a fistula increases the risk of respiratory complications such as pneumonitis and atelectasis due to aspiration of food and secretions (Gardner et al., 2016).

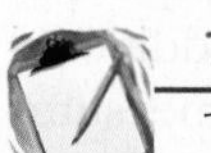

Take Note!

The "three Cs" of choking, coughing, and cyanosis in conjunction with feeding are considered the classic signs of tracheoesophageal fistula and atresia.

Prepare the newborn and parents for radiographic evaluation. Diagnosis is made by x-ray or an ultrasound or MRI, which will demonstrate a gastric tube coiled in the upper esophageal pouch, and air in the gastrointestinal tract indicates the presence of a fistula (Mattson & Smith, 2015). Once a diagnosis of esophageal atresia is established, begin preparations for surgery if the newborn is stable.

Nursing Management

Nursing management focuses on preparing the newborn and parents for surgery and providing meticulous postoperative care.

PROVIDING PREOPERATIVE CARE

Preoperative nursing interventions include the following measures:

- Initiate nothing by mouth (NPO) status.
- Elevate the head of the bed 30 to 45 degrees to prevent reflux and aspiration.
- Monitor hydration status and fluid and electrolyte balance; administer and monitor parenteral IV fluid infusions.
- Assess and maintain the patency of the orogastric tube; monitor the functioning of the tube, which is attached to low continuous suction; and avoid irrigation of the tube to prevent aspiration.
- Have oxygen and suctioning equipment readily available should the newborn experience respiratory distress.
- Assist with diagnostic studies to rule out other anomalies.
- Use comfort measures to minimize crying and prevent respiratory distress; provide nonnutritive sucking.
- Inform the parents about the rationales for the aspiration prevention measures.
- Document frequent observations of the newborn's condition (Kenner & Lott, 2014).

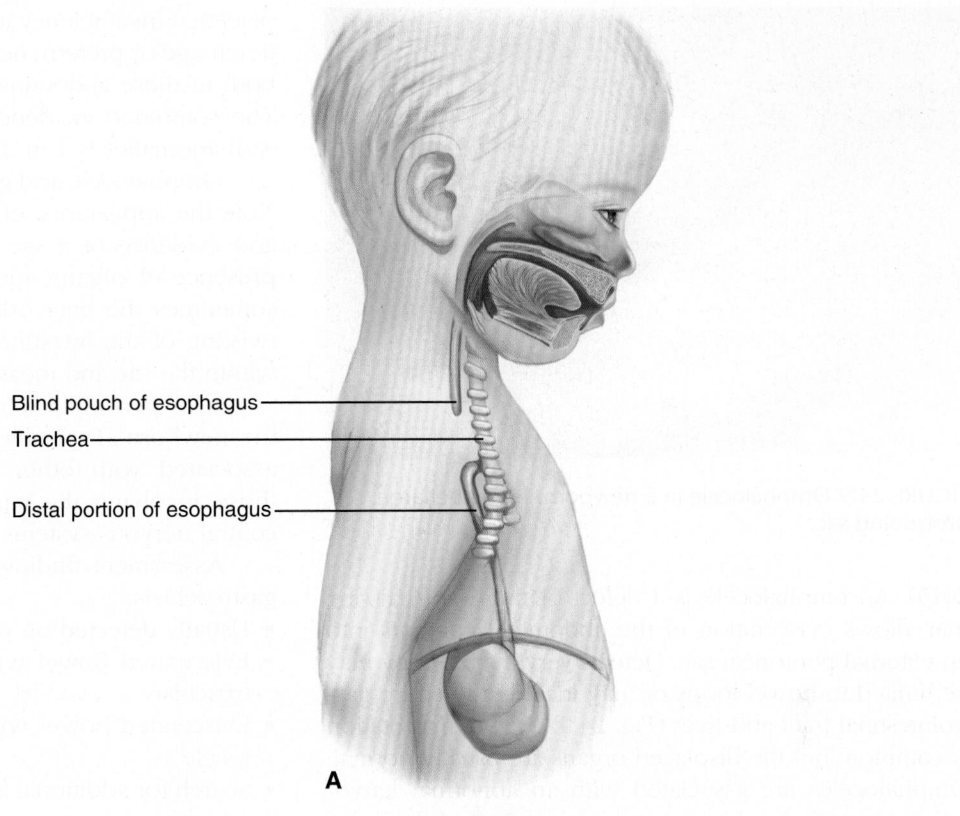

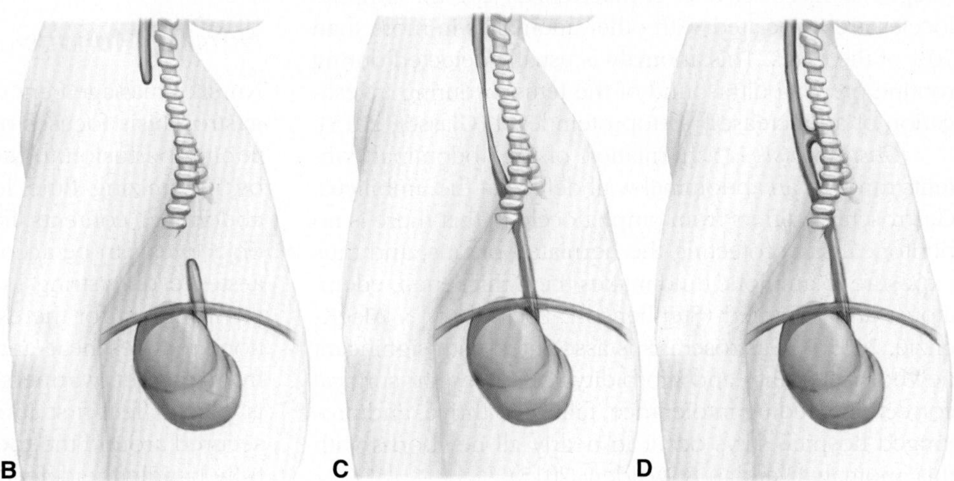

FIGURE 24.8 Esophageal atresia and tracheoesophageal fistula. **A.** The most common type of esophageal atresia, in which the esophagus ends in a blind pouch and a fistula connects the trachea with the distal portion of the esophagus. **B.** The upper and distal portions of the esophagus end in a blind pouch. **C.** The esophagus is one segment, but a portion of it is narrowed. **D.** The upper portion of the esophagus connects to the trachea.

PROVIDING POSTOPERATIVE CARE

Surgery consists of closing the fistula and joining the two esophageal segments. Postoperative care involves closely observing all of the newborn's body systems to identify any complications. Expect to administer TPN and antibiotics until the esophageal anastomosis is proven intact and patent. Then begin oral feedings, usually within a week after surgery (Mahoney & Rosen, 2015). Keep the parents informed of their newborn's condition and progress. Closely assess the newborn during feeding and report any difficulty with swallowing. Provide parent teaching. Demonstrate and reinforce all teaching prior to discharge.

Omphalocele and Gastroschisis

Omphalocele and **gastroschisis** are congenital anomalies of the anterior abdominal wall at or near the umbilicus. Fetal abdominal wall defects result from disturbances in organogenesis during the early embryonic period. Gastroschisis occurs in 1 in 2,000 live births, while omphalocele occurs in 1 in 4,000 live births (Wagner & Lee,

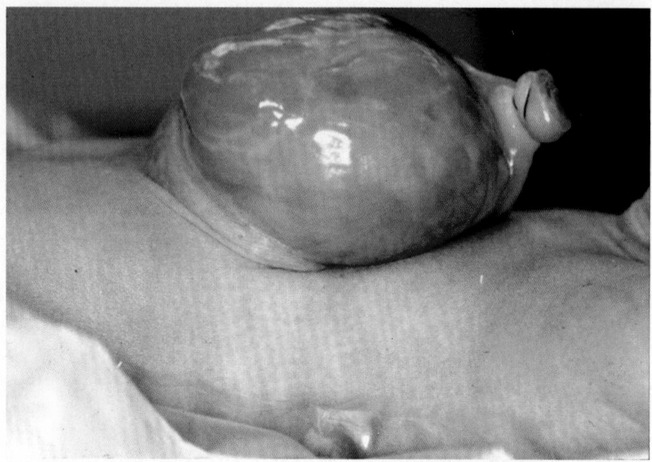

FIGURE 24.9 **Omphalocele in a newborn. Note the large, protruding sac.**

2015). An omphalocele is a defect of the umbilical ring that allows evisceration of the abdominal contents into an external peritoneal sac. Defects vary in size; they may be limited to bowel loops or may include the entire gastrointestinal tract and liver (Fig. 24.9). Bowel malrotation is common, but the displaced organs are usually normal. Omphaloceles are associated with an abnormal karyotype or genetic syndrome in more than 50% of the cases (Stephenson, Lockwood, & MacKenzie, 2015a). Omphaloceles are associated with other anomalies in more than 70% of the cases. This anomaly is usually detected during routine prenatal ultrasound of the fetus or during investigation of an increased -fetoprotein level (Glasser, 2015).

Gastroschisis is a herniation of the abdominal contents through an abdominal wall defect, at the umbilicus. Gastroschisis differs from omphalocele in that there is no peritoneal sac protecting the herniated organs, and thus exposure to amniotic fluid makes them thickened, edematous, and inflamed (Stephenson, Lockwood, & MacKenzie, 2015b). Gastroschisis is associated with significant newborn mortality and morbidity rates. Despite surgical correction, feeding intolerance, failure to thrive, and prolonged hospital stays occur in nearly all newborns with this anomaly (Verklan & Walden, 2015).

Each of these diagnoses requires that a pediatric surgeon be available at delivery to determine the extent of the defect and complications.

Nursing Assessment

Abdominal wall defects are readily diagnosed by prenatal ultrasound, which is helpful in planning for the birth and needed therapy. An early birth may be planned if the ultrasound reveals evidence of progressive bowel distention and thickening. Review the maternal history for factors associated with high-risk pregnancies, such as maternal illness and infection, drug use, smoking, and genetic abnormalities. These factors are also associated with omphalocele and gastroschisis. They contribute to placental insufficiency and the birth of a small-for-gestational-age or preterm newborn, the populations in which both of these abdominal defects most commonly occur. The combined incidence of both congenital abdominal wall anomalies is 1 in 2,000 births (Glasser, 2015).

Omphalocele and gastroschisis are readily observed. Note the appearance of the protrusion on the abdomen and evidence of a sac. Inspect the sac closely for the presence of organs, most commonly the intestines but sometimes the liver. Also inspect the contents for any twisting of the intestines. Note the color of the organs within the sac and measure the size of the omphalocele.

Also perform a complete physical examination of the newborn. Typically these congenital conditions are associated with other congenital anomalies, such as those involving the cardiovascular, genitourinary, and central nervous systems.

Assessment findings summary of omphalocele and gastroschisis:

- Usually detected on prenatal ultrasound examinations
- Eviscerated bowel without peritoneal covering—gastroschisis
- Eviscerated bowel with peritoneal covering—omphalocele
- Search for additional anomalies if omphalocele is diagnosed

Nursing Management

Nursing management of newborns with omphalocele or gastroschisis focuses on preventing hypothermia, maintaining perfusion to the eviscerated abdominal contents by minimizing fluid loss, and protecting the exposed abdominal contents from trauma and infection. These objectives can be accomplished by placing the infant in a sterile drawstring bowel bag that maintains a sterile environment for the exposed contents, allows visualization, reduces heat and moisture loss, and allows heat from radiant warmers to reach the infant. The infant is placed feet-first into the bag and the drawstring is secured around the torso (Mattson & Smith, 2015). Carefully handle the defect utilizing strict sterile technique to prevent contamination of the exposed abdominal contents as well as traumatic damage (Glasser, 2015).

An orogastric tube attached to low suction is used to prevent intestinal distention. IV therapy is administered to maintain fluid and electrolyte balance and provide a route for antibiotic therapy. Monitor the newborn's fluid status frequently. Closely observe the exposed bowel for vascular compromise, such as changes in color or a decrease in temperature, and report these immediately.

PROVIDING POSTOPERATIVE CARE

Surgical repair of both defects occurs after initial stabilization and comprehensive evaluation for any other anomalies. It may have to occur in stages, depending on the defect (Box 24.5).

BOX 24.5

SURGERY TO REPAIR OMPHALOCELE AND GASTROSCHISIS

Surgical repair of gastroschisis is an emergency due to the high risk of intestinal atresia, resulting in obstruction. Primary repair of gastroschisis is usually performed without incident, unless the contents are unable to fit into the abdominal cavity. This occurs more often with a large omphalocele, requiring the surgeon to do a staged closure. This involves covering the defect with a synthetic material that is sequentially squeezed like toothpaste to reduce the defect into the abdominal cavity. After enough of the defect is in the abdominal cavity, a surgical repair is then performed (Glasser, 2015). If damage to the exposed organs occurs, such as necrosis, then the necrotic sections are removed during the repair. If a significant amount of small intestine is lost, then the complication of short bowel syndrome may occur.

Postoperative care involves providing pain management, monitoring respiratory and cardiac status, monitoring intake and output, assessing for vascular compromise, maintaining the orogastric tube to suction, documenting the amount and color of drainage, and administering ordered medications and treatments (Gardner et al., 2016). Also be alert for complications, such as short bowel syndrome (see Chapter 42 for additional information).

PROMOTING PARENT–NEWBORN INTERACTION

The parents need continued support and progress reports on their newborn. They may be distraught at the sight of the anomaly, and they may be frightened to touch their newborn. Encourage the parents to touch the newborn and participate in care as much as possible. Because of the nature of this defect, bonding opportunities will be limited initially. However, strongly encourage frequent visiting. In addition, provide information to the parents about the defect, treatment modalities, and prognosis. After surgery, instruct the parents in care measures and provide them with home care instructions. Anticipate the need for a referral to a home health care agency and community resources for support.

Anorectal Malformations

An imperforate anus is a gastrointestinal system malformation of the anorectal opening and is identified in the newborn period. The rectum may end in a blind pouch that does not connect to the colon, or it may have fistulas (openings) between the rectum and the perineum (the vagina in girls or the urethra in boys) (Fig. 24.10). The malformations occur during early fetal development and may be associated with numerous other congenital anomalies (Rosen, 2014) in other body systems. Refer to Box 24.6 for anomalies associated with anorectal malformations.

Imperforate anus occurs in about 1 of every 3,500 live births (Malcolm, 2015). The defect can be further classified as a high or low type, depending on its level. The level significantly influences the outcome in terms of fecal continence as well as management (Fanaroff & Fanaroff, 2014).

Surgical intervention is needed for both high and low types of imperforate anus. Surgery for a high type

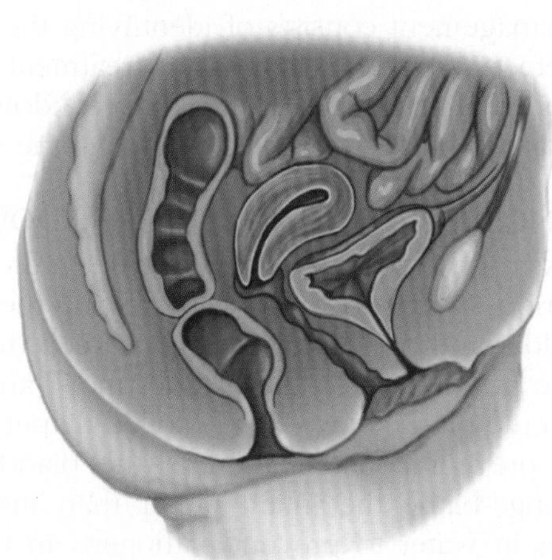

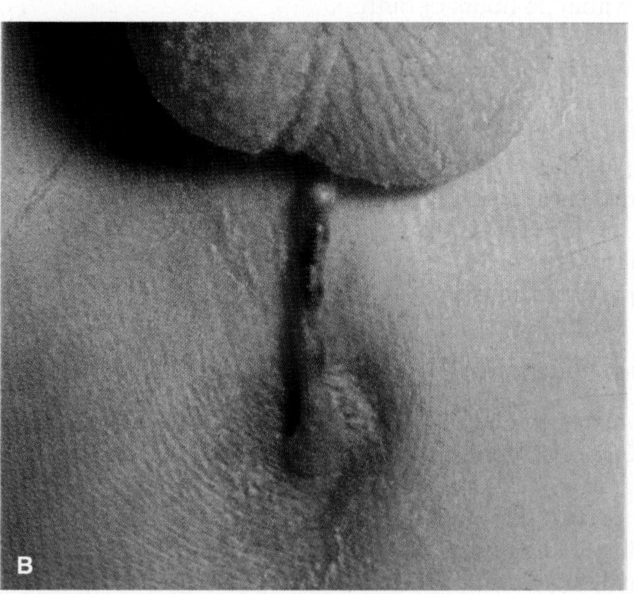

FIGURE 24.10 Image **A** shows an imperforate anus, in which the rectum ends in a blind pouch. Image **B** shows an imperforate anus without fistula. The visible meconium streak along the raphe is consistent with a low imperforate anus. (Courtesy of Kevin P. Lally, MD.)

BOX 24.6

ANOMALIES ASSOCIATED WITH ANORECTAL MALFORMATIONS

VACTERL syndrome: vertebral, anorectal, cardiovascular, tracheoesophageal, renal, and limb
Esophageal atresia
Intestinal atresia
Bowel malrotation
Renal agenesis
Hypospadias
Vesicoureteral reflux
Bladder exstrophy
Cardiac anomalies
Skeletal anomalies

of defect involves a colostomy in the newborn period, with corrective surgery performed in stages to allow for growth. Surgery for the low type of anomaly, which frequently includes a fistula, involves closure of the fistula, creation of an anal opening, and repositioning of the rectal pouch into the anal opening. A major challenge for either type of surgical repair is finding, using, or creating adequate nerve and muscle structures around the rectum to provide for normal evacuation (Malcolm, 2015).

Nursing Assessment

In the newborn, observe for an appropriate anal opening. If the anal opening exists, observe for passage of meconium stool within the first 24 hours of life. Assess urine output to identify genitourinary problems. For the newborn with an imperforate anus, inspection of the perineal area would reveal absence of the usual opening. In addition, meconium generally is not passed or present within 24 hours of birth.

In the infant with suspected imperforate anus, assess for common signs of intestinal obstruction, which may occur as a result of the malformation. These include abdominal distention and bilious vomiting.

Prepare the newborn and family for a perineal ultrasound and an abdominal x-ray that will be ordered to identify the level of defect in the absence of a perineal fistula and also to assess for complications associated with imperforate anus.

Nursing Management

Nursing management focuses on preparing the newborn and parent for surgery and providing postoperative care. Preoperatively, maintain the newborn's NPO status and provide gastric decompression. Administer IV therapy and antibiotic therapy as ordered and monitor the newborn's hydration status. Provide a full explanation of the defect, surgical options, potential complications, typical postoperative course, and long-term care needed to the parents. Make sure they are aware of the available treatment modalities. Prepare them for the possibility that the newborn may require an ostomy. Provide support to the parents and family.

Postoperative care includes ensuring adequate pain relief, maintaining NPO status and gastric decompression until normal bowel function is restored, and providing colostomy care if applicable. Refer to Chapter 42 for additional information related to ostomy care and postoperative care for children undergoing an intestinal pull-through procedure.

Bladder Exstrophy

In classic bladder exstrophy, a midline closure defect occurs during the embryonic period of gestation, leaving the bladder open and exposed outside of the abdomen. The incidence is 1 in 40,000 live births, and happens in males slightly more than females (Glasser, 2015). The bony pelvis may also be malformed, resulting in an opening in the pelvic arch. Bladder exstrophy may be diagnosed by prenatal ultrasound. Complications include UTI from ascending organisms. Treatment of bladder exstrophy involves surgical repair (Fig. 24.11).

Nursing Assessment

On physical examination of the infant or child, note the red appearance to the bladder seen on the abdominal wall. Draining urine will be visible. Note excoriation of abdominal skin around the bladder resulting from contact with urine. A malformed urethra may be present in females, whereas males may have an unformed or malformed penis or a normal penis with an epispadias.

Nursing Management

Nursing management consists of identifying the genitourinary defect at birth so immediate treatment can be initiated, preventing infection and skin breakdown, providing postoperative care, and catheterizing the stoma.

PREVENTING INFECTION AND SKIN BREAKDOWN

Bladder exstrophy requires surgical repair. In the preoperative period, care is focused on protecting the exstrophied bladder and preventing infection. Keep the infant in a supine position; keep the bladder moist and cover it with a sterile plastic bag. Change soiled diapers immediately to prevent contamination of the bladder with feces. Sponge-bathe the infant rather than immersing him or her in water to prevent pathogens in the bath water from entering the bladder. Prevent breakdown of the surrounding abdominal skin by applying protective barrier creams. In some instances it may be necessary to consult the ostomy nurse for further advice (see Chapter 43 for more information).

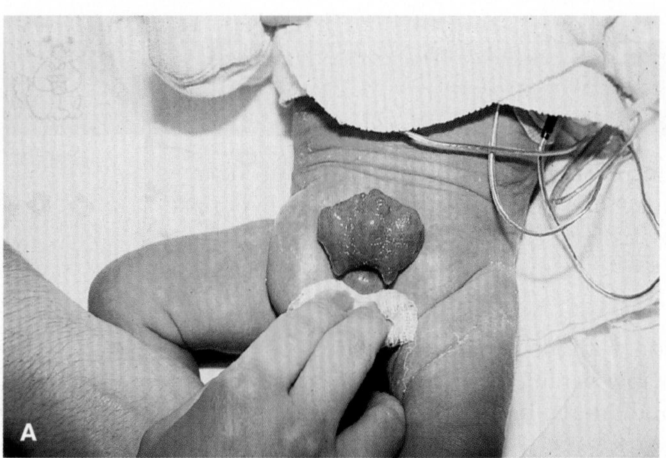

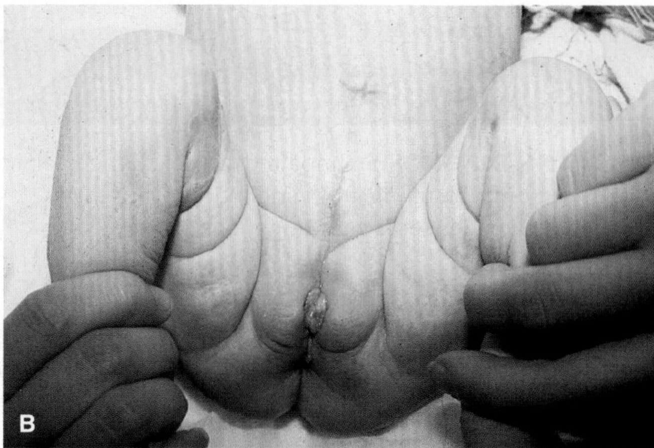

FIGURE 24.11 Bladder exstrophy. **A.** Before surgical repair. **B.** After surgery.

NURSING CARE PLAN 24.1

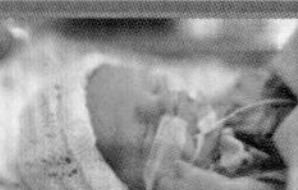

Overview of an Infant of a Diabetic Mother

Jamie, a 38-year-old Hispanic woman, gave birth to a term large-for-gestational-age newborn weighing 10 lb. She had a history of gestational diabetes but had not received any prenatal care. She arrived at the hospital in active labor. Despite macrosomia, the newborn's Apgar scores were 8 and 9 at 1 and 5 minutes, respectively. No resuscitative measures were needed.

One hour after birth, assessment revealed a pale, irritable newborn with sweating and several episodes of apnea. A glucose level obtained at this time via a heel stick was 35 mg/dL. Two hours later, the newborn begins exhibiting signs of respiratory distress—grunting, nasal flaring, retractions, tachypnea (respiratory rate 72 breaths/min), and tachycardia (heart rate 176 bpm).

NURSING DIAGNOSIS: Risk for unstable glucose level related to hypoglycemia secondary to intrauterine hyperinsulin state resulting from maternal gestational diabetes as evidenced by low blood glucose level, irritability, pallor, sweating, and apnea

Outcome Identification and Evaluation

The newborn will exhibit adequate glucose control as evidenced by maintaining blood glucose levels above 40 mg/dL and an absence of clinical signs of hypoglycemia.

Interventions: *Promoting Glucose Control*

- Monitor blood glucose levels hourly for the first 4 hours and then every 3 to 4 hours or as necessary *to detect hypoglycemia, which would be <40 mg/dL.*
- Continue to observe for manifestations of hypoglycemia, such as pallor, tremors, jitteriness, lethargy, and poor feeding, *to allow for early detection and prompt intervention, thereby minimizing the risk of complications associated with hypoglycemia.*
- Monitor temperature frequently and institute measures to maintain a neutral thermal environment *to prevent cold stress, which would increase metabolic demands and further deplete glycogen stores.*
- Initiate early feedings every 2 to 3 hours or as appropriate or administer glucose supplements as ordered *to prevent hypoglycemia caused by the newborn's hyperinsulin state.* Administer IV glucose infusions as ordered *to correct hypoglycemia if glucose levels do not stabilize with feeding.*
- Cluster infant care activities and provide for rest periods *to conserve the newborn's energy and reduce use of glucose and glycogen stores.*
- Reduce environmental stimuli by dimming lights and speaking softly *to reduce energy demands and further utilization of glucose.*
- Explain all events and procedures to the mother *to help alleviate anxiety and promote understanding of the newborn's condition.*

(continued)

NURSING CARE PLAN 24.1

Overview of an Infant of a Diabetic Mother (continued)

NURSING DIAGNOSIS: Impaired gas exchange related to respiratory distress secondary to delayed lung maturity resulting from inhibition of pulmonary surfactant production due to fetal hyperinsulinemia as evidenced by grunting, nasal flaring, retractions, tachypnea, and tachycardia

Outcome Identification and Evaluation

Newborn will demonstrate signs of adequate oxygenation without respiratory distress as evidenced by respiratory rate and vital signs within acceptable parameters, absence of nasal flaring, retractions, and grunting, and oxygen saturation and arterial blood gas levels within acceptable parameters.

Interventions: ***Promoting Oxygenation***

- Monitor newborn's vital signs to establish a baseline and evaluate for changes.
- Assess airway patency and perform gentle suctioning as ordered to ensure patency and allow for adequate oxygen intake.
- Position the newborn prone to optimize respiratory status and reduce stress.
- Assess lung sounds for changes to allow early detection of change in status.
- Continuously monitor oxygen saturation levels via pulse oximetry to determine adequacy of tissue perfusion.
- Assess arterial blood gas results to detect changes indicating acidosis, hypoxemia, or hypercarbia, which would suggest hypoxia. Administer medications as ordered to correct acidosis.
- Administer oxygen as ordered to promote adequate tissue perfusion.
- Assess newborn's skin to identify cyanosis, pallor, and mottling to detect changes indicating compromised oxygenation.
- Administer surfactant replacement therapy as ordered to aid in stabilizing the newborn's lungs until postnatal surfactant synthesis improves.
- Institute measures to maintain normal blood glucose levels and a neutral thermal environment, cluster care activities, and reduce excessive stimuli to reduce oxygen demand and consumption.

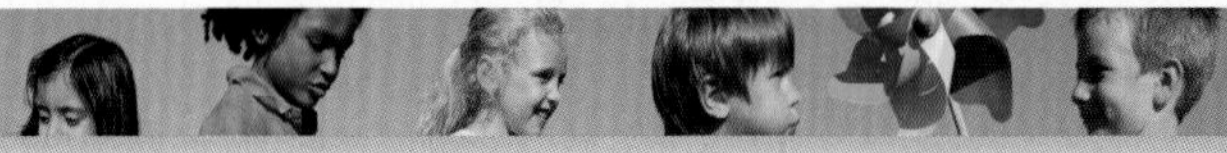

KEY CONCEPTS

- Asphyxia, the most common clinical insult in the perinatal period, results in brain injury and may lead to mental retardation, cerebral palsy, or seizures.
- TTN occurs when the liquid in the lung is removed slowly or incompletely.
- Common risk factors for respiratory distress syndrome (RDS) include young gestational age, perinatal asphyxia regardless of gestational age, cesarean birth in the absence of labor (related to the lack of thoracic squeeze), male gender, and maternal diabetes.
- Meconium aspiration has three major pulmonary effects: airway obstruction, surfactant dysfunction, and chemical pneumonitis.
- The management of PPHN requires meticulous attention to detail, with continuous monitoring of oxygenation, blood pressure, and perfusion.
- Intraventricular hemorrhage is bleeding that usually originates in the subependymal germinal matrix region of the brain with extension into the ventricular system.
- Necrotizing enterocolitis (NEC) is a serious gastrointestinal disease of unknown etiology in newborns that can result in necrosis of a segment of the bowel.
- Infants of diabetic mothers are at risk for malformations most frequently involving the cardiovascular, skeletal, central nervous, gastrointestinal, and genitourinary systems; cardiac anomalies are the most common.

- Factors that place the newborn at risk for birth trauma include cephalopelvic disproportion, maternal pelvic anomalies, oligohydramnios, prolonged or rapid labor, abnormal presentation, fetal prematurity, fetal macrosomia, and fetal abnormalities.
- Women who use drugs during their pregnancy expose their unborn child to the possibility of intrauterine growth restriction, prematurity, neurobehavioral and neurophysiologic dysfunction, birth defects, infections, and long-term developmental sequelae.
- Newborns of women who abuse tobacco, illicit substances, caffeine, and alcohol can exhibit withdrawal behavior.
- Physiologic jaundice is a common, normal newborn phenomenon that appears during the second or third day of life and then declines over the first week after birth. Pathologic jaundice is manifested within the first 24 hours of life when total bilirubin levels increase by more than 5 mg/dL/day and the total serum bilirubin level is higher than 17 mg/dL in a full-term infant.
- Newborn infections are usually classified according to the time of onset and grouped into three categories: congenital infection, acquired in utero by vertical transmission with onset before birth; early-onset neonatal infections, acquired by vertical transmission in the perinatal period, either shortly before or during birth; and late-onset neonatal infections, acquired by horizontal transmission in the nursery.
- Congenital conditions can arise from many etiologies including single-gene disorders, chromosome aberrations, exposure to teratogens, and many sporadic conditions of unknown cause. Congenital structural anomalies may be inherited or sporadic, isolated or multiple, apparent or hidden, and gross or microscopic.
- Esophageal atresia refers to a congenitally interrupted esophagus where the proximal and distal ends do not communicate; the upper esophageal segment ends in a blind pouch and the lower segment ends a variable distance above the diaphragm. Tracheoesophageal fistula is an abnormal communication between the trachea and esophagus.
- Omphalocele and gastroschisis are congenital anomalies of the anterior abdominal wall. An omphalocele is a defect of the umbilical ring that allows evisceration of abdominal contents into an external peritoneal sac. Gastroschisis is a herniation of abdominal contents through an abdominal wall defect, usually to the left or right of the umbilicus.

REFERENCES AND RECOMMENDED READINGS

Adcock, L. M. (2015). *Management and complications of intraventricular hemorrhage in the newborn. UpToDate.* Retrieved from http://www.uptodate.com/contents/management-and-complications-of-intraventricular-hemorrhage-in-the-newborn

Adcock, L. M., & Stark, A. R. (2014). *Systemic effects of perinatal asphyxia.* Retrieved from http://www.uptodate.com/contents/systemic-effects-of-perinatal-asphyxia

American Academy of Pediatrics [AAP]. (2012). Breastfeeding and the use of human milk. *Pediatrics, 129*(3), e827–e841.

American Academy of Pediatrics [AAP], Committee on Drugs. (2012). Neonatal drug withdrawal. *Pediatrics, 129*(2), e540–e560.

American Heart Association [AHA],& American Academy of Pediatrics [AAP]. (2014). *Documentation of neonatal resuscitation.* Retrieved from http://www2.aap.org/nrp/docs/iu/2014_springsummer_iu.pdf

Anderson-Berry, A. L., Bellig, L. L., & Ohning, B. L. (2015). *Neonatal sepsis.* Retrieved from http://emedicine.medscape.com/article/978352-overview

Annibale, D. J. (2014). Periventricular hemorrhage—intraventricular hemorrhage. *eMedicine.* Retrieved from http://emedicine.medscape.com/article/976654-overview

Artigas, V. (2015). Management of neonatal abstinence syndrome in the newborn nursery. *Nursing for Women's Health, 18*(6), 509–514.

Bengtsson, B. O., van Houten, J. P., & Oster, H. A. (2015). Index of suspicion in the nursery. *NeoReviews, 16*(2), e120–e122.

Blackburn, S. T. (2012). *Maternal, fetal and neonatal physiology: A clinical perspective* (4th ed.). St. Louis, MO: Saunders Elsevier.

Blennow, M., & Bohlin, K. (2015). Surfactant and noninvasive ventilation. *Neonatology, 107*(4), 330–336.

Borer, J. G. (2014). *Clinical manifestations and initial management of infants with bladder exstrophy.* Retrieved from http://www.uptodate.com/contents/clinical-manifestations-and-initial-management-of-infants-with-bladder-exstrophy

Centers for Disease Control and Prevention. (2015). *Fetal alcohol spectrum disorders (FASDs).* Retrieved from http://www.cdc.gov/ncbddd/fasd/facts.html

Centers for Disease Control and Prevention. (2016). *Folic acid.* Retrieved from http://www.cdc.gov/ncbddd/folicacid/recommendations.html

Choi, W., Jeong, H., Choi, S. J., Oh, S. Y., Kim, J. S., Roh, C. R., et al. (2015). Risk factors differentiating mild/moderate from severe meconium aspiration syndrome in meconium-stained neonates. *Obstetrics & Gynecology Science, 58*(1), 24–31.

Clark, M. B., & Clark, D. A. (2014). Meconium aspiration syndrome. *eMedicine.* Retrieved from: http://emedicine.medscape.com/article/974110-overview

Cunningham, F. G., Leveno, K. J., Bloom, S. L., Spong, C.Y., Dashe, J. S., Hoffman, B. L., et al. (2014). *Williams obstetrics* (24th ed.). New York, NY: McGraw-Hill.

Deleon, C., Shattuck, K., & Jain, S. K. (2015). Biomarkers of neonatal sepsis. *NeoReviews, 16*(5), e297--e308.

Deshpande, P. G. (2015). Breast milk jaundice. *eMedicine.* Retrieved from http://emedicine.medscape.com/article/973629-overview

Fanaroff, A. A., & Fanaroff, J. M. (2014). *Klaus and Fanaroff's care of the high-risk neonate* (6th ed.). Philadelphia, PA: Elsevier Health Sciences.

Fox, J. R., Thacker, L. R., & Hendricks-Muñoz, K. D. (2015). Early detection tool of intestinal dysfunction: Impact on necrotizing enterocolitis severity. *American Journal of Perinatology, 32*(10), 927–932.

Garcia-Prats, J. A. (2015). Prevention and management of meconium aspiration syndrome. *UpToDate.* Retrieved from http://www.uptodate.com/contents/prevention-and-management-of-meconium-aspiration-syndrome

Gardner, S. L., Carter, B. S., Enzman-Hines, M., & Hernandez, J. A. (2016). *Merenstein & Gardner's handbook of neonatal intensive care* (8th ed.). St. Louis, MO: Mosby Elsevier.

Gaur, K. V., Nimbalkar, S. M., Desai, R., & Ganguly, B. P. (2015). Effect of single dose antenatal steroid for pregnant mothers with high risk of preterm delivery on the respiratory outcome of neonates. *Journal of Clinical Neonatology, 4*(3), 217.

Glasser, J. G. (2015). *Pediatric omphalocele and gastroschisis. eMedicine.* Retrieved from http://emedicine.medscape.com/article/975583-overview

Green, C. J. (2016). *Maternal newborn nursing care plans* (3rd ed.). Burlington, MA: Jones and Bartlett Learning.

Groenendaal, F. (2015). Cooling after perinatal asphyxia. In *Seminars in fetal & neonatal medicine, 20,* 65–66.

Haakonsen Lindenskov, P. H., Castellheim, A., Saugstad, O. D., & Mollnes, T. E. (2015). Meconium aspiration syndrome: Possible pathophysiological mechanisms and future potential therapies. *Neonatology, 107*(3), 225–230.

Hamdan, A. H. (2016). Neonatal abstinence syndrome. *eMedicine.* Retrieved from http://emedicine.medscape.com/article/978763-overview

Hansen, T. W. (2016). Neonatal jaundice. *eMedicine.* Retrieved from http://emedicine.medscape.com/article/974786-overview

Hudson, J. (2015). Facilitating normal physiology in the presence of meconium stained liquor. *The Practicing Midwife, 18*(6), 16–19.

Huybrechts, K. F. (2015). SSRI use in late pregnancy: Small risk of PPHN. *Reactions, 1556,* 11–20.

Ives, N. K. (2015). Management of neonatal jaundice. *Pediatrics and Child Health, 25*(6), 276–281.

Jaecklin, T., Jarreau, P. H., & Kavanagh, B. P. (2015). Ventilator-associated lung injury. In *Pediatric and neonatal mechanical ventilation* (pp. 917–945). Berlin Heidelberg: Springer Publishers.

Jansson, L. M. (2015). Neonatal abstinence syndrome. *UpToDate.* Retrievd from http://www.uptodate.com/contents/neonatal-abstinence-syndrome

Jaques, S. C., & Kennea, N. (2015). Resuscitation of the newborn. *Obstetrics, Gynecology & Reproductive Medicine, 25*(3), 61–67.

Johnson, T. J., Patel, A. L., Bigger, H. R., Engstrom, J. L., & Meier, P. P. (2015). Cost savings of human milk as a strategy to reduce the incidence of necrotizing enterocolitis in very low birth weight infants. *Neonatology, 107*(4), 271–276.

Jones, H. E., & Fielder, A. (2015). Neonatal abstinence syndrome: Historical perspective, current focus, future directions. *Preventive Medicine, 80,* 12–17.

Kenner, C., & Lott, J. W. (2014). *Comprehensive neonatal nursing care* (5th ed.). New York, NY: Springer Publishers.

Kim, H. A., Yang, G. E., & Kim, M. J. (2015). Early neonatal respiratory morbidities in term neonates. *Neonatal Medicine, 22*(1), 8–13.

Kliegman, R. M., Stanton, B., St. Geme, J., Schor, N., & Behrman, R. E. (2015). *Nelson's textbook of pediatrics* (20th ed.). St. Louis: Saunders Elsevier.

Korkmazer, E., Solak, N., & Tokgöz, V. Y. (2015). Gestational diabetes: Screening, management, timing of delivery. *Current Obstetrics and Gynecology Reports, 4*(2), 132–138.

Lauwers, J., & Swisher, A. (2016). *Counseling the nursing mother: A lactation consultant's guide* (6th ed.). Burlington, MA: Jones & Bartlett Learning.

Lee, K. G. (2013). Transient tachypnea—newborn. *MedlinePlus.* Retrieved from http://www.nlm.nih.gov/medlineplus/ency/article/007233.htm

Lim, J. C., Golden, J. M., & Ford, H. R. (2015). Pathogenesis of neonatal necrotizing enterocolitis. *Pediatric Surgery International, 31*(6), 509–518.

Loroia, N. (2015). Birth trauma. *eMedicine.* Retrieved from: http://emedicine.medscape.com/article/980112-overview

Mahoney, L., & Rosen, R. (2015). Feeding difficulties in children with esophageal atresia. *Pediatric Respiratory Reviews,* pii: S1526-0542(15)00040-8.

Malcolm, W. (2015). *Beyond the NICU: Comprehensive care of the high risk infant.* New York, NY: McGraw Hill Education.

March of Dimes. (2015a). *Neonatal abstinence syndrome (NAS).* Retrieved from http://www.marchofdimes.org/baby/neonatal-abstinence-syndrome-(nas).aspx

March of Dimes. (2015b). *Smoking during pregnancy.* Retrieved from http://www.marchofdimes.org/pregnancy/smoking-during-pregnancy.aspx

March of Dimes. (2016a). *Alcohol during pregnancy.* Retrieved from http://www.marchofdimes.org/pregnancy/alcohol-during-pregnancy.aspx

March of Dimes. (2016b). *Birth defects and other health conditions.* Retrieved from http://www.marchofdimes.org/baby/birth-defects.aspx

Martin, R. (2015). Overview of neonatal respiratory distress: Disorders of transition. *UpToDate.* Retrieved from http://www.uptodate.com/contents/overview-of-neonatal-respiratory-distress-disorders-of-transition

Mattson, S., & Smith, J. E. (2015). *Core curriculum for maternal-newborn nursing* (5th ed.). St. Louis, MO: Saunders Elsevier.

Mukhopadhyay, S., & Puopolo, K. M. (2015). Neonatal early-onset sepsis: Epidemiology and risk assessment. *NeoReviews, 16*(4), e221--e230.

Molyneux, E., & Gest, A. (2015). Neonatal sepsis: An old issue needing new answers. *The Lancet Infectious Diseases, 15*(5), 503–505.

Nagtalon-Ramos, J. (2014). *Maternal-newborn nursing care: Best evidence-based practices.* Philadelphia, PA: F. A. Davis Company.

National Institute for Health and Care Excellence [NICE]. (2014). *Jaundice in newborn babies under 28 days.* Retrived from http://www.nice.org.uk/guidance/qs57/chapter/introduction

National Institute on Drug Abuse. (2015). *Substance use while pregnant and breastfeeding.* Retrieved from http://www.drugabuse.gov/publications/research-reports/substance-use-in-women/substance-use-while-pregnant-breastfeeding

Neonatal eHandbook. (2015). *Meconium aspiration syndrome*. Retrieved from https://www2.health.vic.gov.au/hospitals-and-health-services/patient-care/perinatal-reproductive/neonatal-ehandbook/conditions/meconium-aspiration-syndrome

Noori, S., & Seri, I. (2015). Hemodynamic antecedents of peri/intraventricular hemorrhage in very preterm neonates. In *Seminars in fetal and neonatal medicine*. WB Saunders.

Oliver, E., Reagan, P., Slaughter, J., & Buhimschi, I. (2015). Patterns of empiric antibiotic use for presumed early onset neonatal sepsis (EONS). *American Journal of Obstetrics & Gynecology, 212*(1), S384. doi: http://dx.doi.org/10.1016/j.ajog.2014.10.999

Potter, C. F., & Kicklighter, S. D. (2016). Infant of a diabetic mother. *eMedicine*. Retrieved from http://emedicine.medscape.com/article/974230-overview

Pramanik, A. K., Rangaswamy, N., & Gates, T. (2015). Neonatal respiratory distress: A practical approach to its diagnosis and management. *Pediatric Clinics of North America, 62*(2), 453–469.

Pramanik, A. K., & Rosenkrantz, T. (2015). Respiratory distress syndrome. *eMedicine*. Retrieved from http://emedicine.medscape.com/article/976034-overview

Rosen, N. G. (2014). Pediatric imperforate anus. *eMedicine*. Retrieved from http://emedicine.medscape.com/article/929904-overview

Rubarth, L. B., & Quinn, J. (2015). Respiratory development and respiratory distress syndrome. *Neonatal Network, 34*(4), 231–238.

Sachdeva, M., Murki, S., Oleti, T. P., & Kandraju, H. (2015). Intermittent versus continuous phototherapy for the treatment of neonatal non-hemolytic moderate hyperbilirubinemia in infants more than 34 weeks of gestational age: A randomized controlled trial. *European Journal of Pediatrics, 174*(2), 177–181.

Salem, L., & Singer, K. R. (2014). Rh incompatibility. *eMedicine*. Retrieved from http://emedicine.medscape.com/article/797150-overview

Smith, J. R., Donze, A., Wolf, M., Smyser, C. D., Mathur, A., & Proctor, E. K. (2015). Ensuring quality in the NICU: Translating research into appropriate clinical care. *The Journal of Perinatal & Neonatal Nursing, 29*(3), 255–261.

Springer, S. C. & Annibale, D. J. (2014). Kernicterus. *eMedicine*. Retrieved from http://emedicine.medscape.com/article/975276-overview#a5

Springer, S. C. & Annibale, D. J. (2016). Necrotizing enterocolitis. *eMedicine*. Retrieved from http://emedicine.medscape.com/article/977956-overview

Stephenson, C. D., Lockwood, C. J., & MacKenzie, A. P. (2015a). Omphalocele. *UpToDate*. Retrieved from http://www.uptodate.com/contents/omphalocele

Stephenson, C. D., Lockwood, C. J., & MacKenzie, A. P. (2015b). Gastroschisis. *UpToDate*. Retrieved from http://www.uptodate.com/contents/gastroschisis

Substance Abuse & Mental Health Services Administration [SAMHSA]. (n.d.). *Fetal alcohol spectrum disorders*. Retrieved http://www.samhsa.gov/fetal-alcohol-spectrum-disorders-fasd-center

Swanson, J. R., & Sinkin, R. A. (2015). Transition from fetus to newborn. *Pediatric Clinics of North America, 62*(2), 329–343.

Szpecht, D., Szymankiewicz, M., Seremak-Mrozikiewicz, A., & Gadzinowski, J. (2015). Review paper: The role of genetic factors in the pathogenesis of neonatal intraventricular hemorrhage. *Folia Neuropathology, 53*(1), 1–7.

Tewfik, T. L., Karsan, N., & Laberge, J. M. (2015). Congenital malformations of the esophagus. *eMedicine*. Retrieved from http://emedicine.medscape.com/article/837879-overview#a3

U.S. Department of Health and Human Services [USDHHS]. (2016). *Healthy People 2020*. Retrieved from http://healthypeople.gov/2020/default.aspx

Verklan, M. T., & Walden, M. (2015). *Core curriculum for neonatal intensive care nursing* (5th ed.). St. Louis, MO: Saunders.

Wagner, J. P., & Lee, S. L. (2015). Infant born with abdominal wall defect. In *Surgery* (pp. 349–355). New York, NY: Springer Publishers.

Wang, M. (2014). Perinatal drug abuse and neonatal drug withdrawal. *eMedicine*. Retrieved from http://emedicine.medscape.com/article/978492-overview

Whitsett, J. A., Wert, S. E., & Weaver, T. E. (2015). Diseases of pulmonary surfactant homeostasis. *Annual Review of Pathology, 10*, 371.

World Health Organization [WHO]. (2015). *Congenital anomalies*. Retrieved from http://www.who.int/mediacentre/factsheets/fs370/en/

Zanelli, S. A., Kaufman, D. A., & Stanley, D.P. (2015). *Hypoxic-ischemic encephalopathy*. Retrieved from http://emedicine.medscape.com/article/973501-overview

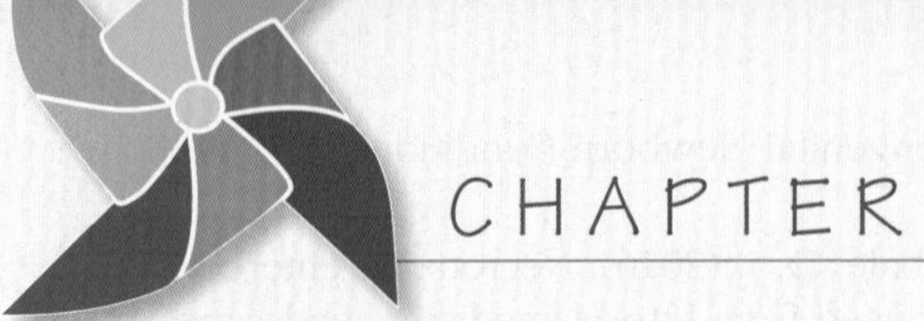

CHAPTER WORKSHEET

MULTIPLE-CHOICE QUESTIONS

1. Which finding would lead the nurse to suspect that a newborn is experiencing respiratory distress syndrome?
   a. Abdominal distention
   b. Acrocyanosis
   c. Depressed fontanels
   d. Nasal flaring

2. When assessing the substance-exposed newborn, which finding would the nurse expect?
   a. Calm facial appearance
   b. Daily weight gain
   c. Increasing irritability
   d. Feeding and sleeping well

3. A newborn with tracheoesophageal fistula is likely to present with which assessment finding?
   a. Subnormal temperature
   b. Absent Moro reflex
   c. Inability to swallow
   d. Drooling from mouth

4. In which of the following infants would the nurse would be most alert for the development of transient tachypnea?
   a. Infant born by cesarean section
   b. Neonate who received no sedation
   c. Newborn of a mother with heart disease
   d. Baby who is small for gestational age

5. The nurse is caring for term neonate who was exposed to cocaine throughout the pregnancy. What effect would this exposure have on the neonate's vital signs?
   a. They would be lower than normal.
   b. They would be higher than normal.
   c. They would not be affected at all.
   d. BP would be lower, pulse would higher.

6. Characteristics of a newborn with fetal alcohol syndrome would include which of the following? Select all that apply:
   a. Hypocalcium and hypokalemia
   b. Malformed ears and cataracts
   c. Microcephaly and thin upper lip
   d. Congenital cardiac defects and SGA
   e. Prominent cheekbones and LGA
   f. Hyperactive behavior and feeding problems

CRITICAL THINKING EXERCISES

1. As the nursery nurse, you receive a newborn from the labor and birth suite and place him under the radiant warmer. The nurse who gives you the report states that the mother couldn't remember when her membranes broke before labor and that she ran a fever during labor for the past few hours. The Apgar scores were good, but the newborn seemed lethargic. As you begin your assessment, you note that he is pale and floppy and has a subnormal temperature; heart rate is 180 bpm and respiratory rate is 70 breaths per minute.
   a. What in the mother's history should raise a red flag to the nurse?
   b. For what condition is this newborn at high risk?
   c. What interventions are appropriate for this condition?

2. Terry, a day-old baby girl, is very fretful, and calming measures don't seem to work. As the nursery nurse you notice that she is losing weight and her formula intake is poor, even though she is manifesting hungry behavior. The mother received no prenatal care and denied drug use, but her drug screen was positive for heroin.
   a. What additional information do you need to obtain from the mother?
   b. What additional laboratory work might be needed for Terry?
   c. What specific measures need to be made for her ongoing care?

3. Baby boy Sims, a term newborn, was brought to the nursery. His mother received no prenatal care, but the newborn's Apgar scores were fine. As the nurse carried out her newborn assessment, she noted an imperforate anus and palpated no testicles in the scrotal sac.
   a. What additional assessments should the nurse complete?
   b. Are anorectal agenesis and genitourinary tract anomalies common?
   c. What diagnostic tests might be ordered? What might be included in the treatment plan for this newborn?

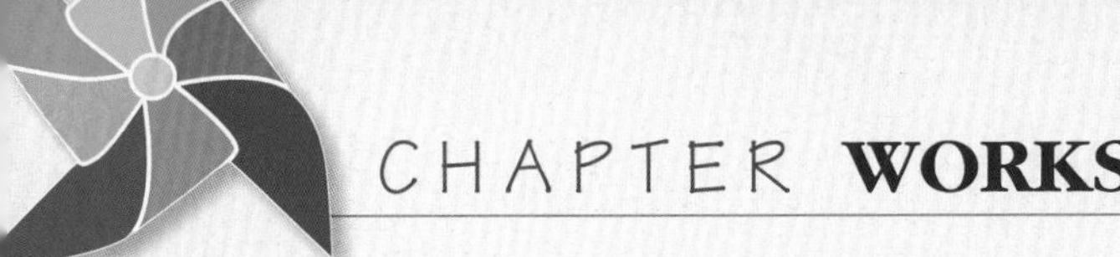

CHAPTER WORKSHEET

STUDY ACTIVITIES

1. Arrange for a tour of a regional NICU to see the nurse's role in caring for sick neonates. Ask the nurse to give a quick history of each newborn's condition. Was the nurse's role like you imagined? What was your impression of the NICU, and how would you describe it to expectant parents?
2. Select a website from the list online at thePoint. What kind of information is given? How helpful would it be for parents with an infant diagnosed with a specific condition?
3. A herniation of a newborn's abdominal contents present at birth describes ____________________.

BRINGING IT ALL TOGETHER: A CASE STUDY

Anna, a Native American, is 17 years old and was diagnosed with type 1 diabetes at the age of 5 years. She presented at the local clinic reporting that she has missed three periods and thinks she could be pregnant. A physical examination supports the possibility and a pregnancy test confirms that she is 12 weeks pregnant.

Go to thePoint to find questions to consider about this case.

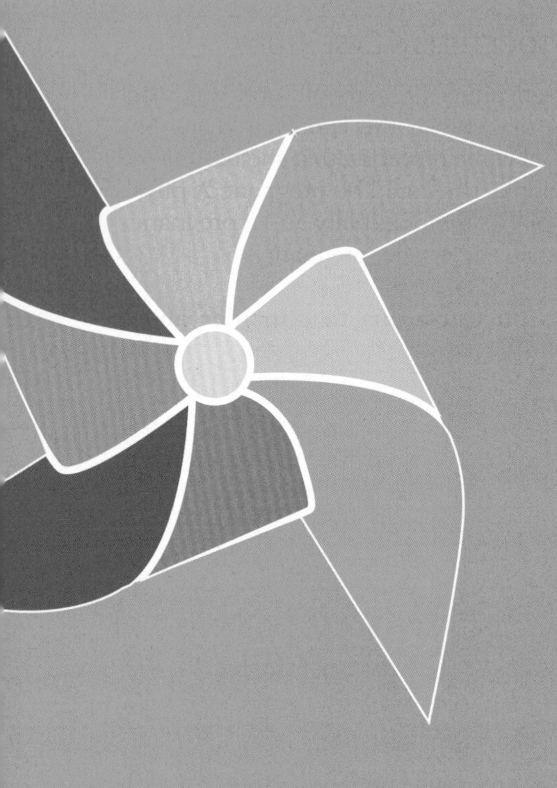

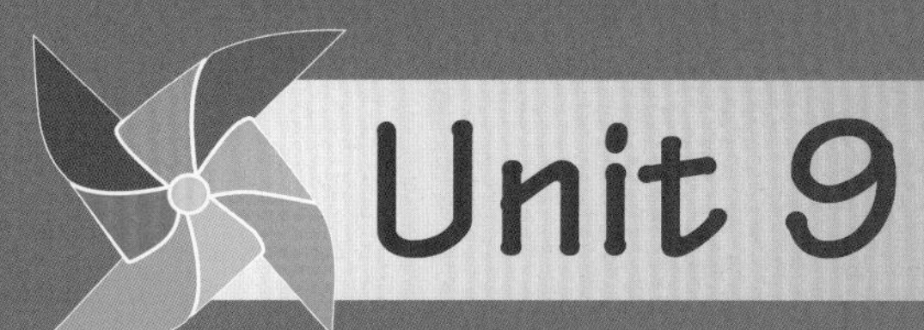

Health Promotion of the Growing Child and Family

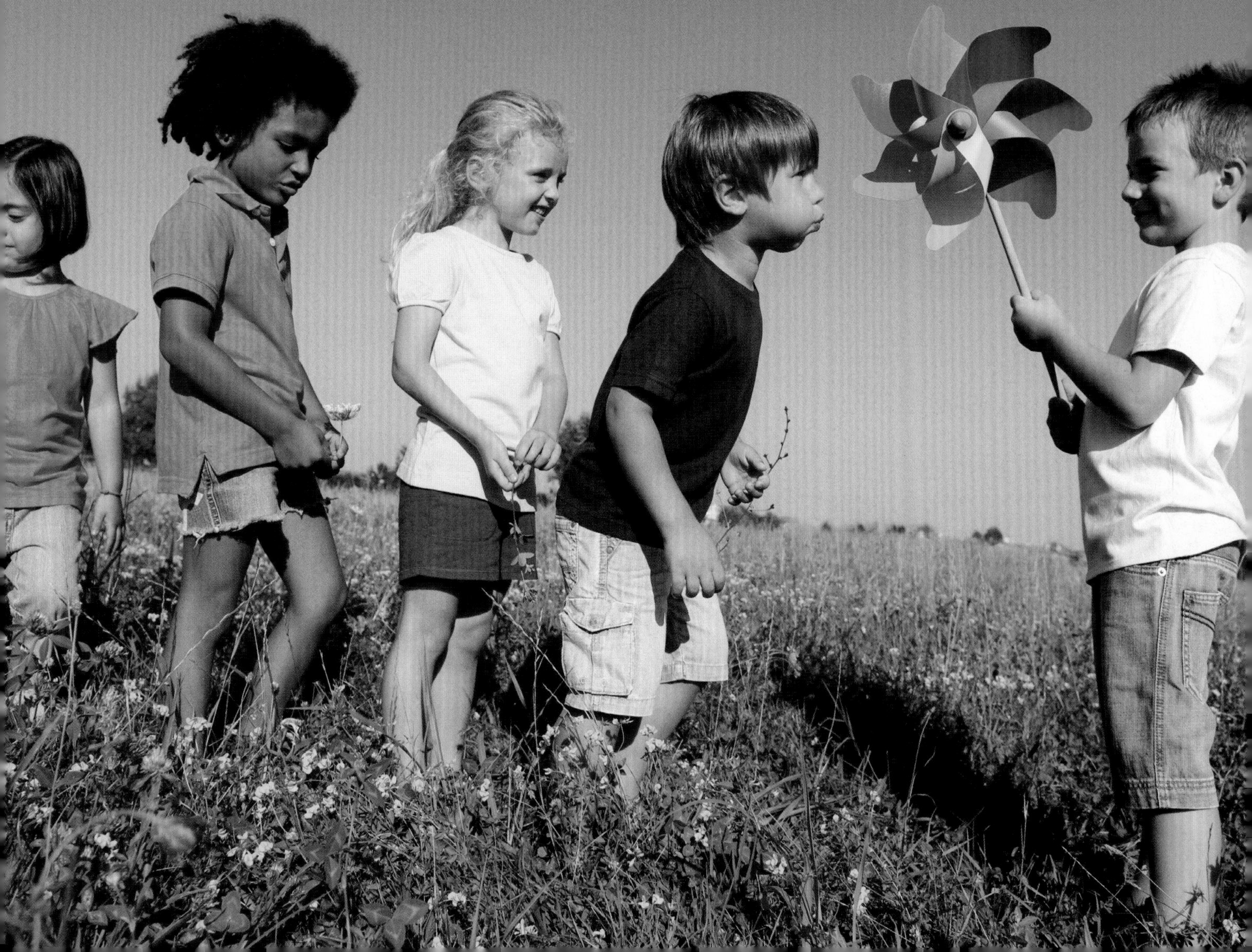

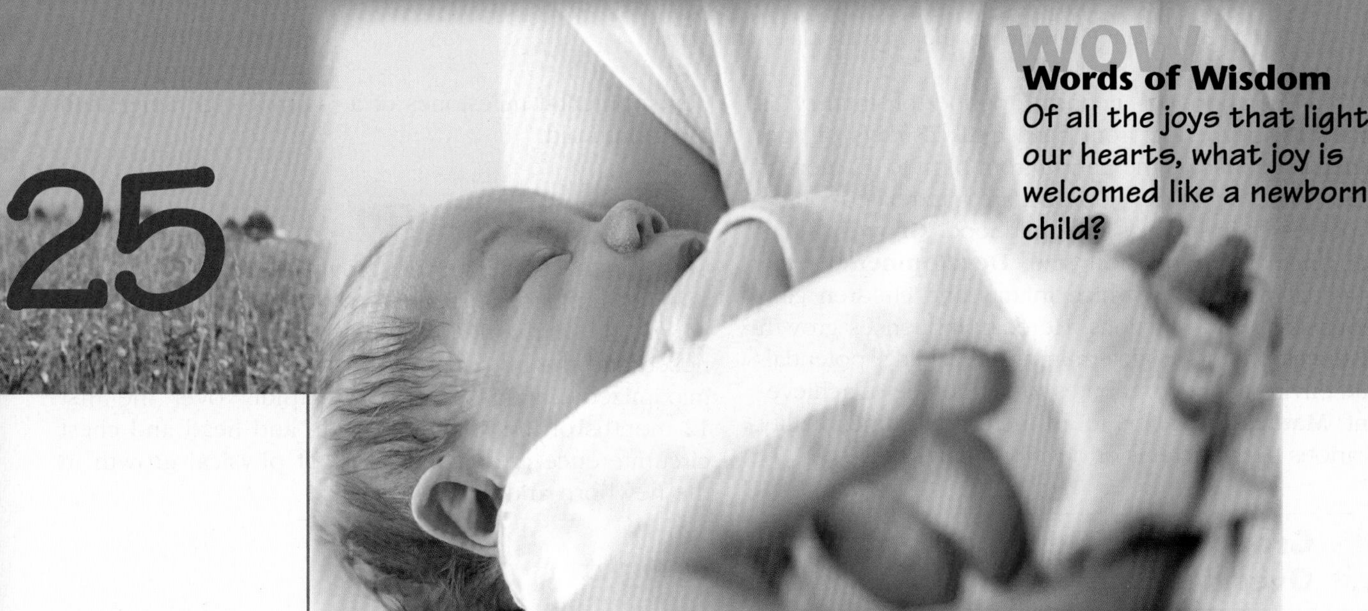

25

Words of Wisdom
Of all the joys that lighten our hearts, what joy is welcomed like a newborn child?

Growth and Development of the Newborn and Infant

KEY TERMS
anticipatory guidance
binocularity
cephalocaudal
colic
colostrum
development
discipline
foremilk
growth
hindmilk
let-down reflex
maturation
object permanence
proximodistal
solitary play
stranger anxiety
temperament

Learning Objectives

Upon completion of the chapter, you will be able to:

1. Identify normal developmental changes occurring in the newborn and infant.
2. Identify the gross and fine motor milestones of the newborn and infant.
3. Express an understanding of language development in the first year of life.
4. Describe nutritional requirements of the newborn and infant.
5. Develop a nutritional plan for the first year of life.
6. Identify common issues related to growth and development in infancy.
7. Demonstrate knowledge of appropriate anticipatory guidance for common developmental issues.

Allison Johnson **is a 6-month-old girl brought to the clinic by her mother and father for her 6-month check-up. As new parents, they have a list of questions and concerns. On assessment you find that Allison's weight is 7.26 kg (16 lb), length 65.41 cm (25¾ inches), and head circumference 43.18 cm (17 inches). As the nurse caring for her, assess Allison's growth and development, and then teach the parents what changes to expect in Allison over the next few months.**

The newborn or neonatal period of infancy is defined as the period from birth until 28 days of age. Infancy is defined as the period from birth to 12 months of age. Growth and development are interrelated, ongoing processes in infancy and childhood. **Growth** refers to an increase in physical size. **Development** is the sequential process by which infants and children gain various skills and functions. Heredity influences growth and development by determining the child's potential, while environment contributes to the degree of achievement. **Maturation** refers to an increase in functionality of various body systems or developmental skills.

Growth and Development Overview

Growth and developmental changes in the first year of life are numerous and dramatic. Physical growth, maturation of body systems, and gross and fine motor skills progress in an orderly and sequential fashion. Though timing may vary from infant to infant, the order in which developmental skills are acquired is consistent. Infants also exhibit vast amounts of learning in the psychosocial and cognitive, language and communication, and social/emotional domains. Adequate growth and development are indicative of health in the infant or young child. Nurses must be familiar with normal developmental milestones so that they can accurately assess the infant's development as well as provide age-appropriate anticipatory guidance to the parents.

Achievement of developmental milestones may be assessed in a variety of ways. While obtaining the health history, the nurse may ask the parent or caregiver if the skill is present and when it was attained. The infant may also demonstrate the skill during the interview or examination, or the nurse may elicit the skill from the infant. A number of screening tools are also used to assess development, such as the Denver II Developmental Screening Test, Prescreening Developmental Questionnaire (PDQ II), Ages and Stages Questionnaire (ASQ), Infant–Toddler Checklist (ITC), and Infant Development Inventory (IDI).

Ill or premature infants may exhibit delayed acquisition of physical growth and developmental skills. When assessing the growth and development of a premature infant, use the infant's adjusted age to determine expected outcomes. To determine adjusted age, subtract the number of weeks that the infant was premature from the infant's chronologic age. Plot growth parameters and assess developmental milestones based on adjusted age. For example, a 6-month-old boy who was born at 28 weeks' gestation was born 12 weeks early (3 months), so subtract 3 months from his chronologic age of 6 months to obtain an adjusted age of 3 months. This infant would demonstrate healthy growth if he were the size of a 3-month-old, and he should be expected to achieve the developmental milestones of a 3-month-old rather than a 6-month-old.

PHYSICAL GROWTH

Ongoing assessments of growth are important so that too-rapid or inadequate growth can be identified early. With early identification, the cause can be diagnosed and the potential for further appropriate growth maximized. Infants grow very rapidly over the first 12 months of life. Weight, length, and head and chest circumference are all indicators of physical growth in the newborn and infant.

Weight

The average newborn weighs 3.400 kg (7.5 lb) at birth, with boys being slightly heavier than girls (Olsson, 2011). Newborns lose up to 10% of their body weight over the first week of life. The average newborn then gains about 30 g per day and regains his or her birth weight by 10 to 14 days of age. Most infants double their birth weight by 4 months of age and triple their birth weight by the time they are 1 year old (Feigelman, 2011).

Height

The average newborn is 50 cm (20 inches) long at birth (Olsson, 2011). The infant grows quickly in length over the first 6 months, than during the second 6 months. By 12 months of age, the infant's length has increased by 50% (Feigelman, 2011).

Head Circumference

The average head circumference of the full-term newborn is 35 cm (14 inches). Similar to the weight and length, the head circumference increases rapidly during the first 6 months. Velocity slows slightly in the 6- to 12-month period, exhibiting an average 10-cm (4-inch) gain from birth to 1 year of age (Feigelman, 2011).

ORGAN SYSTEM MATURATION

The newborn's and infant's organ systems undergo significant changes as the infant grows. Systems that undergo significant change include the neurologic system, the cardiovascular system, the respiratory system, the gastrointestinal (digestive) system, the renal system, the hematopoietic system, the immunologic system, and the integumentary system.

Neurologic System

The infant experiences tremendous changes in the neurologic system over the first year of life. Critical brain growth and continued myelination of the spinal cord occur. Involuntary movement progresses to voluntary control, and immature vocalizations and crying progress to the ability to speak as a result of maturational changes of the neurologic system.

States of Consciousness

The normal term newborn's ability to move sequentially through states of consciousness reassures parents and physicians that the neurologic system, though immature, is intact. A normal newborn will ordinarily move through six states of consciousness:

1. Deep sleep: Sleeping with eyes closed and no movement.
2. Light sleep: Sleeping with eyes closed; rapid eye movements and irregular movements may be noticed.
3. Drowsiness: Eyes may close or be half-lidded; the infant may be dozing.
4. Quiet alert state: The infant's eyes are wide open and the body is calm.
5. Active alert state: The infant's eyes are open; body movements occur.
6. Crying: The infant cries or screams and it is difficult to gain the infant's attention (Brazelton & Nugent, 2011).

Newborns usually progress through these states slowly, rather than going from deep sleep immediately into outright crying.

Brain Growth

The nervous system continues to mature throughout infancy, and the increase in head circumference is indicative of brain growth. The brain undergoes tremendous growth during the first 2 years of life. By 6 months of age the infant's brain weighs half that of the adult brain. At age 12 months, the brain has grown considerably, weighing 2½ times what it did at birth. Usually, the anterior fontanel remains open until 12 to 18 months of age to accommodate this rapid brain growth. However, the fontanel may close as early as 9 months of age, and this is not of concern in the infant with age-appropriate growth and development.

In general, the neurologic system matures a significant amount over the first year of life. Myelination of the spinal cord and nerves continues over the first 2 years. Maturation of the nervous system and continued myelination are necessary for the tremendous developmental skills that are achieved in the first 12 months. During the first few months of life, reflexive behavior is replaced with purposeful action.

Reflexes

Primitive reflexes are subcortical and involve a whole-body response. Selected primitive reflexes present at birth include Moro, root, suck, asymmetric tonic neck, plantar and palmar grasp, step, and Babinski. Except for the Babinski, which disappears around 1 year of age, these primitive reflexes diminish over the first few months of life, giving way to protective reflexes. Protective reflexes (also termed postural responses or reflexes) are gross motor responses related to maintenance of equilibrium. These responses are prerequisites for appropriate motor development and remain throughout life once they are established. The protective reflexes include the righting and parachute reactions. Appropriate presence and disappearance of primitive reflexes, as well as development of protective reflexes, are indicative of a healthy neurologic system. Persistence of primitive reflexes beyond the usual age of disappearance may indicate an abnormality of the neurologic system and should be investigated.

Table 25.1 gives descriptions and illustrations of several primitive and protective reflexes, as well as the timing of appearance and disappearance of these reflexes.

Respiratory System

The respiratory system continues to mature over the first year of life. The respiratory rate slows from an average of 30 to 60 breaths in the newborn to about 20 to 30 in the 12-month-old. The newborn breathes irregularly, with periodic pauses. As the infant matures, the respiratory pattern becomes more regular and rhythmic.

In comparison with the adult, in the infant:

- The nasal passages are narrower.
- The trachea and chest wall are more compliant.
- The bronchi and bronchioles are shorter and narrower.
- The larynx is more funnel shaped.
- The tongue is larger.
- There are significantly fewer alveoli.

These anatomic differences place the infant at higher risk for respiratory compromise. The respiratory system does not reach adult levels of maturity until about 7 years of age. The lack of immunoglobulin A (IgA) in the mucosal lining of the upper respiratory tract also contributes to the frequent infections that occur in infancy.

Cardiovascular System

The heart doubles in size over the first year of life. As the cardiovascular system matures, the average pulse rate decreases from 120 to 140 in the newborn to about 100 in the 1-year-old. Blood pressure steadily increases over the first 12 months of life, from an average of 60/40 in the newborn to 100/50 in the 12-month-old. The peripheral capillaries are closer to the surface of the skin, thus making the newborn and young infant more susceptible to heat loss. Over the first year of life, thermoregulation (the body's ability to stabilize body

(text continues on page 965)

TABLE 25.1 SELECTED PRIMITIVE AND PROTECTIVE REFLEXES IN INFANCY

	Description	Age Reflex Appears	Age Reflex Disappears
Primitive Reflexes			
Root 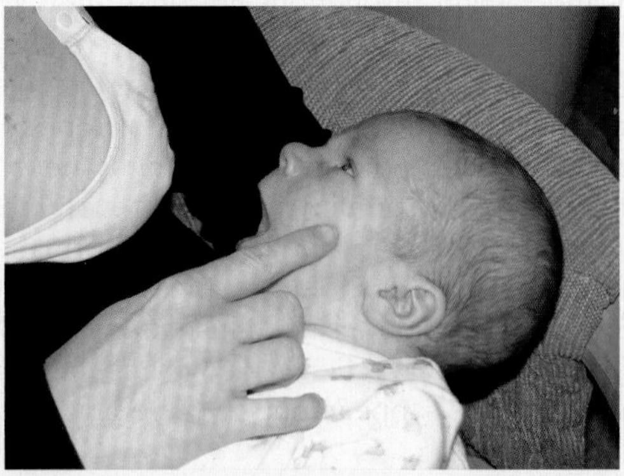	When infant's cheek is stroked, the infant turns to that side, searching with mouth.	Birth	3 months
Suck 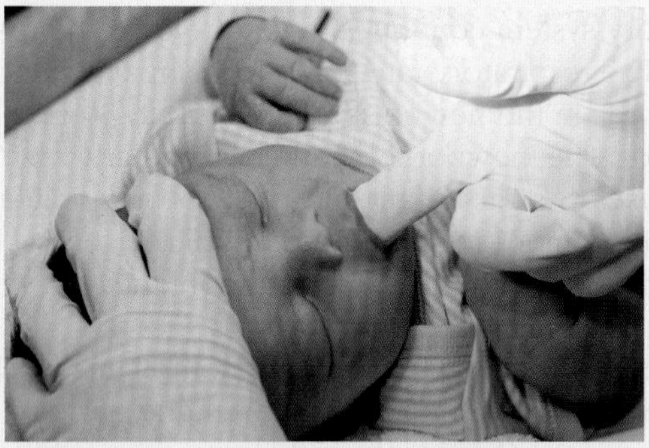	Reflexive sucking when nipple or finger is placed in infant's mouth.	Birth	2–5 months
Moro 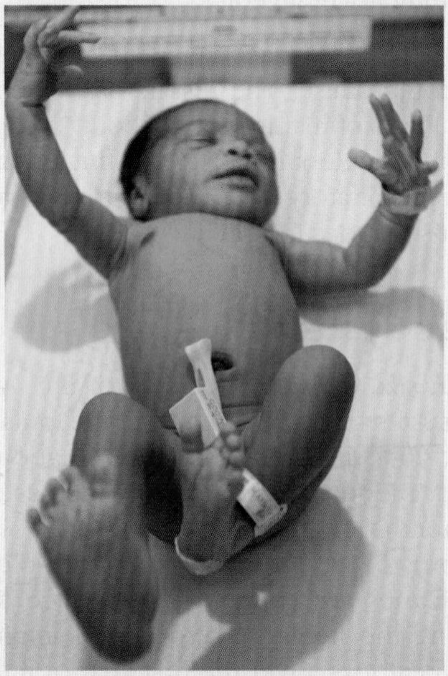	With sudden extension of the head, the arms abduct and move upward and the hands form a "C."	Birth	4 months

TABLE 25.1 SELECTED PRIMITIVE AND PROTECTIVE REFLEXES IN INFANCY (continued)

	Description	Age Reflex Appears	Age Reflex Disappears
Asymmetric tonic neck	While lying supine, extremities are extended on the side of the body to which the head is turned and opposite extremities are flexed (also called the "fencing" position).	Birth	4 months
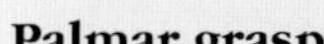 **Palmar grasp** 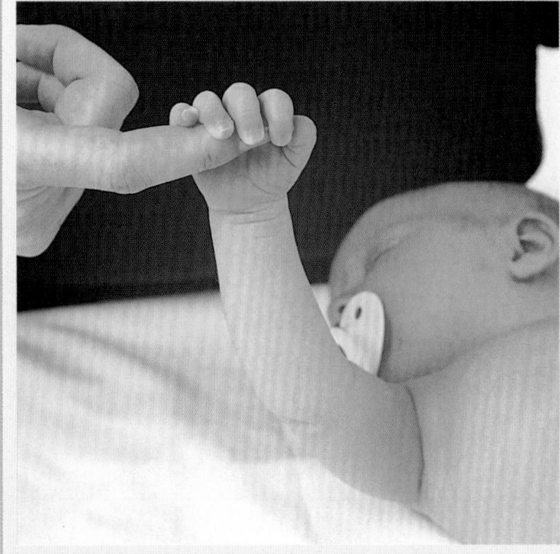	Infant reflexively grasps when palm is touched.	Birth	4–6 months
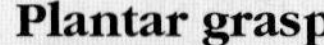 **Plantar grasp** 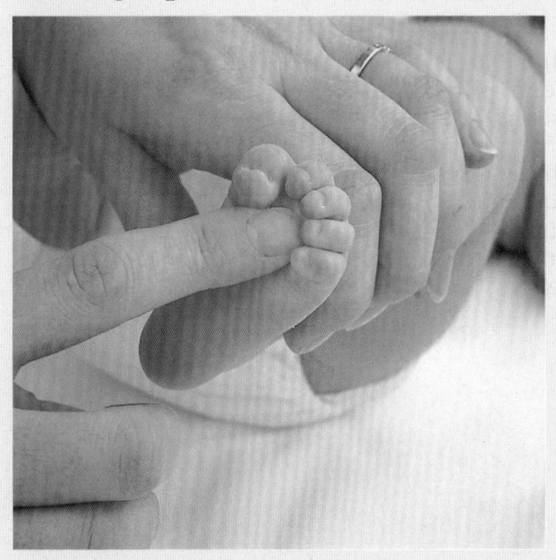	Infant reflexively grasps with bottom of foot when pressure is applied to plantar surface.	Birth	9 months

(continued)

TABLE 25.1 SELECTED PRIMITIVE AND PROTECTIVE REFLEXES IN INFANCY (continued)

	Description	Age Reflex Appears	Age Reflex Disappears
Babinski 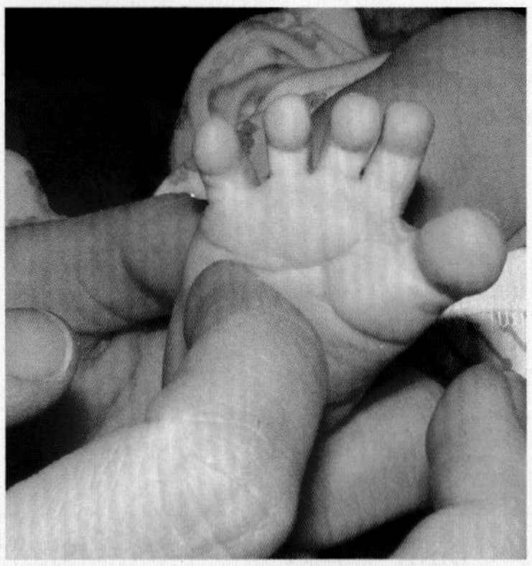	Stroking along the lateral aspect of the sole and across the plantar surface results in fanning and hyperextension of the toes.	Birth	12 months
Step 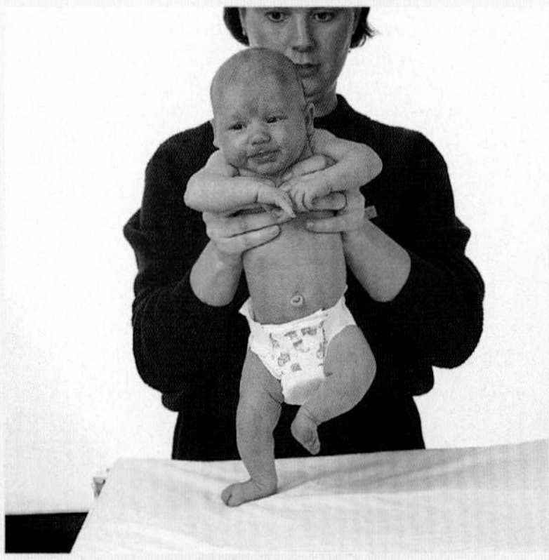	With one foot on a flat surface, the infant puts the other foot down as if to "step."	Birth	4–8 weeks
Protective Reflexes			
Neck righting	Neck keeps head in upright position when body is tilted.	4–6 months	Persists
Parachute (sideways)	Protective extension with the arms when tilted to the side in a supported sitting position.	6 months	Persists
Parachute (forward) 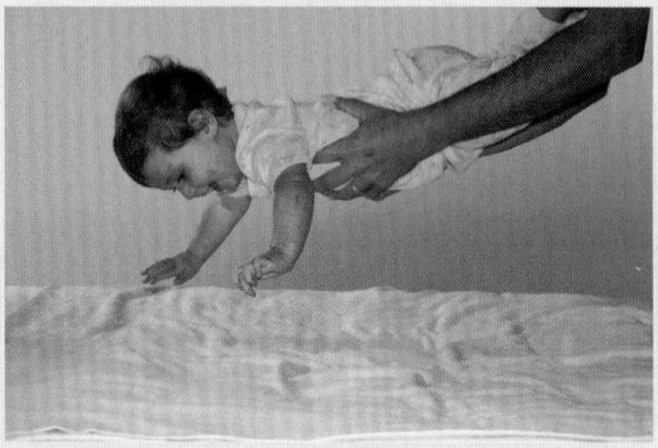	Protective extension with the arms when held up in the air and moved forward. The infant reflexively reaches forward to catch himself or herself.	6–7 months	Persists
Parachute (backward)	Protective extension with the arms when tilted backward.	9–10 months	Persists

temperature) becomes more effective: the peripheral capillaries constrict in response to a cold environment and dilate in response to heat.

Gastrointestinal System

Teeth

Occasionally, an infant is born with one or more teeth (termed natal teeth) or develops teeth in the first 28 days of life (termed neonatal teeth). The presence of natal or neonatal teeth may be associated with other birth anomalies. The vast majority of newborns do not have teeth at birth, nor do they develop them in the first month of life. On average, the first primary teeth begin to erupt between the ages of 6 and 8 months. The primary teeth (also termed deciduous teeth) are lost later in childhood and will be replaced by the permanent teeth. The gums around the emerging tooth often swell. The lower central incisors are usually the first to appear, followed by the upper central incisors (Fig. 25.1). The average 12-month-old has four to eight teeth.

Digestion

The newborn's digestive system is not fully developed. Small amounts of saliva are present for the first 3 months of life and ptyalin is present only in small amounts in the saliva. Gastric digestion occurs as a result of the presence of hydrochloric acid and rennin. The small intestine is about 270 cm long and grows to the adult length over the first few years of life (Liacouras, 2011). The stomach capacity is relatively small at birth, holding about one-half to 1 ounce. However, by 1 year of age the stomach can accommodate three full meals and several snacks per day. In the duodenum, three enzymes in particular are important for digestion. Trypsin is available in sufficient quantities for protein digestion after birth. Amylase (needed for complex carbohydrate digestion) and lipase (essential for appropriate fat digestion) are both deficient in the infant and do not reach adult levels until about 5 months of age.

The liver is also immature at birth. The ability to conjugate bilirubin and secrete bile is present after about 2 weeks of age. Conjugation of medications may remain immature over the first year of life. Other functions of the liver, including gluconeogenesis, vitamin storage, and protein metabolism, remain immature during the first year of life.

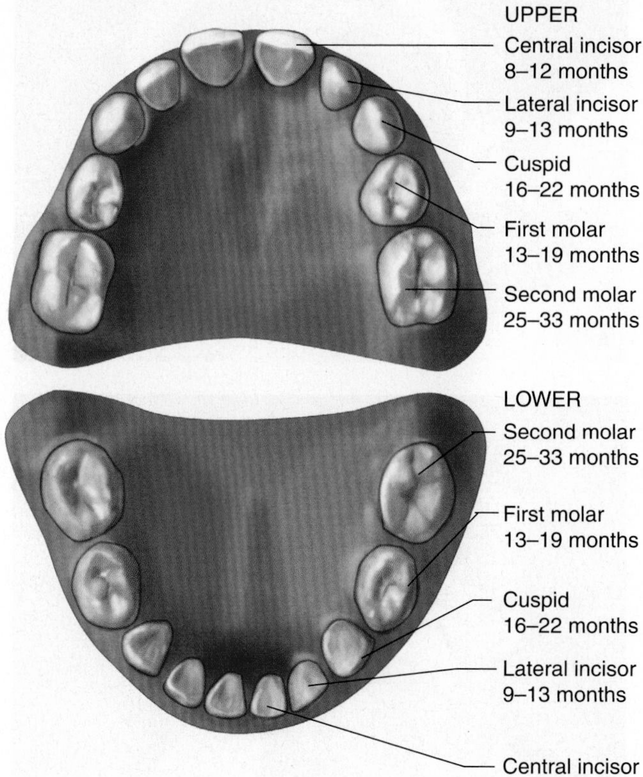

FIGURE 25.1 Sequence and average age of tooth eruption.

Stools

The consistency and frequency of stools change over the first year of life. The newborn's first stools (meconium) are the result of digestion of amniotic fluid swallowed in utero. They are dark green to black and sticky (Fig. 25.2). In the first few days of life the stools become yellowish or tan. Generally, the formula-fed infant has stools the consistency of peanut butter. Breastfed infants' stools are usually looser in texture and appear seedy. Newborns may have as many as 8 to 10 stools per day or as few as one stool every day or two. After the newborn period, the number of stools may decrease, and some infants do not have a bowel movement for several days. Infrequent stooling is considered normal if the bowel movement remains soft. Due to the immaturity of the gastrointestinal system, newborns and young infants often grunt, strain, or cry while attempting to have a bowel movement. This is not of concern unless the stool is hard and dry. Stool color and texture may change depending on the foods that the infant is ingesting. Iron supplements may cause the stool to appear black or very dark green (Swanson, 2016).

Take Note!

Parents should call the primary care provider if the infant's stools are red, white, or black; mucous-like; frequent and watery; frothy or foul-smelling; or hard, dry, formed, or pellet-like; or if the baby is vomiting.

Genitourinary System

In the infant, extracellular fluid (lymph, interstitial fluid, and blood plasma) accounts for about 35% of body weight and intracellular fluid accounts for 40%, compared

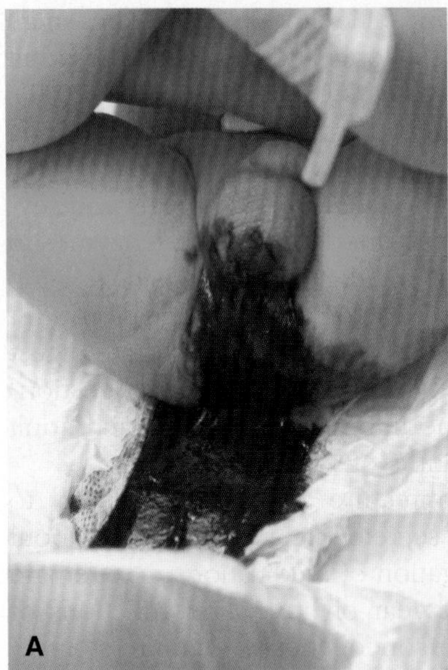

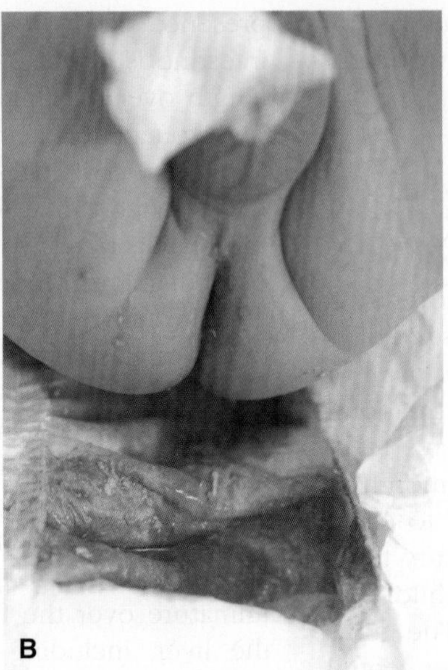

FIGURE 25.2 **(A)** Meconium stool. **(B)** Typical stool after the first few days. Note the yellowish, seedy stool of a breastfed infant.

with the adult quantities of 20% and 40%, respectively (Greenbaum, 2011). Thus, the infant is more susceptible to dehydration. Infants urinate frequently and the urine has a relatively low specific gravity. The renal structures are immature and the glomerular filtration rate, tubular secretion, and reabsorption as well as renal perfusion are all reduced compared with the adult. The glomeruli reach full maturity by 2 years of age.

Integumentary System

In utero, the infant is covered with vernix caseosa, which protects the developing infant's skin. At birth, the infant may be covered with vernix (earlier gestational age) or vernix may be found in the folds of the skin, axilla, and groin areas (later gestational age). Production of vernix ceases at birth. Fine downy hair (lanugo) covers the body of many newborns. Often, this hair is lost over time and is not replaced. Darker-skinned races tend to have more lanugo present at birth than those with light skin.

Acrocyanosis (blueness of the hands and feet) is normal in the newborn; it decreases over the first few days of life (Fig. 25.3). Newborns often experience mottling of the skin (a pink-and-white marbled appearance) because of their immature circulatory system. Mottling decreases over the first few months of life.

The newborn and young infant's skin is relatively thinner than that of the adult, with the peripheral capillaries being closer to the surface. This may cause increased absorption of topical medications.

Hematopoietic System

Significant changes in the hematopoietic system occur over the first year of life. At birth, fetal hemoglobin (HgbF) is present in large amounts. After birth the production of HgbF nearly ceases, and adult hemoglobin (HgbA) is produced in steadily increasing amounts throughout the first 6 months. Since HgbF has a shorter lifespan than HgbA, infants may experience physiologic anemia at age

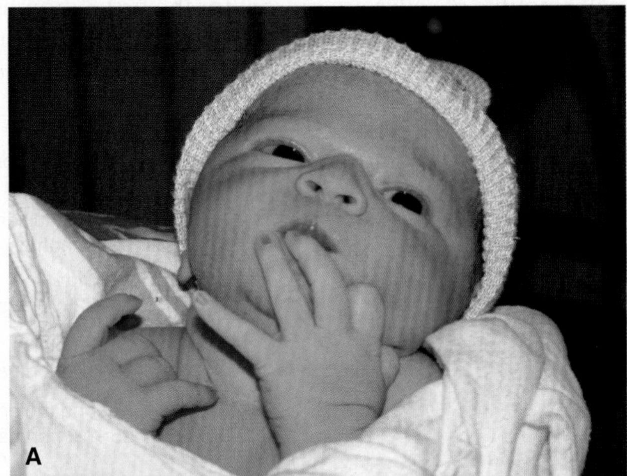

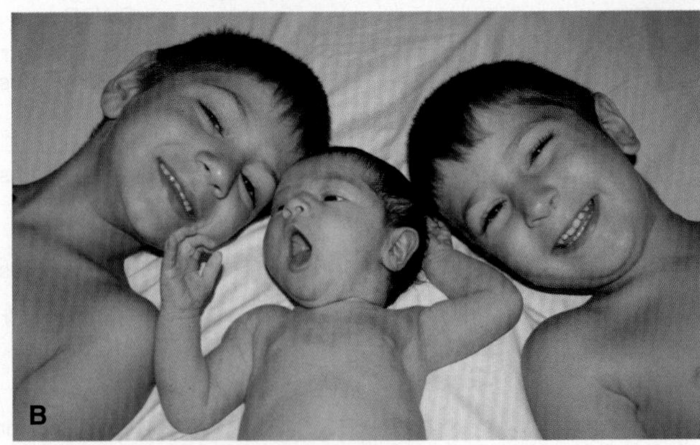

FIGURE 25.3 **(A)** Acrocyanosis. Note blueness of the hands. **(B)** Mottling of the skin in a young infant.

2 to 3 months (Lerner, 2011). During the last 3 months of gestation, maternal iron stores are transferred to the fetus. The newborn typically has 0.3 to 0.5 g of iron stores available. As the high hemoglobin concentration of the newborn decreases over the first 2 to 3 months, iron is reclaimed and stored. These stores may be sufficient for the first 6 to 9 months of life but will become depleted if iron supplementation does not occur. Ongoing iron intake is required throughout the first 15 years of life in order to reach adult levels (Maqbool, Stettler, & Stallings, 2011).

Take Note!

Maternal iron stores are transferred to the fetus throughout the last trimester of pregnancy. Infants born prematurely miss all or at least a portion of this iron store transfer, placing them at increased risk for iron deficiency anemia compared with term infants.

Immunologic System

Newborns receive large amounts of IgG through the placenta from their mothers. This confers immunity during the first 3 to 6 months of life for antigens to which the mother was previously exposed. Infants then synthesize their own IgG, reaching approximately 60% of adult levels at age 12 months (Cherry, Demmler-Harrison, Kaplan, Steinbach, & Hotez, 2014). IgM is produced in significant amounts after birth, reaching adult levels by 9 months of age. IgA, IgD, and IgE production increases very gradually, maturing in early childhood (Cherry et al., 2014).

PSYCHOSOCIAL DEVELOPMENT

Erik Erikson (1963) identifies the psychosocial crisis of infancy as Trust versus Mistrust. Development of a sense of trust is crucial in the first year, as it serves as the foundation for later psychosocial tasks. The parent or primary caregiver can have a significant impact on the infant's development of a sense of trust. When the infant's needs are consistently met, the infant develops this sense of trust. But if the parent or caregiver is inconsistent in meeting the infant's needs in a timely manner, then the infant develops a sense of mistrust. Table 25.2 lists activities that promote a sense of trust in infancy.

TABLE 25.2 DEVELOPMENTAL THEORIES

Theorist	Stage	Activities
Erikson	Trust vs. Mistrust (birth to 1 year)	Caregivers respond to the infant's basic needs by feeding, changing diapers, cleaning, touching, holding, and talking to the infant. This creates a sense of trust in the infant. As the nervous system matures, infants realize they are separate beings from their caregivers. Over time the infant learns to tolerate small amounts of frustration and trusts that although gratification may be delayed, it will eventually be provided.
Piaget	Sensorimotor (birth to 2 years) Substage 1: use of reflexes (birth to 1 month) Substage 2: primary circular reactions (1 to 4 months) Substage 3: secondary circular reactions (4 to 8 months) Substage 4: coordination of secondary schemes (8 to 12 months)	Infant uses senses and motor skills to learn about the world. Reflexive sucking brings the pleasure of ingesting nutrition. Infant begins to gain control over reflexes and recognizes familiar objects, odors, and sounds. Thumb sucking may occur by chance; then the infant repeats it on purpose to bring pleasure. Imitation begins. Object permanence begins. Infant shows affect. Infant repeats actions to achieve wanted results (e.g., shakes rattle to hear the noise it makes). The infant's actions are purposeful but the infant does not always have an end goal in mind. Infants coordinate previously learned schemes with previously learned behaviors. They may grasp and shake a rattle intentionally or crawl across the room to reach a desired toy. Infant can anticipate events. Object permanence is fully present at about 8 months of age. The infant begins to associate symbols with events (e.g., waving goodbye means someone is leaving).
Freud	Oral stage (birth to 1 year)	Pleasure is focused on oral activities: feeding and sucking.

Adapted from Erikson, E. H. (1963). *Childhood and society* (2nd ed.). New York: W. W. Norton and Company; Goldson, E., & Reynolds, A. (2014). Child development and behavior. In W. W. Hay, Jr., M. J. Levin, R. R. Deterding, & M. J. Abzug. (Eds.), *Current diagnosis and treatment: Pediatrics* (22nd ed.). New York, NY: McGraw-Hill Education; and Piaget, J. (1969). *The theory of stages in cognitive development*. New York, NY: McGraw-Hill.

COGNITIVE DEVELOPMENT

The first stage of Jean Piaget's theory of cognitive development is referred to as the sensorimotor stage (birth to 2 years) (Piaget, 1969). Infants learn about themselves and the world through their developing sensory and motor capacities. Infants' development from birth to 1 year of age can be divided into four substages within the sensorimotor stage: reflexes, primary circular reaction, secondary circular reaction, and coordination of secondary schemes. Cause and effect guides most of the cognitive development seen in infancy (Table 25.2).

The concept of **object permanence** begins to develop between 4 and 7 months of age and is solidified by about 8 months of age (Piaget, 1969). If an object is hidden from the infant's sight, he or she will search for it in the last place it was seen, knowing it still exists. This development of object permanence is essential for the development of self-image. By age 12 months the infant knows he or she is separate from the parent or caregiver. Self-image is also promoted through the use of mirrors. By 12 months of age, infants can recognize themselves in the mirror. The 12-month-old will explore objects in different ways, such as throwing, banging, dropping, and shaking. He or she may imitate gestures and knows how to use certain objects correctly (e.g., puts phone to ear, turns up cup to drink, attempts to comb hair) (Piaget, 1969).

MOTOR SKILL DEVELOPMENT

Infants exhibit phenomenal increases in their gross and fine motor skills over the first 12 months of life.

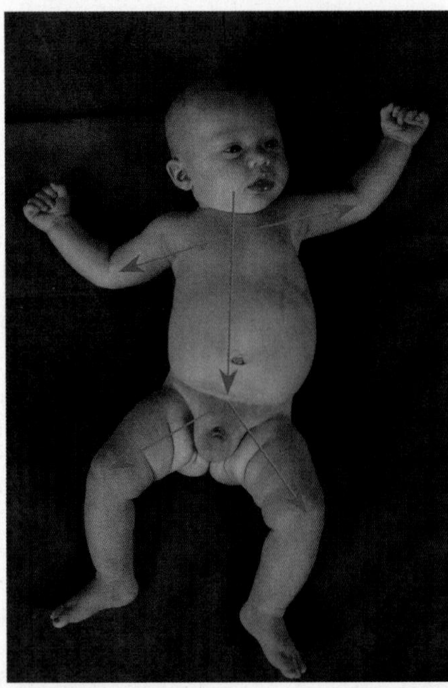

FIGURE 25.4 Gross motor skills develop in a cephalocaudal direction, fine motor skills in a proximodistal fashion.

Gross Motor Skills

The term "gross motor skills" refers to those that use the large muscles (e.g., head control, rolling, sitting, and walking). Gross motor skills develop in a **cephalocaudal** fashion (from the head to the tail) (Fig. 25.4). In other words, the baby learns to lift the head before learning to roll over and sit (Goldson & Reynolds, 2014). At birth, babies have poor head control and need to have their necks supported when being held. They can lift their heads only slightly while in a prone position. Over the next several months the infant's motor skills progress at a dramatic rate. First, the infant achieves head control, then the ability to roll over, sit, crawl, pull to stand, and, usually around 1 year of age, walk independently. Table 25.3 gives details on when the infant develops

TABLE 25.3 DEVELOPMENT OF GROSS MOTOR SKILLS IN INFANCY

Age	Gross Motor Skills
1 month	Lifts and turns head to side in prone position Head lag when pulled to sit Rounded back in sitting
2 months	Raises head and chest, holds position Improving head control
3 months	Raises head to 45 degrees in prone Slight head lag in pull-to-sit
4 months	Lifts head and looks around Rolls from prone to supine Head leads body when pulled to sit
5 months	Rolls from supine to prone and back again Sits with back upright when supported
6 months	Tripod sits
7 months	Sits alone with some use of hands for support
8 months	Sits unsupported
9 months	Crawls, abdomen off floor
10 months	Pulls to stand Cruises
12 months	Sits from standing position Walks independently

Adapted from Feigelman, S. (2011). The first year. In R. M. Kliegman, B. F. Stanton, J. W. St. Geme III, N. F. Schor, & R. E. Behrman (Eds.), *Nelson's textbook of pediatrics* (19th ed.). Philadelphia, PA: Elsevier, Saunders; and Centers for Disease Control and Prevention. (2016). *Developmental milestones*. Retrieved from http://www.cdc.gov/ncbddd/actearly/milestones/index.html

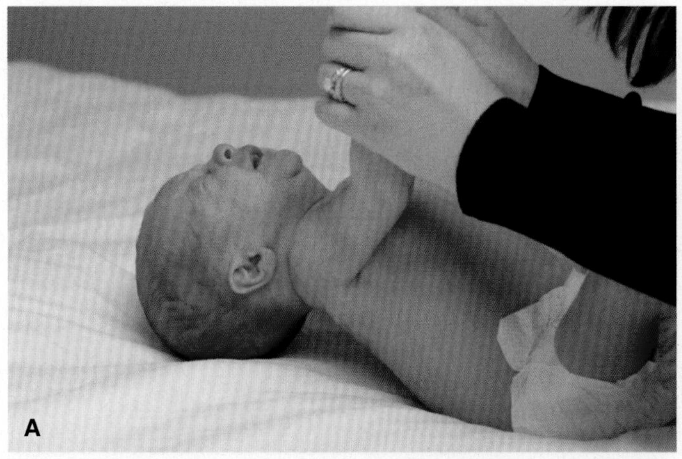

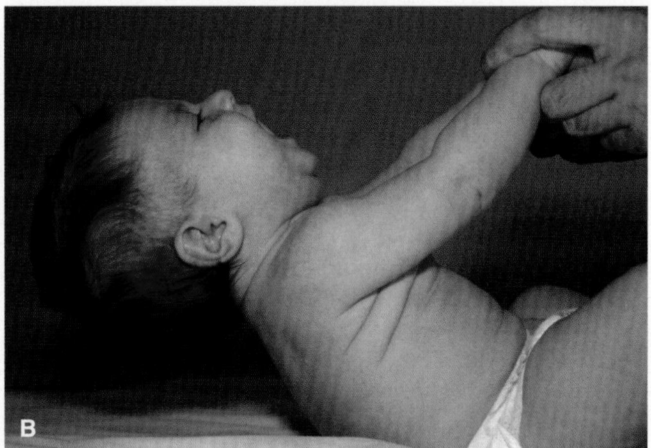

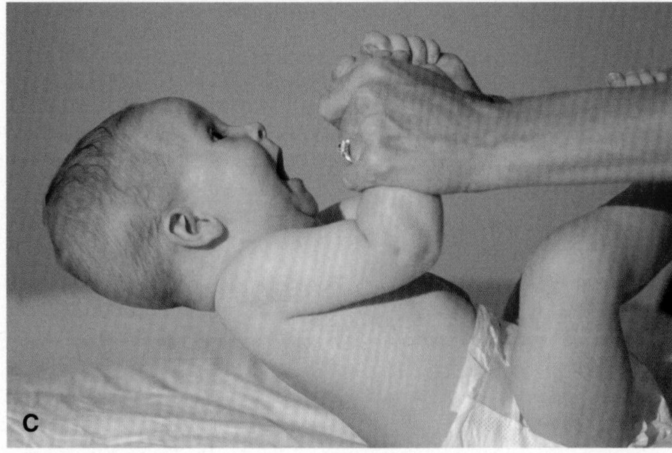

FIGURE 25.5 When pulled to sit, an infant shows **(A)** significant head lag (newborn; 2 or 3 weeks old), **(B)** improving head control (2 months old), and **(C)** no head lag (4 months old).

each specific gross motor skill. Progression of gross motor skills is illustrated in Figures 25.5 through 25.7.

Take Note!

Warning signs that may indicate problems with motor development include the following: arms and legs are stiff or floppy; child cannot support head at 3 to 4 months of age; child reaches with one hand only; child cannot sit with assistance at 6 months of age; child does not crawl by 12 months of age; child cannot stand supported by 12 months of age.

Fine Motor Skills

Fine motor development includes the maturation of hand and finger use. Fine motor skills develop in a **proximodistal** fashion (from the center to the periphery) (Fig. 25.4). In other words, the infant first bats with the whole hand, eventually progressing to gross grasping, before being capable of fine fingertip grasping (Goldson & Reynolds, 2014) (Fig. 25.8). The newborn's hand movements are involuntary in nature, whereas the 12-month-old is capable of feeding himself or herself with a cup and spoon. By 12 months of age the infant should be able to eat with his or her fingers and assist with dressing (e.g., pushing an arm through the sleeve). Table 25.4 gives details on when the infant develops each specific fine motor skill.

SENSORY DEVELOPMENT

Though hearing should be fully developed at birth, the other senses continue to develop as the infant matures. Though they mature at different rates, sight, smell, taste, and touch all continue to develop after birth.

Sight

The newborn is nearsighted, preferring to view objects at a distance of 20 to 38 cm (8 to 15 inches). Newborns prefer the human face to other objects and may even imitate the facial expressions made by those caring for them. In addition to human faces, newborns show a preference for certain objects, particularly those with contrasts such as black-and-white stripes. The newborn's eyes wander and occasionally cross. At 1 month of age the infant can recognize by sight the people he or she knows best. The infant will study objects within his or her visual range closely. The ability to fuse two ocular images into one cerebral picture (**binocularity**) begins to develop at

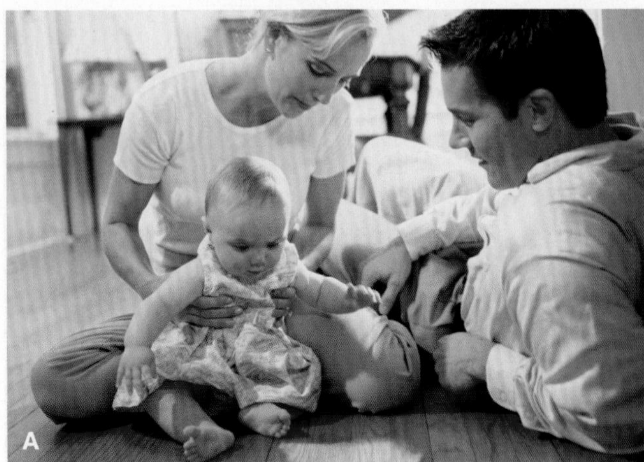

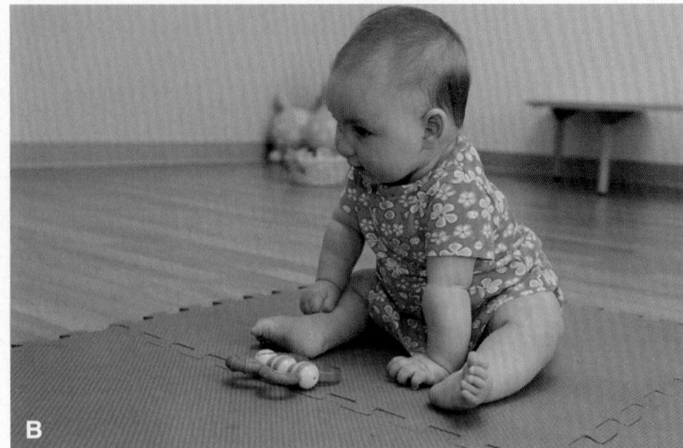

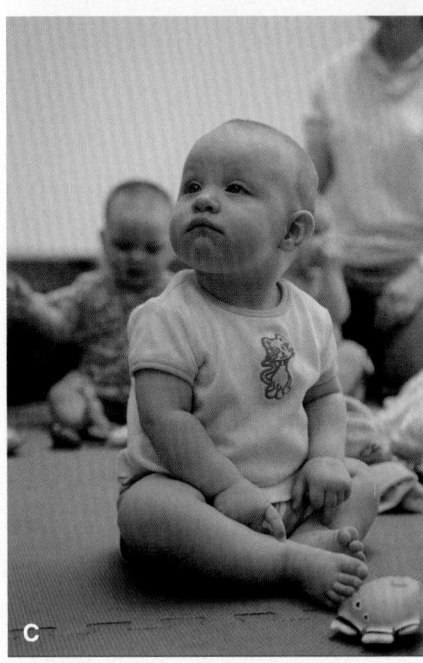

FIGURE 25.6 Development of sitting. **(A)** At 4 months, the infant requires significant support. **(B)** The 6-month-old infant sits in tripod fashion. **(C)** The 8-month-old sits alone.

6 weeks of age and is well established by 4 months of age. Full color vision develops by 7 months of age, as do distance vision and the ability to track objects.

Hearing

The newborn's hearing is intact at birth and as acute as that of an adult. Newborns prefer the sound of human voices to nonhuman sounds. By 1 month of age the infant can recognize the sounds of those he or she knows best.

Smell and Taste

The sense of smell develops rapidly: the 7-day-old infant can differentiate the smell of his or her mother's breast milk from that of another woman and will preferentially turn toward the mother's smell. Newborns prefer sweet tastes to all others. This persists for several months, and eventually the infant will accept nonsweet flavors.

Touch

The sense of touch is perhaps the most important of all the senses for newborn communication. Even the most immature infant responds to soothing stroking. The infant prefers soft sensations to coarse sensations. The infant dislikes rough handling and may cry. Holding, stroking, rocking, or cuddling calms infants when they are upset and makes them more alert when they are drowsy. Infants learn to understand their caregiver's moods by the way they touch them.

Take Note!

Warning signs that may indicate problems with sensory development include the following: young infant does not respond to loud noises; child does not focus on a near object; infant does not start to make sounds or babble by 4 months of age; infant does not turn to locate sound at age 4 months; infant crosses eyes most of the time at age 6 months.

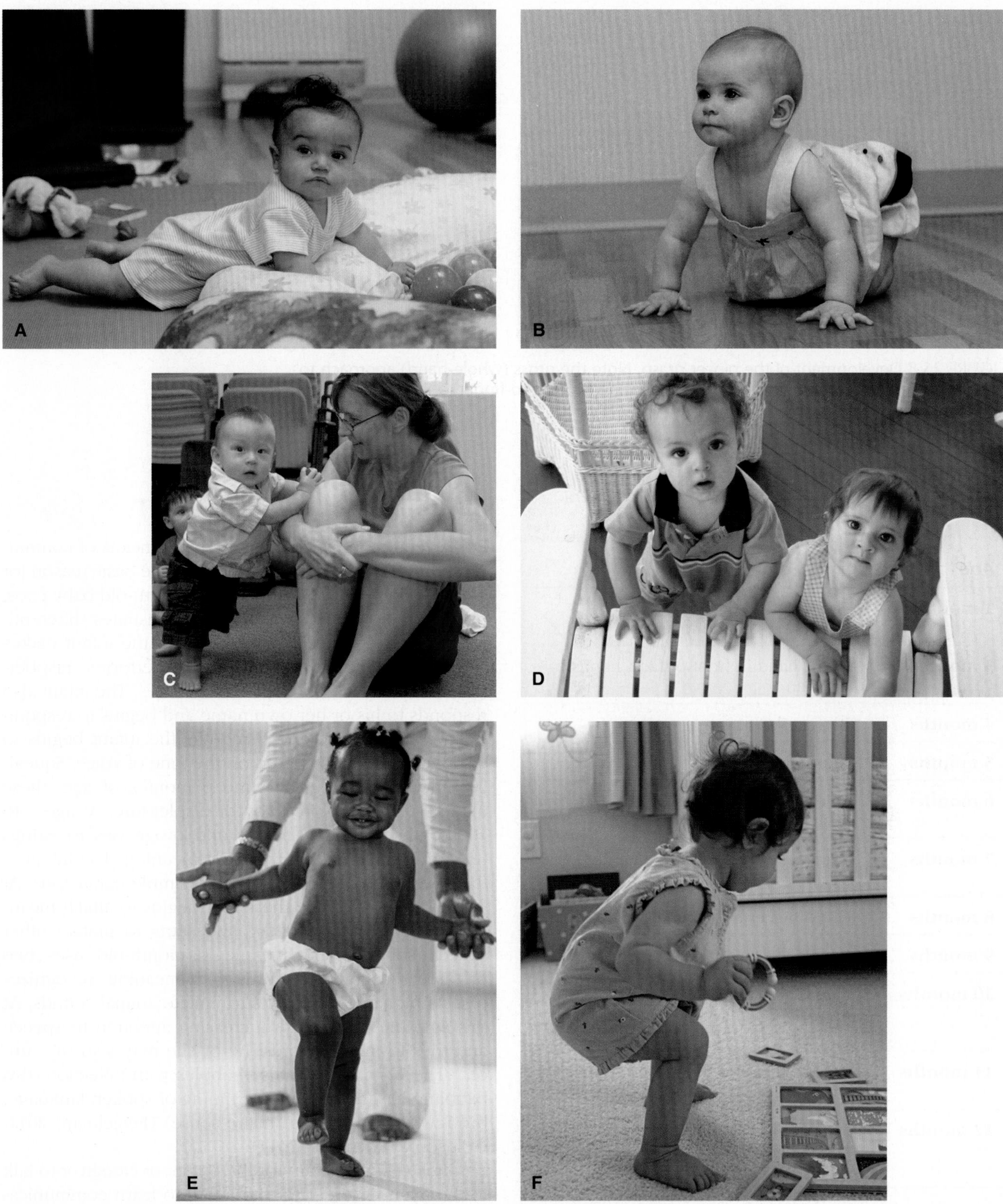

FIGURE 25.7 Development of locomotion. **(A)** At 4 months the infant pushes up from a prone position. **(B)** At 8 months, the infant crawls with the abdomen off the floor. **(C)** The infant pulls to stand by 10 months of age. **(D)** The infant cruises along furniture or **(E)** takes steps with assistance at 10 to 11 months of age. **(F)** The infant independently stands from a crouched position and walks around 12 months of age (plus or minus 3 months).

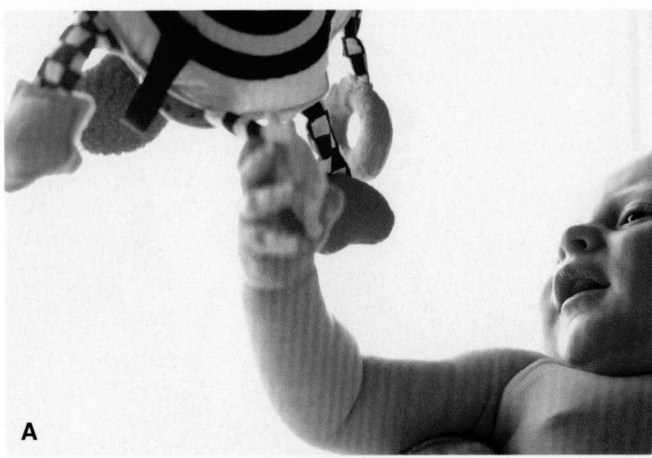

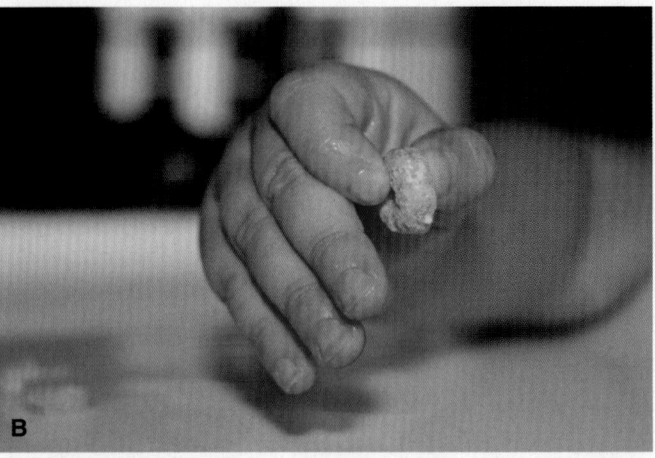

FIGURE 25.8 Development of the pincer grasp. Note the gross (whole-hand) approach to grasping a small object (**A**), compared with the fine (thumb-to-finger) ability (**B**).

TABLE 25.4 DEVELOPMENT OF FINE MOTOR SKILLS IN INFANCY

Age	Fine Motor Skills
1 month	Fists mostly clenched Involuntary hand movements
3 months	Holds hand in front of face, hands open
4 months	Bats at objects
5 months	Grasps rattle
6 months	Releases object in hand to take another
7 months	Transfers object from one hand to the other
8 months	Gross pincer grasp (rakes)
9 months	Bangs objects together
10 months	Fine pincer grasp Puts objects into container and takes them out
11 months	Offers objects to others and releases them
12 months	Feeds self with cup and spoon Makes simple mark on paper Pokes with index finger

Adapted from Feigelman, S. (2011). The first year. In R. M. Kliegman, B. F. Stanton, J. W. St. Geme III, N. F. Schor, & R. E. Behrman (Eds.), *Nelson's textbook of pediatrics* (19th ed.). Philadelphia, PA: Elsevier, Saunders; and Centers for Disease Control and Prevention. (2016). *Developmental milestones*. Retrieved from http://www.cdc.gov/ncbddd/actearly/milestones/index.html

COMMUNICATION AND LANGUAGE DEVELOPMENT

For several months, crying is the only means of communication for the newborn and infant. The basic reason for crying is unmet needs. The 1- to 3-month-old baby coos, makes other vocalizations, and demonstrates differentiated crying. At 4 to 5 months of age, the infant makes simple vowel sounds, laughs aloud, performs "raspberries," and vocalizes in response to voices. The infant also responds to his or her own name and begins to respond to "no." Between 4 and 7 months the infant begins to distinguish emotions based on the tone of voice. Squealing and yelling begin around 6 months of age; these may be used to express joy or displeasure. At age 7 to 10 months, babbling begins and progresses to strings (e.g., mamama, dadada) without meaning. The infant at this age is also able to respond to simple commands. At 9 to 12 months of age the infant begins to attach meaning to "mama" and "dada" and starts to imitate other speech sounds. The average 12-month-old uses two or three recognizable words with meaning, recognizes objects by name, and starts to imitate animal sounds. At this age, the infant pays increasing attention to speech and tries to imitate words; he or she may also say "uh-oh." The 12-month-old also babbles with inflection (this babbling has the rhythm and timing of spoken language, but few of the "words" make sense) (Feigelman, 2011; Goldson & Reynolds, 2014).

It is very important for the parent or caregiver to talk to the infant in order for the infant to learn communication skills. Sometimes regression in language development occurs briefly when the child is focusing energy on other skills, such as crawling or walking. As long as the infant's hearing is normal, language acquisition should continue to progress. Infants in bilingual families may "language mix" (uses some words from each language). This is considered to be a normal progression in language development for these children (Lowry, 2011), but it makes it more difficult for the physician or nurse practitioner to determine delays in communication skills.

Take Note!

Warning signs that may indicate problems in language development are as follows: infant does not make sounds at 4 months of age; infant does not laugh or squeal by 6 months of age; infant does not babble by 8 months of age; infant does not use single words with meaning at 12 months of age (mama, dada).

SOCIAL AND EMOTIONAL DEVELOPMENT

The newborn spends much of the time sleeping, but by 2 months of age the infant is ready to start socializing. The infant exhibits a first real smile at age 2 months. He or she spends a great deal of time while awake watching and observing what is going on around him or her. By about 3 months of age the infant will start an interaction with a caregiver by smiling widely and possibly gurgling. This prompts the caregiver to smile back and talk to the infant. The infant responds with more smiling, cooing, and gurgles as well as moving the arms and legs. The 3- to 4-month-old will also mimic the parent's facial movements, such as widening the eyes and sticking out the tongue. The baby may hesitate at first, but once the other person responds pleasantly to the infant, the infant engages and gets into the interaction. The infant may cry when the pleasant interaction stops. At 6 to 8 months of age the infant may enjoy socially interactive games such as patty-cake and peek-a-boo (Feigelman, 2011; Goldson & Reynolds, 2014).

Stranger Anxiety

Around the age of 8 months the infant may develop **stranger anxiety**. The previously happy and very friendly infant may become clingy and whiny when approached by strangers or people not well known. Stranger anxiety is an indicator that the infant is recognizing himself or herself as separate from others. As the infant becomes more aware of new people and new places, he or she may view an interaction with a stranger as threatening and may start crying, even if the parent is right there. Family members whom the child sees infrequently, as well as others the child does not spend a lot of time with, should approach the infant calmly and slowly, with the parent in sight. Sometimes this will prevent a sudden crying spell (Feigelman, 2011; Goldson & Reynolds, 2014).

Separation Anxiety

Separation anxiety may also start in the last few months of infancy. The infant becomes quite distressed when the parent leaves. The infant will eventually calm down and become engaged with the current caregiver. It is not until the infant is older that cognition and memory are sufficient for him or her to understand that the parent will come back (Feigelman, 2011; Goldson & Reynolds, 2014).

Take Note!

Warning signs of possible problems with social/emotional development include the following: child does not smile at people at 3 months of age; child refuses to cuddle; child does not seem to enjoy people; child shows no interest in peek-a-boo at 8 months of age.

Temperament

Temperament is an individual's nature; it is the child's inborn traits that determine how he interacts with the world (Child Development Institute [CDI], 2015). Temperament ranges from low or moderately active, regular, and predictable to highly active, more intense, and less adaptable. These are all considered normal along a continuum. An infant's innate temperament affects the way he or she responds to the environment. As parents take note of their infant's usual activity level, how intensely he or she reacts with others and the environment, and how stimulated he or she becomes with interactions, they start to learn about their infant's temperament. The parent should note how adaptable and flexible the infant is as well as how predictable and persistent the baby is.

When parents are familiar with how the baby approaches life on a routine basis, they will be better able to recognize when the baby is not acting like himself or herself. Nurses can help parents interpret observations about their infant's temperament and recommend ways to support the infant's individual behavior. Some infants are slower to warm up than others; those infants should be approached slowly and calmly. Some infants exhibit increased levels of activity compared to quieter, more passive babies; those infants generally require more direct play with the parent or caregiver and will be the type of older infant who is in constant motion. Some infants are loud and some are not. The quiet infant may become overwhelmed with excessive stimulation, whereas the very active baby may need additional stimulation to be satisfied. Becoming familiar with the infant's temperament also helps the parents describe the best approach to the infant by others (e.g., child care workers or health care professionals) (CDI, 2015).

CULTURAL INFLUENCES ON GROWTH AND DEVELOPMENT

Many cultural differences have an impact on growth and development. For instance, certain ethnic groups tend to be shorter than others because of their genetic makeup (Sinha, 2015). These children will not grow to be as tall as those of another ethnic background. Cultural feeding practices in some cultures may lead to overweight in some children. Some cultures and certain religions advocate vegetarianism; those children need nutritional assessment to ensure they are getting enough protein intake for adequate growth.

Parenting styles and health promotion behaviors can also be significantly influenced by culture. Parents and extended family are the most significant influences in an infant's life in most cultures. Certain cultures place a high value on independence and may encourage their infants to develop quickly, while other cultures "baby" their infants for longer periods. In most cultures the mother takes primary responsibility for caring for the child, but in some cultures, major health-related decisions may be deferred to the father or grandparents.

Health beliefs are often strongly influenced by an individual's religious or spiritual background. Sometimes this creates conflict in the health care setting when the health providers have a different value system than that of the infant's family.

In some cultures infants and children share a bed with their parents. When an infant or child is hospitalized and is accustomed to sleeping with the parents, it may be difficult and distressing for him or her to try to sleep alone.

The nurse should explore the family's cultural practices related to growth and development. Usually, these practices are not harmful and can be supported by the health care team, but safety must always be considered. The nurse should not make assumptions about a family's cultural practices based on their skin color, accent, or name; rather, the nurse should perform an adequate assessment (Douglas et al., 2011).

Take Note!

Many communities now include people from a variety of cultures, so it is important for nurses to practice transcultural nursing (nursing care that is directed by cultural aspects and that respects the individual's differences). Many nurse researchers are exploring the cultural aspects of health care and the impact that cultural diversity has upon health.

Refer back to Allison Johnson, who was introduced at the beginning of the chapter. What developmental milestones would you expect Allison to have reached by this age? How would this be different if Allison had been born 6 weeks premature?

The Nurse's Role in Newborn and Infant Growth and Development

Growth and development affect every aspect of the infant's life. As infants progress through various stages of development, they do so in a predictable fashion. Growth and development are sequential and orderly, though some children develop at faster rates than others. It is important for the nurse to understand growth and development. Health care visits through infancy often focus primarily on **anticipatory guidance** (educating parents and caregivers about what to expect in the next phase of development). The purpose of anticipatory guidance is to give parents the tools they need to support their infant's development in a safe fashion.

Hospital nurses also need to use their knowledge of growth and development when caring for ill infants. Hospitalization often requires the infant to be confined to the crib or the hospital room. Nurses must support growth and development within the constraints imposed by the child's illness.

NURSING PROCESS OVERVIEW

After the infant's current growth and development status has been assessed, problems related to growth and development may be identified. The nurse may then identify one or more nursing diagnoses, including:

- Ineffective breastfeeding
- Risk for disproportionate growth
- Imbalanced nutrition, less than body requirements
- Risk for impaired parent/infant attachment
- Delayed growth and development
- Risk for caregiver role strain

Nursing care planning for the infant with growth and development issues should be individualized based on the infant's and family's needs. Nursing Care Plan 25.1 (found at the end of the chapter) can be used as a guide in planning nursing care for the infant with a growth and development problem. The nurse may choose the appropriate nursing diagnoses from the plan and individualize them as needed. The nursing care plan is intended to serve as a guide, not as an all-inclusive growth and development care plan.

PROMOTING HEALTHY GROWTH AND DEVELOPMENT

Adding a new person to the family produces both excitement and anxiety. Newborns are completely reliant upon their parents or caregivers to fill every need. It is quite a burden and precious responsibility that new parents are taking on. Many parents read the latest books about caring for newborns, while others rely on information received from family and friends. Newborns and their mothers spend only a short time in the hospital after delivery, so it is very important that parents can care for their newborn and know when to call the primary care provider with concerns.

Periodic screening for adequate growth and development is recommended by the American Academy of Pediatrics (AAP) for all infants and children. The prevention of devastating disease is another priority for infants and children. The AAP and the Advisory Committee on Immunization Practices (ACIP) have made recommendations for immunization schedules. Immunizations are a very important part of the newborn's and infant's health visits. Nurses caring for newborns and infants should be familiar with the recommended infant/child periodic screenings (checkups) as well as the current immunization schedule (see Chapter 31 for further information on immunizations).

Promoting Growth and Development Through Play

Experts in child development and behavior have said repeatedly that play is the work of children. Infants practice their gross and fine motor skills and language through play (Goldson & Reynolds, 2014). Play is a natural way for infants and children to learn. Play is critical to infant development, as it gives infants the opportunity to explore their environment, practice new skills, and solve problems. The newborn prefers interacting with the parent to toys. Parents can talk to and sing to their newborns while participating in the daily activities that infants need, such as feeding, bathing, and changing diapers. Newborns and young infants love to watch people's faces and often appear to mimic the expressions they see.

As infants become older, toys may be geared toward the motor skills or language skills that the child is developing. Parents can promote fine motor development in infants by providing age-appropriate toys. For example, a rattle that a young infant can hold promotes reaching and attaining. The older infant builds fine motor skills by stacking cups or placing smaller toys inside of larger ones. Gross motor skills are reinforced and practiced over and over again when the infant wants to reach something he or she is interested in.

When playing with toys, the infant usually engages in **solitary play**; he or she does not share with other infants or directly play with other infants (Feigelman, 2011; Goldson & Reynolds, 2014). A wide variety of toys are available for infants, but infants often enjoy the most basic ones, such as plastic containers of various shapes and sizes, soft balls, and wooden or plastic spoons.

Books are also very important toys for infants. Reading to all ages of infants is appropriate, and the older infant develops fine motor skills by learning to turn book pages. Table 25.5 lists age-appropriate toys.

TABLE 25.5 APPROPRIATE TOYS FOR NEWBORNS AND INFANTS

Age	Appropriate Toys
Newborn to 1 month	• Mobile with contrasting colors or patterns • Unbreakable mirror • Soft music via tape or music box • Soft, brightly colored toys
1–4 months	• Bright mobile • Unbreakable mirror • Rattles • Singing by parent or caregiver, varied music • High-contrast patterns in books or images
4–7 months	• Fabric or board books • Different types of music • Easy-to-hold toys that do things or make noise (fancy rattles) • Floating, squirting bath toys • Soft dolls or animals
8–12 months	• Plastic cups, bowls, buckets • Unbreakable mirror • Large building blocks • Stacking toys • Busy boxes (with buttons or knobs that make things happen) • Balls • Dolls • Board books with large pictures • Toy telephone • Push–pull toys (older infants)

Promoting Early Learning

Research has shown that reading aloud and sharing books during early infancy are critical to the development of neural networks that are important in the later tasks of reading and word recognition. Reading books increases listening comprehension. Infants demonstrate their excitement about picture books by kicking and waving their arms and babbling when looking at them. At 6 to 12 months, the infant reaches for books and brings them to the mouth. Over time, reading leads to acquisition of language skills. Reading picture books and simple stories to infants starts a good habit that should be continued throughout childhood (Diener, Hobson-Rohrer, & Byington, 2012).

Promoting Safety

Hundreds of children younger than 1 year of age die each year as a result of injury (AAP, 2012b). As infants become more mobile, they risk injury from falls down stairs and off chairs, tables, and other structures. Curiosity leads the infant to explore potentially dangerous items, such as electrical outlets, hot stove or furnace vents, mop buckets, and toilets. Since infants explore so much with their mouths, small objects or hard foods pose a choking hazard. The infant will invariably pick up any accessible object and bring it to the mouth. With increasing dexterity, poisoning from medications, household cleaning products, or other substances also becomes a problem.

Safety in the Car

Motor vehicle accidents are one source of injury, particularly if the infant is improperly restrained. Infants should never be transported in a motor vehicle without proper restraint. Infant car seats should face the rear of the car until the infant is 12 months of age and weighs 9 kg (20 lb) (AAP, 2016). The car seat should be secured tightly in the center of the back seat. The infant should never be placed in a front seat that is equipped with an airbag.

Infants should never be left unattended in a motor vehicle. The temperature rises very quickly inside a closed vehicle, and an infant can suffocate from heat in a closed vehicle in the summer. Even during cooler weather, the heat generated within a closed vehicle can reach three to five times the exterior temperature. Kidnapping is also a concern if the baby is left unattended in a vehicle. Additional information on car safety can be found on thePoint.

Safety in the Home

The baby's crib should have a firm mattress that fits snugly in the crib on a secure support. The distance between crib slats should be no wider than a soda can (6 cm [2⅜ inches] or less) to prevent injury (Safe Kids Worldwide, 2016). All crib edges should be smooth. Only well-fitting crib sheets should be used, not sheets intended for large beds. Crib side rails should always be raised when the parent is not right next to the crib. Additional information about crib and playpen safety can be found on thePoint.

Even before the infant can roll over, he or she wiggles and pushes with the feet. The infant can easily fall from a changing table, sofa, or crib with the side rails down, so the infant should never be left unattended on any surface. If infant seats, bouncy seats, or swings are used, the infant should always be restrained in the seat with the appropriate straps.

The AAP (2012b) does not recommend the use of infant walkers, because the walker may tip over and the baby may fall out of it or the infant may fall down the stairs in it. Walkers allow infants access to things they may not otherwise be capable of reaching until they are able to walk alone, such as hot stoves and items on the edge of the countertop.

As the infant becomes more mobile, learning to crawl and walk, new safety issues arise. Safety gates should be used at the tops and bottoms of stairways. Gates may also be used to block curious infants from rooms that may pose physical danger to them because of sharp-edged furniture or decorative objects. Electrical outlets should be covered with approved safety covers. Cabinets and drawers should be secured with child safety latches. Medications, household cleaning supplies, and other potentially hazardous substances should be stored completely out of reach of infants (AAP, 2012b).

Choking is a risk because infants immediately bring small items to the mouth for exploration. To avoid choking, recommend the following to parents:

- Use only toys recommended for children 0 to 12 months of age.
- Avoid stuffed animals with eyes or buttons that can be dislodged by the persistent infant.
- Keep the floor free of small items (accidentally dropped coins, paper clips, straight pins).
- Avoid feeding popcorn, nuts, carrot slices, grapes, and hot dog pieces to infants.

Suffocation is also a risk for infants. Cribs should not have pillows, comforters, stuffed animals, or other soft items in them. Keep plastic bags of any size away from infants. Avoid the risk of strangulation by keeping window blind and drapery cords out of the infant's reach (AAP, 2012a, 2012b).

Though no safety measure is as effective as close supervision by a watchful parent or caregiver, the aforementioned safety measures can be critical to the infant's well-being.

Safety in the Water

Infants can drown in a very small amount of water. Never leave an infant unattended in the sink, a baby bathtub or standard bathtub, a swimming or wading pool, or any other body of water, even if it is quite shallow. The bathroom door should be kept closed and the toilet lid down. Water should be emptied from tubs, pails, or buckets immediately after use. If the family has a swimming pool, a locked fence or locked screen enclosure should surround it. Exterior doors should be kept locked to prevent the older infant from wandering out to the pool (AAP, 2012b). The AAP recommends that parents use caution when enrolling their infant in an aquatic or swim program. Research has not sufficiently demonstrated that water survival skills taught to infants are effective (AAP, Committee on Injury, Violence, and Poison Prevention, 2010). Completing an aquatic program does not decrease the risk of drowning; vigilant supervision is still always required.

Remember Allison Johnson, the infant described in the beginning of the chapter? What anticipatory guidance related to safety would you provide to Allison's parents?

Promoting Nutrition

Adequate nutrition is essential for growth and development. Breastfeeding and bottle-feeding of infant formula are both acceptable means of nutrition in the newborn and infant. Breast milk or formula supplies all of the infant's daily nutritional requirements until 6 months of age, at which time solid foods may be introduced (AAP, 2012; Stettler, Bhatia, Parish, & Stallings, 2011).

Cultural Factors

Many dietary practices are affected by culture, both in the types of food eaten and in the approach to progression of infant feeding. Some ethnic groups tend to be lactose intolerant (particularly blacks, Native Americans, and Asians); therefore, alternative sources of calcium must be offered. Explore the cultural practices of the family related to infant feeding so that you can support the family's cultural values.

Nutritional Needs

Newborns and infants are experiencing tremendous growth and need diets that support these rapid changes. Table 25.6 compares fluid and caloric needs in the newborn and infant.

TABLE 25.6 NUTRITIONAL REQUIREMENTS

Nutritional Requirements	Newborn	Infant
Fluid	140–160 mL/kg/day	100 mL/kg/day for first 10 kg 50 mL/kg/day for next 10 kg
Calories	105–108 kcal/kg/day	1 to 6 months: 108 kcal/kg 6 to 12 months: 98 kcal/kg

Adapted from Engorn, B., & Flerlage, J. (eds.). (2015). *The Harriett Lane handbook* (20th ed.). Philadelphia, PA: Saunders.

Breastfeeding

The National Association of Pediatric Nurse Practitioners (NAPNAP), the AAP, the American College of Obstetrics and Gynecology, the American Dietetic Association, and the U.S. Breastfeeding Committee of the Department of Health and Human Services all recommend breastfeeding as the natural and preferred method of newborn and infant feeding (NAPNAP, 2013). In their position statement on breastfeeding, NAPNAP (2013), identifies "human milk as superior to all substitute feeding methods." Breast milk provides complete infant nutrition.

Breastfeeding or feeding of expressed human milk is recommended for all infants, including sick or premature newborns (with rare exceptions). The exceptions include infants with galactosemia, maternal use of illicit drugs and a few prescription medications, maternal untreated active tuberculosis, and maternal HIV infection in developed countries.

Data from the Centers for Disease Control and Prevention's (CDC's) *Breastfeeding Report Card—United States, 2014* indicate that 79% of US infants were ever breastfed, 49% of infants were breastfeeding at 6 months of age, and only 27% were still breastfeeding at 1 year of age (CDC, 2014). Even partial breastfeeding is helpful and offers some of the health benefits of breastfeeding. Pediatric nurses in the community and the hospital are in an excellent position to promote and support breastfeeding, thereby contributing to the *Healthy People 2020* goal of increasing the proportion of mothers who breastfeed their babies.

BREAST MILK COMPOSITION

Breast milk includes lactose, lipids, polyunsaturated fatty acids, and amino acids. The ratio of whey to casein protein in breast milk makes it readily digestible. The high concentration of fats and the balance of amino acids are

HEALTHY PEOPLE 2020

Objective	Nursing Significance
Increase the proportion of infants who are breastfed. 2020 target: Ever 81.9% At 6 months 60.5% At 1 year 34.1%	• Encourage breastfeeding in all mothers beginning with the prenatal visit if applicable. • Provide accurate education related to breastfeeding. • Be available for questions or problems related to initiation and continuation of breastfeeding. Consult lactation consultant as needed or available. • Encourage pumping of breast milk when mother returns to work in order to continue breastfeeding. • Refer to local breastfeeding support groups such as La Leche League.

Healthy People Objectives retrieved from http://www.healthypeople.gov

believed to contribute to proper myelination of the nervous system. The concentration of iron in breast milk is less than that of formula, but the iron has increased bioavailability and is sufficient to meet the infant's requirements for the first 4 to 6 months of life.

In addition to complete nutrition, immunologic protection is transferred from mother to infant via breast milk and maternal–infant bonding is promoted. The benefits of breastfeeding are listed in Box 25.1.

BREAST MILK SUPPLY AND DEMAND

Frequent, on-demand breastfeeding of the newborn is necessary to establish an adequate milk supply. After delivery of the placenta, levels of progesterone drop dramatically, which stimulates the anterior pituitary to produce prolactin. Prolactin stimulates the production of milk in the acinar or alveolar cells of the breast. When the infant sucks at the breast, nervous impulses stimulate further production of breast milk.

The first "milk" to be produced by the breasts is termed **colostrum**. It is produced for the first 2 to 4 days after birth. Colostrum is a thin, watery, yellowish fluid that is easy to digest, as it is high in protein and low in sugar and fat. Colostrum is complete nutrition and all that is needed by the newborn for the first 2 to 4 days of life (La Leche League International [LLLI], 2013). Transitional breast milk replaces colostrum on days 2 to 4 after birth. By day 10 after birth, mature breast milk is produced. Mature breast milk has a slightly bluish color and appears thin.

The breastfeeding mother produces milk continually. Called **foremilk**, it collects in the lactiferous sinuses, which are small tubules serving as reservoirs for milk located behind the nipples. The **let-down reflex** is responsible for the release of milk from these reservoirs. When the baby sucks at the breast, oxytocin is released from the posterior pituitary, causing the lactiferous sinuses to contract. This allows milk to "let down" into the nipples, and the infant then sucks the milk. The let-down reflex is triggered not only by suckling at the breast but also by thinking of the baby or by the sound of a baby crying. After the foremilk is let down, new, fattier milk is formed. This **hindmilk** helps the breastfed infant to grow quickly (LLLI, 2013). Mothers should be informed that the production of oxytocin during suckling may also cause uterine contractions and may cause afterpains during breastfeeding.

BOX 25.1

BENEFITS OF BREASTFEEDING

Infant

- Increased bonding with mother
- Immunologic protection
- Breast milk has anti-infective properties
- Decreased incidence and severity of diarrhea
- Decreased incidence of asthma, otitis media, bacterial meningitis, botulism, urinary tract infection
- Possible enhancement of cognitive development
- Decreased incidence of obesity in later childhood

Maternal

- Increased bonding with infant
- Lessens maternal blood loss in the postpartum period
- Decreased risk of ovarian and premenopausal breast cancer
- Reduced incidence of pregnancy-induced, long-term obesity
- Possible delay of return of ovulation in some women
- Always ready; no mixing!
- Economic advantage

Adapted from Lawrence, R. (2011). *Breastfeeding: A guide for the medical professional* (7th ed.). Maryland Heights, MO: Mosby.

BREASTFEEDING TECHNIQUE

Breastfeeding mothers may not have established adequate breastfeeding prior to leaving the hospital after birth of the newborn. The pediatric nurse may encounter an infant–mother dyad experiencing difficulty with breastfeeding for a variety of reasons. Thus, the pediatric nurse must be competent in counseling the breastfeeding mother.

Before each breastfeeding session, mothers should wash their hands. It is not necessary to wash the breast in most cases. The mother should be positioned comfortably. A number of positions are possible, and they should be varied throughout the day (Fig. 25.9). The mother may hold the breast in a "C" position if that is helpful to her (Fig. 25.9C). Stroke the nipple against the baby's cheek (Fig. 25.10). This should stimulate the infant to open the mouth widely. Bring the baby's wide-open mouth to the breast to form a seal around all of the nipple and areola. When the infant is finished feeding, the mother can break the suction by inserting her finger into the baby's mouth, thus releasing the mouth from the nipple (Fig. 25.11). This technique may prevent the infant from pulling on the nipple, which can lead to soreness and cracking.

Watching and listening to the infant feed may assess the adequacy of the baby's latch technique. The infant who is properly latched on to the breast will suck rhythmically, taking most or all of the areola into the mouth. Audible swallowing should be heard as milk is delivered into the infant's mouth. Assess the mother for pain related to breastfeeding. She should not be in pain if the baby is latched on properly.

Establishment of breastfeeding is best achieved if the infant is allowed to feed on demand, whenever he or she is hungry. This may be as often as every 1½ to 3 hours in the neonate. Infants may feed for 10 to 20 minutes on each breast at each feeding, or longer on just one breast, alternating the breast at each feeding. Both methods are acceptable.

The breastfeeding infant does not need supplementation with water or formula even in the first few days of life as long as the newborn continues to wet six to eight

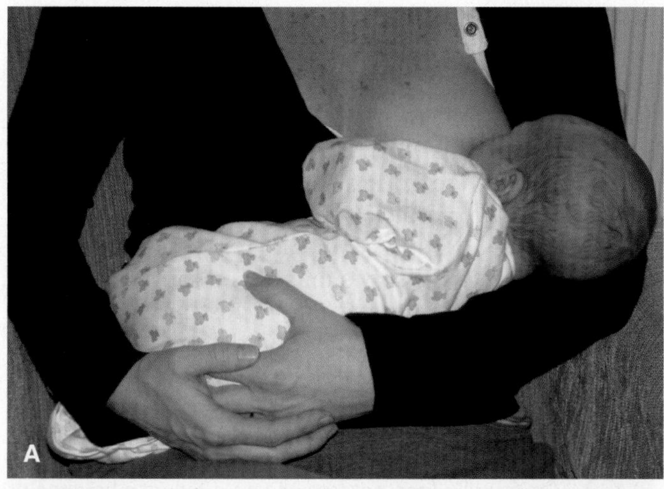

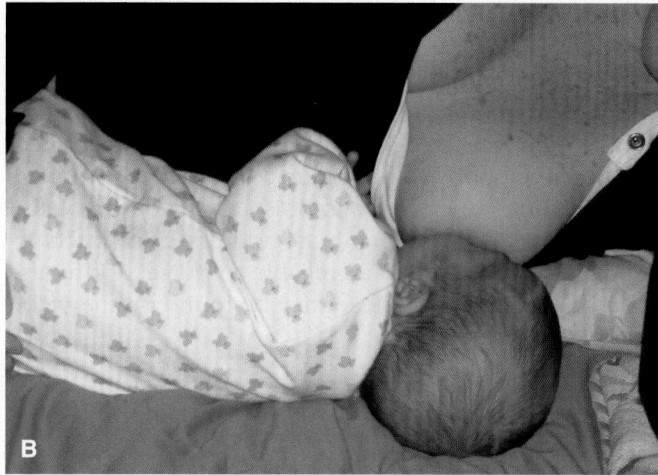

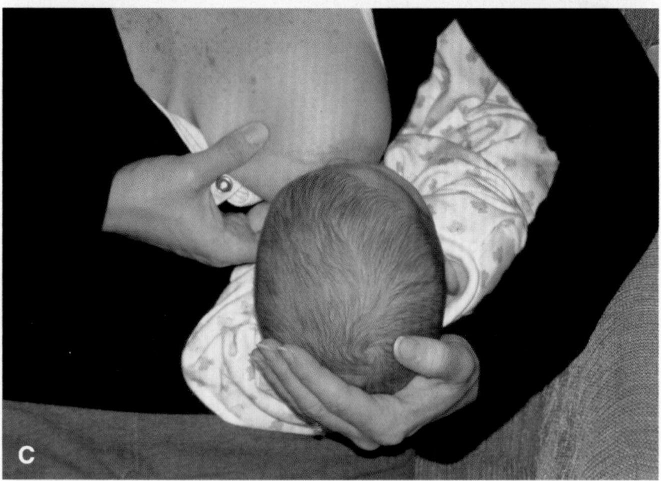

FIGURE 25.9 Various positions may be used during breastfeeding: **(A)** cradle hold, **(B)** side-lying, **(C)** football hold (note the "C" position for holding the breast during latching on).

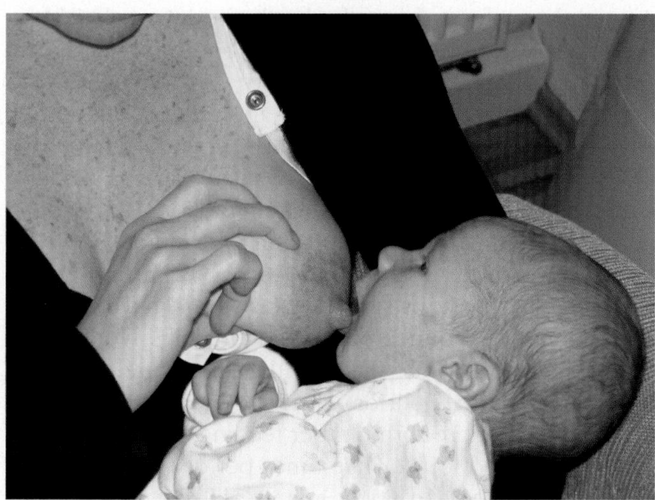

FIGURE 25.10 Stroking the infant's cheek with the nipple will elicit the rooting reflex.

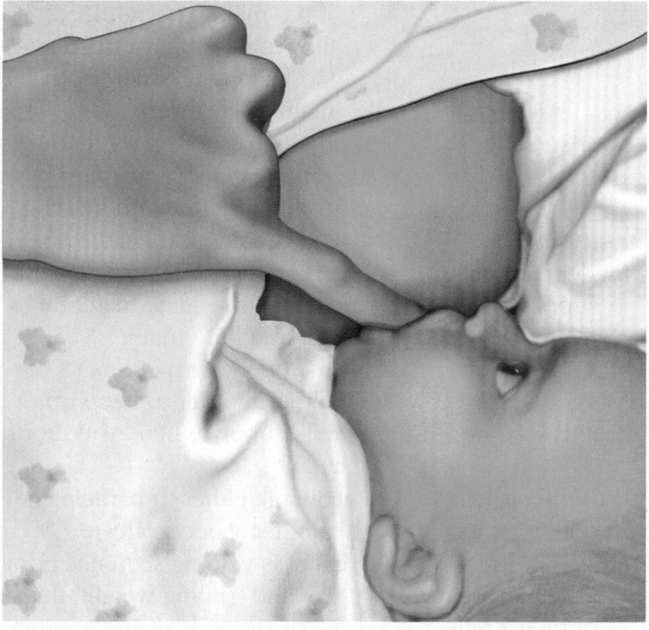

FIGURE 25.11 Inserting the little finger between the areola and the infant's mouth helps to break the suction.

diapers per day. After several days of age, the mother's milk supply should be well established. Adequate urine output and bowel movements, as well as continued weight gain in the infant, indicate the adequacy of breastfeeding. Working mothers in particular may need additional support from the nurse in order to continue breastfeeding if they desire to do so. Common problems occurring with breastfeeding are addressed in Teaching Guidelines 25.1. Additional reliable resources for mothers who desire to breastfeed may be found on the websites listed on the Point.

Teaching Guideline 25.1
PROMOTING BREASTFEEDING

Problem	*Solutions*
Sore nipples	Prevention: encourage appropriate latch-on from the beginning Expose nipples to air between feedings Allow breast milk to dry on nipples Use aloe vera or vitamin E to help heal sore nipples May use medical-grade lanolin or preservative-free lanolin (Lansinoh)
Engorgement	Apply warm compresses or encourage the mother to take a warm shower prior to having the baby latch on (warmth encourages some of the milk to be released, allowing the breast to soften and making it easier for the infant to latch on)
Poor sucking	Feed on cue, not on a schedule Encourage the sleepy infant by stroking the feet, undressing, and rubbing the head
Inadequate milk supply	Decrease maternal stress Encourage adequate maternal diet and fluid intake Instruct working mothers to pump in order to keep up milk supply when away from infant
Father feels left out	Encourage father to participate in other aspects of care
Mother worries about adequacy of breast milk	If infant is voiding six times per day and gaining weight, then he or she is receiving enough milk and appropriate nutrition

BOTTLE-FEEDING

For the mother who does not desire to, or cannot, breastfeed, commercially prepared formulas are available for bottle-feeding. These formulas are designed to imitate human milk. Standard infant formulas based on cow's milk provide 20 kcal/ounce and use lactose as a source for carbohydrates (Stettler et al., 2011). Vegetable oil is used as the source of fat; whey or casein provides protein. Newer cow's milk-based formulas contain long-chain polyunsaturated fatty acids that are thought to improve brain development. Ordinary cow's milk is not recommended for the first year of life.

Take Note!

Cow's milk does not provide an adequate balance of nutrients for the growing infant, especially iron. It may also overload the infant's renal system with inappropriate amounts of protein, sodium, and minerals.

Only formulas that are fortified with iron should be used. Iron stores that the infant received prenatally are depleted by 4 to 6 months of age. To prevent iron deficiency anemia, poor growth patterns, and impaired development, iron-fortified formulas must be used. The AAP recommends that commercial formulas provide 10 to 12 mg of iron per liter (Baker, & Greer; Committee on Nutrition, 2010). Commercial formulas also provide an adequate blend of essential vitamins and minerals.

FEEDING PATTERNS

Infant feeding is an opportune time to establish good eating behaviors. The infant should always be held while being bottle-fed. Cradling in a semi-upright position allows for additional bonding time, as the infant can see the caregiver's face while feeding (Fig. 25.12). Talking or singing during feeding time also increases bonding. As with breastfed infants, the bottle-fed infant should be fed on cue. Overfeeding with the bottle increases the incidence of spitting up and obesity, so families need to learn their baby's cues to hunger and satiety (Hill, 2015).

It is important to feed the baby when he or she displays signs of hunger. Crying is a late sign of hunger; earlier signs include making sucking motions, sucking on hands, or putting the fist to the chin. The infant should be burped two or three times per feeding, when he or she slows feeding or stops sucking. Newborns may only take a half-ounce to 1 ounce per feeding initially, working up to 2 to 3 ounces in the first few days. They need to feed about 6 to 10 times per day. The infant will gradually be able to ingest more formula per feeding. By 6 months of age, babies feed four or five times per day and take 6 to 8 ounces per feeding. Most infants will not require specific amounts per feeding; the infant should be fed until full. To prevent overfeeding, healthy bottle-fed infants

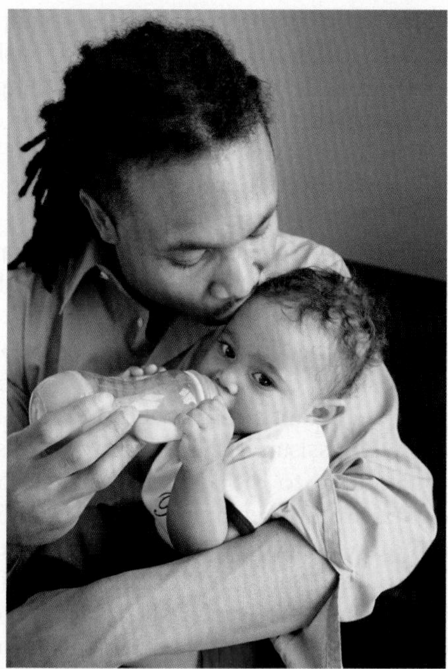

FIGURE 25.12 Technique for bottle-feeding the infant.

BOX 25.2

PREPARATION AND STORAGE OF BOTTLES AND FORMULA

- Wash nipples and bottles in hot soapy water and rinse well OR run nipples and bottles through the dishwasher.
- Store tightly covered ready-to-feed formula can after opening in refrigerator for up to 48 hours.
- After mixing concentrate or powdered formula, store tightly covered in refrigerator for up to 48 hours.
- Do not reheat and reuse partially used bottles. Throw away the unused portion after each feeding.
- Do not add cereal to the formula in the bottle.
- Do not sweeten formula with honey.
- Warm formula by placing bottle in a container of hot water.
- Do not microwave formula.

Adapted from Ben-Joseph, E. P. (2015). *Formula feeding FAQs: Preparation and storage*. Retrieved from kidshealth.org/parent/growth/feeding/formulafeed_storing.html#

should be allowed to self-regulate the amount of formula ingested per feeding. When the baby is satiated, he or she might fall asleep, spit out the nipple or formula, play with the nipple, or lie quietly, only sucking once in a while (Hill, 2015).

TYPES OF FORMULAS AND BOTTLES

Parents may choose to use commercial formulas that are ready to feed or available as a concentrate or as a powder. Parents should follow the instructions for mixing the concentrate or powder to avoid dehydration or fluid and electrolyte imbalances. Ready-to-feed formula should be used as is and never diluted (Stettler, et al., 2011).

A wide variety of baby bottle and nipple types are available for formula feeding, and the choice is purely individual. Few infants require special nipples or bottles. Box 25.2 gives guidelines on preparation and storage of formula and care of bottles.

SPECIAL FORMULAS

Special formulas may be needed for the infant who is allergic to a particular component of standard formula or has a renal, hepatic, metabolic, or intestinal disorder. For example, lactose-free cow's milk formulas are available for the lactose-intolerant child. Formulas using soy as the base ingredient instead of whey or casein are also available. Soy formulas are necessary for infants with a milk allergy, and they may be appealing to the vegetarian family.

These special formulas are designed to meet the nutritional needs of infants, depending on the disorder. Infants who fail to gain weight may be placed on standard infant formula prepared to deliver a higher caloric density per ounce. Preterm infants (those born at less than 36 weeks' gestation) need adequate nutrition to exhibit catch-up growth. Good catch-up growth (quadrupling or even quintupling the birth weight) in the first year or so of life is critical for adequate head growth and avoidance of neurodevelopmental consequences. Premature infant follow-up formulas are designed to provide additional calories, protein, and a particular calcium-to-phosphorus ratio as well as the vitamins and minerals needed for adequate catch-up growth.

Progressing to Solid Foods

After 6 months of age, infants usually require the nutrients available in solid foods in addition to their breast milk or formula. Progressing to feeding solid foods can be exciting and trying. Before solid foods are attempted, the infant should be assessed for readiness to progress. Parents need instruction in choosing appropriate solid foods and support in the progression process.

ASSESSING INFANT READINESS

Several factors contribute to the appropriate timing of solid food introduction. The tongue extrusion reflex is necessary for sucking to be an automatic reaction—that is, when a nipple or other item is placed in the mouth, the tongue extrudes and sucking begins. This reflex disappears at about 4 to 6 months of age (Dietz & Stern, 2012). Introducing solid food with a spoon prior to 4 to 6 months of age will result in extrusion of the tongue. The parent may think that the infant does not want the food and is spitting it out intentionally, but this is not the case;

the infant simply must be mature enough to eat with a spoon (absence of extrusion reflex).

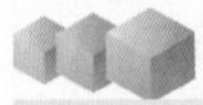

Concept Mastery Alert

Infant Feeding

Cow's milk should never be given to an infant because of its potential to cause an allergic reaction. Parents should avoid adding fruit juice to the infant's diet because the infant needs the protein and fat in breast milk or formula. Fruit juice would displace these important nutrients.

The ability to swallow solid food does not become completely functional until 4 to 6 months of age. Enzymes to appropriately digest food other than breast milk and formula are also not present in sufficient quantities until the age of 4 to 6 months.

Before the introduction of solid foods and the cup, the infant should be able to sit supported in a high chair. Solids should be fed with a spoon, with the infant in an upright position.

CHOOSING APPROPRIATE SOLID FOODS

Iron-fortified rice cereal mixed with a small amount of breast milk or formula is a good choice for the first solid food. The cereal is easily digested and its taste is generally well accepted. The cereal should be quite thin at first; it can be mixed to a thicker consistency as the infant gets older. Once the feeding of cereal with a spoon is successful, other single foods may be introduced. The foods should be puréed to a smooth consistency, whether prepackaged "baby food" or puréed at home.

The introduction of one new food every 3 to 5 days is recommended (Stettler, et al., 2011). This allows for identification of food allergies (Box 25.3). No salt, sugar, or other seasoning should be added to these first foods.

BOX 25.3

FOODS TO AVOID IN INFANCY

- Honey
- Egg yolks and meats (until 10 months of age)
- Excessive amounts of fruit juice
- Foods likely to cause choking
  - Peanuts
  - Popcorn
  - Other small hard foods (e.g., raw carrot chunks)
  - Grapes and hot dog slices (must be cut in smaller pieces)
- Foods likely to result in allergic reaction
  - Citrus
  - Strawberries
  - Wheat
  - Cow's milk
  - Egg whites
  - Peanut butter

Adapted from Brown, J. E. (2014). *Nutrition now* (7th ed.). Belmont, CA: Wadsworth, Cengage Learning.

Generally, by 8 months of age the infant is ready for more texture in his or her foods. Soft, smashed table food without large chunks is appropriate. Finger foods such as Cheerios, soft green bean pieces, or soft peas may also be offered. Avoid hard foods that the infant may choke on. Strained, puréed, or mashed meats may be introduced at 10 to 12 months of age.

The cup should be introduced at 6 to 8 months of age. One ounce of breast milk or formula should be placed in the cup while the infant is learning. This will decrease the amount of mess should the cup be spilled. Old-fashioned sippy cups are generally acceptable for use, though older infants quickly learn to drink from an ordinary cup with assistance when they are thirsty. Older infants are also able to drink from a straw. Newer no-spill sippy cups are not recommended for general home use. They require sucking much like a bottle and do not really encourage the child to learn cup drinking. In addition, the no-spill sippy cup allows for juice or milk to be in constant contact with the baby's teeth increasing the risk of dental caries (American Academy of Pediatric Dentistry [AAPD], 2014a). Fruit juice is unnecessary and should not be introduced until 6 months of age. If juice is given, it should be limited to 2 to 4 ounces per day. Fruit itself is much more nutritious than fruit juice. If infants are allowed to consume larger quantities of juice, it can displace important nutrients from breast milk or formula (Stettler, et al., 2011).

PROMOTING HEALTHY EATING HABITS

Infants and children learn about food within a social context, so the family plays an important role in creating healthy eating habits. Families "model" eating behaviors; infants and children learn about eating through watching others. Lifelong eating patterns are often established in childhood, so it is important to emphasize healthy eating practices beginning in infancy. Parents should not let infants eat whatever they want (permissive feeding style); this will lead to fights over eating in the future. Infants may require as many as 20 exposures to a new food before it is accepted. On the other hand, infants should not be coerced into eating all that is provided (authoritarian feeding style). Forcing an infant to eat when he or she is full sets the child up for overeating in the future and may lead to more power struggles (Dietz & Stern, 2012). Parents need to find a balance between the permissive and authoritarian feeding styles to establish lifelong healthy eating patterns in their children. By providing education about appropriate diet and feeding behaviors, the nurse can help the family accomplish this goal.

Think back to Allison Johnson. What questions should you ask Allison's parents related to her nutritional intake? What anticipatory guidance related to nutrition would be appropriate?

Promoting Healthy Sleep and Rest

Newborns sleep about 20 hours a day, waking frequently to feed and quickly returning to sleep. By 3 months of age, most infants sleep 7 to 8 hours per night without waking. They will continue to take about three naps a day. By 4 months of age the infant is more active and alert and may have more trouble going to sleep in the evening. Night waking may occur, but the infant should be capable of sleeping through the night and does not require a night feeding. By 12 months of age infants sleep 8 to 12 hours per night and take two naps per day (Feigelman, 2011).

Discuss safe sleeping practices with parents of newborns and infants; the baby should sleep on a firm mattress without pillows or comforters. The baby's bed should be placed away from air conditioner vents, open windows, and open heaters. Sudden infant death syndrome (SIDS) has been associated with prone side-lying positioning of newborns and infants, so the infant should be placed to sleep on the back (Moon & Fu, 2012). See Healthy People 2020.

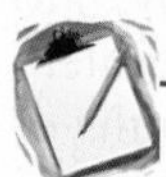

Take Note!

The AAP has determined that side sleeping is not as safe as supine sleeping.

In the newborn period, the primary caregiver should try to sleep when the baby is sleeping. Since newborns need to be fed every 1½ to 3 hours around the clock, parents may become exhausted quickly and are often eager for the infant to sleep through the night. Adding rice cereal to the evening bottle has not been proven to discourage night waking and is not recommended (Nevarez, Rifas-Shiman, Kleinman, Gillman, & Taveras, 2010). Provide support to parents of newborns and educate them on infant sleeping patterns.

It is important to establish a bedtime routine around 4 months of age due to the infant's increased alertness and activity level. The baby who is 4 months or older needs a time of calming and relaxation before going to sleep. A consistent bedtime routine should be established, perhaps a bath followed by rocking, singing, or reading. The infant should fall asleep in his or her own crib rather than being rocked to sleep or held until sleeping and then put in the crib. After 4 months of age, infants must learn to soothe themselves back to sleep following night waking. Older infants may exhibit head banging as a form of self-soothing and use it to fall asleep at night. Night feedings are unnecessary at this age and will create a routine of further night waking that will be difficult to break (Feigelman, 2011). Parents should minimize attention and stimulation provided during a night waking. Briefly checking on the infant to ascertain his or her safety, followed by placing the infant back in a lying position and telling him or her good night, is all that is needed. This may have to be repeated several times before the infant falls back to sleep. It is important to keep interactions brief during the night waking so that the infant learns to fall back to sleep on his or her own. Continued issues with night waking should be discussed with the infant's primary care provider.

What anticipatory guidance should you provide to Allison's parents in relation to sleep?

HEALTHY PEOPLE 2020

Objective	Nursing Significance
Increase the percentage of infants who are put down to sleep on their backs.	• Begin teaching about "back to sleep" at prenatal or newborn visit. • Use each encounter with the young infant as an opportunity to reinforce the supine position for sleep.

Healthy People Objectives retrieved from http://www.healthypeople.gov

Promoting Healthy Teeth and Gums

Healthy teeth and gums require proper oral hygiene and appropriate fluoride supplementation. Children older than 6 months of age who are at risk for developing dental caries and whose drinking water source contains less than 0.3 parts per million may require fluoride supplementation (AAPD, 2014b). Excess fluoride ingestion can result in discoloration of the teeth (fluorosis). Early childhood dental caries can result from pooling of milk or juice around teeth and gums.

Before tooth eruption, parents should clean the child's gums after feeding with a damp washcloth. After teeth have erupted, parents can continue to use a soft cloth for tooth cleaning and then eventually use a small soft-bristled toothbrush. Toothpaste is unnecessary in infancy. Infants should not be allowed to take milk or juice bottles to bed, as the high sugar content of the fluid in contact with the teeth all night leads to dental caries. Weaning from the bottle at age 12 to 15 months may help prevent dental caries. No-spill sippy cups have also been implicated in the development of dental caries and should be avoided. The AAPD recommends that infants receive their first dental visit by the age of 1 year (AAPD, 2014a).

Promoting Appropriate Discipline

Parenting requires ever-changing adaptations to the developing infant's needs. Unconditional love, patience, and compassion must be balanced with the parents' needs. **Discipline** refers to the molding of a child's behavior through instruction, practice, and consistency. Discipline helps build self-esteem in children as well as sets standards for social interactions. The primary goal of discipline is to teach an infant limits. Discipline should be used to help the infant solve problems. The infant's activities are based on the basic needs of food, security, warmth, love, and comfort. Misbehavior is the result of an unmet need, and the parents should respond accordingly.

As the infant is undergoing rapid changes in motor skills, safety needs increase. Nurses should encourage the parents to "childproof" their home so that the infant can develop physical skills without being at risk. In a childproof home, fewer restrictions need to be placed on the infant's behavior, and he or she can explore.

Physical punishment or spanking should never be used in infancy. Infants are at increased risk for physical injury from spanking and cannot make the connection between the spanking and the undesirable behavior. Providing a safe environment, redirection away from undesirable behaviors, and saying "no" in appropriate instances are far more effective. For example, when the infant is in potential danger (e.g., inserting a key into an electrical outlet, attempting to ingest a poisonous substance, or reaching into the toilet), the parent must use a firm but calm and brisk approach. If the infant knows the parent is serious, he or she will usually comply more quickly (AAP, 2015b).

Remaining calm, firm, and consistent is necessary. Immediacy is also an important component of appropriate discipline. The infant cannot make the connection between a subsequent punishment and discussion of behavior with the earlier event itself. Positive reinforcement should be used to support good behavior (NAPNAP, n.d.).

Addressing Child Care Needs

Many mothers work outside the home, there are many single-parent families, and many families live a distance away from relatives. In all of these circumstances, infants may need to be cared for outside the home, often in child care settings or home day care centers.

Parents contemplating child care must consider a number of factors. Do they want a sitter to come to their home? Will they use a traditional day care center or a home care situation with fewer children? How much can they afford? If families choose to use a freestanding day care center or a home-based day care center, they should make sure that the provider is appropriately licensed. Parents should feel comfortable with the caregiver-to-child ratio. Are the caregivers trained in infant cardiopulmonary resuscitation (CPR) and first aid? Families may need to visit or interview several facilities before finding one that meets their requirements.

When an older infant is attending a child care situation for the first time, it may be helpful to visit the center once or twice beforehand so that the infant can get used to the caregivers from the comfort and security of the parent's lap. Warn parents that separation anxiety in late infancy can cause a disturbing crying episode when the parent leaves. Reassure parents that the infant will not suffer harm due to the separation.

ADDRESSING COMMON DEVELOPMENTAL CONCERNS

Parents commonly have multiple concerns during normal infant growth and development. Although most of these issues are not actual disease states or behavior problems, nurses must be aware of these issues to recognize them and to intervene appropriately.

Colic

Colic is defined as inconsolable crying that lasts 3 hours or longer per day and for which there is no physical cause. It may begin as early as 2 weeks of age, and healthy infants cry for a total of about 3 hours daily, 3 to 7 days per week. Crying and fussing are more prevalent in the evenings. Typically, colic resolves by 3 months of age, coinciding with the age at which infants are better able to soothe themselves (e.g., by finger sucking). The cause of colic is thought to be problems in the gastrointestinal or neurologic system (probably system immaturity), temperament, or parenting style of the mother or father. Some parents are overly anxious or overly attentive or, at the other extreme, may not give the infant the attention he or she needs. Any of these may contribute to a baby's fussing and crying.

Prolonged crying leads to increased stress among caregivers. Failure to stop the crying leads to frustration, and crying that prevents the parents from sleeping contributes to the exhaustion they are already experiencing.

Educate parents that normal crying increases by the time the infant is 6 weeks old and diminishes by about 12 weeks. When faced with a colicky baby, parents should develop a stepwise approach to checking that all of the infant's basic needs are met. When these needs are met, attempts at soothing the infant may be used. Reducing stimulation may decrease the length of crying. Carrying the infant more may also be helpful. Some infants respond to the motion of an infant swing or a car ride. Vibration, white noise, or swaddling may also help to decrease fussing in some infants. Pacifiers can be soothing to babies who need additional nonnutritive sucking. Parents should try one intervention at a time, taking care not to stimulate the infant excessively in the process of searching for solutions. Nurses should provide ongoing support to the parents of a colicky infant and reassure them that this is a temporary condition that will resolve in time (Ehrlich, 2014).

Spitting Up

Spitting up (regurgitating small amounts of stomach contents) occurs in all infants, and a significant number of normal infants spit up excessively. Although spitting up after feeding is normal, it can be a cause of great concern to parents. Overfed babies who feed based on a parent-designed schedule and those who burp poorly are more likely to spit up. For some infants, the amount and frequency of spitting up are significant, and those babies should be evaluated by the physician or nurse practitioner (AAP, 2015a).

Teach parents that feeding smaller amounts on a more frequent basis may help to decrease spitting-up episodes. Always burp the baby at least two or three times per feeding. Keep the baby upright for 30 minutes after feeding and do not lay the infant prone after feeding. Avoid bouncing or excess activity immediately after feeding. Positioning in an infant seat compresses the stomach and is not recommended. When placing the baby in bed, position him or her on the back with the head of the bed slightly elevated (AAP, 2015a).

Reassure parents that if the infant is wetting at least six diapers per 24 hours and gaining weight, the spitting up is normal. If the infant vomits one third or more of most feedings, chokes when vomiting, or experiences forceful emesis, the primary care provider should be notified.

Thumb Sucking, Pacifiers, and Security Items

Infants demonstrate a clear need for nonnutritive sucking; even fetuses can be observed sucking their thumbs or fingers in utero. Thumb sucking is a healthy self-comforting activity. Infants who suck their thumbs or pacifiers often are better able to soothe themselves than those who do not. Studies have not shown that sucking either thumbs or pacifiers leads to the need for orthodontic braces unless the sucking continues well beyond the early school-age period. However, pacifier use has been associated with the increased incidence of otitis media, and hygiene is always a concern as pacifiers often fall on the floor (Nelson, 2012).

Infants may also become attached to a doll, stuffed animal, or blanket. Just like thumb sucking, the attachment item gives the infant the security to self-soothe when he or she is uncomfortable.

Families need to explore their feelings and cultural preferences about sucking habits and security items. Parents should not try to break the habit during a stressful time for the infant. When the infant is intensely trying to master a new skill such as sitting or walking, he or she may need the sucking or security item to self-soothe. Pacifiers and security items can be physically taken away at some point, but the thumb is attached. The infant who has become attached to thumb sucking should not have additional attention drawn to the issue, as that may prolong thumb sucking.

Families of infants who use pacifiers may want to wean the infant from the pacifier when the child approaches 1 year of age, as this is the time when the need for additional sucking naturally decreases. Otherwise, weaning from the pacifier should occur by 2 to 3 years of age in order to limit adverse effects upon dentition (Nelson, 2012). Attempts to wean the child from a security blanket or toy should probably be reserved for after infancy (see Evidence-Based Practice 25.1).

Teething

Discomfort is common as the tooth breaks through the periodontal membrane. Infants may drool, bite on hard objects, or increase finger sucking. Some infants may become very irritable, refuse to eat, and not sleep well.

EVIDENCE-BASED PRACTICE 25.1 EVIDENCE AND RECOMMENDATIONS RELATED TO PACIFIER USE

STUDY

The author performed a comprehensive review of research studies related to pacifier usage in order to provide nurses with the highest level of evidence to use when counseling parents about this topic. Studies reviewed included randomized controlled trials (RCTs), meta-analyses of RCTs, and critical literature reviews related to the risks and benefits of pacifier use. The author included only studies performed between 1990 and the present.

Findings

Upon analysis of the various research studies, the author reached several conclusions. Pacifier use has been shown to lower the risk of sudden infant death syndrome (SIDS) when used at the time of sleep. Additional benefits include the calming effect related to nonnutritive sucking and as an adjunct in pain relief. Potential disadvantages include negative effects on breastfeeding if pacifier is used early or extensively; increased incidence of otitis media; and the risks of injury, allergy, and dental malocclusion.

Nursing Implications

In light of the potential risks and benefits of pacifier use, nurses must be prepared to provide parents with accurate information related to the use of pacifiers. Educate parents to avoid introduction of the pacifier until breastfeeding is well established (4 weeks of age), to use pacifiers only during periods of sleep, and to never force a pacifier on an infant or replace a pacifier in a sleeping infant's mouth. In addition, parents should wean the child from the pacifier in late infancy so that it is not used by 2 to 3 years of age to avoid further dental issues.

Adapted from Nelson, A. M. (2012). A comprehensive review of evidence and current recommendations related to pacifier usage. *Journal of Pediatric Nursing, 27*, 690–699.

Fever, vomiting, and diarrhea are generally not considered a sign of teething but rather of illness.

Teething pain results from inflammation. Teach parents that application of cold may be soothing to the gums. The infant may chew on a cold teething ring, or parents can rub an ice cube wrapped in a washcloth on the gums. Over-the-counter topical anesthetics such as baby Orajel may also be helpful. Parents should apply the ointment correctly to the gums, avoiding the lips, as these ointments cause numbing. Occasionally, oral acetaminophen or ibuprofen may be given to relieve pain (Tinanoff, 2011).

Refer back to 6-month-old Allison Johnson. List some common developmental concerns of 6-month-old infants. What anticipatory guidance related to these concerns would you provide to her parents?

NURSING CARE PLAN 25.1

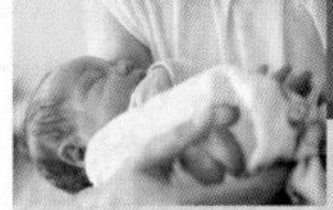

Growth and Development Issues in the Newborn and Infant

NURSING DIAGNOSIS: Breastfeeding, ineffective, related to lack of exposure, misconceptions, or knowledge deficit as evidenced by first baby, mother's verbalization, or nursing observations

Outcome Identification and Evaluation

Mother/infant dyad will experience successful breastfeeding: *infant will latch on, suck and swallow at the breast; mother will not experience sore nipples.*

Interventions: ***Promoting Effective Breastfeeding***

- Educate mother on recognition of and response to infant hunger cues *to promote on-cue breastfeeding, which will establish milk supply.*
- Educate mother on appropriate diet and fluid intake *to ensure ability to manufacture adequate supply of breast milk.*
- Demonstrate breastfeeding positions with infant at the breast *(appropriate positioning increases probability of successful latch).*
- Assess infant's latch technique, sucking motion, and audible swallowing *(an appropriately latched infant will take most of the areola in the mouth, suck in spurts, and demonstrate audible swallowing).*
- Assess infant voiding/stool patterns: *at least six voids per day and passage of stool ranging from one or more per day to one every several days is a normal pattern for breastfed infants.*
- Assess infant weight gain: *gain of 15 to 30 g per day after the second week of life indicates infant is receiving appropriate nutrition.*
- Assess mother's nipples for redness or soreness; *if infant appropriately latches on, nipples will not become sore.*

NURSING DIAGNOSIS: Risk for altered growth pattern (risk factors: caregiver knowledge deficit, first infant, premature infant, or maladaptive feeding behaviors)

Outcome Identification and Evaluation

Infant will demonstrate adequate growth and appropriate feeding behaviors: *steady increases in weight, length, and head circumference; infant feeds appropriately for age.*

Interventions: ***Promoting Adequate Growth***

- Observe mother/infant dyad breastfeeding or bottle-feeding to determine need for further education or identify infant difficulties with feeding.
- Educate mother about appropriate breastfeeding or bottle-feeding so that mother is aware of what to expect in normal feeding pattern.
- When infant is old enough, provide education about addition of solid foods, spoon and cup feeding: after 6 months of age breast milk or formula needs to be supplemented with a variety of foods.

NURSING CARE PLAN 25.1

Growth and Development Issues in the Newborn and Infant (continued)

- Determine need for additional caloric intake if necessary (premature infants and infants with chronic illnesses or metabolic disorders often need adjustments in caloric intake to demonstrate adequate or catch-up growth).
- Obtain daily weights if hospitalized (weekly if outpatient) and weekly length and head circumference to determine whether feeding pattern is sufficient to promote adequate growth.

NURSING DIAGNOSIS: Nutrition, altered, less than body requirements, related to possible ineffective feeding pattern or inadequate caloric intake as evidenced by failure to gain weight or by inadequate increases in weight, length, and head circumference over time

Outcome Identification and Evaluation

Infant will take in adequate nutrients using effective feeding pattern: *infant will demonstrate adequate weight gain (15 to 30 g per day) and steady increases in length and head circumference.*

Interventions: ***Promoting Adequate Nutritional Intake***

- Assess current feeding pattern and daily intake *to determine areas of concern.*
- Increase frequency of breastfeeding or volume of bottle-feeding, *if needed, to meet caloric needs.*
- Introduce solid foods on age-appropriate schedule: *introducing solids at the right time improves the chances that the child will learn to take solid foods.*
- Limit juice intake or discontinue altogether *(juice has little nutritive value and displaces nutrients from breast milk or formula).*
- Use human milk fortifier (if ordered) *to increase caloric density of breast milk.*
- Increase caloric density of formula (if ordered) by mixing to a more concentrated level or with additives (fats or carbohydrates) *to provide increased calories needed to support adequate growth.*
- If infant is taking solids already, choose higher-calorie foods *to maximize nutrient intake.*

NURSING DIAGNOSIS: Parent/infant attachment, altered, risk for (risk factors: premature infant, parental knowledge deficit about normal newborn activity and care, infant with difficult temperament or medical problems)

Outcome Identification and Evaluation

Parent and infant will demonstrate appropriate attachment via *eye contact, parental response to infant cues, parental verbalization of caring for infant, infant response to parent's caretaking behaviors.*

Interventions: ***Encouraging Appropriate Parent–Infant Attachment***

- Assess parent's response to infant cues to determine degree of attachment and level of parent's knowledge about infant care.
- Assess infant's response to parent's caretaking behaviors to determine degree of attachment.
- Determine infant's temperament to counsel parent effectively about responses appropriate for that type of temperament.
- Encourage en face positioning for holding or feeding the young infant to encourage give-and-take response between infant and parent.
- Encourage parent to meet infant's needs promptly and with affection to promote sense of trust in the infant.
- Reinforce parent's attempts at improving attachment with infant (positive reinforcement naturally encourages appropriate behaviors).

(continued)

NURSING CARE PLAN 25.1

Growth and Development Issues in the Newborn and Infant (continued)

NURSING DIAGNOSIS: Growth and development, altered, related to speech, motor, psychosocial, or cognitive concerns as evidenced by delay in meeting expected milestones

Outcome Identification and Evaluation

Development will be maximized: *infant will make continued progress toward attainment of developmental milestones.*

Interventions: ***Maximizing Development***

- Perform developmental evaluation of the infant to determine infant's current level of functioning.
- Offer age-appropriate play, activities, and toys to encourage further development.
- Carry out interventions as prescribed by developmental specialist, physical therapist, occupational therapist, or speech therapist (repeated exposure to the activities or exercises is needed to make developmental progress).
- Provide support to parents of infants with developmental concerns, as developmental progress can be slow and it is difficult for families to stay motivated and maintain hope.

NURSING DIAGNOSIS: Caregiver role strain, risk for (risk factors: first baby, knowledge deficit about infant care, lack of prior exposure, fatigue if premature, ill, or developmentally delayed infant)

Outcome Identification and Evaluation

Parent will experience competence in role: *will demonstrate appropriate caretaking behaviors and verbalize comfort in new role.*

Interventions: ***Preventing Caregiver Role Strain***

- Assess parent's knowledge of newborn/infant care and the issues that arise as a part of normal development *to determine parent's needs.*
- Provide education on normal newborn/infant care *so that parents have the knowledge they need to appropriately care for their new baby.*
- Provide anticipatory guidance related to normal infant development *to prepare parents for what to expect next and how to intervene.*
- Encourage respite for parents *(even a few hours away from the demands of an infant's care can rejuvenate the parents).*

NURSING DIAGNOSIS: Injury, risk for (risk factors: developmental age, infant curiosity, rapidly progressing motor abilities)

Outcome Identification and Evaluation

Infant safety will be maintained: *infant will remain free from injury.*

Interventions: ***Preventing Injury***

- Encourage car seat safety to decrease risk of injury related to motor vehicles.
- Childproof home: as infant becomes more mobile, he or she will want to explore everything, increasing risk of injury.
- Parents should have the Poison Control Center phone number available: should an accidental ingestion occur, Poison Control can give parents the best advice for appropriate intervention.
- Never leave an infant unattended in the sink, bathtub, or swimming pool to prevent drowning.
- Teach parents first aid measures and infant CPR to minimize consequences of injury should it occur.
- Parents should watch the infant at all times (no amount of childproofing can replace the watchful eye of a caring parent).

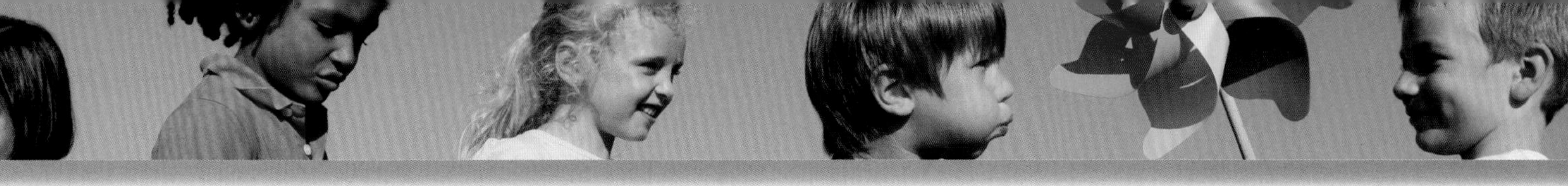

KEY CONCEPTS

- Infancy encompasses the period from birth to age 12 months.
- The infant exhibits tremendous growth, doubling the birthweight by 6 months of age and tripling it by 12 months of age.
- Most organ systems are immature at birth and develop and mature over the first year of life.
- Child development is orderly, sequential, and predictable, progressing in a cephalocaudal and proximodistal fashion.
- The infant is mastering the psychosocial task of Trust versus Mistrust.
- Cognitive development in infancy is sensorimotor; infants use their senses and progressing motor skills to master their environment.
- The 12-month-old babbles expressively and uses two or three words with meaning.
- Promotion of safety is of key importance throughout infancy.
- Breastfeeding is the natural and preferred method for infant feeding.
- Breastfed and bottle-fed infants should both be fed on cue rather than on a parent-designed schedule.
- Solid foods should be introduced at age 4 to 6 months. A spoon should be used to feed the infant, and rice cereal should be the first food. New foods should be introduced no more frequently than every 3 to 5 days.
- The cup may be introduced at 6 months of age. No-spill sippy cups are generally not recommended.
- Spitting up and colic are parts of normal development in the otherwise thriving infant and do not require medical intervention.

REFERENCES AND RECOMMENDED READINGS

American Academy of Pediatrics, Committee on Injury, Violence, and Poison Prevention. (2010). Prevention of drowning. *Pediatrics, 126*(1), 178–185.

American Academy of Pediatrics. (2012). Breastfeeding and the use of human milk. *Pediatrics, 129*(3), e827–e841. doi: 10.1542/peds.2011–3552

American Academy of Pediatrics, The Injury Prevention Program. (2012a). *Safety for your child: Birth to 6 months.* Retrieved from https://www.healthychildren.org/English/ages-stages/baby/Pages/Safety-for-Your-Child-Birth-to-6-Months.aspx

American Academy of Pediatrics, The Injury Prevention Program. (2012b). *Safety for your child: 6 to 12 months.* Retrieved from https://www.healthychildren.org/English/ages-stages/baby/Pages/Safety-for-Your-Child-6-to-12-Months.aspx

American Academy of Pediatric Dentistry. (2014a). *Guideline on infant oral health care.* Retrieved from http://www.aapd.org/media/Policies_Guidelines/G_InfantOralHealthCare.pdf

American Academy of Pediatric Dentistry. (2014b). *Guideline on fluoride therapy.* Retrieved from http://www.aapd.org/media/Policies_Guidelines/G_FluorideTherapy.pdf

American Academy of Pediatrics. (2015a). *Burping, hiccups, and spitting up.* Retrieved from http://www.healthychildren.org/English/ages-stages/baby/feeding-nutrition/pages/Burping-Hiccups-and-Spitting-Up.aspx

American Academy of Pediatrics. (2015b). *Disciplining your child.* Retrieved from http://www.healthychildren.org/English/family-life/family-dynamics/communication-discipline/Pages/Disciplining-Your-Child.aspx

American Academy of Pediatrics. (2016). *Car seats: Information for families.* Retrieved from http://www.healthychildren.org/English/safety-prevention/on-the-go/Pages/Car-Safety-Seats-Information-for-Families.aspx

Baker, R. D., & Greer, F. R.; Committee on Nutrition American Academy of Pediatrics. (2010). Diagnosis and prevention of iron deficiency and iron-deficiency anemia in infants and young children (0–3 years of age). *Pediatrics, 126,* 1040–1050.

Ben-Joseph, E. P. (2015). *Formula feeding FAQs: Preparation and storage.* Retrieved from kidshealth.org/parent/growth/feeding/formulafeed_storing.html#

Brazelton, T. B., & Nugent, J. K. (2011). *Neonatal behavioral assessment scale* (4th ed.). London, UK: Mac Keith Press.

Brown, J. E. (2014). *Nutrition now* (7th ed.). Belmont, CA: Wadsworth, Cengage Learning.

Carpenito-Moyet, L. J. (2013). *Nursing diagnosis: Application to clinical practice* (14th ed.). Philadelphia, PA: Lippincott Williams & Wilkins.

Centers for Disease Control and Prevention. (2014). *Breastfeeding report card United States/2014.* Retrieved from http://www.cdc.gov/breastfeeding/pdf/2014breastfeedingreportcard.pdf

Centers for Disease Control and Prevention. (2016). *Developmental milestones.* Retrieved from http://www.cdc.gov/ncbddd/actearly/milestones/index.html

Cherry, J., Demmler-Harrison, G. J., Kaplan, S. L., Steinbach, W. J., & Hotez, P. (2014). *Feigin and Cherry's textbook of pediatric infectious diseases* (7th ed.). Philadelphia, PA: Elsevier, Saunders.

Child Development Institute. (2015). *Temperament and your child's personality.* Retrieved from http://childdevelopmentinfo.com/child-development/temperament_and_your_child/

Diener, M. L., Hobson-Rohrer, W., & Byington, C. L. (2012). Kindergarten readiness and performance of Latino children participating in Reach Out and Read. *Journal of Community*

Medicine & Health Education, 2(3), 133. doi: 10.4172/jcmhe.1000133

Dietz, W. H., & Stern, L. (2012). *Nutrition: What every parent needs to know* (2nd ed.). Elk Grove Village, IL: American Academy of Pediatrics.

Douglas, M. K., Pierce, J. U., Rosenkoetter, M., Pacquiao, D., Callister, L. C., Hattar-Pollara, M., et al. (2011). Standards of practice for culturally competent nursing care: 2011 update. *Journal of Transcultural Nursing, 22*(4), 317–333.

Ehrlich, S. D. (2014). *Infantile colic.* Retrieved from http://umm.edu/health/medical/altmed/condition/infantile-colic

Engorn, B., & Flerlage, J. (eds.). (2015). *The Harriett Lane handbook* (20th ed.). Philadelphia, PA: Saunders.

Erikson, E. H. (1963). *Childhood and society* (2nd ed.). New York: W. W. Norton and Company.

Feigelman, S. (2011). The first year. In R. M. Kliegman, B. F. Stanton, J. W. St. Geme III, N. F. Schor, & R. E. Behrman (Eds.), (*Nelson's textbook of pediatrics* (19th ed.). Philadelphia, PA: Elsevier, Saunders.

Goldson, E., & Reynolds, A. (2014). Child development and behavior. In W. W. Hay, Jr., M. J. Levin, R. R. Deterding, & M. J. Abzug. (Eds.), *Current diagnosis and treatment: Pediatrics* (22nd ed.). New York, NY: McGraw-Hill Education.

Greenbaum, L. A. (2011). Electrolyte and acid-base disorders. In R. M. Kliegman, B. F. Stanton, J. W. St. Geme III, N. F. Schor, & R. E. Behrman (Eds.), (*Nelson's textbook of pediatrics* (19th ed.). Philadelphia, PA: Elsevier, Saunders.

Hill, D. L. (2015). *Bottle feeding basics.* Retrieved from https://www.healthychildren.org/English/ages-stages/baby/feeding-nutrition/Pages/Bottle-Feeding-How-Its-Done.aspx

La Leche League International. (2013). *The early weeks.* Retrieved from http://www.llli.org/nb/nbearlyweeks.html

Lawrence, R. (2011). *Breastfeeding: A guide for the medical professional* (7th ed.). Maryland Heights, MO: Mosby.

Lerner, N. B. (2011). Physiologic anemia of infancy. In R. M. Kliegman, B. F. Stanton, J. W. St. Geme III, N. F. Schor, & R. E. Behrman (Eds.), (*Nelson's textbook of pediatrics* (19th ed.). Philadelphia, PA: Elsevier, Saunders.

Liacouras, C. A. (2011). Normal development, structure, and function. In R. M. Kliegman, B. F. Stanton, J. W. St. Geme III, N. F. Schor, & R. E. Behrman (Eds.), (*Nelson's textbook of pediatrics* (19th ed.). Philadelphia, PA: Elsevier, Saunders.

Lowry, L. (2011). *Bilingualism in young children: Separating fact from fiction.* Retrieved from http://www.hanen.org/Helpful-Info/Articles/Bilingualism-in-Young-Children–Separating-Fact-fr.aspx

Maqbool, A., Stettler, N., & Stallings, V. A. (2011). Nutritional requirements. In R. M. Kliegman, B. F. Stanton, J. W. St. Geme III, N. F. Schor, & R. E. Behrman (Eds.), (*Nelson's textbook of pediatrics* (19th ed.). Philadelphia, PA: Elsevier, Saunders.

Moon, R. Y., & Fu, L. (2012). Sudden infant death syndrome: An update. *Pediatrics in Review, 33*(7), 314–320.

National Association for the Education of Young Children. (n.d.) *Good toys for young children by age and stage.* Retrieved from http://www.naeyc.org/toys

National Association of Pediatric Nurse Practitioners. (n.d.). *Infant and toddler discipline: Preventing bad behavior.* Retrieved from https://www.napnap.org/sites/default/files/userfiles/membership/No%20Hitting%20Infant%20Revised.pdf

National Association of Pediatric Nurse Practitioners. (2013). NAPNAP position statement on breastfeeding. *Journal of Pediatric Health Care, 27*(1):e13–e15.

Nelson, A. M. (2012). A comprehensive review of evidence and current recommendations related to pacifier usage. *Journal of Pediatric Nursing, 27*, 690–699.

Nevarez, M. D., Rifas-Shiman, S. L., Kleinman, K. P., Gillman, M. W., & Taveras, E. M. (2010). Associations of early life risk factors with infant sleep duration. *Academic Pediatrics, 10*(3), 187–193.

Olsson, J. (2011). The newborn. In R. M. Kliegman, B. F. Stanton, J. W. St. Geme III, N. F. Schor, & R. E. Behrman (Eds.), (*Nelson's textbook of pediatrics* (19th ed.). Philadelphia, PA: Elsevier, Saunders.

Perniciaro, J. (2011). Development, behavior, and mental health. In R. M. Kliegman, B. F. Stanton, J. W. St. Geme III, N. F. Schor, & R. E. Behrman (Eds.) (*Nelson's textbook of pediatrics* (19th ed.). Philadelphia, PA: Elsevier, Saunders.

Piaget, J. (1969). *The theory of stages in cognitive development.* New York: McGraw-Hill.

Safe Kids Worldwide. (2016). *Baby sleep safety and suffocation prevention.* Retrieved from http://www.safekids.org/safetytips/field_age/babies-0%E2%80%9312-months/field_risks/sleep-safety

Sinha, S. (2015). *Short stature.* Retrieved from http://emedicine.medscape.com/article/924411-overview

Stettler, N., Bhatia, J., Parish, A., & Stallings, V. A. (2011). Feeding healthy infants, children, and adolescents. In R. M. Kliegman, B. F. Stanton, J. W. St. Geme III, N. F. Schor, & R. E. Behrman (Eds.), (*Nelson's textbook of pediatrics* (19th ed.). Philadelphia, PA: Elsevier, Saunders.

Swanson, W. S. (2016). *The scoop on poop: What's normal, what's not.* Retrieved from http://www.parents.com/baby/diapers/dirty/baby-bowel-movement/

Tinanoff, N. (2011). The oral cavity. In R. M. Kliegman, B. F. Stanton, J. W. St. Geme III, N. F. Schor, & R. E. Behrman (Eds.), (*Nelson's textbook of pediatrics* (19th ed.). Philadelphia, PA: Elsevier, Saunders.

U.S. Department of Health and Human Services. (2016). *Healthy people 2020.* Retrieved from http://www.healthypeople.gov/2020/default

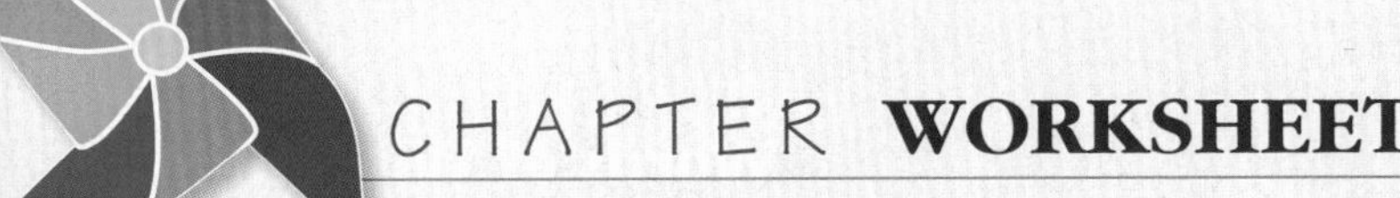

CHAPTER WORKSHEET

MULTIPLE CHOICE QUESTIONS

1. The mother of a 3-month-old boy asks the nurse about starting solid foods. What is the most appropriate response by the nurse?
   a. "It's okay to start puréed solids at this age if fed via the bottle."
   b. "Infants don't require solid food until 12 months of age."
   c. "Solid foods should be delayed until age 6 months, when the infant can handle a spoon on his own."
   d. "The tongue extrusion reflex disappears at age 4 to 6 months, making it a good time to start solid foods."
2. The father of a 2-month-old girl is expressing concern that his infant may be getting spoiled. The nurse's best response is:
   a. "She just needs love and attention. Don't worry; she's too young to spoil."
   b. "Consistently meeting the infant's needs helps promote a sense of trust."
   c. "Infants need to be fed and cleaned; if you're sure those needs are met, just let her cry."
   d. "Consistency in meeting needs is important, but you're right, holding her too much will spoil her."
3. Parents of an 8-month-old girl express concern that she cries when left with the babysitter. How does the nurse best explain this behavior?
   a. Crying when left with the sitter may indicate difficulty with building trust.
   b. Stranger anxiety should not occur until toddlerhood; this concern should be investigated.
   c. Separation anxiety is normal at this age; the infant recognizes parents as separate beings.
   d. Perhaps the sitter doesn't meet the infant's needs; choose a different sitter.
4. The nurse is providing anticipatory guidance to the mother of a 6-month-old infant. What is the best instruction by the nurse in relation to the infant's oral health?
   a. "Start brushing her teeth after all the baby teeth come in."
   b. "Use a washcloth with toothpaste to clean her mouth."
   c. "Clean your baby's gums, then new teeth, with a washcloth."
   d. "Rinse your baby's mouth with water after every feeding."
5. A 9-month-old infant's mother is questioning why cow's milk is not recommended in the first year of life as it is much cheaper than formula. What rationale does the nurse include in her response?
   a. It is permissible to substitute cow's milk for formula at this age as he is so close to 1 year old.
   b. Cow's milk is poor in iron and does not provide the proper balance of nutrients for the infant.
   c. As long as the mother provides whole milk, rather than skim, she can start cow's milk in infancy.
   d. If the mother cannot afford the infant formula, she should dilute it to make it last longer.

CRITICAL THINKING EXERCISES

1. The mother of an 11-month-old boy who was born at 24 weeks' gestation is concerned about his size and motor skills. What information should the nurse provide?
2. An infant's mother thinks there may be something wrong with him because "he spits up so much." What further information should the nurse obtain?
3. If you determine that the infant in the question above is experiencing normal spitting up associated with his developmental age, develop a brief teaching plan to review with the mother.

STUDY ACTIVITIES

1. A mother brings her 9-month-old boy to the clinic for a well-child check-up. She has questions about feeding, speech, and walking. Develop a teaching plan of anticipatory guidance for the 9-month-old infant.
2. Develop a home and car safety plan for the 12-month-old infant.
3. In the clinical setting, observe two infants of the same age, one who is developing appropriately for his or her age and one who is delayed. Note the similarities and differences between the two infants.

BRINGING IT ALL TOGETHER: A CASE STUDY

Mario, a 9-month-old boy, is seen in the clinic for a well-child examination. He has been healthy since birth and now his mother is nervous, as she is considering putting him in day care so she can return to work. She is unsure how she will manage the return to work, as Mario is breastfeeding frequently throughout the day. Mario's grandmother has advised his mother that breast milk is better than baby food, so Mario's mom has not offered him baby food very much. His mother also expresses concern that Mario is not walking yet, because her cousin's baby walked at 9 months.

Go to thePoint to find questions to consider about this case.

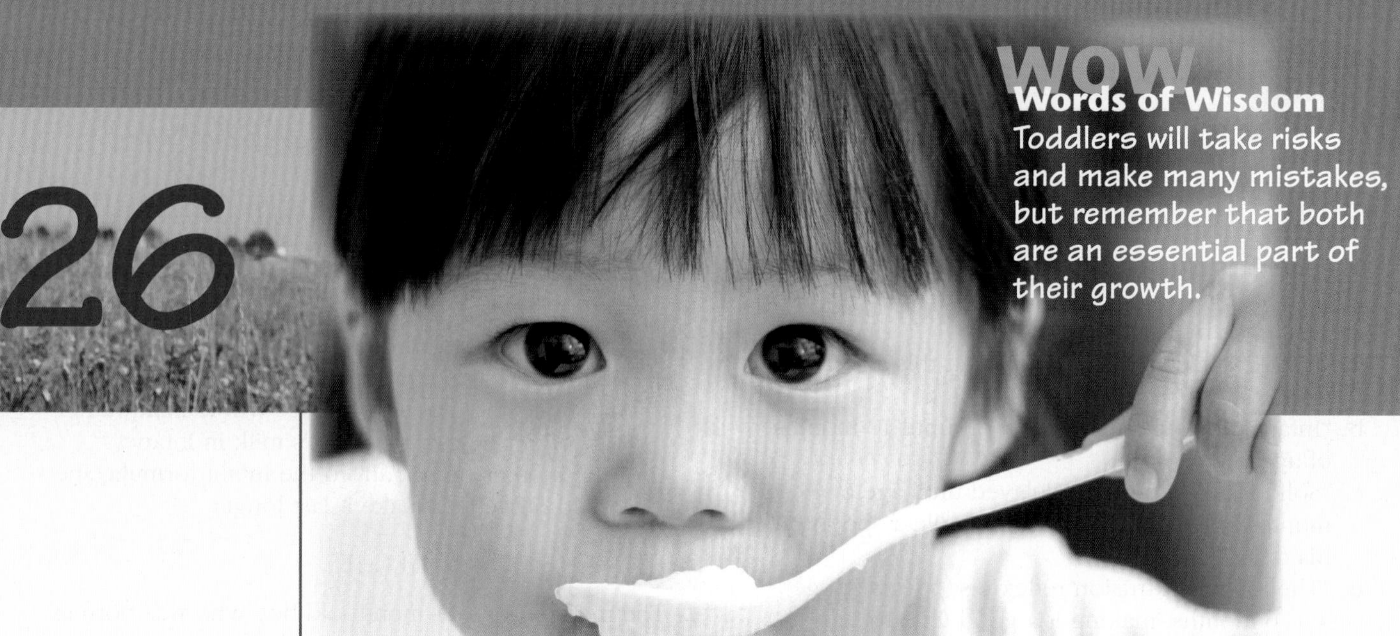
26
WOW
Words of Wisdom
Toddlers will take risks and make many mistakes, but remember that both are an essential part of their growth.

Growth and Development of the Toddler

KEY TERMS
animism
echolalia
egocentrism
expressive language
food jag
individuation
parallel play
physiologic anorexia
receptive language
regression
separation
separation anxiety
sibling rivalry
telegraphic speech

Learning Objectives

Upon completion of the chapter, you will be able to:

1. Explain normal physiologic, psychosocial, and cognitive changes occurring in the toddler.
2. Identify the gross and fine motor milestones of the toddler.
3. Demonstrate an understanding of language development in the toddler years.
4. Discuss sensory development of the toddler.
5. Demonstrate an understanding of emotional/social development and moral/spiritual development during toddlerhood.
6. Implement a nursing care plan to address common issues related to growth and development in toddlerhood.
7. Encourage growth and learning through play.
8. Develop a teaching plan for safety promotion in the toddler period.
9. Demonstrate an understanding of toddler needs related to sleep and rest, as well as dental health.
10. Develop a nutritional plan for the toddler based on average nutritional requirements.
11. Provide appropriate anticipatory guidance for common developmental issues that arise in the toddler period.
12. Demonstrate an understanding of appropriate methods of discipline for use during the toddler years.
13. Identify the role of the parent in the toddler's life and determine ways to support, encourage, and educate the parents about toddler growth, development, and concerns during this period.

Jose Gonzales **is a 2-year-old boy brought to the clinic by his mother and father for his 2-year-old check-up. During your assessment, you find that his weight is 13.6 kg (30 lb), height 83.82 cm (33 inches), and head circumference 49.53 cm (19.5 inches). As the nurse caring for him, assess Jose's growth and development, and then provide appropriate anticipatory guidance to the parents.**

The toddler period encompasses the second 2 years of life, from age 1 year to age 3 years. This period is a time of significant advancement in growth and development for the child. It can also be quite a challenging time for parents. The theme during the toddler years is one of holding on and letting go. Having learned that parents are predictable and reliable, the toddler is now learning that his or her behavior has a predictable, reliable effect on others. The challenge is to encourage independence and autonomy while keeping the curious toddler safe.

Take Note!

As more grandparents are assuming the primary caregiver role for their grandchildren, nurses should be alert to the possibility of increased stress that is placed upon the older caregiver, particularly during the active and sometimes trying years of toddlerhood (Smith & Segal, 2016).

Growth and Development Overview

Infancy is a time of intense growth and development. Both physical growth and acquisition of new motor skills slow somewhat during the toddler years. Refinement of motor skills, continued cognitive growth, and acquisition of appropriate language skills are of prime importance during toddlerhood. The nurse uses the knowledge of normal toddler development as a roadmap for behavioral assessment of the 1- to 3-year-old child.

PHYSICAL GROWTH

The toddler's height and weight continue to increase steadily, though the increase occurs at a slower velocity compared to infancy. Toddler gains in height and weight tend to occur in spurts, rather than in a linear fashion (Fig. 26.1). The average toddler weight gain is 1.36 to 2.27 kg (3 to 5 lb) per year. Length/height increases by an average of 7.62 cm (3 inches) per year. Toddlers generally reach about half of their adult height by 2 years of age. Head circumference increases about 2.54 cm (1 inch) from when the child is between 1 and 2 years of age, then increases an average of 1.27 cm (a half inch) per year until age 5. The anterior fontanel should be closed by the time the child is 18 months old. Head size becomes more proportional to the rest of the body near the age of 3 years (Feigelman, 2011a; Feigelman, 2011b; Goldson & Reynolds, 2014).

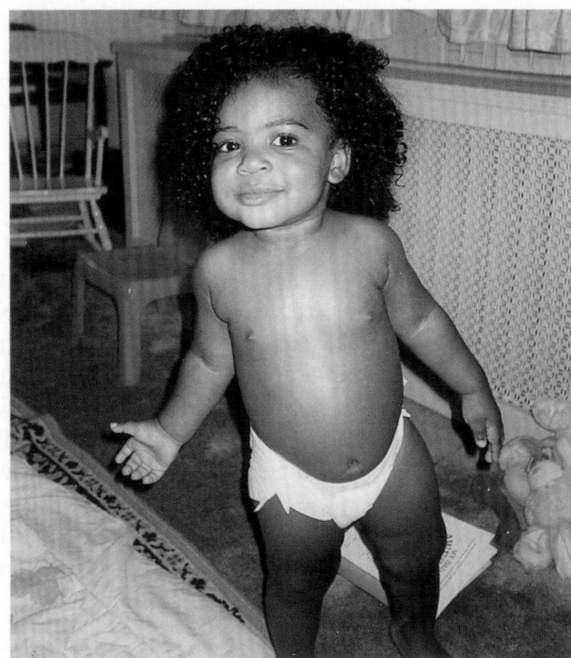

FIGURE 26.1 The typical toddler appearance is that of a rounded abdomen, a slight swayback, and a wide-based stance.

ORGAN SYSTEM MATURATION

Though not as pronounced as the changes occurring during infancy, the toddler's organ systems continue to grow and mature in their functioning. Significant functional changes occur within the neurologic, gastrointestinal, and genitourinary systems. The respiratory and cardiovascular systems undergo changes as well.

Neurologic System

Brain growth continues through toddlerhood, and head circumference (reflective of brain growth) reaches about 90% of its adult size by 2 years of age (Zero to Three, 2016a; Feigelman, 2011b). Myelination of the brain and spinal cord continues to progress and is complete around 24 months of age. Myelination results in improved coordination and equilibrium as well as the ability to exercise sphincter control, which is important for bowel and bladder mastery. Integration of the primitive reflexes occurs in infancy, allowing for the emergence of the protective reflexes near the end of infancy or early in toddlerhood. The forward or downward parachute reflex is particularly helpful when the child starts to toddle. Rapid increase in language skills is evidence of continued progression of cognitive development.

Respiratory System

The respiratory structures continue to grow and mature throughout toddlerhood. The alveoli continue to increase in number, not reaching the adult number until about 7 years of age. The trachea and lower airways continue to grow but remain small compared with the adult. The tongue is relatively large in comparison to the size of the mouth. Tonsils and adenoids are large and the Eustachian tubes are relatively short and straight.

Cardiovascular System

The heart rate decreases and blood pressure increases in toddlerhood. Blood vessels are close to the skin surface and so are compressed easily when palpated.

Gastrointestinal System

The stomach continues to increase in size, allowing the toddler to consume three regular meals per day. Pepsin production matures by 2 years of age. The small intestine continues to grow in length, though it does not reach the maximum length of 2 to 3 m until adulthood. Stool passage decreases in frequency to one or more per day. The color of the stool may change (yellow, orange, brown, or green) depending on the toddler's diet. Since the toddler's intestines remain somewhat immature, the toddler often passes whole pieces of difficult-to-digest food such as corn kernels. Bowel control is generally achieved by the end of the toddler period.

Genitourinary System

Bladder and kidney function reach adult levels by 16 to 24 months of age. The bladder capacity increases, allowing the toddler to retain urine for increased periods of times. Urine output should be about 1 mL/kg/hour. The urethra remains short in both the male and female toddler, making them more susceptible to urinary tract infections compared to adults.

Musculoskeletal System

During toddlerhood, the bones increase in length and the muscles mature and become stronger. The abdominal musculature is weak in early toddlerhood, resulting in a pot-bellied appearance. The toddler appears to have a swayback along with the potbelly. Around 3 years of age, the musculature strengthens and the abdomen is flatter in appearance.

PSYCHOSOCIAL DEVELOPMENT

Erikson defines the toddler period as a time of autonomy versus shame and doubt. It is a time of exerting independence. Since the toddler developed a sense of trust in infancy, he or she is ready to give up dependence and to assert his or her sense of control and autonomy (Erikson, 1963). The toddler is struggling for self-mastery, to learn to do for himself or herself what others have been doing for him or her. Toddlers often experience ambivalence about the move from dependence to autonomy, resulting in emotional lability. The toddler may quickly change from happy and pleasant to crying and screaming. Exertion of independence also results in the toddler's favorite response "no." The toddler will often answer "no" even when he or she really means "yes."

This negativism—always saying "no"—is a normal part of healthy development and is occurring as a result of the toddler's attempt to assert his or her independence. Table 26.1 gives further information related to developing a sense of autonomy.

COGNITIVE DEVELOPMENT

According to Jean Piaget (1969), toddlers move through the last two substages of the first stage of cognitive development, the sensorimotor stage, between 12 and 24 months of age. Young toddlers engage in tertiary circular reactions and progress to mental combinations. Rather than just repeating a behavior, the toddler is able to experiment with a behavior to see what happens. By 2 years of age, toddlers are capable of using symbols to allow for imitation. With increasing cognitive abilities, toddlers may now engage in delayed imitation. For example, they may imitate a household task that they observed a parent doing several days ago.

Piaget identified the second stage of cognitive development as the preoperational stage. It occurs in children between ages 2 and 7 years. During this stage toddlers begin to become more sophisticated with symbolic thought. The thinking of the older toddler is far more advanced than that of the infant or young toddler, who views the world as a series of objects. During the preoperational stage, objects begin to have characteristics that make them unique from one another. Objects are considered large or small, having a particular color or shape, or having a unique texture. This moves beyond the connection of sensory information and physical action. Words and images allow the toddler to begin this process of developing symbolic thought by providing a label for the objects' characteristics (Piaget, 1969).

Toddlers also use symbols in dramatic play. First they imitate life with appropriate toy objects, and then they are able to substitute objects in their play. A bowl may be used to pretend to eat from, but then later it can be used upside down on the head as a hat (Fig. 26.2). Human feelings and characteristics may also be attributed to objects (**animism**) (Papalia & Feldman, 2011). See Table 26.1 for further explanation of cognitive development in toddlerhood.

Take Note!

Mothers who are depressed may not be as sensitive to their children as other mothers. For this reason, maternal depression is a risk factor for poor cognitive development. Be alert to the mental status of a toddler's mother so that appropriate referrals can be made if needed (Giles, Davies, Whitrow, Warin, & Moore, 2011).

TABLE 26.1 DEVELOPMENTAL THEORIES

Theorist	Stage	Activities
Erikson	Autonomy vs. shame & doubt Age 1–3 years	Achieves autonomy and self-control Separates from parent/caregiver Withstands delayed gratification Negativism abounds Imitates adults and playmates Spontaneously shows affection Is increasingly enthusiastic about playmates Cannot take turns in games until age 3 years
Piaget	Sensorimotor Substage 5: tertiary circular reactions Age: 12–18 months Substage 6: Mental combinations Age: 18–24 months Preoperational Age: 2–7 years	Differentiates self from objects Increased object permanence (knows that objects that are out of sight still exist [e.g., cookies in the cabinet]) Uses ALL senses to explore environment Places items in and out of containers Imitates domestic chores (domestic mimicry) Imitation is more symbolic Starting to think before acting Understands requests and is capable of following simple directions Has a sense of ownership (my, mine) Time, space, and causality understanding is increasing Uses mental trial and error rather than physical Makes mechanical toys work Plays make-believe with dolls, animals, and people Increased use of language for mental representation Understands concept of "two" Starting to make connections between an experience in the past and a new one that is currently occurring Sorts objects by shape and color Completes puzzles with four pieces Play becomes more complex
Freud	Anal stage Age: 1–3 years	Focus is on achieving anal sphincter control. Satisfaction and/or frustration may occur as the toddler learns to withhold and expel stool.

Adapted from Erikson, E. H. (1963). *Childhood and society* (2nd ed.). New York: W.W. Norton and Company; Goldson, E., & Reynolds, A. (2014). Child development and behavior. In W. W. Hay, Jr., M. J. Levin, R. R. Deterding, & M. J. Abzug. (Eds.), *Current diagnosis and treatment: Pediatrics* (22nd ed.). New York, NY: McGraw-Hill Education.; and Piaget, J. (1969). *The theory of stages in cognitive development*. New York: McGraw-Hill.

MOTOR SKILL DEVELOPMENT

Toddlers continue to gain new motor skills as well as refine others. Walking progresses to running, climbing, and jumping. Pushing or pulling a toy, throwing a ball, and pedaling a tricycle are accomplished in toddlerhood. Fine motor skills progress from holding and pinching to the ability to manage utensils, hold a crayon, string a bead, and use a computer. Development of eye–hand coordination is necessary for the refinement of fine motor skills. These increased abilities of mobility and manipulation help the curious toddler explore and learn more about his or her environment (Fig. 26.3). As the toddler masters a new task, he or she has confidence to conquer the next challenge. Thus, mastery in motor skill development contributes to the toddler's growing sense of self-esteem. The toddler who is eager to face challenges will likely develop more quickly than one who is reluctant. The senses of sight, hearing, and touch are useful in helping to coordinate gross and fine motor movement.

Gross Motor Skills

As gross motor skills are mastered and then used repeatedly, the large muscle groups in the toddler are strengthened. The "toddler gait" is characteristic of new walkers. The toddler does not walk smoothly and maturely. Instead, the legs are planted widely apart, toes are pointed forward, and the toddler seems to sway from side to side while moving forward (Fig. 26.4). Often, the toddler seems to speed along, be pitching forward, and may appear ready to topple over at any moment. The toddler may fall often, but will use outstretched arms to catch himself or herself (parachute reflex). After

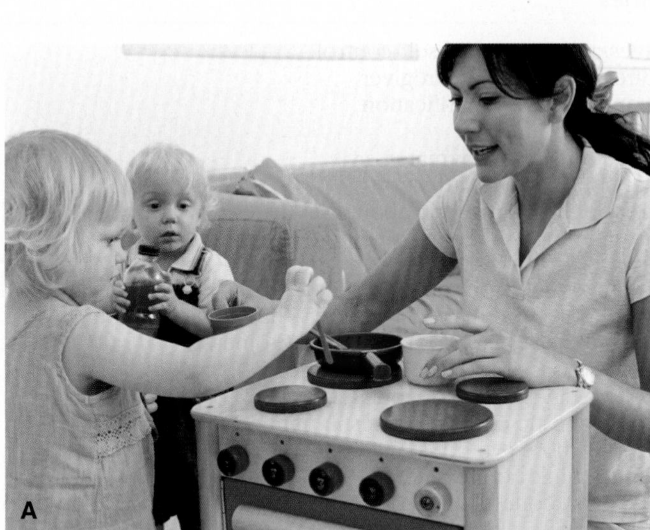

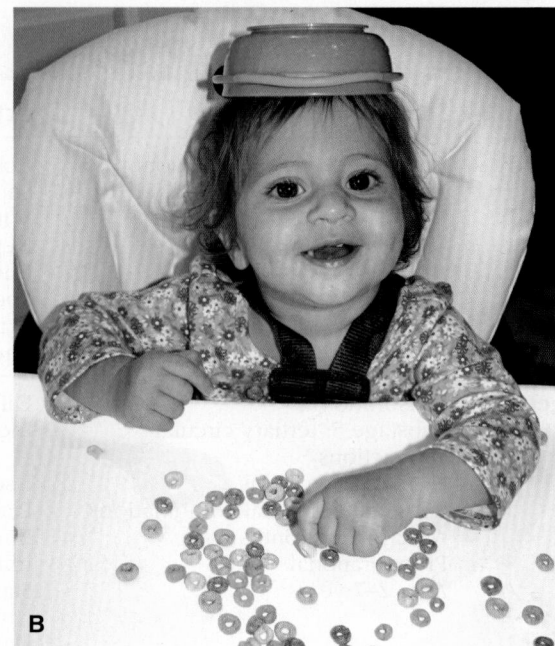

FIGURE 26.2 The toddler will (**A**) pretend with items in the way they are intended to be used as well as (**B**) find other creative uses for them.

about 6 months of practice walking, the toddler's gait is smoother and the feet are closer together. By 3 years of age, the toddler walks in a heel-to-toe fashion similar to that of adults. Toddlers often use physical actions such as running, jumping, and hitting to express their emotions because they are only just learning to express their thoughts and feelings verbally. Table 26.2 lists motor skill expectations in relation to age.

Fine Motor Skills

Fine motor skills in the toddler period are improved and perfected. Holding utensils requires some control and agility, but even more is needed for buttoning and zipping. Adequate vision is necessary for the refinement of fine motor skills because eye–hand coordination is crucial for directing the fingers, hand, and wrist to accomplish

FIGURE 26.3 The toddler's curiosity about the world increases, as does her ability to explore it.

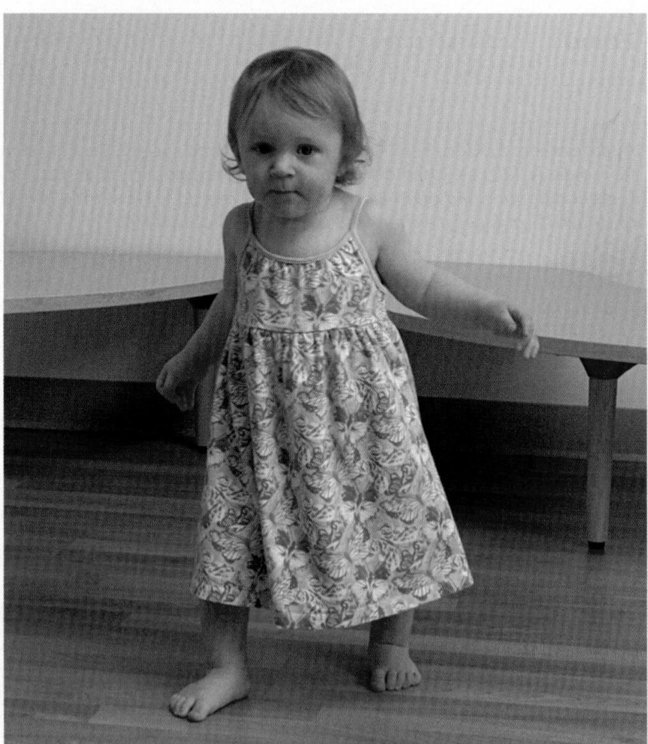

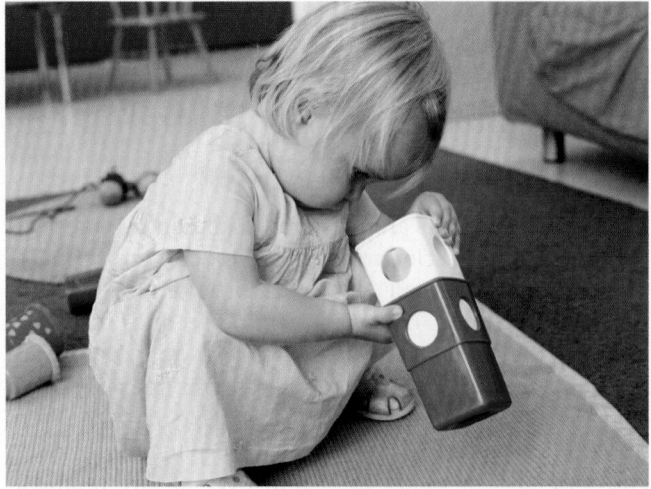

FIGURE 26.4 The young toddler (early walker) walks with a wide-based stance, feet pointing forward and arms akimbo.

TABLE 26.2 MOTOR SKILL DEVELOPMENT

Age	Expected Gross Motor Skill	Expected Fine Motor Skills
12–15 months	Walks independently	Feeds self finger foods Uses index finger to point
18 months	Climbs stairs with assistance Pulls toys while walking	Masters reaching, grasping, and releasing: stacks blocks, puts things in slots Turns book pages (singly with board book, multiple if paper) Removes shoes and socks Stacks four cubes
24 months	Runs Kicks ball Can stand on tiptoe Carries several toys, or a large toy while walking Climbs onto and down from furniture without assistance	Builds tower of six or seven cubes Right- or left-handed Imitates circular and vertical strokes Scribbles and paints Starting to turn knobs Puts round pegs into holes
36 months	Climbs well Pedals tricycle Runs easily Walks up and down stairs with alternate feet Bends over easily without falling	Undresses self Copies circle Builds tower of nine or ten cubes Holds a pencil in writing position Screws/unscrews lids, nuts, bolts Turns book pages one at a time

Adapted from Feigelman, S. (2011a). Preschool years. In R. M. Kliegman, B. F. Stanton, J. W. St. Geme III, N. F. Schor, & R. E. Behrman, (Eds.), *Nelson's textbook of pediatrics* (19th ed.). Philadelphia, PA: Elsevier, Saunders; Feigelman, S. (2011b). The second year. In R. M. Kliegman, B. F. Stanton, J. W. St. Geme III, N. F. Schor, & R. E. Behrman, (Eds.), *Nelson's textbook of pediatrics* (19th ed.). Philadelphia, PA: Elsevier, Saunders; and Goldson, E., & Reynolds, A. (2014). Child development and behavior. In W. W. Hay, Jr., M. J. Levin, R. R. Deterding, & M. J. Abzug. (Eds.), *Current diagnosis and treatment: Pediatrics* (22nd ed.). New York, NY: McGraw-Hill Education.

small muscle tasks such as fitting a puzzle piece or stringing a bead. See Table 26.2 for age expectations for various motor skills.

SENSORY DEVELOPMENT

Toddlers use all of their senses to explore the world around them. Toddlers examine new items by feeling them, looking at them, shaking them to hear what sound they make, smelling them, and placing them in their mouths. Toddler vision continues to progress and should be 20/50 to 20/40 in both eyes. Depth perception also continues to mature. Hearing should be at the adult level, as infants are ordinarily born with hearing intact. The sense of smell continues to mature, and toddlers may comment if they do not care for the scent of something. Though taste discrimination is not completely developed, toddlers may exhibit preferences for certain flavors of foods. The toddler is more likely to try a new food if its appearance or smell is familiar. Lack of complete taste discrimination places the toddler at risk of accidental ingestion.

COMMUNICATION AND LANGUAGE DEVELOPMENT

Language development occurs rapidly during the toddler years. The acquisition of language is a dynamic and complex process. The child's age and social interactions and the types of language to which he or she has been exposed influence language development. **Receptive language** development (the ability to understand what is being said or asked) is typically far more advanced than **expressive language** development (the ability to communicate one's desires and feelings) (Feigelman, 2011b; Goldson & Reynolds, 2014). In other words, the toddler understands language and is able to follow commands far sooner than he or she can actually use the words himself or herself. Language is a very important part of the toddler's ability to organize his or her world and actually make sense of it. Thoughtfully planned use of language can provide behavior guidance and contribute to the avoidance of power struggles. In regard to expressive language development, the young toddler begins to use short sentences and will progress to a vocabulary of 50 words by 2 years of age

(Feigelman, 2011b; Goldson & Reynolds, 2014). **Echolalia** (repetition of words and phrases without understanding) normally occurs in toddlers younger than 30 months of age. "Why" and "what" questions dominate the older toddler's language. Telegraphic speech is common in the 3-year-old. **Telegraphic speech** refers to speech that contains only the essential words to get the point across, much like a telegram. Rather than "I want a cookie and milk," the toddler might say, "Want cookie milk." In telegraphic speech the nouns and verbs are present and are verbalized in the appropriate order (Feigelman, 2011b). Table 26.3 gives an overview of receptive and expressive language development in the toddler.

Early identification and referral of children with potential speech delays is critical. If a delay is identified, early intervention may increase the child's potential to acquire age-appropriate receptive and expressive language skills. Children with pre-existing conditions such as genetic syndromes that are known to have an effect on language development should be referred to a speech–language pathologist as soon as the condition is recognized rather than waiting until the child exhibits a delay.

Of special concern in the toddler years is the development of speech and language in potentially bilingual children. At the age of 1 to 2 years, the potentially bilingual child may blend two languages—that is, parts of the word in both languages are blended into one word. At age 2 to 3 years, the potentially bilingual toddler may mix languages within a sentence. Thus, the

TABLE 26.3 LANGUAGE DEVELOPMENT IN TODDLERS

Age	Receptive Language	Expressive Language
12 months	Understands common words independent of context Follows a one-step command accompanied by gesture	Uses a finger to point to things Imitates or uses gestures such as waving goodbye Communicates desires with word and gesture combinations Vocal imitation First word
15 months	Looks at adult when communicating Follows a one-step command without gesture Understands 100–150 words	Repeats words that he or she hears Babbles in what sound like sentences
18 months	Understands the word "no" Comprehends 200 words Sometimes answers the question, "What's this?"	Uses at least 5–20 words Uses names of familiar object
24 months	Points to named body parts Points to pictures in books Enjoys listening to simple stories Names a variety of objects in the environment Begins to use "my" or "mine"	Vocabulary of 40–50 words Sentences of two or three words ("me up," "want cookie") Asks questions ("what that?") Uses simple phrases Uses descriptive words (hungry, hot) Two thirds of what child says should be understandable Repeats overheard words
30 months	Follows a series of two independent commands	Vocabulary of 150–300 words
36 months	Understands most sentences Understands physical relationships (on, in, under) Participates in short conversations May follow a three-part command	Speech usually understood by those who know the child, about half understood by those outside family Asks "why?" Three- to four-word sentences Talks about something that happened in the past Vocabulary of 1,000 words Can say name, age, and gender Uses pronouns and plurals

Adapted from Feigelman, S. (2011a). Preschool years. In R. M. Kliegman, B. F. Stanton, J. W. St. Geme III, N. F. Schor, & R. E. Behrman, (Eds.), *Nelson's textbook of pediatrics* (19th ed.). Philadelphia, PA: Elsevier, Saunders; Feigelman, S. (2011b). The second year. In R. M. Kliegman, B. F. Stanton, J. W. St. Geme III, N. F. Schor, & R. E. Behrman, (Eds.), *Nelson's textbook of pediatrics* (19th ed.). Philadelphia, PA: Elsevier, Saunders; and Goldson, E., & Reynolds, A. (2014). Child development and behavior. In W. W. Hay, Jr., M. J. Levin, R. R. Deterding, & M. J. Abzug. (Eds.), *Current diagnosis and treatment: Pediatrics* (22nd ed.). New York, NY: McGraw-Hill Education.

assessment of adequate language development is more complicated in bilingual children. There are websites that may be helpful to parents of potentially bilingual children, where they can find support and resources. A list of websites is included on thePoint at http://thePoint.lww.com/Kyle3e.

Take Note!

Young children exposed to more than one language may experience simultaneous acquisition of both languages. The first word may be slightly delayed as compared with single language speakers, but still occurs within the normal range (Lowry, 2011).

EMOTIONAL AND SOCIAL DEVELOPMENT

Emotional development in the toddler years is focused on **separation** and **individuation** (Papalia & Feldman, 2011). Seeing oneself as separate from the parent or primary caregiver is accompanied by forming a sense of self and learning to exert control over one's environment. As this need to feel in control of his or her world emerges, the toddler displays **egocentrism** (focus on self). This need for control results in emotional lability: very happy and pleasant one moment, then overreacting to limit setting with a temper tantrum in the next moment (Brazelton & Sparrow, 2006). As toddlers identify the boundaries between themselves and the parent or primary caregiver, they learn to negotiate a balance between attachment and independence. Toddlers initially rely on the parents' communication and signals in order to initiate appropriate behavior or inhibit undesirable behavior. They have a difficult time choosing between sets of behaviors as they occur in different situations. Power struggles often occur in this age group, and it is important for parents and caregivers to thoughtfully and intentionally develop the rituals and routines that will provide stability and security for the toddler (Feigelman, 2011b). Many toddlers rely on a security item (blanket, doll, or bear) to comfort themselves in stressful situations (Fig. 26.5). This ability to self-soothe is a function of autonomy and is viewed as a sign of a nurturing environment, rather than, as one might suspect, one of neglect.

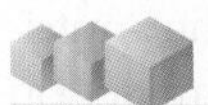

Concept Mastery Alert

Toddler Behavior

When teaching parents interventions appropriate to the emotional development of their toddler, nurses can teach parents that they may offer a toddler limited choices (usually two is sufficient) to assist with control over their environment. Nurses should advise parents that aggressive behavior is normal in the toddler period, so parents should not blame toddlers for the behavior, but should help toddlers understand results of their behavior.

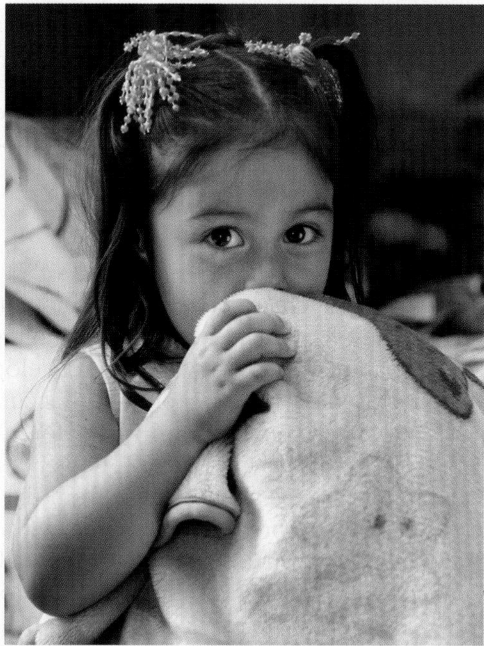

FIGURE 26.5 The toddler may be able to self-soothe and produce a sense of comfort during this stage of establishing autonomy by relying upon a security item such as a doll, bear, or blanket.

Children also begin to learn about gender differences in the toddler years. They observe the differences between male and female body parts if they are exposed to them. Toddlers may question parents about these differences and may begin to explore their own genitals. Toddlers also begin to understand and mimic social gender differences. They make observations about gender-specific behavior dependent upon what they are exposed to.

Aggressive behaviors are typically displayed during the toddler years. Toddlers may hit, bite, or push other children and grab toys. Adults can assist the toddler in building empathy by pointing out when someone is hurt and explaining what happened. Toddlers should not be blamed for their impulsive behavior; rather, they should be guided toward socially acceptable actions in order to foster development of appropriate social judgment. It is particularly important for the parent or caregiver to serve as a role model for appropriate behavior, rather than losing his or her own temper, in order for the toddler to be able to learn how to acceptably handle frustrations. Offering limited choices is one way of allowing toddlers some control over their environment and helping them to establish a sense of mastery. Since toddlers naturally have a short attention span, they tend to dawdle. As the toddlers become more self-aware, they start to develop emotions of self-consciousness such as embarrassment and shame.

Though toddlers are becoming more self-aware, they still do not have clear body boundaries. They do not clearly understand the body's functions, though they are beginning to make appropriate connections. Feces may be viewed as a part of the child, and the toddler may become upset at seeing it disappear in the toilet. The toddler will protect his or her body by resisting intrusive procedures such as temperature or blood pressure measurement.

Separation Anxiety

As toddlers become increasingly skilled at mobility, they realize that if they have the capability of leaving, then so does the parent. As self-awareness develops and conflicts over closeness versus exploration occur, **separation anxiety** may re-emerge in the 18- to 24-month period (Brazelton & Sparrow, 2006). Power struggles may escalate and distress at separating from the parent may increase. Again, a predictable routine with appropriate limit setting may help toddlers to feel safer and more secure during this period. From the age of 24 to 36 months, separation anxiety again eases. The older toddler begins to have a concept of object constancy: he or she has an internal representation of the parent or caregiver and is better able to tolerate separation, knowing that a reunion will occur.

Temperament

Temperament is the biologic basis for personality. It is our emotional and motivational core, around which the personality develops over time (Child Development Institute, 2015). Temperament affects how the toddler interacts with the environment. The easygoing toddler may adapt more easily and not mind changes in routine as much as other toddlers. The easygoing toddler usually sleeps and eats well and has more predictable and regular behaviors. However, the toddler may still express frustration by having a temper tantrum. The "difficult" toddler is more likely to have intense reactions, negative or positive, with temper tantrums being more likely, more frequent, and more intense than in other toddlers. The structure and routine that toddlers need to feel secure are essential for the difficult toddler; otherwise, the child feels insecure and as a result is more likely to behave inappropriately. The difficult toddler is also the most active of the three temperament types. The slow-to-warm-up toddler is more of a loner and may be very shy. He or she may experience more difficulty with separation anxiety. The behavior of the slow-to-warm-up toddler is more passive; the toddler may be very watchful and withdrawn and may take longer to mature. Changes in routine usually do not result in as much upset, since the toddler's natural reaction is one of passivity (Brazelton & Sparrow, 2006).

Based on the toddler's temperament, make suggestions to the parents for interacting with the toddler in various situations. For example, to avoid temper tantrums in the difficult toddler, suggest that the parent should be especially diligent about maintaining structure and routine as well as avoiding tantrum triggers such as fatigue and hunger. Explain to parents that they may need to exercise additional patience with new activities to which the slow-to-warm-up toddler may need extra time becoming accustomed.

Fears

Common fears of toddlers include loss of parents (which contributes to separation anxiety) and fear of strangers. Some toddlers may be very slow to warm up to people they do not know. The nurse caring for a toddler in the outpatient or hospital setting should take the time to establish a relationship with the toddler in order to allay the toddler's fears. Toddlers may be afraid of loud noises and large or unfamiliar animals. Going to sleep may be a scary time for toddlers as they may be afraid of the dark. A nightlight in the toddler's room may be very helpful.

MORAL AND SPIRITUAL DEVELOPMENT

During the toddler years, children may feel comfort from the routine of praying, but they do not understand religious beliefs because of their limited cognitive abilities. Reading simple Bible stories can lay a foundation for later religious teachings. Kohlberg's (1984) description of moral development places the older toddler in the preconventional level. The toddler is only just beginning to learn right from wrong and does not understand the larger concept of morality. The toddler will base his or her actions on the avoidance of punishment and the attainment of pleasure. Older toddlers begin to feel empathy for others.

CULTURAL INFLUENCES ON GROWTH AND DEVELOPMENT

Homelessness or poverty may directly influence the toddler's ability to grow adequately, as resources for the purchase and preparation of appropriate food may be lacking. Appropriate toys (safe ones) may also not be available in those situations. Food customs continue to have an impact on the child's diet and ability to ingest appropriate nutrients. Individual families' value systems have an impact on the toddler's development as well. Some parents desire to keep their child a "baby" for a longer period, thus delaying weaning or continuing to feed the child baby food or puréed food for a longer period. Other families may highly value independence and encourage the toddler to walk everywhere on his or her own rather than carrying the child.

Culture may also affect emotional development. Some families start at a very young age to discourage crying in boys, encouraging them to "act like a big boy" or "be a man." Ridicule for crying at this age may hurt the toddler's self-concept. Educating families about normal growth and development while continuing to value and support cultural practices is important (Papalia & Feldman, 2011).

Remember Jose Gonzales, whom you met at the beginning of the chapter? What developmental milestones would you expect him to have reached at his age?

THE NURSE'S ROLE IN TODDLER GROWTH AND DEVELOPMENT

The toddler's growth and development affects his or her everyday life as well as the family's. Though some toddlers may grow more quickly or reach developmental milestones sooner than others, growth and development remains orderly and sequential. Health care visits throughout toddlerhood continue to focus on growth and development. The nurse must have a good understanding of the changes that occur during the toddler years in order to provide appropriate anticipatory guidance and support to the family.

When the toddler is hospitalized, growth and development may be altered. The toddler's primary task is establishing autonomy, and the toddler's focus is mobility and language development. Hospitalization removes most opportunities for the toddler to learn through exploration of the environment. Isolation for contagious illness further constrains the toddler's ability to find some control over the environment. The nurse caring for the hospitalized toddler must use knowledge of normal growth and development to be successful in interactions with the toddler, promote continued development, and recognize delays (see Chapter 33) (Fig. 26.6).

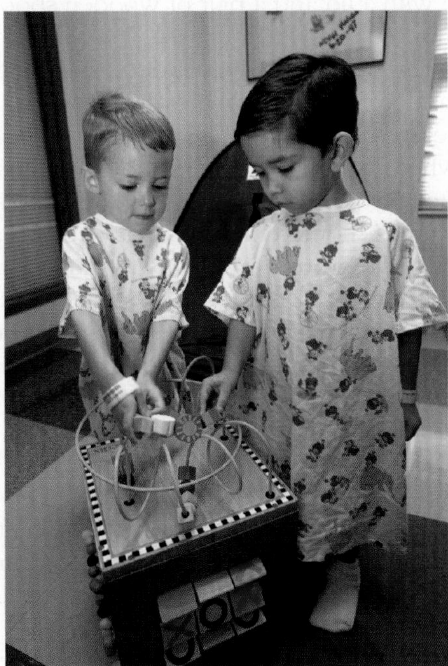

FIGURE 26.6 The hospitalized toddler continues to enjoy developmental tasks appropriate for his or her age, such as playing with manipulative toys.

NURSING PROCESS OVERVIEW

Upon completion of assessment of the toddler's current growth and development status, problems or issues related to growth and development may be identified. The nurse may then identify one or more nursing diagnoses, including but not limited to:

- Delayed growth and development
- Imbalanced nutrition, less than body requirements
- Interrupted family processes
- Readiness for enhanced parenting
- Risk for caregiver role strain
- Risk for delayed development
- Risk for disproportionate growth
- Risk for injury

Nursing care planning for the toddler with growth and development issues should be individualized based on the toddler's and family's needs. The nursing care plan may be used as a guide in planning nursing care for the toddler with a growth or developmental concern. The nurse may choose the appropriate nursing diagnoses from the Nursing Care Plan (found at the end of the chapter) and individualize them as needed. The nursing care plan is intended to serve as a guide only and is not intended to be an inclusive growth and development plan.

PROMOTING HEALTHY GROWTH AND DEVELOPMENT

Parents who give their toddler love and respect regardless of the child's gender, behavior, or capabilities are helping to lay the foundation for self-esteem. Self-esteem is also built through familiarity with the daily routine. Routine and ritual help toddlers develop a conscience. Making expectations known through everyday routines helps to avoid confrontations. If the toddler knows the routine, he or she knows what to expect and how he or she is expected to act. When routine and limits are absent, the toddler develops feelings of uncertainty and anxiety. Limit setting (and remaining consistent with those limits) helps toddlers master their behavior, develop self-esteem, and become successful participants in the family. Children then are able to learn about cooperation throughout the predictable flow of daily life. Nurses

TABLE 26.4 SIGNS OF DEVELOPMENTAL DELAY

Age or Time Frame	Concern
After independent walking for several months	• Persistent tiptoe walking • Failure to develop a mature walking pattern
By 18 months	• Not walking • Not speaking 15 words • Does not understand function of common household items
By 2 years	• Does not use two-word sentences • Does not imitate actions • Does not follow basic instructions • Cannot push a toy with wheels
By 3 years	• Difficulty with stairs • Frequent falling • Cannot build tower of more than four blocks • Difficulty manipulating small objects • Extreme difficulty in separation from parent or caregiver • Cannot copy a circle • Does not engage in make-believe play • Cannot communicate in short phrases • Does not understand simple instructions • Little interest in other children • Unclear speech, persistent drooling

need to be aware of normal developmental expectations in order to determine whether the toddler is progressing appropriately. Table 26.4 lists potential signs of developmental delay. Any toddler with one or more of these concerns should be referred for further developmental evaluation.

Promoting Growth and Development Through Play

Play is the major socializing medium for toddlers. Parents should limit television viewing and encourage creative and physical play instead. Toddlers typically play alongside another child (**parallel play**) rather than cooperatively (Fig. 26.7). The short attention span of the toddler will make him or her often change toys and types of play. It is important to provide a variety of safe toys to allow the toddler many different opportunities for exploring the environment. Toddlers do not need expensive toys; in fact, regular household items sometimes make the most enjoyable toys. Toddlers are egocentric, a normal part of their development (Piaget, 1969). This makes it difficult for them to share. As they are developing a sense of self (who they are as a person), they may see their toys as an extension of themselves. Learning to share occurs in later toddlerhood. Toddlers also like dramatic play and play that recreates familiar activities in the home. Toddlers like to listen to music of all kinds and will often dance to whatever they hear on the radio. Toddlers enjoy drums, xylophones, cymbals, and toy pianos. Musical instruments made at home are also enjoyed. A few pebbles or coins inside an empty water bottle with the top tightly secured is a great music maker; an empty butter tub with a lid and a pair of wooden spoons makes a nice drum.

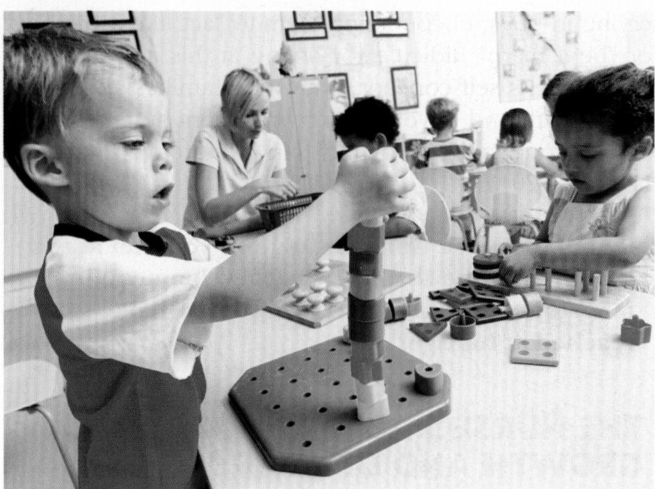

FIGURE 26.7 Parallel play. The toddler usually plays alongside another child rather than cooperatively.

Adequate physical activity is necessary for the development and refinement of movement skills. Toddlers need at least 30 minutes of structured physical activity and anywhere from 1 to several hours of unstructured physical activity per day (Gavin, 2014a). Indoor and outdoor play areas should encourage play activities that use the large muscle groups. The activity must occur within a safe environment. Outdoor play structures should be positioned over surfaces that are soft enough to absorb a fall, such as sand, wood chips, or sawdust (Fig. 26.8). Box 26.1 lists recommended age-appropriate toys.

Promoting Early Learning

The parent–child relationship and the interactions between parent and child form the context for the toddler's early learning.

Promoting Language Development

Talking and singing to the toddler during routine activities such as feeding and dressing provides an environment

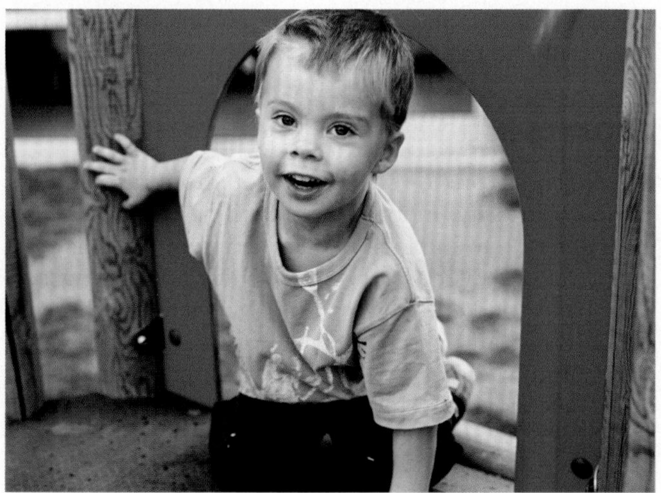

FIGURE 26.8 Toddlers love outdoor physical play, such as climbing on playground equipment. An adult should always supervise toddlers when they are playing outdoors.

that encourages conversation. Frequent, repetitive naming helps the toddler learn appropriate words for objects. The parent or caregiver should be attentive to what the toddler is saying as well as to his or her moods. Using clarification validates the toddler's emotions and ideas. Parents should listen to and answer the toddler's questions. They should sit down quietly with the toddler and gently repeat what the toddler is saying. Encouragement and elaboration convey confidence and interest to the toddler. The toddler needs time to complete his or her thoughts without being interrupted or rushed because he or she is just starting to be able to make the connections necessary to transfer thoughts and feelings into language.

Parents should not overreact to the child's use of the word "no." They can give the toddler opportunities to use the word "no" appropriately by asking silly questions such as, "Can a cat drive a car?" or "Is a banana purple?" When promoting language development, the parent or primary caregiver should teach the toddler appropriate words for body parts and objects and should help the toddler choose appropriate words to label feelings and emotions. Toddlers' receptive language and interpretation of body language and subtle signs far surpass their expressive language, especially at a younger age (Feigelman, 2011b; Goldson & Reynolds, 2014).

Parents should avoid discussing scary or serious topics in the presence of the toddler, since the toddler is very adept at reading emotions.

If the parents speak a foreign language in addition to English, both languages should be used in the home.

BOX 26.1

APPROPRIATE TOYS FOR TODDLERS

- Familiar household items such as plastic bowls and cups of various sizes, large plastic serving utensils, pots and pans, wooden spoons, cardboard boxes and tubes (from paper towel rolls), old magazines, baskets, purses, hats
- Child-size household item toys (kitchen, broom, vacuum cleaner, lawnmower, telephone, and so on)
- Blocks, cars and trucks, plastic animals, trains, plastic figures (family, community helpers), simple dolls, stuffed animals, balls, doll beds and carriages
- Manipulative toys with knobs, wind-ups, and buttons that make things happen; putting large pegs or shapes into matching holes; stringing large beads on shoelaces; blocks and containers that stack; jigsaw puzzles with large pieces; toys that can be taken apart and put back together again
- Gross motor toys: play gym, push and pull toys, wagons, tricycle or other ride-on toys, tunnels
- Tape or CD players for music, various musical instruments
- Chalk, large crayons, finger paint, Play-Doh, washable markers
- Bucket, plastic shovel, and other containers for sand and water play
- Squeaking, floating, and squirting toys for the bath

Adapted from National Association for the Education of Young Children. (n. d.) *Good toys for young children by age and stage.* Retrieved from http://www.naeyc.org/toys

Encouraging Reading

Reading to the toddler every day is one of the best ways to promote language and cognitive development (Fig. 26.9). Toddlers particularly enjoy homemade or purchased books about feelings, family, friends, everyday life, animals and nature, and fun and fantasy. Board books have thick pages that are easier for young toddlers to turn; older toddlers can turn paper pages one at a time. The toddler may also enjoy "reading" the story to the parent. Reach Out and Read, a program designed to

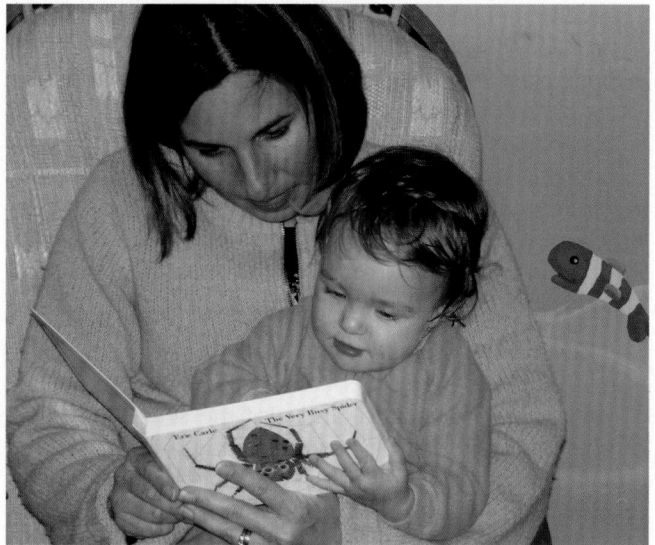

FIGURE 26.9 Reading to a toddler daily is one of the best ways to promote language development and school readiness.

promote early literacy, offers tips for reading with young children (see Teaching Guidelines 26.1).

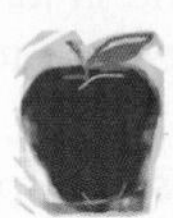

Teaching Guidelines 26.1

TIPS FOR READING WITH YOUNG CHILDREN

- Start at early age.
- Read at least a few minutes every day.
- Encourage your toddler to turn the pages.
- Read stories over and over to help the toddler learn.
- Ask the toddler questions about the book.
- Use voices for the story characters.
- Use body motions during the story.
- Ask questions about the story and about the pictures.
- Read anywhere, at any time.

Adapted from Reach Out and Read. (2013). Reading tips for your young family. Retrieved from http://www.reachoutandread.org/FileRepository/ReadingTips.pdf

Choosing a Preschool

The older toddler may benefit from the structure and socialization provided by attending preschool. Attending preschool will help the toddler become more mature and independent and give the toddler a different source for a sense of accomplishment. At this age, toddlers need supervised play with some direction that fosters their cognitive development. A strict curriculum is not necessary in this age group. When choosing a preschool, the parent or caregiver should look for an environment that has the following qualities:

- Goals and an overall philosophy with which the parents agree (promotion of independence and self-confidence through structured and free play)
- Teachers and assistants trained in early childhood development as well as child cardiopulmonary resuscitation (CPR)
- Small class sizes and an adult-to-child ratio with which the parent feels comfortable
- Disciplinary procedures consistent with the parents' values
- Parents can visit at any time
- School is childproofed inside and out
- Appropriate hygiene procedures, including prohibiting sick children from attending

Teach the parents how to ease the toddler's transition to attending preschool. Encourage parents to talk about going to preschool and visit the school a couple of times. On the first day, parents should calmly and in a matter-of-fact tone tell the toddler that they will return to pick him or her up. If the toddler expresses separation anxiety, the parent should remain calm and follow through with the plan for school attendance. After a few days of attendance, the toddler will be accustomed to the new routine and crying when parting from the parent should be minimal.

Promoting Safety

Safety is of prime concern throughout the toddler period. Curiosity, mobility, and lack of impulse control all contribute to the incidence of unintentional injury in toddlerhood. Even the most watchful and caring parents have toddlers who run into the street, otherwise disappear from parents, and fall down the stairs. Toddlers require direct observation and cannot be trusted to be left alone. A childproof environment provides a safe place for the toddler to explore and learn. Motor vehicle accidents, drowning, choking, burns, falls, and poisoning are the most common injuries suffered by toddlers. Safety and injury prevention focus on these categories.

Safety in the Car

The safest place for the toddler to ride is in the back seat of the car. Parents should use the appropriate size and style of car seat for the child's weight and age as required by state law. At a minimum, toddlers should be in a rear-facing car seat with harness straps and a clip until 2 years of age (American Academy of Pediatrics [AAP], 2016). After age 2 years, a forward-facing seat may be used. A toddler riding in a pickup truck should never ride in the cargo area or truck bed. A full rear seat in the truck is the preferred placement for the toddler car seat. If an appropriate rear seat is unavailable, the air bag should be disarmed and the forward-facing car seat should be secured appropriately in the truck seat. The lower anchor and top tether are additionally required for all forward-facing car seats manufactured since 2002 and are accommodated by motor vehicles manufactured since that time (Fig. 26.10). In older vehicles or car seats, seat belts are utilized for installation. Drivers should avoid using the cell phone or attempting to intervene with the children while they are driving. Excellent resources about car seat safety appropriate for both parents and professionals can be found on thePoint.

Safety in the Home

Key areas of concern for keeping toddlers safe in the home include avoiding exposure to tobacco smoke, preventing injury, and preventing poisoning.

AVOIDING EXPOSURE TO TOBACCO SMOKE

Environmental exposure to tobacco smoke has been associated with increased risk of respiratory disease and infection, decreased lung function, and increased incidence of middle ear effusion and recurrent otitis media. It may also hinder neurodevelopment and may

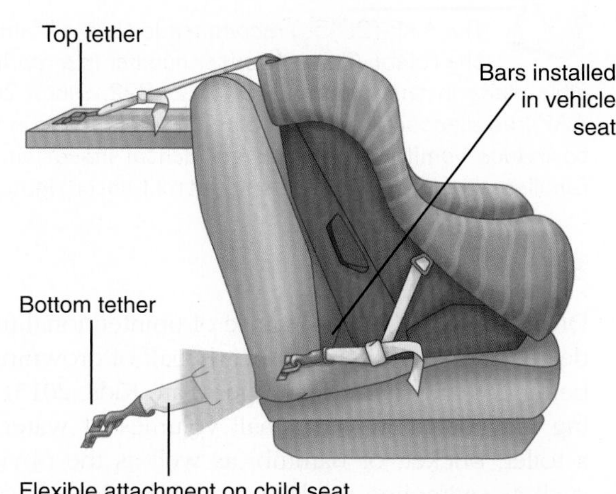

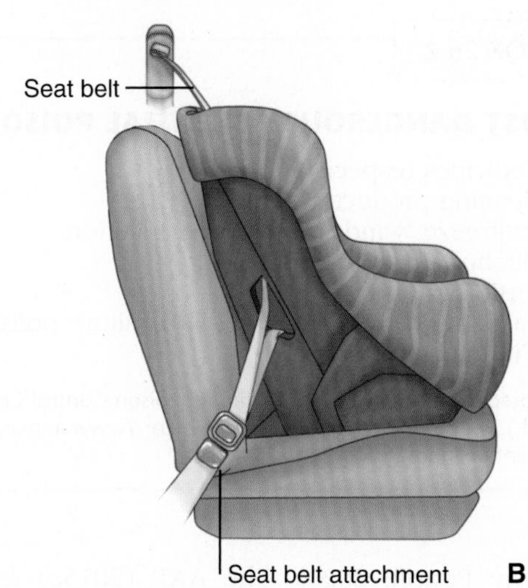

FIGURE 26.10 **(A)** A lower anchor and top tether secure the forward-facing car seat. **(B)** The shoulder safety strap may also be used to secure the toddler seat. (Adapted from American Academy of Pediatrics. (2016). *Car seats: Information for families for 2015.* Retrieved from http://www.healthychildren.org/English/safety-prevention/on-the-go/Pages/Car-Safety-Seats-Information-for-Families.aspx)

be associated with behavior problems (Hwang, Hwang, Moon & Lee, 2012). Parents should avoid cigarette smoking entirely to best protect their children. Even smoking outside of the home is suboptimal because smoke lingers on parents' clothing and children who are often carried (such as younger toddlers) face more exposure. Counsel parents to stop smoking (optimal), but if they continue smoking never to smoke inside the home or car with children present.

PREVENTING INJURY

The toddler is able to open drawers and doors, unlock deadbolts, and climb anywhere he or she wants to go. Toddlers have a limited concept of body boundaries and essentially no fear of danger. Toddlers may fall from any height to which they can climb (e.g., play structures, tables, counters). They may also fall from wheeled toys such as tricycles. As toddlers gain additional height and hand dexterity they are able to reach potentially dangerous items on the counter or stove, leading to an accidental ingestion, burn, or cut.

The AAP advises against having guns in homes with children. If a gun is kept in the home it should be stored unloaded and locked away (AAP, 2013).

To prevent injury in the home, stress the following to parents:

- Never leave a toddler unsupervised out of doors.
- Lock doors to dangerous rooms.
- Install safety gates at the top and bottom of staircases.
- Ensure that window locks are operable; if windows are left opened, then secure all window screens.
- Keep pot handles on the stove turned inward, out of an inquisitive toddler's reach.
- Teach the toddler to avoid the oven, stove, and iron.
- Keep electrical equipment, cords, and matches out of reach.
- Remove firearms from the home, or keep them in a locked cabinet out of the toddler's reach.
- Always require the child to wear a helmet approved by the Consumer Products Safety Commission (CPSC) when riding a wheeled toy. This starts the habit of helmet wearing early, so it can be more easily carried over to the bicycle-riding years of the future.
- Begin teaching the toddler about watching for cars when crossing the street, but always carry or hold the hand of the toddler when crossing the street.
- Teach the toddler to avoid unknown animals (AAP, 2015a, 2015b).

Take Note!

"Bernie Burn," by Sarah Cruz, RN, is a book designed to educate parents and their toddlers about burn prevention while entertaining them. It is endorsed by the American Journal of Nursing. Web link: http://littlebootspublishing.com/bernieburn/index.asp

PREVENTING POISONING

As toddlers become more mobile, they are increasingly able to explore their environment and more easily and efficiently gain access to materials that may be unsafe for them to handle. Their natural curiosity leads them into situations that may place them in danger. Poor taste discrimination in this age group allows for ingestion of chemicals or other materials that older children would find too unpleasant to swallow. Box 26.2 lists most potentially dangerous ingested poisons. Discuss poison prevention in the home at each well-child visit (see

BOX 26.2

MOST DANGEROUS POTENTIAL POISONS

- Medicines (especially iron)
- Cleaning products
- Antifreeze, windshield washer solution
- Alcohol
- Pesticides
- Gasoline, kerosene, lamp oil, furniture polish
- Wild mushrooms

Adapted from American Association of Poison Control Centers. (n. d.). *In the home.* Retrieved from http://www.aapcc.org/prevention/home/

Healthy People 2020). The AAP (2015c) recommends that potentially poisonous substances (e.g., medications, cleaners, hair care products, car care products) be stored out of the toddler's teach, out of the toddler's sight, and in a childproof, locked cabinet.

Encourage all families to take the following safety measures:

- Store all substances in original containers only.
- Never store any liquid other than soda in a soda pop bottle.
- Do not allow toddlers access to baby powder, lotion, cream, or other toddler hygiene products.
- Ensure all medications have child-safety caps.
- Do not leave within the toddler's reach medications such as lozenges or samples that are not packaged in safety bottles.
- Be very careful with medications that are provided in transdermal patch form.
- Do not refer to medicines as candy, as the toddler may mistake pills for candy and ingest them.
- Do not expose toddlers to hazardous vapors such as paints, cleaners, tobacco smoke, and especially street drugs such as crack and marijuana.
- Keep "button" batteries secured and away from a toddler's reach.
- Keep house plants off the floor, remove them from the home, or hang them or place them on a high shelf (American Association of Poison Control Centers, n. d.; AAP, 2015c).

HEALTHY PEOPLE 2020

Objective	Nursing Significance
Prevent an increase in the rate of nonfatal poisonings.	• Use every encounter with the toddler's family as an opportunity to educate about preventing poisonings.

Healthy People Objectives retrieved from http://www.healthypeople.gov

Take Note!

The AAP (2015c) recommends that all families post the Poison Control Center number in a readily accessible place in the home: (800) 222-1222. Since 2003, the AAP has discouraged the use of syrup of ipecac in the home to induce vomiting after an accidental ingestion. Instead, families should call the Poison Control Center right away.

Safety in the Water

Drowning is the leading cause of unintentional injury and death in US children, with nearly half of drowning victims being 4 years old and younger (Safe Kids, 2015). Drowning may occur in very small volumes of water such as a toilet, bucket, or bathtub, as well as the obvious sites such as swimming pools and other bodies of water. Toddlers' large heads in relation to their body size place them at risk for toppling over into a body of water that they are inquisitive about. Toddlers should be supervised at all times when in or around the water. In general, most children do not have the physical and cognitive capabilities necessary to truly learn how to swim until 4 years of age. Parents who want to enroll a toddler in a swimming class should be aware that a water safety skills class would be most appropriate. However, even toddlers who have completed a swimming program still need *constant* supervision in the water (Safe Kids, 2016b). Box 26.3 gives recommendations for the prevention of drowning.

Remember Jose Gonzales, the 2-year-old introduced at the beginning of the chapter? What anticipatory guidance related to safety should you provide to his parents?

Promoting Nutrition

The toddler's ability to chew and swallow is improving, and he or she learns to use utensils effectively to feed

BOX 26.3

PREVENTING DROWNING

- Pools should be fenced with locked gates or screened with locked doors.
- Interior doors should be kept locked.
- Young children should never be left unattended in or near water.
- Water wings or "floaties" are not a substitute for adult supervision or for personal flotation devices.
- US Coast Guard–approved life preservers or personal flotation devices should be available when a young child is in or near a body of water.
- Parents and caregivers should be trained in child cardiopulmonary resuscitation (CPR).

Adapted from Safe Kids. (2016a). *Swimming.* Retrieved from https://www.safekids.org/poolsafety

HEALTHY PEOPLE 2020

Objective	Nursing Significance
Eliminate very low food security among children.	• Counsel families about the appropriate toddler diet. • Refer eligible families to the special supplemental nutrition program for women, infants, and children (WIC).

Healthy People Objectives retrieved from http://www.healthypeople.gov

himself or herself. The early years lay a foundation for the future, and a great deal of parental and societal interest is focused on nutrition and eating. Forming healthy eating habits has its foundation early in life, and diet has significant influence upon the child's future health status. By establishing healthier food choice patterns early in life, the child is better able to continue these healthy choices later in life. The child younger than 2 years of age should not have his or her fat intake restricted, but this does not mean that unhealthy foods such as sweets should be eaten liberally. A diet high in nutrient-rich foods and low in nutrient-poor high-calorie foods such as sweets is appropriate for children of all ages. See Healthy People 2020.

Weaning

The timing of weaning from breastfeeding is influenced by a number of factors such as cultural beliefs, local and regional ethnic beliefs, the mother's work schedule, desired child spacing, or societal feelings about the nature of the mother–infant relationship. The AAP recommends breastfeeding for at least 12 months, then for as long as is mutually agreeable to mother and child (AAP, 2012). Extending breastfeeding into toddlerhood is believed to be beneficial to the child. Extended breastfeeding provides nutritional, immunologic, and emotional benefits to the child. Contrary to popular belief, it is biologically possible to become pregnant while breastfeeding. Breastfeeding a newborn appropriately can occur while continuing to nurse the older sibling.

Weaning from breastfeeding tends to occur earlier in the United States than in countries around the world, despite recommendations on length of breastfeeding by a number of organizations. Most professional organizations recommend breastfeeding for at least 1 year (National Association of Pediatric Nurse Practitioners [NAPNAP], 2013).

Weaning is a highly individualized decision. Educate the mother about the benefits of extended breastfeeding and support her in her decision to wean at a given time.

Weaning from the bottle should occur by 12 to 15 months of age. Prolonged bottle-feeding is associated with the development of dental caries. No-spill "sippy cups" contain a valve that requires sucking by the toddler in order to obtain fluid, thus functioning similar to a baby bottle. Hence, no-spill sippy cups can also be associated with dental caries and are not recommended (American Academy of Pediatric Dentistry [AAPD], 2014). Cups with spouts that do not contain valves are acceptable. The 12- to 15-month-old is developmentally capable of consuming adequate fluid amounts using a cup.

Teaching About Nutritional Needs

Adequate calcium intake and appropriate exercise lay the foundation for proper bone mineralization. The toddler requires an average intake of 500 mg calcium per day (Ross, Taylor, Yaktine, & Del Valle, 2014). Dairy products are considered the primary sources of dietary calcium. One cup of low-fat or whole milk, 8 ounces of low-fat yogurt, and 1½ ounces of cheddar cheese each provide 300 mg of calcium. Broccoli, oranges, sweet potatoes, tofu, and dried beans or legumes are also good sources of calcium (35- to 120-mg calcium per serving).

Take Note!

Though a half-cup of cooked spinach contains 120 mg of calcium, it is essentially nonbioavailable, making spinach a poor source of calcium.

Iron-deficiency anemia in the first 2 years of life may be associated with developmental and psychomotor delays (Baker & Greer; Committee on Nutrition AAP, 2010). Although it is important for toddlers to consume adequate amounts of iron, they tend to have the lowest daily iron intake of any age group. When breastfeeding or formula-feeding ends (most often at 1 year of age), it is often replaced with iron-poor cow's milk. Limiting milk intake to 16 ounces per day, as well as limiting juice intake, can be helpful. Encourage the parents to provide iron-fortified cereals and other foods rich in iron and vitamin C.

Take Note!

Toddlers who consume a strictly vegan diet (no food from animal sources) are at risk for deficiencies in vitamin D, vitamin B_{12}, and iron. Supplementation with these nutrients should occur to promote adequate nutrition and growth (Stettler, Bhatia, Parish, & Stallings, 2011).

Fat or cholesterol intake should not be restricted in children younger than age 2 years. The first 2 years of life require high energy intake because they are a time of very rapid growth and development. To promote healthy cholesterol levels, children older than age 2 years should

BOX 26.4

KEY NUTRIENTS PROVIDED BY FRUITS AND VEGETABLES

Dietary fiber: applesauce, carrots, corn, green beans, mangos, pears
Folate: avocados, broccoli, green peas, oranges, spinach and dark greens, strawberries
Vitamin A: apricots, cantaloupe, carrots, mangos, spinach and dark greens, sweet potatoes
Vitamin C: broccoli, cantaloupe, green peas, oranges, potatoes, strawberries, tomatoes

Adapted from Brown, J. (2011). *Nutrition now* (6th ed.). Florence, KY: Wadsworth Publishing.

consume a diet with a total fat content between 20% and 30% of total calories. Saturated fats should account for less than 10% of total calories (Stettler, et al., 2011). Due to daily variations and the pickiness of the toddler, fat intake should be evaluated over a period of several days. The daily recommended intake of fiber for a 1- to 3-year-old is 19 g. Generally, toddler serving sizes should be about two-thirds that of an older child. Box 26.4 lists common sources of several nutrients.

Parents should encourage toddlers to drink water. Juice intake should be limited to 4 to 6 ounces per day. Milk intake should be limited to 16 to 24 ounces per day. Juice and milk should be served along with meals or snacks. Water should be offered for between-meal drinking. Toddlers should drink from a cup.

Advancing Solid Foods

Parents should offer three full meals and two snacks daily. Portion sizes for toddlers are about one-quarter the size of adult portions. Large portions of a new or different food on the toddler's plate may intimidate the toddler. Normal toddler behaviors of mouthing, handling, tasting, extruding the food from the mouth, and then resampling the food often occur. These behaviors are distasteful to some parents but are a normal part of toddler development. Parents need to understand and tolerate these behaviors rather than scolding the toddler for them (Brazelton & Sparrow, 2006). Toddlers are often afraid to try new things anyway, so the parent or caregiver should be flexible with the toddler's acceptance or rejection of new foods. If the toddler refuses healthy food choices at meal or snack time, parents should not substitute high-fat, high-sugar, processed food just to make sure that the child eats something (Stettler, et al., 2011). This sets the stage for future power struggles. The parent decides which foods will be served or offered. The toddler decides how much will be eaten. The toddler self-regulates the amount of food needed to sustain and allow further growth and development. The toddler may not eat well every day but generally, over the course of several days, will consume the foods he or she needs (Zero to Three, 2016b).

Foods should be served near room temperature. Some of the food on the plate should be soft and moist. Food should always be cut into bite-size pieces. Teaching Guidelines 26.2 gives recommendations on ways to prevent choking.

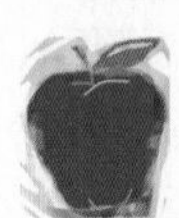

Teaching Guideline 26.2

AVOIDING CHOKING

- Slowly add foods that are more difficult to chew as the toddler becomes more adept at chewing.
- Cut all foods into bite-sized pieces.
- Avoid foods that are hard to chew and may become lodged in the airway, such as:
  - Nuts
  - Gumdrops or other chewy candies
  - Raw carrots
  - Peanut butter (by itself)
  - Popcorn
- Cut hotdogs and grapes into quarters. Cook carrots until soft; if serving raw, then grate them.
- Always supervise the toddler while he or she is eating.

Adapted from Brown, J. (2011). *Nutrition now* (6th ed.). Florence, KY: Wadsworth Publishing.

Promoting Self-Feeding

Toddlers most often eat with their fingers, but they do need to learn to use utensils properly. The following are suggestions for parents:

- Use a child-sized spoon and fork with dull tines.
- Seat the toddler in a high chair or at a comfortable height in a secure chair. The toddler should have his or her feet supported rather than dangling (Fig. 26.11).
- Never leave the toddler unattended while eating.
- Minimize distractions during mealtime. Serve food to the toddler along with the other members of the family (Gavin, 2014b).

Promoting Healthy Eating Habits

Since the toddler's rate of growth has slowed somewhat compared to that in infancy, the toddler requires less caloric intake for his or her size compared to the infant. This results in **physiologic anorexia**: toddlers simply do not require as much food intake for their size as they did in infancy. The toddler will also exhibit **food jags**. During a food jag, the toddler may prefer only one particular food for several days, then not want it for weeks. Again, it is important for the parent to continue to offer healthy food choices during a food jag and not give in by allowing the toddler to eat junk food (Gavin, 2014b).

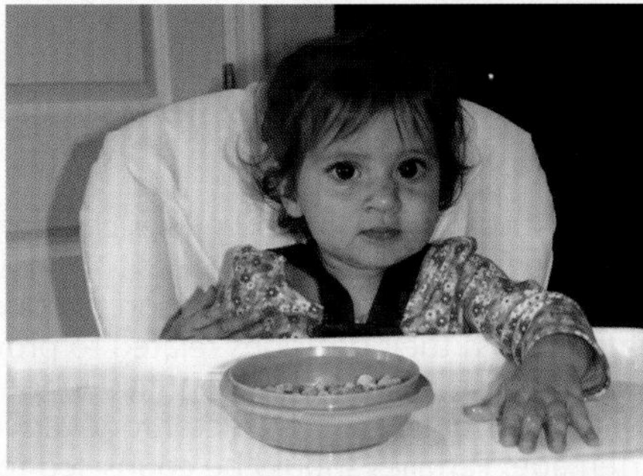
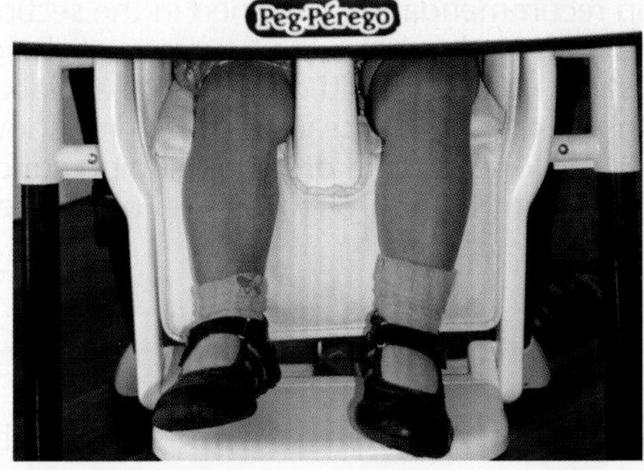

FIGURE 26.11 The toddler should be appropriately and safely seated in the high chair. The safety strap is secure, the toddler's feet are supported, and the tray table is locked in place.

The normal developmental issue of testing limits will also occur for the toddler at mealtime. Since toddlers still have limited ability to express their emotions with words, they use nonverbal behaviors to do so. While eating, the toddler may dislike the taste of a particular food or experience a feeling of fullness but will communicate that feeling by screaming or throwing food. When the child exhibits these behaviors, the parent must remain calm and remove the toddler from the situation. Meals should be eaten in a calm and pleasant environment. Parents should serve as role models for appropriate eating habits, but toddlers may also be willing to try more foods if they are exposed to other children who eat those foods. Praise the child for trying a new food, and never punish the toddler for refusing to try something new. A new food may need to be offered many times in a row before the toddler chooses to try it. Parents should be sure to include foods the child is familiar with and likes to eat at the same meal that the new food is being introduced (Zero to Three, 2016b). Teaching Guidelines 26.3 lists alternative foods that meet nutritional needs and a list of books for parents of the picky eater.

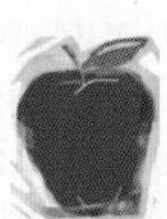

Teaching Guideline 26.3

MEETING NUTRITIONAL NEEDS OF THE PICKY EATER

Alternative Food Choices for the Picky Eater

- Won't drink milk? Obtain calcium through yogurt (frozen or regular), cheese, pudding, and hot cocoa.
- Poor meat intake? Obtain iron through unsweetened iron-fortified cereals or breakfast bars, or raisins; cook with an iron skillet.
- Loves processed white bread? Encourage fiber intake with fresh fruits and vegetables, bran muffins, beans, or peas (can be in soup).
- Refuses vegetables? Encourage vitamin A intake with apricots, sweet potatoes, and vegetable juices.

Books for Parents of the Picky Eater

- *Coping with a Picky Eater: A Guide for the Perplexed Parent* by W. Wilkoff. New York: Simon & Schuster 1998.
- *First Foods* by M. Stoddard. New York: Dorling-Kindersley Publishing, Inc., 1998.
- *How to Get Your Kid to Eat … But Not Too Much* by E. Satter. Boulder, CO: Bull Publishing Co., 1987.
- *The "Everything" Baby's First Food Book* by J. Tarlou. Holbrook, MA: Adams Media Corp., 2001.
- *The Family Nutrition Book* by W. Sears & M. Sears. Boston: Little Brown & Co., 1999.
- *The Healthy Baby Meal Planner* by A. Karmel. New York: Simon & Schuster, 2001.

Preventing Overweight and Obesity

In the child younger than 3 years of age, the greatest risk factor for the development of overweight or obesity is having a parent with a high body mass index (BMI) (Dev, et al., 2013). The nurse can screen for overweight in the child older than 2 years of age by calculating the BMI and plotting the BMI on the standardized age- and gender-appropriate growth charts (see Appendix A for growth charts, and refer to Chapter 32 for BMI calculation instructions). Trends over time may be predictive of the development of overweight or obesity.

Another factor in development of obesity in young children is juice intake (Stettler, et al., 2011). Since most young children like the sweet taste of juice, they may drink excessive amounts of it. Toddlers who drink excess fruit juice and eat well may develop overweight or obesity because of the high sugar content in the juice. On the other end of the spectrum, some children may actually feel full from juice consumption and decrease their intake of solid foods. These children are at risk for malnutrition. Fruit juice intake should be limited to 4 to 6 ounces per day. See Evidence-Based Practice 26.1.

Take Note!

Young children should consume only pasteurized juice, as unpasteurized juice consumption places the toddler at increased risk of *Escherichia coli*, *Salmonella*, and *Cryptosporidium* infection.

EVIDENCE-BASED PRACTICE 26.1 **PREVENTING OVERWEIGHT IN US KINDERGARTNERS**

STUDY

The researchers analyzed results from the Childhood Longitudinal Study-Birth Cohort (CLSBC). The CLSBC was a longitudinal cohort study following a total of 6,800 children from birth through kindergarten. A multitude of factors were analyzed to determine predictors of overweight at kindergarten age.

Findings

A modifiable risk factor identified as predicting kindergarten-age overweight, is having a body mass index (BMI) greater than or equal to the 85th percentile.

Nursing Implications

Overweight and obesity in childhood places children at risk for negative cardiovascular events and obesity ongoing into adulthood. Nurses are in the perfect position to educate and support families in their decisions related to providing nutrition to their young children. As identified in the study, overweight at 2 years of age is a predictor for overweight at kindergarten age. Families should be counseled to follow the nutrition recommendations outlined in the section above. Water or milk should be the beverage of choice with meals, and sugary drinks should generally be avoided. Providing low-nutrient foods at meals or snack time should not routinely occur. Nurses should provide ongoing education to families about nutrition throughout the toddler period.

Data from Flores, G. & Lin, H. (2013). Factors predicting overweight in U. S. kindergartners. *American Journal of Clinical Nutrition, 97*(6), 1178–1187.

Refer back to Jose Gonzales. What questions should you ask his parents related to his nutritional intake? What anticipatory guidance related to nutrition would be appropriate?

Promoting Healthy Sleep and Rest

The 18-month-old requires 13.5 hours of sleep per day, the 24-month-old 13 hours, and the 3-year-old 12 hours (Feigelman, 2011a, 2011b). A typical toddler should sleep through the night and take one daytime nap. Most children discontinue daytime napping at around 3 years of age. The toddler who slept in a crib as an infant will need to move to a youth or toddler bed or even a full-size bed usually sometime in the toddler period. When the crib becomes unsafe (i.e., when the toddler becomes physically capable of climbing over the rails), then he or she must make the transition to a bed.

Consistent bedtime rituals help the toddler prepare for sleep. Choose a bedtime and stick to it as much as possible. The nightly routine might include a bath followed by reading a story. The routine should be a calm period with minimal outside distractions. Toddlers often require a security item to help them get to sleep. Older toddlers may be afraid of the dark, so a nightlight is often helpful.

Night waking is a problem for some toddlers. This may occur as a result of change in routine or as a desire for nighttime attention. Attention during night waking should be minimized so that the toddler receives no reward for being awake at night. The book *Solve Your Child's Sleep Problems,* by Dr. Richard Ferber (2006, New York: Fireside Publishing), is an excellent resource for the family with a toddler who resists bedtime or is a persistent night waker. For some toddlers, night waking is caused by nightmares. As the imagination and capacity for make-believe grow, the toddler may not be able to distinguish between reality and pretend. The parent should hold and comfort the toddler after a nightmare. Limiting television viewing (especially shortly before bedtime) may be helpful in limiting nightmares.

Some families practice "co-sleeping" (when children sleep in the parents' bed). Although some professionals believe that co-sleeping may interfere with the toddler's struggle for independence, this theory has not been proven. The nurse should support the family's choice for sleep arrangements unless the co-sleeping is unsafe either physically or psychologically (SafeBedSharing.org, 2016). Refer to http://www.safebedsharing.org for bed-sharing safety guidelines.

Provide anticipatory guidance to Jose Gonzales' parents in relation to his sleep.

Promoting Healthy Teeth and Gums

By 30 months of age, the toddler should have a full set of primary ("baby") teeth. Parents may not be aware of the importance of preventing cavities in primary teeth since they will eventually be replaced by the permanent teeth. Poor oral hygiene, prolonged use of a bottle or no-spill sippy cup, lack of fluoride intake, and delayed or absent professional dental care may all contribute to the development of dental caries (AAP, n. d.). Cleaning of the toddler's teeth should progress from brushing with simply water to using a very small amount (pea-sized) of fluoridated toothpaste with brushing beginning at 2 years of age (Fig. 26.12). Weaning from the bottle no later than 15 months of age and severely restricting use

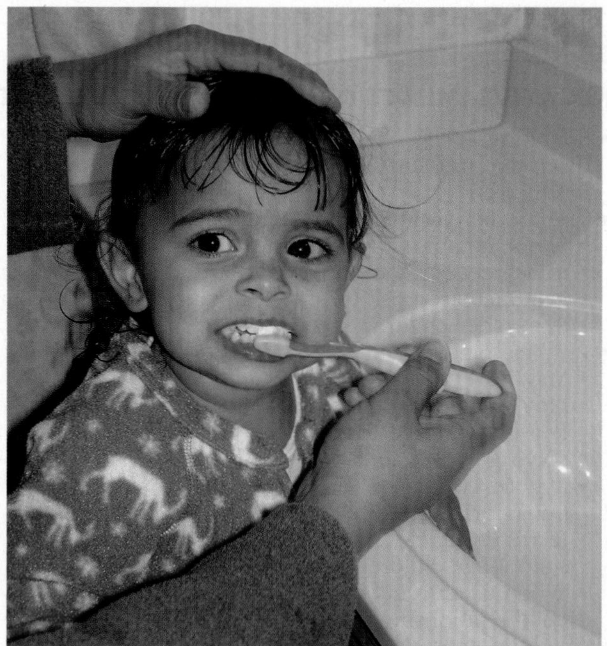

FIGURE 26.12 The parent should brush the toddler's teeth to ensure proper cleaning of the teeth, gums, and tongue. Use only water for brushing before 2 years of age and a pea-sized amount of fluoride-containing toothpaste after age 2 years.

of a no-spill sippy cup (the kind that requires sucking for fluid delivery) is recommended.

At age 1 year, the toddler should have his or her first dentist visit to establish current health of the teeth and gums. Eating should be limited to meal and snack times, as "grazing" throughout the day exposes the teeth to food throughout the day. Carbohydrate-containing foods combined with oral bacteria create a decreased oral pH level that is optimal for the development of dental caries (cavities). See Healthy People 2020.

Public water fluoridation is a public health initiative that ensures that most children receive adequate fluoride intake to prevent dental caries. Table 26.5 gives recommendations regarding fluoride supplementation. If the water supply contains adequate fluoride, no other supplementation is necessary other than brushing with a small amount of fluoride-containing toothpaste after age 2 years. Excess fluoride ingestion should be avoided, as it contributes to the development of fluorosis (mottling of the enamel). Fluorosis occurs most often in the toddler years (AAP, 2012). Risk factors for fluorosis development include:

- High fluoride levels in the local water supply
- Use of fluoride-containing toothpaste prior to age 2 years
- Excessive ingestion of fluoride either in toothpaste or foods
  - Fluoride-containing foods: tea, ready-to-eat infant foods containing chicken, white or purple grape juice, and beverages, processed foods, and cereals that were manufactured with fluoride-containing water

HEALTHY PEOPLE 2020

Objective	Nursing Significance
Reduce the proportion of children with untreated dental decay.	• Encourage weaning from bottle by 15 months of age. • Discourage use of no-spill sippy cups. • Refer any toddler with potential or existing caries to a pediatric dentist.

Healthy People Objectives retrieved from http://www.healthypeople.gov

TABLE 26.5 RECOMMENDATIONS FOR FLUORIDE SUPPLEMENTATION

	Fluoride Ion Level in Drinking Water (ppm)		
Age	*<0.3 ppm*	*0.3–0.6 ppm*	*>0.6 ppm*
Birth to 6 months	None	None	None
6 months to 3 years	0.25 mg/day	None	None
3–6 years	0.50 mg/day	0.25 mg/day	None
6–16 years	1.0 mg/day	0.50 mg/day	None

ppm, parts per million is equivalent to 1 mg/L.

These recommendations are public domain at www.ada.org and were approved by the American Dental Association, the American Academy of Pediatrics, and the American Academy of Pediatric Dentistry.

Promoting Appropriate Discipline

Discipline is a common concern during toddlerhood. The toddler's intense personality and extreme emotional reactions can be difficult for parents to understand and cope with. The toddler needs firm, gentle guidance to learn what the expectations are and how to meet them. The parent's love and respect for the toddler teach the toddler to care about himself or herself and for others. Affection is as important as the guidance aspect of discipline. Having realistic expectations of what the toddler is capable of learning and understanding can help the parent in the disciplinary process. The toddler's intense push for autonomy can often test a parent's limits. The easygoing infant usually becomes more challenging in toddlerhood. The toddler's continual quest for new experiences often places the toddler at risk, and his or her negativism very often taxes the parent's patience.

In an effort to prevent the toddler from experiencing harm and in response to his or her continual testing of limits, parents often resort to spanking. Though commonly accepted, the AAP and the NAPNAP recommend against corporal or physical punishment (American Academy of Child and Adolescent Psychiatry, 2012; NAPNAP, 2011). Recent research points out the dangers inherent in the use of corporal punishment as well as the possibilities for negative effects on the child's future behavior (Box 26.5). Spanking or other forms of corporal punishment lead to a pro-violence attitude, create resentment and anger in some children, and contribute to the cycle of violence (NAPNAP, 2011).

BOX 26.5

NEGATIVE IMPACT OF PHYSICAL PUNISHMENT

- Spanking is less effective than time-out or other discipline measures to reduce undesired behavior in children.
- The toddler younger than 18 months of age:
  - Is not capable of making the appropriate connections between spanking and the undesired behavior
  - Is at increased risk for physical injury from spanking than older children
- Physical punishment:
  - May lead to a pro-violence attitude
  - May create resentment in the toddler
  - Is a poor model for learning effective problem solving
  - May be correlated with antisocial and criminal behavior later in life
  - Leads to increased aggression in preschoolers, school-age children, and adults
  - When used frequently, may weaken the parent–child relationship
- Childhood corporal punishment increases the probability of depression and substance abuse in adulthood.
- Spanking may lead to more severe forms of punishment and to actual child abuse and maltreatment.
- The more frequently children are hit or spanked, the more likely they are to hit their own children and to be involved in spouse abuse as adults.

Adapted from Global Initiative to End All Corporal Punishment of Children. (n. d.). *Global initiative to end corporal punishment.* Retrieved from www.endcorporalpunishment.org; and National Association of Pediatric Nurse Practitioners. (2011). NAPNAP position statement on corporal punishment. *Journal of Pediatric Health Care, 25,* p. e31-e32.

Take Note!

Toddlers younger than 18 months of age should NEVER be spanked, as there is an increased possibility of physical injury in this age group. Also, the infant/young toddler is not capable of linking the spanking with the undesired behavior (Lyness, 2013).

Normal toddler development includes natural curiosity, and this curiosity often results in dangerous or problematic activities for the toddler (Lyness, 2013). Toddlers have a difficult time learning the rules and, in general, do not behave badly intentionally. Providing a childproof environment will allow the toddler to participate in safe exploration, which will meet his or her developmental needs and decrease the frequency of intervention needed on the part of the parents.

Discipline should focus on limit setting, negotiation, and techniques to assist the toddler to learn problem solving. Parents should provide consistency and commit to the limits that are set.

Offering realistic choices helps give the toddler a sense of mastery. Rules should be simple and limited in number. Maintaining the toddler's schedule of meals and rest/sleep will help to prevent conflicts that occur as a result of hunger or fatigue. Toddlers should not be made to share, as this is a concept they do not understand. Parents should encourage simple activities enjoyed by the children involved and avoid confrontation over toys. Parents should offer toddlers appropriate choices to help them develop autonomy, but should not offer a choice when none exists.

Positive reinforcement should be used as much as possible. "Catching" a child being good helps to reinforce appropriate or desirable behaviors. When the toddler is displaying appropriate behavior, the parent should reward the child consistently with praise and physical affection.

"Time-out" can be used effectively at around 2.5 to 3 years of age (refer to Chapter 27 for details). "Extinction" is a particularly useful technique with 2- and 3-year-olds. Extinction involves systematic ignoring of the undesired behavior. Parents sometimes unknowingly contribute to the occurrence of an unwanted behavior simply by the attention they give the toddler (even if it is negative in nature, it is still attention). Parents who want to extinguish an annoying (nondangerous) behavior should resolve to ignore it every time it occurs. When the child withholds the behavior or performs the opposite (appropriate) behavior, they should use compliments and praise. It may be difficult to ignore a difficult behavior, but the results are well worth the effort. Teaching Guidelines 26.4 provides tips on avoiding power struggles and offering appropriate guidance to toddlers.

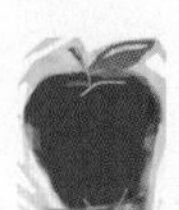

Teaching Guideline 26.4

PROVIDING TODDLERS WITH GUIDANCE

- When giving the toddler instructions, tell the child what to do, NOT what not to do. This allows for a positive focus. If you must say "no," "don't," or "stop," then follow with a direction of what to do instead.
- Offer limited choices, when a choice is truly available. Say, "Do you want to wear your blue hat or your red hat?" NOT "Do you want to put on your hat?" This gives the toddler some, but not all, control.
- Role model appropriate communication, but don't feel like you have to speak nicely all the time. If the situation warrants, use a firm and even tone to get the point across. Avoid yelling.
- Pay attention to the inflection in your voice. A statement or direction should not end in a questioning tone or with "Okay?" Be clear. Statements should sound like statements, and only questions should end in a questioning tone.
- When a toddler behaves aggressively, label the child's feelings calmly, but be firm and consistent with the expectation. For example, "I know you're mad at your friend, but it is not okay to hit."

Adapted from Lyness, D. (2013). Disciplining your toddler. Retrieved from http://kidshealth.org/parent/positive/talk/toddler_tantrums.html# and Sears, W. & Sears, M. (2016b). 8 tools for toddler discipline. Retrieved from http://www.askdrsears.com/topics/parenting/discipline-behavior/8-tools-toddler-discipline

ADDRESSING COMMON DEVELOPMENTAL CONCERNS

Common developmental concerns of the toddler period are toilet teaching, temper tantrums, thumb sucking or pacifier use, sibling rivalry, and regression. An understanding of the normalcy of negativism, temper tantrums, and sibling rivalry will help the family cope with these issues. Prepare parents for these developmental events by giving appropriate anticipatory guidance.

Toilet Teaching

When myelination of the spinal cord is achieved around age 2 years, the toddler is capable of exercising voluntary control over the sphincters. Girls may be ready for toilet teaching earlier than boys. Toddlers are ready for toilet teaching when:

- Bowel movements occur on a fairly regular schedule.
- The toddler expresses knowledge of the need to defecate or urinate. This may be through verbalization, change in activity, or gestures such as:
  - Looks into or grabs diaper
  - Squats
  - Crosses legs
  - Grimaces and/or grunts
  - Hides behind a door or the couch when defecating
- The diaper is not always wet (this indicates the ability to hold the urine for a period of time).
- The toddler is willing to follow instructions.
- The toddler walks well alone and is able to pull down his or her pants.
- The toddler follows caregivers to the bathroom.
- The toddler climbs onto the potty chair or toilet (AAP, 2015d).

Parents should approach toilet teaching with a calm, positive, and nonthreatening manner. Initially it may be helpful to allow the toddler to observe a same-sex family member using the toilet. Start with the toddler fully clothed on the potty chair or toilet while the parent or caregiver talks about what the toilet is used for and when. The toddler will feel most comfortable with a toddler potty chair that sits on the floor (Fig. 26.13). If a potty chair is unavailable, facing toward the toilet tank may make the toddler feel more secure, as the buttocks remain on the front of the seat rather than sinking through the toilet seat opening. After a week or longer, remove a dirty diaper and place the contents in the toilet. Next, try having the toddler sit on the potty chair or toilet without pants or diaper on. The toddler may benefit from watching a caregiver or friend use the toilet. It may also be beneficial to demonstrate using the potty chair with a baby doll that wets.

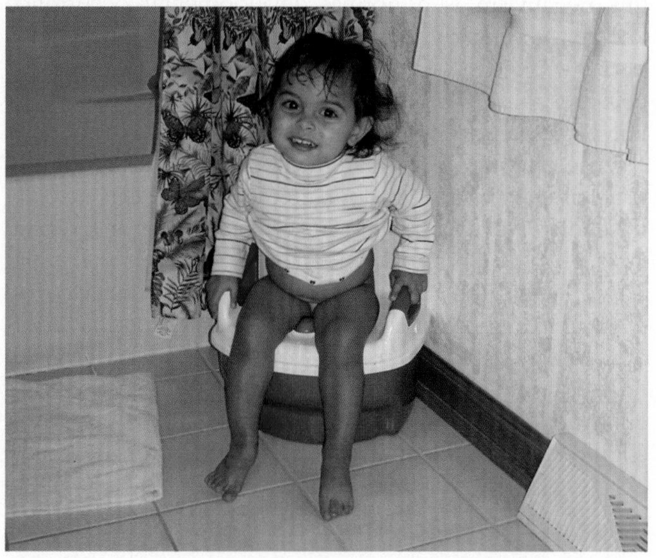

FIGURE 26.13 The toddler will feel most comfortable with a potty chair that sits on the floor.

Parents should always use gentle praise and no reproaches. Usually the best time to achieve success with defecation on the toilet is following a meal. When the toddler has achieved success with bowel control, bladder control will come next. It may be many months before nighttime bladder control is achieved, and the toddler may still require a diaper at night. Parents should use appropriate words for body parts, urination, and defecation, then use those words consistently so the toddler understands what to say and do (AAP, 2015d).

After a couple of weeks of successful toileting, the toddler may start wearing training pants. When toddlers have an accident and do not make it to the toilet, gently remind them about toileting and let them help clean up. Toddlers should never be punished for bowel or bladder "accidents."

With so much attention focused on the genitalia during toilet teaching and the frequency of being without a diaper, it is natural for toddlers to become more focused on their own genitalia. Boys and girls both will explore their genitalia and discover the resulting pleasurable sensation. Masturbation in the toddler often causes a great deal of discomfort in the parent. The parent should not draw attention to the activity, as that may increase its frequency. The parent should calmly explain to the toddler that this is an activity that may only be done in private (Feigelman, 2011b). If the toddler is masturbating excessively or refuses to stop when in public, then there may be additional stressors in the toddler's life that should be explored.

Negativism

Negativism is common in the toddler period (Brazelton & Sparrow, 2006). As the toddler separates from the parent, recognizes his or her own individuality, and exerts autonomy, negativism abounds. Parents should understand that this negativism is a normal developmental occurrence and not necessarily deliberate defiance (though that also occurs). Avoid asking yes-or-no questions, as the toddler's usual response will be "no," whether he or she means it or not. Offering the child simple choices will give the toddler a sense of control. The parent should not ask the toddler if he or she "wants" to do something, if there is actually no choice. "Do you want to use the red cup or the blue cup?" is more appropriate than "Do you want your milk now?" When it is time to go outside, don't ask, "Do you want to put your shoes on?" Instead, state in a matter-of-fact tone that shoes must be worn outside, and give the toddler a choice of type of shoe or color of socks. If the child continues with negative answers, then the parent should remain calm and make the decision for the child.

Temper Tantrums

Even children who displayed an easygoing personality as infants may lose their temper frequently during the toddler years (Fig. 26.14). A toddler who was more intense as an infant may have more temper tantrums. Temper tantrums are a natural result of the frustration that toddlers experience. Toddlers are eager to explore new things, but their efforts are often thwarted (usually for safety reasons). Toddlers do not behave badly on purpose. They need time and maturity to learn the rules and regulations. Some of their frustration may come from lack of language skills to express themselves. Toddlers are just starting to learn how to verbalize feelings and to use alternative actions rather than just "pitching a fit." The temper tantrum may be manifested as a screaming and crying fit or a full-blown episode in which the toddler throws himself or herself on the floor kicking, screaming, and pounding, perhaps even holding the breath. Fatigue or hunger may limit the toddler's coping abilities and promote negative behavior and temper tantrums (Lyness, 2013).

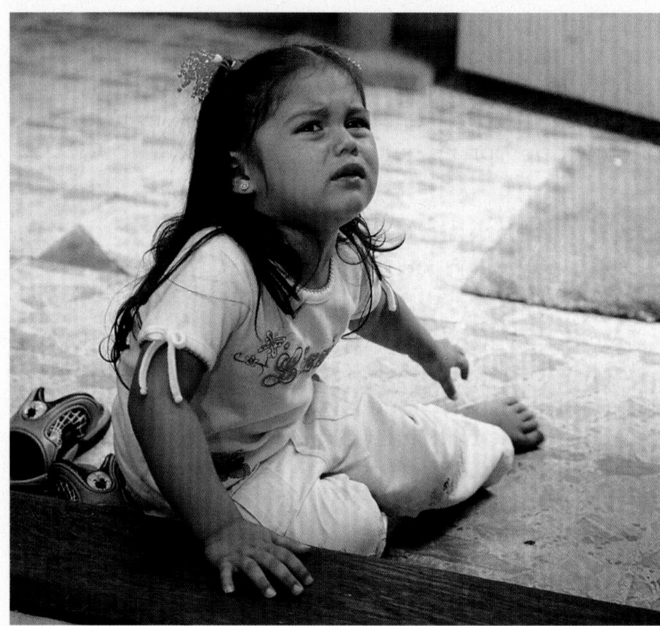

FIGURE 26.14 Tantrums are a normal component of toddler development.

Although tantrums are annoying to parents and caregivers, they are a normal part of the toddler's quest for independence. As toddlers mature, they become better able to express themselves and to understand their environment.

Parents need to learn their toddler's behavioral cues in order to limit activity that is frustrating. When the parent notes the beginnings of frustration, a friendly warning might be given. Intervening early with an activity change might prevent a tantrum. Use distraction, refocusing, or removal from the situation.

When a temper tantrum does occur, the best course of action is to ignore the behavior and ensure that the child is safe during the tantrum. Physical punishment will probably just prolong the tantrum and in fact produce more intense negative behavior. If the tantrum occurs in public, it may be necessary for the parent to immobilize the child with a big bear hug and use a calm voice to soothe the toddler. It is very important for parents to model self-control. Since toddlers' tantrums most often result from frustration, the role-modeled behavior of self-control helps to teach toddlers to control their temper when they can't get what they want (Lyness, 2013).

Thumb Sucking and Pacifiers

Infants bring their hands to their mouths and begin thumb sucking as a form of self-soothing (Sears & Sears, 2016c). This habit may continue into the toddler years and beyond. The pacifier is used for the same reason. Toddlers may calm themselves in a stressful situation by thumb sucking or sucking on a pacifier. Opinions about thumb and finger sucking and pacifier use are significantly affected by family history and culture. For most children there is no need to worry about a sucking habit until it is time for the permanent teeth to erupt. Prolonged and frequent sucking in the withdrawn child is more likely to yield changes to the tooth and jaw structure than sucking that is primarily used for self-soothing. Parents must sort through their own feelings about thumb sucking and pacifier use and then decide how they want to handle the habit.

To ensure safety with pacifier use:

- Use only one-piece pacifiers.
- Replace worn pacifiers with new ones.
- Never tie a pacifier around a toddler's neck.

Parents may want to limit thumb sucking and pacifier use to bedtime, in the car, and in stressful situations. The parent should calmly discuss these limits with the toddler and then remain consistent about enforcing them (Sears & Sears, 2016a, 2016c).

Sibling Rivalry

Many families have subsequent children when their first child is a toddler. The toddler has been accustomed to being the baby and receiving a great deal of attention, both at home and with the extended family. Since toddlers are normally egocentric, bringing a new baby into the home may be quite disruptive. To minimize issues with **sibling rivalry**, parents should attempt to keep the toddler's routine as close to normal as possible. Spend individual time with the toddler on a daily basis. Involve the toddler in the care of the baby. The toddler is capable of fetching a diaper or T-shirt, entertaining the baby with a toy, or helping sing a song to calm the baby (Hirsch, 2013). "Helping" the parent care for the baby gives the toddler a sense of importance (Fig. 26.15). The toddler will need significant support while holding the baby.

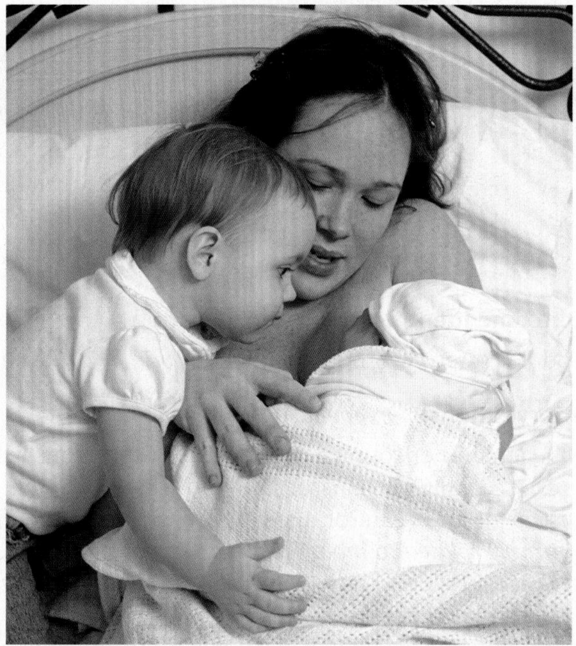

FIGURE 26.15 The toddler may be more likely to accept the new baby in a positive manner if she feels that this is "our baby," not just "mommy's baby." This toddler is meeting her new brother for the first time.

Regression

Some toddlers experience **regression** during a stressful event (e.g., the birth of a sibling, hospitalization). Stress in a toddler's life affects his or her ability to master new developmental tasks. During regression, the toddler may want to go back to an earlier stage. He or she may desire a bottle or pacifier forgotten long ago. The toddler may stop displaying previously achieved language or motor skills. A significant stress in the toddler's life may also disrupt the toilet teaching process (toilet teaching may not be achieved near the time a sibling is born). When regression occurs, parents should ignore the regressive behavior and offer praise for age-appropriate behavior or attainment of skills (Hirsch, 2013).

Refer to Jose Gonzales, the 2-year-old in the case study. List common developmental concerns of the toddler. What anticipatory guidance related to these concerns would the nurse provide to Jose's parents?

NURSING CARE PLAN 26.1

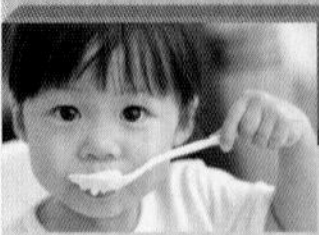

Growth and Development Issues in the Toddler

NURSING DIAGNOSIS: Risk for injury related to curiosity, increased mobility, and developmental immaturity

Outcome Identification and Evaluation

Toddler safety will be maintained: *Toddler will remain free from injury.*

Interventions: ***Preventing Injury***

- Teach and encourage appropriate use of rear-facing car seat until 2 years of age and forward-facing car seat after 2 years of age *to decrease risk of toddler injury related to motor vehicles.*
- Teach toddlers to stay away from the street and provide constant supervision *to prevent pedestrian injury.*
- Require bicycle helmet use while riding any wheeled toy *to prevent head injury and form habit of helmet use.*
- Childproof the home *to provide a developmentally safe environment for the curious and increasingly mobile toddler.*
- Post poison control center phone number *in case of accidental ingestion.*
- Never leave a toddler unattended in a tub or pool or near any body of water *to prevent drowning.*
- Teach parents first-aid measures and child CPR *to minimize consequences of injury should it occur.*
- Provide close observation and keep side rails up on crib/bed in hospital *because toddlers are at particularly high risk for falling or becoming entangled in tubing as they attempt mobility.*

NURSING DIAGNOSIS: Imbalanced nutrition, less than body requirements, related to inappropriate nutritional intake to sustain growth needs (excess juice or milk intake, inadequate food variety intake) as evidenced by failure to attain adequate increases in height and weight over time

Outcome Identification and Evaluation

Toddler will consume adequate nutrients while using an appropriate feeding pattern: *Toddler will demonstrate weight gain and increases in height.*

Interventions: ***Promoting Appropriate Nutrition***

- Assess current feeding schedule and usual intake, as well as methods used to feed, *to determine areas of adequacy versus inadequacy.*
- Determine toddler's ability to drink from cup, finger feed, swallow, and consume textures *to determine if additional exposure is needed or if further interventions such as speech or occupational therapy are required.*
- Weigh toddler daily on same scale if hospitalized, weekly on same scale if at home, and plot growth patterns weekly or monthly as appropriate on standardized growth charts *to determine if growth is improving.*
- Wean from bottle by 15 months of age *to discourage excess milk or juice intake in toddler who can carry bottle around.*
- Limit juice to 4 to 6 ounces per day and milk to 16 to 24 ounces per day *to discourage sense of fullness achieved with excess milk or juice intake, thereby increasing appetite for solid foods.*
- Provide three nutrient-dense meals and at least two healthy snacks per day *to encourage adequate nutrient consumption.*
- Feed toddler on a similar schedule daily, without distractions and with the family: *toddlers respond well to routine and structure and may eat better in the social context of meals, and they become distracted easily (TV should be off).*

NURSING CARE PLAN 26.1

Growth and Development Issues in the Toddler (continued)

NURSING DIAGNOSIS: Delayed growth and development related to motor, cognitive, language, or psychosocial concerns as evidenced by delay in meeting expected milestones

Outcome Identification and Evaluation

Development will be enhanced: *Toddler will make continued progress toward realization of expected developmental milestones.*

Interventions: *Enhancing Growth and Development*

- Screen for developmental capabilities to determine toddler's current level of functioning.
- Offer age-appropriate toys, play, and activities (including gross motor) to encourage further development.
- Perform interventions as prescribed by physical, occupational, or speech therapist: participation in those activities helps to promote function and accomplish acquisition of developmental skills.
- Provide support to families of toddlers with developmental delay (progress in achieving developmental milestones can be slow and ongoing motivation is needed).
- Reinforce positive attributes in the toddler to maintain motivation.
- Model age-appropriate communication skills to illustrate suitable means for parenting the toddler.

NURSING DIAGNOSIS: Risk for disproportionate growth related to excess milk or juice intake, late bottle weaning, and consumption of inappropriate foods or in excess amounts

Outcome Identification and Evaluation

Toddler will grow appropriately and not become overweight or obese: *Toddler will achieve weight and height within the 5th to 95th percentiles on standardized growth charts.*

Interventions: *Promoting Proportionate Growth*

- Wean from bottle and discourage use of no-spill sippy cups by 15 months of age (will keep mobile toddler from carrying around and continually drinking from cup or bottle).
- Provide juice (4 to 6 ounces per day) and milk (16 to 24 ounces per day) from a cup at meal and snack time to encourage appropriate cup drinking and limit intake of nutrient-poor, high-calorie fluids.
- Provide only nutrient-rich foods without high sugar content for meals and snacks; even if the toddler won't eat, it is inappropriate to provide high-calorie junk food just so the toddler eats something.
- Ensure adequate physical activity to stimulate development of motor skills and provide appropriate caloric expenditure. This also sets the stage for forming lifelong habit of appropriate physical activity.

NURSING DIAGNOSIS: Interrupted family processes related to issues with toddler development, hospitalization, or situational crisis as evidenced by decreased parental visitation in hospital, parental verbalization of difficulty with current situation, possible crisis related to health of family member other than the toddler

Outcome Identification and Evaluation

Family will demonstrate adequate functioning: *Family will display coping and psychosocial adjustment.*

(continued)

NURSING CARE PLAN 26.1

Growth and Development Issues in the Toddler (continued)

Interventions: ***Enhancing Family Functioning***

- Assess the family's level of stress and ability to cope to determine family's ability to cope with multiple stressors.
- Engage in family-centered care to provide a holistic approach to care of the toddler and family.
- Encourage the family to verbalize feelings (verbalization is one method of decreasing anxiety levels), and acknowledge feelings and emotions.
- Encourage family visitation and provide for sleeping arrangements for a parent or caregiver to stay in the hospital with the toddler (contributes to family's sense of control of situation).
- Involve family members in toddler's care, giving them a feeling of control and connectedness.

NURSING DIAGNOSIS: Readiness for enhanced parenting related to parental desire for increased skills and success with toddler as evidenced by current healthy relationships and verbalization of desire for improved skills

Outcome Identification and Evaluation

Parent will provide safe and nurturing environment for the toddler.

Interventions: ***Increasing Parenting Skill Set***

- Use family-centered care to provide holistic approach.
- Educate parent about normal toddler development to provide basis for understanding the parenting skills needed in this time period.
- Acknowledge and encourage parent's verbalization of feelings related to chronic illness of child or difficulty with normal toddler behavior to validate the normalcy of the parent's feelings.
- Encourage positive parenting with respect to toddlers and their normal development (helps parents develop approaches to toddlers that can be used in place of anger and frustration).
- Acknowledge and admire positive parenting skills already present to contribute to parents' confidence in their abilities to parent.
- Role model appropriate parenting behaviors related to communicating with and disciplining the toddler (role modeling actually shows rather than just telling the parent what to do).

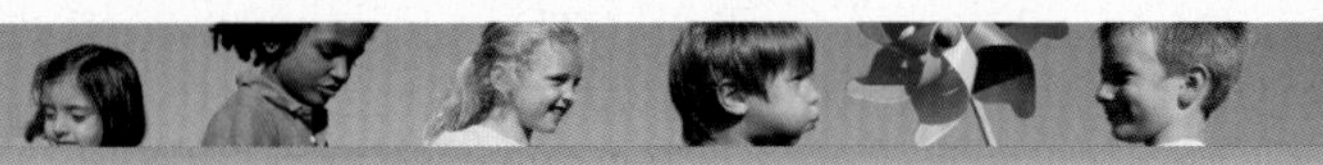

KEY CONCEPTS

- The toddler's organ systems are continuing to mature, and growth slows during this period as compared with infancy.
- The psychosocial task of the toddler years is to attain a sense of autonomy and to experience separation and individuation.
- Cognitive development in toddlerhood progresses from sensorimotor in nature to preoperational.
- The toddler refines gross motor skills after learning to walk and builds fine motor skills through the use of utensils and various manipulative toys.
- The toddler progresses from limited expressive language capabilities to a vocabulary of 900 words by age 3 years.
- Toddlers use all of their senses to explore and learn about their environment.
- Visual acuity progresses to at least 20/50 in the toddler period.

- Negativism abounds in toddlers as they attempt to exert their independence.
- Very ritualistic, toddlers feel safer and more secure when clear limits are enforced and a structured routine is followed.
- The toddler is starting to learn right from wrong and bases actions on punishment avoidance.
- Toddler development may be promoted through active gross motor play, books, music, and block building.
- Safety is a primary concern in the toddler years as the child is more mobile, very curious, and experimenting with autonomy.
- Poisoning in the toddler period may be prevented through proper storage of medications and other potentially poisonous substances and appropriate supervision.
- Consistent bedtime rituals help ease the toddler's transition to sleep.
- All primary teeth are erupted by 30 months of age and may be kept healthy with appropriate tooth brushing and fluoride supplementation.
- The toddler may experience a decrease in appetite as growth slows, yet he or she still needs appropriate nutritional intake for continued development.
- Toilet teaching can be achieved after myelination of the spinal cord is complete, usually around 2 years of age.
- Thumb sucking, pacifier use, security items, and temper tantrums are expected issues in the toddler years.
- Toddler discipline should focus on clear limits and consistency. It should not involve spanking. It should be balanced with a caring and nurturing environment along with frequent praise for appropriate behavior.
- Parental role modeling of appropriate behavior, especially related to dealing with frustration, is beneficial to toddlers.
- Parents play an important role in toddler development, not only by providing a loving environment but also by role modeling appropriate behavior in most areas of daily life.

REFERENCES AND RECOMMENDED READINGS

American Academy of Child and Adolescent Psychiatry. (2012). *Policy statement on corporal punishment.* Retrieved from http://www.aacap.org/aacap/Policy_Statements/2012/Policy_Statement_on_Corporal_Punishment.aspx

American Academy of Pediatrics. (n. d.). *Protecting all children's teeth.* Retrieved from http://www2.aap.org/oralhealth/pact/pact-home.cfm

American Academy of Pediatrics. (2012). Breastfeeding and the use of human milk. *Pediatrics, 129*(3), e827–e841.

American Academy of Pediatric Dentistry. (2014). *Guideline on infant oral health care.* Retrieved from http://www.aapd.org/media/Policies_Guidelines/G_InfantOralHealthCare.pdf

American Academy of Pediatrics. (2013). *Guns safety: Keeping children safe.* Retrieved from https://www.healthychildren.org/English/safety-prevention/all-around/Pages/Gun-Safety-Keeping-Children-Safe.aspx

American Academy of Pediatrics, The Injury Prevention Program. (2015a). *Safety for your child: 1 to 2 years.* Retrieved from http://www.healthychildren.org/english/tips-tools/Pages/Safety-for-Your-Child-1-to-2-Years.aspx

American Academy of Pediatrics, The Injury Prevention Program. (2015b). *Safety for your child: 2 to 4 years.* Retrieved from http://www.healthychildren.org/english/tips-tools/Pages/Safety-for-Your-Child-2-to-4-Years.aspx

American Academy of Pediatrics. (2015c). *Poison prevention.* Retrieved from https://www.healthychildren.org/English/safety-prevention/all-around/Pages/Poison-Prevention.aspx

American Academy of Pediatrics. (2015d). *Toilet training: Which method is best?* Retrieved from https://www.healthychildren.org/English/ages-stages/toddler/toilet-training/Pages/Toilet-Training-Which-Method-is-Best.aspx

American Academy of Pediatrics. (2016). *Car seats: Information for families.* Retrieved from https://www.healthychildren.org/English/safety-prevention/on-the-go/Pages/Car-Safety-Seats-Information-for-Families.aspx

American Association of Poison Control Centers. (n. d.). *In the home.* Retrieved from http://www.aapcc.org/prevention/home/

Baker, R. D., & Greer, F. R.; Committee on Nutrition American Academy of Pediatrics. (2010). Diagnosis and prevention of iron deficiency and iron-deficiency anemia in infants and young children (0–3 years of age). *Pediatrics, 126,* 1040–1050.

Brazelton, T. B., & Sparrow, J. D. (2006). *Touchpoints, birth to 3.* Cambridge, MA: Da Capo Press.

Brown, J. (2011). *Nutrition now* (6th ed.). Florence, KY: Wadsworth Publishing.

Carpenito-Moyet, L. J. (2013). *Nursing diagnosis: Application to clinical practice* (14th ed.). Philadelphia, PA: Lippincott Williams & Wilkins.

Child Development Institute. (2015). *Is your child easy or difficult to raise?* Retrieved from http://childdevelopmentinfo.com/child-development/temperament_and_your_child/

Dev, D. A., McBride, B. A., Fiese, B. H., Jones, B. L., Cho, H. & on behalf of the Strong Kids Research Team. (2013). Risk factors for overweight/obesity in preschool children: An ecological approach. *Childhood Obesity, 9*(5), 399–408.

Erikson, E. H. (1963). *Childhood and society* (2nd ed.). New York: W.W. Norton and Company

Feigelman, S. (2011a). Preschool years. In R. M. Kliegman, B. F. Stanton, J. W. St. Geme III, N. F. Schor, & R. E. Behrman (Eds.), (*Nelson's textbook of pediatrics* (19th ed.). Philadelphia, PA: Elsevier, Saunders.

Feigelman, S. (2011b). The second year. In R. M. Kliegman, B. F. Stanton, J. W. St. Geme III, N. F. Schor, & R. E. Behrman

(Eds.), (*Nelson's textbook of pediatrics* (19th ed.). Philadelphia, PA: Elsevier, Saunders.

Flores, G., & Lin, H. (2013). Factors predicting overweight in U. S. kindergartners. *American Journal of Clinical Nutrition, 97*(6), 1178–1187.

Gavin, M. L. (2014a). *Fitness and your 2- to 3-year-old.* Retrieved from http://kidshealth.org/en/parents/fitness-2-3.html

Gavin, M. (2014b). *Toddlers at the table: Avoiding power struggles.* Retrieved from http://kidshealth.org/en/parents/toddler-meals.html#

Giles, L. C., Davies, M. J., Whitrow, M. J., Warin, M. J., & Moore, V. (2011). Maternal depressive symptoms and child care during toddlerhood relate to child behavior at age 5 years. *Pediatrics, 128*(1), e78–e84.

Global Initiative to End All Corporal Punishment of Children. (n. d.). *Global initiative to end corporal punishment.* Retrieved from www.endcorporalpunishment.org

Goldson, E., & Reynolds, A. (2014). Child development and behavior. In W. W. Hay, Jr., M. J. Levin, R. R. Deterding, & M. J. Abzug (Eds.), *Current diagnosis and treatment: Pediatrics* (22nd ed.). New York, NY: McGraw-Hill Education.

Hirsch, L. (2013). *Birth of a second child.* Retrieved from http://kidshealth.org/en/parents/second-child.html#

Hwang, S., Hwang, J. H., Moon, J. S., & Lee, D. (2012). Environmental tobacco smoke and children's health. *Korean Journal of Pediatrics, 55*(2), 35–41. doi: 10.3345/kjp.2012.55.2.35

Kohlberg, L. (1984). *Moral development.* New York: Harper & Row.

Lowry, L. (2011). *Bilingualism in young children: Separating fact from fiction.* Retrieved from http://www.hanen.org/Helpful-Info/Articles/Bilingualism-in-Young-Children--Separating-Fact-fr.aspx

Lyness, D. (2013). *Disciplining your toddler.* Retrieved from http://kidshealth.org/parent/positive/talk/toddler_tantrums.html#

National Association for the Education of Young Children. (n. d.). *Good toys for young children by age and stage.* Retrieved from http://www.naeyc.org/toys

National Association of Pediatric Nurse Practitioners. (2011). NAPNAP position statement on corporal punishment. *Journal of Pediatric Health Care, 25,* e31–e32.

National Association of Pediatric Nurse Practitioners. (2013). NAPNAP position statement on breastfeeding. *Journal of Pediatric Health Care, 27,* e13–e15.

Papalia, D., & Feldman, R. (2011). *A child's world: Infancy through adolescence* (12th ed.). New York: McGraw-Hill.

Piaget, J. (1969). *The theory of stages in cognitive development.* New York: McGraw-Hill.

Reach Out and Read. (2013). Reading tips for your young family. Retrieved from http://www.reachoutandread.org/FileRepository/ReadingTips.pdf

Ross, C. A., Taylor, C. L., Yaktine, A. L., & Del Valle, H. B. (Eds.). (2014). *DRI dietary reference intakes calcium vitamin D.* Washington, DC: The National Academies Press.

Safe Kids. (2015). *Swimming and boating fact sheet (2015).* Retrieved from https://www.safekids.org/sites/default/files/documents/skw_swimming_fact_sheet_feb_2015.pdf

Safe Kids. (2016a). *Swimming.* Retrieved from https://www.safekids.org/poolsafety

Safe Kids. (2016b). *Water safety at home tips.* Retrieved from https://www.safekids.org/tip/water-safety-home-tips

SafeBedSharing.org. (2016). *Keep it safe.* Retrieved from http://www.safebedsharing.org/safetyguidelines.html

Sears, W., & Sears, M. (2016a). *Choosing and using a pacifier.* Retrieved from http://www.askdrsears.com/topics/parenting/child-rearing-and-development/bringing-baby-home/pacifiers-in-or-out/choosing-using

Sears, W., & Sears, M. (2016b). *8 tools for toddler discipline.* Retrieved from http://www.askdrsears.com/topics/parenting/discipline-behavior/8-tools-toddler-discipline

Sears, W., & Sears, M. (2016c). *Thumbsucking.* Retrieved from http://www.askdrsears.com/topics/parenting/discipline-behavior/bothersome-behaviors/thumbsucking

Smith, M. A., & Segal, J. (2016). *Grandparents as parents: The rewards & challenges of parenting the second time around.* Retrieved from http://www.helpguide.org/articles/grandparenting/grandparents-as-parents.htm

Stettler, N., Bhatia, J., Parish, A., & Stallings, V. A. (2011). Feeding healthy infants, children, and adolescents. In R. M. Kliegman, B. F. Stanton, J. W. St. Geme III, N. F. Schor, & R. E. Behrman (Eds.), (*Nelson's textbook of pediatrics* (19th ed.). Philadelphia, PA: Elsevier, Saunders.

U.S. Department of Health and Human Services. (2016). *Healthy People 2020.* Retrieved from http://www.healthypeople.gov/2020/default.aspx

Zero to Three. (2016a). *Brain development.* Retrieved from https://www.zerotothree.org/early-development/brain-development

Zero to Three. (2016b). *How to handle picky eaters.* Retrieved from https://www.zerotothree.org/resources/ 1072-how-to-handle-picky-eaters

CHAPTER **WORKSHEET**

MULTIPLE CHOICE QUESTIONS

1. The nurse is caring for a hospitalized 30-month-old who is resistant to care, is angry, and yells "no" all the time. The nurse identifies this toddler's behavior as
   a. problematic, as it interferes with needed nursing care.
   b. normal for this stage of growth and development.
   c. normal because the child is hospitalized and out of his routine.
2. The mother of a 15-month-old is concerned about a speech delay. She describes her toddler as being able to understand what she says, sometimes following commands, but using only one or two words with any consistency. What is the nurse's best response to this information?
   a. The toddler should have a developmental evaluation as soon as possible.
   b. If the mother would read to the child, then speech would develop faster.
   c. Receptive language normally develops earlier than expressive language.
   d. The mother should ask her child's physician for a speech therapy evaluation.
3. A 2-year-old is having a temper tantrum. What advice should the nurse give the mother?
   a. For safety reasons, the toddler should be restrained during the tantrum.
   b. Punishment should be initiated, as tantrums should be controlled.
   c. The mother should promise the toddler a reward if the tantrum stops.
   d. The tantrum should be ignored as long as the toddler is safe.
4. What is the best advice about nutrition for the toddler?
   a. Encourage cup drinking and give water between meals and snacks.
   b. Encourage unlimited milk intake, because toddlers need the protein for growth.
   c. Avoid sugar-sweetened fruit drinks and allow as much natural fruit juice as desired.
   d. Allow the toddler unlimited access to the sippy cup to ensure adequate hydration.
5. To gain cooperation from a toddler, what is the best approach by the nurse?
   a. Immediately pick the toddler up from the mother's lap.
   b. Kneel in front of the toddler while he or she is on the mother's lap.
   c. Do the nursing tasks quickly so the toddler can play.
   d. Ask the toddler if it is okay if you begin the needed task.

CRITICAL THINKING EXERCISES

1. Develop a teaching plan about safety to present to a toddler-age preschool class.
2. Construct a 3-day menu for a 2-year-old, one that is realistic and will provide the nutrients needed.
3. Develop a plan for educating the parent of a 34-month-old who has been resistant to toilet teaching. Include assessments the nurse will make as well as the plan for teaching.

STUDY ACTIVITIES

1. Visit a preschool that provides care for special-needs toddlers as well as typical toddlers. Perform a developmental assessment on a typical toddler and one with special needs (both the same age). Compare and contrast your findings.
2. Care for two average 2-year-olds in the clinical setting. Describe each toddler's behavior, response to the parent, and response to the nurse and list strategies used to gain compliance and minimize stress to the toddler.
3. Observe in the toddler classroom of a typical preschool. Choose two toddlers the same age with different temperaments. Record the toddlers' differences and similarities in response to structure and authority, interactions with classmates, attention levels, and language and activity levels.

BRINGING IT ALL TOGETHER: A CASE STUDY

Eva, an 18-month-old girl, comes to be seen in the pediatric office because her mother is concerned that she is not growing well. When Eva's growth measurements are plotted on the growth chart, they indicate she is at the 5th percentile for length and for weight, but at the 25th percentile for head circumference.

Go to thePoint to find questions to consider about this case.

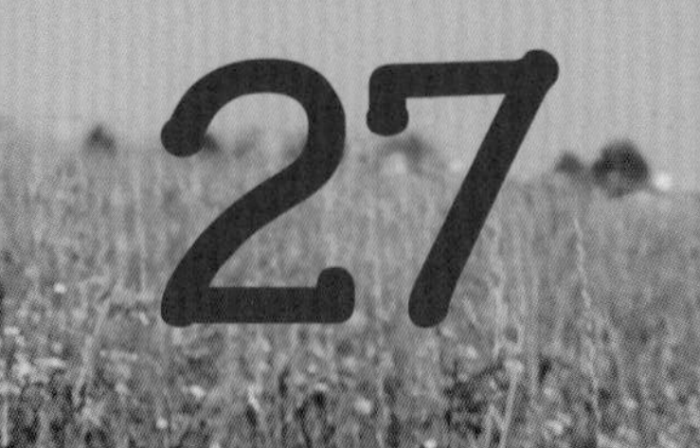

27

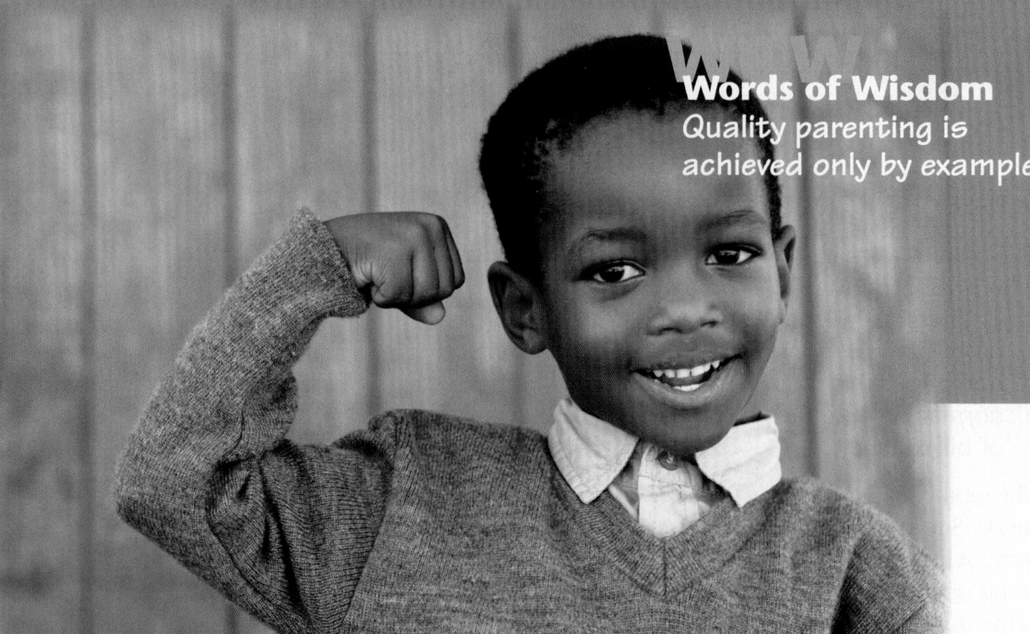

Words of Wisdom
Quality parenting is achieved only by example.

Growth and Development of the Preschooler

KEY TERMS
animism
empathy
imaginary friend
magical thinking
preoperational thought
school readiness
telegraphic speech
transduction

Learning Objectives

Upon completion of the chapter, you will be able to:

1. Identify normal physiologic, cognitive, and psychosocial changes occurring in the preschool-age child.
2. Express an understanding of language development in the preschool years.
3. Implement a nursing care plan that addresses common concerns or delays in the preschooler's development.
4. Integrate knowledge of preschool growth and development with nursing care and health promotion of the preschool-age child.
5. Develop a nutrition plan for the preschool-age child.
6. Identify common issues and concerns related to growth and development during the preschool years.
7. Demonstrate knowledge of appropriate anticipatory guidance for common developmental issues that arise in the preschool period.

Nila Patel **is a 4-year-old girl brought to the clinic by her mother and father for her school check-up. During your assessment you measure her weight to be 20 kg (44 lb) and her height 101.6 cm (40 inches). As the nurse caring for her, assess Nila's growth and development, and then provide appropriate anticipatory guidance to her parents.**

The preschool period is the period between 3 and 6 years of age. This is a time of continued growth and development. Physical growth continues much more slowly compared to earlier years. Gains in cognitive, language, and psychosocial development are substantial throughout the preschool period. Many tasks that began during the toddler years are mastered and perfected during the preschool years. The child has learned to tolerate separation from parents, has a longer attention span, and continues to learn skills that will lead to later success in the school-age period. Preparation for success in school continues during the preschool period because most children enter elementary school by the end of the preschool period.

Growth and Development Overview

The healthy preschooler is slender and agile, with an upright posture. The formerly clumsy toddler becomes more graceful, demonstrating the ability to run more smoothly. Athletic abilities may begin to develop. Major development occurs in the area of fine motor coordination. Psychosocial development is focused on the accomplishment of initiative. Preconceptual thought and intuitiveness dominate cognitive development. The preschooler is an inquisitive learner and absorbs new concepts like a sponge absorbs water.

PHYSICAL GROWTH

The average preschool-age child will grow 6.5 to 7.8 cm (2.5 to 3 inches) per year. The average 3-year-old is 96.2 cm (37 inches) tall, the average 4-year-old is 103.7 cm (40.5 inches) tall, and the average 5-year-old is 118.5 cm (43 inches) tall. Average weight gain during this time period is about 2.3 kg (4 to 5 lb) per year (Feigelman, 2011). The average weight of a 3-year-old is 14.5 kg (32 lb), increasing to an average weight of 18.6 kg (41 lb) by age 5. The loss of baby fat and the growth of muscle during the preschool years give the child a stronger and more mature appearance (Fig. 27.1). The length of the skull also increases slightly, with the lower jaw becoming more pronounced. The upper jaw widens through the preschool years in preparation for the emergence of permanent teeth, usually starting around age 6.

ORGAN SYSTEM MATURATION

Most of the body systems have matured by the preschool years. Myelination of the spinal cord allows for bowel and bladder control to be complete in most children by age 3 years. The respiratory structures are continuing to grow in size, and the number of alveoli continues

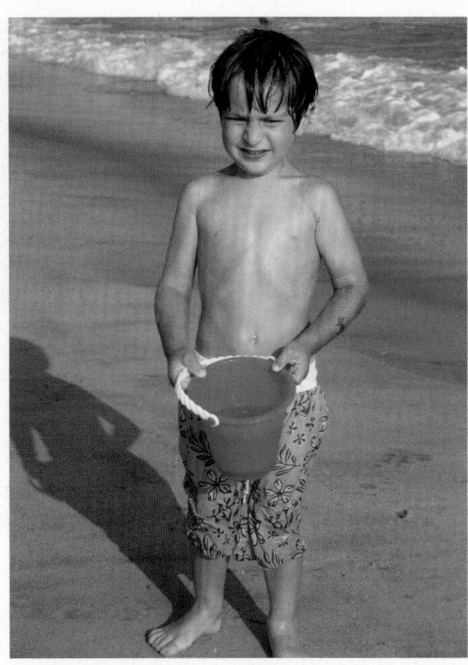

FIGURE 27.1 The preschool child has a more slender appearance and erect posture than the toddler.

to increase, reaching the adult number at about 7 years of age. The eustachian tubes remain relatively short and straight. Heart rate decreases and blood pressure increases slightly during the preschool years. An innocent heart murmur may be heard upon auscultation, and splitting of the second heart sound may become evident. The preschooler should have 20 deciduous teeth present.

The small intestine is continuing to grow in length. Stool passage usually occurs once or twice per day in the average preschooler. The 4-year-old generally has adequate bowel control. The urethra remains short in both boys and girls, making them more susceptible to urinary tract infections than adults. Bladder control is usually present in the 4- and 5-year-old child, but an occasional accident may occur, particularly in stressful situations or when the child is absorbed in an interesting activity.

The bones continue to increase in length and the muscles continue to strengthen and mature. However, the musculoskeletal system is still not fully mature, making the preschooler susceptible to injury, particularly with overexertion or excess activity.

PSYCHOSOCIAL DEVELOPMENT

According to Erik Erikson, the psychosocial task of the preschool years is establishing a sense of initiative versus guilt (Erikson, 1963). The preschooler is an inquisitive learner, very enthusiastic about learning new things. Preschoolers feel a sense of accomplishment when succeeding in activities (Fig. 27.2), and feeling pride in

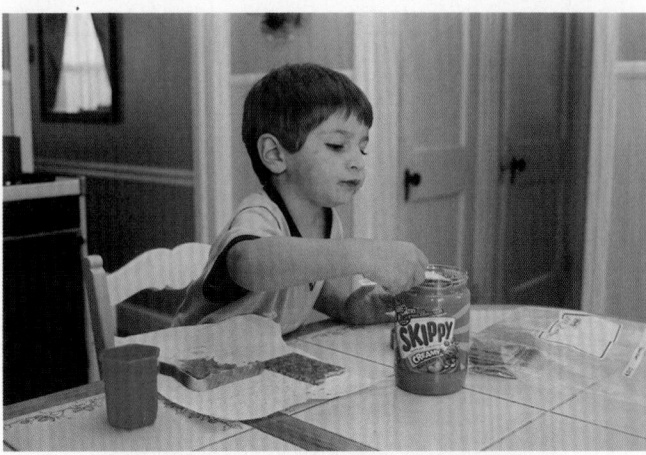

FIGURE 27.2 Allowing the preschooler to assist with simple household tasks such as preparing a sandwich encourages the development of initiative.

one's accomplishment helps the child to use initiative. However, when the child extends himself or herself further than current capabilities allow, he or she may feel a sense of guilt. The superego or conscience development is completed during the preschool period, and this is the basis for moral development (understanding right and wrong). Table 27.1 gives examples illustrating the stage of initiative versus guilt.

COGNITIVE DEVELOPMENT

According to Jean Piaget's theory (1969), the preschool-age child continues in the preoperational stage. **Preoperational thought** dominates during this stage and is based on a self-centered understanding of the world. In the preconceptual phase of preoperational thought, the child remains egocentric and is able to approach a problem from a single point of view only. The young preschooler may understand the concept of counting and begins to engage in fantasy play (Papalia & Feldman, 2011).

Magical thinking is a normal part of preschool development. In magical thinking, the preschooler believes that his or her thoughts are all-powerful. The fantasy experienced through magical thinking allows the preschooler to make room in his or her world for the actual or the real. Through make-believe and magical thinking, preschool-age children satisfy their curiosity about differences in the world around them (Papalia & Feldman, 2011).

The preschooler often has an **imaginary friend** as well (Goldson & Reynolds, 2012). This friend serves as a creative way for the preschooler to sample different activities and behaviors and practice conversational skills. Despite this imagination, the preschooler is able to switch easily between fantasy and reality throughout the day.

The child in the intuitive phase can count 10 or more objects, correctly name at least four colors, and better understand the concept of time, and he or she knows about things that are used in everyday life, such as appliances, money, and food. The preschooler uses **transduction** when reasoning: he or she extrapolates from a particular situation to another, even though the events may be unrelated. The preschooler also attributes life-like qualities to inanimate objects (**animism**) (Papalia & Feldman, 2011). Table 27.1 gives further examples illustrating this developmental stage.

The acquisition of language skills in the toddler period is enhanced in the preschool period. The expansion of vocabulary enables the preschooler to progress further with symbolic thought. At this age, children do not completely understand the concept of death or its permanence: they may ask when their grandparent or pet who died is returning.

MORAL AND SPIRITUAL DEVELOPMENT

The preschool-age child can understand the concepts of right and wrong and is developing a conscience. That inner voice that warns or threatens is developing in the preschool years. Kohlberg identified this stage (between 2 and 7 years) as the preconventional stage, which is characterized by a punishment-and-obedience orientation (Kohlberg, 1984). Preschool children see morality as external to themselves; they defer to power (that of the adult). The child's moral standards are those of their parents or other adults who influence them, not necessarily their own. Preschoolers adhere to those standards to gain rewards or avoid punishment. Since the preschool-age child is facing the psychosocial task of initiative versus guilt, it is natural for the child to experience guilt when something goes wrong.

As the child's moral development progresses, he or she learns how to deal with angry feelings. Sometimes the way the child chooses to deal with those feelings may be inappropriate, such as fighting and biting. Lying begins to occur in the preschool period. Younger preschoolers have difficulty differentiating between reality and their imagination and fantasies, whereas older preschoolers are more aware of right and wrong. Preschoolers also use their limited life experiences to make sense of and help them cope with crises. They need to learn the socially acceptable limits of behavior and are also learning the rewards of manners. The preschool-age child begins to help out in the family and begins to understand the concept of give-and-take in relationships.

During the preoperational phase of cognitive development, the preschooler's concept of faith is intuitive and

TABLE 27.1 DEVELOPMENTAL THEORIES

Theorist	Stage	Activities
Erikson	Initiative vs. Guilt Age 3–6 years	Likes to please parents Begins to plan activities, make up games Initiates activities with others Acts out the roles of other people (real and imaginary) Develops sexual identity Develops conscience May take frustrations out on siblings Likes exploring new things Enjoys sports, shopping, cooking, working Feels remorse when makes wrong choice or behaves badly Cooperates with other children Negotiates solutions to conflicts
Piaget	Preoperational substage: Preconceptual phase Age: 2–4 years	Exhibits egocentric thinking, which lessens as the child approaches age 4 Has short attention span Learns through observing and imitating Displays animism Forms concepts that are not as complete or as logical as the adult's Is able to make simple classifications By age 4 understands the concept of opposites (hot/cold, soft/hard) Reasoning is that of specific to specific Has an active imagination
	Preoperational substage: Intuitive phase Age 4–7 years	Is able to classify and relate objects Has intuitive thought processes; knows if something is right or wrong, though cannot state why Tolerates others' differences but doesn't understand them Is very curious about facts Knows acceptable cultural rules Uses words appropriately but often without true understanding of their meaning Has a more realistic sense of causality May begin to question parents' values
Kohlberg	Punishment–obedience orientation Age 2–7 years (preconventional morality)	Determines good vs. bad dependent upon associated punishment Children may learn inappropriate behavior at this stage if parental intervention does not occur (if the child hits, bites, or is verbally disrespectful but is not punished for these activities, the child will view those behaviors as good and continue to participate in them)
Freud	Phallic stage Age 3–7 years	Child's pleasure centers on genitalia and masturbation. Superego is developing and conscience is emerging. Oedipal stage occurs: jealousy and rivalry toward same-sex parent, with love of the opposite-sex parent. This usually resolves by the end of the preschool years, when the child develops a strong identification with the same-sex parent.

Adapted from Erikson, E. H. (1963). *Childhood and society* (2nd ed.). New York, NY: W. W. Norton and Company; Feigelman, S. (2011). Preschool years. In R. M. Kliegman, B. F. Stanton, J. W. St. Geme III, N. F. Schor, & R. E. Behrman, (Eds.), *Nelson's textbook of pediatrics* (19th ed.). Philadelphia, PA: Elsevier, Saunders; Kohlberg, L. (1984). *Moral development*. New York, NY: Harper & Row; and Piaget, J. (1969). *The theory of stages in cognitive development*. New York, NY: McGraw-Hill.

projective in nature (Keeley, 2010). The preschool-age child's imagination allows for anything to be possible, so he or she does not have a logical view of the world (as adults do). Preschool-age children have limited life experiences, so they may project a feeling onto a new person or situation. They may use this projection to help them understand what is going on around them. Preschoolers may project their parents' or caregiver's feelings or characteristics onto "God": if mommy gets angry, then God is probably also angry.

The family's religious beliefs may affect the child's diet, the mode of discipline that parents use, and even how the parents view their children. Knowing about a family's practices of prayer or meditation is helpful to the pediatric nurse, who can help continue the ritual when the child is ill or hospitalized (Fig. 27.3).

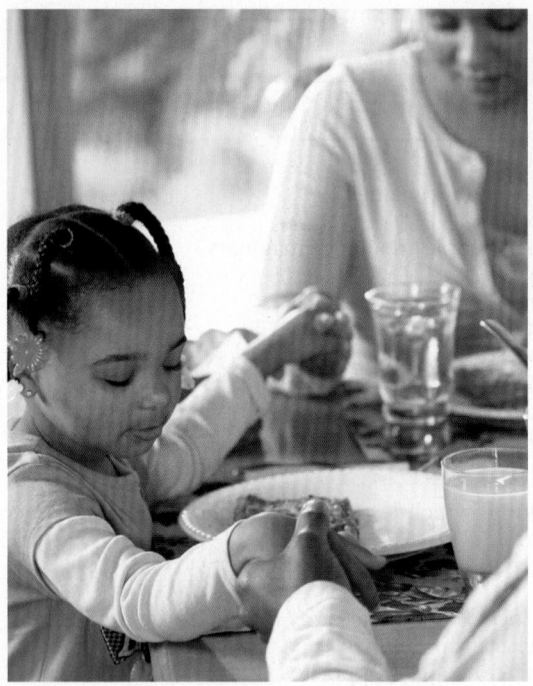

FIGURE 27.3 The preschool child may participate in religious rituals without having full understanding of their meaning.

MOTOR SKILL DEVELOPMENT

As the preschooler's musculoskeletal system continues to mature, existing motor skills become refined and new ones develop. The preschooler has more voluntary control over his or her movements and is less clumsy than the toddler. Significant refinement in fine motor skills occurs during the preschool period (Table 27.2).

Gross Motor Skills

The preschooler is agile while standing, walking, running, and jumping (Fig. 27.4). He or she can go up and down stairs and walk forward and backward easily. Standing on tiptoes or on one foot still requires extra concentration. The preschooler seems to be in constant motion. He or she also uses the body to understand new concepts (such as using the arms in a "chug-chug" motion when describing how the train wheels work).

Fine Motor Skills

The 3-year-old can move each finger independently and is capable of grasping utensils and crayons in adult fashion,

TABLE 27.2 MOTOR SKILL DEVELOPMENT

Age	Expected Gross Motor Skills	Expected Fine Motor Skills
3 years	• Climbs well • Pedals tricycle • Runs easily • Walks up and down stairs with alternate feet • Bends over easily without falling	• Undresses self • Copies circle • Builds tower of 9 or 10 cubes • Holds a pencil in writing position • Screws/unscrews lids, nuts, bolts • Turns book pages one at a time
4 years	• Throws ball overhand • Kicks ball forward • Catches bounced ball • Hops on one foot • Stands on one foot up to 5 seconds • Alternates feet going up and down steps • Moves backward and forward with agility	• Uses scissors successfully • Copies capital letters • Draws circles and squares • Traces a cross or diamond • Draws a person with two to four body parts • Laces shoes
5 years	• Stands on one foot 10 seconds or longer • Swings and climbs well • May skip • Somersaults • May learn to skate and swim	• Prints some letters • Draws person with body and at least six parts • Dresses/undresses without assistance • Can learn to tie laces • Uses fork, spoon, and knife (supervised) well • Copies triangle and other geometric patterns • Mostly cares for own toileting needs

Adapted from Feigelman, S. (2011). Preschool years. In R. M. Kliegman, B. F. Stanton, J. W. St. Geme III, N. F. Schor, & R. E. Behrman, (Eds.), *Nelson's textbook of pediatrics* (19th ed.). Philadelphia, PA: Elsevier, Saunders; Goldson, E., & Reynolds, A. (2012). Child development & behavior. In W. W. Hay, M. J. Levin, R. R., Deterding, et al. (Eds.) *Current diagnosis & treatment: Pediatrics* (21st ed.). New York, NY: McGraw Hill; and Papalia, D., & Feldman, R. (2011). *A child's world: Infancy through adolescence* (12th ed.). New York, NY: McGraw-Hill.

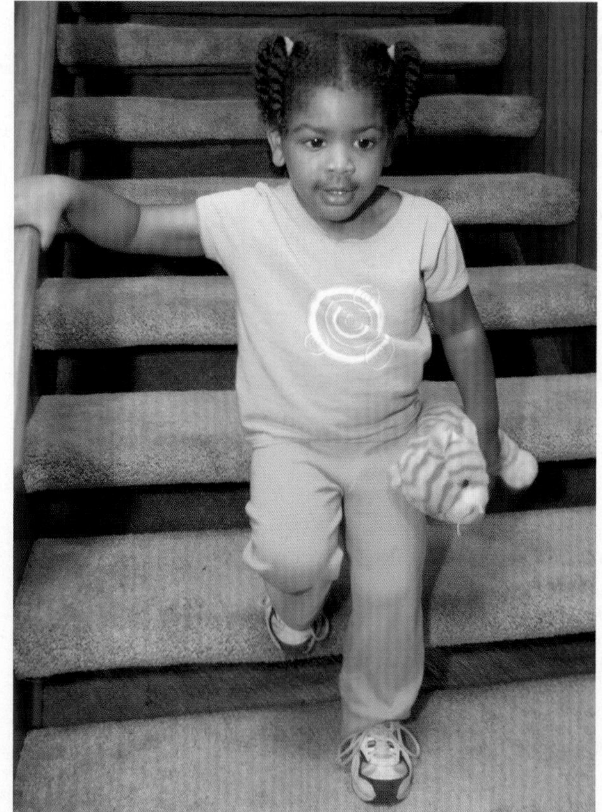

FIGURE 27.4 The preschooler runs well, navigate stairs, and can balance on one foot.

with the thumb on one side and the fingers on the other. He or she can also scribble freely, copy a circle, trace a square, and feed himself or herself without spilling much. These skills become refined over the next 2 years, and by 5 years of age the child can write letters, cut with scissors more accurately, and tie shoelaces (Fig. 27.5).

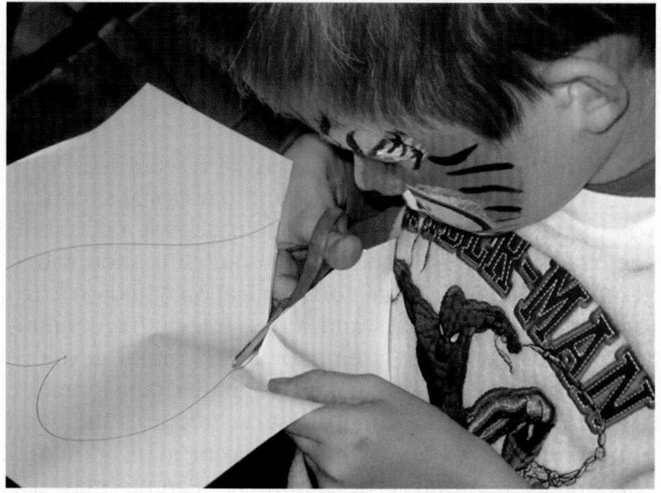

FIGURE 27.5 The 5-year-old has the fine motor dexterity to cut well with scissors.

SENSORY DEVELOPMENT

Hearing is intact at birth and should remain so throughout the preschool years. The senses of smell and touch continue to develop throughout the preschool years. The young preschooler may have a less discriminating sense of taste than the older child, putting him or her at increased risk for accidental ingestion. Visual acuity continues to progress and should be equal bilaterally. The typical 5-year-old has visual acuity of 20/40 or 20/30. Color vision is intact at this age.

COMMUNICATION AND LANGUAGE DEVELOPMENT

The acquisition of language allows the preschool-age child to express thoughts and creativity. The preschool years are a time of refinement of language skills. The 3-year-old exhibits **telegraphic speech**, using short sentences that contain only the essential information. Language development in the preschool years is extensive. At 2 years of age, a child uses 50 to 100 words and by 5 years of age uses about 2,000 words (Feigelman, 2011). By the end of the preschool period, the child is using sentences that are adult-like in structure (Table 27.3).

The 3- to 6-year-old is starting to develop fluency (the ability to smoothly link sounds, syllables, and words when speaking). Initially, the child may exhibit dysfluency or stuttering. Speech may sound choppy, or the child may say repeated consonants or "um." Stuttering usually has its onset in the preschool years and will resolve in 80% of children by age 8 years (Feigelman, 2011). Parents should slow down their speech and should give the child time to speak without rushing or interrupting. Some sounds remain difficult for the preschooler to enunciate properly: "f," "v," "s," and "z" sounds are usually mastered by age 5 years, but some children do not master the sounds of "sh," "l," "th," and "r" until age 6 or later. The potentially bilingual child may lag slightly behind the single-language speaker, but will be able to differentiate and use both languages by the end of the preschool period (Lowry, 2011).

Communication in preschool children is concrete in nature, as they are not yet capable of abstract thought. Despite its concrete nature, the preschooler's communication can be quite elaborate and involved; he or she may talk about dreams and fantasies. In addition to acquiring vocabulary and learning the correct use of grammar, the preschool child's receptive language skills are also becoming refined.

The preschooler is very much in tune with the parent's moods and easily picks up on negative emotions in conversations. If the preschooler hears parents discussing

TABLE 27.3 COMMUNICATION SKILLS IN THE PRESCHOOL CHILD

Age	Communication Abilities
4 years	• Speaks in complete sentences using adult-like grammar • Tells a story that is easy to follow • 75% of speech understood by others outside of family • Asks questions with "who," "how," "how many" • Stays on topic in a conversation • Understands the concepts of "same" and "different" • Asks many questions • Knows names of familiar animals • Names common objects in books and magazines • Knows at least one color • Uses language to engage in make-believe • Follows a three-part command • Can count a few numbers • Vocabulary of 1,500 words
5 years	• Persons outside of the family can understand most of the child's speech • Explains how an item is used • Participates in long, detailed conversations • Talks about past, future, and imaginary events • Answers questions that use "why" and "when" • Can count to 10 • Recalls part of a story • Speech should be completely intelligible, even if the child has articulation difficulties • Speech is generally grammatically correct • Vocabulary of 2,100 words • Says name and address

Adapted from Centers for Disease Control and Prevention. (2016). Developmental milestones. Retrieved from http://www.cdc.gov/ncbddd/actearly/milestones/index.html; Feigelman, S. (2011). Preschool years. In R. M. Kliegman, B. F. Stanton, J. W. St. Geme III, N. F. Schor, & R. E. Behrman, (Eds.), *Nelson's textbook of pediatrics* (19th ed.). Philadelphia, PA: Elsevier, Saunders; and Papalia, D., & Feldman, R. (2011). *A child's world: Infancy through adolescence* (12th ed.). New York, NY: McGraw-Hill.

things that are frightening to the child, the preschooler's imagination may fuel the development of fears and lead to misinterpretation of what the child has heard.

EMOTIONAL AND SOCIAL DEVELOPMENT

By the time a child enters kindergarten, he or she should have developed a useful set of social skills that will help him or her have successful experiences in the school setting as well as in life in general. These skills include cooperation, sharing (of things and feelings), kindness, generosity, affection display, conversation, expression of feelings, helping others, and making friends.

Preschoolers tend to have strong emotions. They can be very excited, happy, and giddy in one moment, then extremely disappointed in the next. The preschool-age child has a vivid imagination, and fears are very real to preschoolers. Most children this age have learned to control their behaviors. They should be able to name the feelings they are having rather than acting on them. Strong feelings may be expressed through outlets such as clay or Play-Doh, water play, drawing or painting, or dramatic play such as with puppets.

Preschoolers are developing a sense of identity. They recognize that they are boys or girls. They know that they belong to a particular family, community, or culture. They take pride in using self-control rather than giving in to their impulses. The preschool-age child is capable of helping others and being involved in routines and transitions.

Parents can encourage and assist preschool-age children with developing the social and emotional skills that will be needed when the child enters school. Preschool-age children thrive on one-to-one communication with a parent. During interactive communication, children learn to express their feelings and ideas. Interactive communication fosters not only emotional and moral development but also self-esteem and cognitive development. Asking the preschool child questions requires the child to think out his or her own intention or motivation and encourages vocabulary development. Parents may use individual communication as a time to explore right and wrong, thus further contributing to moral development. Being listened to while answering parents' questions gives preschoolers a sense that they are valued, that what they think and have to say matters.

Establishing a few simple rules and enforcing them consistently gives preschoolers the structure and security they need while promoting moral development. Parents or caregivers can help the child give a name to the emotion that is being experienced. Fears are very real to preschoolers because of their active imaginations and may result in a variety of emotions. Parents should validate the feeling or emotion, then discuss with the child alternatives for dealing with the emotion.

Preschoolers are developing their sense of identity, and parents should encourage preschoolers to do simple things for themselves, like dressing and washing their hands and face (Fig. 27.6). Parents should give the child the time he or she needs to complete the task. This helps to establish a sense of accomplishment.

At this age, the child may begin to show an interest in basic sexuality (Papalia & Feldman, 2011). The preschooler may want to know why boys' and girls' bodies are different, how the reproductive organs function, and where babies come from. The parent should answer the child honestly and directly, using the correct anatomic terms. Long explanations are not necessary, just simple answers. This curiosity is a normal function of the preschool years, and the curiosity may also involve playing with the genitals (see the section on masturbation later in this chapter).

Friendships

Preschoolers need interactions with friends as well. Learning how to make and keep a friend is an important part of social development. Friends may be other children in the neighborhood or those at preschool or day care. A special friend is someone the preschooler can care about, talk to, and play with (Fig. 27.7). The preschooler is more likely to agree to rules and wants to please friends and be like them. The preschooler loves to sing, dance, and act and will enjoy these activities with friends. Disagreements may occur, but the parent can encourage the children to express their views, discuss and resolve conflicts, and continue being friends.

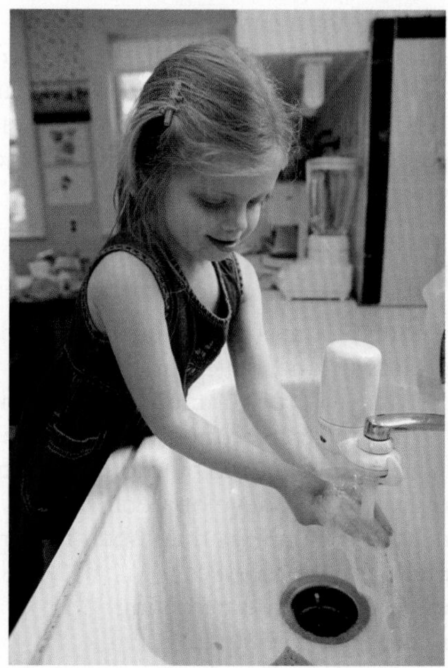

FIGURE 27.6 Encouraging the preschooler to complete simple tasks by himself or herself helps to build self-esteem.

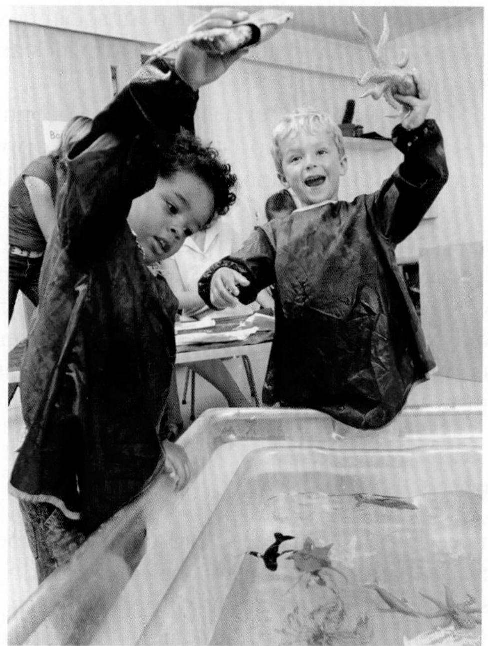

FIGURE 27.7 The preschool child begins to develop friendships.

Temperament

By the time children are 3 years old, they recognize that what they do actually matters. It is helpful for the parent to view the child as an active participant in the parent–child relationship. The child's temperament has become a reliable indicator of how a parent might expect the child to react in a certain situation. When the parent is in tune with the preschooler's temperament, it is easier to find ways to ease transitions and changes for that child. In the area of task orientation, temperament may range from the highly attentive and persistent to the more distractible and active (Child Development Institute, 2015).

A child's social flexibility is also evident by this age. A child who is quite adaptable will handle stimuli from the outside world in an approaching rather than a withdrawing manner. Temperament also determines the extent of reactivity (the child's sensory threshold of responsiveness, high versus low). This determines the quality of the child's mood and the intensity of reactions to stimuli, change, or situations. When the parents are familiar with the child's task orientation, social flexibility, and reactivity, they can better structure activities and situations for the child.

The 4-year-old is better at learning self-control and can use setbacks in appropriate behavior as opportunities for growth. Temper tantrums should ease off by this age, as the child's language skills are more capable of keeping up with complex ideas. The 4-year-old is able to see the rewards of growing up. This awareness of self-power may, however, lead to additional fears. The 5-year-old who has a more vulnerable type of temperament, as opposed to a confident temperament, may be more apt to experience fears.

Fears

With their vivid imaginations, preschoolers experience a variety of fears. Preschoolers may be scared of loud noises such as fire engine sirens or barking dogs. Imaginary monsters may scare the child. Preschoolers are often afraid of people they do not know and of strange people (Santa Claus or people who look or dress very differently from what they are accustomed to). Many preschoolers are afraid of the dark. Preschoolers may also fear insects as well as animals they are not familiar with. The preschooler's memory is long enough that he or she may fear returning to the doctor's office when a painful procedure occurred during the prior visit.

Parents should acknowledge fears rather than minimizing them. They can then collaborate with the child on strategies for dealing with the fear.

CULTURAL INFLUENCES ON GROWTH AND DEVELOPMENT

Children may learn prejudice or bias at home before entering school or day care. The ways that families view other races or cultures may be subtly or overtly demonstrated in routine daily activities. The preschool-age child is developing a conscience, so attitudes of tolerance or bias may influence the child's values. As in the toddler period, the value that the family places on independence will affect the child's development of a healthy self-concept.

Some cultures value reading and education more than others. If reading is not valued in the home, the preschool-age child's first experience with books may not occur until he or she is in school.

Food served in the home is often very specific to the family's ethnic background. As the preschool-age child is exposed to persons of other cultures in school, he or she may or may not like the food that is served. Exploring customs or cultural practices that the family participates in is important so that these practices may be safely incorporated into the child's plan of care.

Refer back to Nila, who was introduced in the beginning of the chapter. What developmental milestones would you expect Nila to have reached at this age? Nila's mother expresses concerns about her child's imaginary friend, Sasha. How would you respond?

The Nurse's Role in Preschool Growth and Development

Growth and development in the preschool-age child remains orderly and sequential. Some preschoolers grow faster than others or reach various developmental milestones sooner than others. Nurses must be aware of the usual growth and development patterns for this age group so that they can assess preschool-age children appropriately and provide guidance to their families. The changes that the preschool-age child is experiencing affect not only the child but also the family. Health care visits throughout the preschool period continue to focus on expected growth and development and anticipatory guidance. An additional concern is the preparation for school entry (**school readiness**).

If the preschooler is hospitalized, growth and development may be altered. Hospitalization hinders the preschool-age child's ability to explore the environment and engage in make-believe play and thus presents a challenge for the curious and inquisitive child. If the child must be isolated for a contagious illness, the opportunities for exploration and experimentation are further restricted. In addition, a sick preschooler may feel a sense of guilt, worrying that maybe he or she caused the illness by negative thoughts or behaviors.

When caring for the hospitalized preschooler, the nurse must use knowledge of normal growth and development to recognize potential delays, promote continued appropriate growth and development, and interact successfully with the preschooler.

NURSING PROCESS OVERVIEW

Upon completion of assessment of the preschool-age child's growth and development status, problems or issues related to growth and development may be identified. The nurse may then identify one or more nursing diagnoses, including but not limited to:

- Delayed growth and development
- Imbalanced nutrition, less than body requirements
- Interrupted family processes
- Readiness for enhanced parenting
- Risk for caregiver role strain
- Risk for delayed development
- Risk for disproportionate growth
- Risk for injury

Planning nursing care for the preschool child with growth and development issues should take into account the preschooler's and family's individual needs. The nursing care plan may be used as a guide in planning nursing care for the preschooler with a growth or developmental concern. The nurse may choose the appropriate nursing diagnoses from the Nursing Care Plan (found at the end of the chapter) and individualize them as needed. The nursing care plan is intended to serve as a guide only and is not intended to be an inclusive growth and development plan.

PROMOTING HEALTHY GROWTH AND DEVELOPMENT

The building of self-esteem continues throughout the preschool period. It is of particular importance during these years, as the preschooler's developmental task is focused on the development of initiative rather than guilt. A sense of guilt will contribute to low self-esteem, whereas a child who is rewarded for his or her initiative will have increased self-confidence. The parent who provides a loving and nurturing environment for the preschooler builds upon the earlier foundation.

Routine and ritual continue to be important throughout the preschool years, as they help the child to develop a sense of time as well as provide the structure for the child to feel safe and secure. Daily routine continues to assist with the development of conscience in the preschooler. As in toddlerhood, making expectations known through everyday routines helps to avoid confrontations. The preschooler is developing the maturity to know how to behave in various situations and is capable of learning manners.

Setting limits (and remaining consistent with those limits) continues to be important in the preschool period. Consistent limits provide the preschooler with expectation and guidance. As the preschooler increasingly participates in fantasy and imagination, the limits of routine and structure help guide his or her behavior and ability to distinguish reality.

Nurses caring for preschoolers should have knowledge of normal developmental expectations so they can determine whether the preschool child is progressing appropriately. Table 27.4 lists potential signs of developmental delay. A preschool child with one or more of these concerns should be referred for further developmental evaluation.

TABLE 27.4 SIGNS OF DEVELOPMENTAL DELAY

Age	Concern
4 years	• Cannot jump in place or ride a tricycle • Cannot stack four blocks • Cannot throw ball overhand • Does not grasp crayon with thumb and fingers • Has difficulty with scribbling • Cannot copy a circle • Does not use sentences with three or more words • Cannot use the words "me" and "you" appropriately • Ignores other children or does not show interest in interactive games • Will not respond to people outside the family; still clings or cries if parents leave • Resists using toilet, dressing, sleeping • Does not engage in fantasy play
By 5 years	• Is unhappy or sad often • Has little interest in playing with other children • Is unable to separate from parent without major protest • Is extremely aggressive • Is extremely fearful or timid, or unusually passive • Cannot build tower of six to eight blocks • Is easily distracted; cannot concentrate on single activity for 5 minutes • Rarely engages in fantasy play • Has trouble with eating, sleeping, or using the toilet • Cannot use plurals or past tense • Cannot brush teeth, wash and dry hands, or undress efficiently

Promoting Growth and Development Through Play

Providing sincere encouragement for the preschool child's efforts and accomplishments helps him or her develop a sense of initiative. Giving children opportunities to decide how and with whom they want to play also helps them develop initiative. Preschool children like to write, color, draw, paint with a brush or their fingers, and trace or copy patterns (Fig. 27.8). They may start small collections that may be sorted. They like using toys for their intended purpose as well as for whatever invented purpose they can imagine.

Preschoolers begin to play cooperatively with one another. Play may be focused around a distinct theme. They define roles, make up rules, and assign jobs. They are able to work together toward a common goal such as building a house or fort with discarded boxes. Cooperative play encourages the preschool child to learn to share, take turns and compromise, listen to others' opinions, consider the feelings of others, and use self-control and overcome fears.

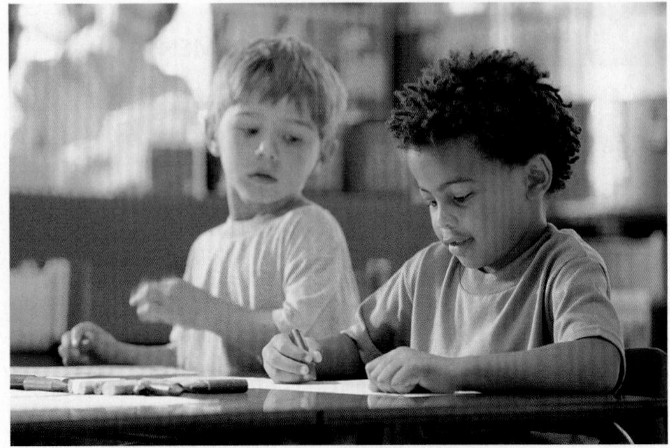

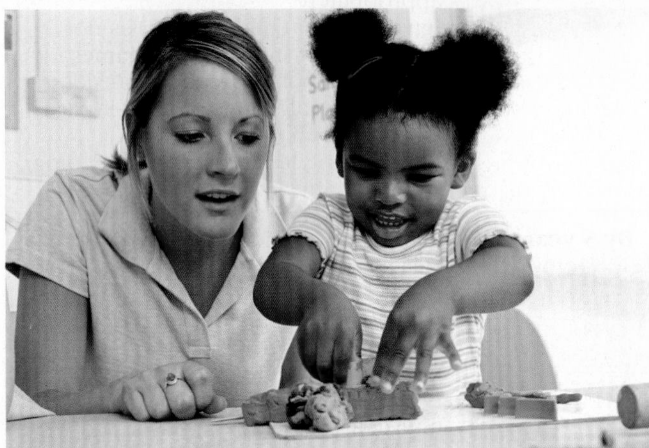

FIGURE 27.8 The preschool child loves to create things, so coloring and molding clay are ideal activities for children this age.

Preschoolers have incredible imaginations and love to play "make-believe" (Fig. 27.9). Encouraging pretend play and providing props for dress-up stimulates curiosity and creativity. Fantasy play is usually cooperative in nature. It encourages the preschooler to develop social skills such as taking turns, communication, paying attention, and responding to one another's words and actions. Fantasy play also allows preschoolers to explore complex social ideas such as power, compassion, and cruelty. Through role playing, children begin to develop their sexual identity as well.

Since preschool children have vivid imaginations, it is important to be careful about what television they watch. The preschooler should be limited to no more than 2 hours per day of quality television (Feigelman, 2011). The violence in some television programs may scare the preschool child or inspire him or her to act out violent behavior. The 2-hour-per-day limit should also include other screen time such as use of the computer or tablet (such as an iPad) for entertainment (American Academy of Pediatrics [AAP], 2013a).

Most preschoolers also engage in dramatic play, fueled by their innate curiosity and vivid imaginations.

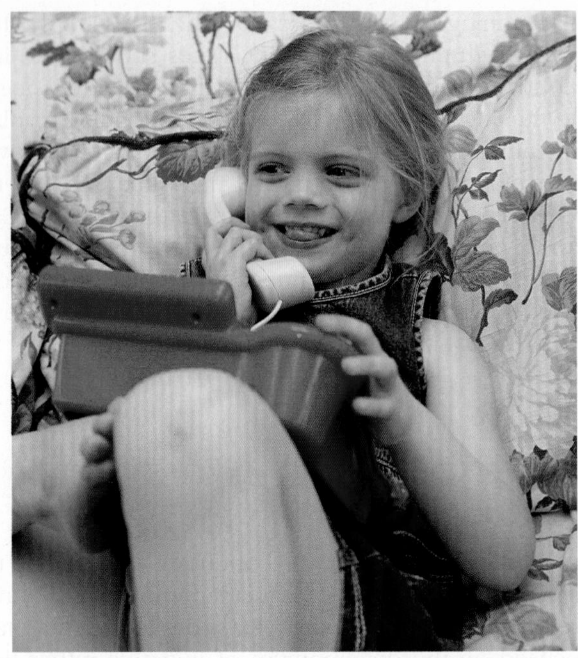

FIGURE 27.9 Preschool children enjoy imitative play.

Three-year-olds may not realize that they are pretending. They run from scary creatures, make plans, and pack their backpacks (never intending to actually leave). Four-year-olds are more sophisticated with dramatic or pretend play: they know they are pretending, and they use dress-up clothes and props to act out more complex roles and scenarios (Fig. 27.10). Five-year-olds are capable of quite complex scenarios. They pretend they are real or fantasy characters. They often use dramatic play to express anxiety, try out negative feelings, or conquer their fears. For example, a child who is afraid of getting a shot at the doctor's office may work through that feeling with pretend play.

Parents should encourage physical activity in the preschool child. Regular physical activity improves gross motor skills, may enhance the child's self-confidence,

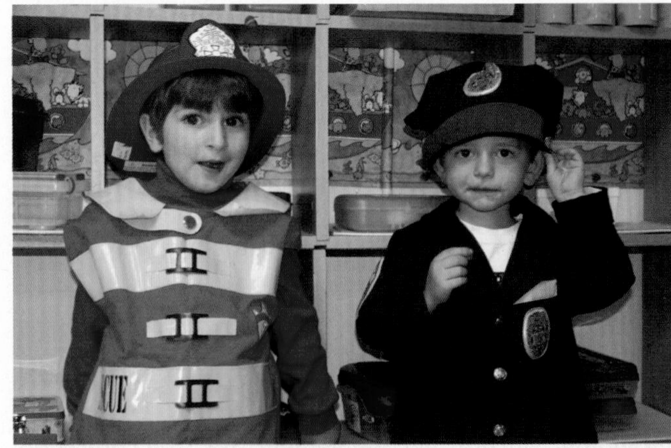

FIGURE 27.10 Preschool children love to dress up and pretend.

BOX 27.1

APPROPRIATE TOYS FOR PRESCHOOLERS

- Blocks, simple jigsaw puzzles (four to six large pieces), pegboards, wooden bead with string
- Supplies for creativity: chalk, large crayons, finger paint, Play-Doh or clay, washable markers, paper, paint and paintbrush, scissors, paste, or glue
- Puppets, dress-up clothes, and props for dramatic play
- Bucket, plastic shovel, and other containers for sand and water play
- Play kitchen with accessories and pretend food (empty food boxes can be recycled for kitchen play)
- Squeaking, floating, squirting toys for the bath
- Sandbox with shovel and various toys for building
- Dolls that can be dressed and undressed (large buttons, zippers, and snaps), doll care accessories (diapers, bottles, carriage, crib)
- Gross motor toys: tricycle or big wheel (with helmet), jungle gym or swing set (with supervision), hula hoop, tunnel, wagon
- Blocks, Legos, cars and trucks, plastic animals, trains, plastic figures (family, community helpers), stuffed animals, balls, sewing cards
- Tape or CD players for music, various musical instruments
- Simple card and board games (older preschooler)
- Dollhouse with furniture and accessories, people, and animals

Adapted from Dowshen, S. (2014). *Smart toys for every age*. Retrieved from http://kidshealth.org/en/parents/smart-toys.html# and National Association for the Education of Young Children. (n.d.) *Good toys for young children by age and stage*. Retrieved from http://www.naeyc.org/toys

and allows the child to expend excess energy. Establishing the habit of daily physical activity in the early years is important in the long-term goal of avoiding obesity. The main goal of organized sports at this age should be fun and enjoyment, although, of course, safety must remain a priority.

Expensive toys that claim to teach the young child are not necessary. Toys that require interactive rather than passive play, and that may include the involvement of the parent, are recommended (Dowshen, 2014 and National Association for the Education of Young Children, [n.d.]). Box 27.1 lists appropriate playthings for the preschool child.

Promoting Early Learning

The family is the foundation for the child's early growth and development. Parents serve as role models for behavior related to education and learning, as well as instilling values in their children. School readiness is a topic that has received a significant amount of national attention in recent years. To succeed in school, children need a safe, responsive home environment that allows them to learn and explore, as well as structure and limits that allow them to learn the socially acceptable behaviors that they will need in school. Language development is critical to the ability to succeed in school and can be encouraged through books and reading. Each of these components is important in readying the child for education in a more formal setting (Child Trends, 2015). Promoting language development, choosing a preschool, and making the transition to kindergarten are discussed in more detail below.

Promoting Language Development

The parent serves as the child's first teacher. The interactions between parent and child in relation to books and other play activities model the types of interactions that the child will later have in school. Asking open-ended questions stimulates the development of thinking as well as language in the preschool child. The preschooler is a great imitator, so the parent should serve as a role model for appropriate language. Parents should avoid swearing, as the child is sure to repeat "bad words" even if he or she does not understand what they mean. Allowing children to pursue interests at their own pace will help them to develop the literacy and numeric skills that will enable them to later focus on academic skills.

Preschoolers enjoy books with pictures that tell stories (Fig. 27.11). Stories with repeated phrases help to keep the child's attention. Children like stories that

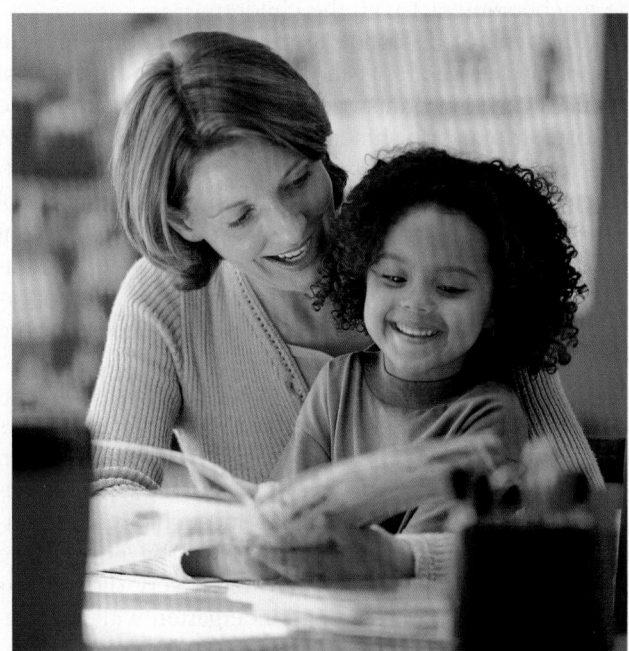

FIGURE 27.11 Preschool children enjoy being read to and looking at the pictures that go along with the story.

describe experiences similar to their own. The preschool child demonstrates early literacy skills by reciting stories or portions of books. He or she also may retell the story from the book, pretend to read books, and ask questions about the story. The preschool child has enough focus and expanded attention to notice when a page is skipped during reading and will call it to the parent's attention.

Take Note!

Risk factors for lack of social and emotional readiness for school include insecure attachment in the early years, maternal depression, parental substance abuse, and low socioeconomic status. Nurses should screen for these factors and make referrals if appropriate.

Choosing a Preschool/ Starting Kindergarten

Many parents choose to enroll their child in preschool. Preschool should be used primarily as an opportunity to foster the child's social skills and accustom him or her to the group environment. When selecting a preschool, the parent may want to consider the accreditation of the school, the teachers' qualifications, and recommendations of other parents. The focus of the school environment is also important: What is the daily schedule of activities? Is the school very structured, or does it have a looser environment? The parents must decide how focused on curriculum they want the school to be. The parent should observe the classroom, evaluating the environment, noise level, and sanitary practices as well as how the children interact with each other and how the teachers interact with the children.

The type of discipline used in the school is also an important factor. Parents should not choose a preschool that uses corporal punishment. The AAP discourages the use of corporal punishment in the school setting (AAP, 2012). Corporal punishment may hurt a child's self-esteem as well as his or her ability to achieve in school (AAP, 2012). It may also lead to disruptive and violent behavior in the classroom. As preschool is the foundation for later education, the child should have the opportunity to build self-esteem and the skills needed for the more formal setting of elementary school.

Whether or not the child attended preschool, kindergarten will be the next big step. Kindergarten hours may be longer than preschool hours, and kindergarten is usually held 5 days per week. This may be a significant change for some children. For most children, the setting and personnel in kindergarten will be new to the child. Rules and expectations are often very different as well. When discussing starting kindergarten with the preschool child, parents should do so in an enthusiastic fashion, keeping the conversation light and positive. Parents should meet with the child's teacher prior to the start of school, if possible, to discuss particular needs or concerns. Parents may want to schedule a tour of the school for the preschooler or attend the school's open house with the child to ease the transition. Practicing the new daily routine prior to the start of school will also be helpful.

Most states require up-to-date immunizations and a health screening of the child before he or she enters kindergarten, so advise parents to plan ahead and schedule these in a timely fashion so that school entrance is not delayed (Centers for Disease Control and Prevention [CDC], 2016a).

Promoting Safety

In the United States, accidental injury remains the leading cause of death for children between the ages of 1 and 14 years (National Center for Injury Prevention and Control, 2010b). Preschoolers are at an ideal age to be taught about safety and safe behaviors. They are cognitively able to absorb concrete information and they desire to master the situations they are in, but they continue to display poor judgment related to safety issues. Their engagement in fantasy is so strong that it makes it difficult for them to master complicated cause-and-effect relationships. The preschool child is capable of learning safe behaviors but may not always be able to transfer those behaviors to a different situation. Parents must continue to closely supervise preschool children to avoid accidental injury during this period.

Safety in the Car

The preschooler up until 4 years of age whose height meets the car seat size requirement should use a forward-facing car seat with harness and top tether. All preschoolers after reaching the car seat height restriction should ride in a booster seat that uses both the lap and shoulder belts (Fig. 27.12). It is recommended that

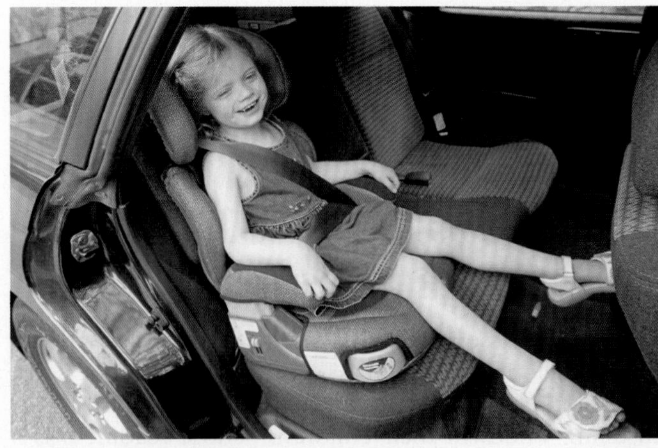

FIGURE 27.12 The older preschool child should be appropriately secured in an approved booster seat.

HEALTHY PEOPLE 2020

Objective	Nursing Significance
Increase age-appropriate vehicle restraint system use in children.	• Encourage car seat and booster seat use until the child is of the appropriate size and age to progress to seat belts.

Healthy People Objectives retrieved from http://www.healthypeople.gov

the booster seat continues to be used until a height of 145 cm (4 feet 9 inches) and age of 8 to 12 years are reached (AAP, 2016). The back seat of the car is always the safest place for a child to ride. If a child younger than 12 years of age must sit in the front seat because there are not enough rear seats available, then the front passenger seat air bag should be deactivated. The National Highway Traffic Safety Administration states that children should never ride in the cargo area of a pickup truck (TN Traffic Safety Resource Service, 2011). See Healthy People 2020.

Take Note!

Although motor vehicle accidents remain a major cause of injury and death in the preschool age group, many families do not use appropriate car seat/seat belt safety with their children. Child passenger safety technicians are available to provide proper installation of car seats. To find one in your area, visit http://cert.safekids.org/ or http://www.seatcheck.org. The National Highway Traffic Safety Administration (NHTSA) Auto Safety Hotline may be reached at (888) 327-4236.

Safety in the Home

Handguns, matches, bodies of water, bicycle riding, and poisons continue to be sources of potential injury during the preschool years. Falls account for the highest percentage of nonfatal injuries among preschoolers. In this age group, motor vehicle accidents are responsible for the most fatal injuries, followed by drowning. A significant number of injuries also occur in or around the home, including burns and poisoning (National Center for Injury Prevention and Control, 2010a).

PREVENTING EXPOSURE TO TOBACCO SMOKE

Parents should protect their preschoolers from secondhand tobacco smoke. Exposure to tobacco smoke is associated with an increased incidence of otitis media and respiratory infections, as well as increased symptoms and medication use in children with asthma. Other effects include decreased lung function and behavioral difficulties (World Health Organization, n.d.). The preschool child should never be in an enclosed space (such as a car) where tobacco smoke is present.

PREVENTING INJURY

The preschool child who runs out into the street is at risk for being struck by a car. Teach preschoolers to stop at the curb and never go into the street without a grown-up. The preschooler may learn to ride a bicycle (with or without training wheels). The child must wear an approved bicycle helmet any time he or she rides the bicycle, even if it is just in the driveway. Requiring helmet use in the early years may lead to the habit of helmet use as the child gets older. Allowing the preschooler to choose his or her own helmet may encourage the child to use the helmet.

Bicycles should be safe for this age group. The size must be correct; the balls of the feet should reach both pedals while the child is sitting on the seat and has both hands on the handlebars. Children younger than 5 years of age have difficulty learning to use hand-operated brakes, so traditional pedal-back brakes are recommended in this age group. Preschoolers are not mature enough to ride a bicycle in the street even if they are riding with adults, so they should always ride on the sidewalk (AAP, 2015b).

It is important to make the inside of the home safe for the preschool child. Parents should install and maintain smoke alarms as well as carbon monoxide detectors in the home. Increased physical dexterity and refinement of motor skills enable the preschooler to strike matches or use a lighter and start a fire. The preschool child is capable of washing his or her hands independently, so the water heater should be set at (49°C) (120°F) or below to prevent scalding (AAP, 2015a).

The preschooler's active imagination and desire to play make-believe may result in a firearm injury. The average preschooler is physically capable of handling and firing a gun, particularly a handgun, which is smaller and lighter. If present in the home, firearms should be kept in a locked cabinet with the ammunition stored elsewhere (AAP, 2015a, AAP, 2015b).

PREVENTING POISONING

Though it is continuing to develop, preschoolers still have unrefined taste discrimination, placing them at risk for accidental ingestion. Parents should never try to coax a child to take a vitamin supplement, tablet, or pill by calling it "candy." Dangerous fluids should be stored in their original containers and should be kept out of reach of preschoolers; they should not be poured into containers that look like ordinary drinking glasses or cups. Potentially dangerous cleaning or personal health and beauty products, gardening and pool chemicals, and automotive materials should be kept out of reach of preschoolers and in a locked cabinet if possible. Medications should have childproof caps and should be kept in a locked cabinet. The Poison Control Center telephone number should be posted on or near the home phone (1-800-222-1222) (American Association of Poison Control Centers, n.d.).

Safety in the Water

Five years of age is an appropriate time for a child to learn to swim (AAP, 2010). Children at this age are physically capable of this activity and have the cognitive maturity to accomplish the task of swimming and basic water safety. Swimming programs should focus on appropriate swim techniques as well as safety measures. Parents and caregivers should be trained in infant/child cardiopulmonary resuscitation (CPR). Homes with swimming pools should have life-saving devices readily accessible. Preschoolers should be taught never to dive into water until an adult has verified its depth. Preschoolers are still too young to be left unattended around any body of water, even if they know how to swim. Preschoolers should never be allowed to swim in a canal or any fast-moving water. Preschoolers who are riding in boats or fishing off riverbanks should wear a personal flotation device. Parents should also be cautioned about close supervision of young children walking, skating, or riding near thin or weak ice. See Healthy People 2020.

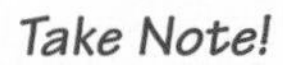

Take Note!

The AAP recommends that all swimming pools be secured by a fence that is at least 5 feet high and has a self-latching gate to protect young children from entering a pool area unattended (AAP, 2010).

Recall Nila Patel, the 4-year-old presented at the beginning of the chapter. What anticipatory guidance related to safety should you provide to her parents?

HEALTHY PEOPLE 2020

Objective	Nursing Significance
Reduce drowning deaths.	• Never leave a young child unattended in or near the water. • Educate families about water safety. • Remind families that the preschooler's ability to swim does not replace the need for constant supervision while in the pool or other body of water.

Healthy People Objectives retrieved from http://www.healthypeople.gov

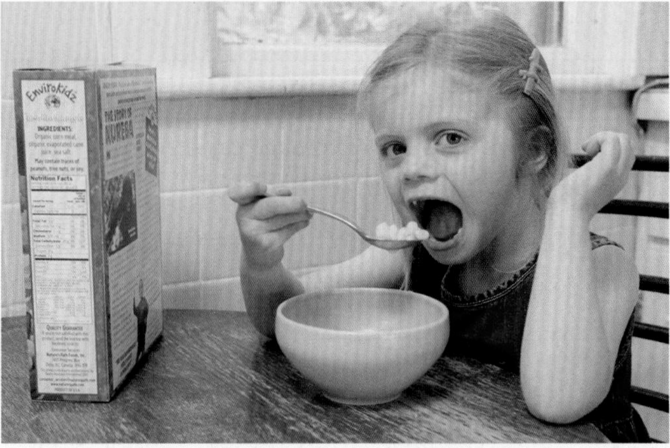

FIGURE 27.13 The preschool child has the manual dexterity to handle utensils appropriately and feed himself or herself independently.

Promoting Nutrition

The preschool child has a full set of primary teeth, is able to chew and swallow competently, and has learned to use utensils fairly effectively to feed himself or herself (Fig. 27.13). As in the toddler years, it is important for the preschool child to continue to learn and build upon healthy eating habits. These habits will last throughout the child's life. A diet high in nutrient-rich foods such as whole grains, vegetables, fruits, appropriate dairy foods, and lean meats is appropriate for the preschooler. Nutrient-poor, high-calorie foods such as sweets and typical fast foods should be offered only in limited amounts.

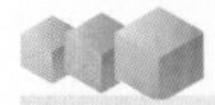

Concept Mastery Alert

Preschool Eating Habits

Preschoolers are erratic eaters and will eat very well one day and then may eat very little the next day. Food jags are not common in the preschooler, but are common in the toddler.

Nutritional Needs

The 3- to 5-year-old requires 700 to 1,000 mg calcium and 7 to 10 mg iron daily (Ross, Taylor, Yaktine, & Del Valle, 2011). Box 27.2 lists calcium and iron sources. Preschoolers should consume a minimum of 19 mg dietary fiber daily (Brown, 2011). The typical preschooler requires about 85 kcal/kg of body weight. Saturated fats should account for less than 10% of total calories. Preschool children's diets should include a daily total fat intake of no less than 20% and not more than 35% of total calories to promote and maintain healthy cholesterol levels (Haemer, Primark, & Krebs, 2012).

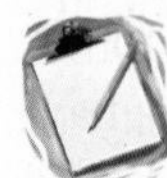

Take Note!

Drinking excess amounts of milk may lead to iron deficiency, as the calcium in milk blocks iron absorption.

BOX 27.2

DAILY CALCIUM AND IRON RECOMMENDATIONS FOR PRESCHOOL CHILDREN

Calcium: 700 mg (3-year-old), 1,000 mg (4- to 8-year-old)

Calcium in Foods

- 8-ounce low-fat or whole milk: 275–300 mg
- 8-ounce low-fat yogurt: 313–415 mg
- 1½-ounce cheddar cheese: 307 mg
- 1-ounce dried white beans (cooked): 75 mg
- ¼ cup tofu: 138–253 mg
- ½ cup raw broccoli: 21 mg

Iron: 7 mg (3-year-old), 10 mg (4- to 8-year-old)

Iron in Foods

- ¾ cup 100% fortified prepared cereal: 18 mg
- 3-ounce beef: 3 mg
- 3-ounce chicken (dark meat): 1.1 mg
- ½ cup cooked lentils: 3 mg
- 3-ounce chicken (white meat): 0.9 mg
- 15.2-cm (6–inch) slice watermelon: 0.7 mg
- ¼ cup fresh cooked spinach: 1.6 mg
- ¼ cup tofu: 1.7 mg
- ¼ cup raisins: 1 mg
- 1 slice enriched bread: 0.8 to 0.9 mg
- ¼ cup frozen spinach, cooked: 0.85 mg

Adapted from National Institutes of Health. (2016a). *Calcium dietary supplement fact sheet.* Retrieved from http://ods.od.nih.gov/factsheets/Calcium-HealthProfessional/#h3 National Institutes of Health. (2016b). *Iron dietary supplement fact sheet.* Retrieved from http://ods.od.nih.gov/factsheets/Iron-HealthProfessional/#h4

Promoting Healthy Eating Habits

Preschool children may be picky eaters. They may eat only a limited variety of foods or foods prepared in certain ways and may not be very willing to try new things. The 3- or 4-year-old may exhibit "food fads," eating only certain foods over a several-day period. As the child gets older, pickiness lessens. By 5 years of age the child is more focused on the social context of eating: table conversation and manners. The 5-year-old is generally more willing to at least try new foods and may like to help with meal preparation and clean-up as appropriate.

If the preschooler is growing well, then the pickiness is not a cause for concern. A larger concern may be the negative relationship that can develop between the parent and child relating to mealtime. The more the parent coaxes, cajoles, bribes, and threatens, the less likely the child is to try new foods or even eat the ones he or she likes that are served. The parent must maintain a positive and patient demeanor at mealtime. The child should be offered a healthy diet, with foods from all groups over the course of the day as recommended by the U.S. Department of Agriculture (USDA) (n.d). Parents may visit the USDA's website at http://www.choosemyplate.gov/PRESCHOOLERS/Plan/index.html to develop a personalized daily food plan for their child based upon age and activity level.

The parent should maintain a matter-of-fact approach, offer the meal or snack, and then allow the child to decide how much of the food, if any, he or she is going to eat. High-fat, nutrient-poor snacks should not be substituted for healthy foods just to coax the child to "eat something." See Healthy People 2020.

Preventing the Development of Overweight and Obesity

Worldwide, over 22 million children younger than 5 years old are obese. In the past 30 years, the number of US children and adolescents who are overweight has doubled. According to the National Health and Nutrition Examination Survey, 8.4% of all 2- to 5-year-olds are either overweight or obese (CDC, 2015). Overweight and obese children are at risk for hypertension, hyperlipidemia, and the development of insulin resistance. Having a high body mass index as a preschooler is consistently associated with adult and central obesity as well as early onset of metabolic syndrome (Graversen et al., 2014). The risk is increased if one or both parents are overweight.

HEALTHY PEOPLE 2020

Objective	Nursing Significance
Increase consumption of calcium in the population aged 2 years and older.	• Screen preschoolers for appropriate dietary intake of calcium. • Educate families about calcium content in foods. • Assist families with choosing a diet that meets calcium needs and is appealing to the young child.

Healthy People Objectives retrieved from http://www.healthypeople.gov

Parents are in an opportune position to exert a positive influence on their preschooler's nutritional intake and activity level. The habits learned in early childhood will likely carry over into the school-age, adolescent, and adult years. Children whose parents take an authoritarian approach to mealtime may learn to overeat, as they are encouraged to finish the entire meal ("Clean your plate!"). If they are offered appropriate, healthy food choices, and access to high-calorie, nutrient-poor food is limited, preschoolers will learn to self-regulate (eat only until full). Food should not be used as either reward or punishment.

Parents should remain positive and patient at mealtime. Mealtimes should continue to be structured. Unstructured meals lead to an increase in fat and calorie consumption. Children who eat nutrient-dense and lower-fat foods are less likely to become overweight (Institute of Medicine, 2011). To limit the chance that overeating will occur, preschoolers should be offered a variety of healthy foods at each meal. This may include one each of a protein source, grain, vegetable, and fruit. The preschool child's serving size is usually one third to one half of the recommended size of an adult serving. The preschool child may imitate the other eaters at the table. Parents have a prime chance to be good role models, setting an example of eating vegetables and fruits.

As with toddlers, fruit juice should be limited to 4 to 6 ounces per day, as excess consumption can lead to excess weight gain (Stettler, Bhatia, Parish, & Stallings, 2011). Preschoolers should be encouraged to drink water.

Limiting television viewing and encouraging physical activity are also important strategies for the prevention of overweight and obesity. See Evidence-Based Practice 27.1

Refer back to Nila Patel, the 4-year-old introduced at the beginning of the chapter. What questions should you ask Nila's parents related to nutritional intake? What anticipatory guidance related to nutrition would be appropriate? Nila's mother expresses concerns regarding obesity. How would you address these?

Promoting Healthy Sleep and Rest

The preschool child needs about 11 to 12 hours of sleep each day (Feigelman, 2011). Some preschool children continue to take a nap during the day. Unless very tired, many preschool children will resist going to bed from time to time. Bedtime rituals continue to be reassuring to children, and it is important to continue them in the preschool years. Having a time of relaxation with a decrease in stimulation will allow the child to fall asleep more easily. Some children continue to need a security item at bedtime or naptime. A nightlight in the bedroom may

EVIDENCE-BASED PRACTICE 27.1 PREVENTING PRESCHOOL OBESITY BY PROMOTING PHYSICAL ACTIVITY

STUDY

One of the most pressing public health issues is the continued rise in the childhood obesity epidemic. Early childhood obesity is associated with immediate health consequences as well as long-term issues such as adult obesity and early-onset metabolic syndrome. Early childhood is a prime time for establishing healthy eating and activity habits that may persist into adulthood.

The authors reviewed 14 recent US studies focusing on children aged 2 to 5 years, and measurement of physical activity as well as perceived factors related to physical activity. Independent reviews were undertaken followed by the authors reconvening and discussing the factors associated with physical activity amongst preschoolers.

Findings

The authors' literature review revealed discrepancies between parents' perceived notions about child physical activity and actual child physical activity. Families perceive their preschoolers to be active throughout the day, but studies show that much of this activity is sedentary in nature. The child's characteristics and personality traits may have an influence on choice of play; children will be more active when engaged in a type of play that they personally enjoy. Parental involvement in physical activities also influences the preschooler's activity level. Perceived safety in the childcare environment or home outdoor setting also affects children's physical activity levels.

Nursing Implications

Parents naturally want what is best for their children, but often need guidance from health care providers to encourage them to move toward healthy habits. Nurses are in a unique position to provide ongoing, repeated education about the importance of physical activity in preschoolers to families wherever they encounter them. Parents may be tired from their busy schedules, but nurses can provide positive reinforcement for even small steps (such as taking a brief walk after the evening meal, while the preschooler rides a bike or skates alongside). Encourage families to discover which physical activities their preschooler prefers, and encourage them to provide opportunities for participation in those activities. Assist families with finding safe parks in their neighborhood and provide consultation with regard to play equipment in child care settings. With continued attention to the need for increased physical activity in preschoolers, an eventual change in a positive direction can be achieved.

Adapted from Hodges, E. A., Smith, C., Tidwell, S. & Berry, D. (2013). Promoting physical activity in preschoolers to prevent obesity: A review of the literature. *Journal of Pediatric Nursing, 28*, 3–19.

be necessary, as many children this age are afraid of the dark. Teaching Guidelines 27.1 gives information about assisting parents to establish a bedtime routine.

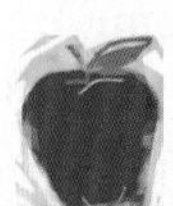

Teaching Guidelines 27.1
BEDTIME ROUTINES

- Establish a bedtime as well as morning wake-up time.
- Avoid sugar or caffeine consumption in the evening.
- Avoid stimulating activities such as roughhousing before bedtime.
- Do not allow television watching in bed.
- Make the child's bedroom an inviting and comfortable area of the home.
- Provide a nightlight in the child's bedroom if he or she is afraid of the dark.
- Conform to a nightly routine.
- Television off at a certain time
- Bath
- Quiet game or story reading/telling
- Bedtime prayer or song
- Maintain quiet in the bedroom and nearby to increase the child's ability to fall asleep.

Adapted from Gupta, R. C. (2014). (2011). Sleep and your preschooler. Retrieved from http://kidshealth.org/parent/general/sleep/sleep_preschool.html; and Goldson, E., & Reynolds, A. (2012). Child development & behavior. In W. W. Hay, M. J. Levin, R. R., Deterding, et al. (Eds.) *Current diagnosis & treatment: Pediatrics* (21st ed.). New York, NY: McGraw Hill.

Nightmares often occur in preschool children as a result of the child's struggle to distinguish what is real from what is not. When a child awakens from a nightmare, he or she is often crying and may be able to recount what the dream was about. Parents should validate the child's fear rather than discounting it (Goldson & Reynolds, 2012). Saying, "Yes, I agree, monsters are scary; it's a good thing they aren't real" is more appropriate than, "Don't be silly: monsters aren't real." Sometimes children benefit from reading stories about dreams. Recommended books include:

- Bedtime for Frances by Russell Hoban
- Ben's Dream by Chris van Allsberg
- In the Night Kitchen by Maurice Sendak
- There's a Nightmare in My Closet by Mercer Mayer

Nightmares should not be confused with night terrors. After a nightmare, the child is aroused and interactive, but night terrors are different: a short time after falling asleep, the child seems to awaken and is screaming. The child usually does not respond much to the parent's soothing, but he or she eventually stops screaming and goes back to sleep. Night terrors are often frightening for parents because the child does not seem to be responding to them. One technique that may help to decrease the incidence of night terrors is to wake the child about 30 to 45 minutes into the sleep cycle. If continued nightly for about a week, the cycle of night terrors may be broken (Cavanaugh, 2011). See Comparison Chart 27.1.

Think back to Nila Patel. What anticipatory guidance would you provide to her parents in relation to sleep during the preschool years?

Promoting Healthy Teeth and Gums

Dental caries prevention continues to be important and can be achieved through daily brushing and flossing.

COMPARISON CHART 27.1 NIGHTMARES VERSUS NIGHT TERRORS

	Nightmare	Night Terror
Definition	Scary or bad dream followed by awakening	Partial arousal from deep sleep
When parents become aware	Child awakens parent after episode is over	Screaming and thrashing during the episode awakens the parent
Timing	Usually in the second half of the night	Usually about an hour after falling asleep
Behavior	Crying, may be scared after awakening	Sits up, thrashes, cries, screams, talks, looks wild-eyed. Sweats, may have racing heartbeat
Responsiveness	Responsive to parent's soothing and reassurances	Child unaware of parent's presence, may scream and thrash more if restrained
Return to sleep	Difficulty going back to sleep if afraid	Rapidly returns to sleep without full awakening
Memory of occurrence	May remember the dream and talk about it later	No memory of event

Adapted from Cavanaugh, K. (2011). Parasomnias. *Advance for NPs & Pas*, 2(2), 21–24.

Parents should use only a pea-sized amount of toothpaste to prevent excess fluoride consumption, which can contribute to fluorosis (Clark & Krol, n. d.). The preschooler may brush his or her own teeth, but the parent must continue to supervise to ensure adequate brushing. Parents must perform flossing because the preschool child cannot perform this task adequately.

Cariogenic foods should be avoided. If sugary foods are consumed, the mouth should be rinsed with water if it is not possible to brush the teeth immediately (American Academy of Pediatric Dentistry, 2014). The preschool child should visit the dentist every 6 months.

Take Note!

Dental caries prevention is important in the primary teeth, because loss of these teeth to caries may affect the proper formation of permanent teeth as well as the width of the dental arch.

Promoting Appropriate Discipline

Successful discipline results from a loving and nurturing environment in which the preschooler's self-esteem is fostered and where limits are well chosen and enforced consistently. Spanking (striking with the open hand) is the least effective discipline practice and is discouraged by the American Academy of Child and Adolescent Psychiatry [AACAP] (2012) and the National Association of Pediatric Nurse Practitioners (2011). Belts, switches, paddles, or other items should never be used to strike a child. The use of physical punishment has been associated with a number of additional problems in adulthood, such as antisocial and criminal behaviors (AACAP, 2012) (see Chapter 26).

If parents are consistent with discipline while encouraging the preschooler's normal growth and development of imagination and make-believe, the child will learn to accept that certain things are not allowed. The sense of initiative can be preserved and guilt avoided if the rules are clear and enforced consistently (Sears & Sears, 2015a).

Take Note!

Corporal punishment not only causes physical and emotional pain, it also decreases learning capacity (AACAP, 2012).

Minimize the occurrence of misbehavior by anticipating conditions likely to lead to the undesired or risky action. When the situation becomes difficult, parents should use distraction to change the preschooler's focus. When discussing the misbehavior, be certain to label the behavior and not the child. This helps to preserve the preschooler's self-esteem. When teaching preschoolers about undesired behavior, be sure they also understand the reason why it is wrong or unacceptable to do it. This helps to encourage the child to use internal controls over behavior. Parents should serve as role models for self-control, including choice of words, the tone they are delivered in, and the actions that accompany them.

Children work harder to obtain praise than to receive punishment, so always reward positive behaviors. Preschool children are becoming capable of understanding the concept of right and wrong. They start to understand each other's feelings (**empathy**) and are cognitively capable of remembering basic rules.

Time-out or time away from the situation can be very effective in this age group. The punishment should be used only for intentional misbehavior (knowing something is forbidden but doing it anyway). It is particularly helpful with dangerous or destructive behavior. The preschooler is given a warning that time-out will occur if the behavior does not stop. The preschooler is removed from the situation and must stay in time-out for a specified period of time. A particular time-out area is helpful; a boring corner of the room without distractions available is a good location. The generally recommended period of time is to require 1 minute of time-out per year of age; thus, a 4-year-old would be in time-out for 4 minutes (Sears & Sears, 2015b). Set the timer so the child will know when the time-out is over. If the child gets up before the prescribed time, replace the child in time-out and restart the timer. Time-out works best if used each and every time the undesirable behavior occurs. Also, praise the child when he or she follows the rules and behaves appropriately.

A simple and clear explanation of the misbehavior should be given to the child; parents should also talk about acceptable alternative strategies that the child can use in the future instead of the undesired behavior. Removal of a privilege such as playing with a favorite toy can be as effective as time-out.

Books and other media that are available to help educate parents about appropriate discipline and to help the child learn self-control are listed in Box 27.3.

ADDRESSING COMMON DEVELOPMENTAL CONCERNS

Common developmental concerns of the preschool period include lying, how to address sex education, and masturbation. Parents often express difficulty in dealing with these issues with their preschool children. Offering appropriate anticipatory guidance may give the parents the support and confidence they need to deal with these issues.

Lying

Lying is common in preschool children. It may occur because the child fears punishment, has gotten carried

BOX 27.3

SELECTED RESOURCES FOR PARENTS AND PRESCHOOLERS

Books for Parents (about discipline)

- How to Talk so Kids Will Listen and Listen so Kids Will Talk by A. Faber & E. Mazlish (Harper Resource)
- Kids Are Worth It: Giving Your Children the Gift of Inner Discipline by B. Colorosos (Harper Collins Publishers)
- Positive Discipline A to Z: 1001 Solutions to Everyday Parenting Problems by J. Nelson, L. Lott, & S. G. Glenn (Three Rivers Press)
- Setting Limits With Your Strong-Willed Child: Eliminating Conflict by Establishing Clear, Firm and Respectful Boundaries by R. MacKenzie (Three Rivers Press)
- The Case Against Spanking: How to Discipline Children Without Hitting by I. A. Hyman (Jossey-Bass)
- The Nurturing Parent: How to Raise Creative, Loving, Responsible Children by J. S. Dacey & A. J. Packer (Fireside)
- Without Spanking or Spoiling: A Practical Approach to Toddler and Preschool Guidance by E. Crary (Parenting Press)

Books for Preschoolers (about dealing with feelings and learning how to behave)

- *Hands Are Not for Hitting* by M. Agassi (Free Spirit Publishing)
- *I Can't Wait* by E. Crary (Parenting Press)
- *I Want It* by E. Crary (Parenting Press)
- *I Want to Play* by E. Crary (Parenting Press)
- *I Was so Mad* by M. Mayer (Golden Books)
- *I Was so Mad* by N. Simon & D. Leder (Albert Whitman & Company)
- *I'm Excited* by E. Crary (Parenting Press)
- *I'm Frustrated* by E. Crary (Parenting Press)
- *I'm Mad* by E. Crary (Parenting Press)
- *I'm Scared* by E. Crary (Parenting Press)
- *Feet Are Not for Kicking* by E. Verdick (Free Spirit Publishing)
- *Teeth Are Not for Biting* by E. Verdick (Free Spirit Publishing)
- *When Sophie Gets Angry ... Really, Really Angry* by M. Bang (Blue Sky Press)
- *Words Are Not for Hurting* by E. Verdick (Free Spirit Publishing)

away with imagination, or is imitating what he or she sees the parent do. The parent should ascertain the reason for the lie before punishing the child. If the child has broken a rule and fears punishment, then the parent must determine the truth. The child needs to learn that lying is usually far worse than the misbehavior itself. The punishment for the misbehavior should be lessened if the child admits the truth. The parent should remain calm and serve as a role model of an even temper. The next time the misbehavior occurs, the child will be more apt to simply tell the truth.

If the child's lying is really just his or her imagination getting carried away, then the parent should guide the child in distinguishing between myth and reality (Sears & Sears, 2015c). The preschooler's imagination is very vivid, and the child needs direction in the use of that faculty. Parents should serve as role models of appropriate behavior for their children to learn it. Children who lie because they hear their parents lying simply must not see or hear their parents do it.

Sex Education

Preschoolers are keen observers but are still not able to interpret all that they see correctly. The child may recognize, but not understand, sexual activity. Preschoolers are very inquisitive and want to learn about everything around them; therefore, they are very likely to ask questions about sex and where babies come from. Before attempting to answer questions, parents should try to find out first what the child is really asking and what the child already thinks about that subject. Then they should provide a simple, direct, and honest answer. The child needs only the information that he or she is requesting. Additional questions will occur in the future and should be addressed as they arise.

Masturbation

The normal curiosity of the preschool years often leads children to explore their own genitals (Feigelman, 2011). This behavior may be upsetting to some parents, but masturbation is a healthy and natural part of normal preschool development if it occurs in moderation. If the parent overreacts to this behavior, then it may occur more frequently. Masturbation should be treated in a matter-of-fact way by the parent. The child needs to learn certain rules about this activity: nudity and masturbation are not acceptable in public. The child should also be taught safety: no other person can touch the private parts unless it is the parent, doctor, or nurse checking to see when something is wrong.

Think back to Nila Patel. What are some developmental concerns that are common during the preschool years? What anticipatory guidance related to these concerns would you provide to Nila's parents?

NURSING CARE PLAN 27.1

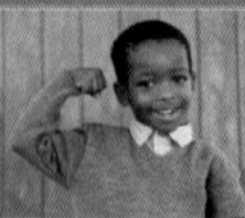

Growth and Development Issues in the Preschool Child

NURSING DIAGNOSIS: risk for (risk factors: developmental age, environment, and motor vehicle travel)

Outcome Identification and Evaluation

Child's safety will be maintained: *Child will remain free from injury.*

Interventions: ***Preventing Injury***

- Teach and encourage appropriate use of forward-facing car seat or booster seat *to decrease risk of injury related to motor vehicles.*
- Teach preschoolers to stay away from street and to cross the street only when holding the hand of an adult *to prevent pedestrian injury.*
- Require bicycle helmet use while riding any wheeled toy *to prevent head injury and form habit of helmet use.*
- Teach the preschooler appropriate safety rules in the home (avoiding electric outlets, etc.): *the preschooler is able to follow simple directions and carry out directives. Limits help him or her to organize the environment.*
- Post Poison Control Center phone number *(in case of accidental ingestion; the preschool child is very curious).*
- Never leave a preschool child unattended in a tub or pool or near any body of water *to prevent drowning.*
- Provide swimming lessons for children age 4 or 5 *to encourage water safety, but not as a replacement for adult supervision.*
- Teach parents first-aid measures and child CPR *to minimize consequences of injury should it occur.*
- Provide close observation and keep side rails up on bed in hospital *because the preschool child continues to be at risk for falling or injuring self on equipment or tubing (because of curiosity).*

NURSING DIAGNOSIS: Imbalanced nutrition, less than body requirements, related to inappropriate nutritional intake to sustain growth needs (excess juice or milk intake, inadequate food variety intake) as evidenced by failure to attain adequate increases in height and weight over time

Outcome Identification and Evaluation

Child will consume adequate nutrients: Child will demonstrate weight gain and increases in height.

Interventions: ***Promoting Appropriate Nutrition***

- Assess current feeding schedule and usual intake, as well as methods used to feed, *to determine areas of adequacy versus inadequacy.*
- Determine if the preschooler is unable to drink from a cup or does not finger feed or use utensils properly, or if the child has difficulty swallowing or tolerating certain textures of foods *to determine if further interventions such as speech or occupational therapy are required.*
- Weigh child daily on same scale if hospitalized, weekly on same scale if at home, and plot growth patterns weekly or monthly as appropriate on standardized growth charts *to determine if growth is improving.*
- Limit juice to 4 to 6 ounces per day, milk to 16 to 24 ounces per day, *to discourage sense of fullness achieved with excess milk or juice intake, thereby increasing appetite for appropriate solid foods.*
- Provide three nutrient-dense meals and at least two healthy snacks per day *to encourage adequate nutrient consumption.*
- Feed child on a similar schedule daily, without distractions and with the family: *preschool children continue to respond well to routine and structure. They are more interested in the social context of meals and are still apt to become distracted easily, so the TV should be off at mealtimes.*

NURSING CARE PLAN 27.1

Growth and Development Issues in the Preschool Child (continued)

NURSING DIAGNOSIS: Delayed growth and development related to motor, cognitive, language, or psychosocial concerns as evidenced by delay in meeting expected milestones

Outcome Identification and Evaluation

Development will be enhanced: Child will make continued progress toward realization of expected developmental milestones.

Interventions: *Enhancing Growth and Development*

- Screen for developmental capabilities to determine child's current level of functioning.
- Offer age-appropriate toys, play, and activities (including gross motor) to encourage further development.
- Perform interventions as prescribed by physical, occupational, or speech therapist: participation in those activities helps to promote function and accomplish acquisition of developmental skills.
- Provide support to families of preschoolers with developmental delay (progress in achieving developmental milestones can be slow and ongoing motivation is needed).
- Reinforce positive attributes in the child to maintain motivation.
- Model age-appropriate communication skills to illustrate suitable means for parenting the preschooler.

NURSING DIAGNOSIS: Disproportionate growth, risk for (risk factors: excess milk or juice intake, consumption of inappropriate foods or in excess amounts)

Outcome Identification and Evaluation

Child will grow appropriately and not become overweight or obese: Child will achieve weight and height within the 5th to 85th percentiles on standardized growth charts.

Interventions: *Promoting Appropriate Growth*

- Discourage use of no-spill sippy cups (they contribute to dental caries and allow unlimited access to fluids, possibly decreasing appetite for appropriate solid foods).
- Provide juice (4 to 6 ounces per day) and milk (16 to 24 ounces per day) from a cup at meal and snack time and water in between to avoid having the child drink excessive juice or milk.
- Provide only nutrient-rich foods without high sugar content for meals and snacks; even if the preschooler is a picky eater, it is inappropriate to provide high-calorie junk food just so the child eats something.
- Teach parents to role model appropriate eating (nutrient-rich, varied diet) to encourage child to try/accept new foods, as well as become familiar with a variety of foods.
- Severely limit the intake of fast foods and foods with high sugar and fat content to decrease intake of nutrient-poor, high-calorie foods.
- Ensure adequate physical activity to stimulate development of motor skills and provide appropriate caloric expenditure. This also sets the stage for forming life-long habit of appropriate physical activity.
- Teach parents to limit entertainment screen time to 1 to 2 hours per day to encourage participation in physical activities.

(continued)

NURSING CARE PLAN 27.1

Growth and Development Issues in the Preschool Child (continued)

NURSING DIAGNOSIS: Interrupted family processes related to issues with preschool child's development, hospitalization, or situational crisis as evidenced by decreased parental visitation in hospital, parental verbalization of difficulty with current situation, possible crisis related to health of family member other than the preschool child

Outcome Identification and Evaluation

Family will demonstrate adequate functioning: Family will display coping and psychosocial adjustment.

Interventions: ***Enhancing Family Functioning***

- Assess the family's level of stress and ability to cope to determine family's ability to cope with multiple stressors.
- Engage in family-centered care to provide a holistic approach to care of the preschooler and family.
- Encourage the family to verbalize feelings (verbalization is one method of decreasing anxiety levels) and acknowledge feelings and emotions.
- Use puppets or dramatic play with the child to elicit the preschooler's feelings about the current situation.
- Encourage family visitation and provide for sleeping arrangements for a parent or caregiver to stay in the hospital with the preschooler; this contributes to family's sense of control in situation.
- Involve family members in preschooler's care, giving them a feeling of control and connectedness.

NURSING DIAGNOSIS: Readiness for enhanced parenting related to parental desire for increased skill level and success with preschool child as evidenced by current healthy relationships and verbalization of desire for improved skills

Outcome Identification and Evaluation

Parent will provide safe and nurturing environment for the preschool child: *Parents will verbalize new skills they will employ in the family.*

Interventions: ***Increasing Parenting Skill Set***

- Use family-centered care to provide holistic approach.
- Educate parent about normal preschool development to provide basis of understanding for parenting skills needed in this time period.
- Acknowledge and encourage parents' verbalization of feelings related to chronic illness of child or difficulty with normal preschool behavior; this validates the normalcy of parents' feelings.
- Encourage positive parenting and respect for preschooler and his or her normal development (helps parents develop approaches to preschoolers that can be used in place of anger and frustration).
- Role model appropriate parenting behaviors related to communicating with and disciplining the child (role modeling actually demonstrates rather than just verbalizes what the parent should strive for).

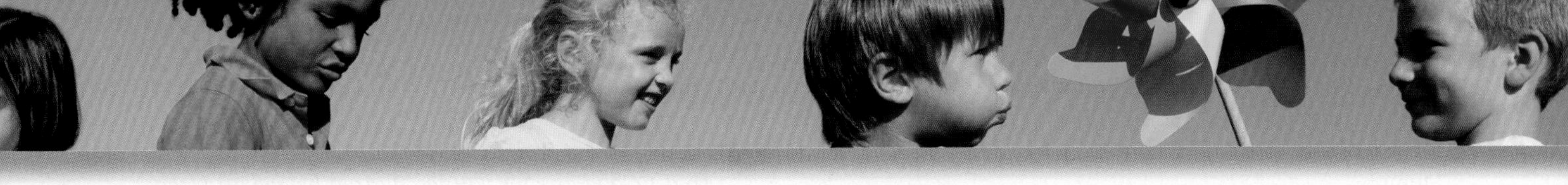

KEY CONCEPTS

- The preschool child grows at a slower rate and takes on a more slender and upright appearance than the toddler.
- The primary psychosocial task of the preschool period is developing a sense of initiative.
- Cognitive development moves from an egocentric approach to the world toward a more empathetic understanding of what happens outside of the self.
- The preschooler gains additional motor skills and displays significant refinement of fine motor abilities.
- Cognitive and language skills that develop in the preschool years help prepare the child for success in school.
- Dysfluency or hesitancy in speech is a normal finding in the preschool period and occurs as a result of the fast pace with which the preschooler is gaining language skills and vocabulary.
- The vocabulary of a preschooler increases to about 2,100 words, and the child speaks in full sentences with appropriate use of tense and prepositions.
- Appropriate growth and development should be maintained in the ill or hospitalized child.
- Recognizing concerns or delays in growth and development is essential so that the appropriate referrals may be made and intervention can begin.
- The preschool child requires a well-balanced diet with fat content between 20% and 30% of calories consumed.
- Adequate physical activity and provision of a nutrient-dense diet (rather than foods high in fat and sugar) are the foundation for obesity prevention in the preschool child.
- Adequate dental care is important for the health of the primary teeth.
- Preschoolers need about 12 hours of sleep per day and benefit from a structured bedtime routine.
- Due to the active imagination of the preschooler, nightmares and night terrors may begin during this period.
- Safety and injury prevention remain a focus in the preschool years.
- Structure, appropriate limit setting, and consistency are the keys for effective discipline in the preschool period.
- Time-out is an effective disciplinary measure for preschoolers.
- Masturbation may occur as the preschooler discovers his or her body. If not excessive, it is considered a normal part of growth and development.

REFERENCES AND RECOMMENDED READINGS

American Academy of Child and Adolescent Psychiatry. (2012). *Policy statement on corporal punishment*. Retrieved from http://www.aacap.org/AACAP/Policy_Statements/2012/Policy_Statement_on_Corporal_Punishment.aspx

American Academy of Pediatric Dentistry. (2014). *Guideline on infant oral health care*. Retrieved from http://www.aapd.org/media/Policies_Guidelines/G_InfantOralHealthCare.pdf

American Academy of Pediatrics. (2012). *Corporal punishment in schools*. Retrieved from http://pediatrics.aappublications.org/content/106/2/343.full?sid=c9b98d4f-a7f3%E2%80%934bfb-a596%E2%80%9305f159c87153

American Academy of Pediatrics. (2013a). Children, adolescents, and the media. *Pediatrics, 132*(5), 958–961.

American Academy of Pediatrics. (2016). *Car safety seats: Information for families*. Retrieved from http://www.healthychildren.org/English/safety-prevention/on-the-go/Pages/Car-Safety-Seats-Information-for-Families.aspx

American Academy of Pediatrics, Committee on Injury, Violence, and Poison Prevention. (2010). Prevention of drowning. *Pediatrics, 126*, 178–185.

American Academy of Pediatrics, The Injury Prevention Program. (2015a). *Safety for your child: 2 to 4 years*. Retrieved from https://www.healthychildren.org/English/ages-stages/toddler/Pages/Safety-for-Your-Child-2-to-4-Years.aspx

American Academy of Pediatrics, The Injury Prevention Program. (2015b). *Safety for your child: 5 years*. Retrieved from https://www.healthychildren.org/English/ages-stages/preschool/Pages/Safety-for-Your-Child-5-Years.aspx

American Association of Poison Control Centers. (n.d.). *Prevention*. Retrieved from http://www.aapcc.org

Brown, J. (2011). *Nutrition now* (6th ed.). Florence, KY: Wadsworth Publishing.

Carpenito-Moyet, L. J. (2013). *Nursing diagnosis: Application to clinical practice* (14th ed.). Philadelphia, PA: Lippincott Williams & Wilkins.

Cavanaugh, K. (2011). Parasomnias. *Advance for NPs & Pas, 2*(2), 21–24.

Centers for Disease Control and Prevention. (2015). *Childhood obesity facts*. Retrieved from http://www.cdc.gov/obesity/data/childhood.html

Centers for Disease Control and Prevention. (2016a). *State vaccination requirements*. Retrieved from http://www.cdc.gov/vaccines/imz-managers/laws/state-reqs.html

Centers for Disease Control and Prevention. (2016b). *Developmental milestones*. Retrieved from http://www.cdc.gov/ncbddd/actearly/milestones/index.html

Child Development Institute. (2015). *Is your child easy or difficult to raise?* Retrieved from http://childdevelopmentinfo.

com/child-development/temperament_and_your_child/temp3

Child Trends. (2015). *Early school readiness*. Retrieved from http://www.childtrends.org/?indicators=early-school-readiness

Clark, M., & Krol, D. (n. d.). Protecting all children's teeth (PACT): A pediatric oral health training program. Retrieved from http://www2.aap.org/ORALHEALTH/pact/pact-home.cfm

Dowshen , S.,(2014). *Smart toys for every age*. Retrieved from http://kidshealth.org/en/parents/smart-toys.html#

Erikson, E. H. (1963). *Childhood and society* (2nd ed.). New York, NY: W. W. Norton and Company.

Feigelman, S. (2011). Preschool years. In R. M. Kliegman, B. F. Stanton, J. W. St. Geme III, N. F. Schor, & R. E. Behrman (Eds.), (*Nelson's textbook of pediatrics* (19th ed.). Philadelphia, PA: Elsevier, Saunders.

Global Initiative to End All Corporal Punishment of Children. (n. d.). *Research on corporal punishment of children*. Retrieved from http://kidshealth.org/en/parents/sleep-preschool.html

Goldson, E., & Reynolds, A. (2012). Child development & behavior. In W. W. Hay, M. J. Levin, R. R, Deterding, et al. (Eds.) *Current diagnosis & treatment: Pediatrics* (21st ed.). New York, NY: McGraw Hill.

Graversen, L., Sørensen, T., Petersen, L., Sovio, U., Kaakinen, M., Sandbaek, A., et al. (2014). Preschool weight and body mass index in relation to central obesity and metabolic syndrome in adulthood. *PLoS ONE, 9*(3), 1–9.

Gupta, R. C. (2014). Sleep and your preschooler. Retrieved from http://kidshealth.org/parent/general/sleep/sleep_preschool.html

Haemer, M., Primark, L. E., & Krebs, N. R. (2012). Normal childhood nutrition and its disorders. In W. W. Hay, M. J. Levin, R. R. Deterding, et al. (Eds.) *Current diagnosis & treatment: Pediatrics* (21st ed.). New York, NY: McGraw Hill.

Hall, J. R. (2013). *Deaths and injuries due to non-fire exposure to gases*. Retrieved from http://www.nfpa.org/research/reports-and-statistics/non-fire-incidents/exposure-to-gases

Hodges, E. A., Smith, C., Tidwell, S., & Berry, D. (2013). Promoting physical activity in preschoolers to prevent obesity: A review of the literature. *Journal of Pediatric Nursing, 28*, 3–19.

Institute of Medicine. (2011). *Early childhood obesity prevention policies*. Retrieved from http://www.iom.edu/Reports/2011/Early-Childhood-Obesity-Prevention-Policies.aspx

Keeley, R. J. (2010). Faith development and faith formation: More than just ages and stages. *Lifelong Faith, 4.3*, 20–27.

Kohlberg, L. (1984). *Moral development*. New York, NY: Harper & Row.

Lowry, L. (2011). *Bilingualism in young children: Separating fact from fiction*. Retrieved from http://www.hanen.org/Helpful-Info/Articles/Bilingualism-in-Young-Children--Separating-Fact-fr.aspx

National Association for the Education of Young Children. (n.d.) *Good toys for young children by age and stage*. Retrieved from http://www.naeyc.org/toys.

National Association of Pediatric Nurse Practitioners. (2011). NAPNAP position statement on corporal punishment. *Journal of Pediatric Health Care, 25*, e31–e32.

National Center for Injury Prevention and Control. (2010a). *10 leading causes of death by age group highlighting unintentional injury deaths, United States – 2010*. Retrieved from http://www.cdc.gov/injury/wisqars/pdf/10LCID_Unintentional_Deaths_2010-a.pdf

National Center for Injury Prevention and Control. (2010b). *10 leading causes of death by age group, United States – 2010*. Retrieved from http://www.cdc.gov/injury/wisqars/pdf/10LCID_All_Deaths_By_Age_Group_2010-a.pdf

National Institutes of Health. (2016a). *Calcium dietary supplement fact sheet*. Retrieved from http://ods.od.nih.gov/factsheets/Calcium-HealthProfessional/#h3

National Institutes of Health. (2016b). *Iron dietary supplement fact sheet*. Retrieved from http://ods.od.nih.gov/factsheets/Iron-HealthProfessional/#h4

Papalia, D., & Feldman, R. (2011). *A child's world: Infancy through adolescence* (12th ed.). New York, NY: McGraw-Hill.

Piaget, J. (1969). *The theory of stages in cognitive development*. New York, NY: McGraw-Hill.

Ross, C. A., Taylor, C. L., Yaktine, A.L., & Del Valle, H. B. (Eds.). (2011). *DRI dietary reference intakes calcium vitamin D*. Washington, DC: The National Academies Press.

Sears, W., & Sears, M. (2015a). *10 techniques to shape children's behavior*. Retrieved from http://www.askdrsears.com/topics/parenting/discipline-behavior/shape-childrens-behavior

Sears, W., & Sears, M. (2015b). *10 time-out techniques*. Retrieved from http://www.askdrsears.com/topics/parenting/discipline-behavior/10-time-out-techniques

Sears, W. & Sears, M. (2015c). *Why do kids lie – what to do*. Retrieved from http://www.askdrsears.com/topics/parenting/discipline-behavior/morals-manners/why-do-kids-lie

Stettler, N., Bhatia, J., Parish, A., & Stallings, V. A. (2011). Feeding healthy infants, children, and adolescents. In R. M. Kliegman, B. F. Stanton, J. W. St. Geme III, N. F. Schor, & R. E. Behrman (Eds.), (*Nelson's textbook of pediatrics* (19th ed.). Philadelphia, PA: Elsevier, Saunders.

TN Traffic Safety Resource Service. (2011). *Kids aren't cargo*. Retrieved from https://tntrafficsafety.org/sites/default/files/kidscargo.pdf

U.S. Department of Agriculture. (n.d.). *Preschoolers: Health and nutrition information*. Retrieved from http://www.choosemyplate.gov/health-and-nutrition-information

U.S. Department of Health and Human Services. (2016). *Healthy People 2020*. Retrieved from https://www.healthypeople.gov/2020/default

World Health Organization. (n.d.). *Passive smoking*. Retrieved from http://www.who.int/tobacco/en/atlas10.pdf

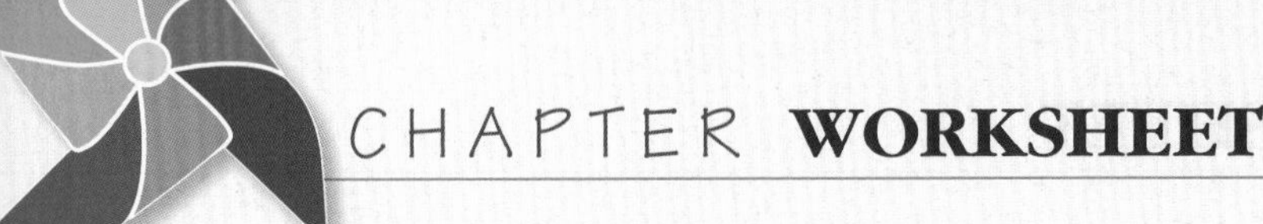

CHAPTER WORKSHEET

MULTIPLE CHOICE QUESTIONS

1. The nurse is caring for a hospitalized 4-year-old who insists on having the nurse perform every assessment and intervention on her imaginary friend first. She then agrees to have the assessment or intervention done to herself. The nurse identifies this preschooler's behavior as:
   a. Problematic; the child is old enough to begin to have a basis in reality.
   b. Normal, because the child is hospitalized and out of her routine.
   c. Normal for this stage of growth and development.
   d. Problematic, as it interferes with needed nursing care.

2. The mother of a 3-year-old is concerned about her child's speech. She describes her preschooler as hesitating at the beginning of sentences and repeating consonant sounds. What is the nurse's best response?
   a. Hesitancy and dysfluency are normal during this period of development.
   b. Reading to the child will help model appropriate speech.
   c. Expressive language concerns warrant a developmental evaluation.
   d. The mother should ask her child's physician for a speech therapy evaluation.

3. The mother of a 4-year-old asks for advice on using time-out for discipline with her child. What advice should the nurse give the mother?
   a. If spanking is not working, then time-out is not likely to be helpful either.
   b. Place the child in time-out for 4 minutes.
   c. Use time-out only if removing privileges is unsuccessful.
   d. The child should stay in time-out until crying ceases.

4. A 5-year-old child is not gaining weight appropriately. Organic problems have been ruled out. What is the priority action by the nurse?
   a. Allow the child unlimited access to the sippy cup to ensure adequate hydration.
   b. Encourage sweets for the extra caloric content.
   c. Teach the mother about nutritional needs of the preschooler.
   d. Assess the child's usual intake pattern at home.

5. The nurse is providing teaching about accidental poisoning to the family of a 3-year-old. The nurse understands that a child of this age is at increased risk of accidental ingestion due to which sensory alteration?
   a. A lack of fully developed hearing.
   b. A less discriminating sense of touch.
   c. Visual acuity that has not fully developed.
   d. A less discriminating sense of taste.

DOSAGE CALCULATION QUESTIONS

1. A child who weighs 33 kg has an order for acetaminophen 10 mg/kg/dose, every 4 hours prn pain or fever.
   a. How many milligrams will the child receive per dose?
   b. Acetaminophen elixir is provided as 160 mg/5 mL. How many milliliters will the nurse administer per dose?

CRITICAL THINKING EXERCISES

1. Teach a preschool class about bicycle and street safety. Be certain to design the content at an appropriate developmental level.
2. Construct a 3-day menu for a picky 4-year-old. Include three daily meals and two snacks. Follow the nutritional guidelines recommended by the USDA.
3. Color or draw with a preschool child. Analyze the drawings and interactions or discussions you have with the child, relating them to psychosocial and cognitive development expected at this age.

STUDY ACTIVITIES

1. Care for two average 3-, 4-, or 5-year-old children in the clinical setting (make sure both are the same age). Describe each child's development level, response to hospitalization, and family dynamics.
2. Visit a preschool that provides care for special needs children as well as typically developing children. Perform a development assessment on a typical child and one with special needs (both the same age). Compare and contrast your findings.

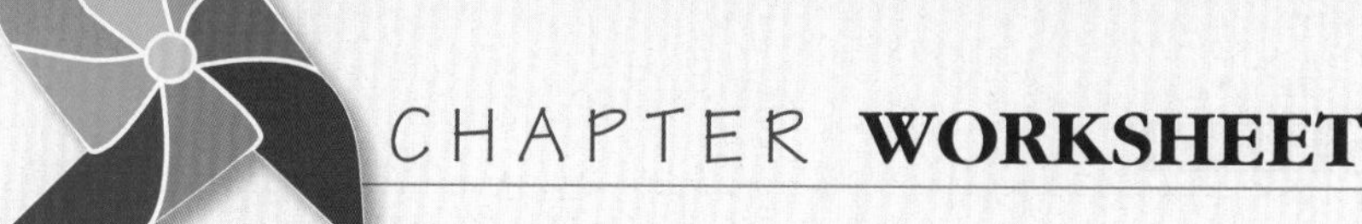

3. Observe in a 3-, 4- or 5-year-old classroom of a typical preschool. Choose two children who are the same age with different temperaments. Record the differences and similarities in their response to structure and authority, interactions with classmates, attention levels, and language and activity levels.

BRINGING IT ALL TOGETHER: A CASE STUDY

Steven, a 4-year-old boy, is seen in the pediatric office for a well-child examination. He is a healthy, active boy who attends extended-day preschool as his mother works long hours. His mother states she has some questions about Steven. She says she is concerned about Steven's growth, his language skills, and disciplining him. Steven's mother tells you that "he seems heavier than my other children did at his age." Upon measuring Steven you note his height to be 98 cm (38.5 inches) and his weight to be 20.9 kg (46 lb). His calculated BMI of 21.76 plots well above the 95th percentile for age. After further discussion with Steven's mother, you determine that he has an excessive daily intake of fruit juice and whole milk, and eats numerous fast food meals weekly.

Go to thePoint **to find questions to consider about this case.**

28

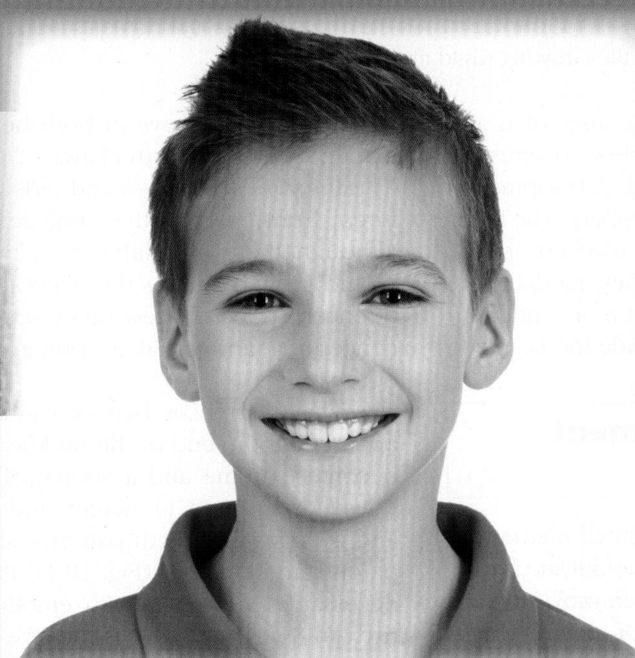

WOW

Words of Wisdom

Always give a hundred percent, and you will never doubt your ability to succeed.

Growth and Development of the School-Age Child

KEY TERMS

bruxism
caries
industry
inferiority
malocclusion
prepubescence
principle of conservation
school-age children
school refusal
temperament
self-esteem

Learning Objectives

Upon completion of the chapter, you will be able to:

1. Identify normal physiologic, cognitive, and moral changes occurring in the school-age child.
2. Describe the role of peers and schools in the development and socialization of the school-age child.
3. Identify the developmental milestones of the school-age child.
4. Identify the role of the nurse in promoting safety for the school-age child.
5. Demonstrate knowledge of the nutritional requirements of the school-age child.
6. Identify common developmental concerns in the school-age child.
7. Demonstrate knowledge of the appropriate nursing guidance for common developmental concerns.

***Lawrence Jones* is a 10-year-old boy brought to the clinic by his mother for his annual school check-up. During your assessment you measure his weight at 28.1 kg (62 lb) and his height at 137.2 cm (54 inches). As the nurse caring for him, assess Lawrence's growth and development, and then provide appropriate anticipatory guidance to his mother.**

School-age children, between the ages of 6 and 12 years, are experiencing a time of slow progressive physical growth, while their social and developmental growth accelerates and increases in complexity. The focus of their world expands from family to teachers, peers, and other outside influences (e.g., coaches, media). The child at this stage becomes increasingly more independent while participating in activities outside the home.

Growth and Development Overview

The school-age years are a time of continued maturation of the child's physical, social, and psychological characteristics. It is during this time that children move toward abstract thinking and seek approval of peers, teachers, and parents. Their eye–hand–muscle coordination allows them to participate in organized sports in school or the community. The school-age child typically values school attendance and school activities. The nurse uses knowledge of normal growth and development of the school-age child to assist the child with coping with disruptions and changes during this time period.

PHYSICAL GROWTH

From 6 to 12 years of age, children grow an average of 6 to 7 cm (2.5 inches) per year, increasing their height by at least 1 foot. An increase of 3 to 3.5 kg (7 lb) per year in weight is expected (Feigelman, 2011a). In the early school-age years, girls and boys are similar in height and weight and appear thinner and more graceful than in previous years. In later school-age years, most girls begin to surpass boys in both height and weight. (See Appendix A for growth charts.)

Preadolescent boys and girls do not want to be different from peers of the same sex or the opposite sex, although there are differences in physical and physiologic growth during the school-age years. These differences, especially secondary sexual characteristics, are concerning and often a source of embarrassment for both sexes.

The differences between girls and boys are more apparent at the end of the middle-school years and may become extreme and a source of emotional problems. These differences in height and weight relationships, and changes in growth patterns, should be explained to parents and children (Fig. 28.1). Physical maturity is not necessarily associated with emotional and social maturity. An 8-year-old who is the size of an 11-year-old will think and act like an 8-year-old. Many times, the expectations placed on these children are unrealistic and can impact the self-esteem and competence of the child. This can work in reverse, to similar effect, for an 11-year-old who is the size of an 8-year-old and is therefore treated as such.

ORGAN SYSTEMS MATURATION

Maturation of organs may differ with age or gender. Maturation of organs remains fairly consistent until late school age. In the late school-age years (10- to 12-year-olds), boys experience a slowed growth in height and increased weight gain, which may lead to obesity. During this time, girls may begin to have changes in the body that soften body lines. Preadolescence is a period of rapid growth, especially for girls.

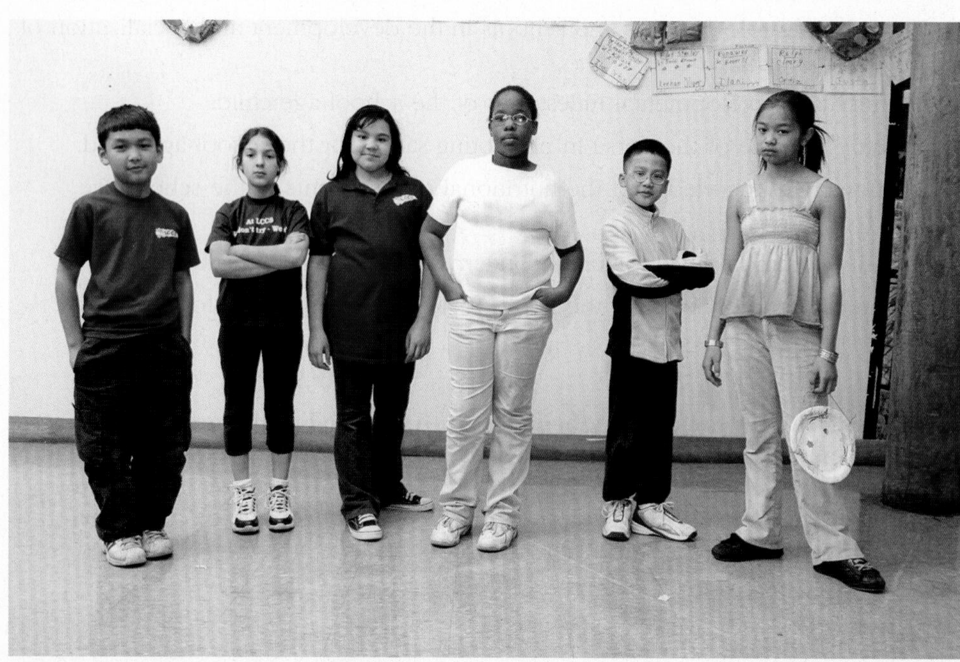

FIGURE 28.1 The different growth rates of school-age children are depicted by these same-age school-age children.

Neurologic System

The brain and skull grow very slowly during the school-age years. Brain growth is complete by the time the child is 10 years of age. The shape of the head is longer and the growth of the facial bones changes facial proportions.

Respiratory System

The respiratory system continues to mature with the development of the lungs and alveoli, resulting in fewer respiratory infections. Respiratory rates decrease, abdominal breathing disappears, and respirations become diaphragmatic in nature. The frontal sinuses are developed by 7 years of age. Tonsils decrease in size from the preschool years, but they remain larger than those of adolescents. The adenoids and tonsils may appear large normally, even in the absence of infection.

Cardiovascular System

The school-age child's blood pressure increases and the pulse rate decreases. The heart grows more slowly during the middle years and is smaller in size in relation to the rest of the body than at any other development stage.

Gastrointestinal System

During the school-age years, all 20 primary deciduous teeth are lost, replaced by 28 of 32 permanent teeth, with the exception of the third molars (commonly known as wisdom teeth). The school-age child experiences fewer gastrointestinal upsets compared with earlier years. Stomach capacity increases, which permits retention of food for longer periods of time. In addition, the caloric needs of the school-age child are lower than in the earlier years.

Genitourinary System

Bladder capacity increases, but varies among individual children. Girls generally have a greater bladder capacity than boys. Urination patterns vary with the amount of fluids ingested, the time they were ingested, and the stress level of the child. The formula for bladder capacity is age in years plus 2 ounces. Therefore, the bladder capacity of the 7-year-old would be 9 ounces. The larger capacity of the bladder allows for the child to experience longer periods between voiding.

Prepubescence

The late school-age years are also referred to as *preadolescence* (the time between middle childhood and the 13th birthday). During preadolescence, **prepubescence** occurs. Prepubescence typically occurs in the 2 years before the beginning of puberty and is characterized by the development of secondary sexual characteristics, a period of rapid growth for girls, and a period of continued growth for boys. There is approximately 2 years' difference in the onset of prepubescence between boys and girls. Sexual development in both boys and girls can lead to a negative perception of physical appearance and lowered self-esteem. Early development in girls can lead to embarrassment, concern over physical appearance, and low self-esteem. Delayed development in boys can lead to a negative self-concept, resulting in substance abuse or reckless use of nonautomobile vehicles. Early development may lead to risk-taking behaviors in both boys and girls. It is important for the nurse and parents to educate the late school-age child about body changes to decrease anxiety and promote comfort with these body changes.

Musculoskeletal System

Musculoskeletal growth leads to greater coordination and strength, yet the muscles are still immature and can be injured easily. Bones continue to ossify throughout childhood, but mineralization is not complete until maturity.

Immune System

Lymphatic tissues continue to grow until the child is 9 years old; immunoglobulins A and G (IgA and IgG) reach adult levels at around 10 years of age. Due to the lymphatic system becoming more competent in localizing infections and producing antibody–antigen responses, school-age children may have fewer infections. They may experience more infections during the first 1 to 2 years of school due to exposure to other children who may have infections.

PSYCHOSOCIAL DEVELOPMENT

Erikson (1963) describes the task of the school-age years to be a sense of **industry** versus **inferiority** (Feigelman, 2011a). During this time, the child is developing his or her sense of self-worth by becoming involved in multiple activities at home, at school, and in the community, which develops his or her cognitive and social skills. The child is very interested in learning how things are made and work. The school-age child's satisfaction from achieving success in developing new skills leads him or her to an increased sense of self-worth and level of competence. It is the role of the parents, teachers, coaches, and nurses of the school-age child to identify areas of competency and to build on the child's successful experiences to promote mastery, success, and self-esteem. If the expectations of adults are set too high, the child will develop a sense of inferiority and incompetence that can affect all aspects of his or her life. See Table 28.1

for a further explanation of psychosocial development in school-age children.

COGNITIVE DEVELOPMENT

Piaget's stage of cognitive development for the 7- to 11-year-old is the period of concrete operational thoughts (Feigelman, 2011a). In developing concrete operations, the child is able to assimilate and coordinate information about his or her world from different dimensions. The child is able to see things from another person's point of view and think through an action, anticipating its consequences and the possibility of having to rethink the action. He or she is able to use stored memories of past experiences to evaluate and interpret present situations. The school-age child also develops the ability to classify or divide things into different sets and to identify their relationships to each other. The school-age child is able to classify members of four generations on a family tree vertically and horizontally, and at the same time see that one person can be a father, son, uncle, and grandson. It is at this time that the school-age child develops an interest in collecting objects. The child starts out collecting multiple objects and becomes more selective as he or she gets older. Also, during concrete operational thinking, the school-age child develops an understanding of the **principle of conservation**—that matter does not change when its form changes. For example, if the child pours a half cup of water into a short, wide glass and into a tall, thin glass, she still only has a half cup of water despite the fact that it looks like the tall, thin glass has more (Fig. 28.2). She learns about conserving matter in a sequence ranging from the simplest to the more complex. See Table 28.1 for further information about cognitive development of school-age children.

TABLE 28.1 DEVELOPMENTAL THEORIES

Theorist	Stage	Activities
Erikson	Industry vs. inferiority	Interested in how things are made and run Success in personal and social tasks Increased activities outside home—clubs, sports Increased interactions with peers Increased interest in knowledge Needs support and encouragement from important people in child's life Needs support when child is not successful Inferiority occurs with repeated failures with little support or trust from those who are important to the child
Piaget	Concrete operational	Learns by manipulating concrete objects Lacks ability to think abstractly Learns that certain characteristics of objects remain constant Understands concepts of time Engages in serial ordering, addition, subtraction Classifies or groups objects by their common elements Understands relationships among objects Starts collections of items Can reverse thought process
Kohlberg	Conventional Stage 3: interpersonal conforming, "good child, bad child," age 7–10 years Stage 4: "law and order," age 10–12 years	An act is wrong because it brings punishment Behavior is completely wrong or right Does not understand the reason behind rules If child and adult differ in opinions, the adult is right Can put self in another person's position Begins to exercise the "golden rule" Acts are judged in terms of intention, not just punishment
Freud	Latency	A time of tranquility between the Oedipal phase of early childhood and adolescence—focuses on activities that develop social and cognitive skills Develops social skills in relating to same-sex friends through joining clubs like Brownies, Girl Scouts, Boy Scouts

Adapted from Erikson, E. (1963). *Childhood and society* (2nd ed.). New York: Norton; Kohlberg, L. (1984). *Moral development*. New York: Harper & Row; Piaget, J. (1969). *The theory of stages in cognitive development*. New York: McGraw-Hill; and Feigelman, S. (2011b). Chapter 6: Overview and assessment variability. In R. M. Kleigman, B. F. Stanton, J. W. St. Geme III, N. F. Schor, & R. E. Behrman (Eds.), *Nelson textbook of pediatrics* (19th ed., pp.26). Philadelphia, PA: Saunders

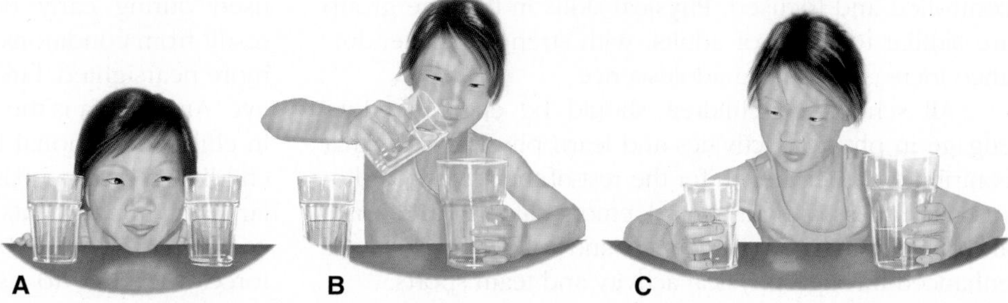
FIGURE 28.2 School-age children understand the theory of conservation (**A**). If you pour an equal amount of liquid into two glasses of unequal shape (**B**), the amount of water you have remains the same despite the unequal appearance in the two glasses (**C**).

MORAL AND SPIRITUAL DEVELOPMENT

During the school-age years, the child's sense of morality is constantly being developed. According to Kohlberg, the school-age child is at the conventional stage of moral development (Kohlberg, 1984). The 7- to 10-year-old usually follows rules out of a sense of being a "good" person. He or she wants to be a good person to parents, friends, and teachers and to himself or herself. The adult is viewed as being right. This is stage 3: interpersonal conformity (good child, bad child), according to Kohlberg. The 10- to 12-year-olds progress to stage 4: the "law and order" stage. At this stage, the child can determine if an action is good or bad based on the reason for the action, not just on the possible consequences of the action. The older school-age child's behavior is guided by his or her desire to cooperate and by his or her respect for others. This leads to the school-age child's ability to understand and incorporate into his or her behavior the concept of the "golden rule," to treat others how you would like to be treated (Feigelman, 2011a). See Table 28.1 for additional information about the moral development of school-age children.

During school age, children may develop a desire to understand more about their religion (Ford, 2007). They are still concrete thinkers and are guided by their family's religious and cultural beliefs. They are comforted by the rituals of their religion, but are just beginning to understand the differences between natural and supernatural. Incorporating religious practices in their lives can assist school-age children in coping with different stressors.

MOTOR SKILL DEVELOPMENT

Gross and fine motor skills continue to mature throughout the school-age years. Refinement of motor skills occurs, and speed and accuracy increase. To assess the motor skills of school-age children, ask questions about participation in sports and after-school activities, band membership, constructing models, and writing skills.

Gross Motor Skills

During the school-age years, coordination, balance, and rhythm improve, facilitating the opportunity to ride a two-wheel bike, jump rope, dance, and participate in a variety of other sports (Fig. 28.3). Older school-age children may become awkward due to their bodies growing faster than their ability to compensate.

School-age children between the ages of 6 and 8 enjoy gross motor activities such as bicycling, skating, and swimming. They are enthralled with the world and are in constant motion. Sometimes fear is limited due to the strong impulses of exploration. Children between 8 and 10 years of age are less restless, but their energy level continues to be high with activities more subdued and directed. These children exhibit greater rhythm and gracefulness of muscular movements, allowing them to participate in physical activities that require longer and more concentrated attention and effort, such as baseball or soccer.

Between the ages of 10 and 12 years (the pubescent years for girls), energy levels remain high but are more

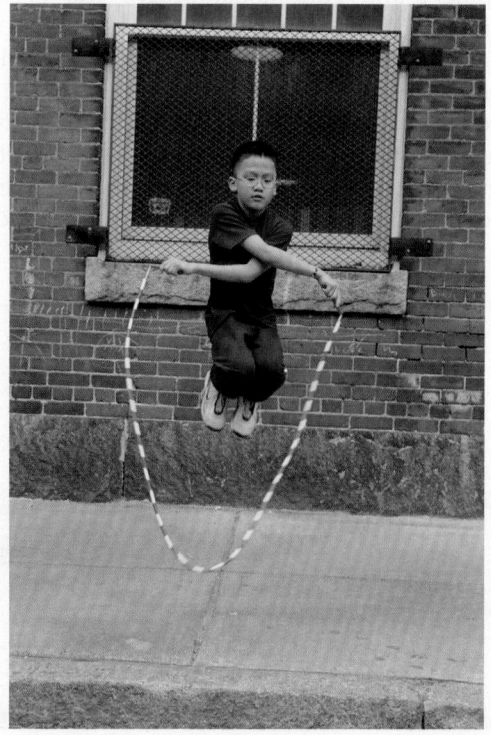
FIGURE 28.3 Jumping rope is an example of the increased development of gross motor skills of the school-age child.

controlled and focused. Physical skills in this age group are similar to those of adults, with strength and endurance increasing during adolescence.

All school-age children should be encouraged to engage in physical activities and learn physical skills that contribute to their health for the rest of their lives. Cardiovascular fitness, weight control, emotional tension release, and development of leadership and following skills are enhanced through physical activity and team sports.

Fine Motor Skills

Myelinization of the central nervous system is reflected by refinement of fine motor skills. Eye–hand coordination and balance improve with maturity and practice. Hand usage improves, becoming steadier and independent and granting an ease and precision that allows these children to write, print words, sew, or build models or other crafts. The child between 10 and 12 years of age begins to exhibit manipulative skills comparable to adults. School-age children take pride in activities that require dexterity and fine motor skills such as playing musical instruments (Fig. 28.4). Talent and practice become the keys to proficiency.

SENSORY DEVELOPMENT

All senses are mature early in the school-age years. The typical school-age child has 20/20 visual acuity (Jarvis, 2012). Good vision is essential to the physical development and educational progression of school-age children. Vision screening programs conducted by school nurses identify problems with vision and result in appropriate referrals when warranted. Some problems frequently identified include amblyopia (lazy eye), uncorrected refractive errors or other eye defects, and malalignment of the eyes (called *strabismus*). Amblyopia is reduced vision in an eye that has not been adequately used during early development. Inadequate use can result from conditions such as strabismus, one eye being more nearsighted, farsighted, or astigmatic than the other eye. Amblyopia is the leading cause of visual impairment in children (National Eye Institute, 2013). If untreated in childhood it can persist into adulthood causing monocular visual impairments (National Eye Institute, 2013). This condition is correctable with glasses or patching which forces the child to use the weaker eye. Recent clinical trials have suggested that older children (7 to 17 years) may benefit from these treatments, which are more commonly used on younger children (National Eye Institute, 2013). Proper screening and referral, as well as notification to parents of the existing condition, are essential to the education and socialization of the school-age child.

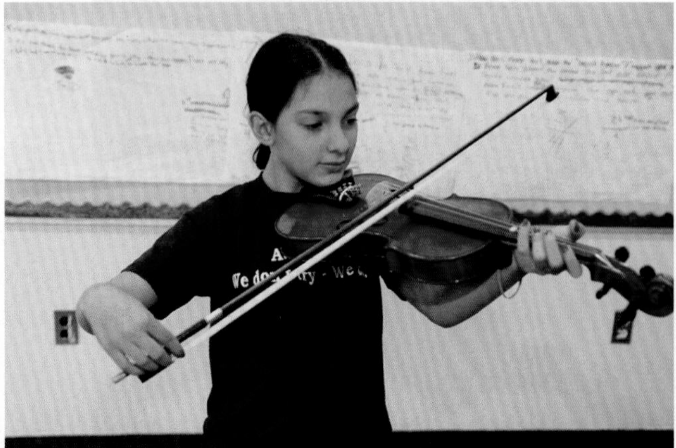

FIGURE 28.4 School-age children improve their fine motor skills so they can play musical instruments well.

Hearing deficits that are severe are usually diagnosed in infancy, but the less severe may not be diagnosed until the child enters school and has difficulty learning or with speech. It is important to screen children for hearing deficits to ensure proper educational and social progression.

The sense of smell is mature and can be tested in the school-age child by using scents that children are familiar with, such as chocolate or other familiar odors. In addition, the school-age child may be tested for the sense of touch with objects to discriminate cold from hot, soft from hard, and blunt from sharp.

COMMUNICATION AND LANGUAGE DEVELOPMENT

Language skills continue to accelerate during the school-age years and vocabulary expands. Culturally specific words are used, with bilingual children speaking English in school and a second language at home. The school-age child learns to read and reading efficiency improves language skills. Reading skills are improved with increased reading exposure. School-age children begin to use more complex grammatical forms such as plurals and pronouns. Also, they develop metalinguistic awareness—an ability to think about language and comment on its properties. This enables them to enjoy jokes and riddles due to their understanding of double meanings and play on words and sounds. They are also beginning to understand metaphors such as "a stitch in time saves nine." School-age children may experiment with profanity and dirty jokes if exposed. This age group tends to imitate parents, family members, or others. Therefore, role modeling is very important.

EMOTIONAL AND SOCIAL DEVELOPMENT

Patterns of temperamental traits identified in infancy may continue to influence behavior in the school-age child.

Analyzing past situations may provide clues to the way a child may react to new or different situations. Children may react differently over time due to their experiences and abilities. **Self-esteem** is the child's view of his or her individual worth. This view is impacted by feedback from family, teachers, and other authority figures.

Temperament

Temperament has been described as the way individuals behave. Three commonly grouped temperaments are the child that is easy and adaptable, the child that is slow to warm up, or the child that is difficult and easily frustrated (Feigelman, 2011b). Variations and combinations of these categories are seen. Not every child can be placed into one of these groups. Understanding a child's temperament can help care providers and parents to understand the child's behavior, actions, and how they relate to the world. For example, the child who is easy may adapt to school entry and other experiences smoothly and with little or no stress. The slow-to-warm child may be slow to adapt to changes. The slow-to-warm school-age child may exhibit discomfort when placed in different or new situations such as school. This child may need time to adjust to the new place or situation, and may demonstrate frustration with tears or somatic complaints. The slow-to-warm child should be allowed time to adjust to new situations and people (such as teachers) within his or her own time frame. All of these factors may impact the younger school-age child upon entering the school environment, with changes in authority and the introduction of many peers. The difficult or easily distracted child may benefit from an introduction to the new experience and people by role-playing, by visiting the site and being introduced to the teachers, and by hearing stories or participating in conversations about the upcoming school experience. These children require patience, firmness, and understanding to make the transition into a new situation or experience such as school. Assessment of temperament by a professional would include a combination of interview, observation, and a standardized questionnaire. Better understanding a child's temperament can assist parents with adjusting their parenting style to better fit their child and may help limit emotional and behavioral problems that occur when these areas are in conflict (Feigelman, 2011b).

Self-Esteem Development

Self-esteem mirrors the child's individual self-worth and consists of both positive and negative qualities. Children strive to achieve internalized goals of attainment, although they continually receive feedback from individuals they perceive as authorities (parent or teacher). By the school-age years, children have received feedback related to their performance or tasks. The direction of this feedback influences the child's opinion of self-worth, which influences self-esteem and self-evaluation.

Children face the process of self-evaluation from a framework of either self-confidence or self-doubt. Children who have mastered the earlier developmental task of autonomy and initiative face the world with feelings of pride rather than shame (Erikson, 1963).

If school-age children regard themselves as worthwhile, they have a positive self-concept and high self-esteem. Significant adults in school-age children's lives can manipulate the environment to facilitate success. This success impacts the self-esteem of the child.

Body Image

Body image is how the school-ager perceives his or her body. School-age children are knowledgeable about the human body but may have different perceptions about body parts. School-age children are very interested in peers' views and acceptances of their body, body changes, and clothing. This age group may model themselves after parents, peers, and persons in movies or on television. It is important for late school-agers to feel accepted by peers. If they feel different and are teased, there may be life-long effects.

School-Age Fears

School-age children are less fearful of harm to their body than in their preschool years, but fear being kidnapped or undergoing surgery. They continue to fear the dark and worry about their past behaviors. They fear death and are fascinated by death and dying. They are less fearful of animals, such as dogs and noises. The school-age child needs reassurance that his or her fears are normal for this developmental age. Parents, teachers, and other caretakers should discuss the fears and answer questions posed by the child (Child Development Institute, 2013). Recognize the child's fears but do not cater to them. Teach the child coping strategies such as positive self-statements such as "I can do this" and relaxation techniques such as deep breathing and visualization (Lyness, 2013).

Peer Relationships

The school-age child's concept of self is shaped not only by his or her parents but also by relationships with others. Peer relationships influence children's independence from parents. Peers play an important role in the approval and critiquing of skills of school-age children. Previously, only adults such as parents and teachers have been authorities; now, peers influence school-age children's perceptions of themselves. Peer relationships help to support the school-age child by providing enough security to risk the parental conflict brought about when establishing independence. School-age children associate with peers of the same sex most of the time. Although games and other activities are shared by both boys and girls, the child's concept of the appropriate sex role is influenced by his or her relationship with peers.

Continuous peer relationships provide the most important social interaction for school-age children. Valuable lessons are learned from interactions with children of their own age. Children learn to respect differing points of view that are represented in their groups (Fig. 28.5). Peer groups establish norms and standards that signify acceptance or rejection. Children may modify behavior to gain acceptance. A characteristic of school-age children is their formation of groups with rules and values. Peer and peer-group identification are important to the socialization of the school-age child (Feigelman, 2011a).

Teacher and School Influences

School serves as a means to transmit values of society and to establish peer relationships. Secondary only to the family, school exerts a profound influence on the social development of the child. Often, school requires changes for the child and parent. The child enters an environment that requires conforming to group activities that are structured and directed by an adult other than the parent. The parent's attitude and support influences the child's transition into the school setting. Parents who are positive and supportive promote a smooth entry into school. Parents who encourage clinging behaviors may delay a successful transition into school.

To facilitate the transition from home to school, the teacher must have the personality and knowledge of development that will allow him or her to meet the needs of young children. Even though the teacher's responsibilities are primarily to stimulate and guide intellectual development, they must share in shaping the child's attitudes and values. The system of awards and punishment administered by teachers affects the self-concept of children and influences their response to school. Teachers and school are important in shaping the socialization, self-concept, and intellectual development of children.

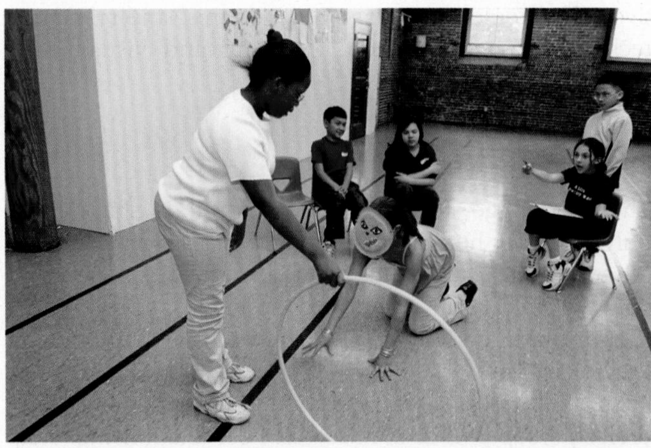

FIGURE 28.5 School-age children like to join clubs. These children, in the acting club at school, are rehearsing for a play.

Family Influences

The school-age years are a time for peer relationships, questioning of parents, and the potential for parental conflict but continued respect for family values. School-age years are the beginning of the time of peer-group influence, with testing of parental and family values. Although the peer group is influential, the family's values usually predominate when parental and peer-group values come into conflict. Even though the school-age child may question the parents' values, the child will usually incorporate the values from parents into his or her values.

Many times in the late school age and preadolescent period, the child may prefer to be in the company of peers and show a decreased interest in family functions. This may require an adjustment for parents. Parents' awareness of this developmental trend and their continuing support for the child are important while they continue to enforce restrictions and control of behaviors. The school-ager is beginning to strive for independence, but parental authority and controls continue to impact choices and values.

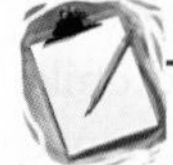

Take Note!

School-age children continue to need parenting. They do not need parents as pals.

CULTURAL INFLUENCES ON GROWTH AND DEVELOPMENT

Culture influences habits, beliefs, language, and values. School-age children thrive on learning the music, language, traditions, holidays, games, values, gender roles, and other aspects of culture. Nurses must be aware of the effects on children of various groups' family structures and traditional values. The school-age child's cultural and ethnic backgrounds must be considered when assessing growth and development, including differences in growth in children of different racial and cultural backgrounds. Cultural implications must be considered for all children and families in order to provide appropriate care.

Refer back to Lawrence Jones, who was introduced at the beginning of this chapter. What developmental milestones would you expect him to have reached by this age?

THE NURSE'S ROLE IN SCHOOL-AGE GROWTH AND DEVELOPMENT

Growth and development in the school-age child occurs in irregular spurts with a wide variation of sizes, shapes, and abilities seen. Nurses must be aware of the usual growth and development patterns for this age group so that they can assess school-age children appropriately and provide guidance to the child and his or her family. This is a time when children compare themselves to peers and self-esteem is a central issue. The school-age child is separating from his or her parents and seeks acceptance from peers and adults outside of his or her family. Health care visits throughout the school-age period continue to focus on expected growth and development and anticipatory guidance. Visits are more infrequent during the school-age years; therefore, the nurse needs to assess the child's functioning not only at home but also at school and within the community.

If the school-age child is hospitalized, growth and development may be altered. The school-age child is able to understand the reason for hospitalization and what will happen. He or she is often worried about pain or changes that may occur to his or her body. It is important for health care providers and family members to be honest and open with the school-age child. The school-age child may miss school and the interactions with his or her peers. The school-age child may regress and exhibit behaviors of a younger child, such as needing special comfort toys or demanding attention from his or her parents. Hospitalization for the school-age child can bring with it a loss of control. The school-age child is used to controlling his or her self-care and making choices about his or her meals and activities.

When caring for the hospitalized school-age child, the nurse must use knowledge of normal growth and development to recognize potential delays, promote continued appropriate growth and development, and interact successfully with the school-age child. Provide opportunities for the school-age child to maintain independence, gain control, and increase self-esteem.

See the Nursing Care Plan at the end of the chapter.

NURSING PROCESS OVERVIEW

Upon completion of assessment of the school-age child's current growth and development status, problems or issues related to growth and development may be identified. The nurse may then identify one or more nursing diagnoses, including:

- Risk for disproportionate growth
- Imbalanced nutrition: more than body requirements
- Delayed growth and development
- Risk for caregiver role strain
- Risk for injury

Nursing care planning for the school-age child with growth and development issues should be individualized based on the school-age child's and family's needs. The nursing care plan can be used as a guide in planning nursing care for the school-age child with a growth and development concern. The nurse may choose the appropriate nursing diagnoses from Nursing Care Plan 28.1 and individualize them as needed. The nursing care plan is intended to serve as a guide, not to be an all-inclusive growth and development care plan.

PROMOTING HEALTHY GROWTH AND DEVELOPMENT

The family plays a critical role in promoting healthy growth and development of the school-age child. Respectful interchange of communication between the parent and child will foster self-esteem and self-confidence. This respect will give the child confidence in achieving personal, educational, and social goals appropriate for his or her age. The nurse should study interactions between parents and school-age children to observe for this respect or lack of respect ("putting the child down"). The nurse can model appropriate behaviors by listening to the child and making appropriate responses. The nurse can be a resource for parents and an advocate for the child in promoting healthy growth and development.

Promoting Growth and Development Through Play

Cooperative play is exhibited by the school-age child. Play for the school-age child includes both organized cooperative activities (such as team sports) and solitary activities. School-age children have the coordination and intellect to participate with other children of their age in sports such as soccer, baseball, football, and tennis. The school-age child comprehends that his or her cooperation with others will lead to a unified whole for the team. In addition, the child learns rules and the value of playing by the rules.

School-age children also enjoy solitary activities including board, card, video, and computer games, and dollhouse and other small-figure play (Fig. 28.6). Many school-agers start collections of stamps, cars, or other valuable or not-so-valuable items. During the school-age years, children may also begin a scrapbook or keep a diary. They may participate in activities such as dance or karate. Girls and boys may join clubs, gangs, or special interest groups.

Active play has decreased in recent years as television viewing and computer games have increased. This trend has resulted in health risks such as obesity, type 2 diabetes, and cardiovascular problems.

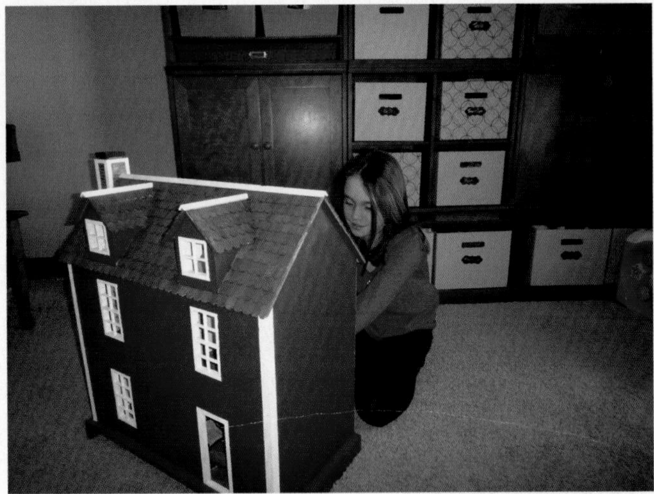

FIGURE 28.6 This school-age girl enjoys solitary play with her dollhouse and dolls.

Promoting Learning

School attendance and learning are very important to the school-age child. Parent–child, child–teacher, and child–peer relationships and activities influence the school-age child's learning.

Formal Education

Most children are excited about starting school and making new friends. They like the notion of getting books, having book bags, and having homework assignments. The reality of the work involved with school and homework may decrease the enthusiasm about school.

Peers are very important within this age group. Both peers and teachers influence children. Attending school may be their first experience interacting with a large number of children of their own age. Through this interaction, children learn cooperation, competition, and the importance of following the rules. Peer approval and influences grow as the child matures. Teachers have significant influences on children. They help to guide the child's intellectual development by rewarding successes and helping the child deal with failures. The student–teacher relationship is a key to success. Teachers play a role in fostering feelings of industry and preventing feelings of inferiority (Fig. 28.7). School-age children also learn skills, rules, values, and other ways to work with peers and other authority figures.

Parental support is important for school adjustment and achievement. Parents must collaborate with teachers and school personnel to ensure that the child is fulfilling the expectations and requirements for this age group in school. Parents must monitor the child's homework assignments and friends, and observe for any changes in behavior that would indicate school or behavioral problems.

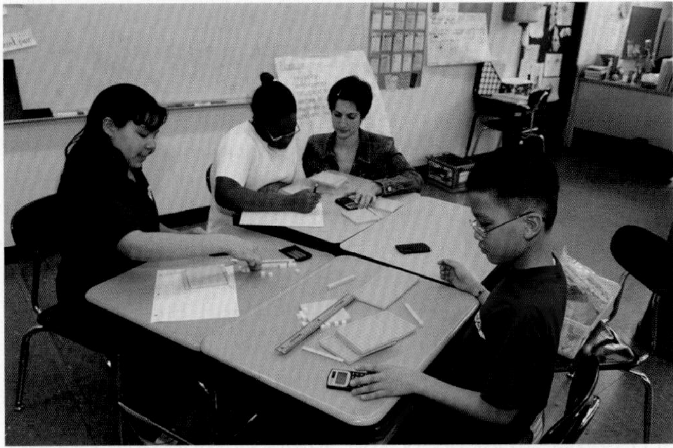

FIGURE 28.7 School is important to the school-age child.

Reading

Encouraging reading is an excellent way to promote learning in the school-age child. Trips to the library and purchasing books help to promote a love of reading. School-age children enjoy being read to as well as reading on their own. Younger school-age children (6 to 8 years) enjoy books that are simple to read with few words on a page, such as the Dr. Seuss books. They enjoy books about animals and trains and simple mysteries. Children 8 to 10 years of age have more advanced reading skills and enjoy those books from early childhood, plus more classic novels and adventures such as the Harry Potter series. Older children enjoy horror stories, mysteries, romances, and adventure stories as well as classic novels. School-age children of all ages benefit from books on topics related to things they may be experiencing, such as a visit to the hospital for a surgical procedure. See Box 28.1 for ideas for parents to promote reading in the school-age child.

BOX 28.1

PROMOTION OF READING IN SCHOOL-AGE CHILDREN

- Read to and with your children
- Ask teachers and librarians for advice on books appropriate for your child
- Choose stories that the child can relate to if the child has difficulty reading
- Choose books with movement if the child has a short attention span
- Take advantage of all reading opportunities (cereal boxes, road signs)
- Provide choices for the child to select a book of interest
- Talk about the text and ask questions to improve understanding
- Keep a record of what the child is reading
- Visit a library, get a library card, and check out books
- Demonstrate role modeling through reading books

Promoting Safety

School-age children become more independent with age. This independence leads to an increased self-confidence and decreased fears, which may contribute to accidents and injuries. School age is a time that the child may walk to school with peers who may influence his or her behavior. Increased independence may also increase exposure to dangerous situations such as the approach of strangers or unsafe streets. Promotion of safe habits during the school-age years is important for parents and nurses. See Teaching Guidelines 28.1 for additional information on safety education for nurses and parents.

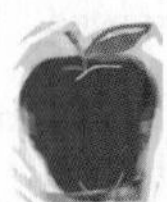

Teaching Guidelines 28.1

SAFETY ISSUES AND INTERVENTIONS OF THE SCHOOL-AGE CHILD

Safety Issue	*Interventions*
Car safety	• Seat belt or age- and weight-appropriate booster seat should be used at all times. The lap belt should lie low and flat on the hips and the shoulder belt should lie on the shoulder not the neck or face (usually when the child is about 144.8 cm [57 inches] tall) • Seat belts should be fastened before car is started • Children under 13 years must sit in back seat • Childproof locks should be used in back seat • Rules of conduct for car rides must be established
Pedestrian safety	• Child should be instructed to stop at the curb and look right, left, then right again before crossing the street; and crossing only at safe crossings • Older children and adults should provide supervision of younger children • Walking should only be done on sidewalks • In parking lots, children should know to watch for cars backing up and not dart out between parked cars • If children are playing outside, drivers should be aware of their presence before backing up
Bike safety: general	• Child should know to wear a properly fitted, CPSC (Consumer Product Safety Commission) or Snell-approved helmet every time he/she rides a bike. • Proper fitting helmet should: sit level, not tilted, and firmly and comfortably on the head; have strong wide Y-shaped straps and when you open your mouth should pull down a bit; not move with sudden pulling or twisting; never be worn over anything else (hat, scarf, etc.) • Bikes should be well maintained and appropriately sized. • Child should be oriented to bike and demonstrate ability to ride bike safely before being allowed to ride on street. • Safe areas for bike riding should be established as well as routes to and from area of activities. • Riding bike barefoot, with someone else on bike, or with clothing that might get entangled in the bike should be prohibited. • Child should know to wear sturdy, well-fitting shoes. • Bike should be inspected often to ensure it is in proper working order. • A basket should be used to carry heavy objects.
Bike safety in traffic	• All traffic signs and signals must be observed. • If riding at night, the bike should have lights and reflectors and the rider should wear light-colored clothes • Child should know to ride on the side of the road traveling with traffic, and keep close to the side of the road in single file • Child should learn to watch and listen for cars • Headphones should not be used while riding a bike • Never hitch a ride on any vehicles
Sports safety	• Sports should be matched to child's ability and desire • Sports program should have warm-up procedure • Coaches should be trained in CPR and first aid • Appropriate protection devices should be used for individual sport

Skateboarding and inline skating safety	• Child should wear helmet, and protective padding on knees, elbows, and wrists • Child should know not to skate in traffic or on streets or highways • Homemade ramps should be assessed for hazards before skating
All-terrain vehicle safety	• Child should be at least 16 years of age to operate vehicle • Helmets must be worn in addition to protective coverings • No night-time riding • Use should be avoided on public roads • Never stand up in the vehicle or ride in a person's lap
Fire safety	• All homes should have working smoke detectors and fire extinguishers. Change the batteries at least twice a year • Have a fire-escape plan • Practice fire-escape plan routinely • Nobody should smoke in the home especially in bed • Teach what to do in case of a fire: use fire extinguisher, call 911, and how to put out clothing fire • Use stove and other cooking facilities under adult supervision • All flammable materials and liquids should be stored safely • Fireplaces should have protective gratings • Teach children to avoid touching wires they might encounter while playing
Water safety	• Teach children how to swim and to never play around or in water without adult supervision • If swimming skill is limited, child must wear life preserver at all times • Child should know never swim alone—if at all possible, swim only where there is a life guard • Understand basic CPR • Teach child to never run or fool around at edge of pool • Drains in pool should be covered with appropriate cover • Life jackets should be worn when on boat • Make sure water is deep enough to support diving
Firearm safety	• Teach child never to touch guns—tell an adult • If have guns in household, need to secure them in a safe place, use gun safety locks, store bullets in a separate place • Never point a gun at a person
Toxin safety	• Teach child the hazards of accepting illegal drugs, alcohol, or dangerous drugs • Store potential dangerous material in a safe place

Adapted from American Academy of Pediatrics, The Injury Prevention Program. (2013a). *Safety for your child: 6 years*. Retrieved from http://www.healthychildren.org/english/tips-tools/Pages/Safety-for-Your-Child-6-Years.aspx; American Academy of Pediatrics, The Injury Prevention Program. (2013b). *Safety for your child: 8 years*. Retrieved from http://www.healthychildren.org/english/tips-tools/Pages/Safety-for-Your-Child-8-Years.aspx; American Academy of Pediatrics, The Injury Prevention Program. (2013c). *Safety for your child: 10 years*. Retrieved from http://www.healthychildren.org/english/tips-tools/Pages/Safety-for-Your-Child-10-Years.aspx; Centers for Disease Control and Prevention (2012a). *Unintentional drowning: Get the Facts*. Retrieved from http://www.cdc.gov/HomeandRecreationalSafety/Water-Safety/waterinjuries-factsheet.html; Dowshen, S (2014). Bike Safety. Retrieved from http://kidshealth.org/teen/safety/safebasics/bike_safety.html#

Unintentional injuries are the leading cause of death in children between 1 and 19 years of age (Gilchrist, Ballesteros, & Parker, 2012). Each year, 9.2 million children seek medical attention for nonfatal unintentional injuries (Centers for Disease Control and Prevention [CDC], 2012b). School-age children are very active at home, in the community, and at school. This increased mobility, activity, and time away from parents increase the risk for unintentional injuries. School-age children continue to need supervision and guidance. They need information and rules about car safety, pedestrian safety, bicycle and other sport safety, fire safety, and water safety.

Car Safety

Motor vehicle accidents are a common cause of injury in the school-age child. While traveling in the car, school-age children should always sit in the rear seat. The front seat is dangerous because of passenger-side airbags in most new-model cars. A school-age child over 18.1 kg (40 lb) (generally 4 to 8 years of age) should use a belt-positioning, forward-facing booster seat using both lap and shoulder belts (American Academy of Pediatrics [AAP], 2013a). School-age children who outgrow the convertible restraint can sit in a booster seat until the vehicle seat belt restraint fits properly over the hips and shoulder, typically when they are 144.8 cm (4 feet 9 inches) or taller, usually between 8 and 12 years of age (AAP, 2013a). The seat belt needs to lie low and flat over the hip bones and across the shoulder not the neck or face. Children younger than 13 years of age should not ride in the front seat of a vehicle with an airbag (AAP, 2013a).

Pedestrian Safety

Every year 51,000 children are injured as pedestrians and 900 pedestrian children are killed (AAP, 2013b). Children younger than 10 years of age should not be unsupervised pedestrians (AAP, 2013b). Young school-age children therefore should walk to school or the bus with an older friend, sibling, or parent. Darting out into the street without looking both ways or from between cars is a common occurrence in the school-age years. Teach children safe street and pedestrian practices.

Bicycle and Sport Safety

Bicycling, riding scooters, skateboarding, and inline skating or roller skating are common activities of school-age children. Laws in some states require helmets for riding bicycles and scooters. In addition, when skating or skateboarding, school-age children should wear a helmet, kneepads, and elbow pads.

Research has shown that head injuries due to bicycle accidents have been reduced by 85% by wearing a well-fitting helmet (Bicycle Helmet Safety Institute, 2012). (see Healthy People 2020). It is important for children to wear helmets that fit and that do not obstruct their vision or hearing. Because school-age children have completed most of their skull growth, a helmet can be worn into adolescence. It is important for the child to have a bicycle that is appropriate for his or her size and age. The child should be able to plant both feet on the ground when sitting on the seat of the bike (Fig. 28.8). It is important to stress to parents the importance of appropriate size and not to get a bike for the child to "grow into." If older school-agers are using the bike for transportation on busy streets, they should be taught to use bike lanes and to give appropriate hand signals for turning. Nonmotorized and motorized scooters also place children at risk for injury, so counsel families about the use of protective gear, including helmets, elbow pads, and kneepads.

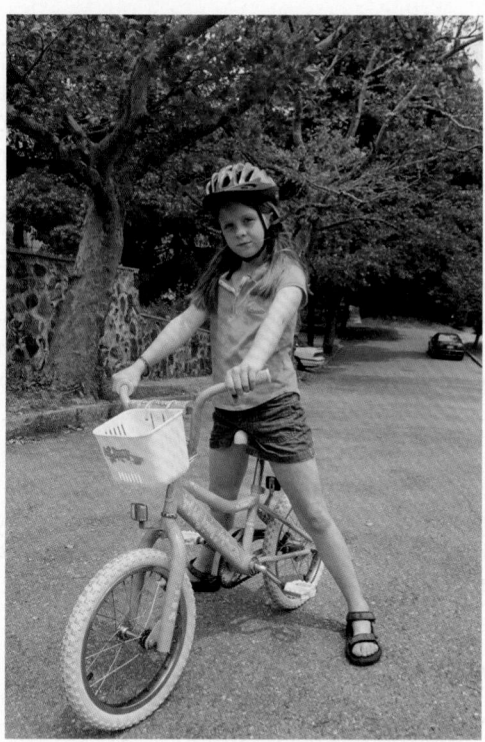

FIGURE 28.8 Wearing the appropriate safety equipment and having an appropriately sized bicycle are important to prevent injuries in school-age children.

HEALTHY PEOPLE 2020

Objective	Nursing Significance
Reduce fatal and nonfatal traumatic brain injuries.	• Provide education to children and their parents about avoiding head injury through helmet use. • Encourage child to choose a helmet that appeals to him or her (one that looks "cool").

Healthy People Objectives retrieved from http://www.healthypeople.gov

Fire Safety

School-age children are eager to help parents with cooking and ironing. They are curious about fire and are drawn to play with fire, matches, and fireworks. Serious burns can occur from any exposure to fire. Educate children about the hazards of fire. In addition, teach children proper behavior around fires at home and outdoors. Always supervise children in the use of matches. In the home setting, parents should develop a fire safety plan with their children, teach children what to do if their clothes catch on fire, and practice evacuating the house in the event of a fire. In the school setting, children should be aware of the appropriate response to fire drills and fire drills should be conducted on a regular basis.

Water Safety

Teach school-age children swim and water safety. An adult should always supervise children when they are swimming to prevent water-related accidents.

Abuse in Children

Child abuse, including physical abuse and sexual abuse, is a common crime of violence against children. An estimated

3.4 million reports of child abuse are made annually to child protective services in the United States (CDC, 2014). Over 686,000 cases were substantiated in 2012, with 78% being victims of neglect, 18% victims of physical abuse, 9% victims of sexual abuse, and 11% victims of other abuse such as emotional or psychological abuse (CDC, 2014). The abusers of children are family, friends, and strangers. It is important for parents to teach children the concept of "good touch" versus "bad touch" prior to school-age years. Whenever the school-age child's behavior yields suspicion of physical or sexual abuse, the nurse should report to the appropriate authorities in his or her state. These topics will be discussed in more depth in Chapter 50.

Remember Lawrence Jones, the 10-year-old presented in the case study? What anticipatory guidance related to safety should you provide to his mother?

Promoting Nutrition

Growth, body composition, and body shape remain constant during late school-age years. Needed calories decrease while the appetite increases. In preparation for adolescence, the body fat composition of school-age children increases. This tendency toward increased body fat occurs earlier in girls than in boys, with the amount of increase greater in girls. Boys have more lean body mass per inch of height than girls.

Diet preferences established in the preschool years continue during the school-age period. As the child grows older, influences of family, media, and peers can impact the eating habits of this age group. Some of these influences are parents' work schedule, outside activities, and exercise level of the child. Decreased exercise levels and poor nutritional choices lead to the mounting problem of obesity seen in this age group. See Box 28.2 for appropriate questions to ask the child and parent regarding nutritional status. Healthy People 2020 provides objectives and actions to improve the nutritional health of children.

BOX 28.2

DIETARY QUESTIONS

Questions for the Child

- How often do you eat together as a family?
- What are the usual mealtimes?
- How often does the family eat out?
- Do you eat breakfast regularly?
- Where do you eat lunch?
- What do you drink/how much?
- What foods do you eat most often?
- What is your favorite food?
- How often do you eat fast foods?
- What type of exercise do you do?

Questions for the Parents

- How would you describe your child's usual appetite?
- Do you have any special cultural/religious practices regarding food?
- Has your child gained or lost weight recently?
- Do you have any concerns about his or her eating behaviors?
- How does your child exercise? Your family?
- Is there a family history of cancer, hypertension, diabetes, obesity, or heart disease?

HEALTHY PEOPLE 2020

Objective	Nursing Significance
Increase the contribution of fruits to the diets of the population aged 2 years and older.	• Educate families about the importance of whole grains, fruits, and vegetables in the diet.
Increase the contribution of total vegetables to the diets of the population aged 2 years and older.	• Encourage the child to choose fruits and vegetables that appeal to him or her.
Increase the contribution of dark green vegetables, orange vegetables, and legumes to the diets of the population aged 2 years and older.	• Provide creative suggestions for vegetable preparation to make them more appealing to children.
Increase the contribution of whole grains to the diets of the population aged 2 years and older.	• Educate families about saturated fat–containing foods.
Reduce consumption of calories from solid fats.	• Offer suggestions for alternative sources of proteins and fats (chicken or fish, olive oil).
Reduce consumption of calories from added sugars.	
Reduce consumption of calories from solid fats and added sugars.	
Reduce consumption of saturated fat in the population aged 2 years and older.	
Reduce consumption of sodium in the population aged 2 years and older.	
Increase consumption of calcium in the population aged 2 years and older.	

Healthy People Objectives retrieved from http://www.healthypeople.gov

Nutritional Needs

The school-age child's calorie needs vary based on age, gender, and activity level. In general, children with higher activity levels and male gender have higher calorie needs (U.S. Department of Agriculture and U.S. Department of Health and Human Services, 2010). Boys and girls 4 to 8 years old who are moderately active will need about 1,400 to 1,600 calories a day (U.S. Department of Agriculture and U.S. Department of Health and Human Services, 2010). Boys 9 to 13 years old who are moderately active need about 1,800 to 2,000 calories a day, while girls this age who are moderately active need about 1,600 to 2,000 calories a day (U.S. Department of Agriculture and U.S. Department of Health and Human Services, 2010). Of these calories, 45% to 65% should come from carbohydrates, 10% to 30% from protein, and 25% to 35% from fat (U.S. Department of Agriculture and U.S. Department of Health and Human Services, 2010). The 4- to 8-year-old child needs 800 to 1,000 mg of calcium, while the 9- to 13-year-old needs 1,300 mg of calcium for maintenance of growth and good nutrition (Krebs, Primark, & Haemer, 2011). Calcium is needed for the development of strong bones and teeth. Milk, yogurt, and cheese provide protein, vitamins, and minerals and are an excellent source of calcium. Meats, poultry, fish, and eggs provide protein, vitamins, and minerals.

Promoting Healthy Eating Habits

School-age children should choose culturally appropriate foods and snacks from the U.S. Department of Agriculture's MyPlate (Appendix D). MyPlate illustrates the five food groups and encourages children to make half of their plate fruits and vegetables, to make half of their grains whole grains, and to choose lean proteins and calcium-rich foods. The website www.choosemyplate.gov/ offers many tools for the child to use including development of personalized goals and menus, online dieting and physical activity assessment tools, games, activities, and tips for parents. School-age children need to limit intake of fat and processed sugars. A prudent diet limits the use of fatty meats, high-fat dairy products, eggs, and hydrogenated shortenings and promotes the consumption of fish and the substitution of polyunsaturated vegetable oils and margarines.

Preventing the Development of Overweight and Obesity

The National Health and Nutrition Examination Survey (NHANES) found that more and more children are overweight. Over the past three decades the number of overweight children has doubled (CDC, 2013a). More than one third of children are overweight or obese (CDC, 2013a). Overweight is classified as a body mass index (BMI) greater than 85% and obese is classified as a BMI greater than 95% (Krebs et al., 2011; U.S. Department of Agriculture and U.S. Department of Health and Human Services, 2010) (see Healthy People 2020).

HEALTHY PEOPLE *2020*

Objective	Nursing Significance
Reduce the proportion of children and adolescents who are considered obese	• Screen all children for the development of overweight as indicated by an increasing BMI for their age
Prevent inappropriate weight gain in youth	• Provide accurate diet counseling • Encourage daily physical activity • Counsel parents to limit television/computer time daily

Healthy People Objectives retrieved from http://www.healthypeople.gov

Obesity occurs when the intake of calories and food exceeds the expenditures. Some factors linked to causing obesity include family role modeling, lack of exercise, unstructured meals, consumption of sugar-sweetened beverages, large portion sizes, television viewing, and video gaming as well as cultural, genetic, environmental, and socioeconomic factors. Some factors that influence lack of exercise include the decreased number of days that school systems offer physical education programs and recess. Also, some children live in unsafe neighborhoods or in a community that lacks sidewalks or parks and have no safe place to play outside; therefore, they spend time doing sedentary activities such as watching TV or playing video or computer games (U.S. Department of Agriculture and U.S. Department of Health and Human Services, 2010). Obese children are at risk for cardiovascular diseases such as high cholesterol and hypertension, type 2 (non–insulin-dependent) diabetes, respiratory complications such as obstructive sleep apnea, mental health issues such as depression, anxiety and eating disorders, and orthopedic problems (Krebs et al., 2011; U.S. Department of Agriculture and U.S. Department of Health and Human Services, 2010). When parents do not have knowledge of nutrition, do not monitor snacks or meals, and have unstructured meals, habits are established that lead to obesity.

Preventing obesity in childhood is important because the fat cells of childhood are carried into adulthood obesity and contribute to disease. Due to the risk of obesity, encourage parents to never use food as a reward. To prevent obesity, establish regular mealtimes and offer healthy foods and snacks. Encourage parents to praise their child's good food choices and to role model appropriate eating and exercise.

Regarding Lawrence Jones, what questions should you ask Lawrence's mother related to nutritional intake? What anticipatory guidance related to nutrition would be appropriate?

Promoting Healthy Sleep and Rest

The number of hours of sleep required for growth and development decreases with age. Children between the ages of 6 and 8 years require about 12 hours of sleep per night, children between 8 and 10 years of age require 10 to 12 hours of sleep per night, and children between 10 and 12 years of age need 9 to 10 hours of sleep per night. Young school-age children may need an occasional brief nap for an energy boost after being in school for most of the day. Bedtime rituals and consistent schedules continue to be important throughout the school-age years. Parents must facilitate the bedtime schedule and quiet time before bed. Bedtime is a special time for parents and children to read together, listen to stories or soothing music, share events of the day, and exchange expressions of affection (AAP, 2013c). Children should have bedtime expectations as well as wake-up times and methods for waking up (alarm, calling by parent, and so forth).

Night terrors or sleepwalking may occur in 6- to 8-year-olds, but should be resolved between the ages of 8 and 10 years. In the older school-age child (11 to 12 years), encourage parents to allow a variation in the sleep schedule on the weekends and a regular schedule on weekdays.

Provide anticipatory guidance to Lawrence Jones's mother in relation to proper sleep for her 10-year-old son.

Promoting Healthy Teeth and Gums

Dental **caries** (tooth decay) remains a leading chronic disease in the United States (CDC, 2012b; The incidence declined from the 1970s to the early 1990s, mostly due to the introduction of fluoride (National Institutes of Dental and Craniofacial Research, National Institutes of Health, 2014). Since then, there has been a small but significant increase in the incidence of dental caries. Recent statistics show that 51% of children between the ages of 6 and 11 have dental caries in their primary teeth, 21% have dental caries in their permanent teeth, and 23% of children 2 to 11 years of age have untreated dental caries (National Institutes of Dental and Craniofacial Research, National Institutes of Health, 2014).

Dental care with emphasis on prevention of caries is important in this age group. School-age children need to brush their teeth two to three times per day for 2 to 3 minutes each time with fluorinated toothpaste (Fig. 28.9). Parents should replace the toothbrush (soft) every 3 to 4 months. Flossing the teeth at least once daily is recommended along with limiting the intake of sugar to aid in the prevention of cavities and improved oral health. Parents must monitor teeth brushing, observe for abnormal alignment of their child's teeth, and schedule regular dental examinations every 6 months to ensure good dental health and prevent dental problems. Children will need help with brushing teeth until they are between 7 and 10 years of age.

Dental sealants are an easy way to protect a child's primary or permanent teeth as children with dental sealants have 60% less decay (CDC, 2013b). The sealant is a plastic coating applied to biting surfaces to seal out tooth decay on back teeth and sometimes to cover deep pits or grooves. In addition, parents should give a fluoride supplement (as directed by the dentist) to their children if fluoride is not in the town's water supply (American Academy of Pediatric Dentistry, 2013). The school-age child should have an established dental home; if not, provide appropriate resources to establish one (AAP, 2014). See the Healthy People 2020 chart.

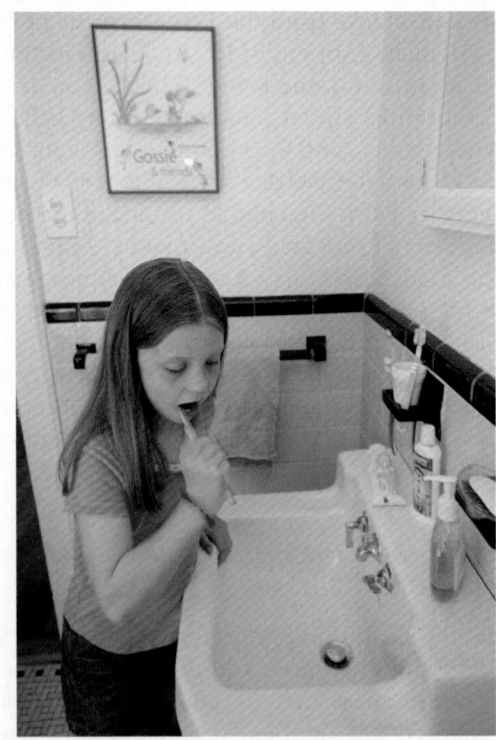

FIGURE 28.9 Using correct technique to brush the teeth is important in the prevention of cavities.

HEALTHY PEOPLE 2020

Objective	Nursing Significance
Reduce the proportion of children and adolescents who have dental caries in their primary or permanent teeth Reduce the proportion of children and adolescents with untreated dental decay Increase the proportion of children who have received dental sealants to their molar teeth	• Encourage appropriate tooth brushing and flossing • Educate child and family about fluoride use • Refer school-age children to dentist for regular check-ups and interventions such as molar sealants • Assist families lacking dental insurance to find resources for the provision of dental care

Healthy People Objectives retrieved from http://www.healthypeople.gov

Proper alignment of teeth is important to tooth formation, speech development, and physical appearance. Many school-age children need braces or other orthodontic devices to correct malocclusion, a condition in which the teeth are crowded, crooked, or misaligned. **Bruxism** or teeth grinding while asleep may continue in the school-age years. Bruxism may result in grinding away of tooth enamel. Teeth grinding may be due to malalignment. A dental evaluation should be scheduled if consistent teeth grinding occurs.

Children wearing braces are more prone to cavities; encourage them to brush their teeth after meals and snacks. School nurses can assist these children with brushing after lunch. In addition, the school nurse should promote dental health through education on dental care and gum problems that result from lack of proper dental care. Diet can play a part in dental health. Limiting sticky, high-sugar, and high-carbohydrate foods will decrease the possibility of cavities.

Promoting Appropriate Discipline

Because of the increasing ability of the school-age child to view situations from different angles, the school-age child should be able to see how his or her actions affect others. The school-age child is aware of the cause and effect of his or her behaviors and realizes that his or her behaviors have consequences. School-age children should be able to express emotions without using violence. Discipline techniques with consequences have both *natural* and *logical* consequences. Natural consequences allow the child to learn the results of his or her actions. For example, if the child throws a toy out of the window, then he or she cannot play with the toy anymore. In logical consequences, if the child does not put away his or her bike, he or she does not get to ride the bike for the rest of the day.

In disciplining children, parents should teach children the rules established by the family, values, and social rules of conduct. Rules should provide the school-age child with guidelines about behavior that is acceptable and unacceptable. School-age children look to their parents for guidance and as role models. Parents should role model appropriate expressions of feelings and emotions and allow the child to express emotions and feelings. Discuss the effects of the child's temperament on his or her behavior, as well as what constitutes age-appropriate behavior. Include how the parents' temperament can influence the child's temperament.

Effective guidance and discipline focus on the development of the child. They can preserve the child's self-esteem and dignity. Discuss with parents guidelines regarding discipline. Explain to parents that they should never belittle the child. Children may view parents and caretakers negatively if they are consistently belittled or insulted. These negative actions can inhibit learning and teach the child to react unkindly to others. Instead, parents should discipline with praise. Positive acknowledgements of progress are likely to encourage healthy development and appropriate behavior (AAP, 2012). Discuss with parents how to be realistic when planning activities so as to not overwhelm the child, resulting in misbehavior. Encourage parents to say "no" only when they mean it, to avoid a negative atmosphere in the home, and to avoid inconsistency.

When misbehaviors occur, the type and amount of discipline are based on different factors:

- Developmental level of both the child and the parents
- Severity of the misbehavior
- Established rules of the family
- Temperament of the child
- Response of the child to rewards

Keep in mind that school-age children should participate in developing a plan of action for their misbehavior. Whatever methods of discipline are chosen, it is important that parents are consistent in providing discipline in a nurturing environment.

ADDRESSING COMMON DEVELOPMENTAL CONCERNS

The developmental task (according to Erikson) of the school-age child is industry (Erikson, 1963; Feigelman, 2011a). The school-age child is busy learning, achieving, and exploring. As the school-age child becomes more independent, forces other than the family such as television, video games, and peers influence him or her. Some of these influences are positive and others are negative.

Some of the common developmental concerns for the school-age child are discussed in the following sections. Guidelines to assist the parents and nurses when encountering these concerns are included in Teaching Guidelines 28.2.

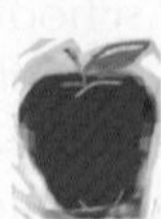

Teaching Guidelines 28.2

ADDRESSING COMMON DEVELOPMENTAL CONCERNS

Television, Video Games, and the Internet

- Limit total screen time, which includes television watching, video game playing, and internet-connected devices to 1 to 2 hours per day
- Monitor television programs and internet activity
- Prohibit television or video games with violence
- Do not put television, video games, or internet-connected devices in children's bedrooms. Place computers in an open area that allows easy monitoring by an adult
- Provide a schedule of accepted television programs for viewing each week
- Co-view television, video games and internet content with the child
- Encourage sports, interactive play, and reading
- Teach your child internet safety, such as to never share personal information or meet a friend you have only met online without parental permission. Never share passwords. Never respond to a message that hurts your feelings or makes you uncomfortable. Never send mean messages over the internet

Obesity

- Provide healthy meals and snacks
- Schedule and encourage daily exercise
- Encourage involvement in sports
- Restrict TV and computer-game use
- Limit the amount of fast-food intake
- Provide education about healthy nutrition
- Never use food as a reward
- Be a good role model

School Refusal

- Return child to school
- Investigate cause of the fear
- Support child
- Collaborate with teachers
- Praise success in school attendance

Latchkey Kids

- Provide rules to follow and expectations, such as:
  - Not answering the door or phone
  - No friends in the house when parents are not home
  - No playing with fire
- Teach child to call a trusted neighbor when help is needed and 911 in the event of emergency
- Post all resource numbers (even numbers you think your child may have memorized), including after-school help lines if available, in a clearly viewable spot. Include pediatrician's number and preferred hospital
- Purchase caller ID for the phone system
- Enroll the child in an after-school program if available
- Discuss limitations of outside play
- Discuss limitations of television viewing and video game use
- Make sure the child knows how to contact the parent
- Set clear homework expectations
- DO NOT keep guns in the home
- Teach the child where first aid supplies are located
- Teach the child household emergency procedures such as circuit breakers and water shut off valves
- Practice with your child. Have a trial run by leaving for a short time but staying close and role playing situations that may occur
- Always check in with your child while you are away

Stealing

- Educate parents about possibility of stealing
- Discuss ways to teach concept of ownership and property rights
- Handle situation openly
- Assist child in developing and enacting a plan to return what was stolen
- Make sure the punishment is appropriate for the action

Lying

- Help parents in understanding why the child is lying
- When the child lies, calmly confront the child and explain why the behavior is not acceptable
- Educate parents that their behavior should reflect what they teach and expect from their child
- Educate parents that too-rigid or severe punishments can decrease the child's sense of worth
- Seek professional help if lying persists in the older school-age child, to rule out underlying problems

Cheating

- Educate parents that the child must be mature enough to understand the concept of rules
- Handle cheating situations openly
- Help parents to understand why their child is cheating and to modify the trigger
- Develop appropriate punishment; inappropriate punishment could undermine the child
- Educate parents that their behavior should reflect what they expect from their child
- Seek professional help if cheating persists in the older school-age child, to rule out underlying problems

Bullying

The Bullied Child

- Educate parents whose children are at risk for being bullied, such as:
  - Children who appear different from the majority
  - Children who act different from the majority
  - Children who have low self-esteem
  - Children with a mental or psychological problem

- Teach parents to role-play different scenarios the child may face at school; show the child different ways to react to being bullied
- Impress upon the child that he or she did not cause the bullying
- Develop ways to increase the child's self-esteem at home
- Discuss the situation with the teacher and develop a plan of care

The Bullying Child

- Educate parents on reasons why it is important to correct the behavior
- Discuss ways the child can appropriately show his or her anger and feelings
- Have parents help the child to see how it feels to be bullied
- Do not allow fighting at home
- Reward settling of conflicts without violence

Tobacco and Alcohol Education

- Inquire about tobacco and alcohol use
- Discuss the physical and social dangers of tobacco and alcohol use
- Urge parents to be good role models
- Limit reading and media materials about alcohol and tobacco use
- Discuss the influences of tobacco and alcohol use by peers
- Educate the child on spit tobacco. Let them know it is just as dangerous as smoking tobacco
- Advocate for a smoke-free environment in the home and other places frequented
- Avoid having tobacco and alcohol products readily available in the home

Television, Video Games, and the Internet

The influence of television, video games, and the internet upon the school-age child is a growing concern for parents and child specialists. Children 8 to 10 years of age in the United States spend about 4 hours a day either watching TV or playing video games and another 2 hours on the computer outside of school work (Dowshen, 2011). During that time, a child by the age of 18 will see 200,000 violent acts (Dowshen, 2011). Although a school-age child can determine what is real from what is fantasy, research has shown that this amount of time in front of a screen—watching it or playing video games—can lead to aggressive behavior, less physical activity, and obesity (Dowshen, 2011) (see Healthy People 2020).

Some television shows, video games, and internet activity can have positive influences on children, but parents should be taught guidelines on the use of TV, video games, and the internet. Parents should set limits on how much screen time the child can have. The AAP recommends 2 hours or less of screen time per day (Dowshen, 2011). The parent should establish guidelines on when the child can watch TV; for example, after homework or when chores are completed (Dowshen, 2011). Television watching, internet activity, or video gaming should not be used as a reward. The parents should be aware of what the child is watching and doing online. This can be accomplished by parents and children watching programs together and parents using that opportunity to discuss the subject matter with the child. There should be no TV during dinner and no TV or internet-connected devices in the child's room. The parents need to set an example for the child by reading instead of watching TV or by doing a physical activity together as a family. If the TV causes fights or arguments, it should be turned off for a period of time.

HEALTHY PEOPLE 2020

Objective	Nursing Significance
Increase the proportion of children and adolescents who do not exceed recommended limits for screen time	• Assist families to identify activities other than television or video games for the child to participate in
Increase the proportion of children and adolescents aged 2 years through 12th grade who view television or videos or play video games for no more than 2 hours a day	• Praise craft, music, and sports participation

Healthy People Objectives retrieved from http://www.healthypeople.gov

Take Note!

According to the AAP age-based guidelines, school-age children need supervision and monitoring when using the internet to ensure they are not exposed to inappropriate material or content (AAP, 2015). Encourage parents of children in this age group to utilize internet safety tools that limit access to content and websites and that provide information on internet activities.

School Refusal

School refusal (also called *school phobia* or *school avoidance*) has been defined as a refusal to attend school or difficulty remaining in school for an entire day. Behaviors include frequent absences, skipping classes, chronically late for school, severe misbehavior before school, or attending school with great fear. School phobia needs to be defined both symptomatically and operationally as the cause for the anxiety. School avoidance occurs in approximately 5% of children (AAP, 2013e).

Some of the fears expressed by school-refusing children include separating from parents, riding the bus, tests, bullying, teacher reprimands, anxieties over toileting in a public bathroom, physical harm, or undressing in the locker room. Due to the emotional distress caused in these children when attending school, they are frequently classified as having school phobia. Young children may complain of stomachache or headache and older children may complain of palpitations or feeling faint.

It is important to investigate specific causes of school refusal/school phobia and take appropriate actions. Many times, school phobia is a symptom of deeper problems. The physician or nurse practitioner should conduct a physical examination of the child to rule out any physical illness. After these measures are taken, the parent, teacher, school counselor, and school administrator may devise a plan to assist the student to overcome a specific fear. In uncomplicated cases, parents must return the child to school as soon as possible. There may be altered schedules (partial days or decreased hours) to help promote a successful transition back to school. Another idea to help desensitize the child may be to have him or her spend part of the day in the counselor's or school nurse's office.

Latchkey Children

With the increasing incidence of both parents in the workforce and many children living with just one parent, often times, children return home alone without adult supervision for a number of hours. Most young children are not capable of handling stress or making decisions on their own before 11 or 12 years of age. However, some school-age children are more mature and can be left alone by 8 to 10 years of age; maturity is the key, not the age. Parents not only need to consider their child's maturity and readiness to be home alone but also must comply with legal requirements if present. Many States offer guidelines of when it is ok to leave a child at home alone and a few States have laws with a minimum age but these vary by State; therefore, the nurse needs to be familiar with the State and local laws in order to assist parents in making decisions about when it is appropriate for their child to be home alone (Child Welfare Information Gateway, 2013). The AAP recommends that a school-age child come home to a parent or another responsible adult (AAP, 2013f).

Despite the level of maturity, children who are unsupervised are more likely to participate in risky behaviors such as smoking, drinking, and doing drugs (AAP, 2013g). In addition, latchkey children may feel anxiety, stress, fear, boredom, loneliness, they miss more days of school, and have lower academic scores (AAP, 2013g).

If children come home to no supervision, they should know the names, addresses, and phone numbers of parents and a neighbor, as well as emergency numbers. They should be given rules about answering the door and the phone. They should tell anyone who comes to the door or who calls that mom is home but busy at this time. Directions as to the handling of the house key and fire safety should be taught and demonstrated (see Teaching Guidelines 28.2).

Stealing, Lying, and Cheating

It is during the school-age years that antisocial behaviors can emerge. Children who were previously well behaved may now exhibit behaviors such as stealing, lying, and cheating (Mannheim, 2012). Parents are usually disturbed by this change in behavior. In turn, they have difficulty in addressing these issues and need help in providing appropriate interventions.

Children between 6 and 8 years old do not fully understand the concept of ownership and property rights. These children may steal things because they like the look of the item. By the age of 9, the child should respect others' possessions and property and understand that stealing is wrong (Roux, 2013). The school-age child may steal because he or she desires the item, feels peer pressure and is trying to impress his or her peers, or has a sense of low self-esteem (Roux, 2013). Stealing becomes a concern if the child steals and does not have remorse or steals continuously, or if stealing is accompanied by other behavior problems (Roux, 2013).

Lying is more common in boys and in children between 5 and 8 years old (Roux, 2013). It is acceptable for these children to tell tall tales, but they should know what truth is and what make-believe is. These younger children typically lie to avoid punishment. However, they do not like others to lie and will tell on them if they lie. Children between 8 and 12 years old typically lie because they are unable to meet expectations of family and peers, they are testing the rules and limits placed on them, or they are unable to explain bad behavior (Roux, 2013). If lying persists in older school-age children, if it is accompanied by other behavior problems, or if the child does not show remorse with lying, parents should discuss the matter with a physician because the lying may be evidence of underlying problems.

The concept of cheating is not well understood until the child is 7 years old. Before this age, the desire to "win" is most important and rigid rules are hard to understand. In children between 8 and 12 years old, the concept of cheating is fully understood and following of rules becomes more important (Roux, 2013). Cheating is usually done because of competition and strong pressure placed on the child to succeed (AAP, 2013h). If cheating persists in older school-age children, parents should discuss the matter with a physician because the behavior may indicate underlying problems.

In dealing with children who exhibit stealing, lying, or cheating behaviors, parents must first realize the importance of their own behaviors in those areas. Parents are role models to the school-age child. Therefore, when

EVIDENCE-BASED PRACTICE 28.1 **BENEFITS OF BULLY-PREVENTION EDUCATION**

STUDY

Bullying and victimization continue to pose a problem in elementary schools. In addition to the behavioral disruption that occurs as a result of bullying and victimization, prior research has demonstrated that child bullies and victims are at increased risk for mental health problems, such as depression, anxiety, low self-esteem, and low social competence. Adverse consequences from bullying have led to prevention programs to decrease peer victimization. This study looked at the effectiveness of one such program, Youth Matters. It used a sample of 876 students in grades 4, 5, and 6. Children were placed in a control or experimental group and bullying and victimization were assessed at four different time points using surveys.

Findings

Upon analysis of the findings, the researchers reported in most cases children who participated in the bullying intervention program transitioned from being part of bullying, victim, or bullying–victim group to uninvolved group. The most positive effect was seen in children in the victim class. Findings support that bully prevention programs can help develop social and emotional skills and can assist in changing perceptions and attitudes to help prevent and help a child handle bullying incidents.

Nursing Implications

Nurses should continue to educate parents and teachers about bullying. Become actively involved in the local elementary school bullying-prevention program and encourage school-wide interventions. When bullies are identified, refer them for education in bullying prevention programs that focus on skill building.

Adapted from Jenson, J. M., Brisson, D., Bender, K. A., & Williford, A. P. (2013). Effects of the Youth Matters Prevention Program on patterns of bullying and victimization in elementary and middle school. *Social Work Research*, 37(4), 361–372. doi: 10.1093/swr/svt030

the child sees or hears that parents lie, steal, or cheat (e.g., parents bragging about cheating on their taxes), they think it is all right to mimic those behaviors. Secondly, parents must directly confront any stealing, lying, or cheating behaviors and discuss (and follow through consistently with) the consequences of such behaviors (see Teaching Guidelines 28.2).

Bullying

Bullying, which is inflicting unwanted, repeated verbal, emotional, or physical abuse upon others, is on the rise (Schuster & Bogart, 2013). Utilizing email, text messages, social networking, and instant messaging, often referred to as cyberbullying, is a growing concern. Bullies often look for victims who appear shy, weak, and defenseless. Children with health issues, such as disabilities, obesity, and food allergies, are at an increased risk of being bullied (Schuster & Bogart, 2013).

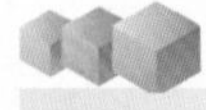

Concept Mastery Alert

Bullying in School Children

Children who bully most often have low self-esteem, poor grades, and poor interpersonal skills. Both boys and girls are bullied but boys tend to bully other boys and more often show force when bullying.

In general, about 10% of all children attending school are frightened and afraid most of the day (American Academy of Child and Adolescent Psychiatry, 2011). About 25% of children have been bullied (Robinson & Segal, 2014). Most of the bullying occurs at school (Augustyn & Zuckerman, 2011). Both boys and girls are bullied and can bully others; however, boys are twice as likely to be bullies and victims of bullying (Augustyn & Zuckerman, 2011). Being bullied can have negative results on children throughout life. These children often have increased episodes of headaches, stomachaches, sleep problems, anxiety, loneliness, depression, and suicidal tendencies (Schuster & Bogart, 2013). After the problem of either being bullied or being the bully has been identified, parents must work with the child, the school, and the physician or nurse practitioner to solve the problem (see Teaching Guidelines 28.2 and Evidence-Based Practice 28.1).

Tobacco and Alcohol Education

School-age children are eager to grow up and be independent. Peers and acceptance are very important at this time. School-age children may be exposed to messages that are in conflict with their parents' values regarding smoking and alcohol. Peers often exert pressure for children to experiment with tobacco and alcohol (see Healthy People 2020).

HEALTHY PEOPLE 2020

Objective	Nursing Significance
Reduce initiation of tobacco use among children and adolescents	• Educate children and families about the dangers of tobacco use

Healthy People Objectives retrieved from http://www.healthypeople.gov

School-age children are ready to absorb information that deals with drugs and alcohol. Information from parents or other adults who are major influences in the child's life is essential at this time to set clear rules and model behaviors for children to embrace. Discussions with children need to be based on facts and focused on the present. Some topics for discussion include:

- What alcohol and drugs are like and how they harm you
- Differences in medical use versus illegal use of drugs
- How to think critically to interpret messages seen in advertising, media, sports, and entertainment personalities

Recall Lawrence Jones, the 10-year-old presented at the beginning of the chapter. List potential developmental problems he may experience. What anticipatory guidance related to these concerns should you provide to his mother?

NURSING CARE PLAN 28.1

Growth and Development Issues of the School-Age Child

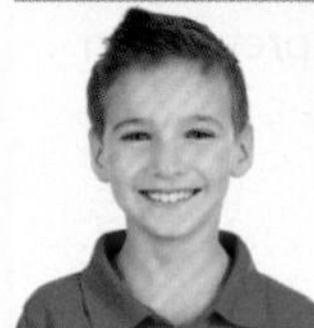

NURSING DIAGNOSIS: Risk for disproportionate growth (risk factors: caregiver knowledge deficit, frequent illnesses)

Outcome Identification and Evaluation

School-age child will demonstrate adequate growth: *appropriate weight gain and increases in height for age and gender*

Interventions: ***Promoting Proportionate Growth***

- Assess parent's knowledge of nutritional needs of school-age children *to determine need for further education.*
- Plot out height, weight, and BMI *to detect possible pattern.*
- Determine need for additional caloric intake if necessary *if very active in sports, if have a chronic illness caloric needs may be altered.*
- Educate primary caregiver about appropriate serving sizes and foods *so that primary caregiver is aware of what to expect for school-age children.*

NURSING DIAGNOSIS: Ineffective health maintenance related to lack of exercise, increased caloric intake, poor food choices

Outcome Identification and Evaluation

School-age child will engage in health maintenance behaviors and lose weight at an appropriate rate: *increase amount of exercise, make appropriate eating choices, decrease caloric intake to appropriate amount for age and gender*

Interventions: ***Promoting Appropriate Health Maintenance Behaviors***

- Assess knowledge of parents and child about nutritional needs of school-age children *to determine deficits in knowledge.*
- Plot out height, weight, and BMI *to detect weight loss or weight gain.*
- Have child keep food and exercise diary for 1 week *to determine current patterns of eating and exercise.*
- Interview parents in relationship to their eating habits and exercise habits *to determine where adjustments might need to be made.*
- Analyze preceding data, and base recommendations for changes on these data.
- Discuss ways to decrease temptation to overeat and to make good meal choices (see Teaching Guidelines 28.2).

NURSING CARE PLAN 28.1

Growth and Development Issues of the School-Age Child (continued)

- Have child assist in meal planning and grocery shopping *to allow him or her some sense of control in process.*
- Incorporate increase in daily exercise, which will stress sense of self-improvement, *to increase caloric expenditure and self-esteem.*
- Decrease TV/computer/device time *to increase caloric expenditure.*
- Develop reward system *to increase self-esteem.*
- Investigate joining weight-loss program for school-age children *to increase self-esteem and to increase awareness that other children have the same problem.*

NURSING DIAGNOSIS: Growth and development, delayed related to speech, motor, psychosocial, or cognitive concerns as evidenced by delay in meeting expected school performances

Outcome Identification and Evaluation

Development will be maximized: *School-age child will make continued progress toward attainment of expected school performances.*

Interventions: ***Promoting Growth and Development***

- Perform scheduled evaluation of the school-age child by school and physician or nurse practitioner *to determine current functioning.*
- Develop realistic multidisciplinary plan *to ensure maximizing resources.*
- Carry out interventions as prescribed by developmental specialist, physical therapist, occupational therapist, or speech therapist at home and at school *to maximize benefit of interventions.*
- Have scheduled evaluation meetings *to be able to adapt interventions as soon as possible.*

NURSING DIAGNOSIS: Caregiver role strain, risk for (risk factors: new sibling in household, knowledge deficit about school-age issues, lack of prior exposure, fatigue, ill or developmentally delayed child)

Outcome Identification and Evaluation

Parent will experience competence in role: *will demonstrate appropriate caretaking behaviors and verbalize comfort in caring for a school-age child*

Interventions: ***Preventing Caregiver Role Strain***

- Assess parents' knowledge of school-age children and the issues that arise as a part of normal development *to determine parents' needs.*
- Provide education on normal issues of school-age children so that parents are armed with the knowledge they need *to appropriately care for their school-age child.*
- Provide anticipatory guidance related to upcoming expected issues related to school-age development *to prepare parents for what to expect next and how to intervene.*

NURSING DIAGNOSIS: Injury, risk for (risk factors: curiosity, increasing cognitive skills and motor abilities)

Outcome Identification and Evaluation

School-age child's safety will be maintained: *will remain free from injury*

(continued)

NURSING CARE PLAN 28.1

Growth and Development Issues of the School-Age Child (continued)

Interventions: ***Preventing Injury***

- Discuss safety measures needed for the following: bikes, scooters, guns, skateboards, cars, water, and playground *to decrease risk of injury related to those areas.*
- Discuss and develop a fire safety plan *to decrease risk of injury related to fire.*
- Discuss appropriate safety equipment needed for each sport *to decrease risk of injury.*
- Discuss appropriate sports to participate in depending on age, sex, and maturity of child *to prevent possible injury and to promote child's self-esteem.*
- Instruct parents to post the Poison Control Center phone number *in the event of accidental ingestion, Poison Control can give parents the best advice for appropriate intervention.*
- Teach parents and child first-aid measures and child cardiopulmonary resuscitation (CPR) *to minimize consequences of injury should it occur.*
- Discuss influence of peers on actions of school-age children *to prevent possible injury due to mimicking behavior.*

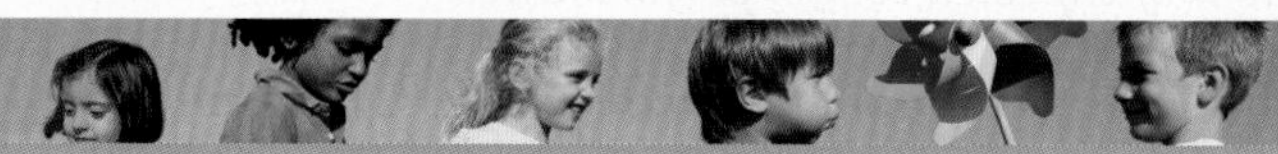

KEY CONCEPTS

- Physical growth is slow and steady, with social and cognitive development progressing rapidly, during the school-age years of 6 to 12. Height increases approximately 6 to 7 cm (2.5 inches) per year and weight gain is 3 to 3.5 kg (7 lb) per year. Boys are taller and heavier than girls during this time period (Feigelman, 2011a).
- With entrance into the school system, school-age children have the influences of peers and teachers.
- With the development of gross motor skills and involvement in sports at school and in the community, safety education and practices are required. Also, with the participation in cooperative sports, injuries occur.
- Visual acuity is reaching maturation and 20/20 vision is expected by 7 years of age (Jarvis, 2012).
- Increased independence leads to increased exposure to safety hazards.
- The school-age child develops the cognitive ability to classify objects and to identify relationships among objects.
- Dental care is very important to prevent dental caries, malocclusion, and other problems. In early school age, the first primary teeth will be lost.
- The onset of puberty may occur by the later school-age years.
- Erikson's (1963) developmental task for the age group is the development of a sense of industry.
- Peers are very important, especially peers of the same sex. School-age children usually have a best friend and belong to clubs. They have collections of nonvaluable items such as rocks, clips, and so forth.
- School-age children are capable of concrete operations, solving problems, and making decisions. They continue to need guidance, rules, and direction from parents.
- The school-age child develops a conscience and knows cultural and social values. He or she can understand and obey rules.
- The school-age child incorporates religious practices into his or her life, which may be a source of comfort during stressful times.
- The nurse's role includes educating parents and school-age children in promoting health and safety.
- Nurses should inform the school-age child about expected developmental changes in the body to promote self-esteem and self-confidence.

REFERENCES AND RECOMMENDED READINGS

American Academy of Child and Adolescent Psychiatry. (2011). *Facts for families: Bullying*. Retrieved from http://www.aacap.org/AACAP/Families_and_Youth/Facts_for_Families/Facts_for_Families_Pages/Bullying_80.aspx

American Academy of Pediatrics. (2010). Policy statement: Prevention of Drowning. *Pediatrics, 126*(1), 178–185. doi: 10.1542/peds.2010–1264

American Academy of Pediatrics. (2012). *Guidance for effective discipline.* Retrieved from http://pediatrics.aappublications.org/content/101/4/723.full

American Academy of Pediatrics. (2013a). *Safety & prevention: Car seats: Information for families for 2013.* Retrieved from http://www.healthychildren.org/English/safety-prevention/on-the-go/pages/Car-Safety-Seats-Information-for-Families.aspx

American Academy of Pediatrics. (2013b). Pedestrian safety. *Pediatrics, 124*(2), 802–812. Retrieved from http://pediatrics.aappublications.org/content/124/2/802.full

American Academy of Pediatrics. (2013c). *Family life: The importance of family routines.* Retrieved from http://www.healthychildren.org/English/family-life/family-dynamics/pages/The-Importance-of-Family-Routines.aspx

American Academy of Pediatrics. (2013d). *Preventing tooth decay in children.* Retrieved from http://www.healthychildren.org/English/healthy-living/oral-health/Pages/Preventing-Tooth-Decay-in-Children.aspx

American Academy of Pediatrics. (2013e). *School avoidance.* Retrieved from http://www.healthychildren.org/English/health-issues/conditions/emotional-problems/pages/School-Avoidance.aspx

American Academy of Pediatrics. (2013f). *Back to school tips.* Retrieved from http://www.aap.org/advocacy/releases/augschool.cfm

American Academy of Pediatrics. (2013g). *Safety & prevention: Is your child ready to stay home alone?* Retrieved from http://www.healthychildren.org/English/safety-prevention/at-home/pages/Is-Your-Child-Ready-To-Stay-Home-Alone.aspx

American Academy of Pediatrics. (2013h). *Family life: Competition and cheating.* Retrieved from http://www.healthychildren.org/English/family-life/family-dynamics/communication-discipline/pages/Competition-and-Cheating.aspx

American Academy of Pediatrics. (2014). *Dental health: Keeping your child's teeth healthy.* Retrieved from http://www.healthychildren.org/English/ages-stages/baby/teething-tooth-care/Pages/Dental-Health-Keeping-Your-Child%27s-Teeth-Healthy.aspx

American Academy of Pediatrics. (2015). *The internet and your family.* Retrieved from http://www.healthychildren.org/English/family-life/Media/Pages/The-Internet-and-Your-Family.aspx

American Academy of Pediatrics, The Injury Prevention Program. (2013a). *Safety for your child: 6 years.* Retrieved from http://www.healthychildren.org/english/tips-tools/Pages/Safety-for-Your-Child-6-Years.aspx

American Academy of Pediatrics, The Injury Prevention Program. (2013b). *Safety for your child: 8 years.* Retrieved from http://www.healthychildren.org/english/tips-tools/Pages/Safety-for-Your-Child-8-Years.aspx

American Academy of Pediatrics, The Injury Prevention Program. (2013c). *Safety for your child: 10 years.* Retrieved from http://www.healthychildren.org/english/tips-tools/Pages/Safety-for-Your-Child-10-Years.aspx

American Academy of Pediatric Dentistry. (2013). *Policy on use of fluoride.* Retrieved from http://www.aapd.org/media/Policies_Guidelines/P_FluorideUse.pdf

Augustyn, M., & Zuckerman, B. (2011). Chapter 36: Impact of violence on children. In R. M. Kleigman, B.F. Stanton, J. W. St. Geme III, N. F. Schor, & R. E. Behrman (Eds.), *Nelson textbook of pediatrics* (19th ed., pp.135). Philadelphia, PA: Saunders.

Bicycle Helmet Safety Institute. (2012). *Pamphlet: A bicycle helmet for my child.* Retrieved from http://www.helmets.org/childpam.htm

Billings, D. M. & Hensel, D. (2014). *Lippincott's Q & A Review for NCLEX-RN* (11th ed.). Philadelphia, PA: Lippincott Williams & Wilkins.

Bright Futures/American Academy of Pediatrics. (2014). *Recommendations for preventive pediatric health care.* Retrieved from http://www.aap.org/en-us/professional-resources/practice-support/Periodicity/Periodicity%20Schedule_FINAL.pdf

Carpenito, L. J. (2013). *Nursing diagnosis: Application to clinical practice* (14th ed.). Philadelphia, PA: Lippincott Williams & Wilkins.

Centers for Disease Control and Prevention. (2014) *Child maltreatment facts at a glance.* Retrieved from http://www.cdc.gov/violenceprevention/pdf/childmaltreatment-facts-at-a-glance.pdf

Centers for Disease Control and Prevention. (2012a). *Unintentional drowning: Get the Facts.* Retrieved from http://www.cdc.gov/HomeandRecreationalSafety/Water-Safety/waterinjuries-factsheet.html

Centers for Disease Control and Prevention. (2012b). *Protect the ones you love: Childhood injuries are preventable: CDC Childhood Injury Report.* Retrieved from http://www.cdc.gov/safechild/child_injury_data.html

Centers for Disease Control and Prevention. (2013a). *Childhood obesity facts.* Retrieved from http://www.cdc.gov/healthyyouth/obesity/facts.htm

Centers for Disease Control and Prevention. (2013b). *Preventing dental caries with community programs.* Retrieved from http://www.cdc.gov/oralhealth/publications/factsheets/dental_caries.htm

Child Development Institute. (2013). *Helping your child deal with fears and phobias.* Retrieved from http://childdevelopmentinfo.com/child-psychology/anxiety_disorders_in_children/fears/

Child Welfare Information Gateway. (2013). *Leaving your child home alone.* Washington, DC: U.S. Department of Health and Human Services, Children's Bureau.

Dowshen, S. (2011). *How TV affects your child.* Retrieved from http://kidshealth.org/parent/positive/family/tv_affects_child.html

Dowshen, S (2014). *Bike Safety.* Retrieved from http://kidshealth.org/teen/safety/safebasics/bike_safety.html#

Erikson, E. (1963). *Childhood and society* (2nd ed.). New York: Norton.

Feigelman, S. (2011a). Chapter 11: Middle childhood. In R. M. Kleigman, B. F. Stanton, J. W. St. Geme III, N. F. Schor, & R. E. Behrman (Eds.), *Nelson textbook of pediatrics* (19th ed., pp.36–39). Philadelphia, PA: Saunders.

Feigelman, S. (2011b). Chapter 6: Overview and assessment variability. In R. M. Kleigman, B. F. Stanton, J. W. St. Geme III, N. F. Schor & R. E. Behrman (Eds.), *Nelson textbook of pediatrics* (19th ed., pp.26). Philadelphia, PA: Saunders.

Ford, G. S. (2007). Hospitalized kids spiritual care at their level. *Journal of Christian Nursing, 24*(3), 135–140.

Gilchrist, J., Ballesteros, M. F., & Parker, E. M. (2012). *Vital signs: Unintentional injury deaths among persons aged 0–19 years—*

United States, 2000–2009. Morbidity and Mortality Weekly Report (MMWR). Retrieved from http://www.cdc.gov/mmwr/preview/mmwrhtml/mm61e0416a1.htm

Jarvis, C. (2012). Chapter 14: Eyes. In C. Jarvis (Eds.) *Physical examination and health assessment* (6th ed. pp. 279–322). St. Louis, MO: Mosby.

Jenson, J. M., Brisson, D., Bender, K. A., & Williford, A. P. (2013). Effects of the Youth Matters Prevention Program on patterns of bullying and victimization in elementary and middle school. *Social Work Research, 37*(4), 361–372. doi: 10.1093/swr/svt030

Kohlberg, L. (1984). *Moral development.* New York: Harper & Row.

Krebs, N. R., Primark, L. E., & Haemer, M. (2011). Normal childhood nutrition & its disorders. In W. W. Hay, M. J. Levin, J. M. Sondheimer, & R. R. Deterding (Eds.), *Current pediatric diagnosis and treatment* (20th ed.). New York: McGraw-Hill.

Lyness, D. (2013). *Anxieties, fears and phobias.* Retrieved from http://kidshealth.org/parent/emotions/feelings/anxiety.html#

Mannheim, J. K. (2012). *School-age children development.* Retrieved from http://www.nlm.nih.gov/medlineplus/ency/article/002017.htm

McDevitt, S., & Carey, W. (1978). The measurement of temperament in 3–7 year old children. *Journal of Child Psychology and Psychiatry, 19,* 245–253.

National Eye Institute. (2013). *Facts about amblyopia.* Retrieved from http://www.nei.nih.gov/health/amblyopia/amblyopia_guide.asp

National Institutes of Dental and Craniofacial Research, National Institutes of Health. (2014). *Dental caries (tooth decay) in children (ages 2 to 11).* Retrieved from http://www.nidcr.nih.gov/DataStatistics/FindDataByTopic/DentalCaries/DentalCariesChildren2to11

Piaget, J. (1969). *The theory of stages in cognitive development.* New York: McGraw-Hill.

Robinson, L., & Segal, J. (2014) *Deal with a bully & overcome bullying helping bullied kids and teens and those who bully them.* HelpGuide.org. Retrieved from http://www.helpguide.org/mental/bullying.htm

Roux, S.L. (2013). *Lying and stealing.* Children's Hospital of Boston Retrieved from http://healthlibrary.childrenshospital.org/Library/Encyclopedia/90,P02241?PrinterFriendly=true

Schuster, M. A., & Bogart, L. M. (2013). Did the ugly duckling have PTSD? Bullying, its effects, and the role of pediatricians. *Pediatrics, 131*(1), e288–e291. doi: 10.1542/peds.2012–3253

Stopbullying.gov. *State anti-bullying laws & policies.* Retrieved from http://www.stopbullying.gov/laws/index.html#listing. Accessed October 22, 2012.

U.S. Department of Agriculture and U.S. Department of Health and Human Services. (2010). *Dietary guidelines for Americans, 2010* (7th ed.). Washington, DC: U.S. Government Printing Office. Retrieved from http://www.cnpp.usda.gov/DGAs2010-PolicyDocument.htm

U.S. Department of Health & Human Services. (2012). *HealthyPeople.gov.* Retrieved at http://www.healthypeople.gov/2020/about/default.aspx

CHAPTER WORKSHEET

MULTIPLE CHOICE QUESTIONS

1. The successful resolution of developmental tasks for the school-age child, according to Erikson, would be identified by:
   a. Learning from repeating tasks
   b. Developing a sense of worth and competence
   c. Using fantasy and magical thinking to cope with problems
   d. Developing a sense of trust
2. Which of the following are reasons that stealing occurs in school-age children? (Choose all that apply.)
   a. To escape punishment
   b. High self-esteem
   c. Low expectations of family/peers
   d. Lack of sense of property
   e. Strong desire to own something
3. Which activities will promote weight loss in an obese school-age child? (Choose all that apply.)
   a. Unlimited computer and TV time
   b. Role modeling by family
   c. Becoming active in sports
   d. Eating unstructured meals
   e. Involving child in meal planning and grocery shopping
   f. Drinking three glasses of water per day
4. As the school nurse conducting screening for vision in a 6-year-old child, you would refer the child to a specialist if the visual acuity in both eyes is:
   a. 20/20
   b. 20/25
   c. 20/30
   d. 20/50
5. The mother of two sons, ages 6 and 9, states they want to play on the same baseball team. As the school nurse, what advice would you give their mother?
   a. Having the boys on the same team will make it more convenient for the mother.
   b. Levels of coordination and concentration differ, so the boys need to be on different teams.
   c. Put the boys on the same team because they are both school-age children.
   d. It is best to avoid putting the boys on the same team to prevent sibling rivalry.

CRITICAL THINKING EXERCISES

1. Ms. Sams brings her 8-year-old son, Frank, to the physician's office for his annual examination. She states that she is concerned about his recent behavior. He went to the grocery store with his friend and his friend's mother and he came home with a Matchbox car. The friend's mother stated she had not purchased the car.
   a. What would be your response to Ms. Sams?
   b. Ms. Sams said she still has the car. What would you advise Ms. Sams to do to make Frank aware of the consequences of his actions?
2. Sally's mother is asking the nurse for advice about purchasing a two-wheeled bike for her 7-year-old. What guidance should the nurse offer this parent?
3. Ms. Shaw brings in her 11-year-old daughter for a well-child check-up. The school-ager says to the nurse, "I look different from my friends. I do not wear bras and my friends are already wearing bras." What would be an appropriate response to this school-ager?
4. Johnny is a 9-year-old whose mother and father both work during the day. He returns home after school. How should the parents prepare Johnny for this experience? What safety rules would be included in the education for Johnny?

STUDY ACTIVITIES

1. Attend a sporting event (such as soccer or baseball) with school-age teams. Describe the coordination and gross motor functioning of this group.
2. Attend a first-grade class. Observe the behaviors exhibited by the school-age children in this class. How do these behaviors compare with normal values for this age group?

BRINGING IT ALL TOGETHER: A CASE STUDY

Grace, a 9-year-old girl, is seen in your clinic for a well-child examination. She is a healthy 3rd grader who enjoys school and activities. Her mother states she has some concerns about Grace. She says "Grace seems tired a lot. I am not sure she is getting enough rest."

Go to thePoint to find questions to consider about this case.

29

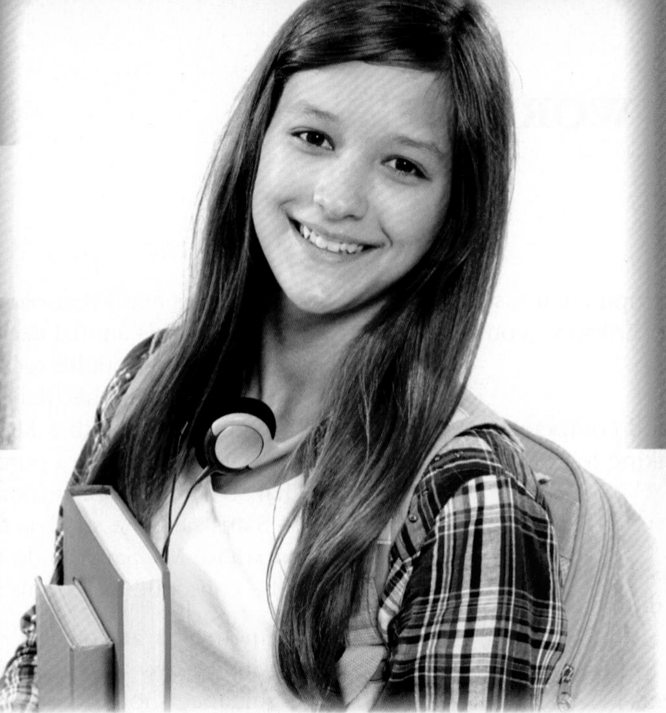

WOW

Words of Wisdom
The only way to grow is to let go ...

Growth and Development of the Adolescent

KEY TERMS
adolescence
menarche
peer groups
puberty
risk-taking behaviors
sexuality
thelarche

Learning Objectives

Upon completion of the chapter, you will be able to:

1. Identify normal physiologic changes, including puberty, occurring in the adolescent.
2. Discuss psychosocial, cognitive, and moral changes occurring in the adolescent.
3. Identify changes in relationships with peers, family, teachers, and community during adolescence.
4. Describe interventions to promote safety during adolescence.
5. Demonstrate knowledge of the nutritional requirements of the adolescent.
6. Demonstrate knowledge of the development of sexuality and its influence on dating during adolescence.
7. Identify common developmental concerns of the adolescent.
8. Demonstrate knowledge of the appropriate nursing guidance for common developmental concerns.

Cho Chung **is a 15-year-old girl brought to the clinic by her mother for her annual school check-up. During your assessment you measure Cho's weight at 49.89 kg (110 lb) and her height at 152.4 cm (60 inches). As the nurse caring for her, assess Cho's growth and development, and then provide appropriate anticipatory guidance to her and her mother.**

Adolescence spans the years of transition from childhood to adulthood, which is usually between the ages of 11 and 20 years. There is some overlap between late school age and adolescence. The adolescent experiences drastic changes in the physical, cognitive, psychosocial, and psychosexual areas. With this rapid growth during adolescence, the development of secondary sexual characteristics, and interest in the opposite sex, the adolescent needs the support and guidance of parents and nurses to facilitate healthy lifestyles and to reduce **risk-taking behaviors** such as drinking, drug use, sexual activity, and participating in reckless behavior or dangerous activities.

Growth and Development Overview

Adolescence is a time of rapid growth with dramatic changes in body size and proportions. The magnitude of these changes is second only to the growth in infancy. During this time sexual characteristics develop and reproductive maturity is achieved. The age of onset and the duration of the physiologic changes vary from individual to individual. Generally, girls enter puberty earlier (at 9 to 10 years of age) than boys (at 10 to 11 years). Adolescents will represent varying levels of identity formation and will offer unique challenges to the nurse (Table 29.1).

PHYSIOLOGIC CHANGES ASSOCIATED WITH PUBERTY

The secretion of estrogen in girls and testosterone in boys stimulates the development of breast tissue in girls, pubic hair in both sexes, and changes in male genitalia. These biologic changes that occur during adolescence are known as **puberty**. Puberty is the result of triggers among the environment, the central nervous system, the hypothalamus, the pituitary gland, the gonads, and the adrenal glands. Gonadotropin-releasing hormone (GnRH), produced by the hypothalamus, travels to the anterior pituitary gland to stimulate the production and secretion of follicle-stimulating hormone (FSH) and luteinizing hormone (LH). The increased levels of FSH and LH stimulate the gonadal response. LH stimulates ovulation in girls and acts on testicular Leydig cells in boys, prompting maturation of the testicles and testosterone production. FSH with LH stimulates sperm production. Estrogen, progesterone, and testosterone and other androgens are released from the gonads and affect biologic changes and changes in various organs, including alterations in muscles, bones, skin, and hair follicles.

Adolescents experience physical development, hormonal changes, and sexual maturation during puberty that correlate to Freud's genital stage of psychosexual development. The genital stage begins with the production of sex hormones and maturation of the reproductive system.

TABLE 29.1 PHYSIOLOGIC CHANGES OF ADOLESCENCE

Stage of Adolescence	Changes in Females	Changes in Males
Early adolescence (10–13 years)	Pubic hair begins to curl and spread over mons pubis; genitalia pigmentation increases Breast bud and areola continue to enlarge; no separation of breasts First menstrual period (average 12 years, normal range 9–16 years)	Pubic hair spreads laterally, begins to curl; pigmentation increases Growth and enlargement of testes in scrotum (scrotum reddish in color) and continued lengthening of penis Leggy look due to extremities growing faster than the trunk
Middle adolescence (14–16 years)	Pubic hair becomes coarse in texture and continues to curl; amount of hair increases Areola and papilla separate from the contour of the breast to form a secondary mound	Pubic hair becomes coarser in texture and takes on adult distribution Testes and scrotum continue to grow; scrotal skin darkens; penis grows in width, and glans penis develops May experience breast enlargement Voice changes; more masculine due to rapid enlargement of the larynx and pharynx as well as lung changes
Late adolescence (17–20 years)	Mature pubic hair distribution and coarseness	Mature pubic hair distribution and coarseness Breast enlargement disappears Adult size and shape of testes, scrotum, and penis; scrotal skin darkening

Adapted from Cromer, B. (2011). Chapter 104: Adolescent development. In R. M. Kleigman, B. F. Stanton, J. W. St. Geme III, N. F. Schor, & R. E. Behrman (Eds.), *Nelson textbook of pediatrics* (19th ed., pp. 649–659). Philadelphia, PA: Saunders.

Girls reach physical maturity before boys and **menarche**, the first menstrual period, usually begins between the ages of 9 and 15 years (average 12.8 years). Breast budding (**thelarche**) occurs at approximately age 9 to 11 years and is followed by the growth of pubic hair.

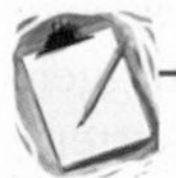

Take Note!

African-American girls on average reach menarche slightly earlier than Caucasian girls (Hirsch, 2011).

The first sign of pubertal changes in boys is testicular enlargement in response to testosterone secretion, usually occurring in Tanner stage 2. As testosterone levels increase, the penis and scrotum enlarge, hair distribution increases, and scrotal skin texture changes. During late puberty, boys will typically experience their first ejaculation, which may occur while they are sleeping (nocturnal emissions). Nurses should provide anticipatory guidance to adolescent males regarding involuntary nocturnal emissions (wet dreams) to assure them that this is a normal occurrence.

Tanner stages 3 to 5 usually occur during adolescence. Refer to Figures 32.28, 32.34, and 32.36 for an illustration of the increase in breast tissue and pubic hair distribution in girls, and scrotal and penile changes as well as hair distribution changes in boys. The nurse should provide guidance to adolescents about the normalcy of the sexual feelings and evolving body changes that occur during puberty.

PHYSICAL GROWTH

Diet, exercise, and hereditary factors influence the height, weight, and body build of the adolescent. Over the past three decades, adolescents have become taller and heavier than their ancestors and the beginning of puberty is earlier. During the early adolescent period, there is an increase in the percentage of body fat and the head, neck, and hands reach adult proportions.

The rapid growth during adolescence is secondary only to that of the infant years and is a direct result of the hormonal changes of puberty. Both girls and boys experience changes in appearance and size. Height in girls increases rapidly after menarche and usually ceases 2 to 2½ years after menarche. Boys' growth spurt occurs later than girls' and usually begins between the ages of 10½ and 16 years and ends sometime between the ages of 13½ and 17½ years. Peak height velocity (PHV) occurs at approximately 12 years of age in girls or at about 6 to 12 months after menarche. Boys reach PHV at about 14 years of age. Peak weight velocity (PWV) occurs about 6 months after menarche in girls and at about 14 years of age in boys. Muscle mass increases in boys and fat deposits increase in girls (Fig. 29.1).

During early adolescence growth is rapid, but it decreases in middle and late adolescence. Height for adolescent boys who are between the 50th and 95th percentile ranges from 132 cm (52½ inches) to 176.8 cm (69½ inches). Weight of boys in these percentiles ranges from 35.3 kg (77¼ lb) to 95.76 kg (211 lb). On average, boys will gain 10 to 30 cm (4 to 12 inches) in height and 7 to 30 kg (15 to 65 lb) in weight.

Height for girls who are between the 50th and 95th percentile ranges from 144.8 cm (57 inches) to 173.6 cm (68½ inches), with weight ranging from 27.24 kg (60 lb) to 82.47 kg (181 lb). On average, girls will gain 5 to 20 cm (2 to 8 inches) in height and 7 to 25 kg (15 to 55 lb) in weight during adolescence. See Appendix A for growth charts for this age group. Refer to Chapter 32,

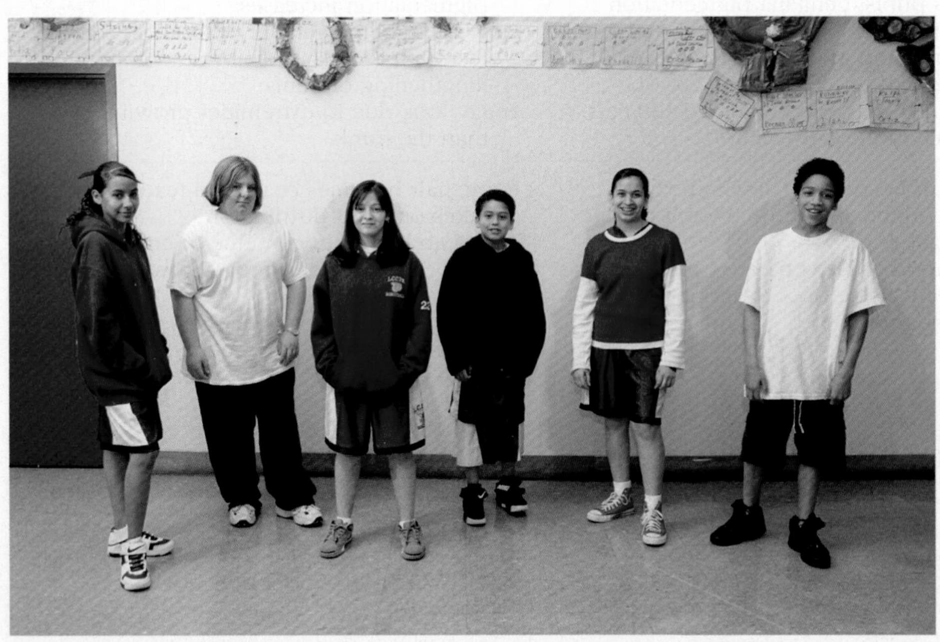

FIGURE 29.1 These adolescents reflect the differences in sizes and shapes seen in adolescents of the same age.

Box 32.1, for instructions for calculating body mass index (BMI).

ORGAN SYSTEM MATURATION

Adolescence is a time of metabolic slowing and of increasing size of some organs. The basal metabolic rate (BMR) reaches the adult level during late adolescence.

Neurologic System

During adolescence there is continued brain growth, although the size of the brain does not increase significantly. Neurons do not increase in number, but growth of the myelin sheath enables faster neural processing.

Respiratory System

The adolescent years see an increase in diameter and length of the lungs. Respiratory rate decreases and reaches the adult rate of 15 to 20 breaths per minute. Respiratory volume and vital capacity increase. Volume and capacity are greater in boys than girls, which may be associated with increased chest and shoulder size in boys. The growth of the laryngeal cartilage, larynx, pharynx, vocal cords, and lungs produces the voice changes experienced in adolescence. These changes in the quality of the child's voice are often preceded with some voice instability where voice cracking is heard. Deepening of both male and female voices occurs but is more pronounced in boys.

Cardiovascular System

There is an increase in size and strength of the heart. Systolic blood pressure increases and heart rate decreases. Blood volume reaches higher levels in boys than girls, which may be due to boys' greater muscle mass.

Gastrointestinal System

The adolescent has a full set of permanent teeth with the exception of the last four molars (wisdom teeth), which may erupt between the ages of 17 and 20 years. The liver, spleen, kidneys, and digestive tract enlarge during the growth spurt in early adolescence, but do not change in function. These systems are mature in early school age.

Musculoskeletal System

The ossification of the skeletal system is incomplete until late adolescence in boys. Ossification is more advanced in girls and occurs at an earlier age. During the growth spurt, muscle mass and strength increase. At similar stages of development, muscle development is generally greater in boys. Estrogen, progesterone, and testosterone (sex steroids) and other androgens are released from the gonads and affect changes in the muscles and bones. Low estrogen levels tend to stimulate skeletal growth, while higher levels inhibit growth. During middle adolescence, shoulder, chest, and hip breadth increase.

Integumentary System

During adolescence the skin becomes thick and tough. Under the influence of androgens, the sebaceous glands become more active, particularly on the face, back, and genitals. Due to the increased levels of testosterone during Tanner stages 4 and 5 in both boys and girls, both sexes may have increased sebum production, which may lead to the development of acne and oily hair.

The exocrine and apocrine sweat glands function at adult levels during adolescence. The exocrine glands are all over the body and they produce sweat that helps to eliminate body heat through evaporation. The apocrine glands are found in the axillae, genital, and anal areas and around the breasts. The apocrine sweat glands produce sweat in response to hair follicles. This sweat is produced continuously and is stored and released in response to emotional stimuli.

PSYCHOSOCIAL DEVELOPMENT

According to Erikson, it is during adolescence that teenagers achieve a sense of identity (Erikson, 1963). As the adolescent is trying out many different roles in regard to his or her relationships with peers, family, community, and society, he or she is developing his or her own individual sense of self. If the adolescent is not successful in forming his or her own sense of self, he or she develops a sense of role confusion or diffusion. The adolescent culture becomes very important to the teenager. It is through his or her involvement with teenage groups that the adolescent finds support and help with developing his or her own identity.

Erikson (1963) believed that during the task of developing his or her own sense of identity, the adolescent revisits each of the previous stages of development. The sense of trust is encountered as the adolescent strives to find out whom and what ideals he or she can have faith in. In revisiting the stage of autonomy, the adolescent is seeking out ways to express his or her individuality in an effective manner. The adolescent would avoid behaviors that would "shame" or ridicule him or her in front of his or her peers. The sense of initiative is revisited as the adolescent develops his or her vision for what he or she might become. And the sense of industry is again encountered as the adolescent makes his or her choice to participate in different activities at school, in the community, at church, and in the workforce.

The ability of the adolescent to successfully form a sense of self is dependent upon how well the adolescent successfully completed the former stages of development. Erikson (1963) believed that if the adolescent has been successful, he or she can develop resources during adolescence to overcome any gaps in previous developmental stages. If the adolescent believes that he or she cannot express himself or herself in any manner due to societal restrictions, he or she will develop role confusion. See Table 29.2 for additional information.

COGNITIVE DEVELOPMENT

According to Piaget, the adolescent progresses from a concrete framework of thinking to an abstract one (Piaget, 1969). It is the formal operational period. During this period, the adolescent develops the ability to think outside of the present; that is, he or she can incorporate into thinking concepts that do exist as well as concepts

TABLE 29.2 DEVELOPMENTAL THEORIES

Theories	Stages	Activities
Erikson (psychosocial)	Identity vs. role confusion or diffusion Early (10–13 years)	Focuses on bodily changes Experiences frequent mood changes Importance placed on conformity to peer norms and peer acceptance Strives to master skills within peer groups Defining boundaries with parents and authority figures Early stage of emancipation—struggles to separate from parents while still desiring dependence upon them Identifies with same-sex peers Takes more responsibility for own behaviors
	Middle (14–16 years)	Continues to adjust to changed body image Tries out different roles within peer groups Need for acceptance by peer group at the highest level Interested in attracting opposite gender Time of greatest conflict with parents/authority figures
	Late (17–20 years)	Able to understand implications of behavior and decisions Roles within peer groups established Feels secure with body image Has matured sexual identity Has idealistic career goals Importance of individual friendships emerges Process of emancipation from family almost complete
Piaget (cognitive)	Formal operations Early (10–13 years)	Limited abstract thought process Egocentrical thinking Eager to apply limited abstract process to different situations and to peer groups
	Middle (14–17 years)	Increased ability to think abstractly or in more idealistic terms Able to solve verbal and mental problems using scientific methods Thinks he or she is invincible—risky behaviors increase Likes making independent decisions Becomes involved/concerned with society, politics
	Late (17–20 years)	Abstract thinking is established Develops critical thinking skills—tests different solutions to problems Less risky behaviors Develops realistic goals and career plans
Kohlberg	Postconventional level III Early (10–13 years)	Morals based on peer, family, church, and societal morals Asks broad, usually unanswerable questions about life
	Middle (14–17 years)	Developing own set of morals—evaluates individual morals in relation to peer, family, and societal morals
	Late (17–20 years)	Internalizes own morals and values Continues to compare own morals and values to those of society Evaluates morals of others

Adapted from Erikson, E. (1963). *Childhood and society* (2nd ed.). New York: Norton; Kohlberg, L. (1984). *Moral development*. New York: Harper & Row; and Piaget, J. (1969). *The theory of stages in cognitive development*. New York: McGraw-Hill.

that might exist. The adolescent's thinking becomes logical, organized, and consistent. He or she is able to think about a problem from all points of view, ranking the possible solutions while solving the problem. Not all adolescents achieve formal operational reasoning at the same time.

In the early stages of formal operational reasoning, the adolescent's thinking is egocentric. The adolescent is very idealistic, constantly challenging the way things are and wondering why things cannot change. These activities lead to the adolescent's feeling of being omnipotent. The adolescent must undergo this way of thinking, even though it can frustrate adults, in his or her quest to reach formal operational reasoning. As the teenager progresses toward middle adolescence, his or her thinking becomes very introspective. He or she assumes others are just as interested in what interests him or her, which leads him or her to feel unique, special, and exceptional. That feeling of "being exceptional" leads to the risk-taking behaviors of which teenagers are well known. Also, the teenager feels very committed to his or her viewpoints. He or she tries very hard to convince others of his or her viewpoints and embraces strongly those causes that support his or her opinions. This idealism can cause the adolescent to reject his or her family, culture, church, and community beliefs, which can cause conflict with his or her family, culture, church, and community. See Table 29.2 for additional information.

MORAL AND SPIRITUAL DEVELOPMENT

It is during the adolescent years that teenagers develop their own set of values and morals. According to Kohlberg, adolescents are experiencing the postconventional stage of moral development (Kohlberg, 1984). It is only because adolescents are developing their formal operational way of thinking that they can experience the postconventional stage of moral development. At the beginning of this stage, teenagers begin to question the status quo. The majority of their choices are based on emotions while they are questioning societal standards. As they progress to developing their own set of morals, adolescents realize that moral decisions are based on rights, values, and principles that are agreeable to a given society. They also realize that those rights, values, and principles can be in conflict with the laws of the given society, but they are able to reconcile the differences. Because adolescents undergo the process of developing their own set of morals at different rates, they might find that their friends view a situation differently. This difference can lead to conflicts and the forming of different friendships. See Table 29.2 for additional information.

Adolescents also may begin to question their formal religious practices or in some cases cling to them (Ford, 2007). As they progress through adolescence, teenagers become more interested in the spiritualism of their religion than in the actual practices of their religion. Adolescents are searching for ideals and may exhibit intense emotions along with introspection (Ford, 2007). Increased spirituality and religious activities are related to increased healthy behaviors and decreased high-risk behaviors (Ford, 2007).

Referring back to Cho Chung, identify the stage of psychosocial development that she should be in according to Erikson. What approaches for assessment and teaching would be most effective based on the stage you identified?

MOTOR SKILL DEVELOPMENT

During adolescence, the teenager refines and continues to develop his or her gross and fine motor skills. Because of this period of rapid growth spurts, teenagers may experience times of decreased coordination and have a diminished ability to perform previously learned skills, which can be worrisome for the teenager.

Gross Motor Skills

It is usually during early adolescence that teenagers begin to develop endurance. Their concentration has increased so they can follow complicated instructions. Coordination can be a problem because of the uneven growth spurts. During middle adolescence, speed and accuracy increase while coordination also improves. Teenagers become more competitive with each other (Fig. 29.2). During late adolescence, the teenager usually narrows his or her areas of interest and concentrates on the needed relevant skills.

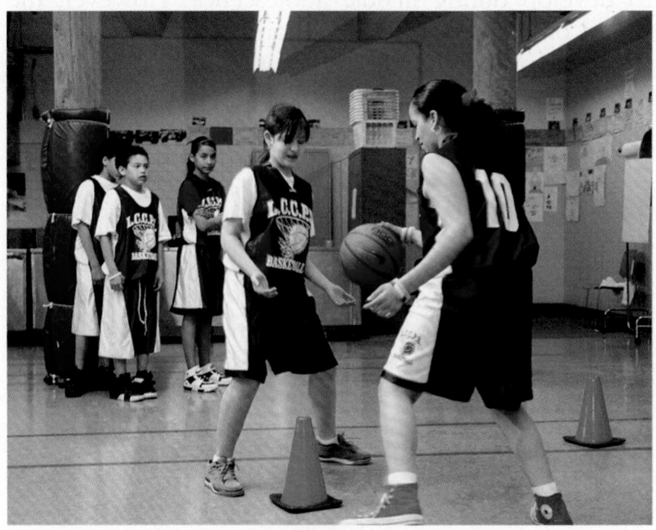

FIGURE 29.2 Adolescents become involved in competitive sports, which draw upon their gross motor skills.

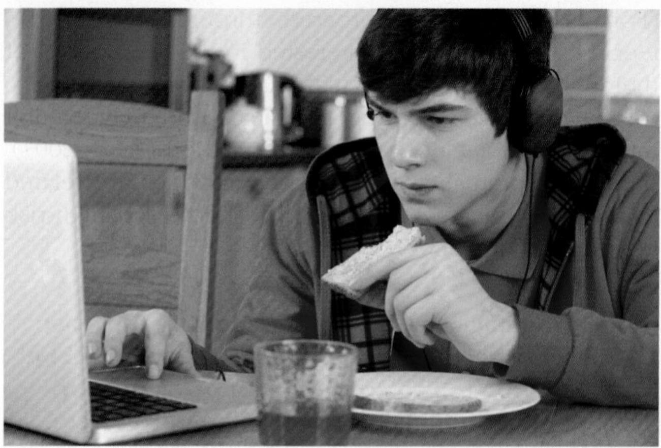

FIGURE 29.3 Using computers has increased the fine motor skills of adolescents.

Fine Motor Skills

The use of computers has greatly increased the fine motor skills of teenagers (Fig. 29.3). In the early adolescent years, the teenager increases his or her ability to manipulate objects. The adolescent's handwriting is neat and he or she increases his or her finger dexterity. The middle adolescent years see the teenager refining his or her dexterity skills. By late adolescence, the teenager has developed precise eye–hand coordination and finger dexterity.

COMMUNICATION AND LANGUAGE DEVELOPMENT

Language skills continue to develop and be refined during adolescence. Adolescents have improved communication skills, using correct grammar and parts of speech. Vocabulary and communication skills continue to develop during middle adolescence. However, the usage of colloquial speech (slang) increases, causing communication with people other than peers to be difficult at times. By late adolescence, language skills are comparable to those of adults.

EMOTIONAL AND SOCIAL DEVELOPMENT

Adolescents undergo a great deal of change in the areas of emotional and social development as they grow and mature into adults. Areas that are affected include the adolescent's relationship with parents; self-concept and body image; importance of peers; and sexuality and dating.

Relationship with Parents

Families and parents of adolescents experience changes and conflict that require adjustments and the understanding of adolescent development. The adolescent is striving for self-identity and increased independence. He or she spends more time with peers and less time with family and attending family functions. Parents sense that they have less influence on the adolescent as the teen questions family values and becomes more mobile. This may lead to a family crisis, and the parents may respond by setting stricter limits or asking questions about the teen's activities and friends. Other parents may drop all rules and assume that the adolescent can manage himself or herself. Both of these responses increase tension in the family.

With the adolescent attempting to establish some level of independence—and the family learning to let go while focusing on aging parents, their marriage, and other children—a state of disequilibrium occurs. The family may experience more stress than at any other time.

Some families have better outcomes with their adolescents than others. Families who listen to and continue to demonstrate affection for and acceptance of their adolescent have a more positive outcome. This does not mean that the family accepts all of the teen's ideas or actions, but they are willing to listen and attempt to negotiate some limits. For tips to improve communication with teenagers, see Box 29.1.

Siblings experience changes in the relationship with the adolescent brother or sister; the older sibling may attempt to parent and the younger sibling may regress in an attempt to avoid the family conflict. Understanding the status of the adolescent–family relationship is essential for the nurse.

Self-Concept and Body Image

Self-concept and self-esteem are often tied to body image. Adolescents who perceive their body as being different than peers or as less than ideal may view themselves

BOX 29.1

WAYS TO IMPROVE COMMUNICATION WITH TEENS

- Set aside appropriate amount of time to discuss subject matter without interruptions
- Talk face to face. Be aware of body language
- Ask questions to see why he or she feels that way
- Ask him or her to be patient as you tell your thoughts
- Choose words carefully so he or she understands you
- Tell him or her exactly what you mean
- Give praise and approval to your teenager often
- Speak to your teenage as an equal—don't talk down to him or her
- Be aware of your tone of voice and body language
- Don't pretend you know all the answers
- Admit that you do make mistakes
- Set rules and limits fairly

negatively. Adolescent girls often are influenced by peers and the media and want to weigh less and have smaller hips, waist, or thighs. Boys tend to view themselves as being too thin or not muscular enough.

Sexual characteristics are important to the adolescent's self-concept and body image. Boys are concerned about the size of their penis and facial hair while girls are concerned about breast size and the onset of menstruation. Larger breasts are considered more feminine and menstruation is considered the right of passage into adulthood. All of these body changes are important to the adolescent's self-concept.

Importance of Peers

Peer groups play an essential role in the identity of the adolescent (Cromer, 2011). Adolescent peer relationships are very important in providing opportunities to learn about negotiating differences; for recreation, companionship, and someone to share problems with; for learning peer loyalty; and for creating stability during transitions or times of stress. Learning to work out differences with peers is a skill that is important throughout life. Peers serve as someone safe to discuss family issues with, as the teen emotionally moves away from the family while trying to find his or her identity. Due to changes that have taken place within family systems in society, peer groups play a significant role in the socialization of adolescents (Fig. 29.4).

Peers serve as credible sources of information, role model social behaviors, and act as sources of social reinforcement. Friends provide an opportunity for fun and excitement. Peers impact teens' appearance, dress, social behavior, and language. Peers can also have positive influences on each other, such as promoting college attendance, or negative influences, such as involvement with alcohol, drugs, or gangs. Early and middle adolescence are periods when teens are prone to join gangs.

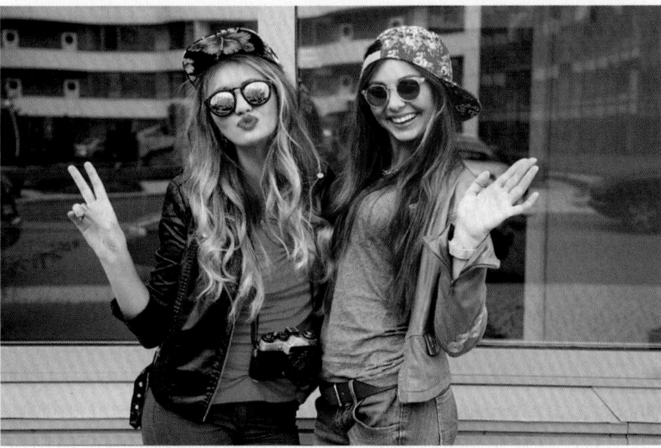

FIGURE 29.4 Peers play an important role in shaping the adolescent's identity.

Peer role modeling and peer acceptance may lead to the formation of a gang that provides a collective identity and gives a sense of belonging. Peer pressure, companionship, and protection are the most frequent reasons given for joining gangs, particularly those associated with criminal activity.

Parents must know their teen's friends and continue to be aware of potential problems while allowing the teen the independence to become his or her own person. Nurses must remind parents of the importance of peers and the impact they have on the teen's decisions and life choices. The transition to greater peer involvement requires guidance and support. Adolescents who do not have parental or adult supervision and opportunities for conversation with adults may be more susceptible to peer influences and at higher risk for poor peer selections.

Sexuality and Dating

Adolescence is a critical time in the development of sexuality. **Sexuality** includes the thoughts, feelings, and behaviors related to the adolescent's sexual identity. Adolescents usually begin experimentation with heterosexual and homosexual behaviors, although these behaviors may occur earlier in some cultures.

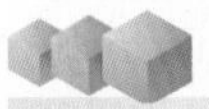

Concept Mastery Alert

Assessment

When providing care to an adolescent who shares information about sexual preferences, the nurse must remember that assessment is the first step in the nursing process.

An interest in romantic partnerships occurs during adolescence (Fig. 29.5). Some of the reasons cited for this developing interest are physical development and body changes, peer-group pressure, and curiosity. During the past couple of decades, the percentage of 8th through 12th graders that have dated has declined (Child Trends, 2013a). It has been found that 34% of 12th graders, 38% of 10th graders, and 53% of 8th graders have never dated (Child Trends, 2013a). The percentage of teens that date frequently increases with age with 7% of 8th graders, 11% of 10th graders, and 18% of 12th graders reporting going on a date one or more times a week (Child Trends, 2013a). Teen dating can range from group dating to single dating to serious relationships. Most early adolescents spend more time in activities with mixed-sex groups, such as dances and parties, than they do dating as a couple. Popular dating activities today include going out to dinner or the movies, "hanging out" at the mall, or visiting each other's home. During early adolescence, teens tend to date for fun and recreation. Also, they may see dating as a way to upgrade social standing by being seen with a popular or attractive boy or girl, for instance.

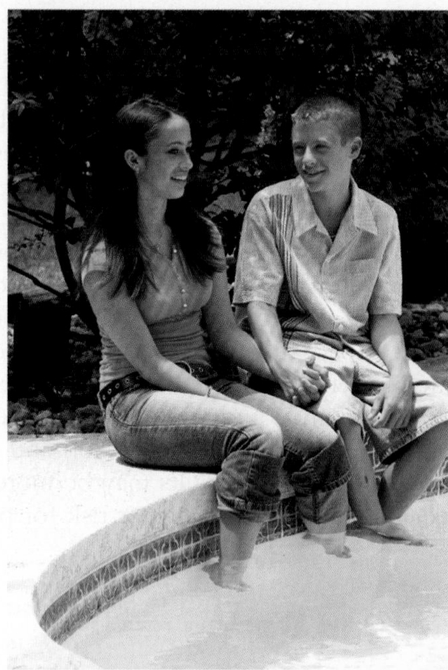

FIGURE 29.5 Dating becomes an important aspect of the teenager's life.

Middle and late adolescents have group and single dates. Romantic relationships are central to the social life of this age group. By 12th grade, 70% of adolescents report being in at least one romantic relationship (Letcher, 2013). Dating or spending time with a potential romantic partner is viewed as a major developmental marker for teens and is one of the most challenging adjustments. Both positive and negative developmental outcomes can result depending on the type of relationship that forms, such as the timing and duration, quality of partner interactions, emotional and cognitive maturity of teens involved, and whether sexual activity is occurring (Child Trends, 2013a). Some teens who date may report slightly higher levels of self-esteem and increased autonomy and perceive themselves as more popular (Child Trends, 2013a). However, other types of dating relationships may result in a teen having lower academic success and motivation, having higher depression rates, and experiencing a higher level of parental conflict.

Trends in dating are changing, but dating remains a developmental milestone for the adolescent. It is a time when they sort through their sexuality. Adolescents may experiment with homosexual behavior, though homosexual behavior as a teen does not necessarily indicate that the adolescent will maintain a homosexual orientation (Lyness, 2013). Gay and lesbian adolescents face many challenges due to society's nonacceptance and peer insensitivity. Teens who self-declare as homosexual during high school are at increased risk for such problems as depression, anxiety, suicide, victimization, school avoidance, and substance abuse (Remafedi, 2011). But many lesbian, gay, and bisexual adolescents will be fully accepted and report feeling happier and experiencing decreased stress once they have declared their sexuality (Lyness, 2013).

Healthy romantic relationships in adolescence can assist the teen in developing a strong sense of self-identity and developing interpersonal skills, such as empathy, and are related to healthy committed relationships in adulthood (Letcher, 2013). The emotional ups and downs that accompany dating can help develop emotional resilience and coping skills. Romantic relationships at this stage are a great source of emotional support. Risks of being involved in unhealthy romantic relationships include dating violence and risky sexual activity such as sexually transmitted infections (STIs) and premature pregnancy. Adolescents do not automatically know what makes for a healthy relationship. They need to be educated on the right and wrong behaviors of dating and what behaviors make up a healthy relationship, such as open communication, honesty, and trust. They need to know the signs of an unhealthy relationship and how to seek help if needed.

Cho Chung's mother states that she is concerned about the changes that have occurred in her and Cho's relationship over the past year. Cho seems much more self-centered, always wants to be with her friends, is very critical of her mother and father, and seems to be constantly in conflict with them. Based on what you know about this stage of development, what guidance, including approaches and techniques, can you discuss with Mrs. Chung to address her concerns?

CULTURAL INFLUENCES ON GROWTH AND DEVELOPMENT

Although the adolescent's culture continues to influence him or her, the desire to be in harmony with peers becomes paramount. That desire can cause conflict with the adolescent's family and culture. Today's adolescents live in a rapidly changing, increasingly culturally diverse world. They are exposed to many different cultures and ethnic groups. In 2012, over 45% of children and adolescents in the United States were minorities (Federal Interagency Forum on Child and Family Statistics, 2013).

Attitudes regarding adolescence vary among different cultures. Certain cultures may have more permissive attitudes toward issues facing adolescents, while others are more conservative (e.g., toward sexuality). Experiencing a rite-of-passage ceremony to signal the adolescent's movement to adult status varies among cultures. The American culture does not universally have a rite of passage for teenagers. Some religious and social groups do have ceremonies that signal a movement toward the maturity of adulthood (e.g., the Jewish bar or bat mitzvah, the Catholic confirmation, and social debuts). In many parts of the world, separate "youth cultures" have developed in an attempt to blend traditional and modern worlds for the adolescent.

It is important for the nurse to recognize the ethnic background of each adolescent. Research has shown that certain ethnic groups are at higher risk for certain diseases. For example, adolescent African Americans are at higher risk for developing hypertension (American Heart Association, 2013). But the major barrier to the adolescent's health and successful achievement of the tasks of adolescence is socioeconomic status. Adolescents at a lower socioeconomic level are at higher risk for developing health care problems and risk-taking behaviors; this may be due to their inability to access health care and to obtain needed services (Seith & Isakson, 2011). In caring for adolescents, recognize the influence of their culture, ethnicity, and socioeconomic level upon them.

The Nurse's Role in Adolescent Growth and Development

Growth and development in the adolescent is rapid. Nurses must be aware of the usual growth and development patterns for this age group so that they can assess the adolescent appropriately and provide guidance to the adolescent and his or her family. (See the Nursing Care Plan at the end of the chapter.)

During adolescence, the teenager faces many challenges. His or her fluctuating relationships with parents and other adult figures may limit the teen from seeking assistance in dealing with the common issues of adolescence. In dealing with adolescents, be aware that they behave unpredictably, are inconsistent with their need for independence, have sensitive feelings, may interpret situations differently from what they are, think friends are extremely important, and have a strong desire to belong. During health care visits the adolescent or parent may have concerns that they are hesitant or uncomfortable talking about in front of each other. Try to provide an opportunity for them to have private time with a health care provider to discuss issues. The adolescent may greatly appreciate the opportunity for time to discuss concerns with a nonjudgmental informed adult.

If the adolescent is hospitalized, growth and development may be altered. The adolescent is concerned about how the illness or injury will affect his or her body and body image. He or she fears pain and loss of privacy. The adolescent may experience anxiety about being separated from friends and loss of control.

When caring for the hospitalized adolescent, the nurse must use knowledge of normal growth and development to recognize potential delays, promote continued appropriate growth and development, and interact successfully with the teen. Provide opportunities for them to maintain independence, participate in decisions, and encourage socialization with friends through phone, e-mail, and visits when possible. The following Nursing Process Overview will address promoting healthy growth and development and dealing with common developmental concerns.

NURSING PROCESS OVERVIEW

Upon completion of assessment of the adolescent's current growth and development status, problems or issues related to growth and development may be identified. The nurse may then identify one or more nursing diagnoses, including:

- Risk for disproportionate growth
- Imbalanced nutrition: more than body requirements
- Delayed growth and development
- Risk for caregiver role strain
- Risk for injury
- Ineffective coping

Nursing care planning for the adolescent with growth and development issues should be individualized based on the adolescent's and family's needs. Nursing Care Plan 29.1 can be used as a guide in planning nursing care for the adolescent with a growth and development concern. The nurse may choose the appropriate nursing diagnoses from this plan and individualize them as needed. The nursing care plan is intended to serve as a guide, not to be an all-inclusive growth and development care plan.

PROMOTING HEALTHY GROWTH AND DEVELOPMENT

It takes multiple groups who address multiple issues to promote healthy growth and development in the adolescent. Some of these groups include sports teams in the school or the community, peers, teachers, band and choir members, and so forth. Also, the family's support and love will influence growth and development.

Promoting Growth and Development Through Sports and Physical Fitness

Many adolescents are involved in team sports that provide avenues for exercise. High levels of physical activity may reduce cardiovascular disease risk factors and provide disease prevention against cancer, obesity, osteoporosis, diabetes, and depression (Centers for Disease Control and Prevention [CDC], 2013a). Also, physical activity may contribute to higher academic performance and achievement (CDC, 2013a). Adolescents probably spend more time and energy participating in sports than any other age group. Participation in sports contributes to the adolescent's development, educational process, and better health. Sports and games provide an opportunity to interact with peers while enjoying socially accepted stimulation and conflict. Competition in sports activities helps the teenager in processing self-appraisal and in developing self-respect and concern for others.

Every sport has some potential for injury. Rapidly growing bones, muscles, joints, and tendons are more vulnerable to unusual strains and fractures. Incidence of concussions (which is considered a mild traumatic brain injury) is a growing concern in all teen athletes. (See Evidence-Based Practice 29.1.) To help prevent injury, parents and coaches need to be aware of early warning signs of fatigue, dehydration, and injury. See Chapter 44 for a discussion of sports injuries.

In relation to youth sports, the role of the nurse is to educate to prevent injuries (Fig. 29.6). This education should include discouraging participation when the teen is tired or has an existing injury, encourage the use of proper well-fitting protective gear, and ensure the adolescent learns how to play a sport before participating in it.

In addition, adolescence is a good time to develop an exercise program. The U.S. Department of Health and Human Services (HHS) recommends that adolescents participate in 60 minutes of moderate to vigorous physical activity each day. Nurses should encourage all adolescents to be physically active daily (CDC, 2013a).

Promoting Learning

School, teachers, family, and peers influence education and learning for the adolescent. Also, activities such as athletics and club membership enhance learning through interactions with peers, coaches, club leaders, and others.

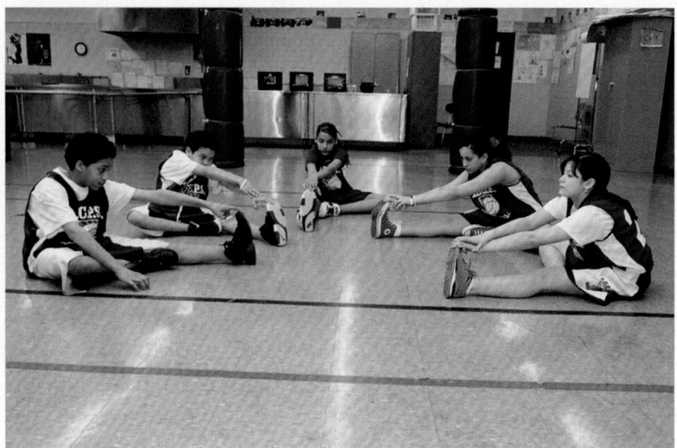

FIGURE 29.6 Stretching before exercise is an important part of exercise.

School

School plays an essential part in preparing adolescents for the future. Completing school prepares the adolescent for college or employment to make an adequate income. Schools in the United States may not meet the developmental needs of all adolescents. Minority students may not be at the appropriate grade level and the dropout rate may be higher than in nonminority students. Dropout rates have declined since the 1970s but still remain a concern. Dropout rates are highest among Hispanic students (Child Trends, 2013b). Those who drop out of school may lack skills needed to function in today's society. They are more likely to be unemployed and have lower income levels and occupational status than those with a high school diploma (Child Trends, 2013b) (see Healthy People 2020). Another

EVIDENCE-BASED PRACTICE 29.1 **DOES COGNITIVE ACTIVITY LEVEL EFFECT LENGTH OF POST CONCUSSION SYMPTOMS?**

STUDY

Concussions in children have been a growing concern for parents, educators, and health care providers. The long-term effects of concussion is not fully understood. Children who have suffered a concussion may have trouble learning new material, difficulty remembering what they learned, and more symptoms and longer recovery due to cognitive activity. Cognitive rest is often recommended in the initial phase of concussion recovery. This prospective cohort study set out to assess the effect of cognitive activity on the duration of concussion symptoms. It tracked 335 people aged 8 to 23 who had suffered a concussion. Participants reported their average level of cognitive activity on a scale. Levels were as follows: complete cognitive rest, minimal cognitive activity (no reading or homework, and less than 20 minutes per day of online activity and video games), moderate cognitive activity (reading less than 10 pages per day, and less than 1 hour total of homework, online activity, and video games), significant cognitive activity (reading less and doing less homework than usual), and full cognitive activity.

Findings

Participants who engaged in the highest quartile of activity took about 100 days to recover while those who participated in the lowest ¾ of cognitive activity took between 20–50 days to recover. Higher level of cognitive activity leads to longer recovery times.

Nursing Implications

Nurses should support academic accommodations that allow for cognitive rest to help speed recovery in a concussed child. Education of school staff may be needed as the child with a concussion typically appears physically well. Nurses should work with a multidisciplinary team which includes medical professionals, school and educational professionals, and the family to develop an individualized plan for the adolescent.

Adapted from Brown, N. J, Mannix, R. C., O'Brien, M. J., Gostine, D., Collins, M. W., & Meehan, W. P. 3rd. (2014). Effect of cognitive activity level on duration of post-concussion symptoms. *Pediatrics*, *133*, e299–e304. doi: 10.1542/peds.2013–2125.

HEALTHY PEOPLE 2020

Objective	Nursing Significance
Increase educational achievement of adolescents.	• Encourage school attendance and completion when encountering teens for well-child or sick visits • Refer children who have difficulty concentrating or learning for further evaluation • Praise school accomplishments

Healthy People Objectives retrieved from http://www.healthypeople.gov

influencing factor is a lack of parental involvement. Due to single-parent families and both parents being in the workforce, parents have less time to devote to involvement in their child's school activities.

There is evidence that the transition from elementary school to middle school at age 12 or 13, and then the transition to high school, both of which occur at the time of physical changes, may have a negative effect on teens. It is important to observe for transition problems into middle or high school, which may be exhibited by failing grades or behavior problems. Also, students who experience difficulties in school, resulting in negative evaluations and failing grades, may feel alienated from school. Students with poor grades and low academic achievement exhibit more emotional behavior such as violence and are more likely to engage in risky behaviors such as early sexual initiation (CDC, 2013b). Schools that support peer-group relationships, promote health and fitness, encourage parental involvement, and strengthen community relationships have better student outcomes. Parents, teachers, and health care providers should provide guidance and support.

Other Activities

Adolescents are involved in many other activities that influence learning. Some of these activities include: school activities such as band, choir, or clubs requiring high achievement; athletic activities in the school and community and sometimes in the state or region; art, sewing, and building classes; and work activities when the late adolescent has a part-time job. These activities all contribute to the growth, development, and education of the adolescent.

Promoting Safety

Unintentional injuries are the leading causes of death in adolescents (HHS, Health Resources and Services Administration, Maternal and Child Health Bureau, 2013). Motor vehicle accidents are the leading cause of injury death followed by poisoning, which includes prescription drug overdose (HHS, Health Resources and Services Administration, Maternal and Child Health Bureau, 2013). Males are more likely than females to die of any type of injury (HHS, Health Resources and Services Administration, Maternal and Child Health Bureau, 2013).

Take Note!

Poisoning is the only unintentional injury rate to increase and death from prescription drug misuse is a growing concern (HHS, Health Resources and Services Administration, Maternal and Child Health Bureau, 2013).

Influencing factors related to the prevalence of adolescent injuries include increased physical growth, insufficient psychomotor coordination for the task, abundance of energy, impulsivity, peer pressure, and inexperience. Impulsivity, inexperience, and peer pressure may place the teen in a vulnerable situation between knowing what is right and wanting to impress peers. On the other hand, teens have a feeling of invulnerability, which may contribute to negative outcomes. Alcohol and other drugs are contributing factors in automobile and firearm accidents among adolescents. Most of the serious or fatal injuries in adolescents are preventable (Fig. 29.7). Nurses must educate parents and adolescents on car, gun, and water safety to prevent unintentional injuries. See Teaching Guidelines 29.1 for information on promoting safety.

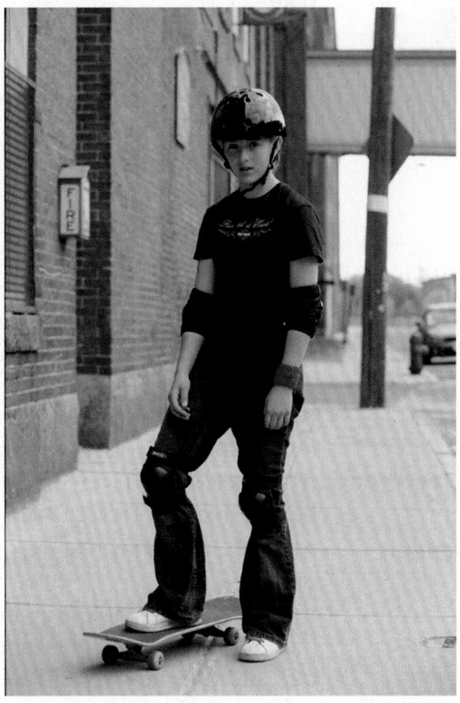

FIGURE 29.7 Wearing appropriate safety equipment can prevent injuries.

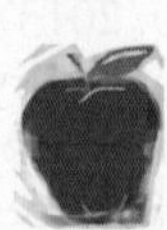

Teaching Guidelines 29.1

PROMOTING SAFETY

Safety Issue	Activity
Motor vehicle	• Wear seat belt at all times. • Do not drive or drive with someone who is impaired. • Take driver-education course. • Establish driving rules between parent and adolescent prior to getting license. • Have all passengers wear seat belts. • Do not use cell phone or text while driving, drink and drive, or drive when tired. • Maintain car in good condition. • Drive with adult supervision for a period of time after receiving license. • Encourage limit on teenage passengers.
Bike: General	• Have a well-maintained and appropriate-size bike for adolescent. • Adolescent should demonstrate his or her ability to ride bike safely before being allowed to ride on street. • Safe areas for bike riding should be established as well as routes to and from area of activities. • Should not ride bike barefoot, with someone else on bike, or with clothing that might get entangled in the bike. • Should wear sturdy, well-fitting shoes and CPSC (Consumer Product Safety Commission) or Snell-approved helmets • Proper fitting helmet should: sit level, not tilted, and firmly and comfortably on the head; have strong wide Y-shaped straps and when you open your mouth should pull down a bit; not move with sudden pulling or twisting; never be worn over anything else (hat, scarf, etc.) • Bike should be inspected often to ensure it is in proper working order. • A basket should be used to carry heavy objects.
Bike: In traffic	• All traffic signs and signals must be observed. • If adolescent is riding at night, the bike should have lights and reflectors and the rider should wear light-colored clothes. • Should ride on the side of the road traveling with traffic and keep close to the side of the road in single file. • Should watch and listen for cars and never hitch a ride on any vehicle. • Should not wear headphones while riding a bike.
All-terrain vehicles	• Should not be operated by an adolescent younger than 16 years of age. • Helmet and protective coverings required. • No nighttime riding. • Not for use on public roads or if teen has been drinking or using drugs. • Do not stand up in the vehicle or ride in a person's lap.
Skateboards/ skates	• Wear helmet, and protective padding on knees, elbows, and wrists. • Do not skate in traffic or on streets or highways. • Skating on homemade ramps could be dangerous—assess ramps for any hazards before skating.
Water safety	• Learn how to swim; if swimming skill is limited, must wear life preserver at all times. • Never swim alone—should, if at all possible, swim only where there is a life guard. • Learn basic cardiopulmonary resuscitation (CPR). • Do not run or fool around at edge of pool. • Drains in pool should be covered with appropriate cover. • Wear life jacket when on boat. • Make sure there is enough water to support diving. • Do not swim if drinking alcohol or using drugs.
Firearms	• If guns are in household, should take firearm safety class, secure guns in safe place, use gun safety locks, and store bullets in separate place. • Never point a gun at a person.
Fire safety	• All homes should have working smoke detectors and fire extinguishers. Change the batteries at least twice a year. • Have a fire-escape plan and practice the plan routinely. • No smoking in bed. • Teach what to do in case of a fire—use fire extinguisher, call 911, how to put out clothing fire.

	• All flammable materials and liquids should be stored safely. • Fireplaces should have protective gratings. • Avoid touching any downed power lines.
Machinery	• Use safety devices. • Receive training on how to use equipment. • Do not use when alone.
Sports	• Match sport to adolescent's ability and desire. • Sports program should have warm-up procedure and hydration policy. • Undergo sports physical before start of activity. • Coaches should be trained in CPR and first aid. • Wear appropriate protection devices for individual sport.
Sun	• Use sunscreen with both ultraviolet A (UVA) and ultraviolet B (UVB) protection. • Apply sunscreen prior to going out and reapply sunscreen often. • Limit sun exposure, especially between 10 AM and 2 PM. • Wear hat and sunglasses while outside.
Personal safety	• Never go with a stranger. • Do not enter a car when the driver has been drinking. • Notify an adult where you are when out after dark. • Keep cell phone fully charged. • Never give out personal information over the internet. • Say "no" to drugs, alcohol, or smoking, or to being touched when you do not want to be touched.
Toxins	• Teach the hazards of accepting illegal drugs, alcohol, dangerous drugs. • Store potential dangerous material in safe place.

Adapted from American Academy of Pediatrics. (2010a). The teen driver. *Pediatrics, 118*(6), 2570–2581. Retrieved from http://pediatrics.aappublications.org/content/118/6/2570.full; Dowshen, S. (2014a). *Bike safety*. Retrieved from http://kidshealth.org/teen/safety/safebasics/bike_safety.html#; Durani, Y. (2011). Water Safety. Retrieved from http://kidshealth.org/teen/safety/safebasics/water_safety.html#

American Academy of Pediatrics, Council on Environmental Health and Section on Dermatology. (2011). Policy statement—ultraviolet radiation: A hazard to children and adolescents. *Pediatrics, 127*(3), 588–597. doi: 10.1542/peds.2010–3501).

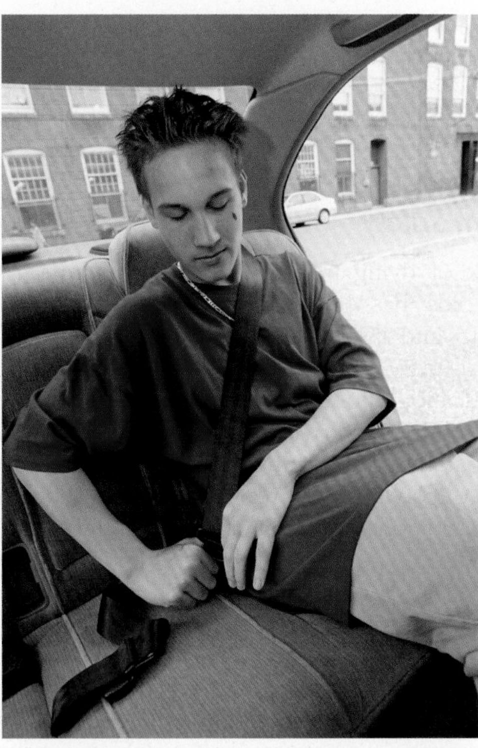

FIGURE 29.8 The use of seat belts has led to fewer fatal injuries in car accidents.

Motor Vehicle Safety

The largest numbers of adolescent injuries are due to motor vehicle crashes. When the adolescent passes his or her driving test, he or she is able to drive legally. However, driving is complex and requires judgments that the teen is often incapable of making. Also, the typical adolescent is opposed to authority and is interested in showing peers and others his or her independence. It is also normal for teens to take risks. These factors coupled with inexperience with driving may lead to underestimating hazardous and dangerous situations. Teenagers are the least likely age group to wear a seat belt, with males less likely than females (CDC, 2012a). Crashes involving adolescents are more likely to involve speeding, driving too fast for conditions, or following too close to the car in front of them (CDC, 2012a). More accidents occur when passengers, mostly other teenagers, are present in the car, during driving at night, or driving under the influence of alcohol or drugs (American Academy of Pediatrics, 2010a).

It is essential to promote driver education, to teach about the importance of wearing seat belts, and to explain laws about teen driving and curfews (Fig. 29.8). See Teaching Guidelines 29.1 for additional information.

Take Note!

Many states have enacted a Graduated Driving License (GDL) program, which allows teens to gain driving experience and limits risky circumstances (such as nighttime driving and driving with passengers) by providing a license in three stages (learners' permit, provisional license, and full license) (CDC, 2012a). Studies have shown this program to be highly effective in reducing teen driver crashes (CDC, 2012a).

Firearm Safety

The risk of dying from a firearm injury among 15- to 19-year-olds has been rising. Eighty-three percent of homicides and 45% of suicides in children and adolescents were caused by a firearm (CDC, 2012b; CDC, 2014a). Provide education about gun safety. Guns in the home must be kept and locked in a safe location, with ammunition kept separately. Parents must teach adolescents about the dangers of playing with firearms. See Teaching Guidelines 29.1 for additional information on gun safety.

Water Safety

Drowning is a needless cause of death in adolescents. Many drownings are a result of risk-taking behaviors. With the independence of the adolescent, many times, adult supervision is not prevalent and the teen takes a risk that results in drowning. Provide water safety education and proper supervision to decrease the incidence of risk taking. Teach about swimming lessons for nonswimmers. See Teaching Guidelines 29.1 for additional information.

Remember Cho Chung, the 15-year-old presented at the beginning of the chapter? What anticipatory guidance related to safety should you provide to Cho and her mother?

Promoting Nutrition

Nutritional needs are increased during adolescence due to accelerated growth and sexual maturation. Adolescents may appear to be hungry constantly and need regular meals and snacks with adequate nutrients to meet the body's needs. Multiple factors influence the adolescent's diet and eating habits (Box 29.2).

According to CDC data, over the past 30 years, the obesity rate in adolescents has more than quadrupled (CDC, 2014b). Poor diet and physical inactivity have led to the mounting problem of obesity in this age group. Obesity in adolescence is associated with obesity in adulthood along with numerous adverse health conditions such as diabetes, heart disease, certain types of cancer, osteoarthritis, and overall poorer health (CDC, 2014b).

BOX 29.2

FACTORS INFLUENCING THE ADOLESCENT'S DIET

- Peer pressure
- Busy schedules
- Concern about weight control
- Convenience of fast food

Nutritional Needs

Teenagers have a need for increased calories, zinc, calcium, and iron for growth. However, the number of calories needed for adolescence depends on the teen's age and activity level as well as growth patterns. Teenage girls who are moderately active require about 2,000 calories per day (U.S. Department of Agriculture [USDA] and HHS, 2010). Teenage boys who are moderately active require between 2,400 and 2,800 calories per day (USDA and HHS, 2010). Of these calories, 45% to 65% should come from carbohydrates, 10% to 30% from protein, and 25% to 35% from fat (USDA and HHS, 2010). Adolescents require about 1,300 mg of calcium each day (Gavin, 2011a). Adolescents should be made aware of foods high in calcium, including milk, white beans, broccoli, cheese, and yogurt. Adolescent males require 11 mg of iron each day and females require 15 mg each day (Gavin, 2012). Advise adolescents about foods high in iron (Box 29.3) (see Healthy People 2020). Protein requirements for adolescent girls, 14 to 18 years of age, are 46 g per day, and for adolescent boys, 14 to 18 years of age, 52 g per day (USDA and HHS, 2010). Some foods high in protein are meats, fish, poultry, beans, and dairy products.

Promoting Healthy Eating Habits

The nurse must understand normal growth and development of the adolescent in order to provide guidance that fits the quest for independence and the need for teens to make their own choices. Assess the eating habits and diet preferences of the adolescent. The assessment should include an evaluation of foods from the different food groups that the adolescent eats each day. Also,

BOX 29.3

FOODS HIGH IN IRON

- Beef, chicken, fish
- Liver
- Peanut butter
- Nuts and seeds
- Green peas, lima beans
- Eggs
- Dark leafy vegetables such as spinach
- Strawberries
- Tomato juice
- Whole-grain bread
- Raisins
- Watermelon

HEALTHY PEOPLE 2020

Objective	Nursing Significance
Reduce iron deficiency among young children and females of child-bearing age.	• Educate parents and teens about iron-containing foods • Encourage adolescent females to consume a diet high in iron-rich foods

Healthy People Objectives retrieved from http://www.healthypeople.gov

assess the number of times that fast foods, snacks, and other junk food are eaten per week. This assessment will help the nurse to guide the adolescent in making better food choices at home and in fast-food establishments. Many fast-food restaurants offer baked chicken sandwiches and salads with fewer calories and less fat. Adolescents may be guided in alternating hamburgers and fries with more nutritious choices. Remember that planning should always include the adolescent.

The USDA provides a personalized food plan called My Daily Food Plan based on an individual's age, sex, weight, height, and amount of physical activity. Refer to Figure 29.9 for an example. At http://www.choosemyplate.gov/myplate/index.aspx, the adolescent can create his or her customized food plan. Table 29.3 outlines daily serving recommendations based on caloric requirements (lower, moderate, or higher). Nurses may use the information in Table 29.3 to help teens plan a healthy diet for themselves. Active teenage girls should eat the number of servings recommended in the "Moderate" column of Table 29.3. Active teenage boys should eat the number of servings recommended in the "Higher" column. Adolescents who are overweight and dieting should base their daily intake on the serving recommendations in the "Lower" column.

My Daily Food Plan

Based on the information you provided, this is your daily recommended amount for each food group.

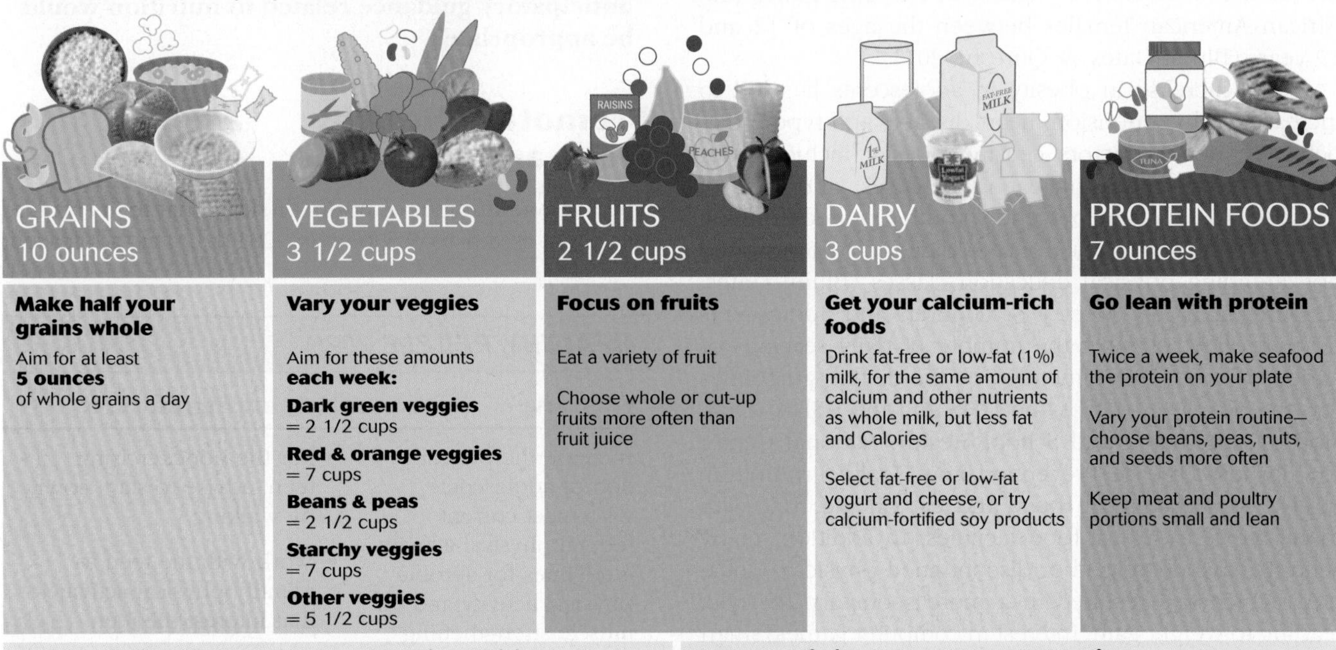

RAISINS
PEACHES
FAT-FREE MILK
1% MILK
TUNA
GRAINS
10 ounces
VEGETABLES
3 1/2 cups
FRUITS
2 1/2 cups
DAIRY
3 cups
PROTEIN FOODS
7 ounces
Make half your grains whole
Aim for at least 5 ounces of whole grains a day
Vary your veggies
Aim for these amounts each week:
Dark green veggies = 2 1/2 cups
Red & orange veggies = 7 cups
Beans & peas = 2 1/2 cups
Starchy veggies = 7 cups
Other veggies = 5 1/2 cups
Focus on fruits
Eat a variety of fruit
Choose whole or cut-up fruits more often than fruit juice
Get your calcium-rich foods
Drink fat-free or low-fat (1%) milk, for the same amount of calcium and other nutrients as whole milk, but less fat and Calories
Select fat-free or low-fat yogurt and cheese, or try calcium-fortified soy products
Go lean with protein
Twice a week, make seafood the protein on your plate
Vary your protein routine—choose beans, peas, nuts, and seeds more often
Keep meat and poultry portions small and lean

Find your balance between food and physical activity

Be physically active for at least **60 minutes** each day.

Know your limits on fats, sugars, and sodium

Your allowance for oils is **8 teaspoons** a day.

Limit Calories from solid fats and added sugars to **400 Calories** a day.

Reduce sodium intake to less than **2300 mg** a day.

Your results are based on a 2800 Calorie pattern. **Name:** ____________________

This Calorie level is only an estimate of your needs. Monitor your body weight to see if you need to adjust your Calorie intake.

FIGURE 29.9 My Daily Food Plan for a 15-year-old boy, 63.5 kg (140 lb), 162.56 cm (5 feet 4 inches), 30 to 60 minutes of exercise daily. Retrieved from http://www.choosemyplate.gov/foodgroups/downloads/results/MyDailyFoodPlan_2800_9to17yr.pdf)

TABLE 29.3 SAMPLE DIET FOR THREE CALORIC LEVELS

Calories for Three Caloric Levels	Lower (About 1,600 Calories)	Moderate (About 2,200 Calories)	Higher (About 2,600 Calories)
Grain group servings	6	6—8	10–11
Vegetable group servings	3–4	4—5	5–6
Fruit group servings	4	4—5	5–6
Milk group servings	2–3	2—3	3
Meat group (ounces)	3–4	6	6

Adapted from U.S. Department of Agriculture and U.S. Department of Health and Human Services (2010). *Dietary guidelines for Americans, 2010* (7th ed.). Washington, DC: U.S. Government Printing Office. Retrieved from http://www.cnpp.usda.gov/DGAs2010-PolicyDocument.htm

Preventing the Development of Overweight and Obesity

Over the past 30 years, the number of overweight adolescents has more than quadrupled from 5% to 21% (CDC, 2014b). Although obesity has increased in all segments of the United States population, there are differences specific to race, ethnicity, and socioeconomic status. The prevalence of obesity is highest in Hispanic males and African American females between the ages of 12 and 19 years (Blum, Gates, & Qureshi, 2011).

This increase in obesity in adolescents has led to increases in hypertension, heart disease, and type 2 diabetes. Influential factors causing obesity include poor food choices, unhealthy eating practices, and lack of exercise. Twenty-nine percent of youth reported drinking sugary beverages at least once a day and 67% reported not attending physical education classes (Blum, Gates, & Qureshi, 2011). Most U.S. children and adolescents do not follow or meet the number of daily servings or variety of foods recommended by the dietary guidelines for Americans set out by the HHS and the USDA (Division of Adolescent and School Health, National Center for Chronic Disease Prevention and Health Promotion, 2011). Adolescents are busy and eat on the run, with many meals from fast-food facilities. In addition, many schools have decreased or discontinued physical education, which has resulted in a more sedentary lifestyle, leading to weight gain. Interest in computer games, smart phones, and television watching at home has decreased physical activity and exercise and further contributed to weight gain and obesity (see Healthy People 2020).

Nurses must make parents and adolescents aware of factors leading to obesity. Nurses should recommend:

- Proper nutrition and healthy food choices
- Good eating habits, including eating a healthy breakfast daily
- Decreased fast-food intake
- Physical activity for at least 60 minutes daily
- Parents/adolescents exercising more at home
- Parents living a healthy lifestyle
- Decreasing nonactive computer and smartphone use and video, DVD, and television viewing

What questions should you ask Cho Chung and her mother related to nutritional intake? What anticipatory guidance related to nutrition would be appropriate?

Promoting Healthy Sleep and Rest

The average number of hours of sleep that teens require per night is 8.5 to 9.5 (Gavin, 2011b). The adolescent

***HEALTHY PEOPLE** 2020*

Objective	Nursing Significance
Increase the proportion of adolescents who meet current federal physical activity guidelines for aerobic physical activity and for muscle-strengthening activity.	• For the nonexercising teen, advise to start slowly by walking • Work with the teen to identify physical activities that interest the teen • Praise efforts to participate in a routine exercise plan • Identify an athletic individual that the teen identifies with and encourage similar activities in the teen

Healthy People Objectives retrieved from http://www.healthypeople.gov

often experiences a change in sleep patterns that leads to feeling more awake at night and the desire to sleep later in the morning (Gavin, 2011b). Also, in this independence-seeking phase of adolescence, the teen may stay up later to do homework or to complete projects and may have difficulty awakening in the morning. Due to early school schedules and activities the teen will often try to make up for needed sleep by sleeping longer hours on the weekend. Rapid growth and increased activities may produce fatigue and the need for more rest. Parents may relate that the teen sleeps all the time and never has the time or energy to help with household chores. Explain to parents the need to discourage late hours on school nights because they may affect school performance. Encourage the teen to go to bed at the same time at night and awaken at the same time in the morning, even on weekends (Gavin, 2011b). Provide advice to teens and parents about having realistic expectations; encourage them to agree on a level of normalcy and adequate rest for the teen so that he or she can still fulfil responsibilities in the home.

Provide anticipatory guidance to Cho Chung and her mother in relation to sleep during the adolescent years.

Promoting Healthy Teeth and Gums

Most permanent teeth have erupted with the possible exception of the third molars (wisdom teeth). These molars may become impacted and require surgical removal. The rate of cavities decreases but the need for routine dental visits every 6 months and brushing two to three times per day is very important. Some of the conditions that occur during adolescence include malocclusion, gingivitis, and tooth avulsion. Malocclusion (a poor bite) occurs from facial and mandibular bone growth that results in misalignment of the top teeth with the bottom teeth. It is the most common reason for referral to an orthodontist. The treatment includes braces and other dental devices. Teach the adolescent to brush the teeth more frequently if he or she has braces or other dental devices. Gingivitis is inflammation of the gums and breakdown of gingival epithelium due to diet and hormonal changes. The use of dental devices/braces makes cleaning more difficult and contributes to gingivitis. Tooth avulsion (knocked-out teeth) may occur during sports and other activities such as falls. The avulsed tooth should be reimplanted as soon as possible. The nurse may see the teen first so it is important that nurses know the proper procedure, which is to reinsert the tooth into its socket if possible or to store it in cool milk or normal saline for transport to the dentist.

Promoting Personal Care

Promotion of personal care during adolescence is an important topic to cover with the adolescent and his or her parents. Topics to discuss include general hygiene tips, caring for body piercings and tattoos, preventing sun-tanning, and promoting a healthy sexual identity.

General Hygiene Tips

Adolescents find that frequent baths and deodorant use are important due to apocrine sweat gland secretory activity. Also, to decrease oily skin due to sex steroids and hormones, teach the adolescent to wash his or her face two to three times per day with plain unscented soap. Vigorous scrubbing should be discouraged because it could irritate the skin and lead to follicular rupture. The hair should be shampooed daily or every other day to remove excess oil from the hair and scalp. Many over-the-counter medications are available for beginning acne or acne with a few lesions. These preparations may cause drying or redness. Discourage adolescents from squeezing acne lesions to prevent further irritation and permanent scarring. If the adolescent has severe acne, encourage him or her to ask a parent to make an appointment with a dermatologist.

Caring for Body Piercings and Tattoos

It is not uncommon for a teen to experiment with body piercing on areas such as the tongue, lip, eyebrow, navel, and nipple (Fig. 29.10). Other sites such as the genitals, chin cleft, knuckles, and even the uvula have been used. Generally, body piercing is harmless, but nurses should caution teens about performing these procedures under nonsterile conditions and should educate them about complications. Qualified personnel using sterile needles should perform the procedure. Teach the adolescent to cleanse the pierced area twice a day and more often at some sites.

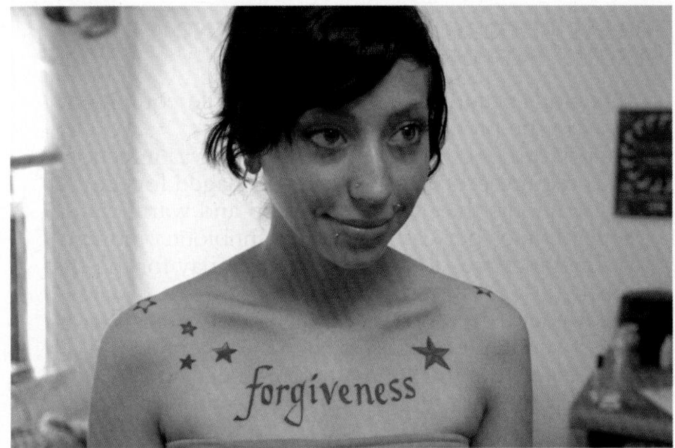

FIGURE 29.10 Having multiple piercings and tattoos can lead to certain health risks.

The complications of body piercing vary by site. Infections from body piercing usually result from unclean tools of the trade. Some of the infections that may occur as a result of unclean tools include hepatitis, tetanus, tuberculosis, and HIV. Also, keloid formation and allergies to metal may occur. The navel is an area prone to infection because it is a moist area that endures friction from clothing. After a navel infection occurs, it may take up to a year to heal. Pierced ear cartilage also heals slowly and is prone to infection. Tongue piercings heal very quickly, usually within 4 weeks, probably due to the antiseptic effects of saliva. Other concerns with tongue piercing include tooth damage from biting on the jewelry or partial paralysis if the jewelry pierces a nerve.

Tattoos are continuing to grow in popularity among adolescents (Gavin, 2013). Tattoos serve to define one's identity and are a form of self-expression (Fig. 29.10). Because of the invasiveness of the tattooing procedure, it should be considered a health-risk situation. Like piercings, tattoos are open wounds predisposing to infection.

Nurses should educate adolescents about the risk of tattooing including blood-borne infections, such as hepatitis B and C, HIV, skin infections, scarring, bleeding, and allergic reactions to dyes used in the tattoo process (American Academy of Pediatrics, 2013). They need to encourage the teen to go to a licensed facility with licensed tattoo artists and to double check that all equipment used is disposable and/or sterilized (American Academy of Pediatrics, 2013). Teach teens to cleanse tattoos with an antibacterial soap and water several times a day and to keep the area moist with an ointment to prevent scab formation. Refer to Box 29.4 for additional information about tattoos.

Preventing Sun-Tanning

Sun-tanning is popular among adolescents and is influenced by the media, which promotes a link between tan skin and beauty. There is no such thing as a good tan (American Skin Association, 2012). Most exposure to ultraviolet rays occurs during childhood and adolescence, thereby putting people at risk for the development of skin cancer. However, it is difficult to convince adolescents that tanning is harmful to their skin and puts them at risk for skin cancer later in life (see Healthy People 2020).

Educate teens about the benefits and effects of different sun protection products. Explain to them that sun damage and skin cancers can be prevented if sunscreens are used as directed on a regular basis. Encourage sunscreen or sunblock use for water sports, beach activities, and participation in outdoor sports. Also, make adolescents aware of allergies to some sunscreen products. See Teaching Guidelines 29.1 for additional information.

BOX 29.4

WHAT ADOLESCENTS NEED TO KNOW ABOUT TATTOOING

- Infections occur as a result of nonsterile equipment used in the procedure
- Tattoos are open wounds predisposing to infection; sites require proper care, keep bandaged for the first 24 hours then wash with soap and warm water several times per day and apply antibiotic ointment or fragrance-free lotion three times a day for the first week
- Do not let the tattoo dry out. Do not expose it to direct sunlight until fully healed and then keep it protected from the sun with sunscreen
- Avoid pools, hot tubs, or long baths/showers until healed
- For most people a tattoo is permanent; new procedures for removal are painful and expensive

HEALTHY PEOPLE 2020

Objective	Nursing Significance
Increase the proportion of persons who participate in behaviors that reduce their exposure to harmful ultraviolet (UV) irradiation and avoid sunburn Reduce the proportion of adolescents in grades 9 through 12 who report using artificial sources of UV light for tanning Increase the proportion of adolescents in grades 9 through 12 who follow protective measures that may reduce the risk of skin cancer	• Encourage female teens to use sunscreen-containing makeup • Discourage teen use of tanning beds • Remind students to use sunscreen during outdoor organized-sports practice • Educate teens and families about the risks associated with sun exposure • Educate teens and their families to avoid the sun between 10 AM and 4 PM, wear sun-protective clothing when exposed to sunlight, use sunscreen with a sun protection factor (SPF) of 15 or higher, and avoid artificial sources of UV light

Healthy People Objectives retrieved from http://www.healthypeople.gov

Promoting a Healthy Sexual Identity

Encourage parents and teens to have discussions about sexuality. In addition, nurses should ensure that adolescents have the knowledge, skills, and opportunities that enable them to make responsible decisions regarding sexual behaviors and sexual orientation. Education for the adolescent should include a discussion about media influences and the use of sexuality to promote products. This discussion should make the adolescent aware of the motives of the media and the need to be an individual and not be influenced by television, magazines, and other forms of advertisement. Encourage parents to be aware of who their adolescents are dating and where they go on their dates. Refer to Teaching Guidelines 29.2 for information on counseling related to adolescent sexuality.

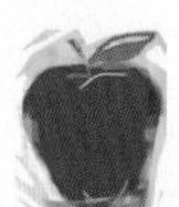

Teaching Guidelines 29.2
ADOLESCENT SEXUALITY

- It should be your choice to engage in sexual relations. Do not be influenced by peers. When you say "no," be firm and clear about your position.
- Pregnancy, sexually transmitted infections, and HIV infection can occur with any sexual encounter without the use of barrier methods of contraception. Use appropriate contraception if sexually active. Discuss abstinence as a contraceptive method.
- Sexual activity in a mature relationship should be pleasurable to both parties. If your sexual partner is not interested in your pleasure, you need to reconsider the relationship.

Promoting Appropriate Discipline

Adolescents naturally misbehave or do not follow the rules of the house, and parents must determine how to respond. Adolescents need to know the rules and expectations. After rules are established, parents must explain to the adolescent the consequences of breaking the rules.

Offer guidance to parents related to disciplining teens. The parent and the teen should collaborate on what the consequences will be if the rules are broken. Parents must acknowledge and offer reinforcement and support when the teen follows the rules. Consistency and predictability are the cornerstones of discipline, and praise is the most powerful reinforcer of learning.

Promoting Proper Media Use

Television, the internet, and other forms of media, such as cell phones, iPads, and social media sites, are a large force in teens lives today. Teenagers spend more than 11 hours a day with a variety of different media (American Academy of Pediatrics, Council on Communications and Media, 2013). Seventy-five percent of teenagers own a cell phone, with almost all teens (88%) sending text messages (O'Keeffe, Clarke-Pearson, & Council on Communications and Media, 2011). With greater technology and media access comes benefits such as enhancing communication skills, increasing social connections, and improving technical skills, but risks also exists, such as cyberbullying, sexting, exposure to inappropriate content, privacy issues, internet addiction, and sleep deprivation. Health care providers need to assess media use and advise parents on ways to decrease media risks. Parents should be advised to evaluate websites their adolescent wants to participate in and verify they are age-appropriate. Parents should talk to their adolescent children daily about online use and activity. They need to discuss the dangers of sharing too much information, posting images or photographs, and the fact that once something is online it is available for others to see and share. Parents need to be educated on the technology their children are using and encourage the development of a family media use plan that involves establishing reasonable rules about use of cell phones, texting, the internet and social media use, such as no media during meals and regular checking of privacy settings and online profiles for inappropriate content (American Academy of Pediatrics, Council on Communications and Media, 2013).

Take Note!

Three key elements have been proposed by researchers to foster healthy internet habits in teens. These are the right balance between online and offline activities, proper set of online boundaries, and regular communication with a trusted adult about their online experiences (Moreno, 2013).

ADDRESSING COMMON DEVELOPMENTAL CONCERNS

Adolescence is a time of rapid growth and development with maturation of sexuality. The adolescent period begins with a child and ends with the expectation of adulthood. There are many developmental concerns that are present during this period, including violence, suicide, homicide, and substance use. The following is an overview of some of these concerns.

Violence

The CDC's Injury Center defines violence as "the intentional use of physical force or power, threatened or actual, against another person or against a group or community that results in or has a high likelihood of resulting in injury, death, psychological harm, maldevelopment, or deprivation" (Dahlberg & Krug, 2002; CDC, 2013c). More than 707,212 adolescents and young adults between 10 and 24 years of age were injured and treated in an emergency department as a result of violence in 2011 (CDC, 2012b). The issue of youth violence is a growing concern in America's communities. The health and well-being of adolescents and society are threatened by this violence. See Box 29.5 for factors contributing to

BOX 29.5

FACTORS CONTRIBUTING TO ADOLESCENT VIOLENCE

- Crowded conditions/housing
- Low socioeconomic status
- Limited parental supervision/involvement
- Single-parent families/both parents in workforce
- History of violent victimization
- Poor family functioning
- Access to guns or cars
- Drug or alcohol use
- Low self-esteem
- Racism
- Peer or gang pressure
- Aggression

adolescent violence. Health care providers need to provide education on the effects and ways to prevent youth violence along with supporting programs developed to curb youth violence.

Homicide

Homicide is the second leading cause of death in children between 15 and 24 years old, with the majority of victims being male and killed by firearms (CDC, 2012b). It is the leading cause of death in African Americans 10 to 24 years old (CDC, 2012b). Refer to Box 29.5 for factors that contribute to violence among adolescents. In a nationwide survey conducted in 2011, 16.6% of youth reported carrying a weapon (gun, club, or knife) on one or more days within the past 30 days (CDC, 2012b) (see Healthy People 2020).

HEALTHY PEOPLE 2020

Objective	Nursing Significance
Reduce homicides, physical fighting, and bullying among adolescents and weapon carrying by adolescents on school property Reduce suicide attempts by adolescents	• Screen teens at all encounters for indications of violent behaviors • Provide education related to decreasing school violence at middle and high schools • Encourage alternative, appropriate methods for dispelling anger • Screen teens at all encounters for indications of depression

Healthy People Objectives retrieved from http://www.healthypeople.gov

BOX 29.6

RISK FACTORS FOR SUICIDE IN ADOLESCENTS

- Depression or other mental illness
- Mental health changes
- History of previous suicide attempt
- Poor school performance
- Family disorganization
- Substance abuse
- Homosexuality
- Giving away valued possessions
- Being a loner/having no close friends
- Changes in behavior
- Incarceration

Suicide

Suicide is the third leading cause of death in youths 10 to 24 years old (CDC, 2014a). In a nationwide CDC study, 16% of adolescents surveyed reported that they had seriously considered suicide within the past 12 months, with 13% creating a plan and 8% attempting to take their own life (CDC, 2014a). Certain factors can put youth at risk for suicide, but having these risk factors does not mean suicide will occur. Refer to Box 29.6 for risk factors for suicide in adolescents (see Healthy People 2020). Most people are not comfortable discussing the topic of suicide and therefore do not communicate openly about it. It is important that health care providers address this important health problem and work to prevent suicide. The National Center for Injury Prevention and Control (NCIPC) is working to create awareness of suicide as a serious public health problem and is developing strategies to reduce injuries and deaths due to suicide.

Dating Violence

Violent behavior that takes place in a context of dating or courtship is not a rare event and can have serious short-term and life-long effects. In a recent survey, approximately 9% of high school students reported dating violence such as being hit, slapped, or physically hurt on purpose by their partner, in the past 12 months (CDC, 2014c). Dating violence in the teen years is a risk factor for continued violence exposure in adulthood. Risk factors for dating violence include inadequate parental supervision, condoning violence, substance use, prior victimization, having violent peers or friends involved in dating violence, depression or anxiety, learning difficulties or problems at school, history of aggression or bullying, and risky sexual practices (CDC, 2014c). Nurses need to assess for and provide interventions to those teens experiencing dating violence or those at risk for being a victim or perpetrator. Education on development of healthy relationships is important.

BOX 29.7

RISK FACTORS FOR GANG INVOLVEMENT

- Delinquency involvement, especially at a young age
- History of or victim of physical violence or aggression
- Precocious sexual activity
- Alcohol and drug use; drug dealing
- Associated with delinquent or aggressive peers
- Poverty/low socioeconomic status
- Family with criminal history, drug or alcohol problems
- Poor parental supervision/involvement
- Poor academic performance
- Living in a community with a large number of troubled youth, access to firearms and drugs

Gangs

Much of youth violence is a result of the behavior of adolescent gangs. Nationwide, there are an estimated 29,900 gangs with 782,500 members (Egley & Howell, 2013). The risk factors for gang involvement are similar to those for aggressive or delinquent behavior. See Box 29.7 for risk factors for adolescent gang involvement. Gang membership occurs in cities and in suburban areas, but may differ in composition. All socioeconomic groups are represented in gang membership. Gang membership may aid in the formation of identity by providing status and a sense of belonging. However, adolescents who are gang members are more likely to commit serious and violent crimes. Identifying those at risk and providing early intervention is important. Research has shown that increasing parental monitoring and improving coping skills to deal with conflict may be beneficial is preventing gang membership (McDaniel, 2012).

Nursing Interventions to Decrease Youth Violence

Nurses working with adolescents should include violence prevention in anticipatory guidance. Violence is a learned behavior. It is often reinforced by the media, television, music, and personal example. Explain to parents, teachers, and peers the importance of being good role models. Parents should monitor video games, music, television, and other media to decrease exposure to violence. Parents need to know who their adolescent's friends are and monitor for negative behaviors and actions. Pediatric nurses play a key role in identifying at-risk youth and developing, planning, implementing, and evaluating interventions to prevent youth violence.

Substance Use

Agents commonly abused by children and adolescents include alcohol, prescribed medications such as Ritalin and OxyContin, hallucinogens, sedatives, analgesics, anxiolytics, steroids, inhalants (inhaling fumes of common household products), stimulants, opiates, and various club drugs such as ecstasy, gamma-hydroxybutyrate (GHB), and lysergic acid diethylamide (LSD). The substance abused is related to its availability and cost. Two common substances that are more accessible and have the highest incidence of use are tobacco and alcohol. A national survey found that 60% or more of teens report drugs are kept, used, or sold at their school (National Center on Addiction and Substance Abuse at Columbia University, 2012). Drug use progresses from beer or wine to cigarettes or hard liquor and then to marijuana, followed by illicit drugs.

Take Note!

One in five 12th graders reports having used a prescription drug without medical supervision. One in nine 8th to 12th graders has inhaled household substances to obtain a high (Murphey, Barry, Vaughn, Guzman, & Terzian, 2013).

Some of the long-term effects and consequences of drug and alcohol use include possibility of overdose and death, unintentional injuries, irrational behaviors, inability to think clearly, unsafe driving and legal consequences, problems with relationships with family and friends, sexual activity and STIs, and health problems such as liver problems (hepatitis) and cardiac problems (sudden death with cocaine). Refer to Table 29.4 for commonly abused drugs and behaviors exhibited (see Healthy People 2020).

(text continues on page 1100)

HEALTHY PEOPLE 2020

Objective	Nursing Significance
Reduce the proportion of adolescents who report that they rode, during the previous 30 days, with a driver who had been drinking alcohol	• Provide education in the office, hospital, or school related to adverse effects of tobacco, alcohol, and illicit substance use
Reduce steroid use among adolescents	• Educate families, teens, and coaches about the negative effects of anabolic steroids
Increase the proportion of adolescents never using substances	
Reduce the past-year nonmedical use of prescription drugs	• Praise teens for abstaining from the above substances and rising above peer pressure
Reduce the proportion of adolescents who use inhalants	

Healthy People Objectives retrieved from http://www.healthypeople.gov

TABLE 29.4 DRUGS COMMONLY ABUSED

Drug	Manifestations	Considerations
Marijuana Street names: "pot," "grass," "herb," "weed," "Mary Jane," "reefer," "skunk," "boom," "gangster," "kif," "chronic," and "ganja."	Red eyes, dry mouth, euphoria, relaxation, decreased motivation, loss of inhibition, appetite stimulation	Considered a gateway drug
Synthetic marijuana Street names: Spice, K-2 most common also called "fake weed," "Bliss," "Black Mamba," "Bombay Blue," "Genie," "Zohai," "Yucatan Fire," "Skunk," and "Moon Rocks")	Laboratory-synthesized liquid chemicals mimic the effect of tetrahydrocannabinol (THC), the psychoactive ingredient in the naturally grown marijuana plant; relaxed feeling, mild changes in perception, extreme paranoia, anxiety, hallucinations	Unpredictable effect; not clear what chemicals are used and how they can harm the body; symptoms reported include increased heart rate, vomiting, agitation, confusion, hallucinations; has been associated with heart attacks
Cocaine and crack Street names: "coke," "Coca," "C," "snow," "flake," "blow," "bump," "candy," "Charlie," "rock," and "toot." (A "speedball" is cocaine or crack combined with heroin, or crack and heroin smoked together.)	Powerful stimulant; Weight loss, euphoria, elation, agitation, increased motor activity, pressured speech, dilated pupils, tachycardia, hypertension, anorexia, insomnia	Psychotic behavior with large doses; if combined with other drugs can be fatal
Heroin Street names: "Smack," "Junk," "H," "Black tar," "Ska," and "Horse."	Elation, euphoria, detachment, drowsiness, constricted pupils, slurred speech, impaired judgment	Self-neglect with malnutrition and dehydration; criminal behaviors to get drugs; infections at injection sites; at risk for acquiring HIV/AIDS and hepatitis; highly addictive; can lead to coma or death
Prescription opiate drugs such as Oxycodone (OxyContin, Percodan, Percocet); Hydrocodone (Vicodin, Lortab, Lorcet); Diphenoxylate (Lomotil); Morphine (Kadian, Avinza, MS Contin); Codeine; Fentanyl (Duragesic); Propoxyphene (Darvon); Hydromorphone (Dilaudid); Meperidine (Demerol); Methadone. Street names: Hillbilly heroin, oxy, OC, oxycotton, percs, happy pills, vikes	Feelings of relaxation and euphoria	Can lead to addiction and drug-seeking behaviors; high doses can lead to breathing complications and death
Methamphetamine Street names: "speed," "meth," "chalk," and "tina." In its smokeable form, it's often called "ice," "crystal," "crank," "glass," "fire," and "go fast."	Euphoria, increased energy and alertness, agitation, weight loss, insomnia, tachycardia, hypertension	Increased risk of HIV/AIDS or hepatitis; risk for arrhythmias and hyperthermia. Repeated use can cause violent behavior and psychosis, possible paradoxical effect of depression in children

TABLE 29.4 DRUGS COMMONLY ABUSED (continued)

Drug	Manifestations	Considerations
MDMA (3,4-methylenedioxymethamphetamine) (Ecstasy and Molly) and other club drugs (LSD, ketamine, PCP) Street names: "E," "XTC," "X," "Adam," "hug," "beans," "clarity," "lover's speed," and "love drug"	Hallucinations, illusions, euphoria, hyperalertness, depersonalization, heightened sensual awareness, dilated pupils, hypertension, increased salivation, distorted perceptions. agitation, violence, antisocial behaviors, loss of sense of time, forceful clenching of the teeth	Panic flashbacks long after use of drugs; psychotic behaviors; can lead to hyperthermia as it interferes with the body's ability to regulate temperature; memory loss with long-term use; high blood levels lead to increased risk of seizures and arrhythmias
Inhalants Street names: "laughing gas" (nitrous oxide), "snappers" (amyl nitrite), "poppers" (amyl nitrite and butyl nitrite), "whippets" (fluorinated hydrocarbons, found in whipped cream dispensers), "bold" (nitrites), and "rush" (nitrites).	Similar effects as alcohol but high only lasts a few minutes, slurred speech, lack of coordination, euphoria, dizziness	Long-term use can breakdown myelin and damage brain cells
Bath salts Street names: "Bloom," "Cloud Nine," "Vanilla Sky," "White Lightning," and "Scarface."	Similar effect as stimulants such as methamphetamines and MDMA; hallucinatory effects	Still a lot unknown about how these substances affect the brain; linked to a high number of emergency room and Poison Control Center visits
Prescription stimulants such as Dextroamphetamine (Dexedrine and Adderall) and Methylphenidate (Ritalin and Concerta Street names: "Skippy," "the smart drug," "vitamin R," "bennies," "black beauties," "roses," "hearts," "speed," "uppers"	Increased alertness, attention, and energy; increased heart rate and blood pressure	High doses increased risk for arrhythmia, hyperthermia, heart failure, and seizures If mixed with antidepressants or over-the-counter cold medicines can lead to dangerously high blood pressure and arrhythmias
Prescription CNS depressants • Mephobarbital (Mebaral); sodium pentobarbital (Nembutal). Street names: Barbs, reds, red birds, phennies, tooies, yellows, or yellow jackets • Diazepam (Valium); Alprazolam (Xanax); Estazolam (ProSom) Street Names Candy, downers, sleeping pills, or tranks • Zolpidem (Ambien); Zaleplon (Sonata); Eszopiclone (Lunesta). Street names: A-minus or zombie pills	Euphoria followed by depression or hostility; impaired judgment; decreased inhibitions; slurred speech; incoordination	Often used with stimulants; may have a paradoxical effect of hyperactivity in children
Dextromethorphan	Taken in very large amounts; effects similar to PCP and ketamine; feelings of being detached from oneself and the environment	Found in over-the-counter cold medicines; can lead to impaired motor function, numbness, nausea, vomiting, increased heart rate and blood pressure; risk for hypoxic brain damage

Adapted from Stager, M. M. (2011). Chapter 108: Substance abuse. In R. M. Kleigman, B. F. Stanton, J. W. St. Geme III, N. F. Schor, & R. E. Behrman (Eds.), *Nelson textbook of pediatrics* (19th ed., pp.671–685). Philadelphia: Saunders; Johnston, L. D., O'Malley, P. M., Miech, R.A., Bachman, J. G., & Schulenberg, J. E. (2014). *Monitoring the future national results on drug use: 1975–2013: Overview, key findings on adolescent drug use*. Ann Arbor, MI: Institute for Social Research, The University of Michigan. Retrieved from http://www.monitoringthefuture.org//pubs/monographs/mtf-overview2013.pdf; NIDA for Teens. (2014). *Drug facts*. Retrieved from http://teens.drugabuse.gov/drug-facts

Take Note!

African Americans have lower rates of most licit and illicit drugs, alcohol and cigarette use than Caucasians (Johnston, O'Malley, Miech, Bachman, & Schulenberg, 2014).

Tobacco

Tobacco use remains the leading preventable cause of death in the United States, causing an estimated 443,000 deaths each year (CDC, 2012d). Long-term consequences of youth smoking are reinforced by the fact that most young people who smoke regularly continue to smoke throughout adulthood. Each day in the United States, approximately 4,000 children younger than 18 years old try their first cigarette, with 1,000 becoming regular smokers; 9 out of 10 adult smokers started smoking before age 18 (American Cancer Society, 2013). One-third of these smokers will die from the effects of smoking (American Cancer Society, 2013). Although the overall rate of smoking has declined since 1999, 18% of high school girls and 23% of high school boys report using some form of tobacco product in the past month (American Cancer Society, 2013). There are many forms of tobacco use, such as flavored cigars, smokeless tobacco, hookahs, pipes, and even electronic cigarettes (American Cancer Society, 2013). Teens who smoke are more likely than nonsmokers to use alcohol and illegal drugs (American Cancer Society, 2013). Smoking is associated with other risky behaviors, including fighting, carrying weapons, mental health problems such as depression, attempting suicide, and engaging in unprotected sex (American Cancer Society, 2013). The short-term health effects of smoking include damage to the respiratory system, addiction to nicotine, and the associated risk of other drug use. Smoking negatively impacts physical fitness and lung growth and increases the potential for addiction in adolescents. Smokeless tobacco may also cause many problems. It can lead to bleeding gums and sores in the mouth that never heal. Smokeless tobacco use leads to discoloration of the teeth and eventually may lead to cancer.

Take Note!

The percentage of adolescents who used electronic cigarettes (also known as vape) doubled from 2011 to 2012 (CDC, 2013d). Teens need to be aware that e-cigarettes are not a safe alternative to smoking. Nicotine, which is highly addictive, and other harmful chemicals are absorbed through the lungs and into the body with the use of e-cigarettes.

Alcohol

A national survey on drug use found that 68% of students have consumed alcohol by the end of high school, with 28% consuming alcohol by the end of 8th grade (Johnston et al., 2014). About half of 12th graders and 12% of 8th graders reported having been drunk at least once (Johnston et al., 2014). The findings revealed that there were no substantial differences among various sociodemographic subgroups with respect to drinking rates, although alcohol use is lowest in African Americans and highest in Caucasians. The incidence of alcohol use increases throughout adolescence. Adolescents who begin drinking before the age of 15 are five times more likely to develop alcohol dependence than those who begin drinking at the age of 21 (CDC, 2013e). Alcohol use in adolescence can lead to prevailing alcohol use in adulthood and contribute to physical health problems. It may also precede other drug abuse.

Illicit Drugs

Adolescents may also experiment with or abuse illicit drugs. Substance abuse remains a widespread problem among American adolescents. Marijuana remains the most widely used illicit drug (Johnston et al., 2014). A national survey on drug use showed the annual prevalence rate for 8th to 12th graders for marijuana use to be 25.8%, amphetamines 5.7%, ecstasy 2.8%, Salvia 2.3%, cocaine 1.8%, LSD 1.6%, inhalants 3.8%, over-the-counter medications (such as cold medicines) 4%, Vicodin 3.7%, OxyContin 2.9%, heroin 0.6%, and steroids 0.9% (Johnston et al., 2014). Half of adolescents reported using an illicit drug by 12th grade (Murphey et al., 2013).

Factors that primarily affect drug use include the psychoactive potential and benefits reported, how risky the drug is to use, how acceptable it is to peer groups, and the accessibility and availability of the drug. The more risky or less accepted a drug is by peers, the less likely the adolescent will use it.

Nursing Interventions to Decrease Substance Use Among Teens

Adolescents' brains are still developing, leaving them particularly vulnerable to the damaging effects of drugs. Substance use in adolescence is related to poorer health outcomes; therefore, it is important that nurses be aware of interventions to decrease these behaviors. Times of life transitions, such as changing schools, moving, or divorce, increase the risk of drug use (Stager, 2011). Therefore, nurses need to target assessments and programs at these critical times. Based on reviews of programs and interventions, it has been found that certain methods work. Programs that reach children and adolescents through a variety of sources such as school, family, community, and media campaigns are more successful. Programs that are culturally competent and address all forms of drug use (alcohol, tobacco, and illicit drugs) tend to work well. Programs that focus on increasing awareness of the risks and health consequences of substance use are important. Certain factors have been found to help teens remain drug free. These include strong connections to parents, family, school, and religion; presence of parents in the home at key times of the day; and limited access to substances such as alcohol, tobacco, and marijuana (Murphey et al, 2013). Programs that focus on decreasing risk factors and increasing protective factors such as enhancing self-esteem, social and parental support, and stress-specific coping skills are beneficial (Stager, 2011). Topics that should be discussed include:

- Short- and long-term effects of alcohol, tobacco, and drugs on health
- Risk factors and implications for unintentional injuries and sexual activity
- Short- and long-term effects of alcohol, tobacco, and drugs on relationships and school performance and progression
- The how and why of chemical dependency
- Impact of substance abuse on society
- Importance of maintaining a healthy lifestyle
- Importance of resisting peer pressure to use drugs and alcohol
- Importance of having confidence in one's own judgment

Think back to Cho, who was introduced at the beginning of the chapter. List common developmental concerns of the adolescent. What anticipatory guidance related to these concerns would you provide?

NURSING CARE PLAN 29.1

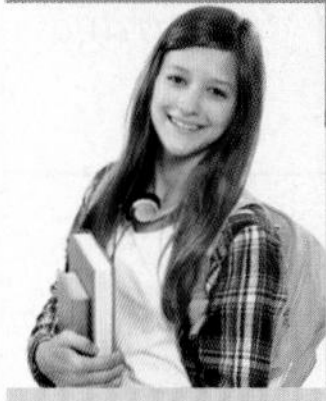

Growth and Development of the Adolescent

NURSING DIAGNOSIS: Risk for disproportionate growth (risk factors: caregiver and adolescent knowledge deficit, low self-esteem, frequent illnesses)

Outcome Identification and Evaluation

Adolescent will demonstrate adequate growth: *appropriate weight gain and increase in height for age and sex*

Intervention: *Promoting Appropriate Physical Growth*

- Assess parents' and adolescent's knowledge of nutritional needs of adolescents *to determine need for further education*
- Educate parents and adolescent about appropriate serving sizes and foods *so that they are aware of what to expect for adolescents*
- Determine need for additional caloric intake if necessary *(if very active in sports, if have a chronic illness)*
- Plot out height, weight, and BMI *to detect possible pattern*
- Assess for risk factors for developing eating disorder *to refer to if needed and plan interventions*

NURSING DIAGNOSIS: Ineffective health maintenance related to lack of exercise, increased caloric intake, poor food choices, and stresses of adolescence

Outcome Identification and Evaluation

Adolescent will engage in health maintenance behaviors and lose weight at an appropriate rate: *increase amount of exercise, make appropriate eating choices, decrease caloric intake to appropriate amount for age and sex*

(continued)

NURSING CARE PLAN 29.1

Growth and Development of the Adolescent (continued)

Intervention: ***Promoting Appropriate Health Maintenance Behaviors***

- Assess knowledge of parents and adolescent about nutritional needs of teenagers *to determine deficits in knowledge*
- Have adolescent keep a detailed food and exercise diary for 1 week *to determine current patterns of eating and exercise*
- Interview family in relationship to their eating habits and exercise habits *to determine where adjustments might need to be made*
- Discuss changes in a positive manner—talk about developing healthy eating habits instead of dieting *to promote compliance*
- Analyze preceding data, and base recommendations for changes on these data *to promote compliance and to prioritize recommendations*
- Discuss ways to decrease temptation to overeat, for example, eat slowly, put down the fork between bites, serve food on smaller plates, and count mouthfuls, *to allow time to realize that you are full*
- Have adolescent create meal plans and grocery shop *to allow him or her some sense of control and decision making*
- Incorporate increase in daily exercise, which will stress sense of self-improvement to *increase caloric expenditure and self-esteem*
- Decrease TV/computer time *to increase caloric expenditure*
- Encourage peer exercise activities *to increase peer interactions and to help teen to realize that others are like him or her*
- Develop reward system *to increase self-esteem*
- Investigate joining weight loss program for adolescents *to increase self-esteem and encourage weight loss*

NURSING DIAGNOSIS: Growth and development, delayed, related to speech, motor, psychosocial, or cognitive concerns as evidenced by delay in meeting expected school performances

Outcome Identification and Evaluation

Development will be maximized: Adolescent will make continued progress toward attainment of expected school performance

Interventions: ***Promoting Growth and Development***

- Perform scheduled evaluation of the adolescent by school and health care provider *to determine current functioning*
- Develop realistic multidisciplinary plan *to ensure maximizing resources*
- Carry out interventions as prescribed by developmental specialist, physical therapist, occupational therapist, or speech therapist at home and at school *to maximize benefit of interventions*
- Have scheduled evaluation meetings *to be able to adapt interventions as soon as possible*

NURSING DIAGNOSIS: Caregiver role strain, risk for (risk factors: knowledge deficit about adolescent issues, lack of prior exposure, fatigue, ill or developmentally delayed child)

Outcome Identification and Evaluation

Parent will experience competence in role: *will demonstrate appropriate caretaking behaviors and verbalize comfort in caring for an adolescent*

Interventions: ***Preventing Caregiver Role Strain***

- Assess parents' knowledge of adolescents and the issues that arise as a part of normal development *to determine parents' needs*
- Provide education on normal issues of adolescence *so that parents are armed with the knowledge they need to appropriately care for their adolescents*
- Provide anticipatory guidance related to upcoming expected issues related to adolescent development *to prepare parents for what to expect next and how to intervene in an appropriate manner*

NURSING CARE PLAN 29.1

Growth and Development of the Adolescent (continued)

NURSING DIAGNOSIS: Injury, risk for (risk factors: increased motor and cognitive skills and feeling of invincibility)

Outcome Identification and Evaluation

Adolescent's safety will be maintained: *will remain free from injury*

Interventions: *Preventing Injury*

- Discuss safety measures needed for the following: bikes, scooters, guns, skateboards, cars, and water *to decrease risk of injury related to those areas*
- Discuss and develop a fire safety plan *to decrease risk of injury related to fire*
- Discuss appropriate safety equipment needed for each sport *to decrease risk of injury*
- Discuss appropriate sports to participate in depending on age, sex, and maturity of adolescent *to prevent possible injury*
- Teach parents and adolescent first-aid measures and cardiopulmonary resuscitation (CPR) *to minimize consequences of injury should it occur*
- Discuss influence of peers upon actions of adolescents *to prevent possible injury due to mimicking behavior*

NURSING DIAGNOSIS: Coping, ineffective (risk factors: low self-esteem, poor relationship with parents and peers, participating in risk-taking behaviors)

Outcome Identification and Evaluation

Adolescent will demonstrate adequate coping abilities *as evidenced by management of stress of adolescence and no evidence of participating in risk-taking behaviors*

Interventions: *Promoting Effective Coping*

- Assess adolescent's knowledge of normal stress-facing teenagers *to determine current knowledge*
- Assess adolescent's present coping skills *to determine areas for improvement/support*
- Encourage parents to accept teenager as a unique individual *to improve self-esteem*
- Discuss with parents and adolescent normal developmental issues facing teens *to give them knowledge needed to cope*
- Provide different situations the teen might be faced with and encourage teen to develop different solutions *to assist teen in developing problem-solving strategies*
- Allow for increasing independence and opportunities to solve own problems *to improve coping skills*
- Encourage parents to provide unconditional love *to improve self-esteem*
- Assess for any evidence of any risk-taking behaviors (drugs, smoking, suicide) *to identify need for early interventions*

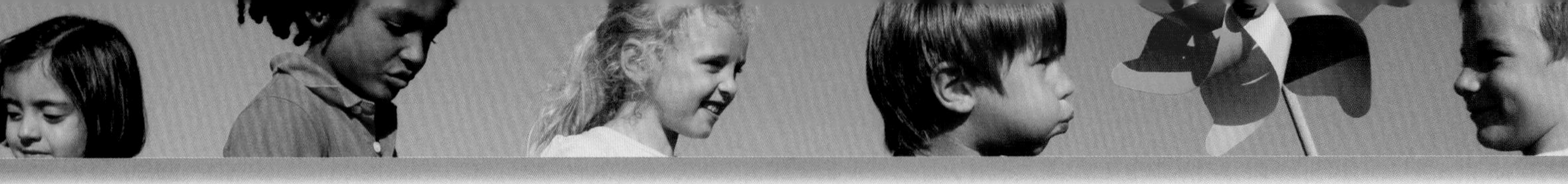

KEY CONCEPTS

- Adolescence is a period of rapid and variable growth in the areas of physical, psychosocial, cognitive, and moral development.
- The adolescent is developing his or her own identity, becoming an abstract thinker, and developing his or her own set of morals and values. Inability to successfully develop an individual identity leads to poor preparation for the challenges of adulthood.
- Relationships with parents fluctuate widely during adolescence. The teenager eventually becomes emancipated from his or her parents.
- Peers become most important—guiding mainly the early and middle adolescent in his or her decisions, while the late adolescent can usually formulate his or her own decisions.
- Adolescence is a critical time in the development of sexuality. Sexuality includes the thoughts, feelings, and behaviors surrounding the adolescent's sexual identity.
- The egocentric and invincible thought processes of the adolescent can lead to injuries. Health care providers must emphasis safety regarding cars, bikes, water, firearms, and fire.
- Motor vehicle accidents are the number one cause of death in adolescents (U.S. Department of Health and Human Services, Health Resources and Services Administration, Maternal and Child Health Bureau, 2013).
- Nutritional habits of the adolescent lead to deficiency in vitamins and minerals needed for the rapid growth during this period.
- Obesity in adolescents is a growing health concern. Health care providers are facing increased numbers of adolescents with hypertension, type 2 diabetes, and hyperlipidemia.
- Substance abuse and experimentation is common during adolescence; it is associated with other risk-taking behaviors such as injuries and sexual activity.
- Health care providers must work collaboratively with the adolescent in the development of interventions to promote health.

REFERENCES AND RECOMMENDED READINGS

American Academy of Pediatrics. (2010a). The teen driver. *Pediatrics, 118*(6), 2570–2581. Retrieved from http://pediatrics.aappublications.org/content/118/6/2570.full

American Academy of Pediatrics. (2010b). Policy statement: Prevention of drowning in infants, children and adolescents. *Pediatrics, 126*(21), 178–185. doi: 10.1542/peds.2010–1264

American Academy of Pediatrics. (2012). *Guidance for effective discipline*. Retrieved from http://pediatrics.aappublications.org/content/101/4/723.full

American Academy of Pediatrics. (2013). *Ages & stages: Tattoos*. Retrieved from http://www.healthychildren.org/English/ages-stages/teen/safety/pages/Tattoos.aspx

American Academy of Pediatrics. (2014). *Cognitive rest after concussion leads to quicker recovery, study finds. target news service*. Retrieved from http://www.aap.org/en-us/about-the-aap/aap-press-room/pages/Cognitive-Rest-After-Concussion-Leads-to-Quicker-Recovery-Study-Finds.aspx

American Academy of Pediatrics, Council on Environmental Health and Section on Dermatology. (2011). Policy statement—ultraviolet radiation: A hazard to children and adolescents. *Pediatrics, 127*(3), 588 -597. doi: 10.1542/peds.2010–3501

American Academy of Pediatrics, Council on Communications and Media. (2013). Policy statement: Children, adolescents, and the media. *Pediatrics, 132*(5), 958–961. doi: 10.1542/peds.2013–2656

American Academy of Pediatric Dentistry. (2013). *Policy on use of fluoride*. Retrieved from http://www.aapd.org/media/Policies_Guidelines/P_FluorideUse.pdf

American Cancer Society. (2013). *Child and teen tobacco use*\. Retrieved from http://www.cancer.org/cancer/cancercauses/tobaccocancer/childandteentobaccouse/child-and-teen-tobacco-use-child-and-teen-tobacco-use

American Heart Association. (2013). *Coronary artery disease-coronary heart disease*. Retrieved from http://www.heart.org/HEARTORG/Conditions/More/MyHeartandStrokeNews/Coronary-Artery-Disease—Coronary-Heart-Disease_UCM_436416_Article.jsp

American Skin Association. (2012). *Sun safety*. Retrieved from http://www.americanskin.org/resource/safety.php

Billings, D. M., & Hensel, D. (2014). *Lippincott's Q & A Review for NCLEX-RN* (11th ed.). Philadelphia, PA: Lippincott Williams & Wilkins.

Blum, R. W., Gates, W. H., & Qureshi, F. (2011). *Morbidity and mortality among adolescents and young adults in the United States: AstraZeneca fact sheet 2011*. Retrieved from http://www.jhsph.edu/research/centers-and-institutes/center-for-adolescent-health/az/_images/US%20Fact%20Sheet_FINAL.pdf

Bright Futures/American Academy of Pediatrics. (2014). *Recommendations for preventive health care*. Retrieved from http://www.aap.org/en-us/professional-resources/practice-support/Periodicity/Periodicity%20Schedule_FINAL.pdf

Brown, N. J., Mannix, R. C., O'Brien, M. J., Gostine, D., Collins, M. W., & Meehan, W. P. 3rd. (2014). Effect of cognitive activity level on duration of post-concussion symptoms. *Pediatrics, 133*, e299–e304. doi: 10.1542/peds.2013–2125

Carpenito, L. J. (2013). *Nursing diagnosis: Application to clinical practice* (14th ed.). Philadelphia, PA: Lippincott Williams & Wilkins.

Centers for Disease Control and Prevention (CDC). (2012a). *Teen drivers: Fact sheet*. Retrieved from http://www.cdc.gov/Motorvehiclesafety/Teen_Drivers/teendrivers_factsheet.html

Centers for Disease Control and Prevention. (2012b). *Youth violence: Facts at a glance*. Retrieved from http://www.cdc.gov/violenceprevention/pdf/yv_datasheet_2012-a.pdf

Centers for Disease Control and Prevention. (2012c). *Understanding youth violence: Fact sheet*. Retrieved from http://www.cdc.gov/violenceprevention/pdf/YV-FactSheet-a.pdf

Centers for Disease Control and Prevention. (2012d). *The burden of tobacco use*. Retrieved from http://www.cdc.gov/chronicdisease/resources/publications/aag/osh.htm

Centers for Disease Control and Prevention. (2013a). *Adolescent and school health: Physical activity facts*. Retrieved from http://www.cdc.gov/healthyyouth/physicalactivity/facts.htm

Centers for Disease Control and Prevention. (2013b). *Adolescent and school health: Health & academics*. Retrieved http://www.cdc.gov/healthyyouth/health_and_academics/index.htm

Centers for Disease Control and Prevention. (2013c). *Youth violence: Definitions*. Retrieved from http://www.cdc.gov/ViolencePrevention/youthviolence/definitions.html

Centers for Disease Control and Prevention. (2013d). *Youth violence: Risk and protective factors*. Retrieved from http://www.cdc.gov/violenceprevention/youthviolence/riskprotectivefactors.html

Centers for Disease Control and Prevention. (2013e). *Alcohol and public health: Fact sheets - Underage drinking*. Retrieved from http://www.cdc.gov/alcohol/fact-sheets/underage-drinking.htm

Centers for Disease Control and Prevention. (2013f). *Press release: e-cigarette use more than doubles among U.S. middle and high school students from 2011–2012*. Retrieved http://www.cdc.gov/media/releases/2013/p0905-ecigarette-use.html

Centers for Disease Control and Prevention. (2014a). *Suicide prevention: Youth suicide*. Retrieved from http://www.cdc.gov/violenceprevention/pub/youth_suicide.html

Centers for Disease Control and Prevention. (2014b). *Childhood obesity facts*. Retrieved from http://www.cdc.gov/healthyyouth/obesity/facts.htm

Centers for Disease Control and Prevention. (2014c). *Understanding teen dating violence*. Retrieved from http://www.cdc.gov/violenceprevention/pdf/teen-dating-violence-2014-a.pdf

Child Trends. (2013a). *Dating*. Retrieved from http://www.childtrends.org/?indicators=dating

Child Trends. (2013b). *High school dropout rates*. Retrieved from http://www.childtrends.org/?indicators=high-school-dropout-rates

Cromer, B. (2011). Chapter 104: Adolescent development. In R. M. Kleigman, B. F. Stanton, J. W. St. Geme III, N. F. Schor & R. E. Behrman (Eds.), *Nelson textbook of pediatrics* (19th ed., pp. 649–659). Philadelphia, PA: Saunders.

Dahlberg, L. L., & Krug, E. G. (2002). Violence: a global public health problem. In E. G. Krug, L. L. Dahlberg, J. A. Mercy, A. B. Zwi, & R. Lozano (Eds.). *World report on violence and health*. Geneva, Switzerland: World Health Organization; 1–21.

Division of Adolescent and School Health, National Center for Chronic Disease Prevention and Health Promotion. (2011). School health guidelines to promote healthy eating and physical activity recommendations and reports. *Morbidity and Mortality Weekly Report (MMWR), 60*(RR05), 1–71. Retrieved from http://www.cdc.gov/mmwr/preview/mmwrhtml/rr6005a1.htm

Dowshen, S. (2013). *Alcohol*. Retrieved from http://kidshealth.org/teen/drug_alcohol/alcohol/alcohol.html#

Dowshen, S. (2014a). *Bike safety*. Retrieved from http://kidshealth.org/teen/safety/safebasics/bike_safety.html#

Dowshen, S. (2014b). *Hygiene basics*. Retrieved from http://kidshealth.org/teen/your_body/take_care/hygiene_basics.html#

Durani, Y. (2011). Water Safety. Retrieved from http://kidshealth.org/teen/safety/safebasics/water_safety.html#

Egley, Jr., A. & Howell, J.S. (2013). Highlights of the 2011 National Youth Gang Survey. *Office of Juvenile Justice and Delinquency Prevention*. Retrieved from http://www.ojjdp.gov/pubs/242884.pdf

Erikson, E. (1963). *Childhood and society* (2nd ed.). New York: Norton.

Federal Interagency Forum on Child and Family Statistics. (2013). *America's children in brief: Key national indicators of well being, 2013*. Washington, DC: U.S. Government Printing Office.

Ford, G. S. (2007). Hospitalized kids spiritual care at their level. *Journal of Christian Nursing, 24*(3), 135–140.

Gavin, M. L. (2011a). *Calcium*. Retrieved from http://kidshealth.org/teen/food_fitness/nutrition/calcium.html#

Gavin, M. L. (2011b). *All about sleep*. Retrieved from http://kidshealth.org/parent/general/sleep/sleep.html

Gavin, M. L. (2012). *Iron*. Retrieved from http://kidshealth.org/parent/growth/feeding/iron.html#

Gavin, M. L. (2013). *Tatoos*. Retrieved from http://kidshealth.org/teen/your_body/beautiful/safe_tattooing.html#

Hagan, J. F., Shaw, J. S., & Duncan, P. (2008). *Bright futures guidelines for health supervision of infants, children, and adolescents* (3rd ed.). Elk Grove Village, IL: American Academy of Pediatrics.

Hirsch, L. (2011). *Menstrual problems*. Retrieved from http://kidshealth.org/parent/growth/growing/menstrual_problems.html

Johnston, L. D., O'Malley, P. M., Miech, R. A., Bachman, J. G., & Schulenberg, J. E. (2014). *Monitoring the future national results on drug use: 1975–2013: Overview, key findings on adolescent drug use*. Ann Arbor, MI: Institute for Social Research, The University of Michigan. Retrieved from http://www.monitoringthefuture.org//pubs/monographs/mtf-overview2013.pdf

Joseph, E. P. B. (2013). *What are E-cigarettes?* Retrieved from http://kidshealth.org/teen/drug_alcohol/tobacco/e-cigarettes.html#

Kohlberg, L. (1984). *Essays on moral development*. San Francisco, CA: Harper & Row.

Letcher, A. (2013). *Dating and your adolescent: part 1*. Retrieved from http://igrow.org/4 h/healthy-living/dating-and-your-adolescent-part-1/

Lyness, D. (2013). *Sexual orientation*. Retrieved from http://kidshealth.org/parent/emotions/feelings/sexual_orientation.html#

McDaniel D. D. (2012). Risk and protective factors associated with gang affiliation among high-risk youth: a public health approach. *Injury Prevention, 18*(4), 253–258. doi:10.1136/injuryprev-2011–040083

Moreno, M. A. (2013). *Sex, drugs'n facebook.* Almeda, CA: Hunter House, Inc

Murphey, D., Barry, M., Vaughn, B. Guzman, L. & Terzian, M. (2013). *Adolescent health highlight: Use of illicit drugs. Child trends.* Retrieved from http://www.childtrends.org/wp-content/uploads/2013/09/Illicit-drug-use-Highlight-9.13.pdf

National Center on Addiction and Substance Abuse at Columbia University. (2012). *National survey of American attitudes on substance abuse XVII: Teens.* Retrieved from http://www.casacolumbia.org/absolutenm/articlefiles/380–2007%20Teen%20Survey%20XII.pdf

NIDA for Teens. (2014). *Drug facts.* Retrieved from http://teens.drugabuse.gov/drug-facts

O'Keeffe, G.S., Clarke-Pearson, K., & Council on Communications and Media. (2011). Clinical report—The impact of social media on children, adolescents, and families. *Pediatrics, 127*(4), 800–804. doi: 10.1542/peds.2011–0054

Piaget, J. (1969). *The theory of stages in cognitive development.* New York: McGraw-Hill.

Rauer, A. J., Pettit, G. S., Lansford, J. E., Bates, J. E., & Dodge, K. A. (2013). Romantic relationship patterns in young adulthood and their developmental antecedents. *Developmental Psychology, 49*(11), 2159–2171. doi: 10.1037/a0031845

Remafedi, G. (2011). Chapter 104.3 adolescent homosexuality. In R. M. Kleigman, B.F. Stanton, J. W. St. Geme III, N.F. Schor & R.E. Behrman (Eds.), *Nelson textbook of pediatrics* (19th ed., pp.658–659). Philadelphia, PA: Saunders.

Seith, D., & Isakson, E. (2011). Who are America's poor children? Examining health disparities among children in the United States. National Center for Children in Poverty. Retrieved from http://www.nccp.org/publications/pdf/text_995.pdf

Stager, M.M. (2011). Chapter 108: Substance abuse. In R. M. Kleigman, B. F. Stanton, J. W. St. Geme III, N. F. Schor, & R. E. Behrman (Eds.), *Nelson textbook of pediatrics* (19th ed., pp. 671–685). Philadelphia: Saunders.

Tanner, J. (1962). *Growth at adolescence* (2nd ed.). Oxford, England: Blackwell Scientific Publications.

Tinanoff, N. (2011). Section 2: The oral cavity. In R. M. Kleigman, B. F. Stanton, J. W. St. Geme III, N. F. Schor, & R. E. Behrman (Eds.), *Nelson textbook of pediatrics* (19th ed., pp. 1249–1261). Philadelphia, PA: Saunders.

U.S. Department of Agriculture and U.S. Department of Health and Human Services. (2010). *Dietary guidelines for Americans, 2010* (7th ed.). Washington, DC: U.S. Government Printing Office. Retrieved from http://www.cnpp.usda.gov/DGAs2010-PolicyDocument.htm

U.S. Department of Health & Human Services. (2012). *Healthypeople.gov.* Retrieved at http://www.healthypeople.gov/2020/about/default.aspx

U.S. Department of Health and Human Services, Health Resources and Services Administration, Maternal and Child Health Bureau. (2013). *Child health USA 2012.* Rockville, MD: U.S. Department of Health and Human. Retrieved from http://mchb.hrsa.gov/chusa12/hs/hsa/pages/am.html

CHAPTER WORKSHEET

MULTIPLE CHOICE QUESTIONS

1. When giving parents guidance for the adolescent years, the nurse would advise the parents to: (Choose all that apply.)
   a. Accept the adolescent as a unique individual
   b. Provide strict, inflexible rules
   c. Listen and try to be open to the adolescent's views
   d. Screen all of his or her friends
   e. Respect the adolescent's privacy
   f. Provide unconditional love

2. In developing a weight-loss plan for an adolescent, which would the nurse include? (Choose all that apply.)
   a. Have parents make all of the meal plans.
   b. Eat slowly and place the fork down between each bite.
   c. Have the family exercise together.
   d. Refer to an adolescent weight-loss program.
   e. Keep a food and exercise diary.

3. Which is associated with early adolescence? (Choose all that apply.)
   a. Uses scientific reasoning to solve problems
   b. Still at times wants to be dependent upon parents
   c. Incorporates own set of morals and values
   d. Is influenced by peers and values memberships in cliques

4. What has the most influence in deterring an adolescent from beginning to drink alcohol?
   a. Drinking habits of parents
   b. Drinking habits of peers
   c. Drinking philosophy of adolescent's culture
   d. Drinking philosophy of adolescent's religion

CRITICAL THINKING EXERCISES

1. During a sports physical examination, Susan, a 16-year-old, tells her health care provider that she is overweight. What additional information would the nurse obtain?

2. The parents of Joe, a 14-year-old, talk to the school nurse about Joe's behavior at home. He is moody, fights with his younger siblings, only wants to be on his computer, and does not want to go on the family vacation. What advice would the nurse give the parents?

3. Jane tells the school nurse that she might be homosexual. What additional information would the nurse obtain?

4. Alicia's parents are worried because all of Alicia's friends wear heavy makeup and have multiple piercings and hair colors. What advice would the nurse give Alicia's parents?

STUDY ACTIVITIES

1. Talk to an early, middle, and late adolescent. Compare and contrast their interactions with you. Identify what psychosocial, cognitive, and moral stage they are in, using examples from their conversations with you.

2. Have an adolescent keep a food and exercise diary for 1 week. Analyze the information. Develop with the adolescent any interventions needed to promote healthy eating and exercise habits.

3. Plan a class on the dangers of smoking for 15-year-olds.

4. Plan a class for parents on how to keep the lines of communication open for adolescents.

5. Go to http://www.choosemyplate.gov/myplate/index.aspx and create and compare a customized meal plan for a healthy adolescent versus an obese adolescent.

BRINGING IT ALL TOGETHER: A CASE STUDY

Ethan, a 15 year old male, is seen in your clinic for his annual examination. After you measure his height, Ethan says to you, "My sister who is 14 years old is 2 inches (5 cm) taller than me."

Go to thePoint to find questions to consider about this case.

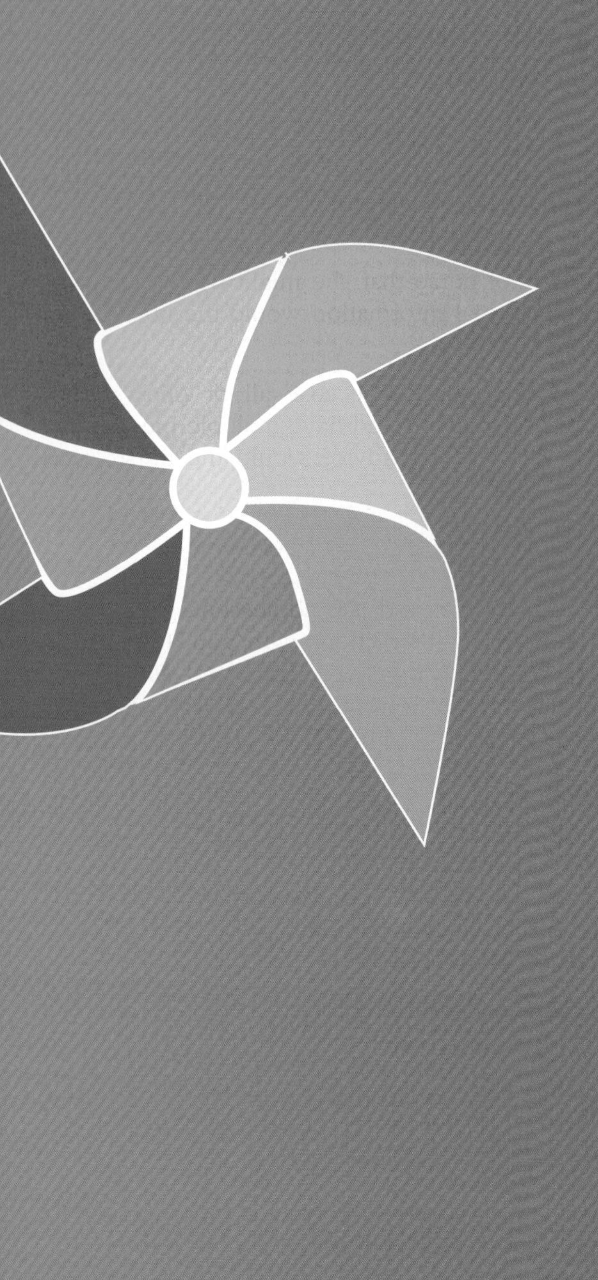

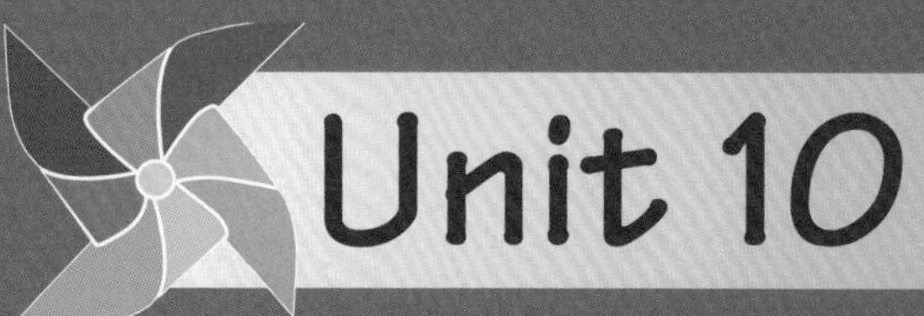

Foundations of Pediatric Nursing

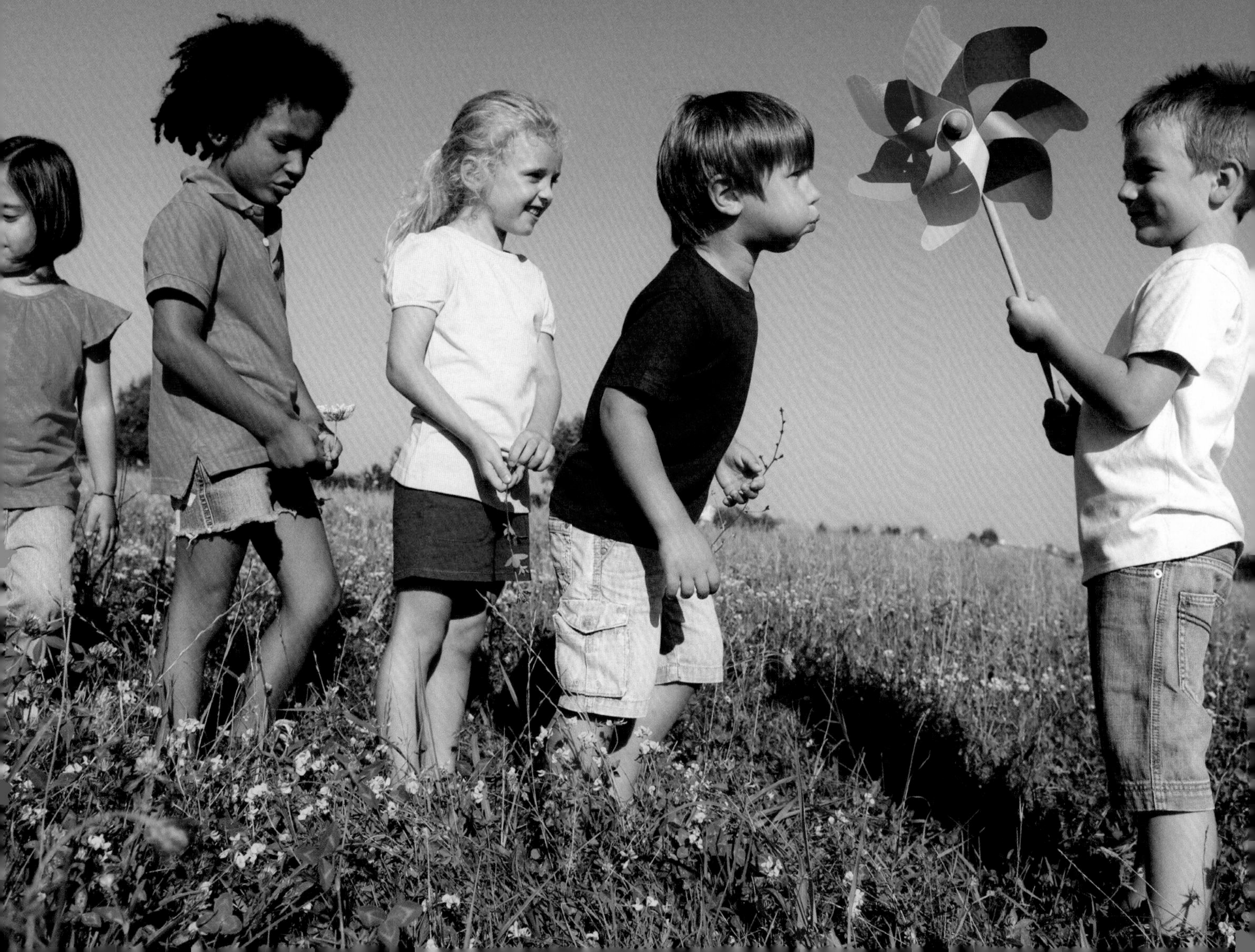

30

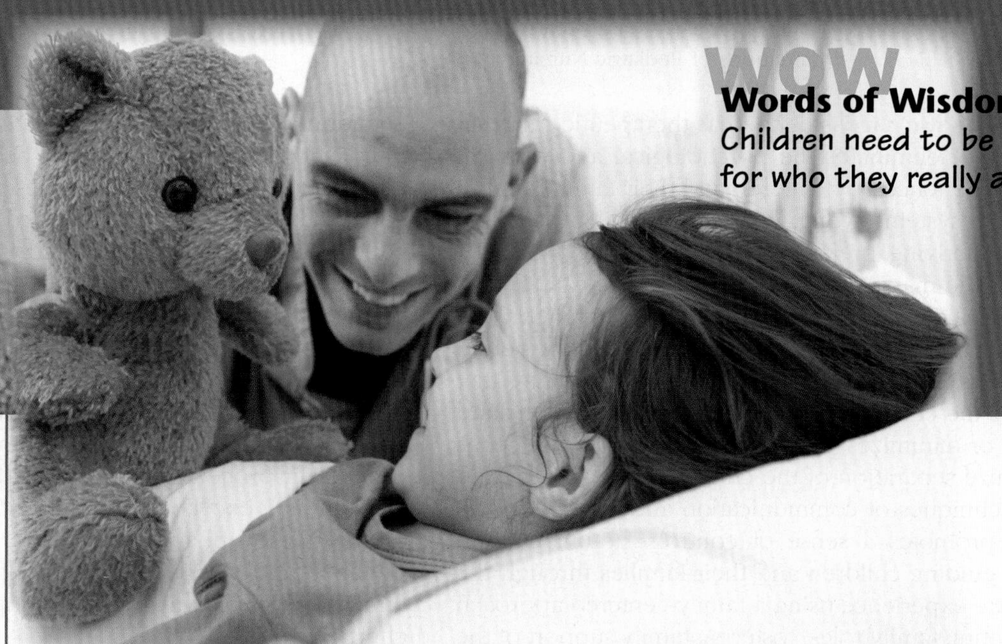

WOW

Words of Wisdom
Children need to be seen for who they really are.

Atraumatic Care of Children and Families

KEY TERMS
atraumatic care
child life specialist
family-centered care
therapeutic hugging

Learning Objectives

Upon completion of the chapter, you will be able to:

1. Describe the major principles and concepts of atraumatic care.
2. Incorporate atraumatic care to prevent and minimize physical stress for children and families.
3. Discuss the major components and concepts of family-centered care.
4. Utilize excellent therapeutic communication skills when interacting with children and their families.
5. Describe the process of health teaching as it relates to children and their families.

***Emma Moore*, 4 years old, is admitted to the pediatric unit with a suspected head injury from a fall. She was playing at a playground with her babysitter and fell from the top of the slide.**

Atraumatic care is defined as therapeutic care that minimizes or eliminates the psychological and physical distress experienced by children and their families in the health care system (Wong, n.d.). This concept is based on the underlying premise of "do no harm." Box 30.1 highlights the major principles of atraumatic care.

Pediatric nurses must be vigilant for any situation that may cause distress and must be able to identify potential stressors. It is important to provide nursing care that decreases the child's exposure to stressful situations and prevents or minimizes pain and bodily injury; take steps to minimize separation of the child from the family; and utilize techniques of communication and provide teaching that promotes a sense of control. Atraumatic care involves guiding children and their families through the health care experience using a family-centered approach by promoting family roles, fostering family support of the child, and providing appropriate information. Help children cope with this experience by using age-appropriate and child-specific interventions. Preparation can help children and their families to adjust to illness and hospitalization. Use appropriate techniques for therapeutic communication (goal-directed, focused, purposeful communication), therapeutic play (type of play that provides an emotional outlet or improves the child's ability to cope with the stress of illness and hospitalization), and education to help the child and family understand the reason for the hospitalization and the necessary tests and procedures. In addition, help the family and other health care personnel to obtain the resources and relationships they need for optimal care.

The best pediatric nursing care encompasses the concepts of atraumatic care. Minimizing physical stressors during procedures, providing family-centered care, and utilizing excellent communication skills on the part of the nurse enhance the health care experience for the child and family. Having an informed and educated family is the best way to provide optimal health care for children.

Table 30.1 gives suggestions for incorporating the principles of atraumatic care into nursing care for the child and family. Look for tips on atraumatic care as it relates to specific topics throughout the text.

BOX 30.1

PRINCIPLES OF ATRAUMATIC CARE

- Prevent or minimize physical stressors, including pain, discomfort, immobility, sleep deprivation, inability to eat or drink, and changes in elimination.
  - Avoid or reduce intrusive and painful procedures, such as injections, multiple punctures, and urethral catheterization.
  - Avoid or reduce other kinds of physical distress, such as noise, smells, shivering, nausea and vomiting, sleeplessness, restraints, and skin trauma.
  - Control pain via frequent assessments and use of pharmacologic and nonpharmacologic interventions.
- Prevent or minimize parent–child separation.
  - Promote family-centered care, treating the family as the patient.
  - Use core primary nursing.
  - Consider research findings related to preferences of parents and children and whether or not to be together.
- Promote a sense of control.
  - Elicit the family's knowledge about the child and his or her health condition, promoting partnerships, empowerment, and enabling.
  - Reduce fear of the unknown through education, familiar articles, and decreasing the threat of the environment.
  - Provide opportunities for control, such as participating in care, attempting to normalize daily schedule, and providing direct suggestions.

Adapted from Wong, D. L. (n.d.). *Innovative approaches for atraumatic cancer care*. RetrievedAugust 25, 2013, from http://www.authorstream.com/presentation/Carolina-48857-op077-INNOVATIVE-APPROACHES-ATRAUMATIC-CANCER-CARE-DEFINITION-SOURCES-PATIENT-FAMILY-STRESSORS-as-Entertainment-ppt-powerpoint/

PREVENTING/MINIMIZING PHYSICAL STRESSORS

The health care facility or hospital is an unfamiliar environment for children and parents and may upset or intimidate them. They may feel anxiety, fear, helplessness, anger, or loss of control. Even health care procedures performed in the home or school may be perceived as threatening to children. To prevent and minimize the physical stress experienced by children and their families in relation to health care, pediatric nurses, child life specialists (CLSs), and other health care professionals recommend the use of atraumatic care.

Utilizing the Child Life Specialist

The **child life specialist** (CLS) is a specially trained individual who provides programs that prepare children for hospitalization, surgery, and other procedures that could be painful (Child Life Council, 2010a). The CLS is a member of the multidisciplinary team and works in conjunction with the health care provider and parents to foster an atmosphere that promotes the child's well-being. Services provided by a CLS include:

- Nonmedical preparation for tests, surgeries, and other medical procedures
- Support during medical procedures
- Therapeutic play
- Activities to support normal growth and development
- Sibling support
- Advocacy for the child and family
- Grief and bereavement support

TABLE 30.1 SUGGESTIONS FOR ATRAUMATIC CARE

Principle	Suggestions for Nursing Care
Preventing or minimizing physical stressors	• For painful injections, blood draws, or IV insertion, use numbing techniques (see Chapter 36). • During painful or invasive procedures, avoid traditional restraint or "holding down" of the child. Use alternative positioning such as "therapeutic hugging." • If the above-mentioned positions are not an option, have the parent stand near the child's head to provide comfort. • Insert a saline lock if the child requires multiple doses of parenteral medications. • Advocate for minimal laboratory blood draws. • Minimize intramuscular or subcutaneous injections. • Provide appropriate pain management (refer to Chapter 36).
Preventing or minimizing child and family separation	• Promote family-centered care. • In the hospital, provide comfortable accommodations for the parent. • Allow the family the choice about whether to stay for an invasive procedure, and support them in their decision.
Promoting a sense of control	• Maintain the child's home routine related to activities of daily living. • In the hospital, use primary nursing. • Encourage the child to have a security item present, if desired. • Involve the child and family in planning care from the moment of the first encounter. • Empower the family and child by providing knowledge. • Allow the child and family choices when they are available. • Make the environment more inviting and less intimidating.

- Emergency room interventions for children and families
- Hospital preadmission tours and information programs
- Outpatient consultation with families (Child Life Council, 2010b)

The goal of the CLS is to decrease the child's anxiety and fear while improving and encouraging the child's understanding and cooperation. The CLS considers the needs of siblings or other children who may be affected by the child's illness or trauma. The CLS provides engaging and uplifting events by coordinating special entertainment and activities. The CLS is an excellent resource and provides education to health care providers and families. The American Academy of Pediatrics recommends child life services because they are "an essential component of quality pediatric health care and are integral to family-centered care and best practice models of health care delivery for children" (American Academy of Pediatrics, 2006, p. 1760).

Minimizing Physical Stress During Procedures

Children undergo numerous diagnostic and therapeutic procedures in a wide range of settings during their development. These procedures may be performed in the community or outpatient setting or in a care facility. Regardless of the procedure and the setting, children, like adults, need thorough preparation before the procedure and support during and after the procedure, to promote the best outcome and to ensure atraumatic care.

Using positions that are comforting to the child during painful procedures is an important aspect of atraumatic care (Fig. 30.1). **Therapeutic hugging** (a holding position that promotes close physical contact between the child and a parent or caregiver) may be used for certain procedures or treatments where the child must remain still. For example, the parent can hold the child in his or her lap snugly to prevent the child from moving during an injection or venipuncture. When using this technique, make sure the parent understands his or her role and knows which body parts to hold still in a safe manner. Alternatively, distraction or stimulation (such as with a toy) can help to gain the child's cooperation. Refer to Box 30.2 for distraction methods. See Figure 30.2.

BOX 30.2

DISTRACTION METHODS

- Have the child point toes inward and wiggle them.
- Ask the child to squeeze your hand.
- Encourage the child to count aloud.
- Sing a song and have the child sing along.
- Point out the pictures on the ceiling.
- Have the child blow bubbles.
- Play music appealing to the child.

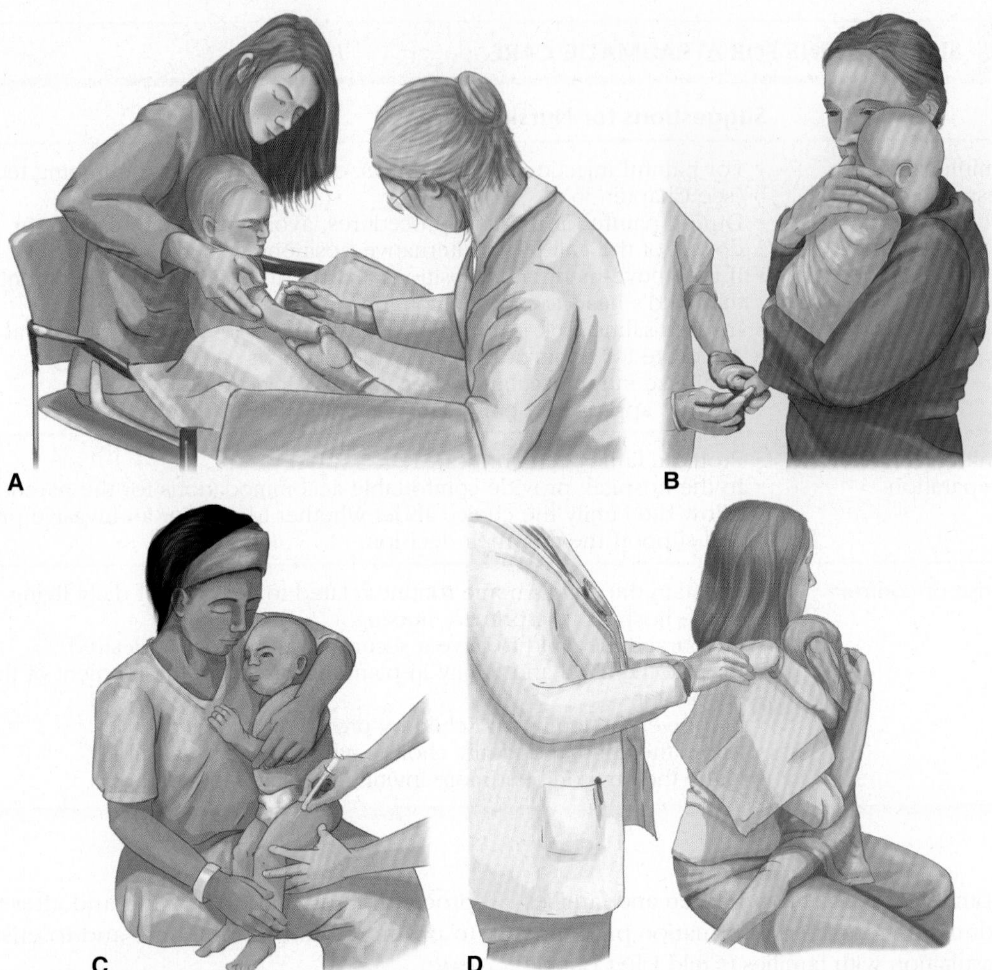

FIGURE 30.1 Positioning a child for comfort during a painful procedure. **(A)** Sitting on the parent's lap while undergoing allergy testing provides this toddler with a sense of comfort. **(B)** Position the infant cuddled over the parent's (preferable) or the nurse's shoulder when obtaining a heelstick. **(C)** Use "therapeutic hugging" to maintain a child's position when the child is receiving an intramuscular injection. **(D)** Use "therapeutic hugging" to position a child while the child is having an IV line inserted.

Before the Procedure

Appropriate preparation for procedures helps to decrease the child's and family's anxiety level, promote the child's cooperation, support the child's and family's coping skills, improve recovery, and increase trust between the child, his or her family, and the physicians health care team (Koller, 2007; Manneheim, 2012). Adequate preparation also helps to encourage long-term coping and improve coping with future medical situations (Koller, 2007).

Preparation may include preparing the child psychologically (including explanation and education) as well as physically. It is very important to employ the concepts of atraumatic care when preparing children for a procedure. General guidelines for preparation include the following:

- Provide a description of and the reason for the procedure using age-appropriate language ("the doctor will look at your blood to see why you are sick").
- Describe where the procedure will occur ("the x-ray department has big machines that won't hurt you; it's a little cold there too").
- Introduce strange equipment the child may see ("you will lie on a special bed that moves in the big machine, but you can still see out").
- Describe how long the procedure will last ("you will be in the x-ray department until lunchtime").
- Identify unusual sensations that may occur during the procedure ("you may smell something different" [e.g., alcohol smell]; "the MRI machine makes loud noises").
- Inform the child if any pain is involved.
- Tell the child it is okay to cry or yell.
- Identify any special care required after the procedure ("you will need to lie quietly for 15 minutes afterward").
- Discuss ways that may help the child stay calm, such as using distraction methods or relaxation techniques ("during the procedure you may want to count from 1 to 100 or sing your favorite song") (Manneheim, 2012).

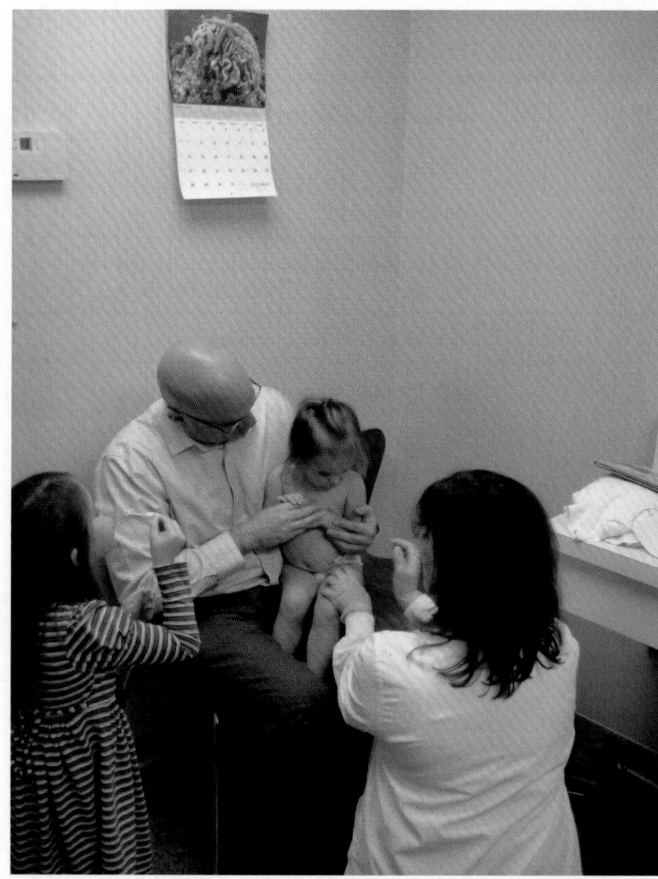

FIGURE 30.2 When possible, allow the caregiver to assist with providing positions of comfort and involve a sibling to assist with distraction techniques such as blowing bubbles, singing, or reading to the child during procedures.

Take Note!

In the hospital, perform all invasive procedures in the treatment room or a room other than the child's room. The child's room should remain a safe and secure area (Leahy, Kennedy, Hesselgrave, et al., 2008).

A major aspect of preparation involves play. Toys and dolls provide an excellent way to demonstrate procedures that will occur. Consider the child's temperament, coping strategies, and previous experiences as well as developmental needs and cognitive abilities. First, gain trust and provide support. Include the child's parents, because parents are usually the greatest source of comfort for the child. Be short, simple, and appropriate in explaining situations at the child's level of development. Explain what is to be done and what is expected of the child. Avoid terms that have double meanings or might be confusing. Table 30.2 lists alternative words or phrases to use for terms that may be confusing or misunderstood. Allow the child time to play with the toy or dolls and medical equipment as appropriate. Watch for signs of anxiety or fears.

During the Procedure

Use a firm, positive, confident approach that provides the child with a sense of security. Encourage cooperation by involving the child in decision making and allowing the child to select from a list or group of appropriate choices. Allow the child to express feelings of anger, anxiety, fear, frustration, or any other emotions. Often, this is how a child communicates and copes with the situation. Remind the child that it is okay to scream or cry, but that it is very important to hold still. Use distraction methods such as those listed in Box 30.2.

Toddlers and preschoolers often resist procedures despite preparation for them. Being held down or restrained is often more traumatizing to the young child than the procedure itself. Use alternative methods (positions that provide comfort for the child) to keep the child still during the procedure (Fig. 30.1). The older child can be held while using a book or story for distraction.

After the Procedure

After the procedure, hold and comfort the child. Cuddle and soothe infants. Encourage children to express their feelings through play, such as dramatic play, or use of puppets. Gross motor activities such as pounding or throwing are also helpful for children to discharge pent-up feelings and energy. School-age children and adolescents may not outwardly demonstrate behavior indicating the need for comforting; however, provide them with opportunities to express their feelings and be comforted. Remember to praise children for appropriate behavior during the procedure and after all interventions are completed.

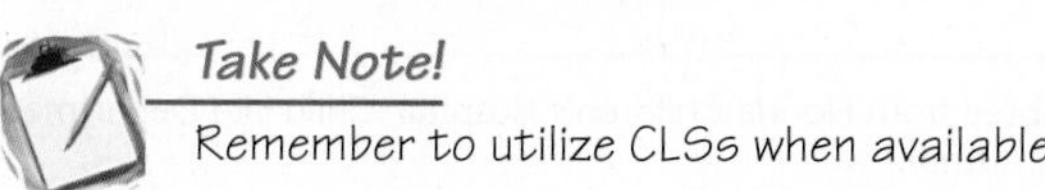

Take Note!

Remember to utilize CLSs when available.

The physician's orders for Emma include starting intravenous (IV) fluids and obtaining blood work upon arrival to the unit. As the admitting nurse, how will you provide atraumatic care?

PREVENTING OR MINIMIZING CHILD AND FAMILY SEPARATION: PROVIDING CHILD- AND FAMILY-CENTERED CARE

Family-centered care involves a partnership between the child, family, and health care providers in planning, providing, and evaluating care (American Academy of Pediatrics, Committee on Hospital Care, Institute for Patient and Family-Centered Care, 2012). It works well for children of any age and in all arenas of health care, from preventive care of the healthy child to long-term

TABLE 30.2 ALTERNATIVES FOR CONFUSING OR MISUNDERSTOOD TERMS

Term to Avoid	How Children Might Interpret It	Use These Terms Instead
Catheter	Too technical	Tube
Deaden	Kill	Make sleepy
Dye	"Die"	Special medicine to help the doctor see _______ (part of the body) better
Electrodes	Too technical	Stickers, ticklers, snaps
ICU	"I see you"	Special room with your own nurse
Incision, cut open, make a hole	Too explicit	Special or small opening
Monitor	Too technical	TV screen
Organ	Like a piano	Special place in the body
Pain	May be too explicit	Child's word for hurt; "boo-boo"
Put to sleep, anesthesia	May confuse with putting a pet to sleep	Special kind of sleep
Shot	Children are scared of shots	Medication under the skin
Stool	Like you sit on	"Poop" or child's word for it
Stretcher or gurney	"Stretch her"	Rolling bed or special bed on wheels
Take your temperature/BP	Where are you going to "take" them	See how warm you are/hug your arm
Test	Like at school (the child will need to perform)	See how your heart is working
Tourniquet	Too technical	Special kind of rubber band
Urine	"You're in"	"Pee" or child's word for it
X-ray	Don't understand	Picture or big camera to take pictures of the inside of your body

Partially adapted from Florida Children's Hospital, Child Life Department. (n.d.). *Suggested vocabulary to use with children.* Orlando, FL: Author.

care of the chronically or terminally ill child. Family-centered care enhances parents' and caregivers' confidence in their own skills and also prepares children and young adults for assuming responsibility for their own health care needs. It is based on the concept that the family is the constant in the child's life and the primary source of strength and support for the child (American Academy of Pediatrics, Committee on Hospital Care, Institute for Patient and Family-Centered Care, 2012; Harrison, 2010).

According to the American Academy of Pediatrics, Committee on Hospital Care, Institute for Patient and Family-Centered Care (2012), family-centered care focuses on several core principles:

- Respect for the child and family
- Recognition of the effects of cultural, racial, ethnic, and socioeconomic diversity on the family's health care experience
- Identification of and expansion of the family's strengths
- Support of the family's choices related to the child's health care
- Maintenance of flexibility
- Provision of honest, unbiased information in an affirming and useful approach
- Assistance with the emotional and other support the child and family require
- Collaboration with families
- Empowerment of families

When children's health care is provided through a family-centered approach, many positive outcomes are possible, including the following.

- Anxiety is decreased.
- Children are calmer and pain management is enhanced.
- Recovery times are shortened.
- Families' confidence and problem-solving skills are improved.

- Communication between the health care team and the family is also improved, leading to greater satisfaction for both health care providers and health care consumers (families).
- A decrease in health care costs is seen and health care resources are used more effectively (American Academy of Pediatrics, Committee on Hospital Care, Institute for Patient and Family-Centered Care, 2012).

Ways to increase collaboration between the family and the health care team may include a family advisory board, a newsletter, conferences, or parent resource notebooks. Methods for increasing communication between the health care team and the family may include the use of mailboxes or dry-erase boards for updating the daily plan of care, including the parents' participation in rounds, or through a daily assessment of health status by the child or family.

Vigilant parents are committed to their child's care and most want to be present for all aspects of their child's care. They want to be part of the decision-making process regarding their child's care; they want to be heard and develop a rapport with the health care professionals caring for their child. They demonstrate resilience in their ability to make it through the emotional upheaval associated with an illness. It is important to be sensitive to the inconveniences that their child's illness may impose on the family. Address the family's emotional and spiritual needs, attend to their concerns, and provide the best accommodations possible (when the child is hospitalized) (Fig. 30.3). Practicing true family-centered care may empower the family, strengthen family resources, and help the child and family feel more secure and supported throughout the process.

Take Note!

Some parents will not know how to advocate or speak up for their child; as a nurse, you must help open this door for them.

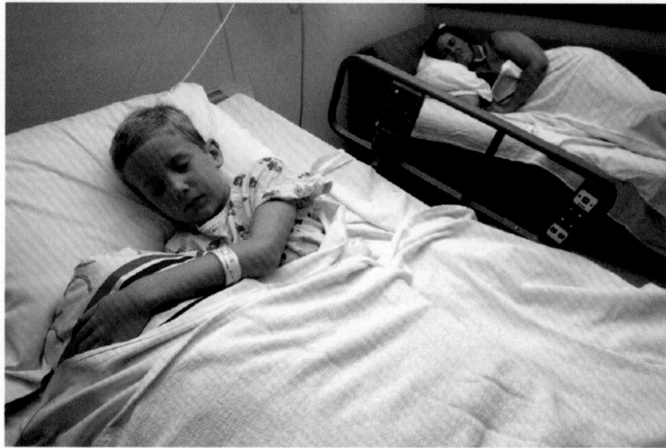

FIGURE 30.3 Providing a comfortable area for the parent to rest is an important component of family-centered care.

How could family-centered care help the Moore family described at the beginning of the chapter?

PROMOTING A SENSE OF CONTROL

During times of illness, hospitalization, or health-related interventions, the child and family can experience an extreme sense of loss of control. Providing effective communication and teaching can help foster feelings of control and improve the child's and family's ability to cope. Assisting the family to obtain necessary information, resources, and relationships contributes to optimal health care for the child and family. Communication and teaching are skills that are used continuously in pediatric nursing, no matter what the setting or the child's state of health.

Enhancing Communication

Effective communication with children and their parents is critical to providing atraumatic quality nursing care. Child- and parent-centered communication enhances child outcomes and child and family satisfaction with nursing care. Effective communication is the foundation of the therapeutic relationship and leads to increased knowledge and health care behaviors on the part of the child and family (Levetown & American Academy of Pediatrics Committee on Bioethics, 2011). Nurses are in an ideal position to improve communication in the health care environment. They need to ensure inclusion of the child and family in health conversations and to clarify misconceptions following medical encounters.

Children are often socialized to be passive participants in health care, doing as they are told, with or without protests. "As pediatric nurses, we have an obligation to listen, to hear, and to feel the voices of the children in our care" (McPherson & Thorne, 2000, p. 28). Children can inform nurses of their experiences in an accurate fashion, and nurses need to be able to discern this information from communication with the child. Children want to be respected, listened to, and understood.

Communication patterns can vary greatly from one child to the next. Some children are very talkative, while others are quiet. Children may be more apt to communicate if they are engaged in another activity. Children often use fewer words than adults and may rely more on nonverbal communication and silence. Communicating in the pediatric setting can be complicated and more difficult than in the adult setting, but remains crucial. The pediatric nurse needs to consider the age of the child, and the child's cognitive and developmental level, as well as communicating at an appropriate level with the parents. Refer to chapter 2 for information on verbal and nonverbal communication.

Developmental Techniques for Communicating With Children

Effective communication with children involves a variety of age-appropriate methods. If the child is shy, talk to the parents first to give the child time to "warm up" to you. Use specific and clear phrases in an unhurried, quiet, yet confident manner. Communicate at the child's eye level (Fig. 30.4A). Spending time and incorporating play with younger children, even just a few moments, may help them feel more at ease with you and help open the door to communication. Instead of direct questioning, use dolls, puppets, or stuffed animals with younger children (Fig. 30.4B). The use of metaphors (e.g., referring to white blood cells as "bad guy fighters") and stories can help to illustrate concepts to young and school-age children.

Older children need privacy. Provide the child or adolescent with honest answers at a developmentally appropriate level. Allow children to express their thoughts and feelings. Offer the child choices when possible, but only when they truly exist. Encourage children to write and draw about their experiences. This may increase their understanding and also draw attention to any misconceptions or fears. Box 30.3 lists requirements for communication with children and adolescents.

Children feel empowered when health care professionals communicate directly with them. Include children in discussions and avoid talking about them in their presence. Children may also desire advice about their health care and reassurance about their health status. To be effective when communicating with children of different developmental stages, the nurse must become familiar with how children of different ages communicate and then use age-appropriate techniques for effective communication.

BOX 30.3

BASICS FOR COMMUNICATING WITH CHILDREN

- Introduce yourself and explain your role.
- Position yourself at the child's level.
- Allow the child to remain near the parent if needed, so the child can remain comfortable and relaxed.
- Smile and make eye contact with the child if culturally appropriate.
- Direct your questions and explanations to the child.
- Listen attentively and pause to allow time for the child to formulate his or her thoughts.
- Use the child's or family's terms for body parts and medical care when possible.
- Speak in a calm, quiet, confident, and unhurried voice.
- Use positive, rather than negative, statements and directions.
- Encourage the child to express his or her feelings and ask questions.
- Observe for nonverbal cues.
- Ask for permission if you need to approach the child to avoid appearing threatening.

- Infants primarily communicate through touch, sight, and hearing. Communication with the infant can occur by cuddling, holding, rocking, and singing to the infant.
- When working with toddlers and preschoolers, allow them time to complete their thoughts. Though language acquisition at this age is exponential, it often takes longer for the young child to find the right words, particularly in response to a question.
- School-age children are very interested in learning and appreciate simple but honest and straightforward responses. When addressed first and allowed to respond, the school-age child may be eager to

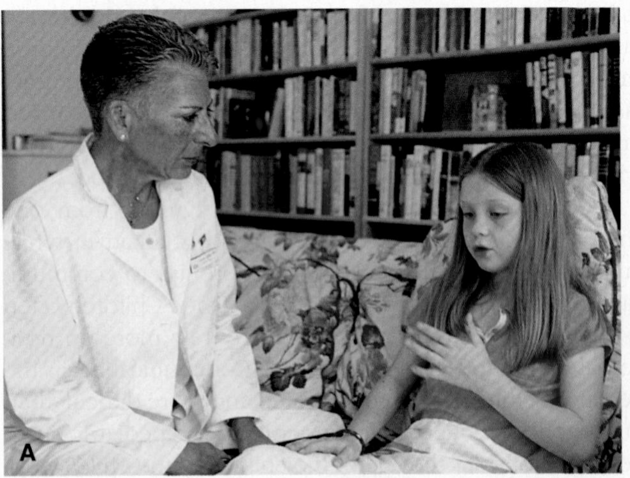

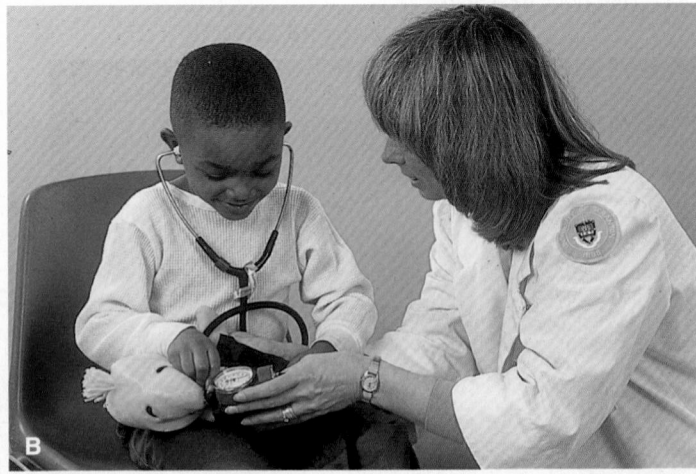

FIGURE 30.4 (A) Sitting at the child's level and allowing the child time for self-expression are steps that improve therapeutic communication. (B) Communication or teaching with dolls may be useful with younger children.

communicate. The school-age child is beginning to utilize more sophisticated language and developing problem solving and critical thinking skills.

- Adolescents tend to experience strong feelings and emotions and perceive situations in extreme terms. Building a trusting, respectful rapport is essential.

For communication tips related to the child's age, see Table 30.3.

Tips for Communicating With Parents

When communicating with parents, be honest. Parents want to feel valued and should be equal partners in the health care team. Allow the parent to express concerns and ask questions. Explain equipment and procedures thoroughly. Help the parents to understand the long-term as well as short-term effects of the treatment. Teach the parents what the child will feel like and how he or she will look during a procedure. Teach and encourage the parent to perform as much of the child's care as is reasonable and permitted. Ask the parent about his or her perception of the child's progress. Allowing the parents to be involved in the care of their child gives them a sense of control and lets them know they are valued by the health care team. Provide parents with positive reinforcement, reassurance, guidance, and support. Refer to chapter 2 for more information on communication across cultures, working with interpreters, and communicating with deaf or hearing impaired children.

In the beginning of the chapter you were introduced to Emma Moore. Discuss ways to facilitate communication with Emma and her family/caregiver.

TABLE 30.3 COMMUNICATING EFFECTIVELY WITH CHILDREN

Age	Techniques
Infants	• Respond to crying in a timely fashion. • Allow the infant time to warm up to you. • Use a soothing and calming tone when speaking to the infant. • Talk to the infant directly. • Communication through play may be helpful with older infants. • Watch for signs of overstimulation such as closing eyes, turning away, yawning, and irritability.
Toddlers	• Approach toddlers carefully; they are often not only fearful but also quite resistant. • Use the toddler's preferred words for objects or actions so he or she is better able to understand. • Toddlers enjoy stories, dolls, and books. • Participate in parallel play to help start communication. • Prepare toddlers for procedures just before they are about to occur.
Preschoolers	• Use play, puppets, or storytelling via a third-party approach. • Speak honestly. • Use simple, concrete terms. • Ask specific questions. • Allow the child to have choices as appropriate. • Participate in imaginative play to help open communication. • Prepare preschoolers about 1 hour prior to a procedure.
School-age children	• Use diagrams, illustrations, books, and videos. • Allow the child to honestly express feelings. • Use third-party stories to elicit desired information (such as "some children feel anxious about...."). • Allow the child to ask questions related to care and treatment. Give the child adequate time for all of the questions to be answered. • Prepare the child a few days in advance for a procedure.
Adolescents	• Always respect the teenager's need for privacy. • Ensure confidentiality. • Remain nonjudgemental. • Listen attentively and speak respectfully. • Use appropriate medical terminology, defining words as necessary. • Use creativity and humor. • Do not force the adolescent to talk as this may shut down communication. • Prepare the teen up to 1 week prior to a procedure.

Teaching Children and Families

Regardless of the type of practice or health care setting, nurses are in a unique position to help families manage the health care needs of their child. Indeed, the family has a right and a responsibility to participate fully in making decisions about health care processes for their child. This is true whether the child is hospitalized with a long-term, devastating illness or needs only health maintenance activities. To accomplish this, families need to be knowledgeable about such things as their child's condition, the health care management plan, and when and how to contact health care providers. With the limited time available in all health care arenas and shortened stays in inpatient facilities, the pediatric nurse must focus on teaching goals and begin teaching at the earliest opportunity.

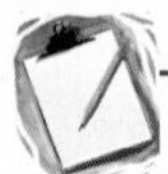

Take Note!

There is no prescription more valuable than knowledge.

—C. Everett Koop, MD, former Surgeon General of the United States (Dhand, 2000).

Patient education occurs when nurses share information, knowledge, and skills with families, thus empowering them to take responsibility for their child's health care. Through patient education, families can overcome feelings of powerlessness and helplessness and gain the confidence and ability to step to the forefront of the health care team. Nurses spend innumerable hours teaching children and families; in fact, on some days in the hospital, more teaching than nursing care is provided. Given the importance of, and the amount of time spent on, child and family education, each nurse should become an expert at basic patient education principles. See Healthy People, 2020.

Goals of Child and Family Education

The goals of child and family education are to:

- Improve the child's and family's health literacy
- Encourage communication with health care providers
- Improve health outcomes and promote healthy lifestyles
- Encourage involvement of the child and family in care and decision making about care
- Improve compliance with care and treatment plan
- Promote a sense of autonomy and control

Overall goals for the child and family include the ability of children and families to make informed decisions, to perform basic health care skills, to recognize when the child has a problem and know how to respond to the problem, and to know how to get answers when questions arise.

HEALTHY PEOPLE 2020

Objective	Nursing Significance
Increase the proportion of persons who report that their physicians have satisfactory communication skills (developmental) Improve the health literacy of the population	• Assess health learning needs of children and their families. • Plan health care education in collaboration with children and their families. • Provide health education at each patient encounter. • Assess for poor health literacy skills.

Healthy People Objectives retrieved from http://www.healthypeople.gov

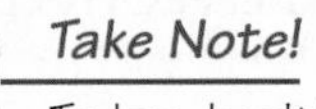

Take Note!

Today health care consumers have information available at their fingertips. It is important to steer children and their families to reliable and credible health care resources. Refer to chapter 2 for information on steps of client and family education.

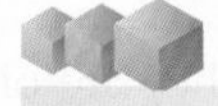

Concept Mastery Alert

Teaching Techniques

When given a diagnosis that will have a significant impact on a family's life, it is important for the nurse to allow the parents time to absorb the information about the disorder. The nurse should give parents only small amounts of information at a time to allow them time to absorb it.

TEACHING CHILDREN AND ADOLESCENTS

Teaching children and adolescents is a vital part of pediatric nursing practice. Children and adolescents have a great need for information about their illness as they attempt to master their anxiety and restore feelings of competency, self-confidence, and hope. As with adults, they learn best when their input is valued and they are actively involved in the learning process. The age and developmental level of the child will determine the amount, format, and timing of the information given. Before beginning to teach a child, it is important to establish rapport and lay the foundation for good communication. Refer to Developmental Techniques for Communicating With Children above and Table 30.3 for additional information related to communicating well with children and adolescents.

TABLE 30.4 GENERAL TEACHING TIPS FOR YOUNG CHILDREN

Teaching Tips	Practical Application
Offer simple, concise, concrete explanations based on the assessed needs, questions, and developmental level of the child.	Use a child's senses and relate what a procedure will look, sound, smell, taste, or feel like ("The MRI machine will sound very loud, like a big train").
Be honest, even when the information you need to convey is not positive. This helps the child to form a bond of trust and confidence with caregivers.	Use the family's words that the child understands; use "soft words" ("This will feel warm" instead of "This will burn").
Time explanations to decrease anxiety and excess worry before the event. Avoid telling unpleasant news close to bedtime.	As a general rule, give toddlers information about procedures, medicines, and other interventions immediately beforehand; give 4- to 7-year-olds information 1 or 2 days in advance.
Parents know their child best. Eliciting information from them about their child's past behaviors and coping skills can often mean the difference between a positive and negative experience for their child.	Teach parents how to coach their child with pain management, visualization, or other methods of distraction when appropriate ("Remember when we went to the beach …").
Provide an active role for the child. This helps to foster a child's sense of self-confidence and control over the situation.	Allow the child to help with simple self-care activities such as holding a dressing or piece of tape. Provide props and dolls to touch and feel as much as possible ("Your job is to keep your hands still").
Children's wishes must be respected when they verbalize or demonstrate that they do not want more information.	Keep explanations short and simple; know when to stop teaching.
Praise the child and let him or her know how much you appreciate his or her help and cooperation.	Use "please" and "thank you" often ("Thank you. I like the way you held still for me").

Teaching Preschool Children. When teaching young children, the nurse or family assumes part or all of the responsibility for what is learned, how it is learned, and when it is learned. Because they have vivid imaginations, young children often attempt to invent pieces of information, or they pick up bits and pieces of misinformation that can lead to false assumptions. Skillfully delivered and timed information can promote trust, calmness, and control in an otherwise apprehensive and uncooperative preschooler. Table 30.4 presents some general guidelines for teaching young children.

Teaching School-Age Children. Unless they are quite ill, school-age children usually want to participate in their care. They have a need to cooperate and achieve. When teaching, speak directly to them and include them in the education plan. Teach the school-age child and parent together, as parents can often learn by observing the care being given and taught to their child. Table 30.5 provides some general guidelines to keep in mind when teaching school-age children.

Teaching Adolescents. Adolescents are particularly sensitive about maintaining body image and feelings of control and autonomy. This is especially important with health care processes and decisions that affect them. Table 30.6 gives guidelines to use when teaching adolescents. Refer to chapter 2 for information on evaluating learning and documenting education.

Consider This!

Elsa is a 5-year-old girl on your unit who was recently diagnosed with diabetes. She is getting ready to be discharged home at the end of the week. Her grandparents are her primary care givers.

What concerns regarding learning would you take into consideration during your assessment?

Describe different teaching strategies you would utilize with Elsa and her family.

How would you evaluate learning with Elsa and her family?

TABLE 30.5 GENERAL GUIDELINES WHEN TEACHING SCHOOL-AGE CHILDREN

Teaching Tips	Practical Application
Allow the child some control and involvement in the decision-making process.	Offer choices whenever possible (taking the medicine with juice or milk), but don't offer choices when there are no alternatives (taking the medicine).
Children can relate present-day happenings to past experiences.	Use examples and past experiences that are familiar to the child ("Remember when you were first learning to swim …").
Achievement and accomplishment are very important to children at this age, so anything they can be actively involved in will help them adjust and learn.	Provide an active role and allow the child to do as much of his or her care as possible. Use props, dolls, games, and computers to enhance learning.
At this age, most children are able to sequence, understand cause and effect, and make sense of time.	Teach children the steps involved and how long it will take ("Today I'm going to teach you how to change your dressing. This will help keep your cut clean. First, wash your hands …").
Gaining control over the situation and preparing mentally are important for their self-confidence.	Provide information 3 to 7 days in advance, depending on the child's age and developmental level.
Praise the child and let him or her know how much you appreciate his or her help and cooperation.	Use "please" and "thank you" often ("Thanks! You did a great job using your inhaler").

TABLE 30.6 GENERAL GUIDELINES WHEN TEACHING ADOLESCENTS

Teaching Tips	Practical Application
Allow teens to be in control and involved in the decision-making process.	Speak directly to teens; consider their input in all decisions about their care and education.
Adolescents can process abstract information and understand how their actions affect long-term outcomes.	Provide reasons why something is important and discuss how their lives will be affected by their decision to take care of their health needs ("If you take your asthma medicine, you'll be better able to play tennis").
Adolescents are very concerned about how they look and how they fit in with peers.	Collaborate with the teen to develop acceptable solutions and strategies for dealing with health issues that affect personal appearance and peer acceptance (e.g., wig vs. head scarves for hair loss from chemotherapy).
Adolescents strive for independence and have personal values and ideologies that may conflict with those of parents and the medical community.	Expect some noncompliance with care, despite your best educational efforts. Work together to achieve win–win outcomes of educational goals.

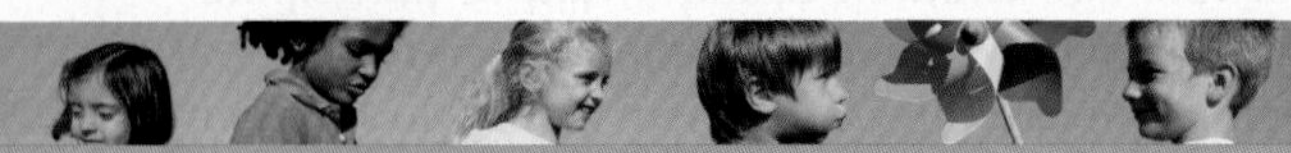

KEY CONCEPTS

- Atraumatic care focuses on minimizing stressors and separation from the family and promoting a sense of control for the child and family.
- Children and families need appropriate explanation and education before a procedure is performed. Preparation may include explaining the procedure as well as physically preparing the child. Appropriate preparation helps to decrease the child's and family's anxiety, promote the child's cooperation, and support the child's and family's coping skills.
- A major aspect of preparation involves play.

- Include the child's parents in preparation because parents are usually the greatest source of comfort for the child.
- Be short, simple, and appropriate in explaining situations at the child's level of development. Explain what is to be done and what is expected of the child.
- Utilize a CLS when available.
- Family-centered care involves a beneficial partnership between the patient, family, and health care providers in planning, providing, and evaluating care.
- Family-centered care is based on the concept that the family is the primary source of strength and support for the child.
- Family-centered care includes: respect for the child and family, recognition of cultural diversity, identification of the family's strengths, assistance with emotional and other support of the family, providing honest and unbiased information, and collaborating and empowering families.
- Maintain open and honest lines of communication with children and their families.
- Therapeutic communication involves the use of open-ended questions, reflection, paraphrasing, acknowledgement of emotions, and active listening.
- To communicate effectively with children, provide information and support on the child's developmental level and utilize age-appropriate methods.
- When communicating with parents, be honest. Parents want to feel valued and should be equal partners in the health care team.
- It is vital for the family to have knowledge about their child's health.
- Patient education begins with the first patient encounter and proceeds through discharge and beyond. Reassessment after each step or change in the process is critical to success.

REFERENCES AND RECOMMENDED READINGS

American Academy of Pediatrics, Child Life Council and Committee on Hospital Care. (2006). Child life services. *Pediatrics, 118*(4), 1757–1763. Retrieved November 14, 2013, from http://pediatrics.aappublications.org/content/118/4/1757 Reaffirmed February 2012

American Academy of Pediatrics, Committee on Hospital Care, Institute for Patient and Family-Centered Care. (2012). *Policy statement: Patient and family-centered care and the pediatrician's role*. Retrieved August 26, 2013, from http://pediatrics.aappublications.org/content/129/2/394.full.pdf+html. doi: 10.1542/peds.2011–3084

American Academy of Pediatrics, Committee on Pediatric Workforce. (2008). *Ensuring culturally effective pediatric care: Implications for education and health policy*. Retrieved August 29, 2013, from http://aappolicy.aappublications.org/cgi/content/abstract/pediatrics;114/6/1677

Bennett, C., & Pflaumer, D. (n.d.). *Positioning & comfort techniques*. Orlando, FL: Florida Children's Hospital.

Child life: Empowering children and families to cope with life's challenges. Retrieved August 25, 2013, from http://www.childlife.org/files/AboutChildLife.pdf

Child Life Council. (2010b). *How a child life specialist can help you*. Retrieved August 25, 2013, from http://www.childlife.org/the%20child%20life%20profession/HowaChildLifeSpecialistCanHelpYou.cfm

Dhand, A. (2000). *The health care and Internet dynamic: A conversation with C. Everett Koop M.D. '37*. Retrieved July 8, 2009, from http://dujs.dartmouth.edu/1999 F/Koop.pdf

Durani, Y. (2011). Preparing your child for surgery. Kids Health from Demours. Retrieved from http://kidshealth.org/parent/system/surgery/hosp_surgery.html#

Florida Children's Hospital, Child Life Department. (n.d.). *Atraumatic care: An age specific approach*. Orlando, FL: Author.

Florida Children's Hospital, Child Life Department. (n.d.). *Suggested vocabulary to use with children*. Orlando, FL: Author.

Harrison, T. M. (2010). Family-centered pediatric nursing care: State of the science. *Journal of Pediatric Nursing, 25*(5), 335–343.

Koller, D. (2007) Child life council evidence-based practice statement preparing children and adolescents for medical procedures. Child Life Council. http://www.childlife.org/files/ebppreparationstatement-complete.pdf

Kolucki, B., & Lemish, D. (2011). *Principles and practices to nurture, inspire, excite, educate and heal communicating with children*. Retrieved on August 29, 2013, at http://www.unicef.org/cwc/files/CwC_Web%282%29.pdf

Leahy, S., Kennedy, R. M., Hesselgrave, J., Gurwitch, K., Barkey, M., & Millar, T. F. (2008). On the front lines: Lessons learned in implementing multidisciplinary peripheral venous access pain-management programs in pediatric hospitals. *Pediatrics, 122*, S161–S170. Retrieved March 31, 2011, from http://pediatrics.aappublications.org/cgi/reprint/122/Supplement_3/S161.pdf

Levetown, M., American Academy of Pediatrics Committee on Bioethics. (2011). Communicating with children and families: From everyday interactions to skill in conveying distressing information. *Pediatrics, 121*(5), e1441–e1460. (doi: 10.1542/peds.2008–0565)

Manneheim, J. K. (2012). *Preschooler test or procedure preparation*. Retreived August 26, 2013, from http://www.nlm.nih.gov/medlineplus/ency/article/002057.htm

McPherson, G., & Thorne, S. (2000). Children's voices: Can we hear them? *Journal of pediatric nursing, 15*(1), 22–29.

Wong, D. L. (n.d.). *Innovative approaches for atraumatic cancer care*. Retrieved August 25, 2013, from http://www.authorstream.com/presentation/Carolina-48857-op077-INNOVATIVE-APPROACHES-ATRAUMATIC-CANCER-CARE-DEFINITION-SOURCES-PATIENT-FAMILY-STRESSORS-as-Entertainment-ppt-powerpoint/

CHAPTER WORKSHEET

MULTIPLE CHOICE QUESTIONS

1. When providing atraumatic care to a child, which action would be the most appropriate?
   a. Applying restraints for any procedure that would be uncomfortable
   b. Keeping the lights on in the child's room throughout the day and night
   c. Limiting the use of topical anesthetics for painful injections
   d. Allowing parents and children an informed choice about being together
2. A 2-year-old boy is scheduled to undergo an endoscopic procedure. His parents are asking when they should tell him about it. Based on the nurse's understanding of the child's developmental stage, when would be the most appropriate time to prepare the child for the procedure?
   a. About 1 week before the scheduled date
   b. A few days in advance of the scheduled date
   c. About 1 hour before the procedure is to occur
   d. Just before the procedure is to be performed
3. When working with children and families, which is a critical strategy for promoting therapeutic communication?
   a. Detailed explanations
   b. Attentive listening
   c. Comforting touch
   d. Closed-ended questions
4. The nurse is caring for a 2-year-old in the hospital, and the mother expresses concern that the toddler will be scared. Which response by the nurse would be most appropriate?
   a. "Don't worry; we practice family-centered and atraumatic care here."
   b. "We will do our best to minimize the stress that your child experiences."
   c. "It will probably be upsetting for you as well, so you should stay home."
   d. "Our practice of atraumatic care will eliminate all pain and stress for your child."
5. When planning education for a child and parents, what is the first step the nurse should take?
   a. Decide which procedures and medications the child will be discharged on.
   b. Determine the child's and family's learning needs and styles.
   c. Ask the family if they have ever performed this type of procedure.
   d. Tell the child and family what the goals of the teaching session are.

CRITICAL THINKING EXERCISES

1. A 5-year-old boy is being admitted to your unit. The physician has ordered IV fluids along with laboratory work including a complete blood count, electrolytes, and a urine culture. As his nurse, how will you prepare him and his family before the procedure and support them during and after the procedure, to promote the best outcome and to ensure atraumatic care?
2. An 8-year-old is admitted to your nursing unit. Please describe the steps the nurse should take to provide health care teaching to this child.

STUDY ACTIVITIES

1. Develop a teaching plan for one of the families that you care for in the clinical setting. Be sure to follow the appropriate steps for providing education.
2. Interview a CLS about the effects that the traditional (not atraumatic) approach to restraining a child for procedures might have on a child of various ages.
3. Research the availability of language interpreters and translators in your local community, compiling a list of the available resources.
4. Describe health education topics that would be appropriate in a school setting for elementary students.

BRINGING IT ALL TOGETHER: A CASE STUDY

Mia, a 5-year-old girl, is admitted to your unit for pneumonia not improving at home on oral antibiotics. Orders for Mia include an IV insertion to begin IV antibiotics.

Go to thePoint to find questions to consider about this case.

31

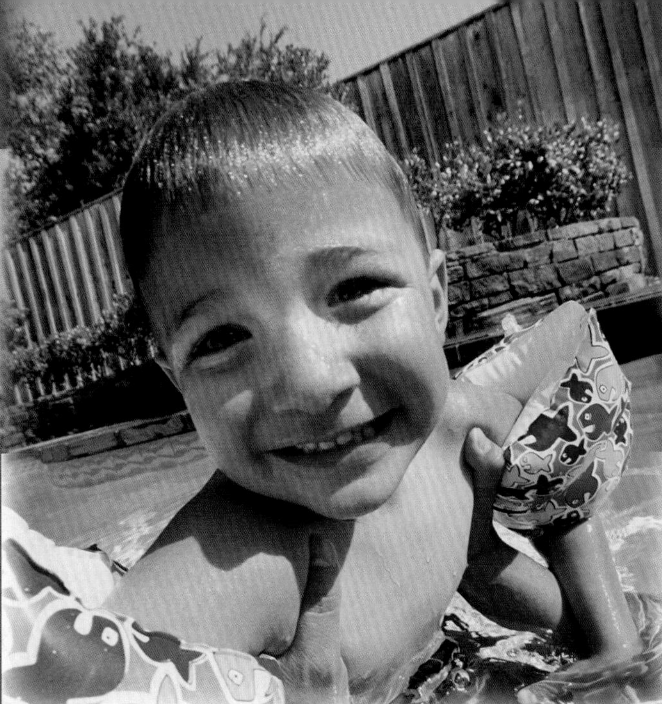

WOW

Words of Wisdom

It is never too late to start prevention. It begins with a genuine desire for health improvement.

Health Supervision

KEY TERMS

active immunity
developmental screenings
developmental surveillance
immunity
medical home
passive immunity
risk assessment
screening tests
selective screening
universal screening

Learning Objectives

Upon completion of the chapter, you will be able to:

1. Describe the principles of health supervision.
2. Identify challenges to health supervision for children with chronic illnesses.
3. List the three components of a health supervision visit.
4. Use instruments appropriately for developmental surveillance and screening of children.
5. Demonstrate knowledge of the principles of immunization.
6. Identify barriers to immunization.
7. Identify the key components of health promotion.
8. Describe the role of anticipatory guidance in health promotion.

***Three-year-old* Maya Randall and 9-month-old Evan Randall are brought to the clinic by their father. Maya was last seen in the clinic when she was 1 year old and Evan has never been seen. The father says that they have both been healthy so they did not need to come to the clinic before this. Maya is complaining of a sore throat, which is what prompted today's visit.**

PRINCIPLES OF HEALTH SUPERVISION

Health supervision involves providing services proactively with the goal of optimizing the child's level of functioning. It ensures the child is growing and developing appropriately and it promotes the best possible health of the child by teaching parents and children about preventing injury and illness (e.g., proper immunizations and anticipatory guidance). This chapter is organized around the three components of health supervision: developmental surveillance and screening; injury and disease prevention; and health promotion. Health supervision of the child begins at birth and continues through adolescence. It is vital to every child and is most effective when the child has a centralized source of health care. Any place publicly accessible by children and families can be an appropriate setting for health supervision services—private physicians' offices, community health departments, sliding-scale clinics, homeless shelters, day care centers, and schools. The framework for the health supervision visit is developed from national guidelines available through the U.S. Department of Health and Human Services (DHHS), the American Medical Association (AMA), and the American Academy of Pediatrics (AAP). These organizations also provide guidelines for children with chronic health problems and services and information regarding unique situations such as the internationally adopted child.

Wellness

The focus of pediatric health supervision is wellness. The health supervision visit provides an opportunity to maximize health promotion for the child, family, and community. Nurses have the ability to promote optimal health during these encounters. Health supervision visits must be viewed as part of a continuum of care, not as the accomplishment of isolated tasks.

Medical Home

A **medical home** is an approach to care that builds a long-term and comprehensive relationship with the family. This continuing relationship promotes trust between the pediatric care team and the family and leads to comprehensive, continuous, coordinated, and cost-effective care. The medical home is the setting that allows the highest level of health supervision. To be effective, the medical home must be accessible, family centered, culturally effective, and community based. It must be integrated into the child's world, not adjacent to it. Characteristics of a medical home are displayed in Box 31.1.

BOX 31.1

CHARACTERISTICS OF A MEDICAL HOME

- Care accessible and in the child's community
- All insurance, including Medicaid, accepted
- Family-centered care provided
- Child or family able to speak directly to the physician when needed
- Partnership based on mutual trust and respect between the family and pediatric care team
  - Preventive care activities provided
  - Ambulatory and inpatient care available 24 hours a day
  - Continuity of care from infancy through adolescence
- Coordinated care with other care providers
- Availability of subspecialty consultation and referrals
- Work with family to meet the nonmedical and medical needs of the child and family
  - Interactive relationships with school and community agencies
  - A centralized database containing all pertinent information
- Concern for the well-being of the child and family expressed
- Respect for family's cultural and religious beliefs

Adapted from American Academy of Pediatrics, National Center for Medical Home Implementation (n.d.). What is a family centered medical home. The medical home. Retrieved from http://www.medicalhomeinfo.org/

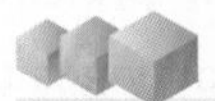
Concept Mastery Alert

Medical Home

A pediatric medical home provides continuity of care from infancy through adolescence. A medical home contains a centralized database that contains all information about a child that pertains to their health status.

Partnerships

The child is the focus of the health supervision visit. However, the child's health is linked to the needs and resources of his or her family and community. For instance, if the family is in turmoil because of divorce, drug abuse, or parental health problems, the child is less likely to receive the attention and energy that he or she needs to thrive. Likewise, a community with high levels of poverty, poor infrastructure, and lack of resources will not be able to provide the support services needed to allow children to reach their full potential. To be effective, the nurse must offer commitment and develop an ongoing partnership with the child, family, and community. These partnerships allow for mutual goal setting, marshalling of resources, and development of optimal health practices.

The partnership between the child and the health supervision team develops over time. In infancy the family is the surrogate for the child in the partnership.

The child's participation in the partnership increases at a rate that is developmentally appropriate. The child's increasing influence in the partnership allows the nurse to tailor health supervision to the child's needs. The partnership allows the child to take increasing responsibility for his or her personal health and optimizes health promotion.

Nurses must validate and enhance the role of family members as they influence and inform the child's concept of wellness. The health care community must involve the family to have a significant impact on a child's health. The family wants the best possible outcome for their child, and health care decisions are based on the knowledge they possess. The nurse can greatly facilitate trust by acknowledging that the family has unique insights to offer on their child's health. Nurses can also strengthen the partnership between the family and the health care community by recognizing the family's healthy practices, addressing their health issues, and strengthening their skills. By contributing to the partnership, both the nurse and the family enhance the chance of success for health care plans, but families are the ones who must implement any health care strategy and know what expected outcomes are reasonable. Their feedback is invaluable to formulating an effective long-term health supervision plan that optimizes their child's wellness.

Take Note!

Observe the parent–child interaction during the health supervision visit. The nurse can learn much about the family dynamic by observing the family for behavioral clues:

- Does the parent make eye contact with the infant?
- Does the parent anticipate and respond to the infant's needs?
- Are parents effective when dealing with a toddler's temper tantrum?
- Do the parents' comments increase the school-age child's sense of self-worth?

Behavioral observations are crucial to the proper assessment of the family's needs and issues.

Partnerships between the community and the health promotion team benefit the community as well as individual children. When nurses develop partnerships with community agencies such as schools, churches, and ancillary health facilities, barriers to care can be overcome. The nurse becomes aware of available resources in the community that can benefit an individual family. With input from community partners, the nurse can perform an assessment of the community's needs. The assessment then provides the foundation for the development of community-based health promotion programs. These programs expand the resources of the community, which in turn enhances the health of its members.

Special Issues in Health Supervision

Special issues in health supervision include cultural influences, community influences, health supervision and the chronically ill child, and health supervision and the internationally adopted child.

Cultural Influences on Health Supervision

A person's definition of health is influenced by his or her culture. Successful interactions result when the nurse is aware of the beliefs and interactive styles that are often present in members of a specific culture. If the goals of the health care plan are not consistent with the health belief system of the family, the plan has little chance for success. Optimal wellness for the child requires the nurse and the family to negotiate a mutually acceptable plan of care. A plan must balance the cultural beliefs and practices of the family with those of the health care establishment. The nurse must possess cultural competence and sensitivity for the partnership to be successful.

Most health promotion and disease prevention strategies in the United States have a future-based orientation, and view the child as an active and controlling agent in his or her own health. This reflects the dominant culture; however, the challenge to the nurse is to develop strategies that are meaningful to children from other cultures. Significant numbers of children belong to cultures with a present-based orientation. These cultures are more concerned about what is going on now. For these children, health promotion activities need shorter-term goals and outcomes to be useful. Children with a fatalistic world view will see any actions on their part as ineffective. They may feel that a god figure or supernatural forces control their fate and that health is a gift to be appreciated, not a goal to be pursued. Certain cultures believe health is the result of being in harmony within oneself and the larger universe. From this viewpoint, taking a medication or receiving a treatment may not be an effective way to restore health because it does not address the problem of being "out of harmony."

However, just because an individual belongs to a certain culture does not guarantee that he or she subscribes to all of its values. The nurse should explore each child's specific beliefs during the health interview.

Community Influences on Health Supervision

The child is a member of a community as well as a family and a culture. Each community has unique strengths, weaknesses, and values. A community can be a contributor to a child's health or be the cause of his or her illnesses. The child's health cannot be totally separated from the health of the surrounding community.

Ideally, the child's medical home is within the family's community. If home and access to medical care are close, barriers such as lack of transportation, expense of travel, and time away from the parents' workplace are reduced. Having the medical home within the community facilitates bonds between the health team and schools, churches, and support services and agencies. Community support and resources are necessary for children with significant problems. A close working relationship between the child's physician and community agencies is an enormous benefit to the child (see the earlier section on partnerships).

The community assessment may reveal problems that are causing or contributing to the child's health problems. A deteriorating infrastructure can contribute to decreased access to care and increased risk of injury or illness. Poverty has been linked to low birthweight and premature birth, among other health problems (Centers for Disease Control and Prevention [CDC], 2012a). Substandard housing can be directly related to lead poisoning and asthma (CDC, 2013d). A thorough knowledge of the family's community is needed before a health surveillance program can be effective.

Health Supervision and the Child With Chronic Illness

Effective health supervision must be responsive to the individual child's situation. The child with a chronic illness needs to be assessed repeatedly to determine his or her health maintenance needs. These assessments determine the frequency of visits and types of interventions needed. The impact of the illness on the child's functional health patterns determines whether standard health supervision visits need to be augmented.

An effective partnership among the child's medical home, family, and community is vital for a child with a chronic illness. Coordination of specialty care, community agencies, and family support networks enhances the quality of life and health of these children. Access to care and services minimizes the risk of injury from the illness. Support groups and community-based resources optimize the family's adaptation to the stressors of chronic illness.

Comprehensive health supervision includes frequent psychosocial assessments. Issues to be covered include:

- Health insurance coverage
- Transportation to health care facilities
- Financial stressors
- Family coping
- School's response to the chronic illness

These are often stressful and emotionally charged issues. The nurse with a trusting and ongoing relationship with the child and family is in the best position to help with these issues. The nurse can assist the family to find financial and medical assistance programs, take advantage of community resources, and participate in support groups. The nurse can also educate school personnel about the child's illness and assist them in maximizing the child's potential for academic success.

Health Supervision and the Child Adopted Internationally

In 2013, approximately 7,090 children were adopted from countries outside the United States, many from areas with a high prevalence of infectious diseases (Intercountry Adoption, Bureau of Consular Affairs, U.S. Department of State, 2014). China, Ethiopia, and Ukraine supplied over half of all international adoptees in 2013, followed by the Democratic Republic of the Congo and Haiti (Intercountry Adoption, Bureau of Consular Affairs, U.S. Department of State, 2014). Health supervision of the internationally adopted child must include comprehensive screening for infectious diseases, disorders of growth and development, along with vision and hearing and any additional testing based on diseases prevalent in their country of origin (Simms & Wilson, 2011) Proper screening is important not only to the child's health but also to the adopting family and the larger community. Screening is recommended within the first few weeks of the child's arrival into the United States.

Intestinal parasites are a common problem and infected children are frequently symptom-free, so a thorough history and physical examination along with universal screening is recommended (Simms & Wilson, 2011).

Universal screening for hepatitis B, C, and A, varicella virus, HIV, syphilis, and tuberculosis infections is recommended (Simms & Wilson, 2011). Due to lack of resources in the home country, screening and treatment for these diseases are sporadic and ineffective. If testing is documented, it is likely to be unreliable. Testing supplies may have been outdated or improperly stored. Also, the test may have been performed before the child's seroconversion occurred.

COMPONENTS OF HEALTH SUPERVISION

Developmental surveillance and screening, injury and disease prevention, and health promotion are the critical components of health supervision for children. Health supervision visits for children without health problems and appropriate growth and development are recommended at birth, within the first week of life, by 1 month, then at 2 months, 4 months, 6 months, 9 months, 12 months, 15 months, 18 months, 24 months, 30 months, and then yearly until age 21 (Bright Futures/American Academy of Pediatrics [AAP], 2014). Children with special needs or concerns will have more frequent and intensive visits. Health supervision visits include assessment of physical health along with intellectual and social development and parent–child interaction.

Each health supervision visit will include (Bright Futures/AAP, 2014):

- A history and physical assessment, including head circumference (until 2 years of age), height, and weight
- Developmental/behavioral assessment
- Sensory screening (vision and hearing)
- Appropriate at-risk screening (such as lead screening, anemia screening, tuberculin test, hypertension screening, cholesterol screening)
- Immunizations
- Health promotion/anticipatory guidance (injury prevention, violence prevention, nutrition counseling)

Disease prevention and health promotion are concepts well established in adult health supervision. Injury prevention and developmental surveillance/screening are additional components of pediatric health supervision visits that help every child achieve his or her optimal state of wellness.

Developmental Surveillance and Screening

Developmental surveillance is an ongoing collection of skilled observations made over time during health care visits. Components include:

- Noting and addressing parental concerns
- Obtaining a developmental history
- Making accurate observations
- Consulting with relevant professionals

Developmental screenings are brief assessment procedures that identify children who warrant more intensive assessment and testing. Developmental screening assessments may be observational or by caregiver report (Fig. 31.1).

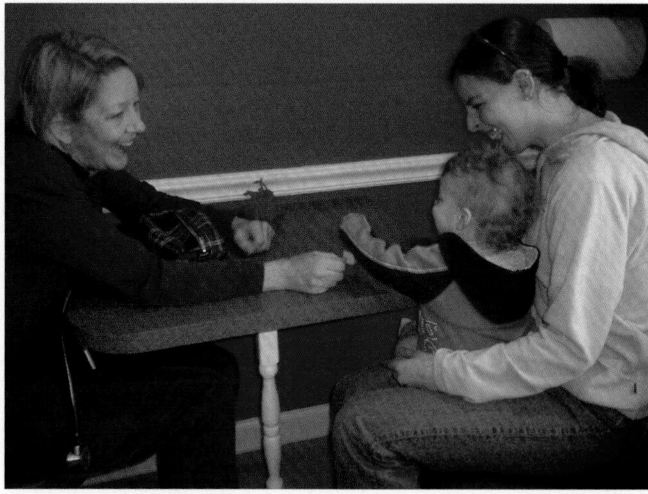

FIGURE 31.1 Developmental screening provides the opportunity for the nurse to identify problems in the child's development.

Development, or the emergence of the child's abilities, is a longitudinal process. Within the trust and security of the medical home, family and physicians can share observations and concerns. In collaboration, the family and the physician observe the child's accomplishments or milestones over time. Data collection for developmental surveillance of infants and young children is performed through developmental questionnaires, physician observations, and a thorough physical examination. School records and test results can provide academic performance data for the older child. Input from teachers, coaches, and other adults involved with the child can give insight into the child's emotional and social development.

When developmental delay is suspected, frequent developmental surveillance is warranted. Re-emphasizing parental roles and responsibilities fosters cooperation and compliance. It is therefore crucial that parents understand the need for frequent assessments. A pattern of developmental delays warrants a formal evaluation.

The pediatric nurse must understand normal growth and development and become proficient at screening for problems related to development. The historical information obtained from the parent or primary caregiver about developmental milestones may indicate warning signs or identify risks for developmental delay (Table 31.1). Factors placing the infant or toddler at risk for developmental problems include:

- Birthweight less than 1.5 kg
- Gestational age less than 33 weeks
- Central nervous system abnormality
- Hypoxic ischemic encephalopathy
- Maternal prenatal alcohol or drug abuse
- Hypertonia
- Hypotonia
- Hyperbilirubinemia requiring exchange transfusion
- Kernicterus
- Congenital malformations
- Symmetric intrauterine growth deficiency
- Perinatal or congenital infection
- Suspected sensory impairment
- Chronic (more than 3 months) otitis media with effusion
- Inborn error of metabolism
- HIV infection
- Lead level above 5 mg/dL
- Inappropriate parental concern about developmental issues (e.g., not allowing a developmentally appropriate 3-year-old feed him- or herself)
- Parent with less than high school education
- Single parent
- Sibling with developmental problems
- Parent with developmental disability or mental illness

TABLE 31.1 EARLY CHILDHOOD DEVELOPMENTAL WARNING SIGNS

Age	Warning Sign
Any age	No response to environmental stimulus
Any age	Persistently up on toes (longer than 30 seconds) in supported standing position
Before 3 months	Rolls over
After 2–3 months	Persistent fisting
After 4 months	Persistent head lag
5 months	Not reaching for toys
6 months	• Lack of tripod sitting • Not smiling • Primitive reflex persistence • Not babbling
9 months	No reciprocal vocalizations or facial expressions
12 months	No spoon or crayon use
15–18 months	• Not walking • No first word
Prior to 18 months	Hand dominance present
By 18 months	• Not walking • Not speaking 15 words • Does not understand function of common household items • No imitative play
After independent walking for several months	• Persistent tiptoe walking • Failure to develop a mature walking pattern
By 2 years	• Does not use two-word sentences • Does not imitate actions • Does not follow basic instructions • Cannot push a toy with wheels • Echolalia (repetitive speech)
By 3 years	• Difficulty with stairs • Frequent falling • Cannot build tower of more than four blocks • Difficulty manipulating small objects • Extreme difficulty in separation from parent or caregiver • Cannot copy a circle • Does not engage in make-believe play • Cannot communicate in short phrases • Does not understand simple instructions • Little interest in other children • Unclear speech, persistent drooling
4 years	• Cannot jump in place or ride a tricycle • Cannot stack four blocks • Cannot throw ball overhand • Does not grasp crayon with thumb and fingers • Difficulty with scribbling • Cannot copy a circle • Does not use sentences with three or more words • Cannot use the words "me" and "you" appropriately • Ignores other children or does not show interest in interactive games • Will not respond to people outside the family; still clings or cries if parents leave • Resists using toilet, dressing, sleeping • Does not engage in fantasy play

TABLE 31.1 EARLY CHILDHOOD DEVELOPMENTAL WARNING SIGNS (continued)

Age	Warning Sign
By 5 years	• Unhappy or sad often • Little interest in playing with other children • Unable to separate from parent without major protest • Is extremely aggressive • Is extremely fearful or timid, or unusually passive • Cannot build tower of six to eight blocks • Easily distracted; cannot concentrate on single activity for 5 minutes • Rarely engages in fantasy play • Trouble with eating, sleeping, or using the toilet • Cannot use plurals or past tense • Cannot brush teeth, wash and dry hands, or undress efficiently

Infants or children with any of these risk factors should be screened carefully for developmental delays. This screening should occur in a prospective manner, with screenings occurring at frequent intervals to identify concerns early.

Take Note!

Any child who "loses" a developmental milestone—for example, the child able to sit without support who now cannot—needs an immediate full evaluation, since this may indicate a significant neurologic problem.

A number of developmental screening tools are available to guide the nurse in assessing development (Table 31.2). Many screening methods assist the nurse in identifying infants and children who may have developmental delays, thus allowing for prompt identification and referral for evaluation. Additional data can be used to determine a school-age child's developmental level, include handwriting samples, ability to draw, school performance, and social skills.

In addition to developmental and behavioral surveillance at every visit, the AAP recommends performing the following additional screening tests. Perform a screening test for autism with a standardized developmental tool at 18 and 24 months or at any point that concerns about autism spectrum disorder (ASD) are raised (see thePoint http://pediatrics.aappublications.org/content/120/5/1183/T3.expansion.html). Also, perform a risk assessment for alcohol and drug use, as well as a depression screening at every visit from 11 to 21 years of age (refer to thePoint for the CRAFFT tool, as well as other AAP-recommended screening tools).

Refer to thePoint to view the full Bright Futures/AAP Periodicity Schedule.

Injury and Disease Prevention

Disease prevention is defined as interventions performed to protect children from a disease or to identify it at an early stage and lessen its consequences. These interventions are determined by the results of the nurse's assessment, nationally accepted practice guidelines, and the family's goals. Components of disease prevention include screening tests and immunizations.

Injury prevention is primarily accomplished through education, anticipatory guidance, and physical changes in the environment. Injuries can be unintentional (poisoning, falls, or drowning) or intentional (child abuse, homicide, or suicide). The types of injuries a child is most likely to encounter vary greatly among age groups. Although aggressive public health initiatives have decreased mortality rates of childhood unintentional injuries significantly in the past 50 years, rates remain high in some populations and continued vigilance and public health action remain necessary (Gilchrist, Ballesteros, & Parker, 2012).The nurse, in partnership with the family and the community, can have an enormous impact on child safety. Specific interventions are discussed in Chapters 25 through 29.

Screening Tests

Screening tests are procedures or laboratory analyses used to identify children with a certain condition. These tests are done to ensure that no child with the disorder is missed. They have a high sensitivity (a high false-positive rate) and a low specificity (a low false-negative rate). If a screening test is positive, follow-up tests with higher specificity are performed. A **risk assessment** is performed by the physician or nurse practitioner in conjunction with the child and includes objective as well as subjective data to determine the likelihood that the child will develop a condition.

In **universal screening**, an entire population is screened regardless of the child's individual risk. This type of screening is performed when a reliable risk assessment procedure is not available. In contrast, **selective screening** is done when a risk assessment

TABLE 31.2 DEVELOPMENTAL SCREENING TOOLS

Age	Screening Tool	Definition	Nursing Implications
Birth–6 years	Child Development Inventory (CDI)	Simple questions about infant, toddler, or preschooler behaviors. Measures social, self-help, gross motor, fine motor, expressive language, language comprehension, letters, numbers, and general development as appropriate	A parental-report screening tool
Birth–6 years	Ages and Stages Questionnaire (ASQ)	Assesses communication, gross motor, fine motor, personal–social, and problem-solving skills	A parental-report screening tool, scored by the nurse after completion to determine child's progress in each of the developmental areas
Birth–8 years	Parents' Evaluation of Developmental Status (PEDS)	Screens for a wide range of developmental, behavioral, and family issues	A parental-report screening tool that can also be used in nurse interview format. Also available in Spanish.
12–96 months	Batelle Developmental Inventory Screening Test	Assesses fine and gross motor, adaptive, personal–social, receptive and expressive language, and cognitive skills	Direct elicitation, parental description, and examiner observation. Requires special training
1–42 months	Bayley Scales of Infant Development II	Provides a mental and motor scale for assessment of cognitive, language, personal–social, and fine and gross motor development. A behavior rating scale is obtained during the testing.	Direct elicitation. Thorough. Requires special training
Birth–3 years	Early Language Milestone Scale	Screens for auditory expressive and receptive, visual components of speech	Requires standardized kit
2½–7 years	Denver Articulation Screening	Screens for articulation disorders	5 minutes to administer. Does not evaluate language ability
5–17 years	Goodenough–Harris Drawing Test	A nonverbal screen for mental ability (intelligence)	Child draws a person, which is analyzed for body parts, clothing, proportion, and perspective.

indicates the child has one or more risk factors for the disorder.

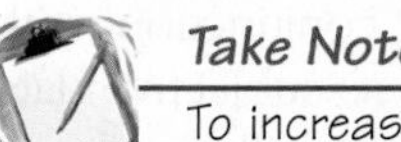

Take Note!

To increase cooperation from young children during screenings, set up a reward system. Easy-to-do rewards include:

- *Stamping the back of the child's hand with a "smiley face"*
- *Making an eye cover by placing two stickers back to back over a tongue blade and letting the child keep the cover after the screening*
- *Copying a design onto a sheet of paper and letting the child take it home to color*
- *Letting the child play with a simple device such as a penlight or stethoscope*

METABOLIC SCREENING

State law determines which metabolic screening tests are mandatory in that state. All states currently require newborn screening for 26 health conditions and some states screen for over 50 disorders (March of Dimes, 2012). In addition to screening for hearing loss, the March of Dimes currently recommends universal newborn metabolic screening tests for 30 disorders for which effective treatment is available (March of Dimes, 2012).

- Amino acid metabolism disorders: phenylketonuria, maple syrup urine disease, homocystinuria, citrullinemia, argininosuccinic acidemia, tyrosinemia type I
- Organic acid metabolism disorders: isovaleric acidemia, glutaric acidemia type I, hydroxymethylglutaric aciduria, multiple carboxylase deficiency, methylmalonic acidemia due to mutase deficiency, methylmalonic acidemia cblA and cblB forms, 3-methylcrotonyl-CoA carboxylase deficiency, propionic acidemia, β-ketothiolase deficiency
- Fatty acid oxidation disorders: medium-chain acyl-CoA dehydrogenase deficiency, very-long-chain acyl-CoA dehydrogenase deficiency, long-chain 3-OH acyl-CoA dehydrogenase deficiency, trifunctional protein deficiency, carnitine uptake defect
- Hemoglobinopathies: sickle cell anemia, HbS/β-thalassemia, HbS/C disease
- Others: congenital hypothyroidism, biotinidase deficiency, congenital adrenal hyperplasia, classical galactosemia, cystic fibrosis, critical congenital heart disease, and severe combined immunodeficiency (SCID)

During the initial health supervision visit, the nurse should confirm that newborn metabolic screening was performed prior to discharge from the birthing unit. If the test was not performed or was performed at younger than 48 hours of age, the screening should be performed at that visit. The metabolic screening results need to be noted in the child's permanent record at the medical home.

HEALTHY PEOPLE *2020*

Objective	Nursing Significance
Increase the proportion of newborns who are screened for hearing loss by age 1 month, have audiologic evaluation by age 3 months, and are enrolled in appropriate intervention services by age 6 months. Increase the proportion of persons who have had a hearing examination on schedule.	• Determine results of newborn hearing screening at first newborn check-up. • Refer any infant with possible hearing deficit for further evaluation. • Ensure infants with hearing impairment receive appropriate augmentation (hearing aids). • Ensure all children and adolescents receive hearing screenings with well-child check-ups as appropriate.

Healthy People Objectives retrieved from http://www.healthypeople.gov

HEARING SCREENING

The AAP recommends hearing screening of all infants. Hearing loss is a common condition in newborns, and even mild hearing loss can cause serious delays in social and emotional development, language acquisition, and cognitive function (Delaney, Meyers, & Ruth, 2012). Identification of hearing loss by 6 months of age is crucial to reduce the impact on the child's development (Delaney, Meyers, & Ruth, 2012). Refer to Healthy People 2020. Targeted screening based on risk factors will identify only 50% of infants with hearing loss, and with reliable screening tests available, universal screening has been implemented (Delaney, Meyers, & Ruth, 2012). Screening should be done before discharge from the birthing unit; if not, the newborn needs to be screened before 1 month of age. Behavioral observations of the infant's response to sounds, such as a ringing bell or clapping hands, are not sensitive enough to preclude mild to moderate hearing loss (Delaney, Meyers, & Ruth, 2012). Accepted methodologies for screening newborn hearing are displayed in Table 31.3.

Screening for hearing loss in older children begins with a history from the primary caregivers. If any problems are noted, audiometry should be performed. When the child is capable of following simple commands reliably, the nurse can perform some basic procedures to screen for hearing loss. The whisper test is easy to perform but to be valid requires a quiet room that is away from distractions. The Weber and Rinne tests are typically performed together and can be used to screen for sensorineural or conductive hearing loss. Refer to Table 31.3 for hearing screening methods.

Universal hearing screening with objective testing is recommended at ages 4, 5, 6, 8, and 10 (Bright Futures/AAP, 2014). At the ages of 7, 9, and 11 through 21 years, age-appropriate risk assessment should be performed (Bright Futures/AAP, 2014). See Box 31.2 for examples of risk assessment. More frequent screening is recommended if there is any behavior that indicates the child's hearing may be impaired. Repeated hearing screenings are recommended if a child has risk factors for acquired hearing loss such as those listed in Box 31.3.

VISION SCREENING

Newborns with ocular structural abnormalities are at high risk for vision impairment. Vision screening is performed at every scheduled health supervision visit. The screening procedures for children younger than 3 years of age or for nonverbal children involve evaluating the child's ability to fixate on and follow objects. The neonate should be able to fixate on an object approximatley 25 to 30 cm (10 to 12 inches) from the face. After

TABLE 31.3 HEARING SCREENING METHODS

Test Name	Age Group	Characteristics	Nursing Implications
Auditory brainstem response (ABR)	Newborn–6 months	Measures electroencephalographic waves; electrodes placed on forehead, mastoid, and nape of neck Click stimulus delivered via earphones Test results may be affected by ear debris	Infant must be quiet (sedation may be needed). Can be conducted in presence of background noise
Otoacoustic emissions (OAEs)	Newborn–6 months or developmentally delayed children at the infant's level of functioning	The machine produces clicks that stimulate cilia in the cochlea and measures the response.	Infant must be quiet. Test results may be inaccurate in first 24 hours of life. Not sufficient to detect neural hearing loss
Visual reinforcement audiometry (VRA)	6 months–2 years	Visual reward is linked to a tone signal. Child looks to the visual reward in response to the tone. Reward is activated, reinforcing the response	Child must be alert and happy for best results Schedule for after sleep/rest period
Tympanometry	Over 7 months	Measures tympanic membrane mobility and determines middle ear pressure	The probe must form a seal with the canal The child must remain still to obtain a valid result
Conditioned play audiometry (CPA)	2–4 years	Similar to VRA except uses "listening games" Child does listening game at the tone and receives social reward May be used when developmental age is 2 years	See Nursing Implications for VRA
Pure-tone (conventional) audiometry	4 years and older	Measures hearing acuity through a range of frequencies and intensities Child must wear earphones Performed in a soundproof room if possible	Teach the child the desired motor response before screening Administer conditioning trials Offer two presentations of stimulus to ensure reliability At a minimum, screen 1,000-, 2,000-, and 4,000-Hz levels at 20 dB
Whisper test	4 years and older	One ear is occluded. Examiner stands behind the child and whispers a word. The child must accurately repeat the whispered word.	The child must be in a quiet room and away from distractions The child should be alert and well rested for accurate results Consider a reward system to increase compliance
Weber test	6 years and older	Place a vibrating tuning fork in the middle of the top of the head. Ask if the sound is in one ear or both ears. The sound should be heard in both ears	The child must understand the instructions and be able to cooperate

TABLE 31.3 HEARING SCREENING METHODS (continued)

Test Name	Age Group	Characteristics	Nursing Implications
Rinne test	6 years and older	Place a vibrating tuning fork on the mastoid process to assess bone conduction. The child signals when the sound is gone Next, place a vibrating tuning fork outside the ear to test air conduction. The child signals when the sound is gone For a passing test, air conduction time should be twice as long as bone conduction time	The child must understand the instructions and be able to cooperate

fixation, the infant should be able to follow the object to the midline. By 2 months of age, the infant should be able to follow the object 180 degrees. The technique of photoscreening can help identify problems such as ocular malalignment, refractive error, and lens and retinal problems.

Take Note!

Use objects with black-and-white patterns when performing vision screening on an infant younger than 6 months of age. The infant's vision at this age is more attuned to high-contrast patterns than to colors. Try checkerboard patterns or concentric circles. Animal figures like pandas and Dalmatians also work well.

After the age of 3 years, a variety of standardized age-appropriate vision screening charts are available. These charts include the "tumbling E" and Allen figures (Fig. 31.2A, B). These charts allow for a more precise vision assessment and aid the nurse in identifying preschool children with visual acuity problems. By age 5 or 6, most children know the alphabet well enough to use the traditional Snellen chart for vision screening (Fig. 31.2C). Refer to Healthy People 2020. Table 31.4 gives further information about vision screening tools.

Screenings should be performed when children are alert, as fatigue and lack of interest can mimic poor vision. When using any vision screening chart, several simple steps need to be followed):

- Place the chart at the child's eye level.
- Make sure there is sufficient lighting.
- Place a mark on the floor approximately 300 to 600 cm (10 to 20 feet) from the chart (distance depends on what the tool is calibrated for).
- Align the child's heels on the mark.
- Have the child read each line with one eye covered and then with the other eye covered. Explain to the child to keep the eye covered but open (Fig. 31.3).
- Have the child read each line with both eyes.

BOX 31.2

HEARING RISK ASSESSMENT

Ages 3 months to 4 years

- Auditory skill monitoring
- Developmental surveillance
- Assessment of parental concerns

Age 4 years

- Difficulty hearing on the telephone
- Difficulty hearing people in a noisy background
- Frequent asking of others to repeat themselves
- Turning the television up too loudly

BOX 31.3

RISK FACTORS FOR HEARING IMPAIRMENT

- Family history of hearing loss
- Prenatal infection
- Anomalies of the head, face, or ears
- Low birthweight (<1.5 kg)
- Hyperbilirubinemia requiring exchange transfusion
- Ototoxic medications
- Low Apgar scores: 4 or less at 1 minute, or 6 or less at 5 minutes
- Mechanical ventilation lasting 5 days
- Syndrome associated with hearing loss
- Head trauma
- Bacterial meningitis
- Neurodegenerative disorders
- Persistent pulmonary hypertension
- Otitis media with effusion for 3 months

Adapted from Delaney, A. M., Meyers, A. D., & Ruth, R. A. (2012). Newborn hearing screening. *eMedicine*. Retrieved from http://emedicine.medscape.com/article/836646-overview#a30

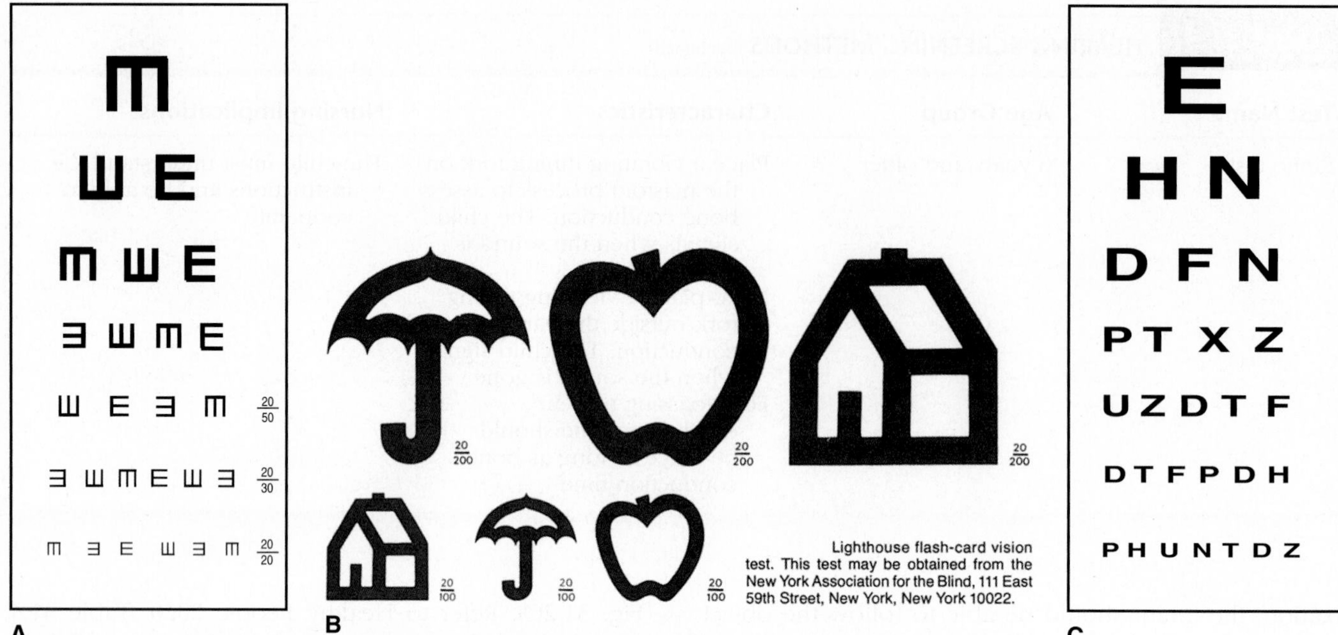
E
H N
D F N
P T X Z
U Z D T F
D T F P D H
P H U N T D Z
20/50
20/30
20/20
20/200
20/100
Lighthouse flash-card vision test. This test may be obtained from the New York Association for the Blind, 111 East 59th Street, New York, New York 10022.
A
B
C

FIGURE 31.2 **(A)** The "tumbling E" chart is appropriate for children who do not yet know the alphabet but who can follow instructions to indicate the direction that the arms of the "E" are pointing. **(B)** A picture chart similar to the Allen object recognition chart is appropriate for vision screening in the preschool-age child. **(C)** The Snellen eye chart may be used for children age 6 or older who know the alphabet. The test can be obtained at www.preventblindness.org/children or by calling 1-800-331-2020.

In addition to visual acuity screening, children should also be screened for color discrimination. Any child with eye abnormalities or who has failed visual screening needs to be evaluated by a specialist appropriately trained to treat children.

IRON-DEFICIENCY ANEMIA SCREENING

Iron deficiency is the leading nutritional deficiency in the United States (CDC, 2011a). Iron deficiency can cause cognitive and motor deficits resulting in developmental delays and behavioral disturbances. The increased incidence of iron-deficiency anemia is directly associated with periods of diminished iron stores, rapid growth, and high metabolic demands. At 6 months of age, the in utero iron stores of a full-term infant are almost depleted (Baker, Greer, & The Committee on Nutrition, 2010). The adolescent growth spurt warrants constant iron replacement. Pregnant adolescents are at even higher risk for iron deficiency due to the demands of the mother's growth spurt and the needs of the developing fetus (CDC, 2011a).

TABLE 31.4 VISION SCREENING TOOLS

Screening Tool	Age	Nursing Implications
Snellen letters or numbers	School-age	The child must know his or her letters or numbers for the test to be valid.
"Tumbling E"	Preschool	The child points in the direction that the "E" is facing.
LEA symbols or Allen figures	Preschool	The child should first identify the pictures with both eyes at a comfortable distance prior to monocular testing to ensure validity of the test.
Ishihara	School-age	Screens for color discrimination (numbers composed of dots, hidden within other dots)
Color Vision Testing Made Easy (CVTME)	Preschool	Uses dot pictures like the Ishihara, but instead of numbers has easily identified shapes imbedded in the dots

HEALTHY PEOPLE 2020

Objective	Nursing Significance
Increase the proportion of preschool children age 5 years and younger who receive vision screening.	• Use a preschool-appropriate vision screening tool to assess vision. • Ensure screening begins at age 3 years.

Healthy People Objectives retrieved from http://www.healthypeople.gov

The AAP recommends assessing for risk factors related to iron-deficiency anemia at 4, 15, 18, and 30 months and then annually and performing a hematocrit or hemoglobin at 12 months. Refer to Box 31.4 for risk factors for iron-deficiency anemia.

LEAD SCREENING

Elevated blood lead levels (5 μg/dL or higher) remains a preventable environmental health threat. Approximately half a million children have blood levels greater than 5 μg/dL, which can lead to a wide variety of symptoms and problems, such as headaches, stomach pain, inattentiveness, irritability, hyperactivity, decreased bone and muscle growth, poor muscle coordination, problems with language and speech, cognitive impairments, hearing problems, and seizures (Durani, 2012; CDC, 2013b). Although the prevalence of elevated lead levels has declined significantly over the past two decades, mainly due to the banning of lead-based paint in 1978, certain communities still possess a high level of lead exposure. Lead poisoning is a problem that affects children younger than 6 years the most because children of this age are crawling on the ground and putting things in their mouths, and their developing neurologic system is more sensitive to the effects of lead. It has also been found that even low blood lead levels can harm children and result in IQ deficits, attention-related behavior problems, and poor academic achievement (Advisory Committee on Childhood Lead Poisoning Prevention [ACCLP], 2012). Studies have also shown that these effects cannot be reversed (ACCLP, 2012). Therefore, a shift to primary prevention is the key. Ensuring that no children spend time or live in homes, buildings, or environments where they are exposed to lead hazards is the key. Educate parents on lead hazards and encourage them to avoid exposure of their children. Lead hazards include homes or buildings built before 1978, contaminated soil and dust, water that flows through old lead pipes or faucets, foods stored in containers that are painted with lead paint (such as lead glazed pottery or lead crystal) or canned food (such as those imported from other countries) that is sealed with lead, toys, or toy jewelry that may be painted with lead paint or have lead components, and folk remedies that contain lead, such as greta and azarcon (United States Environmental Protection Agency, 2014).

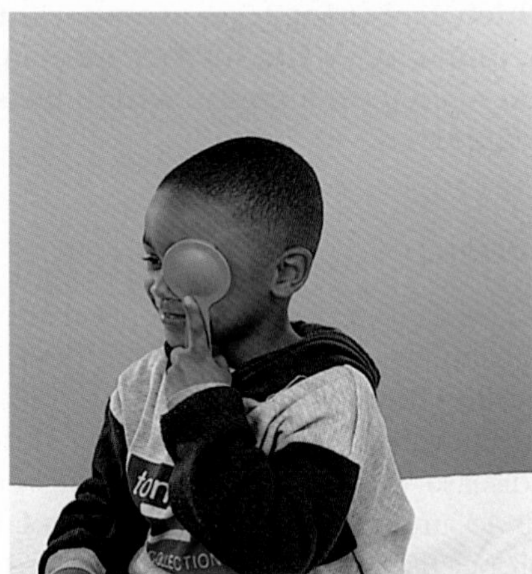

FIGURE 31.3 One eye must be covered while the other is tested in order to detect discrepancies in visual acuity between the two eyes and identify amblyopia early.

BOX 31.4

RISK FACTORS FOR IRON-DEFICIENCY ANEMIA

- Periods of rapid growth
- Low-birthweight or preterm infants
- Low dietary intake of meat, fish, poultry, and ascorbic acid
- Macrobiotic diets
- Inappropriate consumption of cow's milk
- Use of infant formula not fortified with iron
- Exclusive breastfeeding after age 4 months without iron-fortified supplemental foods
- Meal skipping, frequent dieting
- Exposure to lead
- Feeding problems
- Pregnancy or recent pregnancy
- Intensive physical training
- Recent blood loss, heavy/lengthy menstrual periods
- Chronic use of aspirin or nonsteroidal anti-inflammatory drugs
- Parasitic infections

Children at High Risk for Iron-Deficiency Anemia

- Low-income families
- Those eligible for the Special Supplemental Nutrition Program for Women, Infants, and Children (WIC)
- Migrants or recently arrived refugees

Adapted from Baker, R. D., Greer, F. R., & The Committee on Nutrition. (2010). Clinical report. Diagnosis and prevention of iron deficiency and iron-deficiency anemia in infants and young children (0–3 years of age). *Pediatrics, 126*(5), 1040–1050. Retrieved from http://aappolicy.aappublications.org/cgi/content/full/pediatrics;126/5/1040; Centers for Disease Control and Prevention. (2011a). *Nutrition for everyone: Iron and iron deficiency*. Retrieved from http://www.cdc.gov/nutrition/everyone/basics/vitamins/iron.html

Take Note!

A healthy diet that includes calcium, iron, and vitamin C can also help decrease the way the body absorbs lead (Durani, 2012).

The ACCLP recommends that health care providers follow local and state lead screening guidelines (ACCLP, 2012). The AAP Bright Future guidelines recommends performing a risk assessment and, if positive, screen at 6, 9, 12, 18, and 24 months and at 3, 4, 5, and 6 years (Bright Futures/AAP, 2014). Refer to Healthy People 2020.

Take Note!

Many cases of elevated blood lead levels have been reported in children who are recent immigrants, refugees, or international adoptees. The CDC recommends blood lead testing for these children upon entering the United States and a repeat test 3 to 6 months after placement in a permanent residence (CDC, 2013a).

HYPERTENSION SCREENING

Obesity and resulting hypertension have been on the rise in children and can lead to adult cardiovascular disease. Universal hypertension screening for children beginning at 3 years of age is recommended (Bright Futures/AAP, 2014). If the child has risk factors for systemic hypertension, such as preterm birth, very low birthweight, renal disease, organ transplant, congenital heart disease, or other illnesses associated with hypertension, then screening begins when the risk factor becomes apparent (Bright Futures/AAP, 2014).

The guidelines for determining hypertension in children and adolescents utilize body size in order to be more precise. Gender and age are used to determine specific systolic and diastolic blood pressure percentiles. Refer to Appendix B for Blood Pressure Charts for Children and Adolescents. Auscultation is the preferred method of measuring blood pressure in children, and an elevated blood pressure must be confirmed on repeated visits before a diagnosis of hypertension is given. Refer to Box 31.5 for hypertension guidelines. Anticipatory guidance on activity is appropriate for any child and the inclusion of weight management for children with prehypertension, stage 1 or 2 hypertension (National Heart, Lung, and Blood Institute, 2012). Refer to Chapter 41 for additional information on hypertension.

HEALTHY PEOPLE 2020

Objective	Nursing Significance
Eliminate elevated blood lead levels in children.	• Screen for lead exposure. • Ensure that high-risk children have blood lead levels measured.

Healthy People Objectives retrieved from http://www.healthypeople.gov

BOX 31.5

CHILDHOOD HYPERTENSION GUIDELINES

Optimal/normal	<90th percentile for sex, age, and height
Prehypertension	BP at or above 120/80 mm Hg but <95th percentile for sex, age, and height
Stage 1 hypertension	≥95th percentile & <99th percentile + 5 mm Hg for sex, age, and height on three separate occasions
Stage 2 hypertension	≥99th percentile + 5 mm Hg for sex, age, and height on three separate occasions

Adapted from National Heart, Lung, and Blood Institute. (2012). *Expert panel on integrated guidelines for cardiovascular health and risk reduction in children and adolescents. SUMMARY REPORT (NIH Publication No. 12-7486)*. Washington, DC: U.S. Department of Health and Human Services. Retrieved from http://www.nhlbi.nih.gov/guidelines/cvd_ped/peds_guidelines_sum.pdf

HYPERLIPIDEMIA SCREENING

Atherosclerosis has been documented in children, and a link exists between high lipid levels and the development of these lesions. Bright Futures Guidelines recommends universal screening for dyslipidemia once between 9 and 11 years of age and again between 18 and 21 years of age (Bright Futures/AAP, 2014). Performing a risk assessment screening at 24 months and 4, 6, 8, and 12 through 17 years of age is also recommended. Refer to Box 31.6 for details regarding screening for hyperlipidemia.

Remember Maya and Evan, the children introduced at the beginning of the chapter? How would you assess their growth and development? Which screening tests are warranted for them, and why? What further information would you need to determine which tests should be performed?

Immunizations

Immunization is the key disease prevention activity during childhood health supervision visits. The development of effective vaccines, beginning in the 1940s, revolutionized children's health care. Immunization allowed the focus to shift from disease treatment to disease prevention. The nurse needs to understand the principles of immunizations, the proper use of vaccines, and barriers to immunization. Armed with this knowledge, the nurse can partner with families to provide the highest level of disease protection to children (Fig. 31.4). Refer to Healthy People

BOX 31.6

HYPERLIPIDEMIA SCREENING

Screen if parents, grandparents, aunts/uncles, siblings, have/had documented:
- Coronary atherosclerosis
- Myocardial infarction
- Angina pectoris
- Peripheral vascular disease
- Cerebrovascular disease/stroke
- Coronary artery bypass graft/stent/angioplasty at <55 years in males, <65 years in females
- Sudden cardiac death

Screen if a parent's blood cholesterol level is 240 mg/dL or higher.

Screen at physician's discretion:
- Parental history is unobtainable.
- Child has diabetes or hypertension.
- Child has lifestyle risk factors:
  - Cigarette smoking
  - Obesity
  - Sedentary lifestyle
  - High-fat dietary intake

Adapted from National Heart, Lung, and Blood Institute. (2012). *Expert panel on integrated guidelines for cardiovascular health and risk reduction in children and adolescents. SUMMARY REPORT (NIH Publication No. 12-7486)*. Washington, DC: U.S. Department of Health and Human Services. Retrieved from http://www.nhlbi.nih.gov/guidelines/cvd_ped/peds_guidelines_sum.pdf

2020. For information on vaccine-preventable communicable diseases refer Chapter 37.

PRINCIPLES OF IMMUNIZATION

The immune system has the ability to recognize materials present in the body as "self" or "nonself." Foreign materials (nonself) are called antigens. When an antigen is recognized by the immune system, the immune system responds by producing antibodies (immunoglobulins) or directing special cells to destroy and remove the antigen.

***HEALTHY PEOPLE** 2020*

Objective	Nursing Significance
Achieve and maintain effective vaccination coverage levels for universally recommended vaccines among young children.	• Immunize at every opportunity. If a child is due or past due for vaccinations, provide them at a sick visit if not contraindicated. • Educate families about the benefits and risks of immunization.

Healthy People Objectives retrieved from http://www.healthypeople.gov

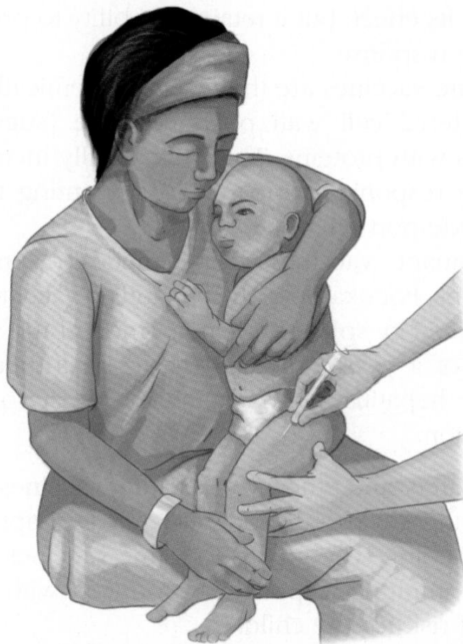

FIGURE 31.4 Nurse administering intramuscular injection into the vastus lateralis of an infant.

Immunity is the ability to destroy and remove a specific antigen from the body. The acquisition of immunity can be active or passive. **Passive immunity** is produced when the immunoglobulins of one person are transferred to another. This immunity lasts only weeks or months. Passive immunity can be obtained by injection of exogenous immunoglobulins. It can also be transferred from mothers to infants via colostrum or the placenta. **Active immunity** is acquired when a person's own immune system generates the immune response. Active immunity lasts for many years or for a lifetime. This long-term protection is the result of immunologic memory. After the initial immune response, specialized cells for that antigen continue to exist. When an antigen returns, these memory cells very rapidly produce a fresh supply of antibodies to re-establish protection. This immunity can occur after exposure to natural pathogens or after exposure to vaccines. Vaccines mimic the characteristics of the natural antigen. The immune system mounts a response and establishes an immunologic memory as it would for an infection.

The classification of vaccines is based on the characteristics of the antigen present. The antigen may be viral or bacterial. It may be live attenuated (weakened) or killed. It may be the whole antigen or a portion of it (fractional).

- Live attenuated vaccines are modified living organisms that are weakened. The organism can produce an immune response but does not produce the complications of the illness.
- Killed vaccines contain whole dead organisms; they are incapable of reproducing, but are capable of producing an immune response.
- Toxoid vaccines contain protein products produced by bacteria called toxins. The toxin is heat-treated to

weaken its effect, but it retains its ability to produce an immune response.

- Conjugate vaccines are the result of chemically linking the bacterial cell wall polysaccharide (sugar-based) portions with proteins. This dramatically increases the immune response compared to presenting the polysaccharide portion alone.
- Recombinant vaccines use genetically engineered organisms. For example, the hepatitis B vaccine (HepB) is produced by splicing a gene portion of the virus into a gene of a yeast cell. The yeast cell is then able to produce hepatitis B surface antigen to use for vaccine production.

The safety and efficacy of existing vaccines are constantly being reviewed, and research to improve vaccines is ongoing. The goal is to refine vaccines so that a maximum immune response is produced with the least amount of risk for the child.

IMMUNIZATION MANAGEMENT

The Advisory Committee on Immunization Practices (ACIP), a branch of the CDC, reviews the recommended immunization schedules at least yearly and updates the schedule to ensure that it reflects current best practices (go to their website at http://www.cdc.gov/vaccines/schedules/hcp/index.html for up-to-date immunizations schedules). In addition to the recommended schedule, the ACIP publishes a "catch-up" schedule for children who have not been adequately immunized. The child's immunization record must be compared with the latest edition of these schedules when assessing the need for immunization.

BOX 31.7

VACCINE ADMINISTRATION ROUTES

Intramuscular	Subcutaneous
DTaP, DT, Tdap	IPV
Hepatitis A, hepatitis B	MMR
Hib	Varicella
Influenza (trivalent)	MPSV4
Pneumococcal conjugate vaccine (PCV)	
HPV	
MCV4	
IPV	

Adapted from Immunization Action Coalition. (2012). *Administering vaccines: Dose, route, site, and needle size*. Retrieved from http://www.immunize.org/catg.d/p3085.pdf. We thank the Immunization Action Coalition.

Take Note!

When obtaining an immunization history from the parent, ask, "When and where did your child receive his (or her) last immunization?" The answer will provide more information than simply asking, "Are your child's immunizations up to date?" The nurse can compare this information with that on the immunization record, discover in what settings the child is getting health care, and use the information as a starting point in a discussion of any reactions to previous immunizations.

Vaccine storage and administration affect the efficacy of a vaccine. Improperly stored or reconstituted vaccines can be ineffective (CDC, 2012c). The vaccine must be given by the correct route; not all vaccines are given intramuscularly (Box 31.7, Table 31.5). The manufacturer's

TABLE 31.5 VACCINE ADMINISTRATION: NEEDLE AND SITE SELECTION

Child	Needle Size	Needle Length (Inches)	Site
Intramuscular			
Birth–28 days	25 gauge	⅝	Anterolateral thigh
1–12 months	23–25 gauge	1	Anterolateral thigh
1–2 years	23–25 gauge	1–1.25 ⅝–1	Anterolateral thigh Deltoid
3–18 years	22–25 gauge	1–1.25 ⅝–1	Anterolateral thigh Deltoid
Subcutaneous			
1–12 months	23–25 gauge	⅝	Fatty tissue over anterolateral thigh
>12 months	23–25 gauge	⅝	Fatty tissue over anterolateral thigh or triceps

A ⅝-length needle should only be used if skin is stretched tight, subcutaneous tissue is not pinched, and a 90-degree angle is used.

Adapted from Immunization Action Coalition. (2012). *Administering vaccines: Dose, route, site, and needle size*. Retrieved from http://www.immunize.org/catg.d/p3085.pdf. We thank the Immunization Action Coalition.

package insert is the best reference source for any vaccine.

Take Note!

Proper vaccine storage is critical to vaccine efficacy. If you suspect that a vaccine was not maintained at the proper storage temperature, do not use it! An ineffective vaccine is of no use in preventing disease.

Any vaccine can have side effects, and the most common ones are mild, such as redness, tenderness, and swelling at the site, low-grade fever, and fussiness. These symptoms usually resolve within a few days. The National Childhood Vaccine Injury Act (NCVIA) requires that Vaccine Information Statements (VISs) (Fig. 31.5) be provided to parents before an immunization is given (CDC, 2013c). These inform about the benefits and risks and discuss specific side effects that may be seen for each immunization. In accordance with the concept of partnership with the parents, allow ample time for them to read the VIS and to discuss their concerns. If the parents do not understand the information presented, they should feel comfortable asking questions. If the parents are illiterate, present the information orally and verify that the parents understand it. If the information in the VIS is not in the parent's native language, have a translator present the information.

At this time, ask the parents about the child's reactions to previous immunizations, and screen for precautions and contraindications for each vaccine to be administered. Before the vaccine is given, the parents must sign consent forms.

Any clinically significant adverse event that occurs after an immunization should be reported to the Vaccine Adverse Event Reporting System (VAERS), which is a cosponsored surveillance program by the CDC and the U.S. Food and Drug Administration (FDA) (VAERS, n.d.). For assistance in obtaining and completing a VAERS form, call 800–822–7967 or visit www.vaers.hhs.gov.

Documentation in the child's permanent record includes the following:

- Date the vaccine was administered
- Name of vaccine (commonly used abbreviation is acceptable)
- Lot number and expiration date of vaccine
- Manufacturer's name
- Site and route by which vaccine was administered (e.g., left deltoid, intramuscularly)
- Edition date of VIS given to the parents
- Name and address of the facility administering the vaccine (where the permanent record will be kept)
- Name of the person administering the immunization

Families should be provided with a copy of the child's immunizations. This reinforces the importance of the procedure and reminds the parents to keep the child's immunizations up to date.

Figure 31.6 shows a typical vaccine administration record.

VACCINE DESCRIPTIONS

This section reviews the most commonly used vaccines. These immunizations are recommended by the ACIP and the AAP. Each state has laws that determine which immunizations are required for school admittance. These requirements can be waived if a contraindication or precaution to the vaccine exists. *Contraindications* are conditions that justify withholding an immunization either permanently or temporarily. The only permanent contraindication to all vaccines is an anaphylactic or systemic allergic reaction to a vaccine component (Kroger, Sumaya, Pickering, & Atkinson, 2011). Children who are severely immunocompromised or women who are pregnant should not receive live vaccines (such as measles, mumps, and rubella [MMR] and varicella) (see below); with pertussis immunization (DTP, DTaP, or TdaP) (see below), encephalopathy without an identified cause within 7 days of the immunization permanently contraindicates further immunization with pertussis-containing vaccine (Kroger et al., 2011). Temporarily postponing vaccinations is recommended for moderate to severe illness, immunosuppression, pregnancy, or recently received blood products or other antibody-containing products (Kroger et al., 2011). Vaccination should not be postponed because of a minor respiratory illness or a low-grade fever (Kroger et al., 2011). *Precautions* are conditions that increase the risk of an adverse reaction or may impair the child's ability to acquire immunity from the vaccine. On an individualized basis, providers must weigh the benefits of immunization against the likelihood of an adverse event.

Diphtheria, Tetanus, and Pertussis Vaccines. Immunization against diphtheria, tetanus, and pertussis diseases is given via a combination vaccine. The vaccine currently used for children younger than age 7 is diphtheria, tetanus, acellular pertussis (DTaP). It contains diphtheria and tetanus toxoids and pertussis cell wall proteins. The older version of this vaccine—diphtheria, tetanus, pertussis (DPT)—contained killed whole cells of pertussis bacteria and caused more frequent and severe adverse reactions than DTaP. Diphtheria and tetanus (DT) vaccine is used for children younger than age 7 who have contraindications to pertussis immunization. Full-strength diphtheria toxoid causes significant adverse reactions in people older than age 7 years. For this group, the TdaP adolescent preparation vaccine is used: it contains tetanus toxoid, reduced diphtheria toxoid, and acellular pertussis vaccine. The lowercase "d" is used to designate the lower dose of diphtheria toxoid. The ACIP recommends that TdaP be used for all tetanus boosters in older children (11 to 12 years) and

(text continues on page 1146)

VACCINE INFORMATION STATEMENT

Hib Vaccine

What You Need to Know

(*Haemophilus Influenzae* Type b)

Many Vaccine Information Statements are available in Spanish and other languages. See www.immunize.org/vis

Hojas de información sobre vacunas están disponibles en español y en muchos otros idiomas. Visite www.immunize.org/vis

1 Why get vaccinated?

Haemophilus influenzae type b (Hib) disease is a serious disease caused by bacteria. It usually affects children under 5 years old. It can also affect adults with certain medical conditions.

Your child can get Hib disease by being around other children or adults who may have the bacteria and not know it. The germs spread from person to person. If the germs stay in the child's nose and throat, the child probably will not get sick. But sometimes the germs spread into the lungs or the bloodstream, and then Hib can cause serious problems. This is called invasive Hib disease.

Before Hib vaccine, Hib disease was the leading cause of bacterial meningitis among children under 5 years old in the United States. Meningitis is an infection of the lining of the brain and spinal cord. It can lead to brain damage and deafness. Hib disease can also cause:

- pneumonia
- severe swelling in the throat, making it hard to breathe
- infections of the blood, joints, bones, and covering of the heart
- death

Before Hib vaccine, about 20,000 children in the United States under 5 years old got Hib disease each year, and about 3% - 6% of them died.

Hib vaccine can prevent Hib disease. Since use of Hib vaccine began, the number of cases of invasive Hib disease has decreased by more than 99%. Many more children would get Hib disease if we stopped vaccinating.

2 Hib vaccine

Several different brands of Hib vaccine are available. Your child will receive either 3 or 4 doses, depending on which vaccine is used.

Doses of Hib vaccine are usually recommended at these ages:

- First Dose: 2 months of age
- Second Dose: 4 months of age
- Third Dose: 6 months of age (if needed, depending on brand of vaccine)
- Final/Booster Dose: 12–15 months of age

Hib vaccine may be given at the same time as other vaccines.

Hib vaccine may be given as part of a combination vaccine. Combination vaccines are made when two or more types of vaccine are combined together into a single shot, so that one vaccination can protect against more than one disease.

Children over 5 years old and adults usually do not need Hib vaccine. But it may be recommended for older children or adults with asplenia or sickle cell disease, before surgery to remove the spleen, or following a bone marrow transplant. It may also be recommended for people 5 to 18 years old with HIV. Ask your doctor for details.

Your doctor or the person giving you the vaccine can give you more information.

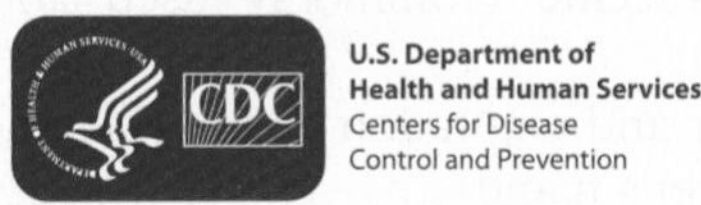

FIGURE 31.5 Federal law mandates the use of Vaccine Information Statements (VISs). These should be given to the parent or primary caregiver for each vaccine the child receives. (Obtained from Centers for Disease Control and Prevention. (2014i). *HIB vaccine: What you need to know*. Retrieved from http://www.cdc.gov/vaccines/hcp/vis/vis-statements/hib.pdf)

3 Some people should not get this vaccine

Hib vaccine should not be given to infants younger than 6 weeks of age.

A person who has ever had a life-threatening allergic reaction after a previous dose of Hib vaccine, OR has a severe allergy to any part of this vaccine, should not get Hib vaccine. *Tell the person giving the vaccine about any severe allergies.*

People who are mildly ill can get Hib vaccine. People who are moderately or severely ill should probably wait until they recover. Talk to your healthcare provider if the person getting the vaccine isn't feeling well on the day the shot is scheduled.

4 Risks of a vaccine reaction

With any medicine, including vaccines, there is a chance of side effects. These are usually mild and go away on their own. Serious reactions are also possible but are rare.

Most people who get Hib vaccine do not have any problems with it.

Mild Problems following Hib vaccine:
- redness, warmth, or swelling where the shot was given
- fever

These problems are uncommon. If they occur, they usually begin soon after the shot and last 2 or 3 days.

Problems that could happen after any vaccine:

Any medication can cause a severe allergic reaction. Such reactions from a vaccine are very rare, estimated at fewer than 1 in a million doses, and would happen within a few minutes to a few hours after the vaccination.

As with any medicine, there is a very remote chance of a vaccine causing a serious injury or death.

Older children, adolescents, and adults might also experience these problems after any vaccine:
- People sometimes faint after a medical procedure, including vaccination. Sitting or lying down for about 15 minutes can help prevent fainting, and injuries caused by a fall. Tell your doctor if you feel dizzy, or have vision changes or ringing in the ears.
- Some people get severe pain in the shoulder and have difficulty moving the arm where a shot was given. This happens very rarely.

The safety of vaccines is always being monitored. For more information, visit: **www.cdc.gov/vaccinesafety/**

5 What if there is a serious reaction?

What should I look for?

- Look for anything that concerns you, such as signs of a **severe allergic reaction**, very high fever, or unusual behavior.

  Signs of a severe allergic reaction can include hives, swelling of the face and throat, difficulty breathing, a fast heartbeat, dizziness, and weakness. These would usually start a few minutes to a few hours after the vaccination.

What should I do?

- If you think it is a severe allergic reaction or other emergency that can't wait, call 9-1-1 or get the person to the nearest hospital. Otherwise, call your doctor.
- Afterward, the reaction should be reported to the Vaccine Adverse Event Reporting System (VAERS). Your doctor might file this report, or you can do it yourself through the VAERS web site at **www.vaers.hhs.gov**, or by calling **1-800-822-7967**.

VAERS does not give medical advice.

6 The National Vaccine Injury Compensation Program

The National Vaccine Injury Compensation Program (VICP) is a federal program that was created to compensate people who may have been injured by certain vaccines.

Persons who believe they may have been injured by a vaccine can learn about the program and about filing a claim by calling **1-800-338-2382** or visiting the VICP website at **www.hrsa.gov/vaccinecompensation**. There is a time limit to file a claim for compensation.

7 How can I learn more?

- Ask your doctor. He or she can give you the vaccine package insert or suggest other sources of information.
- Call your local or state health department.
- Contact the Centers for Disease Control and Prevention (CDC):
  - Call **1-800-232-4636** (**1-800-CDC-INFO**) or
  - Visit CDC's website at **www.cdc.gov/vaccines**

Vaccine Information Statement

Hib Vaccine

4/02/2015

42 U.S.C. § 300aa-26

Office Use Only

FIGURE 31.5 *(continued)*

(Page 1 of 2)

Vaccine Administration Record for Children and Teens

Patient name: Ashley Stebbins

Birthdate: 6/1/2007 Chart number: ______

Clinic name and address
Large Urban Clinic
1234 Any Avenue
Bigville, LM 98765

Before administering any vaccines, give copies of all pertinent Vaccine Information Statements (VISs) to the child's parent or legal representative and make sure he/she understands the risks and benefits of the vaccine(s). Always provide or update the patient's personal record card.

Vaccine	Type of Vaccine[1]	Date given (mo/day/yr)	Funding Source (F,S,P)[2]	Route & Site[3]	Vaccine		Vaccine Information Statement (VIS)		Vaccinator[5] (signature or initials & title)
					Lot #	Mfr.	Date on VIS[4]	Date given[4]	
Hepatitis B[6] (e.g., HepB, Hib-HepB, DTaP-HepB-IPV) Give IM.[3]	HepB	6/2/2007	F	IM/RT	0651M	MRK	7/11/01	6/2/07	JTA
	Pediarix	8/2/2007	F	IM/RT	635A1	GSK	7/18/07	8/2/07	DCP
	Pediarix	10/2/2007	F	IM/RT	712A2	GSK	7/18/07	10/2/07	DCP
	Pediarix	12/2/2007	F	IM/RT	712A2	GSK	7/18/07	12/2/07	DLW
Diphtheria, Tetanus, Pertussis[6] (e.g., DTaP, DTaP/Hib, DTaP-HepB-IPV, DT, DTaP-IPV/Hib, Tdap, DTaP-IPV, Td) Give IM.[3]	Pediarix	8/2/2007	F	IM/RT	635A1	GSK	5/17/07	8/2/07	DCP
	Pediarix	10/2/2007	F	IM/RT	712A2	GSK	5/17/07	10/2/07	DCP
	Pediarix	12/2/2007	F	IM/RT	712A2	GSK	5/17/07	12/2/07	DLW
	DTaP-Hib	9/2/2008	F	IM/RA	P0897AA	PMC	5/17/07	9/2/08	RLV
	DTaP	8/2/2012	F	IM/RA	376-912	PMC	5/17/07	8/2/12	JTA
***Haemophilus influenzae* type b**[6] (e.g., Hib, Hib-HepB, DTaP-IPV/Hib, DTaP/Hib, Hib-MenCY) Give IM.[3]	Hib	8/2/2007	F	IM/RT	635A1	GSK	5/17/07	8/2/07	DCP
	Hib	10/2/2007	F	IM/RT	712A2	GSK	5/17/07	10/2/07	DCP
	Hib	12/2/2007	F	IM/RT	712A2	GSK	5/17/07	12/2/07	DLW
	DTaP-Hib	9/2/2008	F	IM/RA	7172AA	PMC	12/16/98	9/2/08	RLV
Polio[6] (e.g., IPV, DTaP-HepB-IPV, DTaP-IPV/Hib, DTaP-IPV) Give IPV SC or IM.[3] Give all others IM.[3]	Pediarix	8/2/2007	F	IM/RT	635A1	GSK	1/1/00	8/2/07	DCP
	Pediarix	10/2/2007	F	IM/RT	712A2	GSK	1/1/00	10/2/07	DCP
	Pediarix	12/2/2007	F	IM/RT	712A2	GSK	1/1/00	12/2/07	DLW
	IPV	8/2/2012	F	IM/RA	U4569-8	PMC	1/1/00	8/2/12	DCP
Pneumococcal (e.g., PCV7, PCV13, conjugate; PPSV23, polysaccharide) Give PCV IM.[3] Give PPSV SC or IM.[3]	PCV13	8/2/2007	F	IM/LT	7-5095-05A	WYE	9/30/02	8/2/07	DCP
	PCV13	10/2/2007	F	IM/LT	7-5095-05A	WYE	9/30/02	10/2/07	DCP
	PCV13	12/2/2007	F	IM/LT	7-5095-05A	WYE	9/30/02	12/2/07	DLW
	PCV13	9/2/2008	F	IM/LT	7-5095-05A	WYE	9/30/02	9/2/08	RLV
Rotavirus (RV1, RV5) Give orally (po).[3]	RotaTeq	8/2/2007	F	PO	04859	MRK	4/12/06	8/2/07	DCP
	RV5	10/2/2007	F	PO	04859	MRK	4/12/06	10/2/07	DCP
	RotaTeq	12/2/2007	F	PO	04859	MRK	4/12/06	12/2/07	DLW

DTaP-HepB-IPV (Pediarix)

DTaP-Hib (TriHIBit): 2 lot #s, 2 different VISs

DTaP-Hib (TriHIBit): 2 lot #s, 2 different VISs

Example

See page 2 to record measles-mumps-rubella, varicella, hepatitis A, meningococcal, HPV, influenza, and other vaccines (e.g., travel vaccines).

How to Complete This Record

1. Record the generic abbreviation (e.g., Tdap) or the trade name for each vaccine (see table at right).
2. Record the funding source of the vaccine given as either F (federal), S (state), or P (private).
3. Record the route by which the vaccine was given as either intramuscular (IM), subcutaneous (SC), intradermal (ID), intranasal (IN), or oral (PO) and also the site where it was administered as either RA (right arm), LA (left arm), RT (right thigh), or LT (left thigh).
4. Record the publication date of each VIS as well as the date the VIS is given to the patient.
5. To meet the space constraints of this form and federal requirements for documentation, a healthcare setting may want to keep a reference list of vaccinators that includes their initials and titles.
6. For combination vaccines, fill in a row for each antigen in the combination.

Abbreviation	Trade Name and Manufacturer
DTaP	Daptacel (sanofi); Infanrix (GlaxoSmithKline [GSK]); Tripedia (sanofi pasteur)
DT (pediatric)	Generic DT (sanofi pasteur)
DTaP-HepB-IPV	Pediarix (GSK)
DTaP/Hib	TriHIBit (sanofi pasteur)
DTaP-IPV/Hib	Pentacel (sanofi pasteur)
DTaP-IPV	Kinrix (GSK)
HepB	Engerix-B (GSK); Recombivax HB (Merck)
HepA-HepB	Twinrix (GSK), can be given to teens age 18 and older
Hib	ActHIB (sanofi pasteur); Hiberix (GSK); PedvaxHIB (Merck)
Hib-HepB	Comvax (Merck)
Hib-MenCY	MenHibrix (GSK)
IPV	Ipol (sanofi pasteur)
PCV13	Prevnar 13 (Pfizer)
PPSV23	Pneumovax 23 (Merck)
RV1	Rotarix (GSK)
RV5	RotaTeq (Merck)
Tdap	Adacel (sanofi pasteur); Boostrix (GSK)
Td	Decavac (sanofi pasteur); Generic Td (MA Biological Labs)

Technical content reviewed by the Centers for Disease Control and Prevention

For additional copies, visit www.immunize.org/catg.d/p2022.pdf • Item #P2022 (4/14)

This form was created by the Immunization Action Coalition • www.immunize.org • www.vaccineinformation.org

FIGURE 31.6 Sample of a vaccine administration record (Acquired from Immunization Action Coalition. (2011). *Vaccine administration record for children and teens*. Retrieved from http://www.immunize.org/catg.d/p2022.pdf. We thank the Immunization Action Coalition.)

(Page 2 of 2)

Vaccine Administration Record for Children and Teens

Patient name: Ashley Stebbins

Birthdate: 6/1/2007 Chart number: ______

Clinic name and address
Large Urban Clinic
1234 Any Avenue
Bigville, LM 98765

Before administering any vaccines, give copies of all pertinent Vaccine Information Statements (VISs) to the child's parent or legal representative and make sure he/she understands the risks and benefits of the vaccine(s). Always provide or update the patient's personal record card.

Vaccine	Type of Vaccine[1]	Date given (mo/day/yr)	Funding Source (F,S,P)[2]	Route & Site[3]	Vaccine		Vaccine Information Statement (VIS)		Vaccinator[5] (signature or initials & title)
					Lot #	Mfr.	Date on VIS[4]	Date given[4]	
Measles, Mumps, Rubella[6] (e.g., MMR, MMRV) Give SC.[3]	MMRV	6/2/2008	F	SC/RA	0857M	MRK	1/15/03	6/2/08	DLW
	MMRV	8/2/2012	F	SC/LA	0522F	MRK	5/21/10	8/2/12	DCP
Varicella[6] (e.g., VAR, MMRV) Give SC.[3]	MMRV	6/2/2008	F	SC/RA	0857M	MRK	3/13/08	6/2/08	DLW
	MMRV	8/2/2012	F	SC/LA	0522F	MRK	5/21/10	8/2/12	DCP
Hepatitis A[6] (HepA) Give IM.[3]	Havrix	6/2/2008	F	IM/LA	AHAVB944	GSK	3/21/06	6/2/08	DLW
	Vaqta	12/2/2008	F	IM/LA	0634K	MRK	3/21/06	12/2/08	TAA
Meningococcal (e.g., MenACWY-CRM; Men-ACWY-D; Hib-MenCY; MPSV4) Give MenACWY and Hib-MenCY IM[3] and give MPSV4 SC.[3]									
Human papillomavirus[6] (e.g., HPV2, HPV4) Give IM.[3]									
Influenza (e.g., IIV3, trivalent inactivated; IIV4, quadrivalent inactivated; RIV, recombinant inactivated [for ages 18–49 yrs]; LAIV4, quadrivalent live attenuated) Give IIV and RIV IM.[3] Give LAIV IN.[3]	TIV	12/2/2007	F	IM/RT	U097543	PMC	7/16/07	12/2/07	DLW
	Fluzone	9/2/2008	F	IM/LA	U2169MA	PMC	7/24/08	9/2/08	RLV
	TIV-H1N1	11/15/2009	F	IM/RA	UP016AA	PMC	10/2/09	11/15/09	JRM
	LAIV-H1N1	12/29/2009	F	IN	500756P	MED	10/2/09	12/29/09	CJP
	Fluarix	11/12/2010	F	IM/RA	J5G53	GSK	8/10/10	11/12/10	TAA
	Fluvirin	9/2/2011	F	IM/LA	878771P	NOV	7/26/11	9/5/11	DCP
	FluMist	9/25/2012	F	IN	500491P	MED	7/2/12	10/15/12	RLV
Other	Afluria	9/25/2013	F	IM/RA	M50907	CSL	7/26/13	9/25/13	CJP

MMR-VAR (MMRV)

Example

See page 1 to record hepatitis B, diphtheria, tetanus, pertussis, *Haemophilus influenzae* type b, polio, pneumococcal, and rotavirus vaccines.

How to Complete This Record

1. Record the generic abbreviation (e.g., Tdap) or the trade name for each vaccine (see table at right).
2. Record the funding source of the vaccine given as either F (federal), S (state), or P (private).
3. Record the route by which the vaccine was given as either intramuscular (IM), subcutaneous (SC), intradermal (ID), intranasal (IN), or oral (PO) and also the site where it was administered as either RA (right arm), LA (left arm), RT (right thigh), or LT (left thigh).
4. Record the publication date of each VIS as well as the date the VIS is given to the patient.
5. To meet the space constraints of this form and federal requirements for documentation, a healthcare setting may want to keep a reference list of vaccinators that includes their initials and titles.
6. For combination vaccines, fill in a row for each antigen in the combination.

Abbreviation	Trade Name and Manufacturer
MMR	MMRII (Merck)
VAR	Varivax (Merck)
MMRV	ProQuad (Merck)
HepA	Havrix (GlaxoSmithKline [GSK]); Vaqta (Merck)
HepA-HepB	Twinrix (GSK)
HPV2	Cervarix (GSK)
HPV4	Gardasil (Merck)
LAIV (Live attenuated influenza vaccine]	FluMist (MedImmune)
TIV (Trivalent inactivated influenza vaccine); RIV (Recombinant influenza vaccine)	Afluria (CSL Biotherapies); Agriflu (Novartis); Fluarix (GSK); Flublok (Protein Sciences Corp.); Flucelvax (Novartis); FluLaval (GSK); Fluvirin (Novartis); Fluzone, Fluzone Intradermal [for ages 18–64 yrs] (sanofi)
MCV4 or MenACWY, MenACWY-CRM, MenACWY-D; Hib-MenCY	MenACWY-D = Menactra (sanofi pasteur); MenACWY-CRM = Menveo (Novartis); Hib-MenCY (MenHibrix [GSK])
MPSV4	Menomune (sanofi pasteur)

Technical content reviewed by the Centers for Disease Control and Prevention

For additional copies, visit www.immunize.org/catg.d/p2022.pdf • Item #P2022 (4/14)

This form was created by the Immunization Action Coalition • www.immunize.org • www.vaccineinformation.org

FIGURE 31.6 *(continued)*

adolescents because TdaP provides a boost to diphtheria and pertussis immunization.

Haemophilus Influenzae Type B Vaccines. *Haemophilus influenzae* type B is a bacterium that causes several life-threatening illnesses in children younger than 5 years of age. These infections include meningitis, epiglottitis, and septic arthritis. *H. influenzae* type B conjugate vaccines (Hib) have been extremely effective in cutting the rates of these diseases in children. There are several different types of Hib conjugate vaccines. Two or three doses are needed for the primary infant series depending on the vaccine product used (e.g., Pedvax-HIB and Comvax require two doses while ActHib and Pentacel require three doses) (Briere et al., 2014). A booster vaccine is needed at 12 to 15 months. These vaccine products are interchangeable, but if different brands are administered to a child, then a total of three doses is necessary to complete the primary series in infants. Hib vaccine is not routinely given to children 5 years of age or older and is contraindicated in children younger than 6 weeks (CDC, 2014b).

Polio Vaccine. Inactivated polio vaccine (IPV) is the only polio vaccine currently recommended in the United States (ACIP, 2000; CDC, 2009). It is a killed virus vaccine that poses no risk for vaccine-acquired disease. Oral polio vaccine (OPV), a live attenuated virus vaccine, was the preferred polio vaccine until 2000. At that time it became apparent that the only victims of poliomyelitis were people who had acquired it from OPV. The ACIP determined that in this country the risks of OPV outweighed the benefits and withdrew its recommendation of OPV (ACIP, 2000; CDC, 2009).

Measles, Mumps, and Rubella Vaccines. MMR is a live attenuated virus combination vaccine. It is the one most commonly used in childhood immunizations. MMR can be given the same day as other live attenuated virus vaccines such as varicella vaccine (Var). However, if not given on the same day, the immunizations should be spaced at least 28 days apart (Kroger et al., 2011). Anaphylactic reactions are believed to be associated with the neomycin or gelatin components of the vaccine rather than the egg component. The vaccine is not prepared from the allergenic albumen portion of the egg, so egg allergy is no longer a contraindication for measles vaccine (Kroger et al., 2011). Pregnancy in a child's mother is not a contraindication to the vaccination of the child (Kroger et al., 2011).

Hepatitis A Vaccine. Hepatitis A vaccine (HepA) is an inactivated whole virus vaccine. Hepatitis A is spread through close physical contact and by eating or drinking contaminated food or water. It is one of the most frequently reported vaccine-preventable diseases in the United States. Young children are particularly susceptible to hepatitis A because of their close contact with other children, inadequate hygiene practices, and tendency to place everything in their mouth. HepA is recommended to be given to all children at age 12 months, followed by a repeat dose in 6 to 12 months.

Hepatitis B Vaccine. HepB is a recombinant vaccine. Hepatits B virus can result in a serious infection that affects the liver. It is spread through contact with blood and body fluids and can be spread from an infected mother to a newborn at birth. Hepatitis B vaccination is recommended at birth, preferably within the first 12 hours, then at 1 to 2 months and 6 to 18 months (CDC, 2014b). A total of four doses is acceptable when a combination vaccine with hepatitis B is used after birth (CDC, 2014b). Because hepatitis B is a sexually transmitted infection, it is important to verify the immunization status of all adolescents.

Varicella Vaccine. Varicella vaccine is a live attenuated virus vaccine. All children aged 12 to 15 months who have not had varicella (chickenpox) should be immunized. A second dose is recommended at age 4 to 6 years. The vaccine provides effective postexposure prophylaxis if administered within 3 to 5 days after exposure. The ACIP does recommend vaccination even if exposure is greater than 5 days in children without evidence of immunity and eligible for the vaccination (not recommended for children younger than 12 months of age) (CDC, 2012d). Varicella may be given the same day as other live attenuated virus vaccines. However, if not given on the same day, the immunizations should be spaced at least 28 days apart (Kroger et al., 2011). Pregnancy in a child's mother is not a contraindication to the vaccination of the child.

Pneumococcal Vaccines. *Streptococcus pneumoniae* (pneumococcus) is the most common cause of pneumonia, sepsis, meningitis, and otitis media in young children (CDC, 2013e). The two available pneumococcal vaccines are pneumococcal conjugate vaccine (PCV) and pneumococcal polysaccharide vaccine (PPSV). Beginning in 2010, PCV13, which contains 13 strains of *S. pneumoniae,* replaced PCV7, which contained only 7 strains, for use in routine vaccination for children (CDC, 2014b). It stimulates an immune response in infants and is given at 2 months of age as part of the initial immunization series, but can be given as early as 6 weeks of age (CDC, 2014b). PPSV contains 23 strains of *S. pneumoniae.* It does not provoke an immune response in children younger than 2 years of age (CDC, 2014b). PPSV is given to children older than 2 years of age who are at high risk for pneumococcal sepsis. This group includes children with anatomic/functional asplenia; sickle cell disease; chronic cardiac, pulmonary, or renal disease; diabetes mellitus; or HIV infection; children getting or who have cochlear implants; and children with immunosuppression (CDC, 2014b).

Influenza Vaccines. Influenza immunization is recommended yearly for all persons 6 months of age or older. All children 6 months to 8 years of age who are receiving the influenza vaccination for the first time require two doses separated by 4 weeks. Only one dose is needed if the child has received two doses of seasonal influenza in previous years and at least one dose of 2009 H1N1–containing vaccine (Grohskopf et al., 2013). In 2009/2010, in addition to the seasonal influenza vaccinations, the CDC began recommending vaccination against H1N1 influenza due to the influenza pandemic that was occurring worldwide (AAP, 2010; Grohskopf et al., 2013). In the 2010/2011 influenza season, one vaccine was recommended that protected against three strains of influenza, including the 2009 H1N1 (AAP, 2010).

Take Note!

For the first time, during the 2013/2014 influenza season, quadrivalent seasonal influenza vaccine was available which protected against two B virus strains and provided broader protection against influenza (AAP, Committee on Infectious Diseases, 2013).

There are two influenza vaccines available, the live attenuated influenza vaccine (LAIV) and the inactivated influenza vaccine (IIV). LAIV is given intranasally and is indicated for healthy persons between the ages of 2 and 49 years (CDC, 2014b). The virus in LAIV can replicate, and a person who has received LAIV can shed the virus for a week although available data report the risk of transmission to be very low (AAP, Committee on Infectious Diseases, 2013). LAIV should not be given to anyone who will be in contact with an immunosuppressed person requiring a protected environment. It is also contraindicated in children who have large amounts of nasal secretions present at the time of vaccination; children with underlying medical conditions that predispose them to complications from influenza, such as diabetes mellitus; children younger than 5 years of age with a history of recurrent wheezing or medically attended wheezing in the past 12 months; and children who have received another live vaccine in the past 4 weeks, have a known or suspected immunodeficiency, or who are taking aspirin or other salicylates (AAP, Committee on Infectious Diseases, 2013). IIV is suitable for any eligible person aged 6 months or older. IIV is not capable of causing disease and is given by intramuscular injection (AAP, Committee on Infectious Diseases, 2013).

Rotavirus Vaccine. Rotavirus is the most common cause of severe gastroenteritis among young children (CDC, 2014c). The virus is shed in the stool and easily spreads via the fecal–oral route. Severe, watery, crampy diarrhea quickly leads to dehydration in the infected child. The rotavirus vaccine is a live vaccine targeting five strains of rotavirus and is given via the oral route to infants. Two vaccine products are currently available. Rotarix requires two doses (at 2 and 4 months) and RotaTeq requires three doses (at 2, 4, and 6 months) (CDC, 2014b). If RotaTeq was used for any doses or the vaccine product is unknown, a total of three doses should be administered (CDC, 2014b). Administration of rotavirus vaccine is contraindicated in children with SCID or a history of intussusception (CDC, 2014d).

Human Papillomavirus Vaccine. Human papillomavirus (HPV) is a DNA tumor virus transmitted through direct skin-to-skin contact. HPV is contracted most often during vaginal or anal penetrative sexual acts. HPV infection is the most common sexually transmitted infection in the United States (CDC, 2014e). HPV causes genital warts and is responsible for the development of cancer. For these reasons, the ACIP and AAP have recommended that HPV vaccination occur in all preadolescent girls and boys (CDC, 2014b). Two vaccines have been licensed: Cervarix, or HPV2, and Gardasil, or HPV4. The three-vaccine series of either HPV2 or HPV4 is recommended to be given at 11 to 12 years of age over a 6-month period (CDC, 2014b). HPV2 or HPV4 is used for females, while only administration of HPV4 is used for males (CDC, 2014b).

Meningococcal Vaccine. Meningococcal disease may manifest as meningitis, a deadly blood infection (meningococcemia), or bacteremic pneumonia. It is caused by the bacterium *Neisseria meningitidis,* which is spread through direct contact or by air droplets. It develops quickly, usually in healthy children and adolescents, and results in high rates of morbidity and mortality (Cohn et al., 2013). For these reasons, the meningococcal vaccine is recommended for all previously unvaccinated children at age 11 to 12 years with a booster dose at the age of 16 years (CDC, 2014b). Routine vaccination is also recommended for children 2 months or older who are at an increased risk for the disease due to certain medical conditions such as anatomical or functional asplenia or complement component deficiency (Cohn et al., 2013). Special populations such as first-year college students living in residence halls who are unvaccinated or incompletely vaccinated need the immunization. Some colleges and universities have instituted policies requiring the meningococcal vaccination (Cohn et al., 2013). It can also be administered to certain at-risk groups to control an outbreak (Cohn et al., 2013).

Recall the Randall children, introduced at the beginning of the chapter. What immunizations would be appropriate for them to receive? Explain how you would administer the injections, and discuss any contraindications or precautions.

BARRIERS TO IMMUNIZATION

A fully immunized child is protected from the discomforts and complications of many infectious diseases. Disease prevention spares the family the emotional and financial burdens that serious illnesses can cause. Immunization programs prevent devastating epidemics in a community. Health care dollars not spent treating preventable diseases can be used for other urgent issues. Despite the numerous advantages of immunization and improved immunization rates, some communities in this country continue to have high numbers of undervaccinated or unvaccinated children, leaving these communities vulnerable to outbreaks (Black, Yankey, & Kolasa, 2013).

Many factors lead to children not being fully immunized. Parental concerns about vaccine safety are a significant cause of inadequate immunization. A recent survey found that the top parental concerns regarding vaccine safety were too many vaccines given during a single office visit and in the first 2 years of life, along with the perceived link between vaccines and learning problems such as autism (DeStefano, Price, & Weintraub, 2013). See Evidence-Based Practice 31.1. Parents may want to postpone some of the scheduled immunizations because they are concerned about the effects of multiple injections on their child. Postponing a portion of the immunizations puts the child at risk for contracting disease. Disrupting the optimal spacing of the immunizations can decrease the efficacy of vaccine, further putting the child at risk.

Misconceptions of what constitutes a contraindication to vaccination and having more than one physician are major contributors to inadequate immunization status. The more children in a family, the less likely the children are to be fully vaccinated. The costs for vaccines can also deter families from obtaining immunizations.

OVERCOMING BARRIERS TO IMMUNIZATION

The AAP recommends the use of a manufacturer-produced combination vaccine whenever it will reduce the number of injections at a visit (Kroger et al., 2011). These combination vaccines have been studied and approved by the FDA. The nurse should never mix separate vaccines in the same syringe unless expressly permitted in the product insert for all vaccines involved. Examples of combination vaccines are:

- ProQuad: measles, mumps, rubella, varicella
- Comvax: HepB–Hib
- Pediarix: DTaP–Hep B–IPV
- Pentacel: DTaP–IPV/Hib

The Vaccines for Children (VFC) is a federally funded program that was implemented in 1994 in response to the 1989–1991 measles epidemic (CDC, 2014f). Prior to this program, free vaccines were available only through public health agencies. The goal of this program is to improve immunization rates by providing free vaccines to low-income and uninsured families through private physicians who are registered VFC providers. Additional information on the VFC program is available at http://www.cdc.gov/vaccines/programs/vfc/. The Affordable Care Act of 2010 requires new health plans to cover preventative services, including ACIP-approved immunizations, without charging a deductible, copayment, or coinsurance (U.S. Department of Health and Human Services, 2012a). The goal of these programs is to increase access to vaccines.

EVIDENCE-BASED PRACTICE 31.1 ARE VACCINES ASSOCIATED WITH A RISK OF AUTSIM?

STUDY

Concerns about the link between autism and vaccines continue. Most recently, the focus has been on the number of vaccines administered in the first 2 years of life. The number of routine scheduled immunizations is much greater than in the 1990s. This study was a secondary analysis on a previous case control study that investigated the association between exposure to thimerosal-containing injections and autism spectrum disorder (ASD). This study looked at the association between the level of immunologic stimulation received from vaccines in the first 2 years of life and the risk of developing ASD, autistic disorder (AD), and ASD with regression. 252 children with ASD and 752 control children were matched by birth year, sex and managed care organization. Level of immunologic stimulation was determined by adding the antigenic content of each vaccine received.

Findings

In this study, no evidence was found indicating that there is an association to the number of vaccines given over the first 2 years of life or given on a single day and the risk of ASD, AD, or ASD with regression.

Nursing Implications

Parents often have concerns regarding immunizations. Currently, parents' top concerns include too many vaccines being given and the link of immunizations to learning difficulties (including autism). Nurses are in the unique position to educate families and the community that current research findings do not support these concerns. Even though the number of routine immunizations have increased dramatically over the past 2 decades the total number of antigens the child is exposed to is actually less. This is due to the fact that newer vaccines are less crude and less antigenic than before.

Adapted from DeStefano, F., Price, C. S., & Weintraub, E. S. (2013). Increasing exposure to antibody-stimulating proteins and polysaccharides in vaccines is not associated with risk of autism. *The Journal of Pediatrics*, *163*(2), 561–567. doi:10.1016/j.jpeds.2013.02.001

Establishing a medical home for every child will alleviate many of the factors associated with lack of immunization. Parents who have a long-term, trusting relationship with a physician are more likely to have their concerns about vaccine safety discussed and removed. Missed opportunities for immunizations can be reduced by:

- Maintaining a centralized immunization record
- Verifying immunization status at every visit, not just health supervision visits
- Verifying the status of siblings accompanying the child to the appointment
- Providing parents with up-to-date information on vaccines geared to their concerns and needs

Two excellent resources for vaccination recommendations in the United States are the CDC's Vaccines and Immunizations website (http://www.cdc.gov/vaccines/default.htm) and the CDC Hotline (800–232–4636 or 800-CDC-INFO).

Discuss potential barriers to the Randall children being fully immunized. As a nurse, how can you help overcome these barriers?

Health Promotion

Health promotion focuses on maintaining or enhancing the physical and mental health of children. The principal components of health promotion are identifying risk factors for a disease, facilitating lifestyle changes to eliminate or reduce those risk factors, and empowering children at the individual and community level to develop resources to optimize their health. The nurse implements health promotion through education and anticipatory guidance.

Partnership development is the key strategy for success when implementing a health promotion activity. Identifying key stakeholders from the community allows problems to be solved and provides additional venues for disseminating information. Health promotion messages can be reinforced at schools, day care centers, community agencies, and churches. If families have difficulty getting to health care facilities, the community arenas may be the primary source of health promotion.

Providing Anticipatory Guidance

Anticipatory guidance is primary prevention. The nurse partners with the parents to create a "road map" to optimal health for the child. Healthy People 2020 provides a framework for determining health promotion goals. *Bright Futures: Guidelines for Health Supervision of Infants, Children, and Adolescents* (Hagan, Shaw, & Duncan, 2008) is another valuable resource.

The "skeleton" of the guidance provided involves common childhood health problems. The nurse fleshes out that information using the results of risk assessments and screening tests, health concerns unique to the child, and the interests and concerns of the parents. Age-related anticipatory guidance information is provided in Chapters 25 through 29.

Provide appropriate anticipatory guidance for 3-year-old Maya and 9-month-old Evan.

Promoting Oral Health Care

Effective oral health practices are essential to the overall health of children and adolescents. Dental caries are the most common chronic illness seen in children, and 19.5% of children aged 2 to 5 years and about 23% of children aged 6 to 19 years have untreated dental caries (CDC, 2011i). Poor oral health can have significant negative effects on systemic health. Children who suffer from untreated dental caries have an increased incidence of pain and infections and may have problems with eating and playing, difficulty at school, and sleep pattern disturbances (CDC, 2011i). Refer to Healthy People 2020.

Optimal oral health is not limited to the prevention and treatment of dental caries. It includes anticipatory guidance about nonnutritive sucking habits, injury prevention, oral cancer prevention, and tongue and lip piercing. Preventing and treating malocclusion can have a significant benefit for children. Comprehensive health care is not possible if oral health is not a priority in the health delivery system.

Optimizing oral health can benefit the community as well as the individual child. There has been a 60% reduction in early childhood caries over the past 50 years since community water supplies were fluoridated at optimal levels (American Academy of Pediatric Dentistry [AAPD], 2013a). The cost of pediatric oral health care could be reduced by 50% with the proper use of fluoride treatments coupled with other preventive measures (AAPD, 2013a). These health care dollar savings will enhance community resources.

HEALTHY PEOPLE *2020*

Objective	Nursing Significance
Reduce the proportion of children and adolescents who have dental caries in their primary or permanent teeth.	• Teach children and adolescents appropriate tooth brushing and flossing techniques. • Encourage use of fluoride-containing toothpastes. • Encourage routine dental visits.

Healthy People Objectives retrieved from http://www.healthypeople.gov

BOX 31.8

CHARACTERISTICS OF THE DENTAL HOME

- Preventive health program based on risk assessment
- Anticipatory guidance on oral health developmental issues, including dietary counseling related to oral health
- Plans for emergency dental trauma
- Anticipatory guidance on oral hygiene
- Comprehensive dental care (acute and preventative services)
- Comprehensive assessment for oral diseases
- Referral to specialists for care not available at the dental home

Adapted from American Academy of Pediatric Dentistry. (2012). *Policy on the dental home.* Retrieved from http://www.aapd.org/media/Policies_Guidelines/P_DentalHome.pdf

Having a dental home enhances the likelihood that the child will obtain appropriate preventive and routine care. The AAPD adopted the policy of the dental home in 2001 (AAPD, 2012). It is modeled on the AAP medical home policy. The dental home provides the same benefits to the child as the medical home. Characteristics of a dental home are listed in Box 31.8. The AAPD (2012) recommends that the dental home be established by the infant's first birthday.

Promoting Healthy Weight

Childhood obesity is a growing problem. The number of overweight children has doubled since 1980; the rate for teens has quadrupled (CDC, 2014g). The principal causes of this increase in obesity are unhealthy eating habits and decreased physical activity. Weight is best managed by balancing calories with a combination of diet and exercise (U.S. Department of Agriculture and U.S. Department of Health and Human Services, 2010). Nurses can have the maximum effect in promoting healthy weight in children by encouraging activities that address both healthy eating patterns and physical fitness. Children, parents, and communities are all targets for healthy weight promotion by nurses. Refer to Healthy People 2020.

The focus of healthy weight promotion should be health centered, not weight centered. Linking success to numbers on a scale increases the possibility of developing eating disorders, nutritional deficiencies, and body hatred. Instead, emphasizing the benefits of health through an active lifestyle and nutritious eating creates a nurturing environment for the child. This allows the child to maintain his or her self-esteem. In addition, a health-centered orientation also allows the family to develop a lifestyle that incorporates its cultural food patterns and traditions.

Parents who have a healthy eating pattern are likely to maintain and encourage those patterns in their children.

***HEALTHY PEOPLE** 2020*

Objective	Nursing Significance
Reduce the proportion of children and adolescents who are obese.	• Screen all children for the development of overweight as indicated by an increasing body mass index (BMI) for their age. • Provide accurate diet counseling. • Encourage daily physical activity. • Counsel parents to limit television/computer time daily.

Healthy People Objectives retrieved from http://www.healthypeople.gov

The nurse provides parents with anticipatory guidance about age-related eating patterns during each health supervision visit. Parents with toddlers and preschoolers may need training in ways to cope with the child's growing autonomy while providing a variety of nutritious options.

The nurse can begin directly advising the young child on healthy foods. Information and teaching modalities need to be age appropriate. With colorful posters and games, the nurse can teach the preschool child the difference between healthy and unhealthy food choices. As children enter school, group and peer-led activities can be very effective. The nurse must gear material toward the teen's growing autonomy in making self-care decisions.

Before providing education to school-age and teenage children, it is important to obtain nutritional histories directly from them because increasingly they are eating meals away from the family table. As they spend more time away from their parents, they need to develop the ability to make nutritious choices. The goal is to help older children develop strategies for making healthy choices as part of their increasingly independent lifestyle. Detailed anticipatory guidance is provided in Teaching Guidelines 31.1 and in Chapters 25 through 29.

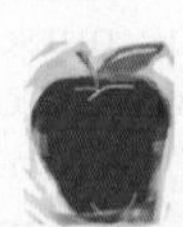

Teaching Guidelines 31.1

HEALTHY EATING

Breakfast

1. Don't skip breakfast. You will not have enough energy to play well later in the day. Skipping breakfast can also lower your grades in school.
2. Avoid eating high-sugar foods at breakfast. They will make you sleepy during the day.

3. Start your breakfast with some fruit. A small glass of juice, berries on your cereal, or a banana is a good choice.
4. Protein is important at breakfast. Milk, either in a glass or on cereal, is a good source of protein; so is yogurt or peanut butter.

Lunch

1. Check the quality of school-provided lunches. If they are high in fat or sugar, bring your lunch. Many schools publish their daily menus in advance. Check the newspaper or ask the school for a copy.
2. Add a variety of healthy alternatives to your lunches.
    a. Try different types of breads. Pitas, wraps, bagels, and taco shells can be a good change of pace in the sandwich routine.
    b. Freeze fruits before putting them in the lunch box. This will keep the lunch items cool and the fruit fresh tasting. Canned pineapple and grapes freeze well; so do bananas.
    c. Try alternatives to high-fat chips. Dried fruits, baked pretzels, and animal crackers are a few examples of tasty, healthy treats.
    d. Low-fat chocolate milk is more nutritious than prepackaged juice boxes, which have high sugar concentrations.

Snacks

1. Limit snacks to after school and bedtime. Light snacks such as yogurt or fruit provide good hunger management. A very hungry child will tend to overeat at meals.
2. Children need to learn to eat only when they are hungry. Children often eat out of boredom. Discourage nonstop grazing by planning activities to occupy the child.
3. A small bedtime snack is OK if the child is hungry but should not become a habit. A light carbohydrate such as graham crackers or a piece of fruit works well.

Dinner

1. Plan your menu a week ahead. Planning ahead reduces the likelihood of eating out or getting take-out food. Restaurant foods are more likely to be high in fats and carbohydrates.
2. Prepare homemade healthy versions of take-out favorites. Top prepared pizza crust with cooked chicken, vegetables, mushrooms, and cheese. Serve the pizza with a salad for a complete and healthy meal. "Make your own tacos" nights, using lean hamburger and low-fat sour cream, can be a lot of fun for children.
3. Don't turn dinner into a battle zone. Forcing children to eat foods they do not like will only deepen their dislike of them. Give them the healthy foods they do enjoy and eventually they will explore more options.
4. Lead by example. Children eventually adopt the eating patterns of their parents. If they see their parents eat vegetables, they will eventually try them.

***HEALTHY PEOPLE** 2020*

Objective	Nursing Significance
Increase the proportion of adolescents who meet current federal physical activity guidelines for aerobic physical activity and for muscle-strengthening activity.	• For the nonexercising teen, advise him or her to start slowly by walking. • Work with the teen to identify physical activities that interest him or her. • Praise efforts to participate in a routine exercise plan. • Identify an athletic individual with whom the teen identifies, and encourage similar activities in the teen.

Healthy People Objectives retrieved from http://www.healthypeople.gov

Promoting Healthy Activity

Healthy physical activity can take many forms. During the preschool years, encourage parents to provide a wide variety of physical activities. This exposure to multiple types of exercise allows the child to find the one that is most enjoyable and increases the chances that he or she will maintain an active lifestyle. The focus should be on noncompetitive, fun activities. When the child enters school, the lure of television and computers can significantly diminish the amount of time spent in physical activity. Parents can encourage their children to stay physically active in several ways. They can limit the amount of time spent in sedentary activities and actively encourage the child to pursue any exercise that he or she enjoys. In addition to verbal encouragement, parents can promote exercise by participating in exercise with the child. A simple family walk can increase physical fitness while providing time for interaction between parent and child. Refer to Healthy People 2020. Teaching Guidelines 31.2 gives additional suggestions for promoting physical activity.

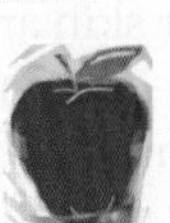

Teaching Guidelines 31.2
HEALTHY ACTIVITY

1. Plan physical activities that your family can do as a group.
2. Write exercise activities on your family's daily schedule.
3. Look for activities that appeal to your child's interest, such as dance, team sports, or swimming.

4. Place value on noncompetitive as well as competitive activities.
5. Show your child you believe exercise is important. Exercise daily yourself.
6. Encourage the community to develop safe areas for spontaneous games and activities.

Take Note!

The U.S. Department of Health and Human Services recommends all children 6 to 17 years of age participate in at least 60 minutes of physical activity every day (CDC, 2014h).

Promoting Personal Hygiene

Hand washing is the first personal hygiene topic that needs to be introduced to children. Hand washing prevents disease by limiting a child's exposure to pathogens. The nurse can introduce the topic to preschool children using cartoons and games. Have the child sing "Twinkle, Twinkle Little Star" while washing his or her hands; this encourages adequate cleansing time. Use soap containers and towels with colorful characters to make the experience more fun. The school-age child can understand the concepts of germs and disease. Slogans such as "Let's drown a germ" can serve as a reminder of the importance of hand washing. The "Glo-germ" program (n.d.) (see websites on thePoint) is very effective in this age group. A nontoxic substance that shines under a black light is placed on the children's hands. The children can follow how germs travel from object to object. After washing their hands, the children can see if they did a good job (Glo-germ program, n.d.).

In response to peer pressure, teenagers are usually stringent about personal hygiene. Young teens may need guidance in dealing with pubescent body changes such as body odor, fungal infections such as tinea pedis (athlete's foot), and acne.

Promoting Safe Sun Exposure

Skin cancer is a significant health problem in the United States. Blistering sunburns in children substantially increase the risk of melanoma and other skin cancers (National Cancer Institute, 2011). People with fair skin are at highest risk for skin cancers, but anyone can become sunburned and develop skin cancer. When teaching children about safe sun exposure, remind them that harmful ultraviolet (UV) rays can reflect off water, snow, sand, and concrete, so being in the shade or under an awning does not guarantee protection. Adequate sun protection requires using sunscreen, avoiding peak sun hours, and wearing proper clothing. Teaching Guidelines 31.3 gives more detailed instructions.

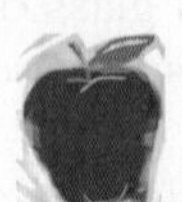

Teaching Guidelines 31.3
SAFE SUN EXPOSURE

Sunscreen

1. Use sunscreen lotions every day. Harmful UV rays penetrate clouds and cause damaging sunburns.
2. Use sunscreens with a sun protection factor (SPF) of 30 or higher and with UVA and UVB protection. An adequate amount for an average-sized child is half an ounce.
3. Apply sunscreens half an hour before sun exposure.
4. Reapply every hour if the child is perspiring heavily.
5. Reapply immediately after swimming.
6. Infants 6 months old or younger should not use sunscreens. Take steps to avoid sun exposure completely with this age group.

Clothing

1. Wear hats. The brim of the hat should be 10.16 cm (4 inches) or more and should shade the ears. Straw hats need to have a sun proof liner to be effective. Children introduced to hats as infants usually accept hats as part of the "outfit."
2. Wear UV-blocking sunglasses. The eye is the second most common site for melanoma.
3. Wear long, loose, and lightweight clothing for maximum sun protection.

Lifestyle

1. Avoid sun exposure between 10 AM and 4 PM. This is when UV rays are the strongest.
2. Ask your physician if your medication will increase your sensitivity to UV rays. If the answer is yes, take extra precautions to reduce sun exposure.
3. Avoid tanning parlors. The devices emit UV rays just like the sun and can cause damage.
4. Check the UV index before going out. The higher the index, the more precautions you should take. UV index figures are available in newspaper, TV, and radio weather reports and on the internet.
5. Advocate for safe-sun scheduling of recreational activities. Talk to others about scheduling outdoor activities before 10 AM, after 4 PM, or in the shade.
6. Consider UV-blocking plastic film for your house and car windows.

Take Note!

Give children the following physical reference when doing health promotion on safe sun exposure. Tell the child, "Play outside only when your shadow is taller than you are." The child's shadow will be "taller" before 10 AM and after 2 PM. The nurse can demonstrate this concept by placing a ruler on end and shining a bright light over it. As the nurse moves the light, the child will see the ruler's shadow lengthen.

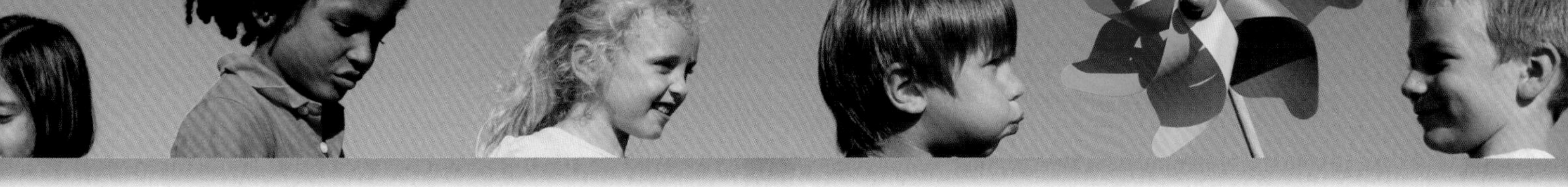

KEY CONCEPTS

- Health supervision for children is a dynamic process. Optimal wellness for the child can only occur if the nurse forms meaningful partnerships with the child, the family, and the community. These partnerships allow for free exchange of information and the establishment of mutually agreed upon goals. The medical home exists when there is a single primary care provider for the child. The medical home establishes a trusting long-term relationship with the child and family. This relationship leads to comprehensive, coordinated, and cost-effective care for the child.
- Children with chronic illnesses have a critical need for comprehensive and coordinated health supervision. Children with chronic illnesses require more frequent health supervision assessments. These children must have a medical home. The location of that medical home may be with a knowledgeable primary physician or at a multidisciplinary specialty facility. The location is determined by the child's needs and the family's preferences.
- The nurse incorporates frequent assessments of the many psychosocial stressors faced by families of children with chronic illnesses when establishing health care plans for them.
- Health supervision has three components: developmental surveillance and screening; injury and disease prevention; and health promotion.
- Developmental surveillance is an ongoing process requiring a skilled observer and interviewer. To be effective, the nurse must understand normal growth and development expectations and be proficient at developmental screening procedures and techniques. Caregivers are most likely to reveal risk factors or warning signs for developmental delay when the nurse has a long-term and trusting relationship with the family.
- Screening tests are part of injury and disease prevention. They are modalities that identify treatable disease in an early or asymptomatic state and allow for cure or lessening of the disease's injury.
- Vision and hearing screening are functional testing modalities that the nurse must be proficient in administering in order for the child's results to be valid.
- Immunizations are a cornerstone of pediatric disease prevention. The nurse increases the effectiveness of immunization by understanding the principles of immunization and applying them to the child's individual circumstances. Adhering to good immunization management practices, as outlined by the ACIP and the AAP, enhances the benefits and reduces the risks of immunization.
- Barriers to full immunization include fragmentation of health care, concerns about vaccine safety, financial constraints, and lack of knowledge. The nurse can be pivotal in ensuring that children and adolescents are fully immunized by serving as child educator and advocate.
- The principal components of health promotion are identifying risk factors for a disease, facilitating lifestyle changes to eliminate or reduce those risk factors, and empowering children at the individual and community level to develop resources to optimize their health.
- The nurse implements health promotion through education and anticipatory guidance.
- Anticipatory guidance provided involves common childhood health problems and seeks to prevent or improve the health of children.
- The nurse uses the results of risk assessments and screening tests, health concerns unique to the child, and the interests and concerns of the parents to develop appropriate anticipatory guidance for each child and family.

REFERENCES AND RECOMMENDED READINGS

Advisory Committee on Immunization Practices. (2000). Recommendations and reports: Poliomyelitis prevention in the United States: Updated recommendations of the Advisory Committee on Immunization Practices (ACIP). *Morbidity and Mortality Weekly Report (MMWR), 49*(RR05), 1–22. Retrieved from http://www.cdc.gov/mmwr/preview/mmwrhtml/rr4905a1.htm

Advisory Committee on Childhood Lead Poisoning Prevention. (2012). *Low Level Lead Exposure Harms Children: A Renewed Call for Primary Prevention.* Retrieved from http://www.cdc.gov/nceh/lead/acclpp/final_document_030712.pdf

American Academy of Pediatric Dentistry. (2012). *Policy on the dental home.* Retrieved from http://www.aapd.org/media/Policies_Guidelines/P_DentalHome.pdf

American Academy of Pediatric Dentistry. (2013a). *Policy on use of fluoride.* Retrieved from http://www.aapd.org/media/Policies_Guidelines/P_FluorideUse.pdf

American Academy of Pediatric Dentistry. (2013b). *Guideline on periodicity of examination, preventive dental services, anticipatory guidance and oral treatment for children.* Retrieved from http://www.aapd.org/media/Policies_Guidelines/G_Periodicity.pdf

American Academy of Pediatrics. (2010). *Policy statement—Recommendations for prevention and control of influenza in children, 2010–2011*. Retrieved from http://pediatrics.aappublications.org/cgi/reprint/peds.2010–2216v1

American Academy of Pediatrics. (2013). *Family life: Well-child care: A check-up for success*. Retrieved from http://www.healthychildren.org/English/family-life/health-management/pages/Well-Child-Care-A-Check-Up-for-Success.aspx

American Academy of Pediatrics (AAP), Committee on Infectious Diseases. (2013). Recommendations for prevention and control of influenza in children. *Pediatrics, 132*(4), 1–16. doi: 10.1542/peds.2013–2377

American Academy of Pediatrics, National Center for Medical Home Implementation. (n.d.). *What is a family centered medical home*. The medical home. Retrieved from http://www.medicalhomeinfo.org/

Baker, R. D., Greer, F. R., The Committee on Nutrition. (2010). Clinical report. Diagnosis and prevention of iron deficiency and iron-deficiency anemia in infants and young children (0–3 years of age). *Pediatrics, 126*(5), 1040–1050. doi: 10.1542/peds.2010–2576

Black, C. L., Yankey, D., & Kolasa, M. (2013). National, state, and local area vaccination coverage among children aged 19–35 months — United States, 2012. *Morbidity and Mortality Weekly Report (MMWR), 62*(36), 733–740.

Briere, E. C., Rubin, L., Moro, P. L., Cohn, A., Clark, T., & Messonnier, N. (2014) Prevention and control of haemophilus influenzae Type b disease: Recommendations of the Advisory Committee on Immunization Practices (ACIP): recommendations and reports. *Morbidity and Mortality Weekly Report (MMWR), 63*(RR01), 1–14.

Bright Futures/American Academy of Pediatrics. (2014). *Recommendations for preventive pediatric health care*. Retrieved from http://www.aap.org/en-us/professional-resources/practice-support/Periodicity/Periodicity%20Schedule_FINAL.pdf healthyhomes.htm

Centers for Disease Control and Prevention. (2009). Updated Recommendations of the Advisory Committee on Immunization Practices (ACIP) regarding routine poliovirus vaccination.*Morbidity and Mortality Weekly Report (MMWR), 58*(30), 829–830.

Centers for Disease Control and Prevention. (2010). Addition of severe combined immunodeficiency as a contraindication for administration of rotavirus vaccine. *Morbidity and Mortality Weekly Report (MMWR), 59*(22), 687–688.

Centers for Disease Control and Prevention. (2011a). *Nutrition for everyone: Iron and iron deficiency*. Retrieved from http://www.cdc.gov/nutrition/everyone/basics/vitamins/iron.html

Centers for Disease Control and Prevention. (2011b). *Untreated dental caries (cavities) in children ages 2–19, United States*. Retrieved from http://www.cdc.gov/Features/dsUntreatedCavitiesKids/

Centers for Disease Control and Prevention. (2012a). *Reproductive and birth outcomes: Premature births and the environment*. Retrieved from http://ephtracking.cdc.gov/showRbPrematureBirthEnv.action

Centers for Disease Control and Prevention. (2012b). *CDC response to advisory committee on childhood lead poisoning prevention recommendations in "Low Level Lead Exposure Harms Children: A Renewed Call of Primary Prevention"*. Retrieved from http://www.cdc.gov/nceh/lead/ACCLPP/CDC_Response_Lead_Exposure_Recs.pdf

Centers for Disease Control and Prevention. (2012c). *Vaccine storage & handling tool kit*. Retrieved from http://www.cdc.gov/vaccines/recs/storage/toolkit/storage-handling-toolkit.pdf

Centers for Disease Control and Prevention. (2012d). *Vaccines and immunizations: Post-exposure varicella vaccination: information for healthcare providers*. Retrieved from http://www.cdc.gov/vaccines/vpd-vac/varicella/hcp-post-exposure.htm

Centers for Disease Control and Prevention. (2013a). *Immigrant and refugee health screening for lead during the domestic medical examination for newly arrived refugees*. Retrieved from http://www.cdc.gov/immigrantrefugeehealth/guidelines/lead-guidelines.html

Centers for Disease Control and Prevention. (2013b). *Lead*. Retrieved from http://www.cdc.gov/nceh/lead/

Centers for Disease Control and Prevention. (2013c). *Vaccine Information Statements (VIS): Facts about VISs*. Retrieved http://www.cdc.gov/vaccines/hcp/vis/about/facts-vis.html

Centers for Disease Control and Prevention. (2013d). *Healthy homes*. Retrieved from http://www.cdc.gov/nceh/lead/

Centers for Disease Control and Prevention. (2013e). *Pneumococcal disease: Types of infection*. Retrieved http://www.cdc.gov/pneumococcal/about/infection-types.html

Centers for Disease Control and Prevention. (2013f). *How can I protect my children from the Sun?* Retrieved from http://www.cdc.gov/cancer/skin/basic_info/children.htm

Centers for Disease Control and Prevention. (2014a). *Birth-18 years & "Catch-up" immunization schedules united states, 2014*. Retrieved from http://www.cdc.gov/vaccines/schedules/hcp/child-adolescent.html.

Centers for Disease Control and Prevention. (2014b). *Vaccine safety: Rotavirus*. Retrieved from http://www.cdc.gov/vaccinesafety/vaccines/rotavsb.html

Centers for Disease Control and Prevention. (2014c). *Vaccines and immunizations: Who should NOT get vaccinated with these Vaccines?* Retrieved from http://www.cdc.gov/vaccines/vpd-vac/should-not-vacc.htm

Centers for Disease Control and Prevention. (2014d). *Human Papillomavirus (HPV): Genital HPV infection - fact sheet*. Retrieved from http://www.cdc.gov/std/HPV/STDFact-HPV.htm

Centers for Disease Control and Prevention. (2014e). *Vaccines for children program (VFC)*. Retrieved from http://www.cdc.gov/vaccines/programs/vfc/about/index.html

Centers for Disease Control and Prevention. (2014f). *Childhood obesity facts*. Retrieved from http://www.cdc.gov/healthyyouth/obesity/facts.htm

Centers for Disease Control and Prevention. (2014g). *Adolescent and school health: Physical activity facts*. Retrieved from http://www.cdc.gov/healthyyouth/physicalactivity/facts.htm

Centers for Disease Control and Prevention. (2014h). *Vaccines and immunizations*. Retrieved from http://www.cdc.gov/vaccines/default.htm

Centers for Disease Control and Prevention. (2014i). *HIB vaccine: What you need to know*. Retrieved from http://www.cdc.gov/vaccines/hcp/vis/vis-statements/hib.pdf

Cohn, A. C., MacNeil, J. R., Clark, T. A., Ortega-Sanchez, I. R., Briere, E. Z., Meissner, H. C., et al. (2013). Prevention and control of meningococcal disease: Recommendations of the Advisory Committee on Immunization Practices (ACIP): Recommendations and reports. *Morbidity and Mortality Weekly Report (MMWR), 62*(RR02);1–22.

Delaney, A. M., Meyers, A. D., & Ruth, R. A. (2012). Newborn hearing screening. *eMedicine*. Retrieved from http://emedicine.medscape.com/article/836646-overview#a30

DeStefano, F., Price, C. S., & Weintraub, E. S. (2013). Increasing exposure to antibody-stimulating proteins and polysaccharides in vaccines is not associated with risk of autism. *The Journal of Pediatrics, 163*(2), 561–567. doi:10.1016/j.jpeds.2013.02.001

Dowshen, S. (2013). *Sun safety*. Retrieved from http://kidshealth.org/parent/firstaid_safe/outdoor/sun_safety.html#

Durani, Y. (2012). *Lead poisoning*. Retrieved from http://kidshealth.org/parent/medical/brain/lead_poisoning.html#

Gilchrist, J., Ballesteros, M. F., & Parker, E. M. (2012). Vital signs: Unintentional injury deaths among persons aged 0–19 Years—United States, 2000–2009. *Morbidity and Mortality Weekly Report (MMWR), 61*, 270–276. Retrieved from http://www.cdc.gov/mmwr/preview/mmwrhtml/mm61e0416a1.htm

Glo-germ program. (n.d.). Retrieved from http://www.glogerm.com

Grohskopf, L. A., Shay, D. K., Shimabukuro, T. T., Sokolow, L. Z., Keitel, W. A., Bresee, J. S., et al. (2013). Prevention and control of seasonal influenza with vaccines: Recommendations of the advisory committee on immunization practices—United States, 2013–2014: Recommendations and reports. *Morbidity and Mortality Weekly Report (MMWR), 62*(RR07), 1–43.

Haddan, J. Jr. (2011). Chapter 329 hearing loss. In R. M. Kleigman, B. F. Stanton, J. W. St. Geme III, N. F. Schor, & R. E. Behrman (Eds.), *Nelson textbook of pediatrics* (19th ed., pp. 2188–2196).

Hagan, J. F., Shaw, J. S., & Duncan, P. M. (Eds.). (2008). *Bright futures: Guidelines for health supervision of infants, children, and adolescents* (3rd ed., rev.). Elk Grove Village, IL: American Academy of Pediatrics. Retrieved from http://brightfutures.aap.org/3rd_Edition_Guidelines_and_Pocket_Guide.html

Immunization Action Coalition. (2011). *Vaccine administration record for children and teens*. Retrieved from http://www.immunize.org/catg.d/p2022.pdf

Immunization Action Coalition. (2012). *Administering vaccines: Dose, route, site, and needle size*. Retrieved from http://www.immunize.org/catg.d/p3085.pdf

Intercountry Adoption, Bureau of Consular Affairs, U.S. Department of State. (2014). *FY 2013 annual report on intercountry adoption*. Retrieved from http://adoption.state.gov/content/pdf/fy2013_annual_report.pdf

Johnson, C. P., Myers, S. M., The Council on Children With Disabilities. (2010). Identification and evaluation of children with autism spectrum disorders. *Pediatrics*. Retrieved http://pediatrics.aappublications.org/content/120/5/1183.full#sec-19

Kroger, A. T., Sumaya, C. V., Pickering, L. K., & Atkinson, W. L. (2011). General recommendations on immunization: Recommendations of the Advisory Committee on Immunization Practices (ACIP). *Morbidity and Mortality Weekly Report (MMWR), 60*(RR02), 1–60. Retrieved from http://www.cdc.gov/mmwr/preview/mmwrhtml/rr6002a1.htm?s_cid = rr6002a1_e

Malani, P. (2013). Vaccination rates for US children remain generally high, but measles outbreaks underscore shortfalls in some regions. *News@JAMA*. Retrieved from http://newsatjama.jama.com/2013/09/16/vaccination-rates-for-us-children-remain-generally-high-but-measles-outbreaks-underscore-shortfalls-in-some-regions/

March of Dimes. (2012). *Newborn screening tests for your baby*. Retrieved from http://www.marchofdimes.com/baby/newborn-screening-tests-for-your-baby.aspx

National Cancer Institute. (2011). *What you need to know about melanoma and other skin cancers: Risk factors*. Retrieved from http://www.cancer.gov/cancertopics/wyntk/skin/page5

National Heart, Lung, and Blood Institute. (2012). *Expert panel on integrated guidelines for cardiovascular health and risk reduction in children and adolescents. SUMMARY REPORT (NIH Publication No. 12–7486)*. Washington, DC: U.S. Department of Health and Human Services. Retrieved from http://www.nhlbi.nih.gov/guidelines/cvd_ped/peds_guidelines_sum.pdf

Simms, M. D., & Wilson, S. L. (2011). Chapter 34: Adoption. In R. M. Kleigman, B. F. Stanton, J. W. St. Geme III, N. F. Schor, & R. E. Behrman (Eds.), *Nelson textbook of pediatrics* (19th ed., pp. 130–134). Philadelphia, PA: Saunders.

U.S. Department of Agriculture and U.S. Department of Health and Human Services. (2010). *Dietary guidelines for Americans, 2010* (7th ed.). Washington, DC: U.S. Government Printing Office. Retrieved from http://www.cnpp.usda.gov/DGAs2010-PolicyDocument.htm

U.S. Department of Health & Human Services. (2012a). *The affordable care act and immunization*. Retrieved from http://www.hhs.gov/healthcare/facts/factsheets/2010/09/The-Affordable-Care-Act-and-Immunization.html

U.S. Department of Health & Human Services. (2012b). *HealthyPeople.gov*. Retrieved at http://www.healthypeople.gov/2020/about/default.aspx

United States Environmental Protection Agency. (2014) *Lead*. Retrieved from http://www2.epa.gov/lead

Vaccine Adverse Event Reporting System. (n.d.). *About the VAERS program*. Retrieved from http://vaers.hhs.gov/index

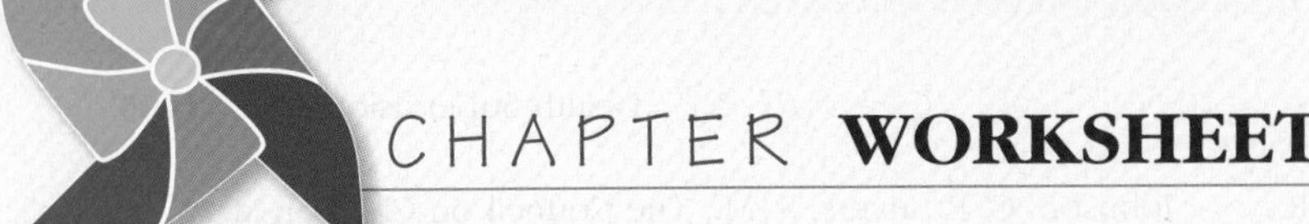

CHAPTER WORKSHEET

MULTIPLE CHOICE QUESTIONS

1. During the health interview, the mother of a 4-month-old says, "I'm not sure my baby is doing what he should be." What is the nurse's best response?
   a. "I'll be able to tell you more after I do his physical."
   b. "Fill out this developmental screening questionnaire and then I can let you know."
   c. "Tell me more about your concerns."
   d. "All mothers worry about their babies. I'm sure he's doing well."

2. An infant boy is at your facility for his initial health supervision visit. He is 2 weeks old and responds to a bell during his examination. You review all his birth records and find no documentation that a newborn hearing screening was performed. What is the best action by the nurse?
   a. Do nothing; responding to the bell proves the infant does not have a hearing deficit.
   b. Schedule the infant immediately for newborn hearing screening.
   c. Ask the mother to observe for signs that the infant is not hearing well.
   d. Screen again with the bell at the infant's 2-month health supervision visit.

3. A 15-month-old girl is having her first health supervision visit at your facility. Her mother has not brought a copy of the child's immunization record but believes she is fully immunized: "She had immunizations 3 months ago at the local health department." Which would be the best action by the nurse?
   a. Ask the mother to bring the records to the 18-month health supervision visit.
   b. Start the "catch-up" schedule because there are no immunization records.
   c. Keep the child at the facility while the mother returns home for the records.
   d. Call the local health department and verify the child's immunization status.

4. A 4-year-old child is having a vision screening performed. Which screening chart would be best for determining the child's visual acuity?
   a. Snellen
   b. Ishihara
   c. Allen figures
   d. CVTME

5. Which facility fulfills the characteristics of a medical home?
   a. An urgent care center
   b. A primary care pediatric practice
   c. A mobile outreach immunization program
   d. A dermatology practice

CRITICAL THINKING EXERCISES

1. During a health supervision visit for a 5-year-old boy, the mother tells you she is worried about his hearing. Your facility has been his medical home since birth. He was the product of a normal pregnancy and delivery. He has had frequent ear infections since the age of 8 months. Six months ago he had a ruptured appendix. He was treated with an aminoglycoside. He has been fully recovered for 4 months.
   a. During the health interview, what information should the nurse elicit from the mother?
   b. What information should the nurse verify from the permanent medical record?
   c. What risk factors for hearing loss does this child have?
   d. What is the best course of action at this time?

2. The nurse is examining a 4-year-old to determine his readiness for school. Describe the developmental, vision, and hearing screening tools that will help the nurse to identify any problems.

STUDY ACTIVITIES

1. Develop an immunization plan for the following well children: a 2-month-old, an 18-month-old who has never been immunized, and a 5-year-old who was current with all immunizations at age 2.

2. This is the first health supervision visit, since arriving in this country 1 week ago, for a 3-year-old international adoptee from Russia. Develop a plan for this visit.

3. Develop a healthy weight program for the following: a preschool class, a family in which the parents and the two school-age children are mildly overweight, and a teenage girl who is of normal weight but fears "getting fat."

BRINGING IT ALL TOGETHER: A CASE STUDY

Fillipa is a 9-month-old who is seen in your clinic for a well-child examination. During the health history, you discover that Fillipa has received no immunizations except her hepatitis B immunization at birth.

Go to thePoint **to find questions to consider about this case.**

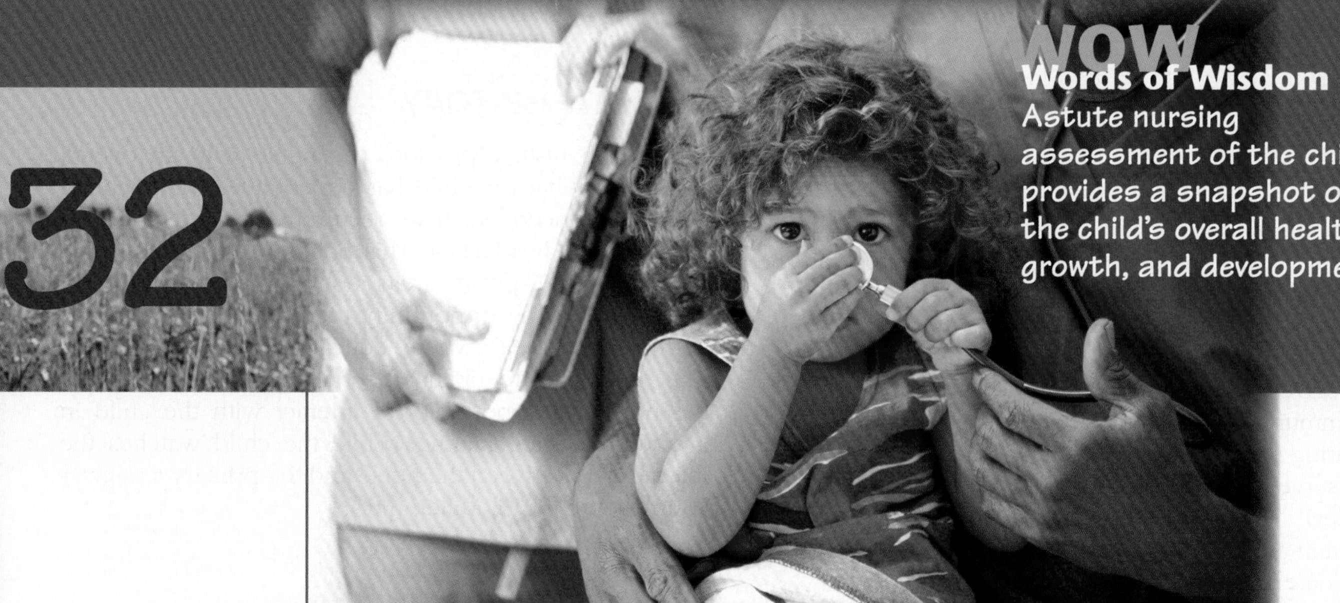
WOW
Words of Wisdom
Astute nursing assessment of the child provides a snapshot of the child's overall health, growth, and development.

32

Health Assessment of Children

KEY TERMS
accommodation
acrocyanosis
body mass index (BMI)
chief complaint
fontanels
lanugo
obligate nose breather
palpation
PERRLA
point of maximal intensity (PMI)
stadiometer
Tanner stages
tympanometer

Learning Objectives

Upon completion of the chapter, you will be able to:

1. Demonstrate an understanding of the appropriate health history to obtain from the child and the parent or primary caregiver.
2. Individualize elements of the health history depending on the age of the child.
3. Discuss important concepts related to health assessment in children.
4. Perform a health assessment using approaches that relate to the age and developmental stage of the child.
5. Describe the appropriate sequence of the physical examination in the context of the child's developmental stage.
6. Distinguish normal variations in the physical examination from differences that may indicate serious alterations in health status.
7. Determine the sexual maturity of females and males based on evaluation of the secondary sex characteristics.

***Elliot Simmons*, 3 years old, is brought to the clinic for his annual examination. His mother states that he is very fearful and anxious about this visit.**

Assessment of the child's health status involves many components: the health interview and history; observation of the parent–child interaction; assessment of the child's emotional, physiologic, cognitive, and social development; and physical examination. The nurse's skills are vital to the success of the assessment process. The nurse must (Treitz, Bunik, & Fox, 2014):

- Establish rapport and trust
- Demonstrate respect for the child and the parent or caregiver
- Communicate effectively by listening actively, demonstrating empathy, and providing feedback
- Observe systematically (especially while the child is quiet)
- Obtain accurate data
- Validate and interpret data accurately

The focus of the assessment process depends on the purpose of the visit and the needs of the child. Assessment is an ongoing process and is repeated to varying degrees at every encounter. The expert nurse is constantly evaluating the children in his or her care, whether directly or indirectly as part of conversation and play. Indeed, some of the subtlest developmental signs may express themselves only during relaxed and casual interaction with a child (Burns, Dunn, Brady, Starr, & Blosser, 2013). The nurse may observe gait while watching a child run down the hall, assess fine motor skills and social adaptation while the child is playing a board game, or observe balance and coordination while the child is bouncing a ball. Playful activities such as tickling a child can give the nurse feedback related to upper body strength when the child attempts to push the nurse's arms away. The nurse must also learn to perform a comprehensive and thorough examination of a child in an efficient manner.

A thorough and thoughtful assessment of a child is the foundation upon which the nurse determines the needs of the child. A comprehensive history, a thorough examination, and developmental or cognitive testing as appropriate will provide practical information about the health of a child and guide the nurse's plan of care (developmental testing is covered in Chapter 31). The history and physical examination also provide a time for health education, teaching about expected growth and development, and discussing healthy lifestyle choices. The nurse uses critical thinking skills to analyze the data and establish priorities for nursing intervention or follow-up care (Burns et al., 2013).

The health assessment may be documented using a number of formats such as a written narrative, a written flow sheet, or an electronic health record. The information should be easily retrievable and available to all members of the child's healthcare team.

HEALTH HISTORY

The health history provides the nurse with an overall picture of what the child has experienced, highlighting areas of concern such as recurrent upper respiratory infections or headaches. This not only helps the nurse to assess those specific areas more comprehensively but also provides the opportunity to ask focused questions and identify areas where education may be needed. The time used to obtain the health history also gives the nurse an opportunity to interact with the child in a nonthreatening manner while the child watches the interactions between the nurse and the primary caregiver (Burns et al., 2013; Miller, n.d.).

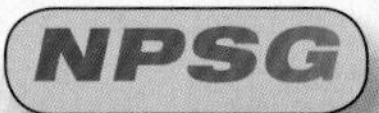

GOAL 3: Improve the Safety of Using Medications

NPSG 03.06.01 Maintain and communicate accurate patient medication information.

Steps: When obtaining the health history, be sure to collect accurate information concerning the child's usual medications.

Joint Commission. (2015). *National patient safety goals effective January 1, 2015.* Retrieved from http://www.jointcommission.org/assets/1/6/2015_NPSG_HAP.pdf

Preparing for the Health History

Appropriate materials and a suitable environment are needed when performing a thorough health history. Take into account family roles and values. Consider the age and developmental stage of the child in order to approach the child appropriately and possibly involve him or her in the health history. Observe the child–parent interaction. Determine the extent of the health history that is needed in a given situation. Being well organized and staying flexible will help ensure success (Burns et al., 2013).

Gathering Materials

Before beginning, make sure the following are available: materials to record the history data (either a computer or chart paper and a pen), a private space with adequate lighting, chairs for adults and the nurse, and a bed or examination table for the child. The space should be safe for the child's developmental stage. Sit down for as much of the history taking as possible to demonstrate a relaxed and welcoming manner (Burns et al., 2013).

Approaching the Parent or Caregiver

Greet the parent or caregiver by name. While interviewing the parent, provide toys or books to occupy the child, allowing the parent to concentrate on the questions. Use open-ended questions and avoid making judgmental comments. Show respect by remaining approachable. Remember that the structure of the family and its roles and dynamics will affect how the family communicates and how they make decisions about health care. Demonstrate patience and help the parent stay on track when there are several children in the family. Throughout the interview, refer to the child by name and use the correct gender when referring to the child, demonstrating interest and competence.

Take Note!

Illness can cause great stress in families and individuals, so nurses must remember to protect themselves from potentially threatening behavior on the part of the family. Sit close to the door, and if uncomfortable with a family member, ask for assistance. The nurse may need to alert security personnel in certain cases (Gillespie, Gates, & Berry, 2013).

Approaching the Child

Show a professional demeanor while still being warm and friendly to the caregivers and child. A white examination coat or all-white uniform may be frightening to children, who may associate the uniform with painful experiences or may associate it with negative emotions such as upset, nervous, or worried (Albert et al., 2013). The nurse can wear a variety of professional-looking outfits, whether colorful uniform tops, aprons, or smocks worn over white uniforms, or everyday clothing, depending on the setting of the nurse's practice. Make eye contact if possible and address the child by name. Use slow deliberate gestures rather than very quick or grand ones, which may be frightening to shy children.

Some young children will warm up when given time to be invisible in the room, such as hiding behind a parent before they tentatively appear. Make physical contact with the child in a nonthreatening way at first. Briefly cuddling a newborn before returning him or her to the caregiver, laying a hand on the head or arm of toddlers and preschoolers, and warmly shaking the hand of older children and teens will convey a gentle demeanor. A joke, a puppet, a silly story, or even a simple magic trick may coax the child into warming up. Being at the same eye level as the child can also be more reassuring than standing over the child (Miller, n.d.). This may require having extra seating for the nurse at the same level as the child and parent/caregiver. Aim to be seen as a trustworthy adult who is the child's partner in feeling better and staying healthy.

Elicit the child's cooperation by allowing him or her control over the pace and order of the health history, or anything else that the child can control while still allowing the nurse to obtain the information needed. All of this establishes a personal relationship with the child and helps gain his or her cooperation (Miller, n.d.).

Communicating with the Child During the Health History

Give the child opportunities to actively participate in the health history and assessment process. For young children, such as toddlers and preschoolers, ask them to point to where it hurts and allow them to answer questions. Validation of the information by the parent/caregiver is essential because of the limited comprehension and language use of children at these ages. The school-aged child can answer more accurately because of his or her increased language skills and maturity level.

Initially, address the child and obtain as much information from him or her as possible. School-aged children should be able to answer questions about interactions with friends and siblings and school and activities they enjoy or in which they are involved. Ask the parent/caregiver if any additional information or observations should be included.

Adolescents may not feel comfortable addressing health issues, answering questions, or being examined in the presence of the parent/caregiver. The nurse must establish a trusting relationship with the adolescent to provide him or her with optimal health care. Ask adolescents whether they would be more comfortable answering questions alone in the examination area or whether they prefer their parents to be present. Either way, the parent/caregiver will have an opportunity to talk with the nurse after the health history and assessment are completed (Burns et al., 2013).

Demonstrate an interest in the teen by asking questions about school, work, hobbies or activities, and friendships. Begin with these topics to make the teen feel comfortable in communicating with the nurse. Communicate honestly with the adolescent and explain the rationale for various aspects of the health history. Teens are very sensitive to nonverbal communication, so be very aware of gestures and expressions (Sass & Kaplan, 2014). Once a rapport has been established, move on to more emotionally charged questions that relate to sexuality, substance use, depression, and suicide.

Always assure the teen that complete confidentiality will be maintained to the extent possible. Current state law will determine the types of information that may be withheld from parents. If the information that the nurse receives indicates that the teen may be in danger, then the nurse must inform the teen that the information will be shared with other providers and/or the parents (Burns et al., 2013).

Take Note!

Do not try to become the adolescent's peer. Remain in the role of the nurse while demonstrating respect and acceptance toward the teen. Clarify the meaning of jargon or slang that the teen uses, but do not use these words yourself; the teen will simply not accept the nurse as a peer.

Observing the Parent–Child Interaction

Observation of the parent–child interaction begins during the focused conversation of the health interview and continues throughout the physical examination. Explore the family dynamics, not only through questions but also by observing the family for behavioral clues. Does the parent make eye contact with the infant? Does the parent anticipate and respond to the infant's needs? Are the parents ineffective when dealing with a toddler's temper tantrum? The plan of care may need to be adjusted to teach appropriate responses to the infant's needs or toddler's behavior. Do the parents' comments increase the school-age child's sense of self-worth? Behavioral observations are crucial to proper assessment of the family's needs (Burns et al., 2013; Columbia University, College of Physicians and Surgeons, n.d).

Further observe the parent–child interaction to determine if the parent appears to be overwhelmed and if his or her behavior seems appropriate (Burns et al., 2013). Monitor the child's behavioral cues. Does the child look at the parent/caregiver before answering? Does the child seem relaxed and happy with the parent/caregiver, or is the child tense? The infant will appear calm and relaxed if his or her needs are generally met. Crying may occur when the baby is ill or frightened, but may also indicate discomfort with the parent or caregiver. Use a calm and comforting voice with the infant. Infants respond well to higher-pitched and soothing voices.

When observing the relationship between the adolescent and the parent/caregiver, does the parent/caregiver allow the adolescent to speak, or does he or she frequently interrupt? Does the parent/caregiver contradict what is being said? Observe the body language of the adolescent: does the teen seem relaxed or tense? Since adolescents are between childhood and adulthood, they have unique needs. They are experiencing a time of multiple physical and emotional changes, many of which they cannot control. They need to know that the nurse is interested in what they have to say (Sass & Kaplan, 2014). The use of open-ended questions allows the adolescent to talk. "Tell me about your. …" or "What have you noticed about … ?" are comfortable phrases to use to elicit the information needed.

Be aware of your own reactions to the adolescent's questions or behaviors, such as nonverbal and facial expressions. Talk with the adolescent using accurate language that is developmentally and age appropriate.

Determining the Type of History Needed

The purpose of the examination will determine how comprehensive the history must be. If the physician or nurse practitioner rarely sees the child or if the child is critically ill, a complete and detailed history is in order, no matter what the setting. The child who has received routine health care and presents with a mild illness may need only a problem-focused history. In critical situations, some of the history taking must be delayed until after the child's condition is stabilized. Evaluate the situation to determine the best timing and the extent of the history (Burns et al., 2013). Also, be sensitive to repetitive interviews in hospital situations, and collaborate with physicians or other members of the healthcare team to ensure that a family already under stress does not need to undergo prolonged or repetitive questioning.

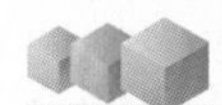

Concept Mastery Alert

Types of Health History

A child in an emergent situation should have a health history that is focused on the child's most immediate need. On the other hand, a comprehensive health history is appropriate for the child who is having his first visit at a pediatrician's office, for example.

Remember Elliot, the 3-year-old being seen for his annual examination? When you enter the room, he is hiding behind his mother's legs. Considering his age and developmental level, how will you proceed with obtaining a health history?

Performing a Health History

The health interview is the foundation of an accurate health assessment. Careful conversation and interview with the child and/or the caregiver will provide important information about the child's health (Burns et al., 2013). Depending on the intent of the health assessment, many of the questions will be direct, and many will require the caregiver or child to answer simply "yes" or "no." In other than emergency situations, though, asking open-ended questions offers an excellent opportunity to learn more about the patient's life. For example, "Are you happy at school?" may elicit a brief nod of the head, whereas "Tell me what it's like on your school playground" may result in a story about the child's friends, the kind of activities the child enjoys, any bullying that goes on, and so forth. These stories will provide the nurse with clues to the child's stage of physical, emotional, and moral development as well as his or her functional status (Burns et al., 2013; Columbia University, College of Physicians and Surgeons, n.d.).

Establish a therapeutic relationship with the child and family. Without the trust that comes from this therapeutic relationship, the family may not reveal vital information due to fear, embarrassment, or mistrust (Treitz, et al., 2014). Use therapeutic communication techniques such as active listening, open-ended questions, and eliminating barriers to communication. Establishing a "medical home" where ongoing health supervision occurs encourages trust through continuity of care and the family's continuing relationships with primary care providers (see Chapter 31).

The structure of the health interview is determined by the nature of the visit. At an initial visit, large amounts of historical data are collected. Having the family fill out a questionnaire can save time, but a questionnaire is not a substitute for the health interview. The questionnaire may serve as a springboard to begin structured conversations between the family and the nurse. At subsequent visits the health interview can focus on the pertinent issues of that visit as well as any health issues that are being monitored.

The health history includes demographics, chief complaint and history of present illness, past health history, review of systems, family health history, developmental history, functional history, and family composition, resources, and home environment.

Take Note!

Any questionnaires used in the healthcare setting should be written at a fifth-grade reading level and be in the primary language of the person completing them (The Joint Commission, 2014).

Demographics

Initially, questions should be simple and nonintrusive; once a rapport between the nurse and patient has started, sensitive questions can be asked. First obtain data such as the child's name, nickname, birth date, and gender. Determine the child's race or ethnicity, the language the child understands, and the language the child speaks. Record the child's address and home telephone number and the parent's or caregiver's work telephone number. Identify who the historian is (the child or the parent or caregiver), and note how reliable this source of information is considered to be. Do not assume that an adult with the child is the child's parent. Establish the relationship of the adult to the child, and ask who cares for the child if that person does not. Determine the composition of the household, including other children and other family members or other persons who live there.

Chief Complaint and History of Present Illness

Next, ask about the **chief complaint** (reason for the visit). The reason may not always be apparent to you. A question such as, "What can I help you with today?" or "What did you notice in your baby/child that you wanted to have checked today?" is very welcoming. The response from the child or parent may be a functional problem, a developmental concern, or a disease. Record the chief complaint in the child's or parent's own words.

Next address the history related to the present illness. For each concern, determine its onset, duration, characteristics, and course (location, signs, symptoms, exposures, and so on), previous episodes in patient or family, previous testing or therapies, what makes it better or worse, and what the concern means to the child and family. Inquire about any exposure to infectious agents.

Past Health History

Ask about the prenatal history (any problems with pregnancy), perinatal history (any problems with labor and delivery), past illnesses, or any other health or developmental problems. Document the child's prior history of illnesses (recurrent, chronic, or serious) and any accidents or injuries in the past. Inquire about any operations or hospitalizations the child has had. Document the child's diet. Note the child's allergies to foods, medications, animals, environmental or contact agents, or latex products. Determine the child's reaction to the allergen as well as its severity. Determine the child's immunization status (refer to Chapter 31 for further information on immunizations). Record any medications the child is taking, the dosage and schedule, as well as when the last dose was given. In preadolescent and adolescent females, determine menstrual history.

Family Health History

Obtaining information about the family's health is a key part of a health interview. Perform a three-generation family health history. This information may be documented in a genogram (Fig. 32.1). Asking about the age and health status of mother, father, siblings, and other family members helps to identify trends and specific health issues (Burns et al., 2013). For example, do the grandparents have early-onset coronary artery disease? If they do, the child may benefit from additional health screening. Siblings may exhibit a genetic disease or carry a trait for the disease. This family health information helps to guide future health planning.

Review of Systems

Inquire about current or past history of problems related to:

- Growth and development
- Skin
- Head and neck
- Eyes and vision
- Ears and hearing

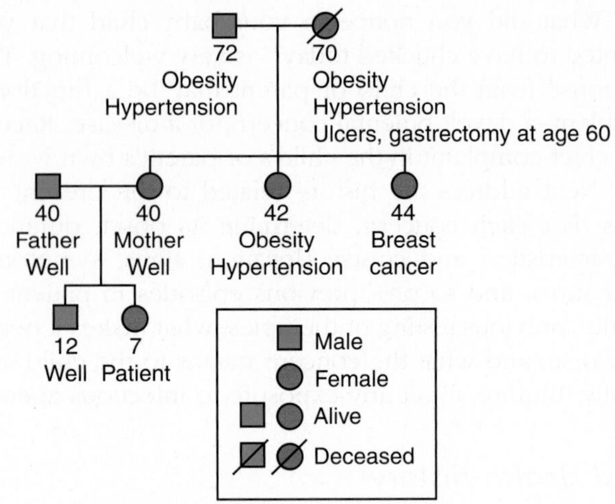

FIGURE 32.1 Genogram.

- Mouth, teeth, and throat
- Respiratory system and breasts
- Cardiovascular system
- Gastrointestinal system
- Genitourinary system
- Musculoskeletal system
- Neurologic system
- Endocrine system
- Hematologic system

Table 32.1 provides specific questions related to each of these systems.

Developmental History

Determine the age when landmarks in gross motor control were achieved, such as sitting, standing, walking, pedaling, and so on. Ask whether the child has attained fine motor skills such as grasping, releasing, pincer grasp, crayon or utensil use, and handwriting skills. Note the child's age and extent of language acquisition. Document speech problems such as a lisp or stuttering. The rate of developmental skill acquisition may vary from child to child, but the sequence of skill attainment should remain the same. Inquire about self-care ability (e.g., tying shoes, dressing, brushing teeth) and, in the younger child, how toilet training is progressing. Question the parents about the child's feeding skills, including how well the child drinks from a cup and uses utensils or whether the child has any special requirements. Inquire about social skills and comfort articles (e.g., blankets, stuffed animals). Note whether the child has a habit of thumb or finger sucking or using a pacifier. Document day care attendance and preschool or school adjustment and achievements.

Functional History

The functional history should contain information about the child's daily routine. Inquire about:

- Safety measures (e.g., car seats and their placement, use of seat belts, smoke detectors, bike helmets)
- Routine health care and dental care (including dates of dental care and what was done)
- Nutrition, including a 24-hour dietary recall or week-long food diary, use of supplements and vitamins, feeding pattern and satisfaction with diet, amount of "junk food" consumed, food likes and dislikes, and the parent's perception of the child's nutrition (refer to Chapters 25 through 29 for nutritional needs at various ages)
- Physical activity, recreation, play, and organized sports
- Television and computer habits
- Sleep behavior and bedtime
- Elimination patterns and any concerns
- Hearing or vision problems (dates of last screenings and results)
- Relationships with other family members and friends, coping and temperament, discipline strategies, attention or school behavior problems
- Religious involvement and other spiritual practices
- Use of adaptive and assistive devices such as eyeglasses or contact lenses, hearing aids, walker, braces, wheelchair
- Sexual practices (Burns et al., 2013)

Family Composition, Resources, and Home Environment

Determine the marital status of the parents. Does the child live with the parents, a stepparent, or other family member? Is the child adopted or in foster care? Are the parents the primary caretakers for the child? If not, the primary caretaker should be included in the interview process if possible. Parents may not know some of the child's routines if the child spends much of the time being cared for by someone else. Working parents may learn about a health or behavior issue only after being alerted by the child's day care center or babysitter. It may be helpful to expand the family history to include the grandparents and their interaction with the child.

Determine the employment status of the parents and their occupations, as this could affect the child's overall well-being; for example, the parents' work schedule may not allow them to spend much time with the child. Assess family income and financial resources, including health insurance and Supplemental Nutrition Assistance Program (SNAP [formerly food stamps]); Aid for Women, Infants, and Children (WIC); or other governmental supplemental income. Major family changes can also affect how the parents and child interact, so evaluate for relationship problems or changes.

Ask about the family's home and its age and environment. Is there a safe outdoor play area? If there is a pool, are safety features in place? Determine whether the home has electricity and an indoor water supply. Also

TABLE 32.1 QUESTIONS FOR THE REVIEW OF SYSTEMS

Systems	Has the Child Experienced
Growth and development	Weight loss or gain, appropriate energy and activity levels, fatigue, behavioral changes such as irritability, nervousness, anger, or increased crying
Skin	Easy bruising or bleeding, rash, lesion, skin disease, pruritus, birthmarks, or change in mole, pigment, hair, or nails
Head and neck	Head injury, headache, dizziness, syncope
Eyes and vision	Pain, redness, discharge, diplopia, strabismus, cataracts, vision changes, reading difficulties, need to sit close to the board at school or close to the TV at home
Ears and hearing	Earache, recurrent ear infection, tubes in eardrums, discharge, difficulty hearing, ringing, excess cerumen
Mouth, teeth, and throat	Swollen gums, pain with teething, caries, tooth loss, toothache, sores, difficulty with chewing or swallowing, hoarseness, sore throat, mouth breathing, change in voice
Respiratory system and breasts	Nasal congestion or discharge, cough, wheeze, noisy breathing, snoring, shortness of breath or other difficulty breathing, problems with or changes in breasts
Cardiovascular system	Murmur, color change (cyanosis), exertional dyspnea, activity intolerance, palpitations, extremity coldness, high blood pressure, high cholesterol
Gastrointestinal system	Nausea, vomiting, abdominal pain, cramping, diarrhea, constipation, stool holding, anal pain or itching
Genitourinary system	Dysuria; polyuria; oliguria; narrow urine stream; dark, cloudy, or discolored urine; difficulty with toilet training; bedwetting *Boys:* undescended testicles, pain in penis or scrotum, sores or lesions, discharge, scrotal swelling when crying, changes in scrotum or penis size, addition of pubic hair *Girls:* vaginal discharge, itching rash, problems with menstruation or menstrual cycle, development of pubic hair
Musculoskeletal system	Joint or bone pain, stiffness, swelling, injury (e.g., broken bones or sprains), movement limitation, decreased strength, altered gait, changes in coordination, back pain, posture changes or spinal curvature
Neurologic system	Numbness, tingling, difficulty learning, altered mood or ability to stay alert, tremors, tics, seizures
Endocrine system	Increased thirst, excessive appetite, delayed or early pubertal changes, problems with growth
Hematologic system	Swelling of lymph nodes, pale color, excessive bruising

Adapted from Burns, C. E., Dunn, A. M., Brady, M. A., Starr, N. B., & Blosser, C. G. (2013). *Pediatric primary care* (5th ed.). Philadelphia, PA: Saunders; and Jarvis, C. (2012). *Physical examination and health assessment* (6th ed.). St. Louis, MO: Saunders.

determine whether the home has heating, air conditioning, and refrigeration. What pets does the family have? How are they housed? Are there infestations of insects or rodents in the home?

Take Note!

Homes or apartments built prior to 1978 may contain lead-based paint, and children who live there are at an increased risk for the development of lead poisoning (CDC, 2015b).

PHYSICAL EXAMINATION

The next step after the health history is the physical examination. It should focus on the chief complaint or any of the systems that engaged the nurse's critical thinking while obtaining the history. The examination will reflect the nurse's general practice style, the developmental stage and age of the child, the temperament of the child and caregiver, and the health status of the child. For example, a very ill child will not waste energy

TABLE 32.2 DEVELOPMENTAL CONSIDERATIONS FOR EXAMINATION

	Newborn	Infant	Toddler	Preschool	School-age	Early Teen	Late Teen
Place to perform examination	May lie on examination table or in caregiver's lap.	In caregiver's lap or on examination table with caregiver right beside infant.	Allow some freedom of movement when possible; child may stand between seated caregiver's legs or sit on the lap.	Some may be willing to sit on examination table with caregiver standing close by with hand on the leg.	Sitting on examination table where they still have eye contact with caregiver.	Some may be willing to have their caregiver wait outside the examination room.	Explain to the caregiver that the teen needs privacy and that he or she should wait outside the examination room.
Examination Direction	Keep up a running dialog with the caregiver, explaining each step as you do it.	Continue to explain each step to the caregiver; address child by name. Perform most invasive parts last.	Introduce yourself to caregiver and child; explain most steps to the child and all steps to caregiver; allow child to handle instruments. Perform most invasive parts last.	Allow child to decide the order of the examination; explain what the instruments do and let the child try them; speak to the caregiver before and after the examination.	Include the child in all parts of the examination; use head-to-toe approach with genital examination last. Speak to the caregiver before and after the examination.	Speak to the child using mature language; appeal to his or her desire for self-care. Use a head-to-toe approach, with genital examination last.	Explain confidentiality to caregiver and teen; allow time talking with them together and separately. Use a head-to-toe approach, with genital examination last.

Adapted from Burns, C. E., Dunn, A. M., Brady, M. A., Starr, N. B., & Blosser, C. G. (2013). *Pediatric primary care* (5th ed.). Philadelphia, PA: Saunders; Miller, S. (n.d.). Pediatric physical exam video. Retrieved from http://www.columbia.edu/itc/hs/medical/clerkships/peds/Student_Information/Reference_Materials/PE_Video.html; and Columbia University, College of Physicians and Surgeons. (n.d.). Points on the pediatric physical exam. Retrieved from http://www.columbia.edu/itc/hs/medical/clerkships/peds/Student_Information/Reference_Materials/Pediatric_PE.html protesting the examination, so the nurse can move quickly in that situation. A healthy child, however, will express his or her normal developmental stage and will show varying degrees of resistance to the examination (Miller, n.d.; Columbia University, College of Physicians and Surgeons, n.d.).

Preparing for the Physical Examination

When performing the physical examination, being prepared and organized ensures that the needed information will be obtained efficiently. The appropriate methods to use and ways to approach the child depend on the child's developmental stage.

Gathering Materials

The examination area should include an examination table or the child's hospital crib or bed. Appropriate lighting is necessary for adequate observation and inspection. Gather the equipment necessary for the examination such as clean gloves, stethoscope, thermometer, sphygmomanometer, tape measure, reflex hammer, penlight, otoscope/ophthalmoscope, tongue depressor, and cotton ball. An infant or adult scale is needed, as well as a **stadiometer** for children capable of standing independently. Young children may be frightened by seeing a large amount of equipment, so take out one piece of equipment at a time. Some children can be very resistant to what they see as a threat or an invasion of their privacy, so it may help to have washable toys in the examination area to use as distractions during the assessment (Burns et al., 2013; Miller, n.d.).

Children and their parents may be able to sense any frustration or anxiety on the part of the examiner, so display a confident and matter-of-fact approach. If the child is not cooperative, do not become discouraged; more time and explanation will usually do the trick.

Regardless of the child's age, if the examination room is cold, the child will be uncomfortable and possibly less cooperative. Provide appropriate covers to ensure the child's comfort, or have the child remain dressed until the time of the examination (Miller, n.d.).

Approaching the Child

Approach the child according to his or her developmental age and stage. Table 32.2 outlines a general approach to the physical examination in each broad developmental category.

If several children are to be seen at the same time, begin with the child who will be most cooperative. If the other children do not see anything scary and realize that their sibling was examined without a problem, it sets the stage for better cooperation from the younger ones.

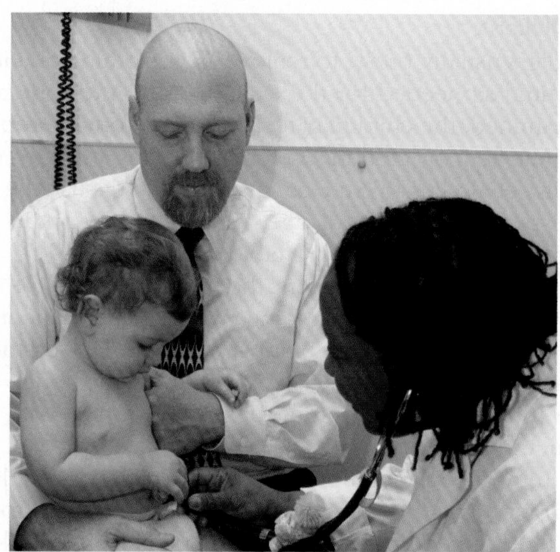

FIGURE 32.2 The infant or toddler may feel more comfortable and secure being examined while sitting in the parent or caregiver's lap.

NEWBORNS AND INFANTS

If the infant is asleep, auscultate the heart, lungs, and abdomen first while the baby is quiet. Count the heart rate and respiratory rate before undressing the baby. Completely undress newborns and infants down to their diaper, removing it just at the end to examine the genitalia, anus, spine, and hips. It is best to examine the infant 1 to 2 hours before a feeding. Having the parent or caregiver hold the child during the examination can help to alleviate fears and anxieties (Fig. 32.2). Allow the parent or caregiver to be a nurturer rather than assisting with painful procedures, unless there are no other choices available (Miller, n.d.).

Perform the assessment in a head-to-toe manner, leaving the most traumatic procedures, such as examination of the ears, nose, mouth, and throat, until last (Burns et al., 2013; Miller, n.d.). Also delay eliciting the Moro reflex until the end of the examination, as the startling sensation may make the infant cry. Use firm, gentle handling while examining the infant. Make sure your hands and the stethoscope are warm. Perform the assessment as quickly and completely as possible. Use a soft and crooning voice, smile, and engage the infant in eye contact. In addition, use brightly colored objects to help distract him or her. If the baby is crying, a pacifier may be useful.

Take Note!

Many older infants demonstrate stranger anxiety as a normal part of development. If the parent is not holding the infant, make sure the parent is within the infant's view; this will increase the baby's comfort and cooperation (Bickley, 2013; Burns et al., 2013; Miller, n.d.).

TODDLERS

Toddlers usually prefer to remove their clothing one item at a time as needed for the examination. After one area is examined, the child may feel more comfortable replacing that item of clothing before removing another one (Treitz, et al., 2014). An examination gown is usually not necessary before school age. Again, make certain the room temperature is comfortable.

When the nurse enters the room, a child of this age is often sitting or standing by the parent. Incorporate play as appropriate during the health assessment. Remember your own facial expressions and tone. Use little touch at the beginning of the encounter with the child and the caregiver.

Introduce the equipment to be used slowly, explaining briefly what is going to happen. Let the child touch and hold the equipment whenever possible, even taking a parent's temperature or putting the blood pressure cuff on a teddy bear (Fig. 32.3). The toddler will prefer to sit on the caregiver's lap. When the toddler must be supine for the abdominal examination, sit in your chair knee-to-knee with the caregiver so the toddler may lie back on the caregiver's and your laps. Praise the child for being cooperative during the examination. "You did such a good job holding still while I listened to your chest" and similar phrases give positive feedback to the child.

If the child is uncooperative, assess as thoroughly as possible and move on to the next area to be assessed. The caregiver may need to place an arm around the toddler's body to provide restraint for invasive procedures. Use short phrases to tell the toddler what you are going to do, rather than asking if it is OK (Miller, n.d.; Nettina, 2014).

Take Note!

Toddlers are egocentric. Telling a toddler how well another child behaved probably will not be helpful in gaining the young child's cooperation.

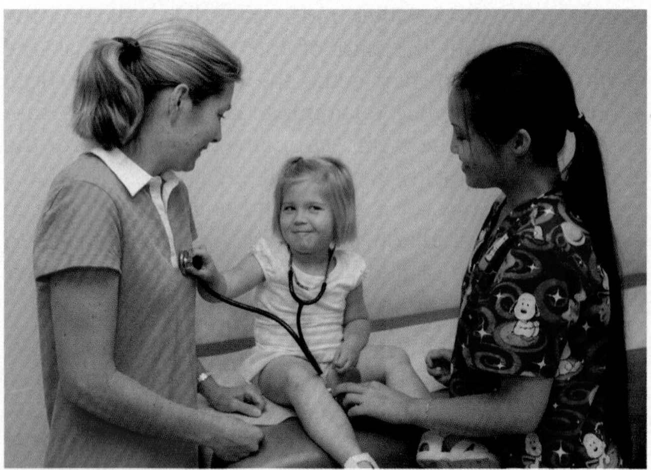

FIGURE 32.3 The preschooler enjoys listening to her mother's heart first.

PRESCHOOLER

The preschooler may fear body invasion and mutilation and will withdraw from any procedure or assessment that is viewed as intrusive. Otherwise, the sense of initiative often leads the preschooler to be cooperative. Use simple explanations to inform the child about each step of the examination, offering reassurance as appropriate. Allow him or her to "help" by holding the stethoscope or penlight. If choices are available, offer them to the child. Again, always compliment the child on his or her cooperation.

Take Note!

Preschoolers like to play games. To encourage deep breathing during lung auscultation, hold up a finger or a lit penlight and instruct the child to "blow it out" (Miller, n.d.).

SCHOOL-AGE CHILDREN

The school-age child's thinking is still very concrete, but he or she can be objective and realistic. Avoid using medical jargon and words that may have a double meaning to a young child. Instead of "take your temperature," "take your blood pressure," "hit your knee," or "test," say, "Let's see how warm you are," "I want to listen to you breathe," and other phrases that describe, in words the child can understand, what you are preparing to do. The school-age child may be very interested in how things work and why certain things need to be done and will be responsive to truthful and simple explanations. Instruments that are colorful or look like toys are very helpful throughout early childhood and the school-age period (Burns et al., 2013; Miller, n.d.).

Always respect a child's desire to avoid pain and insult. Allow children to wear their underpants under the examination gown to provide a sense of security until the genitalia need to be examined. Allow the child to replace his or her clothing as soon as possible. Privacy and respect for the child's feelings are important to children of this age (Treitz, et al., 2014).

Take Note!

Describing and commenting on your findings during the physical examination is interesting to the school-age child, as children of this age like to learn about how the body works (Miller, n.d.).

ADOLESCENTS

Provide privacy while the adolescent is undressing and putting on a gown. Demonstrate an attitude of respect. Perform the assessment in a head-to-toe manner, exposing only the area to be examined. Provide information about physical changes in a matter-of-fact way, such as, "The hair on your legs is what is expected at this time." This provides information related to sensitive areas that the teen may be reluctant to ask about. It also provides the adolescent with information about the sexual development that is normal and expected. Allow opportunities for the teen to ask questions without the caregiver being present. Assure the adolescent that there are no "dumb questions" about the changes being experienced. Teenage girls should remove their bras so that the nurse can perform a breast examination, teach breast self-examination, and check for scoliosis. If the nurse is a male and the patient is an adolescent female, it is appropriate for a female staff member to be present during the breast and genital examination (Sass & Kaplan, 2014).

Steps of the Physical Examination

The physical examination of children, just as for adults, begins with a systematic inspection: checking color, warmth, characteristics, and texture visually and smelling for any odor. **Palpation** follows inspection to validate your observations. Percussion is a useful tool for determining the location, size, and density of organs or masses. Tapping with the reflex hammer elicits deep tendon reflexes. The stethoscope is used to auscultate the heart, lungs, and abdomen.

Performing a Physical Examination

A complete examination includes assessment of the general appearance, vital signs, body measurements, and pain, as well as examination of the head, neck, eyes, ears, nose, mouth and throat, skin, thorax and lungs, breasts, heart and peripheral perfusion, abdomen, genitalia and rectum, musculoskeletal system, and neurologic system. The nurse in most settings will not be assessing the breasts, genitalia, or eyes or ears in detail. Be aware of the role of the nurse in different settings and how the nurse can facilitate the assessment process.

General Appearance

Never discount first impressions. Does the child give an impression of being ill or well? What is the child's expression and energy level? Note lethargy, listlessness, excessive activity, or inappropriate attention span for the child's age. Observe the child's state of alertness and whether he or she is responding appropriately to the stress of the situation. Note the child's posture and positioning:

- The newborn's posture is flexed, with arms and legs tucked in.
- The older infant should have improving head and then trunk control.
- The toddler demonstrates lordosis (swayback) and bowlegs, with a relatively large head and protuberant belly.
- The preschooler is more slender and upright in appearance.
- The school-age child and adolescent should demonstrate an upright, straight, and well-balanced posture.

Note whether the child's development appears appropriate. Observing the child initially may yield a wealth of information about the child's development. Is the child active, moving about the room? Does the child's speech seem appropriate for his or her age? Notice whether the family interacts appropriately with one another and the child. Does the child appear clean and well cared for? Does the child appear well nourished or small for age or obese? Note the scent of tobacco smoke or alcohol on family members. Notice if the baby bottle or pacifier is nearby and whether the child has a toy or transitional object. Assess whether the siblings appear equally well cared for. Observe for tension in the room between adults or children/adolescents. This initial quick assessment of general appearance will serve the nurse well if it is objective; delay interpretation of this assessment until additional data are gathered.

Measurement of Vital Signs

Measure, document, and interpret the vital signs of children using age-appropriate equipment and approaches. The child's age and size, as well as knowledge of underlying health conditions, will affect analysis of the vital signs. Vital signs are the temperature, pulse rate, respiratory rate, and blood pressure. These measurements fluctuate normally in children; assessing vital signs while the child is quiet is most appropriate. Comforting an infant or distracting a young child may be necessary while obtaining vital signs. If the child is crying or otherwise active during the assessment, document that fact. Many acute care settings require continuous measurement of vital signs using specific monitoring equipment. Also assess the child's pain level when assessing the vital signs.

TEMPERATURE

Temperature is measured as it is in adults. Thermometers are available in electronic and digital types. Use the same type of equipment consistently to allow reliable comparisons to be made and to permit tracking of temperatures during the course of illness (Bowden & Greenberg, 2012). No matter which type of thermometer is used, ensure accuracy by carefully following the manufacturer's instructions.

The routes for taking the child's temperature are tympanic, temporal, oral, axillary, and rectal. Numerous research studies have been undertaken to determine the best method for temperature assessment in children. Take the child's temperature using the least invasive method that is best accepted by the child, parent, and physician or nurse practitioner.

Take Note!

Though they may continue to be available in some instances, glass thermometers are not recommended for use due to the mercury they contain (Bowden & Greenberg, 2012).

Choosing a method of measuring temperature depends on what is available at the facility and the child's age and physical condition. Tympanic temperature reflects the pulmonary artery temperature and can be measured with the tympanic thermometer within seconds. The accuracy of a tympanic temperature reading depends on the user's technique and can be safely and effectively used in children 3 months of age and older (Bowden & Greenberg, 2012). Refer to Nursing Procedure 32.1.

Temporal scanning uses infrared scanning on the skin over the temporal artery combined with a mathematical computation to determine the child's arterial temperature. Temporal artery thermometry may be used with any age child except infants younger than 90 days of age who are ill or have a fever (Asher & Northington, 2008). Measure temperature on the exposed side of the head (not the side that has been lying on a pillow or covered by a hat). Depress the sensor button, and slide the sensor tip externally in a horizontal line across the child's forehead, midway between the eyebrows and hairline and ending at the lateral hairline (Fig. 32.4). Continuing to depress the button, lift the sensor from the forehead and then place it on the soft spot behind the ear lobe. Hold it there until the device registers the temperature reading, which usually requires 1 second. Accuracy may be affected by excessive sweating (Exergen Corporation, 2014).

Oral temperature is highly reliable if the child can cooperate. By 5 years of age, the child can hold an electronic oral thermometer in the mouth well enough to obtain a reading. Place the probe under the tongue and ensure the child's mouth remains closed until the device registers the temperature. Oral intake, oxygen administration, and nebulized medications or treatments may affect oral temperature.

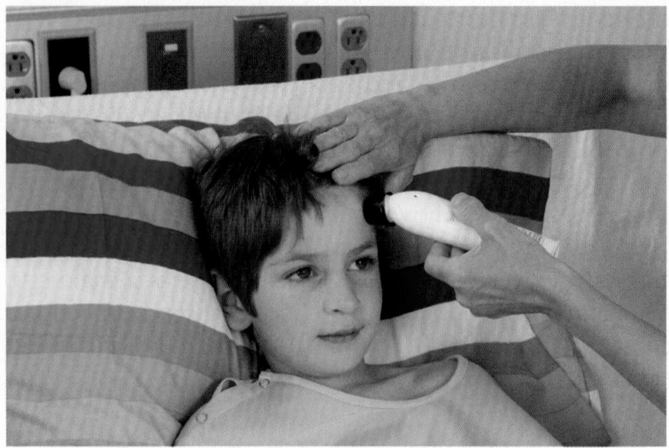

FIGURE 32.4 Temporal artery thermometers are noninvasive and well tolerated by young children. For an accurate reading, move hair to expose forehead and hairline.

The axillary method may be used for children who are uncooperative, neurologically impaired, or immunosuppressed or have injuries or have had surgery to the oral cavity (Bowden & Greenberg, 2012). Place the tip of the electronic or digital thermometer in the axilla to obtain the reading. Make sure the tip is indeed in the axilla and not just between the arm and the child's side. Hold the thermometer parallel rather than perpendicular to the child's side to obtain the most accurate reading. Keep the child's arm pressed

NURSING PROCEDURE 32.1

Measuring Tympanic Temperature

1. Note age of child. If younger than 3 years, pull the earlobe back and down.
2. Insert the tympanic thermometer gently into the ear canal with the infrared sensor beam directed toward the center of the tympanic membrane rather than the sides of the ear canal.
3. Push the button to take the temperature and hold until a reading is obtained. The length of time required for the temperature to register varies per manufacturer but is only a few seconds at most.

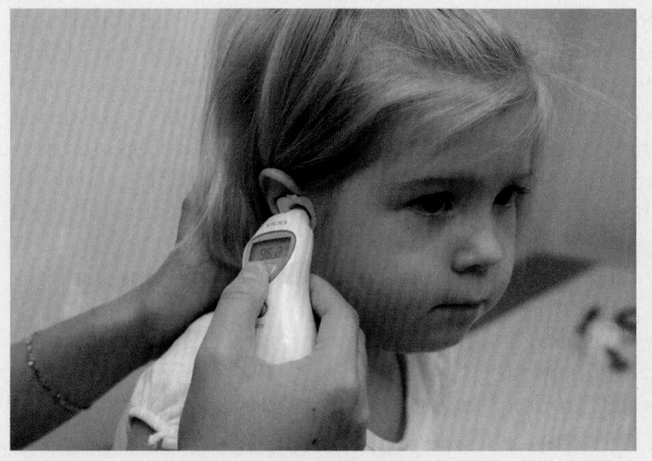

down to the side until the thermometer registers, which will be as little as 10 seconds with certain electronic models but 2 or 3 minutes with digital models commonly used at home.

Though long considered to reflect core temperature, the rectal route is invasive, not well accepted by children or parents, and probably unnecessary with the modern alternative methods now available (El Radhi, 2014). To take the rectal temperature, position the young infant supine with legs flexed. The older infant or child should be prone or side-lying. Small children may lie across the parent's lap for additional comfort. Apply a water-soluble jelly to the covered probe, insert the thermometer past the anal sphincter no more than 1 inch (2.5 cm), and hold it there until the temperature registers (as little as 15 seconds with certain electronic models but longer with digital models).

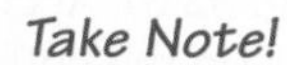

Take Note!

Avoid the rectal route of temperature measurement in the immunosuppressed child as well as the child who has diarrhea, a bleeding disorder, or a history of rectal surgery (Asher & Northington, 2008).

PULSE

Assess the heart rate while the child is resting or sleeping. The heart rate in infants is much faster than in adults. It also varies in infants and children who are anxious, fearful, or crying. As the child grows, the heart rate slows and the range of normal values narrows. Table 32.3 lists heart rate ranges according to the child's age. The radial pulse is difficult to palpate accurately in children younger than 2 years of age because the blood vessels lie close to the skin surface and are easily obliterated (Bickley, 2013). For children younger than 10 years of age, auscultate the apical pulse with the stethoscope for a full minute (Jarvis, 2012). In older children, palpate the radial pulse for a full minute (Fig. 32.5). Note any irregularities in strength or rhythm. Finally, document the method used to obtain pulse measurement as well as any activity of the child during the assessment and any action taken.

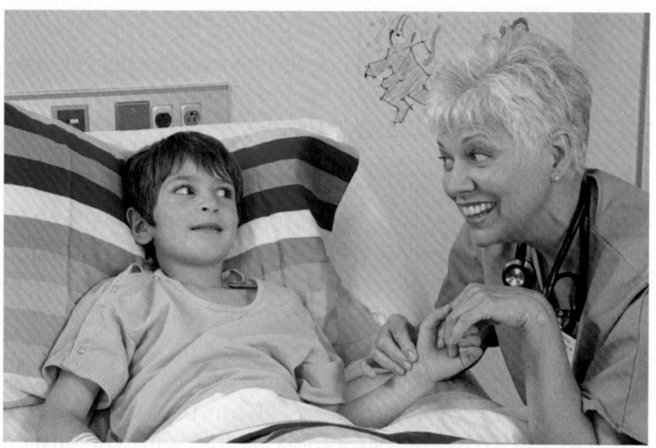

FIGURE 32.5 Assessing the radial pulse of a young child.

Take Note!

In the infant and young child, the heart rate is often quite elevated due to fear or anxiety when the stethoscope is placed on the chest initially. For an accurate heart rate, wait several seconds until the rate slows, and then count for 1 full minute.

RESPIRATORY RATE

Assess respirations when the child is resting or sitting quietly, since respiratory rate often changes when infants or young children cry, feed, or become more active. They also tend to breathe faster when they are anxious or scared. The most accurate respiratory rate is obtained before disturbing the infant or child (Bowden & Greenberg, 2012). This can often be done easily when the parent/caregiver is holding the child before any clothing is removed. Count the respiratory rate for a full minute to ensure accuracy. Infants' respirations are primarily diaphragmatic, so count the abdominal movements. After 1 year of age, count the thoracic movements. Table 32.3 lists ranges of respiratory rate according to the child's age. Document the rate, activity of the child, any deviations from normal, and any action taken.

TABLE 32.3 HEART RATE AND RESPIRATORY RATE RANGES BY AGE GROUP

	Infant	Toddler	Preschooler	School-age	Adolescent
Heart rate	80–150	70–120	65–110	60–100	55–95
Respiratory rate	25–55	20–30	20–25	14–22	12–18

Adapted from Kliegman, R. M., Stanton, B. F, St. Geme III, J. W., Schor N. F., Behrman R. E. (Eds.). (2011). *Nelson textbook of pediatrics* (19th ed.). Philadelphia, PA: Saunders; and Marx, J., Hockberger, R., & Walls, R. (2014). *Rosen's emergency medicine – concepts and clinical practice* (8th ed.). Philadelphia, PA: Saunders.

Take Note!

Infants normally display an uneven or irregular breathing pattern, with short pauses between some breaths. This may be accentuated when they are ill (Bickley, 2013).

MEASURING OXYGEN SATURATION

Since the incidence of respiratory dysfunction is high in ill children, pulse oximetry is often routinely included in the vital signs assessment. This method is reliable and noninvasive. Pulse oximetry determines the oxygen saturation (SaO_2) in blood by using a sensor that measures the absorption of light waves as they pass through highly perfused areas of the body. The pulse rate on the oximeter should coincide with the apical pulse rate to ensure that the oxygen saturation reading is accurate. Nursing Procedure 32.2 details how to use the pulse oximeter. Identify whether pulse oximetry monitoring will be continuous or intermittent (as with vital signs).

A few guidelines to follow when using pulse oximetry are as follows:

- The probe may be placed on the finger, toe, ear, foot, or forehead. Avoid placing the probe on the same extremity with a blood pressure cuff or an intravenous or other type of line.
- Use the physician's or nurse practitioner's orders or healthcare agency guidelines to set parameters for high and low pulse rate as well as high and low oxygen saturation. Never turn off the alarm settings.
- Ensure that the probe is not applied too tightly, as this will prevent venous flow and cause inaccurate readings.
- It is helpful to use the provide cover over the sensor to prevent disruption from ambient light.

Potential sources of errors in pulse oximeter readings include abnormal hemoglobin value, poor perfusion, ambient light interference, motion artifact, and skin breakdown. Falsely low readings may be associated with a nonsecure connection (movement of child's foot or hand), and poor perfusion. Falsely normal readings may be associated with carbon monoxide poisoning and severe anemia (Covidien, 2012).

BLOOD PRESSURE

The National Heart, Lung, and Blood Institute (NHLBI) recommends that children older than 3 years of age have their blood pressure measured at least once during every healthcare episode (U.S. Department of Health and Human Services, National Institutes of Health, National Heart, Lung, and Blood Institute, 2005). Children younger than 3 years old should have blood pressure measured if they have one of the following risk factors:

- History of prematurity, very low birth weight, or other neonatal intensive care complication
- Congenital heart disease
- Recurrent urinary tract infections, hematuria, proteinuria, known renal disease or urologic malformations, family history of congenital renal disease
- Malignancy, bone marrow transplant, or solid organ transplant
- Treatment with medications that raise blood pressure
- Systemic illnesses associated with hypertension such as neurofibromatosis and tuberous sclerosis
- Increased intracranial pressure (U.S. Department of Health and Human Services, National Institutes of Health, National Heart, Lung, and Blood Institute, 2005)

In the hospital or outpatient setting when a child is ill or undergoing surgery or a procedure, the frequency of blood pressure measurement will depend on the child's physical status. Measurement of blood pressure can be frightening to a young child, so include an age-appropriate explanation and perform the procedure after obtaining the pulse rate and respirations (Fig. 32.6). Accuracy of blood pressure measurement depends on the cuff size, as well as the operator's skill and accurate calibration of an electronic device. The NHLBI recommends that the cuff bladder width be at least 40% of the circumference of the upper arm at its midpoint (U.S. Department of Health and Human Services, National Institutes of Health, National Heart, Lung, and Blood Institute, 2005). The cuff bladder length should cover 80% to 100% of the circumference of the upper arm. Various pediatric and infant cuffs are available, as well as larger thigh cuffs that may be used on an arm in an obese adolescent.

Take Note!

Using an accurate cuff size is important: a wider cuff yields a lower reading and a narrower cuff yields a higher reading.

Measure blood pressure in the upper arm, lower arm, thigh, or calf/ankle. The size of the cuff should match the extremity used. The measurement should be taken in the

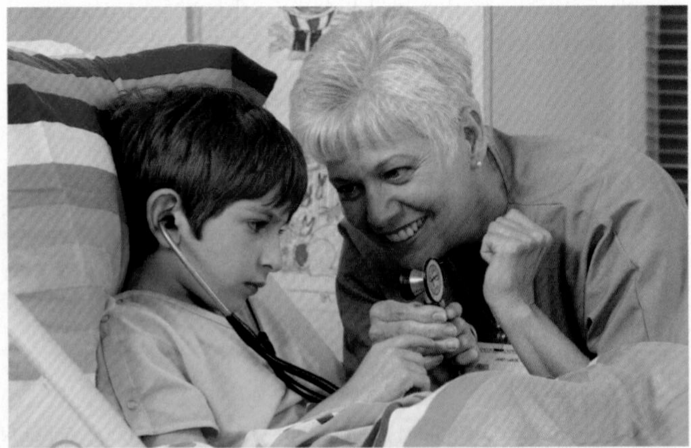

FIGURE 32.6 Allowing children to handle the equipment gives them some control over the situation.

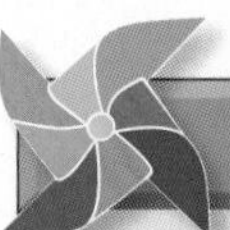

NURSING PROCEDURE 32.2

Pulse Oximetry Monitoring

1. Explain the procedure to the child and family (use a penlight to show how the sensor "looks through the skin").
2. Attach the probe to the child and connect to the monitor.
3. Set the parameters for the alarm if monitoring pulse oximetry continuously.
4. Observe and record pulse rate and oxygen saturation.
5. Record the activity level of the child and the percentage of oxygen in use.
6. Check skin condition and rotate sensor position every few hours if adhesive type used.

Types of sensors

a. Nonadhesive for infants (continuous use)

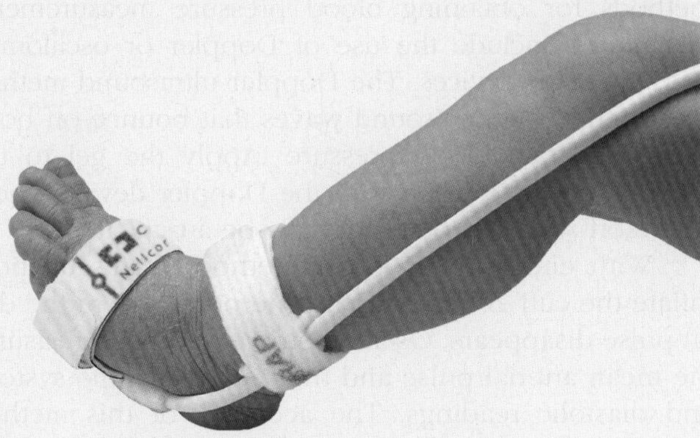

b. Finger adhesive (continuous use)

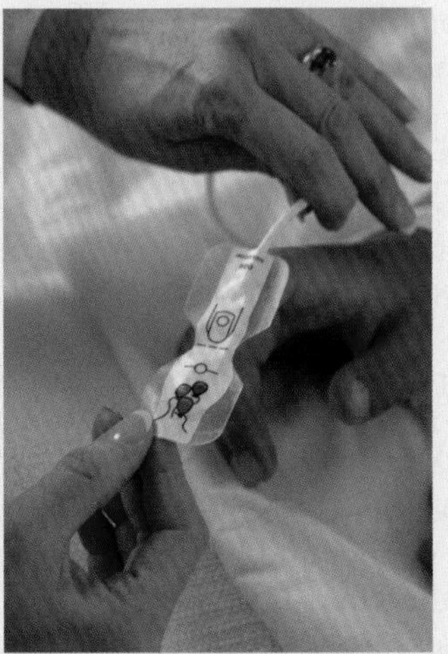

c. Finger reusable (intermittent use)

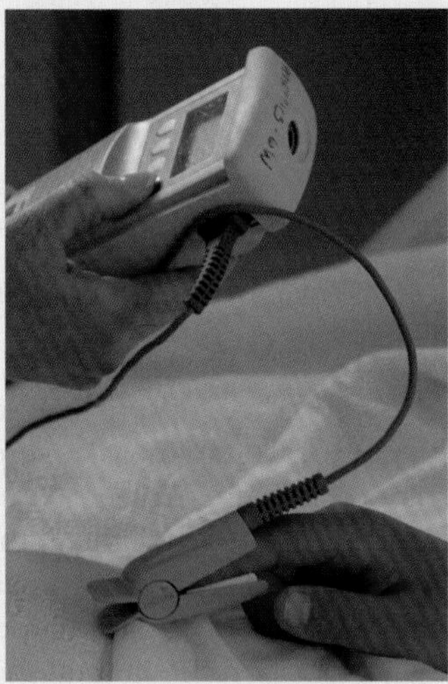

d. Forehead (can be used continuously for 2 days)—especially useful in instances of poor distal perfusion

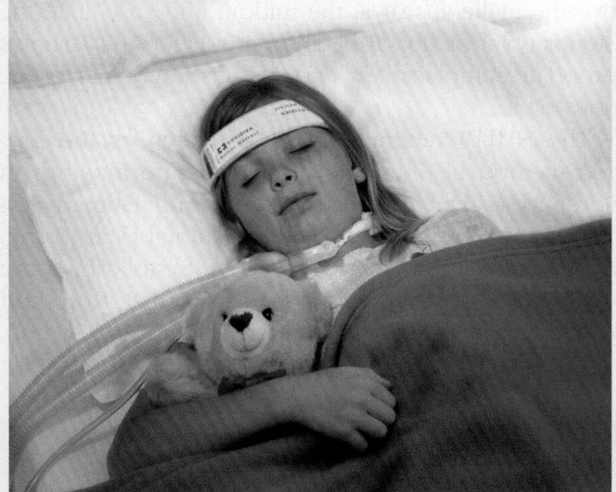

Adapted from Covidien. (2012). *Covidien operator's manual: Nellcor™ bedside spO_2 patient monitoring system*. Mansfield, MA: Author.

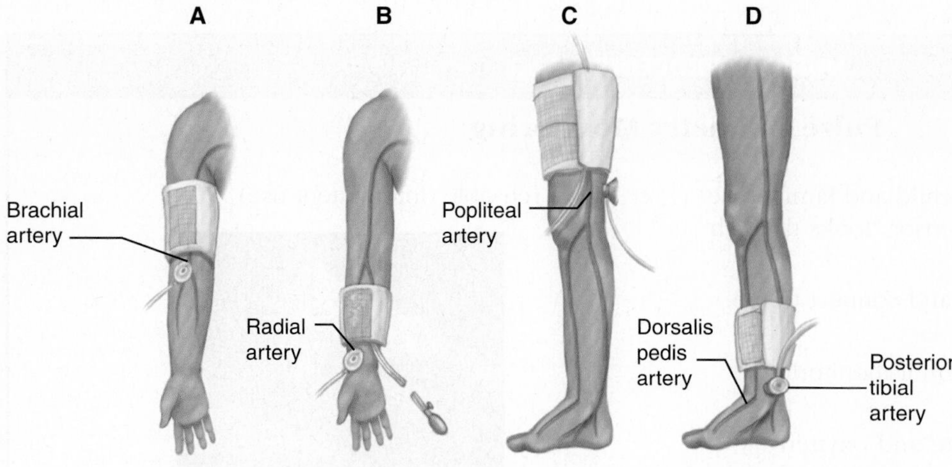

FIGURE 32.7 Various positions of cuff placement and auscultation area for obtaining blood pressure. (**A**) Upper arm. (**B**) Lower arm. (**C**) Thigh. (**D**) Calf/ankle.

same limb, at the same place, and in the same position with each subsequent measurement to ensure consistency in tracking the blood pressure. To measure blood pressure using the upper arm, place the limb at the level of the heart, place the cuff around the upper arm, and auscultate at the brachial artery. When obtaining blood pressure in the lower arm, again, position the limb at the level of the heart, place the cuff above the wrist, and auscultate the radial artery. For measurement in the thigh, place the cuff above the knee and auscultate the popliteal artery. To obtain blood pressure on the calf or ankle, place the cuff above the malleolus or at the midcalf and auscultate the posterior tibial or dorsal pedal artery. Figure 32.7 shows appropriate cuff placement and auscultation points for the various sites.

The NHLBI recommends auscultation as the preferred method of obtaining blood pressure readings in children (U.S. Department of Health and Human Services, National Institutes of Health, National Heart, Lung, and Blood Institute, 2005) (Fig. 32.8). Systolic pressure in children is read at the moment the first Korotkoff sound is heard as the manometer pressure is lowered.

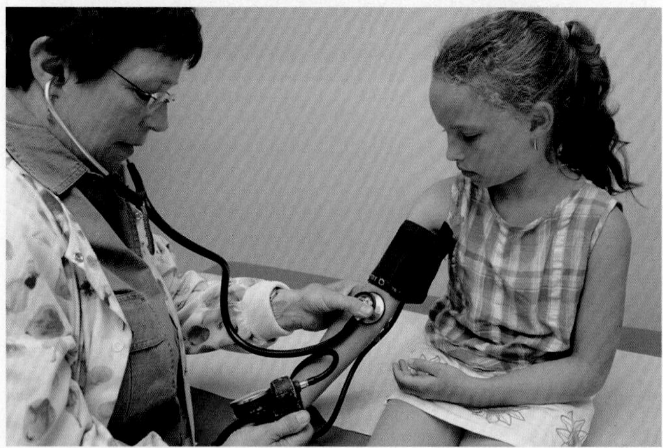

FIGURE 32.8 Auscultation is the preferred method for measuring blood pressure in children.

The point at which the sound disappears is the diastolic pressure. The systolic blood pressure sometimes can be heard to a measurement of zero, so document the reading as systolic pressure over "P" for pulse.

Due to the small arm vessels in infants and young children, it may be very difficult to hear the Korotkoff sounds by auscultation (Jarvis, 2012). Alternative methods for obtaining blood pressure measurements in children include the use of Doppler or oscillometric (Dinamap) devices. The Doppler ultrasound method uses high-frequency sound waves that bounce off body parts to obtain blood pressure. Apply the gel to the Doppler end and listen with the Doppler device where Korotkoff sounds would normally be auscultated.

With either the Doppler method or auscultation, inflate the cuff 20 mm Hg past the point where the distal pulse disappears. Oscillometric equipment measures the mean arterial pulse and then calculates the systolic and diastolic readings. The accuracy of this method depends heavily on ongoing validation and calibration. Also, the cuff inflates to a preset value often far higher than the infant or child's blood pressure, resulting in a tight, uncomfortable cuff being in place for a longer period of time.

Take Note!

If the oscillometric device yields a blood pressure greater than the 90th percentile for gender and height, repeat the reading using auscultation.

In children older than 1 year, the systolic pressure in the thigh tends to be 10 to 40 mm Hg higher than in the arm; the diastolic pressure remains the same. Refer to Appendix B for the NHLBI blood pressure levels based on gender and height. Systolic blood pressure increases if the child is crying or anxious, so measure the blood pressure with the child quiet and relaxed. If the reading is lower in the leg than in the arm, always consider coarctation of the aorta or interference with circulation to the lower extremities. Also pay attention to the pulse pressure (the difference between the systolic and diastolic readings): unusually wide (more than 50 mm Hg) or narrow (less than 10 mm Hg) pulse pressure readings suggest a congenital heart defect (Burns et al., 2013).

Pain Assessment

Pain is considered to be the fifth vital sign (Jarvis, 2012). Use the FLACC pain scale to measure pain in children who are too young to verbally or conceptually quantify their pain, or when there is a language barrier (Manworren & Hynan, 2003). The FLACC pain scale consists of a possible 10 points, with 0, 1, or 2 points given for each of five clinical signs (see Table 36.6).

Children who are older and can express that pain is worsening or improving should use the Pain Faces Scale (see Fig. 36.3). Explain that each face represents a person who is happy or sad, depending on how much or how little pain he has: 0 is for a person who is "very happy because he doesn't hurt at all"; 1 means "it hurts just a little bit"; 2, "it hurts a little more"; 3, "it hurts even more"; 4, "it hurts a whole lot"; and 5, "it hurts as much as you can imagine—but you don't have to be crying to feel this bad." Then ask the child to point to the face that best describes the amount of pain being felt (Wong & Baker, 1988).

For additional information related to pain assessment, refer to Chapter 36.

Body Measurements

Appropriate growth in children is usually an indicator of good health. A child who is not growing well may be in poor health, have inappropriate or inadequate dietary intake, or have a chronic disease (Bickley, 2013). Accurate assessment of growth is a critical skill for the pediatric nurse.

Determine the child's height or length, weight, and weight for length or body mass index (BMI). Measure the head circumference for healthy children younger than age 2. Plot these measurements on a graph so they can be compared with earlier measurements and those of the child's peers. Additional anthropometric measurements used in children may include the chest circumference, mid-upper arm circumference, and skinfold measurement at the triceps, abdomen, or subscapular regions, but these are not performed routinely and are usually used only when a nutritionist consultation is necessary.

The growth chart is a screening tool for nutritional problems as well as a useful screen for chronic illness. Record each measurement in ink with a small dot at the correct location for the child's age and the date of the measurement written above it. Then use a plastic straightedge to connect the previous measurement to the most current one. Children grow at variable rates; in infancy and prepuberty, the growth velocity is normally more rapid. The growth chart allows the nurse to compare the child to other children of the same age and gender while allowing for normal genetic variation. When measurements fall close to the same percentiles over time, growth is normal for that child. Children whose measurements fall within the 5th and 95th percentiles are generally considered within the normal growth range (Reiter, 2011).

Sudden or sustained changes in percentile may indicate a chronic disorder, emotional difficulty, or nutritional intake problem (Bickley, 2013). These findings require further assessment of the physical status of the child as well as other types of evaluations such as dietary intake or serum laboratory measurements.

Appendix A provides growth charts for boys and girls, ages birth to 24 months and 2 to 20 years. The American Academy of Pediatrics and the Centers for Disease Control and Prevention (CDC) recommends the use of these growth charts with all children, though special growth charts are also available for children with specific conditions (CDC, 2015b). Look for a trend over time of healthy growth that is neither too fast nor too slow.

Take Note!

The most valid and reliable growth charts are those supplied by epidemiologists at the Centers for Disease Control and Prevention.

LENGTH OR HEIGHT

Calculate the length of the infant and toddler in a lying position until the age of 24 months. Use a measuring board (Fig. 32.9) or a cloth or paper measuring tape. Stretch out the legs to get a full extension of the body. Marking the examination paper at the child's head and

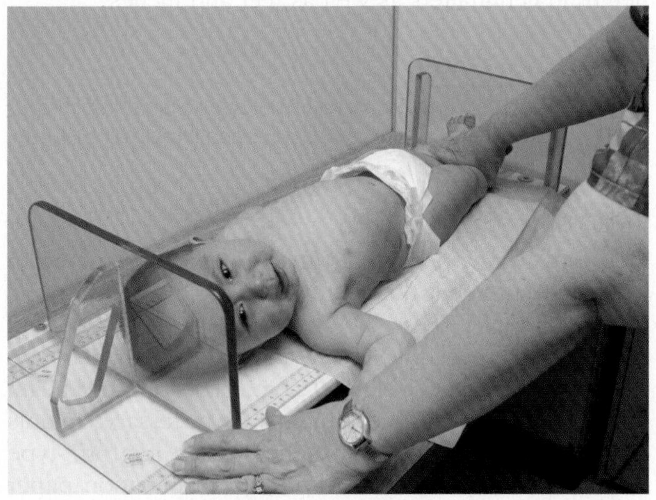

FIGURE 32.9 The recumbent measuring board is the most accurate method for obtaining a length measurement in infants and very young children.

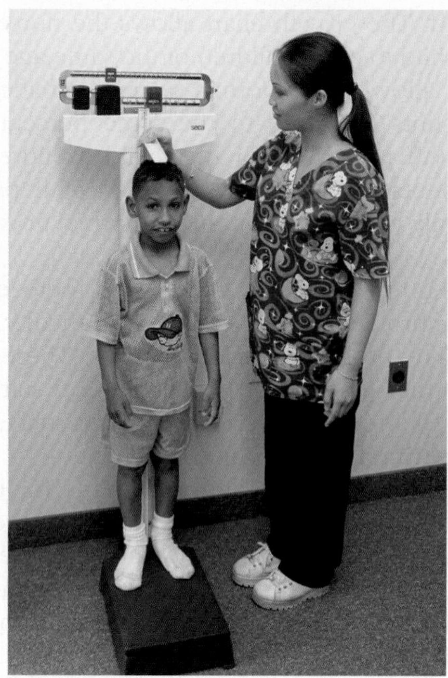

FIGURE 32.10 Standing height is most accurately measured with the stadiometer.

extended foot is an option. Make sure that the growth chart where the measurement is plotted is marked for length and not height, as the two measurements differ. Document the length in centimeters and inches.

Once the child can cooperate and stand independently, begin measuring the standing height. Using a stadiometer is best (Fig. 32.10), but a cloth or paper tape can be used. Ask the child to remove his or her shoes and check that the back, shoulders, buttocks, and heels are against the wall, with the pelvis tucked as much as possible to correct for lordosis. The chin should be parallel to the floor. Plot this measurement on a growth chart marked for height rather than length. Record the height in centimeters as well as feet and inches.

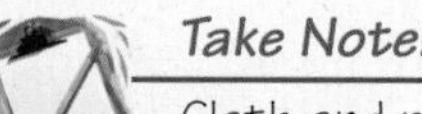

Take Note!

Cloth and paper measuring tapes may stretch over time. Periodically replace or recalibrate all measuring tools.

WEIGHT

Measure weight on a scale that is calibrated between every measurement. Just before placing the child on the electronic scale, press the "zero" or "tare" button and make sure the reading is 0. Calibrate the balance-type scale by setting the weight at zero, observing the beam balance, and making adjustments as necessary. Infants and toddlers should be weighed on a platform-type electronic or balance scale, with an examination paper placed between the child and the scale surface. Calibrate the scale with the examination paper in place. Remove the infant's diaper immediately before placing him or her on the scale. Toddlers may sit on the scale with the nurse or caregiver nearby to avoid falls (Fig. 32.11). Weigh older children and adolescents on a standing scale (Fig. 32.12). They may keep their underpants on and wear a lightweight examination gown.

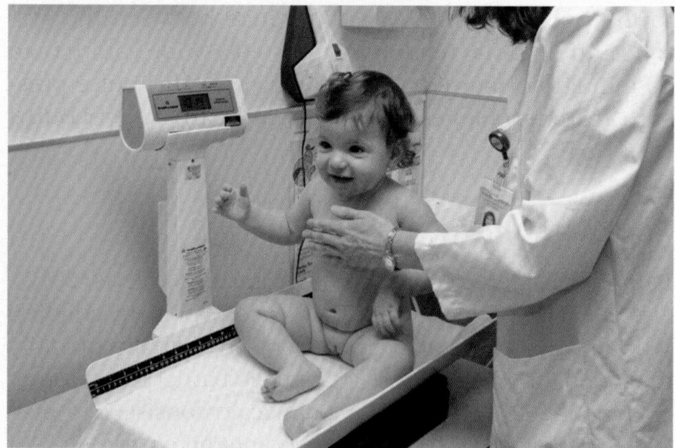

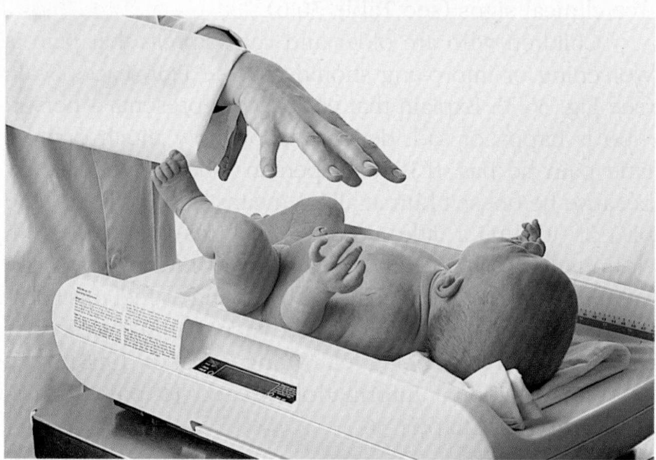

FIGURE 32.11 A nurse or caregiver should remain nearby while weighing the infant or toddler.

An alternate method for obtaining weight, though much less accurate, is to weigh the caregiver initially and then weigh the caregiver holding the child. The difference between the two weights is the child's weight. Regardless of the method used, weigh the infant to the nearest 10 g (or half-ounce) and the toddler and older child to the nearest 100 g (or quarter-pound). Record the weight in kilograms and in pounds.

WEIGHT FOR LENGTH

For children between the ages of newborn and 24 months, plot weight on the growth chart in comparison to the child's length. This allows the nurse to determine whether the child is a healthy weight for how long he or she is. Children placing less than the 5th percentile on the weight-for-length chart are considered underweight. Those placing greater than the 95th percentile are considered to be overweight.

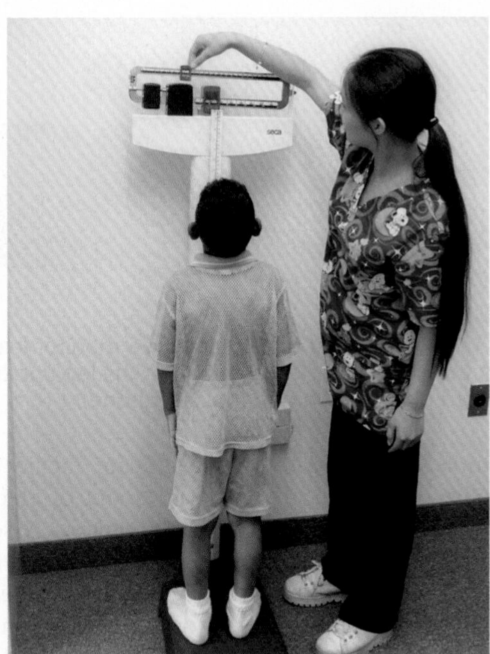

FIGURE 32.12 Children who can stand independently can be weighed on a regular standing balance scale.

BODY MASS INDEX

With the recent increase in obesity in children, BMI is becoming an important measurement. **BMI** is a measure of body fat and is determined by comparing the child's height and weight. Calculate the BMI using the child's weight and height by either the English or metric method. Box 32.1 provides BMI calculation formulas. BMI is included on the charts for children ages 2 to 20 years. Plot the BMI on the growth chart according to the child's age. A child whose BMI for age plots at less than the 5th percentile is considered to be underweight. BMI between the 85th and 95th percentiles indicates risk for overweight. BMI greater than the 95th percentile indicates the child is overweight (CDC, 2015a).

The growth chart can indicate when a child is not growing adequately and can also be used to predict the development of overweight and obesity. Refer to Healthy People 2020.

BOX 32.1

CALCULATION OF BODY MASS INDEX (BMI)

English Formula:

$$\frac{\text{weight in pounds}}{(\text{height in inches}) \times (\text{height in inches})} \times 703$$

Metric Formula:

$$\frac{\text{weight in kilograms}}{(\text{height in meters}) \times (\text{height in meters})} \times 10{,}000$$

HEAD CIRCUMFERENCE

Measure head circumference at well-child visits and upon hospital admission until the third birthday. Then measure it at the annual well-child visit until 6 years old if there are problems such as microcephaly or macrocephaly present at age 3. Measure the largest point across the skull, not including the ears, with a nonstretching cloth or paper tape. Begin at the forehead just above the eyebrows and bring the tape around the head in a taut circle just above the occipital prominence at the back of the head (Fig. 32.13). Plot this measurement in relation to

EVIDENCE-BASED PRACTICE 32.1 PRESCHOOL BODY MASS INDEX ASSOCIATION WITH ADULT OBESITY

STUDY

Overweight and obesity have become significant public health concerns and are acknowledged to be responsible for a significant percentage of chronic disease in the adult population. In this study, a large cohort (4,111 children) was followed into adulthood. The researchers were able to include 2,120 children who had sufficient growth measurements throughout childhood. They analyzed preschool age weight and body mass index, as it compared to body mass index, metabolic syndrome, waist circumference, and other chemical markers at the adult age of 31 years.

Findings

Analysis of the preschool growth measurement data as compared to adult status revealed an important association. High preschool body mass index was consistently associated with adult obesity and early-onset metabolic syndrome. Thus, routine growth measurements throughout the preschool years can help identify children who may benefit from intervention related to decreasing body mass index and preventing adult obesity.

Nursing Implications

Accurate growth measurements are critical for determining overall health in the growing child. Identifying children with slow or inappropriate growth is well known to be important for intervening early to insure adequate growth. Pediatric nurses are also in the ideal position to identify preschoolers who demonstrate higher body mass indexes and heavier weight as noted on standardized growth charts. The nurse may then collaboratively develop a plan with the child and family to insure healthy eating and exercise habits are instilled at this young age, in order to prevent adult obesity and its associated morbidities.

Adapted from Graversen, L., Sørensen, T., Petersen, L., Sovio, U., Kaakinen, M., Sandbaek, A.,... Obel, C. (2014). Preschool weight and body mass index in relation to central obesity and metabolic syndrome in adulthood. *PLoS ONE*, 9(3), 1–9.

HEALTHY PEOPLE 2020

Objective	Nursing Significance
Reduce the proportion of children and adolescents who are considered obese.	• Screen for overweight in all children by plotting weight for length of children younger than 24 months and body mass index for age for children age 2–20 years. • Assess dietary intake and activity level in all children at risk for or overweight. • Provide diet and activity recommendations to attain a healthy weight or BMI. • Refer significantly overweight children to a pediatric endocrinologist.

Healthy People Objectives retrieved from http://www.healthypeople.gov.

the child's age on the appropriate standardized growth chart (usual growth charts include head circumference only up to age 2 years).

Monitoring Equipment

Sometimes children in acute care settings require continuous monitoring of vital signs. This monitoring could be via an apnea monitor or a cardiopulmonary monitor. The apnea monitor measures abnormal or irregular breathing in infants. The cardiopulmonary monitor generally measures heart rate and respiratory rate. Additional equipment on this monitor also allows for blood pressure and temperature monitoring. Set high and low alarm limits according to the healthcare facility's policies. Figure 32.14 indicates the placement of electrodes for the apnea and cardiopulmonary monitors. Assess the skin where the electrodes are placed to ensure there is no skin breakdown. If the alarm sounds, immediately check the child to ensure the leads are not disconnected or the child is not in distress.

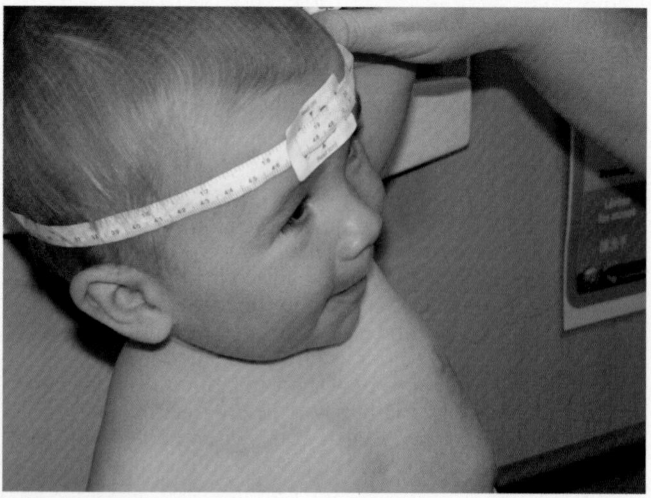

FIGURE 32.13 Measure occipitofrontal head circumference at the largest point.

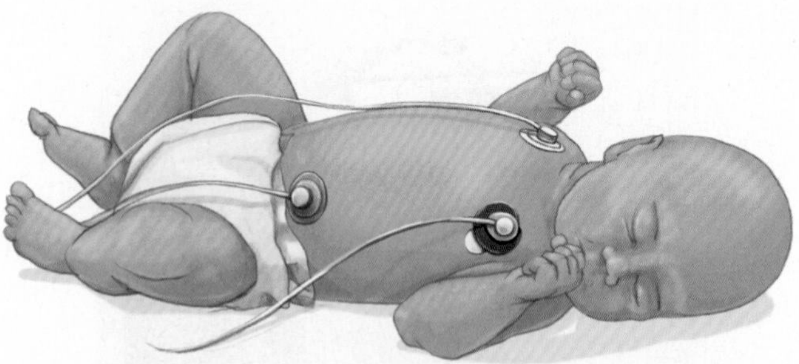

FIGURE 32.14 Placement of cardiac apnea monitor leads: white on the right upper chest, black on the left upper chest, green or red on the abdomen (not over bone).

NPSG

GOAL 6: Reduce the Harm Associated with Clinical Alarm Systems

NPSG.06.01.01 Improve the safety of clinical alarm systems

Steps: Insure alarms on biomedical equipment are properly set according to the child's age, clinical condition, prescribed orders, and facility policy. ALWAYS answer alarms promptly, checking the child first, then attending to the equipment.

Joint Commission. (2015). *National patient safety goals effective January 1, 2015.* Retrieved from http://www.jointcommission.org/assets/1/6/2015_NPSG_HAP.pdf

Skin

The skin is the body's largest organ and reveals information about a child's nutrition, respiratory, cardiac, endocrine, and hydration status at a glance. A careful skin examination provides an invaluable understanding of a child's health (Jarvis, 2012).

INSPECTION

Inspect the color of the skin. The color should be appropriate to the child's racial or ethnic background, with the nail beds, conjunctivae, soles of the feet, and palms of the hands appearing pink. Normal variations include the following:

- Blueness of the hands and feet, known as **acrocyanosis**, is normal in babies up to several days of age and results from an immature circulatory system completing the switch from fetal to extrauterine life (see Fig. 25.3A).
- Cooling or warming the newborn and young infant may produce a vasomotor response that causes a mottling of the skin over the trunk and extremities (see Fig. 25.3B).
- Babies of darkly pigmented Native American, African, and Asian parents will be paler than their parents for

BOX 32.2

VARIATIONS IN SKIN COLOR AND THEIR CAUSES

- **Pallor** (defined as decreased pinkness in light-skinned patients, ashy-gray in dark-skinned) is caused by anemia, shock, fever, or syncope.
- **Central cyanosis** (blueness of the lips, tongue, oral mucosa, trunk) is caused by hypoxia or circulatory collapse.
- Overall yellow color (**jaundice**) may be physiologic in the newborn or related to liver or hematopoietic disease in any age child.
- **Yellowing** of nose, palms, and soles may result from excess intake of yellow vegetables.
- **Redness** of the skin results from blushing, exposure to cold, hyperthermia, inflammation (localized), or alcohol ingestion.
- **Lack of color** in skin, hair, and eyes is related to albinism.

Adapted from Bickley, L. (2013). *Bates' guide to physical examination and history taking* (11th ed.). Philadelphia, PA: Lippincott Williams & Wilkins; and Jarvis, C. (2012). *Physical examination and health assessment* (6th ed.). St. Louis, MO: Saunders.

many months until the melanocytes in the epidermis begin production.

- Dark-skinned infants commonly have hyperpigmented areolas, genitals, and linea nigra.

Other variations related to skin color are discussed in Box 32.2.

Inspect the skin for the presence of **lanugo**. All infants display some degree of lanugo (soft, downy hair on the body, particularly the face and back). Lanugo is more abundant in infants of Hispanic descent and in premature infants and recedes over the first few weeks of life.

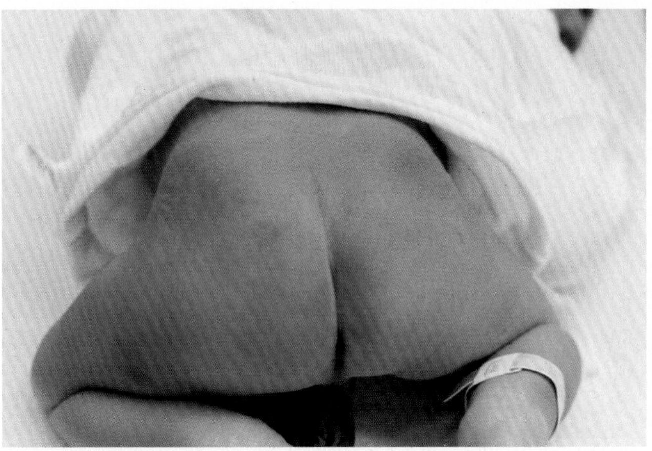

FIGURE 32.15 Transient hyperpigmentation most often occurs in darker-skinned infants.

Inspect the entire body for nevi and vascular and other lesions. Note their location, size, distribution, characteristics, and color. Pigmented nevi (also termed birthmarks) are indicated by a darker patch of skin and generally do not fade over time. Note the presence of hyperpigmented nevi (formerly called Mongolian spots), which appear as blue or gray, variably and irregularly shaped macules (Fig. 32.15). These are a common finding in dark-skinned infants. These nevi fade over months to years as the child's skin pigment darkens. Do not mistake hyperpigmented nevi for bruises. Inspect the skin for vascular lesions. Table 32.4 describes vascular lesions and their significance.

TABLE 32.4 VASCULAR LESIONS AND THEIR SIGNIFICANCE

Description	Significance
Salmon nevi: light pink macule usually on eyelids, nasal bridge, back of neck ("stork bite")	Usually fade over time, but may never go away completely. No complications.
Strawberry nevus: raised reddish papule made of blood vessels (hemangiomas)	Present at or develop after birth; recede over time, usually by the age of 9 years. Usually no complications.
Nevus flammeus: dark purple-red flat patch, grows with the child ("port-wine stain")	May be associated with Sturge–Weber syndrome. May be disfiguring; may be removed with laser therapy.
Ecchymosis: purplish discoloration, changing to blue, brown, black (bruise)	Common on lower extremities in young children. Should correlate with the injury.
Petechiae: pinpoint reddish purple macules that do not blanch when pressed	Broken tiny blood vessels; occur with coughing, bleeding disorders, meningococcemia
Purpura: larger purple macules that do not blanch when pressed	Bleeding under the skin; occur with bleeding disorders, meningococcemia

Adapted from Bickley, L. (2013). *Bates' guide to physical examination and history taking* (11th ed.). Philadelphia, PA: Lippincott Williams & Wilkins; and Jarvis, C. (2012). *Physical examination and health assessment* (6th ed.). St. Louis, MO: Saunders.

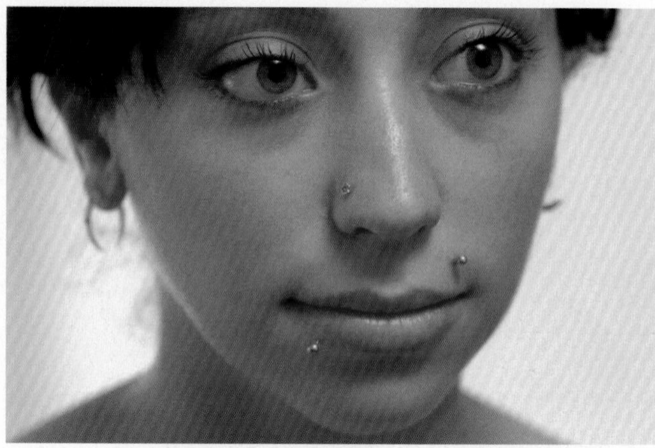

FIGURE 32.16 Adolescent with multiple piercings.

Rashes are common in children and are often associated with communicable diseases. Describe the rash in detail, noting types of lesions, distribution, drying, scabbing, scaling, and any drainage. The newborn and young infant may display milia (small white papules) on the forehead, chin, nose, and cheeks. These recede spontaneously. In adolescents the skin examination may reveal open or closed comedones (pimples or blackheads) across the face, chest, and back. Teens may sport tattoos, brandings, or various body piercings; inspect these areas for signs of infection such as erythema or drainage (Fig. 32.16).

Document the presence of any lacerations, abrasions, or burns. Note the distribution of the injury and whether it seems consistent with the mechanism described in the health history. Be alert to the possibility of child abuse if the type or number of burns, lacerations, or bruises seems unusual for the situation.

Take Note!

Petechiae or ecchymosis may be found over areas traumatized by the birth process; these may take a few weeks to resolve. Certain cultures use "cupping" or "coining" when a child is ill, and these practices may yield bruises or mild burns (International Cupping Therapy Association, 2010).

PALPATION

Palpate the skin for temperature, moisture, texture, turgor, and edema. Use the back of your hand to assess the skin's temperature, comparing the right side of the body to the left and the upper body to the lower. The skin should feel uniformly warm. Cool extremities are associated with environmentally cool temperatures as well as impending circulatory collapse and shock. Warm skin may be associated with fever or sunburn, or locally a burn or infectious process. The skin should feel fairly dry, occasionally moister in the creases. Dry, flaking skin may occur in the young infant, particularly if born postmaturely. Overall skin dryness in the well-hydrated child may occur with excess sun exposure, poor nutrition, or overbathing. Moist skin occurs with perspiration, fever resolution, and shock. The infant's and young child's skin is very soft ordinarily. Older children should continue to have a smooth and even skin texture. The preadolescent and adolescent may have oily-feeling skin on the face, shoulders, or back.

Assess skin turgor by elevating the skin on the abdomen in the infant or on the back of the hand in the older child or teen. The "pinched-up" skin should quickly return to place. Skin that remains tented is strongly suggestive of moderate to severe dehydration. When edema is present, palpate the edematous area to determine its extent. Palpate any lumps or protrusions to determine firmness or tenderness. Palpate lesions or rashes with a gloved hand to document the size and extent of the lesions.

Hair and Nails

Inspect the hair and scalp, noting distribution of hair as well as color, texture, amount, and quality. The young infant's hair may be absent entirely or quite thick; it will be replaced by hair that is of a texture and color closer to what the child will have throughout childhood. Coarse, dry hair at any age may indicate a thyroid disorder or nutritional deficiency. Inspect the scalp thoroughly; it should be free from lesions and infestations. Note the presence of a greasy, scaly plaque on the scalp of infants; termed seborrheic dermatitis or cradle cap, it is benign and easily treated.

Inspect the nails for color, shape, and condition. Full-term infants may have long, papery fingernails that can scratch their skin if not trimmed. Children should have healthy nails. Dry, brittle nails may indicate a nutritional deficiency. Inspect the skin around the nails to ensure that it is intact and without signs of infection. Many children (especially school-age children) have a nervous habit of nail biting or hangnail biting or pulling.

Inspect the school-age child's or adolescent's toenails to ensure they are trimmed in a horizontal fashion. Self-trimming of toenails either too low or in a curved fashion places the child at risk for the development of ingrown nails. Clubbing of the nails indicates chronic hypoxemia related to respiratory or cardiac disease. Nails that curve inward or outward may be hereditary or linked with injury, infection, or iron-deficiency anemia.

Head

Examining the head is critical in the newborn and infant periods but should not be overlooked in older children as an opportunity to check for diseases of the scalp and functional and developmental problems that are reflected in poor hygiene of the head and scalp. Note hair distribution and any bald or thinning areas. Use of gloves may be indicated, depending on the overall scalp cleanliness and chance of infestation by head lice (seen as small grayish specks near the base of hair shafts).

INSPECTION

Examine the head and face for shape and symmetry. In newborns, the head may be temporarily misshapen from uterine positioning or a lengthy vaginal delivery. Some infants have a slight flattening of the back of the head since the recommended sleeping position is supine. Note any irregularities or asymmetry. Observe the infant's head shape by looking down on it from above. Observe whether the head appears centered on the neck or tilts to one side. After 4 months of age, the infant should have achieved enough head control to hold the head erect and in midline when placed in a vertical position. Pull the infant from the supine position into sitting to determine the extent of head lag. To determine the extent of head control in older infants and children, ask the child to turn the head in different directions, either by simple commands or by following a colorful object.

Observe the infant's face when crying, smiling, or babbling for symmetry of muscle movement. In children who are old enough to follow directions, a game of "Simon Says" is a playful way to determine facial symmetry and strength; ask them to puff out their cheeks, make kisses, look surprised, stick out their tongue, and so on (effectively testing function of cranial nerve VII [facial]) (Bickley, 2013).

Take Note!

When you note a flattened occiput in an infant, encourage the parent or caregiver to allow the infant "tummy time" while awake and observed and to change the infant's head position frequently when upright in an infant seat (Shah & Gupta, 2014).

PALPATION

Gently palpate the anterior and posterior **fontanels** (Fig. 32.17). The fontanels are the soft areas on the skull that remain open in infancy to allow for rapid brain growth in the first months of life. Note the size of the fontanels. The anterior fontanel's size is 1 to 4 cm in either direction until it can no longer be felt when it is closed by the age of 9 to 18 months (Rosenberg & Grover, 2014). The posterior fontanel is much smaller and may close any time between shortly after birth and approximately 2 months of age. The fontanels should not be depressed or taut and bulging, though it is not uncommon to see them pulsate or briefly bulge if the baby cries. In an acutely ill infant, assess the fontanels while obtaining the vital signs. Dehydration can cause the fontanels to be sunken; increased intracranial pressure and overhydration can cause them to bulge. Palpate the skull for asymmetry, overriding or open sutures, and lumps or other deformities. Palpate the jaw joints as the child bites down to assess cranial nerve V (trigeminal). Use the fingertips to palpate for occipital, postauricular, preauricular, submental, and submandibular lymph nodes, noting their size, mobility, and consistency (Fig. 32.18).

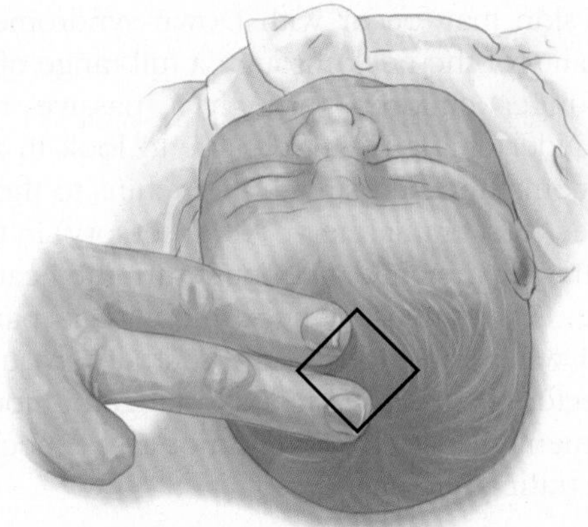

FIGURE 32.17 Note location and size of the fontanels. The anterior fontanel is diamond shaped and closes between the ages of 9 and 18 months.

Take Note!

Large fontanels may be associated with Down syndrome or congenital hypothyroidism. A fontanel that becomes larger over time rather than smaller may indicate the development of hydrocephalus, especially if accompanied by an accelerated increase in head circumference (Bickley, 2013).

Neck

Inspect the neck for symmetry. The infant's neck is short, but by 4 years of age the child's neck should be similar in appearance to the adult's. Webbing or excessive neck skin folds may be associated with Turner syndrome, and

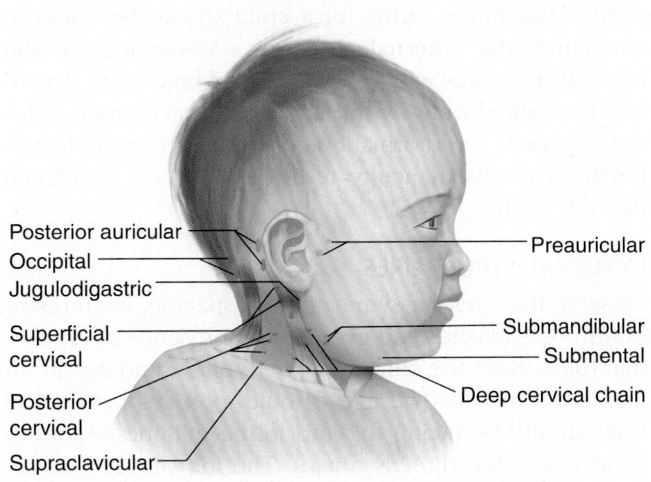

FIGURE 32.18 Location of lymph nodes.

lax neck skin may occur with Down syndrome. Assess the flexibility of the neck through a full range of motion. Take younger children through a passive range of motion. Older children will be able to look in all directions on command and stretch their chins to their chests themselves. Test cranial nerve XI (accessory) in the older child by having the child attempt to turn the head against resistance. Assessment of neck mobility is particularly important when infections of the central nervous system are suspected. Pain or resistance to range of motion may indicate meningeal irritation. Do not assess neck mobility in the trauma victim.

Take Note!

The infant or child who has experienced trauma should have the cervical spine maintained completely immobile until a radiologist has determined that the spinal cord is not damaged.

Palpate the neck for masses and lymph nodes. Palpate the cervical and clavicular lymph nodes with the distal part of the fingers using gentle but firm pressure in a circular motion. Tilt the child's head upward slightly to allow better access. Assess the lymph nodes for swelling, mobility, temperature, and tenderness. In healthy infants and adolescents, the cervical lymph nodes are usually not palpable; in healthy children between 1 and 11 years, the cervical nodes are often found to be small, nontender, and mobile (see Fig. 32.18 for locations of lymph nodes). Enlarged cervical lymph nodes frequently occur in association with upper respiratory infections and otitis media. Report significant enlargement to the physician or nurse practitioner. Palpate the trachea; the thyroid is usually palpable only in older children.

Eyes

Assessment of the eyes includes evaluation of the external and internal structures as well as screening for visual acuity. Any nurse caring for a child should be adept at examining the external structures. Assessment of the internal structures will also be covered below but is usually performed only by the advanced practitioner. Refer to Chapter 31 for information on vision screening. Determination of visual acuity tests the function of cranial nerve II (optic).

EXTERNAL STRUCTURES

Observe the eyes for symmetry and spacing, even distribution of eyelashes and eyelids, and presence of epicanthal folds. Note the child's ability to blink, and report an inability to do so. The eyes should look symmetric and both should be facing forward in the midline when the child is looking directly ahead. The iris should be perfectly round and the sclerae should be clear. The cornea should be uniformly transparent. Inspect the corners of the eye (medial and lateral canthus) and the conjunctiva (lining of the eyelids). They should be free of discharge, inflammation, or swelling. Epicanthal folds may be present in children of Asian descent, children with genetic abnormalities, or those with fetal alcohol spectrum disorder. Using a small penlight or ophthalmoscope, inspect the function and clarity of the pupil by putting your nondominant hand on the child's forehead and moving the light toward and away from each eye. This will elicit the blink reflex. Next observe whether the pupil contracts with the light and expands when the light is removed. Make the same motion with a small toy or object and direct the child to look at it. The eyes demonstrate **accommodation**, or focusing at different distances, if the pupil constricts as the object moves closer. If normal findings are present, report **PERRLA** (pupils are equal, round, reactive to light and accommodation) (Fig. 32.19). This is a particularly important assessment in head and eye injuries, as well as when other neurologic concerns are present. Absence of pupillary reflexive action after age 3 weeks may indicate blindness (Jarvis, 2012).

Take Note!

The normal infant may exhibit intermittent strabismus (crossing of the eyes) until about 3 months of age. However, persistent strabismus at any age or intermittent strabismus after 6 months of age should be evaluated by a pediatric ophthalmologist (Burns et al., 2013).

Check extraocular muscle motility and function of cranial nerves III and IV (oculomotor and abducens) by instructing the child to follow the light through the six cardinal positions of gaze. Infants and very young children will follow an interesting object. Instruct the older child to look downward and inward (testing cranial

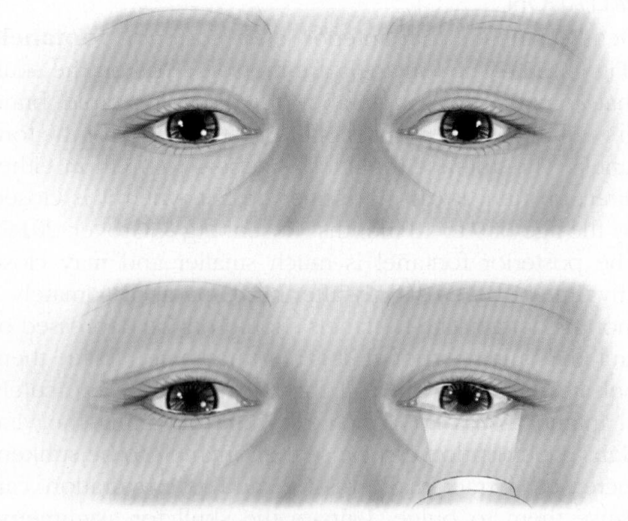

FIGURE 32.19 The pupils should be equal, round, and reactive to light and accommodation (PERRLA).

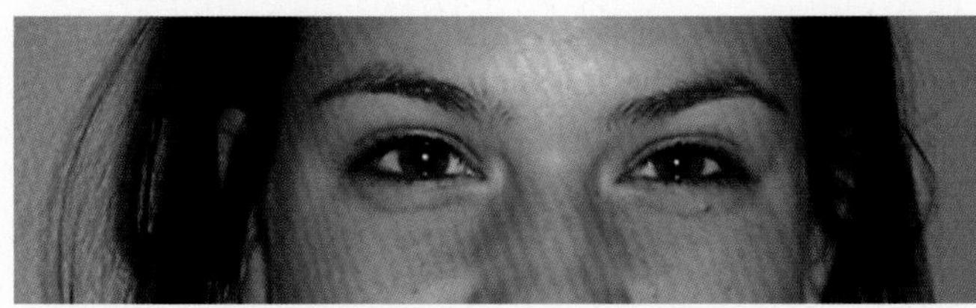

FIGURE 32.20 Note reflected light falling symmetrically on each pupil with the Hirschberg test.

nerve IV [trochlear]). Assess eye muscle strength using two tests. Using the Hirschberg test, bring the penlight to the middle of your face and direct the child to look at it. The small dot of reflected light seen in the iris should be placed symmetrically in each eye (Fig. 32.20). The cover test also assesses eye muscle strength. Cover one of the child's eyes and instruct the child to focus on an interesting object. The eye should not waver. While the child is still focusing with the first eye, remove the cover from the second. Observe the uncovered eye for movement. Report any movement or drift.

To test peripheral vision, have the child focus on a specific point or object directly in front. Bring a finger or a small object from beyond the range of vision into the area of the peripheral vision. When the child sees the object from the side, while still focusing on the object or point in front, the child should say "stop." This also tests cranial nerve II (optic).

INTERNAL STRUCTURES

An advanced practitioner with experience in this type of assessment best accomplishes assessment of the internal structures of the eye. An adequate assessment requires that the child cooperate. Restraint for eye examination does not usually prove fruitful, as movement and tearing of the eyes interfere with the accuracy of the examination. Use the ophthalmoscope to inspect the internal eye structures. Observe the glow of the pupil, which appears red (creamy colored in children with very dark eye color). Inspect the optic disc, macula, fovea, and blood vessels. Refer any child with blurring or bulging of the optic disc or hemorrhage of vessels to a pediatric ophthalmologist for further evaluation.

Take Note!

Immediately report absence of the red reflex in one or both eyes, as this may indicate the presence of cataracts (Bickley, 2013).

Ears

Assessment of the ears includes evaluation of the external and internal structures as well as screening for hearing. Any nurse caring for a child should be adept at examining the external structures. Assessment of the internal structures will also be covered below but is usually performed only by the advanced practitioner. Refer to Chapter 31 for information on hearing screening. Testing of hearing also tests the function of cranial nerve VIII (acoustic).

EXTERNAL STRUCTURES

Assess the placement of the external ears on the head. They should be symmetric and placed no lower than the eyes. The pinna should deviate no more than 10 degrees from an imaginary line that is perpendicular to a line drawn between the outer canthus of the eye and the top of the ear. Low-set ears may be associated with genetic abnormalities or syndromes (Fig. 32.21). Note protrusion or flattening of the ears, which may be normal for that child or may indicate inflammation (protrusion) or persistent side-lying (flattening). Note the presence of pits or skin tags in the preauricular area. Observe the exterior ear canal. A waxy cerumen that is soft and an orangish-brown color is normally found lubricating and protecting the external ear canal and should be left in place or washed gently away when bathing. Note drainage from the ear canal, which is always considered abnormal. Pull on the auricle and palpate the mastoid process, neither of which should result in pain in the healthy child.

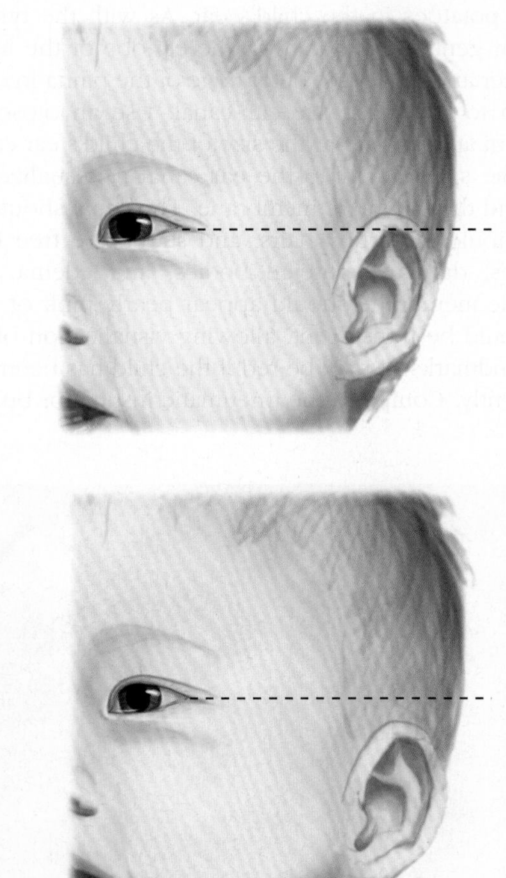

FIGURE 32.21 Low-set ears may be associated with chromosomal or other genetic anomalies.

Take Note!

Impacted and dry cerumen can be softened with a few drops of mineral or cooking oil and then gently irrigated from the canal with an ear syringe and warm water (Nettina, 2014).

INTERNAL STRUCTURES

Use a **tympanometer** to assess the mobility of the eardrum (tympanic membrane). Gently pull down on the earlobe of infants and toddlers and up on the outer edge of the pinna in older children to straighten the ear canal, and press the tip of the tympanometer over the external canal. A reading of air pressure is recorded by the instrument, and this is useful to assess middle ear disease. Many tympanometers record a wave pattern that may be printed to include in the child's chart.

A nurse practitioner or physician generally performs inspection of the ear canal and tympanic membrane with an otoscope (Fig. 32.22). The otoscopic examination is usually performed near the end of the physical assessment for infants and young children, as they are often quite resistant to this intrusive procedure. The infant or toddler may require restraint in the parent's lap for the otoscopic evaluation. The preschooler may cooperate if the nurse uses a game such as looking for pretend puppies or potatoes in the child's ear. As with the tympanometer, gently pull down on the earlobe of the infant or toddler and up on the outer edge of the pinna in older children to straighten the ear canal. Use an otoscopic speculum appropriate to the size of the child's ear canal. Insert the speculum into the ear canal to visualize the canal and the tympanic membrane. The canal should be pink, should have tiny hairs, and should be free from scratches, drainage, foreign bodies, and edema. The tympanic membrane should appear pearly pink or gray and should be translucent, allowing visualization of the bony landmarks. It may be red if the child has been crying recently. Compress the pneumatic insufflator bulb to provide a puff of air; this causes motion of the tympanic membrane when the middle ear is healthy. Note abnormalities such as a fluid level, bubble or pus behind the tympanic membrane, tympanic membrane immobility, holes or perforations in the tympanic membrane, and the presence of tympanostomy tubes, scarring, or vesicles.

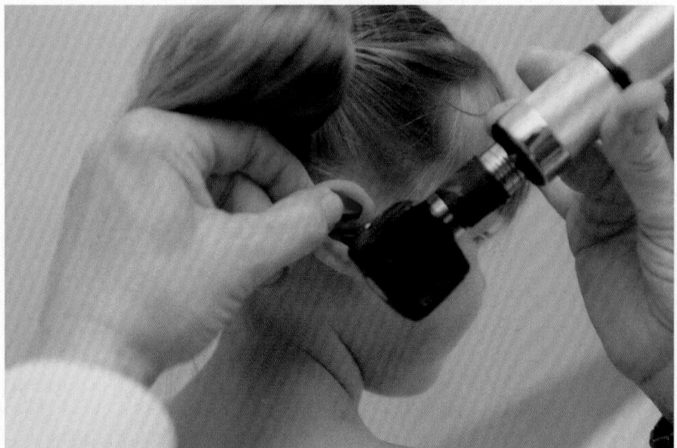

FIGURE 32.22 Otoscopic examination allows visualization of the internal structures of the ear.

Take Note!

Never attempt to flush a foreign object out with water until it has been identified, because small pieces of sponge, clay, or vegetative material like peas or beans swell with water, further obstructing the ear canal (Nettina, 2014).

Nose and Sinuses

The nose, as with all facial features in a child, should be symmetric, but it can be displaced temporarily by birth trauma in newborns. Children of Asian or African descent often display a flattened nasal bridge as a normal variation. Ensure that the nares provide unobstructed airflow by alternately occluding one nostril at a time and observing for air movement through the other nostril. If the child is breathing comfortably, there should be little nostril movement visible. Adolescents may have pierced their nose or nasal septum; ensure that the site is free from infection or loose jewelry that could migrate into the sinuses. Ideally the nose should not be draining, though clear mucus may be present if the child has been crying. Assess the amount, color, thickness, and presence of any odor if drainage is present. Inspect the interior of the nose by tilting the child's head backward and pushing the tip of the nose upward. Direct the beam of a penlight in the nostril. The nasal mucosa should be uniformly firm, pink, and free from edema, excoriation, or masses. Test the older child's sense of smell by having the child close the eyes and identify a familiar scent such as peppermint or coffee (cranial nerve I [olfactory]). Palpate the sinuses for tenderness.

Take Note!

Infants up to 3 to 6 months of age have traditionally been thought to be ***obligate nose breathers*** because of their long soft palate and relatively large tongue, which allows for swallowing without aspiration during breast or artificial nipple feeding. This lessens with age and as the infant becomes better able to breathe through the mouth when necessary (Bickley, 2013).

Mouth and Throat

Wear a powder-free glove to examine the mouth, teeth, and throat. Inspection of the exterior of the mouth may be done at any point in the examination. Infants and young children may find assessment of the mouth and particularly the pharynx and uvula to be quite intrusive, so delay that part of the assessment until the end of the examination, after otoscopic evaluation. Assess the character and quality of the child's voice and the infant's cry. It should be neither too hoarse nor too shrill.

INSPECTION OF THE MOUTH

Observe the lips for color, symmetry, and absence of inflammation or edema. Salivation in infants begins at about 3 months of age; drooling occurs because the infant does not learn to swallow saliva until several months later. Next, inspect the interior of the mouth. The mouth is the first part of the digestive system, and a pink, moist, healthy mucosal lining is indicative of a healthy gastrointestinal tract. In infants, the tongue should lie within the mouth at rest and should be capable of extending over the lower gum line to help the baby feed. The tongue extrusion reflex is normal in infants up until the age of 6 months and allows the infant to suckle easily from birth. Observe movement of the tongue when the infant or young child babbles or cries. Ask the older child to touch the tongue to the roof of the mouth and then stick out the tongue and move it from side to side (testing cranial nerve XII [hypoglossal]). Full movement should be present and the tongue should be free from lesions or exudate. Visualize the hard and soft palate (which should be intact) or palpate with the gloved finger.

Most infants have no teeth before the fifth to sixth month. When the teeth begin to erupt, they usually erupt symmetrically at the rate of about one a month, until toddlers have 20 teeth by 30 months of age. The infant may drool for several months before teething. During teething the gums will be swollen at the location of the impending tooth. In older children, the secondary teeth replace the primary teeth much more slowly and with little discomfort from the 5th to the 20th year. Figure 32.23 shows the usual permanent tooth eruption pattern.

Look for dental caries or alignment problems and inspect the gums for signs of infection. Test cranial nerve IX (glossopharyngeal) by having the child identify taste with the posterior portion of the tongue.

Take Note!

Natal (present at birth) or neonatal (erupting by 30 days of age) teeth should be evaluated by a pediatric dentist for potential extraction, as they may pose an aspiration risk (Bickley, 2013).

INSPECTION OF THE THROAT

Inspect the tonsils, uvula, and oropharynx. Assess the infant's throat during a yawn or cry, as any forcible attempt to depress the tongue with a tongue depressor produces a strong reflex elevation of the base of the tongue that completely blocks the view of the pharynx. The young child will require restraint so that the nurse can depress the tongue and visualize the back of the mouth without injuring the child (Fig. 32.24). Asking the older child to

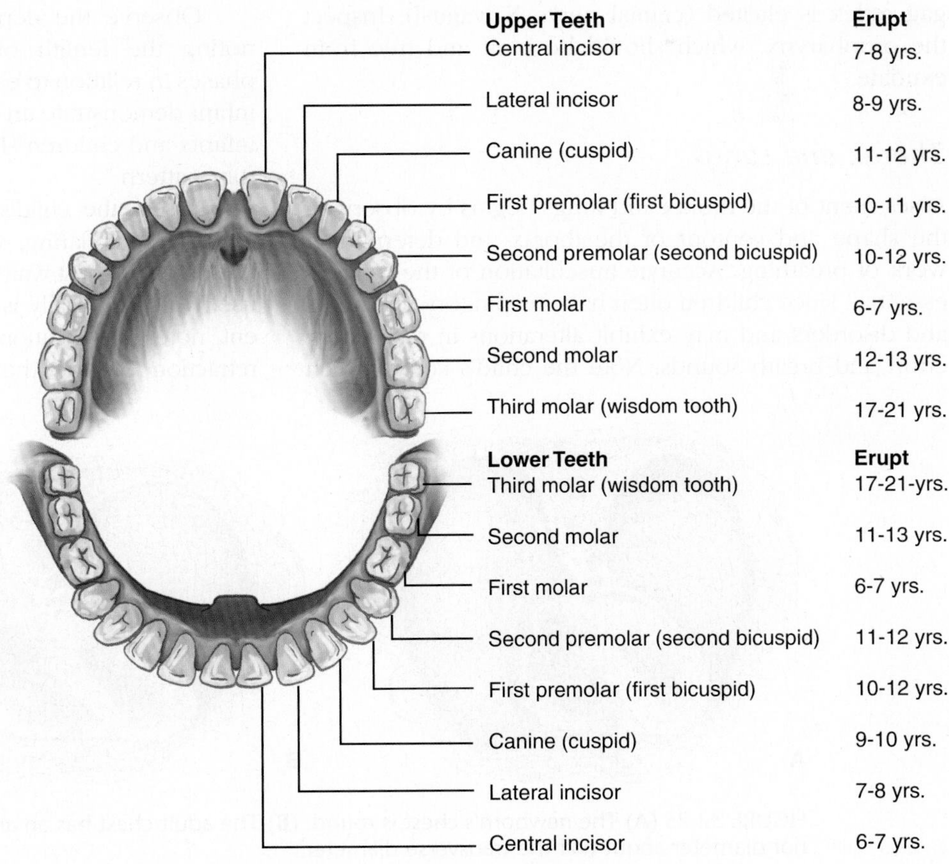

FIGURE 32.23 Usual sequence of permanent tooth eruption.

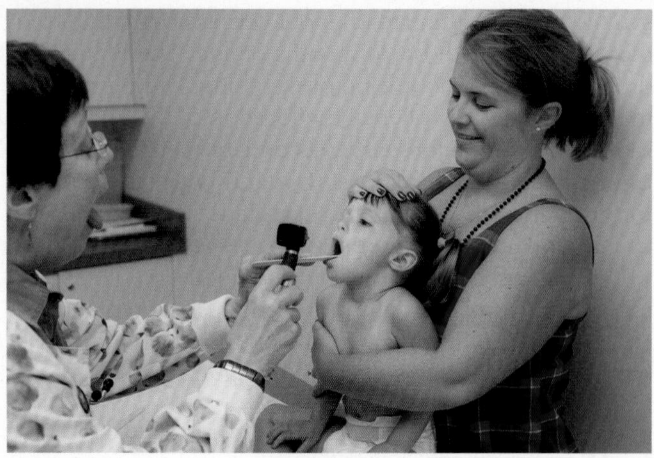

FIGURE 32.24 The young child may need to be restrained so that the throat examination can be done safely.

open wide, stick out the tongue, and say "aaaah" simultaneously will allow for a quick look at the tonsils and pharynx without the need to use a tongue depressor, but the nurse must be very quick because the tongue rises rapidly after those maneuvers are performed.

Tonsils usually cannot be seen in the infant. As the child becomes a toddler, the tonsils become dramatically larger and then begin to decrease in size again by the ninth year. The tonsils should be pink and often have crypts on their surfaces, which are sometimes filled with debris. Ensure that the uvula is midline and rises if the gag reflex is elicited (cranial nerve X [vagus]). Inspect the oropharynx, which should be pink and free from exudate.

Thorax and Lungs

Assessment of the thorax and lungs begins by observing the shape and contour of the thorax and determining work of breathing. Accurate auscultation of the lungs is essential, since children often have respiratory infections and disorders and may exhibit alterations in respiratory effort and breath sounds. Note the child's color, which should be pink; cyanosis indicates hypoxia. Listen for audible stridor (inspiratory high-pitched sound), expiratory grunting or snoring, audible wheezing (heard with the naked ear), or cough. Document type and extent of cough. Observe the nail beds for clubbing, which occurs with diseases inducing chronic hypoxic states.

THORAX

Examine the chest with the head in a midline position to determine size and shape as well as symmetry, movement, and bony landmarks. The newborn's chest should be smooth and round, with the transverse diameter nearly equal to the anterior–posterior diameter. The shape of the chest progresses to that of the adult by the age of 5 to 6 years. At that time the anterior–posterior diameter is about half the transverse diameter (Fig. 32.25). At the point where the xiphoid process and the right and left costal margins meet, the costal angle should measure 90 degrees or less. Inspect for structural deformity such as pectus excavatum (depressed sternum) or pectus carinatum (protuberant sternum) (Fig. 32.26). Note symmetric movement of the chest wall with respiration. Infants and younger children are primarily diaphragmatic breathers, so the abdomen and chest will rise and fall together. Older children, particularly adolescent females, demonstrate thoracic breathing, yet the abdomen and chest should continue to rise and fall together. Asymmetry of chest wall movement is an abnormal finding.

Observe the depth and regularity of respirations, noting the length of the inspiratory and expiratory phases in relation to each other. The newborn and young infant demonstrate an irregular respiratory pattern. Older infants and children should have a more regular respiratory pattern.

Assess the child's respiratory effort by first observing for nasal flaring, which indicates labored breathing. Observe the chest wall and shoulders for accessory muscle use, which normally is not present. If retractions are present, note their location and severity. Typical locations for retraction include the intercostal, subcostal, substernal,

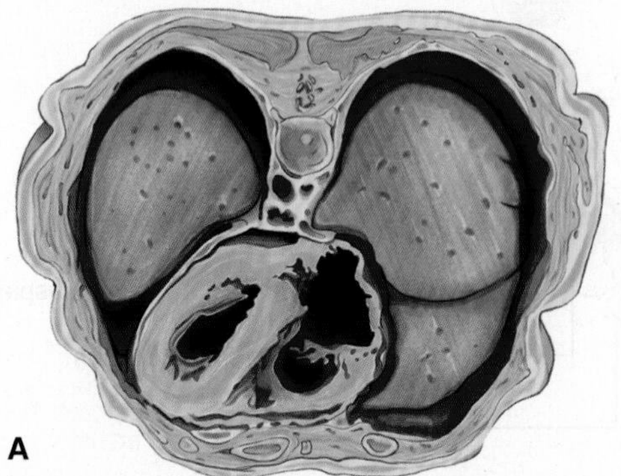

A

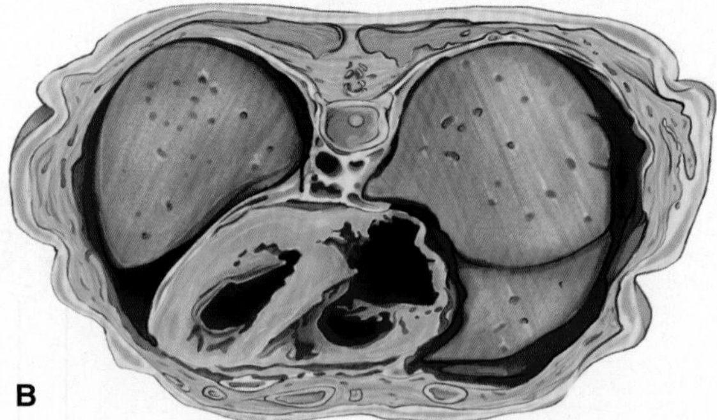

B

FIGURE 32.25 (A) The newborn's chest is round. (B) The adult chest has an anterior–posterior diameter about half the transverse diameter.

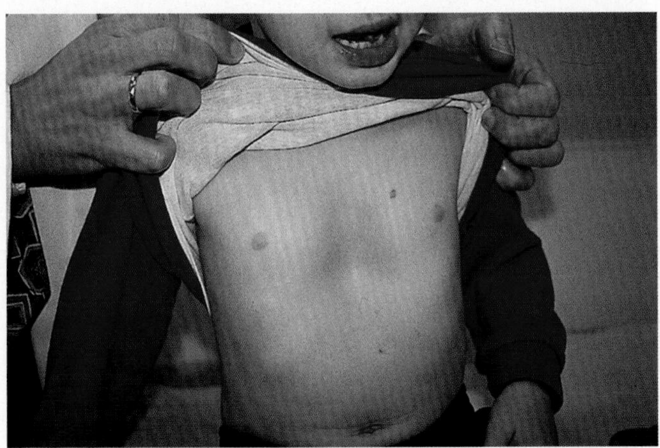

FIGURE 32.26 Pectus excavatum: note depression in xiphoid area.

suprasternal, and clavicular regions (Fig. 32.27). Pay attention to the position the child naturally assumes to breathe comfortably; children in respiratory distress often sit forward and are uncomfortable lying down or talking (Jarvis, 2012).

LUNGS

Experienced examiners may palpate and percuss the lungs before using auscultation to evaluate the breath sounds.

Palpation and Percussion. Palpate for symmetric respiratory excursion by placing the thumbs and fingers together along the costal margin on the chest or back. Movement should be symmetric with each breath. Palpate for the normal presence of tactile fremitus with the palms or fingertips while the infant is crying or the older child says "99." Indirectly percuss the lungs of older children, noting resonance over lung fields. Hyperresonance may be present in conditions resulting in hyperaeration of the lungs, such as asthma.

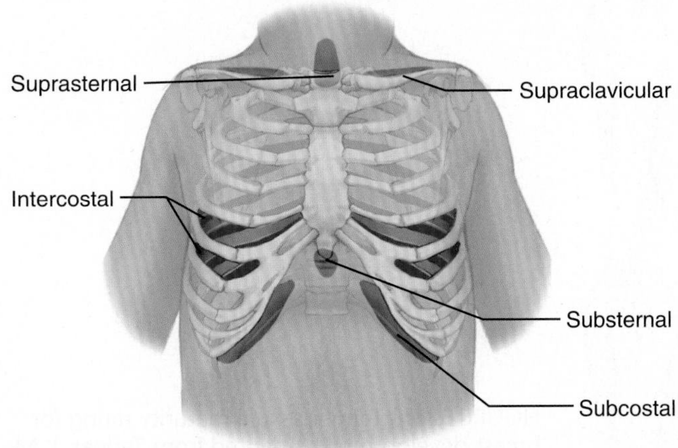

FIGURE 32.27 Location of retractions.

Auscultation. Use the bell of the stethoscope or switch to a small diaphragm to auscultate lung sounds in the infant or child. The adult-sized diaphragm may be used for the adolescent. Auscultate the lung fields with the infant or child in a sitting position, even if that requires propping the infant in a parent's lap. Infants and young children have loud breath sounds because of their thin chest walls. Breath sounds should be clear with adequate aeration throughout all lung fields. Listen to a full inspiration and expiration at the apices of the lungs as well as symmetrically across the entire lung field, systematically comparing the right to the left side. Listen on the anterior chest, on the posterior chest, and in the axillary regions.

Playing games may encourage younger children to cooperate with deep breathing during lung assessment. The child can blow a cotton ball up in the air, blow a pinwheel, or "blow out" the light of the penlight (Miller, n.d.). Older children are capable of deep breathing when instructed to do so.

The child who has a respiratory disorder or who is experiencing respiratory distress may exhibit diminished breath sounds, most often in the lung bases. Diminished breath sounds are softer and quieter than lung sounds demonstrating adequate aeration. In the healthy infant or child, no adventitious sounds should be heard. If noisy breath sounds are heard in the infant or young child, particularly over all lung fields, compare the sound to the noises heard over the trachea or within the nose. Infants and young children with secretions in the nasopharyngeal area may have those sounds transmitted over the lung fields. These sounds usually clear with coughing or airway suctioning; they are not true adventitious sounds. Note adventitious breath sounds such as wheezes or crackles, documenting their location and whether they are present on inspiration, expiration, or both. It is most important to describe the abnormal breath sounds being heard rather than attempting to classify the sounds. Adventitious lung sounds are associated with a variety of disorders, and extensive experience is required to appropriately classify lung sounds. Adventitious breath sounds should be reported for further evaluation.

Breasts

Assess the breasts of children of all ages and both genders. Note the size of the breasts in relation to the age of the child. Palpate the axillary lymph nodes during the breast assessment.

INSPECTION

Observe the breasts for position, shape, size, symmetry, and color. Newborns of both genders may have swollen nipples from the influence of maternal estrogen, but by several weeks of age the nipples should be flat and should continue to be so in all prepubertal children. In children the nipples are located lateral to the midclavicular line, usually between the fourth and fifth ribs. The areola becomes darker in color as the child approaches puberty. Overweight children may appear to have enlarged breasts due to adipose tissue. Note the location of additional (supernumerary) nipples if present (usually located along the mammary ridge); they may appear as darkly pigmented, elevated or nipple-like spots. These are usually of no concern as they do not change over time, but they may be associated with renal disorders.

Inspect the breasts for the current stage of development: widening of the areola, elevation of the nipple, and increase in breast size. Female breast development may begin as early as age 8, but starts by age 13 in most girls. Breast development then continues in a characteristic, but usually asymmetric, pattern, with one breast larger than the other throughout the lifespan. The sexual maturity rating scale developed by Tanner in 1962 is used to describe breast development (**Tanner stages**; Fig. 32.28). Adolescent boys may develop gynecomastia (enlargement of the breast tissue) due to hormonal pubertal changes. When the hormone levels stabilize, male adolescents then have flat nipples. Occasionally gynecomastia is caused by marijuana use, anabolic steroids, or hormonal dysfunction (Jarvis, 2012).

PALPATION

Palpate the breasts in a systematic fashion. A tender nodule palpated just under the nipple confirms pubertal changes. This change may be difficult to assess in girls with excessive adipose tissue. Normal breast tissue should feel smooth, firm, and elastic. Note masses or nodules if present. Palpate for axillary lymph nodes with

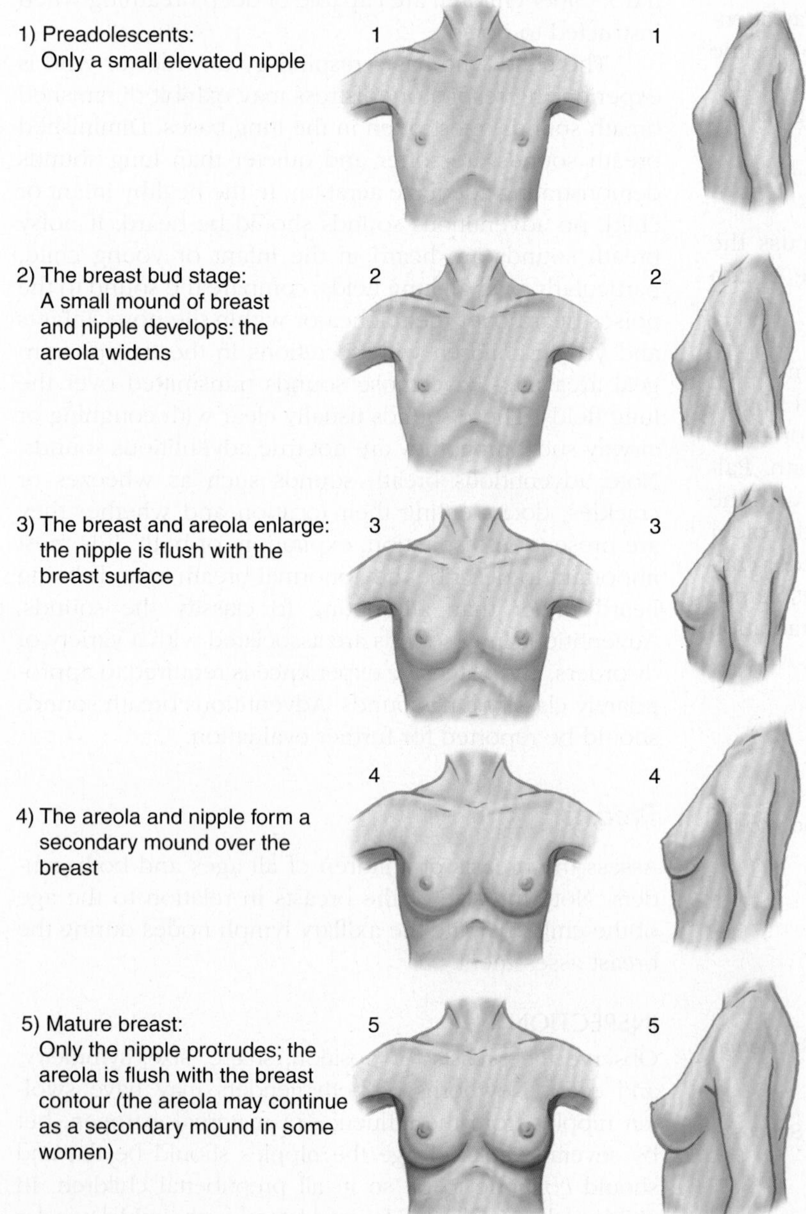

1) Preadolescents:
Only a small elevated nipple
1
1
2) The breast bud stage:
A small mound of breast and nipple develops: the areola widens
2
2
3) The breast and areola enlarge: the nipple is flush with the breast surface
3
3
4) The areola and nipple form a secondary mound over the breast
4
4
5) Mature breast:
Only the nipple protrudes; the areola is flush with the breast contour (the areola may continue as a secondary mound in some women)
5
5

FIGURE 32.28 Tanner sexual maturity rating for breast development. (Adapted from Tanner, J. M. [1962]. *Growth at adolescence*. Oxford, England: Blackwell Scientific Publications.)

the child's arms relaxed at the side but slightly abducted. Note size and texture of nodes if present.

Heart and Peripheral Perfusion

The examination of the heart in children is identical to that of adults except for the focus of the examiner's attention. Congenital heart defects are the most common cause of heart problems in children, and children with these defects present differently than adults with heart disease.

Take Note!

The younger the child, the more responsive the heart rate is to activity changes. It increases with fever, fear, crying, or anxiety and decreases with sleep, sedation, or vagal stimulation (Jarvis, 2012).

INSPECTION

Observe the child's posture. Note the presence of pallor, cyanosis, mottling, or edema, which may indicate a cardiovascular problem. Inspect the anterior chest from the side or at an angle, noting symmetry in shape as well as movement. Observe for the apical impulse, which is visible in about half of children. It occurs at the **point of maximum intensity (PMI)**, which is located at the third to fourth intercostal space just medial of the child's left midclavicular line until the age of 4 years, at the fourth intercostal space at the left midclavicular line in children ages 4 to 6 years, and then lateral to the left midclavicular line at the fifth intercostal space in children ages 7 years and older (Fig. 32.29). Note clubbing of the fingertips or distention of neck veins, both of which may be associated with congenital heart disease.

PALPATION

Using the fingertips, palpate the chest for lifts and heaves or thrills, which are not normal. Palpate the apical pulse in the area of the PMI (Fig. 32.29). Check the pulses and compare the upper body to lower body pulses, as well as left versus right, noting strength and quality (Fig. 32.30). The pedal, brachial, and femoral pulses are usually easily palpated. The radial pulse is very difficult to palpate in children younger than 2 years of age. Note warmth of the distal extremities. To assess capillary refill time, place slight pressure on the nail beds and quickly release it. Observe the length of time required for refill and return to original color. Compare capillary refill time of the fingers to the toes. A capillary refill time of less than 3 seconds indicates adequacy of perfusion.

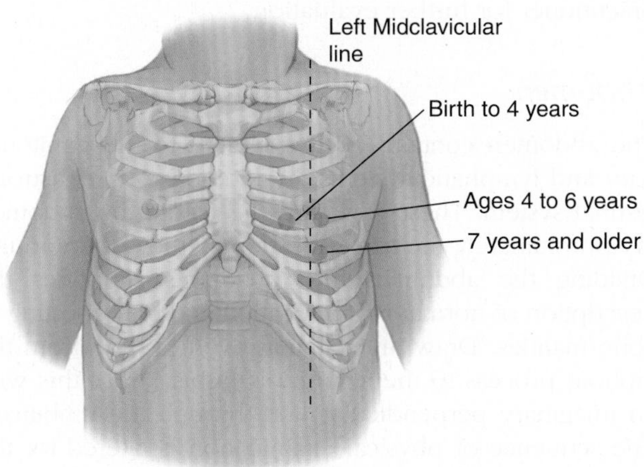

FIGURE 32.29 The point of maximal intensity (PMI) or apical impulse.

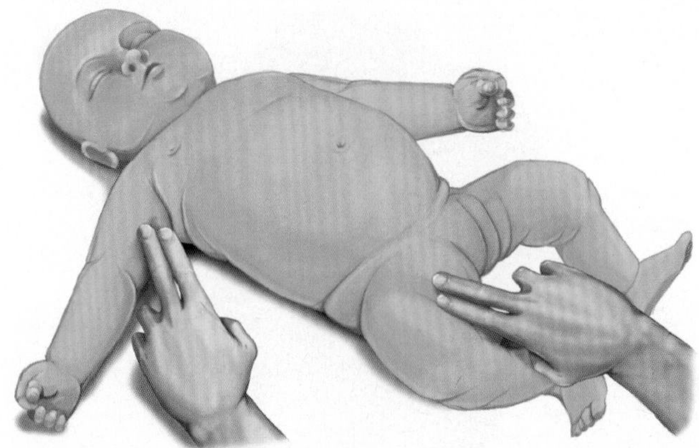

FIGURE 32.30 It is important to assess brachial and femoral pulses simultaneously to determine equality or differences in strength and intensity.

AUSCULTATION

Perform auscultation of the heart with the child in two different positions, upright and reclined (Fig. 32.31). Auscultate the heart rate in the area of the PMI as this is the point on the chest wall where the heartbeat is heard most distinctly (Fig. 32.29). As you begin auscultation, listen first for respirations and note their timing so as not

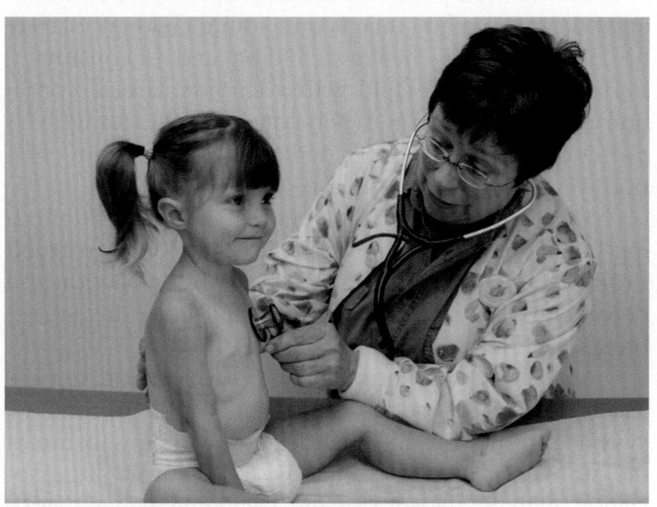

FIGURE 32.31 Auscultating the child's heart.

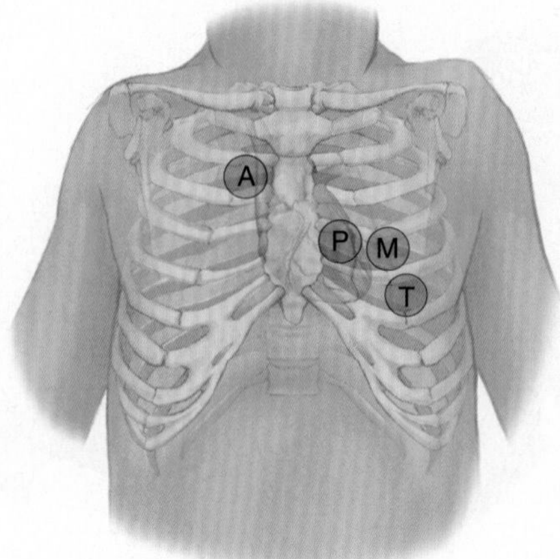

FIGURE 32.32 **Areas where the sounds of heart valves radiate. A: Aortic valve—second intercostal space, just right of sternum. P: Pulmonic valve—second intercostal space, just left of sternum. T: Tricuspid valve—fourth intercostal space, just left of sternum. M: Mitral valve—fourth intercostal space at left midclavicular line.**

to confuse the heart sounds with the lung sounds. A crying infant may help by briefly holding his or her breath between cries. Once you are confident that you are listening to the heart, be sure to listen for 1 full minute because of the irregularity of rhythms in some children. Count the heart rate, which should be consistent with the palpated pulse (either radial or brachial, depending on the child's age).

Develop a systematic approach to auscultation of the heart. Listen over all four valvular areas anteriorly (Fig. 32.32). In the infant or younger child, also auscultate the heart in the axillary region and posteriorly (certain murmurs radiate to these areas). Note S_1, S_2, extra heart sounds, or murmurs. S_1 is usually loudest at the mitral and tricuspid areas and increases in intensity with fever, exercise, and anemia. S_2 is usually most intense at the aortic and pulmonic areas. A split S_2 heard at the apex occurs in many infants and young children. S_3 may be heard in many healthy children and is considered normal, though the child with a chronic cardiac condition may develop an S_3 when congestive heart failure is present. S_4 is usually considered abnormal, most often occurring with cardiac disease.

Sinus arrhythmia is a common and normal finding in children and adolescents. It results in an irregular heart rhythm: the heart rate increases with inhalation and decreases with exhalation. If the child holds his or her breath, the rhythm becomes regular.

Auscultate for murmurs. Note the location (where it is heard best or loudest) and timing of the murmur. A systolic murmur occurs in association with S_1 (closure of the atrioventricular valves), a diastolic murmur in association with S_2 (closure of the semilunar valves). Also note the duration of murmur. Does it occur early or late in diastole or systole? Does it occur all the way across systole (holosystolic)? Note the intensity of the murmur. Table 32.5 discusses grading of murmur intensity.

TABLE 32.5 GRADING HEART MURMURS IN CHILDREN

Grade	Sound
1	Barely audible; sometimes heard, sometimes not. Usually heard only with intense concentration
2	Quiet, soft; heard each time the chest is auscultated
3	Audible, intermediate intensity
4	Audible, with a palpable thrill
5	Loud, audible with edge of the stethoscope lifted off the chest
6	Very loud, audible with the stethoscope placed near but not touching the chest

Adapted from Darst, J. R., Collins, K. K., & Miyamoto, S. D. (2014). Cardiovascular diseases. In W. W. Hay, M. J. Levin, & R. R. Deterding, & M. J. Abzug, (Eds.), *Current pediatric diagnosis and treatment* (22nd ed.). New York, NY: McGraw-Hill.

Innocent murmurs occur frequently in children because of the child's more dynamic circulation, thin chest wall, and angulated vessels (Darst, Collins, & Miyamoto, 2014). An innocent murmur is most often heard at the second or fourth intercostal space, and its timing is systolic. The innocent murmur is usually medium pitched and musical. Often an innocent murmur disappears when the child changes position. A venous hum that is heard in the supraclavicular area and possibly radiating down the chest is considered an innocent murmur. Refer any child with a murmur to an experienced practitioner for further evaluation.

Abdomen

The abdomen contains organs related to the genitourinary and lymphatic systems, in addition to the gastrointestinal system. These structures lie within the abdomen in approximately the same location as they do in adults. Dividing the abdomen into quadrants simplifies the description of normal organ location and the reporting of abnormalities. Draw an imaginary vertical line from the xiphoid process to the symphysis pubis. Cross this with an imaginary perpendicular line through the umbilicus. The sequence of physical examination is altered for the abdominal assessment: auscultation is done before percussion and palpation because manipulation of the lower abdomen may affect the bowel sounds (Bickley, 2013).

INSPECTION

Inspect the abdomen for size, shape, and symmetry. The abdomen in the infant and toddler is rounded and protuberant until the abdominal musculature becomes well developed. Though rounded, the abdomen should not be distended (at any age). By adolescence, the stature is more erect and the abdomen begins to appear flat when standing and concave when supine. The thin skin of a young child may allow the visualization of superficial venous circulation across the abdomen. Inspect the abdomen for movement. At eye level with the abdomen, note abdomen and thorax movement occurring simultaneously. Visible peristaltic waves are abnormal and should be reported immediately.

Inspect the newborn's umbilicus for color, bleeding, odor, and drainage. The umbilical stump should slowly dry, become black and hard, and fall away from the cutaneous navel by the end of the second week of life. Note drainage or granulation at the umbilical site indicating delayed drying of the umbilical stump. Inspect the umbilicus in older infants and young children for the presence of umbilical hernia. Because the umbilicus divides the rectus abdominis muscle, it is not uncommon to see an umbilical hernia protrude through and become larger when the infant or toddler strains or cries. This is a benign finding and will usually disappear as the abdomen becomes stronger. Adolescents may have jewelry piercing the umbilicus.

AUSCULTATION

Auscultate the abdomen using the diaphragm or the bell of the stethoscope pressed firmly against the abdomen. Count the bowel sounds in each of the four quadrants for a full minute. Bowel sounds should be present by a few hours after birth and should remain active throughout life. Note whether bowel sounds are normally active, hyperactive, hypoactive, or absent. Normal bowel sounds can be described as growls, gurgles, and clicking sounds. Hypoactive bowel sounds may occur postoperatively. Hyperactive bowels sounds are common with diarrhea. Classify bowel sounds as absent after listening for 5 full minutes in each area. Absent bowel sounds may indicate ileus or peritonitis.

PERCUSSION

Indirectly percuss all areas of the abdomen. Normal findings include dullness along the costal margins and tympany over the remainder of the abdomen. A full bladder may yield dullness to percussion.

PALPATION

Palpate the abdomen with the child in a supine position. If the child's legs are small enough, the knees may be brought up with the nondominant hand to flex the hips and relax the abdomen. Palpate all four quadrants of the abdomen in a systematic fashion, first lightly and then deeply. Apply light pressure with the fingertips to perform light palpation, assessing for tenderness and muscle tone (Fig. 32.33). Note skin turgor by gently elevating a piece of skin and allowing it to fall back into place. Perform deep palpation to assess the organs and any masses. Place one hand on top of the other and palpate from the lower quadrants to the upper (Fig. 32.33). The edge of the liver may be felt at the right costal margin, and the tip of the spleen can be felt at the left costal margin. The descending colon may be felt in the left lower quadrant as a small column and the bladder as a soft balloon below the umbilicus. The kidneys are rarely palpable. The abdomen should be soft and nontender to palpation. Report firmness, tenderness, or masses. Palpate the inguinal area for the presence of hernia or enlarged lymph nodes.

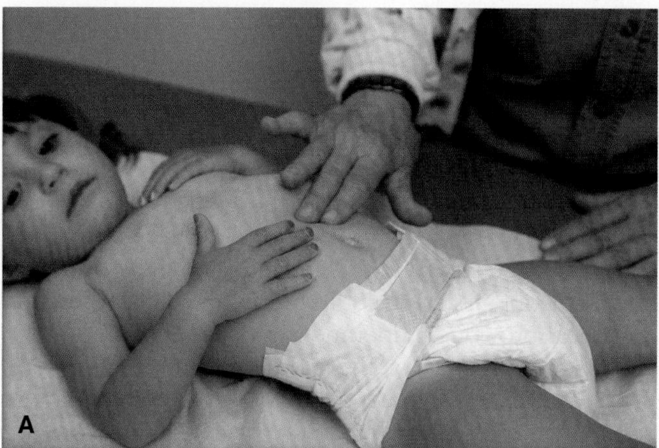

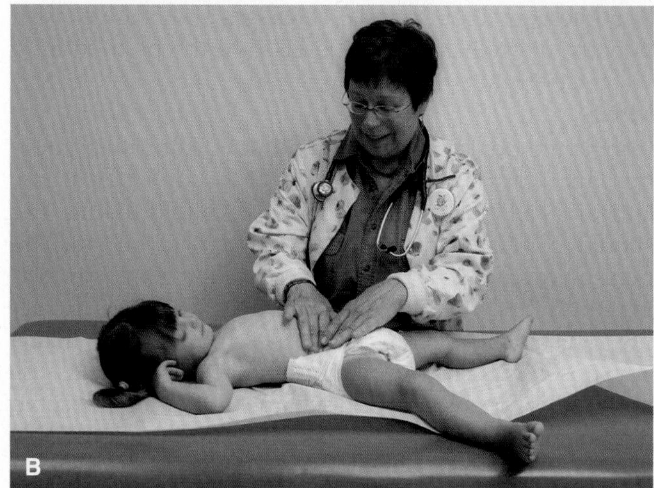

FIGURE 32.33 **(A)** Light and **(B)** deep palpation of the abdomen.

Take Note!

To decrease ticklishness with abdominal palpation, place a flat, warm, still hand on the abdomen while distracting the child before palpation begins. An alternate technique is to first palpate with the child's hand over the examiner's hand.

Genitalia and Anus

Examination of the genitals should immediately follow the abdominal assessment in the younger child and should be reserved for the end of the assessment in the adolescent. Though the anus is part of the gastrointestinal tract, it is best assessed during the genital examination. The American Academy of Pediatrics (2011) recommends that a parent chaperone the genitalia and anus examination of the infant and child. In the case of the adolescent, a medical provider chaperone is recommended.

Ensure privacy for the older child and adolescent. Keep the child covered as much as possible. Use a casual, matter-of-fact approach to place the child or teen at ease. During the genital examination, teach the child or adolescent about normal variations and changes with puberty, as well as issues related to health promotion.

MALE

Inspect the penis and scrotum for size, color, skin integrity, and obvious masses. The obese boy's penis may appear small because of additional skin folds. Penis size should correlate with pubertal stage (Fig. 32.34). The penis may have a foreskin that covers the glans, protecting and lubricating it. If present, do not forcibly retract the foreskin. In circumcised males the urinary meatus is exposed and should be at the tip of the glans. Assess the meatus for absence of discharge. If possible, observe the stream of urine for strength of flow and patency of the urethral orifice. Skin lesions may indicate sexually transmitted infection. A foreskin that cannot be retracted in a boy older than 3 years of age may indicate phimosis. Report abnormal findings.

Take Note!

When you first remove a male infant's diaper, this is the ideal time to assess the force of the urine stream and the erection reflex, as the cool air may make the infant void and briefly experience an erection.

Assess the presence and distribution of pubic hair. Inspect the scrotum for size, slight asymmetry, color, and absence of edema. The scrotum may initially be swollen from birth trauma or maternal hormones, but this swelling should decrease in the first few days of life. The scrotum is ordinarily more deeply pigmented than the rest of the boy's skin. Figure 32.34 illustrates scrotal changes that occur with puberty. Assess the testicles by placing one finger over the inguinal canal and palpating the scrotum with the other. This prevents the retractile testes in a young child from slipping back up the inguinal canal. The testicles should be smooth, of similar sizes, and freely moveable. The infant's testicles may be palpated in the scrotum or in the inguinal canal, where they can be easily moved into the scrotum with gentle pressure from the examiner's nondominant hand (Fig. 32.35). Beyond infancy, allow the boy to sit cross-legged to reduce the cremasteric reflex that retracts the testicles during palpation. An adolescent boy may need to stand for the nurse to fully palpate the scrotum. Document the presence of both testicles in the scrotal sac, if they are retractile, or if they are absent. Report undescended testicle or other abnormal findings.

From top to bottom:
1) No pubic hair and scrotum size and proportion the same as during childhood

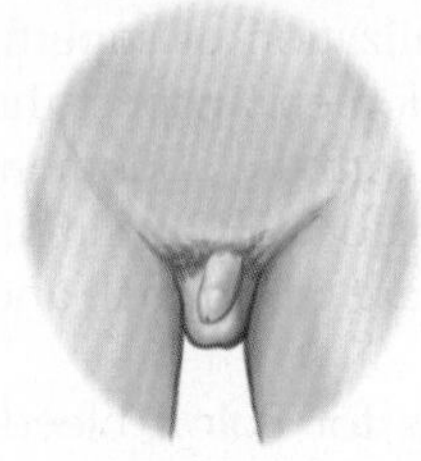
2) Few straight hairs at base of penis, little or no penis enlargement, testes/scrotum begin to enlarge

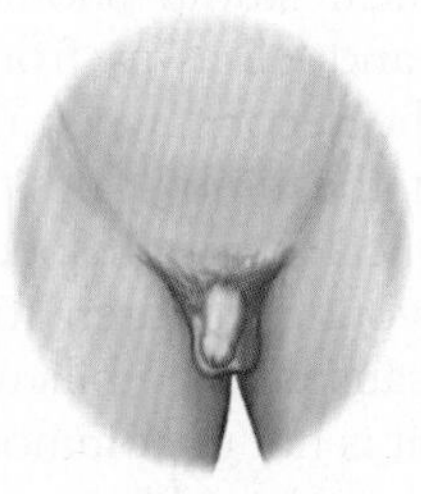
3) Sparse pubic hair growth over entire pubis, penis begins to lengthen, scrotum continues to enlarge

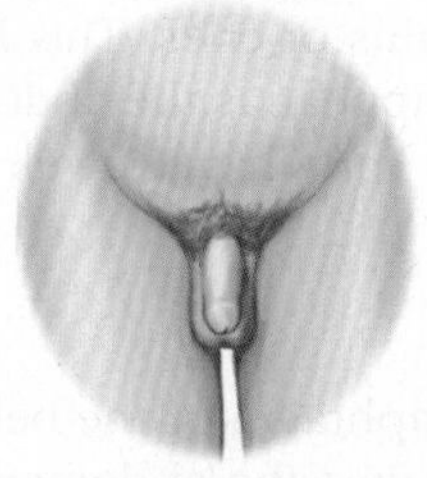
4) Thick pubic hair growth but not on thighs, penis grows in length and diameter, testes almost full grown

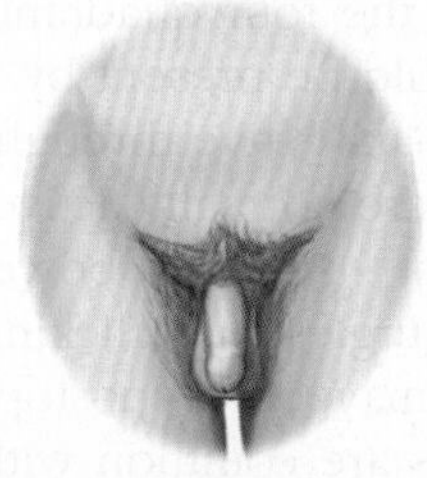
5) Pubic hair growth spread over medial thighs, penis and scrotum are adult size and shape

FIGURE 32.34 Tanner male sexual maturity rating for genitalia and pubic hair. (Adapted from Tanner, J. M. [1962]. *Growth at adolescence*. Oxford, England: Blackwell Scientific Publications.)

FEMALE

In most cases, the female genitalia examination is limited to assessment of the external genitalia. Internal examination is not routinely performed before maturity

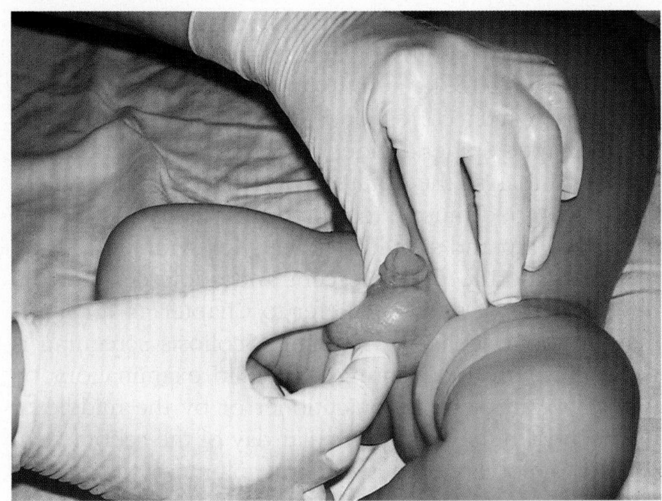

FIGURE 32.35 Placing a digit over the inguinal canal during testicular palpation prevents retraction of the testis into the canal.

unless the adolescent anticipates becoming or is sexually active or requests birth control, or if pathology is suspected. If an internal examination is needed, refer the child or adolescent to the appropriate advanced practitioner or physician.

Position the infant in the parent's lap or on the examination table or crib. The toddler or preschooler should be examined in the parent's lap, in a frog-legged position. The school-age or adolescent girl should lie on the examination table or bed. Provide for privacy by keeping the genital area covered until it is time for the examination.

Perform the assessment of the external genitalia in a systematic fashion. First, determine the presence and distribution of pubic hair. Infants and young girls (particular those of dark-skinned races) may have a small amount of downy pubic hair. Otherwise, the appearance of pubic hair indicates the onset of pubertal changes, sometimes prior to breast changes. Pubic hair generally begins to appear by age 11 years, with age 13 being the latest. Figure 32.36 illustrates the development of pubic hair through puberty in girls.

Inspect the labia majora and minora for size, color, and skin integrity. The newborn's labia minora are swollen from the effects of maternal estrogen but will decrease in size and be hidden by the labia majora within the first weeks of life. Redness or swelling of the labia may occur with infection, sexual abuse, or masturbation. Lesions on the external genitalia may indicate sexually transmitted infection. Gently spread the labia to inspect the clitoris, urethral meatus, and vaginal opening. Some girls may prefer to spread the labia themselves. The urinary meatus and vaginal orifice should be visible and not occluded by the hymen. It is not uncommon to see a hymenal tag. Note clitoral size. Inspect the urinary meatus and vaginal opening for edema or redness, which should not be present. Observe for any vaginal discharge. A small

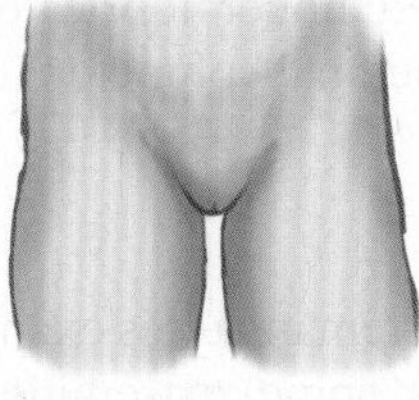

Stage 1 Preadolescents. No pubic hair. Mons and labia covered with fine vellus hair as on abdomen.

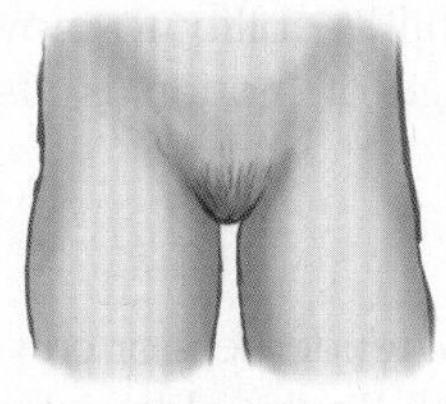

Stage 2 Growth sparse and mostly on labia. Long, downy hair, slightly pigmented, straight or only slightly curly.

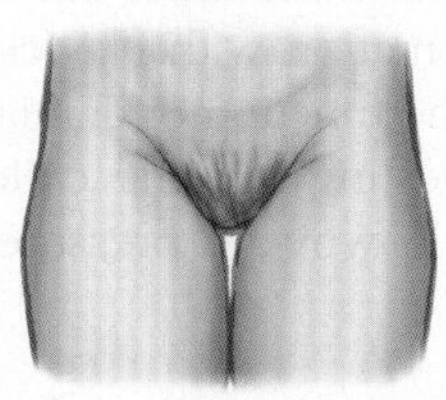

Stage 3 Growth sparse and spreading over mons pubis. Hair darker, coarser, curlier.

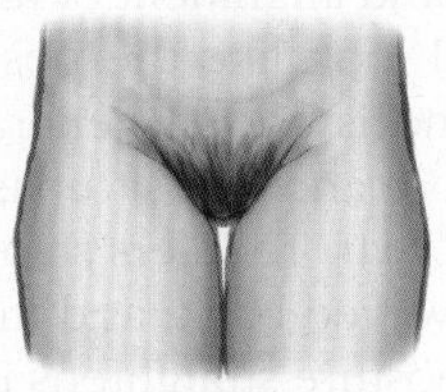

Stage 4 Hair is adult in type but over smaller area; none on medial thigh.

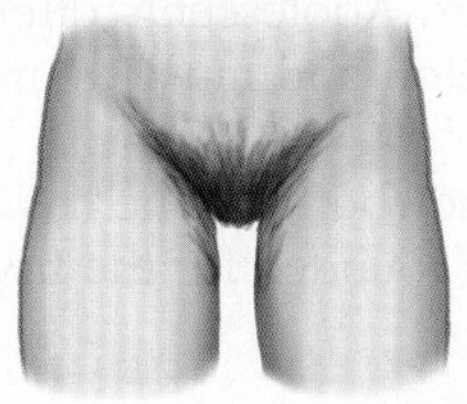

Stage 5 Adult in type and pattern; inverse triangle. Also on medial thigh surface.

FIGURE 32.36 Tanner female sexual maturity rating for pubic hair. (Adapted from Tanner, J. M. [1962]. *Growth at adolescence*. Oxford, England: Blackwell Scientific Publications.)

amount of blood-tinged or mucoid discharge may be noted in the first few weeks of life as a result of maternal hormone exposure. A small amount of clear mucous-like discharge is normal in all females. If present, document labial adhesion or other abnormal findings.

ANUS

Inspect the anal area for fissures, rash, hemorrhoids, prolapse, or skin tags. Examine the infant's anal area while examining the genitalia. The younger child may lie back in the parent's lap and flex the knees to the chest. The older child or adolescent may be prone or in a side-lying position. If the adolescent boy is already standing for the scrotal assessment, have him bend forward so that you can assess the anal area. The anus should appear moist and hairless. Gently stroke the anal area to elicit the anal reflex (quick contraction). If indicated, inspect anal sphincter tone by inserting a gloved finger lubricated with water-soluble jelly just inside the anal sphincter.

Musculoskeletal

Assessment of the musculoskeletal system includes examination of the clavicles and shoulders, spine, extremities, joints, and hips. Determining the child's ability to move all extremities through the full range of motion is also important.

CLAVICLES AND SHOULDERS

Palpate the clavicles. In the newborn, tenderness or crepitus reveals a fracture sustained at birth. In the older infant or child, a bump indicates callus formation with clavicle fracture. Test shoulder strength and the function of cranial nerve XI in the older child by requesting that the child shrug the shoulders while you apply downward pressure.

SPINE

Observe the child's resting posture and alignment of the trunk. The newborn's position will look like the position the baby preferred in utero and is one of general flexion. The older infant moves more and can sit unassisted in the second half of the first year. Toddlers stand with a wide-based gait, a slightly swayed back, and the abdomen slightly protruding. The posture straightens in the preschool and school-age years. Adolescents often demonstrate kyphosis as the skeleton and muscles are both growing rapidly (Fig. 32.37).

Inspect the child's spine. The newborn's spine has a single C-shaped curve and remains rounded for the first 3 months of life. The cervical curve begins to develop around 3 to 4 months of age as the baby gains head control. By 12 to 18 months of age, the lumbar curve develops, which corresponds to the onset of walking. The S-shaped spine in older children and adolescents is similar to that of the adult's. The spine should be flexible, with good muscle tone and no rigidity. Assess the back, and hip and shoulder heights for symmetry.

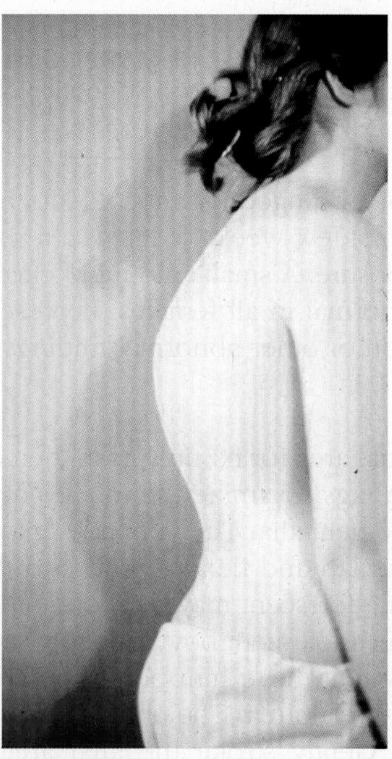

FIGURE 32.37 The teen's posture often demonstrates kyphosis.

Examine the preadolescent and adolescent for the development of scoliosis. Refer to Chapter 44 for information about scoliosis screening. Scoliosis screening is generally performed during well-child examinations by the physician or nurse practitioner or by the middle or high school nurse on a particular day of the school year.

Note mobility of the vertebral column by having the child bend forward and side to side. Flex the neck and move it from side to side. No resistance or pain should occur. Inspect the back for discoloration, tufts of hair, or dimples. A normal pilonidal dimple is sometimes seen at the base of the spine, but there should be no tuft of hair or nevi along the spine. Document and report abnormal findings.

EXTREMITIES

All children, even newborns, should be able to move all extremities spontaneously. Screen the infant younger than 6 months of age for developmental dysplasia of the hip by performing the Ortolani and Barlow maneuvers (refer to Chapter 44 for additional information). These maneuvers are usually best performed by a proficient examiner. Inspect and palpate the child's upper and lower extremities. Assess for symmetry in size, contour, movement, warmth, and color of the extremities. The infant's feet and legs appear bowed secondary to in utero positioning but can be straightened through passive range of motion. Observe the child in a standing position. Bowing of the lower legs (internal tibial torsion) lessens as the toddler begins to bear weight and usually resolves in the second or third year of life as the strength of the muscles and bones increases. When it persists past that time, it is termed genu varum (bow legs). Genu valgum (knock knee) is usually present until the child is 7 years old. Observe the child walking, noting any difficulty with leg position or balance. If the child is reluctant to walk, use play as a way to elicit the behavior. The school-age child should have gait and leg appearance similar to that of the adult.

Note the normal flat foot in the toddler and young child. The arch develops as the child grows and the muscles become less lax, though some children may continue with flexible flat feet; this is considered a normal variation.

Perform passive range of motion of the young infant's extremities. Inability to straighten the foot to midline may indicate clubfoot. Count the fingers and toes, noting abnormalities such as polydactyly (increased number of digits) or syndactyly (webbing of the digits).

Palpate the joints for warmth or tenderness. Check the mobility of the joints of the upper and lower extremities by performing range of motion. Determine lower extremity muscle strength by having the child push against the examiner's hands with the soles of the forefoot. Assess upper extremity strength by having the child squeeze the examiner's crossed fingers and/or push up or down against the examiner's outstretched hands.

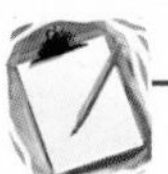

Take Note!

Slight tremors may be noticed in the infant's extremities in the first month of life.

Neurologic

The neurologic examination should include level of consciousness, balance and coordination, sensory function, reflexes, and a developmental screening. Motor function is assessed within the musculoskeletal section. Cranial nerve function is generally tested within other portions of the physical assessment as it applies to that section.

LEVEL OF CONSCIOUSNESS

Note the state of alertness and attentiveness to parents and the environment in the newborn and infant. Older infants become interactive with other people, as do toddlers and preschoolers. Younger children demonstrate orientation by positive interaction with family members and by crying or fussing when they feel threatened. By school age, the child should be oriented to name and place and a few years later should be able to state the date as well (even if only the day of the week).

BALANCE AND COORDINATION

The cerebellum controls balance and coordination. Observe the child's gait to assess balance and coordination. Observe toddlers and older children rising and walking from a seated and supine position. They should be able to stand and balance without straining or holding on to objects. Continue to test cerebellar function by having the younger child skip or hop and requesting that the older child or adolescent walk heel to toe. Further tests of cerebellar function responsible for balance and coordination are discussed in Box 32.3. Demonstrate each test and make sure the child understands your instructions.

BOX 32.3

CEREBELLAR FUNCTION TESTING

- **Romberg:** Ask the school-age or older child to stand still with eyes closed and arms down by the sides. Observe the child for leaning (stand close in case this does occur). This is considered a positive Romberg test, indicating cerebellar dysfunction.
- For the following tests, the child should demonstrate accuracy and smoothness:
- **Heel-to-shin:** Have the child lie in a supine position, place one heel on the opposite knee, and run it down the shin.
- **Rapid alternating movements:** The child pats the thighs with the hands, lifts them, turns them over, pats the thighs with the back of the hands, and repeats the process multiple times. An alternate test is for the child to touch the thumb to each finger of the same hand starting at the index finger, then reverse the direction and repeat.
- **Finger-to-finger:** The child's eyes are open. The child touches the examiner's outstretched finger with the index finger, then touches his or her own nose. The examiner moves the finger to a different spot and the child repeats this process several times.
- **Finger-to-nose:** The child's eyes are closed. The child stretches the arm with the index finger extended, then touches his or her nose with that finger, keeping the eyes closed.

Adapted from Bickley, L. (2013). *Bates' guide to physical examination and history taking* (11th ed.). Philadelphia, PA: Lippincott Williams & Wilkins; and Jarvis, C. (2012). *Physical examination and health assessment* (6th ed.). St. Louis, MO: Saunders.

SENSORY TESTING

Portions of sensory testing related to most of the cranial nerves, vision, hearing, taste, and smell have already been incorporated into other sections as appropriate within the physical assessment. Test cranial nerve V (trigeminal) by lightly touching the child's cheek with a cotton ball. The young infant will root toward the side that is touched. With the child's eyes closed, ask the child to identify other locations where he or she is lightly touched (several different ones) to assess sensation. Ask the child to tell you when he or she is touched. Make a game of this activity to encourage cooperation in younger children. In the older child who knows the definition of sharp and dull, test for these sensations with the child's eyes closed. Use the rounded end of a tongue blade for dull and the broken edge of a tongue blade for the sharp sensation. The child should be able to discriminate the sensations of sharp and dull.

REFLEXES

Assess the infant's primitive and protective reflexes. The primitive reflexes involve a whole-body response and are subcortical in nature. Selected primitive reflexes present at birth include Moro, root, suck, asymmetric tonic neck, plantar and palmar grasp, step, and Babinski. Most of the primitive reflexes diminish over the first few months of life, giving way to protective or postural reflexes. Protective reflexes are motor responses related to maintenance of equilibrium. They are necessary for appropriate motor development and remain throughout life once they are established. The protective reflexes include the righting and parachute reactions.

Place one finger in each of the infant's hands to elicit the palmar grasp reflex (usually disappears by the age of 3 to 4 months). Touch the thumb to the ball of the infant's foot to elicit the plantar grasp reflex. The infant's toes will curl down (this reflex disappears by the age of 8 to 10 months). Refer to Table 25.1 for illustrations and additional explanation of the other reflexes. Appropriate presence and disappearance of primitive reflexes, as well as development of protective reflexes, is indicative of a healthy neurologic system. Primitive reflexes that persist beyond the usual age of disappearance may indicate an abnormality of the neurologic system and should be further investigated (Bickley, 2013).

Assess deep tendon reflexes in all infants and children. Appropriate responses indicate that the reflex arc is intact. Use the reflex hammer in all ages or the curved tips of the two first fingers to elicit the responses in infants. The limb must be relaxed and the muscle partly stretched. Use a snapping motion of the wrist to tap with the fingertips or the reflex hammer. Test the biceps, triceps, patellar, and Achilles reflexes as you would in the adult. It may help to place a finger under the infant's knee to encourage relaxation. Young children who tense up when their reflexes are being tested may relax the area if you have them focus on another area, so have the child clasp the hands while testing the Achilles and patellar reflexes. As the child focuses on the hands, the lower extremities relax (Jarvis, 2012). Distraction may also be helpful.

Grade the strength of the response using the standard scale from 0 to 4+:

- 0: no response
- 1+: diminished or sluggish
- 2+: average
- 3+: brisker than average
- 4+: very brisk, may involve clonus

The newborn's deep tendon reflexes are normally brisk (3+). They decrease to average (2+) usually by 4 months of age. Healthy children should have reflexes of 2+ if the reflex has been elicited properly. Absent, sluggish, or hyperreactive responses usually indicate disease (Bickley, 2013).

DEVELOPMENTAL SCREENING

An important component of the neurologic assessment and a comprehensive child health assessment is developmental screening. Developmental screening may be used to identify children whose developmental status may warrant additional evaluation. Become comfortable with the developmental screening tools used and what the results of the screening mean. Upon completion of the screening, discuss the child's abilities with the parent or caregiver. Developmental screening is often performed separately from the physical examination and is discussed in further detail in Chapter 31.

Refer back to Elliot, the 3-year-old from the beginning of the chapter. What are some important considerations when performing his physical examination?

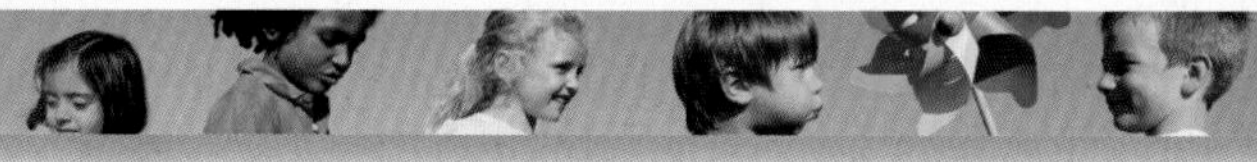

KEY CONCEPTS

- The health history in children includes more than just the chief complaint, history of present illness, and past medical history; it is important to include the perinatal history and developmental milestones.
- Allow the chief complaint to determine which parts of the history require more in-depth investigation.
- The developmental history will warrant more attention in the younger child, while school performance and adjustment will be more important in the school-age child and adolescent.
- Though the parent will provide most of the health history for the infant and young child, allow the young verbal child to answer questions during the health history as appropriate.
- Direct health history questions to the school-age child and adolescent, seeking clarification from the parents as needed.
- Provide confidentiality and privacy for the adolescent during the health history.
- Weight and length or height should be assessed at each well-child visit to determine adequacy of growth.
- Measure head circumference until age 3 years to monitor brain growth.
- Perform hearing and vision screenings for children of all ages.
- BMI can be used to identify children who are overweight or at risk for being overweight.
- The normal range of vital signs varies based on the child's age.

- The sequence of the physical examination in children should be based on the child's developmental age, his or her level of cooperation, and the severity of the illness.
- Obtain heart rate and respiratory rate and auscultate the heart and lungs while the infant or young child is quiet.
- Perform intrusive procedures such as examination of the ears, mouth, and throat last in the infant or young child.
- Perform the health assessment in a head-to-toe fashion in the school-age child or adolescent, reserving the genitalia and anus examination for last.
- Plan the health assessment in such a way as to minimize trauma to the child or adolescent.
- Use age-appropriate measurement tools to assess pain in children.
- Allow the infant or young child to remain in the parent's lap for as much of the assessment as possible so that the child feels secure.
- Use age-appropriate games during the health assessment to gain cooperation in the younger child.
- Having the young boy sit cross-legged for a testicular examination may reduce the cremasteric reflex.
- The newborn may exhibit a wide variety of normal skin variations.
- The infant's fontanels should be soft and flat; report a bulging fontanel immediately.
- Jaundice (outside of the newborn period), pallor, cyanosis, and poor skin turgor indicate illness and may need immediate intervention.
- Heart murmurs should be assessed for intensity, location, and duration. They may be innocent or may indicate a congenital heart defect.
- The infant's chest wall is relatively thin, allowing upper airway sounds to be transmitted throughout the lung fields.
- Substernal or xiphoid retractions indicate that the child is laboring to breathe, whereas a fixed, depressed sternum (pectus excavatum) is a structural abnormality.
- The Tanner stages of sexual maturity provide a basis for assessing pubertal development in boys and girls. Use the breast and pubic hair charts for girls and the pubic hair and penis and scrotum size chart for boys.

REFERENCES AND RECOMMENDED READINGS

Albert, N. M., Burke, J., Bena, J. F., Morrison, S. M., Forney, J., & Krajewski, S. (2013). Nurses' uniform color and feelings/emotions in school-aged children receiving health care. *Journal of Pediatric Nursing, 28*(2), 141–149.

American Academy of Pediatrics. (2011). Use of chaperones during the physical examination of the pediatric patient. *Pediatrics, 127*(5), 991–993.

Asher, C., & Northington, L. K. (2008). Position statement for measurement of temperature/fever in children. *Journal of Pediatric Nursing, 23*(3), 234–236.

Bickley, L. (2013). *Bates' guide to physical examination and history taking* (11th ed.). Philadelphia, PA: Lippincott Williams & Wilkins.

Bowden, V. R., & Greenberg, C. S. (2012). *Pediatric nursing procedures* (3rd ed.). Philadelphia, PA: Lippincott Williams & Wilkins.

Burns, C. E., Dunn, A. M., Brady, M. A., Starr, N. B., & Blosser, C. G. (2013). *Pediatric primary care* (5th ed.). Philadelphia, PA: Saunders.

Centers for Disease Control and Prevention. (2010). *CDC growth charts.* Retrieved from http://www.cdc.gov/growthcharts/cdc_charts.htm

Centers for Disease Control and Prevention. (2015a). *Body mass index (BMI).* Retrieved from http://www.cdc.gov/healthyweight/assessing/bmi/index.html

Centers for Disease Control and Prevention. (2015b). *WHO growth chart training: Using the WHO growth charts to assess growth in the United States among children ages birth to 2 years.* Retrieved from http://www.cdc.gov/nccdphp/dnpao/growthcharts/who/index.htm

Centers for Disease Control and Prevention. (2016). *Lead.* Retrieved from http://www.cdc.gov/nceh/lead/

Columbia University, College of Physicians and Surgeons. (n.d). *Points on the pediatric physical exam.* Retrieved from http://www.columbia.edu/itc/hs/medical/clerkships/peds/Student_Information/Reference_Materials/Pediatric_PE.html

Covidien. (2012). *Covidien operator's manual: Nellcor™ bedside spO2 patient monitoring system.* Mansfield, MA: Author.

Darst, J. R., Collins, K. K., & Miyamoto, S. D. (2014). Cardiovascular diseases. In W. W. Hay, M. J. Levin, R. R. Deterding, & M. J. Abzug, (Eds.), *Current pediatric diagnosis and treatment* (22nd ed.). New York, NY: McGraw-Hill.

El Radhi, A. S. (2014). Determining fever in children: The search for an ideal thermometer. *British Journal of Nursing, 23*(2), 91–94.

Exergen Corporation. (2014). *Exergen temporal artery thermometer instructions for use.* Retrieved from http://www.exergen.com//medical/PDFs/tat2000c%20manual%20818621r5%20artwork.pdf

Gillespie, G. L., Gates, D. M., & Berry, P. (2013). Stressful incidents of physical violence against emergency nurses. *The Online Journal of Issues in Nursing, 18*(1), 2. doi: 10.3912/OJIN.Vol18No01Man02

Graversen, L., Sørensen, T., Petersen, L., Sovio, U., Kaakinen, M., Sandbaek, A., et al. (2014). Preschool weight and body mass index in relation to central obesity and metabolic syndrome in adulthood. *PLoS ONE, 9*(3), 1–9.

International Cupping Therapy Association. (2010). *A word on cupping marks.* Retrieved from http://www.cuppingtherapy.org/pages/discolorations.htm

Jarvis, C. (2012). *Physical examination and health assessment* (6th ed.). St. Louis, MO: Saunders.

Kliegman, R. M., Stanton, B. F, St. Geme III, J. W., Schor N. F., Behrman R. E. (Eds.). (2011). *Nelson textbook of pediatrics* (19th ed.). Philadelphia, PA: Saunders.

Manworren, R., & Hynan, L. (2003). Clinical validation of FLACC: Preverbal patient pain scale. *Pediatric Nursing, 29*(2), 140–146.

Marx, J., Hockberger, R., & Walls, R. (2014). *Rosen's emergency medicine – concepts and clinical practice* (8th ed.). Philadelphia, PA: Saunders.

Miller, S. (n.d.). *Pediatric physical exam video.* Retrieved from http://www.columbia.edu/itc/hs/medical/clerkships/peds/Student_Information/Reference_Materials/PE_Video.html

Nettina, M. S. (Ed.). (2014). *Lippincott manual of nursing practice* (10th ed.). Philadelphia, PA: Lippincott Williams & Wilkins.

Reiter, E. O. (2011). Growth & growth impairment. In C. D. Rudolph, A. M. Rudolph, G. Lister, et al. (Eds.), *Rudolph's pediatrics* (22nd ed.). New York, NY: McGraw-Hill.

Rosenberg, A. A., & Grover, T. (2014). The newborn infant. In W. W. Hay, Jr., M. J. Levin, R. R. Deterding, M. J. Abzug, & J. M. Sondheimer (Eds.), *Current diagnosis and treatment: Pediatrics* (22nd ed.). New York, NY: McGraw-Hill.

Sass, A. E., & Kaplan, D. W. (2014). Adolescence. In W. W. Hay, Jr., M. J. Levin, R. R. Deterding, M. J. Abzug, & J. M. Sondheimer (Eds.), *Current diagnosis and treatment: Pediatrics* (22nd ed.). New York, NY: McGraw-Hill.

Shah, M. N., & Gupta, R. C. (2014). Flat head syndrome (positional plagiocephaly). Retreived from http://kidshealth.org/parent/growth/sleep/positional_plagiocephaly.html#

Tanner, J. M. (1962). *Growth at adolescence.* Oxford, England: Blackwell Scientific Publications.

The Joint Commission. (2014). *Advancing effective communication, cultural competence, and patient- and family-centered care.* Retrieved from http://www.jointcommission.org/Advancing_Effective_Communication/

Treitz, M., Bunik, M., & Fox, D. (2014). Ambulatory & office pediatrics. In W. W. Hay, M. J. Levin, & R. R. Deterding, & M. J. Abzug, (Eds.), *Current pediatric diagnosis and treatment* (22nd ed.). New York, NY: McGraw-Hill.

U.S. Department of Health and Human Services. (2016). *Healthy People 2020.* Retrieved from http://www.healthypeople.gov/2020/default.aspx

U.S. Department of Health and Human Services, National Institutes of Health, National Heart, Lung, and Blood Institute. (2005). *The fourth report on the diagnosis, evaluation, and treatment of high blood pressure in children and adolescents.* (NIH Publication No. 05–5267). Washington, DC: U.S. Department of Health and Human Services.

Willis, M., Merkel, S., Voepel-Lewis, T., & Malviya, S. (2003). FLACC behavioral pain assessment scale: A comparison with the child's self-report. *Pediatric Nursing, 29*(3), 95–198.

Wong, D., & Baker, C. (1988). Pain in children: Comparison of assessment scales. *Pediatric Nursing, 14*, 9–17.

CHAPTER WORKSHEET

MULTIPLE CHOICE QUESTIONS

1. A 5-year-old boy visits the pediatric office with an upper respiratory infection. Which approach would give the nurse the most information about the child's developmental level?
   a. Playing a game with the child.
   b. Talking with the child about the teddy bear next to him.
   c. Using a screening tool during a follow-up office visit.
   d. Asking the 10-year-old sibling about the child.
2. Which statement indicates the best sequence for the nurse to conduct an assessment in a nonemergency situation?
   a. Introduce yourself, ask about any problems, take a history, and do the physical examination.
   b. Perform the physical examination and then ask the family if there are any problems in the child's life.
   c. Do the physical examination while at the same time asking about the child's previous illnesses; then talk about the family's concerns.
   d. Get a complete history of the family's health beliefs and practices, and then assess the child.
3. What approach by the nurse would most likely encourage a child to cooperate with an assessment of physical and developmental health?
   a. Explain to the child what's going to happen when the child asks questions.
   b. Explain what is going to happen in words the child can understand.
   c. Force the child to cooperate by having a parent hold him or her down.
   d. Give the child a sticker before beginning the examination.
4. A sleeping 5-month-old girl is being held by the mother when the nurse comes in to do a physical examination. What assessment should be done initially?
   a. Listening to the bowel sounds
   b. Counting the heart rate
   c. Checking the temperature
   d. Looking in the ears
5. Which assessment finding is considered normal in children?
   a. Irregular respiratory rate and rhythm
   b. Split S_2 and sinus arrhythmia
   c. Decreased heart rate with crying
   d. Genu varum past the age of 5 years
6. A child's weight is 35 pounds, 7 ounces. Convert the weight to kilograms.
7. A child's height is 41 inches. Convert the height to centimeters.

CRITICAL THINKING EXERCISES

1. A soft and muffled heart murmur is heard in a 4-year-old patient. The mother states that she has never heard that the child has a murmur. What should the nurse do?
2. A nurse is helping a new mother breastfeed her 4-day-old baby. The mother notices that the baby has a bluish cast to the skin on his hands and that sometimes the infant has a tremor. She asks the nurse if the baby is cold, though the baby is swaddled and comfortably resting against the mother's skin. How might the nurse help teach this mother?
3. Devise a plan for encouraging cooperation of the toddler or preschooler during various parts of the physical examination.

STUDY ACTIVITIES

1. In the clinical setting, obtain a health history on an infant, child, or adolescent.
2. In the clinical setting, compare the approach you use for the physical examination of a toddler versus a school-aged child or adolescent.
3. No matter how thoughtfully and appropriately you plan your assessment, odds are good that you will have difficulty assessing a 2-year-old. Discuss with your classmates the strategies that you have used for success and brainstorm with them about their ideas for assessing a crying or resistant young child.

BRINGING IT ALL TOGETHER: A CASE STUDY

Isabella is a 6-year-old, typically developing child. She has presented with her mother for an annual well-child check. Though appearing well developed, well nourished, and generally healthy, Isabella has been resistant to the examination. She refuses to hold the thermometer under her tongue appropriately for accurate temperature measurement. In fact, her distress with the thermometer seems to have set the tone for the entire visit.

Go to thePoint to find questions to consider about this case.

33

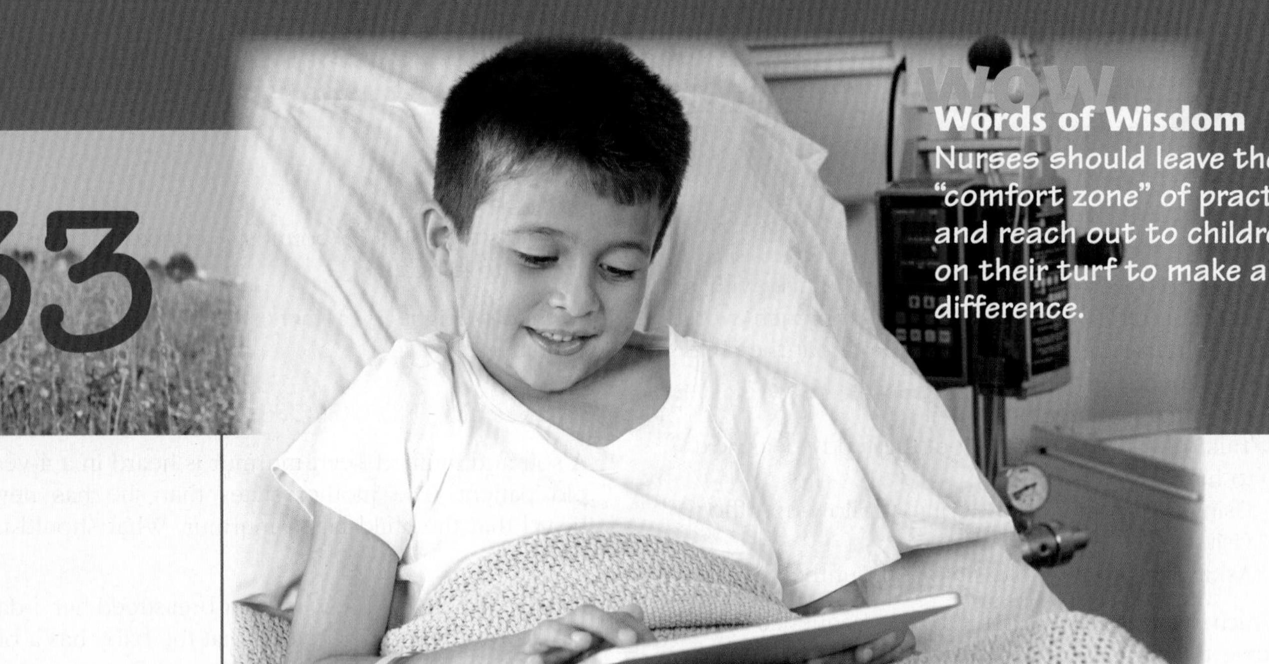
WOW
Words of Wisdom
Nurses should leave their "comfort zone" of practice and reach out to children on their turf to make a difference.

Caring for Children in Diverse Settings

KEY TERMS

Individualized Health Plan
magical thinking
medically fragile child
regression
separation anxiety
therapeutic play

Learning Objectives

Upon completion of the chapter, you will be able to:

1. Identify the major stressors of illness and hospitalization for children.
2. Identify the reactions and responses of children and their families during illness and hospitalization.
3. Explain the factors that influence the reactions and responses of children and their families during illness and hospitalization.
4. Describe the nursing care that minimizes stressors for children who are ill or hospitalized.
5. Discuss the major components of admission for children to the hospital.
6. Discuss appropriate safety measures to use when caring for children of all ages.
7. Review nursing responsibilities related to client discharge from the hospital.
8. Describe the various roles of community and home care nurses.
9. Discuss the variety of settings in which community-based care occurs.
10. Discuss the advantages and disadvantages of home health care.

***Jake Jorgenson*, 8 years old, was brought to the clinic with a history of headaches, vomiting not related to feeding, and changes in his gait. Initial testing leads to a suspected brain tumor. Jake is to be admitted to the neurologic service at a pediatric hospital for further testing and treatment. Up until this point he has been a healthy child with no previous hospitalizations. He lives at home with his parents and two siblings, Jenny, age 11, and Joshua, age 5. As a nurse on this unit, how can you help prepare Jake and his family for this hospitalization?**

Nursing care of the child occurs in a variety of settings, from acute care in a hospital to well and ill care in community settings, such as physicians' offices, schools, churches, health departments, community centers, and even within the child's own home. Within each setting, the nurse incorporates basic nursing care with specific strategies to help promote positive outcomes for the child, family, and community as a whole.

Hospitalization in Childhood

In today's health care environment, children receive much of their care for illnesses in community health settings such as physicians' offices, urgent care settings, or day surgery centers. As a result of this trend, fewer children may actually be admitted to a hospital unit, and those who are hospitalized are generally acutely ill. In addition, hospital stays are often shorter due to economic trends in the health care environment, such as the delivery system of managed care and other factors that attempt to control costs. Acute conditions, trauma, or chronic diseases or illnesses requiring surgical intervention lead to hospitalization for children.

According to *Child Health USA 2012,* diseases of the respiratory system, such as asthma and pneumonia, account for the majority of hospitalizations in children younger than 5 years of age, while diseases of the respiratory system, mental health problems, injuries, and gastrointestinal disorders lead to more hospitalizations in older children (U.S. Department of Health and Human Services, Health Resources and Services Administration, Maternal and Child Health Bureau, 2013). Adolescents between 15 and 19 years of age are often hospitalized because of problems related to pregnancy, childbearing, mental health, and injury (U.S. Department of Health and Human Services, Health Resources and Services Administration, Maternal and Child Health Bureau, 2013).

Other health problems begin before birth or immediately following birth, such as congenital heart disease or gastrointestinal atresia. Just when they are getting used to the idea of having a new child, the family must also deal with illness and possibly extended hospitalizations. Specific genetic or environmental factors also predispose the child to disease and injury, such as the genetic disorder of hemophilia or the environmental situation of homelessness. Many of these factors or situations put the child and family at greater risk for chronic health conditions and long periods of illness, hospitalization, and even death.

Hospitalization is often confusing, complex, and overwhelming for children and their families. Reactions and responses to illness and hospitalization depend on a number of factors, including the child's developmental stage. Nursing strategies are needed to prepare children and their families for this experience while minimizing negative effects. These strategies include identifying the needs of children and families through astute assessment of nonverbal and verbal behaviors, then validating the information with accurate interpretation and providing appropriate responses and interventions.

Although the nurse implements these strategies throughout the interaction with the child and family, a critical time to ensure the best outcome for the child and family is during the admission process. The nurse assesses the learning needs and abilities of the child and family. For the interventions to be successful, the nurse must communicate and teach in the most effective method for the individual child and family. The nurse also evaluates the child's and family's competence in performing specific activities prior to discharge.

Children's Reactions to Hospitalization

In general, children are more vulnerable to the effects of illness and hospitalization because this is a change from their usual state of health and routine. They also have limited understanding and coping mechanisms to assist them in resolving the stressors that might occur during this time. Hospitalization creates a series of traumatic and stressful events in a climate of uncertainty for children and their families, whether it is an elective procedure that is planned in advance or an emergency situation resulting from trauma. The stressors that children experience in relation to hospitalization may result in various reactions. Children react to the stresses of hospitalization before admission, during hospitalization, and after discharge.

Besides the physiologic effects of the health problem, the psychological effects of illness and hospitalization on a child include anxiety and fear related to the overall process and the potential for bodily injury, physical harm, and pain. In addition, children are separated from their homes, families, and friends and what is familiar to them, which may result in **separation anxiety** (distress related to removal from family and familiar surroundings). There is a general loss of control over their lives and sometimes their emotions and behaviors. The result may be feelings of anger and guilt, **regression** (return to a previous stage of development), acting out, and other types of defense mechanisms to cope with these effects. Children's typical coping strategies are tested during this experience.

Anxiety and Fear

For many children, entering the hospital is like entering a foreign world. The result is anxiety and fear. Anxiety often stems from the rapid onset of the illness or injury, particularly when the child has limited experiences with disease or injury. Normal fears of childhood include the fear of separation from their parents and family or guardians, loss of control, and bodily injury, mutilation, or harm. Children's fears are similar to adult fears of the unknown, including fear of unfamiliar environments and losing control.

Therefore, when the child is in the hospital, he or she becomes distressed about the unfamiliar environment; health care procedures, especially the use of needles or associated pain that may occur; and situations such as the strange words being used, ominous-looking equipment, strangers in unusual attire (e.g., surgical caps, masks, gowns), unfamiliar and frightening noises and smells, or the sounds of other children crying. This exposure to people, situations, and procedures that may be new to them and cause them pain leads to increased anxiety and fear (Fig. 33.1). Overall, hospitalization is a difficult experience for children.

Separation Anxiety

Separation anxiety is a major stressor for children of certain ages. Timing of separation anxiety varies among children. It typically begins once a child has developed object permanence (an understanding that things exist even when they are out of sight) which is usually around 4 to 9 months (Swanson, 2014).

James Robertson and John Bowlby described three stages that the infant and child goes through during separation anxiety—protest, despair, and detachment (Robertson & Bowlby, 1952; Hart & Rollins, 2011). The first phase, protest, occurs when the child is separated from the parents or primary caretaker. This phase may last from a few hours to several days. The child reacts aggressively to this separation and exhibits great distress by crying, expressing agitation, and rejecting others who attempt to offer comfort. The child may also display anger and inconsolable grief.

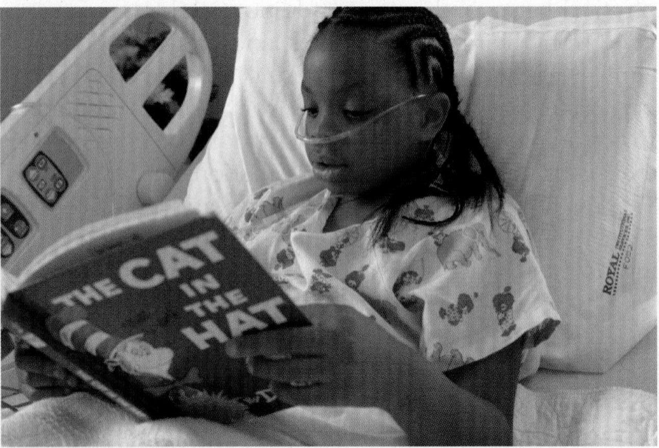

FIGURE 33.1 The presence of familiar objects and home routines normalizes the environment and helps the child cope with hospitalization. Reading a favorite bedtime story can be comforting.

If the parents do not return within a short time, the child exhibits the second phase, despair. The child displays hopelessness by withdrawing from others, becoming quiet without crying, and exhibiting apathy, depression, lack of interest in play and food, and overall feelings of sadness.

Detachment (also known as denial) is the third and final phase of separation anxiety. During this phase the child forms coping mechanisms to protect against further emotional pain. This occurs more often in long-term separations. During this stage, the child shows interest in the environment, starts to play again, and forms superficial relationships with the nurses and other children. If the parents return, the child ignores them. A child in this phase of separation anxiety exhibits resignation, not contentment. It is more difficult to reverse this stage, and developmental delays may occur.

Today, health care providers primarily observe the first and second stages because of the shorter hospital stays and the more common use of a family-centered approach to care.

Loss of Control

When hospitalized, children experience a significant loss of control. This loss of control increases the perception of threat and affects their coping skills. They lose control over routine self-care and their usual tasks and play as well as decisions related to the care of their own bodies. In the hospital, the child's usual routine is disrupted. He or she cannot choose what to do and at what time. The child can no longer accomplish simple tasks independently as he or she does at home or school. Confinement to the bed or crib worsens this loss of control. For example, if connected to tubes or intravenous lines, the child may not even be able to visit the bathroom alone.

Hospitalization also affects the child's control over decisions related to his or her own body. Many of the procedures and treatments that occur in the hospital are invasive or are at least disturbing to children, and much of the time they do not have the option to refuse to undergo them. Adults are presumed to be competent to make health care decisions, but generally, children are not. Though the parents and nurses of hospitalized children have the children's best interest in mind, children often feel powerless when in the hospital, not having their feelings and wishes respected and having minimal control over events.

Take Note!

When advocating for a child, make sure to include the child's voice. Do not assume what his or her wishes may be; ask about them directly.

Factors Affecting Children's Reaction to Hospitalization

Various factors have a great impact on the ability of children to handle illness and hospitalization. These factors may increase or diminish the fears of the child who is ill and hospitalized. Each child responds differently and will perceive the hospital experience differently. Box 33.1 lists the various factors affecting a child's response to illness and hospitalization.

Developmental Level

The child's age, cognitive level, and developmental level will affect his or her perceptions of actual events, and this in turn will affect his or her reaction to illness and hospitalization. Children's responses to the stressors of fear, separation anxiety, and loss of control vary depending on their age and developmental level. Younger children, with their limited life experience and immature intellectual capacities, have a more difficult time comprehending what is happening to them. This can be particularly true for toddlers and preschoolers, who perceive the intactness of their bodies to be exposed during physical intrusions. In addition, they frequently interpret illness as punishment for wrongdoing or hospital procedures as hostile, mutilating acts. Although children are increasingly able to adapt as they grow older, lack of understanding about the need for hospitalization and threatened sense of control can make adaptation difficult.

INFANTS

Newborns and infants are adapting to life outside the womb with rapid growth and development and establishment of a healthy attachment to parents or primary caregivers. They are dependent on others for nurturance and protection. They gain a sense of trust in the world through rhythmic and reciprocal patterns of contact and feeding, resulting in bonding to the primary caregiver. They need a secure pattern of restful sleep, satisfaction of oral and nutritional needs, relaxation of body systems, and spontaneous response to communication and gentle stimuli. The caregiver–infant attachment is critical for psychological health, especially during periods of illness and hospitalization.

Unfortunately, during illness and hospitalization, these critical patterns of feeding, contact, comfort, sleeping, elimination, and stimulation are disrupted, resulting in fear, separation anxiety, and loss of control. By 5 to 6 months of age, infants have developed an awareness of self as separate from mother. As a result, infants of this age are acutely aware of the absence of their primary caregiver and become fearful of unfamiliar persons. Infants may be separated from their parents when hospitalized if the parents cannot room-in because of hospital policy or if they must work or care for other children. This results in separation anxiety.

The infant's oral needs, the basic source of infant satisfaction, are often not met in the hospital due to the condition of the child or the procedures that must be performed. The infant is accustomed to having his or her basic needs met by the parent when he or she cries or gestures. The constraints of hospitalization result in loss of control over the environment, leading to additional anxiety in the infant.

TODDLERS

Toddlers are more aware of self and can communicate their desires. Because their autonomy is developing, toddlers need to master accomplishments to minimize the development of shame and doubt. Control becomes an issue for toddlers. Toddlers also need opportunities to explore, and they need consistent routines. In addition, toddlers are aware of the need for care and protection from others, so they need familiarity and closeness to the primary caregiver. When the toddler is hospitalized, disruption occurs in this development of autonomy.

Toddlers are often fearful of strangers and can recall traumatic events. Simply walking toward the treatment room where a traumatic procedure previously occurred may upset the toddler. Ordinarily, a resurgence in separation anxiety occurs during the toddler years. When the toddler is separated from his or her parents or caregivers in an unfamiliar environment, separation anxiety is compounded. In response to this anxiety, toddlers may demonstrate behaviors such as pleading for the parents to stay, physically trying to go after the parents, throwing temper tantrums, and refusing to comply with usual routines. Restrictions related to mobility and new skill acquisition result in loss of control. Disruption in usual routines also contributes to loss of control, and the toddler feels insecure. As a result, regression in toilet training and refusal to eat are common reactions in toddlers.

BOX 33.1

FACTORS AFFECTING A CHILD'S RESPONSE TO ILLNESS AND HOSPITALIZATION

- Amount of separation from parent/caregiver
- Age
- Developmental level
- Cognitive level
- Previous experience with illness and hospitalization
- Recent life stresses and changes
- Type and amount of preparation
- Temperament
- Innate and acquired coping skills
- Seriousness of the diagnosis/onset of illness or injury (e.g., acute or chronic)
- Support systems available, including the family and health care professionals
- Cultural background
- Parents' reaction to illness and hospitalization

PRESCHOOLERS

The preschooler has better verbal and developmental skills to adapt to various situations, but illness and hospitalization can still be stressful. Preschoolers may understand that they are in the hospital because they are sick, but they may not understand the cause of their illness. Preschoolers fear mutilation and are afraid of intrusive procedures since they do not understand the body's integrity. They interpret words literally and have an active imagination. Therefore, when the nurse says, "I need to take some blood," preschoolers' fantasies may run wild. They may not understand the concept of blood and may think everything will come out of their body. They may think that blood is "taken" the same way a child picks up a toy to take it out of the room. Preschoolers' thinking is egocentric; they believe that some personal deed or thought caused their illness, which can lead to guilt and shame. These feelings may be internalized. Overall, preschoolers' concrete, egocentric, and **magical thinking** (type of thinking that allows for fantasies and creativity) limits their ability to understand, so communication and interventions must be on their level.

Separation anxiety may not be as much of an issue as it is for toddlers since preschoolers may already be spending time away from parents in preschool. They are, however, still acutely aware of the comfort and security that their family provides for them, so disruptions in these relationships lead to challenges. The preschooler may constantly ask for his or her parents or ask to call the parents. He or she may quietly cry, refuse to eat or take medication, or generally be uncooperative.

In addition, the hospitalized preschooler loses control over the environment. The preschooler is naturally curious about his or her surroundings and learns best by observing and working with objects. This might be limited during hospitalization. Because the preschooler cannot participate in typical activities and explore the environment as usual, the child's normal creative, curious nature may give rise to a variety of fantasies that may present challenges.

SCHOOL-AGE

School-age children generally are hospitalized because of long-term illnesses or trauma. The general task of their development stage, to develop confidence through a sense of industry, can be disrupted during hospitalization. Even at this time, they generally want to continue to learn and maintain their skills and abilities. The stress of illness or anxiety related to diagnostic tests and therapeutic interventions may lead to inward or outward expressions of distress. If they have learned various coping skills, this distress may be minimized. After 11 years of age there is an increased awareness of physiologic, psychological, and behavioral causes of illness and injury. Typically, the school-age child has a more realistic understanding of the reasons for the illness and can better comprehend explanations. School-age children are concerned about disability and death, and they fear injury and pain. They want to know why procedures and tests are being performed. They can understand cause and effect and how it relates to their illness. They are uncomfortable with any type of sexual examination.

Separation anxiety is not as much of an issue for school-age children. They are accustomed to periods of separation and may already be experiencing some separation anxiety related to being in school. At the same time, they may be missing school and friends as they try to adjust to the unfamiliar environment. They may feel that friends will forget them if they remain in the hospital for a long time. Some school-age children may regress and become needy, demanding their parents' attention or playing with special "comfort toys" they used at a younger age.

Since school-age children are accustomed to controlling self-care and typically are highly social, they like being involved. They are used to making choices about meals and activities. Hospitalization presents loss of control by limiting their activities, making them feel helpless and dependent. This may result in feelings of loneliness, boredom, isolation, and depression. The key is to give them opportunities to maintain independence, retain a sense of control, enhance self-esteem, and continue to work toward achieving a sense of industry.

ADOLESCENTS

Adolescents fear injury and pain. Since appearance is important to them, they are concerned with how the illness or injury will affect their body image. Anything that changes their perceptions of themselves has a major impact on their response. Typically, adolescents do not like to be different; they like "being cool," which means being in control and not showing how afraid they really are. They also may feel ambivalent about wanting their parents. Adolescents typically do not experience separation anxiety from being away from their parents; instead, their anxiety comes from being separated from friends.

Loss of control is a key factor affecting the behavior of adolescents who are hospitalized. Anger, withdrawal, or general lack of cooperation may occur due to the feelings of loss of control. In addition, their desire to appear confident may lead them to question everything that is being done or that they are asked to do. Their feelings of invincibility may cause them to take risks and be noncompliant with treatment. Overall, adolescents strive for independence, self-assertion, and liberation while developing their identity.

Previous Experiences

In general, children's lack of understanding and experience of illness, hospitalization, and hospital procedures contributes to their anxiety level. However, previous experience with hospitalization and other health-related experiences can either facilitate preparation or impair it if the experiences were perceived as negative. For example, the child who associates the hospital with the birth of a sibling may view this experience as positive. However, the child who associates the hospital with the serious illness or death of a relative or close friend will probably view the experience as negative.

The type of experience may contribute to increased anxiety and fear if the child must be admitted to the hospital. If children have had previous experiences, how the experience unfolded and their response to it will determine many of their reactions to hospitalization. Older children may cling to their parents, kick, or create a scene because of their previous experience.

Recent Stresses and Changes and Individual Coping Skills

The effects of hospitalization on children are influenced by the nature and severity of the health problem, the condition of the child, and the degree to which activities and routines differ from those of everyday life. A lack of sensory stimulation in the hospital environment can lead to listlessness, indifference, unhappiness, and even appetite changes. When the child's motor activity is restricted, anger and hyperactivity may result. Play, recreation, and educational opportunities can provide an outlet to distract the child from the illness, provide pleasant experiences, and help the child understand his or her condition.

The child's ability to work through a situation will also affect his or her responses to illness and hospitalization. This ability depends on the age of the child, his or her perceptions of the event, previous encounters with health care personnel, and support from significant others. Box 33.2 lists various coping skills used by children and suggestions for promoting positive coping.

BOX 33.2

CHILDREN AND COPING

Behavior/Methods for Coping	Suggestions to Promote Coping
Ignore or negate the problem	Breathing techniques such as blowing bubbles, pinwheels, or party noise-makers
Stoicism, passive acceptance	Distraction with books or games
Acting out—yelling, kicking, screaming, crying	Imagery with tapes or scenarios
Anger, withdrawal, rejection	Music
Intellectualizing	Teaching before events or procedures

Parents' Response to Child's Hospitalization

Children take in their parents' anxiety and concern. Even whispers can set off children's imaginations. For example, preschoolers may invent elaborate stories to explain what is happening to them. Parents who do not tell children the truth or do not answer their questions confuse and frighten them and may weaken the child's trust in the parents. It is important for children to believe that someone is in control and that the person can be trusted. Some parents, however, have their own fears and insecurities. Thus, a child's reaction is often related to the parents' reaction to the illness and hospitalization.

The relationship between the family and the hospital staff may either add to or ease the child's stress. This relationship can contribute significantly to the quality of the environment. Hospital personnel must assume responsibility for the care of hospitalized children by maintaining good partnerships with families.

Remember Jake, the 8-year-old with a suspected brain tumor? What responses to hospitalization might you see in him and his family?

Family's Reactions to the Child's Hospitalization

Whether planned or unplanned, hospitalization increases the family's stress and anxiety level. The illness or serious injury of one family member affects all members of the family because the process disrupts the family's usual routines and may alter family roles. Parents and siblings have their own reactions to this experience.

Reactions of Parents

Watching a child in pain is difficult, especially when the parent is assisting with the procedure by holding the child. The parent may feel guilty for not seeking care sooner. Parents may also exhibit other feelings such as denial, anger, depression, and confusion. Parents may deny that the child is ill. They may express anger, especially directed at the nursing staff, another family member, or a higher power, because of their loss of control in caring for the child. Depression may occur because of exhaustion and the psychological and physical requirements of spending long hours in a hospital caring for a child. Confusion may develop because of dealing with an unfamiliar environment or the loss of a parental role. Finally, the parents' marriage may be strained because of dual roles, long separation, and increased stress.

Reactions of Siblings

Siblings of children who are hospitalized may experience jealousy, insecurity, resentment, confusion, and anxiety. They may have difficulty understanding why their sibling is ill or getting all the attention, leaving little for them. They may wonder if their sibling is going to die or ever return home. They may worry that their sibling's illness is going to happen to them. Certain age groups, such as preschoolers, may feel that they caused the illness. Little information or understanding about what is happening, combined with their magical and egocentric thinking, contributes to their fears that they may have caused the illness or injury by their thoughts, wishes, or behaviors. If the family roles or routines change significantly, the siblings may feel insecure or anxious. They may develop changes in behavior or in school performance. See Evidence-Based Practice 33.1.

Take Note!

Research supports the need to provide support and information to the siblings to decrease their stress, anxiety, and confusion and to promote psychological adjustment (Prchal, Graf, Bergstraesser, & Landolt, 2012).

Factors Influencing Family Reactions

The parenting style and the family–child relationship can influence the hospital experience as well as the family members' coping skills. Cultural, ethnic, and religious variations, values, and practices related to illness, general response to stress, and attitudes about the care of a sick child have a significant influence on the family's response. For example, religious beliefs can raise problems or can be a source of strength to the family and child. Families already in crisis or without support systems have a more difficult time dealing with the added stress of hospitalization. Chapter 1 gives further explanations of some of these influences on children and their families.

Jake's parents are very upset that he has to be hospitalized. His mother says to you, "I'm worried how Jake is going to react to all of this. What can we do to help him?" How would you address his mother's concerns?

The Nurse's Role in Caring for the Hospitalized Child

In most instances, the nurse is the primary person involved in the care of a hospitalized child. The nurse is probably the first one to see the child and family and will spend more time with them than other health care personnel. Nurses are part of a medical community that makes decisions in the child's best interest, but the nurse needs to bear in mind the child's rights and must try to minimize the child's distress so that the hospital stay will be as pleasant an experience as possible. When establishing strategies to care for children in the hospital, nurses should examine the general effects of hospitalization on children in each developmental stage and should strive to understand both the reactions of the child and family to

EVIDENCE-BASED PRACTICE 33.1

WHAT IS THE EFFECTIVENESS OF A TWO-SESSION PSYCHOLOGICAL INTERVENTION ON THE SIBLINGS OF A NEWLY DIAGNOSED CHILD WITH CANCER?

Studies show that most siblings of a child with cancer adjust well but some suffer from cancer-related posttraumatic stress symptoms (PTSS) and have a poorer health-related quality of life. Siblings of a child with cancer are at risk for behavioral, emotional, and social problems.

STUDY

In order to test the effectiveness of the psychological interventions on siblings of children with cancer, a randomized control pilot trial was performed. Thirty siblings of a child recently diagnosed with cancer, ages 6 to 17 years, were recruited from two children's hospitals. Siblings assigned to the experimental group received two 50-minute sessions (2 weeks apart) within the first 2 months of diagnosis. Each session had 3 steps which provided medical information, ways to cope with stressful situations, and information for parents. Siblings in the control group received standard psychosocial care.

Findings

The study showed evidence that the psychological intervention had a positive impact on the sibling's psychological well-being, social support, and medical knowledge, but did not affect PTSS or anxiety.

Nursing Considerations

Recognize that siblings of an ill child often experience stress and anxiety. Provide education to the sibling of the ill child. Address the psychosocial and emotional needs of siblings of an ill child. Enlist CLSs to assist with the sibling of an ill child. Educate parents about the needs of siblings of an ill child.

Adapted from Prchal, A., Graf, A., Bergstraesser, E., & Landolt, M. A. (2012). Research: A two-session psychological intervention for siblings of pediatric cancer patients: a randomized controlled pilot trial. *Child and Adolescent Psychiatry and Mental Health, 6*, 3. doi:10.1186/1753-2000-6-3 hospitalization and the factors affecting these reactions. Nursing Care Plan 33.1 (at the end of the chapter) summarizes the nursing care associated with a hospitalized child.

In a study of hospitalized children, Crole and Smith (2002) found that the nursing care for a hospitalized child occurred in four phases: introduction, building a trusting relationship, decision-making phase, and providing comfort and reassurance. These phases remain relevant today. All of these phases are interconnected. For example, if trust is not established, it becomes difficult to move to the next phase.

The introduction phase involves the initial contact with children and their families and it establishes the foundation for a trusting relationship. Use favorite toys and common television shows to establish rapport. Allow the child to participate in the conversation without the pressure of having to comply with requests or undergo any procedures. Next, a trusting relationship can be built by using appropriate language, games, and play such as singing a song during a procedure, preparing the child adequately for procedures, and providing explanations and encouragement. Get down to the child's level and play on his or her terms.

In the decision-making phase, the nurse gives some control over to the child by allowing him or her to participate in making certain decisions. This phase is critical to maintaining the trust the child has developed. For example, it is imperative to decide how much control the child will have during treatment, how much information to share with the child about upcoming events, and whether parents should participate. Reinforce the child's use of coping strategies that lead to healthy outcomes by providing options whenever it is safe to do so. Finally, the comfort and reassurance phase uses techniques such as praising the child and providing opportunities to cuddle with a favorite toy. This phase helps the nurse re-establish trust and provide comfort to the child to increase positive outcomes.

Preparing Children and Families for Hospitalization

When preparing children for hospitalization, be aware of the situations that may create distress in a child and try to minimize or eliminate them. Even the most minor situations may be frightening to young children. Remember, new experiences, unfamiliar sights and sounds, disruption of sleep patterns, and pain associated with procedures and treatments are major causes of stress for the hospitalized child and family. Table 33.1 presents some hospital activities that may seem scary or stressful to a child and gives suggestions for preparing the child and family. Thoughtful preparation for these situations may help relieve stress. Educate children about what to expect so they can cope with their imagination and distinguish reality from fantasy. Describe the intervention and the sequence of steps that will occur, and include sensory information such as how the child will feel.

TABLE 33.1 STRATEGIES TO REDUCE FEAR OF COMMON HOSPITALIZATION SITUATIONS

Situation	Strategies to Reduce Fear
Procedure involving intrusion into the body or use of equipment or technology	Describe the procedure and equipment in terms the child can understand Review the steps of the procedure or steps involved with the use of the equipment Explain what the child's role will be and what is or isn't allowed If appropriate, have the child rehearse with the equipment or role-play
Darkness, such as with radiologic examinations or at night	Keep a light on in the examination area Use a night light in the child's room If possible, allow the child to hold the caregiver's or nurse's hand or a favorite toy
Transport to other areas of the hospital	Allow caregiver to accompany child if possible Inform the child of where he or she is going, about how long he or she will be there, and approximately when he or she will return Introduce the child to the person who will be transporting the child
Numerous personnel in and out of child's room	Identify all staff members working with the child (each shift and each day) Place a small board in the child's room with the name of the nurse caring for the child that shift or day Inform the child how long the nurse will be caring for the child (adapt this information according to the child's cognitive level; for example, instead of saying that you'll be there for 8 hours, say, "I'll be your nurse until just before dinner time" or "I'll be your nurse until you go for your test") Say good-bye to the child when leaving for the day; tell the child about his or her new nurse; inform the child of when you will return

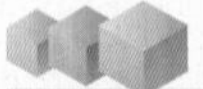
Concept Mastery Alert

Preparing the Child for Hospitalization

To help ease the stress of hospitalization in a child, encourage the parents and child to work with a child-life specialist at the hospital who can give the child a comprehensive preparation for the hospitalization.

Good preparation can reduce the child's fears and increase his or her ability to cope with the hospital experience. Preparation should include exploring the child's perceptions, reviewing previous experiences, and identifying coping strategies. The goal should be to decrease fear and anxiety by allowing the child to better understand what is happening. Useful techniques include the following:

- Perform nursing care on stuffed animals or dolls and allow the child to do the same.
- Avoid the use of medical terms.
- Allow the child to handle some equipment.
- Teach the child the steps of the procedure or inform him or her exactly what will happen during the hospital stay.
- Show the child the room where he or she will be staying.
- Introduce the child to the health care personnel with whom he or she will come in contact.
- Explain the sounds the child may hear.
- Let the child sample the food that will be served.

All techniques used to prepare the child for hospitalization should emphasize the philosophy of atraumatic care. Adapt all information to the cognitive and developmental level of the child. Identify what role the child will play in the situation: it is always helpful for children to have something to do, since it shows them that they are included. A rehearsal of what will occur in the hospital allows the child to become comfortable with the situation. If time permits, provide pamphlets that describe the procedure and suggest preparation activities for the child at home before admission.

The child and family may be able to take a tour of the hospital unit or the surgical facility. Videos or DVDs, photographs, and books on hospitalization and surgery can serve as resources for the family and child. Many institutions offer programs to familiarize children and families with the hospital experience with a guided tour. During the tour, opportunities are provided for role-playing, and during stops along the way the child can see, touch, and feel the equipment that may be used (Fig. 33.2). If the tour guide notes a child or family member is really scared or concerned about something, the pediatric staff can be alerted and therefore address this issue, further leading to improved family-centered care.

The American Society of Anesthesiologists has prepared a coloring book entitled *My Trip to the Hospital* (American Society of Anesthesiologists, 1998). This book is designed to alleviate some of the fears that younger children may have related to the hospital experience. It describes the process from admission (whether it be to the hospital or ambulatory surgery center) through discharge and includes information about preoperative testing, anesthesia, and recovery. The book also includes information for parents. A link to the book's website is listed on thePoint. Several other children's books are available that focus on hospital stays and procedures, such as *My Trip to the Hospital* in the Little Critter Series by Mercer Mayer and *Clifford Visits the Hospital* by Norman Bridwell. A list may be available at the hospital from the child life department.

Parents are instrumental in preparing children by reviewing the materials that are given, answering questions, and being truthful and supportive. Teaching Guidelines 33.1 provides suggestions for parents in preparing their child for hospitalization.

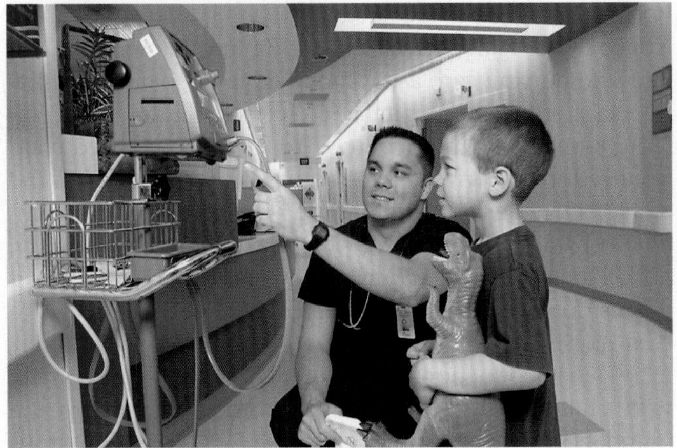

FIGURE 33.2 A child is being prepared for hospitalization by becoming familiar with some of the equipment that might be used.

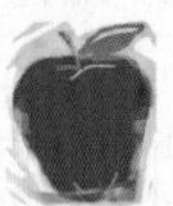

Teaching Guidelines 33.1

PREPARING YOUR CHILD FOR HOSPITALIZATION

- Read stories about experiences with hospitals or surgery.
- Talk about going to the hospital and what it will be like coming home.
- Be honest and encourage the child to ask questions.
- Visit the hospital and go through the preadmission tour if time permits.
- Provide support to the child via your presence, telephone calls, and special items brought from home.
- Encourage the child to draw pictures to express how he or she is feeling.
- Include siblings in the preparation.

Take Note!

Remember to enlist the assistance of the child life specialist (CLS), if possible, to assist with preparing children and families for hospitalization.

Admitting the Child to the Facility

Admitting the child to the facility involves preparing him or her for admission and introducing the child to the unit where he or she will be staying. Use the appropriate hospital forms. Chapter 30 gives general information about communicating with and teaching children and families.

In today's health care environment, the admission process occurs quickly, with little time for extensive preparation; this is why preparation before admission is so important. Of course, the urgency of the child's medical condition may also limit the amount of preparation that can be done in advance.

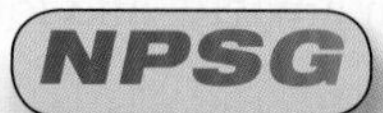

GOAL 3: Improve the Safety of Using Medications

NPSG 03.06.01 Maintain and communicate accurate patient medication information.

Steps: When admitting a child to the facility, be sure to collect accurate information concerning the child's usual medications. Compare this information with ordered medications to check for inconsistencies.

Joint Commission. (2015). *National patient safety goals effective January 1, 2015.* Retrieved from http://www.jointcommission.org/assets/1/6/2015_NPSG_HAP.pdf

TYPES OF ADMISSIONS AND NURSING CARE

The hospital units to which a child may be admitted include:

- General inpatient unit
- Emergency and urgent care department
- Pediatric intensive care unit (PICU)
- Outpatient or special procedures unit
- Rehabilitation unit or hospital

Regardless of the site of care, nursing care must begin by establishing a trusting, caring relationship with the child and family. Smile, introduce yourself, and give your title. Let the child and family know what will happen and what is expected of them. Ask the family and child what names they prefer to be called by. Maintain eye contact at the appropriate level. With a younger child, start with the family first so the child can see that the family trusts you. Communicate with children at age-appropriate levels.

The next step, as the child's medical condition allows, involves an orientation to the hospital unit. Briefly explain policies and routines and the personnel who will be involved in the care of the child.

During the nursing interview that follows, obtain information about the child's history, routines, and reason for admission. Obtain baseline vital signs and height and weight, and perform a physical assessment. Each health care setting has its own policies and procedures for this. Recognize the needs of the family and child during this process. If some of this information already exists, do not ask for it again, except to confirm vital information such as allergies, medications taken at home, and history of the illness. Typically, the information is collected immediately if the child's condition is urgent; otherwise, the information is collected within 8 hours, except for the information that is required for safe care.

General Inpatient Unit Stays. Today, general inpatient unit stays for children are shorter and involve more acute conditions, resulting in little time for admission preparation. Many times the admission procedure and treatment actually occur simultaneously. Sometimes the stay is in a special 23-hour observation unit so the child is in the setting for less than 24 hours. General hospital stays may be in a pediatric hospital, a pediatric unit in a general hospital, or a general unit that occasionally admits children. General units often lack child-oriented services, such as play areas, child-size equipment, and staff familiar with caring for children.

Take Note!

When a child is admitted to a general unit, take extra time to orient and explain the routines and procedures to the child and family. Emphasize that the parents can stay with the child (if institutional policy permits). If possible, place the child in a room close to the nurses' station and order food appropriate for the child's age and developmental level.

Emergency and Urgent Care Departments. A major cause for illness and hospitalization in children is injuries from accidents (U.S. Department of Health and Human Services, Health Resources and Services Administration, Maternal and Child Health Bureau, 2013). Many times a family's first experience with the acute care setting is the urgent care or emergency department. Due to the situation, the child and family may experience increased anxiety, and it may become overwhelming as uncertainties develop and critical decisions must be made. The family may be frightened, insecure, and in a state of shock.

Procedures and tests are performed quickly, with minimal time for preparation. The family is often ill prepared for the visit, having little money or clothing with them. Siblings may be present if the parents did not have time to arrange other child care.

Due to the fast pace of the emergency department, the family may be hesitant to ask questions, so keep the family and child well informed. Allow the family to stay with the child, provide support, and allow the family, and when appropriate the child, to participate in decisions.

Families may have a strong fear of the unknown and may be terrified that the child will die or be permanently disabled. Help the family to identify their concerns and their support systems. Prepare them for what they will experience. Provide comfort such as holding, touching, talking softly, and other appropriate interventions according to age and developmental level.

Pediatric Intensive Care Units. The PICU specializes in caring for children in crisis. The same principles and concepts of general care of children apply to this setting, but everything is intensified. Families will be faced with an unfamiliar, high-tech environment and a large number of staff.

Families must deal with the critical situation that brought them to the PICU. The child will likely experience pain, unusual noises, and increased stimulation and will probably undergo uncomfortable procedures. Parents may face the possibility of losing their child. Sometimes the child cannot talk, eat, or display other appropriate developmental behaviors. Sensory overload (increased stimulation) or sensory deprivation (lack of stimulation) can affect both child and family.

Welcome families (if institutional policy permits) and encourage them to stay with the child and participate in care. Explain everything to the parents and, when appropriate, to the child. Frequently touch the child and encourage the parents to comfort him or her. Listen for clues about what the child and family need during the PICU stay.

Isolation Rooms. Isolation rooms are used for situations involving the risk for infection. When a child is admitted with an infectious disease, or to rule out an infectious disease, or if the child has impaired immune function, isolation will be instituted. Children in this setting may experience sensory deprivation due to the limited contact with others and the use of personal protective equipment such as gloves, masks, and gowns.

Encourage the family to visit often, and help them to understand the reason for the isolation and any special procedures that are required. Introduce yourself before entering the room and allow the child to view your face before applying a mask, if possible. Continue to have contact with the child and hold or touch the child often, especially if the parents are not present.

Rehabilitation Units. The rehabilitation unit provides care for children beyond the initial period of illness or injury. The care involves an interdisciplinary approach that assists the child to reach his or her potential and achieve developmental skills. For example, rehabilitation units help children regain abilities lost due to neurologic injuries or serious burns. The facilities often resemble a home environment, with special services to help children to relearn activities of daily living and to help them deal with the physical or mental challenges associated with the original illness or injury. Typically, families are encouraged to participate and are given support for their child's eventual return home. There is a balance of nurturing and firm discipline while the child reclaims independence.

Addressing the Effects of Hospitalization Developmentally

When addressing the fears, separation anxiety, and loss of control that occur in hospitalized children, the nurse should consider the child's age and cognitive or developmental level. Interventions are then based on how the child experiences these stressors at that age or developmental level. The content, timing, setting, and method of preparation are also based on the child's age and cognitive or developmental level. General guidelines for addressing fear and anxiety, separation anxiety, and loss of control are provided in Box 33.3.

BOX 33.3

GUIDELINES TO ADDRESS THE GENERAL EFFECTS OF HOSPITALIZATION

Minimizing Fear and Anxiety

- Prepare the child and family for hospitalization and procedures.
- Explain everything to the child and their families before it occurs (see Chapter 30).
- Use age-appropriate communication techniques. Include the family in this process so they can help the child cope with fears.
- Allow time for children to play out their fears and concerns.
- Talk to the child and parents using a soft, friendly, comforting tone of voice.
- Have a calm, empathetic approach when caring for the child.

Addressing/Minimizing Separation Anxiety

- Know the stages of separation anxiety and be able to recognize them.
- Remember that behaviors demonstrated during the first stage do not indicate that the child is "bad."
- Encourage the family to stay with the child and always use a family-centered approach to care.
- Help the child cope, and intervene before the behaviors of detachment occur.

Addressing Loss of Control

- Minimize physical restrictions, altered routines and rituals, and dependency issues, because they produce loss of control.
- Allow as much independence as possible within the constraints of the diagnosis.
- Allow the child to participate in care and decisions regarding care whenever possible.

NEWBORNS AND INFANTS

Assess the development or lack of development that is occurring in the infant, and assess the baby's attachment to the parents or primary caregivers. The infant's facial expression is the most consistent indicator of pain or bodily injury. To decrease fear and minimize separation anxiety, avoid separation from the primary caregiver if possible; this will also promote healthy attachment. If the parent or primary caregiver cannot stay with the infant, arrange for volunteers to provide consistent comfort to the baby. Maintaining the infant's home routine related to sleep and feeding helps decrease feelings of loss of control. Weigh the infant daily, at the same time, on the same scale. Monitor intake and output closely. Be alert to signs of discomfort other than crying, such as a furrowed brow or tense body posture. Additional nursing goals related to ensuring safety and promoting growth and development of the infant are presented in Table 33.2.

TODDLERS

Key nursing concerns when caring for toddlers are separation anxiety, growth and development, and autonomy. Establishing a trusting relationship with the toddler through nonthreatening play may decrease the amount of fear the toddler feels. Be alert to subtle, nonverbal indicators of grief or discontent.

Encourage the parent or primary caregiver to stay with the toddler in the hospital to decrease separation anxiety. Maintaining the home routine related to meals and sleep or a nap provides structure and may help decrease the toddler's feelings of loss of control. If indicated, weigh the toddler daily. Closely monitor intake and output. Refer to Table 33.2 for additional nursing considerations related to ensuring safety and promoting growth and development in the hospitalized toddler.

PRESCHOOLERS

Nursing care for hospitalized preschoolers focuses on their special needs, fears, and fantasies. When working with preschoolers, remember that they use magical thinking and fantasy. Be honest and specific, providing information just prior to the intervention to allay the child's fears. As with toddlers, encouraging parental involvement may decrease the amount of separation anxiety the preschooler experiences while in the hospital. Allowing the preschooler to make simple decisions such as which color bandage to use or whether to take medicine from a cup or syringe helps the child to feel some sense of control. Table 33.2 gives specific nursing considerations related to ensuring safety and promoting growth and development for the preschooler in the hospital.

SCHOOL-AGE CHILDREN

Provide honest information using concrete, meaningful words to the school-age child to minimize fear of the unknown. School-age children are still very attached to their parents, so encouraging parental involvement or rooming-in decreases separation anxiety. Involve the child in making simple decisions and planning the schedule as appropriate to give him or her a sense of control. Nursing considerations when caring for hospitalized school-age children include ensuring safety and promoting growth and development (Table 33.2).

ADOLESCENTS

The adolescent may or may not express fears. Educate the teen honestly; younger teens require more concrete explanations, while older teens can process more abstract concepts. Respect the teen's need for privacy. Encourage visits from the adolescent's friends to minimize anxiety related to separation. Prepare a mutually agreeable schedule with the teen, as appropriate, that includes the teen's preferences while incorporating the required nursing care. Collaborating with the adolescent will provide the teen with increased control. Refer to Table 33.2 for additional nursing considerations related to care of the adolescent in the hospital.

Think back to Jake, the 8-year-old from the beginning of the chapter. Discuss nursing care you could provide that will help minimize stressors.

Preparing the Child and Family for Surgery

If the child is to undergo a surgical procedure, whether in the hospital or an outpatient setting, special interventions are necessary. The parents should be allowed to stay with the child until surgery begins. Parents should also be allowed to be with the child when he or she wakes up in the postanesthesia recovery area. Good preparation provides reassurance and comfort to the child and allows him or her to know what will happen and what is expected of him or her.

Preoperative care for the child who is to undergo surgery is similar to that for an adult. The major difference is that the preparation and teaching must be geared to the child's age and developmental level. Table 33.3 discusses strategies for preoperative teaching. Many facilities offer special programs to help prepare children and families for the surgical experience. Preoperative preparation programs allow children and their families to experience a "trial run" in a supportive environment to help reduce anxiety, increase knowledge, increase comfort level, and enhance coping skills (American Academy of Pediatrics, 2012). Books, including the one cited earlier by the American Society of Anesthesiologists, are helpful in preparing the child and family.

Child and family teaching is essential. Like any intervention, adapt the teaching to the child's developmental

TABLE 33.2 NURSING CONSIDERATIONS FOR PROVIDING SAFE, DEVELOPMENTALLY APPROPRIATE CARE

	Ensuring Safety	Promoting Healthy Growth and Development
Infants	• Maintain close supervision of the infant. • Keep one hand on the infant when crib sides are down. • Keep crib rails up all the way when the infant is in the crib. • Avoid leaving small objects that are harmful or that can be swallowed in the crib. • Provide safe and appropriate toys for the infant. • Place infants in rooms close to the nurses' station. • Encourage a family member to stay with the infant at all times.	• Use the en face position when holding newborns. • Smile and talk to the infant during bathing, feeding, and other interactions. • Minimize the number of painful or uncomfortable procedures. • Provide comfort during and after procedures by holding or talking, using soothing tones and movements. • When handling the infant, use smooth, continuous movements. • Use gentle stroking and holding, which may reduce stress. • Serve as a role model for first-time parents. • Encourage the family to maintain home routines while in the hospital, planning nursing care around the usual feeding and sleep times. • Use the pacifier between feedings to satisfy nonnutritive sucking needs.
Toddlers	• Keep crib side rails up with overhead crib protection intact when the toddler is in the crib. • Never leave a toddler alone in the room unless secured in the crib. • Use a bed only for the older toddler who has an adult present in the room at all times. • Avoid leaving small objects that can be swallowed or are harmful in the crib or bed. • Place crib out of reach of cords, equipment, and electrical outlets. • Provide safe and appropriate toys for the toddler. • Place toddlers in rooms close to the nurses' station. • Always have someone with the toddler when ambulating.	• Encourage the parent to stay with the toddler to decrease separation anxiety. • To promote autonomy, allow the toddler to make appropriate choices, such as which juice to take the medicine with. • Encourage active play in the playroom or with push/pull toys in the hallway (accompanied by an adult). • Expect and plan for regression in areas of toilet training, eating, and other behaviors. • Expect increased temper tantrums in general and intense reactions to intrusive procedures. • Maintain home routine while in the hospital, planning nursing care around the usual feeding and sleep times. • Give simple directions with choices appropriate to the hospital situation. • Provide close supervision while encouraging independence.
Preschoolers	• Keep bed in low position with the side rails up when the preschooler is in the bed. • Instruct the child to call the nurse or caregiver for help getting out of bed. • Keep harmful objects out of reach of the child.	• Encourage parents to stay with the preschooler in the room as well as other areas of the hospital. • Encourage the preschooler to be involved in care by providing choices and opportunities for the child to help. • Use play as an opportunity to work through the preschooler's fears. • Explain activities in simple, concrete terms, being cautious with the words you use because of the preschooler's fantasies and magical thinking. • Expect reactions to pain and bodily injury to be verbally aggressive and specific. • Try to maintain home routines while the child is in the hospital, working them into the plan of care when possible.

TABLE 33.2 NURSING CONSIDERATIONS FOR PROVIDING SAFE, DEVELOPMENTALLY APPROPRIATE CARE (continued)

	Ensuring Safety	Promoting Healthy Growth and Development
School-Age Children	• Keep the bed in the low position with the side rails up while the child is in the bed, explaining that this is a hospital rule, not a punishment.	• Provide opportunities for the child to be involved in care. • Allow children to select their meals, assist with treatments, and keep their rooms neat. • Allow visits with other children if the condition allows. • Encourage parents to tell the child when they will return. • Plan care around the child's usual home routines (meals, sleep). • Encourage the child to do schoolwork.
Adolescents	• Be aware of the adolescent's whereabouts. The teen may not wish to stay in the room but may become confused about where the room or unit is located in the hospital.	• Allow teens to interact with others. • Alter hospital routines as possible to allow the teen to sleep in or stay up later at night. • Provide others close to their age as roommates. • Encourage visits from friends. • Provide emotional support for feelings of being alone or away from friends; be alert for regression, which may result in the teen becoming emotional. • Answer questions honestly and with appropriate information. • Give the teen a sense of control by allowing choices. • Be sensitive to concerns about being "different."

level. For example, when teaching a toddler or preschooler about breathing exercises, have the child blow a pinwheel or cotton balls across the table through a straw. The child will enjoy the activity while also reaping the respiratory benefits of the activity.

In preparation for surgery, use items such as stuffed animals or dolls to help children understand what is going to happen to them (Fig. 33.3). Allow the child to role-play various experiences with dolls. Dolls designed to simulate surgical experiences have been developed.

TABLE 33.3 STRATEGIES FOR PREOPERATIVE TEACHING

Developmental Level	Implications for Teaching
Infants and toddlers	Encourage parents to use a soft tone of voice and stroking and secure, comfortable holding positions to promote calm Remind parents to use positive facial expressions Encourage the parent or caregiver to stay with the child as much as possible Use terms that the child and parents can understand For toddlers, provide information as close to the day of surgery as possible to prevent undue anxiety
Preschoolers and school-age children	Provide factual explanations using terms the child and parents can understand Incorporate pictures and other visual aids in explanation Tailor the timing of education to meet the child's learning needs, allowing enough time for the child to ask questions. For preschoolers, provide information 1 to 2 days before surgery. For school-age children, provide information 3 to 5 days before surgery
Adolescents	Provide detailed explanations of the procedure at least 7 to 10 days beforehand Answer questions honestly, ensuring privacy at all times Remain available for questions or concerns arising before or after surgery

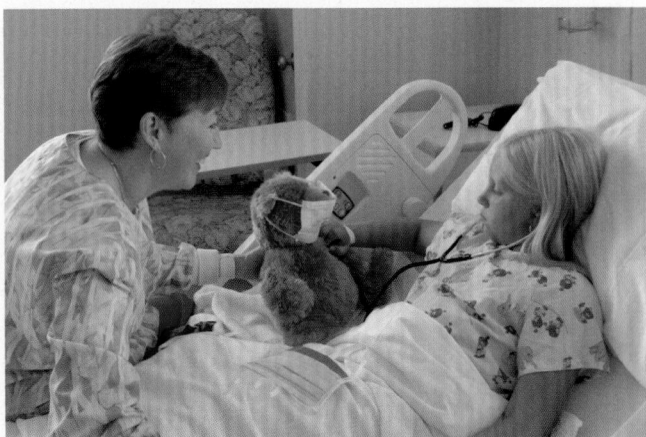

FIGURE 33.3 Using a stuffed animal to explain a surgical procedure to the child.

For example, Shadow Buddies are custom-made dolls that have the same illness or surgery as the child; the doll may have an ostomy, a scar, or a catheter (Shadow Buddies Foundation, 2014). The dolls were developed to help children cope with their illness or disease and send the message that it is okay to be different. These dolls also provide the child with a companion to talk to. Visit thePoint for a link to the Shadow Buddies website.

Maintaining Safety During Hospitalization

Safety is a critical aspect of care of the child in the hospital. Due to their age and developmental level, children are vulnerable to harm. Ensure the child has an identification band in place at all times. Sometimes in implementing interventions an armband is removed, so make sure it is attached to another extremity. Monitor children closely to avoid accidents such as a child pushing the wrong knob, picking up a piece of equipment or supplies left in the bed or room, or climbing out of bed (Fig. 33.4). See Table 33.2, which highlights nursing goals for ensuring safe, developmentally appropriate care for the hospitalized child.

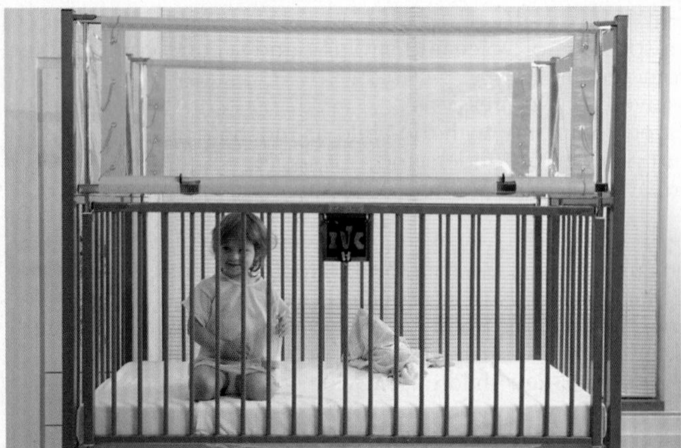

FIGURE 33.4 Safety is an essential aspect of pediatric nursing. A clear plastic cover over the crib prevents the older infant or toddler from climbing out and falling.

USE OF RESTRAINTS

When caring for children, some type of restriction may be necessary. The restriction, often referred to as a restraint, may be needed to ensure the child's safety, allow a therapeutic or diagnostic procedure to be done, immobilize a body part or limit movement, or prevent disruption of prescribed therapy. However, restraints can be overused and are not without risks to the child's safety (Centers for Medicare and Medicaid Services [CMS], 2014). As a result, each facility will have specific procedures and policies in place related to the use of restraints based on standards developed by the Joint Commission, regulations developed by the CMS, state law, and facility requirements. These procedures and policies are designed to safeguard children's physical safety and psychological well-being.

According to these standards, hospitals are required to have a policy in place that specifies the following (CMS, 2014; Disability Rights California, 2014):

- Reason for the restraint
- Client assessment parameters identifying the need for the restraint
- Use of alternative or less restrictive method determined to be ineffective before using a restraint
- Use of the least restrictive type of restraint for the purpose after the decision is made that a restraint is necessary
- Need for a written order by a licensed independent practitioner (LIP) within 1 hour of application of the restraint
- Need for face-to-face evaluation by LIP within 1 hour of application of the restraint
- Documentation of child's response to intervention and rationale for continued use

In addition, the Joint Commission standards and CMS regulations also identify the need for specific staff training and frequent assessment and appropriate discontinuation of use.

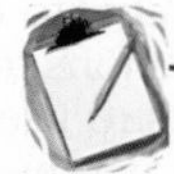

Take Note!

Always refer to your institution's policy regarding restraint use.

Restraints can promote physical distress in a child and be stressful for the parents as well. Children also may view restraints as punishment. Before a restraint is used, other measures need to be considered and alternative attempts or rationale for not using alternatives need to be documented (CMS, 2014).

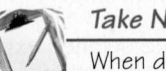

Take Note!

When deciding whether it is necessary to restrain a child, consider the child's age, developmental level, mental status, and threat to others and self.

Explain why the child should not touch the intravenous site or should maintain a certain position so that he or she has a basic understanding of what is necessary. This may be all that is necessary for an older child. One-to-one supervision and behavior modification techniques may be other alternatives to the use of restraints.

Atraumatic Care

Therapeutic hugging should be used for procedures and treatments such as intravenous line insertion for which the child needs to remain still. Refer to Chapter 30 for further information.

If it is determined that a restraint is needed, select the most appropriate, least restrictive type of restraint (Disability Rights California, 2014; CMS, 2014). For example, if the child has an intravenous catheter in the antecubital space that stops flowing when the child bends the arm, an elbow restraint or arm board, rather than a soft wrist restraint or four-point extremity restraint, would be appropriate. Table 33.4 lists the types of restraints and the major issues associated with the use of restraints in children.

Take Note!

When selecting a restraint, the nurse must choose the least restrictive type and apply it for the shortest time necessary (CMS, 2014).

Before applying a restraint, explain the reason for the restraint to the child and the parents. Emphasize that the rationale is to maintain the child's safety; the restraint is not punishment. Having the child and parents state the reason for the restraint demonstrates their understanding.

A written order for the restraint and an evaluation of the child by an LIP must occur within 1 hour of applying the restraint (Disability Rights California, 2014). In addition, the nurse must do the following:

- Ensure that the restraint fits properly.
- Secure the restraints with ties to the bed or crib frame, not the side rails.
- Use a clove-hitch type of knot to secure the restraints with ties (this allows for quick, easy access and release of the restraint).
- Check restraints 15 minutes following initial placement and then every hour for proper placement.
- Assess the temperature of the affected extremities, pulses, and capillary refill, initially after 15 minutes and then every hour after placement.
- Remove the restraint every 2 hours to allow for range of motion and repositioning, with documentation of this process and any findings.
- Encourage parent participation, providing continuous explanations about the reasons for the restraints and tentative time frame for use.
- Offer positive reinforcement to the child and parents.
- Review the criteria for removing the restraints; document removal and continued assessment.

It is important that the nurse is familiar with federal standards and regulations and he or she should always follow facility policy and procedures.

TRANSPORT OF THE CHILD

Children may need to be transported to other units for diagnostic tests or surgery; to different areas in the same unit, such as the playroom or treatment room; or for discharge. When the child is transported to other areas, specific guidelines need to address safety issues, the age and developmental level of the child, the child's physical condition, and the destination. These factors need to be considered before transport so that the appropriate method can be used with the least amount of risk for the child. Various methods to transport children include

TABLE 33.4 TYPES OF RESTRAINTS AND ASSOCIATED SAFETY CONCERNS

Type of Restraint	Purpose	Safety Concerns
Soft limb restraint	Wrist or ankle restraint to prevent range of motion of extremities	Check wrist or ankle for any sign of circulatory, integumentary, or neurologic compromise

(continued)

TABLE 33.4 TYPES OF RESTRAINTS AND ASSOCIATED SAFETY CONCERNS (continued)

Type of Restraint	Purpose	Safety Concerns
Elbow restraint 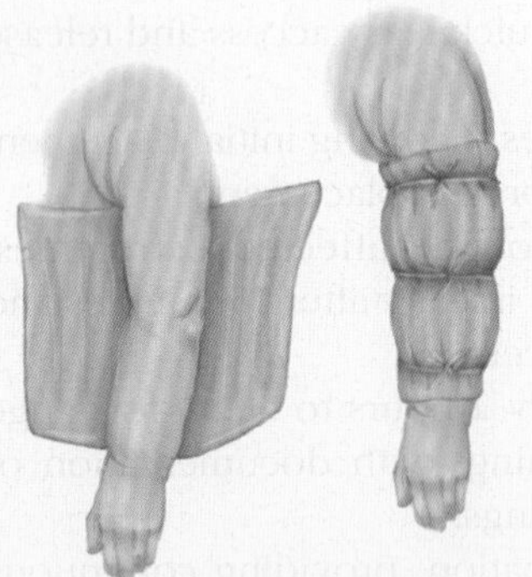	Prevents child from flexing and reaching face, head, IV, and other tubes 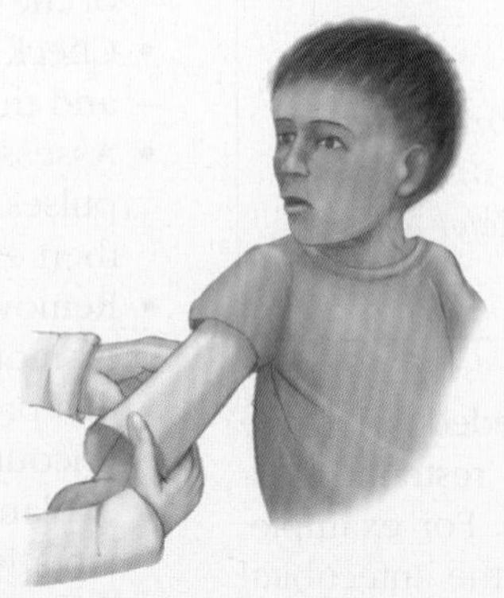	Position the restraint so that it does not rub against axilla. Check pulse, temperature, and capillary refill of the extremity
Mummy restraint 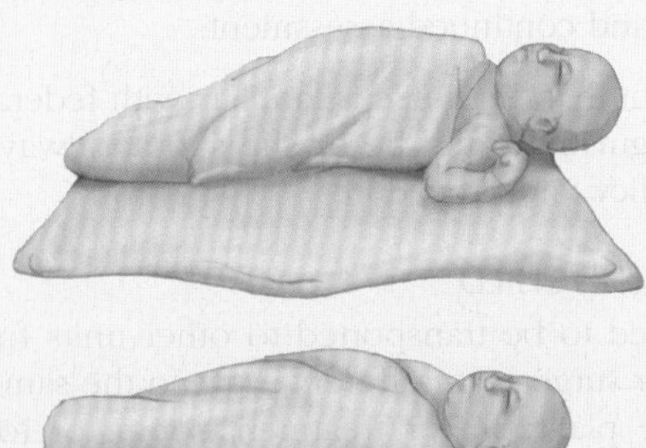	Body restraint using a sheet/blanket folded in a square appropriate to size of infant or young child to secure the whole body of the child or every extremity except for one 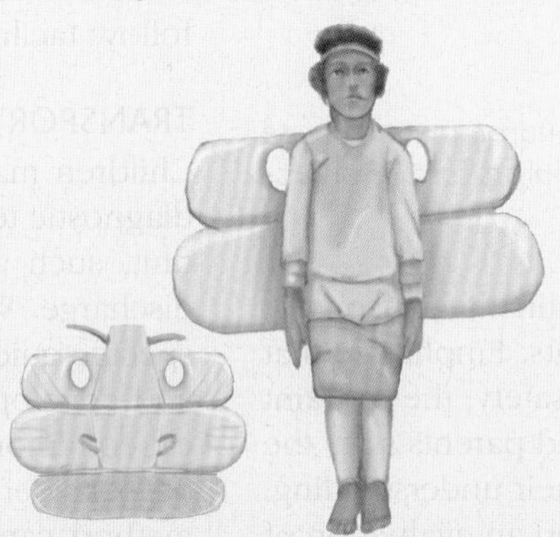	Ensure that all extremities are secured within the sheet Ensure face is not covered or airway restricted
Jacket (vest) restraint 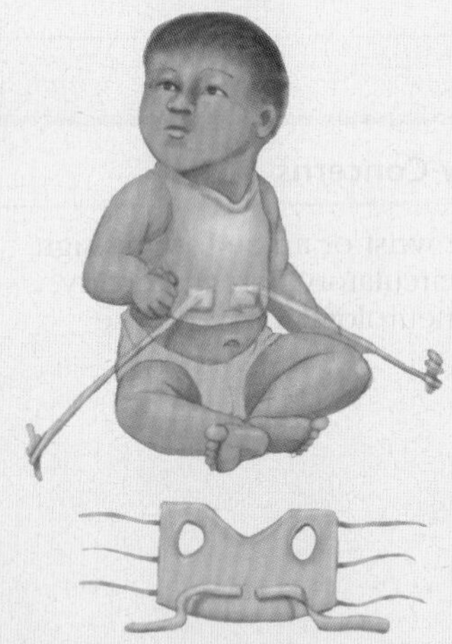	Jacket worn by child with ties attached to the child's back and to side of bed. Used to keep children flat in bed, such as after surgery, or safe in chair	Ensure the child can turn head to side and that the head of the bed is elevated, if possible. Place ties in back so child cannot manipulate them. Ensure attached to nonmovable part of bed frame.

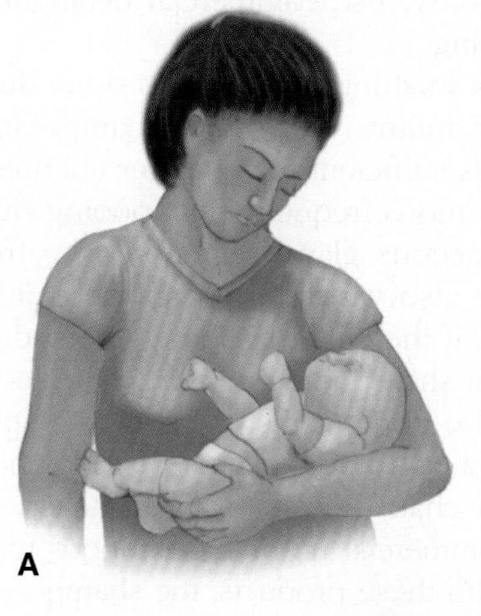

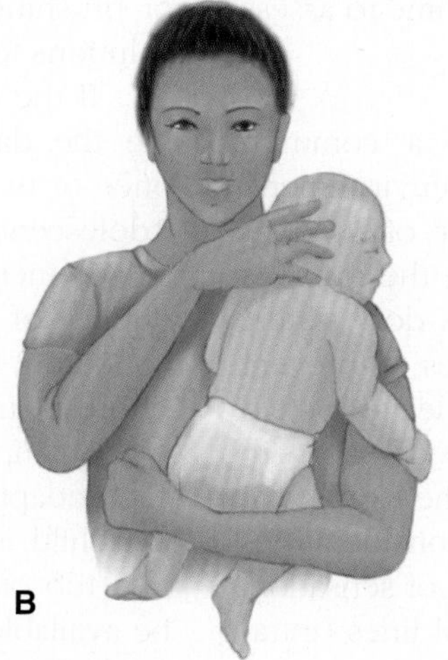

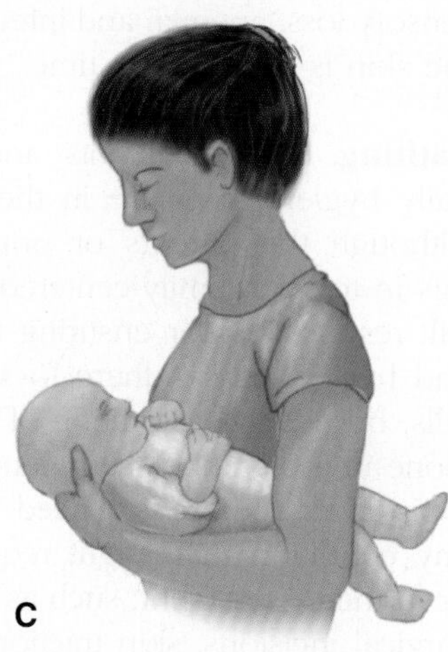

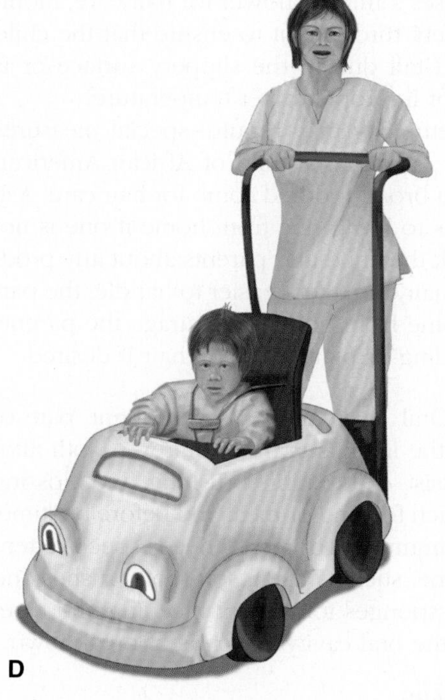

FIGURE 33.5 Methods for transporting the infant or child. **A.** Cradle method for carrying infants up to 3 months of age. One hand grasps the infant's thighs; the other arm supports the infant's head and back. **B.** The "over-the-shoulder" method for carrying infants up to 7 months of age. Support the head if the infant does not have head control. **C.** Football method for carrying infants up to 2 months of age. The forearm and hand support the body and head of the infant. **D.** A wagon with rails and padding is used to transport small children.

carrying the infant and using strollers, wagons, or rolling beds (Fig. 33.5). If possible, the parents should accompany the child to offer support and comfort.

When carrying an infant, good support of the back and head is vital. Rails should be up on all beds and wagons. Use safety belts with strollers and wheelchairs.

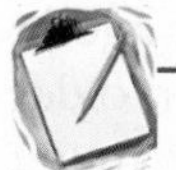

Take Note!

Never leave a child unattended during transport. Keep the child visible at all times during the transport.

Providing Basic Care for the Hospitalized Child

Basic care involves general hygiene measures, including bathing, hair care, oral care, and nutritional care. Young children are dependent on an adult for most, if not all, of their self-care needs. If parents are present, allow them to provide care for the child to decrease the child's stress. Older children may perform hygiene measures themselves but may need some assistance from the nurse.

GENERAL HYGIENE MEASURES

General hygiene measures help to maintain healthy skin, hair, and teeth. Skin is a complex structure; its primary function is to protect the tissues that it encloses and to protect itself. Injury to the child's skin may occur when inserting and maintaining an intravenous line, removing a dressing, positioning a child in bed, changing a diaper, using and removing electrode patches, and maintaining restraints. Risk factors for problems include impaired mobility, protein malnutrition, edema, incontinence, sensory loss, anemia, and infection. A good time to assess the skin is during bath time.

Bathing. Bathing infants and children is a common daily hygiene measure in the health care environment. Although the parents or primary caregiver often does this in today's family-centered environment, the nurse is still responsible for ensuring that bathing is done safely and hygienically. Adhere to safety principles to prevent falls, burns, and aspiration of water. Never leave a child alone in a bathtub. Use a gentle, pH-balanced soap with moisturizer if there is a need to rehydrate the skin. Note any condition that might require special considerations or further assessment, such as paralysis, loss of sensation, surgical incisions, skin traction/cast, external lines (intravenous lines, urinary catheters, or feeding tubes), or other alterations in skin integrity. Pay close attention to the ears, between skin folds, the neck, the back, and the genital area for alterations in skin integrity. Table 33.5 highlights specific developmental considerations for bathing.

Before bathing and performing other hygiene measures, assess the family's preferences and home practices for the child, such as time of day, rituals, special equipment, and allergies to products. This is a good time to assess the amount of assistance that might be required by the parents and to address learning needs related to hygiene. Follow general guidelines in bathing any client with regard to equipment, room temperature, privacy, and use of products such as deodorant and lotion.

Hair Care. Lying in bed can make the hair matted and tangled. Avoid pulling on the child's hair when combing or brushing it. If necessary, use commercial detangling solutions to ease combing.

If the hair requires washing, this is often done during the daily bath for infants. Typically, shampooing once or twice a week is sufficient for younger children. Adolescents may need more frequent shampooing due to the increase in sebaceous gland secretion. The frequency of shampooing also varies based on the child's condition; for example, if the child has experienced diaphoresis, more frequent shampooing may be indicated.

Shampooing may be done at the bedside with specially adapted equipment, at a readily accessible sink while the child is sitting in a chair or lying on a stretcher, or in a tub or shower. Commercial no-rinse shampoos may be available for use. With these products, the shampoo is applied to the hair and then brushed or combed out.

If the child uses a tub or shower for hair care, monitor the child's safety throughout to ensure that the child does not slip and fall due to the slippery surface or is burned because of improper water temperature.

The child's ethnicity may require special measures for hair care. For example, a child of African American descent may use a broad-toothed comb for hair care. Ask the child's parents to bring one from home if one is not available. Also ask the child and parents about any products used on the hair to make it easier to handle; the parents can bring some from home. Encourage the parents to help with braiding or plaiting of the hair if desired.

TABLE 33.5 DEVELOPMENTAL CONSIDERATIONS FOR BATHING

Age of Child	Special Considerations
Infants	Use a sponge bath or tub bath to bathe young infants who cannot sit unaided. Support the infant's body at all times. Ensure appropriate water temperature Avoid use of talcum powder.
Toddlers	Bathe older infants and toddlers at the bedside or in a regular bathtub, depending on their health condition.
School-age children and adolescents	Older children may prefer a shower if available and acceptable for their health condition. Assess whether a shower would be safe. Provide privacy.

Oral Hygiene. Oral hygiene is an important part of basic care. Wipe the infant's gums with a wet cloth after each feeding. Assist children in brushing and flossing their teeth after each feeding or meal and before bedtime. The child who is immunosuppressed needs special attention to oral hygiene, such as using soft toothbrushes and moistened gauze sponges to prevent bleeding and careful inspection of the oral cavity for areas of breakdown.

NUTRITIONAL CARE

Adequate nutrition is necessary for growth and development and tissue repair, so it is an essential component of care for the ill or hospitalized child.

Frequently, the ill or hospitalized child experiences a loss of appetite, which can affect the child's nutritional status. This may be compounded by other problems such as nausea and vomiting and nothing by mouth (NPO) restrictions for testing or surgery. The hospitalized child may adopt feeding habits that do not fit his or her age or stage of development, such as use of a bottle in an older infant/child or a child capable of self-feeding wanting to be fed. Readoption of these feeding habits should be accommodated when possible.

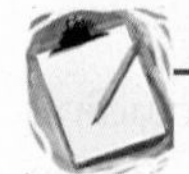

Take Note!

Relieve pain and nausea before meals are served.

If possible, schedule procedures or treatments away from mealtimes. In younger children, refusing to eat may be related to the child's feeling of separation; in others, refusing to eat may reflect the child's attempt to control the situation. Encourage parents to use gentle persuasion instead of force to assist with intake. The use of force can lead to an aversion for food that carries beyond the hospital stay into the home environment. They should give the child choices about what to eat; this reinforces the child's sense of control. Remind parents that the child's appetite will probably improve as his or her condition improves. Teaching Guidelines 33.2 provides tips for promoting nutrition in the hospitalized child. Although geared to parents, nurses can also incorporate these guidelines into the child's plan of care.

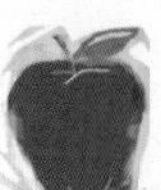

Teaching Guidelines 33.2

PROMOTING NUTRITION FOR YOUR HOSPITALIZED CHILD

- Check with the nurse about any restrictions related to your child's diet. Find out if intake and output are being monitored.
- Encourage your child to eat his or her favorite foods.
- Assist your child with eating or drinking as necessary; be present at mealtimes to promote socialization.
- Frequently offer small cups of fluid and finger foods; avoid giving large quantities at one time.
- Try offering fluids at different temperatures at different times for variety.
- Remember that children can ingest greater amounts of thin liquids (e.g., gelatin or carbonated drinks) than thicker liquids (e.g., cream soups or milkshakes).
- Include ice chips as fluid intake. Ice is approximately equivalent to half the same amount of water (e.g., 1 cup of ice equals a half-cup of water).
- Use straws (unless not allowed) and brightly colored utensils, cups, or dishes to provide contrast and stimulation.
- Offer the child choices; allow the child to choose what he or she wants from the menu.
- Talk with the dietitian to see if any special preferences can be addressed.
- Offer praise to your child for what he or she eats or drinks.
- Never punish the child for not eating or drinking.
- Encourage the older child to help keep track of what he or she eats and drinks.

Providing Play, Activities, and Recreation for the Hospitalized Child

Play is an important component in the child's plan of care. Today, many health care settings providing care for children have playrooms with age-appropriate toys, equipment, and other creative activities (Fig. 33.6). If the facility is large enough, there may even be a separate area for teens where they can listen to music, play video games, and visit with peers.

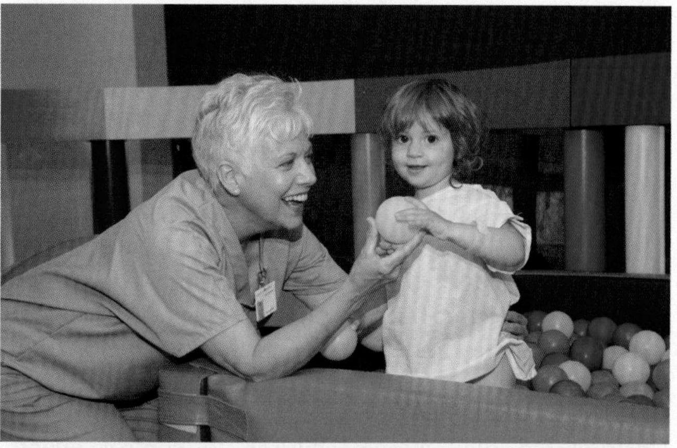

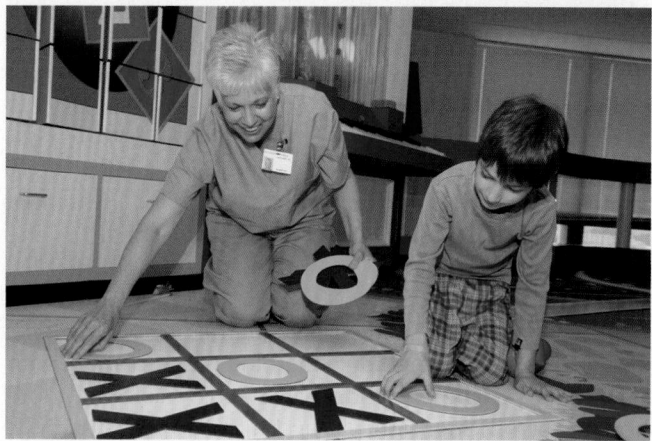

FIGURE 33.6 **Children occupied in a hospital playroom. It is important to provide age-appropriate activities for younger and older children alike.**

Take Note!

Avoid using the term "playroom" when caring for older school-aged children and adolescents. Instead, call it the "activity room" or "social room." Doing so promotes a greater feeling of maturity and makes it more likely that they will use the area.

Obviously, some children will not be able to use these facilities if their activity level is restricted or if isolation is necessary. Children may also play in their rooms. Ensure that opportunities for unstructured play are provided to all children who can engage in play. Therapeutic play may be used to teach children about their health status or to allow them to work through issues in their lives.

Take Note!

Keep the bed or crib and playroom as "safe" places. Perform invasive procedures such as venipunctures in the treatment room if possible. Never perform any nursing interventions in the playroom, no matter how nonthreatening they may appear to the nurse.

The nurse's greatest ally in the hospital in relation to atraumatic care is the CLS. They not only prepare the child for procedures but also provide activities and events to encourage play and normal growth and development.

UNSTRUCTURED PLAY

Unstructured play allows children to control events, ideas, and relationships. Encourage parents to bring small toys and favorite stuffed animals from home to make the child feel more comfortable in the strange environment of the hospital. Children also enjoy receiving small new toys as surprises when they are hospitalized. Many children enjoy diversional activities such as playing board games or electronic games, reading books, and watching TV, videos, or DVDs. Quiet activities appropriate to the child's developmental level provide the opportunity for play and encourage the use and development of fine motor skills even if the child is confined to bed. Infants and toddlers enjoy manipulating blocks and playing with stacking toys. The preschooler may enjoy coloring, dollhouses, or playing with plastic building blocks such as Legos. School-age children and adolescents may enjoy playing video games, putting together a puzzle, or building a model geared toward their developmental level.

PLAY AS PART OF NURSING CARE

Play is also an important part of nursing care. Use play as appropriate while providing routine nursing care to the child. An example of the use of play in nursing care involves the school-age child's love of competition and games. To increase range of motion in a school-age child who is hospitalized for traction due to a fracture, have the child throw a soft sponge ball or beanbag ball into a hoop, and compete against the child. To increase deep breathing, encourage the child to blow bubbles or blow a whistle. To increase intake of fluids, help the child create a graph to chart the number of glasses of fluids he or she drinks over a period of time. Award the child a sticker, baseball card, special pencil, or other small item if he or she reaches a certain level.

When using play as part of nursing care, it is important to evaluate the outcome of play. Play used in the manner described above should enhance the child's outcome. For example, for the child blowing bubbles, determine whether this activity enhanced coughing and deep breathing.

THERAPEUTIC PLAY

Another important aspect of play is therapeutic play. **Therapeutic play** is nondirected and focuses on helping the child cope with feelings and fears. Health care professionals use therapeutic play to help the child deal with the physical and psychological challenges of illness and hospitalization. Supervised play with medical equipment in the hospital environment can help children work through their feelings about what has happened to them (Fig. 33.7). In a large hospital or a children's hospital, the CLS typically coordinates these activities. Goals include maintaining normal living patterns, minimizing psychological trauma, and promoting optimal development of the child. If a CLS is not available, the nurse provides this type of activity. There is a greater emphasis on the developmental and psychosocial implications of illness and hospitalization and validation of the child's voice.

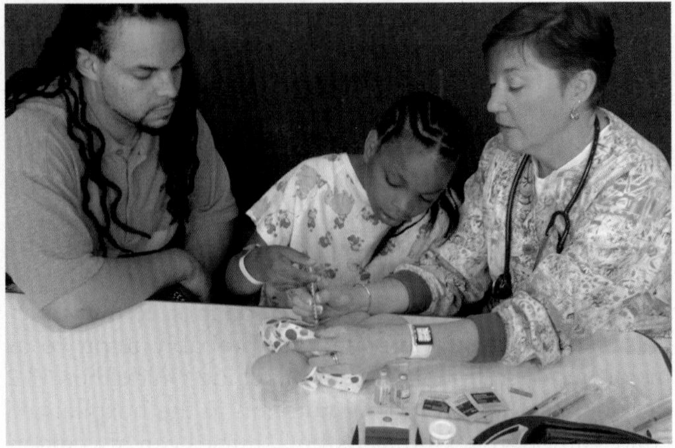

FIGURE 33.7 The nurse supervises play with medical equipment to help the child work through her feelings about being hospitalized.

In emotional outlet play or traumatic play, the child acts out or dramatizes real-life stressors. For example, using a wooden hammer and pegs, a soft sponge ball, or boxing gloves can allow the child to express anger over separation from family and friends. Commercial toys such as anatomically correct dolls and puppets have removable parts so children can see various organs of the body. Sometimes younger children "talk" to puppets and dolls, allowing them to express their feelings to a nonthreatening "person" about a specific situation or what they want from the health care provider. For example, the Shadow Buddies dolls mentioned earlier in the chapter provide a way of coping with a specific condition. The company creates an ostomy buddy who has a stoma, a cancer buddy with thinning hair and a chest catheter for chemotherapy treatments, and a heart buddy who has a chest incision and a repaired heart (Shadow Buddies Foundation, 2014).

Other types of therapeutic play include drawing and supervised "needle play." Drawing is a way for the child to express his or her thoughts and feelings. Supervised "needle play" assists children who must undergo frequent blood work, injections, or intravenous procedures. A doll can receive an injection as the child works out his or her anger and anxiety. Keep in mind safety and the child's growth and development level before planning this type of directed play; an adult must always be present.

Promoting Schoolwork and Education During Hospitalization

Promote schoolwork while the child is in the hospital. Determine the amount of schoolwork that can be done by assessing the child's condition, the availability of teachers, and the family situation. Many children's hospitals have teachers at the hospitals; there may be classrooms too. These teachers work closely with the child's school to continue schoolwork as the child's condition permits. Hospitals without an educational staff will rely on parents to coordinate with the child's school. Parents may bring in schoolbooks and the child's homework for completion while in the hospital. This connection to the child's school helps maintain normalcy for the child and minimizes the disruption of everyday life. Nurses and other health care providers, such as social workers, should help facilitate this process.

Addressing the Needs of Family Members

Assess the factors that may influence the family's reaction to the child's hospitalization and plan the care of the child to accommodate some of these issues. Encourage families to have support systems in place before, during, and after hospitalization. The practice of family-centered care, including good communication and ensuring nursing actions, addresses the child's and family's needs and preferences and increases the child's and parents' satisfaction with the health care setting (American Academy of Pediatrics, Committee on Hospital Care, Institute for Patient and Family-Centered Care, 2012).

PARENTS AND CAREGIVERS

As stated previously, the anxiety level of caregivers greatly affects the anxiety level of the child. Thus, it is important to help the family members work through their feelings. Parents experience many emotions when a child is hospitalized, including disbelief, anger, guilt, fear, anxiety, frustration, and depression. Visiting restrictions, unexpected changes in the child's health status, lack of information or understanding of their child's health condition, changes in their routine and roles, financial stress, and feelings of being undervalued in the care of their child all contribute to their feelings.

The importance of family involvement to the well-being of the child is reflected in the philosophies, policies, procedures, and physical environments where care is delivered. The philosophy of family-centered care places the family at the core of care. The family is the primary and continuing provider of care for the child. Encourage parents to room-in with the child throughout the hospital stay, if possible. Facilities can be designed to welcome family participation. For example, having computer ports, internet, and fax machines available and providing extra meals and beds for the parents can encourage parents to participate in care. View the parents as vital members of the health care team and partners in the care of the ill child.

SIBLINGS

Family-centered care recognizes the need to treat the child in context of the family, including siblings. Important questions that will affect how siblings deal with the hospitalization of their brother or sister include:

- Was the admission an emergency?
- Were there previous admissions, and how did the siblings perceive those hospitalizations?
- How serious is the illness or trauma?
- Is the prognosis known?

Address the siblings' possible feelings of guilt. Use educational materials, allow time for visits, send photographs back and forth between siblings, and allow siblings to talk on the phone.

Providing Child and Family Teaching

Not all experiences with hospitalization are negative; in fact, the experience may enhance the child's and family's coping skills, bolster self-esteem, and provide new socialization experiences. It may allow the child to master self-care skills and provides an opportunity for the child and family to learn new information. Parents may learn more about their child's growth and development skills as well as additional parenting or caregiving skills, resulting in improved parenting abilities. In addition, the child's overall health may be improved because of the hospital stay if the child receives current immunizations and the parents learn more about health care practices.

The overall goals of child and family teaching are to minimize the child's and family's stress, educate them about treatment and nursing care in the hospital, and ensure the family can provide appropriate care at home upon discharge. Providing support before, during, and after hospitalization may minimize stress. Preadmission programs can introduce the child and family to the setting. During the hospital stay, forming partnerships with the child and family, using strategies to promote coping, and providing appropriate preparation for procedures, tests, and surgery serve to decrease stress.

Assess the child's and family's knowledge of the illness and hospital experience. This provides a baseline for teaching. Include hospital rules in child and family teaching. Behavioral changes in hospitalized children often disturb parents or caregivers. Determine the child's usual patterns of behavior and explain to the parents about the child's reaction to hospitalization. Encourage the family to maintain consistent discipline even while in the hospital to provide structure for the child as well as to prevent discipline issues after discharge. Also discuss how siblings may react to the hospitalization, and provide appropriate teaching to the siblings. Every interaction the nurse has with the child or family provides an opportunity for teaching. Explain the purpose of even simple procedures such as vital signs assessment to the child and family. Provide ongoing information about the child's illness or trauma, treatment plan, and expected outcomes. Chapter 30 provides general principles related to teaching children and their families.

Preparing the Child and Family for Discharge

Discharge planning actually begins upon admission. The nurse assesses the family's resources and knowledge level to determine what education and referrals they may need. Upon discharge, children and their parents or caregivers receive written instructions about home care, and a copy is retained in the medical record. These instructions are individualized for the child. Generally, discharge instructions should include:

- Follow-up appointment information
- Guidelines about when to contact the physician or nurse practitioner (e.g., new or worsening symptoms or indications that the child is not improving)
- Diet
- Activity level allowed
- Medications, including dose, times to be given, route, adverse effects, and special instructions; any prescriptions should be included
- Information on additional treatments the child requires at home
- Specific dates for when the child may return to school or day care
- Names and phone numbers of agencies the family has been referred to, such as durable medical equipment providers

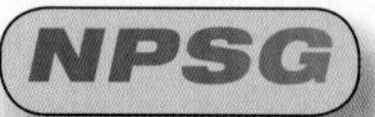

GOAL 3: Improve the Safety of Using Medications

NPSG 03.06.01 Maintain and communicate accurate patient medication information.

Steps: When discharging a child from the facility, be sure to provide accurate information and education concerning the child's medications to be taken at home. Refer to Chapter 35 for further information.

Joint Commission. (2015). *National patient safety goals effective January 1, 2015.* Retrieved from http://www.jointcommission.org/assets/1/6/2015_NPSG_HAP.pdf

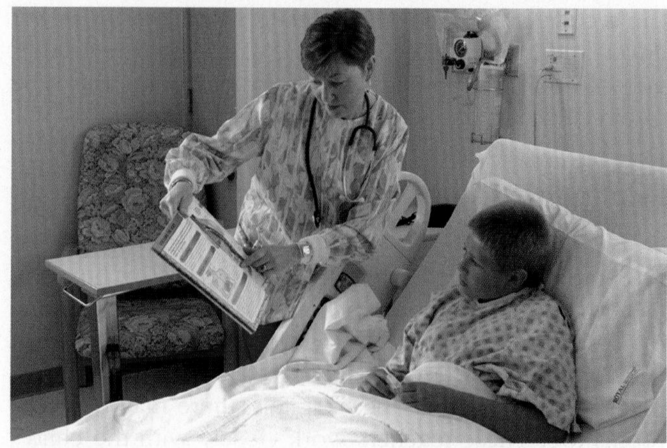

FIGURE 33.8 The nurse uses charts with pictures to perform client teaching before the child goes home.

Provide and review educational booklets that give basic health information or general care for a child with a particular disease (Fig. 33.8). Media such as videos or DVDs may also be used, if available. The ability to watch a procedure over and over is helpful to some families. Explain, demonstrate, and request a return demonstration of any treatments or procedures to be done at home. Provide a written schedule if the child is to receive multiple medications, tube feedings, or other medical treatments. For complicated cases, a written teaching plan may be used to provide continuity of child/family education between various nurses. As the family attempts to perform each task, document whether the caregiver continues to require assistance or prompting with the task or whether he or she can perform the task independently.

Parents of children with multiple medical needs may benefit from a trial period of home care. This occurs while the child is still in the hospital, but the parents or caregivers provide all of the care that the child requires. Support the family and praise their accomplishments during this trial period.

COMMUNITY CARE IN CHILDHOOD

Remember Jake Jorgenson, the boy with suspected brain tumor from the beginning of the chapter? After a long hospital stay and complications resulting from his brain tumor, Jake requires intermittent gastrostomy feedings and has frequent respiratory infections. He has been receiving nursing care at home along with therapies, but is now ready to make the transition to the local elementary school.

Children receive most of their health care, well and ill care, in the community setting. Nurses play an important role in the health and wellness of a community. They not only meet the health care needs of individuals but also go beyond to create interventions that affect the community as a whole. Community health nursing refers to nursing care that strives to improve the health of a specific community as a whole. For example, community health nurses working in the Department of Health and Human Services would strive to make sure that all children in their particular community were up-to-date on immunizations. Community-based nursing focuses more on providing care to the individual or family (which, of course, impacts the community) in settings outside of acute care. For example, a community-based nurse would work in the local public school to care for students' health needs. Nurses practicing in the community promote the health of individuals, families, groups, communities, and populations and promote an environment that supports health. See Chapter 2 for more information on Community Health and Community Based-Nursing. The following section focuses on community based settings where nurses commonly care for children.

Community-Based Nursing Settings

Community-based nursing takes place in a variety of settings, including outpatient and ambulatory care settings, physicians' offices, clinics, health departments, urgent care centers, schools, camps, churches, shelters, and clients' homes. Community-based nurses provide well care, episodic ill care, and chronic care. They work to promote, preserve, and improve the health of children and families in these settings.

OUTPATIENT AND AMBULATORY CARE

Outpatient and ambulatory care is health care provided to individuals who do not require care in an acute setting. Due to advances in medical technology, more medical procedures, such as diagnostic tests, treatments, and surgeries, can be administered on an outpatient basis and do not require clients to be hospitalized. Outpatient and ambulatory care delivers convenient and cost-effective health care to children and their families, many times right within their own community. These settings allow for increased independence and permit children to return to their normal routine as quickly as possible. More and more outpatient and ambulatory care centers are opening, sponsored by health maintenance organizations (HMOs), physicians' groups, community agencies and public health departments, and hospitals.

Outpatient units are used to keep hospital stays short and decrease the cost of hospitalization. Outpatient units may be a part of the hospital or a freestanding facility. The child and family arrive in the morning; the child undergoes the procedure, test, or surgery, and then goes home in the evening. Examples of surgeries and procedures performed in outpatient settings include tympanostomy tube placement, hernia repair, tonsillectomy, cystoscopy, bronchoscopy, blood transfusions, dialysis, and chemotherapy. The advantages of this environment include minimal separation of the child from the family, minimal disruption of the family pattern, decreased risk of infection, and decreased cost. Disadvantages include that the unit does not have the equipment for overnight stays, so if there are complications the child will need to be transported to the hospital.

Many centers offer preoperative health assessment and teaching sessions. These allow the parent and child to ask questions and resolve them before the procedure. On the day of the procedure, parents should be allowed to be with their child until the procedure begins. Parents should also be allowed to be with their child in the postanesthesia recovery unit as quickly as possible. This provides reassurance and comfort to the child while meeting his or her physical and emotional needs.

The role of the nurse in the outpatient or ambulatory setting includes admission and assessment, preoperative teaching and preparation, client assessment and support, postoperative monitoring, case management, discharge planning, and teaching. Before the procedure the nurse reviews with the family the routine to be followed and any special instructions (such as NPO orders), and familiarizes the child with the setting to help alleviate fears. This may occur during the preoperative health assessment.

Take Note!

Encourage the parent to bring one of the child's favorite toys, blankets, or games to make the child feel more comfortable.

The nurse performs any surgical preparation and discusses intraoperative procedures as necessary. The nurse provides postoperative care and assessment of the child. Once the child's condition is stable and he or she meets the discharge criteria of the facility, the nurse reviews with the parent postoperative instructions, including pain management; care of the incision if appropriate; diet; activity, including return to school; necessary follow-up; and when to call the physician or nurse practitioner.

PHYSICIAN'S OFFICE OR CLINIC, HEALTH DEPARTMENTS, AND URGENT CARE CENTERS

Physicians' offices, clinics, health departments, and urgent care centers are used by children and their families for well care, episodic ill care, acute care, and care of chronic conditions. For well care and illness or injury, children are often seen by their primary care physician. They may visit a physician's office or clinic or the health department. In more acute situations or for after-hours issues that cannot wait until clinic operating hours, a child may be seen in an urgent care center or may be referred to the emergency department. The American Academy of Pediatrics discourages children and families from using urgent care centers or the emergency department for routine care, since it is difficult to provide coordinated, comprehensive family-centered care consistent with a "medical home" concept (see Chapter 31 on medical homes) (American Academy of Pediatrics, Committee on Pediatric Emergency Medicine, 2011).

The nurse's role in these settings includes preparing clients, collecting pertinent health information, performing assessments, assisting the physician with diagnostic testing and procedures, administering injections and medications, changing wound dressings, assisting with minor surgery, helping to maintain records, and educating the child and family about home care and when to call the physician or nurse practitioner or return to be seen.

An essential component of primary care practice is telephone triage. Pediatric office nurses often fill this role. When parents feel comfortable with the providers in their child's medical home office, they often call for advice in order to treat their child at home. A telephone triage nurse needs excellent assessment and critical thinking skills along with solid training and education. The triage nurse needs to assess the child's entire situation, including current signs and symptoms, history, and home treatment.

Protocols, standardized policies and procedures, and professional judgment guide the triage nurse in the decision-making process. Pediatric telephone protocols are available for purchase through the American Academy of Pediatrics (http://www.aap.org/). The triage nurse needs to determine whether the child requires emergency care, an office visit, or home management. Good listening and the ability to maintain a calm voice when talking to parents are skills necessary for successful telephone triage. The triage nurse should not discourage parents from bringing the child into the office to be seen; triage is not meant to keep children out of the office, and if a parent is very concerned, that is reason enough to be seen.

Take Note!

Parents often can pick up on subtle problems in their children. They may not be able to accurately describe signs and symptoms, but they know that their child "isn't acting right." Nurses must listen to parents and act on their concerns.

MEDICALLY FRAGILE DAY CARE CENTERS

The **medically fragile child**, recently termed *child with medical complexity,* is defined as a child with "substantial health care needs, one or more chronic conditions, functional limitations often associated with technology assistance, and health care use" (Elias, Murphy, & the Council on Children with Disabilities, 2012 p. 997) The number of medically fragile children is growing. Reasons include improvements in the treatment and care of complex medical conditions, increased sophistication of medical technology, and the increase in premature deliveries (Cohen et al., 2011). For many years these children lived in hospitals their entire lives. Due to concerns about the high cost of long-term hospitalization and the diminished quality of life for these children, alternative care settings in the community, such as medically fragile day care centers, are being developed.

Medically fragile day care centers are specifically designed to meet the needs of these children. Most centers accept children who have complicated medical needs or are dependent on technology. Examples include children with multiple congenital anomalies, children who are ventilator dependent, children with respiratory conditions, children with cardiac conditions, and children with cancer. Some centers accept children with less complicated needs, such as cardiorespiratory monitoring or asthma, and some enroll children without health care needs to promote peer relationships and acceptance. Just as at a regular day care center, the parents or caregivers can drop the child off in the morning and pick the child up in the afternoon. Some centers offer after-school, weekend, or respite services. The centers usually provide needed therapies and have indoor and outdoor play areas, educational activities, and arts and crafts.

Health professionals are present at these centers to provide for the children's medical, emotional, and developmental needs. Nurses trained in pediatric and neonatal care, physical therapists, occupational therapists, speech therapists, CLSs, and social workers staff the centers; some centers have respiratory therapists on site. Children are able to receive all of their prescribed therapies while at the center. Nursing care includes direct care such as administering medication and changing dressings, assessing and evaluating the child's overall condition, identifying potential medical emergencies, determining the need for changes in care or treatment and monitoring, and providing frequent treatments or interventions to maintain life and health.

Most centers are located in the community to help ease transportation issues. Some centers provide transportation to and from home or school. Centers are licensed by the state day care licensing authorities or, in some states, prescribed pediatric extended care (PPEC) agencies. Families may be able to obtain financial assistance from their private insurance or Medicaid. Advantages of community-based services over hospitalization or home care include decreased cost, social isolation, family stress, and rehospitalization rate (Rupert & Host, 2009; Murphy, Carbone, & Council on Children With Disabilities, 2011).

SCHOOLS

School nursing is a specialized practice of professional nursing and focuses on improving students' health and safety to improve their achievement and success. School nurses work to remove or minimize health barriers to learning to provide students with the best opportunity to achieve academic success. The National Association of School Nurses defines school nursing as follows:

"A specialized practice of professional nursing that advances the well-being, academic success, and life-long achievement of students. To that end, school nurses facilitate positive student responses to normal development; promote health and safety; intervene with actual and potential health problems; provide case management services; and actively collaborate with others to build student and family capacity for adaptation, self management, self-advocacy, and learning" (National Association of Nurses, 2010). See Healthy People 2020.

HEALTHY PEOPLE 2020

Objective	Nursing Significance
Increase the proportion of elementary, middle, and senior high schools that provide comprehensive school health education to prevent health problems in the following areas: unintentional injury; violence; suicide; tobacco use and addiction; alcohol or other drug use; unintended pregnancy, HIV/AIDS, and STD infection; unhealthy dietary patterns; and inadequate physical activity	• Provide education and training to school staff in health problem areas • Work with schools to develop appropriate health education with focus on health problem areas • Provide adequate health care services and health education to students
Increase the proportion of elementary, middle, and senior high schools that provide school health education to promote personal health and wellness in the following areas: hand washing or hand hygiene; oral health; growth and development; sun safety and skin cancer prevention; benefits of rest and sleep; ways to prevent vision and hearing loss; and the importance of health screenings and check-ups	
Increase the proportion of elementary, middle, and senior high schools that have a full-time registered school nurse-to-student ratio of at least 1:750	

Healthy People Objectives retrieved from http://www.healthypeople.gov

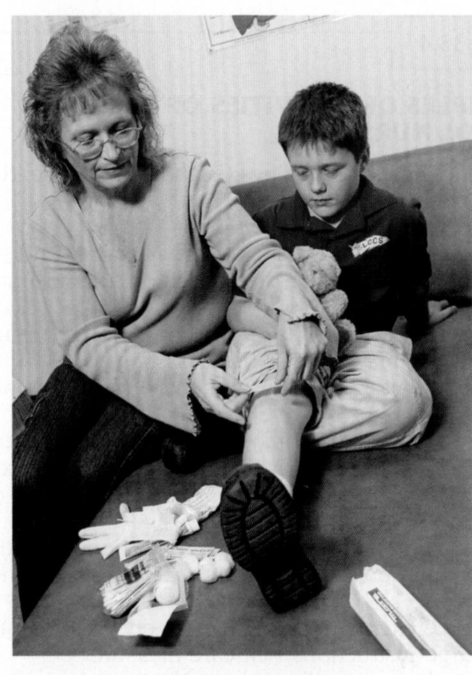

FIGURE 33.9 The school nurse provides nursing assessment as well as health education to students in the school setting.

School nurses provide direct health care to students along with screening and referrals for health conditions. They provide leadership for health services, such as identifying health and safety concerns in the school environment and planning and training for emergencies and disasters. School nurses promote a healthy school environment by supporting healthy food services and promoting proper physical education and sports policies and practices. They promote health education through health counseling and education of students and staff. School nurses coordinate school health programs and link health service programs within the school and community. School nurses carry out a variety of roles in providing health care to children (Fig. 33.9). Box 33.4 lists some of the activities of the school nurse.

The population of students has changed over the years. Access to public schools for children with disabilities is mandated. Due to improvements in technology, children with chronic conditions or special needs live longer and enter school. There has been an increase in the number of children with psychiatric conditions such as depression, attention deficit/hyperactivity disorder, and more serious conditions such as bipolar disorder. All have contributed to an increase in the number of children with diverse and sometimes complex health needs in the school system. The essential role of the school nurse has not changed, but the responsibilities and expectations have. School nurses are challenged to meet the growing needs of the changing school population.

BOX 33.4

EXAMPLES OF ACTIVITIES OF THE SCHOOL NURSE

- Conduct health screenings (such as vision, hearing, and scoliosis)
- Assess growth and development
- Provide emergency first aid, care for acute and chronic illnesses, such as medication administration and diabetes monitoring
- Train and educate staff on cardiopulmonary resuscitation (CPR), first aid, and health issues
- Assess, monitor, and refer students with communicable diseases
- Educate on health promotion and disease prevention (such as immunizations; bike and car safety; decreasing high-risk behaviors, such as smoking, drinking, drug use, and sexual activity)
- Serve as a resource for health issues and education
- Act as a liaison between health care provider and school
- Reinforce client and family health education (such as discharge instructions, self-care measures)
- Monitor long-term illness in students
- Network with community agencies and make necessary referrals

Recall Jake Jorgensen, the 8-year-old boy with history of a brain tumor and resulting complex medical needs? In recent years there have been many more children with special needs attending school than ever before. This brings many challenges for the teachers, staff, and school nurses employed by the school district. The principal of Jake's elementary school tells the school nurse that many of the teachers and staff have expressed concerns that they do not know anything about the health care needs of these children, including Jake. What kinds of interventions might the nurse plan?

Just as nurses in the acute care setting develop nursing care plans, nurses in the school setting develop **Individualized Health Plans** (IHPs). An IHP formalizes the plan of support for a student with complex health care needs. It is a written agreement developed as part of an interdisciplinary collaboration of school staff along with the student, the student's family, and the student's health care provider. The plan describes the student's needs and how the school plans to meet these needs. The nurse plays a critical role in developing these plans. The nurse will use the nursing process and then, based on the nursing assessment and diagnosis, will develop goals and interventions to ensure that the child's needs are being met. Examples of students who may need an IHP are students with asthma, serious allergies, chronic conditions such as type 1 diabetes, physical disabilities, attention deficit/hyperactivity disorder, and medication needs. Figure 33.10 gives an example of an IHP for a child with asthma.

Take Note!

The IHP needs to include directions for care while the child is at school and also must take into account circumstances that may affect the student's health care needs, such as variations in school routine, absence of staff, special outings such as field trips and extracurricular activities, and a plan in case of emergency.

OTHER COMMUNITY SETTINGS

Nurses work in a variety of different settings within the community. Their primary focus continues to be on promoting health, preventing disease and injury, and ensuring a safe environment. Nurses play important roles in child care centers, camps, health department clinics, and shelters. In child care centers, nurses help address infection control issues and assess for a safe environment. They provide education and training to staff members. A camp nurse ensures a safe environment for all campers and provides first-aid and acute illness care as needed. Camps for children with special needs exist, staffed by specially trained nurses. These camps cater to children with complex health care needs, such as diabetes, cancer, head injuries, and physical disabilities, and allow the children the opportunity to experience camp life while providing a safe environment and necessary medical care. Health department and shelter nurses focus on health supervision services and connecting clients to needed community resources.

Take Note!

Nurses have a unique opportunity to give back to their community by volunteering their services in various settings, such as shelters and clinics in medically underserved areas.

HOME HEALTH CARE

Home care provides short- or long-term services for children and their families in the home. It also is used for medically needy and technology-dependent children, such as ventilator-dependent children. Among those who often benefit from home care are children with acute illness, such as a child with osteomyelitis requiring intravenous antibiotics, or chronic health care issues, such as a child with bronchopulmonary dysplasia, who may have required traditional in-hospital care.

Home care is geared toward the needs of the child and family. Private-duty nursing care is used when more extensive care is needed; it may be delivered hourly (several hours per day) or on a full-time, live-in basis. Periodic visiting nurse care is used when the child needs intermittent interventions such as intravenous antibiotic administration, follow-up with child and family teaching, and periodic monitoring, such as bilirubin monitoring. The goals of nursing care in the home setting include promoting, restoring, and maintaining the health of the child. Home care focuses on minimizing the effects of the illness or disability, along with providing the child or family with the means to care for the illness or disability at home. Nurses in the home care setting are direct

Example Individualized Healthcare Plan

Name:

Address:
Home Phone:
Parent/Guardian:
Day/Work Phone:
Healthcare Provider:
Provider's Phone:
IHP Written by:

Birthdate:

School:
Teacher/Counselor:
Grade:
IHP Date:
IEP Date:
Review Dates:
ICD-9 Codes:

Assessment Data	Nursing Diagnosis	Student Goals	Interventions	Outcomes
	Risk for Ineffective Breathing (NANDA 1.5.1.3)		**Airway Management (NIC 2K-3140)** **Activities:**	Symptom Control Behavior (NOC 4Q-1608) Indicators:
12-year-old diagnosed asthma at age 9	Characterized by shortness of breath, coughing, and/or wheezing related to asthma	Student will demonstrate appropriate use of inhaler at the beginning of school year.	Review use of inhaler with student at the beginning of the school year (Nurse).	Recognizes symptom onset **Never** 1 **Rarely** 2 **Sometimes** 3 **Often** 4 **Consistently** 5
Carries Proventil inhaler at all times		Student will initiate treatment when symptoms appear throughout the school year.	At the beginning of the school year, review with teacher, and other appropriate staff, the signs and symptoms of asthma exacerbation and when student should use inhaler (Nurse).	Uses preventative measures **Never** 1 **Rarely** 2 **Sometimes** 3 **Often** 4 **Consistently** 5
Independent in identifying symptoms and need for treatment		Student will keep record of peak flow meter readings if required throughout the school year.	Every two months obtain student's record of inhaler use for documentation in health file. Report increased use of inhaler to parents/physician (Nurse).	Uses relief measures **Never** 1 **Rarely** 2 **Sometimes** 3 **Often** 4 **Consistently** 5
M.D. order normal P.E. program		Student will keep record of use of inhaler for health office throughout the school year.	**Emergency plan:** See STUDENT ASTHMA ACTION CARD located in the classroom, locker room, and health office.	Reports controlling symptoms **Never** 1 **Rarely** 2 **Sometimes** 3 **Often** 4 **Consistently** 5
		Student will avoid having an emergency asthma attack during this school year.		

I have read and approve of the above plan for school healthcare:

Parent signature

Date reviewed by the educational team

Nurse signature

Physician signature (optional)

FIGURE 33.10 Example of an individualized health plan. (Adapted from Arnold, M. J., & Silkworth, C. K. [1999]. *The school nurse's source book of individualized healthcare plans: Issues applications in school nursing practice*, Vol. II. North Branch, MN: Sunrise River Press; and Zentner-Schoessler, S. [1997]. *Computerized version and manual*, Vol. I. North Branch, MN: Sunrise River Press.)

providers of care, child and family educators, child and family advocates, and case managers.

There are some disadvantages to home care. The presence of health care professionals in the home can be an intrusion on family privacy. Also, caring for children with complex medical needs can be overwhelming for some families. Financial issues can become a large burden: families may have higher out-of-pocket costs if their insurance does not reimburse for home care. Having one parent at home full time and not earning an income can contribute to increased financial strain, not to mention social isolation of that parent. All of these can lead to increased stress on family members. The advantages of home care usually outweigh the disadvantages, but nurses need to be aware of these potential disadvantages and provide support and resources as necessary.

Family-Centered Home Care. Family-centered care is a challenging pediatric nursing philosophy and is driven by evidence that a nurturing environment improves the chances of positive outcomes for the child. It places the family in a central position relative to the child and to the child's plan of care. Refer to Chapter 30 for further information regarding family-centered care.

Family-centered home care focuses on increasing support for the emotional and developmental needs of the child. It encourages families to care for their children at home while health care professionals provide the support, empowerment, education, and expertise in caring for the child that they need. In family-centered home care, the family and health care professionals build a partnership of trust to meet the needs of the child. The nurse must value the role of the family and regard family members as the ultimate experts in caring for their child. In home care the family is extensively involved in the child's care, and the home care nurse is there to facilitate this.

Any illness, especially a chronic illness, affects the entire family and can disrupt family structure. There is a change in the role of the parent when he or she has to care for an ill child. These role changes can result in stress for the family members and can affect their participation in the child's care. It is important for home care nurses to seek a partnership role with the family regarding care of the child. This can be difficult for both parties. Many times, nurses set limits on parental involvement and do not consider the parents' perspective. Many nurses are concerned that the parents may not be able to care for the child safely. It is important for nurses to use self-awareness and reflective practice to help them understand and empower families as well as to develop a partnership for care. A communication framework, developed by Berlin & Fowkes (1983), that can assist nurses in the home care setting is the LEARN framework, which can help create cross-cultural collaboration and communication between nurses and families (Box 33.5).

BOX 33.5

LEARN FRAMEWORK

- L: Listen empathetically and with understanding to the family's perception of the situation.
- E: Explain your perception of the situation.
- A: Acknowledge and discuss the similarities as well as differences between the two perceptions.
- R: Recommend interventions.
- N: Negotiate and agree on the interventions.

From Berlin, E. A., & Fowkes, W. C. (1983). A teaching framework for cross-cultural health care—Application to practice. *The Western Journal of Medicine, 139*(6), 934–938.

The Nurse's Role in Home Care. Early discharge planning, teaching, and case management are keys to promoting a successful transition from the hospital setting to home. The environment differs greatly between the acute setting and home setting. In the acute setting the nurse is in control of the environment; in the home setting, the nurse is a guest in the home. It is important for the nurse to establish a trusting relationship with both the child and family (Fig. 33.11). A trusting therapeutic relationship will make all aspects of care more effective. Box 33.6 gives hints on building this relationship.

Nursing in the home care setting can be challenging. The focus is on meeting the child's physical and psychological needs while involving the family. In meeting the child's needs while involving the family, the nurse uses the nursing process. Assessment in the home is similar to that in the acute care setting but involves obtaining first-hand data about the family and the way it functions. The nurse needs to assess the child's growth and development and thoroughly assess the home environment (refer Chapters 26 to 29 and 31 for additional information). The nurse needs to ensure that home offers a safe and nurturing environment for the child. The National Center for Healthy Housing provides online training for community health workers and has developed a

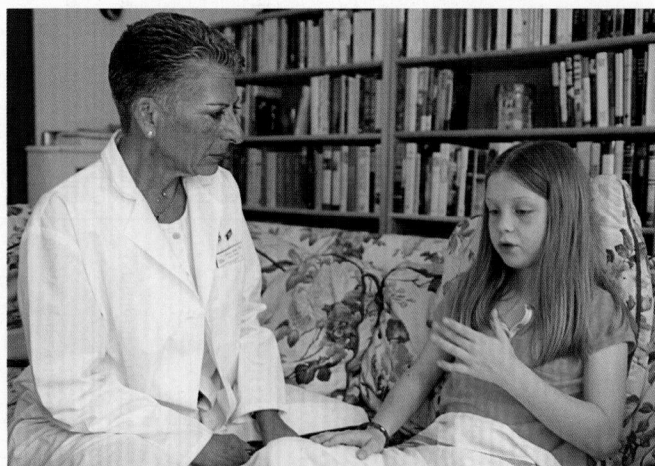

FIGURE 33.11 Listening to the child helps to develop a trusting relationship between the home care nurse and the child and her family.

BOX 33.6

HINTS TO ESTABLISHING A TRUSTING RELATIONSHIP IN HOME CARE

- Include the child in the conversation and make him or her feel a part of the interaction.
- Address caregivers formally unless otherwise instructed.
- Be friendly. Use a soft, calm voice.
- Be interested in the child's activities.
- Have the primary caregiver present at the initial visit.
- Listen to and show respect to the child and the family.

Pediatric Environmental Home Assessment (PEHA) Survey and PEHA nursing care plan to assist in identifying and addressing hazards or potential threats that exist in the child's home (National Center for Healthy Housing, n.d.; National Center for Healthy Housing, 2006). These forms can be accessed from a link on thePoint. The nurse should always individualize these forms to meet the needs and requirements of his or her client and facility.

The nurse also needs to assess availability of resources. This includes necessary equipment such as a hospital bed and oxygen, suitable physical and emotional surroundings (are the family members able to deal with the stress of the situation?), ability to contact emergency services, power backup if needed, and ease of evacuation of the child in case of a fire. The nurse needs to assess whether electricity, sanitary conditions, heat, air conditioning, and telephone access are present. If there is no phone in the home, the family needs to have plans for accessing a phone in case of emergency (perhaps a neighbor's phone or a pay phone near the home). The nurse should identify areas of priority and provide appropriate referrals to resources.

During the assessment phase the nurse identifies the person who is the primary caregiver; this may be the mother, father, grandparent, or older sibling. It is essential to include this person when developing the plan of care, as he or she is the expert on the child and family. The primary caregiver can provide insight into direct care and which strategies will be most effective with this child, taking into account the physical layout of the home, the financial ability of the family, and the way the family functions. The home care nurse must also assess the family's teaching and learning needs.

After the assessment is complete, the nurse develops appropriate nursing diagnoses, outcomes, and goals and implements the plan of care. This will include the frequency and duration of the home visits. The nurse will consider the individual needs of each patient in conjunction with state, federal, and agency policies, certification standards, and payer guidelines from private insurance and/or Medicaid regulations to assist in the development of the plan. The nurse may be the provider of direct care to the child, or the care may be indirect, in which case the nurse plans and supervises the care that is given by others, such as unlicensed personnel and parents.

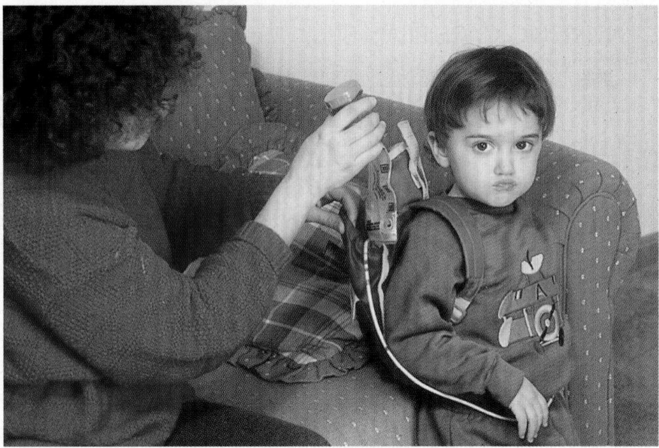

FIGURE 33.12 The home care nurse may have to adjust procedures and equipment use to fit the home setting. Placing a feeding pump in a backpack allows this child to receive feedings continuously while at school.

Nursing care in the home requires excellent critical thinking skills. The nurse has a great deal of independence since there are no other nurses, supervisors, or physicians on site. When complex care is provided in the home, the nurse may need to adjust procedures to fit the setting. For example, feeding schedules may be adjusted to fit a child's school schedule or equipment may be adjusted to allow a child to receive feedings continuously while at school (Fig. 33.12).

An important role of the home care nurse is empowering children and their families through education (refer to Chapter 30 for further information related to teaching). The nurse assesses the learning needs and provides education that is appropriate to the educational and developmental levels of the child and family. The nurse must encourage the family to participate in the child's care. The education goals of home care vary. In many situations parents or caregivers must learn care immediately so the child can be cared for at home, such as a child who needs dressing changes four times a day or a child who is ventilator dependent. A child newly diagnosed with diabetes will have some immediate teaching needs, but as the child grows and his or her condition changes, additional care will need to be taught.

As with any nursing care, the effectiveness of nursing interventions along with changes in the child's or family's status needs to be continuously evaluated and the plan of care altered as needed.

As the home care nurse, what can you do to help with Jake's transition to school? On your last visit, Jake's parents expressed concerns about this transition and the added stress it is causing to the family. They appear tired from the round-the-clock care that Jake requires. What suggestions can you make to help ease their stress and fatigue?

NURSING CARE PLAN 33.1

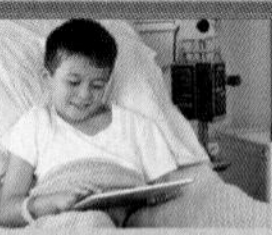

Overview for the Hospitalized Child and Family

NURSING DIAGNOSIS: Anxiety related to hospital situation, fear of injury or bodily mutilation, separation from family or friends, changes in routine, painful procedures and treatments, and unfamiliar events and surroundings as evidenced by crying, fussing, withdrawal, or resistance

Outcome Identification and Evaluation

Child and family will exhibit a decrease in anxiety level as evidenced by positive coping strategies, verbalization or playing out of feelings, appropriate behaviors, positive interactions with staff, child and parent cooperation and participation, and absence of signs and symptoms of increasing anxiety and fear.

Interventions: *Minimizing Anxiety*

- Orient child and family to the unit and the child's room *to familiarize them with the facility.*
- Assess for signs and symptoms of anxiety and fear *to establish a baseline and assess effectiveness of interventions.*
- Place the child in a room with another child of a similar age, developmental level, and condition severity *to promote sharing.*
- Provide atraumatic care *to minimize exposure to distress, which would increase anxiety.*
- Explain all events, treatments, procedures, and activities to the parents and child (at a level the child can understand) in a calm, relaxed manner *to help the child prepare for what is to come and decrease fear of the unknown. A calm, relaxed manner helps to establish rapport and instill trust.*
- Enlist the aid of a CLS *to assist in age-appropriate preparation for all events, treatments, and procedures.*
- Encourage parents to room-in if possible *to provide the child with support;* if parents cannot stay, encourage them to call *to reduce child's fear of being alone.*
- Urge parents to inform the child when they will be leaving and when they are expected to return *to help child cope with their absence and promote trust.*
- Assess child's usual routine at home and attempt to incorporate aspects of usual routine into hospital routine *to ease the transition to the hospital and promote the child's participation in routine.*
- Offer comfort measures such as holding, stroking, and rocking *to relieve distress.*
- Encourage the child to play (unstructured and therapeutic play as necessary) *to allow for expression of feelings and fears and promote energy expenditure.*
- Suggest that parents bring in a special toy or object from home *to promote feelings of security.*
- Provide positive reinforcement for participation in care activities *to foster self-esteem.*
- Assess for regression behaviors and inform parents that such behaviors are common *to alleviate their concerns about this behavior.*
- Provide consistency with care measures *to facilitate trust and acceptance.*

NURSING DIAGNOSIS: Risk for powerlessness (risk factors: lack of control over procedures, treatments, and care, changes in usual routine, continual hospital readmissions)

Outcome Identification and Evaluation

Child and family will demonstrate an increase in control over the situation as evidenced by participation in care activities, identification of needs and choices, and incorporation of appropriate aspects of child's usual routine with that of the hospital routine.

Interventions: *Promoting Control*

- Encourage child and parents to identify areas of concern *to help determine priority needs.*
- Encourage parent and child to participate in care activities *to promote feelings of control.*
- Incorporate aspects of child's routine at home and use terms similar to those used at home *to foster a sense of normalcy.*
- Offer child choices as much as possible, such as options for foods, drinks, hygiene, activities, or clothing (if appropriate) *to promote feelings of individuality and control.*

NURSING CARE PLAN 33.1

Overview for the Hospitalized Child and Family (continued)

- Allow child opportunities for being out of bed or room within limitations as appropriate *to foster independence.*
- Work with child, as age and development allow, and family to set up a schedule *to promote structure and routine.*

NURSING DIAGNOSIS: Deficient diversional activity related to confinement in bed or health care facility, lack of appropriate stimulation from toys or peers, limited mobility, activity restrictions, or equipment as evidenced by verbalization of boredom or lack of participation in play, reading, or schoolwork.

Outcome Identification and Evaluation

Child will participate in diversional activities as evidenced by engagement in unstructured and therapeutic play that is developmentally appropriate and interaction with family, staff, and other children.

Interventions: *Promoting Adequate Diversional Activities*

- Question child and family about favorite types of activities *to establish a baseline for developing appropriate choices during hospitalization.*
- Assist with planning activities within the limits of the child's condition *to maintain muscle tone and strength without overexerting the child.*
- Spend time with the child *to provide stimulation and foster trust.*
- Enlist the aid of a CLS *to provide suggestions for appropriate activities.*
- Encourage interaction with other children *to promote sharing and avoid loneliness.*
- Provide developmentally appropriate opportunities for unstructured and therapeutic play *to facilitate expression of feelings.*
- Encourage short trips to the playroom or activity room *to provide a change of scenery and sensory stimulation.*
- Integrate play activities with nursing care *to achieve therapeutic effect.*

NURSING DIAGNOSIS: Interrupted family processes related to separation from child due to hospitalization, increased demands of caring for an ill child, changes in role function and routine, and effect of hospitalization on other family members such as siblings, as evidenced by parental verbalization of issues, parental presence in hospital, or child's hospitalization requiring parent to miss work.

Outcome Identification and Evaluation

Family will demonstrate positive coping strategies and mutual support for one another as evidenced by visiting frequently and staying with the child as necessary, sharing of family responsibilities, obtaining assistance for relief or respite, and visiting by other members of the child's family and friends.

Interventions: *Maximizing Family Functioning*

- Encourage parents and family members to verbalize concerns about child's illness, diagnosis, and prognosis *to promote family-centered care and identify areas where intervention may be needed.*
- Explain therapies, procedures, child's behaviors, and plan of care to parents *to promote understanding of the child's status and plan of care, which helps to decrease anxiety.*
- Encourage parental involvement in care *to promote feelings of the parents being needed and valued, providing them with a sense of control over their child's health.*
- Identify support system for family and child *to identify resources available for coping.*

(continued)

NURSING CARE PLAN 33.1

Overview for the Hospitalized Child and Family (continued)

- Educate family and child on additional resources available *to promote a wider base of support to deal with the situation.*
- Suggest ways that parents can divide time between child and other siblings *to prevent feelings of guilt.*
- Provide support and positive reinforcement *to promote family coping and foster family strength.*
- Encourage frequent visits by family members, including siblings as appropriate, *to promote ongoing family functioning.*
- Stress the need for adequate rest, sleep, exercise, and nutrition for family members *to promote family health and minimize stress of hospitalization on family.*
- Assist with referrals for resources and help from additional family members and friends as necessary *to allow for respite or relief of care responsibilities.*
- Encourage family to maintain usual routine as much as possible *to minimize the effects of hospitalization on family functioning.*
- Enlist the aid of a CLS to work with any siblings *to provide support and education and to address the needs of a sibling of a hospitalized child.*

NURSING DIAGNOSIS: Self-care deficit related to immobility, activity restrictions, regression, or use of equipment, devices, or prescribed treatments as evidenced by inability to feed, bathe, or dress self or accomplish other activities of daily living.

Outcome Identification and Evaluation

Child will participate in self-care within limitations of condition as evidenced by assisting with bathing and hygiene, feeding, toileting, and dressing and grooming.

Interventions: *Promoting Self-Care*

- Assess child's usual routine for self-care and self-care abilities *to provide a baseline for individualizing interventions.*
- Provide child-sized equipment and devices *to promote child's ability to complete the self-care task.*
- Encourage parents and child to do as much self-care as possible, within limitations of the child's condition and developmental level, *to promote feelings of independence and foster growth and development.*
- Offer praise and encouragement for activities performed *to foster self-esteem, confidence, and competence.*
- Ensure adequate rest periods *to minimize energy expenditure associated with self-care activities.*

NURSING DIAGNOSIS: Risk for delayed development (risk factors: stressors associated with hospitalization, current condition or illness, separation from family, and sensory overload or sensory deprivation).

Outcome Identification and Evaluation

Child will demonstrate developmentally appropriate milestones as evidenced by age-appropriate behaviors and activities.

NURSING CARE PLAN 33.1

Overview for the Hospitalized Child and Family (continued)

Interventions: ***Promoting Growth and Development***

- Assess child's developmental stage *to establish a baseline and determine appropriate strategies.*
- Use unstructured and therapeutic play and adaptive toys *to promote developmental functioning.*
- Provide stimulating environment when possible *to maximize potential for growth and development.*
- Praise accomplishments and emphasize child's abilities *to foster self-esteem and encourage feelings of confidence and competence.*
- Include parents in techniques to foster growth and development *to promote feelings of control in their child's care.*

NURSING DIAGNOSIS: Deficient knowledge related to hospitalization, surgery, treatments, procedures, required care, and follow-up as evidenced by questioning and verbalization, lack of prior exposure.

Outcome Identification and Evaluation

Child and family will demonstrate understanding of all aspects of child's current situation as evidenced by identification of child's and family's needs, verbal statements of understanding and/or need for additional information, return demonstration of procedures and treatments, and verbalization of instructions for follow-up and continued care.

Interventions: ***Providing Child and Family Teaching***

- Assess child's and family's willingness to learn *to ensure effective teaching.*
- Provide family with time to adjust to diagnosis *to facilitate their ability to learn and participate in the child's care.*
- Repeat information *to promote multiple opportunities for child and family to learn.*
- Teach in short sessions *to prevent overloading the child and parents with information.*
- Gear teaching to appropriate level of understanding for the child and the family (depends on age of child, physical condition, memory) *to promote learning.*
- Provide reinforcement and rewards *to facilitate the teaching/learning process.*
- Use multiple modes of learning, such as written information, verbal instruction, demonstrations, and media, when possible *to facilitate learning and retention of information.*
- Provide the child and family with written step-by-step instructions for procedures or care *to provide a reference, if needed, at a later date.*
- Have child and family provide return demonstrations of care procedures *to ensure effectiveness of teaching.*
- Arrange for trial home care during hospitalization and after discharge as appropriate *to ensure understanding and provide opportunities for additional teaching and learning.*

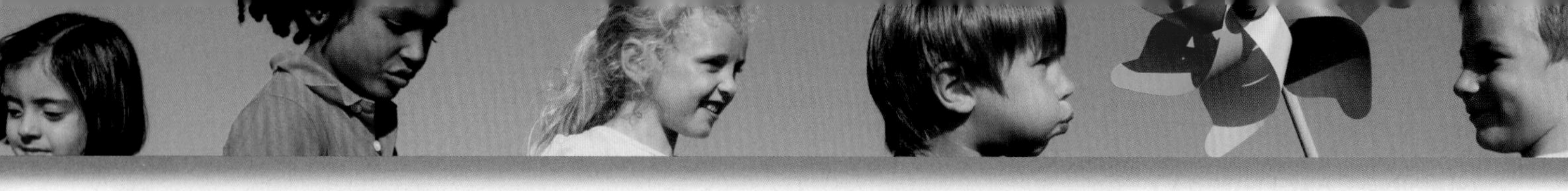

KEY CONCEPTS

- Stressors associated with hospitalization include separation from family and routines; fear of an unknown environment; potential for pain, bodily injury, or mutilation; and loss of control.
- Responses of children to the general stressors of hospitalization include anxiety, fear, anger, guilt, and regression.
- Parents may experience anger or guilt related to the hospitalization of their child.
- The responses of children and families to hospitalization can be influenced by the age and developmental level of the child, their perceptions of the situation, previous experiences, separation from family and peers, coping skills, and the preparation and support provided by the family, facility, and health care providers.
- Play, including therapeutic play, is an important strategy to prepare children for hospitalization and to help them adapt to the effects of illness and hospitalization. It provides an emotional outlet, opportunities for teaching and learning, and the ability to become familiar with a situation and improve physiologic abilities. A CLS is a specially trained individual who is a member of the child's multidisciplinary team. He or she works in conjunction with the child's health care providers and parents to foster an atmosphere that promotes the child's well-being.
- Family-centered care and atraumatic care are philosophies that pay special attention to the concerns of the family and child during hospitalization.
- Providing support to hospitalized children and their families is critical for minimizing stress.
- Whatever the reason for admission, preparation for admission is vital.
- Upon admission to the hospital or outpatient unit, orient the child and family to the unit, discuss unit policies and routines and the personnel who will be involved in the care of the child, and begin child/family teaching.
- Establish a trusting, caring relationship with the child and family. Let the child and family know what will happen and what is expected of them. Obtain information about the child's history, routines, and reason for admission. Obtain baseline vital signs and height and weight, and perform a physical assessment. Each health care setting has its own policies and procedures for this.
- Due to their age and developmental level, children may be vulnerable to harm, and the nurse must use appropriate safety measures in caring for children (e.g., identification of children, use of restraints and transportation, basic hygiene measures). These measures need to address developmental risks, such as that the infants, toddlers, and preschoolers require close supervision and the nurse must avoid leaving small objects within reach.
- Discharge planning begins upon admission. Each interaction with the family is an opportunity for child and family teaching.
- Provide and review discharge instructions with the child and primary caregiver. Use educational booklets or media such as videos or DVDs, that give basic health information or general care for a child with a particular disease.
- Explain, demonstrate, and request a return demonstration of any treatments or procedures to be done at home. Provide a written schedule if the child is to receive multiple medications, tube feedings, or other medical treatments.
- Community-based nurses focus on the practice of nursing that provides personal care to children and families in the community. These nurses focus on promoting and preserving health as well as preventing disease or injury. They help children and their families cope with illness and disease. They are direct providers of care as well as advocates and educators working to minimize and remove barriers to allow the child to develop to his or her full potential.
- Due to the short lengths of stay in acute settings and the shift to home care for children with complex health needs, discharge planning and case management have become important nursing roles. Discharge planning provides a comprehensive plan for the safe discharge of a child from a health care facility and for continuing safe and effective care at home. Case management focuses on coordinating health care services while balancing quality and cost outcomes. Both contribute to improved transitions from hospital to home for children, their families, and the health care team.
- Nursing in the home care setting can be challenging. The focus is on meeting the child's physical and psychological needs while involving the family. Health care professionals provide the support, empowerment, education, and expertise in caring for the child that families need.

- Goals of the nurse in the home care setting include promoting, restoring, and maintaining the health of the child. Home care focuses on minimizing the effects of the illness or disability and providing the child or family with the means to care for the illness or disability at home. Nurses in the home care setting are direct providers of care, child and family educators, child and family advocates, and case managers.
- Community-based nursing takes place in a variety of settings, including physicians' offices, clinics, health departments, urgent care centers, clients' homes, schools, camps, churches, and shelters (such as shelters for abused women, homeless shelters, and disaster shelters). Nurses provide well care, episodic ill care, and chronic care to children and their families in these various settings.
- Advantages of home care include shorter hospital stays and decreased health care costs, but the major advantage of home care is the comfort and family support it provides, promoting an improved quality of life for these children. Caring for children at home not only improves their physical health but also allows for adequate growth and development while keeping them within their family.
- Disadvantages to home care include intrusion on family privacy. Caring for children with complex medical needs can be overwhelming for some families, and financial issues related to home care can become a large burden to families.

REFERENCES AND RECOMMENDED READINGS

American Academy of Pediatrics. (2012). Child life services. *Pediatrics, 130*(1), e248. Retrieved from http://pediatrics.aappublications.org/content/118/4/1757.full

American Academy of Pediatrics, Committee on Hospital Care, Institute for Patient and Family-Centered Care. (2012). Policy statement: Patient and family-centered care and the pediatrician's role. *Pediatrics, 129*(2), 394–404. doi: 10.1542/peds.2011–3084

American Academy of Pediatrics, Committee on Pediatric Emergency Medicine. (2011). Pediatric care recommendations for freestanding urgent care facilities. *Pediatrics, 133*(5), 950–953. Retrieved from http://pediatrics.aappublications.org/content/116/1/258.full

American Society of Anesthesiologists. (1998). *My trip to the hospital coloring book.* Retrieved from https://ftp.asahq.org/p-151-my-trip-to-the-hospital-coloring-book.aspx

Berlin, E. A., & Fowkes, W. C. (1983). A teaching framework for cross-cultural health care—Application to practice. *The Western Journal of Medicine, 139*(6), 934–938.

Bowden, V. R., & Greenberg, C. S. (2011). *Pediatric nursing procedures* (3rd ed.). Philadelphia, PA: Lippincott Williams & Wilkins.

Bretherton, I. (1992). The origins of attachment theory: John Bowlby and Mary Ainsworth. *Developmental Psychology, 28*, 759–775.

Carpenito, L. J. (2013). *Nursing diagnosis: Application to clinical practice* (14th ed.). Philadelphia, PA: Lippincott Williams & Wilkins.

Centers for Medicare and Medicaid Services (CMS). (2014). *State operations manual appendix a-survey protocol, regulations and interpretive guidelines for hospitals.* Retrieved from http://www.cms.gov/Regulations-and-Guidance/Guidance/Manuals/downloads/som107ap_a_hospitals.pdf

Chundamala, J., Wright, J. G., & Kemp, S. M. (2009). An evidence-based review of parental presence during anesthesia induction and parent/child anxiety. *Canadian Journal of Anaesthesia, 56*(1), 57–70.

Cohen, E., Kuo, D. Z., Agrawal, R., Berry, J. G., Bhagat, S. K., Simon, T. D. & Srivastava, R. (2011). Special article: Children with medical complexity: An emerging population for clinical and research initiatives. *Pediatrics, 127*(3), 529-538. doi: 10.1542/peds.2010–0910

Crole, N., & Smith, L. (2002). Examining the phases of nursing care of the hospitalized child. *Australian Nursing Journal, 9*(8), 30–31.

Disability Rights California. (2014). *Compilation of select laws & regulations regarding behavioral restraint & seclusion.* Retrieved from http://www.disabilityrightsca.org/pubs/545701.pdf

Durani, Y. (2011). *Preparing your child for surgery.* Retrieved from http://kidshealth.org/parent/system/surgery/hosp_surgery.html#

Elias, E. R., Murphy, N. A., & the Council on Children with Disabilities. (2012). Clinical report: Home care of children and youth with complex health care needs and technology dependencies. *Pediatrics, 129*(5), 996–1005. doi: 10.1542/peds.2012–0606

Forsner, M., Jansson, L., & Soderberg, A. (2009). Afraid of medical care: School-aged children's narratives about medical fear. *Journal of Pediatric Nursing, 24*(6), 519–528.

Hart, R. & Rollins, J. (2011). Chapter 1: Separation & stranger anxiety. In *Therapeutic activities for children and teens coping with health issues* (pp. 1–22). Hoboken, NJ; John Wiley & Sons, Inc.

Murphy, N. A., Carbone, P. S., & Council on Children With Disabilities. (2011). Parent-provider-community partnerships: optimizing outcomes for children with disabilities. *Pediatrics, 128*(4),795–802. doi: 10.1542/peds.2011–1467

National Association of School Nurses. (2010). *Definition of school nursing.* Retrieved from http://www.nasn.org/RoleCareer

National Association of School Nurses. (2011). *Role of the school nurse.* Retrieved from http://www.nasn.org/portals/0/positions/2011psrole.pdf

National Center for Healthy Housing. (n.d.). *National healthy homes training center and network.* Retrieved from http://www.nchh.org/Training/National-Healthy-Homes-Training-Center.aspx

National Center for Healthy Housing. (2006). *Pediatric environmental home assessment scenario.* Retrieved from http://

www.nchh.org/Portals/0/Contents/CHW_PEHA_Materials_11.24.08.pdf

Prchal, A., Graf, A., Bergstraesser, E., & Landolt, M. A. (2012). Research: A two-session psychological intervention for siblings of pediatric cancer patients: a randomized controlled pilot trial. *Child and Adolescent Psychiatry and Mental Health, 6*, 3. doi:10.1186/1753–2000–6–3

Ralph, S. S., & Taylor, C. M. (2011). *Nursing diagnosis pocket guide*. Philadelphia, PA: Wolters Kluwer/Lippincott Williams & Wilkins.

Robertson, J., & Bowlby, J. (1952). Responses of young children to separation from their mothers II: Observations of the sequences of response of children aged 18 to 24 months during the course of separation. *Courrier du Centre International de l'Enfance, 3*, 131–142.

Rupert, E., & Host, N. (2009). Out-of-home child care and medical day treatment programs. In Section on Home Care, American Academy of Pediatrics (Ed.), *Guidelines for pediatric home health care* (2nd ed., pp. 509–526). Elk Grove Village, IL: American Academy of Pediatrics.

Salmela, M., Salanterä, S., & Aronen, E. (2009). Child-reported hospital fears in 4 to 6 year-old-children. *Pediatric Nursing, 35*(5), 269–278.

Shadow Buddies Foundation. (2014). *Shadow buddies foundation*. Retrieved from http://www.shadowbuddies.org/

Swanson, W. S. (2014). *Ages and stages: How to ease your child's separation anxiety*. Retrieved from http://www.healthychildren.org/English/ages-stages/toddler/pages/Soothing-Your-Childs-Separation-Anxiety.aspx?nfstatus=401&nftoken=00000000–0000–0000–0000–000000000000&nfstatusdescription=ERROR%3 a+No+local+token

U.S. Department of Health and Human Services. (2012). *HealthyPeople.gov*. Retrieved from http://www.healthypeople.gov/2020/about/default.aspx

U.S. Department of Health and Human Services, Health Resources and Services Administration, Maternal and Child Health Bureau. (2013). *Child Health USA 2012*. Rockville, MD: U.S. Department of Health and Human Services.

CHAPTER WORKSHEET

MULTIPLE CHOICE QUESTIONS

1. The nurse is preparing a 5-year-old boy for surgery on his lower leg. His mother is helping him into the hospital gown and the boy fights removal of his underwear. What is the most appropriate nursing action?
   a. Allow the mother to remove the underwear.
   b. Tell the boy he is acting childishly.
   c. Notify the OR that the underwear is on.
   d. Allow the boy to keep his underwear on.
2. A 6-month-old infant requires restraint to prevent removal of his nasogastric tube. What is the priority nursing intervention?
   a. Tie the restraint loosely to prevent skin breakdown.
   b. Leave the baby unrestrained when directly observed.
   c. Position the restrained infant prone to prevent aspiration.
   d. Place the infant in a room near the nurses' station.
3. A 10-year-old child on a regular diet refuses to eat the food on her meal tray. She requests chicken nuggets, French fries, and ice cream. What is the best nursing action?
   a. Ask that the child's desired foods be sent up from the kitchen.
   b. Negotiate with the child to eat at least part of the food on the tray.
   c. Remove a privilege.
   d. Offer the child cereal and milk from stock on the nursing unit.
4. A child is to undergo a tympanostomy tube placement in a freestanding outpatient surgery center. What is the major disadvantage associated with this location?
   a. Increased risk for infection
   b. Increased health care costs
   c. Need to be transferred if overnight stay is required
   d. Increased disruption of family functioning

CRITICAL THINKING EXERCISES

1. Becky, an 8-year-old, is admitted to the pediatric unit for an emergency surgery. She is in third grade and very active in after-school programs. Her mother is with her during the admission process but will have to return to work shortly after Becky returns from surgery to the pediatric unit. Would the nurse expect Becky to show separation anxiety? What are the three top nursing diagnoses for Becky?
2. A 6-year-old is admitted to the general pediatric unit after spending several hours in the emergency department with an acute asthma attack. Her mother and two younger siblings are present, but the mother plans to leave shortly to take the siblings home. The father will visit in about 2 hours, after work. What is the overall goal for this child's care? What could the nurse say to promote coping in this child? What would be the best answer if the mother asks if she should stay?
3. A child with cerebral palsy is discharged from the hospital, where he has been receiving treatment for pneumonia. Home health care nurses, through a local agency, are to help the family administer intravenous antibiotic therapy and to monitor the child's health status.
   a. As the home health nurse assigned to this child, what should your nursing assessment include?
   b. In this situation, what are some nursing interventions that will help ensure family-centered care?
   c. When this child is stable and can go back to school, what will be the role of the school nurse in caring for this child?

STUDY ACTIVITIES

1. Follow a child and family during the admission process, from preadmission to initial time on the unit, to identify the procedures and tasks involved. Examine the response of the child and family and how the nursing staff responds to their needs.
2. Develop a teaching plan to orient a toddler or preschooler and his or her family to a nursing unit. Include the resources, personnel, and techniques to include in the teaching plan.
3. Shadow a nurse working in a community setting, such as a camp, school, shelter, or health department. Identify the role the nurse plays in the health of the children and families in the setting and the community.
4. Spend a day in a medically fragile day care setting. Identify the needs of one child and his or her family, how they may differ from those of a child in a traditional day care setting, and the role of the nurse in meeting those needs.
5. Develop an IHP for a child with diabetes (use the IHP in Fig. 33.10 as a reference).
6. Shadow a nurse working in a home health care setting. Identify ways he or she helps the family to promote the child's growth and development and to ensure that the child has as normal a childhood as possible. Identify interventions that embody the key concepts of family-centered care.

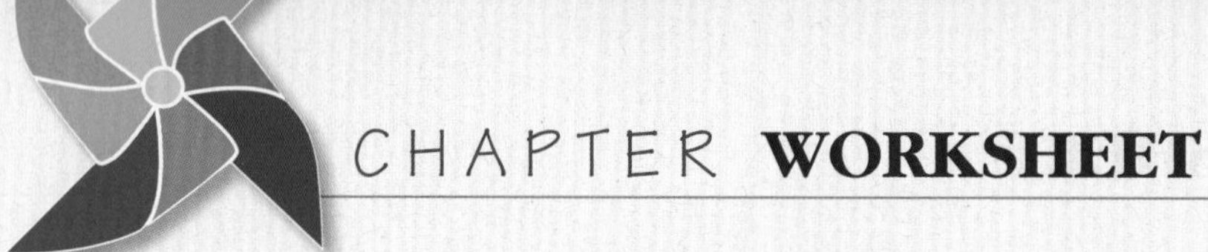

CHAPTER WORKSHEET

BRINGING IT ALL TOGETHER: A CASE STUDY

Nathaniel, a 6-year-old boy, is admitted to your unit for treatment for osteomyelitis. He lives at home with his mom, dad, and two sisters, who are 13 and 10 years old. After getting settled on the unit Nathaniel and his mom go to the playroom. The lab technician, who is new to your hospital, approaches Nathaniel and his mom in the playroom to draw his admission lab work.

Go to thePoint to find questions to consider about this case.

34

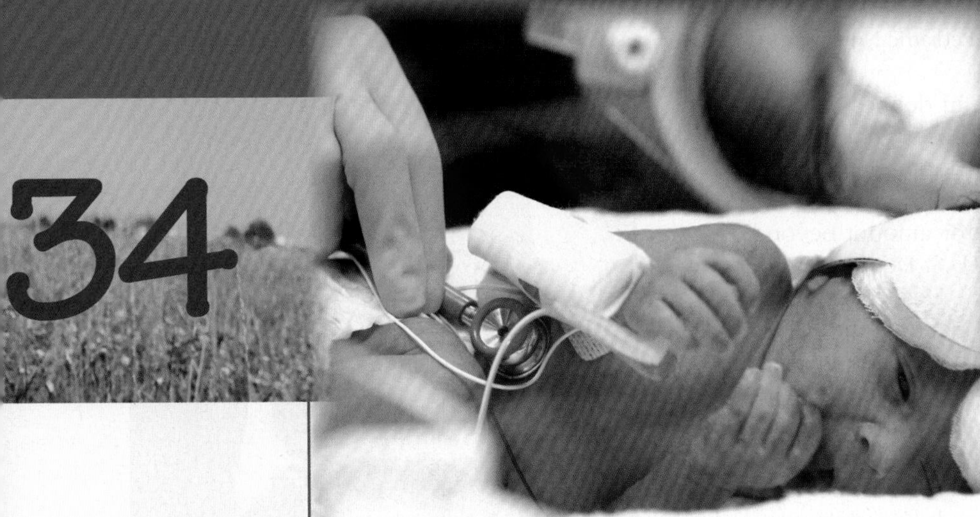

WOW
Words of Wisdom
The touch of a mother's hand and the sound of her voice bring comfort to her special child, and when you bring comfort, you strengthen both of them.

Caring for the Special Needs Child

KEY TERMS
chronic illness
developmental delay
developmental disability
palliative care
respite care
terminal illness

Learning Objectives

Upon completion of the chapter, you will be able to:

1. Analyze the impact that being a child with special needs has on the child and family.
2. Identify anticipated times when the child and family will require additional support.
3. Describe ways that nurses assist children with special needs and their families to obtain optimal functioning.
4. Discuss early intervention and public school education for the special needs child.
5. Plan for transition of the special needs child from the inpatient facility to the home, and from pediatric to adult medical care.
6. Discuss key elements related to pediatric end-of-life care.
7. Differentiate developmental responses to death and appropriate interventions.

***Preet Singh*, a 2-year-old boy who was born at 27 weeks' gestation, is seen in your clinic for the first time. He has a history of hydrocephalus and developmental delay. During the examination, his mother states, "I'm concerned about finding a good, affordable preschool for Preet. His older brother attends public school, but I can't imagine Preet going there." After further discussion with Preet's mother, you realize he has not been involved in an early intervention program.**

The Maternal Child Health Bureau defines children with special health care needs as "those who have or are at risk for a chronic physical, developmental, behavioral, or emotional condition and who also require health and related services of a type or amount beyond that required by children generally" (U.S. Department of Health and Human Services [USDHHS], Health Resources and Services Administration [HRSA], Maternal and Child Health Bureau, 2013). Children who have a terminal illness, or are otherwise dying, also require additional care. Nurses are in a unique position, both in the inpatient and outpatient setting, to have a significant and positive influence on the lives of these children and their families. For children with special needs, in addition to providing direct care, the nurse fills the critical role of child and family advocate and case manager. When a child is dying, nurses not only provide physical care to the child but also strive to meet the emotional needs of the child and family.

THE MEDICALLY FRAGILE CHILD

The numbers of children with **chronic illness** (a long-lasting or recurrent illness) are increasing. Children with special health care needs make up about 15% of the population of children in the United States and, of those children, 27.1% are affected a great deal by their condition (USDHHS, HRSA, Maternal and Child Health Bureau, 2013). Increasing numbers of children are being diagnosed with physical and mental disorders and larger numbers of children are living with the assistance of high-tech treatments and equipment.

Impact of the Problem

Children with special needs may use or need prescription medication, medical care, mental health services, or education services more than other children of their same age. They may be limited in abilities and may need physical, occupational, or speech therapy (Fig. 34.1). Alternatively, they may require ongoing treatment for emotional, developmental, or behavioral problems (USDHHS, HRSA, Maternal and Child Health Bureau, 2013). These children and their families are often insured inadequately, have financial needs and/or unmet family support needs, or have difficulty obtaining the specialty care that the child requires (USDHHS, HRSA, Maternal and Child Health Bureau, 2013). It can be challenging for the family of a child with special needs to navigate the system and obtain all of the services their child requires.

When an infant is born very prematurely, when a child is injured and requires long-term rehabilitation and special care, or when a child is diagnosed with a complex chronic health condition, the parents are often devastated initially. The parents of medically fragile children may feel they must adapt to the risk and protect their

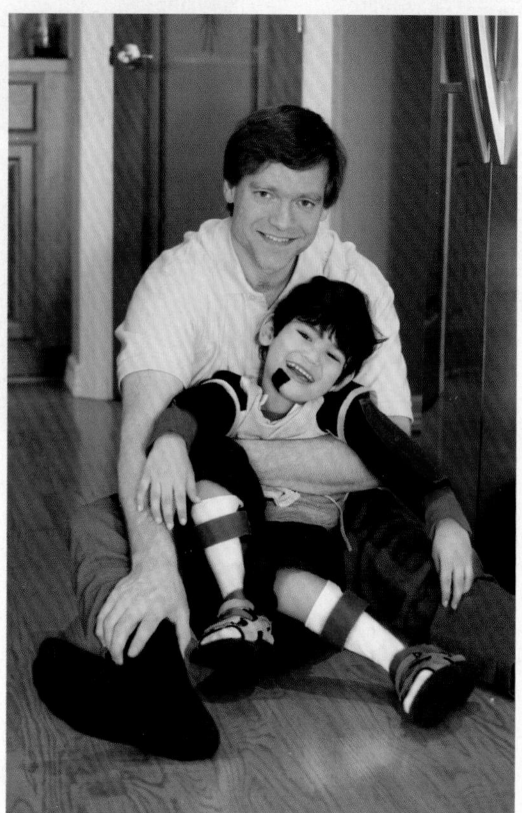

FIGURE 34.1 The special needs child often requires a significant amount of care at home throughout his life.

child. They are interested in preserving their family while compensating for the past, and they cautiously look to the future and become hopeful again. While the infant or child is still in the hospital, nurses can help parents build on their strengths, empowering them to care for their medically fragile infant or special needs child. Education is paramount and should begin as early in the hospitalization as possible (Hewitt-Taylor, 2012). In many situations, particular discharge needs are known early in the course of the infant's or child's hospitalization. Nurses should provide anticipatory guidance about the course of treatment and the expected outcome.

Most children with chronic illness, or those who are dependent on technology, progress through stages of growth and development just as typical children do, though possibly at a slower pace. The exception is the child with significant psychomotor retardation, though some developmental progression may occur. Children with special health care needs desire to be treated as normal, and they want to experience the same events that other children do.

Of particular concern is a growing subset of children with emotional, behavioral, and developmental problems. Children with these needs have even greater difficulty receiving the care and services they require (USDHHS, HRSA, Maternal and Child Health Bureau, 2013). Many children with emotional, behavioral, or developmental

HEALTHY PEOPLE 2020

Objective	Nursing Significance
Reduce the proportion of people with disabilities who report serious psychological distress	• Screen children with special health care needs for depression or sadness. • Refer children and their families to mental health providers as needed.

Healthy People Objectives retrieved from http://www.healthypeople.gov

problems also have health problems. Often, these children's problems are not diagnosed early and treatment is difficult (Horowitz & Marchetti, 2010). Ongoing counseling and therapy is very difficult for some families to obtain. Ultimately, this has a negative impact on the child's physical and mental health and may result in decreased achievement and productivity as the child matures. See Healthy People 2020.

Effects of Special Needs on the Child

When a child is medically fragile or has special needs, the child's coping ability is affected. In addition, the child's ability to cope is significantly affected by the family's response to stressors, which are often numerous in this population. Children with special health care needs experience differing effects of the chronic illness or disability based on their developmental level, which naturally changes over time for most children.

Infants may fail to develop a sense of trust or attach appropriately with the parents because of frequent hospitalizations, often with multiple caregivers involved; lack of consistency in nurturing; or parental detachment or grieving over the child's condition. The infant's ability to learn through sensorimotor exploration may be impaired due to lack of appropriate stimulation, confinement to a crib, or increased contact with painful experiences (Vessey & Sullivan, 2010).

The toddler may experience difficulty developing autonomy because of increased dependency on the parent or overinvolvement by the parent. Motor and language skill development may be delayed if the toddler is not given adequate opportunities to test his or her limits and abilities (Vessey & Sullivan, 2010).

Limited opportunity also reduces the preschooler's development of a sense of initiative. The preschooler may experience limited opportunities for socialization, causing him or her to withdraw or to feel criticized. Body image development may be hindered due to painful exposures and anxiety. In preschoolers, magical thinking may lead to feelings of guilt for having caused their own disease or condition (Vessey & Sullivan, 2010).

The school-age child may have limited opportunities to achieve a sense of industry because of school absence and inability to participate in activities or competitive events. Lack of socialization limits the school-age child's ability to form peer relationships. The ability to learn via concrete operations is affected by the child's physical limitations or possibly the treatments required (Vessey & Sullivan, 2010).

Adolescents may feel as though they are different from their peers because of their lack of skills/abilities or their appearance. This may hinder the teen's ability to form a sense of personal identity. Since the teen with special health care needs often requires significant amounts of support from the parents, it may be difficult for the adolescent to achieve independence. If the earlier stages of cognitive development have been delayed, then reaching the level of abstract thinking may be blocked (Vessey & Sullivan, 2010).

The child with special health care needs may be able to focus on the positive experiences in his or her life as a method of coping, leading to as much independence as possible. Other children may always feel different from their peers (in a negative sense) and withdraw. Irritability and acting out may also occur. Some children may be compliant and/or seek support for themselves. The child's coping pattern may change over time or with certain situations, such as relapse or worsening of the condition. Children with overprotective parents may display marked dependence and may be very fearful. Children whose parents have been overly indulgent may be more independent and defiant. The nurse must assess the child's individual response to the current health care status and intervene as appropriate (Vessey & Sullivan, 2010).

Effects on the Family

Each member of the family experiences effects related to the child's special needs. Family members' experiences and their responses to the child's illness influence each other directly (Fig. 34.2).

Effects on Parents

Raising a child with special needs is generally not the life parents expected to have. Some parents may adapt over time and ultimately accept the child's illness or disability. Others may adapt but do not accept the child's condition and experience the continual fading and re-emergence of chronic sorrow. Denial of their child's problem may prevent parents from progressing through grief, but it also allows them to have hope (Knafl & Santacroce, 2010).

Caring for the special needs child at home (rather than having the child in a facility) may decrease the

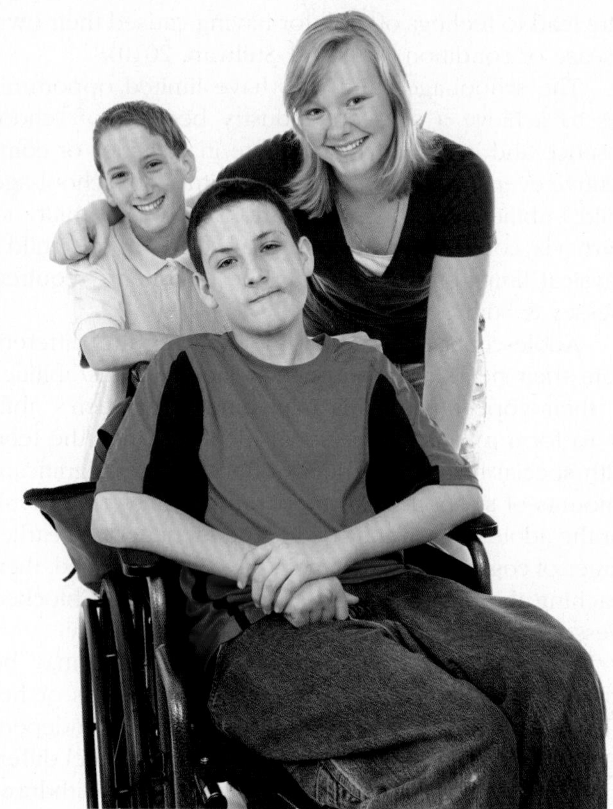

FIGURE 34.2 A wheelchair-bound boy with his younger brother and older sister.

parents' feelings of anxiety and helplessness. As with typically developing children, parents enjoy witnessing the emotional and social growth of the child. Parents of special needs children experience a multitude of emotions and changes in their lives. They worry about their child's and family's well-being, and as experts in their child's care often feel burdened with continual care. They often feel helpless and overwhelmed when their child is discharged from the hospital. Though willing to carry the burden, they may experience fear, anger, sadness, guilt, frustration, or resentment. Many parents experience grief as a result of losing the perfect child of which they dreamed (Knafl & Santacroce, 2010).

STRESSORS OF DAILY LIVING

Families with a child who has special health care needs experience life differently from other families. They may have to change their housing situation to accommodate the child's needs. Their sleep is affected. Constant supervision of the technology-dependent child makes it difficult to carry out other basic household activities. In addition to basic child care and running of the household, medical and technical care must be incorporated into daily life. The family's identity and the parents' employment may be altered radically. Holidays and vacations are affected, as it is difficult to plan activities. Nursing and other health care professional visits are disruptive to family life.

Mothers appear to carry the larger burden of care, though fathers are not unaffected. Somehow, parents eventually take charge, and though they fear failure, they display vigilance, can negotiate and seek information, and become advocates for their child and experts on his or her care. Though parents may feel trapped and isolated and experience a loss of freedom, their need to survive as a family continues to motivate them. Parents may feel a need to be with their child at all times and experience stress related to coping with the heavy load of caregiving.

The extended burden of caregiving can also have adverse health effects on caregivers: only a small percentage of parents of children with special health care needs report that they routinely participate in health-promoting activities for themselves. In addition, parents of children with special health care needs are at increased risk for the development of depression (Knafl & Santacroce, 2010). In addition to the caregiving burden, parents experience role conflicts, financial burdens, and the struggle between independence in providing care and the isolation associated with it. It is very difficult to enjoy spontaneous events outside the home because so much planning is necessary.

The possibility of independence revolves around mobility issues, education, and assistive technology. Though education for all children is federally mandated, parents have anxiety about educational decisions and also find it difficult to obtain the support and educational services the child needs.

Additional stress is associated with transition times in the care of a special needs child. These transition times include:

- Initial diagnosis or change in prognosis
- Increased symptoms
- When the child moves to a new setting (hospital, school)
- During a parent's absence
- During periods of developmental change (Knafl & Santacroce, 2010; Caley, 2012)

VULNERABLE CHILD SYNDROME

Vulnerable child syndrome is a clinical state in which the parents' reactions to a serious illness or event in the child's past continue to have long-term psychologically harmful effects on the child and parents for many years (Chambers, Mahabee-Gittens, & Leonard, 2011).

The parents view the child as being at higher risk for medical, developmental, or behavioral problems. Parents exhibit excessive unwarranted concerns and seek health care for their child very frequently. Risk factors for the development of vulnerable child syndrome include preterm birth, a congenital anomaly, newborn jaundice, a handicapping condition, an accident or illness that the child is not expected to recover from, or crying or feeding problems in the first 5 years of life. The parent has difficulty separating from the child, and the child senses that anxiety and then develops symptoms that reinforce the parent's fears. Alternatively (or in addition), the parents may try to retain control, particularly at times of increasing independence, and fear disciplining the child as they do not want to "upset" the child.

Effects on Siblings

The siblings of children with special health care needs are also affected dramatically. Their relationship with their parents is different from what it would have been if they had a typical brother or sister. Parents often need to spend more time with the child with special needs and have less time with their healthy children. Children exhibit emotional and psychological responses to their sibling's long-term needs (Lane & Mason, 2014). The sibling's knowledge about the illness, the sibling's attitude toward and adjustment to it, the sibling's own self-esteem, how socially supported the sibling is, and the parents' awareness of the sibling's feelings are all related to how well the sibling adjusts.

Nursing Management of the Medically Fragile Child and Family

Family-centered care provides the optimal framework for caring for medically fragile children and their families. Family-centered care minimizes the impact of chronic illness and maximizes the child's developmental potential. To provide the best nursing care for these children and their families, the nurse must first develop a trusting relationship with the family.

To ensure optimal functioning, children with special health care needs require comprehensive and coordinated services from multiple professionals. These professionals should work collaboratively to address the child's health, educational, psychological, and social service needs. In addition to case management and advocacy, nursing management focuses on screening and ongoing assessment of the child, provision of home care, care of the technology-dependent child, education and support of the child and family, and referral for resources.

Developing a Therapeutic Relationship

Raising children is always challenging, but for the parent of a special needs child it is often overwhelming and exhausting. The parents' needs change continuously, so it is best if the family has a permanent relationship with a physician or nurse practitioner. This promotes trust and a more efficient two-way flow of information.

Respect the parents' range of emotions and work with them as a team to manage the child's care. Parents need to be recognized for complying with the treatment plan or for other small gains that are made. Empowering the family strengthens them and gives them self-confidence. Feeling supported and invigorated gives parents strength, energy, and hope. Box 34.1 lists principles related to family involvement.

BOX 34.1

PRINCIPLES RELATED TO FAMILY INVOLVEMENT

Families

- Are the constant in a child's life
- Need to have access to information and training
- Deserve to receive culturally competent care
- Know their strengths, limitations, and fears
- Merit mutual respect and responsibility for outcomes

Adapted from Goode, T. D., Haywood, S. H., Wells, N., & Rhee, K. (2009). Family-centered, culturally, and linguistically competent care: Essential components of the medical home. *Pediatric Annals, 38*(9), 505–512.

Screening and Ongoing Assessment

Nurses should perform screening to identify children with unmet health care needs. A screening tool developed by the Child and Adolescent Health Measurement Initiative may help to identify children with special health care needs. This tool and web links for additional information related to the screening tool can be found on thePoint.

Children with special health care needs may attain developmental milestones more slowly than typically developing children. If the Denver II is used for ongoing developmental surveillance of the young child, then the results should be compared from visit to visit to determine progress rather than using it as a screening tool. Assess special needs children and their families for vulnerable child syndrome.

Promoting Home Care

Home is the most developmentally appropriate environment for all children, even those who are technologically dependent (Hewitt-Taylor, 2012). The child's home provides an emotionally nurturing and socially stimulating environment. Children desire to be cared for at home, and those who are cared for at home display an improved physical, emotional, psychological, and social status.

Technology-dependent children may require supplemental oxygen, assisted ventilation, tracheostomy care, assisted enteral or parenteral feeding, or parenteral medication administration. With advances in technology, children with extensive medical and developmental needs may be cared for at home and it is often assumed that they will be (Mendes, 2013). Early discharge planning is

BOX 34.2

PREPARING FOR HOME CARE BEFORE DISCHARGE

- Promote liaison with community resources. Develop communication between various services. Plan appointments. Set up home nursing care (either private duty or visits).
- Teach skills, encouraging active caregiving in the hospital setting to increase the parents' self-confidence.
- Discuss psychological and emotional issues with parents.
- Obtain/organize equipment and supplies (running out of supplies may cause significant stress on families).
- Refer the family for necessary financial resources.
- Ensure the family's home environment is adequate (enough room for equipment, electricity on, air conditioner for warm weather, heater for cold weather, and refrigeration for food).
- For the baby being discharged from the neonatal intensive care unit (NICU):
  - Teach the parents about the infant's cues and behaviors and the preemie's different sleep–wake patterns.
  - Encourage kangaroo care and infant massage while in the NICU (as the infant's condition allows).
  - Educate the parents about possible effects on short- and long-term neurodevelopment.
  - Refer to local early intervention program.
  - Assist the family with finding a primary care provider who is experienced in the ongoing follow-up of high-risk infants.

Adapted from Stewart, J. (2015). *Discharge planning for high-risk newborns*. Retrieved from http://www.uptodate.com/contents/discharge-planning-for-high-risk-newborns

important, and parents will need detailed instructions and support in caring for the technology-dependent child at home (Hewitt-Taylor, 2012).

EARLY DISCHARGE PLANNING

Early discharge planning and ongoing inclusion and education of the family facilitates continuity of care. Box 34.2 provides information about preparing the medically fragile child for discharge.

CARING FOR THE TECHNOLOGY-DEPENDENT CHILD AT HOME

Home care nurses are often involved in the care of technology-dependent children. Caring for a technology-dependent child at home is a complex process, yet children thrive in the home care setting with appropriate intervention and care. Many parents feel that rearing a technology-dependent child is different only because of the presence of the equipment. Nurses may tend to think that parents treat the technology-dependent child differently from the other children, while parents value normalization and want to raise and provide discipline to all of their children in the same manner. Parents should tell nurses about their childrearing expectations, and nurses need to respect the parents' wishes.

Improved collaboration between parents and home care nurses may decrease the parents' stress and maximize opportunities for appropriate growth and development in the technology-dependent child. Thus, a strong relationship, good communication, and good negotiation skills are assets to the family and child.

Help the family to incorporate the medical regimen into daily life to minimize the child's self-perception of being different from other children. Teach families about the technical issues, such as home and travel oxygen therapy, use of the ventilator, suctioning, chest percussion and postural drainage, tube feedings and care of the feeding tube, and medications. Assist parents with the planning and management of routine care, respiratory treatments, nutritional support, and developmental interventions. Reinforce exercises and techniques as prescribed by developmental therapists. Refer to Chapter 33 for additional information about home care nursing.

Providing Care Coordination

Once a child with special health care needs has been identified and has been discharged to the home setting, the nurse plays a vital role in care coordination. Any child with special health care needs benefits from a medical home. The nurse in the medical home is a critical team member, providing ongoing care coordination and follow-up. If such services are available in the local area, refer the child and family with special needs to an integrated health program that provides interdisciplinary, collaborative care for children requiring complex, coordinated care. Box 34.3 lists nursing interventions for families of children with special health care needs.

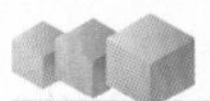
Concept Mastery Alert

Home Care

When coordinating home care for a child with special care need, the nurse can best benefit the family by being available to the family as needed and providing the support they need as they learn how to deal with the child's care needs at home.

Providing Ongoing Follow-Up of the Former Premature Infant

Many former premature infants experience myriad medical and developmental problems throughout infancy, early childhood, and beyond. Upon or following discharge, many former premature infants display one or many of the following medical or developmental problems:

- Chronic lung disease (bronchopulmonary dysplasia)
- Cardiac changes such as right ventricular hypertrophy and pulmonary artery hypertension

BOX 34.3

NURSING INTERVENTIONS FOR FAMILIES OF CHILDREN WITH SPECIAL HEALTH CARE NEEDS

- Develop written health plans.
- Provide care coordination and collaboration with specialists in other disciplines, early intervention, schools, and public agencies.
- Address needs for prior authorization for treatments, medications, or specialist referrals; retain copies in the child's chart of authorization forms and approvals.
- Modify office routines to promote family and child comfort.
- Assist parents with child care decisions.
- Know community resources available to children with special health care needs.
- When the child is hospitalized, encourage high levels of parental participation.
- Provide care coordination across multiple health settings.
- Educate child care providers on child health needs.
- Help parents get involved with parent support networks.

Adapted from Looman, W. S., O'Conner-Von, S., & Lindeke, L. L. (2008). Caring for children with special health care needs and their families: What advanced practice nurses need to know. *Journal for Nurse Practitioners*, *4*(7), 512–518; and McAllister, J. W., Presler, E., Turchi, R., & Antonelli, R. C. (2009). Achieving effective care coordination in the medical home. *Pediatric Annals*, *38*(9), 491–497.

- Growth retardation, poor feeding, anemia of prematurity, other nutrient deficiencies
- Apnea of prematurity, gastroesophageal reflux disease, bradycardia
- Sudden infant death syndrome (SIDS)
- Rickets (osteopenia) of prematurity
- Hydrocephalus, ventriculomegaly, abnormal head magnetic resonance imaging results, ventriculoperitoneal shunt
- Inguinal or umbilical hernias
- Retinopathy of prematurity, strabismus, decreased visual acuity
- Hearing deficits
- Delayed dentition
- Gross motor, fine motor, and language delay; sensory integration issues (Billimoria & Kamat, 2014; Kelly, 2010; Sullivan, Msall, & Miller, 2012)

Over the long term, former premature infants are at higher risk than typical infants of developing cognitive delay, cerebral palsy, attention deficit disorder, learning disabilities, difficulties with socialization, and vulnerable child syndrome (Chambers, Mahabee-Gittens, & Leonard, 2011; Sullivan et al., 2012). In addition, many former premature infants display alterations in muscle tone at or shortly after discharge from the NICU that require physical therapy intervention.

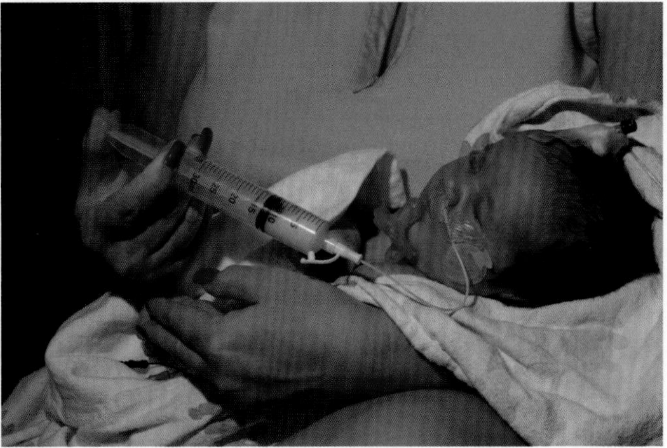

FIGURE 34.3 Parents of an infant discharged from the NICU may need to administer special care, such as feeding.

For these reasons, high-risk infants require special attention and thorough, appropriate assessment to discern subtle changes that may affect their long-term physical, cognitive, emotional, and social outcome. The pediatric nurse should have an understanding of the special concerns that former premature infants and children as well as their families may face (Fig. 34.3).

From the beginning, encourage families to keep a binder that includes all of the infant's pertinent checkup, insurance, and medical and developmental information; this will serve as a resource for the parents, and they will be able to supply complete information when visiting various providers.

PROVIDING ROUTINE WELL-CHILD CARE OF THE FORMER PREMATURE INFANT

Former premature infants require similar well-child care as typical infants do, with additional visits for management of multiple complex medical issues and developmental screening/intervention. Teach families routine newborn care, including bathing, dressing, and avoidance of passive cigarette smoke. All visits for primary care follow-up will be scheduled based on the infant's chronologic age.

Prior to discharge from the NICU, the infant will be tested for oxygen desaturation while seated in the car seat (Kelly, 2010). Clearance will be obtained prior to the infant's discharge. Former preemies require car seat use just as other infants do. Help the parents to find methods of padding the car seat or adding an additional semi-firm cushion inside the seat for the infant to ride in the car safely. Some infants may need to continue cardiac/apnea monitoring while in the car seat.

Since the former premature infant is at increased risk for SIDS compared to the general population, it is critical to teach parents to put the infant on his or her back to sleep (although this is contraindicated with gastroesophageal disease) (Kelly, 2010).

Give immunizations according to the current Centers for Disease Control and Prevention (CDC)-recommended immunization schedule, based on the infant's chronologic age. All former preemies should receive the flu vaccine as recommended after 6 months chronologic age. Respiratory syncytial virus (RSV) prophylaxis is critical for certain groups of premature infants (Billimoria & Kamat, 2014; Kelly, 2010). Therefore, administer palivizumab (Synagis) vaccine according to the recommended schedule (refer to Chapter 40 for additional information about RSV prophylaxis).

ASSESSING GROWTH AND DEVELOPMENT OF THE FORMER PREMATURE INFANT

When assessing growth and development of the infant or child who was born prematurely, determine the child's adjusted or corrected age so that you can perform an accurate assessment. The corrected or adjusted age should be used for evaluating progression in growth as well as development. For example, if a 6-month-old infant was born at 28 weeks' gestation (12 weeks or 3 months early), his growth and development expectations are those of a 3-month-old (corrected age). Continue to correct age for growth and development until the child is 3 years old.

Many former premature infants require special diets to foster catch-up growth (Billimoria & Kamat, 2014; Carey, Russek, & Esposito, 2013). Extra calories are needed for increased growth needs. Additional calcium and phosphorus are required for bone mineralization. For these reasons, former preemies should be fed breast milk fortified with additional nutrients or a commercially prepared formula specific for premature infants. When former preemies demonstrate consistent adequate growth (usually by 6 months corrected age), they may be switched to a "term infant formula" such as Similac or Enfamil, concentrated to a higher caloric density, if needed. Assess the infant's ability to suck efficiently and refer him or her to occupational or speech therapy if the infant is a slow feeder or has difficulty feeding.

All anticipatory guidance related to nutrition is based on the child's corrected age (D'Agostino et al., 2013). In other words, begin solids at 6 months corrected age, not chronologic age, and delay the addition of whole milk until 12 months corrected age, rather than 1 year chronologic age. Signs that the former premature infant may be ready to attempt spoon feeding include interest in feeding, decrease in tongue thrust, and adequate head control.

Early screening and intervention for issues related to development are critical to the attainment of optimal development in the former preemie. The comorbidities that ex-preemies exhibit in the form of prior and current medical problems place these infants at high risk for **developmental delay** (lag in meeting developmental milestones). Even mild developmental delays warrant evaluation and intervention. The Denver II may be used as a screening tool for developmental concerns in the ex-preemie, though it does not always identify children at risk. Parent-report questionnaires demonstrate fairly accurate estimations of developmental problems, and are simple to use. Most importantly, assess the child's development based on corrected age until the child is 3 years old. Refer infants and children early if developmental concerns are suspected.

Identifying and Managing Failure to Thrive and Feeding Disorders in Children with Special Needs

Failure to thrive (FTT) is a term used to describe inadequate growth in infants and children. The child fails to demonstrate appropriate weight gain over a prolonged period of time. Length or height velocity and head circumference growth may also be affected. Typical children may experience FTT, but it is much more common in the child with special needs. Adequate nutrition is critical for appropriate brain growth in the first 2 years of life and obviously for growth in general throughout childhood and adolescence (Starr et al., 2013). FTT is a multifactorial problem. **Developmental disability** (mental or physical or combination impairment resulting in lifelong disability) may contribute to FTT, as the child's ability to consume adequate nutrition is impaired because of sensory or motor delays, such as with cerebral palsy. Other organic causes of FTT include inability to suck and/or swallow correctly, malabsorption, diarrhea, vomiting, or alterations in metabolism and caloric/nutrient needs associated with a variety of chronic illnesses. Infants and children with cardiac or metabolic disease, chronic lung disease (bronchopulmonary dysplasia), cleft palate, or gastroesophageal reflux disease are at particular risk. Feeding disorders or food refusal may occur in infants or children who have required prolonged mechanical ventilation, long-term enteral tube feedings, or an unpleasant event such as a choking episode. Additional causes of FTT include neglect, abuse, behavioral problems, lack of appropriate maternal interaction, poor feeding techniques, lack of parental knowledge, or parental mental illness. Poverty is the single greatest contributing risk factor (Kirkland & Motil, 2015a; Starr et al., 2013).

Screen all children for FTT to identify them early. In addition to poor growth, the infant or child with FTT may present with a history of developmental delay or loss of acquired milestones. Infants or children with feeding problems may display nipple, spoon, or food refusal; difficulty sucking; disinterest in feeding; or difficulty progressing from liquid to puréed to textured food. Perform a detailed dietary history and instruct the parents to complete a 3-day food diary to identify what the child actually eats and drinks. Assess the parent–child interaction, with particular attention to the parent's ability to read and respond to the infant's or child's cues.

BOX 34.4

NURSING INTERVENTIONS DURING THE CHILD'S HOSPITALIZATION FOR FAILURE TO THRIVE

- Observe parent–child interactions, especially during feedings.
- Develop an appropriate feeding schedule.
- Provide feedings as prescribed (usually 120 kcal/kg/day is needed to demonstrate proper weight gain).
- Weigh the child daily and maintain strict records of intake and output.
- Educate parents about proper feeding techniques and volumes.
- Provide extensive support to alleviate parental anxiety related to the child's inability to gain weight.

Adapted from Kirkland, R. T., Motil, K. J., & Duryea, T. K. (2015b). *Failure to thrive (undernutrition) in children younger than two years: Management*. Retrieved from http://www.uptodate.com/contents/failure-to-thrive-undernutrition-in-children-younger-than-two-years-management

Observe feeding, noting the child's oral interest or aversion, oral–motor coordination, and swallowing ability, as well as parent–child interactions before, during, and after the feeding (Kirkland & Motil, 2015b).

Significant FTT may require hospitalization for evaluation and management. Sometimes, enteral tube feedings are necessary in order for children with FTT or feeding disorders to demonstrate adequate growth. Box 34.4 lists nursing interventions for the hospitalized child with FTT.

Take Note!

Infants and children who have experienced maternal neglect may not interact appropriately with their environment or caretaker (lack of eye contact) (Kirkland & Motil, 2015a).

Promoting Growth and Development

When caring for the infant with special health care needs in the hospital, provide consistent caregivers to encourage the infant to develop a sense of trust. Allow and encourage the parent to stay with the infant, providing a comfortable place for the parent to sleep. To promote attachment, emphasize the baby's positive qualities. Encourage developmentally appropriate skills and allow the infant to have pleasurable experiences through all of the senses (Vessey & Sullivan, 2010).

For the toddler, begin developmentally appropriate limit setting and discipline. Encourage independence as the toddler is able. Modify gross motor and sensory activities to accommodate the toddler's limitations. To encourage a sense of control, offer the toddler simple choices. As the preschooler develops, encourage mastery of self-help skills as the child is able. Encourage socialization with same-age peers to develop a sense of friendship. Reinforce to the child that the illness or disability is not a punishment for wrongdoing or the child's fault in any way (Vessey & Sullivan, 2010).

Encourage the school-age child to attend school and make up work that must be missed for medical treatments or appointments. Provide education to the school staff and other students about the child's special needs. Promote involvement in appropriate sports activities; music, drama, or art activities; and clubs such as Boy Scouts or Girl Scouts. Educate the child about the illness or disability and the course of treatment (Vessey & Sullivan, 2010).

Inform parents of teens that those with chronic illness often participate in the same activities as typical teens, such as risk taking, rebelling, and trying out different identities. Assist the teen with coping and interpersonal skills. Promote involvement in activities with other teens with special needs as well as typical adolescents. Ensure that the teen participates in rites of passage as able, such as attending the prom or obtaining a driver's license. Discuss future plans with the teen, such as college or vocation, as well as transition to a nonpediatric physician (Vessey & Sullivan, 2010).

Providing Resources to the Child and Family

Nurses should be familiar with community resources available to children with special health care needs. Educational opportunities for children with special health care needs include early intervention programs and programs offered through the public school system. Financial resources, respite care, and complementary therapies are other areas the nurse should become familiar with.

EDUCATIONAL OPPORTUNITIES FOR THE SPECIAL NEEDS CHILD

The foundation for health and development in children is laid during the first years of life. Children with special health care needs often require multiple developmental interventions and special education in the early years in order to reach their developmental potential later in childhood. Children learn best when they are at the stage of maximal readiness, and the early years must not be missed as an opportunity for development. See Healthy People 2020.

Early intervention programs are intended to enhance the development of infants and toddlers with, or at risk for, disabilities, thereby minimizing educational costs and special education. Early intervention is also directed toward enhancing the capacity of families to meet their child's needs as well as to maximize the likelihood of independent living (Berry, Garzon, & Deloian, 2012).

The Individuals with Disabilities Education Improvement Act of 2004 (formerly called Public Law 99–457) mandates government-funded care coordination and

HEALTHY PEOPLE *2020*

Objective	Nursing Significance
Increase the proportion of children and youth with disabilities who spend at least 80% of their time in regular education programs	• Ensure that children younger than age 3 years who may qualify are referred to the local early intervention program. • Encourage families to advocate for their child's needs on the individualized education plan.

Healthy People Objectives retrieved from http://www.healthypeople.gov

special education for children up to 3 years of age. This early intervention program is administered through each state. Federal law allows each state to define developmental disability differently, but in general, qualified personnel perform an evaluation of the child's physical, language, emotional, and social capabilities to determine eligibility (U. S. Department of Education [USDE], 2011). The law guarantees that eligible children will obtain access to services that will enhance their development. Children who qualify for services receive care coordination, and an individualized family service plan is developed by the service coordinator in conjunction with the family. The service coordinator manages the developmental services and special education that the child requires.

The intent of the program is that the child receives services in a natural environment, so most services occur in the home or day care center. Home visits by the service coordinator and maintenance of regular contact with the family ensure the success of the program.

Refer children suspected of developmental delay to the local early intervention program. For children receiving these services, collaborate with the service coordinator on an ongoing basis, with particular involvement at hospital discharge and when transition of services occurs at age 3 years.

Think back to Preet, the 2-year-old boy with a history of hydrocephalus and developmental delay, from the beginning of the chapter. Discuss with his mother the educational opportunities that are available for Preet. Explain what early intervention is and why it is important for Preet.

Schools may have a profound impact on the child's overall health and development. Some children with special needs do not require additional services to succeed in school. For these children, the nurse's role is to assess for school success or failure and determine the effect of the school environment on the child's health. The Individuals with Disabilities Education Act, reauthorized in 2004, provides for the education of children with special needs through the public school system, from age 3 to 21 years. These services are provided within the public school system.

According to the law, each special needs student is entitled to an individualized education program (IEP), which is a written plan designed to meet the preschool, primary, or secondary school student's individual needs. A committee consisting of the child's parent, a regular teacher, a special education teacher, and various other specialists develops the IEP. Nurses may be called to serve upon this committee. The IEP must include measurable short- and long-term goals. Parents are informed of the student's progress routinely and the IEP is reviewed at least annually (USDE, 2011).

Preschool special education through the local public school system is provided from age 3 to 5 years; access to the curriculum is ensured for all children. A child is eligible for special needs preschool when a significant delay is present in the cognitive, language, adaptive, social-emotional, or motor development domains to the extent that it adversely affects the child's learning ability. The child receives (in the school setting) developmental therapy as needed to augment his or her ability to participate in the education process. The least restrictive environment is preferred, with special needs children participating in classes containing age-appropriate typical peers whenever possible (USDE, n. d.). Special needs preschool services are often offered in the elementary school setting.

FINANCIAL AND INSURANCE RESOURCES

Many special needs children whose families demonstrate financial need may be eligible for Supplemental Security Income (SSI). This program was created in 1972 through Public Law 92–603. SSI is a cash assistance program, and monthly benefits vary per individual. SSI qualification also qualifies the child for state-administered Medicaid. Medicaid benefits vary slightly from state to state, but generally cover medical visits, medication, hospitalization, and limited adjuvant therapies. The State Children's Health Insurance Program (SCHIP) provides low-cost health insurance to eligible children. Eligibility and the extent of benefits provided by SCHIP vary by state (Vessey & Brown, 2010).

Title V programs under the Maternal and Child Health Bureau Block Grant program provides funds to the individual states for administration of services. State Title V programs provide community-based, comprehensive service coordination for children with special needs (Social Security Administration, n. d.).

Online directories providing a wealth of links to resources for special needs children include Children's

Disabilities Information and Special Child. Web links to these sites can be found on thePoint.

RESPITE CARE

Primary caregivers of children with special health care needs must be dedicated, skillful, vigilant, and knowledgeable. Constant care is a stress on the primary caregiver, who needs temporary relief from the daily caregiving demands. **Respite care** provides an opportunity for families to take a break from the daily intensive caregiving responsibilities. Respite care should meet the child's health care needs and offer the child developmental opportunities. Finding and using respite care that the family is comfortable with and trusts may decrease the family's stress and lead to an enhanced quality of life for special needs children and their families. Nurses can facilitate access to respite care, educate respite providers, and ensure quality respite care practices through involvement in community agencies.

COMPLEMENTARY THERAPIES

Families of children with special health care needs often use adjuvant therapies. These may include, among others, homeopathic and herbal medicine, pet therapy, hippotherapy, music, and massage. Many families desire to blend natural or Eastern medicine with traditional allopathic medicine for their special needs child in search of palliation or a cure. When obtaining the health history, ask specifically about homeopathy or herbal medications the child may be taking. Pet therapy may be used to decrease stress or as a component of psychotherapy.

Hippotherapy is also referred to as horseback riding for the handicapped, therapeutic horseback riding, or equine-facilitated psychotherapy. Individuals with almost any cognitive, physical, or emotional disability may benefit from therapeutic riding or other supervised interaction with horses. The unique movement of the horse under the child helps the child with physical disabilities to achieve increased flexibility, balance, and muscle strength. Children with mental or emotional disabilities may experience increased self-esteem, confidence, and patience as a result of the unique relationship with the horse. A physical therapist or psychotherapist (depending on the situation) generally works very closely with specially trained equine staff (Granados & Agis, 2011). Box 34.5 lists chronic medical conditions for which hippotherapy may be beneficial. Additional information may be obtained through the North American Riding for the Handicapped Association or the American Hippotherapy Association. Links to these sites can be found on thePoint.

Music may be used to induce positive behavioral changes, reduce pain or stress, or various other positive effects (American Music Therapy Association, 2016). Massage therapy may be beneficial to a wide variety of children. It may be used to reduce pain, promote relaxation, or demonstrate a specific positive effect related to the child's particular medical condition (Cotton, Luberto, Bogenschutz, et al., 2014).

BOX 34.5

CONDITIONS BENEFITING FROM HIPPOTHERAPY

- Muscular dystrophy
- Cerebral palsy
- Visual impairment
- Down syndrome
- Intellectual disability
- Autism
- Multiple sclerosis
- Brain injury
- Myelomeningocele
- Spinal cord injury
- Amputation
- Attention deficit disorder
- Learning disabilities
- Deafness
- Cerebrovascular accident (stroke)

Adapted fromThe Children's TherAplay Foundation, Inc. (2016). *Hippotherapy*. Retrieved from http://www.childrenstheraplay.org/hippotherapy

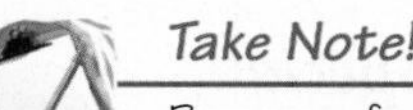

Take Note!

Become familiar with the risks and benefits of homeopathic and herbal medications, as many families use these treatments in an effort to improve their child's quality of life or outcome.

Providing Support and Education

At the time of initial diagnosis, allow and encourage the family to express their feelings. Parents of children with special health care needs require emotional, practical, economic, and social support. Encourage parents to obtain help with daily routines. Encourage stress reduction for the parents through exercise and allowing time for themselves. Be a supportive and encouraging listener, making sure to nurture the whole child, not just his or her special condition.

Parents value peer support groups, sometimes feeling that only other parents of disabled or chronically ill children could understand the heartache, fear, and other emotions they often experience. Pediatric nurses should be proactive in helping families find support systems.

Fathers have the same concerns about their children as mothers do, but they may show these concerns differently. It is important for nurses to involve them in the child's care. Teach skills to both parents, and actively involve fathers by asking about their observations and opinions.

Parents become the experts on their child's needs and care, and they should be recognized as such. Parents want to be taken seriously and do not like being ignored. They should be viewed as having reliable and valuable information about their children. By being an active and reflective listener, the nurse can demonstrate to the parents that their opinion is valued, in addition to finding out what the child really needs. Some parents may hesitate to volunteer information, unsure about which information the nurse needs. Show respect for the parents' knowledge of their child's needs by seeking advice on the child's daily care, medical/physical needs, and current developmental level, no matter what the site of care is.

Families may need additional support from the nurse at times of transition. As the equipment or treatment needs change, adjust the teaching plan. Educate the child and family about the use of adaptive equipment. Ensure that families understand how specific activities must be modified to accommodate the child's needs. Provide anticipatory guidance related to expected developmental changes, including resources and laws related to education. Act as a liaison between the family and the day care center or school. As the child grows and matures, encourage parents to relinquish caregiving tasks to the child as appropriate to encourage independence and promote self-esteem.

Assisting the Adolescent With Special Health Needs Making the Transition to Adulthood

Adolescence is a time of physical changes, psychosocial challenges, and initiation of independence from parents. The adolescent with a chronic illness or one who is technology dependent may experience this period differently from other teens. Puberty is often affected by chronic illness (either delayed or earlier). Chronic illness may lead to isolation from peers at a time when peer interaction is the core of psychosocial development. Teens may struggle to fit in with their peers by hiding their illness or health care needs (ignoring them), complying poorly with treatment regimens, or participating in risky behaviors. At a time when the child should be developing independence from the parents, he or she may be experiencing significant dependence related to the special health condition. For these reasons, the adolescent with special health care needs may require increased amounts of support from the nurse.

Making the transition to adult care for a child with special health care needs can be difficult, and advance planning leads to a smoother transition. Transition planning involves multidisciplinary care coordination; acknowledgement of the changing roles among the youth, family, and health care professionals; and fostering of the youth's self-determination skills. A written plan for transition to adult care should be initiated in mid-adolescence. Have ongoing conversations with the teen about this transition. Issues to be resolved prior to the transition include financial resources for medical care, college or vocational school attendance, living arrangements, and caretaking arrangements (Adolescent Health Transition Project [AHTP], 2012).

The AHTP recommends the following schedule:

- By age 14, ensure that a transition plan is initiated and that the IEP reflects post–high school plans.
- By age 17, explore health care financing for young adults. If needed, notify the local division of vocational rehabilitation by the autumn before the teen is to graduate from high school of the impending transition. Initiate guardianship procedures if appropriate.
- Notify the teen that all rights transfer to him or her at the age of majority. Check the teen's eligibility for SSI the month the child turns 18. Determine if the child is eligible for SSI work incentives.
- If the youth is attending college, contact the college's campus student disability service program.
- By age 21, ensure that the young adult has registered with the Division of Developmental Disabilities for adult services if applicable (AHTP, 2012).

Before moving to adult care (with an adult medical provider), ensure that the adolescent understands the treatment rationale, symptoms of worsening condition, and especially, danger signs. Teach the adolescent about when to seek help from a health professional. Introduce the teen to the medical insurance process. At transition, coordinate a seamless transfer by providing a detailed written plan to the care coordinator or advanced practice nurse (after verbal collaboration).

After the transition, serve as a consultant to the adult office in relation to the teen's needs. Consult with a transition services coordinator or other service agency as available in the local community (AHTP, 2012). See Healthy People 2020.

HEALTHY PEOPLE 2020

Objective	Nursing Significance
(Developmental) Increase the proportion of children with special health care needs whose physician has discussed transition planning from pediatric to adult health care.	• In the primary care setting, assist families with planning for transition beginning in early adolescence. • If available, refer families to multidisciplinary programs for medically complex children.

Healthy People Objectives retrieved from http://www.healthypeople.gov

THE DYING CHILD

The idea that a child may die is simply unimaginable to most people, yet children die daily. Each year, about 45,000 children die in the United States; of those, over 24,500 are infants (Murphy, Xu, & Kochanek, 2013). A child's chronic illness may progress to the point of becoming a **terminal illness** (illness deemed to be noncurable, ultimately leading to death). For example, despite the increased survival rates for children with cancer as a result of improved treatment options and protocols, cancer remains the leading cause of death from disease in all children older than the age of 1 year (Murphy, et al., 2013). Less frequently, other diseases also lead to terminal illness in children, with congenital defects and traumatic injuries being the more common causes. Pediatric nurses will inevitably encounter situations in which a child dies. These situations are extremely difficult for all persons involved, and the nurse plays a key role in caring for the dying child and his or her family. Caring for the dying child is a family-centered, multidisciplinary process. Nurses must respond to the child's and family's physiologic, emotional, and spiritual needs during this difficult time. Children display differing responses to the dying process and impending death depending on their developmental level. Children and their families need significant amounts of support throughout the process of dying.

End-of-Life Decision Making

Parents are obligated not only to protect their children from harm but also to do as much good for them as possible, both from an ethical and a legal standpoint. When the time comes for end-of-life decision making, parents are often torn about the "right" course of action. Parents may be asked to make decisions about stopping treatment, withdrawing treatment, providing palliative care, or consenting to "do not resuscitate" (DNR) orders. Children, parents, and physicians are generally in agreement that continued suffering is not desired for any child with a terminal illness. When all possible curative attempts have been made, then survival is no longer possible (Rushton, 2004).

Nurses involved in this process must examine their own values related to dying and consider the American Nurses Association's code of ethics for nurses as well (2001). The family's feelings must also be acknowledged. During the process of end-of-life decision making, health care providers must assure families that the focus of care is changing and that the child is not being abandoned. Emphasize to parents that no matter what their decision is, the health care team is dedicated to the comfort and expert care of their child (Rushton, 2004).

Ensure that communication is family centered. Quality of life must be taken into consideration when making decisions to continue or withhold treatment. Provide parents facing end-of-life decisions with honest information and education from the time of the diagnosis/prognosis forward. Anticipate that parents may vacillate in the decision-making process. Clarify information for them and allow them private time to discuss the options. Do not make judgments about or question the parents' decision. Be sensitive to any ethnic, spiritual, or cultural preferences during the terminal stage of the illness. Encourage parents to interact with other parents who have a child with a terminal illness (Carter, Levetown, & Friebert, 2013).

Allowing Natural Death

The decision to institute a DNR order is one of the most difficult decisions a family may ever have to make. DNR refers to withholding cardiopulmonary resuscitation should the child's heart stop beating. Parents may initially feel like this means they are giving up on their child. Nurses must educate families that resuscitation may be inappropriate and lead to more suffering than if death were allowed to occur naturally. The parents need to understand that when a palliative care route is chosen, rather than continuing a curative or treatment route, the focus of the child's care is changing but the child and family are not being abandoned. Families may wish to specify a certain extent of resuscitation that they feel more comfortable with (e.g., allowing supplemental oxygen but not providing chest compressions). Some institutions are now replacing the DNR terminology with "allow natural death" (AND), which may be more acceptable to families facing the decision to withhold resuscitation.

Involving the Dying Child in the Decision-Making Process

End-of-life decision making often involves ethical dilemmas for the child, family, and health care team. This is particularly true when the parents' wishes conflict with the child's or adolescent's desires. Children should be involved in decision making to the extent that they are able. Discuss intervention within the context of the child's condition and wishes. Children of sufficient maturity may assent to the continuation or withdrawal of treatment (National Association of Pediatric Nurse Practitioners, 2015). Be available to the older child or adolescent to provide support and information if he or she desires. Talk with the child or adolescent with the parents present, as well as in private. Maintain the child's comfort and dignity. Encourage the child to spend time with other children with a terminal illness. Assure the child that everything will be done to make him or her comfortable. Consult parents about the timing and depth of end-of-life discussions. Just as parents do, the terminally ill child may vacillate in the decision-making process. Remain sensitive, and respect the child's decisions.

Organ or Tissue Donation

With large numbers of organ transplant candidates on waiting lists and the shortage of viable organs, pediatric organ and tissue donation is a priority (Cowl, Cummings, Yager, et al., 2012). For many families, knowing that a child's organs or tissues may save another child's life provides a way to help others despite their own loss. A healthy child who dies unexpectedly is an excellent candidate for organ donation. Many chronic illnesses in children preclude the option of organ or tissue donation, though individual determinations of eligibility should be made.

The discussion of organ donation should be separated from the discussion of impending death or brain death notification. Written consent is necessary for organ donation, so the family must be appropriately informed and educated. Many families who never thought about it before may consider the option of donation if adequately educated about the process. All expenses for organ procurement are borne by the recipient's family, not the donor's. Ask whether the dying child ever expressed a wish to donate organs and whether the parents have considered it.

Families need to know that procurement of the organs does not mar the child's appearance, so that an open casket at the child's funeral is still possible if the family desires. The donating child will not suffer further because of organ donation. The organs or tissues will be harvested in a timely fashion after the declaration of death, so the family need not worry about delay of the wake or funeral. The family's cultural and religious beliefs must be considered, and the team discussing organ donation with the family must do so in a sensitive and ethical manner (Cowl et al., 2012).

Palliative Care of the Dying Child

Appropriate **palliative care** is essential for any child with a life-threatening or progressive incurable condition (Crozier & Hancock, 2012). Whether palliative care is provided in the home, hospital, or hospice setting, the goal is to provide the best quality of life possible at the end of life while alleviating physical, psychological, emotional, and spiritual suffering (Crozier & Hancock, 2012). Palliative care of children should be based upon the following principles:

- Respect for the child's goals, preferences, and choices
- Acknowledgement and addressing of caregiver's concerns
- Provision of a comprehensive, interdisciplinary continuum of care in the community
- Competent and ethical care

Adapted from Association of Pediatric Oncology Nurses (2003). *Precepts of palliative care for children, adolescents and their families.* Retrieved from http://www.apon.org/files/public/last_acts_precepts.pdf and Children's Hospice International. (2005). *Standards of care and practice guidelines.* Retrieved from http://www.chionline.org/standards-of-care-and-practice-guidelines/

Hospice Care

Hospice allows for family-centered care in the child's home or a hospice facility. As with adult hospice care, the comfort of the entire family is important. The goal of pediatric hospice care is enhancement of quality of life for the child and family through an individualized plan of care. The recommended standards for pediatric hospice care allow for palliative care to be given concurrently with potentially curative treatments (this is in contrast to traditional adult hospice), but the model is not yet available in all areas due to funding issues (Klein & Saroyan, 2011). This allows for hope to be maintained and bereavement care provided when that time comes (Children's Hospice International, 2011). Parents are educated on ways to comfort and interact with their dying child, such as massage, movement, or singing. Spiritual support is available through a chaplain, a social worker, or the family's minister. The nurse not only educates the family about the dying process but also assists them with providing basic care and pain management. The decision to withhold nutrition or hydration may be made in certain instances. Pain management is of the utmost importance for the terminally ill child. Adequate pain control has positive impact on families, whereas poor pain management may be associated with complicated grieving (Shaw, 2012). Ongoing bereavement care is also provided to the family by the hospice after the child's death.

Nursing Management of the Dying Child

Though interdisciplinary care is essential for quality care at the end of life, it is the nurse who plays the key role of child/family advocate and who is usually the constant presence throughout the dying process. Nursing management of the dying child focuses on managing pain and discomfort, providing nutrition, providing emotional support to the dying child and family, and assisting the family through the grief process. Throughout the process, it is important to focus on the family as the unit of care.

Managing Pain and Discomfort

Pain management is an essential component of care for the child with a terminal illness. Adequately managing pain may enhance the child's quality of life and minimizes suffering (Crozier & Hancock, 2012). Assess pain using a developmentally appropriate tool (see Chapter 36 for further information). Provide pain medication around

EVIDENCE-BASED PRACTICE 34.1 **INTEGRATIVE THERAPIES FOR PAIN MANAGEMENT IN CHILDREN**

STUDY

Integrative care providers recorded data from 4,749 care visits to 2,404 children. The authors eliminated data from children whose records were incomplete or who were seen as outpatients. The remaining 519 children were included in the study data. Standard pain rating scales (based on developmental age and unit policy) were used to assess pain before and after the integrative treatment.

Findings

Mean pain scores decreased significantly following integrative care interventions. The data demonstrate that integrative care interventions (especially massage and healing touch) contribute to improvement in pain scores and relaxation in pediatric clients.

Nursing Implications

The results suggest that integrative care therapies may improve pain management and relaxation in children. Integrative care therapies continue to be primarily requested by the child or parent, rather than initiating from the health care provider. While the authors concede that additional rigorous studies are needed on this topic, integrative care interventions are not harmful to children and may help with decreasing pain.

Adapted from Cotton, S., Luberto, C. M., Bogenschutz, L. H., Pelley, T. J., & Dusek, J. (2014). Integrative care therapies and pain in hospitalized children and adolescents: A retrospective database review. *The Journal of Alternative and Complementary Medicine*, 20(2), 98–102.

the clock rather than on an "as needed" basis to prevent recurrence or escalation of pain. Determine the child's preferred comfort measures and use them to provide additional relief. Change the child's position frequently but gently to minimize discomfort. Limit nursing care to comfort measures that ease the child's discomfort. Maintain a calm environment, minimizing noise and light. Include integrative care interventions such as massage or healing touch as requested and/or tolerated. See Evidence-Based Practice 34.1.

Providing Nutrition

Since the body naturally requires less nutrition as the child is dying, do not excessively coax the child to eat or drink. Offer frequent small meals or snacks of the child's choosing. Soups and shakes require less energy to eat and so may be desirable. If the child desires a different food, provide that one. Keep strong odors away from the child to decrease nausea. Administer antiemetics as needed. Provide mouth care and keep the lips lubricated to keep the mouth feeling clean and prevent the discomfort associated with chapped lips. Make sure the environment is a pleasant one for eating.

Providing Emotional Support to the Dying Child and Family

Be attuned to the entire family's needs and emotions in order to foster a holistic connection with the child and family. Nurses provide physical care through specific tasks and interventions for the dying child, but they also need to be fully present emotionally with the child and family. In general, people are uncomfortable with the concept of a dying child. Nurses should work through their own feelings about the situation in order to stay fully present with the child and family, attending to their individualized needs. Ask yourself how you can change in order to be fully present with the child and family. (Carter et al., 2013).

Families and dying children benefit from the presence of the nurse, not just the interventions he or she performs. Families report that the simple act of being present with the family is very healing (Carter et al., 2013). Listen to the child and family; be still and silent for a time to accomplish this. Foster respect for the whole child by attending to him or her as such.

Respect the parents of the dying child by helping them honor the commitments they have made to their child. Acknowledge that parents have diverse needs for information and participation in decision making. Allow and encourage family customs or rituals in relation to death and dying. Families may desire the pastor or priest to be present when the child's death is imminent. Certain rituals may be desired, depending on the family's religious or spiritual background. Ensure that these important events occur, and alter nursing care routines as needed to accommodate them. Respect the family's need to participate in these rituals and customs (Carter et al., 2013).

Work collaboratively with the family and health care team to provide for the needs of the child and family. Resources for families of a dying child are listed in Box 34.6. The Make-a-Wish Foundation works to grant the wishes of terminally ill children, giving the child and family an experience of hope, strength, and love. A link to the Make-a-Wish Foundation is included on thePoint.

EASING ANXIETY OR FEARS

Parents may be afraid of their child dying alone or not know what to expect in the death process. This fear may contribute to increased anxiety, which the child

BOX 34.6

RESOURCES FOR FAMILIES OF A DYING CHILD

Websites

- www.joyandhope.org: Project Joy and Hope
- www.chionline.org: Children's Hospice International
- www.compassionatefriends.org: Compassionate Friends

Books

- Gentle Willow: A Story for Children About Dying by Joyce Mills
- 35 Ways to Help a Grieving Child by the Dougy Center for Grieving Children
- Sad Isn't Bad by Michaeline Mundy
- A Child Asks. … What Does Dying Mean? by Lake Pylant Monhollon
- Talking With Children and Young People About Death and Dying: A Workbook by Mary Turner
- The Worst Loss: How Families Heal From the Death of a Child by Barbara Rosof
- I Have No Intention of Saying Goodbye: Parents Share Their Stories of Hope and Healing After a Child's Death by Sandy Fox
- Stars in the Deepest Night: After the Death of a Child by Genesse Gentry
- The Bereaved Parent by Harriet Schiff
- You Are Special by Max Lucado

may sense. Younger children may fear separation from their parents and older children may not want to die alone or experience pain or discomfort associated with dying. Each child and family is individual; discuss their particular fears and anxieties in order to determine the child's and family's needs for education and support (Carter et al., 2013).

Involve the parents and other family members in all phases of the child's care. Explain all aspects of care to the child to minimize anxiety related to nursing interventions. Answer the child's questions honestly. Involve the child in decision making whenever possible. Limit interventions to those related to palliation, rather than treatment, advocating for the child as needed. Remain with the child when a parent or family member is not in the room so the child will not fear dying alone.

MEETING THE DYING CHILD'S NEEDS ACCORDING TO DEVELOPMENTAL STAGE

It is important to provide the type of support and education that the dying child needs according to his or her developmental stage. For the infant, unconditional love and trust are of utmost importance. Ensure that the infant's family is available to the child. The toddler, 1 to 3 years old, thrives on familiarity and routine. Maximize the toddler's time with parents, be consistent, provide favorite toys, and ensure physical comfort. Spirituality in the preschool years focuses on the concept of right versus wrong. The 3- to 5-year-old may see death as punishment for wrongdoing; correct this misunderstanding. Use honest and precise language. Help the parents to teach the child that though the family will miss the child, it will continue to function without him or her (Ethier, 2010).

The school-age child has a concrete understanding of death. Children who are 5 to 10 years old need specific, honest details (as desired). Encourage the child to help make decisions, and help the child to establish a sense of control (Ethier, 2010).

The young adolescent (10 to 14 years old) will benefit from reinforcement of self-esteem, self-respect, and a sense of worth. Respect the child's need for privacy and time alone as well as time requested with peers. Support the need for independence and encourage the child to participate in decision making. The older teen (14 to 18 years of age) has a more adult-like understanding of death and will need further support through honest, detailed explanations and will want to feel truly involved and listened to (Ethier, 2010).

Assisting the Family Through the Grief Process

The family may experience anticipatory grief when the diagnosis of terminal illness is made. Families may deny the prognosis, become angry at the health care system or a higher power, or experience depression. Acute grief is an intense process that occurs around the time of the actual death. Family members may feel short of breath or as though the throat is tight. They may verbalize that the situation is unreal to them or search for reasons why the death was not prevented. Families may also display hostility or restlessness. Each individual will express grief in his or her own manner. Mourning the death of a loved one takes a long time, and families should be supported throughout the process (Carter et al., 2013; Ethier, 2010). Local and national resources are available for grieving parents. Several resources for grieving parents are listed on thePoint. Refer parents to bereavement resources as appropriate.

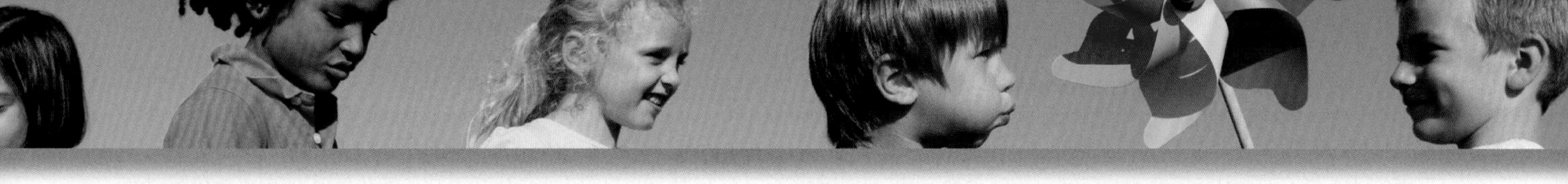

KEY CONCEPTS

- Children with special health care needs are those who have, or are at risk for, a chronic physical, developmental, behavioral, or emotional condition that generally requires more intensive and diverse health services, as well as coordination of those services, than do typical children.
- Most children with chronic illnesses or who are dependent on technology progress through stages of growth and development just as typical children do, though possibly at a slower pace.
- Parents of special needs children experience a multitude of emotions and changes in their lives, often carrying a heavy caregiving burden. They become the experts on their child's care and should be empowered and supported in their efforts.
- The child and family with special needs may require additional support during times of transition, such as at initial diagnosis or change in prognosis, when symptoms increase, when the child moves to a new setting (hospital, school), during periods of developmental change, or during a parent's absence.
- Children with special health care needs are at increased risk for the development of vulnerable child syndrome, which may have psychologically harmful effects on the child and parents for many years.
- Home is the most developmentally appropriate environment for children with special health care needs and those who are technology dependent. Children display an improved physical, emotional, psychological, and social status when they are cared for at home.
- Family-centered care provides the optimal framework for caring for children and families with special needs. Empowering the family strengthens them. A medical home or a permanent relationship with the physician or nurse practitioner benefits the family, as care coordination and advocacy are provided.
- Use adjusted (or corrected) age when assessing growth and development of the infant or child who was born prematurely. Provide early screening and intervention for issues related to development to maximize the former preemie's potential for growth and development.
- Become familiar with the risks and benefits of adjuvant therapies used by some families of children with special health care needs.
- Screen children with special health care needs for failure to thrive or a feeding disorder.
- Screening helps to identify children with unmet health needs so that intervention may begin.
- Early intervention provides care coordination (developmental services and special education), as well as an individualized family service plan for qualifying children and their families.
- Each special needs student is entitled to an IEP, which is a written plan that is designed to meet the preschool, primary, or secondary school student's needs.
- Early discharge planning and ongoing inclusion and education of the family facilitate continuity of care. During midadolescence, initiate a written plan to help the special needs child make the transition to adult care.
- Support the dying child and the family throughout the end-of-life decision-making process, providing facts as desired about palliative care, hospice, and organ donation.
- Younger children who are dying generally need for their families to be close and to trust their needs will be provided for. Older children require honest explanations given at a level appropriate for the child's age or developmental stage.

REFERENCES AND RECOMMENDED READINGS

108th Congress. (2004). *Individuals with disabilities education improvement act of 2004.* Retrieved July 18, 2015, from http://www.gpo.gov/fdsys/pkg/PLAW-108publ446/html/PLAW-108publ446.htm

Adolescent Health Transition Project. (2012). *A resource for adolescents with special health care needs, chronic illnesses, physical or developmental disabilities.* Retrieved from http://depts.washington.edu/healthtr/

American Music Therapy Association. (2016). *What is music therapy?* Retrieved from http://www.musictherapy.org/

American Nurses Association. (2001). *Code of ethics for nurses with interpretive statements.* Washington, DC: Author.

Association of Pediatric Oncology Nurses. (2003). *Precepts of palliative care for children, adolescents and their families.* Retrieved from http://www.apon.org/files/public/last_acts_precepts.pdf

Berry, A. D., Garzon, D. L., & Deloian, B. J. (2012). Developmental management in pediatric primary care. In C. E. Burns, A. M. Dunn, M. A. Brady, N. B. Starr, & C. G. Blosser (Eds.), *Pediatric primary care* (5th ed.). Philadelphia, PA: Elsevier Saunders.

Billimoria, Z. C., & Kamat, D. (2014). A pediatrician's guide to caring for the complex neonatal intensive care unit graduate. *Pediatric Annals, 43*(9), 369–372.

Caley, L. M. (2012). Risk and protective factors associated with stress in mothers whose children are enrolled in early intervention services. *Journal of Pediatric Health Care, 26*(5), 346–355.

Carey, D., Russek, M., & Esposito, P. (2013). Supplementation in preterm and later preterm infants after discharge. *ICAN: Infant, Child, & Adolescent Nutrition, 5*(1), 26–28.

Carter, B. S., Levetown, M., & Friebert, S. E. (2013).*Palliative care for infants, children, and adolescents: A practical handbook* (2nd ed.). Baltimore, MD: Johns Hopkins University Press.

Chambers, P. L., Mahabee-Gittens, E. M., & Leonard, A. C. (2011). Vulnerable child syndrome, parental perception of child vulnerability, and emergency department usage. *Pediatric Emergency Care, 27*(11), 1009–1013.

Child and Adolescent Health Measurement Initiative. (2015). *The children with special health care needs (CSHCN) screener©*. Retrieved from http://www.cahmi.org/projects/children-with-special-health-care-needs-screener/

Children's Hospice International. (2011). *ChiPACC at a glance*. Retrieved from www.chionline.org/chipacc-at-a-glance-2/

Cotton, S., Luberto, C. M., Bogenschutz, L. H., Pelley, T. J., & Dusek, J. (2014). Integrative care therapies and pain in hospitalized children and adolescents: A retrospective database review. *The Journal of Alternative and Complementary Medicine, 20*(2), 98–102.

Cowl, A. S., Cummings, B. M., Yager, P. H., Miller, B., & Noviski, N. (2012). Organ donation after cardiac death in children: Acceptance of a protocol by multidisciplinary staff. *American Journal of Critical Care, 21*(5), 322–327.

Crozier, F., & Hancock, L. E. (2012). Pediatric palliative care. *Pediatric nursing, 38*(4), 198–203, 227.

D'Agostino, J. A., Gerdes, M., Hoffman, C., Manning, M. L., Phalen, A., & Bernbaum, J. (2013). Provider use of corrected age during health supervision visits for premature infants. *Journal of Pediatric Health Care, 27*(3), 172–179.

Ethier, A. M. (2010). Care of the dying child and the family. In D. Tomlinson & N. E. Kline (Eds.), *Pediatric oncology nursing*. New York: Springer.

Goode, T. D., Haywood, S. H., Wells, N., & Rhee, K. (2009). Family-centered, culturally, and linguistically competent care: Essential components of the medical home. *Pediatric Annals, 38*(9), 505–512.

Granados, A. C., & Agis, I. F. (2011). Why children with special needs feel better with hippotherapy sessions: A conceptual review. *The Journal of Alternative and Complementary Medicine, 17*(3), 191–197.

Hewitt-Taylor, J. (2012). Planning the transition of children with complex needs from hospital to home. *Nursing Children and Young People, 24*(10), 28–35.

Horowitz, J. A., & Marchetti, C. M. (2010). Mood disorders. In P. J. Allen, J. A. Vessey, & N. A. Schapiro (Eds.), *Primary care of the child with a chronic condition* (5th ed.). St. Louis, MO: Mosby.

Kelly, M. M. (2010). Prematurity. In P. J. Allen, J. A. Vessey, & N. A. Schapiro (Eds.), *Primary care of the child with a chronic condition* (5th ed.). St. Louis, MO: Mosby.

Kirkland, R. T., Motil, K. J., & Duryea, T. K. (2015a). *Failure to thrive (undernutrition) in children younger than two years: Etiology and evaluation*. Retrieved from http://www.uptodate.com/contents/failure-to-thrive-undernutrition-in-children-younger-than-two-years-etiology-and-evaluation

Kirkland, R. T., Motil, K. J., & Duryea, T. K. (2015b). *Failure to thrive (undernutrition) in children younger than two years: Management*. Retrieved from http://www.uptodate.com/contents/failure-to-thrive-undernutrition-in-children-younger-than-two-years-management

Klein, S. M., & Saroyan, J. M. (2011). Treating a child with a life-threatening condition. *Pediatric Annals, 40*(5), 259–265.

Knafl, K. A., & Santacroce, S. J. (2010). Chronic conditions & the family. In P. J. Allen, J. A. Vessey, & N. A. Schapiro (Eds.), *Primary care of the child with a chronic condition* (5th ed.). St. Louis, MO: Mosby.

Lane, C., & Mason, C. (2014). Meeting the needs of siblings of children with life-limiting illnesses. *Nursing Children & Young People, 26*(3), 16–20.

Looman, W. S., O'Conner-Von, S., & Lindeke, L. L. (2008). Caring for children with special health care needs and their families: What advanced practice nurses need to know. *Journal for Nurse Practitioners, 4*(7), 512–518.

McAllister, J. W., Presler, E., Turchi, R., & Antonelli, R. C. (2009). Achieving effective care coordination in the medical home. *Pediatric Annals, 38*(9), 491–497.

Mendes, M. A. (2013). Parents' descriptions of ideal home nursing care for their technology-dependent children. *Pediatric Nursing, 39*(2), 91–96.

Murphy, S. L., Xu, J., & Kochanek, K. D. (2013). Deaths: Final data for 2010;157(14). Hyattsville, MD: National Center for Health Statistics.

National Association of Pediatric Nurse Practitioners. (2015). NAPNAP position statement on protection of children involved in research studies. *Journal of Pediatric Health Care,* 29, 13A–15A.

Rushton, C. H. (2004). Ethics and palliative care in pediatrics: When should parents agree to withdraw life-sustaining therapy for children? *AJN, 104*(4), 54–63.

Schulman, L. H., Meringolo, D., & Scott, G. (2007). Early intervention: A crash course for pediatricians. *Pediatric Annals, 36*(8), 463–469.

Shaw, T. M. (2012). Pediatric palliative pain and symptom management. *Pediatric Annals, 41*(8), 329–334.

Social Security Administration. (n.d.). *Title V–maternal and child health services block grant*. Retrieved from http://www.ssa.gov/OP_Home/ssact/title05/0500.htm

Starr, N. B., Blosser, C. G., Brady, M. A., Burns, C. E., Dunn, A. M., & Petersen-Smith, A. M. (2013). Gastrointestinal disorders. In C. E. Burns, A. M. Dunn, M. A. Brady, N. B. Starr, & C. G. Blosser. *Pediatric primary care* (5th ed.). Philadelphia, PA: Elsevier Saunders.

Stewart, J. (2015). *Discharge planning for high-risk newborns*. Retrieved from http://www.uptodate.com/contents/discharge-planning-for-high-risk-newborns.

Sullivan, M. C., Msall, M. E., & Miller, R. J. (2012). 17-year outcome of preterm infants with diverse neonatal morbidities: Part 1 – impact on physical, neurological, and psychological health status. *Journal for Specialists in Pediatric Nursing, 17*(3), 1009–1013.

The Children's TherAplay Foundation, Inc. (2016). *Hippotherapy*. Retrieved from http://www.childrenstheraplay.org/hippotherapy

U. S. Department of Education. (n.d.). *Building the legacy: IDEA 2004*. Retrieved from http://idea.ed.gov/

U. S. Department of Education. (2011). *Q and A: Questions and answers on individualized education programs (IEPs), evaluations and reevaluations*. Retrieved from http://idea.ed.gov/explore/view/p/%2Croot%2Cdynamic%2CQaCorner%2C3%2C

U.S. Department of Health and Human Services. (2016). *Healthy people 2020 topics and objectives*. Retrieved from http://www.healthypeople.gov/2020/topicsobjectives2020/default

U.S. Department of Health and Human Services, Health Resources and Services Administration, Maternal and Child Health Bureau. (2013). *The national survey of children with special health care needs chartbook 2009–2010*. Rockville, MD: U.S. Department of Health and Human Services.

Vessey, J. A., & Brown, S. S. (2010). Financing health care for children with chronic conditions. In P. J. Allen, J. A. Vessey, & N. A. Schapiro (Eds.), *Primary care of the child with a chronic condition* (5th ed.). St. Louis, MO: Mosby.

Vessey, J. A., & Sullivan, B. J. (2010). Chronic conditions and child development. In P. J. Allen, J. A. Vessey, & N. A. Schapiro (Eds.), *Primary care of the child with a chronic condition* (5th ed.). St. Louis, MO: Mosby.

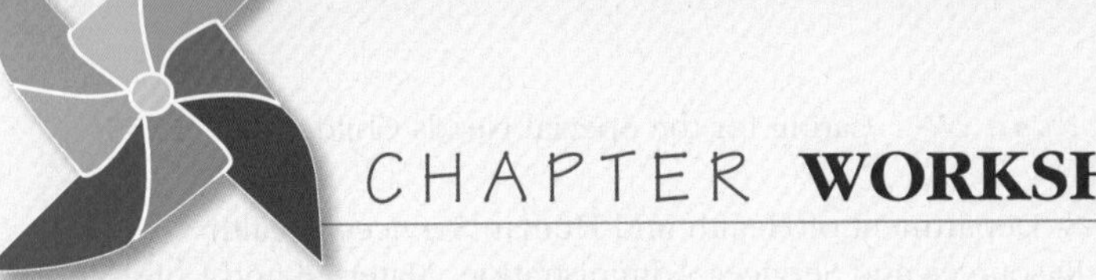

CHAPTER WORKSHEET

MULTIPLE CHOICE QUESTIONS

1. The parents of a 5-year-old with special health care needs talk to the parents of a 10-year-old with a similar condition for quite a while each day. What is the nurse's interpretation of this behavior?
   a. The nurse has not provided enough emotional support for the parents.
   b. This relationship between the children's parents is potentially unhealthy.
   c. Support between parents of special children is extremely valuable.
   d. Confidentiality is a pressing issue in this particular situation.

2. The nurse is caring for a child who has received all possible medical care for cancer, yet continues to experience relapse and metastasis. It is time to make the transition from curative care attempts to palliative care. What is the most important nursing consideration at this time?
   a. The health care professionals should make the decision about the child's care.
   b. The family may lose a sense of hope, so cancer treatments should continue.
   c. Involve the family in the decision-making process about the shift to palliative care.
   d. Palliative care can take place only at home, so the child should be discharged.

3. The nurse is caring for a 3-year-old with a gastrostomy tube and tracheostomy who is on supplemental oxygen and multiple medications. The mother is rooming in during this hospitalization. What is the priority nursing action?
   a. Incorporate the mother's assistance in care when convenient.
   b. Recognize the mother as the expert on her child's needs and care.
   c. Recommend that the mother go home to get some rest.
   d. Provide family-centered care since the mother is there.

4. The nurse is caring for a child with a developmental disability who is starting kindergarten this year. The mother is tearful and doesn't want the child to go to school. What is the best response by the nurse?
   a. "Do you need some time alone to collect yourself?"
   b. "You've known for a while this time would come."
   c. "Can I call your husband or a friend for you?"
   d. "It is normal to feel stressed or sad at this time."

5. The parents of a child with a developmental disability ask the nurse for advice about disciplining their child. What is the best response by the nurse?
   a. "You should choose methods that are most congruent with your values about discipline."
   b. "Children like this really can't follow directions, so they may be very hard to discipline."
   c. "Punish your child only for socially unacceptable or offending behaviors."
   d. "Spanking works well for this type of child, as they really don't like pain."

CRITICAL THINKING EXERCISES

1. A 15-year-old boy is dying of cancer after all medical care options have been exhausted. Describe the plan of care for this child and his family. What strategies should the nurse use to support the child and his family through this difficult process?

2. A 5-month-old infant who was born at 24 weeks' gestation is ready to be discharged from the NICU. She will be going home on oxygen, gastrostomy tube feedings, and eight medications. Develop a teaching plan for the family.

STUDY ACTIVITIES

1. In the clinical setting, care for a child with a terminal illness. Reflect in your clinical journal about the feelings you had during the care of the child, as well as the feelings and behaviors that you noticed in the child, siblings, parents, and nursing staff.

2. Visit a preschool that provides care for developmentally delayed and typical children. Choose two same-age children, one with a disability or impairment and the other a typical healthy child. Perform a Denver developmental screening or developmental assessment on each of the two children. Compare and contrast your findings.

3. Spend the day with a home care nurse providing care for a technology-dependent child. What obstacles has the family overcome to have this child at home? What adjustments does the nurse make to provide family-centered care in the home (as compared to the hospital setting)?

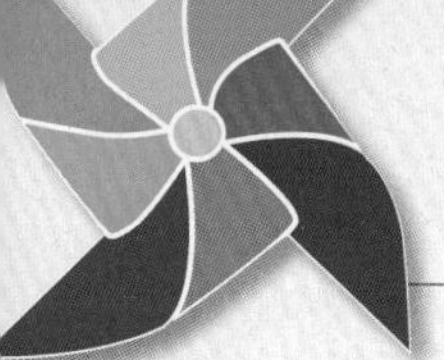

CHAPTER WORKSHEET

BRINGING IT ALL TOGETHER: A CASE STUDY

Trey, a 7-month-old boy, will be receiving private duty nursing 8 hours per day upon his discharge from the NICU. He was born at 24 weeks' gestation and was discharged on oxygen via nasal cannula, a cardiac/apnea monitor, and oral feeding during the day with supplemental gastrostomy tube feedings overnight. In addition to twice-daily nebulized medications, he usually requires additional treatments throughout the day and is also on four additional oral/G-tube medications. His mother has verbalized being overwhelmed by the thought of caring for Trey at home.

Go to thePoint to find questions to consider about this case.

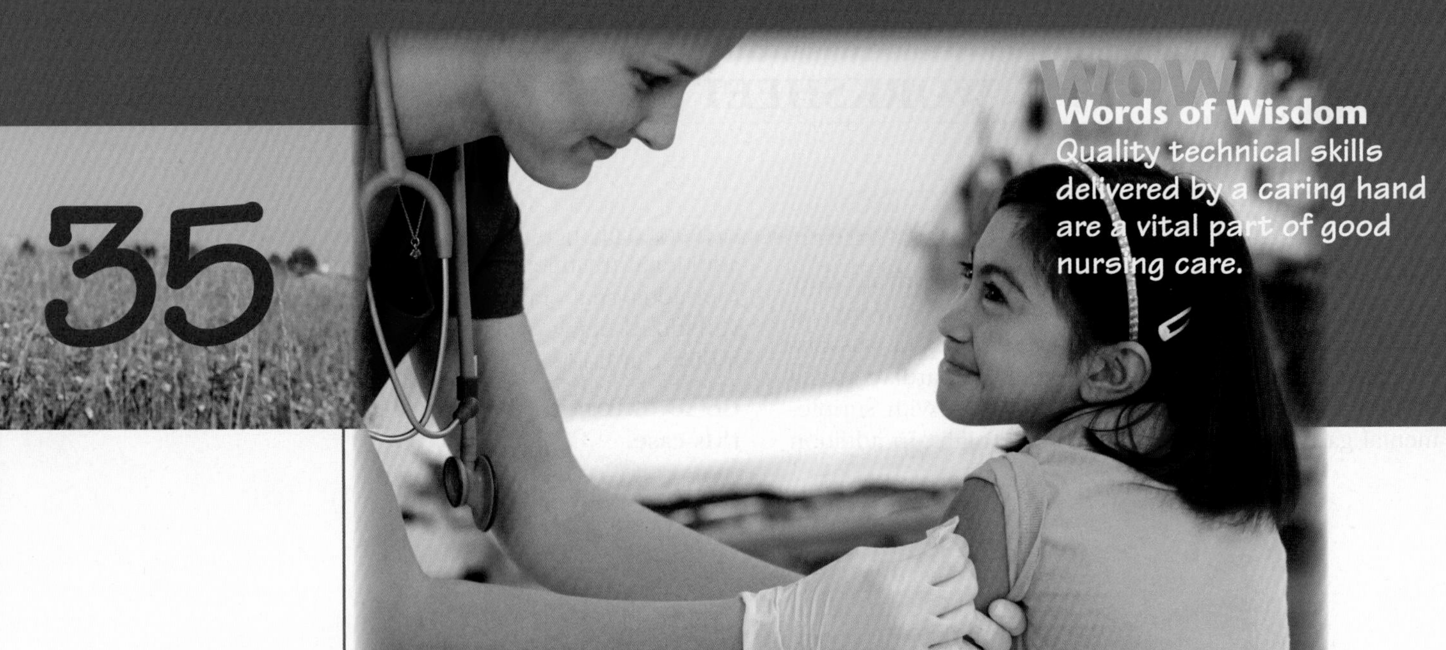

35
Words of Wisdom
Quality technical skills delivered by a caring hand are a vital part of good nursing care.

Key Pediatric Nursing Interventions

KEY TERMS
bolus feeding
enteral nutrition
gastric residual
gastrostomy
gavage feedings
infiltration
parenteral nutrition
pharmacodynamics
pharmacokinetics
total parenteral nutrition

Learning Objectives

Upon completion of this chapter, you will be able to:

1. Describe the "rights" of pediatric medication administration.
2. Explain the physiologic differences in children affecting a medication's pharmacodynamic and pharmacokinetic properties.
3. Accurately determine recommended pediatric medication doses.
4. Demonstrate the proper technique for administering medication to children via the oral, rectal, ophthalmic, otic, intravenous, intramuscular, and subcutaneous routes.
5. Integrate the concepts of atraumatic care in medication administration for children.
6. Identify the preferred sites for peripheral and central intravenous medication administration.
7. Describe nursing management related to maintenance of intravenous infusions in children, as well as prevention of complications.
8. Explain nursing care related to enteral tube feedings.
9. Describe nursing management of the child receiving total parenteral nutrition.

***Lily Kline*, a 9-month-old, is admitted to your unit for failure to thrive. The physician has ordered insertion of a nasogastric tube to begin gavage feedings. The parents are very nervous and upset about this. They ask, "What will this tube do for Lily? It sounds very uncomfortable. What do you have to do to insert it? Will it have to stay in all the time? Won't it move?" How would you address their concerns?**

The ill child often requires medications, intravenous (IV) therapy, or enteral nutrition to restore health. These interventions occur most often in the inpatient setting, but with today's advanced technology many children may receive treatment in the home, day care center, school, physician's office, or other community setting.

This chapter will discuss the key elements of, and guidelines for, care related to medication administration, IV therapy, and nutritional support in children. Child and parent education is emphasized. The chapter will focus on adapting and modifying medication administration and nursing procedures based on the child's growth and development and providing these treatments using a family-centered, atraumatic approach. Refer back to Chapter 30 for an overview of the important aspects of caring for a child who is to undergo a procedure.

MEDICATION ADMINISTRATION

At one time or another, every child will need to receive medication. As with adults, pediatric medication administration is a critical component of safe and effective nursing care. The pediatric nurse must adapt administration principles and techniques to meet the child's needs. Medication administration, regardless of the route, requires a solid knowledge base about the drug and its action. As with medication administration to any person, the nurse must adhere to the "rights" of medication administration (Box 35.1). These rights were developed to ensure patient safety by decreasing the occurrence of medication errors. Some experts have added additional rights, such as right documentation, right to be educated, right to refuse, right form, and right approach. These additional rights are important to consider to increase patient safety and satisfaction.

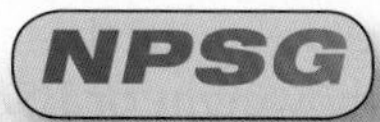

GOAL 1: Improve the Accuracy of Patient identification

NPSG.01.01.01 Use at least two patient identifiers when providing care, treatment, and services.

Steps: When administering medications to a child be sure to use at minimum two patient identifiers that are directly associated with the patient and the medication to be given, such as full name, patient ID number, and birth date.

Joint Commission. (2015). *National patient safety goals effective January 1, 2015.* Retrieved from http://www.jointcommission.org/assets/1/6/2015_NPSG_HAP.pdf

BOX 35.1

RIGHTS OF PEDIATRIC MEDICATION ADMINISTRATION

Right Medication
- Check order and expiration dates.
- Know action of medication and potential side effects (use pharmacy, drug formulary).
- Ensure that the medication provided is the medication that is ordered.

Right Patient
- Confirm child identity by two ways. Children may deny their identity in an attempt to avoid an unpleasant situation, play in another child's bed, or remove ID bracelet.
- Confirm identity each time medication is given.
- Verify child's name with caregiver to provide additional verification.
- Use technology when available (i.e., bar code systems).

Right Time
- Give within 20 to 30 minutes of the ordered time.
- For a medication given on an as-needed (PRN) basis, know when it was last given and how much was given during the past 24 hours.

Right Route of Administration
- Check ordered route and ensure this is the most effective and safest route for this child; clarify any order that is confusing or unclear.
- Give the medication by the route ordered. If there is a need to change route, always check with prescriber (e.g., if a child is vomiting and has an order for an oral medication, the medication may need to be given via the IV or rectal route).

Right Dose
- Calculate the recommended dose according to child's weight and double-check your calculations.
- Always question the pharmacist and/or prescriber if the ordered dose falls outside the recommended dose range.
- Unusually large or small volumes or dosages should always be verified.

Differences in Pharmacodynamics and Pharmacokinetics

Although a drug's mechanism of action is the same in any individual, the physiologic immaturity of some body systems in a child can affect a drug's **pharmacodynamics** (behavior of the medication at the cellular level). As a result, the body may not respond to the drug as intended. The intended effect may be enhanced or diminished, necessitating a change in the dosage to ensure optimal effectiveness without increasing the child's risk for toxicity.

The child's age, weight, body surface area (BSA), and body composition also can affect the drug's **pharmacokinetics** (movement of drugs throughout the body via absorption, distribution, metabolism, and excretion). Drugs are administered to children via many of the same routes that are used for adults. However, this similarity ends once the drug is administered. During the absorption process, drugs move from the administration site into the bloodstream. In infants and young children, the absorption of orally administered medications is affected by slower gastric emptying, increased intestinal motility, a proportionately larger small intestine surface area, higher gastric pH, and decreased lipase and amylase secretion compared with adults. Intramuscular (IM) absorption in infants and young children is affected by the amount of muscle mass, muscle tone and perfusion, and vasomotor instability. Similarly, decreased perfusion alters subcutaneous (SQ) absorption. Absorption by these routes is erratic and may be decreased. In contrast, topical absorption of medications is increased in infants and young children, which can result in adverse effects not seen in adults. Infants and young children have a greater BSA, leading to increased absorption of topical medications. Absorption in infants is also increased due to greater permeability of the infant's skin.

The distribution (movement of a drug from the blood to interstitial spaces and then into cells) of medications is also altered in infants and young children. Medication distribution in children is affected by:

- Higher percentage of body water than adults
- More rapid extracellular fluid exchange
- Decreased body fat
- Liver immaturity, altering first-pass elimination
- Decreased amounts of plasma proteins available for drug binding
- Immature blood–brain barrier, especially in neonates, allowing permeation by certain medications

Metabolism of medications in children is altered because of differences in hepatic enzyme production and the child's increased metabolic rate. Biotransformation (the alteration of chemical structures from their original form, which allows for the eventual excretion of the substance) is affected by the same variations affecting distribution in children. In addition, the immaturity of the kidneys until the age of 1 to 2 years affects renal blood flow, glomerular filtration, and active tubular secretion. This results in a longer half-life and increases the potential for toxicity of drugs primarily excreted by the kidneys.

Developmental Issues and Concerns

Children are constantly growing and developing. The specific psychosocial, cognitive, physical, and motor developmental levels of children are important. Nurses need a solid understanding of growth and development to ensure safe administration of medications to children. Table 35.1 details some growth and development issues related to administering medications to children. Always give developmentally appropriate, truthful explanations before administering medications to children, including:

- Why the drug is needed
- What the child will experience
- What is expected of the child
- How the parents can participate and support their child

Refer to Chapters 25 through 29 for further information about growth and developmental issues.

The child's past experiences with taking medications and the approaches that may have been used will often affect how the child reacts. Always approach children positively; let your manner convey the belief that they can accomplish this needed behavior. Never label the child as "bad" if he or she did not fully cooperate in taking medication. When medications must be administered with a needle (intramuscularly or subcutaneously), assure the child that this method is not a consequence of the child's behavior. Help parents to work through the feelings of frustration that may result from the child's refusal to cooperate with medication administration. Provide parents with facts about growth and developmental issues and children's fears and anxiety related to medication administration. Model alternative ways for the parents to deal with undesirable behavior.

Take Note!

Always administer medications promptly, assist the child in holding still using a comforting position for the child, and reward positive behavior.

Determination of Correct Dose

Administering the correct dose is a key component of medication administration. Children are more vulnerable to medication errors due to the individual dosing necessary for proper medication administration. Incorrect dosing or quantity has been found to be the most commonly reported medication error in the pediatric population (Manias, Kinney, Cranswick, & Williams, 2014). Many drug references list recommended pediatric dosages, and nurses are responsible for checking doses to ensure that they are appropriate for the child. Two common methods for determining pediatric doses are based on the unit of drug per kilogram of body weight or BSA.

Dose Determination by Body Weight

The most common method for calculating pediatric medication doses is based on body weight. The recommended dosage is usually expressed as the amount of drug to be given over a 24-hour period (mg/kg/day) or as a single dose (mg/kg/dose). It is important to differentiate between the 24-hour dosage and the single dose. Use these guidelines to determine the correct dose by body weight:

1. Weigh the child.
2. If the child's weight is in pounds, convert it to kilograms (divide the child's weight in pounds by 2.2).
3. Check a drug reference for the safe dose range (e.g., 10 to 20 mg/kg of body weight).
4. Calculate the low safe dose (Box 35.2).
5. Calculate the high safe dose (Box 35.2).
6. Determine if the dose ordered is within this range.

TABLE 35.1 GROWTH AND DEVELOPMENT ISSUES RELATED TO PEDIATRIC MEDICATION ADMINISTRATION

Stage of Development	Issue/Concern	Nursing Interventions
Infant	Development of trust, which is fostered by consistent care; development of stranger anxiety later in infancy	Involve parents in medication administration to reduce stress for infant Ensure that parents hold and comfort infant during intervention
Toddler	Development of autonomy with displays of negativism; rituals, routines, and choices necessary to maintain some sense of control	Follow routines and rituals from home in giving medications if these are safe and positive approaches Involve parents in medication administration Offer simple choices (e.g., "Do you want Mom or me to give you your medicine?") Allow child to touch or handle equipment as appropriate
Preschooler	Development of initiative, which is fostered when they sense they are helping	Provide an opportunity to play with the equipment and respond positively to explanations and comforting Provide choices that are possible and keep them simple (e.g., "Do you want juice or water with your medication?" or "Which medication do you want to take first?") Do not ask, "Will you take your medicine now?" Involve parents in medication administration Be aware that giving suppositories is particularly upsetting to this age group because of their fears of bodily intrusion and mutilation
School-aged child	Development of industry, benefiting from being a part of their care; generally very cooperative	Explain to child in simple terms the purpose of the medication Seek their assistance, such as putting pills in cup or opening the packet, and allow a broader range of choices Establish a reward system to enhance their cooperation, if necessary
Adolescent	Development of identity, benefiting from much more control over their care	Approach in same manner as adults, with respect and sensitivity to their needs Maintain the adolescent's privacy as much as possible

Take Note!

Pay close attention to ensure if the safe range dose is for 24 hours (mg/day) or a single dose period (mg/dose).

The pediatric dosage should not exceed the minimum recommended adult dosage. Generally, once a child or adolescent weighs 40 to 50 kg or greater, the adult dose is frequently prescribed (Bowden & Greenberg, 2011). However, it remains important to always verify that the dose does not exceed the recommended adult dose.

Dose Determination by Body Surface Area

Calculating the dosage based on BSA takes into account the child's metabolic rate and growth. It is commonly used for chemotherapeutic agents. Some recommended medication doses may read "mg/BSA/dose." To determine the dose using BSA, you will need to know the child's height and weight, which will be plotted on a

BOX 35.2

DOSAGE CALCULATION USING BODY WEIGHT

After converting the child's weight in pounds to kilograms and checking the safe dose range:

- Calculate the low safe dose range (e.g., 10 to 20 mg/kg and the child weighs 30 kg):
  - Set up a proportion using the low safe dose range 10 mg/1 kg = x mg/30 kg
  - Solve for x by cross-multiplying:
    $1 \times x = 10 \times 30$
    $x = 300$ mg
- Calculate the high safe dose range:
  - Set up a proportion using the high safe dose range 20 mg/1 kg = x mg/30 kg
  - Solve for x by cross-multiplying:
    $1 \times x = 20 \times 30$
    $x = 600$
- Compare the safe dose range (for this example, 300 to 600 mg) with the ordered dose. If the dose falls within the range, the dose is safe. If the dose falls outside the range, notify the prescriber.

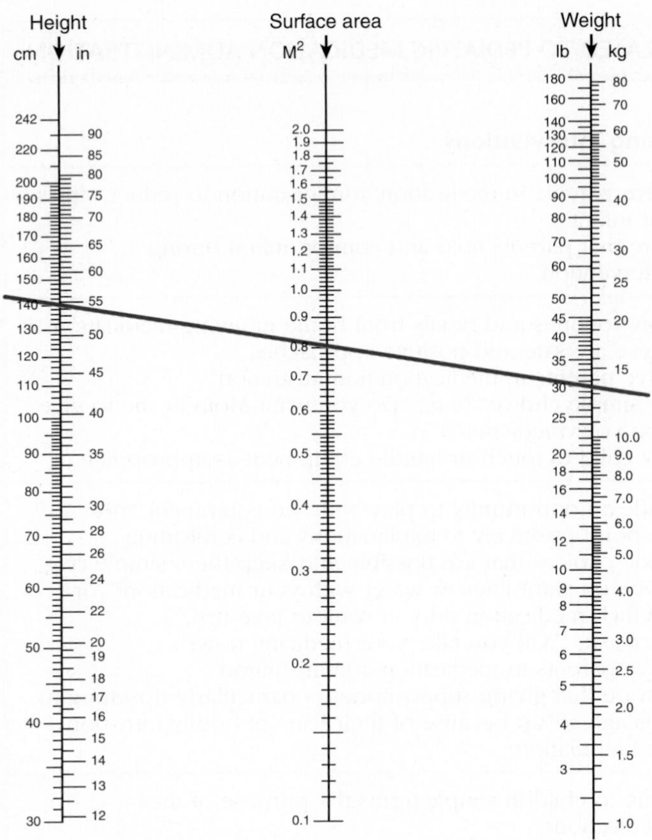

FIGURE 35.1 A nomogram to determine body surface area.

nomogram (Fig. 35.1). A nomogram is a graph divided into three columns: height (left column), surface area (middle column), and weight (right column).

Use these guidelines to determine BSA:

1. Measure the child's height.
2. Determine the child's weight.
3. Using the nomogram, draw a line to connect the height measurement in the left column and the weight measurement in the right column.
4. Determine the point where this line intersects the line in the surface area column. This is the BSA, expressed in meters squared (m^2).

Once you have determined the BSA, use the recommended dosage range to calculate the safe dosage.

Take Note!

Prior to administration of any medication wash hands and don gloves if necessary. Adhere to the rights of medication administration.

Oral Administration

Medications to be given via the oral route are supplied in many forms, including liquids (elixirs, syrups, or suspensions), powders, tablets, and capsules. Generally, children younger than the age of 5 to 6 are at risk for aspiration because they have difficulty swallowing tablets or capsules. Therefore, if a tablet or capsule is the only oral form available, it needs to be crushed or opened and mixed with a pleasant-tasting liquid or a small amount (generally no more than a tablespoon) of a nonessential food such as apple sauce. However, never crush or open an enteric-coated or time-release tablet or capsule. The crushed tablet or inside of a capsule may taste bitter, so never mix it with formula or other essential foods. Otherwise, the child may associate the bitter taste with the food and later refuse to eat it.

Take Note!

Certain drug formulations should not be crushed. Before crushing a pill or opening a capsule, always check that this will not alter the intended effects of the drug. Crushing a time-release medication allows immediate absorption of the entire dose of the medication and can have lethal consequences.

Liquid medications, primarily suspensions, may be less concentrated at the top of the bottle than at the bottom of the bottle. Always shake the liquid to ensure even drug distribution. The key to administering liquid forms of oral medications is to use calibrated equipment such as a medicine cup, spoon, plastic oral syringe, or dropper (Fig. 35.2).

Take Note!

Use the medicine cup or syringe with proper calibration instead of household cups or measuring spoons, since they are not calibrated and may deliver an incorrect dose of medication.

If a dropper is packaged with a certain medication, never use it to administer another medication, since the drop size may vary from one dropper to another. If using a

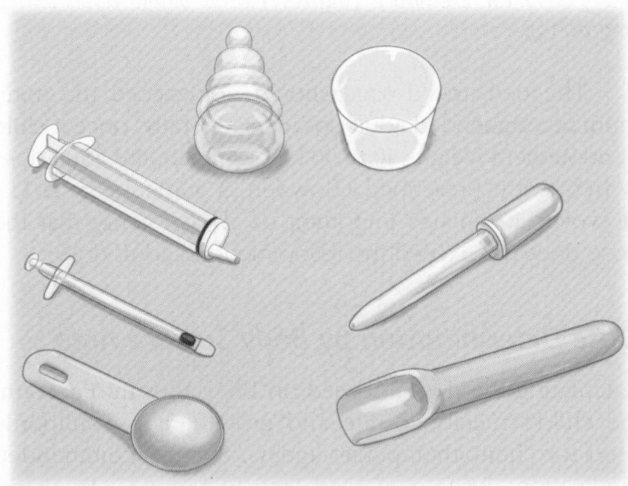

FIGURE 35.2 Devices used to administer oral medications to children.

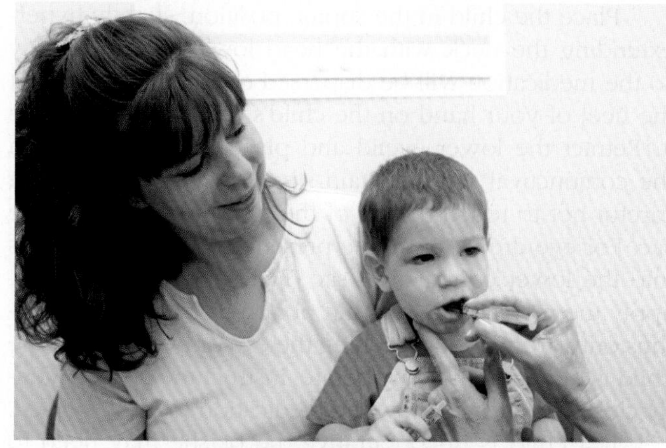

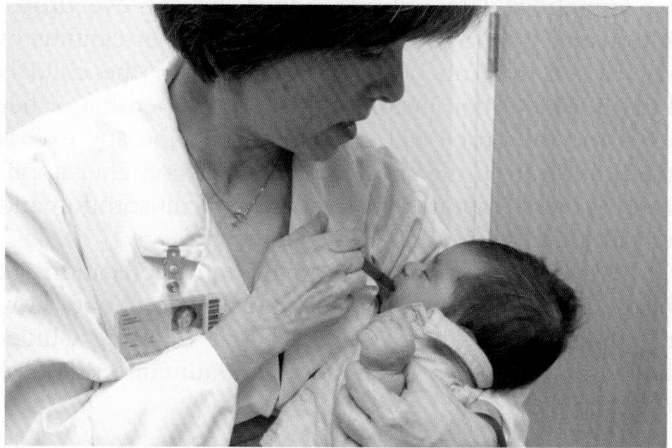

FIGURE 35.3 Position the infant or young child with head elevated for safe medication administration. Holding the child or having a parent hold the child is preferred unless contraindicated.

syringe for oral administration, only use the type intended for oral medications, not the one designed for parenteral administration. When using a dropper or oral syringe (without a needle) for infants or young children, direct the liquid toward the posterior side of the mouth. Give the drug slowly in small amounts (0.2 to 0.5 mL) and allow the child to swallow before more medication is placed in the mouth (Fig. 35.3). A nipple without the bottle attached is sometimes used to administer medication to infants. Place the medication directly in the nipple and keep the nipple filled with medication as the infant sucks so no air is taken in while the infant takes the medication. Always place the infant or young child upright (at least a 45-degree angle) to avoid aspiration. The toddler or young preschooler may enjoy using the oral syringe to squirt the medicine into his or her mouth. Older children can take oral medication from a medicine cup or measured medicine spoon.

Take Note!

Never force an oral medication into a child's mouth or pinch the child's nose. Doing so increases the risk for aspiration and interferes with the development of a trusting relationship.

As children adapt to swallowing tablets or capsules, administration is similar to that of adults. When helping the younger child learn how to swallow medication, the tablet or capsule can be placed at the back of the tongue or in a small amount of food such as ice cream or apple sauce. Always tell children if there is medicine in the food; otherwise, they may not trust you.

When the child has a nasogastric, orogastric, nasojejunal, nasoduodenal, **gastrostomy** (opening into the stomach), or jejunostomy tube, oral medications may be given via these devices. The tube allows for the medication to be placed directly into the stomach or small intestine area. Be aware that not all medications can be placed directly into the duodenum or jejunum. Medication for administration via a tube must be supplied in a liquid form, or a crushed tablet or opened capsule can be mixed with a liquid (Box 35.3). Always check tube placement before administering the medication. After administration, flush the tube to maintain patency.

Take Note!

Parental involvement in medication administration when possible helps decrease stress on the child and provides an opportunity for teaching and evaluating parental techniques.

Rectal Administration

Rectal medications are typically supplied in the form of suppositories. The rectal route is not a preferred route for medication administration in children because the

BOX 35.3

GUIDELINES FOR ADMINISTERING MEDICATIONS VIA GASTROSTOMY OR JEJUNOSTOMY TUBES

Verify correct placement (refer to Box 35.4).

- Give liquid medications directly into the tube. Draw appropriate amount into syringe and clear air.
- Mix powdered medications well with warm water first.
- If medication is in pill form, verify it is OK to crush. Then, crush tablets and mix with warm water to prevent tube occlusion.
- Open up capsules and mix the contents with warm water to dissolve the contents and prevent tube occlusion.
- Label each syringe appropriately.
- Flush the tube with water after administering each medication unless contraindicated to ensure that the entire amount of medication has been given and to prevent tube occlusion.

Adapted from Bowden, V. R., & Greenberg, C. S. (2011). *Pediatric nursing procedures* (3rd ed). Philadelphia, PA: Lippincott Williams & Wilkins; and Cincinnati Children's Hospital Medical Center. (2012). *Gastrostomy Tube (G-tube) home care.* Retrieved from http://www.cincinnatichildrens.org/health/info/abdomen/home/g-tube-care.htm

drug's absorption may be erratic and unpredictable and the method is invasive. The rectal route can be extremely upsetting to the toddler and preschooler because of age-related fears, and may be embarrassing to the school-age child or adolescent. However, the rectal route may be used when the child is vomiting or receiving nothing by mouth (NPO). Use age-appropriate explanations and reassurance. Helping the child to maintain the correct position may be necessary to ensure proper insertion and safety of rectal suppositories.

Lubricate the suppository well with a water-soluble lubricant. With the child in the side-lying position, insert the suppository into the rectum quickly but gently. Use a gloved finger or use a finger cot to insert the suppository. Insert the suppository above the anal sphincter. For an infant or child younger than the age of 3, use the fifth finger for insertion. For an older child, use the index finger. To prevent expulsion of the suppository, hold the buttocks together for several minutes or until the child loses the urge to defecate. If the child has a bowel movement within 10 to 30 minutes after administration of the medication, examine the stool for the presence of the suppository. If it is observed, notify the physician or nurse practitioner to determine if the drug needs to be administered again.

Ophthalmic Administration

Ophthalmic medications are typically supplied in the form of drops or ointment. Many children have a fear of having anything placed in their eyes. Therefore, provide an age-appropriate explanation to gain their cooperation. Also, have the child keep his or her eyes closed until you are ready to administer the medication. Ensure that the medication is at room temperature, as chilled medication may be uncomfortable to the child. Proper positioning of the child is necessary to control the child's head, keep the child's hands from interfering, and prevent injury to the eye. Attempt to administer the medication when the child is not crying to ensure that the medication reaches its intended target area.

Place the child in the supine position, slightly hyperextending the neck with the head lower than the body so the medication will be dispersed over the cornea. Rest the heel of your hand on the child's forehead to stabilize it. Retract the lower eyelid and place the medication in the conjunctival sac; maintain sterile technique by being careful not to touch the tip of the tube or dropper to the sac. For eye drops, place the prescribed number of drops into the lower conjunctival sac (Fig. 35.4). For ointment, apply the medication in a thin ribbon from the inner canthus outward without touching the eye or eyelashes. If the child is old enough to cooperate, instruct the child to gently close the eyes to allow the medication to be dispersed.

If a child is uncooperative, he or she may need to be immobilized in order to administer the eye drops. Alternatively, one or two drops on the inner canthus of the closed eye can be administered while the child is lying supine. Then instruct the child to open his or her eyes and the drops will enter the eye. Wipe any excess medication from the skin. Punctal occlusion after application is also important to slow systemic absorption and ensure that the medicine stays in the eye.

Children often require ophthalmic medications at home. Parents or caregivers need instruction about how to administer this type of medication. Teaching Guidelines 35.1 provides information on administering eye drops and eye ointments.

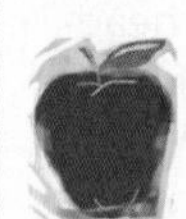

Teaching Guidelines 35.1
APPLYING EYE MEDICATIONS

- Wash your hands with soap and water. Dry them thoroughly using a clean cloth.
- Cleanse the eye. Move from the nose side of the eye outward. Use a clean area of the cloth each time you wipe and a separate cloth for each eye. Use warm water to help clear crusty eye drainage.
- Allow the eye drops or ointment to come to room temperature (if the medication was stored in the

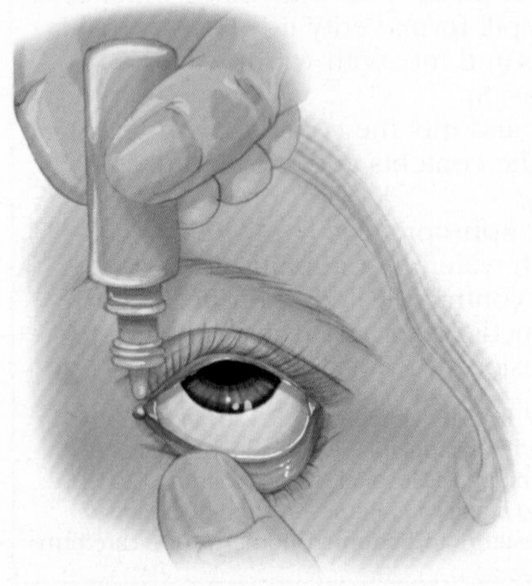

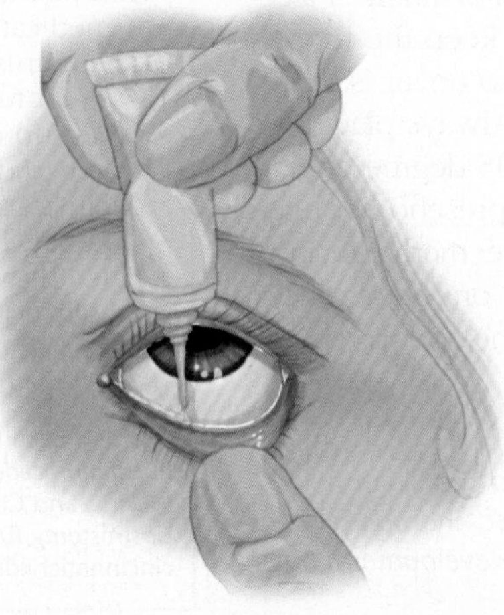

FIGURE 35.4 Administering eye medication: gently press the lower lid down and have the child look up as the medication is instilled into the lower conjunctival sac.

refrigerator). If necessary, warm the eye drops or ointment tube in the palm of your hand. Keep the cap on to avoid any spillage. Make sure medication is well mixed if needed.

- Remove the cap, placing it on a dry, clean surface.
- For young children (3 years or younger), obtain assistance from an additional adult to keep their arms and fingers away during the procedure. If doing this procedure alone, wrap the child in a towel or blanket, keeping the arms inside.
- Have the child look up and to the other side. The eye drops should flow away from the child's nose.
- Place the wrist of the hand you will be using to give the drops against the child's forehead. With the other hand gently pull down the lower eyelid. Have the medication about 1 inch (2.54 cm) away from the eye.
- Gently squeeze the eye drop bottle, dispensing the proper number of drops away from the tear ducts which are in the inner corner of the eye, or gently squeeze the ointment tube, dispensing a small trail (about 2 cm) of ointment into the gap between the lower portion of the eye and the bottom eyelid. Twist or rotate the tube when you reach the outer eye to help disconnect the ointment from the tube.
- Make sure the tip of the bottle or tube does not make contact with the eye or any other surface.
- For eye drops, gently press your finger against the inside corner where the eye meets the nose for about 1 minute, blocking the tears and medication from exiting through the tear duct. This will help the eye retain more of the medication. If the child is old enough, he or she may be able to do this unassisted.
- For ointment, have the child close his or her eye and not rub the area.
- Ask the child not to blink or squeeze the eye shut more than normal, as this may wash away the medication prematurely.
- Gently dab away any tears or excess medication on the face with a clean tissue.
- Wash your hands again and dry them thoroughly.

Adapted from Pediatric Glaucoma & Cataract Family Association. (2013a). How to apply eye drops. Retrieved from http://pgcfa.org/?page_id=160; and Pediatric Glaucoma & Cataract Family Association. (2013b). How to apply eye ointment. Retrieved from http://pgcfa.org/?page_id=155; American Academy of Pediatrics (2013). *Healthy children: Safety & prevention: How to give eye drops and eye ointment.* Retrieved from http://www.healthychildren.org/English/safety-prevention/at-home/medication-safety/Pages/How-to-Give-Eye-Drops-and-Eye-Ointment.aspx; Bowden, V. R., & Greenberg, C. S. (2011). *Pediatric nursing procedures* (3rd ed). Philadelphia, PA: Lippincott Williams & Wilkins.

Otic Administration

Medications for otic administration are typically in the form of ear drops. This route of administration can be upsetting to the child because he or she cannot see what is happening. The child often receives otic drugs for an earache, and he or she may fear that the ear drops will increase the pain. Explain the procedure to the younger child in terms that he or she can understand to help allay these fears. Gain the older child's cooperation by explaining the purpose of the medication and the procedure for administration.

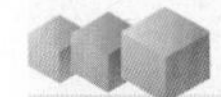

Concept Mastery Alert

Administering Pediatric Ear Drops

When administering pediatric ear drops, pulling the pinna down and back is correct if the child is younger than 3 years of age. To administer ear drops to a child who is 4 years old and older, the nurse should pull the pinna up and back.

Reinforce the need for the child to keep the head still. Younger children may require assistance to do so. Be sure that the ear drops are at room temperature. If necessary, roll the container between the palms of your hands to help warm the drops. Using cold ear drops can cause pain and possibly vertigo or vomit when they reach the eardrum (Bowden & Greenberg, 2011).

Place the child in a supine or side-lying position with the affected ear exposed (Fig. 35.5). Pull the pinna downward and back in children younger than age 3 and upward and back in older children. Instill the prescribed amount of medication using a dropper being careful not to contaminate the tip of the dropper. Then, have the child remain in the same position for several minutes to ensure that the medication stays in the ear canal. Soothe, comfort, and distract the child to allow medication to instill. Massage the area anterior to the affected ear to promote passage of the medication into the ear canal. If necessary, place a piece of cotton or a cotton ball loosely in the ear canal to prevent the medication from leaking.

Nasal Administration

Nasally administered medications are typically drops and sprays. Administering nose drops to infants and young children may be difficult, and additional help may be needed to help maintain the child's position. Ensure medication is at room temperature. Have the child blow his nose or use a bulb syringe to clear nasal passage of secretions. For nose drops, position the child supine with the head hyperextended to ensure that the drops will flow back into the nares. A pillow or folded towel can be used to facilitate this hyperextension. Place the tip of the dropper just at or inside the nasal opening, taking care not to touch the nares with the dropper (Fig. 35.6). Doing so might stimulate the child to sneeze. Although the nasal membranes are not sterile, the drop solution is, and sneezing would contaminate the dropper, leading to contamination of the drop solution when the dropper is returned to the bottle. Once the drops are instilled, maintain the child's head in hyperextension for at least

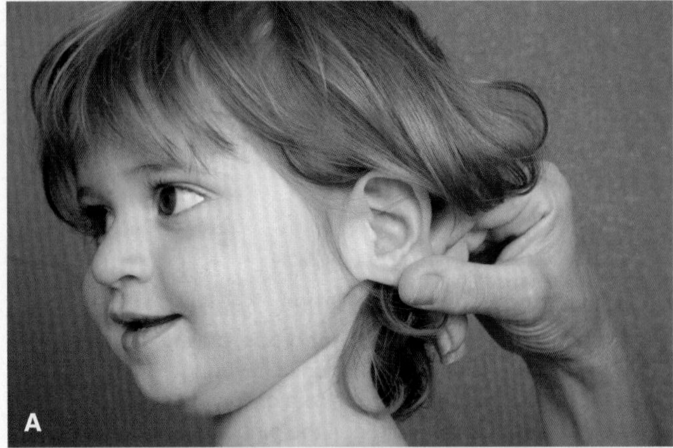

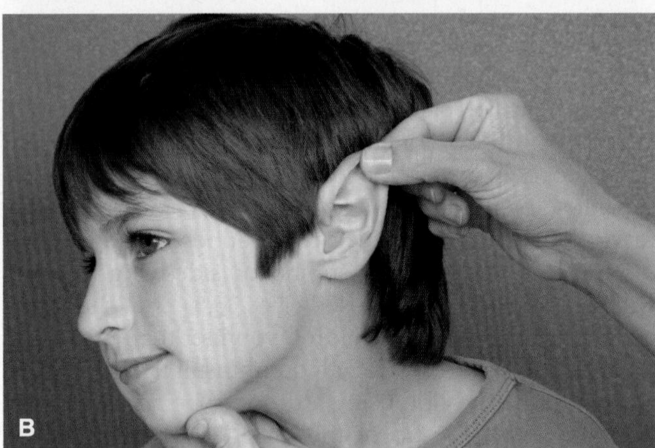

FIGURE 35.5 Administering ear drops. **(A)** For the child younger than 3 years of age, the nurse pulls the pinna of the ear down and back. **(B)** For a child older than age 3 years, the nurse pulls the pinna of the affected ear up and back.

1 minute to ensure that the drops have come in contact with the nasal membranes.

For nasal sprays, position the child upright with head tilted slightly back and place the tip of the spray bottle just inside the nasal opening and tilted toward the back. Hold one nostril closed (or have the child do this if appropriate) and instruct the child to take a deep breath through the nostril while the medication is being administered. Squeeze the container, providing just enough force for the spray to be expelled from the container. Using too great a force can push the spray solution and secretions into the sinuses or eustachian tube.

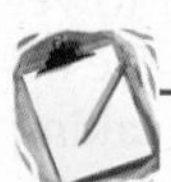

Take Note!

In young infants, instill the medication in one naris at a time, since they are obligate nose breathers.

Intramuscular Administration

IM administration delivers medication to the muscle. In children, this method of medication administration is used as infrequently as possible because it is painful and

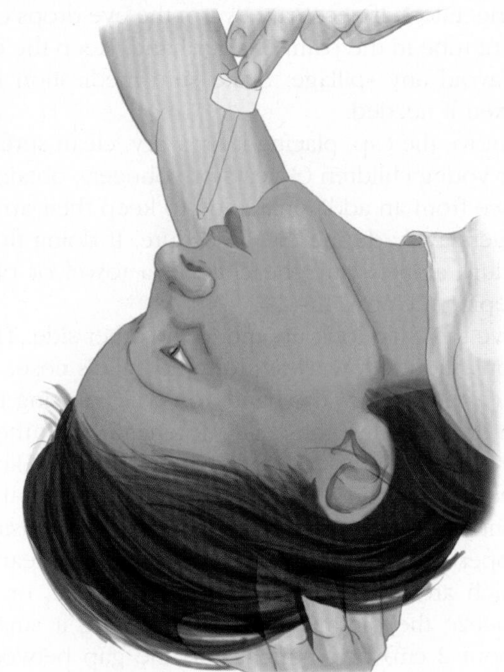

FIGURE 35.6 Administering nose drops. Tilt the head down and back to instill nose drops.

children often lack adequate muscle mass for medication absorption. However, IM administration is used to administer certain medications, such as many immunizations.

Muscle development and the amount of fluid to be injected determine IM injection sites in children. Needle size (gauge and length) is determined by the size of the muscle and the viscosity of the medication. For example, more viscous medications often require a larger-gauge needle. In addition, the needle must be long enough to ensure that the medication reaches the muscle.

The preferred injection site for infants less than 7 months is the vastus lateralis muscle (Immunization Action Coalition, 2012; Bowden & Greenberg, 2011). In infants and children greater than 7 months the ventrogluteal site should be considered (Bowden & Greenberg, 2011). The dorsogluteal site, often used in adults, is not recommended in children younger than 5 years of age (Bowden & Greenberg, 2011). The muscle has not fully developed and the sciatic nerve occupies a larger portion of this area in the young child.

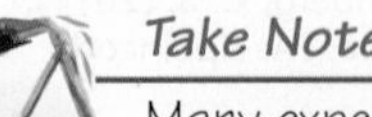

Take Note!

Many experts no longer recommend use of the dorsogluteal site at any age due to the risk of damaging the sciatic nerve (Aschenbrenner & Venable, 2012).

The deltoid muscle is used as an IM injection site in children older than 3 years of age and may be used in toddlers if the muscle mass is sufficient (Immunization Action Coalition, 2012). Figure 35.7 illustrates IM injection sites.

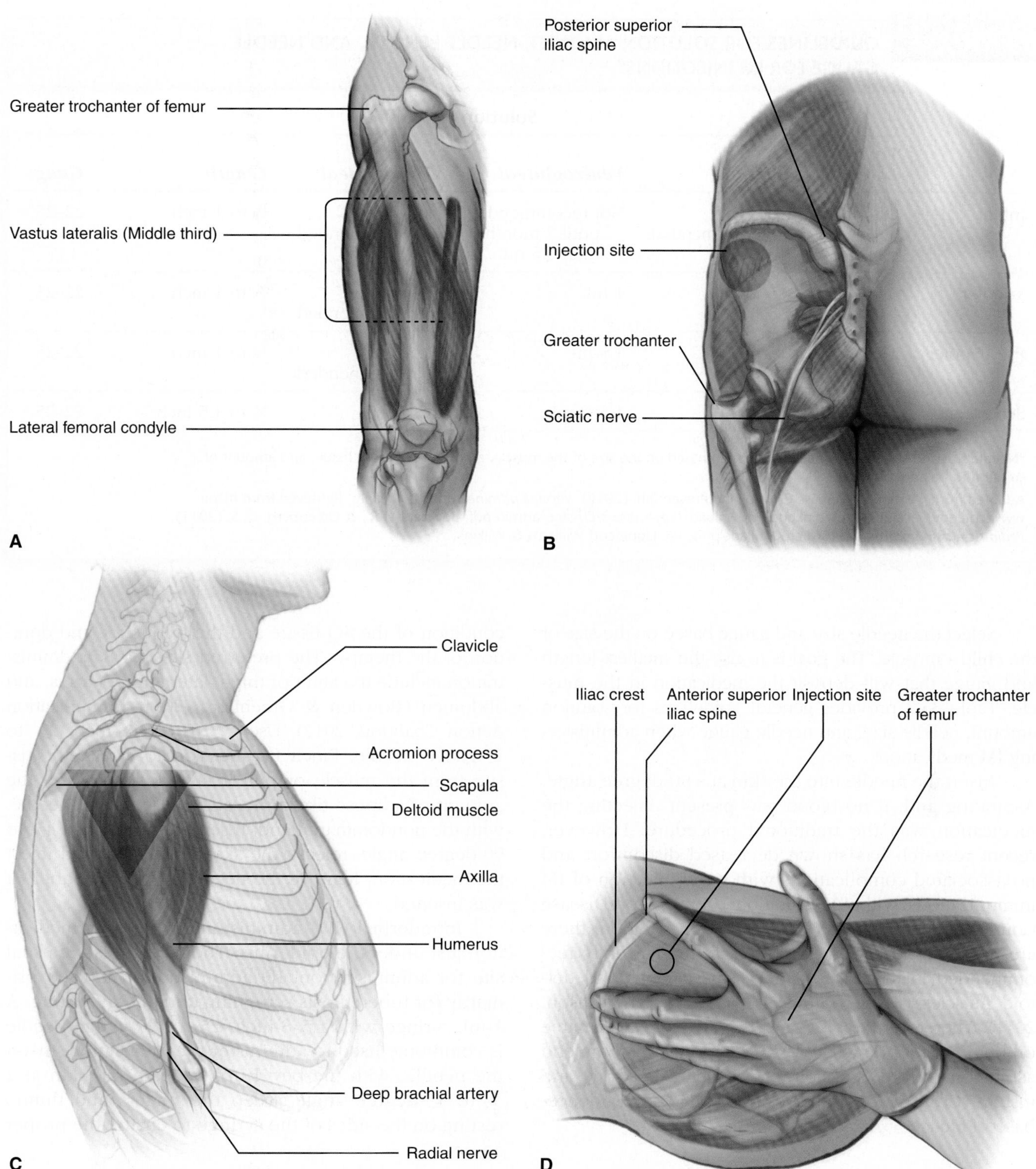

FIGURE 35.7 Locating intramuscular injection sites. (**A**) Vastus lateralis: identify the greater trochanter and the lateral femoral condyle; inject in middle third and anterior lateral aspect. (**B**) Dorsogluteal: place hand on iliac crest and locate the posterosuperior iliac spine; inject in the outer quadrant formed when an imaginary line is drawn between the trochanter and the iliac spine. (**C**) Deltoid: locate the lateral side of the humerus, one to two finger widths below the acromion process. Inject into upper third of muscle. (**D**) Ventrogluteal: place palm of left hand on right greater trochanter so index finger points toward anterosuperior iliac spine, spread middle finger to form a V, and inject in the middle of the V.

TABLE 35.2 GUIDELINES FOR SOLUTION AMOUNT, NEEDLE LENGTH, AND NEEDLE GAUGE FOR IM INJECTIONS[a]

	Solution Amount					
	Vastus Lateralis	***Deltoid***	***Ventrogluteal***	***Dorsogluteal***	***Length***	***Gauge***
Infant	0.5 mL	Not recommended	Not recommended until 7 months; then 0.5 mL	Not recommended	⅝ to 1 inch	22–25
Toddler	0.5–1 mL	0.5 mL	1 mL	Not recommended	⅝ to 1 inch	22–25
Preschooler	1 mL	0.5 mL	1.5 mL	Not recommended	⅝ to 1 inch	22–25
School age	1.5–2 mL	0.5–1 mL	1.5–2 mL	1.5–2 mL	⅝ to 1.5 inch	22–25

[a]Needle size and site need to be individualized based on the size of the muscle, amount of adipose tissue, and amount of solution to be administered.

Adapted from Centers for Disease Control and Prevention. (2012). *Vaccine administration guidelines.* Retrieved from http://www.cdc.gov/vaccines/pubs/pinkbook/downloads/appendices/D/vacc_admin.pdf; Bowden, V. R., & Greenberg, C. S. (2011). *Pediatric nursing procedures* (3rd ed). Philadelphia, PA: Lippincott Williams & Wilkins

Select the needle size and gauge based on the size of the child's muscle. The goal is to use the smallest length and gauge that will deposit the medication in the muscle. Table 35.2 provides general guidelines for solution amount, needle size, and needle gauge when administering IM medications.

Insert the needle into the skin at a 90-degree angle. Aspirating and, if no blood was present, injecting the medication was the traditional procedure. However, recent research has shown decreased discomfort and no associated complications with rapid injection of IM immunizations without aspiration (Centers for Disease Control and Prevention [CDC], 2012). In addition, there are no large blood vessels present in the currently recommended injection sites, the vastus lateralis and deltoid muscles (Kroger, Sumaya, Pickering, & Atkinson, 2011). Therefore, the CDC and the Advisory Committee on Immunization Practices (ACIP) no longer recommend aspiration before injection of vaccines, heparin, and insulin (CDC, 2012; Kroger et al., 2011). See Evidence-based Practice 35.1

Subcutaneous and Intradermal Administration

SQ administration distributes medication into the fatty layers of the body. It is used primarily for insulin administration, heparin, and certain immunizations, such as the MMR. The amount of SQ tissue differs among individuals. Therefore, when selecting a site and needle size, choose the most appropriate based on adequacy and condition of the SQ tissue and the frequency and duration of the therapy. The preferred sites for SQ administration include the anterior thigh, lateral upper arms, and abdomen (Bowden & Greenberg, 2011; Immunization Action Coalition, 2012). Use a 3/8- or 5/8-inch, 23- to 25-gauge needle. Pinch up the skin to isolate the tissue from the muscle or pull it taut depending on the amount of adipose tissue present and length of needle, with the nondominant hand. Insert the needle at a 45- to 90-degree angle, release the skin if pinched, and inject the medication, Remove the needle at the same angle it was inserted.

Intradermal (ID) administration deposits medication just under the epidermis. The forearm is the usual site for administration. ID administration is used primarily for tuberculosis screening and allergy testing. A 1-mL syringe with a 5/8-inch, 25- or 27-gauge needle is commonly used to administer the medication. Insert the needle, with the bevel up, beneath the skin at a 5- to 15-degree angle. Keep the fingers and thumb resting on the sides of the syringe to ensure the proper angle.

Intravenous Administration

IV medication administration is commonly used with children, especially when a rapid response to a drug is desired or when absorption via other routes is difficult due to the child's illness or condition. In some cases, the IV route is the only effective method for administering a medication. Use of the IV route requires that

EVIDENCE-BASED PRACTICE 35.1 **TO ASPIRATE OR NOT PRIOR TO INJECTION?**

The practice of aspirating for blood prior to injection has been a debate for many years. The reason behind aspiration is to ensure that the nurse has not inadvertently penetrated an artery or vein. Critics of this practice state it is nearly impossible for this to occur if the nurse is using proper technique (45- to 90-degree angle) and proper site selection. Current recommended sites are relatively free of blood vessels. They claim aspiration leads to longer injection time and increased pain. A recent study found that rapid injection technique without aspiration leads to decreased pain and increased parent acceptance of immunizations. The AAP, AAFP, ACIP, and WHO all currently recommend not aspirating during injections. This study evaluated the evidence behind the question of many nurses – "Should I aspirate during IM or subcutaneous injection?"

STUDY

An integrative review was performed. The researchers examined evidence that included literature, systematic and integrative reviews.

Findings

No data was found to support the use of aspiration during injection. Recommendations until a standard is established include: No aspiration is indicated for SQ or IM injections of vaccines or immunizations, SQ injections of insulin or heparin, aspiration may be indicated with IM injection of medications such as penicillin (PCN).

Nursing Implications

Nursing care needs to be based on current scientific evidence. Nurses need to continuously question their care practices and review current research and perform research on topics they feel need it. Nurses need to not rely on past practices or go against current evidence due to unfound fears or relying on past practices. Rapid injection technique without aspiration is recommended. Individualize injection technique based on patient, equipment, and medication being given. Always follow agency policy and procedures.

Adapted from Crawford, C. L. & Johnson, J. A. (2012). To aspirate or not: An integrative review of the evidence. *Nursing2012, 42*(3), 20–25.

the child have an IV device inserted, peripherally or centrally. Although insertion of this device is invasive and traumatic for the child, IV medication administration is considered to be less traumatic when compared to the trauma associated with multiple injections. Unfortunately, the veins of a child are small and easily irritated.

Most medications given by the IV route must be given at a specified rate and diluted properly to prevent overdose or toxicity due to the rapid onset of action that occurs with this route. Therefore, when administering medications via the IV route, knowledge of the drug, the amount of drug to be administered, the minimum dilution of the drug, the type of solution for dilution or infusion, the compatibility or various solutions and medications, the length of time for infusion, and the rate of infusion is required. Careful maintenance of the IV site is required to prevent complications.

The primary method for IV medication administration is a syringe pump. This method provides a highly precise rate of infusion. Nursing Procedure 35.1 gives the steps for administering medication via a syringe pump.

If a pump is unavailable, the medication may be administered via a volume control device. The medication is added to the device with a specified amount of compatible fluid and then infused at the ordered rate.

Take Note!

Some facilities have reduced or eliminated the use of volume control devices, especially for medication administration. Concerns include lack of identifying the medication in the volume control device and the potential for interaction or precipitation that may occur when multiple medications are administered using the same volume control device (ISMP, 2009). Be familiar with your facilities policies and procedures and when using a volume control device ensure to label the chamber when medications are added and to check for incompatibilities and potential interaction when multiple medications are given (ISMP, 2009).

Direct IV push medication is typically reserved for emergency situations and when therapeutic blood levels must be reached quickly to achieve the desired effect. Direct IV push administration requires that the drug be diluted appropriately and given at a specified rate, such as over 2 to 3 minutes. Care must be taken to prevent fluid overload, which may occur due to flushing needed to maintain IV patency and prevent drug incompatibilities, and from the administration of multiple drug therapies.

Providing Atraumatic Care

When administering any medication, including oral medications, use the principles of atraumatic care (see Chapter 30 for more information). Children can experience stress and fear or upset when they must take medications. The child may become upset or stressed when he or she must be secured snugly or positioned to minimize movement. The child may experience further discomfort if the medication has an unpleasant taste or results in pain, such as with an injection.

NURSING PROCEDURE 35.1

Administering Medication Via a Syringe Pump

Purpose: To provide accurate and safe administration of IV medication

1. Verify the medication order.
2. Gather the medication and necessary equipment and supplies.
3. Wash hands and put on gloves.
4. Attach the syringe pump tubing to the medication syringe and purge air from the tubing by gently filling the tubing with medication from the syringe.
5. Insert the syringe into the pump according to the manufacturer's directions.
6. Clean the appropriate port on the child's IV access device or tubing, flush the device or tubing if appropriate (e.g., an intermittent infusion device [saline lock or heparin lock]), and attach the syringe tubing to the IV tubing or device.
7. Set the infusion rate on the pump as ordered.
8. When the medication infusion is completed, flush the syringe pump tubing to deliver any medication remaining in the tubing, according to institution protocol.
9. Document the procedure and the child's response to it.

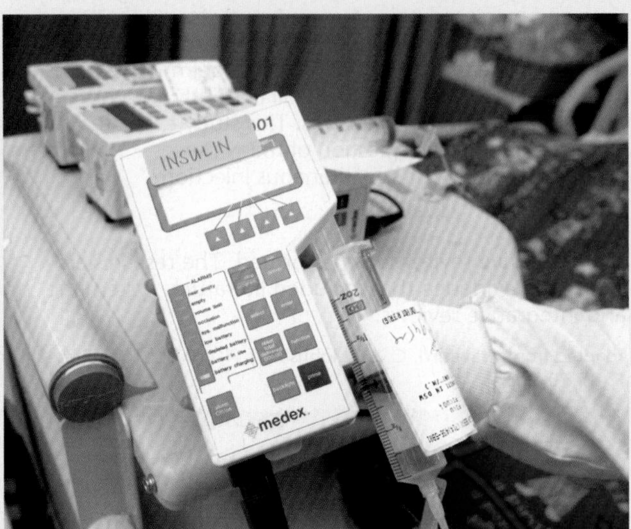

Adapted from Bowden, V. R., & Greenberg, C. S. (2011). *Pediatric nursing procedures* (3rd ed). Philadelphia, PA: Lippincott Williams & Wilkins.

Atraumatic Care

Encourage the child to participate in care and provide the child with developmentally appropriate options, such as which fluid to drink with the medication or which flavor of ice pop to suck on before or after the administration (see Table 35.1).

To decrease discomfort and pain for the child who is to receive an injection, apply a topical anesthetic such as eutectic mixture of local anesthetic (EMLA) cream or vapocoolant spray to the site before injection when possible (Kroger et al., 2011) and inject the most painful medication last (see Chapter 36 for additional information). Also, utilize developmentally appropriate distraction techniques, such as music, books, blowing bubbles or a pinwheel, and deep breathing exercises (see Chapter 30 for additional information).

Ensuring that the child doesn't move is essential to prevent injury when administering an injection. When administering an injection to a young child, at least two adults should hold him or her; this may also be necessary to help an older child to remain still.

Take Note!

Research supports children experience less pain and decreased fear if they are sitting versus lying down when receiving an injection (CDC, 2012).

Atraumatic Care

Use positions that are comforting to the child, such as therapeutic hugging, during injections. Have the child sit on the caregiver's lap with the caregiver holding the child's arms and legs to his or her body. Refer to Chapter 30, Figure 30.1. After administration, encourage the parents or caregivers to hold and cuddle the child and offer praise.

Educating the Child and Parents

Teaching the child and parents or caregivers about medication administration is key. Many medications are given in the home, making the parents or caregivers the persons responsible for administration. They need to know what medications they are giving and why, how to give them, and what to expect from the drug, including adverse effects. Caregivers and parents often incorrectly dose over-the-counter medications and prescription medications or fail to follow prescribed orders, such as missing doses of medications or not completing the full course of medication (Yin et al., 2010; Walsh et al., 2013). Therefore, ensure thorough instruction, including frequency of administration, when the next dose is due, and length of time the medication is to be given. Emphasize the importance of completing the prescribed dose. Demonstrate use with an actual syringe if possible, encourage return demonstration of medication administration, advise against the use of home-measuring devices (such as a spoon), and emphasize the importance of always using the calibrated dispensing device that was given with the medication. If the medication is to be given via injection, parents and caregivers need to learn how to administer the injection properly. Encourage questions or concerns from parents or caregivers.

Parents and caregivers commonly need suggestions about the best ways to administer the medication to their child. Provide them with tips for administration, such as mixing unpleasant-tasting medications with apple sauce or yogurt or offering a favorite liquid as a chaser. Also teach the parents how to properly measure the amount of drug to be given. Teaching Guidelines 35.2 gives pointers about oral medication administration. Refer to Chapter 30 for further information on teaching children and families about medication administration.

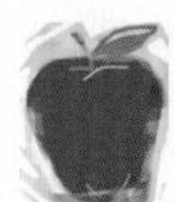

Teaching Guidelines 35.2

ADMINISTERING ORAL MEDICATIONS

- Be firm when telling your child that it is time for his or her medication. State, "It's time for your medicine" instead of asking, "Will you take your medicine?" or "Can you take your medicine for me?"
- Allow your child to choose an appropriate liquid to help swallow the medication or drink after taking it. Limit the choices to two or three.
- Never bribe or threaten your child to take his or her medication.
- Never refer to the medication as "candy."
- Be honest about the taste of the medication. If necessary, mix it with another food such as apple sauce, yogurt, or syrup to help mask the taste.
- Do not mix the medication with formula or baby food.
- Always check with your physician or nurse practitioner and pharmacy about opening capsules or crushing tablets and mixing them with food. Some medications should not be opened or crushed.
- If you are giving a liquid using an oral syringe or dropper, place the medication slowly along the inside of the cheek. Never squirt the medication forcibly to the back of the child's throat. It may cause the child to gag and spit out the medication or aspirate it into his or her lungs.
- Always praise the child after taking the medication and provide comfort and cuddling.

Preventing Medication Errors

The incidence of potentially harmful medication errors may be three times as high in pediatrics compared to adults (Steering Committee on Quality Improvement and Management and Committee on Hospital Care, 2011). This can be related to weight-based dosing calculations, fractional dosing, and the need for the use of decimal points. Children are also more susceptible because many drugs used in pediatrics are formulated and packaged for adults and lack U.S. Food and Drug Administration (FDA) approval and dosing guidelines for children. Recent legislative changes have led to a dramatic increase in pediatric drug trials and improvement in accurate pediatric dosing over the past 5 years (U.S. Food and Drug Administration, 2011).

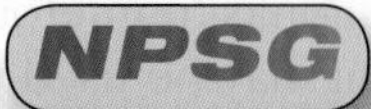

GOAL 3: Improve the Safety of Using Medications

NPSG.03.04.01 Label all medications, medication containers, and other solutions on and off the sterile field in perioperative and other procedural settings. Note: Medication containers include syringes, medicine cups, and basins.

Steps: Label all medications that are removed from the manufacturers package and that are not being given immediately to the child, with pertinent information such as name, dose, and volume.

Joint Commission. (2015). *National patient safety goals effective January 1, 2015.* Retrieved from http://www.jointcommission.org/assets/1/6/2015_NPSG_HAP.pdf

The need for safety takes on even greater importance due to the physiologic, psychological, and cognitive differences inherent in children. Children are more vulnerable to medication errors as they vary in weight, BSA, and organ maturity which effect their ability to metabolize and excrete medications; they depend on others for medication administration, they are often unable to communicate if an adverse reaction is occurring and they need special compound medication formulations (Manias et al., 2014). Confirming the child's identity and double-checking the dosage before administration of any medication are two critical safeguards that play a major role in preventing medication errors. Other ways to prevent medication errors include the following:

- Confirm that the children's weight is accurate.
- Always weigh children in kilograms.

- Double-check medication calculations; utilize another health care provider when possible, especially for high-risk medications.
- If a dose seems unusually small or large, verify the order.
- Utilize medication ordering and dispensing systems, if available.
- Always report medication errors or near-miss errors to help prevent future mistakes.
- Utilize the Joint Commission's official "Do Not Use" list (link to this list is provided on http://www.jointcommission.org/assets/1/18/Do_Not_Use_List.pdf).

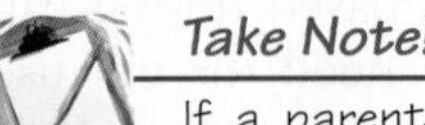

Take Note!

If a parent, caregiver, or child questions whether a medication should be given, listen attentively, answer their questions, and double-check the order.

INTRAVENOUS THERAPY

IV access provides a route for the administration of medications and fluids. It is commonly used for children because it is the quickest, and often the most effective, method of administration. As with adults, numerous sites and various devices and equipment may be used to provide IV therapy over a short or long period of time. When administering IV therapy, safety is crucial. The nurse must have a solid knowledge base about the fluids or medications to be given as well as a thorough understanding of the child's physical and emotional development. Venipuncture can be a terrifying and painful experience for children and their families. Nurses play a crucial role in providing support and education to the child and family before, during, and after the procedure (refer to Chapter 30 for additional information related to provision of atraumatic care with procedures).

Sites

IV therapy may be administered via a peripheral vein or a central vein. Peripheral IV therapy sites commonly include the hands, feet, and forearms (Fig. 35.8). In neonates and young infants, the scalp veins may be used (O'Grady et al., 2011). The scalp veins are easily visualized, being covered only by a thin layer of SQ tissue. These veins do not have valves, so the device may be inserted in either direction, although the preference would be in the direction of blood flow. However, use of a scalp vein requires that that area of the infant's head be cleared of hair to enhance visualization. In addition, use of the scalp veins can be frightening to parents, who may think the fluid is infusing into the infant's brain. Thus, scalp veins are usually used only if attempts at other sites have been unsuccessful (Bergvall & Sawyer, 2012). When used, ensure appropriate education of the parents prior to insertion and, if shaving the child's hair is needed, inquire if parents would like to keep the child's hair.

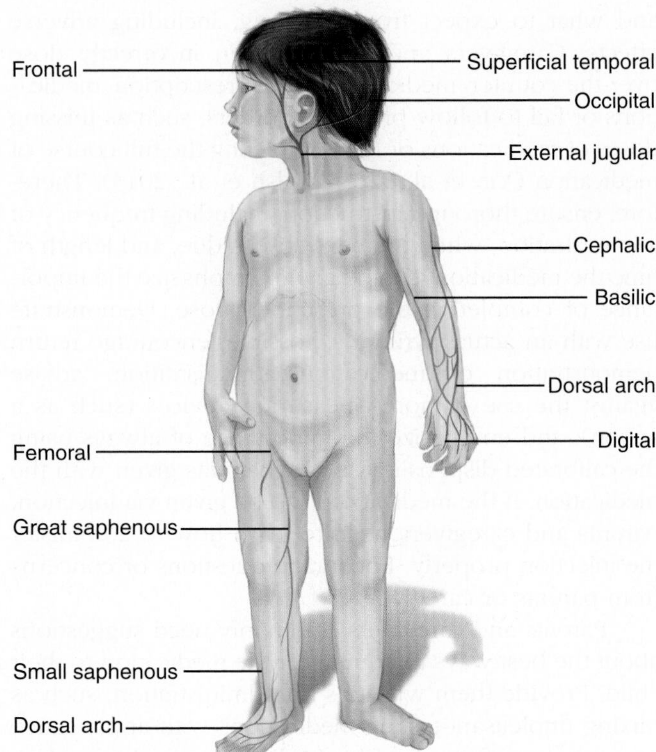

FIGURE 35.8 Preferred peripheral sites for IV insertion.

Take Note!

When selecting an IV site in an extremity, always choose the most distal site. Doing so prevents injury to the veins superior to the site and allows additional access sites should complications develop in the most distal site.

Central IV therapy usually is administered through a large vein, such as the subclavian, femoral, or jugular vein or the vena cava. The tip of the device lies in the superior vena cava just at the entrance to the right atrium. The device is inserted surgically or percutaneously and exits the body typically in the chest area, just below the clavicle. A device can be inserted via a peripheral vein, such as the median, cephalic, or basilic vein, and then threaded into the superior vena cava.

Equipment

The choice of equipment is determined by the solution or medication to be administered, the duration of the therapy, the age and developmental level of the child, the child's status, and the condition of his or her veins. Various types of IV devices are commercially available. In addition, different types of tubing and infusion control devices may be necessary.

Peripheral Access Devices

Devices used for peripheral venous access in a child include over-the-needle catheters or winged-infusion sets, commonly referred to as "butterflies" or scalp vein needles. These devices are inserted into the vein and then connected to the IV solution via tubing to provide a continuous infusion of fluid. These devices can also be inserted for intermittent use if the child does not require a continuous fluid infusion. Typically, the hub of the device is capped or plugged to allow intermittent access, such as for administering medications or obtaining blood specimens. When used in this manner, these devices are termed peripheral intermittent infusion devices or saline or heparin locks.

Needle size on the device also varies. Typically, the needle ranges from 21- to 25-gauge, depending on the child's size. The rule of thumb is to use the smallest-gauge catheter with the shortest length possible to prevent traumatizing the child's fragile veins. Typically, peripheral IV devices are used for short-term therapy, usually averaging 3 to 5 days (O'Grady et al., 2011). Midline catheters are also available, and the CDC recommends the use of midline catheters if therapy is to exceed 6 days (O'Grady et al., 2011). These catheters are longer than peripheral catheters but still remain outside the central veins and can stay in for up to 2 months (Bowden & Greenberg, 2011). They are seated deep in the cephalic or basilic veins, but the tip does not extend past the axilla.

Central Access Devices

Numerous devices for central venous access are available. The type chosen depends on several factors, including the duration of the therapy, the child's diagnosis, the risks to the child from insertion, and the ability of the child and family to care for the device. The device may have one or multiple lumens. Although central venous access devices can be used short term, the majority are used for moderate- to long-term therapy.

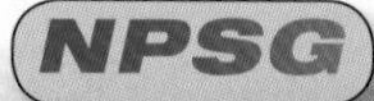

GOAL 7: Reduce the Risk of Health Care–Associated Infections

NPSG.07.04.01 Implement evidence-based practices to prevent central line–associated bloodstream infections. Note: This requirement covers short- and long-term central venous catheters and peripherally inserted central catheter (PICC) lines.

Steps: When caring for a child with a central line ensure to follow evidence-based policies and procedures strictly. Adhere to proper handwashing and aseptic technique.

Joint Commission. (2015). *National patient safety goals effective January 1, 2015.* Retrieved from http://www.jointcommission.org/assets/1/6/2015_NPSG_HAP.pdf

Central venous access devices are indicated when the child lacks suitable peripheral access, requires IV fluid or medication for a prolonged period of time, or is to receive specific treatments, such as the administration of highly concentrated solutions or irritating drugs like chemotherapeutic agents, parenteral nutrition or blood and blood products. Child preference is also a consideration. Central venous access is advantageous because it provides vascular access without the need for multiple IV starts, thus decreasing discomfort and fear. However, central venous access devices are associated with complications such as infection at the site, sepsis due to the direct access to the central circulation, and thrombosis due to partial occlusion of the vessel. Typically, a chest x-ray is performed after a central venous access device is inserted to verify proper placement. No fluids are administered until correct placement is confirmed. Table 35.3 describes the major types of central venous access devices.

Infusion Control Devices

Infants and young children are at increased risk for fluid volume overload compared with adults. Also, malfunction at the IV insertion site, such as infiltration, may result in much greater injury than a similar incident would cause in an adult. Therefore, IV fluids must be carefully administered and monitored. To ensure accurate fluid administration, infusion control devices such as infusion pumps, syringe pumps, and volume control sets may be used.

Infusion pumps used for children are similar to those used for adults. In addition, syringe pumps are often used to deliver fluid and medications to children. These pumps can be programmed to deliver minute amounts of fluid over controlled periods of time (see discussion on syringe pumps in the previous section).

An IV solution bag may be attached to a calibrated volume control set that has been filled with a specified amount of IV solution (Fig. 35.9). The fluid chamber holds a maximum of 100 to 150 mL of fluid that can be infused over a specified period of time as ordered. Usually, a maximum of a 2-hour infusion amount in the chamber avoids accidental fluid overload in the pediatric population. This chamber can be filled every 1 to 2 hours so only small amounts of ordered quantities of fluid can infuse and the child is protected from receiving too much fluid volume. Due to the advances in pump technology and the introduction of "smart pumps" which include dose error reduction systems such as hospital-defined drug libraries (drug lists) with standard drug concentrations, and dose limits, to potentially improve the safety of IV medication administration, the use of volume control devices are less common in practice (Loorand-Stiver, 2011). However, as a safety device for controlling the volume of fluid administered to children

TABLE 35.3 TYPES OF CENTRAL VENOUS ACCESS DEVICES

Device	Description
Peripherally inserted central catheter (PICC)	Short- to moderate-term therapy Insertion via a peripheral vein such as basilic, cephalic, or brachial vein Catheter typically threaded into superior vena cava; distal tip terminates in the superior vena cava, inferior vena cava, or proximal right atrium Insertion via saphenous vein with tip terminating in inferior vena cava above the diaphragm for infants Single or multiple lumens Can be inserted at the bedside; requires additional training and advanced skill
Nontunneled central venous catheter (CVC)	Usually used short term One or more lumens Percutaneous insertion most commonly via the subclavian, internal jugular, or femoral vein with the tip of the catheter at the top of the superior vena cava just above the right atrium Useful for emergency situations Catheter sutured in place at the exit site Increased rate of central line associated blood stream infection than tunneled CVC
Tunneled central venous catheter (e.g., Groshong, Hickman/Broviac)	Usually for long-term use Catheter inserted by a physician via small incision in jugular, femoral, or subclavian vein and tunneled in the subcutaneous tissue under the skin Initially sutured in place to stabilize position; sutures removed after approximately 1 to 2 weeks when cuff on catheter attaches to subcutaneous tissue Single or multiple lumens Some have valves that prevent backflow of blood and air entrance
Implanted ports (e.g., Port-a-Cath, Infus-a-Port, Mediport)	Surgically inserted by a physician Stainless steel port with a polyurethane or silicone catheter attached Catheter tip lying in subclavian or jugular vein; port implanted under skin in a subcutaneous pocket, usually on the upper chest wall Port covered completely by skin and visible only as a slight bulging on the chest; possibly more appealing to the older child and adolescent because there are no visible parts or dressings Access to port via a specially angled, noncoring needle (Huber needle) Site preparation and pain relief measures necessary before accessing the port Lowest risk for central line associated blood stream infection

Adapted from The Joint Commission (2013). Preventing central line–associated bloodstream infections: Useful tools, an international perspective. Retrieved from http://www.jointcommission.org/Topics/Clabsi_toolkit.aspx; & Bowden, V. R., & Greenberg, C. S. (2011). *Pediatric nursing procedures (3rd ed)*. Philadelphia: Lippincott Williams & Wilkins.

they are still available; therefore, nurses should be familiar with how to use them.

Inserting Peripheral IV Access Devices

Peripheral IV devices are used for most IV therapies. Prior to insertion, review the child's diagnosis and medical history for information that may affect therapy, such as site selection or insertion. For example, a child who has a history of chronic illness may have heightened fears and anxieties related to insertion due to his or her previous experiences or difficulty in accessing IV sites. Typically, the nondominant extremity should be used for insertion, but this may not be possible in certain situations, such as if a right-handed child has a cast on his left arm.

Check the orders for the prescribed therapy. Determine the purpose and length of the IV therapy and the type of fluid or medication that is to be administered. This information aids in selecting the best device and insertion site. For example, the device needs to be of an adequate gauge to allow the solution or medication to infuse into the vein while at the same time allowing enough blood flow around the device to promote dilution of the infusion.

Establish rapport with the child and parents. Inform them about IV therapy and what to expect. Be honest with the child. Explain that the venipuncture will hurt but only for a short time. Provide the child with a time

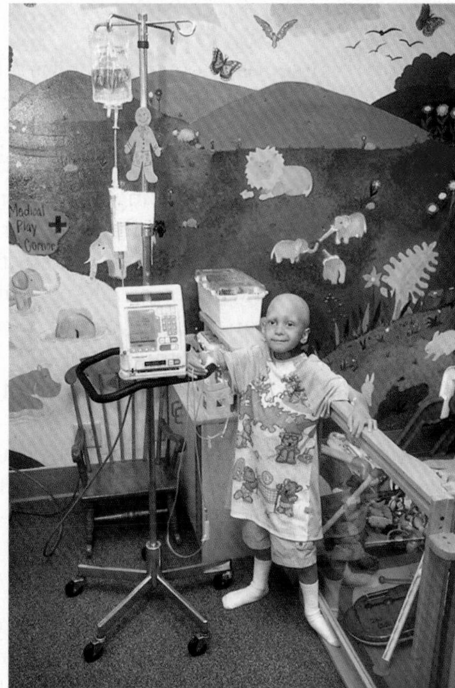

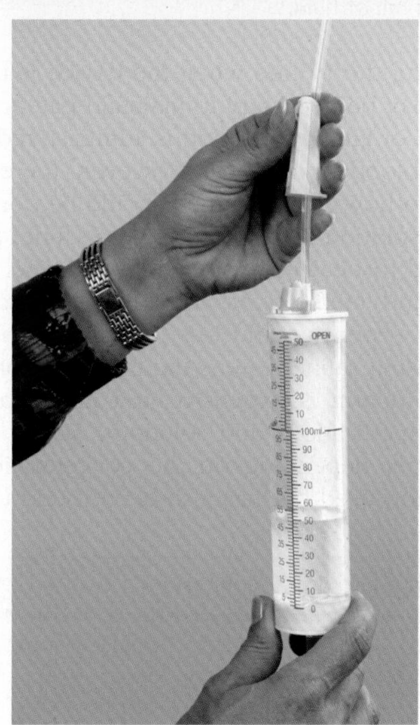

FIGURE 35.9 Volume control infusion device.

frame that he or she can understand, such as the time it takes to brush his or her teeth or eat a snack.

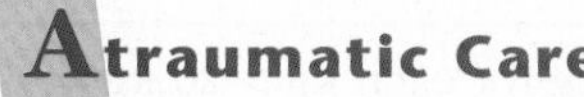

Atraumatic Care

Use therapeutic play to assist the child in preparation and coping for the procedure (see Chapter 33 for more information).

Insertion of an IV therapy device is traumatic. Follow the principles of atraumatic care, including the following:

- Gather all equipment needed before approaching the child.
- If possible, select a site using hand veins rather than wrist or upper arm veins to reduce the risk of phlebitis. Avoid using lower extremity veins and areas of joint flexion if possible because these are associated with an increased risk of thrombophlebitis and other complications (Bowden & Greenberg, 2011).
- Ensure adequate pain relief using pharmacologic and nonpharmacologic methods prior to insertion of the device (see Chapter 36 for more information about management of pain related to procedures).
- Allow the antiseptic used to prepare the site to dry completely before attempting insertion.
- Use a barrier such as gauze or a washcloth or the sleeve of the child's gown under the tourniquet to avoid pinching or damaging the skin.
- If the child's veins are difficult to locate, use a device to transilluminate the vein (utilizes a bright light, which illuminates the vein's size and direction of travel).
- Make only two attempts to gain access; if you are unsuccessful after two attempts, allow another individual two attempts to access a site. If still unsuccessful, evaluate the need for insertion of another device.

Take Note!

Some facilities have policies in place allowing only one stick per nurse with a maximum of two sticks; then the doctor needs to be notified unless the situation is an emergency.

- Encourage parental participation as appropriate in helping to position the child or to provide comfort positioning, such as therapeutic hugging.
- Coordinate care with other departments such as the laboratory for blood specimen collection to minimize the number of venipunctures for the child.
- Secure the IV line using a minimal amount of tape or transparent dressing.
- Protect the site from bumping by using a security device such as the IV house dressing (Fig. 35.10).

IV Fluid Administration

Administering IV fluids to an infant or child requires close attention to the child's fluid status. Typically, the amount of fluid to be administered in a day (24 hours) is determined by the child's weight (in kilograms) using the following formula:

100 mL per kg of body weight for the first 10 kg
50 mL per kg of body weight for the next 10 kg
20 mL per kg of body weight for the remainder of body weight in kilograms

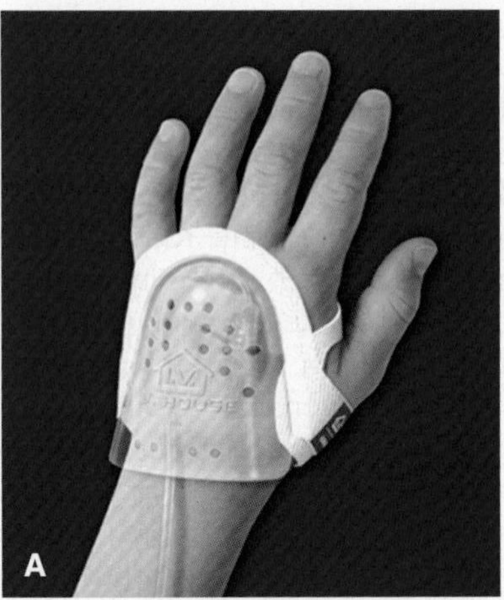

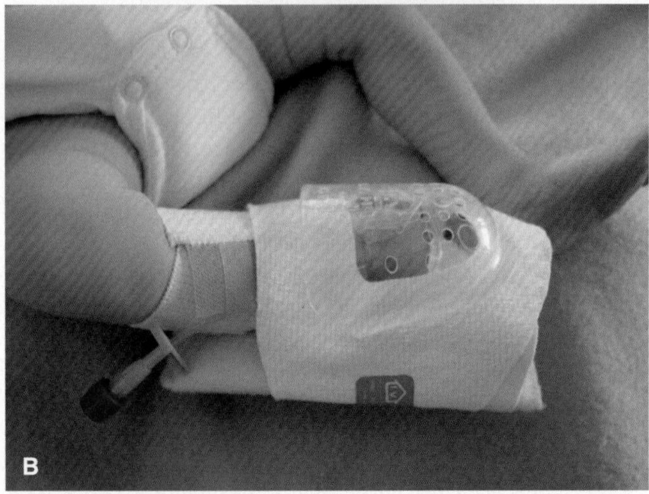

FIGURE 35.10 **(A)** IV house over the IV site on a child's hand. **(B)** IV house over the site on an infant's foot.

Table 35.4 gives examples of calculating a child's fluid requirements using body weight. Once the 24-hour total fluid requirement is determined, this amount is divided by 24 hours to arrive at the correct hourly rate of infusion.

Maintaining IV Fluid Therapy

Throughout the course of therapy, monitor the fluid infusion rate and volume closely, as often as every hour. If a volume control set is used to administer the IV infusion, fill the device with the allotted amount of fluid that the child is to receive in 1 hour. Doing so prevents inadvertent administration of too much fluid. Never assume that just because an infusion pump is in use, the infusion is being administered without problems. Pumps can malfunction. The tubing can become blocked, or the IV device can move out of the vein lumen. Not enough fluid, fluid overload, or infiltration of the solution into the tissues can occur.

In addition to monitoring the fluid infusion, closely monitor the child's output. Expected urine output for children and adolescents is 1 to 2 mL/kg/hour.

Take Note!

When measuring the output of an infant or child who is not toilet trained or who is incontinent, weigh the diaper to determine the output. Remember that 1 g of weight is equal to 1 mL of fluid.

Flushing the IV line when the device is used intermittently may be necessary to maintain patency, such as before and/or after medication is administered and after obtaining blood specimens. However, there is much debate as to how often flushing should be done and the best flush solution to use, heparin or saline. Saline has been found to be more compatible with the numerous solutions and medications administered intravenously, and is less expensive and less irritating to the vein. In addition, using saline lessens the incidence of pain and phlebitis. Heparin is expensive and incompatible with numerous medications and solutions, and it can affect clotting time, depending on the concentration of the flush solution used but has also been found to increase

TABLE 35.4 INTRAVENOUS MAINTENANCE FLUID CALCULATIONS BY BODY WEIGHT

<10 kg in weight	100 mL per kg of weight = # mL for 24 hours Example: A child weighs 7.4 kg 7.4 × 100 = 740 mL (daily requirement) 740/24 = 30.8 or 31 mL/hour
11–20 kg in weight	100 mL per kg of weight for the first 10 kg + 50 mL/kg for the next 10 kg = # mL for 24 hours Example: A child weighs 16 kg (10 × 100 = 1,000) plus (6 × 50 = 300) Total = 1,300 mL (daily requirement) 1,300/24 = 54 mL/hour
>20 kg in weight	100 mL/kg for the first 10 kg + 50 mL/kg for the next 10 kg + 20 mL/kg for each kg > 20 kg = # mL for 24 hours Example: A child weighs 30 kg (10 × 100 = 1,000) plus (10 × 50 = 500) plus (10 × 20 = 200) Total = 1700 mL (daily requirement) 1,700/24 = 70.8 or 71 mL/hour

catheter patency and decrease infusion failures. Evidence appears to support that both heparin and normal saline are effective for maintaining patency of peripheral IV catheters and which fluid used will depend on provider and agency preference. Additional research is needed to determine the best solution, volume and concentration of the flush solution, and interval for flushing. A clinical trial is currently underway that will investigate normal saline versus heparinized solution flush for maintaining patency of peripheral venous catheters in children (ClinicalTrials.gov, 2013). A recent systematic review of randomized control studies did show that continuous infusion of low-dose heparin did result in increased catheter patency and decreased infusion failures while intermittent heparin flushing showed minimal benefits (Kumar, Vandermeer, Bassler & Mansoor, 2013). Flushing solutions and procedure will vary; therefore, it is important to always follow your agency's policy or provider order for flushing IV lines.

If the child is receiving IV therapy via a central venous access device, provide site care using sterile technique and flush the device according to agency policy. Note the exit site for the device and inspect it frequently for signs of infection. If the device has multiple lumens, label each lumen with its use (i.e., blood specimen, medication, or fluid). Always check the compatibilities of solutions and medications being given simultaneously.

Take Note!

When flushing or administering medications through a PICC line, follow the manufacturer's recommended syringe size, because PICC lines are fragile. Using a larger-volume syringe (i.e., 5 mL or larger) exerts less pressure on the PICC, thereby reducing the risk of rupture (Bowden & Greenberg, 2011).

Preventing Complications

IV therapy is an invasive procedure that is associated with numerous complications. Strict aseptic technique is necessary when inserting the device and caring for the site. Adherence to standard precautions is key. Inspect the insertion site every 1 to 2 hours for inflammation or **infiltration** (inadvertent infusion of a nonirritant solution or medication into the surrounding tissue). Note signs of inflammation such as warmth, redness, induration, or tender skin. Check closely for signs of infiltration such as cool, blanched, or puffy skin. Use of a transparent dressing or IV house dressing provides easy access for assessing the IV insertion site. These types of dressings also help to prevent movement of the catheter hub, thus minimizing the risk of mechanical irritation, dislodgement, and complications such as phlebitis or infection (Fig. 35.10).

Typically, in adults, an IV site is changed every 72 to 96 hours and at any time when the integrity of the system has been compromised or contamination is suspected (O'Grady et al., 2011). However, with children, the 72- to 96-hour time frame may need to be adjusted to minimize the child's exposure to the repeated trauma of insertion. Current recommendations include replacement in children only when clinically indicated (O'Grady et al., 2011). Follow the agency's policies and procedures related to site changes. Consider an alternative route for fluid and medication administration or the insertion of an alternative IV device, such as a PICC line. Catheter-related bloodstream infections often can occur with the use of central venous lines. These infections result in increased morbidity and health care costs (O'Grady et al., 2011). Prevention is paramount. Nurses need to practice proper hand hygiene, use maximal barrier protection during insertion, assess the site frequently, provide proper site care using strict sterile technique, and ensure that the child's central venous catheter is removed as soon as it is no longer needed. In children it is important also to prevent the child from touching and playing with the central venous line site or dressing. The CDC and Healthcare Infection Control Practices Advisory Committee (HICPAC) currently recommend changing administration sets that are continuously used no more frequently than 72 to 96 hours but at least every 7 days, except if fluids that increase microbial growth, such as blood, blood products, or parenteral nutrition, have been administered. In these cases changing the administration sets every 24 hours is recommended (O'Grady et al., 2011). Replace administration sets per agency policy. Ensure proper disinfecting of all catheter hubs, needleless connectors, and injection ports before accessing them to minimize contamination.

Take Note!

Chlorhexidine-impregnated sponge (Biopatch) dressings may be used to help prevent infection in children older than 2 months of age (O'Grady et al., 2011). Always follow agency or institution policy and procedures regarding site care.

Discontinuing the IV Device

Prepare the child for removal of the IV device in much the same manner as for insertion. Many children may fear the removal of the device to the same extent that they feared its insertion. Explain what is to occur and enlist the child's help in the removal.

Atraumatic Care

If appropriate, allow the child to assist in removing the tape or dressing. This gives the child a sense of control over the situation and also encourages his or her cooperation.

In addition, practice atraumatic care by doing the following:

- Use water or adhesive remover to help loosen the tape.
- If a transparent dressing is in place, gently lift off the dressing by pulling up opposite corners using a motion parallel to the skin surface.
- Avoid using scissors to cut the tape, but if cutting the tape is necessary, be sure that the child's fingers are clear of the tape and scissors.
- Turn off the infusion solution and pump.
- Once all tape and dressings are removed, gently slide the IV device out using a motion opposite to that used for the insertion.
- Apply pressure to the site with a dry gauze dressing and then cover with a small adhesive bandage. If possible, allow the child to choose the bandage.

Take Note!

If the IV site was in the arm at or near the antecubital space, apply pressure until the bleeding stops. Do not have the child bend his or her arm after removal of the device as this is not sufficient pressure to prevent hematoma formation.

PROVIDING NUTRITIONAL SUPPORT

Adequate nutrition is important for all individuals but especially for children. During the growing years the quality of a child's nutrition affects his or her overall health and development. The presence of a chronic illness, disease, or trauma can increase the child's nutritional demands; if the child cannot meet these even with oral supplementation, other measures may be necessary to provide nutritional support. Such measures may include **enteral nutrition** (delivery of nutrition into the gastrointestinal tract via a tube) and **parenteral nutrition** (IV delivery of nutritional substances). The nutritional plan is determined by the child's age, developmental level, and health status.

Enteral Nutrition

Enteral nutrition, commonly called tube feedings, involves the insertion of a tube, so that feedings can be delivered directly into the child's gastrointestinal tract. The tube may be inserted via the nose or mouth or through an opening in the abdominal area, with the tube ending in the stomach or small intestine. Nasogastric or orogastric tube feedings, a tube from the nose to the stomach or from the mouth to the stomach, respectively, are commonly referred to as **gavage feedings**. Nasoduodenal or nasojejunal feedings involve a tube that is inserted through the nose and ends in either the duodenum or jejunum. Gastrostomy feedings involve the insertion of a gastrostomy tube through an opening in the abdominal wall and into the stomach. Jejunostomy feedings are similar to gastrostomy feedings except that the tube lies in the jejunum.

Enteral nutrition is indicated for children who have a functioning gastrointestinal tract but cannot ingest enough nutrients orally. The child may be unconscious or have a severely debilitating condition that interferes with his or her ability to consume adequate food and fluids. Other conditions that may warrant the use of enteral nutrition include:

- Failure to thrive
- Inability to suck or tiring easily during sucking
- Abnormalities of the throat or esophagus
- Swallowing difficulties or risk for aspiration
- Respiratory distress
- Metabolic conditions
- Severe gastroesophageal reflux disease (GERD)
- Surgery
- Severe trauma

Enteral feedings may be given via nasogastric, orogastric, nasojejunal, nasoduodenal, gastrostomy, or jejunostomy tubes (Fig. 35.11). Table 35.5 provides additional information about these types of feeding tubes. Enteral feedings costs less, are associated with fewer complications, and are considered safer than parenteral feedings. However, tube misplacement is a serious complication.

Inserting a Nasogastric or Orogastric Feeding Tube

Tubes for gavage feeding can be inserted via the nose or mouth. For infants, who are obligate nose breathers,

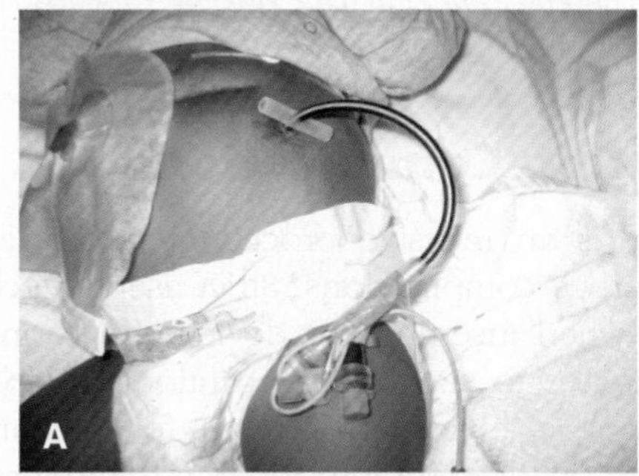

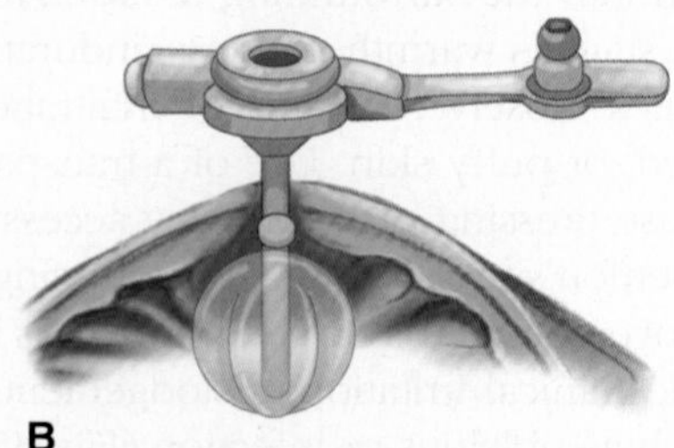

FIGURE 35.11 **(A)** Gastrostomy tube. **(B)** Low-profile (button) gastrostomy tube. The filled balloon keeps the tube in place inside the stomach.

TABLE 35.5 TYPES OF ENTERAL FEEDING TUBES

Type of Tube	Indication	Nursing Implications
Nasogastric (inserted via the nose into the stomach) Orogastric (inserted via the mouth into the stomach)	Short-term enteral feeding Orogastric usually limited to young infants only	• Long-term use or repeated insertion causes irritation and discomfort. • Silicone and polyurethane tubes are very flexible and more comfortable; they require a stylet or guidewire for insertion. • Length of long-term use varies according to the type of tube used and the institution protocol. Periodically, a nasogastric tube is removed and reinserted via the opposite nostril to prevent pressure on the nasal mucosa. • Maintaining orogastric placement between feedings can be difficult due to oral secretions.
Nasoduodenal (inserted via the nose to the duodenum) or nasojejunal (inserted via the nose to the jejunum)	Short-term enteral feeding. Indicated if child has trouble digesting food, cannot use his or her gastrointestinal tract secondary to congenital anomalies or surgery, or is at risk for or has a history of severe reflux or aspiration	• Silicone and polyurethane tubes with weighted tip allow tube to pass from pylorus into small intestines. • Agency may require special training in order to place at bedside; may also be performed in radiology • Length of use same as nasogastric or orogastric tubes
Gastrostomy (surgically inserted through the abdominal wall into the stomach) Jejunostomy (surgically inserted through the abdominal wall into the jejunum)	Long-term enteral feeding or when esophageal atresia or stricture is present Jejunostomy tubes are indicated when gastric feeding is not tolerated.	• The inner section of the tube is below the skin surface with the tip located in the stomach or jejunum (may be balloon, winged, or mushroom shaped). The outer section appears above the skin surface at the insertion site and has an opening or feeding port to which the feeding solution is attached. • Low-profile gastrostomy device (gastrostomy button) is flush with the abdominal surface. The flip-top opening is anchored by a dome that fits against the stomach wall. Less conspicuous, it allows the child to be more active and mobile. • After initial insertion, the tube length is measured from the insertion site to the far end of the tube and recorded. This measurement is checked at least daily to ensure that the tube has not moved. • There are many different devices available. For any gastrostomy or jejunostomy tube, the type and size of tube inserted as well as the amount required to fill the balloon, if present, should be known.

insertion via the mouth may be appropriate. Oral insertion also promotes sucking in the infant. For the older child, nasal insertion is usually the preferred method. If the tube is to remain in place, the nose also is considered to be more comfortable. Nursing Procedure 35.2 gives the steps for inserting a gavage feeding tube.

DETERMINING TUBING LENGTH FOR INSERTION

Traditionally, morphologic methods, measuring from the nose to ear to mid-xiphoid to umbilicus (NEMU) or just nose to ear to mid-xiphoid (NEX), have been used to determine tube length for insertion. Recent research has shown that this way of measurement frequently underestimates the tube length (Cincinnati Children's Hospital Medical Center, 2011; Ellett et al., 2012).

Take Note!

Recent studies have concluded that NEX should no longer be used to determine tubing length for NG/OG tube placement in children due to the significant risk of tube misplacement (Ellett, Cohen, Perkins, et. al, 2012).

Improving the accuracy of predicting tube length will lead to an increase in successful nasogastric tube placements, and therefore, improved outcomes and decreased health care costs.

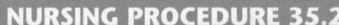

NURSING PROCEDURE 35.2

Inserting a Gavage Feeding Tube

Purpose: To provide a means for delivering nutrition to the child's functioning gastrointestinal tract

1. Verify the order for gavage feeding.
2. Explain the procedure to the child and parents using appropriate language geared to the child's development level.
3. Gather the necessary equipment; remove formula for feeding from refrigerator if appropriate and allow it to come to room temperature.
4. Wash hands and put on gloves.
5. Inspect the child's nose and mouth for deformities that may interfere with passage of the tube.
6. Position the infant supine with the head slightly elevated and with the neck slightly hyperextended so that the nose is pointed upward. If necessary, place a rolled towel or blanket under the neck to help in maintaining this position. Assist the older child to a sitting position, if appropriate. Alternatively, have the parent or another person hold the child to promote comfort and reassurance. Enlist the aid of additional persons, such as a parent or other health care team member, to assist in maintaining the child's position.
7. Determine the tubing length for insertion: Use age-related height based method (see Table 35.6), if possible, or morphologic measurement from the tip of the nose to the earlobe to the middle of the area between the xiphoid process and umbilicus. Mark this measurement on the tube with an indelible pen or with a piece of tape.
8. Lubricate the tube with a generous amount of sterile water (many small-bore feeding tubes have a water-activated lubricant) or water-soluble lubricant to promote passage of the tube and minimize trauma to the child's mucosa.
9. Insert the tube into one of the nares or the mouth. Direct a nasally inserted tube straight back toward the occiput; direct an orally inserted tube toward the back of the throat.
10. Advance the tube slowly to the designated length; encourage the child (if capable) to swallow frequently to assist with advancing the tube.
11. Watch for signs of distress, such as gasping, coughing, or cyanosis, indicating that the tube is in the airway. If these signs develop, withdraw the tube and allow the child to rest before attempting reinsertion.
12. Temporarily secure tube, remove stylet if applicable, and check for proper placement of the tube. Refer to Box 35.4.
13. Document the type of tube inserted; length of tubing inserted; measurement of external tubing length, from nares to end of tube, after insertion; and confirmation of placement.

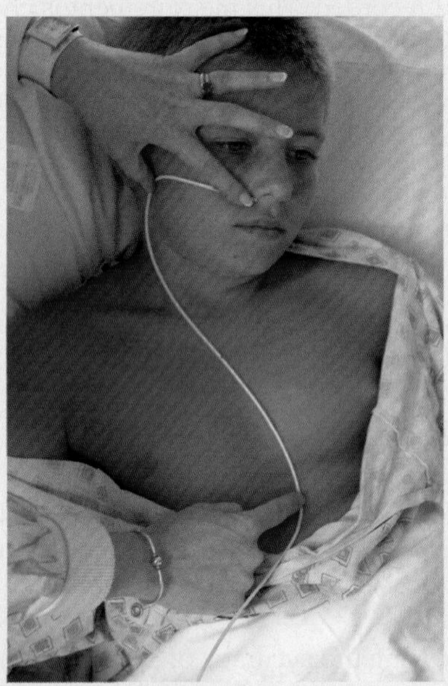

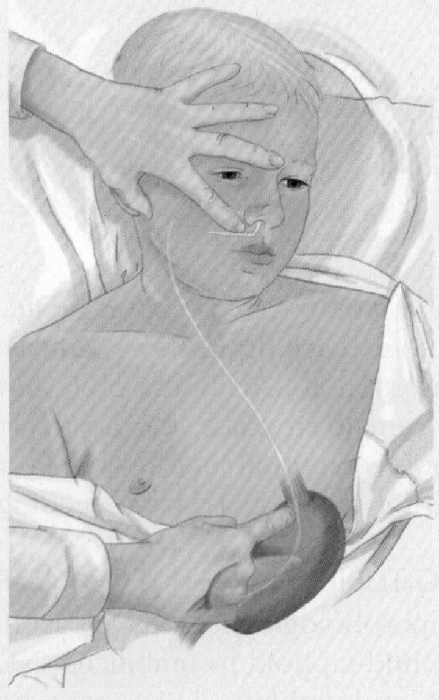

Adapted from Bowden, V. R., & Greenberg, C. S. (2011). *Pediatric nursing procedures* (*3rd ed*). Philadelphia, PA: Lippincott Williams & Wilkins.

TABLE 35.6 AGE-RELATED HEIGHT-BASED (ARHB) EQUATIONS FOR PREDICTING OG/NG TUBE INSERTION LENGTHS

Route	Age Group	Predicted Internal Distance to the Body of the Stomach Determined by:
Oral	Age ≤ 28 months	16.6 + 0.183 (height cm)
	Between ages 28 months and 100 months (8 years 4 months)	20.1 + 0.183 (height cm)
	Between ages 100 months (8 years 4 months) and 121 months (approx. 10 years)	17 + 0.218 (height cm)
	Greater than 121 months (approx. 10 years)	18.5 + 0.218 (height cm)
Nasal	Age < 28 months	17.6 + 0.197 (height cm)
	Between ages 28 months and 100 months (8 years 4 months)	21.1 + 0.197 (height cm)
	Between ages 100 months (8 years 4 months) and 121 months (approx. 10 years)	18.7 + 0.218 (height cm)
	Greater than 121 months (approx. 10 years)	21.2 + 0.218 (height cm)

Adapted from Cincinnati Children's Hospital Medical Center (2011). Best evidence statement (BESt). Confirmation of nasogastric/orogastric tube (NGT/OGT) placement. Cincinnati (OH): Cincinnati Children's Hospital Medical Center. Retrieved from http://www.cincinnatichildrens.org/assets/0/78/1067/2709/2777/2793/9198/ad67ab29–2a71–42a4-b78e-3d0e9710adac.pdf

According to the Agency for Healthcare Research and Quality's National Guideline Clearinghouse (2012), determining tubing length for insertion of a nasogastric tube using age-related height-based (ARHB) methods versus the traditional morphologic, nose–ear–mid-xiphoid–umbilicus method is more accurate for children greater than 2 weeks (National Guideline Clearinghouse, 2012). Refer to Table 35.6 for ARHB equations.

Continue to use traditional morphologic methods in neonates less than 2 weeks, children with short stature, or if unable to obtain an accurate height (Cincinnati Children's Hospital Medical Center, 2011; National Guideline Clearinghouse, 2012).

CHECKING TUBE PLACEMENT

Once the gavage feeding tube is inserted, checking for placement is essential. Tube placement must be confirmed each time the tube is inserted and before each use. Radiologic confirmation of tube placement is considered the most accurate method, but the risks associated with repeated radiation exposure, high costs, and the impractical nature of obtaining a x-ray before feeding tube use make it unrealistic (Cincinnati Children's Hospital Medical Center, 2011). Several methods have been proposed as reliable for checking tube placement, but no single method has been shown to be consistently accurate for continually assessing tube placement.

Take Note!

Instilling air into the tube and then auscultating for the sound is no longer considered a viable, single verification method for checking tube placement (Cincinnati Children's Hospital Medical Center, 2011).

Research has suggested alternative methods such as using measurements of bilirubin, trypsin, and pepsin levels, CO_2 monitoring, transillumination and magnetic detection to enhance assessment of tube placement, but insufficient evidence is available to support these methods. Also, these methods have other limitations such as the cost, the availability of equipment, and the limited availability for bedside testing of these levels.

Refer to Box 35.4 for methods to verify feeding tube placement. However, keep in mind that even with these methods, tube malpositioning can occur. Therefore, nurses need to be vigilant in checking for tube placement using the recommended methods and be cautious and proactive if there is any suspicion that the tube may be misplaced.

Take Note!

If bedside methods are conflicting or the child is at high risk, such as children with swallowing problems, children with altered levels of consciousness, or children in the intensive care unit, radiologic verification is recommended (Cincinnati Children's Hospital Medical Center, 2011).

If the gavage feeding tube is to remain in place, secure it to the child's cheek. Do not tape the tube to the child's forehead, because this could lead to irritation and pressure on, and possible breakdown of, the nasal mucosa. Also, measure the length of the tube extending from the nose or mouth to the end and record this information. Double-check this measurement before administering each intermittent tube feeding to verify that the feeding tube is in the proper position. Once the position

BOX 35.4

METHODS FOR VERIFICATION OF FEEDING TUBE PLACEMENT

- Obtain radiographic confirmation of proper tube placement in children who are considered high risk for aspiration, such as children with neurologic impairment, children obtunded, sedated, unconscious, critically ill, reduced gag reflex or static encephalopathy, or when nonradiologic methods are not feasible or bedside results are conflicting.
- Nonradiologic verification is used in children who are not considered high risk for aspiration, document pH of aspirate; document insertion distance and external length of tube in the chart. Mark and document the tube's exit site from the nose or mouth.
- Use bedside techniques at regular intervals to determine proper tube positioning.
  - Measuring pH
    - Gastric secretions have a pH less than 5. Small intestine secretions will usually have a pH greater than 6, but this does not reliably predict proper tube placement. A pH greater than 6 can occur with respiratory or esophageal placement, with proper tube placement (gastric or intestinal) when feedings are given continuously, or if the child is receiving acid-inhibiting medications. Therefore, if the pH is greater than 5, additional assessment is warranted.
  - Observing appearance of fluid aspirated from tube (can be used in conjunction with pH testing but is not a reliable single verification method)
    - Gastric secretions are usually grassy green or clear and colorless and can have off-white or tan mucous shreds. It may also be brown tinged if blood is present.
    - Intestinal secretions are often bile stained, light golden yellow to brownish green. They tend to be thicker and more translucent than gastric secretions.
    - Respiratory secretions can be white, yellow, straw colored, or clear.
  - Instill air into the tube and then auscultate for the sound (gastric auscultation) (can be used in conjunction with other assessment methods).
  - Check external markings on tube and external tube length (tube remaining from nares to end of tube) to determine if the tube seems to have migrated or been misplaced.
- Continually assess for signs indicative of feeding tube misplacement, such as unexplained gagging, vomiting, or coughing; signs and symptoms of respiratory distress; and decreased oxygen saturations.
- If bedside techniques reveal conflicting results or the child is at high risk, radiologic confirmation is recommended.
- Review routine chest and abdominal x-rays (if obtained) to double-check correct tube position.

Always follow agencies' policy and procedures.

Adapted from Cincinnati Children's Hospital Medical Center (2011). *Best evidence statement (BESt). Confirmation of nasogastric/orogastric tube (NGT/OGT) placement.* Cincinnati (OH): Cincinnati Children's Hospital Medical Center. Retrieved from http://www.cincinnatichildrens.org/assets/0/78/1067/2709/2777/2793/9198/ad67ab29–2a71–42a4-b78e-3d0e9710adac.pdf

of the gavage feeding tube is confirmed, the feeding solution or medication can be administered.

Remember Lily, the 9-month-old infant diagnosed with failure to thrive who is to receive gavage feedings with a nasogastric tube? What equipment will be needed, and what steps will you take to complete the procedure?

Administering Enteral Feedings

Enteral feedings can be given continuously or intermittently, regardless of the type of tube used. Intermittent feedings are commonly called **bolus feedings**. With a bolus feeding, a specified amount of feeding solution is given at specific intervals, usually over a short period of time such as 15 to 30 minutes. Given via a syringe, feeding bag, or infusion pump, bolus feedings most closely resemble regular meals. Continuous feedings are given at a slower rate over a longer period of time. In some cases, the feeding may be given during the night so that the child can be free to move about and participate in activities during the day. For continuous feedings, an enteral feeding pump is used to administer the solution at a prescribed rate.

Checking for tube placement is a priority before administering any intermittent tube feeding and periodically during continuous tube feedings, regardless of the type of tube being used. (Refer to Box 35.4.) For gastrostomy and jejunostomy tubes, ensure that the calibration, if present, has not changed. Measure the length of the tube daily from the exit site on the stomach to the end of the tube. Assess the abdomen for distension and bowel sounds. Also, measure the **gastric residual** (the amount remaining in the stomach; indicates gastric emptying time) by aspirating the gastric contents with a syringe, measuring it, and then replacing the contents. Check the residuals periodically, according to the facility's policy, such as every 4 to 6 hours, and before each intermittent feeding. If the residual volume exceeds the amount specified by the physician's order, hold the feeding and notify the physician or nurse practitioner.

Begin the feeding by placing the child in a supine position with the head and shoulders elevated approximately 30 degrees so that the feeding will remain in the stomach area (Bowden & Greenberg, 2011). Flush the tube with a small amount of water to clear it and prevent occlusion. This is not necessary for a gavage feeding if the tube is being inserted each time a feeding is given. Ensure that the feeding solution is at room temperature. Administer the feeding per the facility's policy.

Feeding solutions may be placed into the barrel of a syringe or into a feeding bag attached to the feeding tube and allowed to flow by gravity. The rate of flow for gravity-assisted feedings can be increased or decreased by raising or lowering the feeding solution container, respectively. Typically, intermittent feedings last from 15 to 30 minutes. A feeding bag also may be attached to a pump to control the rate of flow. Monitor the child's tolerance to the feeding.

Once the feeding is complete, but before the formula completely empties from the container, flush the tube with water. As the water leaves the syringe or tubing, clamp the tube to prevent air from entering the stomach. Then disconnect the syringe or tube-feeding bag from the tube.

Take Note!

If the child vomits during the feeding, stop the feeding immediately and turn the child onto his or her side or sit him or her up.

If the child has a gastrostomy button, open the cap and connect an adaptor or insert extension tubing through the one-way valve. This allows access to the gastric conduit. The feeding solution container is connected to the extension tubing or adaptor and the feeding is given as described previously. After the feeding is completed, the extension tubing or adaptor is flushed with water and the flip-top opening is closed.

Burp the infant during and after any type of tube feeding in the same manner as for an infant who is bottle- or breast-fed. Also, position the child on his or her right side with the head slightly elevated, approximately 30 degrees, for about 1 hour after the feeding to facilitate gastric emptying and reduce the risk of aspiration and regurgitation. Some children have a difficult time with gas and burping on their own after tube placement. Venting, which helps relieve gas, may be ordered by the physician or nurse practitioner. It removes excess air and can be helpful if the child is bloated or the abdomen is distended. Use a catheter-tip syringe with the plunger removed and attach to the end of the tube. Hold the syringe above the child's stomach for a few minutes. Once the air or gas is removed, allow any stomach contents or formula to flow back into the stomach.

Weigh the child daily throughout enteral nutrition therapy to determine the effectiveness of the therapy.

Providing Skin and Insertion Site Care

Skin around the gastrostomy or jejunostomy insertion site may become irritated from movement of the tube, moisture, leakage of stomach or intestinal contents, or the adhesive device holding the tube in place. Keeping the skin clean and dry is important and will help prevent most of these problems.

The skin around a gastrostomy or jejunostomy tube requires cleaning at least once a day. Routine site care includes gentle cleansing with sterile water or saline for newly placed tubes, or for established tubes, soap and water followed by rinsing or cleaning with water alone. To clean under an external disc or bumper, a cotton-tipped applicator may be used. During insertion site care, rotate the gastrostomy tube or button a quarter-turn to prevent skin adherence and irritation. Always follow agency or institution policies and procedures.

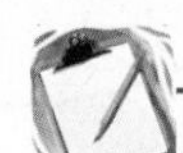

Take Note!

Do not rotate a jejunal or gastrojejunal tube because it can cause kinking (Bowden & Greenberg, 2011).

Assess the insertion site and condition of the surrounding skin for signs and symptoms of infection, such as erythema, induration, foul drainage, or pain. A small amount of clear or tan drainage is normal. If any drainage is present, a dressing can be placed. Use a presplit 2 × 2 gauze and place it loosely around the site. Change this dressing when it is soiled. If no drainage is present, do not place a dressing as it can cause undue pressure and trap moisture, leading to skin irritation.

Preventing movement of the tube also helps reduce skin irritation. Check the volume of the balloon with a balloon-tipped device about once or twice a week and reinflate the balloon to the initial volume if needed. The tube should be able to move slightly in and out of the child's stomach. The plastic disc should be snug against the skin but not tight enough to cause pressure. Tube stabilization methods help prevent the tube from moving around and sliding further into the stomach or jejunum. Stabilize the tube by pulling gently on the tubing and sliding the stabilizer bar or disc snugly against the abdomen.

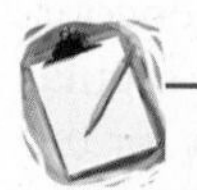

Take Note!

Rotate sites where the tube is secured to the abdomen to prevent tension on the stoma or skin breakdown.

Measure and record the length of the tube from the exit site of the abdominal wall to the end of the tube. All future measurements should be the same unless the tube length is changed. For tubes without a stabilizer bar or disc or for additional stabilization needs, several other methods may be used, including cut baby bottle nipples, taping methods, and commercially available stabilizers (Fig. 35.12). It is always important to follow agency policy.

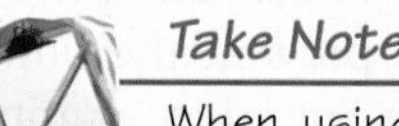

Take Note!

When using the nipple method, make sure to cut several holes in the base of the nipple to allow air circulation and site assessment.

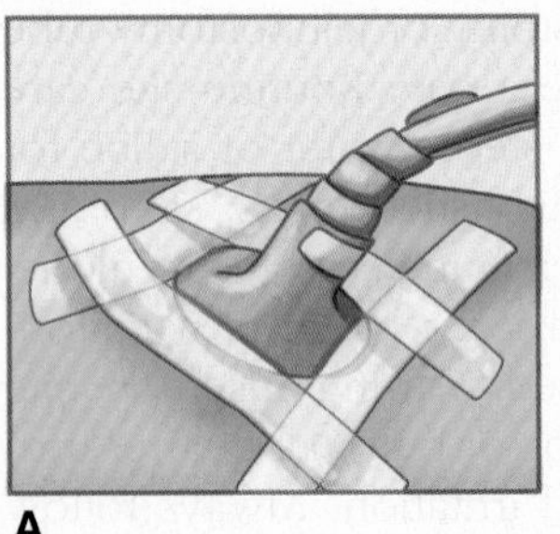

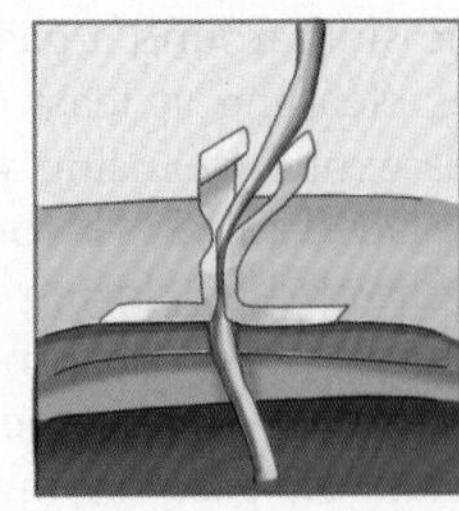

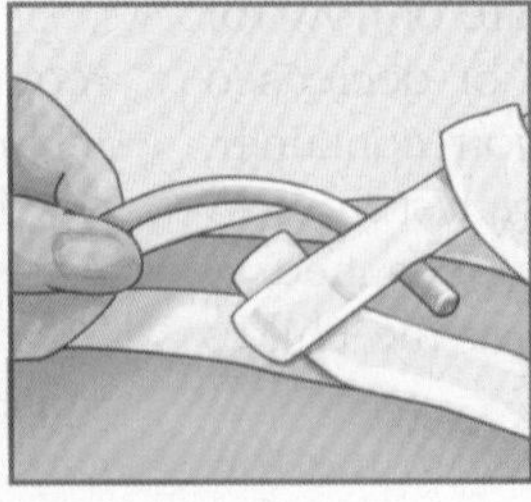

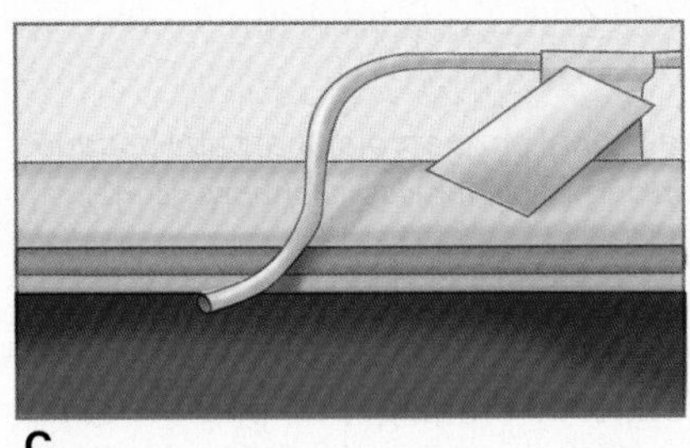

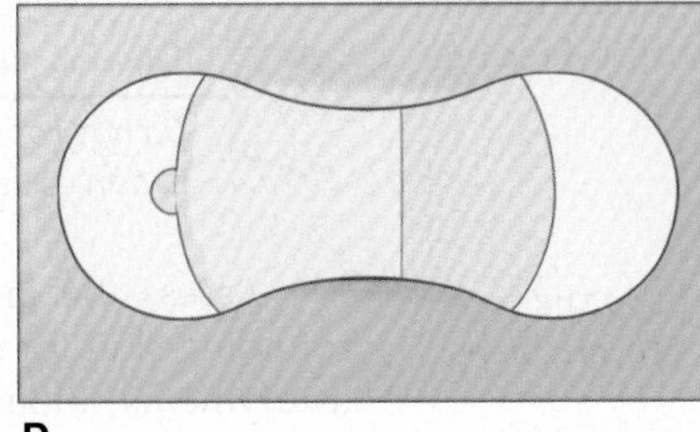

FIGURE 35.12 Methods to stabilize a gastrostomy tube include **(A)** the nipple method, **(B)** taping methods, **(C)** the tension loop method, and **(D)** commercially available stabilizing devices (GripLok®; pictured here).

Promoting Growth and Development

Some children receive all of their nutritional needs through tube feedings, whereas other children use tube feedings as a supplement to eating by mouth. Feeding time is a special time for infants and children. Occasionally, babies who are fed solely through an enteral feeding tube may forget or lose the desire to eat by mouth. Use a pacifier to help avoid this, allowing the infant to associate the nipple in his or her mouth with a feeding (Children's Hospitals and Clinics of Minnesota, 2013). The sucking motion will also exercise the jaw and promote the flow of the feedings. The saliva produced during sucking aids in digestion. Combined with holding the infant and cuddling, rocking, and talking to him or her, this promotes a more normal feeding time.

Talking with children, playing music, or reading a story promotes an active feeding time. At home, encourage parents to include the feeding as a part of regular family mealtime together to provide socialization for the child. Allow the child to participate in the feedings by gathering supplies and administering the actual feeding so that the child may experience independence and adaptation. If the child also eats food by mouth, feed him or her by mouth first and then administer the tube feeding. Children with feeding tubes should be allowed as normal a routine as possible. For example, they can crawl, walk, and jump just like children of the same age and developmental level. However, in some cases, contact sports such as football, hockey, and wrestling should be avoided because of the higher risk of injury. Securing the tubing under the child's clothing will prevent it from becoming accidentally dislodged and prevent the child from pulling and playing with it. Using one-piece outfits, an Ace wrap, or stretchy gauze to cover the tube can help protect it.

Educating the Child and Family

Educate children receiving enteral feedings and their parents thoroughly about this method of nutritional support. Reinforce the reason for the therapy and provide the child and parents with opportunities to verbalize their concerns and ask questions. Ensure that the parents understand the risks and benefits of the therapy and the expected duration.

Provide the child, if developmentally appropriate, and parents with opportunities to participate in the feeding sessions. This helps allay some of their fears and anxieties and promotes a sense of control over the situation. They will also gain valuable practice in learning the skill should the feedings be required at home. Teaching Guidelines 35.3 identifies important topics to include in the teaching plan for a child receiving enteral nutrition at home. Troubleshooting problems at home is an important topic to cover. Refer to Teaching Guidelines 35.4. Education also involves helping the family develop appropriate coping strategies to adapt, solve problems, and access the support and services they will need after discharge.

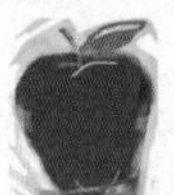

Teaching Guidelines 35.3

TOPICS TO BE COVERED FOR HOME ENTERAL NUTRITION

- Type and size of tube
- Type of nutritional support
- Rationale for therapy
- Expected results from therapy
- Duration of therapy
- Frequency of feedings
- Feeding solution and equipment
- Tube insertion technique (if appropriate)
- Methods to check for correct placement

- Steps for administering the feeding (and medication, if ordered)
- Procedure for flushing tube
- Procedure for venting the tube, if appropriate
- Frequency of weighing the child
- Signs and symptoms of complications and when to notify physician or nurse practitioner
- Troubleshooting problems, such as clogging of the tube or dislodgement (see Teaching Guidelines 35.4)
- Daily tube care (e.g., cleaning the site, rotating tube)
- Site assessment
- Technique for reinsertion/replacement of tube as appropriate
- Equipment suppliers
- Resources for support
- Follow-up visits and referrals

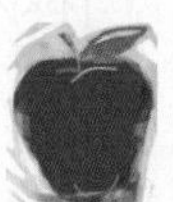

Teaching Guidelines 35.4

TROUBLESHOOTING COMPLICATIONS AT HOME

- If a tube becomes clogged, instruct caregivers to slowly push warm water into the tube. Amount and size of syringe will vary based on child's size and facility policy. Repeat if necessary. Instruct caregivers to never use an object or put anything into the tube. They should call the doctor or nurse if they are unable to unclog the tube. Declogging medications may be prescribed.
- If a tube is inadvertently removed, instruct the caregiver to cover the site with a small clean dressing tape, then to call the physician or nurse immediately; the tube needs to be replaced as soon as possible or the tract will close. Some institutions may instruct the family on how to replace the tube once the tube is more than 6 weeks old and has formed an established G-tube tract.
- If the site is red or irritated, instruct caregivers to continue with routine cleaning and call the physician. An antibiotic or skin barrier cream may be ordered. Assess for leakage and try to minimize, if possible. Check the tube's position and ensure tube is stabilized and secure and not dangling.
- If the tube is leaking, the caregiver needs to keep the dressing clean and dry. Assess tube position and secure the tube to avoid dangling. Assess if leaking is from stoma area or tube valve, if applicable. More frequent venting may help and the physician should be notified.

Always teach following the instructions per agency policy and procedure regarding home care.

Adapted from Bowden, V. R., & Greenberg, C. S. (2011). *Pediatric nursing procedures* (3rd edition). Philadelphia, PA: Lippincott Williams & Wilkins; and Cincinnati Children's Hospital Medical Center. (2012). *Gastrostomy Tube (G-tube) home care.* Retrieved from http://www.cincinnatichildrens.org/health/info/abdomen/home/g-tube-care.htm

Remember Lily from the beginning of the chapter? She is to be discharged home after having a gastrostomy tube inserted to continue feedings at home.

What teaching is needed for her family prior to discharge?

Parenteral Nutrition

Nutritional support can be administered IV through a peripheral or central venous catheter. The concentration and components of the solution determine the type of parenteral nutrition. Parenteral nutrition given via a central venous access device is termed **total parenteral nutrition (TPN)**. Comparison Chart 35.1 gives information about peripheral and central parenteral nutrition.

Administering TPN

Typically, the physician or nurse practitioner determines the concentration and components of the TPN solution based on a thorough assessment of the child's status, including the results of laboratory testing. This information is used as a baseline for evaluating the effectiveness of therapy.

The solution is prepared under sterile conditions in the pharmacy. For TPN, a central venous access device is inserted and secured, if one is not already in place. Use specialized tubing with an in-line filter (to prevent small microparticles from entering the circulation).

TPN solutions may be refrigerated until they are to be used. Once started, a single solution of TPN should hang for no longer than 24 hours (Weinstein & Hagle, 2014). The infusion of the solution is initiated at a slow rate that is gradually increased as ordered based on how the child tolerates the therapy. TPN solutions are highly concentrated glucose solutions that can cause hyperglycemia if given too rapidly. Use of an infusion pump is essential to control the rate of infusion. Fat emulsions are administered periodically to meet the child's need for essential fatty acids. These solutions are given as a piggyback solution into the TPN line, but below the in-line filter.

Throughout TPN therapy, be vigilant in monitoring the infusion rate, and report any changes in the infusion rate to the physician or nurse practitioner immediately. Gradual adjustments may be made to the rate, but only as ordered by the physician or nurse practitioner.

Initially, check blood glucose levels frequently, such as every 4 to 6 hours, to evaluate for hyperglycemia. These levels can be obtained with a bedside glucose meter. Minimize the trauma and discomfort associated with frequent invasive procedures by using the principles of atraumatic care. If blood glucose levels are elevated, SQ administration of insulin may be needed. Once the child's glucose levels stabilize, the frequency of blood

COMPARISON CHART 35.1

PERIPHERAL PARENTERAL NUTRITION VERSUS TOTAL PARENTERAL NUTRITION

	Peripheral Parenteral Nutrition	Total Parenteral Nutrition
Indications/use	Primarily supplemental Short-term use to supply additional calories and nutrients	Provides all nutrients to meet child's needs Enough calories supplied to maintain a positive nitrogen balance[a]
Route	Peripheral vein	Central venous access to allow rapid dilution of hypertonic solution
Child's status	Nutritional status usually within acceptable parameters Oral intake decreased or absent	Child with a nonfunctioning gastrointestinal (GI) tract, such as a congenital or acquired GI disorder Severe failure to thrive Multisystem trauma or organ involvement Preterm newborns
Components	Fluid, electrolytes, and carbohydrates (dextrose); usually no protein or fats Carbohydrate concentration usually limited to 10% or less and osmolarity of <600 mOsm[a]	Highly concentrated solution of carbohydrates, electrolytes, vitamins, and minerals Lipid emulsion to supply need for essential fatty acids Total nutrient admixture (TNA) with components of TPN plus lipids and other additives in one container

[a]Weinstein, S. M. & Hagle, M. E. (2014). *Plumer's principles & practice of infusion therapy* (9th ed.). Philadelphia, PA: Lippincott Williams & Wilkins.

glucose level testing decreases, such as every 8 to 12 hours, based on the facility's policy.

Take Note!

If for any reason the TPN infusion is interrupted or stops, be prepared to begin an infusion of a 5% to 10% dextrose solution at the same infusion rate as the TPN (Bowden & Greenberg, 2011). This helps to prevent rebound hypoglycemia that may occur due to the increased insulin secretion by the child's body in response to the use of the highly concentrated TPN solution.

Perform catheter site care, tubing and filter changes, and dressing changes according to the facility's policy. Inspect the insertion site closely for signs of infection. Also, monitor the child's vital signs, daily weights, and intake and output closely for changes. In addition, review laboratory test results, which can aid in early detection of problems, such as infection or electrolyte excesses or deficits.

TPN can be administered continuously over a 24-hour period, or after initiation it may be given on a cyclic basis, such as over a 12-hour period during the night. When administering cycled TPN, the solution is infused at half the prescribed rate for the first and last hour to prevent hyper- and hypoglycemia.

Preventing Complications

Nurses play a key role in minimizing the risk for complications related to use of central venous access devices and TPN. Box 35.5 describes these complications. Key

BOX 35.5

COMPLICATIONS THAT CAN OCCUR WITH CENTRAL VENOUS ACCESS DEVICES AND TOTAL PARENTERAL NUTRITION (TPN)

- Air embolism from inadvertent entry of air into the system during tubing or cap changes or accidental disconnection
- Cardiac tamponade due to catheter advancement with movement of the arm, neck, or shoulder
- Catheter occlusion from the development of a fibrin sheath or thrombus at the catheter tip, malpositioning or kinking, or the deposition of precipitates or a blood clot
- Venous thrombosis from injury to the vessel wall during insertion or movement of the catheter after insertion or from chemical irritation due to administration of concentrated solutions, vesicants, and other medications through the catheter
- Hyperglycemia, typically with too rapid an infusion of TPN
- Hypoglycemia, which may occur with rapid cessation
- Dehydration as the child's body attempts to rid itself of excess glucose through renal excretion
- Electrolyte imbalance (particularly potassium, sodium, calcium, magnesium, and phosphorus)
- Infection at the skin insertion site, along the catheter pathway, or in the bloodstream. Organisms can arise from the skin, hands of caregivers, or other areas such as wound drainage, droplets from the lungs, or urine. For example, connection sites can be contaminated during tubing or dressing changes.

measures to reduce the risk of complications include the following:

- Monitor the child's vital signs closely for changes.
- Adhere to strict aseptic technique when caring for the catheter and administering TPN.
- Ensure that the system remains a closed system at all times. Secure all connections and clamp the catheter or have the child perform the Valsalva maneuver during tubing and cap changes.
- Use occlusive dressings. Chlorhexidine-impregnated sponge (Biopatch) dressings may be used to help prevent infection. Always follow agency or institution policy and procedures.
- Adhere to agency policy for flushing of the catheter and maintaining catheter patency.
- Assess intake and output frequently.
- Monitor blood glucose levels and obtain laboratory tests as ordered to evaluate for changes in fluid and electrolytes.

Take Note!

Never administer any medication, blood, or other solution through the TPN lumen (Weinstein & Hagle, 2014). Doing so increases the risk for contamination of the system and subsequent infection.

Promoting Growth and Development

Meals are a time for meeting nutritional needs as well as a time for love, comfort, support, and socialization. TPN meets the child's nutritional needs, but the child's need for love and support also must be met. Implement measures similar to those for children receiving enteral nutrition (see discussion earlier in this chapter). Also provide opportunities for holding and cuddling the child. Allow the older child to participate in activities that can help to occupy the time associated with meals. When administering cyclic TPN run the TPN over the night time hours, whenever possible, to allow the child to participate in developmentally appropriate activities during the day. Encourage the child and parents to participate in the care to promote a sense of independence as well as a sense of control over the situation.

Educating the Child and Family

Children who require long-term TPN therapy may receive TPN in the home. Administering TPN at home requires thorough education of the child and parents. This teaching can occur in the health care agency or in the child's home. The amount of information to be taught can be overwhelming, so ensure that ample time is available. Allow time for questions and concerns. Offer emotional support and guidance whenever necessary.

Provide written and verbal instructions about the care involved. Have the child (if appropriate) and parents demonstrate the care needed, including care of the central venous access device. Review with them the measures for obtaining, storing, and handling the solutions and supplies. Develop plans for troubleshooting problems with devices and equipment, and give instructions on how to recognize and treat complications. Also teach them about danger signs and symptoms that require immediate notification. Be sure they have the name and number of a contact person in case of emergency situations.

Initiate the appropriate referrals for support. Specialized home care infusion services are available for follow-up in the home. In addition, social services can be helpful in providing assistance with finances, health insurance reimbursement, scheduling, transportation, emotional support, and community resources.

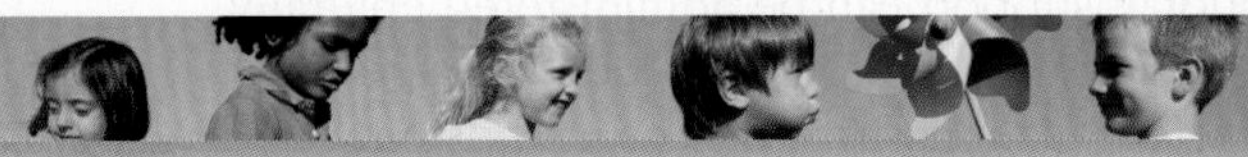

KEY CONCEPTS

- The "rights" of pediatric medication administration are the right drug, right dose, right route, right time, and right patient. Some experts have added additional rights, such as right documentation, right to be educated, right to refuse, right form, and right approach. These additional rights are important to consider to increase patient safety and satisfaction.
- The physiologic immaturity of some body systems in children can affect a drug's pharmacodynamics, leading to differences in the body's response to the drug and thus enhancing or diminishing the drug's effects. The child's age, weight, BSA, and body composition can affect the drug's pharmacokinetics.
- The two most common methods for determining pediatric drug doses involve the use of the child's body weight and BSA.
- Children younger than the age of 5 to 6 are at risk for aspiration when receiving tablets or capsules because they have difficulty swallowing them; liquids may be more appropriate. When administering oral medications to children, always tell them whether a medication is being mixed with food.
- Medication administration via the rectal route is not preferred because the drug's absorption may

be erratic and unpredictable and children find this route extremely upsetting or embarrassing.

- When administering otic medications, pull the pinna downward and back if the child is younger than age 3, and up and back for older children.
- IM administration is used infrequently in children because it is painful and children often lack the adequate muscle mass. When used with infants less than 7 months, the preferred site is the vastus lateralis muscle.
- Administration of medication via the IV route is common with children, especially when a rapid response to the drug is desired or when absorption via other routes is difficult or impossible. The primary method for IV medication administration is via a syringe pump.
- Preferred sites for peripheral IV therapy include the veins of the hands, feet, and forearms. The scalp vein may be used in infants, but only if attempts at other sites have been unsuccessful. The rule of thumb for insertion of any peripheral devices is to use the smallest-gauge catheter for the shortest length of time possible to prevent trauma to the child's fragile veins.
- Central venous therapy usually is administered through a large vein, such as the subclavian, femoral, or jugular vein or vena cava. The tip of the device lies in the superior vena cava just at the entrance to the right atrium. Devices include single- or multiple-lumen short- and long-term catheters, peripherally inserted central catheters, tunneled catheters, and vascular access ports.
- Monitoring intake and output is important when a child is receiving IV therapy. Site inspection, proper care of the site, and proper dressing changes are key to preventing complications.
- Nutritional support can be administered enterally via a nasogastric or orogastric tube (gavage feeding) or via a gastrostomy or jejunostomy device or administered parenterally through a peripheral or central venous access device.
- Enteral nutrition is indicated for children who have a functioning gastrointestinal tract but cannot consume adequate amounts of nutrients orally.
- Prior to any enteral feeding, placement of the feeding tube must be confirmed. The gold standard for confirming placement is with a x-ray. At the bedside, nonradiologic methods are used to confirm placement including checking the color and pH of the aspirate, checking external markings on the tube and verifying external tube length, continually assessing for signs indicative of feeding tube misplacement, such as unexplained gagging, vomiting, or coughing; signs and symptoms of respiratory distress; and decreased oxygen saturations.
- Children receiving TPN require close monitoring of the infusion rate and volume, intake and output, vital signs, and blood glucose levels. Strict aseptic technique is necessary when caring for the central venous access site and TPN infusion.

REFERENCES AND RECOMMENDED READINGS

American Academy of Pediatrics. (2013). *Healthy children: Safety & prevention: How to give eye drops and eye ointment.* Retrieved from http://www.healthychildren.org/English/safety-prevention/at-home/medication-safety/Pages/How-to-Give-Eye-Drops-and-Eye-Ointment.aspx

Aschenbrenner, D. S., & Venable, S. J. (2012). *Drug therapy in nursing* (4th ed.). Philadelphia, PA: Lippincott Williams & Wilkins.

Beckstrand, J., Cirgin Ellett, M. L., & McDaniel, A. (2007). Predicting internal distance to the stomach for positioning nasogastric and orogastric feeding tubes in children. *Journal of Advanced Nursing, 59*(3), 274–289.

Bergvall, E., & Sawyer, T. L. (2012). *Scalp Vein Catheterization.* Retrieved from http://emedicine.medscape.com/article/1348863-overview#a16

Bertolino, G., Pitassi, A., Tinelli, C., Staniscia, A., Guglielmana, B., Scudeller, L., et al. (2012). Intermittent flushing with heparin versus saline for maintenance of peripheral intravenous catheters in a medical department: a pragmatic cluster-randomized controlled study. *Worldviews Evidence Based, 9*(4):221–226. doi: 10.1111/j.1741–6787.2012.00244.x

Bowden, V. R., & Greenberg, C. S. (2011). *Pediatric nursing procedures* (3rd ed). Philadelphia, PA: Lippincott Williams & Wilkins.

Centers for Disease Control and Prevention. (2012). Appendix D: Vaccine administration. In W. Atkinson, S. Wolfe, & J. Hamborsky (Eds.), *Epidemiology and Prevention of Vaccine-Preventable Diseases* (12th ed., second printing). Washington, DC: Public Health Foundation.

Cincinnati Children's Hospital Medical Center. (2011). *Best evidence statement (BESt). Confirmation of nasogastric/orogastric tube (NGT/OGT) placement.* Cincinnati, OH: Cincinnati Children's Hospital Medical Center. Retrieved from http://www.cincinnatichildrens.org/assets/0/78/1067/2709/2777/2793/9198/ad67ab29-2a71-42a4-b78e-3d0e9710adac.pdf

Cincinnati Children's Hospital Medical Center. (2012). *Gastrostomy Tube (G-tube) home care.* Retrieved from http://www.cincinnatichildrens.org/health/info/abdomen/home/g-tube-care.htm

Children's Hospitals and Clinics of Minnesota. (2013). *Patient/family education: Nasogastric tube feeding.* Retrieved from http://www.childrensmn.org/manuals/pfs/homecare/018701.pdf

ClinicalTrials.gov. (2013). *Normal saline versus heparinized solution flush for maintaining patency of peripheral venous catheters in children.* Retrieved from http://clinicaltrial.gov/ct2/show/NCT01794767

Crawford, C. L., & Johnson, J. A. (2012). To aspirate or not: An integrative review of the evidence. *Nursing2012, 42*(3), 20–25.

Ellett, M. L., Cohen, M. D., Perkins, S. M., Croffie, J. M., Lane, K. A., & Austin, J. K. (2012). Comparing methods of determining insertion length for placing gastric tubes in children 1 month to 17 years of age. *Journal for Specialists in Pediatric Nursing, 17*(1):19–32. doi: 10.1111/j.1744–6155.2011.00302.x

Immunization Action Coalition. (2012). *How to administer intramuscular (IM) and how to administer subcutaneous (SC) injections.* Retrieved from http://www.immunize.org/catg.d/p2020.pdf

ISMP. (2009). Medication safety alert! safety briefs. 14(11), Retrieved from file:///C:/Users/Susan/Downloads/ISMP%20Newsletter%20Acute%20Care%206–4–09.pdf

Kroger, A. T., Sumaya, C. V., Pickering, L. K., & Atkinson, W. L. (2011). General recommendations on immunization recommendations of the Advisory Committee on Immunization Practices (ACIP). *Morbidity and Mortality Weekly Report (MMWR), 60*(RR02), 1–60. Retrieved from http://www.cdc.gov/mmwr/preview/mmwrhtml/rr6002a1.htm?s_cid=rr6002a1_e

Kumar, M., Vandermeer, B., Bassler, D., & Mansoor, N. (2013). Low-dose heparin use and the patency of peripheral IV catheters in children: A systematic review. *Pediatrics, 131*, e864–e872. doi: 10.1542/peds.2012–2403

Loorand-Stiver, L. (2011). *Pediatric Intravenous Administration of Drugs and Fluids. Environmental Scan, 21.* Ottawa, ON: Canadian Agency for Drugs and Technologies in Health. Retrieved from http://www.cadth.ca/media/pdf/ES_Ped_IV_Admin_es21_e.pdf

Manias, E., Kinney, S., Cranswick, N., & Williams, A. (2014). Medication errors in hospitalised children. *Journal of Paediatrics and Child Health, 50*(2014), 71–77. doi: 10.1111/jpc.12412

National Guideline Clearinghouse. (2012). *Best evidence statement (BESt). Confirmation of nasogastric tube placement in pediatric patients.* Retrieved from http://www.guideline.gov/content.aspx?id=35117

O'Grady, N. P., Alexander, M., Burns, L. A., Dellinger, E. P., Garland, J., Heard, S. O., et al. (2011). Guidelines for the prevention of intravascular catheter-related infections. *Clinical Infectious Diseases, 52*(1 May), e1–e32.

Pediatric Glaucoma & Cataract Family Association. (2013a). *How to apply eye drops.* Retrieved from http://pgcfa.org/?page_id=160

Pediatric Glaucoma & Cataract Family Association. (2013b). *How to apply eye ointment.* Retrieved from http://pgcfa.org/?page_id=155

Proehl, J. A., Heaton, K., Naccarato, M. K., Crowley, M. A., Storer, A., Moretz, J. D., et al. (2010). *Clinical practice guideline: Gastric tube placement verification: In patients having gastric tubes inserted in the emergency department setting, which bedside technique is best for confirmation of accurate placement immediately after tube insertion compared to x-ray?* Retrieved from http://www.ena.org/practice-research/research/CPG/Documents/GastricTubeCPG.pdf

Potts, A., Mayfield, A., Sinclair-Pingel, J., & Thompson, V. (2011). *Multidisciplinary review of the medication use system results in successful reduction of buretrol use in pediatric patients.* Poster presented at the 20th Annual Pediatric Pharmacy Advocacy Group Meeting Memphis, TN. Retrieved from http://www.mc.vanderbilt.edu/documents/evidencebasedpractice/images/PPAG%20Poster%20Presentations%20Buretrols%202011%20final%20alp.jpg

Steering Committee on Quality Improvement and Management and Committee on Hospital Care. (2011). Policy statement: Principles of pediatric patient safety: Reducing harm due to medical care. *Pediatrics, 127*(6), 1199–1210. doi: 10.1542/peds.2011–0967

The Joint Commission. (2008). *Sentinel event alert: Preventing pediatric medication errors, 39.* Retrieved from http://www.jointcommission.org/sentinel_event_alert_issue_39_preventing_pediatric_medication_errors/

The Joint Commission. (2013). Preventing central line–Associated bloodstream infections: Useful tools, an international perspective. Retrieved from http://www.jointcommission.org/Topics/Clabsi_toolkit.aspx

The Joint Commission. (2014). *Facts about the official "do not use" list.* Retrieved from http://www.jointcommission.org/assets/1/18/Do_Not_Use_List.pdf

U.S. Food and Drug Administration. (2011). *Drug research and children.* Retrieved from http://www.fda.gov/Drugs/ResourcesForYou/Consumers/ucm143565.htm

Walsh, K. E., Roblin, D. W., Weingart, S. N., Houlahan, K. E., Degar, B., Billett, A., et al. (2013). Medication errors in the home: A multisite study of children with cancer. *Pediatrics, 131*(5), e1405–e1414. doi: 10.1542/peds.2012–2434

Weinstein, S. M., & Hagle, M. E. (2014). *Plumer's principles & practice of infusion therapy* (9th ed.). Philadelphia, PA: Lippincott Williams & Wilkins.

Yin, H. S., Mendelsohn, A. L., Wolf, M. S., Parker, R. M., Fierman, A., van Schaick, L., et al. (2010). Parents' medication administration errors role of dosing instruments and health literacy. *Archives of Pediatrics & Adolescent Medicine, 164*(2), 181–186. doi: 10.1001/archpediatrics.2009.269

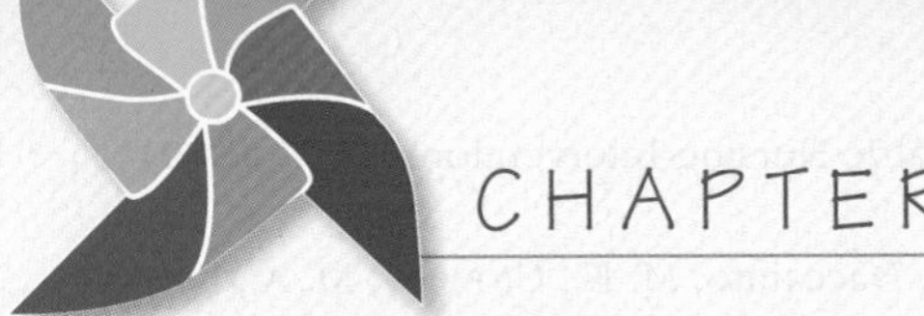

CHAPTER WORKSHEET

MULTIPLE CHOICE QUESTIONS

1. A 3-year-old child is to receive a medication that is supplied as an enteric-coated tablet. What is the best nursing action?
   a. Crush the tablet and mix it with apple sauce.
   b. Dissolve the medication in the child's milk.
   c. Place a pill in the posterior part of the pharynx and tell the child to swallow.
   d. Check with the prescriber to see if an alternative form can be used.

2. The nurse is caring for an infant who weighs 8.2 kg and is NPO and receiving IV fluid therapy. What rate does the nurse calculate as meeting the child's daily fluid requirements?
   a. 82 mL per hour
   b. 41 mL per hour
   c. 34 mL per hour
   d. 22 mL per hour

3. When administering ear drops to a 2-year-old, which action would be most appropriate?
   a. Tell the child that the drops are to treat his infection.
   b. Pull the pinna of the child's ear down and back.
   c. Have the child turn his head to the opposite side after giving the drops.
   d. Massage the child's forehead to facilitate absorption of the medication.

4. An infant is to receive intermittent gavage feedings via a nasogastric tube every 6 hours. The feeding tube was inserted with a previous feeding and remains in place. The nurse is preparing to administer the next scheduled feeding. Place the events in the proper sequence.
   a. Check the placement of the feeding tube.
   b. Position the infant on his right side with the head of the bed slightly elevated.
   c. Allow the feeding to come to room temperature.
   d. Flush the tube with water.
   e. Clamp the tube to prevent air from entering the stomach.
   f. Pour the solution into the barrel of the syringe.

CRITICAL THINKING EXERCISES

1. When reviewing the medical record of a child, the nurse notes that the ordered dose of medication is different from the recommended dose. How should the nurse proceed?
2. While caring for a 5-year-old child who is receiving IV fluid therapy at a rate of 100 mL per hour, the nurse notes that the infusion is running slowly. The insertion site appears slightly reddened and swollen. What should the nurse do next?
3. A school-aged child is to be discharged, continuing TPN therapy at home. The child lives with his parents and two younger siblings. How would the nurse prepare this child and family for discharge? How could the nurse promote growth and development for this child during TPN therapy?

STUDY ACTIVITIES

1. Review the medical records of several children who are on a pediatric unit in your agency. Note the type of medication, route ordered, and what specific interventions are needed for each child related to the medication administration and developmental age of the child, include atraumatic care interventions. Compile a list of the most commonly used routes.
2. Interview several parents about their experiences in giving medications to their children. From these interviews, develop a teaching sheet that provides tips to facilitate oral medication administration to children.
3. Create a chart that compares and contrasts the SQ, intramuscular, and IV methods of medication administration. Include examples of medications given via these routes, onset of action, appropriate sites, and necessary safety measures for each.

BRINGING IT ALL TOGETHER: A CASE STUDY

Fillipia, a 3-year-old, is admitted to your unit with fever and lethargy. She is 36 pounds and 101.6 cm (40 inches) tall. Her current temperature is 101.8 °F, HR 110, RR 22. Her orders include Rocephin 525 mg IM every 12 hours and acetaminophen 2 teaspoons PO every 4 hours as needed for temperature greater than 101.5 °F. The safe dose range for Rocephin is 50 to 75 mg/kg/day and acetaminophen is 15 mg/kg/dose. The concentration for Rocephin is 350 mg/mL and acetaminophen is 160 mg/5 mL.

Go to thePoint to find questions to consider about this case.

36

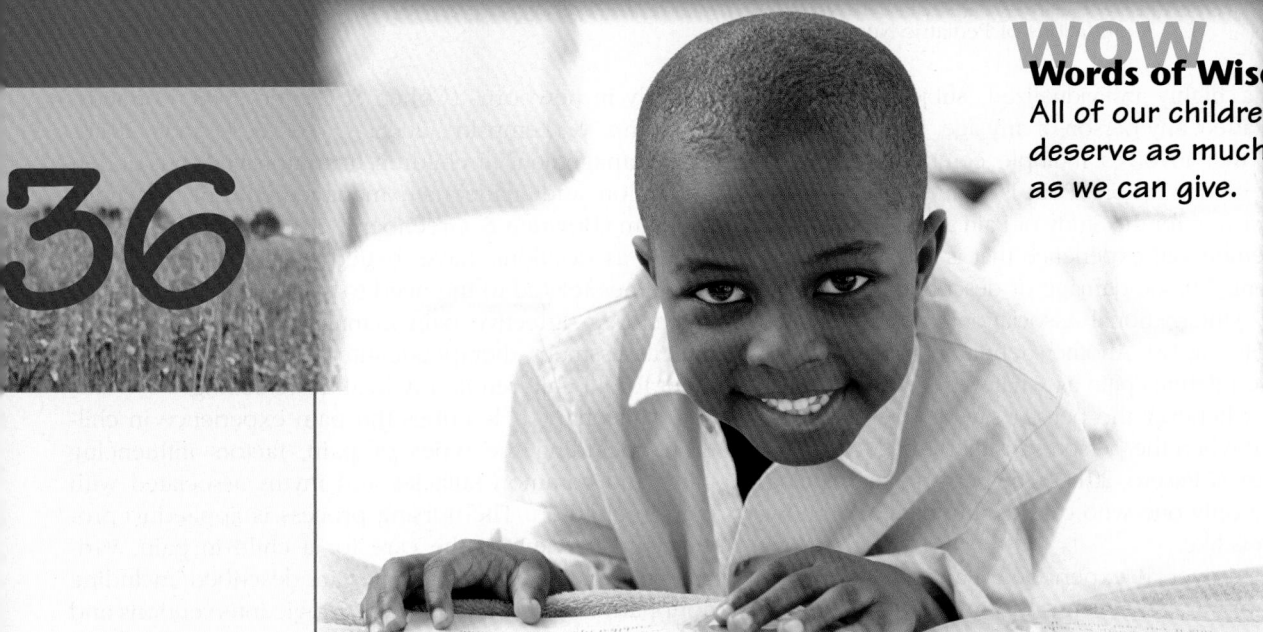

WOW

Words of Wisdom

All of our children in pain deserve as much comfort as we can give.

Pain Management in Children

KEY TERMS

acute pain
chronic pain
drug tolerance
epidural analgesia
moderate sedation
neuromodulators
neuropathic pain
nociceptive pain
nociceptors
pain
pain threshold
patient-controlled analgesia (PCA)
physical dependence
somatic pain
transduction
visceral pain

Learning Objectives

Upon completion of the chapter, you will be able to:

1. Identify the major physiologic events associated with the perception of pain.
2. Discuss the factors that influence the pain response.
3. Identify the developmental considerations of the effects and management of pain in the infant, toddler, preschooler, school-age child, and adolescent.
4. Explain the principles of pain assessment as they relate to children.
5. Understand the use of the various pain rating scales and physiologic monitoring for children.
6. Establish a nursing care plan for children related to management of pain, including pharmacologic and nonpharmacologic techniques and strategies.

Aiden Russell **is a 6-year-old on the pediatric unit admitted for a wound infection. He requires BID dressing changes. In report you are told that Aiden cries and fights during the dressing change but otherwise seems to be playing and not experiencing much pain. The nurse reporting off duty states, "Aiden's mother keeps requesting pain medication for Aiden. She states he's complaining of pain most of the time. I'm not sure if I believe her: when I see Aiden, he's playing Nintendo games or watching television and seems to be fine. I've tried to hold off on his pain medication as long as I can."**

Pain is a highly individualized, subjective experience that can affect any person of any age. It is a complex phenomenon that involves multiple components and is influenced by myriad factors. **Pain** is defined by the International Association for the Study of Pain as "an unpleasant sensory and emotional experience that is associated with actual or potential tissue damage or described in terms of such damage" (International Association for the Study of Pain, 2012;WHO, 2012). Another definition of pain that is commonly used defines pain as whatever the person says it is, existing whenever the person says it does—that is, pain is present when the person says that it is (McCaffery, 1968; McCaffery & Pasero, 2011). The person experiencing the pain is the only one who can identify pain and know what the pain is like.

Pain is a universal experience. Pain affects adults and children of all ages, even preterm infants. Pain can result from numerous causes, including disease processes, injuries, procedures, and surgical interventions. In 1995 the American Pain Society (1995) labeled it "the fifth vital sign." The American Pain Society's goal was to encourage healthcare professionals to assess pain every time that temperature, pulse, respirations, and blood pressure are assessed and to institute measures to manage the pain.

Unlike adults, however, children may lack the verbal capacity to describe their pain accurately. In addition, many caregivers and healthcare providers have misconceptions about pain in children, it is difficult to assess the complex nature of the pain experience, and limited resources and research are available related to pain relief strategies for children. Therefore, pain is a major source of distress for children and their families as well as for healthcare providers.

If left unmanaged, pain in children can lead to serious physical and emotional consequences, such as increased oxygen consumption and alterations in blood glucose metabolism. In addition, the experience of untreated pain early in life may lead to long-term physiologic and psychological consequences for the child (Bowden & Greenberg, 2011). For example, inadequately controlled pain can have long-lasting negative outcomes such as increased distress during later procedures, nonadherence to treatment regimens, inactivity, prolonged bed rest, and the development of chronic pain. Detrimental effects on the course of the disease itself may also be seen with untreated pain. Preterm infants, due to long hospitalizations and numerous painful and invasive procedures, are often at greater risk for experiencing memories of pain (American Academy of Pediatrics, 2010).

All these factors make pain management a critical element in the plan of care for children. Treating pain reduces anxiety during procedures and decreases the need for physical restraints, reduces anxiety regarding subsequent procedures, and prevents short- and long-term consequences of inadequately treated pain, particularly in newborns (Cohen & Baxter, 2008; Kennedy, Luhmann, & Zempsky, 2008; Oakes & D'Arcy, 2011). Pain management in children has improved, but underestimation and inadequate management still remain a problem (Bowden & Greenberg, 2011). Various national health associations have issued position papers and guidelines related to the need to treat pain and suffering in children. Effective pain management involves initial pain assessment, therapeutic interventions, and reassessment for all children in any healthcare setting.

This chapter describes the pain experience in children, including the types of pain, factors influencing pain, and common fallacies and myths associated with pain in children. The nursing process is applied to provide an overview of the care for a child in pain. Various pain management strategies are described, including nonpharmacologic and pharmacologic interventions and measures to address procedure-related and chronic pain.

PHYSIOLOGY OF PAIN

The sensation of pain is a complex phenomenon that involves a sequence of physiologic events in the nervous system. These events are transduction, transmission, perception, and modulation.

Transduction

Peripheral nerve fibers extend from the spinal cord to various locations in and throughout the body's tissues, such as skin, joints, bones, and membranes covering the internal organs. At the end of these fibers are specialized receptors, called **nociceptors**, which become activated when they are exposed to noxious stimuli. The noxious stimuli can be mechanical, chemical, or thermal. Mechanical stimuli may include intense pressure to an area, a strong muscular contraction, or extensive pressure due to muscular overstretching. Chemical stimulation may involve the release of mediators, such as histamine, prostaglandins, leukotrienes, or bradykinin, as a response to tissue trauma, ischemia, or inflammation. Thermal stimuli typically involve extremes of heat and cold. This process of nociceptor activation is called **transduction**.

Transmission

When nociceptors are activated by noxious stimuli, the stimuli are converted to electrical impulses that are relayed along the peripheral nerves to the spinal cord and brain. Specialized afferent nerve fibers are responsible for moving the electrical impulse along. Myelinated A-delta fibers are large fibers that conduct the impulse at very rapid rates. The pain transmitted by these fibers is often referred to as fast pain, most commonly associated with mechanical or thermal stimuli (Bautista & Grossman, 2014). Pain also is transmitted by unmyelinated small C fibers. These fibers transmit the impulse slowly and are often activated by chemical stimuli or continued mechanical or thermal stimuli (Bautista & Grossman, 2014). These fibers carry the impulse to the spinal cord via the dorsal horn. Neurotransmitters are released to facilitate the transmission process to the brain.

Several theories have been proposed in an attempt to explain the process of pain transmission. The best known of these is the gate-control theory. According to this theory, the dorsal horn of the spinal cord contains interneuronal or interconnecting fibers. Large-diameter faster fibers carry nonnociceptive, tactile information, while small nerve fibers carry nociceptive or pain signals. Large fibers, when stimulated, close the gate or pathway to the brain, thereby inhibiting or blocking the transmission of the pain impulse. Subsequently, the impulse does not reach the brain, where it would be interpreted as pain. It is now known that pain modulation is a more complex process but this theory helps explain why some nonpharmacologic therapies, such as massage and pressure, are effective in reducing pain (Bautista & Grossman, 2014).

Perception

Once in the dorsal horn of the spinal cord, the nerve fibers divide and then cross to the opposite side and rise upward to the thalamus. The thalamus responds quickly and sends a message to the somatosensory cortex of the brain, where the impulse is interpreted as the physical sensation of pain. The impulses carried by the fast A-delta fibers lead to the perception of sharp, stabbing localized pain that also commonly involves a reflex response to withdraw from the stimulus. The impulses carried by the slow C fibers lead to the perception of diffuse, dull, burning, or aching pain. The point at which the person first feels the lowest intensity of the painful stimulus is termed the **pain threshold**. In addition to sending a message to the cerebral cortex, the thalamus also sends a message to the limbic system, where the sensation is interpreted emotionally, and to the brain stem centers, where autonomic nervous system responses begin.

Modulation

Research has identified substances called **neuromodulators** that appear to modify the pain sensation. These substances have been found to change a person's perception of pain. Examples of these neuromodulators include serotonin, endorphins, enkephalins, and dynorphins.

Pain perception can be modified peripherally or centrally. In the peripheral nerve fibers, chemical substances are released that either stimulate the nerve fibers or sensitize them. Peripheral sensitization allows the nerve fibers to react to a stimulus that is of lower intensity than would be needed to cause pain. As a result, the person perceives more pain. Actions that block or inhibit

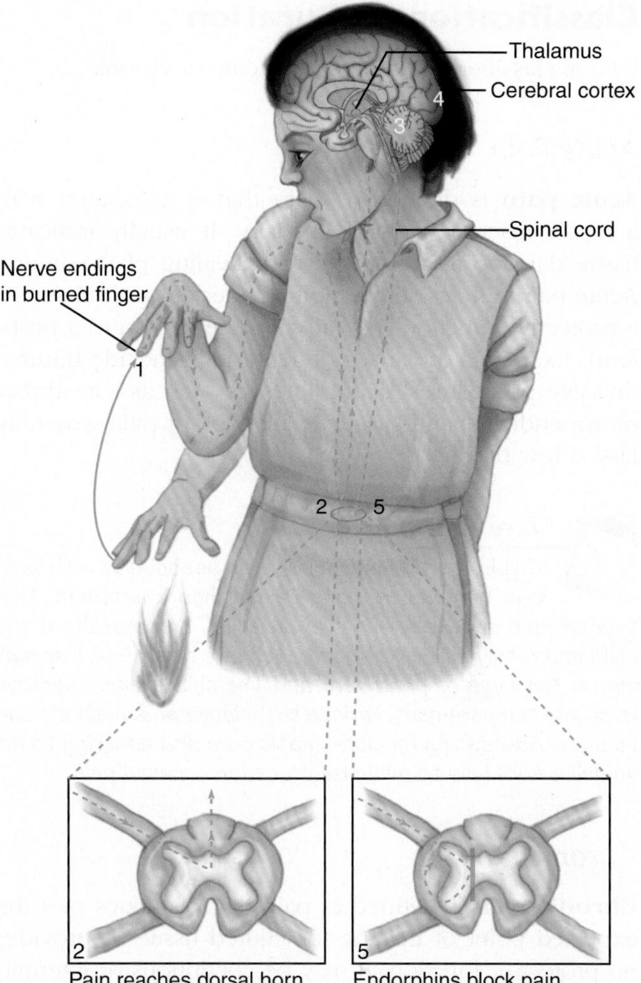

FIGURE 36.1 Physiology of pain. (*1*) Exposure to thermal noxious stimuli results in activation of nociception (transduction). (*2*) Impulses are relayed along the peripheral nerves to the spinal cord through the dorsal horn (transmission). (*3, 4*) This results in the individual feeling the sensation of pain (perception). (*5*) Neurons in the brain stem send signals back down to the dorsal horn, and these fibers release substances such as endorphins, which can inhibit painful impulses in the dorsal horn (modulation). These neurotransmitters are taken back by the body, therefore limiting the analgesic value.

the release of these substances can lead to a decrease in pain perception.

Modification of pain perception can occur centrally in the spinal cord at the dorsal horn. Substances released by the excited interneurons can potentiate the pain sensation. Other neurochemicals, through their binding to specific receptors, can inhibit the perception of pain. Figure 36.1 illustrates the physiology of pain.

TYPES OF PAIN

Many different systems can be used to classify pain. Most commonly, pain is classified based on its duration, etiology, or source or location.

Classification by Duration

Pain is classified by duration as acute or chronic.

Acute Pain

Acute pain is defined as pain that is associated with a rapid onset of varying intensity. It usually indicates tissue damage and resolves with healing of the injury. Acute pain reflects stimulation of nociceptors and serves a protective function (i.e., alerting the person to a problem). Examples of causes of acute pain include trauma, invasive procedures, acute illnesses such as sore throat or appendicitis, and surgery. This type of pain generally lasts a few days.

> *Take Note!*
>
> Children often experience pain associated with various procedures done in healthcare settings. This type of pain is usually short in duration. Preparation of the child and family will help to decrease fears or anxiety. Depending on the type of procedure and the child's age, cognitive level, and temperament, various techniques and methods can be used. Advocating for atraumatic care and adhering to its guidelines will help to minimize procedure-related pain.

Chronic Pain

Chronic pain is defined as pain that continues past the expected point of healing for injured tissue. It provides no protective function. It may be continuous or intermittent, with and without periods of exacerbation or remission. It often interferes with sleep and performance of activities of daily living. It can result in loss of appetite and depression. Thus, chronic pain impairs a person's ability to function. In contrast to acute pain, environmental and psychological factors influence behaviors associated with chronic pain. In children, chronic, recurrent pain is most commonly associated with abdominal pain, nonspecific headache, limb pain, or chest pain. Some conditions, such as sickle cell disease and migraines, have characteristics of both acute and chronic pain (Bautista & Grossman, 2014). Children with chronic pain may not exhibit the same physical or emotional responses as seen with acute pain. As pain becomes prolonged and continuous, the autonomic nervous system response tends to diminish.

Classification by Etiology

Pain can be classified by etiology as nociceptive or neuropathic.

Nociceptive Pain

Nociceptive pain reflects pain due to noxious stimuli that damages normal tissues or has the potential to do so if the pain is prolonged. The pain perceived often correlates closely with the degree or intensity of the stimulus and the extent of real or possible tissue damage. With nociceptive pain, nervous system functioning is intact. Reports of nociceptive pain vary depending on the location of the nociceptors being stimulated. Nociceptive pain ranges from sharp or burning, to dull, aching, or cramping, and to deep aching or sharp stabbing. Examples of conditions that result in nociceptive pain include chemical burns, sunburn, cuts, appendicitis, and bladder distention.

Neuropathic Pain

Neuropathic pain is pain due to malfunctioning of the peripheral or central nervous system. It may be continuous or intermittent and is commonly described as burning, tingling, shooting, squeezing, or spasm-like pain. Examples of neuropathic pain include posttraumatic and postsurgical peripheral nerve injuries, pain after spinal cord injury, metabolic neuropathies, phantom limb pain after amputation, and poststroke pain.

Classification by Source or Location

Pain also may be classified by the source or location of the area involved. It can be somatic pain (superficial and deep) or visceral pain. These classifications typically indicate nociceptive pain.

Somatic Pain

Somatic pain refers to pain that develops in the tissues. It can be further divided into two groups—superficial and deep. Superficial somatic pain, often called cutaneous pain, involves stimulation of nociceptors in the skin, subcutaneous tissue, or mucous membranes. Typically the pain is well localized and described as a sharp, pricking, or burning sensation. Superficial somatic pain may be due to external mechanical, chemical, or thermal injury or skin disorders. Tenderness commonly is present.

Deep somatic pain typically involves the muscles, tendons, joints, fasciae, and bones. It can be localized or diffuse and is usually described as dull, aching, or cramping. Deep somatic pain may be due to strain from overuse or direct injury, ischemia, and inflammation. Tenderness and reflex spasm may be present. In addition, the person may exhibit sympathetic nervous system activation such as tachycardia, hypertension, tachypnea, diaphoresis, pallor, and pupillary dilation.

Visceral Pain

Visceral pain is pain that develops within organs such as the heart, lungs, gastrointestinal tract, pancreas, liver, gallbladder, kidneys, or bladder. It is often produced by disease. It usually is diffuse and poorly localized and is described as a deep ache or sharp stabbing sensation that may be referred to other areas. Visceral pain may be due to distention of the organ, organ muscular spasm, contraction, pulling, ischemia, or inflammation. Tenderness, nausea, vomiting, and diaphoresis may be present.

FACTORS INFLUENCING PAIN

Children, like adults, experience neurologic events that result in the perception of pain. However, research has found that environmental and psychological factors may exert a greater influence on the child's perception of pain (McGrath, 2005). Certain factors such as age, gender, cognitive level, temperament, previous pain experiences, and family and cultural background cannot be changed. However, situational factors involving behavioral, cognitive, and emotional aspects can be modified. These situation-specific factors that affect the child's pain experience include "what the child and parents understand, what they and the healthcare staff do, and how the child and parents feel. Certain situational factors can intensify pain and distress, whereas others can eventually trigger pain episodes, prolong pain-related disability or maintain the repeated pain episodes in recurrent pain syndrome" (McGrath, 2005, p. 437).

Age and Gender

Research has demonstrated that the nervous system structures needed for pain impulse transmission and perception are present before birth (American Medical Association, 2013). Therefore, children of any age, including preterm newborns, are capable of experiencing pain. Early on, children can interpret pain as an unpleasant sensation, but this interpretation is based on their comparison with other sensations. As they get older, they learn to use words to describe their pain more fully.

Gender and sex also may play a role in a child's perception of pain, but most of the research has been performed on adults therefore whether it holds true for children is unclear (Oakes & D'Arcy, 2011). It has been suggested that boys and girls differ in how they perceive, experience, express, and cope with pain and respond to analgesics. This may be influenced by various factors including genetics, hormones, family, and culture. Further research is warranted in this area to allow for more focused care in pain management.

Cognitive Level

Cognitive level is a key factor affecting a child's pain perception and response and usually goes hand in hand with the child's age. Cognitive level typically increases with age, thereby influencing the child's understanding of the pain and its impact and his or her choices for coping strategies. In addition, as the child's cognitive level increases, his or her ability to communicate information about pain increases. However, this increased understanding and ability to communicate with advancing age may not apply to the child experiencing developmental delays. For example, a developmentally delayed school-age child or adolescent may have the cognitive level of a toddler or preschooler. Healthcare providers need to be cognizant of this difference when caring for the child in pain. Numerous research studies have revealed that young children often describe pain in concrete terms, whereas older children use more abstract terms that involve both physical and psychological components (McGrath, 2005).

Temperament

Literature suggests that temperament plays a role in predicting distress and pain levels in a child during painful events (Martin & Cohen, 2012). For example, a child with a "difficult temperament" is more likely to have an increased distress response to pain. Nurses can personalize interventions in the clinical environment and during the pain experience to better fit the child's temperament and other personality traits of the child and family.

Previous Pain Experiences

A child identifies pain based on his or her experiences with pain in the past. The number of episodes of pain, the type of pain, the severity or intensity of the previous pain experience, the effectiveness of treatment of pain, and how the child responded all affect how the child will perceive and respond to the current experience. Research suggests that severe pain experiences in the neonate or young infant can lead to sensory disturbances and altered pain responses lasting into adulthood (Hatfield, Chang, Bittle et al., 2011). Previous pain experiences with inadequate pain control may lead to increased distress during future painful procedures. For example, research studies have demonstrated that neonates who had undergone painful procedures such as circumcision and heel lancing showed a stronger negative response to routine immunizations and venipuncture weeks to months later (Oakes & D'Arcy, 2011).

Family and Culture

The child's cultural and family background will influence how he or she will express and manage pain. Some cultures transmit the standard of accepting pain stoically; others allow outward expression. The parents have a strong influence on the child's ability to cope. For example, if a parent reacts to the child's pain in a positive manner and offers comfort measures, the child may have an easier time coping. If the parent shows anger or disapproval, the pain experience may be intensified for the child.

Situational Factors

Situational factors involve factors or elements that interact with the child and his or her current situation involving the experience of pain. These factors are highly variable and dependent on the specific situation. Situational factors result from the context in which the child is experiencing pain and include cognitive, which is what the child understands and believes about the pain experience; behavioral, which is how the child and family react and what they do about the pain experience; and emotional, which is how the child and family feels about the pain experience (Oakes & D'Arcy, 2011). Due to children's limited experience with pain, situational factors may affect them more than adults (McGrath, 2005). A thorough pain assessment must include assessment for situational factors that may exacerbate pain. Examples of situational factors include:

- Child's lack of understanding of the source of pain
- Child's lack of ability to use coping mechanisms or pain-relieving strategies to decrease pain
- Stress and anxiety in anticipation of pain
- Child's lack of control of cause of pain
- Child's lack of ability to understand what to expect from potentially painful experiences
- Increased anxiety exhibited by the family
- Overly protective behaviors exhibited by the family
- Presence of emotions such as fear, anxiety, frustration, distress, underlying anxiety, and depression (McGrath, 2005; Oakes & D'Arcy, 2011)

DEVELOPMENTAL CONSIDERATIONS

Since children of various developmental ages respond differently to pain and perceive pain in different ways, it is important to review developmental considerations. Refer to Chapters 25 through 29 for a more complete understanding of childhood development. Nurses must understand how children of various ages respond to painful stimuli and what behaviors may be expected on the basis of their developmental level. By understanding these developmental considerations, the nurse can appropriately assess the child's pain and provide effective interventions.

Infants

Research has demonstrated that infants, including preterm infants, experience pain and can distinguish pain from other tactile experiences (American Medical Association, 2013). Much of this research focuses on pain related to invasive procedures, such as heel sticks and intravenous catheter insertion. Research suggests that neonates, especially preterm infants, actually experience pain at a greater intensity than older-age children and adults (American Medical Association, 2013). The belief is related to the immaturity of the inhibitory mechanisms that develop higher in the central nervous system at a later time during fetal development. These mechanisms are more complex and do not become functional until later in gestation.

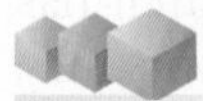 *Concept Mastery Alert*

Levels of Pain

When obtaining a blood sample with a heel stick, the nurse should remember that neonates, and in particular preterm infants, feel pain and feel it with greater intensity than older infants.

In preterm and term newborns, behavioral and physiologic indicators are used for determining pain. Behavioral indicators include facial expression, such as brow contracting and chin quivering; body movements; and crying (American Academy of Pediatrics, 2010). Physiologic signs include changes in heart rate, respiratory rate, blood pressure, oxygen saturation levels, intracranial pressure, vagal tone, palmar sweating, and an increase in plasma cortisol or catecholamine levels (American Academy of Pediatrics, 2010; Naughton & Ikuta, 2013).

In the younger infant, facial expression is the most common response to pain (Fig. 36.2). The brows may

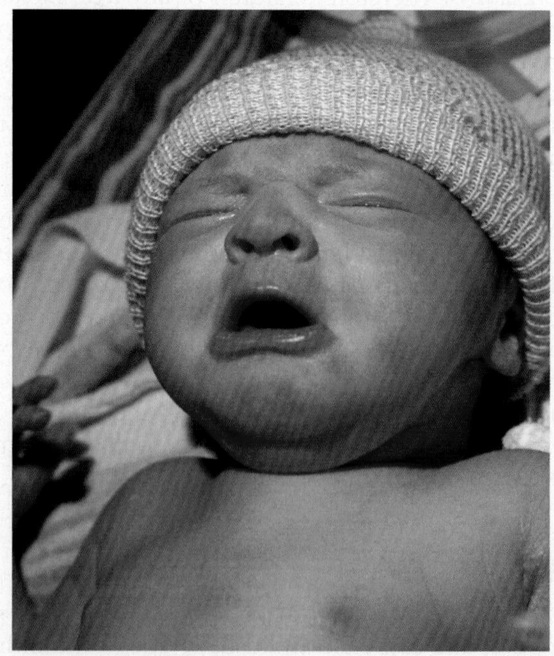

FIGURE 36.2 In the younger infant, facial expression is the most common response to pain.

be lowered and drawn together, with the eyes tightly closed. The mouth is open, often forming a square. The body may be stiff, and thrashing may be seen. When the area is stimulated, the infant may demonstrate a generalized reflex withdrawal. The infant may exhibit a high-pitched, shrill cry.

The older infant often displays similar behavioral manifestations of pain. The older infant may display an angry facial expression, but the eyes are open. He or she often demonstrates a definite withdrawal response when the area is stimulated. The older infant cries loudly and tries to push away the stimulus that is causing the pain. Other manifestations include irritability, restless sleeping, and poor feeding.

Take Note!

Although an infant usually exhibits typical behaviors indicating pain, absence of these manifestations does not indicate a lack of pain; the response to pain is highly variable (Weissman, Aranovitch, Blazer et al., 2009).

Infants also demonstrate physiologic responses to pain. These may include:

- Increased heart rate, usually averaging approximately 10 beats per minute; possibly bradycardia in preterm newborns
- Decreased vagal tone
- Decreased oxygen saturation
- Palmar or plantar sweating (as measured by skin conductivity testing); not reliable in infants before 37 weeks' gestation

Toddlers

Toddlers can react to painless procedures as intensely as painful ones, with intense emotional upset and physical resistance or aggression. They may bite, hit, scream, or kick. Other behaviors may include being very quiet, pointing to where it hurts, or saying such words as "owww." Facial grimacing and teeth clenching may be noted. They may also react with fear and try to hide or leave the room. They often have limited vocabularies, so it may be difficult for them to express pain. It is important to ask about and encourage the child to verbalize his or her pain. Ensure the use of words the toddler understands, such as "owie" or "boo-boo." Toddlers may demonstrate regressive behaviors, such as clinging to the parent or crying loudly.

Take Note!

Young children express pain by using simple words such as "hurt" or "ouchie" or by pointing to the area that hurts. By the age of 2 to 4 years they can express the presence of pain and by 5 years they can usually describe pain and its intensity (WHO, 2012).

Preschoolers

Preschoolers may become quiet or try to withdraw and hide in response to actual or perceived pain. For example, the child may say he or she needs to go to the bathroom or needs to get something from another room. Because of their magical type of thinking, preschoolers may believe pain is a punishment for misbehaving or having bad thoughts. Preschoolers may not verbally report their pain, thinking that pain is something to be expected or that the adults are aware of their pain. They can tell someone where it hurts and can use various tools to describe the severity of pain. However, because they may have limited experience with pain, they may have difficulty distinguishing between types of pain (sharp or dull), describing the intensity of the pain, and determining whether the pain is worse or better.

School-Age Children

School-age children can usually communicate the type, location, and severity of pain. Children older than the age of 8 years can use specific words, such as "sharp as a knife," "burning," or "pulling" to describe their pain. However, they may deny pain in an attempt to appear brave or to avoid further pain related to a procedure or intervention. They may be more concerned with their fear about the illness and its effects rather than the pain. They also may fear being embarrassed by acting-out behaviors in response to pain, such as screaming or thrashing. Thus, a typical response might be to withdraw by staring at the television. Other behaviors that may indicate pain in a school-age child include muscular rigidity, such as clenching the fists, stiffening the body, closing the eyes, wrinkling the forehead, or gritting the teeth.

Adolescents

Adolescents may be concerned primarily about body image and fear losing control over their behavior. This may result in denial or refusal of medications. Their mood and what they think is expected of them will also affect their response to pain. Adolescents often ask numerous questions and pay close attention to how others respond to them. Fearing that their behavior may be viewed as juvenile, they may attempt to remain stoic and not exhibit any emotion. Subtle changes such as increased muscle tension with clenched fists and teeth, rapid breathing, and guarding the affected body part may occur. They may also show lack of interest in everyday activities or a decreased ability to concentrate.

COMMON FALLACIES AND MYTHS ABOUT PAIN IN CHILDREN

In general, children respond to pain based on the type of pain, the extent of pain, and their age and developmental

TABLE 36.1 MYTHS AND MISCONCEPTIONS ABOUT CHILDREN AND PAIN

Myth or Misconception	Fact
Newborns do not feel pain	Newborns, including preterm newborns, do feel pain. The neurologic and hormonal systems needed for the transmission of painful stimuli are sufficiently developed
Exposure to pain at an early age has little to no effect on the child	Prolonged or severe pain can lead to increased newborn morbidity. Infants who have experienced pain during the neonatal period respond differently to subsequent painful events[a]
Infants and small children have little memory of pain	Repeated exposure to painful procedures and events can have long-term consequences Memories of pain may be stored in the child's nervous system, influencing later reactions to painful stimuli[a]
The intensity of a child's behavioral reaction indicates the intensity of the child's pain	Numerous factors affect a child's response to pain. Each child is an individual, with his or her own set of responses
A child who is sleeping or playing is not in pain	Sleep or play may be a coping strategy for the child in pain. Sleep may reflect exhaustion of the child who is coping with pain
Children are truthful when they are asked if they are experiencing pain	Often children deny pain to avoid a painful situation or procedure, embarrassment, or loss of control Children may assume that others know how they are feeling and thus will not verbalize their complaints
Children learn to adapt to pain and painful procedures	Repeated exposure to pain or painful procedures can result in an increase in behavioral manifestations
Children experience more adverse effects of narcotic analgesics than adults do	The risk of adverse effects of narcotic analgesics is the same for children as for adults
Children are more prone to addiction to narcotic analgesics	Addiction to narcotics when used appropriately to treat children's pain is very rare and no more common than in adults[b]

[a]Anand, K. J. S. (2013). Assessment of neonatal pain. UpToDate. Retrieved from http://www.uptodate.com/contents/assessment-of-neonatal-pain?source=search_result&search=neonatal+pain&selectedTitle=2~5#H12

[b]Finley, G. A., Franck, L. S., Grunau, R. E., & von Baeyer, C. L. (2005). Why children's pain matters. International Association for the Study of Pain. Pain: Clinical updates, XIII(4), 1–6. Retrieved from http://iasp.files.cms-plus.com/Content/ContentFolders/Publications2/PainClinicalUpdates/Archives/PCU05–4_1390264071339_24.pdf

Adapted from The Hospital for Sick Children. (2005). *Myths vs facts of children's pain.* Retrieved from http://www.iasp-pain.org/files/Content/ContentFolders/GlobalYearAgainstPain2/20052006PaininChildren/pdfist.pdf; Pawar, D., & Garten, L. (2010). Chapter 34: Pain management in children. In A. Kopf & N. B. Patel (Eds.), *Guide to pain management in low-resource settings* (pp. 255–268). Seattle: International Association for the Study of Pain.

level. Table 36.1 highlights some common myths and misconceptions related to pain in children. Because of these myths, children have been medicated less than adults with a similar diagnosis, leading to inadequate pain management.

NURSING PROCESS OVERVIEW FOR THE CHILD IN PAIN

Nursing care of the child with pain includes nursing assessment, nursing diagnosis, planning, interventions, and evaluation. Each step of this process must be individualized for each child. A general understanding of the physiology of pain, factors that influence pain, and effective pain management techniques can help to individualize the child's plan of care.

Assessment

Assessment of pain in children consists of both subjective and objective data collection. The acronym **QUESTT** is an excellent way to remember the key principles of pain assessment (Baker & Wong, 1987):

- **Q**uestion the child.
- **U**se a reliable and valid pain scale.
- **E**valuate the child's behavior and physiologic changes to establish a baseline and determine the effectiveness of the intervention. The child's behavior and

motor activity may include irritability and protection as well as withdrawal of the affected painful area.

- **S**ecure the parent's involvement.
- **T**ake the cause of pain into account when intervening.
- **T**ake action.

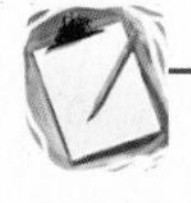

Take Note!

Children do experience pain! Pain management techniques work just as well with children as they do with adults.

Health History

When assessing pain in children, tailor the assessment to the child's developmental level and ask questions geared to the child's cognitive ability. During the health history, determine the child's previous exposure to pain, if any, and how the child responded. This information will provide clues about how the child copes and his or her current response. Attempt to determine what word the child uses to denote pain. Some children may not understand the term "pain" but do understand terms such as "ouchie" or "boo-boo."

The health history also includes questioning the parents about their cultural beliefs related to pain and their child's usual responses. This information aids in planning developmentally and culturally appropriate family-centered care.

QUESTIONING THE CHILD

When questioning the child, phrase the questions in a manner that the child will be able to understand based on his or her developmental level. Some input from the child's family may be helpful in determining where best to focus the questions.

Ask the child what pain means to him or her. Use words that the child may comprehend more easily, such as "hurt," "boo-boo," or "ouch," as appropriate. Inquire about similar experiences in the past and how he or she responded. Determine whether the child let others know that he or she was hurting and how this message was conveyed (e.g., crying, acting out, or pointing to the hurting area).

Review the history of the pain and various influences such as cultural aspects, caregiver attitudes or expectations, previous experiences, and any education or teaching related to pain management. Continue to formulate questions to ascertain the following:

- Location, quality, severity, and onset of the pain, as well as the circumstances in which the child experiences the pain. Have the child point to the area where it hurts or identify the location on a diagram or doll.
- Conditions, if any, that preceded the onset of pain and the conditions that followed the onset of pain.
- Any associated symptoms, such as weight loss, fever, vomiting, or diarrhea, which may indicate a current illness.
- Any recent trauma, including any interventions that were used in an attempt to relieve the pain.

Continue the health history by inquiring about what the child wants others, including the nurse, to do when the child hurts. Conversely, ask the child what he or she doesn't want others to do. Finally, question the child about measures that seem to be most effective in relieving the pain. Ask if there is anything special the child wants to tell the nurse, such as a special pain relief technique or a specific comfort object.

If the child is experiencing chronic or recurrent pain, suggest the child and family record information in a symptom diary. Explain that this will be helpful in identifying the best ways to manage the pain.

QUESTIONING THE PARENTS

Parents play a key role in assessing pain in children. Often it is the parents who provide information about the child's current and past experiences with pain. In addition, parents can provide information about how the child exhibits and responds to pain. Parents may be aware of subtle changes in the child's behavior that may precede the pain, occur with the pain, or indicate relief of pain. Including the parents in this process helps create a positive experience for all involved and promotes feelings of control over the situation.

The questions posed to the parents are similar in focus to those posed to the child. However, more detailed information may be obtained from the parents because they are usually able to describe events more fully or in greater detail due to their higher cognitive level. Parents typically know their child best.

Take Note!

Parents may assume that nurses have greater expertise when it comes to assessing their child's pain and taking appropriate action. Thus, they may not always report when they notice changes suggesting that their child is uncomfortable. Emphasize the important role that parents play in reporting any changes in their child so that pain relief measures can be instituted as soon as possible.

When questioning the parents, use the following examples as a guide for assessing the child's pain:

- Has your child ever been in pain before? If so, what was the cause of the pain? How long did he or she have the pain? Where was the pain located?
- How did your child react to the pain? What did you do to lessen the pain?
- Did your child let you know that he or she was in pain? Did he or she tell you or did you notice something?

- Are there any special signs that let you know that your child is hurting? If so, what are they?
- Is there anything that your child does or that you do when he or she is hurting that helps relieve the pain?
- Does one thing work better than another when your child is hurting?
- Is there any special information that you want to tell me about your child?

USING PAIN RATING SCALES

Various pain assessment, or pain rating, scales are available. These scales allow the child to report his or her pain, and the pain level is quantified. These standardized rating scales provide a greater alignment between the child's pain and the nurse's assessment of the severity of the pain. Self-report is the primary source for the measurement of pain in children (von Baeyer, 2014). Self-report measures should be used in conjunction with observation and discussion with the child and family, especially in children younger than age 5 or in children with cognitive impairments (American Academy of Pediatrics and the American Pain Society, 2001; von Baeyer, 2014). Some studies have found validity in self-report tools used in children as young as 3 years of age, while others have found inconsistent findings when they are used in children younger than 5 years of age (Besenski, Forsyth, & von Baeyer, 2007; Oakes & D'Arcy, 2011). Therefore, it is important to assess young children's ability to perform self-report tasks rather than rely solely on their chronological age (Besenski et al., 2007).

Many healthcare facilities have specific policies and procedures related to pain assessment, including the frequency of assessment, the rating tool to use, and nursing interventions to be instituted on the basis of the rating. For example, many facilities require assessment of the child using a specific tool with documentation at least once a shift and 30 minutes to 1 hour after a nonpharmacologic or pharmacologic pain relief intervention. This process provides a more objective method to determine whether the pain is increasing or decreasing and whether pain relief methods are effective.

Take Note!

Typically, different pain rating scales are appropriate for different developmental levels. However, children may regress when in pain, so a simpler tool may be needed to make sure that the child understands what is being asked. Regardless of the tool used, nurses need to be consistent in using the same tool so that appropriate comparisons can be made and effective interventions can be planned and implemented. Using the most appropriate tool consistently allows the most accurate assessment of the child's pain.

FACES Pain Rating Scale. The FACES pain rating scale (Fig. 36.3) is a self-report tool that can be used by children as young as 3 or 4 years of age (Oakes & D'Arcy, 2011). The scale consists of six illustrations of faces arranged horizontally with expressions ranging from smiling (indicating no hurt) to crying with frowning (indicating hurts worst). Under each face is a short description such as "hurts little bit" and a number. The number scale can be 0, 1, 2, 3, 4, and 5 or 0, 2, 4, 6, 8, and 10. The nurse explains the words associated with each face to the child. Then the nurse asks the child to select the facial expression that best describes the level of pain he or she is feeling. The nurse then documents the number corresponding to the word description and face.

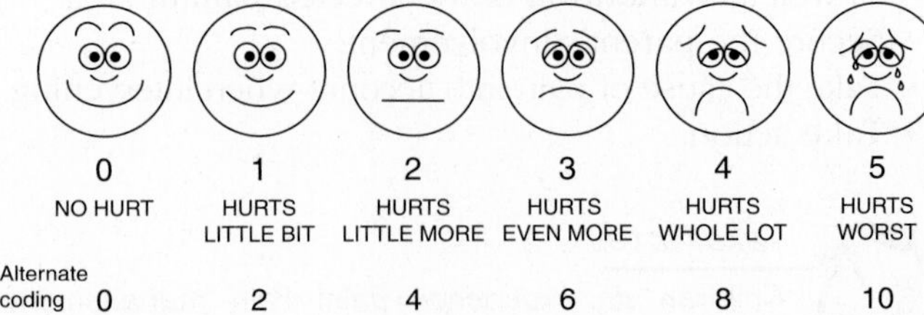

Instructions: Explain to the person that each face is for a person who feels happy because he has no pain (hurt) or sad because he has some or a lot of pain. **Face 0** is very happy because he doesn't hurt at all. **Face 1** hurts just a little bit. **Face 2** hurts a little more. **Face 3** hurts even more. **Face 4** hurts a whole lot. **Face 5** hurts as much as you can imagine, although you don't have to be crying to feel this bad. Ask the person to choose the face that best describes how he is feeling.

FIGURE 36.3 FACES pain rating scale. (From Hockenberry, M. J., & Wilson, D. [2009]. *Wong's essentials of pediatric nursing* [8th ed., p. 162]. St. Louis, MO. Used with permission. Copyright, Mosby.)

Oucher Pain Rating Scale. The Oucher pain rating scale is similar to the FACES scale in that it uses facial expressions to indicate increasing degrees of hurt. However, instead of illustrations, six photographs are used: "no hurt" is placed at the bottom of the arrangement and "most hurt" at the top. Alongside the photos is a scale ranging from 0 to 10 that corresponds to the facial expressions in the photographs (Fig. 36.4). After explaining the photos and numeric scale, the child is asked to point to the number that best describes his or her level of pain (Beyer, Denyes, & Villarruel, 1992).

This scale is useful for self-reporting of pain in children between 3 and 12 years of age (Oakes & D'Arcy, 2011). Different ethnicity versions have been developed for use with Caucasian, Hispanic, Asian, and African American children (Oakes & D'Arcy, 2011).

Poker Chip Tool. The poker chip tool, also known as the pieces of hurt tool, is a self-reporting pain assessment tool that uses four red poker chips to quantify the child's level of pain (American Medical Association,

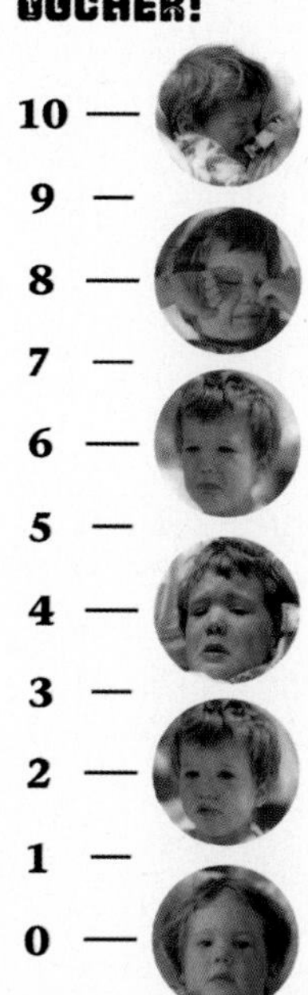

FIGURE 36.4 Oucher pain rating scale. (Used with permission from Beyer, J. E., Denyes, M. J., & Villarruel, A. M. [1992]. The creation, validation, and continuing development of the Oucher: A measure of pain intensity in children. *Journal of Pediatric Nursing, 7*[5], 335–346.)

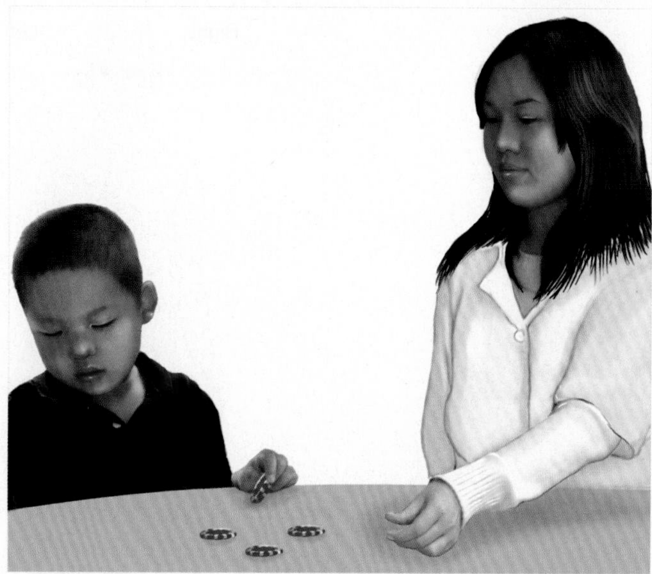

FIGURE 36.5 The poker chip tool. Here the nurse asks the child to identify the number of chips that indicate his degree of "hurt."

2013). The chips are arranged in a horizontal line on a surface in front of the child. Starting with the chip closest to the child's left side, the nurse points to the chip and explains that the first chip means a little hurt, the next chip means more hurt, the third chip means more hurt, and the fourth chip means the worst hurt ever. Then the nurse asks the child how many "pieces of hurt" he or she is having (Fig. 36.5). If the child is not experiencing any pain, typically the child will state that he or she isn't having any. When the child identifies the number of "pieces of hurt," the nurse follows up by asking the child to tell the nurse more about his or her hurt (Hester, 1979).

The poker chip tool is useful for assessing pain in children 4 to 7 years of age (Society of Pediatric Psychology, 2014). Children may view this assessment tool as a game since it involves poker chips. However, the nurse needs to ensure that the child has the cognitive ability to distinguish the numbers.

Take Note!

Toddlers and preschoolers may not be used to being asked questions by strangers, and may not understand quantitative ratings or estimation. Preschoolers will often construct an answer even if they do not understand the question. They also will often use extremes of scales, such as no pain or the worst pain (von Baeyer, 2006).

Visual Analog and Numeric Scales. Visual analog and numeric scales involve a horizontal or vertical line with marked endpoints. With a visual analog scale, the endpoints are identified as no pain and worst pain. A numeric scale typically has endpoints of 0 and 10, reflecting no pain and worst pain, respectively (Fig. 36.6). The nurse explains the scale to the child. With the visual analog scale, the child makes a line that best describes the level of pain. The nurse then measures the distance from the "no pain" endpoint to the child's mark and records this as the pain score. With the numeric scale, the nurse asks the child to pick the number that best describes his or her level of pain.

The visual analog scale can be used in children 8 years or older but some studies report effectiveness in children 5 to 7 years of age (von Baeyer, 2014). The numeric scale can be used with children 8 years or older (von Baeyer, 2014). Even though a younger child

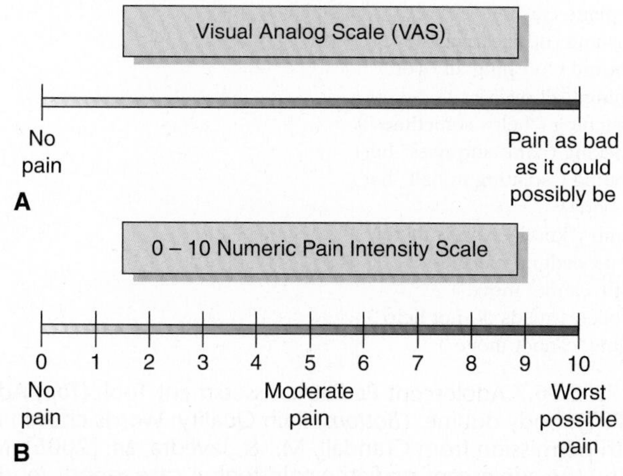

FIGURE 36.6 **(A)** Visual analog scale. **(B)** Numeric scale.

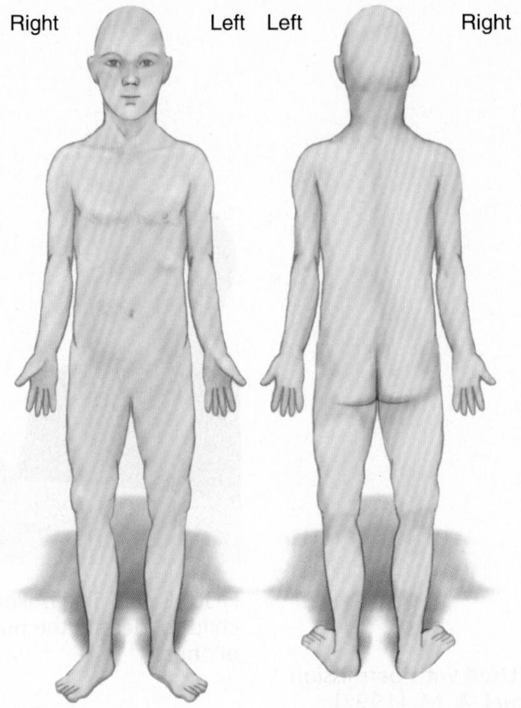

Sensory	Affective	Evaluative	Temporal
Aching ("pain all over")	Awful ("cannot do anything")	Annoying ("cannot sleep")	Always ("pain always there")
Hurting ("pain all over")	Crying ("hurts so bad")	Bad ("cannot stop the hurting")	Comes and goes ("always pain")
Sore ("like a cut")	Frightening ("scared it won't stop")	Miserable ("cannot sleep or do stuff")	Comes on all of a sudden ("no warning")
Beating (procedural pain "spots")	Screaming (afraid of "going to the hospital")	Terrible ("don't like it")	Constant ("never goes away")
Pounding ("gets on your nerves")	Terrifying ("cannot sleep," "really tired," "not going to live")	Uncomfortable ("can't stay in one spot")	Continuous ("pain not going away")
Cutting ("hurts more than a cut")		Uncontrollable ("cannot stop it")	Forever ("never will go away")
Like a sharp knife ("stabbing and sharp")	Dizzy ("don't know where I am")		Once in a while ("in a month sometimes pain; sometimes not")
Sharp (no meaning)			Sneaks up ("don't know when the pain will happen")
Stabbing (no meaning)			Sometimes ("goes away sometimes; sometimes not")
Cramping ("everywhere like a plane crash")			
Crushing (no meaning)			
Pressure ("pushing all over")			
Itching ("all over")			
Scratching ("helps sometimes")			
Shocking (pain "surprises" her)			
Splitting ("splitting in half" her body)			
Numb ("knows pain is there"/ procedural pain)			
Stiff ("cannot move")			
Swollen ("meds do not help")			
Tight ("cannot move")			

FIGURE 36.7 Adolescent Pediatric Assessment Tool. (*Top*) Adolescent Pediatric Pain Tool (APPT): body outline. (*Bottom*) Pain Quality: Words chosen and meaning of words. (Used with permission from Crandall, M., & Savedra, M. [2005]. Multidimensional assessment using the adolescent pediatric pain tool: A case report. *Journal for Specialists in Pediatric Nursing, 10*(3), 115–123.)

may be able to count and give numbers on the scale, they have not yet developed an understanding of the quantitative significance of the numbers.

Adolescent Pediatric Pain Tool. The Adolescent Pediatric Pain Tool is a multidimensional self-report type of tool useful for older children, usually between 8 and 17 years of age (Oakes & D'Arcy, 2011). The tool involves three aspects of assessment. In the first assessment the child identifies the location of the pain on two illustrations of the body—front and back views (Fig. 36.7).

The child is instructed to color the areas where he or she is hurting. The child is also instructed to color the area as big or as small as how much he or she is hurting. For example, if the hurt is mild or moderate, the child would color a moderate area of the location; if the pain is severe, he or she would color a much larger area. The second portion of the tool involves a scale that ranges from "no pain" to "worst possible pain." The nurse instructs the child to identify the severity of his or her pain. The third assessment is a list of words that may be used to describe pain, such as throbbing, pounding, stabbing, or sharp. The nurse asks the child to point to or circle the words that describe the current pain. Children with limited reading skills or vocabulary may have difficulty with some of the words listed to describe pain. Work with the child and encourage the parents to help the child understand the various descriptive words. Parental participation fosters control over the situation and gives the parents some insight into what their child is experiencing (Crandall & Savedra, 2005).

Thinking About Development

Kaylee Cooper is a 4-year-old female with a fractured femur. She has been in traction since arriving in the emergency room last night. When you enter her room at the beginning of your shift you note she is quiet and withdrawn. How will Kaylee's developmental stage affect the use of self-report? What special considerations must the nurse think about when using self-report of pain with Kaylee? What is the most appropriate pain rating scale to be used for Kaylee?

Physical Examination

Physical examination of the child for pain primarily involves the skills of observation and inspection. These skills are used to assess for physiologic and behavioral changes that indicate pain. Auscultation also may be used to assess for changes in vital signs, specifically heart rate and blood pressure.

OBSERVE FOR MANIFESTATIONS OF PAIN

Observe for physical signs and symptoms of pain, keeping in mind the child's developmental level. Look for facial expressions of discomfort, grimacing, or crying. Be alert for movements that may suggest pain. For example, an infant or toddler may pull on the ear when experiencing ear pain. The child may move the head from side to side, suggesting head pain. Typically, children with abdominal pain will lie on one side and draw their knees up to the abdomen. Inspect the child's gait: a limp or avoidance of weight bearing may suggest leg pain. Immobility, guarding of a particular body area, or refusal to move an area may be observed. Inspect the skin for flushing or diaphoresis, possible indicators of pain. Also monitor vital signs for changes. Pulse or heart rate, respiratory rate, and blood pressure may increase. Other physiologic parameters that suggest pain may include elevated intracranial pressure and pulmonary vascular resistance and decreased oxygen saturation levels.

Take Note!

The body responds to acute pain via the sympathetic nervous system, leading to stimulation and a subsequent increase in vital signs. However, if the child has persistent or chronic pain, the body adapts and these changes may be less noticeable (Oakes & D'Arcy, 2011).

The child also may exhibit behavioral changes indicating pain. Be alert for irritability and restlessness. Watch for clenching of teeth or fists, body stiffening, or increased muscle tension. Note any changes in the child's behavior. For example, a child who previously was talkative and playful may become quiet and almost withdrawn in response to pain. Remember, a child in pain may sleep or play in order to cope with the pain. In addition, pay close attention to the child's cultural background and how these beliefs may be affecting the behavioral response to pain.

Each child is an individual with unique responses to pain, so the nurse must ensure that observations of behavior do indeed reflect the child's pain level. To help ensure the accuracy of observations, several physiologic and behavioral assessment tools have been developed to help quantify the observations.

USING PHYSIOLOGIC AND BEHAVIORAL PAIN ASSESSMENT TOOLS

Use of physiologic and behavioral pain assessment tools allows measurement of specific parameters and changes that would indicate that the child is experiencing pain. These measurements aid in determining the intensity of the pain experience. Along with the self-report pain rating scales, measurement of these changes allows the nurse to objectively assess pain and the effectiveness of pain management measures.

TABLE 36.2 THE NEONATAL INFANT PAIN SCALE (NIPS)

Parameter	Finding	Score
Facial expression	Relaxed (restful face; neutral expression) Grimace (tight facial muscles; furrowed brow, chin, or jaw; negative facial expression)	0 1
Cry	No cry (quiet; not crying) Whimper (mild intermittent moaning) Vigorous crying (loud screaming, shrill, continuous)	0 1 2
Breathing patterns	Relaxed Change in breathing (irregular; faster than usual; gagging; breath holding)	0 1
Arms	Relaxed (no muscular rigidity; occasional random movements of arm) Flexed/extended (tense, straight, rigid, or rapid flexion or extension)	0 1
Legs	Relaxed (no muscular rigidity; occasional random movements of leg) Flexed/extended (tense, straight, rigid, or rapid flexion or extension)	0 1
State of arousal	Sleeping/awake (quiet, peaceful; settled) Fussy (alert, restless, thrashing)	0 1

Reproduced with permission from Lawrence, J., Alcock, D., MacGrath, P., Kay, J., MacMurray, S. B., & Dulberg, C. (1993). The development of a tool to assess neonatal pain. *Neonatal Network*, *12*(6), 59–66. Copyright © 1993 Springer Publishing Company, LLC.

Neonatal Infant Pain Scale. The Neonatal Infant Pain Scale (NIPS) is a behavioral assessment tool that is useful for measuring pain in preterm and full-term neonates (Lawrence et al., 1993). Six parameters are measured: facial expression, cry, breathing patterns, arms, legs, and state of arousal (Table 36.2). Each parameter except for cry is scored as 0 or 1; cry is scored as 0, 1, or 2. The scores are then totaled and the maximum score that can be achieved is 7. A higher score indicates increased pain. This scale does not include any physiologic parameters; therefore, it may not detect early pain in neonates who are too ill to respond, who are receiving paralyzing agents, or who are premature (Anand, 2013). In these cases, a falsely low score may be produced.

Riley Infant Pain Scale. The Riley Infant Pain Scale (RIPS) is a behavioral assessment tool useful for infants who lack verbal ability (Schade, Joyce, Gerkensmeyer et al., 1996). Like NIPS, RIPS measures six parameters: facial expression, body movement, sleep, verbal or vocal ability, consolability, and response to movements and touch (Table 36.3). Each parameter is scored as 0, 1, 2, or 3. The score is then totaled and the maximum score that can be achieved is 18. The higher the total score, the more intense the pain.

Pain Observation Scale for Young Children. The Pain Observation Scale for Young Children (POCIS) is a behavioral assessment tool designed for use in children between 1 and 4 years of age (Boelen-van der Loo, Scheffer, de Haan et al., 1999). This tool measures seven parameters: facial expression, cry, breathing, torso, arms and fingers, legs and toes, and state of arousal (Table 36.4). Each parameter is scored as 0 or 1; the maximum score achievable is 7. The higher the score, the greater the pain being experienced by the child.

CRIES Scale for Neonatal Postoperative Pain Assessment. The CRIES scale is a behavioral assessment tool that also includes measures of physiologic parameters (Krechel & Bildner, 1995). It was developed to quantify postoperative pain in the newborn. The tool also may be used to monitor the infant's progress over time during recovery or after interventions. The tool assesses five parameters: cry, oxygen required for saturation levels less than 95%, increased vital signs, facial expression, and sleeplessness (Table 36.5). Each parameter is scored as 0, 1, or 2 and then totaled. As with other assessment tools, the higher the score, the greater the infant's pain.

r-FLACC Behavioral Scale for Pain in Nonverbal Young Children and Children with Cognitive Impairment. The original FLACC behavioral scale is a behavioral assessment tool that is useful in assessing a child's pain when the child cannot report accurately his or her level of pain (Merkel, Voepel-Lewis, Shayevitz et al., 1997). It has been demonstrated to be a reliable tool for children from age 2 months to 7 years of age (Oakes & D'Arcy, 2011). This tool measures five parameters: facial expression, legs, activity, cry, and consolability

TABLE 36.3 THE RILEY INFANT PAIN SCALE

Parameter	Score
Facial expression	
• Neutral/smiling	0
• Frowning/grimacing	1
• Clenched teeth	2
• Full cry expression	3
Body movement	
• Calm, relaxed	0
• Restless, fidgeting	1
• Moderate agitation or mobility; thrashing, flailing, incessant agitation or strong voluntary mobility	2
• Voluntary immobility	3
Sleep	
• Sleeping quietly with easy respirations	0
• Restless while asleep	1
• Sleeping intermittently (sleep/awake)	2
• Sleeping for prolonged periods of time interrupted by jerky movements or inability to sleep	3
Verbal/vocal	
• No cry	0
• Whimpering, complaining	1
• Pain crying	2
• Screaming, high-pitched cry	3
Consolability	
• Neutral	0
• Easy to console	1
• Not easy to console	2
• Inconsolable	3
Response to movement/touch	
• Moves easily	0
• Winces when touched or moved	1
• Cries out when moved or touched	2
• High-pitched cry or scream when touched or moved	3

Used with permission from Schade, J. G., Joyce, B. A., Gerkensmeyer, J., & Keck, J. F. (1996). Comparison of three preverbal scales for postoperative pain assessment in a diverse pediatric sample. *Journal of Pain and Symptom Management*, *12*(6), 348–359.

TABLE 36.4 THE PAIN OBSERVATION SCALE FOR YOUNG CHILDREN (POCIS)

Parameter	Finding	Score
Facial expression	Neutral	0
	Grimace (negative)	1
Cry	No cry	0
	Moan, scream	1
Breathing	Relaxed and regular	0
	Irregular and indrawn	1
Torso	At rest, inactive	0
	Tense, shivering	1
Arms and fingers	At rest, inactive	0
	Tense, restless	1
Legs and toes	At rest, inactive	0
	Tense, restless	1
State of arousal	Calm, sleepy	0
	Fussy	1

Used with permission from Boelen-van der Loo, W. J. C., Scheffer, E., de Haan, R. J., & de Groot, C. J. (1999). Clinimetric evaluation of the pain observation scale for young children in children aged between 1 and 4 years after ear, nose, and throat surgery. *Developmental and Behavioral Pediatrics*, *20*(4), 222–227.

(Table 36.6). Observe the child with the legs and body uncovered. If the child is awake, observe him or her for 1 to 2 minutes; if sleeping, observe the child for 2 minutes or longer. Each parameter is scored as 0, 1, or 2. The scores are totaled, with a maximum achievable score of 10. As with other assessment tools, the higher the score, the greater the pain.

The revised FLACC (r-FLACC) is used in the same manner as the original FLACC but it includes additional descriptors of behaviors most commonly associated with pain that have been validated in children with cognitive impairment (Hauer & Jones, 2014). Refer to Table 36.6. Pain assessment tools are a supplement to pain assessment and are not meant to replace caregiver/parent input. Review the descriptor terms with parents/caregivers and individualize the scale by adding pain-related behaviors that are specific indicators of pain observed in their child in the appropriate categories (Hauer & Jones, 2014).

Nursing Diagnoses, Goals, Interventions, and Evaluation

After assessing the child, the nurse identifies appropriate nursing diagnoses. The most commonly identified nursing diagnosis would be acute or chronic pain. However, the related factors and defining characteristics can vary widely. Nursing diagnoses will focus on the effects of pain on the child, for example, the stress incurred as a result of the pain or the fear or anxiety associated with the pain or events causing the pain. Moreover, pain can affect physiologic functions, such as sleep, nutrition, mobility, and elimination. Examples of common nursing diagnoses may include:

- Acute pain related to repeated need for invasive procedures, surgical experience, recent trauma, or infection
- Chronic pain related to prolonged illness or injury, effects of cancer on surrounding tissues, or treatment-related effects

TABLE 36.5 THE CRIES SCALE FOR NEONATAL POSTOPERATIVE PAIN ASSESSMENT

Assessment	0	1	2
Crying	No	High-pitched, but consolable	High-pitched, inconsolable
Oxygen required for saturation above 95%	No	<30%	>30%
Increased vital signs	Heart rate and blood pressure within 10% of preoperative values	Heart rate or blood pressure 11–20% higher than preoperative values	Heart rate or blood pressure 21% or more above preoperative values
Expression	No grimace	Grimace	Grimace with grunt
Sleepless	No	Waking at frequent intervals	Constantly awake
Total infant score			

Used with permission from Krechel, S. W., & Bildner, J. (1995). CRIES: A new neonatal postoperative pain measurement score. Initial testing of validity and reliability. *Paediatric Anaesthesia*, *5*, 53–61.

- Fear related to the unknown, separation from family, anticipation of invasive procedures, or effects of treatment
- Anxiety related to the stress and uncertainty of the situation
- Deficient knowledge related to current condition and appropriate methods for managing pain
- Sleep deprivation related to inability to manage pain effectively
- Impaired mobility related to increased episodes of pain

TABLE 36.6 FLACC BEHAVIORAL SCALE

	Scoring		
Category	***0***	***1***	***2***
Face	No particular expression or smile	Occasional grimace or frown, withdrawn, disinterested; **appears sad or worried**[a]	Frequent to constant frown, clenched jaw, quivering chin; **distress-looking face: expression of fright or panic**[a]
Legs	Normal position or relaxed	Uneasy, restless, tense; **occasional tremors**[a]	Kicking, or legs drawn up; **marked increase in spasticity, constant tremors or jerking**[a]
Activity	Lying quietly, normal position, moves easily	Squirming, shifting back and forth, tense; **mildly agitated (e.g., head back and forth, aggression); shallow, splinting respirations intermittent sighs**[a]	Arched, rigid, or jerking; **severe agitation, head banging, shivering (not rigors); breath-holding, gasping, or sharp intake of breath; severe splinting**[a]
Cry	No cry (awake or asleep)	Moans or whimpers, occasional complaint; **occasional verbal outburst or grunt**[a]	Crying steadily, screams or sobs, frequent complaints; **repeated outbursts, constant grunting**[a]
Consolability	Content, relaxed	Reassured by occasional touching, hugging, or being talked to, distractible	Difficult to console or comfort; **pushing away caregiver, resisting care, or comfort measures**[a]

Each of the five categories is scored from 0 to 2, which results in a total score between 0 and 10.
[a]Revised descriptors shown in bold.

- Risk for constipation related to potential adverse effects of narcotic analgesic agents

When caring for a child experiencing pain, the ultimate goal is that the child will be free of pain as evidenced by participation in age-appropriate activities of daily living and vital signs within age-appropriate parameters. However, at times, this may be unrealistic, especially if the child is experiencing chronic pain. Therefore, a more appropriate goal would be that the child reports that his or her pain has decreased to a tolerable level. Pain assessment tools can be used to quantify the amount by which the child's pain has decreased. For example, if the child has rated the pain as 7 out of 10, a realistic goal might be that the child reports a pain rating of no more than 4 out of 10. Additional goals would reflect improvement or resolution of the identified problem. For example, a short-term goal for a child experiencing disturbed sleep due to the pain might be that the child sleeps for a minimum of 4 consecutive hours through the night. A long-term goal might be that the child sleeps for 7 to 8 hours undisturbed through the night.

Various interventions can be used for pain management. These interventions include nonpharmacologic and pharmacologic measures. A guiding principle when caring for the child experiencing pain is the provision of atraumatic care (see Chapter 30 for more information). For example, cognitive and behavioral approaches are appropriate for pain management, including pain management related to procedures. In addition to nonpharmacologic measures, pharmacologic measures are appropriate for pain management. For example, apply a topical anesthetic cream to a site early enough before a venipuncture that it becomes effective. Another idea is to use an intermittent infusion device to obtain multiple blood specimen samples rather than performing repeated venipunctures. In addition, it is a good idea to consider the use of sedation for more painful procedures.

Throughout the child's care, be sure to discuss specific goals and interventions with the child and family as appropriate. Include the family in developing appropriate interventions so they can continue to support the child. Education of the child and family about interventions, including various therapies, is key. Ongoing assessment is needed to determine the effectiveness of the pain relief measures in achieving the desired goals.

Take Note!

The National Database of Nursing Quality Indicators were established by the American Nurses Association to evaluate nursing sensitive care. One indicator that can help improve pain management is the pediatric pain assessment, intervention, and reassessment (AIR) cycle (ANA, 2015).

Atraumatic Care

Play therapy may be helpful in allowing the child to express his or her feelings and adapt to the stressors of the current situation.

Nursing Care Plan 36.1 (at the end of the chapter) can be used as a guide in planning nursing care for the child experiencing pain. The nursing care plan should be individualized based on the child's symptoms and needs. Specific information related to pain management and the nurse's role will be discussed later in the chapter.

When you enter Aiden's room, he is crying and says his leg hurts. What will be your initial action? What will be your plan of care to manage Aiden's pain (refer to QUESTT assessment)? How would you address the statements made by the nurse in report? What approaches can you use to change staff behavior about pain management?

MANAGEMENT OF PAIN

Management of pain begins with assessment of the child's comfort level. If pain or the potential for pain, such as during an invasive procedure, is identified, steps must be taken to minimize or treat the pain. Three general principles guide pain management in children:

1. Individualize interventions based on the amount of pain experienced and the child's characteristics, such as developmental level, temperament, previous pain experience, and coping strategies.
2. Use nonpharmacologic and pharmacologic approaches to ease or eliminate the pain.
3. Teach the child and family about pain relief interventions and techniques and discuss with the child and family expectations of pain management.

Specific strategies for pain management include nonpharmacologic interventions such as relaxation, distraction, and guided imagery and pharmacologic interventions such as analgesics, patient-controlled analgesia (PCA), local analgesia, epidural analgesia, and moderate sedation.

Nonpharmacologic Management

Various techniques may be available to assist in managing mild pain in children or to augment the effectiveness of medications for moderate or severe pain. Many of these nonpharmacologic techniques assist children in coping with pain and give them an opportunity to feel a sense of mastery or control over the situation. Two types of techniques are behavioral-cognitive strategies and biophysical strategies. It is important to involve the parents in the process when using these techniques.

Behavioral-Cognitive Strategies

Behavioral-cognitive strategies for pain management involve measures that require the child to focus on a specific area rather than the pain. These strategies help to change the interpretation of the painful stimuli, reducing pain perception or making pain more tolerable. In addition, these strategies help to decrease negative attitudes, thoughts, and anxieties, thereby improving the child's coping mechanisms. Research has shown strong evidence that these strategies reduce pain and distress with needle-related procedures in children (Hsu & Cravero, 2014). Typically, these interventions work well with older children, but younger children also benefit from these techniques if they are adapted to the child's age and developmental level. Common behavioral-cognitive strategies include relaxation, distraction, imagery, biofeedback, thought stopping, and positive self-talk.

RELAXATION

Relaxation aids in reducing muscle tension and anxiety. A wide variety of techniques can be used. Relaxation can be as simple as holding an infant or young child closely while stroking the child or speaking in a soft soothing manner, or having the child inhale and exhale slowly using rhythmically controlled deep breathing. It also can involve more sophisticated techniques such as progressive relaxation. With this technique the child is asked to focus on one area of the body and let that body part go limp. Then in an organized fashion, usually working from the toes to the head or vice versa, the child is asked to focus on another body part, making it go limp. Eventually the exercises work through all body areas, leading to relaxation of the entire body.

DISTRACTION

Distraction involves having the child focus on another stimulus, thereby attempting to shield him or her from pain. Research has shown distraction to be associated with lower parental perception of pain and distress in younger children and decreased situational anxiety in older children (Hsu & Cravero, 2014).

This technique does not eliminate the pain but does help to make it more tolerable. Various methods can be used for distraction, including:

- Counting
- Repeating specific phrases or words, such as "ouch"
- Listening to music or singing
- Playing games, including computer and video games
- Blowing bubbles or blowing pinwheels or party favors
- Listening to favorite stories (Fig. 36.8)

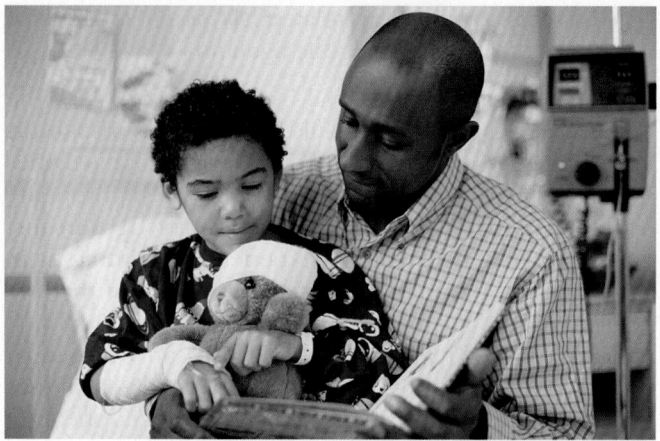

FIGURE 36.8 A child using distraction for pain management.

- Watching cartoons, television shows, or movies
- Visiting with friends
- Humor

Humor has been demonstrated to be an effective distracting technique for pain management. However, make sure that the technique is age appropriate and be sure to determine what or who will make the child laugh. If possible, allow the child and his or her family to choose the materials that they consider humorous.

The type of distraction used depends on the age of the child. For example, a younger child may enjoy blowing pinwheels and blowing bubbles. He or she also will enjoy listening to favorite stories or books. Older children may enjoy computer or video games, listening to favorite music, or visiting with friends.

IMAGERY

Imagery involves the use of the imagination to create a mental image. This mental image usually is a positive, pleasurable image, but it need not be real. The child is encouraged to include details and sensations that are associated with the image, such as specific descriptions of the image, colors, sounds, feelings, and smells. In some instances, the child may write down or record the image. When pain occurs, the child is encouraged to create the mental image or read or listen to the description.

BIOFEEDBACK

Biofeedback involves having the child gain an awareness of his or her body functions and learn ways to modify them voluntarily. The child usually is taught specific skills about how to modify body functions using an apparatus that measures pain-related changes in muscle tone or physiologic data, such as blood pressure or pulse rate. This teaching usually is performed by a specialized healthcare provider and occurs over several sessions, in advance of the pain experience. With practice, the child learns to control the changes without the apparatus. This technique can be used by older children, such as adolescents, who can concentrate for longer periods of time.

THOUGHT STOPPING

Thought stopping involves substituting a pleasurable or positive thought for the painful experience. Examples of positive thoughts might be, "It's only for a short time" or "It's important so I get better." The negative component of the pain is not ignored or suppressed; rather, it is transformed into something positive. Thought stopping also can involve the use of short, positive phrases. For example, the child may repeat "quick stick, feel better go home soon" when he or she anticipates pain or experiences pain.

Thought stopping is a useful method for reducing anxiety before and during events associated with pain. Children can be taught to use this technique any time they experience anxiety related to a painful experience. Doing so helps to promote the child's sense of control over the situation.

POSITIVE SELF-TALK

Positive self-talk is similar to thought stopping in that it involves the use of positive statements. With positive self-talk the child is taught to say positive statements when he or she is experiencing pain. For example, the child may be taught to say, "I will feel better and be able to go home and play with my friends."

Biophysical Interventions

Biophysical interventions focus on interfering with the transmission of pain impulses reaching the brain. The interventions involve some type of cutaneous stimulation near the site of the pain. This stimulation decreases the ability of the A-delta and C fibers to transmit pain impulses. Examples of biophysical interventions include the use of sucking and sucrose, application of heat and cold, massage and pressure, and transcutaneous electrical nerve stimulation (TENS).

SUCKING AND SUCROSE

Sucking is a behavior from which infants derive satisfaction. Therefore, nonnutritive sucking (e.g., sucking a pacifier) can be used to reduce pain behaviors in neonates undergoing painful procedures. In addition, infants show reduced pain behaviors after ingestion of sucrose or other sweet-tasting solutions such as glucose during single-event procedures, such as heel lancing (Anand, 2013). See Evidence-Based Practice 36.1. Optimal dosing for sucrose needs further research and caution must be used in extremely low–birth-weight infants and infants with unstable blood glucose levels.

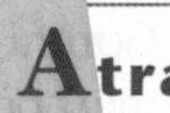

Atraumatic Care

Breastfeeding is also a noninvasive, natural, and feasible way to use sucking to reduce pain in infants.

HEAT AND COLD APPLICATIONS

Heat and cold applications alter physiologic mechanisms associated with pain. Cold results in vasoconstriction and alters capillary permeability, leading to a decrease in edema at the site of the injury. Due to vasoconstriction, blood flow is reduced and the release of pain-producing substances such as histamine and serotonin also is

EVIDENCE-BASED PRACTICE 36.1 **IS COMBINING NONNUTRITIVE SUCKING (NNS) WITH SUCROSE MORE EFFECTIVE AT REDUCING PROCEDURAL PAIN IN NEONATES THAN EITHER INTERVENTION ALONE?**

Neonates who are hospitalized undergo numerous painful experiences. It is well established that neonates feel pain with some research suggesting they have an increased sensitivity to pain. Pain in neonates has been found to have short- and long-term effects on the neonates physical and developmental outcomes. Two common non pharmacologic interventions used to decrease neonatal procedural pain are nonnutritive sucking (NNS) and sucrose.

STUDY

This study was an integrative review of the literature. Ten studies were included to determine if a synergistic effect exists when using NNS and sucrose before and during painful procedures to decrease procedural pain in the neonate.

Findings

The literature review found sufficient evidence to support the effectiveness of combining the use of NNS and sucrose to decrease procedural pain in the neonate.

Nursing Implications

The use of NNS and sucrose together is a safe and effective way to decrease procedural pain in neonates. Nurses should consider making it a standard of care policy in neonatal units. Further research is warranted to determine safe and effective concentration, dosing and dosing intervals of sucrose in the neonatal population.

Adapted from Naughton K. A., & Ikuta, L. (2013). The combined use of sucrose and nonnutritive sucking for procedural pain in both term and preterm neonates: An integrative review of the literature. *Advances in Neonatal Care, 13*(1), 9–19.

decreased. Moreover, transmission of painful stimuli via peripheral nerve fibers is decreased.

Heat results in vasodilation and increases blood flow to the area. It also leads to a decrease in nociceptive stimulation and removal of chemical substances that can stimulate nociceptive fibers. The increase in blood flow alters capillary permeability, leading to a reduction in swelling and pressure on nociceptive nerve fibers. Heat may also trigger the release of endogenous opioids, which mediate the pain response.

MASSAGE AND PRESSURE

Massage and pressure, like other biophysical interventions, are believed to inhibit stimulation of the A-delta and C fibers. These methods are helpful in relaxing muscles and reducing tension. In addition, these techniques can aid in distracting the child. Massage can be as simple as rubbing a body part or pressing on an area such as an injection site for about 10 seconds. It can also be more involved, requiring the use of another person to perform the massage. Lotion or ointment can be used during the massage and may provide a comforting effect. Contralateral pressure or massage of the opposite area may be used, especially if the area of pain cannot be accessed or if the affected area is too painful to touch.

A more formal method of pressure application is acupressure. In acupressure the fingertip, the thumb, or a blunt instrument is used to apply gentle, firm pressure to specifically designated sites to control pain. The pressure may be applied in one motion followed by releasing, in a circular motion for several minutes and then releasing or with a vibrating motion using the fingertips. The motion of applying and then releasing pressure is thought to facilitate the release of endogenous endorphins and enkephalins. The techniques of pressure and massage are easy to learn and use and can be taught to children and parents.

The Nurse's Role in Nonpharmacologic Pain Intervention

The nurse plays a major role in teaching the child and family about nonpharmacologic pain interventions. Help the child and family choose the most appropriate and most effective methods and ensure that the child and parents use the method before pain occurs as well as before the pain increases. Teaching Guidelines 36.1 lists some helpful instructions for the parents and child about nonpharmacologic pain management.

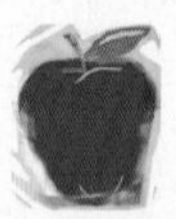

Teaching Guidelines 36.1

TEACHING TO MANAGE PAIN WITHOUT DRUGS

- Review the methods available and choose the method(s) that your child and you find best for your situation.
- Learn to identify the ways in which your child shows pain or demonstrates he or she is anxious about the possibility of pain. For example, does he or she get restless, make a face, or get flushed in the face?
- Begin using the technique chosen before your child experiences pain or when your child first indicates he or she is anxious about, or beginning to experience, pain.
- Practice the technique with your child and encourage the child to use the technique when he or she feels anxious about pain or anticipates that a procedure or experience will be painful.
- Perform the technique with your child. For example, take the deep breath in and out or blow bubbles with him or her; listen to the music or play the computer game with your child.
- Avoid using terms such as "hurt" or "pain" that suggest or cause your child to expect pain.
- Use descriptive terms like "pushing," "pulling," "pinching," or "heat."
- Avoid overly descriptive or judgmental statements such as, "This will really hurt a lot" or "This will be terrible."
- Stay with your child as much as possible; speak softly and gently stroke or cuddle your child.
- Offer praise, positive reinforcement, hugs, and support for using the technique even when it was not effective.

It is also important to assist the child and parents when using the technique in order to make sure that they are using the technique correctly. Offer suggestions for modifications or adaptations as necessary.

Parents are important components of the pain management program. Give them the option to stay with the child, or let them know that someone else will support the child if they opt not to stay. Offer simple, concrete ways to assist and help the child to manage pain. Many of the nonpharmacologic techniques can be done by parents, and children may respond better if their parents demonstrate the technique and encourage them to use it. Invite parents to participate in decisions as well as act as a coach to their child during procedures. Prepare the parents and explain the most appropriate pain management approaches and strategies. Discuss the type and amount of pain expected as well as the potential complications associated with pain management approaches. Ask how the parent predicts the child will react to a painful situation. Finally, offer techniques and strategies to the parents as they act as the coach during these situations.

Take Note!

Although parents want to help their children and some are able to act as coaches, the response of the child to pain and stress and to their parents' distraction interventions is highly variable. Some children appear to be soothed by their parents' distraction actions; others appear to become distressed. Be alert to factors that may influence the child's response, including age, sex, diagnosis, ethnicity, previous experience, temperament, anxiety, and coping style. Also be aware of parental factors, including ethnicity, sex, previous experience, belief in the helpfulness of the intervention, parenting style, and parental anxiety (McCarthy & Kleiber, 2006; McCarthy et al., 2010).

Pharmacologic Management

Pharmacologic interventions involve the administration of drugs for pain relief. Administration may occur using a wide variety of methods. The selection of the method is determined by the drug being administered; the child's status; the type, intensity, and location of the pain; and any factors that may be influencing the child's pain. Research overwhelmingly supports the appropriate use of analgesics to reduce pain perception in children.

Medications Used for Pain Management

Analgesics (medications for pain relief) typically fall into one of two categories—nonopioid analgesics and opioid analgesics. Anesthetics also may be used. Drugs such as sedatives and hypnotics may be used as adjuvant medications to help minimize anxiety or provide or assist with pain relief when typical analgesics are ineffective.

NONOPIOID ANALGESICS

Nonopioid analgesics include acetaminophen and nonsteroidal anti-inflammatory drugs (NSAIDs) such as ibuprofen, ketorolac, naproxen, indomethacin, diclofenac, and piroxicam (Drug Guide 36.1). These agents may be used to treat mild to moderate pain, often for conditions such as arthritis; joint, bone, and muscle pain; headache; dental pain; and menstrual pain. Acetaminophen, probably the most widely known nonopioid analgesic, and ibuprofen are also commonly used to treat fever in children.

Take Note!

Aspirin should not be used in infants or children for analgesic or antipyretic purposes because of the high risk of Reye syndrome.

According to the World Health Organization's (WHO's) recommended 2-step strategy, acetaminophen and NSAIDs are first-line agents for the treatment of pain (WHO, 2012). Nonopioid agents are typically administered orally or rectally. In some cases, such as with postoperative pain, they may be administered intravenously as a continuous infusion or as bolus doses. Administration via intramuscular injection is not recommended because the injection can cause significant pain and the onset of pain relief is not increased.

Acetaminophen is a relatively safe medication and it does not have the same GI or antiplatelet effects of NSAIDs therefore it is useful in children with cancer, with bleeding or clotting disorders or children on anticoagulants. Acetaminophen toxicity and resulting hepatotoxicity can occur with misuse and overdosing. Adverse effects associated with NSAIDs are uncommon but include gastrointestinal irritation, blood clotting problems, and renal dysfunction. Nonopioids are relatively safe, have few incompatibilities with other medications, and do not depress the central nervous system. Unfortunately, they exhibit a ceiling effect for analgesia. That is, after a certain level, they do not provide increasing pain relief even when administered at increased doses. As a result, they may be combined with opioids for more effective pain relief.

OPIOID ANALGESICS

Opioid analgesics are typically used for moderate to severe pain. They are classified as either agonists (when they act as the neurotransmitter at the receptor site) or antagonists (when they block the action at the receptor site). Opioid agents that act as agonists include morphine, fentanyl, meperidine, hydromorphone, oxycodone, and hydrocodone. Opioids that act as mixed agonists–antagonists include pentazocine, butorphanol, and nalbuphine (see Drug Guide 36.1). Opioids can be administered orally, rectally, intramuscularly, or intravenously. In addition, some agents such as fentanyl can be administered transdermally or transmucosally. Morphine is considered the "gold standard" for all opioid agonists; it is the drug to which all other opioids are compared and is the drug of choice for severe pain (Oakes & D'Arcy, 2011; WHO, 2012). Tramadol is an opioid that has been considered for use in treating moderate pain and is associated with a lower risk of respiratory depression and constipation (Oakes & D'Arcy, 2011). Currently the WHO states there is insufficient data to support its effectiveness and safety in children therefore more research is needed (WHO, 2012).

Take Note!

International and national guidelines recommend against the use of codeine in children due to serious safety concerns related to the genetic variability in its metabolism in children (some children are poor metabolizers while others are ultra metabolizers) (Kaiser et al., 2014; WHO, 2012).

Opioid agonists, such as morphine, are associated with numerous adverse effects, resulting primarily from their depressant action on the central nervous system.

DRUG GUIDE 36.1 COMMON DRUGS FOR PAIN MANAGEMENT

Drug	Actions/Indications	Nursing Implications
Acetaminophen (Tylenol)	Possible inhibition of cyclooxygenase in the central nervous system Direct action on hypothalamic heat-regulating center Mild to moderate pain, fever; arthritis, musculoskeletal pain, headache	• Administer orally, rectally, or intravenous. Do not exceed five doses or 60 mg/kg/day intravenous of drug in 24 hours. • Caution parents to read labels of other over-the-counter (OTC) drugs carefully; some may contain acetaminophen and if given in conjunction may lead to overdose and toxicity.
Ibuprofen (Motrin, Advil)	Inhibition of prostaglandin synthesis Mild to moderate pain, fever, treatment of inflammatory diseases	• Administer orally • Give with food or after meals if GI upset occurs. • Assess for easy bruising, bleeding gums, or frank or occult blood in urine or stool. • Monitor for nausea, vomiting, GI upset, diarrhea or constipation, dizziness, or drowsiness. • Caution parents to read labels of OTC medications closely; some may contain ibuprofen or other NSAIDs and if given in conjunction may lead to overdose.
Other NSAIDs: ketorolac (Toradol), diclofenac (Voltaren), indomethacin (Indocin), naproxen (Naprosyn, Aleve)	Inhibition of prostaglandin synthesis Moderate to severe pain	• Administer oral form with food or after meals if GI upset occurs. • Monitor for headache, dizziness, nausea, vomiting, constipation, or diarrhea. • Assess for signs and symptoms of bleeding, such as bruising, epistaxis, gingival bleeding, or frank or occult blood in urine or stool. • Ketorolac: may also be given IV or IM. In children ages 2–16 years, recommended as single dose only • Naproxen: also available in combination products (caution parents to read OTC labels carefully) • Indomethacin: when administering IV, report oliguria or anuria. • Diclofenac: may also be given rectally
Opioid agents: morphine, fentanyl (Sublimaze, Duragesic), hydromorphone (Dilaudid), oxycodone (OxyContin), Methadone	Opioid agonist acting primarily at μ-receptor sites (morphine, fentanyl, hydromorphone, oxycodone, methadone) Moderate to severe acute and chronic pain Morphine: intractable pain, preoperative sedation Fentanyl: pain associated with short procedures such as bone marrow aspiration, fracture reductions, suturing	• Assess respiratory status frequently, noting any decrease in ventilatory rate or changes in breathing patterns; have naloxone readily available in case of respiratory depression (particularly morphine, fentanyl, hydromorphone). • Monitor for sedation dizziness, lethargy, or confusion. • Educate parents and child that the drug may make the child sleepy, drowsy, or lightheaded. • Institute safety measures to prevent injury to the child. • Assess bowel sounds for decreased peristalsis; observe for abdominal distention. • Ensure adequate fiber intake and administer stool softeners as prescribed to minimize risk for constipation. • Monitor urine output for changes and report. • Morphine: may cause itching, particularly facial • Fentanyl: observe for chest wall rigidity, which can occur with rapid IV infusion. • Oxycodone is the opioid component of brand names products such as Tylox, Roxicet, and Percocet.

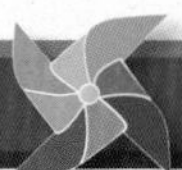

DRUG GUIDE 36.1 COMMON DRUGS FOR PAIN MANAGEMENT (continued)

Drug	Actions/Indications	Nursing Implications
Mixed opioid agonist–antagonist: pentazocine (Talwin), butorphanol (Stadol), nalbuphine (Nubain)	Pentazocine: antagonist at μ-receptor sites, agonist at κ-receptor sites. Butorphanol: high affinity for κ-receptor sites, minimal affinity for κ-receptor sites. Nalbuphine: partial agonist at κ-receptor sites, antagonist at μ-receptor sites Moderate to severe pain Relief of migraine headache (butorphanol) Preoperative analgesia (nalbuphine)	• Monitor the child for sedation. Educate child and parents that the drug may make the child sleepy, drowsy, or lightheaded. • Institute safety measures to prevent injury to the child. • Pentazocine, butorphanol: monitor for diaphoresis, dizziness. Assess for tachycardia and hypertension. • Butorphanol is given intranasally for migraine headaches.

GI, gastrointestinal.
Adapted from Taketokmo, C. K., Hodding, J. H., & Kraus, D. M. (2013). *Lexi-comp's Drug Reference Handbook: Pediatric & Neonatal Dosage Handbook* (20th ed.). Hudson, OH: Lexi-comp, Inc.

Take Note!

When administering parenteral or epidural opioids, always have naloxone (Narcan) readily available to reverse the opioid's effects should respiratory depression occur.

Opioids stimulate the chemoreceptor trigger zone (CTZ), leading to nausea and vomiting. Moreover, **drug tolerance** (increased dosage required for the same pain relief previously achieved with a lower dose) and **physical dependence** (need for continued administration of the drug to prevent withdrawal symptoms) are commonly noted when opioids are given repeatedly. Drug Guide 36.1 gives additional information related to the opioid analgesics.

Take Note!

Drug tolerance occurs when increasing doses are required to manage the pain. Physical dependence can occur after as few as 5 days of continuous use of the drug; symptoms of withdrawal begin if it is suddenly stopped (Oakes & D'Arcy, 2011).

Mixed agonist–antagonists are associated with less respiratory depression than agonists. Unfortunately, like NSAIDs, this group also has a ceiling effect, leading to inadequate pain relief even with increased dosages therefore limiting their use in treating severe pain (Oakes & D'Arcy, 2011).

Take Note!

Meperidine (Demerol), an opioid agonist, is not recommended as a first-choice agent for pain relief in children due to its toxicity on the central nervous system (WHO, 2012).

ADJUVANT DRUGS

Adjuvant drugs are drugs that are used to promote more effective pain relief, either alone or in combination with nonopioids or opioids. Their primary indication is for diagnoses other than pain. These agents are not classified as analgesics but may provide a coanalgesic effect or may treat side effects. Benzodiazepines, such as diazepam and midazolam, help to relieve anxiety. Midazolam also produces amnesia. Anticonvulsants, such as gabapentin, and tricyclic antidepressants, such as amitriptyline and nortriptyline, are used to treat neuropathic pain.

LOCAL ANESTHETICS

Local anesthetics are commonly used to provide analgesia for procedures. They are effective in providing successful pain relief with only minimal risk of systemic adverse effects. However, local anesthetics such as lidocaine historically were not used in children because these drugs need to be injected. The belief was that children feared needles and use of a local anesthetic subjected the child to two needlesticks instead of one. Advances in technology have led to the development of improved methods of delivery such as topical ointments and iontophoresis for administration of local anesthetics, thereby promoting atraumatic care. (For a more detailed discussion, see the next section on drug administration methods and later in the chapter on the nurse's role in managing procedure-related pain.)

Drug Administration Methods

With any medication administered for pain management, the timing of administration is vital. Timing depends on the type of pain. For continuous pain, the current recommendation is to administer analgesia around the clock at scheduled intervals to achieve the necessary effect (Oakes & D'Arcy, 2011; WHO, 2012). Scheduled dosing has been associated with decreased pain intensity ratings for children (Sutters et al., 2010). As-needed or PRN dosing is not recommended for continuous pain. This method can lead to inadequate pain relief because of the delay before the drug reaches its peak effectiveness, and as a result the child continues to experience pain, possibly necessitating a higher dose of analgesic to achieve relief. This then places the child at risk for overmedication and toxic effects.

For pain that can be predicted or considered temporary, such as with a procedure, analgesia is administered so that the peak action of the drug matches the time of the painful event.

There are various methods for administering pain medications to children. The preferred methods are the oral, rectal, intravenous, topical, or local nerve block routes. Epidural administration and moderate sedation also can be used.

ORAL METHOD

The oral method is often preferred because it is simple, easy, and convenient. The medication may be in the form of a pill, capsule, tablet, syrup, or elixir. Oral administration provides relatively steady blood levels of the drug when administered as a scheduled dose. Effectiveness typically occurs 1 to 2 hours after administration. As soon as possible, switch the child to oral dosing from parenteral dosing. However, keep in mind that higher doses of the oral medication may be needed to achieve the same effect.

RECTAL METHOD

The rectal method may be used when the child cannot take the medication orally, such as when he or she has difficulty swallowing or is experiencing nausea and vomiting. It is a viable alternative for drug administration. Some analgesics are available in suppository form. For others that are not, the drug can be compounded into a suppository form. The absorption rate varies with rectal administration, and children may find insertion of a suppository uncomfortable and embarrassing (Bowden & Greenberg, 2011).

INTRAVENOUS METHOD

Intravenous analgesia administration is the method of choice in emergency situations and when pain is severe and quick relief is needed. With intravenous administration, the drug usually takes effect within 5 minutes. Intravenous administration can be accomplished with bolus injections or continuous infusions. Continuous infusions may be preferred over bolus doses because steady blood levels are more easily maintained, thereby enhancing the drug's effect in relieving pain. Typically, opioids such as morphine, hydromorphone, and fentanyl are used due to their short half-life and decreased risk for toxicity.

PATIENT-CONTROLLED ANALGESIA

In **patient-controlled analgesia (PCA)**, a computerized pump is programmed to deliver an infusion of analgesics via a catheter inserted intravenously, epidurally, or subcutaneously. The analgesic may be given as a continuous infusion, as a continuous infusion supplemented by patient-delivered bolus doses, or as patient-delivered bolus doses only. Typically the child presses a button to administer a bolus dose. The pump has a lockout function that is preset with the dose and time interval. If the child presses the button before the preset time, he or she will not receive an overdose of medication. By delivering small, frequent doses of opioids, the child can experience pain relief without the effects of oversedation. The child also experiences a sense of control over the pain experience.

Both the Institute for Safe Medical Practices (ISMP) and the Joint Commission have identified infants and young children as not being good candidates for PCA usage (D'Arcy, 2011; Mann, 2014). However, PCA has been used successfully in children as young as 5 or 6 years old (Oakes & D'Arcy, 2011). It is essential to assess each child individually and consider his or her developmental level and psychosocial factors in determining appropriate PCA use. The child must have the necessary intellect, manual dexterity, and strength to operate the device.

PCA has been used to control postoperative pain and the pain associated with trauma, cancer, and sickle cell crisis. It can be used in acute care settings or in the home. Most commonly, morphine, hydromorphone, and fentanyl are the drugs used with PCA. The dosage is based on the child's response. Dosages for infusions depend on the child's age, the opioid used, and the type of pain. A commonly used range for morphine infusion to treat postoperative pain ranges from 0.01 to 0.04 mg/kg/hr. Higher-dosage ranges have been used to treat the pain associated with sickle cell crisis and cancer.

Serious adverse events, such as oversedation, respiratory depression, and even death, can occur when family members, caregivers, or clinicians who are not authorized administer PCA doses "by proxy" (Cooney et al., 2013; The Joint Commission, 2004). The ISMP recommends developing specific criteria in any situation where authorized agent–activated PCA is being used (Cooney et al., 2013; D'Arcy, 2011). Proper education and instruction are crucial in any situation where someone other than the child may be administering PCA doses. Thorough assessment is necessary to ensure the child's pain is neither undertreated nor overtreated. To ensure safety with PCA use, each institution must have policies and procedures in place, appropriate education of healthcare staff, quality control measures, and quality machines.

LOCAL ANESTHETIC APPLICATION

A local anesthetic may sometimes be used to alleviate the pain associated with procedures such as venipuncture, injections, wound repair, lumbar puncture, or accessing of implanted ports. Local anesthesia is a type of regional analgesia that blocks or numbs specific nerves in a region of the body. Medications called local anesthetics include topical forms, such as creams, agents delivered by iontophoresis, vapocoolants, and skin refrigerants, and injectable forms.

Topical Forms. A common choice for effective, painless local anesthesia is EMLA (eutectic mixture of local anesthetics [lidocaine and prilocaine]). It achieves anesthesia to a depth of 2 to 4 mm, so it reduces pain of phlebotomy, venous cannulation, and intramuscular injections for up to 24 hours after the injection. However, it requires a 60- to 90-minute application time to intact skin using an occlusive dressing for superficial procedures and up to 2 to 3 hours for deeper, more invasive procedures (Box 36.1). EMLA is approved for use in infants 37 weeks' gestation or older (Walden, 2014). Maximum dosage and maximum area of application are based on the child's weight. Parents can be taught how to apply the EMLA at home in preparation for a procedure (Fig. 36.9). Sometimes EMLA is not used due to the expense and the time needed to allow the drug to act. New approaches to EMLA delivery have been developed. Examples include other drug formulations and a patch delivery with a heat-activated system (Synera) that enhances the delivery of lidocaine and prilocaine. Synera is labeled for children older than 3 years of age and needs to be applied only 20 to 30 minutes before the procedure (Taketokmo, Hodding, & Kraus, 2013).

BOX 36.1

APPLYING EMLA

Follow these guidelines when applying EMLA:

- Explain the purpose of the medication to the child and parents, reinforcing that it will help the pain go away.
- Check the scheduled time for the procedure; plan to apply the cream 60 minutes before a superficial procedure such as an intramuscular injection or a venipuncture or 2 to 3 hours before a deeper procedure such as a lumbar puncture or bone marrow aspiration.
- Place a thick layer of the cream on the skin at the intended site of the procedure, making sure that the area where the cream is being applied is free of any breaks. Do not rub the cream in once it is applied to the skin.
- Cover the site with a transparent dressing such as Tegaderm or Op-site and secure it so that the dressing is occlusive. Alternatively, use plastic film wrap and tape the edges to secure the dressing.
- Instruct the child not to touch the dressing once it is secured. If necessary, cover the occlusive dressing with a protection device or a loosely applied gauze or elastic bandage.
- After the allotted time, remove the occlusive dressing and wipe the cream from the skin. Inspect the skin for a change in color (blanching or redness), which indicates that the medication has penetrated the skin adequately.
- Verify that sensation is absent by lightly tapping or scratching the area. Use this technique also to demonstrate to the child that the anesthetic is effective. If sensation is present, reapply the cream.
- Prepare the child for the procedure. Assess the child's pain after the procedure to evaluate for pain and to differentiate pain from fear and anxiety.

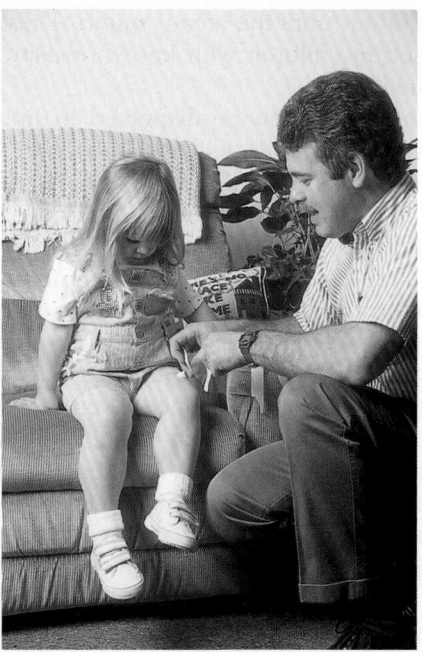

FIGURE 36.9 A parent applies EMLA cream to the child at home in preparation for a procedure.

Take Note!

EMLA is used with caution in children younger than 3 months and other susceptible persons because it may be associated with methemoglobinemia caused by prilocaine toxicity (Oakes & D'Arcy, 2011; Taketokmo, et al., 2013). It is contraindicated in children who have congenital or idiopathic methemoglobinemia (Taketokmo et al., 2013). It must be used cautiously in those younger than age 12 months who are receiving methemoglobin-inducing agents, such as sulfonamides, phenytoin, phenobarbital, and acetaminophen (Taketokmo et al., 2013). Use of these agents in combination with EMLA increases the child's risk for methemoglobinemia, a condition that could lead to cyanosis and hypoxemia.

Other examples of topical anesthetics are TAC (tetracaine, epinephrine, cocaine) and LET (lidocaine, epinephrine, tetracaine). These are commonly used for lacerations that require suturing. The agent is applied directly to the wound with a cotton ball or swab for

20 to 30 minutes until the area is numb. These methods are not used in children with known sensitivity to any of these medications.

Lidocaine can also be dispersed in liposomes to allow for transcutaneous delivery (liposomal lidocaine). Over-the-counter LMX4 (lidocaine 4%), formerly called ELA-Max, is massaged into the skin without the use of an occlusive dressing. Anesthesia to the area is reached in 15 to 30 minutes and lasts about 60 minutes. Recent studies suggest that the analgesic effect may be equal to that of EMLA with the advantage of a shorter onset (American Medical Association, 2013). Research has shown that liposomal lidocaine 4% cream was highly effective in reducing the pain associated with intravenous cannulation (Hsu, 2014; Zempsky, 2008). The researchers cited a short onset of action (30 minutes) and minimal vascular effects as benefits. They found that the liposomal encapsulation protects the anesthetic from being metabolized too quickly (Zempsky, 2008). Study results have shown higher intravenous cannulation success rates, less pain, shorter total procedure time, and minor dermal changes among children (Hsu, 2014; Taddio, Soin, Schuh et al., 2005).

Needle-free powder lidocaine (Zingo or J-tip) is another topical analgesic. It is labeled for use in children 3 to 18 years of age. It is a single-use, prefilled disposable system that provides analgesia in 1 to 3 minutes. Studies have shown it to be safe and well tolerated with a rapid onset and significant reduction in needlestick pain although the degree of relief varied (Hsu, 2014).

Another choice for local anesthesia is iontophoresis. Iontophoretic lidocaine (Numby Stuff) provides a deeper analgesia in a shorter duration (approximately 10 to 25 minutes) and is used over intact skin. A mild electrical current from a small battery-powered generator and two iontophoretic drug-delivery electrodes push drug molecules (lidocaine HCl 2% with epinephrine 1:100,000) into the skin. A mild tingling sensation may be felt during drug delivery, with an increase in tingling noted with higher currents. This type of local anesthesia is not recommended for use in children who have a history of allergy or sensitivity to these drugs, in children who have electrically sensitive equipment such as a pacemaker, or in children who have damaged skin or scar tissue.

Vapocoolant spray, another type of local analgesia, can be sprayed onto the skin or administered using a cotton ball soaked in liquid. The depth of anesthesia is not known, but it appears to provide immediate pain control. It is inexpensive and requires no waiting time. The effect lasts for approximately 1 to 2 minutes. Studies have found it to be an effective analgesic for short-duration procedures (American Medical Association, 2013).

Injectable Forms. Injectable forms of lidocaine or procaine can be administered subcutaneously or intradermally around the procedural area approximately 5 to 10 minutes before the procedure. Common problems with this form of anesthetic include the pain associated with the subcutaneous injection and some burning associated with lidocaine administration, as well as blanching of the skin.

Take Note!

The burning that lidocaine causes on injection may be diminished by buffering lidocaine with sodium bicarbonate, using 10 parts lidocaine and 1 part sodium bicarbonate (1 mL of 1% to 2% lidocaine and 0.1 mL of 8.4% sodium bicarbonate). Then inject 0.1 mL or less of the solution intradermally at the site of venipuncture. Anesthetic action is almost immediate. The solution is stable for only approximately 1 week if not refrigerated.

EPIDURAL ANALGESIA

For **epidural analgesia**, a catheter is inserted in the epidural space usually between the lumbar (L3) and the thoracic (T3) area. The drug, usually fentanyl or morphine, diffuses into the cerebrospinal fluid and crosses the dura mater to the spinal cord. Then it binds with the opioid receptors located at the dorsal horn. The drugs can be administered as bolus injections (a one-time bolus or on an intermittent schedule), a continuous infusion, or PCA. Usually an opioid, such as morphine, fentanyl, or hydromorphone, is given in conjunction with a long-acting local anesthetic such as bupivacaine.

Epidural analgesia is typically used postoperatively, providing analgesia to the lower body for approximately 12 to 14 hours. The small amount of medication used with this type of analgesia causes less sedation, thereby allowing the child to participate more actively in postoperative care activities. This type of analgesia also is effective for children undergoing upper or lower abdominal surgeries because it controls localized intense pain, somatic pain, and visceral pain.

When epidural analgesia is being administered, additional narcotic analgesics are not given in order to prevent complications such as respiratory depression, pruritus, nausea, vomiting, and urinary retention.

Take Note!

Respiratory depression, although rare when epidural analgesia is used, is always a possibility. When it does occur, it usually occurs gradually over a period of several hours after the medication is initiated. This allows adequate time for early detection and prompt intervention.

Constant assessment is essential because insertion of an epidural catheter and epidural analgesia can lead to infection at the site of the insertion, epidural hematoma, arachnoiditis, neuritis, spinal headache (rare) due to a cerebrospinal fluid leak and respiratory depression. Frequent assessment, typically every 1 to 2 hours, of heart rate, respiratory rate, and depth of sedation, and every 2 to 4 hours of blood pressure, pain level, and motor function, is imperative (Oakes & D'Arcy, 2011). Assessing for adverse reactions such as nausea and vomiting and pruritus, checking the tubing and catheter site, and ensuring the occlusive dressing is intact are all important nursing interventions. The dermatome, which is the area of the body associated with supply by a particular nerve, that innervates the diaphragm can become suppressed during continuous epidural analgesia, resulting in respiratory depression. It is important to assess the child's sensory level frequently. Using cool water or an alcohol pad, bilaterally touch the child's body every 2 to 3 cm. The level where the child states he or she feels the temperature change is the level of anesthesia. (Refer to Figure 36.10 for dermatome levels.)

MODERATE (CONSCIOUS) SEDATION

Moderate sedation used to be labeled conscious sedation, but the term "conscious" has been replaced since it can be misleading (Coté & Wilson, and the Work Group on Sedation, 2011). It is a medically controlled state of depressed consciousness that allows protective reflexes to be maintained so the child has the ability to maintain a patent airway and respond to physical or verbal stimulation. Sedation in children is different than in adults as it is often administered to help control behavior in order to complete procedures or diagnostics studies (Coté & Wilson, and the Work Group on Sedation, 2011). Moderate sedation requires adherence to specific protocols, and many regulatory bodies, such as the Joint Commission, and societies, including the American Academy of Pediatrics, American Academy of Pediatric Dentistry, American Society of Anesthesiologists, and American College of Emergency Physicians, have published standards and guidelines to improve patient safety and outcomes. The depressed state is obtained by using various agents such as morphine, fentanyl, midazolam, ketamine, chloral hydrate, diazepam, pentobarbital, nitrous oxide, or propofol. The medication used will depend on the expected degree of pain and discomfort, amount of motion restriction needed and individual factors such as age, ability to cooperate, and medical history.

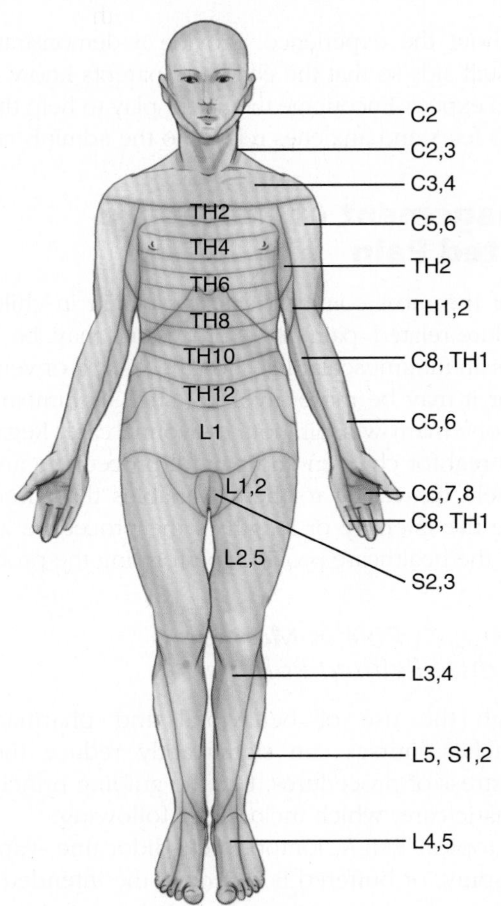

FIGURE 36.10 The level of anesthesia should not go higher than T4, the nipple line, in children.

Moderate sedation is used for procedures that are painful and stressful. For example, moderate sedation is suggested instead of restraints, especially for toddlers and preschool children who are undergoing frightening or invasive procedures and who are manifesting extreme anxiety and behavioral upset. Other indications include situations involving:

- Evidence that the child is experiencing a heightened stress reaction (e.g., attempting to flee, crying inconsolably, or flailing)
- Verbalization by the child that he or she is frightened and does not want to be touched
- Inability to remain immobilized, such as during laceration repair or computed tomography
- Any procedure that is painful and fear provoking

The route of administering the medications for sedation should follow the guidelines of atraumatic care. Oral, topical, or an existing intravenous route should be used. Studies have shown that pediatric clients often pass from the intended level of sedation to a deeper unintended level of sedation therefore personnel administering moderate sedation must be specially trained, with strong resuscitation and advanced pediatric life support skills, and emergency equipment and medications must be readily available (Coté, & Wilson, & the Work Group on Sedation, 2011).

The Nurse's Role in Pharmacologic Pain Management

The nurse plays a major role in providing pharmacologic pain relief. As with any medication, the nurse is responsible for adhering to the rights of medication administration—right drug, right dose, right route, right time, and right patient. In addition, the nurse also adheres to additional rights, such as—the right of the child and parents to be educated, the right of the child to refuse the medication, the right documentation, the right form, and the right approach. The nurse also must have a solid knowledge base about the medications used for pain relief. This knowledge includes information about the drug's pharmacokinetics (absorption, distribution, metabolism, and excretion) and pharmacodynamics (mechanism of action, including adverse effects). Refer to Chapter 35 for further information.

Assessment is crucial when pharmacologic pain interventions are used. An initial assessment of pain provides a baseline from which options for relief can be chosen. Factors that can affect the choice of analgesic, such as the child's age, pain intensity, physiologic status, or previous experiences with pain, also need to be considered. The nurse acts as an advocate for the child and the family to ensure that the most appropriate pharmacologic agent is chosen for the situation.

Assessment is ongoing once the agent is administered. Monitor physiologic parameters such as level of consciousness, vital signs, oxygen saturation levels, and urinary output for changes that might indicate an adverse reaction to the agent. More intensive monitoring is needed when agents are administered intravenously or epidurally or by moderate sedation. For example, if the child is receiving moderate sedation, interventions include:

- Ensuring that emergency equipment is readily available
- Maintaining a patent airway
- Monitoring the child's level of consciousness and responsiveness
- Assessing the child's vital signs (especially heart rate, blood pressure, and respiratory rate)
- Monitoring oxygen saturation levels

Typically, a specially trained healthcare provider is specifically designated to perform these activities during the administration of the sedation. Afterward, the nurse is responsible for ongoing monitoring of the child's status.

Monitor the child closely for evidence of adverse effects. Table 36.7 describes the interventions useful for responding to these adverse effects. Be alert for signs and symptoms of respiratory depression secondary to opioid administration. Have an opioid antagonist such as naloxone (Narcan) and the benzodiazepine antagonist flumazenil (Romazicon) readily available should the child experience respiratory depression.

In addition to assessing physiologic parameters, assess the child's and parents' emotional status before and after the agent is administered. For example, increased anxiety and fear may necessitate a change in method of administration, such as topical application instead of an intradermal injection of a local anesthetic. Use nonpharmacologic methods to help lessen anxiety, thereby promoting more effective relief from the drug.

Nurses also are responsible for ensuring that the child and parents are adequately prepared for the use of the pharmacologic agent. Teach the child and parents about the drug, why it is being used, its intended effects, and possible adverse effects, tailoring the teaching to the child's cognitive level. Provide opportunities for the child and parents to ask questions, offering support and guidance throughout the experience. Provide a demonstration or use visual aids so that the child and parents know exactly what to expect. Encourage the use of play to help the child express fears and anxieties related to the administration.

TABLE 36.7 INTERVENTIONS FOR COMMON OPIOID-INDUCED ADVERSE EFFECTS

Adverse Effect	Nursing Interventions
Constipation	Encourage fluid intake unless contraindicated Ensure intake of high-fiber foods, including fruits, if allowed Encourage activity, including ambulation if possible Obtain order for stool softener and administer laxative as ordered
Pruritus	Apply cool compresses and lotions Administer antihistamine as ordered
Nausea and vomiting	Inform child and parents that these symptoms usually subside in 1 to 2 days Encourage small frequent meals with bland foods Administer antiemetic if ordered Notify physician or nurse practitioner for possible change in pain medication

Management of Procedure-Related Pain

One of the most common causes of pain in children is procedure-related pain. The procedure may be minor, such as an intramuscular injection, heel stick, or venipuncture, or it may be more involved, such as lumbar puncture, bone marrow aspiration, or wound care. Regardless, pain is real for children and painful procedures are often extremely distressing to them. Variables that affect pain include the intensity or length of the procedure and the skill of the healthcare provider performing the procedure.

The Nurse's Role in Managing Procedure-Related Pain

Through the use of behavioral and pharmacologic approaches, nurses can significantly reduce the pain and distress of procedures. Use the guiding principles of atraumatic care, which include the following:

- Use topical EMLA, iontophoretic lidocaine, vapocoolant spray, or buffered lidocaine at the intended site of a skin or vessel puncture.
- Incorporate the use of nonpharmacologic strategies for pain relief in conjunction with pharmacologic methods.

- Prepare the child and parents ahead of time about the procedure and then keep all equipment out of sight until it is ready to be used.
- Use therapeutic hugging (see Chapter 30) to secure the child.
- Use the smallest-gauge needle possible or an automated lancet device to puncture the skin.
- Use an intermittent infusion device or peripherally inserted central catheter (PICC) if multiple or repeated blood samples are necessary. Coordinate care so that several tests can be performed from one sample if possible.
- Opt for venipuncture in newborns instead of heel sticks if the amount of blood needed would require much squeezing.
- Use kangaroo care (skin-to-skin contact) for newborns before and after heel stick.
- Provide nonnutritive sucking, with sucrose solution, if appropriate; pacifier; or breastfeeding for newborns several minutes before the procedure.

Take Note!

Individualize interventions based on the painfulness of the procedure and the child's developmental age and personality. Use behavioral-cognitive approaches and pharmacologic interventions. For example, encouraging the school-age child to assist during painful procedures in age-appropriate ways may actually help ease some of the pain related to a heightened state of anxiety, or at least assist the child in coping with the situation. Always use appropriate pharmacologic treatment especially for the first procedure to provide as painless an experience as possible for the child.

Nursing care for the child with procedure-related pain includes the child as well as the parents. Be sure to prepare them for the procedure using an appropriate developmental approach. Promote environmental comfort, too. Ensure that the child's privacy is maintained and that the lighting is adequate for the procedure but not so bright as to cause the child discomfort.

Painful procedures performed in the child's room can lead to an association of pain or fear with the room or bed. Many hospitals have a special treatment room where procedures can be performed. These rooms are usually equipped with many activities, toys, and decorations to help distract the child. The use of a treatment room may not be feasible or desirable in all situations or for all procedures. The ultimate goal is to do what is best for the child; therefore, the nurse needs to consider the needs of the child, the demands of the procedures, and the conditions that would facilitate the best outcome.

Unless contraindicated, encourage the parents to be present before, during, and after the procedure to provide comforting support to the child. Also encourage the child and parents to use nonpharmacologic methods to help maximize pain relief and reduce anxiety. For example, nonpharmacologic methods that are helpful for the toddler and preschooler may include positioning the child on the lap and hugging the child, distracting the child with toys or interactive books, and blowing bubbles.

Play therapy can be useful when preparing children for painful procedures. Encourage children to make decisions about their care related to pain management if their condition or procedure allows. It is also helpful to anticipate and recognize painful situations and provide pain medication before the actual procedure to ensure comfort. Many nonpharmacologic strategies can be enhanced and better implemented with the help of the child life specialist or play therapist, who have specialized training in these techniques.

Recall Aiden from the beginning of the chapter. What are some interventions that may be helpful prior to, during, and after his dressing change?

Management of Chronic Pain

Typically, pain in children is acute pain, but chronic pain is a significant problem in the pediatric population. Chronic pain is ongoing and recurrent pain that persists beyond the expected healing time, which has been typically defined as 3 to 6 months (American Pain Society, 2012). Chronic pain is the result of a complex interplay of biological, psychological, and socio-cultural factors (American Pain Society, 2012). According to the American Pain Society (2012), children with chronic pain and their families experience significant emotional and social consequences from the pain and disability; also, the experience of chronic pain in childhood may predispose the individual to chronic pain in adulthood.

The Nurse's Role in Managing Chronic Pain

The nurse's role in managing chronic pain in children is similar to that for the child experiencing acute pain or procedure-related pain. Assessment of the child's pain is key and should include a history of the present problem. Questions should focus on the onset of the pain; its intensity, duration, and location; and any factors that alleviate or exacerbate it. In addition, it is important to question the child and parents about the impact of the pain on the child's daily life, such as sleep, play, eating, school, and interactions with peers, other family members, and friends. Also address the impact of the child's chronic pain on the family's life.

Another key area of assessment is determining how the pain affects the child's and family's level of stress. Areas to address include the child's and parents' feelings of hopelessness, anxiety, and depression. Also question the child and parents about what they think has caused the pain and how they have coped with it. In addition, ascertain what methods the child and parents have used to alleviate the pain and the success of these methods. Inquire about any home remedies or alternative therapies that may have been used.

Review past physical examination findings for clues to the underlying problem. Observe the child's overall appearance, gait, and posture. Assess the child's cognitive level and emotional response, especially related to the experience of pain. Expect to complete a neurologic examination and observe for muscle spasms, trigger points, and increased sensitivity to light touch. Abnormal body postures assumed by the child due to chronic pain may result in the development of secondary pain in the muscles and fascia. When children tense their muscles due to fear of examination, somatic pain may occur.

Various nonpharmacologic and pharmacologic strategies are used to manage chronic pain. Often multiple strategies are combined to address pain relief as well as the pain's impact on other areas, such as sleep or school functioning. When pharmacologic agents are used, the oral form is the method of choice. As with any pain management strategy, education of the child and family is paramount. A referral to a pediatric pain specialist may be needed if the child's pain is not controlled effectively.

NURSING CARE PLAN 36.1

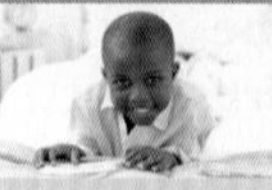

Overview for the Child in Pain

NURSING DIAGNOSIS: Acute pain related to need for invasive procedures, surgery, recent trauma, or infection as evidenced by pain rating scale, facial grimacing, crying, irritability, withdrawal activity, or changes in vital signs

Outcome Identification and Evaluation

Child will achieve adequate comfort level as evidenced by a decrease in rating number on a pain rating scale, quietness, calm resting behaviors, decrease in crying and irritability, and vital signs within acceptable parameters.

Interventions: ***Promoting Pain Relief***

- Assess pain level using a developmentally appropriate pain rating tool *to establish a baseline.*
- Assess for verbal and nonverbal indicators of pain *to help determine child's pain level;* question parents about child's typical behaviors and previous experiences with pain *to determine factors that may be influencing child's response to pain.*
- Institute nonpharmacologic methods for pain control based on the child's age and cognitive level *to help decrease pain;* encourage parental participation in use of methods *to provide additional support and pain relief for the child.*
- Administer pharmacologic agents as ordered using the least traumatic route possible *to alter pain impulse transmission and minimize distress while promoting effective pain relief.*
- Explain the action of the drug and what the child should expect from the medication at a level that the child can understand *to promote trust and reduce fear while providing effective pain relief.*
- Give analgesics around the clock if pain is continuous and can be predicted *to maintain steady blood levels of the drug, thereby maximizing the drug's effect.*
- Perform atraumatic care at all times *to minimize the child's exposure to physical and psychological distress and pain.*
- Anticipate timing of procedures or situations that may lead to pain and provide appropriate analgesic therapy as ordered *to ensure that therapy is most effective at the time of the procedure.*
- Ensure that the child's environment is quiet and conducive to rest, dim the lights, and close the door or curtain *to reduce sensory overload that would increase the child's pain sensation.*
- Encourage the parents to stroke, touch, caress, and hold the child *to reduce discomfort and promote feelings of security.*
- Reassess the child's pain level after use of nonpharmacologic and pharmacologic methods *to determine effectiveness;* anticipate the need to modify or adapt nonpharmacologic methods or adjust analgesic dosage, route, or frequency *to promote maximum pain relief.*
- Perform nursing care activities after administering analgesic *to prevent exacerbating the child's pain.*
- Use diversional activities, distraction, and play appropriate to the child's age and cognitive level *to promote additional pain relief.*

NURSING CARE PLAN 36.1

Overview for the Child in Pain (continued)

NURSING DIAGNOSIS: Anxiety related to stress and uncertainty of the situation, unknown cause of pain, lack of familiarity with procedures, testing, and healthcare facility, and painful procedures, as evidenced by crying, irritability, withdrawal, stoic or aggressive behaviors

Outcome Identification and Evaluation

Child and family will demonstrate a decrease in anxiety level as evidenced by age-appropriate positive coping behaviors, verbalization of feelings, playing out of feelings, child and family cooperation with plan of care, and absence of signs and symptoms associated with escalating anxiety.

Interventions: *Minimizing Anxiety*

- Assess child's and parents' understanding of the situation, including their understanding of what may be causing the pain and the reasons for the procedures and testing, *to provide baseline information about the child's and parents' knowledge and possible clues to anxiety.*
- Spend time with the child and parents discussing what they think might be happening, encouraging the child and parents to talk openly about their feelings, *to facilitate continued expressions and communication.* Allow time for questions and answer questions honestly *to establish rapport and build trust.*
- Approach the child and family in a calm, relaxed manner *to foster trust and communication and decrease anxiety.*
- Allow the child options related to interventions as much as possible, such as fluid to drink or snack to eat, extremity to use for venipuncture (right or left), color of bandage, or holding tape or dressing, *to foster feelings of control.*
- Provide atraumatic care *to reduce exposure to distress, which would exacerbate the child's anxiety level.*
- Explain any procedures, tests, or activities at a level the child can understand *to reduce fear of the unknown.*
- Incorporate aspects of the child's routine at home as much as possible *to reduce feelings of separation and promote feelings of normalcy.*
- Ensure consistency in care *to facilitate trust and acceptance.*
- Encourage parents in the use of comfort measures such as stroking, cuddling, holding, and rocking *to promote feelings of security and minimize stress.*
- Provide positive reinforcement for choices, participation in activities, and use of appropriate coping methods *to foster self-esteem.*
- Encourage the child's participation in play (unstructured and therapeutic play as needed) *to promote expression of feelings and fears.*

NURSING DIAGNOSIS: Deficient knowledge related to current condition and appropriate methods for managing pain as evidenced by crying, irritability, pushing away, and questions and verbalizations about pain and relief methods

Outcome Identification and Evaluation

Child and parents will demonstrate adequate knowledge about the child's current condition and use of pain relief methods as evidenced by statements about the cause of the child's pain, demonstration of chosen nonpharmacologic relief methods, use of pharmacologic agents, and statements related to signs and symptoms of increased and decreased pain.

Intervention: *Providing Child and Family Teaching*

- Assess the child's and parents' knowledge and understanding of the child's current condition and current pain level *to establish a baseline for teaching.*
- Provide time for the child and parents to ask questions; answer questions honestly and in terms they can understand *to promote learning.*
- Explain in simplified terms how the child's condition is associated with pain or the rationale for procedures needed that may contribute to pain *to promote understanding and foster trust.*
- Teach in short sessions *to prevent overloading the child and parents with information.*

(continued)

NURSING CARE PLAN 36.1

Overview for the Child in Pain (continued)

- Provide reinforcement and rewards *to help facilitate the teaching/learning process.*
- Use multiple modes of learning, such as written information, verbal instruction, demonstrations, and media when possible, *to facilitate learning and retention of information.*
- Instruct the parents and child as appropriate in nonpharmacologic methods for pain relief; encourage practice and participation by parents in methods chosen *to foster independence and use of method when necessary.*
- Teach the child as appropriate and parents about pharmacologic methods for pain relief; review specific information about the drug to be used, including action, duration, administration, possible adverse effects, and care necessary when the drug is used, *to promote learning;* have the child and parents report back information or demonstrate administration *to evaluate effectiveness of teaching.*
- Provide parents with written information about pain relief methods for use at home if indicated *to allow for reference at a later date.*

NURSING DIAGNOSIS: Sleep deprivation related to inability to manage pain effectively as evidenced by frequent waking by child during night, signs and symptoms of pain including irritability and restlessness, statements about being tired, pain rating scale remaining the same

Outcome Identification and Evaluation

Child will exhibit increased ability to sleep during the night as evidenced by increasing periods of calm and restfulness (initially starting at 2 hours and gradually increasing to 7 to 8 hours), decreased pain level on pain rating scale, and statements of decreased fatigue.

Intervention: *Promoting Sleep and Rest*

- Assist the child in using nonpharmacologic methods of pain relief, such as imagery, distraction, and muscle relaxation, *to promote relaxation.*
- Administer pharmacologic pain relief as ordered *to minimize pain interfering with sleep;* anticipate a change in drug therapy if pain relief is inadequate.
- Cluster nursing care activities *to minimize energy expenditure and disruptions in the child's ability to rest.*
- Help the child with a nighttime routine similar to one he or she uses at home *to promote feelings of security.*
- Offer the child a back rub, warm bath, or warm liquids; reading a story; or listening to music *to facilitate relaxation;* provide stroking, hugging, cuddling, rocking, and light touch *to promote a sense of security and calm.*
- Dim the lights and close the curtain or door to the room *to provide a quiet, restful environment.*
- Ensure round-the-clock pain relief for the child through the night *to minimize the risk of pain.*

NURSING DIAGNOSIS: Risk for injury related to possible adverse effects of analgesics

Outcome Identification and Evaluation

Child will remain free of any injury related to signs and symptoms of adverse effects of analgesic therapy as evidenced by respiratory rate appropriate for age and no complaints of gastrointestinal (GI) upset, dizziness, or sedation or episodes of constipation, nausea, vomiting, or pruritus.

NURSING CARE PLAN 36.1

Overview for the Child in Pain (continued)

Intervention: ***Promoting Safety***

- Ensure that the child's call light is within reach *to allow for notification of healthcare personnel should problems arise.*
- Administer analgesic exactly as prescribed *to reduce the risk of error and development of adverse effects.*
- Assess the child's respiratory status closely for changes *to allow for early detection of respiratory depression.*
- If an opioid analgesic is being given, have naloxone readily available *to reverse the action of the narcotic if respiratory depression occurs.*
- Monitor appetite and assess bowel sounds for changes; note any abdominal distention or decreased bowel sounds, which would suggest decreased peristalsis, *to allow for early detection of constipation.*
- Ensure adequate fluid and fiber intake *to reduce risk of constipation.*
- Offer small frequent meals and give medication with food *to minimize risk of GI upset.*
- Assess for nausea and vomiting; if necessary, withhold food and fluids *to rest the GI tract* and administer antiemetics until nausea and vomiting resolve *to decrease nausea and vomiting.*
- Instruct the child to remain in bed after receiving analgesic, raise crib or side rails as appropriate, and instruct the child and parents to have someone accompany the child to the bathroom if allowed *to reduce the risk of falls from sedation.*
- Assess for complaints of itching and observe for rash or reddened areas; if pruritus occurs, urge the child not to scratch and expect to administer antihistamine as ordered *to reduce pruritus.*
- Provide the child with distraction *to assist in helping to reduce effects of pruritus.*

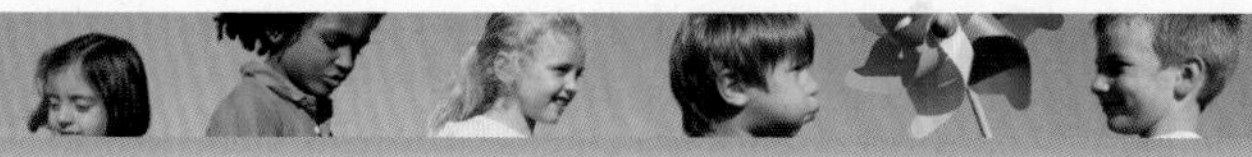

KEY CONCEPTS

- Pain is a highly individualized subjective experience affecting persons of any age. It is a universal experience and is considered the fifth vital sign.
- Pain management is a critical element in a child's plan of care because children may lack the verbal capacity to describe their pain experience; caregivers and healthcare providers often have misconceptions about pain; assessment of the complex nature of the pain experience is difficult; if left unmanaged, pain in children can lead to serious physical and emotional consequences; and available resources and research related to pain relief strategies in children are limited.
- The sensation of pain involves a sequence of physiologic events: transduction, transmission, perception, and modulation.
- Pain can be classified by duration as acute or chronic, by etiology as nociceptive or neuropathic, or by source or location as somatic or visceral.
- Factors influencing a child's perception of pain include age and gender, cognitive level, temperament, previous pain experiences, and family and cultural background, all of which cannot be changed. Situational factors involve behavioral, cognitive, and emotional aspects and can be changed.
- Infants, including preterm infants, experience pain. Behavioral and physiologic indicators are used to assess pain. Toddlers commonly react with intense emotional upset and physical resistance or aggression. Preschoolers may feel that pain is a punishment for misbehaving or having bad thoughts. School-age children can communicate the type, location, and severity of pain but may deny having pain to appear brave or avoid further pain. Adolescents, with their focus on body image and fear of loss of control, often ask numerous questions and may attempt to remain stoic to avoid being viewed as childish.
- Assessment of pain in children includes both subjective and objective data. Nurses need to tailor

the assessment to the child's developmental level and ask appropriate questions geared to the child's cognitive level. Parental questioning during the health history also is important.

- Self-report pain rating scales are valuable assessment tools that allow the child's level of pain to be quantified. Examples include the FACES pain rating scale, the Oucher pain rating scale, the poker chip tool, the visual analog and numeric scales, and the Adolescent Pediatric Pain Tool.
- Different pain rating scales are appropriate for different developmental levels. However, children may regress when in pain, so a simpler tool may be needed to make sure that the child understands what is being asked. Consistency in using the same tool is essential so that appropriate comparisons can be made and effective interventions can be planned and implemented.
- Physical examination of the child for pain primarily involves the skills of observation and inspection. These skills are used to assess for physiologic and behavioral changes that indicate pain. Auscultation also may be used to assess for changes in vital signs, specifically heart rate and blood pressure. Physiologic and behavioral pain assessment tools, such as the Neonatal Infant Pain Scale, Riley Infant Pain Scale, Pain Observation Scale for Young Children, CRIES Scale for Neonatal Postoperative Pain Assessment, and r-FLACC Behavioral Scale, measure specific parameters and changes that would indicate that the child is in pain.
- Nonpharmacologic pain management strategies aim to assist children in coping with pain and to give them a sense of mastery or control over the situation. These strategies may be categorized as behavioral-cognitive, in which the child focuses on a specific area or aspect rather than the pain (e.g., relaxation, distraction, imagery, biofeedback, thought stopping, and positive self-talk), or biophysical, in which the focus is on interfering with the transmission of pain impulses reaching the brain (e.g., heat and cold applications, massage, and pressure).
- The nurse plays a major role in teaching the child and family about available nonpharmacologic pain interventions, helping them choose the most appropriate and most effective methods, and ensuring that the child and parents use the method before the pain occurs as well as before it increases.
- Pharmacologic interventions involve the administration of drugs for pain relief, most commonly nonopioids and opioid analgesics. The selection of the method is determined by the drug being administered; the child's status; the type, intensity, and location of the pain; and any factors that may be influencing the child's pain. The preferred methods for administering analgesics include the oral, rectal, intravenous, or local nerve block routes; epidural administration; and moderate sedation.
- Nonopioid analgesics used to treat mild to moderate pain include acetaminophen and NSAIDs such as ibuprofen, ketorolac, naproxen, and, less commonly, indomethacin, diclofenac, and piroxicam.
- Morphine is considered the "gold standard" for all opioid agonists; it is the drug to which all other opioids are compared and is usually the drug of choice for severe pain (Oakes & D'Arcy, 2011).
- Local anesthetics are commonly used to provide analgesia for procedures. They are effective in providing successful pain relief with only minimal risk of systemic adverse effects. The first choice for the most effective, painless local anesthesia is EMLA (eutectic mixture of local anesthetics [lidocaine and prilocaine]). It achieves anesthesia to a depth of 2 to 4 mm, so it reduces pain of phlebotomy, venous cannulation, and intramuscular injections up to 24 hours after injection.
- Epidural analgesia involves the insertion of a catheter into the epidural space through which drugs can be administered as bolus injections (a one-time bolus or on an intermittent schedule), as a continuous infusion, or as PCA. Usually an opioid, such as morphine, fentanyl, or hydromorphone, is given in conjunction with a long-acting local anesthetic, such as bupivacaine.
- Moderate sedation is a medically controlled state of depressed consciousness that allows protective reflexes to be maintained so the child has the ability to maintain a patent airway and respond to physical or verbal stimulation.
- When providing pharmacologic pain relief, the nurse must adhere to the rights of medication administration and have a solid knowledge base about the medications used for pain relief and the drug's pharmacokinetics (absorption, distribution, metabolism, and excretion) and pharmacodynamics (mechanism of action, including adverse effects). Initial and ongoing assessment is crucial.
- The principles of atraumatic care guide nursing interventions for providing pain relief, especially for procedure-related pain.
- Chronic pain in children can significantly affect the child's daily life and activities as well as the family's life.

REFERENCES AND RECOMMENDED READINGS

American Academy of Pediatrics and the American Pain Society. (2001). Policy statement: The assessment and management of acute pain in infants, children, and adolescents. *Pediatrics, 108*(3), 793–797. Retrieved from http://pediatrics.aappublications.org/content/108/3/793.full

American Academy of Pediatrics, Committee on Fetus and Newborn and Section on Surgery, Section on Anesthesiology and Pain Medicine, Canadian Paediatric Society, Fetus and Newborn Committee. (2010). Policy statement. Prevention and management of pain in the Neonate: An update. *Pediatrics, 118*(5), 2231–2240. Retrieved from http://pediatrics.aappublications.org/content/118/5/2231.full.html

American Medical Association. (2013). *AMA pain management: Module 6 pain management: Pediatric pain management (continuing medical education).* Retrieved from http://www.ama-cmeonline.com/pain_mgmt/printversion/ama_painmgmt_m6.pdf

American Nurses Association (ANA). (2015). *Nursing-sensitive indicators.* Retrieved from http://nursingworld.org/MainMenuCategories/ThePracticeofProfessionalNursing/PatientSafetyQuality/Research-Measurement/The-National-Database/Nursing-Sensitive-Indicators_1

American Pain Society. (1995). *Pain: The fifth vital sign.* Los Angeles: Author.

American Pain Society. (2012). *Assessment and management of children with chronic pain: A position statement from the American pain society.* Retrieved from http://www.americanpainsociety.org/uploads/pdfs/aps12-pcp.pdf

Anand, K. J. S. (2013) *Assessment of neonatal pain.* UpToDate. Retrieved from http://www.uptodate.com/contents/assessment-of-neonatal-pain?source=search_result&search=neonatal+pain&selectedTitle=2~5#H12

Anand, K. J. S. (2014). *Prevention and treatment of neonatal pain.* UpToDate. Retrieved from http://www.uptodate.com/contents/prevention-and-treatment-of-neonatal-pain

Baker, C. M., & Wong, D. L. (1987). Q.U.E.S.T.: A process of pain assessment in children. *Orthopaedic Nursing, 6*(1), 11–21.

Bautista, C., & Grossman, S. (2014) Chapter 18: Somatosensory function, pain and headache. In S. C. Grossman & C. M. Porth (Eds.), *Porth's Pathophysiology: Concepts of altered health states* (9th ed., pp. 422–451). Philadelphia, PA: Wolters Kluwer Health/Lippincott Williams & Wilkins.

Besenski, L. J., Forsyth, S. J., & von Baeyer, C. L. (2007). Commentary: Screening young children for their ability to use self-report pain scales. *Pediatric Pain Letter. Commentaries on pain in infants, children and adolescents, 9*(1), 1–7. Retrieved from http://childpain.org/ppl/issues/v9n1_2007/v9n1_besenski.pdf

Beyer, J. E., Denyes, M. J., & Villarruel, A. M. (1992). The creation, validation, and continuing development of the Oucher: A measure of pain intensity in children. *Journal of Pediatric Nursing, 7*(5), 335–346.

Boelen-van der Loo, W. J., Scheffer, E., de Haan, R. J., & de Groot, C. J. (1999). Clinimetric evaluation of the pain observation scale for young children in children aged between 1 and 4 years after ear, nose, and throat surgery. *Journal of Developmental and Behavioral Pediatrics, 20*(4), 222–227.

Bowden, V. R., & Greenberg, C. S. (2011). *Pediatric nursing procedures* (3rd ed.). Philadelphia, PA: Lippincott Williams & Wilkins.

Buck, M. L. (2010). Promethazine: Recommendations for safe use in children. *Pediatric Pharmacotherapy, 16*(3). Retrieved from http://www.medscape.com/viewarticle/720608

Carpenito, L. J. (2013). *Nursing diagnosis: Application to clinical practice* (14th ed.). Philadelphia, PA: Lippincott Williams & Wilkins.

Cohen, M. R. (2009). *Patient-controlled analgesia: Making it safer for patients.* Retrieved from http://www.ismp.org/profdevelopment/PCAMonograph.pdf

Cohen, L. L., & Baxter, A. L. (2008). *Distraction techniques for procedural pain in children.* Retrieved from http://www.medscape.org/viewarticle/583976

Cooney, M. F., Czarnecki, M., Dunwoody, C., Eksterowicz, N., Merkel, S., Oakes, L., et al. (2013). American Society for Pain Management Nursing position statement with clinical practice guidelines: authorized agent controlled analgesia. *Pain Management Nursing, 14*(3), 176–181. doi: 10.1016/j.pmn.2013.07.003

Coté, C. J., & Wilson, S., & The Work Group on Sedation. (2011). *Guidelines for monitoring and management of pediatric patients during and after sedation for diagnostic and therapeutic procedures: An update.* Retrieved from http://pediatrics.aappublications.org/content/118/6/2587.long

Crandall, M., & Savedra, M. (2005). Multidimensional assessment using the adolescent pediatric pain tool: A case report. *Journal for Specialists in Pediatric Nursing, 10*(3), 115–123.

D'Arcy, Y. (2007). Patient safety issues with patient-controlled analgesia. *Topics in Advanced Practice Nursing eJournal, 7*(1). Retrieved from http://www.medscape.com/viewarticle/557394

D'Arcy, Y. (2011). New thinking about postoperative pain management. *OR Nurse, 5*(6), 28–36. doi: 10.1097/01.ORN.0000406638.19178.07

Finley, G. A., Franck, L. S., Grunau, R. E., & von Baeyer, C. L. (2005). Why children's pain matters. *International Association for the Study of Pain. Pain: Clinical Updates, XIII*(4), 1–6. Retrieved from http://iasp.files.cms-plus.com/Content/ContentFolders/Publications2/PainClinicalUpdates/Archives/PCU05-4_1390264071339_24.pdf

Fernandes, A. M., De Campos, C., Batalha, L., Perdigão, A., & Jacob, E. (2014). Pain assessment using the adolescent pediatric pain tool: A systematic review. *Pain Research & Management, 19*(4), 212–218.

Hand, I. L., Noble, L., Geiss, D., Wozniak, L., & Hall, C. (2010). COVERS neonatal pain scale: development and validation. *International Journal of Pediatrics, 2010*, 1–5. doi: 10.1155/2010/496719

Hatfield, L. A., Chang, K., Bittle, M., Deluca, J., & Polomano, R. C. (2011). The analgesic properties of intraoral sucrose: An integrative review. *Advances in Neonatal Care, 11*(2), 83–92. doi: 10.1097/ANC.0b013e318210d043

Hauer, J., & Jones, B. L. (2014). *Evaluation and management of pain in children.* Retrieved from http://www.uptodate.com/contents/evaluation-and-management-of-pain-in-children?source=search_result&search=r+flacc&selectedTitle=1~2

Hester, N. K. (1979). The preoperational child's reaction to immunization. *Nursing Research, 28*(4), 250–255.

Hockenberry, M. J., & Wilson, D. (2009). *Wong's essentials of pediatric nursing* (8th ed., p. 162). St. Louis: Elsevier Mosby.

Hsu, D. C. (2014). *Topical anesthetics in children.* UpToDateuptodate. Retrieved from http://www.uptodate.com/contents/topical-anesthetics-in-children?source=machineLearning&search=EMLA&selectedTitle=5~49§ionRank=2&anchor=H11#H11

Hsu, D. C., & Cravero, J. P. (2014). Procedural sedation in children outside of the operating room. Retrieved from http://www.uptodate.com/contents/procedural-sedation-in-children-outside-of-the-operating-room?source=see_link&anchor=H1684879#H1684879

International Association for the Study of Pain. (2012). *IASP Taxonomy.* Retrieved from http://www.iasp-pain.org/Education/Content.aspx?ItemNumber=1698#Pain

Kaiser, S. V., Asteria-Penaloza, R., Vittinghoff, E., Rosenbluth, G., Cabana, M. D., & Bardach, N. S. (2014). National patterns of codeine prescriptions for children in the emergency department. *Pediatrics, 133*(5), e1139–e1147. doi: 10.1542/peds.2013–317

Kennedy, R. M., Luhmann, J., & Zempsky, W. T. (2008). Clinical implications of unmanaged needle-insertion pain and distress in children. *Pediatrics, 122*(Suppl 3), S130–S133. doi: 10.1542/peds.2008–1055e

Krechel, S. W., & Bildner, J. (1995). CRIES: A new neonatal postoperative pain measurement score. Initial testing of validity and reliability. *Paediatric Anaesthesia, 5*, 53–61.

Lawrence, J., Alcock, D., McGrath, P., Kay, J., MacMurray, S. B., & Dulberg, C. (1993). The development of a tool to assess neonatal pain. *Neonatal Network, 12*(6), 59–66.

Mann, A. (2014). *Patient-controlled analgesia: This mode of pain control involves careful selection, appropriate dosing and education. ADVANCE for Nurses.* Retrieved from http://nursing.advanceweb.com/article/patient-controlled-analgesia.aspx

Manworren, R. C., & Hynan, L. S. (2003). Clinical validation of FLACC: Preverbal patient pain scale. *Pediatric Nursing, 29*(2), 140–146.

Martin, S., & Cohen, L. L. (2012). Psychological approaches to pediatric pain relief. In A. M. Columbus (Ed.), *Advances in psychology research*, Vol. 89, (pp. 115–130). New York, NY: Nova Science Publishers.

McCaffery, M. (1968). *Nursing practice theories related to cognition, bodily pain and main environment interactions.* Los Angeles: University of California Los Angeles.

McCaffery, M., & Pasero, C. (2011). *Pain assessment and pharmacologic management.* St. Louis: Mosby.

McCarthy, A. M., & Kleiber, C. (2006). A conceptual model of factors influencing children's responses to a painful procedure when parents are distraction coaches. *Journal of Pediatric Nursing, 21*(2), 88–98.

McCarthy A. M., Kleiber, C., Hanrahan, K., Zimmerman, M. B., Westhus, N., & Allen, S. (2010). Factors explaining children's responses to intravenous needle insertions. *Nursing Research, 59*(6), 407–416. doi: 10.1097/NNR.0b013e3181f80ed5

McGrath, P. A. (2005). Children—not simply "little adults." In H. Merskey, J. D. Loeser, & R. Dubner (Eds.), *The paths of pain 1975–2005* (pp. 433–446). Seattle: IASP Press.

Merkel, S. I., Voepel-Lewis, T., Shayevitz, J. R., & Malviya, S. (1997). The FLACC: A behavioral scale for scoring postoperative pain in young children. *Pediatric Nursing, 23*(3), 293–297.

Naughton, K. A., & Ikuta, L. (2013). The combined use of sucrose and nonnutritive sucking for procedural pain in both term and preterm neonates: An integrative review of the literature. *Advances in Neonatal Care, 13*(1), 9–19.

Oakes, L., & D'Arcy, Y. (2011). *Compact clinical guide to infant and child pain management. An evidence-based approach for nurses.* New York, NY: Springer Publishing Company, LLC.

Pawar, D., & Garten, L. (2010). Chapter 34: Pain management in children. In A. Kopf & N. B. Patel (Eds.), *Guide to pain management in low-resource settings,* (pp.255–268). Seattle: International Association for the Study of Pain.

Schade, J. G., Joyce, B. A., Gerkensmeyer, J., & Keck, J. F. (1996). Comparison of three preverbal scales for postoperative pain assessment in a diverse pediatric sample. *Journal of Pain and Symptom Management, 12*(6), 348–359.

Society of Pediatric Psychology. (2014). *Assessment resource sheet: Pediatric pain.* Retrieved from http://www.apadivisions.org/division-54/evidence-based/pain-assessment.aspx

Sutters, K. A., Miaskowski, C., Holdridge-Zeuner, D., Waite, S., Paul, S. M., Savedra, M. C., et al. (2010). A randomized clinical trial of the efficacy of scheduled dosing of acetaminophen and hydrocodone for the management of postoperative pain in children after tonsillectomy. *Clinical Journal of Pain, 26*(2), 95–103.

Taddio, A., Soin, H. K., Schuh, S., Koren, G., & Scolnik, D. (2005). Liposomal lidocaine to improve procedural success rates and reduce procedural pain among children: A randomized controlled trial. *Canadian Medical Association Journal, 172*(13), 1691–1695.

Taketomo, C. K., Hodding, J. H., & Kraus, D. M. (2013). *Lexi-comp's drug reference handbook: pediatric & neonatal dosage handbook* (20th ed.). Hudson, OH: Lexi-comp, Inc.

The Hospital for Sick Children. (2005). *Myths vs facts of children's pain.* Retrieved from http://www.iasp-pain.org/files/Content/ContentFolders/GlobalYearAgainstPain2/20052006PaininChildren/pdfist.pdf

The Joint Commission. (2004). *Sentinel event alert. Patient controlled analgesia by proxy.* Retrieved from http://www.jointcommission.org/assets/1/18/SEA_33.PDF

Vargas-Schaffer, G. (2010). Is the WHO analgesic ladder still valid? Twenty-four years of experience. *Canadian Family Physician, 56*(6), 514–517. Retrieved from http://www.ncbi.nlm.nih.gov/pmc/articles/PMC2902929/

von Baeyer, C. L. (2006). Children's self-reports of pain intensity: Scale selection, limitations, and interpretation. *Pain Research and Management, 11*(3), 157–162.

von Baeyer, C. L. (2014). Chapter 36: Self report: The primary source of assessment after infancy. In P. J. McGrath, B. J. Stevens, S. M. Walker, & W. T. Zempsky (Eds.), *Oxford textbook of paediatric pain* (pp. 370–378). United Kingdom: Oxford University Press.

Walden, M. (2014). Chapter 23: Pain in the newborn and infant. In C. Kenner & J. W. Lott (Eds.), *Comprehensive neonatal nursing care.* (5th ed., pp. 571–586), New York, NY: Springer Publishing Company.

Weissman, A., Aranovitch, M., Blazer, S., & Zimmer, E. Z. (2009). Heel-lancing in newborns: Behavioral and spectral analysis assessment of pain control methods. *Pediatrics, 124*(5), e921–e926. doi: 10.1542/peds.2009–0598

World Health Organization. (2012). *WHO guidelines on the pharmacological treatment of persisting pain in children with medical illnesses*. Retrieved from http://whqlibdoc.who.int/publications/2012/9789241548120_Guidelines.pdf?ua=1

Zeltzer, L. K., & Krane, E. J. (2011). Chapter 71: Pediatric pain management. In R. M. Kleigman, B. F. Stanton, J. W. St. Geme III, N. F. Schor, & R. E. Behrman (Eds.), *Nelson textbook of pediatrics* (19th ed., pp.360–375). Philadelphia, PA: Saunders.

Zempsky, W. T. (2008). Pharmacologic approaches for reducing venous access pain in children. *Pediatrics, 122*, S140–S153. Retrieved from http://pediatrics.aappublications.org/cgi/content/full/122/Supplement_3/S140

Zempsky, W. T., Bean-Lijewski, J., Kauffman, R. E., Koh, J. L., Malviya, S. V., Rose, J. B., et al. (2008). Needle-free powder lidocaine delivery system provides rapid effective analgesia for venipuncture or cannulation pain in children: Randomized, double-blind comparison of venipuncture and venous cannulation pain after fast-onset needle-free powder lidocaine or placebo treatment trial. *Pediatrics, 121*(5), 979–987. Retrieved from http://pediatrics.aappublications.org/cgi/content/abstract/121/5/979

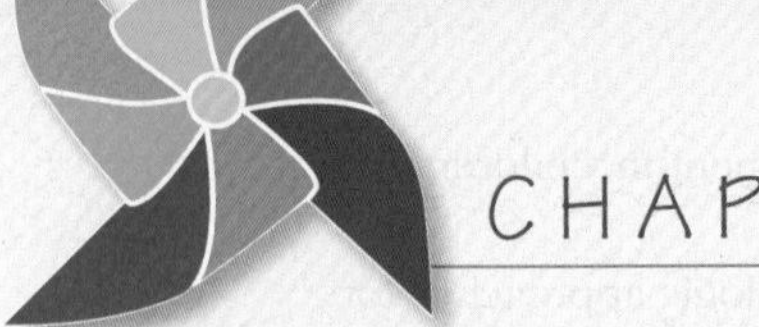

CHAPTER WORKSHEET

MULTIPLE CHOICE QUESTIONS

1. The nurse is preparing to assess the pain of a 3-year-old child who had surgery the day before. Which pain assessment method would be most appropriate for the nurse to use?
   a. FACES pain rating scale and poker chip tool
   b. FACES pain rating scale, observation of the child, and parent report
   c. Asking the parents to rate their child's pain using the word-graphic rating scale
   d. Visual analog scale
2. When developing the plan of care for a child in pain, the nurse identifies appropriate strategies aimed at modifying which factor influencing pain?
   a. Gender
   b. Cognitive level
   c. Previous pain experiences
   d. Anticipatory anxiety
3. An adolescent who is a competitive swimmer comes to the emergency department complaining of localized aching pain in his shoulder. He states, "I've been practicing really hard and long to get myself ready for my meet this weekend." The area is tender to the touch. The nurse determines that the adolescent is most likely experiencing which type of pain?
   a. Cutaneous pain
   b. Deep somatic pain
   c. Visceral pain
   d. Neuropathic pain
4. After teaching a child's parents about the different methods of distraction that can be used for pain management, which statement by the parents indicates a need for additional teaching?
   a. "We'll have her focus on her hand and count each finger slowly."
   b. "We'll read some of her favorite stories to her."
   c. "We'll have her imagine that she's at the beach this summer."
   d. "She likes to play video games, so we'll bring in some from home."
5. A child is scheduled for a bone marrow aspiration at 4 PM. The nurse would plan to apply EMLA cream to the intended site at which time?
   a. 1:30 PM
   b. 3:00 PM
   c. 3:30 PM
   d. 4:00 PM

CRITICAL THINKING EXERCISES

1. The nurse asks a 12-year-old girl if she is having pain. She denies pain, even though she is lying on her left side holding her abdomen with her knees flexed up to it. What might be some underlying factors leading the child to deny her pain? How would the nurse go about assessing this child's pain?
2. The nurse comes into the room of a 6-year-old who is sleeping. His mother states, "He's asleep, so he's not in pain." How should the nurse respond?
3. A child who is receiving ibuprofen is experiencing increased pain. The dosage of ibuprofen is increased but is no longer effective in providing adequate pain relief. What is occurring? What would be most likely to happen next?

STUDY ACTIVITIES

1. Interview nurses who work on a pediatric unit about their experiences with managing pain in children. Ask them how they assess pain in children and the major methods they use to assist the children in managing their pain.
2. Interview families of children with chronic illnesses who deal with pain. Ask the parents how they assess their children's pain level and what methods they have used in assisting their children in managing pain.
3. Compare and contrast the drugs fentanyl and midazolam when used for moderate sedation in terms of onset of action, duration, primary effects, and antidotes.
4. A child is receiving epidural analgesia with morphine. The nurse would be alert for which of the following adverse effects? Select all that apply.
   _____ a. Respiratory depression
   _____ b. Pruritus
   _____ c. Constipation
   _____ d. Vomiting
   _____ e. Amnesia
   _____ f. Hematoma

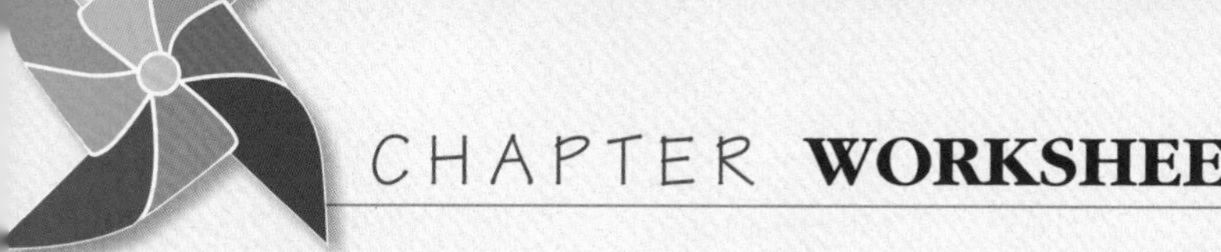

CHAPTER WORKSHEET

DOSAGE CALCULATION

After you have performed your nonpharmacologic interventions, your patient, who is an infant, is exhibiting kicking, is not reaching for toys, and is occasionally crying. There is an order for morphine sulfate 1 mg IV every 3 to 4 hours. The safe dose range for morphine sulfate is 0.1 to 0.2 mg/kg/dose every 3 to 4 hours. Morphine sulfate is supplied as 1 mg/mL.

1. Is this a safe dose?
2. Describe how you will administer this medication and what would you assess for after giving it.

BRINGING IT ALL TOGETHER: A CASE STUDY

You are caring for Chantal, a 7-month-old infant, during the postoperative period. She weighs 17 lb and is 26.5 in long. During your assessment you find her current vital signs are as follows: temperature 37.1°C, heart rate 150, respiratory rate 32. Her behaviors include restlessness, moving a lot around the crib, and looking at her mother when the mother sings to her.

Go to thePoint to find questions to consider about this case.

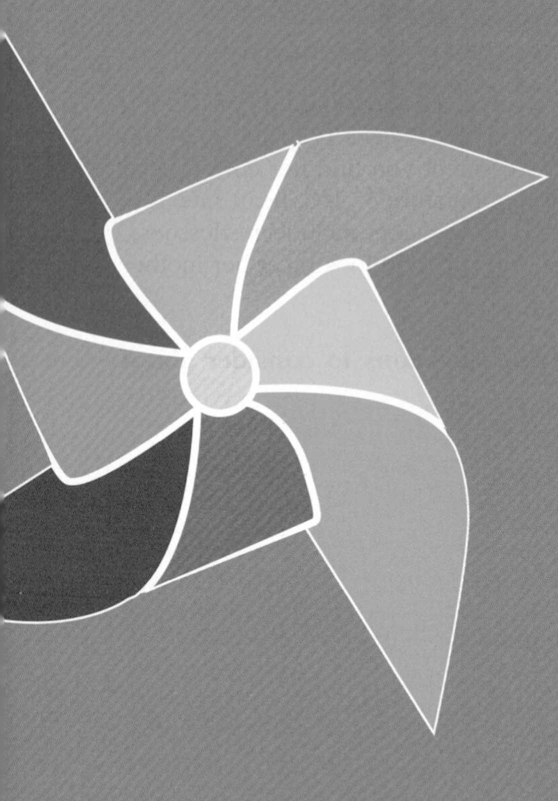

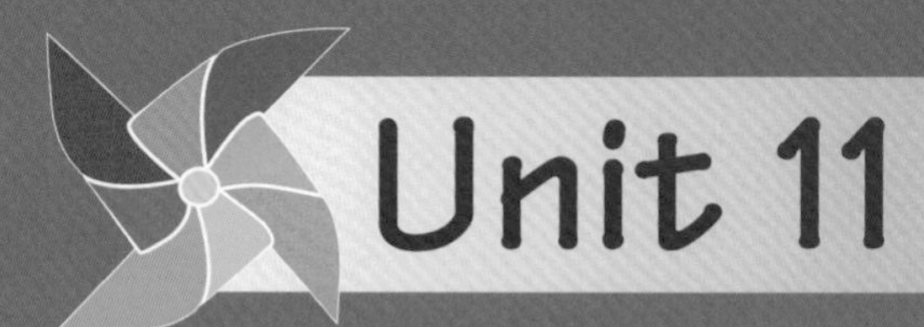

Nursing Care of the Child With a Health Disorder

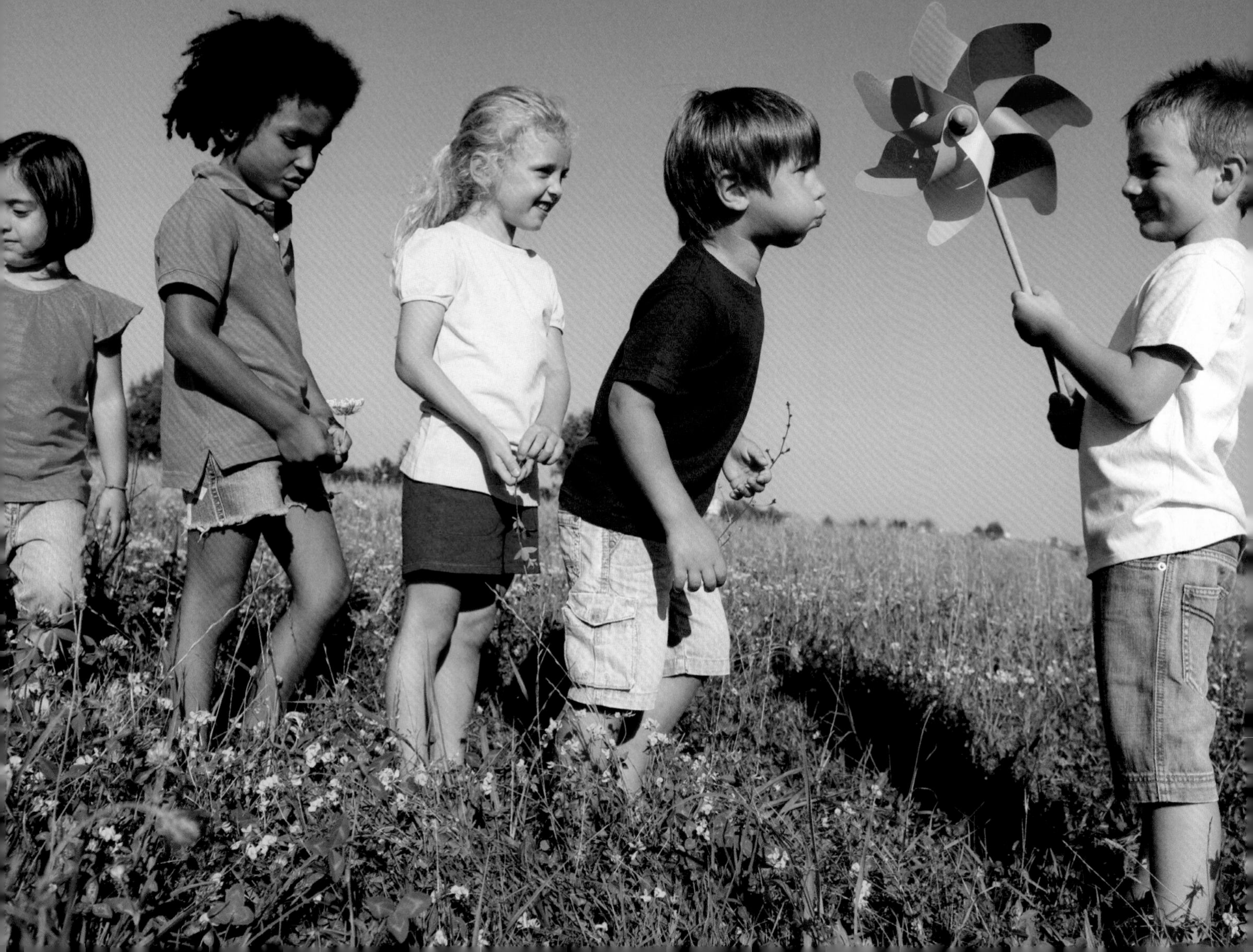

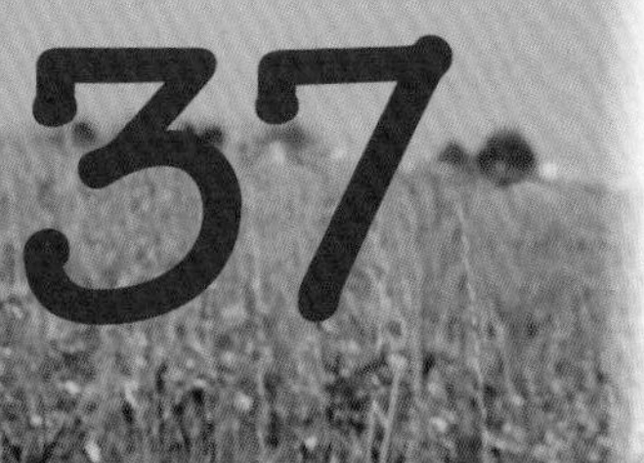

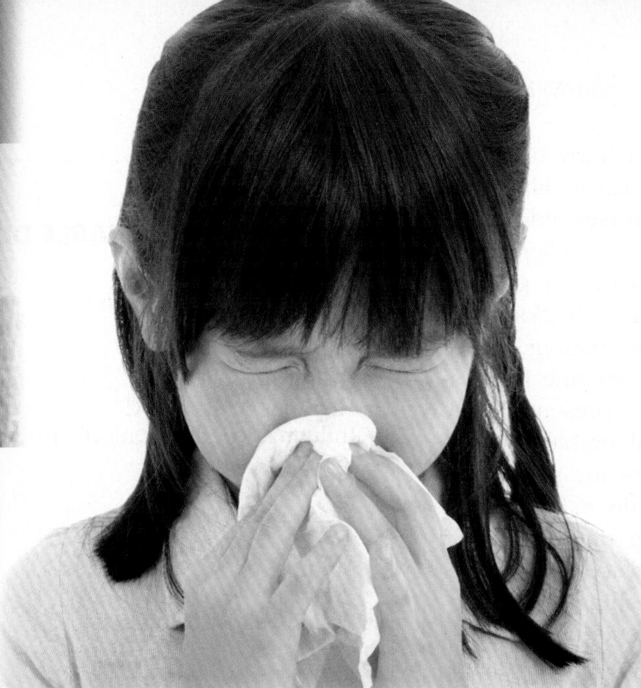

WOW

Words of Wisdom

Complete and lasting freedom from infectious disease remains a dream, but one worth fighting a hard battle for.

37 Nursing Care of the Child With an Infectious or Communicable Disorder

KEY TERMS

antibodies
antigen
chain of infection
communicability
endogenous pyrogens
exanthem
phagocytosis
vector-borne
zoonotic

Learning Objectives

Upon completion of the chapter, you will be able to:

1. Discuss anatomic and physiologic differences in children versus adults in relation to the infectious process.
2. Identify nursing interventions related to common laboratory and diagnostic tests used in the diagnosis and management of infectious conditions.
3. Identify appropriate nursing assessments and interventions related to medications and treatments for childhood infectious and communicable disorders.
4. Distinguish various infectious illnesses occurring in childhood.
5. Devise an individualized nursing care plan for the child with an infectious or communicable disorder.
6. Develop child/family teaching plans for the child with an infectious or communicable disorder.

Mrs. Goldberg **brings her son Samuel, 3 months old, to the clinic. He presents with a history of fever and nasal congestion. His mother tells you, "He's been very irritable and crying more than usual."**

Infection refers to the invasion of body tissue by microorganisms with the potential to cause illness or disease (Pearson Education, 2015). Nurses encounter potential or actual infections in all types of clients and must detect problems and intervene early to prevent life-threatening complications. Infections (infectious and communicable diseases) are one of the leading causes of death worldwide. As the world has become increasingly connected, infectious diseases have presented new challenges. Children are particularly vulnerable to these types of illnesses. Their immune systems are still developing and their natural curiosity, especially in infants and toddlers, leads to wide-range handling of objects and surfaces coupled with a tendency to place their hands and objects in their mouths without washing first. Infectious diseases in children can range in severity from mild with few or no symptoms to serious illness, such as damage to organs, and even death. Infectious and communicable diseases include bacterial infections (e.g., sepsis), viral infections (e.g., viral exanthems and rabies), zoonotic infections, vector-borne infections, parasitic and helminthic infections (e.g., roundworm and pediculosis capitis [head lice]), and sexually transmitted infections (e.g., chlamydia and gonorrhea) (refer to Chapter 5 for information on sexually transmitted infections).

There has been a dramatic decrease in the incidence and severity of infectious and communicable diseases since the advent of vaccines, antibiotics, antiviral drugs, and antitoxins (Interaction, 2013). Some diseases have been effectively controlled, but the vast majority will not be eliminated. New diseases emerge and old diseases are reappearing, sometimes in a drug-resistant form. The Centers for Disease Control and Prevention (CDC) tracks certain infectious diseases. This list of nationally reportable diseases is revised periodically to add new pathogens or remove diseases as their incidence declines. Reporting by each state to the CDC is voluntary. Therefore, slight variations exist from state to state. Box 37.1 lists nationally reportable diseases.

Nurses, particularly those working in schools, child care centers, and outpatient settings, are often the first to see the signs of infectious or communicable diseases in children. These signs are often vague at first (e.g., a sore throat or rash). Therefore, nurses must have accurate assessment skills and be familiar with the signs and symptoms of common childhood infectious diseases so that they can provide prompt recognition, treatment, guidance, and support to families. Identifying the infectious agent is of primary importance to prevent further spread.

Many infectious diseases can be prevented through simple and inexpensive methods such as handwashing, adequate immunization, proper handling and preparation of food, and judicious antibiotic use. Nurses play a key role in educating parents and the community on ways to prevent infectious and communicable diseases.

BOX 37.1

NATIONALLY NOTIFIABLE DISEASES

- Botulism
- *Chlamydia trachomatis*
- Diphtheria
- Ehrlichiosis
- Gonorrhea
- Hepatitis A, B, and C
- Influenza (pediatric mortality)
- Lyme disease
- Malaria
- Measles
- *Meningococcus*
- Mumps
- Pertussis
- Poliomyelitis, paralytic
- Q fever
- Rabies
- Rocky Mountain spotted fever (spotted fever rickettsiosis)
- Rubella
- Streptococcal disease, invasive group A
- Syphilis
- Tetanus
- Tuberculosis
- Varicella (morbidity)
- Varicella (deaths only)

For a complete list of nationally notifiable diseases in the United States, go to http://wwwn.cdc.gov/nndss/conditions/notifiable/2015/infectious-diseases/

INFECTIOUS PROCESS

Infection occurs when an organism enters the body and multiplies, causing damage to the tissues and cells. The body's response to this damage due to infection or injury is inflammation. The body delivers fluid, blood, and nutrients to the area of infection or injury and attempts to eliminate the pathogens and repair the tissues. The body

HEALTHY PEOPLE *2020*

Objective	Nursing Significance
Reduce, eliminate, or maintain elimination of cases of vaccine-preventable diseases	• Educate children and their families on the importance of proper immunizations.
Achieve and maintain effective vaccination coverage levels for universally recommended vaccines among young children	• Assess immunization status at every healthy encounter. • Provide families with a written record of immunizations given.

Healthy People Objectives retrieved from http://www.healthypeople.gov

TABLE 37.1 FUNCTION OF WHITE BLOOD CELLS BY LEUKOCYTE TYPE

Type of White Blood Cell	Function
Granulocytes • Neutrophils (polymorphonuclear leukocytes or PMNs, segs) • Eosinophils • Basophils	Phagocytic cells • First line of defense upon invasion of bacteria, fungus, cell debris, and other foreign substances • Respond to allergic disorders and parasitic infections • Respond to allergic disorders and hypersensitivity reactions; used to study chronic inflammation
Lymphocytes (B lymphocytes, T lymphocytes, and natural killer cells)	Main source of producing an immune response; respond to viral infections (measles, rubella, chickenpox, infectious mononucleosis); tumors
Monocytes	Second line of defense; respond to larger and more severe infections than neutrophils by phagocytosis; leukemias and lymphomas; chronic inflammation

Adapted from Fischbach, F. T., & Dunning III, M. B. (2015). *A manual of laboratory and diagnostic tests* (9th ed., pp. 67–88). Philadelphia, PA: Wolters Kluwer/Lippincott Williams & Wilkins; and Grossman, S. (2014). Chapter 25: Blood cells and the hematopoietic system. In S. Grossman & C. M. Porth (Eds.), *Porth's Pathophysiology: Concepts of altered health states* (9th ed., pp. 638–664). Philadelphia, PA: Wolters Kluwer Health/Lippincott Williams & Wilkins.

does this through vascular and cellular reactions. The vascular response is an initial period of vasoconstriction followed by vasodilatation. This vasodilatation allows for the increase of fluids, blood, and nutrients to the area.

The cellular response involves the arrival of white blood cells (WBCs) to the area. WBCs are the body's defense against infection or injury. The types of WBCs are neutrophils, basophils, eosinophils, lymphocytes, and monocytes. Elevations in certain portions of the WBC count reflect different processes occurring in the body, such as infection, allergic reaction, or leukemia. Table 37.1 explains the function of each type of WBC. Each type is generally present in a balanced state; the types are reported as a percentage of the total WBC count or as the number per certain volume of blood.

WBCs use **phagocytosis** to ingest and destroy the pathogen. If bacteria escape the action of phagocytosis, they enter the bloodstream and lymph system and the immune system is activated. With activation of the immune system, B lymphocytes (humoral immunity) and T lymphocytes (cell-mediated immunity) are matured and activated. B and T cells recognize and attack infectious pathogens. B cells, which mature in the bone marrow, produce specific **antibodies** (specialized immune proteins) that bind to and neutralize a specific offending **antigen** (a substance that the body recognizes as foreign). T cells, which mature in the thymus, attack the antigen directly. Once B and T cells have been exposed to an antigen, some cells will remember the antigen. Therefore, if the particular antigen invades again, the body will act more quickly. A third type of lymphocyte, natural killer cells are a part of the innate immune system and function to destroy foreign material present.

Fever

Infection or inflammation caused by bacteria, viruses, or other pathogens stimulates the release of **endogenous pyrogens** (interleukins, tumor necrosis factor, and interferon). The pyrogens act on the hypothalamus, where they trigger prostaglandin production and increase the body's temperature set point. This triggers the cold response, resulting in shivering, vasoconstriction, and a decrease in peripheral perfusion to help decrease heat loss and allow the body's temperature to rise to the new set point therefore resulting in fever. The definition of fever varies based on the age of the child, the method of temperature measurement, and the presence of any underlying conditions. There is no single value defined for fever due to individual variations but Box 37.2 shows generally accepted guidelines based on measurement route in an otherwise healthy child. Refer to Chapter 32 for further information on measurement of temperature.

Antipyretics are often used to lower fever and increase comfort. They decrease the temperature set point by inhibiting the production of prostaglandins. As

BOX 37.2

GENERAL GUIDELINE OF FEVER BASED ON MEASUREMENT ROUTE

- Oral: >37.8°C (100°F)
- Rectal: >38°C (100.4°F)
- Axillary: >37.2°C (99°F)
- Tympanic: >38°C (100.4°F)
- Temporal: >38°C (100.4°F)

a result, sweating and vasodilation occur and there is heat loss and a drop in temperature.

It is important to distinguish between fever and hyperthermia. Hyperthermia occurs when normal thermoregulation fails, resulting in an unregulated rise in core temperature. Hyperthermia may occur if the central nervous system of the child becomes impaired by disease, drugs, and abnormalities of heat production or thermal stressors, such as being left in a hot automobile or exertional heat stroke. In the absence of hyperthermia and in the normally neurologic child, the body does not allow fever to rise to lethal levels. The body actually produces a natural antipyretic, called cryogen. If there is no hyperthermic insult, it is rare to see a child's temperature rise above 41°C (105.8°F) (Ward, 2015a).

Stages of Infectious Disease

Infectious diseases follow a similar pattern. They progress through certain stages (Table 37.2) in which **communicability** (ability to spread to others) can be predicted. It is important for nurses to understand these stages to help control and manage infectious diseases.

Chain of Infection

The **chain of infection** is the process by which an organism is spread. Behaviors of infants and young children, mainly pertaining to hygiene, increase their risk for infection by promoting the chain of infection. Poor hygiene habits, including lack of handwashing, placing toys and hands in the mouth, drooling, and leaking diapers, all can contribute to the spread of infection and communicable diseases. Table 37.3 reviews the chain of infection and nursing implications related to it.

TABLE 37.2 STAGES OF INFECTIOUS DISEASE

Stage	Explanation
Incubation	Time from entrance of pathogen into the body to appearance of first symptoms; during this time, pathogens grow and multiply
Prodrome	Time from onset of nonspecific symptoms such as fever, malaise, and fatigue to more specific symptoms
Illness	Time during which child demonstrates signs and symptoms specific to an infection type
Convalescence	Time when acute symptoms of illness disappear

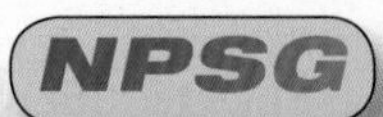

GOAL 7: Reduce the Risk of Healthcare–Associated Infections

NPSG.07.03.01 Implement evidence-based practices to prevent healthcare–associated infections due to multidrug-resistant organisms in acute care hospitals. Note: This requirement applies to, but is not limited to, epidemiologically important organisms such as methicillin-resistant staphylococcus aureus (MRSA), clostridium difficile (CDI), vancomycin-resistant enterococci (VRE), and multidrug-resistant gram-negative bacteria.

Steps: Follow strategies to break the chain of infection and prevent the spread of infection among hospitalized children

Joint Commission. (2015). *National patient safety goals effective January 1, 2015.* Retrieved from http://www.jointcommission.org/assets/1/6/2015_NPSG_HAP.pdf

Preventing the Spread of Infection

Nurses play a key role in breaking the chain of infection and preventing the spread of diseases. It is important to follow infection control and prevention practices. It is also very important to educate parents and children on the measures they can take to prevent the spread of infection.

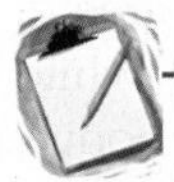

Take Note!

Frequent handwashing is the most important way to prevent the spread of infection.

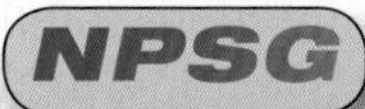

GOAL 7: Reduce the Risk of Healthcare–Associated Infections

NPSG.07.01.01 Comply with either the current Centers for Disease Control and Prevention (CDC) hand hygiene guidelines or the current World Health Organization (WHO) hand hygiene guidelines

Steps: When caring for a child perform proper handwashing before and after all care.

Joint Commission. (2015). *National patient safety goals effective January 1, 2015.* Retrieved from http://www.jointcommission.org/assets/1/6/2015_NPSG_HAP.pdf

Isolation precautions help nurses break the chain of infection and provide strategies to prevent the spread of pathogens among hospitalized children. Guidelines can be found on the CDC website (http://www.cdc.gov/hicpac/2007IP/2007isolationPrecautions.html). Additional guidelines are available from various infection control societies and regulatory agencies such as the Occupational Safety and Health Administration (OSHA) agency. The Joint Commission has also developed infection control standards. This leads to an array of complex guidelines that all health professionals need to be familiar with.

TABLE 37.3 CHAIN OF INFECTION

Chain Link	Explanation	Nursing Implications
Infectious agent	Any agent capable of causing infection; examples: bacteria, viruses, rickettsiae, protozoa, and fungi	Control or eliminate infectious agents through: • Handwashing • Wearing gloves • Cleaning, disinfecting, or sterilizing equipment
Reservoir	A place where the pathogen can thrive and reproduce; examples: human body, animals, insects, food, water, inanimate objects (e.g., stethoscopes)	• Control or eliminate reservoirs. • Control sources of body fluids, drainage, or solutions that may harbor pathogens. • Follow institutional guidelines for disposing of infectious wastes. • Provide proper wound care; change dressings or bandages when soiled. • Assist children to carry out appropriate skin and oral care. • Keep linens clean and dry.
Portal of exit	A way for the pathogen to exit the reservoir; examples: skin and mucous membranes, respiratory tract, urinary tract, gastrointestinal tract, reproductive tract	• Control portals of exit and educate children and families. • Cover mouth and nose when sneezing or coughing. • Avoid talking, coughing, or sneezing over open wounds or sterile fields. • Use personal protective equipment.
Modes of transmission	Direct transmission: body-to-body contact Indirect transmission: transferred by fomite or vector; spread by droplet or air-borne transmission	• Wash hands before and after child contact, invasive procedures, or touching open wounds. • Use personal protective equipment when necessary. • Urge children and family to wash hands frequently, especially before eating or handling food, after eliminating, and after touching infectious material.
Portal of entry	A way for the pathogen to enter the host; examples: skin and mucous membranes, respiratory tract, urinary tract, gastrointestinal tract, reproductive tract	• Use proper sterile technique during invasive procedures. • Provide appropriate wound care. • Dispose of needles and sharps in puncture-resistant containers. • Provide all children with their own personal care items.
Susceptible host	Any person who cannot resist the pathogen	• Protect susceptible host by promoting normal body defenses against infection. • Maintain integrity of the child's skin and mucous membranes. • Protect normal defenses by regular bathing and oral care, adequate fluid intake and nutrition, and proper immunization.

The Hospital Infection Control Practices Advisory Committee (HICPAC) has presented guidelines for hospitalized children that include two tiers (Siegel, Rhinehart, Jackson, Chiarello, & The Healthcare Infection Control Practices Advisory Committee, 2007). Tier 1 is standard precautions, which are designed for the care of all children in the hospital regardless of their diagnosis. Tier 2 is transmission-based precautions, designed for children who are known, or suspected, to be infected with epidemiologically important pathogens. These pathogens can be spread by air-borne, droplet, or contact transmission. Box 37.3 gives an overview of standard and transmission-based precautions.

> ***Take Note!***
>
> *Hand hygiene includes both handwashing with soap and water and the use of alcohol-based products (gels, rinses, foams) that do not require water. If there is no visible soiling of the hands, approved alcohol-based products are preferred because of their superior microbicidal activity, reduced drying of the skin, and convenience (World Health Organization, 2009).*

When caring for children, these guidelines may need to be modified. For instance, diaper changing is routine in the pediatric setting. Since it does not usually soil hands, it is not mandatory to wear gloves (except if

BOX 37.3

STANDARD PRECAUTIONS AND ISOLATION PRECAUTIONS

Standard Precautions (Tier One)

- Apply to all children
- Apply to all body fluids, secretions, and excretions except sweat, nonintact skin, and mucous membranes
- Designed to reduce the risk of transmission of microorganisms from recognized and unrecognized sources
- Techniques include:
  - Proper hand hygiene
  - Use of gloves (clean or sterile) when touching blood, body fluids, secretions or excretions, and contaminated items
  - Masks, eye protection, and face shields when patient care may include splashing or sprays of blood, body fluid secretions, or excretions, and during bronchoscopy, endotracheal intubation, and open suctioning of the respiratory tract
  - Fluid-resistant nonsterile gowns, to protect skin and clothing, when patient care may include splashing or sprays of blood, body fluid secretions, or excretions
  - Patient care equipment handled in a manner that prevents skin or mucous membrane exposure and contamination of clothing
  - All used linen is considered contaminated and needs to be handled and disposed of appropriately
  - Mouthpieces, resuscitation bags with one-way valves, and other ventilation devices should be readily available
  - Cleaning and disinfecting noncritical surfaces in patient care areas
  - Respiratory hygiene/cough etiquette: applies to any person with signs of illness including cough, congestion, rhinorrhea, or increased respiratory secretions that is entering a healthcare facility. It includes education regarding covering the mouth/nose with a tissue; prompt disposal of used tissues, along with surgical masks used by a person who is coughing when appropriate; hand hygiene after contact with respiratory secretions; and separation, ideally greater than 3 ft, of persons with respiratory infections in common waiting areas when possible
  - Safe injection practices: use of sterile single-use disposable needle. When possible use of single-dose vials; precautions used to prevent injury when using, cleaning, or disposing of needles and sharps
  - Use of masks for insertion of catheters or injection into the spinal or epidural space via lumbar puncture procedures

Transmission-Based Precautions (Tier Two)

Designed for children with known or suspected infection with pathogens for which additional precautions are warranted to interrupt transmission

Air-Borne

- Designed to reduce the risk of infectious agents transmitted by air-borne droplet nuclei or dust particles that may contain the infectious agent.
- Examples of such illnesses include measles, varicella, and tuberculosis.
- Techniques include standard precautions as well as:
  - Room with negative air pressure ventilation, with air externally exhausted or high-efficiency particulate air filtered if recirculated; if unavailable, mask the child and place in private room with the door closed.
  - Wear a mask or respirator depending on specific recommendations based on disease, such as if infectious pulmonary tuberculosis is suspected or proven, wear a respiratory protective device, such as an N95 respirator, while in the child's room.
  - Susceptible healthcare personnel should not enter the room of children with measles or varicella zoster infections. Those with proven immunity to these viruses need not wear a mask.

Droplet

- Intended to prevent transmission of pathogens spread through close respiratory or mucous membrane contact with respiratory secretions. Designed to reduce the risk of infectious agents transmitted by contact of the conjunctivae or the mucous membranes of the nose or mouth of a susceptible person with large-particle droplets containing pathogens generated from a person (generally through coughing, sneezing, talking, or procedures such as suctioning) who has a clinical disease or who is a carrier of the disease.
- Examples of such illnesses include diphtheria, pertussis, streptococcal group A, influenza, mumps, rubella, and scarlet fever.
- Techniques include standard precautions as well as:
  - Private room (if unavailable, consider cohorting children with the same disease. If this is not possible, separation of at least 3 ft between other children and visitors should be maintained.)
  - Wear a mask if within 3 ft of the child.

Contact

- Most important and most common route of transmission of healthcare–associated infections
- Designed to reduce the risk of infectious agents transmitted by direct or indirect contact. Direct-contact transmission involves skin-to-skin contact and physical transfer of pathogens between a susceptible host and an infected or colonized person. Examples include patient care activities that involve physical contact such as turning and bathing. Direct-contact transmission also can occur between two children, where one serves as the source of infectious pathogen and the other as a susceptible host. Indirect-contact transmission involves contact of a susceptible host with a contaminated intermediate object, usually inanimate, in the child's environment.
- Examples of such illnesses include diphtheria,[a] pediculosis, scabies, and multidrug-resistant bacteria.

- Techniques include standard precautions as well as:
  - Private room (if unavailable, consultation with infection control personnel is recommended. Consider cohorting children with the same disease. If this is not possible, separation of at least 3 ft between other children and visitors should be maintained.)
  - Gloves (clean or sterile) should be used at all times.
  - Proper hand hygiene after glove removal
  - Use gloves and gowns for all interactions that involve contact with the child or potentially contaminated areas. Don before entering and remove before leaving the child's room.

Prevention standards are applied in all healthcare settings and are modified to meet each setting's unique needs. Healthcare workers must practice within the specific institution's guidelines.

[a]Certain infections require more than one precaution.

Adapted from Siegel, J. D., Rhinehart, E., Jackson, M., Chiarello, L., and the Healthcare Infection Control Practices Advisory Committee. (2007). *Guideline for isolation precautions: Preventing transmission of infectious agents in healthcare settings.* Retrieved from http://www.cdc.gov/hicpac/pdf/isolation/Isolation2007.pdf

gloves are required due to transmission-based precautions). According to the standard precaution guidelines, single rooms are required for those who are incontinent and cannot control bodily excretions. Since the majority of young children are incontinent, obviously this guideline is inappropriate in the pediatric setting. Pediatric units often have common rooms, such as playrooms and schoolrooms. Children placed on transmission-based isolation are not allowed to leave their rooms and therefore are not allowed to use these common rooms.

VARIATIONS IN PEDIATRIC ANATOMY AND PHYSIOLOGY

Normal immune function is an amazing protective response by the body. It involves complex responses including phagocytosis, humoral immunity, cellular immunity, and activation of the complement system. Blood and lymph are responsible for transporting the agents of the immune system. Due to the immature responses of the immune system, infants and young children are more susceptible to infection. The newborn displays a decreased inflammatory response to invading organisms, contributing to an increased risk for infection. Cellular immunity is generally functional at birth, and humoral immunity occurs when the body encounters and then develops immunity to new diseases. Since the infant has had limited exposure to disease and is losing the passive immunity acquired from maternal antibodies, the risk of infection is higher. Young children continue to have an increased risk for infection and communicable disorders because disease protection from immunizations is not complete. (Refer to Chapter 31 for further details.)

COMMON MEDICAL TREATMENTS

A variety of medications and other medical treatments are used to treat infectious disorders in children. Most of these treatments will require a physician's or nurse practitioner's order when the child is in the hospital. The most common treatments and medications are listed in Common Medical Treatments 37.1 and Drug Guide 37.1. The nurse caring for the child with an infectious disorder should be familiar with what the procedures are, how they work, and common nursing implications related to use of these modalities.

NURSING PROCESS OVERVIEW FOR THE CHILD WITH AN INFECTIOUS OR COMMUNICABLE DISORDER

Care of the child with an infectious or communicable disorder includes assessment, nursing diagnosis, planning, interventions, and evaluation. There are a number of general concepts related to the nursing process that may be applied to the care of children with infectious disorders. From a general understanding of the care involved for a child with an infectious disorder, the nurse can then individualize the care based on the child's specifics.

Remember Samuel, the 3-month-old with fever, congestion, and irritability? What additional health history and physical examination assessment information should you obtain?

Assessment

Assessment of the child with a communicable or infectious disorder includes health history, physical examination, and laboratory and diagnostic testing.

Health History

The health history consists of the past medical history, including the mother's pregnancy history; family history; and history of present illness (when the symptoms started and how they have progressed), as well as treatments used at home. The past medical history might be significant for lack of recommended immunizations, prematurity, maternal infection during pregnancy

COMMON MEDICAL TREATMENTS 37.1

Treatment	Explanation	Indications	Nursing Implications
Hydration	Promoting proper fluid balance either orally or intravenously	Child who can't replace insensible loss due to fever, child who is vomiting or has diarrhea	• Encourage oral fluids, if possible. • Offer child preferred fluid; try popsicles or games to promote fluid intake. • If administering IV fluids, ensure proper fluid and rate per order and assess IV site and fluid intake every hour. • Maintain strict record of intake and output.
Fever reduction	Reducing temperature by use of antipyretics or nonpharmacologic interventions	Febrile child who is uncomfortable or who can't keep up with the increased metabolic demands associated with fever	• Administer antipyretics, such as ibuprofen and acetaminophen. • Avoid aspirin use in children and adolescents. • Use nonpharmacologic interventions such as dressing lightly, removing blankets, use of a fan, tepid bath, and cooling blanket. Make sure that nonpharmacologic measures do not induce shivering or discomfort. If they do, they should be stopped immediately.

IV, intravenous.

DRUG GUIDE 37.1 COMMON DRUGS FOR COMMUNICABLE DISORDERS

Medication	Actions/Indications	Nursing Implications
Antibiotics	Kill and prevent the growth of bacteria Used for treatment of bacterial infections such as sepsis	• Check for antibiotic allergies. • Give as prescribed for the length of time prescribed.
Antivirals (e.g., acyclovir)	Kill and prevent the growth of viruses Used for treatment of viral infections such as herpes simplex type 2	• Observe infusion site for signs of tissue damage. • If administering topically, clean and dry area before application and wear gloves. • Give as prescribed for the length of time prescribed.
Antipyretics (acetaminophen, ibuprofen)	Decrease the temperature set point (only in a child with a raised temperature) by inhibiting the production of prostaglandins, leading to heat loss (through vasodilation and sweating) and resulting in a reduction in fever Used to decrease temperature in the febrile child who is uncomfortable or who can't keep up with the increased metabolic demands associated with fever	• Ensure proper dosing, concentration, and dosing interval. • Avoid aspirin use in children and adolescents. • Avoid ibuprofen use in children with a bleeding disorder. • Assess fever and any related symptoms such as tachycardia, shivering, or diaphoresis. • Properly educate caregivers on appropriate dosing, concentration, dosing interval, and use of accurate measuring device.
Antipruritics (usually antihistamines)	Given orally or topically to block the histamine reaction Used to relieve discomfort associated with itching	• When applying topically, wear gloves. • Do not apply to open wounds. • Oral antihistamines may cause drowsiness.

Adapted from Taketokmo, C. K., Hodding, J. H., & Kraus, D. M. (2013). *Lexi-comp's drug reference handbook: Pediatric & neonatal dosage handbook* (20th ed.). Hudson, OH: Lexi-comp, Inc.

or labor, prolonged difficult delivery, or immunocompromise. Family history might be significant for lack of immunization or recent infectious or communicable disease. When eliciting the history of the present illness, inquire about the following:

- Any known exposure to infectious or communicable disease
- Immunization history
- History of having any common childhood communicable diseases
- Fever
- Sore throat
- Lethargy
- Malaise
- Poor feeding or decreased appetite
- Vomiting
- Diarrhea
- Cough
- Rash (in the older child ask for a description [i.e., Is it painful? Does it itch?])

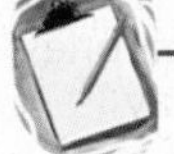

Take Note!

Many childhood infections and communicable diseases involve a rash. Rashes can be difficult to identify. Therefore, it is important to obtain a thorough description and history from the caregiver.

Physical Examination

Physical examination of the child with an infectious disorder includes inspection, observation, and palpation.

INSPECTION AND OBSERVATION

Begin the physical examination with inspection and observation. Assess the child's skin, mouth, throat, and hair for lesions or wounds. Note the color, shape, and distribution of any lesions or wounds. Assess whether there is any exudate from the lesions or wounds. A thorough and accurate description is important to assist in identifying the rash and causative organism. Observe for scratching, restlessness, avoidance of the use of a body part, or guarding of a body part. Observe the child's affect, energy level, and interaction with caregivers. Lethargy can indicate serious infection or sepsis. Observe if there is any discharge from the nose, cough, or respiratory difficulty.

Assess hydration status. Inspect the oral mucosa; dry and pale mucous membranes can indicate dehydration. Observe for other signs of dehydration, such as sunken eyes and no tears with crying.

Assessment of vital signs can provide more information about the child's condition. Elevated temperature can indicate infection. Often tachypnea and tachycardia accompany fever. Hypotension may also occur, but it is usually a late sign with sepsis.

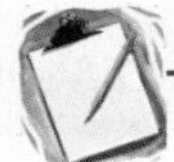

Take Note!

Neonates may not present with fever; some may be hypothermic (Smitherman & Macias, 2015).

PALPATION

Palpate the skin to assess temperature, moisture, texture, and turgor. In a child with an infectious or communicable disease, the skin may be warm and moist due to fever. Turgor may be decreased secondary to dehydration. In infants, palpate the fontanels; if they are sunken, the infant may be dehydrated. Palpate the rash to determine if it is raised or flat. A thorough picture of the presenting rash can help identify the child's illness. Palpate the lymph nodes and note any that are swollen and tender.

Laboratory and Diagnostic Testing

Common Laboratory and Diagnostic Tests 37.1 discusses the tests used most commonly when communicable disorders are suspected. The tests can assist the physician or nurse practitioner in diagnosing the disorder and/or be used as guidelines in determining ongoing treatment. Laboratory or nonnursing personnel obtain some of the tests, while the nurse might obtain others. In either instance the nurse should be familiar with how the tests are obtained, what they are used for, and normal versus abnormal results. This knowledge will also be necessary when providing child and family education related to the testing.

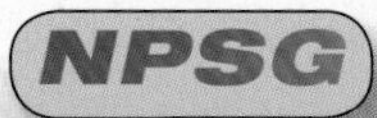

GOAL 2: Improve the Effectiveness of Communication Among Caregivers

NPSG.02.03.01 Report critical results of tests and diagnostic procedures on a timely basis.

Steps: When caring for a child with a potential or actual infectious or communicable disorder notify appropriate healthcare provider with positive culture results, and critical changes to other laboratory values and diagnostic test results.

Joint Commission. (2015). *National patient safety goals effective January 1, 2015.* Retrieved from http://www.jointcommission.org/assets/1/6/2015_NPSG_HAP.pdf

OBTAINING BLOOD SPECIMENS

Giving a blood specimen may be very frightening to children because of the fear of needles, pain, and blood loss. Provide atraumatic care when performing venipunctures and other needlesticks in children (refer to Chapter 30 for further information). Whether the laboratory technician or the nurse is drawing the blood, the procedure should be performed in an area other than the child's bed, such as the treatment room; the child's bed should be kept as a "safe" area. Provide teaching

COMMON LABORATORY AND DIAGNOSTIC TESTS 37.1

Test	Explanation	Indications	Nursing Implications
Complete blood count (CBC)	Evaluate white blood cell count (particularly the percentage of individual white cells)	Detect the presence of inflammation, infection	Normal values vary according to age and gender. • White blood cell count differential is helpful in differentiating source of infection. • May be affected by myelosuppressive drugs
Erythrocyte sedimentation rate (ESR)	Nonspecific test used in conjunction with other tests to determine presence of infection or inflammation	Detect the presence of inflammation, infection	• Send to laboratory immediately; specimens allowed to stand for longer than 3 hours may produce a falsely low result.
C-reactive protein (CRP)	Nonspecific test that measures a type of protein produced in the liver that is present during episodes of acute inflammation or infection Usually used to diagnose bacterial infections; does not consistently rise with viral infections	To detect the presence of infection, CRP is a more sensitive and rapidly responding indicator than ESR.	• Presence of an intrauterine device may cause positive test results because of tissue inflammation. • Exogenous hormones, such as oral contraceptives, may cause increased levels. • Nonsteroidal anti-inflammatories, salicylates, and steroids may cause decreased levels. • Fasting may be required.
Blood culture and sensitivity	Deliberate growing of microorganism in a solid or liquid medium. Once it has grown, it is tested against various antibiotics to determine which antibiotics will kill it.	Detect the presence of bacteria or yeast, which may have spread from a certain site in the body into the bloodstream Determine which antibiotics the bacteria or yeast is sensitive to	• Follow aseptic technique and hospital protocol to prevent contamination. • Two cultures obtained from two different sites are preferred. • Ideally obtain before administering antibiotics; if child is taking antibiotics, notify laboratory and draw specimen shortly before next dose. • Draw below IV line, if possible, to prevent dilution of sample • Deliver specimen to laboratory immediately (within 30 minutes).
Stool culture (including stool for ova and parasites [O&P])	To determine if bacteria or parasite has infected the intestines	Detect pathogens, including parasites or overgrowth of normal flora in the bowel. Indicated for children with diarrhea, fever, or abdominal pain	• Stool must be free of urine, water, and toilet paper. • Do not retrieve out of toilet water. • Deliver to laboratory immediately. • Mineral oil, barium, and bismuth interfere with the detection of parasites; specimen collection should be delayed for 7–10 days. • Often a minimum of three specimens on 3 separate days are required for adequate examination, since many parasites and worm eggs are shed intermittently.

COMMON LABORATORY AND DIAGNOSTIC TESTS 37.1 (continued)

Test	Explanation	Indications	Nursing Implications
Urine culture	Collection of urine to detect the presence of bacteria in the urine	Detect the presence of bacteria in the urinary tract. Indicated for children with fever of unknown origin, dysuria, frequency, or urgency, or if urinalysis suggests infection	• Should be obtained by midstream clean-catch, catheterization, or suprapubic aspiration. Avoid contamination with stool, vaginal secretions, hands, or clothing. • Placing bags on the perineum is not acceptable due to high chance of contamination. • Obtain before antibiotics are administered. • Deliver to laboratory immediately (preferable) or refrigerate.
Wound culture	Allows for microbial growth and identification of specific organism	Identification of specific organism	• Do not take from exudate or eschar. • If moderate to heavy drainage present irrigate the wound with sterile saline. • Specimens taken from wounds can harbor a variety of organisms. Pathogenicity depends of the quantity of organisms present. • Avoid touching intact skin at the wound edges • Culture highly vascular granulation tissue
Throat culture	Vigorous swabbing of the tonsillar area and posterior pharynx to detect the presence of invasive organisms	Most reliable method of detecting group A streptococcal pharyngitis Will also detect *Bordetella pertussis, Corynebacterium diphtheriae* May be performed in those with fever of unknown origin	• Ensure specimen is of secretions in the pharyngeal or tonsillar area. Avoid touching tongue or lips with swab. • When performing on young children, have adult hold child in lap. • Healthcare worker needs to stabilize head by placing hand on the child's forehead.
Nasal swabs (nasopharyngeal)	Insertion of swabs into the nose until reaching the nasopharynx to detect the presence of invasive organisms	Optimal method for detecting Bordetella pertussis. Also used to detect *Corynebacterium diphtheria* and viral illnesses such as *respiratory syncytial virus (RSV), parainfluenza*	• The distance from the child's nose to ear gives an estimate of how far to insert the swab into the nostril to reach the nasopharynx • Insert swab straight back, not up, and leave in nasopharynx for several seconds • When performing on young children, have adult hold child in lap. • Healthcare worker needs to stabilize head as child will likely try to pull away.

Adapted from Fischbach, F. T., & Dunning III, M. B. (2015). *A manual of laboratory and diagnostic tests* (9th ed.). Philadelphia, PA: Wolters Kluwer Health/Lippincott Williams & Wilkins.

about the procedure based on the child's developmental level and readiness to learn. In infants and younger children, additional assistance with positioning and restraint will be needed to perform the procedure safely and to ensure proper collection. Use a topical anesthetic cream or gel, refrigerant spray, or iontophoresis before venipuncture. Refer to Chapter 36 for additional information about decreasing venipuncture-related pain in infants and children.

The usual sites for obtaining blood specimens via venipuncture are the superficial veins of the dorsal surface of the hand or the antecubital fossa, although other locations may also be used. In specific situations, the jugular or femoral vein may be used; in this case either the physician or nurse practitioner will perform the venipuncture.

Capillary puncture of the child's fingertip, the great toe, or the infant's heel may also be used to obtain blood specimens. Fingertip puncture is similar to that in the adult, directed to the sides of the fingertip. Great toe puncture is performed in the same way. Capillary heel puncture must be performed in the proper location to avoid striking the medial plantar artery or periosteum (see Nursing Procedure 37.1). Automatic lancet devices can be used to deliver a more precise puncture depth.

Atraumatic Care

The young infant will benefit from the use of oral sucrose and nonnutritive sucking before and during the capillary puncture (Naughton & Ikuta, 2013).

Occasionally, blood samples may be obtained from an artery rather than a vein or capillary. Blood gases in particular are usually obtained by arterial puncture. Arterial puncture requires additional training and in many institutions is performed only by the respiratory therapist, physician, or nurse practitioner.

Children with indwelling venous access devices may be spared the trauma of puncture for blood specimens. Follow your institution's guidelines for withdrawing blood from peripherally inserted venous catheters or central venous catheters. The initial blood will be discarded to prevent contamination with intravenous fluids or medications such as heparin. The amount discarded depends on the size of the catheter, the weight of the child, and the institution's guidelines. After aspirating the specimen, flush the venous access device with normal saline to prevent clogging. The device may

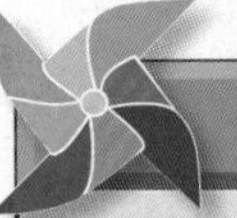

NURSING PROCEDURE 37.1

Capillary Heel Puncture

1. Choose the collection site and apply a commercial heel warmer or warm pack for several minutes prior to specimen collection.
2. Assemble equipment:
   - Gloves
   - Automatic lancet
   - Antiseptic wipe
   - Cotton ball or dry gauze
   - Capillary blood collection tube
   - Band-aid
3. Perform hand hygiene and don gloves. Remove the warm pack.
4. Cleanse the site with antiseptic prep pad and allow to dry.
5. Hold the dorsum of the foot with the nondominant hand; with the dominant hand, pierce the heel with the lancet. Place the extremity in the dependent position.
6. Wipe away the first drop of blood with the cotton ball or dry gauze.
7. Collect the blood specimen with a capillary specimen collection tube. Avoid squeezing the foot during specimen collection if possible, as it may contribute to hemolysis of the specimen.
8. Hold dry gauze over the site until bleeding stops, elevate extremity above the level of the heart, and then apply a Band-aid.

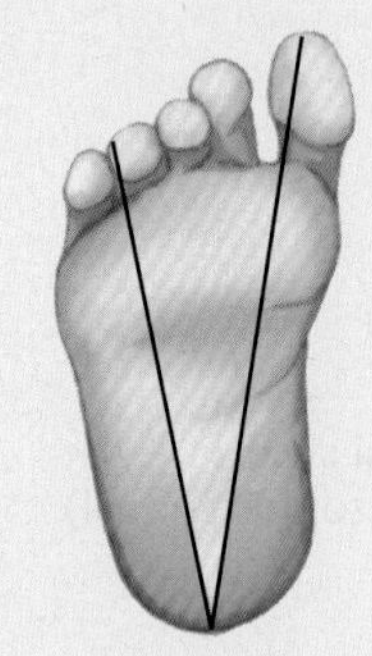

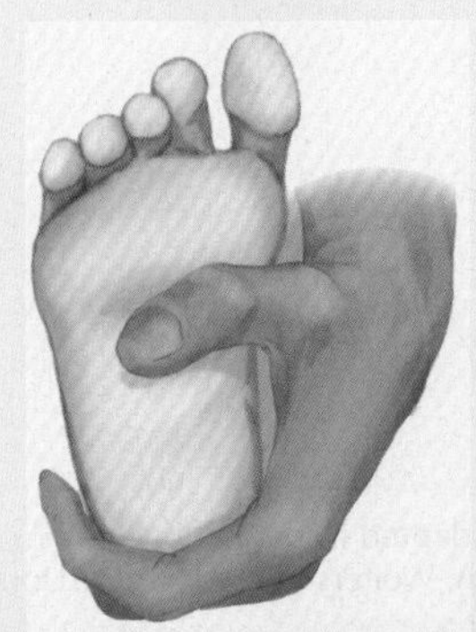

then be reconnected to the intravenous fluid or flushed according to the institution's protocol.

Nursing Diagnoses, Goals, Interventions, and Evaluations

After completing a thorough assessment, the nurse might identify several nursing diagnoses, including:

- Risk for imbalanced body temperature
- Impaired comfort
- Impaired skin integrity
- Risk for infection
- Deficient fluid volume
- Social isolation
- Deficient knowledge (specify)

After completing an assessment of Samuel, you note the following: rectal temperature of 39°C, poor sucking, and lethargy. Based on these assessment findings, what would your top three nursing diagnoses be for Samuel?

Nursing goals, interventions, and evaluation for the child with a communicable or infectious disorder are based on the nursing diagnoses. Nursing Care Plan 37.1 (at the end of the chapter) provides a general guide for planning care for a child with an infectious or communicable disorder. Additional information about nursing management will be included later in the chapter as it relates to specific disorders.

Managing Fever

Fever in their children is one of the most common reasons parents seek medical attention (Sullivan, Farrar, & The AAP's Section on Clinical Pharmacology and Therapeutics, and Committee on Drugs, 2011). Most infections or communicable diseases are accompanied by fever. Many parents have great concerns about fever. For example, they fear febrile seizures, neurologic complications, and a potential serious underlying disease. Many healthcare providers share these fears. This leads to the common recommendation to intervene and reduce fever. These fears and misconceptions about fever can lead to mismanagement of fever, such as inappropriate dosing of antipyretics, awakening the child during sleep to give antipyretics, or inappropriate use of nonpharmacologic treatments such as sponging the child with alcohol or cold water (Sullivan et al., 2011; Ward, 2015b).

It is important to educate parents that fever is a protective mechanism the body uses to fight infection. Evidence exists that an elevated body temperature actually enhances various components of the immune response (Sullivan et al., 2011). Fever can slow the growth of bacteria and viruses and increase neutrophil production and T-cell proliferation (Sullivan et al., 2011). Another concern is that reducing fever may hide signs of serious bacterial illness (Sullivan et al., 2011; Ward, 2015a).

Take Note!

Infants younger than 3 months of age with a rectal temperature greater than 38°C should be seen by a physician or nurse practitioner. They are considered at risk for sepsis until proven otherwise due to their immature immune system and inability to localize or handle infection very well (Nield& Kamat, 2011b).

In infants older than 3 months of age, fever less than 39°C usually does not require treatment (Nield & Kamat, 2011b). Antipyretics provide symptomatic relief but do not change the course of the infection. The major benefits of decreasing fever are increasing comfort in the child and decreasing fluid requirements, which helps to prevent dehydration. Children with certain underlying conditions, such as cardiovascular disease or pulmonary disease, also benefit from treating fever because such treatment decreases demands on the body.

Home Management of Fever

Fever is typically managed at home, so it is important to give guidance and instruction at well-child visits and review this information at subsequent visits. Written and video materials about fever management may be effective in increasing caregivers' knowledge. Parents can refer to the written instructions when needed (see Teaching Guidelines 37.1).

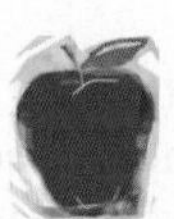

Teaching Guidelines 37.1

FEVER MANAGEMENT

- Fever is a sign of illness, not a disease; it is the body's weapon to fight infection.
- Diurnal variation may allow temperature changes as much as 1°C (1.8°F) over a 24-hour period, peaking in the evening.
- Antipyretics are used if the child demonstrates discomfort. Always check correct doses before administration. Never give aspirin or aspirin-containing products to a child younger than 19 years with a fever due to the risk of Reye syndrome.
- In some children fever can be associated with a seizure or dehydration, but this will not lead to brain damage or death. Discuss the facts about febrile seizures (see Chapter 38 for further information on febrile seizures).
- Watch for the signs and symptoms of dehydration; it is important to provide oral rehydration by increasing fluid intake.

- Dress the child lightly and avoid warm, binding clothing or blankets.
- The use of sponging with tepid water is controversial; if used, encourage the parent to give an antipyretic prior to sponging. Ensure the sponging does not produce shivering (which causes the body to produce heat and maintain the elevated set point), and reinforce the importance of using tepid water, not cold water or alcohol. Instruct the parent to stop if the child experiences discomfort.
- Call the provider for:
  - Any child younger than 3 months of age who has a rectal temperature above 38°C (100.4°F).
  - Any child who is lethargic or listless, regardless of temperature.
  - Fever lasting more than 3–5 days.
  - Fever greater than 40.6°C (105°F).
  - Any child who is immunocompromised by illness, such as cancer or HIV, will need further evaluation and treatment.

The use of acetaminophen or ibuprofen to reduce fever in children has been shown to be safe and effective when the appropriate dose is administered at the appropriate interval (Ward, 2015b). However, some studies have shown that ibuprofen is superior in reducing fever and lasts longer than acetaminophen (Ward, 2015b).

Box 37.4 gives dosing recommendations for both medications.

Take Note!

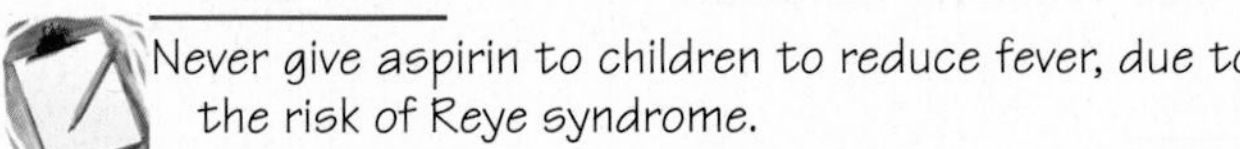

Never give aspirin to children to reduce fever, due to the risk of Reye syndrome.

Acetaminophen is widely used and accepted, with a long track record of safety and efficacy when used according to the label directions, but overdose can lead to toxic reactions (Ward, 2015b). Causes of acetaminophen toxicity include overdosing or incorrect dosing due to failure to read and understand the label instructions, use of an incorrect measuring device or concentration, and coadministration with an over- the-counter fixed-dose combination medication (the parent may not recognize that it has acetaminophen in it).

Another factor that may cause acetaminophen toxicity is the controversial, but common, practice of alternating acetaminophen and ibuprofen to help reduce fever. Studies of the use of alternating acetaminophen with ibuprofen have had conflicting results (Ward, 2015b). This practice can result in overdose or improper administration. It can be hard for parents to keep track of the time each medication is due. Parents may confuse which medication is given every 4 hours and which is given every 6 hours. They may exceed the recommended daily doses or may confuse the strength or dosage of the medicines. See Evidence-Based Practice 37.1.

BOX 37.4

DOSE RECOMMENDATIONS FOR ORAL ACETAMINOPHEN AND IBUPROFEN

Acetaminophen, 10–15 mg/kg/dose
- No more than every 4 hours
- No more than five doses in a 24-hour period

Ibuprofen, 4–10 mg/kg/dose
- Only children older than 6 months of age
- No more than four doses in a 24-hour period

Adapted from Taketomo, C. K., Hodding, J. H., & Kraus, D. M. (2013). *Lexi-comp's drug reference handbook: Pediatric & neonatal dosage handbook* (20th ed.). Hudson, OH: Lexi-comp, Inc.

Dosage Calculation

The nurse is caring for a toddler who is 2 years old and 28 lb. The order reads Ibuprofen 100 mg po every 6 hours as needed for temperature greater than 38°C. Is this a safe and effective dose?

Managing Skin Rashes

Skin rashes accompany many infectious or communicable diseases. These rashes can be very uncomfortable and irritating for the child. Management often occurs at home, so it is important to educate parents on ways to relieve the discomfort and protect and maintain skin integrity. The physician may prescribe antipruritics, including oral medications or topical creams or ointments (see Drug Guide 37.1). Instruct parents on the importance of maintaining skin integrity to prevent infection or scarring. Teach parents to keep their child's fingernails short and hands clean. Explain the importance of discouraging scratching, and discuss distraction techniques they can use with the child. Cool compresses or cool baths can relieve itching. Encourage the child to press on rather than scratch the itchy area; this can relieve discomfort while maintaining skin integrity. Refer to Chapter 45 for more information on managing skin rashes.

Thinking About Development

Lisa Hernandez is a 4-year-old with a history of fever, cold like symptoms and presents currently with an itchy rash. Based on her developmental stage, how will you instruct her and her caregiver on managing her rash at home? How would your instructions change if the child was 12 years old?

EVIDENCE-BASED PRACTICE 37.1 **IS ALTERNATING ACETAMINOPHEN WITH IBUPROFEN MORE EFFECTIVE THAN EITHER ONE ALONE?**

Fever is one of the most common health concerns seen in pediatrics. Alternating paracetamol, also known as acetaminophen, and ibuprofen for fever reduction is a common practice, but there has been limited evidence on its safety or efficacy. It may be a harmful practice due to combined toxicity and potential parental confusion in timing and dosing.

STUDY

This study performed a meta-analysis of randomized controlled trials. A total of six studies were included resulting in 915 enrolled participants. It evaluated the effects and side effects of combining paracetamol (acetaminophen) and ibuprofen or alternating them compared with single antipyretic therapy in treating fever in children.

Findings

Review of the studies suggested that some evidence exists that combining or alternating antipyretics may be more effective at reducing temperature for up to 4 hours than single antipyretic therapy. Evidence supporting whether these practices improve a febrile child's discomfort were inconclusive. No serious side effects were attributed to these practices in these studies.

Nursing Implications

Although this study suggests improved fever reduction with alternating of acetaminophen and ibuprofen, safety concerns remain. Further research with larger sample sizes, longer follow-up and a focus on measuring child's discomfort and safety of combining or alternating antipyretic regimens is warranted. To alleviate some of the concerns that parents have with fever, nurses should consistently educate parents about why fever occurs and fever facts and myths.

Adapted from Wong T., Stang A. S., Ganshorn H., Hartling L., Maconochie I. K., Thomsen A. M., & Johnson D. W. (2013). Combined and alternating paracetamol and ibuprofen therapy for febrile children. *Cochrane Database of Systematic Reviews.* Issue 10: CD009572. doi: 10.1002/14651858.CD009572.pub2; Retrieved from http://www.aub.edu.lb/fm/cri/Documents/Cochrane%20review-Alternating%20antipyretic.pdf

Based on your top three nursing diagnoses for Samuel, describe appropriate nursing interventions.

SEPSIS

Sepsis is a systemic overresponse to infection resulting from bacteria and viruses, which are the most common, fungi, viruses, rickettsia, or parasites. It can lead to septic shock, which results in hypotension, low blood flow, and multisystem organ failure. Septic shock is a medical emergency and children are usually admitted to an intensive care unit (see Chapter 51). The cause of sepsis may not be known, but common causative organisms in infants less than 3 months include *Escherichia coli,* group B *Streptococcus, Staphylococcus aureus,* enteroviruses, and herpes simplex virus, and in older children include *Neisseria meningitidis, Streptococcus pneumoniae,* and *S. aureus* (Pomerantz & Weiss, 2015). Sepsis can affect any age group but infants less than 3 months of age, immunocompromised children, and children with an indwelling vascular catheter are at higher risk (Pomerantz & Weiss, 2015). Neonates and young infants have a higher susceptibility due to their immature immune system, inability to localize infections, and lack of immunoglobulin M (IgM), which is necessary to protect against bacterial infections.

The prognosis for sepsis is variable and depends on the child's age and the cause of the sepsis. The mortality rate ranges from 9% to 35% (Santhanam, 2015). Neonates are at highest risk for a poor outcome. Due to this high mortality rate, when an ill-appearing febrile neonate presents, a full workup is indicated (Nield & Kamat, 2011b). Usually, admission to the hospital to rule out sepsis is the standard of practice.

Pathophysiology

Sepsis results in the systemic inflammatory response syndrome (SIRS) due to infection. The pathophysiology of sepsis is complex. It results from the effects of circulating bacterial products or toxins, mediated by cytokine release, occurring as a result of sustained bacteremia. The pathogens cause an overproduction of proinflammatory cytokines, previously termed endotoxins. These cytokines are responsible for the clinically observable effects of the sepsis. Impaired pulmonary, hepatic, or renal function may result from excessive cytokine release during the septic process.

Therapeutic Management

Therapeutic management of sepsis in infants, especially neonates, is more aggressive than for older children.

Neonates and infants with sepsis or even suspected sepsis are treated in the hospital. The infant is admitted for close monitoring along with antibiotic therapy. Intravenous antibiotics are started immediately after the blood, urine, and cerebrospinal fluid cultures have been obtained. The length of therapy and the specific antibiotic used will be determined based on the source of the positive culture and the results of the culture and sensitivity. If final culture reports are negative and symptoms have subsided, antibiotics may be discontinued (usually after 72 hours of treatment). If the child is not responding to therapy and symptoms worsen, sepsis may be progressing to shock. Management of the child with septic shock is usually done in the intensive care unit.

Nursing Assessment

For a full description of the assessment phase of the nursing process, refer to the assessment section of the Nursing Process Overview earlier in this chapter. Assessment findings pertinent to sepsis are discussed below.

HEALTH HISTORY

Elicit a description of the present illness and chief complaint. Signs of sepsis can vary with each child. Some common signs and symptoms reported during the health history might include:

- Child just does not look or act right
- Crying more than usual, inconsolable
- Fever
- Hypothermia (in neonates and those with severe disease)
- Lethargic and less interactive or playful
- Increased irritability
- Poor feeding or poor suck
- Rash (e.g., petechiae, ecchymosis, diffuse erythema)
- Difficulty breathing
- Nasal congestion
- Diarrhea
- Vomiting
- Decreased urine output
- Hypotonia
- Changes in mental status (confused, anxious, excited)
- Seizures
- Older child may complain of heart racing

Explore the child's current and past medical history for risk factors such as:

- Prematurity
- Lack of immunizations
- Immunocompromise
- Exposure to communicable pathogens

In neonates and young infants, seek pregnancy and labor risk factors such as:

- Premature rupture of membranes or prolonged rupture
- Difficult delivery
- Maternal infection or fever, including sexually transmitted infections
- Resuscitation and other invasive procedures
- Positive maternal group β-streptococcal vaginosis

Sepsis may occur in the hospitalized child. Assess for risk factors such as:

- Intensive care unit stay
- Presence of central line or other invasive lines or tubes
- Immunosuppression

Take Note!

Listen to the parents' descriptions of the neonate's or infant's behavior and appearance, as well as changes they have observed. Many times they are the first to notice when their child is not acting right, even before clinical signs of infection are seen.

PHYSICAL EXAMINATION

Perform a thorough physical examination of the infant or child with proven or suspected sepsis. Specific findings related to inspection and observation are noted below.

Inspection and Observation. Observe the child's general appearance, color, level of arousal, and hydration status. The child with sepsis may appear lethargic and pale and show signs of dehydration. In neonates and infants, observe the quality of their cry and reaction to parental stimulation, noting weak cry, lack of smile or facial expression, or lack of responsiveness. Inspect the skin for petechiae or other skin lesions. Petechiae may indicate a serious bacterial infection (often *N. meningitidis*), and other skin lesion patterns may help identify the cause of the fever. Observe respiratory effort and rate. The infant or child with sepsis may demonstrate tachypnea and increased work of breathing, such as nasal flaring, grunting, and retractions.

Assess vital signs, noting abnormalities. Note elevation in temperature or hypothermia in the young infant. Note tachypnea or tachycardia in the child or apnea or bradycardia in the infant. Document blood pressure. Hypotension, especially when accompanied by signs of poor perfusion, can be a sign of worsening sepsis with progression to shock (refer to Chapter 51).

LABORATORY AND DIAGNOSTIC TESTS

Symptoms of sepsis can be vague in infants. Therefore, laboratory tests play a crucial role in confirming or ruling out sepsis. Common laboratory and diagnostic studies ordered for the assessment of sepsis include:

- Complete blood count: WBC levels will be elevated; in severe cases they may be decreased (this is an ominous sign).
- C-reactive protein: elevated
- Blood culture: positive in septicemia, indicating bacteria is present in the blood

- Urine culture: may be positive, indicating presence of bacteria in the urine
- Cerebrospinal fluid analysis: may reveal increased WBCs and protein and low glucose
- Stool culture: may be positive for bacteria or other infectious organisms
- Culture of tubes, catheters, or shunts suspected to be infected: the fluid inside these tubes may be tested for bacteria.
- Chest x-ray: may reveal signs of pneumonia such as hyperinflation and patchy areas of atelectasis or infiltration

Nursing Management

Monitor the infant or child closely for changes in condition, especially the development of shock. Administer antibiotics as ordered. Refer to Nursing Care Plan 37.1 at the end of the chapter for nursing diagnoses and related interventions. In addition to these interventions, it is important to prevent infection and provide education to the child and family.

PREVENTING INFECTION

Sepsis is a potentially life-threatening illness, and prevention is important. Handwashing is the most effective intervention against nosocomial infection. Nurses play a key role in minimizing environmental sources by cleaning equipment, disposing of soiled linens and dressings properly, and adhering to proper aseptic technique with all invasive procedures. Follow your institution's policies and use evidence-based practice guidelines for interventions such as invasive line dressing changes and intravenous tubing changes to reduce the risk of infection. Encourage immunization as recommended. To reduce group *B. streptococcus* infection in neonates, screen pregnant woman. If the results are positive, administer intrapartum antibiotics.

Take Note!

There has been a dramatic reduction in invasive Haemophilus influenzae type B diseases since the widespread use of the Hib vaccine (Centers for Disease Control and Prevention, 2014b).

EDUCATING THE CHILD AND FAMILY

Early recognition of the signs of sepsis is essential in preventing morbidity and mortality. Educate parents about the significance of fever, especially in neonates and infants younger than 3 months old. Instruct parents to contact their physician or nurse practitioner if their infant or neonate has a fever. A physician or nurse practitioner should see any child with a fever accompanied by lethargy, poor responsiveness, or lack of facial expressions. Signs and symptoms of sepsis can be vague and vary from child to child. Encourage parents to contact their physician or nurse practitioner if they feel their febrile child is "just not acting right."

BACTERIAL INFECTIONS

Bacteria are one-celled organisms that can live, grow, and reproduce. They exist everywhere. Most are completely harmless and some are very useful. Others can lead to disease either because they are in the wrong place in the body or they are designed to invade and cause disease in humans and animals. Children are at a high risk of developing bacterial infections, which can result in life-threatening illness. Fortunately, many bacterial diseases, such as diphtheria, pertussis, and tetanus, can be prevented by immunization (see Chapter 31 for more information on immunizations).

Community-Acquired Methicillin-Resistant *Staphylococcus Aureus*

Community-acquired methicillin-resistant *Staphylococcus aureus* (CAMRSA) is a staphylococcal infection that is resistant to certain antibiotics. Methicillin-resistant *S. aureus* (MRSA) was originally a nosocomial acquired infection with few cases acquired in the community but community-acquired infection, in seemingly healthy individuals, is increasing in occurrence throughout the United States (Kaplan, 2015). These infections range from minor skin rashes to abscesses to serious, complicated, life-threatening infections. Serious and invasive infections, such as sepsis, necrotizing pneumonia, and osteomyelitis, often are secondary to a skin or soft tissue infection.

Transmission occurs through direct person-to-person contact, respiratory droplets, blood, or sharing personal items, such as hair brushes, towels, and sports equipment, and touching surfaces or items contaminated with MRSA. Clusters of MRSA have been found in day care centers and among athletic teams. Staphylococci are resistant to heat and drying and can be found on environmental surfaces months after contamination. Intact skin and mucous membranes, along with proper hand hygiene, are the best barriers to MRSA.

Nursing Assessment

In the child, skin and tissue infections are common infections caused by CAMRSA. Symptoms include a bump or skin area that is red, swollen, painful, and warm to touch. It may also include fever, fluctuance, and purulent drainage. The lesion may have appeared suddenly and be red and raised, resembling an insect bite. Necrotic areas may develop. Abscesses, especially abscessed hair follicles, and pimples are common presentations. Assessment needs to include a thorough past medical history to determine history of recurrent skin infections with or without complete resolution along with assessment for risk factors. Risk factors include frequent skin-to-skin contact; openings in the skin/skin trauma, such as abrasions and cuts; contact with potentially contaminated personal items, equipment and surfaces; poor hygiene; limited access to health care; frequent exposure to antimicrobial agents and crowded living conditions (Kaplan, 2015).

Diagnosis is determined through culture. Diagnostic tests include incision and drainage (I&D), aspiration of the abscess, and culturing the fluid or tissue. Antimicrobial susceptibility along with culture is critical.

Nursing Management

Care of the child with CAMRSA will typically occur at home. Antibiotics with microbial susceptibility will often be prescribed. Comprehensive wound care, which may include I&D, may occur. Follow-up for reassessment is key. Child and family education is crucial. Include the following in the teaching plan:

- Educate the family on the importance of taking the antibiotics as directed and finishing all the medicine. Emphasize that this will help slow the creation of antimicrobial-resistant organisms.
- Teach the child and parents proper hand hygiene and handwashing.
- Discourage family members from sharing personal items.
- Explain the risk factors involved in transmission.
- Explain the importance of keeping cuts and scrapes cleaned and covered.
- Review the signs of MRSA and emphasize the importance of early recognition and treatment.

Scarlet Fever

Scarlet fever is an infection resulting from group A streptococci. It usually occurs with a group A streptococci throat infection (i.e., strep throat) or rarely streptococcal skin infection. However, in the case of scarlet fever, the bacteria produce a toxin that causes a rash. Not all children with a group A streptococci infection will develop the rash of scarlet fever. Only children who are infected with streptococci that produce pyrogenic exotoxins and do not have antitoxin antibodies, making them sensitive to the bacterial toxin, will develop scarlet fever (Gerber, 2011). Scarlet fever is usually seen in children 5 to 12 years of age and is rare in children younger than 2 years old (Centers for Disease Control and Prevention, 2015n; Zabawski, Jr., 2014). Transmission is through droplets and follows contact with respiratory tract secretions. Transmission is facilitated by the type of close contact that occurs in schools and child care centers. Food-borne outbreaks have occurred due to human contamination of food. After exposure, the incubation period is 2 to 5 days (Gerber, 2011). Communicability is highest during acute infection, and the child is no longer contagious 24 hours after the initiation of appropriate antimicrobial therapy (Gerber, 2011).

There has been a dramatic decrease in the mortality rate from scarlet fever due to antibiotic use and scarlet fever today typically follows a benign course (Zabawski, Jr., 2014). Rare but serious complications such as rheumatic fever, glomerulonephritis, skin infections, abscesses of the throat, pneumonia, and arthritis can still occur therefore prompt recognition and proper treatment are important (CDC, 2015n).

Nursing Assessment

Symptoms of scarlet fever begin abruptly. The health history may reveal a fever greater than 101°F, chills, body aches, loss of appetite, nausea, and vomiting. Inspect the pharynx, which is usually very red and swollen. The tonsils may have yellow or white specks of pus, and cervical lymph nodes may be swollen. Inspect the skin for the most striking symptom of scarlet fever, which is an erythematous rash appearing on the face, trunk, and extremities. The rash is typically absent from the palms and soles of the feet. It looks like a sunburn but feels like sandpaper (Fig. 37.1A). The rash lasts approximately 5 days and is followed by desquamation, typically on the fingers and toes. Early in the illness the tongue develops a thick coat with a strawberry appearance. The tongue will later lose the coating and become bright red (Fig. 37.1B).

Diagnosis is made by identification of group A streptococcus on throat culture. Several rapid tests for group A streptococcal pharyngitis are available. The accuracy of these tests depends on the quality of the specimen. It is important that the secretions obtained are pharyngeal or tonsillar (see Common Medical Treatments 37.1 for more information on throat cultures).

Nursing Management

Children with scarlet fever are usually cared for at home. Penicillin V is the antibiotic of choice (Gerber, 2011). In those sensitive to penicillin, erythromycin may be used. Educate the family on the importance of taking the antibiotic as directed and finishing all the medicine.

Encourage fluid intake to maintain adequate hydration due to fever. Teach parents ways to provide comfort for the child. A cool mist humidifier can soothe the child's sore throat. Soft foods, warm liquids like soup, or cold foods like popsicles may also be helpful. If the child is hospitalized, droplet precautions, along with standard precautions, are necessary.

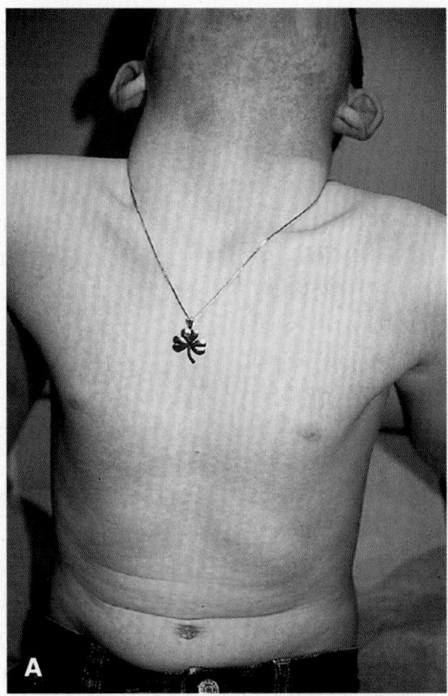

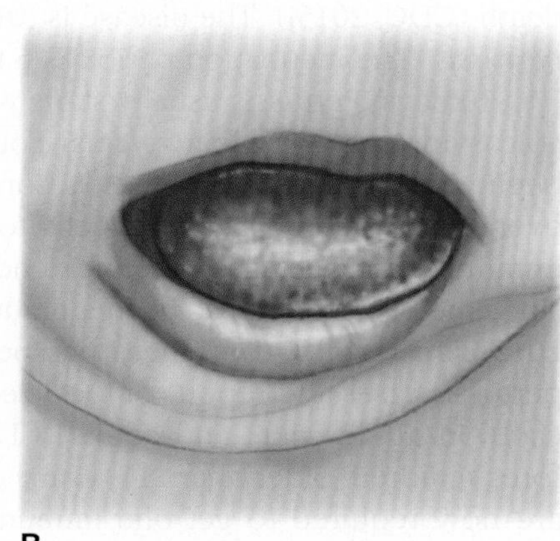

FIGURE 37.1 **(A)** Rash of scarlet fever. **(B)** Strawberry tongue.

Diphtheria

Diphtheria is caused by infection with *Corynebacterium diphtheriae* and may affect the nose, larynx, tonsils, or pharynx. Tonsillar and pharyngeal infections are the most common and will be the focus of this discussion. A pseudomembrane forms over the pharynx, uvula, tonsils, and soft palate (Fig. 37.2). The neck becomes edematous and lymphadenopathy develops. The pseudomembrane causes airway obstruction and suffocation. Diphtheria is rare in the developed countries but is reappearing in some regions and continues to be a serious disease worldwide due to lack of routine immunization (Mayo Clinic Staff, 2015). Risk factors include children and adults who are unimmunized or underimmunized, living in crowded or unsanitary living conditions, having a compromised immune system, and traveling to developing countries where diphtheria remains endemic (Mayo Clinic Staff, 2015). Routine infant immunization can prevent the disease. Therapeutic management involves administration of antibiotics and antitoxin, as well as airway management.

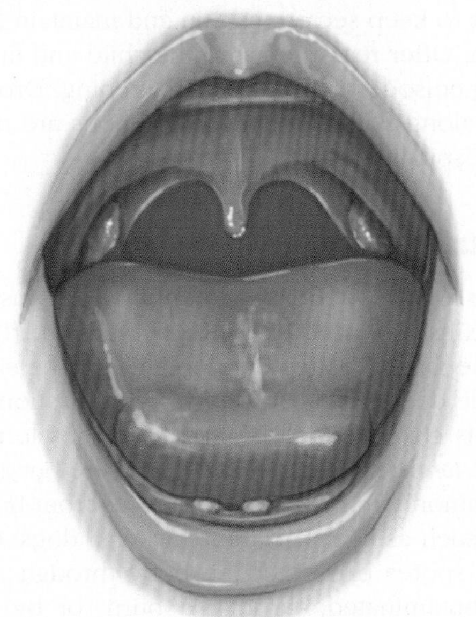

FIGURE 37.2 In diphtheria a pseudomembrane forms over the pharynx, uvula, tonsils, and soft palate.

Nursing Assessment

Children at risk for diphtheria are those who are unimmunized. Note history of sore throat and fever, usually less than 38.9°C. As the pseudomembrane forms, swallowing becomes difficult and signs of airway obstruction become apparent. A specimen of the membrane may be cultured for *C. diphtheriae*.

Nursing Management

Close observation of respiratory status is of utmost importance. Administration of antibiotics and the antitoxin is critical to encourage sloughing of the membrane. The child should remain on strict droplet precautions in addition to standard precautions and should maintain bed rest.

Pertussis

Pertussis is an acute respiratory disorder characterized by paroxysmal cough (whooping cough) and copious secretions. The highest incidence is seen in children younger than 1 year of age, and children younger than 3 months of age are at greatest risk for severe disease and death (CDC, 2015j). The disease is caused by *Bordetella pertussis*. The incubation period is 6 to 21 days, usually 7 to 10 days. Pertussis usually starts with 7 to 10 days of cold symptoms. The paroxysmal coughing spells then begin and can last 1 to 4 weeks. Convalescence occurs over the course of several weeks to months. Initially, immunization decreased the incidence of pertussis, but since the 1980s there has been a gradual increase (CDC, 2015j). In recent years, there has been an increase in pertussis cases and reports of localized outbreaks, especially in adolescents and adults (CDC, 2012a). Therefore, children older than 11 years of age and adults are now required to get one immunization booster of Tdap (tetanus, diphtheria, and pertussis) instead of Td (tetanus and diphtheria) (CDC, 2011, 2012a). Over the last several years an increased incidence of disease in children 7 to 10 years has been reported. The Advisory Committee on Immunization Practices (ACIP) revised their recommendations and currently recommends the use of Tdap in undervaccinated children aged 7 to 10 years (CDC, 2011b; 2012a). Infants and young children continue to be required to get four doses of DTaP (diphtheria, tetanus, and pertussis) at 2 months, 4 months, 6 months, 15 to 18 months, and fifth booster dose 4 to 6 years before entering school. Complications of pertussis include hypoxia, apnea, pneumonia, seizures, encephalopathy, and death.

Therapeutic Management

Therapeutic management of pertussis focuses on eradicating the bacterial infection and providing respiratory support. CDC guidelines recommend antimicrobial treatment (CDC, 2012a). For infants older than 1 month of age, macrolide drugs, including erythromycin, clarithromycin, and azithromycin, are the drugs of choice (CDC, 2015k). For younger infants, azithromycin should be used and erythromycin and clarithromycin avoided (CDC, 2015k). An alternative to macrolides in children older than 2 months is trimethoprim–sulfamethoxazole (TMP-SMZ) (CDC, 2015k). A course of macrolide antibiotics is also recommended to treat all close contacts regardless of age or immunization status (CDC, 2012a, 2015i). Also, all close contacts who are younger than 7 years of age and who are unimmunized or underimmunized should have pertussis immunization initiated or the series completed according to the recommended dosing schedule (CDC, 2012a).

Take Note!

In 2013, the Food and Drug Administration (FDA) issued a warning that azithromycin may cause potentially fatal heart rhythm in some patients because it can lead to abnormal changes in the electrical activity of the heart (U.S. FDA, 2013). Therefore, when treating pertussis in children at risk for cardiovascular events, such as children with prolongation of the QT interval, alternative drugs should be considered.

Nursing Assessment

The most important risk factor for the development of pertussis is lack of immunization. The history may reveal cold and cough symptoms, progressing to paroxysmal coughing spells. During the paroxysms, the child might cough 10 to 30 times in a row, followed by a whooping sound. This might be accompanied by redness in the face, progressive cyanosis, and protrusion of the tongue. Saliva, mucus, and tears flow from the mouth, nose, and eyes. Between the paroxysmal episodes, the child might rest well and appear relatively unaffected. Auscultate the lungs to assess air exchange. The diagnosis may be confirmed by a variety of laboratory tests accompanied by clinical history. Culture is considered the gold standard, but polymerase chain reaction (PCR) is now used by many laboratories due to its increased sensitivity and faster results (CDC, 2012a).

Nursing Management

Nursing care will focus on providing a high-humidity environment and frequent suctioning to mobilize secretions. Observe for signs of airway obstruction. Encourage fluids to keep secretions thin and maintain adequate hydration. Offer reassurance to the child and family; the coughing episodes can be very frightening. Droplet precautions along with standard precautions are necessary for the hospitalized child.

Tetanus

Tetanus is an acute, often fatal neurologic disease caused by the toxins produced by *Clostridium tetani*. Tetanus is rare in the United States but continues to be significant worldwide due to lack of routine immunization (Arnon, 2011). It is characterized by increased muscle tone and spasm. *C. tetani* spores can live anywhere but are found most commonly in soil, dust, and feces from humans or animals, such as sheep, cattle, chickens, dogs, cats, and rats. The spores can enter the body through a wound that is contaminated, through a burn, or by injecting contaminated street drugs. Once it enters the body, an anaerobic environment allows it to multiply and a poisonous toxin is released.

There are four forms of tetanus. Neonatal tetanus is the most common worldwide, affecting newborns in the first week of life secondary to an infected umbilical stump or unsterile surgical technique during circumcision in infants who's mothers were poorly immunized (Arnon, 2011). Most women in the United States have been immunized and will pass the immunity to their fetus. Along with proper hygiene during delivery and adequate cord care, this makes this type rare in the United States, but in underdeveloped countries it remains a significant problem (Sexton, 2015). The second form is local tetanus. This rare form is characterized by local muscle spasms within the area of the wound. The third type is cephalic tetanus, which is associated with recurrent otitis media or head trauma. It is also rare and affects the cranial nerves, especially facial nerves. Generalized tetanus is the most common and severe form and in half of patients will present with trismus (masseter muscle spasm or lockjaw) (Sexton, 2015). Symptoms then progress in a descending fashion with tonic contraction of the skeletal muscles and intermittent intense, painful muscular spasms. The most profoundly affected muscles are those of the neck and back.

In the United States the fatality rate associated with tetanus has declined and cases are rare, but 10% of cases will result in death (CDC, 2012a). The general incubation period is 3 to 21 days, with an average of 8 days. Recovery can be long and difficult, and children with tetanus may have to spend several weeks in the hospital in an intensive care setting. It has been suggested that the shorter the incubation period, the higher the risk of more severe illness and poorer prognosis (CDC, 2012a). Complications associated with tetanus include breathing problems, fractures, elevated blood pressure, dysrhythmias, clotting in the blood vessels of the lung, pneumonia, and coma.

Therapeutic Management

Therapeutic management is directed toward supporting respiratory and cardiovascular function, stopping toxin production, neutralizing unbound toxins, and controlling muscle spasms. Tetanus immunoglobulin may be given as well as the tetanus vaccine. Removal of the offending organism, by debridement of the wound, may occur, and intravenous antibiotics such as metronidazole may be initiated. In severe cases, the child may require intensive nursing care with mechanical ventilation.

Nursing Assessment

Note history of initial signs such as headache, spasms, crankiness, and cramping of the jaw (lockjaw), which are followed by difficulty swallowing and a stiff neck. Tetanus progresses in a descending fashion to other muscle groups, causing spasms of the neck, arms, legs, and stomach; seizures may result. Document the presence of fever along with an elevated blood pressure and tachycardia. Opisthotonos (refer to Fig. 38.13 in Chapter 38) may be noted due to severe spasms of the neck and back. The spasms or muscle contractions in children may be strong enough to result in fractures. The diagnosis of tetanus is based on the clinical findings of the history and physical examination. There is no laboratory test to confirm tetanus.

Nursing Management

Nursing management focuses on observing for signs of respiratory distress. Provide a quiet environment with reduced external stimuli to decrease the incidence of spasms. Appropriately manage pain. Encourage adequate nutrition and hydration. Administer sedatives and muscle relaxants as ordered to reduce the pain associated with the muscle spasms and to prevent seizures. Encourage the parents to stay with their child. The child's mental status is unaffected by the disease, and therefore he or she is aware of what is happening. Efforts need to be made to reduce the child's anxiety and to provide reassuring, sympathetic care to the child and family. Tetanus is not contagious from person to person; therefore, standard precautions are sufficient.

Tetanus is a preventable but potentially fatal disease. Education is essential regarding the importance of receiving this routine immunization (refer to Chapter 31 for immunization information) as well as a booster every 10 years. Instructing parents on proper wound care can also help prevent tetanus. All wounds should be cleaned thoroughly and a proper antiseptic used. If a wound is deep and contamination is suspected, the child should be seen by a physician or nurse practitioner. If it has been more than 5 years since the last tetanus dose, a booster may be needed. This can help to neutralize the poison and prevent it from entering the nervous system.

Botulism

Botulism is a disease that is caused by a toxin produced in the immature intestines of young children resulting from infection with the bacterium *Clostridium botulinum*. It is rare but can cause serious paralytic illness. There are several types of botulism. Food-borne botulism results from ingestion of food contaminated with botulinum toxin. Wound botulism results from wounds infected with *C. botulinum*. Infant botulism is the most common in the United States and results from the ingestion of spores *C. botulinum,* most often from environmental dust. *C. botulinum* is common in soil and can also be found in a variety of foods, such as improperly preserved home-canned foods. It has been associated with feeding honey and corn syrup to infants; thus, these should be avoided in children younger than 1 year of age (Vyas & Zieve, 2013). The disease is not infectious; to become infected, the child must ingest the bacterial spores. These spores then multiply in the intestinal tract and produce the toxin, which is absorbed in the immature intestines of the infant. It is generally not a problem for older children because the bacteria do not grow well in mature intestines due to the presence of the normal intestinal flora. Prognosis is good, but if treatment is not initiated, paralysis of the arms, legs, trunk, and respiratory system can develop. Therapeutic management is usually supportive but may involve administration of botulinum immune globulin or botulism antitoxin.

Nursing Assessment

For a full description of the assessment phase of the nursing process, refer to the assessment section of the Nursing Process Overview earlier in this chapter. Assessment findings pertinent to botulism are discussed below.

HEALTH HISTORY

Elicit a description of the present illness and chief complaint. Signs and symptoms usually occur soon after ingestion of the bacteria. Common signs and symptoms in infants reported during the health history might include:

- Constipation
- Poor feeding
- Listlessness
- Generalized weakness
- Weak cry

Common signs and symptoms in older children reported during the health history might include:

- Double vision
- Blurred vision
- Drooping eyelids
- Difficulty swallowing
- Slurred speech
- Muscle weakness

PHYSICAL EXAMINATION AND LABORATORY AND DIAGNOSTIC TESTS

Assess for a diminished gag reflex, which is indicative of botulism. Diagnostic tests include cultures of stool and serum. Botulism is a rare disease and is difficult to diagnose since its symptoms are similar to those of other neuromuscular diseases. Therefore, assessment may include diagnostic tests to help rule out other diseases, such as Guillain–Barré syndrome, stroke, and myasthenia gravis.

Nursing Management

Treatment is mainly supportive and focuses on maintaining respiratory status and nutritional status. If ordered, administer botulinum immune globulin early in the disease to reduce its severity and progression. Two botulism antitoxins are available in the United States through the State Health Department.

Osteomyelitis

Osteomyelitis is a bacterial infection of the bone and soft tissue surrounding the bone. The long bone metaphysis is the most common location (Haut, 2014). *S. aureus* is the most common infecting organism with methicillin-resistant *S. aureus* (MRSA) infections on the rise (Haut, 2014). Additional causes in infants and children include group A and B streptococcus, *E. coli, S. pneumoniae, Kingella kingae, and Haemophilus influenzae* (which is now rare due to improvements in immunizations) (Haut, 2014; Krogstad, 2014b). Children usually present for evaluation within a few days to a week of onset of symptoms, though some may present later.

Osteomyelitis is acquired hematogenously (spread through the blood). Bacteria from the bloodstream mainly invade the most rapidly growing portion of the bone. The invading bacteria trigger an inflammatory response, formation of pus and edema, and vascular congestion. Small blood vessels thrombose and the infection extends into the metaphyseal marrow cavity. As the infection progresses the inflammation extends throughout the bone and blood supply is disrupted, resulting in death of the bone tissues (Fig. 37.3).

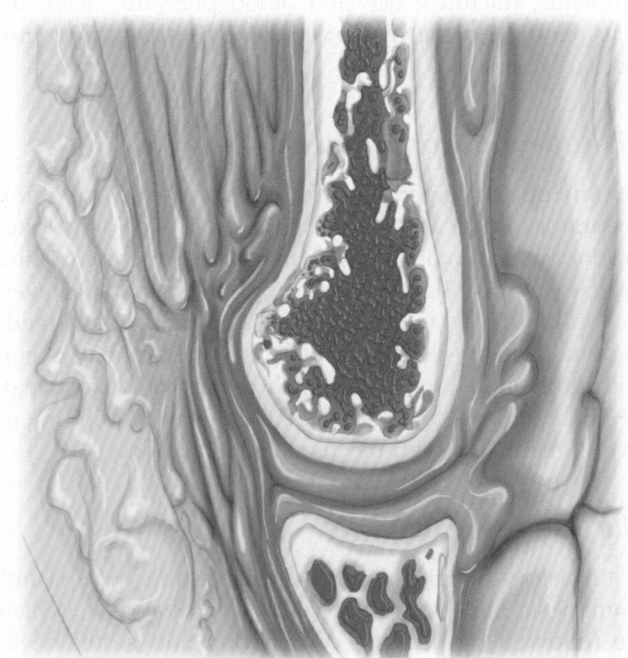

FIGURE 37.3 In osteomyelitis, bacterial invasion leads to infection within the bone.

Therapeutic Management

Aspiration is necessary to confirm diagnosis and identify specific microorganisms. Treatment includes a 4- to 6-week course of antibiotics. Some children may receive 1 to 2 weeks of intravenous antibiotics and then be switched to oral antibiotics for the remainder of the course. Surgical debridement is rarely necessary. Early treatment may prevent the complications of bone destruction, fracture, and growth arrest. Additional complications include recurrent infection, septic arthritis, and systemic infection.

Nursing Assessment

For a full description of the assessment phase of the nursing process, refer to the assessment section of the Nursing Process Overview earlier in this chapter. Assessment findings pertinent to osteomyelitis are discussed here.

Explore the health history for risk factors and symptoms. Risk factors include impetigo, infected varicella lesions, furunculosis, recent trauma, infected burns, and prolonged intravenous line use. Obtain history of current or recent antibiotic therapy and response. Note history of irritability, lethargy, possible fever, and onset of pain or change in activity level. The child usually refuses to walk and demonstrates decreased range of motion in the affected extremity. Inspect the affected extremity for swelling. Palpate for local warmth and tenderness. Note point tenderness over affected bone.

Laboratory and diagnostic testing may reveal:

- Elevated white blood cell count, erythrocyte sedimentation rate, and C-reactive protein level
- Positive blood cultures
- Deep soft tissue swelling on radiography
- Changes on ultrasound, CT scan, or MRI

Nursing Management

Nursing management of the child with osteomyelitis focuses on assessment, pain management, and maintenance of intravenous access for administration of antibiotics. Individualize care based on the child's and family's response to the illness; see Nursing Care Plan 37.1 at the end of the chapter. Maintain bed rest initially to prevent injury and promote comfort. Administer antipyretics as ordered if the child is febrile in the initial stage of the illness. Encourage the use of unaffected extremities by providing developmentally appropriate toys and games. Instruct the child and family on safe and proper use of crutches or walker if prescribed. Some children will be discharged home on intravenous antibiotics, while others will finish an oral antibiotic course. Teach parents proper administration of medications and maintenance of a peripherally inserted central catheter or central line at home if the child is finishing the antibiotic course intravenously.

Septic Arthritis

Acute septic arthritis is a condition in which bacteria invade the joint space, most often the hip or knee. It can occur at any age but usually occurs in children younger than 3 years old (Krogstad, 2014a). Usually bacteria gain access to the joint through the bloodstream but can be due to direct puncture from injections, venipuncture, wound infection, surgery, or injury.

S. aureus is the most common causative organism with community-acquired MRSA on the rise (Krogstad, 2014a). Various streptococci species, *K. kingae, N. meningitidis* (with or without an associated meningitis), *H. influenzae* (in unvaccinated children), and *Neisseria gonorrhoeae* are also responsible organisms (Krogstad, 2014a). Sepsis of the hip joint may cause avascular necrosis of the femoral head due to pressure on blood vessels and cartilage within the joint space. Septic arthritis is considered a medical emergency, as destruction of the joint cartilage may occur within just a few days. Additional complications of septic arthritis include permanent deformity, leg-length discrepancy, and long-term decreased range of motion and disability.

The goals of treatment of septic arthritis are to prevent destruction of the joint cartilage and maintain function, motion, and strength. Septic arthritis is treated rapidly with joint aspiration or arthrotomy, followed by intravenous antibiotic therapy while in the hospital and oral antibiotics at home.

Nursing Assessment

Note a history of predisposing factors such as respiratory infection or otitis media, skin or soft tissue infections, or, in the neonate, traumatic puncture wounds and femoral venipunctures. The history is usually significant for sudden onset of fever and moderate to severe pain.

Upon physical examination, the infant or child appears ill. Note extent of fever, reports of pain, refusal to bear weight or straighten the joint, and limited range of motion (the child usually maintains the joint in flexion and will not allow the leg to be straightened). The child will generally hold the joint in a position of comfort and the child or infant will appear without pain as long as the joint is immobile. Any attempt at passive range of motion will reveal pain. Palpate the affected joint for warmth and swelling.

Laboratory findings may include:

- White blood cell count normal or elevated with elevated neutrophil counts
- Elevated erythrocyte sedimentation rate and C-reactive protein levels
- Fluid from joint aspiration demonstrates elevated white blood cell count; culture determines responsible organism.

- Joint x-ray may show subtle soft tissue changes or increase in the joint space.
- Positive blood culture for the causative organism (15% of cases)

Nursing Management

Refer to Nursing Care Plan 37.1 at the end of the chapter for interventions related to musculoskeletal disorders. Assess aspiration wound for signs of infection. Monitor vital signs for resolution of fever. Pain management with ibuprofen or acetaminophen will be sufficient for some children; others may initially require codeine or morphine. Assess the affected joint for a decrease in swelling, increasing range of motion, and decreasing or absent pain. The child may be discharged after 72 hours of intravenous antibiotics following joint aspiration if he or she is improving and can tolerate oral antibiotics. At discharge, if the child cannot ambulate, physical therapy may be consulted for short-term use of crutches or a wheelchair. Teach families how to assess for signs and symptoms of wound infection, how to administer oral antibiotics and pain medication, and how to assist their child with crutch walking.

VIRAL INFECTIONS

Viruses are very small particles that infect cells. They cannot multiply on their own and require a living host, such as humans, animals, or plants. They can reproduce only by invading and taking over the host cells. Young children are highly sensitive to viruses; their resistance is low and exposure is high. Viruses are hard to destroy without damaging or killing the living cells they infect. Therefore, drugs are not used to control them. However, many viral diseases can be prevented by immunization, such as measles, rubella, varicella, mumps, and poliomyelitis (see Chapter 31 for more information on immunizations).

Viral Exanthems

Many viral infections of the skin in childhood are called viral exanthems. **Exanthem** means rash or skin eruption. Viral exanthems of childhood often present with a distinct rash pattern that assists in the diagnosis of the virus. Table 37.4 discusses common childhood exanthems. Immunizations have led to a decrease in the incidence of certain viral exanthems, such as measles, rubella, and varicella.

Typically, children with viral exanthems are cared for at home, but there are times when a child may be hospitalized or may develop the disease while being hospitalized. Appropriate transmission-based precautions must be taken. Therapeutic management of the viral exanthems focuses on fever management and relief of discomfort.

TABLE 37.4 COMMON VIRAL EXANTHEMS OF CHILDHOOD

Disease	Clinical Manifestations
Rubella (German measles) • Caused by rubella virus • Transmission: by direct or indirect contact with droplets, primarily by nasopharyngeal secretions, but also in blood, stool, and urine. Also transmitted from mother to fetus • Peak incidence: late winter and early spring • Incubation period: 12–23 days (usually 14) • Communicable: 7 days before to 7 days after onset of rash 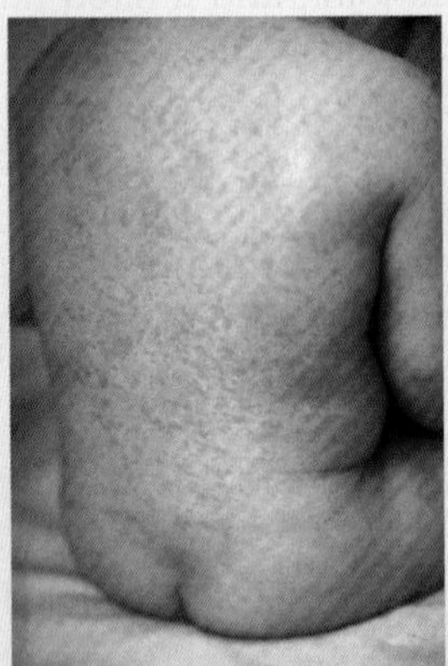 Rubella rash. (Courtesy of CDC. [1966]. Obtained at http://phil.cdc.gov/PHIL_Images/03052002/00002/PHIL_712_lores.jpg)	• Rash usually first sign. Maculopapular rash that begins on face and spreads head to foot; disappears in same order it spread, usually by the third day. On the second day the rash may appear pinpoint. Desquamation is minimal. • In older children: lymphadenopathy (retroauricular, posterior cervical, postoccipital) 24 hours before the onset of the rash; lasting up to 1 week; low-grade fever, malaise, upper respiratory symptoms • Mild pruritus • Polyarthralgia and polyarthritis (rare in children but common in adolescents)

Nursing Assessment

Obtain the history of the present illness, noting the onset of rash in relation to the onset of fever. Note accompanying symptoms such as respiratory complaints. Document known exposure to childhood diseases. Note immunization status. Inspect the skin for rash, noting the distribution, type, and extent of lesions. Table 37.4 describes the rash as well as accompanying symptoms for each of the viral exanthems.

Nursing Management

Nursing management of viral exanthems focuses on fever reduction, relief of discomfort, and protection of skin integrity. Encourage hydration. Administer antipyretics and antipruritics as needed (refer to Drug Guide 37.1). Nonpharmacologic interventions to reduce fever, such as tepid sponging and cool compresses, may be used. Refer to Nursing Care Plan 37.1 at the end of the chapter for additional information. Care should be individualized based on the child's and family's response to the illness.

Take Note!

Trim the child's fingernails or cover hands with mitts, gloves, or socks (which work well with younger infants and children) if the rash itches to help prevent breaks in the skin, which can lead to discomfort and infection.

Mumps

Mumps, a contagious disease caused by Paramyxovirus, is characterized by fever and parotitis (inflammation and swelling of the parotid gland). Mumps is spread via contact with infected droplets. Infected individuals are contagious for 1 to 7 days prior to the onset of symptoms and for 4 to 9 days after parotid swelling begins (CDC, 2012a). About 50% of all infected postpubertal boys also develop orchitis (inflammation of the testicle) (CDC, 2012a). This may lead to some degree of testicular atrophy, but rarely sterility. In about 5% of females oophoritis (ovarian inflammation) occurs with no relationship to infertility (CDC, 2012a). Up to half of people with mumps will have nonspecific or mild respiratory symptoms or no symptoms at all (CDC, 2012a). Complications of mumps include meningitis with or without encephalitis with seizures, pancreatitis, and auditory neuritis, which can result in hearing loss. Therapeutic management is supportive.

Since the recommendation of the two-dose MMR (measles, mumps, rubella) vaccine, the incidence of mumps has declined and made mumps a rare disease seen in the United States (CDC, 2012a). The American Academy of Pediatrics (AAP) and the ACIP recommends immunization against mumps for all children (CDC, 2015m). Current recommendations include first mumps immunization

(text continues on page 1362)

Management/Complications	Nursing Implications
• Usually mild and self-limiting • Treatment is mainly supportive. • Complications: encephalitis and thrombocytopenia (rare) • Maternal rubella during pregnancy can result in miscarriage, fetal death, or congenital malformations.	• Comfort measures such as antipyretics, antipruritics, and analgesics for joint pain

(continued)

TABLE 37.4 COMMON VIRAL EXANTHEMS OF CHILDHOOD (continued)

Disease	Clinical Manifestations
Rubeola (measles) • Caused by measles virus • Transmission: direct or indirect contact with droplets, primarily by nasopharyngeal secretions, but also blood and urine. Highly contagious • Peak incidence: late winter and spring • Incubation period: 10–12 days • Communicable 1–2 days before the onset of symptoms (3–5 days before onset of rash) until 4–6 days after rash has appeared 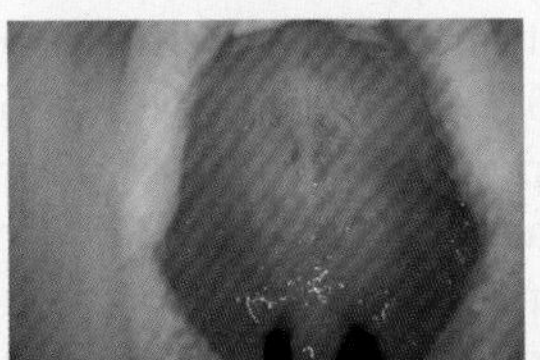 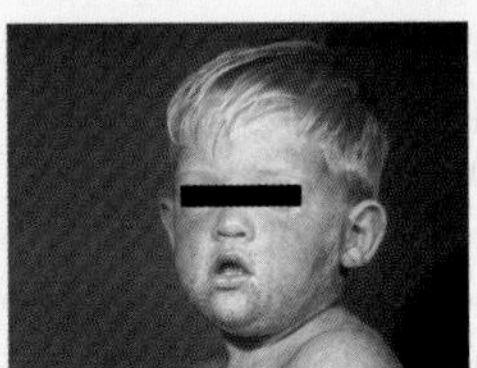 Koplik spots. (Courtesy of CDC/Dr. Heinz F. Eichenwald. [1958]. Obtained at http://phil.cdc.gov/phil/details.asp?pid=3187); Ruboela. (Courtesy of CDC [1963]; Obtained at http://phil.cdc.gov/phil/details.asp?pid=1150)	• Prodromal phase: 2–4 days, consisting of fever, cough, coryza, conjunctivitis • Followed by Koplik spots (bright red spots with blue white centers on mucous membranes, mainly buccal mucosa; look like tiny grains of white sand surrounded by red rings) • Erythematous maculopapular rash appears 3–4 days after the onset of the prodromal phase. Rash gradually proceeds from head downward and outward.
Varicella Zoster (chickenpox) • Caused by varicella zoster virus, human herpes virus 3 • Transmission: direct contact with infected persons' nasopharyngeal secretions or via air-borne spread, to a lesser degree by contact with unscabbed lesions. Highly contagious. Also transmitted from mother to fetus • Peak incidence: late fall, winter, and spring • Incubation period: 10–21 days, usually 14–16 days • Communicable 1–2 days before the onset of rash until all vesicles have crusted over (about 3–7 days after the onset of rash) 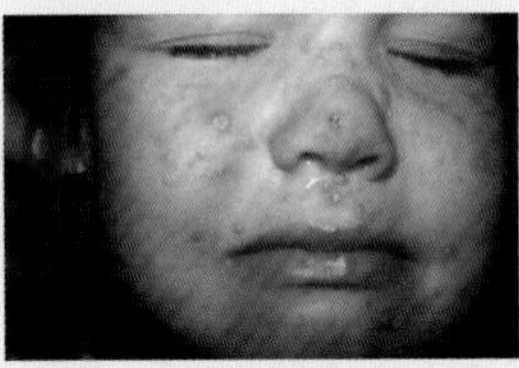 Varicella. (Courtesy of CDC/Dr. John Noble, Jr. [1968]. Obtained at http://phil.cdc.gov/phil/details.asp)	• Prodromal symptoms (fever, malaise, anorexia, headache, mild abdominal pain) may be present 24–48 hours before the onset of the rash. In children, rash is often the first sign of disease. • Lesions often appear first on scalp, face, trunk, then extremities; initially intensely pruritic erythematous macules that evolve to papules and then form clear, fluid-filled vesicles • Vesicles eventually erupt, and then lesions scab and crust. A variety of lesions are present at one time. • More severe in adolescents and adults than in young children
Exanthem Subitum (roseola infantum or sixth disease) • Caused by human herpes virus 6 (HHV-6); less frequently human herpes virus 7 (HHV-7) • Transmission: little is known but suspected to be from saliva of infected person and enters the host through the oral, nasal, or conjunctival mucosa • Peak incidence: age 7–13 months • Incubation period: 5–15 days, average of 10 days • Communicability is unknown, but most likely contagious before symptoms appear 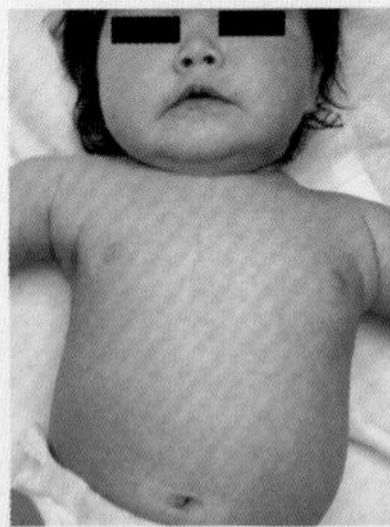 Exanthem subitum (roseola infantum).	• Prodromal phase: usually asymptomatic but may include upper respiratory signs • Clinical illness: high fever ranging from 37.9° to 40°C (101–106°F) for 3–5 days; resolves abruptly; rash appears 12–24 hours later, lasting about 1–3 days. Rash is pinkish red, flat or raised spots that blanch when touched

Management/Complications	Nursing Implications
• Treatment is mainly supportive, including antipyretics, bed rest, and adequate fluid intake. • Possible vitamin A supplementation in children 6 months to 2 years hospitalized for measles or its complications or those with immunodeficiency[a] • Complications: diarrhea, otitis media, and pneumonia, common in young children; acute encephalitis	• Comfort measures, such as antipyretics and antipruritics. • Clean eyes with warm, moist cloth to remove secretions. • Cool mist humidification to alleviate coryza and cough. • Air-borne precautions until 4 days after the onset of rash.
• Usually self-limiting; treatment is mainly supportive: fever reduction, antipruritics, and skin care to prevent infection of lesions. • Antiviral therapy and varicella zoster immune globulin may be used in those considered to be at high risk (immunocompromised, pregnant women, and newborns exposed to maternal varicella). Routine antiviral therapy is not recommended for the treatment of uncomplicated varicella infection in otherwise healthy children. • Complications: bacterial superinfection of skin lesions, thrombocytopenia, arthritis, hepatitis, cerebellar ataxia, encephalitis, meningitis, pneumonia, glomerulonephritis, congenital infection, and life-threatening perinatal infection. • Lifelong latent infection occurs; reactivation results in herpes zoster (shingles), uncommon in childhood.	• Comfort measures, such as antipyretics and antipruritics. • Air-borne and contact precautions in the hospitalized child for a minimum of 5 days after the onset of rash and as long as vesicular lesions are present. • For those with exposure to susceptible persons, air-borne and contact precautions, from 8 to 21 days after exposure. • Children may return to school or child care once lesions have crusted.
• Course is generally benign. • In children who are uncomfortable or irritable or have a history of febrile seizures, antipyretics may be warranted. • Complications: HSV-6 may be responsible for some febrile seizures, encephalitis, and meningoencephalitis (rare).	• Comfort measures, such as antipyretics, antipruritics. • Standard precautions are sufficient in the hospitalized child.

(continued)

TABLE 37.4 COMMON VIRAL EXANTHEMS OF CHILDHOOD (continued)

Disease	Clinical Manifestations
Erythema Infectiosum (fifth disease) • Caused by human parvovirus B19 • Transmitted by large droplet spread from nasopharyngeal viral shedding or percutaneous exposure to blood and blood products. Also transmitted from mother to fetus • Peak incidence late winter and early spring • Incubation period: 4–28 days, average 16–17 days • Communicability is uncertain, but most children are no longer infectious by the time the rash appears and diagnosis is made, so isolation or exclusion from school, once the child is diagnosed, is unnecessary (those with aplastic crisis may be communicable up to 1 week after the onset of symptoms and those who are immunosuppressed with chronic infection and severe anemia may be communicable for months to years). 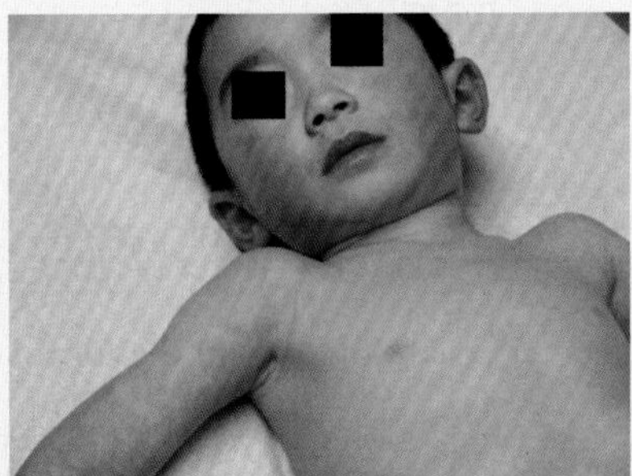 Erythema infectiosum (fifth disease).	• Prodromal phase: mild symptoms, low-grade fever, headache, mild upper respiratory infection • Characteristic rash occurs in three stages: • Begins with erythematous flushing often described as "slapped-cheek" appearance, often with circumoral pallor • Spreads to trunk • Moves peripherally, appearing as a maculopapular, lace-like appearance; often pruritic • Palms and soles are usually spared. Rash fluctuates in intensity and will disappear and reappear with environmental changes such as exposure to sunlight. • Resolves spontaneously over 1–3 weeks • Pain or swelling in joints may be present • Children with pre-existing anemias may develop aplastic crisis (will have fever, malaise, myalgia, but usually no rash).
Hand, Foot, and Mouth Disease, or Herpangina (if only mouth involvement) • Caused by viruses belonging to enterovirus genus. Coxsackie A viruses (especially A16) is the most common. Transmitted by direct contact with infected fecal, oral secretions; spread mostly through saliva • Peak incidence during spring and summer, particularly in children who wear diapers (1- to 4-year-olds) • Incubation period: 3–6 days • Communicable from time of infection until fever resolves; virus is shed for several weeks after the infection begins.	• High fever usually occurs first. • Vesicles on tongue and oral mucosa erode to shallow ulcers; vesicles on hands and feet are football shaped, with erythematous rims. • Extensive mouth lesions may lead to anorexia, dehydration, and drooling.

Adapted from Siegel, J. D., Rhinehart, E., Jackson, M., Chiarello, L., and the Healthcare Infection Control Practices Advisory Committee. (2007). *Guideline for isolation precautions: Preventing transmission of infectious agents in healthcare settings.* Retrieved from http://www.cdc.gov/hicpac/pdf/isolation/Isolation2007.pdf; Centers for Disease Control and Prevention. (2012 a). *Epidemiology and prevention of vaccine-preventable diseases* (12th ed., second printing). Atkinson, W., Wolfe, S., & Hamborsky, J., (Eds.). Washington, DC: Public Health Foundation; Koch, W. C. (2011). Chapter 243: Parvovirus B19. In R. M. Kleigman, B. F. Stanton, J. W. St. Geme III, N. F. Schor & R. E. Behrman (Eds.), *Nelson textbook of pediatrics* (19th ed., pp. 1094–1097). Philadelphia, PA: Saunders; and Centers for Disease Control and Prevention. (2015a). *About Hand, foot and mouth disease (HFMD).* Retrieved from http://www.cdc.gov/hand-foot-mouth/about/index.html; Tremblay, C., & Brady, M. T. (2015). Roseola infantum (exanthem subitum). UpToDate. Retrieved from http://www.uptodate.com/contents/roseola-infantum-exanthem-subitum?source=search_result

Management/Complications	Nursing Implications
• Usually benign and self-limited; supportive treatment is all that is needed. • Blood transfusion may be necessary in children with aplastic crisis. • Complications: arthritis and arthralgia. • May result in fetal loss, hydrops fetalis in pregnant woman.	• Comfort measures, such as antipyretics, antipruritics. • Droplet precautions are required in the hospitalized child. • Inform pregnant women (including healthcare workers) of the potential risks to the fetus and preventive measures to decrease these risks (strict infection control practices, not caring for those likely to be contagious). The CDC does not recommended routine exclusion from a workplace where an outbreak is occurring.
• Usually mild and self-limiting, resolving within 1 week • Treatment is mainly supportive. • Complications: dehydration, meningitis, encephalitis, and pulmonary edema	• Standard precautions and good hand hygiene are necessary. • Encourage oral fluids of preference, such as popsicles. • Provide analgesics as needed.

between 12 and 15 months of age, followed by a second vaccine between 4 and 6 years of age (CDC, 2015m). According to the CDC (2015f), research shows that one dose of MMR prevents 78% of cases and two doses prevent approximately 88% of cases (see Chapter 31 for information on mumps vaccination).

Nursing Assessment

Note history of exposure to infected individuals as well as immunization status. Determine history of low-grade fever and onset and progression of parotid swelling. History may also include malaise, anorexia, headache, and abdominal pain. The parotid swelling is easily observed as swelling of the neck either bilaterally or unilaterally (Fig. 37.4). In boys, note orchitis. The diagnosis is usually based on the history and clinical presentation, but serum may be tested for the presence of mumps IgG or IgM antibody.

Nursing Management

Nursing management of mumps is primarily supportive. Acetaminophen or ibuprofen is used for fever management, and occasionally narcotic analgesics are required for pain management. Oral fluids are encouraged to prevent dehydration. If orchitis is present, ice packs to the testicles and gentle testicular support may be helpful. Hospitalized children should be confined to respiratory isolation to prevent spread of the disease. Infected children are considered no longer contagious 9 days following the onset of parotid swelling (CDC, 2012a).

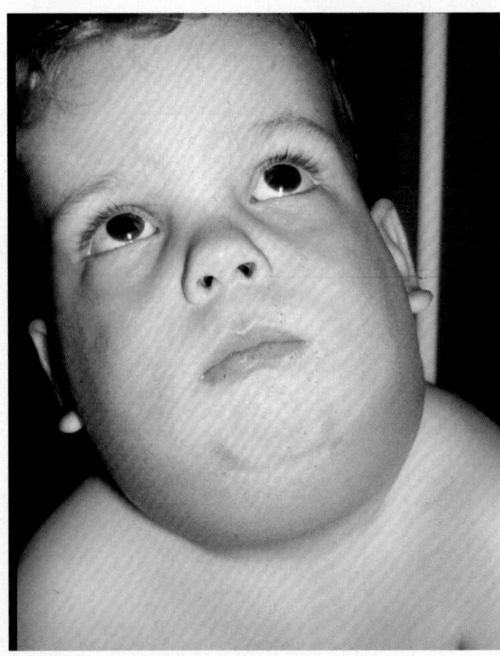

FIGURE 37.4 Parotitis associated with mumps.

Take Note!

In recent years mumps outbreaks have occurred, mainly in settings where prolonged close contact with other people occurs, such as college campuses and camps. The mumps vaccine is not 100% effective, and mumps infection can occur in vaccinated individuals (CDC, 2014d). During an outbreak it is essential to define the population at risk and transmission setting, identify and isolate suspected cases, and identify and vaccinate susceptible individuals.

ZOONOTIC INFECTIONS

Zoonotic and **vector-borne** infections are diseases caused by infectious agents that are transmitted directly or indirectly from animals or vectors, such as ticks, mosquitos, or other insect vectors to humans. Zoonotic infections are responsible for about 75% of emerging infectious diseases, with approximately 60% of all human pathogens originating from animals (Centers for Disease Prevention and Control, 2015g).

Children are at a particular risk for contracting zoonotic or vector-borne diseases. Young children are unaware of the health risks around them and cannot take protective measures. Their immature immune system leads to a decreased capacity to resist zoonotic or vector-borne diseases. These diseases can be severe and even fatal, although most are treatable if identified early. Many times the child presents initially with nonspecific symptoms. Coupled with the fact that there are few definitive diagnostic tests available, this can lead to difficulty in promptly recognizing and treating these diseases. Tick-borne diseases are common vector-borne illnesses in the United States. Determining the incidence of zoonotic and vector-borne diseases is difficult due to the complexity of the transmission cycle and geographic climate variability. Table 37.5 discusses other zoonotic and vector borne diseases. Nurses need to be aware of zoonotic and vector borne diseases common in the area they are practicing as well as the impact of patient travel and the risk of these diseases. Nurses need to tap into state and local resources as well as national and international resources, such as the CDC and WHO.

Take Note!

The CDC lists the current infectious disease outbreaks that are being reported at http://www.cdc.gov/outbreaks/

Cat-Scratch Disease

Cat-scratch disease is a relatively common and occasionally serious disease caused by the bacteria

TABLE 37.5 OTHER ZOONOTIC AND VECTOR-BORNE ILLNESSES

Disease	Causative Organism	Geographic Distribution	Vector of Transmission	Manifestations
West Nile virus	*Flavivirus*	Throughout United States with higher rates found in Great Plains and mountain regions; seasonal epidemic from summer to fall	Mosquito bites Rare cases spread through blood transfusions, transplants, and mother to baby during pregnancy and breastfeeding.	• Symptoms include febrile illness, meningitis, encephalitis, or acute flaccid paralysis. • Children more likely to be asymptomatic or have milder form of disease than adults but children manifest as meningitis more often than adults[a]
Dengue	*Aedes aegypti* *Aedes albopictus*	Tropics and Subtropics Asia, the Pacific, the Americas, Africa, the Carribbean	Mosquito	• Sudden onset high fever, headache, severe pain behind eyes, joint, muscle and bone pain, rash, mild bleeding such as nose or gums bleeding and bruising easily, leukopenia, thrombocytopenia and hemorrhagic manifestations
Anaplasmosis	*Anaplasma phagocytophilum,*	Mostly upper Midwest and northeast United States	Tick	• Headache, fever. malaise, chills, muscle aches, nausea, abdominal pain, cough, and confusion • Rash is rarely seen • Symptoms appear 1–2 weeks after infected tick bite
Ehrlichiosis	Three pathogens: *Ehrlichia chaffeensis, Ehrlichia ewingii, Ehrlichia*	Mostly in southeastern and south-central United States	Tick	• Fever, headaches, fatigue, muscle aches, chills, nausea, vomiting, diarrhea, confusion, red eyes. Clinical signs similar to Rocky Mountain spotted fever. Rash is less commonly associated but is seen in up to 60% of children. • May also present with leukopenia, anemia, and hepatitis.
Malaria	*Plasmodium* (five species exist that infect humans: *P. falciparum, P. vivax, P. ovale, P. malariae, P. knowlesi)*	Endemic in tropical areas of the world Highest incidence in Africa, Asia, and South America. Cases in the United States are usually in travelers and immigrants returning from countries where malaria transmission occurs	Bite of *Anopheles* species of mosquito	• High fever with chills, rigors, sweats, and headache, which may be paroxysmal • Nausea, vomiting, diarrhea, cough, arthralgia, and abdominal and back pain may also occur. • Anemia and thrombocytopenia with pallor and jaundice may be seen. • May occur in a cyclic pattern, and depending on the species fever may occur every other day or every third day.

[a]Centers for Disease Control and Prevention. (2013a). *Anaplasmosis.* Retrieved from http://www.cdc.gov/anaplasmosis/; Centers for Disease Control and Prevention. (2013b). *Ehrlichiosis.* Retrieved from http://www.cdc.gov/ehrlichiosis/; Centers for Disease Control and Prevention. (2015b). *Dengue.* Retrieved from http://www.cdc.gov/Dengue/; Centers for Disease Control and Prevention. (2015p). *West Nile virus.* Retrieved from http://www.cdc.gov/westnile/index.html; and John, C. C., & Krause, P. J. (2011). Chapter 280: Malaria (plasmodium). In R. M. Kleigman, B. F. Stanton, J. W. St. Geme III, N. F. Schor, & R. E. Behrman (Eds.), *Nelson textbook of pediatrics* (19th ed., pp. 1198–1207). Philadelphia, PA: Saunders.

Bartonella henselae. It occurs in both children and adults but is more common in children (Papadopol, 2014). Cats can carry the bacteria in their saliva. In 87% to 99% of cases the child has had a recent interaction with cats and often kittens (Stechenberg, 2011). No evidence exists to support person-to-person transmission (Papadopol, 2015). *B. henselae* is transmitted between cats via the cat flea. The incubation period is 7 to 12 days, with lymphadenopathy appearing in 1 to 4 weeks (Stechenberg, 2011). Therapeutic management is supportive and is aimed at management of symptoms. The disease itself is usually self-limited, resolving on its own in 2 to 4 months. If lymphadenopathy persists or if the child is immunocompromised, antibiotics may be needed. Painful, swollen nodes may be treated with needle aspiration to provide symptom relief.

Nursing Assessment

Note history of headaches, fever, anorexia, and fatigue. The history may also include interaction or rough play with cats or kittens, resulting in a scratch. Document temperature, noting fever. Palpate for enlarged lymph nodes, noting their location. A skin papule or pustule may be present or reported at this site of the bite or scratch. Diagnostic tests are available to detect serum antibodies to antigens of *Bartonella* species.

Nursing Management

Administer antibiotics if ordered. No transmission-based isolation is required; standard precautions are sufficient. Educate the child and family about prevention and control measures. Teach children to avoid rough play with cats and kittens. Teach parents and children to immediately wash any bites or scratches with soap and running water. Explain that cats should never lick open wounds on the child. Control of fleas in cats is important to prevent the spread of *B. henselae*.

Rabies

Rabies is a preventable viral infection of the central nervous system. It is transmitted to other animals and humans through close contact with the saliva of a rabid animal, usually by a bite. It is rare in the United States and Western Europe due to routine vaccination of domestic animals, such as dogs, and the availability of effective postexposure prophylaxis (PEP). Now most cases of rabies in these areas are due to wild animals such as raccoons, skunks, bats, mongooses, and foxes (Willoughby, Jr., 2011). Rabies continues to be a major health problem in other parts of the world, especially in areas where dogs are not controlled.

Most cases of rabies occur in children younger than 15 years of age, and most human deaths occur in Asia and Africa (World Health Organization [WHO], 2014). Children have an increased susceptibility to rabies due to their fearlessness around animals, eagerness to play with animals, shorter stature, and inability to protect themselves. The incubation period for rabies is extremely variable. Typically it is 1 to 3 months but can range from days to years (WHO, 2014). The incubation period tends to be shorter in children. Once symptoms of rabies have developed, the prognosis is poor. Death usually occurs within days of the onset of symptoms. Prevention is of paramount importance, and eliminating infection in animal vectors is essential. Successful animal vaccination and animal control campaigns in the United States have led to a very low rate of human rabies cases. Recently, rabies transmitted from other animals, especially bats, has become a cause for concern (Willoughby, Jr., 2011; WHO, 2014).

It is important to contact the local health department whenever there is an exposure, or suspected exposure, to rabies. Several factors need to be considered when deciding to provide PEP, such as local epidemiology, type of animal involved, availability of the responsible animal for testing or quarantine, and the circumstances of the exposure, such as a provoked versus an unprovoked attack. Algorithms are available to help healthcare providers decide if PEP is warranted (Willoughby, Jr., 2011). In a previously unvaccinated child, PEP should begin with a thorough cleansing of all wounds with soap and water or a virucidal agent, such as povidone–iodine solution. In the United States, concurrent use of passive and active immunoprophylaxis is then recommended. It consists of a regimen of one dose of immune globulin and four doses of human rabies vaccine. Rabies immune globulin and the first dose of rabies vaccine should be given as soon as possible after exposure, ideally within 24 hours. Additional doses of rabies vaccine should be given on days 3, 7, and 14 after the first vaccination. Rabies immune globulin is infiltrated into and around the wound, with any remaining volume administered intramuscularly at a site distant from the vaccine inoculation. Human rabies vaccine is administered intramuscularly into the anterolateral thigh or deltoid, depending on the age and size of the child. Administration into the gluteus muscle should be avoided, since this site has been associated with vaccine failure (Rupprecht et al., 2010; Willoughby, Jr., 2011). Pre-exposure vaccination can be given to prevent rabies in people at high risk, such as veterinarians, laboratory technicians working with the virus, and people exposed to wild animals (Willoughby, Jr., 2011).

Nursing Assessment

Note the history of an animal bite, especially if it was unprovoked, and exposure to bats. Document history of early symptoms of rabies infection, which are nonspecific and flu-like, such as fever, headache, and general malaise. The child may complain of pain, pruritus, and paresthesia at the bite site. As the virus spreads to the central nervous system, encephalitis develops. The disease will have progressive neurologic manifestations, which may include insomnia, confusion, anxiety, changes in behavior, agitation or excitation, hallucinations, hypersalivation, dysphagia, and hydrophobia, which results from aspiration when swallowing liquid or saliva. In some cases progressive paralysis may be present. The child may have periods of lucidity alternating with these neurologic changes.

Laboratory testing may include hair and saliva specimens from which the virus may be isolated. Serum and cerebrospinal fluid can be tested for antibodies to the rabies virus. Direct fluorescent antibody testing can be done to diagnose rabies in a suspected animal. The test can only be done postmortem and requires brain tissue from the potentially rabid animal.

Nursing Management

Few people survive once symptomatic rabies infection develops. Intensive supportive care is required, but recovery is extremely rare. Therefore, it is vital to educate children and families about the importance of seeking medical care after any animal bite to prevent death from rabies infection. Also, teach children to avoid wild animals, stray animals, and any animal with unusual behavior. Teach children not to provoke or attempt to capture wild or stray animals.

Take Note!

There have been three survivors of rabies once symptoms developed using a treatment protocol developed by Dr. Rodney Willoughby called the Milwaukee Protocol at Children's Hospital of Wisconsin (Willoughby, Jr., 2011).

Regardless of whether immunoprophylaxis is initiated, appropriate wound management is necessary in all victims of a bite from a potentially rabid animal. This includes a thorough cleansing of all wounds with soap and water. Irrigation of wounds with large volumes of a virucidal agent, such as povidone–iodine solution, along with avoiding closure of the wound, is recommended (Willoughby, Jr., 2011).

When caring for a child requiring PEP, provide support and education to the child and family. Due to the seriousness and urgency surrounding this disease and treatment, the child and family are often very frightened. Consider comfort measures, such as EMLA (eutectic mixture of local anesthetics) cream and positioning, when giving immunization.

Lyme Disease

Lyme disease, the most common reported vector-borne disease in the United States, is caused by the spirochete *Borrelia burgdorferi* (CDC, 2012b). It is transmitted to humans via the bite of an infected black-legged (deer) tick. Ninety-five percent of reported Lyme disease cases occurred in 14 states, mainly in the northeast (Pennsylvania, New Jersey, New York, Massachusetts, Connecticut, Maryland, New Hampshire, Delaware, Maine, Rhode Island, Vermont, and Virginia) and the upper Midwest (Minnesota and Wisconsin) (CDC, 2015c).

Lyme disease can affect any age group, but the incidence is highest among children between 5 and 9 years of age (Eppes, 2011). The prognosis for recovery in children who are treated is excellent.

Therapeutic Management

In most cases Lyme disease can be cured by antibiotics, especially if they are started early in the illness. Doxycycline is the drug of choice for children older than 8 years (Eppes, 2011). Because of the risk that it can cause permanent discoloration of the teeth, children younger than 8 years should be treated with amoxicillin (Eppes, 2011). For children allergic to penicillin, cefuroxime axetil can be used. Duration of treatment is usually 14 to 28 days, depending on the stage of disease.

Nursing Assessment

The clinical signs of Lyme disease are divided into three stages—early localized, early disseminated, and late disease. Untreated children may progress through the three stages or may present with early disseminated or late disease without having any symptoms of the earlier stages. If children are treated in the early stage, it is uncommon to see them with late disease. Nursing assessment for Lyme disease includes an accurate health history as well as physical examination.

HEALTH HISTORY

Explore the health history for a tick bite. Document onset of rash. In early localized disease, the rash usually occurs 7 to 14 days after the tick bite (though it can appear 3 to 32 days after the bite). In early disseminated disease, the rash usually begins 3 to 5 weeks after the tick bite. Note complaints of fever, malaise, mild neck stiffness, headache, fatigue, myalgia, and arthralgia or pain in the joints. In late disease, note recurrent arthritis of the large joints, such as the knees, beginning weeks to months after the tick bite. The child with late disease may or may not have a history of earlier stages of the disease, including erythema migrans.

PHYSICAL EXAMINATION

Observe for a rash. A ring-like rash at the site of the tick bite (erythema migrans) characterizes early local disease

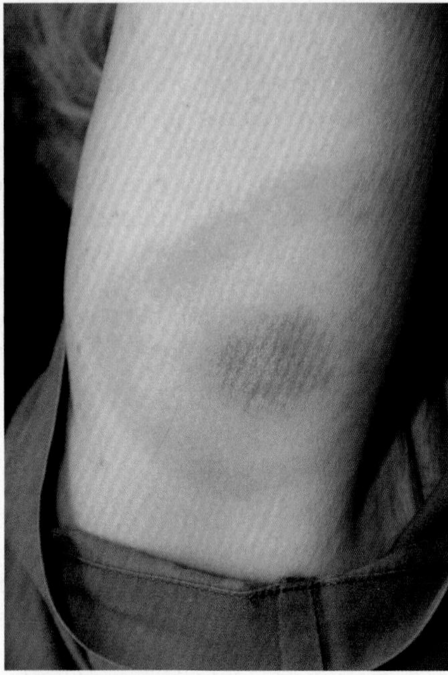

FIGURE 37.5 Erythema migrans, a ring-like rash at the site of the tick bite, occurs in Lyme disease. (Courtesy of CDC/James Gathany. [2007]. Obtained at http://phil.cdc.gov/phil/details.asp?pid=9875)

(Fig. 37.5). If untreated, the rash gradually expands and will remain for 1 to 2 weeks. Suspect early disseminated disease if multiple areas of erythema migrans are found. The multiple lesions are usually smaller than the primary lesions. Note cranial nerve palsies (especially cranial nerve VII), conjunctivitis, or signs of meningeal irritation, which occur in early disseminated disease.

LABORATORY AND DIAGNOSTIC TESTING

Immunoglobulin-specific antibody tests may not be positive in the early stage of the disease but may be useful in the later stages. The CDC recommends a two-step test—a sensitive enzyme immunoassay (EIA) or immunofluorescent assay (IFA), if positive, followed by a Western immunoblot (CDC, 2015d). If these are negative, no further testing is indicated.

Nursing Management

Administer antibiotics as ordered. In the hospitalized child, no transmission-based precautions are necessary. Educate the child and family on the importance of taking the antibiotic as directed and finishing all the medicine. Another important nursing function is educating the child, family, and community on prevention measures (Box 37.5). For infection to occur, typically the tick must be attached for 36 to 48 hours (CDC, 2015e). Therefore, prompt removal of ticks is essential to the prevention of Lyme disease. Teaching Guidelines 37.2 gives information on tick removal.

BOX 37.5

PREVENTION OF TICK-BORNE ILLNESSES

- Wear appropriate protective clothing when entering tick-infested areas. Clothing should fit tightly around wrists, waists, and ankles. Tuck pants into socks if possible.
- After leaving the area, do a full body check for ticks and remove them promptly.
- Examine gear, clothes, and pets for ticks. Tumble dry clothes and appropriate gear on high heat for an hour.
- Insect repellent may provide temporary relief but may produce toxicity, especially in children, if used frequently or in large doses.

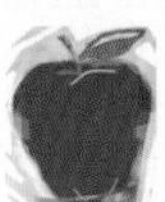

Teaching Guidelines 37.2

TICK REMOVAL

- Use fine-tipped tweezers.
- Protect fingers with a tissue, paper towel, or latex gloves.
- Grasp tick as close to the skin as possible and pull upward with steady, even pressure.
- Do not twist or jerk the tick.
- Once the tick is removed, clean site with soap and water, rubbing alcohol, or iodine scrub and wash your hands.
- Save the tick for identification in case the child becomes sick. Place in a sealable plastic bag and put it in your freezer. Write date of bite on the bag.

Rocky Mountain Spotted Fever

Rocky Mountain spotted fever (RMSF) is the most severe and frequently reported rickettsial illness in the United States and is the second most common vector-borne disease after Lyme disease (Reller & Dumler, 2011). RMSF is caused by the bacteria *Rickettsia rickettsii*. The American dog tick and Rocky Mountain wood tick are the primary vectors, although others have been implicated. RMSF can be fatal without prompt and appropriate treatment (Reller & Dumler, 2011). Most cases occur between April and September (Reller & Dumler, 2011).

RMSF occurs throughout the United States. Its name is derived from the fact that it was discovered in the Rocky Mountain region, though few cases are found there today. RMSF is more common in the coastal Atlantic states, but the highest incidence has been found in North Carolina and Oklahoma. It occurs in all age groups but most frequently in children, with the peak incidence in children greater than 5 years of age (Reller & Dumler, 2011).

Complications of RMSF include noncardiogenic pulmonary edema, cerebral edema, and multiorgan damage. Long-term neurologic involvement, such as partial paralysis of the lower extremities, hearing loss, loss of bladder and bowel control, movement disorders, and language disorders, may be seen, especially in children with severe illness who require long hospital stays.

Therapeutic Management

The fatality rate from RMSF has decreased with the widespread use of antimicrobial therapy (Reller & Dumler, 2011). However, delays in diagnosis and therapy are significant factors associated with severity of disease and death. In most cases RMSF resolves rapidly with appropriate antibiotic therapy, especially if it is started early. Treatments of choice are tetracyclines, such as doxycycline. Doxycycline and other tetracyclines are not normally used in children younger than 8 years due to the risk of teeth staining. However, due to the life-threatening nature of RMSF and the limited course of antibiotic therapy, the American Academy of Pediatrics Committee on Infectious Diseases revised its recommendations and has identified doxycycline as the drug of choice for treating presumed or confirmed RMSF in children of any age (Center for Disease Control and Prevention, 2013f). Length of treatment is typically 7 to 14 days (Center for Disease Control and Prevention, 2013f).

Nursing Assessment

Note history of early signs of RMSF, such as sudden onset of fever, headache, malaise, nausea and vomiting, muscle pain, and anorexia. The incubation period varies from 2 to 14 days, with the average being around 7 days after the tick bite (Reller & Dumler, 2011). Late signs include a rash, usually seen 2 to 5 days after the onset of the fever, abdominal pain, joint pain, and diarrhea. Inspect the skin for a rash, which starts as small, pink, macular, nonitchy, blanchable spots on the wrists, forearms, and ankles. The rash then spreads rapidly over the entire body, including the soles and palms. After several days the rash will appear red, spotted, and petechial or hemorrhagic (Fig. 37.6). Approximately 5% of children with RMSF do not have a rash (Reller & Dumler, 2011). Laboratory findings may include a low leukocyte count, low or decreasing platelet count, and hyponatremia. Biopsy of the rash with immunofluorescent assay and serologic tests may also be used.

Nursing Management

Nursing management is similar to that for Lyme disease. Educate the family about completing the antibiotic course, preventing tick bites, and appropriate tick removal (refer to Box 37.5 and Teaching Guidelines 37.2).

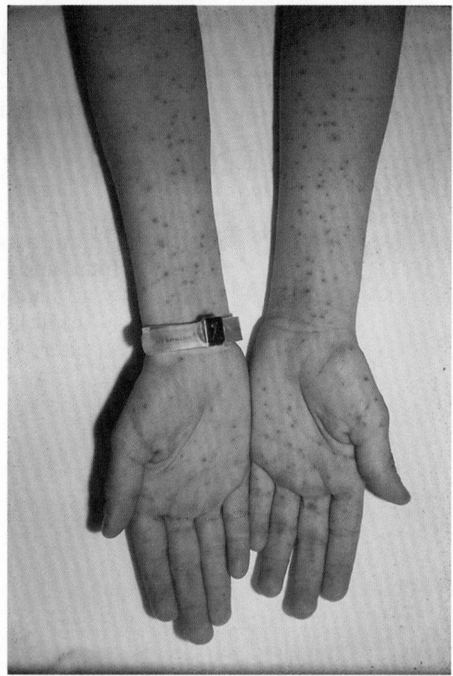

FIGURE 37.6 **Rash associated with Rocky Mountain spotted fever.**

Take Note!

Many folklore remedies exist for tick removal such as use of petroleum jelly or hot matches. These often do little to get the tick to detach and may actually irritate the tick and stimulate it to release more saliva or gut contents, therefore increasing the chance of disease. The goal of tick removal is to detach it as quickly as possible (CDC, 2015o).

PARASITIC AND HELMINTHIC INFECTION

Parasites are organisms larger than yeast or bacteria that can cause infection. They live in or on a host. Parasites receive nourishment from the host without benefiting or killing the host. Parasites frequently seen in children are scabies and head lice. A helminth is a parasitic intestinal worm. Helminthic infections seen in children include pinworms, roundworms, and hookworms. Children are at an increased risk for parasitic or helminthic infections due to poor hygiene practices. For example, children typically are more careless about handwashing and they tend to put things in their mouths and share toys and objects with other children.

Nursing Assessment and Management

Parents are often embarrassed when they find out that their child has a parasitic or helminthic

TABLE 37.6 COMMON PARASITIC INFECTIONS IN CHILDREN

Infection/Causative Organism	Transmission	Clinical Manifestations
Pediculosis capitis (head lice) Caused by *Pediculus humanus capitis* (head louse)	Direct contact with hair of infested people, less commonly with personal belongings, such as combs and hats, of those infested Incubation period from laying of eggs to hatching of nymph is 6–10 days; adult lice will appear 2–3 weeks later	Extreme pruritus is the most common symptom Adult eggs (nits) or lice may be seen, especially behind the ears and at the nape of the neck
Scabies Caused by *Sarcoptes scabiei* 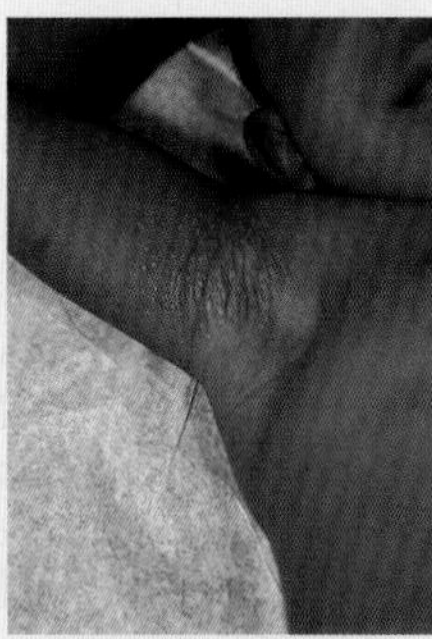 Scabies	Incubation period from laying of eggs to hatching of nymph is 3–4 days; adult lice will appear 2–4 weeks later Incubation period in those without previous exposure is 4–6 weeks. Usually no symptoms are present during this time but transmission to others can occur People who were previously infested can develop symptoms in 1–4 days Transmission usually occurs through prolonged, close personal contact	Intense pruritus (especially at night) with the presence of erythematous, papular rash with excoriations. The lesions are generally distributed but often are concentrated on the hands and feet and in body folds. May be found on head and neck In infants and young children the rash is often heavy on palms, soles and fingers, and it may include vesicles, pustules, or bullous lesions

Adapted from Centers for Disease Control and Prevention. (2013). *Parasites - Lice - Head lice.* Retrieved from http://www.cdc.gov/parasites/lice/head/index.html; Goldstein, B. G. & Goldstein, B. G., & Goldstein, A. O. (2015b). *Scabies.* Retrieved from http://www.uptodate.com/contents/scabies and Siegel, J. D., Rhinehart, E., Jackson, M., Chiarello, L., and the Healthcare Infection Control Practices Advisory Committee. (2007). *Guideline for isolation precautions: Preventing transmission of infectious agents in healthcare settings.* Retrieved from http://www.cdc.gov/hicpac/pdf/isolation/Isolation2007.pdf

infection. Reassure them that these infections can occur in any child. Tables 37.6 and 37.7 give nursing assessment and management information related to specific common parasitic and helminthic infections in children.

Take Note!

The head louse becoming resistant to pediculicides is a growing concern (Goldstein & Goldstien, 2015a). This may lead parents to resort to home remedies, such as covering the head with real mayonnaise or Vaseline. Inform parents that these remedies have not been proven to be effective (Gupta, 2014).

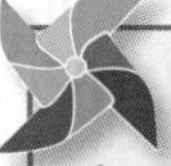

Consider This!

After cheerleading practice I noticed my head was itchy. When I got home I told my mom. She looked at my head and said she found lice. What am I going to do? Am I going to have to cut off all my hair? I love my hair! What are the girls on my cheerleading squad going to say if they find out? How could this happen to me?

Thoughts: Why is this girl so upset?

How does her developmental age affect her reaction to this discover?

How would you respond to her concerns?

Diagnosis/Treatment	Isolation/Control Measures/Concerns
Diagnosis by identification of eggs, nymph, and lice with the naked eye is possible; adult lice are rarely seen Treatment: washing hair with a pediculicide such as permethrin, pyrethrins, lindane, malathion Careful instructions on proper use of any product should be given and strict adherence to application instructions encouraged. Retreatment is usually recommended 9 days after first treatment, depending on treatment used Detection of living lice 24 hours after treatment suggests incorrect use, a very heavy infestation, reinfestation, or resistance to treatment	Contact precautions After treatment check hair and comb nits and lice from hair shafts every 2–3 days to prevent reinfestation Control measures: Household and other close contacts should be examined and if infested treated. Bedmates should be treated prophylactically Head lice do not survive long once they have fallen off. Most children can be treated effectively without treating their clothing and bedding. But to help avoid reinfestation disinfection of clothing, headgear, pillowcases, towels, and other items used by the individual within the past 2 days by washing in hot water and drying on the hot cycle may be helpful Dry-cleaning nonwashable items or simply sealing them in a plastic bag for 10 days is effective Soaking combs and hairbrushes in pediculicide, shampoo, or hot water Lice infestation is not a sign of poor hygiene; all socioeconomic groups are affected
Diagnosis can be made by a history of itching (especially at night), classic rash, and reports of itching in household or sexual contacts Mites can be seen on microscopic examination of skin scrapings to confirm diagnosis Treatment: A scabicide, such as permethrin or lindane, should be applied to the entire body below the head. Treatment of infants and young children should include the head, neck, and body. The cream is left on for a specified time (usually 8–14 hours) depending on the type of scabicide Careful instructions on proper use of any product should be given and strict adherence to application instructions should be urged Itching may not subside for several weeks, even after successful treatment	Contact precautions Prophylactic therapy for household members and sexual contacts Bedding and clothing used by infested person or household, sexual, or close contacts within 4 days before treatment should be laundered in hot water and dried on the hot cycle (mites do not survive more than 3–4 days without skin contact) Avoid direct skin-to-skin contact with person or items used by those infested Room used by an infected person, especially if he or she had crusted scabies, should be thoroughly cleaned and vacuumed

Take Note!

In recent years, three new prescription-only treatments have been approved by the FDA for the treatment of head lice, benzyl alcohol 5% lotion, Spinosad, and ivermectin lotion 5%. Over-the-counter permethrin or pyrethrins remain the first line of treatment but the new medications may be helpful with difficult to get rid of cases or cases of resistant lice (Buck, 2012).

Take Note!

Several tropical diseases including soil-transmitted helminths (hookworm, Ascaris, and whipworm) are often treated through mass drug administrations. The same drug is used to treat several infections and these drugs are safe and inexpensive or donated. Entire risk groups are offered preventive treatment periodically (often yearly) (CDC, 2013c; 2013e).

TABLE 37.7 COMMON HELMINTHIC INFECTIONS IN CHILDREN

Infection/Causative Organism	Clinical Manifestations	Transmission
Ascariasis Caused by *Ascaris lumbricoides,* common in temperate and tropical areas, especially in areas with unsanitary conditions	Most people are asymptomatic, may demonstrate slower growth and weight gain In more severe infections, loss of appetite, nausea, vomiting, and abdominal pain may be seen. Cough and difficulty breathing may be present as immature worms migrate through the lungs In significant infestation, partial or complete intestinal obstruction may occur. The more worms, the worse the symptoms	Human feces are the major source of infected eggs Hand to mouth is the usual route of transmission. The eggs are swallowed due to unclean hands or contaminated food or water. They pass into the intestine; larvae then hatch, penetrate the intestinal wall, enter the circulatory system, and migrate to other body tissues, primarily the lungs first
Hookworm Caused by *Ancylostoma duodenale* (roundworm) and *Necator americanus* (roundworm); common in tropics and subtropics especially in areas with unsanitary conditions; rare in areas with <40 in of annual rain fall	Most often people are asymptomatic until significant worms are established May see pruritic erythematous papular rash at entry site (referred to as ground itch) or pulmonary symptoms as the larvae migrate One of the greatest concerns in chronic infection is anemia (microcytic hypochromic anemia) secondary to blood loss as the worms suck blood and juices from the intestines This can lead to hypoproteinemia, edema, pica, and wasting. The infection may result in physical or intellectual disability in children	Hookworms are found in soil and enter the host through pores, hair follicles, and even intact skin (hands and feet are major sites of entry) The maturing larvae travel through the circulatory system into the lungs and then up the bronchial tree and are swallowed with secretions. They then migrate into the intestinal tract and attach to the wall of the small intestines, where they feed and reproduce
Pinworm Caused by *Enterobius vermicularis* (roundworm); found in temperate climates	Some people are asymptomatic. May cause anal itching (pruritus ani), especially at night Other clinical findings may include restlessness and teeth grinding at night, weight loss, and enuresis	Fecal–oral route directly, indirectly, or inadvertently by contaminated hands or shared toys, bedding, clothing, toilet seats Incubation period is 1–2 months or longer

Adapted from Centers for Disease Control and Prevention. (2013c). *Parasites - ascariasis.* Retrieved from http://www.cdc.gov/parasites/ascariasis/; Centers for Disease Control and Prevention. (2013d). *Parasites - enterobiasis (also known as pinworm infection).* Retrieved from http://www.cdc.gov/parasites/pinworm/; Centers for Disease Control and Prevention. (2013e). *Parasites - hookworm.* Retrieved from http://www.cdc.gov/parasites/hookworm/; and Siegel, J. D., Rhinehart, E., Jackson, M., Chiarello, L., and the Healthcare Infection Control Practices Advisory Committee. (2007). *Guideline for isolation precautions: Preventing transmission of infectious agents in healthcare settings.* Retrieved from http://www.cdc.gov/hicpac/pdf/isolation/Isolation2007.pdf

Diagnosis/Treatment	Isolation/Control Measures
Diagnosis: once female worms are in the intestine, eggs can be visualized by microscopic evaluation of the stool Occasionally a worm may be coughed up and visualized or seen in vomit, stool, or urine Imaging can also be used Treatment is with mebendazole, albendazole, or pyrantel pamoate	Standard precautions are sufficient Sanitary disposal of feces Proper hand hygiene
Diagnosis: through microscopic examination of feces that reveals hookworm eggs Treatment is with albendazole, mebendazole, and pyrantel pamoate Iron supplementation and possible blood transfusion in severe cases	Standard precautions are sufficient. Proper sanitation and disposal of feces Treatment of all known infested people Screening of high-risk individuals Encourage the wearing of shoes and avoiding going barefoot.
Diagnosis: when adult worms are visualized in the perianal region; they are best viewed when the child is sleeping. Very few ova are present in stool, so examination of stool is not recommended Transparent tape pressed to perianal area and then viewed under a microscope may reveal eggs. Three consecutive specimens should be obtained when the child first awakens in the morning Treatment of choice is mebendazole, pyrantel pamoate, and albendazole, usually single doses and repeated in 2 weeks	Standard precautions are sufficient Reinfection occurs easily Infected people should bathe, preferably in a shower, in the morning, which will remove a large portion of the eggs Frequent changing of underclothes and bedding Personal hygiene measures such as keeping fingernails short, avoiding scratching of perianal area and nail biting Good hand hygiene is the most effective preventive measure, especially after using the bathroom and before eating. All family members should be treated since transmission from person to person is very easy

NURSING CARE PLAN 37.1

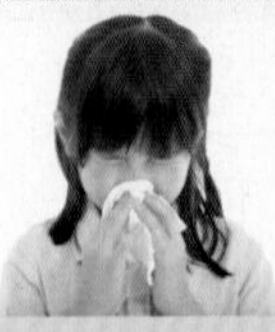

Overview for the Child With an Infectious or Communicable Disorder

NURSING DIAGNOSIS: Risk for imbalanced body temperature: fever related to infectious disease process as evidenced by rectal temperature greater than 38°C or 100.4°F

Outcome Identification and Evaluation

Child will maintain temperature within adaptive levels and be comfortable and remain hydrated. Temperature will be 38°C or 100.4°F or less. Child will verbalize or exhibit signs of comfort during febrile episode; child will demonstrate adequate signs of hydration.

Interventions: *Managing Fever*

- Assess temperature at least every 4 to 6 hours, 30 to 60 minutes after antipyretic is given and with any change in condition: *recognizing the pattern of fever may help identify source.*
- Use same site and device for temperature measurement *to reflect a more accurate trend in temperature, since different sites can result in significant differences in temperature reading.*
- Administer antipyretics per physician order when the child is experiencing discomfort or cannot keep up with the metabolic demands of the fever. *Fever is a protective response of the body to fight infection. Antipyretics provide symptomatic relief but do not change the course of the infection. The major benefits to decreasing fever are increasing comfort in the child and decreasing fluid requirements, helping to prevent dehydration.*
- Notify physician of temperature per institution or specific order guidelines: *increases in temperature may indicate worsening infection and relevant changes in condition.*
- Assess fluid intake and encourage oral intake or administer intravenous fluids per physician order: *increased metabolic rate and diaphoresis related to fever can cause fluid loss and lead to fluid volume deficit.*
- Keep linens and clothing clean and dry: *diaphoresis can leave clothing and linen soaked, increasing discomfort for the child.*
- Use of nonpharmacologic measures such as tepid bath and removal of clothing and blankets is controversial. If used, discontinue if shivering begins.

NURSING DIAGNOSIS: Impaired comfort related to infectious and/or inflammatory process as evidenced by hyperthermia, pruritus, rash or skin lesions, sore throat, or joint pain

Outcome Identification and Evaluation

Pain or discomfort will be reduced to level acceptable to child. Child will verbalize absence or decrease of pain using a pain scale (FLACC, FACES, or linear pain scale), will verbalize decrease in uncomfortable sensations such as itching and aches; infants will exhibit decreased crying and ability to rest quietly.

Interventions: *Improving Comfort*

- Assess pain and response to interventions frequently with use of pain scales or other pain measurement tools: *provides baseline of pain and allows for evaluation of effectiveness of interventions.*
- Administer analgesics and antipruritics as ordered to *relieve pain via interruption of central nervous system (CNS) pathways and to decrease discomfort related to itching.*
- Apply cool compresses to areas of pruritus or provide a cool bath *to decrease inflammation and soothe pruritus.*
- Keep child's fingernails short (use mitts, gloves, or socks over hands if necessary) to prevent injury *to the skin, which leads to increased pain.*

NURSING CARE PLAN 37.1

Overview for the Child With an Infectious or Communicable Disorder (continued)

- Encourage child to press on rather than scratch the area of pruritus: *pressing on the area that itches can soothe the itching and prevent scratching, which can lead to skin injury.*
- Provide fluids frequently and offer warm fluids such as soup or cold foods such as popsicles *to ease the discomfort of a sore throat.*
- Provide cool mist humidification *to ease the discomfort of a sore throat.*
- Dress the child in light clothing: *restrictive clothing and diaphoresis can lead to increased pruritus.*
- Use diversional activities and distraction appropriate to developmental level: *distraction from pain can reduce the need for pharmacologic agents, and distraction from pruritus can minimize scratching.*

NURSING DIAGNOSIS: Impaired skin integrity related to mechanical trauma secondary to infectious disease process as evidenced by rash, pruritus, and scratching

Outcome Identification and Evaluation

Child will maintain or regain skin integrity. Child will not demonstrate increased skin breakdown. Child or parent will be able to describe or demonstrate measures to protect and heal skin and proper care for any lesions.

Interventions: *Promoting Skin Integrity*

- Monitor skin for color changes, temperature, redness, swelling, warmth, pain, signs of infection, or changes in rash lesions, distribution, or size *to help identify problems early and allow for prevention of infection; can also provide information regarding the course of the illness.*
- Encourage fluid intake and proper nutrition *to promote wound healing.*
- Keep child's fingernails short (use mitts, gloves, or socks over hands if necessary) *to prevent injury to the skin, which leads to increased pain.*
- Encourage child to press on rather than scratch the area of pruritus; *pressing on the area that itches can soothe the itching and prevent scratching, which can lead to skin injury.*
- Use antipruritics and topical ointments or creams as ordered *to minimize scratching to prevent injury to skin; can aid in healing.*

NURSING DIAGNOSIS: Risk for infection related to insufficient knowledge regarding measures to avoid exposure to pathogens, increased environmental exposure to pathogens, transmission to others secondary to contagious organism or presence of infectious organisms

Outcome Identification and Evaluation

Child will exhibit no signs or symptoms of local or systemic infection. Child will not spread infection to others. Symptoms of infection will decrease over time; others will remain free of infection. Child and family will demonstrate appropriate hygiene measures using proper technique, such as handwashing, to prevent the spread of infection.

Interventions: *Preventing and Controlling Infection*

- Monitor vital signs: *elevation in temperature may indicate infection.*
- Monitor skin lesions for signs of local infection: redness, warmth, drainage, swelling, and pain at lesions: *can indicate infection.*
- Maintain aseptic technique and practice good handwashing: *to prevent introduction of further infectious agents and prevent transmission to others.*
- Administer antibiotics as prescribed: *to prevent or treat bacterial infection.*

(continued)

NURSING CARE PLAN 37.1

Overview for the Child With an Infectious or Communicable Disorder (continued)

- Encourage nutritious diet and proper hydration according to child's preferences and ability to feed orally: *to assist body's natural defenses against infection.*
- Isolate child as required based on transmission-based precautions: *to prevent nosocomial spread of infection.*
- Teach child and family preventive measures such as good handwashing, covering mouth and nose with cough or sneeze, and proper disposal of used tissues: *to prevent nosocomial or community spread of infection.*

NURSING DIAGNOSIS: Deficient fluid volume, risk for, related to increased metabolic demands and insensible loss due to fever, vomiting, poor feeding, or intake

Outcome Identification and Evaluation

Fluid volume will be maintained and balanced. Oral mucosa is moist and pink, skin turgor is elastic, urine output is at least 1 to 2 mL/kg/hr.

Interventions: ***Promoting Adequate Fluid Balance***

- Administer IV fluids if ordered *to maintain adequate hydration in children who are NPO (nothing by mouth), unable to tolerate oral intake, or unable to keep up with fluid losses.*
- When oral intake is allowed and tolerated, encourage oral fluids *to promote intake and maintain hydration.*
- Assess for signs of adequate hydration such as pink and moist oral mucosa, elastic skin turgor, and adequate urine output *to detect fluid imbalance.*
- Monitor intake and output *to identify fluid imbalance.*
- Assess urine specific gravity, urine and serum electrolytes, blood urea nitrogen, creatinine, and osmolality and daily weights *to monitor fluid status.*

NURSING DIAGNOSIS: Social isolation related to required isolation from peers secondary to transmission-based precautions, as evidenced by disruption in usual play secondary to inability to leave hospital room, activity intolerance, and fatigue

Outcome Identification and Evaluation

Child will participate in stimulating activities. Child is able to verbalize reason for isolation and length of isolation (if developmentally appropriate); child verbalizes interest in activities.

Interventions: ***Preventing Social Isolation***

- Explain reasons for transmission-based precautions and length of time: *this helps increase understanding and decrease anxiety about isolation. Children sometimes mistake isolation as punishment. Explaining length of time gives child an endpoint he or she can work toward.*
- Visit child frequently, at least every hour, and try to spend some uninterrupted time to play and allow child time to verbalize feelings about separation from others: *helps establish a therapeutic relationship and demonstrates caring.*
- Let child see caregiver's face before applying mask if appropriate: *to help child identify and relate to those caring for him or her and minimize anxiety about strangers and the unknown.*
- Consult child life specialist to arrange for stimulating activities child enjoys: *can help child to understand reasons for isolation and minimize feelings of social isolation.*
- Contact volunteers to spend time with child, if appropriate: *gives child attention and support, which will help child to cope and decrease stress.*

NURSING CARE PLAN 37.1

Overview for the Child With an Infectious or Communicable Disorder (continued)

NURSING DIAGNOSIS: Deficient knowledge related to lack of information regarding medical condition, prognosis, and medical needs as evidenced by verbalization, questions, or actions demonstrating lack of understanding regarding child's condition or care

Outcome Identification and Evaluation

Child and family will verbalize accurate information and understanding about condition, prognosis, and medical needs. Child and family demonstrate knowledge of condition and prognosis and medical needs, including possible causes, contributing factors, and treatment measures.

Interventions: *Providing Child and Family Teaching*

- Assess child's and family's willingness to learn: *child and family must be willing to learn in order for teaching to be effective.*
- Provide family with time to adjust to diagnosis: *to facilitate adjustment and ability to learn and participate in child's care.*
- Repeat information: *to give family and child time to learn and understand.*
- Teach in short sessions: *many short sessions are more helpful and facilitate learning compared to one long session.*
- Gear teaching to level of understanding of the child and family (depends on age of child, physical condition, memory) *to ensure understanding.*
- Provide reinforcement and rewards: *to facilitate the teaching/learning process.*
- Use multiple modes of learning involving many senses (provide written, verbal, demonstration, and videos) when possible: *the child and family are more likely to retain information when it is presented in different ways using many senses.*

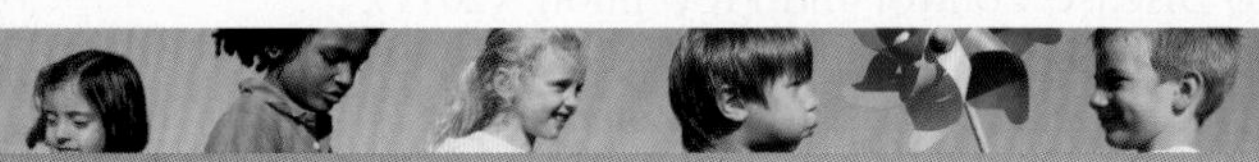

KEY CONCEPTS

- Infants and young children are more susceptible to infection due to their immature immune system. Young children continue to have an increased risk for infections and communicable disorders because disease protection from immunizations is not complete.
- Healthcare providers need to remember to educate parents that fever is a protective mechanism the body uses to fight infection.
- When obtaining blood cultures, follow aseptic technique and hospital protocol to prevent contamination. Obtain the specimen before administering antibiotics.
- When administering antipyretics, proper education must be given to caregivers on appropriate dosing, concentration, dosing interval, and use of proper measuring device.
- Promoting proper fluid balance and reducing temperature in a febrile child are important nursing interventions when caring for a child with an infection or communicable illness.
- Many childhood infectious and communicable diseases involve a rash. Rashes can be difficult to identify, so a thorough description and history from the caregiver is important.
- Sepsis, a systemic overresponse to infection resulting from bacteria, fungi, viruses, or parasites, can lead to septic shock. Any infant younger than 3 months old with a fever or any child with a fever accompanied by extreme lethargy, unresponsiveness, or lack of facial expressions should be seen by a physician or nurse practitioner.
- Many bacterial and viral infections, such as diphtheria, tetanus, pertussis, mumps, measles, rubella, varicella, and poliomyelitis, can be prevented by vaccination.
- Viral exanthems of childhood often present with a distinct rash pattern that assists in the diagnosis of the virus. Common childhood exanthems include exanthem subitum (roseola infantum), rubella (German measles), rubeola (measles), varicella (chickenpox), and erythema infectiosum (fifth disease).

- Nurses play a key role in educating the public on the importance of immunizations.
- Zoonotic infections are diseases caused by infectious agents that are transmitted directly or indirectly from animals to humans. Cat-scratch disease and rabies are types of zoonotic infections.
- Children are at a particular risk for contracting vector-borne diseases, which are diseases transmitted by ticks, mosquitoes, or other insect vectors. Two of the most commonly seen are Lyme disease and Rocky Mountain spotted fever.
- Parasites frequently seen in children are scabies and head lice. Helminthic infections seen in children include pinworms, roundworms, and hookworms.

REFERENCES AND RECOMMENDED READINGS

Arnon, S. S. (2011). Tetanus (Clostridium tetani). In R. M. Kleigman, B. F. Stanton, J. W. St. Geme III, N. F. Schor, & R. E. Behrman (Eds.), *Nelson textbook of pediatrics* (19th ed., pp. 991–994). Philadelphia, PA: Saunders.

Buck, M. L. (2012). New options for eradicating resistant head lice. *Pediatric Pharmacotherapy, 18*(6).

Carpenito, L. J. (2013). *Nursing diagnosis: Application to clinical practice* (14th ed.). Philadelphia, PA: Lippincott Williams & Wilkins.

Centers for Disease Control and Prevention. (2011). Updated recommendations for use of tetanus toxoid, reduced diphtheria toxoid and acellular pertussis (Tdap) vaccine from the Advisory Committee on Immunization. *Morbidity and Mortality Weekly Report (MMWR), 60*(01), 13–15.

Centers for Disease Control and Prevention. (2012a). In W. Atkinson, S. Wolfe, & J. Hamborsky (Eds.), *Epidemiology and prevention of vaccine-preventable diseases* (12th ed., second printing). Washington, DC: Public Health Foundation.

Centers for Disease Control and Prevention. (2012b). *Workplace safety and health topics: Tick-borne diseases*. Retrieved from http://www.cdc.gov/niosh/topics/tick-borne/

Centers for Disease Control and Prevention. (2012c). *Parvovirus B19 and fifth disease*. Retrieved from http://www.cdc.gov/parvovirusB19/index.html

Centers for Disease Control and Prevention. (2013a). *Anaplasmosis*. Retrieved from http://www.cdc.gov/anaplasmosis/

Centers for Disease Control and Prevention. (2013b). *Ehrlichiosis*. Retrieved from http://www.cdc.gov/ehrlichiosis/

Centers for Disease Control and Prevention. (2013c). *Parasites - ascariasis*. Retrieved from http://www.cdc.gov/parasites/ascariasis/

Centers for Disease Control and Prevention. (2013d). *Parasites - enterobiasis (also known as pinworm infection)*. Retrieved from http://www.cdc.gov/parasites/pinworm/

Centers for Disease Control and Prevention. (2013e). *Parasites - hookworm*. Retrieved from http://www.cdc.gov/parasites/hookworm/

Centers for Disease Control and Prevention. (2013f). *Rocky Mountain spotted fever (RMSF): Symptoms, diagnosis and treatment*. Retrieved from http://www.cdc.gov/rmsf/symptoms/index.html

Centers for Disease Control and Prevention. (2014a). *Cat scratch disease (Bartonella henselae infection)*. Retrieved from http://www.cdc.gov/healthypets/diseases/cat-scratch.html

Centers for Disease Control and Prevention. (2014b). *Haemophilus influenzae serotype b (Hib) disease: For clinicians*. Retrieved from http://www.cdc.gov/hi-disease/clinicians.html

Centers for Disease Control and Prevention. (2015a). *About hand, foot and mouth disease (HFMD)*. Retrieved from http://www.cdc.gov/hand-foot-mouth/about/index.html

Centers for Disease Control and Prevention. (2015b). *Dengue*. Retrieved from http://www.cdc.gov/Dengue/

Centers for Disease Control and Prevention. (2015c). *Lyme disease: Data and statistics*. Retrieved from http://www.cdc.gov/lyme/stats/index.html

Centers for Disease Control and Prevention. (2015d). *Lyme disease: Two-step laboratory testing process*. Retrieved from http://www.cdc.gov/lyme/diagnosistesting/LabTest/TwoStep/index.html

Centers for Disease Control and Prevention. (2015e). *Lyme disease: Lyme disease transmission*. Retrieved from http://www.cdc.gov/lyme/transmission/index.html

Centers for Disease Control and Prevention. (2015f). *Mumps Cases and outbreaks*. Retrieved from http://www.cdc.gov/mumps/outbreaks.html

Centers for Disease Control and Prevention. (2015g). *National center for emerging and zoonotic infectious diseases*. Retrieved from http://www.cdc.gov/ncezid/index.html

Centers for Disease Control and Prevention. (2015h). 2015: nationally notifiable infectious conditions. Retrieved from http://wwwn.cdc.gov/nndss/conditions/notifiable/2015/infectious-diseases/

Centers for Disease Control and Prevention. (2015i). *Pertussis (whooping cough): Postexposure antimicrobial prophylaxis*. Retrieved from http://www.cdc.gov/pertussis/outbreaks/pep.html

Centers for Disease Control and Prevention. (2015j). *Pertussis (whooping cough): Surveillance & reporting*. Retrieved from http://www.cdc.gov/pertussis/surv-reporting.html

Centers for Disease Control and Prevention. (2015k). *Pertussis (whooping cough): Treatment*. Retrieved from http://www.cdc.gov/pertussis/clinical/treatment.html

Centers for Disease Control and Prevention. (2015l). *Rabies*. Retrieved from http://www.cdc.gov/rabies/

Centers for Disease Control and Prevention. (2015m). *Recommended immunization schedule for persons aged 0 through 18 years – United States, 2015*. Retrieved from http://www.cdc.gov/vaccines/schedules/downloads/child/0-18yrs-schedule.pdf

Centers for Disease Control and Prevention (CDC). (2015n). *Scarlet fever: A group A streptococcal infection*. Retrieved from http://www.cdc.gov/features/scarletfever/

Centers for Disease Control and Prevention. (2015o). *Ticks. Tick removal.* Retrieved from http://www.cdc.gov/ticks/removing_a_tick.html

Centers for Disease Control and Prevention. (2015p). *West Nile virus.* Retrie

Eppes, S. C. (2011). Chapter 214: Lyme disease (Borrelia burgdorferi). In R. M. Kleigman, B. F. Stanton, J. W. St. Geme III, N. F. Schor, & R. E. Behrman (Eds.), *Nelson textbook of pediatrics* (19th ed., pp.1025–1029). Philadelphia, PA: Saunders.

Fischbach, F. T., & Dunning III, M. B. (2015). *A manual of laboratory and diagnostic tests* (9th ed.). Philadelphia, PA: Wolters Kluwer Health/Lippincott Williams & Wilkins.

Gerber, M. A. (2011). Chapter 176: Group A streptococcus. In R. M. Kleigman, B. F. Stanton, J. W. St. Geme III, N. F. Schor, & R. E. Behrman (Eds.), *Nelson textbook of pediatrics* (19th ed., pp. 914–925). Philadelphia, PA: Saunders.

Goldstein, A. O., & Goldstein, B. G. (2015a). *Pediculosis capitis.* Retrieved from http://www.uptodate.com/contents/pediculosis-capitis

Goldstein, B. G., & Goldstein, A. O. (2015b). *Scabies.* Retrieved from http://www.uptodate.com/contents/scabies

Grossman, S. (2014b). Chapter 25: Blood cells and the hematopoietic system. In S. Grossman, & C. M. Porth (Eds.), *Porth's Pathophysiology: Concepts of altered health states* (9th ed., pp. 638–664). Philadelphia, PA: Wolters Kluwer Health/Lippincott Williams & Wilkins.

Gupta, R. C. (2015). *Head lice.* Retrieved from http://kidshealth.org/parent/infections/common/head_lice.html

Hatfield, L. A., Chang, K., Bittle, M., Deluca, J., & Polomano, R. C. (2011). The analgesic properties of intraoral sucrose: An integrative review. *Advances in Neonatal Care, 11*(2), 83–92. doi: 10.1097/ANC.0b013e318210d043

Haut, C. M. (2014). Chapter 54: Pediatric orthopedic problems. In S. M. Nettina (Ed.), *Lippincott manual of nursing practice* (10th ed., pp. 1743–69). Philadelphia, PA: Wolters/Kluwer Health: Lippincott Williams & Wilkins.

Hirsch, L. (2015). *Questions & answers.* Retrieved http://kidshealth.org/parent/question/general/lice.html

InterAction. (2013). *Global health briefing book.* Retrieved from http://www.globalhealth.org/wp-content/uploads/GlobalHealthBriefingBook_FINAL_web.pdf

John, C. C., & Krause, P. J. (2011). Chapter 280: Malaria (Plasmodium). In R. M. Kleigman, B. F. Stanton, J. W. St. Geme III, N. F. Schor, & R. E. Behrman (Eds.), *Nelson textbook of pediatrics* (19th ed., pp. 1198–1207). Philadelphia, PA: Saunders.

Kaplan, S. L. (2015). *Methicillin-resistant Staphylococcus aureus infections in children: Epidemiology and clinical spectrum.* UpToDate. Retrieved from http://www.uptodate.com/contents/methicillin-resistant-staphylococcus-aureus-infections-in-children-epidemiology-and-clinical-spectrum

Koch, W. C. (2011). Chapter 243: Parvovirus B19. In R. M. Kleigman, B. F. Stanton, J. W. St. Geme III, N. F. Schor & R. E. Behrman (Eds.), *Nelson textbook of pediatrics* (19th ed., pp. 1094–1097). Philadelphia, PA: Saunders.

Krogstad, P. (2014a). *Bacterial arthritis: Epidemiology, pathogenesis, and microbiology in infants and children.* UpToDate. Retrieved from http://www.uptodate.com/contents/bacterial-arthritis-epidemiology-pathogenesis-and-microbiology-in-infants-and-children

Krogstad, P. (2014b). *Hematogenous osteomyelitis in children: Epidemiology, pathogenesis, and microbiology.* Retrieved from http://www.uptodate.com/contents/hematogenous-osteomyelitis-in-children-epidemiology-pathogenesis-and-microbiology

Leder, K. & Weller, P. F. (2014). *Ascariasis.* UpToDate. Retrieved from http://www.uptodate.com/contents/ascariasis

Mayo Clinic Staff. (2015). *Diphtheria.* Retrieved from http://www.mayoclinic.com/health/diphtheria/DS00495/DSECTION=risk-factors

Naughton, K. A., & Ikuta, L. (2013). The combined use of sucrose and nonnutritive sucking for procedural pain in both term and preterm neonates: An integrative review of the literature. *Advances in Neonatal Care, 13*(1), 9–19.

Nield, L. S., & Kamat, D. (2011a). Chapter 169: Fever. In R. M. Kleigman, B. F. Stanton, J. W. St. Geme III, N. F. Schor, & R. E. Behrman (Eds.), *Nelson textbook of pediatrics* (19th ed., p. 896). Philadelphia, PA: Saunders.

Nield, L. S., & Kamat, D. (2011b). Chapter 170: Fever without a focus. In R. M. Kleigman, B. F. Stanton, J. W. St. Geme III, N. F. Schor, & R. E. Behrman (Eds.), *Nelson textbook of pediatrics* (19th ed., pp. 896–902). Philadelphia, PA: Saunders.

Papadopol, R. (2014). *Infections: Cat scratch disease.* Retrieved from http://kidshealth.org/parent/infections/bacterial_viral/cat_scratch.html

Pearson Education. (2015). *Nursing: A concept-based approach to learning, volume I & II* (2nd ed.). Upper Saddle River, NJ: Prentice Hall.

Pegram, P. S., & Stone, S. M. (2015). *Botulism.* UpToDate. Retrieved from http://www.uptodate.com/contents/botulism

Pomerantz, W. J., & Weiss, S. L. (2015). Systemic inflammatory response syndrome (SIRS) and sepsis in children: Definitions, epidemiology, clinical manifestations, and diagnosis. UpToDate. Retrieved from http://www.uptodate.com/contents/systemic-inflammatory-response-syndrome-sirs-and-sepsis-in-children-definitions-epidemiology-clinical-manifestations-and-diagnosis

Reller, M. E., & Dumler, J. S. (2011). Chapter 220: Spotted fever and transitional group rickettsioses. In R. M. Kleigman, B. F. Stanton, J. W. St. Geme III, N. F. Schor, & R. E. Behrman (Eds.), *Nelson textbook of pediatrics* (19th ed., pp. 1038–1045). Philadelphia, PA: Saunders.

Rupprecht, C. E., Briggs, D., Brown, C. M., Franka R., Katz, S. L., Kerr, H. D., & Cieslak, P. R. (2010). Use of a reduced (4-dose) vaccine schedule for postexposure prophylaxis to prevent human rabies. *Morbidity and Mortality Weekly Report (MMWR), 59*(02), 1–9.

Santhanam, S. (2015). *Pediatric sepsis.* Retrieved from http://emedicine.medscape.com/article/972559-overview#a1

Siegel, J. D., Rhinehart, E., Jackson, M., Chiarello, L., and The Healthcare Infection Control Practices Advisory Committee. (2007). *Guideline for isolation precautions: Preventing transmission of infectious agents in healthcare settings.* Retrieved from http://www.cdc.gov/hicpac/pdf/isolation/Isolation2007.pdf

Sexton, D. J. (2015). *Tetanus.* UpToDate. Retrieved from http://www.uptodate.com/contents/tetanus http://www.uptodate.com/contents/evaluation-and-management-of-the-febrile-young-infant-7-to-90-days-of-age

Smitherman, H. F, & Macias, C. G. (2015). *Evaluation and management of the febrile young infant (7 to 90 days of age)*. UpToDate. Retrieved from http://www.uptodate.com/contents/evaluation-and-management-of-the-febrile-young-infant-7-to-90-days-of-age

Stechenberg, B. W. (2011). Chapter 201.2: Cat-scratch disease (Bartonella henselae). In R. M. Kleigman, B. F. Stanton, J. W. St. Geme III, N .F. Schor, & R. E. Behrman (Eds.), *Nelson textbook of pediatrics* (19th ed., pp. 983–986). Philadelphia, PA: Saunders.

Sullivan, J. E., Farrar, H. C., & The AAP's Section on Clinical Pharmacology and Therapeutics, and Committee on Drugs. (2011). Clinical report: Fever and antipyretic use in children. *Pediatrics, 127*(3), 580–587. doi: 10.1542/peds.2010–3852

Taketokmo, C. K., Hodding, J. H., & Kraus, D. M. (2013). *Lexi-comp's drug reference handbook: Pediatric & neonatal dosage handbook* (20th ed.). Hudson, OH: Lexi-comp, Inc.

Tremblay, C., & Brady, M. T. (2015). *Roseola infantum (exanthem subitum)*. Retrieved from http://www.uptodate.com/contents/roseola-infantum-exanthem-subitum

U.S. Department of Health & Human Services. (2015). *HealthyPeople.gov*. Retrieved from http://www.healthypeople.gov/2020/about/default.aspx

U.S. Food and Drug Administration. (2013). *FDA drug safety communication: Azithromycin (Zithromax or Zmax) and the risk of potentially fatal heart rhythms*. Retrieved from http://www.fda.gov/drugs/drugsafety/ucm341822.htm

Vyas, J. M., & Zieve, D. (2013). *Botulism*. Retrieved from http://www.ncbi.nlm.nih.gov/pubmedhealth/PMH0001624/

Ward, M. A. (2015a). *Fever in infants and children: Pathophysiology and management*. UpToDate. Retrieved from http://www.uptodate.com/contents/fever-in-infants-and-children-pathophysiology-and-management

Ward, M. A. (2015b). *Patient information: Fever in children (beyond the basics)*. UpToDate. Retrieved from http://www.uptodate.com/contents/fever-in-children-beyond-the-basics

Weller, P. F., & Leder, K. (2014). *Hookworm*. UpToDate. Retrieved from http://www.uptodate.com/contents/hookworm-infection

Willoughby, Jr., R. E. (2011). Chapter 266: Rabies. In R. M. Kleigman, B. F. Stanton, J. W. St. Geme III, N. F. Schor, & R. E. Behrman (Eds.), *Nelson textbook of pediatrics* (19th ed., pp. 1154–1157). Philadelphia, PA: Saunders.

Wong, T., Stang, A. S., Ganshorn, H., Hartling, L., Maconochie, I. K., Thomsen, A. M. et al. (2013). Combined and alternating paracetamol and ibuprofen therapy for febrile children. *Cochrane Database of Systematic Reviews,* (10), CD009572. doi: 10.1002/14651858.CD009572.pub2.

World Health Organization. (2009). *WHO guidelines on hand hygiene in healthcare*. Retrieved from http://whqlibdoc.who.int/publications/2009/9789241597906_eng.pdf

World Health Organization. (2015). *Rabies*. Retrieved from http://www.who.int/mediacentre/factsheets/fs099/en/

Zabawski, Jr., E. J. (2014). *Scarlet fever*. Retrieved from http://emedicine.medscape.com/article/1053253-overview

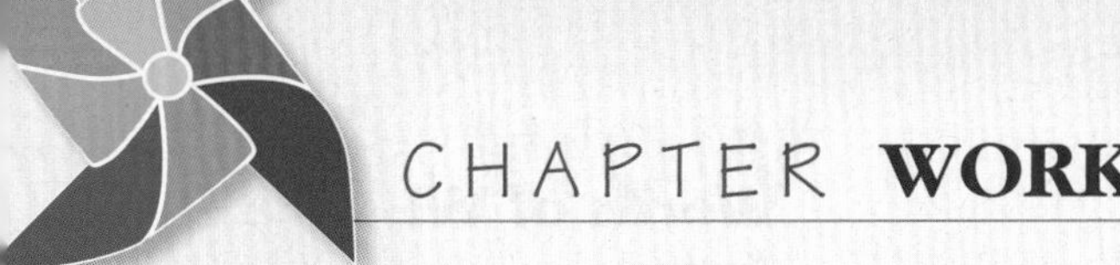

CHAPTER WORKSHEET

MULTIPLE CHOICE QUESTIONS

1. Compared with adults, why are infants and children at an increased risk for infection and communicable diseases?
   a. The infant has had limited exposure to disease and is losing the passive immunity acquired from maternal antibodies.
   b. The infant demonstrates an increased inflammatory response.
   c. Cellular immunity is not functional at birth.
   d. Infants have an increased risk for infection until they receive their first set of immunizations.

2. A mother calls the clinic because her 2-year-old daughter has a rectal temperature of 37.8°C (100°F). She wonders how high a fever should be before she should give medications to reduce it. What is the best response by the nurse?
   a. "All fevers should be treated to prevent seizures."
   b. "Antipyretics should be used with any rise in temperature. They can help change the course of the infection."
   c. "Give your child aspirin when her fever is above 38°C (100.4°F)."
   d. "In a normal healthy child, if your child is not uncomfortable, fevers less than 39°C (102.2°F) do not require medication."

3. A neonate should be evaluated by a physician if which signs and symptoms are present?
   a. Acting fussier than normal
   b. Refusing the pacifier
   c. Rectal temperature above 38°C
   d. Mottling that is present during bathing

4. The public health nurse has been asked to provide information to local child care centers on controlling the spread of infectious diseases. What is the best information the nurse can provide?
   a. The etiology of common infectious diseases
   b. Proper handwashing techniques
   c. The physiology of the immune system
   d. Why children are at a higher risk of infection than adults

DOSAGE CALCULATION QUESTIONS

The nurse is caring for a child who has a rash and is complaining of feeling itchy and is continually scratching. The child weighs 32 lb. The medication order reads: Diphenhydramine 6.25 mg po every 4 to 6 hours as needed for itching. Diphenhydramine is supplied as 12.5 mg/5 mL. How many milliliters will the nurse administer. Round to the nearest tenth.

CRITICAL THINKING EXERCISES

1. A 12-year-old boy presents with a very sore throat and fever. On assessment you find an erythematous rash on his face that feels like sandpaper. You obtain a throat culture, which is positive for group A streptococcus. What instructions would you give the parents regarding his care at home?

2. A 1-month-old infant is admitted to the hospital to rule out sepsis. What would be your priority nursing interventions?

3. A 4-year-old child presents with a fever and rash. What three of the following items should the nurse obtain during the health history?
   _____ a. Immunization history
   _____ b. Any exposure to communicable or infectious diseases
   _____ c. Whether the child takes a daily vitamin
   _____ d. Thorough description and history of the rash
   _____ e. Mother's immunization history

STUDY ACTIVITIES

1. The 4-year-old presented in Question 3 above was diagnosed with varicella zoster virus. Write a nursing care plan for a child with varicella.

2. A child is brought to the school nurse with intense itching. Upon assessment the nurse finds an erythematous, papular rash with excoriations on the child's hands and feet. As suspected, the diagnosis of scabies is confirmed. What teaching is necessary for the parents, family, and classmates of the child?

BRINGING IT ALL TOGETHER: A CASE STUDY

As the nurse in a pediatric clinic, you see a child who comes in because she is having extreme itching, especially at night. The child is diagnosed with scabies. The mother is upset and says to you, "We are clean people! I don't understand how this could happen!"

Go to thePoint to find questions to consider about this case.

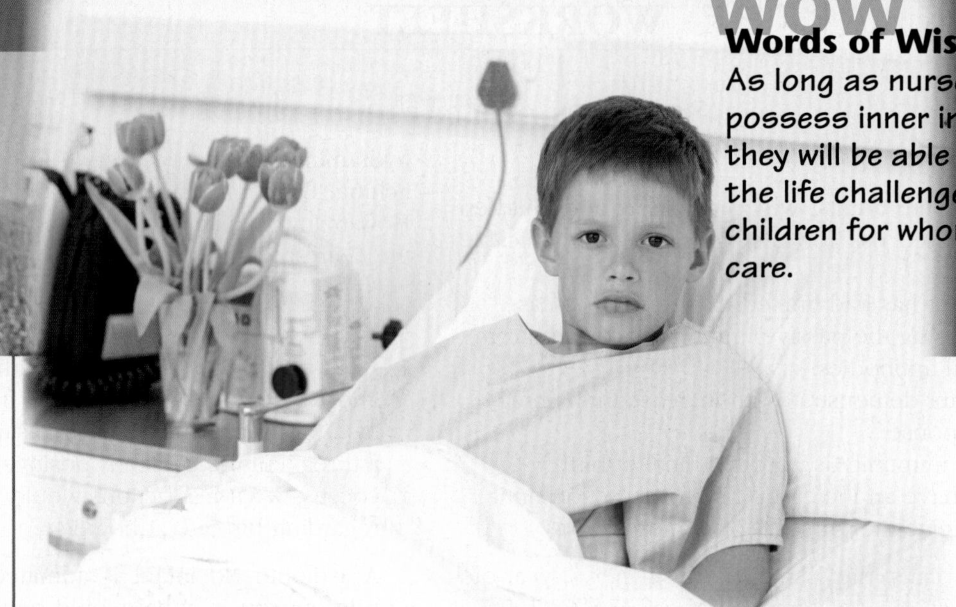

38

WOW

Words of Wisdom

As long as nurses possess inner integrity, they will be able to handle the life challenges of the children for whom they care.

Nursing Care of the Child With an Alteration in Intracranial Regulation/ Neurologic Disorder

KEY TERMS

central nervous system (CNS)
decerebrate posturing
decorticate posturing
head circumference
intracranial pressure (ICP)
lumbar puncture (LP)
myelinization
neural tube
opisthotonic
postictal
status epilepticus
teratogen

Learning Objectives

Upon completion of the chapter, you will be able to:

1. Compare how the anatomy and physiology of the neurologic system in children differs from adults.
2. Identify various factors associated with neurologic disease in infants and children.
3. Discuss common laboratory and other diagnostic tests useful in the diagnosis of neurologic conditions.
4. Discuss common medications and other treatments used for treatment and palliation of neurologic conditions.
5. Recognize risk factors associated with various neurologic disorders.
6. Distinguish among different neurologic illnesses based on the signs and symptoms associated with them.
7. Discuss nursing interventions commonly used for neurologic illnesses.
8. Devise an individualized nursing care plan for the child with a neurologic disorder.
9. Develop child and family teaching plans for the child with a neurologic disorder.
10. Describe the psychosocial impact of chronic neurologic disorders on children.

***Antonio Chapman*, 3 months old, has had increased irritability, poor sucking and feeding, and a fever for the past 24 hours. Today he is lethargic with a weak cry and is vomiting his feeds.**

Intracranial regulation refers to the process that affects equilibrium within the brain and therefore neurologic function (Pellico, 2012). Nurses encounter potential and actual alterations in intracranial regulation in all types of clients and must detect problems and intervene early to prevent life-threatening complications. Alterations in intracranial regulation (neurologic disorders) in children often have a devastating and lasting impact. Neurologic disorders can be divided into several categories, including structural disorders, seizure disorders, infectious disorders, trauma to the neurologic system, blood flow disruption disorders, and chronic disorders.

Nurses must be familiar with neurologic conditions affecting children in order to provide prevention, prompt treatment, guidance, and support to families. Neurologic disorders require acute interventions, but many times have long-lasting implications on the child's health and development. Due to the potentially devastating effects that neurologic disorders can have on children and their families, nurses need to be skilled in assessment and interventions in this area and must be able to provide support throughout the course of the illness and beyond.

VARIATIONS IN PEDIATRIC ANATOMY AND PHYSIOLOGY

Neurologic disorders can result from congenital problems as well as from infections or traumas. Certain neurologic conditions occur in children more often than in adults and these conditions will affect their growth and development. In addition, children are at an increased risk for different neurologic problems compared to adults due to anatomic and physiologic differences.

Brain and Spinal Cord Development

The brain and spinal cord make up the **central nervous system (CNS)**. Development of these structures occurs in the first 3 to 4 weeks of gestation from the **neural tube**. Infection, trauma, **teratogens** (any environmental substance that can cause physical defects in the developing embryo and fetus), and malnutrition during this period can result in malformations in brain and spinal cord development and may affect normal CNS development.

At birth, the cranial bones are not well developed and are not fused. Therefore, there is an increased risk for fracture. The brain is highly vascular, leading to an increased risk for hemorrhage. Premature infants are at greater risk for brain damage; the more premature the infant, the greater the risk. The premature infant has more capillaries in the periventricular area, which is the brain tissue that lines the outside of the lateral ventricles. These capillaries are fragile and at greater risk for rupture, leading to intracranial bleeding. Also, because the cranium is very soft in the preterm infant, external pressure can change its shape and cause increased pressure in areas of the brain and possible hemorrhage.

The sutures and fontanels present in the newborn help make the skull more flexible and help to accommodate for brain growth that continues after birth. Closure of the fontanels too early or too late can be indicative of problems with brain growth. The child's spine is very mobile, especially the cervical spine region, resulting in a high risk for cervical spine injury.

Nervous System

The development of the nervous system is complete but immature at birth. The infant is born with all the nerve cells that he or she will have throughout life. However, **myelinization**, the formation of myelin, which covers and protects the nerves, is incomplete. The speed and accuracy of nerve impulses increases as myelinization increases. This process accounts for the acquisition of fine and gross motor movements and coordination in early childhood. Myelinization proceeds in the cephalocaudal direction. For example, infants are able to control the head and neck before the trunk and extremities.

The immaturity of the CNS in preterm infants can result in delayed development of motor skills. Premature newborns may have difficulty coordinating sucking and swallowing, leading to feeding and growth issues. Also, episodes of apnea can be problematic in the preterm newborn due to the underdevelopment of the nervous system.

Head Size

The head of the infant and young child is large in proportion to the body. The head of an infant accounts for a quarter of the body height; in adults, it accounts for one eighth of the body height (Fig. 38.1). In addition, the infant's and child's neck muscles are not well developed. Both of these differences lead to an increased incidence of head injury from falls. The head is the fastest growing body part during infancy and continues to grow until the child is 5 years old.

COMMON MEDICAL TREATMENTS

A variety of interventions, including medical treatments and medications, are used to treat neurologic illness in children. Most of these treatments will require a physician's or nurse practitioner's order when the child is hospitalized. The most common treatments and medications used for neurologic disorders are listed in Common Medical Treatments 38.1 and Drug Guide 38.1.

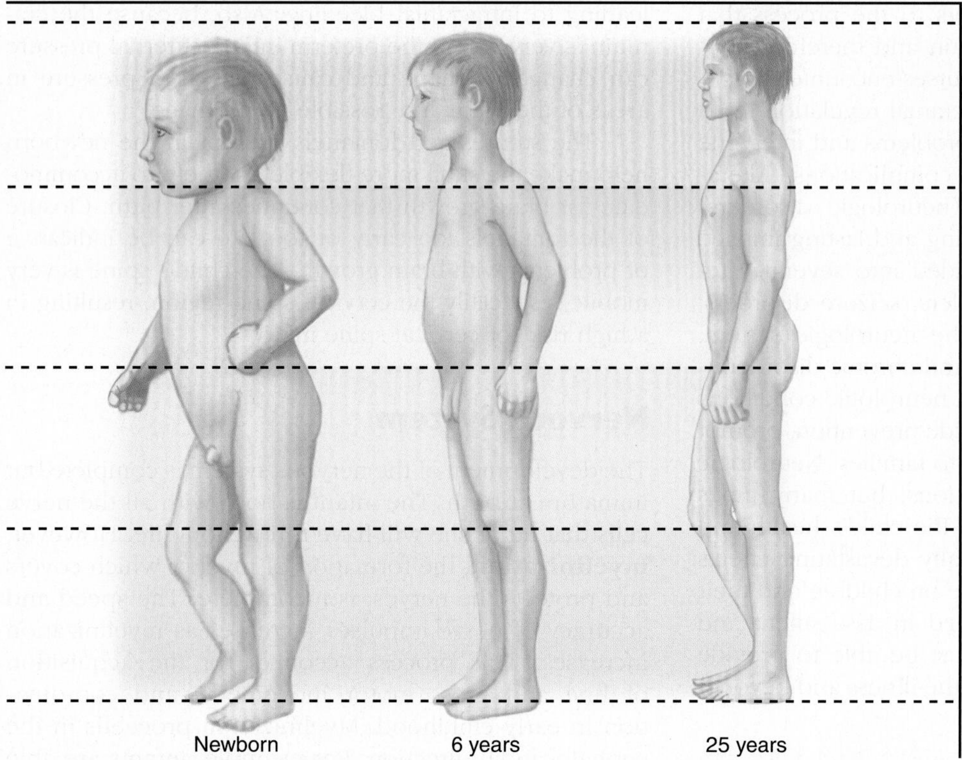

FIGURE 38.1 Proportion of head to body height in the newborn, child, and adult.

NURSING PROCESS OVERVIEW FOR THE CHILD WITH A NEUROLOGIC DISORDER

Care of the child with a neurologic disorder includes assessment, nursing diagnosis, planning, intervention, and evaluation. There are a number of general concepts related to the nursing process that can be applied to the management of neurologic disorders. From a general understanding of the care involved for a child with neurologic dysfunction, the nurse can then individualize the care based on the particular child's specifics.

Remember Antonio, the 3-month-old with lethargy, a weak cry, and vomiting? What additional health history and physical examination assessment information should the nurse obtain?

Assessment

Assessment of neurologic dysfunction in children includes health history, physical examination, and laboratory and diagnostic testing.

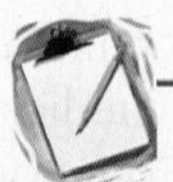

Take Note!

Neurologic assessment should proceed from least invasive to most invasive. The use of toys and familiar objects, as well as incorporating play, will help promote cooperation from the child.

Health History

The health history consists of past medical history, including the mother's pregnancy history, family history, and history of present illness (when the symptoms started and how they have progressed) as well as treatments used at home. The past medical history might be significant for prematurity, difficult birth, infection during pregnancy, nausea, vomiting, headaches, changes in gait, falls, visual disturbances, or recent trauma. Family history might be significant for genetic disorders with neurologic manifestations, seizure disorders, or headaches. When eliciting the history of the present illness, inquire about the following:

- Nausea
- Vomiting
- Changes in gait
- Visual disturbances
- Complaints of headaches
- Recent trauma
- Changes in cognition
- Change in consciousness, including any loss of consciousness
- Poor feeding
- Lethargy
- Increased irritability
- Fever
- Pain
- Altered muscle tonicity
- Delays in growth and development
- Ingestion or inhalation of neurotoxic substances or chemicals

COMMON MEDICAL TREATMENTS 38.1

Treatment	Explanation	Indications	Nursing Implications
Shunt placement	A catheter is placed in the ventricle to pass the CSF to the peritoneal cavity, atrium of the heart, or pleural spaces. (Ventriculoperitoneal shunts are commonly used.)	Hydrocephalus, increased ICP	Monitor: • For signs and symptoms of increased ICP • Neurologic status closely • Level of consciousness and vital signs • For signs and symptoms of infection
Ventilation	Hyperventilation to decrease $PaCO_2$, which will result in vasoconstriction and therefore decrease ICP Adequate oxygenation to prevent hypoxia and further damage to the brain	Increased ICP	Monitor: • Arterial blood gases • For signs and symptoms of increased ICP • Pulse oximetry
PT/OT/ST	Therapies are used to improve motor function and ability of children with neurologic disorders.	Head injury, intellectual disability	Ensure adequate communication exists within the interdisciplinary team.
External ventricular drainage (EVD)	A catheter is temporarily placed in the ventricle and CSF is drained in a closed system to an external reservoir	Most commonly used with shunt infections until CSF is sterile and shunt can be replaced; treats acute-onset hydrocephalus, meningitis, encephalitis, tumors that cause blockage of CSF, closed head injury, subarachnoid hemorrhage, increased ICP; also can be used to monitor ICP	Monitor: • For signs and symptoms of increased ICP • Neurologic status closely • Level of consciousness and vital signs • For signs and symptoms of infection • Level of collection container when drain is unclamped
Ventricular tap	To reduce accumulation of CSF and decrease ICP	Increased ICP	Monitor: • Level of consciousness • Neurologic status
Vagal nerve stimulator	A nerve stimulator is implanted and a lead wire running under the skin is wrapped around the vagus nerve. The stimulator is programmed to provide the appropriate dose of stimulation at preset intervals; additional stimulation can be administered.	Short- and long-term seizure management in children older than 12 years of age	Monitor: • For signs and symptoms of infection • For seizure activity
Ketogenic diet	Diet involving high intake of fats, adequate protein, and a very low intake of carbohydrates, resulting in a ketosis state. Child is kept in a mild state of dehydration.	Prevention, control, and reduction of seizures, in particular for children with difficult-to-control seizures	Monitor: • Input and output closely • For seizure activity • Growth and nutritional status • The diet is time consuming and many children find it unpalatable; therefore, all families and children do not accept it. • Recommended for a minimum of 3 months, maximum of 2 years • Alternative diets include: the medium chain triglyceride diet, modified Atkins diet and a low glycemic index diet

OT, occupational therapy; PT, physical therapy; ST, speech therapy.

DRUG GUIDE 38.1

Medication	Actions/Indications	Nursing Implications
Antibiotics (oral, parenteral, intrathecal)	Treatment of bacterial meningitis and shunt infections; kill and prevent the growth of bacteria	Check for antibiotic allergies. Monitor serum levels to ensure therapeutic dosing, if indicated. Give as prescribed for the length of time prescribed.
Anticonvulsants (oral, parenteral)	Decrease hyperexcitability of nerves Treatment and prevention of seizures	Maintain seizure precautions. Monitor for drug interactions and long-term adverse effects. Monitor and document all seizure activity. Many are used in combination, but need to be aware of interactions and long-term adverse effects. Stopping drug abruptly may precipitate seizures or even status epilepticus.
Benzodiazepines Diazepam (oral, rectal, or parenteral) Lorazepam (parenteral or oral)	Minor sedative that prevents or stops seizures by slowing down the CNS, making abnormal electrical activity unlikely. Treatment for status epilepticus	Diazepam is available in rectal form to stop prolonged seizures in children. Useful for home management; nurses must educate family members on administration and when to call physician or nurse practitioner. Monitor sedation level and for cessation of seizure activity.
Analgesics (acetaminophen, ibuprofen, ketorolac, morphine)	Block pain impulse in response to inhibition of prostaglandin synthesis. Narcotic analgesics (i.e., morphine) act on receptors in the brain to alter perception of pain. Used to treat pain. Used to help avoid increase in ICP	Monitor for improvements in pain. Monitor sedation and respiratory status with narcotics. Monitor neurologic status closely. Used cautiously because loss of accurate neurologic evaluation can occur.
Osmotic diuretics (i.e., mannitol)	Increase plasma osmolality, therefore inducing diffusion back into plasma and extravascular space/reduces ICP	Monitor electrolytes. Monitor I/O closely. Monitor vital signs. Monitor for signs and symptoms of increased ICP.
Corticosteroids (i.e., dexamethasone)	Suppress inflammation and normal immune response/reduce cerebral edema	Give oral doses with food. Dosage must be tapered before discontinuing.

I/O, intake/output.

Adapted from Taketokmo, C. K., Hodding, J. H., & Kraus, D. M. (2013). *Lexi-comp's drug reference handbook: Pediatric & neonatal dosage handbook* (20th ed.). Hudson, OH: Lexi-comp, Inc.

Physical Examination

Physical examination of the nervous system consists of inspection and observation, palpation, and auscultation.

INSPECTION AND OBSERVATION

Specific areas to inspect and observe include:

- Level of consciousness (LOC)
- Vital signs
- Head, face, and neck
- Cranial nerve function
- Motor function
- Reflexes
- Sensory function
- Increased **intracranial pressure (ICP)** (a rise in the normal pressure within the skull)

Level of Consciousness. Begin the physical examination with inspection and observation. Observe the child's LOC, noting a decrease or significant changes. LOC is the earliest indicator of improvement or deterioration of neurologic status. Extreme irritability or lethargy is considered an abnormal finding. Consciousness consists of alertness, which is a wakeful state and includes the ability to respond to stimuli, and cognition, which includes the ability to process stimuli and demonstrate a verbal or motor response. Five different states constitute the levels of consciousness:

1. *Full consciousness* is defined as a state in which the child is awake and alert; is oriented to time, place, and person; and exhibits age-appropriate behaviors.
2. *Confusion* is defined as a state in which disorientation exists. The child may be alert but responds inappropriately to questions.
3. *Obtunded* is defined as a state in which the child has limited responses to the environment and falls asleep unless stimulation is provided.
4. *Stupor* exists when the child only responds to vigorous stimulation.
5. *Coma* defines a state in which the child cannot be aroused, even with painful stimuli.

Take Note!

Lack of response to painful stimuli is abnormal and can indicate a life-threatening condition. Report this finding immediately.

The Pediatric Glasgow Coma Scale is a popular scale used to standardize degree of consciousness. It consists of three parts: eye opening, verbal response, and motor response (Fig. 38.2). When assessing LOC in children, consider that the infant or child may not respond to unfamiliar voices in an unfamiliar environment. Therefore, it may be helpful to have a parent present to elicit the response.

Take Note!

Parents will often be the first to notice changes in their child's LOC. Listen to parents and respond to their concerns.

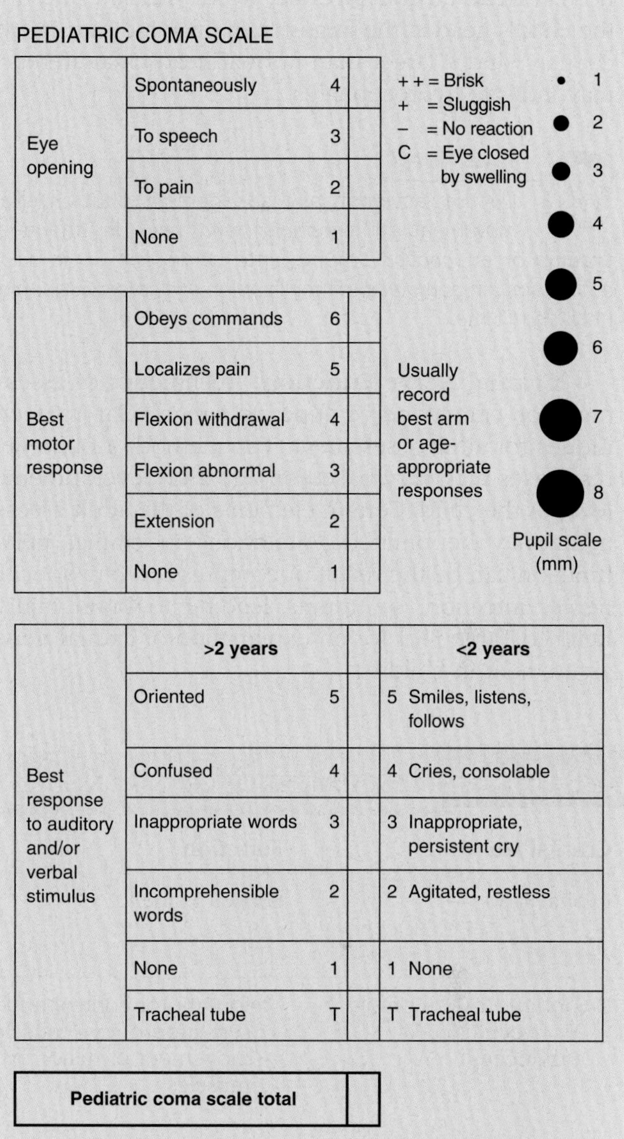
PEDIATRIC COMA SCALE

Eye opening	Spontaneously	4	
	To speech	3	
	To pain	2	
	None	1	
Best motor response	Obeys commands	6	
	Localizes pain	5	
	Flexion withdrawal	4	
	Flexion abnormal	3	
	Extension	2	
	None	1	

	>2 years		<2 years
Best response to auditory and/or verbal stimulus	Oriented	5	5 Smiles, listens, follows
	Confused	4	4 Cries, consolable
	Inappropriate words	3	3 Inappropriate, persistent cry
	Incomprehensible words	2	2 Agitated, restless
	None	1	1 None
	Tracheal tube	T	T Tracheal tube
Pediatric coma scale total			

FIGURE 38.2 Pediatric Glasgow Coma Scale (GCS). The Pediatric GCS provides for developmentally appropriate cues to assess level of consciousness (LOC) in infants and children. Numeric values are assigned to the levels of response and the sum provides an overall picture, as well as an objective measure, of the child's LOC. The lower the score, the less responsive the child.

Vital Signs. Assessment of vital signs can provide probable underlying causes for altered LOC as well as reveal the adequacy of oxygenation and circulation. Certain neurologic conditions like cerebral infections, increased ICP, coma, brain stem injury, or head injuries can cause alterations in the child's vital signs.

Head, Face, and Neck. Inspect and observe the head for size and shape. Abnormal skull shape can result from premature closure or widening of sutures. Inspect and observe the face for symmetry. Asymmetry may occur due to paralysis of certain cranial nerves, position in utero, or swelling caused by trauma. Assess range of motion of the neck. Alterations in range of motion can indicate CNS infections such as meningitis.

The most dramatic increase in brain volume occurs during the last 3 months of fetal development and the first 2 years of life. The relationship between head and brain growth explains why head circumference is a standard assessment made in children younger than 3 years of age. All children younger than 3 years old, and any child whose head size is questionable, should have their head circumference measured and plotted on a growth chart (see Appendix G for growth charts).

Assessment of the growth trend of the head is important in detecting potential neurologic conditions. Report and investigate any variation in head circumference percentiles over time because variations may indicate abnormal brain or skull growth. A smaller than normal **head circumference**, which measures around the child's head at the largest area, may indicate microcephaly, and a larger than normal head circumference may indicate hydrocephalus.

Take Note!

Do not attempt any assessment that involves movement of the head and neck in cases of trauma or suspected trauma until cervical injury is ruled out. Maintain complete immobilization of the cervical spine until that time.

Cranial Nerve Function. Techniques of assessment of cranial nerve function are similar to techniques for adult assessment. The method of obtaining responses may vary based on age and developmental level of the child. Certain elements of the adult assessment may be omitted. Alterations in cranial nerve function can be the result of compression of a specific nerve, infection, or trauma leading to brain injury. Refer to Table 38.1 for an explanation of cranial nerve assessment in children.

Use the doll's eyes maneuver to evaluate cranial nerves III, IV, and VI. This maneuver can be helpful when assessing an infant, uncooperative child, or comatose child. It examines horizontal and vertical eye movements by turning the head in one direction and assessing if the eyes move symmetrically in the other direction. For example, if you suddenly turn the child's head to the right, the child's eyes should look to the left symmetrically. Assess vertical eye movements in a similar manner by flexing or extending the neck. Absence of expected eye movements may indicate increased ICP.

When assessing oculomotor function, be sure to note nystagmus or sunset appearance of the eyes. Observe for nystagmus by looking for involuntary, rapid, rhythmic eye movements that may be present at rest or with eye movement. Horizontal nystagmus may occur with lesions in the brain stem and can be the result of certain medications (phenytoin in particular). Vertical nystagmus indicates brain stem dysfunction. Sunsetting is when the sclera of the eyes is showing over the top of the iris (Fig. 38.3). Sunset eyes may indicate increased ICP as seen in hydrocephalus. Pupillary

TABLE 38.1 ASSESSMENT OF CRANIAL NERVES IN INFANTS AND CHILDREN

Cranial Nerve	Function	Assessment Procedure
I (olfactory)	Sense of smell	Not evaluated in infants and young children. In children, assess child's ability to recognize common smells (i.e., an orange) while eyes are closed.
II (optic), III (oculomotor), IV (trochlear), VI (abducens)	Vision, motor control and sensation of eye muscles, movement of major eye muscles	Assess oculomotor ability by having child follow object (toy or brightly colored object). Assess vision fields and visual acuity in older child. Assess pupil reaction same as adult. May need to talk to child or have parent in visual field while applying light stimulus.
V (trigeminal)	Mastication muscles and facial sensation	Note strength of infant's suck on pacifier, examiner's thumb, or bottle. In children, assess strength of bite and ability to discern light touch on face.
VII (facial)	Facial muscles, salivation, and taste	Note symmetry of facial expressions; in infant, monitor during spontaneous cries or smiles. In older child, test as in adults. Assess taste by asking to discern certain common tastes (salt, sugar).
VIII (acoustic)	Hearing	In infant, note response to voice. In children, use whisper test or Weber or Rinne test.
IX (glossopharyngeal), X (vagus)	Motor impulses to heart and other organs, swallowing, and gag reflex	Gag reflex and swallowing tested as in adults. Check time of last feeding, especially in the infant, to avoid vomiting when gag reflex is tested.
XI (accessory)	Impulses to muscles of shoulders and pharynx	In infants, note symmetry of head position when placed in the sitting position. In children, same as adults.
XII (hypoglossal)	Motor impulses to tongue and skeletal muscles	In infants, note spontaneous tongue movements. In children, same as adults.

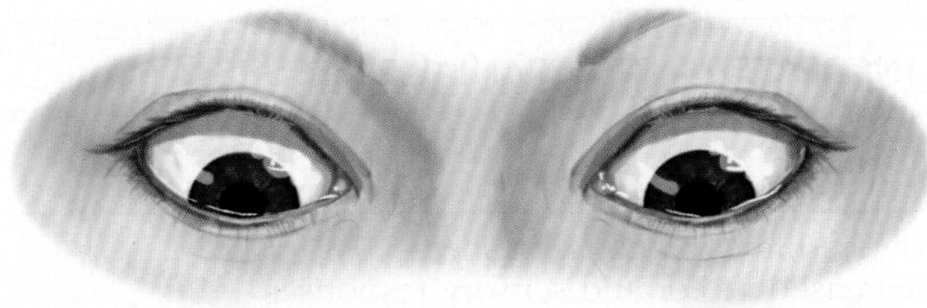

FIGURE 38.3 Sunsetting of the eyes is a sign of increased intracranial pressure.

response is often abnormal when a neurologic disorder is present. Refer to Figure 38.4 for illustrations of varied pupillary responses.

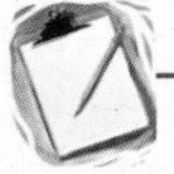

Take Note!

Immediately report the sudden presence of fixed and dilated pupils.

Motor Function. Observe muscle strength, size, and tone in the infant or child. Assess bilaterally and compare. Observe spontaneous activity, posture, and balance and assess for asymmetric movements. In the infant, observe resting posture, which will normally be a slightly flexed posture. The infant should be able to extend extremities to a normal stretch. Alterations in motor function, like changes in gait, muscle tone, or strength, may indicate certain neurologic problems such as increased ICP, head injury, and cerebral infections. Because cortical control of motor function is lost in certain neurologic disorders, postural reflexes reemerge and are directly related to the area of the brain that is damaged. Therefore, it is important to assess for two distinct types of posturing that may occur. **Decorticate posturing** occurs with damage of the cerebral cortex (Fig. 38.5A). **Decerebrate posturing** occurs with damage at the level of the brain stem (Fig. 38.5B). Both types of posturing are characterized by extremely rigid muscle tone.

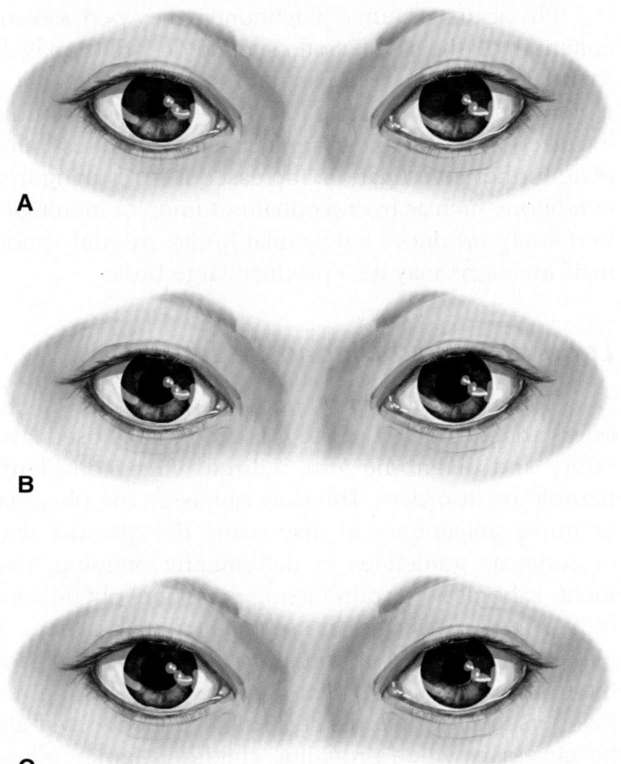

FIGURE 38.4 Assessing pupil size and reaction. **(A)** *Pinpoint* is commonly observed in poisonings, brain stem dysfunction, and opiate use. **(B)** *Dilated but reactive* is seen after seizures. *Fixed and dilated* is associated with brain stem herniation secondary to increased intracranial pressure. **(C)** *One dilated but reactive* is associated with intracranial mass.

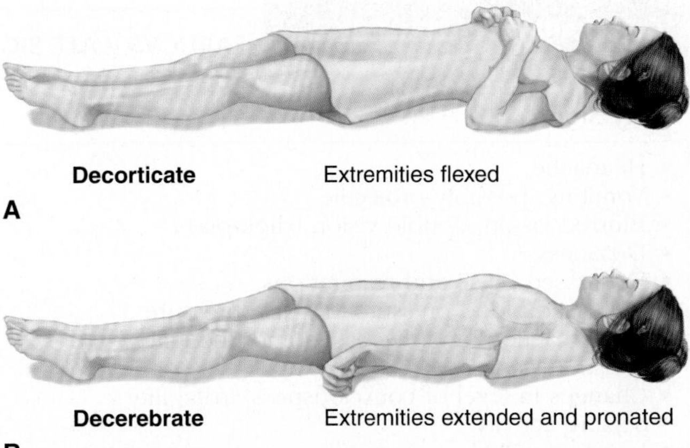

FIGURE 38.5 **(A)** Decorticate posturing occurs with damage of the cerebral cortex and includes adduction of the arms, flexion at the elbows with arms held over chest, and flexion of the wrists with hands fisted. Lower extremities are adducted and extended. **(B)** Decerebrate posturing occurs with damage to the midbrain and includes extension and pronation of the arms and legs.

Reflexes. Testing of deep tendon reflexes is part of the neurologic assessment, just as it is in adults. Testing of primitive and protective reflexes in the infant is important because infants cannot perform tasks on command. The Moro, tonic neck, and withdrawal reflexes are important in assessing neurologic health in infants. Refer to Chapter 25 for a further explanation of primitive and protective reflexes in infants (see Chapter 25, Table 25.1). Absence of certain reflexes, persistence of primitive reflexes after age of normal disappearance, or increases in reflexes may be present in specific neurologic conditions.

Sensory Function. When assessing the child, use techniques similar to those used in the adult assessment. Make sure to explain what you are doing to the child, especially before the pinprick test, to gain continued cooperation. When assessing sensory function,

COMPARISON CHART 38.1 **EARLY VS. LATE SIGNS OF INCREASED INTRACRANIAL PRESSURE**

Early Signs	Late Signs

• Headache
• Vomiting, possibly projectile
• Blurred vision, double vision (diplopia)
• Dizziness
• Decreased pulse and respirations
• Increased blood pressure or pulse pressure
• Pupil reaction time decreased and unequal
• Sunset eyes
• Changes in level of consciousness, irritability
• Seizure activity
• In infant will also see:
  • Bulging, tense fontanel
  • Wide sutures and increased head circumference
  • Dilated scalp veins
  • High-pitched cry
	• Lowered level of consciousness
	• Decreased motor and sensory responses
	• Bradycardia
	• Irregular respirations
	• Cheyne–Stokes respirations
	• Decerebrate or decorticate posturing
	• Fixed and dilated pupils

the child should be able to distinguish between light touch, pain, vibration, heat, and cold. When assessing an infant, limit the examination to responses to touch or pain. The normal response in a 4-month-old infant will be movement away from the stimulus. Alterations in sensory function can result from brain or spinal cord lesions.

Increased Intracranial Pressure. Observe for signs and symptoms associated with increased ICP while caring for a child with a potential or suspected neurologic disorder. Refer to Comparison Chart 38.1 for early versus late signs and symptoms of increased ICP. Increased ICP is a sign that may occur with many neurologic disorders. It may result from head trauma, birth trauma, hydrocephalus, infection, and brain tumors. As ICP increases, LOC decreases and the signs and symptoms will become more pronounced. It is essential to recognize early signs and symptoms of increased ICP and intervene immediately to prevent long-term damage and possible death.

PALPATION

Palpation of the newborn and infant skull and fontanels is an important function of the neurologic examination. Changes in size or fullness of the fontanels may exist in certain neurologic conditions and must be noted. A bulging fontanel can be a sign of increased ICP and is seen in such neurologic disorders as hydrocephalus and head traumas. It is normal for the fontanels to be full or bulging during crying; take this into consideration during assessment.

Note any premature closure of fontanels, which can indicate skull deformities such as craniosynostosis. The posterior fontanel normally closes by 2 months of age and the anterior fontanel normally closes by 12 to 18 months of age. In children with hydrocephalus, widening of the fontanels may be noted, along with a tense appearance and a resulting increase in head circumference.

AUSCULTATION

Physicians or nurse practitioners may perform auscultation of the skull. Soft, symmetric bruits may be found in children younger than 4 years of age or in children with acute febrile illness. A finding of a loud or localized bruit is usually significant and requires immediate further investigation. Increased ICP, resulting from conditions such as hydrocephalus, tumor, or meningitis, frequently produces intracranial bruits. Arterial venous malformations may also produce large bruits.

Laboratory and Diagnostic Testing

Common Laboratory and Diagnostic Tests 38.1 offers an explanation of the most commonly used laboratory and diagnostic tests utilized when considering neurologic disorders. The tests can assist the physician or nurse practitioner in diagnosing the disorder and/or serve as guidelines in determining ongoing treatment. Laboratory or nonnursing personnel obtain some of the tests, while the nurse might obtain others. In either instance, it is important to be familiar with how the tests are obtained, what they are used for, and normal versus abnormal results. This knowledge will also be necessary when providing child and family education related to the testing. Many of these tests, such as lumbar puncture (LP) (Fig. 38.6), can be frightening to parents and the child. Prepare the family and the child and provide support and reassurance during and after the test or procedure.

(text continues on page 1392)

COMMON LABORATORY AND DIAGNOSTIC TESTS 38.1

Test	Explanation	Indications	Nursing Implications
Lumbar puncture (LP)	Withdrawal of cerebrospinal fluid (CSF) from the subarachnoid space for analysis	To diagnose hemorrhage, infection, or obstruction Can obtain measurement of spinal fluid pressure	Assist with proper positioning (Fig. 38.6). Help child maintain position and remain still. Maintain strict asepsis. Assist with collection and transport of specimen. Encourage fluids after procedure, if not contraindicated. Keep child flat for 1 hour if ordered. Apply EMLA cream to puncture site 30–60 minutes before procedure to reduce pain, if ordered.
Head and neck X-ray	Radiographic image of the head and neck will show skull and spine structures	Detects skull and spinal fractures; shows location and course of ventricular catheters; reveals information about increased intracranial pressure (ICP) and skull defects	Children may be afraid. Allow a parent or family member to accompany the child. If the child is unable or unwilling to stay still for the x-ray, restraint may be necessary. The time of restraint should be limited to the amount of time needed for the x-ray.
Fluoroscopy	Radiographic examination that uses continuous x-rays to show live up-to-date images	Can assess cervical spine for instability during movement	Same as head and neck x-rays. Child will need to cooperate with flexion and extension of neck.
Cerebral angiography	X-ray study of cerebral blood vessels. Involves injection of a contrast medium and use of fluoroscopy	Can assess for vessel defects or space-occupying lesions	Same as head and neck x-rays. Assess for allergy to contrast medium. Push fluids following procedure, if not contraindicated, to help flush out contrast medium.
Ultrasound	Use of sound waves to locate the depth and structure within soft tissues and fluid	Used to assess intracranial hemorrhage in newborns, and ventricular size	Better tolerated by nonsedated children than CT or MRI Can be performed portably at bedside
Computed tomography (CT)	Noninvasive x-ray study that looks at tissue density and structures. Images a "slice" of child's tissue	To diagnose congenital abnormalities, such as neural tube defects, hemorrhage, tumors, fractures	Machine is large and can be frightening to children. Procedure can be lengthy and child must remain still. If unable to do so, sedation may be necessary. Can be performed with or without use of contrast medium; if used, assess for allergy. Encourage fluids post procedure, if not contraindicated.
Electroencephalogram (EEG)	Measures electrical activity of the brain	To diagnose seizures and brain death	Must remain still. If unable to do so, sedation may be necessary, but should be avoided if possible because sedatives can alter the EEG reading. Inform technician of what anticonvulsants the child is taking. Morning anticonvulsants may need to be held.

(continued)

COMMON LABORATORY AND DIAGNOSTIC TESTS 38.1 (continued)

Test	Explanation	Indications	Nursing Implications
Magnetic resonance imaging (MRI)	Use of magnetic field to show different tissue compositions	Used to assess tumors and inflammation; used to diagnose congenital abnormalities, such as neural tube defects; shows normal versus abnormal brain tissue	Child may not have any metal devices, internal or external, while undergoing MRI (ensure hospital gown does not have metal snaps). Procedure can be lengthy and child must remain still. Child is placed in long narrow tube and the machine makes a booming noise when it is turned on and off during the procedure; therefore, can be difficult to gain cooperation. If the child is unable to remain still, sedation may be necessary. Can be performed with or without use of a contrast medium. If contrast medium is used, assess for allergy. Encourage fluids post procedure, if not contraindicated.
Positron emission tomography (PET)	Similar to CT or MRI, but radioisotope is added. Measures physiologic function	Provides information on brain functional development. Can assist in identifying seizure foci. Can assess tumors and brain metabolism	Procedure can be lengthy and child must remain still. If unable to do so, sedation may be necessary. Intravenous access will be needed for the procedure. Encourage fluids post procedure, if not contraindicated, to help body eliminate radioisotopes.
Single photon emission computed tomography (SPECT)	Use of radiopharmaceuticals to provide 3-dimensional splices; less expensive and more available than PET	Used to detect brain death, presence of encephalitis, hydrocephalus, to localize epileptic foci, assess metabolic activity, evaluate brain tumors, assessment of childhood development disorders	Similar to PET In uncooperative children do not use sedation until after injection because it may affect brain activity Secure child's head Sudden distractions or loud noises can alter the distribution of radionuclide
Cisternography	Radiopharmaceuticals injected intrathecally during a lumbar puncture to assess flow and reabsorption of CSF	Can assist in selection of type of shunt and pathway to use in treating hydrocephalus	Sterile LP performed and radionuclide injected into cerebrospinal circulation Imaging performed at specified times Child must lie flat after puncture
Intracranial pressure (ICP) monitoring (intraventricular catheter, subarachnoid screw or bolt, epidural sensor, anterior fontanel pressure monitor)	A sensing device is placed in the head that monitors the pressure intracranially.	Used to monitor ICP resulting from hydrocephalus, acute head trauma, and brain tumors. Ventricular catheter also allows for draining of CSF to help reduce ICP.	Usually monitored in critical care setting Monitor for signs and symptoms of increased ICP. Monitor for infection. Keep head of bed elevated 15–30 degrees. Alarms for monitoring device should remain on at all times. Reduce stimulation and avoid interventions that may cause pain or stress and result in an increased ICP.

COMMON LABORATORY AND DIAGNOSTIC TESTS 38.1 (continued)

Test	Explanation	Indications	Nursing Implications
Video EEG	Measures electrical activity of the brain continuously along with recorded video of actions and behaviors	Can help determine precise localization of seizure area before surgery. Assists in diagnosis and management of seizures by correlating behaviors with abnormal EEG activity	Ensure that seizure precautions are in place. Parent or caregiver must be with child at all times. The child's movements are limited and usually confined to the room. When the child changes position, ensure that he or she is still seen by video camera. Boredom can be a problem. Must notify nurse if seizure activity occurs; push the alert button to highlight attack on EEG recoding. Nurse must immediately go to the room, expose as much of the child as possible (remove covers; if at night, turn on light), and avoid blocking the camera. Ask questions (i.e., what is your name, can you raise your left arm, remember the word banana) to help assess responsiveness more accurately. Stay with the child until a full recovery has occurred. Ask the child what word you asked him or her to remember, and document all findings and time of the event.

Adapted from Fischbach, F. T., & Dunning III, M. B. III (2015). *A manual of laboratory and diagnostic tests* (9th ed.). Philadelphia, PA: Wolters Kluwer Health/Lippincott Williams & Wilkins.

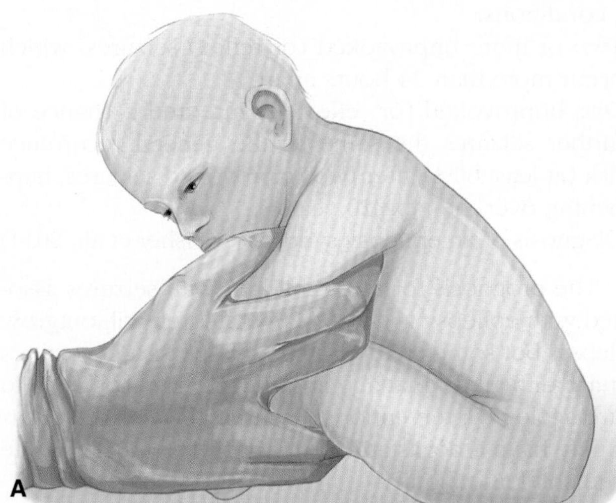

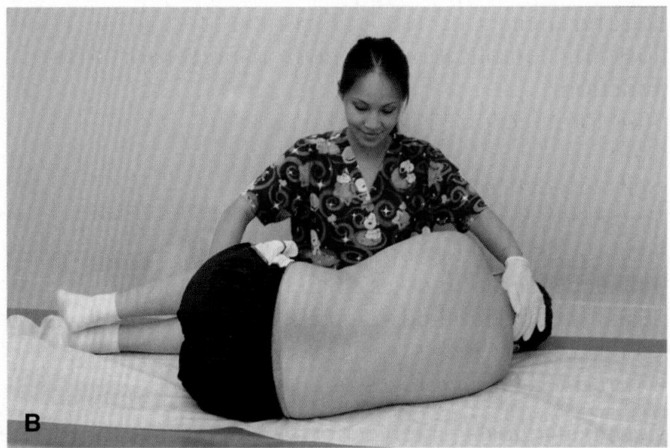

FIGURE 38.6 Proper positioning for a lumbar puncture. (**A**) The newborn is positioned upright with head flexed forward. (**B**) Child or older infant is positioned on the side with head flexed forward and knees flexed to abdomen.

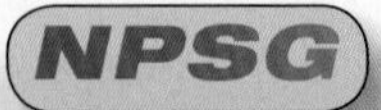

GOAL 2: Improve the Effectiveness of Communication Among Caregivers

NPSG.02.03.01 Report critical results of tests and diagnostic procedures on a timely basis.

Steps: When caring for a child with a potential or actual neurologic disorder notify appropriate health care provider with positive culture results, abnormalities in the CSF, and critical changes to other laboratory values and diagnostic test results.

Joint Commission. (2015). *National patient safety goals effective January 1, 2015.* Retrieved from http://www.jointcommission.org/assets/1/6/2015_NPSG_HAP.pdf

Atraumatic Care

During an LP use distraction techniques that will allow the child to remain in the proper position, such as storytelling or music. Encourage parental involvement and enlist the help of a child life specialist, if possible.

After completing an assessment of Antonio, the nurse noted the following: a full anterior fontanel; when being held, Antonio was inconsolable; when lying still, he was calmer and in the opisthotonic position.

Nursing Diagnoses and Related Interventions

Upon completion of a thorough assessment, the nurse might identify several nursing diagnoses, including:

- Decreased intracranial adaptive capacity
- Risk for ineffective tissue perfusion: cerebral
- Risk for injury
- Risk for complications of neurologic/sensory dysfunction
- Risk for infection
- Pain
- Self-care deficit (specify)
- Impaired physical mobility
- Risk for delayed development
- Imbalanced nutrition: less than body requirements
- Risk for deficient fluid volume
- Deficient knowledge (specify)
- Interrupted family processes

Nursing goals, interventions, and evaluation for the child with a neurologic disorder are based on the nursing diagnoses.

Based on the assessment findings, what would be your top three prioritized nursing diagnoses for Antonio?

Nursing Care Plan 38.1, found at the end of the chapter, may be used as a guide in planning nursing care for the child with a neurologic disorder. It should be individualized based on the child's symptoms and needs. Additional information will be included later in this chapter related to specific disorders.

Based on your top three nursing diagnoses for Antonio, describe appropriate nursing interventions.

SEIZURE DISORDERS

Seizures occur in approximately 4% to 10% of children, with a lifetime incidence of epilepsy being 3%, with half of these starting in childhood (Mikati, 2011). Most seizures are caused by disorders that originate outside of the brain such as a high fever, infection, head trauma, hypoxia, toxins, or cardiac arrhythmias. Seizure disorders discussed below include epilepsy, febrile seizures, and neonatal seizures.

Epilepsy

Epilepsy is a condition in which seizures are triggered recurrently from within the brain. Epilepsy is a common neurologic disorder discovered in childhood, although brain injury or infection can cause epilepsy at any age. The International League Against Epilepsy (ILAE) recently altered the practical definition of epilepsy and it is now defined by the presence of any of the following conditions:

- Two or more unprovoked (or reflex) seizures, which occur more than 24 hours apart
- One unprovoked (or reflex) seizure and a chance of further seizures the same as the general recurrence risk (at least 60%) after two unprovoked seizures, happening over the next 10 years
- Diagnosis of an epilepsy syndrome (Fisher et al., 2014)

The prognosis for most children with seizures associated with epilepsy is good. Many children will outgrow epilepsy, but some children will have persistent seizures that are difficult to manage and may be unresponsive to pharmacologic interventions. Living with a seizure disorder may have a devastating impact on the quality of life of the child and family.

Pathophysiology

Epilepsy is a complex disorder of the CNS in which brain function is affected. Recurrent or unprovoked seizures are the clinical manifestation of epilepsy and result from a disruption of electrical communication among the neurons of the brain. This disruption results from an imbalance between the excitatory and inhibitory mechanisms in the brain, causing the neurons to either fire when they are not supposed to or not fire when they should. Epilepsy has numerous causes. It may be acquired and related to brain injury or it may be a familial tendency, but in many cases the cause is unknown (Centers for Disease Control and Prevention, 2015b).

The ILAE revised their seizure classification system in 2010 related to the technologic and scientific advances, such as improved imaging and genomics, that have led to improved understanding of seizures and epilepsy (Berg et al., 2010; Korff & Wirrell, 2014). International Classification of Epileptic Seizures is used by most neurologists to classify seizure types. There are three categories of seizures—focal (previously known as partial), generalized and unknown seizures (i.e., epileptic spasms). In focal seizures only one hemisphere of the brain is involved, while general seizures involve the entire brain. Focal seizures are seen in 60% of those with epilepsy and are described based on impairment of consciousness, localization, and progression of the seizure (Berg et al., 2010; National Institute of Neurological Disorders and Stroke, 2015). Generalized seizures include absence seizures, tonic, clonic, tonic–clonic seizures, myoclonic seizures, and atonic seizures. Unknown is used for epileptic spasms where it is unclear whether the mode of onset is generalized or focal (Berg et al., 2010). There are many different types of seizures, and the classification of the type of seizure is crucial in assisting with the management and control of seizures. Not all cases are easily classified. The most common seizure types are discussed in Table 38.2.

Therapeutic Management

Management of epilepsy focuses on controlling seizures or reducing their frequency. Another focus of epilepsy management involves helping the child who has recurrent seizures and his or her family to learn to live with the seizures. The primary mode of treatment is the use of anticonvulsants. The goal for every child should be the use of the fewest drugs with the fewest possible side effects for the control of seizures. There have been significant advances in the treatment of epilepsy due to the many new anticonvulsant medications that have become available in recent years (Table 38.3). Most anticonvulsants are taken orally and are often used in combination. Different medications control different types of seizures, which may be due to individual variation. It can take time to find the right combination to best control an individual's seizures.

If seizures remain uncontrolled, another option for managing them is surgery. Depending on the area of the brain that is affected, it may be possible to remove the area that is responsible for the seizure activity or to interrupt the impulses from spreading, and therefore stop or reduce the seizures. The adverse effects of surgery range from mild to severe, depending on the area of the brain that is affected. Other nonpharmacologic treatments that may be considered in children with intractable seizures include a ketogenic diet or placement of a vagal nerve stimulator. Refer to Common Medical Treatments 38.1.

Nursing Assessment

For a full description of the assessment phase of the nursing process, refer to the Assessment section of the Nursing Process Overview earlier in the chapter. Assessment findings pertinent to epilepsy are discussed below.

HEALTH HISTORY

Elicit a description of the present illness and chief complaint, which will usually involve a seizure episode. Gain information to help characterize the episode as a seizure or as a nonepileptic event (see Box 38.1 for a list of nonepileptic events). It is rare to actually observe the child having a seizure; therefore, a complete, accurate, and detailed history from a reliable source is essential. Questions should include:

- Where did the event occur—while sleeping, eating, playing, or just after waking?
- Description of child's behavior during the event—what types of movements, progression, length, respiratory status, apnea?
- How did the child act after the event?
- Have the episodes been recurrent? If so, how frequent?
- Any precipitating factors such as a fever, fall, activity, anxiety, infection, or exposure to strong stimuli such as flashing lights or loud noises?

Explore the child's current and past medical history for risk factors such as:

- Family history of seizures or epilepsy
- Any complications during the prenatal, perinatal, or postnatal periods

(text continues on page 1396)

BOX 38.1

NONEPILEPTIC EVENTS

- Syncope
- Breath holding
- Jitteriness
- Apnea
- Gastroesophageal reflux
- Cardiac conduction abnormalities
- Migraines
- Tics
- Night terrors
- Benign sleep movements

TABLE 38.2 COMMON TYPES OF SEIZURES

Type	Description	Characteristics
Epileptic spasm such as infantile spasms	Mode of seizure onset unknown, whether focal or generalized Type of epileptic spasm seen in infancy Usually seen between 3 and 12 months of age, peak incidence 3 to 7 months and rarely seen after the age of 18 months	Occurs in series or clusters Presents as symmetrical flexing or extending, in variant clinical patterns, of the neck, arms, legs, and trunk May see: • Extension of neck, trunk, arms, and legs • Flexion of neck, trunk, and extremities with contracting of abdominal muscles (may cause body to bend forward, often referred to as "jackknife seizures") • Cry may precede or follow Majority of infants have some brain disorder before seizures begin. The infant seems to stop developing and may lose skills that he or she has already attained after the onset of infantile spasms. Hormonal therapy (mainly corticotropin) and anticonvulsants (most commonly, vigabatrin) are common forms of treatment.
Absence (formerly *petit mal*)	Type of generalized seizure; Uncommon before age 5	Abrupt onset and offset Sudden cessation of motor activity or speech with a blank facial expression or rhythmic twitching of the mouth, eyebrows, chin, eyelids, or other parts of the face Child may experience countless seizures in a day. Not associated with a postictal (after seizure) state May go unrecognized or mistaken for inattentiveness because of subtle change in child's behavior Myoclonic absence seizure consists of jerks of the shoulder and arms may result in lifting of the arms. Eyelid myoclonia brief (6 seconds) jerking of the eyelids with eyeballs rolling back; multiple seizures occur daily
Clonic	Type of generalized seizure that presents with repeated jerking movements	Muscles will spasm, jerk, then relax Spasm/jerking cannot be stopped by restraining or repositioning Clonic seizures alone are rare; may precede a tonic–clonic seizure
Tonic	Type of generalized seizures that present with stiffening of the muscles, typically the back, legs, arms	Consciousness usually preserved Tightening of chest muscles may lead to cyanosis; seen in children with Lennox–Gastaut syndrome
Tonic–clonic (formerly *grand mal*)	Extremely common generalized seizures. Most dramatic seizure type	Associated with an aura Loss of consciousness occurs and may be preceded by a piercing cry. Presents with entire body experiencing tonic contractions followed by rhythmic clonic contractions alternating with relaxation of all muscle groups Cyanosis may be noted due to apnea. Saliva may collect in the mouth due to inability to swallow. Child may bite tongue. Loss of sphincter control, especially the bladder, is common. Postictal phase: child will be semicomatose or in a deep sleep for approximately 30 minutes to 2 hours; usually responds only to painful stimuli Child will have no memory of the seizure; may complain of headache and feeling fatigue Safety of the child is a primary concern. See Teaching Guidelines 38.1.

TABLE 38.2 COMMON TYPES OF SEIZURES (continued)

Type	Description	Characteristics
Myoclonic	Type of generalized seizure that involves the motor cortex of the brain. May occur along with other seizure forms	Sudden, brief, massive muscle jerks that may involve the whole body or one body part Child may or may not lose consciousness.
Atonic	Type of generalized seizure often referred to as "drop attacks." Seen in children with Lennox-Gastaut syndrome	Sudden loss of muscle tone. In children, may only be a sudden drop of the head. Child will regain consciousness within a few seconds to a minute. Can result in injury related to violent fall
Focal seizure without impairment of consciousness (previously referred to as simple partial seizure)	Type of partial seizure that occurs in one part of the brain. The symptoms seen will depend on which area of the brain is affected.	Motor activity characterized by clonic or tonic movements involving the face, neck, and extremities Can include sensory signs such as numbness, tingling, paresthesia, changes in vision and hearing, possible hallucinations, or pain Can include autonomic symptoms such as changes in blood pressure, heart rhythm, bowel function Can include psychic symptoms such as triggering emotions of fear, anxiety, joy, sadness Child remains conscious and may verbalize during the seizure. No postictal state
Focal seizure with impaired consciousness (dyscognitive) previously known as complex partial seizure	Common type of partial seizure May begin with a focal seizure without impaired consciousness, then progress	May or may not have a preceding aura Consciousness will be impaired. Automatisms and complex purposeful movements are common features in infants and children. Infants will present with behaviors such as lip smacking, chewing, swallowing, and excessive salivation; can be difficult to distinguish from normal infant behavior In older children, will see picking or pulling at bed sheets or clothing, rubbing objects, or running or walking in a nondirective and repetitive fashion These seizures can be difficult to control.
Status epilepticus	Common neurologic emergency in children. Can occur with any seizure activity. Febrile seizures are the most common type. In children with epilepsy, it commonly occurs early in the course of epilepsy. Can be life threatening	Prolonged or clustered seizures where consciousness does not return between seizures The age of the child, cause of the seizures, and duration of status epilepticus influence prognosis. Prompt medical intervention is essential to reduce morbidity and mortality. Treatment: • Basic life support—ABCs (airway, breathing, circulation) • Administration of anticonvulsants to cease seizures is crucial. Common medications include benzodiazepines such as lorazepam and diazepam, and fosphenytoin. (see Drug Guide 38.1 and Table 38.3.) • Blood glucose levels and electrolytes along with evaluation of the underlying cause should be initiated.

Adapted from Mikati, M. A. (2011). Chapter 586. Seizures in Childhood. In: R. M. Kleigman, B. F. Stanton, J. W. St. Geme III, N. F. Schor, & R. E. Behrman (Eds.), *Nelson textbook of pediatrics* (19th ed., pp. 2013–39). Philadelphia, PA: Saunders; Zak, M., & Chan, V. W. (2014). Chapter 46: Pediatric neurologic disorders. In S. M. Nettina (Ed.), *Lippincott manual of nursing practice* (10th ed., pp. 1545–1575). Philadelphia, PA: Wolters/Kluwer Health: Lippincott Williams & Wilkins.

TABLE 38.3 COMMON ANTICONVULSANT MEDICATIONS

Medication	Nursing Implications
Phenytoin (IV and PO; IM administration is contraindicated)	Monitor serum levels to ensure therapeutic dosing. Be aware that gingival hyperplasia appears most commonly in children and adolescents. If on prolonged therapy, ensure adequate intake of vitamin D–containing foods. Monitor serum calcium and magnesium levels. IV form given in normal saline to prevent precipitation.
Fosphenytoin (IM or IV only)	Adverse effects are said to be less common than with phenytoin. It does not cause local irritation, but it is a more expensive drug than phenytoin. It is water soluble, therefore allowing faster and easier administration than phenytoin. All dosing is in phenytoin sodium equivalents. It does not precipitate in commonly used IV diluents.
Phenobarbital	Assess for excessive sedation. Monitor serum levels to ensure therapeutic dosing. Monitor for drug interactions. Increase vitamin D–fortified foods or administer supplement, if prescribed. Withdrawal symptoms will occur if drug is stopped abruptly. Valproic acid interferes with this drug, causing increased phenobarbital levels.
Felbamate	Monitor for drug interactions, especially if child is taking phenytoin or carbamazepine.
Valproic acid (divalproex sodium, sodium valproate)	Monitor serum levels to ensure therapeutic dosing. Depakote sprinkles are available and useful for children who are unable to tolerate valproate suspension, tablets, or capsules. The contents can be sprinkled on food that does not require chewing.
Carbamazepine	Monitor serum levels to ensure therapeutic dosing; toxicity can occur even with levels slightly above therapeutic range. Plasma concentration decreased by phenytoin, phenobarbital, and valproic acid
Gabapentin	Do not administer within 2 hours of antacids. Rapidly absorbed in the gastrointestinal tract
Topiramate	Dilantin, Tegretol, and valproic acid decrease concentration of topiramate.
Oxcarbazepine	Monitor phenytoin levels, if administering concurrently. Monitor serum sodium.
Zonisamide	Presence of food will delay absorption. Phenytoin, phenobarbital, and carbamazepine all increase the metabolism of this drug.
Lamotrigine	Valproate inhibits metabolism; therefore, monitor serum blood values and decrease the dose, if necessary.
Levetiracetam	Monitor phenytoin levels, if administering concurrently. Monitor for difficulty with gait or coordination. B-complex vitamin supplementation can help manage side effects.
Ethosuximide	Give with food if GI upset occurs. Monitor closely during periods of dosage adjustment or addition of new medications.

GI, gastrointestinal; IM, intramuscular; IV, intravenous; PO, by mouth.

Adapted from Mikati, M. A. (2011). Chapter 586. Seizures in Childhood. In: R. M. Kleigman, B. F. Stanton, J. W. St. Geme III, N. F. Schor, & R. E. Behrman (Eds.), *Nelson textbook of pediatrics* (19th ed., pp. 2013–39). Philadelphia, PA: Saunders; and Zak, M., & Chan, V. W. (2014). Chapter 46: Pediatric neurologic disorders. In: S. M. Nettina (Ed.), *Lippincott manual of nursing practice* (10th ed., pp. 1545–1575). Philadelphia, PA: Wolters/Kluwer Health: Lippincott Williams & Wilkins

- Changes in developmental status or delays in developmental milestones
- Any recent illness, fever, trauma, or toxin exposure

Children known to have epilepsy are often admitted to the hospital for other health-related issues or complications and treatment of their seizure disorder. The health history should include questions related to:

- Age of onset of seizures
- Seizure control—what medications are the child taking, and has he or she been able to take them; when was his or her last seizure?

- Description and classification of seizures—does the child lose consciousness; does the child become apneic?
- Precipitating factors that may contribute to onset of seizures
- Adverse effects related to anticonvulsant medications
- Compliance with medication regimen

PHYSICAL EXAMINATION

Perform a complete neurologic examination. Careful assessment of the child's mental status, language, learning, behavior, and motor abilities can help provide information about any neurologic deficits. If you observe seizure activity directly, provide a thorough and accurate description of the event. This description needs to include:

- Time of onset and length of seizure activity
- Alterations in behavior such as a cry or changes in facial expression, motor abilities, or sensory alterations before the seizure that may indicate an aura
- Precipitating factors such as fever, anxiety, just waking, or eating
- Description of movements and any progression
- Description of respiratory effort and any apnea noted
- Changes in color (pallor or cyanosis) noted
- Position of mouth, any injury to mouth or tongue, inability to swallow, or excessive salivation
- Loss of bladder or bowel control
- State of consciousness during seizure and **postictal** (after seizure) state—during the seizure, the nurse may ask the child to remember a word; after the seizure, assess if child is able to recall it, to help accurately establish current mental state
- Assess orientation to person, place, and time; motor abilities; speech; behavior; alterations in sensation postictally
- Duration of postictal state

LABORATORY AND DIAGNOSTIC TESTS

Laboratory and diagnostic tests are used to evaluate the cause of, and also aid in identifying the type of, seizure activity (refer to Common Laboratory and Diagnostic Tests 38.1). Common laboratory and diagnostic studies ordered for the diagnosis and assessment of epilepsy include:

- Serum glucose, electrolytes, and calcium—to rule out metabolic causes such as hypoglycemia and hypocalcemia
- LP—to analyze cerebrospinal fluid (CSF) to rule out meningitis or encephalitis
- Skull x-ray examinations—to evaluate for the presence of fracture or trauma
- Computed tomography (CT) and magnetic resonance imaging (MRI) studies—to identify abnormalities and intracranial bleeds and rule out tumors
- Electroencephalographs (EEGs)—EEG findings may be noted with certain seizure types, but a normal EEG does not rule out epilepsy because seizure activity rarely occurs during the actual testing time. EEGs are useful in evaluating seizure type and assisting in medication selection. They can be useful in differentiating seizures from nonepileptic activity.
- Video EEGs—provide the opportunity to see the child's actual behavior on video, accompanied with EEG changes; can improve the chance of catching a seizure because the monitoring is done over a period of time

Nursing Management

Nursing management focuses on preventing injury during seizures, administering appropriate medication and treatments to prevent or reduce seizures, and providing education and support to the child and family to help them cope with the challenges of living with a chronic seizure disorder. See Box 38.2 for a list of basic seizure precautions. In addition to the nursing diagnoses and related interventions discussed in Nursing Care Plan 38.1 at the end of the chapter, interventions common to epilepsy follow.

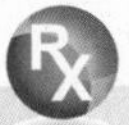

Dosage Calculation

Child's Weight: 9.98 kg (22 lb)

Medication order: Phenobarbital 50 mg PO twice a day

As per the Pediatric Dosage Handbook, the recommended dose is 6 to 8 mg/kg/day in one to two divided doses. Is the ordered dose safe?

Relieving Anxiety

Seizures produce fear and anxiety due to their unpredictable nature along with their uncontrolled, forceful, and, at times, violent appearance. Instruct parents and family members, along with those in the community who may care for the child, on how to respond in case of a seizure (see Teaching Guidelines 38.1). This will help to empower the parents, family, and other caregivers, and, in turn, alleviate some of the anxiety that they may feel.

BOX 38.2

SEIZURE PRECAUTIONS

- Padding of side rails and other hard objects
- Side rails raised on bed at all times when child is in bed
- Oxygen and suction at bedside
- Supervision, especially during bathing, ambulation, or other potentially hazardous activities
- Use of a protective helmet during activity may be appropriate.
- Child should wear a medical alert bracelet.

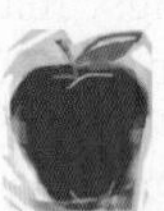

Teaching Guidelines 38.1

HOW TO RESPOND WHEN YOUR CHILD HAS A SEIZURE

Instruct parents and caregivers:

- Remain calm.
- If child is standing or sitting, ease child to the ground, if possible.
- Time seizure episode.
- Tight clothing and jewelry around the neck should be loosened, if possible.
- Place child on one side and open airway, if possible.
- Do not restrain the child.
- Remove hazards in the area.
- Do not forcibly open jaw with a tongue blade or fingers.
- Document length of seizure and movements noted, also cyanosis or loss of bladder or bowel control and any other characteristics.
- Remain with child until fully conscious.
- Call EMS if:
  - The child stops breathing
  - Any injury has occurred
  - Seizure lasts for more than 5 minutes
  - This is the child's first seizure
  - Child is unresponsive to painful stimuli after seizure

MANAGING TREATMENT

Provide child and family teaching and instruction regarding the administration of anticonvulsant therapy and its importance. Included in this discussion should be common adverse effects, the need to continue the medication unless instructed otherwise by the physician or nurse practitioner, and the need to call the physician or nurse practitioner if the child is ill and vomiting and unable to take his or her medication. Encourage parents to discuss unwanted adverse effects with the physician or nurse practitioner so that they can be addressed and noncompliance with the medication regimen can be reduced. A common cause of breakthrough seizures is medication noncompliance.

PROVIDING FAMILY SUPPORT AND EDUCATION

Having a child with a chronic seizure disorder can place stress and anxiety on the family. This stress and anxiety is often due to fears and misconceptions they may have. An important nursing function is to educate not only the child and family but also the community, including the child's teachers and caregivers, on the reality and facts of the disorder. Encourage parents to be involved in the management of their child's seizures, but encourage allowing the child to learn about the disorder and its management as soon as he or she is old enough. Encourage parents to treat the child with epilepsy just as they would treat a child without this disorder. Children who are brought up no differently than children without epilepsy will be more likely to develop a positive self-image and have increased self-esteem. Any activity restrictions, such as limiting swimming or participation in sports, will be based on the type, frequency, and severity of the seizures the child has. Educate parents and children on any restrictions and encourage parents to place only the necessary restrictions on the child.

The needs of the child and family will change as the child grows and develops. The nurse needs to recognize these changes and provide appropriate education and support. Referral to support groups is appropriate. Links to helpful information about epilepsy including foundation information can be found on thePoint.

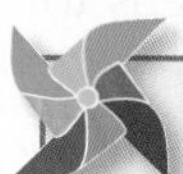

Consider This

I am so worried about having a seizure at school. I think the other kids will tease me and not play with me if they see me having a seizure. I just don't want to go to school.

Thoughts: How would you respond to his concerns? How can you work with the school, family, and child to help ease his concerns?

Febrile Seizures

Febrile seizures are the most common type of seizure seen in children less than 5 years of age, with the peak incidence occurring in children between 12 and 18 months old (American Academy of Pediatrics & Subcommittee on Febrile Seizures, 2011; Millichap & Millichap, 2014). It is rare to see febrile seizures in children younger than 6 months and older than 5 years of age. Febrile seizures are more commonly seen in boys, and there is an increased risk for children who have a family history of febrile seizures (Mikati, 2011). Febrile seizures are associated with a fever that is not the result of an intracranial infection or metabolic imbalance, and are usually related to a viral illness. These seizures are usually benign, but can be very frightening for both the child and family. In most cases the prognosis is excellent. However, febrile seizures may be a sign of a dangerous underlying infection, such as meningitis or sepsis. Though rare, complications associated with febrile seizures include status epilepticus, motor coordination deficits, intellectual disability, and behavioral problems.

Therapeutic Management

Therapeutic management includes determination and treatment of the cause of the fever and interventions to control the fever. The American Academy of Pediatrics does not recommend long-term or intermittent anticonvulsant therapy for the child who has suffered one or more simple febrile seizures (American Academy of Pediatrics, Steering Committee on Quality Improvement and Management, & Subcommittee on Febrile Seizures, 2008; Mikati, 2011). Due to the benign nature of febrile seizures the risks of side effects from the antiepileptic agents outweigh the benefits (Millichap & Millichap, 2014). Rectal diazepam has been shown to be safe and effective in terminating febrile seizures and may be used in children at high risk for febrile seizures or in children whose parents are extremely anxious. Buccal and intranasal midazolam, if available, has also been found to be effective and may be superior (Millichap & Millichap, 2014). Intranasal lorazepam is also an additional option.

Nursing Assessment

A febrile seizure is usually associated with a rapid rise in core temperature to 39°C (102.2°F) or higher. A simple febrile seizure is defined as a generalized seizure lasting less than 15 minutes (usually a few seconds to 10 minutes) that occurs once in a 24-hour period and is accompanied by a fever without any CNS infection present (Mikati, 2011; Millichap & Millichap, 2014). A brief postictal period is often seen when the child appears drowsy. The seizure is likely to have stopped by the time a child receives medical attention. Diagnosis is made based on a thorough history and physical examination, accompanied by a determination of the source of the fever. In some cases an LP and/or neuroimaging may be performed to rule out meningitis or encephalitis. This will be based on the age and the clinical presentation of the child.

Risk factors for recurrence of a febrile seizure include young age at first febrile seizure and family history of febrile seizures and high fever. Children who experience one or more simple febrile seizures have a slightly greater risk of developing epilepsy than the general population (American Academy of Pediatrics, Steering Committee on Quality Improvement and Management, & Subcommittee on Febrile Seizures, 2008; Mikati, 2011; Millichap & Millichap, 2014). No evidence exists that febrile seizures cause structural damage or cognitive declines (American Academy of Pediatrics, Steering Committee on Quality Improvement and Management, & Subcommittee on Febrile Seizures, 2008; Mikati, 2011; Millichap & Millichap, 2014).

Nursing Management

Provide parental support and education regarding febrile seizures. Reassure parents of the benign nature of febrile seizures. Counsel parents on controlling fever, discuss how to keep a child safe during a seizure, and provide instruction and demonstration in the administration of rectal diazepam at the onset of a seizure (if applicable). Instruct parents when to call their physician or nurse practitioner and when to take their child to the emergency room. Reinforce that any recurrent seizure activity will require prompt medical attention.

Neonatal Seizures

There is a high incidence of seizures during the neonatal period. The immature brain is more prone to seizure activity and metabolic, infectious, structural, and toxic diseases are more likely to be seen in this age group (Mikati, 2011). Neonatal seizures are seizures that occur within the first 4 weeks of life and are most commonly seen within the first 10 days. The majority of seizures in newborns are associated with a specific underlying cause such as hypoxic ischemic encephalopathy (most common), metabolic disorders (hypoglycemia and hypocalcemia), neonatal infection (meningitis and encephalitis), cerebral infarction, and intracranial hemorrhage. The prognosis depends mainly on the underlying cause of the seizures and the severity of the insult. There is evidence that neonatal seizures have an adverse effect on neurodevelopment and may predispose the infant to cognitive, behavioral, or epileptic complications later in life (Shellhaas, 2015b). About 20% to 30% of neonates with seizures will go on to develop postnatal epilepsy (Shellhaas, 2015b). Neonatal epileptic syndromes are rare, but are a well recognized cause of neonatal seizures and include benign myoclonic, neonatal convulsions, benign neonatal familial convulsions, early myoclonic encephalopathy, and early infantile epileptic encephalopathy (Shellhaas, 2015b). Our discussion below will focus on the more common symptomatic neonatal seizure related to a specific underlying cause.

Therapeutic Management

Acute neonatal seizures should be treated aggressively because repeated seizure activity may result in injury to the brain. Treatment focuses on addressing the underlying cause, such as correcting metabolic disturbances, treating central nervous system infections, ensuring adequate ventilation and cardiovascular support, and possibly administering anticonvulsant therapy. Phenobarbital is often used in the initial management of neonatal seizures, but efficacy remains uncertain. Anti-epileptic medications may not be effective if the underlying cause is not treated (Shellhaas, 2015c). The dosage of anticonvulsants may be higher in the neonate because neonates metabolize drugs more rapidly than older infants.

Nursing Assessment

Neonatal seizures may be hard to recognize clinically and may be accompanied by a normal EEG, and in some cases, there may be no clinical signs, but only EEG changes (Mikati, 2011). Neonatal seizures have to be distinguished from nonseizure behaviors seen in newborns, such as stretching, sudden random movements, and random sucking movements, coughing, or gagging (Shellhaas, 2015b). Therefore, clinical recognition of newborn seizures is critical. Assessment of neonatal seizures will include a detailed clinical characterization of the seizure activity, including appearance of the neonate; location and involvement of arms, legs, trunk, and face; sequence of clinical changes, and duration and frequency of seizure activity. If seizure activity is not witnessed by a health care provider a detailed history is essential. Once identified, the seizure activity can be classified. The ILAE now proposes that neonatal seizures be classified not as a separate entity, but within the proposed categories (Table 38.2) (Berg et al., 2010). Then, assessment of the cause of the seizure will become a priority.

Laboratory and diagnostic tests including serum testing (e.g., serum glucose, electrolytes, calcium), LP (to analyze CSF), cranial ultrasound, CT, and MRI may be performed to help determine the cause of the seizures. EEGs and video EEGs may assist in the characterization of neonatal seizures and their medical management.

Nursing Management

Nursing management will focus on carrying out interventions to cease seizure activity, monitoring neurologic status closely, recognizing the seizures, preventing injury during seizure activity, and providing support and education to the parents and family.

STRUCTURAL DEFECTS

Due to the sensitivity of the development of the neurologic system in the first weeks of embryonic life, there exists a potential for defects to occur. These structural defects include neural tube defects (NTDs), microcephaly, Chiari malformation, hydrocephalus, intracranial arteriovenous malformation (AVM), and craniosynostosis.

Neural Tube Defects

NTDs account for the majority of congenital anomalies of the CNS (Kinsman & Johnston, 2011). They are the second most common birth defect (the first being cardiac malformations) contributing to infant mortality and disability (Hochberg & Stone, 2015). The incidence in the United States has declined over the past decade, with spina bifida and anencephaly (which account for the majority of NTDs) affecting 0.3 per 1,000 births (Hochberg & Stone, 2015). NTDs are serious birth defects of the spine and the brain and include disorders such as spina bifida occulta, myelomeningocele, meningocele, anencephaly, and encephalocele. The neural tube closes between the third and fourth week in utero. The cause of neural tube defects is not known, but many factors such as drugs, malnutrition, chemicals, and genetics can adversely affect normal CNS development. Strong evidence exists that maternal preconception supplementation of folic acid can decrease the incidence of neural tube defects in pregnancies at risk by 50% (American Academy of Pediatrics & Committee on Genetics, 2012). In 1992, the U.S. Public Health Service recommended that all women of childbearing age who are capable of becoming pregnant take 0.4 mg (400 μg) of folic acid daily (Centers for Disease Control and Prevention, 2015a). Pregnant women with a history of pregnancies affected by NTDs are recommended to take a higher dosage. Prenatal screening of maternal serum for α-fetoprotein (AFP) and ultrasound examination can help identify fetuses at risk. Anencephaly and encephalocele are discussed below. Refer to Chapter 44 for information on spina bifida occulta, meningocele, and myelomeningocele.

Anencephaly

Anencephaly is a defect in brain development resulting in small or missing brain hemispheres, skull, and scalp. It occurs when the cephalic or upper end of the neural tube fails to close during the third to fourth week of gestation. These infants are born without both a forebrain and a cerebrum and the remaining brain tissue may be exposed. The condition is incompatible with life.

NURSING ASSESSMENT

Anencephalic infants have a distinctive appearance, with a large defect noted in the vault of the skull (Fig. 38.7). The mother may have had a difficult labor due to the malformation of the head not allowing it to engage in the cervix. The majority of infants will be stillborn. If not, most anencephalic infants die within hours to several days of birth (Tomita & Ogiwara, 2015). There have been a few cases in which the infant has lived for several months. The infant is usually blind, deaf, unconscious, and unable to feel pain. Some infants born with anencephaly may be born with a brain stem, but due to the lack of a cerebrum there is no possibility of gaining consciousness. Reflex actions such as respirations, reactions to sound and touch, and ability to suck may be present.

NURSING MANAGEMENT

The prognosis is extremely poor. Nursing management is supportive in nature and focuses on comfort measures for the dying infant. Some parents may have been aware of the diagnosis prenatally due to screening tests such as AFP and ultrasounds. Parents and family will need support and understanding from all health care professionals during this difficult time. Fear of what the child will look like may be overwhelming. Use of an infant cap can be helpful and allow parents to feel more comfortable holding

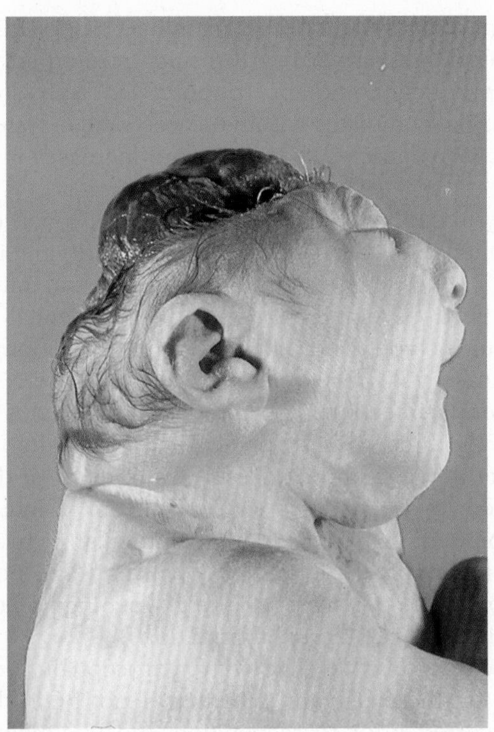

FIGURE 38.7 Anencephalic infant.

and comforting their infant. Assisting with anticipatory grieving and decision making related to end-of-life care will also be key nursing interventions.

Encephalocele

Encephalocele is a protrusion of the brain and meninges through a skull defect. It results from failure of the anterior portion of the neural tube to close. The prognosis, including the extent of complications and cognitive deficits, will depend on the size and location of the encephalocele and involvement of other brain structures. Encephaloceles are often accompanied by craniofacial and other abnormalities such as hydrocephalus, microcephaly, spastic quadriplegia, ataxia, visual problems, developmental delay, mental and growth retardation, and seizures. Some children who are affected may display normal intelligence.

Therapeutic management consists of surgical repair, including placement of tissues back into the skull and removal of the sac; possible shunt placement to correct associated hydrocephalus; and corrective repair of any craniofacial abnormalities.

NURSING ASSESSMENT

Initial assessment after delivery will reveal a visible external sac protruding from the skull area. It occurs most commonly in the occipital region, but can occur elsewhere, such as frontally or nasofrontally. Generally, the lesion is covered by skin, but it may also be open. Therefore, assessment to ensure that the sac covering is intact remains important. Assess neurologic status carefully. Before surgical correction, the infant will be examined thoroughly to determine brain tissue involvement or associated anomalies. Diagnostic procedures such as CT, MRI, and ultrasound may be performed.

NURSING MANAGEMENT

Nursing management will consist of preoperative and postoperative care, along with symptomatic and supportive care. Preoperative and postoperative care will be similar to that for the child with myelomeningocele (refer to Chapter 44), with a focus on preventing rupture of the sac, preventing infection, and providing adequate nutrition and hydration. Infants with an encephalocele are at an increased risk for developing hydrocephalus. Therefore, monitor for signs and symptoms of increased ICP and head circumference.

Microcephaly

Microcephaly is defined as a head circumference that is more than three standard deviations below the mean for the age and sex of the infant (Kinsman & Johnston, 2011). It may be congenital or it may be acquired and develop in the first few years of life. It generally results in intellectual disability due to the lack of functioning brain tissue. There are many causes. Microcephaly can be caused by abnormal development during gestation or follow intrauterine infections such as rubella, toxoplasmosis, and cytomegalovirus. It can also be caused by chromosomal abnormalities or be associated with other syndromes. Acquired microcephaly may occur due to severe malnutrition, perinatal infections, or anoxia in early infancy.

Nursing Assessment

Microcephalic infants will present at birth with a normal or reduced head size. As the child ages, head growth will fail while the face will continue to grow at a normal rate. This results in a small head, a large face, and a loose, often wrinkled, scalp. As the child grows older, this smallness of the skull becomes more pronounced. Development of motor functions and speech may be delayed. The degree of intellectual disability varies, but it is a common occurrence. Convulsions may be present, and motor deficit ranges from clumsiness to spastic quadriplegia.

Nursing Management

There is no treatment. Nursing care will be supportive and focus on determining the extent of neurologic and cognitive deficits, as well as teaching parents how to care for a child with such impairments.

Chiari Malformation

Chiari malformations are classified into different groups and subgroups based on anatomic anomalies of the craniocervical junction along with downward displacement of the cerebellar structures (Khoury, 2015). The most common are type I and type II and are the types discussed here. Type I is usually not associated with hydrocephalus and is the more benign form. The deformity is a result of the cerebellar tonsils displacing into the upper cervical canal (Kinsman & Johnston, 2011). Type II (also referred to as Arnold–Chiari) is the most common and is usually associated with hydrocephalus and myelomeningocele. The deformity results from the cerebellum, the medulla oblongata, and the fourth ventricle displacing into the cervical canal, resulting in an obstruction of the CSF and causing hydrocephalus. The prognosis depends on the extent of the defect. Therapeutic management of the type II Chiari malformation includes surgical decompression.

Nursing Assessment

In type I, symptoms are typically seen in adolescence and adulthood. The client will usually complain of neck pain; recurrent headaches that increase with physical activity or with Valsalva maneuvers such as coughing, laughing, or sneezing; lower extremity spasticity; and urinary frequency (Khoury, 2015). Type II is almost always associated with myelomeningocele; therefore, it is typically detected prenatally or at birth. Symptoms seen in infancy include a weak cry, stridor, and apnea (Kinsman & Johnston, 2011). These symptoms require prompt medical treatment to reduce mortality. Gastrointestinal disturbances along with a history of chronic aspiration, choking, gagging, prolonged feeding times, and weight loss may also be present. In later infancy and childhood, progressive hydrocephalus is a common problem (Khoury, 2015). Assessment of shunt function is extremely important in the infant and older child presenting with type II Chiari malformation and associated hydrocephalus (refer to Hydrocephalus section). An MRI may be performed to help evaluate and diagnose Chiari malformations.

Nursing Management

Nursing management will focus on preoperative and postoperative care, prevention of infection, monitoring of blood loss, improvement of preoperative symptoms in the postoperative period, identification of any signs and symptoms of increased ICP, and identification of any resultant CNS injury.

Hydrocephalus

Hydrocephalus is not a specific illness, but results from underlying brain disorders. It is a frequently seen disorder of the nervous system occurring in 0.5 to 4 per 1,000 live births (Zak & Chan, 2014). It results from an imbalance in the production and absorption of CSF. In hydrocephalus, CSF accumulates within the ventricular system and causes the ventricles to enlarge and increases in ICP to occur.

Hydrocephalus may be congenital or acquired. Congenital hydrocephalus is present at birth and is often due to a genetic disposition or environmental influences during fetal development. Causes of congenital hydrocephalus include abnormal intrauterine development, as is the case with myelomeningocele or other NTDs or intrauterine infections. Acquired hydrocephalus develops at the time of birth or at some point after. It can occur at any age and can result from injury or disease. Acquired hydrocephalus can result from intentional or nonintentional trauma, intraventricular hemorrhage (IVH) in premature infants, neoplasms (e.g., posterior fossa brain tumor), infections (e.g., meningitis), or malformations (e.g., Chiari malformations).

Prognosis for the child with hydrocephalus depends mainly on the cause and whether or not brain damage has occurred prior to recognition and treatment. Children with hydrocephalus are at increased risk for developmental disabilities, visual problems, abnormalities in memory, and reduced intelligence. Long-term follow-up and multidisciplinary care are necessary.

Pathophysiology

CSF is formed primarily in the ventricular system by the choroid plexus. It flows as a result of the pressure gradient that exists between the ventricular system and the venous channels. CSF is absorbed primarily by the arachnoid villi. Hydrocephalus results when there is an obstruction in the ventricular system or obliteration or malfunction of the arachnoid villi. This results in impaired absorption or circulation of the CSF.

Hydrocephalus is classified as obstructive or noncommunicating versus nonobstructive or communicating. Obstructive or noncommunicating hydrocephalus occurs when the flow of CSF is blocked within the ventricular system. This type is more common than communicating hydrocephalus (Zak & Chan, 2014). NTDs, neonatal meningitis, trauma, tumors, or Chiari malformations usually result in this type of hydrocephalus. One of the most common causes of obstructive or noncommunicating hydrocephalus in children is aqueductal stenosis, which results from the narrowing of the aqueduct of Sylvius (a passageway between the third and fourth ventricles in the middle brain) (Kinsman & Johnston, 2011). Nonobstructive or communicating hydrocephalus occurs when the flow of CSF is blocked after it exits from the ventricles. This form of hydrocephalus, in which the CSF can still flow between the ventricles, is most often caused by defective absorption of CSF. Examples include hydrocephalus that results from subarachnoid hemorrhage (most common), certain types of meningitis, and leukemia infiltrates (Kinsman & Johnston, 2011).

Therapeutic Management

Hydrocephalus must be identified early. Treatment needs to be initiated in order to prevent brain tissue damage that can result from the increased ICP that hydrocephalus creates. Specific treatment will depend on the underlying etiology. The goals of treatment include relieving hydrocephalus and managing complications associated with the disorder, such as growth and developmental delay. Most cases of hydrocephalus are treated with the surgical placement of an extracranial shunt. Most often, a ventriculoperitoneal (VP) shunt is placed. See Figure 38.8 for an illustration of a shunt. The shunt will need to be replaced as the child grows. Therefore, the child will undergo shunt revision surgery at various times during his or her life. It is important for health care professionals and parents to be able to recognize when a shunt needs replacing or when complications are occurring, to decrease the possibility of death or disability that may occur due to increased ICP.

Though shunts have been the mainstay of treatment for hydrocephalus, they are not without complications

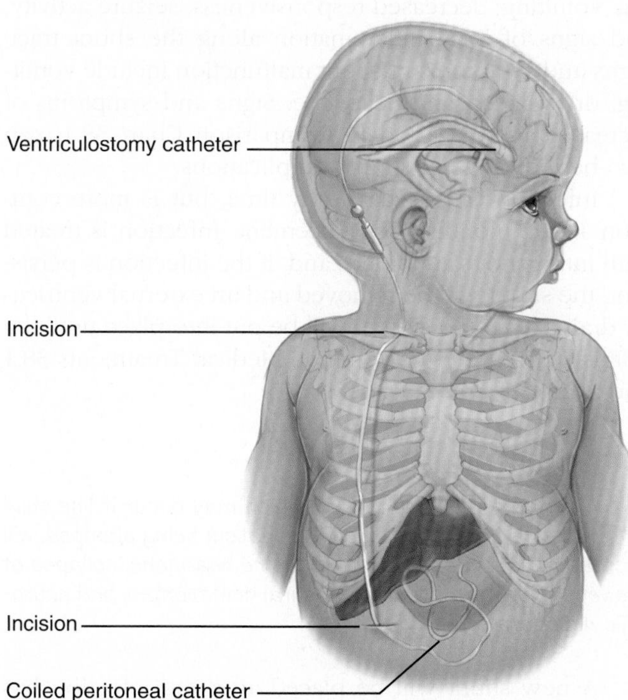

FIGURE 38.8 To treat hydrocephalus, a ventriculoperitoneal (VP) shunt catheter is placed in an enlarged ventricle. The shunt diverts the flow of cerebrospinal fluid (CSF) within the central nervous system to the peritoneum, where CSF is now absorbed across the peritoneal membrane into the body's circulation.

such as infection, obstruction, and need for revision as the child grows. Endoscopic third ventriculostomy is an alternative to shunt placement to treat obstructive hydrocephalus in select children. A small perforation is made in the thinned floor of the third ventricle, which allows for egress of CSF from the ventricle to the subarachnoid space. No permanently implanted hardware is needed.

Nursing Assessment

For a full description of the assessment phase of the nursing process, refer to the assessment section of the Nursing Process Overview earlier in the chapter. Assessment findings pertinent to hydrocephalus are discussed below.

HEALTH HISTORY

Explore the pregnancy history and past medical history for:

- Intrauterine infections
- Prematurity with intracranial hemorrhage
- Meningitis
- Mumps encephalitis

Elicit a description of the present illness and chief complaint. Common signs and symptoms reported during the health history of the undiagnosed child might include:

- Irritability
- Lethargy
- Poor feeding
- Vomiting
- Complaints of headache in older children
- Altered, diminished, or changes in LOC

Children known to have hydrocephalus are often admitted to the hospital for shunt malfunctions or other complications of the disease. The health history should include questions related to:

- Neurologic status—have there been changes or decreases in LOC, changes in personality, or deterioration in school performance?
- Complaints of headache
- Vomiting
- Visual disturbances
- Any other changes in physical or cognitive state

PHYSICAL EXAMINATION

Physical examination of the infant or child with hydrocephalus will include inspection and observation, palpation, and percussion.

Inspection and Observation. Observe general appearance and affect. Pay particular attention to the size of the skull and note any asymmetry. Note LOC and motor

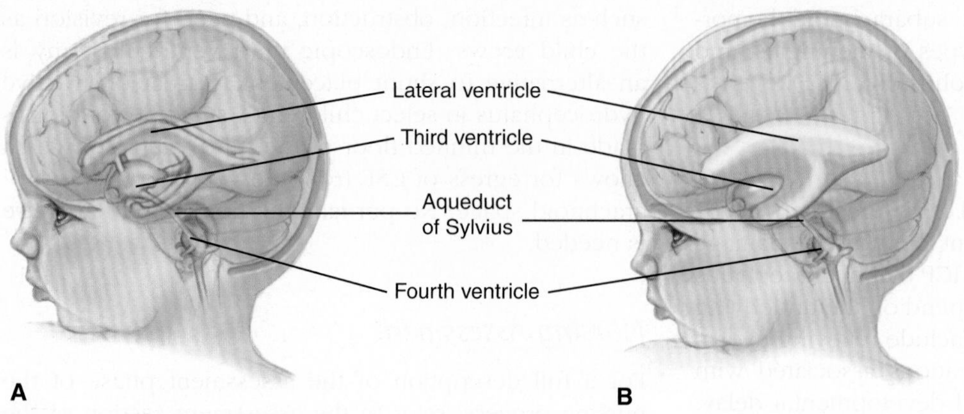

FIGURE 38.9 **(A)** Infant without hydrocephalus. **(B)** Infant with hydrocephalus. Note broadening of the forehead, bulging fontanel, and large head size.

function. Changes or decreases in LOC may be noted along with brisk reflexes and spasticity of the lower extremities. Symptoms seen vary by age, primarily due to the fact that the infant's skull is able to accommodate the buildup of CSF because the sutures have not closed. In the infant, the most obvious indication is often a rapid increase in head circumference (Fig. 38.9). In the older child, loss of development and changes in personality may be seen. Signs and symptoms associated with increased ICP may be seen (refer to Comparison Chart 38.1).

Palpation. In the infant, palpation of the fontanels may reveal wide-open, bulging fontanels. They will be nonpulsatile and feel tense and very full.

Percussion. Upon percussion of the skull, by physicians or nurse practitioners, a positive Macewen sign may be noted. This is when a "cracked pot" sound is heard during percussion and can indicate separation of the sutures.

LABORATORY AND DIAGNOSTIC TESTS

Common laboratory and diagnostic tests ordered for the diagnosis and assessment of hydrocephalus include:

- Skull x-ray studies (may reveal separation of sutures)
- CT
- MRI

CT and MRI are used to evaluate for the presence of hydrocephalus and can also aid in identifying the cause of hydrocephalus. Refer to Common Laboratory and Diagnostic Tests 38.1.

Nursing Management

Nursing management of the child with hydrocephalus will focus on maintaining cerebral perfusion, minimizing neurologic complications, maintaining adequate nutrition, promoting growth and development, and supporting and educating the child and family. In addition to the nursing diagnoses and related interventions discussed in Nursing Care Plan 38.1 at the end of the chapter, interventions common to hydrocephalus are discussed below.

PREVENTING AND RECOGNIZING SHUNT INFECTION AND MALFUNCTION

The major complications associated with shunts are infection and malfunction. Due to the serious nature and potentially devastating effects of shunt infection or malfunction, parents and health professionals need to be aware of the signs and symptoms to provide early recognition and prompt treatment. Signs and symptoms of a shunt infection include elevated vital signs, poor feeding, vomiting, decreased responsiveness, seizure activity, and signs of local inflammation along the shunt tract. Signs and symptoms of shunt malfunction include vomiting, drowsiness, and headache. Signs and symptoms of increased ICP, as listed in Comparison Chart 38.1, can also be indicative of shunt complications.

Infection can occur at any time, but is more common 1 to 2 months after placement. Infection is treated with intravenous antibiotics and, if the infection is persistent, the shunt will be removed and an external ventricular drainage (EVD) system will be put into place until the CSF is sterile (refer to Common Medical Treatments 38.1 and Box 38.3).

Take Note!

Rapid drainage of CSF, which may occur if the child sits up without the EVD system being clamped, will decrease ICP and can lead to extreme headache, collapse of the ventricles, formation of subdural hematomas, and neurologic deterioration.

A new shunt will be placed after the infection has cleared. Intrathecal administration of antibiotics may be performed by the physician or nurse practitioner. Keeping the peritoneal surgical incision free of feces and urine can help prevent infection. In addition, inspect surgical incisions after shunt placement for signs and symptoms of infection and any signs of leaking CSF.

BOX 38.3

NURSING MANAGEMENT OF EXTERNAL VENTRICULAR DRAINAGE (EVD) DEVICE

- Ensure all connections are secure and label line as EVD.
- Regularly check that drip chamber of manometer is set at the height prescribed in relation to the child (i.e., zero at clavicle).
- Clamp the drain in the event of child movement or movement anticipated with care. Rezero and open clamps when done.
- Accurately document volume and color of cerebrospinal fluid (CSF) every hour (CSF is normally clear and colorless; cloudiness indicates infection). Notify physician, nurse practitioner, or charge nurse of any significant increase in amount of drainage (if exceeds 10 mL more than previous volumes).
- If minimal or no drainage, check tubing for kinks, blockage, or closed clamps. Check to see if CSF is oscillating in tubing. If blockage is suspected, notify neurosurgery department immediately.
- Dress the entry site into the skull with a sterile occlusive dressing; change the dressing if it is soiled or nonocclusive.
- Routine CSF samples may be sent for culture and analysis.
- Child may be taking prophylactic antibiotics due to increased risk of infection from the drain.

Malfunction of the shunt can occur due to kinking, clogging, or separation of the tubing. Blockage is the most common reported complication. A shunt that has been placed within the past year is at higher risk of malfunction. Early recognition and operative intervention are essential to prevent neurologic deficits or possible death from occurring.

SUPPORTING AND EDUCATING THE CHILD AND FAMILY

Hydrocephalus is a serious and chronic illness. It will require lifelong follow-up and regular evaluations. It requires early recognition of complications to prevent neurologic damage. Children will require future surgeries and hospitalizations, which can place a strain on the family and its finances. Potential growth and developmental disabilities are an additional strain. The support of the family in establishing realistic goals and helping the child to achieve his or her developmental and educational potential is important.

The family should be involved in the child's care from the time of diagnosis. Initially, parents may be frightened because shunt placement involves entering the brain. Provide parents with accurate information regarding the procedure, and be available to listen to parents' concerns and to answer questions that arise. Ongoing education about the illness and its treatment are important, including signs and symptoms of shunt complications. As the family becomes more comfortable with the diagnosis, treatment, and signs and symptoms of complications, they will become experts on the child's care and will often recognize subtle changes in him or her that may be indicative of shunt complications. Referral to support groups can be helpful for both the family and the child. Links for helpful information about hydrocephalus are provided on thePoint.

Intracranial Arteriovenous Malformation

Intracranial arteriovenous malformation (AVM) is a rare congenital disorder. It is caused by an abnormal development of blood vessels and can occur in the brain, brain stem, or spinal cord. AVMs that hemorrhage can lead to serious neurologic deficits and even death. However, some cases of AVMs never cause problems.

Therapeutic Management

More aggressive treatment strategies are used in children. Treatment options used include surgical excision; endovascular embolization, which involves closing off the vessels of the AVM by injecting glue into them; and radiosurgery, which involves focusing radiation on the AVM. The therapeutic management approach will be based on the age of the child and size and location of the malformation in the brain. The child will usually require at least 24 hours of intensive care monitoring following surgery.

Nursing Assessment

The most common symptoms seen include intracranial hemorrhage (children are more likely to present with hemorrhage than adults), seizures, headaches, and progressive neurologic deficits such as vision problems, loss of speech, problems with memory, and paralysis. In children younger than 2 years of age, presentation may include cardiac failure due to arteriovenous shunting in neonates and infants; a large head secondary to hydrocephalus; and seizure activity. Diagnosis is made using diagnostic imaging procedures such as MRI, CT, and arteriography.

Nursing Management

Nursing management for these children is aimed at supportive care. Monitor for changes in neurologic status, noting any seizure activity, signs or symptoms of increased ICP, or signs and symptoms of intracranial hemorrhage. Hydrocephalus may occur as a result of intracranial hemorrhage secondary to the AVM. An EVD and eventual shunt placement may be necessary (refer to Hydrocephalus section).

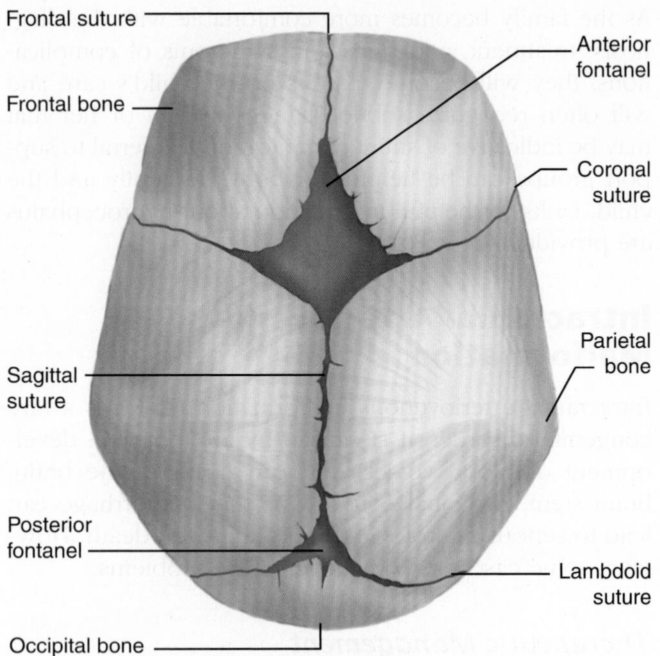

FIGURE 38.10 Skull sutures in the infant.

Craniosynostosis

Craniosynostosis is premature closure of the cranial sutures (Fig. 38.10). Complete closure of all sutures does not normally occur until late in childhood. Premature closure can inhibit brain growth and a distorted skull appearance will be evident. In cases where only one suture is fused, neurologic impairments are rarely seen. When two or more sutures are fused, neurologic complications such as hydrocephalus with increased ICP are more likely to occur. The incidence of craniosynostosis is approximately 1 in 2,000 births (Kinsman & Johnston, 2011). The cause is unknown, but in 10% to 20% of cases a genetic disorder such as Carpenter syndrome or Apert, Crouzon, or Pfeiffer disease is present (Kinsman & Johnston, 2011). There are numerous different types of craniosynostosis; they are listed and illustrated in Table 38.4. The prognosis is good for the majority of infants presenting with craniosynostosis, and normal brain development will occur. Exceptions to this are the infant or child who has associated genetic disorders that involve brain function and development.

Surgical correction may be done and allows for normal expansion of the brain and acceptable appearance of the head and skull. If one suture is fused, the surgical intervention is done mainly for cosmetic reasons. If more than one suture is fused, operative intervention is essential to prevent neurologic complications.

Nursing Assessment

Most cases of craniosynostosis are present at birth. Skull deformity is evident as well as a prominent bony ridge that can be palpated. X-ray studies can confirm fusion of the sutures. It is important that craniosynostosis be detected early if it is not evident at birth because premature closure of the suture lines will inhibit brain development. Therefore, measure head circumference in all children younger than 3 years old and compare findings with normal head circumference parameters as well as past measurements of the infant or child.

Nursing Management

Nursing management focuses on postoperative care. This includes observing hemoglobin and hematocrit levels due to large volumes of blood loss that can occur, and observing for pain, hemorrhage, fever, infection, and swelling. Due to the location of the surgery and incision line, large amounts of facial swelling may be present. This can result in an inability of the child to open his or her eyes for a few days postoperatively. Make sure that parents are aware of this. Encourage the parents to talk to, hold, and comfort their child during this time. Provide support and education to the parents before, during, and after the procedure.

Positional Plagiocephaly

Since the inception of the "back to sleep" program, which recommends placing all infants supine to sleep to decrease the risk of sudden infant death syndrome (SIDS), there has been a dramatic increase in the incidence of positional plagiocephaly (Block, 2012). Positional plagiocephaly refers to asymmetry in head shape without fused sutures. It results from gravitational force exertion on the developing cranium. Torticollis, which is when the neck muscles are too tight, have inadequate tone, or are shorter on one side, can contribute to plagiocephaly. Each condition, plagiocephaly and torticollis, exacerbates the other. Refer to Chapter 44 for further information on torticollis.

Therapeutic management for positional plagiocephaly is generally conservative, such as changing the infant's position, encouraging "tummy time," and avoiding excessive use of the car seat for infant seating outside of the automobile. Some infants may benefit from the use of a molding helmet (Fig. 38.11).

Nursing Assessment

View the infant's head from the top, noting asymmetry ranging from flattening on one side posteriorly to posterior flattening associated with anterior bulging (Fig. 38.12). Assess neck range of motion to determine if torticollis is also present. Palpate the cranial sutures, which will not feel overlapped as they do when they are fused. Skull x-ray examination or head CT scan will rule out craniosynostosis by demonstrating evidence of open sutures.

TABLE 38.4 TYPES OF CRANIOSYNOSTOSIS

Types	Description	Illustration
Sagittal synostosis (scaphocephaly)	Sagittal suture is closed. Head grows long and narrow in anterior–posterior direction. Broad forehead and a prominent occiput are present. Most common form	
Metopic synostosis (trigonocephaly)	Metopic suture is closed. Usually a ridge down the forehead can be seen or felt. Triangular-shaped forehead Eyebrows may appear "pinched" on either side. Eyes may also appear close together.	
Unilateral coronal synostosis (anterior plagiocephaly)	Early closure of one side of the coronal suture Forehead and orbital rim (eyebrow) have a flattened appearance on that side. Eye on affected side has a different shape	
Bicoronal synostosis (brachycephaly)	Very flat, tall, recessed forehead Skull is shortened in the anterior–posterior direction. Wide-shaped head Commonly seen in Apert and Crouzon disease	
Lambdoid (posterior plagiocephaly)	Early closure of one lambdoid suture Flattening of back of head. Similar to shape found in positional molding or positional plagiocephaly	

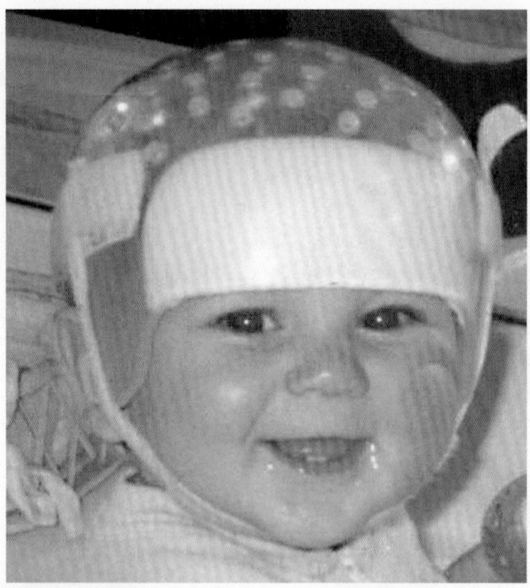

FIGURE 38.11 Molding helmet for positional plagiocephaly.

Nursing Management

Nursing management is directed toward repositioning the infant to decrease time spent with the flattened area in the dependent position. Position the infant so that turning away from the affected side is necessary for him or her to view objects of interest. Place the infant on the abdomen when awake and supervised. Discourage use of the car seat outside of the automobile. Place a rolled washcloth along the affected side of the head to discourage turning the head in that direction. Following these recommendations may prevent positional plagiocephaly in the infant without congenital torticollis.

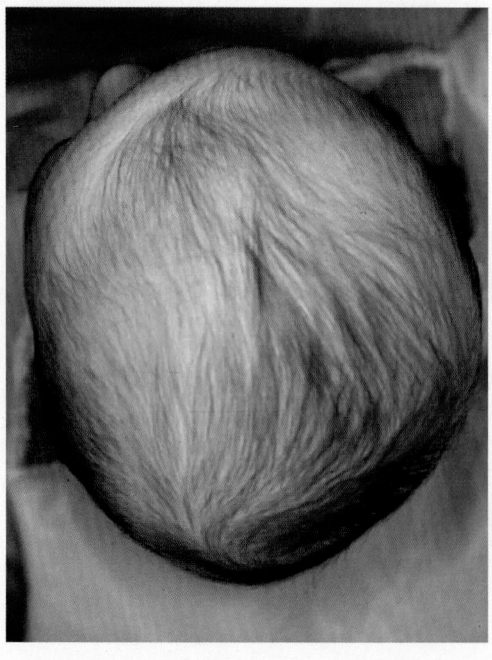

FIGURE 38.12 Note flattening of the right posterior parietal and occipital regions of the skull in this infant with positional plagiocephaly.

INFECTIOUS DISORDERS

Infectious disorders of the neurologic system include bacterial meningitis, aseptic meningitis, encephalitis, and Reye syndrome.

Bacterial Meningitis

Bacterial meningitis is an infection of the meninges, the lining that surrounds the brain and spinal cord. It is a serious illness in children and can lead to brain damage, nerve damage, deafness, stroke, and even death. It requires rapid assessment and treatment. See Table 38.5 for the most common types of meningitis seen in different age groups. In developed countries, disease resulting from *Haemophilus influenzae* type B, once the most common cause of meningitis in children, has decreased dramatically since the introduction of the Hib vaccine. In less developed countries, infection with *H. influenzae* type B still remains a concern.

Pathophysiology

Bacterial meningitis causes inflammation, swelling, purulent exudates, and tissue damage to the brain. It can occur as a secondary infection to upper respiratory infections, sinus infections, or ear infections, and can also be the result of direct introduction through LP; skull fracture or severe head injury; neurosurgical intervention; congenital structural abnormalities, such as spina bifida; or the presence of foreign bodies, such as a ventricular shunt or cochlear implants.

Therapeutic Management

Bacterial meningitis is a medical emergency and requires prompt hospitalization and treatment. Deterioration may be rapid and occur in less than 24 hours, leading to long-term neurologic damage and even death. Intravenous antibiotics will be started immediately after the LP and blood cultures have been obtained if bacterial meningitis is suspected. The length of therapy and specific antibiotic will be determined based on the analysis and the culture and sensitivity of the CSF. Corticosteroids may be ordered to help reduce the inflammatory process. Specific medical treatment varies based on the suspected causative organism and will be determined by the physician or nurse practitioner.

Nursing Assessment

For a full description of the assessment phase of the nursing process, refer to the Assessment section of the

TABLE 38.5 COMMON CAUSES OF MENINGITIS IN DIFFERENT AGE GROUPS

Age Affected	Causative Organism
Newborns and infants (birth to 3 months)	*Escherichia coli; Streptococcus group B; Listeria monocytogenes; pseudomonas aeruginosa; staphylococcus species*
Infants and children (3 months to 6 years)	*Streptococcus pneumonia; Neisseria meningitides (meningococcal meningitis); Haemophilus influenzae type B*
Older children and adolescents (6 years to 16 years)	*Streptococcus pneumonia; Neisseria meningitides (meningococcal meningitis); Mycobacterium tuberculosis*

Adapted from Zak, M., & Chan, V. W. (2014). Chapter 46: Pediatric neurologic disorders. In: S. M. Nettina (Ed.), *Lippincott manual of nursing practice* (10th ed., pp. 1545–1575). Philadelphia, PA: Wolters/Kluwer Health: Lippincott Williams & Wilkins; Centers for Disease Control and Prevention. (2014a). *Meningitis: Bacterial meningiti*. Retrieved from http://www.cdc.gov/meningitis/bacterial.html

Nursing Process Overview earlier in the chapter. Assessment findings pertinent to bacterial meningitis are discussed below.

HEALTH HISTORY

Elicit a description of the present illness and chief complaint. Common signs and symptoms reported during the health history might include:

- Sudden onset of symptoms
- Preceding respiratory illness or sore throat
- Presence of fever, chills
- Headache
- Vomiting
- Photophobia
- Stiff neck
- Rash
- Irritability
- Drowsiness
- Lethargy
- Muscle rigidity
- Seizures

Symptoms in infants can be more subtle and atypical, but the history may reveal:

- Poor sucking and feeding
- Weak cry
- Lethargy
- Vomiting

Explore the child's current and past medical history for risk factors such as:

- Young age: 1 month to 5 years, with most cases in children younger than 1 year of age and young adults 15 to 24 years of age
- Any fever or illness during pregnancy or around delivery (for infants younger than 3 months of age)
- Exposure to ill persons
- Exposure to tuberculosis
- Travel history
- History of maternal illness
- Recent neurosurgical procedure or head trauma
- Presence of a foreign body, such as a shunt or a cochlear implant
- Immunocompromised status
- Close-contact living spaces such as dormitories or military bases
- Day care attendance

PHYSICAL EXAMINATION

Observe the general appearance of the child. The infant with bacterial meningitis may rest in the opisthotonic position (Fig. 38.13), and the older child may complain of neck pain. In the infant a bulging fontanel may be present, which is often a late sign, and the infant may be consolable when lying still as opposed to being held. Presence of positive Kernig and Brudzinski signs can indicate irritation of the meninges (Fig. 38.14). Inspect the child for presence of a rash; a petechial, vesicular, or macular rash may be seen.

Take Note!

Abrupt eruption of a petechial or purplish rash can be indicative of meningococcemia (infection with N. meningitidis). Immediate medical attention is warranted.

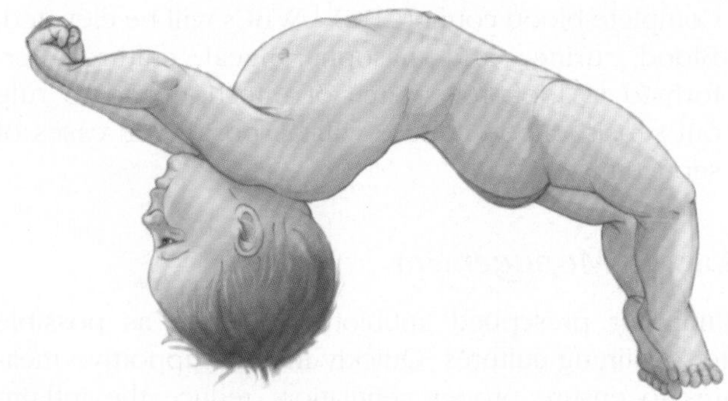

FIGURE 38.13 Infant in **opisthotonic** position: head and neck are hyperextended to relieve discomfort.

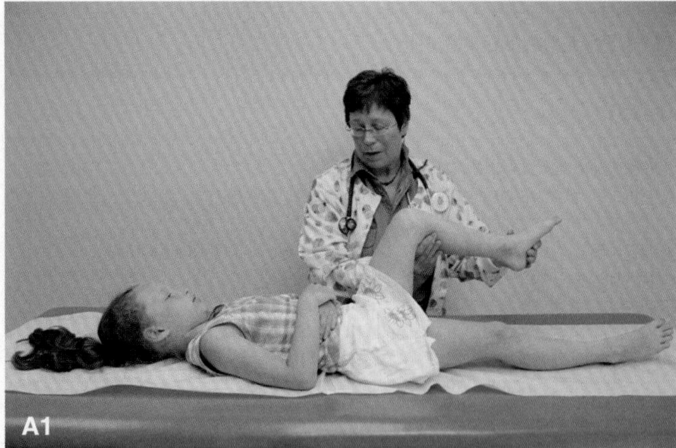

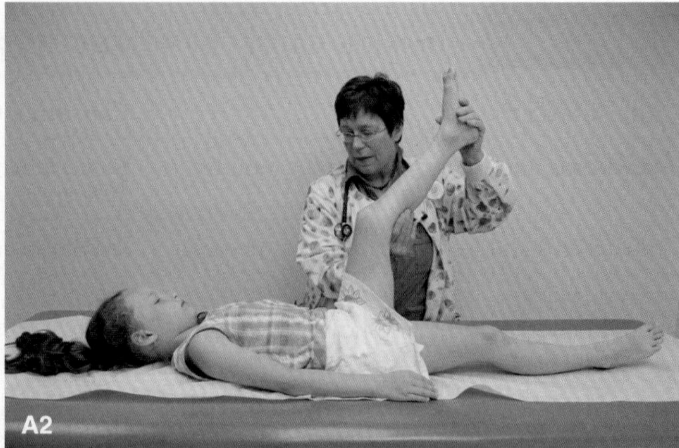

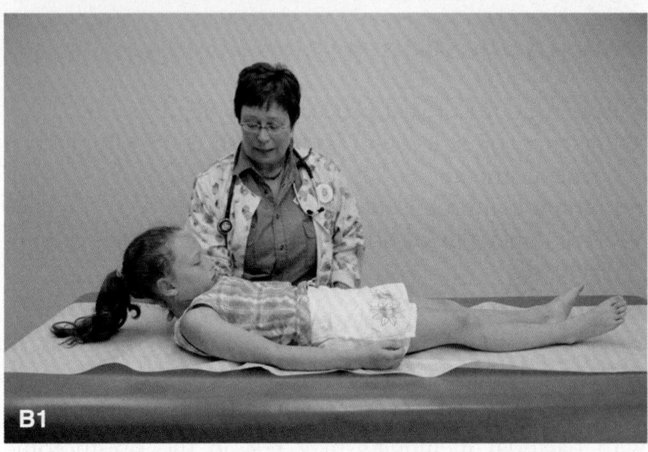

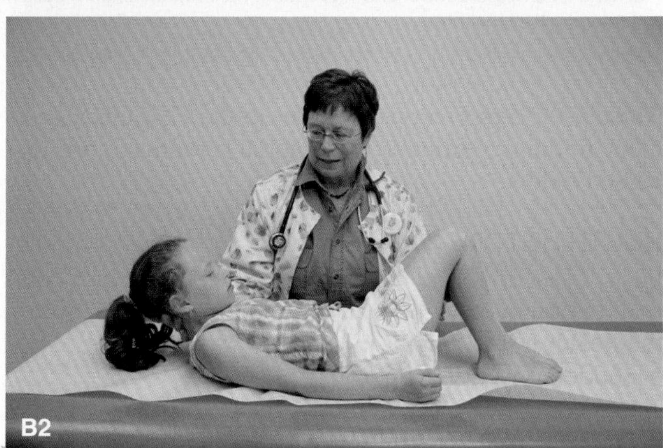

FIGURE 38.14 **(A)** Kernig sign is tested by flexing legs at the hip and knee **(A1)**, then extending the knee **(A2)**. A positive report of pain along the **vertebral** column and/or inability to extend knee is a positive sign and indicates irritation of meninges. **(B)** Brudzinski sign is tested by the child lying supine with the neck flexed **(B1)**. A positive sign occurs if resistance or pain is met. The child may also passively flex hip and knees in reaction, indicating meningeal irritation **(B2)**.

LABORATORY AND DIAGNOSTIC TESTS

Common laboratory and diagnostic studies ordered for the assessment of bacterial meningitis include:

- LP—Fluid pressure will be measured and a sample is obtained for analysis and culture. CSF will be elevated and CSF will reveal increased white blood cells (WBCs) and protein and low glucose (the bacteria present feed on the glucose).
- Complete blood count (CBC)—WBCs will be elevated.
- Blood, urine, and nasopharyngeal culture—Performed to look for source of infection and to rule out sepsis. Blood culture will be positive in cases of septicemia.

Nursing Management

Administer prescribed antibiotics as soon as possible after obtaining cultures. Quickly initiate supportive measures to ensure proper ventilation, reduce the inflammatory response, and help prevent injury to the brain. Interventions are aimed at reducing ICP and maintaining cerebral perfusion along with treating fluid volume deficit, controlling seizures, and preventing injury that may result from altered LOC or seizure activity. Initiate appropriate isolation precautions. In addition to standard precautions, infants and children diagnosed with bacterial meningitis will be placed on droplet isolation until 24 hours of antibiotics have been received to help prevent transmission to others. Refer to Nursing Care Plan 38.1 at the end of the chapter for nursing diagnoses and related interventions. In addition to those diagnoses and interventions, note any measures taken to reduce fever and prevent bacterial meningitis.

REDUCING FEVER

Hyperthermia related to infectious process, increased metabolic rate, and dehydration as evidenced by increased body temperature; warm, flushed skin; and tachycardia may be present. Reducing fever is important to help maintain optimal cerebral perfusion by reducing the metabolic needs of the brain. Administer antipyretics such as acetaminophen and nonsteroidal anti-inflammatory drugs (NSAIDs) such as ibuprofen, per order. Institute nonpharmacologic measures, if needed. Reduce environmental temperature and use cooling blankets, fans, cold compresses, and tepid baths to help reduce fever. Avoid measures that cause shivering because it increases heat production and is therefore counterproductive as well as uncomfortable for the child.

PREVENTING BACTERIAL MENINGITIS

Bacterial meningitis is a serious illness and prevention is important. It is transmitted by direct close contact with respiratory droplets from the nose or throat. Most at risk are those living with the child or anyone with whom the child played or was in close contact. Postexposure prophylaxis and postexposure immunization may be effective. Control measures should be initiated in environments where risk exists. Disinfect toys and other shared objects to decrease transmission of the microorganisms to others.

To reduce group B streptococcus infection in neonates, screen pregnant women. If the screening results are positive, administer intrapartal antibiotics. Vaccines are available for some specific causative organisms, but complete vaccination prevention is not possible at this time. The Hib vaccine is routine starting at 2 months of age and all children should be immunized to continue the reduction of bacterial meningitis caused by *H. influenzae* type B. The pneumococcal vaccine is also routine for all children starting at 2 months of age and should be considered for preschoolers who are at risk. Children at risk include those with immune deficiency; sickle cell disease; asplenia; chronic pulmonary, cardiac, or renal disease; diabetes mellitus; cochlear implants; cerebrospinal leaks; and organ transplants.

During the 1990s, a dramatic increase in the incidence of meningococcal meningitis (and the often fatal blood infection meningococcemia) among adolescents and young adults occurred (CDC, 2000). Living in close quarters, sleeping less than usual, and sharing personal items such as drinking glasses and lip balm contribute to the increase in disease. For these reasons, the American Academy of Pediatrics and ACIP recommendations advise meningococcal vaccination for all children 11 to 12 years of age with a booster at age 16; adolescents who receive their first dose at 13 to 15 years need a booster between 16 and 18 years; vaccination of certain at-risk groups such as all college freshmen living in dormitories; and children who are at high risk, such as children with chronic conditions or immune suppression or those who travel to high-risk areas or live in crowded conditions (American Academy of Pediatrics, 2013; MacNeil & Cohn, 2011). Since the 1990s a dramatic decrease in the incidence of meningococcal meningitis has been seen (MacNeil & Cohn, 2011). Further information and a resource for families are provided on thePoint. (See Healthy People 2020.)

HEALTHY PEOPLE 2020

Objective	Nursing Significance
Reduce meningococcal disease.	• Encourage appropriate immunization as recommended. • Educate families to complete prescribed courses of antibiotics (to avoid progression of minor bacterial infections to meningitis).

Healthy People Objectives retrieved from http://www.healthypeople.gov

Take Note!

Three main serogroups of meningococcal bacteria cause disease, B, C, and Y. In the United States approved routine vaccines protect against C and Y, but not B. Recent outbreaks of serogroup B meningococcal disease have led to the use of a serogroup B meningococcal vaccine licensed in Europe, Canada, and Australia to help control these outbreaks (Centers for Disease Control and Prevention, 2015c).

Aseptic Meningitis

Aseptic meningitis is the most common type of meningitis, and the majority of children affected are younger than 5 years of age (Centers for Disease Control and Prevention, 2014b). If the causative organism can be identified, it is usually a virus. Enteroviruses, such as echovirus and coxsackievirus, account for the majority of cases of aseptic meningitis (Centers for Disease Control and Prevention, 2014b). Less common causes include mumps, herpesvirus, HIV, measles, varicella, influenza, and vector-borne viruses.

Therapeutic Management

Prompt diagnosis and treatment are essential to improve outcomes. The child is treated aggressively as if he or she has bacterial meningitis until the diagnosis is confirmed. Antibiotics are administered and continued until the causative organism is recognized. If the cause is viral, antibiotics may be discontinued and antiviral agents may be started at this time. After diagnosis is confirmed, treatment is mainly supportive in nature and the illness is usually self-limiting, lasting 3 to 10 days.

Nursing Assessment

Elicit a description of the present illness and chief complaint. Common signs and symptoms reported during the health history might include:

- Fever
- General malaise
- Headache
- Photophobia
- Poor feeding
- Nausea
- Vomiting
- Irritability
- Lethargy
- Neck pain
- Positive Kernig and Brudzinski signs

The onset of symptoms may be abrupt or gradual. Assessment is similar to that of the child with bacterial meningitis. Signs and symptoms are similar to those seen in bacterial meningitis, but the child is usually less ill.

Nursing Management

Nursing management is similar to the nursing care of the child with bacterial meningitis and will focus on comfort measures to reduce pain and fever. Aseptic meningitis can be managed successfully at home if the child's neurologic status is stable and he or she is tolerating oral intake.

Encephalitis

Encephalitis is an inflammation of the brain that may also include an inflammation of the meninges. It is a rare complication and can be caused by protozoan, bacterial, fungal, or viral invasion. Viral illness and autoimmune disorders are the most commonly diagnosed cause in children, although in the majority of cases the cause remains unknown (Hardarson, 2015). In the United States, common causative organisms include enteroviruses, such as poliovirus and coxsackievirus; herpes simplex virus 1 and 2; and vector-borne viruses. Recovery from encephalitis can occur in a few days or may be complicated and involve severe neurologic damage with residual effects. Prognosis depends on the age of the child and the causative organism. Prompt diagnosis and treatment are essential. The child suspected of having encephalitis should be hospitalized. Therapeutic management is mainly supportive in nature and focuses on maintaining optimal cerebral perfusion; hydration and nutrition; and injury prevention.

Nursing Assessment

For a full description of the assessment phase of the nursing process, refer to the Assessment section of the Nursing Process Overview earlier in the chapter. Assessment findings pertinent to encephalitis are discussed below.

HEALTH HISTORY

Elicit a description of the present illness and chief complaint. Common signs and symptoms reported during the health history might include:

- Fever
- Flu-like symptoms
- Altered LOC
- Headache
- Lethargy
- Drowsiness
- Generalized weakness
- Seizure activity

Explore the child's current history for risk factors such as:

- Recent travel
- Recreational activities, such as hiking and camping
- Animal contacts

PHYSICAL EXAMINATION

Perform a neurologic examination to distinguish between encephalitis and viral meningitis. In encephalitis, a neurologic examination will reveal changes in sensorium and focal neurologic changes. Neurologic findings vary and reflect the areas of the brain that are involved.

LABORATORY AND DIAGNOSTIC TESTS

An LP may be done and the CSF may show an elevated leukocyte count and elevated protein and glucose levels. However, in some cases, levels may be normal. MRI, CT, and EEG procedures may be performed to help identify early changes and provide useful clues in developing a diagnosis.

Nursing Management

Nursing management is similar to nursing care for the child with meningitis. Specific antiviral therapy may be used for diseases caused by the herpes simplex virus. Teach children and their families how to prevent encephalitis. Encephalitis can result from complications of childhood illnesses such as measles, mumps, or chickenpox. Explain the importance of keeping children up to date in their immunizations. Effective vaccines are available for a few viral pathogens that cause encephalitis (such as rabies virus and Japanese encephalitis virus), but these vaccines are not routine; they are recommended for those at high risk. For example, postexposure rabies vaccines can be administered to a child who was bitten by a suspected rabid animal. Also, those traveling to areas where Japanese encephalitis is endemic, such as India and China, and planning a prolonged stay or extreme outdoor activity should receive the appropriate vaccine.

Vector control and avoiding mosquito and tick bites are the best prevention of vector-borne infection. Preventative measures include:

- Using insect repellent (repellents containing DEET should be used cautiously in children younger than 12 years of age and not at all in children younger than 1 year of age)
- Wearing clothing that covers the arms and legs
- Controlling mosquito populations by eliminating areas of standing water where mosquitoes can breed
- Using insect traps and public measures such as sprayed insecticides to reduce the mosquito population

Reye Syndrome

Reye syndrome is an extremely rare disease that primarily affects children younger than 15 years of age who are recovering from a viral illness. The exact cause of Reye syndrome is unknown. It has been found that Reye syndrome is a reaction that is triggered by the use of salicylates or salicylate-containing products to treat a viral infection. This reaction causes brain swelling, liver failure, and death in hours, if treatment in not initiated. In the 1980s, the adverse effects of salicylates used to treat viral illnesses began to be publicized and the U.S. Food and Drug Administration (FDA) required warning labels to be placed on all salicylate-containing products, such as aspirin. Since then, there has been a dramatic decrease in the occurrence of Reye syndrome.

Nursing Assessment

Elicit a description of the present illness and chief complaint. Common signs and symptoms reported during the health history might include:

- Severe and continual vomiting
- Changes in mental status
- Lethargy
- Irritability
- Confusion
- Hyperreflexia

Explore the child's current and past medical history for risk factors such as:

- A prodromal viral illness, like chickenpox, croup, flu, or an upper respiratory infection
- Ingestion of salicylate-containing products within 3 weeks of the start of the viral illness

Elevated liver function tests and elevated serum ammonia levels can confirm diagnosis.

Nursing Management

Early recognition and treatment are the most important aspects of managing this illness. Nursing management is aimed at maintaining cerebral perfusion, managing and preventing increased ICP, providing safety measures due to changes in LOC and risk for seizures, and monitoring fluid status to prevent dehydration and overhydration.

Education is an important aspect of preventing this disease. Salicylates are found in many products, including many over-the-counter products such as Alka-Seltzer and Pepto-Bismol. A complete list can be found on thePoint. Recovery from Reye syndrome is dependent on the severity of swelling of the brain. Some children will make a full recovery, while others may suffer long-term neurologic damage.

TRAUMA

Trauma or injury is a leading cause of childhood morbidity and mortality in the United States (Child Trends Databank, 2014). The child faces significant risk of trauma to his or her developing neurologic system, often leading to neurologic disorders with life-threatening and lasting effects. Neurologic trauma may include head trauma, nonaccidental head trauma, birth injuries, and near-drowning.

Head Trauma

In the United States, injury causes more death in children than disease (Child Trends Databank, 2014). Of these injuries, head injury is a frequent cause of death and disability in childhood. Common causes of head trauma in children include falls, motor vehicle accidents, pedestrian and bicycle accidents, and child abuse (see next section, Nonaccidental Head Trauma). Many factors make children more susceptible to head trauma than adults. Larger head size in relation to the body, coupled with a higher center of gravity, causes the child to hit his or her head more readily when involved in motor vehicle accidents, bicycle accidents, and falls. Children are also at risk for injury related to psychosocial factors such as their high activity level, curiosity, incomplete motor development, and lack of knowledge and judgment skills.

Head trauma is a broad term that can include specific patterns of injury. Traumatic brain injury (TBI) occurs when a head trauma results in a disruption of the normal function of the brain. Not all head traumas result in a TBI. See Table 38.6 for descriptions of common head injuries seen in children. Head trauma in children is serious because it can cause an immediate threat to the child's life as well as a number of complications that can lead to lifelong impairment of an individual's physical, cognitive, and psychosocial functioning. Prognosis for the child who has suffered a head trauma depends on the extent and severity of the injury as well as any complications (see Healthy People 2020).

TABLE 38.6 COMMON HEAD INJURIES SEEN IN CHILDREN

Types	Description	Characteristics
Skull fractures	A break in the bone surrounding the brain	In infants and children younger than 2 years old, a great deal of force is needed to produce a skull fracture. Due to the flexibility of the immature skull, it is able to withstand a great degree of deformation before a fracture will occur. Can result in little or no brain damage, but may have serious consequences if the underlying brain tissue is injured
Linear skull fracture	A simple break in the skull that follows a relatively straight line	Most common skull fracture. Can result from minor head injuries such as being struck by a rock, stick, or other object; falls; or motor vehicle accidents. Not usually serious unless there is additional injury to the brain
Depressed skull fractures	The bone is locally broken and pushed inward, causing pressure on the brain.	Can result from forceful impact from a blunt object, such as a hammer or another heavy but fairly small object Surgery is often required to elevate the bony pieces and inspect the brain for evidence of injury.
Diastatic skull fracture	A fracture through the skull sutures	Most commonly occurs in the lambdoid sutures (refer to Fig. 38.10 for location of sutures) Usually, treatment is not required, but observation will be necessary.
Compound skull fracture	A laceration of the skin and splintering of the bone	The fracture can be linear or depressed. Generally is the result of blunt force. Usually requires medical intervention and surgery may be necessary
Basilar skull fracture	A fracture of the bones that form the base of the skull	Can result from severe blunt head trauma with significant force. Due to the proximity to the brain stem, this is a serious head injury. Findings include CSF rhinorrhea and otorrhea, bleeding from the ear, and orbital or postauricular ecchymosis (bruising behind ear is referred to as Battle sign), and these children are at increased risk for infection because the fracture may allow a portal of entry into the central nervous system.
Concussion	A type of traumatic brain injury that is caused by a bump, blow, jolt, jarring, or shaking and results in disruption or malfunction of the electrical activities of the brain	Most common head injury. Results from a blow or jolt to the head caused by sports injuries, motor vehicle accidents, and falls. Confusion and amnesia after the head injury are seen. Loss of consciousness may or may not occur. Noted symptoms may include increased distractibility and difficulty with concentration. Treatment includes rest and monitoring for neurologic changes that could indicate a more severe injury, such as increased sleepiness, worsening headache, increased vomiting, worsening confusion, difficulty walking or talking, changes in LOC, and seizures.
Contusion	Bruising of cerebral tissue	Results from a blow to the head from incidents such as a motor vehicle accident, falls, or abuse such as shaken baby syndrome. May cause focal disturbances in vision, strength, and sensation. The signs and symptoms will vary based on the extent of vascular injury and can range from mild weakness to prolonged unconsciousness and paralysis. Treatment includes close monitoring for neurologic changes. Surgery is usually not necessary.

TABLE 38.6 COMMON HEAD INJURIES SEEN IN CHILDREN (continued)

Types	Description	Characteristics
Subdural hematoma	Collection of blood between the dura and cerebrum	Low incidence of fracture. Most common in children younger than 2 years old, especially infants. Results from birth trauma, falls, bicycle injuries, and abuse such as shaken baby syndrome. Usually consists of venous bleeding. Symptoms may occur within 3 days of trauma or as late as 20 days. Symptoms include vomiting, failure to thrive, changes in LOC, seizures, and retinal hemorrhage. Treatment depends on clinical symptoms, size of clot, and area of the brain involved. In some cases, the bleed may be closely monitored for resolution. In other cases, treatment may include subdural taps in infants and surgical evacuation in older children. Close monitoring of neurologic status and for signs of increased ICP is indicated.
Epidural hematoma	Collection of blood located outside the dura but within the skull	Relatively uncommon. Often results from skull fracture. Seen when head trauma is severe. Usually arterial bleeding, therefore brain compression occurs rapidly and can result in impairment of the brain stem and respiratory or cardiovascular function. Symptoms include vomiting, headache, and lethargy. Treatment depends on clinical symptoms, the size of the clot, and the area of the brain involved. Treatment includes prompt surgical evacuation and cauterization of the artery. The earlier the bleed is recognized and treated, the more favorable the outcome. Close monitoring of neurologic status is indicated.

Nursing Assessment

For a full description of the assessment phase of the nursing process, refer to the Assessment section of the Nursing Process Overview earlier in the chapter.

HEALTHY PEOPLE *2020*

Objective	Nursing Significance
Reduce fatal and nonfatal traumatic brain injuries.	• Educate children and families about safety such as helmet use when inline skating, skateboarding, bicycling, and playing football or other sports that may result in head injury. • Encourage appropriate child car seat and seat belt use. • Use every encounter with a child and family as an opportunity to provide education related to injury prevention.

Healthy People Objectives retrieved from http://www.healthypeople.gov

Assessment findings pertinent to head trauma are discussed below.

HEALTH HISTORY

Take a detailed history, including past medical history along with details of the events surrounding the injury such as mental status at the time of the injury, any loss of consciousness, irritability, lethargy, abnormal behavior, vomiting (if so, how many times), any seizure activity, and any complaints of headache, visual changes, or neck pain.

PHYSICAL EXAMINATION

Perform a thorough physical examination. Initial physical assessment will focus on the ABCs (airway, breathing, and circulation) (refer to Chapter 51 for further information on emergency management). All children who experience head trauma need an assessment of their neurologic function as soon as they are seen. This includes LOC, pupillary response, and any seizure activity. Fixed and dilated pupils, fixed and constricted pupils, or sluggish pupillary reaction to light will warrant prompt intervention.

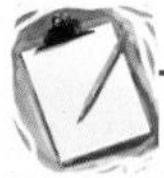

Take Note!

A child's spine must remain stabilized after a head injury until spinal cord injury is ruled out.

LABORATORY AND DIAGNOSTIC TESTS

Diagnostic tests that may be utilized include x-ray examinations of the head and neck and CT and MRI scans. These procedures can assist in providing a more definitive diagnosis of the severity and type of trauma.

Take Note!

If clear liquid fluid is noted draining from the ears or nose, notify the physician or nurse practitioner. If the fluid tests positive for glucose, this is indicative of leaking CSF.

Nursing Management

Nursing management of the child with head trauma depends on the seriousness of the injury. For all head trauma, however, the nurse provides support and education to the family and provides teaching on ways to prevent future head injuries.

CARING FOR THE CHILD WITH MILD TO MODERATE HEAD INJURY

Mild to moderate closed head injury is defined as brain injury without any penetrating injury to the brain, no loss of consciousness, no other injury to the head or body, normal behavior after the injury, and healthy status before the injury. Most children with this type of injury can be cared for and observed at home. Provide parents and caregivers with clear instructions regarding the care of their child at home. Explain that they must seek medical attention if the child's condition worsens at any time during the first several days after injury. See Teaching Guidelines 38.2.

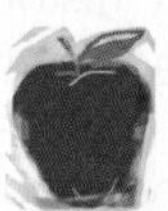

Teaching Guidelines 38.2

MONITORING THE CHILD WITH CLOSED HEAD INJURY AT HOME

Instruct parents and caregivers:

- Stay with the child for the first 24 hours and be ready to take the child to the hospital, if necessary.
- Wake the child every 2 hours to ensure that he or she moves normally, wakes enough to recognize the caregiver, and responds to the caregiver appropriately.
- Closely observe the child for a few days.
- Call the medical provider or bring child to the emergency room if the child exhibits any of the following:
  - Constant headache that gets worse
  - Slurred speech
  - Dizziness that does not go away or happens repeatedly
  - Extreme irritability or other abnormal behavior
  - Vomiting more than two times
  - Clumsiness or difficulty walking
  - Oozing blood or watery fluid from ears or nose
  - Difficulty waking up
  - Unequal-sized pupils
  - Unusual paleness that lasts longer than 1 hour
  - Seizures
- Review signs and symptoms of increased intracranial pressure and provide parents with a number they can call if they have questions or concerns.

Children with mild closed head injury may exhibit some cognitive and behavioral symptoms, such as difficulty paying attention, problems making sense of what has been seen or heard, and forgetting things, in the early days after the injury. The majority make a full recovery. However, some may experience ongoing cognitive and behavioral difficulties, including slow information processing and attention difficulties.

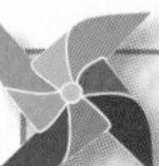

Thinking About Development

Antionio Blackman is an 11-year-old boy who suffered a concussion during his hockey game. Based on his developmental stage, how will you instruct him and his caregivers on managing his head injury at home? How would your instructions change if the child was 5 years old?

CARING FOR THE CHILD WITH SEVERE HEAD INJURY

Severe head injuries can range from a temporary unconsciousness that resolves quickly to children who may remain in a comatose state for a prolonged time. Nursing management of the comatose child is similar to nursing care of the comatose adult.

Children with more severe head injury may require intensive care initially until stabilized. Focus will be on maintaining the child's airway; monitoring breathing, circulation, and neurologic status closely; preventing and ceasing any seizure activity; and treating any other injuries that may have occurred as a result of the trauma. Nursing management will continue to focus on evaluation of neurologic status and assessing for changes in LOC and signs and symptoms of increased ICP. Initiate seizure precautions as ordered.

Individualize care to the specific needs of the child. Maintain a quiet environment to help reduce restlessness and irritability. Manage pain and administer sedation as ordered. Observe the level of sedation closely to ensure that LOC will not become altered, which would hinder the ability to assess adequately for neurologic changes. Monitor for the development of complications, which include hemorrhage, infection, cerebral edema, and herniation.

Take Note!

Parents are extremely helpful resources in evaluating a child's behavior for changes or abnormalities. They can provide insight into whether a behavior seen is normal or abnormal for this child. Examples include the ease at which a child is normally aroused, how much the child normally sleeps during the day, and what is the child's normal visual and hearing acuity.

PROVIDING SUPPORT AND EDUCATION

Provide support and education for the family of a child who has suffered a head trauma. Encourage involvement in the child's care. The extent of residual neurologic damage and recovery may be unclear for the child with a head injury. This can be frustrating and stressful for parents and family. Encourage verbalization of their feelings and concerns. Rehabilitation of the child with permanent brain damage is an essential component of his or her care. It should begin as soon as possible in the hospital setting and may continue for months to years. This can place a strain on the family and its finances. Families need to be involved in the rehabilitation process. The nurse will be a key member in ensuring the parents and family are involved with the interdisciplinary team.

PREVENTING HEAD INJURIES

Prevention of head injuries provides the greatest benefit to children and the community. Nurses play a key role in educating the public on topics such as helmet use with certain sports; bicycle and motorcycle safety; car seat and seat belt use; and providing adequate supervision of children to help prevent injuries and accidents—and resultant head trauma—from occurring (see Healthy People 2020).

HEALTHY PEOPLE 2020

Objective	Nursing Significance
Increase the number of states and the District of Columbia with laws requiring bicycle helmets for bicycle riders.	• Support legislation locally that calls for bicycle helmet laws. • Participate in local "safe kids" activities to demonstrate support for helmet use

Healthy People Objectives retrieved from http://www.healthypeople.gov

Take Note!

Sports related traumatic brain injuries, including concussions, in children and adolescents are a growing concern, particularly related to the long-term effects of these injuries. Increasing education, awareness, and research about concussions will help to improve prevention, recognition, and treatment to this injury among school professionals, parents, coaches, and children and adolescents. See Evidence-Based Practice 38.1

Nonaccidental Head Trauma

In the United States, inflicted or nonaccidental head trauma is the leading cause of traumatic death and morbidity

EVIDENCE-BASED PRACTICE 38.1

DOES THE SLICE (SPORTS LEGACY INSTITUTE COMMUNITY EDUCATORS) CURRICULUM PROVIDE EFFECTIVE EDUCATION TO STUDENT ATHELETES ON CONCUSSIONS?

The high incidence of concussion and the potential for short-term and long-term complications makes concussions in student athletes an important topic. Many states have passed recent legislation addressing concussions in youth sports and recent efforts have provided education on concussions to coaches, athletes, and parents. The need to ensure the provided education is validated and effective is essential.

STUDY

The SLICE concussion workshop was provided to 636 students 9 to 18 years of age. The workshop is presented by trained medical and health-related students. The presentation includes age-specific interactive content such as videos, discussion, audience demonstrations, and case studies. Topics include how student athletes can recognize concussion symptoms and respond to concussions that occur to themselves or teammates. Prepresentation and postpresentation quizzes were given to evaluate effectiveness of learning.

Findings

Significant improvements in quiz scores were seen across all age groups. 34% of students passed the prepresentation quiz, while 80% passed the postpresentation quiz.

Nursing Implications

Education on concussions is one of the most important aspects of concussion prevention. The SLICE curriculum provides an effective model for educating student athletes on concussion. Nurses and nursing students should consider incorporating the SLICE curriculum when providing education to children on concussions.

Adapted from Bagley, A. F., Daniel, H., Daneshvar, D. H., Schanker, B. D., Zurakowski, D., d'Hemecourt, C. A., et al. (2012). Effectiveness of the SLICE Program for Youth Concussion. *Clinical Journal of Sport Medicine, 22*(5), 385–389.

during infancy (Christian & Endom, 2015). Children's dependence on others to care for them places them at a high risk for injuries caused by child abuse.

The infant's large head size and weak neck muscles place him or her at an increased risk for head trauma due to violent shaking or cranial impacts compared to adults. In addition, children younger than 3 years of age have a very mobile spine, especially in the cervical region, along with immature neck muscles. This places them at a higher risk for injury from acceleration/deceleration injuries, which occur when the head receives a blow or is shaken. The sudden acceleration causes deformation of the skull and movement of the brain, allowing brain contents to strike parts of the skull. Bruising of the brain can occur at the point of impact or at that point distant from the impact where the brain collides with the skull. Another result of brain movement is hemorrhages in the brain, which are caused by the shearing forces that may tear small arteries. The child's thin skull places him or her at increased risk for skull fractures and penetrating injuries resulting from head trauma.

Causes of nonaccidental head trauma include violent shaking, referred to as shaken baby syndrome (SBS); blows to the head; and intentional cranial impacts against the wall, furniture, or the floor. The average victim is younger than 9 months of age. SBS is a form of child abuse and a significant number of head traumas result from it. However, it differs from many other forms of child abuse in that frequently there was no intent to harm the child. Shaking happens when the parent or caregiver becomes frustrated or angry because he or she cannot get the baby to stop crying.

The full appearance of neurologic deficits resulting from nonaccidental head trauma may take several years to be identified and recovery can be very slow. Long-term outcomes are not known, but many of these infants and children have poor outcomes and may suffer neurologic defects such as profound intellectual disability, spastic quadriplegia, severe motor dysfunction, and blindness. The majority of children with inflicted head injuries have some impairment of motor and cognitive abilities, language, vision, and behavior. These injuries may also contribute to later problems with education and social attainment.

Nursing Assessment

The infant who has been a victim of nonaccidental trauma can present in many ways. Symptoms and physical findings may be similar to those seen in children with accidental head trauma or increased ICP related to infection. Therefore, many nonaccidental traumas remain unidentified. Nurses are mandatory reporters of abuse (for further information on this, see Chapter 50). Early recognition of suspected child abuse is essential to prevent death and disability from repetitive inflicted head trauma.

HEALTH HISTORY

It is important to review the child's history closely and pay particular attention to the caregivers' explanation of the child's injury. Be alert to any discrepancies between the physical injuries and the history of injury given by the parent, especially if the stories are conflicting, or if the caregivers are unable to give an explanation for the injury. Also, note any previous intracranial or skeletal injuries that cannot be explained.

In less severe cases, common signs and symptoms may include:

- Poor feeding or sucking
- Vomiting
- Lethargy or irritability
- Failure to thrive
- Increased sleeping
- Difficulty arousing

In more severe cases, the symptoms will be more acute and may consist of:

- Seizure activity
- Apnea
- Bradycardia
- Decreased LOC
- Bulging fontanel

PHYSICAL EXAMINATION

External bruising of the head and face may be evident in some inflicted head traumas. However, no evidence of external trauma, but the presence of intracranial or intraocular hemorrhages, is the classic presentation of SBS. Retinal hemorrhages are seen in the majority of cases, which is a rare finding in accidental or nontraumatic events.

LABORATORY AND DIAGNOSTIC TESTS

Diagnostic tests including CT, MRI, ophthalmologic examination to rule out retinal hemorrhages, and skeletal survey x-rays to rule out or confirm other injuries may be performed to help determine the extent and type of injury.

Nursing Management

Treatment and nursing management will be similar to that for the child with accidental head trauma (see earlier section, Head Trauma). Prevention of nonaccidental head trauma, including SBS, is a major concern for all health care professionals. Be aware of risk factors related to the potential for SBS to occur. Recognizing these risk factors will allow appropriate intervention and protection of the child to take place. See Box 38.4 for risk factors related to SBS.

Educating parents and caregivers on appropriate ways to handle stress and ways to cope with a crying infant can help to prevent nonaccidental head trauma (see Teaching Guidelines 38.3). Many parents and caregivers may perceive shaking a child as a less violent way to react than other means of enforcing discipline. They

BOX 38.4

RISK FACTORS ASSOCIATED WITH SHAKEN BABY SYNDROME

- Single parent
- Young parent
- Substance abuse by a parent
- Any external factors present such as financial, social, or physical burdens that place stress on the parent
- Premature or sick infant
- Infant with colic

need to be aware that shaking a baby, even for only a few seconds, can cause serious brain damage and death. Decreasing mortality and morbidity associated with SBS and nonaccidental injury through early preventive education is an essential nursing concern. Information about the dangers of shaking a baby should be a part of prenatal care and standard discharge teaching on postpartum units. In addition, this information should be provided to the community and in health education classes to reach young potential child care providers.

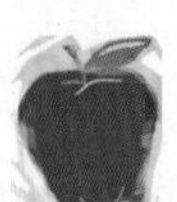

Teaching Guidelines 38.3

TIPS TO CALM A CRYING BABY

Instruct parents and caregivers:

- Try to figure out what is upsetting the baby.
  - Is the baby hungry?
  - Is the baby's diaper dry?
  - Is the baby cold or hot?
  - Is the baby overtired or overstimulated?
  - Is the baby in pain?
  - Is the baby sick or running a fever?
- Try to help the baby relax.
  - Turn down the lights.
  - Swaddle the baby.
  - Walk the baby.
  - Rock the baby.
  - Give the baby a breast, bottle, or pacifier.
  - Shhh, talk to, or sing to the baby.
  - Take the baby for a stroller or car ride.
- Sometimes the baby may continue to cry after all your efforts. If you feel overwhelmed, frustrated, or angry, focus on keeping the baby safe.
  - Stop what you are doing, take a deep breath, and count to 10.
  - Place the baby in a safe place, such as the crib or playpen.
  - Leave the room and shut the door, and find a quiet place for yourself.
  - Check on the baby every 5 to 15 minutes.
  - Do not be afraid to call for help; call a friend, relative, or neighbor.

Near-Drowning

Drowning is the second leading cause of unintentional injury-related death in children between the ages of 1 and 14 years (Centers for Disease Control and Prevention, 2014c). Drowning is a preventable problem that is far too common, especially in children. Those at greatest risk of drowning are children 1 to 4 years of age and adolescent males (Centers for Disease Control and Prevention, 2014c).

Near-drowning is described as an incident in which a child has suffered a submersion injury and has survived for at least 24 hours. Near-drowning events result in a significant number of injured children and can result in long-term neurologic deficits. Children younger than 1 year old most often drown in bathtubs, buckets, or toilets. Children between the ages of 1 and 4 years are more likely to drown or have a near-drowning incident in residential swimming pools (Centers for Disease Control and Prevention, 2014c). In children older than 15 years of age, most drownings occur in natural water settings, such as oceans or lakes (Centers for Disease Control and Prevention, 2014c). Most incidents are accidental and result from inadequately supervising children who are in or near water, lack of use of personal flotation devices while on recreational water apparatus such as boats, and diving accidents.

Nursing Assessment

Hypoxia is the primary problem resulting from near-drowning. Nursing assessment needs to begin with resuscitative measures. The child may be comatose, be hypothermic, lack spontaneous respirations, and present with hypoxia and hypercapnia. Gain information about the site of submersion (was it fresh or salt water?), the water temperature, the time of submersion, and how long it was until the child received interventions such as cardiopulmonary resuscitation (CPR) and emergency medical services (EMS).

Nursing Management

Resuscitative measures should be started as soon as the child is pulled from the water, and the child should be transported to a hospital immediately. Management will be based on the degree of cerebral insult that has occurred. The child who has been successfully resuscitated will usually require intensive nursing care and monitoring. Promotion of oxygenation and monitoring for infection related to aspiration of water are primary nursing concerns. Chronic neurologic damage occurs in many near-drownings secondary to hypoxia. The child may need rehabilitation and long-term follow-up. Provide parents with support and education relating to their child's condition. Educating children, families,

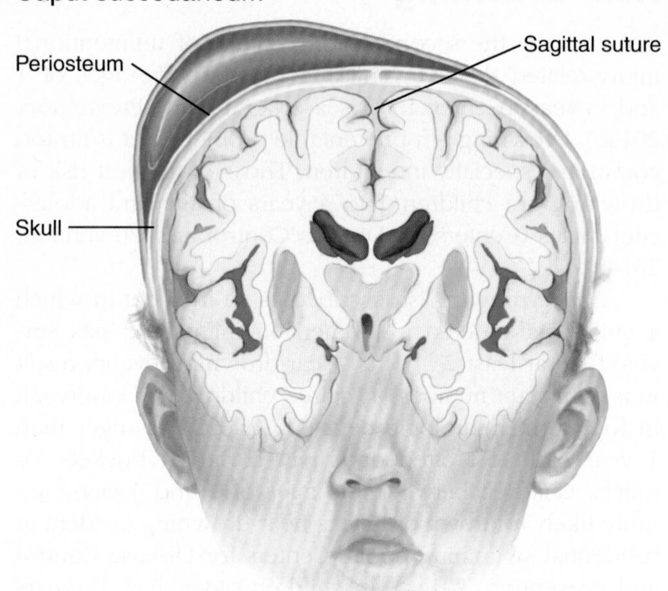

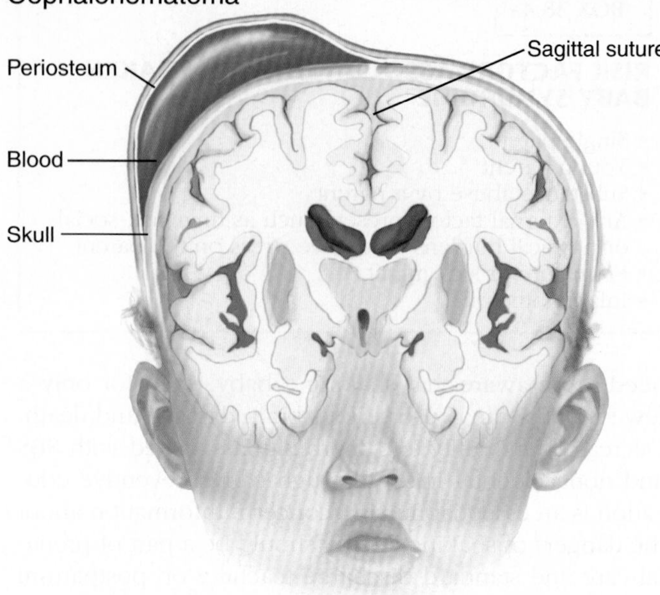

FIGURE 38.15 **(A)** Infant with caput succedaneum. Edema is noted at birth and crosses the suture line. **(B)** Infant with cephalohematoma. Bleeding appears within the first 2 to 3 days of birth and does not cross the suture line.

and the community is an important nursing intervention to help prevent drowning (see Teaching Guidelines 38.4).

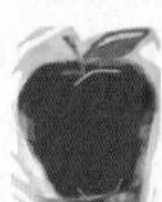

Teaching Guidelines 38.4

TEACHING TO PREVENT DROWNING

Instruct parents and caregivers:

- Install proper pool fencing.
- Start water safety training at a young age.
- Never leave an infant or child without close adult supervision in or near water (this includes bathtubs).
- Empty water from all containers, such as 5-gallon buckets, immediately after use.
- Use proper-fitting, Coast Guard–approved personal flotation devices at all times when near water
- Never allow children to walk, skate, or ride on thinning or thawing ice.
- Learn CPR and keep emergency numbers handy (make sure babysitters are CPR qualified).
- Know the depth of water before permitting a child to jump or dive.

BLOOD FLOW DISRUPTION

Pediatric cerebral vascular disorders occur less often than in adults, but they are still an important cause of mortality and chronic morbidity in children (Smith & Fox, 2015). Many children will develop lifelong cognitive and motor impairments. Childhood cerebral vascular disorders (stroke) are usually seen after the first month of life. Periventricular/intraventricular hemorrhage occurs in preterm infants and in infants up to 1 month of age (see chapter 24).

Cerebral Vascular Disorders (Stroke)

A cerebral vascular disorder is a sudden disruption of the blood supply to the brain. It affects neurologic functioning, such as movement and speech. Two major types of adult cerebral vascular disorders are seen in children—ischemic stroke and hemorrhagic stroke. Ischemic stroke is more common than hemorrhagic stroke in children. In children, there is a wide array of risk factors and causes as compared to adults (see Comparison Chart 38.2), but in many cases the cause remains unidentified. The outcomes reported for cerebral vascular disorders in children vary, but many children will develop some neurologic or cognitive deficit.

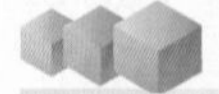

Concept Mastery Alert

Strokes in Children

Children are more likely to experience an ischemic stroke than a hemorrhagic stroke. If a child experiences a stroke, the symptoms are similar to those that an adult experiences.

COMPARISON CHART 38.2 RISK FACTORS AND CAUSES OF STROKE IN CHILDREN AND ADULTS

	Risk Factors and Causes in Children	Risk Factors and Causes in Adults
Ischemic stroke	Cardiac disorders and intracardiac defects (congenital such as ventricular septal defect, atrial septal defect, and aortic stenosis, or acquired such as rheumatic heart disease) Coagulation abnormalities that lead to thrombosis Sickle cell disease Infection, such as meningitis Arterial dissection Genetic disorders	Cardiac disease, including atherosclerosis Diabetes mellitus Hyperlipidemia Hypercoagulability states Polycythemia Sickle cell disease Smoking Increased age Male gender Obesity Excessive alcohol consumption
Hemorrhagic stroke	Vascular malformations such as intracranial arteriovenous malformation (AVM) Aneurysms Warfarin therapy Cavernous malformations Malignancy Trauma Coagulation disorders such as hemophilia Thrombocytopenia Liver failure Leukemia Intracranial tumors such as medulloblastomas	Hypertension Aneurysms Use of anticoagulant medications Smoking Increased age Male gender Obesity Excessive alcohol consumption

Historically, children have been excluded from adult stroke studies. Therefore, many treatments used in children have had to be adapted from adult studies. Acute treatment is supportive and requires intensive care. The exact treatment will depend on the underlying cause.

Nursing Assessment

The clinical presentation will vary according to age, the underlying cause, and the location of the stroke. Signs and symptoms of acute stroke are similar to those seen in the adult and depend on the area of the brain that has been affected. Common signs include:

- Weakness on one side or hemiplegia
- Facial droop
- Slurred speech
- Speech deficits
- Seizures
- Headaches
- Lethargy

Strokes in children are diagnosed in the same manner as strokes in adults. However, further tests may need to be run in the child, such as metabolic studies, coagulation tests, echocardiogram, and LP to help identify the cause of the stroke.

Nursing Management

Nursing management will be similar to that for the adult patient who has suffered a stroke. Care will focus on assessing neurologic status, increasing mobility, providing adequate nutrition and hydration, and encouraging self-care. Rehabilitative care may be initiated, depending on the long-term deficits, to help the child attain optimal function. Parental support and education will be essential in helping them care for a child who has new disabilities.

CHRONIC DISORDERS

Chronic disorders in children necessitate multidisciplinary care. Parents and children are in need of a large amount of education and support from the health care team. Chronic neurologic disorders commonly seen in children include headaches and breath holding.

Headaches

Acute and chronic headaches, including migraines, are common reasons why children miss school, visit their physician or nurse practitioner, and receive subsequent referrals to neurologists. Children with reports or symptoms of headaches need to be examined thoroughly. Headaches may result from sinusitis or eyestrain or can be indicative of more serious conditions such as brain tumors, acute meningitis, or increased ICP. Migraines are a specific type of headache. They are benign, recurrent, throbbing headaches often accompanied by nausea, vomiting, and photophobia. Acute migraines can occur in children as young as 3 to 4 years old. The cause of migraine headaches is not well understood.

After other acute or chronic conditions are ruled out, management will focus on treating the child's pain. Pharmacologic measures may be utilized in the treatment of chronic headaches and migraines. Medications used in children to treat and prevent headaches are similar to the medications used to treat adults. Recent attention has been paid to headaches caused by medication overuse. The child may have a primary headache disorder that is exacerbated by the frequent use of medications. Although medication overuse headaches are common in children, they are frequently underrecognized and underdiagnosed.

Nursing Assessment

Elicit a description of the present illness and chief complaint. Important health history information to obtain is onset of the pain, aggravating and alleviating factors, frequency and duration of the pain, time of day the pain usually occurs, location of the pain, and quality and intensity of the pain.

In young children, symptoms of headache may be hard to recognize. However, common signs and symptoms may include:

- Irritability
- Lethargy
- Head holding
- Head banging
- Sensitivity to sound or light

Assessment also includes a thorough physical examination to rule out any life-threatening illness, such as a brain tumor or increased ICP. A detailed neurologic examination is warranted. Neuroimaging may be performed based on the child's history and physical examination, if needed, to rule out a brain tumor or mass as the cause of the headaches.

Nursing Management

Nursing measures will focus on support and education. After serious illness has been ruled out, reassure the child and family that no serious medical or neurologic disease is present. Because headaches are recurring and the cause may be unknown, pain management can be difficult. Provide education to help the child and parents gain control over the headaches. Teach the child and family to keep very accurate record of headaches and activities surrounding the headaches to help establish a pattern of occurrence and identify triggering factors. Encourage parents and the child to recognize the triggering factors and to avoid them (Box 38.5). Teach the child and family about pain medications and how to use them. Teach other management techniques, which may include exercise, sleep regulation, proper diet with regularly spaced meals, avoiding caffeine, avoiding inadequate hydration, regular attendance at school, use of biofeedback, stress reduction techniques, and possible psychiatric assessment.

BOX 38.5

POTENTIAL HEADACHE TRIGGERS

- Foods, such as chocolate, caffeine, or monosodium glutamate (MSG)-containing foods
- Changes in hormone levels, around menses and ovulation
- Changes in:
  Weather
  Season
  Sleep patterns
  Meal schedule
- Stress
- Intense activity
- Bright or flickering lights
- Odors, such as strong perfumes

Breath Holding

Breath holding is a benign behavior of childhood, although it is extremely frightening for parents. It is normally seen in children 1 to 3 years old and typically is outgrown by 4 to 7 years of age. It is usually triggered by the child becoming angry or stressed after not getting his or her way. It can also occur as a reflexive response to fear, pain, or being startled. The child stops inhaling and exhaling or hyperventilates, the brain becomes anoxic, and the child becomes cyanotic and may pass out. In some cases a change in muscle tone, seizure-like activity, or hypoxic convulsions may be observed. This does not mean the child has a seizure disorder, but it must be ruled out. The spell usually resolves spontaneously. With the loss of consciousness the child will begin breathing on his or her own and will often begin crying, screaming, and trying to catch his or her breath. The spells usually only last 30 to 60 seconds and, as long as the child does not sustain an injury while falling, have no consequences.

If no underlying condition is found, the child needs no therapy. The condition is self-limiting and the child will outgrow it. Iron deficiency may play a role; therefore, iron supplementation may be prescribed (Nguyen, Kaplan, & Wilfong, 2014).

Nursing Assessment

The first time a spell occurs, a primary care provider should evaluate the child because the event could indicate a seizure. Breath holding also has been shown to be aggravated by iron-deficiency anemia and, in rare cases, it could indicate a more serious neurologic condition, and therefore warrants a full evaluation. Elicit a full description of the episode and events leading up to it. Also, collect a thorough past medical history and perform a complete physical examination.

Nursing Management

Nursing management should focus on educating and supporting the parents. Breath holding is a scary event and parents will want information on the effects of the behavior and how to prevent the behavior from recurring. Reinforce that the spells are involuntary and that they should not intervene to stop them. Encourage parents to maintain a safe environment when an episode is occurring, such as holding the child or placing him or her in the side-lying position. Reassure parents that the child will suffer no ill effects from breath holding and that they should not reinforce the breath-holding behavior or give in to the child. Children with breath-holding spells may benefit from structure and consistency to avoid unnecessary frustration and overtiredness.

NURSING CARE PLAN 38.1

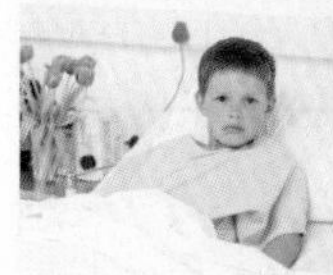

Overview for the Child With a Neurologic Disorder

NURSING DIAGNOSIS: Decreased intracranial adaptive capacity related to compression of brain tissue due to increased CSF or cerebral edema secondary to increased ICP resulting from brain injury, congenital structural defects, brain tumor, decreased reabsorption of CSF, or shunt malfunction as evidenced by vomiting, headache, complaints of visual disturbances, decreased pulse and respirations, elevated blood pressure or pulse pressure, changes in level of consciousness, increased head circumference, or bulging fontanel

Outcome Identification and Evaluation

Child will remain free of signs and symptoms of increased ICP as evidenced by remaining free of headache, vomiting, vision disturbances, vital signs within parameters for age, no signs of altered levels of consciousness, able to maintain effective breathing pattern, free of excessive irritability or lethargy, head circumference within parameters for age.

Interventions: ***Promoting Adequate Intracranial Adaptive Capacity***

- Assess neurologic status closely, and monitor for signs and symptoms of increased ICP: *changes in level of consciousness, signs of irritability or lethargy, and changes in pupillary reaction can indicate changes in ICP.*
- Monitor vital signs: *decreased pulse and respiratory rate and increased blood pressure or pulse pressure can indicate increased ICP.*
- Measure head circumference in children younger than 3 years of age: *increases in head circumference outside parameters for age can indicate increased ICP.*
- Elevate head of bed 15 to 30 degrees: *to facilitate venous return and help to reduce ICP.*
- Minimize environmental stimuli and noise, and avoid pain-producing procedures, if possible: *all can increase ICP.*
- Have emergency equipment ready and available: *increased ICP can result in respiratory or cardiac failure.*
- Notify physician or nurse practitioner immediately if changes in assessment are noted: *early intervention is critical to prevent neurologic damage and death.*

NURSING DIAGNOSIS: Risk for ineffective (cerebral) tissue perfusion related to increased ICP, alteration in blood flow secondary to hemorrhage, vessel malformation, cerebral edema

Outcome Identification and Evaluation

Child will exhibit adequate cerebral tissue perfusion through course of illness and childhood: child will remain alert and oriented with no signs of altered level of consciousness; vital signs will be within parameters for age; motor, sensory, and cognitive function will be within parameters for age; head circumference will remain within parameters for age.

(continued)

NURSING CARE PLAN 38.1

Overview for the Child With a Neurologic Disorder (continued)

Interventions: ***Promoting Adequate Tissue Perfusion***

- Assess neurologic status closely, and monitor for signs and symptoms of increased ICP: *changes in level of consciousness, signs of irritability or lethargy, and changes in pupillary reaction can indicate decreased cerebral tissue perfusion.*
- Monitor vital signs: *decreased pulse and respiratory rate and increased blood pressure or pulse pressure can indicate increased ICP, which can lead to decreased cerebral perfusion.*
- Have emergency equipment ready and available: *decreased cerebral perfusion can result in respiratory or cardiac failure.*
- Notify physician or nurse practitioner immediately if changes in assessment are noted: *early intervention is critical to prevent neurologic damage and death.*

NURSING DIAGNOSIS: Risk for injury related to altered level of consciousness, weakness, dizziness, ataxia, loss of muscle coordination secondary to seizure activity

Outcome Identification and Evaluation

Child will remain free of injury as evidenced by *no signs of aspiration or traumatic injury.*

Interventions: ***Preventing Injury***

- Ensure child has patent airway and adequate oxygenation (have suction, oxygen available at bedside) and place child in side-lying position, if possible: *a child with altered level of consciousness may not be able to manage his or her secretions and is at risk for aspiration and ineffective airway clearance; providing suction and oxygenation can help ensure an open airway and the side-lying position can help secretions drain and prevent obstruction of airway or aspiration.*
- Protect child from hurting self during seizures or changes in level of consciousness by removing environmental obstacles, easing child to lying position, and padding side rails: *helps to keep environment safe.*
- Institute seizure precautions for any child at risk for seizure activity (see Box 38.2) *to help prevent injury that can result from acute seizure activity.*
- With seizure activity do not insert a tongue blade or restrain child: *can lead to injury to caregiver and child.*
- Administer anticonvulsant medications as ordered: *will help to promote cessation and prevention of seizure activity.*
- Assist child with ambulation: *to help prevent injury in child with weakness, dizziness, or ataxia.*
- Allow for periods of rest: *to prevent fatigue and decrease risk of injury.*

NURSING DIAGNOSIS: Risk for complications of neurologic/sensory dysfunction related to presence of neurologic lesion or pressure on sensory or motor nerves secondary to increased ICP, presence of tumor, swelling postoperatively as evidenced by visual disturbances (i.e., reports of double vision), pupillary changes, nystagmus, ataxia, balance disturbances, or loss of response to stimuli

Outcome Identification and Evaluation

Child will be free of changes in sensory perception or will remain at baseline as evidenced by no complaints of double vision, PERRLA (Pupils Equal, Round, Reactive to Light and Accommodation), no disturbances of gait or balance noted, and no increase in loss of responses to stimuli.

NURSING CARE PLAN 38.1

Overview for the Child With a Neurologic Disorder (continued)

Interventions: ***Managing Disturbed Sensory Perception***

- Assess for changes in sensory perception: *provides baseline data and allows nurse to recognize change in sensory perception early.*
- Monitor child for risk of injury secondary to changes in sensory perception: *visual changes and disturbances of gait or balance increase child's risk for injury.*
- Notify physician or nurse practitioner of changes in sensory perception: *can indicate increased ICP and medical emergency.*
- Assist child to learn to use adaptive methods to live with permanent changes in sensory perception (i.e., use of eyeglasses) and maximize the use of intact senses: *adaptive devices can enhance sensory input and intact senses can often compensate for impaired senses.*
- Provide familiar sounds (voices, music): *can help relieve anxiety related to changes in sensory perception, especially visual changes.*

NURSING DIAGNOSIS: Risk for infection related to surgical interventions, presence of foreign body (i.e., shunt), trauma to skull, nutritional deficiencies, stasis of pulmonary secretions and urine, presence of infectious organisms as evidenced by fever, poor feeding, decreased responsiveness, and presence of virus or bacteria on laboratory screening

Outcome Identification and Evaluation

Child will exhibit no signs or symptoms of local or systemic infection and will not spread infection to others: *symptoms of infection will decrease over time; others will remain free of infection.*

Interventions: ***Preventing Infection***

- Monitor vital signs: *elevation in temperature can indicate presence of infection.*
- Monitor incision sites for signs of local infection: *redness, warmth, drainage, swelling, and pain at incision site can indicate presence of infection.*
- Maintain aseptic technique—practice good hand washing and use proper technique when managing postoperative incisions and external shunts: *to prevent introduction of further infectious agents.*
- Administer antibiotics as prescribed: *to prevent or treat bacterial infection.*
- Encourage nutritious diet and proper hydration according to child's preferences and ability to feed orally: *to assist body's natural defenses against infection.*
- Isolate the child as required: *to prevent nosocomial spread of infection.*
- Teach child and family preventive measures such as good hand washing, covering mouth and nose upon cough or sneeze, and adequate disposal of used tissues: *to prevent nosocomial or community spread of infection.*

NURSING DIAGNOSIS: Self-care deficit (specify) related to neuromuscular impairments; cognitive deficits as evidenced by an inability to perform hygiene care and transfer self independently

Outcome Identification and Evaluation

Child will demonstrate ability to care for self within age parameters and limits of disease: *child is able to feed, dress, and manage elimination within limits of disease and age.*

(continued)

NURSING CARE PLAN 38.1

Overview for the Child With a Neurologic Disorder (continued)

Interventions: ***Maximizing Self-Care***

- Introduce child and family to self-help methods as soon as possible: *promotes independence from the beginning.*
- Encourage family and staff to allow child to do as much as possible: *allows child to gain confidence and independence.*
- Teach specific measures for bowel and urinary elimination as needed: *promotes independence and increases self-care abilities and self-esteem.*
- Collaborate with physical therapy, occupational therapy, and speech therapy departments to provide child and family with appropriate tools to modify environment and methods to promote transferring and self-care: *allows for maximum functioning.*
- Praise accomplishments and emphasize child's abilities: *helps improve self-esteem and encourages feeling of confidence and competence.*
- Balance activity with periods to rest *to reduce fatigue and increase energy for self-care.*

NURSING DIAGNOSIS: Impaired physical mobility related to muscle weakness, hypertonicity, impaired coordination, loss of muscle function or control as evidenced by an inability to move extremities, to ambulate without assistance, to move without limitations

Outcome Identification and Evaluation

Child will be able to engage in activities within age parameters and limits of disease: child is able to move extremities, move about environment, and participate in exercise programs within limits of age and disease.

Interventions: ***Maximizing Physical Mobility***

- Encourage gross and fine motor activities: *facilitates motor development.*
- Collaborate with physical therapy, occupational therapy, and speech therapy departments to strengthen muscles and promote optimal mobility: *facilitates motor development.*
- Utilize passive and active range of motion (ROM) and teach child and family how to perform: *prevents contractures and facilitates joint mobility and muscle development (active ROM) to help increase mobility.*
- Praise accomplishments and emphasize child's abilities: *helps improve self-esteem and encourages feeling of confidence and competence.*

NURSING DIAGNOSIS: Risk for delayed development related to physical disability, cognitive deficits, activity restrictions

Outcome Identification and Evaluation

Child will demonstrate developmental milestones within age parameters and limits of disease: child expresses interest in the environment and people around him or her, and interacts with environment age appropriately.

Interventions: ***Maximizing Development***

- Use therapeutic play and adaptive toys: *helps facilitate developmental functioning.*
- Provide stimulating environment when possible *to maximize potential for growth and development.*
- Praise accomplishments and emphasize child's abilities: *helps improve self-esteem and encourages feeling of confidence and competence.*

NURSING CARE PLAN 38.1

Overview for the Child With a Neurologic Disorder (continued)

NURSING DIAGNOSIS: Nutrition, imbalanced: less than body requirements related to vomiting and difficulty feeding secondary to increased ICP; difficulty sucking, swallowing, or chewing; surgical incision pain or difficulty assuming normal feeding position; inability to feed self as evidenced by decreased oral intake, impaired swallowing, weight loss

Outcome Identification and Evaluation

Child will exhibit signs of adequate nutrition: weight will remain within parameters for age, skin turgor will be good, intake/output (I/O) will be within normal limits, adequate calories will be ingested, and vomiting will cease or decrease.

Interventions: *Promoting Adequate Nutrition*

- Monitor height and weight: *insufficient intake will lead to impaired growth and weight gain.*
- Monitor hydration status (moist mucous membranes, elastic skin turgor, adequate urine output): *insufficient intake can lead to dehydration.*
- Use techniques to promote caloric and nutritional intake and teach family (i.e., positioning, modified utensils, soft or blended foods, allow extra time): *these techniques can facilitate intake.*
- Assess respiratory system frequently *to assess for aspiration.*
- Monitor for nausea and vomiting and medicate, if ordered, *to help reduce vomiting and increase intake.*
- Monitor for pain and medicate, if ordered, *to help reduce pain related to surgical incisions and trauma, and increase intake.*
- Assist family to assume as normal a feeding position as possible *to help increase oral intake.*

NURSING DIAGNOSIS: Risk for deficient fluid volume related to vomiting, altered level of consciousness, poor feeding or intake, insensible loss due to fever, failure of regulatory mechanisms (as in diabetes insipidus) as evidenced by dry oral mucosa, decreased skin turgor, sudden weight loss, hypotension, and tachycardia

Outcome Identification and Evaluation

Fluid volume will be maintained and balanced: oral mucosa moist and pink, skin turgor elastic, urine output at least 1 to 2 mL/kg/hour.

Interventions: *Promoting Adequate Fluid Balance*

- Administer intravenous (IV) fluids, if ordered: *to maintain adequate hydration in children who are nothing by mouth (NPO) or unable to tolerate oral intake.*
- When oral intake is allowed and tolerated, encourage oral (PO) fluids: *to promote intake and maintain hydration.*
- Strict intake and output monitoring: *can help identify fluid imbalance and also detect signs of abnormal pituitary secretions resulting in conditions like syndrome of inappropriate antidiuretic hormone secretion (SIADH) and diabetes insipidus (DI) (see Chapter 48 for further information).*
- Maintain minimum hydration and avoid overhydration in children where cerebral edema is a concern: *fluid overload can contribute to cerebral edema.*
- Monitor urine specific gravity, urine and serum electrolytes (especially serum sodium), blood urea nitrogen, creatinine and osmolality, and daily weights as ordered *reliable indicators of fluid status and can also detect signs of abnormal pituitary secretions resulting in conditions like SIADH and DI.*

(continued)

NURSING CARE PLAN 38.1

Overview for the Child With a Neurologic Disorder (continued)

NURSING DIAGNOSIS: Knowledge deficit (specify) related to lack of information regarding complex medical condition, prognosis, and medical needs as evidenced by verbalization, questions, or actions demonstrating lack of understanding regarding child's condition or care

Outcome Identification and Evaluation

Child and family will verbalize accurate information and understanding about condition, prognosis, and medical needs: child and family demonstrate knowledge of condition and prognosis and medical needs including possible causes, contributing factors, and treatment measures.

Interventions: *Providing Child and Family Teaching*

- Assess child's and family's willingness to learn: *child and family must be willing to learn for teaching to be effective.*
- Provide family with time to adjust to diagnosis: *will help facilitate adjustment and ability to learn and participate in child's care.*
- Repeat information: *allows family and child time to learn and understand.*
- Teach in short sessions: *many short sessions are found to be more helpful than one long session.*
- Gear teaching to a level of understanding of the child and also the family (depends on age of child, physical condition, memory): *to ensure understanding.*
- Provide reinforcement and rewards: *helps facilitate the teaching–learning process.*
- Use multiple modes of learning involving many senses (provide written, verbal, demonstration, and videos) when possible: *child and family more likely to retain information when presented in different ways using many senses.*

NURSING DIAGNOSIS: Family processes, interrupted related to child's illness, hospitalization, diagnosis of chronic illness in child, and potential long-term effects of illness as evidenced by family's presence in hospital, missed work, demonstration of inadequate coping

Outcome Identification and Evaluation

Family will maintain functional system of support and demonstrate adequate coping, adaptation of roles and functions, and decreased anxiety: *parents are involved in child's care, ask appropriate questions, express fears and concerns, and are able to discuss child's care and condition calmly.*

Interventions: *Promoting Adequate Family Processes*

- Encourage parents and family members to verbalize concerns related to child's illness, diagnosis, and prognosis: *allows the nurse to identify concerns and areas where further education may be needed; demonstrates family-centered care.*
- Explain therapies, procedures, child's behaviors, and plan of care to parents: *understanding the child's current status and plan of care helps decrease anxiety.*
- Encourage parental involvement in care: *allows parents to feel needed and valued with a sense of control over their child's health.*
- Identify support system for family and child: *helps nurse identify needs and resources available for coping.*
- Educate family and child on additional resources available: *to help them develop a wide base of support.*

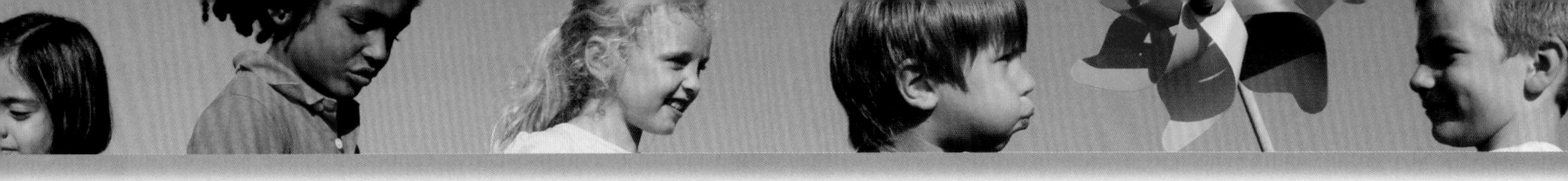

KEY CONCEPTS

- Development of the brain and spinal cord occurs early in gestation, in the first 3 to 4 weeks. Infection, trauma, teratogens, and malnutrition during this period can result in malformations and may affect normal CNS development.
- The brain of the newborn is highly vascular, leading to an increased risk for hemorrhage.
- The head of the infant and young child is large in proportion to the body, and the neck muscles are not well developed, which places the infant at an increased risk of head injury from falls and accidents.
- Neurologic disorders in children can result from congenital problems as well as infections or trauma.
- LP and CSF analysis can be useful in the diagnosis of hemorrhage, infection, or obstruction.
- CT and MRI studies can be useful in diagnosing congenital abnormalities such as neural tube defects, hemorrhage, tumors, fractures, demyelination, or inflammation.
- EEGs measure the electrical activity of the brain and can be used in diagnosing seizures or brain death.
- Antibiotics are utilized in the treatment of bacterial meningitis and shunt infections.
- Anticonvulsants are used in the treatment and prevention of seizures and are often used in combination.
- Corticosteroids are used to reduce cerebral edema and must be tapered before discontinuing.
- Risk factors associated with neurologic disorders include prematurity, difficult birth, infection during pregnancy, family history of genetic disorders with a neurologic manifestation, seizure disorders, and headaches.
- Alterations in motor function, such as changes in gait or muscle tone or strength, may indicate certain neurologic problems such as increased ICP, head injury, and cerebral infections.
- Increased ICP is a sign that may occur with many neurologic disorders. It may result from head trauma, birth trauma, hydrocephalus, infection, and brain tumors. It is essential that the nurse observes for signs and symptoms associated with increased ICP while caring for a child with a potential or suspected neurologic disorder.
- Sunset eyes may indicate increased ICP as seen in hydrocephalus.
- A bulging fontanel can be a sign of increased ICP and is seen in such neurologic disorders as hydrocephalus and head traumas.
- Cortical control of motor function is lost in certain neurologic disorders; postural reflexes re-emerge and are directly related to the area of the brain that is damaged. Decorticate posturing occurs with damage of the cerebral cortex. Decerebrate posturing occurs with damage at the level of the brain stem.
- Nursing management of seizures focuses on preventing injury during seizures, instituting seizure precautions, maintaining a patent airway, administering appropriate medication and treatments to prevent or reduce seizures, and providing education and support to the child and family to help them cope with the challenges of living with a chronic seizure disorder.
- Hydrocephalus results from an imbalance in the production and absorption of CSF. Key assessment findings include a rapid increase in head circumference seen in the infant, or loss of development and changes in personality in the older child. Signs and symptoms associated with increased ICP may be seen.
- Nursing management of the child with hydrocephalus will focus on maintaining cerebral perfusion, minimizing neurologic complications, recognizing and preventing shunt infection and malfunction, maintaining adequate nutrition, promoting growth and development, and supporting and educating the child and family.
- Bacterial meningitis requires rapid assessment and treatment. On assessment, the nurse may find the infant with bacterial meningitis resting in the opisthotonic position, and the older child may complain of neck pain.
- Nursing management of the child with bacterial meningitis will include administration of intravenous antibiotics, reducing ICP, and maintaining cerebral perfusion along with treating fluid volume deficit, controlling seizures, and preventing injury that may result from altered LOC or seizure activity.

- Nurses play a key role in educating the public on topics such as helmet use with certain sports, bicycle and motorcycle safety, car seat and seat belt use, and providing adequate supervision of children to help prevent injuries and accidents and resultant head trauma from occurring.
- Many neurologic disorders affect multiple body systems with lifelong deficits that require long-term rehabilitation. Adjusting to the demands this condition places on the child and family is difficult. Parents may need time to accept their child's condition but as soon as possible they should be involved in the child's care.
- Children with neurologic disorders and their families often need large amounts of education and support throughout the child's lifetime. As the child grows, the needs of the family and child will change. The nurse needs to provide ongoing education and support.
- Some neurologic disorders require complete intensive daily care. Adjusting to these demands can be difficult for the family. Encourage respite care and provide meaningful education programs that emphasize independence for the child in the least restrictive educational environment. Refer caregivers to local resources, including education services and support groups.

REFERENCES AND RECOMMENDED READINGS

American Academy of Pediatrics. (2010). Prevention of drowning. *Pediatrics, 126*(1), 178–185.

American Academy of Pediatrics. (2015). *Meningococcal vaccines: What you need to know.* Healthy Children. Retrieved from http://www.healthychildren.org/English/safety-prevention/immunizations/pages/Meningococcal-Vaccines-What-You-Need-to-Know.aspx?

American Academy of Pediatrics, Committee on Genetics. (2012). Folic acid for the prevention of neural tube defects. *Pediatrics.* Retrieved from http://pediatrics.aappublications.org/content/104/2/325.full

American Academy of Pediatrics, Steering Committee on Quality Improvement and Management, Subcommittee on Febrile Seizures. (2008). Febrile seizures: Clinical practice guideline for the long-term management of the child with simple febrile seizures. *Pediatrics, 121* (6), 1281–1286.

American Academy of Pediatrics, Subcommittee on Febrile Seizures. (2011). Clinical Practice Guideline: Febrile Seizures: Guideline for the Neurodiagnostic Evaluation of the Child With a Simple Febrile Seizure. *Pediatrics, 127*(2), 389–394.

American Heart Association, American Stroke Association. (2013). *FACTS knowing no bounds: Stroke in infants, children and youth.* Retrieved from http://www.heart.org/idc/groups/heart-public/@wcm/@adv/documents/downloadable/ucm_302255.pdf

Bagley, A. F., Daniel, H., Daneshvar, D. H., Schanker, B. D., Zurakowski, D., d'Hemecourt, C. A. et al. (2012). Effectiveness of the SLICE Program for Youth Concussion. *Clinical Journal of Sport Medicine, 22*(5), 385–389.

Bautista, C. (2014). Chapter 20: Disorders of Brain Function. In: S. Grossman, & C. M. Porth (Eds.), *Porth's pathophysiology: Concepts of altered health states* (9th ed., pp. 489–574). Philadelphia, PA: Wolters Kluwer Health/Lippincott Williams & Wilkins.

Berg, A. T., Berkovic, S. F., Brodie, M. J., Buchhalter, J., Cross, J. H., van Emde Boas, W., et al. (2010). Special Report: Revised terminology and concepts for organization of seizures and epilepsies: Report of the ILAE Commission on Classification and Terminology, 2005–2009. *Epilepsia, 51*(4), 676–685.

Block, S. L. (2012). 'Skull-Duggery' and the Management of Positional Plagiocephaly. *Pediatric Annals, 41*(12), 497–501.

Bonthius, D. J., Lee, A. G., Hershey, A. D. (2015). Headache in children: Approach to evaluation and general management strategies. UpToDate. Retrieved from http://www.uptodate.com/contents/headache-in-children-approach-to-evaluation-and-general-management-strategies

Carpenito, L. J. (2013). *Nursing diagnosis: Application to clinical practice* (14th ed.). Philadelphia, PA: Lippincott Williams & Wilkins.

Centers for Disease Control and Prevention (2000). Meningococcal disease and college students. Recommendations of the Advisory Committee on Immunization Practices (ACIP). *MMWR Recommendations and Reports 49 (RR07),* 11–20.

Centers for Disease Control and Prevention. (2014a). *Meningitis: Bacterial meningiti.* Retrieved from http://www.cdc.gov/meningitis/bacterial.html

Centers for Disease Control and Prevention. (2014b). *Meningitis: Viral Meningiti.* Retrieved from http://www.cdc.gov/meningitis/viral.html

Centers for Disease Control and Prevention. (2014c). *Unintentional drowning: Fact sheet.* Retrieved from http://www.cdc.gov/HomeandRecreationalSafety/Water-Safety/waterinjuries-factsheet.html

Centers for Disease Control and Prevention. (2015). *Meningococcal outbreaks.* Retrieved from http://www.cdc.gov/meningococcal/outbreaks/index.html

Centers for Disease Control and Prevention. (2015a). *Folic acid: Recommendations.* Retrieved from http://www.cdc.gov/ncbddd/folicacid/recommendations.html

Centers for Disease Control and Prevention. (2015b). *Epilepsy: Frequently asked questions.* Retrieved from http://www.cdc.gov/epilepsy/basics/faqs.htm#5

Child Trends Databank. (2014). *Unintentional injuries.* Retrieved from http://www.childtrends.org/?indicators=unintentional-injuries

Christian, C., & Endom, E. E. (2015). Child abuse: Evaluation and diagnosis of abusive head trauma in infants and children. UpToDate. Retrieved from http://www.uptodate.com/contents/child-abuse-evaluation-and-diagnosis-of-abusive-head-trauma-in-infants-and-children

Cincinnati Children's. (2015). Health Topics: Endoscopic third ventriculostomy. Retrieved from http://www.cincinnatichildrens.org/health/e/endoscopic/

Fischbach, F. T., & Dunning, M. B. III (2015). *A manual of laboratory and diagnostic tests* (9th ed.). Philadelphia, PA: Wolters Kluwer Health/Lippincott Williams & Wilkins.

Fisher, R. S., Acevedo, C., Arzimanoglou, A., Bogacz, A., Cross, J. H., Elger, C. E., et al. (2014). ILAE Official Report: A practical clinical definition of epilepsy. *Epilepsia, 55*(4):475–482.

Glaze, D. G. (2015). Clinical features and diagnosis of infantile spasms. UpToDate. Retrieved from http://www.uptodate.com/contents/clinical-features-and-diagnosis-of-infantile-spasms

Hardarson, H. S. (2015). Acute viral encephalitis in children and adolescents: Clinical manifestations and diagnosis. UpToDate. Retrieved from http://www.uptodate.com/contents/acute-viral-encephalitis-in-children-and-adolescents-clinical-manifestations-and-diagnosis

Hochberg, L., & Stone, J. (2015). Prenatal screening and diagnosis of neural tube defects. UpToDate. Retrieved from http://www.uptodate.com/contents/prenatal-screening-and-diagnosis-of-neural-tube-defects

International League Against Epilepsy. (2014) Seizure classification. Retrieved from https://www.epilepsydiagnosis.org/seizure/seizure-classification-groupoverview.html

Johnston, M. V. (2011). Chapter 591: Encephalopathies. In: R. M. Kleigman, B. F. Stanton, J. W. St. Geme III, N. F. Schor, & R. E. Behrman (Eds.), *Nelson textbook of pediatrics* (19th ed., pp. 2061–2068). Philadelphia, PA: Saunders.

Khoury, C. (2015). Chiari malformations. UpToDate. Retrieved from http://www.uptodate.com/contents/chiari-malformations

Kinsman, S. L., & Johnston, M. V. (2011). Chapter 585: Congenital anomalies of the central nervous system. In: R. M. Kleigman, B. F. Stanton, J. W. St. Geme III, N. F. Schor, & R. E. Behrman (Eds.), *Nelson textbook of pediatrics* (19th ed., pp. 1998–2013). Philadelphia, PA: Saunders.

Korff, C. M., & Wirrell, E. (2014). ILAE classification of seizures and epilepsy. UpToDate. Retrieved from http://www.uptodate.com/contents/ilae-classification-of-seizures-and-epilepsy

Kossoff, E. H. W. (2014). The ketogenic diet. UpToDate. Retrieved from http://www.uptodate.com/contents/the-ketogenic-diet

MacNeil, J. & Amanda Cohn, A. (2011). Chapter 8: Meningococcal Disease. In: Centers for Disease Control and Prevention. *Manual for the surveillance of vaccine-preventable diseases*. Atlanta, GA: Centers for Disease Control and Prevention.

Mikati, M. A. (2011). Chapter 586. Seizures in childhood. In: R. M. Kleigman, B. F. Stanton, J. W. St. Geme III, N. F. Schor, & R. E. Behrman (Eds.), *Nelson textbook of pediatrics* (19th ed., pp. 2013–2039). Philadelphia, PA: Saunders.

Millichap, J. J., & Millichap, J. G. (2015). Treatment and prognosis of febrile seizures. UpToDate. Retrieved from http://www.uptodate.com/contents/treatment-and-prognosis-of-febrile-seizures

National Institute of Neurological Disorders and Stroke. (2015). *The epilepsies and seizures: Hope through research*. Retrieved from http://www.ninds.nih.gov/disorders/epilepsy/detail_epilepsy.htm

Nguyen, T. T., Kaplan, P. W., & Wilfong, A. (2014). Nonepileptic paroxysmal disorders in infancy. UpToDate. Retrieved from http://www.uptodate.com/contents/nonepileptic-paroxysmal-disorders-in-infancy?source=preview&search=breath+holding+spells+children&selectedTitle=1~13&language=en-US&anchor=H8#H8

Pellico, L. H. (2012). *Focus on adult health: Medical-surgical nursing*. Philadelphia, PA: Lippincott Williams & Wilkins.

Prober, C. G., & Dyner, L. (2011). Chapter 595: Central nervous system infections. In: R. M. Kleigman, B. F. Stanton, J.W. St. Geme III, N. F. Schor, & R. E. Behrman (Eds.), *Nelson textbook of pediatrics* (19th ed., pp. 2086–2098). Philadelphia, PA: Saunders.

Roach, E. S., deVeber, G., Riela, A. R., & Wiznitzer, M. (2011). *Recognition and treatment of stroke in children*. Retrieved from http://www.ninds.nih.gov/news_and_events/proceedings/stroke_proceedings/childneurology.htm

Shellhaas, R. (2015a). *Clinical features, evaluation, and diagnosis of neonatal seizures*. Retrieved from http://www.uptodate.com/contents/clinical-features-evaluation-and-diagnosis-of-neonatal-seizures

Shellhaas, R. (2015b). *Etiology and prognosis of neonatal seizures*. Retrieved from http://www.uptodate.com/contents/etiology-and-prognosis-of-neonatal-seizures

Shellhaas, R. (2015c). *Treatment of neonatal seizures*. Retrieved from http://www.uptodate.com/contents/treatment-of-neonatal-seizures

Smith, S. E. & Fox, C. (2015). Ischemic stroke in children and young adults: Etiology and clinical features. UpToDate. Retrieved from http://www.uptodate.com/contents/ischemic-stroke-in-children-and-young-adults-etiology-and-clinical-features

Taketokmo, C. K., Hodding, J. H., & Kraus, D. M. (2013). *Lexi-comp's drug reference handbook: Pediatric & neonatal dosage handbook* (20th ed.). Hudson, OH: Lexi-comp, Inc.

Tomita, T., & Ogiwara, H. (2015). Anencephaly. UpToDate. Retrieved from http://www.uptodate.com/contents/anencephaly?source=search_result&search=neural+tube+defects&selectedTitle=3~150

U.S. Department of Health & Human Services. (2015). Healthy people 2020. Retrieved at http://www.healthypeople.gov/

Wilfong, A. (2015). Overview of the classification, etiology, and clinical features of pediatric seizures and epilepsy. UpToDate. Retrieved from http://www.uptodate.com/contents/overview-of-the-classification-etiology-and-clinical-features-of-pediatric-seizures-and-epilepsy?

Yadav, Y. R., Parihar, V., Pande, S., Namdev, H., & Agarwal M. (2012). Endoscopic third ventriculostomy. *Journal of Neurosciences in Rural Practice, 3*(2):163–173.

Zak, M., & Chan, V. W. (2014). Chapter 46: Pediatric neurologic disorders. In: S. M. Nettina (Ed.), *Lippincott manual of nursing practice* (10th ed., pp. 1545–1575). Philadelphia, PA: Wolters/Kluwer Health: Lippincott Williams & Wilkins.

CHAPTER WORKSHEET

MULTIPLE CHOICE QUESTIONS

1. When compared with adults, why are infants and children at an increased risk of head trauma?
   a. The head of the infant and young child is large in proportion to the body and the neck muscles are not well developed.
   b. The development of the nervous system is complete at birth but remains immature.
   c. The spine is very immobile in infants and young children.
   d. The skull is more flexible due to the presence of sutures and fontanels.
2. At a well-child visit, hydrocephalus may be suspected in an infant if upon assessment the nurse finds
   a. narrow sutures
   b. sunken fontanels
   c. a rapid increase in head circumference
   d. increase in weight since last visit
3. A 10-year-old child is admitted to the hospital due to history of seizure activity. As his nurse, you are called into the room by his mother, who states he is having a seizure. What would be the priority nursing intervention related to prevention of injury?
   a. Remove the child from his bed.
   b. Place a tongue blade in the child's mouth.
   c. Restrain the child.
   d. Place the child on his side and opening his airway.
4. A 6-month-old infant is admitted to the hospital with suspected bacterial meningitis. She is crying, irritable, and lying in the opisthotonic position. The priority nursing intervention would be:
   a. Educate the family on ways to prevent bacterial meningitis.
   b. Initiate appropriate isolation precautions and begin intravenous antibiotics.
   c. Assess the infant's fontanels.
   d. Encourage the mother to hold the infant and feed her.

DOSAGE CALCULATION QUESTION

The nurse is caring for a child who is in status epilepticus. The child weighs 14.97 kg (33 lb). The medication order reads: Diazepam 3 mg IV push now. Per the Pediatric Dosage Handbook, the recommended dose is 0.1 to 0.3 mg/kg/dose. Diazepam is supplied as 5 mg/mL.

How many milliliters will the nurse administer? Round to the nearest tenth.

CRITICAL THINKING EXERCISES

1. A child is seen in the doctor's office after hitting his head while skateboarding. The child suffered no loss of consciousness, and has no external injuries and no significant past medical history. He is acting appropriately at this time. His only complaint is a dull headache. What instructions would you give the parents regarding his care at home? Include when they should seek further medical care.
2. A 10-year-old child is admitted to the pediatric unit after experiencing a seizure. A complete, accurate, and detailed history from a reliable source is essential. What information would you ask for while obtaining the history?
3. A 6-year-old child is admitted to the hospital because of a possible seizure. The child's mother calls the nurse to the room because the child is "jerking all over" and won't respond when she calls the child's name. List appropriate nursing interventions for this child. Prioritize the list of interventions.
4. Describe the impact of a cerebral vascular accident in the child as compared with the adult. How does it affect the child's future? How will the nurse provide care differently for the child stroke victim as compared with the adult?

STUDY ACTIVITIES

1. A 4-month-old child with a history of hydrocephalus has undergone surgery for placement of a VP shunt. What information would you include in the teaching plan?
2. Develop an example of a "headache log" that could be used by the family for chronicling the child's headaches, including triggers, relieving factors, and precipitating events. Ensure that the log is developed at a 6th-grade reading level to make it practical for low-literacy parents.
3. In the clinical setting, interview the parent of a child who has suffered significant brain trauma or injury (such as head trauma, IVH, or stroke). Talk with the family about the types of care the child requires. Reflect upon this interview in your clinical journal, and compare how the ongoing care for this child compares with that for a typical child.

BRINGING IT ALL TOGETHER: A CASE STUDY

Sandra and Michael Graham have brought their 6-month-old son, Thomas, to the pediatric unit for observation. Thomas's head circumference has increased from the 25th percentile at the 4-month check-up to the 75th percentile at the 6-month check-up. Upon assessment, the nurse notes a bulging anterior fontanel and persistent primitive reflexes.

Go to thePoint to find questions to consider about this case.

39

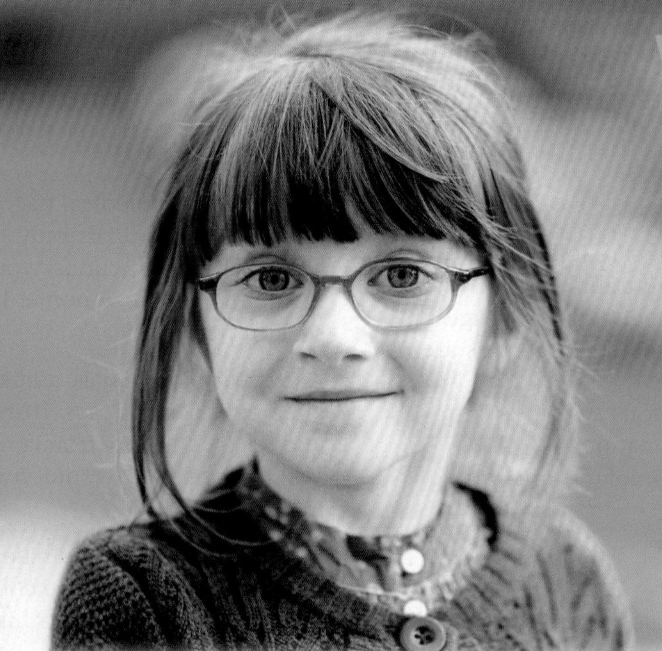

Words of Wisdom
With the help of a nurse's care and healing, the child's senses provide him or her with an antenna to the universe.

Nursing Care of the Child With an Alteration in Sensory Perception/Disorder of the Eyes or Ears

KEY TERMS
acuity
amblyopia
blindness
conductive hearing loss
deafness
decibel
hearing impairment
nystagmus
pressure-equalizing (PE) tubes
ptosis
sensorineural hearing loss
sensory perception
strabismus
tympanometry
tympanostomy
vision impairment

Learning Objectives

Upon completion of the chapter, you will be able to:

1. Differentiate between the anatomic and physiologic differences of the eyes and ears in children as compared with adults.
2. Identify various factors associated with disorders of the eyes and ears in infants and children.
3. Discuss common laboratory and other diagnostic tests useful in the diagnosis of disorders of the eyes and ears.
4. Discuss common medications and other treatments used for treatment and palliation of conditions affecting the eyes and ears.
5. Recognize risk factors associated with various disorders of the eyes and ears.
6. Distinguish between different disorders of the eyes and ears based on the signs and symptoms associated with them.
7. Discuss nursing interventions commonly used in regard to disorders of the eyes and ears.
8. Devise an individualized nursing care plan for the child with a sensory impairment or other disorder of the eyes or ears.
9. Develop child/family teaching plans for the child with a disorder of the eyes or ears.
10. Describe the psychosocial impact of sensory impairments on children.

***Enrique Baxter*, a 9-month-old, is brought to the clinic by his mother. His mother tells you, "Enrique has been fussy and not eating or sleeping well for the past 2 days."**

Sensory perception refers to receiving and interpreting stimuli. Disorders of the eyes or ears may lead to alterations in sensory perception. It is important for nurses to understand how to appropriately intervene for sensory perception alterations as well as other eye and ear disorders.

Children commonly suffer from disorders related to the eyes and ears. Conjunctivitis and otitis media are two very common infectious and inflammatory disorders that affect the child's eyes or ears. Various alterations such as refractive error, strabismus, and amblyopia affect the development of visual **acuity** in children. Any alteration in the ear that contributes to the sensory perception alteration of hearing loss may have a significant impact on the child's language acquisition. It is important for the nurse to understand the impact of eye and ear disorders on the child's development. Some children may be born with anomalies of the eyes or ears that will have a significant impact on vision and hearing, as well as psychomotor development. On the other hand, disorders affecting the eyes or ears, particularly if chronic or recurrent, can have a significant impact on the development of visual acuity or may cause **hearing impairment**.

In addition, the nurse may be caring for a child with another problem who is also either visually or hearing impaired. The nurse must take these developmental differences into account when planning care for these children.

VARIATIONS IN PEDIATRIC ANATOMY AND PHYSIOLOGY

The anatomy of children's eyes and ears differs somewhat from that of adults. In addition, visual acuity develops from birth throughout early childhood. Hearing is intact at birth, but recurrent ear disorders may adversely affect the child's hearing.

Eyes

Light-skinned children are often born with blue eyes. The iris becomes pigmented over time and eye color is determined by 6 to 12 months of age. The newborn's sclera may be slightly bluish tinged but becomes white within weeks. The eyeball of the infant and young child occupies a relatively larger space within the orbit than the adult's does, making it more susceptible to injury (Fig. 39.1).

The spherical shape of the newborn's lens does not allow for distance accommodation, so the newborn sees best at a distance of about 8 to 10 in and a decreased number of cones further contributes to neonatal blurry vision (Bremond-Gignac, Copin, Lapillone, & Milazzo, 2011). The optic nerve is not completely myelinated, so color discrimination is incomplete. Visual acuity develops over the first few years of the child's life. At birth, acuity ranges from 20/100 to 20/400. Visual acuity improves over the first few years of the child's life, with 20/20 achieved by age 6 to 7 years (Weber & Kelley, 2014). The rectus muscles are uncoordinated at birth and mature over time so that binocular vision (the ability to focus with both eyes simultaneously) may be achieved by 4 months of age (Weber & Kelley, 2014). In the very preterm infant, retinal vascularization is incomplete, so visual acuity may be affected (American Academy of Pediatrics [AAP], 2013b; Bremond-Gignac et al., 2011).

Ears

Congenital deformities of the ear are often associated with other body system anomalies and genetic syndromes. The presence of ear anomalies may lead to the search for, and subsequent diagnosis of, the other anomalies or syndromes. The infant's relatively short, wide, and horizontally placed Eustachian tubes allow bacteria and viruses to gain access to the middle ear easily, resulting in increased numbers of ear infections as compared to the adult (Friedman, Scholes, & Yoon, 2014). As the child matures, the tubes assume a more slanted position. Therefore, older children and adults generally have fewer cases of middle ear effusion and infection (Fig. 39.2). Sometimes enlargement of the adenoids contributes to obstruction of the Eustachian tubes, leading to infection.

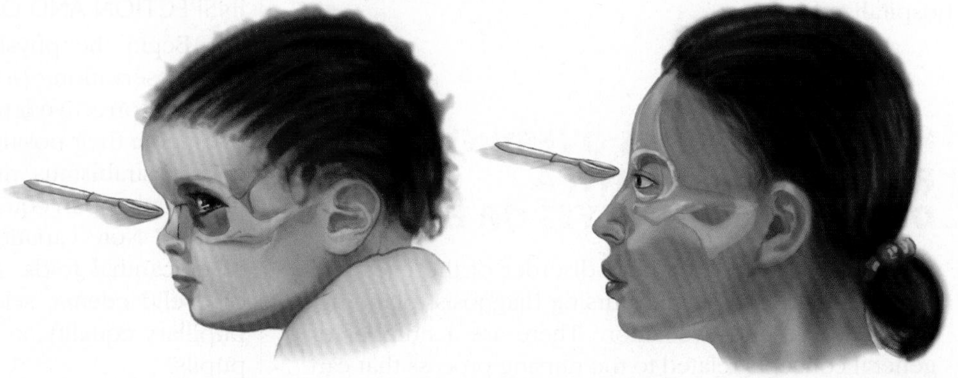

FIGURE 39.1 The relatively larger space that the infant's and young child's eyeball occupies within the orbit makes it more susceptible to injury as compared with the adult's eye.

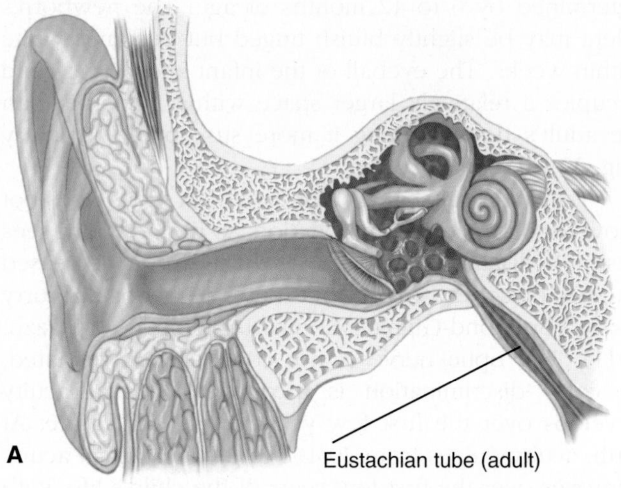

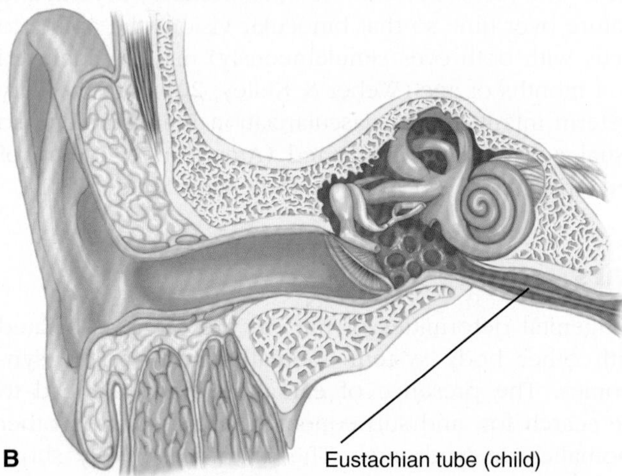

FIGURE 39.2 Note the child's relatively shorter, wider Eustachian tubes and their horizontal positioning (**B**) as compared with the adult's (**A**).

COMMON MEDICAL TREATMENTS

A variety of interventions are used to treat disorders of the eyes and ears in children. The treatments listed in Common Medical Treatments 39.1 and Drug Guide 39.1 usually require a physician's order when a child is hospitalized.

NURSING PROCESS OVERVIEW FOR THE CHILD WITH A DISORDER OF THE EYES OR EARS

Care of the child with a disorder of the eyes and ears includes assessment, nursing diagnosis, planning, interventions, and evaluation. There are a number of general concepts related to the nursing process that can be applied to disorders of the eyes and ears. From a general understanding of the care involved for a child with alterations in the eyes or ears, the nurse can then individualize the care based on child specifics.

Assessment

Assessment of disorders of the eyes and ears in children includes health history, physical assessment, and laboratory or diagnostic testing.

Remember Enrique, the 9-month-old with fussiness and poor feeding who was not sleeping well? What additional health history and physical examination assessment information should you obtain?

Health History

The health history consists of past medical history, family history, history of present illness, and treatments used at home. The past medical history may be significant for prematurity, genetic defect, eye or ear deformities, visual acuity deficit or blindness, hearing impairment or **deafness**, recurrent ear infections, or ear surgeries. Family history might be significant for eye or ear deformities or vision or hearing impairment or may reveal contacts for infectious exposure.

When eliciting the history of the present illness, inquire about its onset and progression and the presence of fever, nasal congestion, eye or ear pain, eye rubbing, ear pulling, headache, lethargy, or behavioral changes. Document if the child has corrective lenses or hearing aids prescribed and to what extent these devices are actually used.

Physical Examination

When assessing the eyes and ears, begin with inspection and observation. In addition, testing of visual activity and hearing may be performed.

INSPECTION AND OBSERVATION

Begin the physical examination with inspection and observation. Note whether the child uses eyeglasses, corrective lenses, or a hearing aid. Observe the eyes: note their positioning and symmetry and the presence of strabismus, nystagmus, and squinting. The eyelids should open equally (failure to open fully is termed **ptosis**). Note variations in eye slant and the presence of epicanthal folds. Assess the eyes for the presence of eyelid edema, sclera color, discharge, tearing, and pupillary equality, as well as the size and shape of the pupils.

COMMON MEDICAL TREATMENTS 39.1

Treatment	Explanation	Indications	Nursing Implications
Warm compress	Warm, moist washcloth	Conjunctivitis	• Use very warm water from the tap (to avoid risk of burning, do not microwave).
Corrective lenses	In eyeglass form or as contact lenses	Correction of astigmatism, refractive error, strabismus	• Use a safety strap to help young children wear their eyeglasses.
Patching	An adhesive patch is applied to the healthier eye for several hours each day.	Strabismus, amblyopia, any other eye condition that results in one eye being weaker than the other	• Inform parents that though difficult to obtain, compliance with patching is critical. • A "pirate patch" may coax preschoolers into compliance.
Eye muscle surgery	Surgical alignment of the eyes	Strabismus	• Protect the operative site with patching. • Use elbow restraints if necessary.
Pressure-equalizing (PE) tubes (tympanostomy tubes)	Tiny plastic tubes inserted in the tympanic membrane	Chronic otitis media with effusion	• Teach parents dry ears precautions if prescribed or preferred by the surgeon. Dry ears can be achieved by placing a cotton ball coated in petroleum jelly over the ear canal, in order to create a watertight seal.
Hearing aids	Amplification device worn in the ear	Hearing impairment	• Ensure appropriate fit and adequate amplification. • Direct families to outfitters that provide loaner aids of various brands and styles to determine best fit and amplification for the child.
Cochlear implants	Surgically inserted electronic prosthetic device	Sensorineural hearing loss	• Inform families that the usual minimum age for this procedure is 12 months.

Adapted from National Institute on Deafness and Other Communication Disorders. (2016). *Cochlear implants.* Retrieved from https://www.nidcd.nih.gov/health/cochlear-implants; and Friedman, N. R., Scholes, M. A., & Yoon, P. J. (2014). Ear, nose, & throat. In W. W. Hay, M. J. Levin, R. R. Deterding, & M. J. Abzug, (Eds.), *Current pediatric diagnosis and treatment* (22nd ed.). New York, NY: McGraw-Hill.

DRUG GUIDE 39.1 COMMON DRUGS FOR EAR AND EYE DISORDERS

Medication	Actions	Indications	Nursing Implications
Antibiotics (oral, otic, ophthalmic)	Treatment of bacterial infections of the eyes and ears	Acute otitis media, otitis externa, conjunctivitis	Teach families to complete the entire course as prescribed. Check for drug allergies prior to administration.
Antihistamines	Block histamine reaction	Allergic conjunctivitis	Topical drops used. Oral agents usually prescribed if allergic rhinitis accompanies the conjunctivitis.
Analgesics	Pain relief	Otitis media, otitis externa, after eye or ear surgery	Narcotic analgesics may be necessary in some instances.

Adapted from Taketomo, C. K., Hodding, J. H., & Kraus, D. M. (2013). *Pediatric & neonatal dosage handbook* (20th ed.). Hudson, OH: Lexicomp.

Take Note!

Though the sclerae are bluish in newborns, they become white in the first few weeks of life. Blue sclerae that persist beyond a few weeks of life may be an indicator of osteogenesis imperfecta type I, an inherited connective tissue disorder (Weber & Kelley, 2014).

Evert the eyelid to inspect the palpebral conjunctivae for redness. Test for extraocular movements and pupillary light response and accommodation. Note the symmetry of the corneal light reflex. Note the presence of the red reflex with an ophthalmoscope. Perform an age-appropriate visual acuity test. Refer to Chapter 31 for more detailed information related to visual acuity testing.

Take Note!

Attempts to inspect the palpebral conjunctivae may be frightening to children. Ask the older, cooperative child to evert the eyelid himself or herself while the nurse inspects the conjunctivae.

Inspect the ears: note their size and shape, position, and the presence of skin tags, dimples, or other anomalies (Fig. 39.3). Upon otoscopic examination, note the presence of cerumen, discharge, inflammation, or a foreign body in the ear canal. Visualize the tympanic membrane and observe its color, landmarks, and light reflex, as well as the presence of perforation, scars, bulging, or retraction. Tympanic membrane mobility may be tested with pneumatic otoscopy. Auditory acuity is tested via the whisper test, audiometry, or other age-appropriate test (refer to Chapter 31 for a more detailed explanation of hearing testing).

PALPATION

Usually, the eyes are not palpated. In the case of injury the upper eyelid may be everted for examination purposes. Palpate the ear for tenderness over the tragus or pinna. Note the presence of tenderness over the mastoid area (tenderness may be present when otitis media progresses to mastoiditis). Palpate for enlarged cervical lymph nodes (this occurs when the eyes or ears are infected).

Laboratory and Diagnostic Testing

Common Laboratory and Diagnostic Tests 39.1 offers an explanation of the laboratory and diagnostic tests most commonly used for disorders of the eyes and ears. These tests can assist the physician or nurse practitioner in diagnosing the disorder and/or can be used as guidelines in determining ongoing treatment. Laboratory or nonnursing personnel obtain some of the tests, while the nurse may obtain others. In either instance be familiar with how the tests are obtained, what they are used for, and normal versus abnormal results. This knowledge will also be necessary when providing child and family education related to the testing.

Nursing Diagnoses and Related Interventions

Upon completion of a thorough assessment, the nurse might identify several nursing diagnoses, including:

- Disturbed sensory perception
- Risk for infection
- Pain
- Delayed growth and development
- Impaired verbal communication
- Deficient knowledge
- Interrupted family processes
- Risk for injury

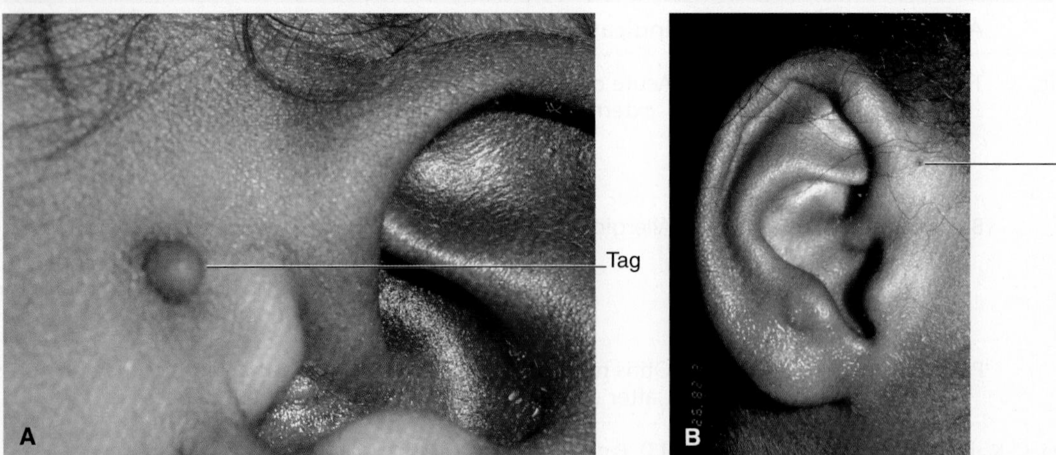

FIGURE 39.3 Note the skin tag **(A)** and preauricular pit **(B)** (in front of the ear).

COMMON LABORATORY AND DIAGNOSTIC TESTS 39.1

Test	Explanation	Indications	Nursing Implications
Culture of eye or ear discharge	Fluid draining from the eye or ear is cultured	To determine specific bacteria present and appropriate antibiotic coverage	Easy to collect, relatively pain-free. If drainage must be removed from within the ear canal, more likely to be painful
Tympanic fluid culture	Culture of fluid aspirated from the middle ear	To determine specific bacteria present and appropriate antibiotic coverage	Painful; usually performed only by specially trained physicians
Tympanometry	Probe in ear canal measures movement of the eardrum	Determines extent of effusion of the middle ear	Quick and easy to perform (seconds). Requires accurate-sized probe for adequate seal of the ear canal

Adapted from Friedman, N. R., Scholes, M. A., & Yoon, P. J. (2014). Ear, nose, & throat. In W. W. Hay, M. J. Levin, & R. R. Deterding, & M. J. Abzug, (Eds.), *Current pediatric diagnosis and treatment* (22nd ed.). New York, NY: McGraw-Hill.

After completing an assessment of Enrique, the nurse noted the following: fever, tugging at his ears, and increased crying when lying down. Based on the assessment findings, what would your top three nursing diagnoses be for Enrique?

Nursing goals, interventions, and evaluation for the child with an eye or ear disorder are based on the nursing diagnoses. Nursing Care Plan 39.1, at the end of the chapter, may be used as a guide in planning nursing care for the child with an eye or ear disorder, but it should be individualized based on the child's symptoms and needs. Refer to Chapter 36 for the nursing care plan for pain management. Additional information will be included later in the chapter as it relates to specific disorders.

Based on your top three nursing diagnoses for Enrique, describe appropriate nursing interventions.

INFECTIOUS AND INFLAMMATORY DISORDERS OF THE EYES

Infectious and inflammatory disorders of the eyes include conjunctivitis, nasolacrimal duct obstruction, eyelid lesions, and periorbital cellulitis.

Conjunctivitis

Inflammation of the bulbar or palpebral conjunctiva is referred to as conjunctivitis. It can be infectious, allergic, or chemical in nature. Viruses or bacteria may cause infectious conjunctivitis. Adenoviruses and influenza account for the bulk of cases of viral conjunctivitis. The most common bacterial cause is *Staphylococcus aureus,* but many cases are also caused by *Streptococcus pneumoniae, Haemophilus influenzae,* and other bacteria (Friedman et al., 2014). In the newborn, *Chlamydia trachomatis* and *Neisseria gonorrhoeae* are more common causes. Infectious conjunctivitis is very contagious, so epidemics are common, particularly in young children. Risk factors for acute infectious conjunctivitis include age younger than 2 weeks; day care, preschool, or school attendance; concomitant viral upper respiratory infection; pharyngitis; or otitis media. Concurrent acute otitis media (AOM) may occur depending on the bacterial cause. Complications from simple infectious conjunctivitis are uncommon. Neonates with chlamydial conjunctivitis may be at risk for the development of chlamydial pneumonia.

Allergic conjunctivitis results from exposure to particular allergens. Allergic conjunctivitis may be a seasonal or year-round complaint. A genetic predisposition to allergic conjunctivitis exists, just as it does for asthma, allergic rhinitis, and atopic dermatitis. Allergic conjunctivitis occurs more frequently in school-age children and adolescents than it does in infants and young children because of repeat exposure to allergens over time. In the case of seasonal allergic conjunctivitis, the severity of symptoms and the number of children affected are directly related to the pollen count in the area.

Pathophysiology

When bacteria or viruses come in contact with the bulbar or palpebral conjunctiva, they are recognized as foreign antigens and an antigen–antibody immune reaction occurs, resulting in inflammation. Allergic conjunctivitis occurs through a different mechanism. Contact with the allergen results in an allergic response (overreaction of the immune response). The mast cell and histamine mediators are then activated, resulting in inflammation.

Therapeutic Management

Therapeutic management of conjunctivitis is prescribed depending on the cause. Bacterial conjunctivitis is generally treated with an ophthalmic antibiotic preparation (drops or ointment). Viral conjunctivitis is a self-limiting disease and does not require topical medication. Eye drops with an antihistamine or mast cell stabilization effect may be helpful in alleviating symptoms of allergic conjunctivitis. If other allergy signs and symptoms are also present, an oral antihistamine may also be prescribed. Table 39.1 compares bacterial, viral, and allergic conjunctivitis.

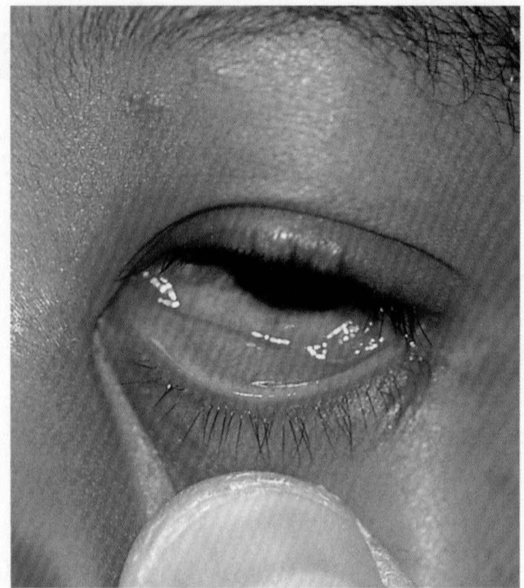

FIGURE 39.4 Note redness of conjunctiva.

Nursing Assessment

Nursing assessment of the child with conjunctivitis, regardless of the cause, is similar. It includes health history, physical examination, and, in rare instances, laboratory testing.

HEALTH HISTORY

Elicit a description of the present illness and chief complaint. Common signs and symptoms reported during the health history might include:

- Redness
- Edema
- Tearing
- Discharge
- Eye pain
- Itching of the eyes (usually with allergic conjunctivitis)

Determine the onset of symptoms and their progression as well as response to treatments used at home. Assess for risk factors for infectious conjunctivitis, such as day care or school attendance. Note any history of an upper respiratory infection, sore throat, or earache. Question parents about possible infectious exposure. Review the health history for risk factors for allergic conjunctivitis, such as a family history and a history of asthma, allergic rhinitis, or atopic dermatitis. Determine seasonality related to the symptoms and whether the symptoms occur after exposure to particular allergens, such as pollen, hay, or animals.

PHYSICAL EXAMINATION

Observe for eyelid swelling or redness. Inspect the conjunctivae for redness (Fig. 39.4). Note quantity, color, and consistency of discharge. Bacterial infections generally result in a thick, colored discharge, whereas a clear or white discharge is generally seen with viral conjunctivitis. Allergic conjunctivitis often results in a watery discharge, sometimes profuse, which is usually present bilaterally. Contact with an allergen rubbed into one of the eyes may result in unilateral symptoms. Observe the child for other signs of allergic or atopic disease, and document the presence of a runny nose or cough as well.

TABLE 39.1 TYPES OF CONJUNCTIVITIS

Type of Conjunctivitis	Conjunctivae	Discharge	Additional Findings	Eyelid Edema	Treatment
Bacterial	Inflamed	Purulent, mucoid	Mild pain	Occasional	Antibiotic drops or ointment
Viral	Inflamed	Watery, mucoid	Lymphadenopathy, photophobia, tearing	Usually present	Symptom relief; antiherpetic agent if cause is herpes
Allergic	Inflamed	Watery or stringy	Itching	Usually present	Antihistamine and/or mast cell stabilizer drops

Adapted from Braverman, R. S. (2014). Eye. In W. W. Hay, M. J. Levin, R. R. Deterding, & M. J. Abzug, (Eds.), *Current pediatric diagnosis and treatment* (22nd ed.). New York, NY: McGraw-Hill.

LABORATORY AND DIAGNOSTIC TESTS

Cases of bacterial, viral, and allergic conjunctivitis are generally diagnosed based on history and clinical presentation. Cases of viral and allergic conjunctivitis do not warrant laboratory testing. If bacterial conjunctivitis is suspected, then a bacterial culture of the eye drainage may be performed to determine the exact causative organism, thus allowing the most appropriate antibiotic to be prescribed.

Nursing Management

Nursing management of the various types of conjunctivitis focuses on alleviating symptoms and, for infectious causes, preventing spread.

ALLEVIATING SYMPTOMS

Teach parents how to apply eye drops or ointment (antibiotic for bacterial causes and antihistamine or mast cell stabilizer for allergic). Warm compresses may be used to help loosen the crust that accumulates on the eyelids overnight when drainage is copious, particularly with bacterial conjunctivitis.

The child with allergic conjunctivitis may experience perennial or seasonal allergies (or both). Encourage the child to avoid perennial allergens once the offending allergen is determined (refer to Chapter 40 for additional information related to education about perennial allergen avoidance). Seasonal allergies may include tree pollen in the winter or spring, grass pollen in the summer, and ragweed or flower pollen in the fall.

It is impossible to completely eliminate seasonal allergic responses, partly because it is important for children to participate in physical activity outdoors. Teach families to minimize seasonal allergens on the child's skin and hair. Educate families to:

- Encourage the child not to rub or touch the eyes.
- Rinse the child's eyelids periodically with a clean washcloth and cool water.
- When the child comes in from outdoors, wash the child's face and hands.
- Ensure that the child showers and shampoos before bedtime.

Take Note!

The itching of allergic conjunctivitis may be relieved with cool compresses. An easy way to accomplish this is to have the child hold a tube of yogurt over the affected eye.

PREVENTING INFECTIOUS SPREAD

Because infectious conjunctivitis is extremely contagious, the parent must wash hands diligently after caring for the child. Teach parents and children about appropriate hand washing and discourage them from sharing towels and washcloths. Children with viral conjunctivitis may return to school or day care when symptoms lessen. When mucopurulent drainage is no longer present (usually after 24 to 48 hours of treatment with a topical antibiotic), the child with bacterial conjunctivitis may safely return to day care or school (Blosser, Brady, & Royal, 2013).

Take Note!

Avoid the use of vasoconstricting eye drops such as Visine to rid the eyes of redness. Rebound vasodilation may occur, and with it the redness returns. This leads to repeated frequent use of the drops to keep the eyes from being red but does not treat the actual cause of the redness (Taketomo, Hodding, & Kraus, 2013).

Talking About Development

Raisa Jordan is a 3-year-old girl who has been diagnosed with bacterial conjunctivitis and prescribed antibiotic eye drops. Based on her developmental stage, how will you assist her caregivers to administer the eye drops? How would this assistance change if the child was 12 years old?

Nasolacrimal Duct Obstruction

Stenosis or simple obstruction of the nasolacrimal duct is a common disorder of infancy, occurring in about 6% to 20% of newborns and infants (Paysse, Coats, & Cassidy, 2015). It is unilateral in about 65% of cases. Chronic tearing occurs and build-up in the lacrimal sac causes a mucoid or mucopurulent drainage. Over 90% of all cases resolve spontaneously by 1 year of age (American Association for Pediatric Ophthalmology and Strabismus [AAPOS], 2016a). No apparent risk factors exist for the development of nasolacrimal duct obstruction or stenosis. Therapeutic management involves a watchful waiting approach. Massage may be prescribed, and if secondary bacterial infection is suspected or confirmed, antibiotic ointment or drops may be ordered. If the obstruction does not resolve by 12 months of age, then the pediatric ophthalmologist may probe the duct to relieve the obstruction (a brief outpatient procedure) (Paysse et al., 2015).

Nursing Assessment

Tearing or discharge from one or both eyes is often first noted at the 2-week checkup. Obtain a thorough history about the eye drainage to distinguish it from neonatal conjunctivitis. Determine the onset and progression of symptoms, as well as the newborn's response to any interventions attempted so far. Upon physical examination, note redness of the lower lid of the affected eye.

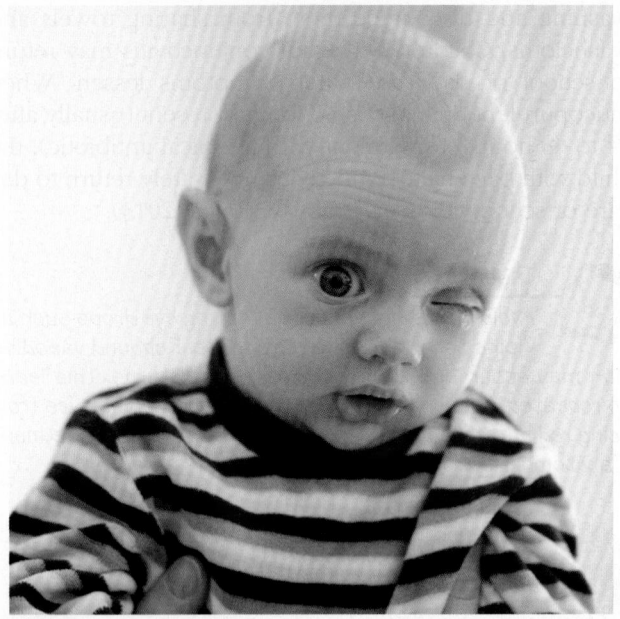

FIGURE 39.5 Mild eyelid redness and crusting are present in the infant with nasolacrimal duct stenosis.

If drainage is present, note its consistency, color, and quantity. Nasolacrimal duct obstruction is usually a diagnosis based on clinical presentation, but culture of the eye drainage may be used to rule out conjunctivitis or secondary bacterial infection (Fig. 39.5).

Nursing Management

As previously stated, the majority of cases of nasolacrimal duct stenosis resolve spontaneously by 12 months of age (AAPOS, 2016a). Nevertheless, the continual tearing and discharge is quite upsetting to the parents. Teach parents to clean the eye area frequently with a moist cloth. In addition, teach parents to massage the nasolacrimal duct, which may change the pressure and cause it to open, allowing drainage to occur. Refer to Teaching Guidelines 39.1 for appropriate nasolacrimal duct massage technique. Ensure that parents are educated about when and how to administer antibiotic eye drops if ordered.

Eyelid Disorders

Disorders of the eyelid include hordeolum (stye), chalazion, and blepharitis. Hordeolum is a localized infection of the sebaceous gland of the eyelid follicle, usually caused by bacterial invasion. Chalazion is a chronic painless infection of the meibomian gland. Blepharitis refers to chronic scaling and discharge along the eyelid margin. Chalazion may resolve spontaneously. Therapeutic management of hordeolum and blepharitis usually involves the use of antibiotic ointment.

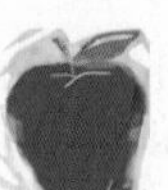

Teaching Guidelines 39.1

NASOLACRIMAL DUCT MASSAGE

- Using the forefinger or little finger, push on top of the bone (the puncta must be blocked).

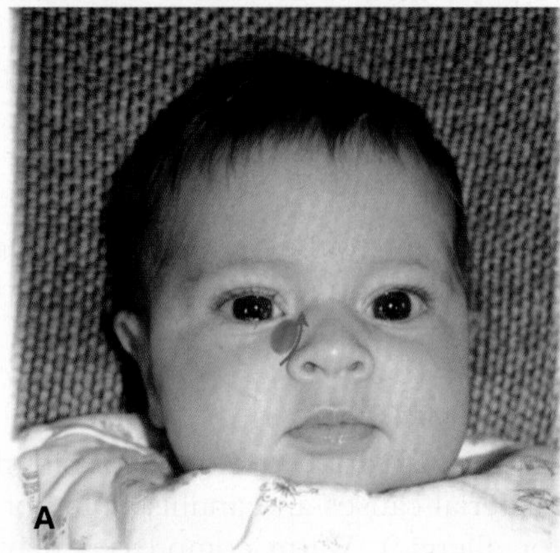

- Gently push in and up.

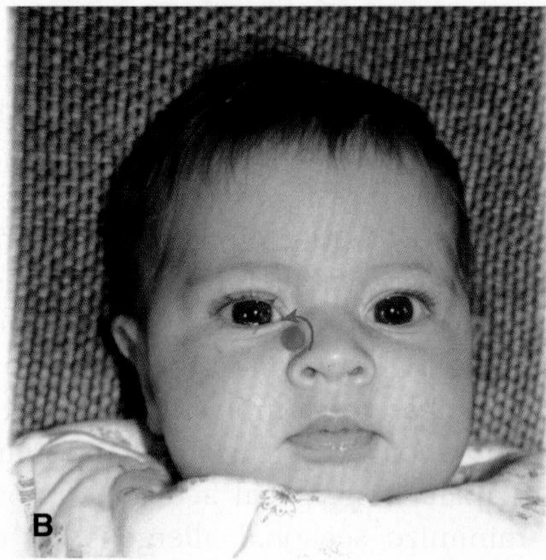

- Then gently push downward along the side of the nose.

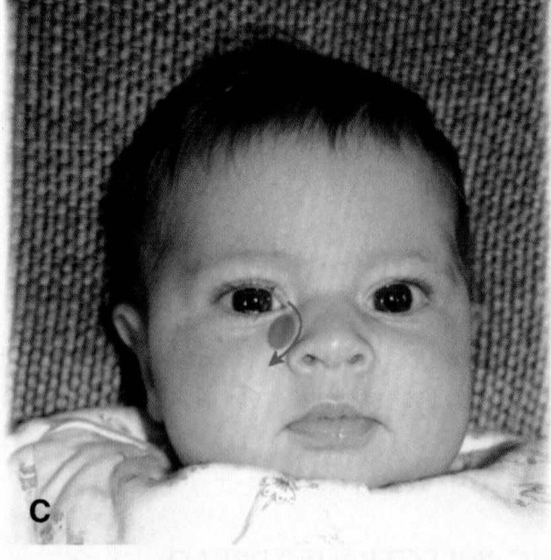

Adapted from American Association for Pediatric Ophthalmology and Strabismus (AAPOS). (2016a). *Nasolacrimal duct obstruction.* Retrieved from http://www.aapos.org/terms/conditions/72

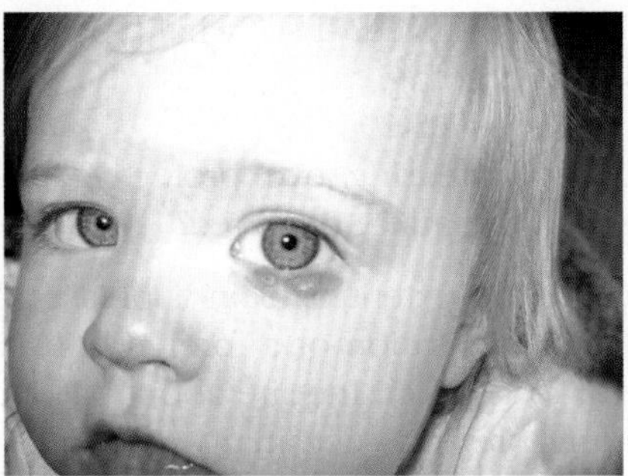

FIGURE 39.6 Hordeolum.

Nursing Assessment

Determine the child's health history, noting onset of symptoms, extent and character of eye discharge, and presence of pain (hordeolum is usually painful). Inspect the eyelids, noting redness along the eyelid margin and presence of eyelid edema (hordeolum, blepharitis). Hordeolum may also be quite visible as an enlarged lesion along the lid margin, with purulent drainage present (Fig. 39.6). Chalazion may be visible as a small nodule on the lid margin. The conjunctivae remain clear with all three of these disorders.

Nursing Management

For hordeolum and blepharitis, instruct parents how to administer antibiotic ointment. Encourage the use of hot, moist compresses. Inform parents that the stye may require several weeks to resolve completely. Also inform parents that chalazion will usually resolve spontaneously; if it does not, it may require minor surgical drainage.

Periorbital Cellulitis

Periorbital cellulitis is a bacterial infection of the eyelids and tissue surrounding the eye. The bacteria may gain entry to the skin via an abrasion, laceration, insect bite, foreign body, or impetiginous lesion. Periorbital cellulitis may also result from a nearby bacterial infection, such as sinusitis. *Staphylococcus aureus, Streptococcus pyogenes,* and *Streptococcus pneumoniae* are the most commonly implicated bacteria. The bacteria produce either an enzyme or endotoxins that initiate the inflammatory response. Redness, swelling, and infiltration of the skin by the inflammatory mediators occur.

Therapeutic management of periorbital cellulitis focuses on intravenous antibiotic administration during the acute phase followed by completion of the course with oral antibiotics. Complications of periorbital cellulitis include bacteremia and progression to orbital cellulitis, which is a more extensive infection involving the orbit of the eye.

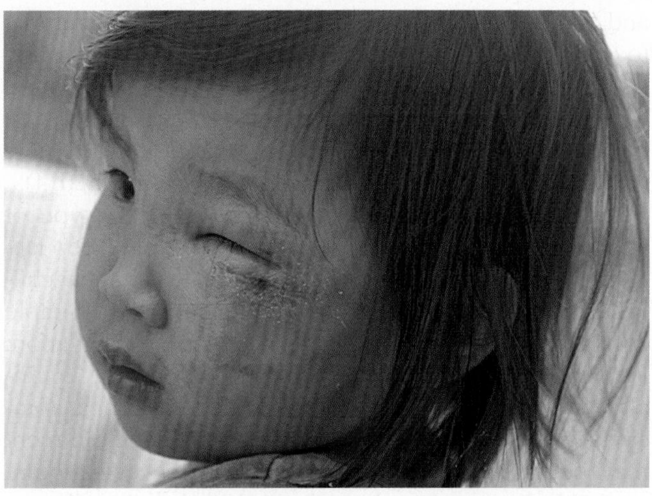

FIGURE 39.7 Periorbital cellulitis.

Nursing Assessment

Note the onset and duration of symptoms, as well as any treatment used so far. Document any history of fever. The child may complain of pain around the eye as well as restricted movement of the eye area. Inspect the eye, noting marked eyelid edema as well as a purplish or red color of the eyelid (Fig. 39.7). Usually the conjunctivae are clear and no discharge is present. If the extent of the edema allows the child to open the eye, assess visual acuity, which should be normal.

> *Take Note!*
>
> Notify the physician or nurse practitioner immediately if any of these signs of progression to orbital cellulitis occur: conjunctival redness, change in vision, pain with eye movement, eye muscle weakness or paralysis, or proptosis.

Nursing Management

Apply warm soaks to the eye area for 20 minutes every 2 to 4 hours. Administer intravenous antibiotics as prescribed. Teach families the importance of completing the entire course of oral antibiotic treatment at home. Instruct parents to call the physician or nurse practitioner or have the child evaluated again if:

- The child is not improving.
- The child reports inability to move the eye.
- Visual acuity changes.
- Proptosis occurs.

EYE INJURIES

As mentioned earlier, infants and young children are more susceptible to eye injuries than adults since the eyeball is relatively larger in relation to the space within the orbit. Developmental maturity may also play a part in eye injuries. For example, as infants and toddlers learn to walk and run, they do not have the awareness and maturity to avert disaster. Older children involved in sports and school science experiments are also at risk for eye injuries. A few of the more common eye injuries are eyelid injuries, contusion, scleral hemorrhage, corneal abrasion, a foreign body in the eye, and chemical injury (Braverman, 2014).

Therapeutic management depends on the type of injury. Eyelid lacerations may require suturing. Deep lacerations may result in ptosis at a later date, so these children should be referred to an ophthalmologist. Simple contusions (black eye) usually need only observation, ice, and analgesics. Scleral hemorrhages resolve gradually without intervention over a few weeks. Corneal abrasions may be allowed to self-heal, or antibiotic ointment may be prescribed. Foreign bodies in the eye require removal to prevent further irritation or abrasion. Chemical injuries require irrigation and vision evaluation.

Nursing Assessment

When a child presents with an eye injury, it is very important to obtain an accurate history related to the injury. Follow the history by performing a focused physical examination, which consists mostly of inspection and observation. It is important to determine whether an eye injury is nonemergent or emergent in order to provide rapid and appropriate treatment in the case of an emergency so that vision may be preserved.

HEALTH HISTORY

Obtain an accurate history. Determine the mechanism of injury and obtain as much detail about the injury as possible. Questions to ask during the health history include:

- When did the injury occur?
- What exactly happened?
- Was an object involved? If so, what type of object, and how fast was it going?
- Was it a splash injury?
- Was the child wearing eye protective gear or eyeglasses when the injury occurred?

Determine the extent of pain if present. Document photosensitivity, sensation of a foreign body in the eye, and blurry or lost vision. Inquire about past medical history, including previous eye injury or surgery or vision problems. Determine the child's immunization status.

PHYSICAL EXAMINATION

Regardless of the type of eye injury, the examination of the child's eye can be quite difficult. The nurse plays an important role in assisting the child and family to cope with the examination. Children with an eye injury often are in acute pain. The area surrounding the eye swells quickly after blunt trauma. Edema and tearing make the eye examination more difficult. Children are very frightened because of the pain and difficulty seeing. Approach the child in a calm and gentle manner. Soothe and coax the child as the eye is examined. Younger children may need to be restrained briefly in order for the examination to proceed safely.

Note the eyelid placement and look for signs of trauma such as bleeding, edema, and eyelid malformation. Evaluate the child's ability to open the eyes. Use a penlight to evaluate the pupils' response to light and accommodation (in the case of nonemergent eye trauma, the pupils should remain equally round and reactive to light and accommodation [PERRLA]). Note redness or irritation of the sclerae and/or conjunctivae. Observe for excessive tearing. Figure 39.8 shows the appropriate technique for eversion and examination of the interior of the eyelid.

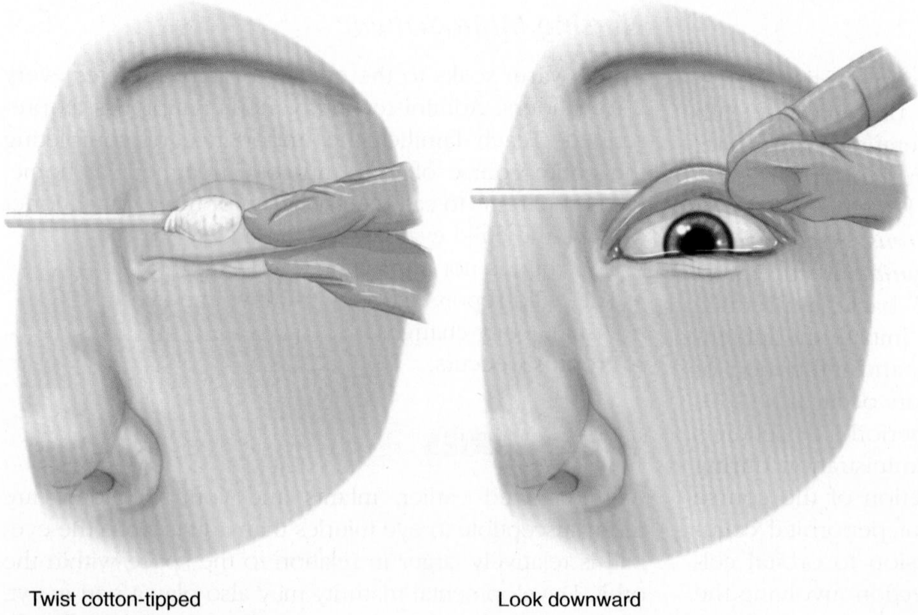

FIGURE 39.8 Eversion of the eyelid for examination. Place a cotton-tipped applicator over the eyelid. Pull the eyelid outward and up over the applicator.

TABLE 39.2 ASSESSMENT OF EYE INJURIES

Description of Injury	Nursing Assessment
Eyelid Injuries: May occur as laceration to the eyelid	• Laceration is noted at any point along the lid • Vision is unaffected
Simple Contusion (Black Eye): Occurs as a result of blunt trauma to the eye area	• Bruising and edema of lids or area surrounding eye • PERRLA • Extraocular movements intact • Visual acuity intact • No diplopia or blurred vision • Pain surrounding eye but not within the eye
Scleral Hemorrhage: Caused by blunt trauma or increased pressure such as with coughing	• Painless • Appears as erythema in the sclera; can be quite large initially • Vision unaffected
Corneal Abrasion: Results from foreign body such as sand, grit, or other small object scratching the cornea	• May have tearing • Eye pain • PERRLA • Vision may be blurry • Photophobia may be present
Foreign Body: May be dirt, glass, or other small particle	• Tearing • Complaint of "something in the eye" • PERRLA • Vision may be blurry

Adapted from Augsburger, J. J., & Correa, C. M. (2011). Ophthalmic trauma. In P. Riordan-Eva & E. T. Cunningham (Eds.), *Vaughan & Asbury's general ophthalmology* (18th ed.). New York, NY: McGraw-Hill.; and Braverman, R. S. (2014). Eye. In W. W. Hay, M. J. Levin, R. R. Deterding, & M. J. Abzug, (Eds.), *Current pediatric diagnosis and treatment* (22nd ed.). New York, NY: McGraw-Hill.

In a nonemergent situation, evaluate visual acuity via the use of an age-appropriate vision-screening tool (refer to Chapter 31 for additional information related to visual acuity screening). Generally, radiologic testing is used only in emergency situations (Augsburger & Correa, 2011). Table 39.2 provides assessment information specific to eyelid laceration, simple contusion, scleral hemorrhage, corneal abrasion, and foreign body in the eye.

Take Note!

If pupillary reaction is abnormal, vision is affected (decreased acuity from the child's norm, diplopia, or blurriness), or extraocular movements are affected, the child should be immediately referred to an ophthalmologist for further evaluation (Braverman, 2014).

Nursing Management

Children with urgent or emergent conditions must be referred to an ophthalmologist immediately to preserve vision. Urgent and emergent conditions include:

- Traumatic hyphema
- Blowout fracture
- Ruptured globe
- Thermal/chemical injury
- Extensive animal bite
- Lid laceration with underlying structural involvement
- Corneal abrasion in which corneal penetration is suspected
- Foreign body embedded in the globe (Augsburger & Correa, 2011; Braverman, 2014)

MANAGING NONEMERGENT EYE INJURIES

Nonemergent eye injuries usually need only simple management. Assist the physician or nurse practitioner with positioning and distraction of the child for eyelid laceration suturing. The child may require sedation or pain medication for this procedure.

To decrease edema in the child with a black eye (simple contusion), instruct the parent to apply an ice pack to the area for 20 minutes, then remove it for 20 minutes, and continue to repeat the cycle as often as possible during the first 24 hours. Tell the parents and child that bruising of the surrounding eye area may take up to 3 weeks to resolve.

The appearance of a scleral hemorrhage may be frightening. Instruct the parents and child about the benign nature of the hemorrhage and its natural history of resolution without intervention over a period of a few weeks.

If the child with a corneal abrasion has pain, analgesics may be helpful. Tell parents that most corneal abrasions heal on their own. If an antibiotic ointment is prescribed, instruct the parents how to administer the ointment appropriately.

Take Note!

Patching of the eye with a small, uncomplicated corneal abrasion or abrasion from a contact lens is not recommended. Patching does not result in decreased pain nor promote faster healing. In addition, it may place the child at risk for injury due to visual field loss while patched (Jacobs, 2015).

Foreign bodies may be removed from the eye by gently everting the eyelid and wiping the foreign body away with a sterile cotton-tipped applicator. Irrigation with normal saline may also wash the foreign body away.

For chemical injury, irrigate the eye with copious amounts of water. Consult ophthalmology for further evaluation and management.

HEALTHY PEOPLE 2020

Objective	Nursing Significance
Increase the use of personal protective eyewear in recreational activities and hazardous situations around the home among children and adolescents aged 6 to 17 years. Increase the proportion of public and private schools that require students to wear appropriate protective gear when engaged in school-sponsored physical activities.	• Educate the family about appropriate use of eye protective equipment during sports, lawn care, chemical use, and other potentially hazardous activities. • Encourage families to provide appropriate supervision of children (particularly young children) to reduce the risk of injury. • Educate families to teach their children safe practices in and around the home (not running with scissors, etc.).

Healthy People Objectives retrieved from http://www.healthypeople.gov

Take Note!

Refer the child with a large foreign body in the eye or one that is embedded in the globe of the eye to the ophthalmologist for appropriate, safe removal.

Eye injuries can be prevented, and nurses play a vital role in educating the public about prevention of eye injuries and use of appropriate safety equipment. See Healthy People 2020 and Evidence-Based Practice 39.1.

VISUAL DISORDERS

Adequate visual development requires appropriate sensory stimulation to both eyes over the first few years of life (Bremond-Gignac et al., 2011). When one or both eyes are deprived of this stimulation, visual development does not progress appropriately, and visual impairment or **blindness** may result. This may occur when the eyes are not aligned properly, visual acuity between the eyes is disparate, or other problems with the eyes exist (Bremond-Gignac et al., 2011). If vision disorders are diagnosed at an early age and treatment is begun, then vision may progress normally. However, when these disorders go untreated, the young child's developing vision may be reduced significantly. Therefore, it is important to appropriately screen children for these disorders.

Common visual disorders in childhood include refractive errors, astigmatism, strabismus, amblyopia, nystagmus, glaucoma, and cataracts.

Refractive Errors

The most common cause of visual difficulties in children is refractive errors. When the light that enters the lens does not bend appropriately to allow it to fall directly on the retina, then a refractive error occurs. Young children naturally have hyperopia (farsightedness) because the depth of the eye globe is not fully developed until about 5 years of age (Braverman, 2014). These children may have blurriness at close range, but by school age this blurriness usually resolves.

When the light entering the eye focuses in front of the retina, it results in myopia (nearsightedness). Children who are nearsighted may see well at close range

EVIDENCE-BASED PRACTICE 39.1 THE EFFECT OF PATCHING FOR CORNEAL ABRASION ON HEALING AND DECREASED PAIN

STUDY

Simple corneal abrasions are a common eye complaint. Eye patching with or without antibiotic ointment has often been used despite a lack of evidence for its use. In addition, patches are difficult to keep on young children and may be associated with corneal erosion. The authors included quasi-randomized and randomized studies evaluating patching versus no patching for treatment of simple corneal abrasion. Eleven trials with a total of 1,014 participants were included in the review.

Findings

The authors found that patching for simple corneal abrasions did not improve healing on day 1, nor did it decrease the amount of pain experienced. In addition, binocular vision is lost when one eye is patched. Based on these results, it is not recommended that patching be used for treatment of simple corneal abrasions.

Nursing Implications

Parents worry significantly when their child experiences even a very mild eye injury. Teach parents about the ability of the cornea to heal quickly from a minor abrasion. Emphasize that nonpatched corneal abrasions have been shown to heal more rapidly than those that are patched.

Adapted from Turner, A., & Rabiu, M. (2007). Patching for corneal abrasion. *The Cochrane Library* 2007. doi: 10.1002/14651858.CD004764.pub2 but have difficulty focusing on the blackboard or other objects at a distance.

Therapeutic management for both hyperopia and myopia is prescription eyeglasses or contact lenses. Generally, a child of 12 years of age can demonstrate the responsibility necessary to wear and care for contact lenses. Contact lenses may be used in younger children but are lost or damaged more readily. Because of the continuing refractive development in the child's vision through adolescence, laser surgery for vision correction is not recommended until 18 to 21 years of age, though it may be done experimentally in some children (Lusby, & Zieve, 2016).

Nursing Assessment

Elicit the health history, noting blurred vision, complaints of eye fatigue with reading, or complaints of eye strain (headache, pulling sensation, or eye burning). Note complaints of difficulty concentrating on or maintaining a clear focus on objects up close, avoidance of up-close work, or poor work performance (hyperopia). Note the risk factor of family history of myopia. Observe for squinting when the child looks at objects at a distance. Observe the hyperopic child for the presence of esotropia. Readily observable physical findings are not noted in the myopic child. Test visual acuity using an age-appropriate screening tool (for more information related to visual acuity screening, refer to Chapter 31). Hyperopia is usually not identified with visual acuity screening alone; it usually requires a retinal examination by an ophthalmologist.

Nursing Management

Nursing management of the child with a refractive error focuses on providing education about corrective lens use and monitoring for the need for new eyeglasses or contact lenses.

EDUCATING ABOUT EYEGLASS USE

Children may or may not be compliant with wearing eyeglasses. Glasses may carry a stigma, and the child may be teased or bullied. However, many children enjoy the improved vision they achieve when wearing their eyeglasses and this can help them overcome the teasing they might suffer. Encourage the child with newly prescribed eyeglasses to wear them by having the parent spend "special time" with the child doing an activity that requires the glasses (such as reading or drawing). Teach the parent and child to remove eyeglasses with both hands and to lay them on their side (not directly on the lens on any surface). Instruct the child and family about cleaning the glasses daily with mild soap and water or a commercial cleansing agent provided by the optometrist. Use a soft cloth to clean the glasses, not paper towels, tissues, or toilet paper.

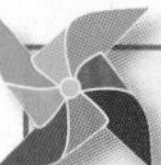

Consider This

I can't believe I have to start wearing glasses! I have heard the other kids mock my classmates and call them 4-eyes. I'm old enough now to start wearing makeup and how will that look with glasses? I'll look like a nerd...

Thoughts: How will you respond to her worries? With this preteen girl, what will your approach be to insure she wears her glasses as prescribed?

EDUCATING ABOUT CONTACT LENS USE

Teach the older child or adolescent how to care for the contact lenses properly, including lens hygiene and lens insertion and removal. Inform the child and parents that protective eyewear should be worn when the child is participating in contact sports. If the eye becomes inflamed, remove the contact lens and wear eyeglasses until the eye is improved. Consult with the child's eye care provider to determine if medications prescribed for an eye problem can be used while the contact lens is in.

MONITORING FOR FIT AND VISUAL CORRECTION

Encourage the family to complete visual assessments as scheduled. Since the child's vision is continuing to develop and refraction is not stable, the corrective lens prescription may change more frequently than it does in an adult. As the young child in particular is continuing to grow at a rapid rate, the head size is also changing (AAPOS, 2015). Eyeglass frames may hurt or pinch the child as the child's head becomes larger. Teach families to check the fit of the glasses monthly. Monitor for signs of ill fit, such as constant removal of the glasses in an older child or rubbing at the glasses or eyes in the very young child. Monitor for squinting, eye fatigue or strain, and complaints of headache or dizziness, which may indicate the need for a change in the lens prescription. See Healthy People 2020.

Astigmatism

In astigmatism the cornea's curvature is uneven, which results in an irregular quality of vision because the light rays are refracted unevenly. Sometimes the lens is irregularly shaped, having the same result.

Nursing Assessment

Explore the health history for symptoms of astigmatism. Children with astigmatism often have blurry vision and difficulty seeing letters as a whole, so their ability to read is affected. They may have headaches or dizziness. Older children may complain of eye fatigue or strain. Children with astigmatism often learn to tilt their heads slightly so that they can focus more effectively. This may lead to "normal" vision screenings, but the headache and dizziness still warrant further examination by an eye specialist

***HEALTHY PEOPLE** 2020*

Objective	Nursing Significance
Increase the proportion of preschool children aged 5 years and under who receive vision screening. Increase the proportion of preschool children aged 5 years and younger who receive vision screening. Reduce uncorrected visual impairment due to uncorrected refractive errors. Reduce blindness and visual impairment in children and adolescents aged 17 years and younger.	• Ensure that visual acuity testing begins with an age-appropriate screening tool by 3 years of age and continues yearly throughout childhood and adolescence. • Refer for an eye evaluation to any children with complaints of difficulty seeing the front of the classroom or complaints of eye strain or difficulty with close work. • Screen infants and children for asymmetric corneal light reflex for early detection of amblyopia.

Healthy People Objectives retrieved from http://www.healthypeople.gov

(Braverman, 2014). The diagnosis of astigmatism requires not only a visual acuity test but also a refractive error evaluation by an optometrist or ophthalmologist.

Nursing Management

Corrective lenses can help to, in effect, smooth out the curvature of the cornea, making the light ray refraction occur smoothly. As with refractive errors, encourage the child who requires corrective lenses for astigmatism to wear the eyeglasses or contact lenses regularly.

Strabismus

Strabismus refers to misalignment of the eyes. It is common and occurs in up to 4% of the population (Coats & Paysse, 2016). The most common types of strabismus are exotropia and esotropia. In exotropia the eyes turn outward; in esotropia they turn inward. Because of this unequal alignment, visual development in each eye may proceed at different rates. Diplopia (double vision) may result, so vision in one eye may be "turned off" by the brain to avoid diplopia. Many infants have strabismus intermittently, but this usually resolves by 3 to 6 months of age. Persistent esotropia that persists past 4 months of age or constant strabismus at any age warrants referral to an ophthalmologist for further evaluation (Coats & Paysse, 2016).

Therapeutic management of strabismus may include patching of the stronger eye or eye muscle surgery. Corrective lenses are also used for strabismus. Complications of strabismus include amblyopia and visual deficits.

Nursing Assessment

Parents may be the first persons to notice that the child's eyes do not face in the same direction. Question parents about the onset of the problem and whether it is continuous or intermittent. If intermittent, does it occur more often when the child is tired? Elicit the health history, noting complaints of blurred vision, tired eyes, squinting or closing one eye in bright sunlight, tilting the head to focus on an object, or a history of bumping into objects (depth perception may be limited).

Observe the child's eyes for obvious exotropia or esotropia. In the absence of an obvious finding, assessment of the symmetry of the corneal light reflex is extremely helpful (Fig. 39.9). The "cover test" is also a useful tool for the identification of strabismus.

True strabismus should not be confused with pseudostrabismus. In pseudostrabismus, the eyes may appear slightly crossed (as in the child with a wide nasal bridge and epicanthal folds), but the corneal light reflex remains symmetric (Weber & Kelley, 2014).

Nursing Management

It is extremely important to treat strabismus appropriately in the developing years so that equal visual acuity may be achieved in both eyes. When patching is prescribed, encourage the family to comply with this modality. Encourage eyeglass wearing if prescribed. Provide appropriate postoperative care by protecting the operative site with eye patching.

Amblyopia

Amblyopia refers to poor visual development in the otherwise structurally normal eye. It develops within the

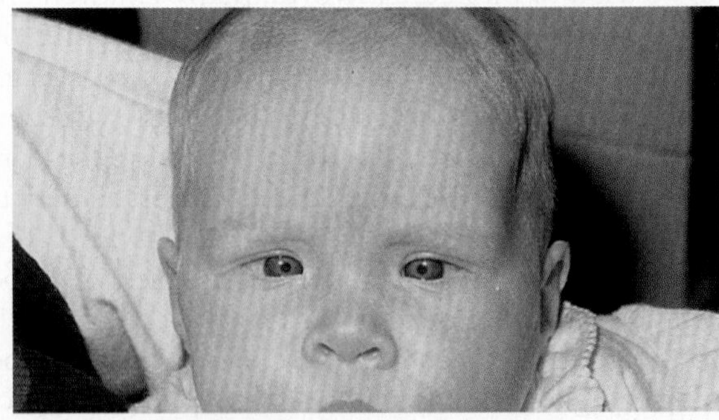

FIGURE 39.9 Esotropia. Test for strabismus by observing symmetry of the corneal light reflex. The reflex falls to the left of one pupil and to the right of the other.

first decade of life and, if left untreated, is the most common cause of vision loss in children and young adults (Coats & Paysse, 2016). Amblyopia occurs in about 1% to 4% of children (Coats & Paysse, 2016). The vision in one eye is reduced because the eye and the brain are not working together properly. While the eyes are fighting to focus differently because of their differences in visual acuity, one eye is stronger than the other. This is why amblyopia is often referred to as "lazy eye."

Amblyopia may be caused by any disorder that affects normal visual development, including strabismus and differences in visual acuity or astigmatism between the two eyes. It may also result from eye trauma, ptosis, or cataract. If untreated, children with amblyopia will have worsening acuity of the poorer eye and strain in the better eye, which may also lead to worsening of acuity in that eye. Eventually blindness will result in one or both eyes.

Therapeutic management of amblyopia focuses on strengthening the weaker eye. This may be achieved through patching for several hours per day, using atropine drops in the better eye (once daily), vision therapy, or eye muscle surgery if the cause is strabismus.

Nursing Assessment

One of the most important functions of the nurse is to identify on screening the preschool child with amblyopia. Begin visual acuity testing using an age-appropriate tool by 3 years of age. Observe for asymmetry of the corneal light reflex in the child of any age. This may be the only sign in the preverbal child.

Nursing Management

It is very important for children with amblyopia to receive appropriate treatment during the early years of visual development. Patching the better eye for several hours each day encourages the eye with poorer vision to be used appropriately and promotes visual development in that eye. The once-daily use of atropine drops in the better eye results in blurring in that eye, similarly encouraging use and development of the weaker eye (Coats & Paysse, 2016). Support and encourage children and parents to comply with the patching protocol or atropine drop use.

Promoting eye safety is extremely important for the child with amblyopia; if the better eye suffers a serious injury, both eyes may become blind.

Nystagmus

Nystagmus refers to a very rapid, irregular eye movement. It is described by some as "bouncing" of the eyes. It may occur in children with congenital cataracts, but the most common cause is a neurologic problem. It is difficult for the brain and eyes to communicate when the eyes are in continuous motion; thus, visual development may be affected. Children with nystagmus must receive further evaluation by an ophthalmologist and possibly a neurologist.

Infantile Glaucoma

Infantile glaucoma is an autosomal recessive disorder that is more common in interrelated marriages or relationships. It is often associated with other genetic disorders. It occurs in about 1 of 10,000 live births (Yeung & Walton, 2012). Infantile glaucoma is characterized by obstruction of aqueous humor flow and increased intraocular pressure that results in large, prominent eyes. Vision loss may occur as a result of corneal scarring, optic nerve damage, or, most commonly, amblyopia.

Unlike adult glaucoma, in which medical management is the first step, therapeutic management of infantile glaucoma is focused on surgical intervention. Infantile glaucoma is treated surgically via goniotomy (removal of obstruction of the aqueous humor). Laser surgery is being used as well. Sometimes several surgeries may be necessary to correct the problem. Ongoing medication therapy may also be required.

Nursing Assessment

Note any family history of infantile glaucoma or other genetic disorders. Elicit the health history, noting history of the infant keeping the eyes closed most of the time or rubbing the eyes. Observe the eye for corneal enlargement and clouding; the eye may appear enlarged. Photophobia may occur, so bright light may bother the infant. Tearing or conjunctivitis and eyelid squeezing or spasm may also occur. The pediatric ophthalmologist may use a tonometer to measure the intraocular pressure during the diagnostic phase.

Nursing Management

The main goal of nursing care for the infant with glaucoma is postoperative care. Family education will also be important.

Providing Postoperative Care

Postoperatively the eye will be patched and the child should be maintained on bed rest. Nursing care focuses on protection of the surgical site. Infants and toddlers may require elbow restraints to prevent them from rubbing the affected eye. These children may be quite anxious with one or both eyes patched, since their ability to see will be affected. Use a calm and soothing approach with these children, as well as distraction and developmentally appropriate play activities.

EDUCATING THE FAMILY

Instruct parents and children to make sure the child avoids roughhousing and contact sports for at least 2 weeks after surgery. Before the first surgery occurs, prepare parents for the possibility that three or four operations may be necessary. Teach families how to administer postoperative medications. Encourage parents to comply with ongoing recommended visual assessments.

Congenital Cataract

A congenital cataract is an opacity of the lens of the eye that is present at birth. Sensory amblyopia will result if the infant goes untreated. Complications include visual developmental delay related to amblyopia. In children younger than 5 years of age, congenital cataract causes more than 10% of the cases of legal blindness (International Council of Ophthalmology (ICP), 2016). Bilateral cataracts may be associated with metabolic or genetic syndromes. Surgery to remove the opaque lens can be done as early as 2 weeks of age. The infant is then fitted with a contact lens. Intraocular lens implants are also being used (Lin & Buckley, 2010). The best visual outcomes occur when cataracts are removed prior to 3 months of age. Glaucoma may occur as a complication after cataract surgery.

Nursing Assessment

Note history of lack of visual awareness. Observe the eyes for apparent cloudiness of the cornea (not always visible). Upon ophthalmoscopic examination, the red reflex will not be observed in the affected eye.

Nursing Management

Postoperative care focuses on protecting the operative site and providing developmentally appropriate activities. Ensure that the protective eye patch is secure. Elbow restraints may be necessary in the older infant to prevent accidental injury to the operative site. Teach families how to administer antibiotic or corticosteroid ophthalmic drops if prescribed for postoperative use. Once the surgical site is healed, the healthy eye may be patched for several hours a day to promote visual development in the eye with the contact or intraocular lens. Regular visual assessments are critical for determining the adequacy of visual development after cataract removal. Instruct parents about the importance of using sunglasses that block ultraviolet rays in the child who has had a lens removed. See Healthy People 2020.

HEALTHY PEOPLE 2020

Objective	Nursing Significance
Reduce visual impairment due to glaucoma. Reduce visual impairment due to cataract.	• Appropriately screen infants and children for glaucoma or cataract. • Refer suspected cases to a pediatric ophthalmologist for further evaluation.

Healthy People Objectives retrieved from http://www.healthypeople.gov

Retinopathy of Prematurity

Retinopathy of prematurity (ROP) is a disorder characterized by rapid growth of retinal blood vessels in the premature infant. In the fetus, retinal vascularization begins at 4 months and progresses until completion at 9 months or shortly after birth. The premature infant is born with incomplete retinal vascularization, yet new vessels continue to grow between the vascularized and nonvascularized retina. Risk factors include low birthweight, early gestational age, sepsis, high light intensity, and hypothermia. Changes in oxygen tension resulting from hypoxia, oxyhemoglobin dissociation curve changes that occur when adult blood is transfused to the premature infant, and the duration/concentration of supplemental oxygen are thought to play an important role in the development of ROP.

Premature infants should have serial examinations by an ophthalmologist until the ROP has regressed and normal vascularization is seen. If ROP continues to progress, laser surgery may be necessary to prevent blindness. Complications of ROP include myopia, glaucoma, and blindness. Strabismus may occur even in cases of regressed (resolved) ROP. Refractive errors and amblyopia may occur as early as 3 months corrected age. In the first year of life, ophthalmologic examinations should occur frequently so that if corrective lenses are needed, they may be prescribed at the earliest possible time. After 1 year corrected age, former premature infants should continue to have yearly ophthalmologic examinations to detect and treat visual deficits early (AAP, 2013b).

Nursing Assessment

Ensure that all former premature infants are routinely screened for visual deficits. Discuss developmental progress with the parents. Observe for the development of strabismus, manifested by an asymmetric corneal light reflex.

Nursing Management

Nursing management of infants with ROP mainly focuses on ensuring that the family is compliant with the ophthalmologist's follow-up recommendations. Recurrent illness or rehospitalization of premature infants may interfere with scheduled eye follow-up appointments. Ensure that these appointments are rescheduled and that the family understands the importance of them. Many children who have regressed ROP or who require cryotherapy have refractive errors, so even when the ROP is considered resolved, these children should still maintain appropriate ophthalmology follow-up.

Visual Impairment

Vision impairment in children refers to acuity between 20/60 and 20/200 in the better eye on examination. "Legal blindness" is a term used to refer to vision of less than 20/200 or peripheral vision less than 20 degrees. In most cases, vision may be augmented with corrective lenses. Some blind children can differentiate light versus dark, while others live in total darkness.

Visual impairment in children may result from a number of different causes. In the United States, visual impairment and blindness are most often caused by refractive error, astigmatism, strabismus, amblyopia, nystagmus, infantile glaucoma, congenital cataract, ROP, and retinoblastoma (ICP, 2016). Factors that increase the risk for developing visual impairment include prematurity, developmental delay, genetic syndrome, family history of eye disease, African-American heritage, previous serious eye injury, diabetes, HIV, and chronic corticosteroid use. Trauma is also an important cause of blindness in children. Visual impairments may also be associated with genetic syndromes.

Children with visual impairments often exhibit motor and cognitive delays as well (Carter, 2015). With one less sense with which to experience their environment, these children may lag behind in developmental milestones.

Take Note!

Laser pointers pose a risk of retinal damage in infants and young children. Damage occurs if the child stares at the red light for longer than 10 seconds. They should not be used as toys (U. S. Food and Drug Administration, 2013).

Nursing Assessment

Nursing assessment for visual impairment includes a careful health history, physical examination, and visual acuity testing.

HEALTH HISTORY

Parents and nurses alike should be alert to signs of potential visual impairment. One of the most important functions of the nurse is to recognize signs of visual impairment as early as possible. These signs may include:

- At any age:
  - Dull, vacant stare
- Infants:
  - Do not "fix and follow"
  - Do not make eye contact
  - Unaffected by bright light
  - Do not imitate facial expression
- Toddlers and older children:
  - Rub, shut, and cover eyes
  - Squinting
  - Frequent blinking
  - Hold objects close or sit close to television
  - Bumping into objects
  - Head tilt or forward thrust

PHYSICAL EXAMINATION

Assess for symmetry or asymmetry of the corneal light reflex. Perform the "cover test." Use an age-appropriate visual acuity screening tool (refer to Chapter 31 for additional information on visual acuity screening).

Nursing Management

Important nursing functions in relation to visual impairment and blindness are supporting the child and family and promoting socialization, development, and education. In addition, when the child with a visual impairment is hospitalized for any reason, the nurse must plan appropriate care for that child, taking into consideration the child's level of disability. Box 39.1 provides tips on working with the visually impaired child. It is important to teach these tips to families.

BOX 39.1

TIPS FOR INTERACTING WITH THE VISUALLY IMPAIRED CHILD

- Use the child's name to gain attention.
- Identify yourself and let the child know you are there before you touch the child.
- Encourage the child to be independent while maintaining safety.
- Name and describe people/objects to make the child more aware of what is happening.
- Discuss upcoming activities with the child.
- Explain what other children or individuals are doing.
- Make directions simple and specific.
- Allow the child additional time to think about the response to a question or statement.
- Use touch and tone of voice appropriate to the situation.
- Use parts of the child's body as reference points for the location of items.
- Encourage exploration of objects through touch.
- Describe unfamiliar environments and provide reference points.
- Use the sighted-guide technique when walking with a visually impaired child.

Adapted from Delta Gamma Center for Children with Visual Impairments. (2011). *Interacting with visually impaired.* Retrieved from http://dgckids.org/resources/interacting-with-visually-impaired/

SUPPORTING THE CHILD AND FAMILY

Provide emotional support to the family with a visually impaired child. Ensure that the child's environment provides familiarity and security. Encourage activities that stimulate development; these activities will vary from child to child depending on whether the child also demonstrates impairment in other areas, such as hearing or motor skills. The blind infant will not provide the eye contact that parents are looking for, so educate the parents about other indicators that the infant is acknowledging the parents' presence, such as:

- Increased motor activity
- Eyelid movement
- Changes in breathing pattern
- Making sounds

Encourage the family of a visually impaired child to display affection through touch and tone of voice. Refer families to support networks and other resources for the blind and visually impaired. Several online resources for families of children who are visually impaired or blind can be found on thePoint.

PROMOTING SOCIALIZATION, DEVELOPMENT, AND EDUCATION

Blind children, since they lack the visual stimulation that children usually receive, may develop self-stimulatory actions in compensation, often called blindisms. Examples of blindisms are eye pressing, rocking, spinning, bouncing, and head banging. These repetitive behaviors may indicate an effort to communicate or alternatively they may interfere with the child's ability to socialize (Hammer, n. d.). Work with the parents to determine whether a strategy for the development of alternative behaviors specific to the individual child would be helpful.

Refer the blind or visually impaired child who is younger than 3 years of age to the local district of Early Intervention to establish case management services for the child's developmental needs. After age 3, state laws provide for public education and related services for children with disabilities. An individualized education plan (IEP) should be developed to maximize the child's learning ability. Nurses may be one of the professionals involved in the development of the IEP.

The severely visually impaired or blind child will need to learn to read Braille and will also need to learn to navigate the environment with the use of a cane or via another method.

INFECTIOUS AND INFLAMMATORY DISORDERS OF THE EARS

Infectious and inflammatory disorders of the ears include otitis externa and types of otitis media. Otitis media is defined as inflammation of the middle ear with the presence of fluid. It can be subdivided into two categories: AOM and otitis media with effusion (OME). AOM refers to an acute infectious process of the middle ear that may produce a rapid onset of ear pain and possibly fever. OME refers to a collection of fluid in the middle ear space without signs and symptoms of infection. Chronic OME is defined as OME lasting longer than 3 months. Otitis externa refers to inflammation of the external ear canal.

Acute Otitis Media

AOM is a common illness in children, resulting from infection (bacterial or viral) of fluid in the middle ear. Increased susceptibility in infants and young children may be partly explained by the short length and horizontal positioning of the Eustachian tube, limited response to antigens, and lack of previous exposure to common pathogens (Friedman et al., 2014). AOM occurs mostly in the fall through spring, with the highest incidence in the winter. AOM often recurs in infants and young children when the fluid in the middle ear becomes reinfected. The most significant risk factors for otitis media are Eustachian tube dysfunction and susceptibility to recurrent upper respiratory infections.

Pathophysiology

An upper respiratory infection frequently precedes AOM. Fluid and pathogens travel upward from the nasopharyngeal area, invading the middle ear space. Fluid behind the eardrum has difficulty draining back out toward the nasopharyngeal area because of the horizontal positioning of the Eustachian tube. A viral upper respiratory infection may cause AOM or may place the child at risk for bacterial invasion. Pathogens gain access to the Eustachian tube, where they proliferate and invade the mucosa. Fever and pain occur acutely. Increased pressure behind the tympanic membrane may result in perforation. This may result in decreased pain and yield drainage in the ear canal. Most perforations heal spontaneously and are completely benign.

AOM is most commonly caused by viral pathogens, *Streptococcus pneumoniae, Haemophilus influenzae,* and *Moraxella catarrhalis.* Viral causes of AOM resolve spontaneously.

After clearance of the infection, fluid remains in the middle ear space behind the tympanic membrane, sometimes for several months (OME). This may occur because of the positioning of the Eustachian tubes, resulting in difficulty in draining fluid back to the nasopharyngeal area. OME may also occur because of the high frequency of upper respiratory infections in infants and young children, which again result in back-up of fluid from the nasopharyngeal area.

The most common complications of AOM include:

- Hearing loss
- Expressive speech delay

- Tympanosclerosis (scarring of the tympanic membrane; usually has no effect on hearing)
- Tympanic membrane perforation (acute with resolution or chronic)
- Chronic suppurative otitis media (chronic drainage via perforation or **tympanostomy** tubes)
- Acute mastoiditis (infection of the mastoid process)
- Intracranial infections, including bacterial meningitis and abscesses

Therapeutic Management

Viral causes of AOM usually resolve spontaneously, but bacterial causes may require treatment with an antibiotic. It is unreasonable to obtain a culture of middle ear fluid with every episode of AOM to determine the specific cause. Scientific studies of fluid obtained via tympanostomy in children with AOM have been performed, and clinical decision making is based on this research. Antibiotic resistance develops due to the overuse of antibiotics (AAP, 2013a). For this reason, clinical practice guidelines have been developed for a number of disorders based on large quantities of research.

Certain diagnosis of AOM is based on:

- Signs of fluid in the middle ear: moderate to severe bulging of the tympanic membrane, or mild bulging of the tympanic membrane with recent (within 48 hours) complaint of ear pain, and presence of middle ear infusion noted on pneumatic otoscopy or tympanometry.

AND

- Signs or symptoms of inflammation in the middle ear: complaint of ear pain or intense erythema of the tympanic membrane

OR

- New onset otorrhea in absence of otitis externa (AAP, 2013a).

The choice of antibiotic will depend on the timing, the child's age, and whether the episode is a first or subsequent infection. The current recommendations by the AAP allow for a period of observation or watchful waiting in certain children. This allows for natural resolution of AOM related to viral causes and decreases the overuse of antibiotics in the pediatric population (AAP, 2013a) (see Dosage Calculation Box 39.1).

Recommendations for AOM treatment in previously healthy children are found in Table 39.3. Pain management is also an important component of AOM treatment, as is appropriate follow-up to ensure disease resolution.

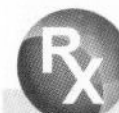

Dosage Calculation Box 39.1

Child's weight: 12 lb, 4 oz
Medication order: cefuroxime 100 mg PO twice a day.
Per the Pediatric Dosage Handbook, the recommended dose is 20–30 mg/kg/day in two divided doses.
Is the ordered dose safe?

TABLE 39.3 TREATMENT RECOMMENDATIONS FOR ACUTE OTITIS MEDIA

Age	Unilateral or Bilateral AOM?	Severe Signs & Symptoms?[a]	Otorrhea Present?	Treatment
6 months to 2 years	Either		Yes	Antibiotics
6 months to 2 years	Either	Yes		Antibiotics
6 months to 2 years	Bilateral	No	No	Antibiotics
6 months to 2 years	Unilateral	No	No	Antibiotics or Observation[b]
>2 years	Either		Yes	Antibiotics
>2 years	Either	Yes		Antibiotics
>2 years	Bilateral	No	No	Antibiotics or Observation[b]
>2 years	Unilateral	No	No	Antibiotics or Observation[b]

[a]Severe illness is defined as temperature 39°C (102.2°F) or higher or moderate to severe otalgia or otalgia for at least 48 hours. Nonsevere illness is defined as mild otalgia for less than 48 hours and fever less than 39°C (102.2°F).

[b]Observation is appropriate when follow-up can be ensured in order that antibiotic therapy may begin if the child fails to improve or worsens within 48 to 72 hours.

Adapted from American Academy of Pediatrics. (2013a). Clinical practice guideline: The diagnosis and management of acute otitis media. *Pediatrics, 131*, e964–e999.

Nursing Assessment

Nursing assessment of the child with AOM consists of health history and physical examination.

HEALTH HISTORY

Elicit a description of the present illness and chief complaint. Note acute, abrupt onset of signs and symptoms. Common signs and symptoms reported during the health history might include:

- Fever (may be low grade or higher)
- Complaints of otalgia (ear pain)
- Fussiness or irritability
- Crying inconsolably, particularly when lying down
- Batting or tugging at the ears (may also occur with teething or OME, or may be a habit)
- Rolling the head from side to side
- Poor feeding or loss of appetite
- Lethargy
- Difficulty sleeping or awakening crying in the night
- Fluid draining from the ear

Determine the child's response to any treatments used thus far. Explore the child's current and past medical history for risk factors such as:

- Young age
- Day care attendance
- Previous history of AOM or OME
- Antecedent or concurrent upper respiratory infection
- Other risk factors (Box 39.2)

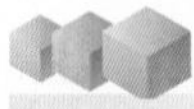

Concept Mastery Alert

Assessment of Otitis Media

Assessment findings in a child with AOM are typically a recent upper respiratory infection fever, loss of appetite, and a dull, opaque, bulging, or red tympanic membrane.

BOX 39.2

RISK FACTORS FOR ACUTE OTITIS MEDIA

- Eustachian tube dysfunction
- Recurrent upper respiratory infection
- First episode of acute otitis media (AOM) before 3 months of age
- Day care attendance (increases exposure to viruses causing upper respiratory infections)
- Previous episodes of AOM
- Family history
- Passive smoking
- Crowding in the home or large family size
- Native American, Inuit, or Australian aborigine ethnicity
- Absence of infant breastfeeding
- Immunocompromise
- Poor nutrition
- Craniofacial anomalies
- Presence of allergies (possibly)

Adapted from American Academy of Pediatrics. (2013a). Clinical practice guideline: The diagnosis and management of acute otitis media. *Pediatrics*, *131*, e964–e999 and Friedman, N. R., Scholes, M. A., & Yoon, P. J. (2014). Ear, nose, & throat. In W. W. Hay, M. J. Levin, & R. R. Deterding, & M. J. Abzug, (Eds.), *Current pediatric diagnosis and treatment* (22nd ed.). New York, NY: McGraw-Hill.

PHYSICAL EXAMINATION AND DIAGNOSTIC TESTING

The child may complain of pain when the ear is examined. On otoscopic examination, the tympanic membrane will have a dull or opaque appearance and is bulging and/or red (Fig. 39.10). Sometimes pus (greenish or yellowish) may be visible behind the eardrum. Upon pneumatic otoscopy, the eardrum will be immobile. (A physician or nurse practitioner usually performs the otoscopic examination.) If the tympanic membrane has become perforated, drainage may be present in the ear canal, but the canal will otherwise appear normal. Palpate for possible cervical lymphadenopathy. **Tympanometry** is used to determine the presence of middle ear effusion (AAP, 2013a).

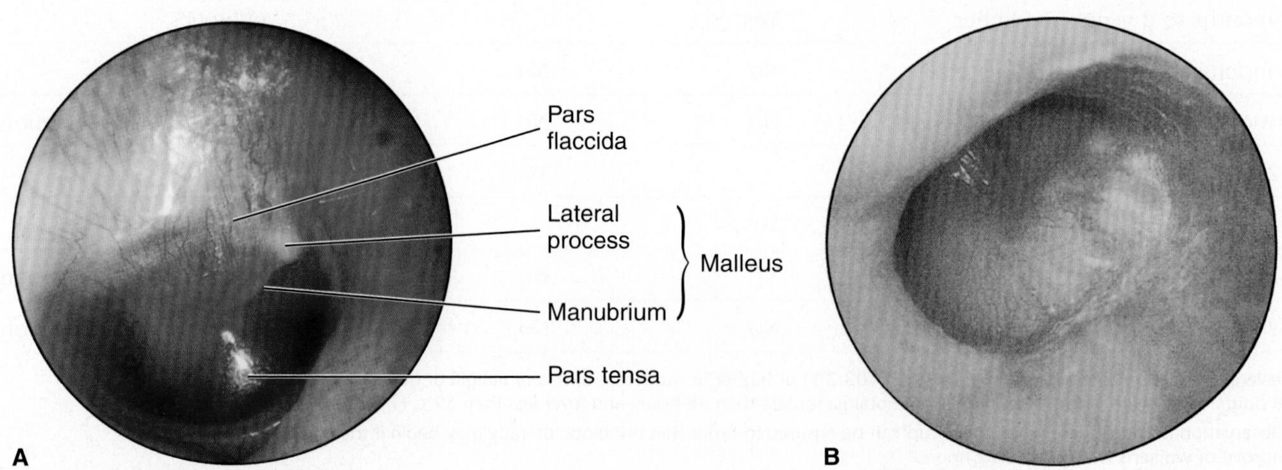

FIGURE 39.10 **(A)** Normal tympanic membrane. **(B)** Acute otitis media: note opacity of the tympanic membrane.

Nursing Management

Nursing management of the child with AOM is mainly supportive in nature. It focuses on pain management, family education, and prevention of AOM.

MANAGING PAIN ASSOCIATED WITH ACUTE OTITIS MEDIA

Analgesics such as acetaminophen and ibuprofen have been shown to be effective at managing mild to moderate pain associated with AOM. They have the added benefit of reducing fever. Occasionally, narcotic analgesics may be prescribed for severe pain. Application of heat or a cool compress may also be helpful. Instruct the family to have the child lie on the affected side with the heating pad or covered ice pack in place to that ear. Numbing eardrops such as benzocaine (Auralgan) may be helpful in the event of acute, severe pain. They should be used in conjunction with analgesics, though, because of the short duration of action (AAP, 2013a).

EDUCATING THE FAMILY

If the treatment selected for AOM is observation or watchful waiting, explain the rationale for this to the family. Ensure that the family understands the importance of returning for re-evaluation if the child is not improving within 48 to 72 hours or if the AOM progresses to severe illness. When antibiotics are prescribed, the family must understand the importance of completing the entire course of antibiotics. Families are tempted to stop giving the antibiotic because the child is usually vastly improved after taking the medication for 24 to 48 hours. Follow-up for resolution of AOM is necessary for all children and the physician or nurse practitioner will determine the timing of that follow-up. Emphasize the importance of follow-up to the parents, educating them about OME and its potential impact on hearing and speech. See Healthy People 2020.

PREVENTING ACUTE OTITIS MEDIA

Breastfed infants have a lower incidence of AOM than formula-fed infants, and breast milk's immunologic benefits are well known (Friedman et al., 2014). Therefore, encourage mothers to breastfeed for at least 6 to 12 months. Instruct families to avoid excess exposure to individuals with upper respiratory infections to decrease the incidence of these infections in their child. Infants and children should not be exposed to second-hand smoke. Encourage parents to stop smoking. If quitting smoking is not possible, then instruct parents not to smoke inside the house or automobile. Encourage the parents to have the child immunized with Prevnar and the influenza vaccine.

Xylitol syrup, a sucrose substitute, may also be protective (Klein & Pelton, 2015). Children who are old enough may chew xylitol-containing gum. Younger children and infants may be given xylitol syrup. Clinical studies are under way to validate the protective effects of xylitol. Care should be taken to avoid excessive dosing, as xylitol can cause diarrhea.

HEALTHY PEOPLE *2020*

Objective	Nursing Significance
Decrease otitis media in children and adolescents.	• Teach children and families the importance of hand washing to avoid the common cold (often a precursor to otitis media). • Teach families the importance of appropriate follow-up for eradication of otitis media. • Educate families about the importance of using antibiotics only for true bacterial infections (in order to decrease the development of resistant organisms, many of which cause otitis media).

Healthy People Objectives retrieved from http://www.healthypeople.gov

Otitis Media with Effusion

OME refers to the presence of fluid within the middle ear space, without signs or symptoms of infection. It may occur independent of AOM or may persist after the infectious process of AOM has resolved. Risk factors for OME include passive smoking, absence of breastfeeding, frequent viral upper respiratory infections, allergy, young age, male sex, adenoid hypertrophy, Eustachian tube dysfunction, and certain congenital disorders (Friedman et al., 2014). Complications of OME include AOM, hearing loss, and deafness.

Nursing Assessment

Nursing assessment of the child with OME includes health history, physical examination, and diagnostic testing.

HEALTH HISTORY

Determine the extent of symptoms. Children may be asymptomatic or may experience a popping sensation or fullness behind the eardrum. Explore the health history for risk factors such as passive smoking, absence of breastfeeding, frequent viral upper respiratory infections, allergy, or recent history of AOM.

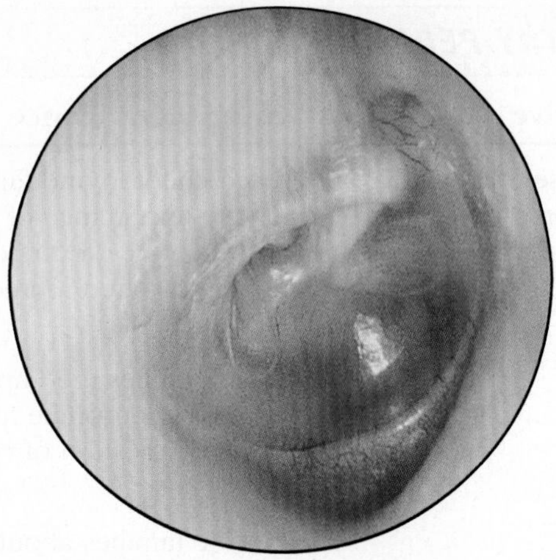

FIGURE 39.11 Otitis media with effusion; note dull white tympanic membrane.

BOX 39.3

CHILDREN AT RISK FOR SPEECH, LANGUAGE, OR LEARNING DIFFICULTIES

- Permanent hearing loss (without otitis media with effusion)
- Speech/language delay (suspected or diagnosed)
- Craniofacial disorder that may interfere with speech
- Any pervasive developmental disorder
- Genetic disorders or syndromes associated with speech or learning problems
- Cleft palate
- Blindness or significant visual impairment

Adapted from American Academy of Pediatrics. (2013a). Clinical practice guideline: The diagnosis and management of acute otitis media. *Pediatrics, 131*, e964–e999.

PHYSICAL EXAMINATION

Otoscopic examination may reveal a dull, opaque tympanic membrane that may be white, gray, or bluish (Fig. 39.11). If the tympanic membrane is not opaque, a fluid level or air bubble may be visualized. Mobility may be absent or diminished upon pneumatic otoscopy. Tympanometry may be used to confirm the diagnosis of OME.

Nursing Management

OME may take several months to resolve. Nursing management during the resolution phase focuses on education and monitoring for hearing loss.

EDUCATING THE FAMILY

Educate the family about the natural history of OME and the anatomic differences in young children that contribute to OME. Inform parents that antihistamines, decongestants, antibiotics, and corticosteroids have not been proven to hasten the resolution of OME and thus are not recommended. OME usually resolves spontaneously, but children should be rechecked every 4 weeks while this resolution is occurring. Teach parents not to feed infants in a supine position and to avoid bottle propping.

MONITORING FOR HEARING LOSS

When OME persists, the primary concern is its effect on hearing. In the infant or toddler who should be experiencing rapid language development, impaired hearing can depress language acquisition significantly (Klein & Pelton, 2016). Children with OME who are at risk for speech, language, or learning problems may be referred for evaluation of hearing earlier than a child with OME who is not at risk (Box 39.3). Children with chronic OME (persistent OME of 3 months' duration or longer) should be referred to a specialist for hearing evaluation (Klein & Pelton, 2016). Children who are not already at risk for speech concerns and are not experiencing difficulty with language acquisition may be reassessed every 3 to 6 months as long as hearing loss is not identified. At-risk children may require treatment earlier.

To communicate more effectively with children with OME who have hearing loss:

- Turn off music or television.
- Position yourself within 3 ft of the child before speaking.
- Face the child while speaking.
- Use visual cues.
- Increase the volume of your speech only slightly.
- Speak clearly.
- Request preferential classroom seating.

Take Note!

Evaluation of hearing is recommended when OME lasts 3 months or more if language delay, hearing loss, or a learning problem is suspected (Klein & Pelton, 2016).

PROVIDING POSTOPERATIVE CARE FOR THE CHILD WITH PRESSURE-EQUALIZING TUBES

The standard treatment for persistent or problematic OME is surgical insertion of **pressure-equalizing (PE) tubes** into the tympanic membrane (via myringotomy). The tubes stay in place for at least several months and generally fall out on their own (Fig. 39.12). The procedure is usually done as an outpatient surgery and the child returns home in the evening. Teach the parents to administer ear drops postoperatively if prescribed. After PE tube placement, the surgeon may recommend avoiding water entry into the ears. If recommended, advise parents to have the child wear earplugs in the bathtub or while swimming.

Placement of the PE tubes allows for adequate hearing, which in turn encourages appropriate speech development. Placement of PE tubes does not prevent middle ear infection. If the middle ear becomes infected with PE tubes in place, the tubes allow infected fluid to drain

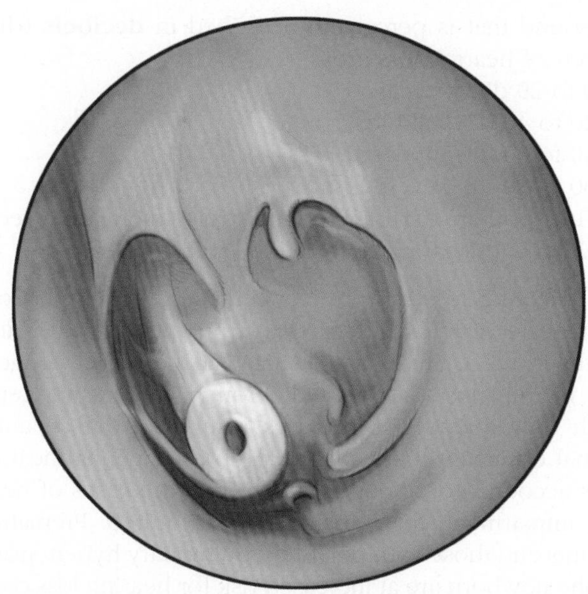

FIGURE 39.12 Pressure-equalizing tube in place in the tympanic membrane.

from the ear. Tell parents to contact their physician or nurse practitioner if drainage from the ear is noted. After PE tubes are placed, young children often have rapid increases in language acquisition, and parents should observe for this (O'Reilly, 2014).

Take Note!

Children with PE tubes who swim in a lake must wear earplugs, as lake water is contaminated with bacteria and entry of that water into the middle ear should be avoided (Cincinnati Children's, 2016).

Otitis Externa

Otitis externa is defined as an infection and inflammation of the skin of the external ear canal. *Pseudomonas aeruginosa* and *Staphylococcus aureus* are typical causative agents, though fungi such as *Aspergillus* and other bacteria also may be implicated. Moisture in the canal contributes to pathogen growth (Friedman et al., 2014). Otitis externa is commonly known as "swimmer's ear" since it occurs more frequently in those who swim often (and thus have wet ear canals). Changing the pH in the ear canal contributes to the inflammatory process.

Nursing Assessment

Nursing assessment of the child with otitis externa focuses on the health history and physical examination.

HEALTH HISTORY

Elicit a description of the present illness and chief complaint. Note history of ear itching or pain, ear drainage, or a feeling of fullness in the ear canal, with possible difficulty hearing. Note onset and progression of symptoms, as well as the child's response to treatments. Explore the child's current and past medical history for risk factors such as previous episodes of otitis externa or history of recent swimming in a pool, lake, or ocean.

Take Note!

The child with otitis externa usually has significant ear pain. Pressure on the tragus should be avoided, as it can worsen the pain.

PHYSICAL EXAMINATION

Typically a white or colored discharge can be seen in the ear canal or running from the ear. On otoscopy, the canal is red and edematous, often too swollen for insertion of the speculum and viewing of the tympanic membrane (Fig. 39.13). Diagnosis is based on clinical findings. Occasionally the ear drainage is cultured for bacteria or fungus, particularly if otitis externa is not improving with treatment.

Nursing Management

The primary goals of nursing management are pain relief, treatment of the infection, and prevention of recurrence.

MANAGING PAIN

Analgesics (often narcotics) may be administered to manage the pain. A warm compress or heating pad to the affected ear is helpful in some children.

TREATING THE INFECTION

Administer antibiotic or antifungal eardrops as prescribed. In some cases a wick is placed in the ear canal. The wick keeps the antibiotic drops in contact with the skin of the ear canal and promotes healing. Wick insertion can be extremely painful, and younger children will need to be restrained during insertion for their safety.

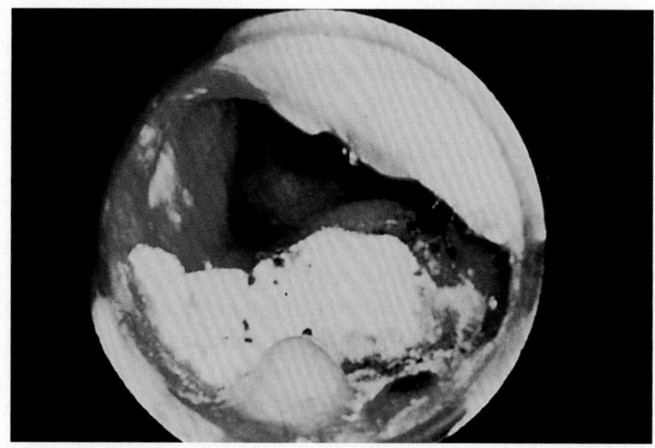

FIGURE 39.13 Note edema and erythema of the ear canal as well as purulent discharge in the child with otitis externa.

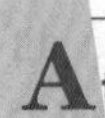

Atraumatic Care

When instilling ear drops in the young child, use distraction (a song, a favorite toy) to decrease perceived trauma to the child.

PREVENTING REINFECTION

Teach children and their parents about prevention of further episodes once the infection has resolved. Since moisture contributes to otitis externa, explain the importance of keeping the ear canals dry. Encourage the child and parents to use one of the methods described in Teaching Guidelines 39.2 after swimming or showering.

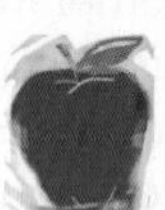

Teaching Guidelines 39.2

PREVENTING OTITIS EXTERNA

1. Avoid the use of cotton swabs, headphones, and earphones.
2. Wear earplugs when swimming.
3. Promote ear canal dryness and alternate pH. Use one or more of the following methods:
   - Dry the ear canals using a hair dryer set on a lower setting.
   - Administer solutions that have a drying effect on the auditory canal skin and change the pH of the canal to discourage organism growth in susceptible children. The following solutions can be used:
   - A few drops of Domeboro solution can be placed in the canal, and then allowed to run out.
   - A mixture of half rubbing alcohol and half vinegar (squirted into the canal and then allowed to run out). The alcohol solution should be used only when the ear canals are healthy. Using it while the canals are inflamed will cause stinging and increased pain.

Adapted from Cook, S. P. & Gupta, R. C. (2016). *Swimmer's ear.* Retrieved from http://kidshealth.org/kid/ill_injure/aches/swimmers_ear.html

HEARING LOSS AND DEAFNESS

Infants are ordinarily born with the sense of hearing fully developed. Language development in infancy and early childhood is dependent upon adequate hearing, and even the fluctuating hearing loss associated with intermittent bouts of AOM can hinder language development (Klein & Pelton, 2015). Hearing loss may be unilateral (involving one ear) or bilateral (involving both ears). The extent of hearing loss is defined based on the softest intensity of sound that is perceived, described in **decibels** (dB). Levels of hearing loss are:

- 0 to 20 dB: normal
- 20 to 40 dB: mild loss
- 40 to 60 dB: moderate loss
- 60 to 80 dB: severe loss
- Greater than 80 dB: profound loss (American Speech-Language-Hearing Association [ASHA], 2016d)

Hearing loss may be congenital or acquired. Congenital hearing loss affects 1 to 6 infants per 1,000 live births in the United States (ASHA, 2016c). Most congenital hearing loss is inherited through a recessive gene, with only about 15% of cases resulting from an autosomal dominant trait (ASHA, 2016b). Congenital hearing loss accounts for about one half of all the cases of hearing impairment; the remainder are acquired. Premature infants and those with persistent pulmonary hypertension of the newborn are at increased risk for hearing loss compared with other infants. Hearing loss commonly occurs with a large number of congenital or genetic syndromes, as well as in association with anomalies of the head and face. A variety of newborn universal hearing screening mandates have been passed by legislation in 43 states, thus allowing for earlier identification of infants with congenital hearing loss (National Center for Hearing Assessment and Management, 2016). See Healthy People 2020.

Delayed-onset (acquired) hearing loss may be conductive, sensorineural, or mixed. **Conductive hearing loss** results when transmission of sound through the middle ear is disrupted, as in the case of OME. When fluid fills the middle ear, the tympanic membrane is unable to move properly, and partial or complete hearing loss occurs. **Sensorineural hearing loss** is caused by damage to the hair cells in the cochlea or along the auditory pathway. This may result from kernicterus, use of ototoxic medication, intrauterine infection with cytomegalovirus or rubella, neonatal or postnatal infection such as meningitis, severe neonatal respiratory depression,

HEALTHY PEOPLE 2020

Objective	Nursing Significance
Increase the proportion of newborns who are screened for hearing loss no later than age 1 month, have an audiologic evaluation by age 3 months, and are enrolled in appropriate intervention services no later than age 6 months.	• Encourage appropriate hearing assessments. • Refer children who are diagnosed with a hearing deficit to local services for the deaf or hearing impaired.

Healthy People Objectives retrieved from http://www.healthypeople.gov

HEALTHY PEOPLE 2020

Objective	Nursing Significance
Increase the use of hearing protection devices. Reduce the proportion of adolescents who have elevated hearing thresholds, or audiometric notches, in high frequencies (3, 4, or 6 kHz) in both ears, signifying noise-induced hearing loss.	• Educate children and families about the dangers of excess noise and its potential for damaging hearing. • Encourage appropriate use of ear protection devices.

Healthy People Objectives retrieved from http://www.healthypeople.gov

or exposure to excess noise. Mixed hearing loss occurs when the cause may be attributed to both conductive and sensorineural problems. See Healthy People 2020.

Regardless of the cause of hearing loss, early intervention can make a difference in the child's ability to communicate. Once the hearing loss has been determined, intervention can begin. Hearing aids, cochlear implants, communication devices, and speech education may enable these children to communicate verbally. Improved communication beginning in infancy and early childhood may also improve the child's school achievement.

Take Note!

Earplugs or covers used to block ambient noise in premature infants in the neonatal intensive care unit may decrease the preemie's risk for hearing loss and improve development outcomes (Turk, Williams, & Lasky, 2009).

Nursing Assessment

Nursing assessment of the child with hearing loss or impairment focuses on the health history, physical examination, and diagnostic hearing testing.

HEALTH HISTORY

Common signs and symptoms reported during the health history might include:

- Infant:
  - Wakes only to touch, not environmental noises
  - Does not startle to loud noises
  - Does not turn to sound by 4 months of age
  - Does not babble at 6 months of age
  - Does not progress with speech development
- Young child:
  - Does not speak by 2 years of age
  - Communicates needs through gestures
  - Does not speak distinctly, as appropriate for his or her age
  - Displays developmental (cognitive) delays
  - Prefers solitary play
  - Displays immature emotional behavior
  - Does not respond to ringing of the telephone or doorbell
  - Focuses on facial expressions when communicating
- Older child:
  - Often asks for statements to be repeated
  - Is inattentive or daydreams
  - Performs poorly at school
  - Displays monotone or other abnormal speech
  - Gives inappropriate answers to questions except when able to view face of speaker
- At any age:
  - Speaks loudly
  - Sits very close to the TV or radio or turns volume up too loud
  - Responds only to moderate or loud voices

Investigate signs of hearing loss as early as possible in order for appropriate intervention to begin.

Explore the child's current and past medical history for risk factors such as congenital anomalies, genetic syndrome, infection, family history, kernicterus, neonatal ventilator use, ototoxic medication, or exposure to excess noise. Note whether newborn hearing screening was done and, if so, what the results were.

PHYSICAL EXAMINATION AND LABORATORY AND DIAGNOSTIC TESTS

Determine the child's level of interaction with the environment. For preschoolers and older children, administer the whisper test, keeping in mind that this is a gross screening test only. Perform the Weber and Rinne tests (refer to Chapter 31 for further explanation). If further evaluation is needed, the nurse may be responsible for administering an otoacoustic emissions test or auditory brain stem evoked response test, either in the hospital or outpatient office.

Nursing Management

The primary goal of nursing care for the child with a hearing impairment is to provide education and support to the family and child. Individualize care for the child with a hearing impairment and the family based on their specific responses to the hearing impairment.

AUGMENTING HEARING

Compliance with hearing aids and communication curriculums is critical so that the child can develop hearing and speech. Teach the child and family that hearing aids should be cleaned daily with a damp cloth. In addition, it is important to change batteries weekly. When inserting the aid, the volume should be turned down, then adjusted to the appropriate level after insertion. As the

HEALTHY PEOPLE 2020

Objective	Nursing Significance
Increase the proportion of persons with hearing impairments who have ever used a hearing aid or assistive listening devices or who have cochlear implants.	• Know resources available in the local area for the deaf and hearing impaired. • Refer children with hearing deficits to these resources and to service providers for augmentative devices.

Healthy People Objectives retrieved from http://www.healthypeople.gov

infant or child grows, the hearing aid will need to be reassessed for proper fit. Many deaf schools and other organizations provide loaner hearing aids so that the best fit and amplification may be determined prior to purchase. Assist the family to explore this type of option in the local community. See Healthy People 2020.

When cochlear implants are used, the nurse focuses on postoperative care of the incision site and pain management.

PROMOTING COMMUNICATION AND EDUCATION

Families and children need to learn how to communicate effectively with one another. If the child learns American Sign Language, for instance, the parents and siblings should as well. Table 39.4 provides information on communication options for hearing-impaired children and their families. Communication may also be enhanced by the use of text telephone service in the home and closed-caption television. Bells and alarms in the home may use lights rather than sound to alert the child. Provide a sign language interpreter for the child at healthcare visits if the parent is not present for interpretation.

ENCOURAGING EDUCATION

Refer the child younger than 3 years of age to the local district of Early Intervention for case management of developmental needs. At 3 years of age and beyond, state laws provide for public education and related services for children with disabilities. An IEP should be developed to maximize the child's learning ability. Nurses may be involved in the development of the IEP.

Some children attend schools specifically geared toward deaf students. The choice of school will depend on the family's preferences and resources.

PROVIDING SUPPORT

The diagnosis of a significant disability can be extremely stressful for the family. Encourage families to express their feelings and provide emotional support. Ensure that the needs of any siblings are also attended to. When the family is ready, encourage them to network with other families who have children with similar needs. Educate the family about the child's prescribed plan of care. Refer families to resources and support groups. Several helpful resources are listed on thePoint.

TABLE 39.4 COMPARING COMMUNICATION OPTIONS FOR THE HEARING IMPAIRED

Spoken Language	
Oral deaf education (auditory-verbal therapy)	Uses technology to boost auditory potential; teaches children to notice sound and give it meaning. Develops oral speech
Cued speech	A system using hand signs to clarify lip-reading; gives the person clues about the sounds the speaker is making
Signed Language	
American Sign Language (ASL)	Entirely communicated through hand signs, gestures, and facial expressions. Has its own grammar and syntax
Combination: Total Communication	Combines auditory training and teaching of spoken language with SEE ("signing exact English"; corresponds to the words and syntax of English)
Augmentative and Alternative Communication (AAC)	
May use gestural communication	Can also include physical devices such as notebooks, communication boards, charts, or computers. Ranges from very low tech to technologically complex

Adapted from American Speech-Language-Hearing Association. (2016b). *Augmentative and alternative communication (AAC).* Retrieved from http://www.asha.org/public/speech/disorders/AAC.htm

NURSING CARE PLAN 39.1

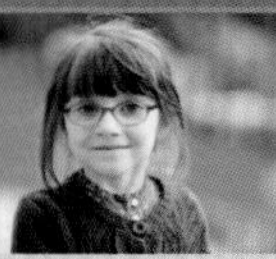

Overview for the Child With a Disorder of Eyes or Ears

NURSING DIAGNOSIS: Disturbed sensory perception (visual) related to visual impairment squinting, holding items close, verbalization of inability to see clearly

Outcome Identification and Evaluation

Child will reach maximal vision potential: *child uses corrective lenses appropriately and is able to participate in play and schoolwork.*

Intervention: ***Improving Vision***

- Encourage corrective lens use *for enhancement of vision.*
- Support the family's efforts at vision therapy and other habilitation programs *to promote vision enhancement.*
- Encourage parents to comply with vision screening appointments *in order to determine visual acuity progression or problems.*

NURSING DIAGNOSIS: Fear related to severe visual impairment or blindness as evidenced by child's behaviors or verbalization

Outcome Identification and Evaluation

Child will experience decreased fear: *child will verbalize comfort with environment or react calmly to interventions.*

Intervention: ***Improving Vision***

- Allow verbal child to share his feelings *to promote coping in the child.*
- For the severely impaired or blind child, identify yourself via voice and name items in environment for the child *so that the child is aware of his or her surroundings.*
- Engage the parents in bedside caregiving *because the parents' voice and presence are reassuring to the child.*

NURSING DIAGNOSIS: Disturbed sensory perception (auditory) related to hearing loss as evidenced by lack of reaction to verbal stimuli, delayed attainment of language milestones

Outcome Identification and Evaluation

Child will reach maximal hearing and speech potential: *child uses aids appropriately and communicates effectively.*

Intervention: ***Improving Hearing***

- Assess hearing ability frequently *because early detection of hearing loss allows for earlier intervention and correction.*
- Assess language development at each visit *to allow for early detection of hearing loss (earlier intervention and correction).*
- Encourage hearing aid use *for amplification of sound.*
- Teach about hearing aid battery safety *to avoid aspiration of battery.*
- Assist child with focusing on sounds in the environment *to encourage listening skills.*
- Refer for and encourage attendance at communication habilitation program *to maximize communication potential.*

(continued)

NURSING CARE PLAN 39.1

Overview for the Child With a Disorder of Eyes or Ears (continued)

NURSING DIAGNOSIS: Risk for infection related to presence of infectious organisms

Outcome Identification and Evaluation

Child will exhibit no signs of secondary infection and will not spread infection to others: *symptoms of infection decrease over time, and others remain free from infection.*

Intervention: ***Reducing Infection Risk***

- Maintain aseptic technique and practice good handwashing *to prevent introduction of further infectious agents.*
- Limit number of visitors, and screen for recent illness, *to prevent further infection.*
- Administer antibiotics if prescribed *to prevent or treat bacterial infection.*
- Encourage nutritious diet according to child's preferences *to assist body's natural infection-fighting mechanisms.*
- Isolate the child as required *to prevent nosocomial spread of infection.*
- Teach child and family preventive measures such as good handwashing, covering mouth and nose when coughing or sneezing, and adequate disposal of used tissues *to prevent nosocomial or community spread of infection.*

NURSING DIAGNOSIS: Delayed growth and development related to sensory impairment as evidenced by delay in attainment of developmental milestones

Outcome Identification and Evaluation

Child will achieve optimum independence for age: *child participates in age-appropriate developmental activities.*

Intervention: ***Encouraging Growth and Development***

- Encourage attainment of developmental milestones with use of assistive devices as needed *for timely developmental achievements.*
- Foster independence in activities of daily living (ADLs) *to promote sense of accomplishment.*
- Encourage participation in play with another child or within a group *to promote socialization.*
- Assist family to set limits and apply discipline *because structure and routine provide a secure environment in which the developing child can grow.*
- Encourage friendships with other children with a sensory impairment *to promote socialization and let the child know that he or she is not the only one with these challenges.*

NURSING DIAGNOSIS: Impaired verbal communication related to hearing loss as evidenced by lack of or inarticulate speech, lack of alternate communication channel

Outcome Identification and Evaluation

The child will communicate effectively with the method chosen by the family (this may be sign language, oral/deaf speech, cued speech, or augmentative alternative communication device).

Intervention: ***Improving Communication***

- Encourage choice of and attendance at communication habilitation program *to promote continued learning.*
- Provide consistency between home and hospital in regard to communication style/devices *to promote continued learning.*
- Support the child's efforts at correct speech *to promote speech development through reinforcement and praise.*
- Encourage family to use spoken language and read books at home *to continue to promote appropriate language development.*

NURSING CARE PLAN 39.1

Overview for the Child With a Disorder of Eyes or Ears (continued)

NURSING DIAGNOSIS: Deficient knowledge related to sensory impairment (vision or hearing) as evidenced by new diagnosis and parents' questions

Outcome Identification and Evaluation

Parents express understanding of diagnosis and care of child: *parents verbalize understanding, demonstrate use of assistive devices, or independently perform medical treatments.*

Intervention: ***Educating the Family***

- Review diagnosis and plan of care with the parents *to promote understanding of the disease process.*
- Refer family to resources available for sensory-impaired children *to provide further education and support to the parents.*
- Demonstrate medical treatments prescribed or use of assistive devices, requiring a return demonstration, *which shows the parents' ability to provide the prescribed care for the child.*
- Encourage exploration of different communication and learning modes available for the sensory-impaired child *to allow the child and family to find the right educational and communication style fit.*

NURSING DIAGNOSIS: Family processes, interrupted, related to child's sensory impairment as evidenced by parent verbalization, nonverbal communication, altered coping

Outcome Identification and Evaluation

Parents demonstrate adequate coping and decreased anxiety: *parents are involved in child's care, ask appropriate questions, and are able to discuss child's care and condition calmly.*

Intervention: ***Encouraging Appropriate Family Interactions***

- Encourage parents' verbalization of grief if child is hearing or vision impaired. *Parents must deal with their own feelings of loss to successfully care for the child with an impairment.*
- Encourage parents' verbalization of concerns related to child's illness: *allows for identification of concerns and demonstrates to the family that the nurse also cares about them, not just the child.*
- Explain therapy, procedures, and child's behavior to parents: *developing an understanding of the child's current status helps decrease anxiety.*
- Encourage parental involvement in care *so that parents may continue to feel needed and valued.*

NURSING DIAGNOSIS: Risk for injury related to vision loss

Outcome Identification and Evaluation

The infant or child will remain free from injury.

Intervention: ***Preventing Injury***

- Orient the child to hospital surroundings *because awareness is the first step to preventing injury.*
- Encourage parent to be at bedside *so that the child feels more comfortable.*
- Encourage use of assistive devise *to promote safety.*

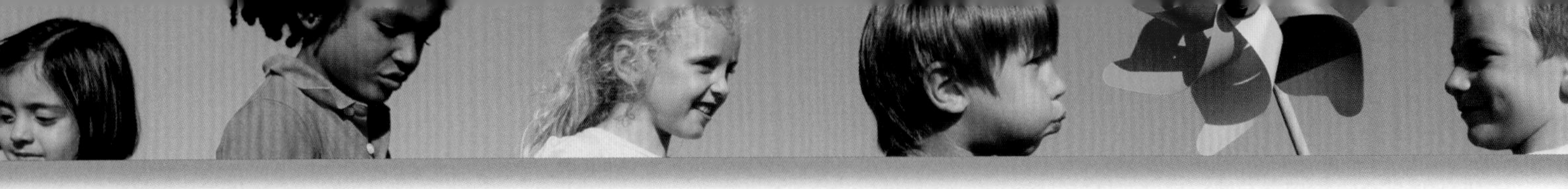

KEY CONCEPTS

- Though hearing is fully developed at birth, visual development continues to progress until about age 7 years.
- Binocular vision develops by age 4 months; visual acuity progresses to 20/50 by age 3 years and usually reaches 20/20 by age 7 years.
- The relatively short and horizontally positioned Eustachian tubes of infants and young children make them more susceptible to otitis media than adults.
- To maximize speech and language development, hearing loss should be identified early and intervention begun immediately.
- Children with genetic syndromes or family history are at increased risk of visual and hearing impairments.
- The corneal light reflex test and cover test are useful tools for identifying strabismus and amblyopia.
- Tympanometry is used to determine the presence of fluid behind the eardrum (such as with otitis media with effusion).
- Topical ophthalmic medications are used to treat certain infectious eye disorders.
- Appropriate hand washing is the single most important factor to reduce the spread of acute viral or bacterial conjunctivitis.
- Systemic antibiotics are used for the treatment of periorbital cellulitis.
- Strabismus, glaucoma, and cataracts may all lead to visual impairment if left untreated.
- Asymmetry of the corneal light reflex occurs with true strabismus.
- Amblyopia must be identified early and treated with patching, corrective lenses, or surgery to prevent visual deterioration and promote appropriate vision development.
- A cloudy cornea indicates the presence of cataract.
- Very premature infants are at high risk of developing visual deficits related to retinopathy of prematurity and are also at increased risk of hearing impairment compared to other infants.
- Eye strain, eye rubbing, and headaches may indicate a visual deficit.
- Children with visual disorders should be encouraged to use prescribed corrective lenses.
- Recurrent episodes of acute otitis media may negatively affect the child's hearing.
- Recurrent or constant nasal congestion contributes to otitis media with effusion.
- Otitis externa can be prevented by keeping the ear canal dry and altering canal pH.
- The fluctuating hearing loss associated with recurrent otitis media and the hearing loss associated with chronic otitis media with effusion can both significantly hinder language development in the infant and toddler.
- The child with hearing loss should receive early intervention with hearing aids or other augmentative devices.

REFERENCES AND RECOMMENDED READINGS

American Academy of Pediatrics (AAP). (2013a). Clinical practice guideline: The diagnosis and management of acute otitis media. *Pediatrics, 131*, e964–e999.

American Academy of Pediatrics (AAP). (2013b). Screening examination of premature infants for retinopathy of prematurity. *Pediatrics, 131*(1), 189–195.

American Association for Pediatric Ophthalmology and Strabismus (AAPOS). (2015). *Glasses fitting for children*. Retrieved from http://www.aapos.org/terms/conditions/53

American Association for Pediatric Ophthalmology and Strabismus (AAPOS). (2016a). *Nasolacrimal duct obstruction*. Retrieved from http://www.aapos.org/terms/conditions/72

American Association for Pediatric Ophthalmology and Strabismus (AAPOS). (2016b). *Photoscreening*. Retrieved from http://www.aapos.org/terms/terms/140

American Speech-Language-Hearing Association. (2016a). *Augmentative and alternative communication (AAC)*. Retrieved from www.asha.org/public/speech/disorders/AAC.htm

American Speech-Language-Hearing Association (ASHA). (2016b). *Hearing loss at birth (congenital hearing loss)*. Retrieved from www.asha.org/public/hearing/congenital-hearing-loss/

American Speech-Language-Hearing Association (ASHA). (2016c). *The prevalence and incidence of hearing loss in children*. Retrieved from www.asha.org/public/hearing/disorders/children.htm

American Speech-Language-Hearing Association (ASHA). (2016d). *Types of hearing loss*. Retrieved from http://www.asha.org/public/hearing/disorders/types.htm

Augsburger, J. J., & Correa, C. M. (2011). Ophthalmic trauma. In P. Riordan-Eva, & E. T. Cunningham (Eds.), *Vaughan & Asbury's general ophthalmology* (18th ed.). New York, NY: McGraw-Hill.

Blosser, C. G., Brady, M. A., & Royal, R. B. (2013). Infectious diseases & immunizations. In C. E. Burns, A. M. Dunn, M. A.

Brady, N. B. Starr, & C. G. Blosser. *Pediatric primary care* (5th ed.). Philadelphia, PA: Saunders.

Braverman, R. S. (2014). Eye. In W. W. Hay, M. J. Levin, R. R. Deterding, & M. J. Abzug, (Eds.), (*Current pediatric diagnosis and treatment* (22nd ed.). New York, NY: McGraw-Hill.

Bremond-Gignac, D., Copin, H., Lapillone, A., & Milazzo, S. (2011). Visual development in infants: Physiological and pathological mechanisms. *Current Opinion in Ophthalmology, 22*(1), S1–S8.

Carpenito-Moyet, L. J. (2013). *Nursing diagnosis: Application to clinical practice* (14th ed.). Philadelphia, PA: Lippincott Williams & Wilkins.

Carter, S. L. (2015). *Sensory impairment.* Retrieved from http://www.pediatrics.emory.edu/divisions/neonatology/dpc/sensory.html

Chiocca, E. (2015). Assessment of the eyes. In E. M. Chiocca (ed.), *Advanced pediatric assessment.* (2nd Ed.). New York, NY: Springer Publishing Company.

Cincinnati Children's. (2016). *Pressure equalizer (PE) tube insertion.* Retrieved from http://www.cincinnatichildrens.org/health/p/pe-tube/

Coats, D. K., & Paysse, E. A., (2016). *Overview of amblyopia.* Retrieved Coats & Paysse, 2015, from http://www.uptodate.com/contents/overview-of-amblyopia?source=search_result&search=amblyopia&selectedTitle=1~150

Cook, S. P. & Gupta, R. C. (2016). *Swimmer's ear.* Retrieved from http://kidshealth.org/kid/ill_injure/aches/swimmers_ear.html

Delta Gamma Center for Children with Visual Impairments. (2011). *Interacting with visually impaired.* Retrieved from http://dgckids.org/resources/interacting-with-visually-impaired/

Friedman, N. R., Scholes, M. A., & Yoon, P. J. (2014). Ear, nose, & throat. In W. W. Hay, M. J. Levin, & R. R. Deterding, & M. J. Abzug, (Eds.), (*Current pediatric diagnosis and treatment* (22nd ed.). New York, NY: McGraw-Hill.

Hammer, E. (n. d.). *Self-stimulation: Dr. Hammer responds.* Retrieved from http://www.nfb.org/images/nfb/Publications/fr/fr17/Issue3/F170308.htm

International Council of Ophthalmology (ICP). (2016). *Childhood blindness.* Retrieved from http://www.icoph.org/dynamic/attachments/resources/childhood-blindness.pdf

Jacobs, D. S. (2015). *Corneal abrasions and corneal foreign bodies: Management.* http://www.uptodate.com/contents/corneal-abrasions-and-corneal-foreign-bodies-management

Klein, J. O., & Pelton, S. (2015). *Acute otitis media: Prevention of recurrence.* Retrieved from http://www.uptodate.com/contents/acute-otitis-media-in-children-prevention-of-recurrence

Klein, J. O. & Pelton, S. (2016). *Otitis media with effusion (serous otitis media) in children: Management.* Retrieved from http://www.uptodate.com/contents/otitis-media-with-effusion-serous-otitis-media-in-children-management

Lin, A. A., & Buckley, E. G. (2010). Update on pediatric cataract surgery and intraocular lens implantation. *Current Opinion in Ophthalmology, 21*(1), 55–59.

Lusby, F. W., & Zieve, D. (2016). LASIK eye surgery. Retrieved from http://umm.edu/health/medical/ency/articles/lasik-eye-surgery

National Center for Hearing Assessment and Management. (2016). *EDHI legislation.* Retrieved from http://www.infanthearing.org/legislation/

National Institute on Deafness and Other Communication Disorders. (2016). *Cochlear implants.* from https://www.nidcd.nih.gov/health/cochlear-implants

Optometrists Network. (2016). *Strabismus.* Retrieved from http://www.strabismus.org/

O'Reilly, R. C. (2014). *Middle ear infections and ear tube surgery.* Retrieved from http://kidshealth.org/en/parents/ear-infections.html

Paysse, E. A., Coats, D. K., & Cassidy, M. (2015). *Nasolacrimal duct obstruction (dacryostenosis) in children and dacrocystocele.* Retrieved from http://www.uptodate.com/contents/congenital-nasolacrimal-duct-obstruction-dacryostenosis-and-dacryocystocele

Taketomo, C. K., Hodding, J. H., & Kraus, D. M. (2013). *Pediatric & neonatal dosage handbook* (20th ed.). Hudson, OH: Lexicomp.

Turk, C., Williams, A. L., & Lasky, R. E. (2009). A randomized clinical trial evaluating silicone earplugs for very low birth weight newborns in intensive care. *Journal of Perinatology, 29*(5), 358–363.

Turner, A., & Rabiu, M. (2007). Patching for corneal abrasion. *The Cochrane Library* 2007, doi: 10.1002/14 August 19, 2015, 651858.CD004764.pub2

U. S. Food and Drug Administration. (2015). *FDA safety notification: Risk of eye and skin injuries from high-powered, hand-held lasers used for pointing or entertainment.* Retrieved from http://www.fda.gov/MedicalDevices/Safety/AlertsandNotices/ucm237129.htm

U. S. Department of Health and Human Services. (2016). *Healthy people 2020.* Retrieved from http://www.healthypeople.gov/2020/default.aspx

Weber, J., & Kelley, J. H. (2014). *Health assessment in nursing* (5th ed.). Philadelphia, PA: Lippincott Williams & Wilkins.

Yeung, H., & Walton, D. S. (2012). Recognizing childhood glaucoma in the primary pediatric setting. *Contemporary Pediatrics, 29*(5), 32–40.

CHAPTER WORKSHEET

MULTIPLE CHOICE QUESTIONS

1. Which situation would cause the nurse to become concerned about possible hearing loss?
   a. 12-month old who babbles incessantly, making no sense
   b. 8-month old who says only "da"
   c. 3-month old who startles easily to sound
   d. 3-year old who drops the letter "s"
2. A 4-year old complains of extreme pain when the tragus is touched. Though not diagnostic, this sign is most indicative of which disorder?
   a. acute otitis media
   b. acute tympanic effusion
   c. otitis interna
   d. otitis externa
3. The nurse is caring for an infant who has undergone surgery for infantile glaucoma. What is the priority nursing intervention?
   a. Place the child prone postoperatively for comfort.
   b. Teach the family use of the contact lens.
   c. Place elbow restraints on the infant.
   d. Provide a mobile for optical stimulation.
4. A 2-year old has been prescribed eye patching for strabismus 6 hours per day. What teaching does the nurse provide for the mother?
   a. Try to patch 6 hours per day, but if you miss some it is OK.
   b. Patching is necessary to strengthen vision in the weaker eye.
   c. Patching will keep the eye from turning in.
   d. Since the child is so young, patching can be delayed until school age.

DOSAGE CALCULATION QUESTION

1. The nurse is caring for a child with acute otitis media. The child weighs 22 lb. The medication order reads: amoxicillin 160 mg PO every 8 hours. Amoxicillin is supplied as 200 mg/5 mL. How many milliliters will the nurse administer? Round to the nearest whole number.

CRITICAL THINKING EXERCISES

1. A 16-month-old toddler is being seen for his sixth ear infection. What particular information about his growth and development must the nurse ask about? Be specific about the questions you would ask.
2. How would you distinguish allergic conjunctivitis from acute bacterial conjunctivitis?
3. A 13-month old has been diagnosed with severe visual impairment. Develop a list of sample nursing diagnoses for this situation.

STUDY ACTIVITIES

1. Develop a sample plan for teaching a low-literacy parent about the etiology, treatment, and complications of recurrent acute otitis media.
2. While in the pediatric clinical setting, compare the play styles of a sighted child with those of a visually impaired child.
3. Research hearing and vision resources in your local community.

BRINGING IT ALL TOGETHER: A CASE STUDY

Bryn Carle, a 6-year old, is brought to the clinic by her mother. She presents with redness of the left eye, edema, and drainage. What other assessment information would be helpful? Based on the history and clinical presentation, Bryn is diagnosed with conjunctivitis. What education will be necessary for the family to assist in alleviating symptoms and preventing infectious spread?

Go to thePoint to find questions to consider about this case.

40

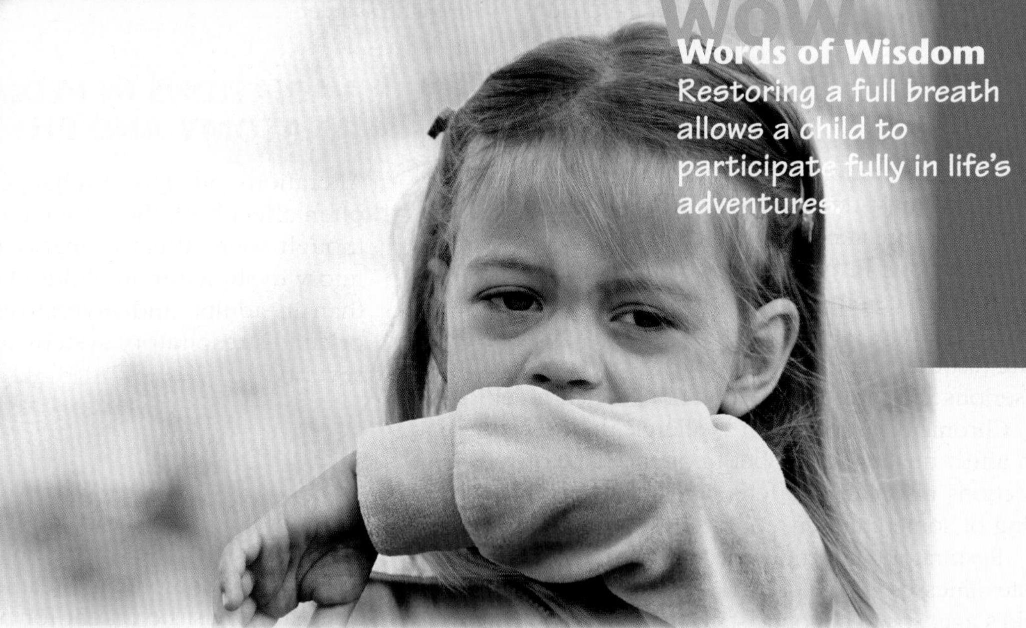
WOW
Words of Wisdom
Restoring a full breath allows a child to participate fully in life's adventures.

Nursing Care of the Child With an Alteration in Gas Exchange/ Respiratory Disorder

KEY TERMS

atelectasis
atopy
clubbing
coryza
cyanosis
hypoxemia
hypoxia
infiltrates
oxygenation
pulse oximetry
rales
retractions
rhinorrhea
stridor
suctioning
tachypnea
tracheostomy
ventilation
wheezing
work of breathing

Learning Objectives

Upon completion of the chapter, you will be able to:

1. Distinguish differences between the anatomy and physiology of the respiratory system in children versus adults.
2. Identify various factors associated with respiratory illness in infants and children.
3. Discuss common laboratory and other diagnostic tests useful in the diagnosis of respiratory conditions.
4. Describe nursing care related to common medications and other treatments used for management and palliation of respiratory conditions.
5. Recognize risk factors associated with various respiratory disorders.
6. Distinguish different respiratory disorders based on their signs and symptoms.
7. Discuss nursing interventions commonly used for respiratory illnesses.
8. Devise an individualized nursing care plan for the child with a respiratory disorder.
9. Develop child/family teaching plans for the child with a respiratory disorder.
10. Describe the psychosocial impact of chronic respiratory disorders on children.

***Alexander Roberts*, 4 months old, is brought to the clinic by his mother. He has a cold and has been coughing a great deal for 2 days. Today he has had difficulty taking his bottle and is breathing very quickly. Mrs. Roberts says he seems tired.**

Gas exchange refers to the process by which oxygen is transported to cells and carbon dioxide is transported from cells (Giddens, 2013). Nurses encounter potential and actual alterations in gas exchange in all types of clients and must detect problems and intervene early to prevent life-threatening complications.

Alterations in gas exchange (respiratory disorders) are the most common causes of illness and hospitalization in children. These illnesses range from mild, nonacute disorders (such as the common cold or sore throat) to serious life-threatening conditions (such as epiglottitis). Chronic disorders, such as allergic rhinitis or asthma, can affect quality of life, but frequent acute or recurrent infections also can interfere significantly with the well-being of some children.

Respiratory infections account for the majority of acute illnesses in children (Federico et al., 2014). The child's age, socioeconomic status, and general health status can influence both the development of respiratory disorders and the course of the illness. For example, low-income children have a higher risk for increased severity or increased frequency of respiratory disease (Sato et al., 2013). Infants and younger children are more likely to deteriorate quickly from a respiratory illness, and children with chronic disorders such as diabetes, congenital heart disease, sickle cell anemia, cystic fibrosis, and cerebral palsy tend to be more severely affected with respiratory disorders.

In addition, the season of the year can influence the development of respiratory disorders and the course of the illness. For example, certain viruses are more prevalent in the winter, whereas allergen-related respiratory diseases are more prevalent in the spring and fall.

Parents may have difficulty determining the severity of their child's condition and might either seek care very early in the course of the illness (when it is still very mild) or wait, presenting to the healthcare setting when the child is very ill. Nurses must be familiar with respiratory conditions affecting children so that they can provide guidance and support to families. Difficulty with breathing can be very frightening for both the child and parents. Nurses must be able to ask questions that can help establish the severity of the child's illness and determine whether the family should seek care at a healthcare facility.

Since respiratory illnesses account for the majority of pediatric admissions to general hospitals, nurses caring for children need to have expert assessment and intervention skills in this area. Detection of worsening respiratory status early in the course of deterioration allows for timely treatment and the chance to prevent a minor problem from becoming a critical illness. Nurses are also in a unique position to provide education about respiratory illnesses and to promote efforts to prevent these illnesses.

VARIATIONS IN PEDIATRIC ANATOMY AND PHYSIOLOGY

Alterations in gas exchange/respiratory conditions often affect both the upper and lower respiratory tract, though some affect primarily one or the other. Respiratory dysfunction in children tends to be more severe than in adults, and several differences in the infant's or child's respiratory system account for this increased severity.

Nose

Newborns are obligatory nose breathers until at least 4 weeks of age. The young infant cannot automatically open his or her mouth to breathe if the nose is obstructed. The nares must be patent for breathing to be successful while feeding. Newborns breathe through their mouths only while crying.

The upper respiratory mucus serves as a cleansing agent, yet newborns produce very little mucus, making them more susceptible to infection. However, the newborn and young infant have very small nasal passages, so when excess mucus is present, airway obstruction is more likely.

Infants are born with maxillary and ethmoid sinuses present. The frontal sinuses (most often associated with sinus infection) and the sphenoid sinuses develop by age 6 to 8 years. Therefore, younger children are less apt to acquire sinus infections compared to adults.

Throat

The tongue of the infant relative to the oropharynx is larger than in adults. Posterior displacement of the tongue can quickly lead to severe airway obstruction. Through early school age, children tend to have enlarged tonsillar and adenoidal tissue even in the absence of illness. This can contribute to an increased incidence of airway obstruction.

Trachea

The airway lumen is smaller in infants and children than in adults. The infant's trachea is approximately 4 mm wide compared with the adult width of 20 mm. When edema, mucus, or bronchospasm is present, the capacity for air passage is greatly diminished. A small reduction in the diameter of a child's airway (resulting from the presence of edema or mucus) will result in an exponential increase in resistance to airflow (Fig. 40.1). Increased **work of breathing** (effort or labor associated with respiration) then occurs.

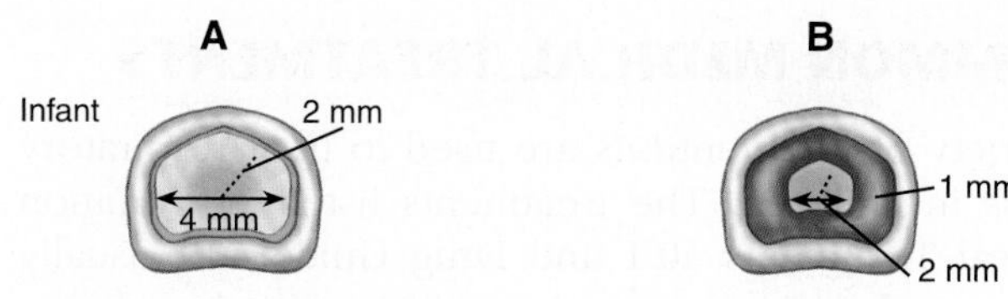

1 mm circumferential edema causes 50% reduction of diameter and radius, increasing pulmonary resistance by a factor of 16.

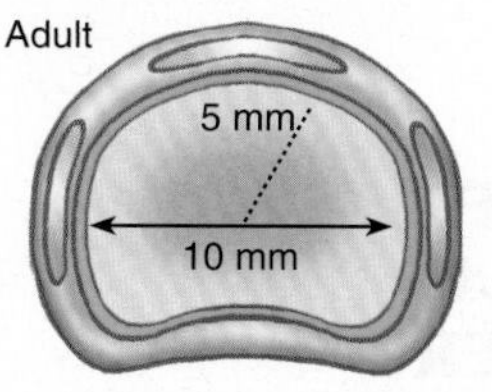

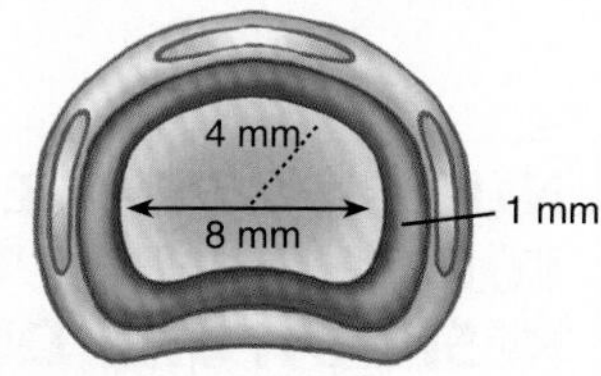

1 mm circumferential edema causes 20% reduction of diameter and radius, increasing pulmonary resistance by a factor of 2.4.

FIGURE 40.1 **(A)** Note the smaller diameter of the child's airway under normal circumstances. **(B)** With 1 mm of edema present, note the exponential decrease in airway lumen diameter as compared with the adult.

In teenagers and adults the larynx is cylindrical and fairly uniform in width. In infants and children younger than 10 years old, the cricoid cartilage is underdeveloped, resulting in laryngeal narrowing (Tewfik & Alghonaim, 2013). Thus, in infants and children, the larynx is funnel shaped. In addition, the larynx and glottis are located higher in the neck, increasing the chance of aspiration of foreign material into the lower airways. Congenital laryngomalacia occurs in some infants and results in the laryngeal structure being weaker than normal, yielding greater collapse on inspiration. Box 40.1 discusses congenital laryngomalacia.

BOX 40.1

CONGENITAL LARYNGOMALACIA

- Inspiratory stridor is present and is intensified with certain positions.
- Suprasternal retractions may be present, but the infant exhibits no other signs of respiratory distress.
- Congenital laryngomalacia is generally a benign condition that improves as the cartilage in the larynx matures. It usually disappears by age 1 year.
- The crowing noise heard with breathing can make parents very anxious. Reassure parents that the condition will improve with time.
- Parents become very familiar with the "normal" sound their infant makes and are often able to identify intensification or change in the stridor. Airway obstruction may occur earlier in infants with this condition, so intensification of stridor or symptoms of respiratory illness should be evaluated early by the physician or nurse practitioner.

The child's airway is highly compliant, making it quite susceptible to dynamic collapse in the presence of airway obstruction (American Heart Association [AHA], 2011). The muscles supporting the airway are less functional than those in the adult. Children have a large amount of soft tissue surrounding the trachea, and the mucous membranes lining the airway are less securely attached as compared with adults. This increases the risk for airway edema and obstruction. Upper airway obstruction resulting from a foreign body, croup, or epiglottitis can result in tracheal collapse during inspiration.

Lower Respiratory Structures

The bifurcation of the trachea occurs at the level of the third thoracic vertebra in children, compared to the level of the sixth thoracic vertebra in adults (Tewfik & Alghonaim, 2013). This anatomic difference is important when suctioning children and when endotracheal intubation is required (see Chapter 51 for further discussion). This difference in placement also contributes to risk for foreign material aspiration. The bronchi and bronchioles of infants and children are narrower in diameter than the adult's, placing them at increased risk for lower airway obstruction (see Fig. 40.1). Lower airway obstruction during exhalation often results from bronchiolitis or asthma or is caused by foreign body aspiration into the lower airway.

Alveoli develop at approximately 24 weeks' gestation. Term infants are born with about 50 million alveoli. After birth, alveolar growth slows until 3 months of age and then progresses until the child reaches 7 or 8 years of age, at which time the alveoli reach the adult number of around 300 million (Moore, Persaud, & Torchia, 2013). Alveoli make up most of the lung tissue and are the major sites for gas exchange. Oxygen moves from the alveolar air to the blood, while carbon dioxide moves from the blood into the alveolar air. Smaller numbers of alveoli, particularly in the premature and/or young infant, place the child at a higher risk of **hypoxemia** (deficiency in the concentration of oxygen in arterial blood) and carbon dioxide retention.

Chest Wall

In older children and adults, the ribs and sternum support the lungs and help keep them well expanded. The movement of the diaphragm and intercostal muscles alters volume and pressure within the chest cavity, resulting in air movement into the lungs. Infants' chest walls are highly compliant (pliable) and fail to support the lungs adequately. Functional residual capacity can be greatly reduced if respiratory effort is diminished. This lack of lung support also makes the tidal volume of infants and toddlers almost completely dependent upon movement of the diaphragm. If diaphragm movement is impaired (as in states of hyperinflation, such as asthma), the intercostal muscles cannot lift the chest wall and respiration is further compromised.

Metabolic Rate and Oxygen Need

Children have a significantly higher metabolic rate than adults. Their resting respiratory rates are faster and their demand for oxygen is higher. Adult oxygen consumption is 3 to 4 liters per minute, while infants consume 6 to 8 L per minute. In any situation of respiratory distress, infants and children will develop hypoxemia more rapidly than adults (AHA, 2011). This may be attributed not only to the child's increased oxygen requirement but also to the effect that certain conditions have on the oxyhemoglobin dissociation curve.

Normal oxygen transport relies on binding of oxygen to hemoglobin in areas of high partial pressure of oxygen (pO_2) (pulmonary arterial beds) and release of oxygen from hemoglobin when the pO_2 is low (peripheral tissues). Normally, a pO_2 of 95 mm Hg results in an oxygen saturation of 97%. A decrease in oxygen saturation results in a disproportionate (much larger) decrease in pO_2 (Fig. 40.2). Thus, a small decrease in oxygen saturation reflects a larger decrease in pO_2. Conditions such as alkalosis, hypothermia, hypocarbia, anemia, and fetal hemoglobin cause oxygen to become more tightly bound to hemoglobin, resulting in the curve shifting to the left. Common pediatric conditions such as acidosis, hyperthermia, and hypercarbia cause hemoglobin to decrease its affinity for oxygen, further shifting the curve to the right.

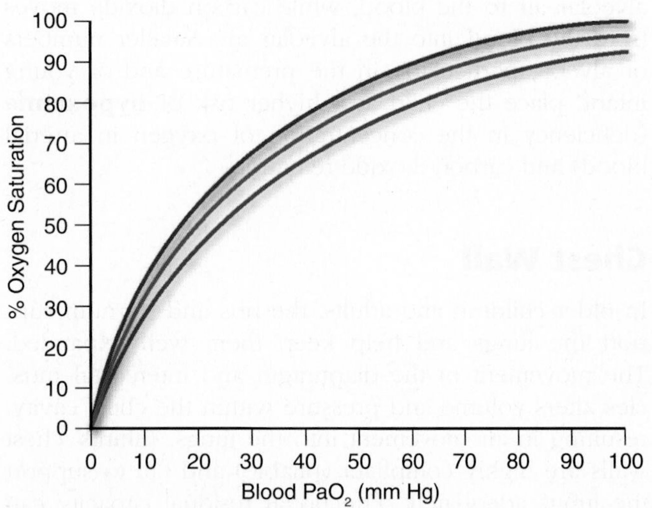

FIGURE 40.2 Normal hemoglobin dissociation curve (*green*), shift to the right (*red*), and shift to the left (*blue*).

COMMON MEDICAL TREATMENTS

A variety of interventions are used to treat respiratory illness in children. The treatments listed in Common Medical Treatments 40.1 and Drug Guide 40.1 usually require a physician or nurse practitioner's order when a child is hospitalized.

NURSING PROCESS OVERVIEW FOR THE CHILD WITH A RESPIRATORY DISORDER

Care of the child with a respiratory disorder includes assessment, nursing diagnosis, planning, interventions, and evaluation. There are a number of general concepts related to the nursing process that can be applied to respiratory disorders. From a general understanding of the care involved for a child with an alteration in gas exchange, the nurse can then individualize the care based on specifics for the particular child.

Assessment

Assessment of respiratory dysfunction in children includes health history, physical examination, and laboratory or diagnostic testing.

Remember Alexander, the 4-month-old with the cold, cough, fatigue, feeding difficulty, and fast breathing? What additional health history and physical examination assessment information should the nurse obtain?

Health History

The health history consists of the past medical history, family history, and history of present illness (when the symptoms started and how they have progressed), as well as treatments used at home. Ascertain immunization history. The past medical history might be significant for recurrent colds or sore throats, **atopy** (such as asthma or atopic dermatitis), prematurity, respiratory dysfunction at birth, poor weight gain, or history of recurrent respiratory illnesses or chronic lung disease. Family history might be significant for chronic respiratory disorders such as asthma or might reveal contacts for infectious exposure. When eliciting the history of the present illness, inquire about onset and progression; fever; nasal congestion; noisy breathing; presence and description of cough; rapid respirations; increased work of breathing; ear, nose, sinus, or throat pain; ear pulling; headache; vomiting with coughing; poor

COMMON MEDICAL TREATMENTS 40.1 RESPIRATORY DISORDERS

Treatment	Explanation	Indications	Nursing Implications
Oxygen	Supplemented via mask, nasal cannula, hood, or tent or via endotracheal or nasotracheal tube	Hypoxemia, respiratory distress	Monitor response via work of breathing and pulse oximetry.
High humidity	Addition of moisture to inspired air	Common cold, croup, tonsillectomy	Infant may require extra blankets with cool mist, and frequent changes of bedclothes under oxygen hood or tent as they become damp.
Suctioning	Removal of secretions via bulb syringe or suction catheter	Excessive airway secretions (common cold, flu, bronchiolitis, pertussis)	Should be done carefully and only as far as recommended for age or tracheostomy tube size, or until cough or gag occurs.
Chest physiotherapy (CPT) and postural drainage	Promotes mucus clearance by mobilizing secretions with the assistance of percussion or vibration accompanied by postural drainage	Bronchiolitis, pneumonia, cystic fibrosis, or other conditions resulting in increased mucus production. Not effective in inflammatory conditions without increased mucus	May be performed by respiratory therapist in some institutions, by nurses in others. In either case, nurses must be familiar with the technique and able to educate families on its use.
Saline gargles	Relieves throat pain via salt water gargle	Pharyngitis, tonsillitis	Recommended for children old enough to understand the concept of gargling (to avoid choking).
Saline lavage	Normal saline introduced into the airway, followed by suctioning	Common cold, flu, bronchiolitis, any condition resulting in increased mucus production in the upper airway	Very helpful for loosening thick mucus; child may need to be in semi-upright position to avoid aspiration.
Chest tube	Insertion of a drainage tube into the pleural cavity to facilitate removal of air or fluid and allow full lung expansion	Pneumothorax, empyema	Should tube become dislodged from container, the chest tube must be clamped immediately or the open end placed into a container of sterile water to avoid further air entry into the chest cavity.
Bronchoscopy	Introduction of a bronchoscope into the bronchial tree for diagnostic purposes. Also allows for bronchiolar lavage.	Removal of foreign body, cleansing of bronchial tree	Watch for postprocedure airway swelling, complaints of sore throat.

feeding; and lethargy. Also inquire about exposure to second-hand smoke. Children exposed to environmental smoke have an increased incidence of respiratory illnesses such as asthma, bronchitis, and pneumonia (World Health Organization, n. d.). See Healthy People 2020.

***HEALTHY PEOPLE** 2020*

Objective	Nursing Significance
Reduce the proportion of nonsmokers (children and adolescents) exposed to second-hand smoke.	• Educate the family about the effects that passive smoking has on children. • Encourage families to join smoking cessation programs.

Healthy People Objectives retrieved from http://www.healthypeople.gov

Physical Examination

Physical examination of the respiratory system includes inspection and observation, auscultation, percussion, and palpation.

(text continues on page 1474)

DRUG GUIDE 40.1 COMMON DRUGS FOR RESPIRATORY DISORDERS

Medication	Actions/Indications	Nursing Implications
Expectorant (guaifenesin)	Reduces viscosity of thickened secretions by increasing respiratory tract fluid Used for the common cold, pneumonia, and other conditions requiring mobilization and subsequent expectoration of mucus	Encourage deep breathing before coughing in order to mobilize secretions Maintain adequate fluid intake Assess breath sounds frequently
Cough suppressants (dextromethorphan, codeine, hydrocodone)	Relieve irritating, nonproductive cough by direct effect on the cough center in the medulla, which suppresses the cough reflex Used for the common cold, sinusitis, pneumonia, bronchitis	Should be used only with nonproductive coughs in the absence of wheezing
Antihistamines	Treatment of allergic conditions such as allergic rhinitis, asthma	May cause drowsiness or dry mouth
Antibiotics (oral, parenteral)	Treatment of bacterial infections of the respiratory tract such as pharyngitis, tonsillitis, sinusitis, bacterial pneumonia, cystic fibrosis, empyema, abscess, tuberculosis	Check for antibiotic allergies. Should be given as prescribed for the length of time prescribed
Antibiotics (inhaled)	Treatment of bacterial infections of the respiratory tract in children with cystic fibrosis	Can be given via nebulizer
β_2-Adrenergic agonists (short acting) (i.e., albuterol, levalbuterol, pirbuterol)	Relax airway smooth muscle, resulting in bronchodilation Used for acute and chronic treatment of wheezing and bronchospasm in asthma, bronchiolitis, cystic fibrosis, chronic lung disease. Also used to prevent wheezing in exercise-induced asthma	Administered via inhalation Can be used for acute relief of bronchospasm May cause nervousness, tachycardia, and jitteriness Inhaled agents result in fewer systemic side effects
β_2-Adrenergic agonists (long acting) (i.e., formoterol, salmeterol)	Long-acting bronchodilator used in chronic asthma management and for prevention of exercise-induced asthma Long-term control in chronic asthma Prevention of exercise-induced asthma	Administered via inhalation Used only for long-term control or for exercise-induced asthma. Not for relief of bronchospasm in an acute wheezing episode
Racemic epinephrine	Produces bronchodilation Indicated for croup	Assess lung sounds and work of breathing Observe for rebound bronchospasm
Anticholinergic (ipratropium)	Produces bronchodilation in asthma or chronic lung disease	In children, generally used as an adjunct to β_2-adrenergic agonists for treatment of bronchospasm
Antiviral agents (oral: amantadine, rimantadine, oseltamivir: inhaled zanamivir)	Treatment and prevention of influenza A	Amantadine, rimantadine: monitor for confusion, nervousness, and jitteriness. Oseltamivir, zanamivir: well tolerated but expensive
Antiviral (specific to RSV) (Ribavirin)	Treatment of severe lower respiratory tract infection with RSV, usually reserved for ventilated children	Administer via aerosol with the small-particle aerosol generator (SPAG). Suction children on assisted ventilation every 2 hours; monitor pulmonary pressures every 2 to 4 hours. May cause blurred vision and photosensitivity. Pregnant women should not be exposed to drug due to teratogenic effects.

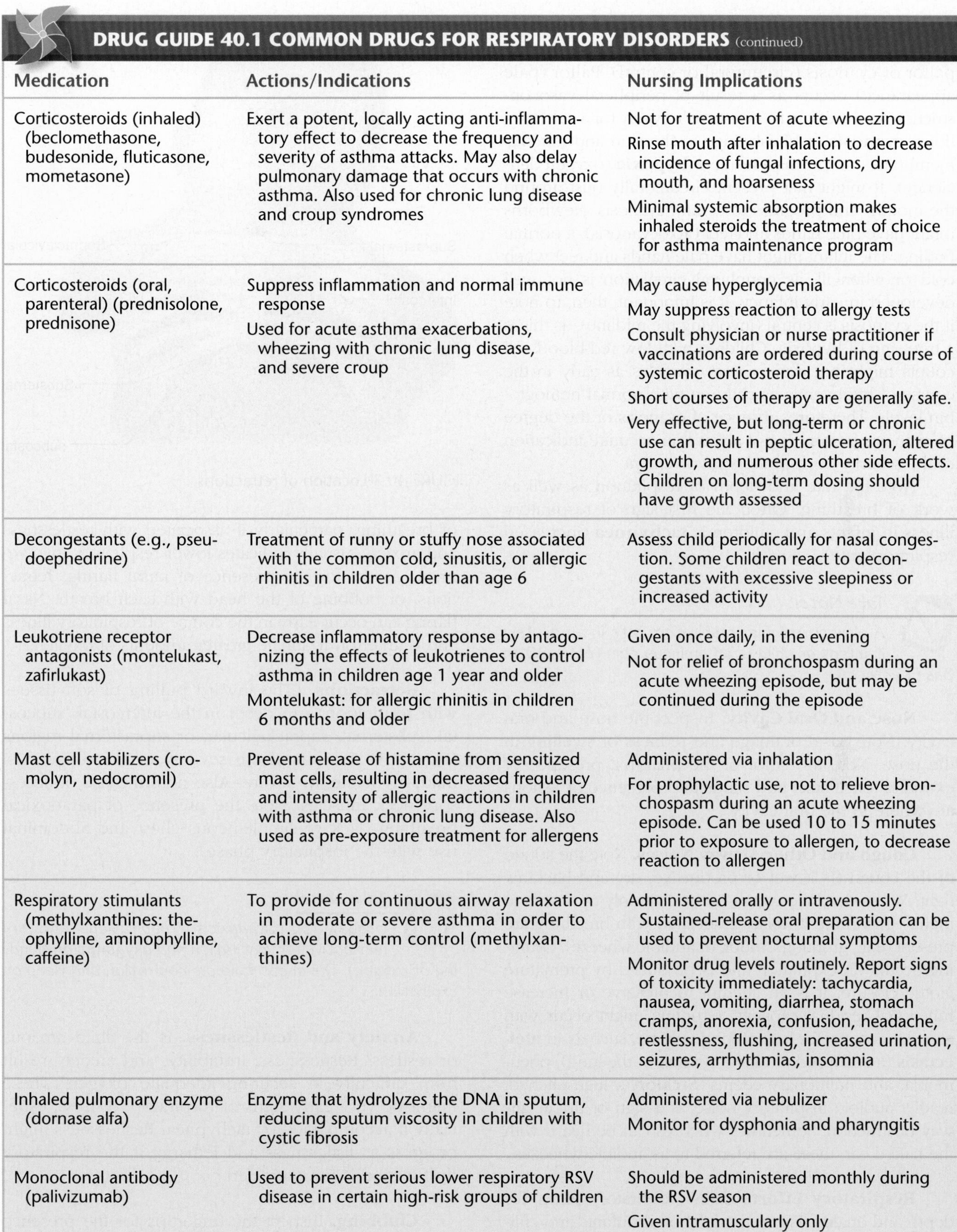

DRUG GUIDE 40.1 COMMON DRUGS FOR RESPIRATORY DISORDERS (continued)

Medication	Actions/Indications	Nursing Implications
Corticosteroids (inhaled) (beclomethasone, budesonide, fluticasone, mometasone)	Exert a potent, locally acting anti-inflammatory effect to decrease the frequency and severity of asthma attacks. May also delay pulmonary damage that occurs with chronic asthma. Also used for chronic lung disease and croup syndromes	Not for treatment of acute wheezing Rinse mouth after inhalation to decrease incidence of fungal infections, dry mouth, and hoarseness Minimal systemic absorption makes inhaled steroids the treatment of choice for asthma maintenance program
Corticosteroids (oral, parenteral) (prednisolone, prednisone)	Suppress inflammation and normal immune response Used for acute asthma exacerbations, wheezing with chronic lung disease, and severe croup	May cause hyperglycemia May suppress reaction to allergy tests Consult physician or nurse practitioner if vaccinations are ordered during course of systemic corticosteroid therapy Short courses of therapy are generally safe. Very effective, but long-term or chronic use can result in peptic ulceration, altered growth, and numerous other side effects. Children on long-term dosing should have growth assessed
Decongestants (e.g., pseudoephedrine)	Treatment of runny or stuffy nose associated with the common cold, sinusitis, or allergic rhinitis in children older than age 6	Assess child periodically for nasal congestion. Some children react to decongestants with excessive sleepiness or increased activity
Leukotriene receptor antagonists (montelukast, zafirlukast)	Decrease inflammatory response by antagonizing the effects of leukotrienes to control asthma in children age 1 year and older Montelukast: for allergic rhinitis in children 6 months and older	Given once daily, in the evening Not for relief of bronchospasm during an acute wheezing episode, but may be continued during the episode
Mast cell stabilizers (cromolyn, nedocromil)	Prevent release of histamine from sensitized mast cells, resulting in decreased frequency and intensity of allergic reactions in children with asthma or chronic lung disease. Also used as pre-exposure treatment for allergens	Administered via inhalation For prophylactic use, not to relieve bronchospasm during an acute wheezing episode. Can be used 10 to 15 minutes prior to exposure to allergen, to decrease reaction to allergen
Respiratory stimulants (methylxanthines: theophylline, aminophylline, caffeine)	To provide for continuous airway relaxation in moderate or severe asthma in order to achieve long-term control (methylxanthines)	Administered orally or intravenously. Sustained-release oral preparation can be used to prevent nocturnal symptoms Monitor drug levels routinely. Report signs of toxicity immediately: tachycardia, nausea, vomiting, diarrhea, stomach cramps, anorexia, confusion, headache, restlessness, flushing, increased urination, seizures, arrhythmias, insomnia
Inhaled pulmonary enzyme (dornase alfa)	Enzyme that hydrolyzes the DNA in sputum, reducing sputum viscosity in children with cystic fibrosis	Administered via nebulizer Monitor for dysphonia and pharyngitis
Monoclonal antibody (palivizumab)	Used to prevent serious lower respiratory RSV disease in certain high-risk groups of children	Should be administered monthly during the RSV season Given intramuscularly only

Adapted from Taketomo, C. K., Hodding, J. H., & Kraus, D. M. (2013). *Pediatric & neonatal dosage handbook* (20th ed.). Hudson, OH: Lexicomp.

INSPECTION AND OBSERVATION

Color. Observe the child's skin color, noting pallor or cyanosis (circumoral or central). Pallor (pale appearance) occurs as a result of peripheral vasoconstriction in an effort to conserve oxygen for vital functions. **cyanosis** (a bluish tinge to the skin and mucous membranes) occurs as a result of **hypoxia** (oxygen deficiency). It might first present circumorally (just around the mouth) and progress to central cyanosis. Newborns might have blue hands and feet (acrocyanosis), a normal finding. The infant might have pale hands and feet when cold or when ill, as peripheral circulation is not well developed in early infancy. It is important, then, to note if the cyanosis is central (involving the midline), as this is a true sign of hypoxia. Children with low red blood cell counts might not demonstrate cyanosis as early in the course of hypoxemia as children with normal hemoglobin levels. Therefore, absence of cyanosis or the degree of cyanosis present is not always an accurate indication of the severity of respiratory involvement.

Note the rate and depth of respiration as well as work of breathing. Often the first sign of respiratory illness in infants and children is **tachypnea** (increased respiratory rate).

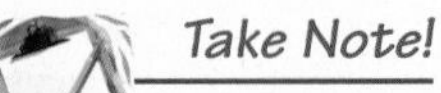

Take Note!

A slow or irregular respiratory rate in an acutely ill infant or child is an ominous sign (AHA, 2011). See Chapter 51.

Nose and Oral Cavity. Inspect the nose and oral cavity. Note nasal drainage and redness or swelling in the nose. Note the color of the pharynx, presence of exudate, tonsil size, and status and presence of lesions anywhere in the oral cavity.

Cough and Other Airway Noises. Note the sound of the cough (Is it wet or productive, dry and hacking, tight? When does the cough occur? Is it only or mainly at night?). Also note if noises associated with breathing are present (e.g., grunting, stridor, or audible wheeze). Grunting occurs on expiration and is produced by premature glottic closure. It is an attempt to preserve or increase functional residual capacity. Grunting might occur with alveolar collapse or loss of lung volume, such as in **atelectasis** (a collapsed or airless portion of the lung), pneumonia, and pulmonary edema. **Stridor**, a high-pitched, readily audible inspiratory noise, is a sign of upper airway obstruction. Sometimes wheezes can be heard with the naked ear; these are referred to as audible wheezes.

Respiratory Effort. Assess respiratory effort for depth and quality. Is breathing labored? Infants and children with significant nasal congestion may have tachypnea, which usually resolves when the nose is cleared of mucus. Mouth breathing may occur when a large amount of nasal congestion is present. Increased work of breathing, particularly if associated with restlessness and anxiety, usually indicates lower respiratory involvement. Assess for the presence of nasal flaring, retractions, or bobbing of the head with each breath. Nasal flaring can occur early in the course of respiratory illness and is an effort to inhale greater amounts of oxygen.

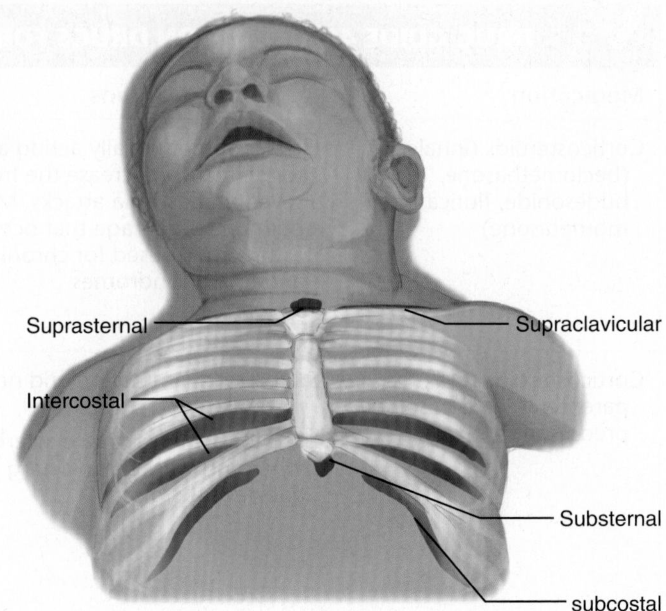

FIGURE 40.3 Location of retractions.

Retractions. (The inward pulling of soft tissues with respiration) can occur in the intercostal, subcostal, substernal, supraclavicular, or suprasternal regions (Fig. 40.3). Document the severity of the retractions: mild, moderate, or severe. Also note the use of accessory neck muscles. Note the presence of paradoxical breathing (lack of simultaneous chest and abdominal rise with the inspiratory phase).

Take Note!

Seesaw (or paradoxical) respirations are very ineffective for ventilation and **oxygenation** (binding of oxygen). The chest falls on inspiration and rises on expiration.

Anxiety and Restlessness. Is the child anxious or restless? Restlessness, irritability, and anxiety result from difficulty in securing adequate oxygen. These might be very early signs of respiratory distress, especially if accompanied by tachypnea. Restlessness might progress to listlessness and lethargy if the respiratory dysfunction is not corrected.

Clubbing. Inspect the fingertips for the presence of **clubbing**, an enlargement of the terminal phalanx of the finger, resulting in a change in the angle of the nail to the fingertip (Fig. 40.4). Clubbing might occur in children with a chronic respiratory illness. It is the result

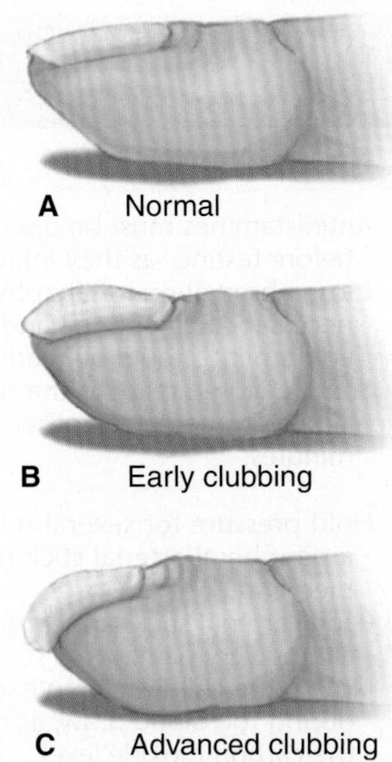

FIGURE 40.4 **(A)** Normal fingertip. Early clubbing **(B)** may progress eventually to advanced clubbing **(C)** as a result of chronic hypoxemia.

of increased capillary growth as the body attempts to supply more oxygen to distal body cells.

Hydration Status. Note the child's hydration status. Palpate the infant's fontanels to determine if sunken. Assess the oral mucosa for color and moisture. Note skin turgor, presence of tears, and adequacy of urine output. The child with a respiratory illness is at risk for dehydration. Pain related to sore throat or mouth lesions may prevent the child from drinking properly. Nasal congestion interferes with the infant's ability to suck effectively at the breast or bottle. Tachypnea and increased work of breathing interfere with the ability to safely ingest fluids.

Auscultation

Assess lung sounds via auscultation. Evaluate breath sounds over the anterior and posterior chest, as well as in the axillary areas. Note the adequacy of aeration. Breath sounds should be equal bilaterally. The intensity and pitch should be equal throughout the lungs; document diminished breath sounds. In the absence of concurrent lower respiratory illness, the breath sounds should be clear throughout all lung fields. During normal respiration, the inspiratory phase is usually softer and longer than the expiratory phase. Prolonged expiration is a sign of bronchial or bronchiolar obstruction. Bronchiolitis, asthma, pulmonary edema, and an intrathoracic foreign body can cause prolonged expiratory phases.

Infants and young children have thin chest walls. When the upper airway is congested (as in a severe cold), the noise produced in the upper airway might be transmitted throughout the lung fields. When upper airway congestion is transmitted to the lung fields, the congested sounding noise heard over the trachea is the same type of noise heard over the lungs but is much louder and more intense. To ascertain if these sounds are truly adventitious lung sounds or if they are transmitted from the upper airway, auscultate again after the child coughs or his or her nose has been suctioned. Another way to discern the difference is to compare auscultatory findings over the trachea to the lung fields to determine if the abnormal sound is truly from within the lung or is actually a sound transmitted from the upper airway.

Note adventitious sounds heard on auscultation. **Wheezing**, a high-pitched sound that usually occurs on expiration, results from obstruction in the lower trachea or bronchioles. Wheezing that clears with coughing is most likely a result of secretions in the lower trachea. Wheezing resulting from obstruction of the bronchioles, as in bronchiolitis, asthma, chronic lung disease, or cystic fibrosis, does not clear with coughing. **Rales** (crackling sounds) result when the alveoli become fluid filled, such as in pneumonia. Note the location of the adventitious sounds as well as the timing (on inspiration, expiration, or both). Tachycardia might also be present. An increase in heart rate often initially accompanies hypoxemia.

Percussion

When percussing, note sounds that are not resonant in nature. Flat or dull sounds might be percussed over partially consolidated lung tissue, as in pneumonia. Tympany might be percussed with a pneumothorax. Note the presence of hyperresonance (as might be apparent with asthma).

Palpation

Palpate the sinuses for tenderness in the older child. Assess for enlargement or tenderness of the lymph nodes of the head and neck. Document alterations in tactile fremitus detected on palpation. Increased tactile fremitus might occur in a case of pneumonia or pleural effusion. Fremitus might be decreased in the case of barrel chest, as with cystic fibrosis. Absent fremitus might be noted with pneumothorax or atelectasis.

Compare central and peripheral pulses. Note the quality of the pulse as well as the rate. With significant respiratory distress, perfusion often becomes compromised. Poor perfusion might be reflected in weaker peripheral pulses (radial, pedal) when compared to central pulses.

Laboratory and Diagnostic Testing

Common Laboratory and Diagnostic Tests 40.1 explains the laboratory and diagnostic tests most

(text continues on page 1478)

COMMON LABORATORY AND DIAGNOSTIC TESTS 40.1 ALTERATIONS IN GAS EXCHANGE/ RESPIRATORY DISORDERS

Test	Explanation	Indications	Nursing Implications
Allergy skin testing	Suggested allergen is applied to skin via scratch, pin, or prick. A wheal response indicates allergy to the substance	Allergic rhinitis, asthma	Antihistamines must be discontinued before testing, as they inhibit the test. Close observation for anaphylaxis is necessary. Epinephrine and emergency equipment should be readily available. Some children react to the skin test almost immediately; others take several minutes.
Arterial blood gases	Invasive method (requires blood sampling) of measuring arterial pH, partial pressure of oxygen and carbon dioxide, and base excess in blood	Usually reserved for severe illness, the intubated child, or suspected carbon dioxide retention	Hold pressure for several minutes after a peripheral arterial stick to avoid bleeding. Radial arterial sticks are common and can be very painful. Note if the child is crying excessively during the blood draw, as this affects the carbon dioxide level.
Chest x-ray	Radiographic image of the expanded lungs: can show hyperinflation, atelectasis, pneumonia, foreign body, pleural effusion, abnormal heart or lung size	Bronchiolitis, pneumonia, tuberculosis, asthma, cystic fibrosis, bronchopulmonary dysplasia	Children may be afraid of the x-ray equipment. If a parent or familiar adult can accompany the child, often the child is less afraid. If the child is unable or unwilling to hold still for the x-ray, restraint may be necessary. Restraint should be limited to the amount of time needed for the x-ray.
Fluorescent antibody testing	Determines presence of respiratory syncytial virus (RSV), adenovirus, influenza, parainfluenza, or *Chlamydia* in nasopharyngeal secretions	Bronchiolitis, pneumonia	To obtain a nasopharyngeal specimen, instill 1 to 3 mL of sterile normal saline into one nostril, aspirate the contents using a small sterile bulb syringe, place the contents in sterile container, and immediately send them to the lab.
Fluoroscopy	Radiographic examination that uses a fluorescent screen—"real-time" imaging	Identification of masses, abscesses	Requires the child to lie still. Equipment can be frightening. Children may respond to presence of parent or familiar adult.
Gastric washings for AFB	Determines presence of AFB (acid-fast bacilli) in stomach (children often swallow sputum)	Tuberculosis	Nasogastric tube is inserted and saline is instilled and suctioned out of the stomach to obtain the specimen.
Peak expiratory flow	Measures the maximum flow of air (in L/s) that can be forcefully exhaled in 1 second	Daily use can indicate adequacy of asthma control	It is important to establish the child's "personal best" by taking twice-daily readings over a 2-week period while well. The average of these is termed "personal best." Charts based on height and age are also available to determine expected peak expiratory flow.
Pulmonary function tests	Measure respiratory flow and lung volumes	Asthma, cystic fibrosis, chronic lung disease	Usually performed by a respiratory therapist trained to do the full spectrum of tests. Spirometry can be obtained by the trained nurse in the outpatient setting.

COMMON LABORATORY AND DIAGNOSTIC TESTS 40.1 ALTERATIONS IN GAS EXCHANGE/ RESPIRATORY DISORDERS (continued)

Test	Explanation	Indications	Nursing Implications
Pulse oximetry	Noninvasive method of continuously (or intermittently) measuring oxygen saturation	Can be useful in any situation in which a child is experiencing respiratory distress	Probe must be applied correctly to finger, toe, foot, hand, forehead, or ear in order for the machine to appropriately pick up the pulse and oxygen saturation.
Rapid flu test	Rapid test for detection of influenza A or B	Influenza	Should be done in first 24 hours of illness so that medication administration can begin. Have the child gargle with sterile normal saline and then spit into a sterile container. Send immediately to the lab.
Rapid strep test	Instant test for presence of streptococcus A antibody in pharyngeal secretions	Pharyngitis, tonsillitis	Results in 5 to 10 minutes. Negative tests should be backed up with throat culture.
RAST (radioallergosorbent test)	Measures minute quantities of immunoglobulin E in the blood Carries no risk of anaphylaxis but is not as sensitive as skin testing	Asthma (food allergies)	Blood test that is usually sent out to a reference laboratory.
Sinus x-rays, computed tomography (CT), or magnetic resonance imaging (MRI)	Radiologic tests that may show sinus involvement	Sinusitis, recurrent colds	X-ray results are usually received more quickly than CT or MRI results.
Sputum culture	Bacterial culture of invasive organisms in the sputum	Pneumonia, cystic fibrosis, tuberculosis	Must be true sputum, not mucus from the mouth or nose. Child can deep breathe, cough, and spit, or specimen may be obtained via suctioning of the artificial airway.
Sweat chloride test	Collection of sweat on filter paper after stimulation of skin with pilocarpine Measures concentration of chloride in the sweat	Cystic fibrosis	May be difficult to obtain sweat in a young infant.
Throat culture	Bacterial culture (minimum of 24 to 48 hours required) to determine presence of streptococcus A or other bacteria	Pharyngitis, tonsillitis	Can be obtained on separate swab at same time as rapid strep test to decrease trauma to the child (swab both applicators at once). Do not perform immediately after the child has had medication or something to eat or drink.
Tuberculin skin test	Mantoux test (intradermal injection of purified protein derivative)	Tuberculosis, chronic cough	Must be given intradermally; not a valid test if injected incorrectly.

Adapted from Beckton Dickinson and Company. (2016). *Product center.* Retrieved from http://www.bd.com/ds/productCenter/index.asp; Corbett, J. A. & Banks, A. D. (2013). *Laboratory tests and diagnostic procedures with nursing diagnoses* (8th ed.). Upper Saddle River, NJ: Pearson Education Inc., and Fouzas, S., Priftis, K. N., & Anthracopoulos, M. B. (2011). Pulse oximetry in pediatric practice. *Pediatrics*, *128*, 740–752.

commonly used for a child with a respiratory disorder. The tests can assist the physician or nurse practitioner in diagnosing the disorder and/or be used as guidelines in determining ongoing treatment. Laboratory or nonnursing personnel obtain some of the tests, while the nurse might obtain others. In either instance it is important for the nurse to be familiar with how the tests are obtained, what they are used for, and normal versus abnormal results. This knowledge will also be necessary when providing child and family education related to the testing.

Take Note!

Ambient light may interfere with pulse oximetry readings. When the pulse oximeter probe is placed on the infant's foot or the young child's toe, covering the probe and foot with a sock may help to ensure an accurate measurement (Fouzas, Priftis, & Anthracopoulos, 2011).

Nursing Diagnoses, Goals, Interventions, and Evaluation

Upon completion of a thorough assessment, the nurse might identify several nursing diagnoses, including:

- Ineffective airway clearance
- Ineffective breathing pattern
- Impaired gas exchange
- Risk for infection
- Pain
- Risk for fluid volume deficit
- Altered nutrition, less than body requirements
- Activity intolerance
- Fear
- Altered family processes

After completing an assessment of Alexander, the nurse notes the following: lots of clear secretions in the airway, child appears pale, respiratory rate 68, retractions, nasal flaring, wheezing, and diminished breath sounds. Based on these assessment findings, what would your top three nursing diagnoses be for Alexander?

Nursing goals, interventions, and evaluation for the child with a respiratory disorder are based on the nursing diagnoses. Nursing Care Plan 40.1 (at the end of the chapter) can be used as a guide in planning nursing care for the child with a respiratory disorder. The nursing care plan should be individualized based on the child's symptoms and needs; refer to Chapter 36 for detailed information on pain management. Additional information will be included later in the chapter as it relates to specific disorders.

Based on your top three nursing diagnoses for Alexander, describe appropriate nursing interventions.

Providing Oxygen Supplementation

Oxygen may be delivered to the child by a variety of methods (Fig. 40.5). Since oxygen administration is considered a drug, it requires a physician or nurse practitioner's order, except when following emergency protocols outlined in a healthcare facility's policies and procedures. Many healthcare settings develop specific guidelines for oxygen administration that are often coordinated by respiratory therapists, yet the nurse still remains responsible for ensuring that oxygen is administered properly.

Oxygen sources include wall-mounted systems as well as cylinders. The supply of oxygen available from a wall-mounted source is limitless, but use of a wall-mounted source restricts the child to the hospital room. Cylinders are portable oxygen tanks; the D-cylinder holds a little less than 400 L of oxygen and the E-cylinder holds about 650 L of oxygen. Cylinders turn on with a gauge attached to the top of the tank. The cylinder is useful for the child on low-flow oxygen because it allows for mobility.

The tank empties relatively quickly if the child requires a high flow of oxygen, so this is not the best oxygen source in an emergency. Respiratory therapists usually maintain the respiratory equipment that is found in the emergency room or hospital. However, in an outpatient setting the nurse may be responsible for maintaining respiratory equipment and checking the level of oxygen in the office's oxygen tanks each day.

Take Note!

Oxygen is highly flammable, so use safety precautions. Post signs ("Oxygen in Use"); inform the family to avoid matches, lighters, and flammable or volatile materials; and use only facility-approved equipment.

The efficiency of oxygen delivery systems is affected by several variables, including the child's respiratory effort, the liter flow of oxygen delivered, and whether the equipment is being used appropriately. In general, oxygen facemasks come in infant, child, and adult sizes. Select the mask that best fits the child. In addition, ensure that the mask is sealed properly to decrease the amount of oxygen that escapes from the mask. Ensure that the liter flow is set according to the manufacturer's recommendations for use with that particular delivery method. The oxygen flow rate or concentration is usually determined by the physician or nurse practitioner's order. Whichever method of delivery is used, provide humidification during oxygen delivery to prevent drying of nasal passages and to assist with liquefying secretions. Table 40.1 provides details on oxygen delivery methods.

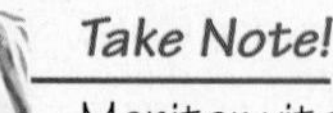

Take Note!

Monitor vital signs, color, respiratory effort, pulse oximetry, and level of consciousness before, during, and after oxygen therapy to evaluate its effectiveness.

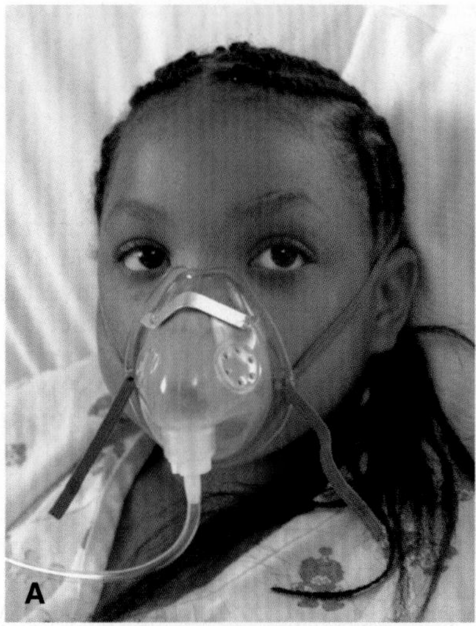

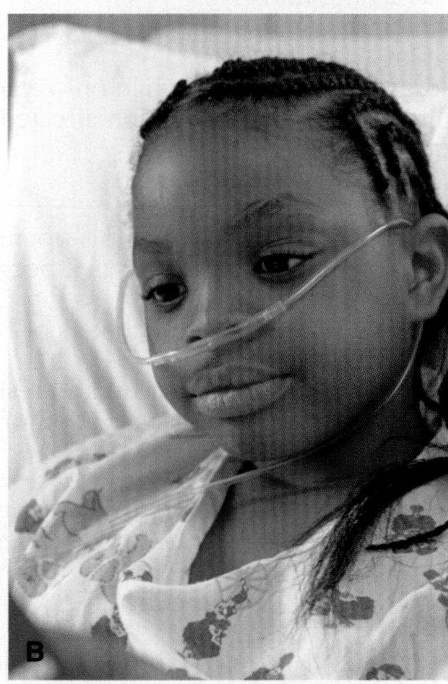

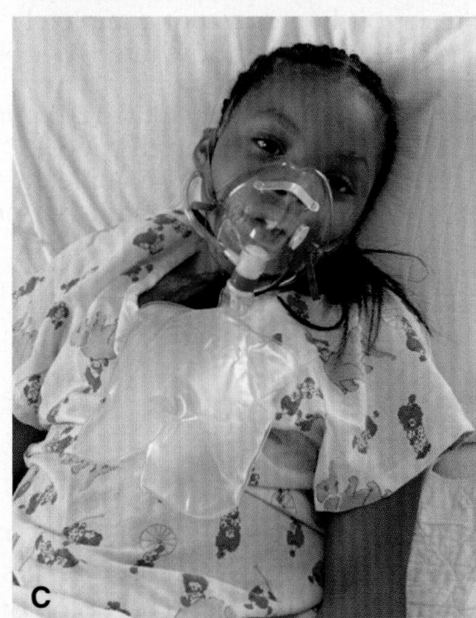

FIGURE 40.5 **(A)** Simple oxygen mask provides about 40% oxygen. **(B)** The nasal cannula provides an additional 4% oxygen per 1 L of oxygen flow (i.e., 1 L will deliver 25% oxygen). **(C)** The nonrebreather mask provides 80% to 100% oxygen.

ACUTE INFECTIOUS DISORDERS

Acute infectious disorders include the common cold, sinusitis, influenza, pharyngitis, tonsillitis, laryngitis, croup syndromes, respiratory syncytial virus (RSV), pneumonia, and bronchitis.

Common Cold

The common cold is also referred to as a viral upper respiratory infection (URI) or nasopharyngitis. Colds can be caused by rhinoviruses, parainfluenza, RSV, enteroviruses, adenoviruses, and human metapneumovirus. Viral particles spread through the air or from person-to-person contact. Colds occur more frequently in the winter. They affect children of all ages and have a higher incidence among children who attend day care and school-age children (Scholes, & Yoon, 2014). It is not unusual for a child to have six to nine colds per year. Spontaneous resolution of the common cold occurs after about 7 to 10 days. Potential complications include secondary bacterial infections of the ears, throat, sinuses, or lungs.

Therapeutic management of the common cold is directed toward symptom relief. Nasal congestion may be relieved via humidity and use of normal saline nasal wash or spray followed by suctioning. Antihistamines are not indicated, as they dry secretions further. Over-the-counter cold preparations are available singly and in combinations. These preparations have not been proven to reduce the length or severity of the cold but may offer symptomatic relief in some children older than 6 years of age (they are not recommended in children younger than the age of 4 due to side effects) (Friedman, et al., 2014). See Healthy People 2020.

HEALTHY PEOPLE 2020

Objective	Nursing Significance
Reduce the number of courses of antibiotics prescribed for the sole diagnosis of the common cold.	• Appropriately educate families that the cause of the common cold is a number of viruses and that antibiotics are inappropriate for the treatment of viral infections. • Encourage families to use measures such as normal saline nasal washes to decrease symptoms associated with the common cold more quickly.

Healthy People Objectives retrieved from http://www.healthypeople.gov

TABLE 40.1 OXYGEN DELIVERY METHODS

Delivery Method	Description	Nursing Implications
Simple mask	Provides 35–60% oxygen with a flow rate of 6 to 10 L/min. Oxygen delivery percentage is affected by respiratory rate, inspiratory flow, and adequacy of mask fit.	• Must maintain oxygen flow rate of at least 6 L/min to maintain inspired oxygen concentration and prevent rebreathing of carbon dioxide • Mask must fit snugly to be effective but should not be so tight as to irritate the face.
Venturi mask	Provides 24–50% oxygen by using a special gauge at the base of the mask that allows mixing of room air with oxygen flow	• Set oxygen flow rate according to percentage of oxygen desired as indicated on the gauge/dial. • As with simple mask, must fit snugly.
Nasal cannula	Provides low oxygen concentration (22–44%)	• Must be used with humidification to prevent drying and irritation of airways. • Can provide very small amounts of oxygen (as low as 25 mL/min). • Maximum recommended liter flow in children is 4 L/min. • Children can eat or talk while on oxygen. • Inspired oxygen concentration affected by mouth breathing. • Requires patent nasal passages.
Oxygen tent	Provides high-humidity environment with up to 50% oxygen concentration	• Oxygen level drops when tent is opened. • Must change linen frequently as it becomes damp from the humidity. • Secure edges of tent with blankets or by tucking edges under mattress. • Young children may be fearful and resistant. • Mist may interfere with visualization of child inside tent.
Oxygen hood	Provides high concentration (up to 80–90%) for infants only. Allows easy access to chest and lower body.	• Liter flow must be set at 10 to 15 L/min. • Good method for infant but need to remove for feeding. • Can and should be humidified.
Partial rebreathing mask	Simple facemask with an oxygen reservoir bag. Provides 50–60% oxygen concentration	• Must set liter flow rate at 10 to 12 L/min to prevent rebreathing of carbon dioxide. • The reservoir bag does not completely empty when child inspires if flow rate is set properly.
Nonrebreathing mask	Simple facemask with valves at the exhalation ports and an oxygen reservoir bag with a valve to prevent exhaled air from entering the reservoir. Provides 95% oxygen concentration	• Must set liter flow rate at 10 to 12 L/min to prevent rebreathing of carbon dioxide. • The reservoir bag does not completely empty when child inspires if flow rate is set properly.

Adapted from American Heart Association. (2011). *Pediatric advanced life support provider manual*. Dallas, TX: Author; and Bowden, V. R., & Greenberg, C. S. (2012). *Pediatric nursing procedures* (3rd ed.). Philadelphia, PA: Lippincott Williams & Wilkins.

Take Note!

In 2007, over-the-counter cold preparations containing decongestants intended for use in infants and toddlers were removed from the market. Several research studies have not shown the preparations to be effective and they are known to have potentially serious side effects (Yust & Slattery, 2012). Safety of these products in children 2 to 11 years of age remains under review by the Food and Drug Administration.

Nursing Assessment

The child may have either a stuffy or runny nose. Nasal discharge is usually thin and watery at first but may become thicker and discolored. The color of nasal discharge is not an accurate indicator of viral versus bacterial infection. The child may be hoarse and complain of a sore throat. Cough usually produces very little sputum. Fever, fatigue, watery eyes, and appetite loss may also

COMPARISON CHART 40.1 **CAUSES OF NASAL CONGESTION**

Sign or Symptom	Allergic Rhinitis	Common Cold	Sinusitis
Length of illness	Varies; may have year-round symptoms	10 days or less	Longer than 10 to 14 days
Nasal discharge	Thin, watery, clear	Thick, white, yellow, or green; can be thin	Thick, yellow or green
Nasal congestion	Varies	Present	Present
Sneezing	Varies	Present	Absent
Cough	Varies	Present	Varies
Headache	Varies	Varies	Varies
Fever	Absent	Varies	Varies
Bad breath	Absent	Absent	Varies

occur. Symptoms are generally at their worst over the first few days and then decrease over the course of the illness.

Assess for risk factors such as day care or school attendance. Inspect for edema and vasodilation of the mucosa. Diagnosis is based on clinical presentation rather than laboratory or x-ray studies. Comparison Chart 40.1 differentiates causes of nasal congestion.

Nursing Management

Nursing management of the child with a common cold consists of promoting comfort, providing family education, and preventing spread of the cold.

PROMOTING COMFORT

Nursing care of the common cold is aimed at supportive measures. Nasal congestion may be relieved with the use of normal saline nose drops, followed by bulb syringe suctioning in infants and toddlers. Older children may use a normal saline nose spray to mobilize secretions. A cool mist humidifier also helps with nasal congestion. Generally, other over-the-counter nose sprays are not recommended for use in children, but they are sometimes prescribed for very short-term use. Promotion of adequate oral fluid intake is important to liquefy secretions.

Educate parents about the use of cold and cough medications. Although they may offer some symptomatic relief, they have not been proven to shorten the length of cold symptoms. Counsel parents to use the appropriate product depending on the symptom relief desired, rather than a combination product. Products containing acetaminophen combined with other "cold symptom" medications may mask a fever in the child who is developing a secondary bacterial infection. As with all viral infections in children, teach parents that aspirin use should be avoided because of its association with Reye syndrome (Clute, 2014).

PROVIDING FAMILY EDUCATION

Currently there are no medications available to treat the viruses that cause the common cold, so symptomatic treatment is all that is necessary. Antibiotics are not indicated unless the child also has a bacterial infection. See Evidence-Based Practice 40.1. Explain to parents the importance of reserving antibiotic use for appropriate illnesses. Provide education about the use of normal saline nose drops and bulb suctioning to clear the infant's nose of secretions. Normal saline nasal wash using a bulb syringe to instill the solution is also helpful for children of all ages with nasal congestion. Though normal saline for nasal administration is available commercially, parents can also make it at home (Box 40.2). Teaching Guidelines 40.1 gives instructions on use of the bulb syringe.

Counsel parents about how to recognize complications of the common cold, which includes:

- Prolonged fever
- Increased throat pain or enlarged, painful lymph nodes
- Increased or worsening cough, cough lasting longer than 10 days, chest pain, difficulty breathing
- Earache, headache, tooth or sinus pain
- Unusual irritability or lethargy
- Skin rash

BOX 40.2

HOMEMADE SALT WATER NOSE DROPS

Mix 8 oz distilled water, a half-teaspoon sea salt, and a quarter-teaspoon baking soda. Keep for 24 hours in the refrigerator, but should be allowed to come to room temperature prior to use.

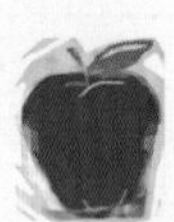

Teaching Guidelines 40.1

USING THE BULB SYRINGE TO SUCTION NASAL SECRETIONS

1. Hold the infant on your lap or on the bed with the head tilted slightly back.

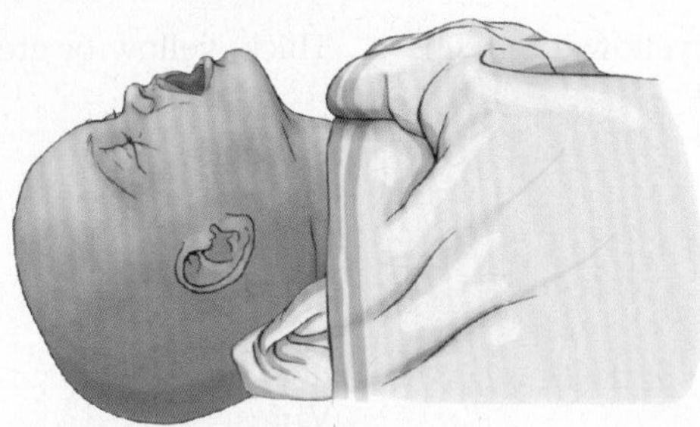

2. If using saline, instill several drops of saline solution in one of the infant's nostrils.

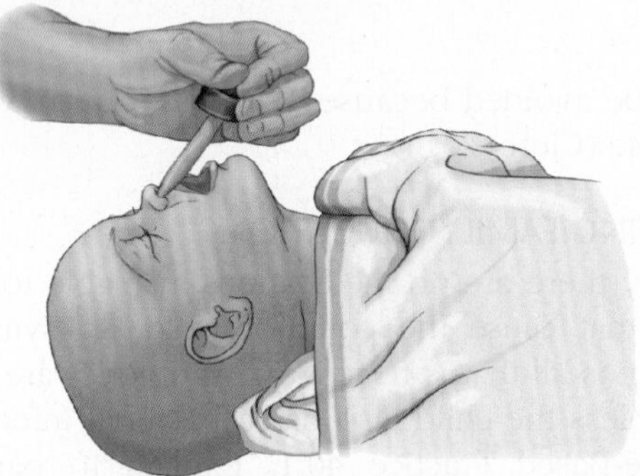

3. Compress the sides of the bulb syringe completely. Use only a rubber-tipped bulb syringe. Place the rubber tip in the infant's nose.

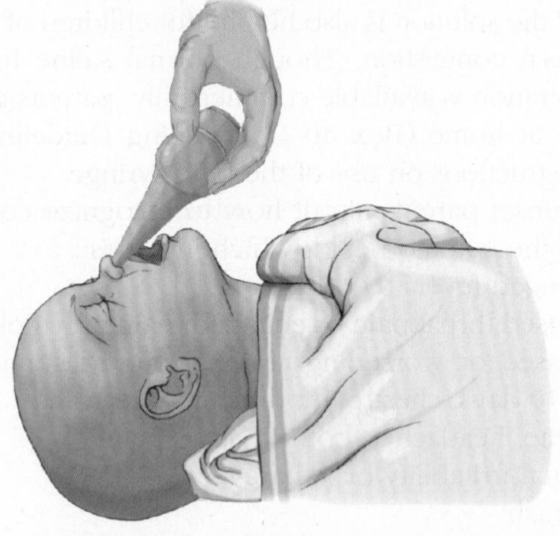

4. Release pressure on the bulb.

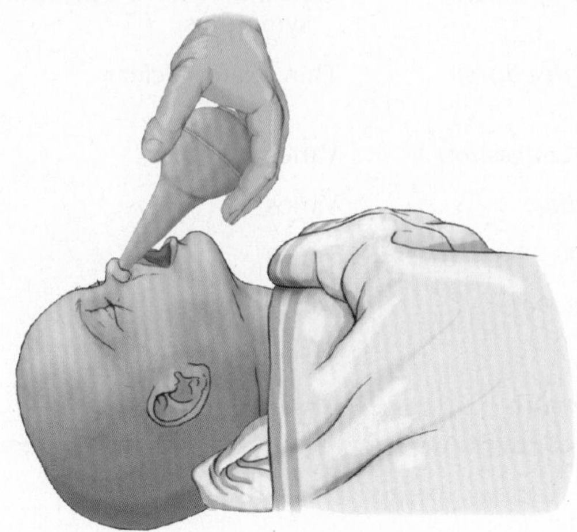

5. Remove the syringe and squeeze bulb over tissue or the sink to empty it of secretions.

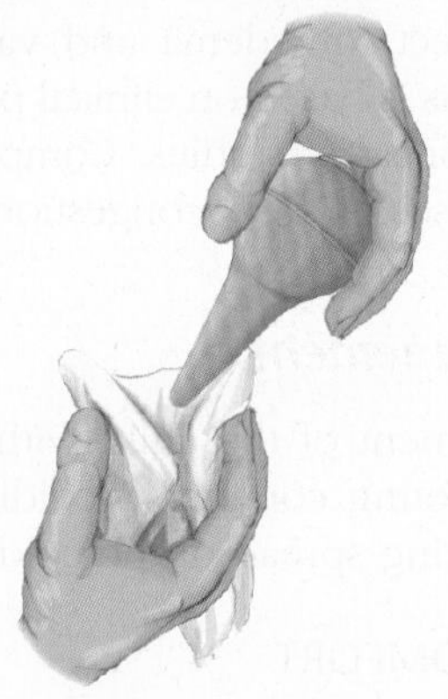

6. Repeat on other nostril if necessary. Using a bulb syringe prior to bottle-feeding or breastfeeding may relieve congestion enough to allow the infant to suck more efficiently.
7. Clean the bulb syringe thoroughly with warm water after each use and allow to air dry.

If complications do occur, tell parents to notify the physician or nurse practitioner for further instructions or reassessment.

PREVENTING THE COMMON COLD

Teaching about ways to prevent the common cold is a vital nursing intervention. Explain that frequent hand washing helps to decrease the spread of viruses that cause the common cold. Teach parents and family to avoid second-hand smoke as well as crowded places, especially during the winter. Avoid close contact with individuals known to have a cold. Encourage parents and families to consume a healthy diet and get enough rest.

EVIDENCE-BASED PRACTICE 40.1 **ANTIBIOTICS FOR THE COMMON COLD AND ACUTE PURULENT RHINITIS**

STUDY

Though the common cold is known to be viral in origin, antibiotics continue to be prescribed for colds and purulent rhinitis as treatment or for prophylaxis against development of a bacterial infection. Overuse of antibiotics is known to contribute to the problem of antibiotic resistance. The review included 11 randomized controlled trials evaluating the effectiveness of antibiotics versus placebo in the common cold or acute purulent rhinitis.

Findings

Use of antibiotics for the common cold and acute purulent rhinitis is not effective. In the studies reviewed, use of antibiotics did not contribute to cure, nor did it decrease persistence of symptoms as compared with placebo.

Nursing Implications

Nurses should consider the results of this review. With antibiotic resistance continuing to rise, it is important to support non-use of antibiotics in the instance of viral infections. Teach families about the difference between viral and bacterial illness. Provide support and insure that families understand the natural history of the common cold and that when symptoms persist rather than improve over time, they should reconnect with their physician or nurse practitioner.

Adapted from: Kenealy T. & Arroll B. (2013). Antibiotics for the common cold and acute purulent rhinitis. *Cochrane Database of Systematic Reviews*, 6. Art. No.: CD000247. doi: 10.1002/14651858.CD000247.pub3.

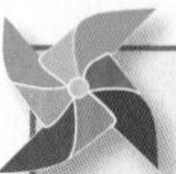

Consider This

Corey Davis, a 3-year-old, is brought to the clinic by her mother. She presents with a runny nose, congestion, and a nonproductive cough. Her mother says, "She's miserable." "I just don't know what to do." "Ever since I put her in day care she gets sick every few weeks." "This is all my fault."

How should the nurse respond? How would you feel if your child was healthy until entering day care? What type of support can the nurse provide to Corey's mother?

Sinusitis

Sinusitis (also called rhinosinusitis) generally refers to a bacterial infection of the paranasal sinuses. The disease may be either acute or chronic in nature. Approximately 5% of upper respiratory infections are complicated with acute sinusitis (Brook, 2013). In young children the maxillary and ethmoid sinuses are the main sites of infection. After age 10 years, the frontal sinuses may be more commonly involved (Friedman et al., 2014). Mucosal swelling, decreased ciliary movement, and thickened nasal discharge all contribute to bacterial invasion of the nose. Nasal polyps also place the child at risk for bacterial sinusitis. Complications include orbital cellulitis and intracranial infections, such as subdural empyemas.

Symptoms lasting less than 30 days generally indicate acute sinusitis, whereas symptoms persisting longer than 4 to 6 weeks usually indicate chronic sinusitis. Sinusitis is managed with antibiotic treatment. The therapeutic management approach varies with chronicity. The course of treatment is usually 14 days. Naturally, chronic sinusitis requires a longer course of treatment than acute sinusitis. Surgical therapy may be indicated for children with chronic sinusitis, particularly if it is recurrent or if nasal polyps are present.

Nursing Assessment

The most common presentation of sinusitis is persistent signs and symptoms of a cold. Rather than improving after 7 to 10 days, nasal discharge persists. Explore the history for:

- Cough
- Fever
- In preschoolers or older children, halitosis (bad breath)
- Facial pain may or may not be present, so is not a reliable indicator of disease
- Eyelid edema (in the case of ethmoid sinus involvement)
- Irritability
- Poor appetite

Assess for risk factors such as a history of recurrent cold symptoms or a history of nasal polyps.

On physical examination, note eyelid swelling, extent of nasal drainage, and halitosis. Inspect the throat for postnasal drainage. Inspect the nasal mucosa for erythema. Palpate the sinuses, noting pain with mild pressure. The diagnosis may be made based on the history and clinical presentation. The use of x-ray, computed tomography scan, or magnetic resonance imaging is not necessary as they are not specific and do not distinguish viral from bacterial infection (Brook, 2013). (Refer to Comparison Chart 40.1, which differentiates the causes of nasal congestion.)

Nursing Management

Normal saline nose drops or spray, cool mist humidifiers, and adequate oral fluid intake are recommended for children with sinusitis. Teach families the importance of continuing the full course of antibiotics to eradicate the cause of infection. Also educate the family that the use of decongestants, antihistamines, and intranasal steroids as adjuncts in the treatment of sinusitis has not been shown to be beneficial (Brook, 2013). Normal saline nose spray or nasal washes may promote drainage.

Influenza

Influenza viral infection (known commonly as the "flu") occurs primarily during the winter. It is spread through inhalation of droplets or contact with fine-particle aerosols. Infected children shed the virus for 1 to 2 days before symptoms begin and may continue shedding the virus in increased amounts (as compared to adults) for as long as 2 weeks. Average annual infection rates in children range from 20% to 50% (Wright, 2011). Influenza viruses primarily affect the upper respiratory epithelium but can cause systemic effects as well. Children with chronic heart or lung conditions, diabetes, chronic renal disease, or immune deficiency are at higher risk for more severe influenza infection compared to other children.

Bacterial infections of the respiratory system commonly occur as complications of influenza infection, severe pneumococcal pneumonia in particular. Otitis media occurs in 18% to 40% of all influenza cases (Wright, 2011). Less common complications include Reye syndrome and acute myositis. Reye syndrome is an acute encephalopathy that has been associated with aspirin use in the influenza-infected child (Clute, 2014). Acute myositis is particular to children. A sudden onset of severe pain and tenderness in both calves causes the child to refuse to walk. Due to the potential for complications, a prolonged fever or a fever that returns during convalescence should be investigated.

> *Take Note!*
>
> Current recommendations are for all children older than 6 months of age to be immunized yearly against influenza (Centers for Disease Control and Prevention [CDC], 2016a).

Nursing Assessment

Children who attend day care or school are at higher risk for influenza infection than those who are routinely at home. Note the presence of risk factors for severe disease, such as chronic heart or lung disease (such as asthma), diabetes, chronic renal disease, or immune deficiency or children with cancer receiving chemotherapy. School-age children and adolescents experience the illness similarly to adults. Abrupt onset of fever, facial flushing, chills, headache, myalgia, and malaise are accompanied by cough and **coryza** (nasal discharge). About half of infected individuals have a dry or sore throat. Ocular symptoms such as photophobia, tearing, burning, and eye pain are common.

Infants and young children exhibit symptoms similar to other respiratory illnesses. Fever greater than 39.5°C is common. Infants may be mildly toxic in appearance and irritable and have a cough, coryza, and pharyngitis. Wheezing may occur, as influenza also can cause bronchiolitis. An erythematous rash may be present and diarrhea may also occur. The diagnosis may be confirmed by a rapid assay test.

Nursing Management

Nursing management of influenza is mainly supportive. Symptomatic treatment of cough and fever and maintenance of hydration are the focus of care. Antiviral drugs can reduce the symptoms associated with influenza if they are started within the first 24 to 48 hours of the illness (Wright, 2011).

Pharyngitis

Inflammation of the throat mucosa (pharynx) is referred to as pharyngitis. A sore throat may accompany nasal congestion and is often viral in nature. A bacterial sore throat most often occurs without nasal symptoms. Group A streptococci account for 15% to 30% of cases, with the remainder being caused by other viruses or bacteria (John & Brady, 2013b).

Suppurative complications of group A streptococcal infection include peritonsillar or retropharyngeal abscess. Peritonsillar abscess may be noted by asymmetric swelling of the tonsils, shifting of the uvula to one side, and palatal edema. Retropharyngeal abscess may progress to the point of airway obstruction, hence requiring careful evaluation and appropriate treatment. Additional complications include acute rheumatic fever (see Chapter 41) and acute glomerulonephritis (see Chapter 43).

Viral pharyngitis is usually self-limited and does not require therapy beyond symptomatic relief. Group A streptococcal pharyngitis requires antibiotic therapy. If either the rapid diagnostic test or throat culture (described below) is positive for group A streptococci, penicillin is generally prescribed. Appropriate alternative antibiotics include amoxicillin and, for those allergic to penicillin, macrolides, and cephalosporins.

> *Take Note!*
>
> A "strep carrier" is a child who has a positive throat culture for streptococci when asymptomatic. Strep carriers are not at risk for complications from streptococci, as are those who are acutely infected with streptococci and are symptomatic (Hayden & Turner, 2011).

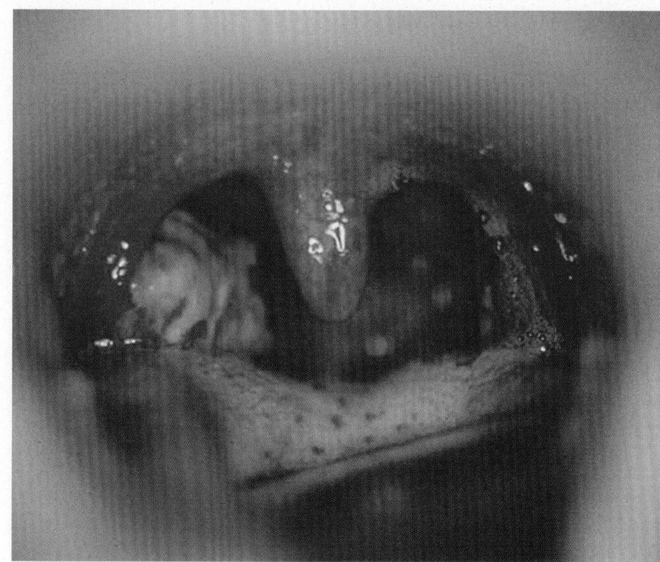

FIGURE 40.6 **Note the redness of the pharynx, tonsillar exudate, and white strawberry tongue coating.**

Nursing Assessment

Onset of pharyngitis is often quite abrupt. The history may include a fever, sore throat and difficulty swallowing, headache, and abdominal pain. Inquire about recent incidence of viral or strep throat in the family, day care center, or school.

Inspect the pharynx and tonsils, which may demonstrate varying degrees of inflammation (Fig. 40.6). Exudate may be present but is not diagnostic of bacterial infection. Note the presence of petechiae on the palate. Inspect the tongue for a strawberry appearance. Palpate for enlargement and tenderness of the anterior cervical nodes. Inspect the skin for a fine, red, sandpaper-like rash (called scarlatiniform), particularly on the trunk or abdomen, a common finding with streptococcus A infection.

The nurse may obtain a throat swab for rapid diagnostic testing and throat culture. The rapid strep test is a sensitive and reliable measure, rarely resulting in false-positive readings (John & Brady, 2013b). If the rapid strep test is negative, the second swab may be sent for a throat culture.

Atraumatic Care 40.1

When obtaining two swabs for rapid strep testing and throat culture, swab the applicators simultaneously to decrease perceived trauma to the child.

Nursing Management

Nursing management of the child with pharyngitis focuses on promoting comfort and providing family education.

PROMOTING COMFORT

Saline gargles (made with 8 oz of warm water and a half teaspoon of table salt) are soothing for children old enough to cooperate. Analgesics such as acetaminophen and ibuprofen may ease fever and pain. Sucking on throat lozenges or hard candy may also ease pain. Cool mist humidity helps to keep the mucosa moist in the event of mouth breathing. Encourage the child to ingest popsicles, cool liquids, and ice chips to maintain hydration.

PROVIDING FAMILY EDUCATION

Parents may be accustomed to "sore throats" being treated with antibiotics. However, in the case of a viral cause antibiotics will not be necessary and the pharyngitis will resolve in a few days. For the child with streptococcal pharyngitis, urge parents to have the child complete the entire prescribed course of antibiotics. After 24 hours of antibiotic therapy, instruct the parents to discard the child's toothbrush to avoid reinfection. Children may return to day care or school after they have been receiving antibiotics for 24 hours; they are considered noncontagious at that point.

Tonsillitis

Inflammation of the tonsils often occurs with pharyngitis and, thus, may also be viral or bacterial in nature. Viral infections require only symptomatic treatment. Treatment for bacterial tonsillitis is the same as for bacterial pharyngitis. Occasionally surgical intervention is warranted. Tonsillectomy (surgical removal of the palatine tonsils) may be indicated for the child with recurrent streptococcal tonsillitis or massive tonsillar hypertrophy or for other reasons. When hypertrophied adenoids obstruct breathing, then adenoidectomy (surgical removal of the adenoids) may be indicated.

Nursing Assessment

Note whether fever is present currently or by history. Inquire about the history of recurrent pharyngitis or tonsillitis. Note if the child's voice sounds muffled or hoarse. Inspect the pharynx for redness and enlargement of the tonsils. As the tonsils enlarge, the child may experience difficulty breathing and swallowing. When tonsils touch at the midline ("kissing tonsils" or 4+ in size), the airway may become obstructed. Also, if the adenoids are enlarged, the posterior nares become obstructed. The child may breathe through the mouth and may snore. Palpate the anterior cervical nodes for enlargement and tenderness. Rapid test or culture may be positive for streptococcus A.

Nursing Management

Tonsillitis that is medically treated requires the same nursing management as pharyngitis. Nursing care for the child after tonsillectomy is described below.

PROMOTING AIRWAY CLEARANCE

Until fully awake, place the child in a side-lying or prone position to facilitate safe drainage of secretions. Once alert, the child may prefer to sit up or have the head of the bed elevated. Suctioning, if necessary, should be done carefully to avoid trauma to the surgical site. Dried blood may be present on the teeth and the nares, with old blood present in emesis. Since the presence of blood can be very frightening to parents, alert them to this possibility.

MAINTAINING FLUID VOLUME

Hemorrhage is unusual postoperatively but may occur any time from the immediate postoperative period to as late as 10 days after surgery. Inspect the throat for bleeding. Mucus tinged with blood may be expected, but fresh blood in the secretions indicates bleeding. Early bleeding may be identified by continuous swallowing of small amounts of blood while awake or sleeping. Other signs of hemorrhage include tachycardia, pallor, restlessness, frequent throat clearing, and emesis of bright red blood.

To avoid trauma to the surgical site, discourage the child from coughing, clearing the throat, blowing the nose, and using straws. Upon discharge, instruct the parents to immediately report any sign of bleeding to the physician or nurse practitioner. To maintain fluid volume postoperatively, encourage children to take any fluids they desire; popsicles and ice chips are particularly soothing. Citrus juice and brown or red fluids should be avoided: the acid in citrus juice may irritate the throat, and red or brown fluids may be confused with blood if vomiting occurs.

RELIEVING PAIN

For the first 24 hours after surgery, the throat is very sore. Adequate pain relief is essential to establish adequate oral fluid intake. An ice collar may be prescribed, as well as analgesics with or without narcotics. Counsel parents to maintain pain control upon discharge from the facility, not only for the child's sake, but also to enable the child to continue to drink fluids.

Infectious Mononucleosis

Infectious mononucleosis is a self-limited illness caused by the Epstein–Barr virus. It is characterized by fever, malaise, sore throat, and lymphadenopathy. Mononucleosis is commonly called the "kissing disease" since it is transmitted by oropharyngeal secretions. It can occur at any age but is most often diagnosed in adolescents and young adults (Blosser, Brady, & Royal, 2013). Some infected individuals may have concomitant streptococcal pharyngitis. Complications include splenic rupture, Guillain–Barré syndrome, and aseptic meningitis.

Nursing Assessment

Note any history of exposure to infected individuals. Determine history of fever and onset and progression of sore throat, malaise, and other complaints. Observe for periorbital edema. Inspect the pharynx and tonsils for inflammation and patches of gray exudate. Petechiae may be present on the palate. Palpate for bilateral nontender enlargement of the posterior cervical lymph nodes. After 3 to 5 days of illness, the pharynx may become edematous and the tonsillar exudate more extensive. Lymphadenopathy may progress to include the anterior cervical nodes, which may become tender. Palpate the abdomen for splenomegaly or hepatomegaly. An erythematous maculopapular rash may appear as the illness progresses. Definitive diagnosis may be made by Monospot or Epstein–Barr virus titers.

Take Note!

The Monospot is usually negative if obtained within the first 7 to 10 days of illness with infectious mononucleosis. Epstein–Barr virus titer is reliable at any point in the illness (Blosser et al., 2013).

Nursing Management

Nursing management of mononucleosis is primarily symptomatic. The throat may be very sore, so analgesics and salt-water gargles are recommended. Bed rest should be encouraged while the child is febrile. Frequent rest periods may be necessary for several weeks after the onset of illness, as fatigue may persist as long as 6 weeks. During the acute phase, if tonsillar or pharyngeal edema threatens to obstruct the airway, then corticosteroids may be given to decrease the inflammation. In the presence of splenomegaly or hepatomegaly, strenuous activity and contact sports should be avoided. Appearance of rash or jaundice should be reported to the physician or nurse practitioner.

Laryngitis

Inflammation of the larynx is termed laryngitis. It may occur alone or in conjunction with other respiratory symptoms. It is characterized by a hoarse voice or loss of the voice (so soft as to make it difficult to hear). Oral fluids might offer relief, but resting the voice for 24 hours will allow the inflammation to subside. Laryngitis alone requires no further intervention.

Croup

Children between 3 months and 3 years of age are the most frequently affected with croup, though croup may affect any child (John & Brady, 2013b). Croup is also referred to as laryngotracheobronchitis because inflammation

COMPARISON CHART 40.2 **CROUP VS. EPIGLOTTITIS**

	Spasmodic Croup	Epiglottitis
Preceding illness	None or minimal coryza	None or mild upper respiratory infection
Age group usually affected	3 months to 3 years	1–8 years
Onset	Usually sudden, often at night	Rapid (within hours)
Fever	Variable	High
Barking cough, hoarseness	Yes	No
Dysphagia	No	Yes
Toxic appearance	No	Yes
Cause	Viral	*Haemophilus influenzae type B*

and edema of the larynx, trachea, and bronchi occur as a result of viral infection. Parainfluenza is responsible for the majority of cases of croup (John & Brady, 2013b). Other causes include adenovirus, influenza virus A and B, RSV, and rarely measles virus or *Mycoplasma pneumoniae*. The inflammation and edema obstruct the airway, resulting in symptoms. Mucus production also occurs, further contributing to obstruction of the airway. Narrowing of the subglottic area of the trachea results in audible inspiratory stridor. Edema of the larynx causes hoarseness. Inflammation in the larynx and trachea causes the characteristic barking cough of croup.

Symptoms occur most often at night, presenting suddenly, with resolution of symptoms in the morning. Croup is usually self-limited, lasting only about 3 to 5 days. Complications of croup are rare but may include worsening respiratory distress, hypoxia, or bacterial superinfection (as in the case of bacterial tracheitis).

Croup is usually managed on an outpatient basis, with affected children rarely requiring hospitalization. Corticosteroids (usually a single dose) are used to decrease inflammation, and racemic epinephrine aerosols demonstrate the α-adrenergic effect of mucosal vasoconstriction, helping to decrease edema. Children with croup may be hospitalized if they have significant stridor at rest or severe retractions after a several-hour period of observation. Comparison Chart 40.2 compares croup to epiglottitis.

Nursing Assessment

Note the age of the child; children between 3 months and 3 years of age are most likely to present with viral croup (laryngotracheobronchitis). History may reveal a cough that developed during the night (most common presentation) and that sounds like barking (or a seal). Inspect for the presence of mild URI symptoms. Temperature may be normal or elevated mildly. Listen for inspiratory stridor and observe for suprasternal retractions. Auscultate the lungs for adequacy of breath sounds. Croup is usually diagnosed based on history and clinical presentation, but a lateral neck x-ray may be obtained to rule out epiglottitis.

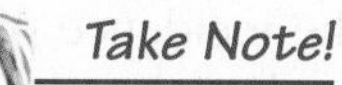

Take Note!

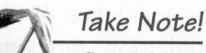

The child with fever, a toxic appearance, and increasing respiratory distress despite appropriate croup treatment may have bacterial tracheitis. Notify the physician or nurse practitioner of these findings in a child with croup (John & Brady, 2013b).

Nursing Management

If the child's care is being managed at home, advise parents about the symptoms of respiratory distress and instruct them to seek treatment if the child's respiratory condition worsens. Teach parents to expose their child to humidified air (via a cool mist humidifier or steamy bathroom). Though never clinically proven, use of humidified air has long been recommended for alleviating coughing jags and anecdotally has been reported as helpful (particularly exposure to cooler air). Administer dexamethasone if ordered or teach parents about home administration. Explain to parents that the effects of racemic epinephrine last about 2 hours and the child must be observed closely as occasionally a child will worsen again, requiring another aerosol. Teaching Guidelines 40.2 provides information about home care of croup.

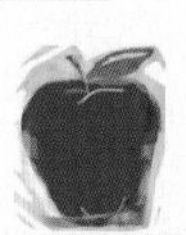

Teaching Guidelines 40.2

HOME CARE OF CROUP

- Keep the child quiet and discourage crying.
- Allow the child to sit up (in your arms).

- Encourage rest and fluid intake.
- If stridor occurs, take the child into a steamy bathroom for 10 minutes.
- Administer medication (corticosteroid) as directed.
- Watch the child closely. Call the physician or nurse practitioner if:
  - The child breathes faster, has retractions, or has any other difficulty breathing
  - The nostrils flare or the lips or nails have a bluish tint
  - The cough or stridor does not improve with exposure to moist air
  - Restlessness increases or the child is confused
  - The child begins to drool or cannot swallow

Adapted from Durani, Y. (2012). *Croup*. Retrieved from http://kidshealth.org/parent/infections/lung/croup.html

Epiglottitis

Epiglottitis (inflammation and swelling of the epiglottis) is most often caused by *Haemophilus influenzae* type b. Extensive use of the Hib vaccine since the 1980s has resulted in a significant decrease in the incidence of epiglottitis (John & Brady, 2013b). Though now rare, epiglottitis most often occurs in children between the ages of 2 and 7 years and can be life-threatening (John & Brady, 2013b). Respiratory arrest and death may occur if the airway becomes completely occluded. Additional complications include pneumothorax and pulmonary edema. Therapeutic management focuses on airway maintenance and support. Intravenous antibiotic therapy is necessary. The child will be managed in the intensive care unit. See Comparison Chart 40.2 for information comparing croup to epiglottitis.

Nursing Assessment

Carefully assess the child with suspected epiglottitis. Note sudden onset of symptoms and high fever. The child has an overall toxic appearance. He or she may refuse to speak or may speak only with a very soft voice. The child may refuse to lie down and may assume the characteristic position: sitting forward with the neck extended. Drooling may be present. Note anxiety or a frightened appearance. Note the child's color. Cough is usually absent. A lateral neck x-ray may be performed to determine whether epiglottitis is present. This is done cautiously, so as not to induce airway obstruction with changes in position of the child's neck.

Take Note!

Do not under any circumstance attempt to visualize the throat: reflex laryngospasm may occur, precipitating immediate airway occlusion (John & Brady, 2013b).

Nursing Management

Do not leave the child unattended. Keep the child and parents as calm as possible. Allow the child to assume a position of comfort. Do not place the child in a supine position, as airway occlusion may occur. Provide 100% oxygen in the least invasive manner that is acceptable to the child. If the child with epiglottitis experiences complete airway occlusion, an emergency tracheostomy may be necessary. Ensure that emergency equipment is available and that personnel trained in intubation of the pediatric occluded airway and percutaneous tracheostomy are notified of the child's presence in the facility.

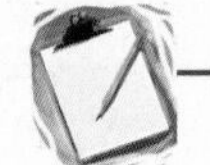

Take Note!

Epiglottitis is characterized by dysphagia, drooling, anxiety, irritability, and significant respiratory distress. Prepare for the event of sudden airway occlusion.

Bronchiolitis

Bronchiolitis is an acute inflammatory process of the bronchioles and small bronchi. Nearly always caused by a viral pathogen, RSV accounts for the majority of cases of bronchiolitis, with adenovirus, parainfluenza, and human meta-pneumovirus also being important causative agents. This discussion will focus on RSV bronchiolitis.

The peak incidence of bronchiolitis is in the winter and spring, coinciding with RSV season. RSV season in the United States and Canada generally begins in September or October and continues through April or May, with the exception of Florida which experiences a near year-round RSV season. Virtually all children will contract RSV infection within the first few years of life. RSV bronchiolitis occurs most often in infants and toddlers, with a peak incidence around 6 months of age (DeNicola, Maraqa, Udeani, & Custodio, 2016). The severity of disease is related inversely to the age of the child. The frequency and severity of RSV infection decrease with age. Repeated RSV infections occur throughout life but are usually localized to the upper respiratory tract after toddlerhood.

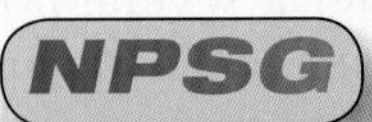

GOAL 6: Reduce the Harm Associated with Clinical Alarm Systems

NPSG.06.01.01 Improve the safety of clinical alarm systems

Steps: Insure alarms on biomedical equipment are properly set according to the child's age, clinical condition, prescribed orders, and facility policy. ALWAYS answer alarms promptly, checking the child first, then attending to the equipment.

Joint Commission. (2015). *National patient safety goals effective January 1, 2015.* Retrieved from http://www.jointcommission.org/assets/1/6/2015_NPSG_HAP.pdf

Pathophysiology

RSV is a highly contagious virus and may be contracted through direct contact with respiratory secretions or from particles on objects contaminated with the virus. RSV invades the nasopharynx, where it replicates and then spreads down to the lower airway via aspiration of upper airway secretions. RSV infection causes necrosis of the respiratory epithelium of the small airways, peribronchiolar mononuclear infiltration, and plugging of the lumens with mucus and exudate. The small airways become variably obstructed; this allows adequate inspiratory volume but prevents full expiration. This leads to hyperinflation and atelectasis. Serious alterations in gas exchange occur, with arterial hypoxemia and carbon dioxide retention resulting from mismatching of pulmonary **ventilation** (gas exchange within the lungs) and perfusion. Hypoventilation occurs secondary to markedly increased work of breathing.

Therapeutic Management

Management of RSV focuses on supportive treatment. Supplemental oxygen, nasal and/or nasopharyngeal suctioning, oral or intravenous hydration, and inhaled bronchodilator therapy (racemic epinephrine or albuterol/levalbuterol) are used. Many infants are managed at home with close observation and adequate hydration. Hospitalization is required for children with more severe disease. The infant with tachypnea, significant retractions, poor oral intake, or lethargy can deteriorate quickly, to the point of requiring ventilatory support, and thus warrants hospital admission.

Nursing Assessment

For a full description of the assessment phase of the nursing process, refer to Nursing Process Overview section earlier in the chapter. Assessment findings pertinent to RSV bronchiolitis are discussed below.

HEALTH HISTORY

Elicit a description of the present illness and chief complaint. Common signs and symptoms reported during the health history might include:

- Onset of illness with a clear runny nose (sometimes profuse)
- Pharyngitis
- Low-grade fever
- Development of cough 1 to 3 days into the illness, followed by a wheeze shortly thereafter
- Poor feeding

Explore the child's current and past medical history for risk factors such as:

- Young age (younger than 2 years old), more severe disease in a child younger than 6 months old
- Prematurity
- Multiple births
- Birth during April to September
- History of chronic lung disease (bronchopulmonary disease)
- Cyanotic or complicated congenital heart disease
- Immunocompromise
- Male gender
- Exposure to passive tobacco smoke
- Crowded living conditions
- Day care attendance
- School-age siblings
- Low socioeconomic status
- Lack of breastfeeding

PHYSICAL EXAMINATION

Examination of the child with RSV involves inspection, observation, and auscultation.

Inspection and Observation. Observe the child's general appearance and color (centrally and peripherally). The infant with RSV bronchiolitis might appear air-hungry, exhibiting various degrees of cyanosis and respiratory distress, including tachypnea, retractions, accessory muscle use, grunting, and periods of apnea. Cough and audible wheeze might be heard. The infant might appear listless and uninterested in feeding, surroundings, or parents.

Auscultation. Auscultate the lungs, noting adventitious sounds and determining the quality of aeration of the lung fields. Earlier in the illness, wheezes might be heard scattered throughout the lung fields. In more serious cases, the chest might sound quiet and without wheeze. This is due to significant hyperexpansion with very poor air exchange.

LABORATORY AND DIAGNOSTIC TESTS

Common laboratory and diagnostic studies ordered for the assessment of RSV bronchiolitis include:

- Pulse oximetry: oxygen saturation might be decreased significantly
- Chest x-ray: might reveal hyperinflation and patchy areas of atelectasis or infiltration
- Blood gases: might show carbon dioxide retention and hypoxemia
- Nasal-pharyngeal washings: positive identification of RSV can be made via enzyme-linked immunosorbent assay (ELISA) or immunofluorescent antibody (IFA) testing

Nursing Management

RSV infection is usually self-limited, and nursing diagnoses, goals, and interventions for the child with bronchiolitis are aimed at supportive care. Children with less severe disease might require only antipyretics, adequate hydration, and close observation. They can often be successfully managed at home, provided the primary caregiver is reliable and comfortable with close observation. Teach parents or caregivers to watch for signs of worsening and to seek care quickly should the child's condition deteriorate.

Hospitalization is required for children with more severe disease, and children admitted with RSV bronchiolitis warrant close observation. In addition to the nursing diagnoses and related interventions discussed in Nursing Care Plan 40.1 at the end of the chapter for respiratory disorders, interventions common to bronchiolitis follow.

Take Note!

Currently no safe and effective antiviral drug is available for definitive treatment of RSV. Aerosolized ribavirin is recommended only for the highest-risk, most severely ill children. Routine antibiotic use is discouraged in RSV bronchiolitis treatment because the secondary bacterial infection rate of the lower airway is very low (DeNicola et al., 2016).

MAINTAINING PATENT AIRWAY

Infants and young children with RSV tend to have copious secretions. Position the child with the head of the bed elevated to facilitate an open airway. These children often require frequent assessment and suctioning to maintain a patent airway. Use a Yankauer or tonsil-tip suction catheter to suction the mouth or pharynx of older infants or children, rinsing the catheter after each suctioning. Nasal bulb suctioning may be sufficient to clear the airway in some infants, while others will require nasopharyngeal suctioning with a suction catheter. Nursing Procedure 40.1 gives further information. Adjust the pressure ranges for suctioning infants and children between 60 and 100 mm Hg (40 and 60 mm Hg for premature infants).

PROMOTING ADEQUATE GAS EXCHANGE

Infants and children with RSV bronchiolitis might deteriorate quickly as the disease progresses. In the child ill enough to require oxygen, the risk is even greater. Assessment should include work of breathing, respiratory rate, and oxygen saturation. The percentage of inspired oxygen (FiO_2) should be adjusted as needed to maintain oxygen saturation within the desired range. Positioning the infant with the head of the bed elevated may also improve gas exchange. Frequent assessment is necessary for the hospitalized child with bronchiolitis.

Take Note!

In the tachypneic infant, slowing of the respiratory rate does not necessarily indicate improvement: often, a slower respiratory rate is an indication of tiring, and carbon dioxide retention may soon be followed by apnea (AHA, 2011).

NURSING PROCEDURE 40.1

Nasopharyngeal or Artificial Airway Suction Technique

1. Make sure the suction equipment works properly before starting.
2. After washing your hands, assemble the equipment needed:
   - Appropriate-size sterile suction catheter
   - Sterile gloves
   - Supplemental oxygen
   - Sterile water-based lubricant
   - Sterile normal saline if indicated
3. Don sterile gloves, keeping dominant hand sterile and nondominant hand clean.
4. Preoxygenate the infant or child if indicated.
5. Apply lubricant to the end of the suction catheter.
6. If indicated for loosening of secretions, instill sterile saline.
7. Maintaining sterile technique, insert the suction catheter into the child's nostril or airway.
   - Insert only to the point of gagging if inserting via the nostril.
   - Insert only 0.5 cm further than the length of the artificial airway.
8. Intermittently apply suction for no longer than 10 seconds while twisting and removing the catheter.
9. Supplement with oxygen after suctioning.

REDUCING RISK FOR INFECTION

Since RSV is easily spread through contact with droplets, isolate inpatients according to hospital policy to decrease the risk of nosocomial spread to other children. Children with RSV can be safely cohorted. Attention to hand washing is necessary, as droplets might enter the eyes, nose, or mouth via the hands.

PROVIDING FAMILY EDUCATION

Educate parents so they can recognize signs of worsening distress. Tell parents to call the physician or nurse practitioner if the child's breathing becomes rapid or more difficult or if the child cannot eat secondary to tachypnea. Children who are younger than 1 year of age or who are at higher risk (those who were born prematurely or who have chronic heart or lung conditions) might have a longer course of illness. Instruct parents that cough can persist for several days to weeks after resolution of the disease, but infants usually act well otherwise.

PREVENTING RESPIRATORY SYNCYTIAL VIRUS DISEASE

Strict adherence to hand washing policies in day care centers and when exposed to individuals with cold symptoms is important for all age groups. Though generally benign in healthy older children, RSV can be devastating in young infants or children with preexisting risk factors. Palivizumab (Synagis) is a monoclonal antibody that can prevent severe RSV disease in those who are most susceptible (Ohler & Pham, 2013). It is given as an intramuscular injection once a month throughout the RSV season. Though quite costly, it is covered by most insurance policies and Medicaid for those who qualify. It is generally indicated for use in certain qualifying children younger than 2 years of age. Qualifying factors include:

- Prematurity
- Chronic lung disease (bronchopulmonary dysplasia) requiring medication or oxygen
- Certain congenital heart diseases
- Certain neuromuscular disorders (Taketomo, Hodding, & Kraus, 2013)

Links to additional information related to palivizumab are located on thePoint.

HEALTHY PEOPLE 2020

Objective	Nursing Significance
Reduce invasive pneumococcal infections.	• Provide accurate information to families about pneumococcal disease. • Encourage pneumococcal immunization per recommendations.

Healthy People Objectives retrieved from http://www.healthypeople.gov

Pneumonia

Pneumonia is an inflammation of the lung parenchyma. It can be caused by a virus, bacteria, *Mycoplasma,* or a fungus. Respiratory viruses are the most common cause of pneumonia in younger children and the least common cause in older children. Viral pneumonia is usually better tolerated in children of all ages. Children with bacterial pneumonia are more apt to present with a toxic appearance, but they generally recover rapidly if appropriate antibiotic treatment is instituted early. *Streptococcus pneumoniae* is a common cause of bacterial pneumonia in all ages of children, and *M. pneumoniae* is a common causative agent in the school-age child and adolescent. Fungal infection may also result in pneumonia. Aspiration pneumonia may result from aspiration of foreign material into the lower respiratory tract. Pneumonia occurs more often in winter and early spring. It is common in children but is seen most frequently in infants and young toddlers.

Take Note!

Community-acquired pneumonia (CAP) refers to pneumonia in a previously healthy person that is contracted outside of the hospital setting (Barson, 2016).

Pneumonia is usually a self-limited disease. A child who presents with recurrent pneumonia should be evaluated for chronic lung disease such as asthma or cystic fibrosis. Potential complications of pneumonia include bacteremia, pleural effusion, empyema, lung abscess, and pneumothorax. Excluding bacteremia, these complications are often treated with thoracentesis and/or chest tubes as well as antibiotics if appropriate. Pneumatoceles (thin-walled cavities developing in the lung) might occur with certain bacterial pneumonias and usually resolve spontaneously over time.

Therapeutic management of children with less severe disease includes antipyretics, adequate hydration, and close observation. Even bacterial pneumonia can be successfully managed at home if the work of breathing is not severe and oxygen saturation is within normal limits. However, hospitalization is required for children with more severe disease. The child with tachypnea, significant retractions, poor oral intake, or lethargy might require hospital admission for the administration of supplemental oxygen, intravenous hydration, and antibiotics. See Healthy People 2020.

Nursing Assessment

For a full description of the assessment phase of the nursing process, refer to page 1470. Assessment findings pertinent to pneumonia are discussed below.

HEALTH HISTORY

Elicit a description of the present illness and chief complaint. Note onset and progression of symptoms. Common signs and symptoms reported during the health history include:

- Antecedent viral URI
- Fever
- Cough (note type and whether productive or not)
- Increased respiratory rate
- History of lethargy, poor feeding, vomiting, or diarrhea in infants
- Chills, headache, dyspnea, chest pain, abdominal pain, and nausea or vomiting in older children

Explore the child's past and current medical history for risk factors known to be associated with an increase in the severity of pneumonia, such as:

- Prematurity
- Malnutrition

- Passive smoke exposure
- Low socioeconomic status
- Day care attendance
- Underlying cardiopulmonary, immune, or nervous system disease (John & Brady, 2013a)

PHYSICAL EXAMINATION

Physical examination consists of inspection, auscultation, percussion, and palpation.

Inspection. Observe the child's general appearance and color (centrally and peripherally). Cyanosis might accompany coughing spells. The child with bacterial pneumonia may appear ill. Assess work of breathing. Children with pneumonia might exhibit substernal, subcostal, or intercostal retractions. Tachypnea and nasal flaring may be present. Describe cough and quality of sputum if produced.

Auscultation. Auscultation of the lungs might reveal wheezes or rales in the younger child. Local or diffuse rales may be present in the older child. Document diminished breath sounds.

Percussion and Palpation. In the older child, percussion might yield local dullness over a consolidated area. Percussion is much less valuable in the infant or younger child. Tactile fremitus felt upon palpation may be increased with pneumonia.

LABORATORY AND DIAGNOSTIC TESTS

Common laboratory and diagnostic studies ordered for the assessment of pneumonia include:

- Pulse oximetry: oxygen saturation might be decreased significantly or within normal range
- Chest x-ray: varies according to child age and causative agent. In infants and young children, bilateral air trapping and perihilar **infiltrates** (collection of inflammatory cells, cellular debris, and foreign organisms) are the most common findings. Patchy areas of consolidation might also be present. In older children, lobar consolidation is seen more frequently
- Sputum culture: may be useful in determining causative bacteria in older children and adolescents
- White blood cell count: might be elevated in the case of bacterial pneumonia

Nursing Management

Nursing diagnoses, goals, and interventions for the child with pneumonia are primarily aimed at providing supportive care and education about the illness and its treatment. Prevention of pneumococcal infection is also important. Children with more severe disease will require hospitalization. Refer to Nursing Care Plan 40.1 at the end of the chapter for nursing diagnoses and related interventions. In addition to the interventions listed there, the following should be noted.

PROVIDING SUPPORTIVE CARE

Ensure adequate hydration and assist in thinning of secretions by encouraging oral fluid intake in the child whose respiratory status is stable. In children with increased work of breathing, intravenous fluids may be necessary to maintain hydration. Allow and encourage the child to assume a position of comfort, usually with the head of the bed elevated to promote aeration of the lungs. If pain due to coughing or pneumonia itself is severe, administer analgesics as prescribed. Provide supplemental oxygen to the child with respiratory distress or hypoxia as needed.

PROVIDING FAMILY EDUCATION

Educate the family about the importance of adhering to the prescribed antibiotic regimen. Antibiotics may be given intravenously if the child is hospitalized. Oral antibiotics are used upon discharge or if the child is managed on an outpatient basis.

Teach the parents of a child with bacterial pneumonia to expect that following resolution of the acute illness. For 1 to 2 weeks the child might continue to tire easily and the infant might continue to need small, frequent feedings. Cough may also persist after the acute recovery period but should lessen over time.

If the child is diagnosed with viral pneumonia, parents might not understand that their child does not require an antibiotic. Pneumonia is often perceived by the public as a bacterial infection, so most parents will need an explanation related to treatment of viral infections. As with bacterial pneumonia, the child may experience a week or two of weakness or fatigue following resolution of the acute illness.

The young child is at risk for the development of aspiration pneumonia. Parents need to understand that the child might be at risk for injury related to his or her age and developmental stage. To prevent recurrent or further aspiration, teach the parents the safety measures in Teaching Guidelines 40.3.

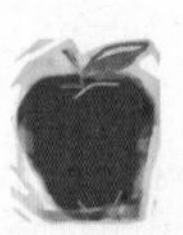

Teaching Guidelines 40.3
PREVENTING ASPIRATION

- Keep toxic substances such as lighter fluid, solvents, and hydrocarbons out of reach of young children. Toddlers and preschoolers cannot distinguish safe from unsafe fluids due to their developmental stage.
- Avoid oily nose drops and oil-based vitamins or home remedies to avoid lipid aspiration into the lungs.

- Avoid oral feedings if the infant's respiratory rate is 60 or greater to minimize the risk of aspiration of the feeding.
- Discourage parents from "force-feeding" in the event of poor oral intake or severe illness to minimize the risk of aspiration of the feeding.
- Position infants and ill children on their right side after feeding to minimize the risk of aspirating emesis or regurgitated feeding.

PREVENTING PNEUMOCOCCAL INFECTION

Children at high risk for severe pneumococcal infection should be immunized against it. This includes all children between 0 and 23 months of age, as well as children between 24 and 59 months of age who either never received the vaccine before age 2 or did not receive a booster dose between 12 and 23 months of age. In addition, children between 24 and 59 months of age with certain conditions such as immune deficiency, sickle cell disease, asplenia, chronic cardiac conditions, chronic lung problems, cerebrospinal fluid leaks, chronic renal insufficiency, diabetes mellitus, and organ transplants should receive the vaccine (CDC, 2016b). For additional information on immunization, refer to Chapter 31.

Bronchitis

Bronchitis is an inflammation of the trachea and major bronchi. It is often associated with a URI. Bronchitis is usually viral in nature, though *M. pneumoniae* and other bacterial organisms are causative in about 10% of cases (Carolan & Bye, 2015). Recovery usually occurs within 5 to 10 days. Therapeutic management involves mainly supportive care. Expectorant administration and adequate hydration are important. If bacterial infection is the cause, antibiotics are indicated.

Nursing Assessment

The illness might begin with a mild URI. Fever develops, followed by a dry, hacking cough that might become productive in older children. The cough might wake the child at night. Auscultation of the lungs might reveal coarse rales. Respirations remain unlabored. The chest x-ray might show diffuse alveolar hyperinflation and perihilar markings.

Nursing Management

Nursing management is aimed at providing supportive care. Teach parents that expectorants will help loosen secretions and antipyretics will help reduce the fever, making the child more comfortable. Encourage adequate hydration. Antibiotics are prescribed only in cases believed to be bacterial in nature. Discourage the use of cough suppressants: it is important for accumulated sputum to be raised.

Tuberculosis

Tuberculosis (TB) is a highly contagious disease caused by inhalation of droplets of *Mycobacterium tuberculosis* or *Mycobacterium bovis*. Children usually contract the disease from an immediate household member. Homeless and impoverished children are at higher risk, as are those exposed to an adult with TB infection (Batra & Ang, 2015). After exposure to an infected individual, the incubation period is 2 to 10 weeks. The inhaled tubercle bacilli multiply in the alveoli and alveolar ducts, forming an inflammatory exudate. The bacilli are spread by the bloodstream and lymphatic system to various parts of the body. Though pulmonary tuberculosis is the most common, children may also have infection in other parts of the body, such as the gastrointestinal tract or central nervous system.

In the case of drug-sensitive tuberculosis, the American Academy of Pediatrics recommends a 6-month course of oral therapy. The first 2 months consist of isoniazid, rifampin, and pyrazinamide given daily. This is followed by twice-weekly isoniazid and rifampin; administration must be observed directly (usually by a public health nurse). In the case of multidrug-resistant tuberculosis, ethambutol or streptomycin is given via intramuscular injection (Pickering, 2012). See Healthy People 2020.

HEALTHY PEOPLE 2020

Objective	Nursing Significance
Reduce tuberculosis. Increase treatment completion rate of all children with tuberculosis who are eligible to complete therapy. Increase the treatment completion rate of contacts to sputum smear–positive cases who are diagnosed with latent tuberculosis infection (LTBI) and started LTBI treatment.	• Assess the health history of all infants, children, and adolescents for risk factors for tuberculosis infection. • Provide tuberculosis screening as recommended. • Refer all tuberculosis infections to the local public health department. • Educate families about the importance of completing medication therapy as prescribed for active and latent tuberculosis, and the need for appropriate follow-up and retesting for tuberculosis infection.

Healthy People Objectives retrieved from http://www.healthypeople.gov

Nursing Assessment

Routine screening for tuberculosis infection is not recommended for low-risk individuals, but children considered to be at high risk for contracting tuberculosis should be screened using the Mantoux test. Children considered to be at high risk are those who:

- Are infected with HIV
- Are incarcerated or institutionalized
- Have a positive recent history of latent tuberculosis infection
- Are immigrants from or have a history of travel to endemic countries
- Are exposed at home to HIV-infected or homeless persons, illicit drug users, persons recently incarcerated, migrant farm workers, or nursing home residents

The presentation of tuberculosis in children is quite varied. Children can be asymptomatic or exhibit a broad range of symptoms. Symptoms may include fever, malaise, weight loss, anorexia, pain and tightness in the chest, and rarely hemoptysis. Cough may or may not be present and usually progresses slowly over several weeks to months. As tuberculosis progresses, the respiratory rate increases and the lung on the affected side is poorly expanded. Dullness to percussion might be present, as well as diminished breath sounds and crackles. Fever persists and pallor, anemia, weakness, and weight loss are present. Diagnosis is confirmed with a positive Mantoux test, positive gastric washings for acid-fast bacillus, interferon-gamma release assay (IGRA), and/or a chest x-ray consistent with tuberculosis.

Nursing Management

Hospitalization of children with tuberculosis is necessary only for the most serious cases. Nursing management is aimed at providing supportive care and encouraging adherence to the treatment regimen. Most nursing care for childhood tuberculosis is provided in outpatient clinics, schools, or a public health setting. Supportive care includes ensuring adequate nutrition and adequate rest, providing comfort measures such as fever reduction, preventing exposure to other infectious diseases, and preventing reinfection.

PROVIDING CARE FOR THE CHILD WITH LATENT TUBERCULOSIS INFECTION

Children who test positive for tuberculosis but who do not have symptoms or radiographic/laboratory evidence of disease are considered to have latent infection. These children should be treated with isoniazid for 9 months to prevent progression to active disease. Follow-up and appropriate monitoring can be achieved via the child's physician or nurse practitioner or local health department.

PREVENTING INFECTION

Tuberculosis infection is prevented by avoiding contact with the tubercle bacillus. Thus, hospitalized children with tuberculosis must be isolated according to hospital policy to prevent nosocomial spread of tuberculosis infection. Promotion of natural resistance through nutrition, rest, and avoidance of serious infections does not prevent infection. Pasteurization of milk has helped to decrease the transmission of *M. bovis*. Administration of bacille Calmette–Guérin (BCG) vaccine can provide incomplete protection against tuberculosis, and it is not widely used in the United States (Pickering, 2012).

ACUTE NONINFECTIOUS DISORDERS

Acute noninfectious disorders include epistaxis, foreign body aspiration, acute respiratory distress syndrome, and pneumothorax.

Epistaxis

Epistaxis (a nosebleed) occurs most frequently in children before adolescence. Bleeding of the nasal mucosa occurs most often from the anterior portion of the septum. Epistaxis may be recurrent and idiopathic (meaning there is no cause). The majority of cases are benign, but in children with bleeding disorders or other hematologic concerns, epistaxis should be further investigated and treated.

Take Note!

The child with recurrent epistaxis or epistaxis that is difficult to control should be further evaluated for underlying bleeding or platelet concerns.

Nursing Assessment

Explore the child's history for initiating factors such as local inflammation, mucosal drying, or local trauma (usually nose picking). Inspect the nasal cavity for blood.

Nursing Management

The presence of blood often frightens children and their parents. The nurse and parents should remain calm. The child should sit up and lean forward (lying down may allow aspiration of the blood). Apply continuous pressure to the anterior portion of the nose by pinching it closed. Encourage the child to breathe through the mouth during this portion of the treatment. Ice or a cold cloth applied to the bridge of the nose may also be helpful. The bleeding usually stops within 10 to 15 minutes. Apply water-soluble gel to the nasal mucosa with a cotton-tipped applicator to moisten the mucosa and prevent recurrence.

Foreign Body Aspiration

Foreign body aspiration occurs when any solid or liquid substance is inhaled into the respiratory tract. It is common in infants and young children and can present in a life-threatening manner. The object may lodge in the upper or lower airway, causing varying degrees of respiratory difficulty. Small, smooth objects such as peanuts are the most frequently aspirated, but any small toy, article, or piece of food smaller than the diameter of the young child's airway can be aspirated.

Take Note!

Items smaller than 1.25 in (3.2 cm) can be aspirated easily. A simple way for parents to estimate the safe size of a small item or toy piece is to gauge its size against a standard toilet paper roll, which is generally about 1.5 in in diameter (Safe Kids, 2016).

Foreign body aspiration occurs most frequently in children between 6 months and 4 years of age (John & Brady, 2013b). Children this age are growing and developing rapidly. They tend to explore things with their mouths and can easily aspirate small items.

The child often coughs out foreign bodies from the upper airway. If the foreign body reaches the bronchus, then it may need to be surgically removed via bronchoscopy. Postoperative antibiotics are used if an infection is also present. Complications of foreign body aspiration include pneumonia or abscess formation, hypoxia, respiratory failure, and death.

Nursing Assessment

The infant or young child might present with a history of sudden onset of cough, wheeze, or stridor. Stridor suggests that the foreign body is lodged in the upper airway. Sometimes the onset of respiratory symptoms is much more gradual. When the item has traveled down one of the bronchi, then wheezing, rhonchi, and decreased aeration can be heard on the affected side. A chest x-ray will demonstrate the foreign body only if it is radiopaque (Fig. 40.7).

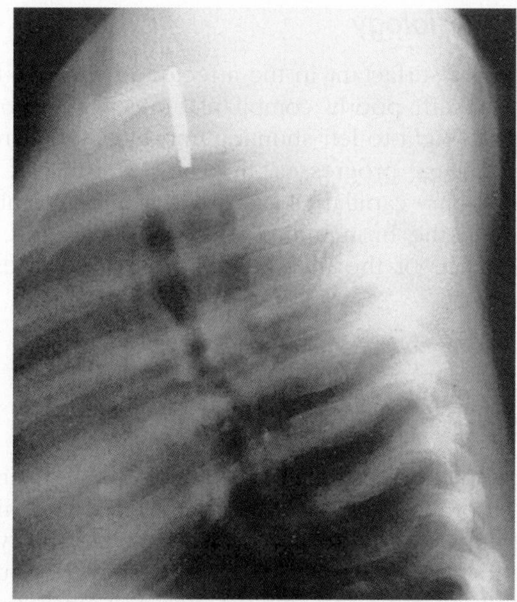

FIGURE 40.7 Foreign body is noted in the bronchus on a chest x-ray.

Nursing Management

The most important nursing intervention related to foreign body aspiration is prevention. Anticipatory guidance for families with 6-month-olds should include a discussion of aspiration avoidance. Repeat this information at each subsequent well-child visit through age 5. Tell parents to avoid letting their child play with toys with small parts and to keep coins and other small objects out of the reach of children. Teach parents not to feed peanuts and popcorn to their child until he or she is at least 3 years old (Gavin, 2013). When children progress to table food, teach parents to chop all foods so that they are small enough to pass down the trachea should the child neglect to chew them up thoroughly. Carrots, grapes, and hot dogs should be cut into small pieces. Harmful liquids should be kept out of the reach of children.

Take Note!

Prevent young children from playing with latex balloons. When popped, small pieces pose an aspiration danger (Gavin, 2013).

Respiratory Distress Syndrome

Respiratory distress syndrome (RDS) is a respiratory disorder that is specific to neonates. It results from lung immaturity and a deficiency in surfactant, so it is seen most often in premature infants. Other infants who might experience RDS include infants of diabetic mothers, those delivered via cesarean section without preceding labor, and those experiencing perinatal asphyxia (Thilo & Rosenberg, 2012). It is believed that each of these conditions has an impact on surfactant production, thus resulting in RDS in the term infant.

Pathophysiology

The lack of surfactant in the affected newborn's lungs results in stiff, poorly compliant lungs with poor gas exchange. Right-to-left shunting and hypoxemia result. As the disease progresses, fluid and fibrin leak from the pulmonary capillaries, causing a hyaline membrane to form in the bronchioles, alveolar ducts, and alveoli. Presence of the membrane further decreases gas exchange.

Acute Respiratory Distress Syndrome

Acute respiratory distress syndrome (ARDS) occurs following a primary insult such as sepsis, viral pneumonia, smoke inhalation, or near drowning. Respiratory distress and hypoxemia occur acutely within 72 hours of the insult in infants and children with previously healthy lungs (Cornfield, 2012). The alveolar–capillary membrane becomes more permeable and pulmonary edema develops. Hyaline membrane formation over the alveolar surfaces and decreased surfactant production cause lung stiffness. Mucosal swelling and cellular debris lead to atelectasis. Gas diffusion is impaired significantly. Some children have residual lung disease and some recover completely. However, ARDS can progress to respiratory failure and death.

Therapeutic management is aimed at improving oxygenation and ventilation. Mechanical ventilation is used, with special attention to lung volumes and positive end-expiratory pressure (PEEP). Newer treatment modalities show promise for improving outcomes of ARDS (see Table 40.2 for additional information on alternative methods of mechanical ventilation).

Nursing Assessment

Tachycardia and tachypnea occur over the first few hours of the illness. Significantly increased work of breathing with nasal flaring and retractions develops. Auscultate the breath sounds, which might range from normal to high-pitched crackles throughout the lung fields. Hypoxemia develops. Bilateral infiltrates can be seen on a chest x-ray.

Nursing Management

Nursing care of the child with ARDS is mainly supportive and occurs in the intensive care unit. Closely monitor respiratory and cardiovascular status. Comfort measures such as hygiene and positioning as well as pain and anxiety management, maintenance of nutrition, and prevention of infection are also key nursing interventions. The acute phase of worsening respiratory distress can be frightening for a child of any age, and the nurse can be instrumental in soothing the child's fears. As the disease worsens and progresses, especially when ventilatory support is required, it is especially important to provide psychological support of the family as well as education about the intensive care unit procedures.

Pneumothorax

A collection of air in the pleural space is called a pneumothorax. It can occur spontaneously in an otherwise healthy child or as a result of chronic lung disease, cardiopulmonary resuscitation, surgery, or trauma. Trapped air consumes space within the pleural cavity, and the affected lung suffers at least partial collapse.

TABLE 40.2 ALTERNATIVES TO TRADITIONAL MECHANICAL VENTILATION

Mode	Description	Additional Information
High-frequency ventilators (high-frequency, oscillating, or jet)	Provide very high respiratory rates (up to 1,200 breaths per min) and very low tidal volumes	May decrease risk of barotrauma associated with ventilator pressures
Nitric oxide	Causes pulmonary vasodilation, helping to increase blood flow to alveoli	Safe; no long-term developmental risks
Liquid ventilation	Perfluorocarbon liquid acts as a surfactant. Provides an effective medium for gas exchange and increases pulmonary function	Virtually no reported physiologic sequelae
Extracorporeal membrane oxygenation (ECMO)	Blood is removed from body via catheter, warmed and oxygenated in the ECMO machine, and then returned to infant.	Labor-intensive. Risk of bleeding is great.

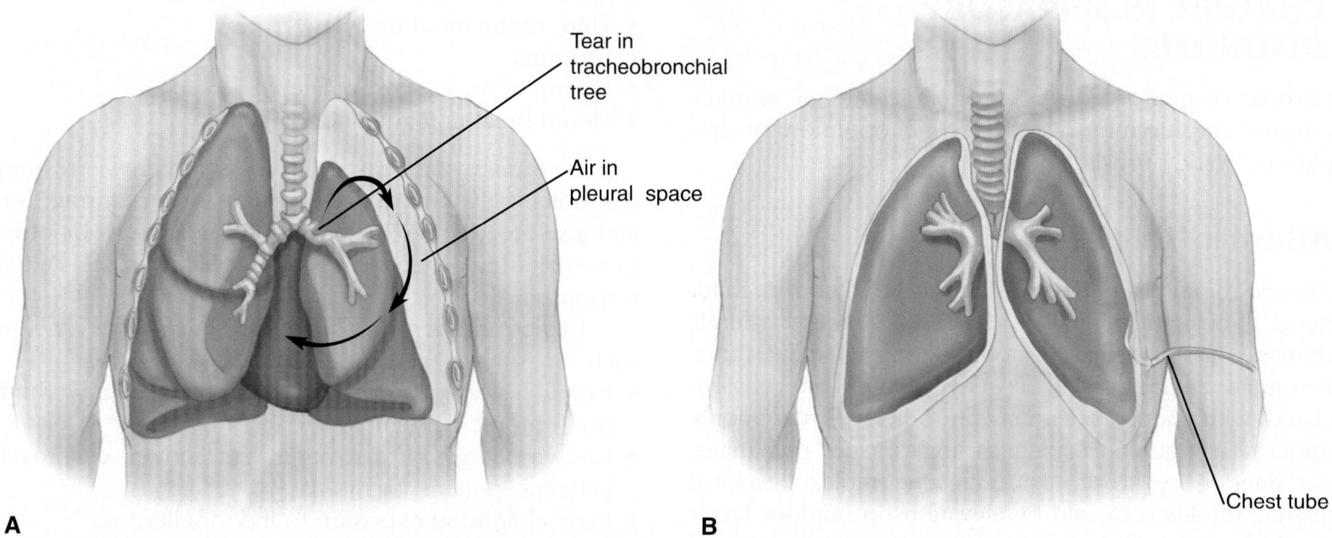

FIGURE 40.8 **(A)** Pneumothorax. **(B)** Note reinflation of the lung when the chest tube is present.

Needle aspiration and/or placement of a chest tube are used to evacuate the air from the chest. Some small pneumothoraces resolve independently, without intervention.

Nursing Assessment

Primary pneumothorax (spontaneous) occurs most often in adolescence (Winnie & Lossef, 2011). The infant or child with a pneumothorax might have a sudden or gradual onset of symptoms. Chest pain might be present as well as signs of respiratory distress such as tachypnea, retractions, nasal flaring, or grunting. Assess risk factors for acquiring a pneumothorax, including chest trauma or surgery, intubation and mechanical ventilation, or a history of chronic lung disease such as cystic fibrosis. Inspect the child for a pale or cyanotic appearance. Auscultate for increased heart rate (tachycardia) and absent or diminished breath sounds on the affected side. The x-ray reveals air within the thoracic cavity (Fig. 40.8).

Nursing Management

The child with a pneumothorax requires frequent respiratory assessments. Pulse oximetry might be used as an adjunct, but clinical evaluation of respiratory status is most useful. In some cases, administration of 100% oxygen hastens the reabsorption of air, but it is generally used only for a few hours (Winnie & Lossef, 2011). If a chest tube is connected to a dry suction or water seal apparatus, provide care of the drainage apparatus as appropriate (Fig. 40.9). A pair of hemostats should be kept at the bedside to clamp the tube should it become dislodged from the drainage container or the open end may be placed in a container of sterile water. The dressing around the chest tube is occlusive and is not routinely changed. If the tube becomes dislodged from the child's chest, apply Vaseline gauze and an occlusive dressing, immediately perform appropriate respiratory assessment, and notify the physician or nurse practitioner or nurse practitioner.

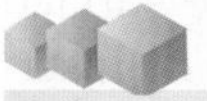

Concept Mastery Alert

Use of Oxygen With a Pneumothorax

In a child with a pneumothorax, the nurse would administer 100% oxygen to hasten air reabsorption. This treatment is only used for a short period of time early in the course of treatment. Although it does help to prevent hypoxemia during administration, this is not the primary reason it is administered.

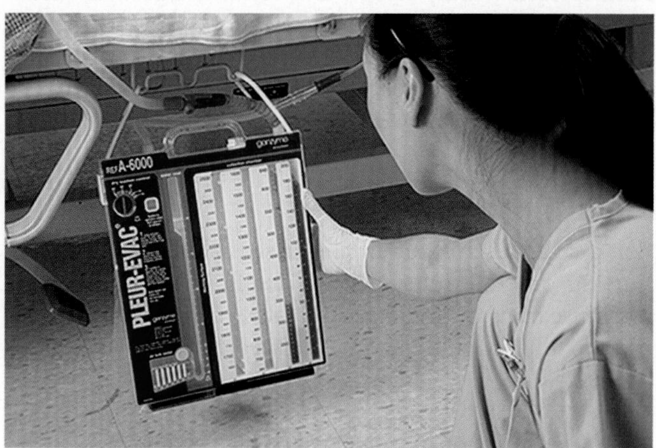

FIGURE 40.9 The chest tube is connected to a suction or water seal via a drainage container.

CHRONIC RESPIRATORY DISORDERS

Chronic respiratory disorders include allergic rhinitis, asthma, chronic lung disease (bronchopulmonary dysplasia), cystic fibrosis, and apnea.

Allergic Rhinitis

Allergic rhinitis is a common chronic condition in childhood, affecting a significant number of children. Allergic rhinitis is associated with atopic dermatitis and asthma. Perennial allergic rhinitis occurs year-round and is associated with indoor environments. Allergens commonly implicated in perennial allergic rhinitis include dust mites, pet dander, cockroach antigens, and molds. Seasonal allergic rhinitis is caused by elevations in outdoor levels of allergens. It is typically caused by certain pollens, trees, weeds, fungi, and molds. Complications from allergic rhinitis include exacerbation of asthma symptoms, recurrent sinusitis and otitis media, and dental malocclusion.

Pathophysiology

Allergic rhinitis is an intermittent or persistent inflammatory state that is mediated by immunoglobulin E (IgE). In response to contact with an airborne allergen protein, the nasal mucosa mounts an immune response. The antigen (from the allergen) binds to a specific IgE on the surface of mast cells, releasing the chemical mediators of histamine and leukotrienes. The release of mediators results in acute tissue edema and mucus production. Late-phase mediators are released and more inflammation results. IgE binds to receptors on the surfaces of mast cells and basophils, creating the sensitization memory that causes the reaction with subsequent allergen exposures. Allergen exposure then results in mast cell degranulation and release of histamine and other chemotactic factors. Histamine and other factors cause nasal vasodilation, watery **rhinorrhea** (runny nose), and nasal congestion. Irritation of local nerve endings by histamine produces pruritus and sneezing (Milgrom & Leung, 2011). Treatment of allergic rhinitis is aimed at decreasing response to these allergic mediators as well as treating inflammation.

Nursing Assessment

For a full description of the assessment phase of the nursing process, refer to the Nursing Process Overview section earlier in the chapter. Assessment findings pertinent to allergic rhinitis are discussed below.

HEALTH HISTORY

Elicit a description of the present illness and chief complaint. Common signs and symptoms reported during the health history might include:

- Mild, intermittent to chronic nasal stuffiness
- Thin, runny nasal discharge
- Sneezing
- Itching of nose, eyes, palate
- Mouth breathing and snoring

Determine the seasonality of symptoms. Are they perennial (year-round) or do they occur during certain seasons only? What types of medications or other treatments have been used, and what was the child's response?

Explore the history for the presence of risk factors such as:

- Family history of atopic disease (asthma, allergic rhinitis, or atopic dermatitis)
- Known allergy to dust mites, pet dander, cockroach antigens, pollens, or molds
- Early childhood exposure to indoor allergens
- Early introduction to foods or formula in infancy
- Exposure to tobacco smoke
- Environmental air pollution
- Recurrent viral infections (Milgrom & Leung, 2011)

Nonwhite race and higher socioeconomic status have also been noted as risk factors.

PHYSICAL EXAMINATION

Physical examination of the child with allergic rhinitis includes inspection, observation, and auscultation.

Inspection and Observation. Observe the child's facies for red-rimmed eyes or tearing, mild eyelid edema, "allergic shiners" (bluish or grayish cast beneath the eyes), and "allergic salute" (a transverse nasal crease between the lower and middle thirds of the nose that results from repeated nose rubbing) (Fig. 40.10). Inspect the nasal cavity. The turbinates may be swollen and gray/blue. Clear mucoid nasal drainage may be observed. Inspect the skin for rash. Listen for nasal phonation with speech.

Auscultation. Auscultate the lungs for adequate aeration and clarity of breath sounds. In the child who also has asthma, exacerbation with wheezing often occurs with allergic rhinitis.

LABORATORY AND DIAGNOSTIC TESTS

The initial diagnosis is often made based on the history and clinical findings. Common laboratory and diagnostic studies ordered for the assessment of allergic rhinitis may include:

- Nasal smear (positive for eosinophilia)
- Positive allergy skin test
- Positive radioallergosorbent test (RAST)

To distinguish between the causes of nasal congestion, refer to Comparison Chart 40.1.

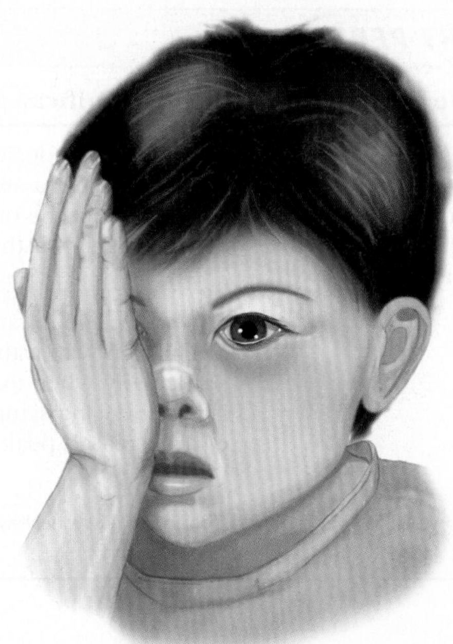

FIGURE 40.10 Allergic shiners beneath the eyes and allergic salute across the nose.

Nursing Management

In addition to the nursing diagnoses and related interventions discussed in Nursing Care Plan 40.1 at the end of the chapter for disorders of the nose, mouth, and throat, interventions common to allergic rhinitis follow.

MAINTAINING PATENT AIRWAY

The constant nasal obstruction that occurs with allergic rhinitis can be very problematic for some children. Performing nasal washes with normal saline may keep the nasal mucus from becoming thickened. Thickened, immobile secretions often lead to a secondary bacterial infection. The nasal wash also decongests the nose, allowing for improved nasal airflow. Anti-inflammatory (corticosteroid) nasal sprays can decrease the inflammatory response to allergens. A mast cell stabilizing nasal spray such as cromolyn sodium may decrease the intensity and frequency of allergic responses. Oral antihistamines are now available in once-daily dosing, providing convenience for the family. Some children may benefit from a combined antihistamine/nasal decongestant if nasal congestion is significant. Leukotriene modifiers such as montelukast may also be beneficial for some children. See Dosage Calculation Box 40.1.

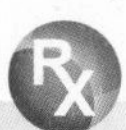

Dosage Calculation Box 40.1

Child's weight: 30 lb
Medication order: cetirizine 2.5 mg PO every morning.
Cetirizine is supplied as 5 mg/5 mL.
How many milliliters will the nurse administer? Round to the nearest tenth.

PROVIDING FAMILY EDUCATION

One of the most important tools in the treatment of allergic rhinitis is learning to avoid known allergens. Teaching Guidelines 40.4 gives information on educating families about avoidance of allergens. Children may be referred to a specialist for allergen desensitization (allergy shots). Products helpful with control of allergies are available from a number of vendors. Links to such vendors can be found on thePoint.

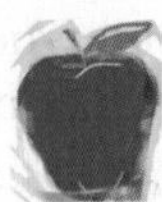

Teaching Guidelines 40.4

CONTROLLING EXPOSURE TO ALLERGENS

Tobacco

- Avoid all exposure to tobacco smoke.
- No parental smoking inside the home or car.

Dust Mites

- Use pillow and mattress covers.
- Wash bed linens once a week in 130°F water.
- Use blinds rather than curtains in bedroom.
- Remove stuffed animals from bedroom or minimize number and wash weekly.
- Reduce indoor humidity to <50%.
- Remove carpet from bedroom.
- Clean solid-surface floors with wet mop each week.

Pet Dander

- Remove pets from home permanently.
- If unable to remove them, keep them out of bedroom and off carpet and upholstered furniture.

Cockroaches

- Keep kitchen very clean.
- Avoiding leaving food or drinks out.
- Use pesticides if necessary but ensure that the asthmatic child is not inside the home when the pesticide is sprayed.

Indoor Molds

- Repair water leaks.
- Use dehumidifier to keep basement dry.
- Reduce indoor humidity to <50%.

Outdoor Molds, Pollen, and Air Pollution

- Avoid going outdoors when mold and pollen counts are high.
- Avoid outdoor activity when pollution levels are high.

Adapted from National Asthma Education and Prevention Program. (2007). *Expert panel report 3: Guidelines for the diagnosis and management of asthma* (NIH Publication No. 07–4051). Bethesda, MD: National Institutes of Health, National Heart, Lung and Blood Institute; and Ratcliffe, M. M., & Kieckhefer, G. M. (2010). Asthma. In P. J. Allen, J. A. Vessey, & N. A. Schapiro (Eds.), *Primary care of the child with a chronic condition* (5th ed.). St. Louis, MO: Mosby.

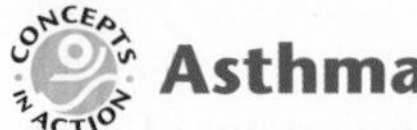

Asthma

Asthma is a chronic inflammatory airway disorder characterized by airway hyperresponsiveness, airway edema, and mucus production. Airway obstruction resulting from asthma might be partially or completely reversed. Severity ranges from long periods of control with infrequent acute exacerbations in some children to the presence of persistent daily symptoms in others. It is the most common chronic illness of childhood with more than 10 million American children diagnosed before age 18 years (Lynch, 2011). A small percentage of children with asthma account for a large percentage of healthcare use and expense. In school-age children who have experienced one asthma attack, the average school days missed per year is 10.5 and asthma accounts for 3 billion dollars in healthcare costs per year (Lynch, 2011). The incidence and severity of asthma are increasing; this might be attributed to increased urbanization, increased air pollution, and more accurate diagnosis. See Healthy People 2020.

Severity ranges from symptoms associated only with vigorous activity (exercise-induced bronchospasm) to daily symptoms that interfere with quality of life. Table 40.3 discusses classification of asthma severity. Though uncommon, childhood death related to asthma is also on the rise worldwide. Air pollution, allergens, family history, and viral infections might all play a role in asthma (John & Brady, 2013a). Many children with asthma also have gastroesophageal disease, though the relationship between the two diseases is not clearly understood.

A significant long-term complication, chronic airway remodeling, may result from recurrent asthma exacerbation and inflammation. Children with asthma

HEALTHY PEOPLE 2020

Objective	Nursing Significance
Reduce asthma deaths, hospitalizations for asthma, and hospital emergency department visits for asthma.	• Appropriately educate children with asthma and their families about the ongoing management of asthma. • Provide appropriate education and triage to families of children with asthma, particularly when the child is experiencing symptoms or a decreased peak flow rate.

Healthy People Objectives retrieved from http://www.healthypeople.gov

TABLE 40.3 ASTHMA SEVERITY CLASSIFICATION IN CHILDREN NOT TAKING LONG-TERM CONTROL MEDICATIONS

Classification	Symptoms	Lung Function	Interference With Normal Activity	Short-Acting β_2-Agonist Use for Symptom Control
Intermittent	• 1 or 2 times a week • Nighttime symptoms 1 or 2 times a month	FEV 80% or more of predicted	None	1 or 2 days per week
Mild persistent	• Symptoms more than twice a week but less than once a day • Nighttime symptoms 3 or 4 times a month	FEV 80% or more of predicted, variability	Minor limitation	Greater than twice per week, but not more than once a day
Moderate persistent	• Daily symptoms • Nighttime symptoms >1 time a week, but not nightly	FEV 60–80% of predicted	Some limitation	Daily
Severe persistent	• Throughout the day • Nighttime symptoms often 7 times per week	FEV <60% of predicted	Extremely limited	Several times per day

FEV, forced expiratory volume.

Adapted from National Asthma Education and Prevention Program. (2007). *Expert panel report 3: Guidelines for the diagnosis and management of asthma* (NIH Publication No. 07–4051). Bethesda, MD: National Institutes of Health, National Heart, Lung and Blood Institute.

are more susceptible to serious bacterial and viral respiratory infections (John & Brady, 2013a). Acute complications also include status asthmaticus and respiratory failure.

Pathophysiology

In asthma, the inflammatory process contributes to increased airway activity. Thus, control or prevention of inflammation is the core of asthma management. Asthma results from a complex variety of responses in relation to a trigger. When the process begins, mast cells, T lymphocytes, macrophages, and epithelial cells are involved in the release of inflammatory mediators. Eosinophils and neutrophils migrate to the airway, causing injury. Chemical mediators such as leukotrienes, bradykinin, histamine, and platelet-activating factor also contribute to the inflammatory response. The presence of leukotrienes contributes to prolonged airway constriction. Autonomic neural control of airway tone is affected, airway mucus secretion is increased, mucociliary function changes, and airway smooth muscle responsiveness increases. As a result, acute bronchoconstriction, airway edema, and mucus plugging occur (Fig. 40.11).

In most children, this process is considered reversible and until recently it was not considered to have long-standing effects on lung function. Current research and scientific thought, however, recognize the concept of airway remodeling (Sirivimonpan, 2013). Airway remodeling occurs as a result of chronic inflammation of the airway. Following the acute response to a trigger, continued allergen response results in a chronic phase. During this phase, the epithelial cells are denuded and the influx of inflammatory cells into the airway continues. This results in structural changes of the airway that are irreversible, and further loss of pulmonary function might occur. The irreversible changes include thickening of the sub-basement membrane, subepithelial fibrosis, airway smooth muscle hypertrophy and hyperplasia, blood vessel proliferation and dilation, and mucous gland hyperplasia and hypersecretion (Sirivimonpan, 2013). In some individuals with poorly controlled asthma, these changes may be permanent, resulting in decreased responsiveness to therapy.

Therapeutic Management

Current goals of medical therapy are avoidance of asthma triggers and reduction or control of inflammatory episodes. The most recent recommendations by the National Asthma Education and Prevention Program (NAEPP) suggest a stepwise approach to medication management as well as control of environmental factors (allergens) and comorbid conditions that affect asthma. The NAEPP guidelines stress periodic assessment of asthma control. Treatment decisions may then be made based on the individual's level of asthma control, rather than on the severity at diagnosis. See Healthy People 2020.

The stepwise approach to asthma treatment involves increasing medications as the child's condition worsens, then backing off treatment as he or she improves (Box 40.3).

Short-acting bronchodilators may be used in the acute treatment of bronchoconstriction and long-acting forms may be used to prevent bronchospasm. Exercise-induced bronchospasm may occur in any child with asthma or as the only symptom in the child with mild intermittent asthma. Most children may avoid exercise-induced bronchospasm by using a longer warm-up period prior to vigorous exercise and, if necessary, inhaling a short-acting bronchodilator just prior to exercise. Long-term prevention usually involves inhaled steroids.

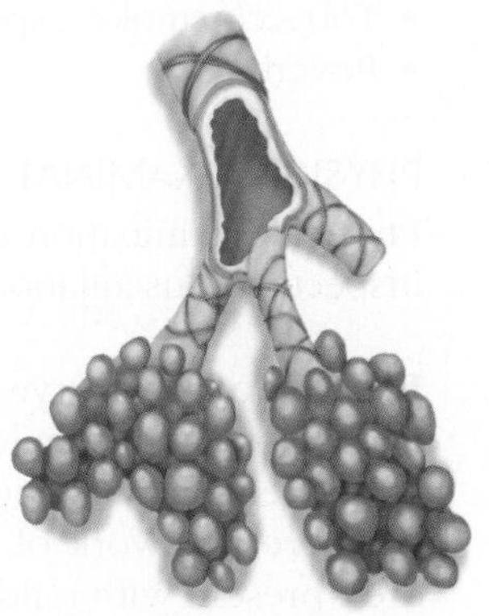

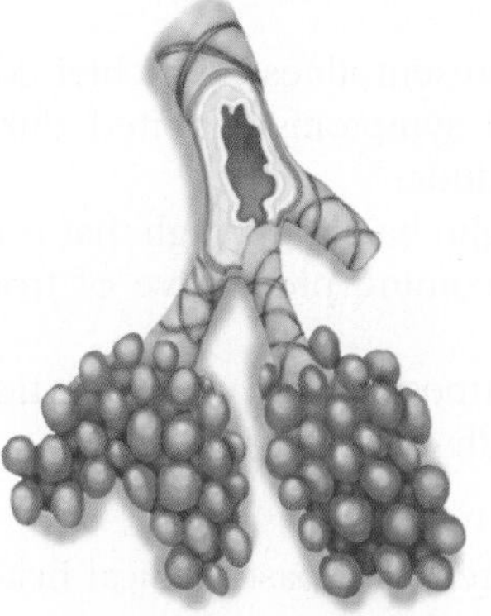

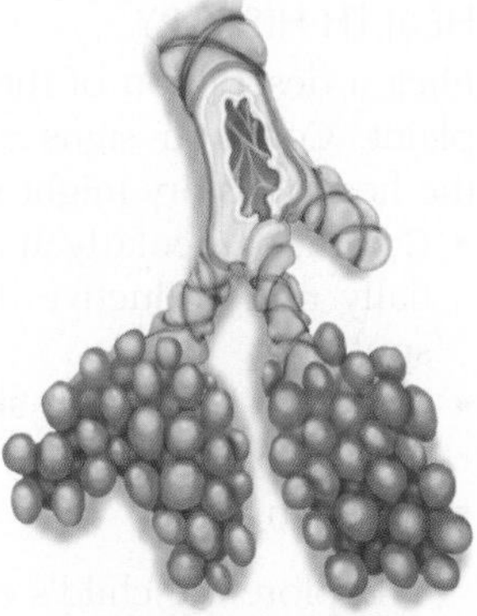

FIGURE 40.11 Note airway edema, mucus production, and bronchospasm occurring with asthma.

HEALTHY PEOPLE 2020

Objective	Nursing Significance
Reduce activity limitations among persons with current asthma.	• Encourage appropriate physical activity in children with asthma.
Reduce the proportion of persons with asthma who miss school or work days.	• Provide extensive education to children and families about peak flow meter use and its meaning, maintenance and rescue medications, symptoms of asthma exacerbation, and a written plan for how to "step up" and "step down" asthma management.
Increase the proportion of persons with current asthma who receive formal patient education.	• Refer children and their families to local or Internet resources and support groups.
	• Refer families to formal classes on asthma education.

Healthy People Objectives retrieved from http://www.healthypeople.gov

Leukotriene modifiers may be used as an alternative but are not preferred for mild persistent asthma (NAEPP, 2007).

BOX 40.3

STEPWISE APPROACH TO ASTHMA MANAGEMENT

All children: child education, environmental control, and management of comorbidities at each step. Consider referral to asthma specialist at step 3. (Step 2 and above are persistent asthma.)

Step 1 (intermittent asthma)
Preferred: short-acting β_2-agonist PRN

Step 2
Preferred: low-dose inhaled corticosteroid
Alternative: cromolyn or leukotriene modifier

Step 3
Preferred: medium-dose inhaled corticosteroid (all ages) OR low-dose inhaled corticosteroid and leukotriene modifier or long-acting β_2-agonist (children older than 4 years)

Step 4
Preferred: medium-dose inhaled corticosteroids and long-acting β_2-agonist (can use leukotriene modifier in children younger than 4 years)

Step 5
Preferred: high-dose inhaled corticosteroids and long-acting β_2-agonist (or leukotriene modifier or theophylline)

Step 6
Preferred: high-dose inhaled corticosteroids, long-acting β_2-agonist, and oral systemic corticosteroids

Adapted from National Asthma Education and Prevention Program. (2007). *Expert panel report 3: Guidelines for the diagnosis and management of asthma* (NIH Publication No. 07–4051). Bethesda, MD: National Institutes of Health, National Heart, Lung and Blood Institute. These recommendations are intended to be used as a guide in individualized asthma care.

Nursing Assessment

For a full description of the assessment phase of the nursing process, refer to the Nursing Process Overview section earlier in the chapter. Assessment findings pertinent to asthma are discussed below.

HEALTH HISTORY

Elicit a description of the present illness and chief complaint. Common signs and symptoms reported during the health history might include:

- Cough, particularly at night: hacking cough that is initially nonproductive, becoming productive of frothy sputum
- Difficulty breathing: shortness of breath, chest tightness or pain, dyspnea with exercise
- Wheezing

Explore the child's current and past medical history for risk factors such as:

- History of allergic rhinitis or atopic dermatitis
- Family history of atopy (asthma, allergic rhinitis, atopic dermatitis)
- Recurrent episodes diagnosed as wheezing, bronchiolitis, or bronchitis
- Known allergies
- Seasonal response to environmental pollen
- Tobacco smoke exposure
- Poverty

PHYSICAL EXAMINATION

Physical examination of the child with asthma includes inspection, auscultation, and percussion.

Inspection. Observe the child's general appearance and color. During mild exacerbations, the child's color might remain pink, but as the child worsens, cyanosis might result. Work of breathing is variable. Some children present with mild retractions, while others demonstrate significant accessory muscle use and eventually head bobbing if not treated effectively. The child may appear anxious and fearful or may be lethargic and irritable. An audible wheeze might be present. Children with persistent severe asthma may have a barrel chest and routinely demonstrate mildly increased work of breathing.

Auscultation and Percussion. A thorough assessment of lung fields is necessary. Wheezing is the hallmark of airway obstruction and might vary throughout the lung fields. Coarseness might also be present. Assess the adequacy of aeration. Breath sounds might be diminished in the bases or throughout. A quiet chest in an asthmatic child can be an ominous sign. With severe airway obstruction, air movement can be so poor that wheezes might not be heard upon auscultation. Percussion may yield hyperresonance.

LABORATORY AND DIAGNOSTIC TESTS

Laboratory and diagnostic studies commonly ordered for the assessment of asthma include:

- Pulse oximetry: oxygen saturation may be decreased significantly or normal during a mild exacerbation
- Chest x-ray: usually reveals hyperinflation
- Blood gases: might show carbon dioxide retention and hypoxemia
- Pulmonary function tests (PFTs): can be very useful in determining the degree of disease but are not useful during an acute attack. Children as young as 5 or 6 years might be able to comply with spirometry.
- Peak expiratory flow rate (PEFR): is decreased during an exacerbation
- Allergy testing: skin test or RAST can determine allergic triggers for the asthmatic child

Nursing Management

Initial nursing management of the child with an acute exacerbation of asthma is aimed at restoring a clear airway and effective breathing pattern as well as promoting adequate oxygenation and ventilation (gas exchange). Refer to Nursing Care Plan 40.1 at the end of the chapter. Additional considerations are reviewed below.

> **Atraumatic Care 40.2**
>
> *When caring for a young child who must receive a nebulizer treatment by mask, play make-believe about the mask and utilize other distraction techniques such as reading a book. Making activities into games, and utilizing distraction both help to minimize trauma when providing necessary care to young children.*

EDUCATING THE CHILD AND FAMILY

Asthma is a chronic illness and needs to be understood as such. Teach families of children with asthma, and the children themselves, how to care for the disease. Symptom-free periods (often very long) are interspersed with episodes of exacerbation. Parents and children often do not understand the importance of maintenance medications for long-term control. They may view the episodes of exacerbation (sometimes requiring hospitalization or emergency room visits) as an acute illness and are simply relieved when they are over. Frequently during the periods between acute episodes, children are viewed as disease-free and long-term maintenance schedules are abandoned. The prolonged inflammatory process occurring in the absence of symptoms, primarily in children with moderate to severe asthma, can lead to airway remodeling and eventual irreversible disease.

Each child should have a management plan in place to determine when to step up or step down treatment. Figure 40.12 provides an example of an action plan that may be helpful to families in the management of asthma. The action plan should also be kept on file at the child's school, and relief medication should be available to the child at all times. Children who experience exercise-induced bronchospasm may still participate in physical education or athletics, but may need to be allowed to use their medicine before the activity. Provide appropriate education to the child and family based on the child's individualized stepwise treatment plan. Stress the concept of maintenance medications for the prevention of future serious disease in addition to controlling or preventing current symptoms.

Educate families and children on the appropriate use of nebulizers, metered-dose inhalers, spacers, dry-powder inhalers, and Diskus, as well as the purposes, functions, and side effects of the medications they deliver. Require return demonstrations of equipment use to ensure that children and families can use the equipment properly (Teaching Guidelines 40.5).

> **Take Note!**
>
> The NAEPP (2007) recommends use of a spacer or holding chamber with metered-dose inhalers to increase the bioavailability of medication in the lungs (John & Brady, 2013a).

In children who have more severe asthma, the NAEPP (2007) recommends the use of the PEFR to determine daily control. PEFR measurements obtained via a home peak flow meter can be very helpful as long as the meter is used appropriately (John & Brady, 2013a); Teaching Guidelines 40.6 gives instructions on peak flow meter

(text continues on page 1507)

AAAAI
AMERICAN ACADEMY OF ALLERGY ASTHMA & IMMUNOLOGY
www.aaaai.org

ASTHMA ACTION PLAN

Name: ____ Date: ____
Emergency Contact: ____ Relationship: ____
Cell phone: ____ Work phone: ____
Health Care Provider: ____ Phone number: ____
Personal Best Peak Flow: ____

GREEN ZONE:
Doing Well
✓ No coughing, wheezing, chest tightness, or difficulty breathing
✓ Can work, play, exercise, perform usual activities without symptoms
OR
✓ Peak flow ___ to ___
(80% to 100% of personal best)

Take these medicines every day for control and maintenance:

Medicine	How much to take	When and how often

YELLOW ZONE:
Caution/Getting Worse
✓ Coughing, wheezing, chest tightness, or difficulty breathing
✓ Symptoms with daily activities, work, play, and exercise
✓ Nighttime awakenings with symptoms
OR
✓ Peak flow ___ to ___
(50% to 80% of personal best)

CONTINUE your Green Zone medicines PLUS take these quick-relief medicines:

Medicine	How much to take	When and how often

Call your doctor if you have been in the Yellow Zone for more than 24 hours.

Also call your doctor if: ____

RED ZONE:
Alert!
✓ Difficulty breathing, coughing, wheezing not helped with medications
✓ Trouble walking or talking due to asthma symptoms
✓ Not responding to quick relief medication
OR
✓ Peak flow is less than ___
(50% of personal best)

FOR EXTREME TROUBLE BREATHING/SHORTNESS OF BREATH GET IMMEDIATE HELP!

Take these quick-relief medicines:

Medicine	How much to take	When and how often

CALL your doctor NOW.
GO to the hospital/emergency department or CALL for an ambulance NOW!

This information is for general purposes and is not intended to replace the advice of a qualified health professional. For more information on asthma, visit www.aaaai.org.

FIGURE 40.12 Asthma action plan. (*Used with permission from American Academy of Allergy, Asthma and Immunology,* http://www.aaaai.org/professionals/asthma-action-plan.pdf)

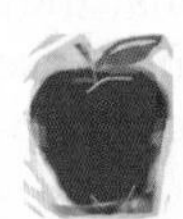

Teaching Guidelines 40.5

USING ASTHMA MEDICATION DELIVERY DEVICES

Nebulizer

1. Plug in the nebulizer and connect the air compressor tubing.

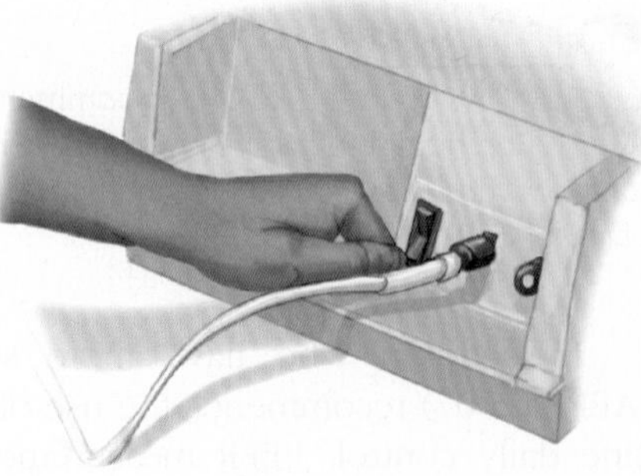

2. Add the medication to the medicine cup.

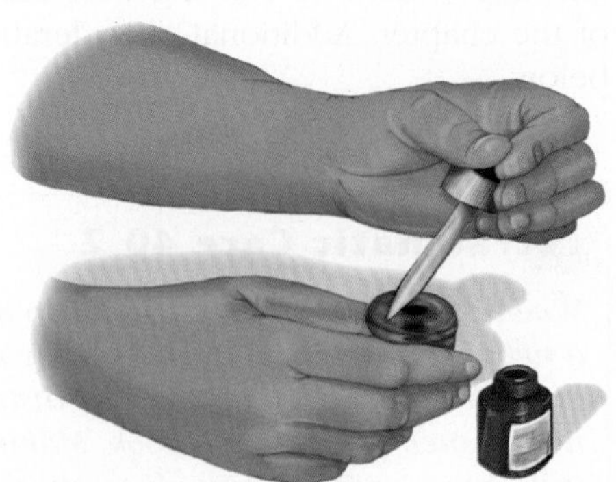

3. Attach the mask or the mouthpiece and hose to the medicine cup.

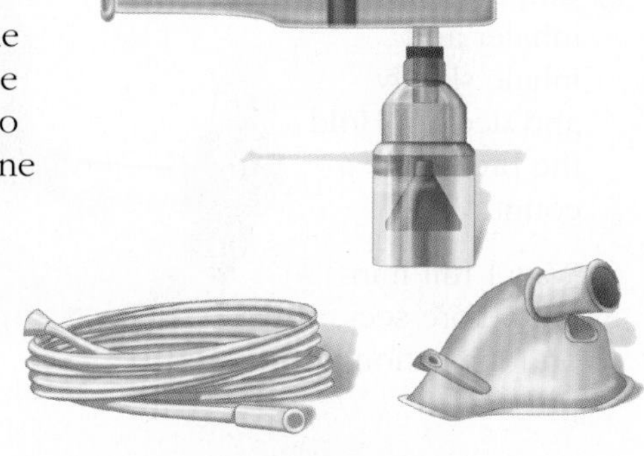

4. Place the mask on the child *or* (see step 5)

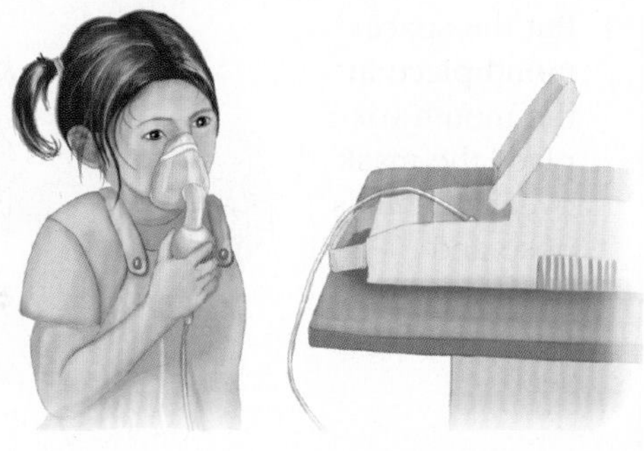

5. Instruct the child to close the lips around the mouthpiece and breathe through the mouth.

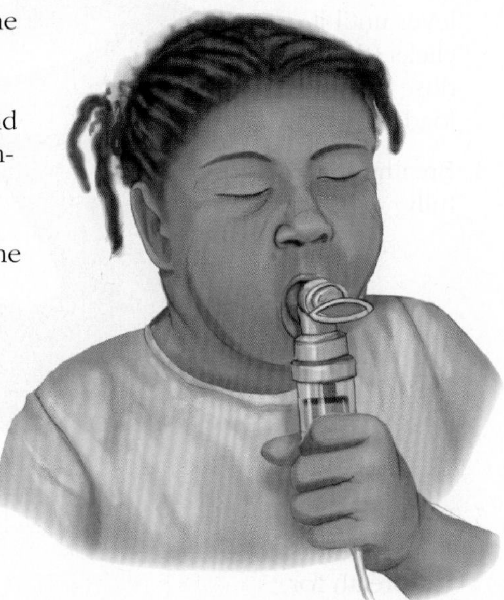

6. After use, wash the mouthpiece and medicine cup with water and allow to air dry.

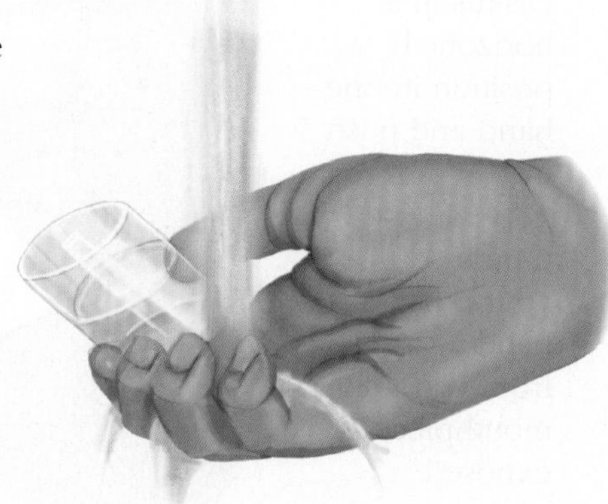

Metered-Dose Inhaler

1. Shake the inhaler and take off the cap.

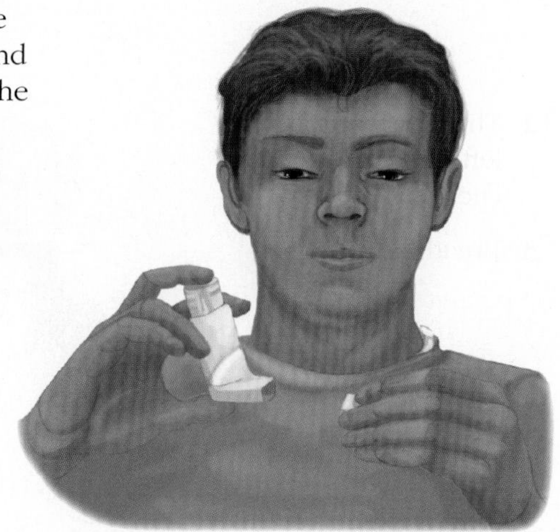

2. Attach the inhaler to the spacer or holding chamber.
3. Breathe out completely.

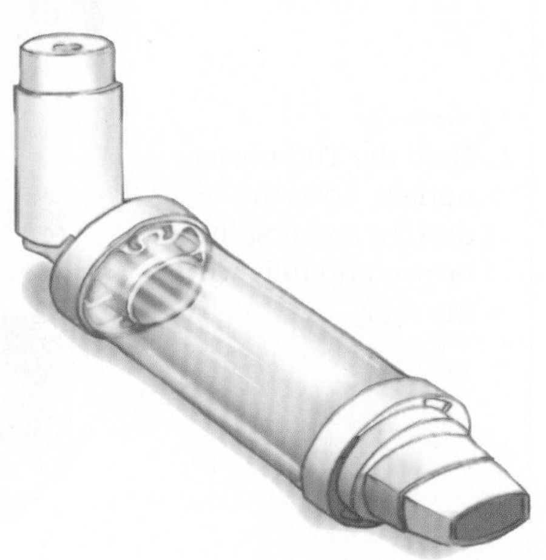

(continued)

4. Put the spacer mouthpiece in the mouth (or place the mask over the child's nose and mouth, ensuring a good seal).

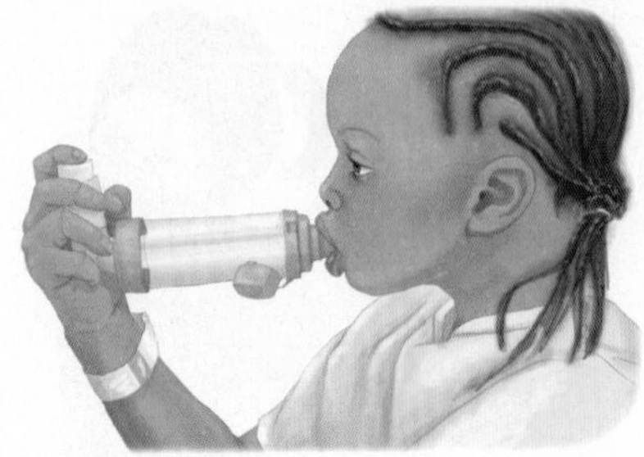

5. Compress the inhaler and inhale slowly and deeply. Hold the breath for a count of 10.
6. Wait 1 full minute before second inhalation, if prescribed.

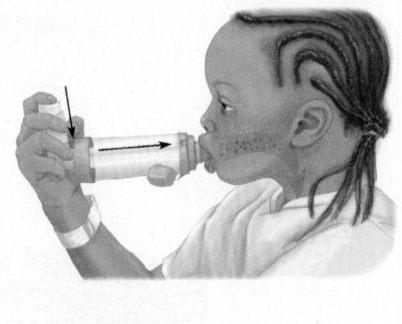

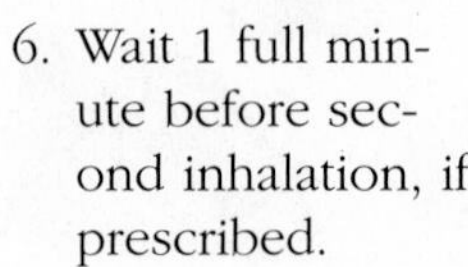

Diskus

1. Hold the Diskus in a horizontal position in one hand and push the thumb grip with the thumb of your other hand away from you until mouthpiece is exposed.

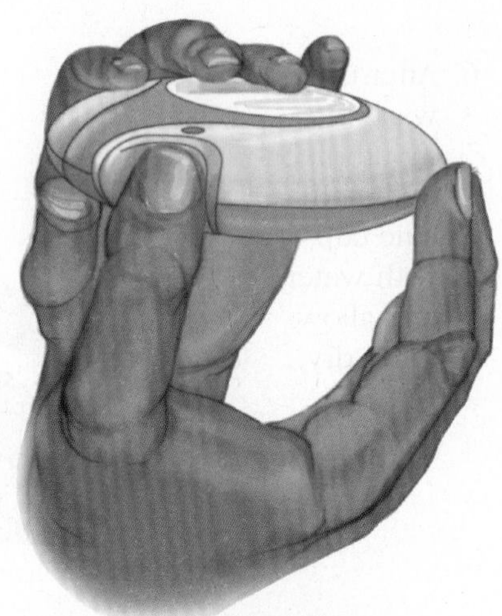

2. Push the lever until it clicks (the dose is now loaded).
3. Breathe out fully.

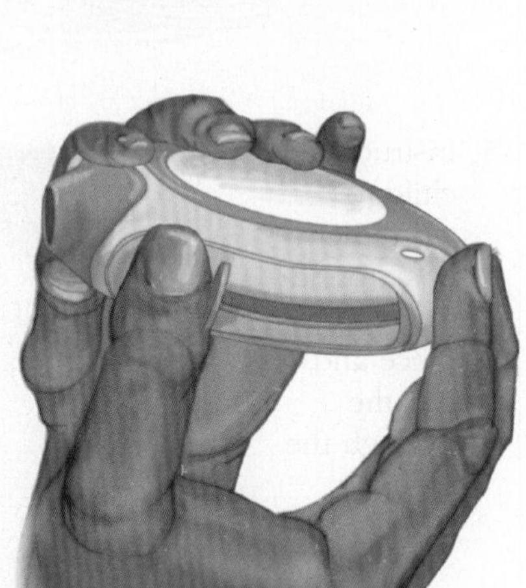

4. Place your mouth securely around the mouthpiece then inhale.

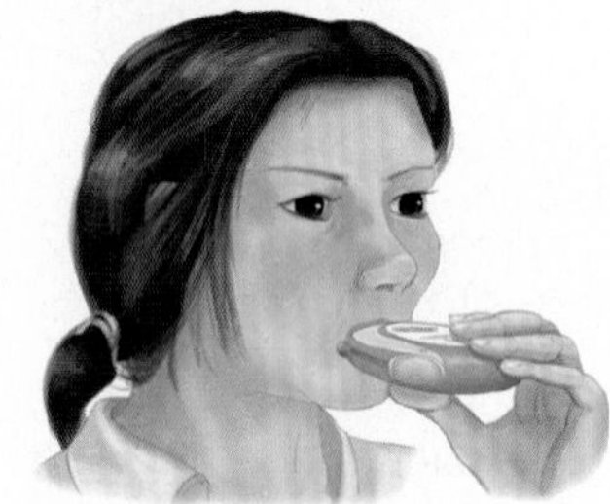

5. Remove the Diskus, hold the breath for 10 seconds, and then breathe out.

Turbuhaler

1. Hold the Turbuhaler upright. Load the dose by twisting the brown grip fully to the right.

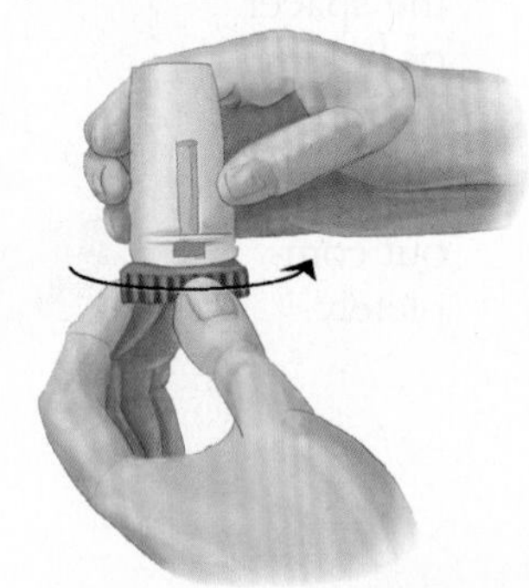

2. Then twist it to the left until you hear it click.
3. Breathe out fully.

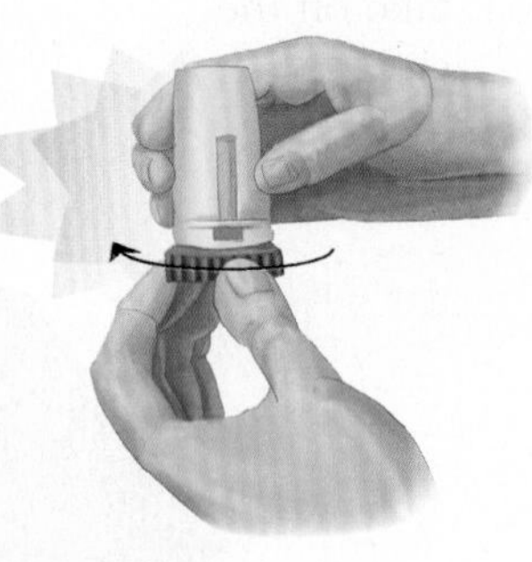

4. Holding the Turbuhaler horizontally, place the mouth firmly around the mouthpiece and inhale deeply and forcefully.

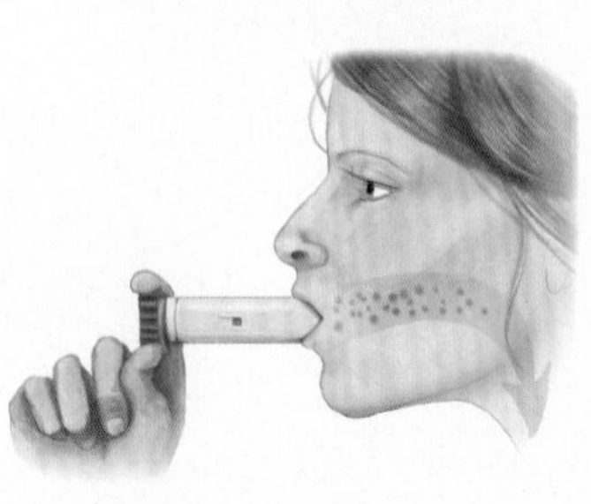

5. Remove the Turbuhaler from the mouth and then breathe out.

TABLE 40.4 ASSESSMENT OF PEAK EXPIRATORY FLOW RATE (PEFR)

Zone[a]	PEFR	Symptoms	Action
Green: Good control	>80% personal best	None	Take usual medications.
Yellow: Caution	50–80% personal best	Possibly present	Take short-acting inhaled β_2-agonist right away. Talk to your physician or nurse practitioner.
Red: Medical alert	<50% personal best	Usually present	Take short-acting inhaled β_2-agonist right away. Go to office or emergency department.

[a]The National Asthma Education and Prevention Program recommended the "traffic light" approach for educating individuals on PEFRs and management plans.

Adapted from National Asthma Education and Prevention Program. (2007). *Expert panel report 3: Guidelines for the diagnosis and management of asthma* (NIH Publication No. 07–4051). Bethesda, MD: National Institutes of Health, National Heart, Lung and Blood Institute.

use. The child's "personal best" is determined collaboratively with the physician or nurse practitioner during a symptom-free period. PEFR is measured daily at home using the peak flow meter. The asthma management plan then gives specific instructions based on the PEFR measurement (Table 40.4).

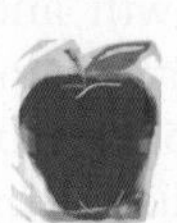

Teaching Guidelines 40.6

USING A PEAK FLOW METER

- Slide the arrow down to "zero."
- Stand up straight.
- Take a deep breath and close the lips tightly around the mouthpiece.
- Blow out hard and fast.
- Note the number the arrow moves to.
- Repeat three times and record the highest reading.
- Keep a record of daily readings, being sure to measure peak flow at the same time each day.

Adapted from John, R. M. & Brady, M. A. (2013a). Atopic and rheumatic disorders. In C. E. Burns, A. M. Dunn., M. A. Brady, N. B. Starr, & C. G. Blosser (Eds.), *Pediatric primary care* (5th ed.). Philadelphia, PA: Elsevier Saunders.

Take Note!

Young children with asthma receiving inhaled medications via a nebulizer should use a snugly fitting mask to ensure accurate deposition of medication to the lungs. Discourage "blow-by" via nebulizer, as medication delivery is variable and unreliable (NAEPP, 2007).

Avoidance of allergens is another key component of asthma management. Avoiding known triggers helps to prevent exacerbations as well as long-term inflammatory changes. This can be a difficult task for most families, particularly if the affected child suffers from several allergies. Refer to Teaching Guidelines 40.4 for strategies of allergen avoidance.

Take Note!

Teach the child and family that exposure to cigarette smoke increases the need for medications in children with asthma as well as the frequency of asthma exacerbations. Both indoor air quality and environmental pollution contribute to asthma in children (John & Brady, 2013a).

Asthma education is a critical component for ensuring optimal health in children with asthma. This education is not limited to the hospital or clinic setting. Nurses can become involved in community asthma education: community-centered education in schools, churches, and day care centers or through peer educators has been shown to be effective. Education should include pathophysiology, asthma triggers, and prevention and treatment strategies. With such a large number of children affected with this chronic disease, community education has the potential to make a broad impact.

School nurses must also become experts in asthma management as well as being committed to ongoing education of the child and family. Resources for schools include:

- Open airways for schools: an educational program presented by the American Lung Association or its local chapter, focusing on increasing asthma awareness and compliance with asthma action plans and decreasing asthma emergencies. Contact the local lung association or call 1-800-LUNG-USA.
- Indoor air repair at school: a kit available from Allergy and Asthma Network Mothers of Asthmatics (AANMA);

and Healthy School Environments Assessment Tool. Links to these and other helpful resources are provided on thePoint.

PROMOTING THE CHILD'S SELF-ESTEEM

Fear of an exacerbation and feeling "different" from other children can harm a child's self-esteem. In qualitative research studies, children have made such statements as "my body shuts down" and "I feel like I'm going to die" (Yoos, Kitzman, McMullen, Sidora-Arcoleo, & Anson, 2005). The fatigue and fear associated with chronic asthma may reduce the child's confidence and sense of control over his or her body and life. In addition to coping with a chronic illness, the asthmatic child often also has to cope with school-related issues. Moodiness, acting out, and withdrawal correlate with increases in school absence, which can contribute to poor school performance. To live in fear of an exacerbation or to be unable to participate in activities affects the child's self-esteem (Yoos et al., 2005).

Through education and support, the child can gain a sense of control. Children need to learn to master their disease. Accurate evaluation of asthma symptoms and improvement of self-esteem may help the child to experience less panic with an acute episode. Improved self-esteem might also help the child cope with the disease in general and with being different from his or her peers. The school-age child has the cognitive ability to begin taking responsibility for asthma management, with continued involvement on the part of the parents. Transferring control of asthma care to the child is an important developmental process that will increase the child's feeling of control over the illness.

PROMOTING FAMILY COPING

Parent denial is an issue in many families. The family, through education and encouragement, can become the experts on the child's illness as well as advocates for the child's well-being. The resilient child is better able to cope with the challenges facing him or her, including asthma. Cohesiveness and warmth in the family environment can improve a child's resiliency as well as contribute to family hardiness. Parents need to be allowed to ask questions and voice their concerns. A nurse who understands the family's issues and concerns is better able to plan for support and education. Provide culturally sensitive education and interventions that focus on increasing the family's commitment to, and control of, asthma management. As the child and parents become confident in their ability to recognize asthma symptoms and cope with asthma and its periodic episodes, the family's ability to cope will improve.

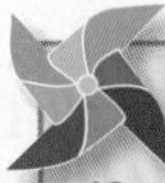

Thinking About Development

Ryan Jennings is a 13-year-old male with a history of moderate asthma. He has been prescribed a long-term control medication to be taken routinely and a rescue medicine to be used as needed and before exercise. He is a talented pitcher and would like to participate with his school's baseball team.

How will Ryan's developmental stage affect self-care related to his asthma? What is the most appropriate approach for the nurse to take to educate Ryan about his medications and disease process?

How will the nurse foster compliance in Ryan?

Chronic Lung Disease

Chronic lung disease (formerly termed bronchopulmonary dysplasia) is often diagnosed in infants who have experienced RDS and continue to require oxygen at 28 days of age. It is a chronic respiratory condition seen most commonly in premature infants. It results from a variety of factors, including pulmonary immaturity, acute lung injury, barotrauma, inflammatory mediators, and volutrauma. Epithelial stretching, macrophage and polymorphonuclear cell invasion, and airway edema affect the growth and development of lung structures. Cilia loss and airway lining denudation reduce the normal cleansing abilities of the lung. The number of normal alveoli is reduced by one third to one half. Lower birth weights, white race, and male gender pose increased risk for development of chronic lung disease. Complications include pulmonary artery hypertension, cor pulmonale, congestive heart failure, and severe bacterial or viral pneumonia.

Anti-inflammatory inhaled medications are used for maintenance, and short-acting bronchodilators are used as needed for wheezing episodes. Supplemental long-term oxygen therapy may be required in some infants.

Nursing Assessment

Tachypnea and increased work of breathing are characteristic of chronic lung disease. After discharge from the neonatal intensive care unit (NICU), these symptoms can continue. Exertion such as activity or oral feeding can cause dyspnea to worsen. Failure to thrive might also be evident. Auscultation might reveal breath sounds that are diminished in the bases. These infants have reactive airway episodes, so wheezing might be present during times of exacerbation. If fluid overload develops, rales may be heard.

Nursing Management

If the infant is oxygen dependent, provide education to the parents about oxygen tanks, nasal cannula use, pulse oximetry use, and nebulizer treatments. Often these children require increased calorie formulas to grow adequately. Fluid restrictions and/or diuretics are necessary in some infants. Follow-up echocardiograms might be used to determine resolution of pulmonary artery hypertension prior to weaning from oxygen. Encourage developmentally appropriate activities. It might be difficult for the oxygen-dependent infant or toddler to reach gross motor milestones or explore the environment because the length of the oxygen tubing limits him or her.

Parental support is also a key nursing intervention. After a long and trying period of ups and downs with their newborn in the intensive care unit, parents find themselves exhausted caring for their medically fragile infant at home.

Cystic Fibrosis

Cystic fibrosis is an autosomal recessive disorder that affects 30,000 children and adults in the United States (Cystic Fibrosis Foundation [CFF], n. d.). A deletion occurring on the long arm of chromosome 7 at the cystic fibrosis transmembrane regulator (CFTR) is the responsible gene mutation. DNA testing can be used prenatally and in newborns to identify the presence of the mutation. The American College of Obstetrics and Gynecology currently recommends screening for cystic fibrosis to any person seeking preconception or prenatal care. At present, all states include testing for cystic fibrosis as part of newborn screening (CFF, n. d.).

Cystic fibrosis is the most common debilitating disease of childhood among those of European descent. Medical advances in recent years have greatly increased the length and quality of life for affected children, with median age for survival being the late 30s (CFF, n. d.). Complications include hemoptysis, pneumothorax, bacterial colonization, cor pulmonale, volvulus, intussusception, intestinal obstruction, rectal prolapse, gastroesophageal reflux disease, diabetes, portal hypertension, liver failure, gallstones, and decreased fertility.

Pathophysiology

In cystic fibrosis, the CFTR mutation causes alterations in epithelial ion transport on mucosal surfaces, resulting in generalized dysfunction of the exocrine glands. The epithelial cells fail to conduct chloride, and water transport abnormalities occur. This results in thickened, tenacious secretions in the sweat glands, gastrointestinal tract, pancreas, respiratory tract, and other exocrine tissues. The increased viscosity of these secretions makes them difficult to clear. The sweat glands produce a larger amount of chloride, leading to a salty taste of the skin and alterations in electrolyte balance and dehydration. The pancreas, intrahepatic bile ducts, intestinal glands, gallbladder, and submaxillary glands become obstructed by viscous mucus and eosinophilic material. Pancreatic enzyme activity is lost and malabsorption of fats, proteins, and carbohydrates occurs, resulting in poor growth and large, malodorous stools. Excess mucus is produced by the tracheobronchial glands. Abnormally thick mucus plugs the small airways, and then bronchiolitis and further plugging of the airways occur. Secondary bacterial infection with *Staphylococcus aureus, Pseudomonas aeruginosa,* and *Burkholderia cepacia* often occurs. This contributes to obstruction and inflammation, leading to chronic infection, tissue damage, and respiratory failure. Nasal polyps and recurrent sinusitis are common. Boys have tenacious seminal fluid and experience blocking of the vas deferens, often making them infertile (Hazle, 2010). In girls, thick cervical secretions might limit penetration of sperm. Table 40.5 gives further details of the pathophysiology and resulting respiratory and gastrointestinal clinical manifestations of cystic fibrosis.

Therapeutic Management

Therapeutic management of cystic fibrosis is aimed toward minimizing pulmonary complications, maximizing lung function, preventing infection, and facilitating growth. All children with cystic fibrosis who have pulmonary involvement require chest physiotherapy with postural drainage several times daily to mobilize secretions from the lungs. Physical exercise is encouraged. Recombinant human DNase (Pulmozyme) is given daily using a nebulizer to decrease sputum viscosity and help clear secretions. Inhaled bronchodilators and anti-inflammatory agents are prescribed for some children. Aerosolized antibiotics are often prescribed and may be given at home as well as in the hospital. Choice of antibiotic is determined by sputum culture and sensitivity results. Pancreatic enzymes and supplemental fat-soluble vitamins are prescribed to promote adequate digestion and absorption of nutrients and optimize nutritional status. Increased-calorie, high-protein diets are recommended, and sometimes supplemental high-calorie formula, either orally or via feeding tube, is needed. Some children require total parenteral nutrition to maintain or gain weight. Lung transplantation has been successful in some children with cystic fibrosis.

Nursing Assessment

For a full description of the assessment phase of the nursing process, refer to the Nursing Process Overview section earlier in the chapter. Assessment findings pertinent to cystic fibrosis are discussed below.

HEALTH HISTORY

Elicit a description of the present illness and chief complaint. Common signs and symptoms reported during the health history in the undiagnosed child might include:

- A salty taste to the child's skin (resulting from excess chloride loss via perspiration)

TABLE 40.5 PATHOPHYSIOLOGY OF CYSTIC FIBROSIS AND RESULTANT RESPIRATORY AND GASTROINTESTINAL CLINICAL MANIFESTATIONS

Defect in the CFTR Gene Effects	Pathophysiology	Clinical Manifestations
Respiratory tract	• Infection leads to neutrophilic inflammation. • Cleavage of complement receptors and immunoglobin G leads to opsonophagocytosis failure. • Chemoattractant interleukin-8 and elastin degradase contribute to inflammatory response. • Thick, tenacious sputum that is chronically colonized with bacteria results. • Air trapping related to airway obstruction occurs. • Pulmonary parenchyma is eventually destroyed.	• Airway obstruction • Difficulty clearing secretions • Respiratory distress and impaired gas exchange • Chronic cough • Barrel-shaped chest • Decreased pulmonary function • Clubbing • Recurrent pneumonia • Hemoptysis • Pneumothorax • Chronic sinusitis • Nasal polyps • Cor pulmonale (right-sided heart failure)
Gastrointestinal tract	• Decreased chloride and water secretion into the intestine (causing dehydration of the intestinal material) and into the bile ducts (causing increased bile viscosity). • Reduced pancreatic bicarbonate secretion. • Hypersecretion of gastric acid. • Insufficiency of pancreatic enzymes (amylase, lipase, pancrease) necessary for digestion and absorption. • Pancreas secretes thick mucus.	• Meconium ileus • Retention of fecal matter in distal intestine, resulting in vomiting, abdominal distention and cramping, anorexia, right lower quadrant pain • Sludging of intestinal contents may lead to fecal impaction, rectal prolapse, bowel obstruction, and intussusception. • Obstructive cirrhosis with esophageal varices, and splenomegaly • Gallstones • Gastroesophageal reflux disease (compounded by postural drainage with chest physiotherapy) • Inadequate protein absorption • Altered absorption of iron and vitamins A, D, E, and K • Failure to thrive • Hyperglycemia and development of diabetes later in life

Adapted from Federico, M. J., Halbower, S., Kerby, G. S., Sagel, S. D., Stillwell, P., Zemanick, E. T.,… Deterding, R. R. (2014). Respiratory tract & mediastinum. In W. W. Hay, M. J. Levin, R. R. Deterding, M. J. Abzug, and J. M. Sondheimer (Eds.), *Current pediatric diagnosis and treatment* (21st ed.). New York, NY: McGraw-Hill; and Hazle, L. A. (2010). Cystic fibrosis. In P. J. Allen, J. A. Vessey, & N. A. Schapiro (Eds.), *Primary care of the child with a chronic condition* (5th ed.). St. Louis, MO: Mosby.

- Meconium ileus or late, difficult passage of meconium stool in the newborn period
- Abdominal pain or difficulty passing stool (infants or toddlers might present with intestinal obstruction or intussusception at the time of diagnosis)
- Bulky, greasy stools
- Poor weight gain and growth despite good appetite
- Chronic or recurrent cough and/or upper or lower respiratory infections

Children known to have cystic fibrosis are often admitted to the hospital for pulmonary exacerbations or other complications of the disease. The health history should include questions related to:

- Respiratory status: has cough, sputum production, or work of breathing increased?
- Appetite and weight gain
- Activity tolerance
- Increased need for pulmonary or pancreatic medications
- Presence of fever
- Presence of bone pain
- Any other changes in physical state or medication regimen

PHYSICAL EXAMINATION

The physical examination includes inspection, auscultation, percussion, and palpation.

Inspection. Observe the child's general appearance and color. Check the nasal passages for polyps. Note respiratory rate, work of breathing, use of accessory muscles, position of comfort, frequency and severity of cough, and quality and quantity of sputum produced. The child with cystic fibrosis often has a barrel chest

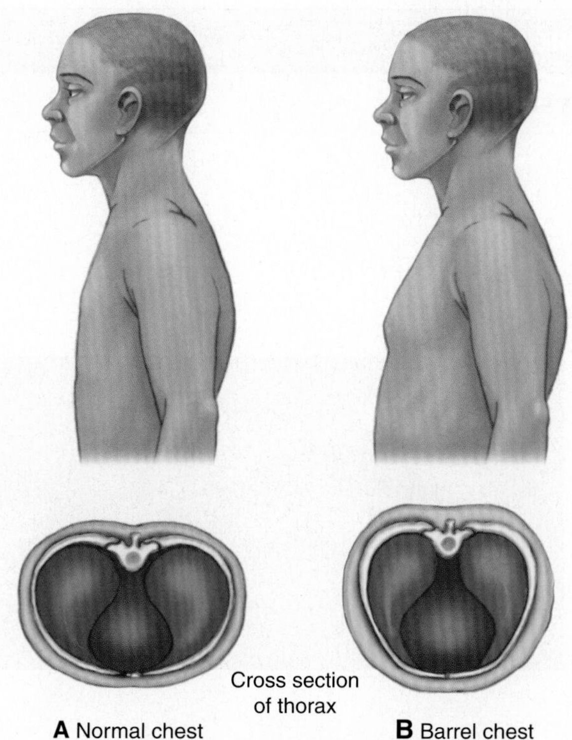

FIGURE 40.13 **(A)** Normal chest shape—transverse diameter is greater than anterior–posterior diameter. **(B)** Barrel chest—transverse diameter equals anterior–posterior diameter.

(anterior–posterior diameter approximates transverse diameter) (Fig. 40.13). Clubbing of the nail beds might also be present. Note whether rectal prolapse is present. Does the child appear small or thin for his or her age? The child might have a protuberant abdomen and thin extremities, with decreased amounts of subcutaneous fat. Observe for the presence of edema (sign of cardiac or liver failure). Note distended neck veins or the presence of a heave (signs of cor pulmonale).

Auscultation. Auscultation may reveal a variety of adventitious breath sounds. Fine or coarse crackles and scattered or localized wheezing might be present. With progressive obstructive pulmonary involvement, breath sounds might be diminished. Tachycardia might be present. Note the presence of a gallop (might occur with cor pulmonale). Note the adequacy of bowel sounds.

Percussion. Percussion over the lung fields usually yields hyperresonance due to air trapping. Diaphragmatic excursion might be decreased. Percussion of the abdomen might reveal dullness over an enlarged liver or mass related to intestinal obstruction.

Palpation. Palpation might yield a finding of asymmetric chest excursion if atelectasis is present. Tactile fremitus may be decreased over areas of atelectasis. Note if tenderness is present over the liver (might be an early sign of cor pulmonale).

LABORATORY AND DIAGNOSTIC TESTS

Common laboratory and diagnostic studies ordered for the diagnosis and assessment of cystic fibrosis include:

- Sweat chloride test: considered suspicious if the level of chloride in collected sweat is above 50 mEq/L and diagnostic if the level is above 60 mEq/L
- Pulse oximetry: oxygen saturation might be decreased, particularly during a pulmonary exacerbation
- Chest x-ray: may reveal hyperinflation, bronchial wall thickening, atelectasis, or infiltration
- Pulmonary function tests: might reveal a decrease in forced vital capacity and forced expiratory volume, with increases in residual volume

Nursing Management

Management of cystic fibrosis focuses on minimizing pulmonary complications, promoting growth and development, and facilitating coping and adjustment by the child and family. In addition to the nursing diagnoses and related interventions discussed in Nursing Care Plan 40.1, at the end of the chapter, for respiratory disorders, interventions common to cystic fibrosis follow.

MAINTAINING PATENT AIRWAY

Chest physiotherapy is often used as an adjunct therapy in respiratory illnesses, but for children with cystic fibrosis it is a critical intervention. Chest physiotherapy involves percussion, vibration, and postural drainage, and either it or another bronchial hygiene therapy must be performed several times a day to assist with mobilization of secretions. Nursing Procedure 40.2 gives instructions on the chest physiotherapy technique.

For older children and adolescents, the flutter-valve device, positive expiratory pressure therapy, or a high-frequency chest compression vest may also be used. The flutter valve device provides high-frequency oscillation to the airway as the child exhales into a mouthpiece that contains a steel ball. Positive expiratory pressure therapy involves exhaling through a flow resistor, which creates positive expiratory pressure. The cycles of exhalation are repeated until coughing yields expectoration of secretions. The vest airway clearance system provides high-frequency chest wall oscillation to increase airflow velocity to create repetitive cough-like shear forces and to decrease the viscosity of secretions. Breathing exercises are also helpful in promoting mucus clearance. Encourage physical exercise, as it helps to promote mucus secretion as well as provides cardiopulmonary conditioning. Ensure that Pulmozyme is administered, as well as inhaled bronchodilators and anti-inflammatory agents if prescribed.

PREVENTING INFECTION

Vigorous pulmonary hygiene for mobilization of secretions is critical to prevent infection. Aerosolized antibiotics can be given at home as well as in the hospital. Children

(text continues on page 1514)

NURSING PROCEDURE 40.2

Performing Chest Physiotherapy

May be preceded by an inhalation treatment; should not be performed after eating.

1. Provide percussion via a cupped hand or an infant percussion device. Appropriate percussion yields a hollow sound, not a slapping sound.

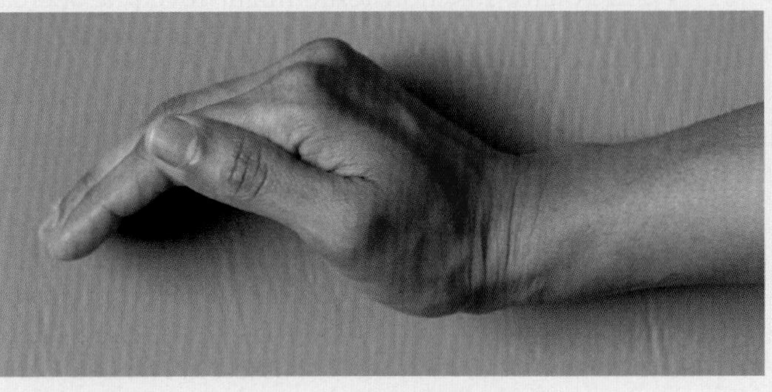

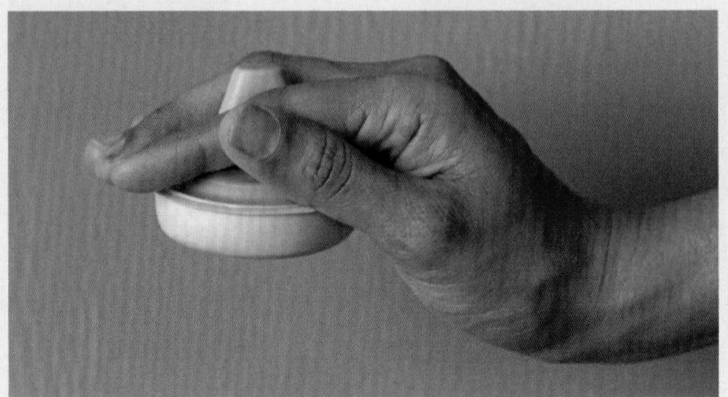

2. Percuss each segment of the lung for 1 to 2 minutes.

POSITION #1
UPPER LOBES, Apical segments

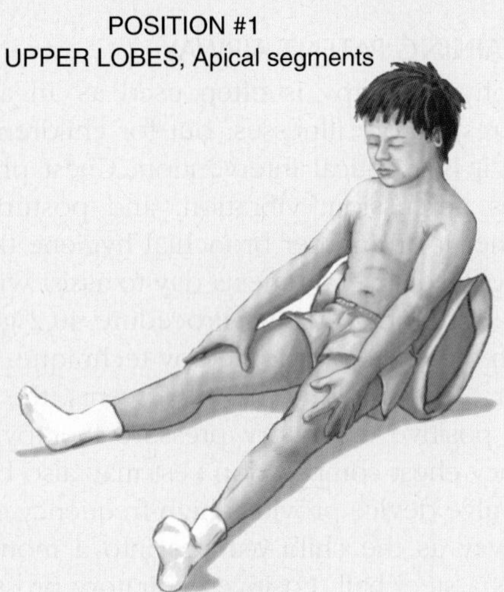

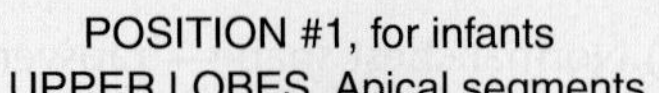

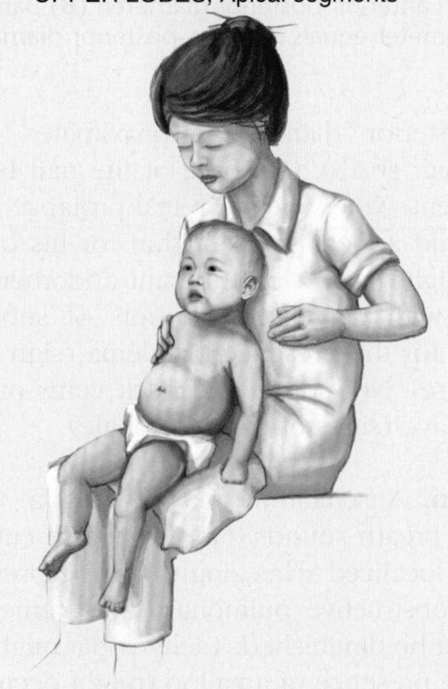

POSITION #2
UPPER LOBES, Posterior segments

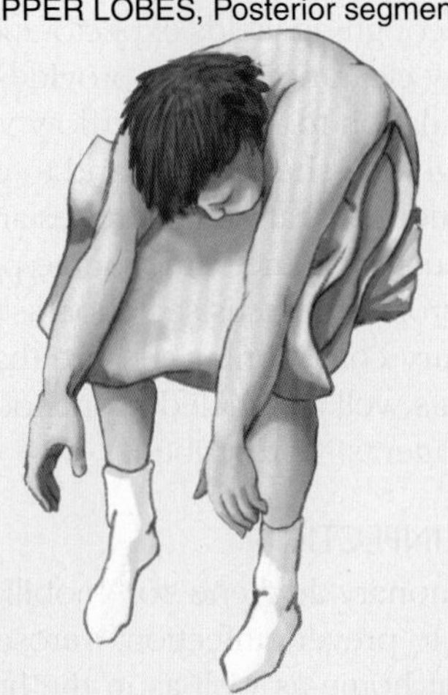

POSITION #3
UPPER LOBES, Anterior segments

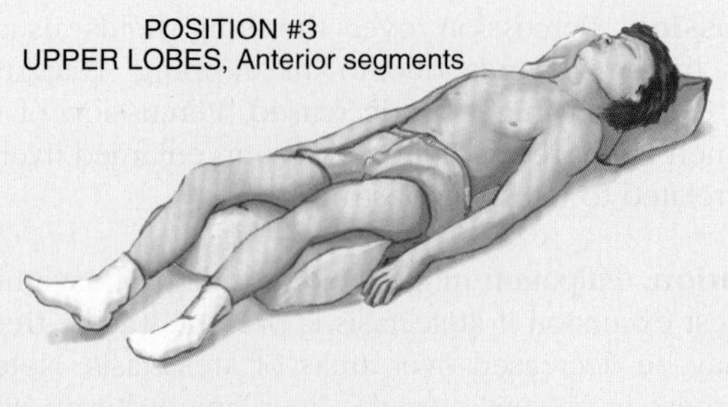

NURSING PROCEDURE 40.2

Performing Chest Physiotherapy (continued)

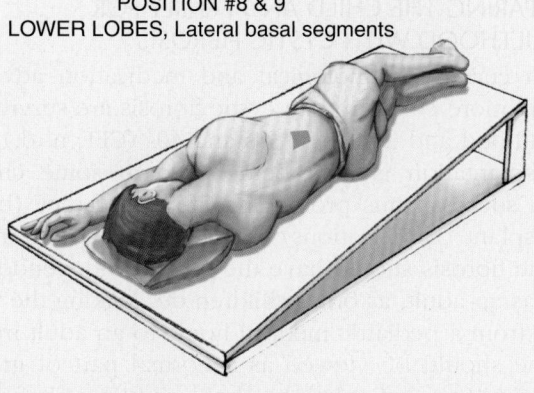

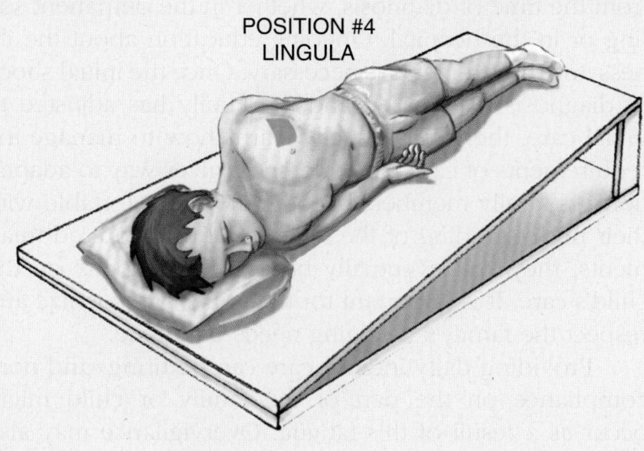

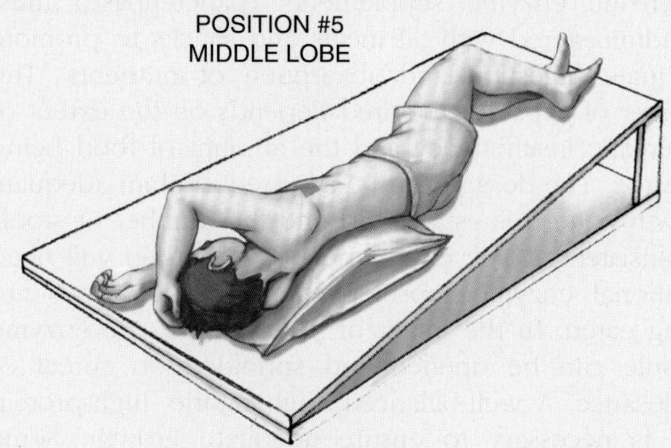

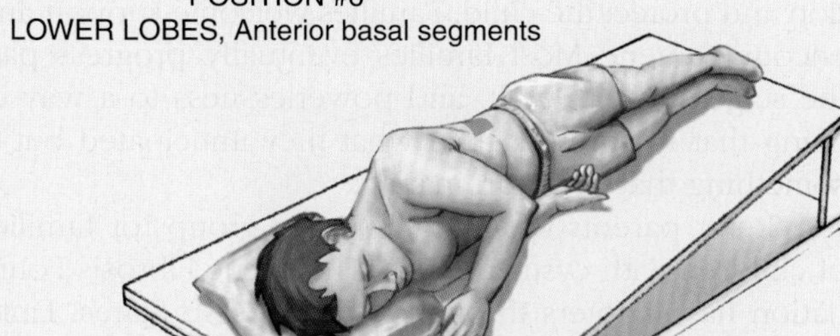

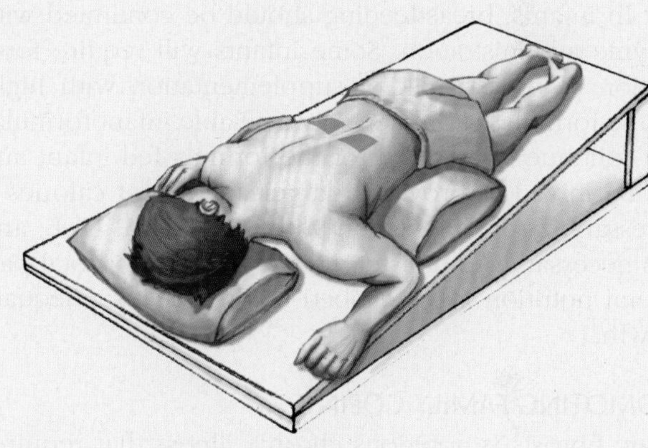

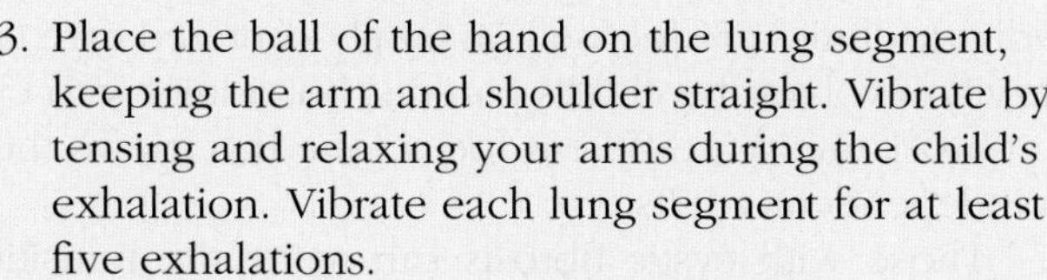

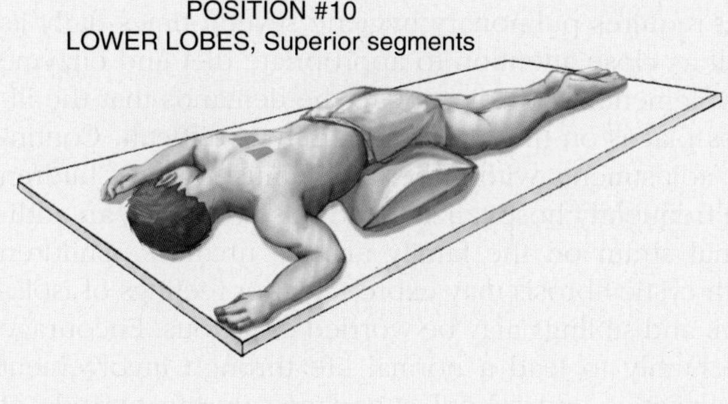

3. Place the ball of the hand on the lung segment, keeping the arm and shoulder straight. Vibrate by tensing and relaxing your arms during the child's exhalation. Vibrate each lung segment for at least five exhalations.
4. Encourage the child to deep breathe and cough.
5. Change drainage positions and repeat percussion and vibration.

with frequent or severe respiratory exacerbations might require lengthy courses of intravenous antibiotics.

MAINTAINING GROWTH

Pancreatic enzyme supplements (pancrelipase) must be administered with all meals and snacks to promote adequate digestion and absorption of nutrients. The number of capsules required depends on the extent of pancreatic insufficiency and the amount of food being ingested. The dosage can be adjusted until an adequate growth pattern is established and the number of stools is consistent at one or two per day. Children will need additional enzyme capsules when high-fat foods are being eaten. In the infant or young child, the enzyme capsule can be opened and sprinkled on cereal or applesauce. A well-balanced, high-calorie, high-protein diet is necessary to ensure adequate growth. Some children require up to one and a half times the recommended daily allowance of calories for children their age. A number of commercially available nutritional formulas and shakes are available for diet supplementation.

In infants, breastfeeding should be continued with enzyme administration. Some infants will require fortification of breast milk or supplementation with high-calorie formulas. Commercially available infant formulas can continue to be used for the formula-fed infant and can be mixed to provide a larger amount of calories if necessary. Supplementation with vitamins A, D, E, and K is necessary. Administer gavage feedings or total parenteral nutrition as prescribed to provide for adequate growth.

PROMOTING FAMILY COPING

Cystic fibrosis is a serious chronic illness that requires daily interventions. It can be hard to maintain a schedule that requires pulmonary hygiene several times daily as well as close attention to appropriate diet and enzyme supplementation. Adjusting to the demands that the illness places on the child and family is difficult. Continual adjustments within the family must occur. Children are frequently hospitalized, and this may place an additional strain on the family and its finances. Children with cystic fibrosis may express fear or feelings of isolation, and siblings may be worried or jealous. Encourage the family to lead a normal life through involvement in activities and school attendance during periods of wellness.

Take Note!

Children 6 and older who have the G551D, G1244E, G1349D, G178R, G551 S, S1251 N, S1255P, S549 N, or S549R mutation of the cystic fibrosis gene may be prescribed ivacaftor. Use of ivacaftor results in thinning of lung mucous, resulting in easier airway clearance via coughing. It is the first drug to act directly on the defective gene (Vertex Pharmaceuticals, 2015).

Starting at the time of diagnosis, families often demonstrate significant stress as the severity of the diagnosis and the significance of disease chronicity become real for them. The family should be involved in the child's care from the time of diagnosis, whether in the outpatient setting or in the hospital. Ongoing education about the illness and its treatments is necessary. Once the initial shock of diagnosis has passed and the family has adjusted to initial care, the family usually learns how to manage the requirements of care. Powerlessness gives way to adaptation. As family members become more comfortable with their understanding of the illness and the required treatments, they will eventually become the experts on the child's care. It is important for the nurse to recognize and respect the family's changing needs over time.

Providing daily intense care can be tiring, and noncompliance on the part of the family or child might occur as a result of this fatigue. Overvigilance may also occur as parents attempt to control the difficult situation and protect the child. Families welcome support and encouragement. Most families eventually progress past the stages of fear, guilt, and powerlessness to a way of living that is different than what they anticipated but is something that they can manage.

Refer parents to a local support group for families of children with cystic fibrosis. The Cystic Fibrosis Foundation has chapters throughout the United States. Links to The Cystic Fibrosis Foundation and other helpful resources can be found on thePoint.

Parents of children with a terminal illness might face the death of their child at an earlier age than expected. Assisting with anticipatory grieving and making decisions related to end-of-life care are other important nursing interventions.

PREPARING THE CHILD AND FAMILY FOR ADULTHOOD WITH CYSTIC FIBROSIS

With current technological and medication advances, many more children with cystic fibrosis are surviving to adulthood and into their 30s and 40s (CFF, n. d.). Lung transplantation is now being used in some children with success, thus prolonging life expectancy (barring transplant complications) (Hazle, 2010). Children with cystic fibrosis should have the goal of independent living as an adult, as other children do. Making the transition from a pediatric medical home to an adult medical home should be viewed as a normal part of growing up, similar to completing school or finding a first job. Pediatric clinics are focused on family-centered care that heavily involves the child's parents, but adults with cystic fibrosis need a different focus, one that views them as independent adults.

Those with cystic fibrosis can make the transition from pediatric to adult care with thoughtful preparation and coordination. They desire and deserve a smooth transition in care that will result in appropriate ongoing medical management of cystic fibrosis in an environment that is geared toward adults rather than children.

Adults with cystic fibrosis are able to find rewarding work and pursue relationships. Most men with cystic fibrosis are capable of sexual intercourse, though unable to reproduce. Females might have difficulty conceiving, and when they do they should be cautioned about the additional respiratory strain that pregnancy causes. All children of parents with cystic fibrosis will be carriers of the gene.

Apnea

Apnea is defined as absence of breathing for longer than 20 seconds; it might be accompanied by bradycardia. Sometimes apnea presents in the form of an acute life-threatening event (ALTE), an event in which the infant or child exhibits some combination of apnea, color change, muscle tone alteration, coughing, or gagging. Apnea may also occur acutely at any age as a result of respiratory distress. This discussion will focus on apnea that is chronic or recurrent in nature or that occurs as part of an ALTE.

Apnea in infants may be central (unrelated to any other cause) or may occur with other illnesses such as sepsis and respiratory infection. Apnea in newborns might be associated with hypothermia, hypoglycemia, infection, or hyperbilirubinemia. Apnea of prematurity occurs secondary to an immature respiratory system. Apnea should not be considered a predecessor to sudden infant death syndrome (SIDS). Current research has not proven this theory, and SIDS generally occurs in otherwise healthy young infants (American Academy of Pediatrics [AAP], 2011). Box 40.4 gives more information about SIDS and its prevention.

Therapeutic management of apnea varies depending on the cause. When apnea occurs as a result of another disorder or infection, treatment is directed toward that cause. In the event of apnea, stimulation may trigger the infant to take a breath. If breathing does not resume, rescue breathing or bag-valve-mask ventilation is necessary. Infants and children who have experienced an ALTE or who have chronic apnea may require ongoing cardiac/apnea monitoring. Caffeine or theophylline is sometimes administered, primarily in premature infants, to stimulate respirations (Kelly, 2010).

BOX 40.4

SUDDEN INFANT DEATH SYNDROME (SIDs)

Definition

Sudden death of a previously healthy infant younger than 1 year of age

Prevention

- Place all infants in the supine position to sleep (even side-lying is not as safe and is not recommended by the AAP).
- Provide a firm sleep surface and avoid soft bedding, excess covers, pillows, and stuffed animals in the crib.
- Avoid maternal prenatal smoking and exposure of the infant to second-hand smoke.
- Ensure the infant sleeps separately from the parents.
- Avoid overbundling or overdressing the infant.
- Encourage pacifier use during naps and at bedtime if the infant is receptive to it (AAP, 2011).

Support and Information

- Association for SIDS and Infant Mortality Program: www.asip1.org
- National Sudden Infant Death Resource Center: www.sidscenter.org
- SIDS Alliance: www.sidsalliance.org
- Sudden Infant Death Syndrome Network, Inc.: http://sids-network.org/

Nursing Assessment

Question the parents about the infant's position and activities preceding the apneic episode. Did the infant experience a color change? Did the infant self-stimulate (breathe again on his or her own), or did he or she require stimulation from the caretaker? Assess risk factors for apnea, which may include prematurity, anemia, and history of metabolic disorders. Apnea may occur in association with cardiac or neurologic disturbances, respiratory infection, sepsis, child abuse, or poisoning.

In the hospitalized infant, note absence of respiration, position, color, and other associated findings, such as emesis on the bedclothes. If an infant who is apneic fails to be stimulated and does not breathe again, pulselessness will result.

Nursing Management

When an infant is noted to be apneic, gently stimulate him or her to take a breath again. If gentle stimulation is unsuccessful, then rescue breathing or bag-valve-mask ventilation must be started.

To avoid apnea in the newborn, maintain a neutral thermal environment. Avoid excessive vagal stimulation and taking rectal temperatures (the vagal response can cause bradycardia, resulting in apnea) (Jarvis, 2012). Administer caffeine or theophylline if prescribed and teach families about the use of these medications.

Infants with recurrent apnea or ALTE may be discharged on a home apnea monitor (Fig. 40.14). Provide education on use of the monitor, guidance about when to notify the physician or nurse practitioner or monitor service about alarms, and training in infant cardiopulmonary resuscitation (CPR). The monitor is usually discontinued after 3 months without a significant event of apnea or bradycardia. In some ways the monitor gives parents peace of mind, but in others it can make them more nervous about the well-being of their child. Parents often

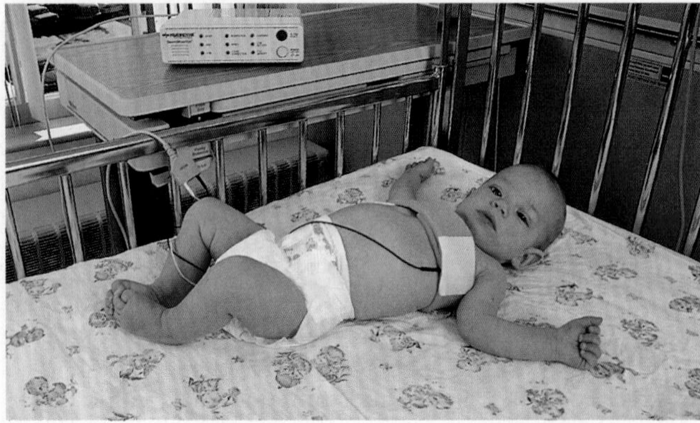

FIGURE 40.14 The home apnea monitor uses a soft belt with a Velcro attachment to hold two leads in the appropriate position on the chest.

experience disrupted sleep and some may display negative coping patterns (Scollan-Koliopoulos & Koliopoulos, 2010). Providing appropriate education to the parents about the nature of the child's disorder as well as action to take in the event of apnea may give the family a sense of mastery over the situation, thus decreasing their anxiety. Refer families to local support groups such as those offered by Parent to Parent and Parents Helping Parents.

TRACHEOSTOMY

A **tracheostomy** is an artificial opening in the airway; usually a plastic tracheostomy tube is in place to form a patent airway. Tracheostomies are performed to relieve airway obstruction, such as with subglottic stenosis (narrowing of the airway sometimes resulting from long-term intubation). They are also used for pulmonary hygiene and in the child who requires chronic mechanical ventilation. The tracheostomy facilitates secretion removal, reduces work of breathing, and increases the child's comfort. In some cases the tracheostomy facilitates mechanical ventilation weaning. It may be permanent or temporary, depending on the indication. The tracheostomy tube varies in size and type depending on the child's airway size and health and the length of time the child will require the tracheostomy. Silastic tracheostomy tubes are soft and flexible; they are available with a single lumen or may have an outer and inner lumen. Both types have an obturator (the guide used during tube changes). Uncuffed tubes are used more often in the pediatric population (Deutsch, 2010). Figure 40.15 shows various types of tracheostomy tubes.

Complications immediately after surgery include hemorrhage, air entry, pulmonary edema, anatomic damage, and respiratory arrest. At any point in time the tracheostomy tube may become occluded, which compromises ventilation. Complications of chronic tracheostomy include infection, cellulitis, and formation of granulation tissue around the insertion site.

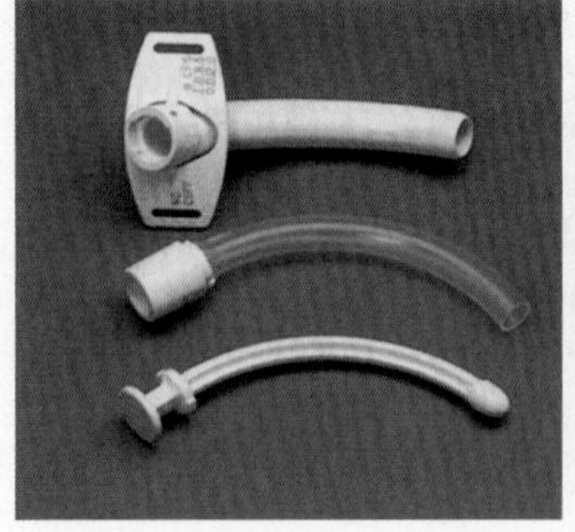

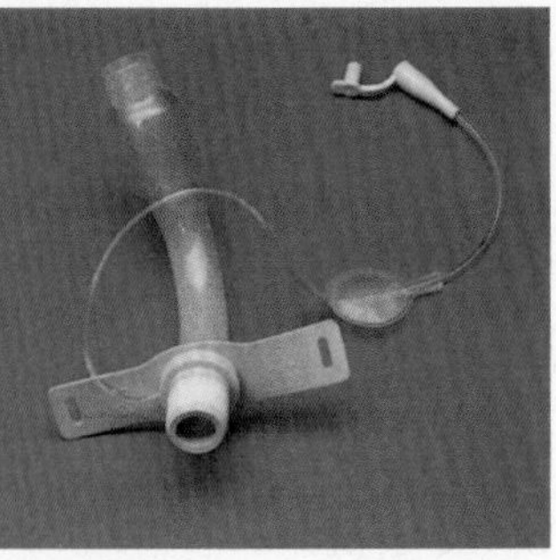

FIGURE 40.15 Note smaller size and absence of inner cannula on particular brands of pediatric tracheostomy tubes.

Nursing Assessment

When obtaining the history for a child with a tracheostomy, note the reason for the tracheostomy, as well as the size and type of tracheostomy tube. Inspect the site. The stoma should appear pink and without bleeding or drainage. The tube itself should be clean and free from secretions. The tracheostomy ties should fit securely, allowing one finger to slide beneath the ties. Inspect the skin under the ties for rash or redness. Observe work of breathing.

When caring for the infant or child with a tracheostomy, whether in the hospital, home, or community setting, a thorough respiratory assessment is necessary. Note presence of secretions and their color, thickness, and amount. Auscultate for breath sounds, which should be clear and equal throughout all lung fields. Measure pulse oximetry. When infection is suspected or secretions are discolored or have a foul odor, a sputum culture may be obtained.

Take Note!

Keep small toys (risk of aspiration), plastic bibs or bedding (risk of airway occlusion), and talcum powder (risk of inhalation injury) out of reach of the child with a tracheostomy.

Nursing Management

In the immediate postoperative period the infant or child may require restraints to avoid accidental dislodgment of the tracheostomy tube. Infants and children who have had a tracheostomy for a period of time become accustomed to it and usually do not attempt to remove the tube. Since air inspired via the tracheostomy tube bypasses the upper airway, it lacks humidification, and this lack of humidity can lead to a mucous plug in the tracheostomy and resultant hypoxia. Provide humidity to either room air or oxygen via a tracheostomy collar or ventilator, depending on the child's need (Fig. 40.16). Box 40.5 lists the equipment that should be available at the bedside of any child who has a tracheostomy.

Tracheostomies require frequent suctioning to maintain patency. The appropriate length for insertion of the suction catheter depends on the size of the tracheostomy and the child's needs. Place a sign at the head of the child's

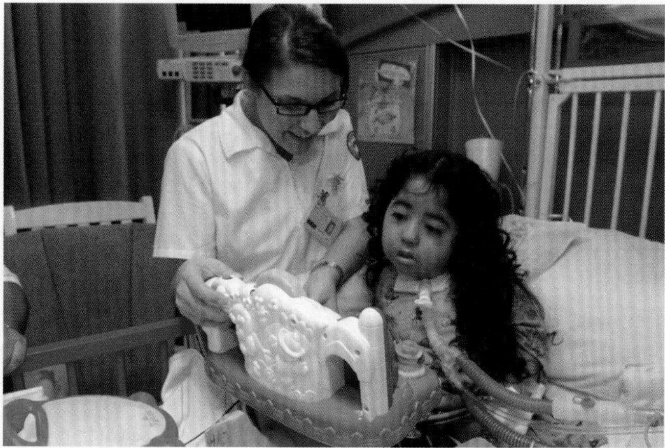

FIGURE 40.16 The trach collar allows for humidification of inspired air or supplemental oxygen.

bed indicating the suction catheter size and the length (in centimeters) that it should be inserted for suctioning. Keep an extra tracheostomy tube of the same size and one size smaller at the bedside in the event of an emergency.

Many pediatric tracheostomy tubes do not have an inner cannula that requires periodic removal and cleaning, so periodic removal and replacement of the chronic tracheostomy tube is required. Clean the removed tracheostomy tube with half-strength hydrogen peroxide and pipe cleaners. Rinse with distilled water and allow it to dry. The tracheostomy tube can be reused many times if adequately cleaned between uses.

Perform tracheostomy care every 8 hours or per institution protocol. Change the tracheostomy tube only as needed or per institution protocol. Nursing Procedure 40.3 gives information about tracheostomy care. Always change tracheostomy ties with an assistant to avoid accidental dislodgement of the tube.

If the older child or teen has a tracheostomy tube with an inner cannula, care of the inner cannula is similar to that of an adult. Involve parents in care of the tracheostomy and begin education about caring for the tracheostomy tube at home as soon as the child is stable. The child with a tracheostomy often qualifies for a Medicaid waiver that will provide a certain amount of home nursing care. Refer the family to local support groups. Links for additional helpful resources can be found on thePoint.

BOX 40.5

EMERGENCY EQUIPMENT (AVAILABLE AT BEDSIDE)

- Two spare tracheostomy tubes (one the same size and one a size smaller)
- Suction equipment
- Stitch cutter (new tracheostomy)
- Spare tracheostomy ties
- Lubricating jelly
- Bag-valve-mask device
- Call bell within child's/parent's reach

NURSING PROCEDURE 40.3

Tracheostomy Care

1. Gather the necessary equipment:
   - Cleaning solution
   - Gloves
   - Precut gauze pad
   - Cotton-tipped applicators
   - Clean tracheostomy ties
   - Extra tracheostomy tube in case of accidental dislodgement
2. Position the infant/child supine with a blanket or towel roll to extend the neck.
3. Open all packaging and cut tracheostomy ties to appropriate length if necessary.
4. Cleanse around the tracheostomy site with prescribed solution (half-strength hydrogen peroxide or acetic acid, normal saline or soap and water if at home) and cotton-tipped applicators, working from just around the tracheostomy tube outward.
5. Rinse with sterile water and cotton-tipped applicator in similar fashion.
6. Place the precut sterile gauze under the tracheostomy tube.
7. With the assistant holding the tube in place, cut the ties and remove from the tube.
8. Attach the clean ties to the tube and tie or secure in place with Velcro (Fig. 40.17).

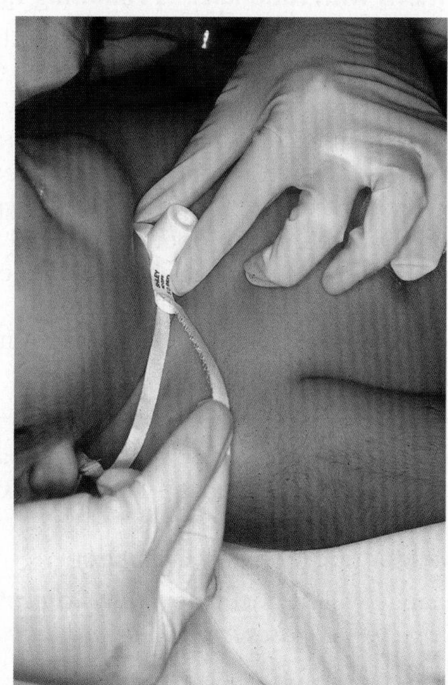

FIGURE 40.17 Trach ties are attached to the tube and secured in place with Velcro.

NURSING CARE PLAN 40.1

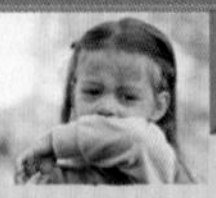

Overview for the Child With a Respiratory Disorder

NURSING DIAGNOSIS: Ineffective airway clearance related to inflammation, increased secretions, mechanical obstruction, or pain as evidenced by presence of secretions, productive cough, tachypnea, and increased work of breathing

Outcome Identification and Evaluation

Child will maintain patent airway, *free from secretions or obstruction, easy work of breathing, respiratory rate within parameters for age.*

Interventions with rationale: ***Maintaining a Patent Airway***

- Position with airway open (sniffing position if supine) and/or elevate head of bed *to allow for adequate ventilation.*
- Humidify oxygen or room air and ensure adequate fluid intake (intravenous or oral) *to liquefy secretions for ease in clearance.*
- Suction with bulb syringe or via nasopharyngeal catheter as needed, particularly prior to bottle-feeding, *to promote clearance of secretions.*
- If tachypneic, maintain nothing by mouth (NPO) status *to avoid aspiration.*
- In older child, encourage expectoration of sputum with coughing *to promote airway clearance.*
- Perform chest physiotherapy if ordered *to mobilize secretions.*
- Ensure emergency equipment is readily available *to avoid delay should airway become unmaintainable.*

NURSING DIAGNOSIS: Ineffective breathing pattern related to inflammatory or infectious process as evidenced by tachypnea, increased work of breathing, nasal flaring, retractions, diminished breath sounds

Outcome Identification and Evaluation

Child will exhibit adequate ventilation: *respiratory rate within parameters for age, easy work of breathing (absence of retractions, accessory muscle use, grunting), clear breath sounds with adequate aeration, oxygen saturation >94% or within prescribed parameters.*

Interventions with rationale: ***Promoting Effective Breathing Patterns***

- Assess respiratory rate, breath sounds, and work of breathing frequently to ensure progress with treatment and so that deterioration can be noted early.
- Use pulse oximetry to monitor oxygen saturation in the least invasive manner to note adequacy of oxygenation and ensure early detection of hypoxemia.
- Position for comfort with open airway and room for lung expansion (usually with head of bed elevated). Use pillows or padding if necessary to maintain position to ensure optimal ventilation via maximum lung expansion.
- Administer supplemental oxygen and/or humidity as ordered to improve oxygenation.
- Allow for adequate sleep and rest periods to conserve energy.
- Administer antibiotics as ordered: may be indicated in the case of bacterial respiratory infection.
- Encourage incentive spirometry and coughing with deep breathing (can be accomplished through play) to maximize ventilation (play enhances the child's participation).

NURSING DIAGNOSIS: Gas exchange, impaired, related to airway plugging, hyperinflation, atelectasis, as evidenced by cyanosis, decreased oxygen saturation, and alterations in arterial blood gases

Outcome Identification and Evaluation

Gas exchange will be adequate: *pulse oximetry reading on room air is within normal parameters for age, blood gases within normal limits, absence of cyanosis.*

NURSING CARE PLAN 40.1

Overview for the Child With a Respiratory Disorder (continued)

Interventions with rationale: ***Promoting Adequate Gas Exchange***

- Administer oxygen as ordered *to improve oxygenation.*
- Monitor oxygen saturation via pulse oximetry *to detect alterations in oxygenation.*
- Encourage clearance of secretions via coughing, expectoration, chest physiotherapy, and suctioning *to improve gas exchange.*
- Administer bronchodilators if ordered (albuterol, levalbuterol, and racemic epinephrine) *to treat bronchospasm and improve gas exchange.*
- Provide frequent contact and support to the child and family *to decrease anxiety, which increases the child's oxygen demands.*
- Assess and monitor mental status (confusion, lethargy, restlessness, combativeness): *hypoxemia can lead to changes in mental status.*

NURSING DIAGNOSIS: Risk for infection related to presence of infectious organisms

Outcome Identification and Evaluation

Child will exhibit no signs of secondary infection and will not spread infection to others: *symptoms of infection decrease over time; others remain free from infection.*

Interventions with rationale: ***Preventing Infection***

- Maintain aseptic technique, practice good hand washing, and use disposable suction catheters *to prevent introduction of further infectious agents.*
- Limit number of visitors and screen them for recent illness *to prevent further infection.*
- Administer antibiotics if prescribed *to prevent or treat bacterial infection.*
- Encourage nutritious diet according to child's preferences and ability to feed orally *to assist body's natural infection-fighting mechanisms.*
- Isolate the child as required *to prevent nosocomial spread of infection.*
- Teach child and family preventive measures such as good hand washing, covering mouth and nose when coughing or sneezing, and proper disposal of used tissues *to prevent nosocomial or community spread of infection.*

NURSING DIAGNOSIS: Fluid volume deficit, risk for, related to decreased oral intake, insensible losses via fever, tachypnea, or diaphoresis

Outcome Identification and Evaluation

Fluid volume will be maintained: oral mucosa moist and pink, skin turgor elastic, urine output at least 1 to 2 mL/kg/hour.

Interventions with rationale: ***Maintaining Adequate Fluid Volume***

- Administer intravenous fluids if ordered *to maintain adequate hydration in NPO state.*
- When allowed oral intake, encourage oral fluids. Popsicles, favorite fluids, and games can be used *to promote intake.*
- Assess for signs of adequate hydration (flat fontanels, elastic skin turgor, moist mucosa, adequate urine output).
- Monitor intake and output *to identify fluid imbalance.*
- Monitor urine specific gravity, urine and serum electrolytes, blood urea nitrogen, creatinine, and osmolality *to determine fluid status.*

(continued)

NURSING CARE PLAN 40.1

Overview for the Child With a Respiratory Disorder (continued)

NURSING DIAGNOSIS: Nutrition, altered: less than body requirements related to difficulty feeding as evidenced by poor oral intake, tiring with feeding

Outcome Identification and Evaluation

Child will maintain adequate nutritional intake: *weight is gained or maintained. Child consumes adequate diet for age.*

Interventions with rationale: ***Promoting Adequate Nutritional Intake***

- Weigh on same scale at same time daily *so that measurements are consistent.*
- Perform calorie counts over a 3-day period *to determine whether caloric intake is sufficient.*
- Encourage child to choose higher-calorie, protein-rich foods *to optimize growth potential.*
- Coax young children to eat better by playing games and offering favorite foods *to improve intake.*

NURSING DIAGNOSIS: Activity intolerance related to high respiratory demand as evidenced by increased work of breathing and need for frequent rest when playing

Outcome Identification and Evaluation

Child will resume normal activity level: *activity is tolerated without difficulty breathing. Pulse oximetry readings and vital signs are within parameters for age and activity level.*

Interventions with rationale: ***Increasing Activity Tolerance***

- Provide rest periods balanced with periods of activity, and group nursing activities and visits *to allow for sufficient rest.*
- Provide small, frequent meals *to prevent overtiring (energy is expended while eating).*
- Encourage quiet activities that do not require exertion *to prevent boredom.*
- Allow gradual increase in activity as tolerated, keeping pulse oximetry reading within normal parameters, *to minimize risk for further respiratory compromise.*

NURSING DIAGNOSIS: Fear related to difficulty breathing, unfamiliar personnel, procedures, and environment (hospital), as evidenced by clinging, crying, fussing, verbalization, or lack of cooperation

Outcome Identification and Evaluation

Fear/anxiety will be reduced: *decreased episodes of crying or fussing, happy and playful at times.*

Interventions with rationale: ***Relieving Fear***

- Establish trusting relationship with child and family *to decrease anxiety and fear.*
- Utilize play *to gain child's cooperation and trust.*
- Explain procedures to child at developmentally appropriate level *to decrease fear of unknown.*
- Provide favorite blanket or bear as well as comfort measures preferred by child such as rocking or music *for added security.*
- Involve parents in care *to give child reassurance and decrease fear.*

NURSING CARE PLAN 40.1

Overview for the Child With a Respiratory Disorder (continued)

NURSING DIAGNOSIS: Family processes, altered, related to child's illness or hospitalization as evidenced by family's presence in hospital, missed work, demonstration of inadequate coping

Outcome Identification and Evaluation

Parents demonstrate adequate coping and decreased anxiety: *parents are involved in child's care, ask appropriate questions, and are able to discuss child's care and condition calmly.*

Interventions with rationale: ***Promoting Adequate Family Processes***

- Encourage parents to discuss their concerns related to child's illness to identify concerns and show parents that the nurse also cares about them, not just the child.
- Explain therapy, procedures, and child's behavior to parents to decrease their anxiety.
- Encourage parents to be involved in care so they feel needed and valued.

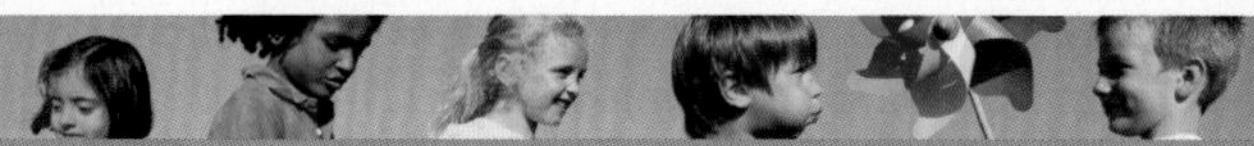

KEY CONCEPTS

- Respiratory infections account for the majority of acute illnesses in children.
- The upper and lower airways are smaller in children than adults, making them more susceptible to obstruction in the presence of mucus, debris, or edema.
- Newborns are obligatory nose breathers.
- The child's highly compliant airway is quite susceptible to dynamic collapse in the presence of airway obstruction.
- Because they have fewer alveoli, children have a higher risk for hypoxemia than adults.
- Generally, disorders of the nose and throat do not result in increased work of breathing or affect the lungs. Thus, if the lungs are involved, lower respiratory disease must be considered.
- Wheezing may be associated with a variety of lower respiratory disorders, such as asthma, bronchiolitis, and cystic fibrosis.
- Pulse oximetry is a useful tool for determining the extent of hypoxia. Findings should be correlated with the child's clinical presentation.
- Rapid streptococcus and rapid influenza tests are very useful for the quick diagnosis of strep throat or influenza so that appropriate treatment may be instituted early in the illness.
- Supplemental oxygen is often necessary in the child who is hospitalized (particularly with lower respiratory disease). Oxygen should be humidified to prevent drying of secretions.
- Suctioning, whether with a bulb syringe or suction catheter, is very effective at maintaining airway patency, especially in the younger child or infant.
- Normal saline nasal wash is an inexpensive, simple, and safe method for decongesting the nose in the case of the common cold, allergic rhinitis, and sinusitis.
- Infants who were born prematurely; children with a chronic illness such as diabetes, congenital heart disease, sickle cell anemia, or cystic fibrosis; and children with developmental disorders such as cerebral palsy tend to be more severely affected with respiratory disorders.
- Passive cigarette smoke exposure increases the infant's and child's risk for respiratory disease.
- Continual swallowing while awake or asleep is an indication of bleeding in the postoperative tonsillectomy child.
- Positioning to ease work of breathing and maintaining a patent airway are priorities for the child with a respiratory disorder.
- To avoid Reye syndrome, aspirin should not be given to treat fever or pain in the infant or child with a viral infection.
- Infants and children at high risk for serious RSV disease should be immunized with palivizumab each RSV season. Children older than 6 months of age should be immunized against influenza yearly.

- Children at high risk for exposure to tuberculosis should be screened for infection.
- Promoting airway clearance and maintenance, effective breathing patterns, and adequate gas exchange is the priority focus of nursing intervention in pediatric respiratory disease.
- Children with any degree of respiratory distress require frequent assessment and early intervention to prevent progression to respiratory failure.
- Avoidance of allergens is critical in the treatment plan for the child with allergic rhinitis.
- Avoidance of allergic triggers, control of the inflammatory process, and education of the child and family are the focus of asthma management.
- Chest physiotherapy is extremely useful for mobilizing secretions in any condition resulting in an increase in mucus production and is required in children with cystic fibrosis.
- Children with chronic respiratory disorders and their families often need large amounts of education and psychosocial support: children often experience fear and isolation, while families must learn to balance care of the chronically ill child with other family life.

REFERENCES AND RECOMMENDED READINGS

Allergy and Asthma Network Mothers of Asthmatics. (2014). *Indoor AIRepair at home, school, and play*. Vienna, VA: Author.

American Academy of Allergy, Asthma and Immunology. (2011). *Asthma action plan*. Retrieved from http://www.aaaai.org/Aaaai/media/MediaLibrary/PDF%20Documents/Libraries/NEW-WEBSITE-LOGO-asthma-action-plan_HI.pdf

American Academy of Pediatrics, Task Force on Sudden Infant Death Syndrome. (2011). Policy statement: SIDS and other sleep-related deaths: Expansion of recommendations for a safe infant sleeping environment. *Pediatrics, 128*(5), 1030–1039.

American Heart Association (AHA). (2011). *Pediatric advanced life support provider manual*. Dallas, TX: Author.

Barson, W. J. (2016). *Outpatient treatment of community-acquired pneumonia in children*. Retrieved from http://www.uptodate.com/contents/outpatient-treatment-of-community-acquired-pneumonia-in-children

Batra, V., & Ang, J. Y. (2015). *Pediatric tuberculosis*. Retrieved from emedicine.medscape.com/article/969401-overview.

Beckton Dickinson and Company. (2016). *Product center.* Retrieved from http://www.bd.com/ds/productCenter/index.asp.

Blosser, C. G., Brady, M. A., & Royal, R. B. (2013). Infectious diseases and immunizations. In C. A. Burns, A. M. Dunn, M. A. Brady, N. B. Starr, & C. G. Blosser (Eds.), *Pediatric primary care* (5th ed.). Philadelphia, PA: Elsevier Saunders.

Bowden, V. R., & Greenberg, C. S. (2012). *Pediatric nursing procedures* (3rd ed.). Philadelphia, PA: Lippincott Williams & Wilkins.

Brook, I. (2013). Acute sinusitis in children. *Pediatric Clinics of North America, 60*, 409–424.

Carolan, P. L. & Bye, M. R. (2015). *Pediatric bronchitis.* Retrieved from http://emedicine.medscape.com/article/1001332-overview#aw2aab6b2b3aa

Carpenito-Moyet, L. J. (2013). *Nursing diagnosis: Application to clinical practice* (14th ed.). Philadelphia, PA: Lippincott Williams & Wilkins.

Centers for Disease Control and Prevention. (2016a). *Key facts about seasonal flu vaccine*. Retrieved from http://www.cdc.gov/flu/protect/keyfacts.htm

Centers for Disease Control and Prevention. (2016b). *Pneumococcal vaccination*. Retrieved from http://www.cdc.gov/vaccines/vpd-vac/pneumo/default.htm

Clute, J. L. (2014). *Reye syndrome*. Retrieved from http://kidshealth.org/parent/infections/bacterial_viral/reye.html#

Corbett, J. A., & Banks, A. D. (2013). *Laboratory tests and diagnostic procedures with nursing diagnoses* (8th ed.). Upper Saddle River, NJ: Pearson Education Inc.

Cornfield, D. N. (2013). Acute respiratory distress syndrome in children: Physiology and management. *Current Opinion in Pediatrics, 25*(3), 338–343.

Cystic Fibrosis Foundation. (n. d.). *About cystic fibrosis.* Retrieved from https://www.cff.org/What-is-CF/About-Cystic-Fibrosis/

Denicola, L. K., Maraqa, N. F., Udeani, J. & Custodio, H. T. (2016). *Bronchiolitis*. Retrieved from http://emedicine.medscape.com/article/961963-overview

Deutsch, E. S. (2010). Tracheostomy: Pediatric considerations. *Respiratory Care, 55*(8), 1082–1090.

Durani, Y. (2012). *Croup* Retrieved from http://kidshealth.org/parent/infections/lung/croup.html

Environmental Protection Agency. (2016). *Healthy schools, healthy kids*. Retrieved from http://www2.epa.gov/schools

Federico, M. J., Baker, C. D., Balasubramaniam, V., Deboer, E. M., Deterding, R. R., Halbower, S., Zemanick, E. T. (2014). Respiratory tract & mediastinum. In W. W. Hay, M. J. Levin, R. R. Deterding, and M. J. Abzug, (Eds.), *Current pediatric diagnosis and treatment* (22nd ed.). New York, NY: McGraw-Hill.

Fouzas, S., Priftis, K. N., & Anthracopoulos, M. B. (2011). Pulse oximetry in pediatric practice. *Pediatrics, 128*, 740–752.

Gavin, M. L. (2013). *Preventing choking*. Retrieved from http://kidshealth.org/parent/firstaid_safe/home/safety_choking.html

Giddens, J. F. (2013). *Concepts for nursing practice*. St. Louis, MO: Elsevier

Hayden, G. F, & Turner, R. B. (2011). Acute pharyngitis. In R. M. Kliegman, B. M. D. Stanton, J. St. Geme, N. F. Schor, & R. E. Behrman (Eds.), *Nelson textbook of pediatrics* (19th ed.). Philadelphia, PA: Elsevier Saunders.

Hazle, L. A. (2010). Cystic fibrosis. In P. J. Allen, J. A. Vessey, & N. A. Schapiro (Eds.), *Primary care of the child with a chronic condition* (5th ed.). St. Louis, MO: Mosby.

Hill-Rom, Inc. (2016). The Visi-Vest system™. Retrieved from https://respiratorycare.hill-rom.com/en/patients/products/the-visivest-system/

Isaacson, G. (2012). Tonsillectomy care for the pediatrician. *Pediatrics, 130*(2), 324–334.

Jarvis, C. (2012). *Physical examination and health assessment* (6th ed.). St. Louis, MO: Saunders.

John, R. M., & Brady, M. A. (2013a). Atopic and rheumatic disorders. In C. E. Burns, A. M. Dunn, M. A. Brady, N. B. Starr, & C. G. Blosser (Eds.), *Pediatric primary care* (5th ed.). Philadelphia, PA: Elsevier Saunders.

John, R. M., & Brady, M. A. (2013b). Respiratory disorders. In C. E. Burns, A. M. Dunn, M. A. Brady, N. B. Starr, & C. G. Blosser (Eds.), *Pediatric primary care* (5th ed.). Philadelphia, PA: Elsevier Saunders.

Kelly, M. M. (2010). Prematurity. In P. J. Allen, J. A. Vessey, & N. A. Schapiro (Eds.), *Primary care of the child with a chronic condition* (5th ed.). St. Louis, MO: Mosby.

Kenealy T., & Arroll B. (2013). Antibiotics for the common cold and acute purulent rhinitis. *Cochrane Database of Systematic Reviews, 6*, CD000247. doi: 10.1002/14651858.CD000247.pub3

Lynch, P. (2011). Asthma education for children: Basic strategies can make a big difference. *Advance for NPs and PAs, 2*(7), 18–22.

Milgrom, H., & Leung, D. Y. M. (2011). Allergic rhinitis. In R. M. Kliegman, B. M. D. Stanton, J. St. Geme, N. F. Schor, & R. E. Behrman (Eds.), *Nelson textbook of pediatrics* (19th ed.). Philadelphia, PA: Elsevier Saunders.

Moore, K. L., Persaud, T. V. N., & Torchia, M. G. (2013). *The developing human: Clinically oriented embryology.* Philadelphia, PA: Elsevier Saunders.

National Asthma Education and Prevention Program. (2007). *Expert panel report 3: Guidelines for the diagnosis and management of asthma (NIH Publication No. 07–4051).* Bethesda, MD: National Institutes of Health, National Heart, Lung and Blood Institute.

Ohler, K. H., & Pham, J. T. (2013). Comparison of the timing of initial prophylactic palivizumab dosing on hospitalization of neonates for respiratory syncytial virus. *American Journal of Health-System Pharmacy, 70*, 1342–1346.

Pickering, L. K. (Ed.). (2012). *Red book: 2012 report of the committee on infectious diseases* (29th ed.). Elk Grove Village, IL: American Academy of Pediatrics.

Ratcliffe, M. M., & Kieckhefer, G. M. (2010). Asthma. In P. J. Allen, J. A. Vessey, & N. A. Schapiro (Eds.), *Primary care of the child with a chronic condition* (5th ed.). St. Louis, MO: Mosby.

Safe Kids. (2016). *Choking and strangulation.* Retrieved from https://www.safekids.org/safetytips/field_risks/choking-and-strangulation

Sato, A. F., Koppel, A. J., Quaid, E. L., Seiner, R., Esteban, C., Coutinho, M. T., et al. (2013). The home environment and family asthma management among ethnically diverse urban youth with asthma. *Families, Systems, & Health, 31*(2), 156–170.

Schechter, M. S. (2007). Airway clearance applications in infants and children. *Respiratory Care, 52*(10), 1382–1391.

Scollan-Koliopoulos, M., & Koliopoulos, J. S. (2010). Evaluation and management of apparent life-threatening events in infants. *Pediatric Nursing, 36*(2), 77–83.

Sirivimonpan, S. (2013). *Airway remodeling in asthma.* Retrieved from http://www.slideshare.net/AllergyChula/airway-remodeling-in-asthma

Taketomo, C. K., Hodding, J. H., & Kraus, D. M. (2013). *Pediatric & neonatal dosage handbook* (20th ed.). Hudson, OH: Lexicomp.

Tewfik, T. L., & Alghonaim, Y. (2015). *Trachea anatomy.* Retrieved from http://emedicine.medscape.com/article/1949391-overview

U.S. Department of Health and Human Services. (2016). *Healthy people 2020.* Retrieved from http://www.healthypeople.gov/2020/default.aspx

U.S. Food and Drug Administration. (2015). *OTC cough and cold products: Not for infants and children under 2 years of age.* Retrieved from http://www.fda.gov/forconsumers/consumerupdates/ucm048682.htm

Vertex Pharmaceuticals. (2015). *Kalydeco.* Retrieved from http://www.kalydeco.com.

Winnie, G. B., & Lossef, S. V. (2011). Pneumothorax. In R. M. Kliegman, B. M. D. Stanton, J. St. Geme, N. F. Schor, & R. E. Behrman (Eds.), *Nelson textbook of pediatrics* (19th ed.). Philadelphia, PA: Elsevier Saunders.

World Health Organization. (n.d.). *Passive smoking.* Retrieved from http://www.who.int/tobacco/en/atlas10.pdf

Wright, P. F. (2011). Influenza viruses. In R. M. Kliegman, B. M. D. Stanton, J. St. Geme, N. F. Schor, & R. E. Behrman (Eds.), *Nelson textbook of pediatrics* (19th ed.). Philadelphia, PA: Elsevier Saunders.

Yoon, P. J., Kelley, P. E., & Friedman, N. R. (2012). Ear, nose, & throat. In W. W. Hay, M. J. Levin, J. R. R. Deterding, M. J. Abzug, & M. Sondheimer (Eds.), *Current pediatric diagnosis and treatment* (21st ed.). New York, NY: McGraw-Hill.

Yoos, H. L., Kitzman, H., McMullen, A., Sidora-Arcoleo, K., Anson, E. (2005). The language of breathlessness: Do families and health care providers speak the same language when describing asthma symptoms? *Journal of Pediatric Health Care, 19*(4), 197–205.

Yust, E. & Slattery, A. (2012). Cold and cough medications for children. *Clinical Pediatric Emergency Medicine, 13*(4), 292–299.

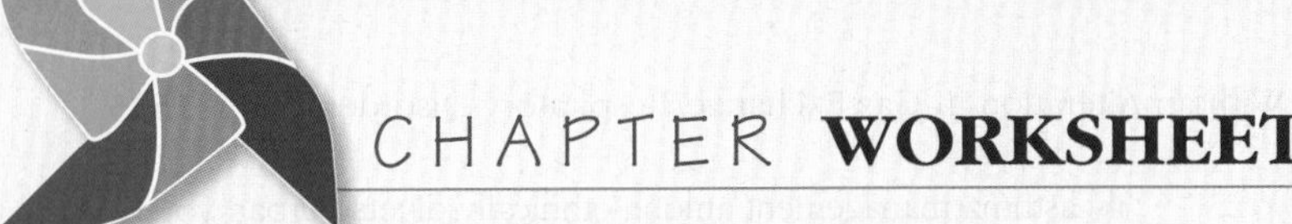

CHAPTER WORKSHEET

MULTIPLE CHOICE QUESTIONS

1. A 5-month-old infant with RSV bronchiolitis is in respiratory distress. The baby has copious secretions, increased work of breathing, cyanosis, and a respiratory rate of 78. What is the most appropriate initial nursing intervention?
   a. Attempt to calm the infant by placing him in his mother's lap and offering him a bottle.
   b. Alert the physician or nurse practitioner to the situation and ask for an order for a stat chest x-ray.
   c. Suction secretions, provide 100% oxygen via mask, and anticipate respiratory failure.
   d. Bring the emergency equipment to the room and begin bag-valve-mask ventilation.
2. A toddler has moderate respiratory distress, is mildly cyanotic, and has increased work of breathing, with a respiratory rate of 40. What is the priority nursing intervention?
   a. Airway maintenance and 100% oxygen by mask
   b. 100% oxygen and pulse oximetry monitoring
   c. Airway maintenance and continued reassessment
   d. 100% oxygen and provision of comfort
3. The nurse is caring for a child with cystic fibrosis who receives pancreatic enzymes. Which statement by the child's mother indicates an understanding of how to administer the supplemental enzymes?
   a. "I will stop the enzymes if my child is receiving antibiotics."
   b. "I will decrease the dose by half if my child is having frequent, bulky stools."
   c. "Between meals is the best time for me to give the enzymes."
   d. "The enzymes should be given at the beginning of each meal and snack."
4. Which of these factors contributes to infants' and children's increased risk for upper airway obstruction as compared with adults?
   a. Underdeveloped cricoid cartilage and narrow nasal passages
   b. Small tonsils and narrow nasal passages
   c. Cylinder-shaped larynx and underdeveloped sinuses
   d. Underdeveloped cricoid cartilage and smaller tongue
5. Which is the most appropriate treatment for epistaxis?
   a. With the child lying down and breathing through the mouth, apply pressure to the bridge of the nose.
   b. With the child lying down and breathing through the mouth, pinch the lower third of the nose closed.
   c. With the child sitting up and leaning forward, apply pressure to the bridge of the nose.
   d. With the child sitting up and leaning forward, pinch the lower third of the nose closed.

DOSAGE CALCULATION QUESTION

1. The nurse is caring for a child with allergic cute asthma. The child weighs 37 ½ pounds. The medication order reads: methylprednisolone 20 mg IV twice a day. The Pediatric Dosage Handbook provides a recommended dose for acute asthma of 1–2 mg/kg/day in 2 divided doses. Is the ordered dose safe?

CRITICAL THINKING EXERCISES

1. A 10-month-old girl is admitted to the pediatric unit with a history of recurrent pneumonia and failure to thrive. Her sweat chloride test confirms the diagnosis of cystic fibrosis. She is a frail-appearing infant with thin extremities and a slightly protuberant abdomen. She is tachypneic, has retractions, and coughs frequently. Based on the limited information given here and your knowledge of cystic fibrosis, choose three of the categories below as priorities to focus on when planning her care:
   a. Prevention of bronchospasm
   b. Promotion of adequate nutrition
   c. Education of the child and family
   d. Prevention of pulmonary infection
   e. Balancing fluid and electrolytes
   f. Management of excess weight gain
   g. Prevention of spread of infection
   h. Promoting adequate sleep and rest
2. A boy with asthma is admitted to the pediatric unit for the fourth time this year. The mother expresses frustration that he is getting sick so often. Besides information about onset of symptoms and events leading up to this present episode, what other types of information would you ask for while obtaining the history?

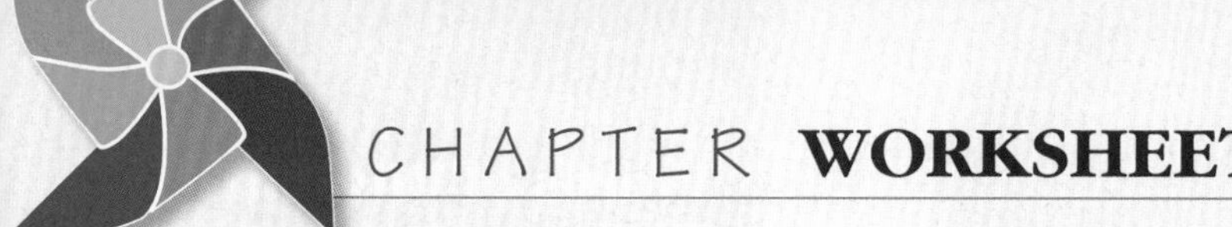

CHAPTER WORKSHEET

3. The mother of the boy in the previous question tells you that she smokes (but never around the boy), the family has a cat that comes inside sometimes, and she always gives her son the medication prescribed. She gives salmeterol and budesonide as soon as he starts to cough. When he is not having an episode, she gives him albuterol before his baseball games. Diphenhydramine helps his runny nose in the springtime. Based on this new information, what advice/ instructions would you give the mother?
4. A 7-year-old presents with a history of recurrent nasal discharge. He sneezes every time he visits his cousins, who have pets. He lives in an older home that is carpeted. Tobacco smokers live in the home. His mother reports that he snores and is a mouth breather. She says he has symptoms nearly year-round, but they are worse in the fall and the spring. She reports that diphenhydramine is somewhat helpful with his symptoms, but she doesn't like to give it to him on school days because it makes him drowsy. Based on the history above, develop a teaching plan for this child.
5. The nurse is caring for a 4-year-old girl who returned from the recovery room after a tonsillectomy 3 hours ago. She has cried off and on over the past 2 hours and is now sleeping. What areas should the nurse assess and focus on for this child?

STUDY ACTIVITIES

1. While caring for children in the pediatric setting, compare the signs and symptoms of a child with asthma to those of an infant with bronchiolitis. What are the most notable differences? How does the history of the two children differ?
2. A child with asthma has been prescribed Advair (fluticasone and salmeterol), albuterol, and prednisone. Develop a sample teaching plan for the child and family. Include appropriate use of the devices used to deliver the medications, as well as important information about the medications (uses and adverse effects).
3. While caring for children in the pediatric setting, compare the signs and symptoms and presentation of a child with the common cold to those of a child with either sinusitis or allergic rhinitis.
4. While caring for children in the pediatric setting review the census of children and identify those at risk for severe influenza and thus those who would benefit from annual influenza vaccination.
5. Compare the differences in oxygen administration between a young infant and an older child.

BRINGING IT ALL TOGETHER: A CASE STUDY

Bradley is a 5-year-old with a history of moderate asthma who was started on oral steroids yesterday after visiting his pediatrician for an asthma exacerbation. In addition, he has been receiving aerosol treatments every 4 hours since yesterday. He received his last levalbuterol nebulizer treatment 3 hours ago. His mother has brought him back to the office because she is concerned that he does not seem to be getting any better.

Go to thePoint to find questions to consider about this case.

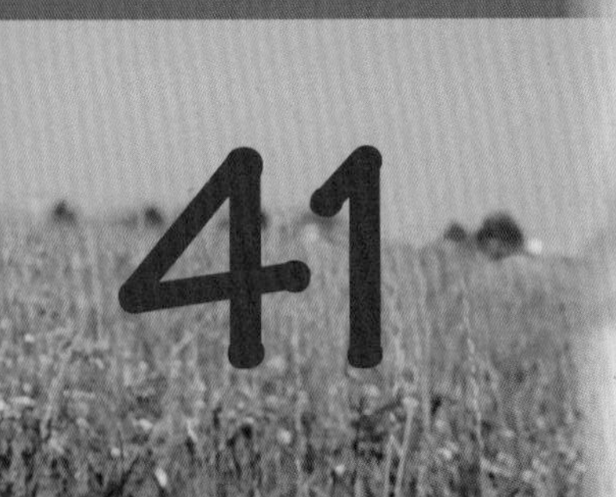

41

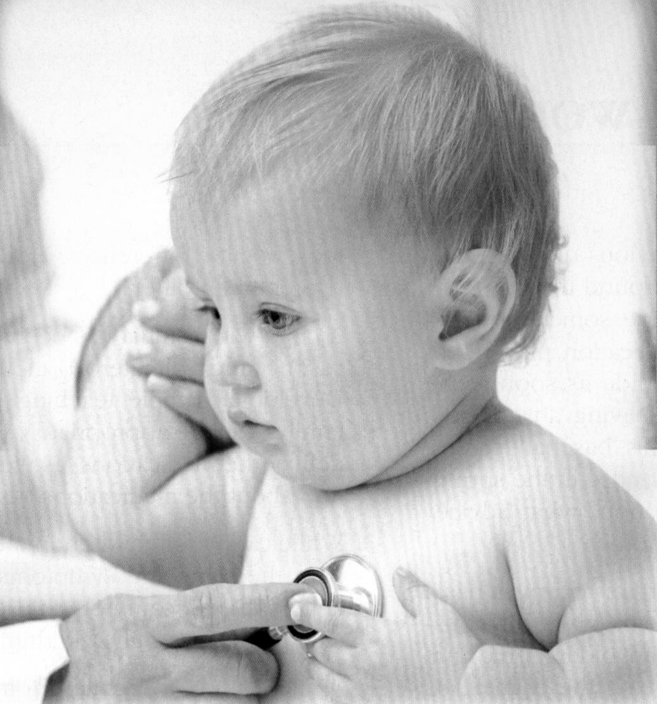

WOW

Words of Wisdom

The heart of the matter is healing the child's heart so he or she can embrace life to its fullest.

Nursing Care of the Child With an Alteration in Perfusion/Cardiovascular Disorder

KEY TERMS

arrhythmia
cardiomegaly
clubbing
echocardiography
electrocardiogram (ECG)
heart failure
orthotopic
polycythemia

Learning Objectives

Upon completion of the chapter, you will be able to:

1. Compare anatomic and physiologic differences of the cardiovascular system in infants and children versus adults.
2. Describe nursing care related to common laboratory and diagnostic tests used in the medical diagnosis of pediatric cardiovascular conditions.
3. Distinguish cardiovascular disorders common in infants, children, and adolescents.
4. Identify appropriate nursing assessments and interventions related to medications and treatments for pediatric cardiovascular disorders.
5. Develop an individualized nursing care plan for the child with a cardiovascular disorder.
6. Describe the psychosocial impact of chronic cardiovascular disorders on children.
7. Devise a nutrition plan for the child with cardiovascular disease.
8. Develop child/family teaching plans for the child with a cardiovascular disorder.

***Logan Bernstein*, 6 weeks old, is brought to the clinic by his mother. He presents with poor feeding. His mother states, "Logan falls asleep while feeding, and he's always very sweaty during feedings."**

Perfusion refers to the mechanisms that facilitate blood through tissue. Nurses may encounter alterations in perfusion in children and should be familiar with various cardiovascular disorders that children experience. Alterations in perfusion, or cardiovascular disease is a significant cause of chronic illness and death in children. Typically cardiovascular disorders in children are divided into two major categories—congenital heart disease (CHD) and acquired heart disease.

CHD is defined as structural anomalies that are present at birth, though they are often not diagnosed until later in life. CHD accounts for the largest percentage of all birth defects. About 32,000 babies are born annually with a congenital heart defect (American Heart Association [AHA], 2015b).

Acquired heart disease includes disorders that occur after birth. These disorders develop from a wide range of causes, or they can occur as a complication or long-term effect of CHD. Over 100 genes have been identified that may be involved in the development of CHD (Cunningham et al., 2014). Additional noncardiac anomalies occur in about 28% of children with CHD. CHD is also commonly associated with chromosomal abnormalities (Marian, Brugada, & Roberts, 2011). Many congenital heart defects result in heart failure and chronic cyanosis, leading to failure to thrive.

The diagnosis of a cardiovascular disorder in any person can be extremely frightening and overwhelming. Early on, children learn that the heart is necessary for life, so knowing that there is a heart problem can promote feelings of dread. These feelings are compounded by the child's age, the view of the child as being vulnerable and defenseless, and the stressors associated with the disorder itself. The child and parents need much support and reassurance (Cook & Higgins, 2010).

Nurses need to have a sound knowledge base about cardiovascular conditions affecting children so that they can provide appropriate assessment, intervention, guidance, and support to the child and family. Cardiovascular disorders require acute interventions that often have long-term implications for the child's health and growth and development. Due to the potentially overwhelming and devastating effects that cardiovascular disorders can have on children and their families, nurses need to be skilled in assessment and interventions in this area and able to provide support throughout the course of the illness and beyond.

VARIATIONS IN PEDIATRIC ANATOMY AND PHYSIOLOGY

The cardiovascular system undergoes numerous changes at birth. Structures that were vital to the fetus are no longer needed. Circulation via the umbilical arteries and vein is replaced with the child's own closed independent circulation. Changes in the size of the heart, pulse rate, and blood pressure (BP) also occur.

Circulatory Changes From Gestation to Birth

The fetal heart rate is present on about postconceptual day 17. The four chambers of the heart and arteries are formed during gestational weeks 2 through 8, with maturation of the structures occurring throughout the remainder of gestation. During fetal development, oxygenation of the fetus occurs via the placenta; the lungs, though perfused, do not perform oxygenation and ventilation. The foramen ovale, an opening between the atria, allows blood flow from the right to the left atrium. The ductus arteriosus allows blood flow between the pulmonary artery and the aorta, shunting blood away from the pulmonary circulation (Cunningham et al., 2014). Figure 41.1 illustrates fetal circulation.

With the newborn's first breath, several changes occur in the cardiopulmonary system that enable the newborn to make the transition from fetal circulation to normal circulation. As the newborn breathes for the first time, the lungs inflate, reducing pulmonary vascular resistance to blood flow. As a result, pulmonary artery pressure drops. Subsequently, pressure in the right atrium decreases. Blood flow to the left side of the heart increases the pressure in the left atrium. This change in pressure leads to closure of the foramen ovale. The drop in pressure of the pulmonary artery promotes closure of the ductus arteriosus, which is located between the aorta and pulmonary artery. The ductus venosus, located between the left umbilical vein and the inferior vena cava, closes because of a lack of blood flow and vasoconstriction. The closed ductus arteriosus and ductus venosus eventually become ligaments. With the lack of blood flow to the umbilical arteries and vein, these structures atrophy (Cunningham et al., 2014).

Structural and Functional Differences

The structure and function of the infant's and child's cardiovascular system differ from those of adults, depending on age. In infants and children younger than 7 years of age, the heart lies more horizontally, resulting in the apex lying higher in the chest, below the fourth intercostal space. As the lungs grow over time, the heart is displaced downward. Between ages 1 and 6 years, the heart is four times the birth size. Between 6 and 12 years of age, the child's heart is 10 times the size it was at birth. However, the heart is smaller proportionally at this time than at any other stage in life. During the school-age years, the heart grows more vertically within the thoracic

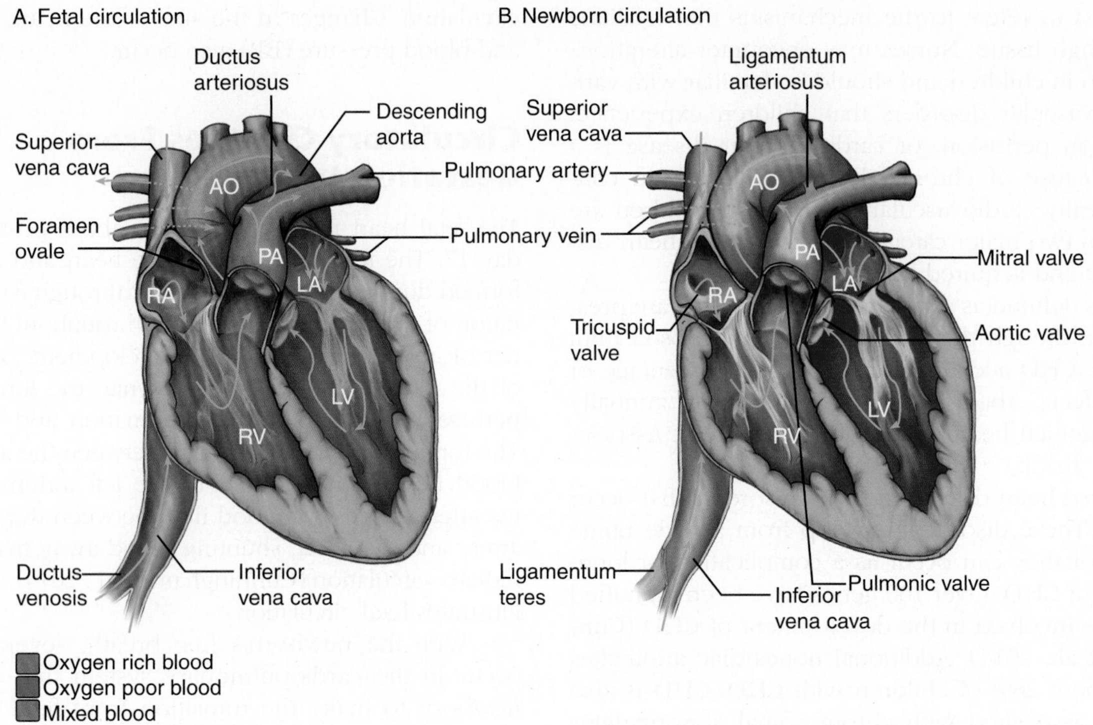

FIGURE 41.1 Fetal and newborn circulation.

cavity. During adolescence, the heart continues to grow in relation to the teen's rapid growth.

At birth, the ventricle walls are similar in thickness, but with time the left ventricular wall thickens. The immature myocytes of the infant's heart are thinner and less compliant than those of the adult. Right ventricular function dominates at birth, and over the first few months of life, left ventricular function becomes dominant. The infant's heart at rest exhibits a greater resting tension than the adult's, so volume loading or increased stretch may actually lead to decreased cardiac output. The infant's sarcoplasmic reticulum is less well organized than the adult's, making the infant dependent on serum calcium for contraction. Inotropic response to calcium in the actin and myosin (contractile proteins) increases with age.

The normal heart rate is higher in infancy than in adulthood, limiting the infant's ability to increase cardiac output by increasing the heart rate. The heart's efficiency increases as the child ages and the heart rate drops over time. The normal infant heart rate ranges from 90 to 160 beats per minute (bpm), the toddler's or preschooler's is 80 to 115 bpm, the school-age child's and the adolescent's ranges from 60 to 100 bpm. Innocent murmurs and physiologic splitting of heart sounds may be noted in infancy or childhood. These findings are related to the change in the size of the heart in relation to the thoracic cavity. The infant's and child's blood vessels widen and increase in length over time. The average infant's BP is about 80/55 mm Hg; BP is usually lower in the younger infant, and can be slightly higher in the older infant. The BP increases over time to the adult level. The toddler or preschooler's BP averages 90 to 110/55 to 75 mm Hg, the school-age child's 100 to 120/60 to 75 mm Hg, and the adolescent's 100 to 120/70 to 80 mm Hg (Engorn & Flerlage, 2015).

COMMON MEDICAL TREATMENTS

A variety of medications as well as other medical treatments and surgical procedures are used to treat cardiovascular problems in children. Most of these treatments will require a physician's order when the child is in the hospital. The most common treatments and medications are listed in Common Medical Treatments 41.1 and Drug Guide 41.1. The nurse caring for the child with a cardiovascular disorder should be familiar with what the procedures and medications are and how they work as well as common nursing implications related to use of these modalities.

Take Note!

Give digoxin at regular intervals, every 12 hours, such as at 8 AM and 8 PM, 1 hour before or 2 hours after a feeding. If a digoxin dose is missed and more than 4 hours have elapsed, withhold the dose and give the dose at the regular time; if less than 4 hours have elapsed, give the missed dose. If the child vomits digoxin, do not give a second dose. Monitor potassium levels, as a decrease enhances the effects of digitalis, causing toxicity (Taketokmo, Hodding, & Kraus, 2013).

COMMON MEDICAL TREATMENTS 41.1

Treatment	Explanation	Indications	Nursing Implications
Oxygen	Supplemented via mask, nasal cannula, hood, tent, or endotracheal/nasotracheal tube	Hypoxemia, respiratory distress, heart failure	Monitor response via work of breathing and pulse oximetry.
Chest physiotherapy (CPT) and postural drainage	Promotes mucous clearance by mobilizing secretions with the assistance of percussion or vibration accompanied by postural drainage (refer to Chapter 40 for additional information related to CPT and postural drainage)	Mobilization of secretions, particularly in postoperative period or with heart failure	May be performed by respiratory therapist in some institutions, by nurses in others. In either case, nurses must be familiar with the technique and able to educate families on its use.
Chest tube	Drainage tube is inserted into the pleural cavity to facilitate removal of air or fluid and allow full lung expansion	After open heart surgery, pneumothorax	If tube becomes dislodged from container, the chest tube must be clamped immediately to avoid further air entry into the chest cavity. Alternatively, the end may be immediately placed into a container of sterile water or saline to create a water seal.
Pacing	External wiring connected to a small generator used to electrophysiologically correct cardiac arrhythmias or heart block (temporary). Permanent pacing achieved with an implantable internal pacemaker	Bradyarrhythmias, heart block, cardiomyopathy, sinoatrial or atrioventricular node malfunction	Provide close observation of the child, pacing unit, and ECG. Maintain asepsis at pacing lead insertion site. Explain to child and family that the permanent pacemaker may be felt under the skin. Advise against participation in contact sports.[a]

[a]Skippen, P., Sanatina, S., Froese, N., & Gow, R. M. (2010). Pacemaker therapy of postoperative arrhythmias after pediatric cardiac surgery. *Pediatric Critical Care Medicine*, 11, 113–138.

Dosage Calculation Box 41.1

Child's weight: 12 lb 12 oz

Medication order: digoxin 60 μg by mouth every 12 hours.

Per the Pediatric Dosage Handbook, the recommended dose is 10–15 μg/kg/day in 2 divided doses.

Is the ordered dose safe?

NURSING PROCESS OVERVIEW FOR THE CHILD WITH A CARDIOVASCULAR DISORDER

Care of the child with a cardiovascular disorder includes all steps of the nursing process: assessment, nursing diagnosis, planning, interventions, and evaluation. There are a number of general concepts related to the nursing process that may be applied to any child with a cardiovascular disorder. The nurse should be knowledgeable about the procedures, treatments, and medications as well as familiar with the nursing implications related to these interventions. With an understanding of these concepts, the nurse can individualize the care based on the child's and family's needs.

Remember Logan, the 6-week-old with poor feeding? What additional health history and physical examination assessment information should the nurse obtain?

Assessment

When assessing a child with a cardiovascular disorder, expect to obtain a health history, perform a physical examination, and prepare the child for laboratory and diagnostic testing.

DRUG GUIDE 41.1

Medication	Actions/Indications	Nursing Implications
Alprostadil (prostaglandin)	Direct vasodilation of the ductus arteriosus smooth muscle Indicated for temporary maintenance of ductus arteriosus patency in infants with ductal-dependent congenital heart defects	• Apnea occurs in 10– 20% of neonates within first hour of infusion. • Monitor arterial BP, respiratory rate, heart rate, ECG, temperature, and pO_2; watch for abdominal distention. • Fresh IV solution required every 24 hours. • Reposition catheter if facial or arm flushing occurs. • Use with caution in neonate with bleeding tendency. • Contraindicated in respiratory distress syndrome or persistent fetal circulation.
Digoxin (cardiac glycoside, antiarrhythmic agent)	Increases contractility of the heart muscle by decreasing conduction and increasing force Used for heart failure, atrial fibrillation, atrial flutter, supraventricular tachycardia	• Prior to administering each dose, count apical pulse for 1 full minute, noting rate, rhythm, and quality. Withhold if apical pulse is <60 in an adolescent, <90 in an infant. • Avoid giving oral form with meals, as altered absorption may occur. • Monitor serum digoxin levels (therapeutic range: 0.8–2 ng/mL). • Notes signs of toxicity: nausea, vomiting, diarrhea, lethargy, and bradycardia. • Ginseng, hawthorn, and licorice intake increases risk for drug toxicity. • Note contraindications (ventricular fibrillation and hypersensitivity to digitalis). • Avoid rapid IV administration, as this may lead to systemic and coronary artery vasoconstriction.
Furosemide (loop diuretic)	Inhibits resorption of sodium and chloride Used to manage edema associated with heart failure, and hypertension in combination with antihypertensives	• Administer with food or milk to decrease GI upset. • Monitor BP, renal function, electrolytes (particularly potassium), and hearing. • May cause photosensitivity.
Heparin (anticoagulant)	Interferes with conversion of prothrombin to thrombin, preventing clot formation Indicated for the prophylaxis and treatment of thromboembolic disorders, especially after cardiac surgery	• Administer SQ, not IM. • Dose is adjusted according to coagulation test results. • Monitor for signs of bleeding, platelet counts. • Ensure that the antidote, protamine sulfate, is available. • Do not administer with uncontrolled bleeding or if subacute bacterial endocarditis is suspected.
Indomethacin (nonsteroidal anti-inflammatory agent)	Inhibits prostaglandin synthesis in order to close patent ductus arteriosus	• Monitor heart rate, BP, ECG, and urine output; monitor for murmur. • Monitor serum sodium, glucose, platelet count, BUN, creatinine, potassium, and liver enzymes. • May mask signs of infection. • Note development of edema.
Spironolactone (potassium sparing diuretic)	Competes with aldosterone to result in increased water and sodium excretion (spares potassium) Used to manage edema due to heart failure and for treatment of hypertension	• Administer with food. • Monitor serum potassium, sodium, and renal function. • May cause drowsiness, headache, and arrhythmia. • May cause false elevations in digitalis level. • Teach children to avoid high-potassium diets, salt substitutes, and natural licorice. • Contraindicated in hyperkalemia, renal failure, and anuria.

DRUG GUIDE 41.1 (continued)

Medication	Actions/Indications	Nursing Implications
Antibiotics		
Penicillin G benzathine Penicillin V potassium	Inhibits bacterial wall synthesis in susceptible organisms Indicated in mild to moderate infections, for prophylaxis of endocarditis and rheumatic fever	• Contraindications include hypersensitivity to penicillins. • Report hypersensitivity reactions (chills, fever, wheezing, pruritus, anaphylaxis) immediately. • PCN-G: administer IM. • Pen-VK: administer orally on empty stomach 1 hour prior to or 2 hours after a meal.
Erythromycin (macrolide)	Inhibits RNA transcription in susceptible organisms Used in children with penicillin allergy, mild to moderate infections, or endocarditis, and for rheumatic fever prophylaxis	• Contraindicated in pre-existing liver disease. • IV administration may result in CV abnormalities. • Abdominal distress common with oral use. • Fever, dizziness, and rash may occur.
Antihypertensive Drugs		
Angiotensin-converting enzyme (ACE) inhibitors (captopril, enalapril)	Competitive inhibition of ACE for management of hypertension Heart failure management in conjunction with digitalis and diuretics	• Monitor BP, renal function, WBC count, and serum potassium. • Discontinue if angioedema occurs. • Captopril: administer orally on empty stomach 1 hour before or 2 hours after meals. • Enalapril: may administer orally without regard to food.
β-Adrenergic blockers (propranolol, atenolol, sotalol)	Competitively block response to β-adrenergic stimulation, decreasing heart rate and force of contraction Used for management of hypertension, arrhythmias, and prevention of myocardial infarction	• Monitor ECG and BP. • Propranolol: administer with food. • Atenolol, sotalol: administer without regard to food. Do not stop drug abruptly. • May result in bradycardia, dizziness, nausea and vomiting, dyspnea, and hypoglycemia (propranolol). • Contraindications: heart block, uncompensated heart failure, cardiogenic shock, asthma, or hypersensitivity.
Hydralazine (vasodilator)	Direct vasodilation of arterioles to manage moderate to severe hypertension, heart failure	• Monitor heart rate and BP. • Closely monitor BP with IV use. • Administer oral dose with food. • May cause palpitations, flushing, tachycardia, dizziness, nausea, and vomiting. • Notify physician or nurse practitioner if flu-like symptoms occur. • Contraindicated in rheumatic valvular disease.

BUN, blood urea nitrogen; CV, cardiovascular; GI, gastrointestinal; IM, intramuscularly; pO_2, partial pressure of oxygen; SQ, subcutaneously; WBC, white blood cell.

Adapted from Taketomo, C. K., Hodding, J. H., & Kraus, D. M. (2013). *Pediatric & neonatal dosage handbook* (20th ed.). Hudson, OH: Lexicomp.

Health History

The health history consists of a history of the present illness, past medical history, and family history. Depending on his or her age, the child should be included in the health history interview; the child's age will determine the degree of involvement and the terminology used. Table 41.1 gives examples of typical questions that can be used when obtaining the child's health history.

HISTORY OF PRESENT ILLNESS

Elicit the history of the present illness, which addresses when the symptoms started and how they

TABLE 41.1 EXAMPLES OF QUESTIONS FOR OBTAINING A CHILD'S HEALTH HISTORY

Questions	Provides Information About
• What types and amounts (dosages) of medications has the child received? What were they used for?	• Possible underlying conditions that may be related to the child's current status
• Who prescribed them?	• Other healthcare personnel involved in the child's care as well as the parents' healthcare beliefs and patterns
• Were they effective? Did the child experience any adverse effects?	• How the medications may be affecting the child's health
• To whom does the child go for medical evaluation? How often? Were the visits for regular health check-ups or for situational problems? Were there previous hospitalizations? What for?	• The child's health status and the parents' healthcare knowledge, practices, and beliefs
• Has the child experienced any growth delay? Does the child have any problems with activity and coordination?	• Problems that may result from impaired cardiac output, adequacy of tissue oxygenation, and concomitant disorders associated with heart disease
• Does the child's skin color change when crying? If so, what color do you see?	• Effectiveness of tissue oxygenation. A blue or gray skin color may be due to cyanosis
• Does the child stop frequently during play to sit or squat?	• The child's exercise tolerance and tissue oxygenation
• Does the child have feeding difficulty? Does the child tire easily or sleep excessively?	• The child's energy expenditure, ability to tolerate activity, and tissue oxygenation
• Does the child frequently develop strep throat?	• The child's risk for developing rheumatic fever and heart disease

Adapted from Park, M. K. (2014). *Park's pediatric cardiology for practitioners* (6th ed.). St. Louis, MO: Mosby.

have progressed. Inquire about any treatments and medications used at home. Ask parents about history of orthopnea, dyspnea, easy fatigability, growth delays, squatting, edema, dizziness, and/or frequent occurrences of pneumonia, which can be significant signs of pediatric heart disease. The history of present illness may reveal a history of poor feeding, including fatigue, lethargy, and/or vomiting, or failure to thrive, even with adequate caloric intake. The parents may report diaphoresis, which is often seen in early heart failure. The parent or caregiver may also report delays in gross motor development, cyanosis (possibly reported by the parents as more of a gray color than blue), and tachypnea (indicative of heart failure).

PAST MEDICAL HISTORY

The past medical history includes information about the child as well as the mother's pregnancy history. Assess the child's past medical history for:

- Problems occurring after birth (history of the child's condition after birth may reveal evidence of an associated congenital malformation or other disorder)
- Frequent infections
- Chromosomal abnormalities
- Prematurity
- Autoimmune disorders
- Use of medications, such as corticosteroids

Assess the mother's pregnancy, labor, and delivery history. Be sure to include information about the status of the neonate at birth. Also inquire about maternal use of medications, including illicit or over-the-counter drugs and alcohol; exposure to radiation; presence of hypertension; and maternal viral illnesses such as coxsackievirus, cytomegalovirus, influenza, mumps, or rubella. A history of significant problems related to labor and delivery is also important: stress or asphyxia at birth may be related to cardiac dysfunction and pulmonary hypertension in the newborn.

Assess for additional risk factors such as:

- Family history of heart disease or CHD (investigate the history further if heart disease occurred in a first-degree relative)
- Hyperlipidemia
- Diabetes mellitus
- Obesity
- Inactivity
- Stress
- High-cholesterol diet

Physical Examination

Physical examination of the child with a cardiovascular condition consists of inspection, palpation, and auscultation. In addition, obtain the child's vital signs and measure the child's height and weight. Plot this information on a standard growth chart to evaluate nutritional status and growth. If the child is younger than 3 years of age, measure and plot the head circumference also.

INSPECTION

Assess the child's overall appearance. Inspect the color of the skin, noting cyanosis. Inspect the skin for edema. In infants, peripheral edema occurs first in the face, then the presacral region, and then the extremities. Edema of the lower extremities is characteristic of right ventricular heart failure in older children.

Take Note!

Suspect CHD in the cyanotic newborn who does not improve with oxygen administration (American Academy of Pediatrics [AAP] & American Heart Association [AHA], 2011).

Inspect the fingers and toes for **clubbing**. Clubbing (which usually does not appear until after 1 year of age) implies chronic hypoxia due to severe CHD. The first sign of clubbing is softening of the nail beds, followed by rounding of the fingernails, followed by shininess and thickening of the nail ends (see Fig. 40.5 in Chapter 40).

Obtain the child's temperature; fever would suggest infection. Assess respirations, including rate, rhythm, and effort. Note location and severity of retractions if present. Inspect the chest configuration, noting any prominence of the precordial chest wall, which is often seen in infants and children with **cardiomegaly** (abnormal heart enlargement). Note visible pulsations, which may indicate increased heart activity. Also inspect the neck veins for engorgement or abnormal pulsations. Note abdominal distention.

Take Note!

Children with cardiac conditions resulting in cyanosis will often have baseline oxygen saturations that are relatively low because of the mixing of oxygenated with deoxygenated blood.

PALPATION

Palpate the right and left radial or brachial pulse to assess cardiac rate and rhythm. Throughout infancy and childhood, the rate may vary. Palpate the femoral pulse; it should be readily palpable and equal in amplitude and strength to the brachial or radial pulse. A femoral pulse that is weak or absent in comparison to the brachial pulse is associated with coarctation of the aorta. Significant variations in pulse occur with activity, so the most accurate heart rate may be determined during sleep. In older children, exercise and emotional factors may influence the heart rate. A bounding pulse is characteristic of patent ductus arteriosus (PDA) or aortic regurgitation. Narrow or thready pulses may occur in children with heart failure or severe aortic stenosis (Cassidy, Allen, & Phillips, 2013). Note tachycardia, bradycardia, rhythm irregularities, diminished peripheral pulses, or thready pulse. Palpate the child's abdomen for hepatomegaly, a sign of right-sided heart failure in the infant and child.

AUSCULTATION

Auscultate the apical pulse for a full minute to determine heart rate and rhythm. Note irregularities in rhythm, tachycardia, or bradycardia. Auscultate the heart for murmurs. Many children have functional or innocent murmurs, but all murmurs must be evaluated on the basis of the following characteristics:

- Location
- Relation to the heart cycle and duration
- Intensity: grade I, soft and hard to hear; grade II, soft and easily heard; grade III, loud without thrill; grade IV, loud with a precordial thrill; grade V, loud, with a precordial thrill, audible with a stethoscope partially off chest; grade VI, very loud, audible with a stethoscope or with the naked ear
- Quality: harsh, musical, or rough; high, medium, or low pitch
- Variation with position (sitting, lying, standing) (Cassidy et al., 2013)

Auscultate for the character of heart sounds. Note distinct, muffled, or distant heart sounds. Abnormal splitting or intensifying of S_2 sounds occurs in children with major heart problems. Ejection clicks, which are high pitched, are related to problems with dilated vessels and/or valve abnormalities. Heard throughout systole, they can be early, moderate, or late. Clicks on the upper left sternal border are related to the pulmonary area. Aortic clicks are best heard at the apex and can be mitral or aortic in origin. A mild to late ejection click at the apex is typical of a mitral valve prolapse. The S_3 heart sound may be heard in children and is associated with cardiac abnormalities. The S_4 heart sound is not normally heard and is always associated with cardiac abnormalities (Lorts, Krawczeski, & Marino, 2013).

Auscultate the BP in the upper extremities and lower extremities and compare the findings; there should be no major differences between the upper and lower extremities. Determine the pulse pressure by subtracting the diastolic pressure from the systolic pressure. The pulse pressure is less than 50 mm Hg, or less than half the systolic pressure. A widened pulse pressure, which usually is accompanied by a bounding pulse, is associated with PDA, aortic insufficiency, fever, anemia, or complete heart block. A narrowed pulse pressure is associated with aortic stenosis. Note hypotension or hypertension.

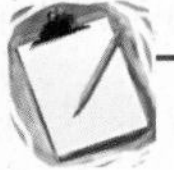

Take Note!

Alert children and parents if a heart murmur is detected, even if it is benign.

Laboratory and Diagnostic Testing

Common Laboratory and Diagnostic Tests 41.1 explains the laboratory and diagnostic tests most commonly used when considering cardiovascular disorders in children. The tests can assist the physician in diagnosing the disorder or can be used as guidelines in

COMMON LABORATORY AND DIAGNOSTIC TESTS 41.1

Test	Explanation	Indications	Nursing Implications
Arteriogram (angiogram: visualization of arteries or veins)	Radiopaque contrast solution is injected through a catheter and into the circulation. x-rays are then taken to visualize the structure of the heart and blood vessels	To observe blood flow to parts of body and detect lesions; to confirm a diagnosis. Catheters can be used to remove plaques	• Make sure the parent signs a consent form. • Administer premedication as ordered. • Obtain child's weight to determine amount of dye needed. • Keep the child NPO before the procedure according to institutional protocol. • After the procedure, maintain the child on bed rest. • Observe the puncture site for bleeding. • Monitor vital signs frequently and check the pulse distal to the site.
Ambulatory electrocardiographic monitoring (Holter)	Monitoring of the heart's electrical patterns for 24 hours using a portable compact unit	To identify and quantify arrhythmias in a 24-hour period during normal daily activities	• Instruct the child and parent to push the "event button" whenever chest pain, syncope, or palpitations occur. • Normal daily activities should be carried out during the testing period. • Having the child wear a snug undershirt over the leads helps to keep them in place.
Chest x-ray	A radiographic film of the chest area; will determine size of the heart and its chambers and pulmonary blood flow	Serves as a baseline for comparison with films taken after surgery; used to identify abnormalities of the lungs, heart, and other structures in the chest	• Instruct child not to wear jewelry or any metal around neck or on the hospital gown. • Explain to the child and family that no pain or discomfort should result. • If a portable x-ray at bedside is done, remove electrodes temporarily.
Echocardiogram	Noninvasive ultrasound procedure used to assess heart wall thickness, size of heart chambers, motion of valves and septa, and relationship of great vessels to other cardiac structures	Specific diagnosis of structural defects; determines hemodynamics and detects valvular defects	• Assure the child that the echo does not hurt. • Instruct the child about ECG lead placement and use of gel on the scope's wand during the procedure. • Encourage the child to lie still throughout the test.
Electrocardiogram (ECG)	A graphic record produced by an electrocardiograph (device used to record the electrical activity of the myocardium to detect transmission of the cardiac impulse through the conductive tissues of the muscle). Facilitates evaluation of the heart rate, rhythm, conduction, and musculature	To detect heart rhythm and chamber overload; also serves as a baseline for measuring postoperative complications	• Assure the child that monitoring is a painless procedure. • Place electrodes in the appropriate location. • The child must lie still during the ECG recording period (usually about 5 minutes). • Wipe electrode paste or jelly off after procedure.

COMMON LABORATORY AND DIAGNOSTIC TESTS 41.1 (continued)

Test	Explanation	Indications	Nursing Implications
Exercise stress test	Monitoring of heart rate, blood pressure, ECG, and oxygen consumption at rest and during exercise	Quantifies exercise tolerance; can be used to provoke symptoms or arrhythmias	• Child should be NPO for 4 hours prior to test. • Obtain baseline ECG and vital signs. • Instruct child to verbalize symptoms during testing. • Usually takes about 45 minutes.
Hemoglobin (Hgb) and hematocrit (Hct)	Measures the total amount of hemoglobin in the blood and indirectly measures the red blood cell number and volume	To detect anemia or polycythemia (may occur with CHD resulting in cyanosis)	• False elevations occur with dehydration. • May be obtained quickly via capillary puncture. • Normal values vary with age.
Partial pressure of oxygen (pO_2)	Measures the amount of oxygen in the blood	To determine the presence and degree of hypoxia	• Most accurate result is with arterial specimen (venous and capillary specimens demonstrate lower levels). • Observe child for cyanosis. • Supplement with oxygen per protocol.

Adapted from Abdallah, H. (2016). *About the Children's Heart Institute*. Retrieved from www.childrenheartinstitute.org/testing/testhome.htm; and Corbett, J. A. & Banks, A. D. (2013). *Laboratory tests and diagnostic procedures with nursing diagnoses* (8th ed.). Upper Saddle River, NJ: Pearson Education Inc.

determining ongoing treatment. Laboratory or nonnursing personnel obtain some of the tests, while the nurse might obtain others. In either instance the nurse should be familiar with how the tests are obtained, what they are used for, and normal versus abnormal results. This knowledge will also be necessary when providing child and family education related to the testing.

CARDIAC CATHETERIZATION

Cardiac catheterization is the definitive study for infants and children with cardiac disease and thus deserves special attention in this section on assessment of cardiovascular disorders. Cardiac catheterization has become almost a routine diagnostic procedure and may be performed on an outpatient basis. However, it is highly invasive and not without risks, especially in sick infants and children. Indications for cardiac catheterization include:

- Cardiovascular disease causing cyanosis in infants: these infants need to be catheterized as soon as they are in a reasonably stable condition
- Severe heart failure or progressive problems such as pulmonary edema
- Questionable anatomic or physiologic abnormalities
- Planned cardiac surgery
- Progressive monitoring related to pulmonary hypertension
- Periodic assessment after repair of a cardiac defect
- Therapeutic interventions such as septostomy or balloon valvotomy

Cardiac catheterization may be categorized as diagnostic, interventional, or electrophysiologic. Diagnostic cardiac catheterization typically is used to identify structural defects. Interventional cardiac catheterization is used as a treatment measure to dilate occluded or stenotic structures or vessels or close some defects. Electrophysiologic cardiac catheterization involves the use of electrodes to identify abnormal rhythms and destroy sites of abnormal electrical conduction. The type of catheterization performed varies based on the individual needs of the child. The procedure lasts from 1 to 3 hours (Park, 2014).

PERFORMING CARDIAC CATHETERIZATION

In cardiac catheterization, a radiopaque catheter is inserted into a blood vessel and is then guided through the vessel to the heart with the aid of fluoroscopy. For a right-sided catheterization, the catheter is threaded to the right atrium via a major vein such as the femoral vein. With a left-sided catheterization, the catheter is threaded to the aorta and heart via an artery. Once the tip of the catheter is in the heart, contrast material is injected via the catheter and radiographic images are taken.

While the catheter is in the heart, several procedures can be performed. The BPs, changes in cardiac output or stroke volume, and oxygen saturation in each heart chamber and major blood vessels are recorded. With the injection of contrast material, information is revealed about the heart anatomy, ventricular wall motion and ejection fraction, intracardiac pressures and hemodynamic parameters, cardiac valve function, and structural abnormalities. The movement of the contrast material is filmed so that the details of the cardiac procedure are recorded. Samples of heart tissue to evaluate for infection, muscular dysfunction, or rejection after a transplant may also be obtained (Park, 2014).

NURSING MANAGEMENT OF CARDIAC CATHETERIZATION

For children and parents or guardians, cardiac catheterization can be a source of much anxiety. Therefore, the nurse needs to educate the parents and, if appropriate for age, the child about all aspects of the procedure. The procedure is commonly performed on an outpatient basis, but some physicians or nurse practitioners require the child to be admitted for an overnight stay for observation. Nursing management of the child undergoing cardiac catheterization includes preprocedure nursing assessment and preparation of the child and family, postprocedural nursing care, and discharge teaching.

Before the Procedure. A thorough history and physical examination are necessary to establish a baseline. Obtain vital signs. Note fever or other signs and symptoms of infection, which may necessitate rescheduling the procedure. Obtain the child's height and weight to aid in determining medication dosages. Assess the child for any allergies, especially to iodine and shellfish, because some contrast materials contain iodine as a base. Review the child's medications: medications such as anticoagulants are typically withheld for several days or longer prior to the procedure to reduce the child's risk for bleeding. Check the results of any laboratory tests, such as hemoglobin and hematocrit levels.

Perform a complete physical examination. Pay particular attention to assessing the child's peripheral pulses, including pedal pulses. Use an indelible pen to mark the location of the child's pedal pulses so they can be easily assessed after the procedure. Document the location and quality in the child's medical record.

Teach the parents and child, if appropriate, about the procedure. Include information about what the procedure involves, how long it will take, and any special instructions from the physician or nurse practitioner. Use a variety of teaching methods as appropriate, such as videotapes, books, and pamphlets. Adapt these teaching methods to the child's developmental stage. For example, introduce the younger child to equipment through play therapy. For school-age and older children and their parents, offer a tour of the cardiac catheterization laboratory. Mention sounds and sights they may experience during the procedure. Explain the use of intravenous fluid therapy, sedation, and, if ordered, anesthesia to the child and parents. Tell the child that he or she may feel a sensation of the heart racing when the catheter is inserted. Also warn the older child that he or she may experience a feeling of warmth or stinging when the contrast material is injected. Encourage the child to use familiar ways to help him or her relax. If necessary, teach the child simple relaxation measures.

Typically, food and fluid are withheld for 4 to 6 hours before the procedure. Prescribed medications may be taken with a sip of water. On the day of the procedure, check to ensure that a signed informed consent form is on the child's medical record and that all necessary assessment data have been included. Just before the procedure, ask the child to void and administer a sedative, as ordered. If appropriate and permitted, allow the parents to accompany the child to the catheterization area.

Teach the child and family what to expect after the procedure is completed. Inform the parents of the possible complications that might occur, such as bleeding, low-grade fever, loss of pulse in the extremity used for the catheterization, and development of **arrhythmia** (abnormal heart rhythm). Explain to the child that he or she will have a dressing over the catheter site and that he or she will need to keep the leg straight for several hours after the procedure. Teach the child and parent that frequent monitoring will be required after the procedure.

Take Note!

In order to decrease the risk for catheterization-induced arrhythmia, an order for digitalis to be held the night before and morning of the catheterization may be written (Park, 2014).

After the Procedure. Throughout the postprocedure period, closely monitor the child for complications of bleeding, arrhythmia, hematoma, and thrombus formation and infection. After the procedure, evaluate the child's vital signs, the neurovascular status of the lower extremities, and the pressure dressing over the catheterization site every 15 minutes for the first hour and then every 30 minutes for 1 hour. Vital signs should remain within acceptable parameters. Hypotension may signify hemorrhage due to perforation of the heart muscle or bleeding from the insertion site. Expect to monitor cardiac rhythm and oxygen saturation levels via pulse oximetry for the first few hours after the procedure to help identify possible complications.

Assess the child's distal pulses bilaterally for presence and quality. The pulse of the affected extremity may be slightly less than that of the other extremity in the initial postprocedure period, but it should gradually return to baseline. Also assess the color and temperature of the extremity; pallor or blanching would indicate an obstruction in blood flow. Check capillary refill and sensation to evaluate blood flow to the area.

Maintain bed rest in the immediate postprocedure period. Ensure that the child maintains the extremity in a straight position for approximately 4 to 8 hours, depending on the approach used and the facility's policy. Inspect the pressure dressing frequently. Check to make sure that it is dry and intact, without evidence of bleeding. Reinforce the dressing as necessary and report any evidence of drainage on the dressing. If there is a risk of the dressing becoming soiled or wet, cover it with plastic.

Take Note!

If bleeding occurs after a cardiac catheterization, apply pressure 1 in above the site to create pressure over the vessel, thereby reducing the blood flow to the area.

Monitor the child's intake and output closely to ensure adequate hydration. The contrast material has a diuretic effect, so assess the child for signs and symptoms of dehydration and hypovolemia. Typically, the child resumes oral intake as tolerated, beginning with sips of clear liquids and progressing to his or her preprocedure diet. Continue intravenous fluids as ordered and encourage oral fluid intake as allowed and ordered to promote elimination of the contrast material.

Allow the child to talk about the experience and how and what he or she felt. Provide positive reinforcement for the child's actions.

Provide child and family education before the child is discharged home (see Teaching Guidelines 41.1). Areas to address include site care, signs and symptoms of complications (especially within 24 hours after the catheterization, such as fever, bleeding or bruising at the catheterization site, or changes in color, temperature, or sensation in the extremity used), diet, and activity level.

Teaching Guidelines 41.1

PROVIDING CARE AFTER A CARDIAC CATHETERIZATION

- Change the pressure dressing on the day after the procedure. Apply a dry sterile dressing or adhesive bandage for the next several days. Keep the dressing dry; cover it with plastic if there is a chance that the dressing could become wet or soiled.
- When changing the dressing, inspect the insertion site for redness, irritation, swelling, drainage, and bleeding. Report any of these to the physician or nurse practitioner.
- Check the temperature, color, sensation, and pulses on the child's extremities and compare. Report any changes to the physician or nurse practitioner.
- Resume the child's usual diet after the procedure; report any nausea or vomiting.
- Check the child's temperature at least once a day for approximately 3 days after the procedure. Report any temperature elevation of 100.4°F or greater.
- Avoid giving the child a tub bath for approximately 3 days after the procedure; use sponge baths or showers instead.
- Discourage strenuous exercise or activity for approximately 3 days after the procedure.
- Watch for changes in the child's appearance, such as changes in skin color, reports of the heart "fluttering" or "skipping a beat," fever, or difficulty breathing.
- Give acetaminophen (Tylenol) or ibuprofen (Motrin) for complaints of pain.
- Schedule a follow-up appointment with the physician or nurse practitioner in the time specified.

Adapted from Children's Healthcare of Atlanta. (2010). *Your child's heart catheterization*. Retrieved from www.choa.org/Childrens-Hospital-Services/Cardiac/Testing-and-Treatments/Heart-Testing/~/media/CHOA/Documents/Services/Cardiac/Your-Childs-Heart-Cath.pdf; and The University of Chicago Medicine Comer Children's Hospital (2016). *Heart catheterization in children*. Retrieved from www.uchicagokidshospital.org/specialties/heart/patient-education/cath-guide.html

Thinking About Development

Jeremy Titus is a 2-year-old male with congenital heart disease. He is having a cardiac catheterization today. How will the nurse encourage Jeremy to stay in bed and keep his leg straight for several hours following the catheterization? What types of activities would be appropriate for occupying Jeremy while he is confined to bed? How would the nurse's approach differ if Jeremy were an older child?

Nursing Diagnoses and Related Interventions

Upon completion of a thorough assessment, the nurse might identify several nursing diagnoses. These may include but are not limited to:

- Decreased cardiac output
- Ineffective tissue perfusion
- Imbalanced nutrition, less than body requirements
- Risk for delayed growth and development

- Risk for infection
- Excess fluid volume
- Interrupted family processes
- Activity intolerance
- Pain

After completing Logan's assessment, the nurse noted the following: poor weight gain, tachypnea with occasional nasal flaring, crackles heard on auscultation, and edema noted in the face, presacral area, and extremities. Based on these assessment findings, what would your top three nursing diagnoses be for Logan?

Nursing goals, interventions, and evaluation for the child with a cardiovascular disorder are based on the nursing diagnoses. Nursing Care Plan 41.1, at the end of the chapter, can be used as a guide in planning nursing care for the child with a cardiovascular disorder. The nursing care plan overview should be individualized based on the child's symptoms and needs. Refer to Chapter 36 for detailed information about pain assessment and management. Additional information will be included later in the chapter as it relates to specific disorders.

Based on your top three nursing diagnoses for Logan, describe appropriate nursing interventions.

CONGENITAL HEART DISEASE

In North America, more than 1% of newborn infants have CHD resulting from numerous causes. The prevalence of CHD ranges from 6 to 13 per 1,000 live births; premature infants have a higher rate (Altman, 2015). Many chromosome defects are associated with CHD, including Down syndrome, velocardiofacial syndrome, Turner syndrome, trisomy 13, trisomy 18, Williams syndrome, Prader–Willi syndrome, and cri-du-chat (Marian et al., 2011). About one third of infants with CHD will have disease serious enough to result in death or will require cardiac catheterization or cardiac surgery within the first year of life. Complications of CHD include heart failure, hypoxemia, growth retardation, developmental delay, and pulmonary vascular disease. Children with severe anomalies frequently experience failure to thrive.

With advances in palliative and corrective surgery in the past 20 years, many more children are now able to survive into adulthood. As many as 85% of children with CHD grow to be adults, yet many have problems related to education, insurance, and employment (Abdoulhosn & Child, 2011). Hypothermia, cardiopulmonary bypass required during cardiac surgery for CHD, and episodes of hypoxemia may have a long-term impact on the child's cognitive ability and academic function (Brown & Fulton, 2011). Due to the potential long-term effects that CHD may have on these children, nurses must be expertly equipped to care for them.

Pathophysiology

The exact cause of CHD is unknown. However, the belief is that it results from interplay of several factors, including genetics (e.g., chromosomal alterations) and maternal exposure to environmental factors (e.g., toxins, infections, chronic illnesses, and alcohol).

Congenital heart defects result from some interference in the development of the heart structure during fetal life. Subsequently, the septal walls or valves may fail to develop completely, or vessels or valves may be stenotic, narrowed, or transposed. Structures that formed to allow fetal circulation may fail to close after birth, altering the pressures necessary to maintain adequate blood flow.

After birth, with the change from fetal to newborn circulation, pressures within the chambers of the right side of the heart are less than those of the left side and pulmonary vascular resistance is less than that for the systemic circulation. These normal pressure gradients are necessary for adequate circulation to the lungs and the rest of the body. However, these pressure gradients become disrupted if a structure has failed to develop, a fetal structure has failed to close, or a narrowing, stenosis, or transposition of a vessel has occurred. For example, blood typically flows from an area of higher pressure to lower pressure. If the ductus arteriosus fails to close, blood will move from the aorta to the pulmonary artery, ultimately increasing right atrial pressure. With this shunting of blood, highly oxygenated blood can mix with less oxygenated blood, interfering with the amount available to the tissues via the systemic circulation. Some of the defects may result in significant hypoxemia, the sequelae of which include clubbing, polycythemia, exercise intolerance, hypercyanotic spells, brain abscess, and cerebrovascular accident (CVA) (Brown & Fulton, 2011).

Congenital heart defects are categorized based on hemodynamic characteristics (blood flow patterns in the heart):

- Disorders with decreased pulmonary blood flow: tetralogy of Fallot and tricuspid atresia
- Disorders with increased pulmonary blood flow: PDA, atrial septal defect (ASD), and ventricular septal defect (VSD)
- Obstructive disorders: coarctation of the aorta, aortic stenosis, and pulmonary stenosis
- Mixed disorders: transposition of the great vessels (TGV), total anomalous pulmonary venous return (TAPVR), truncus arteriosus, and hypoplastic left heart syndrome (HLHS)

Therapeutic Management

Prenatal education about avoiding certain substances or preventing infection is essential to promote optimal outcomes for the fetus. Encourage parents of children with CHD to receive genetic counseling because of the probability of having subsequent children with a congenital heart defect. Children with small septal defects are urged to lead a normal life and often require no medical intervention. Therapeutic management of other forms of CHD focuses on palliative care or a surgical corrective approach necessary for most of the defects. In newborns and very young infants with severe cyanosis (tricuspid atresia, TGV), a prostaglandin infusion will maintain patency of the ductus arteriosus, improving pulmonary blood flow. Definitive correction of structural disorders requires surgical intervention. Table 41.2 describes the surgical procedures used for the various congenital heart defects and the relevant nursing measures. Nursing management for the child with CHD will be provided following the disorders section. See Evidence-Based Practice 41.1.

Disorders with Decreased Pulmonary Blood Flow

Defects involving decreased pulmonary blood flow occur when there is some obstruction of blood flow to the lungs. As a result of the obstruction, pressure in the right side of the heart increases and becomes greater than that of the left side of the heart. Blood from the higher-pressure right side of the heart then shunts to the lower-pressure left side through a structural defect. Subsequently, deoxygenated blood mixes with oxygenated blood on the left side of the heart. This mixed blood, which is low in oxygen, is pumped via the systemic circulation to the body tissues.

Defects with decreased pulmonary blood flow are characterized by mild to severe oxygen desaturation. Typically, the child exhibits oxygen saturation levels ranging from 50% to 90%, which can produce severe cyanosis. To compensate for low blood oxygen levels, the kidneys produce the hormone erythropoietin to stimulate the bone marrow to produce more red blood cells (RBCs). This increase in RBCs is called **polycythemia**. Polycythemia can lead to an increase in blood volume and possibly blood viscosity, further taxing the workload of the heart. Although the number of RBCs increases, there is no change in the amount of blood that reaches the lungs for oxygenation. Disorders within this classification include tetralogy of Fallot and tricuspid atresia.

Tetralogy of Fallot

Tetralogy of Fallot is a congenital heart defect composed of four heart defects: pulmonary stenosis (a narrowing of the pulmonary valve and outflow tract, creating an obstruction of blood flow from the right ventricle to the pulmonary artery), VSD, overriding aorta (enlargement of the aortic valve to the extent that it appears to arise from the right and left ventricles rather than the anatomically correct left ventricle), and right ventricular hypertrophy (the muscle walls of the right ventricle increase in size due to continued overuse as the right ventricle attempts to overcome a high-pressure gradient). Surgical intervention is usually required during the first year of life (Brown & Fulton, 2011; Darst, Collins, & Miyamoto, 2014).

PATHOPHYSIOLOGY

With pulmonary stenosis, the blood flow from the right ventricle is obstructed and slowed, resulting in a

EVIDENCE-BASED PRACTICE 41.1

EFFECTS OF CHRONIC OR INTERMITTENT HYPOXIA ON COGNITION IN CHILDREN

STUDY

It is well known that significant hypoxia demonstrates an adverse effect on cognition, yet little is known about the effects of chronic or intermittent hypoxia on cognition in children. Many children with congenital heart disease (CHD) suffer either chronic or intermittent hypoxia. The authors performed a systematic literature review to study this question. Fifty-five studies were included, and a significant proportion of them addressed hypoxia with CHD.

Findings

About 80% of the studies reported adverse effects on cognition in children who suffered chronic or intermittent hypoxia, including developmental and academic achievement. Adverse effects were noted at all childhood age levels except premature infants. The effects were noted even with mild oxygen desaturation.

Nursing Implications

It is critical that the developing child be afforded the opportunity to develop optimal cognition. Know the child's normal oxygen saturation so that decreases may be quickly acted upon. Use supplemental oxygen judiciously and within the physician order parameters. Since many children experience improved oxygenation after CHD repair, encourage adequate nutrition so that, in turn, the infant or child will demonstrate growth adequate for safe surgical intervention.

Adapted from Bass, J. L., Corwin, M., Gozal, D., Moore, C., Nishida, H., Parker, S., et al. (2004). The effect of chronic or intermittent hypoxia on cognition in childhood: A review of the evidence. *Pediatrics, 114*(3), 805–816.

TABLE 41.2 COMMON SURGICAL PROCEDURES AND NURSING MEASURES FOR CONGENITAL HEART DEFECTS

Disorder	Surgical Procedure	Nursing Measures
Tetralogy of Fallot	Palliation with systemic-to-pulmonary anastomoses: • Blalock–Taussig shunt: an end-to-side anastomosis (or connection with a small Gore-Tex tube) of the subclavian artery and the pulmonary artery. • Waterston shunt: anastomosis of the ascending aorta and the pulmonary artery. • Definitive correction involves patch closure of the ventricular septal defect and repair of the pulmonary valve and right ventricular outflow tract.	• Avoid BP measurements and venipunctures in the affected arm after a Blalock–Taussig shunt. Pulse will not be palpable in that arm because of use of the subclavian artery for the shunt. • Monitor for ventricular arrhythmias after corrective repair.
Tricuspid atresia	• Palliation with Blalock–Taussig shunt or pulmonary artery banding may be performed. • At 3–6 months of age, the superior vena cava is detached from the heart and connected to the pulmonary artery (Glenn procedure). • By age 2–5 years, a modified Fontan procedure may be performed. Systemic venous return is redirected to the pulmonary artery directly.	• Monitor for atrial arrhythmias, left ventricular dysfunction, and protein-losing enteropathy. • Some children may eventually require a pacemaker.
Atrial septal defect (ASD)	• If small, the defect may be sutured closed. Larger defects may require a patch of pericardium or synthetic material. • Ostium secundum ASD may be repaired percutaneously via cardiac catheterization with a Gore Helex septal occluder (other brands are also available).	• Monitor for atrial arrhythmias (lifelong) after surgical closure. • With the Gore Helex device, strenuous activity should be avoided for 2 weeks after the procedure.[a]
Ventricular septal defect (VSD)	• If surgical closure is required, it should be performed before permanent pulmonary vascular changes develop. • Surgical closure may be in the form of suture closure of the VSD, transcatheter placement of a device in the defect, or Dacron patch closure.	• Monitor for ventricular dysrhythmias or AV block. • With the clamshell occluding or Amplatzer device, strenuous activity should be avoided for 1 month after the procedure.[b]
Atrioventricular canal defect	• Pulmonary artery banding as palliation in very young infants. • Surgical correction by 3–18 months of age • Patch closure of the septal defects and suturing of the valve leaflets or valve reconstruction are performed.	• Monitor for complete heart block postoperatively. • Teach parents that mitral regurgitation is a long-term complication and may require valve replacement.
Patent ductus arteriosus (PDA)	• PDA is closed by coil embolization or device via cardiac catheterization. • May also be surgically ligated.	• Monitor for bleeding and laryngeal nerve damage.
Coarctation of the aorta	• Balloon angioplasty via cardiac catheterization is possible in some children. • Most common surgical repair is resection of the narrowed portion of the aorta, followed by end-to-end reanastomosis.	• Preoperatively, administer prostaglandin medications as ordered to relax the ductal tissue. • Postoperatively, measure and compare BP in all four extremities and quality of upper vs. lower pulses.

TABLE 41.2 COMMON SURGICAL PROCEDURES AND NURSING MEASURES FOR CONGENITAL HEART DEFECTS (continued)

Disorder	Surgical Procedure	Nursing Measures
Aortic stenosis	• Balloon dilatation is accomplished via the umbilical artery in the newborn or the femoral artery via cardiac catheterization in the older child.	• Provide routine postcatheterization care. • Teach parents that long-term aortic regurgitation requiring valve replacement may occur.
Pulmonary stenosis	• Balloon dilation valvuloplasty is performed via cardiac catheterization to dilate the valve. This is effective in all but the most severe of cases, which will require surgical valvotomy.	• Provide routine postcatheterization care for balloon dilation. • Explain to parents that prognosis is excellent.
Transposition of the great vessels (arteries)	• Balloon atrial septotomy is usually done as soon as the diagnosis is made. A balloon-tipped catheter is passed through the atrial septum to enlarge the atrial septum. • Surgical correction involves switching the arteries into their normal anatomic positions.	• Administer prostaglandin to maintain the open state of the ductus arteriosus, which will allow the mixing of poorly oxygenated blood with well-oxygenated blood. • Monitor for rapid respirations and cyanosis. • Administer oxygen as needed preoperatively.
Total anomalous pulmonary venous return	The pulmonary vein is repositioned to the back of the left atrium and the ASD is closed.	• Monitor for dysrhythmias, heart block, and persistent heart failure.
Truncus arteriosus	VSD repair, separation of the pulmonary arteries from the aorta, with subsequent connection to the right ventricle with a valve conduit.	• Preoperatively, administer prostaglandin infusion to prevent closing of the ductus arteriosus.
Hypoplastic left heart syndrome	• Heart transplantation is the treatment of choice. • Palliative staged treatment. First: Norwood procedure, reconstruction of the aorta and pulmonary arteries includes a cardiac transplant. Second: bidirectional Glenn procedure, connection of the superior vena cava to the right pulmonary artery to increase the blood flow to the lungs. Third: modified Fontan procedure	• Preoperatively, administer prostaglandin infusion to prevent closing of the ductus arteriosus. • After palliative repairs, monitor for dysrhythmias or worsening ventricular function.
Valve disorders	• The incompetent valve is replaced with valve prosthesis.	• Lifelong anticoagulation therapy is necessary with prosthetic valves. • Monitor prothrombin times. • Monitor heart sounds for alterations.

[a]W. L. Gore & Associates, Inc. (2010). Instructions for use: Gore® Helex septal occluder. Retrieved from www.fda.gov/ucm/groups/fdagov-public/@fdagov-afda-adcom/documents/document/ucm304933.pdf

[b]AGA Medical Corporation. (2014). *Amplatzer™ muscular VSD occluder: Instructions for use.* Plymouth, MN: Author.

Adapted from Brown, D. W., & Fulton, D. R. (2011). Congenital heart disease in children and adolescents. In V. Fuster, R. A. Walsh, & R. A. Harrington (Eds.), *Hurst's the heart* (13th ed.). New York, NY: McGraw-Hill Companies, Inc. ; and Darst, J. R., Collins, K. K., & Miyamoto, S. D. (2014). Cardiovascular diseases. In W. W. Hay, M. J. Levin, & R. R. Deterding, & M. J. Abzug (Eds.), *Current pediatric diagnosis and treatment* (22nd ed.). New York, NY: McGraw-Hill.

decrease in blood flow to the lungs for oxygenation and a decrease in the amount of oxygenated blood returning to the left atrium from the lungs. The obstructed flow also increases the pressure in the right ventricle. This blood, which is poorly oxygenated, is then shunted across the VSD into the left atrium. Poorly oxygenated blood also travels through the overriding aorta (if it extends to both ventricles). In some cases when the VSD is large, the pressure in the right ventricle may be equal to that of the left ventricle. In this case, the path of blood shunting depends on which circulation is exerting the higher pressure, pulmonary or systemic.

Regardless of which way shunting occurs, a mixing of oxygenated and poorly oxygenated blood occurs, with this blood ultimately being pumped into the systemic circulation. The oxygen saturation of the blood in the systemic circulation is reduced, leading to cyanosis. The degree of cyanosis depends on the extent of the pulmonary stenosis, the size of the VSD, and the vascular resistance of the pulmonary and systemic circulations.

Tetralogy of Fallot is usually diagnosed during the first weeks of life due to the presence of a murmur and/or cyanosis. Some newborns may be acutely cyanotic, while others may exhibit only mild cyanosis that gradually becomes more severe, particularly during times of stress as the child grows older. Most often, infants with tetralogy of Fallot have a PDA at birth, providing additional pulmonary blood flow and thereby decreasing the severity of the initial cyanosis. Later, as the ductus arteriosus closes, such as within the first days of life, more severe cyanosis can occur (Fig. 41.2) (Brown & Fulton, 2011; Darst et al., 2014).

NURSING ASSESSMENT

Nursing assessment consists of the health history, physical examination, and laboratory and diagnostic tests.

Health History and Physical Examination

Obtain the health history, noting a history of color changes associated with feeding, activity, or crying. Determine if the infant or child is demonstrating hypercyanotic spells. Hypercyanosis develops suddenly and is manifested as increased cyanosis, hypoxemia, dyspnea, and agitation. If the infant's oxygen demand is greater than the supply, such as with crying or during feeding, then the spell progresses to anoxia. When the degree of cyanosis is severe and persistent, the infant may become unresponsive. As the infant gets older, he or she may use specific postures, such as bending at the knees or assuming the fetal position, to relieve a hypercyanotic spell. The walking infant or toddler may squat periodically. These positions improve pulmonary blood flow by increasing systemic vascular resistance. Ask the parents if they have noticed any of these unusual positions. Note history of irritability, sleepiness, or difficulty breathing.

During the physical examination, observe the skin color and note any evidence of cyanosis. Also observe for changes in skin color with positional changes, and inspect the fingers for clubbing. Note if the child has a hypercyanotic spell during the assessment. Count the

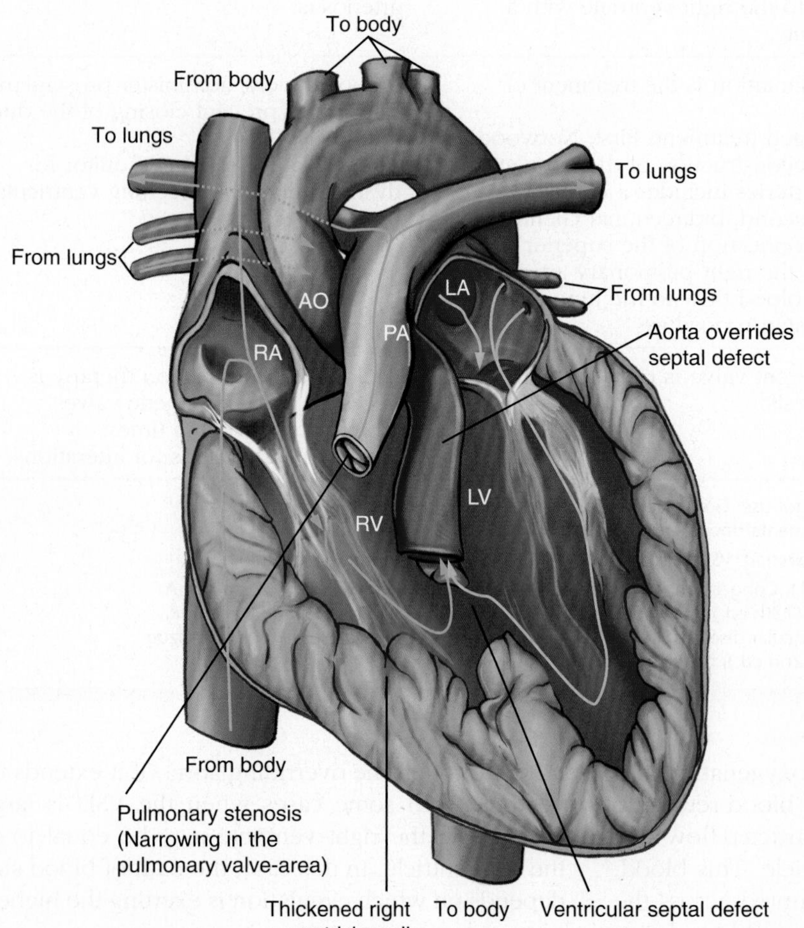

FIGURE 41.2 Tetralogy of Fallot.

child's respiratory rate and observe work of breathing, noting retractions, shortness of breath, or noisy breathing. Document oxygen saturation via pulse oximetry; it will likely be decreased. Auscultate the chest for adventitious breath sounds, which may suggest the development of heart failure. Auscultate the heart, noting a loud, harsh murmur characteristic of this disorder.

Laboratory and Diagnostic Tests

Note increased hematocrit, hemoglobin, and RBC count associated with polycythemia. Additional testing may include:

- **Echocardiography** (ultrasound study of structure and motion of heart), possibly revealing right ventricular hypertrophy, decreased pulmonary blood flow, and reduced size of the pulmonary artery
- Electrocardiogram (ECG), indicating right ventricular hypertrophy
- Cardiac catheterization and angiography, which reveal the extent of the structural defects

> **Consider This!**
>
> Ava Gardener, 2 weeks old, is brought to the clinic by her mother. She presents with trouble feeding. Her mother states, "When Ava eats, she seems to have trouble breathing, and a couple of times she has looked a little bluish." As the nurse takes Ava into her arms, Ava has a hypercyanotic spell.
>
> Ava is to be admitted to the hospital secondary to suspected tetralogy of Fallot. Ava's mother is very upset about the diagnosis. She says "my poor baby; she'll never ever be able to run and play like a normal child."
>
> How should the nurse respond? How would you feel if your young baby was diagnosed with a serious disorder? What type of support can the nurse provide to Ava's mother?

Tricuspid Atresia

Tricuspid atresia is a congenital heart defect in which the valve between the right atrium and right ventricle fails to develop. As a result, there is no opening to allow blood to flow from the right atrium to the right ventricle and subsequently through the pulmonary artery into the lungs (Brown & Fulton, 2011; Darst et al., 2014).

Pathophysiology

In tricuspid atresia, blood returning from the systemic circulation to the right atrium cannot directly enter the right ventricle due to agenesis of the tricuspid valve. Subsequently, deoxygenated blood may pass through an opening in the atrial septum (patent foramen ovale)

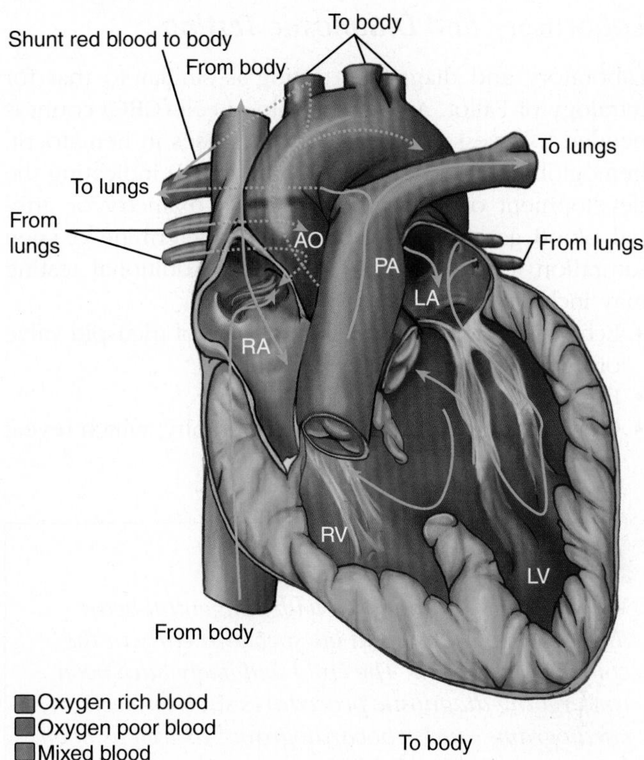

FIGURE 41.3 Tricuspid atresia.

into the left atrium, never entering the pulmonary vasculature. Thus, deoxygenated blood mixes with oxygenated blood in the left atrium. The blood then travels to the lungs through a PDA. Most cases of tricuspid atresia are associated with a VSD and the newborn receives inadequately oxygenated blood (Fig. 41.3) (Darst et al., 2014).

Nursing Assessment

Nursing assessment consists of the health history, physical examination, and laboratory and diagnostic tests.

Health History and Physical Examination

Note the infant's history since birth. Document history of cyanosis either at birth or a few days later when the ductus arteriosus closed. Note history of rapid respirations and difficulty with feeding. Inspect the skin for cyanosis or a pale gray color. Observe the apical impulse, noting overactivity. Evaluate the baby's sucking strength (will usually have a weak or poor suck). Count the respiratory rate, noting tachypnea. Note increased work of breathing. Auscultate the lungs, noting crackles or wheezes if heart failure is beginning to develop. Auscultate the heart, noting a murmur. Palpate the skin, noting coolness and clamminess of the extremities. Document the presence of clubbing in the older infant or child.

Laboratory and Diagnostic Testing

Laboratory and diagnostic testing is similar to that for tetralogy of Fallot. A complete blood cell (CBC) count is needed to assess compensatory increases in hematocrit, hemoglobin, and erythrocyte count (RBC) indicating the development of polycythemia. Pulse oximetry or arterial blood gas tests may be used to determine oxygen saturation levels (typically reduced). Additional testing may include:

- Echocardiography, revealing absence of tricuspid valve or underdeveloped right ventricle
- ECG, indicating possible heart failure
- Cardiac catheterization and angiography, which reveal the extent of the structural defects

Atraumatic Care

When a child is diagnosed with congenital heart disease, involve the child life specialist early in the course of treatment. The child will likely have been undergoing diagnostic procedures such as electrocardiograms, and echocardiograms, as well as open heart surgery. The child life specialist can be very helpful with providing atraumatic care.

Disorders with Increased Pulmonary Flow

Most congenital heart defects involve increased pulmonary blood flow. Normally, the left side of the heart has a higher pressure than the right side. Defects with connections involving the left and right sides will shunt blood from the higher-pressure left side to the lower-pressure right side. Even a small pressure gradient such as a 1- to 3-mm difference between the left and right sides will produce a movement of blood from the left to the right. In turn, the increase of blood on the right side of the heart will cause a greater amount of blood to move through the heart. If the amount of blood flowing to the lungs is large, the child may develop heart failure early in life. In addition, right ventricular hypertrophy may result. Sometimes with ventricular hypertrophy the right side of the heart pumps so forcefully that left-to-right shunting is reversed to right-to-left shunting. If this occurs, deoxygenated blood mixes with oxygenated blood, thereby lowering the overall blood oxygen saturation level.

Excessive blood flow to the lungs can produce a compensatory response such as tachypnea or tachycardia. Tachypnea increases caloric expenditure; poor cellular nutrition from decreased peripheral blood flow leads to feeding problems. Subsequently, the infant experiences poor weight gain, which retards overall growth and development. Increased pulmonary blood flow results in decreased systemic blood flow, so sodium and fluid retention may occur. Increased pulmonary blood flow also places the child at higher risk for pulmonary infections. As the child grows, the continuous increased pulmonary blood flow will cause vasoconstriction of the pulmonary vessels, actually decreasing the pulmonary blood flow. This may lead to pulmonary hypertension. For children with congenital defects with increased pulmonary blood flow, oxygen supplementation is not helpful. Oxygen acts as a pulmonary vasodilator. If pulmonary dilation occurs, pulmonary blood flow is even greater, causing tachypnea, increasing lung fluid retention, and eventually causing a much greater problem with oxygenation. Over time, continuous increased pulmonary blood flow may cause pulmonary vasoconstriction and pulmonary hypertension. Therefore, preventing the development of pulmonary disease via early surgical correction is essential.

Examples of defects with increased pulmonary blood flow are ASD, VSD, atrioventricular canal defect, and PDA.

Atrial Septal Defect

An ASD is a passageway or hole in the wall (septum) that divides the right atrium from the left atrium (Fig. 41.4). Three types of ASDs are identified based on the location of the opening:

- Ostium primum (ASD1): the opening is at the lower portion of the septum.
- Ostium secundum (ASD2): the opening is near the center of the septum.
- Sinus venosus defect: the opening is near the junction of the superior vena cava and the right atrium.

When the ASD is small, as many as 80% of infants may have a spontaneous closure within the first 18 months of life. If it does not spontaneously close by age 3, the child will most likely need corrective surgery (Brown & Fulton, 2011; Darst et al., 2014).

Pathophysiology

With ASD, blood flows through the opening from the left atrium to the right atrium due to pressure differences. The shunting increases the blood volume entering the right atrium. This, in turn, leads to increased blood flow into the lungs. If untreated, the defect can cause problems such as pulmonary hypertension, heart failure, atrial arrhythmias, or stroke (Brown & Fulton, 2011; Darst et al., 2014).

Nursing Assessment

Most children with ASDs are asymptomatic. However, a very large defect can cause increased blood flow, leading to heart failure, which results in shortness of breath, easy fatigability, or poor growth.

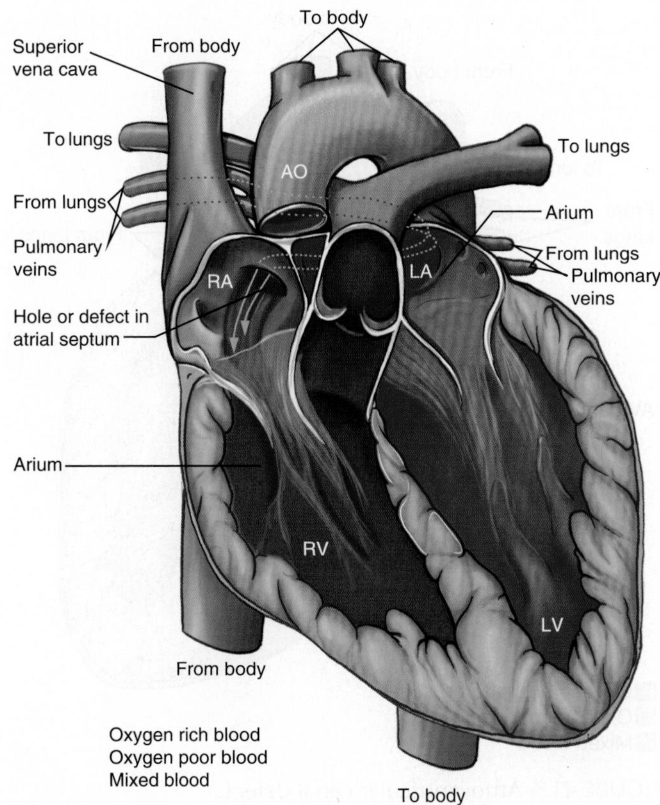

FIGURE 41.4 Atrial septal defect; note the opening between the two atria.

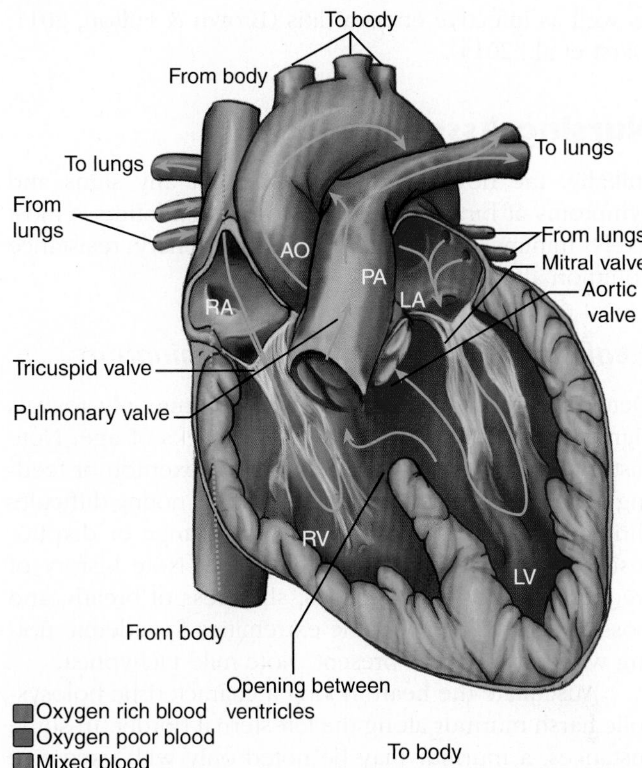

FIGURE 41.5 Ventricular septal defect; note the opening between the ventricles.

Health History and Physical Examination

Obtain the health history, noting poor feeding as an infant, decreased ability to keep up with peers, or history of difficulty growing. Observe the child's chest, noting a hyperdynamic precordium. Auscultate the heart, noting a fixed split second heart sound and a systolic ejection murmur, best heard in the pulmonic valve area. Palpate along the left sternal border for a right ventricular heave.

Laboratory and Diagnostic Tests

Echocardiography is done to confirm the diagnosis. An **electrocardiogram (ECG)** (graphic recording of the heart's electrical activity) may show normal sinus rhythm or prolonged PR intervals. The chest x-ray may show enlargement of the heart and increased vascularity of the lungs.

Ventricular Septal Defect

A VSD is an opening between the right and left ventricular chambers of the heart (Fig. 41.5). It is one of the most common congenital heart defects and accounts for about 30% of all congenital heart defects. Spontaneous closure of small VSDs occurs in about half of children by age 2 years. Long-term outcomes for surgically repaired VSDs are good. Repair of larger defects by 2 years of age is recommended to prevent the development of pulmonary disease (Brown & Fulton, 2011; Darst et al., 2014).

Pathophysiology

In VSD, there is an abnormal opening between the right and left ventricles. The opening varies in size, from as small as a pinhole to a complete opening between the ventricles so that the right and left sides are as one. Children with small VSDs may remain asymptomatic. In other children, blood shunts across the opening in the septum. Pulmonary vascular resistance and systemic vascular resistance determine the direction of blood flow. A left-to-right shunt results when pulmonary vascular resistance is low. Increased amounts of blood flowing into the right ventricle are then pumped to the pulmonary circulation, eventually causing an increase in pulmonary vascular resistance. Increased pulmonary vascular resistance leads to increased pulmonary artery pressure (pulmonary hypertension) and right ventricular hypertrophy. When the pulmonary vascular resistance exceeds the systemic vascular resistance, right-to-left shunting of blood across the VSD occurs, resulting in Eisenmenger syndrome (pulmonary hypertension and cyanosis). Heart failure commonly occurs in children with moderate to severe unrepaired VSDs. Children with VSDs are also at risk for the development of aortic valve regurgitation as well as infective endocarditis (Brown & Fulton, 2011; Darst et al., 2014).

Nursing Assessment

Initially, the newborn may not exhibit any signs and symptoms at birth because left-to-right shunting is most likely minimal due to the high pulmonary resistance common after birth.

Health History and Physical Examination

Determine the health history, which commonly reveals signs of heart failure around 4 to 8 weeks of age. Note history of tiring easily, particularly with exertion or feeding. Document the child's growth history, noting difficulty thriving. Ask the parent about color change or diaphoresis with nipple feeding in the infant. Note history of frequent pulmonary infections, shortness of breath, and possibly edema. Inspect the extremities for edema, noting whether pitting is present. Note mild tachypnea.

Auscultate the heart, noting a characteristic holosystolic harsh murmur along the left sternal border. In some instances, a murmur may be noted only with excessive blood flow across the opening. Adventitious lung sounds may be auscultated if the child is experiencing heart failure. Palpate the chest for a thrill.

Laboratory and Diagnostic Tests

Magnetic resonance imaging (MRI) or echocardiogram with color flow Doppler may reveal the opening as well as the extent of left-to-right shunting. These studies also may identify right ventricular hypertrophy and dilation of the pulmonary artery resulting from the increased blood flow. Cardiac catheterization may be used to evaluate the extent of blood flow being pumped to the pulmonary circulation and to evaluate hemodynamic pressures.

Atrioventricular Canal Defect

Atrioventricular canal defect (atrioventricular septal defect [AVSD], AV canal, or endocardial cushion defect) accounts for 3.5% of CHD. Forty-five percent of children with Down syndrome and CHD have this defect (Brown & Fulton, 2011).

Pathophysiology

AV canal defect occurs as a result of failure of the endocardial cushions to fuse (Fig. 41.6). These cushions are needed to separate the central parts of the heart near the tricuspid and mitral (AV) valves. The complete AV canal defect involves ASDs and VSDs as well as a common AV orifice and a common AV valve. Partial and transitional

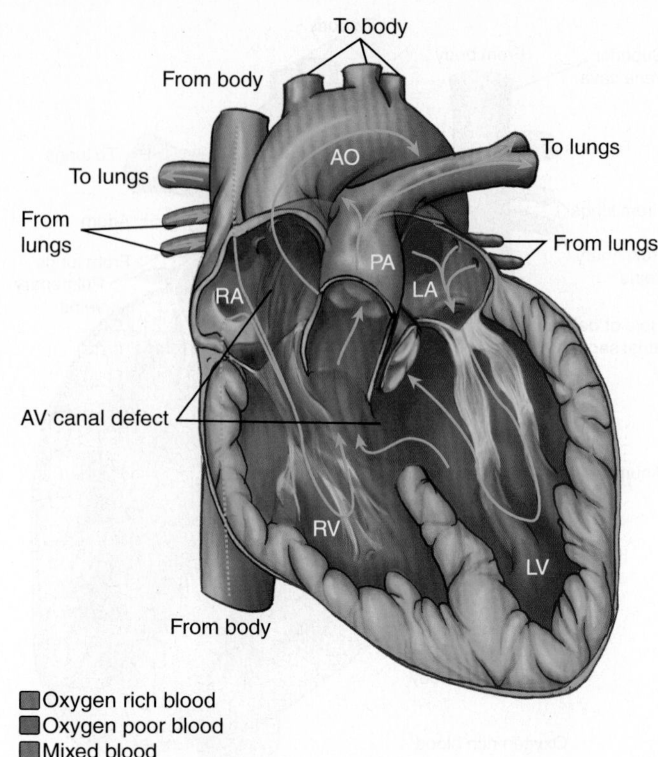

FIGURE 41.6 Atrioventricular canal defect.

forms of AV canal defect also occur, involving variations of the complete form.

The complete AV canal defect permits oxygenated blood from the lungs to enter the left atrium and ventricle, crossing over the atrial or ventricular septum and returning to the lungs via the pulmonary artery. This recirculation problem, which typically involves a left-to-right shunt, is inefficient because the left ventricle must pump blood back to the lungs and also meet the body's peripheral demand for oxygenated blood. Subsequently, the left ventricle must pump two to three times more blood than in a normal heart. Therefore, this specific type of cardiac defect causes a large left-to-right shunt; an increased workload of the left ventricle; and high pulmonary arterial pressure, resulting in an increased amount of blood in the lungs and causing pulmonary edema (Brown & Fulton, 2011; Darst et al., 2014).

Nursing Assessment

The infant with a complete AV canal defect commonly exhibits moderate to severe signs and symptoms of heart failure. However, for infants with partial or transitional AV canal defects, the signs and symptoms will be subtler.

Health History and Physical Examination

Obtain the health history, noting frequent respiratory infections and difficulty gaining weight. Ask the parent if the infant has been experiencing difficulty feeding or increased work of breathing.

Inspect the skin, fingernails, and lips for cyanosis. Observe for retractions, tachypnea, and nasal flaring. Auscultate the lungs and heart, noting rales and a loud murmur. The murmur is commonly noted within the first 2 weeks of life. Infants with partial or transitional AV canal defects may display more subtle signs.

Laboratory and Diagnostic Tests

Echocardiography will reveal the extent of the defect and shunting as well as right ventricular hypertrophy. ECG may indicate right ventricular hypertrophy and possible first-degree heart block due to impulse blocking before reaching the AV node.

Patent Ductus Arteriosus

PDA is failure of the ductus arteriosus, a fetal circulatory structure, to close within the first weeks of life (Fig. 41.7). As a result, there is a connection between the aorta and pulmonary artery. PDA is the second most common congenital heart defect and accounts for 10% of CHD cases (Darst et al., 2014). PDA occurs much more frequently in premature than in term infants and in infants born at high altitudes compared with those born at sea level. Infants with other CHDs that result in right-to-left shunting of blood and cyanosis may additionally display a PDA. In these infants, the PDA allows for some level of oxygenated blood to reach the systemic circulation (Brown & Fulton, 2011; Darst et al., 2014).

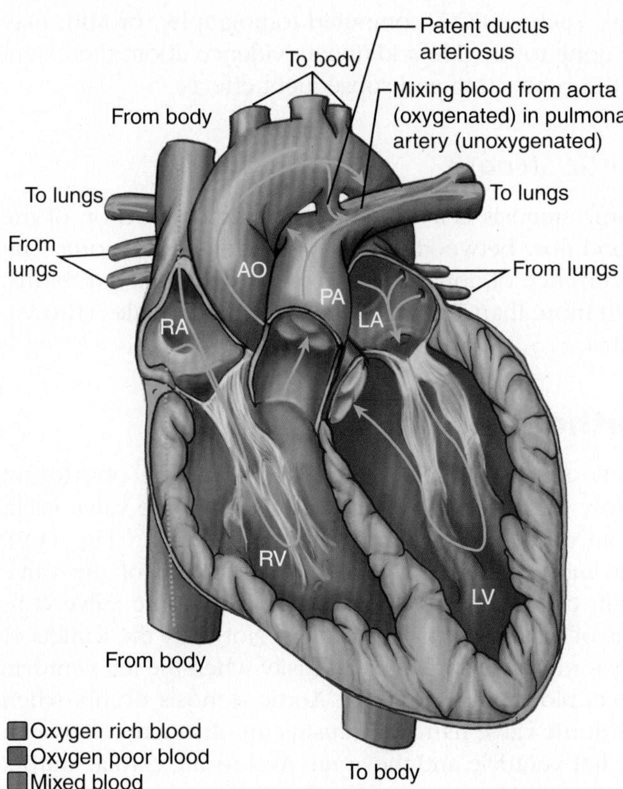

FIGURE 41.7 Patent ductus arteriosus.

Pathophysiology

Failure of the ductus arteriosus to close leads to continued blood flow from the aorta to the pulmonary artery. Blood returning to the left atrium passes to the left ventricle, enters the aorta, and then travels to the pulmonary artery via the PDA instead of entering the systemic circulation. This altered blood flow pattern increases the workload of the left side of the heart. Pulmonary vascular congestion occurs, causing an increase in pressure. Right ventricular pressure increases in an attempt to overcome this increase in pulmonary pressure. Eventually, right ventricular hypertrophy occurs (Brown & Fulton, 2011; Darst et al., 2014).

Nursing Assessment

The symptoms of PDA depend on the size of the ductus arteriosus and the amount of blood flow it carries. If it is small, the infant may be asymptomatic. Some infants demonstrate signs and symptoms of heart failure.

Health History and Physical Examination

Determine the health history, which may reveal frequent respiratory infections, fatigue, and poor growth and development. On physical examination, note tachycardia, tachypnea, bounding peripheral pulses, and a widened pulse pressure. The diastolic BP typically is low due to the shunting. Auscultate the lungs and heart, noting rales if heart failure is present. Note a harsh, continuous, machine-like murmur, usually loudest under the left clavicle at the first and second intercostal spaces.

Laboratory and Diagnostic Tests

Echocardiogram reveals the extent of the defective opening and confirms the diagnosis. ECG may be normal or it may indicate ventricular hypertrophy, especially if the defect is large. Chest radiography demonstrates cardiomegaly.

Obstructive Disorders

Another group of congenital heart defects is classified as obstructive disorders. These disorders involve some type of narrowing of a major vessel, interfering with the ability of the blood to flow freely through the vessel. As a result, peripheral circulation or blood flow to the lungs is affected. Increased pressure backing up toward the heart causes an increased workload on the heart. Examples

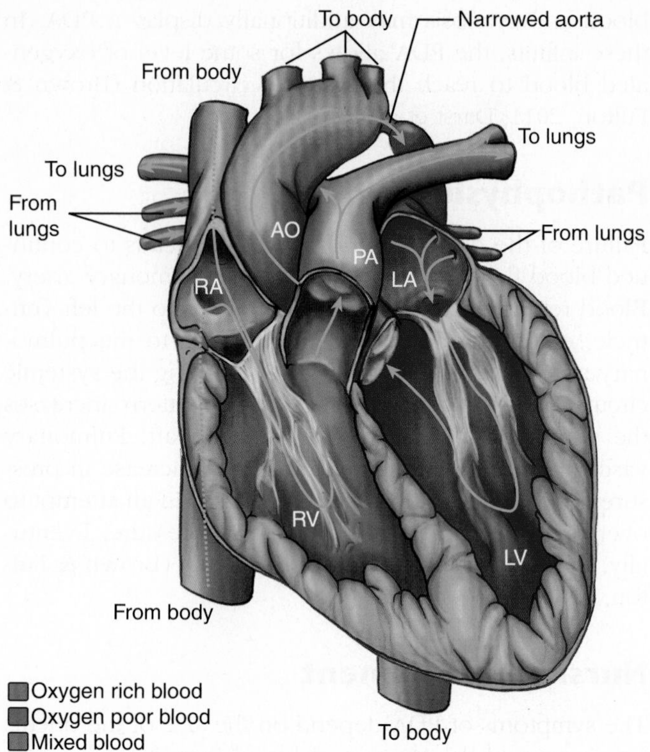

FIGURE 41.8 Coarctation of the aorta.

of defects in this group include coarctation of the aorta, aortic stenosis, and pulmonic stenosis.

Coarctation of the Aorta

Coarctation of the aorta is narrowing of the aorta, the major blood vessel carrying highly oxygenated blood from the left ventricle of the heart to the rest of the body (Fig. 41.8). It accounts for 4.2% to 6% of congenital heart defects and occurs three times more often in males than in females (Brown & Fulton, 2011; Darst et al., 2014).

Pathophysiology

Coarctation of the aorta occurs most often in the area near the ductus arteriosus. The narrowing can be preductal (between the subclavian artery and ductus arteriosus) or postductal (after the ductus arteriosus). As a result of the narrowing, blood flow is impeded, causing pressure to increase in the area proximal to the defect and to decrease in the area distal to it. Thus, BP is increased in the heart and upper portions of the body and decreased in the lower portions of the body. Left ventricular afterload is increased, and in some children this may lead to heart failure. Collateral circulation also may develop as the body attempts to ensure adequate blood flow to the descending aorta. Due to the elevation in BP, the child is also at risk for aortic rupture, aortic aneurysm, and CVA (Brown & Fulton, 2011; Darst et al., 2014).

Nursing Assessment

The extent of the symptoms depends on the severity of the coarctation. Some children with coarctation of the aorta grow well into the school-age years before the defect is discovered.

Health History and Physical Examination

Determine the health history, noting problems with irritability and frequent epistaxis. In older children, there also may be reports of leg pain with activity, dizziness, fainting, and headaches. Assess pulses throughout, noting full, bounding pulses in the upper extremities with weak or absent pulses in the lower extremities. Determine BP in all four extremities. BP in the upper extremities may be 20 mm Hg or higher than that in the lower extremities. Inspect the school-age child's chest, noting notching of the ribs. Auscultate the heart for a soft or moderately loud systolic murmur, most often heard at the base of the heart (on the back or in the left axilla) (Darst et al., 2014).

Laboratory and Diagnostic Tests

Diagnosis of coarctation of the aorta is based primarily on the history and physical examination. In addition, an echocardiogram may disclose the extent of narrowing and evidence of collateral circulation. Chest radiography may reveal left-sided cardiac enlargement and rib notching indicative of collateral arterial enlargement. Other tests, such as ECG, computed tomography, or MRI, may be done to provide additional evidence about the extent of the coarctation and subsequent effects.

Aortic Stenosis

Aortic stenosis is a condition causing obstruction of the blood flow between the left ventricle and the aorta. The occurrence of aortic stenosis is 3.8 per 1,000 live births, with more than 75% of cases occurring in males (Brown, 2016).

Pathophysiology

Aortic stenosis can be caused by a muscle obstruction below the aortic valve, an obstruction at the valve itself, or an aortic narrowing just above the valve (Fig. 41.9). The most common type is an obstruction of the valve itself, called aortic valve stenosis. The aortic valve consists of three very pliable leaflets. Normally the leaflets of the aortic valve spread open easily when the left ventricle ejects blood into the aorta. Aortic stenosis occurs when the aortic valve narrows, causing an obstruction between the left ventricle and the aorta. As a result, cardiac output decreases. When the aortic valve does not function properly, the left ventricle must work harder to pump blood

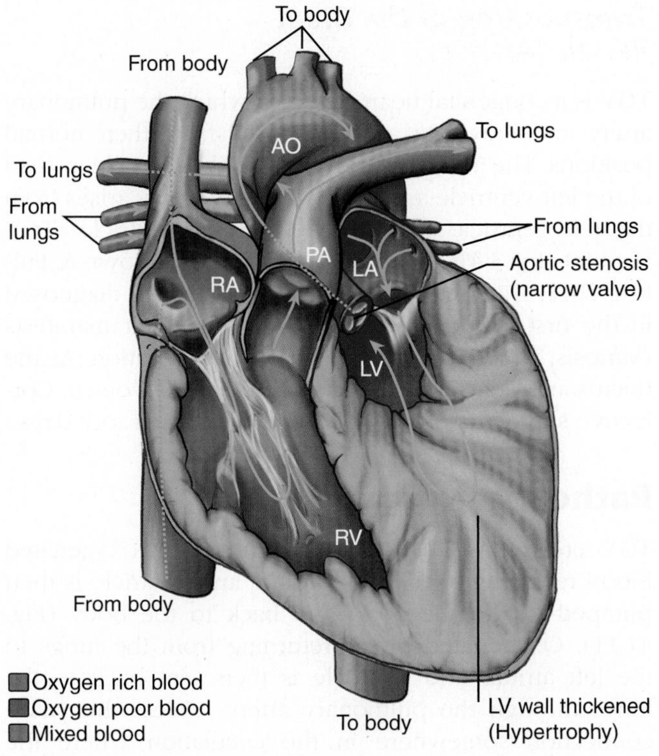

FIGURE 41.9 Aortic stenosis.

into the aorta. Because of the increased workload, the left ventricular muscle hypertrophies. If this continues, left ventricular failure can occur, leading to a backup of pressure in the pulmonary circulation and pulmonary edema. Heart failure may occur, but this is more commonly seen in the infant (Brown, 2016; Brown & Fulton, 2011).

Nursing Assessment

Typically, the child with aortic stenosis is asymptomatic. However, it is important to obtain an accurate health history and perform a physical examination.

Health History and Physical Examination

Obtain the child's health history, noting easy fatigability or complaints of chest pain similar to anginal pain when active. Dizziness with prolonged standing also may be reported. In the infant, note difficulty with feeding. Palpate the child's pulse; if aortic stenosis is severe, the pulses may be faint. Palpate the child's chest, noting a thrill at the base of the heart. Auscultate the heart, noting a systolic murmur best heard along the left sternal border with radiation to the right upper sternal border.

Laboratory and Diagnostic Tests

The echocardiogram is the most important noninvasive test to identify aortic stenosis. An ECG may be normal in children with mild to moderate forms of aortic stenosis. For children with severe aortic stenosis, left ventricular hypertrophy may be determined from the ECG. For children experiencing easy fatigability and chest pain, an exercise stress test may be done to evaluate the degree of cardiac compromise.

Pulmonary Stenosis

Pulmonary stenosis is a condition that causes an obstruction in blood flow between the right ventricle and the pulmonary arteries. Pulmonary stenosis occurs in 0.6 to 0.8 per 1,000 live births (Peng & Perry, 2016). It is often associated with other heart anomalies and with genetic syndromes. Children may be asymptomatic, although some children with severe stenosis may exhibit dyspnea and fatigue with exertion (demonstrating hypercyanotic spells similar to those in children with tetralogy of Fallot) (Peng & Perry, 2016).

Pathophysiology

Pulmonary stenosis may occur as a muscular obstruction below the pulmonary valve, an obstruction at the valve, or a narrowing of the pulmonary artery above the valve (Fig. 41.10). Valve obstruction is the most common form of pulmonary stenosis. Normally the pulmonary valve is constructed with three thin and pliable

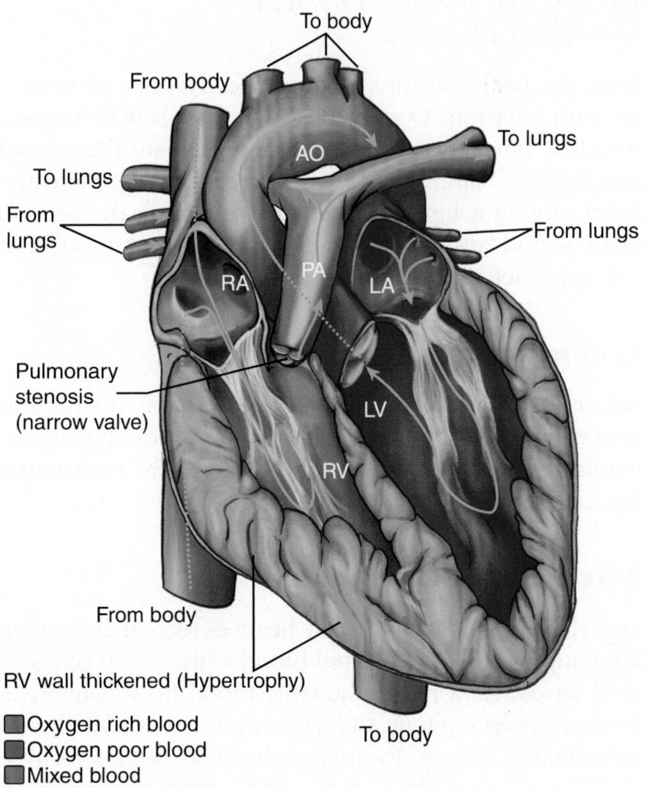

FIGURE 41.10 Pulmonary stenosis.

valve leaflets; they spread apart easily, allowing the right ventricle to eject blood freely into the pulmonary artery. The most common problem causing pulmonary stenosis is that the pulmonary valve leaflets are thickened and fused together along their separation lines, causing the obstruction to blood flow. The right ventricle has an additional workload, causing the muscle to thicken, resulting in right ventricular hypertrophy and decreased pulmonary blood flow. When the pulmonary valve is severely obstructed, the right ventricle cannot eject sufficient blood into the pulmonary artery. As a result, pressure in the right atrium increases, which could lead to a reopening of the foramen ovale. If this occurs, deoxygenated blood would pass through the foramen ovale into the left side of the heart and would then be pumped to the systemic circulation. In some cases, a PDA may be present, thus allowing for some compensation by shunting blood from the aorta to the pulmonary circulation for oxygenation (Brown & Fulton, 2011; Peng & Perry, 2016).

Nursing Assessment

The child with pulmonary stenosis may be asymptomatic or may exhibit signs and symptoms of mild heart failure. If the stenosis is severe, the child may demonstrate cyanosis. Therefore, it is important for the nurse to obtain an accurate health history and physical examination.

Health History and Physical Examination

Elicit the health history, noting mild dyspnea or cyanosis with exertion. Document the child's growth history, which is typically normal. Carefully palpate the sternal border for a thrill (not always present). Auscultate the heart, noting a high-pitched click following the second heart sound and a systolic ejection murmur loudest at the upper left sternal border.

Laboratory and Diagnostic Tests

An echocardiogram reveals the extent of obstruction present at the valve, as well as right ventricular hypertrophy. An ECG also helps to detect right ventricular hypertrophy.

Mixed Defects

Mixed defects are congenital heart defects that involve a mixing of well-oxygenated blood with poorly oxygenated blood. As a result, systemic blood flow contains a lower oxygen content. Cardiac output is decreased, and heart failure occurs. Examples of mixed defects include TGV, total anomalous pulmonary venous connection (TAPVC), truncus arteriosus, and HLHS.

Transposition of the Great Vessels (Arteries)

TGV is a congenital heart defect in which the pulmonary artery and the aorta are transposed from their normal positions. The aorta arises from the right ventricle instead of the left ventricle and the pulmonary artery arises from the left ventricle instead of the right ventricle. TGV accounts for 3.4% to 5% of all CHD cases (Brown & Fulton, 2011; Darst et al., 2014). It is most often diagnosed in the first few days of life when the infant manifests cyanosis, which indicates decreased oxygenation. As the ductus arteriosus closes, the symptoms will worsen. Corrective surgery is usually performed by age 4 to 7 days.

Pathophysiology

TGV creates a situation in which poorly oxygenated blood returning to the right atrium and ventricle is then pumped out to the aorta and back to the body (Fig. 41.11). Oxygenated blood returning from the lungs to the left atrium and ventricle is then sent back to the lungs through the pulmonary artery. Unless there is a connection somewhere in the circulation where the oxygen-rich and oxygen-poor blood can mix, all the organs of the body will be poorly oxygenated. Often the ductus arteriosus remains patent, allowing for some mixing of blood. Similarly, if a VSD is also present, mixing of blood may occur and cyanosis will be delayed. However, these associated defects can lead to increased

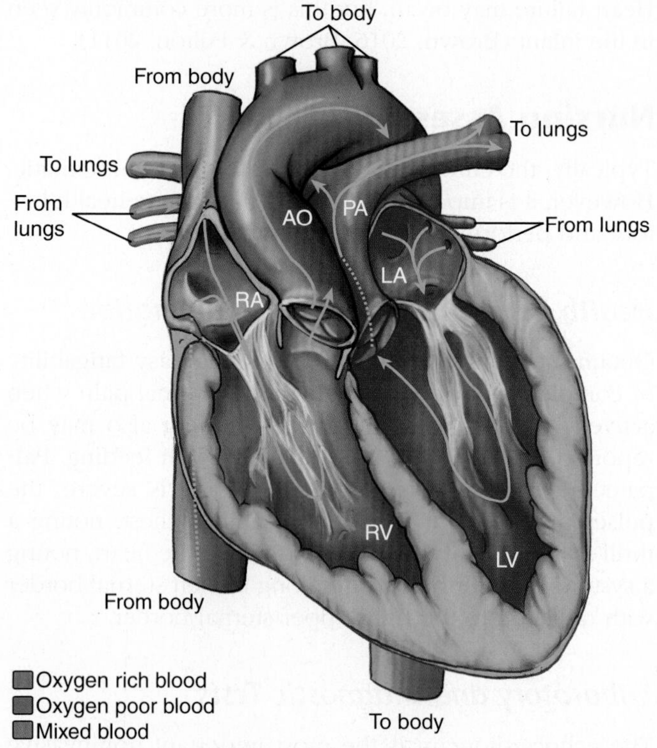

FIGURE 41.11 Transposition of the great vessels.

pulmonary blood flow that increases pressure in the pulmonary circulation. This predisposes the child to heart failure (Brown & Fulton, 2011; Darst et al., 2014).

Nursing Assessment

Significant cyanosis without a murmur in the newborn period is highly indicative of TGV. In some infants, cyanosis will not develop until several days of age as the PDA closes. In infants with septal defects, cyanosis may be further delayed.

Health History and Physical Examination

Elicit the health history, noting onset of cyanosis with feeding or crying. Observe the infant for cyanosis while active and at rest. Observe the chest, noting a prominent ventricular impulse. Auscultate the heart, noting a loud second heart sound. A murmur may be heard if the ductus remains open or a septal defect is present. If heart failure is present, note edema, tachypnea, and adventitious lung sounds.

Laboratory and Diagnostic Tests

Echocardiography clearly reveals evidence of the transposition. Cardiac catheterization may be performed to determine whether oxygen saturation levels are low due to the mixing of the blood.

Total Anomalous Pulmonary Venous Connection

TAPVC is a congenital heart defect in which the pulmonary veins do not connect normally to the left atrium. Instead, they connect to the right atrium, often by way of the superior vena cava. Relatively rare, it occurs in about 1 in 17,000 live births (Brown & Fulton, 2011).

Pathophysiology

Oxygenated blood that would normally enter the left atrium now enters the right atrium and passes to the right ventricle. As a result, the pressure on the right side of the heart increases, leading to hypertrophy. TAPVC is incompatible with life unless there is an associated defect present that allows for shunting of blood from the highly pressured right side of the heart. A patent foramen ovale or an ASD is usually present. Since none of the pulmonary veins connect normally to the left atrium, the only source of blood to the left atrium is blood that is shunted from the right atrium across the defect to the left side of the heart (Fig. 41.12). The highly oxygenated blood from the lungs completely mixes with the poorly oxygenated blood returning from the systemic circulation. This causes an overload of the right atrium and right ventricle. The increased blood volume going into the lungs can lead to pulmonary hypertension and pulmonary edema (Brown & Fulton, 2011; Darst et al., 2014).

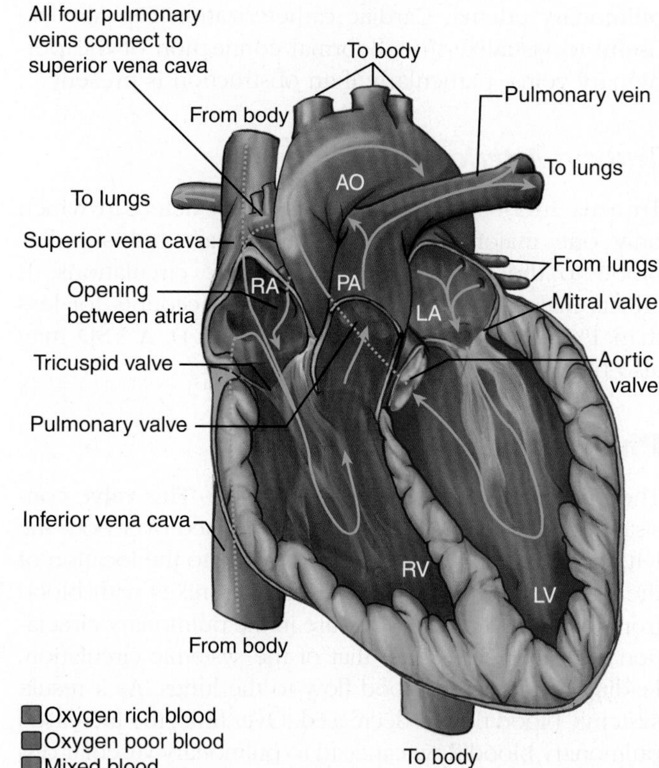

FIGURE 41.12 Total anomalous pulmonary venous connection.

Nursing Assessment

The degree of cyanosis present with TAPVC depends on the extent of the associated defects. For example, if the foramen ovale closes or the ASD is small, significant cyanosis will be present. The physical examination findings will vary depending on the type of TAPVC the infant has, whether obstruction is present, and whether other associated cardiac anomalies are present.

Health History and Physical Examination

Note history of cyanosis, tiring easily, and difficulty feeding. Observe the chest for prominence of the right ventricular impulse and retractions with tachypnea. Auscultate the heart, noting fixed splitting of the second heart sound and a murmur. Palpate the abdomen for hepatomegaly.

Laboratory and Diagnostic Tests

An echocardiogram will reveal the abnormal connection of the pulmonary veins, enlargement of the right atrium and right ventricle, and an ASD if present. The chest x-ray will demonstrate an enlarged heart and pulmonary edema. Cardiac catheterization can also be useful to visualize the abnormal connection of the pulmonary veins, particularly if an obstruction is present.

Truncus Arteriosus

Truncus arteriosus is a congenital heart defect in which only one major artery leaves the heart and supplies blood to the pulmonary and systemic circulations. It affects males and females equally and accounts for less than 1% all CHD cases (Darst et al., 2014). A VSD may also be present.

Pathophysiology

The one great vessel contains one valve. This valve consists of two to five leaflets and is positioned over both the left and right ventricles (Fig. 41.13). Due to the location of the valve, blood from the left ventricle mixes with blood from the right ventricle. Pressure in the pulmonary circulation typically is less than that of the systemic circulation, leading to increased blood flow to the lungs. As a result, systemic blood flow is decreased. Over time, the increased pulmonary blood flow can lead to pulmonary vascular disease (Brown & Fulton, 2011; Darst et al., 2014).

Nursing Assessment

Typically, the infant demonstrates cyanosis in varying degrees, depending on the extent of compromise in the systemic circulation. Obtain an accurate health history and perform a physical examination.

Health History and Physical Examination

Elicit the health history, noting history of cyanosis that increases with periods of activity such as feeding. Also note history of tiring easily, difficulty in feeding, and poor growth. Count the respiratory rate, which may be elevated. Observe for nasal flaring, grunting or noisy breathing, retractions, and restlessness. Auscultate the lungs, noting adventitious breath sounds, and the heart, noting a murmur associated with a VSD.

Laboratory and Diagnostic Tests

An echocardiogram will confirm the presence of truncus arteriosus as the anatomy of the great vessels, the single truncal valve, and the VSD will be seen. On rare occasions a cardiac catheterization may be done to determine pressures in the pulmonary arteries.

Hypoplastic Left Heart Syndrome

HLHS is a congenital heart defect in which all of the structures on the left side of the heart are severely underdeveloped (Fig. 41.14). The mitral and aortic valves are completely closed or very small. The left ventricle is nonfunctional. Thus, the left side of the heart is completely

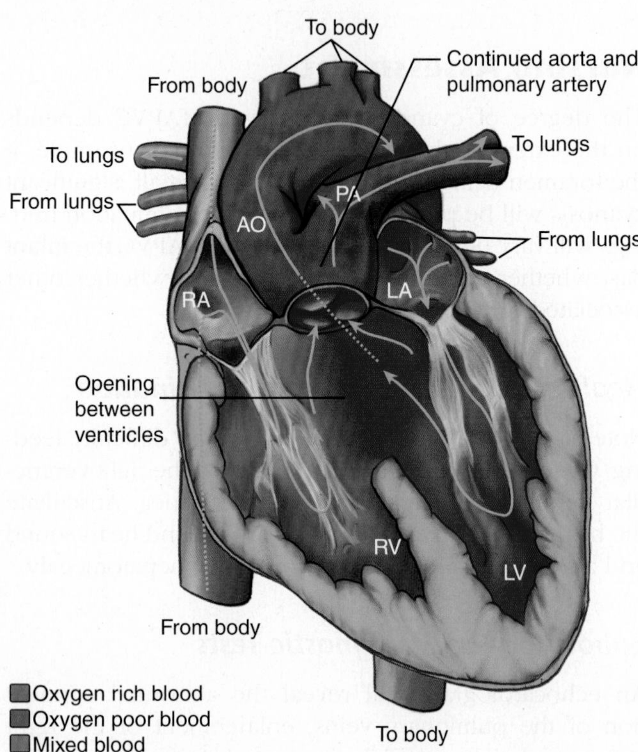

FIGURE 41.13 Truncus arteriosus.

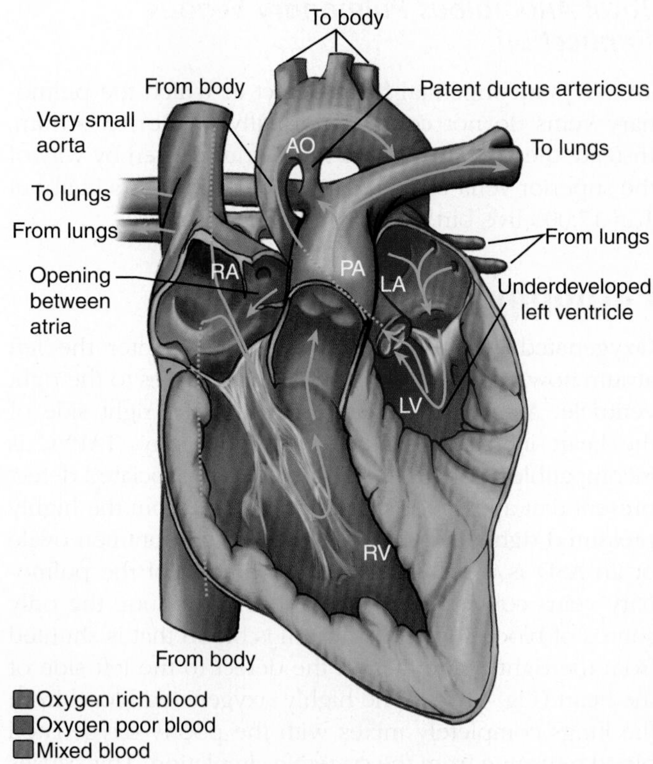

FIGURE 41.14 Hypoplastic left heart syndrome.

unable to supply blood to the systemic circulation. HLHS is the fourth most common congenital heart defect. It appears to have a multifactorial and autosomal recessive inheritance pattern and occurs in 1.4% to 3.8% of cases of CHD (Darst et al., 2014). The options for treatment include palliative care, cardiac transplantation within the first few weeks of life, or palliative reconstructive surgery consisting of three stages, beginning within days to weeks of birth.

Pathophysiology

With HLHS, the right side of the heart is the main working part of the heart. Blood returning from the lungs into the left atrium must pass through an ASD to the right side of the heart. The right ventricle must then pump blood to the lungs and also to the systemic circulation through the PDA. A few days after birth, when the ductus arteriosus closes, the heart cannot pump blood into the systemic circulation, causing poor perfusion of the vital organs and shock. Death will occur rapidly without intervention (Brown & Fulton, 2011; Darst et al., 2014).

Nursing Assessment

Initially after birth, the newborn may be asymptomatic because the ductus arteriosus is still patent. However, as the ductus begins to close at a few days of age, the newborn will begin to exhibit cyanosis. Some infants may present with circulatory collapse (shock) and must be resuscitated emergently.

Health History and Physical Examination

Obtain the health history, noting onset of cyanosis. Note poor feeding and history of tiring easily. Evaluate the vital signs, noting tachycardia, tachypnea, and hypothermia. Observe for increased work of breathing and gradually increasing cyanosis. Note pallor of the extremities and decreased oxygen saturation via pulse oximetry. Auscultate the heart and lungs. Note adventitious breath sounds, a gallop rhythm, a single second heart sound, and a soft systolic ejection or holosystolic murmur.

Laboratory and Diagnostic Tests

Prenatally, a fetal echocardiogram can diagnose this syndrome, as can a maternal ultrasound. After birth, the echocardiogram illustrates the defect.

Nursing Management of the Child with Congenital Heart Disease

The child with a congenital heart defect has multiple needs and requires comprehensive, multidisciplinary care. Nurses play a key role in helping the child and family during this intensely stressful time. Nursing care focuses on improving oxygenation, promoting adequate nutrition, assisting the child and family with coping, providing postoperative nursing care, preventing infection, and providing child and family education. An important component of education involves preparing the child and parents for discharge. In addition to the nursing management presented below, refer to Nursing Care Plan 41.1 for additional interventions appropriate for the child with CHD. Individualize nursing care specific to the child's needs.

Improving Oxygenation

Due to the hemodynamic changes accompanying the underlying structural defect, oxygenation is key. Provide frequent ongoing assessment of the child's cardiopulmonary status. Assess airway patency and suction as needed. Position the child in the Fowler or semi-Fowler position to facilitate lung expansion. Monitor vital signs, especially heart and respiratory rates. Monitor the child's color and oxygen saturation levels closely, using these to guide oxygen administration. Observe for tachypnea and other signs of respiratory distress, such as nasal flaring, grunting, and retractions. Auscultate the lungs for adventitious sounds. Provide humidified supplemental oxygen as ordered, warming it to prevent wide temperature fluctuations. Anticipate the need for assisted ventilation if the child has difficulty maintaining the airway or experiences deterioration in oxygenation capacity. Box 41.1 lists interventions related to relief of hypercyanotic spells.

Promoting Adequate Nutrition

Adequate nutrition is critical to foster growth and development as well as to reduce the risk for infection. Children with congenital heart defects typically have

BOX 41.1

RELIEVING HYPERCYANOTIC SPELLS

- Use a calm, comforting approach.
- Place the infant or child in a knee-to-chest position.
- Provide supplemental oxygen.
- Administer morphine sulfate (0.1 mg/kg IV, IM, or SQ).
- Supply IV fluids.
- Administer propranolol (0.1 mg/kg IV).

IM, intramuscularly; SQ, subcutaneously.

Adapted from Doyle, T., Kavanaugh-McHugh, A., & Fish, F. A. (2016). *Management and outcome of tetralogy of Fallot*. Retrieved from www.uptodate.com/contents/management-and-outcome-of-tetralogy-of-fallot

increased nutritional needs due to the increased energy expenditure associated with increased cardiac and respiratory workloads. In addition, many of the defects lead to heart failure, which may affect the child's fluid balance status, further increasing the child's energy expenditure.

Nutrition may be provided orally, enterally, or parenterally. For example, for the newborn or infant, nutrition via breast milk or formula may be provided orally or via gavage feedings. Breastfeeding is usually associated with decreased energy expenditure during the act of feeding, yet some infants in intensive care are not stable enough to breastfeed. Gavage with breast milk is possible, and the use of human milk fortifier (either with breastfeeding or added to the gavage feed) adds additional calories that the infant requires. Formula-fed infants may also require increased-calorie formula, which may be achieved by more concentrated mixing of the formula or through the use of additives such as Polycose or vegetable oil. Consult the nutritionist to determine the individual infant's caloric needs and prescription of appropriate feeding.

Cutting a large hole in the nipple or "cross-cutting" the nipple decreases the work of feeding for some infants. Generally, nipple feedings should be limited to a 20-minute duration, as feeding for longer periods results in excess caloric expenditure. Many infants may feed orally for 20 minutes, receiving the remainder of that feeding via orogastric or nasogastric tube. Offer older children small, frequent feedings to reduce the amount of energy required to feed or eat and to prevent overtiring the child. When needed, administer and monitor total parenteral nutrition as prescribed.

Take Note!

Breastfeeding a child before and after cardiac surgery may boost the infant's immune system, which can help fight postoperative infection. If breastfeeding is not possible, mothers can pump milk and the breast milk may be given via bottle, dropper, or gavage feeding.

Assisting the Child and Family to Cope

The diagnosis of CHD is especially overwhelming for the child and the parents. The numerous examinations, diagnostic tests, and procedures are sources of stress for the infant or child regardless of age and for the parents. The parents may fear long-term disability or death or may worry that allowing the child to engage in any activity will worsen his or her status. Thus, the parents may tend to overprotect the child. It is important for the parents to continue parenting the child, even when the child requires extended hospitalizations or intensive care. Explain all that is happening with the child, using language the parents and child can understand. Allow the parents and child to voice their feelings, concerns, or questions. Provide ample time to address these questions and concerns. Encourage the parents and the child, as developmentally appropriate, to participate in the child's care.

If the child is a newborn or infant, encourage attachment and bonding. Emphasize the child's positive attributes, including the normal aspects of the infant. Help the parents to experience the joy of a new infant and see the beauty of the child, no matter how ill the infant is. Urge the parents to touch, stroke, pat, and talk to the infant. Encourage them to hold the infant close, using kangaroo care as appropriate. If the child is older, offer suggestions as to how the parents can meet the child's emotional needs. For example, encourage them to bring a favorite toy or object from home while the child is hospitalized.

Provide developmentally appropriate explanations to the child. Encourage play therapy to help the child understand what is happening.

Preventing Infection

Teach parents proper hand hygiene. Provide appropriate dental care. Make sure the child receives prophylaxis for infective endocarditis as needed. Ensure that children 24 months or younger who have hemodynamically significant heart defects receive respiratory syncytial virus (RSV) prophylaxis as recommended during RSV season (Ralston et al., 2014).

Providing Care for the Child Undergoing Cardiac Surgery

Cardiac surgery may be necessary to correct a congenital defect or to provide symptomatic relief. The surgery may be planned as an elective procedure or done as an emergency. Open heart surgery involves an incision of the heart muscle to repair the internal structures. This may require cardiopulmonary bypass. Closed heart surgery involves structures related to the heart but not the heart muscle itself and may be performed with or without cardiopulmonary bypass.

PROVIDING PREOPERATIVE CARE

The preoperative nursing assessment complements the history and physical examination and provides important baseline information for comparison during the postoperative period. Establish a relationship with the child and parents. Identify problems that may require particular nursing interventions during the postoperative period. Before cardiac surgery, interview the parents and, if age appropriate, the child. Focus the interview on the history of the present illness, cardiac risk factors, the child's present physical and functional status, additional medical problems, current medications and drug allergies, the child's and family's understanding of the illness and planned procedure, and the family support system.

The preoperative physical assessment includes:

- Temperature and weight measurements
- Examination of extremities for peripheral edema, clubbing, and evaluation of peripheral pulses
- Auscultation of the heart (rate, rhythm, heart sounds, murmurs, clicks, and rubs)
- Respiratory assessment, including respiratory rate, work of breathing, and auscultation of the lungs for breath sounds

Obtain any necessary laboratory and diagnostic tests to establish a baseline. In addition, review the results of any tests done previously. Testing may include CBC count, electrolyte levels, clotting studies, urinalysis, cultures of blood and other body secretions, renal and hepatic function tests, chest radiography, ECG, echocardiogram, and cardiac catheterization.

In most nonemergent cases, preoperative assessment is performed in an outpatient setting and the child is admitted to the hospital on the day of surgery. Nursing care during this phase focuses on thorough child and parent education. If the surgery is an emergency, teaching must be done quickly, emphasizing the most important elements of the child's care (Beke, Braudis, & Lincoln, 2005).

Child and parent education typically includes the following topics:

- Heart anatomy and its function, including what area is involved with the defect that is to be corrected
- Events before surgery, including any testing or preparation such as a skin scrub
- Location of the child after surgery, such as a pediatric intensive care unit, which may include a visit to the unit if appropriate and explanation of the sights and sounds that may be present
- Appearance of the child after surgery (equipment or devices used for monitoring, such as oxygen administration, ECG leads, pulse oximeter, chest tubes, mechanical ventilation, or intravenous lines)
- Approximate location of the incision and coverage with dressings
- Postoperative activity level, including measures to reduce the risk of complications, such as coughing and deep-breathing exercises, incentive spirometry, early ambulation, and leg exercises
- Nutritional restrictions, such as nothing by mouth for a specified time before surgery and use of intravenous fluids
- Medications, such as anesthesia, sedation, and analgesics as well as medications the child is taking now that need to be continued or withheld (Beke et al., 2005)

Prepare and educate the child at an age- and developmentally appropriate level. Advise parents to read books with their child about CHD and hospitalization such as:

- *Clifford Visits the Hospital* by N. Bridwell, 2000 (Scholastic Inc.)
- *Franklin Goes to the Hospital* by P. Bourgeois, 2000 (Scholastic Paperbacks)
- *Pump the Bear* by G. O. Whittingon, 2000 (Brown Books)
- *Blue Lewis and Sasha the Great* by C. D. Newell, 2005 (Cally Press)
- *Cardiac Kids: A Book for Families Who Have a Child with Heart Disease* by V. Elder, 1994 (Dayton Area Heart and Cancer Association)
- *When Molly Was in the Hospital: A Book for Brothers and Sisters of Hospitalized Children* by D. Duncan, 1994 (Rayve Productions) (siblings)
- *A Night Without Stars* by J. Howe, 1993 (Camelot) (older children)

In addition, parents may order *It's My Heart,* a parent resource book, free of charge from the Children's Heart Foundation, a link to which is provided on thePoint.

Parents may also help their child by buying a small thrift-store suitcase, spray-painting it, and allowing the child to decorate it with his or her name, pictures of family, stickers, or favorite story characters. This will be the child's "hospital suitcase" that the child may pack with toys and videos to bring to the hospital. Hospital tours are appropriate for school-age children and older children and teens may benefit from an intensive care unit tour before surgery.

Instruct parents to stop food and liquids at the designated time, depending on the child's age, and to give all medications as directed. Some medications may be withheld before surgery. If the child's nutritional status is poor or questionable, nutritional supplementation may be ordered for a period of time preoperatively to ensure that the child has the best possible nutritional status before surgery. When it is time for the child to be transported to the surgical area, allow the parents to accompany the child as far as possible, depending on the institution's policy. Also reinforce with the child that his or her parents will be present at the bedside when he or she awakens from surgery (Beke et al., 2005).

PROVIDING POSTOPERATIVE CARE

The child will usually be transported from the operating room to the intensive care unit. Depending on the child's age, postoperative stability, and type of surgery, the child may stay in the intensive care unit for several hours up to several days. Vigilant nursing care aids in the transition of the child and parents after surgery and reduces the risk of complications.

During the postoperative period the nurse should do the following:

- Assess vital signs frequently, as often as every 1 hour, until stable.

- Assess the color of the skin and mucous membranes, check capillary refill, and palpate peripheral pulses.
- Observe cardiac rate and rhythm via electronic monitoring and auscultate heart rate and rhythm and heart sounds frequently.
- Monitor hemodynamic status via arterial and/or central venous lines (left and right atrial and pulmonary artery pressures, pulmonary artery oxygen saturation).
- Provide site care and tubing changes according to the institution's policy.
- Auscultate lungs for adventitious, diminished, or absent breath sounds.
- Assess oxygen saturation levels via pulse oximetry and arterial blood gases as well as work of breathing and level of consciousness frequently.
- Administer supplemental oxygen as needed.
- Monitor mechanical ventilation and suction as ordered.
- Inspect chest tube functioning, noting amount, color, and character of drainage.
- Inspect the dressing (incision and chest tube) for drainage and intactness. Reinforce or change the dressing as ordered.
- Assess the incision for redness, irritation, drainage, or separation.
- Monitor intake and output hourly.
- Maintain accurate intravenous infusion rate; restrict fluids as ordered to prevent hypervolemia.
- Assess for changes in level of consciousness. Report restlessness, irritability, or seizures.
- Obtain ordered laboratory tests, such as CBC count, coagulation studies, cardiac enzyme levels, and electrolyte levels. Report abnormal results.
- Administer medications, such as digoxin or inotropic or vasopressor agents, as ordered, watching the child closely for possible adverse effects.
- Encourage the child to turn, cough, deep breathe, use the incentive spirometer, and splint the incisional area with pillows.
- Assess the child's pain level and administer analgesics as ordered. Allow time for the child to rest and sleep.
- Assist the child to get out of bed as soon as possible and as ordered.
- Assess daily weights.
- Administer small, frequent feedings or meals when oral intake is allowed.
- Position the child in a comfortable position, one that maximizes chest expansion. Change position frequently.
- Assess the child for complications (Box 41.2).
- Provide emotional and physical support to the child and family, making appropriate referrals such as to social services for assistance.
- Prepare the child and family for discharge (Beke et al., 2005).

BOX 41.2

POSSIBLE COMPLICATIONS AFTER CARDIAC SURGERY

- Atelectasis
- Bacterial endocarditis
- Cardiac arrhythmias
- Cardiac tamponade
- Cerebrovascular accident
- Heart failure
- Hemorrhage
- Pleural effusion
- Pneumonia
- Pneumothorax
- Postperfusion syndrome
- Postcardiac surgery syndrome
- Pulmonary edema
- Seizures
- Wound infection

Adapted from Bacha, E. A., Cooper, D., Thiagarajan, R., et al. (2008). Cardiac complications associated with the treatment of patients with congenital cardiac disease: Consensus definitions from the Multi-Societal Database Committee for Pediatric and Congenital Heart Disease. *Cardiology in the Young, 18*(Suppl. 2), 196–201.

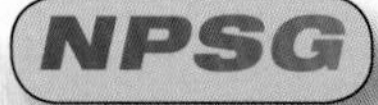

Take Note!

Abrupt cessation of chest tube output accompanied by an increase in heart rate and increased filling pressure (right atrial) may indicate cardiac tamponade (Beke et al., 2005).

NPSG

GOAL 3: Improve the Safety of Using Medications (Use Medicines Safely)

NPSG 03.05.01 Reduce the likelihood of patient harm associated with the use of anticoagulant therapy

Steps: Follow the facility's protocol for starting and continuing anticoagulant therapy, including assessment of laboratory tests. For children, use pre-filled syringes ONLY if specifically designed for pediatric use. Provide family education related to compliance, follow-up monitoring, drug–food interactions, drug–drug interactions, and adverse drug reactions.

Joint Commission. (2015). *National patient safety goals effective January 1, 2015.* Retrieved from www.jointcommission.org/assets/1/6/2015_NPSG_HAP.pdf

Providing Child and Family Education

Provide child and family education throughout the child's stay. Initially, teaching focuses on the underlying defect and measures to treat or control the problem. If the child requires surgery, teaching shifts to preoperative and postoperative events. Emphasize discharge teaching for each admission. Teaching Guidelines 41.2 highlights the major areas to be addressed in child and family education.

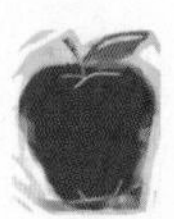

Teaching Guidelines 41.2

CARING FOR THE CHILD WITH A CONGENITAL HEART DISEASE

- Give medications, if ordered, exactly as prescribed.
- Weigh the child at least once a week or as ordered, at approximately the same time of the day with the same scale, and wearing the same amount of clothing.
- Allow the child to engage in activity as directed. Provide time for the child to rest frequently throughout the day to prevent overexertion.
- Provide a nutritious diet, taking into account any restrictions for fluids or foods.
- Use measures to prevent infection, such as frequent hand washing, prophylactic antibiotics, and skin care.
- Adhere to schedule for follow-up diagnostic tests and procedures.
- Support the child's growth and development needs.
- Use available community support services.
- Notify the physician or nurse practitioner if the child has increasing episodes of respiratory distress, cyanosis, or difficulty breathing; fever; increased edema of the hands, feet, or face; decreased urinary output; weight loss or difficulty eating or drinking; increased fatigue or irritability; decreased level of alertness; or vomiting or diarrhea.

Adapted from Cook, E. H., & Higgins, S. S. (2010). Congenital heart disease. In P. J. Allen, J. A. Vessey, & N. A. Schapiro (Eds.), *Primary care of the child with a chronic condition* (5th ed.). St. Louis: Mosby.

ACQUIRED CARDIOVASCULAR DISORDERS

Acquired cardiovascular disorders occur in children as a result of an underlying cardiovascular problem or may refer to other cardiac disorders that are not congenital. The most common type of acquired cardiovascular disorder in children is heart failure. Other acquired disorders include rheumatic fever, cardiomyopathy, infective endocarditis, hyperlipidemia, hypertension, and Kawasaki disease.

Heart Failure

Heart failure occurs most often in children with CHD and is the most common reason for admission to the hospital for children with CHD. Most cases of heart failure in children with CHD occur by 6 months of age (Darst et al., 2014). Heart failure also occurs secondary to other conditions such as myocardial dysfunction following surgical intervention for CHD, cardiomyopathy, myocarditis, fluid volume overload, hypertension, anemia, or sepsis or as a toxic effect of certain chemotherapeutic agents used in the treatment of cancer. **Heart failure** refers to a set of clinical signs and symptoms that reflect the heart's inability to pump effectively to provide adequate blood, oxygen, and nutrients to the body organs and tissues (Francis, Wilson Tang, & Walsh, 2011; Darst et al., 2014).

The child experiencing heart failure requires a multidisciplinary approach to care. Collaboration is necessary to achieve improved cardiac function, restored fluid balance, decreased cardiac workload, and improved oxygen delivery to the tissues.

Pathophysiology

Cardiac output is controlled by preload (diastolic volume), afterload (ventricular wall tension), myocardial contractility (inotropic state), and heart rate. Protracted alterations in any of these factors may lead to heart failure. In the event of reduced cardiac output, multiple compensatory mechanisms are activated. When the ventricular contraction is impaired (systolic dysfunction), reduced ejection of blood occurs, and therefore cardiac output is reduced. Diminished ability to receive venous return (diastolic dysfunction) occurs when high venous pressures are required to support ventricular function. As a result of decreased cardiac output, the renin–angiotensin–aldosterone system is activated as a compensatory mechanism. Fluid and sodium retention as well as improved contractility and vasoconstriction then occur. Initially BP is supported and organ perfusion is maintained, but increased afterload worsens systolic dysfunction. As the heart chambers dilate, myocardial oxygen consumption increases and cardiac output is limited by excessive wall stretch. Over time, the capacity of the heart to respond to these compensatory mechanisms fails, and cardiac output is further decreased (Francis et al., 2011; Darst et al., 2014). Figure 41.15 shows the clinical manifestations that occur related to the mechanisms of heart failure.

Therapeutic Management

Management of heart failure is supportive. Promotion of oxygenation and ventilation is of utmost importance. Digitalis, diuretics, inotropic agents, vasodilators, antiarrhythmics, and antithrombotics have been widely used in children for palliation of symptoms. Many children with heart failure require management in the intensive care unit until they are stabilized. Augmenting nutrition and ensuring adequate rest are also key components of management.

Nursing Assessment

For a full description of the assessment phase of the nursing process, refer to the Assessment section of the Nursing Process Overview earlier in the chapter. Specific assessment findings related to heart failure are discussed below.

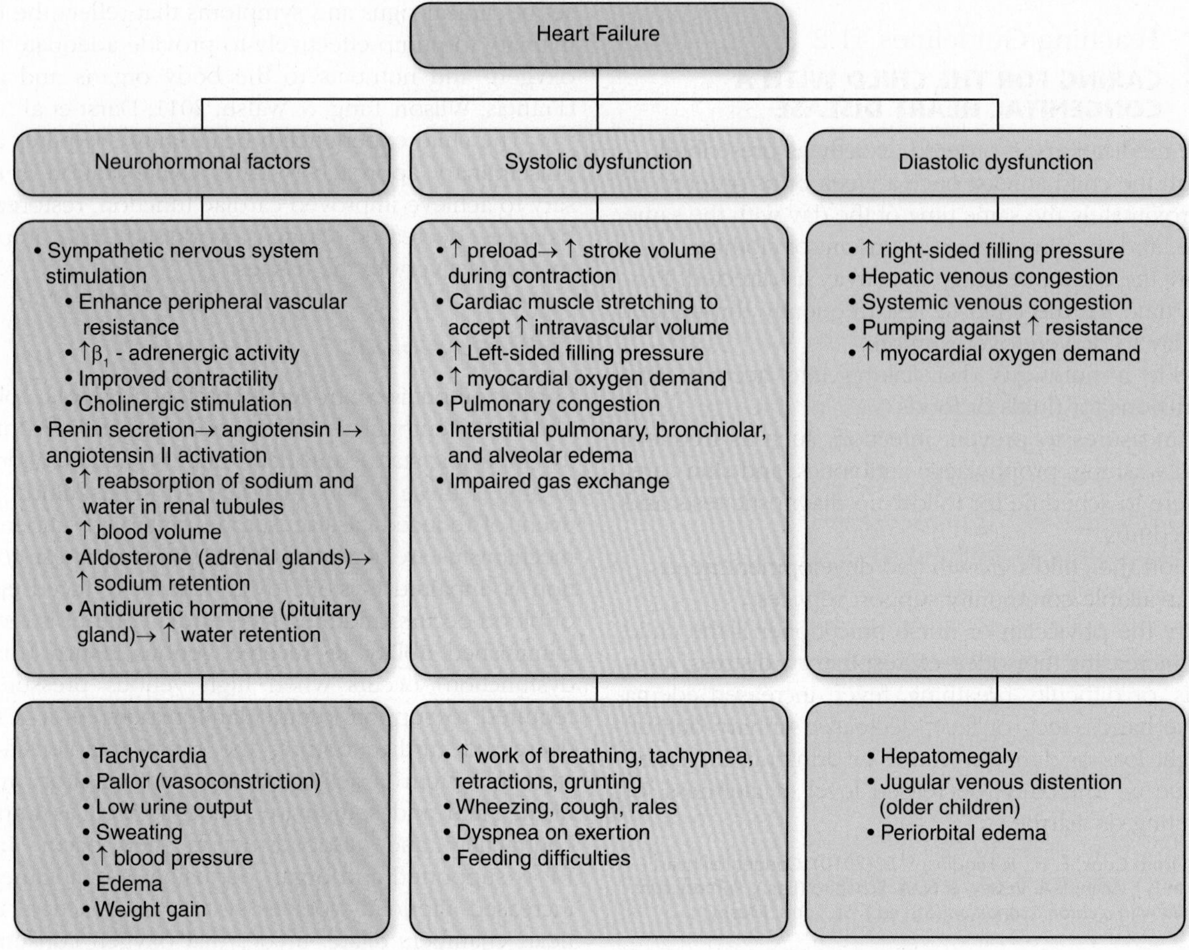

FIGURE 41.15 Pathophysiology of heart failure. (Adapted from Francis, G. S., Wilson Tang, W. H., & Walsh, R. A. (2011). Pathophysiology of heart failure. In V. Fuster, R. A. Walsh, & R. A. Harrington (Eds.), *Hurst's the heart* (13th ed.). New York, NY: McGraw-Hill Companies, Inc.)

Health History

When obtaining the health history, elicit a description of the present illness and chief complaint. Common complaints reported during the health history might include:

- Failure to gain weight or rapid weight gain
- Failure to thrive
- Difficulty feeding
- Fatigue
- Dizziness, irritability
- Exercise intolerance
- Shortness of breath
- Sucking and then tiring quickly
- Syncope
- Decreased number of wet diapers

Infants with heart failure often display subtle signs such as difficulty feeding and tiring easily. Pay close attention for reports of these problems from the parents. Also be alert for statements such as "The baby drinks a small amount of breast milk (or formula) and stops, but then wants to eat again very soon afterwards"; "The baby seems to perspire a lot during feedings"; or "The baby seems to be more comfortable when he's sitting up or on my shoulder than when he's lying flat." In addition, the parents may report episodes of rapid breathing and grunting.

The child's current and past medical history also provide additional clues. Question the parents about any history of congenital heart defects and treatments such as surgery to repair the defect. Determine the current medication regimen. Also ask about any recent or past infections, such as streptococcal infections or fever.

Physical Examination

Weigh the child and note recent rapid weight gain or lack of weight gain. Obtain the child's vital signs, noting tachycardia or tachypnea. These findings are often the first indicators of heart failure in an infant or older child. Measure the BP in the upper and lower extremities, comparing the findings for differences. Note decreased BP, which may be due to impaired cardiac muscle function. Inspect the skin color, noting pallor or cyanosis. Also observe for diaphoresis (profuse sweating). Inspect the face, hands, and lower extremities for edema. Observe for increased work of breathing, such as nasal flaring or retractions. Note the presence of a cough, which may be productive with bloody sputum. Auscultate the apical pulse, noting its location and character. Listen for a murmur, which may suggest a congenital heart defect, a gallop rhythm, or an accentuated third heart sound, suggesting sudden ventricular distention. Auscultate the lungs, noting crackles or wheezes suggestive of pulmonary congestion. Palpate the peripheral pulses, noting weak or thready pulses. Note the temperature and color of the extremities; they may be cool, clammy, and pale.

Assess the child's abdomen, looking for distention indicative of ascites. Gently palpate the abdomen to identify hepatomegaly or splenomegaly.

Laboratory and Diagnostic Tests

The diagnosis of heart failure is based on the child's signs and symptoms and is confirmed with several laboratory and diagnostic tests. These include:

- Chest x-ray, revealing an enlarged heart and/or pulmonary edema
- Electrocardiogram, indicating ventricular hypertrophy
- Echocardiogram, revealing the underlying cause of heart failure, such as a congenital heart defect

Other tests may be done to support the diagnosis. For example, the CBC count may show evidence of anemia or infection. Electrolyte levels may reveal hyponatremia secondary to fluid retention and hyperkalemia secondary to tissue destruction or impaired renal function. Arterial blood gas results may demonstrate respiratory alkalosis in mild heart failure or metabolic acidosis. Tissue hypoxia may be evidenced by increased lactic acid and decreased bicarbonate levels.

Nursing Management

Nursing management of the child with heart failure focuses on promoting oxygenation, supporting cardiac function, providing adequate nutrition, and promoting rest.

Promoting Oxygenation

Position the infant or child in a semi-upright position to decrease work of breathing and lessen pulmonary congestion. Suction as needed. Chest physiotherapy and postural drainage may also be beneficial. Administer supplemental oxygen as ordered and monitor oxygen saturation via pulse oximetry. Oxygen also serves the function of vasodilator and decreases pulmonary vascular resistance. Occasionally, the infant or child with heart failure may require intubation and positive-pressure ventilation to normalize blood gas tension.

Take Note!

In a child with a large left-to-right shunt, oxygen will decrease pulmonary vascular resistance while increasing the systemic vascular resistance, which leads to increased left-to-right shunting. Monitor the child carefully and use oxygen only as prescribed.

Supporting Cardiac Function

Administer digitalis, angiotensin-converting enzyme (ACE) inhibitors, and diuretics as prescribed. Digoxin therapy begins with a digitalizing dose divided into several doses (oral or intravenous [IV]) over a 24-hour period to reach maximum cardiac effect. During digitalization, monitor the ECG for a prolonged PR interval and decreased ventricular rate. Doses are then administered every 12 hours. Monitor the child for signs of digoxin toxicity. Measure BP before and after administration of ACE inhibitors, holding the dose and notifying the physician if the BP falls more than 15 mm Hg. Observe for signs of hypotension such as lightheadedness, dizziness, or fainting. Weigh the child daily to determine fluid loss. Maintain accurate records of intake and output, restricting fluid intake if ordered. Carefully monitor potassium levels, administering potassium supplements if prescribed. Sodium intake is not usually restricted in the child with heart failure.

Providing Adequate Nutrition

Due to the increased metabolic rate associated with heart failure, the infant may require as much as 150 calories/kg/day. Older children will also require higher caloric intake than typical children. Offer small, frequent feedings if the child can tolerate them. During the acute phase of heart failure, many infants in particular will require continuous or intermittent gavage feeding to maintain or gain weight. Concentrate infant formula to 24 to 28 calories/ounce as instructed by the nutritionist.

Promoting Rest

Minimize metabolic needs to decrease cardiac demand. The infant or older child with heart failure will usually limit activities based on energy level. Ensure adequate time for sleep and attempt to limit disturbing interventions. Provide age-appropriate activities that can be performed quietly or in bed, such as books, coloring or drawing, and video or board games. The older child or adolescent with significant heart failure may require home schooling. As the child improves, a rehabilitation program may be helpful for maximizing activity within the child's cardiovascular status limits.

INFECTIVE ENDOCARDITIS

Infective endocarditis is a microbial infection of the endothelial surfaces of the heart's chambers, septum, or valves (most common). Children with congenital heart defects (septum or valve defects) or prosthetic valves are at increased risk of acquiring bacterial endocarditis, which is potentially fatal in these children. Other risk factors for endocarditis include central venous catheters and intravenous drug use. Infective endocarditis occurs when bacteria or fungi gain access to a damaged epithelium. Turbulence in blood flow associated with narrowed or incompetent valves or with a communication between the systemic and pulmonary circulation leads to damage of the endothelium. Thrombi and platelets then adhere to the endothelium, forming vegetations. When a microbe gains access to the bloodstream, it colonizes the vegetation, using the thrombi as a breeding ground. Clumps may separate from the vegetative patch and travel to other organs of the body, causing significant damage (septic emboli). Fungi or more commonly bacteria (particularly α-hemolytic streptococcus or *Staphylococcus aureus*) are frequently implicated in infective endocarditis (Brusch & Bronze, 2015; Darst et al., 2014).

Complete antibiotic or antifungal treatment of the causative organism is necessary, and treatment generally lasts 4 to 6 weeks. Prevention of infective endocarditis in the susceptible child with CHD or a valvular disorder is of the utmost importance (Brusch & Bronze, 2015; Darst et al., 2014).

Nursing Assessment

For a full description of the assessment phase of the nursing process, refer to page 1529. Assessment findings related to endocarditis are discussed below.

Health History

Obtain the health history, noting intermittent, unexplained low-grade fever. Document history of fatigue, anorexia, weight loss, or flu-like symptoms (e.g., arthralgia, myalgia, chills, night sweats). Note history of CHD, valve disorder, or heart failure.

Physical Examination

Measure the child's temperature, noting low-grade fever. Observe for edema if heart failure is also present. Note petechiae on the palpebral conjunctiva, the oral mucosa, or the extremities. Inspect for signs of extracardiac emboli:

- Roth spots: splinter hemorrhages with pale centers on sclerae, palate, buccal mucosa, chest, fingers, or toes
- Janeway lesions: painless, flat, red or blue hemorrhagic lesions on the palms or the soles
- Osler nodes: small, tender nodules on the pads of the toes or fingers
- Black lines (splinter hemorrhages) under the nails (Brusch & Bronze, 2015; Darst et al., 2014)

Evaluate the ECG for a prolonged PR interval or dysrhythmias. Auscultate the heart for a new or changing murmur. Auscultate the lungs for adventitious breath sounds. Palpate the abdomen for splenomegaly.

Laboratory and Diagnostic Tests

Diagnosis is usually based on the clinical presentation. Laboratory tests may reveal:

- Blood culture: bacteria or fungus
- CBC count: anemia, leukocytosis
- Urinalysis: microscopic hematuria
- Echocardiogram: cardiomegaly, abnormal valve function, area of vegetation

Nursing Management

Nursing management focuses on maintaining IV access for at least 4 weeks to appropriately administer the antibiotic or antifungal course of therapy. Monitor the child's temperature and subsequent blood culture results.

Ideally, infective endocarditis in children should be prevented. Children at increased risk for the development of infective endocarditis include those with:

- Prosthetic cardiac valve or prosthetic material used for cardiac valve repair
- Previous endocarditis
- Unrepaired cyanotic CHD
- Completely repaired congenital heart defect with prosthetic material or device within the first 6 months after the procedure
- Repaired CHD with residual defects at the site or adjacent to the site of a prosthetic patch or prosthetic device
- Cardiac transplantation recipients who develop cardiac valve abnormalities (Brusch & Bronze, 2015)

Children at high risk should practice good oral hygiene, including regular tooth brushing and flossing. Instruct parents or the older child to carry emergency medical identification at all times. A wallet card is available from the American Heart Association and a direct link is provided on thePoint. The card may be presented to any physician or nurse practitioner and includes the recommended antibiotic prophylactic regimen (AHA, 2014). Instruct the parents to notify the primary care provider or cardiologist if the child develops flu-like symptoms or a fever.

High-risk children (as noted above) who are undergoing dental procedures should receive prophylaxis as recommended by the American Heart Association.

Antibiotics typically used for prophylaxis may include ampicillin, amoxicillin, gentamicin, or vancomycin.

ACUTE RHEUMATIC FEVER

Acute rheumatic fever (ARF) is a delayed sequela of group A streptococcal pharyngeal infection. In the United States this disease occurs more often in school-age children between 5 and 15 years of age in areas where streptococcal pharyngitis is more prevalent, especially during the colder months. It usually develops 2 to 4 weeks after the initial streptococcal infection. Current understanding of the disease process of ARF is that the child develops an antibody response to surface proteins of the bacteria. The antibodies then cross-react with antigens in cardiac muscle and neuronal and synovial tissues, causing carditis, arthritis, and chorea (involuntary random, jerking movements). ARF affects the joints, central nervous system, skin, and subcutaneous tissue and causes chronic, progressive damage to the heart and valves. Most attacks of ARF last 6 to 12 weeks and then are resolved, but rheumatic fever may recur with subsequent streptococcal infections (Gibofsky, 2015).

Diagnosis of ARF is based on the modified Jones criteria (Box 41.3). Therapeutic management is directed toward managing inflammation and fever, eradicating the bacteria, preventing permanent heart damage, and preventing recurrences. A full 10-day course of penicillin therapy (or equivalent) is used along with corticosteroids and nonsteroidal anti-inflammatory drugs. Children without valvular disease will receive continued prophylaxis with monthly intramuscular injections of penicillin G benzathine or daily oral doses of penicillin or erythromycin following the initial illness in order to prevent a new streptococcal infection and recurrent ARF. Prophylaxis is continued until adulthood (Gibofsky, 2015).

BOX 41.3

MODIFIED JONES CRITERIA (AMERICAN HEART ASSOCIATION)

Diagnosis of acute rheumatic fever requires the presence of either two major criteria or one major plus two minor criteria.

Major Criteria

- Carditis
- Migratory polyarthritis
- Subcutaneous nodules
- Erythema marginatum
- Sydenham chorea

Minor Criteria

- Arthralgia
- Fever
- Elevated erythrocyte sedimentation rate or C-reactive protein
- Prolonged PR interval

Adapted from Darst, J. R., Collins, K. K., & Miyamoto, S. D. (2014). Cardiovascular diseases. In W. W. Hay, M. J. Levin, & R. R. Deterding, & M. J. Abzug, (Eds.), *Current pediatric diagnosis and treatment* (22nd ed.). New York, NY: McGraw-Hill.

Nursing Assessment

Elicit a description of the present illness and chief complaint, noting fever and joint pain. Explore the child's recent medical history for risk factors such as documented streptococcal infection or sore throat within the past 2 to 3 weeks, or for past history of ARF. Observe the child for Sydenham chorea, a movement disorder of the face and upper extremities. Inspect the skin for evidence of the classic rash, erythema marginatum, a maculopapular red rash with central clearing and elevated edges. Auscultate the heart, noting a murmur. Palpate the surfaces of the wrist, elbows, and knees for firm, painless, subcutaneous nodules. Note prolonged PR interval on the ECG. Throat culture will provide definitive diagnosis of current streptococcal infection, while streptococcal antibody tests may yield evidence of recent infection. Echocardiogram is required to determine if carditis is present.

Nursing Management

Nursing management of the child with ARF focuses on ensuring compliance with the acute course of antibiotics as well as prophylaxis following initial recovery from ARF. Allow the child to verbalize the frustration he or she may be feeling in relation to chorea symptoms. Offer support for dealing with the abnormal movements. Educate the child and others that the sudden jerky movements of chorea will eventually disappear, though they may last as long as several months. Some children may require a neuroleptic agent such as haloperidol (Haldol) for management of chorea. Administer corticosteroids or nonsteroidal anti-inflammatory agents for control of joint pain and swelling.

CARDIOMYOPATHY

Cardiomyopathy is a condition in which the myocardium cannot contract properly. The incidence of cardiomyopathy among children is increasing; it occurs at a rate of 1 per 100,000 (AHA, 2015). Cardiomyopathy may occur in children with genetic disorders or congenital heart defects, as a result of an inflammatory or infectious process or hypertension, or after cardiac transplantation or surgery, but most commonly it is idiopathic. Cardiomyopathy occurs predominately in clusters in infancy and adolescence. Three types of cardiomyopathy exist—restrictive, dilated, and hypertrophic. Restrictive cardiomyopathy is rare in children and results in atrial relaxation. Dilated cardiomyopathy is the most common type in childhood and may result in heart failure because of ventricular dilatation with decreased contractility (Kantor, Abraham, Dipchand, Benson, & Redington, 2010). There is some familial tendency toward dilated cardiomyopathy, and it is also associated with Duchenne and Becker muscular dystrophy (Marian et al., 2011). Children with dilated cardiomyopathy may present with heart failure (Kantor et al., 2010). Hypertrophic cardiomyopathy is more common in adolescence and results in hypertrophy of the heart muscle, particularly the left ventricle, affecting the heart's ability to fill. About two thirds of all cases of hypertrophic cardiomyopathy are familial, with some inherited in an autosomal dominant fashion (Marian et al., 2011).

There is no cure for cardiomyopathy, meaning that, currently, heart muscle function cannot be restored. Therapeutic management is directed toward improving heart function and BP. Mechanical ventilation and vasoactive medications are needed in many children. ACE inhibitors, beta blockers, or calcium channel blockers may be used. Pacemakers or surgery is helpful in some children. For severely affected children, heart transplantation is the only viable long-term treatment option (Kantor et al., 2010).

Nursing Assessment

Explore the health history for risk factors such as:

- Congenital heart defect, cardiac transplantation, or surgery
- Duchenne or Becker muscular dystrophy
- History of myocarditis, HIV infection, or Kawasaki disease
- Hypertension
- Drugs, alcohol, or radiation exposure
- Connective tissue, autoimmune, or endocrine disease
- Maternal diabetes
- Familial history of sudden death

Inquire about a history of respiratory distress, fatigue, poor growth (dilated), chest pain, dizziness, or syncope (hypertrophic). Observe the child for extremity edema and abdominal distention. Note increased work of breathing. Auscultate the heart, noting tachycardia and irregular rhythm. Evaluate heart rhythm via ECG, noting dysrhythmias or indications of left ventricular hypertrophy.

Chest radiography may reveal cardiomegaly or congested lungs. Echocardiogram demonstrates increased heart size, poor contractility, decreased ejection fraction, or asymmetric septal hypertrophy. Cardiac catheterization is usually performed to aid in the diagnosis.

Nursing Management

Many children with cardiomyopathy require intensive care initially. Monitor for complications such as blood clots or arrhythmias, which could lead to cardiac arrest. Refer to the previous section on heart failure for nursing interventions related to heart failure, which may be present with dilated cardiomyopathy. Administer vasoactive and other medications as prescribed, monitoring the child closely for response to these therapies as well as for complications. Support the child in choosing activities that fit within the prescribed restrictions. Provide extensive emotional support to the child and family, who may experience significant stress as they realize the severity of this illness.

HYPERTENSION

Hypertension has seen a rise in prevalence among children and adolescents. It has been found to be independently associated with body mass index and waist circumference. Childhood/adolescent hypertension often leads to long-term health consequences such as cardiovascular disease and left ventricular hypertrophy (Mattoo, 2016a). In children, acceptable BP values are based on gender, age, and height. Hypertension is defined as BP persistently greater than the 95th percentile for gender, age, and height. Prehypertension refers to BP that is persistently between the 90th and 95th percentiles. BP is considered normal when the systolic and diastolic values are less than the 90th percentile for gender, age, and height (Mattoo, 2016a).

Childhood hypertension may be further defined as primary or secondary. Primary hypertension in children is found more commonly in postpubertal children, African Americans, and children who are overweight or obese (Mattoo, 2016a). Secondary hypertension in children most frequently occurs with an underlying medical problem such as renal or cardiac disease (Mattoo, 2016a). Mild to moderate hypertension in childhood is usually asymptomatic and usually is determined only upon BP screening during a well-child visit or during follow-up for known risk factors. Refer to Table 31.5 in Chapter 31, for a synopsis of childhood hypertension guidelines.

It is important to screen for and treat prehypertension and hypertension in children and adolescents, as they are more likely to experience hypertension as adults progressing to further cardiovascular disease (Mattoo, 2016b). Therapeutic management depends on the extent of the hypertension and the length of time it has existed. Weight reduction, appropriate diet (including sodium restriction in some children), and increased physical activity are important components of management of prehypertensive and asymptomatic hypertensive children. Some children are candidates for, and require, antihypertensive medications or diuretics (Mattoo, 2016b).

Pathophysiology

The balance between cardiac output and vascular resistance determines the BP. An increase in either of these variables, in the absence of a compensatory decrease in the other, increases the mean BP. Factors regulating cardiac output and vascular resistance include changes in electrolyte balance, particularly sodium, calcium, and potassium.

Nursing Assessment

Nursing assessment consists of the health history, physical examination, and laboratory and diagnostic tests.

Health History

Elicit the health history, determining the presence of risk factors for hypertension such as:

- Family history
- Obesity
- Hyperlipidemia
- Renal disease (including frequent urinary tract infections)
- Systemic lupus erythematosus
- CHD
- Neurofibromatosis, Turner syndrome, and other genetic disorders
- Prematurity
- Prolonged neonatal ventilation
- Umbilical artery catheterization
- Diabetes mellitus
- Increased intracranial pressure
- Malignancy
- Solid organ transplant
- Medications known to raise BP

Signs and symptoms reported during the health history might include:

- Growth retardation (with certain chronic medical conditions)
- Obesity
- Signs and symptoms seen particularly in older children
- Headache
- Subtle behavioral or school performance changes
- Fatigue
- Blurred vision
- Nosebleed
- Bell palsy

Physical Examination

Determine the child's weight and height/length. Plot these growth parameters on the gender-appropriate chart for the child's age. Note the percentile for height/length, as it will be used to determine the BP percentile (see Appendix B: Blood Pressure Charts for Children and Adolescents). Measure the BP in all four extremities (to rule out coarctation of the aorta). Ensure that the child is relaxed and sitting or reclined. Refer to Chapter 32 for specific information related to accurate BP measurement in children.

Inspect the skin for:

- Acne, hirsutism, or striae (associated with anabolic steroid use)
- Café-au-lait spots (associated with neurofibromatosis)
- Malar rash (associated with lupus)
- Pallor, diaphoresis, or flushing (associated with pheochromocytoma)

Observe the extremities for edema (renal disease) or joint swelling (lupus). Inspect the chest for apical heave (ventricular hypertrophy) or wide-spaced nipples (Turner syndrome). Auscultate heart sounds, noting tachycardia (associated with primary hypertension) or murmur (associated with coarctation of the aorta). Palpate the abdomen for a mass or enlarged kidney.

Laboratory and Diagnostic Testing

Though diagnosis of hypertension is based on BP measurements, additional laboratory or diagnostic tests may be used to evaluate the underlying cause of secondary hypertension, including:

- Urinalysis, blood urea nitrogen, and serum creatinine: may determine the presence of renal disease
- Renal ultrasound or angiography: may reveal kidney or genitourinary tract abnormalities
- Echocardiogram: may show left ventricular hypertrophy
- Lipid profile: determines the presence of hyperlipidemia

Nursing Management

Salt restriction and potassium or calcium supplements have not been scientifically shown to decrease BP in children. However, obese children may benefit from salt restriction, as those children seem to be sensitive to salt intake. Assist the child and family to develop a plan for weight reduction if the child is overweight or obese. Encourage the child and family to control portion sizes, decrease the intake of sugary beverages and snacks, eat more fresh fruits and vegetables, and eat a healthy breakfast. Consult the nutritionist for additional assistance with meal planning. To increase physical activity, encourage the child to find a sport or type of exercise in which he or she is interested. Aerobic activities involving running, walking, or cycling are particularly helpful. When a child requires antihypertensive therapy, teach the child and family how to administer the medication. Caution the parents about side effects related to antihypertensives. Teach the parent to measure the child's BP as determined by the physician or nurse practitioner, as well as to keep appointments for BP follow-up. See Healthy People 2020.

HEALTHY PEOPLE 2020

Objective	Nursing Significance
Reduce the proportion of children and adolescents with hypertension.	• To prevent development of hypertension and encourage children to maintain a healthy weight and participate in regular exercise.

Healthy People Objectives retrieved from www.healthypeople.gov

KAWASAKI DISEASE

Kawasaki disease is an acute systemic vasculitis occurring mostly in children 6 months to 5 years of age. It is the leading cause of acquired heart disease among children and occurs more often in the winter and summer, affecting 20 per 100,000 children (Sundel, 2016b). Although Kawasaki disease affects all ethnic groups, it occurs more frequently in those of Asian or Pacific descent. It is a self-limited syndrome but can cause cardiovascular complications such as coronary artery aneurysm and cardiomyopathy, among others (Sundel, 2016a).

Therapeutic management of acute Kawasaki disease focuses on reducing inflammation in the walls of the coronary arteries and preventing coronary thrombosis. Chronic management of children developing aneurysms during the initial phase is directed toward preventing myocardial ischemia. In the acute phase, high-dose aspirin in four divided doses daily and a single infusion of intravenous immunoglobulin (IVIG) are used. It appears that the best response occurs if IVIG is given within the first 7 to 10 days of the illness (Sundel, 2016c).

Pathophysiology

Though the etiology is still unknown, current thought is that some infectious organism (as yet unidentified) causes disease in genetically susceptible people. Kawasaki disease appears to be an autoimmune response mediated by cytokine-induced endothelial cell surface antigens that leads to vasculitis. Neutrophils, followed by mononuclear cells, T lymphocytes, and immunoglobulin A–producing plasma cells, infiltrate the vessels. Then elastin and collagen fibers fragment and the structural integrity of the vessel wall are impaired. Generalized systemic vasculitis occurs in the blood vessels throughout the body due to the inflammation and edema and can lead to coronary dilatation or aneurysm. Some children never develop coronary artery changes, while others develop an aneurysm in either the acute phase or as a long-term sequela (Sundel, 2016a).

Nursing Assessment

Nursing assessment consists of determining the health history, physical examination, and laboratory and diagnostic testing.

Health History

Elicit the health history, noting any of the following:

- Fever
- Chills
- Headache
- Malaise
- Extreme irritability
- Vomiting
- Diarrhea
- Abdominal pain
- Joint pain

Of particular note is a history of high fever (39.9°C) of at least 5 days' duration that is unresponsive to antibiotics.

Physical Examination

Observe for significant bilateral conjunctivitis without exudate. Inspect the mouth and throat for dry, fissured lips; strawberry (cracked and reddened) tongue; and pharyngeal and oral mucosa erythema. Note hyperdynamic precordium. Evaluate the skin for:

- Diffuse, erythematous, polymorphous rash
- Edema of the hands and feet
- Erythema and painful induration of the palms and soles
- Desquamation (peeling) of the perineal region, fingers, and toes, extending to the palms and soles
- Possible jaundice

Palpate the neck for cervical lymphadenopathy (usually unilateral) and the joints for tenderness. Palpate the abdomen for liver enlargement. Auscultate the heart, noting tachycardia, gallop, or murmur.

Laboratory and Diagnostic Testing

The CBC count may reveal mild to moderate anemia, an elevated white blood cell count during the acute phase, and significant thrombocytosis (elevated platelet count [500,000 to 1 million]) in the later phase. The erythrocyte sedimentation rate (ESR) and the C-reactive protein (CRP) level are elevated. Echocardiogram is performed as soon as possible after the diagnosis is confirmed to provide a baseline of a healthy heart or to evaluate for coronary artery involvement. Echocardiograms may be repeated during the illness and as part of long-term follow-up. Occasionally cardiac involvement warrants cardiac catheterization.

Nursing Management

In addition to the administration of aspirin and immunoglobulin, nursing management of the child with Kawasaki disease focuses on monitoring cardiac status, promoting comfort, and providing family education.

Monitoring Cardiac Status

Administer intravenous and oral fluids as ordered, evaluating intake and output carefully. Prepare the child for the echocardiogram. Assess frequently for signs of developing heart failure such as tachycardia, gallop, decreased urine output, or respiratory distress. Evaluate quality and strength of pulses. Provide cardiac monitoring as ordered, reporting arrhythmias.

Promoting Comfort

Provide acetaminophen for fever management and apply cool cloths as tolerated. Keep the environment quiet and cluster nursing care activities to decrease stimulation and hence irritability. Teach parents that irritability is a prominent feature of Kawasaki disease, and support their efforts to console the child. Apply petrolatum jelly or another lubricating ointment to the lips. Encourage the older child to suck on ice chips; the younger child may suck on a cool, moist washcloth. Popsicles are also soothing. Provide comfortable positioning, particularly if the child has joint pain or arthritis.

Providing Child and Family Education

Teach parents to continue to monitor the child's temperature after discharge until the child has been afebrile for several days. Children with prolonged or recurrent fever may require a second dose of IVIG. Inform parents that irritability may last for up to 2 months after initial diagnosis with Kawasaki disease. Report any toxic effects of aspirin therapy, such as headache, confusion, dizziness, or tinnitus to the physician or nurse practitioner. It is important to avoid nonsteroidal anti-inflammatory agents while aspirin therapy is ongoing. For children with continued arthritis (which resolves in several weeks), range-of-motion exercises with a morning bath may help to decrease stiffness. Instruct parents to avoid measles and varicella vaccination for 11 months after high-dose IVIG administration. It is critical that the family comply with regularly scheduled cardiology follow-up appointments to determine development or progression of coronary artery ectasia or aneurysm. If the child has severe cardiac involvement, teach the parents about infant and/or child cardiopulmonary resuscitation before discharge from the hospital.

HYPERLIPIDEMIA

Hyperlipidemia refers to high levels of lipids (fats/cholesterol) in the blood. High lipid levels are a risk factor for the development of atherosclerosis, which can result in coronary artery disease, a serious cardiovascular disorder occurring in adults. Children with high lipid levels, though remaining asymptomatic, are likely to have high levels as adults, which increases their risk for coronary artery disease. Therefore, detection, screening, and early intervention are important, especially if there is a family tendency toward heart disease (Schuman, 2013).

Pathophysiology

Cholesterol is a building block for hormones and cell membranes. It occurs naturally in foods derived from animals such as eggs, dairy products, meat, poultry, and seafood. Cholesterol is also manufactured in the body. Together, cholesterol and triglycerides are known as lipids. Very low–density lipoprotein (VLDL) is a lipoprotein composed mainly of triglycerides with only small amounts of cholesterol, phospholipid, and protein. VLDLs are easily converted to low-density lipoproteins (LDLs). Cholesterol is expressed in terms of LDL cholesterol or high-density lipoprotein (HDL) cholesterol. LDLs contain relatively more cholesterol and triglycerides than they do protein. HDLs contain about 50% protein, with the rest being cholesterol, triglyceride, and phospholipid. High levels of cholesterol and triglycerides place a person at risk for atherosclerosis. Elevated VLDL and LDL levels and decreased HDL levels produce a particular increase in the risk for atherosclerosis (Darst et al., 2014).

Therapeutic Management

Screening children for hyperlipidemia is of prime importance for early detection, intervention, and subsequent prevention of adult atherosclerosis.

Bright Futures Guidelines recommend universal screening for dyslipidemia between 9 and 11 years of age and again between 18 and 21 years of age (Bright Futures/American Academy of Pediatrics, 2016). Performing a risk assessment screening at 24 months and at 4, 6, 8, and 12 through 17 years of age is also recommended. Selectively screening of children at high risk for hyperlipidemia can reduce their lifelong risk of coronary artery disease. The risk assessment focuses on the child's family history. Screen if parents, grandparents, aunts and uncles, or siblings, have or have had documented:

- Coronary atherosclerosis
- Myocardial infarction
- Angina pectoris
- Peripheral vascular disease
- Cerebrovascular disease/stroke

- Coronary artery bypass graft/stent/angioplasty at less than 55 years of age in males and less than 65 years in females
- Sudden cardiac death
- Blood cholesterol level of 240 mg/dL or higher

The child should be screened at the healthcare provider's discretion if the parental history is unobtainable, the child has diabetes or hypertension, or if the child has any lifestyle risk factors (cigarette smoking, obesity, sedentary lifestyle, or high-fat dietary intake) (National Heart, Lung, and Blood Institute, 2012).

All children should eat a diet with the appropriate amount of fats (see the section on nursing management below) and should participate in physical activity. When diet and exercise are not enough to lower cholesterol to appropriate levels, medications such as resins, fibric acid derivatives, statins, or niacin may be used (Schuman, 2013).

Nursing Assessment

Elicit the health history, noting risk factors such as family history of hyperlipidemia, early heart disease, hypertension, diabetes or other endocrine abnormality, cerebral vascular accident, or sudden death. Note prior lipid levels if available. Measure the child's height and weight, plotting them on standardized growth charts. Note if the child is overweight or obese, as these are risk factors associated with hyperlipidemia. Typically, there are no other particular physical findings associated with hyperlipidemia. Table 41.3 gives details about the interpretation of cholesterol levels.

Nursing Management

Instruct families that the child must fast for 12 hours before lipid screening (initially and on follow-up samples). Dietary management is the first step in the prevention and management of hyperlipidemia in children older than 2 years of age. The diet should consist primarily of fruits, vegetables, low-fat dairy products, whole grains, beans, lean meat, poultry, and fish. As in adults, fat should account for no more than 30% of daily caloric intake. Fat intake may vary over a period of days, as many young children are picky eaters. Limit saturated fats by choosing lean meats, removing skin from poultry before cooking, and avoiding palm, palm kernel, and coconut oils as well as hydrogenated fats. Teach families to read nutrition labels to determine the content of the food. Limit intake of processed or refined foods as well as high-sugar drinks; these products provide minimal nutrition and significant calories. Children older than 2 years of age should have 60 minutes per day of vigorous play or physical activity (McCord & Lee, 2011). Refer parents to "Healthy Habits for Healthy Kids—A Nutrition and Activity Guide for Parents" published by the American Dietetic Association. (See thePoint for a direct link.)

If medications are required, teach the child and family about the dose, administration, and possible adverse effects. Assist the family to develop a medication-dosing plan that is compatible with school and work schedules to increase compliance.

TABLE 41.3 INTERPRETATION OF CHOLESTEROL LEVELS FOR CHILDREN AGE 2–19 YEARS

Total Cholesterol (mg/dL)	LDL (mg/dL)	Interpretation
<170	<110	Acceptable
170–199	100–129	Borderline
≥200	≥130	Elevated

Adapted from National Heart, Lung, and Blood Institute. (2012). *Expert Panel on Integrated Guidelines for Cardiovascular Health and Risk Reduction in Children and Adolescents*. SUMMARY REPORT (NIH Publication No. 12–7486). Washington, DC: U.S. Department of Health and Human Services.

HEART TRANSPLANTATION

Heart transplantation is indicated in children with end-stage heart disease related to cardiomyopathy or inoperable CHD. Over 500 children receive a heart transplant each year (Chinnock & Ohye, 2014). The 1-year survival rate is 80% to 90%, 5-year survival rate is 70% to 80%, and although 20-year survival has been achieved, many children require a second transplantation (Chinnock & Ohye, 2014). While awaiting transplantation, about 30% of young infants and 20% of children over 6 months of age die (Lankin, 2012).

A comprehensive evaluation is performed to determine whether the child is a candidate for heart transplant. The evaluation includes:

- Chest x-ray, ECG, echocardiogram, exercise stress test, cardiac catheterization, and pulmonary function tests
- CBC count with differential, prothrombin and partial thromboplastin time, serum chemistries and electrolytes, blood urea nitrogen, and creatinine
- Urinalysis and urine creatinine clearance
- Blood, throat, urine, stool, and sputum cultures for bacteria, viruses, fungi, and parasites
- Epstein–Barr virus, cytomegalovirus, varicella, herpes, hepatitis, and HIV titers
- HLA typing and panel reactive antibody typing and titer
- Computed tomography or MRI scan and electroencephalogram

- Consults with neurology, psychology, genetics, social work, nutritionist, physical and occupational therapy, and financial coordinator or case manager (Dipchand, Bastardi, & Dupuis, 2013)

Children with irreversible lung, liver, kidney, or central nervous system disease; recent malignancy (past 5 years); or chronic viral infection may be excluded as candidates.

Once candidacy is determined, the transplant center registers the child as a potential recipient with the United Network for Organ Sharing (UNOS). Blood type, body size, length of time on the waiting list, and medical urgency are used to evaluate compatibility. Children awaiting transplantation may need continuous or intermittent hospitalization. Coordination of organ procurement and the transplantation procedure is essential.

Surgical Procedure and Postoperative Therapeutic Management

Most transplantation procedures are **orthotopic**, which means that the recipient's heart is removed and the donor heart is implanted in its place in the normal anatomic position. Cardiopulmonary bypass and hypothermia are used to maintain circulation, protect the brain, and oxygenate the recipient during the procedure. Postoperatively, the child may have near-normal heart function and capacity for exercise and may be able to return to school.

Immunosuppressive therapy is necessary for the rest of the child's life to avoid rejection of the transplanted heart. Usually a three-drug regimen is used that includes calcineurin inhibitors (cyclosporine, tacrolimus), cell toxins (mycophenolate mofetil, azathioprine), and corticosteroids. The cardiologist and transplant surgeon provide ongoing follow-up. Complications of heart transplantation include infection, pulmonary hypertension, arrhythmia, heart failure, hypertension, renal dysfunction, and organ rejection. Neoplasm may occur as a result of chronic immunosuppression.

Nursing Management

Preoperative nursing care for the child undergoing a heart transplant is similar for children undergoing other types of heart surgery. In addition, the nurse should assist with the comprehensive pretransplant evaluation. Care for the child in the posttransplant period is intense and complex. Evaluate the family's ability to perform the tasks that will be necessary. Teach families about the evaluation and transplantation process, as well as the waiting period. In the immediate preoperative period, perform a thorough history and physical examination and obtain last-minute blood work. Provide preoperative teaching similar to other cardiac surgeries. Older children, adolescents, and parents may enjoy the book *Future Conditional* by J. Hatton (1996, Yorkshire Art Circus), which was written by one of the first heart transplant survivors.

Postoperatively, provide frequent assessments and routine care for cardiac surgery children. In addition, monitor the child closely for infection or signs of rejection. Acute rejection may be indicated by low-grade fever, fatigue, tachycardia, nausea, vomiting, abdominal pain, and decreased activity tolerance, though some children will be asymptomatic. Maintain strict hand washing techniques and isolate the child from other children with infections. Though live vaccines are contraindicated in immunosuppressed children, inactivated vaccines should be given as recommended (Centers for Disease Control and Prevention, 2016). Teach children and families that the child may return to school and usual activities about 3 months after the transplant. Provide emotional support to the child related to body image changes such as hair growth, gum hyperplasia, weight gain, moon facies, acne, and rashes that occur due to long-term immunosuppressive therapy.

NURSING CARE PLAN 41.1

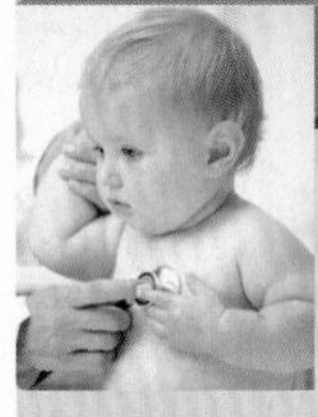

Overview for the Child With a Cardiovascular Disorder

NURSING DIAGNOSIS: Decreased cardiac output related to structural defect, congenital anomaly, or ineffective heart pumping as evidenced by arrhythmias, edema, murmur, abnormal heart rate, or abnormal heart sounds

Outcome Identification and Evaluation

Child or infant will demonstrate adequate cardiac output: will have elastic skin turgor, brisk capillary refill, demonstrate pink color, pulse and BP within normal limits for age, regular heart rhythm, adequate urinary output.

Interventions: *Increasing Cardiac Output*

- Monitor vital signs closely, especially BP and heart rate, *to detect increases or decreases.*
- Monitor cardiac rhythm via cardiac monitor *to detect arrhythmias quickly.*
- Observe for signs of hypoxia such as tachypnea, cyanosis, tachycardia, bradycardia, dizziness, and/or restlessness *to identify this change early.*
- Administer oxygen as needed *to correct hypoxia.*
- Place child in knee-to-chest or squatting position as needed *to increase systemic vascular resistance.*
- Administer antiarrhythmics, vasopressors, ACE inhibitors, beta blockers, corticosteroids, or diuretics as prescribed *to improve cardiac output.*
- Monitor for signs of thrombosis such as restlessness, seizure, coma, oliguria, anuria, edema, hematuria, or paralysis *to identify this condition early.*
- Administer adequate hydration *to decrease possibility of thrombosis formation.*
- Cluster nursing care and other activities *to allow adequate periods of rest.*
- Anticipate child's needs *to decrease the child's stress, thereby decreasing oxygen consumption requirement.*

NURSING DIAGNOSIS: Excess fluid volume related to ineffective cardiac muscle function as evidenced by weight gain, edema, jugular vein distention, dyspnea, shortness of breath, abnormal breath sounds, or pulmonary congestion

Outcome Identification and Evaluation

Child will attain appropriate fluid balance, will lose weight (fluid), edema or bloating will decrease, lung sounds will be clear, and heart sounds normal.

Interventions: *Encouraging Fluid Loss*

- Weigh daily on same scale in similar amount of clothing: in children weight is the best indicator of changes in fluid status.
- Monitor location and extent of edema (measure abdominal girth daily if ascites is present): decrease in edema indicates positive increase in oncotic pressure.
- Protect edematous areas from skin breakdown: edema leads to increased risk for alterations in skin integrity.
- Auscultate lungs carefully to identify crackles, indicating pulmonary edema.
- Assess work of breathing and respiratory rate: increased work of breathing is associated with pulmonary edema.
- Assess heart sounds for gallop: presence of S_3 may indicate fluid overload.
- Maintain fluid restriction as ordered to decrease intravascular volume and workload on the heart.
- Strictly monitor intake and output to quickly note discrepancies and provide intervention.
- Provide sodium-restricted diet as ordered: restricting sodium intake allows better renal excretion of extra fluid.
- Administer diuretics as ordered and monitor for adverse effects. Diuretics encourage excretion of fluid and elimination of edema, reduce cardiac filling pressures, and increase renal blood flow. Adverse effects include electrolyte imbalance as well as orthostatic hypotension.

NURSING CARE PLAN 41.1

Overview for the Child With a Cardiovascular Disorder (continued)

NURSING DIAGNOSIS: Imbalanced nutrition, less than body requirements, related to increased energy expenditure and fatigue as evidenced by weight loss or height and weight below accepted standards

Outcome Identification and Evaluation

Child will improve nutritional intake resulting in steady increase in weight and length/height and will feed without tiring easily.

Interventions: *Promoting Adequate Nutrition*

- Determine body weight and length/height norm for age *to determine goal to work toward.*
- Assess child for food preferences that fall within dietary restrictions: *child will be more likely to consume adequate amounts of foods that he or she likes.*
- Weigh child daily or weekly (according to physician order or institutional standard) and measure length/height weekly *to monitor for increased growth.*
- Offer highest-calorie meals at the time of day when the child's appetite is the greatest *to increase likelihood of increased caloric intake.*
- Provide increased-calorie shakes or puddings within diet restriction: *high-calorie foods increase weight gain.*
- Consult with the pediatric dietician *to provide optimal caloric intake within dietary restrictions.*
- Provide small, frequent feedings *to discourage tiring with feeding.*
- Feed infants with special nipple as needed *to decrease amount of energy expended for sucking.*
- Administer vitamin and mineral supplements as prescribed *to attain/maintain vitamin and mineral balance in the body.*

NURSING DIAGNOSIS: Ineffective tissue perfusion related to inadequate cardiac function or cardiac surgery as evidenced by pallor, cyanosis, edema, changes in mental status, prolonged capillary refill, clubbing, or diminished pulses

Outcome Identification and Evaluation

Child will demonstrate adequate tissue perfusion: child will be alert, not restless or lethargic, will have pink color, decrease in edema, normal perfusion, and strong pulses.

Interventions: *Promoting Tissue Perfusion*

- Assess level of consciousness, pulse, BP, peripheral perfusion, and skin color frequently *to determine baseline and ongoing improvement.*
- Administer cardiac glycosides or vasodilators as ordered *to promote cardiac output necessary for proper perfusion.*
- Monitor pulse oximetry and arterial blood gas results *to assess ability to appropriately oxygenate.*
- Supplement oxygen as needed *to provide oxygen to organs for proper functioning.*
- Monitor hemoglobin and hematocrit *to identify blood loss.*
- Strictly assess intake and output *to determine adequacy of renal perfusion.*
- Position with head of bed elevated *to decrease blood volume returning to heart.*
- Change position every 2 to 4 hours *to promote circulation and avoid skin breakdown in areas of poor perfusion.*

(continued)

NURSING CARE PLAN 41.1

Overview for the Child With a Cardiovascular Disorder (continued)

NURSING DIAGNOSIS: Risk for delayed development related to effects of cardiac disease and necessary treatments, inadequate nutrition, or frequent separation from caregivers secondary to illness

Outcome Identification and Evaluation

Child will display development appropriate for age: will display evidence of cognitive and motor function within normal limits (individualized for each child).

Interventions: ***Promoting Appropriate Development***

- Promote adequate caloric intake to stimulate growth and provide adequate energy.
- Provide age-appropriate developmental activities to stimulate development.
- Consult with the physical or occupational therapist or child life specialist to determine activities most appropriate for the child within the constraints of the child's illness.
- Schedule daily activities to allow for essential rest periods for energy conservation.
- Encourage parents, teachers, and playmates to be sensitive to child's self-image, using positive comments, to improve the child's self-concept.
- As energy allows, encourage participation in all activities as feasible to allow the child to feel normal.

NURSING DIAGNOSIS: Risk for infection related to need for multiple invasive procedures or cardiac surgery

Outcome Identification and Evaluation

Child will remain free from infection: vital signs will be within normal limits, white blood cell count normal, and cultures negative. Child will exhibit no signs or symptoms of infection.

Interventions: ***Preventing Infection***

- Maintain strict hand hygiene to prevent spread of infectious organisms to the child.
- Assess temperature to detect elevation early in course of infection.
- Avoid contact with persons with known infections to prevent risk of becoming ill.
- Ensure appropriate immunization, including pneumococcal and influenza vaccinations, to prevent development of common childhood illness.
- Administer prophylactic antibiotics prior to all dental procedures, surgery, and many invasive procedures to prevent subacute bacterial endocarditis.
- Encourage good dental hygiene to reduce the risk of endocarditis.

NURSING DIAGNOSIS: Interrupted family processes related to crisis associated with heart disease, frequent need for testing and hospitalizations, or stresses associated with care demands, as evidenced by inadequate parental coping, frequent separations of parent and child, or inadequate support

Outcome Identification and Evaluation

Family will maintain functional system of support and will demonstrate adequate coping, adaptation of roles and functions, and decreased anxiety: *parents are involved in child's care, ask appropriate questions, express fears and concerns, and can discuss child's care and condition calmly.*

NURSING CARE PLAN 41.1

Overview for the Child With a Cardiovascular Disorder (continued)

Interventions: ***Promoting Family Processes***

- Provide ongoing support to the child and family *to help them cope.*
- Encourage parents and family members to verbalize concerns related to child's illness, diagnosis, and prognosis: *allows the nurse to identify concerns and areas where further education may be needed and demonstrates family-centered care.*
- Allow families to grieve over the loss of a "perfect" child: *parents must work through those grief feelings so they can be fully "present" for this chronically ill child.*
- Explain therapies, procedures, child's behaviors, and plan of care to parents: *understanding the child's current status and plan of care helps decrease anxiety.*
- Encourage parents to be involved in care: *allows parents to feel needed and valued and gives them a sense of control over their child's health.*
- Identify support system for family and child: *helps nurse identify needs and resources available for coping.*
- Educate family and child on additional resources available *to help them develop a wide base of support.*
- Encourage parents to seek genetic counseling *to provide them with the information required to make an informed decision about having another child.*

NURSING DIAGNOSIS: Activity intolerance related to ineffective cardiac muscle function, increased energy expenditure, or inability to meet increased oxygen or metabolic demands as evidenced by squatting positions, shortness of breath, cyanosis, or fatigue

Outcome Identification and Evaluation

Child will increase activity level as tolerated: child participates in play and activities (specify particular activities and level as individualized for each child).

Interventions: ***Promoting Activity***

- Assess level of fatigue and activity tolerance *to determine baseline for comparison.*
- Note extent of dyspnea, oxygen requirement, or color change with exertion *to provide baseline for comparison.*
- Cluster care activities, allowing rest periods in between, *to conserve child's energy.*
- Work with the parent and child to determine a mutually satisfactory daily schedule *to allow adequate rest and energy conservation.*
- Instruct family and child in prescribed activity restrictions *to prevent fatigue while allowing some activity.*
- In the infant, avoid long periods of crying or prolonged nipple feeding: *expends excessive calories.*
- Provide neutral thermal environment *to avoid increased oxygen and energy needs associated with excessive heat or cold.*

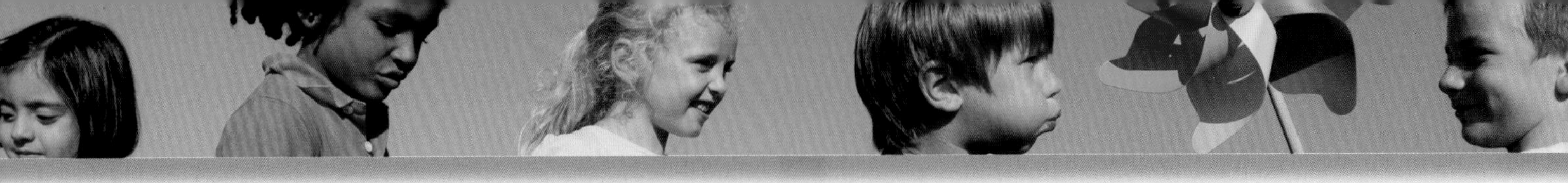

KEY CONCEPTS

- At birth, when the umbilical cord is cut and the neonate's first breath occurs, the ductus venosus closes with the foramen ovale and the ductus arteriosus closes shortly thereafter. Pulmonary vascular resistance decreases and systemic vascular resistance increases.
- The infant's heart rate averages 120 to 130 bpm and decreases throughout childhood, reaching the adult rate in adolescence. Conversely, the infant's and child's BP is significantly lower than the adult's, increasing as the child ages.
- Check the infant's apical pulse prior to digoxin administration and hold the dose if the heart rate is less than 90.
- Poor weight gain, failure to thrive, and increased fatigability commonly occur with congestive heart failure.
- Clubbing of the fingernails occurs as a result of chronic hypoxia in the child with severe CHD.
- Children with cardiac conditions resulting in cyanosis often have baseline oxygen saturations that are relatively low, because of the mixing of oxygenated with deoxygenated blood.
- Document the presence of a murmur by grading its intensity (I through IV), describing where it occurs within the cardiac cycle, and noting the location where the murmur is best heard.
- CHD should be suspected in the cyanotic newborn who does not improve with oxygen administration.
- Cardiac catheterization postprocedure care focuses on evaluation of the child's vital signs and condition of the pressure dressing, as well as assessment of the distal pulses bilaterally for presence and quality.
- Congenital heart disorders resulting in decreased pulmonary blood flow (tetralogy of Fallot, tricuspid atresia) result in cyanosis.
- Disorders with increased pulmonary blood flow (PDA, ASD, and VSD) may result in pulmonary edema if the defect is severe.
- A decrease in the lower extremity pulses or BP as compared with the upper extremities may be indicative of coarctation of the aorta.
- It is important to remain calm when an infant or child demonstrates a hypercyanotic spell. Place the child in a knee-chest position, administer oxygen and/or morphine or propranolol, and supply intravenous fluids.
- Children with certain congenital heart defects and/or heart failure require additional calories in order to display adequate growth.
- Children with hypertrophic cardiomyopathy, certain congenital heart defects, valve dysfunction, or prosthetic valves require prophylaxis for infective endocarditis when undergoing procedures or invasive dental work.
- Hypertension in the child or adolescent often leads to long-term health consequences such as cardiovascular disease and left ventricular hypertrophy.
- Kawasaki disease may result in severe cardiac sequelae, so these children need ongoing cardiac follow-up to screen for development of problems.
- It is important to screen for hyperlipidemia in high-risk children.
- Abrupt cessation of chest tube output, accompanied by an increase in the heart rate and increased filling pressure, may indicate cardiac tamponade.

REFERENCES AND RECOMMENDED READINGS

Abdallah, H. (2016). *About the Children's Heart Institute.* Retrieved from www.childrenheartinstitute.org/testing/testhome.htm

Abdoulhosn, J. A., & Child, J. S. (2011). Congenital heart disease in adults. In: V. Fuster, R. A. Walsh, & R. A. Harrington (Eds.), *Hurst's the heart* (13th ed.). New York, NY: McGraw-Hill Companies, Inc.

AGA Medical Corporation. (2014). *Amplatzer™ muscular VSD occluder: Instructions for use.* Plymouth, MN: Author.

Altman, C. A. (2015). *Identifying newborns with critical congenital heart disease.* Retrieved from www.uptodate.com/contents/identifying-newborns-with-critical-congenital-heart-disease

American Academy of Pediatrics and American Heart Association. (2011). *Textbook of neonatal resuscitation* (6th ed.). Elk Grove Village, IL: American Academy of Pediatrics.

American Heart Association. (2014). *Infective (bacterial) endocarditis wallet card.* Retrieved from www.heart.org/HEARTORG/Conditions/More/ToolsForYourHeartHealth/Infective-Bacterial-Endocarditis-Wallet-Card_UCM_311659_Article.jsp

American Heart Association. (2015a). *Pediatric cardiomyopathies.* Retrieved from www.heart.org/HEARTORG/Conditions/More/CardiovascularConditionsofChildhood/Pediatric-Cardiomyopathies_UCM_312219_Article.jsp#.Vz3aOZErLNM

American Heart Association. (2015b). *Understand your risk for congenital heart defects.* Retrieved from www.heart.org/

HEARTORG/Conditions/CongenitalHeartDefects/UnderstandYourRiskforCongenitalHeartDefects/Understand-Your-Risk-for-Congenital-Heart-Defects_UCM_001219_Article.jsp

Bacha, E. A., Cooper, D., Thiagarajan, R., et al. (2008). Cardiac complications associated with the treatment of patients with congenital cardiac disease: Consensus definitions from the Multi-Societal Database Committee for Pediatric and Congenital Heart Disease. *Cardiology in the Young, 18*(Suppl 2), 196–201.

Bass, J. L., Corwin, M., Gozal, D., Moore, C., Nishida, H., Parker, S., et al. (2004). The effect of chronic or intermittent hypoxia on cognition in childhood: A review of the evidence. *Pediatrics, 114*(3), 805–816.

Beke, D. M., Braudis, N. J., & Lincoln, P. (2005). Management of the pediatric postoperative cardiac surgery patient. *Critical Care Nursing Clinics of North America, 17*(4), 405–416.

Bright Futures/American Academy of Pediatrics. (2016). Recommendations for Preventive Pediatric Health Care. Retrieved from https://pediatriccare.solutions.aap.org/DocumentLibrary/Periodicity%20Schedule_FINAL.pdf

Brown, D. (2016). *Valvar aortic stenosis in children.* Retrieved from www.uptodate.com/contents/valvar-aortic-stenosis-in-children

Brown, D. W., & Fulton, D. R. (2011). Congenital heart disease in children and adolescents. In: V. Fuster, R. A. Walsh, & R. A. Harrington (Eds.), *Hurst's the heart* (13th ed.). New York, NY: McGraw-Hill Companies, Inc.

Brusch, J. L. & Bronze, M. S. (2015). *Infective endocarditis.* Retrieved from http://emedicine.medscape.com/article/216650-overview

Carpenito-Moyet, L. J. (2013). *Nursing diagnosis: Application to clinical practice* (14th ed.). Philadelphia, PA: Lippincott Williams & Wilkins.

Cassidy, S. C., Allen, H. D., & Phillips, J. R. (2013). History and physical examination. In: H. D. Allen, D. J. Driscoll, R. E. Shaddy, & T. F. Feltes (Eds.), *Moss and Adams' heart disease in infants, children, and adolescents: Including the fetus and young adult.* Philadelphia, PA: Lippincott Williams and Wilkins.

Centers for Disease Control and Prevention. (2016). *Who should not get vaccinated with these vaccines?* Retrieved from www.cdc.gov/vaccines/vpd-vac/should-not-vacc.htm#mmr

Children's Healthcare of Atlanta. (2010). *Your child's heart catheterization.* Retrieved from www.choa.org/Childrens-Hospital-Services/Cardiac/Testing-and-Treatments/Heart-Testing/~/media/CHOA/Documents/Services/Cardiac/Your-Childs-Heart-Cath.pdf

Chinnock, R. E., & Ohye, R. G. (2014). *Pediatric heart transplantation.* Retrieved from http://emedicine.medscape.com/article/1011927-overview

Cook, E. H., & Higgins, S. S. (2010). Congenital heart disease. In: P. J. Allen, J. A. Vessey, & N. A. Schapiro (Eds.), *Primary care of the child with a chronic condition* (5th ed.). St. Louis, MO: Mosby.

Corbett, J. A., & Banks, A. D. (2013). *Laboratory tests and diagnostic procedures with nursing diagnoses* (8th ed.). Upper Saddle River, NJ: Pearson Education Inc.

Cunningham, F. G., Leveno, K. J., Bloom, S. L., Spong, C. Y., Dashe, J. S., Hoffman, B. L., et al. (2014). *Williams obstetrics* (24th ed.). New York, NY: McGraw-Hill Education.

Darst, J. R., Collins, K. K., & Miyamoto, S. D. (2014). Cardiovascular diseases. In: W. W. Hay, M. J. Levin, R. R. Deterding, & M. J. Abzug, (Eds.), (*Current pediatric diagnosis and treatment* (22nd ed.). New York, NY: McGraw-Hill.

Dipchand, A. I., Bastardi, H., & Dupuis, J. (2013). *Pediatric heart transplants: A guide for patients and families.* Birmingham, AL: Pediatric Heart Transplant Study Foundation.

Doyle, T., Kavanaugh-McHugh, A., & Fish, F. A. (2016). *Management and outcome of tetralogy of Fallot.* Retrieved from www.uptodate.com/contents/management-and-outcome-of-tetralogy-of-fallot

Engorn, B., & Flerlage, J. (2015). *The Harriet Lane handbook* (20th ed.). Philadelphia, PA: Saunders.

Francis, G. S., Wilson Tang, W. H., & Walsh, R. A. (2011). Pathophysiology of heart failure. In: V. Fuster, R. A. Walsh, & R. A. Harrington (Eds.), *Hurst's the heart* (13th ed.). New York, NY: McGraw-Hill Companies, Inc.

Gibofsky, A. (2015). *Clinical manifestations and diagnosis of acute rheumatic fever.* Retrieved from www.uptodate.com/contents/clinical-manifestations-and-diagnosis-of-acute-rheumatic-fever

Kantor, P. F., Abraham, J. R., Dipchand, A. I., Benson, L. N., & Redington, A. N. (2010). The impact of changing medical therapy on transplantation-free survival in pediatric dilated cardiomyopathy. *Journal of the American College of Cardiology, 55*(13), 1377–1384.

Lankin, K. (2012). Pediatric heart transplantation. In: Hazinski, M. F. (Ed.), *Nursing care of the critically ill child* (3rd ed.). St. Louis, MO: Elsevier, Mosby.

Lorts, A., Krawczeski, C. D., & Marino, B. S. (2013). Cardiology. In: B. S. Marino, & K. S. Fine (Eds.), *Blueprints: Pediatrics* (6th ed.). Philadelphia, PA: Lippincott Williams & Wilkins.

Marian, A. J., Brugada, R., & Roberts, R. (2011). Cardiovascular disease due to genetic abnormalities. In: V. Fuster, R. A. Walsh, & R. A. Harrington (Eds.), *Hurst's the heart* (13th ed.). New York, NY: McGraw-Hill Companies, Inc.

Mattoo, T. K. (2016b). *Treatment of hypertension in children and adolescents.* Retrieved from www.uptodate.com/contents/treatment-of-hypertension-in-children-and-adolescents

Mattoo, T. K. (2106a). *Epidemiology, risk factors, and etiology of hypertension in children and adolescents.* Retrieved from www.uptodate.com/contents/epidemiology-risk-factors-and-etiology-of-hypertension-in-children-and-adolescents

McCord, M. E., & Lee, L. E. (2011). Dyslipidemia in children: Nonpharmacologic approaches for early intervention. *Advance for NPs & PAs, 1*(3), 24–29.

National Heart, Lung, and Blood Institute. (2012). *Expert Panel on Integrated Guidelines for Cardiovascular Health and Risk Reduction in Children and Adolescents.* SUMMARY REPORT (NIH Publication No. 12–7486). Washington, DC: U.S. Department of Health and Human Services.

Park, M. K. (2014). *Park's pediatric cardiology for practitioners* (6th ed.). Philadelphia, PA: Saunders.

Peng, L. F., & Perry, S. (2016). *Pulmonic stenosis (PS) in neonates, infants, and children.* Retrieved from www.uptodate.com/contents/pulmonic-stenosis-ps-in-neonates-infants-and-children

Ralston, S. L., Lieberthal, A. S., Meissner, C., Alverson, B. K., Baley, J. E., Gadomski, A. M., et al. (2014). Clinical practice guideline: The diagnosis, management, and prevention of bronchiolitis. *Pediatrics, 134*, e1474-e1502.

Schuman, A. J. (2013). Making a difference. *Contemporary Pediatrics, 30*(4), 38–41.

Skippen, P., Sanatina, S., Froese, N., & Gow, R. M. (2010). Pacemaker therapy of postoperative arrhythmias after pediatric cardiac surgery. *Pediatric Critical Care Medicine, 11*, 113–138.

Sundel, R. (2016a). *Kawasaki disease: Clinical features and diagnosis*. Retrieved from www.uptodate.com/contents/kawasaki-disease-clinical-features-and-diagnosis

Sundel, R. (2016b). *Kawasaki disease: Epidemiology and etiology*. Retrieved from www.uptodate.com/contents/kawasaki-disease-epidemiology-and-etiology

Sundel, R. (2016c). *Kawasaki disease: Initial treatment and prognosis*. Retrieved from www.uptodate.com/contents/kawasaki-disease-initial-treatment-and-prognosis

Taketomo, C. K., Hodding, J. H., & Kraus, D. M. (2013). *Pediatric & neonatal dosage handbook* (20th ed.). Hudson, OH: Lexicomp.

The University of Chicago Medicine Comer Children's Hospital. (2016). *Heart catheterization in children*. Retrieved from www.uchicagokidshospital.org/specialties/heart/patient-education/cath-guide.html

U.S. Department of Health and Human Services. (2016). *Healthy people 2020*. Retrieved from www.healthypeople.gov/2020/default

W. L. Gore & Associates, Inc. (2010). Instructions for use: Gore Helex septal occluder. Retrieved from www.fda.gov/ucm/groups/fdagov-public/@fdagov-afda-adcom/documents/document/ucm304933.pdf

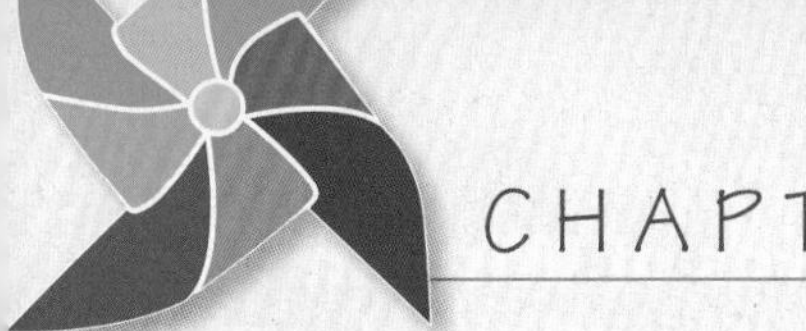

CHAPTER WORKSHEET

MULTIPLE CHOICE QUESTIONS

1. The nurse is caring for a 5-year-old child with a congenital heart anomaly causing chronic cyanosis. When performing the history and physical examination, what is the nurse least likely to assess?
   a. obesity from overeating
   b. clubbing of the nail beds
   c. squatting during play activities
   d. exercise intolerance
2. A 2-day-old infant was just diagnosed with aortic stenosis. What is the most likely nursing assessment finding?
   a. gallop and rales
   b. blood pressure discrepancies in the extremities
   c. right ventricular hypertrophy on ECG
   d. heart murmur
3. Sam, age 11, has a diagnosis of rheumatic fever and has missed school for a week. What is the most likely cause of this problem?
   a. previous streptococcal throat infection
   b. history of open heart surgery at 5 years of age
   c. playing too much soccer and not getting enough rest
   d. exposure to a sibling with pneumonia
4. The nurse is caring for a child after a cardiac catheterization. What is the nursing priority?
   a. Allow early ambulation to encourage activity participation.
   b. Check pulses above the catheter insertion site for strength and quality.
   c. Assess extremity distal to the insertion site for temperature and color.
   d. Change the dressing to evaluate the site for infection.
5. While assessing a 4-month-old infant, the nurse notes that the baby experiences a hypercyanotic spell. What is the priority nursing action?
   a. Provide supplemental oxygen by face mask.
   b. Administer a dose of IV morphine sulfate.
   c. Begin cardiopulmonary resuscitation.
   d. Place the infant in a knee-to-chest position.

DOSAGE CALCULATION QUESTION

The nurse is caring for an infant with a ventricular septal defect who has heart failure. The infant weighs 11 lb. The medication order reads: spironolactone 5 mg PO every 12 hours. Spironolactone is provided by the pharmacy in a solution of 2.5 mg/1 mL. How many milliliters will the nurse administer? Round to the nearest whole number.

CRITICAL THINKING EXERCISES

1. A baby boy was born at 26 weeks' gestation to 15-year-old unmarried parents who abuse drugs. The infant weighed 1.5 kg at birth and was diagnosed with AV canal defect and Down syndrome. Discuss some of the major issues in planning for care. Include a care plan and a list of teaching needs for the family.
2. A 4-year-old boy has parents with little education, and the child has Medicaid coverage. Another child is 7 years old and has well-educated parents with private insurance coverage. Both of these children need a heart transplant, and a heart is available that is a very good match for both children. Discuss some of the issues involved in deciding which child should receive the heart.
3. A 13-year-old boy was diagnosed with hypertension over 2 years ago. He is noncompliant with his antihypertensive medication regimen. He is 5 ft tall and weighs 170 lb. His favorite activity is video games. Develop a teaching plan for this teen, providing creative approaches at the appropriate developmental level.

STUDY ACTIVITIES

1. Teach a class of sixth graders about healthy activities to prevent high cholesterol levels, hypertension, and heart disease. Use visual materials.
2. Spend the day with a nurse practitioner in the pediatric cardiology clinic. Report to the clinical group your observations about the children's quality of life, growth, and development.
3. Observe in the pediatric cardiothoracic intensive care unit or telemetry unit. Note the different cardiac rhythms displayed by children with a variety of cardiovascular disorders.

BRINGING IT ALL TOGETHER: A CASE STUDY

Mitchell Ryder, 4 months old, is brought to the hospital by his mother. He presents with difficulty gaining weight. His mother states, "He just gets so tired when he eats, and sometimes when he is nursing he has a bluish color around his lips."

Go to thePoint to find questions to consider about this case.

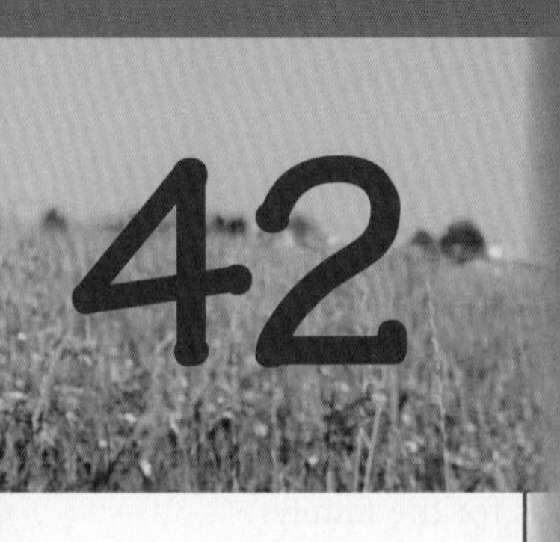

42

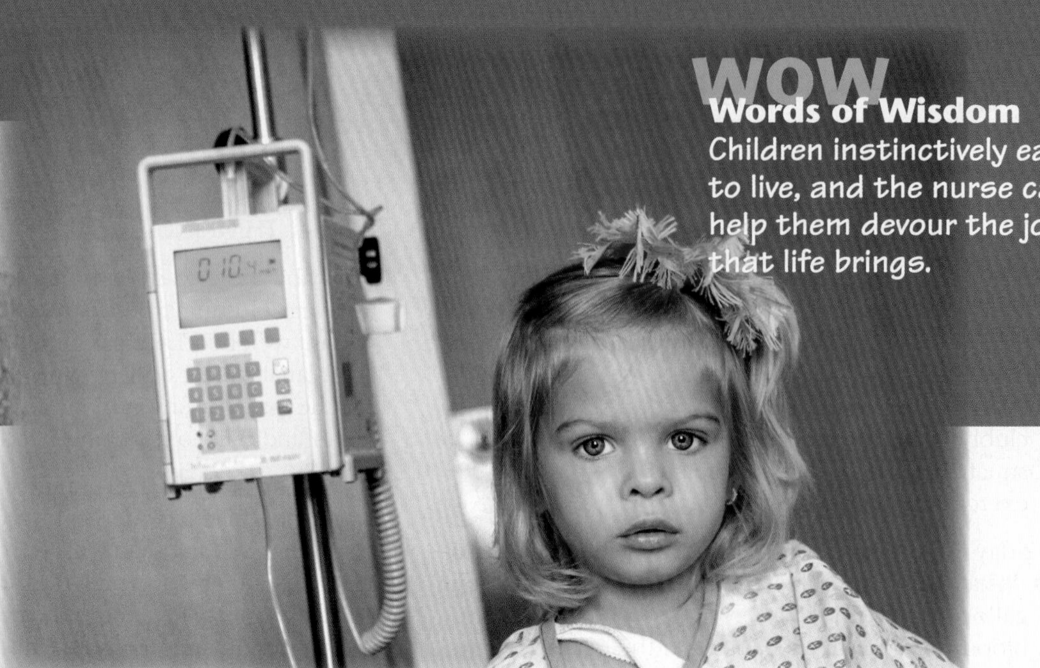

WOW
Words of Wisdom
Children instinctively eat to live, and the nurse can help them devour the joys that life brings.

Nursing Care of the Child With an Alteration in Bowel Elimination/ Gastrointestinal Disorder

KEY TERMS
atresia
cholestasis
cirrhosis
cleft
dysphagia
fecal impaction
guarding
icteric
lethargy
protuberant
rebound tenderness
regurgitation
steatorrhea

Learning Objectives

Upon completion of the chapter, you will be able to:

1. Compare the differences in the anatomy and physiology of the gastrointestinal system between children and adults.
2. Discuss common medical treatments for infants and children with alterations in bowel elimination (gastrointestinal disorders).
3. Discuss common laboratory and diagnostic tests used to identify disorders of the gastrointestinal tract.
4. Discuss medication therapy used in infants and children with alterations in bowel elimination (gastrointestinal disorders).
5. Recognize risk factors associated with various gastrointestinal illnesses.
6. Differentiate between acute and chronic gastrointestinal disorders.
7. Distinguish common gastrointestinal illnesses of childhood.
8. Discuss nursing interventions commonly used for gastrointestinal illnesses.
9. Devise an individualized nursing care plan for infants/children with an alteration in bowel elimination/gastrointestinal disorder.
10. Develop teaching plans for family/child education for children with gastrointestinal illnesses.
11. Describe the psychosocial impact that chronic gastrointestinal illnesses have on children.

***Ethan Richardson*, 2 months old, is brought to the clinic by his mother. He has been vomiting for the past 3 days. His mother states that she switched formula to see if that would help, but the vomiting worsened. Since last night she has attempted to feed him only Pedialyte. Mrs. Roberts says, "He can't keep anything down and he's very irritable." His weight at birth was 8 lb 9 oz, length 21 in, and head circumference 37 cm. At his 2-month check-up last week he weighed 13 lb.**

Bowel elimination refers to the secretion and excretion of body waste through the intestinal system. Nurses may encounter children with alterations in bowel elimination should be familiar with various gastrointestinal disorders that children experience. Alterations in bowel elimination, or gastrointestinal (GI) disorders affect children of all ages. GI illnesses range from acute to chronic and from non–life-threatening to life-threatening problems. However, even acute, non–life-threatening illnesses (e.g., diarrhea or vomiting) can become life-threatening without proper nursing assessment and interventions. The most common result of a GI illness is dehydration, requiring fluid therapy at home or, in more extreme cases, in a hospital setting. It is important to take all GI disorders seriously until symptoms are well controlled.

Child and family education related to the treatment of GI disorders is key to preventing the illness from progressing to an emergency situation. Therefore, the nurse's knowledge of the disorders that affect the GI system is crucial. Most often, the parents or child, if the child is older, will contact the physician or nurse practitioner in an outpatient setting to seek help. The nurse is usually the person to triage the phone call to determine the next step in the situation, which may be determining whether the child should be managed at home, brought to the office for assessment, or sent directly to an emergency room for evaluation. The majority of GI disorders can be handled in an outpatient setting to avoid unnecessary hospitalizations. However, some life-threatening problems (e.g., bowel obstruction) require emergency care in the hospital. Again, the knowledge base of the nurse is instrumental in obtaining the proper information by taking a thorough and accurate health history from the parents or child (if the child is older).

VARIATIONS IN PEDIATRIC ANATOMY AND PHYSIOLOGY

The GI tract includes all of the structures from the mouth to the anus. The primary functions of the GI system are the digestion and absorption of nutrients and water, elimination of waste products, and secretion of various substances required for digestion. Babies are born with immature GI tracts that are not fully mature until age 2. Due to this immaturity, there are many differences between the digestive tract of the young child and that of the older child or adult.

Mouth

The mouth is highly vascular, making it a common entry point for infectious invaders. In addition, the infant and young child repeatedly bring objects to their mouths and explore them in that fashion. This behavior increases the infant's and young child's risk for contracting infectious agents via the mouth.

Esophagus

The esophagus provides a passageway from the mouth to the stomach for food. The lower esophageal sphincter (LES) prevents **regurgitation** (backflow) of stomach contents up into the esophagus and/or oral cavity. The muscle tone of the LES is not fully developed until age 1 month, so infants younger than 1 month of age frequently regurgitate after feedings. Many children younger than 1 year of age continue to regurgitate for several months, but this usually disappears with age. If edema or narrowing of the esophagus occurs in a child with undeveloped esophageal muscle tone, **dysphagia** (difficult or painful swallowing) may occur.

Stomach

Newborns have a stomach capacity of only 10 to 20 mL. At 2 months of age an infant has the capacity to hold up to 200 mL, though most young infants cannot tolerate 200-mL feedings. By age 16, the stomach capacity is 1,500 mL; by adulthood it is 2,000 to 3,000 mL. Hydrochloric acid, which is found in gastric contents to aid in digestion, reaches the adult level by the time the child is 6 months old.

Intestines

The small intestine is not functionally mature at birth. A full-term infant has approximately 250 cm of small intestine; an adult has up to 600 cm. Infants who have small bowel loss during early infancy have more problems with absorption and diarrhea than adults who have the same amount of small bowel loss.

Biliary System

The liver is relatively large at birth, allowing for the smooth edge of the liver to be easily palpated in infancy, as much as 2 cm below the costal margin. The pancreatic enzymes continue to develop postnatally, reaching adult levels around 2 years of age.

Fluid Balance and Losses

Compared with adults, children exhibit differences in how fluid volume is maintained. These differences are evident in body fluid balance and insensible fluid losses.

Body Fluid Balance

Infants and children have a proportionately greater amount of body water than do adults. Infants and young children require a larger relative fluid intake than adults and excrete a relatively greater amount of fluid. This places them at increased risk for fluid loss with illness compared to adults. Until age 2 years, the extracellular fluid, with its larger proportion of sodium and chloride, makes up about half of the child's total body water. Therefore, when potential fluid-loss states occur, water loss occurs more rapidly and in larger amounts than in adults.

Insensible Fluid Losses

Fever increases fluid loss at a rate of about 7 mL/kg/24-hour period for every sustained 1°C rise in temperature. Since children become febrile with illness more readily and their fevers are higher than those of adults, infants and young children are more apt than adults to experience insensible fluid loss with fever when ill.

Fluid loss via the skin accounts for about two thirds of insensible fluid loss. Infants have a relatively larger body surface area (BSA) relative to their body mass as compared to older children and adults. The newborn's BSA ratio to body mass is about two or three times greater than the adult's, and the preterm infant's is about five times greater than the adult's. This places infants, especially young infants, at increased risk of insensible fluid loss as compared to older children and adults.

The basal metabolic rate in infants and children is higher than that of adults in order to support growth. This higher metabolic rate, even in states of wellness, accounts for increased insensible fluid losses and increased need for water for excretory functions. The young infant's renal immaturity does not allow the kidneys to concentrate urine as well as in older children and adults. This puts infants at particular risk for dehydration or overhydration, depending on the circumstances.

COMMON MEDICAL TREATMENTS

There are many different forms of medical treatment for GI disorders. In the hospital setting, most medical treatments will require a physician's order. The most common treatments and medications used for GI disorders are listed in Common Medical Treatments 42.1 and Drug Guide 42.1. Both tables provide essential information about medical treatments and medications used in pediatric GI disorders. Refer to these tables as needed while completing the remainder of the chapter.

NURSING PROCESS OVERVIEW FOR THE CHILD WITH AN ALTERATION IN BOWEL ELIMINATION OR GASTROINTESTINAL DISORDER

Nursing care of the child with a GI disorder or alteration in bowel elimination includes nursing assessment, nursing diagnosis, planning, interventions, and evaluation. It is important to individualize each step of this process for each child. A general understanding of the GI tract and the most common disorders can help the nurse to individualize the nursing care plan.

Remember Ethan, the 2-month-old with vomiting and irritability? What additional health history and physical examination assessment information should you obtain?

Assessment

The assessment of the child with a GI disorder includes a health history, physical examination, and laboratory and diagnostic testing.

Health History

A thorough health history is very important in the assessment of a child with a GI disorder. The health history includes past history (previous illnesses/surgeries), past family history, present illness (when the symptoms began and how this differs from the child's normal status), and how the child's symptoms have been managed up to this point (relevant medical records/home treatments). Detailed knowledge of the past medical and surgical history of the child may reveal bowel resection, previous intestinal infections, and dietary issues and problems.

The child's growth patterns can also be an instrumental part of the health history and may help to generate a timeline for when the current problems appeared. The family history is also extremely important in identifying common genetic or familial GI symptoms or disorders such as irritable bowel syndrome (IBS), inflammatory bowel disease, or food allergies. The history of the present illness and symptoms can often distinguish chronic problems from acute disorders. All of these pieces of the health history require descriptive questions and answers from both the nurse and the child, or the child's family. The person providing the history must be able to provide accurate details of the health history.

Physical Examination

Perform the physical examination of the child from the least invasive part of the examination to the most invasive. It is important for the child to remain as relaxed as possible during this part of the assessment.

INSPECTION AND OBSERVATION

Inspect and observe the child's color, hydration status, abdominal size and shape, and mental status.

Color. First observe the child's skin, eye, and lip color. Pale skin or lips in a child with a GI disorder

COMMON MEDICAL TREATMENTS 42.1 GASTROINTESTINAL DISORDERS

Treatment	Explanation	Indications	Nursing Implications
Cleansing enema	Insertion of fluid into the rectum to soften the stool and stimulate bowel activity	Fecal impaction, severe constipation	Explain procedure to child prior to enema. With multiple enemas, observe for electrolyte imbalances.
Bowel preparation	Use of highly osmotic fluids to induce severe diarrhea to cleanse the entire bowel	Preparation for colonoscopy or bowel surgery	Some children may need to have a nasogastric tube placed so they can consume the needed amounts of fluids. Observe for signs and symptoms of dehydration/electrolyte imbalance.
Feeding tubes	Flexible tubes used for enteral feeding when the infant or child is incapable of swallowing safely or for augmenting nutrition. May be orogastric, nasogastric, gastrostomy, or jejunostomy	Feeding difficulties, failure to thrive, gastroesophageal reflux disease, chronic illness	Orogastric and nasogastric tubes must be checked for placement prior to each use. If required long-term, use a softer, flexible tube intended for long-term use. Stomahesive or Duoderm applied to the cheek may decrease risk of skin breakdown from tape. Gastrostomy tubes vary in type. Keep insertion site clean and dry.
Intravenous therapy	Administration of fluids via a catheter that delivers electrolytes and fluids into the venous system	Dehydration, bowel rest, NPO status	Monitor intravenous site for redness, swelling, and pain. Assess urine output to evaluate hydration status.
Ostomy	A portion of the intestine is brought to the level of the skin to allow passage of stool.	Imperforate anus, gastroschisis, omphalocele, Hirschsprung disease, necrotizing enterocolitis, Crohn disease, ulcerative colitis	Ostomy contents may be acidic and irritate the skin. Use Stomahesive or Duoderm under the pouch to avoid tape irritation to the skin. Pouch should fit the stoma correctly. Assess stoma for pinkness and moist appearance.
Oral rehydration therapy	Administration by mouth of fluids that contain certain amounts of electrolytes and glucose to prevent dehydration and/or promote rehydration	Diarrhea, acute gastroenteritis, vomiting	Fluid administration should begin prior to the onset of dehydration. Urine output should be monitored to evaluate hydration status.
Probiotics (lactobacillus, acidophilus)	Food supplement containing dormant bacteria that when activated may alter the intestinal microflora	Treatment/prevention of diarrhea	Particularly helpful in prevention of or decreasing incidence of antibiotic-induced diarrhea.
Total parenteral nutrition (TPN)	Intravenous complete nutrition. Provides glucose, protein, lipids, vitamins, and minerals	Long-term NPO status, swallowing difficulties, difficulties tolerating enteral feeding (short bowel syndrome, necrotizing enterocolitis)	Higher glucose and protein concentrations and solutions containing calcium require central venous access. Monitor blood glucose levels with initiation, rate changes, and discontinuation. Blood chemistries should be monitored on a regular basis.

DRUG GUIDE 42.1 COMMON DRUGS FOR GI DISORDERS

Classification	Actions/Indications	Nursing Implications
Histamine-2 blockers (ranitidine, famotidine, cimetidine, nizatidine)	Decrease histamine production, thereby reducing gastric acid secretion Used for heartburn, esophagitis, GERD, benign duodenal or gastric ulcers	May cause drowsiness or dizziness.
Proton pump inhibitors (omeprazole, lansoprazole, esomeprazole, pantoprazole, rabeprazole)	Block the pump that produces gastric acids Indicated for erosive esophagitis, symptomatic GERD, *H. pylori* eradication	Adverse effects include headache, nausea, abdominal pain, or diarrhea.
Prokinetics (metoclopramide, cisapride)	Stimulate GI motility to help empty the stomach faster and promote intestinal motility	Metoclopramide may have central nervous system adverse effects. Cisapride available only in limited-access protocol studies.
Antibacterials/antibiotics (metronidazole, vancomycin)	Treatment of bacterial infections of the GI tract Used for suspected or proven bacterial infections of the GI tract, such as *Clostridium difficile* or parasitic infections	May cause GI upset, diarrhea. Very important to finish entire course of treatment.
Immunosuppressants (6-mercaptopurine, azathioprine)	Suppress the immune system to keep autoimmune disorders in remission such as Crohn disease, ulcerative colitis, autoimmune hepatitis	Drug levels should be checked to determine drug metabolite levels and potential for hepatotoxicity or bone marrow suppression.
Stimulants (senna, docusate sodium)	Stimulate peristalsis in the large intestine to produce a bowel movement Used to relieve constipation	May cause cramping or diarrhea. Stool patterns should be constantly assessed.
Laxatives (polyethylene glycol, milk of magnesia, lactulose)	Soften the stool to allow for easier passage through the colon Used to relieve constipation	Stool patterns should be monitored. Doses may need to be readjusted frequently to find the correct dose for the child.
Antidiarrheals (loperamide, diphenoxylate/atropine)	Decrease peristalsis, thus prolonging transit time of stool through the intestines Indicated to treat diarrhea related to short bowel syndrome, chronic nonspecific diarrhea, irritable bowel syndrome	May cause drowsiness or constipation.
Corticosteroids (prednisone)	Act systemically to reduce inflammation and suppress the normal immune response Used in inflammatory bowel disease, autoimmune disorders	Systemic adverse effects include hirsutism, osteoporosis, GI upset, cushingoid appearance, increased intraocular pressure, irritability, and personality changes. Should be taken as directed. Stopping the medication suddenly may cause adrenal insufficiency.
Antiemetics (promethazine, metoclopramide)	Act on the central nervous system transmitters to prevent nausea and vomiting	May have central nervous system adverse effects, such as drowsiness or irritability.
Anticholinergic/antispasmodics (hyoscyamine, dicyclomine, glycopyrrolate)	Used to control abdominal spasms and cramping associated with irritable bowel syndrome, functional bowel disorders	May cause excessive thirst or dizziness. Encourage plenty of fluids while taking these medications.
Anti-inflammatories (mesalamine, balsalazide, hydrocortisone enemas/suppositories, olsalazine, sulfasalazine)	Reduce inflammation in the colon associated with ulcerative colitis, proctitis	Stool output should be monitored to assess for presence of oral medications (indicating poor absorption).

Adapted from Taketomo, C. K., Hodding, J. H., & Kraus, D. M. (2013). *Pediatric & neonatal dosage handbook* (20th ed.). Hudson, OH: Lexicomp.

may be a sign of anemia or dehydration. During liver dysfunction, the bilirubin levels can rise, causing the skin to look jaundiced (yellow). The sclerae can also become **icteric** (yellowed in color), further indicating that the liver is not functioning correctly. Inspect the abdomen for distended veins, which can indicate abdominal or vascular obstruction or distention. As in any part of a physical assessment, watch for areas of ecchymosis (bruising), which may be a sign of abuse.

Hydration Status. The child's hydration status often indicates how severe the current GI illness is. Dehydration can occur rapidly in children, especially in infants and young children. The oral mucosa should be pink and moist. Skin turgor should be elastic. Decreased turgor and tenting indicate dehydration. During crying, especially in infants, the absence of tears may indicate dehydration. Assess the amount of urine output the child has had in the past 24 hours.

Abdominal Size and Shape. Inspect the size and shape of the abdomen while the child is standing and while the child is lying supine. The abdomen should be flat when the child is supine. An especially **protuberant** (bulging outward) abdomen suggests the presence of ascites, fluid retention, gaseous distention, or even a tumor. However, many children (toddlers in particular) have a prominent "pot-bellied" abdomen as a normal variation of their anatomy (Weber & Kelley, 2014). A depressed or concave abdomen could indicate a high abdominal obstruction or dehydration. Inspect the umbilicus for color, odor, discharge, inflammation, and herniation.

Mental Status. Perform a brief mental status examination of all children with GI complaints. Mental status changes can occur in many instances, such as during severe dehydration, with anaphylactic reactions to foods or medicines, when ammonia levels are elevated with severe liver disease, and with other metabolic disorders. Irritability and restlessness are usually the early signs of mental status changes. **Lethargy** (sluggishness or abnormal drowsiness) and listlessness can occur much more rapidly in children than in adults. It is important to identify this promptly and treat it emergently.

AUSCULTATION

As with all children, auscultate bowel sounds in all four quadrants. Hyperactive bowel sounds may be noted in children with diarrhea or gastroenteritis. Hypoactive or absent bowel sounds may signify an obstructive process. The nurse can determine absence of bowel sounds after a 5-minute period of auscultation. This can be extremely difficult to perform with children and infants, who may be uncooperative during the examination. Immediately report hypoactive or absent bowel sound findings to the physician or nurse practitioner.

PERCUSSION

Dullness or flatness is normally found along the right costal margin and 1 to 3 cm below the costal margin of the liver. The area above the symphysis pubis may be dull in young children with full bladders, which is a normal finding. Percussion of the remainder of the abdomen should reveal tympany. Note abnormal findings.

PALPATION

Reserve palpation for last in the sequence of abdominal examination. First, lightly palpate the abdomen to assess for areas of tenderness, lesions, muscle tone, turgor, and cutaneous hyperesthesia (a finding in acute peritonitis). Then perform deep palpation from the lower quadrants upward to best feel the liver edge, which should be firm and smooth. In infants and children, palpate the liver during inspiration below the right costal margin. The tip of the spleen may be palpated also during inspiration; it should be 1 to 2 cm below the left costal margin. Palpable kidneys, except in neonates, may indicate tumor or hydronephrosis. The sigmoid colon can be palpated in the left lower quadrant. The cecum may be felt in the right lower quadrant as a soft mass. Areas of firmness or masses may indicate tumor or stool in the abdomen.

Tenderness in the abdomen is not a normal physical finding. Right upper quadrant tenderness could indicate liver enlargement. Right lower quadrant pain, including **rebound tenderness** (pain upon release of pressure during palpation), can be a warning sign of appendicitis; immediately report any positive findings to a physician. Palpate the external inguinal canals for the presence of inguinal hernias, often elicited by having the child turn the head and cough, or blow up a balloon.

Laboratory and Diagnostic Testing

Common Laboratory and Diagnostic Tests 42.1 gives information about the tests most often ordered by physicians for children with GI illnesses. Some of these tests are ordered in the hospital setting; others are done on an outpatient basis. Typically, the nurse is involved directly in specimen collection while a specifically trained person performs the diagnostic tests. Regardless of who performs the test, nurses must be familiar with preparation guidelines for the child, how each test is performed, and normal and abnormal findings and their significance in order to provide appropriate child and family education. Teaching Guidelines 42.1 gives tips on collecting stool specimens.

(text continues on page 1584)

COMMON LABORATORY AND DIAGNOSTIC TESTS 42.1

Test	Explanation	Indications	Nursing Implications
Abdominal ultrasonography	Visualizes abdominal organs and related vessels	Abdominal pain, vomiting, pregnancy, abnormal liver tests, abdominal mass, enlarged organs on palpation	Barium decreases visualization of organs on ultrasound.
Abdominal x-ray (KUB)	Plain x-ray of the abdomen without contrast media	Constipation, abdominal pain, abdominal distention, ascites, foreign body, palpable mass	Usually ordered as flat and upright to allow for free air and fluid levels in the bowel to be detected.
Amylase (serum)	An enzyme that changes starch to sugar, which enters the blood with inflammation of the pancreas	Acute pancreatitis, pancreatic trauma, acute cholecystitis	Increased levels are seen after 3–6 hours of the onset of abdominal pain.
Barium enema	After instillation of barium, fluoroscopically allows visualization of the colon	Constipation, rectal prolapse, bleeding, suspected intussusception	Bowel preparation prior to examination may be ordered. Stool will be light colored due to barium for a few days.
Electrolytes (serum)	Sodium, potassium, CO_2, chloride, blood urea nitrogen (BUN), creatinine	To determine extent of dehydration	BUN and creatinine may be elevated with dehydration. Sodium, potassium, chloride, and CO_2 levels can be greatly affected with dehydration.
Barium swallow/upper GI series	Visualizes the form, position, mucosal folds, peristaltic activity, and motility of the esophagus, stomach, and upper GI tract	Foreign body ingestion, abdominal pain, vomiting, dysphagia, malrotation	Females of reproductive age must be screened for pregnancy. Infants may need to be given barium via syringe.
Small bowel series	Done in conjunction with upper GI series to visualize the small intestine contour, position, and motility	Suspected inflammatory bowel disease (bowel wall thickening), intussusception	Very important to encourage large amounts of water/fluids after test to avoid barium-induced constipation.
Endoscopic retrograde cholangiopancreatography (ERCP)	A fiberoptic endoscope is used to view the hepatobiliary system by instilling contrast to outline the pancreatic and common bile ducts.	Pancreatitis, jaundice, pancreatic tumors, common duct stones, biliary tract disease	Monitor for infection, urinary retention, cholangitis, or pancreatitis after the procedure. Done only occasionally in children.
Esophageal manometry	Tests the esophagus for normal contractile activity and effectiveness of swallowing by measurement of intraluminal pressures and acid sensors	Abnormal esophageal muscle function, dysphagia, chest pain of unknown cause, esophagitis, vomiting	Often done in conjunction with pH probe. The manometric catheter is placed through the nose into the esophagus. May cause nasal irritation/sore throat.
Esophageal pH probe	A single- or double-channeled probe placed into the esophagus to monitor the pH of the contents that are regurgitated into the esophagus from the stomach	Vomiting, gastroesophageal reflux, correlation of symptoms to gastroesophageal reflux events and high risk for problems, as in asthma, apparent life-threatening event, sinusitis, or choking/gagging episodes	24-hour study is most accurate. Special diet during study is often used. Accurate diary of symptoms and feedings during the study is essential. May cause nasal irritation/sore throat.

COMMON LABORATORY AND DIAGNOSTIC TESTS 42.1 (continued)

Test	Explanation	Indications	Nursing Implications
Gastric emptying scan	Assesses the rate at which the stomach empties food into the small intestine by adding isotopes to food and visualizing with scans	Unexplained nausea, vomiting, diarrhea, abdominal cramping	Medications may alter gastric emptying times. Crying or stress during the examination may cause delay in emptying and should be documented.
Hemoccult	Checks for occult blood in the stool	Crohn disease, ulcerative colitis, malabsorption syndromes, diarrhea, abdominal pain	Indicates bleeding in the GI tract.
Hepatobiliary scan (HIDA scan)	Visualizes the gallbladder and determines patency of the biliary system by use of a radionuclide. The amount of radionuclide ejected from the gallbladder (ejection fraction) is calculated.	Differentiate between biliary atresia and neonatal hepatitis; assess liver trauma, right upper quadrant pain, and congenital malformations	Intravenous line will be established to give radionuclide. Pain during injection should be assessed and documented.
Lactose tolerance test	After ingesting lactose, this tests the hydrogen levels in the breath, which will increase with lactose build-up in the intestines.	Postprandial diarrhea, gassiness, bloating, abdominal pain	May produce similar symptoms during the test itself. A positive test will require diet modification and education regarding lactose intolerance.
Lipase (serum)	An enzyme that changes fat to fatty acids and glycerol appearing in the blood with pancreatic change	Pancreatitis, pancreatic carcinoma, cholecystitis, peritonitis	Lipase levels stay elevated longer with acute pancreatitis.
Liver biopsy	A test done to evaluate the microscopic hepatic structures	Hyperbilirubinemia, jaundice, chronic liver disease, hepatitis	Monitor after procedure for bleeding complications; must maintain strict bed rest for up to 8 hours.
Liver function tests (LFTs) (AST/ALT/GGT)	Enzymes that have high concentrations in the liver	Elevations may indicate the severity of liver disease.	May be affected by drugs or viral illnesses.
Lower endoscopy (colonoscopy)	Allows visualization and biopsies of the lower GI tract from the anus to the terminal ileum with a fiberoptic instrument	Rectal bleeding, lower abdominal pain, suspected tumors or strictures, foreign body removal	The child must undergo a bowel cleansing prior to the examination. Encourage fluids to prevent dehydration. Conscious sedation or anesthesia care; monitor for possible complications of perforation, bleeding, and increased abdominal pain.
Meckel scan	A gamma camera is used to identify gastric mucosa seen in the distal portion of the ileum after injection of radiopharmaceuticals.	Rectal bleeding, anemia, used only to identify a Meckel diverticulum	Gloves are worn by nurse during and after scan when radiopharmaceuticals are given.
Oropharyngeal motility study (OPMS)	A study done with different textures to evaluate the dynamics of swallowing and reveal transient abnormalities	Dysphagia, recurrent aspiration	Usually done in combination with therapists and nutritionist.

(continued)

COMMON LABORATORY AND DIAGNOSTIC TESTS 42.1 (continued)

Test	Explanation	Indications	Nursing Implications
Rectal suction biopsy	Biopsy is taken of the rectum at different levels to assess for the presence of ganglion cells.	Absence of ganglion cells indicates Hirschsprung disease.	Infants/children should be assessed for rectal bleeding after examination.
Stool culture	Stool is smeared on culture medium and assessed for growth of bacteria over a period of days.	To determine bacterial cause of diarrhea	Requires minimum of 48 hours for growth, several days to weeks in some cases. Can be done with a small amount of stool
Stool for ova and parasites (O&P)	Checks for the presence of parasites or their eggs in the stool	To determine cause of diarrhea or abdominal pain	Requires about 2 tablespoons of stool.
Upper endoscopy (EGD)	Allows visualization and biopsies of the upper GI tract (mouth to upper jejunum) with a fiberoptic instrument	Dysphagia, foreign body removal, epigastric/abdominal pain, suspected celiac disease	Conscious sedation or anesthesia care; monitor for complications of perforation/bleeding.
Urea breath test	Used to detect the presence of *H. pylori* in the exhaled breath	*H. pylori* infection	Child must not take proton pump inhibitors for 5 days, all antibiotic therapy and Pepto-Bismol for 14 days.

Adapted from Corbett, J. A. & Banks, A. D. (2013). *Laboratory tests and diagnostic procedures with nursing diagnoses* (8th ed.). Upper Saddle River, NJ: Pearson Education Inc.; and Dowshen, S. (2014). *Stool tests*. Retrieved from http://www.kidshealth.org/parent/general/sick/labtest8.html

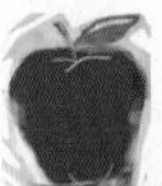

Teaching Guidelines 42.1

STOOL SPECIMEN COLLECTION VARIATIONS

- If the child is in diapers, use a tongue blade to scrape a specimen into the collection container.
- If the child has runny stool, a piece of plastic wrap in the diaper may catch the stool specimen. Very liquid stool may require application of a urine bag to the anal area to collect the stool.
- The older ambulatory child may first urinate in the toilet, and then the stool specimen may be retrieved from the new or clean collection container that fits under the seat at the back of the toilet.
- For the bedridden child, collect the stool specimen from a clean bedpan (do not allow urine to contaminate the stool specimen).
- Send the specimen to the laboratory immediately for accuracy of results.

Nursing Diagnoses, Goals, Interventions, and Evaluation

Upon completion of a thorough assessment, the nurse might identify several nursing diagnoses, including:

- Risk for deficient fluid volume
- Diarrhea
- Constipation
- Risk for impaired skin integrity
- Imbalanced nutrition: less than body requirements
- Pain
- Ineffective breathing pattern
- Risk for caregiver role strain
- Disturbed body image

After completing an assessment on Ethan, you note the following: weight 10 lb, length 23.5 in, head circumference 40.75 cm. Head is round with sunken anterior fontanel, eyes appear sunken, mucous membranes are dry, heart rate 158, breath sounds clear with respiratory rate of 42, positive bowel sounds in all four quadrants, difficulty palpating abdomen due to crying. Based on these assessment findings, what would your top three nursing diagnoses be for Ethan?

Nursing goals, interventions, and evaluation for the child with a GI disorder are based on the nursing diagnoses. Nursing Care Plan 42.1, at the end of the chapter, can be used as a guide in planning nursing care for the child with a GI disorder. Individualize the nursing care plan based on the child's symptoms and needs. Refer to Chapter 36 for detailed information about pain management. Additional information will be included later in the chapter as it relates to specific disorders.

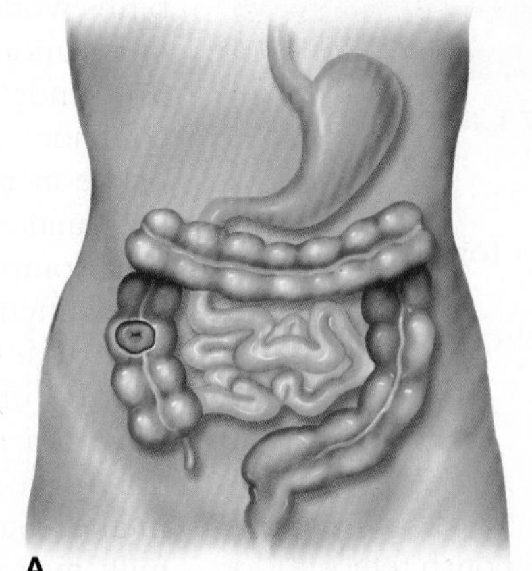

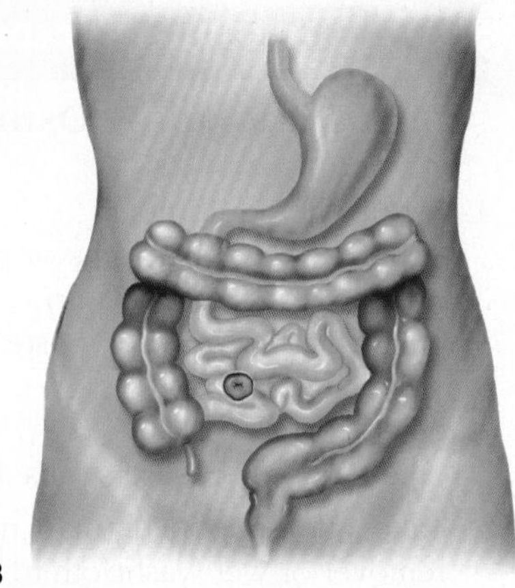

FIGURE 42.1 (**A**) A colostomy is a stoma from the colon; (**B**) an ileostomy is a stoma from the ileum.

Based on your top three nursing diagnoses for Ethan, describe appropriate nursing interventions.

Stool Diversions

Children may undergo stool diversions for a variety of GI disorders. Surgical procedures involve the creation of an ostomy, primarily an *ileostomy* or *colostomy,* by bringing a portion of the small or large intestine to the surface of the abdomen (Fig. 42.1).

Ostomy pouches are worn over the ostomy site to collect stool. The pouch must be of an appropriate size and it should fit around the stoma properly (Fig. 42.2). The pouch may be tucked inside the diaper or underwear or angled to fit outside of the diaper/underwear. Contemporary pouches cannot be seen under most clothing because they are designed to lie flat against the body. Avoid tight or constricting clothing around the stoma site. Teach families to store ostomy supplies in a cool, dry place. Educate parents to inform school staff that the child should be allowed to use the water fountain and the bathroom without restriction, and the school nurse should have extra ostomy supplies available.

Ostomy care for a child can be challenging due to the child's normal growth and development as well as activity. Empty the ostomy pouch and measure for stool output several times per day. The stool may be semisolid to very liquid in consistency depending on the location of the stoma. Liquid stool output can be acidic, causing irritation and severe burn-like areas on the surrounding skin, so special attention to skin care around the ostomy site is essential. Products such as powders and pastes are available to help protect the skin.

The stoma should be moist and pink or red, demonstrating proper circulation to the intestine (Fig. 42.3). Immediately notify the provider if the stoma is not moist and pink or red. Also notify the provider if the volume of stool output is greatly increased, or if the stoma is prolapsed or retracted.

Perform ostomy care as needed; pouches usually need to be changed every 1 to 4 days. Refer to Nursing Procedure 42.1 for an explanation of the steps for changing an ostomy pouch.

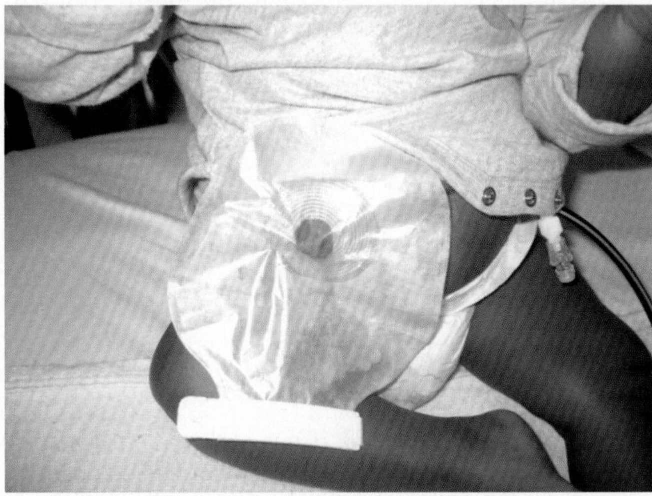

FIGURE 42.2 Ensure that the ostomy pouch fits closely around the stoma to prevent irritation of the surrounding skin.

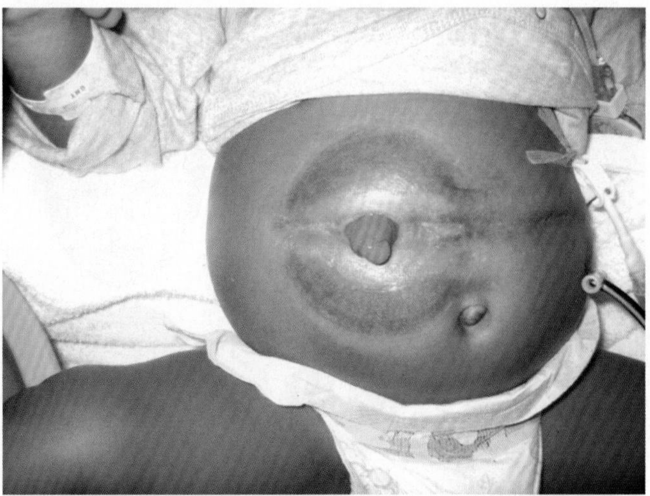

FIGURE 42.3 The healthy stoma is pink and moist.

NURSING PROCEDURE 42.1

Performing Ostomy Care

1. Set up the equipment:
   - Warm, wet washcloths or paper towels
   - Clean pouch and clamp
   - Skin barrier powder, paste, and/or sealant
   - Pencil or pen
   - Scissors
   - Pattern to measure stoma size
2. Take off the pouch (may need to use adhesive remover or wet washcloth to ease pouch removal).
3. Observe the stoma and surrounding skin. Clean the stoma and skin as needed, allowing it to dry thoroughly.
4. Measure the stoma, mark the new pouch backing, and cut the new backing to size.
5. Apply the new pouch.

Adapted from University of California, San Francisco. (2016). *Colostomy.* Retrieved from http://pedsurg.ucsf.edu/conditions–procedures/colostomy.aspx.

STRUCTURAL ANOMALIES OF THE GASTROINTESTINAL TRACT

Structural anomalies of the GI tract include cleft lip and palate, omphalocele and gastroschisis, hernias (inguinal and umbilical), and anorectal malformations. Omphalocele, gastroschisis, and anorectal malformations are discussed in chapter 24.

Cleft Lip and Palate

Cleft lip and palate (Fig. 42.4) is the most common congenital craniofacial anomaly, occurring once in every 700 births worldwide. It occurs frequently in association with other anomalies and has been identified in more than 350 syndromes (Curtin & Boekelheide, 2010). The most common anomalies associated with cleft lip and cleft palate include heart defects, ear malformations, skeletal deformities, and genitourinary abnormality.

Complications of cleft lip and palate include feeding difficulties, altered dentition, delayed or altered speech development, and otitis media. The infant with cleft lip may have difficulty forming an adequate seal around a nipple in order to create the necessary suction for feeding and may also experience excessive air intake. Gagging, choking, and nasal regurgitation of milk may occur in babies with cleft palate. Excessive feeding time, inadequate intake, and fatigue contribute to insufficient growth. Primary or permanent teeth may be missing, malformed, or unusually positioned. Children with cleft palate may have a nasal quality to the speech as well as delays in speech development. Optimally, speech articulation should be clear by 4 years of age, or additional surgical intervention may be necessary (Curtin & Boekelheide, 2010). The opening in the cleft palate contributes to build-up of fluid in the middle ear (otitis media with effusion), which can lead to an acute infection (acute otitis media). Long-lasting otitis media with effusion leads to temporary and sometimes permanent hearing loss (Curtin & Boekelheide, 2010).

Pathophysiology

Development of the **cleft** occurs early in pregnancy. The tissue that forms the lip ordinarily fuses by 5 to 6 weeks of gestation, and the palate closes between 7 and 9 weeks of gestation. Therefore, if either the lip or palate does not fuse, then the infant is born with a cleft. Cleft lip or cleft palate may occur in isolation from one another, but 50% of infants born with cleft lip also have cleft palate (Curtin & Boekelheide, 2010). The cleft

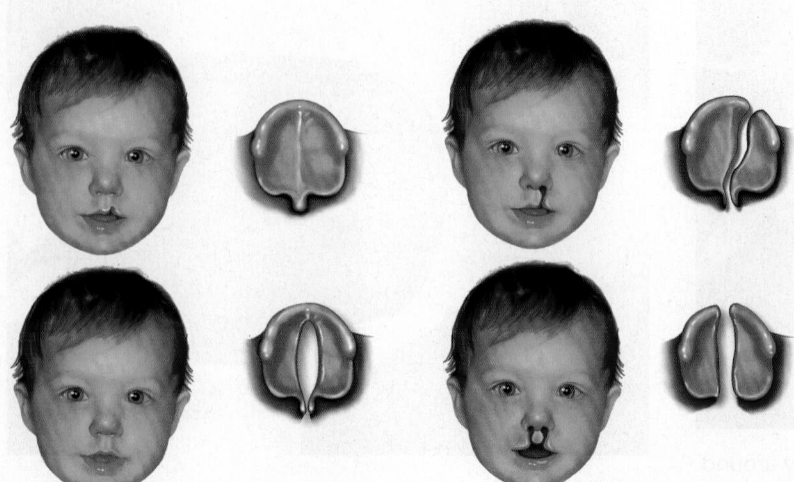

FIGURE 42.4 The cleft lip may extend all the way through the vermilion border and up into the nostril, or it may be significantly smaller. The cleft palate may be a small opening or may involve the entire palate.

may be unilateral (the left side is affected more often) or bilateral.

Therapeutic Management

Babies with cleft lip and cleft palate are usually managed by a specialized team that may include a plastic surgeon or craniofacial specialist, oral surgeon, dentist or orthodontist, prosthodontist, psychologist, otolaryngologist, nurse, social worker, audiologist, and speech-language pathologist. Many children's hospitals offer these services in one location, such as a craniofacial specialty center. Historically, cleft lip has been repaired surgically around the age of 2 to 3 months and cleft palate at 6 to 9 months. Early repair of the cleft lip restores a normal appearance to the child's face and may improve parent–infant bonding. Regardless of the timing of the surgical repair, however, surgical revision of the palate may be required as the child grows.

Nursing Assessment

For a full description of the assessment phase of the nursing process, refer to the Assessment section of the Nursing Process Overview earlier in the chapter. Assessment findings pertinent to cleft lip and palate are discussed below.

HEALTH HISTORY

For the newborn, explore pregnancy history for risk factors for development of cleft lip and cleft palate, which include:

- Maternal smoking
- Prenatal infection
- Advanced maternal age
- Use of anticonvulsants, steroids, and other medications during early pregnancy

When an infant or child with cleft lip or palate returns for a clinic visit or hospitalization, inquire about feeding difficulties, respiratory difficulties, speech development, and otitis media.

PHYSICAL EXAMINATION

Observe the infant for the presence of the characteristic physical appearance of cleft lip. The cleft may involve the lip only or extend up into the nostril (Fig. 42.5). Cleft palate may be visualized on examination of the mouth. Palpate with a gloved finger to discover mild clefts.

LABORATORY AND DIAGNOSTIC TESTS

Cleft lip may be diagnosed by prenatal ultrasound, but it is diagnosed most commonly at birth by the classic physical appearance.

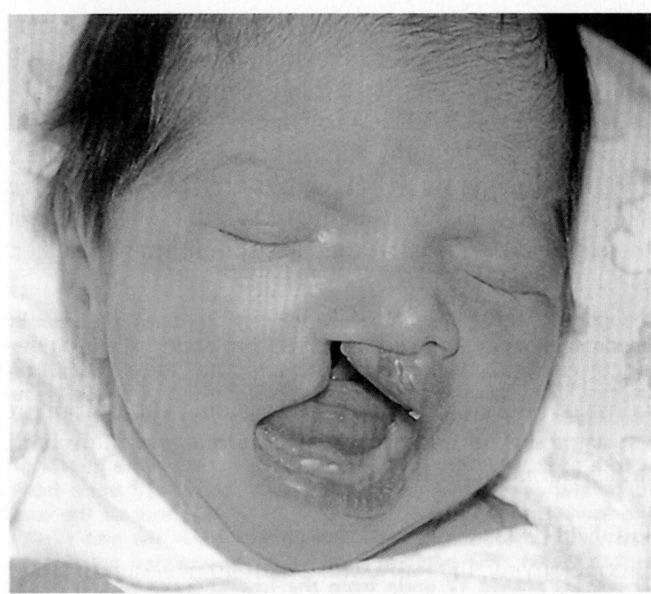

FIGURE 42.5 Cleft lip.

Consider This

The nurse is caring for a 2-week-old infant with a cleft lip who presents for a well-child check. The mother states, "I can't believe she looks like this; I always wanted a perfect baby girl. I feel like I can't go anywhere with her, other people will look at her like she's a monster. And after her surgery she's going to have an ugly scar over her lip." She then begins crying.

How will you respond as the nurse? Are you concerned about anything other than the mother's feelings in the situation? What would feel like if you had a baby with a facial deformity? Think about the best ways to respond to this mother in a therapeutic manner.

Nursing Management

Refer to Nursing Care Plan 42.1 at the end of the chapter for nursing diagnoses and interventions related to airway maintenance, fluid balance promotion, and restoration of family processes, and to Chapter 36 for pain management. These should be individualized for the particular situation. In addition to the nursing diagnoses and related interventions discussed in Nursing Care Plan 42.1, interventions common to cleft lip and cleft palate follow.

PREVENTING INJURY TO THE SUTURE LINE

It is critical to prevent injury to the facial suture line or to the palatal operative sites. Do not allow the infant to rub the facial suture line. To prevent this, position the infant in a supine or side-lying position. It may be necessary to use arm restraints to stop the hands from touching the face or entering the mouth. Clean the suture line as ordered by the surgeon. Possible care options include using petroleum jelly on the facial suture line or a lip-protective device such as a Logan bow (curved thin metal apparatus) or a butterfly adhesive, both of which protect and maintain the suture line. Protect the palate operative site. Avoid putting items in the mouth that might disrupt the sutures (e.g., suction catheter, spoon, straw, pacifier, or plastic syringe).

Prevent vigorous or sustained crying in the infant, because this may cause tension on either suture line. Ways to prevent crying include administering medications as needed for pain and providing other comfort or distraction measures, such as cuddling, rocking, and anticipation of needs.

PROMOTING ADEQUATE NUTRITION

Preoperatively, the baby with a cleft lip may demonstrate enhanced growth patterns if breastfed. The contour and softness of the breast against the lip may allow for a better seal to be maintained for adequate sucking in some infants (Donovan, 2012). Some infants will be fed with a special cleft lip nipple (Fig. 42.6). Parent and surgeon preference will determine the method of feeding. Burp the infant well to expel excess air taken in during difficulty with sucking.

The infant with unrepaired cleft palate is at risk for aspiration with oral feeding. In some instances a prosthodontic device may be created to form a false palate covering. This device may prevent breast milk or formula from being aspirated. Breastfeeding may be effective in the infant with cleft palate due to the pliability of the breast and the fact that soft breast tissue may cover the opening in the palate. Postoperatively, some surgeons allow breastfeeding to be resumed almost immediately (Donovan, 2012). In the bottle-fed infant special nipples or feeders may have to be used. When the suture line is healed, ordinary feeding may resume.

ENCOURAGING INFANT–PARENT BONDING

For some parents, the appearance of a cleft lip is appalling (Curtin & Boekelheide, 2010). Encourage parents to hold the medically stable infant immediately after delivery to encourage bonding. Acknowledge normal feelings of guilt, anger, and sadness. Support the parents in providing care for the infant, particularly feeding, which is viewed as a significant nurturing function. Provide education about the anticipated surgical procedure and eventual normal appearance of the infant's lip.

PROVIDING EMOTIONAL SUPPORT

Many families will benefit from support in addition to that received from the craniofacial team. Refer parents to the Cleft Palate Foundation or a parent-to-parent support network, links to which can be found on thePoint. See Healthy People 2020.

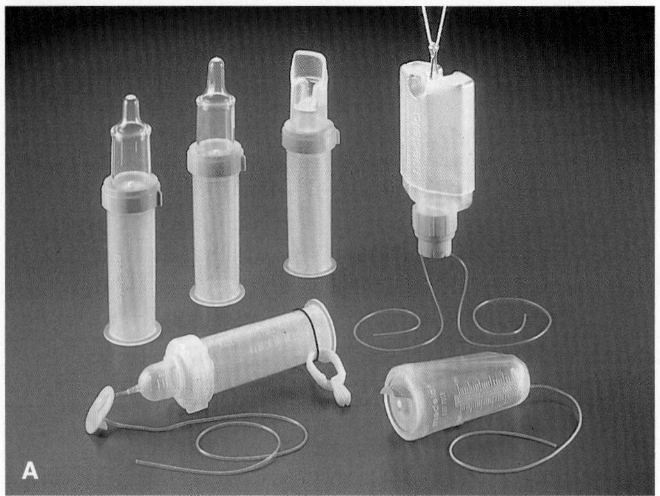

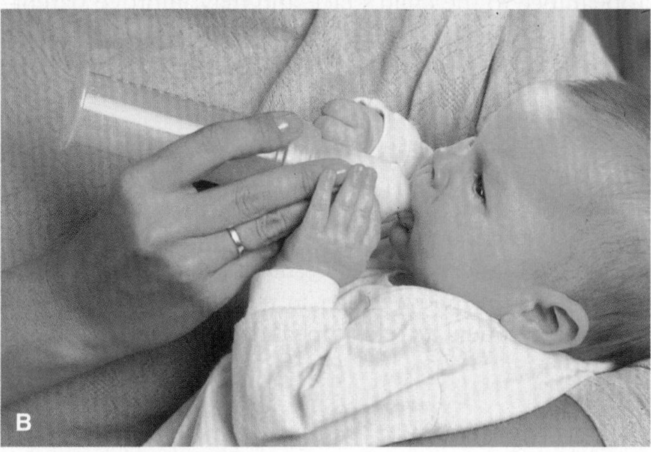

FIGURE 42.6 **(A)** Specialty feeding devices used for infants with cleft lip and cleft palate. **(B)** An infant uses a Haberman feeder.

Anorectal Malformations

Imperforate anus is a congenital malformation of the anorectal opening. Refer to chapter 24 for information related to the incidence and etiology of anorectal malformations, as well as nursing care in the neonatal period. Other congenital anomalies may be associated with imperforate anus in 50% of cases (Hoffenberg et al., 2014) (Box 42.1).

HEALTHY PEOPLE 2020

Objective	Nursing Significance
Increase the number of states and the District of Columbia that have a system for referral for cleft lips and cleft palates to rehabilitative teams.	• Ensure that your office, clinic, or hospital participates in such a system. • If it does not, advocate for such participation.

Healthy People Objectives retrieved from http://www.healthypeople.gov

BOX 42.1

ANOMALIES ASSOCIATED WITH ANORECTAL MALFORMATIONS

- VACTERL syndrome: vertebral, anorectal, cardiovascular, tracheoesophageal, renal, and limb
- Esophageal atresia
- Intestinal atresia
- Malrotation
- Renal agenesis
- Hypospadias
- Vesicoureteral reflux
- Bladder exstrophy
- Cardiac anomalies
- Skeletal anomalies

The nurse may encounter the infant with imperforate anus and an ostomy when the child is admitted to the hospital at several months of age for corrective surgery. Infants often require a staged repair in which the bowel is connected to the anal opening or an anal opening is created. When the final repair is achieved, the stoma will be closed and the infant will pass stool through the anal opening.

Surgical intervention is needed for both high and low types of imperforate anus. Surgery for a high type of defect involves a colostomy in the newborn period, with corrective surgery performed in stages to allow for growth. Surgery for the low type of anomaly, which frequently includes a fistula, involves closure of the fistula, creation of an anal opening, and repositioning of the rectal pouch into the anal opening. After repair, only about 30% with a high defect will achieve continence (Hoffenberg et al., 2014). A major challenge for either type of surgical repair is finding, using, or creating adequate nerve and muscle structures around the rectum to provide for normal evacuation.

Nursing Assessment

In the newborn, observe for an appropriate anal opening. If the anal opening exists, observe for passage of meconium stool within the first 24 hours of life (generally not passed in the infant with imperforate anus). Assess urine output to identify accompanying genitourinary problems. Assess for signs of intestinal obstruction, which may occur as a result of the malformation. These include abdominal distention and bilious vomiting. Refer to chapter 24 for information related to nursing assessment in the newborn period. In the older infant, noted condition of the stoma, as well as quantity and quality of stoma output.

Nursing Management

Nursing management focuses on preparing the infant for surgery and providing postoperative care. It is important to provide the parents with a full explanation of the typical postoperative course, and long-term care needed. Provide support to the parents and family.

Postoperative care includes ensuring adequate pain relief, maintaining NPO status and gastric decompression until normal bowel function is restored, and providing colostomy care, if applicable. After the intestinal pull-through procedure is completed, it will be the first time that stool has passed through the anal sphincter. The stool may be quite loose depending on the severity of the imperforate anus. The perianal skin is at significant risk for breakdown. Therefore, use a barrier cream on the area and clean it once daily with soap and water. Otherwise, wipe liquid stool off the barrier cream with mineral oil and cotton balls. Most of the barrier cream will remain intact, protecting the infant's perianal area.

Take Note!

To decrease the drying associated with frequent cleaning, avoid baby wipes and frequent use of soap and water.

Meckel Diverticulum

Meckel diverticulum is the result of an incomplete fusion of the omphalomesenteric duct during embryonic development. This causes a fibrous band to connect the small intestine to the umbilicus, known as a Meckel diverticulum. It is the most common congenital anomaly of the GI tract, occurring in 1.5% of the population (Hoffenberg et al., 2014). Complications associated with Meckel diverticulum include bleeding, anemia, and intestinal obstruction such as volvulus and intussusception, half of which occur within the first 2 years of life (Hoffenberg et al., 2014). Surgical correction of the Meckel diverticulum is necessary in children who have complications. The surgery is usually done to remove the diverticulum itself. At times, ileal resection is necessary.

Nursing Assessment

For a full description of the assessment phase of the nursing process, refer to page 1578. Assessment findings pertinent to Meckel diverticulum are discussed below.

HEALTH HISTORY

Elicit a description of the present illness and chief complaint. Common signs and symptoms reported during the health history might include:

- Bleeding
- Anemia
- Severe colicky abdominal pain (in children with associated intestinal obstruction)

PHYSICAL EXAMINATION

Assess the child for an acute abdomen. Observe for abdominal distention, auscultate for hypoactive bowel sounds, and then palpate for an abdominal mass, **guarding** (tensing of the abdominal wall muscles), and rebound tenderness.

LABORATORY AND DIAGNOSTIC TESTS

Common laboratory and diagnostic tests ordered for assessment of Meckel diverticulum include:

- Abdominal x-rays to rule out an acute obstructive process
- Meckel scan (conclusive)
- Stool tests for color, consistency, and occult blood (usually positive in Meckel diverticulum)
- Complete blood count (CBC) to assess for anemia

Nursing Management

If anemia is significant, administer ordered blood products (packed red blood cells) to stabilize the child before surgery. Administer intravenous fluids and maintain NPO status for symptomatic children while further evaluation is being performed. Immediately report an acute abdomen to a physician or nurse practitioner. Postoperative care will vary depending on the surgery that was performed. Provide child and family education as necessary to relieve anxiety related to the diagnosis and surgical intervention. Refer to the Nursing Care Plan 42.1 at the end of the chapter for additional information.

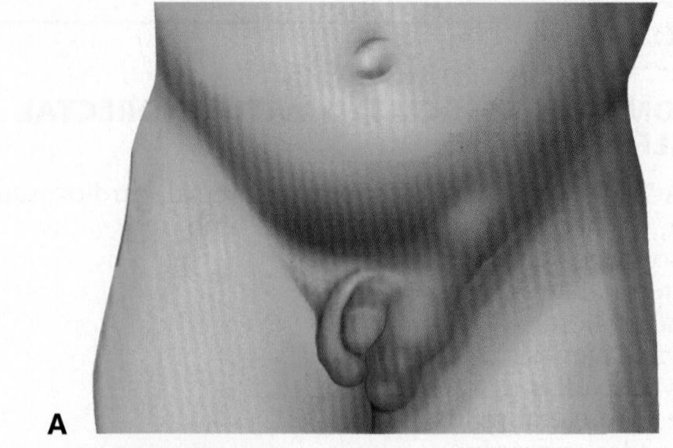

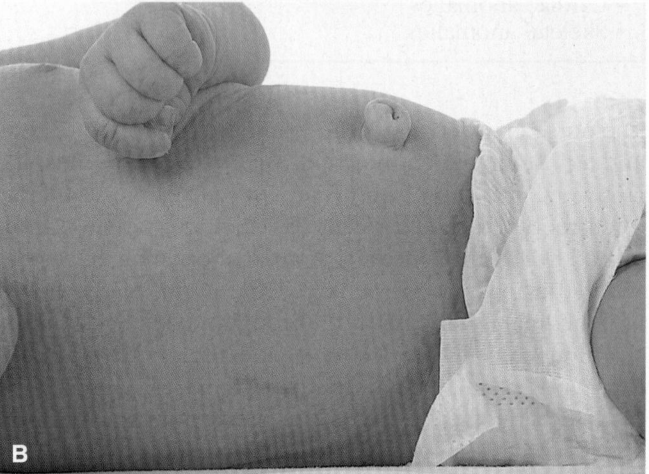

FIGURE 42.7 **(A)** Inguinal hernia: note the bulge in the inguinal (groin) area. **(B)** Umbilical hernia: note the protrusion in the umbilical area.

Inguinal and Umbilical Hernias

Inguinal and umbilical hernias are defects that occur during fetal development. Either may be visible at birth, and inguinal hernias may be noted later in life (Hoffenberg et al., 2014).

Inguinal Hernia

When the processus vaginalis fails to close completely during embryonal development, an inguinal hernia may occur. This allows the abdominal or pelvic viscera to travel through the internal inguinal ring into the inguinal canal The hernia sacs that develop most often contain bowel in males and fallopian tubes or ovaries in females. Boys are more likely than girls to develop inguinal hernia and premature infants demonstrate an increased incidence overall (Hoffenberg et al., 2014). Surgical correction of the inguinal hernia is usually performed when the infant is several weeks old and has been thriving.

NURSING ASSESSMENT

Assess infants and children with an inguinal hernia for the presence of a bulging mass in the lower abdomen or groin area (Fig. 42.7). It may be possible to visualize the mass, but often the mass is seen only during crying or straining, making it difficult to actually identify in the clinic setting.

NURSING MANAGEMENT

If a mass is felt upon palpation, the physician or nurse practitioner may attempt to reduce the hernia by pushing it back through the external inguinal ring. The physician or nurse practitioner may ask the nurse to assist in a reduction, most likely helping to hold the child in a position that will allow the physician or nurse practitioner to reduce the hernia. If reduction is not possible even with sedation, the hernia could be incarcerated (Hoffenberg et al., 2014). An incarcerated hernia could eventually lead to bowel strangulation.

Reduction is only a temporary method of managing inguinal hernias; they must be corrected surgically. The hernia should be manually reduced as needed until the time of the surgery, so teach the family how to reduce the hernia. Instruct the family to contact the surgeon immediately if the hernia becomes irreducible. Provide routine pre- and postoperative care during inguinal hernia surgical repair, including child and family education to relieve anxiety.

Take Note!

Tell the parents that if the child's inguinal hernia becomes hard, discolored, or painful (evidenced by inconsolable crying), they should immediately call the physician or nurse practitioner to determine the next course of action (office visit or emergency room visit).

Umbilical Hernia

Umbilical hernia occurs commonly in preterm infants and much more frequently in African Americans compared to Caucasians (Hoffenberg et al., 2014). An umbilical hernia is caused by an incomplete closure of the umbilical ring, allowing intestinal contents to herniate through the opening. Unlike inguinal hernias, most umbilical hernias are not corrected surgically. Most children will have spontaneous closure of the umbilical hernia by 4 years of age (Hoffenberg et al., 2014). Surgical correction is necessary only for the largest umbilical hernias that have failed to close by the time the child is 4 years old.

NURSING ASSESSMENT

Assess whether the hernia can be reduced. Notify the surgeon if the hernia will not reduce. Incarceration is extremely rare, but when it does occur, the child will report abdominal pain, tenderness, or redness at the umbilicus (Fig. 42.7).

NURSING MANAGEMENT

Since operative repair is not as likely with umbilical hernias as with inguinal hernias, the aim of nursing management is education. Teach the child and family how to reduce the hernia. The child may have some self-esteem issues related to the large protrusion of the unrepaired umbilical hernia. Teach the child coping skills to help relieve anxiety.

Take Note!

The use of home remedies to reduce an umbilical hernia should be discouraged because of the risk of bowel strangulation. This includes taping a quarter over a reduced umbilical hernia and the use of "belly bands" (American Academy of Pediatrics, 2015).

ACUTE GASTROINTESTINAL DISORDERS

Acute GI disorders include dehydration, vomiting, diarrhea, oral candidiasis, oral lesions, hypertrophic pyloric stenosis, necrotizing enterocolitis, intussusception, malrotation and volvulus, and appendicitis.

Dehydration

Dehydration occurs more readily in infants and young children than it does in adults. The risk is increased in infants and young children because they have an increased extracellular fluid percentage and a relative increase in body water compared to adults. Increased basal metabolic rate, increased ratio of BSA to body mass, immature renal function, and increased insensible fluid loss through temperature elevation also contribute to the increased risk for dehydration in infants and young children as compared to adults. Dehydration left unchecked leads to shock, so early recognition and treatment of dehydration is critical to prevent progression to hypovolemic shock. The goals of therapeutic management of dehydration are to restore appropriate fluid balance and to prevent complications.

Nursing Assessment

For a full description of the assessment phase of the nursing process, refer to page 1578. Assessment findings pertinent to dehydration are discussed below.

HEALTH HISTORY

Elicit a description of the present illness and chief complaint. Common signs and symptoms reported during the health history are included in Comparison Chart 42.1, which compares the clinical manifestations of mild, moderate, and severe dehydration.

Explore the child's current and past medical history for risk factors for dehydration such as:

- Diarrhea
- Vomiting
- Decreased oral intake
- Sustained high fever
- Diabetic ketoacidosis
- Extensive burns

Take Note!

Nurses must be able to assess a child's hydration status accurately and intervene quickly. Children are at higher risk than adults for hypovolemic shock. Dehydrated children may deteriorate very quickly and experience shock.

PHYSICAL EXAMINATION AND LABORATORY AND DIAGNOSTIC TESTS

Assess the child's hydration status, including heart rate, blood pressure, skin turgor, fontanels, oral mucosa, eyes, temperature and color of extremities, mental status, and urine output. Children usually compensate well initially; their heart rate increases in moderate dehydration, but blood pressure remains normal until it decreases in severe dehydration.

COMPARISON CHART 42.1 DEHYDRATION

	Mild	Moderate	Severe
Mental status	Alert	Alert to listless	Alert to comatose
Fontanels	Soft and flat	Sunken	Sunken
Eyes	Normal	Mildly sunken orbits	Deeply sunken orbits
Oral mucosa	Pink and moist	Pale and slightly dry	Dry
Skin turgor	Elastic	Decreased	Tenting
Heart rate	Normal	May be increased	Increased, progressing to bradycardia
Blood pressure	Normal	Normal	Normal, progressing to hypotension
Extremities	Warm, pink, brisk capillary refill	Delayed capillary refill	Cool, mottled or dusky, significantly delayed capillary refill
Urine output	May be slightly decreased	<1 mL/kg/hr	Significantly <1 mL/kg/hr

Adapted from Engorn, B., & Flerlage, J. (2015). *The Harriet Lane handbook* (20th ed.). Philadelphia, PA: Saunders; and Ford, D. M. (2014). Fluid, electrolyte, and acid-base disorders & therapy. In W. W. Hay, M. J. Levin, & R. R. Deterding, & M. J. Abzug (Eds.), *Current pediatric diagnosis and treatment* (22nd ed.). New York, NY: McGraw-Hill.

Nursing Management

Nursing goals for the infant or child with dehydration are aimed at restoring fluid volume and preventing progression to hypovolemia. Provide oral rehydration to children for mild to moderate states of dehydration (see Teaching Guidelines 42.2). Children with severe dehydration should receive intravenous fluids. Initially, administer 20 mL/kg of normal saline or lactated Ringer, and then reassess the hydration status (refer to Chapter 51 for further specifics regarding hypovolemic shock).

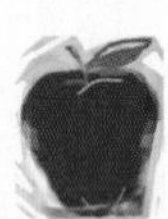

Teaching Guidelines 42.2

ORAL REHYDRATION THERAPY

- Oral rehydration solution (ORS) should contain 75 mmol/L sodium chloride and 13.5 g/L glucose (standard ORS solutions include Pedialyte, Infalyte, and Ricelyte).
- Tap water, milk, undiluted fruit juice, soup, and broth are NOT appropriate for oral rehydration.
- Children with mild to moderate dehydration require 50–100 mL/kg of ORS over 4 hours.
- After reevaluation, oral rehydration may need to be continued if the child is still dehydrated.
- When rehydrated, the child can resume a regular diet.

Adapted from Freedman, S. (2016). *Oral rehydration therapy*. Retrieved from http://www.uptodate.com/contents/oral-rehydration-therapy

Once initial fluid balance is restored, the physician or nurse practitioner may order intravenous fluids at the maintenance rate or as much as 1.5 times maintenance. Maintenance fluid requirements refer to the amount needed under conditions of normal hydration. Maintenance fluid requirements may be determined with the use of the formula found in Box 42.2. In the example provided in Box 42.2, a 23-kg child will need maintenance fluid equivalent to 65 mL/hr.

The same anatomic and physiologic differences that make infants and young children susceptible to dehydration also make them susceptible to overhydration. Thus, continuously evaluate hydration status and be aware of the appropriateness of intravenous fluid orders.

BOX 42.2

FORMULA FOR FLUID MAINTENANCE

- 100 mL/kg for first 10 kg
- 50 mL/kg for next 10 kg
- 20 mL/kg for remaining kg
- Add together for total mL needed per 24-hour period.
- Divide by 24 for mL/hr fluid requirement.

Thus, for a 23-kg child:

- $100 \times 10 = 1{,}000$
- $50 \times 10 = 500$
- $20 \times 3 = 60$
- $1{,}000 + 500 + 60 = 1{,}560$

$1{,}560/24 = 65$ mL/hr

Adapted from Engorn, B., & Flerlage, J. (2015). *The Harriet Lane handbook* (20th ed.). Philadelphia, PA: Saunders.

Vomiting

Vomiting is the forceful expulsion of gastric contents through the mouth. It occurs as a reflex with three different phases:

- Prodromal period: nausea and signs of autonomic nervous system stimulation
- Retching
- Vomiting

Vomiting in infants and children has many different causes and is considered to be a symptom of some other condition. Table 42.1 lists common causes of vomiting.

Therapeutic management of vomiting most often involves slow oral rehydration and at times may require administration of antiemetics.

Nursing Assessment

For a full description of the assessment phase of the nursing process, refer to page 1578. Assessment findings pertinent to vomiting are discussed below.

HEALTH HISTORY

Elicit a description of the present illness and chief complaint. Note onset and progression of symptoms. The assessment of an infant or child with vomiting should include a history of the vomiting events, including:

- Contents/character of the emesis
- Effort and force of vomiting episodes
- Timing (in relation to meals, as well as time of day)

Contents and character of the vomitus may give clues to the cause of vomiting. Bilious vomiting is never considered normal and suggests an obstruction, whereas bloody emesis can signify esophageal or GI bleeding (Hoffenberg et al., 2014). Assess the effort and force of vomiting to identify whether the episodes are effortful and projectile, as with pyloric stenosis, or effortless, as is often seen in gastroesophageal reflux (GER). The timing of the vomiting also is helpful in determining the cause. Vomiting that occurs several hours past meals could signify delayed gastric emptying. When vomiting occurs upon waking or in the middle of the night, particularly if it is associated with headaches, an intracranial lesion or tumor may be suspected.

Note any events associated with the vomiting, such as diarrhea or pain. Diarrhea may occur with viral gastroenteritis or food poisoning. Pain in the epigastric area could signify peptic ulcer disease (PUD), pancreatitis, or cholecystitis.

Assess the child's past medical history to identify preexisting illnesses, drug abuse, trauma, prescribed medications, and previous abdominal surgery. Risk factors for vomiting include exposure to viruses, certain medication use, and overfeeding in an infant.

PHYSICAL EXAMINATION

Perform a physical examination, noting the child's general appearance. Note hydration status, as well as mental status changes. Note the quality of bowel sounds upon auscultation. Palpate the abdomen for the presence of abdominal masses, tenderness, or signs of trauma.

TABLE 42.1 CAUSES OF VOMITING BY TEMPORAL PATTERN

Category	Acute	Chronic	Cyclic
Infectious	Gastroenteritis, otitis media, pharyngitis, sinusitis (acute), hepatitis, pyelonephritis, meningitis	*H. pylori*, *Giardia*, sinusitis (chronic)	Chronic sinusitis
GI	Intussusception, malrotation with volvulus, appendicitis, cholecystitis, pancreatitis	GERD, gastritis, peptic ulcer disease	GERD, malrotation with volvulus
Genitourinary	Ureteropelvic junction obstruction, pyelonephritis	Pregnancy, pyelonephritis	Hydronephrosis
Endocrine/metabolic	Diabetic ketoacidosis	Adrenal hyperplasia	Diabetic ketoacidosis, Addison disease, acute intermittent porphyria
Neurologic	Concussion, subdural hematoma, brain tumor	Brain tumor, Arnold–Chiari malformation	Migraines, Arnold–Chiari malformation, brain tumor
Other	Food poisoning, toxic ingestion	Bulimia, rumination	Cyclic vomiting syndrome

LABORATORY AND DIAGNOSTIC TESTS

Laboratory studies may be ordered to assess the child's hydration status or to rule out certain causes of vomiting, such as urinary tract infection, pancreatitis, or an acute infectious process. Common laboratory and diagnostic tests ordered for assessment of the cause of vomiting include:

- Abdominal ultrasound
- Upper GI series
- Plain abdominal x-rays

Nursing Management

Nursing management focuses on promoting fluid and electrolyte balance. Oral rehydration is accomplished successfully in most outpatient cases of simple vomiting. Teach the primary caregiver about oral rehydration (refer to Teaching Guidelines 42.2). In the child with mild to moderate dehydration resulting from vomiting, withhold oral feeding for 1 to 2 hours after emesis, after which time oral rehydration can begin. Give the infant or child 0.5 to 2 oz of oral rehydration solution every 15 minutes, depending on the child's age and size. Most infants and children can retain this small amount of fluid if fed the restricted amount every 15 minutes. As the child improves, larger amounts will be tolerated.

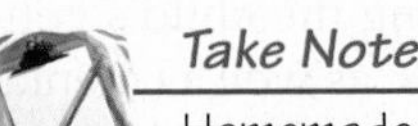

Take Note!

Homemade oral rehydration solution can be made by combining 1 quart of water (can be water poured from cooking rice if desired), 8 teaspoons sugar, and 1 teaspoon salt.

If oral rehydration is not possible due to continued nausea and vomiting, intravenous fluids will likely be ordered. In some cases, antiemetics may be used to help control the vomiting. Some antiemetics can cause drowsiness or other side effects and should not be used until a definitive diagnosis is made or severe pathologic processes can be excluded (Hoffenberg et al., 2014). Educate the family regarding the prevention of vomiting and use of antiemetic therapy.

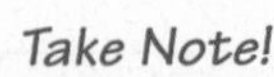

Take Note!

Ginger capsules, ginger tea, and candied ginger are generally useful in reducing nausea, are safe for use in children over age 2 years, and usually produce no side effects (University of Maryland Medical Center, 2016).

Diarrhea

Diarrhea is either an increase in the frequency or a decrease in the consistency of stool. Diarrhea in children can either be acute or chronic. In the developed world, viruses account for most diarrhea cases leading to more than 1.5 million office visits and 200,000 hospitalizations each year (Fleisher, 2014).

Pathophysiology

Acute diarrhea in children is most commonly caused by viruses, but it may also be related to bacterial or parasitic enteropathogens. Viruses injure the absorptive surface of mature villous cells, resulting in decreased fluid absorption and disaccharidase deficiency. Bacteria produce intestinal injury by directly invading the mucosa, damaging the villous surface, or releasing toxins. Acute diarrhea may be bloody or nonbloody. The viral, bacterial, and parasitic causes of acute infectious diarrhea are discussed in Box 42.3. Diarrhea may also occur in relation to antibiotic use. Risk factors for acute diarrhea include recent ingestion of undercooked meats, foreign travel, day care attendance, and well water use.

Since most cases of diarrhea are acute and viral in nature, therapeutic management of diarrhea is usually supportive (maintaining fluid balance and nutrition). Probiotic supplementation may decrease the length and extent of diarrhea in otherwise healthy children (Hoffenberg et al., 2014).

Though most cases of diarrhea in children are of acute origin, diarrhea may also occur chronically. Chronic diarrhea is diarrhea that lasts for more than 2 weeks. This type of diarrhea is not usually caused by serious illnesses. The causes of chronic diarrhea are listed according to age groups in Box 42.4.

Nursing Assessment

For a full description of the assessment phase of the nursing process, refer to the Assessment section of the Nursing Process Overview earlier in the chapter. Assessment findings pertinent to diarrhea are discussed below.

HEALTH HISTORY

Elicit a description of the present illness and chief complaint. Important information related to the course of the diarrhea includes:

- Number and frequency of stools
- Duration of symptoms
- Stool volume
- Associated symptoms (abdominal pain, cramping, nausea, vomiting, fever)
- Presence of blood or mucus in the stool

Explore the child's current and past medical history for risk factors such as:

- Likelihood of exposure to infectious agents (well water, farm animals, day care attendance)
- Dietary history
- Family history of similar symptoms
- Recent travel
- Child's age (to identify common etiology for that age group)

BOX 42.3

ACUTE INFECTIOUS DIARRHEA

Causes	Manifestations	Distinguishing Features	Treatment
Viruses: rotavirus, adenovirus, norovirus, parvovirus, pestivirus, calicivirus, astrovirus, cytomegalovirus	Loose, watery stools, fever, vomiting	Rotavirus most common, especially in young children. Norovirus more common in older children.	Supportive care: oral rehydration, electrolyte replacement in some cases, early refeeding of diet. Antidiarrheals are not effective.
Bacteria: *Salmonella, Shigella, Escherichia coli* 0157:H7, *Campylobacter, Clostridium difficile, Yersinia enterocolitica*	Stools may be bloody or mucousy	*Salmonella* may be shed for a year. *E. coli* 0157: H7 causes hemolytic anemia. *Clostridium difficile* results from antibiotic use	Rehydration, early refeeding of diet. Some but not all cases require antibiotic therapy.
Parasites: *Giardia lamblia, Entamoeba histolytica, Cryptosporidium*	Fever, watery stools	Oral–fecal transmission, *Cryptosporidium* spread by farm animals	Some cases require antiparasitic therapy.

Adapted from Hoffenberg, E., Brumbaugh, D., Furuta, G. T., Kobak, G., Liu, E., Soden, J., & Kramer, R. (2014). Gastrointestinal tract. In W. W. Hay, M. J. Levin, & R. R. Deterding, & M. J. Abzug (Eds.), *Current pediatric diagnosis and treatment* (22nd ed.). New York, NY: McGraw-Hill; and Gilger, M. A. (2016). *Pathogenesis of acute diarrhea in children*. Retrieved from http://www.uptodate.com/contents/pathogenesis-of-acute-diarrhea-in-children

PHYSICAL EXAMINATION

Inspection. Assess the child with diarrhea for dehydration. Observe the child's general appearance and color. In mild dehydration, the child may appear normal. In moderate dehydration, the eyes may have decreased tear production or sunken orbits. Mucous membranes may also be dry. Mental status may be compromised with moderate to severe dehydration, as evidenced by listlessness or lethargy. Skin may be nonelastic or exhibit tenting, signifying lack of proper hydration. Abdominal distention or concavity may be present. Urine output may also be decreased if the child is dehydrated. Stool output may be available to assess for color and consistency. Inspect the anal area for presence of redness or rash related to increased stool volumes and increased frequency.

Auscultation. Auscultate bowel sounds to assess for the presence of hypoactive or hyperactive bowel sounds. Hypoactive bowel sounds may indicate obstruction or peritonitis. Hyperactive bowel sounds may indicate diarrhea/gastroenteritis.

Percussion. Percuss the abdomen. Note any abnormalities. The presence of abnormalities on examination for a diagnosis of acute or chronic diarrhea would indicate a pathologic process.

Palpation. Tenderness in the lower quadrants may be related to gastroenteritis. Rebound tenderness or pain should not be found on palpation. If found, it could indicate appendicitis or peritonitis.

BOX 42.4

CAUSES OF CHRONIC DIARRHEA BY AGE

Infants	Toddlers	School-Age Children
Intractable diarrhea of infancy	Chronic nonspecific diarrhea	Inflammatory bowel disease
Milk and soy protein intolerance	Viral enteritis	Appendiceal abscess
Infectious enteritis	*Giardia*	Lactase deficiency
Hirschsprung disease	Tumors (secretory diarrhea)	Constipation with encopresis
Nutrient malabsorption	Ulcerative colitis	
	Celiac disease	

LABORATORY AND DIAGNOSTIC TESTS

Common laboratory and diagnostic studies ordered for the assessment of diarrhea include:

- Stool culture: may indicate presence of bacteria
- Stool for ova and parasites (O&P): may indicate the presence of parasites
- Stool viral panel or culture: to determine the presence of rotavirus or other viruses
- Stool for occult blood: may be positive if inflammation or ulceration is present in the GI tract
- Stool for leukocytes: may be positive in cases of inflammation or infection
- Stool pH/reducing substances: to see if the diarrhea is caused by carbohydrate intolerance
- Electrolyte panel: may indicate dehydration
- Abdominal x-rays (KUB): presence of stool in colon may indicate constipation or **fecal impaction** (hardened immobile bulk of stool); air–fluid levels may indicate intestinal obstruction

Nursing Management

Nursing management of the child with diarrhea focuses on restoring fluid and electrolyte balance and providing family education.

RESTORING FLUID AND ELECTROLYTE BALANCE

Continue the child's regular diet if the child is not dehydrated. Initial nursing management of the dehydrated child with diarrhea is focused on fluid and electrolyte balance restoration. Refer to Nursing Care Plan 42.1 on page 1622–1625. Probiotic supplementation while a child is taking antibiotics for other disorders may reduce the incidence of antibiotic-related diarrhea (Hoffenberg et al., 2014) (see Common Medical Treatments 42.1 and Evidence-Based Practice 42.1). After rehydration is achieved, it is important to encourage the child to consume a regular diet to maintain energy and growth.

Take Note!

Avoid prolonged use of clear liquids in the child with diarrhea because "starvation stools" may result. Also avoid fluids high in glucose, such as fruit juice, gelatin, and soda, which may worsen diarrhea (Fleisher, 2014).

PROVIDING FAMILY EDUCATION

Teach the parents the importance of oral rehydration therapy (see Teaching Guidelines 42.2). The physician may order medication therapy. In such instances, teach the importance of finishing all prescribed antibiotic therapy. After the cause of the diarrhea is known, teach the child and family how to prevent further occurrences. As most cases of acute diarrhea are infectious, provide education about proper hand-washing techniques and transmission route. Chronic diarrhea is often a result of excessive intake of formula, water, or fruit juice, so teach the parents about appropriate fluid intake.

Oral Candidiasis (Thrush)

Oral candidiasis (thrush) is a fungal infection of the oral mucosa. It is most common in newborns and infants. Children at risk for thrush include those with immune disorders, those using corticosteroid inhalers, and those receiving therapy that suppresses the immune system (e.g., chemotherapy for cancer). Antibiotic use may also contribute to thrush. In addition, fungal infection may be transmitted between the infant and the breastfeeding mother.

Therapeutic management includes treatment with oral antifungal agents such as Nystatin or fluconazole.

Nursing Assessment

Assess for risk factors for oral candidiasis such as young age, immune suppression, antibiotic use, use of corticosteroid inhalers, or presence of fungal infection in

EVIDENCE-BASED PRACTICE 42.1 PROBIOTICS FOR TREATING ACUTE INFECTIOUS DIARRHOEA

STUDY

Diarrhea (more than three loose, watery stools in a 24-hour period) occurs frequently in children, and is an important cause of dehydration. Most cases of diarrhea are caused by viruses, and symptomatic treatment is the only available therapy. The authors reviewed 63 randomized controlled studies that included a total of over 8,000 participants, most of which were infants and young children. The studies evaluated the use of probiotics as compared with placebo or no treatment in relation to the severity and length of diarrhea.

Findings

A variety of probiotics were noted to reduce stool frequency in infants and children as well as adults, as well as shortening the course of diarrhea. The results were statistically significant, leading the authors to determine that probiotic therapy during acute diarrhea may be beneficial.

Nursing Implications

Probiotics are available as supplements: capsules or powder that may be sprinkled on food. In addition, live culture yogurt contains probiotics. Recommend these additions to the diet of older infants or children with acute diarrhea.

Adapted from Allen, S. J., Martinez, E. G., Gregorio, G. V, & Dans, L. F. (2010). Probiotics for treating acute infectious diarrhoea (review). *The Cochrane Library 2007,* 12. Indianapolis, IN: John Wiley & Sons.

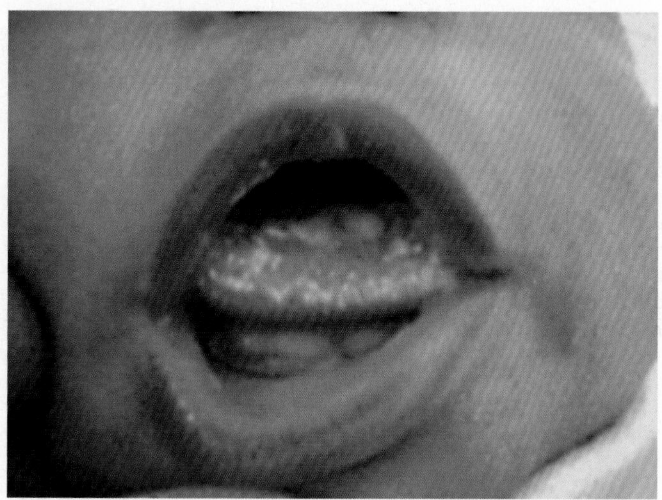

FIGURE 42.8 Thick white patches in the infant with oral candidiasis (thrush).

the mother. Inspect the oral mucosa. Thrush appears as thick white patches on the tongue, mucosa, or palate, resembling curdled milk (Fig. 42.8). Unlike milk retained in the mouth, the patches do not easily wipe off with a swab or washcloth. Also assess for the presence of candidal diaper rash (beefy-red rash with satellite lesions). Determine the extent to which the presence of the lesions is interfering with the infant's ability to feed. The lesions may cause significant discomfort.

Diagnosis is usually based on clinical presentation. However, a careful scraping of the lesions can be sent out for fungal culture.

Nursing Management

Nursing management of the child with thrush includes administering medications and providing family education.

ADMINISTERING MEDICATIONS

Ensure appropriate administration of oral antifungal agents. Administer nystatin suspension four times per day following feeding to allow the medication to remain in contact with the lesions. In the younger infant, apply nystatin to the lesions with a cotton-tipped applicator. The older infant or child can easily swallow the pleasantly flavored suspension. An advantage of fluconazole is its once-daily dosing, but monitor infants and children receiving it for hepatotoxicity. Unlike nystatin, it is important to administer fluconazole with food to decrease the side effects of nausea and vomiting.

EDUCATING THE FAMILY

If the mother is also infected, she must receive antifungal treatment as well. Fungal infection of the breast can cause the mother a great deal of pain with nursing, but if appropriately treated breastfeeding can continue without interruption. Stress appropriate hand washing. It is important to keep bottle nipples and pacifiers clean. Infants and young children often mouth their toys, so it is important to clean them appropriately. Explain to parents of infants with thrush the importance of reporting diaper rash because fungal infections in the diaper area often occur concomitantly with thrush and also need to be treated.

Take Note!

Geographic tongue is a benign, noncontagious condition. A reduction in the filiform papillae (bumps on the tongue) occurs in patches that migrate periodically, thus giving a map-like appearance to the tongue, with darker and lighter, higher and lower patches. Do not confuse the lighter patches of geographic tongue with the thick white plaques that form on the tongue with thrush.

Oral Lesions

A number of oral lesions may affect infants and children. A few of the most common are aphthous ulcers, gingivostomatitis (from herpes simplex virus [HSV]), and herpangina. Table 42.2 lists the causes of common oral lesions. Regardless of type, oral lesions are often painful and can interfere with the child's ability to eat. Therapeutic management of oral lesions varies depending on the cause.

Nursing Assessment

Explore the health history for the presence of risk factors such as immune deficiency, cancer chemotherapy treatment, exposure to infectious agents, trauma, stress, or celiac or Crohn disease. Note the onset of the lesion(s) and progression over time. Question the parent or child about the presence of sore throat or dysphagia (occurs with herpangina). Inspect the oral cavity, including the tongue, buccal mucosa, palate, and hypoglossal area. Note the presence of lesions and their distribution. Refer to Table 42.2 for descriptions and illustrations of various oral lesions. Inspect the pharynx, which may be red with herpangina. Generally the diagnosis is based on the history and clinical presentation, but occasionally oral lesions are cultured for HSV.

Nursing Management

The primary concerns with oral lesions are pain management and maintenance of hydration. A corticosteroid-containing dental paste used for aphthous ulcers is formulated to "stick" to mucous membranes, so the lesion area should be as dry as possible prior to application of the paste. Children do not care for having the paste applied and will often resist. Older children with herpangina or stomatitis can "swish and spit" various formulations of "magic mouthwash" (typically a combination of liquid diphenhydramine, liquid acetaminophen,

TABLE 42.2 ORAL LESIONS

	Aphthous Ulcers	Gingivostomatitis	Herpangina
Cause	Trauma, vitamin deficiency, celiac disease, Crohn disease	Herpes simplex virus	Enterovirus (Coxsackie)
Appearance	Erythematous border, often yellow appearance to the ulcer, anywhere on oral mucosa or lips	Vesicular lesions on erythematous base, anywhere in oral cavity, including lips	Bright-red ulcers, generally in posterior oral cavity
Fever	Generally absent	May have high fever with initial outbreak	Abrupt onset of high fever (up to 39.4–40.6°C), lasting 1–4 days
Length of illness	Generally heal within 7–14 days; may recur	10–12 days initially; may recur with stress, febrile illness, or intense sunlight exposure (as virus lies dormant in system)	Generally resolves within 5–7 days
Therapeutic management	Topical corticosteroid in dental paste may help.	Acyclovir	Supportive treatment only

Adapted from Ben-Joseph, E. P. (2013). *Canker sores*. Retrieved from http://kidshealth.org/parent/general/aches/canker.html#; Keels, M. A. & Clements, D. A. (2015). *Herpetic gingivostomatitis in young children*. Retrieved from http://www.uptodate.com/contents/herpetic-gingivostomatitis-in-young-children; and Romero, J. R. (2015). *Hand, foot, and mouth disease and herpangina: An overview*. Retrieved from http://www.uptodate.com/contents/hand-foot-and-mouth-disease-and-herpangina-an-overview

and milk of magnesia); they may offer some pain relief. Common over-the-counter medications such as Anbesol, Oragel, and Kank-A may be helpful for topical pain relief, though oral analgesics are often necessary.

The child with herpangina is typically an infant or young child (Romero, 2015). It may be very difficult to coach a young child to drink fluids when his or her mouth is hurting. Playing games and offering favorite fluids and popsicles may encourage adequate oral intake. It is important to avoid carbonated beverages and citrus juices when oral lesions are present as they can cause further stinging and burning.

Take Note!

Viscous lidocaine should be used with caution in younger children as a topical treatment for numbing the lesions or as a swish-and-spit treatment because they may swallow the lidocaine (Taketomo, Hodding, & Kraus, 2013).

Hypertrophic Pyloric Stenosis

In hypertrophic pyloric stenosis, the circular muscle of the pylorus becomes hypertrophied, causing thickness in the luminal side of the pyloric canal (Fig. 42.9). This thickness creates a gastric outlet obstruction, causing nonbilious vomiting that presents between weeks 3 and 6 of life. The vomiting becomes more frequent and forceful as time goes on and is often projectile. The incidence is 2 to 3.5 per 1,000 live births, occurring more often in males than females, with 30% to 40% being in first-born infants (Olivé & Endom, 2016). The cause of pyloric stenosis is probably multifactorial.

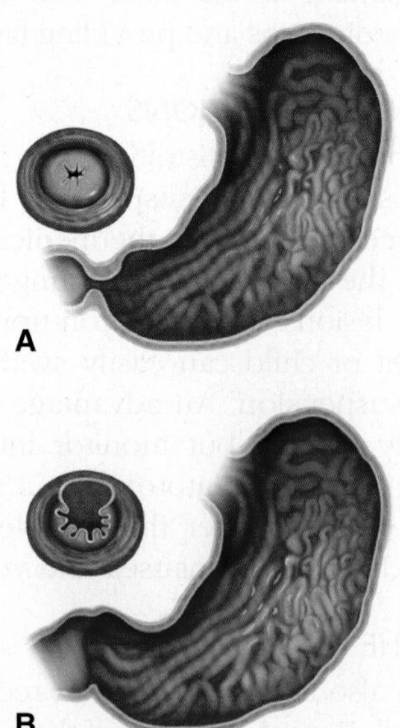

FIGURE 42.9 **(A)** Hypertrophied pylorus muscle and narrowed stomach outlet. **(B)** In pyloromyotomy, the pylorus is incised, thus increasing the diameter of the pyloric outlet.

Pyloric stenosis requires surgical intervention. A pyloromyotomy is performed to cut the muscle of the pylorus and relieve the gastric outlet obstruction (Fig. 42.9). Postoperative complications are rare.

Nursing Assessment

For a full description of the assessment phase of the nursing process, refer to the Assessment section in the Nursing Process Overview earlier in the chapter. Assessment findings pertinent to hypertrophic pyloric stenosis are discussed below.

HEALTH HISTORY

Elicit a description of the present illness and chief complaint. Common signs and symptoms reported during the health history might include:

- Forceful, nonbilious vomiting, unrelated to feeding position
- Hunger soon after vomiting episode
- Weight loss due to vomiting
- Progressive dehydration with subsequent lethargy
- Possible positive family history

PHYSICAL EXAMINATION AND LABORATORY AND DIAGNOSTIC TESTS

Palpate for a hard, moveable "olive" in the right upper quadrant (hypertrophied pylorus). If an easily palpable mass is felt, no further testing is necessary and a surgical consult is called. If no mass is identified, a pyloric ultrasound may be ordered to identify a thickened hypoechoic ring in the region of the pylorus. An upper GI series may identify pyloric stenosis as well, but an ultrasound is less invasive and is considered more diagnostic of pyloric stenosis. Assess laboratory values to determine if the infant has metabolic alkalosis resulting from dehydration.

Take Note!

It may be difficult to examine the infant's abdomen when pyloric stenosis is suspected because of the infant's extreme irritability. A pacifier or nipple dipped in glucose water may soothe the infant long enough to perform the abdominal examination.

Nursing Management

Preoperative management of infants with pyloric stenosis is aimed at fluid management and correcting abnormal electrolyte values. Family anxiety is high during this time because of the impending surgery for an otherwise healthy infant. Provide emotional support to the family. Teach them about the surgical procedure and what to expect postoperatively. After surgery, infants usually resume oral feedings after 1 to 2 days.

Intussusception

Intussusception is a process that occurs when a proximal segment of bowel "telescopes" into a more distal segment, causing edema, vascular compromise, and, ultimately, partial or total bowel obstruction (Fig. 42.10). In children younger than 2 years of age, intussusception is the most common cause of intestinal obstruction (Galloway & Seguias, 2013). A lead point (i.e., pathologic point) may cause the telescoping. Examples of lead points are Meckel diverticulum, duplication cysts, polyps, hemangiomas, tumors, or the appendix.

A barium enema is successful at reducing a large percentage of intussusception cases; other cases are reduced surgically. If surgical reduction is unsuccessful or bowel necrosis has occurred, a portion of the bowel must be resected.

Nursing Assessment

For a full description of the assessment phase of the nursing process, refer to the Assessment section in the Nursing Process Overview earlier in the chapter. Assessment findings pertinent to intussusception are discussed below.

HEALTH HISTORY

Elicit a description of the present illness and chief complaint. Common signs and symptoms reported during the health history might include:

- Sudden onset of intermittent, crampy abdominal pain
- Severe pain (children usually draw up their knees and scream)
- Vomiting
- Diarrhea
- Currant-jelly stools, gross blood, or hemoccult-positive stools
- Lethargy

Typically, symptoms flare and then regress. Between episodes, children may have no symptoms of

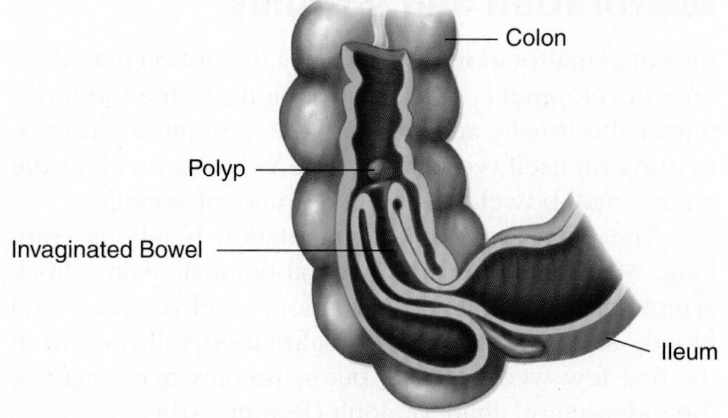

FIGURE 42.10 In intussusception, the intestine telescopes upon itself.

intussusception. This return to a normal state is due to the intussusception reducing on its own. The child may be asymptomatic and may appear well when presenting to the physician or nurse practitioner or emergency room. Again, this may be a sign that the bowel has reduced spontaneously. Assess the severity of pain, length of time the symptoms have been present, presence of vomiting, and stool patterns and color. Immediately report the presence of bilious vomiting, which occurs only in an obstructive situation. Also assess for signs and symptoms of acute peritonitis. Explore the child's current and past medical history for risk factors, such as cystic fibrosis or celiac disease.

PHYSICAL EXAMINATION

Palpate the abdomen for the presence of a sausage-shaped mass in the upper midabdomen; this is a hallmark sign of intussusception. Note any mental status changes.

LABORATORY AND DIAGNOSTIC TESTS

Intussusception is usually diagnosed with an air or barium enema. Use of an enema may show the intussusception and also may reduce it, making the enema therapeutic. A pediatric surgeon should be available at the time the enema is given in case the enema is unsuccessful or perforation (rare) occurs. White blood cell elevation may occur and electrolytes may show signs of dehydration.

Nursing Management

Administer intravenous fluids and antibiotics before the diagnostic laboratory and x-ray studies are performed. Refer to Nursing Care Plan 42.1, at the end of the chapter, for nursing management of the postoperative child.

The parents may be very fatigued after dealing with a crying infant. They are often quite anxious about surgery in an otherwise healthy child. Offer emotional support and provide appropriate preoperative and postoperative education to the family.

Malrotation and Volvulus

Intestinal malrotation results from a disruption in embryonic development. When malrotation occurs, the intestine is abnormally attached and the mesentery narrows, twisting on itself (volvulus). If the volvulus involves the entire small bowel, it is termed a midgut volvulus.

The main symptom of malrotation is bilious vomiting. Many children also have abdominal pain, shock symptoms, abdominal distention, tachycardia, and bloody stools. Most cases of malrotation will present in the first few weeks of life, but symptoms may occur in the older infant, child, or adult (Brandt, 2014).

Therapeutic management of malrotation and volvulus is accomplished surgically. A Ladd procedure is performed, during which the intestine is straightened out and bands contributing to the misalignment are divided. If bowel necrosis has occurred (rare), then an ostomy may be necessary.

Nursing Assessment

For a full description of the assessment phase of the nursing process, refer to the Assessment section in the Nursing Process Overview earlier in the chapter. Assessment findings pertinent to malrotation and volvulus are discussed below.

HEALTH HISTORY

Elicit a description of the present illness and chief complaint. Common signs and symptoms reported during the health history might include vomiting and abdominal pain. Since obstruction can occur with resulting necrosis of the bowel, immediately inform the physician if obstruction is suspected.

PHYSICAL EXAMINATION AND DIAGNOSTIC AND LABORATORY TESTS

Observe for severity of pain, auscultate for hypoactive bowel sounds, and palpate for abdominal guarding or rebound tenderness. Common laboratory and diagnostic studies ordered for the assessment of malrotation and volvulus include:

- KUB to reveal obstruction
- Upper GI series to identify the location of the duodenojejunal junction and corkscrew appearance of the twisted bowel

Nursing Management

When diagnostic testing reveals malrotation/volvulus, administer ordered intravenous fluids and intravenous antibiotics. Often a nasogastric tube is placed to decompress the stomach. Surgery is performed as soon as possible. After surgery, provide postoperative care of the child (see Nursing Care Plan 42.1 at the end of the chapter). Provide continuous emotional support and family education.

Appendicitis

Appendicitis, an acute inflammation of the appendix, is the most common cause of emergent abdominal surgery in children (Hoffenberg et al., 2014). It occurs in all age groups; the median age in the pediatric population is 4 to 15 years (Wall & Albanese, 2015).

Pathophysiology

Appendicitis is due to a closed-loop obstruction of the appendix (Fig. 42.11). It is thought that the obstruction is

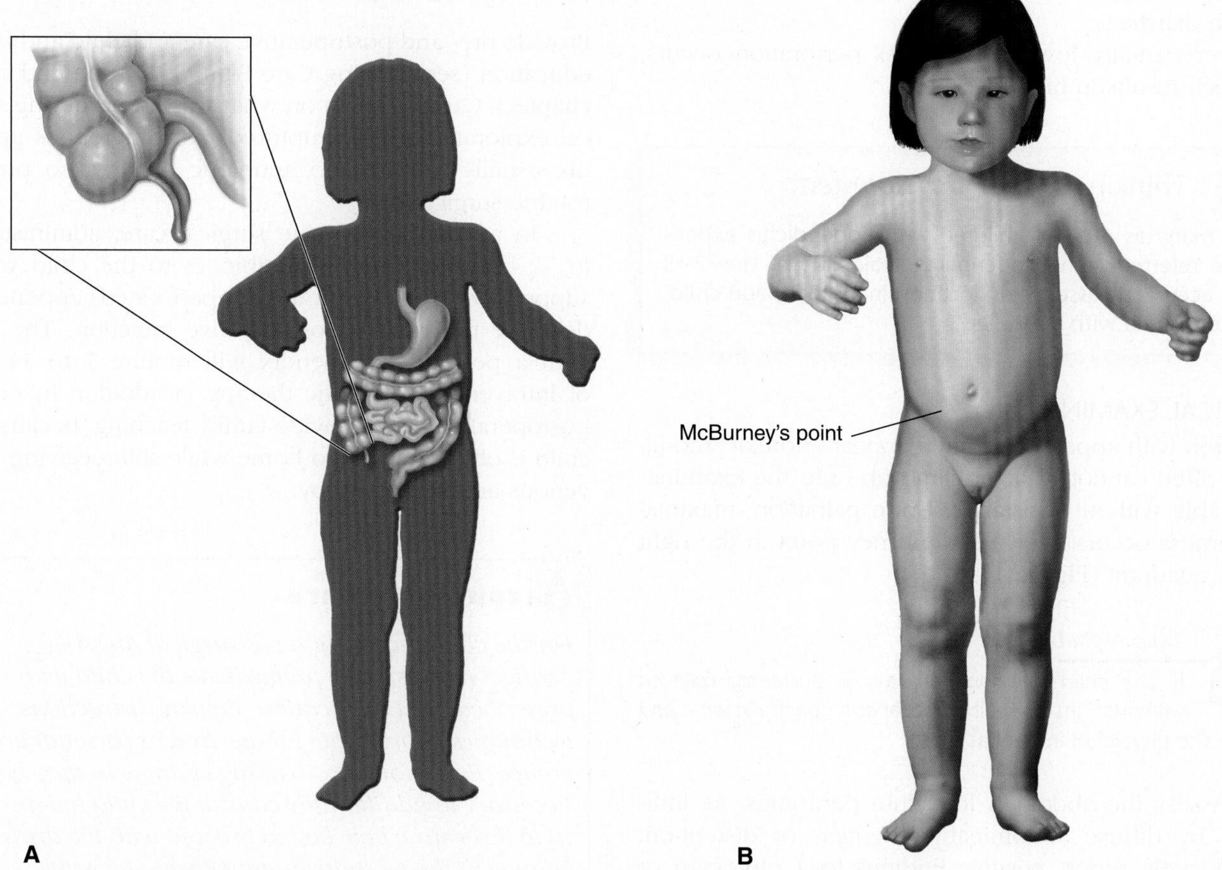

FIGURE 42.11 **(A)** In appendicitis, the lumen of the appendix is obstructed, resulting in edema and compressed blood vessels. **(B)** As appendicitis progresses, pain may become localized at McBurney's point (a point midway between the anterior superior iliac crest and the umbilicus).

due to fecal material impacted into the relatively narrow appendix, though other causes such as ingested foreign bodies may exist. This causes a subsequent increase in the intraluminal pressure of the appendix, resulting in mucosal edema, bacterial overgrowth, and eventual perforation. The rate of perforation is high in children, especially those under 2 years old (Hoffenberg et al., 2014). Due to the fecal material in the appendix, perforation causes inflammatory fluid and bacterial contents to leak into the abdominal cavity, resulting in peritonitis. Diffuse peritonitis is more likely in younger children. Older children and adolescents have a more developed omentum, which walls off the inflamed or perforated appendix, often causing a focal abscess.

Therapeutic Management

Appendicitis is considered a surgical emergency because if left uncorrected, the appendix may perforate. Surgical removal of the appendix is necessary and is often accomplished via a minimally invasive laparoscopic technique. In the case of perforation, an open surgical procedure is usually required, and lavage of the abdominal cavity may be performed to cleanse it of the infected fluid released from the appendix.

Nursing Assessment

Early diagnosis and intervention are the key elements to avoid perforation. For a full description of the assessment phase of the nursing process, refer to the Assessment section in the Nursing Process Overview earlier in the chapter. Assessment findings pertinent to appendicitis are discussed below.

HEALTH HISTORY

Elicit a description of the present illness and chief complaint. Appendicitis may be gradual, but symptoms usually do not come and go; they remain persistent and intensify. Common signs and symptoms reported during the health history might include:

- Vague abdominal pain in the initial stages, localizing to the right lower quadrant over a few hours
- Nausea and vomiting (which usually develop after the onset of pain)

- Small-volume, frequent, soft stools, often confused with diarrhea
- Fever (usually low grade unless perforation occurs, which results in high fever)

Thinking About Development

As many as 40% of children with appendicitis experience referred pain (Hoffenberg et al., 2014). How will you accurately assess pain location in a school-age child, as compared with a toddler?

PHYSICAL EXAMINATION

Children with appendicitis often appear anorexic and ill. They often cannot walk or climb up onto the examination table without assistance. Upon palpation, maximal tenderness occurs over the McBurney point in the right lower quadrant (Fig. 42.11).

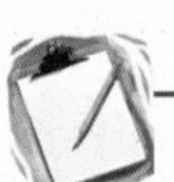

Take Note!

If the child's abdominal pain is suddenly relieved without intervention, suspect perforation and notify the physician immediately.

Assess the abdomen for acute peritonitis, as indicated by diffuse abdominal tenderness or distention. Immediately report positive findings to a physician or nurse practitioner.

LABORATORY AND DIAGNOSTIC TESTS

Common laboratory and diagnostic studies ordered for the assessment of appendicitis include:

- Abdominal computed tomography (CT) scan: performed to visualize the appendix for further evaluation
- Laboratory testing: may reveal an elevated white blood cell count
- C-reactive protein: may be elevated

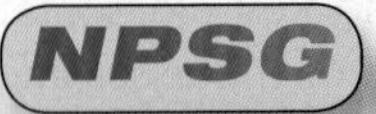

UNIVERSAL: Protocol for Preventing Wrong Site, Wrong Procedure, and Wrong Person Surgery™ (Prevent mistakes in surgery)

UP 01.01.01 Conduct a pre-procedure verification process.

Steps: Ascertain patient identity usually via bracelet which include the appropriate patient identifiers as determined by the facility.

UP 01.02.01 Mark the procedure site.

Steps: Insure the procedure site is appropriately marked prior to the procedure. Involve the patient's parent/caregiver in the marking verification process.

Joint Commission. (2015). *National patient safety goals effective January 1, 2015.* Retrieved from http://www.jointcommission.org/assets/1/6/2015_NPSG_HAP.pdf

Nursing Management

Provide pre- and postoperative care and child and family education (see Nursing Care Plan 42.1 at the end of the chapter). Care depends on what was found during surgical exploration. A nonruptured, nongangrenous appendix usually requires no antibiotic therapy, so provide routine surgical care.

In addition to routine surgical care, administer 48 to 72 hours of ordered antibiotics to the child with a suppurative or gangrenous (nonperforated) appendix to decrease the risk of postoperative infection. The child with a perforated appendix will require 7 to 14 days of intravenous antibiotic therapy in addition to normal postoperative care. Provide family teaching, because the child is often discharged home while still receiving intravenous antibiotic therapy.

Atraumatic Care

For the child requiring a postsurgical dressing change, make sure to premedicate the child with prescribed pain medication. Employ distractions techniques appropriate for age and/or personal preference. For a complex dressing change, in may be necessary to additionally consult the child life specialist to determine how best to proceed with the dressing change in the most atraumatic fashion possible.

CHRONIC GASTROINTESTINAL DISORDERS

Chronic GI disorders include GER, PUD, constipation/encopresis, Hirschsprung disease, short bowel syndrome, inflammatory bowel disease, celiac disease, functional abdominal pain, failure to thrive, and chronic feeding problems.

Gastroesophageal Reflux

GER is passage of gastric contents into the esophagus. It is considered a normal physiologic process that occurs in healthy infants and children. However, when complications develop from the reflux of gastric contents back into the esophagus or oropharynx, it becomes more of a pathologic process known as gastroesophageal reflux disease (GERD). GER occurs frequently during the first year of life, is considered benign, and usually resolves by 12 to 18 months of age (Hoffenberg et al., 2014). GER is particularly common in premature infants. Other possible diagnoses that can be mistaken for GER include food allergies, formula enteropathies, gastric outlet obstruction, malrotation, cyclic vomiting, and central nervous system lesions.

Pathophysiology

The process of GER occurs during episodes of transient relaxation of the LES, which can occur during swallowing, crying, or other Valsalva maneuvers that increase intra-abdominal pressure. Delayed esophageal clearance and gastric emptying, highly acidic gastric contents, hiatal hernia (protrusion of the stomach upward into the mediastinal cavity through the esophageal hiatus of the diaphragm), or neurologic disease may also be contributing factors associated with reflux.

The signs and symptoms of GERD are often seen as a result of the damaging components of the refluxate (the pH of the gastric contents, bile acids, and pepsin). The longer the pH of the refluxate is below 4, the higher the suspicion of GERD, but results must be correlated with the child's clinical presentation (Winter, 2015). Symptoms of GERD in infants and children are listed below in the health history section.

GERD may cause esophagitis, esophageal stricture, Barrett esophagus (a precancerous condition), or anemia from chronic esophageal erosion. In addition, complications such as laryngitis, recurrent pneumonia, or asthma may occur.

Therapeutic Management

Conservative medical management begins with appropriate positioning, such as elevating the head of the bed and keeping the infant or child upright for 30 minutes after feeding. Smaller, more frequent feedings may be helpful. If reflux does not improve with these measures, medications are prescribed to decrease acid production and stabilize the pH of the gastric contents. Also, prokinetic agents may be used to help empty the stomach more quickly, minimizing the amount of gastric contents in the stomach that the child can reflux (Winter, 2016a; 2016b) (Dosage Calculation Box 42.1).

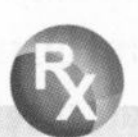

Dosage Calculation Box 42.1

Infant's weight: 11 lb, 8 oz

Medication order: omeprazole 4 mg PO once a day.

Per the Pediatric Dosage Handbook, the recommended dose is 0.7 mg/kg/dose.

Is the ordered dose safe?

If the GERD cannot be medically managed effectively or requires long-term medication therapy, surgical intervention may be necessary. A Nissen fundoplication is the most common surgical procedure performed for antireflux therapy. The gastric fundus is wrapped around the lower 2 to 3 cm of the esophagus (Fig. 42.12). Laparoscopic fundoplications are being performed as a way to minimize the recovery period and reduce potential complications.

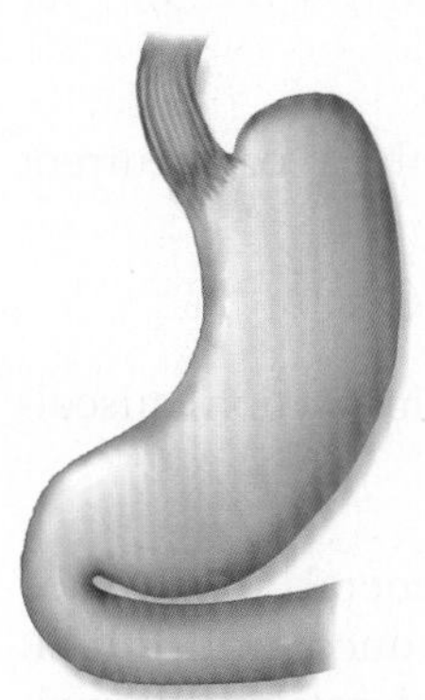
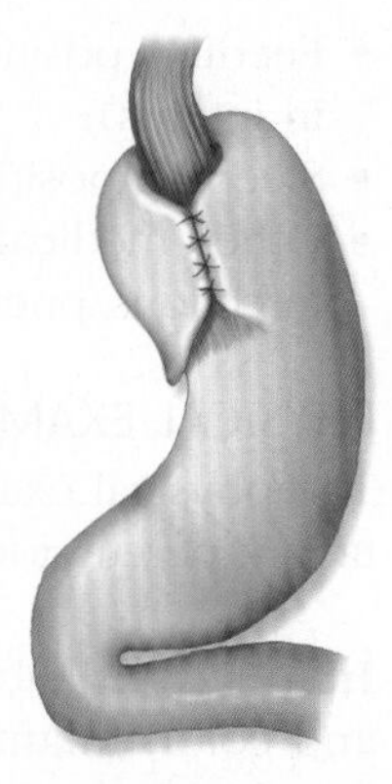

FIGURE 42.12 In the Nissen fundoplication, the fundus (upper portion of the stomach) is wrapped around the lower segment of the esophagus.

Nursing Assessment

For a full description of the assessment phase of the nursing process, refer to the Assessment section in the Nursing Process Overview earlier in the chapter. Assessment findings pertinent to GER are discussed below.

HEALTH HISTORY

Elicit a description of the present illness and chief complaint. Note onset and progression of symptoms. Common signs and symptoms reported during the health history include:

- Recurrent vomiting or regurgitation
- Weight loss or poor weight gain
- Irritability in infants
- Respiratory symptoms (chronic cough, wheezing, stridor, asthma, apnea)
- Hoarseness/sore throat
- Halitosis (mostly in older children)
- Heartburn or chest pain
- Abdominal pain
- Abnormal neck posturing (Sandifer syndrome)
- Hematemesis
- Dysphagia or feeding refusal
- Chronic sinusitis, otitis media
- Poor dentition (caused by acid erosion)

Explore the child's current and past medical history for risk factors such as:

- Prematurity, noting prolonged ventilator use or chronic lung disease
- Dietary habits (e.g., chocolate, coffee, spicy or fatty foods, caffeine, formula-fed or breastfed, overeating or overfeeding)
- Current medications
- Smoking/alcohol use (older children)
- Food allergies
- Other GI disorders (gastric outlet dysfunction/hiatal hernia) or congenital abnormalities

- Feeding positions and patterns (especially important in infants)
- Sleeping positions/patterns
- Other medical history, such as asthma or recurrent infections/pneumonia

PHYSICAL EXAMINATION

The physical examination consists of inspection, auscultation, percussion, and palpation.

Inspection. Observe the child's general appearance and color. Infants and children with uncontrolled GER for a period of time may appear underweight or malnourished. Infants may be irritable due to painful regurgitation/reflux events. Note breathing patterns, because reflux-induced asthma may have developed. Acute life-threatening events (ALTEs) and apnea have been associated with severe GERD (Hoffenberg et al., 2014). Observe the child for cyanosis, altered mental status, and alterations in tone. Inspect emesis for blood or bile.

Auscultation. Evaluate the lung fields for the presence of complications related to GERD, such as wheezing or pneumonia. No further pathologic findings related to GERD should be auscultated on examination.

Percussion. Perform routine abdominal percussion, noting any abnormalities. No specific findings should be noted.

Palpation. Use caution when palpating the abdomen, especially with infants with GERD, because it may induce vomiting. No abnormalities should be palpated.

Take Note!

Not all infants with GERD actually vomit. Some may only demonstrate irritability associated with feeding or posturing (arching back during or after feeding [termed Sandifer syndrome]) and grimacing. Episodes of GERD often cause bradycardia, so if the above signs occur, they should be reported to the physician or nurse practitioner, even if the baby is not vomiting (Winter, 2016).

LABORATORY AND DIAGNOSTIC TESTS

Common laboratory and diagnostic studies ordered for the assessment of GER include:

- Upper GI series: though not sensitive or specific to GER, may show some reflux; studies are used to narrow down the differential diagnosis
- Esophageal pH probe study: quantifies GER episodes as they correlate to symptoms
- Esophagogastroduodenoscopy (EGD): shows esophageal and gastric tissue damage from GERD
- Complete blood count: may demonstrate anemia if chronic esophagitis or hematemesis is present
- Hemoccult: may be positive if chronic esophagitis is present

Nursing Management

As with most GI disorders, initial nursing management is aimed at restoring proper fluid balance and nutrition. Refer to Nursing Care Plan 42.1 at the end of the chapter. Additional considerations are reviewed below.

PROMOTING SAFE FEEDING TECHNIQUES AND POSITIONING

Feeding adjustments are an essential part of reflux management. Give infants smaller, more frequent feedings using a nipple that controls flow well. Frequently burp the infant during feeds to control reflux. Thickening of the formula with products such as rice or oatmeal cereal can significantly help keep the formula and gastric contents down. Positioning after feedings is important. Keep infants upright for 30 to 45 minutes after feeding by holding them and/or elevating the head of the crib 30 degrees. Placing in infant seats or swings is not recommended as this increases intra-abdominal pressure (Winter, 2016a). For older children, elevate the head of the bed as much as possible and restrict meals for several hours before bedtime.

MAINTAINING A PATENT AIRWAY

GERD symptoms often involve the airway. Maximize reflux precautions to keep the risk of airway involvement to a minimum. In rare instances, GERD causes apnea or an ALTE (Hoffenberg et al., 2014). In these cases, use an apnea or bradycardia monitor to monitor for such episodes. The monitor requires a physician's order and can be ordered through a home health company. Teach parents how to deal with these episodes, as their anxiety is very high. Provide cardiopulmonary resuscitation (CPR) instruction to all parents whose children have had an ALTE previously.

EDUCATING THE FAMILY AND CHILD

The goals for the infant and child with GER are a decrease in symptoms, a decrease in the frequency and duration of reflux episodes, healing of the injured mucosa, and prevention of further complications of GERD. Teach the parents the signs and symptoms of complications. Explain that reflux is usually limited to the first year of life, though in some cases it persists. If medications are prescribed, thoroughly explain their use and their side effects (see Drug Guide 42.1).

PROVIDING POSTOPERATIVE CARE

If the child requires fundoplication, a gastrostomy tube is often placed for use in the immediate postoperative period or for long-term feeding. In the immediate postoperative period, assess for pain, abdominal distention, and return of bowel sounds. If a gastrostomy tube is placed, it is often open to straight drain for a period of time postoperatively to keep the stomach empty and allow for the internal incision to heal. When bowel sounds have returned and the infant or child is stable, introduce feedings slowly (typically via the gastrostomy tube). Assess for tolerance of feedings (absence of abdominal distention or pain, minimal residual, and passage of stool). If the abdomen does become distended or the child has discomfort, open the gastrostomy tube to air to decompress the stomach. Assess the insertion site of the gastrostomy tube for redness, edema, or drainage. Keep the site clean and dry per surgeon or hospital protocol. Teach the parents how to care for the gastrostomy tube and insertion site and how to use the tube for feeding.

PROMOTING FAMILY AND CHILD COPING

Parents may experience a great deal of anxiety. Teach the family about all aspects of GERD to help promote coping. School-age children often have reflux episodes exhibited by postprandial vomiting, which can be very embarrassing for the children. Notify the school about the medical issues related to GER to minimize the situations for the child.

Peptic Ulcer Disease

PUD is a term used to describe a variety of disorders of the upper GI tract that result from the action of gastric secretions (Fig. 42.13). Mucosal inflammation and subsequent ulceration occur as a result of either a primary or a secondary factor. In children, duodenal ulcers are more common than gastric ulcers (Hoffenberg et al., 2014). Primary peptic ulcers are usually associated with *Helicobacter pylori,* a gram-negative organism that causes mucosal inflammation and in some cases more severe disease (Hoffenberg et al., 2014). *H. pylori* is found mostly in the duodenum.

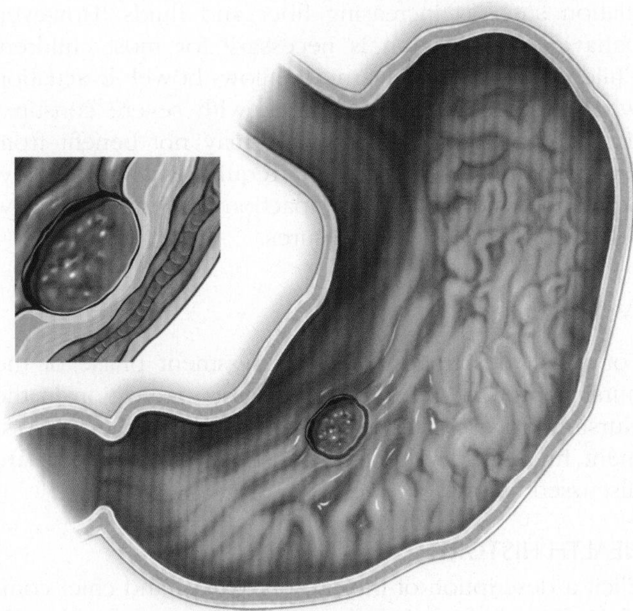

FIGURE 42.13 Peptic ulcer disease.

Secondary peptic ulcers may occur as a result of an identifiable factor, such as excess acid production, stress, medications, or the presence of other underlying conditions. Secondary ulcers tend to be gastric in location as opposed to duodenal.

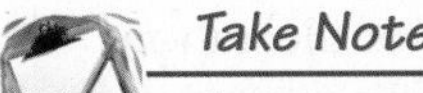

Take Note!

Severe stress, such as burns or another illness necessitating critical care, can contribute to the development of a peptic ulcer in children (Hoffenberg et al., 2014).

Therapeutic Management

PUD may be treated with antibiotics (if *H. pylori* is verified), histamine agonists, and/or proton pump inhibitors. If the child presents with a severe esophageal or gastric hemorrhage, a nasogastric tube may be placed to decompress the stomach. The child may require intravenous infusion of a histamine-2 receptor antagonist or a proton pump inhibitor initially until the bleeding has stopped and the disease is stabilized.

Nursing Assessment

For a full description of the assessment phase of the nursing process, refer to the Assessment section in the Nursing Process Overview earlier in the chapter. Assessment findings pertinent to PUD are discussed below.

HEALTH HISTORY

Elicit a description of the present illness and chief complaint. Common signs and symptoms reported during the health history might include:

- Abdominal pain
- GI bleeding
- Vomiting

Abdominal pain is the most common complaint of children with PUD. It is important to characterize the abdominal pain, as many other digestive disorders may mimic PUD. The pain tends to be dull and vague, mostly epigastric or periumbilical. Most often, children with PUD have pain that worsens after meals, and the pain may wake them at night. Vomiting may be noted in preschool- and school-age children.

Explore the child's current and past medical history for risk factors such as a family history of PUD or other GI diseases, or chronic salicylate or prednisone use.

Take Note!

Adolescents at increased risk for the development of PUD include those who smoke, and/or use alcohol (Vakil, 2014).

PHYSICAL EXAMINATION AND LABORATORY AND DIAGNOSTIC TESTS

Palpate the abdomen for the location of the pain, which is usually epigastric or periumbilical. Note the presence of blood in emesis or stools, as GI bleeding may occur. Common laboratory and diagnostic studies ordered for the assessment of PUD include the following:

- Laboratory studies: to identify anemia or *H. pylori* antibodies
- Urea breath test: to identify *H. pylori* gastritis
- Upper GI series: to detect presence of ulcerations
- Upper endoscopy: the definitive diagnostic test to look for ulceration and nodularity in the upper GI tract
- Biopsies: to assess for *H. pylori,* granulomas, eosinophils, or corrosive agents to identify the primary cause of PUD

Nursing Management

Hemodynamic stabilization should be the focus of nursing management if significant GI bleeding occurs. Once children are stabilized and tolerating oral feeds, they may be discharged to home. Provide discharge instructions on the following topics:

- Medications
- Dietary management (especially when allergic gastroenteropathy is found)
- Safety precautions (in cases of ingested substances)
- Stressors
- Prevention of disease recurrence

Constipation and Encopresis

Constipation is a very common problem among children, affecting about 30% of the pediatric population, and accounting for 3% to 5% of all pediatric outpatient visits (Sood, 2016). It may be defined as failure to achieve complete evacuation of the lower colon. Term newborns should pass a meconium stool within the first 24 hours of life. If this does not occur, the newborn is at risk for developing an underlying GI disorder. Breastfed infants may produce a stool with each feeding, though some will skip a few days between stools. Most bottle-fed babies will produce a stool one or two times per day, but they may go 2 to 3 days without producing a stool. The bowel habits of both infants and children vary widely, so assess and treat each child on an individual basis.

Functional constipation occurs commonly in preschool-age children (Sood, 2016). It may be defined by the presence of at least two of the following over the course of 2 months:

- Less than three bowel movements weekly
- At least one episode of fecal incontinence weekly
- Stool withholding behavior (retentive posturing)
- Hard or painful bowel movements
- Large fecal rectal mass
- Stool passage of a volume to clog the toilet (Dunn, 2013; Sood, 2016)

Encopresis is a term used to describe soiling of fecal contents into the underwear beyond the age of expected toilet training (4 to 5 years of age). Encopresis is often seen as a result of chronic constipation and withholding of stool. As stool is withheld in the rectum, the rectal muscle can stretch over time, and this stretching of the rectum causes fecal impactions. Children who have a stretched rectal vault may experience liquid stool leakage around a fecal mass. This is often an embarrassing issue that occurs with school-age children, and the child may hide his or her underwear to avoid punishment. Many psychological issues arise from chronic constipation and encopresis as the child may experience ridicule and shame (Dunn, 2013).

Pathophysiology

As stool passes through the colon, water is reabsorbed into the colon, resulting in a formed stool by the time it reaches the rectum. At this point, the anal sphincter relaxes to allow the passage of stool from the anus. In constipation, however, this relaxation does not occur.

Most causes of constipation are functional in nature (inorganic) (Sood, 2016). Children with functional constipation usually present with this problem during the toilet-training years. Children have a painful experience during defecation, which in turn creates a fear of defecation, resulting in further withholding of stool. Organic causes of constipation rarely occur in children. When they do occur, they may be a sign of a disease such as spina bifida or sacral agenesis. The causes of pediatric constipation are discussed in Table 42.3.

Therapeutic Management

Once any organic process is ruled out as a cause, constipation may initially be managed with dietary manipulation such as increasing fiber and fluids. However, behavior modification is necessary for most children. Children need to relearn to allow bowel evacuation when stool is present. Children with severe constipation and withholding behaviors may not benefit from dietary management and may require laxative therapy. Sometimes mechanical disimpaction is required initially, followed by the above measures.

Nursing Assessment

For a full description of the assessment phase of the nursing process, refer to the Assessment section in the Nursing Process Overview earlier in the chapter. Assessment findings pertinent to constipation/encopresis are discussed below.

HEALTH HISTORY

Elicit a description of the present illness and chief complaint. Note the onset of symptoms as described by the

TABLE 42.3 CAUSES OF PEDIATRIC CONSTIPATION BY AGE

Newborn/Infant	Toddler and Ages 2–4 Years	School Age	Adolescent	Any Age
• Meconium plug • Hirschsprung disease • Cystic fibrosis • Congenital anorectal malformations • Pseudo-obstruction • Endocrine: hypothyroidism • Metabolic: diabetes insipidus, renal tubular acidosis • Withholding • Dietary changes	• Anal fissures • Withholding • Toilet refusal • Short-segment Hirschsprung disease • Neurologic disorders • Spinal cord: meningomyelocele, tumors, tethered cord	• Toilet or bathroom access limited or unavailable • Limited ability to recognize physiologic cues, preoccupation with other activities • Tethered cord • Withholding	• Spinal cord injury (accidents, trauma) • Dieting • Anorexia • Pregnancy • Idiopathic slow transit constipation, particularly in females • Laxative abuse • Irritable bowel syndrome, constipation variant	• Medication side effect, dietary, post-operative state • Previous anorectal surgery • Withholding and overflow from chronic rectal distention • Relatively rapid change to sedentary state, dehydration • Hypothyroidism

Adapted from Dunn, A. (2013). Elimination patterns. In C. Burns, A. Dunn, M. Brady, N. B. Starr, & C. Blosser (Eds.), *Pediatric primary care* (5th ed.). Philadelphia, PA: Saunders; and Hoffenberg, E., Brumbaugh, D., Furuta, G. T., Kobak, G., Liu, E., Soden, J., & Kramer, R. (2014). Gastrointestinal tract. In W. W. Hay, M. J. Levin, & R. R. Deterding, & M. J. Abzug (Eds.), *Current pediatric diagnosis and treatment* (22nd ed.). New York, NY: McGraw-Hill.

parent/child. Common signs and symptoms reported during the health history may include:

- Altered stooling patterns (size, frequency, amount, and color)
- Pain with defecation
- Withholding behaviors (postures to try to withhold the stool, such as crossing the legs, squatting or hiding in a corner, or "dancing")
- Complaints of abdominal pain and cramping and poor appetite
- Diarrhea leakage
- Soiling of undergarments

It is important to note the duration of the symptoms to determine an acute onset versus a chronic disorder. Explore the child's past and current medical history for risk factors such as:

- Family history of GI disorders
- History of rectal bleeding or anal fissures
- Report of first meconium stool after 24 hours of age
- History of sexual abuse

It is important to take an accurate dietary history as well as a history of fluid intake. Also explore current medication or laxative use.

PHYSICAL EXAMINATION

Physical examination of the child with constipation consists of inspection, auscultation, percussion, and palpation.

Inspection. Observe the child's general appearance. Note whether the abdomen appears distended or rounded. Observe the lower back for a deep pilonidal dimple with hair tuft, which is suggestive of spina bifida occulta. Flat buttocks may be suggestive of sacral agenesis. Inspect the anus for signs of fissures or soiling. Inspect the child's underwear for stains or smears, which are indicative of soiling.

Auscultation. Auscultate bowel sounds to determine the possibility of an obstruction (hypoactive or absent bowel sounds) in the child with an acute case of constipation.

Percussion. Percuss the abdomen to reveal dullness, which would indicate a fecal mass.

Palpation. Palpate the abdomen for any tenderness or masses. The nurse may assist the physician or nurse practitioner with the performance of a rectal examination to assess for rectal tone and rectal vault size.

LABORATORY AND DIAGNOSTIC TESTS

Laboratory and diagnostic tests are not routine with the diagnosis of functional constipation, but if an organic cause is suspected, the following laboratory and diagnostic tests would be ordered:

- Stool for occult blood: the presence of blood could indicate some other disease process
- Abdominal x-ray: large quantities of stool may be seen in the colon
- Sitz marker study: to detect colonic dysmotility
- Barium enema: to rule out a stricture or Hirschsprung disease
- Rectal manometry: to evaluate rectal musculature dysfunction
- Rectal suction biopsy: to rule out Hirschsprung disease

Nursing Management

Nursing management for the infant or child with constipation is aimed at educating the child and family and promoting child and family coping. Refer to Nursing Care Plan 42.1 at the end of the chapter. Additional considerations are reviewed below.

EDUCATING THE FAMILY AND CHILD

Teach parents how to assess for signs of constipation and withholding behaviors. Also provide guidelines on scheduling and supervising bowel habits in reconditioning the child to use the toilet regularly. Teach parents to use positive reinforcement techniques. For example, when the child produces an adequate-volume bowel movement, reward him or her with stickers, extra playtime or television time, and so on thePoint.

Dietary changes may help some children. High-fiber diets help to regulate bowel activity. Increasing fluid intake may also aid in bringing extra water into the bowel, thereby softening the stool. Infants and toddlers with constipation may be experiencing constipation from formula or milk changes. Therefore, manipulating the formula or milk may result in better bowel habits.

Educate families about the importance of compliance with medication use, if medication is ordered. Parents often are very anxious about the use of these medications, but stress to them that compliance is essential. Assess for improper laxative use based on the history of stool patterns.

Many children present to their physician or nurse practitioner with fecal impaction or partial impaction. Teach parents how to disimpact their children at home; this often requires an enema or stimulation therapy. Nursing Procedure 42.2 gives instructions on enema administration in children. Explain the procedure to the child in developmentally appropriate terms. Enema administration can be uncomfortable, but calming measures, such as distraction and praise, provide a comforting environment. After the impaction is removed, promote regular bowel habits to keep the impaction from recurring.

PROMOTING CHILD AND FAMILY COPING

Childhood constipation can be a very stressful process for both the child and family. Behavior modification is necessary for many children. To facilitate daily bowel evacuation, the child should sit on the toilet twice a day (after breakfast and dinner) for 5 to 15 minutes. Instruct the family to keep a "star" or reward chart to encourage compliance. Parents should award the star for compliance with time sitting on the toilet and should not reserve rewards for successful bowel movements only. Weeks to months may be required to change the stooling pattern (Dunn, 2013).

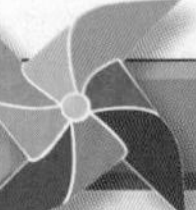

NURSING PROCEDURE 42.2

Administering an Enema

1. Gather supplies (enema bag, lubricant, enema solution).
2. Wash hands and apply gloves.
3. Position the child:
   - Infant or toddler on abdomen with knees bent
   - Child or adolescent on left side with right leg flexed toward chest
4. Clamp the enema tubing, remove the cap, and apply lubricant to the tip.
5. Insert the tube into the rectum:
   - 2.5–4 cm (1–1.5 in) in the infant
   - 5–7.5 cm (2–3 in) in the child
6. Unclamp the tubing and administer the prescribed volume of enema solution at a rate of about 100 mL per minute. Recommended volumes:
   - 250 mL or less for the infant
   - 250–500 mL for the toddler or preschooler
   - 500–1,000 mL for the school-age child
7. Hold the child's buttocks together if needed to encourage retentiaon of the enema for 5–10 minutes.

Adapted from Cincinnati Children's. (2016). *Enema administration.* Retrieved from http://www.cincinnatichildrens.org/health/e/enema/

Many parents seek counselors to help the entire family deal with the issues. Counseling is geared toward allaying the fears of a child who is afraid to defecate due to pain. Also, children who are older may have behavioral issues that need to be addressed. Psychological evaluation and possible behavioral therapy may need to be implemented if constipation becomes a power struggle.

Hirschsprung Disease (Congenital Aganglionic Megacolon)

Hirschsprung disease is a movement disorder of the intestinal track resulting in obstruction (Wesson, 2015) (Fig. 42.14). The disease is most commonly characterized by failure to pass a stool (meconium) within the first 24 hours of life. This is due to a lack of ganglion cells in the bowel, which causes inadequate motility in part of the intestine. These ganglion cells can be absent from the rectosigmoid colon all the way into the small intestine. Hirschsprung disease occurs in 1 of every 5, 000 live

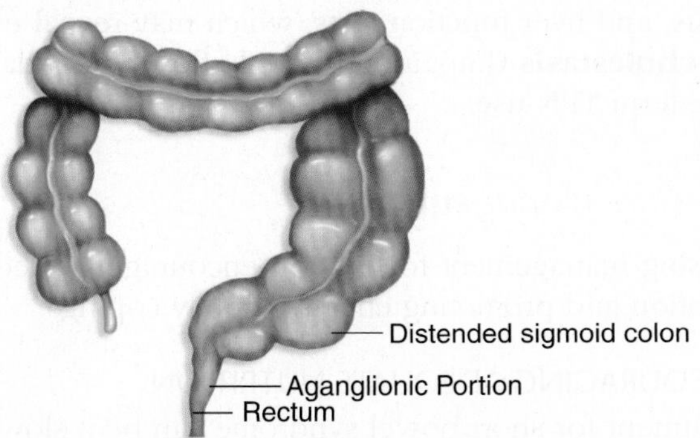

FIGURE 42.14 Enlarged megacolon of Hirschsprung disease.

births, being about four times more common in boys than in girls (Hoffenberg et al., 2014; Wesson, 2015).

Therapeutic Management

Surgical resection of the aganglionic bowel and reanastomosis of the remaining intestine are necessary to promote proper bowel function. There are several types of surgical procedures to correct this, usually performed in stages. The surgical resection requires the child to have an ostomy to divert the stool through a stoma on the abdomen. This allows the area of the resected bowel and anastomosis to heal before it is used. The ostomy is closed at a later date.

Nursing Assessment

For a full description of the assessment phase of the nursing process, refer to the Assessment section in the Nursing Process Overview earlier in the chapter. Assessment findings pertinent to Hirschsprung disease are discussed below.

HEALTH HISTORY

Elicit a description of the present illness and chief complaint. Newborn stool patterns are a key element in recognizing this diagnosis. Assess whether the newborn passed a meconium stool; most children with Hirschsprung disease do not pass a meconium stool within the first 24 to 48 hours of life. Also, newborns who required rectal stimulation to pass their first meconium stool or who passed a meconium plug should be evaluated for Hirschsprung disease.

Explore the child's current and past medical history for risk factors such as a family history of Hirschsprung disease or Down syndrome, or intestinal **atresia** (lack of a normal opening) (Wesson, 2015).

PHYSICAL EXAMINATION

Inspect and palpate the abdomen. The abdomen is typically distended, and, often, it is possible to palpate stool masses in the abdomen. Perform a rectal examination to assess for rectal tone and the presence of stool in the rectum. Often with Hirschsprung disease, no stool is present in the rectum. However, at the end of the rectal examination, when the finger is being withdrawn, a child with Hirschsprung disease may have a forceful expulsion of fecal material.

LABORATORY AND DIAGNOSTIC TESTS

Common laboratory and diagnostic studies ordered for the assessment of Hirschsprung disease include:

- Barium enema: to look for a narrowing of the intestine
- Rectal suction biopsy: to demonstrate an absence of ganglion cells (definitive diagnosis)

Nursing Management

Nursing management includes providing postoperative care, performing ostomy care, and providing child and family education.

PROVIDING POSTOPERATIVE AND OSTOMY CARE

Provide routine postoperative care and observe for the possible complication of enterocolitis (see Nursing Care Plan 42.1 at the end of the chapter).

The child with Hirschsprung disease may have either a colostomy or ileostomy, depending on the extent of disease in the intestine. In either case, perform proper ostomy care to avoid skin breakdown. Accurately measure stool output to assess the child's fluid volume status.

Observe for the following signs and symptoms of enterocolitis:

- Fever
- Abdominal distention
- Chronic diarrhea
- Explosive stools
- Rectal bleeding
- Straining

If any of the above symptoms are noted, immediately notify the physician or nurse practitioner, maintain bowel rest, and administer intravenous fluids and antibiotics to prevent the development of shock and possibly death.

PROVIDING CHILD AND FAMILY EDUCATION

The family may be anxious and fearful about upcoming surgeries and possible complications. Help to relieve their anxiety by providing information about the diagnosis and the stages of surgical procedures the child will undergo. Provide postoperative teaching to educate parents on proper stoma care as well as medication management (to avoid dehydration, most children with Hirschsprung disease will be prescribed medications to slow stool output). Arrange for the family to consult with a wound care nurse to help them deal with the anxieties and care of newly placed stomas. Provide education about possible postsurgical problems, emphasizing the importance of prompt medical treatment for signs of enterocolitis.

Short Bowel Syndrome

Short bowel syndrome is a clinical syndrome of nutrient malabsorption and excessive intestinal fluid and electrolyte losses that occurs following massive small intestinal loss or surgical resection. The degree of malabsorption is usually related to the extent of resection of small bowel (Hoffenberg et al., 2014). The most common causes of short bowel syndrome are necrotizing enterocolitis, small intestinal atresia, gastroschisis, malrotation with volvulus, and trauma to the small intestine. The extent of malabsorption experienced by an individual child is dependent upon the extent of duodenal, ileal, and/or jejunal loss and the length of small intestine lost, as well as the type. If the terminal ileum is lost, vitamin B_{12} deficiency and bile salt malabsorption may occur. If the ileocecal valve is lost, small bowel bacterial overgrowth is likely to occur, as well as poor intestinal motility.

Therapeutic Management

The child with short bowel syndrome is at risk for chronic complications. The goals of therapeutic management are to minimize bacterial overgrowth and to maximize the child's nutritional status. Antibiotics may be used to control bacterial overgrowth. Vitamin and mineral supplementation is necessary because the small intestine is usually where fat-soluble vitamins, calcium, magnesium, and zinc are absorbed. Antidiarrheal agents such as loperamide and gastric acid–suppressive medications may be used to decrease stool output. Many children with short bowel syndrome require TPN for extended periods to achieve adequate growth. Progression to enteral feeding may occur extremely slowly, depending on the intestine's response. Despite a markedly improved prognosis for these children, some will not do as well and may ultimately require intestinal and liver transplantation due to irreversible liver damage from long-term use of TPN.

Nursing Assessment

Elicit the health history, noting diarrhea, which is the primary symptom of short bowel syndrome. Note past history of bowel loss or resection as noted above. Assess the child's hydration state. Inspect the stool for consistency, color, odor, and volume. Review laboratory results, particularly chemistries, to evaluate hydration status, and liver function tests, which may reveal evolving **cholestasis** (impairment of bile flow) secondary to long-term TPN use.

Nursing Management

Nursing management focuses on encouraging adequate nutrition and promoting effective family coping.

ENCOURAGING ADEQUATE NUTRITION

Treatment for short bowel syndrome can be a slow and tedious process. Most children will require TPN until they can tolerate enteral feeds without significant malabsorption. TPN is usually required for a lengthy time, so most children will require long-term intravenous access. Long-term intravenous access places the child at high risk for infection and resulting sepsis. Therefore, closely monitor for signs and symptoms of infection. Immediately report to the physician or nurse practitioner any fevers or redness or drainage at the intravenous site.

When started, enteral feeding must be administered very slowly to avoid further malabsorption. Usually the feeding is started continuously, 24 hours per day, via a feeding pump. Most children have long-term feeding tubes, usually gastrostomy tubes. Most of these children will require special formulas to promote absorption. Assess for feeding tube residuals and abdominal distention or discomfort. Strictly monitor intake and output to avoid dehydration. Assess the stool for signs of carbohydrate malabsorption. Administer vitamin and mineral supplementation, antidiarrheals, and antibiotics as ordered. Teach the family about use of enteral feeding tubes, feeding pumps, and medication administration.

PROMOTING EFFECTIVE FAMILY COPING

Children with short bowel syndrome are considered to be medically fragile for a lengthy period. There is much anxiety related to the initial bowel resection that resulted in short bowel. Long-term hospitalization is almost always required, causing parents to miss work and cutting down on the time they have to spend with other children. This can lead to even more anxiety about finances and relationships. Encourage families to become the experts on their child's needs and condition via education and participation in care. Provide teaching so that the family is better able to care for the child in an outpatient setting. Education focuses on information about TPN and central line care, enteral feedings, assessing for hydration status, and managing medications.

Take Note!

Maintaining long-term central venous access for TPN in infants can present a challenge. One-piece clothing with the central venous line (CVL) tubing exiting and secured on the back of the outfit can help discourage the infant from pulling on (and subsequently dislodging) the line.

Inflammatory Bowel Disease

Crohn disease and ulcerative colitis are the two major idiopathic inflammatory bowel diseases of children. The causes are unknown. However, they may be due to an abnormal or uncontrolled genetically determined immunologic or inflammatory response to an environmental antigenic trigger, possibly a virus or bacterium (Judge, Giordano, & English, 2014). The features of Crohn disease and ulcerative colitis are listed in Comparison Chart 42.2.

Therapeutic Management

Medication is used to control inflammation and symptoms. Medications commonly used include 5-aminosalicylates, antibiotics, immunomodulators, immunosuppressives, and anti–tumor necrosis antibody therapy. Dietary manipulation is also very important.

Failure to respond to medical therapy may result in surgical intervention. Many children with ulcerative colitis eventually undergo a total proctocolectomy, with resulting ostomy, as a curative measure. Children or adolescents with Crohn disease may require surgery to relieve obstruction, drain an abscess, or relieve intractable symptoms.

Nursing Assessment

For a full description of the assessment phase of the nursing process, refer to the Assessment section in the Nursing Process Overview earlier in the chapter. Assessment findings pertinent to Crohn disease and ulcerative colitis are discussed below.

HEALTH HISTORY

Elicit a description of the present illness and chief complaint. Common signs and symptoms reported during the health history include:

- Abdominal cramping
- Nighttime symptoms, including waking due to abdominal pain or urge to defecate
- Fever
- Weight loss
- Poor growth
- Delayed sexual development

Children may be reluctant or unwilling to talk about their bowel movements, so explain the importance of doing so. Assess stool pattern history, including frequency, presence of blood or mucus, and duration of symptoms.

Explore the child's current and past medical history for risk factors, such as:

- Family history of inflammatory bowel disease
- Family history of colon cancer
- Family history of immunologic disorders

PHYSICAL EXAMINATION

Assess the child's growth using growth charts to identify any poor growth patterns. Perform a full abdominal examination, noting tenderness, masses, or fullness. Inspect the perianal area to look for skin tags or fissures, which would be highly suspicious for Crohn disease. Assist the physician in performing a rectal examination to further assess the rectal area for blood or other lesions.

LABORATORY AND DIAGNOSTIC TESTS

Laboratory test results may be normal. Results for children with Crohn disease and ulcerative colitis are found in Comparison Chart 42.2. Common laboratory and diagnostic studies ordered for the assessment of inflammatory bowel disease include:

- Radiologic studies such as upper GI series with small bowel series: may identify evidence of intestinal inflammation, estimate distribution and extent of disease, and help distinguish between Crohn disease and ulcerative colitis
- CT scan: to rule out suspected abscess
- Colonoscopy: to diagnose inflammatory bowel disease
- Upper endoscopy: to rule out affected mucosal tissue between the mouth and anus in children with upper abdominal complaints

Nursing Management

Nursing management focuses on teaching about disease management, teaching about nutritional management, teaching about medication therapy, and promoting family and child coping.

TEACHING ABOUT DISEASE MANAGEMENT

The diagnosis of Crohn disease or ulcerative colitis can be very difficult for the child and family to comprehend. Provide teaching about the disease process and medication therapy to help the child and family understand the seriousness of the disease. The physician may discuss surgical options during uncontrolled flare-ups, but the nurse may be the person to whom the family members or child address their questions regarding surgery. Provide the family with information to help answer some of their questions and allay fears.

TEACHING ABOUT NUTRITIONAL MANAGEMENT

Teach the child and family about nutritional management of the disease. For example, adequate nutrition with a high-protein and high-carbohydrate diet may be recommended. When the disease is active, lactose may be tolerated poorly, and vitamin and iron supplements will most likely be recommended. Explain that in severe cases enteral feeding tubes or TPN may be needed; this is rare but often induces remission.

COMPARISON CHART 42.2 FEATURES OF CROHN DISEASE AND ULCERATIVE COLITIS

Feature	Crohn Disease	Ulcerative Colitis
Age at onset	10–20 years	10–20 years
Incidence	4–6 per 100,000	3–15 per 100,000
Area of bowel affected	Oropharynx, esophagus, and stomach, rare: small bowel only, 25–30%; colon and anus only, 25%; ileocolitis, 40%; diffuse disease, 5%	Total colon, 90%; proctitis, 10%
Distribution	Segmental; disease-free skip areas common	Continuous; distal to proximal
Pathology	Full-thickness, acute, and chronic inflammation; noncaseating granulomas (50%), extraintestinal fistulas, abscesses, stricture, and fibrosis may be present	Superficial, acute inflammation of mucosa with microscopic crypt abscess
Radiography findings	Segmental lesions; thickened, circular folds; cobblestone appearance of bowel wall secondary to longitudinal ulcers and transverse fissures; fixation and separation of loops; narrowed lumen; "sting sign"; fistulas	Superficial colitis; loss of haustra; shortened colon and pseudopolyps (islands of normal tissue surrounded by denuded mucosa) are late findings
Intestinal symptoms	Abdominal pain, diarrhea (usually loose with blood if colon involved), perianal disease, enteroenteric or enterocutaneous fistula, abscess, anorexia	Abdominal pain, bloody diarrhea, urgency, tenesmus
Extraintestinal symptoms:		
Arthritis/arthralgia	15%	9%
Fever	40–50%	40–50%
Stomatitis	9%	2%
Weight loss	90% (mean 5.7 kg)	68% (mean 4.1 kg)
Delayed growth and sexual development	30%	5–10%
Uveitis, conjunctivitis	15% (in Crohn colitis)	4%
Sclerosing cholangitis	—	4%
Renal stones	6% (oxalate)	6% (urate)
Pyoderma gangrenosum	1–3%	5%
Erythema nodosum	8–15%	4%
Laboratory findings	High erythrocyte sedimentation rate; microcytic anemia; low serum iron and total iron-binding capacity; increased fecal protein loss; low serum albumin; antineutrophil cytoplasmic antibodies present in 10–20%; Saccharomyces cerevisiae antibodies positive in 60%	High erythrocyte sedimentation rate; microcytic anemia; high white blood cell count with left shift; antineutrophil cytoplasmic antibodies present in 80%

Adapted from Haas-Beckert, B., & Heyman, M. B. (2010). Inflammatory bowel disease. In P. J. Allen, J. A. Vessey, & N. A. Schapiro (Eds.) *Primary care of the child with a chronic condition* (5th ed.). St. Louis, MO: Mosby; and Hoffenberg, E., Brumbaugh, D., Furuta, G. T., Kobak, G., Liu, E., Soden, J., & Kramer, R. (2014). Gastrointestinal tract. In W. W. Hay, M. J. Levin, & R. R. Deterding, & M. J. Abzug (Eds.), *Current pediatric diagnosis and treatment* (22nd ed.). New York, NY: McGraw-Hill.

TEACHING ABOUT MEDICATION THERAPY

Medications are extremely important in controlling inflammatory bowel disease. Provide information about the following common medications used to control the disease:

- 5-Aminosalicylates (5-ASA): used to prevent relapse (usually used in ulcerative colitis)
- Antibiotics (usually metronidazole and ciprofloxacin): typically used in children who have perianal Crohn disease
- Immunomodulators (usually 6-mercaptopurine [6-MP] or azathioprine): used to help maintain remission. Monitor children for neutropenia and hepatotoxicity.
- Cyclosporine or tacrolimus: used occasionally in conjunction with 6-MP or azathioprine to maintain remission in fulminant ulcerative colitis
- Methotrexate: sometimes used to manage severe Crohn disease
- Anti–tumor necrosis antibody therapy: widely used for children with Crohn disease; occasionally used for children with ulcerative colitis

PROMOTING FAMILY AND CHILD COPING

Inflammatory bowel disease is a chronic and often debilitating illness. Many children with this diagnosis can lead normal lives, but frequent illnesses can cause school absences, which in turn add stress to the situation. Because schools have become much less tolerant of absences and tardiness, it may be necessary to write letters to the school explaining the frequent absences or in-school needs. Bathroom privileges should be very flexible for children during flare-ups. Children tend to be of small stature due to the illness itself and steroid use, which stunts growth; this may cause psychological issues, especially for older boys (Haas-Beckert & Heyman, 2010). Children with ostomies as a result of surgical resection may have self-esteem issues related to the presence and care of the ostomy. Arrange for counseling for both the child and family to discuss fears and anxiety related to a chronic disease.

Celiac Disease

Celiac disease, also known as celiac sprue, is an immunologic disorder in which gluten, a product most commonly found in grains, causes damage to the small intestine. The villi of the small intestine are damaged due to the body's immunologic response to the digestion of gluten. The function of the villi is to absorb nutrients into the bloodstream. When the villi are blunted or damaged, malnutrition occurs.

Celiac disease is one of the most common chronic disorders in Europe and the United States, affecting about 1% of the general population and up to 2% of Caucasians (Swanson & John, 2013). Increased incidence occurs in those with a family history of celiac disease and in persons with autoimmune or genetic disorders (Swanson & John, 2013).

The only current treatment for celiac disease is a strict gluten-free diet. Eliminating gluten will cause the villi of the intestines to heal and function normally, with subsequent improvement of symptoms. Even very small amounts of gluten introduced back into the diet can cause damage to the villi, so the child must adhere to the diet throughout life (Swanson & John, 2013).

Nursing Assessment

For a full description of the assessment phase of the nursing process, refer to the Assessment section in the Nursing Process Overview earlier in the chapter. Assessment findings pertinent to celiac disease are discussed below. The child with symptoms of celiac disease often presents for evaluation by age 2.

HEALTH HISTORY

Elicit a description of the present illness and chief complaint. The symptoms of celiac disease are very broad and are easily confused with other GI disorders. The classic symptoms of children with celiac disease are:

- Diarrhea
- **Steatorrhea** (fatty stools)
- Constipation
- Failure to thrive or weight loss
- Abdominal distention or bloating
- Poor muscle tone
- Irritability and listlessness
- Dental disorders
- Anemia
- Delayed onset of puberty or amenorrhea
- Nutritional deficiencies

Explore the child's current and past medical history for risk factors such as Caucasian European descent and a family history of celiac disease.

PHYSICAL EXAMINATION

Assess for the typical appearance of children with celiac disease: distended abdomen, wasted buttocks, and very thin extremities (Fig. 42.15).

LABORATORY AND DIAGNOSTIC TESTS

Common laboratory and diagnostic studies ordered for the assessment of celiac disease include autotissue transglutaminase IgA, intestinal biopsy, and genetic testing. Autotissue transglutaminase IgA is a first-line test, and the most sensitive; yet if the result is negative, the anti-endomysium IgA test is 100% specific for celiac disease (Swanson & John, 2013). A small bowel biopsy reveals partial or subtotal villous atrophy or blunting of the villi of the small intestine. Genetic testing for celiac disease includes DQ2 and/or DQ8 human leukocyte antigen (HLA) haplotypes (Denham, 2014).

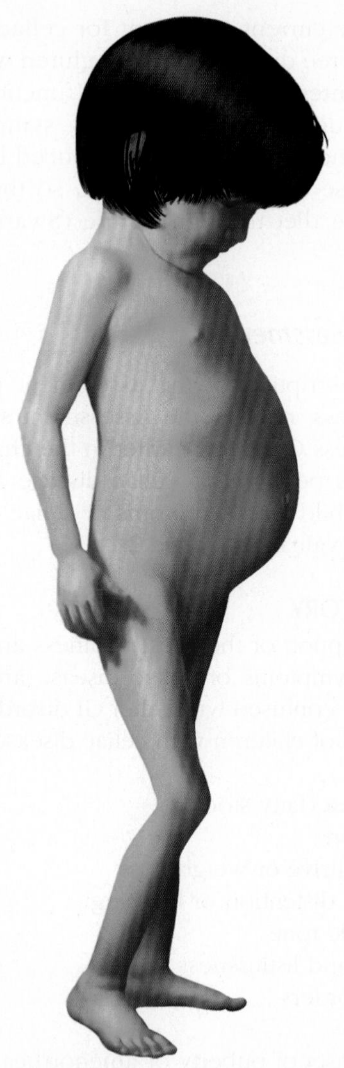

FIGURE 42.15 The child with celiac disease typically displays a distended abdomen and wasted extremities.

Nursing Management

Providing child and family education is the key nursing role in managing children with celiac disease. The child must adhere to a strict gluten-free diet for his or her entire life. This is often very challenging, because gluten is found in most wheat products, rye, barley, and possibly oats. Encourage the parents and child to maintain this gluten-free diet. Often, families consult a dietitian to learn about the gluten-free diet (Teaching Guidelines 42.3).

Provide educational materials and resources to the parents. Many resources are available today about celiac disease because it is becoming more commonly diagnosed. Links to several resources are located on thePoint. These resources can offer information on all aspects of celiac disease, including dietary guidelines and resources for food shopping and eating in restaurants. A reading source appropriate for school-age children is *Gluten-free Friends: An Activity Book for Kids* by Nancy Patin Falini.

Functional Abdominal Pain

Functional abdominal pain is a common GI complaint of children and adolescents. It affects children of all ages, and about 2% to 4% of all pediatric outpatient visits are related to functional abdominal pain (Hofenberg et al., 2014). The etiology remains unclear. The Rome Committee is a group of specialists who are focusing on the identification, management, and treatment of both adults and children with functional GI disorders. Functional abdominal pain in children should not be confused with IBS. Box 42.5 outlines the Rome Committee's criteria for IBS and information on treatment of IBS.

Pathophysiology

The etiology of functional abdominal pain is likely multifactorial (Starr et al., 2013). It is thought that the autonomic nervous system, which controls the body's response to emotions and stress, and intestinal motility are the two mechanisms. Symptoms may result from an alteration in the transmission of messages between the enteric nervous system and the central nervous system, leading to visceral hypersensitivity. Information from the GI tract is transmitted through bidirectional nerve pathways to the brain. Most neurotransmitters are found in both the brain and the gut, suggesting the potential for integrated effects of pain modulation. As different possibilities exist for the pathophysiology of functional abdominal pain, it is clear that there are no structural or biochemical abnormalities that are identifiable. Therapeutic management most often focuses on increasing the child's coping skills (Starr et al., 2013).

BOX 42.5

ROME COMMITTEE CRITERIA FOR IRRITABLE BOWEL SYNDROME

All of the following occur least once per week minimum for at least 2 months before diagnosis:

- Abdominal pain relieved 25% of the time by defecation
- Onset of discomfort associated with a change in frequency of stool
- Onset of discomfort associated with a change in appearance of the stool
- No structural, neoplastic, inflammatory, or metabolic explanation for this abdominal pain

TREATMENT OF IBS

For some children, dietary manipulation or medications may help to control diarrhea.

Adapted from Starr, N. B., Blosser, C. G., Brady, M. A., Burns, C. E., Dunn, A. M., & Petersen-Smith, A. M. (2013). Gastrointestinal disorders. In C. Burns, A. Dunn, M. Brady, N. B. Starr, & C. Blosser (Eds.), *Pediatric primary care* (5th ed.). Philadelphia, PA: Saunders.

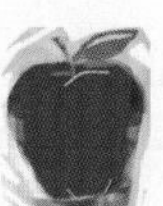

Teaching Guidelines 42.3

DIETARY CONSIDERATIONS IN A GLUTEN-FREE DIET

Foods Allowed	Foods to Avoid
Potato, soy, rice, or bean flour; rice bran, cornmeal, arrowroot, corn or potato starch, sago, tapioca, buckwheat, millet, flax, teff, sorghum, amaranth, quinoa	All wheat products; rye, triticale, barley, oats, or oat bran; graham, gluten, spelt, or durum flour, bulgur, farina, or kamut; malt extract; hydrolyzed vegetable protein
Plain, fresh, frozen, or canned vegetables made with allowed ingredients	Any creamed or breaded vegetables, canned baked beans, some French fries
All fruits and fruit juices	Some commercial fruit pie fillings and dried fruit
All milk and milk products except those made with gluten additives, aged cheese	Malted milk, flavored or frozen yogurt
All meat, poultry, fish, and shellfish; dried peas and beans, nuts; peanut butter; soybean; cold cuts, frankfurters or sausage without fillers	Any meats or poultry prepared with wheat, rye, oats, barley, gluten stabilizers, or fillers for meats; canned meats; self-basting turkey; some egg substitutes
Butter, margarine, salad dressings, sauces, soups, and desserts with allowable ingredients; sugar, honey, jelly, jam, hard candy, plain chocolate, coconut, molasses, marshmallows, meringues, pure instant or ground coffee, tea, carbonated drinks, wine (from the United States)	Commercial salad dressings, prepared soups, condiments, sauces, and seasonings made with avoided products; nondairy cream substitutes, flavored instant coffee, alcohol distilled from cereals, licorice

Adapted from Celiac Disease Foundation. (2016). *Gluten-free diet.* Retrieved from http://celiac.org/live-gluten-free/glutenfreediet/

Nursing Assessment

For a full description of the assessment phase of the nursing process, refer to the Assessment section of the Nursing Process Overview earlier in the chapter. Assessment findings pertinent to functional abdominal pain are discussed below.

HEALTH HISTORY

The diagnosis of functional abdominal pain is made on a symptom-based approach. Elicit a description of the present illness and chief complaint. The symptom reported mostly commonly during the health history is abdominal pain. The child may have difficulty providing a good description of the pain. It is usually periumbilical and is usually described as attacks of pain. It is uncommon for the child to wake up in the middle of the night with this type of pain. Because diet may play a large role in the symptoms, obtain a dietary history. Take a detailed medication history, because abdominal pain may be an adverse effect of some medications. Identifying social and school stressors is essential.

PHYSICAL EXAMINATION

Note the child's body positioning and facial expressions. Interactions with family members during the interview may provide more details regarding social stressors. Palpate the abdomen for tenderness.

LABORATORY AND DIAGNOSTIC TESTS

Common laboratory and diagnostic studies ordered for the assessment of functional abdominal pain include:

- Complete blood count: to rule out organic causes of abdominal pain
- Erythrocyte sedimentation rate: to rule out organic causes of abdominal pain
- Urinalysis: to rule out organic causes of abdominal pain
- Complete metabolic panel (CMP): to rule out organic causes of abdominal pain
- Stool studies: to assess for routine pathogens

Nursing Management

Once the diagnosis of functional abdominal pain with no organic cause is made, the majority of the nursing management is focused on promoting coping skills. Often the physician or nurse practitioner performs a battery of tests to rule out organic causes, especially when child and family anxiety is high. After these tests are complete, teach the family about the factors that exacerbate the pain and how to deal with these factors.

Diet changes may need to be implemented. High-fiber diets help with bowel regulation by keeping motility regular.

Medications may be used to relieve abdominal cramps. Occasionally pain modulators and antidepressants are used to help block the neurotransmitters in the brain–gut connection that cause pain. Encourage compliance with the medication regimen; compliance is needed to achieve beneficial results with many of these medications (Almadhoun, 2012).

Arrange for counseling, if necessary, for children with social stressors. Children with functional abdominal pain may become so debilitated that they cannot function in school, possibly requiring homebound instruction. Provide education to the school, with parental permission, regarding the child's illness and how to best deal with it. Explain that this recurrent abdominal pain is a true pain that children feel and is not "in their minds."

HEPATOBILIARY DISORDERS

Hepatobiliary disorders include pancreatitis, gallbladder disease, jaundice, biliary atresia, hepatitis, cirrhosis and portal hypertension, and liver transplantation.

Pancreatitis

Pancreatitis is increasingly being recognized as a childhood problem (Sokol, Narkewicz, Sundaram, & Mack, 2014). It is classified into two categories—acute and chronic. Acute pancreatitis is an acute inflammatory process that occurs within the pancreas, with variable involvement of localized tissues and remote organ systems. Most common causes of acute pancreatitis include abdominal trauma, drugs and alcohol (though probably rare in children), multisystem disease (such as inflammatory bowel disease or systemic lupus erythematosus), infections (usually viruses such as cytomegalovirus or hepatitis), congenital anomalies (ductal or pancreatic malformations), obstruction (most likely gallstones or tumors in children), or metabolic disorders. Chronic pancreatitis is defined based on the structural and/or functional permanent changes that occur in the pancreas.

When pancreatitis is suspected, the child is placed on immediate bowel rest (NPO). Often, a nasogastric tube placed for suction will be needed to keep the stomach decompressed. Serial monitoring of serum amylase levels will determine when oral feeding may be restarted.

Nursing Assessment

For a full description of the assessment phase of the nursing process, refer to the Assessment section of the Nursing Process Overview earlier in the chapter. Assessment findings pertinent to pancreatitis are discussed below.

HEALTH HISTORY

Elicit a description of the present illness and chief complaint. Common signs and symptoms reported during the health history include:

- Acute onset of persistent midepigastric and periumbilical abdominal pain, often with radiation to the back or chest
- Vomiting, especially after meals
- Fever

Explore the child's current and past medical history for risk factors such as:

- Cystic fibrosis
- History of gallstones
- Traumatic injury
- Family history of hereditary pancreatitis

PHYSICAL EXAMINATION

On abdominal assessment, the bowel sounds may be diminished, suggesting peritonitis. The abdomen may be tender, and distention may occur in younger children and infants. In severe cases, jaundice, ascites, or pleural effusions may occur. Bluish discoloration around the umbilicus or flanks is seen in the most severe cases of pancreatitis when hemorrhage is present.

LABORATORY AND DIAGNOSTIC TESTS

Common laboratory and diagnostic studies ordered for the assessment and monitoring of pancreatitis include:

- Serum amylase and/or lipase: levels three times the normal values are extremely indicative of pancreatitis
- Liver profile: often done to check for increased liver functions and/or bilirubin levels
- Blood work: leukocytosis is common with acute pancreatitis. Hyperglycemia and hypocalcemia may also be noted.
- C-reactive protein: levels may be elevated

Diagnostic imaging studies performed to identify malformations or cysts on the pancreas include:

- Plain abdominal x-ray: may show a localized ileus
- Ultrasound: allows direct visualization of the pancreas and the surrounding structures. This is used most frequently with children, as it is less invasive than a CT scan. A CT scan is usually used when there is difficulty in determining the cause of the pancreatitis during ultrasonography.
- Endoscopic retrograde cholangiopancreatography (ERCP): used in some children who may have ductal anomalies, usually with chronic pancreatitis, though complications from this procedure may occur

Nursing Management

Maintain NPO status and nasogastric tube suction and patency. Administer intravenous fluids to keep the child hydrated and correct any alterations in fluid and electrolyte balance. Pain management is crucial in children with pancreatitis. If hemorrhagic pancreatitis has occurred, blood products and/or intravenous antibiotics may be needed. Oral feedings are restarted only after the serum amylase level has returned to normal (usually in 2 to 4 days). Often, pancreatic enzymes are given with oral feedings if pain occurs after oral feeds are restarted.

Surgery is rarely needed in children with pancreatitis, except in those with severe abdominal trauma or major ductal abnormalities.

Though chronic pancreatitis is rare in children, provide child and family education regarding the signs and symptoms of recurrence and complications.

Gallbladder Disease

Cholelithiasis is the presence of stones in the gallbladder. Cholesterol stones are usually associated with hyperlipidemia, obesity, pregnancy, birth control pill use, or cystic fibrosis (Schwarz, 2015). They are seen more often in females than males, and increased risk occurs with age and onset of puberty (Schwarz, 2015). These stones occur in the gallbladder and may be found in the common bile duct. Pigment stones are found in prepubertal children and occur about equally in males and females. They are usually found in the common bile duct (associated with bacterial or parasitic infections) or the gallbladder itself (associated with hemolytic anemia or liver cirrhosis).

Cholecystitis is an inflammation of the gallbladder that is caused by the chemical irritation due to the obstruction of bile flow from the gallbladder into the cystic ducts. This inflammation is typically associated with gallstones in children. The most common complication in children with gallstone disease is pancreatitis.

If cholelithiasis results in symptomatic cholecystitis, then surgical removal of the gallbladder (cholecystectomy) will be necessary. This is often accomplished laparoscopically.

Nursing Assessment

For a full description of the assessment phase of the nursing process, refer to the Assessment section of the Nursing Process Overview earlier in the chapter. Assessment findings pertinent to gallbladder disease are discussed below.

HEALTH HISTORY

Elicit a description of the present illness and chief complaint. Common signs and symptoms reported during the health history include:

- Right upper quadrant pain, often radiating substernally or to the right shoulder
- Nausea and vomiting
- Jaundice and fever (with cholecystitis)

Document a detailed diet history as it relates to the presenting symptoms. Pain episodes usually occur after meals (postprandially), especially after the ingestion of fatty or greasy foods. Younger children may present with more nonspecific symptoms, most often due to their lack of ability to communicate their symptoms to others. Explore the child's current and past medical history for risk factors such as chronic TPN use or sickle cell disease.

PHYSICAL EXAMINATION

Palpate the abdomen for tenderness. If cholecystitis is present, the gallbladder becomes inflamed, often to the point of causing localized tenderness upon palpation. Assess skin and sclerae color for jaundice. Note presence of fever.

LABORATORY AND DIAGNOSTIC TESTS

Common laboratory and diagnostic studies ordered for the assessment of cholecystitis include:

- Liver function tests, bilirubin, and C-reactive protein: values may be elevated if ductal stones are present
- CBC: may reveal leukocytosis
- Amylase and lipase: may be elevated if pancreatitis is also present
- Plain abdominal x-rays: may reveal radiopaque stones
- Ultrasound of the gallbladder and surrounding structures: to assess the intraluminal contents of the gallbladder as well as any anatomic alterations
- ERCP: to rule out ductal stones
- Hepatobiliary iminodiacetic acid (HIDA) scan: to evaluate the function of the gallbladder

Nursing Management

The child with symptomatic cholecystitis will usually be hospitalized. Administer intravenous fluids, maintain NPO status and gastric decompression, and administer pain medications. If ordered, administer intravenous antibiotics to treat clinically worsening symptoms of cholecystitis, such as persistent fever. Provide routine postoperative care after cholecystectomy is performed. Provide pre- and postoperative teaching for families of children undergoing gallbladder removal.

Biliary Atresia

Biliary atresia is an absence of some or all of the major biliary ducts, resulting in obstruction of bile flow. The ensuing obstruction to bile flow causes cholestasis resulting in jaundice and eventual progressive fibrosis with end-stage cirrhosis of the liver. Biliary atresia affects 1 in

12,000 infants (Sokol et al., 2014). The etiology of biliary atresia is unknown, but there are several theories, including infectious, autoimmune, or ischemic causes.

Therapeutic Management

If there is a high suspicion of biliary atresia, the infant will undergo exploratory laparotomy. If biliary atresia is found, a Kasai procedure (hepatoportoenterostomy) is performed to connect the bowel lumen to the bile duct remnants found at the porta hepatis. This procedure is most successful for infants up to 45 days of age, as bile flow restoration after this age is minimal (Sokol et al., 2014). Infants who are not identified early enough or those who have failed to respond to the Kasai procedure will need to undergo liver transplantation, (Sokol et al., 2014).

Nursing Assessment

For a full description of the assessment phase of the nursing process, refer to the Assessment section of the Nursing Process Overview earlier in the chapter. Assessment findings pertinent to biliary atresia are discussed below.

HEALTH HISTORY

Elicit a description of the present illness and chief complaint. Persistent or recurring jaundice is the most common symptom reported during the health history.

PHYSICAL EXAMINATION

In the initial assessment of an infant with cholestasis of unknown origin, assess the stool character. In biliary atresia, stools will be acholic (chalky and white due to the lack of bile pigment). Note jaundice of the skin and sclerae (yellow discoloration caused by bile pigment deposition). Palpate the abdomen; the liver will feel enlarged and hardened. Splenomegaly may occur. In the absence of other congenital malformations, the infant will otherwise appear healthy.

LABORATORY AND DIAGNOSTIC STUDIES

Common laboratory and diagnostic studies ordered for the assessment of biliary atresia include:

- Serum bilirubin, alkaline phosphatase, liver enzymes, γ-glutamyl transferase (GGT): elevated
- Ultrasound: to identify anomalies
- Biliary scan: to distinguish whether the cholestasis is intrahepatic or extrahepatic
- Liver biopsy: to confirm the diagnosis

Nursing Management

Nursing management of infants who have biliary atresia will focus on vitamin and caloric support. Administer fat-soluble vitamins A, D, E, and K. Special formulas containing medium-chain triglycerides are used because significant fat malabsorption occurs when cholestasis is present. Administer feedings via nasogastric tube as needed to ensure increased caloric intake. Identify infections as quickly as possible and administer intravenous antibiotics as ordered. Manage ascites with diuretics and dietary restrictions. Preoperative management before a Kasai procedure is focused on preparation for surgery; infants who have suspected biliary atresia require immediate surgery to optimize outcomes.

Parents and family members of these infants will have extreme anxiety due to the implications of the diagnosis and outcomes. Focus education on the diagnosis and postoperative care. Nursing Care Plan 42.1, at the end of the chapter, gives information about routine postoperative care.

Hepatitis

Hepatitis is an inflammation of the liver that is caused by a variety of agents, including viral infections, bacterial invasion, metabolic disorders, chemical toxicity, and trauma. The most common viral causes of hepatitis are listed in Table 42.4. Other viruses that may cause hepatitis are cytomegalovirus (CMV), Epstein–Barr virus (EBV), and adenovirus. Fulminant hepatitis is thought to be caused by a non-A, non-B, non-C virus. Children who present with fulminant hepatitis have acute massive hepatic necrosis. The disease progresses rapidly to severe jaundice, coagulopathy, elevated ammonia levels, significantly elevated liver enzyme levels (aspartate aminotransferase [AST] and alanine aminotransferase [ALT]), and progressive coma, resulting in death without liver transplantation. Autoimmune hepatitis is a chronic disorder, affecting mostly adolescent females. The clinical presentation of a child with autoimmune hepatitis includes hepatosplenomegaly, jaundice, fever, fatigue, and right upper quadrant pain.

Therapeutic Management

Acute hepatitis is treated with rest, hydration, and nutrition. Control of bleeding may also be necessary. Chronic hepatitis often eventually requires liver transplantation. Corticosteroids and immunosuppressants may be used for autoimmune hepatitis. The child with fulminant hepatitis usually requires intensive care with cardiorespiratory support. See Healthy People 2020.

Nursing Assessment

For a full description of the assessment phase of the nursing process, refer to the Assessment section of the Nursing Process Overview earlier in the chapter. Assessment findings pertinent to hepatitis are discussed below.

TABLE 42.4 HEPATITIS VIRUSES A–E

	Hepatitis A (HAV)	Hepatitis B (HBV)	Hepatitis C (HCV)	Hepatitis D (HDV)	Hepatitis E (HEV)
Transmission route	Oral–fecal route, poor sanitation, waterborne	Sexual, intravenous drug use, blood transfusion, perinatally transmitted from mother to infant	Blood product transfusion, intravenous drug use	Same as HBV; HBV markers in serum must be present	Oral–fecal
Incubation period	15–30 days	50–150 days	30–160 days	50–150 days	15–65 days
Signs and symptoms	Flu-like symptoms Preicteric phase: headache, fatigue, fever, anorexia Icteric phase: jaundice, dark urine, tender liver (right upper quadrant pain)	Some cases are asymptomatic; others present with anorexia, abdominal pain, and fatigue, rash, slight fever, visible jaundice, enlarged liver	Chronic cases usually present asymptomatically; others with flu-like symptoms, jaundice, hepatosplenomegaly	Same as HBV	Same as HAV, more severe in pregnant women
Prognosis	Rarely develops into fulminant liver failure; 95% of children recover without sequelae	Chronic disease state likely; increased risk of hepatic cancer	Many will develop chronic hepatitis and cirrhosis	Same as HBV, but increased likelihood of chronic active hepatitis and cirrhosis	Same as HAV; high mortality in pregnant women

Adapted from Sokol, R. J., Narkewicz, M. R., Sundaram, S. S., & Mack, C. L. (2014). Liver & pancreas. In W. W. Hay, M. J. Levin, & R. R. Deterding, & M. J. Abzug (Eds.), *Current pediatric diagnosis and treatment* (22nd ed.). New York, NY: McGraw-Hill.

HEALTHY PEOPLE 2020

Objective	Nursing Significance
Reduce hepatitis A and hepatitis B. Reduce chronic hepatitis B virus infections in infants and young children.	• Educate families about hepatitis B and its transmission. • Encourage routine infant and childhood vaccination against hepatitis A and hepatitis B as recommended. • For hepatitis A prevention, educate families about appropriate hygiene and hand washing.

Healthy People Objectives retrieved from http://www.healthypeople.gov

The nursing assessment for any child who presents with suspected hepatitis should be the same.

HEALTH HISTORY

Elicit a description of the present illness and the chief complaint. Common signs and symptoms reported during the health history include:

- Jaundice
- Fever
- Fatigue
- Abdominal pain

Explore the child's current and past medical history for risk factors such as:

- Recent foreign travel
- Sick contacts
- Medication use
- Abdominal trauma
- Sexual activity
- Intravenous drug use
- Blood product transfusion

Document onset of symptoms as well as all signs and symptoms the child has been experiencing.

PHYSICAL EXAMINATION

Observe the skin for jaundice and the sclerae for icterus. Palpate the abdomen to reveal abnormal liver and spleen size or tenderness.

LABORATORY AND DIAGNOSTIC STUDIES

Common laboratory and diagnostic studies ordered for the assessment of hepatitis include:

- Liver enzymes, GGT: elevated
- Prothrombin time (PT)/partial thromboplastin time (PTT): prolonged
- Ammonia: elevated in the presence of encephalopathy
- Autoimmune studies, such as antinuclear antibodies, anti–smooth muscle antibodies, and liver–kidney microsomal antibodies: may be used to diagnose autoimmune hepatitis
- Viral studies: to identify viral causes of hepatitis, such as hepatitis A to E antigens and antibodies, CMV, and EBV
- Ultrasound: to assess liver or spleen abnormalities
- Liver biopsy: to determine the type of hepatitis and to assess for damage that has already been done to the liver

Nursing Management

Acute hepatitis requires rest, hydration, and nutrition. If the child develops vomiting, dehydration, elevated bleeding times (PT/PTT), or mental status changes (encephalopathy), hospitalization may be required. When caring for children with infectious hepatitis, provide education about transmission and prevention, including proper hygiene, safe sexual activity, careful hand-washing techniques, and blood/bodily fluid precautions.

Fulminant hepatitis treatment is aggressive and will require NPO status, nasogastric tube administration of lactulose to decrease ammonia levels that lead to encephalopathic conditions, TPN administration, vitamin K injections to help with coagulopathies, and, ultimately, liver transplantation. Fear and anxiety of the child and parents will likely be very high. Teach the child and family about the diagnosis and what to expect during treatment. Provide immunoglobulin therapy and vaccinations to close contacts of children with infectious hepatitis.

Cirrhosis and Portal Hypertension

Cirrhosis of the liver occurs as a result of the destructive processes that occur during liver damage, leading to the formation of nodules. These nodules can be small (micronodular [less than 3 mm]) or large (macronodular [greater than 3 mm]) and distort the vasculature of the liver, leading to further complications. Causes of cirrhosis in children include biliary malformations, α_1-antitrypsin deficiency, Wilson disease, galactosemia, tyrosinemia, chronic active hepatitis, and prolonged TPN use (Sokol et al., 2014).

Major complications may exist due to cirrhosis of the liver, including portal hypertension. In portal hypertension, the blood flow to, through, or from the liver meets resistance, causing portal blood flow pressures to rise. As these pressures rise, collateral veins form between the portal and systemic venous circulations. The most significant complication of portal hypertension is GI bleeding, from shunting to submucosal veins (varices) in the stomach and esophagus. Esophageal varices may be treated with sclerotherapy during endoscopy to stop acute bleeding. Often blood product administration and vasopressive drugs are needed. In the long term, the only cure for cirrhosis is liver transplantation.

Nursing Assessment

For a full description of the assessment phase of the nursing process, refer to the Assessment section of the Nursing Process Overview earlier in the chapter. Assessment findings pertinent to cirrhosis and portal hypertension are discussed below.

HEALTH HISTORY

Elicit a description of the present illness and chief complaint. Common signs and symptoms reported during the health history include:

- Nausea and vomiting
- Jaundice
- Weakness
- Swelling
- Weight loss

Explore the child's current and past medical history for risk factors such as hepatitis, cystic fibrosis, Wilson disease, hematochromatosis, and biliary atresia. Assess the past medical history to identify possible causes for liver disease.

PHYSICAL EXAMINATION

Inspect for jaundice, ascites, spider angiomas, and palmar erythema. Gynecomastia is often seen in males. Palpate the liver; typically it is enlarged and hard, but occasionally it is small and shrunken. Evaluate mental status to determine the presence of hepatic encephalopathy.

LABORATORY AND DIAGNOSTIC STUDIES

Laboratory and diagnostic testing will be similar to that of a child with hepatitis. Common laboratory and diagnostic studies ordered for the assessment of cirrhosis or portal hypertension include:

- Liver biopsy: reveals regenerating nodules and surrounding fibrosis
- Upper endoscopy: reveals varices and bleeding

Nursing Management

Nursing management is very similar to the care of the child with hepatitis. In cases of cirrhosis causing portal hypertension and bleeding varices, GI bleeding must be controlled. This is usually done by replacing blood loss and providing vasopressive therapy to constrict the shunted blood flow. As with all liver disorders and GI bleeding, address and manage family and child anxiety. Be honest about the child's treatment plan and prognosis. Involve the family in the care of the child and educate them as needed.

Liver Transplantation

Hepatobiliary disorders that result in failure of the liver to function result in the need for liver transplantation. Liver transplantation in children has become increasingly successful in the past several years due to advances in immunosuppression, better selection of transplant candidates, and improvements in surgical techniques and postoperative care (Sokol et al., 2014). Transplant centers now offer both cadaveric and living-related liver transplants for children. Rejection of the transplanted liver is the most significant complication. Most children will require immunosuppressive therapy for a lifetime, putting them at risk for infections.

Nursing Assessment

Many children will be admitted to a transplant center for a preoperative workup to determine the best possible tissue and blood match for the child. There is much anxiety among family members when a cadaveric transplant is the only possibility for survival. This puts a child on a waiting list that is prioritized based on several criteria. Because there are a limited number of pediatric liver transplant centers throughout the country, there may be many issues regarding transportation, finances, job loss, and lodging. Assess the need for social work intervention; a social worker is almost always involved with these children. A liver transplant coordinator will assist with coordinating the care for pre- and posttransplant children.

Nursing Management

Preoperatively, assist with the transplant workup and teach the child and family what to expect during and after the liver transplantation. Postoperatively, the child will be in the intensive care unit for several days until he or she is stabilized from the actual surgery (see Nursing Care Plan 42.1 at the end of the chapter). After the child is sent to a regular unit in the hospital, monitor the child for several days to weeks for signs and symptoms of rejection and infection, including fever, increasing liver function test results and GGT, and increasing pain, redness, and swelling at the incision site.

Child and family education is an important element of nursing management in the posttransplant child. Assess and reassess medication knowledge throughout the entire hospitalization, as these children usually require medications for a lifetime.

NURSING CARE PLAN 42.1

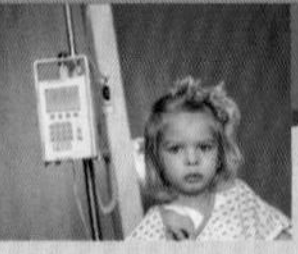

Overview for the Child With a Gastrointestinal Disorder

NURSING DIAGNOSIS: Fluid volume, risk for deficit: risk factors may include excessive losses through vomiting or diarrhea, inadequate oral intake, possible NPO status (particularly in the surgical child)

Outcome Identification and Evaluation

Child will maintain adequate fluid volume as evidenced by elastic skin turgor; moist, pink oral mucosa; presence of tears; urine output 1 mL/kg/hr or more.

Interventions: ***Maintaining Fluid Balance***

- Maintain IV line and administer IV fluid as ordered *to maintain fluid volume.*
- Offer small amounts of oral rehydration solution frequently *to maintain fluid volume. Small amounts are usually well tolerated by children with diarrhea and vomiting.*
- When symptoms have lessened or resolved, reintroduce regular diet *to reduce number of stools, provide adequate nutrition, and shorten duration of effects of illness.*
- Avoid high-carbohydrate fluids such as Kool-aid and fruit juice, *as they are low in electrolytes, and increased simple carbohydrate consumption can decrease stool transit time.*
- Assess hydration status (skin turgor, oral mucosa, presence of tears) every 4 to 8 hours *to evaluate maintenance of adequate fluid volume.*
- Assess adequacy of urine output *to assess end-organ perfusion.*
- Maintain strict intake and output record and weigh child daily *to evaluate effectiveness of rehydration.*
- Weigh child daily: *accurate weight is one of the best indicators of fluid volume status in children.*
- Discourage milk products and fluids that contain high levels of sugar during the acute phase of illness, *as these products may worsen diarrhea.*

NURSING DIAGNOSIS: Diarrhea; may be related to inflammation of small intestines, presence of infectious agents or toxins, possibly evidenced by loose liquid stools, hyperactive bowel sounds, or abdominal cramping

Outcome Identification and Evaluation

Child will experience decrease in diarrhea: *will have bulkier stool as per normal routine.*

Interventions: ***Relieving Diarrhea***

- Maintain clear liquid diet no longer than 24 hours, as prolonged clear liquids will result in continued liquid ("starvation") stools.
- Avoid milk products until diarrhea improves: temporary poor absorption from villus injury follows viral diarrhea.
- Encourage complex carbohydrate foods to bulk up the stools.
- Add fat to carbohydrates to increase intestinal transit time to encourage water absorption (bulks up stool).

NURSING DIAGNOSIS: Constipation, related to GI obstructive lesions, pain on defecation, diagnostic procedures, inadequate toileting, or behavioral stool holding, possibly evidenced by change in character or frequency of stools, feeling of abdominal or rectal fullness or pressure, changes in bowel sounds, and abdominal distention

Outcome Identification and Evaluation

Child will experience improvement in constipation by passing daily soft bowel movement without pain or straining.

NURSING CARE PLAN 42.1

Overview for the Child With a Gastrointestinal Disorder (continued)

Intervention: ***Relieving Constipation***

- Palpate for abdominal distention, percuss for dullness, and auscultate for bowel sounds *to assess for signs of constipation.*
- Encourage adequate fluid intake *to soften the stool.*
- Administer medications as ordered *to keep stool moving on daily basis.*
- Encourage activity as tolerated: *immobility contributes to constipation.*
- The child with stool withholding should sit on the toilet twice daily, preferably after breakfast and dinner, *to maximize chances for successful stool passage by taking advantage of the gastrocolic reflex.*
- For behavioral stool holding, use rewards or stickers *to encourage appropriate toileting.*

NURSING DIAGNOSIS: Skin integrity, risk for impaired: risk factors include frequent loose stools, poor nutritional status, presence of stoma, acidic gastric contents contact with skin if gastrostomy present

Outcome Identification and Evaluation

Infant's skin will remain intact: *buttocks skin will be free from rash, excoriation.* In the child with an ostomy: skin surrounding stoma will remain intact: *free from redness, rash, excoriation.*

Intervention: ***Maintaining Skin Integrity***

- Change diapers frequently to limit acidic stool content contact with skin.
- Use barrier diaper cream to protect skin.
- Assess skin integrity at every diaper change to recognize skin changes early so that corrective measures can begin.
- Leave diaper area open to air several times a day if redness is present so that air can circulate and skin healing can be facilitated.
- Use plain water or only mild soap to cleanse the skin with diaper changes to avoid pH changes that contribute to diaper area skin breakdown.
- Avoid diaper wipes that contain fragrance or alcohol if the skin is red or has a rash, as both alcohol and perfume cause stinging if used on nonintact skin and can worsen skin breakdown.

For the child with an ostomy:

- Ensure proper fit of the ostomy appliance/pouch *to avoid acidic stool contact with skin.*
- Use a barrier wafer (e.g., Stomahesive or Duoderm) to attach appliance: *avoids repeated pulling of adhesive tape from skin.*
- If redness occurs, use barrier/healing cream or paste on skin around stoma *to promote healing and prevent further skin breakdown.*
- Consult enterostomal therapy nurse as needed *to provide additional support.*

NURSING DIAGNOSIS: Nutrition: imbalanced, less than body requirements; may be related to inability to ingest, digest, or absorb nutrients; intestinal pain after eating; decreased transit time through bowel; or psychosocial factors, possibly evidenced by lack of appropriate weight gain or growth, weight loss, aversion to eating, poor muscle tone, or observed lack of intake

Outcome Identification and Evaluation

Nutritional status will be maximized: child will maintain or gain weight appropriately.

Intervention: ***Maintaining Appropriate Nutrition***

- Encourage favorite foods (within prescribed diet restrictions if present) *to maximize oral intake.*
- Administer enteral tube feedings as ordered *to maximize caloric intake.*
- Add butter, gravy, or cheese as appropriate to foods (if allowed within diet restrictions) *to increase caloric intake.*

(continued)

NURSING CARE PLAN 42.1

Overview for the Child With a Gastrointestinal Disorder (continued)

- Encourage high-quality, high-calorie snacks between meals, *so as not to interfere with meal intake.*
- Document response to feeding *to determine feeding tolerance.*
- Limit intake of calorie-free beverages: *beverages should contain nutrients and calories.*
- Consult nutritionist *for appropriate diet supplementation recommendations.*

NURSING DIAGNOSIS: Breathing pattern, ineffective, related to postoperative immobility, abdominal pain interfering with breathing, use of narcotic analgesics as evidenced by increased work of or shallow breathing, tachypnea, decreased lung aeration

Outcome Identification and Evaluation

Child will demonstrate effective breathing pattern: respiratory rate normal for age, absence of accessory muscle use, adequate aeration with clear breath sounds throughout all lung fields.

Intervention: *Promoting Effective Breathing Patterns*

- Turn, cough, and deep breathe every 2 hours *to encourage adequate aeration and discourage fluid pooling in lungs.* In the infant or toddler, turn every 2 hours and use percussor or chest physiotherapy *to prevent pooling of secretions.*
- Play games to encourage deep breathing (blow out penlight, blow cotton ball across bedside table with straw, etc.): *children are more likely to cooperate with interventions if play is involved.*
- In the developmentally able child, encourage incentive spirometer use every 2 hours *to improve lung aeration.*
- Demonstrate/encourage use of pillow splinting with coughing *to decrease abdominal pain and stress on incision.*

NURSING DIAGNOSIS: Caregiver role strain, risk for: risk factors may include infant with congenital defect, child with chronic illness, marginal caregiver coping patterns, long-term stress, complexity and quantity of care child requires

Outcome Identification and Evaluation

Caregiver will exhibit emotional health: verbalizes concerns calmly, participates in child's care, and demonstrates knowledge of resources.

Intervention: *Easing Caregiver Role Strain*

- Assess parental behavior *to identify role strain.*
- Provide emotional support and encourage talking about feelings, fears, and concerns *to promote trust in nurse as a source of emotional support.*
- Arrange for and/or encourage respite care for child: *provides parent with time away from continual care.*
- Consult social services *to identify community resources available for caregiver support (home health, support group, etc.).*
- Encourage parent to meet own needs and find personal time *to increase energy level and self-esteem, ultimately enhancing the quality of care given.*

NURSING CARE PLAN 42.1

Overview for the Child With a Gastrointestinal Disorder (continued)

NURSING DIAGNOSIS: Body image disturbance; may be related to presence of stoma, loss of control of bowel elimination, scars from multiple surgical procedures, or effects of treatment regimen, possibly evidenced by verbalization of negative feelings about body, refusal to look at stoma or participate in care

Outcome Identification and Evaluation

Child or teen will demonstrate acceptance of change in body image by verbalization of adjustment; looking at, touching, and caring for body; and returning to previous social involvement.

Intervention: ***Promoting Proper Body Image***

- Observe child's coping mechanisms to reinforce their use in times of stress.
- Acknowledge denial, anger, and other feelings as normal to support child/teen through difficult transition.
- Allow child gradual introduction to stoma to ease transition.
- Encourage child/teen to participate in care, as this sense of control will contribute to positive self-esteem.

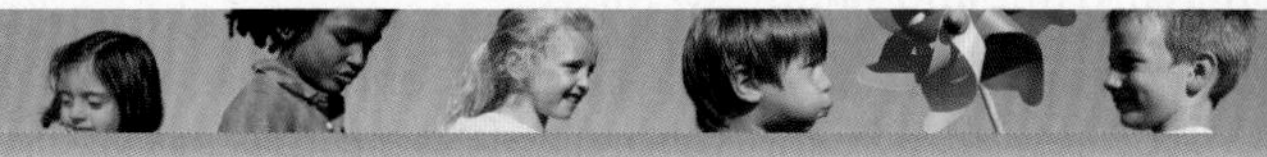

KEY CONCEPTS

- The esophagus of the young child exhibits underdeveloped muscle tone compared with the adult.
- A major difference between children and adults is the reduced stomach capacity in the child and the significantly shorter length of the small intestine (250 cm in the child vs. 600 cm in the adult).
- Infants and children have a proportionately greater amount of body water than adults, resulting in a relatively greater fluid intake requirement than adults and placing infants and children at higher risk for fluid loss as compared with adults.
- The most common result of GI illnesses in infants and children is dehydration.
- The mildly or moderately dehydrated child must be identified and receive rehydration therapy to prevent progression to hypovolemic shock.
- Rehydration is a key medical treatment for dehydration as a result of many different GI disorders. Oral rehydration is most common, but in cases requiring hospitalization intravenous fluid therapy is key.
- Promotion of adequate nutrition is another significant treatment component. The child with a chronic GI disorder may require intravenous TPN or enteral tube feedings to exhibit appropriate growth.
- Surgical intervention is necessary for many acute or congenital GI disorders, such as pyloric stenosis, cleft lip and palate, appendicitis, Hirschsprung disease, and intestinal malrotation.
- Monitoring the blood count, electrolyte levels, and liver function tests is necessary in many pediatric GI disorders.
- Histamine-2 blockers, proton pump inhibitors, and prokinetic agents are used to treat disorders in which gastric acid is a problem, such as esophagitis, GERD, and ulcers.
- Close monitoring for infection is important in children with inflammatory bowel disease, autoimmune hepatitis, or liver transplant who are being treated with immunosuppressants and/or corticosteroids.
- GI stimulants and laxatives may be necessary for treating constipation and encopresis.

- Diarrhea, vomiting, decreased oral intake, sustained high fever, diabetic ketoacidosis, and extensive burns place the infant or child at risk for the development of dehydration.
- Risk factors for vomiting include exposure to viruses, use of certain medications, and overfeeding in the infant.
- Risk factors for acute diarrhea include recent ingestion of undercooked meats, foreign travel, day care attendance, and well water ingestion.
- Vomiting is a symptom and should be characterized in terms of volume, color, relation to meals, duration, and associated symptoms.
- Bleeding may occur as a result of a GI disorder, particularly from the intestine with Meckel diverticulum and from esophageal varices with portal hypertension.
- Acute GI disorders are those that usually have a rapid onset and a short course, which at times may be severe. Examples include dehydration, vomiting, diarrhea, hypertrophic pyloric stenosis, and appendicitis.
- Chronic GI disorders are those that are long lasting or recur over time. Examples include constipation, GER, inflammatory bowel disease, functional abdominal pain, and failure to thrive.
- Right lower quadrant pain and rebound tenderness of the abdomen found on physical examination are telltale signs of appendicitis, which is considered a surgical emergency.
- Bilious vomiting is the main symptom of conditions resulting in bowel obstruction, such as malrotation with volvulus.
- The focus of nursing management of the child with diarrhea or vomiting is restoring proper fluid and electrolyte balance through oral rehydration therapy or intravenous fluids if necessary.
- Reduction of inguinal and umbilical hernias should be attempted; if reduction of the hernia is impossible, immediately notify the physician.
- Small, frequent, and thickened feedings and proper positioning after feedings are key elements in the treatment of GER.
- A crucial nursing intervention related to cleft lip and palate repair is protection of the surgical site while it is healing.
- Palpation of the abdomen should be the last part of the physical examination of an infant or child.
- A key element of nursing care for the child with a GI disorder is promotion of appropriate bowel elimination.
- Maximizing nutritional status is a critical nursing function for the child with a GI disorder.
- For the child who has undergone surgical repair for correction of a GI disorder, promoting effective breathing patterns and managing pain are important nursing goals.
- Counseling families about how to manage the child with vomiting or diarrhea at home, including oral rehydration therapy, is a key component of child/family education.
- Education of the child and family regarding the importance of medication compliance for management of inflammatory bowel disease is critical.
- Behavioral therapy and counseling may be necessary for children who have functional constipation and stool withholding.
- The child or adolescent with ineffective bowel control, poor growth, or an ostomy may have poor self-esteem and body image.

REFERENCES AND RECOMMENDED READINGS

Allen, S. J., Martinez, E. G., Gregorio, G. V, & Dans, L. F. (2010). *Probiotics for treating acute infectious diarrhoea (review). The Cochrane Library 2007, 12.* Indianapolis, IN: John Wiley & Sons.

Almadhoun, O. (2012). Managing chronic abdominal pain in children: Understanding physical and behavioral components of functional abdominal pain. *Contemporary Pediatrics, 29*(3), 18–23.

American Academy of Pediatrics. (2015). *Umbilical cord care.* Retrieved from http://www.healthychildren.org/English/ages-stages/baby/bathing-skin-care/Pages/Umbilical-Cord-Care.aspx

Ben-Joseph, E. P. (2013). *Canker sores.* Retrieved from http://kidshealth.org/en/parents/canker.html#

Brandt, M. (2014). *Intestinal malrotation.* Retrieved from http://www.uptodate.com/contents/intestinal-malrotation

Celiac Disease Foundation. (2016). *Gluten-free diet.* Retrieved from http://celiac.org/live-gluten-free/glutenfreediet/

Cincinnati Children's. (2016). *Enema administration.* Retrieved from http://www.cincinnatichildrens.org/health/e/enema/

Corbett, J. A. & Banks, A. D. (2013). *Laboratory tests and diagnostic procedures with nursing diagnoses* (8th ed.). Upper Saddle River, NJ: Pearson Education Inc.

Curtin, G., & Boekelheide, A. (2010). Cleft lip and cleft palate. In P. J. Allen, J. A. Vessey, & N. A. Schapiro (Eds.), *Primary care of the child with a chronic condition* (5th ed.). St. Louis, MO: Mosby.

Denham, J. M. (2014). *Non-celiac gluten sensitivity.* Presented at meeting of the Florida Chapter of the National Association of Pediatric Nurse Practitioners, Orlando, FL.

Donovan, K. (2012). Breastfeeding the infant with cleft lip and palate. *ICAN: Infant, Child, & Adolescent Nutrition, 4*(4), 194–198.

Dowshen, S. (2014). *Stool tests*. Retrieved from http://www.kidshealth.org/parent/general/sick/labtest8.html

Dunn, A. (2013). Elimination patterns. In C. Burns, A. Dunn, M. Brady, N. B. Starr, & C. Blosser (Eds.), *Pediatric primary care* (5th ed.). Philadelphia, PA: Saunders.

Engorn, B., & Flerlage, J. (2015). *The Harriet Lane handbook* (20th ed.). Philadelphia, PA: Saunders.

Fleisher, G. R., (2014). *Evaluation of diarrhea in children*. Retrieved from http://www.uptodate.com/contents/evaluation-of-diarrhea-in-children

Ford, D. M. (2014). Fluid, electrolyte, and acid-base disorders & therapy. In W. W. Hay, M. J. Levin, R. R. Deterding, & M. J. Abzug (Eds.), *Current pediatric diagnosis and treatment* (22nd ed.). New York, NY: McGraw-Hill.

Freedman, S. (2016). *Oral rehydration therapy*. Retrieved from http://www.uptodate.com/contents/oral-rehydration-therapy

Galloway, A., & Seguias, L. (2013). A 7-year-old Hispanic boy with acute onset of abdominal pain. *Pediatric Annals, 42*(12), 491–493.

Gilger, M. A. (2016). *Pathogenesis of acute diarrhea in children*. Retrieved from http://www.uptodate.com/contents/pathogenesis-of-acute-diarrhea-in-children

Haas-Beckert, B., & Heyman, M. B. (2010). Inflammatory bowel disease. In P. J. Allen, J. A. Vessey, & N. A. Schapiro (Eds.), *Primary care of the child with a chronic condition* (5th ed.). St. Louis, MO: Mosby.

Hoffenberg, E., Brumbaugh, D., Furuta, G. T., Kobak, G., Liu, E., Soden, J., et al. (2014). Gastrointestinal tract. In W. W. Hay, M. J. Levin, R. R. Deterding, & M. J. Abzug (Eds.), *Current pediatric diagnosis and treatment* (22nd ed.). New York, NY: McGraw-Hill.

Judge, J., Giordano, B. P., & English, J. (2014). Crohn's disease masquerading as an acute abdomen. *Journal of Pediatric Health Care, 28*(5), 444–450.

Keels, M. A., & Clements, D. A. (2015). *Herpetic gingivostomatitis in young children*. Retrieved from http://www.uptodate.com/contents/herpetic-gingivostomatitis-in-young-children

Olivé, A. P., & Endom, E. E. (2016). *Infantile hypertrophic pyloric stenosis*. Retrieved from http://www.uptodate.com/contents/infantile-hypertrophic-pyloric-stenosis

Romero, J. R. (2015). *Hand, foot, and mouth disease and herpangina: An overview*. Retrieved from http://www.uptodate.com/contents/hand-foot-and-mouth-disease-and-herpangina-an-overview

Rosenberg, A. A., & Grover, T. (2014). The newborn infant. In W. W. Hay, M. J. Levin, R. R. Deterding, & M. J. Abzug (Eds.), *Current pediatric diagnosis and treatment* (22nd ed.). New York, NY: McGraw-Hill.

Schwarz, S. M. & Hebra, A. (2015). *Pediatric cholecystitis*. Retrieved from http://emedicine.medscape.com/article/927340-overview

Sokol, R. J., Narkewicz, M. R., Sundaram, S. S., & Mack, C. L. (2014). Liver & pancreas. In W. W. Hay, M. J. Levin, R. R. Deterding, & M. J. Abzug (Eds.), *Current pediatric diagnosis and treatment* (22nd ed.). New York, NY: McGraw-Hill.

Sood, M. R. (2016). *Constipation in infants and children: Evaluation*. Retrieved from http://www.uptodate.com/contents/constipation-in-infants-and-children-evaluation

Starr, N. B., Blosser, C. G., Brady, M. A., Burns, C. E., Dunn, A. M., & Petersen-Smith, A. M. (2013). Gastrointestinal disorders. In C. Burns, A. Dunn, M. Brady, N. B. Starr, & C. Blosser (Eds.), *Pediatric primary care* (5th ed.). Philadelphia, PA: Saunders.

Swanson, J. & John, R. M. (2013). Does celiac disease ever travel alone? *ICAN: Infant, Child, & Adolescent Nutrition, 5*(4), 236–247.

Taketomo, C. K., Hodding, J. H., & Kraus, D. M. (2013). *Pediatric & neonatal dosage handbook* (20th ed.). Hudson, OH: Lexicomp.

University of California, San Francisco. (2016). *Colostomy*. Retrieved from http://pedsurg.ucsf.edu/conditions--procedures/colostomy.aspx

University of Maryland Medical Center. (2016). *Ginger*. Retrieved from http://umm.edu/health/medical/altmed/herb/ginger

U.S. Department of Health and Human Services. (2016). *Healthy people 2020*. Retrieved from http://www.healthypeople.gov/2020/default

Vakil, N. B. (2014). *Epidemiology and etiology of peptic ulcer disease*. Retrieved from http://www.uptodate.com/contents/epidemiology-and-etiology-of-peptic-ulcer-disease

Wall, J., & Albanese, C. T. (2015). Pediatric surgery. In G. M. Doherty (Ed.), *Current diagnosis and treatment: Surgery* (14th ed.). New York, NY: McGraw-Hill.

Weber, J. R., & Kelley, J. H. (2014). *Health assessment in nursing* (5th ed.). Philadelphia, PA: Lippincott Williams & Wilkins.

Wesson, D. E. (2015). *Congenital aganglionic megacolon (Hirschsprung disease)*. Retrieved from http://www.uptodate.com/contents/congenital-aganglionic-megacolon-hirschsprung-disease

Winter, H. S. (2015). *Clinical manifestations and diagnosis of gastroesophageal reflux disease in children and adolescents*. Retrieved from http://www.uptodate.com/contents/clinical-manifestations-and-diagnosis-of-gastroesophageal-reflux-disease-in-children-and-adolescents

Winter, H. S. (2016a). *Gastroesophageal reflux in infants*. Retrieved from http://www.uptodate.com/contents/gastroesophageal-reflux-in-infants

Winter, H. S. (2016b). *Management of gastroesophageal reflux disease in children and adolescents*. Retrieved from http://www.uptodate.com/contents/management-of-gastroesophageal-reflux-disease-in-children-and-adolescents

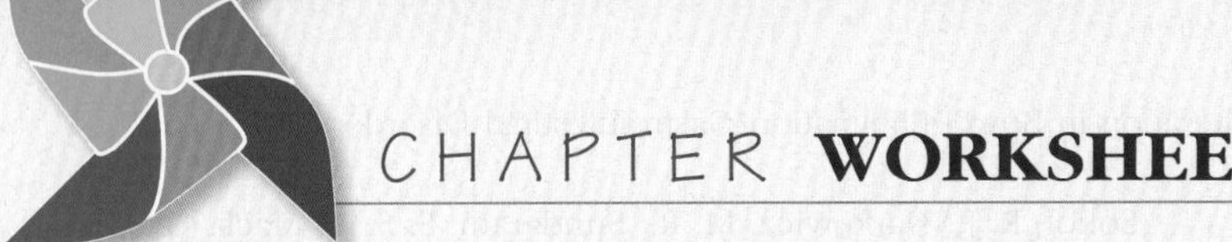

CHAPTER WORKSHEET

MULTIPLE CHOICE QUESTIONS

1. A mother brings her 6-month-old infant to the clinic. The child has been vomiting since early morning and has had diarrhea since the day before. His temperature is 38°C, pulse 140, and respiratory rate 38. He has lost 6 oz since his well-child visit 4 days ago. He cries before passing a bowel movement. He will not breastfeed today. What is the priority nursing diagnosis?
   a. thermoregulation alteration
   b. pain (abdominal) related to diarrhea
   c. fluid volume deficit related to excessive losses and inadequate intake
   d. alteration in nutrition, less than body requirements, related to decreased oral intake
2. A child presents with a 2-day history of fever, abdominal pain, occasional vomiting, and decreased oral intake. Which finding would the nurse prioritize for immediate reporting to the physician?
   a. temperature 101.9°F
   b. rebound tenderness and abdominal guarding
   c. Parents will be leaving the child alone in the hospital.
   d. Child can tolerate only sips of fluid without nausea.
3. A 3-day-old infant presenting with physiologic jaundice is hospitalized and placed under phototherapy. Which response indicates to the nurse that the parent needs more teaching?
   a. "My infant is at risk for dehydration."
   b. "My infant needs to stay under the lights, except during feeding time."
   c. "My infant can continue to breastfeed during this time."
   d. "My infant has a serious liver disease."
4. A 3-month-old infant presents with a history of vomiting after feeding. The plan for the infant is to rule out GER. What information from the history would lead the nurse to believe that this infant may need further intervention?
   a. poor weight gain
   b. small "spits" after feeding
   c. sleeps through the night
   d. difficult to burp
5. The nurse is caring for a child who has had diarrhea and vomiting for the past several days. What is the priority nursing assessment?
   a. Determine the child's weight.
   b. Ask if the family has traveled outside of the country.
   c. Assess circulation and perfusion.
   d. Send a stool specimen to the lab.

DOSAGE CALCULATION QUESTION

A child is NPO during the preoperative period and requires IV fluid maintenance. The child weighs 31 lb 4 oz. What is the child's recommended hourly IV fluid rate?

CRITICAL THINKING EXERCISES

1. A 6-month-old baby is brought to the physician's office with a history of diarrhea. She has had six watery stools in the past 18 hours. She is vomiting her formula. Her mother states that she has had no fever.
   a. Upon completion of the history and physical examination, what signs and symptoms would you expect to find that would indicate that the baby is experiencing mild dehydration?
   b. What is the priority nursing diagnosis for this infant?
   c. Identify a plan for this nursing diagnosis; include a teaching plan for the mother.
2. A 14-kg child with moderate dehydration has received two boluses of normal saline in the emergency room prior to being admitted to the pediatric nursing unit. The physician orders D5 ½ NS @ 1½ maintenance.
   a. What would the intravenous fluid rate be?
   b. What will the nurse assess for to determine whether the child is becoming overhydrated?
3. An infant requires a temporary colostomy. What discharge instructions would you provide to the parents about how to take care of the colostomy and when to call their child's physician or nurse practitioner?

STUDY ACTIVITIES

1. In the clinical setting, compare the growth records of a child with celiac disease to those of a similar-aged child without disease.
2. While caring for children in the clinical setting, compare and contrast the medical history, signs and symptoms of illness, and prescribed treatment for a child with Crohn disease and one with ulcerative colitis.
3. In the clinical setting, observe the behavioral responses of an infant or young child with inorganic failure to thrive.

BRINGING IT ALL TOGETHER: A CASE STUDY

Jung Kim, 4 years old, is brought to the clinic by his parents with abdominal pain and a poor appetite. His mother states, "He cries when I put him on the toilet."

Go to thePoint to find questions to consider about this case.

43

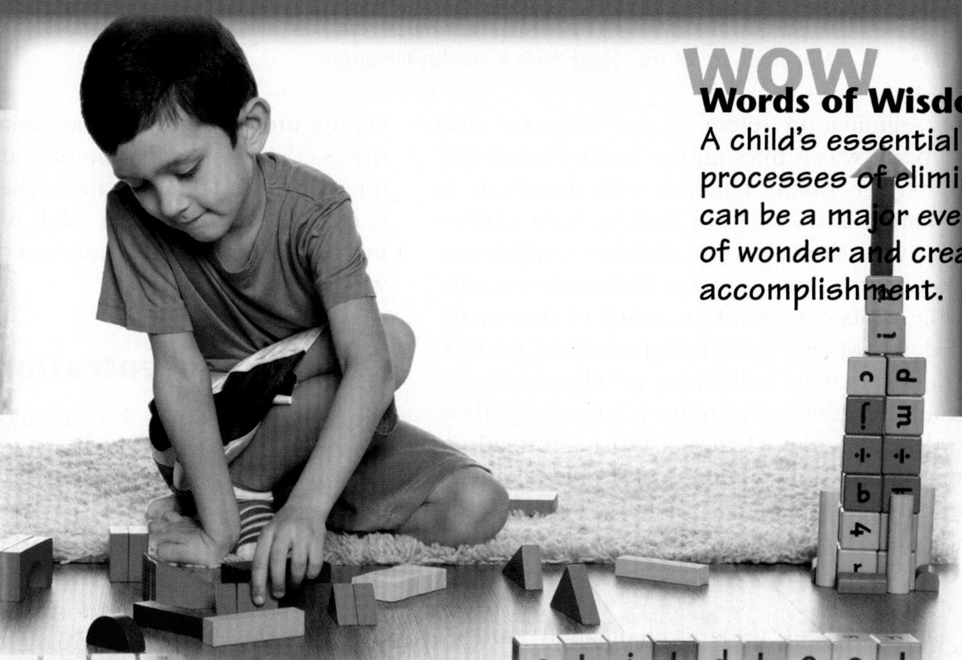

WOW

Words of Wisdom

A child's essential bodily processes of elimination can be a major event of wonder and creative accomplishment.

Nursing Care of the Child With an Alteration in Urinary Elimination/ Genitourinary Disorder

KEY TERMS

amenorrhea
anasarca
anuria
bacteriuria
dysmenorrhea
dysuria
enuresis
hematuria
menorrhagia
oliguria
proteinuria
urgency
urinary frequency

Learning Objectives

Upon completion of the chapter, you will be able to:

1. Compare anatomic and physiologic differences of the genitourinary system in infants and children versus adults.
2. Describe nursing care related to common laboratory and diagnostic testing used in the medical diagnosis of pediatric genitourinary conditions.
3. Distinguish alterations in urinary elimination and genitourinary disorders common in infants, children, and adolescents.
4. Identify appropriate nursing assessments and interventions related to medications and treatments for alterations in urinary elimination and pediatric genitourinary disorders.
5. Develop an individualized nursing care plan for the child with an alteration in urinary elimination or genitourinary disorder.
6. Describe the psychosocial impact of chronic genitourinary disorders on children.
7. Devise a nutrition plan for the child with renal insufficiency.
8. Develop child/family teaching plans for the child with an alteration in urinary elimination or genitourinary disorder.

***Corey Bond*, 5-years old, is brought to the clinic by her mother. She presents with fever and lethargy for the past 24 hours. Her mother states, "Corey has had a few accidents in her pants over the past few days, which is unusual for her. She also has been getting up at night more often to use the bathroom."**

Urinary elimination refers to the secretion and excretion of body waste through the urinary/renal system. Nurses may encounter children with alterations in urinary elimination and should be familiar with various genitourinary (GU) disorders that children experience. Alterations in urinary elimination, or GU disorders in children and adolescents may occur as a result of abnormalities in fetal development, infectious processes, trauma, neurologic deficit, genetic influences, or other causes.

Congenital disorders account for a large proportion of GU disorders in infants. External GU malformations are easily identified at birth, but internal structural defects may not be identified until later in infancy or childhood when symptoms or complications arise. Enuresis and urinary tract infection (UTI) also occur in a significant number of children.

Some alterations in urinary elimination directly involve the kidney from the outset, while others involve other parts of the urinary tract and may have a long-term effect on the kidneys and renal function, particularly if left untreated or treated inadequately.

Disorders affecting the reproductive organs often require early diagnosis and management to preserve future reproductive capabilities.

Nurses must be knowledgeable about pediatric GU conditions to provide prompt recognition, nursing care, education, and support to children and their families. Though some disorders are acute and resolve quickly, many have a long-term effect on quality of life and will require more intense, extended support.

Management of acute or common pediatric GU disorders may be provided in the pediatric or family practice outpatient setting, while specialists such as pediatric nephrologists or urologists usually manage chronic or involved GU disorders.

VARIATIONS IN PEDIATRIC ANATOMY AND PHYSIOLOGY

Though all of the urinary tract and reproductive organs are present at birth, their functioning is immature initially. The infant or child is at increased risk for the development of certain urinary elimination alterations because of the anatomic and physiologic differences between children and adults.

Structural Differences

The kidney is large in relation to the size of the abdomen until the child reaches adolescence. Due to this increased size, the kidneys of the child are less well protected from injury by the ribs and fat padding than they are in the adult. The urethra is naturally shorter in all ages of females compared to males, placing them at increased risk for the entrance of bacteria into the bladder via the urethra. In the female infant or young child, this risk is compounded by the physical proximity of the urethral opening to the rectum. The young male's urethra is much shorter than the adult male's, placing the male infant or young child at increased risk of UTI compared with the adult male.

Urinary Concentration

Blood flow through the kidneys (glomerular filtration rate [GFR]) is slower in the infant and young toddler compared with the adult (Lum, 2014). The kidney is less able to concentrate urine and reabsorb amino acids, placing the infant and young toddler at increased risk for dehydration during times when fluid loss or decreased fluid intake occurs. The normal range for serum blood urea nitrogen (BUN) and creatinine of the healthy infant or young toddler is usually less than the older child's or adult's. The renal system usually reaches functional maturity at around 2 years of age.

Urine Output

Bladder capacity is about 30 mL in the newborn; it increases to the usual adult capacity of about 270 mL by 1 year of age. The expected urine output in the infant and child is 0.5 to 2 mL/kg/hour, with the average 1-year old voiding about 400 to 500 mL per day. The average urine output for a teenager is about 800 to 1400 mL per day. The infant and toddler may void as often as 9 or 10 times per day. By age 3 the average number of voids per day is the same as the adult's (three to eight).

Reproductive Organ Maturity

The reproductive organs are also immature at birth. The gonads are not mature until adolescence in most children. The hormonal changes that occur with puberty account for some of the reproductive concerns, particularly for female adolescents.

COMMON MEDICAL TREATMENTS

A variety of medications as well as other medical treatments and surgical procedures are used to treat urinary elimination alterations and GU problems in children. Most of these treatments will require a physician's or nurse practitioner's order when the child is in the hospital. The most common treatments and medications are listed in Common Medical Treatments 43.1 and Drug Guide 43.1. The nurse caring for the child with a GU disorder should be familiar with what the procedures are, how the treatments and medications work, and common nursing implications related to use of these modalities.

COMMON MEDICAL TREATMENTS 43.1 GENITOURINARY DISORDERS

Treatment	Explanation	Indications	Nursing Implications
Urinary diversion	Surgical diversion of ureters to the abdominal wall. Continent diversion uses a piece of intestine to create a bladder that can be catheterized. Noncontinent diversion involves a stoma on the abdominal wall that requires use of an ostomy pouch.	Any situation in which the bladder needs to be removed or does not function correctly (bladder exstrophy or prune belly)	Meticulous skin care is necessary to prevent breakdown around stoma. Teach families how to care for ostomy pouch or how to catheterize continent stoma. Expect mucus in urine if intestine is used for urinary reservoir. Monitor for signs of urinary tract infection.
Foley catheter	An indwelling urinary catheter stays in place by means of an inflated balloon.	Usually used only during the postoperative period	Monitor for urethral drainage or irritation. Keep area clean and dry. Monitor color, consistency, clarity, and amount of urine in drainage bag. Monitor for infection, checking results of urinalysis and urine cultures.
Ureteral stent	A thin catheter temporarily placed in the ureter to drain urine. Removed via cystoscopy when it is time for discontinuation	Urinary tract anomalies	Monitor urine output carefully. Check for bleeding postoperatively.
Nephrostomy tube	Tube placed directly into the kidney to drain urine externally to a bag	Urinary tract anomalies	Monitor urine output carefully.
Suprapubic tube	Catheter placed in the bladder via the abdominal wall above the symphysis pubis	Postoperative urine drainage with reconstructive surgeries	Monitor for blood in urine, adequate urine output. Minimize manipulation of suprapubic tube to avoid triggering bladder spasms.
Vesicostomy	Stoma in the abdominal wall to the bladder	Urinary tract anomalies, neurogenic bladder	Constant urine drainage requires diaper use. Monitor urine output. Assess skin around stoma for breakdown.
Appendicovesicostomy (Mitrofanoff procedure)	Uses appendix to create a stoma on the abdominal wall that allows for catheterization of the bladder	Urinary tract anomalies, neurogenic bladder	Allows for urinary continence, which improves the child's self-esteem. Teach family and child how to catheterize stoma.
Bladder augmentation	Uses a piece of stomach or intestine to enlarge bladder capacity	Decreased bladder capacity	Since a portion of the GI tract is used, urine is often mucus-like.

NURSING PROCESS OVERVIEW FOR THE CHILD WITH AN ALTERATION IN URINARY ELIMINATION OR GENITOURINARY DISORDER

Care of the child with an alteration in urinary elimination or GU disorder includes assessment, nursing diagnosis, planning, interventions, and evaluation. There are a number of general concepts related to the nursing process that may be applied to GU disorders. From a general understanding of the care involved for a child with urinary, renal, or reproductive dysfunction, the nurse can then individualize the care based on specifics for that child.

Assessment

Assessment of urinary tract, renal, or reproductive dysfunction includes health history, physical examination, and laboratory and diagnostic testing.

DRUG GUIDE 43.1 COMMON DRUGS FOR GU DISORDERS

Medication	Actions/Indications	Nursing Implications
Anticholinergic agents (oxybutynin, propantheline bromide, belladonna & opium suppository)	Cause smooth muscle relaxation of the bladder, used for urinary tract spasms or contractions related to surgical procedure or use of catheters. Control of nocturnal enuresis	Increase fluid intake (limit to during the day in the child with nocturnal enuresis) Avoid use in febrile child
Antibiotics (oral, parenteral)	Kill bacteria or arrest their growth. Used for urinary tract infection	Check for antibiotic allergies Should be given as prescribed for the length of time indicated
Desmopressin	Antidiuretic hormone effects by causing renal tubule to absorb more water, decreasing volume of urine in children with nocturnal enuresis	Nasal spray may cause nasal irritation, nausea, flushing, or headache Administer at bedtime; alternate nares. Associated with a high relapse rate
Human chorionic gonadotropin (hCG)	Stimulates production of gonadal steroids to precipitate testicular descent	Monitor for signs of precocious puberty if used long term.
Corticosteroids	Anti-inflammatory and immunosuppressive action to induce remission and promote diuresis in nephrotic syndrome. High-dose intravenous therapy used when nephrotic syndrome is resistant to conventional doses	Administer with food to decrease GI upset May mask signs of infection Do not stop treatment abruptly, or acute adrenal insufficiency may occur Monitor for Cushing syndrome
Cytotoxic drugs (cyclophosphamide and chlorambucil)	Interfere with normal function of DNA by alkylation. Used to induce prolonged remission in nephrotic syndrome	Doses may be tapered over time Monitor for hypertension during infusion Causes bone marrow suppression. Monitor for signs of infection Cyclophosphamide: administer in the morning; provide adequate hydration; have child void frequently during and after infusion to decrease risk of hemorrhagic cystitis Chlorambucil: administer with nonspicy, nonacidic foods; rarely seizures occur
Immunosuppressant drugs (cyclosporine A [CyA], azathioprine, tacrolimus, mycophenolate)	Cause immune suppression to prevent rejection of renal transplants. CyA and tacrolimus may be used for steroid-dependent nephrotic syndrome	Monitor complete blood count, serum creatinine, potassium, and magnesium Monitor blood pressure and observe for signs of infection Blood levels should be drawn prior to morning dose CyA: do not give with grapefruit juice Azathioprine and mycophenolate: give on empty stomach; do not open capsule or crush tablet Tacrolimus: give on empty stomach; assess for development of hyperglycemia Relapse of nephrotic syndrome may occur after withdrawal of CyA or tacrolimus therapy
Muromonab-CD3	Removal of all CD3 molecules from T-lymphocyte surface so it has inability to act. Used for treatment of acute renal transplant rejection	Monitor for development of pulmonary edema First-dose effect may cause fever, chills, chest tightness, wheezing, nausea, and vomiting

DRUG GUIDE 43.1 COMMON DRUGS FOR GU DISORDERS (continued)

Medication	Actions/Indications	Nursing Implications
Angiotensin-converting enzyme (ACE) inhibitors (captopril, enalapril)	Potent vasoconstrictor, prevent conversion of angiotensin I to angiotensin II. Used to treat renal causes of hypertension	Monitor blood pressure frequently. May cause cough, hyperkalemia Captopril: administer on empty stomach Enalapril: administer without regard to food
Imipramine (tricyclic antidepressant)	Increases the synaptic concentration of serotonin and/or norepinephrine. Treatment of enuresis	Monitor for urinary retention. May cause decreased appetite
Diuretics: furosemide, hydrochlorothiazide	Inhibit resorption of sodium and chloride leading to increased excretion of water and electrolytes. Used in nephrotic syndrome, acute glomerulonephritis, hemolytic-uremic syndrome, or other instances of fluid overload with renal sufficiency	Administer with food or milk to decrease GI upset Monitor blood pressure, renal function, and electrolytes (particularly potassium) May cause photosensitivity
Vasodilators: hydralazine, minoxidil	Direct vasodilation of arterioles, resulting in decreased systemic resistance. Used to treat renal causes of hypertension	May cause fluid retention Hydralazine: administer with food. Monitor heart rate and blood pressure (closely with intravenous use) Minoxidil: may be administered without regard to food. May cause dizziness
Calcium channel blocker: nifedipine	Prevents calcium from entering voltage-sensitive channels, resulting in coronary vasodilation. Used to treat renal causes of hypertension	Administer with food; avoid grapefruit juice Insoluble shell of extended-release tablet may pass in stool Use caution when administering liquid-filled capsule sublingually or by bite-and-swallow method, as significant hypotension may occur
Albumin (intravenous)	Increases intravascular oncotic pressure, resulting in movement of fluid from interstitial to intravascular space. Indicated for fluid volume excess associated with nephrotic syndrome	May require a filter depending on brand used Rapid infusion can result in vascular overload Monitor vital signs; observe for pulmonary edema and cardiac failure

Adapted from Taketomo, C. K., Hodding, J. H., & Kraus, D. M. (2013). *Pediatric & neonatal dosage handbook* (20th ed.). Hudson, OH: Lexicomp.

Remember Corey, the 5-year old with fever and lethargy? What additional health history and physical examination assessment information should you obtain?

Health History

The health history consists of the past medical history, including the mother's pregnancy history; family history; and history of present illness (when the symptoms started and how they have progressed), as well as medications and treatments used at home. The past medical history may be significant for maternal polyhydramnios, oligohydramnios, diabetes, hypertension, or alcohol or cocaine ingestion. Neonatal history may include the presence of a single umbilical artery or an abdominal mass, chromosome abnormality, or congenital malformation. Document past medical history of UTI or other problems with the GU tract. Family history may be significant for renal disease or uropathology, chronic UTIs, renal calculi, or a history of parental enuresis. Determine age of successful toilet training, pattern of incontinent episodes (having "accidents"), and toileting hygiene self-care routines. Note myelomeningocele or other spinal disturbance that may affect the child's ability to urinate. Note previous urologic surgeries or ongoing renal interventions (e.g., dialysis). For the adolescent girl, obtain a thorough menstrual history, including sexual behavior and pregnancy history.

When determining the history of the present illness, inquire about the following:

- Burning on urination
- Changes in voiding patterns
- Foul-smelling urine
- Vaginal or urethral discharge
- Genital pain, irritation, or discomfort
- Blood in the urine
- Edema
- Masses in the groin, scrotum, or abdomen
- Flank or abdominal pain
- Cramps
- Nausea and/or vomiting
- Poor growth
- Weight gain
- Fever
- Infectious exposure (particularly *Streptococcus* A or *Escherichia coli*)
- Trauma

Record medications used for acute or chronic conditions, or for contraception.

Physical Examination

Physical examination of the GU system includes inspection and observation, auscultation, percussion, and palpation.

INSPECTION AND OBSERVATION

Observe the child's general appearance, noting growth retardation or unusual weight gain. Inspect the skin for the presence of pruritus, edema (generalized or periorbital), or bruising. Note pallor of the skin or dysmorphic features (associated with genetic conditions). Document the presence of lethargy, fatigue, rapid respirations, confusion, or developmental delay. Observe the external genitalia area for infant diaper rash, constant urine dribble, displaced urethral opening, reddened urethral opening, or discharge. In females, note vaginal irritation or labial fusion. In males, observe the scrotal sac for enlargement or discoloration. Note the condition of a urinary stoma or diversion if present. With the child lying flat, observe the abdomen for distention, ascites, or slack abdominal musculature.

AUSCULTATION

Listen carefully to heart sounds, as a flow murmur may be present in the anemic child with a renal disorder (Klein, 2010). Note elevated heart rate. Auscultate blood pressure with the appropriate-size cuff, noting elevation or depression. In the edematous child, carefully auscultate the lungs, noting the presence of adventitious sounds. Note the absence of bowel sounds, as this may indicate peritonitis. In the child who receives chronic hemodialysis, auscultate the fistula for the presence of a bruit (desired normal finding).

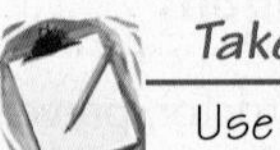

Take Note!

Use the bell of the stethoscope when auscultating the infant's or child's blood pressure so that you can hear the softer Korotkoff sounds more accurately.

PERCUSSION

Percuss the abdomen. Note unusual dullness or flatness (dullness is usually heard over the spleen at the right costal margin, over the kidneys, and 1 to 3 cm below the left costal margin). A full bladder may yield dullness above the symphysis pubis.

PALPATION

Palpate the abdomen. Note the presence of palpable kidneys (indicating enlargement or mass, as they are usually difficult to palpate in the older infant or child). Note the presence of abdominal masses or a distended bladder. Document tenderness to palpation or along the costovertebral angle. Palpate the scrotum for the presence of descended testicles, masses, or other abnormalities. Note whether the foreskin, if present, can be retracted. In the child who receives chronic hemodialysis, palpate the fistula or graft for the presence of a thrill (desired normal finding).

Laboratory and Diagnostic Testing

Common Laboratory and Diagnostic Tests 43.1 offers an explanation of the most commonly used laboratory and diagnostic tests for a child suspected of having a GU disorder. The test results can help the physician or nurse practitioner to diagnose the disorder or to determine treatment. Laboratory or nonnursing personnel obtain some of the tests, while the nurse might obtain others. In either instance the nurse should be familiar with how the tests are obtained, what they are used for, and normal versus abnormal results. This knowledge will also be necessary when providing child and family education related to the tests and results.

Urine specimens may be collected using a variety of different methods in infants and children. Suprapubic aspiration is a useful method for obtaining a sterile urine specimen from the neonate or young infant. A sterile needle is inserted into the bladder through the anterior wall of the abdomen and the urine is then aspirated. The physician or nurse practitioner generally performs this method. Infants and toddlers who are not toilet trained may require a urine bag for urine collection. A sterile urine bag is required for a urine culture, a clean bag for routine urinalysis. A 24-hour urine collection bag is also available. Nursing Procedure 43.1 gives details on the use of the urine bag.

COMMON LABORATORY AND DIAGNOSTIC TESTS 43.1 GENITOURINARY DISORDERS

Test	Explanation	Indications	Nursing Implications
Complete blood count	Evaluate hemoglobin and hematocrit, white blood cell count, and platelet count	Any condition in which anemia, infection, or thrombocytopenia is suspected	Normal values vary according to age and gender. White blood cell count differential is helpful in evaluating source of infection.
Blood urea nitrogen (BUN) (serum)	Indirect measurement of renal function and glomerular filtration in the presence of adequate liver function	Nephrotic syndrome, hemolytic-uremic syndrome, renal failure, acute glomerulonephritis, or other renal diseases	BUN may be elevated with high-protein diet or dehydration, may be decreased with overhydration or malnutrition.
Creatinine (serum)	A more direct measurement of renal function, only minimally affected by liver function. Generally, doubling of the creatinine level is suggestive of a 50% reduction in glomerular filtration rate.	Used to diagnose impaired renal function	A diet high in meat may cause a transient though not pronounced increase in creatinine. There are also slight diurnal variations in levels. Draw at same time each day if serial evaluations are ordered.
Creatinine clearance (urine and serum)	A 24-hour urine collection is evaluated for the presence of creatinine, then compared with the serum creatinine level to determine creatinine clearance.	Used to diagnose impaired renal function	Discard the first void and then begin the 24-hour urine collection. Keep the specimen on ice during the collection period. Collect ALL urine passed in the 24-hour period. Ensure that a venous blood sample is drawn during the 24-hour period. The urine specimen should be sent promptly to the laboratory at the end of the 24-hour period.
Potassium (serum)	Measures the concentration of potassium in the blood	Any suspected renal disease; followed routinely in renal failure	Avoid hemolysis and allowing child to open and close the hand with a tourniquet in place, as these can cause elevation in potassium levels. Evaluate the child with increased or decreased potassium levels for cardiac arrhythmias. Immediately notify physician or nurse practitioner of critically high potassium levels.
Total protein, globulin, albumin (serum)	Protein electrophoresis separates the various components into zones according to their electrical charge.	Used to diagnose, evaluate, and monitor chronic renal disease	Significantly low levels of albumin contribute to extent of edema, as albumin is necessary in the blood to maintain colloidal osmotic pressure.
Calcium (serum)	Measurement of calcium level in the blood; half of all calcium is protein-bound, so the level will decrease with hypoalbuminemia.	Renal diseases associated with hypoalbuminemia and edema	Avoid prolonged tourniquet use during blood draw, as this may falsely increase the calcium level.
Phosphorus (serum)	Measurement of phosphate level in the blood. Phosphorus levels are inversely related to calcium levels (they increase when calcium levels decrease).	Renal disease, ongoing monitoring, particularly in the child with hypocalcemia	Child should be NPO past midnight prior to the morning of the blood draw. Avoid hemolysis, as it can falsely elevate the phosphate level.

(continued)

COMMON LABORATORY AND DIAGNOSTIC TESTS 43.1 GENITOURINARY DISORDERS (continued)

Test	Explanation	Indications	Nursing Implications
Urinalysis (urine)	Evaluates color, pH, specific gravity, and odor of urine. Also assess for presence of protein, glucose, ketones, blood, leukocyte esterase, red and white blood cells, bacteria, crystals, and casts.	Reveals preliminary information about the urinary tract. Useful in children with fever, dysuria, flank pain, urgency, or hematuria. Proteinuria may be noted in renal disorders.	Be aware of the many drugs affecting urine color and notify laboratory if child is taking one. Notify laboratory if female is menstruating. Refrigerate specimen if not processed promptly. While proteinuria may occur with various renal disorders, it may also occur as either transient or orthostatic proteinuria, both of which are benign events.
Cystoscopy	Endoscopic visualization of the urethra and bladder	Evaluate hematuria, recurrent urinary tract infection; determine ureteral reflux; measure bladder capacity	Encourage fluids. Monitor vital signs. Child may feel burning with voiding after procedure. Pink tinge to urine is common after procedure.
Urine culture and sensitivity	Urine is plated in the laboratory and evaluated every day for the presence of bacteria. A final report is usually issued after 48 to 72 hours. Sensitivity testing is performed to determine the best choice of antibiotic.	Used to diagnose urinary tract infection	Obtain culture specimen prior to starting antibiotics if at all possible. Avoid contamination of the specimen with stool. May be obtained by catheterization, clean-catch specimen, or sterile U-bag. In some institutions, suprapubic tap is performed in neonates and young infants by the physician or nurse practitioner.
Urodynamic studies	Measure the urine flow during micturition via a urine flow meter	Dysfunctional voiding	The child must have a full bladder. The child then urinates into the urine flow meter. There is no discomfort associated with the test.
Voiding cystourethrogram (VCUG)	The bladder is filled with contrast material via catheterization. Fluoroscopy is performed to demonstrate filling of the bladder and collapsing after emptying.	Hematuria, urinary tract infections, vesicoureteral reflux, suspected structural anomalies	Just prior to the test, insert the Foley catheter. Ensure that the adolescent female is not pregnant. After the test, encourage the child to drink fluids to prevent bacterial accumulation and aid in dye elimination.
Intravenous pyelogram (IVP)	Radiopaque contrast material is injected intravenously and filtered by the kidneys. X-ray films are obtained at set intervals to show passage of the dye through the kidneys, ureters, and bladder.	Urinary outlet obstruction, hematuria, trauma to the renal system, suspected kidney tumor	Contraindicated in children allergic to shellfish or iodine. If the dye infiltrates at the intravenous site, hyaluronidase may be used to speed absorption of the iodine. Ensure adequate hydration before and after the test. Some institutions require enema or laxative evacuation of the bowel prior to the study to ensure adequate visualization of the urinary tract.
Renal biopsy	Usually a percutaneous specimen is obtained by inserting a needle through the skin and into the kidney. The sample of kidney tissue obtained is then microscopically examined.	Diagnosis of renal disease or assessment of renal transplant rejection	After the biopsy, carefully assess for signs or symptoms of bleeding: increased heart rate, pale color, flank pain or backache, shoulder pain, lightheadedness. Inspect urine for gross hematuria. Child will be on bed rest, preferably supine for 24 hours.
Renal ultrasound	Reflected sound waves allow visualization of the kidneys, ureters, and bladder.	Useful in determining kidney size (as with hydronephrosis and polycystic kidney), presence of cysts or tumors, or rejection of kidney transplant	No fasting is required prior to the procedure. Does not require contrast material. The child should feel no discomfort during the ultrasound.

Adapted from Corbett, J. A. & Banks, A. D. (2013). *Laboratory tests and diagnostic procedures with nursing diagnoses* (8th ed.). Upper Saddle River, NJ: Pearson Education Inc.

NURSING PROCEDURE 43.1

Applying The Urine Bag

1. Cleanse the perineal area well and pat dry (Figure A). If a culture is to be obtained, cleanse the genital area with povidone–iodine (Betadine) or per institutional protocol.
2. Apply benzoin around the scrotum or the vulvar area to aid with urine bag adhesion.
3. Allow the benzoin to dry.
4. Apply the urine bag.
   - For boys: Ensure that the penis is fully inside the bag; a portion of the scrotum may or may not be inside the bag, depending on scrotal size.
   - For girls: Apply the narrow portion of the bag on the perineal space between the anal and vulvar areas first for best adhesion, and then spread the remaining adhesive section (Figure B).
5. Tuck the bag downward inside the diaper to discourage leaking.
6. Check the bag frequently for urine (Figure C).

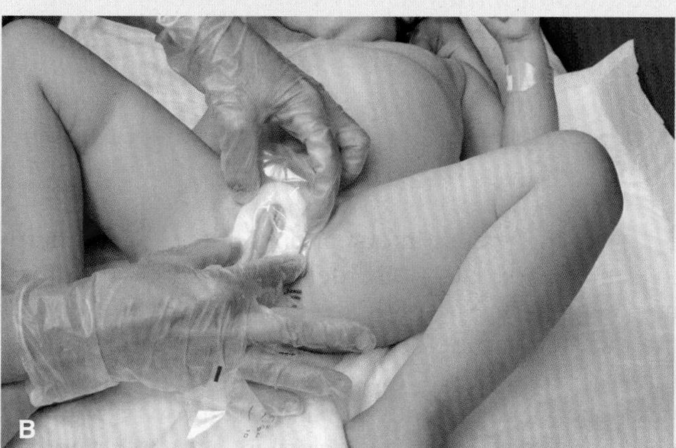

B

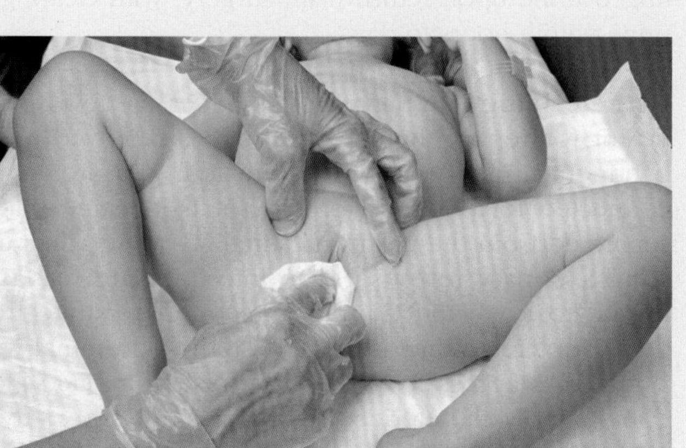

A

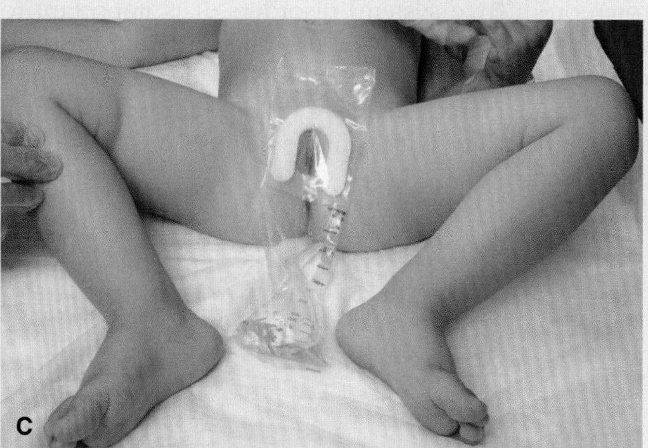

C

Atraumatic Care

When examining the genital area or performing urinary catheterization of the young female, allow the girl to sit with her mother on the examination table to decrease anxiety. Have the girl lie back on her mother's chest, seated on the table between the mother's legs. Encourage the mother to console and hug the girl while the invasive examination or procedure is being performed.

- Sterile urinary catheterization is performed like that in adults. The size of the catheter varies depending on the size of the child. General size recommendations are:
  - 6 French: Birth to 2 years old
  - 6 to 8 French: 2 to 5 years old
  - 8 to 10 French: 5 to 10 years old
  - 10 to 12 French: 10 to 16 years old (Bowden & Greenberg, 2012)

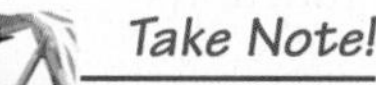

Take Note!

Use familiar terms such as "pee-pee," "tinkle," or "potty" to explain to the child what is needed and to gain his or her cooperation.

Nursing Diagnoses and Related Interventions

Upon completion of a thorough assessment, the nurse might identify several nursing diagnoses, such as:

- Impaired urinary elimination
- Fluid volume excess
- Imbalanced nutrition, less (or more) than body requirements

- Risk for infection
- Deficient knowledge of the child or family
- Urinary retention
- Activity intolerance
- Interrupted family processes
- Disturbed body image

After completing an assessment of Corey, you note the following: foul-smelling urine, abdominal tenderness, redness in her perineal area, and slightly blood-tinged, cloudy urine. Based on these assessment findings, what would your top three nursing diagnoses be for Corey?

Nursing goals, interventions, and evaluation for the child with a GU disorder are based on the nursing diagnoses. Nursing Care Plan 43.1, at the end of the chapter, can be used as a guide in planning nursing care for the child with a GU disorder. The care plan overview includes nursing diagnoses and interventions for urinary tract disorders as well as genital (or reproductive system) disorders. It is important to individualize it based on the child's symptoms and needs. Refer to Chapter 36 for detailed information about pain management. Additional information will be included later in the chapter as it relates to specific disorders.

Based on your top three nursing diagnoses for Corey, describe appropriate nursing interventions.

URINARY TRACT AND RENAL DISORDERS

The urinary tract and renal disorders discussed below include structural disorders, UTI, enuresis, and acquired disorders that result in altered renal function.

Structural Disorders

Numerous urologic conditions are congenital (present at birth) and occur as a result of altered fetal development. Many of these defects are apparent at birth, yet some are not recognized until later in infancy or childhood when symptoms or complications arise.

Bladder Exstrophy

Bladder exstrophy is a congenital defect resulting in the bladder being open and exposed outside of the abdomen. Refer to Chapter 24 for additional information as well as nursing assessment. Nursing management consists of preventing infection and skin breakdown (covered in Chapter 24) as well as providing postoperative care and catheterizing the stoma.

Providing Postoperative Care. Nursing management in the postoperative period focuses on preventing infection. Keep the infant supine and quickly change soiled diapers to prevent contamination of the incision with stool. Surgical reconstruction of the bladder within the pelvic cavity and reconstruction of a urethra are done if enough bladder tissue is present. An indwelling urethral catheter or suprapubic tube will allow urinary drainage, allowing the bladder to rest in the initial postoperative period. Ensure that catheters drain freely and do not become kinked. Sometimes tubes or catheters used in the postoperative period require irrigation. Refer to the institution's policy and the surgeon's orders for specifics related to urinary catheter irrigation.

Manage bladder spasms with oxybutynin or belladonna and opioid suppositories as ordered. Note blood-tinged urine upon return from surgery, with clearing of urine within hours to days.

Catheterizing the Stoma. If bladder tissue is insufficient for repair, then the bladder is removed and a continent urinary reservoir is created. The ureters are connected to a portion of the small intestine that is separated from the gastrointestinal (GI) tract, thus creating a urinary reservoir. The intestines are reanastomosed to leave the GI tract intact and separate from the GU tract. A stoma is created on the abdominal wall; it provides access to the urinary reservoir (Fig. 43.1). The stoma is catheterized about four times per day to empty the reservoir of urine. Urine from an intestine-based urinary reservoir tends to be mucus-like and is

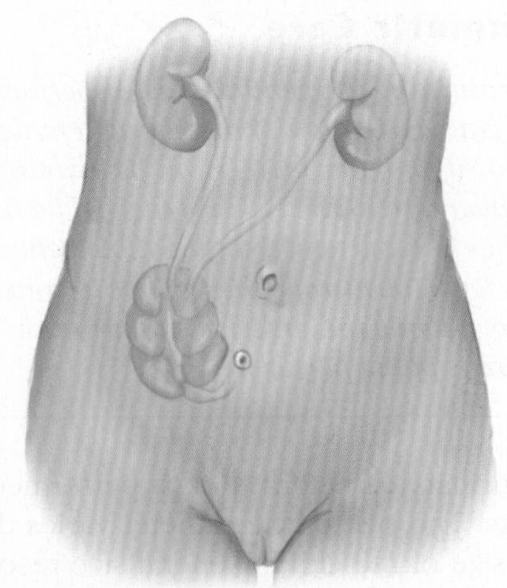

FIGURE 43.1 The abdominal stoma allows for urinary continence and requires catheterization.

often cloudier than urine from a urinary bladder. Teach parents the procedure for catheterizing the urinary reservoir and instruct them to call the child's urologist or physician or nurse practitioner if signs or symptoms of UTI occur.

Take Note!

Children with congenital urologic malformations are at high risk for the development of latex allergy (Hamilton, 2015). Latex allergy can result in anaphylaxis. Primary prevention of latex allergy is warranted in all children with urologic malformations, so use latex-free gloves, tubes, and catheters in these children.

Hypospadias/Epispadias

Hypospadias is a urethral defect in which the opening is on the ventral surface of the penis rather than at the end of the penis (Fig. 43.2). Epispadias is a urethral defect in which the opening is on the dorsal surface of the penis. In either case, the opening may be near the glans of the penis, midway along the penis, or near the base. If left uncorrected, the boy may not be capable of appropriately aiming a urinary stream from a standing position. In addition, the abnormal placement of the urethral opening may interfere with the deposition of sperm during intercourse, leaving the man infertile. Also, if left uncorrected, the boy's self-esteem and body image may be damaged by the abnormal appearance of his genitalia (Pfeil & Lindsay, 2010). For these reasons, the defect is usually repaired sometime after about 1 year of age. The goal of surgical correction for either condition is to provide for an appropriately placed meatus that allows for normal voiding and ejaculation. The meatus is moved to the glans penis and the urethra is reconstructed as needed. Most repairs are accomplished in one surgery. More extensive reconstructions may require two stages.

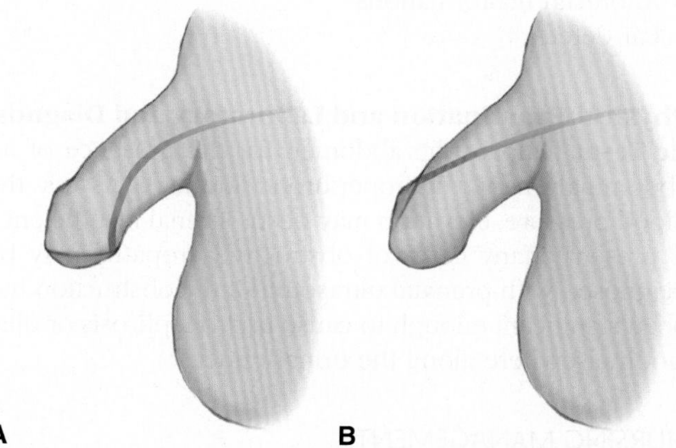

FIGURE 43.2 **(A)** Hypospadias: the urethral opening is located on the ventral side of the penis. **(B)** Epispadias: the urethral opening is located on the dorsal side of the penis.

NURSING ASSESSMENT

Note history of an unusual urine stream. Inspect the penis for placement of the urethral meatus: it may be slightly off center of the glans or may be present somewhere along the shaft of the penis. Inspect for chordee, a fibrous band causing the penis to curve downward. Palpate for the presence or absence of testicles in the scrotal sac, because cryptorchidism (undescended testicles) often occurs with hypospadias, as do hydrocele and inguinal hernia.

NURSING MANAGEMENT

The newborn with hypospadias or epispadias should not undergo circumcision until after surgical repair of the urethral meatus. In more extreme cases, the surgeon may need to use some of the excess foreskin while reconstructing the meatus. Nursing management of the infant who has undergone a hypospadias or epispadias repair focuses on providing routine postoperative care and parent education.

Providing Postoperative Care. Postoperatively, assess urinary drainage from the urethral stent or drainage tube, which allows for discharge of urine without stress along the surgical site. Ensure that the urinary drainage tube remains carefully taped with the penis in an upright position to prevent stress on the urethral incision. The penile dressing is usually a compression type, used to decrease edema and bruising. Administer antibiotics if prescribed. Assess for pain, which is usually not extensive, and administer analgesics or antispasmodics (oral oxybutynin or B & O suppository) as needed for bladder spasms. Bladder spasms may also be managed effectively through the use of epidural analgesia. See Dosage Calculation Box 43.1.

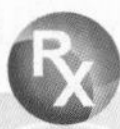

Dosage Calculation Box 43.1

Child's weight: 17 lb, 12 oz

Medication order: oxybutynin 1.6 mg PO three times a day.

Per the Pediatric Dosage Handbook, the recommended dose is 0.2 mg/kg/dose two to three times daily.

Is the ordered dose safe?

Double diapering is a method used to protect the urethra and stent or catheter after surgery; it also helps keep the area clean and free from infection. The inner diaper contains stool and the outer diaper contains urine, allowing separation between the bowel and bladder output. Nursing Procedure 43.2 details the double-diapering technique. Change the outside (larger) diaper when the child is wet; change both diapers when the child has a bowel movement.

NURSING PROCEDURE 43.2

Double Diapering

1. Cut a hole or a cross-shaped slit in the front of the smaller diaper.
2. Unfold both diapers and place the smaller diaper (with the hole) inside the larger one.
3. Place both diapers under the child.
4. Carefully bring the penis (if applicable) and catheter/stent through the hole in the smaller diaper and close the diaper.
5. Close the larger diaper, making sure the tip of the catheter/stent is inside the larger diaper.

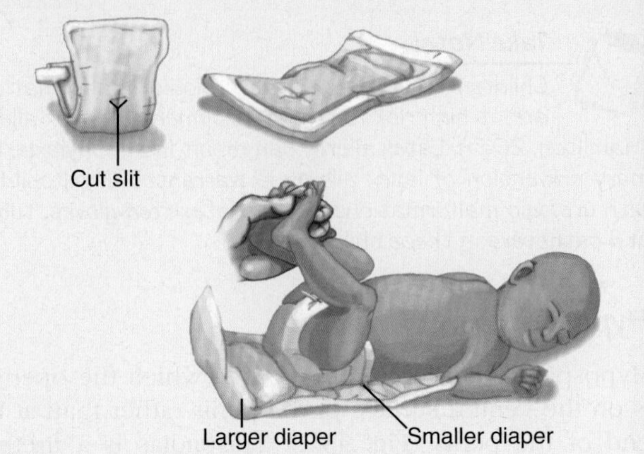

Pictures and text adapted from Mount Nittany Medical Center. (2013). *When your son needs surgery for hypospadias*. Retrieved from http://www.mountnittany.org/articles/healthsheets/11970

Educating the Family. If the child is to be discharged with the urinary catheter in place (which is common), teach the parents how to care for the catheter and drainage system. Have parents demonstrate their ability to irrigate the catheter should a mucus plug occur. Tub baths are generally prohibited until it is time to remove the penile dressing. Roughhousing, ride-on toys, or any activity involving straddling is not allowed for 2 to 3 weeks.

Obstructive Uropathy

Obstructive uropathy is an obstruction at any level along the upper or lower urinary tract. This discussion will focus on congenital structural defects, though obstruction can also occur as a result of other disease processes (acquired obstructive uropathy). The most common sites of obstruction are listed in Table 43.1. The defect may be unilateral or bilateral and can cause partial or complete obstruction of urine flow, resulting in dilation of the affected kidney (hydronephrosis). Complications include recurrent UTI, renal insufficiency, and progressive damage to the kidney resulting in renal failure.

NURSING ASSESSMENT

For a full description of the assessment phase of the nursing process, refer to the Assessment section of the Nursing Process Overview earlier in the chapter. Assessment findings pertinent to obstructive uropathy are discussed below.

Health History. Elicit a description of the present illness and chief complaint. Common signs and symptoms reported during the health history might include:

- Recurrent UTI
- Incontinence
- Fever
- Foul-smelling urine
- Flank pain
- Abdominal pain
- Urinary frequency (needing to void often)
- Urinary urgency (urge to void immediately)
- Dysuria (difficulty or pain with voiding)
- Hematuria (blood in the urine)

Explore the child's current and past medical history for risk factors such as:

- "Prune belly" syndrome
- Chromosome abnormalities
- Anorectal malformations
- Ear defects

Physical Examination and Laboratory and Diagnostic Tests. Palpate the abdomen for the presence of an abdominal mass (hydronephrotic kidney). Assess the blood pressure; elevation may occur if renal insufficiency is present. Many cases of obstructive uropathy may be diagnosed with prenatal ultrasound if the obstruction has been significant enough to cause hydronephrosis or dilatation elsewhere along the urinary tract.

NURSING MANAGEMENT

Surgical correction is specific to the type of obstruction and generally consists of removal of the obstruction, reimplantation of the ureters as necessary, and, occasionally, creation of a urinary diversion. Postoperatively,

TABLE 43.1 COMMON SITES OF OBSTRUCTIVE UROPATHY

Disorder	Site	Illustration
Ureteropelvic junction (UPJ) obstruction	Junction of the upper ureter with the pelvis of the kidney	Urinary tract with unilateral hydronephrosis and narrowing of the UPJ on that side Renal pelvis; Site of obstruction; Kidney; Ureter; Bladder
Ureterovesical junction (UVJ) obstruction	Junction of the lower ureter and the bladder	Urinary tract with unilateral hydronephrosis and dilated ureters with narrowing of the UVJ on that side Kidney; Bladder; Ureter; Obstruction
Ureterocele	Ureter swells into the bladder	Bladder with cystic pouch where ureters insert (unilateral) Hydroureter; Ureterocele
Posterior urethral valves (males only)	Flaps of tissue in the proximal urethra	Distended proximal urethra, bladder, ureters, and hydronephrosis Kidney; Renal pelvis; Ureter; Thickened bladder walls with dilated bladder; Posterior valves

Adapted from Gaylord, N. M., & Petersen-Smith, A. M. (2013). Genitourinary disorders. In C. Burns, A. Dunn, M. Brady, N. B. Starr, & C. Blosser (Eds.), *Pediatric primary care* (5th ed.). Philadelphia, PA: Saunders; and Lum, G. M. (2014). Kidney & urinary tract. In W. W. Hay, M. J. Levin, R. R. Deterding, & M. J. Abzug, (Eds.), *Current pediatric diagnosis and treatment* (22nd ed.). New York, NY: McGraw-Hill.

assess urine output via vesicostomy, nephrostomy, suprapubic tube, or urethral catheter for color, clots, clarity, and amount. Encourage fluids once the child can tolerate them orally. Administer analgesics and/or antispasmodics as needed for bladder spasms. Teach parents care of vesicostomy or drainage tubes, with which the child may be discharged.

Take Note!

Upon return from surgery, most children have intravenous fluids without added potassium infusion. Potassium is withheld from the intravenous fluid until adequate urine output is established postoperatively to avoid the development of hyperkalemia should the kidneys fail to function properly (Browne, Flanigan, McComiskey, & Pieper, 2013).

Hydronephrosis

Hydronephrosis is a condition in which the pelvis and calyces of the kidney are dilated (Fig. 43.3). Hydronephrosis may occur as a congenital defect, as a result of obstructive uropathy, or secondary to vesicoureteral reflux (VUR). Congenital hydronephrosis may be revealed on prenatal ultrasound. Complications of hydronephrosis include renal insufficiency, hypertension, and eventually renal failure.

NURSING ASSESSMENT

For a full description of the assessment phase of the nursing process, refer to the Assessment section of the Nursing Process Overview earlier in the chapter. Assessment findings pertinent to hydronephrosis are discussed below.

Health History. Elicit a description of the present illness and chief complaint. The infant may be asymptomatic, but signs and symptoms reported during the health history might include:

- Failure to thrive
- Intermittent hematuria
- Presence of an abdominal mass
- Signs and symptoms associated with a UTI such as fever, vomiting, poor feeding, and irritability

Explore the child's current and past medical history for risk factors such as:

- Maternal oligohydramnios or polyhydramnios (congenital hydronephrosis)
- Elevated levels of serum α-fetoprotein (congenital hydronephrosis)

Physical Examination and Diagnostic and Laboratory Tests. Monitor the blood pressure of infants and children suspected of having hydronephrosis. Palpation of the abdomen may reveal enlarged kidney(s) or a distended bladder. A voiding cystourethrogram (VCUG) will be performed to determine the presence of a structural defect that may be causing the hydronephrosis. Other diagnostic tests, such as a renal ultrasound or an intravenous pyelogram, may also be performed to clarify the diagnosis.

NURSING MANAGEMENT

Teach the parents signs and symptoms of UTI and sepsis, as these complications may occur. Explain to the parents that they should observe the child for adequacy of urine output and hydration status. Teach the parents to perform appropriate perineal hygiene and to avoid using irritants in the genital area. The infant or child with hydronephrosis will need follow-up with a pediatric nephrologist or urologist.

Vesicoureteral Reflux

VUR is a condition in which urine from the bladder flows back up the ureters. This reflux of urine occurs during bladder contraction with voiding (Fig. 43.4). Reflux may occur in one or both ureters. If reflux occurs when the

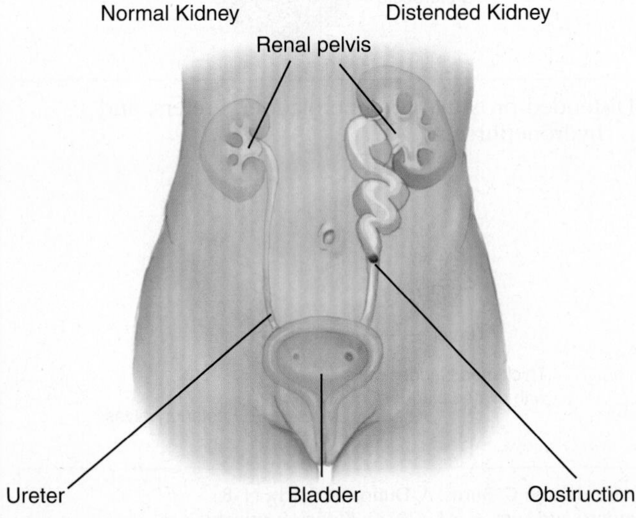

FIGURE 43.3 Hydronephrosis.

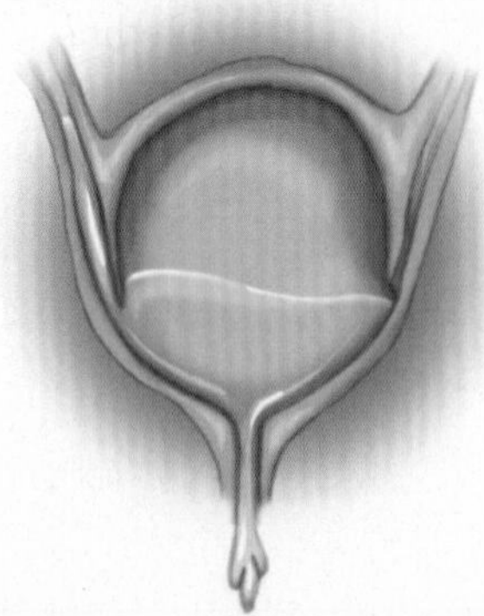

FIGURE 43.4 Note retrograde flow of urine up the ureter upon bladder contraction.

urine is infected, the kidney is exposed to bacteria and pyelonephritis may result. The increased pressure placed upon the kidney with reflux can cause renal scarring and lead to hypertension later in life and, if severe, renal insufficiency or failure.

Primary VUR results from a congenital abnormality at the vesicoureteral junction that results in incompetence of the valve. Secondary VUR is related to other structural or functional problems such as neurogenic bladder, bladder dysfunction, or bladder outlet obstruction. As many as 70% of all children diagnosed with UTI have VUR (Nelson & Koo, 2014).

VUR is graded according to its severity, from grade I, which is characterized by minor dilatation of the proximal ureter, to grade V, which is characterized by severe dilatation of the ureter and pelvis of the kidney. Grade I and II VUR cases usually resolve spontaneously, but grade III through V cases are generally associated with recurrent UTIs, hydronephrosis, and progressive renal damage (Nelson & Koo, 2014).

The goal of therapeutic management of VUR is prevention of pyelonephritis and subsequent renal scarring, which may contribute to the development of hypertension later in life (Nelson & Koo, 2014). Management continues to include antibiotic prophylaxis though evidence is nonconclusive as to whether prophylaxis is actually beneficial (Worcester, 2014). Additionally, hygiene and voiding practices are used to assist with prevention of UTI. Serial urine cultures are used to determine recurrence of UTI. Biannual, annual, or biennial radionuclide VCUGs are performed to determine the status of VUR.

Grade III, IV, and V cases usually warrant surgical intervention. The ureters are resected from the bladder and reimplanted elsewhere in the bladder wall to regain functionality.

Take Note!

The keys to prevention of long-term sequelae such as hypertension in children with urologic conditions are early diagnosis and intervention, prevention of infection, and close clinical follow-up. Nurses play a key role in monitoring and education.

NURSING ASSESSMENT

For a full description of the assessment phase of the nursing process, refer to the Assessment section of the Nursing Process Overview earlier in the chapter. Assessment findings pertinent to VUR are discussed below.

Health History. Elicit a description of the present illness and chief complaint. Common signs and symptoms reported during the health history might include:

- Fever
- Dysuria
- Frequency or urgency
- Nocturia
- Hematuria
- Pain in the back, abdomen, or flank

Explore the child's current and past medical history for risk factors such as:

- Recurrent UTI in the female
- Single episode of UTI in the male
- Congenital defect
- Family history of VUR

For the child who is receiving ongoing follow-up for VUR, determine whether UTIs have occurred since the last visit, as well as the name and dose of prophylactic antibiotic.

Physical Examination. Monitor the blood pressure for elevation. Palpate the abdomen for presence of a mass (if hydronephrosis is present). VCUG may be used to diagnose VUR.

NURSING MANAGEMENT

Nursing management for the child with VUR includes preventing infection and providing postoperative care.

Preventing Infection. When VUR is present, the goal is to avoid urine infection so that infected urine cannot gain access to the kidneys. Initially, most cases of VUR are managed medically. Teach the child to empty the bladder completely. Teach the child and parents appropriate perineal hygiene as well as toileting hygiene to prevent recurrence of UTI. Teach parents about the antibiotic therapy prescribed; the child will be maintained on a low daily dose to prevent UTI. The drug is most effective when given at bedtime because of urinary stasis overnight. Inform parents of the schedule for serial urine cultures and follow-up VCUG.

Providing Postoperative Care. If VUR is severe or if UTI is recurrent, surgical correction will be necessary. In the first 24 to 48 hours after surgery, maintain the intravenous fluid rate at 1.5 times maintenance to encourage a high urinary output. Monitor urine output via the Foley catheter; urine should be bloody initially, clearing within 2 to 3 days. If ureteral stents are present, monitor urine output from those as well. Administer analgesics for incisional pain relief and antispasmodics or B & O suppositories as needed for bladder spasms. Encourage ambulation and advancement of diet as ordered to promote return of appropriate bowel function. Teach parents that prophylactic antibiotics will be given until 1 to 2 months after surgery, when the VCUG demonstrates absence of reflux.

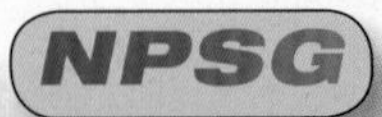

GOAL 7: Reduce the Risk of Healthcare-Associated Infections. (Prevent infection)

NPSG 07.06.01 Use proven guidelines to prevent infections of the urinary tract that are caused by catheters.

Steps: Insure aseptic technique utilized for indwelling catheter insertion and ongoing catheter care provided according to facility policy. Maintain urine drainage by providing unobstructed flow and securing catheter.

Joint Commission. (2015). *National patient safety goals effective January 1, 2015.* Retrieved from http://www.jointcommission.org/assets/1/6/2015_NPSG_HAP.pdf

Take Note!

When caring for the child who has undergone urologic surgery, avoid manipulating the Foley or suprapubic catheter: catheter manipulation contributes to bladder spasms.

Urinary Tract Infection

UTI is an infection of the urinary tract, most commonly affecting the bladder. UTI occurs most often as a result of bacteria ascending to the bladder via the urethra. About 8% of girls and 2% of boys will experience at least one UTI during childhood (Lum, 2014). One explanation for the more common occurrence in females is that the female's shorter urethra allows bacteria to have easier access to the bladder. The urethra is also located quite close to the vagina and anus in females, allowing spread of bacteria from those areas. The sexually active female adolescent is at risk for the development of UTI, as bacteria may be forced into the urethra by pressure from intercourse. The adolescent male may be somewhat protected from UTI by the antibacterial properties of prostate secretions.

UTI presents differently in infants than it does in children. Infants may exhibit fever, irritability, vomiting, failure to thrive, or jaundice. Children may also experience fever and vomiting, but also may have dysuria, frequency, hesitancy, urgency, and/or pain.

PATHOPHYSIOLOGY

E. coli most commonly causes UTI, as it is usually found in the perineal and anal region, close to the urethral opening. Other organisms include *Klebsiella, Staphylococcus aureus, Proteus, Pseudomonas,* and *Haemophilus*. Numerous factors may contribute to bacterial proliferation. Urinary stasis contributes to the development of a UTI once the bacteria have gained entry. Urine that remains in the bladder after voiding allows bacteria to grow rapidly. A decreased fluid intake also contributes to bacterial growth, as the bacteria become more concentrated. If the urine is alkaline, bacteria are better able to flourish. Untreated bladder infection may allow reflux of infected urine up the ureters to the kidneys and result in pyelonephritis, a more serious infection.

THERAPEUTIC MANAGEMENT

UTIs are treated with either oral or intravenous antibiotics, depending on the severity of the infection. Urine culture and sensitivity determines the appropriate antibiotic. A 7- to 14-day course of antibiotics is often prescribed, though 2- to 5-day courses may be as effective. Adequate fluid intake is necessary to flush the bacteria from the bladder. Fever management may also be needed.

NURSING ASSESSMENT

For a full description of the assessment phase of the nursing process, refer to the Assessment section of the Nursing Process Overview earlier in the chapter. Assessment findings pertinent to UTI are discussed below.

Health History. Elicit a description of the present illness and chief complaint. Common signs and symptoms reported during the health history might include:

- Fever
- Nausea or vomiting
- Chills
- Abdomen, back, or flank pain
- Lethargy
- Jaundice (in the neonate)
- Poor feeding or "just not acting right" (in the infant)
- Urinary urgency or frequency
- Burning or stinging with urination (the infant may cry with urination, the toddler may grab the diaper)
- Foul-smelling urine
- Poor appetite (child)
- Enuresis or incontinence in a previously toilet-trained child
- Blood in the urine

Explore the child's current and past medical history for risk factors such as:

- Previous UTI
- Obstructive uropathy
- Inadequate toileting hygiene (often occurs with preschool girls)
- VUR
- Constipation
- Urine holding or dysfunctional voiding
- Neurogenic bladder
- Uncircumcised male
- Sexual intercourse
- Pregnancy
- Chronic illness

Physical Examination. In the neonate or young infant, observe for jaundice or increased respiratory rate.

In infants and children, inspect the perineal area for redness or irritation. Observe the urine for visible blood, cloudiness, dark color, sediment, mucus, or foul odor. Note pallor, edema, or elevated blood pressure. Palpate the abdomen. Note distended bladder, abdominal mass, or tenderness, particularly in the flank area.

Laboratory and Diagnostic Tests. Common laboratory and diagnostic studies ordered for the assessment of UTI include:

- Urinalysis (clean-catch, suprapubic, or catheterized): may be positive for blood, nitrites, leukocyte esterase, white blood cells, or bacteria (**bacteriuria**)
- Urine culture: will be positive for infecting organism
- Renal ultrasound: may show hydronephrosis if child also has a structural defect
- VCUG: not usually performed until the child has been treated with antibiotics for at least 48 hours, as infected urine tends to reflux up the ureters anyway. VCUG performed once the urine has regained sterility may be positive for VUR.

Renal ultrasound, or VCUG may be indicated in certain populations. The physician or nurse practitioner will determine the need for radiologic testing.

NURSING MANAGEMENT

Goals for nursing management include eradicating infection, promoting comfort, and preventing recurrence of infection.

Eradicating Infection. The child who can tolerate oral intake will be prescribed an oral antibiotic. The child who has protracted vomiting related to the UTI or who has suspected pyelonephritis will require hospitalization and intravenous antibiotics. Children younger than 3 months, and those with dehydration, a toxic appearance, or sepsis should also be hospitalized for administration of intravenous antibiotics (Lum, 2014). Administer oral or intravenous antibiotics as prescribed. Urge the parent to complete the entire course of oral antibiotic at home, even though the child is feeling better. Administer intravenous fluids as ordered or encourage generous oral fluid intake to help flush the bacteria from the bladder.

Promoting Comfort. Administer antipyretics such as acetaminophen or ibuprofen to reduce fever. A heating pad or warm compress may help relieve abdomen or flank pain. If the child is afraid to urinate due to burning or stinging, encourage voiding in a warm sitz or tub bath.

Preventing Recurrence of Infection. Encourage the parents to return as ordered for a repeat urine culture after completion of the antibiotic course to ensure eradication of bacteria. Teaching Guidelines 43.1 gives further information on preventing UTI.

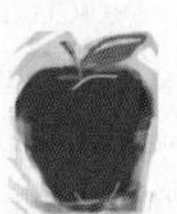

Teaching Guidelines 43.1

PREVENTING URINARY TRACT INFECTION IN FEMALES

- Drink enough fluid (to keep urine flushed through bladder).
- Drink cranberry juice to acidify the urine.
- Avoid colas and caffeine, which irritate the bladder.
- Urinate frequently and do not "hold" urine (to discourage urinary stasis).
- Avoid bubble baths (they contribute to vulvar and perineal irritation).
- Wipe from front to back after voiding (to avoid contaminating the urethra with rectal material).
- Wear cotton underwear (to decrease the incidence of perineal irritation).
- Avoid wearing tight jeans or pants.
- Wash the perineal area daily with soap and water.
- While menstruating, change sanitary pads frequently to discourage bacterial growth.
- Void immediately after sexual intercourse.

Enuresis

Enuresis is continued incontinence of urine past the age of toilet training. Box 43.1 gives further definitions related to enuresis. Nocturnal enuresis generally subsides by 6 years of age; if it does not, further investigation and treatment may be warranted. Occasional daytime wetting or dribbling of urine is usually not a cause for concern, but frequent daytime wetting concerns both the child and the parents. Nocturnal enuresis may persist in some children into late childhood and adolescence, causing significant distress for the affected child and family.

In some children, enuresis may occur secondary to a physical disorder such as diabetes mellitus or insipidus, sickle cell anemia, ectopic ureter, or urethral obstruction. Other causes common to both diurnal and nocturnal enuresis include a urine-concentrating defect, UTI, constipation, and emotional distress (sometimes serious). The most frequent cause of daytime enuresis is dysfunctional voiding or holding of urine, though giggle

BOX 43.1

DEFINITIONS RELATED TO ENURESIS

- **Primary enuresis:** enuresis in the child who has never achieved voluntary bladder control
- **Secondary enuresis:** urinary incontinence in the child who previously demonstrated bladder control over a period of at least 3 to 6 consecutive months
- **Diurnal enuresis:** daytime loss of urinary control
- **Nocturnal enuresis:** nighttime bedwetting

incontinence and stress incontinence also occur. Nocturnal enuresis may be related to a high fluid intake in the evening, obstructive sleep apnea, sexual abuse, a family history of enuresis, or inappropriate family expectations. Physical causes of enuresis must be treated; further management of the disorder focuses on behavioral training, which may be augmented with the use of enuresis alarms or medications.

NURSING ASSESSMENT

Elicit a description of the present illness and chief complaint. Determine the age of toilet training and when or if the child achieved successful daytime and nighttime dryness. Inquire about urine-holding behaviors such as squatting, dancing, or staring as well as rushing to the bathroom (diurnal enuresis). Inquire about the amount and types of fluid the child typically consumes before bedtime (nocturnal enuresis). Assess for risk factors such as:

- Family disruption or other stressors
- Chronic constipation (carefully assess bowel movement patterns)
- Excessive family demands related to toileting patterns
- History of being difficult to arouse from sleep
- Family history of enuresis

Assess the child's cognitive status: developmentally delayed children may take significantly longer to achieve urine continence than their typical same-age peers. Assess for short stature or elevated blood pressure, as these may occur when renal abnormalities are present.

NURSING MANAGEMENT

For the child with diurnal enuresis, encourage him or her to increase the amount of fluid consumed during the day in order to increase the frequency of the urge to void. Set a fixed schedule for the child to attempt to void throughout the day. These practices will usually be sufficient to retrain the child's voiding patterns. The child with nocturnal enuresis without a physiologic cause for bedwetting may require a varied approach (Dunn, 2013). (See Evidence-Based Practice 43.1.)

Educating the Child and Family About Nocturnal Enuresis. Teach the family that the child is not lazy, nor does he or she wet the bed intentionally. Encourage the child and family to read books such as *Dry All Night: The Picture Book Technique That Stops Bedwetting* by Alison Mack or *Waking Up Dry: A Guide to Help Children Overcome Bedwetting* by Dr. Howard Bennett. Encourage the parents to limit intake of bladder irritants such as chocolate and caffeine. Teach parents to limit fluid intake after dinner and ensure that the child voids just before going to bed. Waking the child to void at 11 PM may also be helpful. Teach the parents to use bed pads and to make the bed with two sets of sheets and pads to decrease the workload in the middle of the night. When sleeping at home, the child should wear his or her usual underwear or pajamas. If away on a family vacation, pull-ups may decrease the stress on both the child and the parents.

Providing Support and Encouragement. It is important for the child to understand that he or she is not alone. Depending on the child's developmental level, explain that as many as 5 million people have enuresis (this can be done in terms the child can relate to, such as a proportion within a school or 100 times the number of children in one school, etc.). It is not only "little kids" who wet the bed, and all kids who wet the bed need help overcoming this problem. Parents

EVIDENCE-BASED PRACTICE 43.1 BEHAVIORAL INTERVENTIONS FOR ENURESIS

STUDY

Nocturnal enuresis (bedwetting) may affect the child's psychosocial well-being. Lowered self-esteem, sibling teasing, and social problems may occur in the child or adolescent who experiences bedwetting. The authors included 16 randomized and quasi-randomized trials with a total of 1,643 child participants. Most of the studies were single (and often differing) intervention trials, yielding the evidence slightly less reliable.

Findings

The authors did not note an individual treatment that was more effective than another. Simple treatments such as star charts for dry nights (e.g., with star charts), lifting (parental lifting of the sleeping child from the bed to urinate elsewhere), waking the child to urinate, and structured bladder training were noted to be more effective than no treatment.

Nursing Implications

Simple behavioral interventions are inexpensive and do not have side effects nor safety concerns. They should be implementing first in the treatment of nocturnal enuresis and nurses play a key role in educating and supporting the family using these simple strategies.

Adapted from Caldwell, P. H., Nankivell, G., & Sureshkumar, P. (2013). Simple behavioural interventions for nocturnal enuresis in children. *The Cochrane Library* 2013, 7. Indianapolis, IN: John Wiley & Sons.

should include the child in plans for nighttime urinary control; this helps to increase the child's motivation to become dry. Parents should set up a reward system for dry nights. Parents should include the child in bed linen changes when he or she does wet the bed, but should do so in a matter-of-fact manner rather than in a punitive way; in fact, it is important to always avoid punishment for bedwetting.

With patience, consistency, and time, dryness will be achieved. Provide ongoing emotional support and positive reinforcement to the child and family.

Decreasing Nighttime Voiding. Teach the family using an enuresis alarm system how to use the alarm as well as the previously mentioned techniques (Fig. 43.5). (Also see links to resources on thePoint.) Most of these devices work by sounding an alarm when the first few drops of urine appear; the child then awakens and stops the urine flow. Over time the child becomes conditioned to either awaken when the bladder is full or stop the urine flow when sleeping.

When behavioral and motivational therapies are unsuccessful, particularly in the older child, medications may be prescribed. Teach the child and parents about the use of medications such as oxybutynin, imipramine, and desmopressin if these are prescribed (refer to Drug Guide 43.1).

Take Note!

Enuresis is a source of shame and embarrassment for children and adolescents. It affects the child's life emotionally, behaviorally, and socially. The family's life is also significantly affected. Enuresis is associated with childhood and adolescent low self-esteem (Dunn, 2013).

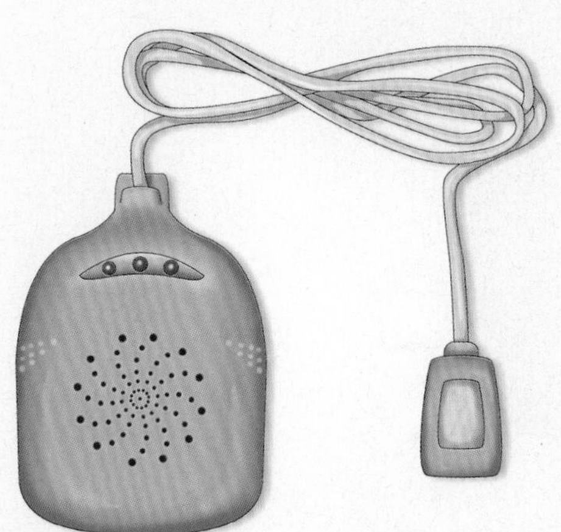

FIGURE 43.5 Some children and families find great success with the use of an enuresis alarm. The alarm wakes the child at the first sign of wetness. Over time, the child learns to awaken at night in response to the sensation of a full bladder.

Acquired Disorders Resulting in Altered Renal Function

A number of acquired disorders are responsible for alterations in renal function. They may occur as an autoimmune response or in relation to a bacterial infection. Renal dysfunction may also occur as a result of obstructive disorders or repeated VUR, as discussed earlier. Left untreated, these disorders may lead to renal failure. Even when treated appropriately, sometimes the appropriate response is not achieved and acute or chronic renal failure develops. Renal disorders are the most frequent cause of hypertension in children.

Take Note!

Severe hypertension (blood pressure higher than the 99th percentile for age and sex) may lead to damage of the eye or vital organs (kidney, brain, or heart), or even death (Mattoo, 2016). Nurses must be adept at accurately measuring blood pressure in children.

Nephrotic Syndrome

Nephrotic syndrome occurs as a result of increased glomerular basement membrane permeability, which allows abnormal loss of protein in the urine. Nephrotic syndrome generally occurs in three forms—congenital, idiopathic, and secondary.

Congenital nephrotic syndrome is an inherited disorder; it is rare and occurs primarily in families of Finnish descent. The prognosis is poor, though some success has occurred with early, aggressive treatment and with the advances in kidney transplantation in infants (Lum, 2014). Nephrotic syndrome may also occur secondary to another condition such as systemic lupus erythematosus, Henoch–Schönlein purpura, or diabetes.

Idiopathic nephrotic syndrome is the most commonly occurring type in children and is also called minimal change nephrotic syndrome (MCNS). MCNS most often has its onset in children by age 6 years (Lum, 2014). This discussion will focus primarily on MCNS. Complications of nephrotic syndrome include anemia, infection, poor growth, peritonitis, thrombosis, and renal failure.

PATHOPHYSIOLOGY

Increased glomerular permeability results in the passage of larger plasma proteins through the glomerular basement membrane. This results in excess loss of protein (albumin) in the urine (**proteinuria**) and decreased protein and albumin (hypoalbuminemia) in the bloodstream. Protein loss in nephrotic syndrome tends to be almost exclusively albumin. Hypoalbuminemia results in a change in osmotic pressure, and fluid shifts from the bloodstream into the interstitial tissue (causing edema). This decrease in blood volume triggers the kidneys to respond by conserving sodium and water, leading to further edema. The liver senses the protein loss and increases production of lipoproteins. Hyperlipidemia then develops as the excess lipids cannot be excreted in the urine. Hyperlipidemia associated with nephrotic syndrome may be quite severe, yet cholesterol levels may decrease when the nephrotic syndrome is in remission, only to rise significantly again with a relapse.

Children with nephrotic syndrome are at increased risk for clotting (thromboembolism) because of the decreased intravascular volume. They are also at increased risk for the development of serious infection, most commonly pneumococcal pneumonia, sepsis, or spontaneous peritonitis. Steroid-resistant nephrotic syndrome may result in acute renal failure.

THERAPEUTIC MANAGEMENT

Medical management of MCNS usually involves the use of corticosteroids. Intravenous albumin may be used in the severely edematous child. Diuretics are also required in the edematous phase. Long-term therapy is usually required to induce remission. The nephrologist will determine the length of therapy based on the child's response. Children who have steroid-responsive MCNS generally have a favorable prognosis. Some children with MCNS exhibit a minimal response to steroid therapy or experience remissions and the MCNS is steroid resistant (Lum, 2014). Immunosuppressive therapy such as cyclophosphamide, cyclosporine A, or mycophenolate mofetil may be necessary.

NURSING ASSESSMENT

For a full description of the assessment phase of the nursing process, refer to the Assessment section of the Nursing Process Overview earlier in the chapter. Assessment findings pertinent to MCNS are discussed below.

Health History. Elicit a description of the present illness and chief complaint. Common signs and symptoms reported during the health history might include:

- Nausea or vomiting (may be related to ascites)
- Recent weight gain
- History of periorbital edema upon waking, progressing to generalized edema throughout the day
- Weakness or fatigue
- Irritability or fussiness

Explore the child's current and past medical history for risk factors such as:

- Intrauterine growth retardation
- Young age (younger than 3 years)
- Male sex

Physical Examination. The physical assessment of the child with nephrotic syndrome includes inspection and observation, auscultation, and palpation.

Observe the child for edema (periorbital, generalized [**anasarca**], or abdominal ascites). As the disease progresses, the edema also progresses to become more generalized, eventually becoming severe. Inspect the skin for a stretched, tight appearance; pallor; or skin breakdown related to significant edema (Fig. 43.6). Document height (or length) and weight. Note increased respiratory rate or increased work of breathing related to ascites and edema.

Note the blood pressure; it may be elevated in the child with nephrotic syndrome, though it is most often either normal or decreased unless the child is progressing to renal failure. Auscultate heart and lung sounds, noting abnormalities related to fluid overload. Palpate the skin, noting tautness. Palpate the abdomen and document the presence of ascites.

Laboratory and Diagnostic Tests. Urine dipstick will reveal marked proteinuria. Infrequently, mild hematuria is also present. Serum protein and albumin levels will be low (often markedly so). Serum cholesterol and triglyceride levels are elevated. With continued nephrotic syndrome, creatinine and BUN may become elevated.

NURSING MANAGEMENT

Goals for nursing management include promoting diuresis, preventing infection, promoting adequate nutrition, and educating the parents about ongoing care at home. As with other chronic disorders, provide ongoing emotional support to the child and family.

Promoting Diuresis. Administer corticosteroids as ordered. Tapering or weaning doses are required when the time comes to stop corticosteroid therapy. Administer diuretics if ordered, usually furosemide. Children may develop hypokalemia because of potassium loss as an adverse effect of furosemide. Those children may require potassium supplementation or a diet higher in

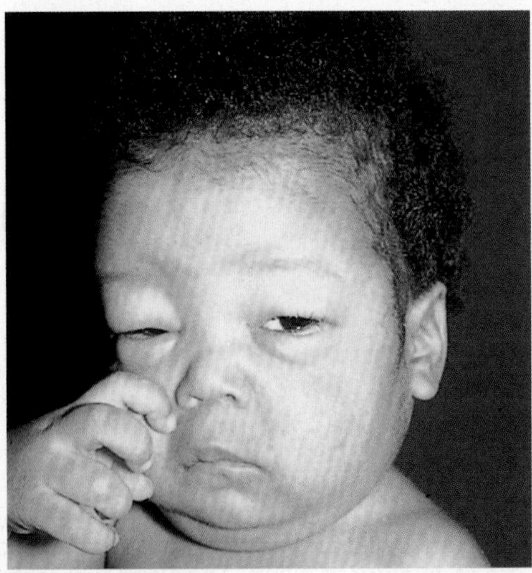

FIGURE 43.6 Note marked edema associated with nephrotic syndrome.

potassium-containing foods. Monitor urine output and the amount of protein in the urine (by dipstick). Weigh the child daily on the same scale either naked or wearing the same amount of clothing. Assess for resolution of edema. Measure pulse rate and blood pressure every 4 hours to detect hypovolemia resulting from excessive fluid shifts. Enforce oral fluid restrictions if ordered.

In cases of severe hypoalbuminemia, intravenous albumin may be administered. Increases in the serum albumin level cause fluid to shift from the subcutaneous spaces back into the bloodstream. A diuretic such as furosemide administered immediately after the albumin infusion allows for optimal diuresis and prevents fluid overload. Refer to Drug Guide 43.1 for the nursing implications related to use of these medications.

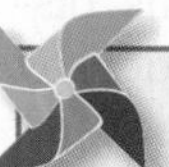

Consider This

Thirteen-year-old Jimmy Sanderson has a history of steroid-responsive nephrotic syndrome. In the clinic today he tells you, "I am not going to take those steroids any more!" "I am shorter than everyone in my class, my 11-year-old brother is taller than me." "It's just not fair, I'll never get a girlfriend, if I'm a shorty."

Think back to when you were an adolescent. How would you have felt if you had a chronic illness and your necessary medications stunted your growth? As the nurse, how can you help Jimmy in this situation?

Preventing Infection. Monitor the child's temperature. Administer pneumococcal vaccine as prescribed (see Chapter 31 for information on immunizations). Administer prophylactic antibiotics, if prescribed. Delay administering live vaccines until at least 2 weeks after corticosteroid or other immunosuppressive medication therapy ceases. Teach parents that if the child is unimmunized and is exposed to chickenpox, the parents should notify the child's pediatrician, nurse practitioner, or nephrologist immediately so that the child may receive varicella zoster immunoglobulin.

Encouraging Adequate Nutrition and Growth. Encourage a nutrient-rich diet within prescribed restrictions. Fluid restriction is reserved for children with massive edema. Sodium intake may be restricted in the edematous child in an effort to prevent further fluid retention. Consultation with the dietitian is often helpful in meal planning because many of the foods that children like are high in sodium. Encourage protein-rich snacks. Consult with the child and family in planning meals and snacks that the child likes and will be likely to consume. Use of nutritional supplement shakes may be helpful for some children.

Educating the Family. Teach parents how to give medications and monitor for adverse effects. Demonstrate the urine dipstick technique for detecting protein, and encourage the family to keep a chart of dipstick results. The child may return to school but should avoid contact with sick playmates. If the child is exposed to another child with an infectious illness, explain to the parents that they should monitor temperature and urine dipstick results more frequently to identify a relapse in nephrotic syndrome early so that treatment can begin.

Providing Emotional Support. Nephrotic syndrome is often a chronic condition, and children who are responsive to steroid treatment may enter remission only to experience relapse. This cycle of relapse and remission takes an emotional toll on the child and family. Frequent hospitalizations require the child to miss school and the parents to miss work; this creates further stress for the family. The child may experience social isolation because he or she must avoid exposure to infections or because of self-esteem problems. The child may be dissatisfied with his or her appearance because of edema and weight gain, short stature, and the classic "moon face" associated with chronic steroid use.

Provide emotional support to the child and family. Encourage them in their efforts to maintain the treatment plan. Introduce the child to other youngsters with chronic renal conditions. Refer families to the National Kidney Foundation, a link to which can be found on thePoint, for information about local support groups and resources.

Acute Post-streptococcal Glomerulonephritis

Acute post-streptococcal glomerulonephritis (APSGN) is a condition in which immune processes injure the glomeruli. Immune mechanisms cause inflammation, which results in altered glomerular structure and function in both kidneys. It often occurs following an infection, usually an upper respiratory or skin infection. APSGN is caused by an antibody–antigen reaction secondary to an infection with a nephritogenic strain of group A β-hemolytic streptococcus. APSGN occurs more frequently in males than females and more frequently between the ages of 5 and 12 years (Gaylord & Petersen-Smith, 2013). The most serious complication is progression to uremia and renal failure (either acute or chronic).

There is no specific medical treatment for APSGN. Treatment is aimed at maintaining fluid volume and managing hypertension. If there is evidence of a current streptococcal infection, antibiotic therapy will be necessary.

NURSING ASSESSMENT

For a full description of the assessment phase of the nursing process, refer to the Assessment section of the

Nursing Process Overview earlier in the chapter. Assessment findings pertinent to acute glomerulonephritis are discussed below.

Health History. Elicit a description of the present illness and chief complaint. Common signs and symptoms reported during the health history might include:

- Fever
- Lethargy
- Headache
- Decreased urine output
- Abdominal pain
- Vomiting
- Anorexia

Assess the child's current and past medical history for risk factors such as a recent episode of pharyngitis or other streptococcal infection, age older than 2 years, or male sex.

Physical Examination and Laboratory and Diagnostic Tests. Assess the child's blood pressure for elevation, which is common. Note the presence of mild edema. Observe for signs of cardiopulmonary congestion such as increased work of breathing or cough. Auscultate the lungs for crackles and the heart for gallop. The urine dipstick test will reveal proteinuria as well as hematuria. Inspect the urine for gross hematuria, which will cause the urine to appear tea colored, cola colored, or even a dirty green color. Serum creatinine and BUN may be normal or elevated, the serum complement level is depressed, and the erythrocyte sedimentation rate is elevated. Laboratory findings specific to streptococcus include an elevated antistreptolysin O (ASO) titer and an elevated DNAase B antigen titer.

NURSING MANAGEMENT

Administer antihypertensives such as labetalol or nifedipine and diuretics as ordered. Monitor blood pressure frequently. Maintain sodium and fluid restrictions as prescribed during the initial edematous phase. Weigh the child daily on the same scale wearing the same amount of clothing. Monitor increasing urine output and note improvement in the urine color. Document resolution of edema. Provide a careful neurologic evaluation, as hypertension may cause encephalopathy and seizures. Children with APSGN generally are fatigued and choose bed rest during the acute phase. Provide the child with age-appropriate activities and cluster care to allow rest periods.

Some children may be managed at home if edema is mild and they are not hypertensive. Teach the family to monitor urine output and color, take blood pressure measurements, and restrict the diet as prescribed. The child cared for at home should not participate in strenuous activity until proteinuria and hematuria are resolved. If renal involvement progresses, dialysis may become necessary.

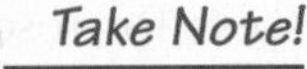

Take Note!

Avoid use of nonsteroidal anti-inflammatory drugs (NSAIDs) in children with questionable renal function, as the antiprostaglandin action of NSAIDs may cause a further decrease in the glomerular filtration rate (Solomon, 2015).

Hemolytic-Uremic Syndrome

Hemolytic-uremic syndrome (HUS) is defined by three features—hemolytic anemia, thrombocytopenia, and acute renal failure. Typical HUS features an antecedent diarrheal illness. Other causes of HUS include idiopathic, inherited, drug-related, association with malignancies, transplantation, and malignant hypertension. This discussion will focus on typical HUS, the type preceded by a diarrheal illness. Watery diarrhea progresses to hemorrhagic colitis, then to the triad of HUS. The features of HUS, as well as effects on other organs, are caused primarily by microthrombi and ischemic changes within the organs. The thrombotic events in the small blood vessels of the glomerulus lead to occlusion of the glomerular capillary loops and glomerulosclerosis, resulting in renal failure.

A verotoxin-producing strain of *E. coli,* O157:H7, causes the majority of cases, though *Streptococcus pneumoniae, Shigella dysenteriae,* and other bacteria may also be the cause (Tan & Silverberg, 2015). It is thought that antibiotic treatment for the bacteria may contribute to release of the verotoxin. Undercooked ground beef accounts for most cases of *E. coli* O157:H7 infection, but it is also transmitted via the feces of numerous animals as well as unpasteurized dairy and fruit products. Transmission also occurs via human feces, and cases have been linked to public swimming pools. HUS occurs most often in children age 6 months to 4 years (Tan & Silverberg, 2015). Complications include chronic renal failure, seizures and coma, pancreatitis, intussusception, rectal prolapse, cardiomyopathy, congestive heart failure, and acute respiratory distress syndrome.

Therapeutic management of HUS is directed toward maintaining fluid balance; correcting hypertension, acidosis, and electrolyte abnormalities; replenishing circulating red blood cells; and providing dialysis if needed.

NURSING ASSESSMENT

For a full description of the assessment phase of the nursing process, refer to the Assessment section of the Nursing Process Overview earlier in the chapter. Assessment findings pertinent to HUS are discussed below.

Health History. Elicit a description of the present illness and chief complaint. Common signs and symptoms reported during the health history might include watery diarrhea accompanied by cramping and sometimes vomiting. After several days, the diarrhea becomes bloody and eventually improves.

Explore the child's current and past medical history for risk factors such as ingestion of ground beef, visits to a water park or to a petting zoo before the onset of the diarrheal illness, or use of antidiarrheal medications or antibiotics.

Physical Examination. Observe the child for pallor, toxic appearance, edema, **oliguria** (decreased urine output), or **anuria** (absent urine output). Assess for elevated blood pressure and tenderness in the abdomen. Assess the child for neurologic involvement, which may include irritability, altered level of consciousness, seizures, posturing, or coma.

Laboratory and Diagnostic Tests. Urinalysis may reveal the presence of blood, protein, pus, and/or casts. Serum laboratory abnormalities are numerous and may include:

- Elevated BUN and creatinine
- Moderate to severe anemia (with the presence of Burr cells, schistocytes, spherocytes, or helmet cells), mild to severe thrombocytopenia
- Increased reticulocyte count
- Increased bilirubin and lactic dehydrogenase (LDH) levels
- Negative Coombs test (except in cases of *Streptococcus pneumoniae* infection)
- Leukocytosis with left shift
- Hyponatremia
- Hyperkalemia
- Hyperphosphatemia
- Metabolic acidosis

NURSING MANAGEMENT

Nursing management of the child with HUS focuses on close observation and monitoring of the child's status. Institute and maintain contact precautions to prevent spread of *E. coli* O157:H7 to other children (bacteria are shed for up to 17 days after resolution of the diarrhea). Close attention must be paid to fluid volume status. Prevention of HUS is also an important nursing function.

Maintaining Appropriate Fluid Volume Balance. Maintain strict intake and output monitoring and recording to evaluate the progression toward renal failure. Carefully monitor intravenous infusions and blood chemistries. Administer diuretics as ordered. Assess blood pressure frequently and report elevations to the physician or nurse practitioner. Administer antihypertensives as ordered and monitor their effectiveness. Encourage adequate nutritional intake within the constraints of prescribed dietary restrictions. Monitor for bleeding as well as for fatigue and pallor. Follow the institutional protocol for transfusion of packed red blood cells and/or platelets (platelets are usually transfused only if active bleeding or severe thrombocytopenia occurs). Report progressive deterioration in laboratory findings to the physician or nurse practitioner. Some children with HUS will require dialysis for at least several days.

Preventing Hemolytic-Uremic Syndrome. Proper hand washing is necessary. Teach children to wash their hands after using the bathroom, before eating, and after petting farm animals. Encourage the use of "swim diapers," which contain feces, for children who are not toilet trained. Teach parents to thoroughly cook all meats to a core temperature of 155°F, or until the meat is gray or brown throughout and the juices from the meat are clear rather than pink. Wash all fruits and vegetables thoroughly. Ensure that drinking water and water used for recreation are treated appropriately. Avoid unpasteurized dairy products and fruit juices (including cider).

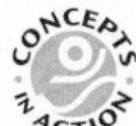 Renal Failure

Renal failure is a condition in which the kidneys cannot concentrate urine, conserve electrolytes, or excrete waste products. As in adults, renal failure in children may occur as an acute or chronic condition. Some cases of acute renal failure resolve without further complications, while dialysis is necessary in other children. When acute renal failure continues to progress, it becomes chronic (also known as end-stage renal disease [ESRD]). Dialysis and kidney transplantation are treatment modalities used for ESRD.

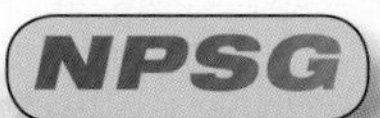

GOAL 2: Improve the Effectiveness of Communication Among Caregivers. (Improve staff communication)

NPSG.02.03.01 Report critical results of tests and diagnostic procedures on a timely basis.

Steps: When caring for a child with a renal disorder notify appropriate healthcare provider with critical lab values (often-times potassium), and critical changes to other laboratory values.

Joint Commission. (2015). *National patient safety goals effective January 1, 2015.* Retrieved from http://www.jointcommission.org/assets/1/6/2015_NPSG_HAP.pdf

Acute Renal Failure

Acute renal failure is defined as a sudden, often reversible, decline in renal function that results in the accumulation of metabolic toxins (particularly nitrogenous wastes) as well as fluid and electrolyte imbalance. Fluid overload may lead to hypertension, pulmonary edema, and congestive heart failure. Additional complications include hyperkalemia, metabolic acidosis, hyperphosphatemia, and uremia. In children, acute renal failure most commonly occurs as a result of decreased renal perfusion, as occurs in hypovolemic or septic shock. It may also occur in children with hemolytic anemia or as a result of nephrotoxicity from medications. Complications include anemia, hyperkalemia, hypertension, pulmonary edema, cardiac failure, and altered level of consciousness or seizures. In addition, acute renal failure may also progress to a chronic state.

Therapeutic management is aimed at treating the underlying cause, managing the fluid and electrolyte disturbances, and decreasing blood pressure.

Take Note!

Medications commonly used in children can reduce renal function. Cephalosporins may cause a transient increase in BUN and creatinine. Truly nephrotoxic drugs often used in children include aminoglycosides, sulfonamides, vancomycin, and NSAIDs. Make sure that potentially nephrotoxic drugs are administered according to published safe guidelines (dosage, frequency, rate of administration) (Taketomo, Hodding, & Kraus, 2013).

NURSING ASSESSMENT

For a full description of the assessment phase of the nursing process, refer to the Assessment section of the Nursing Process Overview earlier in the chapter. Assessment findings pertinent to acute renal failure are discussed below.

Health History. Elicit a description of the present illness and chief complaint. Common signs and symptoms reported during the health history might include:

- Nausea
- Vomiting
- Diarrhea
- Lethargy
- Fever
- Decreased urine output

Assess the child's current and past medical history for risk factors such as history of shock, trauma, burns, urologic abnormalities, renal disease, use of nephrotoxic medications, or severe blood transfusion reaction.

Physical Examination and Laboratory and Diagnostic Tests. Note decreased skin elasticity, dry mucous membranes, or edema. Auscultate the lungs for crackles, which may occur with pulmonary edema. Document tachypnea. Note cardiac rhythm disturbances. Evaluate the child's level of consciousness. Laboratory tests will reveal increased serum creatinine levels and possible electrolyte disturbances, such as hyperkalemia or hypocalcemia. Urinalysis may reveal proteinuria or hematuria.

Take Note!

Monitor the infant or child with renal failure carefully for signs of congestive heart failure, such as edema accompanied by bounding pulse, presence of an S_3 heart sound, adventitious lung sounds, and shortness of breath.

NURSING MANAGEMENT

Nursing care focuses on managing hypertension, restoring fluid and electrolyte balance, and educating the family.

Managing Hypertension. Carefully monitor the child's blood pressure. Administer antihypertensives as prescribed. When a fast-acting drug such as nifedipine (Procardia) sublingually or labetalol intravenously is used, stay with the child and frequently monitor blood pressure. Immediately notify the physician or nurse practitioner if high blood pressure is resistant to medication and the blood pressure remains elevated.

Restoring Fluid and Electrolyte Balance. Monitor vital signs frequently and assess urine specific gravity. Maintain strict records of intake and output. Administer diuretics as ordered. When urine output is restored, diuresis may be significant. Monitor for signs of hyperkalemia (weak, irregular pulse; muscle weakness; abdominal cramping) and hypocalcemia (muscle twitching or tetany). Administer polystyrene sulfonate as ordered orally, rectally, or through a nasogastric tube to decrease potassium levels. polystyrene sulfonate removes potassium primarily by exchanging sodium for it, which is then eliminated in the feces. Administer packed red blood cell transfusions as ordered (may need to be followed by a dose of diuretic). Dialysis may become necessary if oliguria is sustained and leads to significant fluid overload, the electrolyte imbalance reaches dangerous levels, or uremia results in depression of the central nervous system.

Providing Family Education. Educate the family about the plan of care and the need for fluid restriction, if ordered. Instruct the family to save all voids for observation and measurement by the nurse. Provide education about the use of dialysis if relevant.

End-Stage Renal Disease

ESRD is chronic renal failure requiring long-term dialysis or renal transplantation. Chronic renal failure in children most often results from congenital structural defects such as obstructive uropathy (Klein, 2010). It may also be caused by an inherited condition such as familial nephritis or may result from an acquired problem such as glomerulonephritis; it may follow an infectious process such as pyelonephritis or HUS (Klein, 2010). This is in contrast to chronic renal failure in adults, which primarily results from diabetes or hypertension.

Uremia, hypocalcemia, hyperkalemia, and metabolic acidosis occur. Complications of ESRD are many. Uremic toxins deplete erythrocytes and the failing kidneys cannot produce erythropoietin, so severe anemia results. Hypertension is common and heart failure may occur. Hypocalcemia results in renal rickets (brittle bones). Growth is retarded and sexual maturation may be delayed or

HEALTHY PEOPLE 2020

Objective	Nursing Significance
Reduce the rate of new cases of end-stage renal disease (ESRD).	• Encourage compliance with medical regimens related to urinary tract disorders in order to prevent progression to chronic renal failure

Healthy People Objectives retrieved from http://www.healthypeople.gov

absent. Many children with ESRD experience depression, anxiety, impaired social interaction, and poor self-esteem (Klein, 2010). See Healthy People 2020.

NURSING ASSESSMENT

For a full description of the assessment phase of the nursing process, refer to the Assessment section of the Nursing Process Overview earlier in the chapter. Assessment findings pertinent to ESRD are discussed below.

Health History. Explore the health history for low birthweight (associated with kidney dysfunction and anatomic alterations), poor growth (weight, length/height, and head circumference), and regimen of dialysis. Note decreased appetite or energy level, dry or itchy skin, or bone or joint pain.

Physical Examination and Laboratory and Diagnostic Tests. Perform a thorough physical assessment, noting any abnormalities (may vary from child to child). If present, assess the peritoneal catheter site for absence of drainage, bleeding, or redness. If the child undergoes hemodialysis, assess the fistula or graft site for the presence of a bruit and a thrill. Laboratory tests may reveal low hemoglobin and hematocrit, increased serum phosphorus and potassium levels, and decreased sodium, calcium, and bicarbonate levels. BUN, uric acid, and creatinine levels will be elevated. A 24-hour urine creatinine clearance test will show increased amounts of creatinine in the urine, reflecting decreasing kidney function.

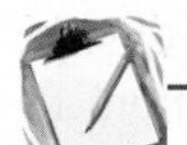

Take Note!

Carefully assess children with ESRD for worsening uremia or metabolic acidosis. Uremia may result in central nervous system symptoms such as headache or coma, or gastrointestinal or neuromuscular disturbances. Metabolic acidosis causes lethargy, dull headache, and confusion.

NURSING MANAGEMENT

Nursing goals for the child with ESRD include promoting growth and development, removing waste products and maintaining fluid balance via dialysis, encouraging psychosocial well-being, and supporting and educating the family.

Promoting Growth and Development. Encourage the child to choose foods he or she likes that are within the imposed dietary restrictions. Daily protein requirements for adequate growth range from 0.9 to 1.5 g of protein per kilogram of weight. Sodium and/or potassium restrictions may also be necessary. Enforce fluid restrictions if prescribed. Administer medications such as erythropoietin, growth hormone, and vitamin and mineral supplements to augment nutritional status and promote growth. Table 43.2 lists medications and supplements used to support growth.

Encouraging Psychosocial Well-Being. The child with chronic renal failure and particularly ESRD often suffers from depression and anxiety. Refer children and their families to the hospital social worker or counselor as needed for depression or anxiety issues. The chronic need for dialysis (daily with peritoneal dialysis or three or

TABLE 43.2 MEDICATIONS AND SUPPLEMENTS COMMONLY USED TO TREAT ESRD COMPLICATIONS

Medication or Supplement	Purpose
Vitamin D and calcium	Correction of hypocalcemia and hyperphosphatemia
Ferrous sulfate	Treatment of anemia
Bicitra or sodium bicarbonate tablets	Correction of acidosis
Multivitamin	Augment nutritional status
Erythropoietin injections	Stimulate red blood cell growth
Growth hormone injections	Stimulate growth in stature

Adapted from Klein, M. S. (2010). Kidney disease, chronic. In P. J. Allen, J. A. Vessey, and N. A. Schapiro (Eds.), *Primary care of the child with a chronic condition* (5th ed.). St. Louis, MO: Mosby.

four times per week with hemodialysis) confers long-term stress on the child and family. The child usually demonstrates poor growth and often suffers from body image disturbance. Frequent medical appointments and hospitalizations interfere with the child's scholastic achievements. Introduce the child to other children with ESRD (this often happens anyway at the hemodialysis center).

Ensure that the family is aware of financial and support resources within the community and refer them to the National Kidney Foundation. Also suggest the American Kidney Fund, which provides financial aid and access to summer camps for children with renal problems. Links to both of these resources are located on thePoint. Camp is an excellent way for children to demonstrate that they have mastered some of the loss-of-control issues related to their disease.

Several websites provide forums for children and teens with kidney failure or transplantation so they can learn about their disease, access resources, and/or communicate with other children. Links to such websites are available on thePoint.

Dialysis and Transplantation

Peritoneal dialysis or hemodialysis is required on a long-term basis for children with chronic renal failure or ESRD. Once the child has progressed to ESRD, kidney transplantation is needed in order for the child to progress with normal growth and development.

Peritoneal Dialysis

Peritoneal dialysis uses the child's abdominal cavity as a semipermeable membrane to help remove excess fluid and waste products (Figs. 43.7 and 43.8). The parent or caregiver performs peritoneal dialysis at home after completing a training course. The process is either completed overnight with the use of a machine (continuous cyclic peritoneal dialysis) or in increments throughout the day for a total of 4 to 8 hours (continuous ambulatory peritoneal dialysis). Comparison Chart 43.1 compares these two methods of peritoneal dialysis.

BOX 43.2

RISKS ASSOCIATED WITH PERITONEAL DIALYSIS

- Hypertension and other cardiac complications
- Seizures
- Obstructed catheter
- Dialysate leakage
- Hyperglycemia
- Increased triglyceride levels
- Increased protein loss
- Parental stress and burnout related to repetitive nature of daily intervention

The advantages of peritoneal dialysis over hemodialysis include improved growth as a result of more dietary freedom, increased independence in daily activities, and a steadier state of electrolyte balance. However, the risk for infection (peritonitis and sepsis) is a continual concern with peritoneal dialysis (Klein, 2010). Dialysate exchange protocols, care of the catheter in the abdomen, and dressing changes must all be performed using sterile technique to avoid introducing microorganisms into the peritoneal cavity. Box 43.2 lists additional risks associated with peritoneal dialysis.

Hemodialysis

Hemodialysis removes toxins and excess fluid from the blood by pumping the child's blood through a hemodialysis machine and then reinfusing the blood into the child. Needles to remove and reinfuse the blood are inserted into an arteriovenous fistula or graft, usually located in the child's arm (Figs. 43.9 and 43.10).

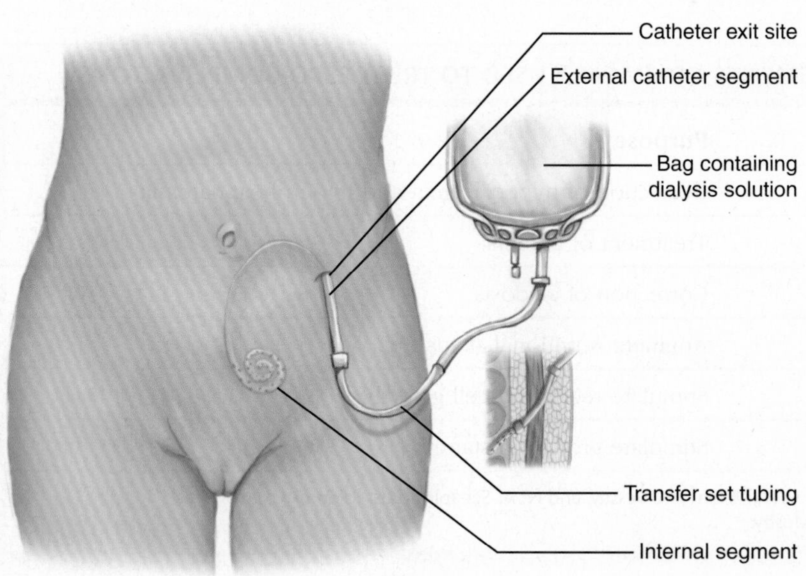

FIGURE 43.7 The peritoneal dialysis catheter is tunneled under the skin into the peritoneal cavity.

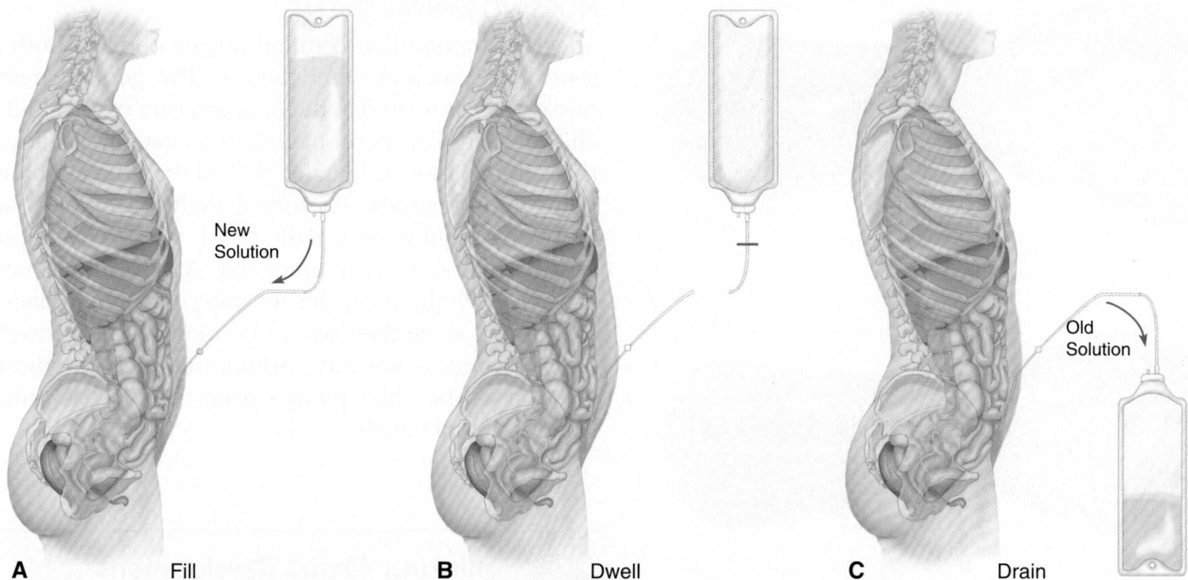

FIGURE 43.8 (**A**) During the "fill" phase of peritoneal dialysis, dialysate fluid is instilled into the peritoneal cavity. (**B**) During the "dwell" phase, the child may be up out of bed with the empty dialysate bag folded up with the tubing under his clothing. (**C**) During the "drain" phase, the old dialysate is drained from the peritoneum by gravity, bringing with it waste products and excess fluid. The dialysate bags are weighed prior to filling and after draining to determine the amount of fluid removed from the child.

Hemodialysis frees the parent from the need to perform daily dialysis, but the procedure, which takes 3 to 6 hours, must be done two to four times per week (usually three) at a pediatric hemodialysis center. This requires time away from school and other activities for the child and from work and other family responsibilities for the parent. Since hemodialysis is usually performed only every other day, larger amounts of waste products build up in the child's blood (uremia), placing the child at higher risk for seizures. The access site may become infected, and occlusion is also possible. The child must follow a stricter diet between hemodialysis treatments, though dietary restrictions are usually lifted while the child is actually undergoing the treatment.

NURSING ASSESSMENT

Refer to the section on nursing assessment of the child with chronic renal failure/ESRD, as it is similar to assessment of the child undergoing dialysis. Assess for alterations in blood pressure and laboratory values following dialysis. Monitor for signs and symptoms of infection.

Assess the child receiving peritoneal dialysis for toleration of the fluid volume instilled within the peritoneum. The abdomen will remain distended while the fluid is indwelling and will be significantly flatter when the fluid is drained. Assess the Tenckhoff catheter site for signs of infection. Monitor the child's temperature. Inspect the dialysate effluent for fibrin or cloudiness, which may indicate

COMPARISON CHART 43.1 METHODS OF PERITONEAL DIALYSIS

	Continuous Ambulatory Peritoneal Dialysis (CAPD)	Continuous Cyclic Peritoneal Dialysis (CCPD)
When performed	Throughout the day, with exchanges every 3 to 6 hours. Fluid is usually allowed to dwell overnight to allow child to sleep	Usually overnight while child is sleeping
Method	Manual instillation and draining and changing of dialysate bags with each exchange	Automated via CCPD machine; bags and tubing are attached when started, then disconnected in the morning
Dwell time	3 to 6 hours	Usually 30 minutes to 1 hour
Mobility	Allows for mobility and permits child to participate in activities between exchanges	Child is confined to bed during the night while CCPD is ongoing but completely mobile while off CCPD during the day

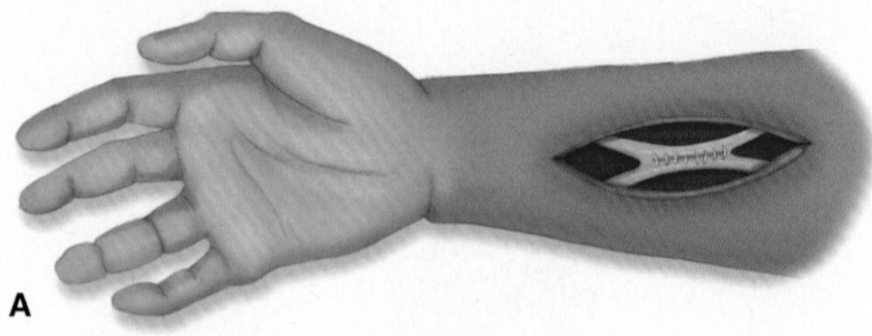

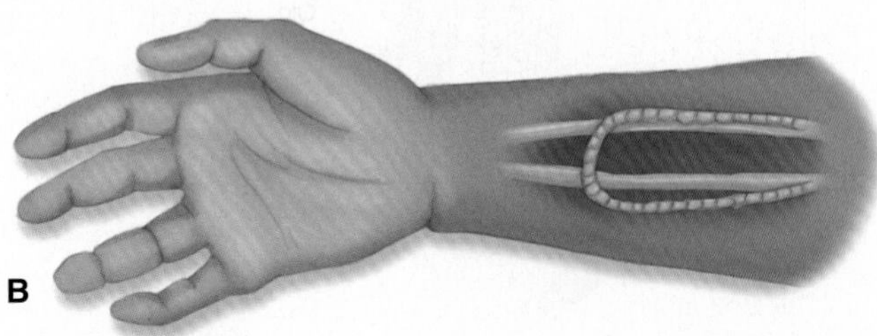

FIGURE 43.9 **(A)** Arteriovenous fistula. **(B)** Arteriovenous graft.

infection. Weigh the child daily (in the drain phase if on peritoneal dialysis).

For the child who receives hemodialysis, assess the arteriovenous fistula or graft site with each set of vital signs. Auscultate the site for the presence of a bruit and palpate for the presence of a thrill. Notify the physician or nurse practitioner immediately if either is absent.

Take Note!

Avoid taking blood pressure, performing venipuncture, or using a tourniquet in the extremity with the arteriovenous fistula or graft; these procedures may cause occlusion and subsequent malfunction of the fistula or graft. Teach parents and children to inform all healthcare providers they come in contact with about the presence of the fistula or graft.

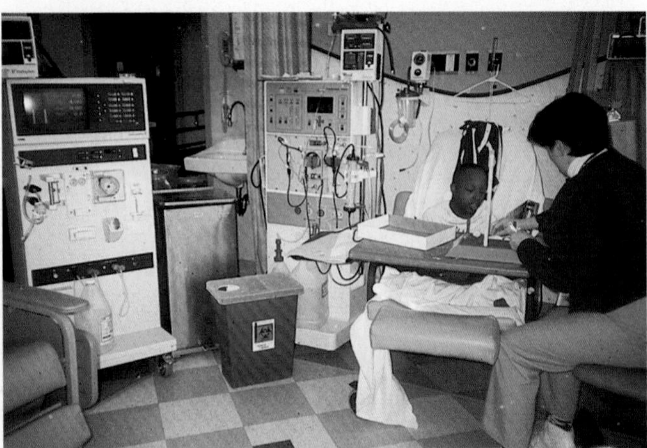

FIGURE 43.10 Pediatric hemodialysis.

NURSING MANAGEMENT

Specially trained and certified nurses perform both peritoneal dialysis and hemodialysis. The general pediatric nurse's role is related to the ongoing care of the child. The child undergoing peritoneal dialysis usually is allowed a more liberal diet and intake of fluid than the child undergoing hemodialysis. Peritoneal dialysis removes waste and excess fluids on a daily basis, whereas hemodialysis occurs about every other day. Most routine medications are withheld on the morning that hemodialysis is scheduled, since they would be filtered out through the dialysis process anyway. Administer these medications as soon as the child returns from the dialysis unit. See Healthy People 2020.

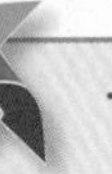

Thinking About Development

Trevon Smith is a 17-year-old male football player who was on track for a college scholarship. Following an episode of acute glomerulonephritis, Trevon has progressed to chronic renal failure and is dependent upon hemodialysis. He is listed for a kidney transplant.

How will Trevon's developmental stage affect his desire to comply with the medical regimen? What types of psychosocial issues might Trevon be experiencing and how can the nurse best support Trevon at this time?

How will the nurse educate Trevon about self-care?

HEALTHY PEOPLE 2020

Objective	Nursing Significance
Increase the proportion of new hemodialysis patients who use arteriovenous fistulas as the primary mode of vascular access. Increase the proportion of dialysis patients registered on the waiting list for transplantation.	• Educate families about the benefits of an arteriovenous fistula over other methods of hemodialysis access. • Advocate for the child to obtain an arteriovenous fistula. • Educate families about transplantation, and if no living-related match is available, encourage the family to seek placement on the organ transplant waiting list.

Healthy People Objectives retrieved from http://www.healthypeople.gov

Renal Transplantation

Renal transplantation is the optimal treatment for ESRD and offers the best opportunity for the child to live a normal life. Vigilant medication administration is necessary after the transplant to prevent organ rejection. The child achieves improved renal function with the transplant and may demonstrate improved growth, enhanced cognitive development, and improved psychosocial development and quality of life.

Kidneys are obtained from a cadaver (a patient declared brain-dead who had previously given consent to organ donation) or from a blood relative (living-related). The transplanted kidney must match the child's blood type and the child's human leukocyte antigens (HLAs). The cadaver kidney or living-related kidney is implanted surgically in the abdomen and the blood vessels are anastomosed to the aorta and superior vena cava.

Generally, living-related transplants have a decreased rejection rate compared to cadaver transplants (Klein & Martin, 2010). Living-related kidney donation and subsequent transplantation can be planned ahead and scheduled in advance. In contrast, cadaver kidneys become available suddenly, leaving less time for preoperative preparation. For either type, last-minute blood tissue typing is required before the final decision is made to move forward with transplantation. Often the child's native kidneys are removed before or at the time of the renal transplant because of their association with hypertension in the child (Klein & Martin, 2010).

Take Note!

Cadaver kidneys are allocated to potential recipients based on the age of the child with renal failure, the time that he or she has been awaiting a transplant, blood type, HLA antibody matching, panel reactive antibodies, and region of the country (so that the donated kidney can be received expeditiously).

NURSING ASSESSMENT

A thorough physical assessment is warranted for any child undergoing renal transplant, whether in the initial postoperative period, at a clinic visit, or when admitted to the hospital, to rule out transplant rejection. Note recent health history, medications and their doses, and any symptoms the child has been having. In the initial postoperative period, assess the incision for redness, edema, or drainage. If any of these signs of infection or rejection occur, notify the transplant surgeon and nephrologist immediately. Monitor blood pressure and other vital signs closely. Document resolution of edema. Record intake and output accurately. Assess for signs and symptoms of transplant rejection such as malaise, fever, unexplained weight gain, or pain over the transplant area.

NURSING MANAGEMENT

Postoperative care focuses on preventing rejection, monitoring renal function, maintaining fluid and electrolyte balance, and educating the child and family.

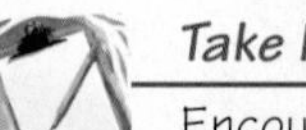

Take Note!

Encourage the child with a renal transplant to wear a medical alert necklace or bracelet, and urge the parents to inform community emergency services of the child's transplant status.

Preventing Rejection and Promoting Renal Function. Administer immunosuppressants accurately and in a timely fashion. Obtain and monitor serum levels of these medications per protocol. Immediately report significant alterations in vital signs or edema at the surgical site, as they may indicate transplant rejection. Maintain strict documentation of intake and output. Once adequate urine output is established, intake is usually liberalized.

Educating the Child and Family. Develop a schedule to cluster care so that the child may receive the rest needed for recovery despite the many and frequent assessments and interventions. With the family, develop a medication schedule that will be compatible with the family's life at home as well as the restrictions related to some medications. Begin teaching with the family as soon as the child's condition is stable. Accurate medication administration and home monitoring are necessary to prevent rejection. The child may return to school when discharged from the hospital, but the family will need to communicate closely with the school nurse about the child's immunosuppressed status. The American Nephrology Nurses Association has developed a renal transplant fact sheet that can be shared with the school nurse. A link to the association's website is located on thePoint.

Take Note!

Tell the parents to inform their child's physician or nurse practitioner about the child's long-term corticosteroid use and/or immunosuppressed status, as the child should not receive any live vaccines.

REPRODUCTIVE ORGAN DISORDERS

A number of disorders may occur within the female or male genitalia and internal reproductive organs in children. These problems may be structural or infectious.

Female Disorders

Disorders of the female reproductive organs that occur in children and adolescents include structural disorders, infectious disorders, and menstrual disorders.

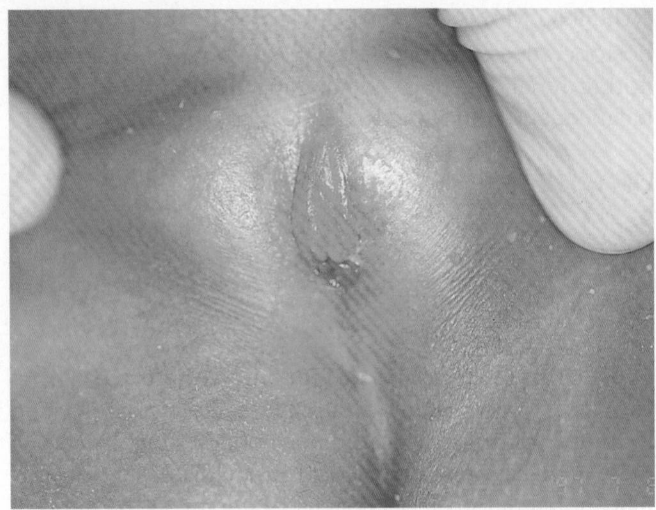

FIGURE 43.11 Labial adhesions. Note fusion of the labia minora. Copyrighted 2011. UBM Medica LLC.82486:1111JM

Labial Adhesions

Labial adhesion or labial fusion is partial or complete adherence of the labia minora (Fig. 43.11). UTI may result from urinary stasis behind the labia; if the adhesions are left untreated, the vaginal orifice may become inaccessible, presenting difficulty with sexual intercourse in the future.

NURSING ASSESSMENT

Younger girls have a higher risk of adhesions (3 months to 6 years) (Gerlt & Starr, 2013). Assess the history for dysuria or urinary frequency. Inspect the genitalia for fusion or adherence of the labia minora.

NURSING MANAGEMENT

Administer topical estrogen cream as prescribed, usually once or twice daily. Teach the parents to continue cream application until the labia separate. Encourage use of petroleum jelly daily for 1 month following labial separation to prevent recurrence of adhesion.

Vulvovaginitis

Vulvovaginitis is inflammation of the vulva and vagina. Inflammation may occur as a result of bacterial or yeast overgrowth or from chemical factors such as bubble bath, soaps, or perfumes found in personal care products. Poor hygiene may also cause vulvovaginitis. Tight clothing may cause a heat rash in the perineal area. Persistent scratching of the irritated area may result in the complication of superficial skin infection.

NURSING ASSESSMENT

Elicit a description of the present illness and chief complaint. Common signs and symptoms reported during the health history may include itching or burning in the perineal area. Explore the child's current and past medical history for risk factors, which may include:

- Young age (toilet-trained preschooler)
- Poor hygiene
- Sexual activity
- Immune disorders
- Diabetes mellitus

Inspect the perineum for redness, edema, irritation, rash, or vaginal discharge (note color, consistency, and odor).

NURSING MANAGEMENT

Teach appropriate hygiene (daily and toileting). Girls (or their parents) should wash the genital area thoroughly on a daily basis with mild soap and water. Rinse the area well. Encourage girls to wipe after urinating and after bowel movements to wipe in a front-to-back motion. The girl should wear cotton underwear and should change it at least once a day. Administer topical or oral medications as ordered. Table 43.3 lists treatments related to specific types of vulvovaginitis.

Inflammatory Disease

Pelvic inflammatory disease (PID) is an inflammation of the upper female genital tract and nearby structures. The fallopian tubes, ovaries, or peritoneum may be involved, and endometriosis may also be present. PID results from bacterial invasion through the cervix and vagina, ascending into the uterus and fallopian tubes. The most common causes of PID are *Chlamydia trachomatis* and *Neisseria gonorrhoeae,* although other bacteria and normal vaginal flora may be implicated. PID may result in fever, abdominal pain, pain with intercourse, **dysmenorrhea** (painful menstrual cycles), and abnormal uterine bleeding. Long-term complications include chronic pelvic pain, ectopic pregnancy, and infertility related to scarring.

NURSING ASSESSMENT

For a full description of the assessment phase of the nursing process, refer to the Assessment section of the Nursing Process Overview earlier in the chapter.

When discussing any problem related to the reproductive organs or menstruation with the preteen or teen, it is necessary to discuss sexuality. The girl may be reluctant to share this information with the nurse. Approaches to discussing sexuality with the adolescent that may increase the likelihood of obtaining a truthful history include:

- Discuss the girl's general health, menarche, and menstrual cycle first, and then work toward discussing sexual behavior.
- Start with questions about the girl's friends and social life, moving the conversation toward sexual behavior.

TABLE 43.3 VULVOVAGINITIS: TYPES AND TREATMENTS

Cause	Assessment Findings	Treatment
Unhygienic practices	Irritation of labia and vaginal opening May have foul brownish-green discharge if infected with bacteria from rectum	Good hygiene Sometimes a mild anti-inflammatory cream is prescribed. Assess for signs and symptoms of UTI, which may occur as a complication
Candida albicans	Red bumpy perineal rash in infants White cottage-cheese–like discharge Intense itching	Antifungal cream or vaginal suppository Prevent by ingesting probiotics (found in yogurt and kefir) daily and supplementing with a probiotic such as Lactinex when taking antibiotics
Bordetella, Gardnerella	Thin gray vaginal discharge with fishy odor	Metronidazole orally.
Trichomonas vaginalis	Foul yellow-gray or green vaginal discharge	Metronidazole orally. Sexually transmitted, so can be prevented with the use of condoms.

Adapted from Neinstein, L. S., Gordon, C. M., Katzman, D. K., Rosen, D. S., & Woods, E. R. (2009). *Handbook of adolescent health care*. Philadelphia, PA: Lippincott Williams & Wilkins.

- Always discuss sexual behavior one on one with the adolescent (without the parent present), and then ask the adolescent's permission to discuss concerns with the parent. If the adolescent does not consent to parental involvement, then confidentiality must be maintained.

Assessment findings pertinent to PID are discussed below.

Health History. Elicit a description of the present illness and chief complaint. Common signs and symptoms reported during the health history might include:

- Abdominal pain (ranging from mild to severe)
- Prolonged or increased menstrual bleeding
- Dysmenorrhea
- Dysuria
- Painful sexual intercourse
- Nausea
- Vomiting

Explore the girl's current and past medical health history for risk factors such as:

- Multiple sexual partners
- Lack of consistent condom use
- Lack of contraceptive use
- History of prior sexually transmitted infection
- Douching
- Prostitution
- Alcohol or drug use (particularly if associated with sexual activity)

Physical Examination. Inspect for fever (usually over 101°F) or vaginal discharge. Palpate the abdomen, noting tenderness over the uterus or ovaries. An elevated C-reactive protein level and an elevated erythrocyte sedimentation rate indicate an inflammatory process. Cervical culture reveals the causative bacterial organism.

NURSING MANAGEMENT

PID is often treated in the outpatient setting with intramuscular or oral antibiotic regimens. If the adolescent is severely ill or has a very high fever or protracted vomiting, then she may be hospitalized. Antibiotics are needed to eradicate the infection. Maintain hydration via intravenous fluids if necessary and administer analgesics as needed for pain. Semi-Fowler positioning promotes pelvic drainage. A key element to treatment of PID is education to prevent recurrence (see Healthy People 2020 and Teaching Guideline 43.2).

HEALTHY PEOPLE 2020

Objective	Nursing Significance
Reduce the proportion of females who have ever required treatment for pelvic inflammatory disease (PID).	• Educate teens that abstinence is the only way to completely avoid contracting a sexually transmitted infection. • Encourage teens to always use condoms if participating in any sexual act. • Provide an open and confidential environment so teen girls will report symptoms and seek treatment earlier.

Healthy People Objectives retrieved from http://www.healthypeople.gov

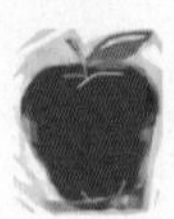

Teaching Guidelines 43.2
PREVENTING PELVIC INFLAMMATORY DISEASE

- Insist that sexual partners use condoms.
- Do not use a vaginal douche routinely, as this may lead to bacterial overgrowth.
- Get screened regularly for sexually transmitted infections.
- Make sure that each sexual partner also receives antibiotic treatment.

Menstrual Disorders

Menstruation begins in most girls about 2 years after breast development starts, around the time of Tanner stage 4 breast and pubic hair development and on average at around 12 to 13 years of age. Menstruation has many effects on girls and women, including emotional and self-image issues. Adolescents may suffer from a variety of menstrual disorders, including premenstrual syndrome and several different disorders related to menstrual bleeding and cramping (Table 43.4).

TABLE 43.4 COMMON MENSTRUAL DISORDERS

Disorder	Definition	Cause
Primary amenorrhea	Lack of menarche within 2 years of reaching Tanner stage 4 breast development, or by 16 years of age	• Imperforate hymen • Agenesis of vulva or vagina • Turner syndrome • Chronic illness associated with delayed pubertal development (e.g., cystic fibrosis, Crohn disease, sickle cell disease) • Suppressed levels of follicle-stimulating hormone (FSH) or luteinizing hormone (LH), as occurs with eating disorders, intense athletics, severe psychological stress, or extreme weight loss
Secondary amenorrhea	Absence of menses for 6 months in the girl who has been menstruating regularly	• Pregnancy (most common cause) • Anovulation (resulting from lack of hypothalamic-pituitary axis maturity) • Polycystic ovary syndrome (PCOS) • Suppressed levels of FSH or LH, as occurs with eating disorders, intense athletics, severe psychological stress, or extreme weight loss
Mittelschmerz	Abdominal pain, usually unilateral, that varies from a few sharp cramps to several hours of crampy pain	• Usually occurs midway through the menstrual cycle, around the time of ovulation; is thought to be a result of egg release from the ovary
Dysmenorrhea	Pain associated with menstruation, usually abdominal cramps ranging from mild to severe	• Prostaglandin release is responsible for the smooth muscle contraction of the uterus during menstruation (primary) • Fibroids, adenomyosis, endometriosis, scar tissue (secondary)
Menorrhagia	Excessive menstrual bleeding	• Anovulatory cycles • Endometriosis • Blood dyscrasias, bleeding disorders, or use of anticoagulants • Reproductive system neoplasms
Metrorrhagia	Bleeding between menstrual periods	• Improper use of oral contraceptives • Intrauterine device • Endometriosis • Reproductive system neoplasms • Miscarriage or ectopic pregnancy

Adapted from Sass, A. E., & Kaplan, D. W. (2014). Adolescence. In W. W. Hay, M. J. Levin, R. R. Deterding, & M. J. Abzug, (Eds.), *Current pediatric diagnosis and treatment* (22nd ed.). New York, NY: McGraw-Hill.

In healthy girls, the menstrual period varies in the heaviness of flow. Periods may occur irregularly for up to 2 years after menarche (the onset of menstruation), but after that the regular menstrual cycle should be established. The normal cycle can vary from 21 to 45 days in length, with the period usually lasting 2 to 7 days. Girls who take oral contraceptives usually have very regular 28-day cycles, with lighter bleeding than those who do not take contraceptives.

PATHOPHYSIOLOGY

Premenstrual syndrome is a collection of physical and/or affective symptoms that occur predictably during the luteal phase of the menstrual cycle. Symptoms begin 5 to 10 days before each period and usually resolve by the time the period begins or shortly thereafter (the timing may vary by adolescent but is consistent with each cycle). Disorders of bleeding and cramping are summarized in Table 43.4.

NURSING ASSESSMENT

For a full description of the assessment phase of the nursing process, refer to the Assessment section of the Nursing Process Overview earlier in the chapter. When girls present for evaluation of menstrual concerns, a focused yet thorough nursing assessment is necessary.

Health History. Obtain a thorough and accurate menstrual history; determine age at menarche, usual length of menstrual period, usual menstrual flow, number of pads or tampons used per day, date of last normal menstrual period, premenstrual symptoms, and any pain related to the menstrual cycle. Obtain a description of the pain, what relief measures have been tried, and what the success of those measures has been. If pain occurs with menstrual periods, assess for associated symptoms such as nausea, vomiting, dizziness, or loose stools. Explore the history for symptoms of bloating, water retention, weight gain, headache, muscle aches, abdominal pain, food cravings, or breast tenderness. Determine the extent of emotional symptoms related to the menstrual cycle, such as anxiety, insomnia, mood swings, tension, crying spells, or irritability. Note the timing of these symptoms within the menstrual cycle.

Note past medical history, including any chronic illnesses and family history of gynecologic concerns. Elicit a sexual behavior history, including the type of sexual activity (oral, anal, or vaginal), number and gender of sexual partners, frequency and most recent sexual contact, history of molestation or sexual abuse, and use of contraceptives (noting type) and/or condoms.

Take a medication history, including prescription medications and contraceptives, and determine whether the girl uses anabolic steroids, tobacco, or marijuana, cocaine, or other illegal drugs.

Physical Examination. The physical assessment related to menstrual disorders includes inspection and observation, auscultation, and palpation. The bimanual pelvic examination and Papanicolaou (Pap) smear are usually indicated only for more severe menstrual disorders and are usually performed by the physician or nurse practitioner.

Inspect the breasts and pubic hair distribution to determine Tanner stage. Observe the external genitalia for vaginal discharge, redness, or irritation. Note pallor or weight gain. Document presence and extent of clots in menstrual flow. Measure orthostatic blood pressure and orthostatic pulse; decreases with position change may occur in girls with anemia. Palpate the abdomen, noting distention or tenderness.

Laboratory and Diagnostic Tests. Common laboratory and diagnostic studies ordered for the assessment of menstrual disorders include:

- Complete blood count: to determine presence of anemia with **menorrhagia** (excess menstrual flow) or metrorrhagia
- Human chorionic gonadotropin: to assess for pregnancy with **amenorrhea** (absence of menses)

NURSING MANAGEMENT

Nursing goals for the girl with a menstrual disorder focus on normalizing menstrual flow and restoring blood volume, providing comfort, and encouraging independence in self-care.

Normalizing Menstrual Flow and Restoring Blood Volume. For the girl with mild anemia related to menorrhagia, administer iron supplements as ordered. For moderate menorrhagia, oral contraceptives may also be prescribed, since altering hormone levels decrease menstrual flow. If the contraceptive contains a high dose of estrogen, the girl may experience nausea. Administer antiemetics as ordered and encourage the girl to eat small, frequent meals to alleviate nausea. Adolescents with severe anemia may require hospitalization and blood transfusion.

Providing Comfort. Provide a heating pad or warm compress to help alleviate menstrual cramps. Administer NSAIDs such as ibuprofen or naproxen to inhibit prostaglandin synthesis, which contributes to menstrual cramps. Advise girls that beginning NSAID therapy at the first sign of menstrual discomfort is the best way to minimize discomfort. If NSAIDs are unsuccessful, oral contraceptives may be ordered; teach the girl appropriate use of oral contraceptives.

The adolescent experiencing premenstrual syndrome should keep a diary of her symptoms, their severity, and when they occur in the menstrual cycle. Like all adolescents, girls with premenstrual syndrome should eat a balanced diet that includes nutrient-rich foods so they can avoid hypoglycemia and associated mood swings. Encourage adolescent girls to participate in aerobic exercise three times a week to promote a sense of well-being, decrease fatigue, and reduce stress. Administer calcium (1200 to 1600 mg per day), magnesium (400 to 800 mg per day), and vitamin B6 (50 to 100 mg per day) as prescribed. In some studies, these nutrients have been shown to decrease the intensity of premenstrual symptoms (Moreno, Giesel, Rogers, & Clark, 2012). NSAIDs may be useful for painful physical symptoms, and spironolactone may help reduce bloating and water retention. Herbs such as chasteberry or ginkgo may be recommended.

Take Note!

Adolescents who experience more extensive emotional symptoms with premenstrual syndrome should be evaluated for premenstrual dysphoric disorder, as they may require antidepressant therapy (Moreno et al., 2012).

Encouraging Independence in Self-Care. Establishing a trusting relationship with the adolescent may make education about self-care more successful. Some girls have open relationships with their mothers and can discuss issues related to menses and sexuality with them, but many others cannot discuss such "embarrassing" issues with their mothers, and the nurse or other healthcare provider may be the only source of reliable information. Provide the adolescent with accurate information about menstruation and sexuality. Educate her about normal menstruation, the menstrual cycle, and the risk for pregnancy if sexual intercourse occurs. Refer the teen for contraception if sexually active. Refer girls to reliable websites if they are not comfortable with receiving information from the nurse. Links to several websites are available on thePoint. Encourage the girl to call or visit the office if she has additional questions.

Male Disorders

Male reproductive disorders include structural disorders and disorders caused by infection or inflammation. Circumcision will also be discussed below.

Phimosis and Paraphimosis

In phimosis, the foreskin of the penis cannot be retracted. Although this is normal in the newborn, it can be pathologic later. Over time, the prepuce (foreskin) naturally becomes retractable. Local irritation, balanitis, or UTI may occur if urine is retained within the foreskin after voiding. Paraphimosis (Fig. 43.12) is a more serious disorder characterized by retraction of the phimotic prepuce, which causes a constricting band behind the glans of the penis and results in incarceration if left untreated.

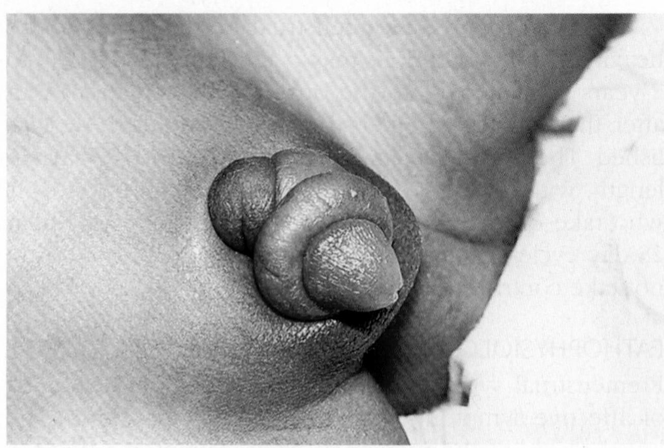

FIGURE 43.12 Paraphimosis: note the swollen prepuce. Copyrighted 2011. UBM Medica LLC. 82486:1111JM

Topical steroid cream applied twice a day for 1 month may be prescribed for phimosis. Paraphimosis requires reduction of the prepuce or a small dorsal incision to release the foreskin. Circumcision may be used to treat either condition.

NURSING ASSESSMENT

Elicit a description of the present illness and chief complaint. Common signs and symptoms reported during the health history might include:

- Irritation or bleeding from the opening of the prepuce (phimosis)
- Dysuria (phimosis)
- Pain (paraphimosis)
- Swollen penis (paraphimosis)

Determine the onset of symptoms and inspect the penis for irritation, erythema, edema, or discharge.

Take Note!

A swollen, reddened penis (paraphimosis) is a medical emergency and can quickly result in necrosis of the tip of the penis if left untreated.

NURSING MANAGEMENT

Apply topical steroid medication as prescribed for phimosis, following gentle retraction to stretch the foreskin back. Topical vitamin E cream may also help to soften the phimotic ring. When surgical intervention is necessary, provide routine postprocedural care and pain management (refer to the section on circumcision below). Teach the parents and uncircumcised boy proper hygiene, which will help to prevent phimosis and paraphimosis (Teaching Guidelines 43.3).

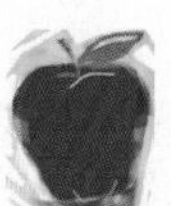

Teaching Guidelines 43.3

HYGIENE IN THE UNCIRCUMCISED MALE

- The foreskin does not normally retract in the newborn boy, so do not force it to do so.
- Change the diaper frequently and wash the penis daily with water and mild soap.
- When the infant is older and the foreskin easily retracts, gently retract the foreskin and clean around the glans with water and mild soap once a week.
- Dry the area prior to replacing the foreskin.
- Always replace the foreskin after retraction.
- Teach the preschool-age boy to retract the foreskin and clean the penis during each bath or shower.

Circumcision

Circumcision is the removal of the excess foreskin of the penis. Some newborn boys are circumcised shortly after birth before going home from the hospital. Some parents elect not to have their newborn boy circumcised at that time but may desire it later. Neonatal circumcision may be performed in the newborn nursery, hospital unit treatment room, or outpatient office. Circumcision is indicated later for the conditions of phimosis and paraphimosis. Circumcision done after the newborn period usually requires general anesthesia.

The benefits of circumcision include a decreased incidence of UTI, sexually transmitted diseases, AIDS, and penile cancer, and in female partners a decreased occurrence of cervical cancer. Complications of circumcision are rare and include bleeding, penile adhesions, imperfect amount of foreskin removal, and meatal stenosis. (American Academy of Pediatrics [AAP], 2012).

Whether to circumcise or not is a personal decision and often based on religious beliefs or social or cultural customs. Nurses should support and educate the parents in either case.

NURSING ASSESSMENT

Prior to the procedure, assess for normal placement of the urinary meatus on the glans penis (in boys with hypospadias, circumcision should be delayed until evaluation by the pediatric urologist). After the circumcision, assess for redness, edema, or active bleeding. Note signs of infection, such as purulent drainage. Assess pain level.

NURSING MANAGEMENT

Nursing care of the boy undergoing circumcision focuses on managing pain, providing postprocedural care, and educating the parents.

Managing Pain. Whether circumcision is performed in the obstetric area of the hospital before newborn discharge or in the outpatient setting at a few days of age, pain management during the procedure must not be neglected. Advocate for appropriate pain management for the infant undergoing circumcision. The American Academy of Pediatrics recommends using a subcutaneous ring block with lidocaine, local anesthetic with lidocaine/prilocaine, or a dorsal nerve block to the penis (AAP, 2012). Playing calming music during the procedure may also help to soothe the infant, providing distraction. A sucrose-dipped pacifier may also be used as adjuvant therapy for pain management.

Atraumatic Care

Restrain the infant in a padded circumcision chair with blankets covering the legs and upper body to provide a sense of comfort. If a padded restraint chair is not available, provide atraumatic care by padding the circumcision board and covering the infant as previously described.

Providing Postprocedural Care. Usual care after circumcision depends on the type of appliance used (Gomco or Mogen clamp or Plastibell apparatus). Cleanse the penis with clear water for the first few days and avoid using alcohol-containing wipes. To avoid irritation to the penis, fasten diapers loosely. Notify the physician or nurse practitioner if excessive redness, active bleeding, or purulent discharge occurs. Assess for the first void following the procedure, or if performed in the outpatient setting instruct parents to call the physician or nurse practitioner if the infant has not voided by 6 to 8 hours after the circumcision. Apply antibiotic ointment or petroleum jelly to the penile head with each diaper change as prescribed, based on the circumcision method used and the preference of the physician or nurse practitioner.

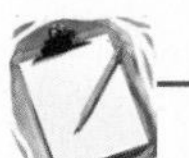

Take Note!

If excess bleeding occurs after the circumcision, apply direct pressure and notify the physician or nurse practitioner immediately.

Educating the Parents. Instruct parents to give sponge baths until the circumcision is healed. Describe the normal granulation tissue that will be present during the healing process. Teach parents to apply ointment or petroleum jelly if indicated. Instruct the parents to call the physician or nurse practitioner if any of the following occur:

- The infant does not urinate within 6 to 8 hours after the procedure.

- Heavy bleeding occurs (more than small spots on the diaper or bleeding that requires direct pressure to stop it).
- There is purulent or serous drainage from the circumcised area.
- There is redness or swelling of the penile shaft.

Take Note!

If the Plastibell is used, teach parents NOT to use petroleum jelly, as it may cause the ring to be dislodged. A yellowish crust may form that should be allowed to fall off on its own after several days.

Cryptorchidism

Cryptorchidism (also known as undescended testicles) occurs when one or both testicles do not descend into the scrotal sac. Ordinarily the testes, which in the fetus develop in the abdomen, make their descent into the scrotal sac during the seventh month of gestation. The cause for this failure to descend may be mechanical, hormonal, chromosomal, or enzymatic. The disorder may occur unilaterally or bilaterally. Up to 3% of term male infants exhibit cryptorchidism (Ashley, Barthold, & Kolon, 2010).

Complications associated with cryptorchidism that is allowed to progress into the school-age years include sterility and an increased risk for testicular cancer in adolescence or the young adult years. Therapeutic management is surgical. An orchiopexy is performed to release the spermatic cord, and the testes are then pulled into the scrotum and tacked into place.

NURSING ASSESSMENT

Explore the health history for risk factors such as:

- Prematurity
- First-born child
- Cesarean birth
- Low birthweight
- Hypospadias

Palpate for the presence (or absence) of both testes in the scrotal sac.

Take Note!

A retractile testis is one that may be brought into the scrotum, remains for a time, and then retracts back up the inguinal canal. This should not be confused with true cryptorchidism.

NURSING MANAGEMENT

If the testes are not descended by 6 months of age, the infant should be referred for surgical repair (Ashley et al., 2010). Postoperatively, observe the incision for signs of bleeding or infection.

Hydrocele and Varicocele

Hydrocele (fluid in the scrotal sac) is usually a benign and self-limiting disorder. It is usually noted early in infancy and often resolves spontaneously by 1 year of age. Varicocele (a venous varicosity along the spermatic cord) is often noted as a swelling of the scrotal sac. Complications of varicocele include low sperm count or reduced sperm motility, which can result in infertility.

NURSING ASSESSMENT

Elicit a description of the present illness and chief complaint. The boy with hydrocele will have an enlarged scrotum that may decrease in size when he is lying down. Inspect the scrotum for a fluid-filled appearance.

The boy with varicocele will have a mass on one or both sides of the scrotum and bluish discoloration. Inspect the scrotum for masses; the spermatic vein feels worm-like on palpation. The boy with varicocele may have pain.

NURSING MANAGEMENT

Both hydrocele and painless varicocele require watchful waiting, as these conditions will usually resolve spontaneously. If they do not resolve, or if the difference in testicular volume is marked in the boy with varicocele, refer the child to a urologist, as surgery may be indicated. Reassure parents that hydrocele is not associated with the development of infertility. Varicocele may lead to infertility if left untreated, so instruct parents to seek care if pain occurs or if there is a large difference in testicular size. Either condition may be surgically corrected on an outpatient basis. Provide routine postoperative care following either surgery.

Testicular Torsion

In testicular torsion, a testicle is abnormally attached to the scrotum and twisted. It requires immediate attention because ischemia can result if the torsion is left untreated, leading to infertility. Testicular torsion may occur at any age but most commonly occurs in boys aged 12 to 18 years (Brenner & Ojo, 2015).

NURSING ASSESSMENT

Elicit a description of the present illness and chief complaint. Signs and symptoms of testicular torsion include sudden, severe scrotal pain. Inspect the affected side for significant swelling, which may appear hemorrhagic or blue-black.

NURSING MANAGEMENT

Surgical correction is necessary immediately. Administer pain medication prior to surgery. Reassure the child and family that surgery will alleviate the problem and is performed to restore adequate blood flow to the testicle. After surgical repair, provide routine postoperative care.

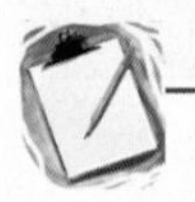

Take Note!

Testicular torsion is considered a surgical emergency, as necrosis of the testis may occur and gangrene may set in.

Epididymitis

Epididymitis (inflammation of the epididymis) is caused by infection with bacteria. It is the most common cause of pain in the scrotum. It rarely occurs before puberty, but if it does it may occur as a result of a urethral or bladder infection related to a urogenital anomaly. Therapeutic management is directed toward eradicating the bacteria. If left untreated, a scrotal abscess, testicular infarction, or infertility may occur.

NURSING ASSESSMENT

Note history of painful swelling of the scrotum, which may be gradual or acute. If the boy is sexually active, explore history of sexual encounters prior to the onset of symptoms. Document history of dysuria or urethral discharge. Note fever, which may last from days to weeks. On inspection, note edema and erythema of the scrotum. Gently palpate the scrotum for a hardened and tender epididymis. Note urethral discharge if present. Palpate the inguinal lymph nodes for enlargement. Urinalysis may be positive for bacteria and white blood cells. The culture of urethral discharge may be positive for a sexually transmitted infection such as gonorrhea or *Chlamydia*. The complete blood count may reveal an elevated white blood cell count.

NURSING MANAGEMENT

Encourage the boy to rest in bed with the scrotum elevated. Ice packs to the scrotum may help with pain relief. Administer pain medications such as NSAIDs or other analgesics as needed.

Administer antibiotics as prescribed. Educate the boy and his family to complete the entire course of antibiotics as prescribed to eradicate the infection. Advise the child and family to notify the physician or nurse practitioner if the condition is not improving or if the pain and swelling worsen.

NURSING CARE PLAN 43.1

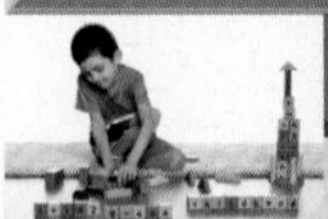

Overview for the Child With a Genitourinary Disorder

NURSINGS DIAGNOSIS: Activity intolerance related to generalized edema, anemia, or generalized weakness as evidenced by verbalization of weakness or fatigue; elevated heart rate, respiratory rate, or blood pressure with activity; complaint of shortness of breath with play or activity

Outcome Identification and Evaluation

Child will display increased activity tolerance, desire to play without developing symptoms of exertion.

Intervention: ***Promoting Activity***

- Encourage activity or ambulation per physician's or nurse practitioner's orders: *early mobilization results in better outcomes.*
- Observe child for symptoms of activity intolerance such as pallor, nausea, lightheadedness, or dizziness or changes in vital signs *to determine level of tolerance.*
- If child is on bed rest, perform range-of-motion exercises and frequent position changes, *as negative changes to the musculoskeletal system occur quickly with inactivity and immobility.*
- Cluster nursing care activities and plan for periods of rest before and after exertional activities *to decrease oxygen need and consumption.*
- Refer the child to physical therapy *for exercise prescription to increase skeletal muscle strength.*

(continued)

NURSING CARE PLAN 43.1

Overview for the Child With a Genitourinary Disorder (continued)

NURSING DIAGNOSIS: Excess fluid volume related to decreased protein in the bloodstream, decreased urine output, sodium retention, possible inappropriate fluid intake, or altered hormone levels inducing fluid retention as evidenced by edema, bloating, weight gain, oliguria, azotemia, or changes in heart and lung sounds

Outcome Identification and Evaluation

Child will attain appropriate fluid balance, will lose weight (fluid), edema or bloating will decrease, lung sounds will be clear and heart sounds normal.

Intervention: *Encouraging Fluid Loss*

- Weigh child daily on same scale in similar amount of clothing: *in children, weight is the best indicator of changes in fluid status.*
- Monitor location and extent of edema (measure abdominal girth daily if ascites present): *decrease in edema indicates positive increase in oncotic pressure.*
- Auscultate lungs carefully to determine presence of crackles *(indicating pulmonary edema).*
- Assess work of breathing and respiratory rate: *increased work of breathing is associated with pulmonary edema.*
- Assess heart sounds for presence or absence of gallop: *presence of S_3 may indicate fluid overload.*
- Maintain fluid restriction as ordered *to decrease intravascular volume and workload on the heart.*
- Strictly monitor intake and output *to quickly note discrepancies and provide intervention.*
- Provide sodium-restricted diet as ordered: *restricting sodium in the diet allows for better renal excretion of extra fluid.*
- Administer diuretics as ordered and monitor for side effects of those medications. *Diuretics encourage excretion of fluid and elimination of edema, reduce cardiac filling pressures, and increase renal blood flow. Side effects include electrolyte imbalance as well as orthostatic hypotension.*

NURSING DIAGNOSIS: Imbalanced nutrition: less than body requirements related to anorexia and protein loss as evidenced by weight, length/height, and/or BMI below average for age

Outcome Identification and Evaluation

Child will improve nutritional intake, resulting in steady increase in weight and length/height.

Intervention: *Promoting Adequate Nutrition*

- Determine body weight and length/height norm for age *to determine goal to work toward.*
- Assess child for food preferences that fall within dietary restrictions, *as the child will be more likely to consume adequate amounts of foods that he or she likes.*
- Weigh daily or weekly (according to physician or nurse practitioner's order or institutional standard) and measure length/height weekly *to monitor for increased growth.*
- Offer highest-calorie meals at the time of day when the child's appetite is the greatest *to increase likelihood of increased caloric intake.*
- Provide increased-calorie shakes or puddings within diet restriction: *high-calorie foods increase weight gain.*
- Administer vitamin and mineral supplements as prescribed *to attain/maintain vitamin and mineral balance in the body.*

NURSING CARE PLAN 43.1

Overview for the Child With a Genitourinary Disorder (continued)

NURSING DIAGNOSIS: Imbalanced nutrition: more than body requirements related to increased appetite secondary to steroid therapy as evidenced by weight greater than 95th percentile for age or recent increase in weight

Outcome Identification and Evaluation

Child will demonstrate balanced nutritional intake, will maintain current weight or steadily lose excess weight.

Intervention: ***Encouraging Appropriate Nutritional Intake***

- Determine ideal body weight and body mass index for age *to determine goal to work toward.*
- Consult dietitian *for guidance in planning nutrient-rich diet in context of restrictions.*
- Evaluate for emotional/psychological reasons for overeating *to address these concerns.*
- Formulate a contract with the child *to involve him or her in the planning process and encourage compliance with the plan.*
- With the child, plan for daily exercise/activity to expend excess calories: *it is important to involve the child in planning, in order to increase compliance.*
- Instruct the child/parent about appropriate nutrient-rich foods to choose within the constraints of diet and fluid restrictions *to provide basis for ongoing diet management at home.*
- Weigh child twice weekly on same scale *to determine progress toward goal.*

NURSING DIAGNOSIS: Impaired urinary elimination related to urinary tract infection, anatomic obstruction, sensory motor impairment, or dysfunctional voiding as evidenced by urinary retention or incontinence, dribbling, urgency, or dysuria

Child's bladder will empty adequately, according to pre-established quantities and frequencies individualized for the child (usual urine output is 0.5 to 2 mL/kg/hr).

Intervention: ***Promoting Adequate Urinary Elimination and Successful Bladder Emptying***

- Assess the child's usual voiding pattern and success within that pattern *to determine baseline.*
- Assess child's ability to adequately empty bladder via history focused on character and duration of lower urinary symptoms *to determine baseline.*
- Develop a schedule for bladder emptying *to decrease bladder overdistention and to encourage voiding in the toilet.*
- Maintain adequate hydration, *to avoid irritating effects of dehydration on the bladder.*
- Avoid constipation, encopresis, or fecal impaction *as alterations in bowel elimination may have a negative impact on urinary elimination.*
- Assess for bladder distention by palpation or urinary retention by postvoid residual obtained via catheterization or bladder ultrasound *to determine extent of retention.*
- Teach parents to restrict child's fluid intake after dinner *to avoid bedwetting.*
- Ensure child voids prior to going to bed *to avoid bedwetting.*
- Teach bladder-stretching exercises as prescribed per physician or nurse practitioner *to increase bladder capacity.*
- In the child with significant urinary retention, teach parents/child the technique of clean intermittent catheterization, *which allows for regular complete bladder emptying.*

(continued)

NURSING CARE PLAN 43.1

Overview for the Child With a Genitourinary Disorder (continued)

NURSING DIAGNOSIS: Disturbed body image related to anatomic differences, short stature, or effects of long-term corticosteroid use as evidenced by verbalization of dissatisfaction with the child's or adolescent's looks

Outcome Identification and Evaluation

Child or adolescent will display appropriate body image, will look at self in mirror and participate in social activities.

Intervention: ***Promoting Body Image***

- Acknowledge feelings of anger over body changes and illness: *venting feelings is associated with less body image disturbance.*
- Support the child's or teen's choices of comfortable, fashionable clothing *that may disguise anatomic abnormalities and dialysis tubing.*
- Involve the child and especially the teen in the decision-making process, *as a sense of control of his or her own body will improve body image.*
- Encourage children or teens to spend time with others of their own age who have short stature or other effects of renal disorders: *a peer's opinions are often better accepted than those of persons in authority, such as parents or healthcare professionals.*

NURSING DIAGNOSIS: Deficient knowledge related to lack of information regarding complex medical condition, prognosis, and medical needs as evidenced by verbalization, questions, or actions demonstrating lack of understanding regarding child's condition or care

Outcome Identification and Evaluation

Child and parents will verbalize accurate information and understanding about condition, prognosis, and medical needs: *child and parents demonstrate knowledge of condition and medications and will demonstrate therapeutic procedures the child requires.*

Intervention: ***Educating the Child and Parents***

- Assess child's and parents' willingness to learn: *child and parents must be open to learning for teaching to be effective.*
- Provide parents with time to adjust to diagnosis: *will facilitate adjustment and ability to learn and participate in child's care.*
- Teach in short sessions: *many short sessions are found to be more helpful than one long session.*
- Repeat information: *allows parents and child time to learn and understand.*
- Individualize teaching to the parents' and child's level of understanding (depends on age of child, physical condition, memory) *to ensure understanding.*
- Provide reinforcement and rewards *to facilitate the teaching/learning process.*
- Use multiple modes of learning involving many senses (written, verbal, demonstration, and videos) when possible: *child and parents are more likely to retain information when it is presented in different ways using many senses.*

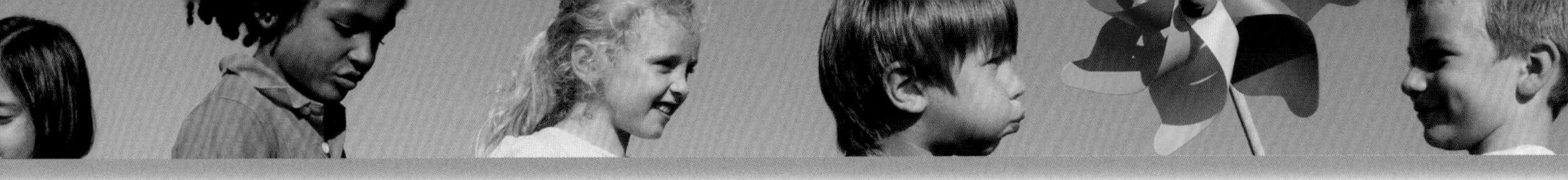

KEY CONCEPTS

- Though present at birth, the reproductive organs do not reach functional maturity until puberty.
- The short length of the urethra in girls and its proximity to the vagina and anus place the young girl at higher risk for the development of urinary tract infections compared with the adult.
- The urinary tract is immature in infants and young children, with a slower glomerular filtration rate and a decreased ability to concentrate urine and reabsorb amino acids compared with the adult.
- The expected urine output in the infant and child is 0.5 to 2 mL/kg/hr.
- Obtaining a clean or sterile urine specimen is necessary for accurate urine culture results.
- A urinary catheter must be inserted just prior to the voiding cystourethrogram.
- Close monitoring of serum blood counts and electrolytes is a critical component of nursing care related to renal disorders.
- Certain congenital urologic anomalies may require multiple surgeries as well as urinary diversion; urine drains through a stoma on the abdominal wall that is either pouched or catheterized.
- The treatment for nocturnal enuresis may include the use of desmopressin nasal spray and/or an enuresis alarm to train the child to awaken to the sensation of a filling bladder.
- Nephrotic syndrome results in significant proteinuria and edema.
- Acute glomerulonephritis most often follows a group A streptococcal infection and commonly results in hematuria, proteinuria, and hypertension.
- The most common cause of hemolytic-uremic syndrome is infection with *E. coli* O157:H7. It can be prevented by adequately cooking ground meat, washing hands and produce well, and making sure that an appropriate chemical balance is maintained in public recreational water sources such as swimming pools and water parks.
- Corticosteroids can cause gastrointestinal upset. If used on a long-term basis, they should be tapered rather than discontinued abruptly to avoid adrenal crisis.
- In children, chronic kidney disease is most often the result of congenital structural defects, or infectious, inflammatory, or immune processes that damage the kidney, whereas in adults it usually results from hypertension or diabetes.
- Children taking immunosuppressants for nephrotic syndrome or for renal transplant are at increased risk for the development of overwhelming infection.
- Peritoneal dialysis may be accomplished at home by the parent. Close attention to sterile technique is needed.
- Hemodialysis requires an arteriovenous fistula or graft that is accessed with needles three or four times per week at a hemodialysis center. This is disruptive to the child's academic, social, and family lives.
- Renal transplantation is the best option for the treatment of end-stage renal disease in children, but vigilant medication administration is needed to prevent organ rejection.
- Children with renal failure experience anemia, poor growth, depression, anxiety, and low self-esteem.
- The diet for a child with a renal disorder must be individualized according to prescribed sodium, fluid, and/or protein restrictions.
- Postoperative care for the child undergoing urologic surgery includes pain management, avoidance or treatment of bladder spasms, and monitoring of urine output.

REFERENCES AND RECOMMENDED READINGS

American Academy of Pediatrics. (2012). Technical report: Male circumcision. *Pediatrics, 130*(3), e756–e3785.

American Academy of Pediatrics. (2015). *Care for an uncircumcised penis*. Retrieved from https://www.healthychildren.org/English/ages-stages/baby/bathing-skin-care/Pages/Care-for-an-Uncircumcised-Penis.aspx

American Nephrology Nurses' Association. (2013). *Pediatric ESRD renal transplant fact sheet*. Pitman, NJ: Author.

Ashley, R. A., Barthold, J. S., & Kolon, T. F. (2010). Cryptorchidism: Pathogenesis, diagnosis, treatment and prognosis. *Urologic Clinics of North America, 37*(2), 183–193.

Bowden, V. R., & Greenberg, C. S. (2012). *Pediatric nursing procedures* (3rd ed.). Philadelphia, PA: Lippincott Williams & Wilkins.

Brenner, J. S., & Ojo, A. (2015). *Causes of scrotal pain in children and adolescents*. Retrieved from http://www.uptodate.com/contents/causes-of-scrotal-pain-in-children-and-adolescents

Browne, N. T., Flanigan, L. M., McComiskey, C. A., & Pieper, P. (2013). *Nursing care of the pediatric surgical patient* (3rd ed.). Burlington, MA: Jones & Bartlett Learning.

Caldwell, P. H., Nankivell, G., & Sureshkumar, P. (2013). *Simple behavioural interventions for nocturnal enuresis in children* (review). The Cochrane Library 2013, 7. Indianapolis, IN: John Wiley & Sons.

Carpenito-Moyet, L. J. (2013). *Nursing diagnosis: Application to clinical practice* (14th ed.). Philadelphia, PA: Lippincott Williams & Wilkins.

Centers for Disease Control and Prevention (CDC). (2016). *Pelvic inflammatory disease (PID)—CDC fact sheet.* Retrieved from http://www.cdc.gov/std/PID/STDFact-PID.htm

Corbett, J. A., & Banks, A. D. (2013). *Laboratory tests and diagnostic procedures with nursing diagnoses* (8th ed.). Upper Saddle River, NJ: Pearson Education Inc.

Dunn, A. (2013). Elimination patterns. In C. Burns, A. Dunn, M. Brady, N. B. Starr, & C. Blosser (Eds.), *Pediatric primary care* (5th ed.). Philadelphia, PA: Saunders.

Gaylord, N. M., & Petersen-Smith, A. M. (2013). Genitourinary disorders. In C. Burns, A. Dunn, M. Brady, N. B. Starr, & C. Blosser (Eds.), *Pediatric primary care* (5th ed.). Philadelphia, PA: Saunders.

Gerlt, T., & Starr, N. B. (2013). Gynecologic disorders. In C. Burns, A. Dunn, M. Brady, N. B. Starr, & C. Blosser (Eds.), *Pediatric primary care* (5th ed.). Philadelphia, PA: Saunders.

Hamilton, R. G. (2015). *Latex allergy: Epidemiology, clinical manifestations, and diagnosis.* Retrieved from http://www.uptodate.com/contents/latex-allergy-epidemiology-clinical-manifestations-and-diagnosis

Klein, M. S. (2010). Kidney disease, chronic. In P. J. Allen, J. A. Vessey, & N. A. Schapiro (Eds.), *Primary care of the child with a chronic condition* (5th ed.). St. Louis, MO: Mosby.

Klein, M. S., & Martin, K. (2010). Organ transplantation. In P. J. Allen, J. A. Vessey, & N. A. Schapiro (Eds.), *Primary care of the child with a chronic condition* (5th ed.). St. Louis, MO: Mosby.

Lum, G. M. (2014). Kidney & urinary tract. In W. W. Hay, M. J. Levin, R. R. Deterding, & M. J. Abzug, (Eds.), (*Current pediatric diagnosis and treatment* (22nd ed.). New York, NY: McGraw-Hill.

Mattoo, T. K. (2016). *Treatment of hypertension in children and adolescents.* Retrieved from http://www.uptodate.com/contents/treatment-of-hypertension-in-children-and-adolescents?source=see_link

Moreno, M. A., Giesel, A. E., Clark, L. R., & Rogers, C. B. (2015). *Premenstrual syndrome.* Retrieved from http://emedicine.medscape.com/article/953696-overview

Mount Nittany Medical Center. (2013). *When your son needs surgery for hypospadias.* Retrieved from http://www.mountnittany.org/articles/healthsheets/11970

Neinstein, L. S., Gordon, C. M., Katzman, D. K., Rosen, D. S., & Woods, E. R. (2009). *Handbook of adolescent health care.* Philadelphia, PA: Lippincott Williams & Wilkins.

Nelson, C. P., & Koo, H. P. (2014). *Pediatric vesicoureteral reflux.* Retrieved from http://emedicine.medscape.com/article/1016439-overview

Pfeil, M., & Lindsay, B. (2010). Hypospadias repair: An overview. *International Journal of Urological Nursing, 4*(1), 4–12.

Sass, A. E., & Kaplan, D. W. (2014). Adolescence. In W. W. Hay, M. J. Levin, R. R. Deterding, & M. J. Abzug, (Eds.), (*Current pediatric diagnosis and treatment* (22nd ed.). New York, NY: McGraw-Hill.

Solomon, D. H. (2015). *Patient information: Nonsteroidal anti-inflammatory drugs (NSAIDs) (beyond the basics).* Retrieved from http://www.uptodate.com/contents/nonsteroidal-antiinflammatory-drugs-nsaids-beyond-the-basics

Taketomo, C. K., Hodding, J. H., & Kraus, D. M. (2013). *Pediatric & neonatal dosage handbook* (20th ed.). Hudson, OH: Lexicomp.

Tan, A. J., & Silverberg, M. A. (2015). *Hemolytic uremic syndrome in emergency medicine.* Retrieved from http://emedicine.medscape.com/article/779218-overview

Tews, M., & Singer, J. I. (2014). *Paraphimosis: Definition, pathophysiology, and clinical features.* Retrieved from http://www.uptodate.com/contents/paraphimosis-definition-pathophysiology-and-clinical-features

Tullus, K. (2013). A review of guidelines for urinary tract infections in children younger than 2 years. *Pediatric Annals, 42*(3), 111.

Worcester, S. (2014). Debate continues on antibiotic prophylaxis for UTIs with VUR. *Pediatric News, 48*(8), 3.

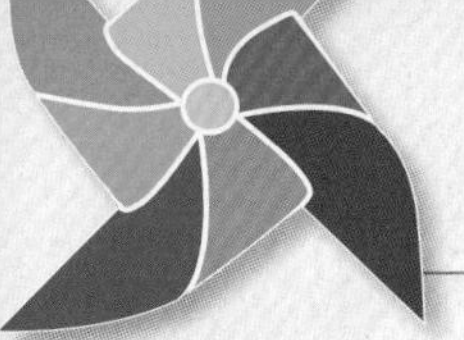

CHAPTER WORKSHEET

MULTIPLE CHOICE QUESTIONS

1. The nurse is performing education for the parents of an infant with bladder exstrophy. Which statement by the parents would indicate an understanding of the child's future care?
   a. "Care will be no different than that of any other infant."
   b. "My infant will only need this one surgery."
   c. "My child will wear diapers all his life."
   d. "We will need to care for the urinary diversion."

2. A 4-year-old girl presents with recurrent urinary tract infection. A prior workup did not reveal any urinary tract abnormalities. What is the priority nursing action?
   a. Obtain a sterile urine sample after completion of antibiotics.
   b. Teach appropriate toileting hygiene.
   c. Prepare the child for surgery to reimplant the ureters.
   d. Administer antibiotics intramuscularly.

3. A 5-year old who had a renal transplant 9 months ago and has no history of chickenpox presents to the pediatric clinic for his vaccinations. Which is the most appropriate set to give?
   a. DTaP, IPV
   b. DTaP, IPV, MMR, varicella
   c. DTaP, IPV, varicella
   d. IPV only

4. When the nurse is caring for a child with hemolytic-uremic syndrome or acute glomerulonephritis and the child is not yet toilet trained, which action by the nurse would best determine fluid retention?
   a. Test urine for specific gravity.
   b. Weigh child daily.
   c. Weigh the wet diapers.
   d. Measure abdominal girth daily.

DOSAGE CALCULATION QUESTION

1. The nurse is caring for a child who has had a renal transplant. The child weighs 47 lb. The medication order reads: cyclosporine 96 mg PO every 12 hours. Cyclosporine is supplied as 100 mg/mL. How many milliliters will the nurse administer? Round to the nearest whole number.

CRITICAL THINKING EXERCISES

1. Devise a meal plan for a 5-year-old child with a renal disorder that requires a 2-g sodium restriction per day. Keep in mind the child's developmental level and feeding idiosyncrasies at this age.

2. Develop a discharge teaching plan for a 3-year old with nephrotic syndrome who will be taking corticosteroids long term.

3. Devise a developmental stimulation plan for an 11-month old who has had significant urinary tract reconstruction surgery and is facing a prolonged period of confinement to the crib.

STUDY ACTIVITIES

1. In the clinical setting, compare the growth and development of two children of the same age, one with chronic renal failure and one who has been healthy.

2. While caring for children in the clinical setting, compare and contrast the medical history, signs and symptoms of illness, and prescribed treatments for a child with nephrotic syndrome and one with acute glomerulonephritis.

3. Observe peritoneal dialysis in the hospital or hemodialysis in a hospital or outpatient center. Record observations about the children's psychosocial and developmental status.

BRINGING IT ALL TOGETHER: A CASE STUDY

Antonio Cruise, a 7-year-old boy, is brought to the clinic by his mother for his annual examination. During your assessment the mother brings up concerns that Antonio continues to wet the bed at night. She states, "I was hoping this would end on its own, but now I'm concerned that there is a problem."

Go to thePoint to find questions to consider about this case.

44

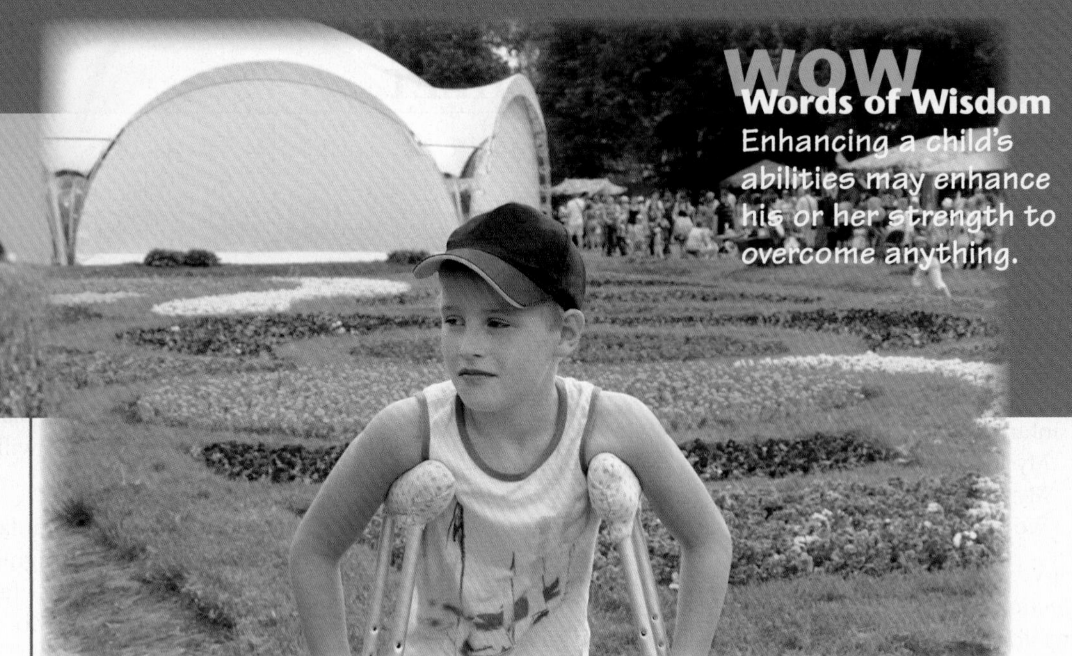
WOW
Words of Wisdom
Enhancing a child's abilities may enhance his or her strength to overcome anything.

Nursing Care of the Child With an Alteration in Mobility/Neuromuscular or Musculoskeletal Disorder

KEY TERMS

ataxia
clonus
contracture
epiphysis
external fixation
hypertonia
hypotonia
neurogenic bladder
spasticity
kyphosis
lordosis
ossification
traction
Trendelenburg gait

Learning Objectives

Upon completion of the chapter, you will be able to:

1. Compare differences between the anatomy and physiology of the neuromuscular and musculoskeletal systems in children versus adults.
2. Identify nursing interventions related to common laboratory and diagnostic tests used in the diagnosis and management of neuromuscular and musculoskeletal conditions.
3. Identify appropriate nursing assessments and interventions related to medications and treatments used for childhood neuromuscular and musculoskeletal conditions.
4. Distinguish various neuromuscular and musculoskeletal disorders occurring in childhood.
5. Devise an individualized nursing care plan for the child with a neuromuscular and musculoskeletal disorder.
6. Develop child/family teaching plans for the child with a neuromuscular and musculoskeletal disorder.
7. Describe the psychosocial impact of chronic neuromuscular and musculoskeletal disorders on the growth and development of children.

***Frederick Stevens*, 4 years old, seems to be falling often and has started to have difficulty climbing the stairs on his own. His mother states, "Recently he hasn't been able to keep up with his 6-year-old sister when we're playing at the park. He usually ends up sitting on the bench with me." She is concerned about the changes she has seen in her son.**

Mobility refers to mechanisms that facilitate or impair a person's ability to move (Herzing University—Orlando, 2014). Nurses encounter potential or actual alterations in mobility in all types of clients and must detect problems and intervene early to prevent complications. A variety of alterations in mobility (neuromuscular or musculoskeletal disorders) may affect children, but the result of each is muscular and/or skeletal dysfunction. Some of the disorders result from a neurologic insult such as trauma or hypoxia to the brain or spinal cord. Others occur as a result of genetic dysfunction or structural abnormality that is present from birth but may not be identified until later in childhood or adolescence. Infants and young children have resilient soft tissue, so sprains and strains are less common in this age group. Older school-age children and adolescents often participate in sports, resulting in an increased risk of injuries such as sprains, fractures, and torn ligaments.

The immobility associated with most neuromuscular and musculoskeletal disorders may affect the child's development and acquisition of motor skills, leading to motor dysfunction. Many neuromuscular and musculoskeletal disorders are chronic, lasting the child's entire life and resulting in handicaps.

The nurse caring for a child with altered mobility plays an important role in the management of these disorders. Not only must the nurse provide direct intervention in response to health alterations that result, but also the nurse is often part of the larger multidisciplinary team and may serve as the coordinator of many specialists or interventions. Understanding the most common responses to these disorders gives the nurse the foundation required to plan care for any child with any neuromuscular or musculoskeletal disorder.

VARIATIONS IN PEDIATRIC ANATOMY AND PHYSIOLOGY

The neuromuscular system is the combination of the nervous system and the muscles working together to create movement. The musculoskeletal system provides the body with form, support, stability, protection, and the ability to move. It is made up of bones, muscles, cartilage, tendons, ligaments, joints, and connective tissue. Anatomic and physiologic differences in infants and children, such as the immaturity of the neurologic and musculoskeletal systems, place them at increased risk for the development of a neuromuscular and musculoskeletal disorder and may hinder the child's growth and movement.

Brain and Spinal Cord Development

Early in gestation, around 3 to 4 weeks, the neural tube of the embryo begins to differentiate into the brain and spinal cord. If the fetus suffers infection, trauma, malnutrition, or teratogen exposure during this critical period of growth and differentiation, brain or spinal cord development may be altered. The premature infant's central nervous system is less mature than the term newborn's. Such immaturity in the preterm infant places him or her at a higher risk of central nervous insult within the neonatal period, which may result in delayed motor skill attainment or cerebral palsy. Compared with the adult, the child's spine is very mobile, especially the cervical spine region, resulting in a higher risk for cervical spine injury.

Myelinization

Though development of the structures of the nervous system is complete at birth, myelinization is incomplete. Myelinization continues to progress and is complete by about 2 years of age. Myelinization proceeds in a cephalocaudal and proximodistal fashion, allowing the infant to gain head and neck control before becoming able to control the trunk and the extremities. As myelinization proceeds, the speed and accuracy of nerve impulses increase. Primitive reflexes are replaced with voluntary movement.

Muscular Development

The muscular system, including tendons, ligaments, and cartilage, arises from the mesoderm in early embryonic development. At birth (term or preterm), the muscles, tendons, ligaments, and cartilage are all present and functional. The newborn infant is capable of spontaneous movement but lacks purposeful control. Full range of motion is present at birth. Healthy infants and children demonstrate normal muscle tone; **hypertonia** (increased muscle tone) or **hypotonia** (low muscle tone) is an abnormal finding. Deep tendon reflexes are present at birth and are initially brisk in the newborn and progress to average over the first few months. Sluggish deep tendon reflexes indicate an abnormality. As the infant matures and becomes mobile, the muscles develop further and become stronger. The infant's muscles account for approximately 25% of total body weight, as compared with the adult's muscle mass, which accounts for about 40% of total body weight (Carroll & Kerr, 2013). Muscles grow rapidly in adolescence; this contributes to clumsiness, which places the teen at increased risk for injury. In response to testosterone release, the adolescent boy experiences a growth spurt, particularly in the trunk and legs, and develops bulkier muscles. Female infants tend to have laxer ligaments than male infants, possibly due to the presence of female hormones, placing them at increased risk for developmental dysplasia of the hip (DDH) (Sankar, Horn, Wells, & Dormans, 2011).

Skeletal Development

The infant's skeleton is not fully ossified at birth. The infant and young child's bones are more flexible and more porous and have a lower mineral content than the adult's. These structural differences of a young child's bones allow for greater shock absorption, so the bones will often bend rather than break when an injury occurs. The thick, strong periosteum of the child's bones allows for a greater absorption of force than is seen in adults. As a result, the cortex of the bone does not always break, sometimes buckling or bending only. The skeleton contains increased amounts of cartilage compared with adolescents and adults. **Ossification**, the conversion of cartilage to bone, continues throughout childhood and is complete at adolescence.

During fetal development the spine displays **kyphosis**, an outward curvature. Cervical **lordosis**, inward curvature, develops as the infant starts to hold the head up. When the infant or toddler assumes an upright position, the primary and secondary curves of the spine begin to develop. The balance of the curves allows the head to be centered over the pelvis. During the toddler years, the period of early walking, lumbar lordosis may be significant (also termed toddler lordosis), and the toddler appears quite swaybacked and potbellied. As the child develops, the spine takes on more adult-like curves. During adolescence thoracic kyphosis may become evident. This is most often a postural effect, and as the teen matures, the posture appears similar to that of an adult.

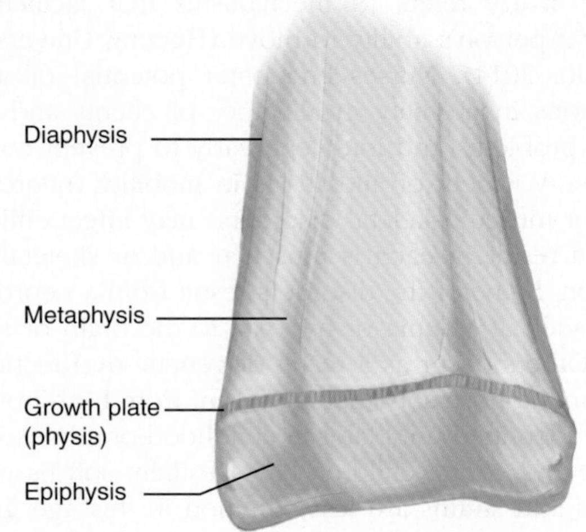

FIGURE 44.1 Anatomic areas of growing bone.

Growth Plate

The ends of the bones in young children are composed of the **epiphysis**, the end of a long bone, and the physis, in combination termed the growth plate. In infants, the epiphyses are cartilaginous and ossify over time. In children, the epiphysis is the secondary ossification center at the end of the bone. The physis is a cartilaginous area between the epiphysis and the metaphysis. Growth of the bones occurs primarily in the epiphyseal region. This area is vulnerable and structurally weak. Traumatic force applied to the epiphysis during injury may result in fracture in that area of the bone. Epiphyseal injury may result in early, incomplete, or partial closure of the growth plate, leading to deformity or shortening of the bone. Epiphyseal growth continues until skeletal maturity is reached during adolescence. Production of androgens in adolescence gradually causes the growth plates to fuse, and thus long bone growth is complete (Fig. 44.1).

Bone Healing

The child's bones have a thick, strong periosteum with an abundant blood supply. Bone healing occurs in the same fashion as in the adult, but because of the rich nutrient supply to the periosteum, it occurs more quickly in children. Children's bones produce callus more rapidly and in larger quantities than do adults. As new bone cells quickly form, a bulge of new bone growth occurs at the site of the fracture. The younger the child, the more quickly the bone heals. Also, the closer the fracture is to the growth plate (epiphysis), the more quickly the fracture heals. The capacity for remodeling (the process of breaking down and forming new bone) is increased in children as compared with adults. This means that straightening of the bone over time occurs more easily in children.

Positional Alterations

The lower extremities of the infant tend to have a bowed appearance, attributed to in utero positioning. In utero, the fetus' hips are usually flexed, abducted, and externally rotated, with the knees also flexed and the lower limbs inwardly rotated. This normal developmental variation is termed internal tibial torsion. The legs straighten with passive motion, and internal tibial torsion should not be confused with "bowlegs" (Fig. 44.2). Internal tibial torsion usually resolves independently some time in the second or third year of life as the toddler bears weight and the lower extremity muscles and bones mature. The bowlegged appearance is sometimes also referred to as genu varum. As internal tibial torsion or genu varum resolves, physiologic genu valgum occurs. Children usually demonstrate symmetric genu valgum (knock-knees) by the age of 2 to 3 years. In genu valgum, when the knees are touching, the ankles are significantly separated, with the lower portion of the legs angled outward (Fig. 44.3). By age 7 or 8 years, genu valgum gradually resolves in most children.

The newborn's feet also display in-toeing (metatarsus adductus) as a result of in utero positioning (see Fig. 44.2).

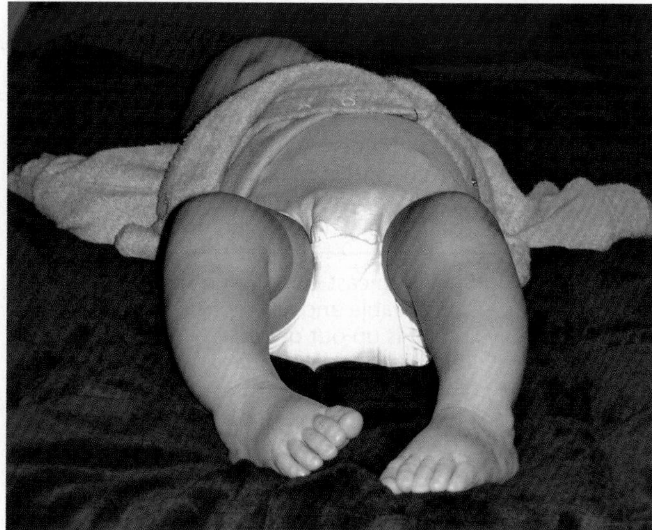

FIGURE 44.2 Internal tibial torsion with metatarsus adductus—normal findings in the infant.

The feet remain flexible and may be passively moved to midline and in a straight position. This also resolves as the infant's musculoskeletal system matures. Pes planus (flat feet) is noted in infants when they begin to walk. The long arch of the foot is not yet developed and makes contact with the floor, resulting in a medial bulge. As the child grows and the muscles become less lax, the arch generally develops. Some children may continue with flexible flat feet, and this is considered a normal variation.

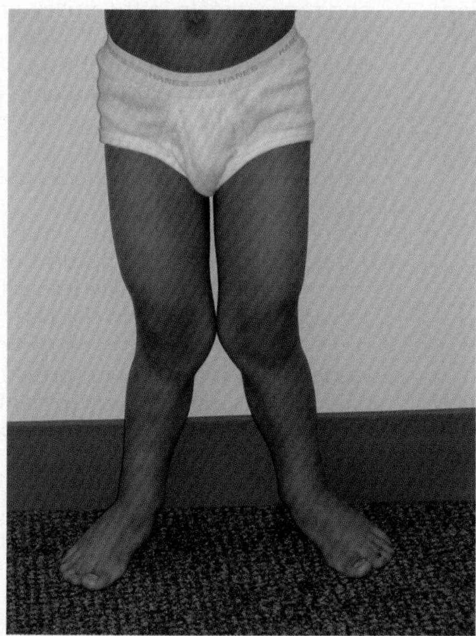

FIGURE 44.3 Genu valgum (knock-knees): note knees touching at midline and outward angle of the lower half of the legs.

Take Note!

Fractures are rare in children younger than 1 year of age. Carefully evaluate the infant who presents with a fracture for child abuse or an underlying musculoskeletal disorder (Haut, 2014).

COMMON MEDICAL TREATMENTS

A variety of medications as well as other medical treatments are used to treat neuromuscular and musculoskeletal disorders in children. Most of these treatments will require a physician's or nurse practitioner's order when the child is in the hospital. The most common treatments and medications are listed in Common Medical Treatments 44.1 and Drug Guide 44.1. The nurse caring for the child with a neuromuscular or musculoskeletal disorder should become familiar with what these procedures are and how they work as well as common nursing implications related to use of these modalities. The treatment of musculoskeletal disorders often involves immobilization via casting, bracing, splinting, or traction to allow healing with the bones in appropriate alignment. The length of treatment with these immobilization methods varies from weeks to months depending on the type of disorder being treated and its severity. Complications related to casting and traction include neurovascular compromise, skin integrity impairment, soft tissue injury, compartment syndrome, and, with skeletal traction, pin site infection or osteomyelitis.

Casts

Casts are used to immobilize a bone that has been injured or a diseased joint. When a fracture has occurred, a cast serves to hold the bone in reduction, thus preventing deformity as the fracture heals. Casts are constructed of a hard material, traditionally plaster but now more commonly fiberglass. The hard nature of the cast keeps the bone aligned so that healing may occur more quickly. In a fracture that would heal on its own without specific immobilization, a cast may be used to reduce pain and to allow the child increased mobility. The choice of cast material and type of cast will be determined by the physician or nurse practitioner or orthopedic surgeon. Figure 44.4 shows selected casts used in children.

Take Note!

Gore-Tex is a special material that can be used to line casts and make them waterproof. These casts can get completely wet in the bath, in the shower, or during swimming. These casts cannot be used for all types of fractures, fractures where skin pins are in place under the cast, or recently manipulated fractures (Cincinnati's Children's, 2013). These casts also have an increased cost that may not be covered by insurance.

(text continues on page 1679)

COMMON MEDICAL TREATMENTS 44.1

Treatment	Explanation	Indications	Nursing Implications
Casting	Application of plaster or fiberglass material to form a rigid apparatus to immobilize a body part	Fracture reduction, dislocations, correction of deformities	Assess frequently for neurovascular compromise, skin impairment at cast edges. Protect cast from moisture. Teach family how to care for cast at home.
Splinting	Temporary stiff support of injured area	Temporary fracture reduction, immobilization and support of sprains	Similar to cast care. Some splints are removable and are replaced when the child is up out of bed. Teach family appropriate use of splints.
Fixation	Surgical reduction of a fracture or skeletal deformity with an internal or external pin or fixation device	Fractures, skeletal deformities	No additional care for internal fixation External fixation: perform pin care as prescribed by the surgeon. Assess for excess drainage or pin slippage, notifying physician or nurse practitioner if this occurs. Velcro or snaps on sleeves and pant legs help with dressing.
Cold therapy	Application of ice bags, commercial cold packs, or cold compresses	Most often used in acute injuries to cause vasoconstriction, thereby decreasing pain and swelling	Apply for 20–30 minutes, then remove for 1 hour, and then reapply for 20–30 minutes. Discontinue when numbness occurs. Place a towel between the cold pack and the skin to prevent thermal injury.
Crutches	Ambulatory devices that transfer body weight from lower to upper extremities	Used whenever weight bearing is contraindicated	Top of crutch should reach 2–3 fingerbreadths below the axillae to prevent nerve palsy. Teach child appropriate ambulation with crutches or reinforce teaching if performed by physical therapist.
Skeletal or cervical traction	Traction is an application of a pulling force on an extremity or body part.	To minimize or prevent trauma to the spinal cord; Fracture reduction, dislocations, correction of deformities	To maintain even, constant traction: • Ensure weights hang free at all times and ropes remain in the pulley grooves. • Keep weights out of child's reach. • Maintain prescribed weight. • Elevate head or foot of bed only with physician order. Monitor for complications: • Perform neurovascular checks at least every 4 hours. • Monitor neurologic status closely. • Assess for signs and symptoms of infection or impaired skin integrity. • Provide appropriate pin site care.
Physical therapy, occupational therapy, or speech therapy	Physical therapy focuses on attainment or improvement of gross motor skills. Occupational therapy focuses on refinement of fine motor skills, feeding, and activities of daily living. Speech therapy is warranted for the child with a speech impairment or feeding difficulty related to oral muscular issues.	Cerebral palsy, spina bifida, spinal cord injury, muscular dystrophy, spinal muscular atrophy; Restore function after injury or surgery; promote developmental activities when limb use is compromised, as in limb deficiency.	Provide follow-through with prescribed exercises or supportive equipment. Success of therapy is dependent upon continued compliance with the prescribed regimen. Ensure that adequate communication exists within the interdisciplinary team.

COMMON MEDICAL TREATMENTS 44.1 (continued)

Treatment	Explanation	Indications	Nursing Implications
Orthotics, braces	Adaptive positioning devices specially fitted for each child by the physical or occupational therapist or orthotist. Used to maintain proper body or extremity alignment, improve mobility, and prevent contractures	Cerebral palsy, spinal cord injury, spina bifida, muscular dystrophy, spinal muscular atrophy; Used to immobilize a body part or prevent deformity through positioning. Used to treat developmental dysplasia of the hip and scoliosis; also may be used for a period of time after cast removal.	Provide frequent assessments of skin covered by the device to avoid skin breakdown. Cotton undergarment worn under the brace helps to maintain skin integrity. Follow the therapist's schedule of recommended "on" and "off" times. Encourage families to comply with use.

DRUG GUIDE 44.1 COMMON DRUGS FOR NEUROMUSCULAR DISORDERS

Medication	Actions/Indications	Nursing Implications
Benzodiazepines (diazepam, lorazepam)	Anticonvulsant; enhance the inhibition of GABA Used adjunctively for relief of skeletal muscle spasm associated with cerebral palsy, paralysis resulting from spinal cord injury, traction, and casting	Monitor sedation level. May cause dizziness Paradoxical excitement may occur. Assess for improvements in spasticity.
Baclofen (oral or intrathecal)	Central-acting skeletal muscle relaxant; precise mechanism unknown Used to treat painful spasms and decrease spasticity in children with motor neuron lesions, such as cerebral palsy and spinal cord injury	Assess motor function. Monitor for a decrease in spasticity. Observe for mental confusion, depression, or hallucinations. Dosage must be tapered before discontinuing because withdrawal symptoms may occur.
Corticosteroids	Anti-inflammatory and immunosuppressive action Duchenne muscular dystrophy, myasthenia gravis, dermatomyositis	Administer with food to decrease GI upset. May mask signs of infection Do not stop treatment abruptly or acute adrenal insufficiency may occur. Monitor for Cushing syndrome. Dosage may be tapered over time.
Botulin toxin	Neurotoxin produced by *Clostridium botulinum* that blocks neuromuscular conduction Relief of spasticity in cerebral palsy, occasionally for torticollis	Injected into the muscle by an advanced provider. May cause dry mouth
Acetaminophen	Blocks pain impulses in response to inhibition of prostaglandin synthesis. Relief of mild pain if used alone, moderate or severe pain if used with a narcotic analgesic	Often combined with a narcotic such as codeine or oxycodone for increased analgesic effect Monitor pain levels and response to medication.
Narcotic analgesics	Act on receptors in the brain to alter perception of pain. Relief of moderate to severe pain associated with injuries, orthopedic procedures	Assess pain location, quality, intensity, and duration. Assess respiratory rate prior to and periodically after administration. Monitor sedation level. May cause nausea, vomiting, constipation, pupil constriction

(continued)

DRUG GUIDE 44.1 COMMON DRUGS FOR NEUROMUSCULAR DISORDERS (continued)

Medication	Actions/Indications	Nursing Implications
Nonsteroidal anti-inflammatory drugs (NSAIDs: ibuprofen, ketorolac)	Inhibit prostaglandin synthesis, having a direct inhibitory effect on pain perception. Relief of mild to moderate pain, treatment of Legg-Calvé-Perthes disease	Monitor for nausea, vomiting, diarrhea, and constipation. Administer with water or food to decrease GI upset.
Bisphosphonate: IV—pamidronate, zoledronic acid; oral—alendronate, risedronate	Increase bone mineral density, decrease incidence of fractures in moderate to severe osteogenesis imperfecta.	IV: given at 4-month intervals, causes a decrease in serum calcium level, influenza-like reaction with first IV dose Oral: side effects include heartburn, regurgitation, and upper abdominal discomfort.

GABA, γ-aminobutyric acid; GI, gastrointestinal; IV, intravenously.

Adapted from Taketokmo, C. K., Hodding, J. H., & Kraus, D. M. (2013). *Lexi-comp's Drug Reference Handbook: Pediatric & Neonatal Dosage Handbook* (20th ed.). Hudson, OH: Lexi-comp, Inc.

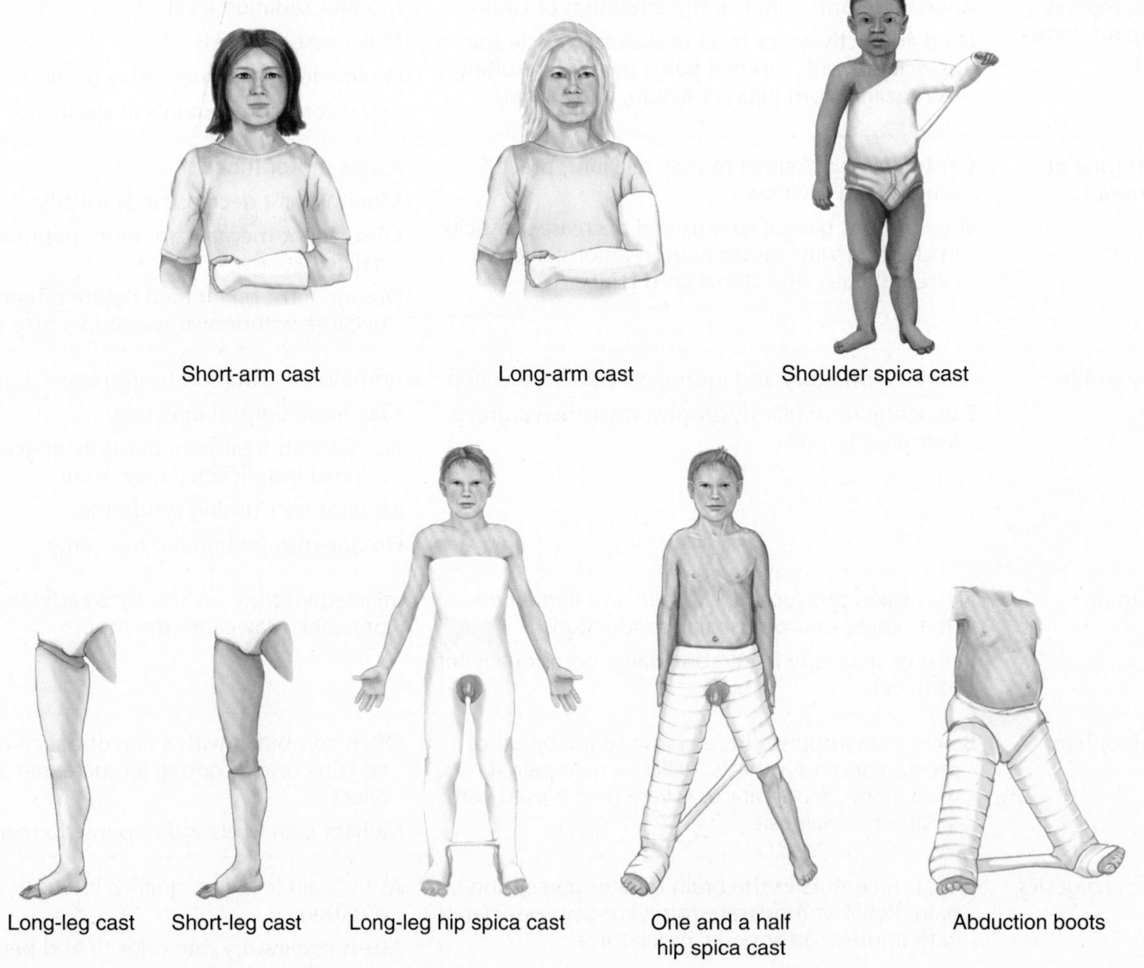

FIGURE 44.4 Selected casts used in children.

COMPARISON CHART 44.1 SKIN VERSUS SKELETAL TRACTION

	Skin Traction	Skeletal Traction
Application of force	To the skin via strips or tapes secured with Ace bandages or traction boots	To the body part directly by fixation into or through the bone
Length of treatment	Usually limited	Allows for longer periods of traction
Amount of force	Less	More

Traction

Traction, another common method of immobilization, may be used to reduce and/or immobilize a fracture, to align an injured extremity, and to allow the extremity to be restored to its normal length. Traction may also reduce pain by decreasing the incidence of muscle spasm. In running traction, the weight pulls directly on the extremity in only one plane. This may be achieved with either skin or skeletal traction. In balanced suspension traction, additional weights are used to provide a counterbalance to the force of traction. This allows for constant pull on the extremity even if the child changes position somewhat. Comparison Chart 44.1 discusses skin versus skeletal traction.

External Fixation

External fixation may be used for complicated fractures, especially open fractures with soft tissue damage. A series of pins or wires are inserted into bone and then attached to an external frame. The fixator apparatus may be adjusted as needed by the physician or nurse practitioner. Once the desired level of correction is achieved, no further adjustment occurs and the bone is allowed to heal. Advantages of external fixation include increased comfort for the injured child and improved function of muscles and joints when complicated fracture occurs.

NURSING PROCESS OVERVIEW FOR THE CHILD WITH A NEUROMUSCULAR OR MUSCULOSKELETAL DISORDER

Care of the child with a neuromuscular or musculoskeletal disorder includes assessment, nursing diagnosis, planning, interventions, and evaluation. There are a number of general concepts related to the nursing process that may be applied to neuromuscular and musculoskeletal dysfunction in children. From a general understanding of the care involved for a child with a neuromuscular or musculoskeletal disorder, the nurse can then individualize the care based on specifics particular for that child. The nursing care of immobilized children is similar to that of adults, yet developmental and age-appropriate effects must be taken into account. Prevention of complications is a key nursing function. Nursing Care Plan 44.1, at the end of the chapter, gives interventions related to prevention of complications. Particular care related to casts, traction, and fixators is discussed below.

Assessment

Assessment of neuromuscular and musculoskeletal dysfunction in children includes health history, physical examination, and laboratory and diagnostic testing.

Remember Frederick, the 4-year-old who has been falling and having difficulty climbing stairs and who seems to tire easily when playing with his sister? What additional health history and physical examination assessment information should the nurse obtain?

Health History

The health history consists of the past medical history, including the mother's pregnancy history, family history, and history of present illness (when the symptoms started and how they have progressed), as well as treatments used at home. The past medical history might be significant for prematurity, difficult birth, infection during pregnancy, changes in gait, falls, delayed development, poor growth, musculoskeletal congenital anomaly or orthopedic injury during the birthing process. Breech delivery may be associated with developmental dysplasia of the hip. Inquire about the child's usual level of physical activity, participation in sports, and use of protective equipment. Family history might be significant for neuromuscular disorders that are genetic or orthopedic problems. Determine the child's history of attainment of developmental milestones. Note the age that milestones such as sitting, crawling, and walking were attained, and determine whether the pace of attainment of milestones has decreased. Some children may progress normally at first and then demonstrate decreased velocity of development of achievements or even loss of abilities. Obtain a clear description of weakness; is it fatigue, or is the child truly not as strong as he or she was in the past?

When eliciting the history of the present illness, inquire about the following:

- Changes in gait or limp
- Recent trauma (determine the mechanism of injury)
- Recent strenuous exercise
- Poor feeding
- Lethargy
- Fever
- Weakness
- Alteration in muscle tone
- Areas of redness or swelling

Physical Examination

Physical examination of the nervous and musculoskeletal systems consists of inspection, observation, and palpation. It should also include auscultation of the heart and lungs, as the function of these organs may be affected by certain neuromuscular conditions.

INSPECTION AND OBSERVATION

Observe the infant or child playing with toys, crawling, or walking to obtain significant information about cranial nerve, cerebellar, and motor function. Observe the child's general appearance, noting any asymmetry in muscle development. Observe the child's posture and alignment of the trunk. Inspect the extremities for symmetry and positioning and for absence, duplication, or webbing of any digits. Note any obvious extremity deformity or limb-length discrepancy. When extremities are not used, muscular atrophy develops, so a shortened limb may indicate chronic hemiparesis. Observe gait in the child who has achieved the developmental skill of walking. Note refusal to walk, limping, in-toeing, out-toeing, or foot slap. Inspect injured joints for ecchymosis or swelling. In the injured extremity, note the color of the fingertips or toes. Observe spontaneous range of motion. Perform scoliosis screening to determine spinal alignment. Note symmetry of thigh folds. Note symmetry of spontaneous movement of extremities as well as facial muscles. Determine cranial nerve function (refer back to Chapter 38 for a complete description of assessment of cranial nerves). Inspect the skin for redness, warmth, bruises, and puncture sites. Inspect the spine for cutaneous abnormalities such as dimples or hair tufts, which may be associated with spinal cord abnormalities. Observe the child's level of consciousness (LOC), noting a decrease or significant changes. Note the presence of lethargy. Refer to Chapter 38 for a complete description of evaluation of LOC.

Motor Function. Observe spontaneous activity, posture, and balance, and assess for asymmetric movements. In the infant, observe resting posture, which will normally be a slightly flexed posture. The infant should be able to extend extremities to a normal stretch. Note position of comfort of the infant's or child's neck.

Reflexes. Note sluggish or brisk deep tendon reflexes. Note persistence of primitive reflexes in the older infant or child, such as Moro or tonic neck. Assess for development of protective reflexes, which is often delayed in infants with motor disorders.

Sensory Function. Alterations in sensory function accompany many neuromuscular disorders. Assess sensory function in a similar fashion to that used in the adult. The sensory functions of light touch, pain, vibration, heat, and cold are distinguishable by a child. In the infant, assess for response to light touch or pain. The usual response to pain will be withdrawal from the stimulus. Always prepare the child for the sensory examination in order to gain cooperation. The pinprick test may be particularly frightening, but most children will cooperate if educated appropriately.

PALPATION

Assess muscle strength and tone in the infant or child. Compare strength and tone bilaterally. Evaluate neck tone by pulling the infant from a supine position to a sitting position (Fig. 44.5). By 4 to 5 months the infant should be able to maintain the head in a neutral position. Perform passive range of motion of the neck. Alterations in range of motion may indicate a neuromuscular disorder or torticollis. Note trunk tone in the infant by holding the infant under the axillae and palpating for trunk tone. The hypotonic infant will

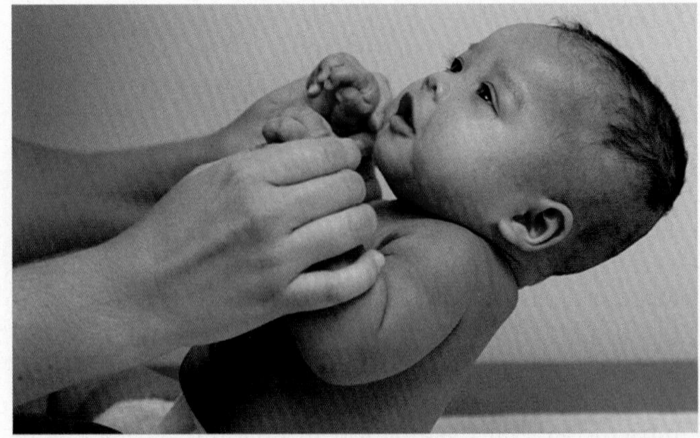

FIGURE 44.5 Assessing neck tone in an infant.

feel as though he or she is slipping through the examiner's hands. Generalized hypotonia is a common sign of neuromuscular disease in the infant and young child (Sarant, 2011a). The hypertonic infant will feel rigid, extending the trunk and legs. Assess leg tone in the infant by placing the infant in the vertical position with the feet on a flat surface; the 4-month-old infant should be able to momentarily support his or her weight (Fig. 44.6). Assess the strength of the infant or young child by noting ability to move the muscles against gravity. In older children, have the child push against the examiner's hand with the sole of the foot to determine muscle strength (Fig. 44.7). Note any hypertonia or **spasticity**, which is involuntary muscle contractions that are not coordinated with other muscles (e.g., when you stretch out your forearm the triceps contract and the biceps stretch; in spasticity they both contract at the same time). These may be an early indication of cerebral palsy or another neuromuscular disorder.

Take Note!

In cases of trauma or suspected trauma, do not perform any assessment that involves movement of the head and neck until cervical injury is ruled out. Maintain complete immobilization of the cervical spine until that time.

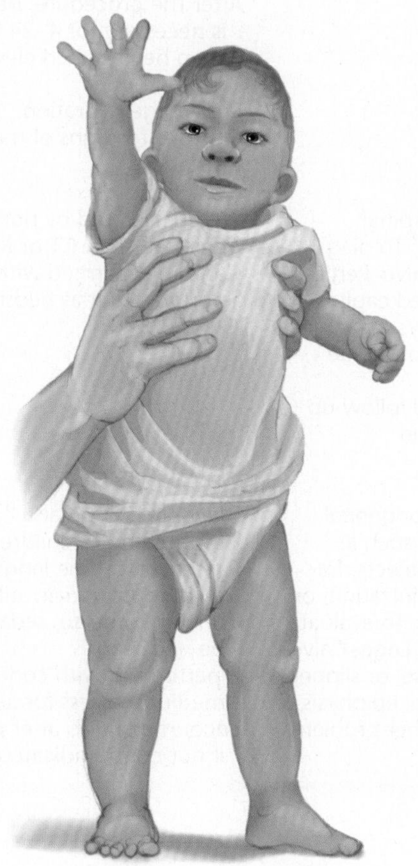

FIGURE 44.6 Assessing leg tone in an infant.

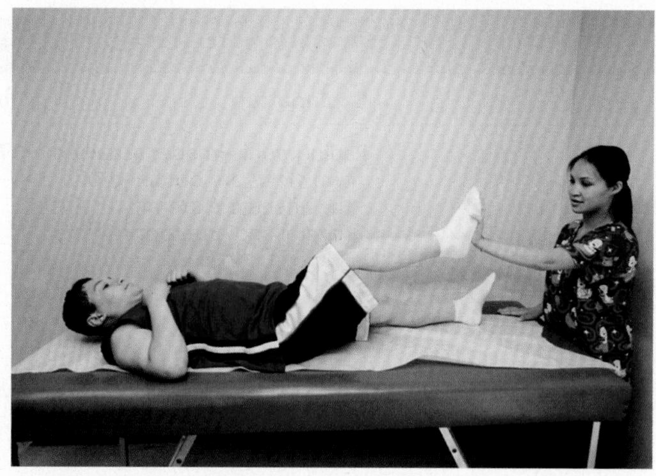

FIGURE 44.7 Assessing leg strength of the child.

Palpate the clavicles in the newborn or young infant for tenderness or a bump that indicates callus formation with clavicle fracture. Perform active range of motion to determine if a joint position is fixed (e.g., clubfoot). Palpate the affected joint or extremity to detect warmth or tenderness. In the injured child or the child with a cast or splint, thoroughly assess the neurovascular status of the affected extremities. Palpate the fingers or toes for warmth. Determine the capillary refill time. Note the presence of sensation or motion. Evaluate muscle strength. Palpate pulses distal to the injury, noting their strength and quality. Perform the Ortolani and Barlow maneuvers (see section on developmental dysplasia of the hip later in this chapter) to assess for developmental dysplasia of the hip.

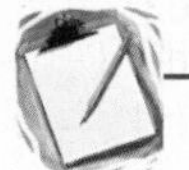

Take Note!

Assess the injured site last, and do so gently.

AUSCULTATION

Auscultate the child's lungs; adventitious sounds are often present when respiratory muscle function is impaired.

Laboratory and Diagnostic Testing

Common Laboratory and Diagnostic Tests 44.1 offers an explanation of the laboratory and diagnostic tests most commonly used in neuromuscular and musculoskeletal disorders. The tests can assist the physician or nurse practitioner in diagnosing the disorder and/or be used as guidelines in determining ongoing treatment. Laboratory or nonnursing personnel perform some of the tests, while the nurse might perform others. In either instance the nurse should be familiar

(text continues on page 1684)

COMMON LABORATORY AND DIAGNOSTIC TESTS 44.1

Test	Explanation	Indications	Nursing Implications
X-rays	Radiographic image; usually two views are obtained of the affected extremity (lateral and anteroposterior)	To detect fractures and other anomalies	Child must cooperate and hold still. Enlist the family's help in calming the child. In the trauma victim, the cervical spine should remain immobilized until cleared after cervical spine x-rays.
Fluoroscopy	Radiographic examination that uses continuous x-rays to show live, real-time images	Assessment of cervical spine instability during movement	Children may be afraid of the x-ray machine but will need to cooperate with flexion and extension of the neck. Allow a parent or family member to accompany the child.
Myelography	X-ray study of the spinal cord allowing visualization of the cord, nerve roots, and surrounding meninges	Detection of space-occupying lesions of the spinal cord; visualization of neural tube defects; evaluation of traumatic injury	Involves injection of contrast medium into the CSF via lumbar puncture. Most common contrast used is water-soluble iodine, but there is also oil and air contrast. Postprocedure interventions vary based on type of contrast medium; therefore, determine which one was used. After the procedure, bedrest is necessary for 4–24 hours; keep head of bed elevated for several hours. Encourage hydration. Observe for signs of meningeal irritation.
Ultrasound	Use of sound waves to locate the depth and structure within soft tissues and fluid	Assessment of spinal abnormalities; To diagnose Legg–Calvé–Perthes disease, slipped capital femoral epiphysis, fractures, ligament or soft tissue injuries Monitoring and follow-up of fractures and remodeling	Better tolerated by nonsedated children than CT or MRI Can be performed with a portable unit at bedside
Computed tomography (CT)	Noninvasive x-ray study that looks at tissue density and structures. Images a "slice" of tissue	Evaluation of congenital abnormalities such as neural tube defects, fractures, demyelinization, or inflammation; To evaluate the extent of, Legg–Calvé–Perthes disease, or slipped capital femoral epiphysis or to rule out other problems	Machine is large and can be frightening to children. Procedure can be lengthy and child must remain still. If unable to do so, sedation may be necessary. If performed with contrast medium, assess for allergy. Encourage fluids after procedure if not contraindicated.

COMMON LABORATORY AND DIAGNOSTIC TESTS 44.1 (continued)

Test	Explanation	Indications	Nursing Implications
Magnetic resonance imaging (MRI)	Based on how hydrogen atoms behave in a magnetic field when disturbed by radiofrequency signals. Does not require ionizing radiation. Provides a 3D view of the body part being scanned	Assessment of inflammation, congenital abnormalities such as neural tube defects; To assess hard and soft tissue, as well as bone marrow; to evaluate extent of Legg–Calvé–Perthes disease, or slipped capital femoral epiphysis; or to rule out other problems	Remove all metal objects from the child. Child must remain motionless for entire scan; parent can stay in room with child. Younger children will require sedation in order to be still. A loud thumping sound occurs inside the machine during the procedure, which can be frightening to children.
Creatine kinase	Reflects muscle damage: it leaks from muscle into plasma as muscles deteriorate.	Diagnosis of muscular dystrophy, spinal muscular atrophy	Draw sample before electromyogram or muscle biopsy, as those tests may lead to release of creatine kinase.
Electromyography (EMG)	A recording electrode is placed in the skeletal muscle and electrical activity is recorded.	Differentiates muscular disorders from those that are neurologic in origin	Requires insertion of short needles into the muscles. Sedation or analgesia may be ordered.
Nerve conduction velocity	Measures the speed of nerve conduction. Patch-like electrodes are attached to the skin at various nerve locations	Differentiation of muscular disorders	Feels like mild electric shocks EMG often performed at same time
Muscle biopsy	Removal of a piece of muscular tissue either by needle or by open biopsy	Determination of type of muscular dystrophy or spinal muscular atrophy	Postbiopsy care is similar to that for other types of biopsy. Involves a small incision with one or two sutures
Complete blood count	Evaluates hemoglobin and hematocrit, white blood cell count, platelet count	To evaluate hemoglobin and hematocrit with fracture with potential bleeding. To determine infection toxic synovitis	Normal values vary according to age and gender. White blood cell count differential is helpful in evaluating for infection. May be affected by myelosuppressive drugs
Arthrography	Multiple radiographic images of a joint after direct injection with a radiopaque substance	To assess ligaments, muscles, tendons, and cartilage, particularly after injury	Should not be performed if joint infection is present. The joint should be rested for 12 hours. Apply cold therapy afterward and assess for swelling and pain. Crepitus may be present in the joint for 1–2 days after procedure.
Genetic testing	Tests for presence of the gene for the disease or for carrier status	Determination of disease or carrier status of inherited muscular disorder	Entire family should be tested, even those unaffected, because carrier status should be determined and genetic counseling related to reproduction provided.

Adapted from Fischbach, F. T. & Dunning III, M. B. (2015). *A manual of laboratory and diagnostic tests* (9th ed.). Philadelphia, PA: Wolters Kluwer Health/Lippincott Williams & Wilkins.

with how the tests are performed, what they are used for, and normal versus abnormal results. This knowledge will also be necessary when providing child and family education related to the testing.

Nursing Diagnoses, Goals, Interventions, and Evaluations

Upon completion of a thorough assessment, the nurse might identify several nursing diagnoses, including:

- Pain (see Chapter 36)
- Impaired physical mobility
- Imbalanced nutrition: less than body requirements
- Urinary retention
- Risk for constipation
- Self-care deficit (specify)
- Risk for impaired skin integrity
- Chronic sorrow
- Risk for injury
- Deficient knowledge (specify)
- Family processes, interrupted

After completing an assessment of Fredrick, the nurse noted the following: he started walking at 2 years of age, he has difficulty jumping, his gait has a waddling appearance, and he does not rise from the floor in the usual fashion. Based on these assessment findings, what would your top three nursing diagnoses be for Fredrick?

Nursing goals, interventions, and evaluation for the child with neuromuscular and musculoskeletal dysfunction are based on the nursing diagnoses (see Nursing Care Plan 44.1 at the end of the chapter). The nursing care plan may be used as a guide in planning nursing care for the child with a neuromuscular or musculoskeletal disorder. The care plan includes many nursing diagnoses that are applicable to the child or adolescent. Children's responses to neuromuscular or musculoskeletal dysfunction and its treatment will vary, and nursing care should be individualized based on the child's and family's responses to illness; see Healthy People 2020. The nursing care of immobilized children is similar to that of adults, but developmental and age-appropriate effects must be taken into account. Prevention of complications is a key nursing function. Refer to Nursing Care Plan 44.1 at the end of the chapter for interventions related to prevention of complications. Additional information about nursing care related to certain disorders will be included later in the chapter as it relates to specific disorders. Refer to Chapter 36 for nursing interventions related to pain management. Particular care related to casts, traction, and external fixation is discussed below.

HEALTHY PEOPLE 2020

Objective	Nursing Significance
Increase the proportion of children with special health needs who have access to a medical home.	• Educate the family that specialist care (though often consisting of frequent and multiple visits) does not replace primary care through the medical home. • Encourage families to find a physician or nurse practitioner with whom they feel comfortable for well-child check-ups and routine childhood illnesses.

Healthy People Objectives retrieved from http://www.healthypeople.gov

Based on your top three nursing diagnoses for Fredrick, describe appropriate nursing interventions.

Assisting with Cast Application

Before cast or splint application, perform baseline neurovascular assessment for comparison after immobilization. Include:

- Color (note cyanosis or other discoloration)
- Movement (note inability to move fingers or toes)
- Sensation (note whether loss of sensation is present)
- Edema
- Quality of pulses

Enlist the cooperation of the child and reduce his or her fear by showing the child the cast materials and using an age-appropriate approach to describe cast application. Premedicate as ordered to reduce pain when manual traction is applied to align the bone. Use distraction throughout cast application and assist with application of the cast or splint (Fig. 44.8).

Take Note!

Modern fiberglass cast materials are available in a variety of colors, as well as a few patterns. Allowing the child to choose the color will increase the child's cooperation with the procedure.

After the cast or splint is applied, drying time will vary based on the type of material used. Splints and fiberglass casts usually take only a few minutes to dry and will cause a very warm feeling inside the cast, so warn the child that it will begin to feel very warm. Plaster requires

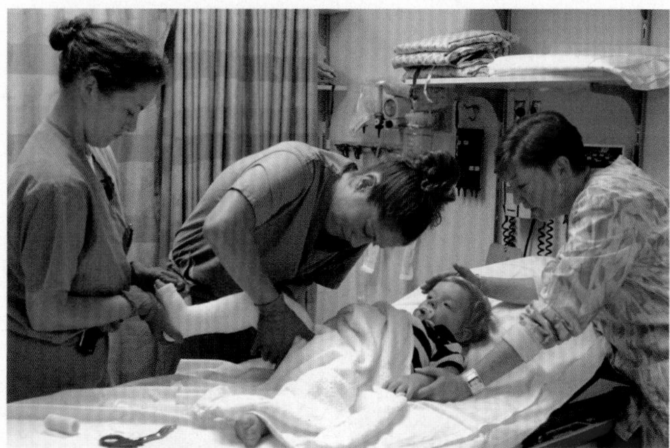

FIGURE 44.8 Assist with cast application by distracting or comforting the child.

24 to 48 hours to dry. Take care not to cause depressions in the plaster cast while drying, as those may cause skin pressure and breakdown. Instruct the child and family to keep the cast still, positioning it with pillows as needed.

Caring for the Child with a Cast

Perform frequent neurovascular checks of the casted extremity to identify signs of compromise early. These signs include:

- Increased pain
- Increased edema
- Pale or blue color
- Skin coolness
- Numbness or tingling
- Prolonged capillary refill
- Decreased pulse strength (or absence of pulse)

Notify the physician or nurse practitioner of changes in neurovascular status or odor or drainage from the cast.

Fiberglass casts usually have a soft fabric edge, so they usually do not cause skin rubbing at the edges of the cast. On the other hand, plaster casts require special treatment of the cast edge to prevent skin rubbing. This may be accomplished through a technique called petaling: cut rounded-edge strips of moleskin or another soft material with an adhesive backing and apply them to the edge of cast, as shown in Figure 44.9.

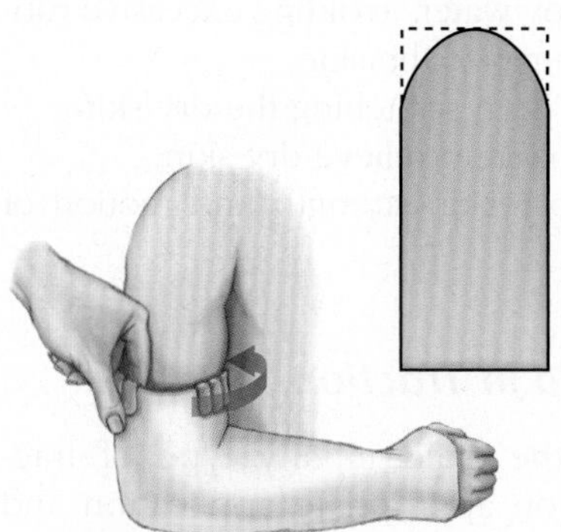

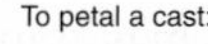

To petal a cast:
1. Cut several strips of adhesive tape or moleskin three to four inches in length. Use one inch tape for smaller areas (e.g., infant's foot) and two inch tape for larger areas (e.g., adolescent's waist).
2. Round one end of each strip to keep the corners from rolling.
3. Apply the first strip by tucking the straight end inside the cast and by bringing the rounded end over the cast edge to the outside.
4. Repeat the procedure, overlapping each additional strip, until all rough edges are completely covered.

FIGURE 44.9 Petaling the cast.

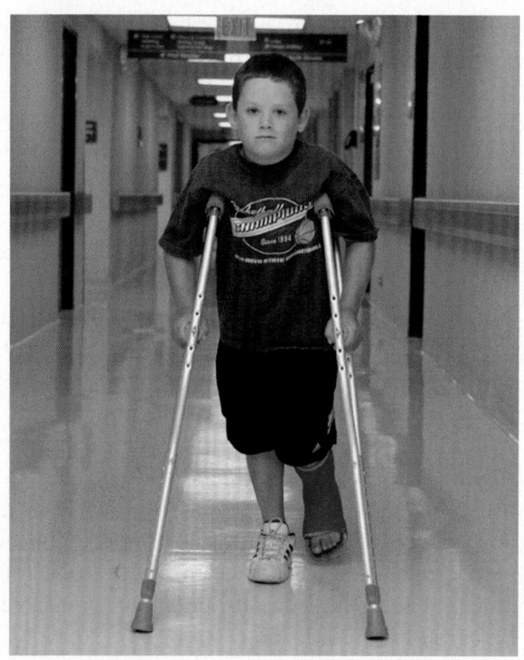

FIGURE 44.10 Reinforce appropriate crutch walking for children with lower extremity immobilization.

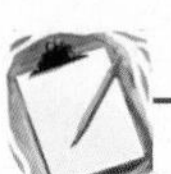

Take Note!

If a cast is lined with Gore-Tex, do not petal it.

Position the child with the casted extremity elevated on pillows. Ice may be applied during the first 24 to 48 hours after casting if needed. Teaching the child to use crutches is an important nursing intervention for any child with lower extremity immobilization so that the child can maintain mobility (Fig. 44.10). Provide home care instructions to the family about cast care. (See Teaching Guidelines 44.1.)

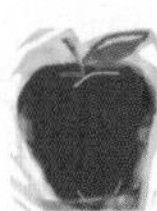

Teaching Guidelines 44.1
HOME CAST CARE

- For the first 48 hours, elevate the extremity above the level of the heart and apply cold therapy for 20 to 30 minutes, then off 1 to 2 hours, and repeat.
- Take your prescribed pain medication.
- Assess for swelling, and have the child wiggle the fingers or toes hourly.
- For itching inside the cast:
  - Never insert anything into the cast for the purposes of scratching.

  - Blow cool air in from a hair dryer set on the lowest setting or tap lightly on the cast.
  - Do not use lotions or powders.
- Do not pull padding out from the inside of the cast.
- Protect the cast from wetness.
  - Apply a plastic bag around cast and tape securely for bathing or showering. Continue to avoid placing the cast directly in water (unless it is Gore-Tex lined).
  - Waterproof cast covers are available through medical supply stores (still remain cautious about submerging cast with water).
  - Cover it when your child eats or drinks.
  - If a cast become soiled it can be wiped clean with a slightly damp clean cloth.
  - If the cast gets wet, dry it with a blow dryer on the cold setting (if warm setting is used the child could get burned). Use of a vacuum cleaner with a hose attachment to pull air through may speed drying-be careful to avoid skin.
- If the child has a large cast, change position every 2 hours during the day and while sleeping change position as often as possible.
- Check the skin for irritation.
  - Press the skin back around edges of the cast.
  - Use a flashlight to look for reddened or irritated areas.
  - Feel for blisters or sores.
- Call the physician or nurse practitioner if:
  - The casted extremity is cool to the touch, pale, blue, or very swollen.
  - The child cannot move the fingers or toes.
  - Severe pain occurs when the child attempts to move the fingers or toes.
  - Persistent numbness or tingling occurs.
  - Drainage or a foul smell comes from under the cast.
  - Severe itching occurs inside the cast.
  - The child runs a fever greater than 101.5°F for longer than 24 hours.
  - Skin edges are red and swollen or exhibit breakdown.
  - Child complains of rubbing or burning under cast.
  - The cast gets wet and does not dry or is cracked, split, or softened.

Adapted from Bowden, V. R., & Greenberg, C. S. (2012). *Pediatric nursing procedures* (3rd ed.). Philadelphia, PA: Lippincott Williams & Wilkins; Schweich, P. (2014). Patient information: Cast and splint care (Beyond the Basics). UpToDate. Retrieved from http://www.uptodate.com/contents/cast-and-splint-care-beyond-the-basics?source=see_link

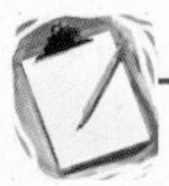

Take Note!

Persistent complaints of pain may indicate compromised skin integrity under the cast.

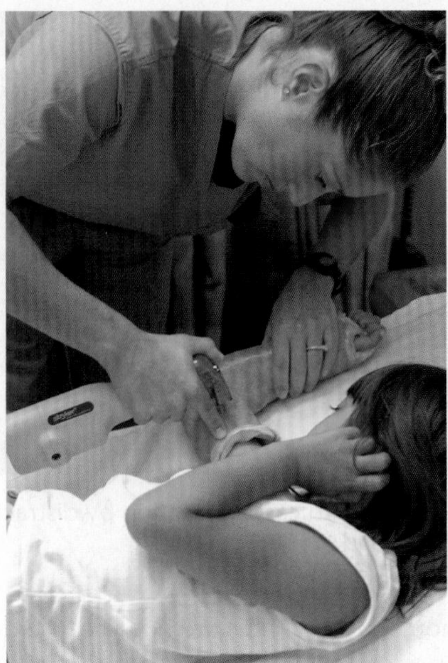

FIGURE 44.11 The loud noise of the cast saw may frighten the child.

Assisting with Cast Removal

Children may be frightened by cast removal. Prepare the child using age-appropriate terminology:

- The cast cutter will make a loud noise (Fig. 44.11).
- The skin or extremity will not be injured (demonstrate by touching the cast cutter lightly to your palm).
- The child will feel warmth or vibration during cast removal.

Teaching Guidelines 44.2 gives instructions related to skin care after cast removal.

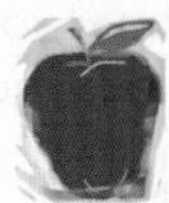

Teaching Guidelines 44.2
SKIN CARE AFTER CAST REMOVAL

- Brown, flaky skin is normal and occurs as dead skin and secretions accumulate under the cast.
- New skin may be tender.
- Soak with warm water daily.
- Wash with warm soapy water, avoiding excessive rubbing, which may traumatize the skin.
- Discourage the child from scratching the dry skin.
- Apply moisturizing lotion to relieve dry skin.
- Encourage activity to regain strength and motion of extremity.

Caring for the Child in Traction

Nursing care of the child in any type of traction focuses not only on appropriate application and maintenance of traction but also on promoting normal growth and development and preventing complications (see Table 44.1). Apply skin traction over intact skin

TABLE 44.1 TYPES OF TRACTION AND NURSING IMPLICATIONS

Type of Traction	Description	Nursing Implications
Bryant traction Knees slightly flexed Buttocks slightly elevated and clear of bed	Both legs are extended vertically, with child's weight serving as countertraction. Skin traction is applied to both legs. Used to reduce femur fracture in children younger than 2 years or with developmental dysplasia of the hip.	Maintain appropriate position. Ensure heels and ankles are free from pressure. Assess condition and position of elastic bandages every shift and rewrap elastic bandages as ordered.
Russell traction	Skin traction for femur fracture, hip, and specific types of knee injuries or contractures. Uses a knee sling. In split Russell traction, a portion of the traction weight may be redistributed via a pulley from the sling to the head of the bed (used for femur fracture, Legg–Calvé–Perthes disease, slipped capital femoral epiphysis).	Wrap bandages from ankle to thigh on children younger than age 2 years, from ankle to knee on children older than 2 years. Use a foot support to prevent foot drop. Ensure heel is free from bed. Assess popliteal region for skin breakdown from the sling. Mark leg to ensure proper replacement of sling.
Buck traction	Skin traction for hip and knee contractures, Legg–Calvé–Perthes disease, slipped capital femoral epiphysis. Used to rest an injured limb or to prevent spasms of injured muscles or joints Traction force delivered in straight line	Remove traction boot every 8 hours to assess skin. Leg may be slightly abducted.
Cervical skin traction	Skin traction applied with a skin strap (head halter). Used for neck sprains/strains, torticollis, or nerve trauma	Ensure that head halter or skin strap does not place pressure on ears or throat. Limit of 5 to 7 lb of weight
Side-arm 90–90	Skin traction for humerus fractures and injuries in or around the shoulder girdle.	Maintain elbow flexed at 90 degrees. Fingers and hand may feel cool because of elevation. Child may turn to affected side only.

(continued)

TABLE 44.1 TYPES OF TRACTION AND NURSING IMPLICATIONS (continued)

Type of Traction	Description	Nursing Implications
Dunlop side-arm 00–90	Skeletal traction through an olecranon screw or pin in distal humerus. Lower arm is held in balanced suspension.	See side-arm 90–90. In addition, provide appropriate pin site care.
90–90 traction	For femur fracture reduction when skin traction is inadequate. Skeletal traction with force applied through pin in distal femur	A foam boot may be used for suspension of the lower leg. Force of traction applied to femur via the pin. The amount of weight used is just enough to hold lower limb suspended.
Cervical skeletal tongs	Tongs attached to skull via pins. Used with fractures or dislocations of the cervical or high thoracic vertebrae	Assess frequently for increased pain, respiratory distress, and spinal cord, cranial nerve, or brachial plexus injury. Place on Stryker frame or specially equipped bed to ease positioning without disruption of alignment.
Halo traction	Metal halo attached to skull via pins. Used for cervical or high thoracic vertebrae fracture or dislocation and for postoperative immobilization following cervical fusion	Refer to nursing implications for cervical tongs. Tape small wrench to front of brace so that front panel can be quickly removed in an emergency. May become ambulatory in this type of traction; will be top-heavy so may need assistance with balance Assess pin sites and provide pin care as ordered.
Balanced suspension traction 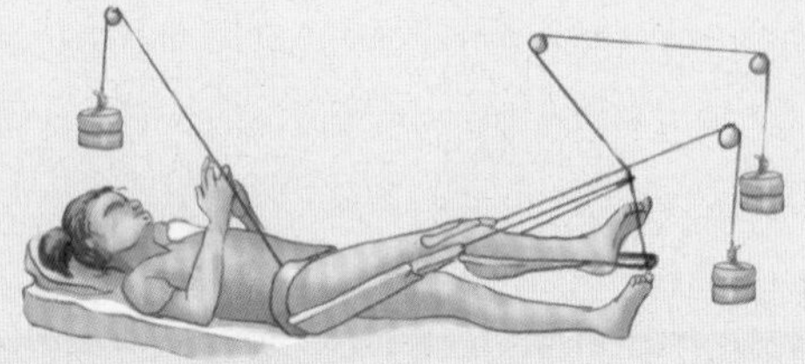	Used for femur, hip, or tibial fracture. Thomas splint suspends the thigh while the Pearson attachment allows knee flexion and supports the leg below the knee.	Avoid pressure to popliteal area.

only so that the pull of the traction is effective. Prepare the skin with an appropriate adhesive before applying the traction tapes to ensure that the tapes adhere well, preventing skin friction. After application of the traction tapes, apply the elastic bandage or use the foam boot. Attach the traction spreader block and then apply the prescribed amount of weight via a rope attached to the spreader block. Ensure that the rope moves without obstruction and that the weights hang freely without touching the floor.

In skeletal traction, apply weight via ropes attached to the skeletal pins. Treat the pin sites as surgical wounds (see section on pin site care). Protect the exposed ends of the pins to avoid injury. Whether skin or skeletal traction is used, be sure that constant and even traction is maintained.

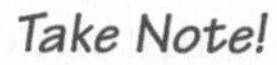

Take Note!

Avoid sudden bumping or movement of the bed: this can disturb traction alignment and cause additional pain to the child as the weights are jostled.

Preventing Complications

Refer to Nursing Care Plan 36.1 for interventions related to pain management and refer to Nursing Care Plan 44.1 for interventions related to prevention of complications of immobility such as skin integrity impairment. To prevent contractures and atrophy that may result from disuse of muscles, ensure that unaffected extremities are exercised. Assist the child to exercise the unaffected joints and to use the unaffected extremity if this does not disrupt traction alignment. Promote use of a trapeze if not contraindicated to involve the child in repositioning and assist with movement. Encourage deep-breathing exercises to prevent the pulmonary complications of long-term immobilization.

Promote normal growth and development by:

- Placing age-appropriate toys within the child's reach
- Encouraging visits from friends
- Providing diversional activities such as drawing, coloring, or video games (Fig. 44.12)

Take Note!

Ongoing, careful neurovascular assessments are critical in the child with a cast or in skeletal traction. Notify the physician or nurse practitioner immediately if these signs of compartment syndrome occur: extreme pain (out of proportion to the situation), pain with passive range of motion of digits, distal extremity pallor, inability to move digits, or loss of pulses.

Caring for the Child with an External Fixator

Care of an external fixator involves maintaining skin integrity, preventing infection, and preventing injury. Routine neurovascular and skin assessment is essential. Skin care is similar to a child in skeletal traction and includes pin care daily. Elevation of the extremity can help prevent swelling. The fixator may be moved by grasping the frame, as the fixator can tolerate ordinary movement. Encourage weight bearing as prescribed. Provide appropriate education to the child and family. Encourage the child to look at the apparatus. Teach the child not to pick or manipulate the pins. Baggy or loose clothing can be worn over the device. Velcro sewn into the seams can be helpful and allows clothes to slip over the device.

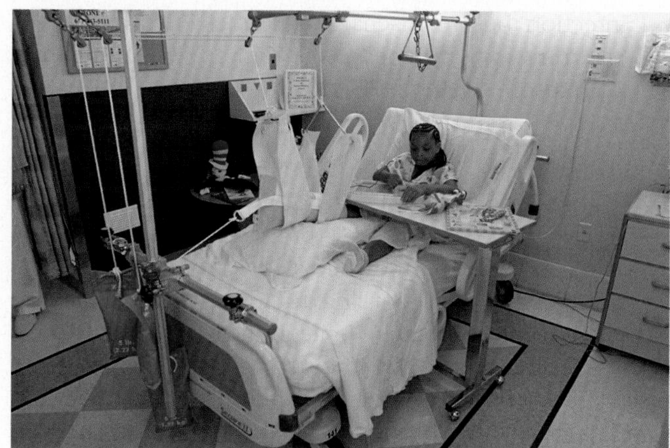

FIGURE 44.12 Provide age-appropriate diversional activities and schoolwork for children confined to bed in traction.

Providing Pin Care

Whether pins are inserted for skeletal traction or as part of an external fixator (see section on fractures), keeping the pin sites clean is important to prevent infection. Cleaning of the pin sites prevents infection by promoting comfort and preventing healing skin from adhering to the metal pin. Notify the orthopedic surgeon if signs of pin site infection are present or if pin slippage occurs.

Thus far, there is insufficient evidence that supports a particular strategy of pin care. More randomized trials are needed. The National Association of Orthopaedic Nurses and the Royal College of Nursing have published minimal guidelines, which include:

- Perform pin care weekly after the first 48 to 72 hours. Perform earlier if large amounts of drainage is present, dressing becomes wet, or infection is suspected.
- The most effective solution for pin site care may be chlorhexidine 2 mg/mL in alcohol. If child has sensitivity to this, use normal saline.
- Use a nonshedding material for cleaning.
- Cover pin sites with a nonshedding dressing.
- Teach children and their families pin site care along with instructions on the signs and symptoms of

infection before discharge (Holmes, Brown, & Pin Site Care Expert Panel, 2005; Timms, Vincent, Santy-Tomlinson, & Hertz, 2011).

Since the research available is minimal, these recommendations are made tentatively (Holmes et al., 2005; Lethaby, Temple, & Santy-Tomlinson, 2013). Therefore, interventions for pin care need to be individualized based on the child's condition and response to treatment and according to institutional policy or the physician's or nurse practitioner's orders. Certain physicians or nurse practitioners prefer the site to be cleaned with normal saline; others choose a solution with antibacterial properties. Some institutions recommend removal of all crusts formed on the skin around the pin; others do not. The rationale for crust removal is to promote free drainage and prevent the surrounding skin from adhering to the pin. A keyhole dressing may be necessary around the pin if drainage is present. No matter which procedure is ordered or preferred, perform pin care as necessary to prevent infection at the pin site. The Ilizarov fixator uses wires that are thinner than ordinary pins, so simply cleansing by showering is usually sufficient to keep the pin site clean. If drainage is present, cleanse the skin around the wires with a dry gauze pad.

When caring for children in the hospital, particularly those with complex medical needs, follow their home care routines as much as possible.

CONGENITAL AND DEVELOPMENTAL DISORDERS

Several disorders with neuromuscular and musculoskeletal effects are congenital in nature. These include neural tube defects and genetic neuromuscular disorders. The structural disorders are spina bifida occulta, meningocele, and myelomeningocele (neural tube defects). Congenital anomalies of the musculoskeletal system are usually readily identified at birth. Congenital structural anomalies involving the skeleton include pectus excavatum, pectus carinatum, limb deficiencies, polydactyly or syndactyly, metatarsus adductus, congenital clubfoot, and osteogenesis imperfecta. A developmental anomaly that may be diagnosed at birth or later in life is DDH. A muscular condition, torticollis, most often presents as a congenital condition but may also develop after birth. Tibia vara is a developmental disorder affecting young children. Rarely, a developmental positional alteration such as genu varum, genu valgum, or pes planus will persist past the usual age of resolution or cause the child pain. If those situations occur, bracing, orthotics, or surgical correction may become necessary. The genetic neuromuscular disorders include the various types of muscular dystrophy and spinal muscular atrophy (SMA). These disorders are not always recognized at birth because signs and symptoms are not evident until months or even years after birth. However, they are still considered to be congenital as they have a genetic basis.

Neural Tube Defects

Neural tube defects account for the majority of congenital anomalies of the central nervous system. The neural tube closes between the third and fourth week of gestation. The cause of neural tube defects is not known, but many factors, such as drugs, malnutrition, chemicals, and genetics, can hinder normal central nervous system development. Strong evidence exists that maternal preconception supplementation of folic acid can decrease the incidence of neural tube defects in pregnancies by 50% or more (American Academy of Pediatrics, 2012). Beginning in 1992 and continuing until today, the U.S. Public Health Service along with the Centers for Disease Control and Prevention (CDC) recommends that all women of childbearing age who are capable of becoming pregnant take 0.4 mg (400 mcg) of folic acid daily (Centers for Disease Control and Prevention, 2015). Pregnant women who had a previous child with a neural tube defect are recommended to take a higher dosage and should consult with their physician or nurse practitioner (American Academy of Pediatrics, 2012). Prenatal screening of maternal serum for α-fetoprotein (AFP) and ultrasound examination can help identify fetuses at risk. Neural tube defects primarily affecting spinal cord development include spina bifida occulta, meningocele, and myelomeningocele (Fig. 44.13). Neural tube defects primarily affecting brain development are discussed in Chapter 38.

Spina Bifida Occulta

Spina bifida is a term that is often used to refer to all neural tube disorders that affect the spinal cord. This can be confusing and a cause of concern for parents. There are well-defined degrees of spinal cord involvement, and it is important for healthcare professionals to use the correct terminology.

Spina bifida occulta is a defect of the vertebral bodies without protrusion of the spinal cord or meninges. This defect is not visible externally and in most cases has no adverse affects (see Fig. 44.13). Spina bifida occulta is a common anomaly. It is estimated that it affects 10% to 20% of otherwise healthy people (National Institute of Neurological Disorders and Stroke, 2015c). Children with spina bifida occulta need no immediate medical intervention. Complications are rare, but may include more

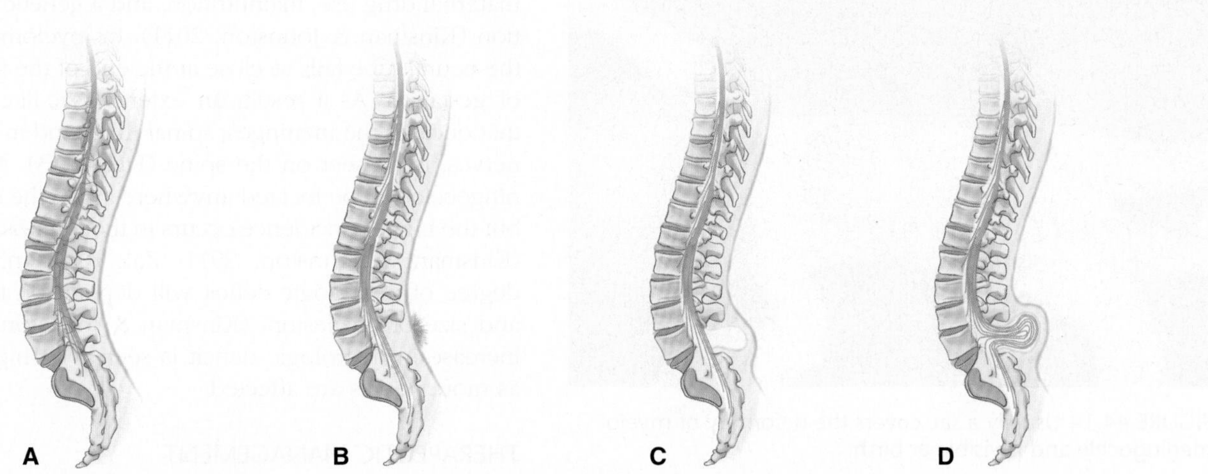

FIGURE 44.13 **(A)** Normal spine. **(B)** Spina bifida occulta. **(C)** Meningocele. **(D)** Myelomeningocele.

significant abnormalities of the spinal cord such as tethered cord, syringomyelia, or diastematomyelia.

NURSING ASSESSMENT

In most cases, spina bifida occulta is benign and asymptomatic and produces no neurologic signs. The defect, which is usually present in the lumbosacral area, often goes undetected. However, there may be noticeable dimpling, abnormal patches of hair, or discoloration of skin at the defect site. If so, further investigation, including magnetic resonance imaging (MRI), may be warranted.

NURSING MANAGEMENT

Nursing care will focus on educating the family. Inform parents of its presence and what the diagnosis means. Many times parents will confuse this diagnosis with spina bifida cystica, a much more serious defect. Occasionally, children with spina bifida occulta eventually need surgical intervention due to degenerative changes or involvement of the spine and nerve roots resulting in complications such as tethered cord, syringomyelia, or diastematomyelia. When these associated problems occur, the condition is often termed "occult spinal dysraphism" to avoid confusion.

Meningocele

Meningocele, the less serious form of spina bifida cystica, occurs when the meninges herniate through a defect in the vertebrae. The spinal cord is usually normal and there are typically minor or no associated neurologic deficits. Treatment for meningocele involves surgical correction of the lesion (see Fig. 44.13).

NURSING ASSESSMENT

Initial assessment after delivery will reveal a visible external sac protruding from the spinal area. It is most often seen in the lumbar region but can be anywhere along the spinal canal. Most are covered with skin and pose no threat to the child. However, assessment to ensure that the sac covering is intact remains important. Assess neurologic status carefully. Before surgical correction the infant will be thoroughly examined to determine whether there is any neural involvement or associated anomalies. Diagnostic procedures such as computed tomography (CT), MRI, and ultrasound may be performed.

NURSING MANAGEMENT

If the skin covering the sac is intact and the child has normal neurologic functioning, surgical correction may be delayed (Kinsman & Johnston, 2011). However, as in a child with myelomeningocele, immediately report any evidence of leaking cerebrospinal fluid (CSF) to ensure prompt intervention to prevent infection. Nursing management will be supportive. Provide preoperative and postoperative care similar to the child with myelomeningocele to prevent rupture of the sac, to prevent infection, and to provide adequate nutrition and hydration. Monitor for symptoms of constipation or bladder dysfunction that may result due to increasing size of the lesion. Resulting hydrocephalus has been associated with some cases of meningocele (Kinsman & Johnston, 2011). Therefore, monitor head circumference and watch for signs and symptoms of increased intracranial pressure (ICP).

Myelomeningocele

Myelomeningocele, the most severe form of neural tube defect, occurs in approximately 1 in 1,500 births (Committee on Obstetric Practice, 2013). Myelomeningocele is a type of spina bifida cystica, and clinically the term "spina bifida" is often used to refer to myelomeningocele. It may be diagnosed in utero via ultrasound. Otherwise

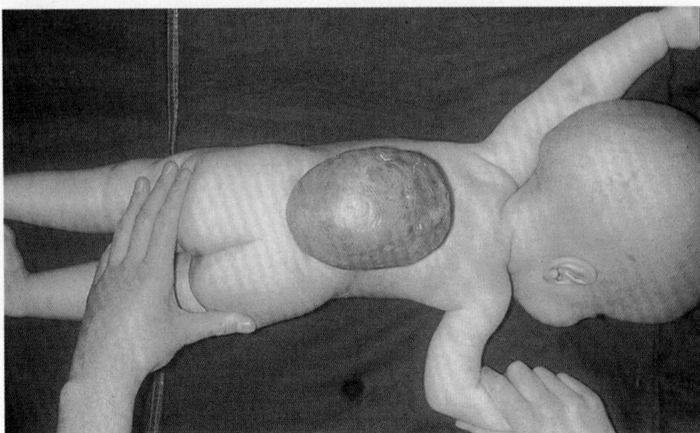

FIGURE 44.14 Usually a sac covers the deformity of myelomeningocele and is visible at birth.

it is visually obvious at birth. The newborn with myelomeningocele is at increased risk for meningitis, hypoxia, and hemorrhage.

In myelomeningocele, the spinal cord often ends at the point of the defect, resulting in absent motor and sensory function beyond that point (see Fig. 44.14). Therefore, the long-term complications of paralysis, orthopedic deformities, and bladder and bowel incontinence are often seen in children with myelomeningocele. The presence of neurogenic bladder and frequent catheterization puts the child at an increased risk for urinary tract infections, pyelonephritis, and hydronephrosis, which may result in long-term renal damage if managed inappropriately. Accompanying hydrocephalus associated with type II Chiari defect is seen in 90% of children with myelomeningocele (Zak & Chan, 2014). Due to the improper development and the downward displacement of the brain into the cervical spine, CSF flow is blocked, resulting in hydrocephalus. The lower the deformity is on the spine, the lower the risk of developing hydrocephalus (Kinsman & Johnston, 2011).

Children with myelomeningocele usually require multiple surgical procedures. In addition, due to frequent catheterizations, these children are at an increased risk of developing a latex allergy (Kinsman & Johnston, 2011; Zak & Chan, 2014). Learning problems and seizures are common in these children, but the majority of those surviving with myelomeningocele have average intelligence (Kinsman & Johnston, 2011; Zak & Chan, 2014). Ambulation is possible for some children, depending on the level of the lesion. Due to advances in medical treatment, research and improved services, the life expectancy of children with this disorder has increased and the quality of life has been improved (Zak & Chan, 2014).

PATHOPHYSIOLOGY

The cause of myelomeningocele is unknown, but risk factors are consistent with other neural tube defects, such as maternal drug use, malnutrition, and a genetic predisposition (Kinsman & Johnston, 2011). In myelomeningocele, the neural tube fails to close at the end of the fourth week of gestation. As a result, an external sac-like protrusion that encases the meninges, spinal fluid, and in some cases nerves, is present on the spine (Fig. 44.13). A myelomeningocele can be located anywhere along the spinal cord, but the highest incidence occurs in the lumbosacral region (Kinsman & Johnston, 2011; Zak & Chan, 2014).The degree of neurologic deficit will depend on the location and size of the lesion. (Kinsman & Johnston, 2011). An increase in neurologic deficit is seen with higher lesions as more nerves are affected.

THERAPEUTIC MANAGEMENT

Surgical closure will be performed as soon as possible after birth, especially if a CSF leak is present or if there is a danger of the sac rupturing. The goal of early surgical intervention is to prevent infection and to minimize further loss of function, which can result from the stretching of nerve roots as the meningeal sac expands after birth. A new option is becoming available but remains experimental. In utero fetal surgery to repair the myelomeningocele has been performed in the United States, with the first randomized trial showing improved outcomes for the fetuses but is not without risks to the mother and fetus (Robinson, 2011; Committee on Obstetric Practice, 2013). Ongoing management of this disorder remains complex. A multidisciplinary approach is needed, involving specialists in neurology, neurosurgery, urology, orthopedics, therapy, and rehabilitation along with intense nursing care. The chronic nature of this disorder necessitates lifelong follow-up.

NURSING ASSESSMENT

For a full description of the assessment phase of the nursing process, refer to the Assessment section of the Nursing Process Overview earlier in the chapter. Assessment findings pertinent to myelomeningocele are discussed below.

Health History. High-risk deliveries should be identified. Explore the pregnancy history and past medical history for risk factors such as:

- Lack of prenatal care
- Lack of preconception and/or prenatal folic acid supplementation
- Previous child born with neural tube defect or family history of neural tube defects
- Maternal consumption of certain drugs that antagonize folic acid, such as anticonvulsants (carbamazepine and phenobarbital)

The older infant or child with a history of myelomeningocele requires numerous surgical procedures and lifelong follow-up. In an infant or child returning for a clinic visit or hospitalization, the health history should include questions related to:

- Current mobility status and any changes in motor abilities
- Genitourinary function and regimen
- Bowel function and regimen
- Signs or symptoms of urinary infections
- History of hydrocephalus with presence of shunt
- Signs or symptoms of shunt infection or malfunction (refer to section on hydrocephalus in Chapter 38)
- Latex sensitivity
- Nutritional status, including changes in weight
- Any other changes in physical or cognitive state
- Resources available and used by the family

Physical Examination. Initial assessment after delivery will reveal a visible external sac protruding from the spinal area (Fig. 44.14). Observe the baby's general appearance and assess whether the sac covering is intact. Assess neurologic status and look for associated anomalies. Assess for movement of extremities and anal reflex, which will help determine the level of neurologic involvement. Flaccid paralysis, absence of deep tendon reflexes, lack of response to touch and pain stimuli, skeletal abnormalities such as club feet, constant dribbling of urine, and a relaxed anal sphincter may be found.

In the older infant or child, perform a thorough physical examination and focus on the functional assessment. Note the level of paralysis or paresthesia. Inspect skin for breakdown. Determine the child's motor capabilities.

Laboratory and Diagnostic Tests. A myelomeningocele may be detected prenatally around 16 to 18 weeks' gestation by ultrasound, by a blood test that detects AFP increases, or by analysis of amniotic fluid for AFP increases. Common laboratory and diagnostic studies ordered for the assessment of myelomeningocele include:

- MRI
- CT
- Ultrasound
- Myelography

These diagnostic tests are used to evaluate brain and spinal cord involvement (refer to Common Laboratory and Diagnostic Tests 44.1).

NURSING MANAGEMENT

Initial nursing management of the child with myelomeningocele involves preventing trauma to the meningeal sac and preventing infection before surgical repair of the defect. Refer to the Nursing Care Plan Overview in this chapter. Additional considerations are reviewed below.

Preventing Infection. Risk for infection related to the presence of the meningeal sac and potential for rupture is a central nursing concern in the newborn with myelomeningocele. Until surgical intervention occurs, the goal is to prevent rupture or leakage of CSF from the sac. Keeping the sac from drying out is important, as is preventing trauma or pressure on the sac. Use sterile saline-soaked nonadhesive gauze or antibiotic-soaked gauze to keep the sac moist. Immediately report any seepage of clear fluid from the lesion, as this could indicate an opening in the sac and provide a portal of entry for microorganisms. Position the infant in the prone position or supported on the side to avoid pressure on the sac. To keep the infant warm, place the infant in a warmer or isolette to avoid the use of blankets, which could exert too much pressure on the sac. Pay special attention while the infant is in a warmer or isolette because the radiant heat can cause drying and cracking of the sac.

Keep the lesion free of feces and urine to help avoid infection. Position the infant so that urine and feces flow away from the sac (e.g., prone position, or place a folded towel under the abdomen) to help prevent infection. Placing a piece of plastic wrap below the meningocele is another way of preventing feces from coming into contact with the lesion. After surgery, position the infant in the prone or side-lying position to allow the incision to heal. Continue with precautions to prevent urine or feces from coming into contact with the incision.

Promoting Urinary Elimination. Children with myelomeningocele often have bladder incontinence, though some children may achieve normal urinary continence. The level of the lesion will influence the amount of dysfunction. Myelomeningocele remains one of the most common causes of neurogenic bladder in children. Therefore, evaluation of renal function by a pediatric urologist should be performed on each child with myelomeningocele.

Neurogenic bladder refers to the failure of the bladder to either store urine or empty itself of urine. Children with neurogenic bladder have loss of control over voiding. The spastic type of neurogenic bladder is hyperreflexive and yields frequent release of urine, but with incomplete emptying. The hypotonic neurogenic bladder is flaccid and weak and becomes stretched out; it can hold very large amounts of urine, resulting in continuous dribbling of urine from the urethra. Urinary stasis and retention occur in both types, placing the child at risk for urinary tract infection as well as reflux of bladder contents back up into the ureters and kidneys, resulting in renal scarring and insufficiency.

The goals of neurogenic bladder management are to promote optimal urinary continence and prevent renal complications. Interventions for neurogenic bladder include clean intermittent catheterization to promote bladder emptying; medications such as oxybutynin chloride (Ditropan) to improve bladder capacity; prompt recognition and treatment of infections; and in some children surgical interventions such as a continent urinary reservoir or vesicostomy to facilitate urinary elimination. Clean intermittent catheterization is addressed below. In the child with a spastic or rigid bladder, teach parents how to administer antispasmodic medications such as oxybutynin. Teach the parents that the medication is used to increase the bladder capacity and reduce the potential for reflux. Refer to Chapter 43 for additional information on nursing care related to the surgical procedures.

Assessing Urinary Function. Determine the child's pattern and success of toilet training, both for bladder and bowel. Assess the child's cognitive/developmental level. Observe the genital area for dribbling of urine from the urethra, noting odor of urine if present. Note redness of the urethra or excoriation in the diaper area. Inspect the abdomen for scars from prior surgeries and the presence of urinary diversion or continent stoma. Palpate the abdomen for presence of distended bladder, fecal mass, or enlarged kidneys. Determine the child's level of paralysis or paresthesia.

Performing Clean Intermittent Catheterization. Depending on the level of paralysis at birth in the child with myelomeningocele, clean intermittent catheterization may be started at that time. In other children with spina bifida and in children who suffer spinal cord injury, catheterization may be started at a later age. Teach parents the technique of clean intermittent catheterization via the urethra, unless a urinary diversion or continent stoma has been created (Teaching Guidelines 44.3). See Evidence-Based Practice 44.1.

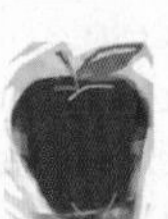

Teaching Guidelines 44.3

CLEAN INTERMITTENT CATHETERIZATION

- Wash hands with soap and water or use waterless antibacterial cleanser.
- Have supplies within reach and place child on his or her back, on toilet, or in wheelchair.
- Clean genitalia with a washcloth or disposable wipe (on girls separate labia and wipe front to back; on boys clean the tip of the penis; if uncircumcised, pull back foreskin so tip of penis is visible).
- Apply generous amount of water-based lubricant to catheter.
- Perform catheterization. Insert catheter only as far as needed to obtain urine flow (about 2 to 3 inches for females, about 4 to 6 inches for males). Hold catheter there until urine flow stops. Move catheter slightly, press on lower abdomen, or have child lean forward to tense abdominals to ensure no more urine is in the bladder.
- Wash reusable catheter after use with soapy water inside and out; rinse well (a syringe can be used to flush the catheter) and allow to dry.
- When dry, store in zip-top plastic bag or other clean storage container.
- Sterilize daily (time frames and procedure may vary based on institution policy and procedures); soak the catheter in a 1:1 vinegar and water solution for about 30 minutes, rinsing well before next use, or place the catheter in boiling water for 10 minutes. Allow to dry very well before storing.
- Replace the catheter when it becomes cloudy, stiff, rough, cracked, or damaged.
- Teach the child to self-catheterize when he or she is developmentally ready.

Adapted from Bozic, D., & Daniels, C. (2009a). *AboutKidsHealth clean intermittent catheterization (CIC): Step by step instructions for boys*. Retrieved from http://www.aboutkidshealth.ca/en/healthaz/testsandtreatments/medicaldevices/pages/clean-intermittent-catheterization-cic-step-by-step-instructions-for-boys.aspx

Bozic, D., & Daniels, C. (2009b). *AboutKidsHealth clean intermittent catheterization (CIC): Step by step instructions for girls*. Retrieved from http://www.aboutkidshealth.ca/En/HealthAZ/TestsAndTreatments/MedicalDevices/Pages/Clean-Intermittent-Catheterization-CIC-Step-By-Step-Instructions-for-Girls.aspx

Teaching the parents the techniques of clean intermittent catheterization is an important step in preserving renal functioning, preventing infection, and helping the family gain some control over the child's physical condition. Until the child is able to self-catheterize, the parents will be responsible for this procedure. Children with normal intelligence and upper extremity motor skills usually learn to self-catheterize at the age of 6 or 7 years (Zak & Chan, 2014). Urinary incontinence is associated with poor self-esteem, particularly as the child gets older. Educating the child to self-catheterize the urethra or stoma as appropriate empowers the child, gives him or her a sense of control, and allows for appropriate urinary elimination when the child is away from the parents (e.g., at school).

Offer support and appropriate referrals to the child and family. Refer families to vendors in the local area for catheterization supplies.

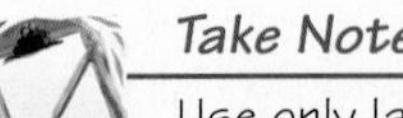

Take Note!

Use only latex-free catheters and gloves for catheterization of children with myelomeningocele and/or neurogenic bladder, as these children exhibit a high incidence of latex allergy.

Promoting Bowel Elimination. Children with myelomeningocele often have bowel incontinence as well; the level of the lesion affects the amount of dysfunction. Many children with myelomeningocele can achieve

EVIDENCE-BASED PRACTICE 44.1

SELF-INTERMITTENT CATHETERIZATION AMONG FEMALE CHILDREN WITH MYELOMENINGOCELE AND THE POTENTIAL FOR INCREASED COMPLICATIONS

STUDY

This study was a comparative cross-over trial on children performing clean intermittent catheterization (CIC). It compared the incidence of symptomatic urinary tract infection (UTI) and presence of bacteriuria in 40 children, aged 2–16, who reused catheters for 1 week versus 3 weeks. For the first 9 weeks the children changed CIC catheters once every 3 weeks and for the second 9 weeks they changed catheters weekly.

Findings

The occurrence of bacteriuria was 74% during the every 3 week catheter changed and dropped to 34% during the weekly changes. No episodes of UTI occurred during the study.

Nursing Implications

There are few complications occurring in females with myelomeningocele who self-catheterize using clean technique. Encourage the use of large-size noncoated polyvinyl catheters. Teach females when developmentally capable to perform self-CIC. This function is safe and yields greater independence in this special population.

Bacteriuria is common in children with neurogenic bladder. Children who require clean intermittent catheterization may reuse their catheters multiple times. There is limited data or guidelines on how often these catheters need to be replaced. This study found that reusing a catheter for up to 3 weeks increased in incidence of bacteriuria but did not increase the occurrence of UTIs. This finding supports the idea that bacteria colonization of the urinary tract may actually provide protection against invasion of more virulent bacteria. These authors conclude that reusing catheters for up to 3 weeks is safe and 3 week catheter changes may provide some protection against UTIs.

Adapted from Kanaheswari Y., Kavitha R., & Rizal A.M. (2014). Urinary tract infection and bacteriuria in children performing clean intermittent catheterization with reused catheters. *Spinal Cord, 53*, 209–212.

some degree of bowel continence. Bowel training with the use of timed enemas or suppositories along with diet modifications can allow for defecation at predetermined times once or twice a day. Although bowel incontinence can be difficult for children as they grow older due to social concerns and self-esteem and body image disturbances, it does not pose the same health risks as urinary incontinence.

Promoting Adequate Nutrition. The risk for altered nutrition, less than body requirements, related to the restrictions on positioning of the infant before and after surgery is another nursing concern. Assist the family in assuming as normal a feeding position as possible. Preoperatively, the risk of rupture may be too high to warrant holding. Therefore, the infant's head can be turned to the side or the infant can be placed in the side-lying position to facilitate feeding. If the infant is held, special care needs to be taken to avoid pressure on the sac or postoperative incision. Encourage the parents to interact as much as possible with the infant by talking to and touching the infant during feeding to help promote intake. If the mother was planning on breastfeeding the infant, assist her in meeting this goal, if possible. If the infant can be held, encourage her to do this, or assist her in pumping and saving breast milk to be given to the infant via bottle until the infant is able to be held. Feeding an infant in an unusual position can be difficult, and it is the nurse's role to provide support, education, and modeling for the parents and family when needed.

Preventing Latex Allergic Reaction. Sensitivity to latex or natural rubber is very common among children with myelomeningocele. They are at an increased risk of developing an allergy to latex related to the multiple exposures to latex products during surgical procedures and bladder catheterizations. A latex-free environment should be created for all procedures performed on children with myelomeningocele to prevent latex allergy. Also, children with a known latex allergy must be identified and managed in a latex-free environment. The nurse must ensure that these children do not come into direct contact with latex or equipment and supplies that contain latex. Be familiar with those products and equipment at your facility that contain latex and those that are latex-free. The Food and Drug Administration (FDA) now requires that all medical supplies be labeled if they contain latex (FDA, 2014), but this is not the case for consumer products. Many resources exist that list products that are latex-free, and each hospital should have such a list readily available to healthcare professionals. For an updated list of latex-containing products and other helpful information for parents regarding consumer products, contact the Spina Bifida Association of America, a link to which can be found on thePoint.

Children who are at a high risk for latex sensitivity should wear medical alert identification. Education programs regarding latex sensitivity and ways to prevent it need to be directed at those who care for high-risk children, including teachers, school nurses, relatives, babysitters, and all healthcare professionals.

Maintaining Skin Integrity. Address the risk for altered skin integrity related to the infant's prone position and impaired mobility. The prone position puts constant pressure on the knees and elbows, and it may be difficult to keep the infant clean of urine and feces. Diapering may be contraindicated preoperatively to avoid pressure on the sac. Therefore, ensure that the infant is kept as clean and dry as possible. This is made more difficult by the constant dribbling of stool and urine that may be present. Placing a pad beneath the diaper area and changing it frequently is important. Perform meticulous skin care. Place the infant on a special care mattress and place synthetic sheepskin under the infant to help reduce friction. Special attention to the infant's legs needs to occur when positioning them, since paralysis may be present. Using a folded diaper between the legs can help reduce pressure and friction from the legs rubbing together.

Educating and Supporting the Child and Family. Myelomeningocele is a serious disorder that affects multiple body systems and produces varying degrees of deficits. It is a disorder that has lifelong effects. Thanks to medical advances and technology most children born with myelomeningocele can expect to live a normal life, but challenges remain for the family and child as they learn to cope and live with this physical condition. Adjusting to the demands this condition places on the child and family is difficult. Parents may need time to accept their infant's condition, but as soon as possible they should be involved in the infant's care.

Teaching should begin immediately in the hospital. Teaching should include positioning, preventing infection, feeding, promoting urinary elimination through clean intermittent catheterization, preventing latex allergy, and identifying the signs and symptoms of complications such as increased ICP. Due to the chronic nature of this condition, long-term planning needs to begin in the hospital. These children usually require multiple surgical procedures and hospitalizations, and this can place stress on the family and their finances. The nurse has an important role in providing ongoing education about the illness and its treatments and the plan of care. As the family becomes more comfortable with the condition, they will become the experts in the child's care. Respect and recognize the family's changing needs. Providing intense daily care can take its toll on a family, and continual support and encouragement are needed. Referral to the Spina Bifida Association and a local support group for families of children with myelomeningocele is appropriate. See Healthy People 2020.

HEALTHY PEOPLE 2020

Objective	Nursing Significance
Increase the proportion of children and youth with disabilities who spend at least 80% of their time in regular education programs.	• Become familiar with local schools' offerings and capabilities so that you can refer families to an educational site appropriate for their child.

Healthy People Objectives retrieved from http://www.healthypeople.gov

Consider This

After learning that our new baby will be born with spina bifida I felt so alone. I feel scared and sad, I am angry too. I wish I knew how this could happen.

Thoughts: How would you respond to her concerns? What local resources could you refer her to?

Pectus Excavatum

Pectus excavatum and pectus carinatum are anterior chest wall deformities. Pectus excavatum, a funnel-shaped chest, accounts for greater than 90% of all congenital chest wall deformities (Boas, 2011). A depression that sinks inward is apparent at the xiphoid process (Fig. 44.15). Pectus carinatum, a protuberance of the chest wall, accounts for only 5% to 15% of anterior chest wall deformities (Boas, 2011). The remainder are mixed deformities. Male predominance is evident in both types (Boas, 2011).

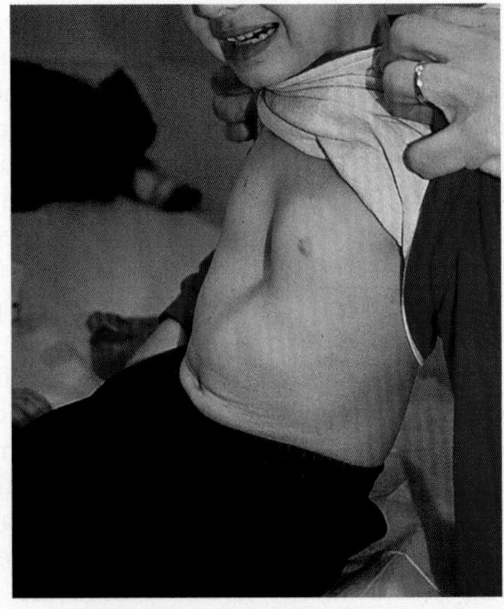

FIGURE 44.15 Pectus excavatum: note the depression in the chest wall at the xiphoid process.

Pectus excavatum does not resolve as the child grows; rather, it progresses with growth. The chest depression may be minimal or marked. When the pectus is more pronounced, cardiac and pulmonary compression occurs. Symptoms of this compression most often present during puberty, when the pectus quickly worsens. Children may complain of shortness of breath, withdraw from physical activities, and have a poor body image.

Therapeutic Management

Therapeutic management of pectus excavatum is based on the severity and physiologic compromise. Options include observation, use of physical therapy to work on musculoskeletal compromise, and surgical correction, preferably before puberty, when the skeleton is more pliable. Various surgical techniques may be used and generally involve either the placement of a surgical steel bar or using a piece of bone in the rib cage to lift the depression. This discussion will focus on care of the child who undergoes surgical steel bar placement for pectus correction.

Nursing Assessment

Elicit the health history, noting progression of the defect and effects on the child's cardiopulmonary function. Note shortness of breath, exercise intolerance, or chest pain. Observe the child's chest for anterior wall deformity, noting depth and severity. Auscultate the lungs to determine the adequacy of aeration. X-rays, CT, or MRI may be used to determine the extent of the anomaly and compression of inner structures.

Nursing Management

Prepare the child preoperatively by allowing a tour of the surgical area and the pediatric intensive care unit. Introduce the child to the pain scale that will be used in the postoperative period.

Postoperatively, nursing management focuses on assessment, protection of the surgical site, and pain management. Auscultate lung sounds frequently to determine the adequacy of aeration and to monitor for development of the complication of pneumothorax. Assess for signs of wound infection that would necessitate removal of the curved bar. During the first few postoperative days positioning is challenging; do not allow the child to roll in bed, lie on either side, or rotate or flex the spine (these positions may disrupt the bar's position). Administer analgesics as needed either intravenously or via the epidural catheter. Teach families that the child will not be allowed to lie on his or her side at home for 4 weeks after the surgery to ensure that the band does not shift. Encourage aerobic activity at home after being cleared by the surgeon (this will increase the child's vital capacity, previously hindered by the pectus). The bar will be removed 2 to 4 years after the initial placement.

Limb Deficiencies

Limb deficiencies, either complete absence of a limb or a portion of it or deformity, occur as the fetus is developing. The limb either fails to form normally or does not form at all. The cause is unknown. Certain behaviors and exposures can increase the risk of limb deficiencies such as exposure to certain chemicals, viruses, medications, and possible maternal exposure to tobacco smoke (Centers for Disease Control and Prevention, 2014). These defects can be attributed to an amniotic band constricting the limb, resulting in either incomplete development or amputation of the limb. Many children born with limb deformities also have congenital anomalies such as craniofacial abnormalities, cardiac and abdominal wall defects (Centers for Disease Control and Prevention, 2014).

Therapeutic management is aimed at improving the child's functional ability. Physical therapy and occupational therapy may be helpful. Adaptive equipment such as a prosthesis may also be prescribed.

Nursing Assessment

Note the extent of limb deformity, providing an accurate description of the presence or absence of a portion of the arm or leg, or missing fingers or toes. Assess the child's ability to use the extremity as a helper (arms) or in ambulation (legs). Determine status of acquisition of developmental skills.

Nursing Management

Reinforce prescribed activities that are meant to improve the child's function. Provide activities in which the child is capable of participating. If the limb deficiency is significant, refer the infant to the local early intervention office as soon as possible after birth. Early intervention, available in all 50 states, is designed to promote development from birth to age 3 years. Absence of a limb or a significant portion of a limb will have a considerable impact on the child's ability to meet developmental milestones as expected.

Polydactyly/Syndactyly

Polydactyly is the presence of extra digits on the hand or foot (Fig. 44.16). One third of the time, polydactyly occurs in both the hand and foot (Hosalkar, Spiegel, & Davidson, 2011). It usually involves digits at the border of the hand or foot, but can also occur by a central digit (Hosalkar et al., 2011). Syndactyly is webbing of the fingers and toes. Both polydactyly and syndactyly

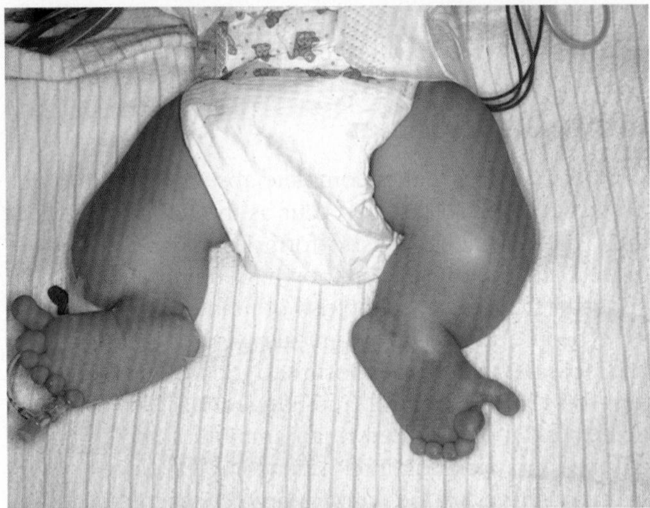

FIGURE 44.16 Note additional digits (toes) of polydactyly.

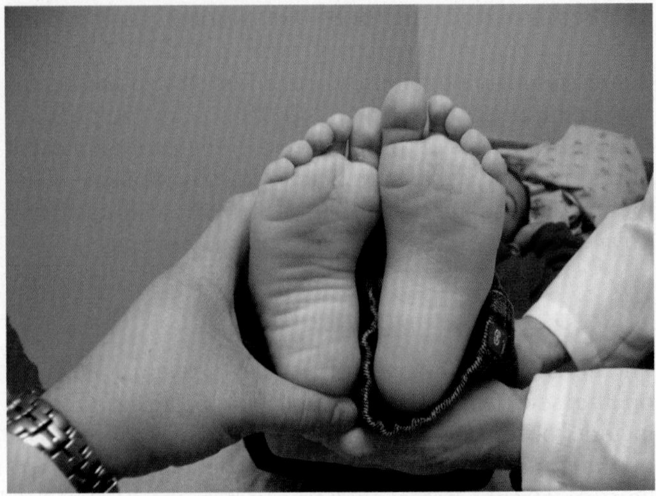

FIGURE 44.17 Metatarsus adductus: note medial deviation of the forefoot.

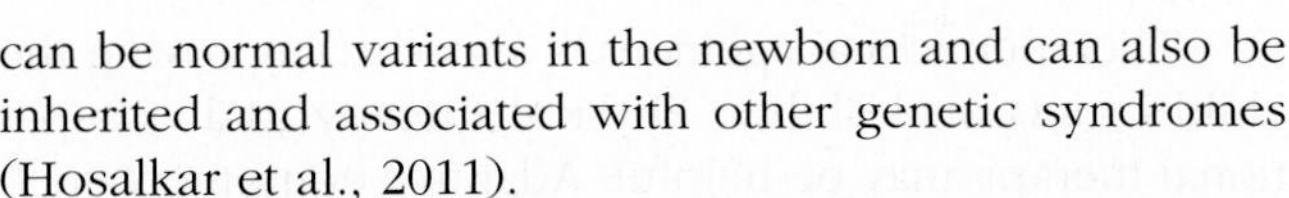

can be normal variants in the newborn and can also be inherited and associated with other genetic syndromes (Hosalkar et al., 2011).

Therapeutic management includes surgical removal of the digit. No treatment is usually required for syndactyly, though surgical repair is sometimes performed for cosmetic reasons.

Nursing Assessment

Inspect the hands and feet for the presence of extra digits. Note whether the additional digits are soft (without bone) or are full or partial digits with bone present. Note location of webbing.

Nursing Management

When surgical removal is necessary, provide routine pre- and postoperative care as appropriate.

Metatarsus Adductus

Metatarsus adductus, a medial deviation of the forefoot, is one of the most common foot deformities of childhood (Fig. 44.17). It occurs most commonly as a result of in utero positioning (Hosalkar et al., 2011). Half of all cases occur bilaterally (Hosalkar et al., 2011). The degree of flexibility is important and determines treatment. If the forefoot is flexible past neutral manipulation passively, observation is often sufficient. If the forefoot is flexible only to neutral manipulation, stretching exercises may be beneficial. If the forefoot is rigid and is not flexible to neutral manipulation, serial casting, preferably before the age of 8 months, may be required (Hosalkar et al., 2011). Surgical intervention is rarely needed.

Nursing Assessment

The deformity is usually noted at birth. Note inward deviation of the forefoot with the hindfoot remaining in normal position. The great and second toes might be separated. Determine forefoot flexibility. Range of motion of the ankle, hindfoot, and midfoot is normal.

Nursing Management

Most cases will resolve without treatment and nursing care is aimed at education and reassurance of the parents. Nursing care for the child with severe metatarsus adductus is similar to that of the child with clubfoot (see below).

Congenital Clubfoot

Congenital clubfoot (also termed congenital talipes equinovarus) is a congenital anomaly that occurs in about 1 of 1,000 live births (Hosalkar et al., 2011). Clubfoot consists of:

- Talipes varus (inversion of the heel)
- Talipes equinus (plantarflexion of the foot; the heel is raised and would not strike the ground in a standing position)
- Cavus (plantarflexion of the forefoot on the hindfoot)
- Forefoot adduction with supination (the forefoot is inverted and turned slightly upward)

The foot resembles the head of a golf club (Fig. 44.18). Half of all cases occur bilaterally and males are affected more frequently than females (Hosalkar et al., 2011). The exact etiology of clubfoot is unknown.

Clubfoot may be classified into four categories: postural, neurogenic, syndromic, and idiopathic. Postural

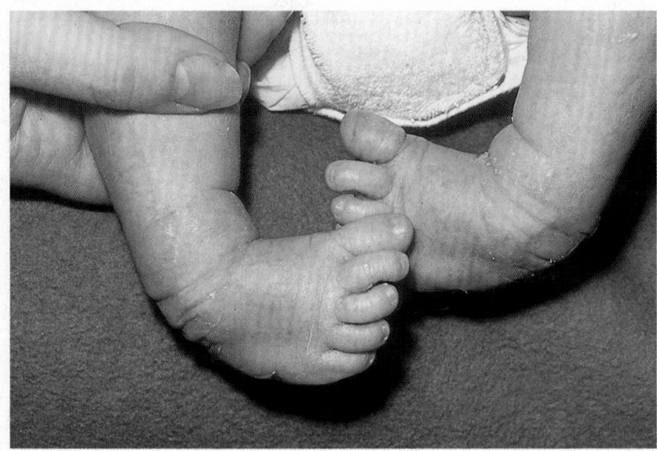

FIGURE 44.18 Note inverted heel, ankle equinus, and forefoot adduction in this infant with bilateral clubfoot.

clubfoot often resolves with a short series of manipulative casting. Neurogenic clubfoot occurs in infants with myelomeningocele. Clubfoot in association with other syndromes (syndromic) is often resistant to treatment. Idiopathic clubfoot occurs in otherwise normal healthy infants. The approach to treatment is similar regardless of the classification.

Therapeutic Management

The goal of therapeutic management of clubfoot is achievement of a functional foot; treatment starts as soon after birth as possible. Weekly manipulation with serial cast changes is performed; later, cast changes occur every 2 weeks. Other infants require corrective shoes or bracing. In some infants surgical release of soft tissue may be necessary. Following surgery, the foot is immobilized with a cast for up to 12 weeks, and then ankle–foot orthoses or corrective shoes are used for several years.

Complications of clubfoot and its treatment include residual deformity, rocker-bottom foot, awkward gait, weight bearing on the lateral portion of the foot if uncorrected, and disturbance to the epiphysis.

Nursing Assessment

Note family history of foot deformities and obstetric history of breech position. Inspect the foot for position at rest. Perform active range of motion, noting inability to move foot into normal positioning at midline. X-rays are obtained to determine bony abnormality and note progress during treatment.

Nursing Management

Perform neurovascular assessment and cast care for infants requiring casting. Provide emotional support, as treatment often begins in the newborn period and families may have a difficult time adjusting to the diagnosis and treatment required for their new baby. Teach families cast care and about the use of orthotics or braces as prescribed.

Osteogenesis Imperfecta

Osteogenesis imperfecta is a genetic bone disorder that results in low bone mass, increased fragility of the bones, and other connective tissue problems such as joint hypermobility, resulting in instability of the joints. All of these contribute to fracture occurrence. Dentinogenesis imperfecta may also occur. This is characterized by the tooth enamel wearing easily and brittle and discolored teeth.

The disorder usually occurs as a result of a defect in the collagen type 1 gene, usually through an autosomal dominant inheritance pattern but some types are inherited in a recessive manner (Grossman, 2014). The types of osteogenesis imperfecta range from mild to severe connective tissue and bone involvement (Table 44.2). Subtypes A and B exist depending on (A) the absence or (B) the presence of dentinogenesis imperfecta (Marini, 2011). In children with moderate to severe disease, fractures are more likely to occur, and short stature is common. In addition to multiple fractures, additional complications include early hearing loss, acute and chronic pain, scoliosis, and respiratory problems.

Take Note!

Blue/gray sclera is not diagnostic of osteogenesis imperfecta, but it is a common finding (Grossman, 2014). However, there are some individuals with blue sclerae who do not have osteogenesis imperfecta. Keep in mind that the sclerae of newborns tend to be bluish, progressing to white over the first few weeks of life.

Therapeutic Management

The goal of medical and surgical management is to decrease the incidence of fractures and maintain mobility. Bisphosphonate administration is used for moderate to severe disease. Fracture care is often required. Physical therapy and occupational therapy prevent contractures and maximize mobility. Standing with bracing is encouraged. Lightweight splints or braces may allow the child to bear weight earlier. Severe cases may require surgical insertion of rods into the long bones.

Nursing Assessment

Elicit a health history, which may reveal a family history of osteogenesis imperfecta, a pattern of frequent fractures, or screaming associated with routine care and handling of the newborn. Inspect the eyes for sclerae

TABLE 44.2 CLASSIFICATION OF OSTEOGENESIS IMPERFECTA

Classification	Characteristics
I	Mild Accounts for 50% of OI cases[a] Blue sclera Hearing loss Frequent shoulder and elbow dislocations Recurrent fractures in childhood After growth is complete incidence of fractures diminishes dramatically. Average or slightly shorter stature compared to family members Gross motor development delays
II	Most severe form Lethal in perinatal period or die within first year of life Low birthweight, very short limbs, small chest, and soft skull Intrauterine fractures evident Very dark blue/gray sclera
III	Most severe nonlethal form Sclera ranges from white to blue Fractures in utero and at birth with progressive deformity Bone fragility and fracture rate vary Results in significant disability Marked short stature
IV	Moderately severe Sclera may be light blue in infancy and lighten to white during childhood Fragile bones May present at birth with in utero fractures or bowing of lower long bones Height may be less than average for age
V and VI	Clinically within type IV but microscopic studies reveal distinct bone patterns; do not involve deficits of type I collagen Moderate in severity Similar to type IV in degree of fractures and skeletal deformity Type VI is extremely rare
VII and VIII	Recessive inheritance patterns Type VII resembles type IV or III, except infants have white sclera: stature is short. Type VIII resembles type II or III, except for white sclera; growth deficiency is severe.

[a]Osteogenesis Imperfecta Foundation. (2015). *Types of OI.* Retrieved from http://www.oif.org/site/PageServer?pagename=AOI_Types

Adapted from Marini, J. C. (2011). Chapter 692: Osteogenesis imperfecta. Osteogenesis imperfecta. In: R. M. Kleigman, B. F. Stanton, J. W. St. Geme III, N. F. Schor, & R. E. Behrman (Eds.), *Nelson textbook of pediatrics* (19th ed., pp. 2437–2440). Philadelphia, PA: Saunders.

that have a blue, purple, or gray tint. Note abnormalities of the primary teeth. Inspect skin for bruising and note joint hypermobility with active range of motion. Laboratory tests may include a skin biopsy (which reveals abnormalities in type 1 collagen) or DNA testing (locating the genetic mutation).

Nursing Management

Handle the child carefully and teach the family to avoid trauma (Teaching Guidelines 44.4). Refer families to the Osteogenesis Imperfecta Foundation (a link to which can be found on thePoint), which provides access to multiple resources as well as clinical trials. The site includes an online store with excellent books and booklets.

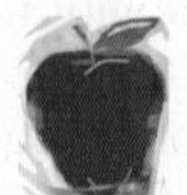

Teaching Guidelines 44.4

PREVENTING INJURY IN CHILDREN WITH OSTEOGENESIS IMPERFECTA

- Never push or pull on an arm or leg.
- Do not bend an arm or leg into an awkward position.
- Lift a baby by placing one hand under the legs and buttocks and one hand under the shoulders, head, and neck.

- Do not lift a baby's legs by the ankles to change the diaper.
- Do not lift a baby or small child from under the armpits.
- Provide supported positioning.
- If fracture is suspected, handle the limb minimally.

Encourage safe mobility. Reinforce physical and occupational therapists' recommendations for promotion of fine motor skills and independence in activities of daily living, as well as use of adaptive equipment and appropriate promotion of mobility. Adapted physical education is important to promote mobility and maintain bone and muscle mass. If the child is ambulatory, even with adaptive equipment use, walking is a good form of exercise. Swimming and water therapy are appropriate, allowing independent movement with little fracture risk.

Take Note!

Use caution when inserting an intravenous line or taking a blood pressure measurement, as pressure on the arm or leg can lead to bruising and fractures.

Developmental Dysplasia of the Hip (DDH)

DDH refers to abnormalities of the developing hip that include dislocation, subluxation, and dysplasia of the hip joint. In DDH, the femoral head has an abnormal relationship to the acetabulum. Frank dislocation of the hip may occur, in which there is no contact between the femoral head and acetabulum. Subluxation is a partial dislocation, meaning that the acetabulum is not fully seated within the hip joint. Dysplasia refers to an acetabulum that is shallow or sloping instead of cup shaped. DDH may affect just one or both hips. The dysplastic hip may be provoked to subluxation or dislocated and then reduced again (Fig. 44.19).

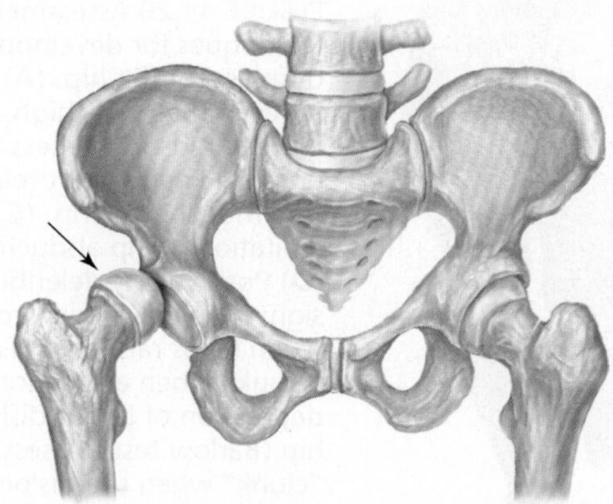

FIGURE 44.19 Developmental dysplasia of the hip.

Pathophysiology

While dislocation may occur during a growth period in utero, the laxity of the newborn's hip allows dislocation and relocation of the hip to occur. The hip can develop normally only if the femoral head is appropriately and deeply seated within the acetabulum. If subluxation and periodic or continued dislocation occur, then structural changes in the hip's anatomy occur. Continued dysplasia of the hip leads to limited abduction of the hip and contracture of muscles. DDH is more common in females, probably due to the greater susceptibility of the female newborn to maternal hormones that contribute to laxity of the ligaments (Sankar et al., 2011). Mechanical factors such as breech positioning or the presence of oligohydramnios also contribute to the development of DDH. Genetic factors also play a role: there is an increased incidence of DDH among persons of Native American and Eastern Europe descent, with very low rates among people of African or Chinese heritage (Sankar et al., 2011). Complications of DDH include avascular necrosis of the femoral head, loss of range of motion, recurrently unstable hip, femoral nerve palsy, leg-length discrepancy, and early osteoarthritis.

Therapeutic Management

The goal of therapeutic management is to maintain the hip joint in reduction so that the femoral head and acetabulum can develop properly.

Treatment varies based on the child's age and the severity of DDH. Infants younger than 6 months of age may be treated with a Pavlik harness, which reduces and stabilizes the hip by preventing hip extension and adduction and maintaining the hip in flexion and abduction (Sankar et al., 2011; Grossman, 2014). The Pavlik harness is successful in the treatment of DDH in the majority of infants younger than 6 months of age if it is used on a full-time basis and applied properly (Sankar et al., 2011). Children from 4 months to 2 years of age often require closed reduction (Sankar et al., 2011). Skin or skeletal traction may be used first to gradually stretch the associated soft tissue structures. Closed reduction occurs under general anesthesia, with the hip being gently maneuvered back into the acetabulum. A spica cast worn for 12 weeks maintains reduction of the hip. After the cast is removed, the child may wear an abduction brace full time (except for baths) (Sankar et al., 2011). Then the brace is worn at night and during naps until development of the acetabulum is normal. Children older than 2 years of age or those who have failed to respond to prior treatment require an open surgical reduction followed by a period of casting (Sankar et al., 2011). Follow-up continues until the age of skeletal maturity.

Nursing Assessment

Nursing assessment of children with DDH includes obtaining a health history and inspecting, observing, and palpating for findings common to DDH.

HEALTH HISTORY

Assess the health history for risk factors such as:

- Family history of DDH
- Female gender
- Oligohydramnios or breech birth
- Native American or Eastern European descent
- Associated lower limb deformity, metatarsus adductus, hip asymmetry, torticollis, or other congenital musculoskeletal deformity

Previously undiagnosed older children may complain of hip pain.

PHYSICAL ASSESSMENT

The physical examination for DDH includes inspection, observation, and palpation. Since DDH is a developmental process, ongoing screening assessments are required throughout at least the first several months of the infant's life.

Inspection and Observation. Ensure that the infant is on a flat surface and is relaxed. Note asymmetry of thigh or gluteal folds with the infant in a prone position. Document shortening of the affected femur observed as limb-length discrepancy. Older children may exhibit **Trendelenburg gait**, due to the weakness of the hip abductors the childs trunk in shifted over the affected hip during ambulation. Figure 44.20 illustrates these assessments.

Palpation. Note limited hip abduction while performing passive range of motion. Abduction should ordinarily occur to 75 degrees and adduction to within 30 degrees with the infant's pelvis stabilized. Perform Barlow and Ortolani tests, feeling for, or noting, a "clunk" as the femoral head dislocates (positive Barlow) or reduces (positive Ortolani) back into the acetabulum. Force is not necessary when performing the Barlow and Ortolani maneuvers (Fig. 44.20 and Nursing Procedure 44.1).

Take Note!

A higher-pitched "click" may occur with flexion or extension of the hip. When assessing for DDH, do not confuse this benign, adventitial sound with a true "clunk."

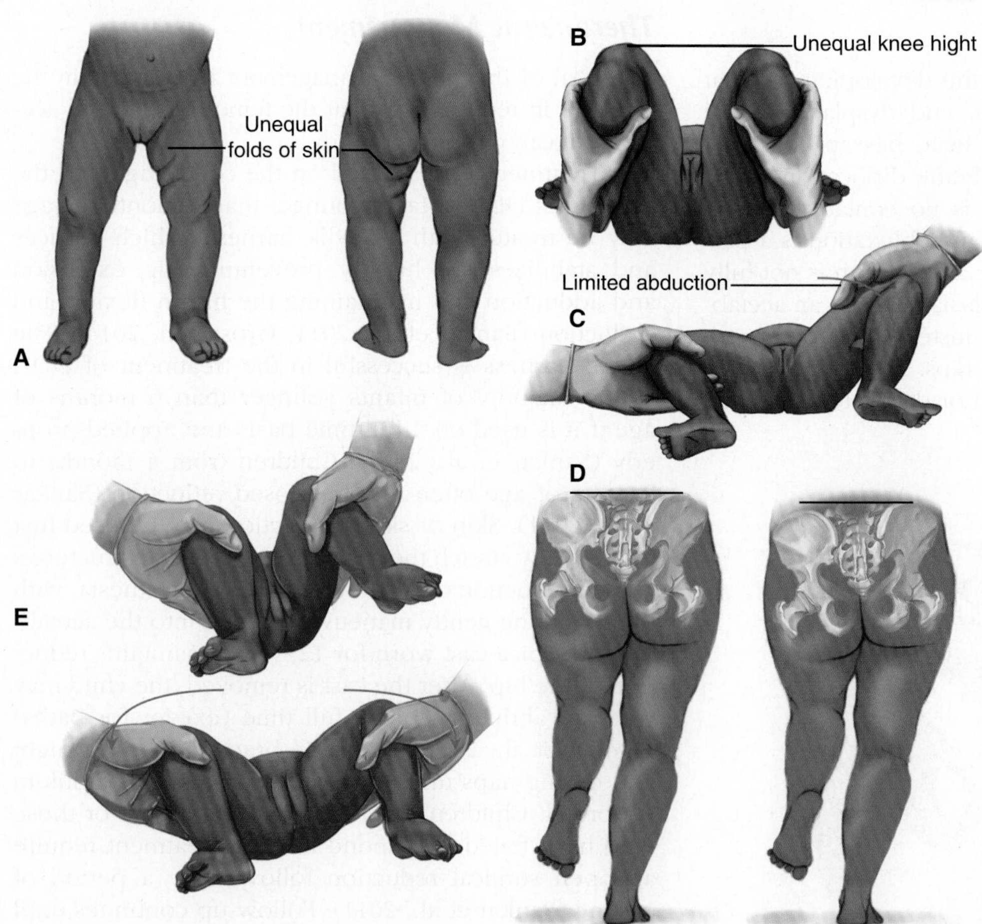

FIGURE 44.20 Assessment techniques for developmental dysplasia of the hip. (**A**) Assess for asymmetry of thigh and gluteal folds. (**B**) Assess for unequal knee height related to femur shortening. (**C**) Note limitation in hip abduction. (**D**) Positive Trendelenburg sign: note pelvis/hip drops when leg is raised. (**E**) Feel for "clunk" when adduction and depression of femur dislocates hip (Barlow test). Assess for "clunk" when the dislocated hip is abducted and relocated (Ortolani sign).

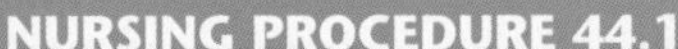

NURSING PROCEDURE 44.1

Performing Ortolani and Barlow Maneuvers

Purpose: To Detect Congenital Developmental Dysplasia of the Hip

Ortolani Maneuver

1. Place the newborn in the supine position and flex the hips and knees to 90 degrees at the hip.
2. Grasp the inner aspect of the thighs and abduct the hips (usually to approximately 180 degrees) while applying upward pressure.

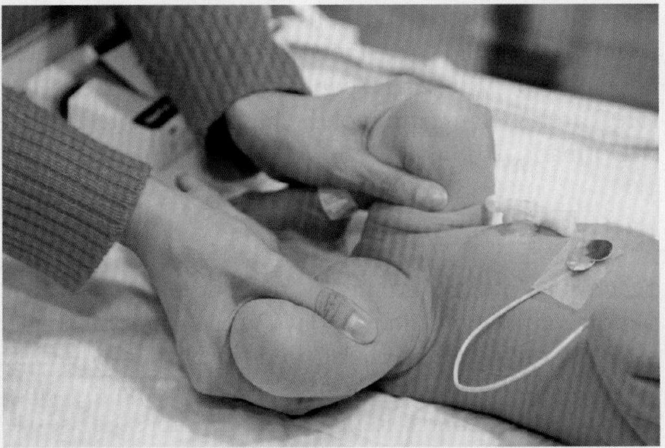

3. Listen for any sounds during the maneuver. There should be no "clunk" heard or felt when the legs are abducted. Such a sound indicates the femoral head hitting the acetabulum as the femoral head re-enters the area. This suggests developmental hip dysplasia.

Barlow Maneuver

1. With the newborn still lying supine and grasping the inner aspect of the thighs (as just mentioned), adduct the thighs while applying outward and downward pressure to the thighs.

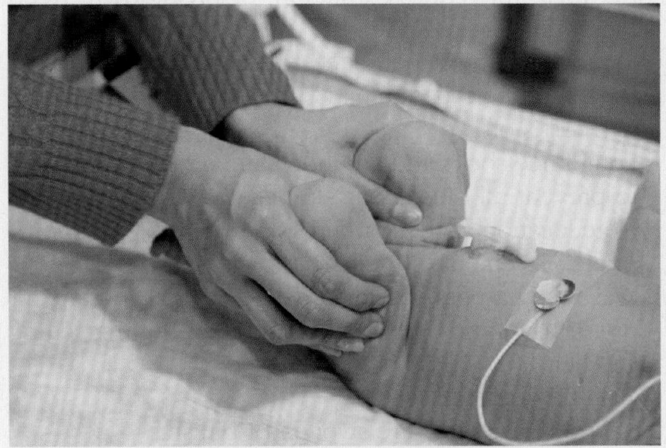

2. Feel for the femoral head slipping out of the acetabulum; also listen and feel for a "clunk."

LABORATORY AND DIAGNOSTIC TESTING

Ultrasound of the hip allows for visualization of the femoral head and the outer edge of the acetabulum. Plain hip x-rays may be used in the infant or child older than 6 months of age.

Nursing Management

Earlier recognition of hip dysplasia with earlier harness use results in better correction of the anomaly. Excellent assessment skills and reporting of any abnormal findings are critical. Initially, the infant will need to wear the Pavlik harness continuously (Fig. 44.21). The physician or nurse practitioner makes all appropriate adjustments to the harness when applied so that the hips are held in the optimal position for appropriate development. Teach parents use of the harness and assessment of the baby's skin. If started early, harness use usually continues for about 3 months (Teaching Guidelines 44.5). Breastfeeding can continue throughout the harness treatment period, but creative positioning of the infant may be needed.

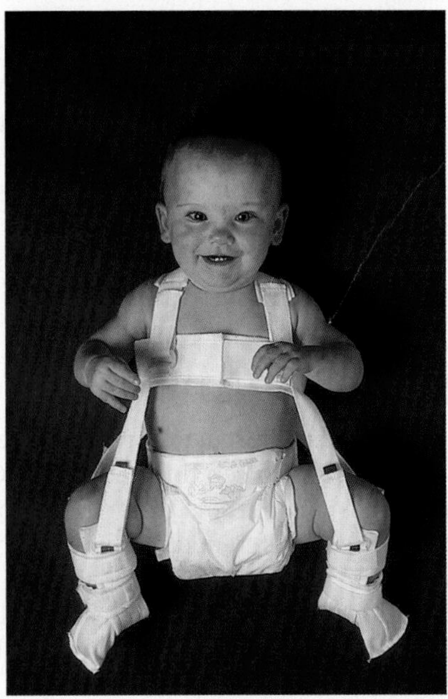

FIGURE 44.21 Pavlik harness used to keep the knees flexed and hips abducted to allow the hips to grow normally in a child with developmental dysplasia of the hip.

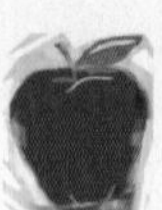

Teaching Guidelines 44.5

CARING FOR A CHILD IN A PAVLIK HARNESS

- Do not adjust the straps without checking with the physician or nurse practitioner first.
- Until your physician or nurse practitioner instructs you to take the harness off for a period of time each day, it must be used continuously (for the first week or sometimes longer).
- Change your baby's diaper while he or she is in the harness.
- Place your baby to sleep on his or her back.
- Check skin folds, especially behind the knees and diaper area, for redness, irritation, or breakdown. Keep these areas clean and dry.
- Once the baby is permitted to be out of the harness for a short period, you may bathe your baby while the harness is off.
- Long knee socks and an undershirt are recommended to prevent rubbing of the skin against the brace.
- Note location of the markings on the straps for appropriate placement of the harness.
- Wash the harness with mild detergent by hand and air dry. If using the dryer, use *only* the air fluffing setting (no heat).
- Call the doctor if:
  - Your baby's feet are swollen or bluish.
  - The harness appears too small.
  - Skin is raw or a rash develops.
  - Your baby is unable to actively kick his or her legs.

For infants or children diagnosed later than 6 months of age or those who do not improve with harness use, surgical reduction may be performed (Sankar et al., 2011). Postoperative casting followed by bracing or orthotic use is common. Caring for the child in the postoperative period is similar to care of any child in a cast. Pain management and monitoring for bleeding are priority activities. Teach families care of the cast at home.

Torticollis

Torticollis is a painless muscular condition presenting in infants or in children with certain syndromes. Congenital muscular torticollis may result from in utero positioning or difficult birth. Preferential turning of the head to one side while in the supine position after birth may also lead to torticollis. Torticollis results from tightness of the sternocleidomastoid muscle, resulting in the infant's head being tilted to one side.

Therapeutic management involves passive stretching exercises. These exercises should be effective in 90% of cases of congenital torticollis, especially if treatment is started within the first 3 months of life (Spiegel & Dormans, 2011a). Physical therapy may be prescribed and a tubular orthosis for torticollis (TOT) collar may also be used. Surgery is not common but may be done in the preschool years if other methods have been unsuccessful. Plagiocephaly may result from the continued pressure on the side of the skull to which the neck is turned.

Nursing Assessment

Note history of head tilt and infant's lack of desire to turn the head in the opposite direction. Observe the infant for wryneck (tilting of the head to one side; Fig. 44.22). Note limited movement of the neck while performing passive range of motion. Palpate the neck, noting a mass in the sternocleidomastoid muscle on the affected side. Examine the head for evidence of plagiocephaly. Accompanying hip dysplasia is seen in 7% to 9% of cases. Therefore, careful examination of the hips is warranted (Spiegel & Dormans, 2011a).

Nursing Management

Teach parents gentle neck-stretching exercises to be performed several times a day. While immobilizing the shoulder on the affected side, gently sustain a side-to-side stretch toward the unaffected side, holding the stretch for 10 to 30 seconds. Repeat 10 to 15 times per session.

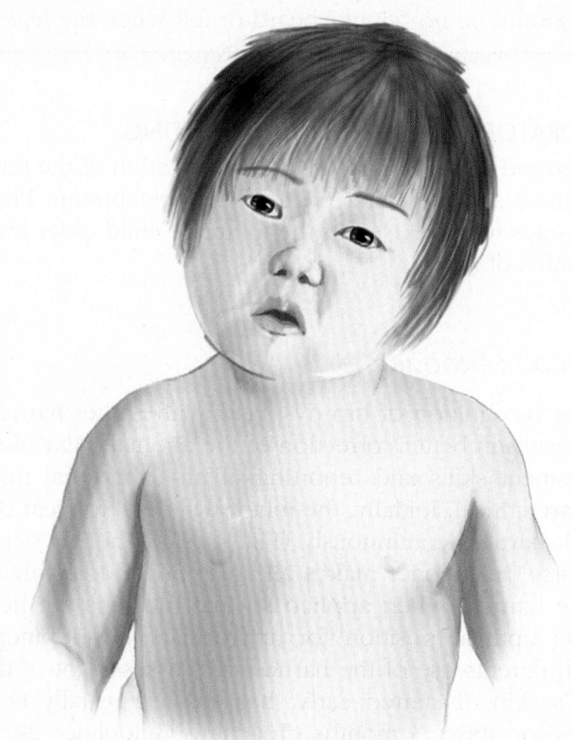

FIGURE 44.22 Note wryneck or head tilt in the infant with torticollis.

Perform an ear-to-shoulder stretch in a similar fashion. To prevent the development of torticollis in the unaffected infant, prevent positional plagiocephaly. Prevent flatness of one side of the head by varying the infant's head position, and do not always turn the infant's head to one side while he or she is in the infant seat, in the swing, or lying supine. Refer families to the Infant Torticollis Organization, a parent support network, and Torticollis Kids, links to which can be found on thePoint.

Tibia Vara (Blount Disease)

Tibia vara (Blount disease) is a developmental disorder affecting young children. There are three types: infantile (1 to 3 years), juvenile (4 to 10 years), and adolescent (11 years or older) (Wells & Sehgal, 2011). Infantile is the most common and is discussed here (Wells & Sehgal, 2011). The normal physiologic bowing or genu varum becomes more pronounced in the child with tibia vara. The cause of tibia vara is unknown, but it is considered to be a developmental disorder because it occurs most frequently in children who are early walkers. Most cases occur in African-American females and both extremities are affected (Wells & Sehgal, 2011). In addition to early walking, obesity is also a risk factor. If left untreated, the growth plate of the upper tibia ceases bone production. Asymmetric growth at the knee then occurs and the bowing progresses. Severe degenerative arthritis of the knee is an additional long-term complication.

Therapeutic management is aimed at stopping the progression of the disease through bracing or surgical treatment. Medical or surgical treatment should begin early, before 4 years of age.

Nursing Assessment

Elicit a health history and determine the age at which the child started walking. Assess growth parameters to determine whether the risk factor of obesity is present. Note significant bowing of the legs while the child is standing and ambulating (see Fig. 44.23).

Nursing Management

Bracing may include a modified knee–ankle–foot orthosis that relieves the compression forces on the growth plate, allowing bone growth resumption and correction of bowlegs. To be successful, bracing must be continued for months to years and the brace must be worn 23 hours per day. Compliance is the most significant barrier to successful treatment. Parents have a difficult time forcing their toddler to stay in a brace that inhibits mobility for the bulk of the day (particularly a bilateral brace). Support parents by encouraging and praising their compliance with bracing. Teach parents to assess for potential skin impairment from brace rubbing.

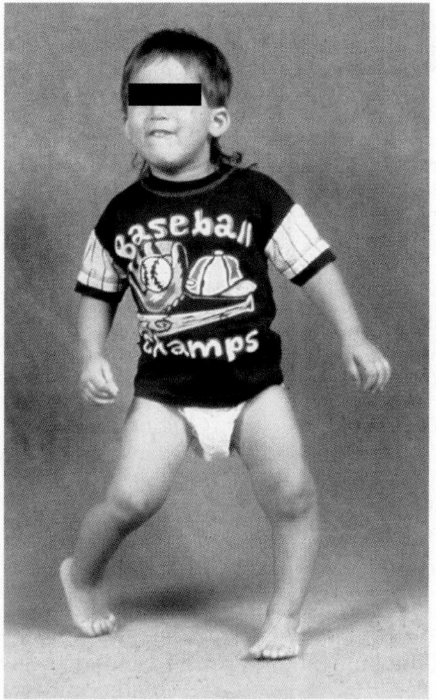

FIGURE 44.23 Note extreme bowing of the legs in tibia vara.

When surgical treatment is required, the leg(s) will be immobilized in a long-leg bent knee or spica cast after the osteotomy is performed. Perform routine cast care. Refer to Nursing Care Plan 44.1 for additional interventions related to care of the immobilized child.

Muscular Dystrophy

Muscular dystrophy refers to a group of inherited conditions that result in progressive muscle weakness and wasting. The muscles affected are primarily the skeletal (voluntary) muscles. Nine types of muscular dystrophy exist. All include muscle weakness over the lifetime; it is progressive in all cases but more severe in others. The various muscular dystrophies are most often diagnosed in childhood and affect a variety of muscle groups. The inheritance pattern for muscular dystrophy differs for each type but may be X-linked, autosomal dominant, or recessive. The genetic mutation in muscular dystrophy results in absence or decrease of a specific muscle protein that prevents normal function of the muscle. The skeletal muscle fibers are affected, yet there are no structural abnormalities in the spinal cord or the peripheral nerves. Table 44.3 gives specifics related to the various types of muscular dystrophy.

Duchenne muscular dystrophy, the most common neuromuscular disorder of childhood, is universally fatal (usually by age 20 to 25) (Zak & Chan, 2014). Due to advances in medical care, such as improvements in noninvasive mechanical ventilation, better management of cardiac dysfunction using angiotensin-converting

TABLE 44.3 TYPES OF MUSCULAR DYSTROPHY

Type	Onset	Inheritance	Muscle Involvement
Duchenne (pseudohypertrophic)	Early childhood (usually 3–6 years)	X-linked recessive (affects only males)	Generalized weakness, muscle wasting; limb and trunk first
Becker	2–16 years	X-linked recessive (affects only males)	Similar but less severe than Duchenne
Congenital	At birth	Most forms are autosomal recessive (primarily affects males)	Generalized muscular weakness, possible joint deformities
Emery–Dreifuss	Childhood to early teens (usually by 10 years)	Most often X-linked recessive (primarily affects males)	Weakness, wasting of shoulder, upper arm, and shin muscles
Limb-girdle	late teen to middle age	Most often autosomal recessive but may be dominant (primarily affects males)	Weakness, wasting of shoulder and pelvic girdles first
Facioscapulohumeral	Late childhood to early adulthood (usually by age 20)	Autosomal dominant (affects males and females)	Facial muscles weaken first, then shoulders and upper arms
Myotonic	Teen or adult years	Autosomal dominant (affects males and females)	Generalized weakness, wasting of face, feet, hands, and neck first Delayed relaxation of muscles after contraction

Adapted from Zak, M., & Chan, V. W. (2014). Chapter 46: Pediatric neurologic disorders. In S. M. Nettina (Ed.), *Lippincott manual of nursing practice* (10th ed., pp. 1545–1575). Philadelphia, PA: Wolters Kluwer Health: Lippincott Williams & Wilkins; Sarant, H. B. (2011b). Chapter 601: Muscular dystrophies. In R. M. Kleigman, B.F. Stanton, J.W. St. Geme III, N.F. Schor, & R.E. Behrman (Eds.), *Nelson textbook of pediatrics* (19th ed., pp. 2119–2129). Philadelphia, PA: Saunders.

enzymes (ACE) inhibitors and the use of steroids, survival into their 30s, with some cases into their 40s or 50s, is becoming more common (Passamano et al., 2012; Muscular Dystrophy Association, 2014). The incidence is about 1 in 3,500 live male births (Zak & Chan, 2014). For these reasons, this discussion will focus on Duchenne muscular dystrophy.

Pathophysiology

The gene mutation in Duchenne muscular dystrophy results in the absence of dystrophin, a protein that is critical for maintenance of muscle cells. The gene is X-linked recessive, meaning that mainly boys are affected and they receive the gene from their mothers (women are carriers but have no symptoms). Absence of dystrophin leads to generalized weakness of voluntary muscles, and the weakness progresses over time. The hips, thighs, pelvis, and shoulders are affected initially; as the disease progresses, all voluntary muscles as well as cardiac and respiratory muscles are affected.

Boys with Duchenne muscular dystrophy are often late in learning to walk. As toddlers, they may display pseudohypertrophy (enlarged appearance) of the calves. During the preschool years they fall often and are quite clumsy. The affected child has difficulty climbing stairs and running and cannot get up from the floor in the usual fashion. The school-age child walks on the toes or balls of the feet with a rolling or waddling gait. Balance is disturbed significantly, and the child's belly may stick out when the shoulders are pulled back to stay upright and keep from falling over. During the school-age years it also becomes difficult for the child to raise his or her arms. Sometime between the ages of 7 and 12 years nearly all boys with Duchenne muscular dystrophy lose the ability to ambulate, and by the teen years any activity of the arms, legs, or trunk requires assistance or support (Muscular Dystrophy Association, 2011). Most boys with Duchenne muscular dystrophy have normal intelligence, but many may exhibit a specific learning disability (Sarant, 2011b).

Therapeutic Management

There is no cure for Duchenne muscular dystrophy. However, the use of corticosteroids may slow the progression

HEALTHY PEOPLE 2020

Objective	Nursing Significance
Reduce the proportion of children and adolescents with disabilities who are reported to be sad, unhappy, or depressed.	• Use every encounter with the child or adolescent with a disability as an opportunity to screen for mental health concerns. • Refer these children and teens as appropriate for mental health assessment and intervention.

Healthy People Objectives retrieved from http://www.healthypeople.gov

of the disease (Muscular Dystrophy Association, 2011; Zak & Chan, 2014). It is thought that prednisone helps by protecting muscle fibers from damage to the sarcolemma (defective in the absence of dystrophin). Numerous studies have shown that boys treated with prednisone demonstrate improved strength and function (Muscular Dystrophy Association, 2011). The side effects of corticosteroids are many, including weight gain, osteoporosis, and mood changes (Sarant, 2011b; Muscular Dystrophy Association, 2011). Calcium supplements and vitamin D are prescribed to prevent osteoporosis, and antidepressants may be helpful when depression occurs related to the chronicity of the disease and/or as an effect of corticosteroid use (Muscular Dystrophy Association, 2011); see Healthy People 2020. Medications to decrease the workload of the heart, such as beta-blockers and ACE inhibitors may be prescribed.

Take Note!

Researchers continue to search for a way to stop or reverse this disease. Gene therapy clinical trials for the treatment of Duchenne muscular dystrophy are in progress (Muscular Dystrophy Association, 2011).

Braces or orthoses and mobility and positioning aids are necessary. As the muscles deteriorate, joints may become fixated, resulting in **contractures**. Contractures restrict flexibility and mobility and cause discomfort. Sometimes contractures require surgical tendon release. Spinal curvatures result over time. The boy with Duchenne muscular dystrophy who can still walk may develop lordosis. More frequently, scoliosis or kyphosis develops with this disorder. Surgical spinal fixation with rod implantation is often required by adolescence (Muscular Dystrophy Association, 2009). Additional complications include pulmonary, urinary, or systemic infections; depression; learning or behavioral disorders; aspiration pneumonia (as oropharyngeal muscles become affected); cardiac dysrhythmias; and, eventually, respiratory insufficiency and failure (as weakness of the chest muscles and diaphragm progresses).

Nursing Assessment

For a full description of the assessment phase of the nursing process, refer to the Assessment section of the Nursing Process Overview earlier in the chapter. Assessment findings pertinent to Duchenne muscular dystrophy are discussed below.

HEALTH HISTORY

Examine the health history for a family history of neuromuscular disorders. Note pregnancy and delivery history, as this information may be useful in ruling out a pregnancy problem or birth trauma as a cause for the motor dysfunction. Determine status of developmental milestone achievement. Boys with Duchenne muscular dystrophy learn to walk but over time become unable to do so. If the child was previously diagnosed with muscular dystrophy, determine progression of disease. Inquire about functional status and need for assistive or adaptive equipment such as braces or wheelchairs. Determine skills related to activities of daily living. Note history of cough or frequent respiratory infections, which occur as the respiratory muscles weaken. While talking with the child and family, determine whether psychosocial issues such as decreased self-esteem, depression, alterations in socialization, or altered family processes might be present.

PHYSICAL EXAMINATION

Perform a thorough physical examination on the child with suspected muscular dystrophy or the child with known history of the disorder. Particular findings related to inspection, observation, auscultation, and palpation are presented below.

Inspection and Observation. Observe the child's ability to rise from the floor. A hallmark finding of Duchenne muscular dystrophy is the presence of the Gowers sign: the child cannot rise from the floor in standard fashion because of increasing weakness (Fig. 44.24). Observe the child's gait. Determine effectiveness of cough.

Auscultation and Palpation. Auscultate the heart and lungs. Note tachycardia, which develops as the heart muscle weakens. Note adequacy of breath sounds, which may diminish with decreasing respiratory function. Note muscle strength with resistance testing. Palpate muscle tone.

LABORATORY AND DIAGNOSTIC TESTS

Electromyography (EMG) demonstrates that the problem lies in the muscles, not in the nerves. Serum creatine kinase levels are elevated early in the disorder, when

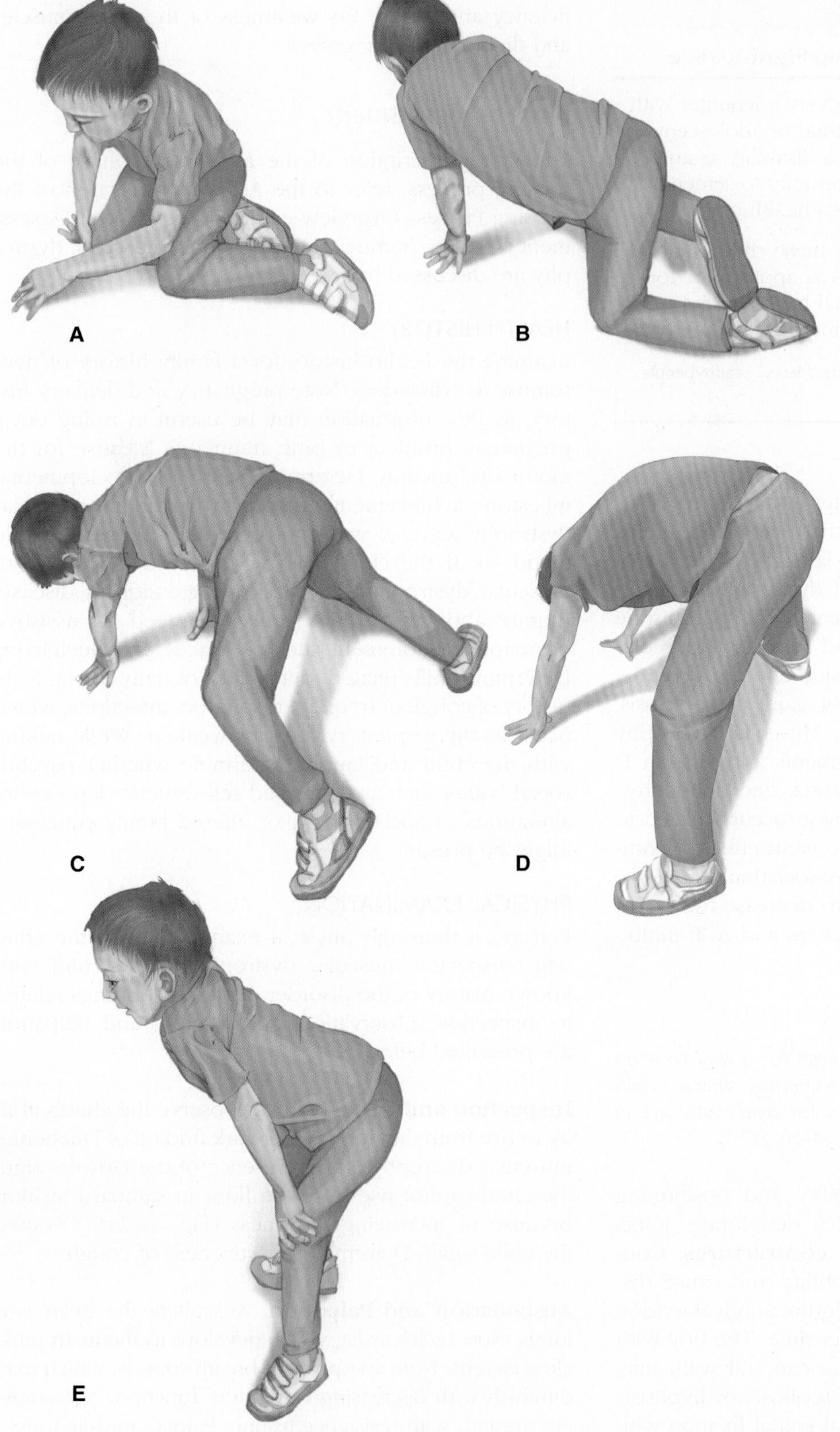

FIGURE 44.24 The Gower sign. (**A**) First the child must roll onto his hands and knees. (**B**) Then he must bear weight by using his hands to support some of his weight, while raising his posterior. (**C–E**) The boy then uses his hands to "walk" up his legs to assume an upright position.

significant muscle wasting is actively occurring. Muscle biopsy provides definitive diagnosis, demonstrating the absence of dystrophin. DNA testing reveals the presence of the gene.

Nursing Management

Nursing management is aimed at promoting mobility, maintaining cardiopulmonary function, preventing complications, and maximizing quality of life. Interventions directed at maintaining mobility and cardiopulmonary function also help to prevent complications. Refer to Nursing Care Plan 44.1, at the end of the chapter, and individualize nursing care based on the child's and family's response to the illness. Additional specifics related to care of the child with muscular dystrophy are discussed below.

PROMOTING MOBILITY

Administer corticosteroids and calcium supplements as ordered. Encourage at least minimal weight bearing in a standing position to promote improved circulation, healthier bones, and a straight spine. Boys with Duchenne muscular dystrophy may use a standing walker or standing frame to maintain an upright position. Perform passive stretching or strengthening exercises as recommended by the physical therapist. These exercises preserve mobility and may help to prevent muscle atrophy. Use orthotic supports such as hand braces or ankle–foot orthoses (AFOs) to prevent contractures of joints. Schedule activities during the part of the day when the child has the most energy. Teach parents the use of positioning, exercises, orthoses, and adaptive equipment. Use of a wheelchair full time typically occurs by age 12 (Muscular Dystrophy Association, 2011).

> **Thinking about Development**
>
> You are caring for a 6-year-old boy with Duchenne muscular dystrophy. How can you best help him meet developmental milestones? How would this differ if he was a 12-year-old?

MAINTAINING CARDIOPULMONARY FUNCTION

Assess respiratory rate, depth of respirations, and work of breathing. Auscultate the lungs to determine whether aeration is sufficient and to assess clarity of breath sounds. Position the child for maximum chest expansion, usually in the upright position. Teach the child and family deep-breathing exercises to strengthen or maintain respiratory muscles and encourage coughing to clear the airways. Perform chest physical therapy or assist with chest percussion. Monitor the results of pulmonary function testing. Use of intermittent positive-pressure ventilation and mechanically assisted coughing will become necessary in the teen years for some boys, possibly later for others. Teach parents monitoring of respiratory status and use of these modalities in conjunction with the respiratory therapist. Monitor cardiac status closely to identify heart failure early. Assess for edema, weight gain, or crackles. Strictly monitor fluid intake and output.

MAXIMIZING QUALITY OF LIFE

Long periods of bed rest may contribute to further weakness. Work with the family and child to develop a schedule for diversional activities that provide appropriate developmental stimulation but avoid overexertion or frustration (related to inability to perform the activity). Periods of adequate rest must be balanced with activities. Walking or riding a stationary bike is appropriate for the child who has upper extremity involvement. For the child with lower extremity involvement, a wheelchair may become necessary for mobility, and the child may participate in crafts, drawing, and computer activities. Participating in the Special Olympics may be appropriate for some children. Visit thePoint for a link to the Special Olympics website. Do not place limits on the child but encourage activities he or she is interested in that can be modified as needed to fit his or her abilities.

Provide emotional support to the child and family. Long-term direct care is stressful for families and becomes more complex as the child gets older. Families often need respite from continual caregiving duties. When a child is hospitalized, the caregiver may feel comfortable allowing nurses and other healthcare professionals to assume more of the child's daily care; this can be an opportunity for the caregiver to obtain respite from daily care. Respite care may also be offered in the home by various community services, so explore these resources with families.

Assess the child's educational status. Some children attend school; others may opt for home schooling. Administer antidepressants as ordered; managing depression may increase the child's desire to participate in activities and self-care. Refer the child and family to the Muscular Dystrophy Association (a link to which is located on thePoint), which provides multidisciplinary care via clinics located throughout the United States. The association is also a clearinghouse for resources for individuals with muscular dystrophy. Ensure that families receive genetic counseling for family planning purposes as well as determining which family members may be carriers for muscular dystrophy.

Spinal Muscular Atrophy

SMA is a genetic motor neuron disease that affects the spinal nerves' ability to communicate with the muscles. It is inherited via an autosomal recessive mechanism. The motor neuron protein survival of motor neurons (SMNs)

TABLE 44.4 FEATURES OF SPINAL MUSCULAR ATROPHY

Features	Type 1 SMA (Werdnig–Hoffman Disease, Infantile SMA)	Type 2 SMA (Intermediate SMA)	Type 3 SMA (Kugelberg–Welander Disease, Juvenile SMA)
Onset	Before birth to 6 months of age	6–18 months of age	After 18 months of age; child has started walking or has taken at least five independent steps
Symptoms	• Generalized weakness; cannot sit without support • Weak cry • Difficulty sucking, swallowing, and breathing	• Proximal muscles are more affected; that is, thighs are weaker than lower legs; legs tend to be weaker than arms. • Respiratory muscles may be involved. • Scoliosis may occur.	• Weakness that is most severe in the shoulders, hips, thighs, and upper back • Respiratory muscles may be involved. • Scoliosis may occur.
Progression	Rapidly progresses to early childhood death. Use of ventilators and gastrostomy feeding tubes may prolong life expectancy but typically death occurring by age 2.	Slower progression. Life expectancy related to age of onset (the younger the onset the more severe the disease and the shorter the life expectancy) Survival into adulthood common if respiratory status maintained appropriately	Slow progression. Life span usually unaffected. Walking ability maintained until at least adolescence; may need wheelchair later in life

Adapted from Muscular Dystrophy Association. (2009c). *Facts about spinal muscular atrophy (SMA)*. Retrieved from http://www.mda.org/publications/PDFs/FA-SMA.pdf; National Institute of Neurological Disorders and Stroke (2015b). NINDS Spinal Muscular Atrophy Information Page. Retrieved from http://www.ninds.nih.gov/disorders/sma/sma.htm

is deficient as a result of a faulty gene on chromosome 5. The motor neurons are located mostly in the spinal cord. Without adequate SMN, the signals from the neurons to the muscles instructing them to contract are ineffective, so the muscles lose function and over time atrophy. The proximal muscles, those closer to the body's center, are usually more affected than the distal muscles. The heart, emotional and mental development as well as sensation are unaffected by the disease (Sarant, 2011c).

There are several types of SMA, including type 1 (Werdnig–Hoffmann disease, infantile SMA), type 2 (intermediate), and type 3 (Kugelberg–Welander disease or juvenile SMA). Their usual progression and prognosis are compared in Table 44.4.

Respiratory muscle weakness may occur with all types of SMA and is usually the cause of death in type 1 SMA. Upper respiratory tract infections and aspiration related to dysphagia or gastroesophageal reflux often develop into pneumonia and eventual respiratory failure, as the affected child cannot effectively cough independently in order to clear the airway. Many children with severe type 1 SMA are ventilator dependent. Pectus excavatum develops in children with type 1 and type 2 SMA who exhibit paradoxical breathing (use of the diaphragm without intercostal muscle support). The chest becomes funnel shaped and the xiphoid process is retracted (pectus excavatum), further restricting respiratory development. Inability to appropriately suck and swallow leads to difficulty feeding in the child with type 1 SMA. Weak back muscles affect the developing spine, resulting in the complication of scoliosis, kyphosis, or both.

Therapeutic management of SMA is supportive, aimed at promoting mobility, maintaining adequate nutrition and pulmonary function, and preventing complications. Spinal fusion may be performed in older children with significant scoliosis. Since the discovery of the disease-causing gene for SMA, further research and improved diagnostic techniques have occurred. The International Standard of Care Committee for SMA published guidelines for care of the child with SMA in 2007 due to the wide variation of care and clinical outcomes seen in children with SMA (Wang et al., 2007). The guidelines discussed diagnostic testing and care of the child with newly diagnosed SMA, consensus on pulmonary care, consensus on gastrointestinal and nutritional care, consensus on orthopedic care, and rehabilitation and palliative care issues (Wang et al., 2007).

Nursing Assessment

Note history of attainment of developmental milestones, as well as loss of milestones. SMA should be suspected

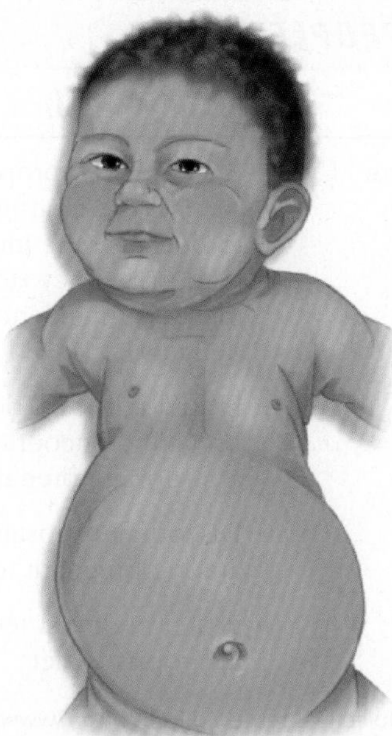

FIGURE 44.25 Note the very narrow chest, beginning xiphoid depression, and relatively enlarged appearance of the abdomen in this infant with type 1 spinal muscular atrophy (SMA).

in a child showing symmetric weakness that is more proximal than distal and greater in the legs than arms, diminished or absent tendon reflexes, and preserved sensation (Wang et al., 2007). In the infant or child with known SMA, assess for recent hospitalizations or respiratory illness. Determine the respiratory support regimen used at home (if any). Note level of motor ability, and identify the orthoses or adaptive equipment used. Elicit history related to feeding patterns at home. Assess for floppy appearance in the infant with SMA. Note decreased ability to initiate spontaneous muscle movement. In the infant or young child with SMA, note narrow chest with decreased excursion, relatively protuberant abdomen, and paradoxical breathing pattern (Fig. 44.25). Observe the chest for formation of pectus excavatum. Auscultate the lungs for diminished or adventitious breath sounds. Monitor laboratory testing, which may include:

- Creatine kinase (CK): elevated when muscular damage is occurring
- Genetic testing: identifies presence of gene for SMA
- Muscle biopsy: shows the muscle abnormality
- Nerve conduction velocity test and electromyelogram: to determine extent of involvement

Nursing Management

Nursing management of type 2 and type 3 SMA focuses on promoting mobility, maintaining pulmonary function, and preventing complications. Children with type 1 SMA need additional interventions related to prevention of complications from immobility and assistance with nutrition. Refer to Nursing Care Plan 44.1 at the end of the chapter for interventions related to these areas. Individualize the nursing plan of care based on the individual child's responses to the disorder.

Promote mobility through the use of range-of-motion exercises, lightweight orthotics, standing frames, and wheelchair use as appropriate. Support parents in their efforts to comply with physical and occupational therapy regimens. Older children may exercise with assistance in a warm pool. Position the child in a fashion that maintains appropriate body alignment.

Provide airway clearance techniques such as manual or mechanical cough assistance, chest percussion, and postural drainage to assist with clearance of secretions. In collaboration with respiratory therapy, teach families the use of noninvasive ventilation support, in which positive pressure is delivered to the lungs through a mask or mouthpiece (Fig. 44.26). Provide routine tracheostomy care if the child has a tracheostomy (refer to tracheostomy section of Chapter 40).

Administer gastrostomy tube feedings if ordered, and teach families gastrostomy tube care. Use bracing as prescribed to prevent spinal curvature. Make frequent inspections for skin breakdown in areas affected by bracing.

Cerebral Palsy

Cerebral palsy is a term used to describe a range of nonspecific clinical symptoms characterized by abnormal motor pattern and postures caused by nonprogressive

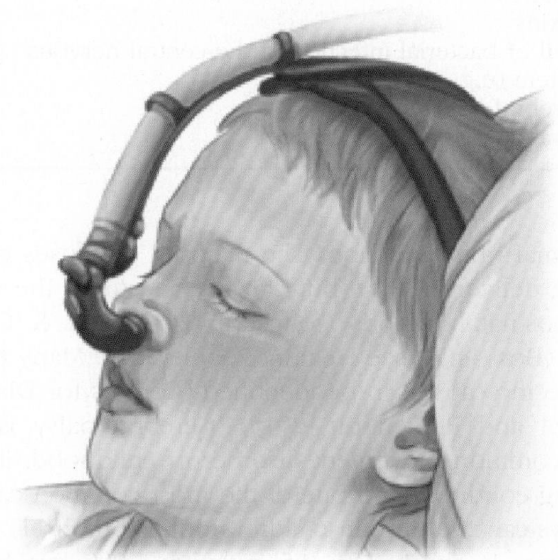

FIGURE 44.26 Use of noninvasive positive-pressure monitoring via nasal prongs can maximize respiration and may help prevent pulmonary complications.

BOX 44.1

CAUSES OF CEREBRAL PALSY

Prenatal

- Congenital malformation
- Hypoxia
- Maternal fever
- Maternal seizures
- Maternal bleeding
- Exposure to radiation
- Environmental toxins
- Genetic abnormalities
- Metabolic disorders
- Intrauterine growth restriction
- Intrauterine infection, such as cytomegalovirus and toxoplasmosis
- Nutritional deficits
- Preeclampsia
- Multiple births
- Prematurity
- Low birthweight
- Malformation of brain structure
- Abnormalities of blood flow to the brain
- Abdominal insults

Perinatal

- Prematurity (<32 weeks)
- Asphyxia
- Hypoxia
- Abnormal fetal presentation
- Sepsis or central nervous system infection
- Placental complications
- Electrolyte disturbance
- Cerebral hemorrhage
- Chorioamnionitis (infection of the placental tissues and amniotic fluid)

Postnatal

- Kernicterus (a type of brain damage that may result from neonatal hyperbilirubinemia)
- Asphyxia
- Head trauma (e.g., motor vehicle accidents, abuse)
- Seizures
- Toxins
- Viral or bacterial infection of the central nervous system (e.g., meningitis)
- Cerebral infarcts
- Intraventricular hemorrhage

abnormal brain function. The majority of causes occur before delivery (80%), but can also occur in the natal and postnatal periods (Johnston, 2011; Zak & Chan, 2014) (Box 44.1); see Healthy People 2020. Many times no specific cause can be identified (Centers for Disease Control and Prevention, 2015). Cerebral palsy is the most common movement disorder of childhood; it is a lifelong condition and one of the most common causes of physical disability in children (Johnston, 2011). The incidence is about 2 to 2.5 in every 1,000 live births (Zak & Chan, 2014). The incidence is higher in premature and low-birthweight infants (Johnston, 2011; Zak & Chan, 2014).

***HEALTHY PEOPLE** 2020*

Objective	Nursing Significance
Reduce preterm births.	• Encourage appropriate birth control use among adolescents to decrease the incidence of teen pregnancy (teens have an increased incidence of preterm delivery). • If an adolescent does become pregnant, encourage early appropriate prenatal care. • Discourage substance use among pregnant teens. • Teach pregnant teens about an appropriate diet.

Healthy People Objectives retrieved from http://www.healthypeople.gov

Most affected children will develop symptoms in infancy or early childhood. There is a large variation in symptoms and disability. For some children it may be as mild as a slight limp; for others it may result in severe motor and neurologic impairments. Primary signs include motor impairments such as spasticity, muscle weakness, and **ataxia**, which is lack of coordination of muscle movements during voluntary movements such as walking or picking up objects. Complications include mental impairments, seizures, growth problems, impaired vision or hearing, abnormal sensation or perception, and hydrocephalus. Most children can survive into adulthood, but function and quality of life can vary from near normal to substantial impairments (NINDS, 2015a).

Pathophysiology

Cerebral palsy is a disorder caused by abnormal development of, or damage to, the motor areas of the brain, resulting in a neurologic lesion. It is difficult to establish an exact location of the neurologic lesion, but it causes a disruption in the brain's ability to control movement and posture. The lesion itself does not change over time; thus, the disorder is considered nonprogressive since the brain injury does not progress. However, the clinical manifestations of the lesion change as the child grows. Some children may improve, but many either plateau in their attainment of motor skills or demonstrate worsening of motor abilities because it is difficult to maintain the ability to move over time.

Cerebral palsy is classified in several ways. One common way is by the type of movement disturbance (Table 44.5).

TABLE 44.5 CLASSIFICATION OF CEREBRAL PALSY

Types	Description	Characteristics
Spastic	Hypertonicity and permanent contractures; different types based on which limbs are affected: • Hemiplegia: both extremities on one side • Quadriplegia: all four extremities • Diplegia or paraplegia: lower extremities	• Most common form • Poor control of posture, balance, and movement • Exaggeration of deep tendon reflexes • Hypertonicity of affected extremities • Continuation of primitive reflexes • In some children, failure to progress to protective reflexes
Athetoid or dyskinetic	Abnormal involuntary movements	• Infant is limp and flaccid. • Uncontrolled, slow, worm-like writhing or twisting movements • Affects all four extremities and possible involvement of face, neck, and tongue • Movements increase during periods of stress • Dysarthria and drooling may be present
Ataxic	Affects balance and depth perception	• Rare form • Poor coordination • Unsteady gait • Wide-based gait
Mixed	Combination of the above	Most common is spastic and athetoid.

Therapeutic Management

Management of cerebral palsy involves multiple disciplines, including a primary physician, specialty physicians such as a neurologist and an orthopedic surgeon, nurses, physical therapists, occupational therapists, speech therapists, dietitians, psychologists, counselors, teachers, and parents. There is no standard treatment for all children. The overall focus of therapeutic management will be to assist the child to gain optimal development and function within the limits of the disease. Treatment is mainly preventative, symptomatic, and supportive. Spasticity management will be a primary concern and will be determined by clinical findings.

Medical management is focused on promoting mobility through the use of therapeutic modalities and medications. Surgical management is often required and is used to correct deformities related to spasticity.

PHYSICAL, OCCUPATIONAL, AND SPEECH THERAPY

The use of therapeutic modalities such as physical therapy, occupational therapy, and speech therapy will be essential in promoting mobility and development in the child with cerebral palsy. The earlier the treatment begins, the better chance the child has of overcoming developmental disabilities (NINDS, 2015a).

Physical therapists work with children to assist in the development of gross motor movements such as walking and positioning, and they help the child develop independent movement. They also assist in preventing contractures, and they instruct children and caregivers in the use of assistive devices such as walkers and wheelchairs. Occupational therapists may be responsible for fashioning orthotics and splints. AFOs are the most common orthotic used by children with cerebral palsy (Fig. 44.27) (Cervasio, 2011). AFOs help prevent deformity from conditions such as contractures and help reduce the effects of existing deformities. They can help improve a child's mobility by assisting in control of alignment and helping to increase the efficiency of the child's gait. Spinal orthotics such as braces are used in young children with cerebral palsy to combat scoliosis that develops due to spasticity. These braces are used to delay surgical management of the scoliosis until the child reaches skeletal maturity. Splinting is used to maintain muscle length. Serial casting may also be used to increase muscle and tendon length.

Occupational therapy also assists in the development of fine motor skills and will help the child to perform optimal self-care by working on skills such as activities of daily living. Speech therapy assists in the development of receptive and expressive language and addresses the use of appropriate feeding techniques in the child who has swallowing problems. Speech therapists may teach augmented communication strategies to children who are nonverbal or who have articulation problems. Many children may not communicate verbally but can use alternative means such as communication books or boards and computers with

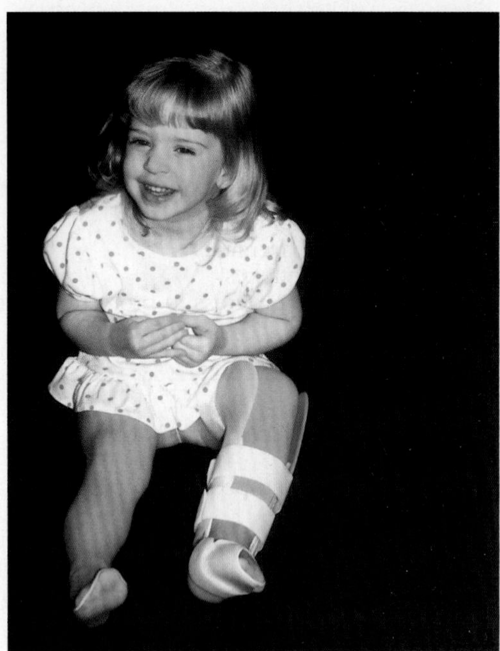

FIGURE 44.27 The child with cerebral palsy may benefit from wearing ankle–foot orthotics (AFOs) to provide support needed for independent or assisted walking.

voice synthesizers to make their desires known or to participate in conversation.

PHARMACOLOGIC MANAGEMENT

Various pharmacologic options are available to manage spasticity (see Drug Guide 44.1). Oral medications used to treat spasticity include baclofen, dantrolene sodium, and diazepam. Children with athetoid cerebral palsy may be given anticholinergics to help decrease abnormal movements. Anticholinergic agents, such as scopolamine (also known as hyoscine) or glycopyrrolate decrease saliva and are used to help control drooling.

> **Take Note!**
>
> *Pathologic drooling is a problem for many children with cerebral palsy. It can lead to dehydration, dental enamel erosion, and maceration of the skin, and an odor can result, along with social stigmatization. Recent research has shown that intraglandular injection of botulinum toxin type A can improve drooling with few side effects in children with neurologic disorders (Fairhurst & Cockerill, 2011; Miller, 2015).*

> **Dosage Calculation Box**
>
> Child's weight: 87 lb
>
> Medication order: Glycopyrrolate 0.8 mg per gastrostomy tube three times a day.
>
> Per the Pediatric Dosage Handbook, the recommended dose is 20 mcg/kg/dose three times daily and may titrate to a maximum dose of 100 mcg/kg/dose three times daily (not to exceed 1500–3000 mcg/dose)
>
> Is this ordered dose safe?

Parenterally administered medications such as botulin toxins and baclofen are also used to manage spasticity. Botulinum toxin is injected into the spastic muscle to balance the muscle forces across joints and to decrease spasticity. It is useful in managing focal spasticity in which the spasticity is interfering with function, producing pain, or contributing to a progressive deformity. Botulin toxin injection is performed by the physician or nurse practitioner and can be done in the clinic or outpatient setting.

Intrathecal administration of baclofen has been shown to decrease tone, but it must be infused continuously due to its short half-life. Surgical placement of a baclofen pump will be considered in children with general spasticity that is limiting function, comfort, activities of daily living, and endurance. To test whether it is a suitable option, an intrathecal test dose of baclofen will be administered. If the trial is successful, a baclofen pump will be implanted. Once inserted, delivery of the drug can be individualized to meet the child's unique needs. The pump needs to be replaced every 5 to 7 years and must be refilled with medication approximately every 3 months, depending on the type of pump. Complications with baclofen pump placement include infection, rupture, dislodgement, or blockage of the catheter.

Medications are also used to treat seizure disorders in children with cerebral palsy (refer to Chapter 38 for information related to seizure management).

SURGICAL MANAGEMENT

Many children will require surgical procedures to correct deformities related to spasticity. Multiple corrective surgeries may be required; they usually are orthopedic or neurosurgical. Surgery may be used to correct contractures that are severe enough to cause movement limitations. Common orthopedic procedures include tendon lengthening procedures, correction of hip and adductor muscle spasticity, and fusion of unstable joints to help improve locomotion, correct bony deformities, decrease painful spasticity, and maintain, restore, or stabilize a spinal deformity. Neurosurgical interventions may include placement of a shunt in children who have developed hydrocephalus, or surgical interventions to decrease spasticity. Selective dorsal root rhizotomy is used to decrease spasticity in the lower extremities by reducing the amount of stimulation that reaches the muscles via the nerves.

Nursing Assessment

For a full description of the assessment phase of the nursing process, refer to the Assessment section of the Nursing Process Overview earlier in the chapter. Assessment findings pertinent to cerebral palsy are discussed below.

HEALTH HISTORY

Elicit a description of the present illness and chief complaint. Obtain a detailed account of gestational and perinatal events (refer to Box 44.1). Common signs and symptoms reported during the health history of the undiagnosed child might include:

- Intrauterine infections
- Prematurity with intracranial hemorrhage
- Difficult, complicated, or prolonged labor and delivery
- Multiple births
- History of possible anoxia during prenatal life or birth
- History of head trauma
- Delayed attainment of developmental milestones
- Muscle weakness or rigidity
- Poor feeding
- Hips and knees feel rigid and unbending when pulled to a sitting position
- Seizure activity
- Subnormal learning
- Abnormal motor performance, scoots on back instead of crawling on abdomen, walks or stands on toes

Children known to have cerebral palsy are often admitted to the hospital for corrective surgeries or other complications of the disease, such as aspiration pneumonia and urinary tract infections. The health history should include questions related to:

- Respiratory status: Has a cough, sputum production, or increased work of breathing developed?
- Motor function: Has there been a change in muscle tone or increase in spasticity?
- Presence of fever
- Feeding and weight loss
- Any other changes in physical state or medication regimen

PHYSICAL EXAMINATION

Observe general appearance. Pay close attention to the neurologic assessment and motor assessment. Assess for delayed development, size for age, and sensory alterations such as strabismus, vision problems, and speech disorders. Abnormal postures may be present. While lying supine, the infant may demonstrate scissor crossing of the legs with plantar flexion. In the prone position the infant may raise his or her head higher than normal due to arching of the back, or the opisthotonic position may be noted. The infant may also abnormally flex the arms and legs under the trunk. Primitive reflexes may persist beyond the point at which they disappear in a healthy infant. Evolution of protective reflexes may be delayed. Watch the infant or child play, crawl, walk, or climb to determine motor function and capability. Note any movement disorder. Infants with cerebral palsy may demonstrate abnormal use of muscle groups such as scooting on their back instead of crawling or walking.

Assess active and passive range of motion. Pay particular attention to muscle tone. Though an increased or decreased resistance may be noted with passive movements, hypertonicity is most often seen. Increased resistance to dorsiflexion and passive hip abduction are the most common early signs. Sustained **clonus** (muscular spasm) may be present after forced dorsiflexion. Lift the child by placing your hands in the infant's or child's axillary area to assess shoulder girdle function and tone. Infants with cerebral palsy often demonstrate prolonged standing on their toes when supported in an upright standing position in this fashion. Lift the young child off the ground while the child holds your thumbs to test hand strength. Observe for presence of limb deformity, as decreased use of an extremity (as in the case of hemiparesis) may result in shortening of the extremity compared to the other one.

LABORATORY AND DIAGNOSTIC TESTS

A complete history, physical examination, and ancillary investigations are the primary modality for establishing a diagnosis of cerebral palsy. The following laboratory and diagnostic tests will help determine whether cerebral palsy is the likely cause or whether another condition may be the cause of the child's symptoms. These tests also will be important in evaluating the severity of the child's physical disabilities. Common supplementary laboratory and diagnostic tests ordered for the diagnosis and assessment of cerebral palsy include:

- Electroencephalogram: usually abnormal but the pattern is highly variable
- Cranial x-rays or ultrasound: may show cerebral asymmetry
- MRI or CT: may show area of damage or abnormal development but may be normal
- Screening for metabolic defects and genetic testing may be performed to help determine the cause of cerebral palsy.

Nursing Management

In addition to the nursing diagnoses and related interventions discussed in the Nursing Care Plan 44.1, at the end of the chapter, nursing management focuses on promoting growth and development by promoting mobility and maintaining optimal nutritional intake. Providing support and education to the child and family is also an important nursing function.

PROMOTING MOBILITY

Mobility is critical to the development of the child with cerebral palsy. Treatment modalities to promote mobility include physiotherapy, pharmacologic management, and surgery. Surgical procedures are discussed above. Physical or occupational therapy as well as medications may be used to address musculoskeletal abnormalities, to facilitate range of motion, to delay or prevent deformities such as contractures, to provide joint stability, to maximize activity, and to encourage the use of adaptive devices. The nurse's role in relation to the various therapies is to provide ongoing follow-through with prescribed exercises, positioning, or bracing.

When casting, splinting, or orthotics are used, assess skin integrity frequently. Pain management may also be necessary. Nursing management of children receiving botulin toxin focuses on assisting with the procedure and providing education and support to the child and family. Nursing interventions related to baclofen include assisting with the test dose and providing preoperative and postoperative care if a pump is placed, as well as providing support and education to the child and family. Teaching Guidelines 44.6 gives information related to baclofen pump insertion.

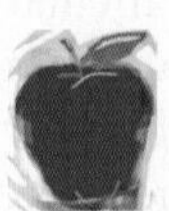

Teaching Guidelines 44.6

BACLOFEN PUMP: CHILD/FAMILY EDUCATION

- Check the incisions daily for redness, drainage, or swelling.
- Notify the physician or nurse practitioner if the child has a temperature greater than 101.5°F, or if the child has persistent incision pain.
- Avoid tub baths for 2 weeks.
- Do not allow the child to sleep on the stomach for 4 weeks after pump insertion.
- Discourage twisting at the waist, reaching high overhead, stretching, or bending forward or backward for 4 weeks.
- When the incisions have healed, normal activity may be resumed.
- Wear loose clothing to prevent irritation at the incision site.
- Carry implanted device identification and emergency information cards at all times.

PROMOTING NUTRITION

Children with cerebral palsy may have difficulty eating and swallowing due to poor motor control of the mouth, tongue, and throat. This may lead to poor nutrition and problems with growth. The child may require a longer time to eat because of poor motor control. Special diets, such as soft or puréed, may make swallowing easier. Proper positioning during feeding is essential to facilitate swallowing and reduce the risk of aspiration. Speech or occupational therapists can assist in working on strengthening swallowing muscles as well as assisting in developing accommodations to facilitate nutritional intake. Consult a dietitian to ensure adequate nutrition for children with cerebral palsy. In children with severe swallowing problems or malnutrition, a feeding tube such as a gastrostomy tube may be placed.

PROVIDING SUPPORT AND EDUCATION

Cerebral palsy is a lifelong disorder that can result in severe physical and cognitive disability. In some cases disability may require complete intensive daily care of the child. Adjusting to the demands of this multifaceted illness is difficult. Children are frequently hospitalized and need numerous corrective surgeries, which places strain on the family and its finances. From the time of diagnosis, the family should be involved in the child's care. It is important to include parents in the planning of interventions and care of this child. In most cases they are the primary caregivers and will assist the child in development of functioning and skills as well as providing daily care. They will provide essential information to the healthcare team and will be advocates for their child throughout his or her life. It is important that nurses provide ongoing education for the child and family.

As the child grows, the needs of the family and child will change. Recognize and respect these needs. Providing daily intense care can be demanding and tiring. When a child with cerebral palsy is admitted to the hospital, this may serve as a time of respite for family and primary caregivers. Encourage respite care and provide support and encouragement. Because cerebral palsy is a lifelong condition, children will need meaningful education programs that emphasize independence in the least restrictive educational environment. Refer caregivers to local resources, including education services and support groups. Links to United Cerebral Palsy, a national organization, and Easter Seals, an organization that helps children with disabilities and special needs and provides support to families, can be accessed on thePoint.

Refer children younger than age 3 years to the local early intervention service. Early intervention provides case management of developmental services for children with special needs. Each state has a coordinator for early intervention. The office of the early intervention coordinator can then direct the healthcare professional to the local or district early intervention office. The website MyChild (a link to which is available on thePoint) provides information, resources, and support.

Additional links to resources for families of young children with special needs are available on thePoint. For additional reading, recommend the book *Children With Cerebral Palsy: A Parent's Guide* by E. Geralis (published by Woodbine House).

ACQUIRED DISORDERS

A number of neuromuscular and musculoskeletal disorders may be acquired during childhood or adolescence. These include disorders resulting from nutritional deficits or malabsorption of fats which may lead to rickets. Slipped capital femoral epiphysis (SCFE) and Legg–Calvé–Perthes disease which affect mainly school-age and adolescent boys. Transient synovitis of the hip is a common cause of hip pain or limp in children. Spinal curvature may occur as a result of a neuromuscular disorder or idiopathically.

Injuries throughout childhood are inevitable. Trauma or unintentional injury is a leading cause of childhood morbidity and mortality in the United States (Child Trends Databank, 2014). The child is at increased risk for trauma based on the developmental factors of physical and emotional immaturity; additionally, adolescents often display belief of invincibility. The developing neuromuscular system, if injured, may be irreparable, so the injury may result in life-threatening or lifelong effects. Neuromuscular trauma includes spinal cord injury and birth trauma. Birth trauma is discussed in Chapter 24. Younger children tend to suffer contusions, sprains, and simple upper extremity fractures; adolescents more frequently experience lower extremity trauma. As the number of children participating in youth sports increases and the intensity of training and the level of competition also increase, the incidence of injury is also likely to increase. Many types of musculoskeletal injuries exist. This discussion will focus on fractures, sprains, overuse syndromes, and dislocated radial head.

Rickets

Rickets is a condition in which there is softening or weakening of the bones. Childhood rickets may occur as a result of nutritional deficiencies such as inadequate consumption of calcium or vitamin D or limited exposure to sunlight (required for adequate production of vitamin D). Rickets caused by vitamin D deficiency is a preventable condition but cases continue to be reported in infants, children, and adolescents (Wagner, Greer, & the Section on Breastfeeding and Committee on Nutrition, 2008; Misra, 2015). Rickets may also occur if the body cannot regulate calcium and phosphorus in the appropriate balance, such as in chronic renal disease. Gastrointestinal disorders in which fat absorption is altered (e.g., Crohn disease, celiac disease, and cystic fibrosis) may lead to rickets, as vitamin D is a fat-soluble vitamin.

Calcium is primarily laid down in the bones of the fetus during the third trimester. Premature infants miss this period of calcium accumulation and also suffer from inadequate calcium intake in the neonatal period. Thus, premature infants often demonstrate rickets of prematurity. Regardless of the underlying cause, rickets is most likely to occur during periods of rapid growth.

Vitamin D regulates calcium absorption from the small intestine and levels of calcium and phosphate in the bones. When calcium and phosphate levels in the blood are imbalanced, then calcium is released from the bones into the blood, resulting in loss of the supportive bony matrix.

Therapeutic Management

Treatment of rickets is aimed at correcting the calcium imbalance so that the skeleton may develop properly and without deformity. Calcium and phosphorus supplements are given, and some children also require vitamin D supplements. If rickets is not corrected while the child is still growing, permanent skeletal deformities and short stature may result.

Take Note!

The Academy of Pediatrics currently recommends all infants and children, including adolescents, have a minimum daily intake of 400 IU of vitamin D beginning soon after birth (Wagner et al., 2008).

Nursing Assessment

Obtain a health history, determining risk factors such as:

- Limited exposure to sunlight
- Strict vegetarian diet or lactose intolerance (either one without milk product ingestion)
- Exclusive breastfeeding by a mother who has a vitamin D deficiency
- Dark-pigmented skin
- Prematurity
- Malabsorptive gastrointestinal disorder
- Chronic renal disease

Note history of fractures or bone pain. Observe for dental deformities and bowlegs. Decreased muscle tone may also be present. Note low serum calcium and phosphate levels and high alkaline phosphatase levels. X-rays may show changes in the shape and structure of the bone.

Nursing Management

Administer calcium and phosphorus supplements at alternate times to promote proper absorption of both of these supplements. Encourage exposure to moderate amounts of sunlight and administer vitamin D supplements as prescribed. Teach families that good dietary sources of vitamin D are fish, liver, and processed milk.

Slipped Capital Femoral Epiphysis (SCFE)

SCFE is a condition in which the femoral head dislocates from the neck and shaft of the femur at the level of the epiphyseal plate. The epiphysis slips downward and backward. The left hip is more often affected (Haut, 2014). The exact cause is unknown, but it is thought that during the teenage growth spurt the femoral growth plate weakens and becomes less resistant to stressors. Hormonal alterations during this period may also play a role.

SCFE is classified based on its severity and whether the slip is acute or chronic. Chronic SCFE may lead to shortening of the affected leg and thigh atrophy.

Therapeutic Management

Promptly refer the child with SCFE to an orthopedic surgeon, as early surgical intervention will decrease the risk of long-term deformity. The goals of therapeutic management are to prevent further slippage, minimize deformity, and avoid the complications of cartilage necrosis (chondrolysis) and avascular necrosis of the femoral head. Surgical intervention may include in situ pinning, in which a pin or screw is inserted percutaneously into the femoral head to hold it in place. Osteotomy may be used for more severe cases. Osteoarthritis may be a long-term complication of SCFE.

Nursing Assessment

Elicit a health history, determining the onset and extent of pain. In acute SCFE, the pain is usually sudden in onset and results in inability to bear weight. Chronic SCFE may present with an insidious onset of pain and limp. Note risk factors for SCFE, including age 9 to 16 years, African-American or Polynesian race, sedentary lifestyle, rapid growth spurt, and being overweight or obese (Haut, 2014; Sankar et al., 2011). Observe ambulation, noting Trendelenburg gait. Assess for pain that is in the hip or that is referred to the groin, medial thigh, or knee. Note decreased range of motion in the affected hip with external rotation. X-rays will be obtained to confirm the diagnosis (anteroposterior and lateral frog-leg views of hips). Bone scan can rule out avascular necrosis, and CT scan helps define the extent of slippage.

Take Note!

Do not attempt to perform passive range of motion to determine the extent of limitation in the child with SCFE; this may cause worsening of the condition.

Nursing Management

Enforce bed rest and activity restriction. If traction is used for a period before surgery, perform routine traction care and neurovascular assessments. If surgery is performed, provide routine preoperative and postoperative care. Assess pain and administer analgesics as needed. After in situ pinning, assist the child with crutch walking. Teach the family that weight bearing is usually resumed about a week after the surgery and that the pin will be removed later. Prolonged immobility may isolate the adolescent from usual peer interactions, so encourage phone calls and visits with friends. Provide books, games, electronic devices, and magazines for distraction during the period of immobility. Provide education and support to the child and family.

Legg–Calvé–Perthes Disease

Legg–Calvé–Perthes disease is a self-limiting condition that involves avascular necrosis of the femoral head. It most often affects children between 4 and 8 years of age, but it can occur as early as 18 months and up until skeletal maturity (Sankar et al., 2011; Haut, 2014). The disease affects males more often (Sankar et al., 2011; Haut, 2014). The etiology is unknown, but interruption of the blood supply to the femoral head results in bone death, and the spherical shape of the femoral head may be lost. Swelling of the soft tissues around the hip may occur. As new blood vessels develop, the area is supplied with circulation, allowing bone resorption and deposition to take place. During this period of revascularization, which takes 18 to 24 months, the bone is soft and more likely to fracture. Over time, the femoral head reforms.

Therapeutic Management

The goal of therapeutic management is to maintain normal femoral head shape and to restore appropriate motion. Treatment of Legg–Calvé–Perthes disease includes anti-inflammatory medication to decrease muscle spasms around the hip joint and to relieve pain. Activity limitation may be prescribed, and sometimes bracing, casting, or traction is recommended to contain the femoral head. Serial x-ray follow-up determines progress of the disease. If surgery becomes warranted, which is rarely done, then osteotomy may be performed. Complications include joint deformity, early degenerative joint disease, persistent pain, loss of hip motion or function, and gait disturbance.

Nursing Assessment

Explore the health history for short stature, delayed bone maturation, related trauma, or a family history of Legg–Calvé–Perthes disease. Note painless limp, which may be intermittent over a period of months. Mild hip pain may result and may be referred to the knee or the thigh. Pain may be aggravated by exercise. Observe the child walking and note Trendelenburg gait. Perform range of motion, noting internal rotation of the hip and limited abduction. Muscle spasm may result with hip extension and rotation. Hip x-rays are obtained to evaluate the extent of epiphyseal involvement. MRI or bone scan may also be used to differentiate Legg–Calvé–Perthes disease from other disorders. Ultrasound and arthrograms may also be useful.

Nursing Management

Nursing care of Legg–Calvé–Perthes disease is highly variable and depends on the stage of the disease and its severity. Administer anti-inflammatory medications, noting their effect on pain. If activities are restricted, exercise the unaffected body parts. Assist families with use of the brace if prescribed. The brace may be wiped with a damp cloth if it becomes dirty. Some children will be prescribed no treatment other than avoidance of contact or high-impact sports. Swimming and bicycle riding help to maintain range of motion with little risk. If mobility equipment is needed, educate the child and family on its use. If osteotomy is performed, provide routine postoperative care, including education and support of the child and family.

Transient Synovitis of the Hip

Transient synovitis of the hip (also termed toxic synovitis) is a common cause of hip pain and limping in children in the United States (Nigrovic, 2015). It typically occurs in children between 3 and 8 years old (Nigrovic, 2015). Boys are affected more than girls (Nigrovic, 2015). The exact cause is unclear, but it is thought to be associated with recent or active infection, trauma, or allergic hypersensitivity (Nigrovic, 2015). It is a self-limiting disease and most cases resolve within a week, but it may last as long as 4 weeks. Usually septic arthritis and osteomyelitis must be excluded before diagnosis can be confirmed.

Therapeutic management involves nonsteroidal anti-inflammatory medications, analgesics, and bed rest to relieve weight bearing on the affected hip joint.

Nursing Assessment

Explore the health history for risk factors such as antecedent trauma, concurrent or recent upper respiratory tract infection, pharyngitis, or otitis media. Note sudden acute onset of moderate to severe pain of one hip. Sometimes pain is referred to the anterior thigh or knee. Pain is usually the worst upon arising in the morning, and the child refuses to walk; pain then decreases throughout the day. Temperature usually will be normal or low grade (less than 38°C). Observe for a limp or for refusal to bear weight. Observe position of the affected hip: it will be held in a flexed and externally rotated position. Note restricted range of motion for abduction and internal rotation.

Nursing Management

Nursing care focuses on educating the family including instructions on administering nonsteroidal anti-inflammatory medications, analgesics, and bed rest. Parents are very concerned when their child refuses to walk; therefore, provide significant support and reassure the child and family of the self-limiting nature of the disease.

TABLE 44.6 TYPES OF SCOLIOSIS

Type	Associated Factors
Idiopathic	Unknown cause Infantile: occurs in the first 3 years of life Juvenile: diagnosed between age 4 and 10 years, or prior to adolescence Adolescent: age 11–17 years
Neuromuscular	Associated with neurologic or muscular disease such as cerebral palsy, myelomeningocele, spinal cord tumors, spinal muscular atrophy, muscular dystrophies
Congenital	Results from anomalous vertebral development

Scoliosis

Scoliosis is a lateral curvature of the spine that exceeds 10 degrees. It may be congenital, associated with other disorders, or idiopathic. Table 44.6 explains the types of scoliosis. Idiopathic scoliosis, with the majority of cases occurring during adolescence, is the most common scoliosis (Spiegel & Dormans, 2011b). Hence, this discussion will focus on adolescent idiopathic scoliosis. The etiology of idiopathic scoliosis is not known, but genetic factors, growth abnormalities, and bone, muscle, disc, or central nervous system disorders may contribute to its development. Early screening and detection of scoliosis result in improved outcomes.

Pathophysiology

In the rapidly growing adolescent, the involved vertebrae rotate around a vertical axis, resulting in lateral curvature. The vertebrae rotate to the convex side of the curve, with the spinous processes rotating toward the concave side. Wedge-shaped vertebral bodies and discs develop because growth is suppressed on the concave side of the curve (Haut, 2014). As the curve progresses, the shape of the thoracic cage changes and respiratory and cardiovascular compromise may occur (the main complications of severe scoliosis).

Therapeutic Management

Treatment of scoliosis is aimed at preventing progression of the curve and decreasing the impact on pulmonary and cardiac function. Treatment is based on the age of the child, expected future growth, and severity of the curve. Observation with serial examinations and spine

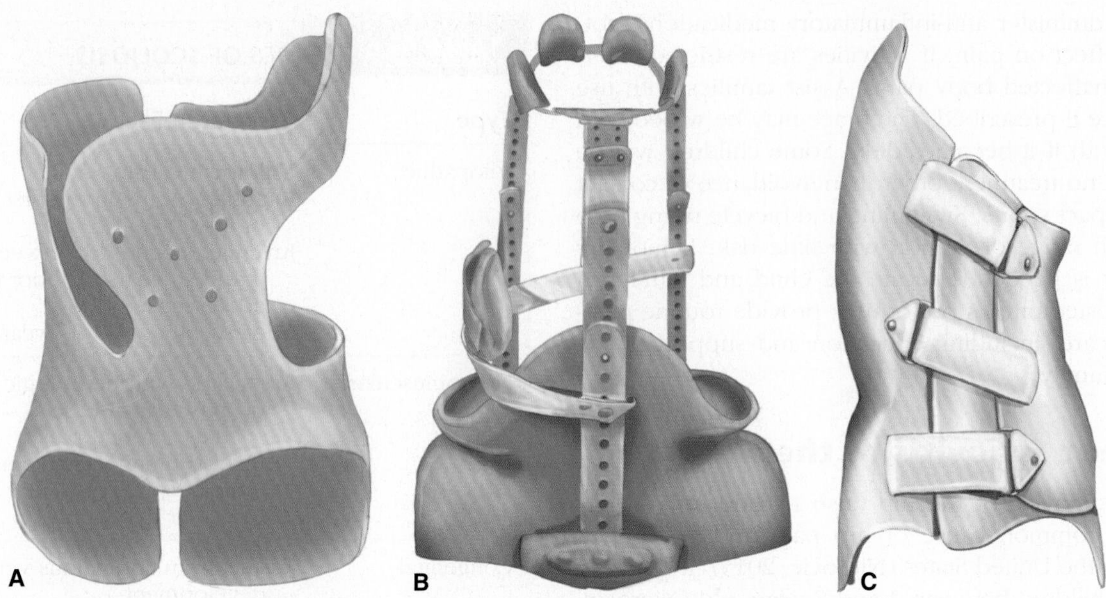

FIGURE 44.28 **(A)** Boston brace. **(B)** Milwaukee brace. **(C)** Nighttime bending brace.

x-rays is used to monitor curve progression. For curves of 25 to 40 degrees, bracing may be sufficient to decrease progression of the curve (Haut, 2014). Box 44.2 describes types of scoliosis braces and Figure 44.28 shows examples of braces. The choice of brace will depend on the location and severity of the curve. Some curves will progress despite appropriate bracing and compliance.

Surgical correction is often required for curves greater than 45 degrees; it is achieved with rod placement and bone grafting (Spiegel & Dormans, 2011b). Partial spinal fusion accompanies many of the corrective surgeries. Multiple surgical approaches and techniques with various instrumentation methods exist for fusion and rod placement. The surgical approach may be anterior, posterior, or both. Traditional rod placement (Harrington rod) involves a single rod fused to the vertebrae, resulting in curve correction but also a flat-backed appearance. Newer rod instrumentations allow for scoliosis curve correction with maintenance of normal back curvature. The rods are shorter, and several are wired or grafted to the appropriate vertebrae to achieve correction. Figure 44.29 shows one example of surgical rod instrumentation.

BOX 44.2

TYPES OF BRACES USED TO TREAT SCOLIOSIS

- Underarm (thoracolumbosacral orthosis [TLSO], Boston, Wilmington): for low thoracic and thoracolumbar curves; less conspicuous, no visible neckpiece
- Milwaukee: for thoracic or major double curves; traditional, standard, has a visible neckpiece with chin rest
- Nighttime bending (Charleston): creates a curve so severe that walking is not possible, so can be worn only at night

Nursing Assessment

For a full description of the assessment phase of the nursing process, refer to the Assessment section of the Nursing Process Overview earlier in the chapter. Assessment findings pertinent to scoliosis are discussed below.

HEALTH HISTORY

Determine why the child is presenting for evaluation of scoliosis. Commonly the child or adolescent will not report back pain; only mild discomfort is associated with idiopathic scoliosis until the curve becomes severe. Often the family recognizes asymmetry in the hips or

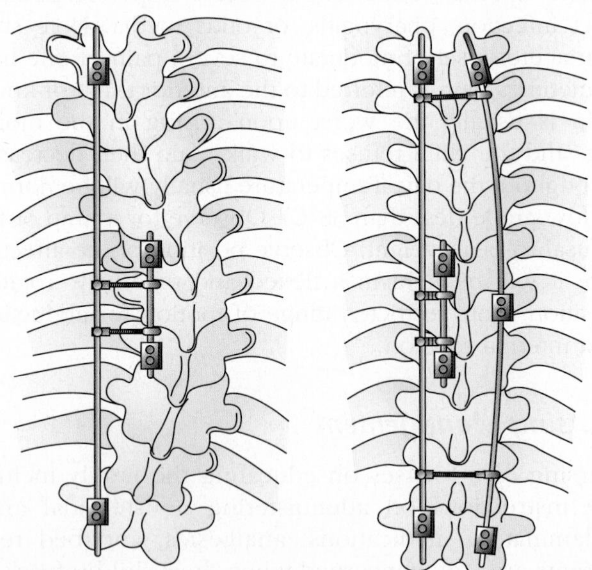
FIGURE 44.29 **Rods are fused to the vertebrae and connected to a distracting rod to rotate the vertebral column (Cotrel–Dubousset method is shown).**

shoulders or the child is screened for scoliosis at school and determined to be at risk. Explore the child's current and past medical history for risk factors such as:

- Family history of scoliosis
- Recent growth spurt
- Physical changes related to puberty

Determine the age of development of secondary sex characteristics and the age of menarche, as these signs of pubertal development indicate the expected velocity and length of remaining growth.

PHYSICAL EXAMINATION

The physical assessment of a child with possible or actual scoliosis involves mainly inspection and observation. Auscultate the heart and lungs to determine compromise related to severe curvature.

Observe the child at rest, sitting, and standing for evidence of poor posture. Inspect the child's back in a standing position. Note asymmetries such as shoulder elevation, prominence of one scapula, uneven curve at the waistline, or a rib hump on one side. Measure shoulder levels from the floor to the acromioclavicular joints. Note the difference between the height of the high and low shoulder in centimeters. Measure heights of anterior and posterior iliac spines and note the difference in centimeters. View the child from the side, noting abnormalities in the spinal curve. With the child bending forward, arms hanging freely, note asymmetry of the back (pronounced hump on one side). Figure 44.30 shows scoliosis noted upon visual inspection. Note leg-length discrepancy if present. During the neurologic examination, balance, motor strength, sensation, and reflexes should all be normal.

LABORATORY AND DIAGNOSTIC TESTS

Full-spine x-rays are necessary to determine the degree of curvature. The radiologist will determine the extent of the curve based on specific formulas and techniques of measurement.

Nursing Management

Nursing Care Plan 44.1, at the end of the chapter, lists general interventions. Tailor nursing care based on the adolescent's response to the disease and its treatment. Additional nursing interventions specific to scoliosis are discussed here.

ENCOURAGING COMPLIANCE WITH BRACING

Bracing is intended to prevent progression of the curve but does not correct the current curve. Although modern braces display an improved appearance, with no visible neckpiece, and can be worn under clothes, many adolescents are not compliant with brace wear. The brace must be worn 23 hours per day to prevent curve progression. Many factors may contribute to noncompliance, including the discomfort associated with brace wear such as pain, heat, and poor fit. The family environment may not be conducive to compliance with brace wear, and teenagers are very concerned about body image.

Inspect the skin for evidence of rubbing by the brace that may impair skin integrity. Teach families appropriate skin care and recommend they check the brace daily for fit and breakage. Encourage the teen to shower during 1 hour per day that the brace is off and to ensure that the skin is clean and dry before putting the brace

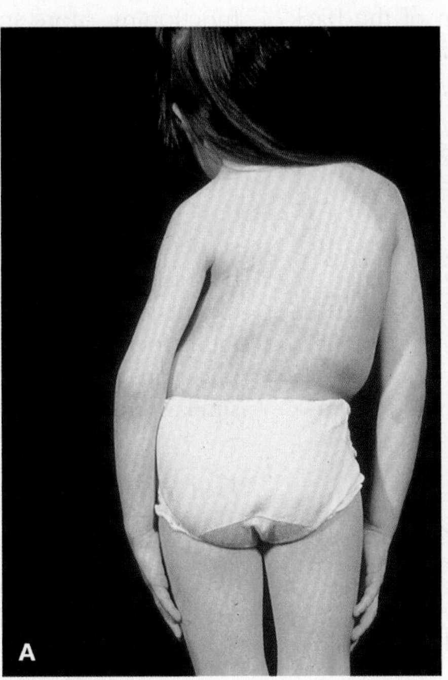

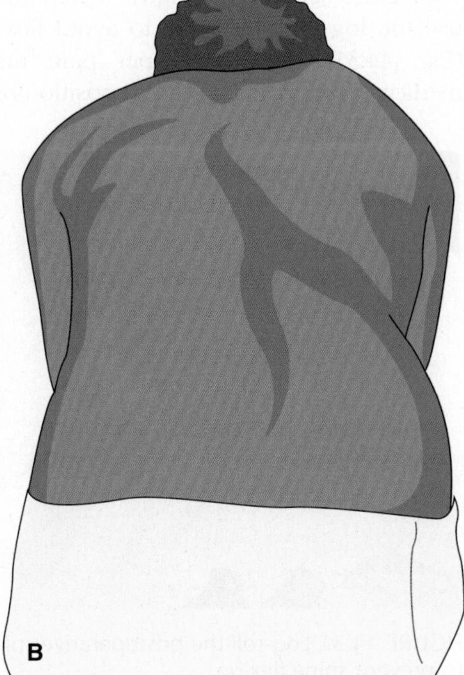

FIGURE 44.30 **(A)** Note right shoulder, scapula, and hip elevation as well as discrepancy in waist curvature. **(B)** Note right upper back hump.

back on. Wearing a cotton T-shirt under the brace may decrease some of the discomfort associated with brace wear. Exercises to strengthen back muscles may prevent muscle atrophy from prolonged bracing and maintain spine flexibility.

PROMOTING POSITIVE BODY IMAGE

Encourage the teen to express his or her feelings or concerns about wearing the brace. Give the teen ways to explain scoliosis and its treatment to his or her peers. Wearing stylish baggy clothes may help the teen to conceal the brace if desired. Refer teens and their families to the National Scoliosis Foundation for additional support. A link to the National Scoliosis Foundation is provided on thePoint.

PROVIDING PREOPERATIVE CARE

If the curve progresses despite bracing or causes pulmonary or cardiac compromise, surgical intervention will be warranted. In the preoperative period, teach the teen the importance of turning, coughing, and deep breathing in the postoperative period. Explain the tubes and lines that will be present immediately after the surgery. Review positioning guidelines: back flexion or extension will not be allowed. Introduce the child to the patient-controlled analgesia pump and explain pain scales. There is a high risk for significant blood loss with spinal fusion and instrumentation, so if possible arrange for preoperative autologous blood donation.

PROVIDING POSTOPERATIVE CARE

The goal of nursing management in the postoperative period after spinal fusion with or without instrumentation is to avoid complications. Perform neurovascular checks with each set of vital signs. When turning the child, use the log-roll technique to avoid flexion of the back (Fig. 44.31). Provide proper pain management and medicate for pain before repositioning and ambulation. Administer prophylactic intravenous antibiotics if ordered. Assess for drainage from the operative site and for excess blood loss via the Hemovac or other drainage tube. Maintain Foley patency, as the child will be confined to bed for the first couple of days. Maintain strict recording of fluid intake and output. Administer transfusions of packed red blood cells if ordered. Ambulation, once ordered, should be done slowly to avoid orthostatic hypotension. Assist the family with arrangements to continue the teen's schoolwork while hospitalized and/or arrange for home tutoring during the several-week recovery period.

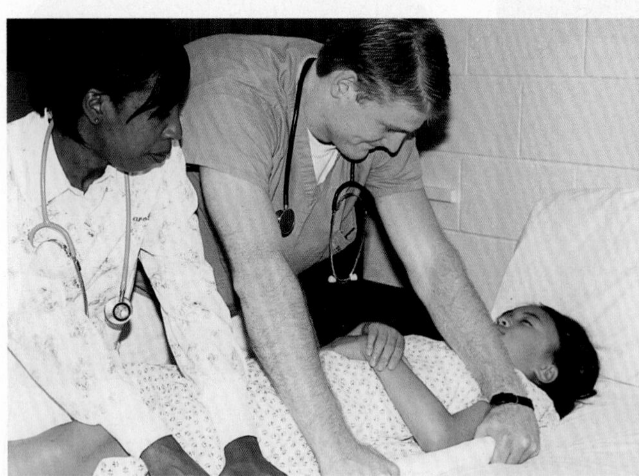

FIGURE 44.31 Log-roll the postoperative spinal fusion child to prevent spine flexion.

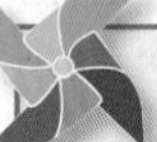

Consider This

I have been diagnosed with scoliosis and the doctor told me I have to wear a brace at night. How did this happen? I will never be able to go to another sleep over, all the other kids will laugh at me.

Thoughts: How would you respond to her concerns? What education will be necessary and how can you promote compliance?

What local resources could you refer her to?

Spinal Cord Injury

Spinal cord injury is damage to the spinal cord that results in loss of function. Frequent causes are trauma, such as car accidents, falls, diving into shallow water, gunshot or stab wounds, sports injuries, child abuse, or birth injuries. Spinal cord injuries are relatively uncommon in children, but when they do occur they have a devastating impact on the child's physical and functional status, social and emotional development, and family functioning. More spinal cord injuries are seen in people 16 to 30 years of age due to their increased incidence of accidents, particularly motor vehicle accidents (Mayo Clinic Staff, 2014).

Spinal cord injury is a medical emergency and immediate medical attention is required. Cervical traction is often used initially and surgical intervention is sometimes necessary. Ongoing medical treatment will be based on the child's age and overall health and the extent and location of the injury. Therapeutic management focuses on rehabilitation and prevention of complications. Spinal cord injury in children is managed similarly to that in adults.

Nursing Assessment

Symptoms vary based on the location and severity of the injury. Common signs and symptoms associated with spinal cord injury include:

- Inability to move or feel extremities
- Numbness

- Tingling
- Weakness

Paralysis depends on the location of the injury to the spinal cord; the higher the injury in the spinal cord, the more extensive the damage and the greater the loss of function. High cervical injury will result in damage to the phrenic nerve, which innervates the diaphragm. Damage to this nerve will leave the child unable to breathe without assistance.

The diagnosis of spinal cord injury is made by clinical signs and diagnostic tests, which may include x-rays, CT scans, and MRI.

Nursing Management

Any child who requires hospitalization due to trauma should be considered at risk for a spinal cord injury. Immobilization of the spine is essential until full evaluation of the injury is complete and spinal cord damage is ruled out. Nursing management will be similar to management of the adult with a spinal cord injury and will focus on optimizing mobility, promoting bladder and bowel management, promoting adequate nutritional status, preventing complications associated with extreme immobility such as contractures and muscle atrophy, managing pain, and providing support and education to the child and family. Refer to the myelomeningocele section of this chapter for information related to urinary and bowel elimination.

The nurse plays an important role not only in the acute care of children with spinal cord injury but also during rehabilitation. Recovery from a spinal cord injury requires long-term hospitalization and rehabilitation. An interdisciplinary team of physicians, nurses, therapists, social workers, and case managers will work to manage the child's complex and long-term needs. Promoting communication among the interdisciplinary team is essential and will be a key nursing function. Rehabilitation will need to focus on the ever-changing developmental needs of the child as he or she grows.

Prevention of spinal cord injuries is an important nursing consideration. Educate the public on vehicular safety, including seat belt use and the proper use of age-appropriate safety seats. Additional education topics include bicycle, sports, and recreation safety; prevention of falls; violence prevention including gun safety; and water safety, including the risk of diving. This education can help decrease the incidence of spinal cord injury in children.

Fracture

Fractures occur frequently in children and adolescents; 42% of boys and 27% of girls will suffer a fracture during childhood (Haut, 2014). The most common fractures in children occur in the forearm and wrist (Haut, 2014). Most pediatric fractures heal well with minimal treatment (Wells, Sehgal, & Dormans, 2011). Midclavicular, humerus, or femur fractures can occur as a result of birth trauma. They typically heal well but may require limiting mobility or splinting.

Fractures in children result most frequently from accidental trauma (Haut, 2014). Nonaccidental trauma (child abuse) and other disease processes are the other causes of fractures. In children younger than 2 years, most fractures that occur are the result of another person causing the injury (Haut, 2014).

Take Note!

Fracture in the newborn (with the exception of birth trauma) or infant should raise a high index of suspicion for abuse, as fractures are very unusual in children who cannot yet walk.

Pathophysiology

The growth plate is the most vulnerable portion of the child's bone and is frequently the site of injury. The Salter–Harris classification system is used to describe fractures involving the growth plate (Table 44.7). The thicker, more elastic periosteum in children yields to the force encountered with trauma, resulting more frequently in nondisplaced fractures in children. The increased vascularity and decreased mineral content make the child's bones more flexible. Plastic or bowing deformities and buckle and greenstick fractures are the result. Complete fractures do occur in children, but they tend to be more stable than in the adult, resulting in improved healing and function. Spiral, pelvic, and hip fractures are rare in children. Table 44.8 explains common types of fractures in children.

Fractures in children heal more rapidly and result in less disability and deformity than adults. The younger the child, the more quickly the bone heals. However, plastic deformity and Salter–Harris type IV fractures may result in an angular deformity. Though healing of fractures is usually quick and without incident in children, delayed union, nonunion, or malunion can occur. Additional complications include infection, avascular necrosis, bone shortening from epiphyseal arrest, vascular or nerve injuries, fat embolism, reflex sympathetic dystrophy, and compartment syndrome, which is an orthopedic emergency. Later in life, osteoarthritis may occur as a long-term complication from childhood fracture (Haut, 2014).

Take Note!

Any type of fracture can be the result of child abuse but spiral femur fractures, rib fractures, and humerus fractures, particularly in the child younger than 2 years of age, should always be thoroughly investigated to rule out the possibility of abuse (Wells, Sehgal, & Dormans, 2011).

TABLE 44.7 THE SALTER–HARRIS CLASSIFICATION SYSTEM

Type	Description	Illustration
I	Fracture is through the physis, widening it.	
II	Fracture is partially through the physis, extending into the metaphysis.	
III	Fracture is partially through the epiphysis, extending into the epiphysis.	

(continued)

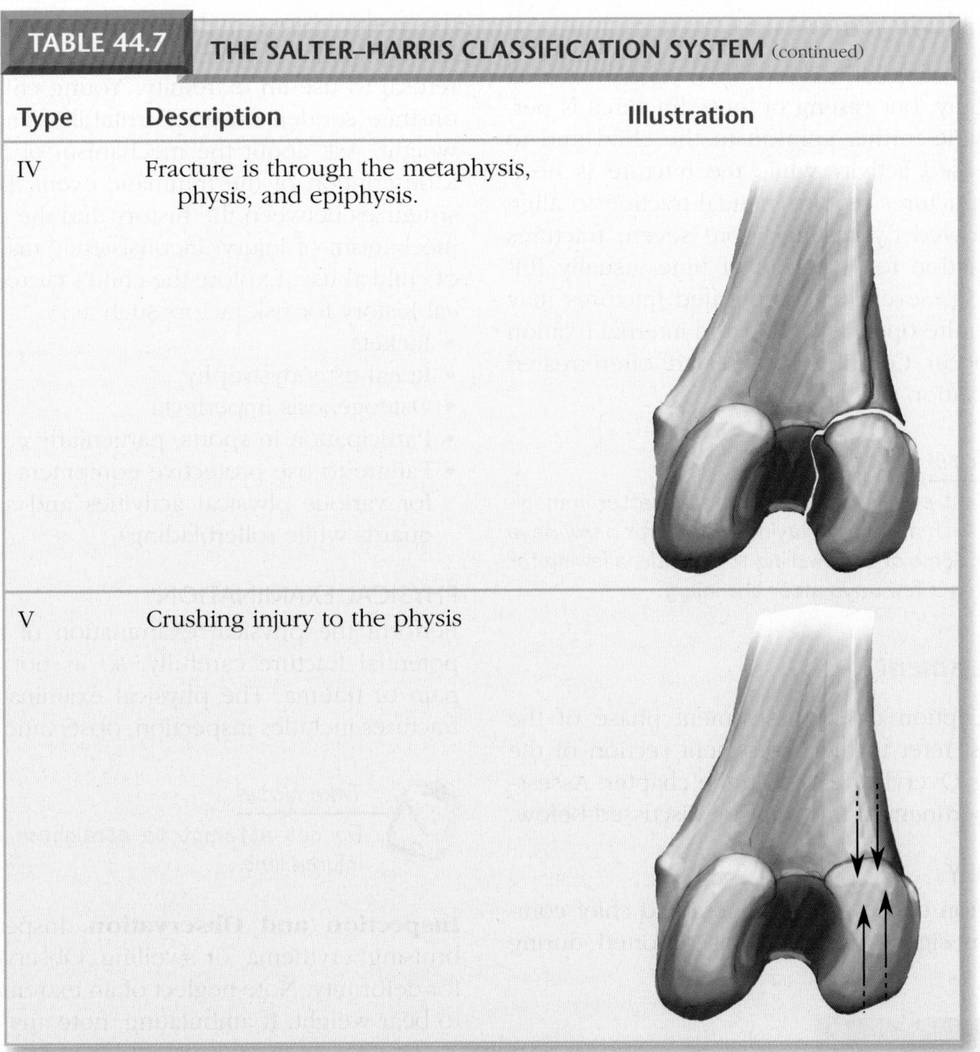

TABLE 44.7 THE SALTER–HARRIS CLASSIFICATION SYSTEM (continued)

Type	Description	Illustration
IV	Fracture is through the metaphysis, physis, and epiphysis.	
V	Crushing injury to the physis	

TABLE 44.8 TYPES OF FRACTURES IN CHILDREN

Fracture Type	Description	Illustration
Plastic or bowing deformity	Significant bending without breaking of the bone	A
Buckle fracture	Compression injury; the bone buckles rather than breaks.	B
Greenstick fracture	Incomplete fracture of the bone	C
Complete fracture	Bone breaks into two pieces.	D

Therapeutic Management

The vast majority of childhood fractures would heal well with splinting only, but casting of these fractures is performed to provide further comfort to the child and to allow for increased activity while the fracture is healing. Displaced fractures require manual traction to align the bones, followed by casting. More severe fractures may require traction for a period of time, usually followed by casting. Severe or complicated fractures may alternatively require open reduction and internal fixation for healing to occur. Complex fractures are often treated with external fixation (Fig. 44.32).

Take Note!

Significant swelling may occur initially after immobilization with a splint. Delaying casting for a few days provides time for some of the swelling to subside, allowing for successful casting a few days after the injury.

Nursing Assessment

For a full description of the assessment phase of the nursing process, refer to the Assessment section of the Nursing Process Overview earlier in the chapter. Assessment findings pertinent to fractures are discussed below.

HEALTH HISTORY

Elicit a description of the present illness and chief complaint. Common signs and symptoms reported during the health history might include recent injury, trauma, or fall; complaint of pain; difficulty bearing weight; limp; or refusal to use an extremity. Young children often demonstrate sudden onset of irritability and refusal to bear weight. Ask about the mechanism of injury and obtain a description of the traumatic event. Be alert to inconsistencies between the history and the clinical picture or mechanism of injury; inconsistency may be an indicator of child abuse. Explore the child's current and past medical history for risk factors such as:

- Rickets
- Renal osteodystrophy
- Osteogenesis imperfecta
- Participation in sports, particularly contact sports
- Failure to use protective equipment as recommended for various physical activities and sports (e.g., wrist guards while rollerblading)

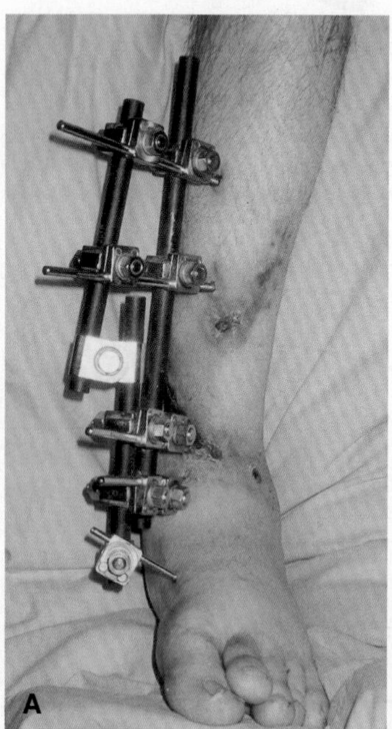

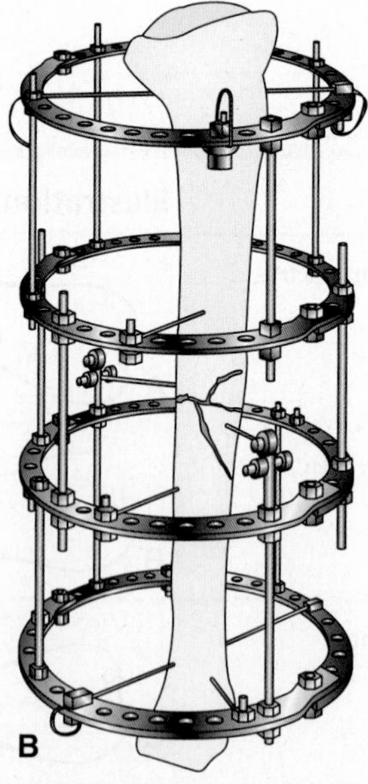

FIGURE 44.32 **(A)** External fixation is required for complicated fractures. **(B)** The Ilizarov fixator is a circular apparatus usually used for complicated lower extremity fractures. The pins are smaller in diameter, more like wires, than those used in other fixators.

PHYSICAL EXAMINATION

Perform the physical examination of the child with a potential fracture carefully, so as not to cause further pain or trauma. The physical examination particular to fractures includes inspection, observation, and palpation.

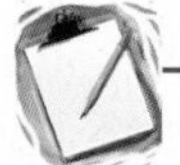

Take Note!

Do not attempt to straighten or manipulate an injured limb.

Inspection and Observation. Inspect the skin for bruising, erythema, or swelling. Observe the extremities for deformity. Note neglect of an extremity or an inability to bear weight. If ambulating, note any limp.

Palpation. Carefully palpate the joint or injured part. Distract the young child with a toy or activity while palpating. Note point tenderness, which is a reliable indicator of fracture in children. Assess neurovascular status, noting distal extremity temperature, spontaneous movement, sensation, numbness, capillary refill time, and quality of pulses. The neurovascular assessment is critical to providing a baseline so that any changes associated with compartment syndrome can be identified quickly.

LABORATORY AND DIAGNOSTIC TESTS

Usually plain x-ray films are all that is required to identify a simple fracture. Complicated fractures that require surgical intervention may require further evaluation with CT or MRI.

Nursing Management

Immediately after the injury, immobilize the limb above and below the site of injury in the most comfortable position with a splint. Use cold therapy to reduce swelling in the first 48 hours after injury. Elevate the injured extremity above the level of the heart. Perform frequent neurovascular checks.

Take Note!

Assess the injured, splinted, or casted extremity frequently for the "5 Ps," which may indicate compartment syndrome: pain (increased out of proportion), pulselessness, pallor, paresthesia, and paralysis. Report these findings immediately.

Assess pain level and administer pain medications as needed. Utilize nonpharmacologic methods of pain relief as needed. Administer tetanus vaccine in the child with an open fracture if he or she has not received a tetanus booster within the past 5 years. Additional nursing interventions include providing family education and teaching on fracture prevention.

PROVIDING FAMILY EDUCATION

Unless bed rest is prescribed, children with upper extremity casts and "walking" leg casts can resume increased levels of activity as the pain subsides. Children who require crutches while in a cast may return to school, but those in spica casts will be at home for several weeks. Providing distraction and finding ways to keep up with school work are important. Teach families to care for the cast (see Teaching Guidelines 44.1).

PREVENTING FRACTURES

Discourage risky behavior such as climbing trees and performing tricks on bicycles. Provide appropriate supervision, particularly with outdoor activity. Encourage appropriate use of protective equipment, such as wrist guards with rollerblading and shin guards with soccer. Ensure that playground equipment is in good working order and intact; there should not be protruding screws or unbalanced portions of equipment, which may increase the risk for falling.

Sprains

Sprains result from a twisting or turning motion of the affected body part. The tendons and ligaments stretch excessively and may tear slightly. They are uncommon in young children as their growth plates are weaker than their muscles and tendons, making them more prone to fracture. They may occur at any joint, but the most common are ankle and knee sprains. Therapeutic management of sprains includes rest, ice, compression, and elevation (RICE). Other treatment options may include activity restrictions, splints or casts, crutches or wheelchair, and physical therapy. On initial evaluation, sprains need to be differentiated from torn ligaments and meniscal tears, as those conditions are more serious and may require surgical intervention.

Nursing Assessment

Elicit a health history, determining the mechanism of injury (whether it occurred during sports or simply a misstep or fall). Determine what treatment the family has used so far. Inspect the affected body part for edema, which is frequently present, and bruising, which sometimes occurs. Note limp or inability to bear weight. Do not attempt to perform passive range of motion on the affected body part. Assess neurovascular status distal to the injury (usually normal).

Nursing Management

Instruct the child and family in appropriate treatment of sprains, which includes:

- Rest: limit activity.
- Ice: apply cold packs for 20 to 30 minutes, remove for 1 hour, and repeat (for the first 24 to 48 hours).
- Compression: apply an Ace wrap or other elastic bandage or brace; check skin for alterations when rewrapping.
- Elevation: elevate the injured extremity above the level of the heart to decrease swelling (Fig. 44.33).

The child may require instruction in crutch walking as well. Teach families that to prevent sprains during sports, it is important for the child to perform appropriate stretching and warm-up activities.

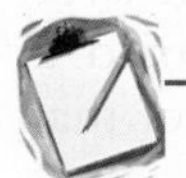

Take Note!

If the child's fingers or toes become increasingly swollen or discolored, remove the Ace wrap immediately.

Overuse Syndromes

The term "overuse syndrome" refers to a group of disorders that result from repeated force applied to normal tissue. The connective tissues fail in response to repetitive stress, leading to a small amount of tissue breakdown. They develop over the course of weeks to months. There is usually no identifiable injury associated with overuse syndromes. Pain is usually associated with the activity and worsens with continued participation in the activity. The incidence of overuse injuries in the young athlete has increased as participation of youths in organized sports has grown along with children today participating in sports year-round and sometimes in multiple sports simultaneously (Brenner & the Council on Sports Medicine and Fitness, 2014). The young athlete is at risk for more serious overuse injuries due to the following:

- The growing bones of the young athlete cannot handle as much stress as mature bones in adults.

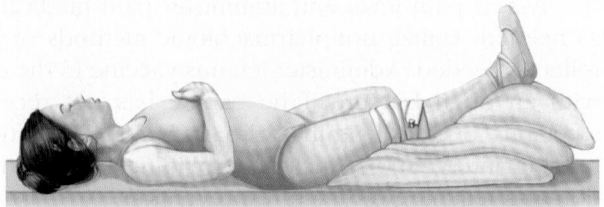

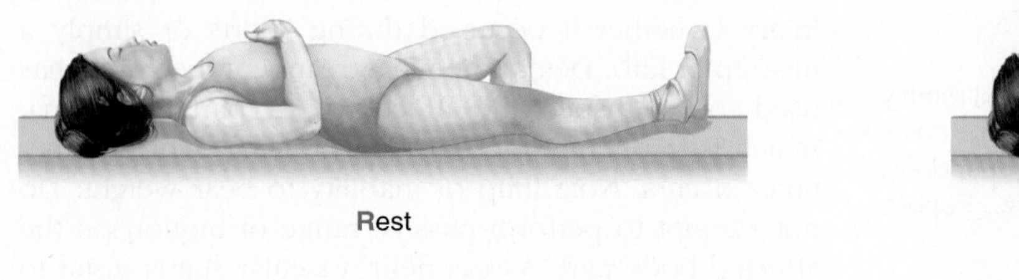

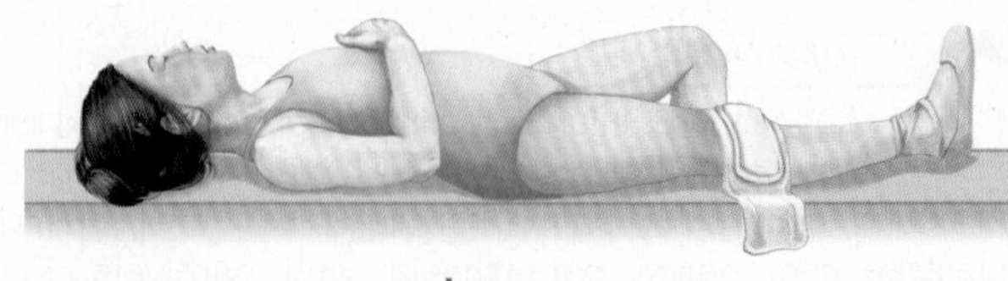

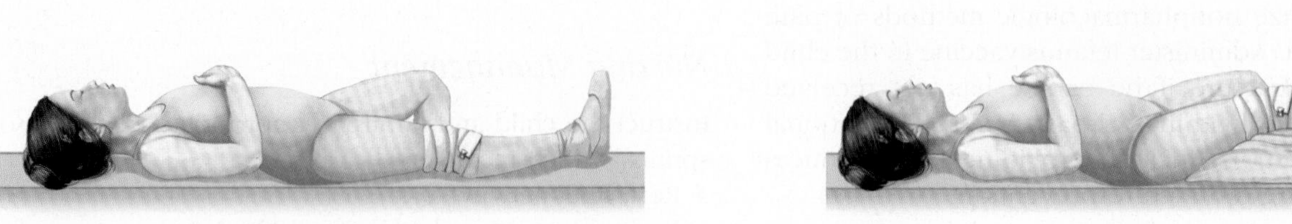

FIGURE 44.33 RICE (rest, ice, compression, elevation) is the appropriate treatment for sprains.

- The child is just learning the proper mechanisms for skills, such as throwing a baseball.
- The child is unable to recognize vague signs of injury such as fatigue and poor performance (Brenner & the Council on Sports Medicine and Fitness, 2014).

Table 44.9 gives details on several common overuse syndromes. Therapeutic management is aimed at reassurance, pain management, and limiting rather than eliminating activity.

Nursing Assessment

Elicit a health history to determine the extent of involvement in sports. Note onset of pain, duration, intensity, aggravating factors, and treatments used at home. Examine the painful part, noting findings similar to those noted for each syndrome in Table 44.9.

Nursing Management

Initially, apply ice when pain is severe. Anti-inflammatory medications such as ibuprofen may be helpful. Encourage the child to limit exercise and participate in a different activity. After a few weeks, most overuse syndromes resolve; at that point, the athlete may resume the prior activity. Osgood–Schlatter disease is the exception and may require 6 to 18 months to resolve (Kienstra & Macias, 2014). Using pads or braces that are appropriate to the painful body part is also helpful. Supporting the arm with a sling may relieve stress on the proximal humerus when epiphysiolysis occurs. Heel cups used in athletic shoes help relieve stress on the heels associated with Sever disease. To prevent overuse syndromes, encourage athletes to perform appropriate stretching exercises during a 20- to 30-minute warm-up period before each practice or game. Also encourage several weeks of conditioning training before the season begins.

There is currently limited research pertaining to overuse injuries in the young athlete. The American Academy of Pediatrics has developed some guidelines to help prevent these injuries such as the following: encourage 1 to 2 days off per week of competitive athletics, sports training, and competitive practice; encourage 2 to 3 months away from a specific sport during the year; and educate to increase weekly training time, number of repetitions, or total distance by no more than 10% a week; participation in sports should be about fun, skill acquisition, sportsmanship, and safety (Brenner & the Council on Sports Medicine and Fitness, 2014).

Take Note!

"Energy healing" such as therapeutic touch and Reiki may provide a nonpharmacologic adjunct to pain management for musculoskeletal injuries.

Radial Head Subluxation

Subluxation of the radial head ("nursemaid's elbow") occurs when a pulling motion on the arm causes the annular ligament surrounding the radial head to stretch

TABLE 44.9 OVERUSE DISORDERS

Disorder	Anatomic Area Affected	Most Commonly Occurs in	Symptoms
Osgood–Schlatter disease	Partial avulsion of the ossification center of the tibial tubercle	Active adolescents, most often boys. Most frequently during periods of rapid growth	• Mild to moderate pain, activity related • Tibial tubercle is tender when palpated • Painful swelling or prominence of the anterior portion of the tibial tubercle
Epiphysiolysis of proximal humerus	Proximal humerus (widening of growth plate)	Occurs with rigorous upper extremity activity, such as baseball pitching	• Tenderness in the shoulder or proximal humerus • Pain with active internal rotation • Full shoulder range of motion continues
Epiphysiolysis of distal radius	Distal radius (widening of growth plate)	Occurs with overuse of the distal radius, such as in gymnasts	• Wrist pain that worsens with activity
Sever disease (calcaneal apophysitis)	Calcaneus (heel)	Usually in 9- to 14-year olds	• Pain over the posterior aspect of the calcaneus • Limited active and passive dorsiflexion of foot
Shin splints	Refer to a variety of overuse syndromes associated with the shin (stress fracture, tibial stress, muscular issues)	Occur with activities that place repeated exertion on the lower leg, as in runners, ballerinas, elite soccer players	• Exercise-induced pain of the anterior aspect of the middle part of the lower leg • May be sharp pain • Worsens with exercise • With stress fracture, may have a limp that worsens with activity

or tear, therefore displacing the radial head. The ligament becomes entrapped within the joint, preventing spontaneous reduction. It usually occurs in children younger than 5 years of age (Carrigan, 2011). In most cases a parent, sibling, or caregiver inadvertently injures the child while holding or pulling on a pronated upper extremity. Radiologic examination may be done, especially if the mechanism of injury is not clear, to rule out fracture or dislocation. To reduce the injury, the elbow is flexed to 90 degrees and then the forearm is fully and firmly supinated, causing the ligament to snap back into place. With appropriate reduction of the radial head, no complications result.

Nursing Assessment

Elicit a health history to help determine the mechanism of injury. Common precipitators of this injury include pulling on the child's arm while leading him or her in one direction, helping the child up the stairs, a child dropping or falling to the ground while an adult is holding the hand, or swinging or lifting the child by the hands. Assess neurovascular status and examine the extremity. The child will hold the arm slightly flexed at the side or across the abdomen and refuse to move it. When the arm is still, the child apparently has no discomfort. Neurovascular status is normally intact with no bruising or swelling present.

Nursing Management

After treatment, usually hyperpronation to reduce the dislocation, assess the child's ability to use the arm without pain. Typically after reduction the child will demonstrate less pain almost immediately. Educate parents that once a radial head subluxation occurs it may recur. Teach parents to avoid excessive pulling or pulling up on the child's arm, particularly in an abrupt jerking fashion, to prevent recurrence. Encourage parents and caregivers to always lift the child under the arms.

NURSING CARE PLAN 44.1

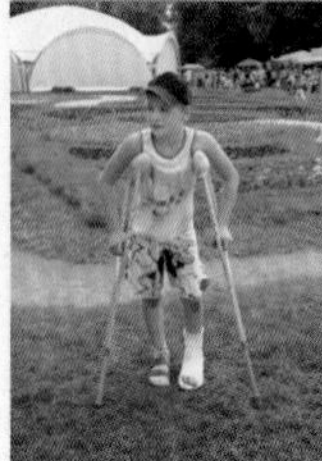

Overview for the Child With a Neuromuscular or Musculoskeletal Disorder

NURSING DIAGNOSIS: Impaired physical mobility related to injury, pain, muscle weakness, hypertonicity, impaired coordination, loss of muscle function or control as evidenced by an inability to move extremities, to ambulate without assistance, to move without limitations

Outcome Identification and Evaluation

Child will be able to engage in activities within age parameters and limits of injury or disease: child is able to move extremities, move about environment, assist with transfers and positioning in bed and/or participate in exercise programs within limits of age and disease.

Interventions: *Maximizing Physical Mobility*

- Assess child's ability to move based on injury or disease and within limits of prescribed treatment *to determine baseline.*
- Prior to prescribed exercise or major position changes, ensure that pain medication is given: *relief of pain increases child's ability to tolerate and participate in activity.*
- Encourage gross and fine motor activities *to facilitate motor development.*
- Collaborate with physical therapy, occupational therapy, and speech therapy to strengthen muscles and promote optimal mobility. Support therapy activities by using same equipment and technique *to help rehabilitate musculoskeletal deficits, improve mobility, facilitate motor development, and allow for maximum functioning.*
- Use passive and active range-of-motion (ROM) exercises and teach child and family how to perform them *to prevent contractures, facilitate joint mobility and muscle development (active ROM), and help increase mobility.*
- Praise accomplishments and emphasize child's abilities *to improve self-esteem and encourage feeling of confidence and competence.*
- Teach child and family necessary care related to mobility issues *so the family can continue with these measures at home.*

NURSING DIAGNOSIS: Nutrition, imbalanced, less than body requirements, related to difficulty feeding secondary to deficient sucking, swallowing, or chewing; difficulty assuming normal feeding position; inability to feed self as evidenced by decreased oral intake, impaired swallowing, weight loss, or plateau

Outcome Identification and Evaluation

Child will exhibit signs of adequate nutrition as evidenced by appropriate weight gain, intake and output within normal limits, and adequate ingestion of calories.

Intervention: *Promoting Adequate Nutrition*

- Monitor height and weight: *insufficient intake will lead to impaired growth and weight gain.*
- Monitor hydration status (moist mucous membranes, elastic skin turgor, adequate urine output): *insufficient intake can lead to dehydration.*
- Use techniques to promote caloric and nutritional intake and teach family about these techniques (e.g., positioning, modified utensils, soft or blended foods, allowing extra time) *to facilitate intake.*
- Assess respiratory system frequently *to assess for aspiration.*
- Assist family to help child assume as normal a feeding position as possible *to help increase oral intake.*

NURSING CARE PLAN 44.1

Overview for the Child With a Neuromuscular or Musculoskeletal Disorder (continued)

NURSING DIAGNOSIS: Urinary retention related to sensory motor impairment as evidenced by dribbling, inadequate bladder emptying

Outcome Identification and Evaluation

Child's bladder will empty adequately, according to pre-established quantities and frequencies individualized for the child (usual urine output is 0.5 to 2 mL/kg/hour).

Intervention: ***Promoting Successful Bladder Emptying***

- Assess child's ability to empty bladder via history focused on character and duration of lower urinary symptoms *to establish baseline.*
- Assess for history of fecal impaction or constipation, *as alterations in bowel elimination may hinder urinary elimination.*
- Assess for bladder distention by palpation or urinary retention by postvoid residual obtained via catheterization or bladder ultrasound *to determine extent of retention.*
- Maintain adequate hydration *to avoid irritating effects that dehydration has on the bladder.*
- Schedule voiding *to decrease bladder overdistention.*
- Teach the family (and the child if old enough) with significant urinary retention the technique of clean intermittent catheterization *to allow regular, complete bladder emptying.*

NURSING DIAGNOSIS: Risk for constipation related to immobility, loss of sensation, and/or use of narcotic analgesics

Outcome Identification and Evaluation

Child will demonstrate adequate stool passage: will pass soft, formed stool every 1 to 3 days without straining or other adverse effects.

Intervention: ***Promoting Appropriate Bowel Elimination***

- Assess usual pattern of stooling *to determine baseline and identify potential problems with elimination.*
- Palpate for abdominal fullness and auscultate for bowel sounds *to assess for bowel function and presence of constipation.*
- Encourage fiber intake *to increase frequency of stools.*
- Ensure adequate fluid intake *to prevent formation of hard, dry stools.*
- Encourage activity within child's limits or restrictions: *even minimal activity increases peristalsis.*
- Administer medications or enemas as ordered *to promote bowel training/evacuation (especially in child with myelomeningocele or spinal cord injury).*

NURSING DIAGNOSIS: Self-care deficit related to neuromuscular impairments, cognitive deficits, immobility as evidenced by an inability to perform hygiene care and transfer self independently

Outcome Identification and Evaluation

Child will demonstrate ability to care for self within age parameters and limits of injury or disease: *child is able to feed, dress, and manage elimination within limits of injury, disease and age.*

Intervention: ***Maximizing Self-Care***

- Introduce child and family to self-help methods as soon as possible *to promote independence from the beginning.*
- Encourage family and staff to allow child to do as much as possible *to allow child to gain confidence and independence.*

(continued)

NURSING CARE PLAN 44.1

Overview for the Child With a Neuromuscular or Musculoskeletal Disorder (continued)

- Teach specific measures for bowel and urinary elimination as needed *to promote independence and increase self-care abilities and self-esteem.*
- Collaborate with physical therapy, occupational therapy, and speech therapy to provide child and family with appropriate tools to modify environment and methods to promote transferring and self-care *to allow for maximum functioning.*
- Praise accomplishments and emphasize child's abilities *to improve self-esteem and encourage feelings of confidence and competence.*
- Balance activity with periods of rest *to reduce fatigue and increase energy for self-care.*

NURSING DIAGNOSIS: Risk for impaired skin integrity related to immobility, casting, traction, use of braces or adaptive devices

Outcome Identification and Evaluation

Child's skin will remain intact, without evidence of redness or breakdown.

Intervention: *Promoting Skin Integrity*

- Monitor condition of entire skin surface at least daily *to provide baseline and allow for early identification of areas at risk.*
- Avoid excessive friction or harsh cleaning products *that may increase risk of breakdown in child with susceptible skin.*
- Keep child's skin free from stool and urine *to decrease risk of breakdown.*
- Keep linen clean, dry, and free from food crumbs and wrinkles *to prevent pressure areas from forming.*
- Change child's position frequently *to decrease pressure to susceptible areas.*
- Monitor skin condition affected by braces or adaptive equipment frequently *to prevent skin breakdown related to poor fit.*

For the child in traction:

- Pad bony prominences with cotton padding before applying traction *to protect skin from injury.*
- Gently massage child's back and sacrum with lotion *to stimulate circulation.*

For the child in a spica cast:

- Apply plastic wrap to the perineal edges of the cast to prevent soiling of cast edges, *which can contribute to cast breakdown.*
- Use a fracture bedpan *to facilitate toileting without soiling cast.*
- For the child still in diapers, tuck a smaller diaper under the perineal edges of cast and cover with a larger diaper *to prevent cast soiling.*

NURSING DIAGNOSIS: Chronic sorrow related to presence of chronic disability as evidenced by child's or family's expression of sadness, anger, disappointment, or feeling overwhelmed

Outcome Identification and Evaluation

Child and/or family will accept situation: child/family will appropriately identify feelings, function at a normal developmental level, and plan for the future.

Intervention: *Easing Sorrow*

- Assess degree of sorrow *to provide baseline for intervention.*
- Identify problems with eating or sleeping, *often affected when grief or sorrow is present.*
- Spend time with the child and family: *an empathetic presence is valued by suffering families.*
- Encourage the use of positive coping techniques: *taking action, expressing feelings, and intentional attempts at coping are helpful techniques.*
- Refer to appropriate support groups: *can be helpful to talk to others in similar situations.*
- Refer for spiritual counseling as desired: *many families experience grief resolution in a more timely fashion if spiritual needs are addressed.*

NURSING CARE PLAN 44.1

Overview for the Child With a Neuromuscular or Musculoskeletal Disorder (continued)

NURSING DIAGNOSIS: Risk for injury related to muscle weakness

Outcome Identification and Evaluation

Child will remain free from injury: child will not fall or experience other injury.

Intervention: ***Preventing Injury***

- Ensure that side rails of bed are elevated when caregiver is not directly at bedside *to prevent fall from bed.*
- Use appropriate safety restraints with adaptive equipment and wheelchairs *to prevent fall or slipping from equipment.*
- Do not leave child unattended in tub *as weakness may cause the child to slip under the water.*
- Avoid restraint use if at all possible: *close observation is more appropriate.*

NURSING DIAGNOSIS: Deficient knowledge related to cast care, activity restrictions, lack of information regarding complex medical condition, prognosis, and medical needs as evidenced by verbalization, questions, or actions demonstrating lack of understanding regarding child's condition or care

Outcome Identification and Evaluation

Child and family will verbalize accurate information and understanding about condition, prognosis, and medical needs: child and family demonstrate knowledge of condition and prognosis and medical needs, including possible causes, contributing factors, and treatment measures through verbalization and return demonstration.

Intervention: ***Providing Child and Family Teaching***

- Assess child's and family's willingness to learn: *child and family must be willing to learn for teaching to be effective.*
- Provide family with time to adjust to diagnosis *to facilitate adjustment and ability to learn and participate in child's care.*
- Repeat information *to allow family and child time to learn and understand.*
- Teach in short sessions: *many short sessions are more helpful than one long session.*
- Gear teaching to the level of understanding of the child and family (depends on age of child, physical condition, memory) *to ensure understanding.*
- Provide reinforcement and rewards *to facilitate the teaching/learning process.*
- Use multiple modes of learning involving many senses (provide written, verbal, demonstration, and videos) when possible: *child and family are more likely to retain information when it is presented in different ways using many senses.*

NURSING DIAGNOSIS: Family processes, interrupted, related to child's illness, hospitalization, diagnosis of chronic illness in child, and potential long-term effects of illness as evidenced by family's presence in hospital, missed work, demonstration of inadequate coping

Outcome Identification and Evaluation

Family will maintain functional system of support and demonstrate adequate coping and adaptation of roles: parents are involved in child's care, ask appropriate questions, express fears and concerns, and are able to discuss child's care and condition calmly.

(continued)

NURSING CARE PLAN 44.1

Overview for the Child With a Neuromuscular or Musculoskeletal Disorder (continued)

Intervention: ***Promoting Appropriate Family Functioning***

- Encourage parents and family to verbalize concerns related to child's illness, diagnosis, and prognosis: *allows the nurse to identify concerns and areas where further education may be needed; demonstrates family-centered care.*
- Explain therapies, procedures, child's behaviors, and plan of care to parents: *understanding of the child's current status and plan of care helps decrease anxiety.*
- Encourage parental involvement in care *to allow parents to feel needed and valued and to have a sense of control over their child's health.*
- Identify support system for family and child: *support system is often needed by stressed families to assist with coping.*
- Educate family and child on additional resources available *to help them develop a wide base of support.*

NURSING DIAGNOSIS: Risk for delayed development related to immobility, alterations in extremities

Outcome Identification and Evaluation

Development will be enhanced: child will make continued progress toward developmental milestones and will not show regression in abilities.

Intervention: ***Promoting Development***

- Screen for developmental capabilities *to determine child's current level of functioning.*
- Offer age-appropriate toys, play, and activities (including gross motor) *to encourage further development.*
- Perform exercises or interventions as prescribed by physical or occupational therapist: *repeat participation in those activities helps to promote function and acquisition of developmental skills.*
- Provide support to child and families: *immobility and extremity deficits may lead to slow progress in achieving developmental milestones, so ongoing motivation is needed.*

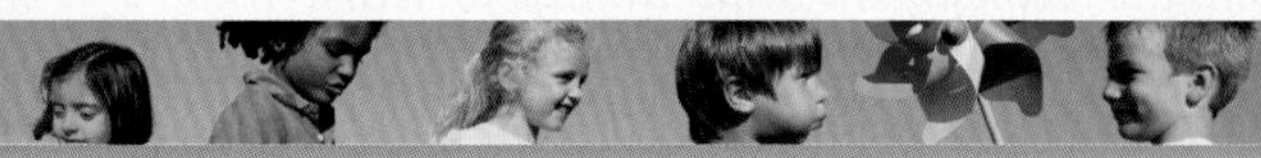

KEY CONCEPTS

- Muscles, tendons, ligaments, and cartilage are all present and functional at birth, though intentional, purposeful movement develops only as the infant matures.
- The spine is very mobile in the newborn and infant, especially the cervical spine region, resulting in a high risk for cervical spine injury.
- Rapid muscle growth in the adolescent years places the teenager at increased risk for injury compared with other age groups.
- The bones of the infant and young child are more flexible and have a thicker periosteum and more abundant blood supply than the adult's; as a result, bending occurs more frequently than breaking of the bone, and the fractured bone heals more quickly.
- The epiphysis of long bones is the growth center of the bones in children. Injury to this area may result in long-term extremity deformity.
- The nurse's role in laboratory and diagnostic testing for neuromuscular or musculoskeletal disorders is mainly that of educating the child and family about and preparing the child for the test or procedure.
- Plain x-rays are usually sufficient for diagnosing injuries in children. If CT or MRI scans are

required, the nurse may need to help the child stay calm and still during the procedure.

- Apply a pressure dressing following joint aspiration to prevent hematoma formation or fluid recollection.
- Perform frequent assessments of pain status and the effect of pain medication in the child with a musculoskeletal disorder.
- Diazepam (Valium) may be helpful in relieving muscle spasm associated with traction.
- Maintain traction and the appropriate amount of weight as ordered.
- The bulk of cast care occurs in the home. Teach the family of a child with a cast to perform neurovascular assessments, prevent the cast from getting wet, and care for the skin appropriately.
- Assessment of range of motion and muscle tone is critical in the child with a neuromuscular disorder. Hypertonia or hypotonia is an abnormal finding in the infant or child.
- Assessment of neurovascular status is an essential component of care for a child with a musculoskeletal disorder.
- Determining attainment of developmental milestones and subsequent progression or loss of those milestones is useful in distinguishing various neuromuscular disorders.
- The nurse reinforces and carries out the exercise plans and adaptive equipment use as prescribed by the physical or occupational therapist in order to maintain neuromuscular and musculoskeletal function and to prevent complications.
- Nursing management of a child with myelomeningocele focuses on preventing infection, promoting bowel and urinary elimination, promoting adequate nutrition, preventing latex allergy reaction, maintaining skin integrity, providing education and support to the family, and recognizing complications, such as hydrocephalus or increased ICP, associated with the disorder.
- Cerebral palsy may result in significant motor impairment. Children with cerebral palsy require ongoing physical therapy as well as nutritional intervention.
- Boys with Duchenne muscular dystrophy initially learn to walk but later lose this ability.
- Respiratory compromise occurs in muscular dystrophy and spinal muscular atrophy and eventually leads to death.
- Children with chronic disorders such as osteogenesis imperfecta may demonstrate slower or lesser growth than other children and may also be unable to participate in certain activities because of bone fragility.
- Congenital or developmental disorders such as DDH or clubfoot require bracing or casting for correction and to prevent deformity later in life.
- Torticollis may be treated by teaching the family to perform daily neck muscle stretching exercises.
- To prevent complications after a spinal fusion for scoliosis correction, use the log-roll method for turning the child so that back flexion is avoided.
- Children with spinal cord injury require intense nursing management and lengthy rehabilitation to maintain or regain function.
- Children with neuromuscular disorders often suffer depression related to the chronic nature of the disorder.
- School attendance and participation in activities such as the Special Olympics are important for children with neuromuscular dysfunction.
- Fractures may occur as a result of unintentional or intentional injury, or because the bones are fragile, as in rickets or osteogenesis imperfecta.
- Sprains, fractures, and overuse syndromes occur frequently in young athletes. Appropriate warm-up and stretching may help prevent some of these injuries.
- Rest, ice, compression, and elevation is the appropriate treatment for sprains.

REFERENCES AND RECOMMENDED READINGS

American Academy of Pediatrics, Committee on Genetics. (2012). Folic acid for the prevention of neural tube defects. *Pediatrics*. Retrieved from http://pediatrics.aappublications.org/content/104/2/325.full

Boas, S. R. (2011). Chapter 411: Skeletal diseases influencing pulmonary function. In: R. M. Kleigman, B. F. Stanton, J. W. St. Geme III, N. F. Schor, & R. E. Behrman (Eds.), *Nelson textbook of pediatrics* (19th ed., pp. 1516–1519). Philadelphia, PA: Saunders.

Bonner S. (2009). Pinning quality care on OR nurses. *OR Nurse 2015, 3*(1), 32–37.

Bowden, V. R., & Greenberg, C. S. (2012). *Pediatric nursing procedures* (3rd ed). Philadelphia, PA: Lippincott Williams & Wilkins.

Bozic, D., & Daniels, C. (2009a). *AboutKidsHealth clean intermittent catheterization (CIC): Step by step instructions for boys.* Retrieved from http://www.aboutkidshealth.ca/en/healthaz/testsandtreatments/medicaldevices/pages/clean-intermittent-catheterization-cic-step-by-step-instructions-for-boys.aspx

Bozic, D., & Daniels, C. (2009b). *AboutKidsHealth clean intermittent catheterization (CIC): Step by step instructions for girls.* Retrieved from http://www.aboutkidshealth.ca/En/HealthAZ/TestsAndTreatments/MedicalDevices/Pages/Clean-Intermittent-Catheterization-CIC-Step-By-Step-Instructions-for-Girls.aspx

Brenner, J. S., & The Council on Sports Medicine and Fitness. (2014). Overuse injuries, overtraining, and burnout in child and adolescent athletes. *Pediatrics, 119*(6), 1242–1245.

Carpenito, L. J. (2013). *Nursing diagnosis: Application to clinical practice* (14th ed.). Philadelphia, PA: Lippincott Williams & Wilkins.

Carrigan, R. B. (2011). Chapter 673: The upper limb. In: R. M. Kleigman, B. F. Stanton, J. W. St. Geme III, N. F. Schor, & R. E. Behrman (Eds.), *Nelson textbook of pediatrics* (19th ed., pp. 2383–2387). Philadelphia, PA: Saunders.

Carroll, K. L., & Kerr, L. M. (2013). Chapter 45: Alterations in musculoskeletal function in children. In: K. L. McCance, & S. E. Huether (Eds.), *Pathophysiology: The biologic basis for disease in adults and children* (7th ed., pp. 1591–1615). St Louis, MO: Elsevier/Mosby.

Centers for Disease Control and Prevention. (2004). Use of vitamins containing folic acid among women of childbearing age—United States [electronic version]. *MMWR. Morbidity And Mortality Weekly Report, 53*(36), 847–850.

Centers for Disease Control and Prevention. (2015). *Folic acid: Recommendations.* Retrieved from http://www.cdc.gov/ncbddd/folicacid/recommendations.html

Centers for Disease Control and Prevention. (2015). Cerebral Pasly (CP). Causes and Risk Factors of Cerebral Palsy. Retrieved from http://www.cdc.gov/ncbddd/cp/causes.html

Centers for Disease Control and Prevention. (2014). Facts about Upper and Lower Limb Reduction Defects. Retrieved from http://www.cdc.gov/ncbddd/birthdefects/UL-LimbReductionDefects.html

Cervasio, K. (2011). Lower extremity orthoses in children with spastic quadriplegic cerebral palsy: Implications for nurses, parents, and caregivers. *Orthopaedic Nursing, 30*(3), 155–159.

Child Trends Databank. (2014). *Unintentional injuries.* Retrieved from http://www.childtrends.org/?indicators=unintentional-injuries

Cincinnati's Children's. (2013). Cast Care. Retrieved from http://www.cincinnatichildrens.org/health/c/cast-care/

Committee on Obstetric Practice. (2013). Committee Opinion Number 550: Maternal–Fetal Surgery for Myelomeningocele. Retrieved from http://www.acog.org/Resources-And-Publications/Committee-Opinions/Committee-on-Obstetric-Practice/Maternal-Fetal-Surgery-for-Myelomeningocele

Emory University School of Medicine, Department of Pediatrics. (2015). *Baclofen Information.* Retrieved from http://www.pediatrics.emory.edu/divisions/neurology/baclofen/

Fairhurst, C. B. R., & Cockerill, H. (2011). Management of drooling in children. *Archives of Diseases in Childhood Education & Practice, 96*(1), 25–30.

Fischbach, F. T., & Dunning, M. B. III. (2015). *A manual of laboratory and diagnostic tests* (9th ed.). Philadelphia, PA: Wolters Kluwer Health/Lippincott Williams & Wilkins.

Food and Drug Administration. (2014). *Latex labeling required for medical devices.* Retrieved from http://www.fda.gov/ForPatients/Illness/HIVAIDS/Prevention/ucm126385.htm

Grossman, S. (2014). Chapter 58: Disorders of musculoskeletal function: Developmental and metabolic disorders. In: S. Grossman, & C. M. Porth (Eds.), *Porth's Pathophysiology: Concepts of altered health states* (9th ed., pp. 489–574). Philadelphia, PA: Wolters Kluwer Health/Lippincott Williams & Wilkins.

Haut, C. M. (2014). Chapter 54: Pediatric orthopedic disorders. In: S. M. Nettina (Ed.), *Lippincott manual of nursing practice* (10th ed., pp. 1743–1769). Philadelphia, PA: Wolters/Kluwer Health: Lippincott Williams & Wilkins.

Healthy Children. (2015). *Clean intermittent catheterization.* Retrieved from http://www.healthychildren.org/English/health-issues/conditions/chronic/Pages/Clean-Intermittent-Catheterization.aspx

Herzing University—Orlando. (2014). *ASN/BSN concept definitions.* Winter Park, FL: Author.

Holmes, S. B., Brown, S. J., & Pin Site Care Expert Panel. (2005). Skeletal pin site care: National Association of Orthopaedic Nurses guidelines for orthopaedic nursing. *Orthopaedic Nursing, 24*(2), 99–107.

Hosalkar, H. S., Spiegel, D. A., & Davidson, R. S. (2011). Chapter 666: The foot and toes. In: R. M. Kleigman, B. F. Stanton, J. W. St. Geme III, N. F. Schor, & R. E. Behrman (Eds.), *Nelson textbook of pediatrics* (19th ed., pp. 2335–2344). Philadelphia, PA: Saunders.

Johnston, M. V. (2011). Chapter 591: Encephalopathies. In: R. M. Kleigman, B. F. Stanton, J. W. St. Geme III, N. F. Schor, & R. E. Behrman (Eds.), *Nelson textbook of pediatrics* (19th ed., pp. 2061–2069). Philadelphia, PA: Saunders.

Kanaheswari, Y., Kavitha, R., & Rizal, A. M. (2014). Urinary tract infection and bacteriuria in children performing clean intermittent catheterization with reused catheters. *Spinal Cord, 53*, 209–212.

Kienstra, A. J., & Macias, C. G. (2014). Osgood-Schlatter disease (tibial tuberosity avulsion). UpToDate. Retrieved from http://www.uptodate.com/contents/osgood-schlatter-disease-tibial-tuberosity-avulsion

Kinsman, S. L., & Johnston, M. V. (2011). Chapter 585: Congenital anomalies of the central nervous system. In: R. M. Kleigman, B. F. Stanton, J.W. St. Geme III, N. F. Schor, & R. E. Behrman (Eds.), *Nelson textbook of pediatrics* (19th ed., pp. 1998–2013). Philadelphia, PA: Saunders.

Lethaby, A., Temple, J., & Santy-Tomlinson, J. (2013). Pin site care for preventing infections associated with external bone fixators and pins. *Cochrane Database of Systematic Reviews, 12*(CD004551). Retrieved from http://onlinelibrary.wiley.com/doi/10.1002/14651858.CD004551.pub3/epdf

Marini, J. C. (2011). Chapter 692: Osteogenesis imperfecta. In: R. M. Kleigman, B. F. Stanton, J. W. St. Geme III, N. F. Schor, & R. E. Behrman (Eds.), (*Nelson textbook of pediatrics* (19th ed., pp. 2437–2440). Philadelphia, PA: Saunders.

Mayo Clinic Staff. (2014). *Spinal cord injury*. Retrieved from http://www.mayoclinic.com/health/spinal-cord-injury/DS00460

Miller, G. (2015). Management and prognosis of cerebral palsy. UpToDate. Retrieved from http://www.uptodate.com/contents/management-and-prognosis-of-cerebral-palsy

Misra, M. (2015). Vitamin D insufficiency and deficiency in children and adolescents. UpToDate. Retrieved from http://www.uptodate.com/contents/vitamin-d-insufficiency-and-deficiency-in-children-and-adolescents

Muscular Dystrophy Association. (2009). *Facts about spinal muscular atrophy (SMA)*. Retrieved from http://www.mda.org/publications/PDFs/FA-SMA.pdf

Muscular Dystrophy Association. (2011). *Facts about Duchenne and Becker muscular dystrophies*. Retrieved from http://www.mda.org/publications/PDFs/FA-DMD.pdf

Muscular Dystrophy Association. (2014). *Duchenne muscular dystrophies (DMD) overview*. Retrieved from http://mda.org/disease/duchenne-muscular-dystrophy/overview

Muscular Dystrophy Association. (n.d.). Diseases: Select a Muscle Disease. Retrieved from http://www.mdausa.org/disease/

National Institute of Neurological Disorders and Stroke. (2015c). Spina Bifida Fact Sheet. Retrieved from http://www.ninds.nih.gov/disorders/spina_bifida/detail_spina_bifida.htm

National Institute of Neurological Disorders and Stroke. (2015b). NINDS Spinal Muscular Atrophy Information Page. Retrieved from http://www.ninds.nih.gov/disorders/sma/sma.htm

National Institute of Neurological Disorders and Stroke (NINDS). (2015a). *NINDS cerebral palsy information page*. Retrieved from http://www.ninds.nih.gov/disorders/cerebral_palsy/cerebral_palsy.htm#What_research_is_being_done

Nigrovic, P. A. (2015). Overview of hip pain in childhood. UpToDate. Retrieved from http://www.uptodate.com/contents/overview-of-hip-pain-in-childhood

Ong, L. C., Wong, S. W., & Hamid, H. A. (2009). Treatment of drooling in children with cerebral palsy using ultrasound guided intraglandular injections of botulinum toxin A. *Journal of Pediatric Neurology, 7*(2), 141–146.

Osteogenesis Imperfecta Foundation. (2015). Types of OI. Retrieved from http://www.oif.org/site/PageServer?pagename=AOI_Types

Passamano, L., Taglia A., Palladino A., Viggiano E., D'Ambrosio P., Scutifero M, et al. (2012). Improvement of survival in Duchenne Muscular Dystrophy: Retrospective analysis of 835 patients. *Acta Myologica, 31*(2), 121–125.

Robinson, R. (2011). Prenatal surgery to correct spina bifida found to improve fetal outcomes. *Neurology Today, 11*(6), 1, 6, 7.

Sankar, W. N., Horn, B. D., Wells, L., & Dormans, J. P. (2011). Chapter 670: The hip. In: R. M. Kleigman, B. F. Stanton, J. W. St. Geme III, N. F. Schor, & R. E. Behrman (Eds.), *Nelson textbook of pediatrics* (19th ed., pp. 2355–2365). Philadelphia, PA: Saunders.

Sarant, H. B. (2011a). Chapter 599: Neuromuscular disorders. In: R. M. Kleigman, B. F. Stanton, J. W. St. Geme III, N. F. Schor, & R. E. Behrman (Eds.), *Nelson textbook of pediatrics* (19th ed., pp. 2109–2122). Philadelphia, PA: Saunders.

Sarant, H. B. (2011b). Chapter 601: Muscular dystrophies. In: R. M. Kleigman, B. F. Stanton, J. W. St. Geme III, N. F. Schor, & R. E. Behrman (Eds.), *Nelson textbook of pediatrics* (19th ed., pp. 2119–2129). Philadelphia, PA: Saunders.

Sarant, H. B. (2011c). Chapter 604: Disorders of neuromuscular transmission and of motor neuron. In: R. M. Kleigman, B. F. Stanton, J. W. St. Geme III, N. F. Schor, & R. E. Behrman, (Eds.), (*Nelson textbook of pediatrics* (19th ed., pp. 2132–2138). Philadelphia, PA: Saunders.

Schweich, P. (2014). Patient information: Cast and splint care (Beyond the Basics). UpToDate. Retrieved from http://www.uptodate.com/contents/cast-and-splint-care-beyond-the-basics

Spiegel, D. A., & Dormans, J. P. (2011a). Chapter 672.1 Torticollis. In: R. M. Kleigman, B. F. Stanton, J. W. St. Geme III, N. F. Schor, & R. E. Behrman (Eds.), *Nelson textbook of pediatrics* (19th ed., pp. 2377–2379). Philadelphia, PA: Saunders.

Spiegel, D. A., & Dormans, J. P. (2011b). Chapter 671: The spine. In: R. M. Kleigman, B. F. Stanton, J. W. St. Geme III, N. F. Schor, & R.E. Behrman (Eds.), *Nelson textbook of pediatrics* (19th ed., pp. 2365–2377). Philadelphia, PA: Saunders.

Spina Bifida Association. (2015). *Latex in the Hospital Environment*. Retrieved from http://spinabifidaassociation.org/infosheets/latex-hospital/

Taketokmo, C. K., Hodding, J. H., & Kraus, D. M. (2013). *Lexi-comp's Drug Reference Handbook: Pediatric & Neonatal Dosage Handbook* (20th ed.). Hudson, OH: Lexi-comp, Inc.

Timms, A., Vincent, M., Santy-Tomlinson, S., & Hertz, K. (2011). Guidance on pin site care. Report and recommendations from the 2010 Consensus Project on Pin Site Care. Royal College of Nursing. Retrieved from http://www.rcn.org.uk/__data/assets/pdf_file/0009/413982/004137.pdf

U.S. Department of Health & Human Services. (2015). HealthyPeople.gov. Retrieved from, at http://www.healthypeople.gov/2020/About-Healthy-People

Wagner, C. L., Greer, F. R., & The Section on Breastfeeding and Committee on Nutrition. (2008). Prevention of rickets and vitamin D deficiency in infants, children, and adolescents. *Pediatrics, 122*(5), 1142–1115. doi: 10.1542/peds. 2008–1862

Wang, C. H., Finkel, R. S., Bertini, E. S., Schroth, M., Simonds, A., Wong, B., et al. (2007). Consensus statement for standard of care in spinal muscular atrophy. *Journal of Child Neurology, 22*(8), 1027–1049.

Wells, L., & Sehgal, K. (2011). Chapter 667.4: Coronal plane deformities. In: R. M. Kleigman, B. F. Stanton, J.W. St. Geme III, N. F. Schor, & R. E. Behrman (Eds.), *Nelson textbook of pediatrics* (19th ed., pp. 2348–2351). Philadelphia, PA: Saunders.

Wells, L., Sehgal, K., & Dormans, J. P. (2011). Chapter 675: Common fractures. In: R. M. Kliegman, R. E. Behrman, H. B. Jenson, & B. F. Stanton. *Nelson's textbook of pediatrics* (19th ed., pp. 2387–2394). Philadelphia, PA: Saunders.

Zak, M., & Chan, V. W. (2014). Chapter 46: Pediatric neurologic disorders. In: S. M. Nettina (Ed.), *Lippincott manual of nursing practice* (10th ed., pp. 1545–1575). Philadelphia, PA: Wolters/Kluwer Health: Lippincott Williams & Wilkins.

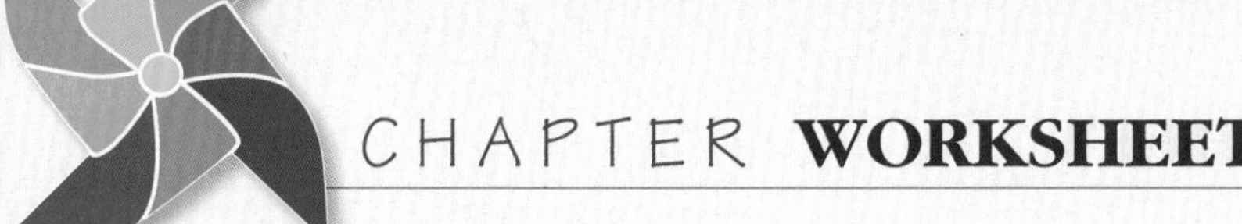

CHAPTER WORKSHEET

MULTIPLE CHOICE QUESTIONS

1. A boy with Duchenne muscular dystrophy is admitted to the pediatric unit. He has an ineffective cough. Lung auscultation reveals diminished breath sounds. What is the priority nursing intervention?
   a. Apply supplemental oxygen.
   b. Notify the respiratory therapist.
   c. Monitor pulse oximetry.
   d. Position for adequate airway clearance.
2. A 7-year-old child with cerebral palsy has been admitted to the hospital. Which information is most important for the nurse to obtain in the history?
   a. Age that the child learned to walk
   b. Parents' expectations of the child's development
   c. Functional status related to eating and mobility
   d. Birth history to identify cause of cerebral palsy
3. The nurse is caring for a 2-year-old with myelomeningocele. When teaching about care related to neurogenic bladder, what response by the parent would indicate that additional teaching is required?
   a. "Routine catheterization will decrease the risk of infection from urine staying in the bladder."
   b. "I know it will be important for me to catheterize my child for the rest of her life."
   c. "I will make sure that I always use latex-free catheters."
   d. "I will wash the catheter with warm soapy water after each use."
4. The nurse is caring for a child with cerebral palsy who requires a wheelchair to attain mobility. Which intervention would help the child achieve a sense of normality?
   a. Encourage follow-through with physical therapy exercises.
   b. Restrict the child to a special needs classroom.
   c. Encourage after-school activities within the limits of the child's abilities.
   d. Ensure the school is aware of the child's capabilities.
5. The nurse is caring for orthopedic children who are in the postoperative period following spinal fusion. What is the most appropriate activity to delegate to unlicensed assistive personnel?
   a. Ambulate the children twice daily to promote mobility.
   b. Encourage commode use to promote bowel function.
   c. Provide diversionary activities, as the children must stay flat on their backs.
   d. Assist with log-rolling the children every 2 hours.

DOSAGE CALCULATION EXERCISE

The nurse is caring for a child who is experiencing painful spasms. The child is 6 years old and weighs 42 lb. The medication order reads: Baclofen 25 mg per GT every 8 hours. Baclofen is supplied as 5 mg/mL.

How many milliliters will the nurse administer. Round to the nearest tenth.

CRITICAL THINKING EXERCISES

1. A 5-year-old girl, diagnosed with myelomeningocele, is admitted to the hospital for a corrective surgical procedure. Choose four questions from below that the nurse should ask when obtaining the health history that would assist in planning the child's care.
   a. What is the child's current mobility status?
   b. Is there a family history of myelomeningocele?
   c. What is the child's genitourinary and bowel function and regimen?
   d. Does this child have a history of hydrocephalus with presence of shunt?
   e. Does she have known latex sensitivity?
   f. Were there any complications during the pregnancy or birth of this child?
   g. Did the mother take prenatal folic acid supplementation?
2. Based on the case in the above question, develop a nursing care plan for the child with myelomeningocele.
3. A 5-year-old child is admitted to the pediatric unit with a history of cerebral palsy sustained at birth. The child is admitted for a scheduled tendon lengthening procedure. Based on your knowledge about the effects of cerebral palsy, list three priorities to focus on when planning her care. Compare this to a child admitted for surgical correction of a broken femur with no significant past medical history.
4. Develop a discharge teaching plan for a 2-year old who will be in a hip spica cast for 10 more weeks at home.
5. Devise a developmental/education plan for a child who will be confined to traction for 6 weeks. Choose a child in the clinical area whom you have cared for or choose a particular age group and develop the plan.

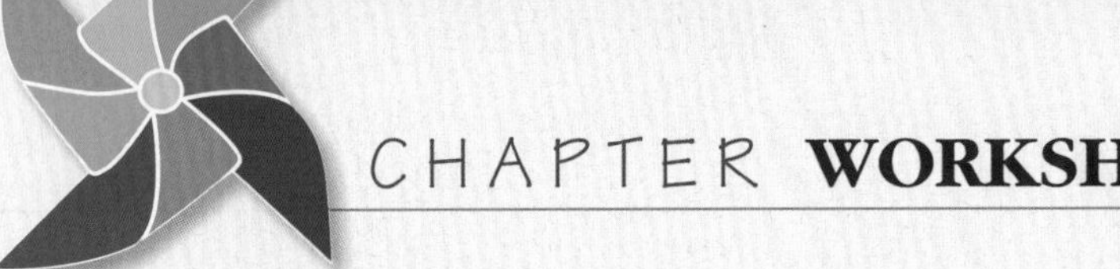

CHAPTER WORKSHEET

STUDY ACTIVITIES

1. In the clinical setting, compare the growth of a child with muscular dystrophy, spinal muscular atrophy, or cerebral palsy to the growth of a similar-age child who has been healthy. What differences or similarities do you find? What are the explanations for your findings?
2. Identify the role of the registered nurse in the multidisciplinary care of the child with a debilitating neuromuscular disorder.
3. In the clinical setting, interview the parent of a child with Duchenne muscular dystrophy, myelomeningocele, spinal muscular atrophy, or severe cerebral palsy. Determine the parent's feelings about the ongoing care that he or she is responsible for. Reflect upon this interview in your clinical journal.
4. In the clinical setting, compare the cognitive abilities of two children with a severe neuromuscular disorder. What are the reasons for the similarities or differences that you find?

BRINGING IT ALL TOGETHER: A CASE STUDY

Turner Wilson was just born with an obvious defect on his spine. Upon assessment, the nurse notes flaccid extremities and a distended bladder. The parents are devastated.

Go to thePoint to find questions to consider about this case.

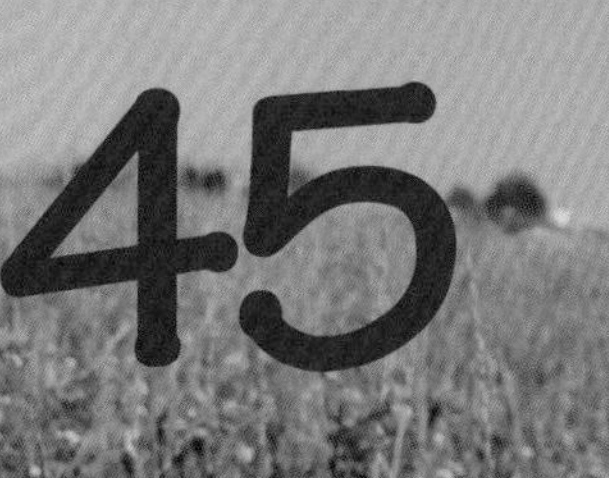

45

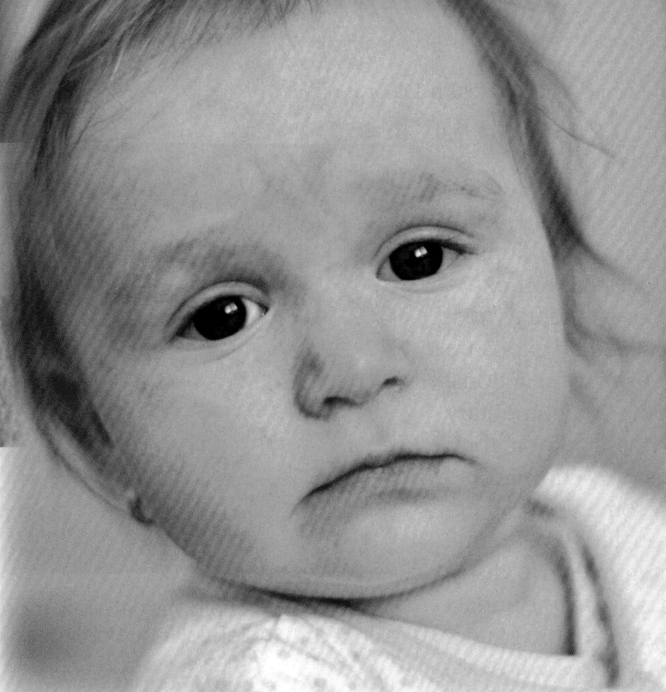

WOW

Words of Wisdom

To a nurse the child's skin is life's gift-wrapping, but to the child the skin is the space suit for life.

Nursing Care of the Child With an Alteration in Tissue Integrity/Integumentary Disorder

KEY TERMS
annular
dermatitis
erythema
macule
papule
pruritus
scaling
vesicle

Learning Objectives

Upon completion of the chapter, you will be able to:

1. Compare anatomic and physiologic differences of the integumentary system in infants and children versus adults.
2. Describe nursing care related to common laboratory and diagnostic tests used in the medical diagnosis of integumentary disorders/alterations in tissue integrity in infants, children, and adolescents.
3. Distinguish alterations in tissue integrity/integumentary disorders common in infants, children, and adolescents.
4. Identify appropriate nursing assessments and interventions related to pediatric integumentary disorders/alterations in tissue integrity.
5. Develop an individualized nursing care plan for the child with an alteration in tissue integrity integumentary disorder.
6. Describe the psychosocial impact of a chronic integumentary disorder on children or adolescents.
7. Develop child/family teaching plans for the child with an integumentary disorder/tissue integrity alteration.

***Eva Lopez*, 1-year old, is brought to the clinic by her mother, who states, "Eva has dry patches of skin, her wrists bleed from her scratching, and she's having trouble sleeping at night."**

Tissue integrity refers to the ability of body tissues to maintain normal physiologic processes (Herzing University—Orlando, 2014). Nurses may encounter children with alterations in tissue integrity should be familiar with various integumentary disorders that children experience. Alterations in tissue integrity or integumentary disorders occur often in children and are caused by exposure to infectious microorganisms, hypersensitivity reactions, hormonal influences, and injuries. Some integumentary disorders are as mild and self-limited as a minor abrasion. Others, such as atopic dermatitis, are chronic and must be managed consistently. Finally, some tissue integrity alterations can be severe and even life-threatening, such as full-thickness burns. If the integumentary disorders are chronic or severe, they can have a major impact on the child's physiologic or psychological status (Magin, Adams, Heading, Pond, & Smith, 2008). Nurses who care for children need to be familiar with common skin disorders of infancy, childhood, and adolescence so they can effectively intervene with children and their families.

VARIATIONS IN PEDIATRIC ANATOMY AND PHYSIOLOGY

Skin is the largest organ of the body and serves to protect the underlying tissues from trauma and invasion by microorganisms. The skin's health reflects the internal well-being of the body (Vernon, Brady, Starr, & Petersen-Smith, 2013). The skin is also important for the perception of pain, heat, and cold and for the regulation of body temperature.

Differences in the Skin Between Children and Adults

The infant's epidermis is thinner than the adult's, and the blood vessels lie closer to the surface because there is a decreased amount of subcutaneous fat. Thus, the infant loses heat more readily through the skin's surface than the older child or adult does. The thinness of the infant's skin also allows substances to be absorbed through the skin more readily than they would be in an adult. Bacteria can gain access via the infant's and younger child's skin more readily than they can through the adult's skin. The infant's skin contains more water than the adult's, and the epidermis is loosely bound to the dermis. This means that friction may easily cause separation of the layers, resulting in blistering or skin breakdown. The infant's skin is also less pigmented than that of the adult (in all races), placing the infant at increased risk of skin damage from ultraviolet radiation. Over time, the infant's skin toughens and becomes less hydrated and thus is less susceptible to microorganism invasion. The skin thickness and characteristics reach adult levels in the late teenage years.

Differences in Dark-Skinned Children

Children with dark skin tend to have more pronounced cutaneous reactions compared to children with lighter skin. Hypopigmentation or hyperpigmentation in the affected area following healing of a dermatologic condition is common in dark-skinned children. This change in pigmentation may be temporary (a few months following a superficial skin disorder) or permanent (following a more involved skin condition). Dark-skinned children tend to have more prominent **papules** (rounded, nonpustular elevation on the skin), follicular responses, lichenification, and vesicular or bullous reactions than lighter-skinned children with the same disorder. Hypertrophic scarring and keloid formation (Fig. 45.1) occur more often in dark-skinned children (Vernon et al., 2013).

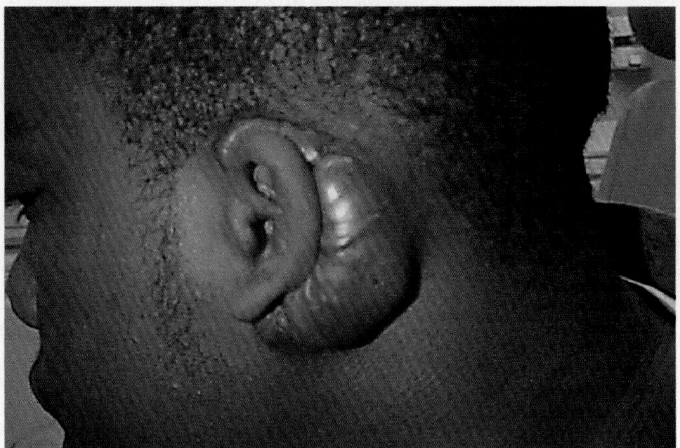

FIGURE 45.1 Keloid formation is more common in dark-skinned than light-skinned children.

Sebaceous and Sweat Glands

Sebaceous glands function immaturely at birth. The sebum secreted serves to lubricate the skin and hair. Sebum production increases in the preadolescent and adolescent years, which is why acne develops at that time. The infant's eccrine sweat glands are somewhat functional and will produce sweat as a response to emotional stimuli and heat. They become fully functional in the middle childhood years. Until that time, temperature regulation is less effective compared to older children and adults. The apocrine sweat glands are small and nonfunctional in the infant. They mature during puberty, at which time body odor develops in response to the fluid secreted by these glands.

COMMON MEDICAL TREATMENTS

A variety of medications as well as other medical treatments are used to treat integumentary disorders in children. Most of these treatments will require a physician's or nurse practitioner's order when the child is in the hospital. The most common treatments and medications are listed in Common Medical Treatments 45.1 and Drug Guide 45.1. The nurse caring for the child with an integumentary disorder should be familiar with the procedures

COMMON MEDICAL TREATMENTS 45.1

Treatment	Explanation	Indications	Nursing Implications
Wet dressing	Dressing moistened with lukewarm water (sterile water may be required in certain cases)	In the presence of itching, crusting, or oozing—helps to remove crusts	May use Burow, Domeboro, or saline solutions in certain cases Provide atraumatic care by giving premedication before dressing change
Sunscreen	Lotion, gel, or cream with a sun-protective factor (SPF)	All children older than 6 months of age	Use a fragrance-free, para-aminobenzoic acid (PABA)–free preparation with an SPF of 15 or higher Apply at least 30 minutes prior to sun exposure. Reapply at least every 2 hours while exposed (every 60 to 80 minutes while in the water) Sweat- and water-resistant preparations are available yet still require reapplication as noted above Use daily in summer and in warm climates, even on overcast and cloudy days
Bathing	Use of lukewarm water (with or without soap) to bathe	Itchy and irritating skin conditions	Recommend fragrance-free, dye-free soaps such as Dove, Aveeno, Basis, Lubriderm Colloid (oatmeal baths) are especially helpful Pat the child dry; do not rub the skin. Leave the child moist before applying medication, dressing, or moisturizer

DRUG GUIDE 45.1 COMMON DRUGS FOR INTEGUMENTARY DISORDERS

Medication	Actions/Indications	Nursing Implications
Antibiotics (topical)	Decrease skin colonization with bacteria Indicated for mild acne vulgaris, impetigo, folliculitis	Apply as prescribed to clean skin or a cleansed wound Be alert for neomycin allergy
Antibiotics (systemic)	Bactericidal or bacteriostatic against a variety of organisms, depending on the preparation Used for moderate to severe acne vulgaris, extensive impetigo, cellulitis, scalded skin syndrome	Check for medication allergies prior to administration Teach families to finish entire course of antibiotics
Corticosteroids (topical)	Anti-inflammatory effect in atopic dermatitis and certain kinds of contact dermatitis	Do not use moderate- or high-potency corticosteroid preparations on the face or genitals Do not cover with an occlusive dressing Absorption is increased in the young infant
Antifungals (topical)	Fungicidal used to treat tinea, candidal diaper rash	Apply a thin layer as prescribed Comply with length of treatment as prescribed to prevent reemergence of the rash
Antifungals (systemic): griseofulvin, ketoconazole	Kill fungus; bind to human keratin, making it resistant to fungus Indicated for tinea capitis and severe or widespread fungal skin infections	Griseofulvin: give with fatty food to increase absorption. Requires minimum 4-week course Monitor liver function tests and CBC. May cause photosensitivity Ketoconazole: administer with food to decrease GI upset

(continued)

DRUG GUIDE 45.1 COMMON DRUGS FOR INTEGUMENTARY DISORDERS (continued)

Medication	Actions/Indications	Nursing Implications
Benzoyl peroxide	Decreases colonization of *P. acnes* in mild acne vulgaris	Available in combination with topical antibiotics Apply sparingly. Shake before application Avoid contact with eyes and mucous membranes
Retinoids (topical): tretinoin, adapalene, tazarotene	Anticomedogenic activity in moderate to severe acne vulgaris	Adverse effects: dryness, burning, photosensitivity Instruct child to use SPF 15 or higher sunscreen
Topical immune modulators (tacrolimus, pimecrolimus)	Inhibit T-lymphocyte action at the skin level Used for moderate to severe atopic dermatitis, or in conditions resistant to topical steroids	Use only in children older than 2 years old Avoid sunlight exposure May cause burning, pruritus, flu-like symptoms, or headache
Antihistamines (diphenhydramine, chlorpheniramine, hydroxyzine)	Antihistaminic effect, results in sedation Indicated for hypersensitivity reactions, atopic dermatitis or contact dermatitis that is severely pruritic	May give three or four times a day unless sedation effect interferes with activities of daily living or school
Systemic corticosteroids (prednisone, dexamethasone, methylprednisolone)	Anti-inflammatory and immunosuppressive action Used in severe contact dermatitis	Administer with food to decrease GI upset May mask signs of infection Monitor blood pressure, urine for glucose Do not stop treatment abruptly or acute adrenal insufficiency may occur Monitor for Cushing syndrome Doses may be tapered over time
Isotretinoin	Reduces sebaceous gland size, decreases sebum production, and regulates cell proliferation and differentiation Indicated for cystic acne or severe acne that is resistant to 3 months of treatment with oral antibiotics	Ensure that the adolescent girl is not pregnant and does not become pregnant Monitor CBC, lipid profiles, liver function tests, and β-human chorionic gonadotropin monthly Monitor for suicide risk
Coal tar preparations	Antipruritic and anti-inflammatory effect Useful in psoriasis, atopic dermatitis	May stain fabrics; strong and unpleasant odor Apply at bedtime and rinse off in the morning to improve compliance
Silver sulfadiazine 1%	Bactericidal against gram-positive and gram-negative bacteria and yeasts Indicated for burns	Cover with occlusive dressing Apply twice daily Do not use in children with sulfa allergy Forms a gel on the burn that is painful to remove May cause transient neutropenia Do not use on the child's face or on an infant younger than 2 months of age

CBC, complete blood count; GI, gastrointestinal.

Adapted from Taketomo, C. K., Hodding, J. H., & Kraus, D. M. (2013). *Pediatric & neonatal dosage handbook* (20th ed.). Hudson, OH: Lexicomp.

and medications, how they work, and common nursing implications related to their use.

NURSING PROCESS OVERVIEW FOR THE CHILD WITH AN INTEGUMENTARY DISORDER

Nursing management of the child with an alteration in tissue integrity/integumentary disorder requires astute assessment skills, development of accurate nursing diagnoses and expected outcomes, implementation of appropriate interventions, and evaluation of the entire process. Many skin rashes may be associated with other, often serious illnesses, so the nurse must use comprehensive and excellent assessment skills when evaluating rashes in children. Certain integumentary conditions are chronic and require ongoing care related to health maintenance, education, and psychosocial needs.

Assessment

Nursing assessment of the child with an integumentary disorder/tissue integrity alteration includes obtaining the health history and performing a physical examination. Assisting with or obtaining laboratory tests may also be necessary.

Remember Eva, the 1-year old with the dry patches, itching, and trouble sleeping? What additional health history and physical examination assessment information should the nurse obtain?

Health History

Determine the child's or parent's chief complaint, which is most often related to pruritus, **scaling** (dry, flaky skin), or a cosmetic disruption. Document the history of the present illness, noting onset, location, duration, characteristics, other symptoms, and relieving factors, particularly as related to a rash or lesion. Also ask about the quantity and quality of any discharge from the rash or lesions. Document accompanying symptoms. Note the child's general state of health, history of chronic medical conditions, recent surgeries, hospitalizations, medications, or immunizations. Has there been a recent change in the child's food intake or environment? Is there a family history of chronic or acute skin conditions? Does anyone in the home have a similar concern at this time? Does the family have pets that go outdoors? Does the child play in the woods or garden? Note usual skin care routines, as well as types of soaps, cosmetics, or other skin care products used. Determine the amount of daily sun exposure and whether the child consistently uses sunscreen.

Physical Examination

Perform a complete physical examination, noting any abnormalities. Perform a focused and thorough examination of the skin. The best lighting for examination of the skin is natural daylight. Look at the skin in general, noting distribution of any obvious rashes or lesions. Inspect the mucous membranes, noting and describing lesions if present. Examine all surfaces of the skin and scalp carefully. Note temperature, moisture, texture, and fragility of the skin. If a rash or lesions are present, note their location and provide a detailed description of them. Describe whether a rash is macular, papular, pustular, or vesicular.

Provide a description of vascular lesions if present. If lesions are present on the scalp, has hair loss in that region occurred? Describe lesions according to the following criteria:

- Linear: in a line
- Shape: are the lesions round, oval, or **annular** (ring around central clearing)?
- Morbilliform: a rosy, maculopapular rash
- Target lesions: like a bull's eye

If drainage is present, describe it as clear, purulent, honey colored, or otherwise. Note scaling or lichenification of the skin. Palpate for regional lymphadenopathy.

Laboratory and Diagnostic Testing

Common Laboratory and Diagnostic Tests 45.1 details the laboratory and diagnostic tests most commonly used when considering integumentary disorders. The tests can assist the physician or nurse practitioner in diagnosing the disorder or can be used as guidelines in determining ongoing treatment. Some of the tests are obtained by laboratory or nonnursing personnel, while others might be obtained by the nurse. In either instance the nurse should be familiar with how the tests are obtained, what they are used for, and normal versus abnormal results. This knowledge will also be necessary when providing child and family education related to the testing.

Nursing Diagnoses and Related Interventions

Upon completion of a thorough assessment, the nurse might identify several nursing diagnoses, such as:

- Impaired skin integrity
- Pain
- Risk for infection
- Disturbed body image
- Risk for fluid volume deficit
- Altered nutrition

COMMON LABORATORY AND DIAGNOSTIC TESTS 45.1

Test	Explanation	Indications	Nursing Implications
Complete blood count (CBC) with differential	Evaluate hemoglobin and hematocrit, WBC count (particularly the percentage of individual WBCs), and platelet count	Infection or inflammatory process	Normal values vary according to age and gender WBC differential is helpful in evaluating source of infection May be affected by myelosuppressive drugs Eosinophils may be elevated in the child with atopic dermatitis
Erythrocyte sedimentation rate (ESR)	Nonspecific test used to detect presence of infection or inflammation	Infection or inflammatory process	Send sample to laboratory immediately; if allowed to stand for longer than 3 hours, may result in falsely low result.
Potassium hydroxide (KOH) prep	Reveals branching hyphae (fungus) when viewed under microscope	To identify fungal infection	Place skin scrapings on a microscope slide and add KOH 20% drop
Culture of wound or skin drainage	Allows for microbial growth and organism identification	Identification of specific organism	Note sensitivities
Immunoglobulin E (IgE)	Measurement of serum IgE	Atopic dermatitis	Often elevated in allergic or atopic disease, though this is a nonspecific finding. May be increased if the child takes systemic corticosteroids
Patch or skin testing	Needle prick testing with allergens	Atopic or contact dermatitis	Have emergency equipment available in the event of anaphylaxis (rare)

Adapted from Corbett, J. A. & Banks, A. D. (2013). *Laboratory tests and diagnostic procedures with nursing diagnoses* (8th ed.). Upper Saddle River, NJ: Pearson Education Inc.

After completing an assessment of Eva, the nurse noted the following: hypopigmentation of the skin behind her knees, dry patches on her wrists and face, and slight wheezing heard bilaterally on auscultation. Based on these assessment findings, what would your top three nursing diagnoses be for Eva?

Desired outcomes and interventions are based on the nursing diagnoses. Nursing Care Plan 45.1, found at the end of the chapter, can be used as a guide in planning nursing care for the child with an integumentary disorder. Individualize the plan of care based on the child's and family's responses to the health alteration. See Chapter 36 for information about pain management. Additional information will be included later in the chapter as it relates to specific disorders.

Based on your top three nursing diagnoses for Eva, describe appropriate nursing interventions.

INFECTIOUS DISORDERS

Infectious disorders of the skin include those caused by viral, bacterial, or fungal infection. The viral exanthems are discussed in Chapter 37. Bacterial and fungal infections of the skin are discussed below.

Bacterial Infections

Bacterial infections of the skin include bullous and nonbullous impetigo, folliculitis, cellulitis, and staphylococcal scalded skin syndrome. These bacterial skin infections are often caused by *Staphylococcus aureus* and group A β-hemolytic streptococcus, which are ordinarily normal flora on the skin. Impetigo, folliculitis, and cellulitis are usually self-limited disorders that rarely become severe.

Impetigo is a readily recognizable skin rash (Fig. 45.2). Nonbullous impetigo generally follows some type of skin trauma or may arise as a secondary bacterial infection of another skin disorder, such as atopic dermatitis. Bullous impetigo demonstrates a sporadic occurrence pattern and develops on intact skin, resulting from toxin production by *S. aureus*.

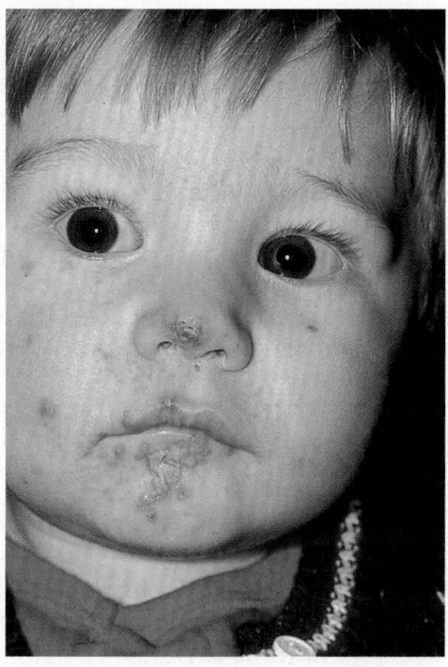

FIGURE 45.2 Note honey-colored crusting with impetigo.

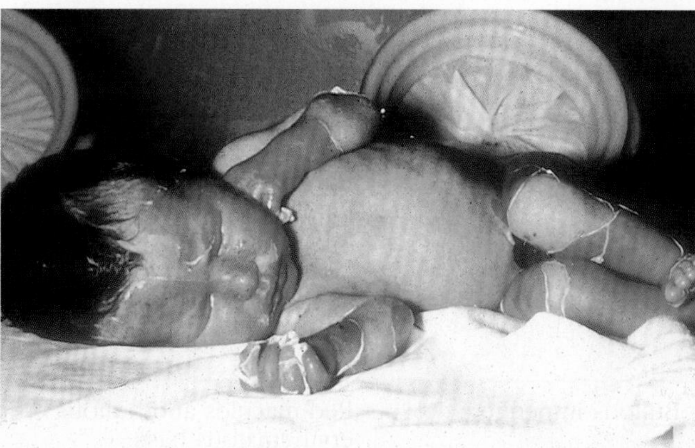

FIGURE 45.4 Staphylococcal scalded skin syndrome (SSSS) with ruptured bullae. (Used with permission from Goodheart, H. P. *Goodheart's photoguide to common skin disorders: Diagnosis and management* (3rd ed.). Philadelphia, PA: Lippincott Williams & Wilkins, 2009.)

Folliculitis, infection of the hair follicle, most often results from occlusion of the hair follicle. It may occur as a result of poor hygiene, prolonged contact with contaminated water, maceration, a moist environment, or use of occlusive emollient products.

Cellulitis is a localized infection and inflammation of the skin and subcutaneous tissues and is usually preceded by skin trauma of some sort (Fig. 45.3).

Staphylococcal scalded skin syndrome results from infection with *S. aureus* that produces a toxin, which then causes exfoliation. It has an abrupt onset and results in diffuse **erythema** (reddening of the skin) and skin tenderness (Fig. 45.4). Scalded skin syndrome is most common in infancy and rare beyond 5 years of age (Vernon et al., 2013).

Of particular concern are community-acquired bacterial skin infections caused by methicillin-resistant *S. aureus* (CA-MRSA) (Baddour, 2015). CA-MRSA most commonly occurs as a skin or soft tissue infection, such as cellulitis or an abscess. Risk factors for CA-MRSA are turf burns, towel sharing, participation in team sports, or attendance at day care or outdoor camps. If the child presents with a moderate to severe skin infection or with an infection that is not responding as expected to therapy, it is important to culture the infected area for MRSA.

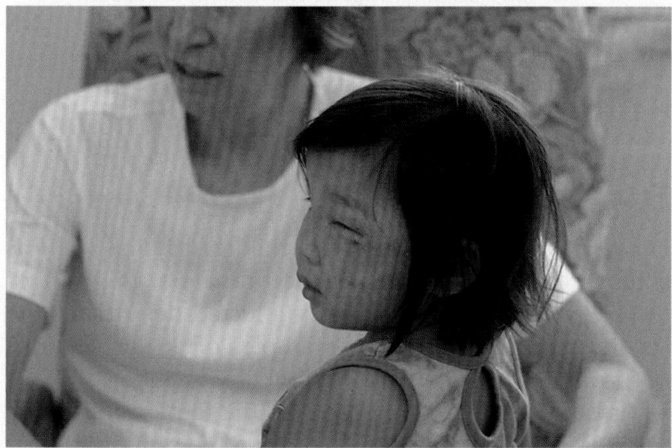

FIGURE 45.3 Note erythema and edema associated with cellulitis.

Therapeutic management of bacterial skin infections includes topical or systemic antibiotics and appropriate hygiene (see Table 45.1).

Nursing Assessment

Obtain the history as noted in the nursing process overview section. Note history of skin disruption such as a cut, scrape, or insect or spider bite (nonbullous impetigo and cellulitis). Note body piercing in the adolescent, which can lead to impetigo or cellulitis. Measure the child's temperature. Fever may occur with bullous impetigo or cellulitis and is common with scalded skin syndrome. Inspect the skin, noting abnormalities, documenting their location and distribution, and describing drainage if present. Table 45.1 gives specific clinical manifestations of the various bacterial skin infections. Palpate for regional lymphadenopathy, which may be present with impetigo or cellulitis. Blood cultures are indicated in the child with cellulitis with lymphangitic streaking and in all cases of periorbital or orbital cellulitis.

Nursing Management

Administer antibiotics topically or systemically as prescribed. Teach the family about antibiotic administration and care of the lesions or rash. Soak impetiginous lesions with cool compresses or Burow solution to remove

TABLE 45.1 BACTERIAL SKIN INFECTIONS

Disorder	Skin Findings	Usual Treatment
Nonbullous impetigo	• **Papules** progressing to vesicles, then painless pustules with a narrow erythematous border • Honey-colored exudate when the vesicles or pustules rupture, which forms a crust on the ulcer-like base (see Fig. 45.2)	• Limited amount: treat topically with mupirocin ointment. • If numerous lesions, oral first-generation cephalosporin is indicated. • Clindamycin may be needed for MRSA. • Remove honey-colored crust with cool compresses twice daily.
Bullous impetigo	• Red macules and bullous eruptions on an erythematous base • Size may be from a few millimeters to several centimeters	• Oral first-generation cephalosporin. • Good hygiene.
Folliculitis	• Red, raised hair follicles	• Treat with aggressive hygiene: warm compresses after washing with soap and water several times a day. • Topical mupirocin is indicated; occasionally oral antibiotics are required.
Cellulitis	• Localized reaction: **erythema**, pain, edema, warmth at site of skin disruption (see Fig. 45.3)	• Mild cases are usually treated with cephalexin or amoxicillin/clavulanic acid. • More severe cases and periorbital or orbital cellulitis require IV cephalosporins.
Staphylococcal scalded skin syndrome	• Flattish bullae that rupture within hours • Red, weeping surface is left, most commonly on face, groin, neck, and axillary region (see Fig. 45.4)	• Mild to moderate cases are treated with oral cephalexin, dicloxacillin, or amoxicillin/clavulanic acid. • Severe cases are managed similar to burns with aggressive fluid management and IV oxacillin or clindamycin.

Adapted from Morelli, J. G., & Prok, L. D. (2014). Skin. In W. W. Hay, M. J. Levin, & R. R. Deterding, & M. J. Abzug, (Eds.), *Current pediatric diagnosis and treatment* (22nd ed.). New York, NY: McGraw-Hill; and Baddour, L. M. (2015). *Impetigo*. Retrieved from http://www.uptodate.com/contents/impetigo

crusts before applying topical antibiotics. Though impetigo is considered a contagious disorder among vulnerable populations, removal from school or day care is not necessary unless the condition is widespread or actively weeping. Prevent transmission of nosocomial MRSA by appropriately isolating children according to the institution's policy when the child is hospitalized. In children with scalded skin syndrome, reduce the risk of scarring by minimal handling, avoiding corticosteroids, and applying soothing ointments as the skin heals.

Educate the family about prevention of bacterial skin infections. Stress the importance of cleanliness and hygiene. Teach the family to keep the child's fingernails cut short and to clean the nails with a nail brush at bath time. When a skin disruption such as a cut, scrape, or insect bite occurs, teach the family to clean the area well to prevent the development of cellulitis. Folliculitis may be prevented with diligent hygiene and avoidance of occlusive emollients. Table 45.1 gives additional information about specific treatments for bacterial skin infections. See Dosage Calculation Box 45.1.

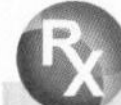

Dosage Calculation Box 45.1

Child's weight: 13 lb, 3 oz

Medication order: cephalexin 125 mg/5 mL, 4 mL PO every 6 hours.

Per the Pediatric Dosage Handbook, the recommended dose is 25–50 mg/kg/day divided every 6 to 8 hours daily.

Is the ordered dose safe?

Fungal Infections

Fungi also cause infections on children's skin. *Tinea* is a fungal disease of the skin occurring on any part of the body. The part of the body affected determines the second word in the name. Examples of tinea infections occurring on various parts of the body include:

- Tinea pedis: fungal infection on the feet
- Tinea corporis: fungal infection on the arms or legs
- Tinea versicolor: fungal infection on the trunk and extremities

- Tinea capitis: fungal infection on the scalp, eyebrows, or eyelashes
- Tinea cruris: fungal infection on the groin

The three organisms most often responsible for tinea are *Epidermophyton, Microsporum,* and *Trichophyton,* though *Malassezia furfur* causes tinea versicolor. *Candida albicans* may cause an infection of the skin, particularly in a warm, moist area such as the diaper area. All fungal skin infections may occur year-round, but tinea versicolor is more common in warm weather.

Therapeutic management of fungal infections involves appropriate hygiene and administration of an antifungal agent. Table 45.2 gives further information about treatment.

Nursing Assessment

Elicit the health history, noting exposure to another person with a fungal infection or exposure to a pet (fungi are often carried by pets). Note onset of the rash and whether it is itchy. Determine if the child has recently visited the barber (tinea capitis). Note contact with damp areas such as locker rooms and swimming pools, use of nylon socks or nonbreathable shoes, or minor trauma to the feet (tinea pedis). Document a history of wearing tight clothing or participating in a contact sport such as wrestling (tinea cruris). Inspect the skin and scalp, noting the location, description, and distribution of the rash or lesions (Figs. 45.5 to 45.9). Table 45.2 describes the clinical findings associated with various types of tinea.

Scraping and KOH preparation show branching hyphae. For tinea capitis, the Wood lamp will fluoresce yellow-green if it is caused by *Microsporum,* but not with *Trichophyton*. A fungal culture of a plucked hair is more reliable for diagnosis of tinea capitis.

Nursing Management

Maintain appropriate hygiene and administer antifungal agents as prescribed (see Table 45.2). Additional

TABLE 45.2 MANAGEMENT OF FUNGAL INFECTIONS

Disorder	Skin Findings	Usual Treatment
Tinea corporis (ringworm)	• Annular lesion with raised peripheral scaling and central clearing (looks like a ring) (Fig. 45.5)	• Topical antifungal cream is required for at least 4 weeks.
Tinea capitis	• Patches of scaling in the scalp with central hair loss • Risk of kerion development (inflamed, boggy mass that is filled with pustules) (Fig. 45.6)	• Oral griseofulvin for 4–6 weeks. • Selenium sulfide shampoo may be used to decrease contagiousness (adjunct only). • No school or day care for 1 week after treatment initiated.
Tinea versicolor	• Superficial tan or hypopigmented oval scaly lesions, especially on upper back and chest and proximal arms • More noticeable in the summer with tanning of unaffected areas (Fig. 45.7)	• Apply selenium sulfide shampoo all over body (from face to knees) and allow to stay on skin overnight, rinsing in the morning, once a week for 4 weeks (this may cause skin irritation). • Topical antifungals in the imidazole family may be used instead.
Tinea pedis (athlete's foot)	• Red, scaling rash on soles and between the toes (Fig. 45.8)	• Topical antifungal cream, powder, or spray. • Appropriate foot hygiene.
Tinea cruris	• Erythema, scaling, maceration in the inguinal creases and inner thighs (penis/scrotum spared)	• Topical antifungal preparation for 4–6 weeks.
Diaper candidiasis (also called monilial diaper rash)	• Fiery red lesions, scaling in the skin folds, and satellite lesions (located further out from the main rash) (Fig. 45.9)	• Topical nystatin with diaper changes for several days. • See section on diaper dermatitis for additional information.

Adapted from Morelli, J. G., & Prok, L. D. (2014). Skin. In W. W. Hay, M. J. Levin, & R. R. Deterding, & M. J. Abzug, (Eds.), *Current pediatric diagnosis and treatment* (22nd ed.). New York, NY: McGraw-Hill.

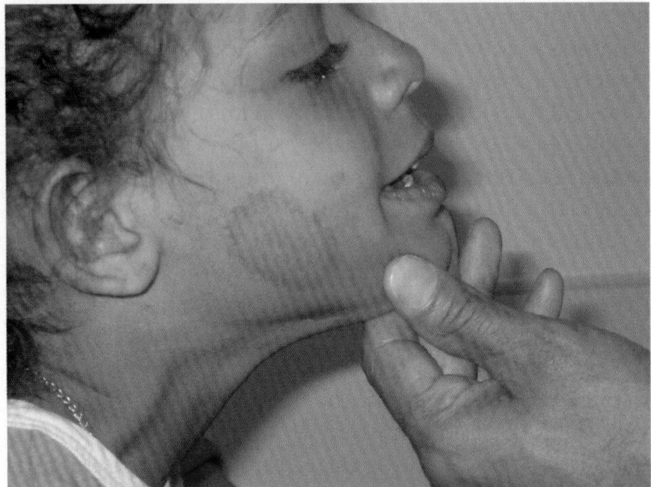

FIGURE 45.5 Tinea corporis: note raised scaly border with clearing in center.

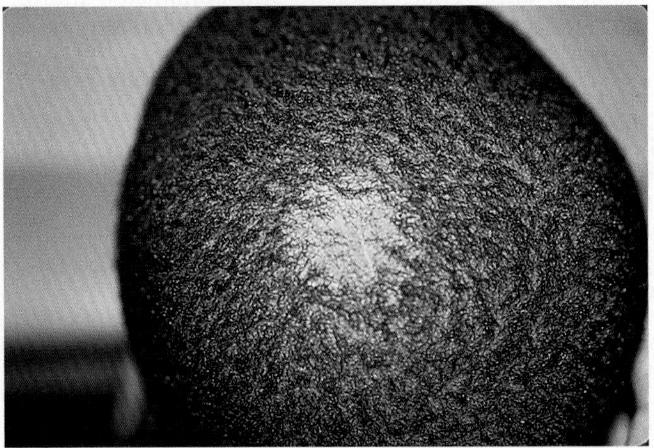

FIGURE 45.6 Note hair breakage and loss with tinea capitis.

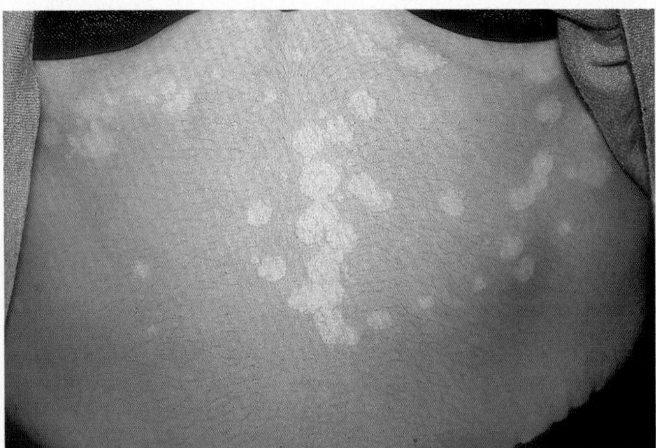

FIGURE 45.7 Tinea versicolor. Hypopigmented scaly lesions on the back of a darkly pigmented adolescent. (Used with permission from Goodheart, H. P. *Goodheart's photoguide to common skin disorders: Diagnosis and management* (3rd ed.). Philadelphia, PA: Lippincott Williams & Wilkins, 2009.)

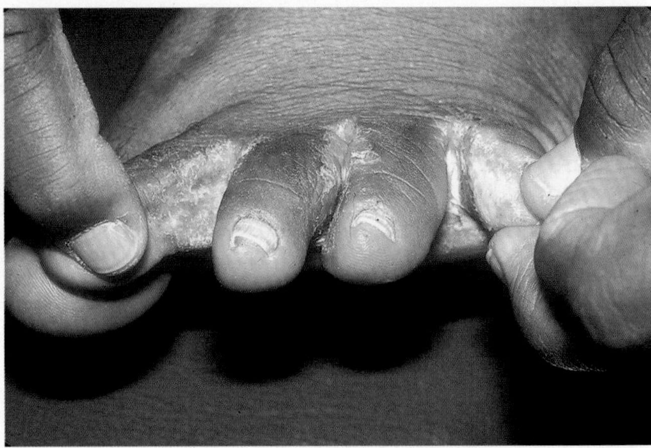

FIGURE 45.8 Tinea pedis. The interdigital pattern of tinea pedis is common. (Used with permission from Goodheart, H. P. *Goodheart's photoguide to common skin disorders: Diagnosis and management* (3rd ed.). Philadelphia, PA: Lippincott Williams & Wilkins, 2009.)

specifics related to the individual fungal disorders are as follows:

- Tinea corporis is contagious, but the child may return to day care or school once treatment has begun. Identify and treat family members or other contacts.
- Counsel the child with tinea capitis and parents that hair will usually regrow in 3 to 12 months. Wash sheets and clothes in hot water to decrease the risk of the infection spreading to other family members.
- Instruct the child with tinea pedis to keep the feet clean and dry. Rinse feet with water or a water/vinegar mixture and dry them well, especially between the toes. Encourage the child to wear cotton socks and shoes that allow the feet to breathe. Going barefoot at home is allowed, but flip-flops should be worn around swimming pools and in locker rooms.
- Inform the child with tinea versicolor that return to normal skin pigmentation may take several months.

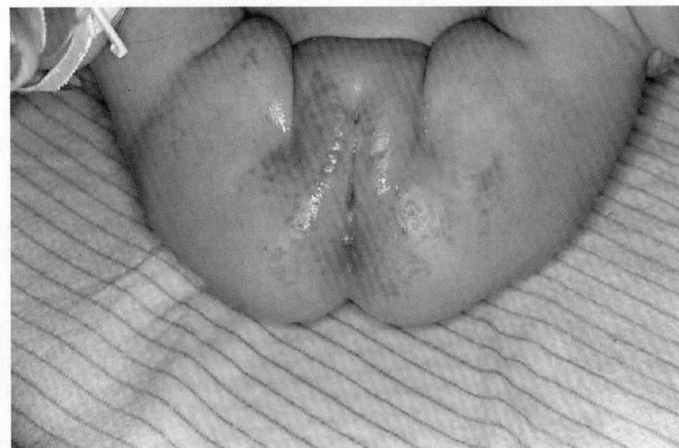

FIGURE 45.9 A bright red rash with satellite lesions occurs with diaper candidiasis.

- Counsel the child or adolescent with tinea cruris to wear cotton underwear and loose clothing. It is important to maintain good hygiene, particularly after sports practice or a sporting event.
- For management of diaper candidiasis, follow the suggestions listed below in the section on diaper dermatitis.

INFLAMMATORY SKIN CONDITIONS

Inflammatory skin conditions may be either acute or chronic. Acute hypersensitivity reactions may cause diaper dermatitis, contact dermatitis, erythema multiforme, and urticaria. Atopic dermatitis is a chronic hypersensitivity disorder. Seborrhea and psoriasis are chronic inflammatory skin disorders that do not occur as a result of hypersensitivity.

Diaper Dermatitis

Dermatitis refers to an inflammatory reaction of the skin. Diaper dermatitis refers to an inflammatory reaction of the skin in the area covered by a diaper. It is a nonimmunologic response to a skin irritant that results in skin cell hydration disturbance. Prolonged exposure to urine and feces may lead to skin breakdown (Fig. 45.10). Diaper wearing increases the skin's pH, activating fecal enzymes that further contribute to skin maceration.

Nursing Assessment

Determine from the history whether the infant or child wears diapers. Ask about the onset and progression of the rash, as well as any treatments and response. Inspect the skin in the diaper area for erythema and maceration (see Fig. 45.10). Ordinary diaper dermatitis does not usually result in a bumpy rash, but starts as a flat red rash in the convex skin creases. It may appear red and shiny and may or may not also have papules. Untreated, it may become more widespread or severe. Some cases of diaper dermatitis are caused by overgrowth of *C. albicans* (see Fig. 45.9 and the section on fungal infections).

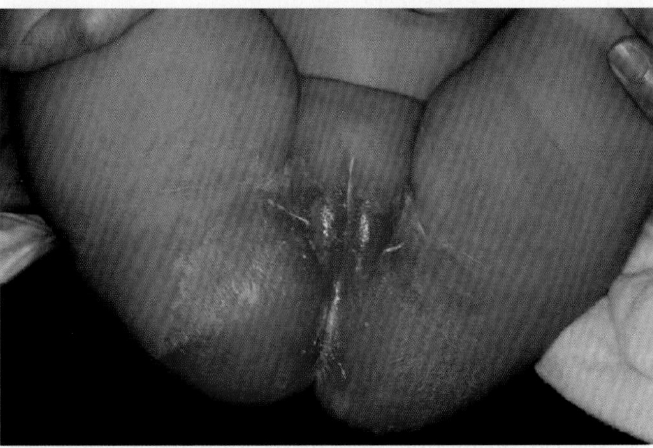

FIGURE 45.10 Diaper dermatitis.

Nursing Management

Prevention is the best management of diaper dermatitis. Topical products such as ointments or creams containing vitamins A, D, and E; zinc oxide; or petrolatum are helpful to provide a barrier to the skin. Teaching Guidelines 45.1 gives further information on prevention and management of diaper dermatitis. See above for treatment of diaper rash caused by *C. albicans* infection.

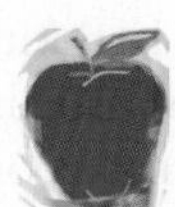

Teaching Guidelines 45.1

PREVENTION AND MANAGEMENT OF DIAPER DERMATITIS

- Change diapers frequently. Change stool-soiled diapers as soon as possible.
- Avoid rubber pants.
- Gently wash the diaper area with a soft cloth, avoiding harsh soaps.
- Use baby wipes in most children, but avoid wipes that contain fragrance or preservatives.
- Once a rash has occurred, follow all the prevention tips above and add the following:
  - Allow the infant or child to go diaperless for a period of time each day to allow the rash to heal.
  - Blow-dry the diaper area/rash area with the dryer set on the warm (not hot) setting for 3 to 5 minutes.

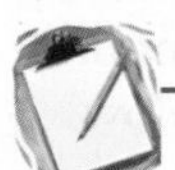

Take Note!

Discourage parents from using any type of baby powder to avoid the risk of aspiration; inhalation of talcum-containing powders may result in pneumonitis (Garlich & Nelson, 2011).

Atopic Dermatitis

Atopic dermatitis (eczema) is one of the disorders in the atopy family (along with asthma and allergic rhinitis). Atopic dermatitis affects 10% to 12% of U.S. children and up to 95% of children with atopic dermatitis develop symptoms before 5 years of age (John & Brady, 2013). About 30 to 35% of children who have atopic dermatitis will also develop allergic rhinitis and/or asthma (John & Brady, 2013).

The chronic itching associated with atopic dermatitis causes a great deal of psychological distress. The child's self-image may be affected, particularly if the rash is extensive. Difficulty sleeping may occur because of the itching. The child is irritable and has difficulty concentrating, and family life is disrupted. Parents' stress related to the child's condition may increase the child's anxiety and lead to an increase in itching and scratching. The child may outgrow atopic dermatitis, its severity may decrease as the child approaches adulthood, or the child may continue to have difficulties into the adult years. Bacterial superinfection may occur as a complication.

Therapeutic management includes good skin hydration, application of topical corticosteroids or immune modulators, oral antihistamines for sedative effects, and antibiotics if secondary infection occurs.

Pathophysiology

Atopic dermatitis is a chronic disorder characterized by extreme itching and inflamed, reddened, and swollen skin. It has a relapsing and remitting nature. The skin reaction occurs in response to specific allergens, usually food (especially eggs, wheat, milk, and peanuts) or environmental triggers (e.g., molds, dust mites, and cat dander). Other factors, such as high or low ambient temperatures, perspiring, scratching, skin irritants, or stress, may contribute to flare-ups. When the child encounters a triggering antigen, antigen-presenting cells stimulate interleukins to begin the inflammatory process. The skin begins to feel pruritic and the child starts to scratch. The sensation of itchiness comes first, and then the rash becomes apparent. The scratching causes the rash to appear. Sweating causes atopic dermatitis to worsen, as does excessively humid or dry environments.

Nursing Assessment

For a full description of the assessment phase of the nursing process, refer to the Assessment section of the Nursing Process Overview earlier in the chapter. Assessment findings pertinent to atopic dermatitis are discussed below.

HEALTH HISTORY

Elicit a description of the present illness and chief complaint. Common signs and symptoms reported during the health history might include:

- Wiggling or scratching
- Dry skin
- Scratch marks noticed by the parents
- Disrupted sleep
- Irritability

Explore the child's current and past medical history for risk factors such as:

- Family history of atopic dermatitis, allergic rhinitis, or asthma
- Child's history of asthma or allergic rhinitis
- Food or environmental allergies

Determine the onset of the rash; its location, progression, and severity; and response to treatments used so far. Note medications used to treat the rash, as well as other medications the child may be taking.

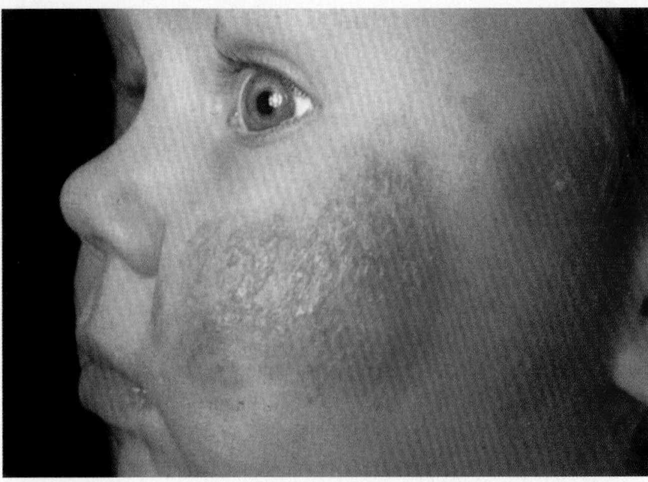

FIGURE 45.11 Atopic dermatitis rash is red, dry, and scaly.

PHYSICAL EXAMINATION

Physical examination consists of inspection and observation and auscultation.

Inspection and Observation. Observe whether the infant is wiggling or the child is actively scratching. Carefully inspect the skin. Document dry, scaly, or flaky skin, as well as hypertrophy and lichenification (Fig. 45.11). If lesions are present they may be dry lesions or weepy papules or **vesicles** (fluid-filled lesions). In children younger than 2 years old, the rash is most likely to occur on the face, scalp, wrists, and extensor surfaces of the arms or legs. In older children it may occur anywhere on the skin, but is found more commonly on the flexor areas. Note erythema or warmth, which may indicate associated secondary bacterial infection. Document areas of hyperpigmentation or hypopigmentation, which may have resulted from a prior exacerbation of atopic dermatitis or its treatment. Inspect the eyes, nose, and throat for symptoms of allergic rhinitis.

Auscultation. Auscultate the lungs for wheezing (commonly found in the associated condition of asthma).

LABORATORY AND DIAGNOSTIC TESTS

Serum immunoglobulin E (IgE) levels may be elevated in the child with atopic dermatitis. Skin prick allergy testing may determine the food or environmental allergen to which the child is sensitive.

Nursing Management

Nursing management of the child with atopic dermatitis focuses on promoting skin hydration, maintaining skin integrity, and preventing infection.

PROMOTING SKIN HYDRATION

First and foremost, avoid hot water and any skin or hair product containing perfumes, dyes, or fragrance. Bathe the child twice daily in warm (not hot) water. Use a mild soap to clean only the dirty areas. Recommended mild soaps or cleansing agents include:

- Unscented Dove or Dove for sensitive skin
- Tone
- Caress
- Oil of Olay
- Cetaphil
- Aquanil

Slightly pat the child dry after the bath, but do not rub the skin with the towel. Leave the child moist. Apply prescribed topical ointments or creams to the affected area. Apply fragrance-free moisturizer over the prescribed topical medication and all over the child's body. Recommended moisturizers include:

- Eucerin, Moisturel, Curel (cream or lotion)
- Aquaphor
- Vaseline
- Crisco

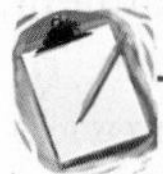

Take Note!

Vaseline or generic petrolatum is an inexpensive, readily available moisturizer.

Apply moisturizer multiple times throughout the day. Avoid clothing made of synthetic fabrics or wool. Avoid triggers known to exacerbate atopic dermatitis.

Taking evening primrose oil and other essential fatty acids as an oral supplement may result in a reduction in redness and scaling (Ehrlich, 2015b). If not initially recommended by the physician or nurse practitioner, the parent should consult with him or her first before starting these supplements. Headache and nausea are rare adverse effects of these supplements and, if they occur, are usually mild. Chamomile preparations for topical use may also be effective and are generally considered safe.

MAINTAINING SKIN INTEGRITY AND PREVENTING INFECTION

Cut the child's fingernails short and keep them clean. Avoid tight clothing and heat. Use 100% cotton bed sheets and pajamas. In addition to keeping the child's skin well moisturized, it is extremely important to prevent the child from scratching. Scratching causes the rash to appear and further scratching may lead to secondary infection. Antihistamines given at bedtime may sedate the child enough to allow him or her to sleep without awakening because of itching.

During the waking hours, behavior modification may help to keep the child from scratching. Have the parent keep a diary for 1 week to determine the pattern of scratching. Help the parent to determine specific strategies that may raise the child's awareness of scratching. A handheld clicker or counter may help to identify the scratching episode for the child, thus raising awareness. The use of diversion, imagination, and play may help to distract the child from scratching. The parent and child may create a game together that results in the child participating in a behavior rather than scratching. Pressing the skin or clenching the fist may replace scratching. It is important for the child to stay active to distract his or her mind from the itching. It is important for the parent to positively reinforce and reward the desired behaviors.

Contact Dermatitis

Contact dermatitis is a cell-mediated response to an antigenic substance exposure. The first exposure is the sensitization phase. The antigen attaches to cells that migrate to regional lymph nodes and have contact with T lymphocytes, where recognition of antigen is developed. During the second phase, elicitation, contact with the antigen results in T-lymphocyte proliferation and release of inflammatory mediators. An allergic response occurs within 24 to 48 hours after contact with the substance.

Contact dermatitis may occur as a result of allergy to nickel or cobalt found in clothing hardware and dyes, and chemicals found in many hygiene products and cosmetics. One of the more common causes of contact dermatitis in children results from exposure to highly allergenic plants such as *Toxicodendron radicans* (poison ivy), *Toxicodendron quercifolium* (Eastern poison oak), *Toxicodendron diversilobum* (Western poison oak), and *Toxicodendron vernix* (poison sumac).

Direct or indirect contact with the plant's oleoresin found in the leaves, stems, and roots results in an allergic reaction. Even contact with dormant plants or plants perceived to be dead may cause an allergic response. The rash is extremely pruritic and may last for 2 to 4 weeks; lesions continue to appear during the illness. Contact dermatitis is not contagious and does not spread either to other parts of the affected child's skin or to other people. Scratching does not spread the rash, but it may cause skin damage or secondary infection. Complications of contact dermatitis include secondary bacterial skin infections and lichenification or hyperpigmentation, particularly in dark-skinned people.

Therapeutic management is directed toward management of itching and the use of topical corticosteroids. Moderate-potency topical glucocorticoid cream or ointment is used for mild to moderate contact dermatitis, and high-potency preparations are used for more severe cases. Some severe cases of contact dermatitis may require the use of systemic steroids.

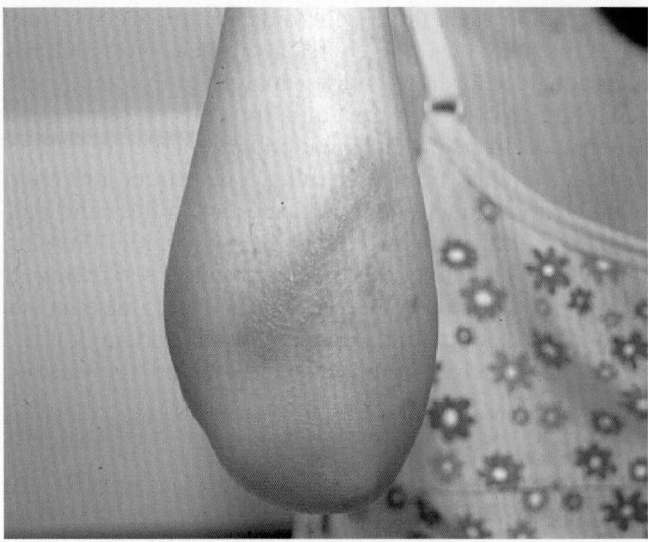

FIGURE 45.12 Note vesicular rash in linear formation characteristic of poison ivy.

Nursing Assessment

Elicit the health history, noting onset, description, location, and progression of the rash, which may be intensely pruritic and vesicular if caused by allergenic plant exposure (see Fig. 45.12). Rashes caused by other allergic exposure may be quite variable in their appearance and intensity of pruritus. Document treatment used thus far, and the child's response to it. Examine the skin, noting rash that may vary from maculopapular in nature to an erythematous papulovesicular rash at the site of contact. Some lesions may be weeping; others may erupt and form a crust. The lesions are often distributed in an asymmetric linear pattern on exposed body parts if caused by allergenic plant exposure. If the child's shirt came in contact with the plant and then the shirt was removed by pulling it over the head, there may be widespread lesions over both sides of the face. Lesions near the eyes often cause significant eyelid edema.

Take Note!

Nickel dermatitis may occur from contact with jewelry, eyeglasses, belts, or clothing snaps. Infants may display a small red circle with scaling at the site of contact with sleeper snaps.

Nursing Management

Contact dermatitis may be prevented by avoiding contact with the allergen. When the condition does occur, nursing management focuses on relieving the discomfort associated with the rash. Administer topical or systemic corticosteroids as prescribed and teach the family about use of the medications. Teaching Guidelines 45.2 gives more information about the treatment and prevention of contact dermatitis.

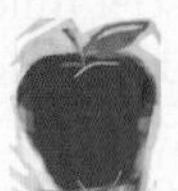

Teaching Guidelines 45.2

PREVENTION AND TREATMENT OF CONTACT DERMATITIS

Prevention

- Wear long sleeves and long pants on outings in the woods.
- Identify and remove offending plants in the yard by using a commercial weed or underbrush killer.
- Vinyl gloves (not rubber or latex) are an effective barrier.
- The plant's oil residue may be on clothes, pets, garden and sports equipment, and toys; wash those well with soap and water.
- If contact occurs, wash vigorously with soap and water within 10 minutes of contact.
- Zanfel and Tecnu Oak-N-Ivy Outdoor Skin Cleanser (both soap mixtures) may prevent rash if used to wash the skin soon after exposure.
- Ivy Block (an organoclay) is the only U.S. Food and Drug Administration–approved preventive treatment for contact dermatitis related to poison ivy, oak, or sumac. (Visit thePoint for web links that will provide additional information.) It is applied to the skin before possible exposure.

Treatment

- Wash lesions daily with mild soap and water.
- Mildly debride crusted lesions.
- Tepid baths (colloidal oatmeal such as Aveeno) are helpful to decrease itching.
- Avoid hot baths or showers, as they aggravate itching.
- Apply corticosteroid preparations topically as directed (if using high-potency preparations, do not cover with an occlusive dressing).
- Weeping lesions may be wrapped lightly; avoid occlusion.
- Burow or Domeboro solutions with a dressing applied twice daily for 20 minutes may help to dry weepy lesions.
- Over-the-counter preparations such as calamine lotion or Ivy Rest may reduce itching and help the lesions to dry.
- Do not use topical antihistamines, benzocaine, or neomycin because of the potential for sensitization.

Erythema Multiforme

Erythema multiforme, though uncommon in children, is an acute, self-limiting hypersensitivity reaction. It may occur in response to viral infections, such as adenovirus or Epstein–Barr virus; *Mycoplasma pneumoniae* infection; or a drug (especially sulfa drugs, penicillins,

BOX 45.1

STEVENS–JOHNSON SYNDROME AND TOXIC EPIDERMAL NECROLYSIS

- High fever and flu-like symptoms for 1 to 3 days prior to rash appearing
- Rash is characteristic of erythema multiforme with the addition of inflammatory bullae on at least two types of mucosa (lips, oral mucosa, bulbar conjunctivae, or anogenital region)
- Stevens–Johnson syndrome results in skin detachment of 10% or less, while toxic epidermal necrolysis involves 30% skin detachment
- Mortality rate of 10% (Nirken, High, & Roujeau, 2015).
- Treatment: hospitalization, isolation, fluid and electrolyte support, treatment of secondary infection of the lesions
- Ophthalmologic consult to determine if corneal ulceration, keratitis, uveitis, or panophthalmitis is present

or immunizations) or food reaction. Stevens–Johnson syndrome and toxic epidermal necrolysis are the most severe forms of erythema multiforme and most often occur in response to certain medications or to *Mycoplasma* infection (Box 45.1). Therapeutic management of erythema multiforme is generally supportive because it resolves on its own.

Nursing Assessment

Note history of fever, malaise, and achiness (myalgia). Determine onset and progression of rash, and presence of **pruritus** (itchiness) and burning. Document the child's temperature upon assessment. Inspect the skin for lesions, which most commonly occur over the hands and feet and extensor surfaces of the extremities, with spread to the trunk. Lesions progress from erythematous **macules** (flat reddened areas) to papules, plaques, vesicles, and target lesions over a period of days (hence the name *multiforme*) (Fig. 45.13).

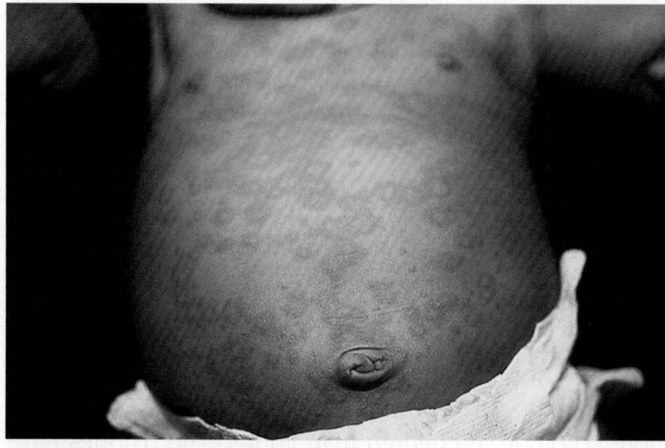

FIGURE 45.13 Erythema multiforme.

Nursing Management

Discontinue the medication or food if it is identified as the cause. Ensure that treatment for *Mycoplasma* is instituted if present. Encourage oral hydration. Administer analgesics and antihistamines as needed to promote comfort. If oral lesions are present, encourage soothing mouthwashes or use of topic oral anesthetics in the older child or teen. Oral lesions may be debrided with hydrogen peroxide.

Urticaria

Urticaria, commonly called hives, is a type I hypersensitivity reaction caused by an immunologically mediated antigen–antibody response of histamine release from mast cells. Vasodilation and increased vascular permeability result, and erythema and wheals then occur. Urticaria usually begins rapidly and may disappear in a few days or may take up to 6 to 8 weeks to resolve. The most common causes of this reaction are foods, drugs, animal stings, infections, environmental stimuli (e.g., heat, cold, sun, tight clothes), and stress. Therapeutic management focuses on identifying and removing the cause as well as providing antihistamines or steroids.

Nursing Assessment

Obtain a detailed history of new foods, medications, symptoms of a recent infection, changes in environment, or unusual stress. Inspect the skin, noting raised, edematous hives anywhere on the body or mucous membranes (Fig. 45.14). The hives are pruritic, blanch when pressed, and may migrate. Angioedema may also be present and is identifiable as subcutaneous edema and warmth, occurring most frequently on the extremities, face, or genitalia.

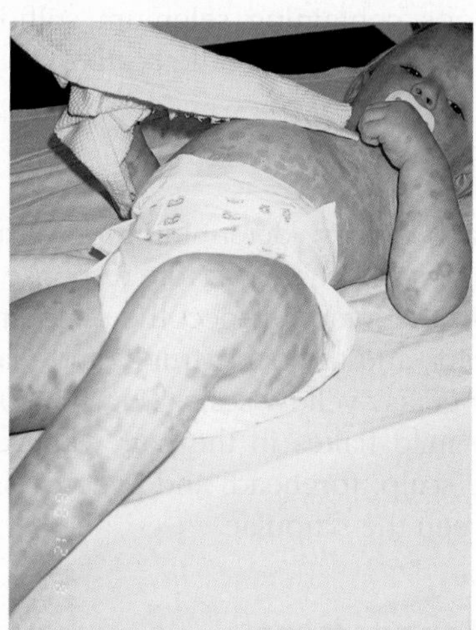

FIGURE 45.14 Ill-appearing child with urticaria. (Used with permission from Fleisher GR, Ludwig S, Baskin MN. *Atlas of pediatric emergency medicine*. Philadelphia, PA: Lippincott Williams & Wilkins, 2004:88).

Carefully assess airway and breathing, as hypersensitivity reactions may affect respiratory status.

Nursing Management

Identify and remove the offending trigger. Discontinue antibiotics. Administer antihistamines, corticosteroids, and topical antipruritics as prescribed. Inform the child and family that the episode should resolve within a few days. If it lasts up to 6 weeks, the child should be reevaluated (Vernon et al., 2013). Advise the family to obtain a medical alert bracelet for the child if the reaction is severe.

Take Note!

In an emergency situation when airway and breathing are compromised, subcutaneous epinephrine followed by intravenous (IV) diphenhydramine and corticosteroids is necessary.

Seborrhea

Seborrhea is a chronic inflammatory dermatitis that may occur on the skin or scalp. In infants it occurs most often on the scalp and is commonly referred to as cradle cap. Infants may also manifest seborrhea on the nose or eyebrows, behind the ears, or in the diaper area. It usually resolves over a period of weeks to months (Sasseville, 2015). Adolescents manifest seborrhea on the scalp (dandruff) and on the eyebrows and eyelashes, behind the ears, and between the shoulder blades.

It is thought that seborrhea is an inflammatory reaction to the fungus *Pityrosporum ovale* and is worsened by sebaceous involvement related to maternal hormones in the infant and androgens in the adolescent.

Therapeutic management includes treating the skin lesions with corticosteroid creams or lotions. Antidandruff shampoos containing selenium sulfide, ketoconazole, or tar are used to treat the scalp.

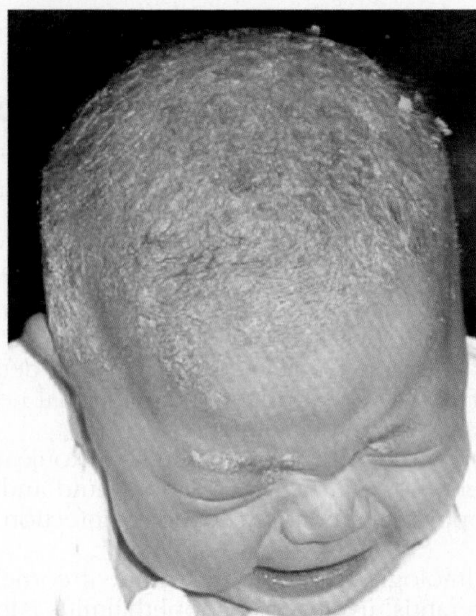

FIGURE 45.15 Severe cradle cap (yellow, greasy-appearing plaques).

Nursing Assessment

Elicit the health history, determining onset and progression of skin and scalp changes. Note response to treatment used so far. In the infant, inspect the scalp and forehead, behind the ears, and the neck, trunk, and diaper area for thick or flaky greasy yellow scales (Fig. 45.15). In the adolescent, note mild flakes in the hair with yellow greasy scales on the scalp, forehead, and eyebrows; behind the ears; or between the scapulae.

Nursing Management

Wash or shampoo the affected areas with a mild soap. Apply anti-inflammatory cream to skin lesions if prescribed. In the infant, apply mineral oil to the scalp, massage it well with a washcloth, and then shampoo 10 to 15 minutes later, using a brush to gently lift the crusts; do not forcibly remove the crusts. If needed, selenium sulfide shampoo may safely be used on the infant, following the aforementioned procedure. The adolescent may require daily shampooing with an antidandruff shampoo.

Psoriasis

Psoriasis is a chronic inflammatory skin disease with periods of remission and exacerbation; control is possible with conscientious therapy. It is an immune-mediated disorder occurring in persons with a genetic predisposition. About 30% of all psoriasis cases are diagnosed in childhood (Vernon et al., 2013).

Hyperproliferation of the epidermis occurs, with a rash developing at sites of mechanical, thermal, or physical trauma. Therapeutic management includes skin hydration with emollient creams, use of tar preparations, topical steroids, and ultraviolet light, among others. Narrow-band ultraviolet light has been used with some success in children with severe psoriasis.

Nursing Assessment

Note family history of psoriasis. Determine onset and progression of rash, as well as treatments used and the response to treatment. Question the child about pruritus, which is usually absent with psoriasis. Inspect the skin for erythematous papules that coalesce to form plaques, most frequently found on the scalp, elbows, genital area, and knees (Fig. 45.16). Facial plaques may also occur and are more common in children than adults. The plaques have a silvery or yellow-white scale and sharply demarcated

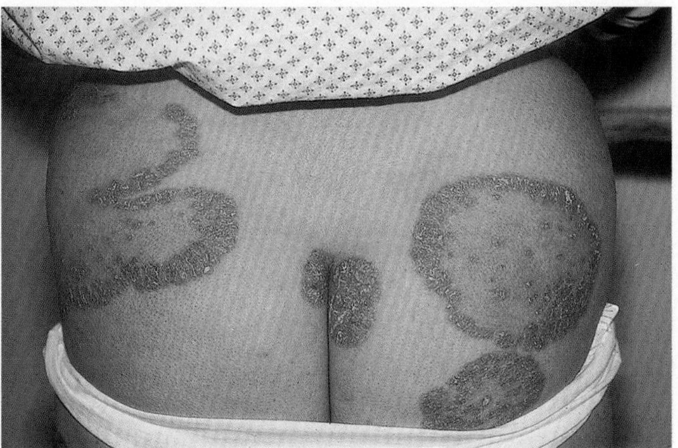

FIGURE 45.16 Psoriasis. (Used with permission from Goodheart, H. P. *Goodheart's photoguide to common skin disorders: Diagnosis and management* (3rd ed.). Philadelphia, PA: Lippincott Williams & Wilkins, 2009.)

borders. Layers of scale may be present, which, when removed, result in pinpoint bleeding (referred to as the Auspitz sign). Plaques on the scalp may result in alopecia. Examine the palms and soles, noting fissures and scaling. Skin biopsy, though rarely needed for diagnosis, will show hyperplastic epidermis, with thinning of the papillary dermis.

Nursing Management

Exposure to sunlight may promote healing, but take care not to allow the child to become sunburned. Apply skin moisturizers or emollients daily to prevent dry skin and flare-ups. Apply topical anti-inflammatory creams as prescribed during flare-ups. Apply tar shampoos or skin preparations. Use mineral oil and warm towels to soak and remove thick plaques.

> **Thinking About Development**
>
> Emily Wilson is a 15-year-old female with a history of moderate psoriasis. She experiences significant scaling along her hairline, forehead, scalp, and arms. Hypopigmentation and striae are beginning to occur on her arms as a result of topical medication use. She is a talented ballerina but expresses increasing concerns about her skin alterations showing while she is performing.
>
> How does Emily's developmental stage affect self-care related to her psoriasis?
>
> What is the most appropriate approach for the nurse to take to educate Emily about control of her psoriasis?
>
> How will the nurse best promote an appropriate body image for Emily?

ACNE

Acne, the most common skin condition occurring in childhood (Morelli & Prok, 2014), is a disorder that affects the pilosebaceous unit. It affects males and females, as well as all ethnic groups. Overall, males tend to have more severe disease than females, probably because of the androgen influence (Morelli & Prok, 2014). Acne that persists past the usual course of time for infantile or adolescent acne may be caused by endocrine abnormalities. It may also occur in response to the use of certain types of drugs such as corticosteroids, androgens, phenytoin, and others. The usual presentation and nursing management of acne neonatorum and acne vulgaris is presented below.

Acne Neonatorum

Acne neonatorum occurs as a response to the presence of maternal androgens or to transient androgen production in the newborn. It affects about 20% of newborns (Vernon et al., 2013). Usually no treatment is necessary, but in severe cases there is a risk of scarring, so a topical preparation may be prescribed.

Nursing Assessment

Note oily face or scalp. Examine the face (especially the cheeks), upper chest, and back for inflammatory papules and pustules. Document absence of fever.

Nursing Management

Instruct parents to avoid picking or squeezing the pimples; to do so places the infant at risk for secondary bacterial infection and cellulitis. Teach parents to wash the affected areas daily with clear water. Avoid using fragranced soaps or lotions on the area with acne. Inform the parents that as the newborn's hormones stabilize over time, the acne usually resolves without additional intervention.

Acne Vulgaris

Acne vulgaris affects 50% to 85% of adolescents between the ages of 12 and 16 years, and endogenous androgens play a role in its development (Morelli & Prok, 2014). It occurs most frequently on the face, chest, and back. Risk factors for the development of acne vulgaris include preadolescent or adolescent age, male gender (due to the presence of androgens), an oily complexion, Cushing syndrome, or another disease process resulting in increased androgen production.

Pathophysiology

The sebaceous gland produces sebum and is connected by a duct to the follicular canal that opens on the skin's surface. Androgenous hormones stimulate sebaceous gland proliferation and production of sebum. These hormones exhibit increased activity during the pubertal years. Abnormal shedding of the outermost layer of the skin (the stratum corneum) occurs at the level of the follicular opening, resulting in a keratin plug that fills the follicle. The sebaceous glands increase sebum production. Bacterial overgrowth of *Propionibacterium acnes* occurs because the presence of sebum and keratin in the follicular canal creates an excellent environment for growth. Inflammation occurs as the follicular wall perforates, allowing the contents to leak into nearby tissue.

Therapeutic Management

Therapeutic management focuses on reducing *P. acnes,* decreasing sebum production, normalizing skin shedding, and eliminating inflammation. Teach the adolescent to cleanse the skin gently twice a day. Medication therapy may include a combination of benzoyl peroxide, salicylic acid, retinoids, and topical or oral antibiotics. Isotretinoin may be used in severe cases. Drug Guide 45.1 gives further information on these medications. In girls, oral contraceptives may help lessen acne by decreasing the effects of androgens on the sebaceous glands. Diode laser or blue ultraviolet light therapy may also be used. CO_2 lasers and dermabrasion may be used to treat pitted scarring.

Nursing Assessment

Note history of onset of acne lesions, as well as family history of acne. Determine medication use; certain medications may hasten the onset of acne or worsen it when already present. In particular, note use of corticosteroids, androgens, lithium, phenytoin, and isoniazid. Document history of an endocrine disorder, particularly one that results in hyperandrogenism. In girls, note worsening of acne 2 to 7 days before the start of the menstrual period. Inspect the skin for lesions (particularly on the face and upper chest and back, which are the areas of highest sebaceous activity). Note presence, distribution, and extent of noninflammatory lesions, such as open and closed comedones, as well as inflammatory lesions such as papules, pustules, nodules, or cysts (open comedones are commonly referred to as blackheads and closed comedones as whiteheads; see Fig. 45.17). Examine the skin for hypertrophic scarring resulting from inflammatory lesions. Table 45.3 explains the acne classification. Note oily skin and oily hair, which result from increased sebum production. Determine remedies that have been used and the extent of success of those treatments. Assess the child's or teen's feelings about the disorder.

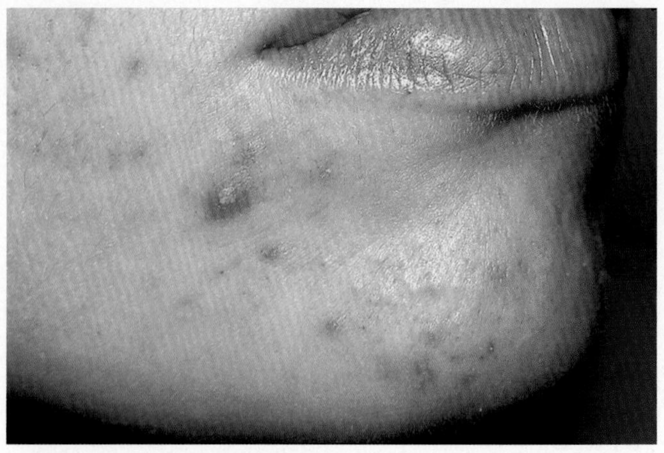

FIGURE 45.17 Acne vulgaris.

Nursing Management

Avoid oil-based cosmetics and hair products, as their use may block pores, contributing to noninflammatory lesions. Look for cosmetic products labeled as noncomedogenic. Headbands, helmets, and hats may exacerbate the lesions by causing friction. Dryness and peeling may occur with acne treatment, so encourage the child to use a humectant moisturizer. Mild cleansing with soap and water twice daily is appropriate. Avoid excessive scrubbing and harsh chemical or alcohol-based cleansers. Avoid picking or squeezing the lesions. Using a noncomedogenic sunscreen with an SPF of 30 or higher may reduce the risk of postinflammatory discoloration from acne lesions (Vernon et al., 2013). Teach adolescents that the prescribed topical medications must be used daily and that it may take 4 to 6 weeks to see results. Avoid the use of over-the-counter preparations because they are irritating and aggravate the drying effect of prescription acne treatments. Instruct boys to shave gently and avoid using dull razors, so as not to further irritate

TABLE 45.3 CLASSIFICATION OF ACNE

Classification	Manifestations
Mild acne	Primarily noninflammatory lesions (comedones)
Moderate acne	Comedones plus inflammatory lesions such as papules or pustules (localized to face or back)
Severe acne	Lesions similar to moderate acne, but more widespread, and/or presence of cysts or nodules. Associated more frequently with scarring

BOX 45.2

DECREASING RISK OF FETAL EXPOSURE TO ISOTRETINOIN: iPLEDGE

- As of 2006, physicians, pharmacists, and patients are required to register in the iPLEDGE program before they prescribe, dispense, or receive isotretinoin.
- The iPLEDGE program is a central registry requiring monthly input as noted below in order to continue isotretinoin treatment.
- Monthly input includes the following:
  - Females of childbearing age are using two forms of contraception.
  - Pregnancy test results are negative.
  - Isotretinoin users do not donate blood during treatment or for 1 month after completion of treatment.
  - Additional information available at https://www.ipledgeprogram.com/

Adapted from Vernon, P., Brady, M. A., Starr, N. B., & Petersen-Smith, A. M. (2013). Dermatologic disorders. In C. Burns, A. Dunn, M. Brady, N. B. Starr, & C. Blosser (Eds.), *Pediatric primary care* (5th ed.). Philadelphia, PA: Saunders.

the condition. Adolescent girls taking isotretinoin who are sexually active must be on a pregnancy prevention program because the drug causes defects in fetal development (Vernon et al., 2013) (Box 45.2).

Adolescents interested in complementary medicine approaches may try topical use of a tea tree oil preparation. Fewer adverse effects may occur with tea tree oil preparations than with benzoyl peroxide preparations, but local reactions may still occur (Berman, 2015).

If the acne is severe, depression may occur as a result of body image disturbances. Provide emotional support to adolescents undergoing acne therapy. Refer teens for counseling if necessary.

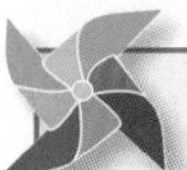

Take Note!

Chocolate, skim milk, and French fries have not been proven to contribute to the incidence or severity of acne. However, advise teens to wash their hands after eating greasy finger foods to avoid spreading additional oil to the surface of the face (Morelli & Prok, 2014).

Consider This

Paxton Herman, age 16, comes to the clinic with complaints of acne on his face and back. He states, "I hate the way my face looks." "I'll never get a date looking like this." "I don't even want to take my shirt off at the beach, because there's bumps on my back."

Think back to when you were an adolescent. How would you have felt if you had a skin condition that altered the way your face looked? As the nurse, how can you help Paxton in this situation?

INJURIES

Children, by their inquisitive natures, developmental immaturity, and skin's properties, are prone to experience a variety of skin injuries. Pressure ulcers are most likely to occur in hospitalized or otherwise immobile children. Typical healthy, active children are likely to suffer cuts, abrasions, foreign body penetration, burns and other thermal injuries, bites, and stings.

Pressure Ulcers

Skin breakdown involves changes in intact skin, which may range from blanchable erythema to deep pressure ulcers. The term pressure ulcer refers to damage to the skin resulting in skin loss and development of a crater that may range from mild to deep. The incidence of pressure ulcers in critically ill children is 18% to 27% (Schindler et al., 2011). Pressure ulcers develop from a combination of factors, including immobility or decreased activity, decreased sensory perception, increased moisture, impaired nutritional status, inadequate tissue perfusion, and the forces of friction and shear. Common sites of pressure ulcers in hospitalized children include the occiput and toes, while children who require wheelchairs for mobility have pressure ulcers in the sacral or hip area more frequently.

Nursing Assessment

Note history of immobility (chronic, related to a condition such as paralysis) or lengthy hospitalization, particularly in intensive care. Inspect the skin for areas of erythema or warmth. Note ulceration of the skin. Use the facility's wound assessment scale to document the extent of the ulcer. Take a photo of the ulcer if possible.

Nursing Management

Position the child to alleviate pressure on the area of the ulcer. Use specialized beds or mattresses to prevent further pressure areas from developing. Perform prescribed wound care meticulously, noting the formation of granulation tissue as the ulcer begins to heal. Prevent pressure ulcers in the child who is hospitalized for long periods of time by turning the child frequently, assessing the entire surface of the child's skin at least every shift, using pressure-alleviating beds and mattresses, and maintaining the child's nutritional status. See Evidence-Based Practice 45.1.

Minor Injuries

Children suffer minor injuries very frequently. Because of their developmental immaturity and inquisitive nature, children often attempt tasks they are not yet capable of

EVIDENCE-BASED PRACTICE 45.1 **PEDIATRIC SKIN INTEGRITY PRACTICE GUIDELINE**

STUDY

Immobility in the pediatric critical care unit places the child at increased risk of the development of pressure ulcers or other alterations in tissue integrity. About ¾ of children in critical care units have a Braden Q score of 16 or less, indicating increased risk for skin breakdown. The researchers undertook a study to determine the effect of implementation of a pediatric skin integrity practice guideline on skin breakdown in intubated children. Over a 6-month period, 200 charts were reviewed.

Findings

Children admitted to the unit prior to implementation of the guideline were 1.35 times more likely to develop alterations in skin integrity, than those cared for after the pediatric skin integrity practice guideline implementation.

Nursing Implications

Following practice guidelines that address assessment and interventions related to skin, device use, and pressure relief such as the guideline used in this study, may result in decreased tissue integrity alterations such as skin breakdown and pressure ulcers in immobile children. The study was small, involving one institution only, so should be replicated for further demonstration of effectiveness. Nurse should pay close attention to skin assessments and interventions designed to decrease the incidence of tissue integrity alteration, in order to best preserve immobile children's skin integrity.

Adapted from Kiss, E. A., & Heiler, M. (2014). Pediatric skin integrity practice guideline for institutional use: A quality improvement project. *Journal of Pediatric Nursing, 29*, 362–357.

or take risks that an adult would not, often resulting in a fall or other accident. Minor injuries include minor cuts and abrasions, as well as skin penetration of foreign bodies such as splinters or glass fragments. The break in the skin allows an entry point for bacteria, and the complication of cellulitis may occur. Treatment is directed at cleaning the wound and preventing infection.

Nursing Assessment

Obtain the history from the child or caregiver to determine whether dirt or a foreign object may be present in the wound. Inspect the wound, noting depth of injury, a foreign body, and bleeding.

Nursing Management

Cleanse the wound with mild soap and water or with an antibacterial cleanser. Wet gauze helps to scrub away fine and large sand particles. Remove pieces of loose skin with sterile scissors, foreign particles with sterile forceps, and road tar with petrolatum. Small abrasions and minor, well-approximated cuts may be left open to the air. Apply a small amount of antibacterial ointment and cover large abrasions with a loose dressing. Change the dressing 12 hours later and redress after cleaning the wound. Leave it open to air after 23 hours have passed from the time of injury.

Calendula preparations are presumed to be safe for topical use and may speed wound healing. Chamomile may help to dry a weeping wound, and allergic reactions to the herb are rare (Ehrlich, 2015a). Assess the wound daily for signs of infection, which include purulence, warmth, edema, increasing pain, and erythema that extends past the margin of the cut or abrasion.

Burns

Burns are a common preventable mechanism of injury among children and adolescents. Young children are at highest risk for burns and the mortality rate from burns is highest in children younger than 5 years of age (Joffe, 2015). Specifically, burns are the fourth leading cause of death from unintentional injury in children between 1 and 4 years of age (Centers for Disease Control and Prevention, 2016). Most pediatric burn-related injuries do not result in death, but injuries from burns often cause extreme pain and extensive burns can result in serious disfigurement. The majority of children younger than 4 years of age experience scald burns (Myers, 2011). Fires in the home are often related to cooking, cigarette or other smoking materials (Myers, 2011). Carbon monoxide poisoning often occurs in conjunction with burns as a result of smoke inhalation, and infants and children are at greater risk for carbon monoxide poisoning than adults. See Healthy People 2020.

HEALTHY PEOPLE *2020*

Objective	Nursing Significance
Reduce residential fire deaths. Increase functioning residential smoke alarms.	• Question all families about smoke detectors and if they are working. • Provide families with resources related to fire prevention.

Healthy People Objectives retrieved from http://www.healthypeople.gov

Great advances have been made in the care of children with serious burns. As a result of improved burn care, children who in the past would have died as a result of burns over large body surface areas have a much greater chance of survival (Quilty, 2010).

Conventional wisdom is that children with severe burns should be transferred to a specialized burn unit. The American Burn Association has developed the following criteria for referral of burned persons to a specialized burn unit:

- Partial thickness burns greater than 10% of total body surface area
- Burns that involve the face, the hands and feet, genitalia, perineum, or major joints
- Full-thickness burns of any size
- Chemical or electrical burns (including lightning injury)
- Inhalation injury
- Burn injury in children who have pre-existing conditions that might affect their care
- Persons with burns and traumatic injuries
- Persons who will require special social, emotional, or long-term rehabilitative care
- Burned children in a hospital without qualified personnel or equipment for the care of children (Myers, 2011)

The old terms used to describe the depth of burns as first, second, and third degree have been replaced by contemporary terminology. Burns are now classified according to the extent of injury and the terminology used to describe each type includes superficial, partial thickness, deep partial thickness, and full thickness (Garzon, Degolier, & Brehm, 2013). Superficial burns involve only epidermal injury and usually heal without scarring or other sequelae within 4 to 5 days. In partial-thickness burns, injury occurs not only to the epidermis but also to portions of the dermis. These burns usually heal within about 2 weeks and carry a minimal risk of scar formation. Deep partial-thickness burns take longer to heal, may scar, and result in changes in nail and hair appearance as well as sebaceous gland function in the affected area. They may require surgical intervention. Full-thickness burns result in significant tissue damage as they extend through the epidermis, dermis, and hypodermis. Extensive scarring results, as hair follicles and sweat glands are destroyed. Full-thickness burns require a significant time to heal. If underlying tendons and/or bone are involved, the burn may be termed fourth degree. Contractures and limited function may occur as a complication of full-thickness burns. Skin grafting is usually necessary. Full or partially circumferential burns may result in ischemia from loss of blood flow related to progressive swelling of the area.

Pathophysiology

Burned tissue begins to coagulate after the injury, and direct coagulation and microvascular reactions in the adjacent dermis may extend the burn. The blood vessels demonstrate increased capillary permeability, resulting in vasodilatation. This leads to increased hydrostatic pressure in the capillaries, causing water, electrolytes, and protein to leak out of the vasculature and result in significant edema. Edema forms very rapidly in the first 18 hours after the burn, peaking at around 48 hours. Capillary permeability then returns to normal between 48 and 72 hours after the burn and the lymphatics can reabsorb the edema fluid. Diuresis occurs, ridding the body of the excess fluid. Fluid loss from burned skin occurs at an amount that is 5 to 10 times greater than that from undamaged skin, and this fluid loss continues until the damaged surface is healed or grafted.

Initially, the severely burned child experiences a decrease in cardiac output, with a subsequent hypermetabolic response during which cardiac output increases dramatically. During this heightened metabolic state, the child is at risk for insulin resistance and increased protein catabolism. Children who are burned during an indoor or chemical fire are at an increased risk of respiratory injury. Children who have aspirated hot liquids are particularly at risk for airway-altering edema.

Therapeutic Management

Therapeutic management of burns focuses on fluid resuscitation, wound care, prevention of infection, and restoration of function. Burn infections are treated with antibiotics specific to the causative organism. If invasive burn damage occurs, surgery may be necessary.

Nursing Assessment

For a full description of the assessment phase of the nursing process, refer to the Assessment section of the Nursing Process Overview earlier in the chapter. Upon arrival, evaluate the child with burns to determine if he or she will require intensive management. Remove any smoldering clothing. Obtain a brief history of the burn circumstances while you are assessing the child and providing care.

HEALTH HISTORY

If the burn is severe or there is a potential for respiratory compromise, obtain a brief history while simultaneously evaluating the child and providing emergency care. If the burn does not appear to pose an immediate life-threatening risk, obtain an in-depth history. Elicit a description of how the burn occurred, noting date, time, and cause. Determine if smoke inhalation or an associated fall may have occurred. Document treatment that the parent or caregiver has provided to the child's burn so far. Note the child's recent health status, current medications, recent or chronic illness, and immunization status, in particular noting the date of the most recent tetanus vaccination.

Determine whether the history being given sounds consistent with the type of burn injury that has occurred. Inquire about what caused the burn and if the event was witnessed by anyone. Spatter-type burns resulting from the child pulling a source of hot fluid onto himself or herself usually yield a nonuniform, asymmetric distribution of injury. In contrast, intentional scald injuries usually yield a uniform "stocking" or "glove" distribution when the child's extremity is held under very hot water as punishment (Diamond, Abdoo, Brady, & Dunn, 2013). It is important for the nurse to pick up on clues in the health history that may indicate that the burn is a result of child abuse, rather than an accident (Box 45.3). Children are also burned by curling irons, gasoline, fireworks, room heaters, ovens, and ranges. Obtain a detailed history about the circumstances surrounding these types of burns. Ask the parent what the home hot water heater temperature is.

PHYSICAL EXAMINATION

Emergency examination of the burned child consists of a primary survey followed by a secondary survey. The primary survey includes evaluation of the child's airway, breathing, and circulation. The secondary survey focuses on evaluation of the burns and other injuries. Box 45.4 gives information about emergency assessment of the burned child. Inspect the child's skin, noting erythema, blistering, weeping, or eschar (charred skin).

Classify the burn according to its severity. Superficial burns are painful, red, dry, and possibly edematous (Fig. 45.18). Partial-thickness and deep partial-thickness burns are very painful and edematous and have a wet appearance or blisters (Fig. 45.19). Full-thickness burns may be very painful or numb or pain-free in some areas. They appear red, edematous, leathery, dry, or waxy and may display peeling or charred skin (Fig. 45.20). Note

BOX 45.3

SIGNS OF CHILD ABUSE–INDUCED BURNS

- Inconsistent history given when caregivers are interviewed separately
- Delay in seeking treatment by caregiver
- Uniform appearance of the burn, with clear delineation of burned and nonburned area (as with a hot object applied to the skin)
- In the case of a scald-induced burn, lack of spattering of water but evidence of so-called "porcelain-contact sparing," where the portion of the child's skin that was in contact with the tub or sink is not burned (commonly seen with a forced immersion in extremely hot water used as punishment)
- Flexor-sparing burns or burns that involve the dorsum of the hand
- A stocking/glove pattern on the hands or feet (circumferential ring appearing around the extremity, resulting from a caregiver forcefully holding the child under extremely hot water)

Adapted from Diamond, J. S., Abdoo, D. C., Brady, M. A., & Dunn, A. M. (2013). Role relationships. In C. Burns, A. Dunn, M. Brady, N. B. Starr, & C. Blosser (Eds.), *Pediatric primary care* (5th ed.). Philadelphia, PA: Saunders.

BOX 45.4

EMERGENCY ASSESSMENT OF THE BURNED CHILD

Primary Survey

- Assess the child's airway, noting whether it is patent, maintainable, or unmaintainable.
- Suspect airway injury from burn or smoke inhalation if any of the following are present: burns around the mouth, nose, or eyes; carbonaceous (black-colored) sputum; hoarseness or stridor.
- Evaluate the child's skin color, respiratory effort, symmetry of breathing, and breath sounds.
- Determine the pulse strength, perfusion status, and heart rate. Note extent and location of edema.

Secondary Survey

- Determine burn depth.
- Estimate burn extent by determining the percentage of body surface area affected. Use a chart for estimation (see Fig. 45.21) or rapidly estimate by using the child's palm size, which is equivalent to about 1% of the child's body surface area.
- Inspect the child for other traumatic injuries (children who have jumped or fallen from a house fire may suffer cervical spine or internal injuries).

Adapted from Joffe, M. D. (2015). Emergency care of moderate and severe thermal burns in children. Retrieved from http://www.uptodate.com/contents/emergency-care-of-moderate-and-severe-thermal-burns-in-children and Myers, T. (2011). When to treat or refer a burn-injured patient. *Clinical Advisor, 14*(7), 31–36.

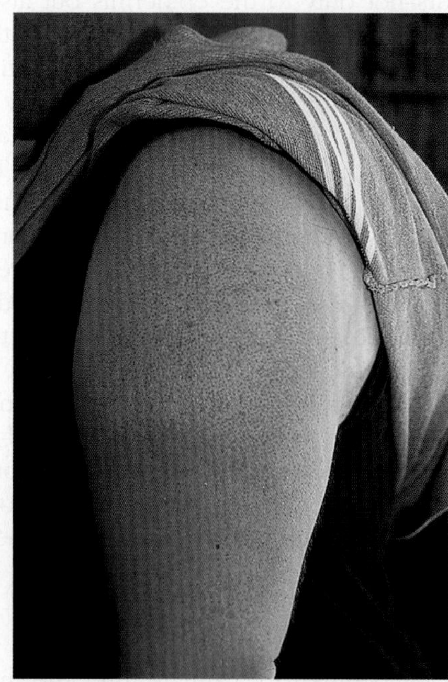

FIGURE 45.18 Superficial burn—painful but without blisters.

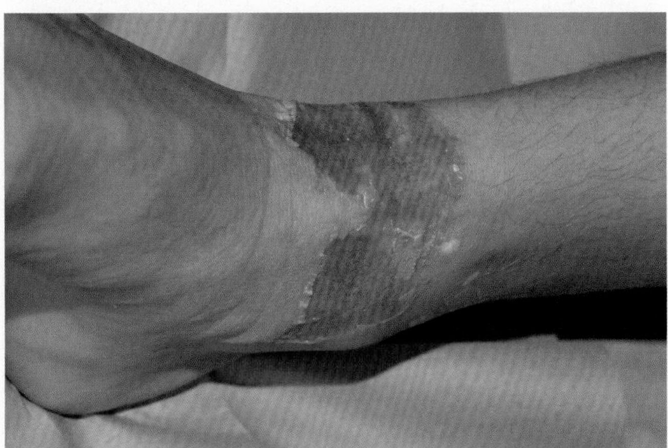

FIGURE 45.19 Partial-thickness burn—very painful, with blistering.

whether the burn is circumferential (encircling a body part) or partially circumferential.

Take Note!

Due to overlying blistering, it is difficult to accurately distinguish between partial- and full-thickness burns. In addition, in the case of third-degree burns, it is difficult to estimate burn depth during the initial evaluation.

LABORATORY AND DIAGNOSTIC TESTS

In the child with more extensive burns, electrolytes and complete blood count are used to measure fluid and electrolyte balance and to determine the possibility of infection, respectively. If wound infection is suspected, culture of the drainage will determine the particular bacteria. Nutritional indices such as albumin, transferrin, carotene, retinol, copper, cholesterol, calcium, thiamine, riboflavin, pyridoxine, and iron may be evaluated when the child has severe or extensive burns. Pulmonary status may be evaluated via pulse oximetry and end-tidal CO_2 monitoring, arterial blood gases, carboxyhemoglobin levels, and chest radiography. Fiberoptic bronchoscopy and xenon ventilation–perfusion scanning may be used to evaluate inhalation injury. Electrocardiographic monitoring is important for the child who has suffered an electrical burn to identify cardiac arrhythmias, which can be noted for up to 72 hours after a burn injury.

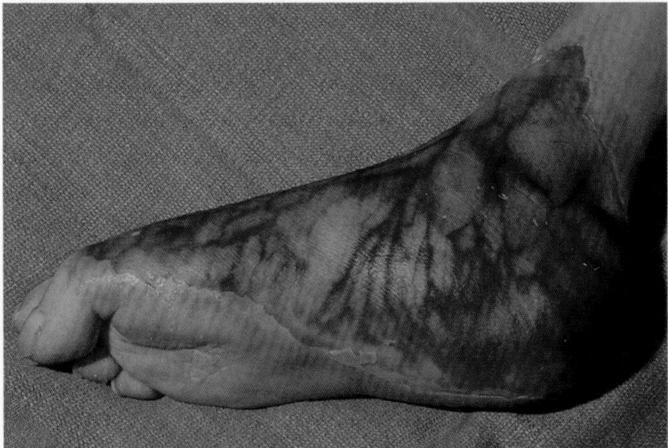

FIGURE 45.20 Full-thickness burn—color ranges from red to charred, or white, minimal pain, marked edema.

Nursing Management

Nursing management of the child who has been burned focuses first on stabilizing the child. Place the child on a cardiac/apnea monitor, measure the child with the Broselow tape, monitor pulse oximetry, and apply an end-tidal CO_2 monitor if the child is ventilated. Further management focuses on cleansing the burn, pain management, and prevention and treatment of infection. Fluid status and nutrition are important components of burn care, particularly in the early stages. Rehabilitation of the child with severe burns is also an important nursing function. Providing child and family education about the prevention of burns as well as care of burns at home is critical. Nursing Care Plan 45.1, at the end of the chapter, gives additional interventions related to fluid and nutritional management.

PROMOTING OXYGENATION AND VENTILATION

Institute emergency airway management as needed. If the child requires intubation, make sure that the tracheal tube is taped in a very secure manner, as reintubation in these children will become increasingly difficult as the edema spreads. The burned child's respiratory status warrants vigilant evaluation and reevaluation, as airway edema that is secondary to a burn may not become evident until 2 days after the injury. Administer 100% oxygen via nonrebreather mask or bag–valve–mask ventilation to all children with severe burns. Continue to reassess the child's pulmonary status, adjusting the interventions as necessary (refer to Chapter 51 for further information about respiratory emergency care).

Take Note!

High levels of carboxyhemoglobin as a result of smoke inhalation may contribute to falsely high pulse oximetry readings (Mechem, 2016).

RESTORING AND MAINTAINING FLUID VOLUME

Several formulas are available for the calculation of resuscitative fluids in children. Most experts recommend that pediatric burn therapy include:

- Fluid calculation based on the body surface area burned (Fig. 45.21)
- Use of a crystalloid (Ringer lactate) during the first 24 hours; in smaller children, a small amount of dextrose may be added

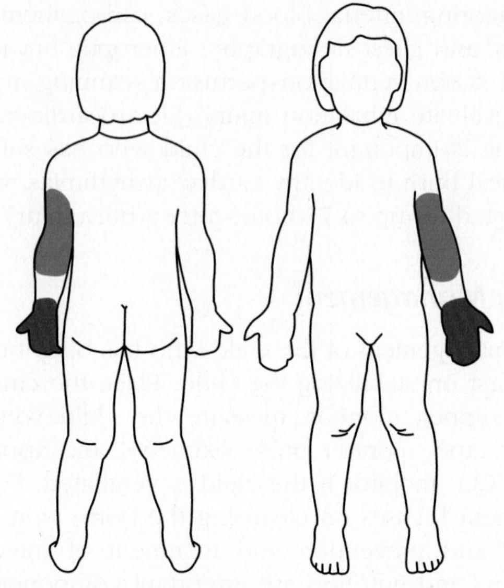

EXAMPLE

Calculating TBSA By Age (Total Body Surface Area)

Color Code
Red - 3° (full thickness)
Blue - 2° (partial thickness)

Area	Birth 1 yr	1-4 yrs	5-9 yrs	10-14 yrs	15 yrs	Adult	2	3	Total
Head	19	17	13	11	9	7	—	8	8.0
Neck	2	2	2	2	2	2	—	1	1.0
Ant.Trunk	13	13	13	13	13	13	1	12	13.0
Post. Trunk	13	13	13	13	13	13	—	—	—
R. Buttock	2 1/2	2 1/2	2 1/2	2 1/2	2 1/2	2 1/2	—	—	—
L. Buttock	2 1/2	2 1/2	2 1/2	2 1/2	2 1/2	2 1/2	—	—	—
Genitalia	1	1	1	1	1	1	—	—	—
R.U. Arm	4	4	4	4	4	4	—	3.5	3.5
L.U. Arm	4	4	4	4	4	4	1	2.5	3.5
R.L. Arm	3	3	3	3	3	3	—	3	3
L.L. Arm	3	3	3	3	3	3	—	3	3
R. Hand	2 1/2	2 1/2	2 1/2	2 1/2	2 1/2	2 1/2	—	2.5	2.5
L. Hand	2 1/2	2 1/2	2 1/2	2 1/2	2 1/2	2 1/2	—	2.5	2.5
R. Thigh	5 1/2	6 1/2	8	8 1/2	9	9 1/2	1	2	3
L. Thigh	5 1/2	6 1/2	8	8 1/2	9	9 1/2	—	2	2
R. Leg	5	5	5 1/2	6	6 1/2	7	—	—	—
L. Leg	5	5	5 1/2	6	6 1/2	7	—	—	—
R. Foot	3 1/2	3 1/2	3 1/2	3 1/2	3 1/2	3 1/2	—	—	—
L. Foot	3 1/2	3 1/2	3 1/2	3 1/2	3 1/2	3 1/2	—	—	—
						Total	3%	42%	45%

FIGURE 45.21 Calculate total body surface area (TBSA) affected by using the child's age and the area affected, as well as whether the burned area is second degree (partial thickness) or third degree (full thickness).

- Administration of most of the volume during the first 8 hours (amounts and timing of fluid volume resuscitation will vary from child to child)
- Reassessment of the child and adjustment of the fluid rate accordingly; fluid requirements greatly decrease after 24 hours and should be adjusted to reflect this.
- Administration of a colloid fluid later in therapy once capillary permeability is less of a concern
- Monitoring of the child's urine output as part of ongoing assessment of response to therapy, expecting at least 1 mL/kg/hr
- Daily weights obtained at the same time each day (the best indicator of fluid volume status)
- Monitoring of electrolyte levels (particularly sodium and potassium) for their return to normal levels

PREVENTING HYPOTHERMIA

Due to the loss of the protective dermis, children who are burned are at high risk for hypothermia and secondary infection. Therefore, take care to keep the child warm. Warm intravenous fluids before administration. Maintain a neutral thermal environment and monitor the child's temperature frequently.

CLEANSING THE BURN

Initially, it is very important to stop the burning. Therefore, remove charred clothing. Wash and rinse the burn thoroughly with mild soap and cool water from the tap. Never apply ice. Children who are burned with tar require special care. Remove tar with cool water and mineral oil. Do not routinely remove blisters because they provide a protective barrier; however, debridement is recommended in certain cases where large blisters impede wound care. Wounds that are open require debridement. Debridement involves the removal of loose skin and eschar (dead, charred skin). This procedure is usually performed with sterile scissors and a pair of forceps or with a gauze sponge. Gently cleanse the burned area; there is no advantage to aggressive scrubbing, and this technique only makes the pain more intense for the child. Wear a gown, mask, head covering, and gloves during dressing changes. Debridement is a necessary, but often excruciatingly painful, procedure. Thus, pain management needs of the child are of utmost importance (refer to the pain management section below).

When children return for evaluation of a wound that was previously seen in your facility, remove the dressing. Soak the dressing in lukewarm tap water to ease the removal of gauze, which may be stuck to the wound. The nurse plays an important role in ensuring that the dressing change goes smoothly. Be sure to:

- Have all dressing supplies ready.
- Provide pain medication as ordered.
- Promote good infection control technique among your colleagues.
- Assist with restraining young children, using the positions of comfort previously discussed in relation to atraumatic care.
- Encourage participation by the child's parents.
- Talk soothingly to the child, explain what you are going to do, and provide distraction during the procedure.

PREVENTING INFECTION

Prevention of infection is critical to successful outcomes for burned children. If the child's immunization status is unknown or if it has been 5 years or longer since the last tetanus vaccine, administer the tetanus vaccine (Garzon et al., 2013). If the child has never received tetanus vaccination, also give 250 units tetanus human immunoglobulin intravenously. Apply antibiotic ointment in conjunction with burn dressing changes. Refer to Drug Guide 45.1 for information about topical antibiotics. Membrane dressings such as biosynthetic, hydrocolloid, and antibiotic-impregnated foam dressings are alternatives to topical antibiotics and sterile dressings. Evaluate the child's wound during dressing changes, looking for wound redness, swelling, odor, or drainage. Strictly adhere to infection control procedures and hand hygiene to decrease the risk of burn infection. Maximize the child's nutritional status to decrease his or her susceptibility to a burn infection. Monitor the child's temperature for the development of fever. Upon discharge, instruct the parents about the signs of a wound infection.

MANAGING PAIN

Pain management is of the utmost importance, and several options are available for the treatment of burn-related pain. Local anesthesia, sedatives, and systemic analgesics are commonly used. Children who have less severe burns that are managed at home can be given oral medications such as acetaminophen with codeine 30 to 45 minutes before dressing changes. In burns that result in more severe pain, the child should be hospitalized and given intravenous pain control with medications such as morphine sulfate. Midazolam (a sedative) may be used in conjunction with pain medication for pain reduction during dressing changes.

Pain may also occur at any time of the day or night, not just in relation to dressing changes. Assess the child's pain status frequently using an age-appropriate pain assessment scale. Administer pain medications as prescribed and/or use nonpharmacologic techniques to alleviate or decrease the child's perception of pain.

Atraumatic Care

Immersion in virtual reality computer games before and during burn dressing changes provides an exceptionally powerful form of cognitive distraction. (Li, Montano, Chen, & Gold, 2011).

TREATING INFECTED BURNS

The potential for burn infection increases if the child has a large, open burn wound and if there are other sources of infection, such as multiple intravenous lines. In addition, children who are immunocompromised have an increased risk of burn infection. In burn wound cellulitis, the area around the burn becomes increasingly red, swollen, and painful early in the course of burn management. With invasive burn cellulitis, the burn develops a dark brown, black, or purplish color, with a discharge and foul odor. Burn impetigo is characterized by multifocal small superficial abscesses. Burn impetigo causes marked destruction of skin-grafted areas. Extensive infected burns may also become infected with a fungus.

When an infection is suspected, antibiotics are usually started, pending wound culture results. Administer antibiotics as prescribed or antifungals if necessary.

PROVIDING BURN REHABILITATION

Children who have suffered a significant burn injury face myriad physical and psychological challenges that extend well beyond the acute injury phase. Burned children most often exhibit anxiety and attention or behavioral problems (Pardo, Garcia, & Gomez-Cia, 2010). Skin grafting or special burn dressings are required for some children (Box 45.5). Children who have suffered extensive burns often require multiple skin-grafting surgeries. Figures 45.22 and 45.23 show healed skin grafts. Extensive burns may also result in the need for pressure garments to decrease the risk of extensive scarring. Pressure garments are not comfortable and they must be worn

BOX 45.5

SPECIAL BURN CARE AND SKIN GRAFTING

- To prevent infection and promote healing:
  - Biosynthetic skin coverings such as Biobrane (silicone film bonded to flexible nylon fabric and purified collagen peptides) and Mepilex Ag (soft silicone soaked with silver)
  - Kaltostat (calcium alginate dressing) is a brown seaweed extract that is spun into a fiber that is highly absorbent. It reacts with exudate on the wound to form a protective gel.
- Autograft allows for permanent coverage of a deep partial-thickness or full-thickness burn.
  - Consists of child's own skin
  - Split thickness consists of epidermis and superficial layers of dermis. The donor site heals completely.
  - Full thickness consists of full dermal thickness. Cover the donor site with fine-mesh gauze or synthetic wound coverings to allow the site to heal.

Adapted from Quilty, J. (2010, May). *Pediatric burn management.* Presented at meeting of the Florida Chapter of the National Association of Pediatric Nurse Practitioners, Orlando, FL.

continuously for at least 1 year, sometimes 2, but they have been shown to be very effective in reducing hypertrophic scarring resulting from significant burn injury.

Physical therapy will usually be initiated in the critical care setting and will continue long after hospital discharge, sometimes throughout life. Positioning, exercise, and range of motion are necessary to maintain joint flexibility.

Nurses play a key role in smoothing the transition from the acute care phase of life-saving interventions and frequent dressing changes to normal activities such as school and play. Body image considerations may have a significant impact on the child when he or she returns to school and should be addressed. Children with altered body image as a result of a burn might benefit from regular counseling and group therapy.

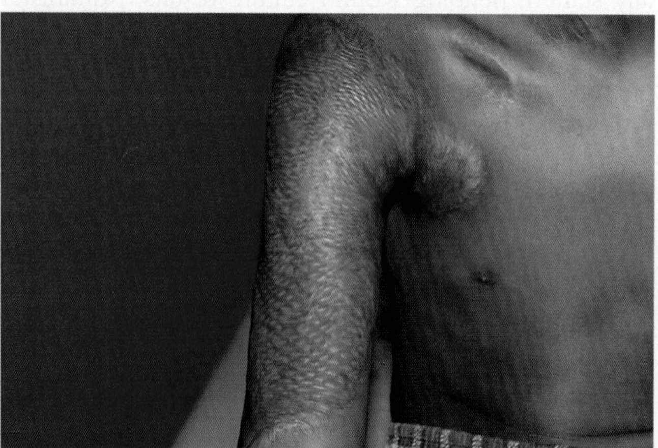

FIGURE 45.22 Healed mesh graft.

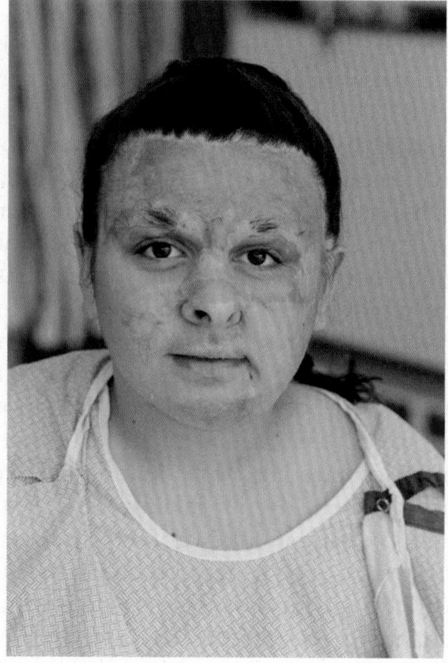

FIGURE 45.23 Extensive grafting to the face.

Parents often need assistance with the behavioral challenges of caring for a child who is recovering from a burn injury. Various websites are available for support of persons who are burned. Links to websites are available on thePoint.

Navigating through life after suffering a serious burn injury can be difficult for the child and family, and a skilled nurse can provide valuable assistance to families during the equally important, but less acute, phase of the journey.

PREVENTING BURNS AND CARBON MONOXIDE POISONING

Instruct parents about prevention of burns. Explain that all homes should have working smoke detectors, and batteries should be changed yearly. Instruct families that all homes should be equipped with fire extinguishers, and adults and older teenagers should be taught how to operate them. Explain that children should sleep in fire-retardant sleepwear, parents should not smoke in the house or the car, and parents should keep lighters and matches out of children's reach. Young children are particularly susceptible to burns that occur in the kitchen, such as scalds from hot liquids and foods and burns from contact with hot burners or oven doors. Caution parents about the extreme danger that fireworks present to children. Teaching Guidelines 45.3 gives additional information for parents related to burn prevention. The booklet "Burn Prevention Tips," which includes a coloring book, is available from the Shriners Hospitals for Children. A link to their website is provided on thePoint.

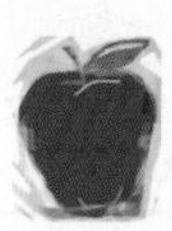

Teaching Guidelines 45.3
BURN PREVENTION

- Keep hot water heater temperature lower than 120°F.
- Test bath water temperature before bathing children.
- Keep children away from open flames, stoves, and candles.
- Cook with pots on the inside of the stove with the handles turned in.
- Keep children away from the stove while cooking.
- Place hot liquids out of reach of children.
- Avoid drinking hot beverages while holding a child.
- Keep curling irons out of reach of children.
- Teach older children how to safely get out of the house in case of fire.
- Practice fire drills.
- Teach children to "stop, drop, and roll" if their clothes catch on fire.

Children are at significant risk for burns related to hot water. Scald burns can occur when hot water comes into contact with the child's skin, even for a relatively short time. Since hot water presents such a serious risk to children, the temperature on all hot water heaters should be 120°F or lower. Figure 45.24 is a graph that shows how long a child can be exposed to water of various temperatures before a burn occurs. For example:

- If the water is 150°F, a child can receive a third-degree burn within 2 seconds.
- If the water is 140°F, it takes 6 seconds of exposure to cause a significant burn.
- If the water is 130°F, a child can be burned significantly in only 30 seconds.
- At 120°F, the recommended maximal home hot water heater temperature, it takes as long as 5 minutes of exposure to burn a person (plenty of time to get out of the tub!) (Accurate Building Inspectors, 2016).

Instruct parents about prevention of carbon monoxide poisoning. All homes should have working carbon monoxide detectors, and batteries should be changed yearly. Teach parents the signs of carbon monoxide poisoning: headaches, dizziness, disorientation, and nausea. If the carbon monoxide detector sounds, turn off any potential sources of combustion, if possible, and evacuate all occupants immediately. Do not attempt to reenter the home until a qualified professional repairs the source of the carbon monoxide leak.

PROVIDING BURN CARE AT HOME

Teach parents about proper burn care in the home. Seek medical attention for burns when:

- The child has a second- or third-degree burn.
- Burns result from a fire, an electrical wire or socket, or chemicals.
- The child has a burn on the face, scalp, hands, feet, or genitals or over the joints.

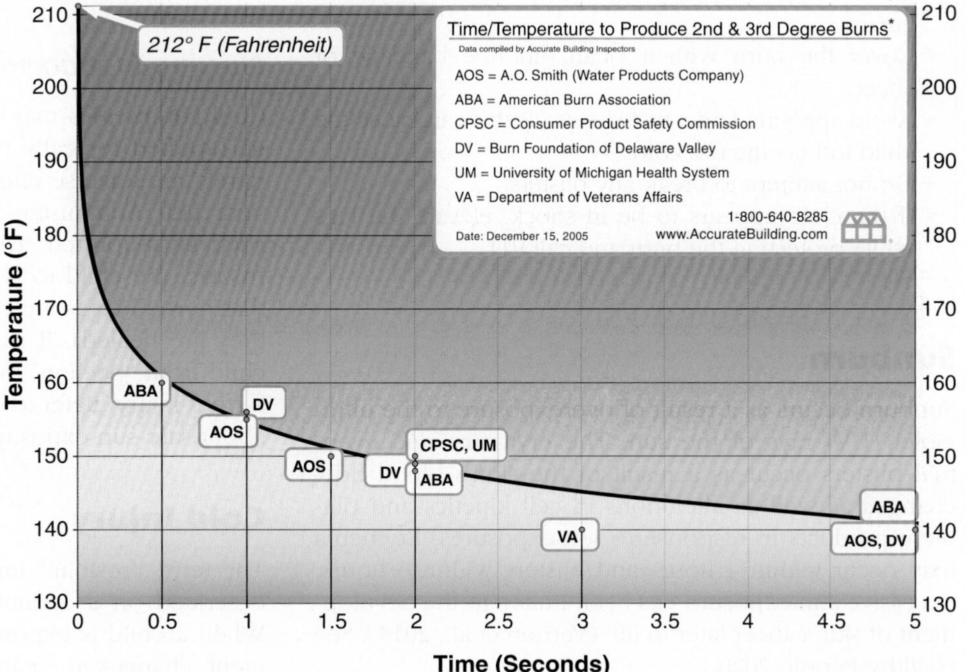

FIGURE 45.24 Length of hot water exposure that results in significant burns based on water temperature. (Used with permission from Accurate Building Inspectors. (2016). *Water temperature thermometry*. Retrieved from http://www.accuratebuilding.com/services/legal/charts/hot_water_burn_scalding_graph.html)

- The burn appears to be infected.
- The burn is causing prolonged and significant pain.
- Concern exists that the burn was a result of abuse.

If the burn is very extensive, even if it appears to be a first-degree burn, seek medical attention immediately. Teaching Guidelines 45.4 gives specific information about burn care at home.

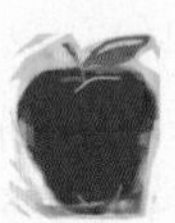

Teaching Guidelines 45.4
PROVIDING BURN CARE AT HOME

For First-Degree (Superficial) Burns

- Run cool water over the burned area until the pain lessens.
- Do not apply ice to the skin.
- Do not apply butter, ointment, or cream.
- Cover the burn lightly with a clean, nonadhesive bandage.
- Administer acetaminophen or ibuprofen for pain.
- Have the child seen by the physician or nurse practitioner within 24 hours.
- Ongoing care: clean in tub or shower with fragrance-free mild soap; pat or air dry.
  - Apply a thin layer of antibiotic ointment.
  - Cover with a nonadherent dressing such as Adaptic, and then cover with dry gauze.

For More Extensive Burns

- Remove clothing only if it comes off easily or if it is still smoldering.
- Check the child's ABCs (airway, breathing, and circulation) and perform cardiopulmonary resuscitation (CPR) if necessary.
- Do not apply butter, ointment, or any other type of cream.
- Cover the burn with a clean, lint-free bandage or sheet.
- Avoid applying large, wet sheets, as this can cause the child to become too cold.
- Do not attempt to break any blisters.
- If the child appears to be in shock, elevate the legs while protecting the burn and call 911.

Sunburn

Sunburn occurs as a result of overexposure to the ultraviolet (UV) rays of the sun. The erythema and eventual blisters occur as a result of the skin's blood flow changes as well as alterations in cell kinetics and pigment products in response to UV exposures. Erythema may occur within 4 hours and blisters within 6 hours. Excessive sun exposure has been linked to the development of skin cancer later in life (Vernon et al., 2013). See Healthy People 2020.

HEALTHY PEOPLE 2020

Objective	Nursing Significance
(Developmental) Increase the proportion of adolescents in grades 9 through 12 who follow protective measures that may reduce the risk of skin cancer.	• Encourage use of sunscreen in all children older than 6 months of age, to form a lifelong habit. • Discourage sun exposure between 10 AM and 2 PM • Inform teens of the hazards of ultraviolet light (even artificial) and discourage the use of tanning beds.

Healthy People Objectives retrieved from http://www.healthypeople.gov

Sunburn is usually treated with cool compresses, cooling lotions, and oral nonsteroidal anti-inflammatory agents.

Nursing Assessment

Obtain the health history, noting recent sun exposure. Determine length of exposure and whether any type of sunscreen or sun block product was used. Note redness of the skin on the exposed areas. More severe areas will have a darker red, slightly purple hue. Blisters may be noted with more severe sunburn.

Nursing Management

Cool compresses may help to cool the burn. Aloe vera gel applied topically may provide significant soothing. Rarely are adverse effects reported with the use of aloe vera gel. Administer a nonsteroidal anti-inflammatory such as ibuprofen. Discourage hot showers or baths. Instruct the child to wear loose clothing and to ensure that burned areas are covered when going outside (until they are healed). If skin flaking occurs, discourage the child from "peeling" the flaked skin in order to prevent further injury. Refer to Chapter 31 for further information about safe sun exposure.

Cold Injury

The term "frostbite" implies freezing of the tissues. It is described on a continuum from first to fourth degree. When a child is exposed to an extremely cold environment, changes in cutaneous circulation help to maintain the core body temperature. Because circulation is shunted to the core, the most peripheral body parts are those at highest risk for frostbite. Local damage occurs when the tissue temperature drops to 32°F (0°C). Initially skin sensation is lost, the vasculature constricts, and plasma leakage occurs. Ice crystals develop in the extracellular fluid, and eventually vascular stasis leads to endothelial cell damage, necrosis, and sloughing of dead tissue.

Nursing Assessment

Note history of cold exposure. Inquire about pain or numbness. Examine the skin for indications of frostbite. First-degree frostbite results in superficial white plaques with surrounding erythema. Second-degree frostbite demonstrates blistering with erythema and edema. In third-degree frostbite, hemorrhagic blisters occur, progressing to tissue necrosis and sloughing in fourth-degree frostbite.

Nursing Management

Remove wet or tight clothing. Avoid vigorous massage to decrease the chance of damaging the skin further. Immerse the affected part in 104°F water for 15 to 30 minutes. Thawing may cause significant pain, so administer analgesics. Keep the thawed part loosely covered, warm, and dry. Splinting may be used to help decrease associated edema. Consult the wound care specialist or plastic surgeon for further management.

Prevent frostbite by:

- Dressing warmly in layers, and keeping warm and dry
- Avoiding exertion
- Not playing outside when wind chill advisories are in effect, and locking doors with high locks to prevent toddlers from going outside

Human and Animal Bites

Yearly, significant emergency room visits occur as a result of bites from mammals. Dog bites account for the majority of injuries, but children may be bitten by other children, cats, or rodents (Hansen & Ahmed, 2010). The hand and face are common locations for animal bites. A dog is most often provoked to bite a child when the child is playing with the dog or when the child hits, kicks, hugs, grabs, or chases the dog.

Therapeutic management involves cleansing and irrigating the wound, wound suturing or stapling if necessary, and administering topical and/or systemic antibiotic therapy. Rabies prophylaxis is indicated if the rabies status of the dog is unknown. Secondary bacterial infection of the bite wound with streptococci, staphylococci, or *Pasteurella multocida* may occur. Cat and human bites are the most likely to become infected (Hansen & Ahmed, 2010).

Nursing Assessment

Determine the history of the attack and whether it was provoked. Determine the child's tetanus vaccination status. Inspect the bite to determine the extent of laceration, avulsion, or crushing injury.

Nursing Management

Provide rabies immunoprophylaxis and a tetanus booster vaccination if indicated. Thoroughly cleanse the wound with soap and water or a povidone–iodine solution. Irrigate the wound well with normal saline after cleansing. If the animal may be rabid, cleanse the wound for at least 10 minutes with a virucidal agent such as povidone–iodine solution. Administer antibiotics as prescribed.

Prevention of animal bites is important. Teach children the following:

- Never provoke a dog with teasing or roughhousing.
- Get adult permission before interacting with a dog, cat, or other animal that is not your pet.
- Do not bother an eating, sleeping, or nursing dog.
- Avoid high-pitched talking or screaming around dogs.
- Display a closed fist first for the dog to sniff.
- Keep ferrets away from the face.
- If a cat hisses or lashes out with the paw, leave it alone

Never leave a child younger than 5 years of age alone with a dog (American Veterinary Medical Association, 2016). Contact the local humane society for a dog bite prevention program that is appropriate for school-age children.

Children may suffer significant emotional distress after being bitten. Nightmares and increased anxiety are common (National Health Service, 2016). Help children through this period by talking about the incident or reading books about this type of event.

Insect Stings and Spider Bites

Members of the Hymenoptera class of insects sting. This class includes bees, wasps, ants, yellow jackets, and hornets. Spiders inject their venom when they bite. Stings and bites usually result in a local reaction. A systemic or anaphylactic reaction to a Hymenoptera sting may also occur, possibly resulting in airway compromise (refer to Chapter 47 for additional information on anaphylaxis). Serious reactions may occur with brown recluse or black widow spider bites. This discussion will focus on local reactions.

Local reactions to insect stings and spider bites include pruritus, pain, and edema. A hypersensitivity reaction thought to be mediated by IgE occurs in response to the venom. This may be a physiologic response to the antigens present in the insect's or spider's saliva and other fluids that are transmitted during stinging or biting. Bacterial superinfection may occur as a complication and as a result of scratching. Therapeutic management includes antihistamines to decrease itching and in some cases corticosteroids to decrease inflammation and swelling.

Nursing Assessment

Obtain the history of the bite or sting. Children are usually acutely aware when they have been stung by an insect, but spiders are generally not observed before the bite. Inspect the bite or sting, noting an urticarial wheal or papular reaction. A large local reaction may be mistaken for cellulitis. Note whether a stinger remains present. Assess the child's work of breathing to determine if a systemic reaction or anaphylaxis is occurring (refer to Chapter 47 http://www.nhs.uk/Conditions/Bites-human-and-animal/Pages/Introduction.aspx).

Nursing Management

Remove jewelry or constrictive clothing if the sting is on an extremity. Cleanse the wound with mild soap and water. If the stinger is present, scrape it away with your fingernail or a credit card. Apply ice intermittently to decrease pain and edema. Administer diphenhydramine as soon as possible after the sting in an attempt to minimize the reaction.

Prevent insect stings and spider bites by wearing protective clothing and shoes when outdoors. Use insect repellants (with a maximum concentration of 30% *n,n*-diethyl-meta-toluamide [DEET] in infants and children older than 2 months) (U.S. Food and Drug Administration, 2014). Teach children never to disturb a bee or wasp nest or an ant hill.

NURSING CARE PLAN 45.1

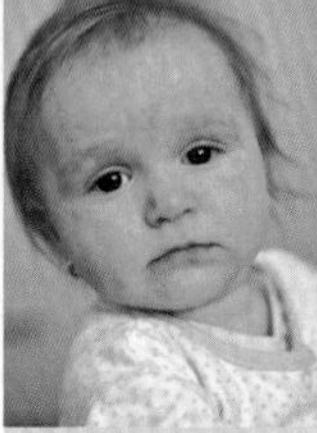

Overview for The Child With an Alteration in Tissue Integrity/Integumentary Disorder

NURSING DIAGNOSIS: Impaired skin integrity related to infectious process, hypersensitivity reaction, injury, or mechanical factors as evidenced by rash, inflammation, abrasion, laceration, or disrupted epidermis

Outcome Identification and Evaluation

Integrity of skin surface will be restored: rash, abrasion, laceration, or other skin disruption will heal.

Interventions: ***Restoring Skin Integrity***

- Assess site of skin impairment to determine extent of involvement and plan care.
- Monitor skin impairment every shift for changes in color, warmth, redness, or other signs of infection to identify problems early.
- Determine the child's and family's skin care practices to establish need for education related to skin care.
- Individualize the child's skin care regimen depending on the child's particular skin condition to most appropriately care for skin in light of the child's disorder.
- In the immobile child, use a risk assessment tool (such as a modified Norton or Braden Q scale) to identify risk for skin breakdown.
- Position the child on the opposite side of the skin impairment to avoid further skin breakdown.
- Encourage appropriate nutritional intake as adequate nutrients are necessary for appropriate immune function and skin healing.
- Consult the wound and ostomy care nurse specialist to determine the best approach for individualized wound care.
- Provide dressing change and wound care as prescribed to promote wound or burn healing.

NURSING DIAGNOSIS: Risk for infection related to disruption in protective skin barrier

Outcome Identification and Evaluation

Child will remain free from local or systemic infection, will remain afebrile, *without additional redness or warmth at skin disruption site.*

NURSING CARE PLAN 45.1

Overview for The Child With an Alteration in Tissue Integrity/Integumentary Disorder (continued)

Interventions: ***Preventing Infection***

- Use appropriate hand hygiene to decrease transmission of infectious organisms.
- Assess the skin impairment site for increased warmth, redness, discharge, or new purulence to identify infection early.
- Assess temperature every 4 hours or more frequently if needed, as children develop fever quickly in response to infection.
- Note white blood cell (WBC) count and culture results, reporting unexpected values to the physician or nurse practitioner so that appropriate treatment may be started.
- Follow prescribed therapies for skin alteration to maintain skin moisture and prevent further breakdown, which may lead to infection.
- Encourage appropriate nutritional intake as adequate nutrients are necessary for appropriate immune function and skin healing.

NURSING DIAGNOSIS: Disturbed body image related to chronic skin changes caused by disease process, burns, or other skin alteration as evidenced by child's verbalization, reluctance to participate in activities, or social withdrawal

Outcome Identification and Evaluation

Child will verbalize or demonstrate acceptance of alteration in body, *will return to previous level of social involvement.*

Interventions: ***Promoting Appropriate Body Image***

- Assess child or teen for feelings about alteration in skin *to determine baseline.*
- Acknowledge feelings of anger or depression related to skin changes *to provide an outlet for feelings.*
- Encourage the child or teen to participate in skin care *to give some sense of control over what is occurring.*
- Help the child or teen to accept self *as the perception of self is tied to knowing oneself and identifying what the self values.*

NURSING DIAGNOSIS: Risk for deficient fluid volume related to burns

Outcome Identification and Evaluation

Fluid volume status will be balanced, *child will maintain urine output of 1 to 2 mL/kg/hr, oral mucosa will be moist and pink, heart rate will remain within age- and situation-specific parameters.*

Interventions: ***Promoting Fluid Balance***

- Assess fluid volume status at least every shift, more frequently if disrupted, *to obtain baseline for comparison.*
- Strictly monitor intake and output *to detect imbalance or need for additional fluid intake.*
- Weigh the child daily on the same scale, at the same time, in the same amount of clothing *as changes in weight are an accurate indicator of fluid volume status in children.*
- Provide intravenous fluid resuscitation in initial period, followed by encouragement of oral fluid intake in the burned child, *to compensate for fluid loss through burned areas.*

(continued)

NURSING CARE PLAN 45.1

Overview for The Child With an Alteration in Tissue Integrity/Integumentary Disorder (continued)

NURSING DIAGNOSIS: Imbalanced nutrition, less than body requirements, related to increased metabolic state (burns) as evidenced by poor wound healing, difficulty gaining or maintaining body weight

Outcome Identification and Evaluation

Child will demonstrate balanced nutritional state, *will maintain or gain weight as appropriate for situation, will demonstrate improvement in wound healing.*

Interventions: ***Promoting Nutrition***

- Assess the child's food preferences and ability to eat *to provide a baseline for planning nursing care.*
- Consult the nutritionist *because nutritional needs are increased related to altered metabolic state as a result of burns.*
- Collaborate with the nutritionist, child, and parents to plan meals that appeal to the child *to increase the child's intake.*
- Administer vitamin and mineral preparations as prescribed *to supplement nutrients.*
- Provide smaller, more frequent meals and snacks *to promote increased intake.*
- Weigh the child daily *to determine progress.*

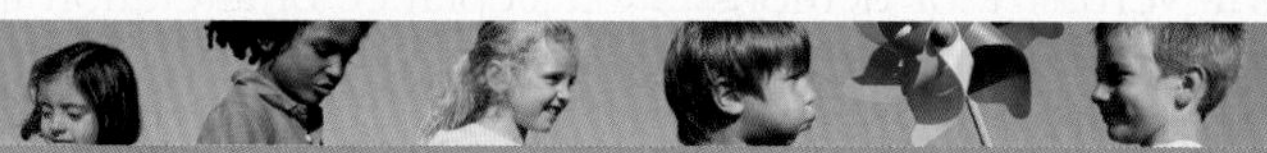

KEY CONCEPTS

- The infant's epidermis is thinner, loses heat more readily, absorbs substances more easily, and is more accessible to bacterial invasion than the skin of the adult. The increased water content of the infant's skin compared with the adult's places the infant at increased risk of blister development and other skin alterations.
- The child's skin thickness and characteristics reach adult levels in the late teenage years.
- Children with dark skin tend to have more pronounced cutaneous reactions than children with lighter skin.
- Sebum production increases in the preadolescent and adolescent years, contributing to the development of acne at that time.
- Most bacterial skin infections are caused by *Staphylococcus aureus* and group A β-hemolytic streptococcus.
- Skin scrapings placed on a slide and prepared with potassium chloride may be evaluated microscopically to determine the presence of fungus.
- Fungal skin infections, referred to collectively as tinea, may require up to several weeks of treatment.
- Contact dermatitis and atopic dermatitis both present as pruritic rashes, whereas psoriasis is generally nonpruritic.
- Hypersensitivity responses may result in erythema multiforme or urticaria.
- Scaling may occur with atopic dermatitis and psoriasis, whereas honey-colored crusting is common with impetigo. Erythema is a common finding with many skin disorders in children.
- Burns may result in significant weeping and fluid loss.
- Keeping the skin well moisturized is a key intervention in the management of atopic dermatitis and psoriasis.
- Appropriate hygiene is of particular importance in integumentary disorders.
- Pain management, prevention of infection, and rehabilitation are the focus of nursing management for the burned child.
- The constant itch–rash–itch cycle of atopic dermatitis may have a considerable impact on the child's sleep, school functioning, and self-esteem.
- Acne vulgaris, particularly if moderate or severe, may have a significant negative effect on the teen's self-esteem.

- Teach children with chronic disorders such as atopic dermatitis, psoriasis, and acne (and their parents) to cleanse and moisturize the skin properly, avoid particular skin irritants, and use medications appropriately.
- Many skin disorders are preventable. Teach families how to prevent contact dermatitis, burns, sunburn, frostbite, and bites and stings.
- Educate children and families about the importance of good soap-and-water cleansing of all minor skin injuries.

REFERENCES AND RECOMMENDED READINGS

Accurate Building Inspectors. (2016). *Water temperature thermometry*. Retrieved from http://www.accuratebuilding.com/services/legal/charts/hot_water_burn_scalding_graph.html

American Veterinary Medical Association. (2016). *Dog bite prevention*. Retrieved from https://www.avma.org/public/Pages/Dog-Bite-Prevention.aspx

Baddour, L. M. (2015). *Impetigo*. Retrieved from http://www.uptodate.com/contents/impetigo

Barron, S. (2015). *Burns*. Retrieved from http://kidshealth.org/en/parents/burns.html

Berman, K. (2015). *Acne*. Retrieved from http://umm.edu/health/medical/ency/articles/acne

Carpenito-Moyet, L. J. (2013). *Nursing diagnosis: Application to clinical practice* (14th ed.). Philadelphia, PA: Lippincott Williams & Wilkins.

Centers for Disease Control and Prevention. (2016). *Ten leading causes of death and injury*. Retrieved from http://www.cdc.gov/injury/wisqars/leadingcauses.html

Corbett, J. A., & Banks, A. D. (2013). *Laboratory tests and diagnostic procedures with nursing diagnoses* (8th ed.). Upper Saddle River, NJ: Pearson Education Inc.

Diamond, J. S., Abdoo, D. C., Brady, M. A., & Dunn, A. M. (2013). Role relationships. In C. Burns, A. Dunn, M. Brady, N. B. Starr, & C. Blosser (Eds.), *Pediatric primary care* (5th ed.). Philadelphia, PA: Saunders.

Edlich, R. F., Long, W. B., & Gubler, K. D. (2016). *Cold injuries*. Retrieved from http://emedicine.medscape.com/article/1278523-overview

Ehrlich, S. D. (2015a). *Calendula*. Retrieved from http://umm.edu/health/medical/altmed/herb/calendula

Ehrlich, S. D. (2015b). *Evening primrose oil*. Retrieved from http://umm.edu/health/medical/altmed/herb/evening-primrose-oil.

Garlich, F. M., & Nelson, L. S. (2011). Inhalation of baby powder. *Emergency Medicine, 43*(1), 17–20.

Garzon, D. L., Degolier, S. D., & Brehm, C. B. (2013). Common injuries. In C. Burns, A. Dunn, M. Brady, N. B. Starr, & C. Blosser (Eds.), *Pediatric primary care* (5th ed.). Philadelphia, PA: Saunders.

Hansen, J. J., & Ahmed, A. (2010). Emergent management of bite wounds. *Emergency Medicine, 42*(6), 6–11.

Herzing University—Orlando. (2014). *ASN/BSN concept definitions*. Winter Park, FL: Author.

Joffe, M. D. (2015). Emergency care of moderate and severe thermal burns in children. Retrieved from http://www.uptodate.com/contents/emergency-care-of-moderate-and-severe-thermal-burns-in-children

John, R. M., & Brady, M. A. (2013). Atopic and rheumatic disorders. In C. Burns, A. Dunn, M. Brady, N. B. Starr, & C. Blosser (Eds.), *Pediatric primary care* (5th ed.). Philadelphia, PA: Saunders.

Kiss, E. A., & Heiler, M. (2014). Pediatric skin integrity practice guideline for institutional use: A quality improvement project. *Journal of Pediatric Nursing, 29*, 362–357.

Li, A., Montano, Z., Chen, V. J., & Gold, J. I. (2011). Virtual reality and pain management: Current trends and future directions. *Pain Management, 1*(2), 147–157.

Magin, P., Adams, J., Heading, G., Pond, D., & Smith, W. (2008). Experiences of appearance-related teasing and bullying in skin disease and their psychological sequelae: Results of a qualitative study. *Scandinavian Journal of Caring Sciences, 22*(3), 430–435.

Mechem, C. C. (2016). *Pulse oximetry in adults*. Retrieved from http://www.uptodate.com/contents/pulse-oximetry.

Morelli, J. G., & Prok, L. D. (2014). Skin. In W. W. Hay, M. J. Levin, R. R. Deterding, & M. J. Abzug (Eds.), (*Current pediatric diagnosis and treatment* (22nd ed.). New York, NY: McGraw-Hill.

Myers, T. (2011). When to treat or refer a burn-injured patient. *Clinical Advisor, 14*(7), 31–36.

National Health Service. (2016). *Animal and human bites*. Retrieved from http://www.nhs.uk/Conditions/Bites-human-and-animal/Pages/Introduction.aspx

Nirken, M. H., High, W. A., & Roujeau, J. C. (2015). *Stevens-Johnson syndrome and toxic epidermal necrolysis: Pathogenesis, clinical manifestations, and diagnosis*. Retrieved from http://www.uptodate.com/contents/stevens-johnson-syndrome-and-toxic-epidermal-necrolysis-pathogenesis-clinical-manifestations-and-diagnosis

Pardo, G. D., Garcia, I. M., & Gomez-Cia, T. (2010). Psychological effects observed in child burn patients during the acute phase of hospitalization and comparison with pediatric patients awaiting surgery. *Journal of Burn Care & Research, 31*(4), 569–578.

Quilty, J. (2010, May). *Pediatric burn management*. Presented at meeting of the Florida Chapter of the National Association of Pediatric Nurse Practitioners, Orlando, FL.

Sasseville, D. (2015). *Cradle cap and seborrheic dermatitis in infants*. Retrieved from http://www.uptodate.com/contents/cradle-cap-and-seborrheic-dermatitis-in-infants.

Schindler, C. A., Mikhailov, T. A., Kuhn, E. M., Christopher, J., Conway, P., Ridling, D., et al. (2011). Protecting fragile skin: Nursing interventions to decrease development of pressure ulcers in pediatric intensive care. *American Journal of Critical Care, 20*(1), 26–35.

Taketomo, C. K., Hodding, J. H., & Kraus, D. M. (2013). *Pediatric & neonatal dosage handbook* (20th ed.). Hudson, OH: Lexicomp.

U.S. Food and Drug Administration. (2016). *Insect repellant use and safety in children*. Retrieved from http://www.fda.gov/Drugs/EmergencyPreparedness/ucm085277.htm

Vernon, P., Brady, M. A., Starr, N. B., & Petersen-Smith, A. M. (2013). Dermatologic disorders. In C. Burns, A. Dunn, M. Brady, N. B. Starr, & C. Blosser (Eds.), *Pediatric primary care* (5th ed.). Philadelphia, PA: Saunders.

CHAPTER WORKSHEET

MULTIPLE CHOICE QUESTIONS

1. The nurse is teaching about skin care for atopic dermatitis. Which statement by the parent indicates that further teaching may be necessary?
   a. "I will use Vaseline or Crisco to moisturize my child's skin."
   b. "A hot bath will soothe my child's itching when it is severe."
   c. "I will buy cotton rather than wool or synthetic clothing for my child."
   d. "I will apply a small amount of the prescribed cream after the bath."
2. The nurse is caring for a child who has received significant partial-thickness burns to the lower body. What is the priority assessment in the first 24 hours after injury?
   a. fluid balance
   b. wound infection
   c. respiratory arrest
   d. separation anxiety
3. The nurse is caring for a child in the emergency department who was bitten by the family dog, who is fully immunized. What is the priority nursing action?
   a. Administer rabies immunoglobulin.
   b. Refer the child to a counselor.
   c. Assess the depth and extent of the wound.
   d. Administer a tetanus booster.
4. The nurse is caring for an infant on the pediatric unit who has a very red rash in the diaper area, with red lesions scattered on the abdomen and thighs. What is the priority nursing intervention?
   a. Administer griseofulvin with a fatty meal.
   b. Institute contact isolation precautions.
   c. Apply topical antibiotic cream.
   d. Apply topical antifungal cream.
5. A varsity high-school wrestler presents with a "rug burn" type of rash on his shoulder that is not healing as expected, despite use of triple antibiotic cream. Two other wrestlers on his team have a similar abrasion. What infection should the nurse be most concerned about, based on the history?
   a. tinea cruris
   b. MRSA
   c. impetigo
   d. tinea versicolor

DOSAGE CALCULATION QUESTION

1. The nurse is caring for a child who has tinea corporis. The child weighs 18 lb 11 oz. The medication order reads: griseofulvin 85 mg PO every day. Griseofulvin is supplied as 125 mg/5 mL. How many milliliters will the nurse administer? Round to the nearest tenth.

CRITICAL THINKING EXERCISES

1. A 4-year-old presents with his mother for evaluation of a yellowish, runny sore on his head. What questions would be most appropriate to ask the mother when taking the history? Should this child be placed in isolation? If so, why?
2. An 11-month-old comes to the primary care office with his mother for evaluation of a significant flaking red rash on both cheeks. The child is diagnosed with atopic dermatitis. What additional information should be obtained in the health history? What information should be included in the teaching plan for this family?

STUDY ACTIVITIES

1. Plan an educational activity:
   a. For parents of babies about the treatment and prevention of diaper dermatitis
   b. For parents of school-age children about prevention of contact dermatitis (related to poison ivy)
2. During your clinical rotation, spend a day with the wound and ostomy care nurse in a children's hospital. Report to the clinical group about what you learned that day.
3. Talk to teenagers with severe acne, atopic dermatitis, or psoriasis about their feelings about their skin's appearance. Reflect on this information in your clinical journal.

BRINGING IT ALL TOGETHER: A CASE STUDY

Mary Stillman, a 3-year-old girl, is brought to the clinic by her mother for worsening of her atopic dermatitis. During your assessment the mother states that even though the doctor told her that milk makes Mary's skin worse, she likes it so much, she just can't take it away from her.

Go to thePoint to find questions to consider about this case.

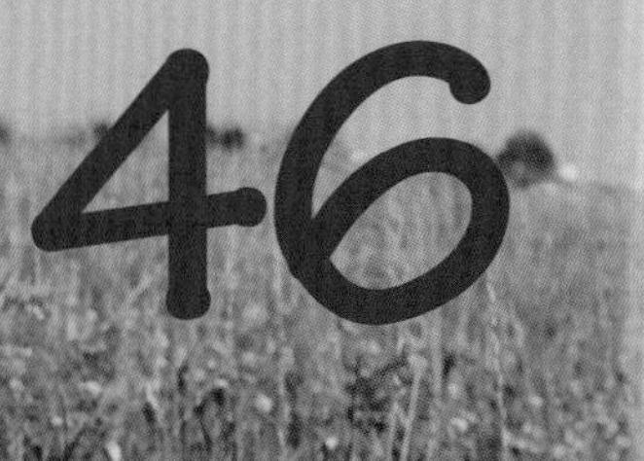

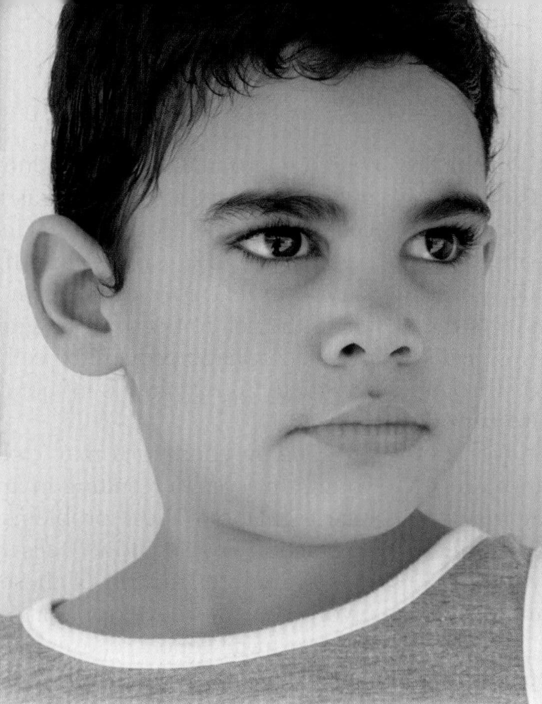

46

WOW

Words of Wisdom

Be inspired by the courage of a child with cancer and reflect it in the care you provide.

Nursing Care of the Child With an Alteration in Cellular Regulation/Hematologic or Neoplastic Disorder

KEY TERMS

anemia
anisocytosis
biopsy
chelation therapy
chemotherapy
clinical trial
extravasation
hematocrit
hemoglobin
hemosiderosis
hypochromic
macrocytic
malignant
metastasis
microcytic
neoplastic
petechiae
platelet count
platelets
poikilocytosis
polycythemia
purpura
red blood cell (RBC)
splenomegaly
staging
white blood cell (WBC)

Learning Objectives

Upon completion of the chapter, you will be able to:

1. Identify major hematologic disorders that affect children.
2. Compare childhood and adult cancers.
3. Identify types of cancer common in infants, children, and adolescents.
4. Determine priority assessment information for children with alterations in cellular regulation/hematologic and neoplastic disorders.
5. Analyze laboratory data and describe nursing care related to common laboratory and diagnostic testing used in alterations in cellular regulation/hematologic and neoplastic disorders.
6. Develop an individualized nursing care plan for the child with cancer or a hematologic disorder.
7. Identify priority interventions for children with alterations in cellular regulation.
8. Develop a teaching plan for the family of children with hematologic disorders or cancer.
9. Devise a nutrition plan for the child with cancer.
10. Describe the psychosocial impact of cancer on children and their families.
11. Identify resources for children and families with hematologic disorders, nutrition deficits, or cancer.

***Shaun O'Malley*, 10 months old, is being admitted to the pediatric unit after being brought to the clinic by his father for a small laceration that he thought needed stitches. His father states, "I didn't think the cut was very deep. I was surprised by how long it bled."**

Cellular regulation is the process by which cells replicate, proliferate, and grow. The hematologic system is integrally involved in the process of cellular regulation. The hematologic system consists of the blood and blood-forming tissues of the body. These typically function together in a balance that affects the metabolism of the body. The three categories of cells are erythrocytes, or **red blood cells (RBCs)**; thrombocytes, or platelets; and leukocytes, or **white blood cells (WBCs)**. RBCs are responsible for transporting nutrients and oxygen to the body tissues and waste products from the tissues. The platelets are responsible for clotting. WBCs are responsible for fighting infection. WBCs are further divided into granulocytes (neutrophils, eosinophils, and basophils) and agranulocytes (lymphocytes and monocytes).

All blood cells originate from a single type of cell called a multipotent stem cell, which goes on to differentiate into the various types of blood cells. Thrombopoietin (TPO) and interleukin-7 (IL-7) act on the cell and differentiate the cell into either myeloid or lymphoid progenitor cells. The lymphoid cells either, under the influence of IL-6, become B lymphocytes or change directly into T lymphocytes. The myeloid cells are differentiated in one of two ways, either by the action of erythropoietin (EPO) or granulocyte–monocyte colony-stimulating factor (GM-CSF). When the cell is acted upon by EPO, which is produced by the kidneys, the cell becomes the megakaryocyte, also known as the erythroid progenitor cell. The megakaryocyte is acted on by either EPO, to become the RBC, or TPO and IL-11, to become a megakaryocyte that goes on to form platelets. GM-CSF influences the cell to become the granulocyte, also known as the macrophage progenitor cell. These cells further differentiate under various influences to become the WBCs (Fig. 46.1).

Certain conditions may cause problems to develop within this system resulting in an alteration in blood cellular regulation. These problems are related to either the production of the blood cells (too much or too little) or loss and destruction of these cells. Many factors are involved in the development of hematologic disorders, ranging from genetic causes to disorders resulting from injury, infection, or nutritional deficit.

Neoplastic (referring to cells that abnormally proliferate) disorders are also alterations in cellular regulation. **Cancer** results from an alteration in cellular regulation resulting in out-of-control cell growth. Cancer accounts for the most deaths from disease in children older than 1 year of age. Cure has been achieved in some children with childhood leukemia and other cancers, but there is no universal long-term cure available for any of the childhood cancers. However, the 5-year survival rate for all cancers in children is 80% (Baggott, 2010).

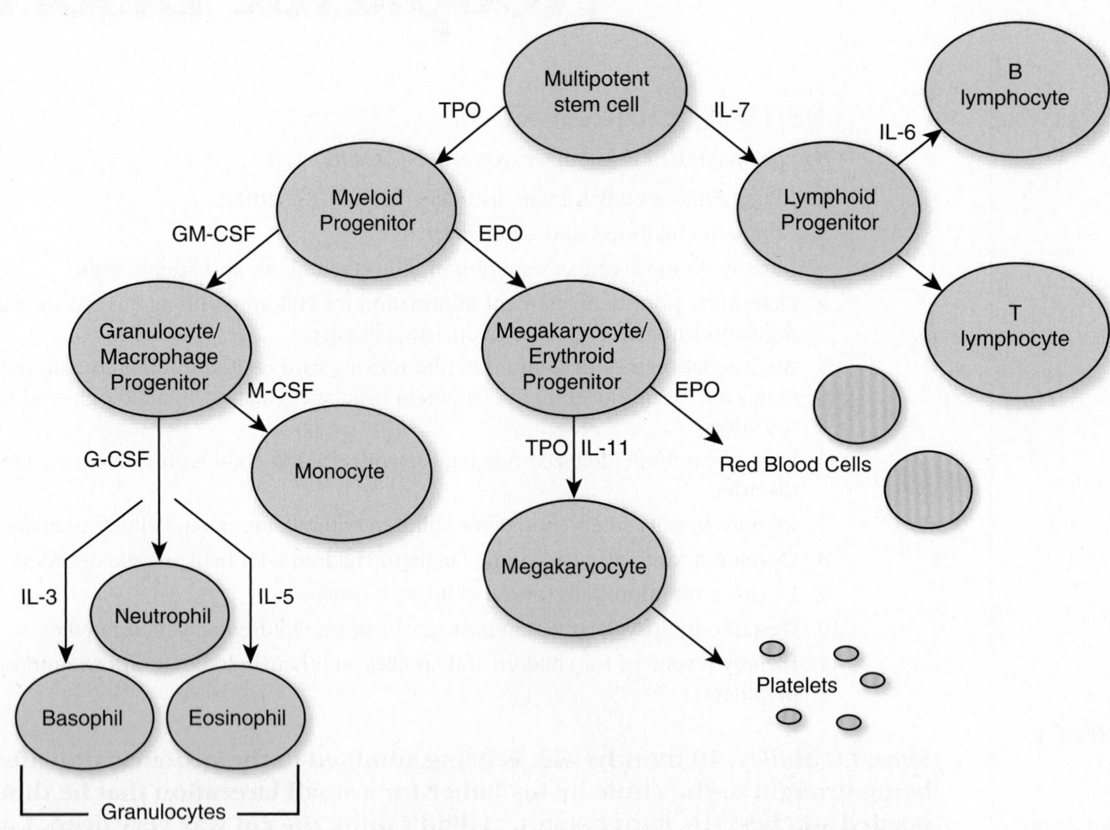

FIGURE 46.1 Process of blood cell formation.

Cancer is a life-threatening illness that involves emotional distress, fear of the unknown, and changes in life priorities for the child and family. Initial and ongoing diagnostic testing and the adverse effects of treatment for cancer, including chemotherapy, radiation, surgery, or other treatments, are often painful as well. Management of cancer also has a significant psychosocial impact on the child or adolescent. Children with cancer are at risk for distress because they have a life-threatening illness and must undergo frequent and stressful tests and treatments (National Cancer Institute, 2016). In addition, the child often feels isolated from his or her peers, and the adolescent may have difficulty achieving independence, which is the core developmental task of the teenage years. Children and teens with cancer often demonstrate poorer school performance compared to healthy peers.

Nursing care for the child with a hematologic disorder is often multifaceted. A child who has iron-deficiency anemia requires adequate oxygenation and may require packed red blood cells (PRBCs); a child with hemophilia requires factor replacement and monitoring for safety. Nursing care for the child with cancer is also complex. Nurses caring for children with cellular regulation alterations such as cancer and hematologic disorders need not only be knowledgeable about the medical treatment of the disease (including adverse effects) but must also be able to effectively intervene with these children. Nurses need to be particularly aware of the psychosocial and emotional impact of cancer or a chronic hematologic disorder on the child and family.

VARIATIONS IN PEDIATRIC ANATOMY AND PHYSIOLOGY

In the absence of a congenital defect, the hematologic system is intact and functional at birth. RBC and hemoglobin production as well as iron stores undergo changes in the first few months of life; after this time, hematologic function is stable.

Red Blood Cell Production

The production of blood cells in the embryo begins by 8 weeks' gestation. In the embryo, blood cells primarily form in the liver; this continues until a few weeks before delivery. Some cell production, lymphoid cells in particular, takes place in the spleen of the embryo, and the thymus is a site for some transient lymphocyte production. EPO, the hormone that regulates RBC production, is derived primarily from the liver in the fetus, and after birth the kidneys take over this production.

Hemoglobin

Three types of normal **hemoglobin** (Hgb) are present at any given time in the blood: Hgb A, Hgb F or fetal, and Hgb A_2. After 6 months of age, Hgb A is the predominant type. In the neonatal period, the largest difference is with the RBCs. Fetal hemoglobin, which has a much shorter cell life, is present in higher quantities, putting the infant at risk for anemia and leading to problems with the oxygen-carrying capacity of the blood. As the production of the cells transfers from the liver to the bone marrow of the long and flat bones, the balance between oxygenation and production is affected.

Iron

The fetus receives iron through the placenta from the mother. The preterm infant misses out on the final weeks or months of transplacental iron transfer, putting him or her at increased risk for anemia (Cunningham et al., 2014). In the term infant, a period of physiologic anemia occurs between the age of 2 and 6 months. This is due to the fact that the infant demonstrates rapid growth and an increase in blood volume over the first several months of life, and maternally derived iron stores are depleted by 4 to 6 months of age. Sufficient iron intake is critical for the appropriate development of hemoglobin and RBCs. Therefore, the infant must ingest adequate quantities of iron either from breast milk or from iron-fortified formula in early infancy and other food sources in later infancy (Bryant, 2010). Adolescence is also a time of rapid growth, and intake of iron must increase.

CHILDHOOD CANCER VERSUS ADULT CANCER

Cancers in children differ greatly from cancers in adults. Pediatric cancers most often arise from primitive embryonal (mesodermal) and neuroectodermal tissues, resulting in leukemias, lymphomas, sarcomas, or central nervous system (CNS) tumors (American Cancer Society, 2015). This is in direct contrast to adult cancers, which mostly arise from epithelial cells, resulting in carcinomas. The most common childhood cancers, in order of frequency, are leukemia, CNS tumors, lymphoma, neuroblastoma, rhabdomyosarcoma, Wilms tumor, bone tumors, and retinoblastoma. Comparison Chart 46.1 explains how cancer is different in children versus adults.

In children, warning signs of cancer are most often related to changes in blood cell production or as a result of compression, infiltration, or obstruction caused by the tumor. Changes in blood cell production may result in fatigue, pallor, frequent or severe infection, or easy bruising. Infiltration, obstruction, or compression by a tumor may result in bone or abdominal pain, pain in other parts of the body, swelling, or unusual discharge.

COMPARISON CHART 46.1 CHILDHOOD CANCER VERSUS ADULT CANCER

	Childhood Cancer	Adult Cancer
Cancer usually affects	Tissues	Organs
Histologic type	Embryonal, leukemia, lymphoma	Epithelial in origin
Most common sites	Blood, lymph, brain, bone, kidney, muscle	Breast, lung, prostate, bowel, bladder
Environmental and lifestyle factors	Only a small amount of environmental influence proven	Strong influence on cancer development
Cancer prevention	Little known	80% preventable
Detection	Usually incidental or accidental	Very early detection possible if screening recommendations followed
Latent period	Relatively short	Can be very long (20 years or greater)
Extent of disease	Metastasis often present at diagnosis	Metastasis less often present at diagnosis
Response to treatment	Very responsive	Less responsive

Adapted from American Cancer Society. (2015). *Cancer in children*. Retrieved from http://www.cancer.org/acs/groups/cid/documents/webcontent/002287-pdf.pdf

COMMON MEDICAL TREATMENTS

Various medications as well as other medical treatments are used to treat hematologic and neoplastic disorders in children. Most of these treatments will require a physician's or nurse practitioner's order when the child is in the hospital. Deciding on a course of medical treatment for cancer in a developing child is complicated. Some of the treatments can impair the child's growth and development. Many pediatric oncologists and cancer treatment centers are active members of the Children's Oncology Group (COG), a National Cancer Institute–supported group that approves and administers clinical trials devoted exclusively to childhood and adolescent cancer research. A **clinical trial** is a carefully designed research study that assesses the effectiveness of a treatment as well as its acute and long-term effects on the child. Current cancer care in children is a result of the knowledge gained through clinical trials. A clinical trial may include existing medications or treatments in combination with new drugs or may involve a different approach to sequencing or dosing of medications and treatment (Dzolganovski, 2010).

To provide optimal outcomes, the child with cancer should be treated at an institution with multidisciplinary cancer care specialists that can provide the most advanced care available. Each case of pediatric cancer should be considered individually, with the oncology healthcare team and the family reaching treatment decisions together, whether the treatment plan is standard or involves enrollment in a clinical trial.

In the child with cancer, particularly advanced disease, the decision to provide treatment ("let's do everything we can") or to withhold treatment in the event of an extremely poor prognosis is extraordinarily challenging in an ethical sense. A mature older child or adolescent may have a strong desire to continue or discontinue treatment, and sometimes this desire conflicts with the parents' desires or choices. The American Academy of Pediatrics (AAP) Committee on Bioethics (2011) recommends that decision making for older children and adolescents should include the assent of the older child or adolescent (Box 46.1).

HEALTHY PEOPLE 2020

Objective	Nursing Significance
Increase the proportion of persons who participate in behaviors that reduce their exposure to harmful ultraviolet (UV) irradiation and avoid sunburn.	• Educate families to start skin protection from the sun in childhood to reduce the risk of skin cancer as an adult. • Teach parents to use PABA-free sunscreen (formulated specifically for children) after age 6 months with an SPF of 15 or greater and to reapply sunscreen frequently while the child is out of doors. • Advocate for schools to encourage a sun-safe environment.

Healthy People Objectives retrieved from http://www.healthypeople.gov

BOX 46.1

AMERICAN ACADEMY OF PEDIATRICS COMMITTEE ON BIOETHICS RECOMMENDATIONS REGARDING PEDIATRIC ASSENT

- Give consideration to each child's developmental capacity, rationality, and autonomy.
- Help each child to achieve a developmentally appropriate understanding of the illness.
- Tell the child what he or she can expect regarding testing procedures and treatments.
- Assess the child's understanding of the situation and how he or she is responding.
- Note if there is inappropriate pressure to assent to testing or treatment.
- Seriously solicit the child's expression of willingness to accept the proposed plan of care.

American Academy of Pediatrics, Committee on Bioethics. (2011). *Informed consent, parental permission, and assent in pediatric practice*. Retrieved from http://pediatrics.aappublications.org/content/95/2/314

Hospice or palliative care may be needed for the child with cancer. Children facing the end of life experience the same symptoms that adults do, including pain, fatigue, nausea, and dyspnea. Standards for end-of-life care are still in development, but all dying children have the right to die comfortably and with palliation of symptoms, as has been well established in adult hospice programs. Children's Hospice International (CHI) has demonstration models in several U.S. states that focus on enhancing the quality of life of children with life-threatening conditions. Formerly, only children with a life expectancy of less than 6 months had access to hospice care, and they were required to forego curative care to enroll in hospice. CHI's goal is to provide a comprehensive, interdisciplinary continuum of care to the child and family from the time of diagnosis with a life-threatening condition through the time of death, if cure is not achieved (CHI, 2011). For further information related to nursing care of the dying child, refer to Chapter 34.

Commonly, chemotherapy and radiation therapy are used to treat childhood cancers. In some instances, hematopoietic stem cell transplantation is used. The nurse caring for the child with cancer should be familiar with the procedures, how the treatments and medications work, and common nursing implications related to use of these modalities. The most common treatments and medications are listed in Common Medical Treatments 46.1 and Drug Guide 46.1. The nurse caring for the child with a hematologic disorder or cancer should be familiar with the procedures used, how the medications work, and common nursing implications related to their use.

(text continues on page 1786)

COMMON MEDICAL TREATMENTS 46.1

Treatment	Explanation	Indications	Nursing Implications
Blood product transfusion	Intravenous administration of whole blood, packed red blood cells (PRBCs), platelets, or plasma	PRBCs: severe anemia, thalassemia, sickle cell disease Whole blood: acute hemorrhage or trauma Fresh-frozen plasma: hemophilia Platelets: thrombocytopenia	Follow institution's transfusion protocol Double-check blood type and product label with a second nurse Use only leukodepleted, CMV-negative blood products in the child with a hemoglobinopathy or cancer Monitor vital signs and assess child frequently to detect adverse reaction to blood transfusion If adverse reaction is suspected, immediately discontinue transfusion, run normal saline IV, reassess the child, and notify the physician Some children require premedication with diphenhydramine and/or acetaminophen before receiving blood products
Leukapheresis	Whole blood is removed from the body, the WBCs are extracted, and then the blood is retransfused into the child	Hyperviscosity with leukemia (WBC >100,000)	Performed by specially trained personnel Monitor blood pressure and other vital signs

(continued)

COMMON MEDICAL TREATMENTS 46.1 (continued)

Treatment	Explanation	Indications	Nursing Implications
Hematopoietic stem cell transplantation	Bone marrow transplant: transfer of healthy bone marrow into a child with disease; the transplanted cells can then develop into functional cells Stem cell transplant: Peripheral stem cells are removed from the donor via apheresis, or stem cells are retrieved from the umbilical cord and placenta. The stem cells are then transplanted into the recipient	Leukemia, lymphoma, other cancers, sickle cell disease, aplastic anemias, thalassemia	Maintain medical asepsis and protective isolation to prevent infection Monitor closely for graft-versus-host disease Provide meticulous oral care Avoid taking rectal temperatures and inserting suppositories Encourage appropriate nutrition Administer immunosuppressive medications as ordered
Supplemental oxygen	Administration of oxygen via mask, cannula, or blow-by	Hypoxia associated with sickle cell crisis or severe anemia	Frequently monitor work of breathing, oxygen saturation via pulse oximetry, cardiopulmonary status, and level of consciousness
Biopsy	A small piece of the tumor is removed with a needle or via an open incision	Solid tumors	Monitor for bleeding at the needle biopsy site Provide routine incision care for open biopsy site
Splenectomy	Surgical removal of the spleen	Life-threatening or recurrent splenic sequestration of sickle cell disease; thalassemia	Provide immunization against the following organisms, because they place the child at risk for overwhelming infection: *Streptococcus pneumoniae*, *Neisseria meningitidis*, and *Haemophilus influenzae* type B Monitor carefully for signs of infection Administer prophylactic antibiotics Instruct child or teen to wear medical alert bracelet Teach families to seek medical treatment at first sign of infection or fever
Surgical removal of tumor	The tumor is completely or partially resected surgically	Solid tumors	Provide routine postoperative nursing care based on the location of the tumor excision
Radiation therapy	Ionizing radiation (high-energy x-ray) is delivered to the cancerous area. The radiation damages all cells in the locally treated area (normal and cancerous), but the normal cells are able to repair themselves. Usually administered several times a week for several weeks (a short rest between treatments allows the normal cells time to regenerate). The lowest possible dose of radiation is used and it is directed to a specific area	Solid tumors, before or after surgical resection, leukemia, lymphoma	Do not wash off radiation marking Keep skin clean and dry Fatigue is a common side effect Skin at the site of radiation may become red, dry, or pruritic or may peel; eventually may become moist and red Mucositis, dry mouth, and loss of taste may occur if head or neck radiated Radiation may also have adverse effects on the organ irradiated, such as the brain; monitor for changes

COMMON MEDICAL TREATMENTS 46.1 (continued)

<table>
<tr><th>Treatment</th><th>Explanation</th><th>Indications</th><th>Nursing Implications</th></tr>
<tr><td>Central venous catheter (see image A)</td><td>IV catheters are inserted into the central circulation for the purpose of administering medications, total parenteral medication, or blood products
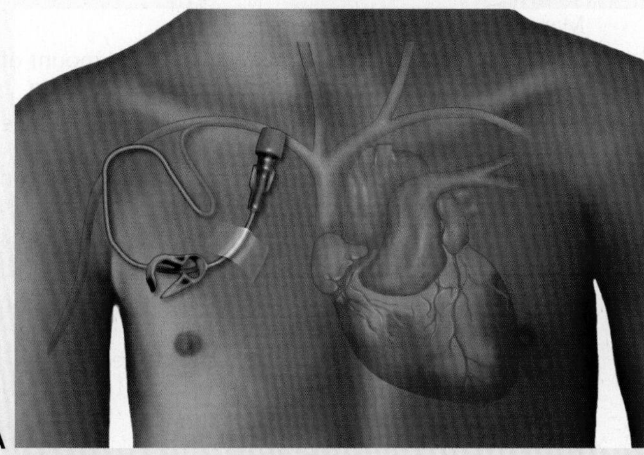
A
Image A: The central venous access catheter is tunneled under the skin and secured with a cuff</td><td>Any child with cancer who will require long-term IV medications or parenteral nutrition</td><td>Complaints of shortness of breath or chest pain may indicate air entry into the central venous catheter. Have child lie on left side, and notify physician immediately
Keep dressing clean and dry. Perform sterile dressing change per institution policy or physician order
Monitor for fever
Monitor insertion site for erythema or drainage
Maintain sterile technique when accessing line, performing dressing change, or administering any fluid through catheter</td></tr>
<tr><td>Implanted port (see image B)</td><td>A needle-accessible port is implanted under the skin, usually on the chest. The port has a thin catheter exiting it that is tunneled under the skin into the superior vena cava or subclavian vein</td><td>Any child with cancer who will require long-term IV medications or parenteral nutrition</td><td>Flush nonaccessed port with prescribed heparin dose per institution policy
Use sterile technique to access port with Huber needle
Monitor port site for erythema or warmth</td></tr>
<tr><td colspan="4">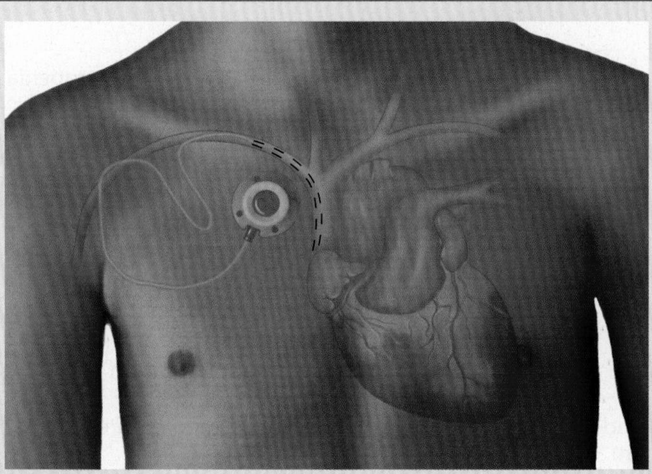
B
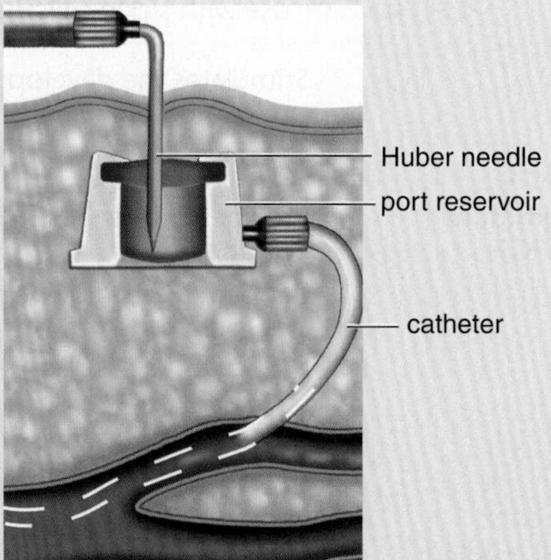

Image 2: The implanted port consists of a reservoir under the skin for ready access. The catheter exiting the port is threaded into the subclavian vein or right atrium. Image 3: A 90-degree Huber needle is used to access the port</td></tr>
<tr><td colspan="4">Adapted from Baggott, C. (2010). Cancer. In P. J. Allen, J. A. Vessey, & N. A. Schapiro (Eds.), Primary care of the child with a chronic condition (5th ed.). St. Louis, MO: Mosby; and D. Tomlinson & N. E. Kline (Eds.). (2010). Pediatric oncology nursing. New York, NY: Springer.</td></tr>
</table>

DRUG GUIDE 46.1 COMMON DRUGS FOR HEMATOLOGIC AND NEOPLASTIC DISORDERS

Medication	Actions/Indications	Nursing Implications
Iron supplements (ferrous sulfate, ferrous fumarate)	Supplemental iron in deficient child Iron-deficiency anemia	Dosage is based on milligrams of elemental iron Give with vitamin C–containing foods to increase absorption Do not administer with milk or milk products May color stools and urine black Liquid can stain the teeth; mix with a small amount of juice; drinking with straw decreases tooth staining May cause constipation; increase fiber and fluid intake
Deferasirox	Binds with iron, which is removed in the feces Iron toxicity (as in children chronically transfused)	Oral agent, should be taken at the same time daily, on an empty stomach Do not chew or swallow whole pills; disperse completely in orange juice, apple juice, or water Monitor iron level, CBC, creatinine, hearing and vision
Deferoxamine	Binds with iron, which is removed via the kidneys Iron toxicity (as in children chronically transfused)	Rotate subcutaneous injection sites to decrease local reactions Apply corticosteroid cream to irritation
Factor (VIII or IX) replacement	Replaces deficient clotting factors Hemophilia	Use filter needle to draw up medication Administer IV when bleeding occurs
Penicillin VK	Kills susceptible bacteria Prophylaxis of infection in asplenia	Determine whether penicillin allergy is present Monitor renal and hematologic function during prolonged use
Folic acid	Replaces the vitamin Folic acid deficiency; questionable use with sickle cell anemia	Administer without regard to meals Monitor hematologic function
Hydroxyurea	Stimulates the development of hemoglobin F in sickle cell anemia	Monitor for mild GI discomfort, modest neutropenia, hyperpigmentation of the skin and nails
Intravenous immune globulin (IVIG)	Provides exogenous IgG antibodies Idiopathic thrombocytopenic purpura	Do not mix with IV medications or with other IV fluids Do not give IM or SQ Monitor vital signs and watch for adverse reactions frequently during infusion. Child may require antipyretic or antihistamine to prevent chills and fever during infusion Have epinephrine available during infusion
Chelating agents: dimercaprol, edetate calcium disodium, succimer	Remove lead from soft tissues and bone, allowing for its excretion via the renal system Used for blood lead levels >45 µg/dL	Monitor intake and output closely to ensure adequacy of renal system Encourage adequate oral hydration or provide IV hydration if required Follow lead levels as prescribed Ensure that lead is being removed from the child's home
Allopurinol	Decreases production of uric acid Use to treat secondary hyperuricemia occurring during leukemia or tumor treatment	Give PO after meals with plenty of food Cardiovascular adverse effects may occur with IV administration Maintain adequate hydration

DRUG GUIDE 46.1 COMMON DRUGS FOR HEMATOLOGIC AND NEOPLASTIC DISORDERS (continued)

Medication	Actions/Indications	Nursing Implications
Antibiotics (oral, parenteral)	Treatment of documented bacterial infections Also used as prophylaxis of *Pneumocystis jirovecii* and in the neutropenic child	Check for antibiotic allergies Should be given as prescribed for the length of time prescribed Start IV antibiotics as soon as possible in the neutropenic child admitted with fever
Antiemetics: promethazine, metoclopramide, ondansetron	Act on the CNS transmitters to prevent vomiting	May cause CNS side effects, such as drowsiness or irritability Ondansetron: may cause dry mouth
Antifungal agents: nystatin, amphotericin B (conventional and lipid complex)	Invade fungal cell wall, enabling its destruction Indicated for mucositis, or systemic fungal infection	Nystatin: administer after meals Amphotericin B: may cause fever, chills, rigors, cardiovascular adverse effects; monitor child closely throughout infusion; note dose differences between conventional and lipid complex
Immunosuppressant drugs: cyclosporine A (CyA), mycophenolate, tacrolimus	Inhibition of production and release of interleukin-2 (CyA) Inhibition of T- and B-cell proliferation (mycophenolate). Inhibition of T-cell activation (tacrolimus) Used for treatment of GVHD after HSCT	Monitor CBC, serum creatinine, potassium, and magnesium Monitor blood pressure and for signs of infection Draw blood levels prior to morning dose CyA: do not give with grapefruit juice Mycophenolate: give on empty stomach; do not open capsule or crush tablet Tacrolimus: give on empty stomach; monitor for anaphylaxis with first IV dose
Mesna	Binds with and detoxifies cyclophosphamide and ifosfamide metabolites in the urinary bladder to prevent hemorrhagic cystitis	Maintain adequate hydration Administer concurrently and after cyclophosphamide or ifosfamide May cause hypotension
Methotrexate antidote: leucovorin	Reduces toxic effects of methotrexate	May cause skin disturbances, wheezing, thrombocytosis Dose depends on methotrexate level Dose increased with increased creatinine levels
Biotherapy		
Colony-stimulating factors: darbepoetin alfa, epoetin alfa, filgrastim, sargramostim	Stimulate production of red blood cells (epoetin) or granulocytes (filgrastim, sargramostim) Used to counteract myelosuppressive effects of chemotherapy	Administer SQ or IV Filgrastim, sargramostim: may cause bone pain Sargramostim may cause hypotension and a first-dose reaction
Interleukins: aldesleukin	Recombinant DNA interleukin-2 product that recruits T, B, and natural killer cells Indicated for non-Hodgkin lymphoma	Adverse effects are dose dependent May cause capillary leak syndrome within 2–12 hours of start of treatment: hypotension and decreased organ perfusion result
Tumor necrosis factor (protein cytokine)	Increases effectiveness of immune cells, stops cancer cells from dividing, damages tumor blood vessels Used in a variety of cancer protocols	May cause fever, chills, rigors, nausea, vomiting

(continued)

DRUG GUIDE 46.1 COMMON DRUGS FOR HEMATOLOGIC AND NEOPLASTIC DISORDERS (continued)

Medication	Actions/Indications	Nursing Implications
Monoclonal antibodies: rituximab, gemtuzumab	Bind to CD20 antigen on B lymphocytes Indicated in CD20-positive non-Hodgkin lymphoma, posttransplant lymphoproliferative disorder	Monitor blood pressure for hypotension Monitor for anaphylaxis and infusion-related reaction Have epinephrine, antihistamines, and steroids available at bedside for treatment of reaction
Interferons: α, γ	Alter cancer cell proliferation (α), stimulate macrophage production to fight bacteria and fungus (γ) Indicated in a variety of cancer protocols	May cause flu-like symptoms Maintain adequate hydration
Chemotherapy		
Alkylating agents: busulfan, carboplatin, cisplatin, ifosfamide, temozolomide, thiotepa Nitrosoureas: carmustine, lomustine Nitrogen mustard: chlorambucil, cyclophosphamide, mechlorethamine, melphalan	Interfere with DNA replication and RNA transcription by alkylation (replacing the hydrogen ion with an alkyl group), cross-link DNA Cell cycle nonspecific The nitrosoureas are highly lipid soluble and easily cross the blood–brain barrier Used in a variety of cancer protocols	Causes myelosuppression, nausea, vomiting, alopecia, mucositis Monitor for signs of infection Provide adequate hydration Cyclophosphamide, ifosfamide: administer in the morning, provide adequate hydration, and have child void frequently during and after infusion to decrease risk of hemorrhagic cystitis Cisplatin, mechlorethamine, melphalan: avoid **extravasation** (leakage into surrounding tissues, potentially damaging them) Temozolomide: avoid opening capsules Thiotepa: if contact with skin occurs, wash thoroughly with soap and water
Antitumor antibiotics: bleomycin, dactinomycin, daunorubicin, doxorubicin, idarubicin, mitomycin, mitoxantrone	Interfere with cellular metabolism, causing disruptions in DNA and/or RNA synthesis Cell cycle nonspecific Indicated in a variety of cancer protocols	May cause alopecia, nausea, vomiting, myelosuppression Bleomycin: fever and chills may occur 20 hours after infusion Dactinomycin, mitomycin: avoid extravasation Daunorubicin, doxorubicin, idarubicin: may turn urine red-orange, monitor for arrhythmias, congestive heart failure; avoid extravasation Mitoxantrone: may color urine, sweat, tears, skin, sclera blue-green; monitor for arrhythmias, congestive heart failure
Antimetabolites: cladribine, cytarabine, fludarabine, fluorouracil, mercaptopurine, methotrexate, thioguanine	Substitute for a natural metabolite in the molecule, altering the cell's function and ability to replicate Cell cycle specific (S phase); cladribine is cell cycle nonspecific Used in a variety of cancer protocols	May cause alopecia, nausea, vomiting, mucositis, and myelosuppression Cladribine: monitor for fever Cytarabine: use corticosteroid eye drops to prevent conjunctivitis with high doses Fludarabine: monitor for visual changes and neurotoxicity; maintain adequate hydration Fluorouracil: maintain adequate hydration; may cause photosensitivity Mercaptopurine: do not give oral doses with meals; may cause drug fever; avoid extravasation Methotrexate: intensive hydration with high doses; may cause photosensitivity Thioguanine: maintain hydration; administer on empty stomach

DRUG GUIDE 46.1 COMMON DRUGS FOR HEMATOLOGIC AND NEOPLASTIC DISORDERS (continued)

Medication	Actions/Indications	Nursing Implications
Antimicrotubulars: paclitaxel	Inhibit mitotic cellular function in late G2 and M phases of cell cycle Indicated for refractory leukemia, recurrent Wilms tumor	May cause alopecia, nausea, vomiting, mucositis, myelosuppression May cause drowsiness Avoid extravasation
Miscellaneous: asparaginase, pegaspargase	Inhibit protein synthesis by depriving tumor cells of the essential amino acid asparagine Used in acute lymphocytic leukemia, lymphomas	May cause alopecia, nausea, vomiting, and myelosuppression Monitor for vital signs during infusion and for signs of anaphylaxis Have emergency equipment, oxygen, epinephrine, antihistamines, and steroids available at bedside
Miscellaneous: dacarbazine, procarbazine	Inhibit DNA and RNA synthesis via cross-linking or suppression of mitosis Indicated in a variety of cancer protocols	May cause alopecia, nausea, vomiting, myelosuppression Monitor for flu-like symptoms Dacarbazine: photosensitivity may occur; avoid extravasation
Mitotic inhibitors: etoposide, vinblastine, vincristine	Inhibit mitotic activity by inhibiting DNA topoisomerase (etoposide) Cause metaphase arrest by binding to the mitotic spindle (vinblastine, vincristine) Used in a variety of cancer protocols	May cause alopecia, nausea, vomiting, myelosuppression (only minimal with vincristine) Etoposide: monitor for anaphylaxis; have emergency equipment, oxygen, epinephrine, antihistamines, and steroids available at bedside Vinblastine, vincristine: maintain hydration; administer allopurinol; avoid extravasation
Topoisomerase inhibitors: irinotecan, topotecan	Bind to DNA complex, preventing religation of single-strand DNA breaks Indicated for refractory solid tumors	May cause alopecia, nausea, vomiting, myelosuppression, severe diarrhea (irinotecan), hypotension (topotecan) Maintain hydration Avoid extravasation Monitor blood pressure during topotecan infusion
Corticosteroids: prednisone, dexamethasone	Suppress immune system by decreasing lymphatic activity and volume. Also decrease edema caused by tumor or tumor necrosis Indicated for leukemia and some other cancers	Administer with food to decrease GI upset May mask signs of infection Monitor blood pressure; monitor urine for glucose Do not stop treatment abruptly or acute adrenal insufficiency may occur Monitor for Cushing syndrome Doses may be tapered over time

GI, gastrointestinal; IM, intramuscularly; SQ, subcutaneously.

Adapted from Baggott, C. (2010). Cancer. In P. J. Allen, J. A. Vessey, & N. A. Schapiro (Eds.), *Primary care of the child with a chronic condition* (5th ed.). St. Louis, MO: Mosby; Taketomo, C. K., Hodding, J. H., & Kraus, D. M. (2013). *Pediatric & neonatal dosage handbook* (20th ed.). Hudson, OH: Lexicomp; and D. Tomlinson, & N. E. Kline (Eds.). (2010). *Pediatric oncology nursing*. New York, NY: Springer.

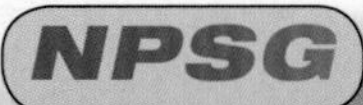

GOAL 7: Reduce the Risk of Healthcare-Associated Infections. (Prevent Infection)

NPSG.07.04.01 Implement evidence-based practices to prevent central line–associated bloodstream infections. Note: This requirement covers short- and long-term central venous catheters and peripherally inserted central catheter (PICC) lines.

Steps: When caring for a child with a central line ensure to follow evidence-based policies and procedures strictly. Adhere to proper handwashing and aseptic technique.

Joint Commission. (2015). *National patient safety goals effective January 1, 2015.* Retrieved from http://www.jointcommission.org/assets/1/6/2015_NPSG_HAP.pdf

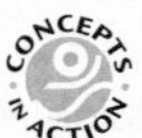

Chemotherapy

To understand how **chemotherapy** works to destroy cancer cells, it is necessary to review the normal cell cycle, through which all cells progress (Fig. 46.2). The cell cycle consists of five phases:

- G0 phase: the resting phase; lasts from a few hours to a few years; cells have not started to divide
- G1 phase: cell makes more protein in preparation for dividing; lasts 18 to 30 hours
- S phase: chromosomes are copied so that newly formed cells have the appropriate DNA; lasts 18 to 20 hours
- G2 phase: just before the cell splits into two cells; lasts 2 to 10 hours
- M phase: mitosis, the actual splitting of the cell into two new cells; lasts 30 minutes to 1 hour

Chemotherapy drugs work in two different ways in relation to the cell cycle. Cell cycle–specific agents exert their actions during a specific phase of the cell cycle. Cell cycle–nonspecific drugs exert their effect on the cells regardless of which phase the cell is in. Chemotherapy protocols often call for a combination of drugs that act on different phases of the cell cycle, thus maximizing the destruction of cancer cells.

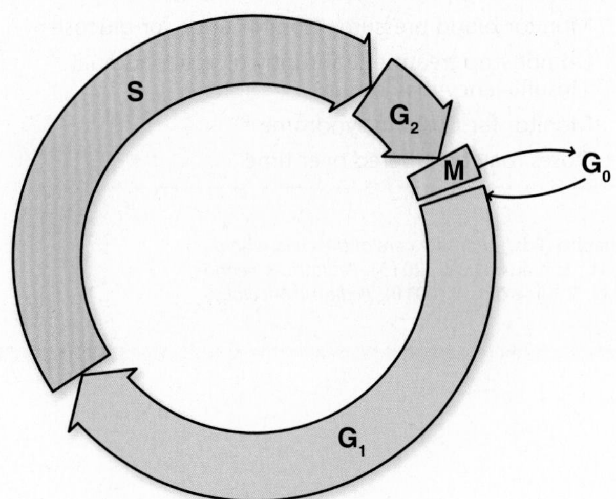

FIGURE 46.2 Phases of the cell cycle.

Chemotherapy drugs are divided into classes that exert slightly different actions and have an effect on different portions of the cell cycle. Drug Guide 46.1 gives further explanation about the different classes of chemotherapy drugs.

Unfortunately, chemotherapeutic medications disrupt the cell cycle of not only cancer cells but also normal rapidly dividing cells. This results in a significant number of adverse effects. The cells most likely to be affected by chemotherapy are those in the bone marrow, the digestive tract (especially the mouth), the reproductive system, and hair follicles.

Adverse effects common to chemotherapeutic drugs include immunosuppression, infection, myelosuppression, nausea, vomiting, constipation, oral mucositis, alopecia, and pain. Long-term complications include microdontia and missing teeth as a result of damage to developing permanent teeth; hearing and vision changes; hematopoietic, immunologic, or gonadal dysfunction; endocrine dysfunction, including altered growth and precocious or delayed puberty; various alterations of the cardiorespiratory, gastrointestinal, and genitourinary systems; and development of a second cancer as an adolescent or adult (Chordas & Graham, 2010).

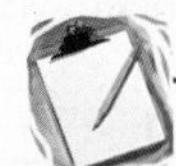

Take Note!

Acupuncture as an adjunct therapy may help to decrease nausea, vomiting, and aversion to chemotherapy.

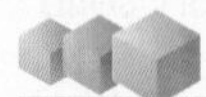

Concept Mastery Alert

Cell Cycle–Specific Agents versus Noncell Cycle–Specific Agents

Chemotherapeutic drugs that act as cell cycle–specific agents are classified as antimetabolites. Alkylating agents are not cell cycle–specific agents.

Radiation Therapy

Radiation therapy uses high-energy radiation to damage or kill cancer cells. Radiant energy in either a gamma or particle form is emitted during the treatment. Radiation affects not only cancer cells but also any rapidly growing cells with which they are in contact. It may be used as a curative, adjuvant, or palliative treatment, either alone or in combination with chemotherapy. Radiation therapy is also used to shrink a tumor prior to surgical resection. The area to be treated is marked carefully to minimize damage to normal cells.

Adverse effects of radiation therapy include fatigue, nausea, vomiting, oral mucositis, myelosuppression, and alterations in skin integrity at the site of irradiation. Long-term complications are related to the area of the body that was irradiated and include alterations in growth; hormone dysfunction; hearing and vision alterations; learning problems; cardiac dysfunction; pulmonary fibrosis; hepatic, sexual, or renal dysfunction; osteoporosis; and development of secondary cancer (particularly at the site of irradiation) (Loch & Khorrami, 2010).

Hematopoietic Stem Cell Transplantation

Hematopoietic stem cell transplantation (HSCT), also called bone marrow transplantation, is a procedure in which hematopoietic stem cells are infused intravenously into the child. This follows a period of purging of abnormal cells in the child that is accomplished through high-dose chemotherapy or irradiation. The use of high-dose chemotherapy and total body irradiation kills the tumor cells but also destroys the child's bone marrow. The transplanted cells migrate to the empty spaces in the child's bone marrow and reestablish normal hematopoiesis in the child.

HSCT is used for a variety of childhood cancers, including leukemia, lymphoma, brain tumors, neuroblastoma, and other solid tumors. For most pediatric cancers, it is not the first line of treatment but is used for refractory or advanced disease.

Autologous HSCT is achieved through harvest and treatment of the child's own bone marrow, followed by infusion of the treated stem cells. Risk for relapse of the original disease is highest in autologous HSCT. Allogenic HSCT refers to transplantation using stem cells from another individual that are harvested from the bone marrow, peripheral blood, or umbilical cord blood. Allogenic HSCT requires human leukocyte antibody (HLA) matching for antigen-specific sites on the leukocytes. Closely matched HLA donors may be difficult to find from a donor listing, and sibling donors are often the closest match. The degree of match is inversely related to the risk for graft rejection and the development of graft-versus-host disease (GVHD). In other words, the lesser the degree of HLA matching in the donor, the higher the risk for graft rejection and GVHD. GVHD occurs to at least some extent in 11% to 85% of all allogenic HSCT recipients (Kristovich & Callard, 2010).

In addition to graft rejection and GVHD, additional initial complications of HSCT are infection, electrolyte imbalance, bleeding, and organ, skin, and mucous membrane toxicities. Long-term complications include impaired growth and fertility related to endocrine dysfunction, developmental delay, cataracts, pulmonary and cardiac disease, avascular necrosis of the bone, and development of secondary cancers.

NURSING PROCESS OVERVIEW FOR THE CHILD WITH AN ALTERATION IN CELLULAR REGULATION (HEMATOLOGIC DISORDER OR CANCER)

Care of the child with a hematologic disorder or cancer includes assessment, nursing diagnosis, planning, interventions, and evaluation. There are a number of general concepts related to the nursing process that may be applied to hematologic dysfunction and neoplasia in children.

Development of a plan of care will depend on which component of the blood is altered in the hematologic disorder. A decrease in hemoglobin will necessitate evaluation of oxygen-carrying capacity and effects of hypoxia on the tissues. A reduction in platelet production will lead the nurse to evaluate for prolonged bleeding, hemorrhage, and shock. An elevation in WBCs would require an evaluation for infection.

From a general understanding of the care involved for a child with cancer, the nurse can then individualize the care based on specifics for the particular child. Children with cancer often suffer many physical effects as a result of the disease and its treatment. The nurse must be diligent when assessing for these effects and should involve the parents as a reliable source for reporting the child's physical symptoms.

Remember Shaun, the 10-month-old with the laceration and prolonged bleeding? What additional health history and physical examination assessment information should you obtain?

Assessment

Signs of changes in the hematologic system are often insidious and overlooked. Children with cancer often demonstrate similar signs. Skin color changes such as pallor, bruising, and flushing are often the first signs that a problem is developing. Changes in mental status such as lethargy can indicate a decrease in Hgb and a decreased amount of oxygen being delivered to the brain. Nursing assessment must include a thorough approach.

Health History

Elicit the birth and maternal history, noting low birth weight or gestational diabetes and ascertaining whether vitamin K was given after birth. The past medical history might be significant for recent illnesses that may contribute to a change in blood cell distribution. Determine the child's sleep/wake patterns and bowel elimination patterns, which may be affected by alterations in circulating blood volume or changes in oxygenation. Explore the family history for inherited disorders such as hemophilia, sickle cell disease, thalassemia, or history of cancer. Determine the presence of risk factors such as previous malignancy and treatment; synthetic chemical exposures; parental exposure to radiation, chemicals, or chemotherapeutic agents; and a family history of malignancy (especially childhood), immune disorders, or genetic disorders such as neurofibromatosis or Down syndrome. Evaluate the child's typical diet for nutritional deficits. Determine risk for lead exposure based on the use of a standard questionnaire. Determine current medical history. When eliciting the history of the present illness, inquire about:

- Fatigue or malaise
- Pallor of the skin
- Unusual bruising or petechiae
- Excessive bleeding or difficulty stopping bleeding
- Pain: location, onset, duration, quality, and relieving factors
  - recurrent fever or frequent infections
  - early-morning headache with nausea or vomiting
  - gait or behavior changes
  - visual disturbances
  - history of bone fractures unrelated to trauma

Physical Examination

A child's general appearance gives great insight into his or her health and can indicate problems such as malnutrition or lead poisoning. A complete physical examination should be performed on any child with, or suspected of having, cancer or a hematologic disorder. Note particular findings as discussed below. Physical examination of the child with a hematologic or neoplastic disorder includes inspection and observation, palpation, and auscultation.

INSPECTION AND OBSERVATION

Observe the child's overall appearance and energy level. Note a thin or frail appearance, fatigue, or altered level of consciousness. Measure weight and height (or length) and plot on standardized growth charts. Examine the oral cavity for bleeding gums or pale mucous membranes. Document visible masses or asymmetry of the face, thorax, abdomen, or extremities. Observe the nail beds, palms, and soles for pallor. Evaluate the fingertips for clubbing, which occurs with chronic hypoxemia. Document the location and extent of bruises, petechiae, or purpura. Count the respiratory rate and observe for work of breathing. Obtain a pulse oximeter reading to determine oxygen saturation of tissues. Note conjunctival color as well as color and moisture of oral mucosa. Determine urinary output, which may be altered with decreases in circulatory blood volume or inadequate oxygenation. Note the child's responsiveness to stimuli and movement of extremities. Observe the child's gait, noting ataxia or limp. Note rectal bleeding or vaginal discharge.

AUSCULTATION

Auscultate breath sounds, noting adequacy of air movement and depth of respiration. Note adventitious sounds or absence of breath sounds (which would occur in an area of the lung filled with blood). Auscultate heart sounds, listening closely for murmurs (which can develop with changes in blood viscosity and volume). Note the rate and rhythm of the heart tones. Auscultate bowel sounds, noting presence and normalcy.

PERCUSSION

Percuss the abdomen, noting dullness over a mass if present.

PALPATION

Measure blood pressure, which may change with alterations in blood volume. Palpate the peripheral pulses for strength and equality. Palpate for lymphadenopathy; in particular, note nontender or firm lymph nodes. Determine capillary refill time, which may be prolonged when the circulating blood volume is decreased. Carefully palpate the abdomen for tenderness, hepatomegaly, **splenomegaly** (increased spleen size) or presence of a mass. Palpate any unusual area of swelling anywhere on the body, noting size and absence of tenderness. Note temperature of the skin. Determine elasticity of skin, noting decreased turgor. Palpate the joints for tenderness and determine if range of motion is limited.

Psychosocial Assessment

Assess the child's and family's psychosocial status, using open-ended questions. It is particularly important to determine the child's self-esteem, level of anxiety or stress, and coping mechanisms. Determine the spiritual status of the child and family. Ongoing medical procedures and the fear of dying take a toll on the child and family when cancer is present. Ask the child how things are going at home; how does he or she get along with brothers, sisters, and parents? If the child is school age, ask how school is going. Does the child have friends with whom he or she gets to spend time? Ask the child what he or she does in his spare time; are there any hobbies? These types of queries will provide the nurse with information about how well the child is coping. Assess the parents' status as well. Ask about the marital relationship and how other children in the family are doing. Determine whether certain stressors may need to be addressed.

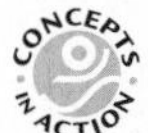

Laboratory and Diagnostic Testing

The nurse must understand the main elements of the complete blood count (CBC; hemogram) to recognize critical values and intervene as appropriate. The components of the CBC are:

- RBC count: the actual number of counted RBCs in a certain volume of blood
- Hemoglobin (Hgb): measure of the protein made up of heme (iron surrounded by protoporphyrin) and globin, α- and β-polypeptide chains, primarily responsible for the transport of nutrients and oxygen to the tissues
- **Hematocrit (Hct):** an indirect measure of red blood cells (number and volume)
- RBC indices
  - Mean corpuscular volume (MCV): average size of the RBC
  - Mean corpuscular hemoglobin (MCH): a calculated value of the oxygen-carrying capacity of the Hgb in the RBCs
  - Mean corpuscular hemoglobin concentration (MCHC): a calculated value that reflects the concentration of Hgb inside the RBC
  - Red cell distribution width (RDW): a calculated value that is a measure of the width of RBCs
- WBC count: actual count of the number of WBCs in a volume of blood
- **Platelet count**: number of platelets per blood volume
- Mean platelet volume (MPV): a measurement of the size of the platelets

Tables 46.1 and 46.2 provide age-related values for the CBC and leukocyte count. When evaluating the CBC, the nurse must take into account the presenting clinical picture of the child. For instance, the RBC count may be truly elevated (erythrocytosis or **polycythemia**) in certain diseases or in the case of dehydration from diarrhea or burns. When anemia is present, the RBC count is low. When the MCV is elevated, the RBCs are larger than normal (**macrocytic**). When the MCV is decreased, the RBCs are smaller than normal (**microcytic**). A decrease in the MCHC means that the Hgb is diluted in the cell and less of the red color is present (**hypochromic**). When the Hgb concentration is increased in the RBC, then the pigmentation (red color) is increased (hyperchromic). Alterations in these RBC indices assist the physician or nurse practitioner with diagnosis.

WBCs are the body's defense against infection or injury. The specific types of WBCs are discussed in Chapter 37. **Platelets** are necessary for clot formation, and if changes occur, problems may develop. Elevations in platelet levels can indicate an increase in clotting, while decreases can put the child at risk for increased bleeding. Decreases can result if the platelets are being used up when bleeding is present, if an inherited disorder is present, or if the spleen holds them, as in hypersplenism. Platelets are larger when they are new; thus, an elevation in the mean platelet volume indicates that an increased number of platelets are being produced in the bone marrow.

Common Laboratory and Diagnostic Tests 46.1 explains the most commonly used laboratory and diagnostic tests for children with hematologic and neoplastic disorders. The tests can assist the physician or nurse practitioner in diagnosing the disorder and/or be used as guidelines in determining ongoing treatment. Laboratory or nonnursing personnel obtain some of the tests, while the nurse might obtain others. In either instance the nurse should be familiar with how the tests are obtained, what they are used for, and normal versus abnormal results. This knowledge will also be necessary when providing child and family education related to the testing.

Nursing Diagnoses, Goals, Interventions, and Evaluation

Upon completion of a thorough assessment, the nurse might identify several nursing diagnoses, including:

- Fatigue
- Pain
- Impaired physical mobility
- Ineffective health management
- Anxiety
- Ineffective family coping
- Risk for infection
- Impaired oral mucous membranes
- Nausea
- Imbalanced nutrition
- Constipation
- Diarrhea
- Risk for impaired skin integrity
- Activity intolerance
- Disturbed body image
- Situational low self-esteem
- Compromised family coping
- Grieving

You have finished assessing Shaun and your findings include the following. The health history revealed he bled with all four of the teeth he has cut. Upon physical examination numerous bruises are noted. Based on the assessment findings, what would your top three nursing diagnoses be for Shaun?

Nursing goals, interventions, and evaluation for the child with hematologic dysfunction or cancer are based

(text continues on page 1793)

TABLE 46.1 NORMAL HEMOGRAM VALUES

Age	WBC ($\times10^3$/mm^3)	RBC ($\times10^6$/mm^3)	Hgb (g/dL)	Hct (%)	MCV (fL)	MCH (pg/cell)	MCHC (g/dL)	Platelets ($\times10^3$/mm^3)	RDW (%)	MPV (fL)
Birth–2 weeks	9.0–30.0	4.1–6.1	14.5–24.5	44–54	98–112	34–40	33–37	150–450	—	—
2–8 weeks	5.0–21.0	4.0–6.0	12.5–20.5	39–59	98–112	30–36	32–36	—	—	—
2–6 months	5.0–19.0	3.8–5.6	10.7–17.3	35–49	83–97	27–33	31–35	—	—	—
6 months–1 year	5.0–19.0	3.8–5.2	9.9–14.5	29–43	73–87	24–30	32–36	—	—	—
1–6 years	5.0–19.0	3.9–5.3	9.5–14.1	30–40	70–84	23–29	31–35	—	—	—
6–16 years	4.8–10.8	4.0–5.2	10.3–14.9	32–42	73–87	24–30	32–36	—	—	—
16–18 years	4.8–10.8	4.2–5.4	11.1–15.7	34–44	75–89	25–31	32–36	—	—	—
>18 years (males)	5.0–10.0	4.5–5.5	14.0–17.4	42–52	84–96	28–34	32–36	140–400	11.5–14.5	7.4–10.4
>18 years (females)	5.0–10.0	4.0–5.0	12.0–16.0	36–48	84–96	28–34	32–36	140–400	11.5–14.5	7.4–10.4

Adapted from Fischbach, F. T., & Dunning, M. B. (2014). *A manual of laboratory and diagnostic tests* (9th ed.). Philadelphia, PA: Lippincott Williams & Wilkins.

TABLE 46.2 NORMAL DIFFERENTIAL FOR LEUKOCYTES (WHITE BLOOD CELL DIFFERENTIAL)

Age	Bands/Stab (%)	Segs/Polys (%)	Eos (%)	Basos (%)	Lymphs (%)	Monos (%)
Birth–1 week	10–18	32–62	0–2	0–1	26–36	0–6
1–2 weeks	8–16	19–49	0–4	0	38–46	0–9
2–4 weeks	7–15	14–34	0–3	0	43–53	0–9
4–8 weeks	7–13	15–35	0–3	0–1	41–71	0–7
2–6 months	5–11	15–35	0–3	0–1	42–72	0–6
6 months–1 year	6–12	13–33	0–3	0	46–76	0–5
1–6 years	5–11	13–33	0–3	0	46–76	0–5
6–16 years	5–11	32–54	0–3	0–1	27–57	0–5
16–18 years	5–11	34–64	0–3	0–1	25–45	0–5
>18 years	3–6	50–62	0–3	0–1	25–40	3–7

Adapted from Fischbach, F. T., & Dunning, M. B. (2014). *A manual of laboratory and diagnostic tests* (9th ed.). Philadelphia, PA: Lippincott Williams & Wilkins.

COMMON LABORATORY AND DIAGNOSTIC TESTS 46.1

Test	Explanation	Indications	Nursing Implications
α-Fetoprotein (AFP)	Produced by the fetal liver and yolk sac; normally decreases to very low levels by 1 year of age	May be elevated in Hodgkin disease and other cancers. Used to determine tumor burden	No food or fluid restriction required
Blood type and cross-match	Determines ABO blood type as well as presence of antigens. Cross-match is performed on RBC-containing products to avoid transfusion reaction	Trauma victim or any person in whom blood loss is suspected, in preparation for transfusion	Avoid hemolysis of specimen Appropriately sign and date specimen. Apply "type and cross" or "blood band" to child at the time of blood draw if indicated by the institution Most type and cross-match specimens expire after 48–72 hours
Bone marrow aspiration and biopsy	A needle is inserted through the cortex of the bone into the bone marrow (most often the iliac spine), bone marrow is aspirated, and the cells are evaluated	Evaluation for leukemia or metastasis of other cancers to bone marrow	Use EMLA or lidocaine to decrease pain with procedure Often performed under conscious sedation Apply a pressure dressing to arrest bleeding Assess for tenderness or erythema May require mild analgesia for postprocedure pain
Bone scan	Administration of IV radionuclide material, which is taken up by the bone and is visible on the scans	Identify metastasis to bone	Requires patent IV for injection Encourage fluid intake after injection to increase uptake of injected radionuclide Scan will be performed 1–3 hours after injection

(continued)

COMMON LABORATORY AND DIAGNOSTIC TESTS 46.1 (continued)

Test	Explanation	Indications	Nursing Implications
Chest radiography	X-ray of the chest	Identify tumor or metastasis in the thorax	Chest must be held stationary for a brief time
Clotting studies	Prothrombin time (PT), partial thromboplastin time (PTT), activated partial thromboplastin time (aPTT), international normalized ratio (INR)	Evaluation of common pathway in clotting mechanism PT, INR: evaluation of extrinsic system PTT, aPTT: evaluation of intrinsic system	Apply pressure to venipuncture site Assess for bleeding (gums, bruising, blood in urine or stool)
Coagulating factor concentration	Measures concentration of specific coagulating factors in the blood	Hemophilia, DIC	Apply pressure to venipuncture site Assess for bleeding (gums, bruising, blood in urine or stool) Deliver specimen to laboratory as soon as possible (unstable at room temperature).
Complete blood count (CBC) with differential	Evaluates hemoglobin and hematocrit, WBC count (particularly the percentage of individual WBCs), and platelet count	Anemia, infection, bleeding disorder, clotting disorder, immunosuppression, to determine neutropenia in myelosuppression	Normal values vary according to age and gender WBC differential is helpful in evaluating source of infection May be affected by certain medications
Computed tomography (CT) scan	Multiple films taken in successive layers to provide a 3D view of the body part being scanned	Identify tumor location or metastasis	Some CT scans are done with oral or IV contrast (notify physician if child has iodine or shellfish allergy) May require a several-hour period of NPO if contrast is used (contrast may cause nausea). Encourage fluid intake after scan to facilitate excretion of contrast dye
Hemoglobin electrophoresis	Measures percentage of normal and abnormal hemoglobin in the blood	Sickle cell anemia, thalassemia	Blood transfusions within the previous 12 weeks may alter test results
Iron	Evaluates iron metabolism	Iron-deficiency anemia, hemosiderosis with chronic transfusion or hemoglobinopathies	Recent blood transfusions increase level Child should fast for 12 hours before the test Avoid hemolysis (will falsely elevate result)
Lead	Measures level of lead in blood	Lead poisoning	Normal amount in blood is zero.
Lumbar puncture (LP)	A needle is placed in the subarachnoid space of the spinal column, below the base of the cord, and cerebrospinal fluid is withdrawn for analysis	Evaluation of tumor or metastasis to brain or spinal cord. Also used to administer intrathecal medications	Use EMLA before the procedure to decrease pain. May be performed under conscious sedation. Position child appropriately Use distraction techniques in the older child or teen Encourage child to recline for up to 12 hours after LP

COMMON LABORATORY AND DIAGNOSTIC TESTS 46.1 (continued)

Test	Explanation	Indications	Nursing Implications
Magnetic resonance imaging (MRI)	Based on how hydrogen atoms behave in a magnetic field when disturbed by radiofrequency signals. Does not require ionizing radiation. Provides a 3D view of the body part being scanned	Identify extent of tumor or metastatic spread	Remove all metal objects from the child Child must remain motionless for entire scan; parent can stay in room with child. Younger children will require sedation to keep still A loud thumping sound occurs inside the machine during the scan procedure; this can be frightening to children
Reticulocyte count	Measures the amount of reticulocytes (immature RBCs) in the blood	Indicates bone marrow's ability to respond to anemia with production of RBCs	Rises quickly in response to iron supplementation in the iron-deficient child
Serum ferritin	Measures the level of ferritin (the major iron storage protein) in the blood	Most sensitive test for determining iron-deficiency anemia	Elevated in hemolytic disease and if transfused recently Iron supplementation increases ferritin levels
Urine catechol amines (VMA, HVA)	Catabolism of catecholamines causes elevated levels in urine	Diagnosis of neuroblastoma (produces catecholamines)	24-hour urine collection Levels may be altered with certain foods and drugs or vigorous exercise
Ultrasound	High-frequency sound waves are directed at internal organs and structures, and an image is made of the waves as they are reflected back through the tissues	Identify tumor presence, especially in abdomen or on kidney	Fasting for a few hours may be required when certain organs are to be visualized

Adapted from Corbett, J. A., & Banks, A. D. (2013). *Laboratory tests and diagnostic procedures with nursing diagnoses* (8th ed.). Upper Saddle River, NJ: Pearson Education Inc.

on the nursing diagnoses. Nursing Care Plan 46.1, found at the end of the chapter, may be used as a guide in planning nursing care for the child with a hematologic disorder. Refer to Chapter 36 for additional information related to pain management. Children's responses to alterations in cellular regulation and their treatments will vary, and nursing care should be individualized based on the child's and family's responses to illness. Other conditions may contribute to these nursing diagnoses and must also be considered when prioritizing care. Additional information about nursing management will be included later in the chapter as it relates to specific disorders.

Based on your top three nursing diagnoses for Shaun, describe appropriate nursing interventions.

CARING FOR THE CHILD WITH CANCER

Providing Education

Provide education to families of all children with cancer as outlined in Teaching Guidelines 46.1.

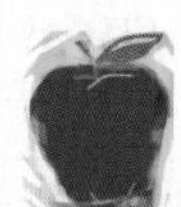

Teaching Guidelines 46.1

EDUCATION FOR FAMILIES OF CHILDREN WITH CANCER

- Obtain a printed or written copy of the child's treatment plan
- Keep a calendar of all appointment times, blood count lab draw days, and phone numbers of all physicians and nurse practitioners, home care companies, the laboratory, and the hospital

- Seek medical care IMMEDIATELY if the child's temperature is 38.3°C (101°F) or higher
- Call the oncologist or seek medical care if any of the following occur:
  - Cough or rapid breathing
  - Increased bruising, bleeding or petechiae, pallor, or increased levels of fatigue
  - Earache, sore throat, nuchal rigidity
  - Blisters, rashes, ulcers
  - Red, irritated skin on the child's buttocks
  - Abdominal pain, difficulty or pain with eating, drinking, or swallowing
  - Constipation or diarrhea
  - For children with central venous catheters:
    - Pus, redness, or swelling at the site
    - Breakage of the catheter
- Do not give the child aspirin

Adapted from Kline, N. E. (2014). *Essentials of pediatric oncology nursing: A core curriculum* (4th ed.). Chicago, IL: Association of Pediatric Hematology/Oncology Nurses.

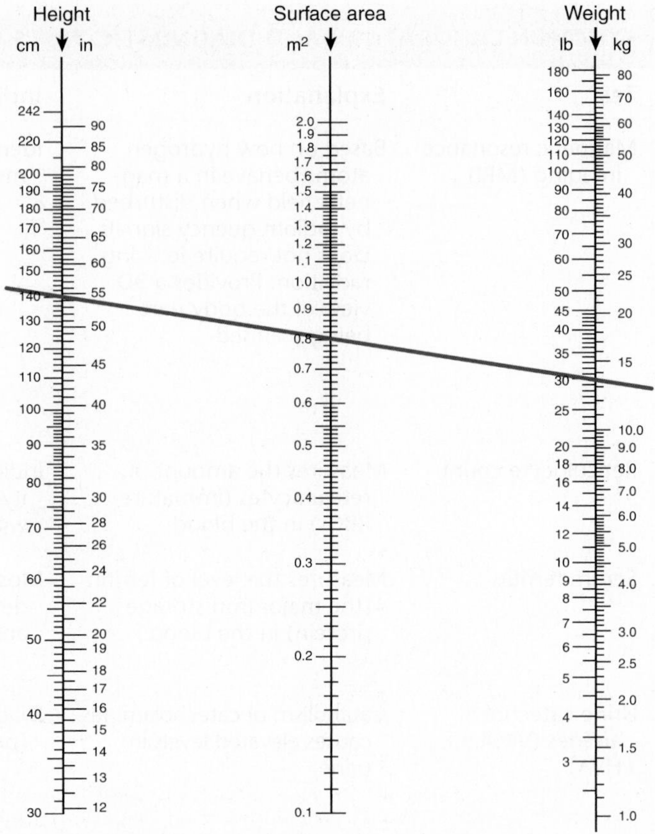

FIGURE 46.3 A child who weighs 13.2 kg and is 140 cm tall has a body surface area (BSA) of 0.80 m^2.

Administering Chemotherapy

All chemotherapy medications have the potential to cause toxicities in the child as well as the persons handling or preparing the medication. General guidelines related to the preparation and administration of chemotherapy include:

- Chemotherapy should be prepared and administered only by specially trained personnel.
- Personal protective equipment (PPE) in the form of double gloves and nonpermeable gowns should be worn when preparing or administering chemotherapy. If splashing is possible or a spill occurs, then a face shield and/or mask may also be necessary.
- Dispose of all equipment used in chemotherapy preparation and administration in a puncture-resistant container (Chordas & Graham, 2010).

It is critical to calculate the chemotherapy dose correctly. Chemotherapy medication doses in children are based on body surface area (BSA). A nomogram is a commonly used device for determining BSA. To use the nomogram, draw a straight line between the child's height on the left and the child's weight on the right. The point at which the straight line crosses the center is the child's BSA expressed in meters squared (Fig. 46.3).

An alternative to using the nomogram is to use the following formula: BSA (m^2) = the square root of (height [in centimeters] × weight [in kilograms] divided by 3,600) (Chordas & Graham, 2010). For example, for a child 140 cm tall and weighing 30 kg: 140 × 30 = 4,200; 4,200/3,600 = 1.167; and the square root of 1.167 is 1.08. The BSA would be 1.08.

Managing Adverse Effects of Chemotherapy

Chemotherapy can result in multiple adverse effects. Myelosuppression leads to low blood counts in all cell lines, placing the child at risk for infection, hemorrhage, and anemia. Nausea, vomiting, and anorexia may hinder the child's growth. Alopecia and facial changes may affect the child's self-esteem (Fig. 46.4). Nursing interventions

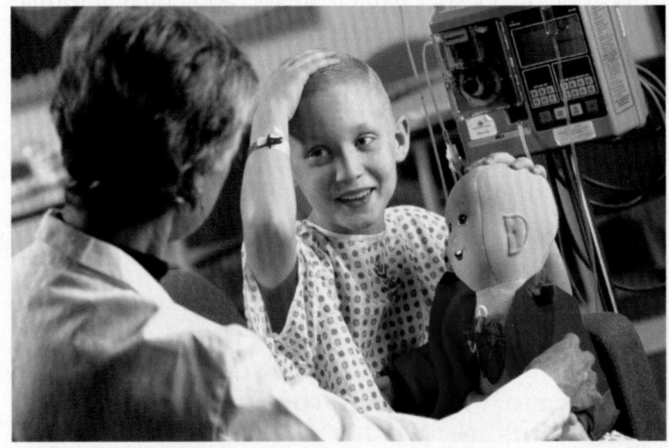

FIGURE 46.4 Chemotherapy often causes alopecia.

related to the effects of myelosuppression, nausea, vomiting, and anorexia are discussed below. Refer to Nursing Care Plan 46.1, at the end of the chapter, for nursing interventions related to altered body image.

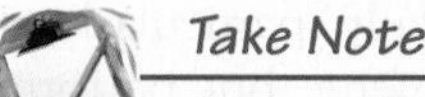

Take Note!

Cooling the scalp during chemotherapy administration with the use of a cooling cap may decrease hair loss (Tomlinson & Kline, 2010).

Preventing Infection

Many chemotherapeutic drugs cause significant bone marrow suppression and decreased amounts of circulating mature neutrophils ("segs," or segmented neutrophils). Administer granulocyte colony–stimulating factor (GCSF) as ordered to promote neutrophil growth and maturation (Brundige, 2010). Administer varicella zoster immunoglobulin (VZIG) within 72 hours of exposure to active chickenpox. If the child is actively infected with chickenpox, administer intravenous acyclovir as ordered. Children receiving treatment for acute lymphoblastic leukemia (ALL) are at risk for opportunistic infection with *Pneumocystis jirovecii,* as most children are colonized with this fungus. Administer prophylactic antibiotics as ordered and teach the parents to administer them at home (Tomlinson & Kline, 2010). Teaching Guidelines 46.2 gives further information about infection prevention at home.

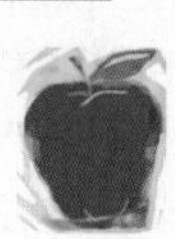

Teaching Guidelines 46.2

PREVENTING INFECTION IN CHILDREN RECEIVING CHEMOTHERAPY FOR CANCER

- Practice meticulous hygiene (oral, body, perianal).
- Avoid known ill contacts, especially persons with chickenpox.
- Immediately notify the physician or nurse practitioner if exposed to chickenpox.
- Avoid crowded areas.
- Do not let the child receive live vaccines.
- Do not take the child's temperature rectally or give medications by the rectal route.
- Administer twice-daily trimethoprim–sulfamethoxazole for 3 consecutive days each week as ordered for prevention of *Pneumocystis* pneumonia.

Adapted from Baggott, C. (2010). Cancer. In P. J. Allen, J. A. Vessey, & N. A. Schapiro (Eds.), Primary care of the child with a chronic condition (5th ed.). St. Louis, MO: Mosby; and D. Tomlinson & N. E. Kline (Eds.). (2010). *Pediatric oncology nursing.* New York, NY: Springer.

As neutrophils are the primary means of fighting bacterial infection, when the neutrophil count is low, the chance for developing an overwhelming bacterial infection is high. Each drug that causes bone marrow suppression has a point of nadir. *Nadir* is the time after administration of the drug when bone marrow suppression is expected to be at its greatest and the neutrophil count is expected to be at its lowest (neutropenia). Nadir is individual for each drug and ranges from 7 to 28 days after dosing. An absolute neutrophil count (ANC) below 500 places the child at greatest risk, although an ANC below 1,500 usually warrants evaluation (Brundige, 2010). Refer to Box 46.2 for information related to calculating the absolute neutrophil count.

BOX 46.2

CALCULATING THE ABSOLUTE NEUTROPHIL COUNT (ANC)

- Add together the percentage of banded and segmented neutrophils reported on the complete blood count with differential (CBC with diff).
- Multiply the total number of white blood cells reported on the CBC by the sum above. This yields the ANC (total number of neutrophils present).

Example: Bands 5%, Segs 15%, WBCs 2,500

5% + 15% = 20% (0.20)

2,500 × 0.20 = 500

ANC = 500

Adapted from Brundige, K. (2010). Neutropenia. In D. Tomlinson & N. E. Kline (Eds.), *Pediatric oncology nursing.* New York, NY: Springer.

Depending on institutional policy, precautions for neutropenia will be followed if the ANC is depressed. Precautions related to neutropenia generally include:

- Place the child in a private room.
- Perform hand hygiene before and after contact with each child.
- Monitor vital signs every 4 hours.
- Assess for signs and symptoms of infection at least every 8 hours.
- Avoid rectal suppositories, enemas, or examinations; urinary catheterization; and invasive procedures.
- Restrict visitors with fever, cough, or other signs/symptoms of infection.
- Do not permit raw fruits or vegetables or fresh flowers or live plants in the room.
- Place a mask on the child when he or she is being transported outside of the room.
- Perform dental care with a soft toothbrush if the platelet count is adequate.

Children with neutropenia and fever must be started on intravenous broad-spectrum antibiotics without delay to avoid overwhelming sepsis (Brundige, 2010).

Preventing Hemorrhage

Assess for petechiae, purpura, bruising, or bleeding. Determine changes from baseline that warrant intervention. Encourage quiet activities or play to avoid trauma.

Avoid rectal temperatures and examinations to avoid rectal mucosal damage that results in bleeding. Post a sign at the head of the bed stating "no rectal temperatures or medications." Avoid intramuscular injections and lumbar puncture if possible to decrease the risk of bleeding from a puncture site. If bone marrow aspiration must be performed, apply a pressure dressing to the site to prevent bleeding. For active or uncontrolled bleeding, transfuse platelets as ordered to control bleeding.

Preventing Anemia

To maintain blood volume, limit blood draws to the minimum volume required. Encourage the child to eat an appropriate diet that includes adequate iron. Administer EPO injections as ordered. Teach families to give the injections at home if prescribed.

Managing Nausea, Vomiting, and Anorexia

Many chemotherapeutic drugs produce the adverse effect of nausea and vomiting, which often leads to anorexia. The cycle of nausea, vomiting, and anorexia is difficult to break once it begins. In addition, taste alterations are common in children who have received chemotherapy. During or after chemotherapy, children may develop an aversion to a food that was previously their favorite (Tomlinson & Kline, 2010). Provide foods the child desires or asks for in order to increase the likelihood of eating.

Prevent nausea by administering antiemetic medications prior to the administration of chemotherapy and on a routine schedule around the clock for the first 1 to 2 days rather than on an as-needed (PRN) basis. Herbal or complementary therapies may provide another option for management of nausea.

Take Note!

Ginger capsules, ginger tea, and candied ginger have been used as a nausea remedy for centuries (ginger ale is usually artificially flavored, so it would not have the same effect). Though ginger is considered safe, instruct families to check with the oncologist before using this remedy.

Bright lights and noise may worsen nausea. Therefore, keep the child's environment dimly lit and calm. Relaxation therapy and guided imagery may also be helpful in preventing or treating nausea and vomiting. Refer to Nursing Care Plan 46.1 at the end of the chapter for additional interventions.

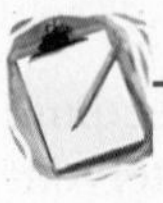

Take Note!

Foot massage may decrease the nausea and pain associated with chemotherapy (Post-White & Ladas, 2010).

Monitoring the Child Receiving Radiation Therapy

Radiation causes damage to the cells in a localized area, which may include normal cells in addition to the cancerous ones. Assess the child's skin daily, particularly at the treatment site. Provide good hygiene, but perform this care gently. Encourage moisture retention in the skin by applying aqueous creams or moisturizers. Do not apply deodorants or perfumed lotions on the radiation treatment site. Avoid the use of heat or ice packs at the site. Instruct the child and family that clothing should fit loosely so as not to irritate the site (Loch & Khorrami, 2010). During, and for 8 weeks after, the radiation treatment, the skin will be more photosensitive. Explain the importance of protecting the skin with a high-SPF (30 or above) sunscreen.

Providing Care to the Child Undergoing Hematopoietic Stem Cell Transplantation

Stem cell transplantation is performed at limited specialty medical centers in the United States. In addition, special training is required for all personnel caring for the child who undergoes a stem cell transplant. The intent of this discussion is to provide only a brief introduction to, and overview of, nursing management related to HSCT.

Care for the child undergoing HSCT may be divided into three phases—the pretransplant phase, the posttransplant phase, and the lengthy supportive care phase. Nursing management of each phase is briefly discussed below.

Pretransplant Phase

In the pretransplant phase, the child is being prepared to receive the transplant. The child's own bone marrow cells are eradicated through high-dose chemotherapy and total body irradiation. This phase usually occurs over 7 to 10 days. The child will be hospitalized because he or she is at extreme risk for serious infection. Maintain protective isolation in a positive-pressure room and limit visitors. Administer gammaglobulin, acyclovir, or antibiotics as ordered to prevent or treat infection. Lymphohematopoietic rescue occurs with infusion of the donor or autologous cells (Norville & Tomlinson, 2010).

Posttransplant Phase

The posttransplant phase is also a time of high risk for the child. Monitor closely for symptoms of GVHD such as severe diarrhea and maculopapular rash progressing to redness or desquamation of the skin (especially palms or soles) (Fig. 46.5). If GVHD occurs, administer immunosuppressive drugs such as cyclosporine, tacrolimus, or

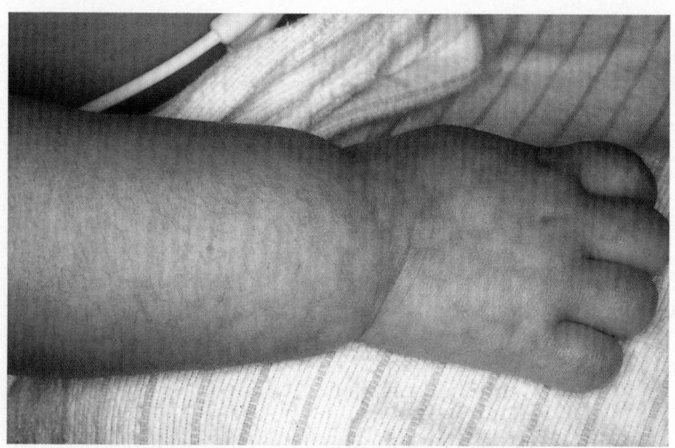

FIGURE 46.5 The first sign of graft-versus-host disease (GVHD) may be a maculopapular rash. (Courtesy of Mary L. Brandt, MD)

mycophenolate (which place the child at further risk for infection) (Norville & Tomlinson, 2010).

Supportive Care

During the supportive care phase, which lasts several months after the transplant, continue to monitor for and prevent infection. Administer PRBCs or platelets and granulocyte colony-stimulating factor as needed.

Families and children who undergo HSCT need prolonged and extensive emotional and psychosocial support. A medical social worker and psychologist or counselor are usually members of the transplant team and are excellent resources for these families' needs (Norville & Tomlinson, 2010).

Promoting a Normal Life

Children and teens want to be normal and to experience the things that other children their age do. The child should attend school when he or she is well enough and the WBC counts are not dangerously low. Children, their families, and their teachers should be aware that cancer and its treatment can affect scholastic abilities. Learning disabilities, difficulty with memory, attention disorders, and cognitive deficits can occur (Tomlinson & Kline, 2010).

Maintain other activities if the child is able and if platelet counts are within normal limits. Special camps are available for children with cancer. These camps offer an opportunity for children and adolescents to experience a variety of activities safely and to network with other children who are experiencing similar physical and emotional challenges. The Children's Oncology Camping Association and the American Childhood Cancer Foundation provide lists of camps throughout the United States and Canada and internationally for children and teens with cancer. Links to these resources are provided on thePoint.

Promoting Growth

Promote growth in children with cancer by encouraging an appropriate diet and preventing nausea and vomiting and also by addressing concerns such as diarrhea and constipation. Chronic diarrhea related to radiation therapy may prevent the child from gaining weight and growing properly (see Nursing Care Plan 46.1 at the end of the chapter). The use of vinca alkaloids and opioids, as well as the decreased activity level of the child with cancer, may contribute to constipation. Constipation increases the pain experience, contributes to the child's malaise, and decreases quality of life. It directly affects the child's ability to grow by increasing anorexia, nausea, and vomiting (Tomlinson & Kline, 2010). Nursing Care Plan 46.1 details interventions related to preventing and managing constipation.

Preventing and Treating Oncologic Emergencies

Oncologic emergencies may occur as an effect of the disease process itself or from cancer treatment. As progress is made in chemotherapy and radiation treatment, children with cancer have an increased survival rate, but they still face the risk of developing an oncologic emergency. Nurses caring for children with cancer need to be familiar with signs and symptoms of oncologic emergencies as well as with their treatment. All of these problems warrant careful, frequent monitoring of respiratory, cardiovascular, neurologic, and renal status. Table 46.3 provides information about oncologic emergencies.

Caring for the Dying Child

Among children in the United States diagnosed with cancer, close to 2,000 will die from the disease each year (CureSearch, n. d.). A "do not resuscitate" (DNR) order for the child with progressive cancer is obtained in many situations. This order helps to optimize care in the terminal phase of cancer. Nurses serve as child and family advocates, clarifying terminology and providing support as needed during the discussion of DNR orders and throughout the rest of the terminal phase.

Children with terminal cancer often experience a great deal of pain, particularly when death is imminent. Pain is often accompanied by agitation and dyspnea, which further contribute to the child's discomfort. Whether the child has a DNR order or his or her status remains that of "full code," pain management is central to the nursing care of the child who is dying from cancer. The Association of Pediatric Hematology Oncology Nurses' position paper entitled "Pain Management

TABLE 46.3 ONCOLOGIC EMERGENCIES

Emergency	Associated With	Signs and Symptoms	Laboratory or Diagnostic Test Findings	Management
Sepsis	Neutropenia resulting from bone marrow suppression due to chemotherapy	• Fever or low temperature • Respiratory distress • Poor perfusion • Altered level of consciousness	• ANC <500 • Positive blood culture • Increased BUN, creatinine, potassium, clotting times • Decreased platelet count • Metabolic acidosis	• Airway and ventilation maintenance • Fluid volume resuscitation • Inotropic support • Broad-spectrum antibiotics and antifungals • Dialysis if needed
Tumor lysis syndrome	ALL, lymphoma, neuroblastoma	• Nausea, vomiting, diarrhea, anorexia • Lethargy • Increased heart rate and blood pressure • Decreased or absent urine output • Altered level of consciousness	• Hyperuricemia • Hyperkalemia • Hyperphosphatemia • Hypocalcemia • Hypoxia	• Prevent by giving allopurinol for several days prior to chemotherapy (also treat with allopurinol) • Double IV fluid maintenance • Sodium bicarbonate
Typhlitis (neutropenic enterocolitis)	Inflammatory process of GI tract occurring with induction phase of leukemia chemotherapy	• Acute abdominal pain • Nausea, vomiting • Bloody diarrhea and emesis • Fever • Anorexia	• KUB: scarcity of bowel gas, possibly ileus • CT (abdominal): inflammation, bowel wall thickening, peritoneal fluid	• Bowel rest (NPO status) • IV nutrition • Assess for bowel perforation/shock • Broad-spectrum antibiotics and antifungals • Comfort measures
Superior vena cava (SVC) syndrome	Compression on the SVC by NHL or other mediastinal mass, such as neuroblastoma	• Dyspnea and cyanosis • Large cervical lymph nodes • Wheezing, diminished breath sounds	• Chest x-ray or CT shows mediastinal mass • Pleural effusion	• Intubation and ventilation • Comfort measures • Treat cause (usually surgical removal of mass)
Spinal cord compression	Tumor or metastasis compresses spinal cord.	• Back, neck, or leg pain • Sensory or autonomic dysfunction • Extremity weakness or paralysis	• MRI reveals location of tumor or metastasis to epidural space	• Dexamethasone • Careful assessment • Radiation therapy • Comfort measures
Increased intracranial pressure	Brain tumor or metastasis to brain causing compression of brain; may result in herniation	• Headache, visual disturbances • Morning vomiting • Infants: increased head circumference • Altered level of consciousness • Cushing triad • Seizure activity	• Head CT or MRI reveals extent of mass	• Frequent, careful neurologic assessment • Limit fluids • Dexamethasone • Anticonvulsants • Tumor resection, radiation, or chemotherapy • Comfort measures

TABLE 46.3 ONCOLOGIC EMERGENCIES (continued)

Emergency	Associated With	Signs and Symptoms	Laboratory or Diagnostic Test Findings	Management
Massive hepatomegaly	Obstruction caused by neuroblastoma filling a large portion of the abdominal cavity	• Distended, enlarged abdomen • Respiratory distress, hypoxia • Poor perfusion • Tachycardia, hypotension	• Abdominal CT reveals extent of tumor • Coagulopathy	• Tumor resection or debulking • Mechanical ventilation, inotropic support • Nasogastric decompression • Position to minimize abdominal pressure • Blood transfusions • Comfort measures

GI, gastrointestinal; KUB, kidney, ureters, and bladder scan; NPO, nothing by mouth.
Adapted from Graham, D. K., Craddock, J. A., Quinones, R. R., Keating, A. K., Maloney, K. Foreman, N. K., Giller, R. H., & Greffe, B. S. (2014). Neoplastic disease. In W. W. Hay, M. J. Levin, R. R. Deterding, & M. J. Abzug (Eds.), *Current pediatric diagnosis and treatment* (22nd ed.). New York, NY: McGraw-Hill; and D. Tomlinson & N. E. Kline (Eds.). (2010). *Pediatric oncology nursing*. New York, NY: Springer.

for the Child With Cancer in End-of-Life Care" outlines the following recommendations for managing children's pain at the end of life:

- Prevention and alleviation of pain is a primary goal of care in the child dying of cancer.
- Children and parents are equal partners with members of the healthcare team in managing the child's pain.
- Children dying of cancer may require aggressive dosing of analgesics. Medications that do not have a dose maximum should be escalated, sometimes rapidly, to achieve adequate pain control or to maintain pain control when tolerance has occurred.
- The nurse's role in caring for children who are in pain at the end of life includes assessment, identifying expected outcomes, and planning, performing, and evaluating interventions (Hooke, Hellsten, Stutzer, & Forte, 2002).

Interventions related to pain management may be found in Nursing Care Plan 46.1, at the end of the chapter. Further discussion related to care of the dying child is found in Chapter 34.

ANEMIA

Anemia is a condition in which levels of RBCs and Hgb are lower than normal. Hgb levels vary throughout childhood. Therefore, it is important to monitor them to ensure that adequate growth and development will be achieved. Anemia may develop as a result of decreased production of RBCs or loss and destruction of RBCs. The loss of production can be related to lack of dietary intake of the nutrients needed to produce the cells, alterations in the cell structure, or malfunctioning tissues (e.g., bone marrow). Anemia related to nutritional deficiency includes iron deficiency, folic acid deficiency, and pernicious anemia. Anemia may also result from toxin exposure (lead poisoning) or as an adverse reaction to a medication (aplastic anemia). Blood loss may result from surgery or trauma. Alteration or destruction of cells occurs in certain genetic and cellular development disorders (Bryant, 2010).

Anemia caused by the alteration or destruction of the RBCs is termed hemolytic anemia. There are several types of hemolytic anemia, such as sickle cell disease and thalassemia; these two disorders are discussed under the section on hemoglobinopathies.

Anemia related to insufficient intake of specific nutrients is the most common type of anemia in children. Nutrient intake may be reduced in children due to food dislikes or conditions that produce malabsorption.

Iron-Deficiency Anemia

Iron-deficiency anemia occurs when the body does not have enough iron to produce Hgb. In the United States, iron-deficiency anemia has a peak prevalence in children between the ages of 6 and 24 months, and again at the age of puberty (Ambruso, Nuss, & Wang, 2014). Cow's milk consumption contributes to iron-deficiency anemia in older infants and young children due to its poor iron availability (Bryant, 2010).

The heme portion of Hgb consists of iron surrounded by protoporphyrin. When not enough iron is available to the bone marrow, Hgb production is reduced. Adequate dietary intake of iron is required for the body to make enough Hgb. As Hgb levels decrease, the oxygen-carrying capacity of the blood is decreased, resulting in weakness and fatigue. In addition to delayed growth, iron-deficiency anemia has been associated with cognitive delays and behavioral changes.

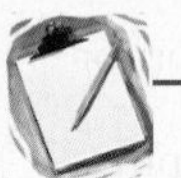

Take Note!

For appropriate growth to occur in adolescence, increased amounts of iron must be consumed and absorbed.

Therapeutic Management

Iron supplements are usually provided in the form of ferrous sulfate or ferrous fumarate and are available over the counter. The recommended dose is 3 mg of elemental iron once or twice daily (Mahoney, 2015b).

In more severe cases, blood transfusions may be indicated. Transfusion of PRBCs is reserved for the most severe cases (Bryant, 2010). When PRBC administration is warranted, follow specific blood bank guidelines for administration. Monitor subsequent laboratory results for improvement.

Nursing Assessment

For a full description of the assessment phase of the nursing process, refer to the Assessment section of the Nursing Process Overview earlier in the chapter. Assessment findings pertinent to iron-deficiency anemia are discussed below.

HEALTH HISTORY

Elicit a description of the current illness and chief complaint. Common signs and symptoms reported during the health history may include irritability, headache, dizziness, weakness, shortness of breath, pallor, and fatigue. Other symptoms may be subtle and difficult for the clinician to identify; these include difficulty feeding, pica, muscle weakness, or unsteady gait.

Explore the health history for risk factors such as:

- Maternal anemia during pregnancy
- Poorly controlled diabetes during pregnancy
- Prematurity, low birth weight, or multiple birth
- Cow's milk consumption before 12 months of age
- Excessive cow's milk consumption (greater than 24 oz a day)
- Infant consumption of low-iron formula
- Lack of iron supplementation after age 6 months in breast-fed infants
- Excessive weight gain
- Chronic infection or inflammation
- Chronic or acute blood loss
- Restricted diets
- Use of medication interfering with iron absorption, such as antacids
- Low socioeconomic status
- Recent immigration from a developing country (Bryant, 2010; Mahoney, 2015a)

Evaluate the child's diet for adequate intake of iron-rich foods. Recommended dietary daily intake for iron in children is:

- 0 to 6 months: 0.27 mg
- 6 to 12 months: 3 mg
- 1 to 3 years: 7 mg
- 4 to 8 years: 11 mg
- 9 to 13 years: 8 mg
- Boys 14 to 18 years: 11 mg
- Girls 14 to 18 years: 15 mg (Haemer, Primark, & Krebs, 2014)

PHYSICAL EXAMINATION

Observe the child for fatigue and lethargy. Inspect the skin, conjunctivae, oral mucosa, palms, and soles for pallor. Note spooning of the nails (concave shape) (Fig. 46.6). Obtain a pulse oximeter reading. Evaluate the heart rate for tachycardia. Auscultate the heart for a flow murmur. Palpate the abdomen for splenomegaly.

LABORATORY AND DIAGNOSTIC TESTS

Laboratory evaluation will reveal decreased Hgb and Hct, decreased reticulocyte count, microcytosis, hypochromia, decreased serum iron and ferritin levels, and an increased free erythrocyte protoporphyrin (FEP) level.

Nursing Management

Nursing management of the child with iron deficiency focuses on promoting safety, ensuring adequate iron intake, and educating the family.

PROMOTING SAFETY

The child with anemia is at risk for changes in neurologic functioning related to the decreased oxygen supply to the brain. This can lead to fatigue and inability to eat enough. Neurologic effects may be manifested when the child's ability to sit, stand, or walk

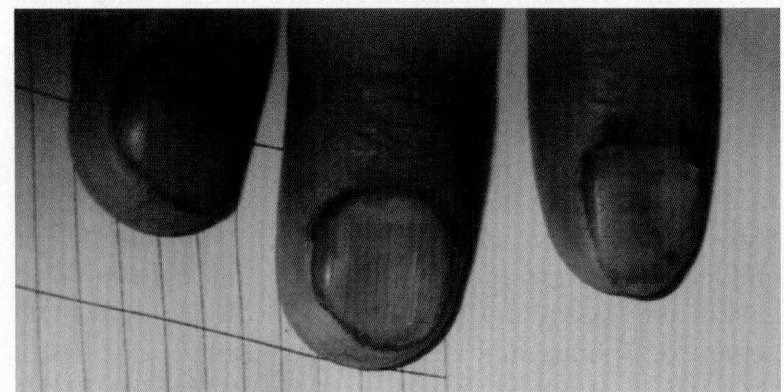

FIGURE 46.6 Note the concave shape of nails ("spooning") that occurs with iron-deficiency anemia.

is impaired. Provide close observation of the anemic child. Assist the older child with ambulation. Educate the parents on how to protect the child from injury due to an unsteady gait or dizziness.

PROVIDING DIETARY INTERVENTIONS

Ensure that iron-deficient infants are fed only formulas fortified with iron. Interventions for breast-fed infants include beginning iron supplementation around the age of 4 or 5 months. Iron supplementation may range from adding iron-fortified cereals to the child's diet to giving iron-containing drops. Encourage breastfeeding mothers to increase their dietary intake of iron or take iron supplements when breastfeeding so that the iron may be passed on to the infant. For children over 1 year of age, limit cow's milk intake to 24 oz per day. Limit fast-food consumption and encourage intake of iron-rich foods such as red meats (iron from red meat is the easiest for the body to absorb), tuna, salmon, eggs, tofu, enriched grains, dried beans and peas, dried fruits, leafy green vegetables, and iron-fortified breakfast cereals.

Teach the parents about dietary intake of iron. Encourage parents to provide a variety of foods for iron support and vitamins and other minerals necessary for growth. A big problem for toddlers is their picky eating. This often becomes a means of control for the child, and parents should guard against getting involved in a power struggle with their child. Referring parents to a developmental specialist who can assist them in their approach to diet may prove beneficial. Refer families who meet the financial limits and who have children age 5 and younger to the Women, Infants, and Children (WIC) program, which provides for supplementation of infants' and children's diets.

HEALTHY PEOPLE 2020

Objective	Nursing Significance
Reduce iron deficiency among young children and females of child-bearing age	• Encourage use of iron-fortified formulas and infant cereal. • Encourage iron supplementation in the second half of infancy for the breast-fed infant. • Educate parents about iron-containing foods. • Encourage adolescent females to consume a diet high in iron-rich foods.

Healthy People Objectives retrieved from http://www.healthypeople.gov

Take Note!

Parents are often concerned that a diagnosis of iron-deficiency anemia or referral to the WIC program may lead to interventions from children's services. Assure the family that as long as appropriate measures are taken to address the anemia, referrals of this nature are not generally made.

TEACHING ABOUT IRON SUPPLEMENT ADMINISTRATION

The use of iron supplements in infants begins with the use of formula fortified with iron in the formula-fed infant. Oral supplements may also be necessary if the baby's iron levels are extremely low. Oral supplements or multivitamin formulas that contain iron are often dark in color because the iron is pigmented. Teach parents to precisely measure the amount of iron to be administered. Parents should place the liquid behind the teeth, as iron in liquid form can stain the teeth. Iron supplementation can also cause constipation. In some cases reducing the amount of iron can resolve this problem, but stool softeners may be necessary to control painful or difficult-to-pass stools. Encourage parents to increase their child's fluid intake and include adequate dietary fiber to avoid constipation.

Take Note!

Teach parents to keep iron-containing supplements out of the reach of young children in order to prevent accidental ingestion leading to overdose or poisoning.

Other Nutritional Causes of Anemia

Other forms of anemia related to nutritional deficit include folic acid deficiency and pernicious anemia. Comparison Chart 46.2 discusses the causes, assessment, and management of these disorders.

Lead Poisoning

Elevated lead levels are found annually in nearly 500,000 U.S. children between 1 and 5 years of age (Centers for Disease Control and Prevention [CDC], 2016). Lead exerts toxic effects on the bone marrow, erythroid cells, nervous system, and kidneys. The presence of lead in the bloodstream interferes with the enzymatic processes of the biosynthesis of heme. The process results in hypochromic, microcytic anemia, and children may exhibit classic signs of anemia. Risk factors for lead poisoning are related to lead exposure in the home, school, or local environment. Sources of lead include:

- Paint in homes built before 1978, at which time lead was banned as an additive to paint used in houses

COMPARISON CHART 46.2 FOLIC ACID DEFICIENCY VERSUS PERNICIOUS ANEMIA

	Folic Acid Deficiency	Pernicious Anemia
Cause	Low dietary intake of green leafy vegetables, liver, and citrus Malabsorption from medication such as phenytoin (Dilantin) or parasitic infection	Deficiency in vitamin B_{12}
Assessment	Determine risk factors such as prematurity, low socioeconomic status, and history of malabsorption disease. Determine dietary history, noting dislike of fresh vegetables or fruit, ingestion of overcooked foods, or lack of family purchase of fruits and vegetables. Note history of fatigue, headache, poor growth, anorexia, or diarrhea. Inspect the skin for pallor or jaundice, and note presence of a sore on the mouth or tongue	Note history of anorexia, irritability, or chronic diarrhea. Observe the skin or conjunctivae for pallor and the tongue for smooth texture and bright-red color
Laboratory analysis	RBC, Hgb, Hct	RBC, Hgb, Hct, low vitamin B_{12} level
Management	Encourage parents to include green leafy vegetables, liver, and citrus in diet. Ensure that parents comply with dietary changes	Administer monthly injections of vitamin B_{12}. Inform parents injections will be required throughout the child's life. Provide emotional support related to the chronic nature of this disorder

- Soil where cars that used leaded gas have been in the past (lead was removed from all gasoline in the United States as of 1996)
- Glazed pottery
- Stained glass products
- Lead pipes supplying water to the home
- On the clothing of parents who work in certain manufacturing jobs (battery makers, cable makers)
- Certain folk remedies, such as *greta or arzacon*
- Old painted toys or furniture (Lee & Hurwitz, 2016)

Complications of lead poisoning include behavioral problems and learning difficulties and, with higher lead levels, encephalopathy, seizures, and brain damage.

Therapeutic management for high blood levels of lead involves **chelation therapy** (removal of heavy metals from the body via chelating agents), either orally or intravenously. Drug Guide 46.1 gives further information on chelating agents.

Nursing Assessment

Explore the health history for subtle signs such as anorexia, fatigue, or abdominal pain. Determine whether behavioral problems, irritability, hyperactivity, or lack of ability to meet developmental milestones have occurred in recent months. Screen children for risk of exposure to lead in the home. Refer to Chapter 31 for a simple screening questionnaire that can be used to determine the need for lead screening in young children. Blood levels of lead greater than 10 μg/dL require conscientious follow-up. Note pallor of the skin.

Nursing Management

Prevention of elevated lead levels is critical. Screen children for lead exposure risk. The American Academy of Pediatrics Bright Future guidelines recommends performing a risk assessment and if positive screen at 6, 9, 12, 18, and 24 months, and 3, 4, 5, and 6 years. Table 46.4 gives recommendations for appropriate follow-up depending on lead levels.

Removing old paint is the best way to eliminate the most significant source of lead exposure for a large number of children. If the family rents or lives in public housing, the landlord or owner is responsible for following the guidelines set forth by local and state governmental agencies to correct the problem.

Educate families about how to prevent exposure to lead, particularly in young children. Additional resources for families are located on thePoint.

If the child is undergoing chelation therapy, ensure adequate fluid intake and monitor intake and output closely. Refer children with elevated lead levels and developmental or cognitive deficits to developmental centers. These children may need an early intervention program for further evaluation and treatment of developmental delays.

Aplastic Anemia

Aplastic anemia (failure of the bone marrow to produce cells) is characterized by bone marrow aplasia and pancytopenia (decreased numbers of all blood cells). Most cases are acquired, but there are a few rare types of

TABLE 46.4 INTERVENTIONS BASED ON BLOOD LEAD LEVEL

Blood Lead Level (in mcg/dL)	Recommended Action
<5	Repeat test annually or sooner if <2 years old.
5–14	Confirm with repeat test in 1 month and educate parents to decrease lead exposure. Repeat test within 3 months.
15–19	Confirm with repeat test in 1 month and educate parents to decrease lead exposure. Report to local health authorities for surveillance. Repeat test within 2 months.
20–44	Confirm with repeat test within 1 week and educate parents to decrease lead exposure. Refer to local health department for investigation of home for lead reduction, with referrals for support services.
45–69	Confirm with repeat test within 2 days and educate parents to decrease lead exposure. Begin chelation therapy and refer to health department as above.
>70	Hospitalize child and begin chelation therapy. Ensure lead is removed from the home.

Adapted from Hurwitz, R. L., & Lee, D. A. (2016). *Childhood lead poisoning: Management*. Retrieved from http://www.uptodate.com/contents/childhood-lead-poisoning-management

inherited aplastic anemias (Bryant, 2010). The inherited types present as congenital bone marrow failure; the best known is Fanconi anemia, an autosomal recessive disorder. Acquired aplastic anemia is thought to be an immune-mediated response. Most cases are idiopathic, meaning the trigger remains unidentified. Other causes include exposure to environmental toxins, viruses, myelosuppressive drugs, or radiation.

Aplastic anemia may be classified as severe or nonsevere. In the severe form, the granulocyte count is less than 500, the platelet count is less than 20,000, and the reticulocyte count is less than 1%. In nonsevere aplastic anemia, the granulocyte count is about 500, the platelet count is over 20,000, and the reticulocyte count is over 1% (Ambruso et al., 2014). Complications of aplastic anemia include severe overwhelming infection, hemorrhage, and death. Therapeutic management of aplastic anemia in children involves hematopoietic stem cell transplantation from a human leukocyte antigen (HLA)–matched sibling donor; if one is not available, immunosuppressive therapy or high-dose cyclophosphamide can be given.

HEALTHY PEOPLE 2020

Objective	Nursing Significance
Eliminate elevated blood lead levels in children.	• Appropriately screen infants and young children for lead exposure at each healthcare visit.

Healthy People Objectives retrieved from http://www.healthypeople.gov

Nursing Assessment

Determine history of exposure to myelosuppressive medications or radiation therapy. Obtain a detailed family, environmental, and infectious disease history. Note history of epistaxis, gingival oozing, or increased bleeding with menstruation. Anemia may lead to headache and fatigue. On physical examination, note ecchymoses, petechiae or purpura, oral ulcerations, tachycardia, or tachypnea. In addition to suppression of all blood cells, laboratory and diagnostic testing may reveal:

- Guaiac-positive stool
- Blood in the urine
- Severe decrease in or the absence of hematopoietic cells on bone marrow aspiration

Nursing Management

Safety is of the utmost concern in children with aplastic anemia. It is important to prevent injury in order to avoid hemorrhage. Stool softeners may be used to prevent anal fissures associated with constipation. Administer only irradiated and leukocyte-depleted PRBCs or platelet transfusions as necessary. This limits exposure to HLA antigens should the child require bone marrow transplantation in the future. If the child requires hematopoietic stem cell transplantation, refer to the section earlier in this chapter for additional nursing management information.

Refer families whose child has only mild or moderate disease to the Aplastic Anemia and Myelodysplastic Syndrome International Foundation, a link to which can be found on thePoint.

Hemoglobinopathies

Hemoglobinopathy is a condition in which abnormal hemoglobin is present. A large percentage of the newborn's hemoglobin is fetal hemoglobin (Hgb F). Hgb F can exchange oxygen molecules at lower oxygen tensions compared to adult hemoglobin. Over the first several months of life, Hgb F levels fall as it is replaced with Hgb A (adult hemoglobin). The healthy older infant then displays Hgb AA. In hemoglobinopathies, this normal hemoglobin configuration is disturbed. Causes of hemoglobinopathies are genetic and include sickle cell anemia, hemoglobin SC disease, α-thalassemia, and β-thalassemia. This discussion will focus on sickle cell disease and β-thalassemia (Cooley anemia).

Sickle Cell Disease

Sickle cell disease is a group of inherited hemoglobinopathies in which the RBCs do not carry the normal adult hemoglobin, but instead carry a less effective type. In the United States, the most common types of sickle cell disease are hemoglobin SS disease (sickle cell anemia), hemoglobin SC disease, and hemoglobin sickle–β-thalassemia. Among the sickle cell diseases, sickle cell anemia is the most common and will be the focus of this discussion (Bryant, 2010).

Sickle cell anemia is a severe chronic blood disorder that occurs once in every 2,000 newborns in the United States each year (Chandrakason & Kamat, 2013). It is most common in individuals of African, Mediterranean, Middle Eastern, and Indian decent. One in 400 African Americans has sickle cell anemia (Ambruso et al., 2014). Instead of Hgb AA, individuals with sickle cell anemia have Hgb SS. In hemoglobin S, glutamic acid is replaced with valine in the hemoglobin molecule. This results in an elongated RBC with a shortened life span. The elongated cell is more rigid than a normal cell and becomes sickled in shape (Fig. 46.7). Persons with heterozygous representation (Hgb AS) are said to have sickle cell trait and are carriers for the disorder; about 8% of African Americans have sickle cell trait (Ambruso et al., 2014). Generally, persons with sickle cell trait have only minimal health problems.

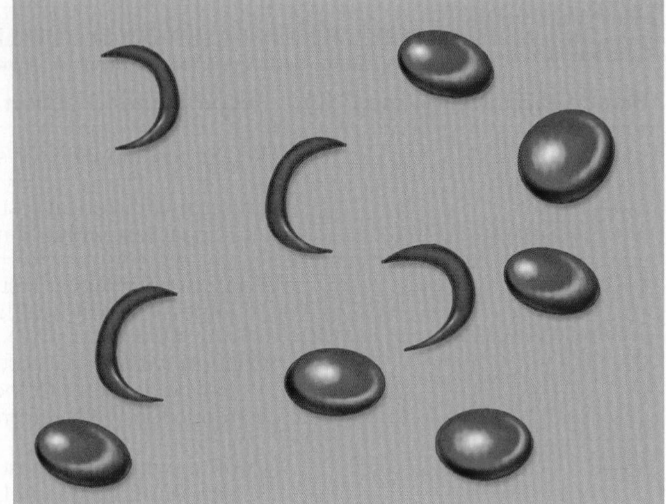

FIGURE 46.7 This peripheral blood smear demonstrates the elongated sickle-shaped red blood cell seen in sickle cell disease.

The recessive genes for sickle cell are passed on from both parents who have the gene or trait. Each parent has the gene Hgb AS. Hgb A refers to normal adult hemoglobin and Hgb S refers to sickle hemoglobin. These recessive genes for sickle cell may be passed on to the child. The risk for developing Hgb SS is one in four, or 25%, in each child from this union. With each pregnancy the risk is 25% that the child will have disease, 25% that the child will have normal hemoglobin, and 50% that the child will have the trait (Hgb AS) and will be a carrier (Pitts & Record, 2010). Figure 46.8 illustrates the inheritance probability. Infants with sickle cell anemia are usually asymptomatic until 3 to 4 months of age because Hgb F protects against sickling.

Complications of sickle cell anemia include recurrent vaso-occlusive pain crises, stroke, sepsis, acute chest syndrome, splenic sequestration, reduced visual acuity related to decreased retinal blood flow, chronic leg ulcers, cholestasis and gallstones, delayed growth and development, delayed puberty, and priapism (the sickled cells prevent blood from flowing out of an erect penis). Children with sickle cell anemia have an increased incidence of enuresis because the kidneys cannot concentrate urine effectively (Pitts & Record, 2010). As children reach adulthood, multiple organ dysfunction is common.

PATHOPHYSIOLOGY

Significant anemia may occur when the RBCs sickle. Sickling may be triggered by any stress or traumatic event, such as infection, fever, acidosis, dehydration, physical exertion, excessive cold exposure, or hypoxia

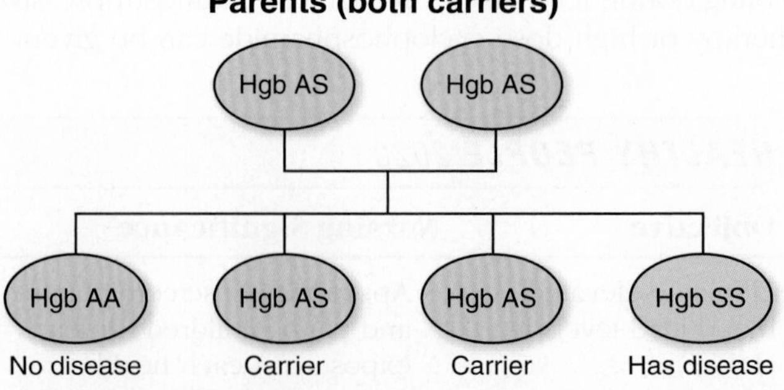

FIGURE 46.8 Simplified genetic scheme for sickle cell disease. *A* denotes adult hemoglobin; *S* denotes sickle hemoglobin. Hemoglobin AA, normal hemoglobin; hemoglobin AS, sickle cell trait; hemoglobin SS, sickle cell disease.

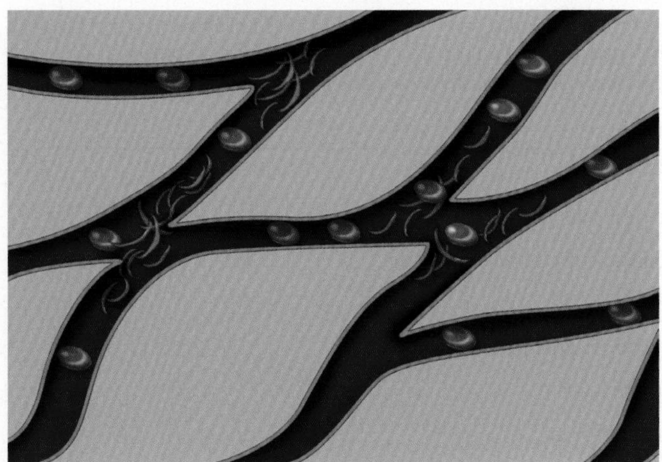

FIGURE 46.9 Clumping of sickle-shaped cells.

(Ambruso et al., 2014). As the cells sickle, the blood becomes more viscous because the sickled cells clump together and prevent normal blood flow to the tissues of that area. The sickle-shaped RBCs cannot pass through the smaller capillaries and venules of the circulatory system (Fig. 46.9). This vaso-occlusive process leads to local tissue hypoxia followed by ischemia and may result in infarction. Pain crisis results as circulation is decreased to the area. Pain can occur in any part of the body but is most common in the joints. Pain causes increased metabolic need by resulting in tachycardia and sometimes tachypnea, which leads to further sickling. Clumping of cells in the lungs (acute chest syndrome [ACS]) results in decreased gas exchange, producing hypoxia, which leads to further sickling. ACS is the most common cause of death in children with sickle cell disease (Abbas, Kahale, Hosn, & Inati, 2013). Sequestration of blood in the spleen leads to splenomegaly and abdominal pain. Hemolysis follows sickling and leads to further anemia. The increased activity of the spleen related to RBC hemolysis leads to splenomegaly, then fibrosis and atrophy. Functional asplenia may develop as early as 6 months of age, and occurs by age 9 years in 90% of children with sickle cell disease (Pitts & Record, 2010).

THERAPEUTIC MANAGEMENT

The therapeutic management of children with sickle cell anemia focuses on preventing sickling crisis and infection as well as other complications. Prevention of infection is critical because the child with sickle cell anemia is at increased risk for serious infection related to alterations in splenic function. Functional asplenia (decrease in the ability of the spleen to function appropriately) places the child at significant risk for serious infection with *Streptococcus pneumoniae* or other encapsulated organisms. Prophylactic antibiotics in the young child and appropriate immunization in all children with sickle cell anemia can reduce the risk of serious infection (Pitts & Record, 2010).

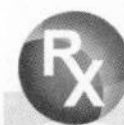

Dosage Calculation Box 46.1

Child's weight: 50 lb

Medication order: hydroxyurea 450 mg oral daily.

Per the Pediatric Dosage Handbook, the recommended dose is 20 mg/kg/dose, once daily

Is the ordered dose safe?

Treatment of sickle cell crisis focuses on pain control. Oxygen administration is necessary during episodes of crisis to prevent additional cell sickling. Adequate hydration with intravenous fluids is critical. Close monitoring of Hgb, Hct, and reticulocytes determines the point at which transfusion of PRBCs becomes necessary. Electrolyte analysis is also necessary to ensure that appropriate amounts of electrolytes are present in the serum. When RBCs are administered, there is the potential for hemolysis of the cells, thus increasing the potassium level in the serum. Antibiotic therapy is necessary when infection is present. Box 46.3 describes additional medical treatments that are needed in some children.

NURSING ASSESSMENT

Children with sickle cell anemia experience a significant number of acute and chronic manifestations of the condition (Comparison Chart 46.3). For a full description of the assessment phase of the nursing process, refer to the Assessment section in the Nursing Process Overview earlier in the chapter. Assessment findings pertinent to sickle cell anemia are discussed below.

Health History. Elicit the health history, noting growth and development, frequency and extent of vaso-occlusive

BOX 46.3

ADDITIONAL MEDICAL TREATMENTS FOR SOME CHILDREN WITH SICKLE CELL ANEMIA

- Cholecystectomy may become necessary if gallstones develop.
- Splenectomy may be performed to prevent recurrence of splenic sequestration if it is life-threatening.
- Considered investigational, administration of hydroxyurea may increase the percentage of fetal hemoglobin; a large clinical trial in children is ongoing.
- Blood transfusions, though not routinely given to children with sickle cell disease, are indicated in children with prolonged or widespread pain, aplastic crisis, or splenic sequestration.
- Partial exchange transfusion may be used to rapidly lower the circulating amount of Hgb SS in the event of stroke or acute chest syndrome.
- Hematopoietic stem cell transplantation is usually reserved for children with an identical HLA-matched sibling (risk of death and incidence of graft-versus-host disease is high) (Pitts & Record, 2010).

COMPARISON CHART 46.3

ACUTE VERSUS CHRONIC MANIFESTATIONS OF SICKLE CELL ANEMIA

Acute	Chronic
[a]Acute chest syndrome	Anemia
[a]Aplastic crisis	Avascular necrosis of the hip
[a]Bacterial sepsis or meningitis	Cardiomegaly, functional murmur
Bone infarction	Cholelithiasis
Dactylitis	Delayed growth and development
Hematuria	Delayed puberty
Recurrent pain episodes	Functional asplenia
Pain crisis	Hyposthenuria (low urine specific gravity) and enuresis
[a]Splenic sequestration	Jaundice
[a]Stroke	Leg ulcers
Priapism	Proteinuria
	[a]Pulmonary hypertension
	[a]Restrictive lung disease
	Retinopathy

[a]Often life-threatening.

crises, past hospitalizations, and treatment for pain crises. Note history of immunizations, including pneumococcal, flu, and meningococcal vaccinations. Determine history of blood transfusions. Document the current medication regimen. Note history of recurrent infections. Determine history of the present illness that results in a precipitating event, such as hypoxia, infection, or dehydration. Note onset, character, and quality of pain, as well as relieving factors.

Physical Examination. Perform a thorough physical examination, because sickling, hypoxia, and tissue ischemia affect most areas of the body (Fig. 46.10). Note the physical findings discussed below that may be detected using inspection, observation, auscultation, and palpation.

Inspection and Observation. Inspect the conjunctivae, palms, and soles for pallor and the skin for pallor, lesions, or ulcers. Note jaundice of the skin or scleral icterus. Document color and moisture of oral mucosa. Measure temperature to evaluate for infection (which can precipitate a sickling crisis). Note blood pressure, which may be decreased with severe anemia or increased with sickle cell nephropathy. Determine baseline mental status. Perform a neurologic assessment frequently, as about 11% of children with sickle cell anemia will experience an overt stroke (Ambruso et al., 2014).

Auscultation. Auscultate heart sounds for a murmur. The heart rate is often elevated with pain, hyperthermia, or dehydration. Listen to breath sounds, noting the rate and depth of respiration as well as the adequacy of aeration. Adventitious breath sounds may be present if a respiratory infection has triggered the sickle cell crisis or in the case of ACS. About half of the cases of ACS occur in the child already hospitalized for a pain crisis.

Palpation. Palpate the joints for warmth, tenderness, and range of motion. Palpate the abdomen for areas of tenderness. Note hepatomegaly or splenomegaly.

Take Note!

Immediately report symmetric swelling of the hands and feet in the infant or toddler. Termed dactylitis, aseptic infarction occurs in the metacarpals and metatarsals. (Fig. 46.11).

Laboratory and Diagnostic Testing. Newborn screening for sickle cell anemia is required by law or rule in all of the 50 United States (National Newborn Screening and Genetics Resource Center, 2014). Screening by Sickledex or sickle cell prep does not distinguish between sickle cell disease and sickle cell trait. If the screening test result indicates the possibility of sickle cell anemia or sickle

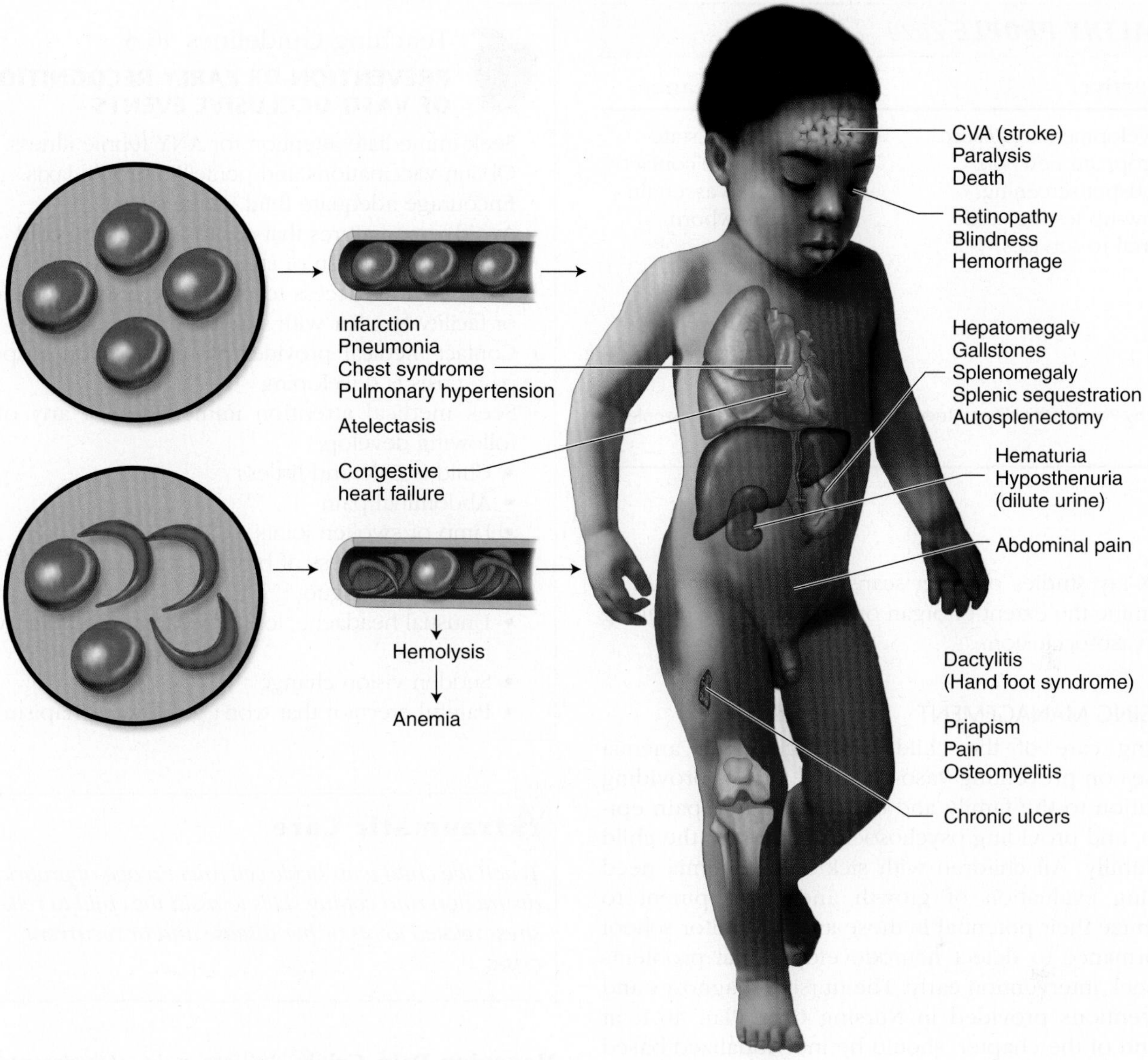

FIGURE 46.10 Effects of sickle cell anemia on various parts of the body.

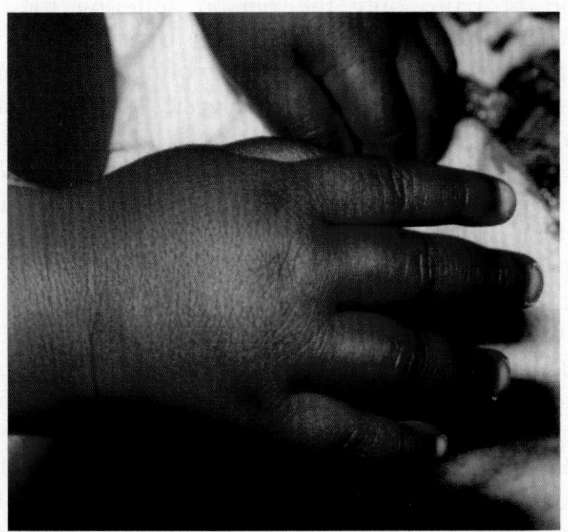

FIGURE 46.11 Swelling of the hands (dactylitis) in a toddler.

cell trait, Hgb electrophoresis is performed promptly to confirm the diagnosis. Hgb electrophoresis is the only accurate test for sickle cell disease. Hgb electrophoresis will demonstrate the presence of Hgb S and Hgb F only in the young infant; in the older infant or child, the result will be Hgb SS.

Common laboratory and diagnostic studies ordered for the assessment of sickle cell anemia include:

- Hemoglobin: baseline is usually 7 to 10 mg/dL; will be significantly lower with splenic sequestration, acute chest syndrome, or aplastic crisis
- Reticulocyte count: greatly elevated
- Peripheral blood smear: presence of sickle-shaped cells and target cells
- Platelet count: increased
- Erythrocyte sedimentation rate: elevated
- Abnormal liver function tests with elevated bilirubin

HEALTHY PEOPLE 2020

Objective	Nursing Significance
(Developmental) Ensure appropriate newborn bloodspot screening, follow-up testing, and referral to services.	• Follow-up with state agencies at first contact with infant to ascertain results of newborn screening. • If screening was not done at birth, ensure Hgb electrophoresis is obtained.

Healthy People Objectives retrieved from http://www.healthypeople.gov

X-ray studies or other scans may be performed to determine the extent of organ or tissue damage resulting from vaso-occlusion.

NURSING MANAGEMENT

Nursing care of the child with sickle cell anemia focuses on preventing vaso-occlusive crises, providing education to the family and child, managing pain episodes, and providing psychosocial support to the child and family. All children with sickle cell anemia need ongoing evaluation of growth and development to maximize their potential in those areas. Monitor school performance to detect neurodevelopmental problems and seek intervention early. The nursing diagnoses and interventions provided in Nursing Care Plan 46.1, at the end of the chapter, should be individualized based on the child's and family's response to the disorder. Specifics related to sickle cell disease are discussed below.

Educating the Family and Child. Begin child and family education immediately after the diagnosis of sickle cell anemia is confirmed. Initially, teach the family about the genetics of the disease and encourage family members to be tested for carrier status. Educate families about the disease process. Emphasize the importance of regularly scheduled health maintenance visits and immunizations. Teach families how to administer prophylactic penicillin. Encourage families to seek medical evaluation urgently for any febrile illness. Educate families about how to prevent and recognize vaso-occlusive events (Teaching Guidelines 46.3). Discuss complications such as delayed growth and development, delayed puberty, stroke, cholelithiasis, retinopathy, avascular necrosis, priapism, and leg ulcers.

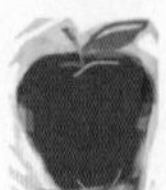

Teaching Guidelines 46.3
PREVENTION OR EARLY RECOGNITION OF VASO-OCCLUSIVE EVENTS

- Seek immediate attention for ANY febrile illness.
- Obtain vaccinations and penicillin prophylaxis.
- Encourage adequate fluid intake daily
- Avoid temperatures that are too hot or too cold
- Avoid overexertion or stress
- Have 24-hour access to physician, nurse practitioner, or facility familiar with sickle cell care
- Contact medical provider promptly if you suspect a pain crisis is developing.
- Seek medical attention immediately if any of the following develop:
  - Child is pale and listless
  - Abdominal pain
  - Limp or swollen joints
  - Cough, shortness of breath, chest pain
  - Increasing fatigue
  - Unusual headache, loss of feeling, or sudden weakness
  - Sudden vision change
  - Painful erection that won't go down (priapism)

Atraumatic Care

Teach the child with sickle cell anemia age-appropriate distraction and coping skills to assist the child to relieve stress related to his or her disease and/or recurrent crises.

Managing Pain Crisis. Initiate pain assessment with a standardized pain scale upon admission. Provide frequent evaluations of pain. Always believe the child's report of pain; only the person suffering the pain knows what it feels like. Moderate to severe pain usually requires opioid medication. To bring the pain under control, initially administer analgesics routinely rather than on an "as needed" (PRN) basis. Once the pain is better managed, medications may be moved to PRN status. Monitor patient-controlled analgesia (PCA) in the child or adolescent. Addiction to narcotics is rarely a concern in the child with sickle cell anemia if the narcotic is used to alleviate severe pain (Pitts & Record, 2010). Nonsteroidal anti-inflammatory medications and acetaminophen are often used for less severe pain. Adequate pain management helps to decrease the child's stress level; elevated stress may contribute to further sickling and additional pain. Use nonpharmacologic pain management techniques such as relaxation or hypnosis, music, massage, play, guided imagery, therapeutic

BOX 46.4

ABCS OF MANAGING SICKLE CELL PAIN

A. Assess the pain (use a pain assessment tool)
B. Believe the child's report of pain
C. Complications or cause of pain (look for complications)
D. Drugs and distraction: pain medication (opiates and NSAIDs, if no contraindications); use fixed dosing; give on a timed schedule; no PRN dosing for pain medications; distraction with music, TV, and relaxation techniques
E. Environment (rest in quiet area with privacy)
F. Fluids (hypotonic—D_5W or D_5 with 0.25% normal saline solution)

Adapted from Platt, A., Eckman, J. R., Beasley, J., & Miller, G. (2002). Treating sickle cell pain: An update from the Georgia Comprehensive Sickle Cell Information Center. *Journal of Emergency Nursing, 28*(4), 297–303, with permission.

touch, or behavior modification to augment the pain medication regimen. Box 46.4 provides a summary of sickle cell pain management.

Take Note!

Avoid repeated use of meperidine for pain management during sickle cell crises because it has been associated with an increased risk of neurotoxicity when used in children with sickle cell anemia (National Heart, Lung, and Blood Institute, 2014).

Managing Sickle Cell Crisis. Treat any underlying conditions such as infection or injury. Deficient fluid volume occurs as a result of decreased intake, increased fluid requirements during sickle cell crisis, and the kidney's inability to concentrate urine. Increasing fluid intake will dilute the blood and decrease its viscosity. To promote hemodilution, provide 150 mL/kg of fluids per day or as much as double maintenance, either orally or intravenously. Maintain appropriate electrolyte and pH balance.

Risk for ineffective tissue perfusion related to the effects of RBC sickling and infarction of tissues is another concern. Frequently evaluate respiratory and circulatory status. Administer supplemental oxygen if the pulse oximetry reading is 92% or less to promote adequate oxygenation (SCIC, 2011). Supplementation with oxygen in the absence of hypoxia is unnecessary and may inhibit erythropoiesis. Monitor level of consciousness and immediately report changes.

Take Note!

Maintain the child's temperature as close to normal as possible without the use of cooling mattresses, as sudden temperature change can further precipitate sickling of the red blood cells (National Heart, Lung, and Blood Institute, 2015).

***HEALTHY PEOPLE** 2020*

Objective	Nursing Significance
Reduce stroke deaths	• Educate families appropriately to decrease incidence of vaso-occlusive episodes in children with sickle cell anemia.

Healthy People Objectives retrieved from http://www.healthypeople.gov

Preventing Infection. To prevent severe infection in the child with sickle cell anemia, a variety of interventions are necessary. By 2 months of age, begin administration of oral penicillin V potassium as prophylaxis against pneumococcal infection. In the penicillin-allergic child, erythromycin may be used. Continue prophylaxis until at least age 5 years. Administer childhood immunizations according to the currently recommended schedule. To prevent overwhelming sepsis or meningitis as a result of infection with *S. pneumoniae,* the child should receive not only the 7-valent pneumococcal vaccine series in infancy but also the 23-valent pneumococcal conjugate vaccine annually after age 2 years. Meningococcal vaccination is also warranted (refer to Chapter 31 for additional information on these vaccines). Provide influenza immunization annually before the onset of flu season (after 6 months of age) (Pitts & Record, 2010).

Supporting the Family and Child. As with any chronic illness, families of children with sickle cell anemia need significant support. They often feel guilty or responsible for the disease. Reassure the family and provide education. Refer families to a regional sickle cell disease center for multidisciplinary care. See Evidence-Based Practice 46.1. Web links for additional resources for families are included on thePoint.

Thalassemia

Thalassemia is a genetic disorder that most often affects those of African descent, but it also affects individuals of Caribbean, Middle Eastern, South Asian, and Mediterranean descent (Bryant, 2010). The genetics of thalassemia are similar to those of sickle cell disease in that it is inherited via an autosomal recessive process. Children with thalassemia have reduced production of normal hemoglobin.

There are two basic types of thalassemia, α and β. In α-thalassemia, synthesis of the α chain of the hemoglobin

EVIDENCE-BASED PRACTICE 46.1

WIRELESS TECHNOLOGY TO FACILITATE PROVIDER COMMUNICATION IN PATIENTS WITH SICKLE CELL DISEASE

Children with sickle cell disease require ongoing medical care. Often, their parents provide primary communicators with the provider. Wireless communications between the child or adolescent, directly with the provider have the potential to improve ongoing health care of the patient with sickle cell disease.

STUDY

In a small study, children and adolescents used a web-based electronic diary twice daily via text messaging to communicate with their nurse practitioners. Preprogrammed parameters determined alert messages, and the nurse practitioner responded to all messages.

Findings

As a result of the text message interchanges, collaboration (screening and referring), and coaching (informing and supporting) occurred. The children and adolescents communicated directly with the nurse practitioner (NP) and experienced an ongoing relationship with the NP. Children and teens reluctant to enter the hospital were able to voice their concerns about their health and receive ongoing education and support.

Nursing Implications

Nurses are in an optimal position to educate and support children and adolescents with sickle cell disease. Utilizing wireless devices to communicate with these patients has the potential to transform the way primary health care is delivered for the pediatric sickle cell population.

Adapted from Jacob, E., Pavlish, C., Duran, J., Stinson, J., Lewis, M. A., & Zeltzer, L. (2013). Facilitating pediatric patient-provider communications using wireless technology in children and adolescents with sickle cell disease.

protein is affected. Problems with the β chain occur more often, and the condition β-thalassemia can be divided into three subcategories based on severity:

- Thalassemia minor (also called β-thalassemia trait): leads to mild microcytic anemia; often no treatment is required.
- Thalassemia intermedia: child requires blood transfusions to maintain adequate quality of life.
- Thalassemia major: to survive the child requires ongoing medical attention, blood transfusions, and iron removal (chelation therapy).

The focus of this discussion will be on β-thalassemia major (Cooley anemia).

In β-thalassemia major, the β-globulin chain in hemoglobin synthesis is reduced or entirely absent. A large number of unstable globulin chains accumulate, causing the RBCs to be rigid and hemolyzed easily. The result is severe hemolytic anemia and chronic hypoxia. In response to the increased rate of RBC destruction, erythroid activity is increased. The increased activity causes massive bone marrow expansion and thinning of the bony cortex. Growth retardation, pathologic fractures, and skeletal deformities (frontal and maxillary bossing) result.

Hemosiderosis (excessive supply of iron) is an additional complication of significant concern. It occurs as a result of rapid hemolysis of RBCs, the decrease in hemoglobin production, and the increased absorption of dietary iron in response to the severely anemic state. The excess iron is deposited in the body's tissues, causing bronze pigmentation of the skin, bony changes, and altered organ function, particularly in the cardiac system. Additional complications include splenomegaly, endocrine abnormalities, osteoporosis, liver and gallbladder disease, and leg ulcers.

Left untreated, β-thalassemia major is fatal, but the use of blood transfusions and chelation therapy has increased the life expectancy of these children to beyond their teen years (Ambruso et al., 2014).

THERAPEUTIC MANAGEMENT

The therapeutic management for children with β-thalassemia includes monitoring hemoglobin and hematocrit and transfusing PRBCs at regular intervals. Blood iron levels are also monitored and iron chelation therapy is provided.

NURSING ASSESSMENT

Infants are usually diagnosed by 1 year of age and have a history of pallor, jaundice, failure to thrive, and hepatosplenomegaly (Ambruso et al., 2014). Determine the history of the present illness or whether the child is presenting for a routine blood transfusion. Note medications taken at home and any concerns that have arisen since the last visit. Inspect the skin, oral mucosa, conjunctivae, soles, and/or palms for pallor. Note icteric sclerae or jaundice of the skin. Measure weight and height (or length) and plot on an appropriate growth chart. Observe the child for bony deformities and frontal bossing (prominent forehead) (Fig. 46.12). Measure oxygen saturation via pulse oximetry. Evaluate neurologic status, determining level of consciousness and developmental abilities.

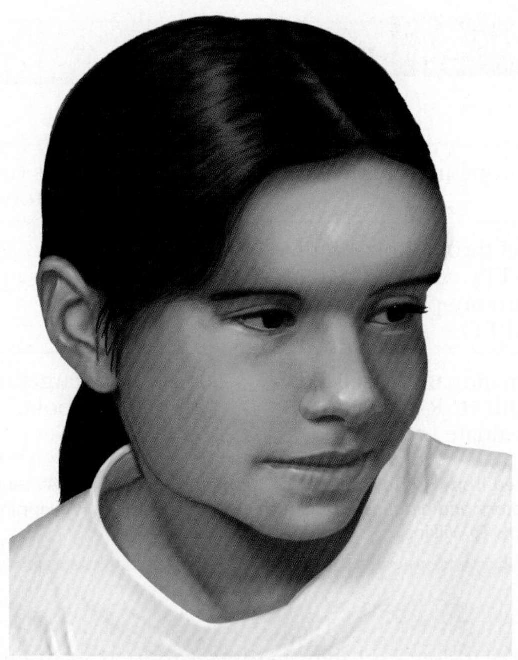

FIGURE 46.12 Iron overload related to thalassemia leads to bony changes such as frontal bossing and maxillary prominence.

Laboratory testing may reveal the following:

- Hemoglobin and hematocrit are significantly decreased.
- Peripheral blood smear shows prominence of target cells, hypochromia, microcytosis, and extensive **anisocytosis** and **poikilocytosis** (variation in the size and shape of the RBCs, respectively).
- Bilirubin levels are elevated.
- Hgb electrophoresis shows the presence of Hgb F and Hgb A_2 only.
- Iron level is elevated.

NURSING MANAGEMENT

The nursing care of the child with thalassemia is primarily aimed at supporting the family and minimizing the effects of the illness. This includes administering blood transfusions and educating the family.

Administering Packed Red Blood Cell Transfusions. Administer PRBC transfusions as prescribed to maintain an adequate level of hemoglobin for oxygen delivery to the tissues and to suppress erythrocytosis in the bone marrow. Monitor for reactions to the transfusions.

Excess iron (hemosiderosis) is removed by chelation therapy. Administer the chelating agent deferoxamine with the transfusion. Deferoxamine binds to the iron and allows it to be removed through the stool or urine. Oral deferasirox may also be prescribed and is generally well tolerated, with minimal gastrointestinal side effects.

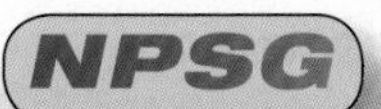

GOAL 1: Improve the Accuracy of Patient Identification. (Identify Patients Correctly)

NPSG 01.03.01 Eliminate transfusion errors related to patient misidentification.

Steps: Always match the blood component to the order. Use a two-person verification process as determined by facility policy to match the patient to the blood component.

Joint Commission. (2015). *National patient safety goals effective January 1, 2015.* Retrieved from http://www.jointcommission.org/assets/1/6/2015_NPSG_HAP.pdf

Educating the Family. Educate the child and family about the recommended regimen. Ensure that families understand that adhering to the prescribed blood transfusion and chelation therapy schedule is essential to the child's survival. Chelation therapy must be maintained at home to continuously decrease the iron levels in the body. Teach family members to administer deferoxamine subcutaneously with a small battery-powered infusion pump over a several-hour period each night (usually while the child is sleeping). If oral deferasirox is prescribed, instruct the family to dissolve the tablet in juice or water and administer it once daily.

Refer the family for genetic counseling and family support as needed. A good resource for families of children with thalassemia is the Cooley's Anemia Foundation, a link to which can be found on thePoint. A group of young adults with Cooley anemia started the Thalassemia Action Group (TAG) (a subgroup of the Cooley's Anemia Foundation) to provide a forum for communication and information, promote a positive outlook on living with the disease, and raise awareness of the importance of continuing therapy for the disease. TAG is part of the Cooley anemia website and more information about the group can be found by calling (510) 409–9664.

Atraumatic Care

When a child is receiving blood transfusion every few weeks, he or she must experience at least two venipunctures each time, one for the type and cross-match and other relevant laboratory tests on the day before transfusion, and the intravenous (IV) insertion for the actual transfusion. Minimize trauma by teaching the parent to apply EMLA (eutectic mixture of local anesthetic) cream at home just before leaving for the blood draw or transfusion appointment.

Glucose-6-Phosphate Dehydrogenase Deficiency

Glucose-6-phosphate dehydrogenase (G6PD) is an enzyme that is responsible for maintaining the integrity of RBCs by protecting them from oxidative substances. G6PD deficiency is an X-linked recessive disorder that occurs when the RBCs have insufficient G6PD, or the enzyme is abnormal and does not function properly. The RBCs are then affected by oxidative stress more easily. Triggers that may result in oxidative stress and hemolysis include bacterial or viral illness or exposure to certain substances such as medications (e.g., sulfonamides, sulfones, malaria-fighting drugs [such as quinine], or methylene blue [for treating urinary tract infections]), naphthalene (an agent in mothballs), or fava beans.

G6PD deficiency occurs most commonly in children of African, Mediterranean, or Asian descent (Ambruso et al., 2014). Complications include prolonged neonatal jaundice and life-threatening acute episodes of hemolysis. Therapeutic management is primarily aimed at avoiding triggers that cause oxidative stress.

NURSING ASSESSMENT

Note health history, including fatigue. Determine the parents' understanding of the disorder and the medications and foods to avoid. Inspect the skin for pallor or jaundice. Evaluate neurologic status, which may also be affected. Measure heart rate and respiratory rate, noting elevations. Determine oxygen saturation via pulse oximeter or blood gas analysis. Note tea-colored urine. Palpate the abdomen for splenomegaly. Laboratory studies will reveal anemia.

NURSING MANAGEMENT

Administer oxygen and treat the symptoms. Once the triggering agent is removed or the child recovers from an illness, the child will improve. Provide further education to the child and family about triggers and advise them that the child should avoid contact with these agents.

CLOTTING DISORDERS

Clotting of blood is a process that occurs after injury. The blood clotting system requires certain factors in the blood and platelets to perform adequately. Individuals with deficiencies of these factors or platelets tend to bleed; they do not bleed more easily than people without these conditions, but it is just more difficult for the clot to form, and bleeding cannot be stopped easily. Factors that are most often involved in problems with clotting include factor VIII, factor IX, and factor XI. Each plays a role in clot formation. Platelets also play a role in the clotting cascade and are necessary for clot formation. Some processes can lead to destruction of the platelets and may lead to a reduction in clotting. Bleeding times are prolonged when a clotting disorder is present. Table 46.5 provides usual values for clotting studies.

TABLE 46.5 CLOTTING STUDIES

Test	Measure
Prothrombin time (PT)	11.0–13.0 seconds (may vary by laboratory)
Partial thromboplastin time (PTT), activated partial thromboplastin time (aPTT)	21–35 seconds
International normalized ratio (INR) (used to evaluate coagulation)	2.0–3.0 usual target in thromboembolic conditions

Adapted from Fischbach, F. T., & Dunning, M. B. (2014). *A manual of laboratory and diagnostic tests* (9th ed.). Philadelphia, PA: Lippincott Williams & Wilkins.

Conditions affecting clotting include idiopathic thrombocytopenia purpura, Henoch–Schönlein purpura, disseminated intravascular coagulation (DIC), and factor deficiencies such as hemophilia A (factor VIII deficiency), von Willebrand disease (vWD), hemophilia B (Christmas disease, factor IX deficiency), and hemophilia C (factor XI deficiency). Table 46.6 reviews the proteins involved in coagulation.

Idiopathic Thrombocytopenia Purpura

Idiopathic thrombocytopenia purpura (ITP) is thought to be an immune response following a viral infection that produces antiplatelet antibodies. These antibodies destroy platelets, which then lead to the development of petechiae, purpura, and excessive bruising. **Petechiae** are pinpoint hemorrhages that occur anywhere on the body and do not blanch to pressure (Fig. 46.13). **Purpura** are larger areas of hemorrhage in which blood collects under the tissues; they are purplish (see Fig. 46.13). ITP usually develops a few weeks after a viral infection and is most common in young children (Ambruso et al., 2014). Within a few months, most children will recover spontaneously (Ambruso et al., 2014). Complications include severe hemorrhage and bleeding into vital organs and intracranial hemorrhage, although these rarely occur.

For children with platelet counts below 10,000/mm^3, corticosteroids may be administered for 2 to 3 weeks. In acute or chronic ITP, intravenous immunoglobulin (IVIG) may be used as an adjunct and is infused for 1 to

TABLE 46.6 SELECT PROTEINS INVOLVED IN COAGULATION (FACTORS)

Protein	Synonym	Concentration in Plasma (mg/dL)	Function
Fibrinogen	Factor I	200–400	Converts fibrin along with platelets to form clot
Factor II	Prothrombin	10–15	Converted to thrombin (Iia), splits fibrinogen into fibrin
Factor V	Proaccelerin; labile factor	0.5–1.0	Supports Xa activation of II to Iia
Factor VII	Stable factor; proconvertin	0.2	Activates X
Factor VIIIC	Antihemophilic factor (AHF); platelet cofactor I	1.0–2.0	Supports IXa activation of X
Factor IX	Christmas factor; plasma thromboplastin component (PTC)	0.3–0.4	Activates X
Factor X	Stewart–Prower factor (AVTD prothrombin III)	0.6–0.8	Activates II
Factor XI	Plasma thromboplastin antecedent (antihemophilic factor C)	0.4	Activates XII and prekallikrein
Factor XII	Hageman factor	2.9	Activates XI and prekallikrein
Factor XIII	Fibrin-stabilizing factor; Laki-Lorand factor	2.5	Cross-links fibrin and other proteins
von Willebrand factor	Factor VIII–related antigen (VIII: VWD)	1.0	Stabilizes VIII, mediates platelet adhesion

Adapted from Fischbach, F. T., & Dunning, M. B. (2014). *A manual of laboratory and diagnostic tests* (9th ed.). Philadelphia, PA: Lippincott Williams & Wilkins.

2 days (Ambruso et al., 2014). Platelet transfusions are not indicated unless life-threatening bleeding is present. Refer the child for follow-up care with a pediatric hematologist. ITP is usually self-limiting, but if it persists for a year or longer, splenectomy may be indicated.

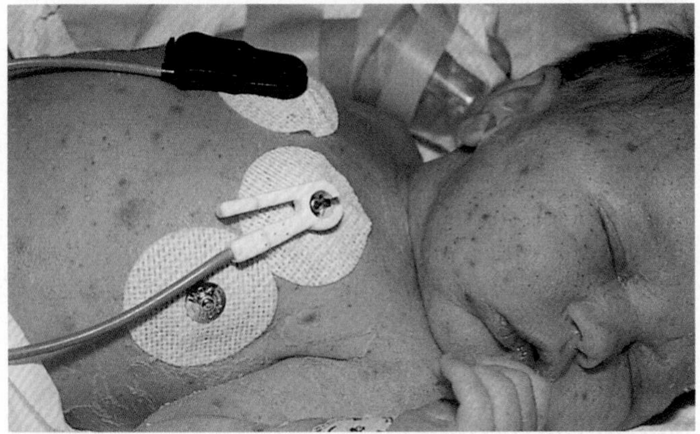

FIGURE 46.13 Pinpoint hemorrhages (petechiae) and large purplish areas of discoloration (purpura) in an infant with idiopathic thrombocytopenia purpura (ITP).

Nursing Assessment

Elicit the child's health history (usually a previously healthy child who recently has developed increased bruising, epistaxis, or bleeding of the gums). Note history of blood in the stool. Note risk factors such as recent viral illness, recent MMR immunization, or ingestion of medications that can cause thrombocytopenia. Inspect for petechiae, purpura, and bruising, which may progress rapidly within the first 24 to 48 hours of the illness. Document the size and location of each lesion. Inspect the lips and buccal mucosa for petechiae. The remainder of the physical examination is usually within normal limits.

Usual laboratory findings include an extremely low platelet count (less than 50,000), normal WBC count and differential, and normal hemoglobin and hematocrit unless hemorrhage has occurred (this is rare). Bone marrow aspiration may be performed to rule out leukemia.

Nursing Management

Many children require no medical treatment except observation and reevaluation of laboratory values.

Educate the family about avoiding aspirin, nonsteroidal anti-inflammatory drugs (NSAIDs), and antihistamines because these medications may precipitate the development of anemia in these children. The use of acetaminophen for pain control is more appropriate when necessary. Teach the family to prevent trauma by avoiding activities that may cause injury, such as contact sports. Instead, encourage activities, such as swimming, that provide physical activity with less risk of trauma. Explain to parents the signs and symptoms of serious bleeding and whom to call if it is suspected.

Henoch–Schönlein Purpura

Henoch–Schönlein purpura is a condition that, in children, develops in association with a viral or bacterial infection (most often respiratory) (Ambruso et al., 2014). The classic presentation is vasculitis with immunoglobulin A (IgA)–dominant immune deposits affecting small vessels. These small vessels are generally in the skin, gut, and kidney. In most children the course of the disease is benign and the prognosis is good. In a few children, however, ongoing nephrotic syndrome may occur as a result of renal injury, and those children may have hypertension. Pulmonary, cardiac, and neurologic complications can also occur.

No specific treatment exists for Henoch–Schönlein purpura, since most of the cases resolve without treatment. Treatment with corticosteroids, such as prednisone, may be helpful in children with severe joint or gastrointestinal manifestations (Ambruso, et al., 2014). If renal injury occurs, children may require renal function testing, and evaluation for hypertension and treatment when present.

Nursing Assessment

Note history of viral or bacterial infection. Determine the onset of the complaint and how it has progressed or changed. Note history of joint or abdominal pain. Measure blood pressure. Inspect the skin for a purpuric palpable rash, and document the size and location of lesions. Palpate the rash to determine its extent (Fig. 46.14). Gently palpate the joints for tenderness. Palpate the abdomen for tenderness. Note visible or occult blood in the stool. Note cherry- or tea-colored urine, indicating the presence of blood in the urine; urinalysis can verify the amount of blood present in the urine. Serum IgA levels may be elevated.

Nursing Management

Treatment of the symptoms is the focus. In children with severe joint or abdominal pain, administer analgesics as prescribed and note the response to pain medications. If the child has normal renal function, maintaining hydration is the most important intervention. Monitor intake and output. Note the color of urine. Administer corticosteroids and anticoagulants, alone or together, if ordered to reduce renal impairment. Teach the child and family about the therapy, such as management of hypertension with medications, and sodium restriction. Teach them about signs of renal injury, such as blood in the urine and changes in weight, as well as frequency and volume of urine output.

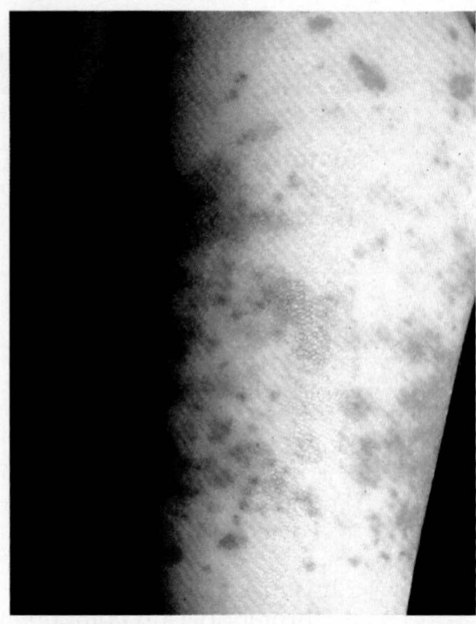

FIGURE 46.14 Palpable purpura on an adolescent's arm.

Disseminated Intravascular Coagulation

DIC is a complex condition that leads to activation of coagulation; it usually occurs in critically ill children. Common triggers of DIC include septic shock, presence of endotoxins and viruses, tissue necrosis or injury, and cancer treatment (Ambruso et al., 2014). In DIC, thrombin is generated, fibrin is deposited in the circulation, and platelets are consumed. Deficiencies of coagulation and anticoagulation pathways occur. Hemorrhage and organ tissue damage result and can be irreversible if not recognized and treated immediately.

Therapeutic management of children with DIC requires careful consideration of the etiology. Initial treatment focuses on treating the underlying cause. For example, if DIC occurs secondary to an infection, appropriate antibiotics would be used to treat the infection. Heparin is also used at lower doses to counteract the deficiency in the coagulation/anticoagulation pathway. Heparin reduces consumption of the platelets, resulting in improved platelet counts. Since heparin is an anticoagulant, there is an increased risk of bleeding.

Nursing Assessment

Because DIC occurs as a secondary condition, it may occur in a child hospitalized for any reason. DIC may affect any body system, so a thorough physical examination is warranted. Inspect for signs of bleeding such as petechiae or purpura, blood in the urine or stool, or persistent oozing from venipuncture or from the umbilical cord in the newborn. Evaluate respiratory status and determine the level of tissue oxygenation via pulse oximetry. Perform a complete circulatory assessment and note signs of circulatory collapse such as poor perfusion, tachycardia, prolonged capillary refill, and weak distal pulses. Note altered level of consciousness and decreased urine output. Careful abdominal palpation may reveal hepatomegaly or splenomegaly.

Laboratory testing may reveal prolonged prothrombin time (PT), partial thromboplastin time (PTT), activated partial thromboplastin time (aPTT), bleeding time, and thrombin time and decreased levels of fibrinogen; platelets; clotting factors II, V, VIII, and X; and antithrombin III. Increases will be noted in levels of fibrinolysin, fibrinopeptide A, positive fibrin split products, and D-dimers.

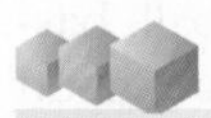
Concept Mastery Alert

DIC Diagnostic Testing

Diagnostic tests that indicate the development of DIC include increased fibrinogen/fibrin degradation products, decreased antithrombin III, increased fibrinopeptide A level, and an increased D-dimer assay.

Nursing Management

Continue to provide nursing care related to the triggering event. Assess the child's status frequently. If bleeding is observed, apply pressure to the area along with cold compresses. Elevate the affected body part if this does not affect the child's overall stability. If neurologic deficits are assessed, report the findings immediately so that treatment to prevent permanent damage can be started. Administer anticoagulation therapy (even though hemorrhage is a concern) to interrupt the coagulation process that is present in this condition. Provide ventilatory support as needed and provide continuous cardiac monitoring. Administer clotting factors, platelets, and cryoprecipitate as prescribed to prevent severe hemorrhage. Report changes in laboratory values to the physician or nurse practitioner. Changes can occur rapidly, and vigilance is necessary to prevent further tissue damage to the affected system.

Hemophilia

Hemophilia is a group of X-linked recessive disorders that result in deficiency in one of the coagulation factors in the blood. X-linked recessive disorders are transmitted by carrier mothers to their sons, so usually only males are affected by hemophilia. The coagulation factors in the blood are essential for clot formation either spontaneously or from an injury, and when factors are absent bleeding will be difficult to stop. There are several types of hemophilia, including factor VIII deficiency (hemophilia A), factor IX deficiency or Christmas disease (hemophilia B), and factor XI deficiency (hemophilia C). The most common, hemophilia A, will be the focus of this discussion (Karp & Riddell, 2010). Hemophilia A occurs when there is a deficiency of factor VIII in an individual. Factor VIII is essential in the activation of factor X, which is required for the conversion of prothrombin into thrombin, resulting in an inability of the platelets to be used in clot formation.

Hemophilia is classified according to the severity of the disease, ranging from mild to severe. The more severe the disease, the more likely it is that there will be bleeding episodes. When bleeding occurs the vessels constrict and a platelet plug forms, but because of the deficient factor the fibrin will not solidify, and thus bleeding continues.

Therapeutic Management

The primary goal of managing hemophilia is to prevent bleeding. This is best accomplished by instructing the child to avoid activities with a high potential for injury (e.g., football, riding motorcycles, skateboarding). Instead, encourage the child to participate in activities with the least amount of contact (e.g., swimming, running, tennis). Limiting activities does not mean the child should do nothing; activities that promote health without increased exposure to injury are best.

If bleeding or injury occurs, factor administration is prescribed; this practice has been common in outpatient facilities or the child's home for many years. Once the deficient factor is replaced, clotting factors return to fairly normal levels for a period of time. Factor replacement should be given before any surgeries or other procedures that can lead to bleeding, such as intramuscular injections and dental care.

Nursing Assessment

For a full description of the assessment phase of the nursing process, refer to the Assessment section of the Nursing Process Overview earlier in the chapter. Assessment findings pertinent to hemophilia in children are discussed below.

HEALTH HISTORY

Elicit the health history, determining the nature of the bleeding episode or bruise. Include in the history any hemorrhagic episodes in other systems, such as the gastrointestinal tract (e.g., black tarry stools, hematemesis)

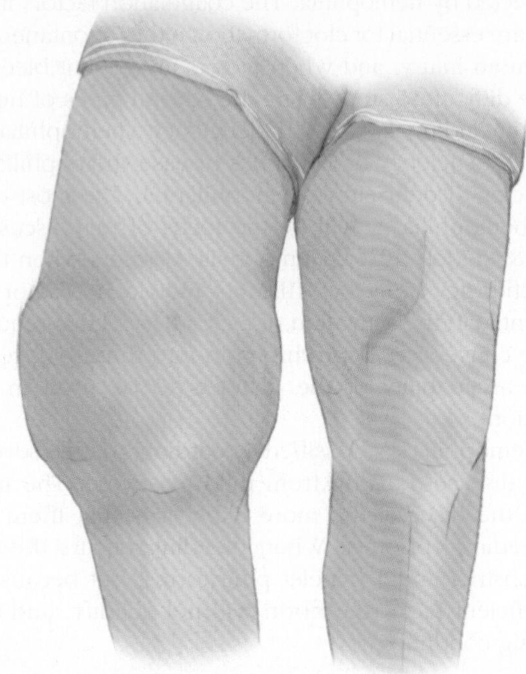

FIGURE 46.15 Significant swelling and discoloration associated with a bleeding episode in a hemophiliac's knee.

or as a result from injury resulting in joint hemorrhage, or hematuria (Fig. 46.15). Inquire about length of bleeding and amount of blood loss. Because hemophilia A results in difficulty with clotting, the child may bleed for a longer period when injury occurs.

PHYSICAL EXAMINATION

Focus the physical examination on identification of any bleeding. This is of particular concern after injury, but a nosebleed or other spontaneous bleed can occur if factor levels are extremely low. Assess circulation by evaluating pulses and heart sounds if severe or prolonged bleeding is identified. Without intervention, hypovolemia could follow, leading to shock. Note chest pain or abdominal pain, which may indicate internal bleeding. Report these findings immediately so that the underlying condition can be diagnosed and treated rapidly.

LABORATORY AND DIAGNOSTIC TESTING

Laboratory findings may include decreased hemoglobin and hematocrit if bleeding is prolonged or severe. Factor levels may be quantified with blood testing.

Nursing Management

Nursing management includes preventing bleeding episodes, managing bleeding episodes, and providing education and support.

PREVENTING BLEEDING EPISODES

All children with hemophilia should attempt to prevent bleeding episodes. Major bleeds into the joints may limit range of motion and function, eventually decreasing physical abilities and crippling some boys (Karp & Riddell, 2010). Teach children and families that regular physical activity or exercise helps to keep the muscles and joints stronger, and children with stronger joints and muscles have fewer bleeding episodes (see Teaching Guidelines 46.4). Refer the child with moderate to severe hemophilia to a pediatric hematologist and/or a comprehensive hemophilia treatment center.

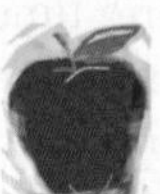

Teaching Guidelines 46.4

PREVENTING BLEEDING IN THE CHILD WITH HEMOPHILIA

- Protect toddlers with soft helmets, padding on the knees, carpets in the home, and softened or covered corners.
- Children should stay active: swimming, baseball, basketball, and bicycling (wearing a helmet) are good physical activities.
- Avoid intense contact sports such as football, wrestling, soccer, and high diving.
- Avoid trampoline use and riding all-terrain vehicles (ATVs).
- Arrange premedication with Amicar if oral surgery is indicated.

MANAGING A BLEEDING EPISODE

Administer factor VIII replacement as prescribed. Factor replacement is pooled from multiple blood donors, so families may be concerned about transmission of viruses via the product (specifically hepatitis and HIV). Several methods of viral inactivation (solvent detergent, dry heat, and monoclonal purification) have been used to treat factors VIII and IX since 1986, so since that time there has been no risk of HIV transmission via factor infusion (National Hemophilia Foundation, 2009).

Administer factor replacement by slow IV push. Document the product name, number of units, lot number, and expiration date. Doses are based on the severity of the bleeding and the weight of the child. Specific dosing guidelines can be obtained from the product insert. In mild cases of hemophilia A, desmopressin may be effective in stopping bleeding (see below in the nursing management section of VWD for additional information).

If external bleeding develops, apply pressure to the area until bleeding stops. If it is inside a joint, apply ice or cold compresses to the area and elevate any injured extremities, except when contraindicated by further injury.

Make sure that all cases of bleeding are followed up to identify whether factor replacement is necessary.

PROVIDING EDUCATION

Inform the family that the child should wear a medical alert bracelet. Families should notify the school nurse and teachers of the child's diagnosis and share precautions with them. Instruct all school personnel to call the parent immediately if the child sustains a head, abdominal, or orbit injury at school. Teach parents and caregivers how to administer the intravenous infusion of factor VIII. Administration in the home is the preferred method for factor infusion, as the child will be able to receive treatment in the most timely and efficient manner when a bleeding episode occurs. Alternatives to the parent giving the infusion are to arrange for a home care nursing visit or for the family to keep their own supply of factor VIII that they take to the local emergency room for infusion if bleeding occurs.

Involve children as developmentally appropriate in the infusion process. Young children may hold and apply the Band-Aid; older children may assist with dilution and mixing of the factor. Teach teenagers to administer their own factor infusions.

Children with severe hemophilia may need factor infusions so often that implantation of a central venous access port is warranted. Teach the family access, care, and flushing of the implanted port.

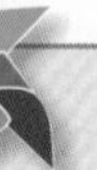

Thinking About Development

Toby Henderson is an 18-month-old male with a history of moderate hemophilia. He is a very active child; his mother calls him a "typical boy."

Considering Toby's developmental stage, how will his diagnosis impact his ability to accomplish toddler developmental milestones?

Develop a teaching plan for Toby's parents related to safety for Toby. Incorporate age-appropriate activities that would be safe for Toby in the plan.

How would the safety plan be different if Toby were 13 years old?

PROVIDING SUPPORT

Children with hemophilia may be able to lead a fairly normal life, with the exception of avoiding a few activities. However, accepting the diagnosis of a bleeding disorder in their child is very difficult for parents. They fear the worst (bleeding that won't stop) as well as complications such as infection with blood-borne viruses. Reassure parents that since 1986, when factor replacement began to be treated with heat, there have been no reports of virus transmission from factor infusion (National Hemophilia Foundation, 2009). Educate and support the parents. Factor replacement is expensive and bleeding episodes often cause parents to miss work, both of which create financial strains. Refer families to the National Hemophilia Foundation and NHF Youthworld, which offer support, education, youth leadership, scholarships, and a directory of camps for children with hemophilia and other bleeding disorders. Links to these and other helpful resources are located on thePoint.

Von Willebrand Disease

Von Willebrand Disease (vWD) is a genetically transmitted bleeding disorder that may affect both genders and all races. The disorder is a deficiency in von Willebrand factor (vWF). Under ordinary circumstances vWF serves two functions: to bind with factor VIII, protecting it from breakdown, and to serve as the "glue" that attaches platelets to the site of injury. Deficiency in this factor results in a mild bleeding disorder. Children with vWD bruise easily, have frequent nosebleeds (epistaxis), and tend to bleed after oral surgery. Pubescent girls often have menorrhagia.

Therapeutic management of vWD is similar to that of hemophilia. Prevention of injury is important. When bleeding or injury does occur, vWF is administered. Desmopressin may also be used to release the factors necessary for clotting. Desmopressin raises the plasma level from stores in the endothelium of blood vessels; this releases factor VIII and vWF from these stores into the bloodstream. These may also be administered before dental work or surgery.

Nursing Assessment

Nursing assessment of the child with vWD is similar to the assessment of the child with hemophilia, though severe bleeding occurs much less frequently.

Nursing Management

Nursing management is also similar to the management of the child with hemophilia. The major difference is the administration of desmopressin. Administer desmopressin nasal spray as prescribed when a bleeding episode occurs. Desmopressin may also be given via an intravenous infusion or subcutaneously (less common). Stimate is the only brand of desmopressin nasal spray that is used for controlling bleeding; the other brands are used for homeostasis and enuresis. Desmopressin is an antidiuretic hormone, so closely monitor fluid balance. Twenty-four hours should lapse between doses, as lessening of the response (tachyphylaxis) occurs with more frequent use (Karp & Riddell, 2010). vWD may also be treated with intravenous infusion of vWF, similar to factor

VIII infusion for hemophilia A. Teach children and their families how to avoid or minimize bleeding episodes (see Teaching Guidelines 46.4).

LEUKEMIA

Leukemia accounts for about one third of all childhood cancers (Zupanec & Tomlinson, 2010). It is a primary disorder of the bone marrow in which the normal elements are replaced with abnormal WBCs. Normally, lymphoid cells grow and develop into lymphocytes, and myeloid cells grow and develop into RBCs, granulocytes, monocytes, and platelets. Leukemia may develop at any time during the usual stages of normal lymphoid or myeloid development.

Leukemia may be classified as acute or chronic, lymphocytic or myelogenous. Acute leukemias are rapidly progressive diseases affecting the undifferentiated or immature cells; the result is cells without normal function. Chronic leukemias progress more slowly, permitting maturation and differentiation of cells so that they retain some of their normal function. Acute leukemias, including ALL and acute myelogenous leukemia (AML), make up a significant majority of all cases of leukemia in children and adolescents (Zupanec & Tomlinson, 2010). Therefore, they will be the focus of the discussion below.

Complications of leukemia include **metastasis** (spread of cancer to other sites) to the blood, bone, CNS, spleen, liver, or other organs and alterations in growth. Late effects include problems with neurocognitive function and ocular, cardiovascular, or thyroid dysfunction. With advances in treatment over the past 50 years, most cases of childhood leukemia are curable. However, children who experience relapse or present with advanced disease have a poorer prognosis (Zupanec & Tomlinson, 2010).

Acute Lymphoblastic Leukemia

Acute lymphoblastic leukemia is the most common form of cancer in children. Eighty-five percent of cases of ALL occur in children between 2 and 10 years of age (Graham et al., 2014). It is more common in white children than in other races. ALL is classified according to the type of cells involved—T cell, B cell, early pre-B cell, or pre-B cell. Most children will achieve initial remission if appropriate treatment is given. The overall cure rate of ALL is over 70% (Graham et al., 2014).

Prognosis is based on the WBC count at diagnosis, the type of cytogenetic factors and immunophenotype, the age at diagnosis, and the extent of extramedullary involvement. Generally, the higher the WBC count at diagnosis, the worse the prognosis. Children between 1 and 9 years of age and with a WBC count less than 50,000 at diagnosis have the best prognosis. When a child experiences a relapse, the prognosis becomes poorer. Complications include infection, hemorrhage, poor growth, and CNS, bone, or testicular involvement.

Take Note!

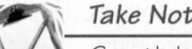

Growth hormone replacement therapy using recombinant human growth hormone may improve the long-term growth of children with leukemia (Zupanec & Tomlinson, 2010).

Pathophysiology

The exact cause of ALL remains unknown. Genetic factors and chromosome abnormalities may play a role in its development. In ALL, abnormal lymphoblasts abound in the blood-forming tissues. The lymphoblasts are fragile and immature, lacking the infection-fighting capabilities of the normal WBC. The growth of lymphoblasts is excessive and the abnormal cells replace the normal cells in the bone marrow. The proliferating leukemic cells demonstrate massive metabolic needs, depriving normal body cells of needed nutrients and resulting in fatigue, weight loss or growth arrest, and muscle wasting. The bone marrow becomes unable to maintain normal levels of RBCs, WBCs, and platelets, so anemia, neutropenia, and thrombocytopenia result. As the bone marrow expands or the leukemic cells infiltrate the bone, joint and bone pain may occur. The leukemic cells may permeate the lymph nodes, causing diffuse lymphadenopathy, or the liver and spleen, resulting in hepatosplenomegaly. With spread to the CNS, vomiting, headache, seizures, coma, vision alterations, or cranial nerve palsies may occur (Zupanec & Tomlinson, 2010).

Take Note!

Changes in behavior or personality, headache, irritability, dizziness, persistent nausea or vomiting, seizures, gait changes, lethargy, or altered level of consciousness may indicate CNS infiltration with leukemic cells. Immediately report these findings to the pediatric oncologist.

Therapeutic Management

Therapeutic management of the child with ALL focuses on giving chemotherapy to eradicate the leukemic cells and restore normal bone marrow function. Treatment is divided into three stages. CNS prophylaxis is provided at each stage; without CNS prophylaxis, leukemia would spread to the CNS in up to 50% of children with ALL (Zupanec & Tomlinson, 2010). The length of treatment and choice of medications are based on the child's age, risk category, and subtype determined by bone marrow analysis. Table 46.7 discusses the stages of leukemia treatment. For relapsed or less responsive leukemia, HSCT may be necessary.

Nursing Assessment

For a full description of the assessment phase of the nursing process, refer to page 1787. Assessment findings pertinent to ALL are discussed below.

TABLE 46.7 STAGES OF LEUKEMIA TREATMENT

Stage	Purpose	Length	Usual Medications
Induction	Rapid induction of complete remission	3–4 weeks	Oral steroids, IV vincristine, IM L-asparaginase, daunomycin (high risk)
Consolidation (intensification)	Strengthen remission, reduce leukemic cell burden	Varies	High-dose methotrexate, 6-mercaptopurine; possibly cyclophosphamide, cytarabine, asparaginase, thioguanine, epipodophyllotoxins
Maintenance	Eliminate all residual leukemic cells	2–3 years	Low dose: daily 6-mercaptopurine, weekly methotrexate, intermittent IV vincristine, and oral steroids
CNS prophylaxis	Reduce risk of development of CNS disease	Given periodically in all stages	Intrathecal chemotherapy; cranial radiation is used infrequently

Adapted from Graham, D. K., Craddock, J. A., Quinones, R. R., Keating, A. K., Maloney, K. Foreman, N. K., Giller, R. H., & Greffe, B. S. (2014). Neoplastic disease. In W. W. Hay, M. J. Levin, R. R. Deterding, & M. J. Abzug (Eds.), *Current pediatric diagnosis and treatment* (22nd ed.). New York, NY: McGraw-Hill; and Zupanec, S., & Tomlinson, D. (2010). Leukemia. In D. Tomlinson & N. E. Kline (Eds.), *Pediatric oncology nursing*. New York, NY: Springer.

HEALTH HISTORY

Elicit a description of the present illness and chief complaint. Common signs and symptoms reported during the health history might include:

- Fever (may be persistent or recurrent, with unknown cause)
- Recurrent infection
- Fatigue, malaise, or listlessness
- Pallor
- Unusual bleeding or bruising
- Abdominal pain
- Nausea or vomiting
- Bone pain
- Headache (Zupanec & Tomlinson, 2010)

Explore the child's current and past medical history for risk factors such as:

- Male gender
- Age 2 to 5 years
- Caucasian race
- Down syndrome, Shwachman syndrome, or ataxia-telangiectasia
- X-ray exposure in utero
- Previous radiation-treated cancer (Zupanec & Tomlinson, 2010)

Determine the child's history of varicella zoster immunization or disease. Chickenpox infection in the leukemic child may lead to disseminated, overwhelming infection.

PHYSICAL EXAMINATION

Take the child's temperature (fever may be present), and look for petechiae, purpura, or unusual bruising (due to decreased platelet levels). Inspect the skin for signs of infection. Auscultate the lungs, noting adventitious breath sounds, which may indicate pneumonia (present at diagnosis or due to immunosuppression during treatment). Note location and size of enlarged lymph nodes. Palpate the liver and spleen for enlargement. Document tenderness on abdominal palpation.

LABORATORY AND DIAGNOSTIC TESTS

Common laboratory and diagnostic studies ordered for the assessment of ALL include:

- Complete blood counts: abnormal findings include low hemoglobin and hematocrit, decreased RBC count, decreased platelet count, and elevated, normal, or decreased WBC count
- Peripheral blood smear may reveal blasts.
- Bone marrow aspiration: stained smear from bone marrow aspiration will show greater than 25% lymphoblasts. Bone marrow aspirate is also examined for immunophenotyping (lymphoid vs. myeloid, and level of cancer cell maturity) and cytogenetic analysis (determines abnormalities in chromosome number and structure). Immunophenotyping and cytogenetic analysis are used in the classification of the leukemia, which helps guide treatment.
- Lumbar puncture will reveal whether leukemic cells have infiltrated the CNS.
- Liver function tests and blood urea nitrogen (BUN) and creatinine levels determine liver and renal function, which, if abnormal, may preclude treatment with certain chemotherapeutic agents.
- Chest radiography may reveal pneumonia or a mediastinal mass.

Atraumatic Care

The child with leukemia undergoes frequent implantable port accesses for blood draws and chemotherapy, bone marrow aspirations for assessment of blood cell status, and lumbar punctures for laboratory studies and intrathecal medication administration. To decrease trauma produced by these repetitive painful procedures, utilize EMLA (eutectic mixture of local anesthetics) cream appropriately. Teach the child's primary caregiver to apply the cream to the implantable port site 30 minutes to 1 hour prior to the child's clinic appointment time. Apply EMLA cream to the posterior hip or lumbar spine, 1 to 3 hours prior to bone marrow aspiration or lumbar puncture.

Nursing Management

Nursing care of children with ALL focuses on managing disease complications such as infection, pain, anemia, bleeding, and hyperuricemia and the many adverse effects related to treatment. Many children require blood product transfusion for the treatment of severe anemia or low platelet levels with active bleeding.

Individualize nursing care based on the diagnoses, interventions, and outcomes presented in Nursing Care Plan 46.1 (at the end of the chapter), depending on the child's response to the disease and chemotherapy. Refer to the nursing process overview section for further information related to managing the adverse effects of chemotherapy.

Take Note!

Blood products administered to children with any type of leukemia should be irradiated, cytomegalovirus (CMV) negative, and leukodepleted. This treatment of blood products before transfusion will decrease the amount of antibodies in the blood, an important factor in preventing GVHD should HSCT become necessary at a later date (Nixon, 2010).

REDUCING PAIN

Children and teens with leukemia suffer pain related to the disease as well as the treatment. Chemotherapy drugs commonly used in leukemia may cause peripheral neuropathy and headache. Lumbar puncture and bone marrow aspiration, which are periodically performed throughout the course of treatment, also cause pain. The most common areas of pain are the head and neck, legs, and abdomen (probably from protracted vomiting with chemotherapy). Use distraction techniques, such as listening to music, watching TV, or playing games, to help take the child's mind off the pain. Administer mild analgesics such as acetaminophen for acute episodes of pain. Using EMLA cream prior to venipuncture, port access, lumbar puncture, and bone marrow aspiration may decrease procedure-related pain events. In addition, applying heat or cold to the painful area is usually acceptable. Administer narcotic analgesics, as prescribed, for episodes of acute severe pain or for palliation of chronic pain (Simon, 2010).

Acute Myelogenous Leukemia

AML is the second most common type of leukemia in children (Zupanec & Tomlinson, 2010). Its incidence peaks during the adolescent years (Zupanec & Tomlinson, 2010). AML affects the myeloid cell progenitors or precursors in the bone marrow, resulting in **malignant** (invasive and fast-growing) cells. The French–American–British (FAB) classification system identifies eight subtypes of AML (M0 to M7), depending on myeloid lineage involved and the degree of cell differentiation. These subtypes are useful for determining treatment. The long-term survival rate for childhood AML is about 50% (Graham et al., 2014). Complications include treatment resistance, infection, hemorrhage, and metastasis. The induction phase of AML requires intense bone marrow suppression and prolonged hospitalization because AML is less responsive to treatment than ALL. Toxicity from treatment is more common in AML and is likely to be more serious than with ALL. Empiric broad-spectrum antibiotics and prophylactic platelet transfusions may be prescribed. After remission is achieved, children require intensive chemotherapy to prolong the duration of remission. HSCT is often required in children with AML, depending on the subtype (Zupanec & Tomlinson, 2010).

Take Note!

At the time of diagnosis, some children with AML present with a WBC count above 100,000 (hyperleukocytosis); this results in venous stasis and backup of blast cells in small vessels, causing hypoxia, hemorrhage, and lung or brain infarction. Hyperleukocytosis is a medical emergency. These children require leukapheresis to decrease hyperviscosity by quickly decreasing the number of circulating blasts (Graham et al., 2014).

Nursing Assessment

Explore the health history for common signs and symptoms, including recurrent infections, fever, or fatigue. Explore the medical history for risk factors, such as Hispanic race, previous chemotherapy, and genetic abnormalities such as Down syndrome, Fanconi anemia, neurofibromatosis type I, Shwachman syndrome, Bloom syndrome, and familial monosomy 7.

Perform a thorough physical examination. Note skin pallor and salmon-colored or blue-gray papular lesions. Palpate the skin for subcutaneous rubbery nodules. Palpate for lymphadenopathy. Note headache, visual disturbance, or signs of increased intracranial pressure, such as vomiting, which may indicate CNS involvement. Upon diagnosis of AML, the child's WBC count is typically extremely elevated. Bone marrow aspiration will reveal greater than 20% blast cells (Zupanec & Tomlinson, 2010).

Nursing Management

Nursing management of the child with AML is similar to that of the child with ALL. Nursing interventions focus on managing the adverse effects of treatment and preventing infection. Refer to the nursing process overview section and to Nursing Care Plan 46.1, at the end of the chapter, for appropriate interventions.

LYMPHOMAS

Lymphomas, or tumors of the lymph tissue (lymph nodes, thymus, spleen), account for about 10% to 15% of cases of childhood cancer (Graham et al., 2014). Lymphomas may be divided into two categories—Hodgkin disease (or Hodgkin lymphoma) and non-Hodgkin lymphoma (NHL), which includes more than a dozen types. Hodgkin disease tends to affect lymph nodes located closer to the body's surface, such as those in the cervical, axillary, and inguinal areas, whereas NHL tends to affect lymph nodes located more deeply inside the body.

Hodgkin Disease

In Hodgkin disease, malignant B lymphocytes grow in the lymph tissue, usually starting in one general area of lymph nodes. The presence of Reed–Sternberg cells (giant transformed B lymphocytes with one or two nuclei) differentiates Hodgkin disease from other lymphomas. As the cells multiply, the lymph nodes enlarge, compressing nearby structures, destroying normal cells, and invading other tissues. The cause of Hodgkin disease is still being researched, but there appears to be a link to Epstein–Barr virus infection (Zupanec, 2010). Hodgkin disease is rare in children younger than 5 years of age and is most common in adolescents and young adults; in children 14 years and younger, it is more common in boys than girls (Zupanec, 2010).

In addition to the traditional **staging** (I through IV, depending on the amount of spread; Table 46.8), Hodgkin is also classified as A (asymptomatic) or B (presence of symptoms of fever, night sweats, or weight loss of 10% or more). Prognosis depends on the stage of the disease, tumor bulk, and A or B classification (disease classified as A generally carries a better prognosis). Overall, children with Hodgkin disease have a 75% 20-year survival rate (Graham et al., 2014). Complications of Hodgkin disease include liver failure and secondary cancer such as acute nonlymphocytic leukemia and NHL.

TABLE 46.8 STAGING OF HODGKIN DISEASE

Stage	Clinical Findings
I	One group of lymph nodes is affected.
II	Two or more groups on the same side of the diaphragm are affected.
III	Groups of lymph nodes above and below the diaphragm are affected.
IV	Metastasis to organs such as the liver, bone, or lungs
A or B suffix	A—Absence of systemic symptoms at diagnosis B—Systemic symptoms present at diagnosis (fever, night sweats, weight loss)

Adapted from Zupanec, S. (2010). Lymphoma. In D. Tomlinson & N. E. Kline (Eds.), *Pediatric oncology nursing*. New York, NY: Springer.

Chemotherapy, usually with a combination of drugs, is the treatment of choice for children with Hodgkin disease. Radiation therapy may also be necessary. In the child with disease that does not go into remission or in the child who experiences relapse, HSCT may be an option.

Nursing Assessment

Explore the health history for common signs and symptoms, which may include recent weight loss, fever, drenching night sweats, anorexia, malaise, fatigue, or pruritus. Elicit the health history, determining risk factors such as prior Epstein–Barr virus infection, family history of Hodgkin disease, genetic immune disorder, or HIV infection.

Evaluate respiratory status, as the presence of a mediastinal mass may compromise respiration. Palpate for enlarged lymph nodes; they may feel rubbery and tend to occur in clusters (most common sites are cervical and supraclavicular) (Fig. 46.16). Palpate the abdomen for hepatomegaly or splenomegaly, which may be present with advanced disease. The chest x-ray may reveal a mediastinal mass. The complete blood count may be normal or reflect anemia. Tissue sampling will reveal Reed–Sternberg cells.

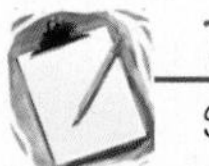

Take Note!

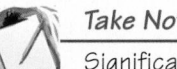

Significant pain in the affected lymph nodes has sometimes been noted after alcohol ingestion (Zupanec, 2010).

Nursing Management

Nursing management of the child with Hodgkin lymphoma focuses on addressing the adverse effects of

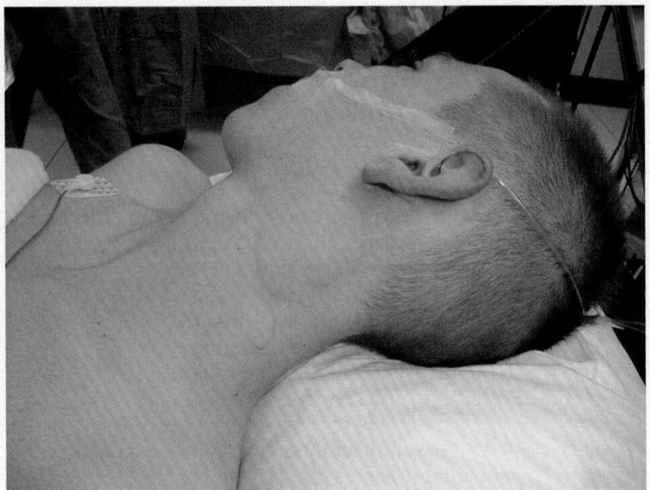

FIGURE 46.16 Hodgkin lymphoma. Large, fixed cervical masses in a 14-year-old with weight loss. (Used with permission from Chung, E. K., Atkinson-McEvoy, L. R., Boom, J. A., & Matz, P. S. (2010). *Visual diagnosis and treatment in pediatrics* (2nd ed.). Philadelphia, PA: Lippincott Williams & Wilkins.)

chemotherapy or radiation. Refer to the Nursing Process Overview section and Nursing Care Plan 46.1 to develop an individualized nursing care plan based on the child's response to treatment.

Non-Hodgkin Lymphoma

NHL results from mutations in the B and T lymphocytes that lead to uncontrolled growth. NHL tends to affect lymph nodes located more deeply within the body. NHL spreads by the bloodstream and in children is a rapidly proliferating, aggressive malignancy that is very responsive to treatment. Prognosis depends on the cell type involved and the extent of the disease at diagnosis. Ninety percent of children with localized NHL have disease-free long-term survival after treatment (Graham et al., 2014). Complications include metastasis and the development of a secondary malignancy later in life.

Remission is induced with chemotherapy and followed with a maintenance phase of chemotherapy lasting about 2 years. NHL tends to spread easily to the CNS, so CNS prophylaxis similar to that used in leukemia is warranted (Zupanec, 2010). Autologous bone marrow transplantation may be used in some children.

Nursing Assessment

Children with NHL are usually symptomatic for only a few days or a few weeks before diagnosis because the disease progresses so quickly. Note onset and location of pain or lymph node swelling. Document history of abdominal pain, diarrhea, or constipation. Explore the health history for risk factors such as congenital or acquired immune deficiency.

Observe for increased work of breathing, facial edema, or venous engorgement (mediastinal mass). Palpate for the presence of lymphadenopathy and palpate the abdomen for the presence of a mass. Lymph node biopsy and bone marrow aspiration determine the diagnosis. Computed tomography (CT) scan, chest radiography, and bone marrow results may be used to determine the extent of metastasis.

Take Note!

Cough, dyspnea, orthopnea, facial edema, or venous engorgement may indicate mediastinal disease in the child with NHL. This is an emergency requiring rapid treatment (Graham et al., 2014).

Nursing Management

As with Hodgkin lymphoma, nursing management of NHL is directed toward managing the adverse effects of chemotherapy. Refer to the nursing process overview section and Nursing Care Plan 46.1 to plan nursing care for the child and family based on the responses they exhibit.

BRAIN TUMORS

Brain tumors are the most common form of solid tumor and the second most common type of cancer in children (Graham et al., 2014). Slightly more than half of brain tumors arise in the posterior fossa (infratentorial); the rest are supratentorial in origin. The cause of brain tumors in children is unknown. Some tumors are localized (low grade), while others are of higher grade and more invasive. The prognosis depends on the location of the tumor and extent of tumor. Low-grade tumors and those that are fully resectable have a better prognosis than tumors that are located deeper within the brain or are more invasive, making them difficult to resect (Kline & O'Hanlon-Curry, 2010). There are many different types of childhood brain tumors; Table 46.9 explains the most common ones.

Complications of brain tumors include hydrocephalus, increased intracranial pressure, brain stem herniation, and negative effects of radiation such as neuropsychological, intellectual, and endocrinologic sequelae (Graham et al., 2014; Kline & O'Hanlon-Curry, 2010).

Pathophysiology

Though the cause of brain tumors is generally not known, the effects of brain tumors are predictable. As the tumor grows within the cranium, it exerts pressure on the brain tissues surrounding it. The tumor mass may compress vital structures in the brain, block cerebrospinal fluid flow, or cause edema in the brain. The result

TABLE 46.9 CHILDHOOD BRAIN TUMORS

Tumor	Location	Characteristics
Medulloblastoma (most common)	Cerebellum	Invasive, highly malignant, grows rapidly. Less favorable outcome with disseminated disease. Progresses quickly to increased intracranial pressure, seeds on CNS pathways. Half occur in children younger than 6 years old.
Brain stem glioma	Brain stem	Aggressive, difficult to resect, resistant to chemotherapy. Spreads widely within the brain stem but rarely extends outside of brain stem area. Affects cranial nerve function.
Ependymoma	Frequently arises from floor of fourth ventricle	Varying speed of growth. Often causes hydrocephalus. Usually diagnosed before it spreads to other parts of the brain or spinal cord.
Astrocytoma	Cerebellum, cerebral hemispheres, thalamus, hypothalamus	Slow course with insidious onset. Responsive to chemotherapy, often resectable. Causes slowly increasing intracranial pressure. Low-grade tumor may be removed completely. High-grade tumors have poor prognosis.

Adapted from Kline, N. E. (2008). *Essentials of pediatric oncology nursing: A core curriculum* (3rd ed.). Glenview, IL: Association of Pediatric Hematology/Oncology Nurses; and Graham, D. K., Craddock, J. A., Quinones, R. R., Keating, A. K., Maloney, K. Foreman, N. K., Giller, R. H., & Greffe, B. S. (2014). Neoplastic disease. In W. W. Hay, M. J. Levin, R. R. Deterding, & M. J. Abzug (Eds.), *Current pediatric diagnosis and treatment* (22nd ed.). New York, NY: McGraw-Hill.

is an increase in intracranial pressure. Presenting symptoms vary according to location and type of tumor.

Therapeutic Management

The type of tumor may be identified at the time of surgery. The location of the tumor within the brain will determine the extent to which it can safely be resected. Children with hydrocephalus may require a ventriculoperitoneal shunt (see Chapter 38 for further information on hydrocephalus). Radiation is reserved for children older than age 2 years because it can have long-term neurocognitive effects (Graham et al., 2014). Chemotherapy is being used increasingly in the treatment of pediatric brain tumors in an attempt to avoid the use of radiation therapy.

Nursing Assessment

For a full description of the assessment phase of the nursing process, refer to the Assessment section of the Nursing Process Overview earlier in the chapter. Assessment findings pertinent to CNS tumors are discussed below.

HEALTH HISTORY

Elicit a description of the present illness and chief complaint. Common signs and symptoms reported during the health history might include:

- Nausea or vomiting
- Headache
- Unsteady gait
- Blurred or double vision
- Seizures
- Motor abnormality or hemiparesis
- Weakness, atrophy
- Swallowing difficulties
- Behavior or personality changes
- Irritability, failure to thrive, or developmental delay (in very young children)

Explore the child's current and past medical history for risk factors such as history of neurofibromatosis, tuberous sclerosis, or prior treatment for CNS leukemia.

PHYSICAL EXAMINATION

Inspection and Observation. Observe for strabismus or nystagmus, "sunsetting" eyes, head tilt, alterations in coordination, gait disturbance, or alterations in sensation. Note alteration in gag reflex, cranial nerve palsy, lethargy, or irritability. Note the child's posture. Check pupillary reaction, noting size, equality, reaction to light, and accommodation.

Palpation. Measure blood pressure, which may decrease with increasing intracranial pressure. In the infant, palpate the anterior fontanel for bulging. Assess deep tendon reflexes, noting hyperreflexia.

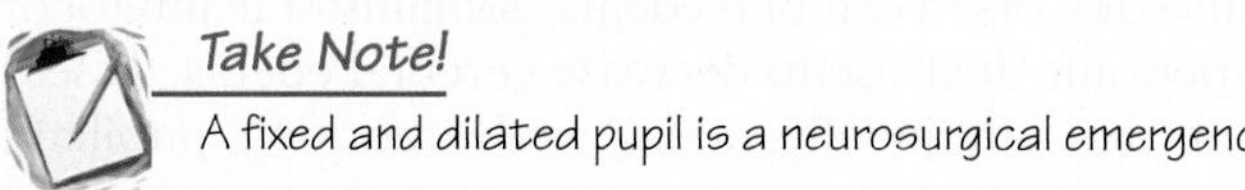
Take Note!
A fixed and dilated pupil is a neurosurgical emergency.

LABORATORY AND DIAGNOSTIC TESTS

Common laboratory and diagnostic studies ordered for the assessment of CNS tumors include:

- CT, magnetic resonance imaging (MRI), or positron emission tomography (PET) will demonstrate evidence of the tumor and its location within the intracranial cavity.
- Lumbar puncture with cerebrospinal fluid cell evaluation may show tumor markers or the presence of α-fetoprotein or human chorionic gonadotropin, which may assist in the diagnosis.

Nursing Management

Nursing management of the child with a brain tumor includes preoperative and postoperative care, as well as interventions to manage adverse effects related to chemotherapy and radiation. Refer to the nursing process overview section for a discussion of nursing interventions related to chemotherapy adverse effects. Nursing Care Plan 46.1 provides additional interventions that may be individualized depending on the child's response to the brain tumor and its treatment.

PROVIDING PREOPERATIVE CARE

Preoperatively, care focuses on monitoring for additional increases in intracranial pressure and avoiding activities that cause transient increases in intracranial pressure. Administer dexamethasone as prescribed to decrease intracranial inflammation. Prevent straining with bowel movements by use of a stool softener. Assess the child's pain level as well as level of consciousness, vital signs, and pupillary reaction to determine subtle changes as soon as possible. Provide a tour of the intensive care unit, which is where the child will wake up after the surgery. Instruct the child and family about the possibility of intubation and ventilation in the postoperative period. If a ventriculoperitoneal shunt will be placed for the treatment of hydrocephalus caused by the tumor, provide education about shunts to the child and family (see Chapter 38).

Shave the portion of the head as determined by the neurosurgeon. Some children may choose to have the entire head shaved. Sometimes children with long hair may feel better about losing it if they donate it to Locks of Love, an organization that provides hairpieces for financially disadvantaged children who have long-term medical hair loss. A link to this resource is provided on thePoint.

PROVIDING POSTOPERATIVE CARE

Regulate fluid administration, as excess fluid intake may cause or worsen cerebral edema. Administer mannitol or hypertonic dextrose to decrease cerebral edema. Assess vital signs frequently, along with checking pupillary reactions and determining level of consciousness. Extreme lethargy or coma may be present for several days postoperatively. Increases in temperature may indicate infection or may be caused by cerebral edema or disturbance of the hypothalamus. Treat hyperthermia with antipyretics such as acetaminophen and with sponge baths, as increases in temperature increase metabolic need. Reduce the temperature slowly.

Monitor for signs of increased intracranial pressure. Headache is common in the postoperative period. Assess pain level and provide analgesics as prescribed. Minimize environmental stimuli, providing a calm and quiet atmosphere. Check the head dressing for cerebrospinal fluid drainage or bleeding. Assess for and document the extent of head, face, or neck edema. Administer eye lubricant if edema prevents complete closure of the eyelids. Apply cool compresses to the eyes to decrease swelling.

As the child begins to regain consciousness, he or she may be confused or combative. Restrain the child if needed to keep him or her in bed and prevent dislodging of tubes and lines.

POSITIONING THE CHILD IN THE POSTOPERATIVE PERIOD

Position the child on the unaffected side with the head of the bed flat or at the level prescribed by the neurosurgeon. Side positioning is usually preferred, as the child may have difficulty handling oral secretions if the level of consciousness is decreased. Do not elevate the foot of the bed, as this may increase intracranial pressure and contribute to bleeding. When changing the child's position, maintain the head in alignment with the remainder of the body. Children with paralyzed or spastic extremities will need additional positioning support.

Take Note!

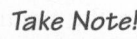

Observe preoperatively and postoperatively for signs of brain stem herniation such as opisthotonos (see Fig. 38.13 in Chapter 38), nuchal rigidity, head tilt, sluggish pupils, increased blood pressure with widening pulse pressure, change in respirations, bradycardia, irregular pulse, and changes in body temperature.

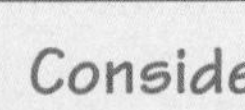

Consider This

Alice Tice, 8 years old, is scheduled to receive chemotherapy for a brain tumor. Alice states, "I'm scared!" A moment later she cries out, "And I don't want to go bald!" Think about when you were a school age child—what things were important to you then? As the nurse caring for her, how can you prepare Alice for this?

NEUROBLASTOMA

Neuroblastoma, a tumor that arises from embryonic neural crest cells, is the most common extracranial solid tumor in children (Hendershot, 2010). It most frequently occurs in the abdomen, mainly in the adrenal gland, but it may occur anywhere along the paravertebral sympathetic chain in the chest or retroperitoneum (Hendershot, 2010). By the time of diagnosis, the neuroblastoma has usually already metastasized. Neuroblastoma is the second most frequently occurring solid tumor in children; 90% of cases are diagnosed before the age of 5 years (Graham et al., 2014).

Staging of the tumor at diagnosis determines the course of treatment and prognosis. Table 46.10 discusses the staging of neuroblastomas. Survival rates range from about 40% to 90%, depending on the staging of the tumor (Hendershot, 2010). Prognosis depends on the tumor stage, age at diagnosis, location of tumor, and location of metastasis. Infants younger than 12 months of age and children with stage I disease have the best survival rates (Graham et al., 2014). Children with tumors above the diaphragm tend to have a better prognosis than those with abdominal tumors. Metastasis to the bone is a worse prognostic factor than metastasis to the skin, liver, or bone marrow. Children who relapse after initial treatment also tend to have a dismal prognosis. In addition to metastasis, complications may include nerve compression, resulting in neurologic deficits.

The neuroblastoma must be removed surgically. Radiation and chemotherapy are administered to all children with neuroblastoma except those with stage I disease, in whom the tumor is completely resected.

TABLE 46.10 STAGING OF NEUROBLASTOMA

Stage	Clinical Findings
I	Tumor confined to organ or structure of origin
II	Tumor extends beyond organ or structure, not beyond midline ("A" negative lymph nodes, "B" regional nodes on same side involved)
III	Tumor invasively extends beyond the midline with bilateral lymph node involvement
IV	Metastasis to bone, bone marrow, other organs, distant lymph nodes
IV-S	Tumor would have been considered a stage I or II, but remote metastasis to one or more sites (liver, skin, or bone marrow) has occurred without metastasis to the bone

Adapted from Hendershot, E. (2010). Solid tumors. In D. Tomlinson & N. E. Kline (Eds.), *Pediatric oncology nursing*. New York, NY: Springer; and Graham, D. K., Craddock, J. A., Quinones, R. R., Keating, A. K., Maloney, K. Foreman, N. K., Giller, R. H., & Greffe, B. S. (2014). Neoplastic disease. In W. W. Hay, M. J. Levin, R. R. Deterding, & M. J. Abzug (Eds.), *Current pediatric diagnosis and treatment* (22nd ed.). New York, NY: McGraw-Hill.

Nursing Assessment

For a full description of the assessment phase of the nursing process, refer to the Assessment section of the Nursing Process Overview earlier in the chapter. Assessment findings pertinent to neuroblastoma are discussed below.

HEALTH HISTORY

Presenting signs and symptoms of neuroblastoma depend on the location of the primary tumor and the extent of metastasis. Often parents are the first to notice a swollen or asymmetric abdomen. Elicit the health history, documenting bowel or bladder dysfunction, especially watery diarrhea, neurologic symptoms (brain metastasis), bone pain (bone metastasis), anorexia, vomiting, or weight loss.

PHYSICAL EXAMINATION

Note neck or facial swelling, bruising above the eyes, or edema around the eyes (metastasis to skull bones). Inspect the skin for pallor or bruising (bone marrow metastasis) and document cough or difficulty breathing. Auscultate the lungs for wheezing. Palpate for lymphadenopathy, especially cervical. Palpate the abdomen, noting a firm, nontender mass. Palpate for and note hepatomegaly or splenomegaly if present.

LABORATORY AND DIAGNOSTIC TESTING

Laboratory and diagnostic testing may reveal the following:

- CT scan or MRI to determine site of tumor and evidence of metastasis
- Chest x-ray, bone scan, and skeletal survey to identify metastasis
- Bone marrow aspiration and biopsy to determine metastasis to the bone marrow
- 24-hour urine collection for homovanillic acid (HVA) and vanillylmandelic acid (VMA); levels will be elevated.

Nursing Management

Postoperative nursing care depends on the site of tumor removal, which is most often the abdomen. Provide routine care after abdominal surgery. Refer to the nursing process overview section and Nursing Care Plan 46.1 at the end of the chapter for nursing care related to the effects of chemotherapy and radiation. Provide emotional support and possible referrals to help children and families cope with a potentially poor prognosis (due to the fact that the disease has often metastasized significantly by the time of diagnosis).

Atraumatic Care

The child with cancer often undergoes a large number of painful procedures related to laboratory specimens and treatment protocols. To assist the child to cope with these procedures, provide distraction in the form of reading a favorite book or playing a favorite movie or musical selection.

BONE AND SOFT TISSUE TUMORS

Bone and soft tissue tumors are common solid tumors in children. Bone tumors are most often diagnosed in adolescence, whereas soft tissue tumors tend to occur in younger children (Hendershot, 2010). This discussion will focus on the most common bone and soft tissue tumors occurring in childhood. The most common bone tumors in children are osteosarcoma and Ewing sarcoma (Hendershot, 2010). These bone tumors often initially go undiagnosed, as adolescents frequently seek care for traumatic events and the pain suffered with a bone tumor may initially be attributed to trauma. Rhabdomyosarcoma is the most common soft tissue tumor in childhood (Hendershot, 2010).

Osteosarcoma

Osteosarcoma is the most common malignant bone cancer in children, occurring most frequently in adolescents at the peak of the growth spurt (Graham et al., 2014). Osteosarcoma occurs slightly more often in males and Caucasians (Hendershot, 2010). It presumably arises from the embryonic mesenchymal tissue that forms the bones. The most common sites are in the long bones, particularly the proximal humerus, proximal tibia, and distal femur. Complications include metastasis, particularly to the lungs and other bones, and recurrence of disease within 3 years, primarily affecting the lungs.

Surgical removal of the tumor is necessary. Chemotherapy is often administered before surgery to decrease the size of the tumor; it is usually administered after surgery to treat or prevent metastasis. The type of surgery performed depends on the tumor size, extent of disease outside of the bone, distant metastasis, and skeletal maturity. Radical amputation may be performed, but often teens undergo a limb salvage procedure. Radical amputation may include the entire extremity or the entire affected bone. Limb-sparing surgery entails removing only the affected portion of the bone, replacing it with either an endoprosthesis or cadaver bone (Abed & Grimer, 2010).

Nursing Assessment

Obtain the health history, ascertaining when pain, limp, or limitation of motion was first noticed. Dull bone pain may be present for several months, eventually progressing to limp or gait changes.

Inspect the affected limb for erythema and swelling. Palpate the affected area for warmth and tenderness and to determine the size of the soft tissue mass, if also present. As with other pediatric cancers, a thorough physical examination is warranted to detect other abnormalities that may indicate metastasis.

Laboratory and diagnostic testing may include:

- CT scan or MRI to determine the extent of the lesion and to identify metastasis
- Bone scan to determine the extent of malignancy

Nursing Management

The adolescent will generally be quite anxious about the possibility of amputation and even about the limb salvage procedure. Present preoperative teaching at the adolescent's developmental level and ensure that he or she is included in planning treatment. Regardless of the type of surgery performed, provide routine orthopedic postoperative care. Educate the adolescent and parents on the care of the stump, if amputation is necessary, and ensure that the teen becomes competent in crutch walking. A prosthesis may be ordered. The adolescent will need time to adjust to these significant body image changes and may benefit from talking with another teen who has undergone a similar procedure. Support the teen in choosing clothing that may camouflage the prosthesis while still allowing the teen to appear fashionable. Provide emotional support, as the teen's maturity level allows him or her to understand the severity of the disease. Peer support groups are often helpful, as teens value their peers' opinions and enjoy being part of a group. Examples of comprehensive online support groups are Melissa's Living Legacy Foundation/Helping Teens Live with Cancer and The Wellness Community. Links to these resources are provided on thePoint.

Ewing Sarcoma

Ewing sarcoma is a highly malignant bone tumor. It is rarer than osteosarcoma, accounting for only about 10% of childhood bone tumors (Graham et al., 2014). It occurs most frequently in the pelvis, chest wall, vertebrae, and long bone diaphyses (midshaft). About 25% of children demonstrate metastasis; the lungs, bone, and bone marrow are the most common sites (Graham et al., 2014).

The prognosis for Ewing sarcoma depends on the extent of metastasis.

Radiation, chemotherapy, and surgical excision are usually used in combination. Treatment varies depending on the site of the primary tumor and the extent of metastasis at diagnosis. Myeloablative chemotherapy (which destroys the child's marrow) may be used for metastatic disease, followed by a stem cell rescue transplant.

Nursing Assessment

Explore the history for intermittent pain that progressively worsens. Note a possible history of fever. Eventually the pain becomes constant and severe, sometimes interrupting sleep.

Note the presence of swelling or erythema at the tumor site. CT scan or MRI of the affected area will reveal the extent of the tumor. Biopsy is necessary to establish the diagnosis. CT scan of the chest, bone scan, and bilateral bone marrow aspiration with biopsy determine the extent of metastasis.

Nursing Management

Before treatment begins, discourage active play or weight bearing on the affected extremity to avoid pathologic fracture at the tumor site. Nursing management focuses on addressing the adverse effects of treatment (refer to the nursing process overview section). Give honest and direct answers to teens with Ewing sarcoma who ask questions about their disease. These children will undergo intensive therapy and spend a great deal of time in the hospital. Depending on the age of the child, fantasy play, art or pet therapy, drama, writing, humor, and/or music may help the child to work through the psychological impact of this disease. Refer to Nursing Care Plan 46.1 for additional interventions, which should be individualized depending on the child's and family's response to the disease process and treatment.

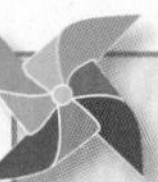

Thinking About Development

Serena Jameson is a 14-year-old cheerleader with newly diagnosed Ewing sarcoma. Her prescribed treatment protocol involves several medications known to cause severe alopecia. Considering Serena's developmental stage, how will this impact her ability and/or willingness to participate in future cheerleading exhibitions? Develop a list of ideas for assisting Serena to cope with the anticipated changes to her body image.

Rhabdomyosarcoma

Rhabdomyosarcoma is a soft tissue tumor that usually arises from the embryonic mesenchymal cells that would ordinarily form striated muscle. The most common locations for the tumor are the head and neck, genitourinary tract, and extremities (Fig. 46.17). The tumor is highly malignant and spreads via local extension or through the venous or lymphatic system, with the lung being the most common site for metastasis. Diagnosis is usually made between 2 and 5 years of age, with 70% of all rhabdomyosarcomas diagnosed by age 10 years (Graham et al., 2014). The prognosis is based on the stage of the disease at diagnosis. Box 46.5 explains the staging of rhabdomyosarcoma. Prognosis is generally favorable for stage I disease, but 3-year survival occurs in only 39% of children with metastatic disease (Graham et al., 2014). Complications of rhabdomyosarcoma include metastasis to lung, bone, or bone marrow and direct extension into the CNS, resulting in brain stem compromise or cranial nerve palsy.

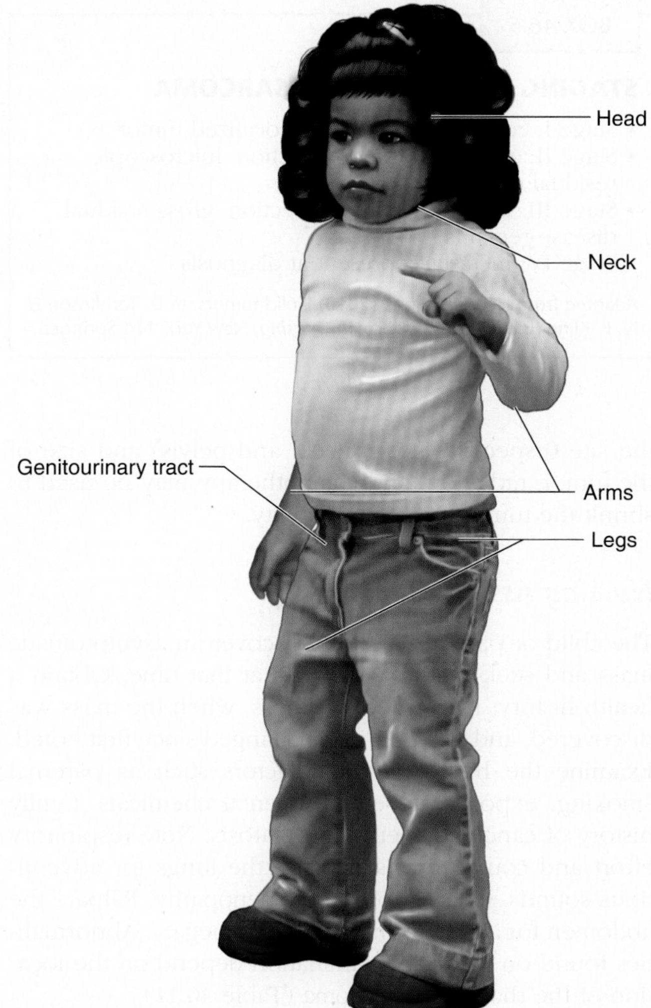

FIGURE 46.17 The most common sites of rhabdomyosarcoma.

Surgical removal of the primary tumor is generally performed. At the time of the surgery, the lesion is biopsied and the stage of disease determined. Depending on

BOX 46.5

STAGING OF RHABDOMYOSARCOMA

- Stage I: completely resectable localized tumor
- Stage II: after local tumor resection, microscopic residual disease remains
- Stage III: after local tumor resection, gross residual disease remains
- Stage IV: metastasis present at diagnosis

Adapted from Hendershot, E. (2010). Solid tumors. In D. Tomlinson & N. E. Kline (Eds.), *Pediatric oncology nursing*. New York, NY: Springer.

the site (especially head, neck, and pelvis) and size of the tumor, radiation, and chemotherapy may be used to shrink the tumor to avoid disability.

Nursing Assessment

The child or parent will often discover an asymptomatic mass and seek medical attention at that time. Obtain a health history, noting recent illness, when the mass was discovered, and whether it has changed since first noted. Examine the history for risk factors such as parental smoking, exposure to environmental chemicals, family history of cancer, or neurofibromatosis. Note respiratory effort and cough, and auscultate the lungs for adventitious sounds. Palpate for lymphadenopathy. Palpate the abdomen for a mass or hepatosplenomegaly. Abnormalities found on physical examination depend on the location of the rhabdomyosarcoma (Table 46.11).

Laboratory and diagnostic testing may include:

- CT scan or MRI of primary lesion and the chest for metastasis
- Open biopsy of the primary tumor for definitive diagnosis
- Bone marrow aspiration and biopsy, bone scan, and skeletal survey to determine metastasis

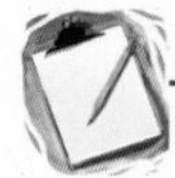

Take Note!

Primary tumors arising in the neck region may compress the child's airway. Assess work of breathing and lung sounds.

Nursing Management

Provide routine postoperative care, depending on the site of surgery. Assess for adverse effects of high-dose radiation, which is generally used to treat the primary tumor as well as metastatic sites. Administer chemotherapy as ordered and assess for adverse effects. Refer to the nursing process overview section and Nursing Care Plan 46.1 to determine an individualized plan of care based on the child's response to the treatment.

WILMS TUMOR

Wilms tumor is the most common renal tumor and the fourth most common solid tumor in children (Hendershot, 2010). Peak incidence occurs between the ages of 2 and 3 years (Hendershot, 2010). It usually affects only one kidney (Fig. 46.18). The etiology is unknown,

TABLE 46.11 PRESENTING SIGNS AND SYMPTOMS RELATED TO LOCATION OF RHABDOMYOSARCOMA

Location of Tumor	Presenting Signs and Symptoms
Orbit	Proptosis
Middle ear	Drainage, pain, facial nerve palsy
Sinuses	Discharge, pain, sinusitis, facial swelling
Nasopharynx	Pain, epistaxis, dysphagia, nasal quality to speech, airway obstruction
Neck	Dysphagia, hoarseness
Thorax, testicle, extremities	Enlarging mass, painless
Retroperitoneum	Gastrointestinal and urinary tract obstruction, pain, weakness, paresthesia
Bladder, prostate	Hematuria, urinary obstruction
Vagina	Mass, vaginal bleeding or chronic discharge

Adapted from Hendershot, E. (2010). Solid tumors. In D. Tomlinson & N. E. Kline (Eds.), *Pediatric oncology nursing*. New York, NY: Springer; and Graham, D. K., Craddock, J. A., Quinones, R. R., Keating, A. K., Maloney, K. Foreman, N. K., Giller, R. H., & Greffe, B. S. (2014). Neoplastic disease. In W. W. Hay, M. J. Levin, R. R. Deterding, & M. J. Abzug (Eds.), *Current pediatric diagnosis and treatment* (22nd ed.). New York, NY: McGraw-Hill.

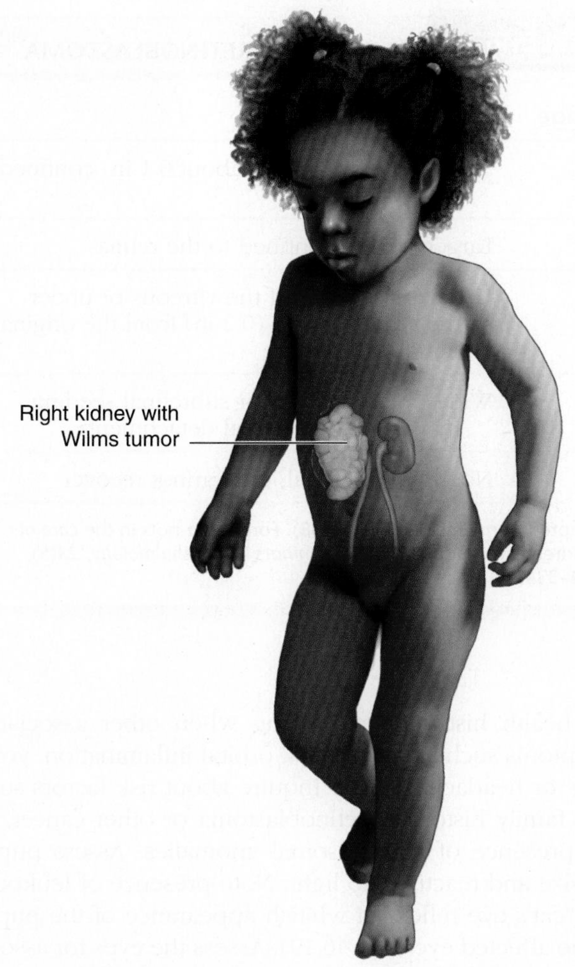

FIGURE 46.18 Wilms tumor is usually unilateral.

but some cases occur via genetic inheritance. Associated anomalies may occur with Wilms tumor. Wilms tumor demonstrates rapid growth and is usually large at diagnosis. Metastasis occurs via direct extension or through the bloodstream. Wilms tumor most commonly metastasizes to the perirenal tissues, liver, diaphragm, lungs, abdominal muscles, and lymph nodes. The prognosis depends on staging at diagnosis and the extent of metastasis (Box 46.6). The overall survival rate is about 90% (Hendershot, 2010). Complications include metastasis or complications from radiation therapy such as liver or renal damage, female sterility, bowel obstruction, pneumonia, or scoliosis.

Therapeutic Management

Surgical removal of the tumor and affected kidney (nephrectomy) is the treatment of choice and also allows for accurate staging and assessment of tumor spread. Radiation or chemotherapy may be administered either before or after surgery.

BOX 46.6

STAGING OF WILMS TUMOR

- Stage I: unilateral, limited to kidney, completely resectable
- Stage II: unilateral, tumor extends beyond kidney but is completely resectable
- Stage III: unilateral, tumor has spread outside of kidney, located in abdominal cavity only, not fully removed
- Stage IV: unilateral with metastasis in liver, lung, bone, or brain
- Stage V: bilateral kidney involvement

Nursing Assessment

For a full description of the assessment phase of the nursing process, refer to the Assessment section of the Nursing Process Overview earlier in the chapter. Assessment findings pertinent to Wilms tumor are discussed below.

HEALTH HISTORY

Parents typically initially observe the abdominal mass associated with Wilms tumor and then seek medical attention. Elicit the health history, noting when the mass was discovered. Note abdominal pain, which may be related to rapid tumor growth. Document history of constipation, vomiting, anorexia, weight loss, or difficulty breathing. Determine risk factors such as hemihypertrophy of the spine, Beckwith–Wiedemann syndrome, genitourinary anomalies, absence of the iris, or family history of cancer.

PHYSICAL EXAMINATION

Measure blood pressure; hypertension occurs in 25% of children with Wilms tumor (Graham et al., 2014). Inspect the abdomen for asymmetry or a visible mass. Observe for associated anomalies as noted above. Auscultate the lungs for adventitious breath sounds associated with tumor metastasis. Palpate for lymphadenopathy.

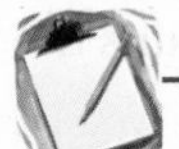

Take Note!

Avoid palpating the abdomen after the initial assessment preoperatively. Wilms tumor is highly vascular and soft, so excessive handling of the tumor may result in tumor seeding and metastasis.

LABORATORY AND DIAGNOSTIC TESTING

Laboratory and diagnostic testing may include:

- Renal or abdominal ultrasound to assess the tumor and the contralateral kidney
- CT scan or MRI of the abdomen and chest to determine local spread to lymph nodes or adjacent organs, as well as any distant metastasis
- Complete blood count, BUN, and creatinine: usually within normal limits

- Urinalysis: may reveal hematuria or leukocytes
- 24-hour urine collection for HVA and VMA to distinguish the tumor from neuroblastoma (levels will not be elevated with Wilms tumor)

Nursing Management

Postoperative care of the child with Wilms tumor resection is similar to that of children undergoing other abdominal surgery. Assessment of remaining kidney function is critical. The child may have adverse effects related to chemotherapy or radiation. Refer to the nursing process overview section and Nursing Care Plan 46.1 to individualize care for the child based on the child's response to therapy.

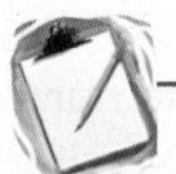

Take Note!

To avoid injuring the remaining kidney, children with a single kidney should not play contact sports.

RETINOBLASTOMA

Retinoblastoma is a congenital, highly malignant tumor that arises from embryonic retinal cells. It accounts for 5% of cases of blindness in children (Graham et al., 2014). Most children are diagnosed by age 5, and the 5-year survival rate is 90% (Graham et al., 2014). Retinoblastoma may be hereditary or nonhereditary. Nonhereditary retinoblastoma may be associated with advanced paternal age and always presents with unilateral involvement. Hereditary retinoblastoma is inherited via the autosomal dominant mode. These cases may be unilateral or bilateral. The tumor may grow forward into the vitreous cavity of the eye or extend into the subretinal space, causing retinal detachment. The tumor may extend into the choroid, the sclera, and the optic nerve.

Complications include spread to the brain and the opposite eye, as well as metastasis to lymph nodes, bone, bone marrow, and liver. Secondary tumors, most often sarcomas, may also occur in children who have been treated for retinoblastoma. Table 46.12 explains the staging of retinoblastoma.

TABLE 46.12 STAGING OF RETINOBLASTOMA

Stage	Clinical Findings
A	Small tumors (<3 mm; about 0.1 in) confined to the retina
B	Larger tumors confined to the retina
C	Localized seeding of the vitreous or under the retina <6 mm (0.2 in) from the original tumor
D	Widespread vitreous or subretinal seeding, may have total retinal detachment
E	No visual potential, eye cannot recover

Adapted from Shields, C. L. (2008). Forget-me-nots in the care of children with retinoblastoma. *Seminars in Ophthalmology, 23*(5), 324–334.

The goals of treatment are to eradicate the tumor, preserve vision, and provide a good cosmetic outcome. Retinoblastoma may be treated with radiation, chemotherapy, laser surgery, cryotherapy, or a combination of these treatments. Moderate vision may be preserved for most children without advanced disease. In advanced disease or in the case of a massive tumor with retinal detachment, enucleation (removal of the eye) is necessary.

Nursing Assessment

Parents are often the first to notice the "cat's eye reflex" or "whitewash glow" to the child's affected pupil. Obtain the health history, determining when other associated symptoms such as strabismus, orbital inflammation, vomiting, or headache began. Inquire about risk factors such as a family history of retinoblastoma or other cancer, or the presence of chromosomal anomalies. Assess pupils for size and reactivity to light. Note presence of leukocoria ("cat's eye reflex," a whitish appearance of the pupil) in the affected eye (Fig. 46.19). Assess the eyes for associated signs, which may include erythema, orbital inflammation, or hyphema.

Diagnostic evaluation includes an ophthalmologic examination under anesthesia. CT, MRI, or ultrasound of the head and eyes will help to visualize the tumor. The infant or toddler may also undergo lumbar puncture and

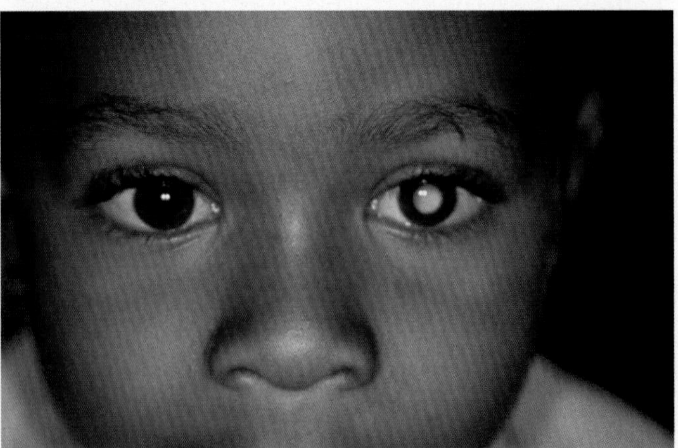

FIGURE 46.19 Note the whitish appearance of this child's pupil (leukocoria). (Used with permission from Rubin, E., & Farber, J. L. (1999) *Pathology* (3rd ed.). Philadelphia, PA: Lippincott Williams & Wilkins.)

bone marrow aspiration to determine the presence and extent of metastasis.

Nursing Management

Provide routine postoperative care to the infant or toddler. If the eye is enucleated, observe the large pressure dressing on the eye socket for bleeding. Dressing changes to the socket may include sterile saline rinses and/or antibiotic ointment application. If disease occurs outside of the eye or if metastasis is present, inform the parents that chemotherapy will be necessary. Monitor for side effects of chemotherapy (see the nursing process overview section). Follow-up will include eye examinations every 3 to 6 months until age 6 and then annually to check for further tumor development. If the eye is enucleated, a prosthetic eye will be fitted several weeks after removal. Teach families use of the prosthetic eye; it does not require daily removal.

Provide parents with support and encouragement. Refer the family for genetic counseling. Children with a family history of retinoblastoma need ophthalmologic examination shortly after birth and routinely until age 5 to 6 years (Kaufman, Kim, & Berry, 2016). Children with the heritable form of retinoblastoma should have genetic counseling as they reach puberty because of the risk of bilateral disease in their offspring (Kaufman et al., 2016).

Take Note!

Educate parents about protecting vision in the remaining eye: routine eye check-ups, protection from accidental injury, use of safety goggles during sports, and prompt treatment of eye infections. Generally, children with one eye should not participate in contact sports.

SCREENING FOR REPRODUCTIVE CANCERS IN ADOLESCENTS

Increasingly, reproductive cancers are being diagnosed in adolescents. Cervical cancer and testicular cancer may be discovered early with appropriate screening, and earlier discovery leads to better outcomes. Starting screening in the teenage years may also instill a lifelong healthy habit in the adolescent.

Cervical Cancer

Risk factors for cervical cancer include young age at first intercourse, infection with a sexually transmitted disease, and a history of multiple sex partners. More and more teenagers are presenting with these risk factors. Cervical cancer is most commonly attributed to human papillomavirus (HPV) (AAP, 2016). HPV vaccine (Gardasil) is recommended to be given as a three-vaccine series to all girls and boys beginning at age 11 to 12 years (AAP, 2016). Despite the availability of the vaccine, not all girls and boys will receive it. Counsel all sexually active adolescents to seek reproductive care, which is available without parental consent in most states. The screening Papanicolaou (Pap) smear is efficient and reliable at determining abnormal cervical cells and is a key part of screening for cervical cancer (if cancer is present, the parent will have to be notified). Cervical cancer has a very high response to therapy and rate of cure if treated in its early stages. Therefore, encourage teenage girls to be responsible for their sexual health by seeking appropriate examination and screening.

HEALTHY PEOPLE 2020

Objective	Nursing Significance
Increase the proportion of women who receive a cervical cancer screening based on the most recent guidelines.	• When an adolescent girl makes the decision to become sexually active, counsel her about the importance of getting annual Pap smears, which should begin within 3 years of becoming sexually active.

Healthy People Objectives retrieved from http://www.healthypeople.gov

Testicular Cancer

Although uncommon in teens, testicular cancer is the most frequently diagnosed cancer in males between 20 and 34 years of age (National Cancer Institute, n. d.). It is one of the most curable cancers if diagnosed

HEALTHY PEOPLE 2020

Objective	Nursing Significance
Reduce the overall cancer death rate. Increase the proportion of cancer survivors who are living 5 years or longer after diagnosis	• Teach adolescent boys testicular self-examination. • Reinforce the importance of this self-screening measure at subsequent visits.

Healthy People Objectives retrieved from http://www.healthypeople.gov

early. To get into the habit of screening for testicular lumps, encourage adolescent boys to begin performing testicular self-examinations monthly (Teaching Guidelines 46.5).

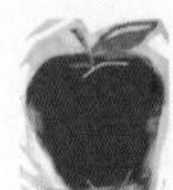

Teaching Guidelines 46.5

TESTICULAR SELF-EXAMINATION

- Perform the examination once a month, after a shower.
- Be familiar with the size and weight of your testicles.
- Roll the testicle between your fingers. The small rope-like structure is the epididymis; this is normal.
- Report any lump, swelling, or heaviness of one testicle to your physician or nurse practitioner.

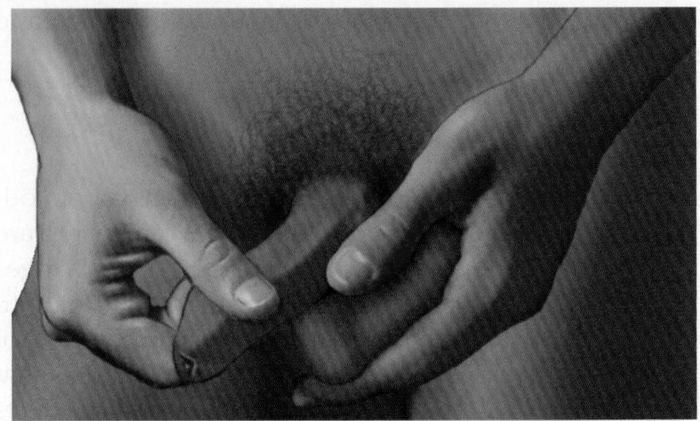

Adapted from Figueroa, T. E. (2012). *How to perform a testicular self-examination*. Retrieved from http://kidshealth.org/teen/sexual_health/guys/tse.html

NURSING CARE PLAN 46.1

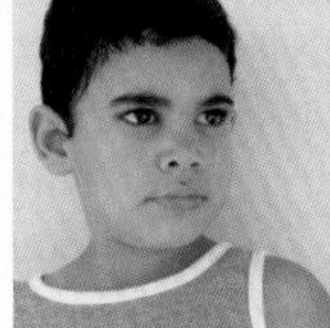

Overview for the Child With an Alteration in Cellular Regulation

NURSING DIAGNOSIS: Fatigue related to decreased oxygen supply in the body as evidenced by lack of energy, increased sleep requirements, or decreased interest in play

Outcome Identification and Evaluation

Child will display increased endurance, desire to play without developing symptoms of exertion.

Intervention: ***Decreasing Fatigue***

- Cluster nursing care activities and plan for periods of rest before and after exertion *to decrease oxygen need and consumption.*
- Encourage activity or ambulation per physician's orders: *early mobilization results in better outcomes.*
- Observe child for signs of activity intolerance such as pallor, nausea, lightheadedness, or dizziness or changes in vital signs *to determine level of tolerance.*
- If child is on bed rest, perform range-of-motion exercises and frequent position changes: *negative changes to the musculoskeletal system occur quickly with inactivity and immobility.*
- Refer the child to physical therapy *for exercise prescription to increase skeletal muscle strength.*

NURSING DIAGNOSIS: Impaired physical mobility related to pain from sickle cell crisis or acute bleeds or imposed activity restrictions, as evidenced by guarding of painful extremity, resistance to activity

Outcome Identification and Evaluation

Child will be able to engage in activities within age parameters and limits of disease: *child is able to move extremities, move about environment, and participate in exercise programs within limits of age and disease.*

NURSING CARE PLAN 46.1

Overview for the Child With an Alteration in Cellular Regulation (continued)

Interventions: ***Promoting Physical Mobility***

- Encourage gross and fine motor activities as able within constraints of pain/bleed *to facilitate motor development.*
- Collaborate with physical therapy to strengthen muscles and promote mobility *to facilitate motor development.*
- Use passive and active range-of-motion (ROM) exercises and teach the child and family how to perform them *to prevent contractures and facilitate joint mobility and muscle development (active ROM) to help increase mobility.*
- Praise accomplishments and emphasize child's abilities *to improve self-esteem and encourage feelings of confidence and competence.*

NURSING DIAGNOSIS: Ineffective health management related to knowledge and skill acquisition regarding nutritional and medical treatment of anemia, prevention of infection, home administration of intravenous clotting factors, or protection from injury as evidenced by new diagnosis and inability to verbalize appropriate treatment regimen or demonstrate medication administration skills

Outcome Identification and Evaluation

Child's health will be maintained: child will receive supplements, medications as prescribed and will eat an appropriate diet.

Intervention: ***Educating Parents About Effective Health Maintenance***

- Educate the family about iron-rich foods to be promoted in the child with iron-deficiency anemia and limited in the child with thalassemia.
- Limit cow's milk intake in the child with iron-deficiency anemia *to decrease risk of microscopic gastrointestinal (GI) bleeding and increase appetite for other foods.*
- Provide ongoing evaluation of nutritional intake *to ensure that appropriate dietary restrictions are followed.*
- Ensure that parents can verbalize understanding of home medication regimen: iron or folic acid supplementation for anemia, prophylactic antibiotics for sickle cell anemia, chelation for thalassemia, and factor replacement for hemophilia.
- Have parents provide return demonstration of subcutaneous infusion of deferoxamine or intravenous factor as appropriate *to ensure accuracy and independence in the home environment.*
- Educate families about when to call or visit physician or nurse practitioner *to ensure timely intervention when signs and symptoms develop.*

NURSING DIAGNOSIS: Anxiety related to diagnostic testing as evidenced by parent verbalization, child resistance, or crying with procedures

Outcome Identification and Evaluation

Child's anxiety will be minimized: child will verbalize less fear, experience less pain with procedures.

Intervention: ***Relieving Anxiety***

- Use topical anesthetic creams or agents for nonemergency laboratory draws to decrease stress related *to needlesticks or venipunctures.*
- Maintain a quiet and calm environment *to reduce the child's stress.*
- Educate the child, as appropriate, and the family regarding the need for laboratory specimens *to alleviate anxiety related to the unknown.*
- Identify the need for the specific test and explain the procedure before obtaining the specimen *to decrease the anxiety and time required for the procedure.*
- Provide developmentally appropriate activities for the child: *activities can reduce stress and also provide stimulus for children; serves as a model for the family.*

(continued)

NURSING CARE PLAN 46.1

Overview for the Child With an Alteration in Cellular Regulation (continued)

NURSING DIAGNOSIS: Ineffective family coping related to hospitalization of child or chronic, possibly life-threatening genetic disorder as evidenced by excessive tearfulness or denial statements, withdrawal, or verbalization of inadequate coping skills

Outcome Identification and Evaluation

Child and/or family will demonstrate adequate coping skills, *will verbalize feeling supported and demonstrate healthy family interactions.*

Intervention: ***Promoting Effective Family Coping***

- Provide emotional support to the child and family *to improve coping abilities.*
- Actively listen to the child's and family's concerns *to validate their feelings and establish trust.*
- Encourage parents to talk about their child and the illness *to bring feelings out in the open.*
- Validate feelings of guilt, shock, frustration, resentment, or depression *to promote trust and begin appropriate coping.*
- Provide open communication with the child and siblings: *children appreciate honesty about their illness, and coping is improved.*
- Refer families to community resources such as parent support groups and grief counseling *to improve coping abilities.*
- Encourage role-playing and play activities *to identify the child's fears and work through feelings.*

NURSING DIAGNOSIS: Risk for injury related to alteration in peripheral sensory perception, decreased platelet count, deficient coagulation factor, or excessive iron load

Outcome Identification and Evaluation

Child will not experience hemorrhage: *will experience decreased bruising or episodes of prolonged bleeding.*

Intervention: ***Preventing Injury***

- Assess for petechiae, purpura, bruising, or bleeding *to provide baseline data for comparison; if present, may warrant intervention.*
- Encourage quiet activities or play *to avoid trauma with active play.*
- Avoid rectal temperatures and examinations. Post sign at head of bed "no rectal temperatures or medications" *to avoid rectal mucosa damage resulting in bleeding.*
- Avoid intramuscular injections and lumbar puncture if possible *to decrease risk of bleeding from a puncture site.*
- If bone marrow aspiration must be performed, apply pressure dressing to site *to prevent bleeding.*
- Teach families about preferred physical activities for the child with idiopathic thrombocytopenia purpura (ITP) or hemophilia *to provide safe physical activities and decrease risk for injury.*

NURSING DIAGNOSIS: Risk for infection related to neutropenia and immunosuppression

Outcome Identification and Evaluation

Child will not experience overwhelming infection: *will be free from infection or able to recover if he or she becomes infected.*

Interventions: ***Preventing Infection***

- Assess for fever, pain, cough, tachypnea, adventitious breath sounds, skin ulceration, stomatitis, and perirectal fissures *to identify potential infection.*
- Administer antibiotics for temperature greater than 38.4°C *to decrease likelihood of overwhelming sepsis.*

NURSING CARE PLAN 46.1

Overview for the Child With an Alteration in Cellular Regulation (continued)

- Maintain meticulous hand-washing procedures (including family, visitors, staff) *to minimize spread of infectious organisms.*
- Maintain isolation as prescribed *to minimize exposure to infectious organisms.*
- Avoid rectal temperatures and examinations, intramuscular injections, and urinary catheterization when child is neutropenic *to decrease possibility of introducing microorganisms.*
- Educate family and visitors that child should be restricted from contact with known infectious exposures (in hospital and at home) *to encourage cooperation with infection control.*
- Strictly observe medical asepsis *to avoid unintentional introduction of microorganisms.*
- Promote nutrition and appropriate rest *to maximize body's potential to heal.*
- Inform family to contact the physician or nurse practitioner if child has known exposure to chickenpox or measles *so that preventive measures (e.g., varicella zoster immunoglobulin [VZIG]) can be taken.*
- Administer vaccines (not live) as prescribed (after clearance with oncologist) *to prevent common childhood communicable diseases.*
- Teach family to monitor for fever at home and report temperature elevations to oncologist immediately *so that antibiotic therapy may be instituted as soon as possible.*

NURSING DIAGNOSIS: Pain related to invasive diagnostic testing, surgical procedure, neuropathy, disease progression, or adverse effects of treatment as evidenced by verbalization of pain, elevated pain scale ratings, guarding, withdrawal from play or refusal to participate in activities of daily living, or physiologic indicators such as elevated heart rate, diaphoresis, muscle tension or rigidity

Outcome Identification and Evaluation

Child will demonstrate pain relief *in amount sufficient to allow participation in play, activities of daily living, or therapeutic interventions. Use the age-appropriate pain scale to set the goal and set a time frame for achievement of the goal.*

Interventions: *Promoting Comfort*

- Determine level of pain using child interview, pain scale, and assessment of physiologic variables *to determine baseline.*
- Document location, intensity, and description of pain to *determine baseline.*
- Discuss with the child and parent techniques that have helped alleviate pain in the past *to incorporate successful interventions into the plan of care.*
- Administer acetaminophen for mild pain: *avoid salicylate and NSAIDs due to increased risk for bleeding.*
- Administer medications as ordered using the least invasive method possible *to avoid pain (intramuscular, subcutaneous, and rectal route should be avoided in the child with thrombocytopenia).*
- Monitor frequently for adverse effects (particularly respiratory effects) of opioid analgesics, *as opioids reduce responsiveness of carbon dioxide receptors in the brain's respiratory center.*
- Use nonpharmacologic measures such as play therapy, games, TV, guided breathing, imagery, hypnosis, or meditation as appropriate: *distracts child's attention from the pain.*
- Use massage, positioning, or heat *to relieve pain in a particular area.*
- Use EMLA before needlesticks and conscious sedation with lumbar puncture and bone marrow aspiration *to reduce recurrent acute painful episodes associated with frequent blood draws and diagnostic/treatment procedures.*
- Have the child lie flat for 30 minutes after a lumbar puncture and increase fluid intake for 24 hours after the procedure *to decrease incidence of headache.*

(continued)

NURSING CARE PLAN 46.1

Overview for the Child With an Alteration in Cellular Regulation (continued)

NURSING DIAGNOSIS: Impaired oral mucous membranes related to chemotherapy, radiation therapy, immunocompromise, decreased platelet count, malnutrition, or dehydration as evidenced by oral lesions, ulcers, plaques, hyperemia or bleeding, difficulty eating or swallowing, or complaint of oral discomfort

Outcome Identification and Evaluation

Child will maintain intact, moist mucosa *free from redness, ulceration, or debris.*

Interventions: *Restoring Healthy Oral Mucosa*

- Frequently assess oral cavity for redness, lesions, ulcers, plaques, or bleeding *to provide baseline for comparison and identify alterations early.*
- Offer ice chips frequently while child is NPO *to maintain hydration of mucosa.*
- Use only a soft toothbrush or toothette for dental care, avoiding excessive pressure with brushing, *to decrease incidence of bleeding with mouth care.*
- Keep lips lubricated with petroleum jelly or fragrance-free lip balm *to maintain moist, hydrated lips.*
- Rinse with salt solution or mouthwash every 1 to 2 hours *to keep oral cavity clean and moist.*
- Administer glutamine and/or β-carotene supplements, *which have been shown to decrease the incidence and severity of mucositis.*
- Have child swish and spit 1:1 Benadryl/Maalox solution *to decrease pain.*
- Administer antifungal solution *to prevent or treat oral candidiasis.*
- Avoid spicy, acidic, or very hot or very cold foods *to decrease pain.*
- Administer pain medication (usually acetaminophen or codeine) as ordered *to decrease pain.*

NURSING DIAGNOSIS: Nausea related to adverse effects of chemotherapy or radiation therapy as evidenced by verbalization of nausea, increased salivation, swallowing movements, or vomiting

Outcome Identification and Evaluation

Child will experience decreased nausea: *will verbalize symptom relief and will be free from vomiting.*

Interventions: *Alleviating Nausea and Vomiting*

- Administer antiemetics prior to chemotherapy and as needed thereafter *to decrease frequency of nausea.*
- Assess frequency of vomiting and level of hydration *to provide baseline data and recognize alterations early.*
- Offer frequent, smaller meals or snacks: *smaller amounts are less likely to be vomited.*
- Avoid spicy foods *to avoid stomach upset.*
- Allow bubbles to dissipate from carbonated beverages before they are ingested: *carbonation may contribute to nausea.*
- Remove cover from meal tray before entering child's room: *this will allow the food odor to dissipate outside of the room; food odors may trigger nausea and vomiting.*

NURSING DIAGNOSIS: Imbalanced nutrition: less than body requirements related to anorexia, nausea, vomiting, or mucosal irritation associated with chemotherapy or radiation as evidenced by decreased oral intake and weight, length/height, and/or body mass index (BMI) below average for age or individual child's usual measures

Outcome Identification and Evaluation

Child will improve nutritional intake, resulting in *steady increase in weight and length/height.*

NURSING CARE PLAN 46.1

Overview for the Child With an Alteration in Cellular Regulation (continued)

Interventions: ***Promoting Adequate Nutrition***

- Determine body weight and length/height norm for age or find out what the child's pretreatment measurements were *to determine goal to work toward.*
- Determine child's food preferences and provide favorite foods as able *to increase the likelihood that the child will consume adequate amounts of foods.*
- Administer antiemetics as ordered *to increase the likelihood that the child will retain the food he or she ingests.*
- Weigh child daily or weekly (according to physician order or institutional standard) and measure length/height weekly *to monitor for growth.*
- Offer highest-calorie meals at the time of day when the child's appetite is the greatest *to increase likelihood of increased caloric intake.*
- Provide increased-calorie shakes or puddings within diet restriction: *high-calorie foods increase weight gain.*
- Administer vitamin and mineral supplements as prescribed *to attain/maintain vitamin and mineral balance in the body.*
- Administer total parenteral nutrition and intravenous lipids as ordered *to provide adequate nutrition for healing.*

NURSING DIAGNOSIS: Constipation related to effects of vinca alkaloids, opioid use, decreased activity, and dietary changes as evidenced by hard stool or stool that is difficult to pass

Outcome Identification and Evaluation

Child's bowel function will return to usual pattern: *child will pass a formed, soft stool every day (or modify this criterion according to child's usual pattern).*

Interventions: ***Preventing or Managing Constipation***

- Ensure that child increases fluid intake *to provide enough water in the intestines for soft stool formation.*
- Increase fiber in the diet *to provide bulk for stool formation.*
- Administer stool softeners such as mineral oil or docusate sodium: *these help soften the stool, aiding in passage.*
- Provide motivator laxatives such as magnesium hydroxide, lactulose, or sorbitol *to stimulate stool passage.*
- Use stimulant laxatives such as senna or bisacodyl only intermittently rather than on a daily basis *to avoid dependency and diarrhea.*

NURSING DIAGNOSIS: Diarrhea related to effects of radiation therapy as evidenced by loose or watery stools, possibly frequent

Child's bowel function will return to usual pattern: child will pass a formed, soft stool daily (or modify this criterion according to child's usual pattern).

Interventions: ***Managing Diarrhea***

- Assess frequency of diarrhea and level of hydration *to provide data about severity.*
- Obtain weight daily on same scale *to determine extent of fluid loss.*
- Maintain accurate intake and output records *to determine extent of fluid loss.*
- Administer oral rehydration solutions or intravenous fluids as ordered *to maintain or restore adequate hydration.*

(continued)

NURSING CARE PLAN 46.1

Overview for the Child With an Alteration in Cellular Regulation (continued)

- Restrict roughage and residue in diet *to decrease likelihood of diarrhea.*
- Avoid milk products during acute diarrheal phase: *lactose often worsens diarrhea.*
- Provide an elemental diet to relieve symptoms: *absorbed in the upper small bowel.*
- Provide meticulous perineal care *to avoid skin breakdown related to frequent or loose stools.*
- Administer antidiarrheal medications if ordered *to decrease frequency of stools.*
- If severe and related to radiation therapy, a 3- to 4-day rest period from radiation may be required *to begin recovery of normal absorptive capabilities of bowel.*

NURSING DIAGNOSIS: Risk for impaired skin integrity related to radiation therapy

Outcome Identification and Evaluation

Child's skin will remain intact: *areas of redness in radiation field will not progress to desquamation.*

Interventions: ***Promoting Skin Integrity***

- Assess skin frequently for erythema, erosions, ulcers, or blisters *to provide baseline data and intervene early if skin is impaired.*
- Use a mild soap for cleansing and pat dry rather than rubbing *to avoid skin irritation.*
- Use aloe vera lotion *to moisturize the skin.*
- Avoid perfumed lotions, soaps, heat, cold, or sun, *as these will further irritate the skin in the irradiated area.*
- Do not scrub ink from marked radiation field, and avoid adhesive tape in that area, *to avoid further skin irritation.*
- Administer diphenhydramine or apply hydrocortisone 1% cream *to reduce itching and urge to scratch.*
- For areas of desquamation related to radiation, apply Silvadene cream once or twice a day *to hasten skin repair.*

NURSING DIAGNOSIS: Activity intolerance related to treatment adverse effects, anemia, or generalized weakness as evidenced by verbalization of weakness or fatigue; elevation of heart rate, respiratory rate, or blood pressure with activity; complaint of shortness of breath with play or activity

Outcome Identification and Evaluation

Child will display increased activity tolerance: desire to play without developing symptoms of exertion.

Interventions: ***Promoting Activity***

- Encourage activity or ambulation per physician's orders: *early mobilization results in better outcomes.*
- Observe child for symptoms of activity intolerance such as pallor, nausea, lightheadedness or dizziness, or changes in vital signs *to determine level of tolerance.*
- If child is on bed rest, perform range-of-motion exercises and frequent position changes: *negative changes to the musculoskeletal system occur quickly with inactivity and immobility.*
- Cluster nursing care activities and plan for periods of rest before and after exertion *to decrease oxygen need and consumption.*
- Refer the child to physical therapy *for exercise prescription to increase skeletal muscle strength.*

NURSING CARE PLAN 46.1

Overview for the Child With an Alteration in Cellular Regulation (continued)

NURSING DIAGNOSIS: Disturbed body image related to hair loss as evidenced by verbalization of dissatisfaction with appearance

Outcome Identification and Evaluation

Child or adolescent will display appropriate body image: *will look at self in mirror and participate in social activities.*

Interventions: ***Promoting Body Image***

- Acknowledge the child's feelings of anger over body changes and illness: *venting feelings is associated with less body image disturbance.*
- Encourage the child or teen to choose a wig or hats and scarves *to involve the child in making decisions about appearance.*
- Support the child's or teen's choices of comfortable, fashionable clothing *to disguise weight loss or scarring while promoting self-esteem.*
- Involve the child in the decision-making process, *as a sense of control will improve body image.*
- Encourage the child to spend time with peers who have experienced hair, limb, or weight loss, *as peers' opinions are often better accepted than those of persons in authority, such as parents or healthcare professionals.*

NURSING DIAGNOSIS: Risk for situational low self-esteem related to loss of control and inability to progress with quest for independence (adolescents)

Outcome Identification and Evaluation

Adolescent will maintain or increase self-esteem: *will display increased coping responses and verbalize control as appropriate as well as discuss plans for future.*

Interventions: ***Promoting Self-Esteem***

- Identify the adolescent's positive abilities *to promote self-esteem.*
- Give genuine and honest positive feedback, *as the child or adolescent desires honesty.*
- Explore strengths and weaknesses with the adolescent: *helps the teen to see similarities and differences with healthy peers of the same age.*
- Encourage the teen to perform self-care as possible *to promote independence.*
- Offer emotional support: *reduces psychological distress and increases coping abilities.*
- Encourage participation in a support group *to allow teens to discuss body changes and the reactions they perceive in others.*
- When the adolescent is physically able, encourage attendance at camp or an adventure/wilderness event: *these programs have been shown to improve mental health and coping skills.*

NURSING DIAGNOSIS: Compromised family coping related to potentially life-threatening illness and stressors involved with cancer treatment

Outcome Identification and Evaluation

Child and/or family will demonstrate adequate coping skills: will verbalize feeling supported and demonstrate healthy family interactions.

(continued)

NURSING CARE PLAN 46.1

Overview for the Child With an Alteration in Cellular Regulation (continued)

Interventions: ***Promoting Child and Family Coping***

- Provide emotional support to the child and family: *improves coping abilities.*
- Actively listen to the child's and family's concerns: *validates their feelings and establishes trust.*
- Provide open communication with the child and siblings: *children appreciate honesty about their illness, and coping is improved.*
- Refer families to community resources such as parent support groups and grief counseling: *such support improves coping abilities.*
- Give terminally ill children permission to discuss their feelings about their illness, *allowing them to conquer fears and express love for their family and friends.*
- Encourage families to be honest with siblings about the treatment and prognosis of the child with cancer: *children often sense what is going on and cope better when they are prepared and are given an honest explanation of events.*
- Prepare siblings for the death of the child with cancer, using the child life specialist and chaplain as necessary: *the bereavement period is eased when siblings are prepared.*

NURSING DIAGNOSIS: Grief related to diagnosis of cancer in a child and impending loss of child as evidenced by crying, disbelief of diagnosis, and expressions of grief

Outcome Identification and Evaluation

Family will express feelings of grief: *seek help in dealing with feelings, plan for future one day at the time.*

Intervention: ***Supporting the Grieving Family***

- Use therapeutic communication with open-ended questions to encourage an open and trusting relationship for better communication.
- Actively listen to the family's expression of grief: just being present and listening conveys support.
- Encourage the family to cry and express feelings away from the child to work through feelings while not upsetting the child.
- Assess for spiritual distress and refer the family to the hospital chaplain or clergy of choice for support.
- Educate the family about the child's condition honestly: knowing what is going on, what is to be expected, and what the treatment plan is gives the family a sense of control.
- Support the family through discussions with the child about anticipated death when the illness is deemed terminal.

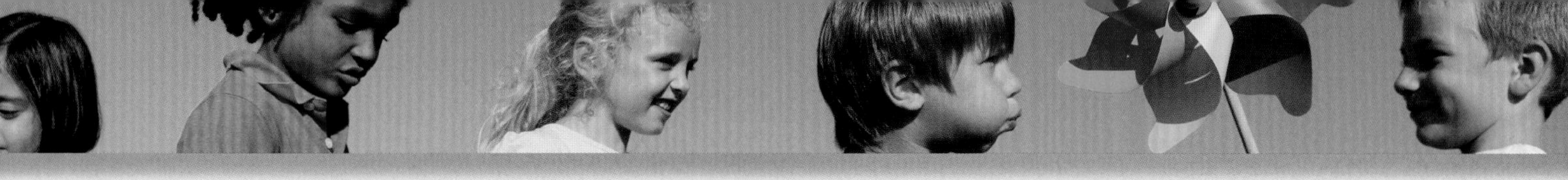

KEY CONCEPTS

- The major forms of anemia affecting children are iron-deficiency anemia, lead poisoning, folic acid deficiency, pernicious anemia, sickle cell anemia, thalassemia, and G6PD deficiency.
- The major bleeding disorders affecting children are idiopathic thrombocytopenic purpura, Henoch–Schönlein purpura, DIC, and hemophilia and vWD.
- Childhood cancer tends to develop from embryonal tissue; in general, it is more responsive to therapy than adult cancers, which tend to be derived from epithelial tissue.
- In adults, cancer is influenced to a large extent by environmental factors. Cancer in children is most often not attributed to environmental factors, so generally there are no routine screening measures or prevention strategies for childhood cancer.
- The pain associated with lumbar puncture or bone marrow aspiration may be minimized with the use of topical anesthetics or conscious sedation.
- CT scans and MRI are used extensively in the diagnosis and follow-up of childhood cancer. The young child may have difficulty holding still for these scans and may need short-term sedation.
- Assess for hypoxia, fatigue, and pallor in the child with anemia.
- Nursing assessment for the child with a bleeding disorder focuses on determining its extent and severity.
- Supplementation with iron is the key intervention for the child with iron-deficiency anemia.
- All young children should be screened for lead exposure.
- Prevention of infection and vaso-occlusive episodes takes priority in children with sickle cell anemia.
- Multimodal pain management and astute physical assessment for serious complications are critical in the nursing care of the child having a sickle cell crisis.
- The priority intervention for management of thalassemia is chronic transfusion of PRBCs and chelation of iron.
- Idiopathic thrombocytopenic purpura and Henoch–Schönlein purpura are usually self-limiting diseases.
- Administration of factor VII or desmopressin is the key nursing intervention when a bleeding episode occurs in the child with hemophilia or vWD.
- Significant anemia may result in hypoxia to the tissues.
- Prolonged bleeding times place the child at risk for hemorrhage.
- Prevention of injury is key for all children with hematologic disorders. Leukemia often presents in children with a history of fever, infection, and fatigue. Bone pain or CNS symptoms may be present if metastasis to the bone or brain has occurred.
- Lymphomas in children present similarly to those in adults, often with an enlarged, nontender lymph node.
- Symptoms of brain tumors depend on the location of the tumor; commonly they present with signs and symptoms of increased intracranial pressure, such as headache, nausea, and vomiting.
- Neuroblastoma has often significantly metastasized at diagnosis. It most commonly presents as a mass in the abdomen.
- Shortness of breath or chest pain in the child with cancer is a medical emergency; it may indicate superior vena cava syndrome or a tumor in the mediastinal region.
- Retinoblastoma may be identified by the presence of leukocoria in one or both eyes. Retinoblastoma occurs in early infancy up until early childhood.
- Bone cancer does not necessarily require amputation; it may be treated with a combination of limb salvage procedure, radiation, and chemotherapy.
- The symptoms of rhabdomyosarcoma depend on the location of the tumor.
- Avoid abdominal palpation preoperatively in the child with Wilms tumor; palpation may cause seeding of the tumor and metastasis.
- Radiation therapy may result in fatigue, nausea and vomiting, and long-term cognitive sequelae (if directed to the cranium).
- Nursing care of the child receiving treatment for cancer focuses on preventing or treating adverse effects such as fatigue, nausea, vomiting, alopecia, mucositis, and infection.
- The neutropenic child with fever should receive medical attention as soon as possible so that intravenous antibiotics may be started immediately.

- Cancer is a significant stressor for children and families. Families need support and education throughout the diagnostic process, treatment and cure, or palliative care.
- The child with cancer should lead as near normal a life as possible. When physically able and cleared by the oncologist, the child should resume usual activities such as school. Camps for children with cancer provide an excellent opportunity for children to enjoy everyday activities and meet children experiencing similar alterations in their lives.
- Nutrition may be optimized for children with cancer by managing nausea and vomiting with antiemetics, providing favorite foods, and possibly using total parenteral nutrition.
- Child and family teaching for anemias resulting from nutritional deficiencies focuses on promotion of a diet high in the deficient nutrients.
- Child and family teaching for bleeding disorders focuses on the prevention of injury.
- Numerous nationwide and local resources are available to children with hematologic disorders or nutritional deficits. These organizations offer a wide range of services, including education, support, multidisciplinary care (as appropriate), and financial assistance in caring for the disease.
- Teach adolescents appropriate screening techniques for reproductive cancers.
- Educate the child and family about the adverse effects of cancer treatments.
- Teach parents how to avoid infection in the child receiving chemotherapy, the signs and symptoms of infection, and when to seek medical treatment.

REFERENCES AND RECOMMENDED READINGS

Abed, R., & Grimer, R. (2010). Surgical modalities in the treatment of bone sarcoma in children. *Cancer Treatment Reviews, 36*(4), 342–347.

Abbas, H. A., Kahale, M., Hosn, M. A., & Inati, A. (2013). A review of acute chest syndrome in pediatric sickle cell disease. *Pediatric Annals, 42*(3), 115–120.

Ambruso, D. R., Nuss, R., & Wang, M. (2014). Hematologic disorders. In W. W. Hay, M. J. Levin, R. R. Deterding, & M. J. Abzug (Eds.), *Current pediatric diagnosis and treatment* (22nd ed.). New York, NY: McGraw-Hill.

American Academy of Pediatrics. (2016). *HPV (Gardasil®): What you need to know*. Retrieved from http://www.healthychildren.org/english/safety-prevention/immunizations/pages/Human-Papilomavirus-HPV-Vaccine-What-You-Need-to-Know.aspx

American Academy of Pediatrics, Committee on Bioethics. (2011). *Informed consent, parental permission, and assent in pediatric practice*. Retrieved from http://pediatrics.aappublications.org/content/95/2/314

American Cancer Society. (2015). *Cancer in children*. Retrieved from http://www.cancer.org/acs/groups/cid/documents/webcontent/002287-pdf.pdf

Baggott, C. (2010). Cancer. In P. J. Allen, J. A. Vessey, & N. A. Schapiro (Eds.), *Primary care of the child with a chronic condition* (5th ed.). St. Louis, MO: Mosby.

Bright Futures/American Academy of Pediatrics. (2016). *Recommendations for preventive pediatric health care*. Retrieved from https://pediatriccare.solutions.aap.org/DocumentLibrary/Periodicity%20Schedule_FINAL.pdf

Brundige, K. (2010). Neutropenia. In D. Tomlinson & N. E. Kline (Eds.), *Pediatric oncology nursing*. New York, NY: Springer.

Bryant, R. (2010). Anemias. In D. Tomlinson & N. E. Kline (Eds.), *Pediatric oncology nursing*. New York, NY: Springer.

Centers for Disease Control and Prevention. (2016). *Lead*. Retrieved from http://www.cdc.gov/nceh/lead/

Chandrakasan, S., & Kamat, D. (2013). An overview of hemoglobinopathies and the interpretation of newborn screening results. *Pediatric Annals, 42*(12), 502–508.

Children's Hospice International. (2011). *ChiPacc*. Retrieved from http://www.chionline.org/chipacc-model/

Chordas, C., & Graham, K. (2010). Chemotherapy. In D. Tomlinson & N. E. Kline (Eds.), *Pediatric oncology nursing*. New York, NY: Springer.

Corbett, J. A., & Banks, A. D. (2013). *Laboratory tests and diagnostic procedures with nursing diagnoses* (8th ed.). Upper Saddle River, NJ: Pearson Education Inc.

Cunningham, F. G., Leveno, K. J., Bloom, S. L., Spong, C. Y., Dashe, J. S., Hoffman, B. L., et al. (2014). *Williams obstetrics* (24th ed.). New York, NY: McGraw Hill.

CureSearch. (n. d.). *Childhood cancer deaths per years*. Retrieved from http://curesearch.org/Childhood-Cancer-Deaths-Per-Year

Dzolganovski, B. (2010). Clinical trials. In D. Tomlinson & N. E. Kline (Eds.), *Pediatric oncology nursing*. New York, NY: Springer.

Figueroa, T. E. (2012). *How to perform a testicular self-examination*. Retrieved from http://kidshealth.org/teen/sexual_health/guys/tse.html

Fischbach, F. T., & Dunning, M. B. (2014). *A manual of laboratory and diagnostic tests* (9th ed.). Philadelphia, PA: Lippincott Williams & Wilkins.

Graham, D. K., Craddock, J. A., Quinones, R. R., Keating, A. K., Maloney, K. Foreman, N. K. (2014). Neoplastic disease. In W. W. Hay, M. J. Levin, R. R. Deterding, & M. J. Abzug (Eds.), *Current pediatric diagnosis and treatment* (22nd ed.). New York, NY: McGraw-Hill.

Haemer, M., Primark, L. E., & Krebs, N. R. (2014). Normal childhood nutrition & its disorders. In W. W. Hay, M. J. Levin, R. R. Deterding, & M. J. Abzug (Eds.), *Current pediatric diagnosis and treatment* (22nd ed.). New York, NY: McGraw-Hill.

Hendershot, E. (2010). Solid tumors. In D. Tomlinson & N. E. Kline (Eds.), *Pediatric oncology nursing*. New York, NY: Springer.

Herdman, T. H., & Kamitsuru, S. (Eds.). (2014). *NANDA International nursing diagnoses: Definitions & classifications 2015–2017* (10th ed.). West Sussex, UK: John Wiley & Sons, Ltd.

Hooke, C., Hellsten, M. B., Stutzer, C., & Forte, K. (2002). Pain management for the child with cancer in end-of-life: APON position paper. *Journal of Pediatric Oncology Nursing, 19,* 43–47.

Hurwitz, R. L., & Lee, D. A. (2016). *Childhood lead poisoning: Management.* Retrieved from http://www.uptodate.com/contents/childhood-lead-poisoning-management

Jacob, E., Pavlish, C., Duran, J., Stinson, J., Lewis, M. A., & Zeltzer, L. (2013). Facilitating pediatric patient-provider communications using wireless technology in children and adolescents with sickle cell disease. *Journal of Pediatric Health Care : Official Publication of National Association of Pediatric Nurse Associates & Practitioners, 27*(4), 284–292.

Karp, S., & Riddell, J. P. (2010). Bleeding disorders. In P. J. Allen, J. A. Vessey, & N. A. Schapiro (Eds.), *Primary care of the child with a chronic condition* (5th ed.). St. Louis, MO: Mosby.

Kaufman, P. L., Kim, J., & Berry, J. L. (2016). *Overview of retinoblastoma.* Retrieved from http://www.uptodate.com/contents/overview-of-retinoblastoma

Kline, N. E. (2014). *Essentials of pediatric oncology nursing: A core curriculum* (4th ed.). Chicago, IL: Association of Pediatric Hematology/Oncology Nurses.

Kline, N. E., & O'Hanlon-Curry, J. (2010). Central nervous system tumors. In D. Tomlinson & N. E. Kline (Eds.), *Pediatric oncology nursing.* New York, NY: Springer.

Kristovich, K. M., & Callard, E. (2010). Bone marrow transplantation. In P. J. Allen, J. A. Vessey, & N. A. Schapiro (Eds.), *Primary care of the child with a chronic condition* (5th ed.). St. Louis, MO: Mosby.

Lee, D. A., & Hurwitz, R. L. (2016). Childhood lead poisoning: Exposure and prevention. Retrieved from http://www.uptodate.com/contents/childhood-lead-poisoning-exposure-and-prevention.

Loch, I., & Khorrami, J. (2010). Radiotherapy. In D. Tomlinson & N. E. Kline (Eds.), *Pediatric oncology nursing.* New York, NY: Springer.

Mahoney, D. H. (2015). *Iron deficiency in infants and young children: Treatment.* Retrieved from http://www.uptodate.com/contents/iron-deficiency-in-infants-and-young-children-treatment

Mahoney, D. H. (2016). Iron deficiency in infants and young children: Screening, prevention, clinical manifestations, and diagnosis. Retrieved from http://www.uptodate.com/contents/iron-deficiency-in-infants-andyoung-children-screening-prevention-clinical-manifestations-and-diagnosis

National Cancer Institute. (n. d.). *SEER stat fact sheets: Testis cancer.* Retrieved from http://seer.cancer.gov/statfacts/html/testis.html

National Cancer Institute. (2016). *Pediatric supportive care (PDQ®)-health professional version.* Retrieved from http://www.cancer.gov/types/childhood-cancers/pediatric-care-hp-pdq#section/all

National Heart, Lung, and Blood Institute. (2014). *Evidence-based management of sickle cell disease: Expert panel report, 2014.* Bethesda, MD: Author.

National Heart, Lung, and Blood Institute. (2015). *Living with sickle cell disease.* Retrieved from https://www.nhlbi.nih.gov/health/health-topics/topics/sca/livingwith

National Hemophilia Foundation. (2009). *Fast facts.* Retrieved from http://www.hemophilia.org/walk/docs/FastFacts.pdf

National Newborn Screening and Genetics Resource Center. (2014). *National newborn screening status report.* Retrieved from http://genes-r-us.uthscsa.edu/sites/genes-r-us/files/nbsdisorders.pdf

Nixon, C. (2010). Blood transfusion therapy. In D. Tomlinson & N. E. Kline (Eds.), *Pediatric oncology nursing.* New York, NY: Springer.

Norville, R., & Tomlinson, D. (2010). Hematopoietic stem cell transplantation. In D. Tomlinson & N. E. Kline (Eds.), *Pediatric oncology nursing.* New York, NY: Springer.

Pitts, R. H., & Record, E. O. (2010). Sickle cell disease. In P. J. Allen, J. A. Vessey, & N. A. Schapiro (Eds.), *Primary care of the child with a chronic condition* (5th ed.). St. Louis, MO: Mosby.

Platt, A., Eckman, J. R., Beasley, J., & Miller, G. (2002). Treating sickle cell pain: An update from the Georgia Comprehensive Sickle Cell Center. *Journal of Emergency Nursing, 28*(4), 297–303.

Post-White, J., & Ladas, E. (2010). Complementary and alternative medicine. In D. Tomlinson & N. E. Kline (Eds.), *Pediatric oncology nursing.* New York, NY: Springer.

Shields, C. L. (2008). Forget-me-nots in the care of children with retinoblastoma. *Seminars in Ophthalmology, 23*(5), 324–334.

Simon, C. (2010). Pain in children with cancer. In D. Tomlinson & N. E. Kline (Eds.), *Pediatric oncology nursing.* New York, NY: Springer.

Taketomo, C. K., Hodding, J. H., & Kraus, D. M. (2013). *Pediatric & neonatal dosage handbook* (20th ed.). Hudson, OH: Lexicomp.

Tomlinson, D., & Kline, N. E. (Eds.). (2010). *Pediatric oncology nursing.* New York, NY: Springer.

United States Environmental Protection Agency. (2016). *Lead.* Retrieved from http://www2.epa.gov/lead

Zupanec, S. (2010). *Lymphoma.* In D. Tomlinson & N. E. Kline (Eds.), *Pediatric oncology nursing.* New York, NY: Springer.

Zupanec, S., & Tomlinson, D. (2010). Leukemia. In D. Tomlinson & N. E. Kline (Eds.), *Pediatric oncology nursing.* New York, NY: Springer.

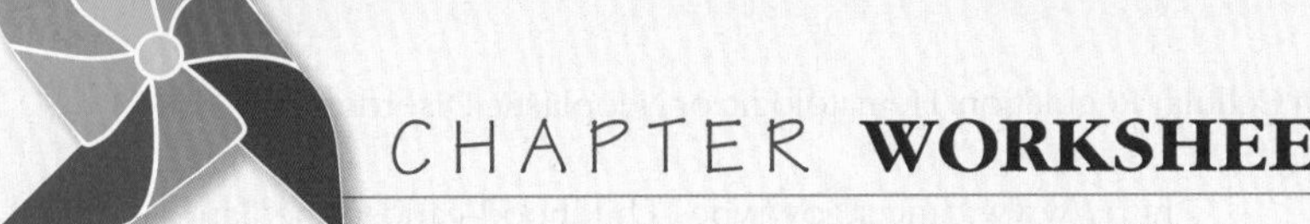

CHAPTER WORKSHEET

MULTIPLE CHOICE QUESTIONS

1. A child on the pediatric unit has morning laboratory results of Hgb 10.0, Hct 30.2, WBC 24,000, and platelets 20,000. What is the priority nursing assessment?
   a. Assess for pallor, fatigue, and tachycardia.
   b. Monitor for fever.
   c. Assess for bruising or bleeding.
   d. Determine intake and output.
2. A child with hemophilia fell while riding his bicycle. He was wearing a helmet and did not lose consciousness. He has a mild abrasion on his knee that is not oozing. He is complaining of abdominal pain. What is the priority nursing assessment?
   a. Perform neurologic checks.
   b. Assess ability to void frequently.
   c. Carefully assess his abdomen.
   d. Examine his knee frequently.
3. A 14-year-old with thalassemia asks for your assistance in choosing her afternoon snack. Which choice is the most appropriate?
   a. peanut butter with rice cake
   b. small spinach salad
   c. apple slices with cheddar cheese
   d. small burger on wheat bun
4. The nurse is caring for a child who has just been admitted to the pediatric unit with sickle cell crisis. He is complaining that his right arm and leg hurt. What is the priority nursing intervention?
   a. Administer pain medication every 3 hours intravenously until pain is controlled.
   b. Perform passive range of motion of the arm and leg to maintain function.
   c. Try acetaminophen for pain first, moving up to opioids only if needed.
   d. Use narcotic analgesics and warm compresses as needed to control the pain.
5. A 5-year-old has been diagnosed with Wilms tumor. What is the priority nursing intervention for this child?
   a. Educate the parents about dialysis, as the kidney will be removed.
   b. Measure abdominal girth every shift.
   c. Avoid palpating the child's abdomen.
   d. Monitor BUN and creatinine every 4 hours.
6. A child with leukemia has the following AM laboratory results: Hgb 8.0, Hct 24.2, WBC 8,000, platelets 150,000. What is the priority nursing assessment?
   a. Monitor for fever.
   b. Assess for bruising or bleeding.
   c. Determine intake and output.
   d. Assess for pallor, fatigue, and tachycardia.
7. A child with leukemia received chemotherapy about 10 days ago. She presents today with a temperature of 100.4°F, an absolute neutrophil count of 500, and mild bleeding of the gums. What is the priority nursing intervention?
   a. Administer IV antibiotics as ordered.
   b. Provide vigorous oral care frequently with a firm toothbrush.
   c. Monitor pulse and blood pressure for changes.
   d. Administer packed red blood cell transfusion.
8. A child with cancer is receiving chemotherapy, and his mother is concerned that the nausea and vomiting associated with chemotherapy are reducing his ability to eat and gain weight appropriately. What is the most appropriate nursing action?
   a. Administer an antiemetic at the first hint of nausea.
   b. Offer the child's favorite foods to encourage him to eat.
   c. Start antiemetic drugs prior to the chemotherapy infusion.
   d. Maintain IV fluid infusion to avoid dehydration.

DOSAGE CALCULATION QUESTION

1. The nurse is caring for a 4-year-old with acute lymphoblastic leukemia. The child weighs 38 lb. The medication order reads: ondansetron 2.6 mg IV every 8 hours for chemotherapy-related nausea/vomiting. Ondansetron is supplied as 4 mg/2 mL. How many milliliters will the nurse administer? Round to the nearest tenth.

CRITICAL THINKING EXERCISES

1. Develop a discharge teaching plan for the parent of a toddler who has just been diagnosed with hemophilia and received factor infusion treatment for a bleeding episode.
2. An 8-year-old girl has been diagnosed with iron-deficiency anemia. Formulate a nutrition plan for this child.
3. A 5-year-old with β-thalassemia is resistant to nightly chelation therapy at home. Devise a developmentally appropriate teaching plan for this child.
4. Develop a nursing care plan for a child with sickle cell disease who experiences frequent vaso-occlusive crises.
5. Develop a discharge teaching plan for a child who has just completed the induction phase of chemotherapy for acute lymphocytic leukemia.

CHAPTER WORKSHEET

6. A 17-year-old girl has recently been diagnosed with osteosarcoma. She is worried about how treatment will affect her plans for college, marriage, and children. How will you respond to her concerns?
7. A 3-year-old is going to be starting chemotherapy for rhabdomyosarcoma. Develop an age-appropriate teaching plan for this child.
8. Develop a nursing care plan for an adolescent with cancer who is undergoing radiation and chemotherapy and experiencing a significant number of adverse effects from his treatment.

STUDY ACTIVITIES

1. Visit your local WIC office. Meet with the staff and learn about the services offered for prevention of and nutritional support for anemia. Provide a written report of your learning experience or provide a presentation to your classmates.
2. In the clinical setting, compare the growth and development of a child with sickle cell disease to that of a similarly aged child who has been healthy.
3. Talk to a teenager with hemophilia about his life experiences and feelings about his disease and his health. Reflect upon this conversation in your clinical journal.
4. Visit a public health clinic that provides primary care to children. Spend time with the registered nurse, the advanced practice nurse, and the unlicensed assistive personnel. Write a summary of the roles of the registered nurse in screening for and managing hematologic disorders in children, noting roles that are reserved for the advanced practice nurse and activities that the RN would delegate to unlicensed assistive personnel.
5. While in the clinical area, care for a young child who has undergone therapy for a brain tumor. Compare this child's growth and development to those of a healthy similar-age child who you know or have cared for.
6. During your clinical rotation, care for a child who has received several chemotherapy treatments. After establishing a therapeutic relationship, talk with the child about his or her understanding of the disease and the experience the child has had with diagnosis and treatment thus far. If time allows, ask the child to draw a picture describing this experience. Record your observations in your clinical journal and reflect on the emotions you feel about this experience.
7. Attend the pediatric oncology clinic. Determine the role of the advanced practice nurse (nurse practitioner or clinical nurse specialist) compared to the role of the registered nurse in the outpatient care of children with cancer. Determine which activities the nurse appropriately delegates to unlicensed assistive personnel in that setting.
8. Talk to the hospital chaplain about his or her experiences with dying children. Reflect on this conversation in your clinical journal.

BRINGING IT ALL TOGETHER: A CASE STUDY

John Shaw, 7 years old, is brought to the clinic by his parents with a fever. His father states, "John seems to get fevers and colds more often than our other children. He's also very tired these days. He hardly ever wants to go out and play with his friends. He complains of headaches frequently and just doesn't really seem like himself."

Go to thePoint to find questions to consider about this case.

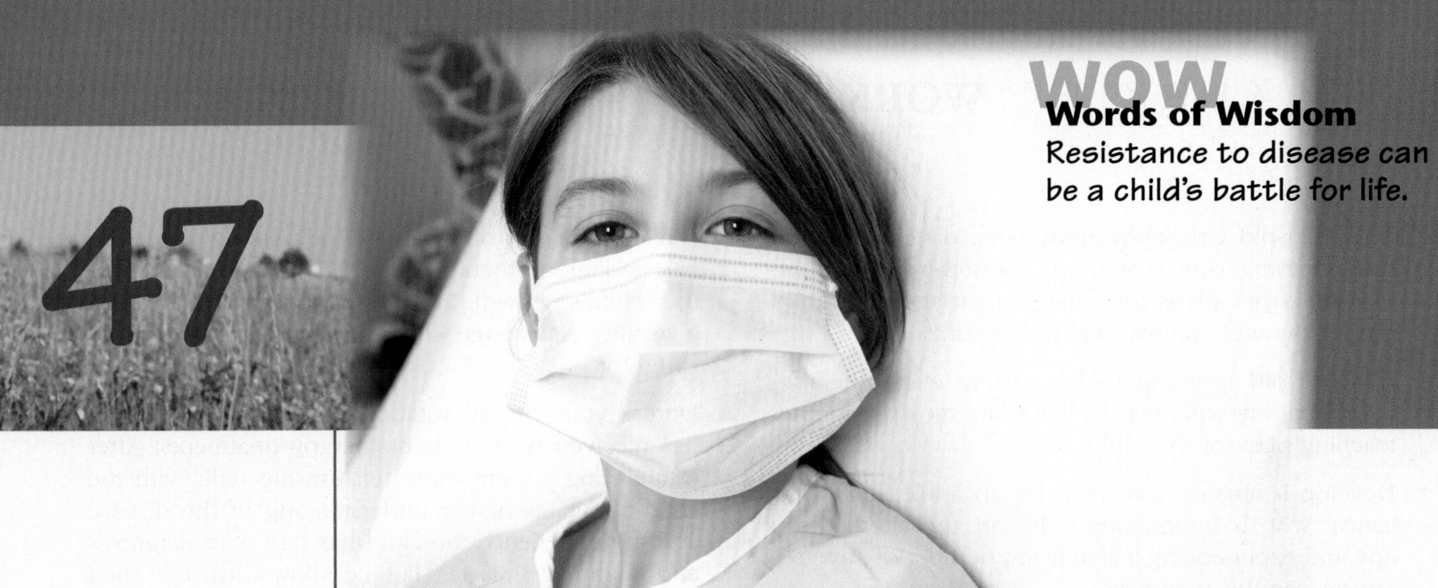

WOW
Words of Wisdom
Resistance to disease can be a child's battle for life.

47

Nursing Care of the Child With an Alteration in Immunity or Immunologic Disorder

KEY TERMS

antibodies
antigen
autoantibodies
cellular immunity
chemotaxis
graft-versus-host disease
humoral immunity
immunodeficiency
immunoglobulins
immunosuppressive
opsonization
phagocytosis

Learning Objectives

Upon completion of the chapter, the learner will be able to:

1. Explain anatomic and physiologic differences of the immune system in infants and children versus adults.
2. Describe nursing care related to common laboratory and diagnostic testing used in the medical diagnosis of pediatric immune and autoimmune disorders.
3. Distinguish immune, autoimmune, and allergic disorders common in infants, children, and adolescents.
4. Identify appropriate nursing assessments and interventions related to medications and treatments for pediatric immune, autoimmune, and allergic disorders.
5. Develop an individualized nursing care plan for the child with an immune or autoimmune disorder.
6. Describe the psychosocial impact of chronic immune disorders on children.
7. Devise a nutrition plan for the child with immunodeficiency.
8. Develop child/family teaching plans for the child with an immune or autoimmune disorder.

***Lakeisha Harris*, 15 years old, is brought to the clinic by her mother. She presents with complaints of pain and swelling in her joints, weight gain, and fatigue. Lakeisha states, "I'm just very tired all the time, and my knees and ankles ache."**

Immunity refers to natural or induced resistance to infection. Nurses may encounter children with alterations in immunity and should be familiar with various immunologic disorders that children experience. **Immunodeficiency** (incapacity to mount an appropriate immune response), autoimmune, and allergic disorders have a significant impact on the lives of affected children. Infants and children are exposed to many infectious microorganisms and allergens and thus need a functional immune system to protect themselves. Temporary immune deficiencies may follow a common viral infection, surgery, or blood transfusion, and may also be caused by malnutrition or the use of certain medications (Atkinson, Wolfe, & Hamborsky, 2012). Temporary immune depression resolves over a period of time. Primary or secondary immune deficiencies are the focus of this discussion, along with allergy and anaphylaxis. These immune disorders are chronic, and affected children have more infections compared with healthy children. Recurrent viral or bacterial infections may cause the child to miss significant amounts of school or playtime with other children. Many immunodeficiencies require chronic and frequent clinic visits as well as daily medications. This can be a stress on the family as well. Autoimmune disorders are also chronic, causing significant disruption to the child's and family's life. Allergic disorders in some children may cause significant stress for the child and family. Nurses who care for children need to be familiar with common immunodeficiencies, autoimmune disorders, and allergies to intervene effectively with children and their families.

VARIATIONS IN PEDIATRIC ANATOMY AND PHYSIOLOGY

Normal immune function is a complex process involving **phagocytosis** (process by which phagocytes swallow up and break down microorganisms), **humoral immunity** (immunity mediated by antibodies secreted by B cells), **cellular immunity** (cell-mediated immunity controlled by T cells), and activation of the complement system. The lymphatic system and the white blood cells (WBCs) are the primary players in the immune response. Though these structures and cells are present at birth, the healthy full-term infant's immune system is still immature. The newborn exhibits a decreased inflammatory response to invading organisms, and this increases his or her susceptibility to infection. Cellular immunity is generally functional at birth, and as the infant is exposed to various substances over time, humoral immunity develops. Comparison Chart 47.1 provides more information on humoral and cellular immunity.

Lymph System

Lymph nodes in the newborn are relatively small, soft, and difficult to palpate. As the infant is exposed to various germs or illnesses, the lymph system passively filters plasma for bacteria or other foreign material before returning it to the bloodstream and back to the heart. As WBCs infiltrate the lymph nodes to attack the foreign substance, the nodes enlarge. Young children have frequent episodes of localized enlarged lymph nodes because of their repeated exposure to viral illnesses (Tosi, 2014). The spleen is functional at birth and also filters the blood for foreign cells. The thymus, responsible for the production of lymphocyte T cells as well as for the development and maturation of peripheral lymphoid tissue, is quite enlarged at birth and remains so until about 10 years of age. It then involutes slowly throughout adulthood. The tonsils are also often enlarged throughout early childhood. The bone marrow is functional at birth, producing stem cells capable of differentiating into various blood cells.

Phagocytosis

Under conditions of stress, the newborn and infant exhibit decreased phagocytic activity. The complement system, which is responsible for **opsonization** (process of making microorganisms more susceptible to phagocytosis) and **chemotaxis** (movement of neutrophils

COMPARISON CHART 47.1 HUMORAL VERSUS CELLULAR IMMUNITY

Humoral Immunity (Antibody Protection)	Cellular Immunity (Cell-Mediated Immune Response)
• Lymphocytes: B cells	• Lymphocytes: T cells
• Secrete antibodies to viruses and bacteria	• Do not recognize antigens
• Recognize antigens	• Direct and regulate immune response (helper T cells)
• Antibodies mark the antigen cell for destruction	• Attack infected or foreign cells (killer T cells and natural killer cells)
• Do not destroy the foreign cell	• Do not cross the placenta
• Crosses the placenta in the form of IgG	

toward microorganisms), is immature in the newborn but reaches adult levels of activity by 3 to 6 months of age. The infant's phagocytic cells (neutrophils and monocytes) demonstrate decreased chemotaxis, reaching adult levels when the child is several years old. With complement levels being only 50% to 75% of adult levels in the full-term infant, decreased opsonization may be responsible for decreased phagocytic activity compared with adults.

Cellular Immunity

Maternal T cells do not cross the placenta, so the fetal thymus begins production of T cells early in gestation, and the newborn demonstrates a relative lymphocytosis compared with the adult, probably due to increased amounts of T-cell lymphocytes. Though cellular immunity does not cross the placenta, the fetal T cells may become sensitized to antigens that do cross the placenta. Viral infection, hyperbilirubinemia, and drugs taken by the mother late in pregnancy may contribute to depressed T-cell function in the newborn. Since delayed hypersensitivity reactions are mediated by T cells rather than antibodies, skin test responses (such as purified protein derivative [PPD] for tuberculosis detection) are diminished until about 1 year of age, probably due to the infant's decreased ability to mount an inflammatory response.

Humoral Immunity

The newborn's B cells do not respond as well to infection as do adults. B cells are responsible for the formation of **antibodies** (specific immunity). The antibodies bind to the **antigen** (substance stimulating an immune response), thus disabling the specific toxin. The fetus is normally in an antigen-free environment and so produces only trace amounts of **immunoglobulins** (Ig; gammaglobulin antibody proteins), specifically IgM. Most of the newborn's IgG is acquired transplacentally from the mother. Hence, the newborn exhibits passive immunity to antigens to which the mother had developed antibodies. These antibodies wane over the first months of life as the transplacental IgG is catabolized, having a half-life of only about 25 days.

The newborn begins to make IgG but ordinarily experiences a physiologic hypogammaglobulinemia between 2 and 6 months of age until self-production of IgG reaches higher levels. The breastfed infant will acquire passive transfer of maternal immunity via the breast milk and will be better protected during the physiologic hypogammaglobulinemia phase. By 1 year of age IgG is 50% of the adult level, and by 7 years of age it reaches the average adult level.

IgA, IgD, IgE, and IgM do not cross the placenta; they require an antigenic challenge for production. IgD and IgE constitute a very small percentage of the immunoglobulins in all ages. IgA increases slowly to about 30% of the adult level at 1 year of age, reaching the adult level by age 113 years. IgM is close to the adult level by 1 year of age (Mayo Foundation, 2016).

COMMON MEDICAL TREATMENTS

A variety of medications and other medical treatments are used to treat immune deficiencies and autoimmune problems in children. Most of these treatments will require a physician's or nurse practitioner's order when the child is in the hospital. The most common treatments and medications are listed in Common Medical Treatments 47.1 and Drug Guide 47.1. The nurse caring for

COMMON MEDICAL TREATMENTS 47.1

Treatment	Explanation	Indications	Nursing Implications
Immunizations	Killed or modified microorganisms, or components of them, cause the immune system to develop antibodies to the microorganism without developing disease	Prevention of certain viral and bacterial infections	Do not administer live vaccines to immunosuppressed persons Refer to the individual vaccine for method of administration and contraindications Report adverse reactions via the vaccine adverse reaction (VAR) reporting system
Bone marrow or stem cell transplantation	Bone marrow transplant: transfer of healthy bone marrow into the bones of a person with immune malfunction; the transplanted cells can then develop into functional B and T cells Stem cell transplant: peripheral stem cells are removed from the donor via apheresis or stem cells are retrieved from the umbilical cord and placenta. The stem cells are then transplanted into the recipient	Wiskott–Aldrich syndrome, SCID	Administer immunosuppressive medications as ordered Maintain medical asepsis and protective isolation to prevent infection Monitor closely for graft-versus-host disease Provide meticulous oral care. Avoid rectal temperatures and suppositories Encourage appropriate nutrition

DRUG GUIDE 47.1 COMMON DRUGS FOR IMMUNOLOGIC DISORDERS

Medication	Actions/Indications	Nursing Implications
Intravenous immune globulin (IVIG)	Provides exogenous IgG antibodies Indicated for primary immune deficiencies, HIV infection, myasthenia gravis	Do not mix with IV medications or with other IV fluids Do not give IM or SQ Monitor vital signs and watch for adverse reactions frequently during infusion May require antipyretic or antihistamine to prevent chills and fever during infusion Have epinephrine available during infusion
Nucleoside analog reverse transcriptase inhibitors (NRTIs): abacavir, lamivudine, zidovudine	Inhibit reverse transcription of the viral DNA chain For treatment of HIV-1 infection as part of a three-drug regimen. Zidovudine is also used to prevent perinatal transmission of HIV	Notify physician of muscle weakness, shortness of breath, headache, insomnia, rash, or unusual bleeding. Give IV zidovudine over 1 hour. Fatal hypersensitivity reaction may occur with abacavir
Nonnucleoside analog reverse transcriptase inhibitors (NNRTIs): efavirenz, nevirapine	Bind to HIV-1 reverse transcriptase, blocking DNA polymerase activity and disrupting the virus life cycle. Used for treatment of HIV-1 infection as part of a three-drug regimen	*Nevirapine:* Avoid St. John's wort Shake suspension gently before administration Observe for symptoms of Stevens–Johnson syndrome *Efavirenz:* May cause drowsiness
Protease inhibitors: amprenavir, atazanavir, indinavir, lopinavir, nelfinavir, ritonavir, saquinavir	Inhibit protease activity in the HIV-1 cell, resulting in immature, noninfectious viral particles. Used for treatment of HIV-1 infection as part of a three-drug regimen	Multiple drug interactions. Review specific medication for adverse effects and administration implications
Nonsteroidal anti-inflammatory drugs (NSAIDs): diclofenac, ibuprofen, naproxen, others	Inhibit prostaglandin synthesis, anti-inflammatory action Indicated for juvenile idiopathic arthritis	Administer with food to decrease GI upset May cause gastric bleeding, increased liver enzymes, decreased renal function Monitor liver enzymes Do not crush or chew extended-release or timed-release preparations
Neuromuscular blocking agent: pyridostigmine	Cholinergic for myasthenia gravis—inhibits destruction of acetylcholine	Note muscle strength, heart rate, respirations Overdose may result in a cholinergic crisis. Monitor for sweating, salivation, urinary incontinence
Corticosteroids	Anti-inflammatory and immunosuppressive action. Used for juvenile idiopathic arthritis, SLE, myasthenia gravis, and immunosuppression in children with bone marrow or stem cell transplants	Administer with food to decrease GI upset May mask signs of infection Monitor blood pressure, urine for glucose Do not stop treatment abruptly or acute adrenal insufficiency may occur Monitor for Cushing syndrome Doses may be tapered over time *Intravenous pulse:* Monitor for hypertension during infusion

(continued)

DRUG GUIDE 47.1 COMMON DRUGS FOR IMMUNOLOGIC DISORDERS (continued)

Medication	Actions/Indications	Nursing Implications
Cytotoxic drugs (cyclophosphamide)	Interfere with normal function of DNA by alkylation. For treatment of severe SLE	Cause bone marrow suppression. Monitor for signs of infection *Cyclophosphamide:* Administer in the morning Provide adequate hydration and have child void frequently during and after infusion to decrease risk of hemorrhagic cystitis
Immunosuppressant drugs (cyclosporine A [CyA], azathioprine)	Inhibition of production and release of interleukin II (CyA) Antagonize purine metabolism (azathioprine). Used for severe steroid-resistant autoimmune disease	Monitor CBC, serum creatinine, potassium, and magnesium Monitor blood pressure and watch for signs of infection Draw blood levels before morning dose *CyA:* Do not give with grapefruit juice
Antimalarial drugs: hydroxychloroquine sulfate	Impair complement-dependent antigen–antibody reactions to prevent flares in SLE and juvenile arthritis	Funduscopic eye examination and visual field testing every year
Disease-modifying antirheumatic drugs (DMARDs): methotrexate, etanercept	Methotrexate: antimetabolite that depletes DNA precursors, inhibits DNA and urine synthesis Etanercept: binds to tumor necrosis factor (TNF), rendering it ineffective. Used for severe polyarticular juvenile arthritis	*Methotrexate:* Do not give oral form with dairy products. Approximate time to benefit in treatment of arthritis is 3–6 weeks Salicylates may delay clearance Protect IV preparation from light Monitor CBC, renal and liver function, and symptoms of infection *Etanercept:* Monitor closely for infection Do not give live vaccines Give SQ, twice weekly; effect in 1 week to 3 months

CBC, complete blood count; GI, gastrointestinal; IM, intramuscularly; SQ, subcutaneously.
Adapted from Taketomo, C. K., Hodding, J. H., & Kraus, D. M. (2013). *Pediatric & neonatal dosage handbook* (20th ed.). Hudson, OH: Lexicomp.

the child with an immune deficiency or autoimmune disorder should be familiar with what the procedures and medications are, how they work, and common nursing implications related to use of these modalities.

Atraumatic Care

When a child requires repeat injections related to an immune or allergic disorder, use a local anesthetic such as EMLA (eutectic mixture of local anesthetic) cream or a numbing spray to reduce the amount of associated pain.

NURSING PROCESS OVERVIEW FOR THE CHILD WITH AN IMMUNOLOGIC DISORDER

Care of the child with an immunologic or allergic disorder includes assessment, nursing diagnosis, planning, interventions, and evaluation. There are a number of general concepts related to the nursing process that may be applied to immunodeficiencies and autoimmune disorders. From a general understanding of the care involved for a child with immune dysfunction, the nurse can then individualize the care based on the particular child's specifics.

Assessment

Assessment of children with immunodeficiency, autoimmune disorders, or allergy includes health history, physical examination, and laboratory and diagnostic testing.

Remember Lakeisha, the 15-year-old with joint pain and swelling, fatigue, and weight gain? What additional health history and physical examination assessment information should you obtain?

Health History

The health history consists of past medical history, including the mother's pregnancy history; family history; and history of present illness (when the symptoms started and how they have progressed), as well as medications and treatments used at home. The past medical history may be significant for:

- Maternal HIV infection
- Frequent, recurrent infections such as otitis media, sinusitis, or pneumonia
- Chronic cough
- Recurrent low-grade fever
- Two or more serious infections in early childhood
- Recurrent deep skin or organ abscesses
- Persistent thrush in the mouth
- Extensive eczema
- Growth failure

Family history may be positive for primary immune deficiency or autoimmune disorder. Document history of known allergy. Note the response that occurs when the child encounters the allergen.

Physical Examination

Physical examination of the child with immunodeficiency or autoimmune disorder includes inspection and observation, auscultation, percussion, and palpation.

INSPECTION AND OBSERVATION

Plot weight and length or height on appropriate growth charts. Inspect the oropharynx for tonsillar size. Note eczematous or other skin lesions, which may occur with allergic diseases or Wiskott–Aldrich syndrome. Document the presence of thrush, which occurs frequently in children with immunodeficiency. Observe gait for unexplained ataxia (neurologic alterations occur with HIV infection).

AUSCULTATION, PERCUSSION, AND PALPATION

Auscultate the lungs for adventitious sounds, which may be present with a concurrent respiratory infection. Note any wheezing that may occur with an allergic reaction. Percuss the abdomen and determine liver span. Palpate for unusually enlarged lymph nodes, particularly in nonadjacent locations. Palpate the abdomen for an enlarged spleen or liver.

Laboratory and Diagnostic Testing

Common Laboratory and Diagnostic Tests 47.1 explains the laboratory and diagnostic tests most commonly used when considering immune disorders. Results of these tests may assist the physician or nurse practitioner in diagnosing the disorder and/or be used as guidelines in determining ongoing treatment. Laboratory or nonnursing personnel obtain some of the tests, while the nurse might obtain others. In either instance it is important for the nurse to be familiar with how the tests are obtained, what they are used for, and normal versus abnormal results. This knowledge will also be necessary when providing child and family education related to the testing.

Nursing Diagnoses and Related Interventions

Upon completion of a thorough assessment, the nurse might identify several nursing diagnoses. These may include:

- Ineffective protection
- Imbalanced nutrition, less than body requirements
- Pain
- Impaired skin integrity
- Activity intolerance
- Delayed growth and development

After completing an assessment of Lakeisha, you note the following: alopecia, abdominal tenderness, and oral ulcers. Based on these assessment findings, what would your top three nursing diagnoses be for Lakeisha?

Nursing goals, interventions, and evaluation for the child with an immunologic disorder are based on the nursing diagnoses. Nursing Care Plan 47.1 can be used as a guide in planning nursing care for the child with an immunologic disorder, autoimmune disorder, or allergic response. It should be individualized based on the child's symptoms and needs. Refer to Chapter 36 for thorough information related to pain management. Additional information will be included later in the chapter as it relates to specific disorders.

Based on your top three nursing diagnoses for Lakeisha, describe appropriate nursing interventions.

COMMON LABORATORY AND DIAGNOSTIC TESTS 47.1

Test	Explanation	Indications	Nursing Implications
Complete blood count (CBC) with differential	Evaluates hemoglobin and hematocrit, WBC count (particularly the percentage of individual WBCs), and platelet count	Infection, inflammatory process, immunosuppression	Normal values vary according to age and gender WBC count differential is helpful in evaluating source of infection May be affected by myelosuppressive drugs
Immunoglobulin electrophoresis	Determines level of individual immunoglobulins (IgA, IgD, IgE, IgG, IgM) in the blood	Immune deficiency, autoimmune disorders	Normal levels vary with age IVIG administration and steroids alter levels
IgG subclasses	Measure the levels of the four subclasses of IgG (1, 2, 3, and 4)	Determine immune deficiency	Normal levels vary with age IVIG administration and steroids alter levels
Lymphocyte immunophenotyping T-cell quantification	Measures level of T cells (T helper [CD4], T suppressor [CD8]), B cells, and natural killer cells in the blood	Ongoing monitoring of progressive depletion of CD4 T lymphocytes in HIV disease	Do not refrigerate specimen Steroids may elevate and immunosuppressive drugs may depress lymphocyte levels
Delayed hypersensitivity skin test	Measures the presence of activated T cells that recognize certain substances	Immune disorders	Administered intradermally Read and document size of reaction at 48–72 hours (tuberculosis, mumps, Candida, tetanus)
HIV antibodies	Used to detect antibodies to HIV	Determining HIV infection when suspected	ELISA method detects only antibodies, so may remain negative for several weeks up to 6 months (false-negative). False-positive may result with autoimmune disease. Requires serial testing. HIV test results are confidential.
Virologic Assay (HIV RNA and DNA nucleic acid and polymerase chain reaction tests)	Used to detect HIV RNA and DNA	Diagnosis of HIV infection in children older than 2 weeks of age and ongoing monitoring of viral load	Sensitive and specific for presence of HIV in blood Sequential testing needed to determine perinatal transmission
CD4 Count	Measures the number of CD4 T lymphocytes in the blood	Used in HIV-infected persons to determine response to antiretroviral therapy	Normal is $\geq$1,500/mm^3 in the infant, $\geq$1,000/mm^3 in the 1–5-year-old, $\geq$500/mm^3 in children 6 years and older
Complement assay (C3 and C4)	Measures the level of total complement in the blood, as well as levels of C3 and C4	Monitor SLE. Determine complement deficiency	Send to laboratory immediately (unstable at room temperature) Usually sent out to a reference laboratory
Erythrocyte sedimentation rate (ESR)	Nonspecific test used to determine presence of infection or inflammation	Immune disorder initial workup, ongoing monitoring of autoimmune disease	Send to laboratory immediately; if allowed to stand >3 hours, falsely low result may occur
Rheumatoid factor (RF)	Determines the presence of RF in the blood	Juvenile idiopathic arthritis, SLE	Positive RF is also sometimes seen in chronic infectious disorders

COMMON LABORATORY AND DIAGNOSTIC TESTS 47.1 (continued)

Test	Explanation	Indications	Nursing Implications
Antinuclear antibody (ANA)	Tests for presence of autoantibodies that react against cellular nuclear material	SLE	Check for signs of infection at venipuncture site Steroid use can cause false-negative result May be weakly positive in about 20% of healthy individuals
RAST (radioallergosorbent test)	Measures minute quantities of IgE in the blood Carries no risk of anaphylaxis but is not as sensitive as skin testing	Asthma (food allergies)	Blood test that is usually sent out to a reference laboratory
Allergy skin testing	Suggested allergen is applied to skin via scratch, pin, or prick. A wheal response indicates allergy to the substance. Carries risk of anaphylaxis. (Nursing note: Antihistamines must be discontinued before testing, as they inhibit the test.)	Allergic rhinitis, asthma	Close observation for anaphylaxis is necessary. Epinephrine and emergency equipment should be readily available Some children react to the skin test almost immediately; others take several minutes
Food-specific IgE antibody testing	Measures IgE antibody to specific food allergens	Accurately determine specific food allergy	IVIG administration and steroids alter levels

Adapted from Corbett, J. A., & Banks, A. D. (2013). Laboratory tests and diagnostic procedures with nursing diagnoses (8th ed.). Upper Saddle River, NJ: Pearson Education Inc.

PRIMARY IMMUNODEFICIENCIES

Many primary immunodeficiencies have been identified. They are mostly hereditary or congenital. Primary immunodeficiencies may be related to humoral deficiencies, cellular immunity deficiencies, or a combination of the two; phagocytic system defects; or complement deficiencies. This discussion will focus on a few of the more common and/or severe primary immunodeficiencies in children. Box 47.1 lists 10 warning signs that a child may need further evaluation for the possibility of primary immunodeficiency.

Hypogammaglobulinemia

Hypogammaglobulinemia refers to a variety of conditions in which the child does not form antibodies appropriately. It results in low or absent levels of one or more of the immunoglobulin classes or subclasses. Table 47.1 provides an overview of several types of hypogammaglobulinemia. Therapeutic management of most types of hypogammaglobulinemia is periodic administration of intravenous immunoglobulin (IVIG).

BOX 47.1

TEN WARNING SIGNS OF PRIMARY IMMUNODEFICIENCY

- Four or more new episodes of acute otitis media in 1 year
- Two or more episodes of severe sinusitis in 1 year
- Treatment with antibiotics for 2 months or longer with little effect
- Two or more episodes of pneumonia in 1 year
- Failure to thrive in the infant
- Recurrent deep skin or organ abscesses
- Persistent oral thrush or skin candidiasis after 1 year of age
- History of infections requiring IV antibiotics to clear
- Two or more serious infections such as sepsis
- Family history of primary immunodeficiency

Adapted from Jeffrey Modell Foundation. (2013). *10 warning signs of primary immunodeficiency*. Retrieved from http://downloads.info4pi.org/pdfs/General10WarningSignsFINAL.pdf and Varadhi, A., Hageman, J. R., & Yu, K. O. A. (2013). The 'five fingers' of the diagnostic evaluation for suspected immunodeficiency, *Pediatric Annals*, *42*(5), 210–215.

TABLE 47.1 TYPES OF HYPOGAMMAGLOBULINEMIA

Type	Definition	Characteristics	Treatment
Selective IgA deficiency	Serum IgA <7 mg/dL, normal IgG and IgM	May be asymptomatic Child is more prone to allergies due to lack of the mucosal protection that IgA offers. Recurrent infections of respiratory, gastrointestinal, and genitourinary tracts, development of autoimmune disorders	No specific gammaglobulin treatment available Treat infections or autoimmune disorders. Severe anaphylactic reaction can occur if child receives transfusion of blood containing IgA and IgA antibodies
X-linked agammaglobulinemia	Markedly reduced or absent IgG, IgM, and IgA. Absence of B cells	Males only Recurrent respiratory and gastrointestinal infections	Routine IVIG infusions Treat infections
X-linked hyper-IgM syndrome	Defect in protein found on T-cell surface, resulting in decreased IgG and IgA levels with significant increase in IgM levels	Males only Recurrent respiratory infections, diarrhea, malabsorption Neutropenia, autoimmune disorders	Routine administration of IVIG Subcutaneous granulocyte colony-stimulating factor (G-CSF) when neutropenic Bone marrow transplantation Treatment of autoimmune disorders
IgG subclass deficiency	Low levels of one or more of the subclasses of IgG	Recurrent respiratory infections. Some children outgrow this condition	Treatment of respiratory infections Administration of IVIG is helpful in some children

Nursing Assessment

Note history of recurrent respiratory, gastrointestinal, or genitourinary infections. Palpate for enlarged lymph nodes and spleen in the child with X-linked hyper-IgM syndrome. In children presenting for routine administration of IVIG, determine whether any infections have occurred since the previous infusion.

Nursing Management

Nursing management of hypogammaglobulinemia involves IVIG administration and the provision of education and support to the child and family.

ADMINISTERING INTRAVENOUS IMMUNOGLOBULIN

Determine the amount of IVIG to be given and reconstitute the product according to the manufacturer's directions (available on the package insert). Some IVIG preparations are provided as a solution, requiring no reconstitution (Fig. 47.1). Others are packaged as two vials, one of IVIG powder and one of sterile diluent. After the diluent is added to the powder, gently roll the vial between your hands to mix. Reconstituted IVIG may be refrigerated overnight but should be brought to room temperature prior to infusion. Assess baseline serum blood urea nitrogen (BUN) and creatinine, as acute renal insufficiency may occur as a serious adverse reaction. Though less common in children than adults, assess for risk factors associated with an increased risk for a thromboembolic event, such as history of atherosclerosis, hyperviscosity or hypercoagulability, stroke, hypertension, hypercholesterolemia, impaired cardiac output, immobility (Taketokmo, Hodding, & Kraus, 2013).

Take Note!

Do not shake the IVIG, as this may lead to foaming and may cause the immunoglobulin protein to degrade (Taketokmo et al., 2013).

Ensure that the child is well hydrated before the infusion to decrease the risk for rate-related reactions and aseptic meningitis after the infusion. Premedication with diphenhydramine or acetaminophen may be indicated in children who have never received IVIG, have not had an infusion in more than 8 weeks, have had a recent bacterial infection, have a history of serious infusion-related adverse reactions, or are diagnosed with agammaglobulinemia or hypogammaglobulinemia (Taketokmo et al., 2013).

The rate for infusion of IVIG is generally prescribed as milligrams of IVIG per kilogram of body weight per minute. Carefully calculate the infusion rate. Obtain a baseline physical assessment and set of vital signs. Begin the infusion slowly, increasing to the prescribed rate as tolerated (see Fig. 47.1). Assess vital signs and check for adverse reactions every 15 minutes for the first hour, then every 30 minutes throughout the remainder of the infusion (the frequency of assessments may vary according to institutional protocol). IVIG is a plasma product, so observe closely for signs of anaphylaxis such as headache, facial flushing, urticaria, dyspnea, shortness of breath, wheezing, chest pain, fever, chills, nausea, vomiting, increased anxiety, or hypotension. If these symptoms occur, discontinue the infusion and notify the physician or nurse practitioner. The infusion may be restarted after the symptoms have subsided. Have oxygen and emergency medications such as epinephrine, diphenhydramine, and intravenous corticosteroids available in case of anaphylactic reaction. If the child complains of discomfort at the intravenous site, a cold compress may be helpful.

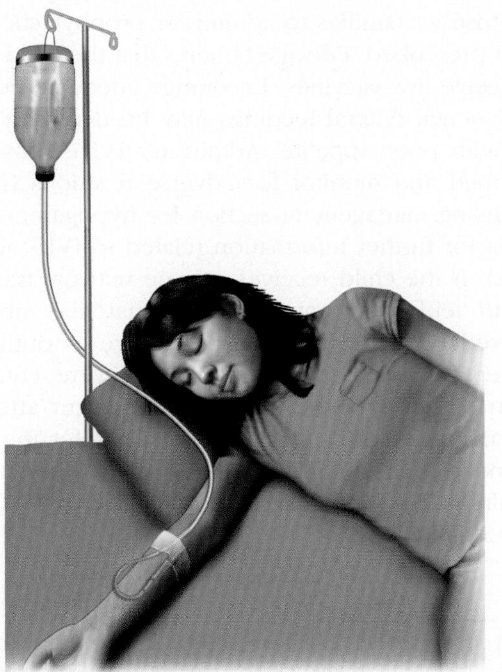

FIGURE 47.1 Intravenous administration of exogenous immunoglobulin every several weeks can decrease the frequency and severity of infections in children with various forms of hypogammaglobulinemia.

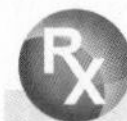

Dosage Calculation Box 47.1

Child's weight: 33 lb

Medication order: intravenous immunoglobulin 6,000 mg IV today.

Per the Pediatric Dosage Handbook, the recommended dose is 300 to 600 mg/dose, IV, every 3 to 4 weeks. Infuse at 0.5 mL/kg/hr for first 30 minutes, increasing rate every 30 minutes as tolerated, not to exceed 5 mL/kg/hr.

Is the ordered dose safe?

Intravenous immunoglobulin is provided as 100 mg/mL. If the dose is safe, what will the infusion rate be for the first 30 minutes?

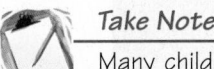

Take Note!

Many children who have had previous reactions to IVIG can tolerate the infusion without reaction if they are premedicated and if the infusion is given at a slower rate (Taketokmo et al., 2013).

PROVIDING EDUCATION AND SUPPORT

Provide education and support to the child and family. An excellent book for children with an immune deficiency is *Our Immune System* (1993) by Sara le Bien (available from the Immune Deficiency Foundation, a link to which can be found on thePoint).

Wiskott–Aldrich Syndrome

Wiskott–Aldrich syndrome is an X-linked genetic disorder that results in immunodeficiency, eczema, and thrombocytopenia. It affects males only. The defective gene responsible for this disorder is called the Wiskott–Aldrich syndrome protein (WASp). Complications include autoimmune hemolytic anemia, neutropenia, skin or cerebral vasculitis, arthritis, inflammatory bowel disease, and renal disease (Ochs, 2015).

Autoimmune disease may require high-dose steroids, azathioprine, or cyclophosphamide. Splenectomy may be performed to correct thrombocytopenia. The only cure is hematopoietic cell transplantation, though gene therapy is currently under investigation.

Nursing Assessment

Note history of petechiae, bloody diarrhea, or bleeding episode in the first 6 months of life. Note any history of hematemesis or intracranial or conjunctival hemorrhages. Observe the skin for eczema, which usually worsens with time and tends to become secondarily infected (Fig. 47.2). Laboratory findings include low IgM concentration, elevated IgA and IgE concentrations, and normal IgG concentrations.

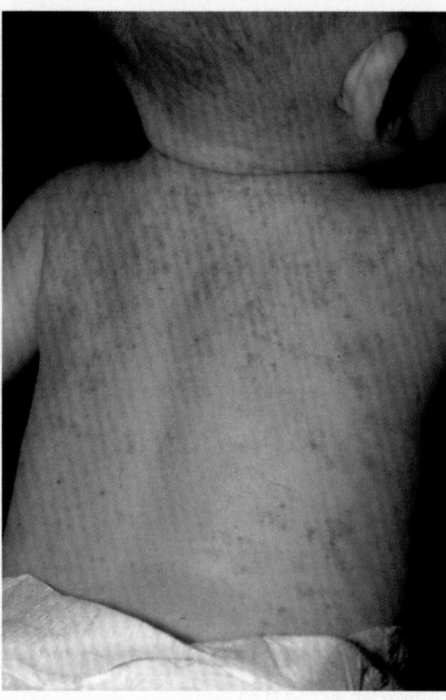

FIGURE 47.2 Boys with Wiskott–Aldrich syndrome often have worsening of eczema over time.

Take Note!

An episode of prolonged bleeding, such as at the umbilical stump or after circumcision, may be the first sign of Wiskott–Aldrich syndrome in the newborn (Ochs, 2015).

Nursing Management

Administer IVIG as ordered to help decrease the frequency of bacterial infections. Perform good skin care and frequently assess eczematous areas to detect secondary infection (refer to Chapter 45 for care of eczema). If the child undergoes splenectomy, in addition to providing routine postoperative care, be aware of the additional risk for development of infection in the asplenic child. Refer to Chapter 46 for information related to hematopoietic cell transplantation.

Severe Combined Immune Deficiency

Severe combined immune deficiency (SCID) is a rare X-linked or autosomal recessive disorder; it can occur in girls or boys. SCID is characterized by absent T-cell and B-cell function. There are at least five types of SCID, classified according to the exact genetic defect. SCID is a potentially fatal disorder requiring emergency intervention at the time of diagnosis. Gene therapy provides some promise for the future treatment of SCID, but until then hematopoietic cell transplantation is necessary (Bonilla, 2015).

Take Note!

Use only cytomegalovirus (CMV)-negative, irradiated blood or platelets if transfusion is necessary in the infant with SCID. CMV-positive blood could cause an infection in the infant, and T lymphocytes in blood products may cause fatal graft-versus-host disease to occur (Norville & Tomlinson, 2010).

IVIG infusions may help decrease the number of infections until bone marrow or stem cell transplantation can be done (Bonilla, 2015). Certain children with SCID (adenosine deaminase enzyme deficiency) may benefit from lifelong subcutaneous adenosine deaminase enzyme replacement. In addition, long-term antibiotic therapy helps to contain chronic infections in some children with SCID.

Nursing Assessment

Note history of chronic diarrhea and failure to thrive. Note history of severe infections beginning early in infancy. Inspect the mouth for persistent thrush. Auscultate the lungs, noting adventitious sounds related to pneumonia. Laboratory findings include very low levels of all of the immunoglobulins.

Nursing Management

Preventing infection is critical. Teach the family to practice good hand washing. The child must not be exposed to persons outside the family, particularly young children. Instruct families to administer prophylactic antibiotics if prescribed. Educate families that the child should not receive live vaccines. Encourage adequate nutrition; supplemental enteral feedings may be necessary in the child with poor appetite. Administer IVIG infusions as prescribed and monitor for adverse reactions (refer to the nursing management section for hypogammaglobulinemia for further information related to IVIG administration). If the child receives a bone marrow transplant (human leukocyte antigen [HLA]–matched sibling is preferred), provide posttransplant care as outlined in Chapter 46. Teach the family that severe cutaneous human papillomavirus infection may occur after stem cell transplantation (even years later). Refer the family for genetic counseling. Provide ongoing support; this is a difficult disease for families to cope with and the therapy required is lifelong.

Take Note!

Monitor the child who had a bone marrow or stem cell transplant closely for a maculopapular rash that usually starts on the palms and soles; this is an indication that **graft-versus-host disease** (GVHD) is developing. GVHD is a life-threatening condition in which donor cells attack host cells (Norville & Tomlinson, 2010).

SECONDARY IMMUNODEFICIENCIES

Secondary immunodeficiency may occur as a result of chronic illness, malignancy, use of **immunosuppressive** (lowering the immune response) medication, malnutrition or protein-losing state, prematurity, or HIV infection. This discussion will focus on HIV infection.

HIV Infection

Worldwide, 3.2 million children younger than 18 years old are living with HIV infection and about 650 become infected with HIV each day (UNAIDS, 2014). Children acquire HIV either vertically or horizontally. Vertical transmission refers to perinatal (in utero or during birth) transmission or via breast milk. Vertical transmission may also be referred to as mother to child transmission. Horizontal transmission refers to transmission via nonsterile needles (as in intravenous drug use or tattooing) or via intimate sexual contact. With nationwide screening of blood products, HIV transmission via transfused blood products has become rare (Fahrner & Romano, 2010; McFarland, 2014). HIV infection in children may be further classified depending on severity of immune suppression. This classification may serve to guide healthcare planning.

Infants primarily become infected through their mothers, whereas adolescents primarily contract HIV infection through sexual activity or intravenous drug use (Fahrner & Romano, 2010). In the United States, perinatal transmission of HIV infection has declined dramatically due to improved maternal detection and treatment, as well as newborn treatment (McFarland, 2014). Current United States data indicate that the rate of new diagnosis of HIV infection in children less than 13 years of age is 164 per 100,000 (Centers for Disease Control and Prevention, 2015). Currently, there is no cure for HIV infection, though survival has improved since the advent of highly active antiretroviral therapy (HAART) (see Evidence-Based Practice 47.1). In addition to improved survival, improved growth, neurodevelopment, and immune function occur with HAART (Fahrner & Romano, 2010).

Pathophysiology

HIV affects immune function via alterations mainly in T-cell function, but it also affects B cells, natural killer cells, and monocyte/macrophage function. HIV infects the CD4 (T-helper) cells. The virus replicates itself via the CD4 cell and renders the cell dysfunctional. Immune deficiency results as the number of normal, functioning CD4 cells drops. Initially, as CD4 counts decrease, the T-suppressor (CD8) counts increase, but as the disease progresses, CD8 counts also fall. The helper T-cell function declines even in asymptomatic infants and children who have not experienced significant decreases in the CD4 cell count. The T cells lose response to recall antigens, and this loss is associated with an increased risk of serious bacterial infection (McFarland, 2014).

B-cell defects also occur in HIV-infected children, contributing to high rates of serious bacterial infections. The B cells demonstrate impaired response to mitogens and antigens. They also exhibit defective antibody production in response to antigen exposure or vaccination. Also, infants lack a pool of memory B cells for recall antigens (simply from lack of exposure). Natural killer cells also are affected by HIV infection, as they are dependent on cytokines secreted by the CD4 cells for development of functionality. Functional killer cells play a role in fighting viruses and are critical to immunity in the newborn while the T-cell line develops. Decreased function of the natural killer cells then contributes to increased severity of viral infection in the HIV-infected child or infant. Though the virus does not destroy monocytes and macrophages, their function is affected. Macrophages in the HIV-infected child exhibit

EVIDENCE-BASED PRACTICE 47.1 **DOES TEXT MESSAGING PROMOTE ADHERENCE TO ANTIRETROVIRAL THERAPY FOR HIV INFECTION?**

STUDY

The key determinant of degree and length of viral suppression in HIV infection is high adherence to antiretroviral therapy. Conversely, poor adherence leads to treatment failure. Children potentially have a significant number of years of life for which they will need to remain compliant with antiretroviral therapy. The authors evaluated 17 randomized controlled trials that examined the effect of text messaging on improving antiretroviral adherence.

Findings

Weekly text messaging reminders to patients and/or their caregivers (of infants and children) were found to be effective in improving antiretroviral adherence.

Nursing Implications

Antiretroviral adherence is critical to the potential life of an HIV-infected child. Implementing a weekly text message reminder system related to antiretroviral therapy has the potential to improve adherence.

Adapted from Horvath, T., Azman, H., Kennedy, G. E., & Rutherford, G. W. (2012). Mobile phone text messaging for promoting adherence to antiretroviral therapy in patients with HIV infection. *The Cochrane Library 2012, 3*. Indianapolis, IN: John Wiley & Sons.

decreased chemotaxis and the antigen-presenting capability of the monocytes is defective.

Without appropriate T-cell, B-cell, natural killer cell, monocyte, and macrophage function, the infant's or child's immune system cannot fight infections it ordinarily could. Recurrent infection with ordinary organisms occurs more frequently in children with HIV infection, and the infections are more severe than in noninfected children. Opportunistic infections also occur in HIV-infected children, similar to those in adults with HIV infection. Current guidelines related to opportunistic infection prevention emphasize antiretroviral therapy for prevention as well as insuring appropriate immunization and antibiotic prophylaxis for certain organisms (Siberry, Abzug, & Nachman, 2013).

HIV rapidly invades the central nervous system in infants and children and is responsible for progressive HIV encephalopathy. As a result of encephalopathy, acquired microcephaly, motor deficits, or loss of previously achieved developmental milestones may occur. In children with progressive HIV encephalopathy, neurologic symptoms may present before immune suppression.

Therapeutic Management

Current recommendations for treatment of HIV infection in children include the use of a combination of antiretroviral drugs (McFarland, 2014). Medication therapy ranges from single-drug therapy in the asymptomatic HIV-exposed newborn to highly active antiretroviral therapy, consisting of a combination of antiretroviral drugs. Medications are prescribed based on the severity of the child's illness. One of the goals of HAART is to prevent or arrest progressive HIV encephalopathy (Fahrner & Romano, 2010).

Nursing Assessment

For a full description of the assessment phase of the nursing process, refer to the Assessment section of the Nursing Process Overview earlier in the chapter. Assessment findings pertinent to HIV infection in children are discussed below.

HEALTH HISTORY

Elicit a description of the present illness and chief complaint. Common signs and symptoms reported during the health history might include:

- Failure to thrive
- Recurrent bacterial infections
- Opportunistic infections
- Chronic or recurrent diarrhea
- Recurrent or persistent fever
- Developmental delay
- Prolonged candidiasis

These signs and symptoms may be present in either the child who is undergoing initial diagnosis or the child with known HIV infection. Explore the child's current and past medical history for risk factors such as maternal HIV infection or AIDS, receipt of blood transfusions in a developing country (without adequate screening measures), adolescent or childhood sexual abuse, substance use or abuse (including intravenous drug use), or participation in vaginal or anal sex without the use of a condom. Document who the primary caregiver is, as many children with HIV have lost their parents to the disease. In addition, for the child with known HIV infection, determine the child's medications and dosages as well as the outcome of any recent healthcare visits or hospitalizations.

PHYSICAL EXAMINATION

Perform a thorough and complete physical examination on the child with suspected or known HIV infection.

Inspection and Observation. Note presence of fever. Measure weight, height or length, and head circumference (in children younger than 3 years old) and plot this information on standard growth charts, noting whether the measurements fall within the average or below the lower percentiles. Perform a developmental screening test to detect developmental delay. Inspect the oral cavity for candidiasis. Observe work of breathing (may be increased if pneumonitis or pneumonia is present). Determine level of consciousness (may be depressed if HIV encephalopathy is present).

Auscultation and Palpation. Auscultate the lungs, noting adventitious breath sounds associated with pneumonia or pneumonitis. Palpate for the presence of enlarged lymph nodes (lymphadenopathy) or swollen parotid glands. Palpate the abdomen, noting hepatosplenomegaly.

LABORATORY AND DIAGNOSTIC TESTS

Common laboratory and diagnostic studies ordered for the assessment of HIV infection include:

- Reverse transcriptase—polymerase chain reaction (PCR) test: positive in infected infants older than 1 month of age. RT-PCR is the preferred test to determine HIV infection in infants and to exclude HIV infection as early as possible. Box 47.2 gives information on testing.
- Enzyme-linked immunosorbent assay (ELISA) test: positive in infants of HIV-infected mothers because of transplacentally received antibodies. These antibodies may persist and remain detectable up to 24 months of age, making the ELISA test less accurate at detecting HIV infection in infants and toddlers than the PCR.
- CD4 counts (low in HIV infection)

Nursing Management

Nursing care of the child with HIV infection is directed at avoiding infection, promoting compliance with the

BOX 47.2

VIROLOGIC ASSAY TESTING FOR HIV-EXPOSED INFANTS

- 14 to 21 days of age
- 1 to 2 months of age
- 4 to 6 months of age
- In the nonbreastfed infant, 2 or more negative tests (one at ≥1 month of age and one at ≥4 months of age) determine absence of HIV infection

From Panel on Antiretroviral Therapy and Medical Management of HIV-Infected Children. (2016). *Guidelines for the use of antiretroviral agents in pediatric HIV infection*. Retrieved from http://aidsinfo.nih.gov/contentfiles/lvguidelines/pediatricguidelines.pdf

medication regimen, promoting nutrition, providing pain management and comfort measures, educating the child and caregivers, and providing ongoing psychosocial support. Children with HIV infection may access health services through funding provided by the Ryan White Comprehensive AIDS Resources Emergency Act (Health Resources and Services Administration, the HIV/AIDS Program, n. d.). This federal funding provides for primary health care and other services to persons with HIV infection. Nursing Care Plan 47.1, found at the end of the chapter, lists appropriate nursing diagnoses and interventions. In addition, nursing management specific to HIV infection is covered below.

PREVENTING HIV INFECTION IN CHILDREN

It is important to offer all pregnant women routine HIV counseling and voluntary testing. Depending on the stage of pregnancy, the mother should be treated with an antiretroviral drug if she is HIV positive. Children born to HIV-positive mothers should receive a 6-week course of zidovudine (ZDV) therapy (McFarland, 2014). Discourage breastfeeding in the HIV-infected mother and instruct her about safe alternatives to breastfeeding. Early recognition of infection is crucial so that treatment can begin, HIV encephalopathy may be prevented, and progression to acquired immune deficiency syndrome can be prevented. Educate sexually active adolescents about HIV transmission and urge them to use condoms. Counsel teens about the increased risk of HIV transmission with all forms of sexual activity, explaining that vaginal and anal sex are even riskier than oral sex. Urge teens to limit the number of sexual partners. Discourage substance use, as the effects of drugs and alcohol often impair the teen's ability to make wise choices about sexual conduct. Warn teens of the risk of contracting HIV infection via shared needles (as with intravenous drug use or via unclean needles used in tattooing). See Healthy People 2020.

HEALTHY PEOPLE 2020

Objective	Nursing Significance
Reduce the number of perinatally acquired HIV and AIDS cases. (Developmental) Increase the proportion of pregnant females screened for sexually transmitted diseases (including HIV infection and bacterial vaginosis) during prenatal health-care visits, according to recognized standards.	• Encourage sexually active adolescents to seek appropriate reproductive health care and screening. • For the pregnant adolescent, encourage HIV testing to determine status. • Encourage the HIV-positive pregnant adolescent to comply with HIV treatment as prescribed.

Healthy People Objectives retrieved from http://www.healthypeople.gov

PROMOTING COMPLIANCE WITH ANTIRETROVIRAL THERAPY

Before HAART was available as a treatment option, progressive HIV encephalopathy was inevitably fatal, usually within 2 years of diagnosis (Fahrner & Romano, 2010). To prevent progression of HIV disease and prevent encephalopathy, compliance with the HAART regimen is required. Educate the family about the importance of complying with the medication regimen. Help the caregivers develop a schedule for medication administration that is compatible with the family's home routine. See Healthy People 2020.

HEALTHY PEOPLE 2020

Objective	Nursing Significance
Reduce the number of new cases of HIV infection and diagnoses among adolescents and adults.	• Discourage intravenous illicit drug use. Educate teens about the risk of contaminated tattoo needles.
Reduce the number of new AIDS cases among adolescent and adult heterosexuals, males who have sex with males, and those who inject drugs.	• Encourage abstinence in adolescents. • If adolescents are sexually active, educate about the risks of HIV transmission; encourage condom use with all sexual activity.

Healthy People Objectives retrieved from http://www.healthypeople.gov

HEALTHY PEOPLE 2020

Objective	Nursing Significance
Reduce deaths from HIV infection Increase the proportion of HIV-infected adolescents and adults who receive HIV care and treatment consistent with current standards	• Educate families about the importance of complying with medication therapy (highly active antiretroviral therapy [HAART]) and receiving regularly scheduled medical evaluations.

Healthy People Objectives retrieved from http://www.healthypeople.gov

REDUCING RISK FOR INFECTION

In the newborn whose mother is infected with tuberculosis, syphilis, toxoplasmosis, cytomegalovirus, hepatitis B or C, or herpes simplex virus, provide testing and treatment. To prevent infection with *Pneumocystis jirovecii,* administer prophylactic antibiotics as prescribed in any HIV-exposed infant in whom HIV infection has not yet been excluded. Provide tuberculosis screening and childhood immunization in accordance with national guidelines.

Thinking About Development

Jasmine Smith is a 5-year-old female with HIV infection. She fights taking her antiretroviral medications because of the nausea and vomiting associated with them. Lucy Panco is a 15-year-old female also with HIV infection. She is noncompliant with her antiretroviral medications, also because of the associated nausea and vomiting.

How will the nurse teach Jasmine about the medications? How will she foster compliance in Jasmine?

What is the most appropriate approach for the nurse to take to educate Lucy about compliance with medications?

How will the approaches to education and encouragement of compliance be different for these two children? How will they be similar?

Take Note!

Do not administer live vaccines to the immunocompromised child without the express consent of the infectious disease or immunology specialist. Immunosuppression is a contraindication to vaccination with live vaccines (Atkinson et al., 2012).

PROMOTING NUTRITION

For the infant, provide increased-calorie formula as tolerated. For the child, provide high-calorie, high-protein meals and snacks. Supplements may be added to milkshakes to increase the protein intake. Ensure that the child is able to choose foods that he or she prefers from the hospital menu. Document growth through weekly measurements of weight and height/length.

PROMOTING COMFORT

Children with HIV infection experience pain from infections, encephalopathy, adverse effects of medications, and the numerous procedures and treatments that are required, such as venipuncture, biopsy, or lumbar puncture. Refer to Chapter 36 for detailed information about pain assessment and management.

Take Note!

Family-centered care of the HIV-exposed child and HIV-infected mother may involve a multidisciplinary approach and can result in improved outcomes for both the mother and the child (Fahrner & Romano, 2010).

PROVIDING FAMILY EDUCATION AND SUPPORT

Educate caregivers about the medication regimen, the ongoing follow-up that is needed, and when to call the infectious disease provider. Families of HIV-infected children experience a significant amount of stress from many sources: the diagnosis of an incurable disease, financial difficulties, multiple family members with HIV, HIV-associated stigmas, desire to keep HIV infection confidential, and multiple medical appointments and hospitalizations. Parents of HIV-infected children often die of AIDS themselves, leaving care of the child to another relative or foster parent. The day care center or school that the child attends will need education about HIV, which can be provided only if the parent or caretaker consents to divulging the child's diagnosis to that agency. Provide education to the school or day care center about how the infection is transmitted (i.e., not through casual contact).

Disclosure of the diagnosis of HIV to the child is another source of stress for the family. The timing of this disclosure will vary considerably depending on the child's and family's situation. Generally, children older than 6 years of age will eventually need to have their diagnosis disclosed to them in an age-appropriate manner. They begin to ask questions and often seem to sense that something is going on other than what they've been told so far. When made aware of the diagnosis and educated about the disease, the child may exhibit a variety of reactions. Anger, depression, or school problems may occur. The child may experience a spiritual dilemma. Adolescents with perinatal HIV infection reported that disclosure of the diagnosis resulted in significant stress in their lives (De Santis, Garcia, Chaparro, & Beltron, 2014). The nurse should continue to provide emotional support to the child

BOX 47.3

RESOURCES FOR HIV-INFECTED CHILDREN AND THEIR FAMILIES

- www.pedaids.org: Elizabeth Glaser Pediatric AIDS Foundation—resources for HIV-infected children and their families
- www.vachss.com/help_text/hiv_aids_ped.html: Pediatric HIV infection and AIDS resources
- www.womenchildrenhiv.org/: Women, Children, and HIV—resources for prevention and treatment

and family. If the disclosure results in significant emotional turmoil, refer the child and caregivers to a counselor, social worker, or psychologist. Anticipatory grieving also may occur. Parents or caregivers may express guilt or anger over the diagnosis of HIV infection. At the other end of the spectrum, families may use denial as their method for coping. Use therapeutic communication with open-ended questions to discover the family's thoughts and fears. Provide emotional support and allow for crying and verbalization. If needed, refer the caregivers to the appropriate professional for additional psychological and emotional intervention.

Many children with HIV have psychosocial, emotional, and cognitive problems. These contribute to a lower quality of life. They are affected by the stigma of their diagnosis and often by the social isolation associated with it. Adolescents with HIV infection note that this stigma has a profound impact on coping their coping abilities (De Santis et al., 2014). They may suffer multiple losses within the family related to deaths caused by HIV infection. Children with HIV infection need significant psychosocial support and intervention. Resources for families of HIV-infected children are listed in Box 47.3.

AUTOIMMUNE DISORDERS

Autoimmune disorders result from the immune system's malfunction. The body manufactures T cells and antibodies against its own cells and organs (**autoantibodies**). The development of an autoimmune disorder is thought to be multifactorial. Potential influencing factors include heredity, hormones, self-marker molecules, and environmental influences such as viruses and certain drugs.

Systemic Lupus Erythematosus

Systemic lupus erythematosus (SLE) is a multisystem autoimmune disorder that affects both humoral and cellular immunity. SLE can affect any organ system, so the onset and course of the disease are quite variable. SLE is usually diagnosed after age 5 years (usually between 15 and 45 years of age), but onset can occur at any age. The peak incidence for diagnosis is in the preadolescent years (Mattingly, 2011). The female-to-male ratio for persons affected by SLE is 4:1 in childhood and 8:1 in adolescence (Lehman, 2015). SLE is more common in non-Caucasians, and typically African-American and Hispanic children and adolescents experience more severe effects from SLE than other racial or ethnic groups (Lehman, 2015).

Pathophysiology

In SLE, autoantibodies react with the child's self-antigens to form immune complexes. The immune complexes accumulate in the tissues and organs, causing an inflammatory response resulting in vasculitis. Injury to the tissues and pain occur. Since SLE may affect any organ system, the potential for alterations or damage to tissues anywhere in the body is significant. In some cases, the autoimmune response may be preceded by a drug reaction, an infection, or excessive sun exposure. In children, the most common initial symptoms are hematologic, cutaneous, and musculoskeletal in origin. The disease is chronic, with periods of remission and exacerbation (flares). Common complications of SLE include ocular or visual changes, cerebrovascular accident (CVA), transverse myelitis, immune complex–mediated glomerulonephritis, pericarditis, valvular heart disease, coronary artery disease, seizures, and psychosis.

Therapeutic Management

Therapeutic management focuses on treating the inflammatory response. Nonsteroidal anti-inflammatory drugs (NSAIDs), corticosteroids, and antimalarial agents are often prescribed for the child with mild to moderate SLE. The child with severe SLE or frequent flare-ups of symptoms may require high-dose (pulse) corticosteroid therapy or immunosuppressive drugs. When end-stage renal failure develops as a result of glomerulonephritis, dialysis becomes necessary.

Nursing Assessment

For a full description of the assessment phase of the nursing process, refer to the Assessment section of the Nursing Process Overview earlier in the chapter. Assessment findings pertinent to SLE in children are discussed below.

HEALTH HISTORY

Elicit a description of the present illness and chief complaint. Common signs and symptoms reported during the health history are history of fatigue, fever, weight changes, pain or swelling in the joints, numbness, tingling or coolness of extremities, or prolonged bleeding. Assess for risk

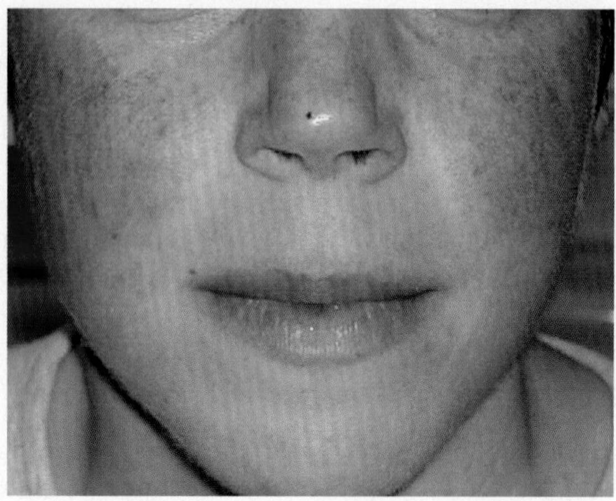

FIGURE 47.3 The malar or butterfly rash (erythema over the cheeks in the shape of a butterfly) is typical in systemic lupus erythematosus (SLE).

factors, which include female sex; family history; African, Native American, or Asian descent; recent infection; drug reaction; or excessive sun exposure.

PHYSICAL EXAMINATION

Measure temperature and document the presence of fever. Observe the skin for malar rash (a butterfly-shaped rash over the cheeks); discoid lesions on the face, scalp, or neck; changes in skin pigmentation; or scarring (Fig. 47.3). Document alopecia. Inspect the oral cavity for painless ulcerations and the joints for edema.

Measure blood pressure, as hypertension may occur with renal involvement. Auscultate the lungs; adventitious breath sounds may be present if the pulmonary system is involved. Palpate the joints, noting tenderness. Palpate the abdomen and note areas of tenderness (abdominal involvement is more common in children with SLE than in adults). Box 47.4 lists common clinical findings in SLE.

BOX 47.4

MOST COMMON CLINICAL MANIFESTATIONS OF SYSTEMIC LUPUS ERYTHEMATOSUS

- Alopecia
- Anemia
- Arthralgia
- Arthritis
- Fatigue
- Lupus nephritis
- Photosensitivity
- Pleurisy
- Raynaud phenomenon
- Seizures
- Skin rashes, including malar rash
- Stomatitis
- Thrombocytopenia

LABORATORY AND DIAGNOSTIC FINDINGS

Laboratory findings may include decreased hemoglobin and hematocrit, decreased platelet count, and low WBC count. Complement levels, C3 and C4, will also be decreased. Though not specific to SLE, the antinuclear antibody (ANA) is usually positive in children with SLE.

Nursing Management

Nursing management of the child or adolescent with SLE is long term and supportive. Management focuses on preventing and monitoring for complications. Educate the child and family about the importance of a healthy diet, regular exercise, and adequate sleep and rest. Administer NSAIDs, corticosteroids, and antimalarial agents as ordered for the child with mild to moderate SLE and pulse corticosteroid therapy or immunomodulators to the child with severe SLE or frequent flare-ups. Dealing with a chronic illness can be difficult for the child and family. In addition, adolescents struggle with body image and independence (Mattingly, 2011). Refer families to support services such as the Lupus Alliance of America and the Lupus Foundation of America, links to which can be found on thePoint.

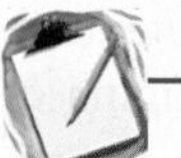

Take Note!

Counsel adolescents with SLE about the risk of autoantibody transmission to the fetus should they become pregnant. This antibody transmission can result in lupus in the newborn (Johnson, 2014).

PREVENTING AND MONITORING FOR COMPLICATIONS

Teach families to apply sunscreen (minimum SPF 15) to their child's skin daily to prevent rashes resulting from photosensitivity. Instruct the child and family to protect against cold weather by layering warm socks and wearing gloves when outdoors in the winter. If the child is outside for extended periods during the winter months, inspect the fingers and toes for discoloration. Watch for the development of nephritis by evaluating blood pressure, serum BUN and creatinine levels, and urine output and monitoring for hematuria or proteinuria. Ensure that yearly vision screening and ophthalmic examinations are performed to preserve visual function should changes occur.

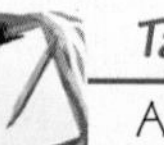

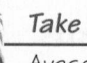

Take Note!

Avascular necrosis (lack of blood supply to a joint, resulting in tissue damage) may occur as an adverse effect of long-term or high-dose corticosteroid use. Teach families to report new onset of joint pain, particularly with weight bearing, or limited range of motion to their physician or nurse practitioner (Tofferi, 2015).

TABLE 47.2 TYPES OF JUVENILE IDIOPATHIC ARTHRITIS

Type	Definition	Nonjoint Manifestations	Complications
Pauciarticular (oligoarticular)	Involvement of four or fewer joints; quite often the knee is involved. Most common type	Eye inflammation, malaise, poor appetite, poor weight gain	Iritis, uveitis, uneven leg bone growth
Polyarticular	Involvement of five or more joints; frequently involves small joints and often affects the body symmetrically	Malaise, lymphadenopathy, organomegaly, poor growth	Often a severe form of arthritis; rapidly progressing joint damage, rheumatoid nodules
Systemic	In addition to joint involvement, fever and rash may be present at diagnosis	Enlarged spleen, liver, and lymph nodes; myalgia; severe anemia	Pericarditis, pericardial effusion, pleuritis, pulmonary fibrosis

Adapted from Jones, K. B., & Higgins, G. C. (2010). Juvenile rheumatoid arthritis. In P. J. Allen, J. A. Vessey, & N. A. Schapiro (Eds.), *Primary care of the child with a chronic condition* (5th ed.). St. Louis, MO: Mosby; and Stanley, L. C., & Ward-Smith, P. (2011). The diagnosis and management of juvenile idiopathic arthritis. *Journal of Pediatric Health Care, 25*(3), 191–194.

Juvenile Idiopathic Arthritis

Juvenile idiopathic arthritis is an autoimmune disorder in which the autoantibodies mainly target the joints. Inflammatory changes in the joints cause pain, redness, warmth, stiffness, and swelling. Stiffness usually occurs after inactivity (as in the morning, after sleep). Some forms also affect the eyes or other organs. Table 47.2 explains the three types. Juvenile idiopathic arthritis is a chronic disease; the child may experience healthy periods alternating with flare-ups. In some children the disease resolves as they approach adolescence or adulthood, while others will have more severe disease that continues throughout the adult years (Jones & Higgins, 2010). Juvenile idiopathic arthritis was formerly termed "juvenile rheumatoid arthritis," but unlike adult rheumatoid arthritis, few types of juvenile arthritis actually demonstrate a positive rheumatoid factor.

Therapeutic management focuses on inflammation control, pain relief, promotion of remission, and maintenance of mobility. NSAIDs, corticosteroids, and antirheumatic drugs such as methotrexate and etanercept are prescribed, depending on the type and severity of the disease. NSAIDs are helpful with pain relief, but disease-modifying (antirheumatic) drugs are necessary to prevent disease progression.

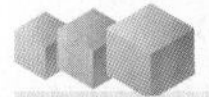
Concept Mastery Alert

Juvenile Idiopathic Arthritis

Prednisone is used to decrease the inflammatory process in children with juvenile idiopathic arthritis. Methotrexate is used to prevent disease progression.

Nursing Assessment

Note history of irritability or fussiness, which may be the first sign of this disease in the infant or very young child. Note complaints of pain, though children do not always communicate this. Document history of withdrawal from play or difficulty getting the child out of bed in the morning (joint stiffness after inactivity). Inquire about history of fever (above 39.5°C for 2 weeks or more in systemic disease).

Measure temperature (fever is present with systemic disease). Inspect skin for evanescent, pale red, nonpruritic macular rash, which may be present at diagnosis of systemic disease. Observe the gait, noting limping or guarding of a joint or extremity. Document growth, which may be delayed. Inspect and palpate each joint for edema, redness, warmth, and tenderness (Fig. 47.4). Note positioning of joints (usually flexed in position of comfort). Mild to moderate anemia and an elevated erythrocyte sedimentation rate are common. Young children with the pauciarticular form may demonstrate a positive antinuclear antibody, and adolescents with polyarticular disease may have a positive rheumatoid factor.

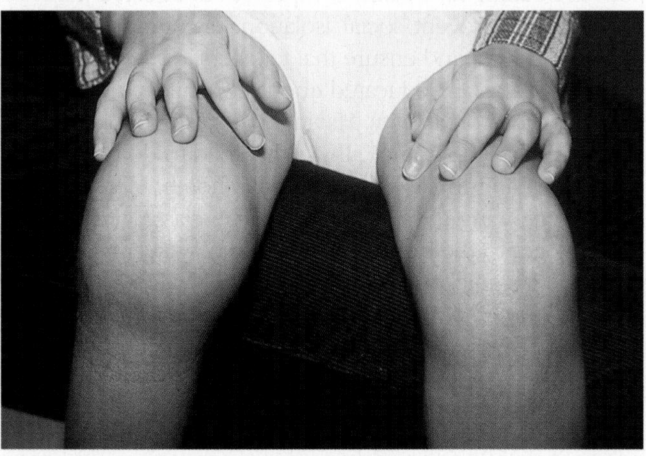

FIGURE 47.4 Note the swollen, reddened joints of this child with juvenile arthritis.

Nursing Management

Nursing management focuses on managing pain, maintaining mobility, and promoting a normal life. Refer the child to a pediatric rheumatologist to ensure that he or she receives the most up-to-date treatment. Disease-modifying medications approved for use in children may produce better long-term outcomes than were possible in the past. Clinical research trial information is available through the Childhood Arthritis & Rheumatology Research Alliance. Encourage regular eye examinations and vision screening to allow for early treatment of visual changes and to prevent blindness.

MANAGING PAIN AND MAINTAINING MOBILITY

Administer medications as prescribed to control inflammation and prevent disease progression. Refer to Drug Guide 47.1 for information related to NSAIDs, corticosteroids, and disease-modifying antirheumatic drugs. Maintain joint range of motion and muscle strength via exercise (physical or occupational therapy). Swimming is a particularly useful exercise to maintain joint mobility without placing pressure on the joints. Teach families appropriate use of splints prescribed to prevent joint contractures. Monitor for pressure areas or skin breakdown with splint or orthotic use.

PROMOTING NORMAL LIFE

Chronic pain and decreased mobility may impact the child's psychological and emotional status significantly, during both childhood and adulthood. Providing adequate pain relief and promoting compliance with the disease-modifying medication regimen may allow the child to have a more normal life in the present as well as in the future. In addition to measures described in the previous section, encourage adequate sleep. Sleep disturbance contributes to daytime sleepiness and fatigue which interferes with the child's ability to cope with symptoms and with school function (Ward et al., 2014). Sleep may be promoted by a warm bath at bedtime and warm compresses to affected joints or massage. To prevent social isolation, encourage the child to attend school and ensure that teachers, the school nurse, and classmates are educated about the child's disease and any limitations on activity. Having two sets of books (one at school and one at home) allows the child to do homework without having to carry heavy books home. Modifications such as allowing the child to leave the classroom early in order to get to the next class on time may seem small but can have a significant impact on the child's life.

Encourage children and families to become involved with local support groups so they can see that they are not alone. Assist children to set and achieve goals to increase their sense of hopefulness. Special summer camps for children with juvenile arthritis allow the child to socialize and belong to a group and have been shown to promote self-esteem in the child with chronic illness. Encourage appropriate family functioning and refer the family to support groups such as those sponsored by the American Juvenile Arthritis Organization.

Guillain–Barré Syndrome

Guillain–Barré syndrome (GBS) (also called acute immune-mediated polyneuropathies) is a diverse group of syndromes with several forms. The disorder occurring most often is a one in which an immune response within the body attacks the peripheral nervous system but does not usually affect the brain or spinal cord. Guillain–Barré syndrome results in inflammation and demyelinization of the peripheral nerves. Weakness and paralysis occur in a progressive fashion. Progression is usually complete in 2 to 4 weeks, followed by a stable period leading to the recovery phase, which lasts for a few weeks to months in most cases but can take years. Severity of the disorder ranges from mild weakness to total paralysis.

Though not fully understood, it is believed to be an autoimmune condition that most commonly is triggered by a previous viral or bacterial infection, usually described as an upper respiratory tract infection or an acute gastroenteritis with fever. In rare cases it has occurred after the child has had an immunization or surgery. GBS is more commonly seen in adults than in children (Curse, 2014).

Therapeutic Management

Treatment of Guillain–Barré syndrome is symptomatic and focuses on lessening the severity and speeding recovery. Management may include plasma exchange and administration of intravenous immunoglobulins, especially in severe cases. The goal of treatment is to keep the body functioning until the nervous system recovers. Guillain–Barré syndrome is a life-threatening condition, and some children will die during the acute phase due to respiratory failure. Most children will make a full recovery, but a few may have residual damage.

Nursing Assessment

Early diagnosis and prompt treatment are essential since the disorder can quickly lead to respiratory failure and death from muscle paralysis. For a full description of the assessment phase of the nursing process, refer to the Assessment section of the Nursing Process Overview earlier in the chapter. Assessment findings pertinent to Guillain–Barré syndrome are discussed below.

HEALTH HISTORY

Elicit a description of the present illness and chief complaint. The clinical presentation of Guillain–Barré syndrome is fairly similar in children and adults. Note onset of symptoms within a few days or weeks after the causative infection or event. Determine presence of muscle weakness and paresthesias such as numbness and tingling which have a quick onset. Classically Guillain–Barré syndrome initially affects the legs and progresses in an ascending manner, but occasionally it affects the arms or face first and proceeds in a descending manner. Note paralysis if present.

In children, pain, especially of the lower extremities, as the initial presentation preceding motor involvement has been reported. Other symptoms which may be present during the course of the illness ataxia and sensory disturbances.

PHYSICAL EXAMINATION AND LABORATORY AND DIAGNOSTIC TESTS

Physical examination findings may include decreased or absent tendon reflexes. Facial weakness or difficulty swallowing may be noted. Diagnosis is usually based on clinical findings of paralysis. Cerebrospinal fluid (CSF) analysis may reveal an increased level of protein, but this may not be evident until after the first week of the illness. Electrodiagnostic studies, such as electromyelogram (EMG) and nerve conduction velocity, can assist in the diagnosis of GBS.

Take Note!

Tickling may be a successful technique for assessing the level of paralysis in the child with Guillain–Barré syndrome, either initially or in the recovery phase.

Nursing Management

Nursing management is supportive. In severe cases the child may require intensive nursing care along with mechanical ventilation. Observe the child closely for the extent of paralysis and monitor for respiratory involvement. Nursing care focuses on the same concerns as in any child with extreme immobility or paralysis.

Prevention of complications associated with immobility is a central concern and involves maintaining skin integrity, preventing respiratory complications and contractures, maintaining adequate nutrition, and managing pain. Interventions include turning and repositioning every 2 hours, assessing the skin for redness or breakdown, performing range-of-motion exercises, keeping the skin clean and dry, encouraging intake of fluids to maintain hydration status, and encouraging coughing and deep breathing every 2 hours and as needed. Enteral feeding or parenteral nutrition may be indicated if swallowing becomes impaired. Physical therapy may be helpful in preventing complications and promoting motor skill recovery. Provide support and education to the parent and child. The rapid onset and long recovery can be difficult and can cause strain on the family and its finances. If residual disability occurs, the family will need help adjusting and caring for their child.

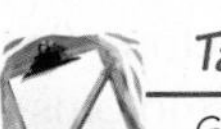

Take Note!

Serial measurement of tidal volumes may reveal respiratory deterioration in the child with Guillain–Barré syndrome.

Myasthenia Gravis

Myasthenia gravis is an autoimmune disease that may be inherited as a rare genetic disease (congenital), may be acquired by infants born to mothers with myasthenia gravis (neonatal), or may develop later in childhood (juvenile). The most common form seen is juvenile myasthenia gravis and will be covered here. See Comparison Chart 47.2 for further information on the less common forms, neonatal myasthenia gravis and congenital myasthenia gravis. Juvenile myasthenia gravis is a relatively rare autoimmune disorder (Liew & Kang, 2013). The child's antibodies attack the acetylcholine receptor and other proteins at the neuromuscular junction, inhibiting normal neuromuscular transmission. The result is progressive weakness and fatigue of the skeletal muscles.

There is no cure for myasthenia gravis. Symptoms can be controlled, but it is a lifelong condition, with early detection being the key to managing the disorder successfully. The disease may be aggravated by stress, exposure to extreme temperatures, and infections,

COMPARISON CHART 47.2 TYPES OF MYSATHENIA GRAVIS

	Neonatal Mysathenia Gravis	Congenital Mysathenia Gravis
Definition	Transient form resulting from transplacental transfer of maternal antibodies that interfere with neuromuscular junction	A group of disorders resulting from a genetic mutation of components of the neuromuscular junction resulting in neuromuscular junction failure
Characteristics	Present within a few hours after birth. Generalized weakness and hypotonia. Bulbar and respiratory weakness leads to poor suck and swallow, weak cry, and possible respiratory failure. Neonate will be very ill. Prompt diagnosis and treatment is essential. Recovery usually within a few weeks	Apparent at birth. Frequently have ptosis, ophthalmoplegia, bulbar, and respiratory muscle weakness. Fluctuating generalized weakness and hypotonia, life-threatening apnea. Typically improves with age but spontaneous exacerbations seen. Exacerbations also during periods of stress, increased activity, or febrile illness are seen. Management depends on specific type

resulting in a myasthenic crisis. Myasthenic crisis is a medical emergency with symptoms including sudden respiratory distress, dysphagia, dysarthria, ptosis, diplopia, tachycardia, anxiety, and rapidly increasing weakness.

Therapeutic management generally involves the use of anticholinesterase medications such as pyridostigmine, which blocks the breakdown of acetylcholine at the neuromuscular junction and enhances neuromuscular transmission. If weakness is not controlled, additional medications may include corticosteroids and other immunosuppressants. Other treatments include plasmapheresis, which removes antibodies from the blood; intravenous immunoglobulin, and thymectomy (however, the role of the thymus gland in the disease process is unclear; therefore, this procedure may or may not improve the child's symptoms).

Nursing Assessment

Note history of fatigue and weakness; difficulty chewing, swallowing, or holding up the head; or pain with muscle fatigue. In the verbal child, note complaints of double vision. Observe the child for ptosis (droopy eyelids) or altered eye movements from partial paralysis. Note increased work of breathing. Laboratory testing may involve the edrophonium (Tensilon) test, in which a short-acting cholinesterase inhibitor is used. Acetylcholine receptor (AchR) antibodies may be present in elevated quantities in the serum.

Nursing Management

The goals of nursing management include prevention of respiratory problems and providing adequate nutrition. Administer anticholinergic or other medications as ordered, teaching children and families about the use of these drugs. Anticholinergic drugs should be given 30 to 45 minutes before meals, on time and exactly as ordered. Encourage families to seek prompt medical treatment for suspected infections. Encourage appropriate stress management and avoidance of extreme temperatures. Teach families that physical activities should be performed during times of peak energy; rest periods are needed for energy conservation. Teach families to call their neurologist immediately if signs and symptoms of myasthenic crisis or cholinergic crisis, which results from overmedication with anticholinergic medications, appear. Myasthenic crisis and cholinergic crisis have a similar presentation: rapidly increasing muscle weakness with resultant respiratory distress. Encourage children to wear a medical alert bracelet.

Take Note!

Signs and symptoms of myasthenic crisis include severe muscle weakness, respiratory difficulty, tachycardia, and dysphagia. Signs and symptoms of cholinergic crisis include severe muscle weakness, sweating, increased salivation, bradycardia, and hypotension.

Dermatomyositis

Juvenile dermatomyositis is an autoimmune disease that results in inflammation of the muscles or associated tissues. It occurs more often in girls and is generally diagnosed between the ages of 5 and 10 years (Hutchinson & Feldman, 2016a). The cause remains unclear but it may be an autoimmune response triggered by exposure to a virus or to certain medications (Hutchinson & Feldman, 2016a). As with other autoimmune diseases, a genetic predisposition is present. The inflammatory cells of the immune system cause a vasculitis that affects the skin, muscles, kidneys, retinas, and gastrointestinal tract.

Therapeutic management involving the use of high-dose glucocorticoid or other immunosuppressants is necessary to prevent the complications of painful calcium deposits under the skin, as well as joint contractures. Methotrexate, IVIG, and cyclosporine may also be used. With appropriate treatment, children may recover completely, though some children experience relapses (Hutchinson & Feldman, 2016b).

Nursing Assessment

Elicit a health history, which commonly includes fever, fatigue, and rash, usually followed by muscle pain and weakness. Determine onset and progression of muscle weakness. Inspect the skin for the presence of rash involving the upper eyelids and extensor surfaces of the knuckles, elbows, and knees. The rash is initially a reddish-purplish color, and then progresses to scaling with resulting roughness of the skin. Test muscle strength, particularly noting weakness in the pelvic and shoulder girdles. Laboratory and diagnostic testing may include muscle enzyme levels, a positive antinuclear antibody (ANA) test, and an electromyelogram to distinguish muscular weakness from other causes.

Nursing Management

Administer medications as ordered and teach families about their use; instruct them to monitor for side effects. Educate the family about the importance of maintaining the medication regimen in order to prevent calcinosis (calcium deposits) and joint deformity in the future. Encourage compliance with physical therapy regimens. Ensure that children are excused from physical education classes while the disease is active.

ALLERGY AND ANAPHYLAXIS

Allergy is an immune-mediated response resulting in an adverse physiologic event or reaction and affects up to 25% of population in developed countries (Covar, Fleischer, Cho, & Boguniewicz, 2014). The extent of the allergic response is determined by the duration, rate, and amount of exposure to the allergen as well as environmental and host factors. IgE-mediated allergy will be the focus of this discussion. This type of allergic response is mediated by antigen-specific IgE antibodies. When the antibody is exposed to the antigen (allergen), rapid cell activation occurs and potent mediators and cytokines are released, resulting in changes in the blood vessels, bronchi, and mucus-secreting glands. In addition to the atopic diseases (asthma, allergic rhinitis, and atopic dermatitis), urticaria, digestive allergy, and systemic anaphylaxis are also IgE mediated. Though any allergen has the potential to trigger an anaphylactic response, food and insect sting allergies are most common (Sloand & Caschera, 2010).

Food Allergies

A true food hypersensitivity or allergy is defined as an immunologic reaction resulting from the ingestion of a food or food additive. This type of reaction is an IgE-mediated response to a particular food. Food allergy affects approximately 8% of children and can lead to significant medical complications (Covar et al., 2014). During the first few years of life, the most common food allergens are milk, eggs, peanuts, tree nuts, fish and shellfish, wheat, and soy. Typically, allergies to these foods are acquired in childhood. For most children only allergies to peanuts, tree nuts, and fish and shellfish persist into adulthood (Covar et al., 2014). Most reactions occur within minutes of exposure, but they may occur up to 2 hours after ingestion. Signs and symptoms of a food allergy reaction include hives, flushing, facial swelling, mouth and throat itching, and runny nose. Many children also have a gastrointestinal reaction, including vomiting, abdominal pain, and diarrhea. In extreme cases, swelling of the tongue, uvula, pharynx, or upper airway may occur. Wheezing can be an ominous sign that the airway is edematous. Rarely, cardiovascular collapse occurs. Though the risk for anaphylaxis is small, parents, caregivers, and physicians and nurse practitioners should be vigilant when caring for children with food allergies.

Therapeutic Management

Therapeutic management involves verifying the food allergy, avoiding the allergen, and treating the reaction with medications, including antihistamines and epinephrine (in the case of an anaphylactic reaction).

Discerning a true food allergy from intolerance to certain foods is an important part of therapeutic management. "Food intolerance" is a general term that describes an abnormal physiologic response to an ingested food or food additive that has not been proven to be immunologic. Often a milk allergy is confused with lactose intolerance. Therefore, a detailed dietary history is important when distinguishing a true allergy versus intolerance. To prevent the development of food allergies, infants should be breastfed for at least the first 6 months of life.

Nursing Assessment

It is important to accurately assess children with food allergy reactions. In the initial nursing assessment, immediately assess the child for airway, breathing, or circulation problems (see Chapter 51). If the child's condition is stable, finish the assessment. Make sure that the health history includes a detailed food history and documentation of the reaction, including the food suspected of causing the reaction, the quantity of food ingested, the length of time between ingestion and development of symptoms, the symptoms, what treatment has been administered, and the subsequent response. Note gastrointestinal symptoms such as:

- Burning in the mouth or throat
- Bloating
- Nausea
- Diarrhea

Assess for risk factors such as previous exposure to the food, history of poorly controlled asthma, or an increase in atopic dermatitis flare-ups in relation to food intake.

Inspect the skin for color, rash, hives, or edema. Auscultate the heart and lungs to determine heart rate and to assess for wheezing.

Allergy skin-prick tests and radioallergosorbent blood tests (RASTs) are used widely by physicians and nurse practitioners to look for allergic reactions. However, these tests may have false-positive results, and children may need to avoid many foods unnecessarily (Sloand & Caschera, 2010). Food-specific IgE testing is recommended if the child has a history of food allergy. If the child has episodic symptoms, an oral challenge in a controlled setting may be appropriate. For an oral challenge, the child slowly eats a serving of the offending food over the period of 1 hour. Record vital signs and note the presence or absence of allergic symptoms.

If symptoms are chronic, a trial elimination diet may be indicated. If symptoms resolve without the food, true allergy may be present. On an elimination diet, the child should stop eating all suspicious foods for 1 to 2 weeks and then retry the foods one at a time, over a period of several days, to see whether a similar reaction occurs. Oral challenge testing and retrying of foods after an elimination diet are often done in the physician's or nurse practitioner's office or hospital setting if severe reactions have occurred in the past. If a similar reaction to a previous reaction to a certain food or foods occurs with the oral challenge or elimination diet testing, it is very suggestive of a food allergy. Food avoidance is recommended for those who have a highly predictive reaction to testing or a history of anaphylactic response.

Nursing Management

Initial nursing management is aimed at stabilizing the child's condition if an acute reaction to a food allergen

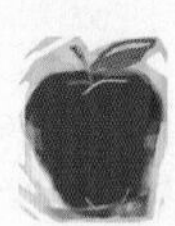

Teaching Guidelines 47.1
ALLERGENS HIDDEN IN FOOD

If Child is Allergic to	Teach Families to Avoid	Unexpected Locations of Common Ingredients
Milk	Artificial butter flavor, casein, lactalbumin, nougat, pudding, whey, yogurt, ghee	Some deli meats and hot dogs, nondairy products, coffee whiteners
Wheat	Cereal extract, couscous, durum, semolina, spelt	Some imitation crab meat and wheat flour shaped to look like shrimp, beef, or pork especially in Asian dishes
Eggs	Albumin, globulin, ovalbumin	Some egg substitutes and foam toppings for drinks, commercially cooked pastas
Peanuts	Fast food cooked in peanut oil, many Asian foods, baked goods with nuts, or foods processed on equipment that also processes peanuts	Brown gravy, barbeque sauce, meat sauce, egg rolls, enchilada sauce, hot chocolate

Adapted from Kids with Food Allergies. (2016). *Allergen avoidance lists*. Retrieved from http://www.kidswithfoodallergies.org/page/top-food-allergens.aspx

is present (see Chapter 51). As stated above, medications used in the treatment of a food allergy reaction include histamine blockers and, in anaphylactic reactions, epinephrine. Teach the child (if appropriate) and the parents how and when to use these medications during an allergic reaction. The child who has been prescribed an EpiPen should carry the pen with him or her at all times. Since these reactions can be so sudden (unknown ingestion of allergen) and severe, it is helpful for the family to have a written emergency plan in case of a reaction.

MANAGING THE CHILD'S DIET

Aim dietary teaching at educating the child and family on how to avoid the offending foods. Families should be extremely careful when reading food labels. A dietitian may be helpful in this teaching process. Teaching Guidelines 47.1 gives information about hidden allergens in food. Teach the parents what "safe" foods can be substituted for offensive ones (Box 47.5). Children with peanut allergy should also avoid tree nuts.

Having a child with a food allergy can be very anxiety producing for parents; they often live in fear that the child may accidentally ingest an allergen. Educate the child and family about allergic reactions to help decrease their anxiety. Teach the child and family how to recognize the signs and symptoms of an allergic reaction. It may be necessary to provide information to day care providers as well as schoolteachers, staff, and camp counselors. Refer families to the Food Allergy & Anaphylaxis Network. A link to this website can be found on thePoint.

BOX 47.5

FOOD SUBSTITUTIONS

- Replace milk with water, fruit juice, rice milk, or soymilk.
- Replace each egg with 1.5 tablespoons each of water and oil and 1 teaspoon baking powder; OR 1 packet plain gelatin with 2 tablespoons warm water added at time of use; OR 1 teaspoon yeast and a quarter-cup warm water.
- Replace peanuts or tree nuts with raisins, dates, or crispy cereal.

Adapted from Winkels, K. (2015). *Allergy-free substitutes*. Retrieved from http://www.eatingwithfoodallergies.com/allergyfreesubstitutes.html

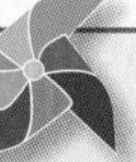

Consider This

The mother of Mina Stepelman (6 years old) is very distraught about the significance of Mina's peanut allergy. She has been prescribed an EpiPen and is comfortable with when and how to use. Mina's mom says tearfully, "I'm just so scared she'll eat the wrong thing when she's not with me. I'm never letting her go to a party alone, or spend the night at someone's house. Even though I've talked to her school nurse, I'm even scared about what she'll eat at school."

Think about if you or your child had this type of significant allergy how would you feel? How would you deal with this perceived risk?

As a nurse, how should respond to Mina's mother?

Anaphylaxis

Anaphylaxis is an acute IgE-mediated response to an allergen that involves many organ systems and may be life-threatening. In addition to nuts, shellfish, eggs, and bee or wasp stings, drugs such as penicillin and NSAIDs, radiopaque dyes, and latex are the leading causes of anaphylaxis (Covar et al., 2014). The reaction is severe and usually starts within 5 to 10 minutes of exposure, though delayed reactions are possible. Histamines and secondary mediators are released from the mast cells and eosinophils in response to contact with an allergen. Cutaneous, cardiopulmonary, gastrointestinal, and neurologic symptoms occur. Vasodilation results in a rapid decrease in plasma volume, leading to the risk of circulatory collapse. Prolonged resuscitation may be needed, and death may occur.

Therapeutic management focuses on assessment and support of the airway, breathing, and circulation. Epinephrine is usually required, and intramuscular or intravenous diphenhydramine is used secondarily. Late-onset reactions can be prevented with corticosteroids.

Nursing Assessment

Assess patency of the airway and adequacy of breathing. Determine if circulation is sufficient. Note level of consciousness. Obtain a brief history, inquiring specifically about allergen exposure. Determine whether the child has received any medication (e.g., epinephrine or diphenhydramine) since the onset of the reaction and what effect the medication had on the symptoms. Table 47.3 gives additional signs and symptoms of anaphylaxis.

TABLE 47.3 CLINICAL MANIFESTATIONS OF ANAPHYLAXIS

Body Area or System	Manifestation
Oral	• Lip, tongue, or palate pruritus • Lip or tongue edema
Cutaneous	• Urticaria (hives), flushing, pruritus, angioedema
Respiratory	• Nasal pruritus, congestion, sneezing, rhinorrhea • Stridor, tightness in the throat, dysphagia, dysphonia, hoarseness • Shortness of breath, dyspnea, tight chest, wheeze
Cardiovascular	• Tachycardia, chest pain, arrhythmia, hypotension
Neurologic	• Syncope, feeling faint, aura of doom, lethargy, disorientation
Gastrointestinal	• Bloating, abdominal pain, diarrhea, vomiting

Adapted from Covar, R. A., Fleischer, D. M., Cho, C., & Boguniewicz, M. (2014). Allergic disorders. In W. W. Hay, M. J. Levin, R. R. Deterding, & M. J. Abzug (Eds.), *Current pediatric diagnosis and treatment* (22nd ed.). New York, NY: McGraw-Hill; and Wagner, C. W. (2013). Anaphylaxis in the pediatric patient: Optimizing management and prevention. *Journal of Pediatric Health Care, 27*(2 S), S5–S17.

Nursing Management

Nursing management initially focuses on supporting the airway, breathing, and circulation. Provide supplemental oxygen by mask or bag-valve-mask ventilation. Administer epinephrine as ordered to reverse the allergic process. Ensure that bronchodilator inhalation treatment (albuterol) is given if bronchospasm is present. Administer intravenous fluids to provide volume expansion. Observe the child for at least 2 hours in case of recurrent attack (Wagner, 2013).

PREVENTING AND MANAGING FUTURE EPISODES

It is critical to educate the family about preventing and managing future episodes. Teach the family how to use injectable epinephrine in case of subsequent allergen exposure. Intramuscular epinephrine may be given via the EpiPen or EpiPen Jr. Dosage is based on the child's weight. The child should carry the pen with him or her at all times. Explain to the child and family that the gray safety release on the EpiPen should never be removed until just before use. In addition, teach the child and family that the thumb, fingers, or hand should not be placed over the black tip. Nursing Procedure 47.1 gives further instructions related to EpiPen use. Instruct the child and family to call 911 and seek immediate medical attention after using the EpiPen. Warn the child that the epinephrine may make him or her feel as if the heart is racing.

Day care providers, school nurses, teachers, and staff who interact with the child must know how to recognize an anaphylactic event. In 2004, Public Law No. 108–377, Asthmatic Schoolchildren's Treatment and Health Management Act, was passed by the U.S. Congress. This law is intended to ensure that students with severe allergies can carry prescribed medications (i.e., EpiPen) with them. All children with allergies should have an action plan in place at the school or day care center. Advise the child to wear a medical ID alert bracelet or necklace at all times.

Teach children and families to avoid known food allergens. Avoid stings from bees and wasps (Hymenoptera) by being alert when eating outdoors, wearing long sleeves and pants when in fields, and having bee and wasp hives or nests removed from areas near the family's home. Immunotherapy (allergy shots) may be indicated in children with a hypersensitivity to stinging insects. Avoid use of cephalosporins in children with severe penicillin allergy. Desensitization is available for children with severe penicillin allergy. Desensitization involves administration of increasingly larger doses of penicillin over a period of hours to days in an intensive care setting.

NURSING PROCEDURE 47.1

Using the Epipen or Epipen JR.

1. Grasp the EpiPen or EpiPen Jr. with the black tip pointing downward, forming a fist (Fig. 1).

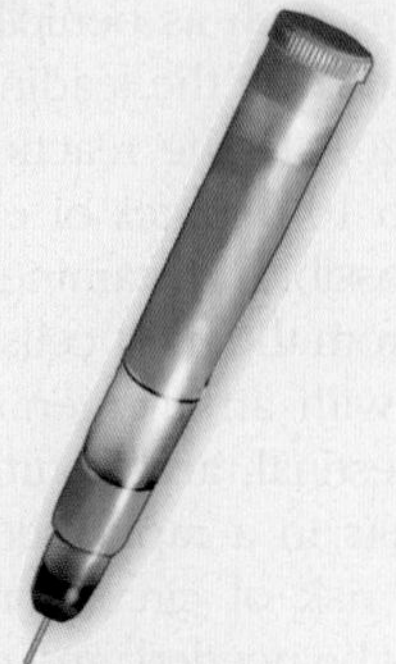

2. With the other hand, pull off the gray safety release.
3. Swing and jab the EpiPen firmly into the outer thigh at a 90-degree angle and hold firmly there for 10 seconds (Figs. 2 and 3).

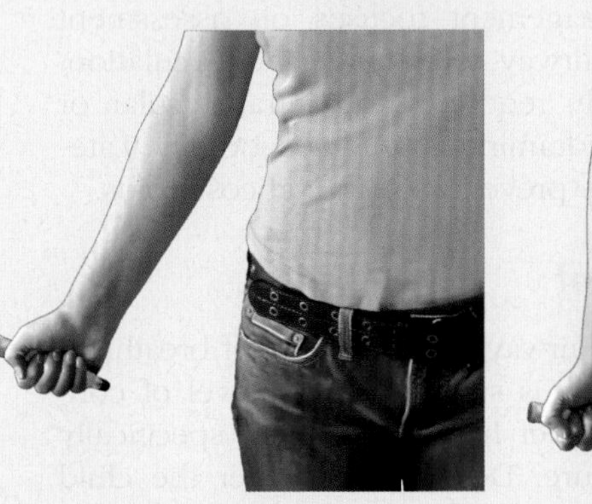

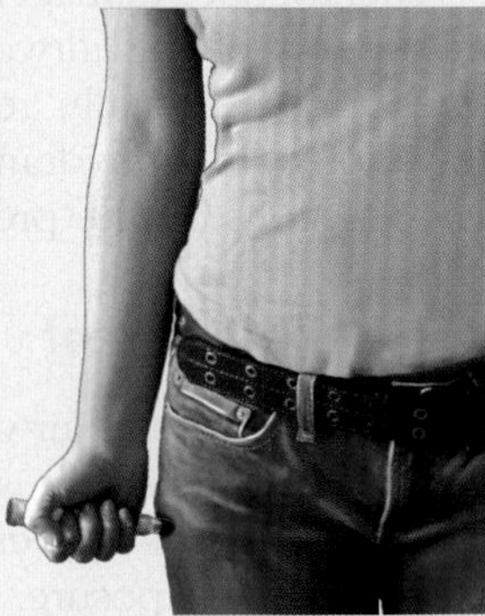

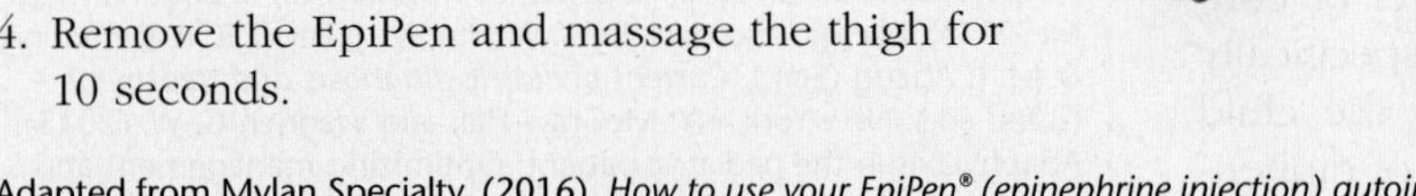

4. Remove the EpiPen and massage the thigh for 10 seconds.

Adapted from Mylan Specialty. (2016). *How to use your EpiPen® (epinephrine injection) autoinjector.* Retrieved from http://www.epipen.com/how-to-use-epipen

Latex Allergy

Latex allergy is an IgE-mediated response to exposure to latex, a natural rubber product used in many common items (especially gloves in the healthcare setting). The pathophysiology of latex allergy is similar to that of food allergy. Avoidance of latex products is recommended for those who are allergic to it. An immediate allergic reaction may occur if a latex-allergic child comes into contact with latex. Latex allergy can also result in anaphylaxis (refer to section above on anaphylaxis).

Nursing Assessment

Screen all children who visit a healthcare facility of any kind for latex allergy. Ask if the child is allergic to rubber gloves or has ever developed hives after exposure to them. Ask the parent if the child has symptoms such as coughing, wheezing, or shortness of breath after glove exposure. Has the child ever had swelling in the mouth or complained that the mouth itched after a dental examination? Determine whether the child has ever had allergic symptoms after eating foods with a known cross-reactivity to latex, such as pear, peach, passion fruit, plum, pineapple, kiwi, fig, grape, cherry, melon, nectarine, papaya, apple, apricot, banana, chestnut, carrot, celery, avocado, tomato, or potato. For the child who has come into contact with latex, assess for symptoms of a reaction such as hives; wheeze; cough; shortness of breath; nasal congestion and rhinorrhea; sneezing; nose, palate, or eye pruritus; or hypotension.

Nursing Management

Nursing management of latex allergy focuses on preventing exposure to latex products. Instruct children and their families to avoid foods with a known cross-reactivity to latex such as those listed above. If the child is exposed to latex, remove the irritating substance and cleanse the area with soap and water. Assess for the need for resuscitation and perform it if needed. Become familiar with your institution's latex allergy policy. Know which products contain latex and which do not. Document latex allergy on the chart, the child's identification band, the medication administration record, and the physician's order sheet. Refer families to resources for persons with latex allergy. Some helpful links are provided on thePoint.

NURSING CARE PLAN 47.1

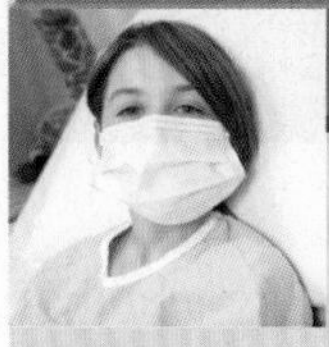

Overview for The Child With an Immunologic Disorder

NURSING DIAGNOSIS: Ineffective protection related to inadequate body defenses, inability to fight infection as evidenced by deficient immunity

Outcome Identification and Evaluation

Child will not experience overwhelming infection: *will be infection-free or able to recover if he or she becomes infected.*

Intervention: ***Preventing Infection***

- Maintain meticulous hand-washing procedures (include family, visitors, staff) *to minimize spread of infectious organisms.*
- Maintain isolation as prescribed *to minimize exposure to infectious organisms.*
- Clean frequently touched surfaces with an appropriate cleanser *to minimize spread of infectious organisms.*
- Educate family and visitors that child should be restricted from contact with known infectious exposures (in hospital and at home) *to encourage cooperation with infection control.*
- Strictly observe medical asepsis *to avoid unintentional introduction of microorganisms.*
- Promote nutrition and appropriate rest *to maximize body's potential to heal.*
- Educate family to contact physician or nurse practitioner if child has known exposure to chickenpox or measles *so that preventive measures (e.g., varicella zoster immunoglobulin [VZIG]) can be taken.*
- Administer vaccines (not live) as prescribed *to prevent common childhood communicable diseases.*
- Administer prophylactic antibiotics as prescribed *to prevent infection with opportunistic organisms.*

NURSING DIAGNOSIS: Imbalanced nutrition, less than body requirements, related to poor appetite, chronic illness, debilitated state, concurrent illness as evidenced by poor growth, weight gain and stature increases less than expected, poor head growth

Outcome Identification and Evaluation

Child will consume adequate intake: *will demonstrate appropriate weight gain and growth of length/height and/or head circumference.*

Intervention: ***Promoting Adequate Nutritional Intake***

- Monitor growth (weight and height/length weekly) *to determine progress toward goal.*
- Determine realistic goal for weight gain for age (consulting dietitian if necessary) *to have a specific outcome to work toward.*
- Observe child's physical ability to eat *(if pain from candidiasis or motor impairment is present, will need additional interventions).*
- Provide nutrient-rich meals and snacks *to maximize caloric intake.*
- Supplement milkshakes with protein powder or other additives *to maximize caloric intake.*
- Provide child's favorite foods *to encourage increased intake.*
- Provide smaller, more frequent meals *to reduce sensation of fullness and increase overall intake.*
- If vomiting is an issue, administer antiemetics as ordered prior to meals *to provide optimal state for success at mealtime.*

NURSING DIAGNOSIS: Impaired skin integrity related to disease process or photosensitivity as evidenced by skin rash or alopecia

Outcome Identification and Evaluation

Skin integrity will be maintained: *secondary infection will not occur, rash will not increase.*

(continued)

NURSING CARE PLAN 47.1

Overview for The Child With an Immunologic Disorder (continued)

Intervention: ***Preventing Skin Impairment***

- Assess and monitor extent and location of rash *to provide baseline information and evaluate success of interventions.*
- Keep skin clean and dry *to prevent secondary infection.*
- For the child with eczema, apply topical medications as ordered *to decrease inflammatory response.*
- For the child with limited mobility, turn frequently and use specialty mattress or bed *to prevent pressure ulcers.*
- Implement a written plan of care directed toward topical treatment of skin integrity impairment *to provide consistency of care and documentation.*
- Educate child and family to limit direct sun exposure and use sunscreen *to prevent sun damage.*

NURSING DIAGNOSIS: Activity intolerance related to joint pain, fatigue or weakness, concurrent illness as evidenced by dyspnea, lack of desire to participate in play, inability to maintain usual routine

Outcome Identification and Evaluation

Child will participate in activities: *will demonstrate easy work of breathing and participate in daily routine and play.*

Intervention: ***Promoting Activity***

- Cluster care *to decrease disturbances and allow for longer uninterrupted rest periods.*
- Pace activities and encourage regular rest periods *to conserve energy.*
- Administer early morning warm bath *to ease a.m. stiffness (juvenile arthritis).*
- Use assistive devices such as splints and orthotics *to improve physical function.*
- Plan developmentally appropriate activities that the child can participate in while in bed *to encourage play and continued development.*
- Schedule activities for the time of day the child usually has the most energy *to encourage successful participation.*

NURSING DIAGNOSIS: Delayed growth and development related to physical effects of chronic illness, or physical disability (juvenile arthritis) as evidenced by delay in meeting expected milestones

Outcome Identification and Evaluation

Development will be enhanced: *child will make continued progress toward expected developmental milestones.*

Intervention: ***Enhancing Growth and Development***

- Screen for developmental capabilities *to determine child's current level of functioning.*
- Offer age-appropriate toys, play, and activities (including gross motor) *to encourage further development.*
- Encourage peer contact through telephone, e-mail, or letters *to promote/continue socialization.*
- Perform interventions as prescribed by physical or occupational therapist: *repeat participation in those activities helps child improve function and acquire developmental skills.*
- Provide support to families of children with developmental delay: *progress in achieving developmental milestones can be slow, and ongoing motivation is needed.*
- Encourage child to continue schoolwork *so that child will not fall behind.*
- Reinforce positive attributes in the child *to maintain motivation.*

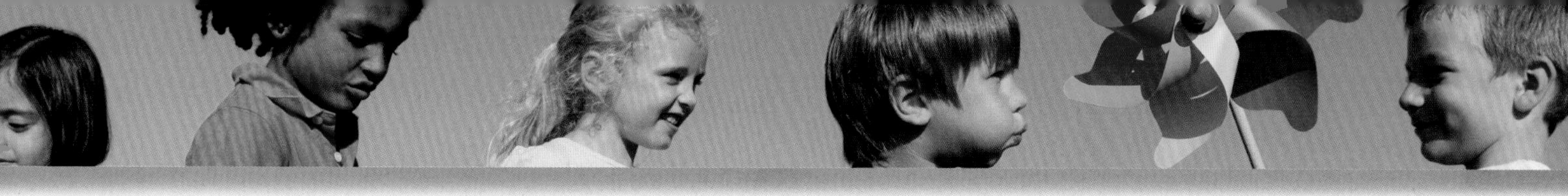

KEY CONCEPTS

- Waning of maternal antibodies in early infancy while humoral immunity is developing leads to physiologic hypogammaglobulinemia, placing the young infant at risk for overwhelming infection.
- Infants and young children have large lymph nodes, tonsils, and thymus compared with adults.
- Infants have decreased phagocytic activity, placing them at higher risk for serious infection.
- Children with immune disorders often show a decreased or absent response to delayed hypersensitivity skin testing (e.g., the tuberculosis test).
- The ELISA test for HIV detects only antibodies to HIV (which in the infant may be maternal in origin), whereas the PCR test for HIV tests for HIV genetic material, making it the more accurate test for HIV infection in infants and young children.
- Primary immune deficiencies such as SCID and Wiskott–Aldrich syndrome are congenital and serious; they can be cured only by bone marrow or stem cell transplantation.
- SLE is a chronic autoimmune disorder that can affect any organ system, primarily causing vasculitis.
- Juvenile idiopathic arthritis results in chronic pain and affects growth and development as well as school performance.
- Nasal, palatal, or throat pruritus and difficulty breathing may indicate an anaphylactic reaction.
- Various forms of hypogammaglobulinemia may be treated with exogenous immunoglobulin administered intravenously every several weeks, allowing children to lead a healthier life with fewer infections.
- Children with severe allergy or previous anaphylactic episodes must avoid contact with allergens.
- Nursing management of lupus focuses on preventing flare-ups and complications.
- Managing pain, maintaining mobility, and administering disease-modifying medications are key nursing interventions in the management of juvenile idiopathic arthritis.
- HIV infection may be prevented in infants by prenatal screening and maternal treatment, as well as postnatal treatment with zidovudine.
- HIV infection in children often results in encephalopathy and developmental delay.
- Spread of HIV infection can be prevented in adolescence by avoiding high-risk behaviors.
- For children with immune deficiency or autoimmune disease, prevention of infection is a primary nursing concern.
- A chronic illness such as immune deficiency, SLE, or juvenile arthritis has a significant impact on the family as well as the child.
- When planning care for the child with an immune deficiency or autoimmune disorder, the nurse should include the child and the family.
- To promote proper growth, encourage the child with an immune or autoimmune disorder to eat a balanced diet.
- Teach families of children with immune deficiencies about infection prevention.
- Teach the family of the child with juvenile arthritis about ways to decrease pain while increasing or maintaining the child's mobility.
- Teach families of children with severe allergy how to avoid allergens and how to use the EpiPen. Make sure that staff at the child's school or day care center are aware of the allergy.
- Explain to the child with severe allergy the importance of wearing a medical ID alert bracelet or necklace.

REFERENCES AND RECOMMENDED READINGS

Atkinson, W., Wolfe, S., & Hamborsky, J. (Eds.). (2012). *Epidemiology and prevention of vaccine-preventable diseases* (12th ed.). Washington, DC: Public Health Foundation.

Blaese, R. M., Bonilla, F. A., Stiehm, E. R., & Younger, M. E. (Eds.). (2013). *Patient and family handbook for primary immune deficiency diseases* (5th ed.). Towson, MD: Immune Deficiency Foundation.

Bonilla, F. A. (2015). *Severe combined immunodeficiency (SCID): An overview.* Retrieved from http://www.uptodate.com/contents/severe-combined-immunodeficiency-scid-an-overview

Carpenito-Moyet, L. J. (2013). *Nursing diagnosis: Application to clinical practice* (14th ed.). Philadelphia, PA: Lippincott Williams & Wilkins.

Centers for Disease Control and Prevention. (2015). *HIV surveillance report, 2013; vol. 25.* Atlanta, GA: Author.

Corbett, J. A., & Banks, A. D. (2013). *Laboratory tests and diagnostic procedures with nursing diagnoses* (8th ed.). Upper Saddle River, NJ: Pearson Education Inc.

Covar, R. A., Fleischer, D. M., Cho, C., & Boguniewicz, M. (2014). Allergic disorders. In W. W. Hay, M. J. Levin, R. R. Deterding, & M. J. Abzug (Eds.), *Current pediatric diagnosis and treatment* (22nd ed.). New York, NY: McGraw-Hill.

Cruse, R. P. (2014). *Epidemiology, clinical features, and diagnosis of Guillain-Barré syndrome in children*. Retrieved from http://www.uptodate.com/contents/epidemiology-clinical-features-and-diagnosis-of-guillain-barre-syndrome-in-children.

De Santis, J. P., Garcia, A., Chaparro, A., & Beltran, O. (2014). Integration versus disintegration: A grounded theory study of adolescent and young adult development in the context of perinatally-acquired HIV infection. *Journal of Pediatric Nursing, 29*, 422–435.

Fahrner, R., & Romano, S. (2010). HIV infection and AIDS. In P. J. Allen, J. A. Vessey, & N. A. Schapiro (Eds.), *Primary care of the child with a chronic condition* (5th ed.). St. Louis, MO: Mosby.

Hauk, P. J., Johnston, R. B., & Liu, A. H. (2014). Immunodeficiency. In W. W. Hay, M. J. Levin, R. R. Deterding, & M. J. Abzug (Eds.), *Current pediatric diagnosis and treatment* (22nd ed.). New York, NY: McGraw-Hill.

Health Resources and Services Administration, the HIV/AIDS Program. (n.d.). *About the Ryan White HIV/AIDS program*. Retrieved from http://hab.hrsa.gov/abouthab/aboutprogram.html

Horvath, T., Azman, H., Kennedy, G. E., & Rutherford, G. W. (2012). *Mobile phone text messaging for promoting adherence to antiretroviral therapy in patients with HIV infection. The Cochrane Library 2012, 3*. Indianapolis, IN: John Wiley & Sons.

Hutchinson, C., & Feldman, B. M. (2016a). *Juvenile dermatomyositis and polymyositis: Epidemiology, pathogenesis, and clinical manifestations*. Retrieved from http://www.uptodate.com/contents/juvenile-dermatomyositis-and-polymyositis-epidemiology-pathogenesis-and-clinical-manifestations

Hutchinson, C., & Feldman, B. M. (2016b). *Juvenile dermatomyositis and polymyositis: Treatment, complications, and prognosis*. Retrieved from http://www.uptodate.com/contents/juvenile-dermatomyositis-and-polymyositis-treatment-complications-and-prognosis

Jeffrey Modell Foundation. (2013). *10 warning signs of primary immunodeficiency*. Retrieved from http://downloads.info4pi.org/pdfs/General10WarningSignsFINAL.pdf

Johnson, B. (2014). Overview of neonatal lupus. *Journal of Pediatric Health Care, 28*(4), 331–341.

Jones, K. B., & Higgins, G. C. (2010). Juvenile rheumatoid arthritis. In P. J. Allen, J. A. Vessey, & N. A. Schapiro (Eds.), *Primary care of the child with a chronic condition* (5th ed.). St. Louis, MO: Mosby.

Kids with Food Allergies. (2016). *Allergen avoidance lists*. Retrieved from http://www.kidswithfoodallergies.org/page/top-food-allergens.aspx

Lehman, T. J. A. (2015). Systemic lupus erythematosus (SLE) in children: Clinical manifestations and diagnosis. Retrieved from http://www.uptodate.com/contents/systemic-lupus-erythematosus-sle-in-children-clinical-manifestations-and-diagnosis

Lierl, M. B. (2011). Allergen immunotherapy: Shots for asthma, wheezing, and bee sting. *Pediatric Annals, 40*(4), 192–199.

Liew, W. K., & Kang, P. B. (2013). Update on juvenile myasthenia gravis. *Current Opinion in Pediatrics, 25*(6), 694–700.

Mattingly, E. (2011). Lupus in adolescents. *Advance for NPs & PAs, 2*(4), 27–32.

Mayo Foundation. (2016). *Pediatric test reference values*. Retrieved from http://www.mayomedicallaboratories.com/test-info/pediatric/refvalues/reference.php

McFarland, E. J. (2014). Human immunodeficiency virus infection. In W. W. Hay, M. J. Levin, R. R. Deterding, & M. J. Abzug (Eds.), *Current pediatric diagnosis and treatment* (22nd ed.). New York, NY: McGraw-Hill.

Mylan Specialty. (2016). *How to use your EpiPen® (epinephrine injection) autoinjector*. Retrieved from http://www.epipen.com/how-to-use-epipen

Norville, R., & Tomlinson, D. (2010). Hematopoietic stem cell transplantation. In D. Tomlinson & N. E. Kline (Eds.), *Pediatric oncology nursing: Advanced clinical handbook* (2nd ed.). New York, NY: Springer.

Ochs, H. D. (2015). *Wiskott-Aldrich syndrome*. Retrieved from http://www.uptodate.com/contents/wiskott-aldrich-syndrome

Panel on Antiretroviral Therapy and Medical Management of HIV-Infected Children. (2016). *Guidelines for the use of antiretroviral agents in pediatric HIV infection*. Retrieved from http://aidsinfo.nih.gov/contentfiles/lvguidelines/pediatricguidelines.pdf

Siberry, G. K., Abzug, M. J., & Nachman, S. (2013). Executive summary: 2013 update of the guidelines for the prevention and treatment of opportunistic infections in HIV-exposed and HIV-infected children. *Pediatric Infectious Disease Journal, 32*(12), 1303–1307.

Soep, J. B. (2014). Rheumatic diseases. In W. W. Hay, M. J. Levin, R. R. Deterding, & M. J. Abzug (Eds.), *Current pediatric diagnosis and treatment* (22nd ed.). New York, NY: McGraw-Hill.

Sloand, E., & Caschera, J. (2010). Allergies. In P. J. Allen, J. A. Vessey, & N. A. Schapiro (Eds.), *Primary care of the child with a chronic condition* (5th ed.). St. Louis, MO: Mosby.

Stanley, L. C., & Ward-Smith, P. (2011). The diagnosis and management of juvenile idiopathic arthritis. *Journal of Pediatric Health Care, 25*(3), 191–194.

Taketomo, C. K., Hodding, J. H., & Kraus, D. M. (2013). *Pediatric & neonatal dosage handbook* (20th ed.). Hudson, OH: Lexicomp.

Tofferi, J. K. (2015). *Avascular necrosis*. Retrieved from http://emedicine.medscape.com/article/333364-overview

Tosi, M. F. (2014). Normal and impaired immunologic responses to infection. In J. Cherry, G. J. Demmler-Harrison, S. L. Kaplan, W. J. Steinbach, & P. Hotez (Eds.), *Feigin & Cherry's textbook of pediatric infectious disease* (7th ed.). Philadelphia, PA: Saunders.

UNAIDS. (2014). *Children and HIV fact sheet*. Geneva, Switzerland: World Health Organization.

U.S. House of Representatives. (2004). *Public law No. 108–377 asthmatic schoolchildren's treatment and health management act of 2004*. Washington, DC: Library of Congress.

Varadhi, A., Hageman, J. R., & Yu, K. O. A. (2013). The 'five fingers' of the diagnostic evaluation for suspected immunodeficiency. *Pediatric Annals, 42*(5), 210–215.

Wagner, C. W. (2013). Anaphylaxis in the pediatric patient: Optimizing management and prevention. *Journal of Pediatric Health Care, 27*(2S), S5–S17.

Ward, T. M., Sonney, J., Ringold, S., Stockfish, S., Wallace, C.A., & Landis, C. A. (2014). Sleep disturbances and behavior problems in children with and without arthritis. *Journal of Pediatric Nursing, 29*, 321–328.

Winkels, K. (2015). *Allergy-free substitutes*. Retrieved from http://www.eatingwithfoodallergies.com/allergyfreesubstitutes.html

Woo, C. K., & Bahna, S. L. (2011). Evaluation of the child with immunodeficiency disorder. *Pediatric Annals, 40*(4), 205–211.

CHAPTER WORKSHEET

MULTIPLE CHOICE QUESTIONS

1. The nurse is caring for a 6-year-old with juvenile idiopathic arthritis. The mother states that she has trouble getting her daughter out of bed in the morning and believes the girl's behavior is due to a desire to avoid going to school. What is the best advice by the nurse?
   a. Refer the girl to a psychologist for evaluation of school phobia related to chronic illness.
   b. Administer a warm bath every morning before school.
   c. Give the child her prescribed NSAIDs 30 minutes before getting out of bed.
   d. Allow her to stay in bed some mornings if she wants.
2. A 14-year-old with systemic lupus erythematosus wants to know how to care for her skin. What should the nurse teach this adolescent?
   a. Careful sun tanning will give her skin an attractive color.
   b. No special skin care is needed.
   c. Use sunscreen daily to avoid rashes.
   d. Use makeup to camouflage the butterfly rash on her face.
3. The mother of a child with hypogammaglobulinemia reports that her child had a fever and slight chills with an intravenous gammaglobulin infusion last month. She wants to know what other course of treatment might be available. What is the best response by the nurse?
   a. Administration of acetaminophen or diphenhydramine prior to the next infusion may decrease the incidence of fever or chills.
   b. Giving the gammaglobulin intramuscularly is recommended to prevent a reaction.
   c. Talk to her physician or nurse practitioner about alternative medications that may be used to boost the gammaglobulin level in the blood.
   d. If the child is no longer experiencing frequent infections, then the IV infusions may not be necessary.
4. A 4-month-old infant born to an HIV-infected mother is going into foster care because the mother is too ill to care for the child. The foster mother wants to know if the infant is also infected. What is the best response by the nurse?
   a. "It's too early to know; we have to wait until the infant has symptoms."
   b. "Since the mother is so ill, it's likely the child is also infected with HIV."
   c. "The ELISA test is positive, so the child is definitely infected."
   d. "The PCR test is positive; this indicates HIV infection, which may or may not progress to AIDS."
5. A mother has received instructions about avoiding wheat and soy allergens. Which response by the mother would indicate that further education is needed?
   a. "I will not feed my child any breads made with wheat flour."
   b. "I will allow my child to eat semolina pasta, the kind he loves."
   c. "I will not feed my child shakes made with soy protein."
   d. "I will read labels to be sure I am avoiding wheat and soy."
6. What is the priority nursing intervention for the child recently admitted with Guillain–Barré syndrome?
   a. Perform range-of-motion exercises.
   b. Take temperature every 4 hours.
   c. Monitor respiratory status closely.
   d. Assess skin frequently.

DOSAGE CALCULATION QUESTION

1. The nurse is caring for a term newborn born to a mother with HIV infection. The infant weighs 6 lb 5 oz. The medication order reads: zidovudine 25 mg PO twice daily. Zidovudine is supplied as 50 mg/5 mL. How many milliliters will the nurse administer? Round to the nearest tenth.

CRITICAL THINKING EXERCISES

1. Develop a discharge teaching plan for a 14-year-old with systemic lupus erythematosus who will be taking corticosteroids long term.
2. Devise a developmental stimulation plan for a 22-month-old with HIV infection and encephalopathy with developmental delay (to the level of a 9-month-old).
3. Determine an appropriate nursing plan of care for an infant who has undergone bone marrow transplantation for SCID.
4. Develop a prioritized list of nursing diagnoses for a child with HIV infection, candidiasis, poor growth, and pneumonia requiring oxygen.
5. A child with recurrent infections is being evaluated. Other than information about onset of symptoms and events leading up to this present episode, what other types of information would the nurse ask while obtaining the history?

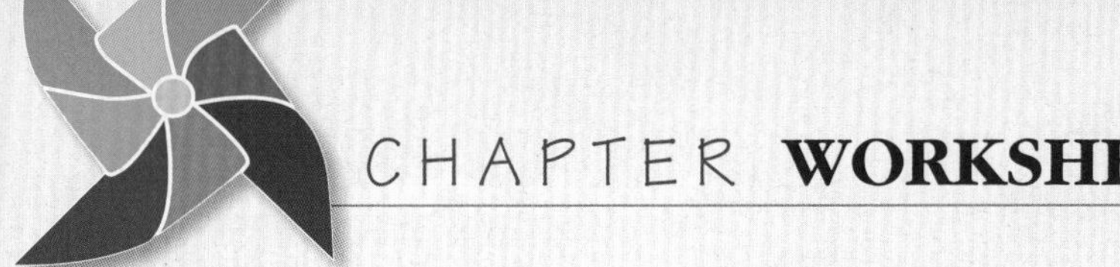

CHAPTER WORKSHEET

STUDY ACTIVITIES

1. In the clinical setting, compare the growth and development of two children the same age, one with HIV infection and one who has been healthy.
2. Attend an outpatient clinic that provides care to children with HIV infection. Observe the physician or nurse practitioner during office visits and attend a multidisciplinary planning meeting. Identify the role of the registered nurse in providing family education, coordination of care, and referrals.
3. Conduct an Internet search to determine the educational material available to children and their families related to immune deficiencies, autoimmune disorders, or allergies.
4. Research your clinical institution's policies related to latex allergy, alternative products available at the institution, and how to obtain them for a child with latex allergy. Provide a presentation to your clinical group about your findings.

BRINGING IT ALL TOGETHER: A CASE STUDY

Jake Reddington, a 2-year-old diagnosed with HIV infection, is brought to the clinic by his aunt for his regular check-up. His aunt has recently taken over the care of Jake since his mother is too ill with HIV infection to care for him.

Go to thePoint **to find questions to consider about this case.**

48

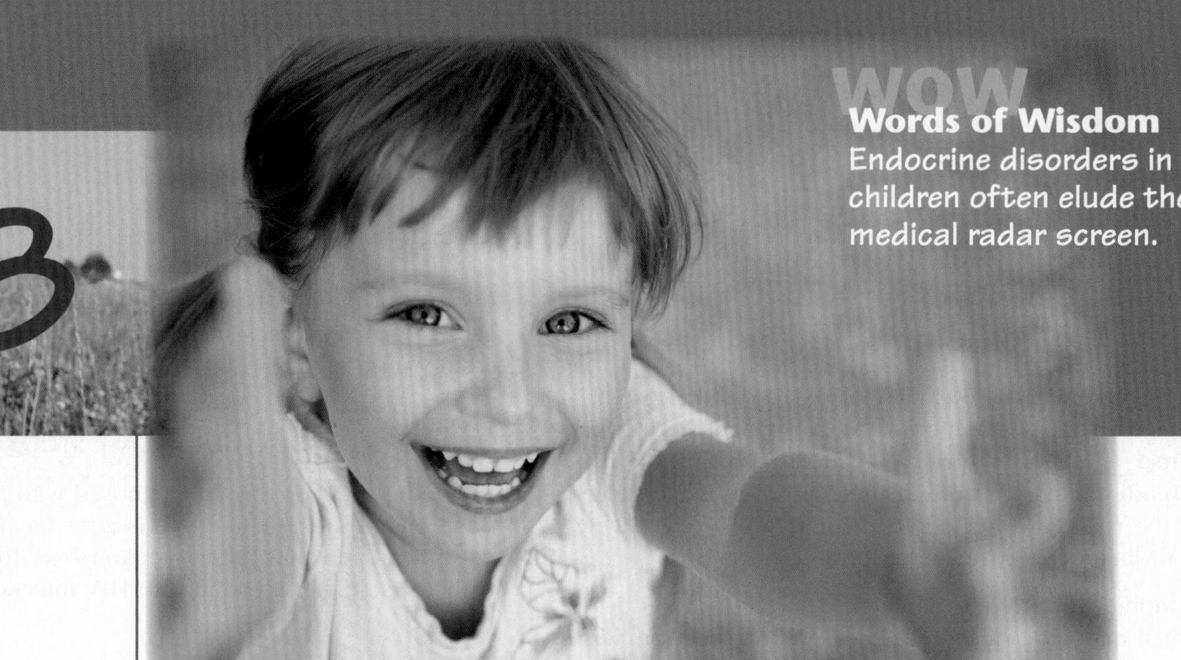
WOW
Words of Wisdom
Endocrine disorders in children often elude the medical radar screen.

Nursing Care of the Child With an Alteration in Metabolism/Endocrine Disorder

KEY TERMS

adrenarche
constitutional delay
diabetic ketoacidosis (DKA)
exophthalmos
goiter
hemoglobin A1C
hirsutism
hormone
hyperfunction
hypofunction
menarche
polydipsia
polyuria

Learning Objectives

Upon completion of the chapter, the learner will be able to:

1. Describe the major components and functions of a child's endocrine system.
2. Differentiate between the anatomic and physiologic differences of the endocrine system in children versus adults.
3. Identify the essential assessment elements, common diagnostic procedures, and laboratory tests associated with the diagnosis of endocrine disorders in children.
4. Identify the common medications and treatment modalities used for palliation of endocrine disorders in children.
5. Distinguish specific disorders of the endocrine system affecting children.
6. Link the clinical manifestations of specific disorders in the endocrine system of a child with the appropriate nursing diagnoses.
7. Establish the nursing outcomes, evaluative criteria, and interventions for a child with specific disorders in the endocrine system.
8. Develop child/family teaching plans for the child with an endocrine disorder.

***Carlos Rodriguez*, 12 years old, is seen in the clinic today with complaints of weakness, fatigue, blurred vision, and headaches. His mother states, "Carlos' teacher has noticed mood changes and is concerned about his behavior at school. He's always been a good boy. I'm not sure what's going on."**

Metabolism refers to all physical and chemical reaction occurring in the body's cells that are necessary to sustain life (Herzing University - Orlando, 2014). Nurses encounter potential and actual alterations in metabolism in all types of clients and must detect problems and intervene early to prevent life threatening or long-term complications. The endocrine system consists of various glands, tissues, or clusters of cells that produce and release hormones. **Hormones** are chemical messengers that stimulate and/or regulate the actions of other tissues, organs, or other endocrine glands that have specific receptors to a hormone. Along with the nervous system, the endocrine milieu influences all physiologic effects such as growth and development, metabolic processes related to fluid and electrolyte balance and energy production, sexual maturation and reproduction, and the body's response to stress. The release patterns of the hormones vary, but the level in the body is maintained within specified limits to preserve health.

Alterations in metabolism develop in the endocrine system when there is a deficiency (**hypofunction**) or excess (**hyperfunction**) of a specific hormone. In children, alterations in metabolism/endocrine conditions often develop insidiously and result from an insufficient production of hormones. If the problem is not diagnosed and treated early, delayed growth and development, cognitive impairments, or death may result. Generally, the treatment plan involves correction of the underlying reason for the dysfunction, such as surgical removal of a tumor, and supplementation of missing hormones or adjustment of specific hormone levels. This allows most children to live normal lives.

VARIATIONS IN ANATOMY AND PHYSIOLOGY

The organs or tissues of the endocrine system include the hypothalamus, pituitary gland, thyroid gland, parathyroid glands, adrenal glands, gonads, and islets of Langerhans located in the pancreas. Figure 48.1 shows the location of the organs or tissues involved in the endocrine system. Typically, most endocrine glands begin to develop during the first trimester of gestation, but their development is incomplete at birth. Thus, complete hormonal control is lacking during the early years of life, and the infant cannot appropriately balance fluid concentration, electrolytes, amino acids, glucose, and trace substances.

Hormone Production and Secretion

The hypothalamic–pituitary axis produces a number of releasing and inhibiting hormones that regulate the function of many of the other endocrine glands, including the thyroid gland, the adrenal glands, and the male and female gonads. Some glands regulate their function in connection with the nervous system, such as the islets of Langerhans in the pancreas and the parathyroid glands. Many other cells in the body secrete hormones such as the pineal gland, the scattered epithelial cells in the gastrointestinal tract, and the thymus. Disorders related to these other cells are discussed in other chapters in this textbook.

Figure 48.1 shows the major glands, the hormones produced by the glands, and the effect each hormone has on the target cell, tissue, or organ. The process of hormone production and secretion involves the principle of feedback control. One gland produces a hormone that affects another endocrine gland. Once the physiologic effect is achieved, this gland, known as the target organ, inhibits the further release of the original hormone. The reverse occurs when the first gland detects low levels of the target gland hormone. If the original gland does not release enough of the hormone, the inhibition process stops so that the gland increases the production of the hormone. The endocrine system and the nervous system work closely together to maintain an optimal internal environment for the body, known as homeostasis.

COMMON MEDICAL TREATMENTS

Primarily, the treatment of endocrine disorders involves decreasing hormone production (in cases of hypersecretion) or replacing the hormones (in cases of hypofunction). The first step in treating many of these disorders is to screen for potential problems, especially when familial patterns are present. Since the proper functioning of the endocrine system is critical to growth and development, the child's growth is affected by endocrine dysfunction and lack of treatment may lead to serious problems, such as intellectual disability or even death. Early treatment is often associated with better prognosis and prevention of long-term problems. The next step in treatment involves identifying underlying causes for the dysfunction (e.g., a tumor or growth that requires surgical removal or irradiation). The use of supplemental hormone in cases of hypofunction is generally successful in children, as is the use of inhibiting substances in cases of hyperfunction.

Common Medical Treatments 48.1 describes the common treatments used in children with endocrine disorders. The table explains and gives indications for each treatment as well as relevant nursing implications. Advances in technology and our understanding of molecular biology continue to increase our knowledge of these disorders and the modalities needed to prevent them or improve quality of life for affected children. These advances are vital, since the whole body is influenced by the endocrine milieu.

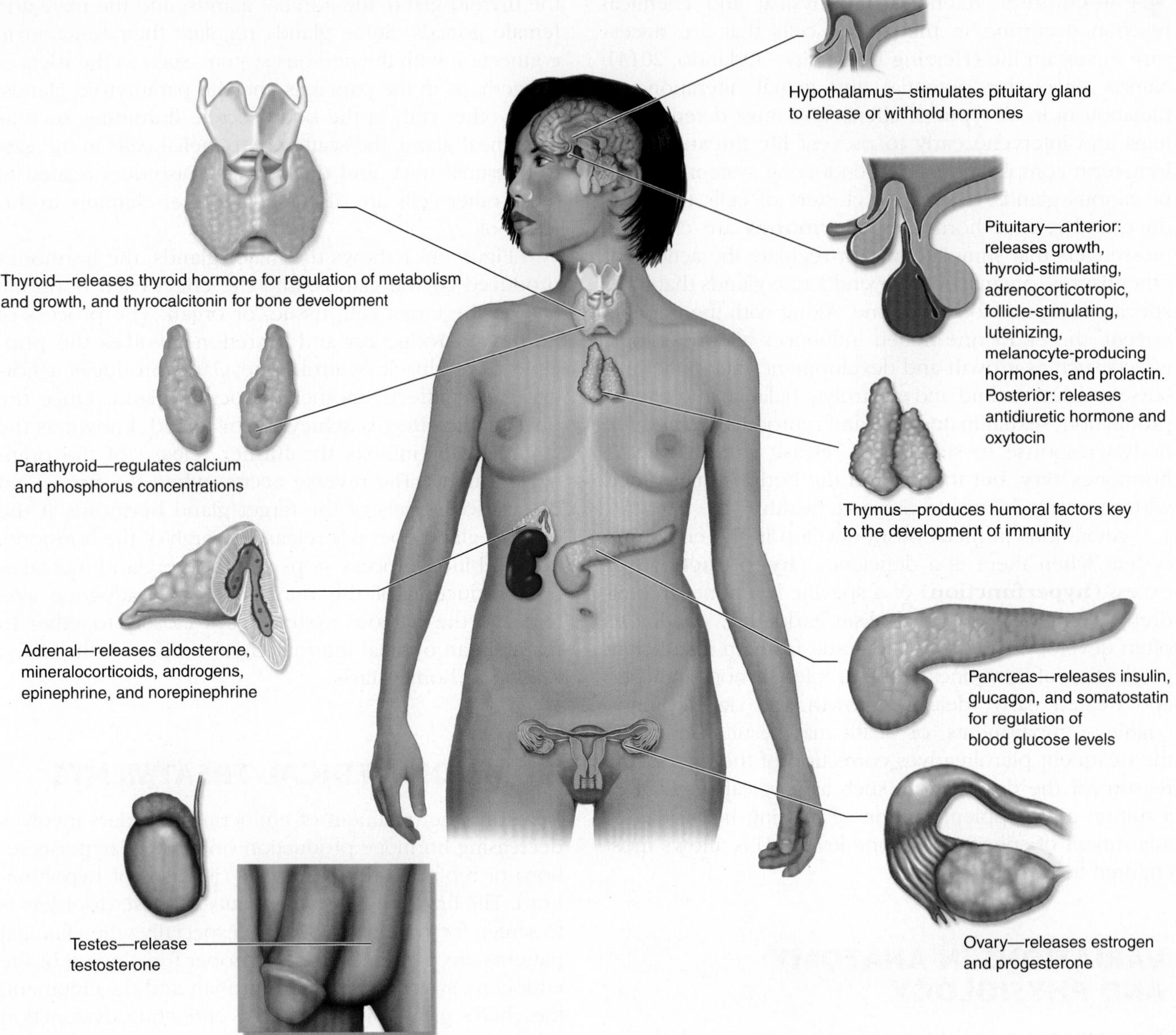
Hypothalamus—stimulates pituitary gland to release or withhold hormones
Pituitary—anterior: releases growth, thyroid-stimulating, adrenocorticotropic, follicle-stimulating, luteinizing, melanocyte-producing hormones, and prolactin. Posterior: releases antidiuretic hormone and oxytocin
Thyroid—releases thyroid hormone for regulation of metabolism and growth, and thyrocalcitonin for bone development
Thymus—produces humoral factors key to the development of immunity
Parathyroid—regulates calcium and phosphorus concentrations
Adrenal—releases aldosterone, mineralocorticoids, androgens, epinephrine, and norepinephrine
Pancreas—releases insulin, glucagon, and somatostatin for regulation of blood glucose levels
Testes—release testosterone
Ovary—releases estrogen and progesterone

FIGURE 48.1 **Location of the endocrine glands in the body, with the major effects of the glands listed.**

Drug Guide 48.1 lists the medications most commonly used to treat endocrine disorders. The table gives the actions and indications of each drug, as well as pertinent nursing implications. Many of the medications are synthetic preparations of the actual hormones. It is important to maintain specific blood levels of the drugs to mimic the actual hormone in the body. Nurses must monitor for side effects of too little or too much of the hormone in the child's system. Most endocrine disorders in children require treatment and follow-up with a pediatric endocrinologist as well as a multidisciplinary team that includes a registered nurse who specializes in this area.

NURSING PROCESS OVERVIEW FOR THE CHILD WITH AN ENDOCRINE DISORDER

The nursing care of the child with an endocrine disorder requires astute assessment skills, accurate nursing diagnoses and expected outcomes, skilled interventions, and evaluation of the entire process. Children, especially very young ones, easily develop imbalances such as fluid and electrolyte disturbances that can cause further problems. Most of the endocrine disorders are chronic conditions that require ongoing care related to health maintenance, education, developmental issues,

COMMON MEDICAL TREATMENTS 48.1

Treatment	Explanation	Indications	Nursing Implications
Surgery	Surgical removal of tumors or cysts	Any endocrine malfunction caused by the presence of a mass	• Provide routine preoperative and postoperative care, depending on location and extent of surgery. • Keep family informed of choices.
Irradiation/radioactive iodine	Radiation is used to influence the hormone secretion of a gland; it is less invasive than surgery.	Hyperfunction of an endocrine gland; may be used when surgery is not possible	• Prepare child for specific procedures following protocols. • Explain the procedure. • Check to ensure child has no sensitivity to iodine preparations.
Glucose monitoring	Fingerstick blood sample several times per day	Monitoring of glucose control	• Teach family appropriate procedure. • Refer family to sources for equipment and supplies. • Assist family to develop a system of record keeping that works for them.
Dietary interventions (medical nutrition therapy)	Restriction or manipulation of dietary intake	Diabetes mellitus	• Refer family to a dietitian specializing in pediatric diabetes mellitus. • Reinforce teaching related to special diets.

DRUG GUIDE 48.1 COMMON DRUGS FOR ENDOCRINE DISORDERS

Medication	Actions/Indications	Nursing Implications
Insulin	Used for DM to replace body's natural insulin, which is necessary for proper glucose use. Indicated for DM type 1 and, sometimes, DM type 2	• Monitor vital signs and blood glucose levels. • Educate child and family on proper techniques, actions, and adverse effects. • Rotate site of injections to prevent adipose hypertrophy.
Oral hypoglycemic drugs (glipizide, glyburide, metformin)	Assist body's production of insulin by stimulating β cells to secrete more insulin Indicated for DM type 2	• Monitor vital signs and glucose levels. • Administer with food to minimize gastric upset. • Instruct child and family on use of drug and adverse effects. • Warn family that some over-the-counter or other drugs may increase hypoglycemic effect.
Growth hormone (GH)/somatropin (Humatrope)	Stimulates linear bone, skeletal muscle, and organ growth Used for GH deficiency, growth failure related to inadequate pituitary hormone	• Monitor blood sugar and electrolyte levels. • Administer before epiphyses are fused. • Monitor growth with accurate measurements. • Instruct child and family on appropriate route and method of administration. • Periodic thyroid function tests will be needed. • May interact with glucocorticoid therapy. • Monitor for limping or complaints in knee or hip related to slipped epiphysis.
Octreotide acetate (Sandostatin)	Suppresses GH release Indicated for acromegaly	• Monitor for biliary tract abnormalities, glucose tolerance, and hypothyroidism. • Give subcutaneous injections between meals to decrease gastric effects.

(continued)

DRUG GUIDE 48.1 COMMON DRUGS FOR ENDOCRINE DISORDERS (continued)

Medication	Actions/Indications	Nursing Implications
Corticosteroids (dexamethasone or hydrocortisone)	Cortisol replacement in congenital adrenal hyperplasia, absence of adrenal glands. Also used to close epiphyseal plates in hyperpituitarism.	• Give with milk or food. • May need to increase dose if child is ill or runs fever • Monitor for edema, weight gain, glycosuria, signs of infection, and symptoms of peptic ulcer development. • Do not decrease dose or abruptly stop drug to avoid adrenal crisis.
Desmopressin acetate (DDAVP)	Synthetic antidiuretic hormone that promotes reabsorption of water by action on renal tubules Used to control diabetes insipidus	• Monitor for water intoxication, signs and symptoms of hyponatremia, and adverse effects such as nasal irritation, headache, nausea, and increased blood pressure. • Record fluid intake and output and weigh child daily. • Titrate dose until appropriate fluid output is obtained. • Instruct child and family in proper intranasal administration. • Avoid over-the-counter cough/hay fever preparations, as they may decrease the drug response. • Store in refrigerator.
Levothyroxine (Synthroid)	Thyroid hormone replacement for hypothyroidism	• Check blood pressure and pulse before each dose. • Monitor fluid intake and output, daily weights, and thyroid function tests. • Watch for thyroid storm. • Report irritability or anxiety. • Instruct child and family to avoid over-the-counter preparations with iodine or foods such as soybeans, iodized salt, tofu, and turnips. • Administer at same time each day.
Methimazole, propylthiouracil	Antithyroid drug; blocks synthesis of T_3 and T_4 Indicated for hyperthyroidism	• Check pulse and blood pressure before each dose. • Monitor input and output, daily weights, serum T_3 and T_4 levels; watch for edema, leukopenia, thrombocytopenia, or agranulocytosis. • Administer with meals to decrease gastric upset. • Give at the same time each day. • Store in light-resistant container. • Instruct child and family to report sore throat, mouth lesions, unusual bleeding, or bruising. • Signs of overdose: periorbital edema, cold intolerance, mental depression • Signs of inadequate dose: tachycardia, diarrhea, fever, or irritability
Mineralocorticoid (Florinef)	Promotes reabsorption of Na and K, water from distal renal tubules Used in adrenal insufficiency	• Monitor daily weights, blood pressure, and intake and output. • Observe for potassium depletion. • Titrate dose to lowest effective dose. • Adverse effects include flushing, sweating, headache, and increased blood pressure.

Adapted from Taketokmo, C. K., Hodding, J. H., & Kraus, D. M. (2013). *Lexi-comp's Drug Reference Handbook: Pediatric & Neonatal Dosage Handbook* (20th ed.). Hudson, OH: Lexi-comp, Inc.

and psychosocial needs. These conditions are sometimes complex and range from mild to profound. Early diagnosis and treatment can improve the long-term outcomes for these children.

Remember Carlos, the 12-year-old with weakness, fatigue, blurred vision, headaches, and mood changes? What additional health history and physical examination assessment information should the nurse obtain?

Assessment

Nursing assessment of a child with endocrine dysfunction includes obtaining a thorough health history, performing a physical assessment, and assisting with or obtaining laboratory and diagnostic tests. The clinical manifestations of endocrine disorders occur as a result of the altered control of the bodily processes normally regulated by the gland or hormone. These manifestations present in many areas of the body because of the diverse functions associated with the endocrine system.

Health History

The health history should include questions regarding any family history of an endocrine disorder or growth and development difficulties. Use a genogram or family tree to detail the information about the family history in a clear and concise manner.

Discuss prenatal history, including any maternal factors that may affect growth and development such as substance abuse, use of tobacco or alcohol, and Graves disease; birth history, such as trauma during delivery, birth size, feeding difficulties, and neonatal screening and results; past medical history, such as any chronic childhood disease, treatment for any endocrine problems, recent gastroenteritis or viral syndrome, or exposures to exogenous steroids or gonadotropins; and growth and development patterns, including presence of any delays, learning disabilities, and early or late development of secondary sexual characteristics.

Discuss present complaints or illness. Note onset of symptoms, whether gradual or sudden. Endocrine disorders often cause problems in normal growth and development as well as behavioral changes. Question the parent or caregiver about prior growth patterns, achievement of developmental milestones, and the child's behavior. Inquire about recent increases or decreases in weight and height, changes in physical appearance, sleep patterns, muscle weakness, cramps, twitching, or headaches. Have the child and family describe the child's activities on a typical day, including school performance, to identify subtle variations in the child's behavior or moods. For example, a child who is typically quiet might ordinarily be less active than average children of that age, and the child with decreased endocrine function also often displays inactivity and fatigue. By having the family and child describe a typical day, the nurse can distinguish between what is appropriate for that child and what may be a change related to endocrine dysfunction.

In addition, obtain a history of dietary and elimination habits. Note extreme thirst, excessive appetite, vomiting, or frequent voiding. Children with endocrine disorders may have some of these symptoms.

Physical Examination

Physical examination of the child with an endocrine disorder includes inspection and observation, auscultation, percussion, and palpation. Table 48.1 lists key physical examination findings that may be present in the child with endocrine dysfunction.

INSPECTION AND OBSERVATION

Note a fatigued appearance, poor muscle tone, sweatiness, faintness, nervousness, or confusion. Inspect the head and face, and note hair texture and growth, a protuberant tongue, drooping eyelids, or **exophthalmos** (protrusion of the eyeballs). Plot the child's height and weight on growth charts to determine abnormal growth velocity, which occurs in many of these disorders.

AUSCULTATION

Auscultate the heart and lungs. Note heart rate and rhythm. During auscultation of the lungs, note labored respiratory effort, such as Kussmaul breathing, which occurs in diabetic ketoacidosis. Document blood pressure.

PERCUSSION AND PALPATION

Percuss and then palpate the abdomen. Dull (nontympanic) sounds or the presence of masses may indicate constipation or a tumor of the ovaries.

Laboratory and Diagnostic Testing

Common Laboratory and Diagnostic Tests 48.1 describes the diagnostic tests and procedures frequently used in identifying and monitoring endocrine disorders in children. Serum and urine hormone and other levels are used to determine whether amounts are adequate, deficient, or excessive. Radiographic studies are used to evaluate bone maturation and growth potential as well as density or tissue calcification. Genetic studies may be used to determine enzyme deficiencies or chromosome defects. Stimulation studies provide a more accurate or definitive test for identifying the disorder after preliminary serum levels are abnormal. Serial blood sampling

(text continues on page 1887)

TABLE 48.1 KEY PHYSICAL EXAMINATION FINDINGS RELATED TO ENDOCRINE PROBLEMS

Height and weight	Below 3rd percentile or above 90th percentile (pituitary, thyroid, adrenal, or diabetes mellitus)
Hair	Coarse, brittle, excessive (hypothyroidism) Abnormal distribution (adrenal disorders)
Face	Round with hair growth (Cushing syndrome) Deformities or abnormal features (hypoparathyroidism)
Eyes	Blurred or changes in vision (diabetes mellitus, pituitary tumors, precocious puberty)
Mouth	Delayed dentition (hypocalcemia, hypopituitarism) Fruity breath (ketoacidosis)
Neck	Goiter (hyperthyroidism)
Skin	Cool to touch, dry (hypothyroidism) Changes in color or texture (pituitary disorders) Easy bruising, striae (Cushing syndrome)
Chest	Tachycardia (hyperthyroidism) Palpitations, sweating (thyroid disorders) Deep, labored breathing (ketoacidosis) Hypertension (Cushing syndrome)
Abdomen	Extreme weight loss (diabetes mellitus) Extreme fat (Cushing syndrome) Changes in bowel habits (SIADH, diabetes insipidus, diabetes mellitus)
Fingers	Trembling (hyperthyroidism, parathyroid disorders)
Genitals	Excessive growth (adrenogenital syndrome) Early growth (precocious puberty) Delayed growth (hypopituitarism)

COMMON LABORATORY AND DIAGNOSTIC TESTS 48.1

Diagnostic Test or Procedure	Explanation	Indications	Nursing Implications
Newborn metabolic screening programs (refer to Chapter 31 for further information)	Newborn blood testing to identify certain harmful or potentially fatal disorders that are otherwise not apparent at birth. Disorders tested vary by state	Identify newborns so that treatment can begin early to prevent impact of disorder, such as severe cognitive impairment or death	• Refer to each state's protocol for fetal/newborn screening for endocrine disorders. • Explain to family the rationale and procedure. • Collect blood sample accurately. • Collect prior to blood transfusion if possible. • Ensure screening is done for early discharges. • Screening typically between 24 and 48 hours[a] after birth. • If collected before 24 hours of age, a repeat test is needed within 14 days. Some states now require a repeat screen at 2 weeks of age[b]

COMMON LABORATORY AND DIAGNOSTIC TESTS 48.1 (continued)

Diagnostic Test or Procedure	Explanation	Indications	Nursing Implications
Random serum hormone levels	Serum levels of various hormones; immunoassay measures levels with very small amounts of blood.	High or low levels are used to evaluate the function of the specific gland.	• May need to draw specimens at specific times. • Keep child NPO after midnight before test if ordered. • Diurnal variations and episodic secretion of many hormones may require special directions or further testing.
Self-monitoring blood glucose (SMBG)	Fingerstick (monitors that utilize alternative sites, such as the forearm, are available); blood sample several times per day Noninvasive methods are being developed.[c]	Monitor glucose level and effectiveness of treatment	• Teach family appropriate procedure. • Refer family to sources for equipment and supplies. • Assist family to develop a system of record keeping that works for them. • Refer to Teaching Guideline 48.2.
Fasting plasma glucose	Fasting forces the body to produce glucagon, which causes the release of glucose. In a healthy child the body will respond by releasing insulin, therefore lowering blood glucose and preventing hyperglycemia	Detect hyperglycemia related to diabetes or other conditions such as Cushing syndrome or liver or kidney disease Can detect prediabetes	• Child may not have had any caloric intake for at least 8 hours. • Draw sample prior to insulin or oral diabetic medications. • Normal value in children 2–18 years of age 60–100 mg/dL; in children 0–2 years of age 60–110 mg/dL; impaired fasting glucose or prediabetes is between 100 and 125 mg/dL; diabetes is considered with a result greater than or equal to 126 mg/dL on two separate occasions.
2-hour plasma glucose test (2-h PG)	Oral glucose tolerance test Oral glucose is ingested and in a healthy child insulin will respond and return blood glucose to normal levels.	Usually performed to detect diabetes, often gestational diabetes Can also detect prediabetes	• Child should not have taken any insulin or oral diabetic medication before the test. • Time of oral glucose ingestion needs to be noted. • Specimen to be drawn at specified time interval from ingestion. • May have limited value in diagnosing children.[c]
Urine or serum ketone testing	Ketones are the result of the metabolism of fat and in a healthy child are present in insignificant amounts	Screening for ketones in urine is regularly performed in children, people with diabetes, hospitalized patients, preoperatively, and in pregnant women In children, ketones found in urine during routine urinalysis can detect undiagnosed diabetes In children with diabetes, the presence of ketones in serum or urine is a sign that their diabetes is not well controlled and can be an early sign of diabetic ketoacidosis (DKA)	• Urine ketone testing can be performed using dipsticks at the bedside and at home (follow manufacturer's directions; time reaction accurately and compare the strip to the control chart on the bottle). • Encourage testing for ketones when blood glucose is elevated, when therapy regimen is changing, or during times of stress or illness.

(continued)

COMMON LABORATORY AND DIAGNOSTIC TESTS 48.1 (continued)

Diagnostic Test or Procedure	Explanation	Indications	Nursing Implications
Hemoglobin A1C (glycated hemoglobin)	Glycated hemoglobin reflects the percentage of hemoglobin to which glucose is attached. In the case of hyperglycemia an increase in glycohemoglobin leads to an increase in hemoglobin A1C. This test shows the average blood glucose level for the past 2–3 months.	Diagnose diabetes Indicated for children with diabetes. Provides information regarding long-term glycemic control and effectiveness of therapy	• Elevated levels seen in newly diagnosed diabetes or poorly controlled diabetes. • Levels can be elevated in nondiabetic children with certain conditions such as blood loss, hemolysis, iron-deficiency anemia, sickle cell disease, and lead toxicity.
Genetic testing	Tests for the presence of the gene for disease or carrier status	Determine genetic involvement of any disorder	• Explain procedure and the expense involved. • Refer for genetic counseling if needed.
Serum chemistry levels	Serum blood urea nitrogen (BUN), creatinine, sodium, potassium, glucose, calcium, phosphorus, alkaline phosphatase, etc.	Rule out chronic renal failure or other chronic illnesses; monitor effects of treatment	• BUN levels may be elevated with high-protein diet or dehydration, and may be decreased with overhydration or malnutrition. • A diet high in meat may cause a transient but not pronounced increase in creatinine. There are also slight diurnal variations in levels. • Avoid hemolysis of specimen, as this may cause elevation in potassium levels. • Calcium and phosphorus: avoid prolonged tourniquet use during blood draw, as this may falsely increase levels. Child should be NPO past midnight prior to the morning of the blood draw.
Growth hormone stimulation	Stimulate release of GH in response to administration of insulin, arginine, clonidine, or glucagon	Evaluate and diagnose GH deficiency	• Keep child NPO for specified time. • Limit stress and physical activity at least 30 minutes before test. • Obtain serial blood samples at specific times. • Monitor blood glucose levels during study. • Observe for signs of hypoglycemia, diaphoresis, and somnolence. • Provide a snack, such as cookies and juice at end of test.
Water deprivation study	Child is deprived of fluids for several hours, and serum sodium and urine osmolality are monitored.	Diagnose diabetes insipidus and distinguish between types of DI	• Stop test if child exhibits extreme weight loss or changes in vital signs or neurologic status. • Weigh child before, during, and after test. • Rehydrate child after test. • Monitor for orthostatic hypotension.

COMMON LABORATORY AND DIAGNOSTIC TESTS 48.1 (continued)

Diagnostic Test or Procedure	Explanation	Indications	Nursing Implications
Bone age x-ray	Radiographic study of wrist or hand to determine bone maturation compared to national standards	Determine if bone age is consistent with chronologic age to rule out GH deficiency or excess or hypothyroidism	• Explain procedure to child because child must hold still for the x-ray. • Allow family to accompany child. Enlist the family's help if needed to calm child during radiography.
Other nuclear medicine studies	Contrast media uptake is assessed with serial x-rays	Visualize an ectopic, enlarged, absent, or nodular gland	• Assess child for allergy to iodine or shellfish. • Explain procedure to child.
Computed tomography (CT)	Noninvasive x-ray study that looks at tissue density and structures. Images a "slice" of tissue	Evaluate presence of tumors, cysts, or structural abnormalities that may affect specific gland or structure	• Machine is large and can be frightening to children. • Scan may be lengthy and the child must remain still, so sedation may be necessary. • If contrast medium is to be used, assess for allergy. • Encourage fluids after procedure if not contraindicated.
Magnetic resonance imaging (MRI)	Based on how hydrogen atoms behave in a magnetic field when disturbed by radiofrequency signals. Does not require ionizing radiation. Provides a 3D view of the body part being scanned	Evaluate presence of tumors, cysts, or structural abnormalities that may affect specific gland or structure	• Remove all metal objects from the child. • Child must remain motionless for entire scan; parent can stay in room with child. Younger children will require sedation in order to be still. • A loud thumping sound occurs inside the machine during the procedure, which can be frightening to children.
Ultrasonography	Noninvasive sound waves are used to visualize structures such as thyroid or pelvic region	Evaluate presence of tumors or cysts in specific gland, such as the adrenal glands or ovaries, to rule out disorders	• Requires full bladder if in pelvic region. • Better tolerated by nonsedated children than CT or MRI. • Can be performed with a portable unit at bedside.

[a]March of Dimes. (2012). *Newborn screening.* Retrieved from http://www.marchofdimes.org/baby/newborn-screening-tests-for-your-baby.aspx

[b]Centers for Disease Control and Prevention (2014a). Newborn Screening: Importance of Newborn Screening. Retrieved from http://www.cdc.gov/ncbddd/newbornscreening/

[c]Fischbach, F. T., & Dunning III, M. B. (2015). *A manual of laboratory and diagnostic tests* (9th ed.). Philadelphia, PA: Wolters Kluwer Health/Lippincott Williams & Wilkins.

Adapted from Fischbach, F. T., & Dunning III, M. B. (2015). *A manual of laboratory and diagnostic tests* (9th ed.). Philadelphia, PA: Wolters Kluwer Health/Lippincott Williams & Wilkins.

identifies peak or trough levels of hormones. Computed tomography (CT) scans, magnetic resonance imaging (MRI), nuclear medicine studies, and ultrasonography are used to look for tumors, cysts, or structural defects.

Nursing Diagnoses, Goals, Interventions, and Evaluation

After completing the assessment, the nurse identifies nursing diagnoses with related goals/outcomes, interventions, and evaluations. The nursing diagnoses for a child with endocrine dysfunction may include:

- Delayed growth and development
- Disturbed body image
- Deficient knowledge (specify)
- Interrupted family processes
- Imbalanced nutrition: less than or more than body requirements
- Deficient or excess fluid volume
- Noncompliance

After completing an assessment of Carlos, the nurse noted the following: history reveals Carlos has had episodes of bedwetting over the past month and has had polydipsia and polyphagia. His weight continues to be greater than the 95th percentile on the growth chart. Based on these assessment findings, what would your top three nursing diagnoses be for Carlos?

Because of the gradual, insidious onset of many of these disorders, the child may first be seen in an acute situation. It may be easier for the child and family to work with short-term goals until they accept the chronic situation. A major goal will be to achieve compliance with medical management. The goals for the child with a disorder of the endocrine system generally include reestablishing homeostasis, promoting adequate growth and development, establishing appropriate body image, promoting health-seeking behaviors, and providing education so the family can manage the condition.

Nursing Care Plan 48.1, found at the end of the chapter, can be used as a guide in planning care for the child with a disorder of the endocrine system. Of course, this plan will need to be individualized based on the child's symptoms, needs, and disorder as well as the family's requirements. A key element to include in any care plan for the child with an endocrine disorder involves preparing the child, based on his or her developmental needs, for invasive procedures and tests. Provide an opportunity for the family and child to express their concerns and fears during diagnosis and treatment. Reinforce realistic expectations for treatment and prospects for improvement with the family and child. The care plan also needs to address developmental, acute, chronic, and home care issues as well as child and family education. Families will need assistance with managing the condition from a multidisciplinary team.

Based on your top three nursing diagnoses for Carlos, describe appropriate nursing interventions.

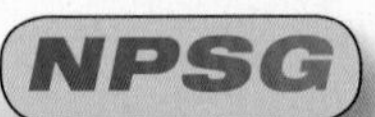

GOAL 2: Improve the Effectiveness of Communication Among Caregivers

NPSG.02.03.01 Report critical results of tests and diagnostic procedures on a timely basis.

Steps: When caring for a child with a potential or actual endocrine disorder notify appropriate healthcare provider with positive newborn screen results, and critical changes to other laboratory values and diagnostic test results.

Joint Commission. (2015). *National patient safety goals effective January 1, 2015.* Retrieved from http://www.jointcommission.org/assets/1/6/2015_NPSG_HAP.pdf

PITUITARY DISORDERS

Because of the close anatomic and functional relationships between the hypothalamus and pituitary gland, we will discuss them together. The hypothalamus affects the pituitary by releasing and inhibiting hormones and may be the cause of pituitary disorders. In general, disorders of the pituitary fall into two major groups: the anterior pituitary hormones and the posterior pituitary hormones. Anterior pituitary primary disorders in children include growth hormone (GH) deficiency, hyperpituitarism, and precocious puberty. Posterior pituitary disorders include diabetes insipidus (DI) and syndrome of inappropriate antidiuretic hormone secretion.

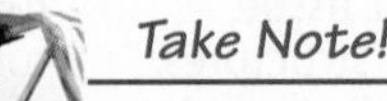

Take Note!

Infants with congenital defects of the pituitary gland or hypothalamus may present as a neonatal emergency. The symptoms include apnea, cyanosis, severe hypoglycemia with possible seizures, and prolonged jaundice (Parks & Felner, 2011).

Growth Hormone Deficiency

GH deficiency, also known as hypopituitarism or dwarfism, is characterized by poor growth and short stature. GH is vital for postnatal growth. It is released throughout the day, with most secreted during sleep. GH stimulates linear growth, bone mineral density, and growth in all body tissues.

GH deficiency occurs in approximately 1 in 4,000 children (Nelson-Tuttle, 2014). Often this condition is first identified when the physician or nurse practitioner assesses growth patterns. Children may start with a normal birth weight and length, but within a few years the child is less than the third percentile on the growth chart.

Possible complications related to GH deficiency and its treatment include altered carbohydrate, protein, and fat metabolism; hypoglycemia; glucose intolerance/diabetes; slipped capital femoral epiphysis; pseudotumor cerebri; leukemia; recurrence of central nervous system (CNS) tumors; infection at the injection site; edema; and sodium retention.

Pathophysiology

GH deficiency is generally a result of the failure of the anterior pituitary or hypothalamic stimulation on the pituitary to produce sufficient GH. This lack of GH impairs the body's ability to metabolize protein, fat, and carbohydrates.

Primary causes of GH deficiency include injury to, or destruction of, the anterior pituitary gland or hypothalamus. Causes include a tumor (e.g., craniopharyngioma), infection, infarction, CNS irradiation, abnormal formation of these organs in utero, or damage or trauma during birth or after. It may also be part of a genetic syndrome, such as Prader–Willi syndrome or Turner syndrome, or the result of a genetic mutation or deletion.

In some cases the cause may be idiopathic, such as nutritional deprivation or psychosocial issues, and reversible. Psychosocial dwarfism results from emotional deprivation that causes suppression of production of the pituitary hormones, resulting in decreased growth hormone. The child is withdrawn, has bizarre eating and drinking habits such as drinking from toilets, and has primitive speech. The treatment involves removing the child from the dysfunctional environment and providing normal dietary intake. With normalized eating and behavioral habits, pituitary secretion is restored and the child dramatically catches up in growth parameters.

Therapeutic Management

Treatment of primary GH deficiency involves the use of supplemental GH. Secondary GH deficiency requires removal of any tumors that might be the underlying problem, followed by GH therapy. Biosynthetic GH, derived from recombinant DNA, is given by subcutaneous injection. The weekly dosage is 0.2 to 0.3 mg/kg, divided into equal doses given daily for best growth (Nelson-Tuttle, 2014). Treatment continues until near final height is achieved. This can be determined by the child deciding he or she is tall enough, a growth rate of less than 1 inch/year, or bone age greater than 16 years in boys and greater than 14 years in girls (Parks & Felner, 2011).

Take Note!

Reports have found no evidence linking GH therapy to higher risk of leukemias or brain tumors (Parks & Felner, 2011).

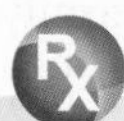

Dosage Calculation Box 48.1

Child's weight: 30 lb

Medication order: Somatropin 0.5 mg subcutaneously once a day

Per the Pediatric Dosage Handbook, the recommended dose is 0.18 to 0.3 mg/kg weekly divided into 6 to 7 doses.

Is the ordered dose safe?

Nursing Assessment

The focus of the evaluation for GH deficiency is to rule out chronic illnesses such as renal failure, liver disorders, and thyroid dysfunction. For a full description of the assessment phase of the nursing process, refer to the Assessment section of the Nursing Process Overview earlier in the chapter. Assessment findings pertinent to GH deficiency are discussed below.

HEALTH HISTORY

The health history may reveal a familial pattern of short stature or a prenatal history of maternal disorders such as malnutrition. The past history may be significant for birth history of intrauterine growth retardation or past history of severe head trauma or a brain tumor such as craniopharyngioma. Evaluate previous and current growth patterns. Note history of chronic illness such as cardiac, kidney, or intestinal disorders that may contribute to a decreased growth pattern. Assess the child's feelings about being short.

PHYSICAL EXAMINATION

In addition to the linear height being at or below the third percentile on standard growth charts, the physical assessment findings may show that the child has a higher weight-to-height ratio (Fig. 48.2). Other physical findings may include prominent subcutaneous deposits of abdominal fat; a child-like face with a large, prominent forehead; a high-pitched voice; delayed sexual maturation (e.g., micropenis and undescended testes in boys); delayed dentition; delayed skeletal maturation; and decreased muscle mass.

Take Note!

Growth measurements are often inaccurate and unreliable in children. Improved accuracy, especially in performing linear measurements, could yield earlier detection and diagnosis of growth disorders (Foote et al., 2011). Evidence-based clinical practice guidelines on linear growth measurement of children have been developed and have been endorsed by the Pediatric Endocrinology Nursing Society (PENS, 2014). A link to these and other helpful resources are provided on thePoint.

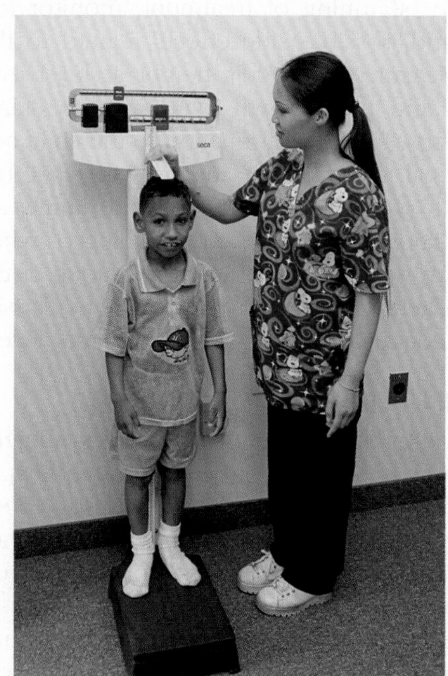

FIGURE 48.2 The child with growth hormone deficiency displays short stature.

LABORATORY AND DIAGNOSTIC TESTING

The child will undergo laboratory tests to rule out chronic illnesses such as renal failure or liver and thyroid dysfunction. Laboratory and diagnostic tests used in children with suspected GH deficiency include:

- Bone age (as shown by x-rays) will be two or more deviations below normal.
- CT or MRI scans rule out tumors or structural abnormalities.
- Pituitary function testing confirms the diagnosis. This test consists of providing a GH stimulant such as glucagon, clonidine, insulin, arginine, or L-dopa to stimulate the pituitary to release a burst of GH. Peak GH levels below 7 to 10 ng/mL in at least two tests confirm the diagnosis.

Nursing Management

Nursing management for the child with GH deficiency focuses on promoting growth, enhancing the child's self-esteem related to short stature, and providing appropriate education about the disorder.

PROMOTING GROWTH

The goal of growth promotion is for the child to demonstrate an improved growth rate, as evidenced by at least 3 to 5 inches in linear growth in the first year of treatment without complications. With early diagnosis and treatment, the child has a better prognosis for reaching a normal adult height. Growth is usually excellent in the first year of therapy compared to later years (Parks & Felner, 2011). Treatment stops when the epiphyseal growth plates fuse.

At the beginning of treatment, monitor for height increase and possible side effects related to the medications. Measure the child's height at least every 3 to 6 months and plot growth over time on standardized growth charts. Provide information to the child and family about normal development and growth rates, bone age, and growth potential. Explore with the family and child the expectations and their understanding of what is normal so they will have realistic expectations of treatment. Consult a dietitian if the child and family need assistance in providing adequate nutrition for growth and development.

ENHANCING THE CHILD'S SELF-ESTEEM

The child with GH deficiency often has younger-looking features and is shorter than his or her peers. Encourage the child to express positive feelings about his or her self-image, as shown by comments during healthcare visits as well as involvement with peers. Encourage the child to voice concerns. Emphasize the child's strengths and assets. Provide information about community support groups or websites related to GH deficiency. Evaluate for long-term learning problems that may develop if the child had a tumor and surgery or irradiation to remove it. Unidentified learning problems can have a negative impact on the child's self-esteem. Treat and communicate with the child in an age-appropriate manner even though he or she may appear younger.

EDUCATING THE FAMILY

GH is available as a powder that is mixed with packaged diluents. Recently, pen delivery systems and autoinjectors have become available, with some systems not requiring reconstitution (Kremidas, 2013). Explain how to prepare the medication and give the correct dosage. Encourage rotation of sites in the subcutaneous tissue to prevent skin irritation. Have the family provide a return demonstration to make sure they understand correct dilution and administration of GH. Continue to provide periodic evaluation and ongoing support.

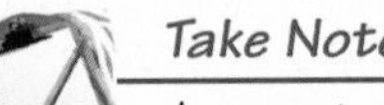

Take Note!

A recent study found that suboptimal treatment outcomes remain a concern due to nonadherence to the treatment plan, and they can often be attributed to the administration burden of the medication, such as the need for refrigeration storage, reconstitution, and discomfort and bruising from injection of the medication. Providing the child and caregivers with choices regarding medication delivery systems may lead to increased adherence to treatment plan and better clinical outcomes (Kremidas, 2013).

Instruct the family to report headaches, rapid weight gain, increased thirst or urination, or painful hip or knee joints as possible adverse reactions. Explain to the family that the child will need to visit the pediatric endocrinologist every 3 to 6 months to monitor for growth, for potential adverse effects, and for compliance with therapy. Stress the importance of complying with the GH replacement therapy and frequent supervision by a pediatric endocrinologist. Educate the family about the financial costs of therapy, which may be high; the family may need help in obtaining assistance and require referral to social services.

Guide the family and child in setting realistic goals and expectations based on age, personal abilities and strengths, and the effectiveness of the GH replacement therapy. For example, the family may want to encourage the child to choose sports that are not dependent on height. Encourage the family to dress the child according to age, not size. Refer the child and family to counseling if indicated. Inform families about support groups such as the Short Stature Foundation, the Human Growth Foundation, and the Magic Foundation. Links and additional information about these groups are provided on thePoint.

Precocious Puberty

In precocious puberty, the child develops sexual characteristics before the usual age of pubertal onset. Puberty, also known as sexual maturation, occurs when the gonads produce increased amounts of sex hormones. Typically, this occurs around 10 to 12 years of age for girls and 11 to 14 years of age for boys. In precocious puberty, secondary sex characteristics develop in girls before the age of 8 years and in boys younger than 9 years (Saenger, 2013). The disorder is more common in females and the majority of the time the cause is unknown in females while in males the majority of the time a structural CNS abnormality is present (Garibaldi & Chemaitilly, 2011). Other causes include benign hypothalamic tumor, brain injury or radiation, a history of infectious encephalitis, meningitis, congenital adrenal hyperplasia (CAH), and tumors of the ovary, adrenal gland, pituitary gland, or testes.

Pathophysiology

Central precocious puberty, the most common form, develops as a result of premature activation of the hypothalamic–pituitary–gonadal axis that results in the production of gonadotropin-releasing hormone (GnRH), which stimulates the pituitary to produce luteinizing hormone (LH) and follicle-stimulating hormone (FSH). These hormones in turn stimulate the gonads to secrete the sex hormones (estrogen or testosterone). The child develops sexual characteristics, shows increased growth and skeletal maturation, and has reproductive capability.

Peripheral precocious puberty presents with no early secretion of gonadotropin or maturation of gonads but rather early overproduction of sex hormones. The condition results in increased end-organ sensitivity to low levels of circulating sex hormones and leads to premature pubic hair and breast development. If left untreated, the child may become fertile. In addition, the hormones stimulate rapid growth. Therefore, the child may appear taller than peers but will reach skeletal maturity and closure of the epiphyseal plates early, which results in overall short stature.

Therapeutic Management

The clinical treatment for precocious puberty first involves determining the cause. For example, if the etiology is a tumor of the CNS, the child undergoes surgery, radiation, or chemotherapy. The treatment for central precocious puberty involves administering a GnRH analog. This is available as a subcutaneous injection given daily, an intranasal compound given two or three times each day, a depot injection given every 3 to 4 weeks, a depot injection given quarterly, or a subcutaneous implant yearly. This analog stimulates gonadotropin release initially but when given on a long-term basis will suppress gonadotropin release. With this treatment, the growth rate slows and secondary sexual development stabilizes or regresses. Medroxyprogesterone injections (Depo-Provera) or tablets (Cycrin) reduce secretion of gonadotropins and prevent menstruation. When treatment is discontinued, puberty resumes according to appropriate developmental stages. The overall aim of treatment is to halt or even reverse sexual development and rapid growth as well as promote psychosocial well-being.

Nursing Assessment

For a full description of the assessment phase of the nursing process, refer to the Assessment section of the Nursing Process Overview earlier in the chapter. Pertinent assessment findings related to precocious puberty are discussed below.

HEALTH HISTORY

The health history may reveal complaints of headaches, nausea, vomiting, and visual difficulties due to the circulating hormones. The psychosocial development is typical for the child's age, but the child may show emotional lability, aggressive behavior, and mood swings. Information from the child and family may also reveal risk factors such as exposure to exogenous hormones, history of CNS trauma or infection, or a family history of early puberty.

PHYSICAL EXAMINATION

Physical examination may reveal acne and an adult-like body odor. The child will present with an accelerated rate of growth. The Tanner staging of breasts, pubic hair, and genitalia reveals advanced maturation for the child's age, but the child does not typically display sexual behavior.

LABORATORY AND DIAGNOSTIC TESTING

Radiologic examinations and pelvic ultrasound identify advanced bone age, increased uterus size, and development of ovaries consistent with the diagnosis of precocious puberty. Laboratory studies include screening radioimmunoassays for LH, FSH, estradiol, or testosterone. The child's response to GnRH stimulation confirms the diagnosis of central precocious puberty versus gonadotropin-independent puberty. This test involves administering synthetic GnRH intravenously and drawing serial blood levels, about every 2 hours, of LH, FSH, and estrogen or testosterone. A positive result is defined as pubertal or adult levels of these hormones in response to the GnRH administration. CT, MRI, or skull radiography reveals any lesions in the CNS or tumors or cysts present in the abdomen, pelvic area, or testes.

Nursing Management

In general, nursing management of the child with precocious puberty focuses on educating the child and family about the physical changes the child is experiencing and how to correctly use the prescribed medications and helping the child to deal with self-esteem issues related to the accelerated growth and development of secondary sexual characteristics. Goals of nursing management include appropriate physical development and pubertal progression appropriate for age. Refer to Nursing Care Plan 48.1, at the end of the chapter, and individualize care based on the child's and family's response to this disorder.

PROVIDING EDUCATION

Nursing care involves assessing and documenting the physical changes the child is experiencing and administering medications. Demonstrate correct administration of medication and observe for potential adverse effects (teach this information to the family as well). Encourage the family to comply with follow-up appointments, which typically occur every 6 months and include scheduled stimulation tests. Inform families that pharmacologic intervention stops when the child reaches the age appropriate for pubertal development. Provide appropriate sex education. Reassure parents that precocious puberty does not always involve precocious sexual behavior, but that it may be seen, especially in boys (Dowshen, 2012a).

DEALING WITH SELF-ESTEEM ISSUES

Often these children develop self-esteem issues and anxiety related to body image disturbances and impaired social interactions (Dowshen, 2012a). The goal is for the child to exhibit normal psychosocial development and understand the physical and emotional changes that occur with early onset of puberty. Communicate with the child on an age-appropriate level, even when physical characteristics make the child appear older. Maintain a calm, supportive atmosphere and provide for privacy during examinations. Refer the child and family for counseling as needed. Since the child may have issues with self-image and may be self-conscious, encourage him or her to express his or her feelings about the changes, and use role-playing to show the child how to handle teasing from other children. Let the child know that everyone develops sexual characteristics in time.

Delayed Puberty

Delayed puberty is a condition of delayed secondary sexual development. In girls, it exists if the breasts have not developed by age 12, pubic hair has not appeared by age 14, or **menarche** (first menstrual period) has not occurred by age 15 (Children's Hospital of Pittsburgh, 2014; Nelson-Tuttle, 2014). In boys, it exists when no testicular enlargement or scrotal changes have occurred by age 14 or pubic hair has not appeared by age 15 followed by testicular enlargement (Children's Hospital of Pittsburgh, 2014; Nelson-Tuttle, 2014).

The most common cause for delayed puberty is a hereditary pattern of growth and development known as **constitutional delay** (or a "late bloomer") (Dowshen, 2011). In these cases there is a family pattern of late-onset puberty. These teens will usually develop normally, just at a later time than their peers. Hypogonadism also may result when there is decreased stimulation of the gonads due to dysfunction or tumors in the hypothalamus or pituitary gland. Other causes include irradiation, infection, trauma, or genetic syndromes such as Turner or Klinefelter syndrome. Another common cause is a chronic condition such as anorexia or cystic fibrosis.

Therapeutic management involves administering testosterone (males) or estradiol conjugated estrogen (females) in low dosages if there is no underlying situation to address. This is usually necessary for only a short time to get puberty started.

Nursing Assessment

Assessment involves obtaining a health history to identify the indications for this condition. Assessment of the growth pattern using correct techniques and standards for comparison is essential. On physical assessment, note absence of secondary sex characteristics as noted above. Laboratory and diagnostic testing rules out other causes for delayed puberty. Blood levels of reproductive hormones may also be evaluated.

Nursing Management

In addition to the general interventions presented in Nursing Care Plan 48.1 (at the end of the chapter), instruct the child and family about the medication therapy. Educate the child and family about the different stages of puberty. Help the family develop a home management schedule for the administration of medication. Answer the family's questions about the condition or potential complications (e.g., infertility), depending on the cause of the condition.

Diabetes Insipidus

DI can be classified into two types—nephrogenic DI and central DI. Nephrogenic DI can be transmitted genetically (e.g., sex-linked, autosomal dominant, or autosomal recessive forms) or be acquired due to chronic renal disease, hypercalcemia, hypokalemia, or use of certain drugs such as lithium, amphotericin, methicillin, and rifampin (Breault & Majzoub, 2011a). This variant of DI is not associated with the pituitary gland and is related to decreased renal sensitivity to antidiuretic hormone (ADH). Therapeutic management for nephrogenic DI involves diuretics, high fluid intake, restricted sodium intake, and a high-protein diet. Desmopressin acetate (DDAVP) is usually ineffective in the treatment of nephrogenic DI.

Central DI is a disorder of the posterior pituitary gland and is the most common form of DI (Children's Hospital of Boston, 2012). Therefore, central DI will be the focus of the remainder of this discussion. Central DI is characterized by excessive thirst (**polydipsia**) and excessive urination (**polyuria**) that is not affected by decreasing fluid intake. Typically, this disorder occurs in children as a result of complications from head trauma or after cranial surgery to remove hypothalamic–pituitary tumors such as craniopharyngioma. Other causes include genetic mutations, granulomatous disease, infections such as meningitis or encephalitis, vascular anomalies, congenital malformations, infiltrative disease such as leukemia, or administration of certain drugs that are associated with inhibition of vasopressin release, such as phenytoin (Breault & Majzoub, 2011a). However, 10% of central DI cases in children are idiopathic (Breault & Majzoub, 2011a). Some cases can be hereditary.

DI is usually permanent and requires treatment throughout life.

Pathophysiology

Central DI results from a deficiency in the secretion of ADH. This hormone, also known as vasopressin, is produced in the hypothalamus and stored in the pituitary gland. ADH is involved in concentrating the urine from the kidneys by stimulating reabsorption of water in the renal collecting tubules through increased membrane permeability. This conserves water and maintains normal osmolality. With a deficiency in ADH, the kidney loses massive amounts of water and retains sodium in the serum.

Therapeutic Management

Unless a tumor is present (in which case it is removed by surgery), the usual treatment of central DI involves a low solute diet (low sodium and low protein), daily replacement of ADH, and/or use of a thiazide diuretic (Bichet, 2013a). The drug of choice for home treatment is DDAVP, a long-acting vasopressin analog (Breault & Majzoub, 2011a; Nelson-Tuttle, 2014). In children, it is typically given intranasally. However, it can also be administered subcutaneously or orally. The drug is given every 8 to 12 hours. The dose depends on the child's age, urine output, and urine-specific gravity. Treatment of DI and the use of DDAVP in infants and small children is challenging and complicated due to their inability to access fluids and articulate thirst (Bichet, 2013a). In neonates and young infants, the treatment is often solely fluid therapy due to their large volume requirements of nutritive fluid (i.e., the drive behind an infant's fluid intake is hunger rather than thirst) (Breault & Majzoub, 2011a). However, research has shown that subcutaneously administered DDAVP may be more effective than oral or intranasal therapy in infants and small children related to variable absorption and the challenge of administering accurate doses via these routes (Bichet, 2013a).

In the hospital, the child may receive aqueous vasopressin, 8-arginine vasopressin (Pitressin), intravenously (Breault & Majzoub, 2011a). This is a short-acting drug, so the dosage can be adjusted quickly.

Both the long-acting and short-acting forms of the medication decrease urinary output and thirst, and the dosages of both forms of these drugs need to be titrated to achieve the desired effect.

Take Note!

A metered nasal spray form of DDAVP is available, but the prescribed dose must be greater than 10 μg/0.1 mL in order for the child to use the spray (Bichet, 2013a).

Nursing Assessment

For a full description of the assessment phase of the nursing process, refer to the Assessment section of the Nursing Process Overview earlier in the chapter. Assessment findings pertinent to DI are discussed below.

HEALTH HISTORY

Nursing assessment involves obtaining a history of any conditions that led to the development of the disorder. This review includes information about the neonatal period as well as a current history of infections such as meningitis, diseases such as leukemia, or familial patterns. Although most symptoms of endocrine disorders develop slowly, the onset of this disorder is abrupt. The health history usually elicits the cardinal symptoms as well as complaints representing the early signs of dehydration.

The most common initial symptoms reported are polyuria and polydipsia (Breault & Majzoub, 2011a; Bichet, 2013b). Except for unconscious children, the child typically maintains adequate perfusion by drinking water. The parent or child may report frequent trips to the bathroom, nocturia, or enuresis. When the child cannot compensate for the excessive loss of water by increasing fluid intake, other symptoms will be reported, such as weight loss or signs of dehydration. For example, irritability may be due to the early signs of dehydration or the frustration the child feels at being unable to quench his or her thirst. Other signs may be intermittent fever, vomiting, and constipation.

PHYSICAL EXAMINATION

Observation and inspection may reveal weight loss or failure to thrive in the young infant. Inspection may also reveal signs of dehydration, such as dry mucous membranes or decreased tears. The child may excrete greater than 3 L/m^2 of urine per day. On auscultation, tachycardia or increased respiratory rate may be signs of compensation for the decrease in fluid volume. Palpation reveals slightly depressed fontanels or decreased skin turgor.

LABORATORY AND DIAGNOSTIC TESTING

Diagnostic tests used to evaluate DI include:

- Radiographic studies such as CT scan, MRI, or ultrasound of the skull and kidneys can determine whether a lesion or tumor is present.
- Urinalysis: urine is dilute, osmolarity is less than 3,000 mOsm/L, specific gravity is less than 1.005, and sodium is decreased.
- Serum osmolarity is greater than 300 mOsm/L.
- Serum sodium is elevated.
- Fluid deprivation test measures vasopressin release from the pituitary in response to water deprivation. Normal results will show decreased urine output, increased urine-specific gravity, and no change in serum sodium.

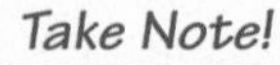

Take Note!

During a fluid deprivation test, the child may be irritable and frustrated because fluid is being withheld. Don't drink in front of the child.

Nursing Management

Refer to Nursing Care Plan 48.1 at the end of the chapter and individualize the plan of care based on the child's and family's response to the illness. Specific interventions related to nursing care of the child with DI are discussed below.

PROMOTING HYDRATION

The goal of treatment is to achieve hourly urine output of 1 to 2 mL/kg and urine-specific gravity of at least 1.010.

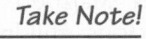

Take Note!

Notify the physician or nurse practitioner if the urine output is greater than 1,000 mL per hour for two consecutive voids.

Maintain fluid intake regimens as ordered. Monitor fluid status by measuring vital signs, fluid intake and output, and daily weights (using the same scale at the same time of day). If fluids are stopped too soon, the child may become hypernatremic, which can lead to seizures. Feed infants more frequently, since they excrete more dilute urine, consume larger volumes of free water, and secrete lower amounts of vasopressin than older children. Monitor for signs and symptoms of dehydration during the fluid deprivation test as well as when starting the treatment regimen.

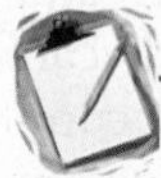

Take Note!

Monitor blood pressure closely when initiating vasopressin.

If the child is unconscious or has brain injury, maintain hydration and nutrition with nasogastric or gastrostomy feedings.

PROMOTING ACTIVITY

Establish appropriate activity for the child, and allow time for him or her to regain strength and the desire to increase level of activity. Assess the child's abilities daily, schedule frequent bathroom breaks, keep fluids the child likes available at all times, and fit the treatment plan to the child's daily activities.

EDUCATING THE FAMILY

Involve the family in development of the fluid intake regimens. A journal or daily log is essential in maintaining the fluid regimen and identifying problems. Children with intact thirst centers can self-regulate their need for fluids, but if this is not the situation, help the family develop a plan for 24-hour fluid replacement. This may require instruction on nasogastric or gastrostomy feedings. Infants will need fluid intake at night. Educate the family about the symptoms of water intoxication (drowsiness, listlessness, headache, confusion, sudden weight gain, and anuria) and dehydration. Help the family develop a plan to inform the school and other individuals in the child's life about the need for liberal bathroom privileges and extra fluids to prevent accidents or dehydration. Teaching Guidelines 48.1 gives tips on educating the family about the medication regimen. Recommend that the family obtain a medical ID alert bracelet or necklace for the child. Encourage compliance with follow-up appointments, which will probably be every 6 months.

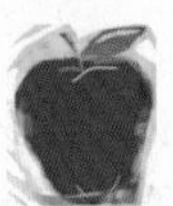

Teaching Guidelines 48.1

DDAVP INTRANASAL ADMINISTRATION

- Keep DDAVP in the refrigerator at all times (if directed, some products no longer require refrigeration, refer to product insert).
- Clear the nostrils (the medication may be poorly absorbed if the child has nasal congestion).
- Insert the measuring tube into the bottle.
- Fill to proper dosage and hold the top of the tube closed while inserting the medication-filled end into the nostril.
- Blow the liquid out of the tubing into the nostril.
- When using metered nasal spray, spray must be primed before first use.
- If the child sneezes, repeat the dosage.
- Measure urine-specific gravity to monitor effectiveness of the drug.
- Monitor for signs and symptoms of overdosage such as confusion, headache, drowsiness, and rapid weight gain due to fluid retention.

Syndrome of Inappropriate Antidiuretic Hormone

Syndrome of inappropriate antidiuretic hormone (SIADH) occurs when ADH (vasopressin) is secreted in the presence of low serum osmolality because the feedback mechanism that regulates ADH does not function properly. ADH continues to be released, and this leads to water retention, decreased serum sodium due to hemodilution, and extracellular fluid volume expansion. SIADH can be caused by CNS infections such as meningitis, head trauma, brain tumors, intracranial surgery, and certain medications such as analgesics, barbiturates, or chemotherapy. SIADH is rare in children (Breault & Majzoub, 2011b). However, when seen, it is often related to excessive administration of vasopressin during the treatment of DI (Breault & Majzoub, 2011b).

Therapeutic management of SIADH includes correcting the underlying disorder in addition to fluid restriction and intravenous sodium chloride administration to correct hyponatremia and increase serum osmolality.

Nursing Assessment

Obtain a health history, noting history of a CNS infection or tumor, intracranial surgery, head trauma, use of the above-mentioned medications, or a history of DI. Note symptoms such as decreased urine output and weight gain, or gastrointestinal symptoms such as anorexia, nausea, and vomiting. Assess neurologic status, noting lethargy, behavioral changes, headache, altered level of consciousness, seizure, or coma. Neurologic signs develop as the sodium level decreases. Diagnostic tests reveal low serum sodium and osmolality, as well as decreased urea, creatinine, uric acid, and albumin levels. Urine samples demonstrate elevated osmolality, high sodium concentrations, and specific gravity greater than 1.030. Adrenal, thyroid, and renal function studies may be used to rule out other causes of hyponatremia.

Comparison Chart 48.1 lists the differences between DI and SIADH.

Nursing Management

Nursing goals focus on restoring fluid balance and preventing injury. Institute safety precautions if altered level of consciousness, confusion, or seizures are present. Notify the physician or nurse practitioner if headache or irritability is present. Monitor fluid intake and output and weigh the child daily. An indwelling urinary catheter may be needed to allow for hourly monitoring of urine volume and specific gravity. Help the child cope with fluid restriction by offering sugarless candy, a wet washcloth, or, perhaps, ice chips. Administer electrolyte replacement as necessary to correct imbalances.

DISORDERS OF THYROID FUNCTION

Disorders of the thyroid gland are seen in infancy and childhood and are broadly classified as hypothyroidism and hyperthyroidism (Nelson-Tuttle, 2014). These disorders can be serious because thyroid hormones are important for growth and development; they regulate metabolism of nutrients and energy production.

Congenital Hypothyroidism

Congenital hypothyroidism, also known as cretinism, usually results from failure of the thyroid gland to migrate during fetal development (Lafranchi, 2011). This results in malformation or malfunction of the thyroid gland, which leads to insufficient production of the thyroid hormones that are required to meet the body's metabolic and growth and development needs. Congenital hypothyroidism leads to low concentrations of circulating thyroid hormones (triiodothyronine [T_3] and thyroxine [T_4]).

Congenital hypothyroidism occurs in 1 in 4,000 live births (Nelson-Tuttle, 2014). It occurs over a wide range of ethnic groups, though less among African Americans, and is more common in girls than boys (Lafranchi, 2011). Complications include intellectual disability if untreated,

COMPARISON CHART 48.1 DIABETES INSIPIDUS VERSUS SIADH

Diabetes Insipidus	Syndrome of Inappropriate Antidiuretic Hormone
• "High and dry"	• "Low and wet"
• Increased urination	• Decreased urination
• Hypernatremia	• Hyponatremia
• Serum osmolality >300 mOsm/kg	• Serum osmolality <280 mOsm/kg
• Urine-specific gravity <1.005	• Urine-specific gravity >1.030
• Decreased urine osmolality	• Increased urine osmolality
• Dehydration, thirst	• Fluid retention, weight gain, and hypertension

short stature, growth failure, and delayed physical maturation and development (Nelson-Tuttle, 2014). Congenital hypothyroidism is one of the most common preventable causes of intellectual disability. The later it is diagnosed the greater the disability is (LaFranchi, 2014a). Most newborns have few if any symptoms and the occurrence is sporadic not typically hereditary therefore most cases of congenital hypothyroidism are detected via newborn screening programs.

Pathophysiology

Congenital hypothyroidism is due to a defect in the development of the thyroid gland in the fetus due to a spontaneous gene mutation, an inborn error of thyroid hormone synthesis resulting from an autosomal recessive trait, pituitary dysfunction, or failure of the CNS–thyroid feedback mechanism to develop. Transient primary hypothyroidism may also occur; it results from transplacental transfer of maternal medications, maternal thyroid-blocking antibodies, iodine deficiency, and fetal or neonatal exposure to excessive iodines (such as use of iodine antiseptics during delivery or procedures or excess ingestion of iodine by the mother) (Lafranchi, 2014a).

Therapeutic Management

To prevent intellectual disability and restore normal growth and motor development, thyroid hormone replacement with sodium L-thyroxine (synthroid, synthetic thyroxine, or levothroid) is given. The recommended starting dosage is 10 to 15 μg/kg per day; infants and younger children typically require a higher dosage per unit of body weight (American Academy of Pediatrics, 2011). There are no adverse effects with physiologic doses, but thyroid function tests are performed initially every 2 weeks to closely monitor for effects and to ensure proper dosing. Since thyroid hormone is vital to the infant's developing CNS, the goal is to normalize thyroid function as quickly as possible. This treatment will be needed lifelong to maintain normal metabolism and promote normal physical and mental growth and development.

Nursing Assessment

Nursing assessment of the child with congenital hypothyroidism includes health history, physical examination, and laboratory testing.

HEALTH HISTORY

Inquire whether the neonatal metabolic screening test was performed and results obtained. Determine if the test was done less than 24 to 48 hours after birth. If so a repeat test may be warranted (see Laboratory and Diagnostic Testing below). Inquire about maternal history that may indicate a connection to hypothyroidism, such as maternal exposure to iodine. Additional history findings may include sensitivity to cold, constipation, feeding problems, or lethargy. Since parents like babies to sleep well, the parents may not complain that the baby is sleeping too much; rather, they may remark that it is difficult to keep the baby awake.

PHYSICAL EXAMINATION

Most infants are asymptomatic until the first month, when they begin to develop clinical signs. Inspection and observation reveal a lethargic baby or a child with hypotonia, hypoactivity, and a dull expression. A combination of lethargy and irritability may exist, with an overall delayed mental responsiveness. Measurements of weight and height may reveal delayed growth. Other findings may include a persistent open posterior fontanel, coarse facies with short neck and limbs, periorbital puffiness, enlarged tongue, and poor sucking response (Fig. 48.3). The skin may appear pale with mottling or yellow from prolonged jaundice, or it may be cool, dry, and scaly to the touch, with sparse hair development on the older child. Auscultation of the chest might reveal bradycardia. Signs of respiratory distress and decreased pulse pressure may also be present. On palpation of the abdomen, there may be evidence of an umbilical hernia or a mass due to constipation.

LABORATORY AND DIAGNOSTIC TESTING

Every infant should have a newborn screen for thyroid hormone levels before discharge from the hospital or 2 to 4 days after birth (American Academy of Pediatrics, 2011). When the test is performed within the first 24 to 48 hours along with other metabolic screenings, the result may be inaccurate because of the immediate increase in thyroid-stimulating hormone (TSH) shortly after birth (Nelson-Tuttle, 2014; American Academy of Pediatrics, 2011). Radioimmunoassay is used to measure levels of T_4, which accurately reflects the child's thyroid

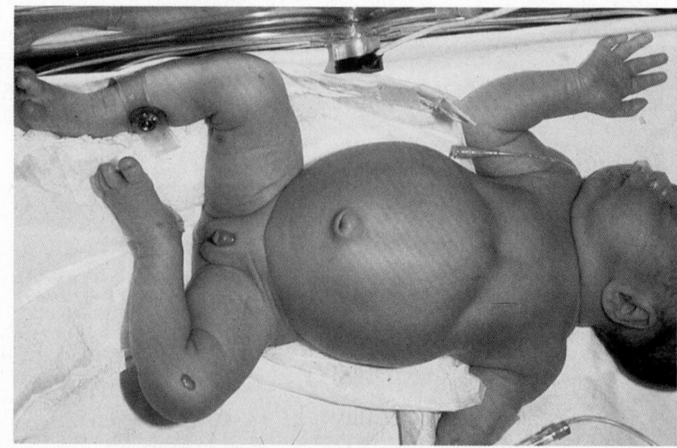

FIGURE 48.3 Newborn with congenital hypothyroidism.

status. If the T_4 level is low then a second confirming laboratory test is performed, as well as determining whether the TSH is elevated. A thyroid scan may also be used to check for the absence or ectopic placement of the gland. In addition to serum measurement of T_4, other diagnostic tests include serum T_3, radioiodine uptake, thyroid-bound globulin, and ultrasonography.

Nursing Management

The overall goal of nursing management of the infant or child with congenital hypothyroidism is to establish a normal growth pattern without complications such as intellectual disability or failure to thrive. Individualize the nursing care plan based on the infant's responses to the illness.

PROMOTING APPROPRIATE GROWTH

Measure and record growth at regular intervals. Thyroid levels are measured at recommended intervals, such as every 2 weeks until the target range is reached on a stabilized dose of medication, then every 1 to 3 months until the child is 1 year old, every 2 to 3 months until the child is 3 years old, and becoming less frequent as the child gets older (Lafranchi, 2014b). A trial off the medication may be performed around the age of 3, under physician or nurse practitioner supervision, to confirm the diagnosis (Nelson-Tuttle, 2014). Monitor for signs of hypo- or hyperfunction, including changes in vital signs, thermoregulation, and activity level. Provide adequate rest periods and meet thermoregulation needs. If the infant's tongue is unusually large, observe feeding ability, prevent airway obstruction, and position the infant on the side. Fluid restrictions or a low-salt diet may be ordered.

> **Take Note!**
>
> Observe for signs of thyroid hormone overdose (irritability, rapid pulse, dyspnea, sweating, and fever) or ineffective treatment (fatigue, constipation, and decreased appetite).

EDUCATING THE FAMILY

Since many infants are asymptomatic, the diagnosis may be unexpected, so reassure and convey realistic expectations to the family. Developmental screening may be required if the child showed any symptoms initially or as the child gets older to ensure that drug therapy is appropriate. Educate the family about the disorder, the medication and method of administration, and adverse effects such as increased pulse rate (which may indicate an overdose of thyroid hormone).

L-Thyroxine is an oral medication and is not available in a liquid form. The pill form must be crushed for infants and young children. It can be mixed with a small amount of formula or breastmilk and placed in the nipple, but it should not be placed in a full bottle of formula or breastmilk because the infant will not ingest all the medication if he or she does not finish the bottle. The medication can also be mixed with a small amount of liquid and given with a dropper. Medication absorption is affected by soy-based formulas, fiber, and iron preparations (American Academy of Pediatrics, 2011; LaFranchi, 2014b). Therefore, carefully evaluate the formula the infant is on before administering L-thyroxine.

Inform the family that this medication will be needed throughout the child's life. Explain that missed doses may lead to developmental delays and poor growth. Tell them that frequent blood tests will be needed to evaluate thyroid function and the child's growth rate; genetic counseling may be needed. Clinical examination, including growth and development assessment, should occur every few months until the child is 3 years old. Serum T_4 and TSH should be evaluated often, and more frequent monitoring may be needed if noncompliance occurs, if abnormal values occur, or with any changes in medication dosage or treatment regimen. The nurse may need to help the family to find a laboratory nearby or to handle financial issues related to the therapy. Educate the family about infant stimulation programs if the child shows cognitive problems, retarded physical growth, or slow intellectual development. Some information may need to be reinforced during school-age or adolescent stages of development. Finally, encourage the family to obtain a medical ID bracelet or necklace for the child.

> **Consider This**
>
> Asha Virani, 1 week old, is brought to the clinic. Her newborn screening test was positive for hypothyroidism. Her parents are shocked and upset by the news. Her mother states, "My daughter's been doing so well since she came home from the hospital. She seems to be doing everything she should be. I just can't believe anything's wrong with her. I felt so blessed to have a baby that slept so much but she could have died. What kind of mother will I be?"
>
> Thoughts: How would you respond to this mother?

Acquired Hypothyroidism

Hypothyroidism also occurs as an acquired condition. This disorder most commonly results from an autoimmune chronic lymphocytic thyroiditis (Lafranchi, 2011, 2013). As a genetic condition, antibodies develop against the thyroid gland, causing the gland to become inflamed, infiltrated, and progressively destroyed. It occurs more often in girls during childhood and adolescence (Lafranchi, 2011, 2013). Less common etiologies include hypothyroidism associated with pituitary or hypothalamic dysfunction or exposure to drugs or substances such as lithium and amiodarone that interfere with thyroid hormone synthesis, radiation, thyroidectomy, hemiangiomas, and iodine deficiency (LaFranchi, 2011, 2013).

Therapeutic management is the same as for congenital hypothyroidism. Management involves oral sodium L-thyroxine, which is given at 2 to 5 μg/kg per day to maintain T_4 in the upper half of the normal range and to suppress TSH.

Nursing Assessment

Interview the family and child to determine activity tolerance and behavior changes. The symptoms may develop over a period of time and may be subtle. Note vague complaints of fatigue, weakness, weight gain, cold intolerance, constipation, and dry skin. The severity of symptoms depends on the length of time that the hormone deficiency has existed and its extent. Reviewing the growth pattern may reveal a slowed or arrested growth rate (height) and increased weight.

Physical examination may reveal a **goiter** (enlargement of the thyroid gland). Deep tendon reflexes may be sluggish and the face, eyes, and hands may be edematous. Note thinning or coarse hair, muscle hypertrophy with muscle weakness, and signs of delayed or precocious puberty. The diagnostic evaluation involves serum thyroid function studies (TSH, T_3, and T_4) as well as serum thyroid antibodies to confirm autoimmune thyroiditis. MRI and a thyroid uptake test and scan may also be necessary.

Nursing Management

Work with the family to establish a daily schedule for administering L-thyroxine, which should be taken 30 to 60 minutes before a meal for optimal absorption. Explain to the family that growth is related to the child's response to the treatment, and there are no specific strategies to aid in this growth. The family should understand the diagnosis, should be able to recognize signs and symptoms of thyroid hypo- and hyperfunction, and should know when to notify the physician or nurse practitioner. The family and child may need assistance in accepting the therapy as well as the experience of catch-up growth that may occur at the beginning of therapy. The child with chronic or severe hypothyroidism may be at risk for adverse effects such as restlessness, insomnia, or irritability. The child's thyroid levels should be evaluated at recommended intervals such as every 3 to 6 months by a pediatric endocrinologist.

Hyperthyroidism

Hyperthyroidism is the result of hyperfunction of the thyroid gland. This leads to excessive levels of circulating thyroid hormones. This condition is uncommon in children. The peak incidence in children occurs in adolescence as a result of Graves disease (LaFranchi, 2011). Graves disease is an autoimmune disorder that causes excessive amounts of thyroid hormone to be released in response to human thyroid stimulator immunoglobulin (TSI). It occurs five times more often in girls than in boys (Lafranchi, 2011). A goiter usually develops in this condition. There is a genetic marker in individuals affected by Graves disease, with the majority of children having a positive family history of autoimmune thyroid problems (LaFranchi, 2011). A congenital form of hyperthyroidism, neonatal thyrotoxicosis, occurs in infants of mothers with Graves disease. This neonatal condition, which can be life-threatening, is a self-limiting disorder lasting 2 to 4 months. Less common causes of hyperthyroidism are thyroiditis, thyroid hormone–producing tumors, and pituitary adenomas.

Therapeutic management is aimed at decreasing thyroid hormone levels. Current treatment involves antithyroid medication, radioactive iodine therapy, and subtotal thyroidectomy. First-line treatment involves propylthiouracil (PTU) or methimazole (MTZ, Tapazole), which blocks the production of T_3 and T_4. Adjunct therapy with β-adrenergic blockers (such as propranolol or atenolol) may also be used if the child has marked symptoms. Radioactive iodine therapy is becoming acceptable for children greater than 10 years as a long-term therapy (LaFranchi, 2011). This therapy is administered orally and results in tissue damage and destruction of the thyroid gland within 6 to 18 weeks, but it can result in hypothyroidism. Subtotal thyroidectomy is used when drug therapy is not possible or other treatments have failed. Risks include hypothyroidism, hypoparathyroidism, or laryngeal nerve damage.

Nursing Assessment

Initially, symptoms of hyperthyroidism are mild and often overlooked. Many children with hyperthyroidism are first seen in the outpatient setting with a history of a problem with sleep, school performance, and distractibility. They become easily frustrated, overheated, and fatigued during physical education class. The child may complain of diarrhea, excessive perspiration, and muscle weakness. The history may also reveal hyperactivity, heat intolerance, emotional lability, and insomnia.

Physical examination of the older child may reveal an increased rate of growth; weight loss despite an excellent appetite; hyperactivity; warm, moist skin; tachycardia; fine tremors; an enlarged thyroid gland or goiter; and ophthalmic changes (exophthalmos, which is less pronounced in children; proptosis; lid lag and retraction; staring expression; periorbital edema; and diplopia) (Fig. 48.4). Elevated pulse and blood pressure may also be noted. Laboratory and diagnostic tests

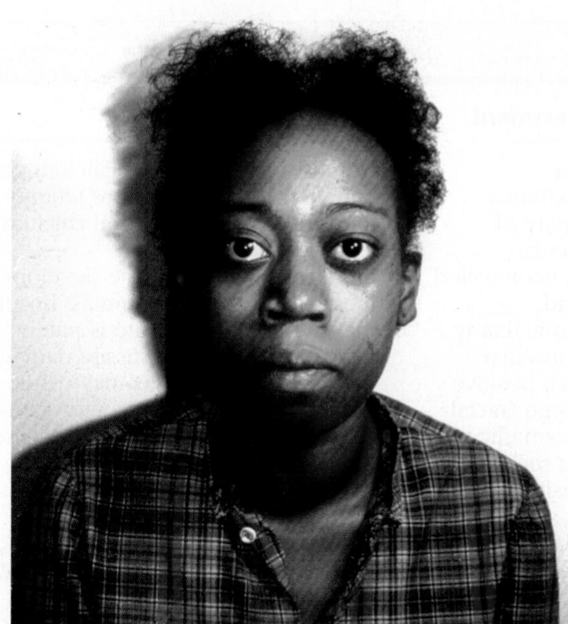

FIGURE 48.4 Adolescent with Graves disease.

reveal that serum T_4 and T_3 levels are markedly elevated while TSH levels are suppressed.

Take Note!

The sudden release of high levels of thyroid hormones results in thyroid storm, which progresses to heart failure and shock. Immediately report the signs of thyroid storm, which include sudden onset of severe restlessness and irritability, fever, diaphoresis, and severe tachycardia (Lafranchi, 2011).

Nursing Management

Once the treatment plan is initiated, educate the family and child about the medication and potential adverse effects, the goals of treatment, and possible complications. Monitor for adverse drug effects such as rash, mild leukopenia, loss of taste, sore throat, gastrointestinal disturbances, and arthralgia. If the medication is given two or three times a day, teach the family to use a pill dispenser and alarm clock. Inform the family of the need for routine blood tests and follow-up visits with the pediatric endocrinologist every 2 to 4 months until normal levels are reached; then visits may be decreased to once or twice a year. Instruct the parents to contact the physician or nurse practitioner if the child has tachycardia or extreme fatigue.

Help the child and family to cope with symptoms such as heat intolerance, emotional lability, or eye problems. Explain these symptoms to the school or day care personnel and make sure that they understand that the child should take more frequent rest breaks in a cool environment, and should avoid physical education classes until normal hormone levels are attained. Encourage the family to have the child consume a healthy diet with an appropriate level of calories; the child may need to eat five or six meals a day. Provide community referrals such as to the National Graves' Disease Foundation, a link to which can be found on thePoint. Encourage the family to obtain a medical ID bracelet or necklace.

If surgical intervention is chosen, provide appropriate preoperative teaching and postoperative care. Provide supportive measures such as fluid maintenance, nutritional support, and electrolyte correction. Monitor red blood cell count and liver function tests. Close monitoring for signs and symptoms of hypothyroidism is important.

Comparison Chart 48.2 compares hypothyroidism and hyperthyroidism.

DISORDERS RELATED TO PARATHYROID GLAND FUNCTION

The parathyroid glands secrete parathyroid hormone (PTH). This hormone, along with vitamin D and calcitonin, regulates calcium/phosphate homeostasis by increasing osteoclastic activity, absorption of calcium and excretion of phosphate by the kidneys, and absorption of calcium in the gastrointestinal tract. The two disorders associated with parathyroid gland dysfunction are hypoparathyroidism and hyperparathyroidism. Both of these disorders are rare in children. Refer to Table 48.2.

COMPARISON CHART 48.2 HYPOTHYROIDISM VERSUS HYPERTHYROIDISM

Hyperthyroidism	Hypothyroidism
• Nervousness/anxiety	• Tiredness/fatigue
• Diarrhea	• Constipation
• Heat intolerance	• Cold intolerance
• Weight loss	• Weight gain
• Smooth, velvety skin	• Dry, thick skin; edema of face, eyes, and hands
	• Decreased growth

TABLE 48.2 **PARATHYROID DISORDERS**

Parathyroid Disorder	Cause	Nursing Assessment	Nursing Management
Hypoparathyroidism (deficiency of PTH)	Most common is accidental removal or destruction of the parathyroid gland during thyroidectomy or radial neck dissection; may also be congenital (result of aplasia or hypoplasia of the parathyroid gland)	Hypocalcemia Hyperphosphatemia Hyperexcitability of neuromuscular function, uncontrolled spasms, and hypocalcemic tetany (general muscular hypertonia); positive Chvostek sign (facial muscle spasm elicited by tapping the facial nerve); positive Trousseau sign (carpopedal spasm that results from oxygen deficiency) Laryngeal spasm, stridor Poor eating Lethargy	• Administer intravenous calcium gluconate for acute or severe tetany, then intramuscular or oral calcium as prescribed. • Monitor the child for the development of cardiac arrhythmias. Ensure that the intravenous site is patent; if extravasation occurs, tissue damage or cardiac arrhythmias may result. • Monitor fluid and electrolyte status, weigh the child daily, and measure urinary calcium excretion to prevent nephrocalcinosis. • Institute seizure precautions and reduce environmental stimuli (e.g., loud or sudden noises, bright lights, or stimulating activities). • Observe for signs and symptoms of laryngospasm (e.g., stridor, hoarseness, or a feeling of tightness in the throat). Teach the child and family about the need for continuous daily administration of calcium salts and vitamin D. Have the family observe for vitamin D toxicity by observing for signs such as weakness, fatigue, lassitude, headache, nausea and vomiting, and diarrhea.
Hyperparathyroidism (hypersecretion of PTH)	Parathyroid adenoma is the most common cause; secondary hyperparathyroidism is primarily due to renal failure	Hypercalcemia Hypophosphatemia Depression of neuromuscular function, child may trip and drop objects, general fatigue, failure to thrive, headaches, poor school performance, and irritability, somnolence, stupor, or difficulty concentrating. Irregular heart rate, possibly related to cardiac dysrhythmias. Skeletal pain, fractures, formation of bone tumors, or flank pain related to renal calculi	• Administer IV fluids and diuretics as prescribed to increase urinary excretion of calcium in children not in renal failure. • Administer prescribed medication to treat hypercalcemia, such as oral phosphate (antihypercalcemic agent), pamidronate, calcitonin, or etidronate disodium (by inhibiting bone resorption of calcium). • Increase the child's fluid intake to minimize renal calculi formation. Provide fruit juices to maintain low urinary pH, acidity of body fluids, and calcium absorption. Strain the urine for renal casts. • Dietary calcium is restricted. • Monitor for safety by assessing the child's level of muscular weakness, preventing falls or injury, and checking for fractures. • If the child develops renal rickets (osteodystrophy), long-term braces may be required, so provide family education and encourage compliance. • Surgery may be performed to remove abnormal parathyroid tumor. • Keep the diet low in phosphorus and watch for hypocalcemia and onset of tetany after surgery.

DISORDERS RELATED TO ADRENAL GLAND FUNCTION

Disorders of the adrenal gland include acute and chronic adrenal insufficiency (hypofunction) and disorders of hyperfunction, such as Cushing syndrome. The adrenal cortex is the site of production of glucocorticoids (for blood glucose regulation), mineralocorticoids (for sodium retention), and androgenic and estrogenic steroid compounds (for phallic and secondary sex development). The adrenal medulla is the site of production of the catecholamines (dopamine, norepinephrine, and epinephrine) and is under neuroendocrine control. When production of these compounds is altered, disease results. Pediatric adrenocortical insufficiency is similar to adults with the exception of congenital adrenal hyperplasia CAH, which will be discussed below. Refer to Table 48.3 for an overview of other disorders of the adrenal gland.

TABLE 48.3 OTHER DISORDERS OF THE ADRENAL GLAND

Disorder	Cause	Nursing Assessment	Nursing Management
Addison disease (deficiency in the adrenal steroids, glucocorticoids [cortisol], and mineralocorticoids [aldosterone])	It results from damage or destruction of the adrenal glands caused by infections such as tuberculosis, fungal infections, or HIV-related infections; hemorrhage or surgical removal of both glands; or dysfunction of the hypothalamus or pituitary gland. Generally, the etiology in children is an autoimmune process that is familial or sporadic[a]	Hyponatremia Hyperkalemia Water loss, dehydration, muscular weakness, fatigue, weight loss, anorexia, syncope, nausea, vomiting, and diarrhea Hypoglycemia Hypotension Hyperpigmentation of skin Adrenal crisis, also referred to as addisonian crisis, can occur (refer to section on CAH for more information)	• Similar to that of congenital adrenal insufficiency
Cushing syndrome (excess levels of one or all the hormones [glucocorticoids, mineralocorticoids, and adrenal androgens] but most commonly glucocorticoid excess)	Usually this condition is due to a small ACTH-producing pituitary adenoma. The most common cause in older children is prolonged or excessive use of corticosteroid therapy[a]	Note history of rapid weight gain, decreased velocity of linear growth, muscle weakness, fatigue, irritability, sleep disturbance, and hypertension History of long-term corticosteroid use, water retention, poor wound healing, frequent infections, and in teenage girls, missed menstrual periods Refer to Figure 48.5 Skin may be thin and fragile; acne may be present	• Management varies depending on the cause. • The goal is to restore hormone balance and reverse Cushing syndrome. • If the cause is an adrenal or pituitary tumor, then surgical removal of the tumor alone or the entire adrenal gland is performed. • If the cause is long-term steroid therapy, then the corticosteroid dose is reduced to the lowest dose that is effective in treating the underlying disorder. • Cortisol synthesis–inhibiting medications may be used. • Counsel the family that the cushingoid appearance is reversible with appropriate treatment. • Be alert for signs of adrenal insufficiency if the child has surgery or if corticosteroid withdrawal occurs quickly.

[a]White, P. C.(2011). Section 4: Disorders of the adrenal glands. In R. M. Kleigman, B.F. Stanton, J. W. St. Geme III, N. F. Schor, & R. E. Behrman (Eds.), *Nelson textbook of pediatrics* (19th ed., pp. 1923–1943). Philadelphia, PA: Saunders.

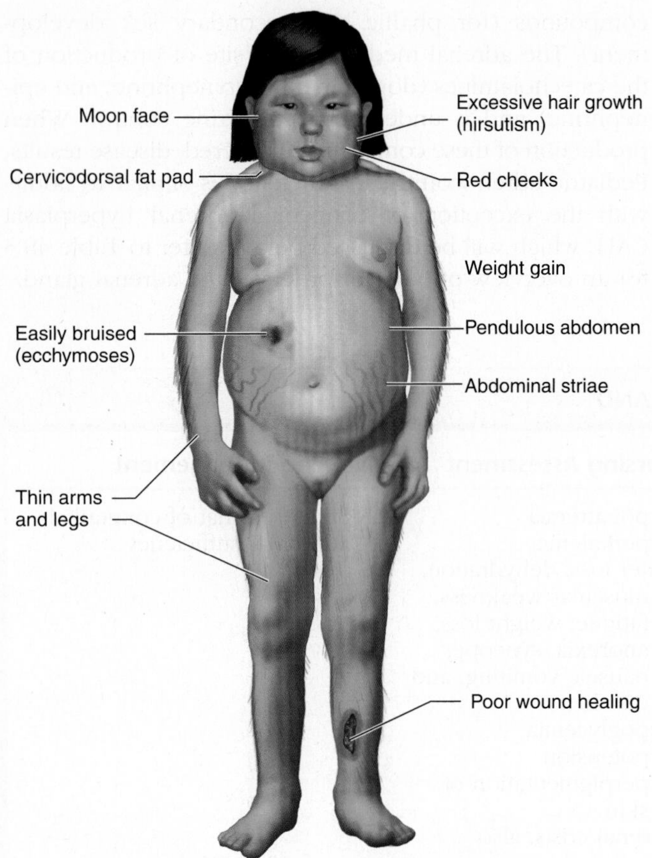

FIGURE 48.5 Newborn with ambiguous genitalia.

Congenital Adrenal Hyperplasia

CAH is a group of autosomal recessive inherited disorders in which there is an insufficient supply of the enzymes required for the synthesis of cortisol and aldosterone. It is the most common type of adrenocortical insufficiency seen in children with an incidence of about 1 in 15,000 to 20,000 live births (White, 2011). More than 90% of the cases of CAH are caused by a deficiency of 21-hydroxylase (21-OH) enzyme (Nelson-Tuttle, 2014; White, 2011). Therefore, our discussion will focus on this type. This condition can be life-threatening and requires prompt diagnosis and treatment after birth (Nelson-Tuttle, 2014). Complications of CAH include hyponatremia, hyperkalemia, hypotension, shock, hypoglycemia, short adult stature, and adult testicular tumor in males.

Pathophysiology

21-OH enzyme deficiency results in blocking the production of adrenal mineralocorticoids and glucocorticoids. A reduction of cortisol occurs, which leads to increased adrenocorticotropic hormone (ACTH) production by the anterior pituitary to stimulate adrenal gland production. Prolonged oversecretion of ACTH causes enlargement or hyperplasia of the adrenal glands and excess production of androgens, leading to male characteristics appearing early or inappropriately.

In males, the enzyme deficiency of 21-OH with excessive androgen secretion leads to a slightly enlarged penis, which may become adult-sized by school age, and a hyperpigmented scrotum. Males do not have obvious signs at birth but may enter puberty by 2 to 3 years of age. The female fetus develops male secondary sexual characteristics; thus, CAH causes ambiguous genitalia in girls (Nelson-Tuttle, 2014). The clitoris is enlarged and may resemble the penis, the labia have a rugated appearance, and the labial folds are fused, but the internal reproductive organs, including the ovaries, fallopian tubes, and uterus, are normal.

A milder form of 21-OH deficiency becomes evident later (genitals are normal at birth), in the toddler or preschool years, with premature **adrenarche** (early sexual maturation), pubic hair development, accelerated growth velocity, advanced bone age, early closure of the epiphyseal plates resulting in short stature as an adult, acne, and **hirsutism** (excessive body hair growth). Males usually have normal fertility while females may have lower fertility.

Aldosterone insufficiency also leads to fluid and electrolyte imbalances, such as hyponatremia, hyperkalemia, and hypotension due to depletion of extracellular fluid. Cortisol insufficiency leads to hypoglycemia.

Therapeutic Management

The goal of treatment is to stop excessive adrenal secretion of androgens while maintaining normal growth and development. Most children with 21-OH deficiency will take a glucocorticoid such as hydrocortisone and the mineralocorticoid fludrocortisone (Florinef) for life. Infants may also require sodium supplementation. When the medications are taken at physiologic doses there are no adverse effects, but if the drug levels become elevated, hypertension, growth impairment, and acne become a problem. Regular follow-up care and appropriate titration maintain the dose at appropriate levels to allow normal growth and development.

Usually when girls are born with ambiguous genitalia, standard medical treatment is to correct the external genitalia and establish adequate sexual functioning. Gender can be determined by karyotyping chromosomes. Typically, a reduction of the clitoris and opening of the labial folds is done within 2 to 6 months of life, with further surgeries at puberty (White, 2011). Some argue that surgery should be delayed until the child is old enough to decide what kind of correction (if any) should be performed (White, 2011). The decision to intervene immediately or to delay treatment is a complex one that raises many concerns for the family. Further long-term follow-up research is needed to determine risks and benefits of early versus delayed treatment (White, 2011).

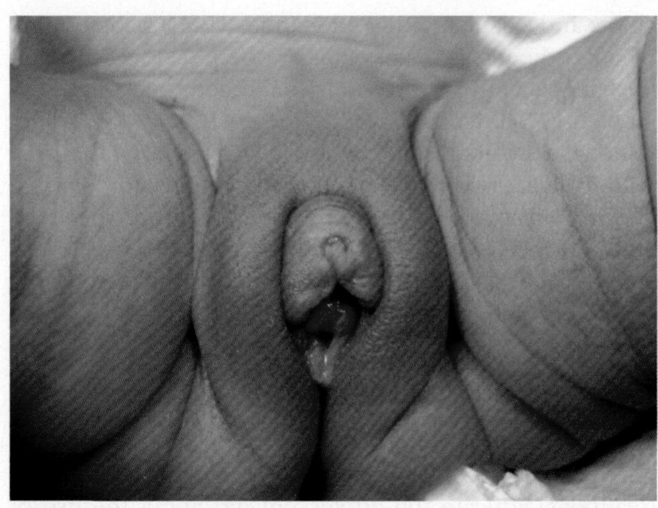

FIGURE 48.6 Cushing syndrome.

Nursing Assessment

Nursing assessment of the child with CAH includes health history, physical examination, and laboratory and diagnostic testing. Specific findings related to CAH are presented below.

HEALTH HISTORY AND PHYSICAL EXAMINATION

Obtain the health history, noting history of abnormal genitalia at birth in the infant. In the toddler or preschooler, note history of accelerated growth velocity and signs of premature adrenarche. Upon inspection of the infant's genitalia, note a large penis in the boy and ambiguous genitalia in the girl (Fig. 48.6). When observing the toddler or preschooler, note pubic hair development, acne, and hirsutism.

LABORATORY AND DIAGNOSTIC TESTING

The most common type of CAH, 21-OH enzyme deficiency, is detected by newborn metabolic screening. See Healthy People 2020. If this test has not been done or the results are unavailable, obtain random hormone levels or levels associated with ACTH stimulation. X-rays reveal advanced bone age and premature closure of epiphyseal plates of the long bones.

Nursing Management

In addition to the common interventions associated with endocrine disorders in childhood (see Nursing Care Plan 48.1 at the end of the chapter), nursing management of the infant or child with CAH focuses on preventing and monitoring for acute adrenal crisis, helping the family to understand the disease, providing education to the child and family about the importance of maintaining hormone supplementation, and providing emotional support to the family.

HEALTHY PEOPLE 2020

Objective	Nursing Significance
Increase appropriate newborn blood-spot screening and follow-up testing.	• Follow up with state agencies at first contact with infant to ascertain results of newborn screening.

Healthy People Objectives retrieved from http://www.healthypeople.gov

PREVENTING AND MONITORING FOR ACUTE ADRENAL CRISIS

Providing ongoing assessment of the ill or hospitalized child with a history of CAH is crucial in order to recognize the development of life-threatening acute adrenal crisis. Signs and symptoms of acute adrenal crisis include persistent vomiting, dehydration, hyponatremia, hyperkalemia, hypotension, tachycardia, and shock. Monitor children with CAH closely and notify the physician or nurse practitioner if adrenal crisis is suspected. If signs and symptoms of adrenal crisis develop, the child will receive intravenous steroids, such as hydrocortisone, and aggressive fluid resuscitation, often using 5% dextrose in normal saline (D5NS), to correct electrolyte imbalances.

Take Note!

Adrenal crisis in the newborn is often unrecognized. It presents within the first few days to weeks of life with vomiting, lethargy, and feeding difficulties.

EDUCATING THE FAMILY ABOUT THE MEDICATION REGIMEN

Medication will be required throughout the child's life because cortisone is necessary to sustain life. Teach the family the appropriate oral dosages of hydrocortisone and fludrocortisone. It is critical to maintain tight control over the levels of these medications in the bloodstream. Either underdosing or overdosing may lead to short adult stature. Low levels of the hormones may also result in adrenal crisis (as discussed above). These drugs are usually given orally but in some instances will need to be given via intramuscular injections. Teach families how to give hydrocortisone intramuscularly if the child is vomiting and cannot keep down oral medication. If the child becomes ill, is under stress, or needs surgery, additional doses of medications may be required. Encourage the family to obtain a medical ID bracelet or necklace for the child.

Take Note!

Families must keep extra steroids in an injectable form, such as Solu-Cortef or Decadron, at home to give during an emergency.

PROVIDING FAMILY SUPPORT

Make sure the family of a newborn with ambiguous genitalia feels comfortable asking questions and exploring their feelings. There are many issues to consider, such as whether the family will reassign the child's sex or raise the child with the original assignment at birth. The birth certificate may pose a problem if the state requires identification of sex. Cultural attitudes, the parents' expectations, and the extent of family support influence the family's response to the child and the decision-making process related to sex assignment and surgical correction. If corrective surgery is immediately decided upon, then typical surgical concerns for newborns will need to be addressed.

In general, laypeople do not understand adrenal function and what this diagnosis may mean to the family. Provide families with privacy to discuss these issues, and offer emotional support. When referring to the infant, use terms such as "your baby" instead of the pronouns "he," "she," or "it" and describe the genitals as "sex organs" instead of "penis" or "clitoris." Refer families to the CARES Foundation (Congenital Adrenal Hyperplasia Research, Education, and Support) and the Magic Foundation for additional support and resources. Links to these resources are provided on thePoint. Local parent-to-parent support groups are also helpful.

POLYCYSTIC OVARY SYNDROME

Polycystic ovary syndrome (PCOS), also referred to as functional ovarian hyperandrogenism or ovarian androgen excess, is an endocrine disorder that produces a variety of symptoms in adolescent girls and women. The exact cause is unknown. Testosterone production by the ovaries and adrenal cells is excessive, causing hirsutism, balding, acne, increased muscle mass, and decreased breast size. Polycystic ovaries may or may not be present. There is a genetic predisposition for PCOS along with nonhereditary factors, the most common being insulin resistance and obesity. (Rosenfield, 2014).

Complications of excess androgen production in women include infertility, insulin resistance, and hyperinsulinemia, leading to diabetes mellitus, increased risk for endometrial carcinoma, and cardiovascular disease. Therapeutic management involves the administration of oral contraceptives for their hormonal effects, as well as insulin-sensitizing medications such as metformin (Glucophage).

Nursing Assessment

Explore the health history for oligomenorrhea (irregular, infrequent periods) or amenorrhea. Symptoms typically emerge at or soon after puberty but often go undiagnosed. Note weight in relation to standardized growth charts and calculate body mass index (BMI) to determine whether the girl is overweight or obese. Inspect the skin for acne, acanthosis nigricans (darkened, thickened pigmentation, particularly around the neck or in the axillary region), and hirsutism (excess body hair growth). Assist with collection of timed blood specimens for glucose and insulin levels (which will often show unexpectedly elevated insulin levels in relation to the glucose level). Laboratory tests may show elevated levels of free testosterone and other androgenic hormones.

Nursing Management

One of the most important functions of the nurse in relation to PCOS is to assist with early recognition and treatment. Educate the adolescent girl about the use of oral contraceptives to normalize hormone levels, which will decrease androgenic effects. Support the teen in her efforts to diet and exercise to lose weight. Oral insulin-sensitizing drugs such as metformin (Glucophage) may be prescribed. Encourage the teen to comply with the medication regimen. Routinely measure weight to determine progress with weight loss. Measure blood pressure to screen for hypertension, which may develop as a complication of PCOS. Online support groups and education are available. Links to several resources are provided on thePoint.

DIABETES MELLITUS

Diabetes mellitus (DM) is a common chronic disease seen in children and adolescents. In DM, carbohydrate, protein, and lipid metabolism are impaired. The cardinal feature of DM is hyperglycemia. The major forms of diabetes are classified as:

- Type 1, which is caused by a deficiency of insulin secretion due to pancreatic β-cell damage
- Type 2, which is a consequence of insulin resistance that occurs at the level of skeletal muscle, liver, and adipose tissue with different degrees of β-cell impairment (Alemzadeh & Ali, 2011)
- Other types of diabetes secondary to certain conditions such as cystic fibrosis, glucocorticoid use (as in Cushing syndrome), infections, and certain genetic syndromes such as Down syndrome, Klinefelter syndrome, and Turner syndrome (Alemzadeh & Ali, 2011)
- Gestational diabetes (diabetes during pregnancy)

The discussion for this chapter will focus on type 1 and type 2 diabetes as these are the most common types seen in children. However, clinical presentation and disease progression of DM can vary considerably. Therefore, in some cases children cannot be clearly defined as having type 1 or type 2 (American Diabetes Association, 2014).

Every year approximately 18,000 children and adolescents are diagnosed with type 1 DM and approximately

HEALTHY PEOPLE 2020

Objective	Nursing Significance
Reduce the annual number of new cases of diagnosed diabetes in the population.	• Screen all children periodically for the development of overweight and obesity using body mass index on the Centers for Disease Control and Prevention growth charts. • Educate families about appropriate diet and exercise beginning in toddlerhood in order to prevent the development of obesity.

Healthy People Objectives retrieved from http://www.healthypeople.gov

5,000 with type 2 DM (Center for Disease Control and Prevention, 2014b). Historically, childhood DM was assumed to be type 1 and type 2 DM occurred mostly in adults. However, in recent years, type 2 DM has been reported in U.S. children and adolescents at an increasing rate (Dabelea et.al, 2014). Some studies report that between 20% and 50% of children with newly diagnosed diabetes have type 2 (Dabelea et al., 2014). This increase in incidence of type 2 DM among children and adolescents may be attributed to the rise in obesity and decreased physical activity in young people along with exposure to diabetes in utero (Dabelea et al., 2014). Many children with type 2 DM have a relative with type 2 DM and/or are overweight. Certain minority ethnic groups, such as Hispanic and African-American children, have a higher rate of type 2 DM (Dabelea et al., 2014). See Healthy People 2020.

Care of children with diabetes differs from that of adults due to physiologic and developmental differences. In children insulin sensitivity varies as the child grows and goes through sexual maturation. Children are dependent on others for their care, and self-management ability varies among children based on age, developmental level, and individual differences. Care will be needed in a variety of settings such as school, day care, and extracurricular activities. Therefore, teaching and education will need to involve parents and other caregivers throughout childhood and adolescence. Refer to Table 48.4, which discusses developmental issues related to diabetes mellitus.

Pathophysiology

Type 1 DM is an autoimmune disorder that occurs in genetically susceptible individuals who may also be exposed to one of several environmental or acquired factors, such as chemicals, viruses, or other toxic agents implicated in the development process. As the genetically susceptible individual is exposed to environmental factors, the immune system begins a T-lymphocyte–mediated process that damages and destroys the β cells of the pancreas, resulting in inadequate insulin secretion. This deficiency of insulin leads to an inability of cells to take up glucose. The end result is hyperglycemia, glucose accumulation in the blood, and the body's inability to use its main source of fuel efficiently. The kidneys try to lower blood glucose, resulting in glycosuria and polyuria, and protein and fat are broken down for energy. The metabolism of fat leads to a build-up of ketones and acidosis (see discussion of diabetic ketoacidosis below).

In type 2 DM the pancreas usually produces insulin but the body is resistant to the insulin or there is an inadequate insulin secretion response (the body can produce insulin but not enough to meet the body's needs). Eventually, insulin production decreases (resulting from the pancreas working overtime to produce insulin), with a result similar to type 1 DM.

If DM goes unrecognized or is inadequately treated (especially type 1 DM), **diabetic ketoacidosis (DKA)** or fat catabolism develops (a deficiency or ineffectiveness of insulin results in the body using fat instead of glucose for energy), resulting in anorexia, nausea and vomiting, lethargy, stupor, altered level of consciousness, confusion, decreased skin turgor, abdominal pain, Kussmaul respirations and air hunger, fruity (sweet-smelling) or acetone breath odor, presence of ketones in urine and blood, tachycardia, and, if left untreated, coma and death.

Take Note!

DKA is a medical emergency. It requires early recognition and prompt intervention. Be alert to the increased chance of DKA during times of stress such as illness, infection, and surgery, as hormones produced by the body in times of stress result in decreased insulin sensitivity and increased glucose production.

Prolonged exposure to high blood glucose levels results in damage to blood vessels and nerves. Long-term complications of DM include failure to grow, delayed sexual maturation, poor wound healing, recurrent infections (especially of the skin), retinopathy, neuropathy, vascular complications, nephropathy, cerebrovascular disease, peripheral vascular disease, and cardiovascular disease. Consistent, well-controlled blood glucose levels can prevent these complications from developing for many years. On the other hand, poorly controlled DM can lead to complications much earlier.

Therapeutic Management

Treatment for DM must occur as part of a multidisciplinary healthcare team, with the family and child as a

TABLE 48.4 DEVELOPMENTAL ISSUES RELATED TO DIABETES MELLITUS

Age Group	Child and Family Implications	Nursing Implications
Infants	Management falls on parents/caretakers. Infant is unable to communicate hypo-/hyperglycemic symptoms; signs and symptoms are sometimes difficult to assess. Increased risk of hypoglycemia due to inconsistent feeding times and amounts. Developing brain may experience adverse consequences to severe hypo-/hyperglycemia	Prevent extreme fluctuations in blood glucose. Prevent hypoglycemia and, if present, treat promptly. Attempt to achieve consistent dietary intake. Establish rituals/routines with home management. Provide support for parents and caregivers
Toddlers	Management falls on parents/caretakers. Increased risk of hypoglycemia due to inconsistent food intake (picky eaters). Developing brain may experience adverse consequences to severe hypo-/hyperglycemia. Discipline and temper tantrums common in this age group; may be hard to distinguish between normal toddler behavior and hypoglycemia symptoms Parents may be overcautious and hinder child's ability to explore and develop normally	Prevent hypoglycemia and if present treat promptly. Assist parents in managing a picky eater. Let toddler choose foods. Get toddler to find a word or phrase to use to describe feelings when hypoglycemic Help parents to provide appropriate discipline and protection while continuing to promote normal development Establish rituals/routines with home management
Preschoolers	Increased motor maturity. Widening social circle, so the child will notice that he or she is "different." Magical thinking presents some issues. Developing brain may experience more adverse consequences to severe hypo-/hyperglycemia than older children. Preschooler wants to be an active participant in diabetes care but may lack some of the developmental skills (such as fine motor and cognitive skills). Some children can begin to perform blood glucose testing with the newer devices. Increased risk of hypoglycemia due to varied food intake and activity	Prevent hypoglycemia and if present treat promptly. Use simple explanations and play therapy when instructing or preparing for a procedure. Encourage child's participation as appropriate
School-age children	Can begin to participate in more of the daily diabetes care; may be able to perform self-monitoring blood glucose testing, record glucose levels, choose injection sites and give injections, perform ketone testing, count carbohydrates, recognize need to eat, and treat for hypoglycemia. Beginning to rely on others (such as school nurse, child care provider, teacher) to provide diabetes care. Children may feel different from their peers and struggle socially. Must incorporate management into school day, and plan for field trips	Use concise and concrete terms when instructing. Allow child to proceed at his or her own rate. Assist family to incorporate the testing and injections into school day and plan for field trips. Involve the school nurse in helping with the school plan Encourage the child's participation but emphasize importance of continued adult supervision Encourage regular attendance at school and participation in extracurricular activities. Assist in the development of a care schedule that is flexible enough to allow for participation in school activities Assist with education of other care providers as needed
Adolescents	Undergoing rapid physical, emotional and cognitive growth. Working toward separate identity from parents and the demands of diabetic care can hinder this. This struggle for independence can lead to nonadherence of diabetic care regimen. Conflicts develop with self-management, body image, and peer group acceptance. They acquire the skills to perform tasks related to diabetic care but may lack decision-making skills needed to adjust treatment plan. Teens do not always foresee the consequences of their activity	Slowly care is turned over to the adolescent with minor supervision from the family Encourage parents and teen to find the right balance of shared management. Encourage parents to continue to provide guidance and supervision and be actively involved in the plan of care. Assess adherence to diabetic care regimen Assess for signs/symptoms of depression, eating disorders, or evidence of risky behaviors In later adolescence assist teen in transitioning to independent self-management and adult diabetes physician or nurse practitioner

central part of that team. In the past the child would be admitted to the hospital for 3 to 5 days for stabilization and education, but today the trend is toward treating children on an outpatient basis. Established glucose control is essential in reducing the risk of long-term complications associated with DM. Therefore, general goals for therapeutic management include:

- Achieving normal growth and development
- Promoting optimal serum glucose control, including fluid and electrolyte levels and near-normal **hemoglobin A1C** or glycosylated hemoglobin (which is hemoglobin that glucose is bound to and it monitors long-term control of blood sugars and diabetes) levels
- Preventing complications
- Promoting positive adjustment to the disease, with ability to self-manage in the home

The key to success is to educate the child and family so they can self-manage this chronic condition. Therapeutic management involves blood glucose monitoring; daily injections of insulin and/or administration of oral hypoglycemic medications; a realistic and well-balanced diet; an exercise program; and self-management and decision-making skills.

Research is ongoing to develop alternative medications, including alternative routes for insulin administration and therapies to monitor and treat diabetes. The FDA recently approved the use of a rapid acting inhaled insulin in adults to be used before meals (U.S. Food and Drug Administration, 2014a).

Monitoring Glycemic Control

Consistent glycemic control leads to fewer long-term diabetes-related complications. Two important methods for monitoring glycemic control include blood glucose monitoring and monitoring hemoglobin A1C levels.

BLOOD GLUCOSE MONITORING

Blood glucose monitoring evaluates short-term glycemic control. It allows for tight glucose control because supplemental insulin can be used to correct or prevent hyperglycemia; it also enables children and their parents and their physicians or nurse practitioners to provide better management of the disease. (Refer to Common Laboratory and Diagnostic Tests 48.1). The frequency of blood glucose monitoring is based on the goals for each particular child. Children who are in the hospital for management of their DM or are on insulin therapy require blood glucose monitoring before meals and at bedtime if not more frequently. Additional glucose checks may be necessary if glycemic control has not occurred, during times of illness, during episodes of hypoglycemic or hyperglycemic symptoms, or when there are changes in therapy. Children receiving noninsulin therapy may check their blood glucose less frequently but it can remain a useful guide to their therapy and its effectiveness. The procedure for glucose monitoring will vary based on equipment used but often involves a fingerstick, a reagent strip, and a glucometer.

Self-monitoring of blood glucose (SMBG) at home is essential to improve glycemic control, to provide self-management of this disease, and to help to prevent complications such as severe hypo-/hyperglycemia. The child and caregiver need to be aware of the importance of checking blood glucose regularly and more frequently when needed. Documenting blood glucose values is necessary to provide information on glucose control. This allows their physician or nurse practitioner to evaluate the effectiveness of their treatment regimen. Accuracy of SMBG is dependent on proper user technique; therefore, assessment of technique and education reinforcement are important at each visit (see Teaching Guidelines 48.2).

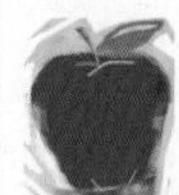

Teaching Guidelines 48.2

BLOOD GLUCOSE MONITORING

- Obtain glucose levels before meals and bedtime snacks.
- Perform monitoring more often during prolonged exercise, if you are ill, if you have eaten more food than usual, or if you suspect nighttime hypoglycemia.
- Use the manufacturer's recommendations and perform quality control measures as directed.
- Look for patterns. For example, 3 to 4 days of a consistent pattern of glucose values above 200 mg/dL before dinner indicates a need to adjust the insulin dose.
- Blood glucose measurements are the best way to determine daily insulin dosages.
- Normal levels are as follows: nondiabetics: 70 to 110 mg/dL; toddlers and children with type 1 DM younger than 6 years old: before meals 100 to 180 mg/dL, at bedtime 110 to 200 mg/dL; children with type 1 DM ages 6 to 12: before meals 90 to 180 mg/dL, at bedtime 100 to 180 mg/dL; adolescents 13 to 19 years of age, before meals 90 to 130 mg/dL, at bedtime 90 to 150 mg/dL (American Diabetes Association, 2014).

The FDA recently approved a continuous glucose monitoring system for pediatric use. This may be helpful in children with hypoglycemic unawareness or frequent hypoglycemic episodes. A sensor is placed under the skin that measures interstitial glucose. These monitors must be used in conjunction with a blood glucose meter and treatment decisions, such as insulin dosing should continue to be made based on blood glucose meter readings (U.S. Food and Drug Administration, 2014b).

MONITORING HEMOGLOBIN A1C LEVELS

Hemoglobin A1C (HbA1C) provides the physician or nurse practitioner with information regarding the long-term control of glucose levels (refer to Common Laboratory and Diagnostic Tests 48.1). In adults the goal is to achieve a near-normal HbA1C. However, in children, especially infants and children younger than 3 years, hypoglycemia poses some unique risks and can be hard to recognize. Therefore the HbA1C goals in children need to take into account the risks of severe hypoglycemia and glycemic control goals need to be individualized (American Diabetes Association, 2014) (refer to Table 48.1). The American Association of Diabetes (2014) has developed standards related to HbA1C goals in children with type 1 diabetes. These include:

- Infants and young children 0 to 6 years: HbA1C less than 8.5% and less than 8.0% if this can be achieved without excessive hypoglycemia
- Children 6 to 12 years: less than 8%
- Children and adolescents 13 to 19 years: less than 7.5%

Take Note!

HbA1C levels may vary in different races/ethnicities. Recent studies have questioned the validity of HbA1C in the pediatric population, especially ethnic minorities. Further research is needed to investigate these issues. At the current time the American Diabetes Association continues to recommend its use in the pediatric population (American Diabetes Association, 2014).

Insulin Replacement Therapy

Insulin replacement therapy is the cornerstone of management of type 1 DM. Insulin is administered daily by subcutaneous injections into adipose tissue over large muscle masses using a traditional insulin syringe or a subcutaneous injector (Fig. 48.7). U-100 insulin may also be administered using a portable insulin pump (see discussion below). The frequency, dose, and type of insulin are based on how much the child needs to achieve a normal, average blood glucose concentration and to prevent hypoglycemia. Typically, two to four daily injections are commonly used, with dosage depending on the needs of the child. The dose may need to be increased during the pubertal growth spurt as well as during times of illness or stress.

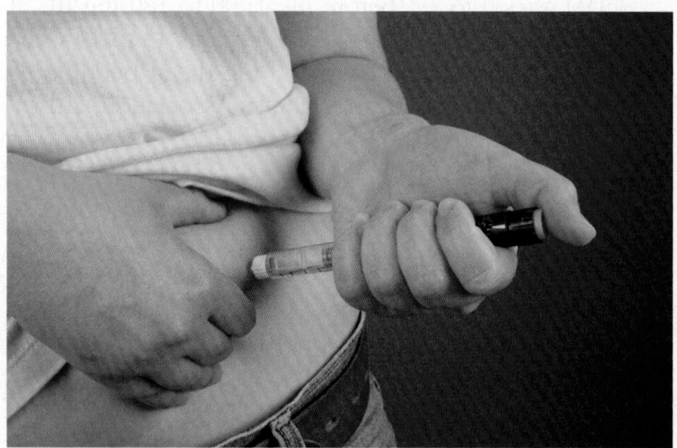

FIGURE 48.7 The subcutaneous injector uses pressure jets to deliver insulin safely and accurately.

An insulin pump is a device that administers a continuous infusion of rapid-acting insulin. These devices have been increasing in usage and studies have found them to be a safe and effective way to improve glycemic control and reduce episodes of severe hypoglycemia in young people (Johnson, Cooper, Jones, & Davis, 2013). See Evidence-Based Practice 48.1. It consists of a computer, a reservoir of rapid-acting insulin, thin tubing through which the insulin is delivered, and a small needle inserted into the abdomen. Insulin pumps attempt to mimic the physiologic insulin release by delivering small continuous infusions of insulin with additional bolus units administered at mealtimes, for planned carbohydrate intake, and if glucose testing results show it is needed. Advantages of this kind of therapy include:

- There are fewer injections and less trauma.
- Children's food intake can be unpredictable, so insulin delivery can occur after a meal and be adjusted based on actual intake.
- Children can be sensitive to insulin and require only minute doses, which the pump can deliver with precision.
- The pumps can store different basal rates for different times during the day and days of the week. For example, a higher basal rate may be needed in the morning when the child is sitting at his or her desk and a lower rate may be necessary during the afternoon when the child is more active with recess and physical education classes. In addition, rates can be programmed differently for school days versus weekend days, when the child may sleep later and have differing activity levels.

The use of an insulin pump does require a commitment from the child and caregiver in order to achieve success and improved glycemic control. The child and caregiver must be able to count carbohydrates, monitor glucose levels frequently, and work closely with the physician or nurse practitioner.

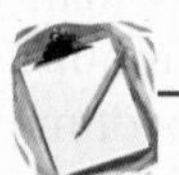

Take Note!

Some insulin pumps have a built-in sensor to monitor blood glucose continuously.

Types of insulin include rapid acting, short acting, intermediate acting, and long acting (Table 48.5). Each type works at a different pace and most children will use more than one type. In some cases premixed

EVIDENCE-BASED PRACTICE 48.1 **WHAT IS THE LONG-TERM IMPACT OF INSULIN PUMP THERAPY IN CHILDREN?**

STUDY

A case-control design study was performed to assess the impact insulin pump therapy has on long-term glycemic control, BMI, rate of severe hypoglycemia and diabetes ketoacidosis. Three hundred and forty-five children on pump therapy were matched with 345 children on injection therapy. The average age was 11.4 years (+ or −3.5), average duration of diabetes at the time pump was started was 4.1 years (+ or −3.0) and the average duration of follow-up was 3.5 years (+ or −2.5).

Findings

The mean hemoglobin A1C in the pump group decreased by 0.6% and remained significant throughout the 7-year follow-up. No significant change in BMI was found between the two groups. Severe hypoglycemia was reduced in the pump group and was increased in the injection group. The rate of hospitalization due to diabetic ketoacidosis was lower in the pump group versus the injection group.

Nursing Implications

The use of insulin pump therapy improves glycemic control over a sustained period of time and was accomplished with a reduction in severe hypoglycemia and diabetic ketoacidosis and without an increase in BMI. Children with poor glycemic control were found to have the biggest improvements in hemoglobin A1C levels with the use of insulin pump therapy. Nurses need to recognize the success of insulin pump therapy use in children as evidenced by this long-term study.

Adapted from Johnson, S. R., Cooper, M. N., Jones, T. W., & Davis, E. A. (2013). Long-term outcome of insulin pump therapy in children with type 1 diabetes assessed in a large population-based case–control study. *Diabetologia, 56*(11), 2392–2400. doi: 10.1007/s00125-013-3007-9

combinations of intermediate and short or rapid acting, such as 70% NPH and 30% regular, may be used. Again, this depends on the needs of the child. Insulin can be kept at room temperature (insulin that is administered cold may increase discomfort with injection) but should be discarded 1 month after opening even if refrigerated. Any extra, unopened vials should be stored in the refrigerator.

Take Note!

Lantus is usually given in a single dose at bedtime. Do not mix Lantus with other insulins.

Oral Diabetic Medications

Oral diabetic medications, also referred to as hypoglycemic, antidiabetic, or antihyperglycemic medications, are used in DM type 2 if glycemic control cannot be achieved by diet and exercise. Oral diabetic medications work in a variety of ways. Sulfonylureas such as glipizide [Glucotrol] and glyburide [DiaBeta]), meglitinides (such as repaglinide [Prandin]), and nateglinide (Starlix) stimulate insulin secretion by increasing the response of β cells to glucose. Another group, the biguanides, reduces glucose production from the liver. Metformin is an example of a biguanide and is an effective initial

TABLE 48.5 INSULIN TYPE, ACTION, AND DURATION

Type	Generic (Brand) Name	Onset	Peak	Duration (hours)
Rapid acting	Aspart/(NovoLog) Lispro/(Humalog) Glulisine/(Apidra)	Within 15 minutes	30–90 minutes	3–5
Short acting	Regular (Humulin R, Novolin R)	30–60 minutes	2–4 hours	5–8
Intermediate acting	NPH (Humulin N, Novolin N)	1–3 hours	4–10 hours	10–16
Long acting	Glargine (Lantus) Detemir (Levemir)	1–2 hours	No clear peak, offer continuously steady coverage	6–24

Adapted from National Diabetes Information Clearinghouse (NDIC). (2012). *What I need to know about diabetes medicines: Types of Insulin*. Retrieved from http://diabetes.niddk.nih.gov/dm/pubs/medicines_ez/insert_C.aspx

therapy unless significant liver or kidney impairment is present. Insulin sensitizers are used to help decrease insulin resistance and improve the body's ability to use insulin in the liver and skeletal tissues. α-Glucosidase inhibitors are used to slow digestion of starch in the small intestines so that glucose from the starch enters the bloodstream more slowly and can be matched more effectively with the impaired insulin response of the body. Combination agents are also available.

Common adverse effects of these oral diabetic medications include headache, dizziness, flatulence and gastrointestinal (GI) distress, edema, and liver enzyme elevation. If the oral hypoglycemics fail to maintain a normal glucose level, then insulin injections will be required to manage type 2 DM.

Diet and Exercise

Other therapies involve diet and exercise protocols. Medical nutrition therapy (MNT) can be initiated to prevent type 2 diabetes in children showing signs of prediabetes, to help glycemic control in existing diabetes, and to help slow the development of complications associated with diabetes (Gerard, 2014). MNT can be complex and must be individualized to each child incorporating the child's food preferences, activity level, cultural preferences, and family habits and schedule. Enlisting the help of a registered dietician who has expertise in diabetic management is recommended (American Diabetes Association, 2014).

The appropriate diet for a child or adolescent with diabetes is a balanced, healthy diet that meets the child's growth and development needs. The child and family need to understand the effect that food has on the child's glucose levels. Monitoring carbohydrate intake is an important component of diet management and assists with glycemic control. Nutritional recommendations for a child with diabetes or prediabetes include the following: limit sweets, ensure consistent food intake (eat often and try to avoid skipping meals), monitor carbohydrate intake, eat whole grains and plenty of fruits and vegetables, and limit fat.

It has been shown that regular exercise can improve glycemic control and can prevent the development of type 2 diabetes (American Diabetes Association, 2014). Also, exercise has an important influence on the hypoglycemic effects of insulin (by causing the release of glucagon, which will result in increased blood glucose). Therefore, it is important for the child to maintain or increase his or her activity levels. If the child is taking insulin, the family must know how to change the medication dosage or add food to maintain blood glucose control. Children with type 2 DM are often overweight, so the exercise plan is very important in helping the child to lose weight as well as assisting with the hypoglycemic effects of the medications.

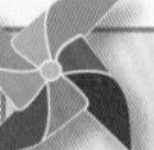

Thinking About Development

Jayda Jones is a 12-year-old girl recently diagnosed with type 2 diabetes.

Based on her developmental age, how will you instruct her and her caregivers on ways to manage her diabetes at home?

How would your instructions change is she was 16 years old?

Management of Complications

Another important aspect of therapeutic management includes monitoring and managing complications. The American Diabetes Association (2014) has developed recommendations for standards of medical care to help monitor complications and reduce risk. These include:

- Retinopathy:
  - Type 1 diabetes: eye examination by ophthalmologist (with expertise in diabetes) once child is 10 and has had diabetes for 3 to 5 years; annual examinations unless different recommendation by professional
  - Type 2 diabetes: eye examination by ophthalmologist (with expertise in diabetes) shortly after diagnosis; annual examinations unless different recommendation by professional
- Nephropathy:
  - Type 1 diabetes: annual screening for microalbuminuria (which occurs when the kidneys leak small amounts of albumin into the urine) once child is 10 and has had diabetes for 5 years
  - Type 2 diabetes: annual screening for microalbuminuria shortly after diagnosis
- Dyslipidemia: in children older than 2 years with a family history of high cholesterol or cardiovascular disease or unknown family history, obtain a lipid profile at time of diagnosis (once glucose level has been stabilized); otherwise, obtain lipid panel at puberty.
- Hypertension: Blood pressure measured at each routine visit.
- In addition, children with type 1 diabetes should be screened for celiac disease and hypothyroidism every 1 to 2 years (once glucose levels are stabilized) since both are commonly associated with diabetes.

Nursing Assessment

Assessment involves understanding the ever-changing needs of children as they grow and develop. The first phase of assessment involves identifying the child who may have DM. The second phase involves identifying problems that might develop in the child with DM. It is important to always be aware of this when observing the child for possible complications or management problems. In addition, always be alert for opportunities to provide education that will expand the understanding and skills related to management of DM of the child and family.

Health History and Physical Examination

During the initial diagnosis of DM, obtain a detailed history of family patterns and problems in school related to some of the mental and behavior changes that may occur in a hyperglycemic state (e.g., weakness, fatigue, and mood changes). The child or parent may report unusual or excessive thirst (polydipsia) coupled with frequent urination (polyuria). The child may also complain of blurred vision, headaches, or bedwetting. The child with type 1 DM may have a history of poor growth. Comparison Chart 48.3 gives information about common history and physical examination findings in children with type 1 DM versus type 2 DM. Type 1 DM typically presents with acute symptoms and hyperglycemia, while type 2 DM can frequently go undiagnosed until complications appear (American Diabetes Association, 2014).

In the child who is known to have DM, the health history includes any problems with hyperglycemia or hypoglycemia, diet, activity and exercise patterns, types of medications (insulin or oral diabetic medications) and dose and times of administration, ability to monitor blood glucose levels, and ability to administer insulin. Perform a thorough physical examination, noting any abnormal findings.

Laboratory and Diagnostic Testing

The American Diabetes Association (2014) currently recommends the use of fasting plasma glucose levels, 2-hour postprandial glucose levels, and/or hemoglobin A1C as reliable sources to diagnose diabetes (refer to Common Laboratory and Diagnostic Tests 48.1). A fasting glucose level greater than or equal to 126 mg/dL, a 2-hour plasma glucose level greater than or equal to 200 mg/dL during an oral glucose tolerance test, a random glucose level greater than or equal to 200 mg/dL (accompanied by typical symptoms of diabetes), or a hemoglobin A1C greater than 6.5% are laboratory criteria for the diagnosis of DM (American Diabetes Association, 2014). With each of these tests, if hyperglycemia is not explicit, the results should be confirmed with a repeat test on a different day (American Diabetes Association, 2014). Other laboratory and diagnostic tests include serum measurements of islet cell antibodies. Serum levels of urea nitrogen, creatinine, calcium, magnesium, phosphate, and electrolytes such as potassium and sodium may be drawn. Additional tests include a complete blood count, urinalysis, and immunoassay to measure levels of C peptides after a glucose challenge to verify endogenous insulin secretion.

COMPARISON CHART 48.3 **TYPE 1 VERSUS TYPE 2 DIABETES MELLITUS**

History and Physical Findings Usually Present at Diagnosis	Type 1	Type 2
Family history	Less tendency than type 2	Yes
Prone ethnic groups	All	Native American, African American, Hispanic/Latino, Asian/Pacific Island descent
Polydipsia, polyuria, polyphagia	Yes	Yes, may be mild or absent
Weight	Possibly weight loss	Usually obese
Age of onset	Usually younger children	Usually pubertal children
Incidental finding on screening urinalysis	Rare	Common
Antecedent flu-like illness/symptoms	Common	Possible
Autoimmune antibodies	Yes	No
Diabetic ketoacidosis	Common	Possible
Hypertension	No	Common
Acanthosis nigricans	No	Common
Dyslipidemia	No	Common

Adapted from Alemzadeh, R., & Ali, O. (2011). Section 6: Diabetes mellitus in children. In R. M. Kleigman, B. F. Stanton, J. W. St. Geme III, N. F. Schor, & R. E. Behrman (Eds.), *Nelson textbook of pediatrics* (19th ed., pp. 1968–1997). Philadelphia, PA: Saunders.

The American Diabetes Association (2014) recommends screening for type 2 DM if a child presents with being overweight or obese and also has any two of the following risk factors:

- Family history: a parent or relative with type 2 DM
- Ethnic background: Native American, African American, Latino, Asian American, or Pacific Islander
- Conditions associated with insulin resistance such as acanthosis nigricans, hypertension, dyslipidemia, or PCOS
- History of maternal diabetes or mother with gestational diabetes when child was in utero
- Age older than 10 years or onset of puberty before age 10 (American Diabetes Association, 2014)

Nursing Management

Individualize the general nursing care discussed in Nursing Care Plan 48.1, at the end of the chapter, based on the child's and family's response to illness. Additional nursing care topics related to DM are discussed below, including regulating glucose control, monitoring for complications, providing education to the child and family, and supporting the child and family.

Regulating Glucose Control

Consistent and established glucose control can reduce the risk of long-term complications associated with diabetes. Therefore, regulating glucose is a very important nursing function.

Typically, in children with type 1 DM and sometimes in cases of type 2 DM, glucose is regulated by subcutaneous injections of insulin. Often, the regimen consists of three injections of intermediate-acting insulin, with the addition of rapid-acting insulin before breakfast and dinner or three injections of a short-acting insulin with a long-acting injection at bedtime. Insulin doses are typically ordered on a sliding scale related to the serum glucose level and how the insulin works. Insulin doses and frequency are based on the needs of the child utilizing information gained from blood glucose testing. Regulating glucose can be challenging in children due to continual growth, onset of puberty, varying activity levels with unpredictable schedules, unpredictable eating habits, and the inability to always verbalize the way they are feeling. Thus, close monitoring of changing glucose levels through SMBG is essential in determining adjustments needed in insulin therapy, food intake, and activity level. Adjustment of insulin dosing based on carbohydrate intake is essential to manage blood sugar levels. The use of carbohydrate counting can help children enjoy more freedom to choose their type or amount of food and can allow them to vary their meal and snack times. It allows them to predict the rise in blood sugar that will occur after eating a specific amount or type of carbohydrate and allows them to take into account recent or expected activity level. It requires knowledge of carbohydrate amounts and calculations with each dose of short-acting insulin. Each scale will vary per child as the insulin per carbohydrate serving is calculated on an individual basis. See the Dosage Calculation Box on the Chapter Worksheet for an example. Parents will need extensive education and continual follow-up in order to ensure successful use of this method.

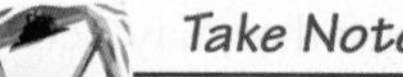

Take Note!

Blood sugar level should never be the only factor considered when calculating insulin dosing. Food intake and recent or expected activity/exercise must be factored.

Teach the child and family to use proper subcutaneous injection techniques to avoid injecting into muscle or vascular spaces. Figure 48.8 shows appropriate sites for subcutaneous injection of insulin. Teach the child and family to rotate sites to avoid adipose hypertrophy (fatty lumps that absorb insulin poorly). If the child is using an insulin pump, additional education will be needed.

Atraumatic Care

Children with diabetes experience numerous fingerpricks and injections. Providing atraumatic care remains important. Allow the child to choose the prick or injection site when possible. Use positioning that is comforting to the child. Encourage participation in care as developmentally appropriate.

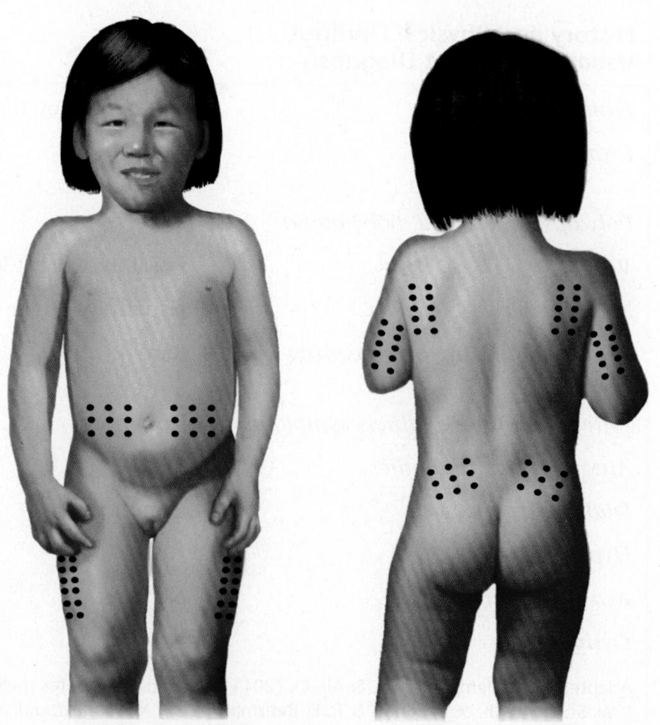

FIGURE 48.8 Insulin injection sites.

Take Note!

When giving a combination of short- and long-acting insulin, draw up the clear (short-acting) insulin first to prevent contamination with the long-acting insulin.

In children with type 2 diabetes, glucose levels can be controlled by the use of oral diabetic medications, diet, and exercise or a combination of all three.

Monitoring for and Managing Complications

While the child is in the hospital, monitor for signs of complications such as acidosis, coma, hyperkalemia or hypokalemia, hypocalcemia, cerebral edema, or hyponatremia. Assess for the development of hypoglycemia or hyperglycemia every 2 hours (Comparison Chart 48.4). Monitor the child's status closely during peak times of insulin action. Perform blood glucose testing as ordered or as needed if the child develops symptoms.

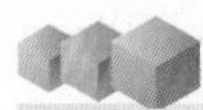

Concept Mastery Alert

Manifestations of Hypoglycemia Versus Hyperglycemia

Manifestations of hypoglycemia include behavioral changes, confusion, slurred speech, diaphoresis, tremors, palpitations, and tachycardia. In contrast, manifestations of hyperglycemia are blurred vision; dry, flushed skin; and a fruity odor to the breath.

If the child has a severe hypoglycemic reaction, administer glucagon (a hormone produced by the pancreas and stored in the liver) either subcutaneously or intramuscularly. Children under 20 kg receive 0.5 mg; children over 20 kg receive 1 mg (Alemzadeh & Ali, 2011). Dextrose (50%) may be given intravenously if needed. If the child is not having a severe reaction and is coherent, glucose paste or tablets may be used. Offer 10 to 15 g of a simple carbohydrate such as orange juice if the child feels some symptoms of low blood glucose and glucose monitoring indicates a drop in blood glucose level. Follow this with a more complex carbohydrate such as peanut butter and crackers to maintain the glucose level.

The child with severe hyperglycemia resulting in DKA is usually treated in the pediatric intensive care unit. In the case of a child presenting with DKA to the hospital, monitor the glucose level hourly to prevent it from falling more than 100 mg/dL per hour. A too-rapid decline in blood glucose predisposes the child to cerebral edema. Fluid therapy is given to treat dehydration, correct electrolyte imbalances (sodium and potassium due to osmotic diuresis), and improve peripheral perfusion. Administration of regular insulin, given intravenously, is preferred during DKA (only regular insulin may be given intravenously [IV]). A bolus dose of 0.1 unit/kg is given, followed by a continuous infusion of 0.1 unit/kg per hour (Nelson-Tuttle, 2014).

Any child exhibiting signs and symptoms of hyperglycemia requires insulin. The dosage is usually based on a sliding scale or determined after consultation with the physician or nurse practitioner.

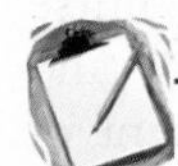

Take Note!

Double check all insulin doses against the order sheet and with another nurse to ensure accuracy.

Educating the Family

Education is the priority intervention for DM because it will enable the child and family to self-manage this chronic condition. Allow the child and family time to adjust to the diagnosis of a chronic illness that will require self-management. DM is a lifelong condition that requires regular follow-up visits (three or four times a year) to a diabetes specialty clinic. Because approximately 208,000 children and adolescents younger than the age of 20 have diabetes, this becomes a health issue for the community, especially for the schools (Centers for Disease Control and Prevention, 2014b). Daily management

COMPARISON CHART 48.4 HYPOGLYCEMIA VERSUS HYPERGLYCEMIA

Hypoglycemia	Hyperglycemia
Behavioral changes (tearfulness, irritability, naughtiness), confusion, slurred speech, belligerence	Mental status changes, fatigue, weakness
Diaphoresis	Dry, flushed skin
Tremors	Blurred vision
Palpitations, tachycardia	Abdominal cramping, nausea, vomiting, fruity breath odor

HEALTHY PEOPLE 2020

Objective	Nursing Significance
Increase the proportion of persons with diabetes who receive formal diabetes education Increase the proportion of persons with diagnosed diabetes who receive formal diabetes education	• Begin diabetes education with child and family upon knowledge of diagnosis. • Use developmentally appropriate education with children. • Increase the self-management skills taught as the child progresses in age and cognitive development.

Healthy People Objectives retrieved from http://www.healthypeople.gov

of the child with DM is complex and dynamic. It will require frequent monitoring of blood glucose levels, medications (including oral diabetic medications and insulin injections), and individual meal plans, including snacks, while the child is at school. The school nurse will be a principal contact person for both staff and family. With appropriate management, involvement of the community, and confidence and compliance by the family, the child can maintain a happy, productive life. See Healthy People 2020.

Challenges related to educating children with DM include:

- Children lack the maturity to understand the long-term consequences of this serious chronic illness.
- Children do not want to be different from their peers; having to make lifestyle changes may result in anger or depression.
- Poor families may not be able to afford appropriate food, medication, transportation, and telephone service.
- Families may demonstrate unhealthy behaviors, making it difficult for the child to initiate change because of the lack of supervision or role modeling.
- Family dynamics are affected because management of diabetes must occur all day, every day.

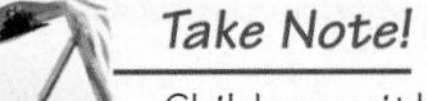

Take Note!

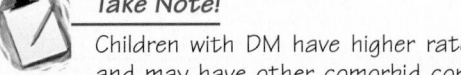

Children with DM have higher rates of depression and may have other comorbid conditions, such as eating disorders, adjustment disorders, or anxiety disorders (Alemzadeh & Ali, 2011).

The initial goal of education is for the family to develop basic management and decision-making skills. Assess the family's ability to learn the basic concepts and offer psychological support. Teach about specific topics in sessions lasting 15 to 20 minutes for the children and 45 to 60 minutes for the caregivers. Teaching must be geared toward the child's level of development and understanding (refer to Table 48.4).

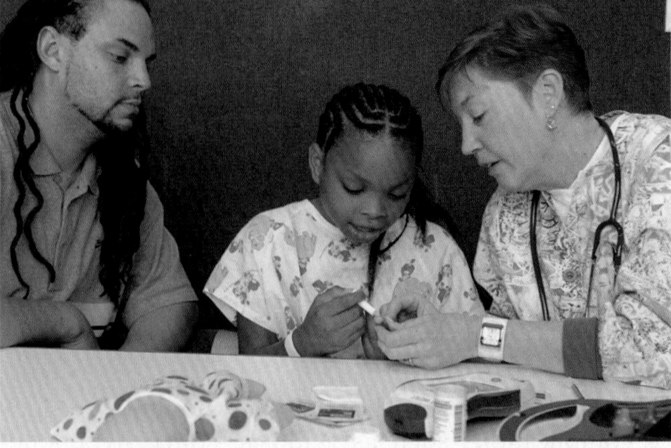

FIGURE 48.9 The school-age child has developed the psychomotor skills needed for blood glucose monitoring and insulin injection.

Among the topics to include when teaching children and their families about diabetes management are:

- Self-measurement of blood glucose (Fig. 48.9)
- Urine ketone testing
- Medication use (Fig. 48.10)
  - Oral diabetic agents
  - Subcutaneous insulin injection or insulin pump use
  - Subcutaneous site selection and rotation
  - When to alter insulin dosages
  - Use of glucagon to treat severe hypoglycemia
- Signs and symptoms of hypoglycemia and hyperglycemia (refer to Comparison Chart 48.4)
- Treatment for hypoglycemia and hyperglycemia at home or other setting such as school
- Monitoring for and managing complications (see above)

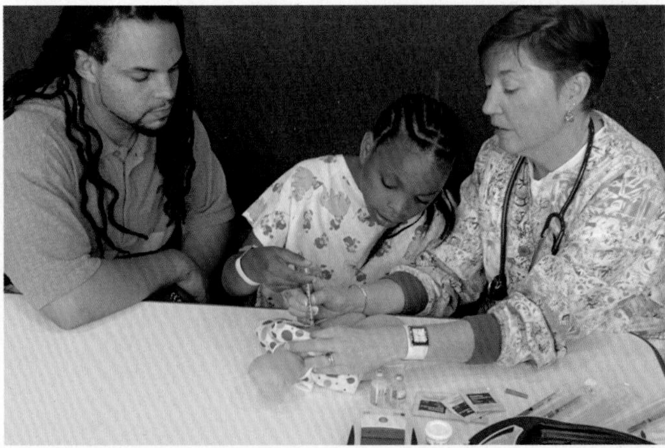

FIGURE 48.10 The school-age child may first practice insulin injections on a doll.

- Sick-day instructions
- Laboratory testing and follow-up care
- Diet and exercise as part of DM management (see above)

Teaching Guidelines 48.2 presents information to cover when teaching the family about self-monitoring of blood glucose. Teach families how to give insulin, how to use the insulin pump, and how to rotate injection sites (see above).

Good glucose control is dependent on accurate monitoring and medication administration by the child or caregiver. Assessment of the child's or parent's technique and review of procedure and instructions should occur with each visit. Treatment of hypoglycemia and hyperglycemia may have to occur at home or in another setting such as school. In either case, someone that is trained and able to check the child's blood glucose level needs to be available. In the case of hypoglycemia, early recognition is key. Therefore, all caregivers need to be educated on the causes of hypoglycemia (such as increased physical activity, delayed meals or snacks, insulin, oral diabetic medication, illness, stress, and hormonal fluctuations) along with the signs and symptoms. The child also needs access to glucose tablets or a rapidly absorbing carbohydrate such as orange juice as well as a snack with complex carbohydrates and protein within 30 to 60 minutes of the hypoglycemic episode. Injectable glucagon needs to be available in the case that the hypoglycemia is severe and the child is unconscious. In the event of hyperglycemia, the child needs immediate access to rapid-acting insulin injection.

Sick-day instructions may include the following:

- Contact the physician or nurse practitioner.
- Perform SMBG more often.
- Check for ketones in the urine, especially if blood glucose is elevated.
- Use a sliding scale to calculate the insulin dosage.

A dietitian can help the family with detailed meal planning and dietary guidelines. Review basic nutritional information with the child and family and provide sample meals. Encourage the child and family to keep a food diary. For the child who needs to lose weight, suggest low-carbohydrate snacks. Encourage all children with DM to incorporate physical activity daily (Teaching Guidelines 48.3).

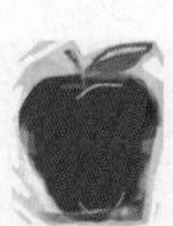

Teaching Guidelines 48.3

DIET AND EXERCISE FOR CHILDREN WITH DIABETES MELLITUS

- Provide sufficient calories and good nutrition for normal growth and development. The diet should be low in saturated fats and concentrated carbohydrates.
- Learn to identify carbohydrate, protein, and fat foods.
- Make adjustments during periods of rapid growth and for issues such as travel, school parties, and holidays.
- Consult a dietitian with expertise in diabetes education as needed.
- Provide three meals per day and midafternoon and bedtime snacks. Consistency of intake can help prevent complications and maintain near-normal blood glucose levels.
- Encourage the child to exercise routinely to help the body use insulin efficiently, thus reducing the insulin requirement.
- Encourage the child to participate in age-appropriate sports.
- When exercising, monitor insulin dose and nutritional and fluid intake, and observe for hypoglycemic reactions. Add an extra snack containing 15 to 30 g carbohydrate for each 45 to 60 minutes of exercise. Avoid exercising excessively when insulin is peaking.

Supporting the Child and Family

Children with DM and their families may have difficulty coping if they lack confidence in their self-management skills. Assess the ability of the child and family to handle situations. Role-play specific situations related to symptoms or complications to help them see different ways to solve problems. Work with the child and family to enhance their conflict resolution skills. Provide opportunities for them to express their feelings. Observe for signs of depression, especially in adolescents.

To enhance the child's confidence and promote feelings of mastery and inclusion, refer him or her to a special camp for children with DM. Also refer families to local support groups, parent-to-parent networks, or one of many national support resources and foundations. Links to camps for children as well as support groups, parent-to-parent networks, and national foundations are provided on thePoint.

NURSING CARE PLAN 48.1

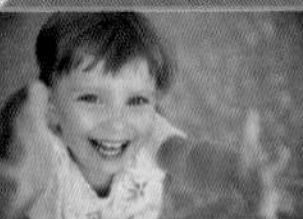

Overview for the Child With an Endocrine Disorder

NURSING DIAGNOSIS: Delayed growth and development related to hypo- or hyperfunction of gland/hormone as evidenced by weight and/or height less than expected for age, failure to meet expected age-appropriate developmental milestones

Outcome Identification and Evaluation

Nutritional status will be maximized and development will be enhanced: *child will maintain or gain weight appropriately and will make continued progress toward expected developmental milestones.*

Interventions: *Enhancing Growth and Development*

- Monitor growth parameters using standard growth charts: *to establish baseline and monitor growth trend.*
- Encourage favorite foods (within prescribed diet restrictions if present) *to maximize oral intake.*
- Consult dietitian *for appropriate diet supplementation recommendations.*
- Encourage compliance with hormone supplementation *to enhance ability to achieve appropriate growth.*
- Provide care related to any complications of dysfunction *such as correcting fluid and electrolyte imbalances or diarrhea.*
- Screen for developmental capabilities *to determine child's current level of functioning.*
- Offer age-appropriate toys, play, and activities (including gross motor) *to encourage further development.*
- Provide support to families of children with developmental delay: *progress in achieving developmental milestones can be slow and ongoing motivation is needed.*
- Reinforce positive attributes in the child *to maintain motivation.*

For the child with diabetes mellitus:

- Provide a calorie-appropriate, nonrestricted, well-balanced diet *to maintain appropriate growth.*
- Encourage three meals with two or three snacks with consistent carbohydrates *to maintain appropriate blood glucose levels and promote growth.*

NURSING DIAGNOSIS: Disturbed body image related to abnormal growth and development/changes in physical appearance due to hormone dysfunction as evidenced by verbalization of dissatisfaction with the child's or adolescent's looks

Outcome Identification and Evaluation

Child demonstrates appropriate self-esteem in relation to body image: *expresses positive feelings about self and participates in social activities.*

Interventions: *Promoting Healthy Body Image*

- Provide opportunities for child to explore feelings related to appearance: *venting feelings is associated with less body image disturbance.*
- Relate to child on age level, not appearance level: *"babying" a child who looks younger due to his or her small size reduces self-image.*
- Involve the child and especially the teen in the decision-making process: *a sense of control will improve body image.*
- Encourage the child to spend time with peers who have similar endocrine disorders: *peers' opinions are often better accepted than those of persons in authority, such as parents or healthcare professionals.*
- Refer to counseling or support groups *to further support the child.*

NURSING CARE PLAN 48.1

Overview for the Child With an Endocrine Disorder (continued)

NURSING DIAGNOSIS: Deficient knowledge related to therapeutic regimen as evidenced by questions about endocrine disorder and self-management

Outcome Identification and Evaluation

Child and family will demonstrate sufficient understanding and skills for self-management: *verbalize information about disorder, complications/adverse effects, home care regimen, and long-term needs, and provide return demonstrations of medication administration or other procedures.*

Interventions: ***Promoting Knowledge Required for Self-Management***

- Assess child's developmental level and family's ability to absorb instruction *to determine how to approach teaching sessions.*
- Establish teaching plan with child and family *to gain cooperation and involvement.*
- Teach and give printed instructions on disorder, complications, home care, and follow-up requirements *so family has a source to refer to at home.*
- Evaluate teaching with return demonstrations *to determine whether child/family is skilled enough for home management of the disorder.*

For the child with diabetes mellitus:

- First teach "survival skills" (e.g., glucose and urine testing, administering insulin, record keeping, food guidelines, when to call physician) *to provide initial base of knowledge for self-management.*
- Implement second-phase home management program with more extensive instruction: *providing additional teaching over time is necessary for management of a significant chronic illness.*
- Monitor outcomes of teaching with every contact *to ensure progress with child/family education.*

NURSING DIAGNOSIS: Interrupted family processes or adjustment issues related to lifestyle changes required to manage chronic illness and possible lifestyle changes as evidenced by family's presence in the hospital, missed work, demonstration of inadequate coping

Outcome Identification and Evaluation

Family will maintain functional system of support; demonstrate adequate coping, adaptation of roles and functions, and decreased anxiety: *parents are involved in child's care, ask appropriate questions, express fears and concerns, identify needs, seek appropriate resources and support, can discuss child's care and condition calmly.*

Interventions: ***Encouraging Healthy Family Processes***

- Encourage parents and family members to verbalize concerns related to child's illness, diagnosis, and prognosis: *allows the nurse to identify concerns and areas where further education may be needed.*
- Explain treatments, medications, procedures, child's behaviors, and plan of care to parents: *understanding of the child's current status and plan of care helps decrease anxiety.*
- Identify support system for family and child: *helps nurse identify needs and resources available for coping.*
- Provide family with information about support groups, financial resources, and special clinics in the area for the particular type of disorder *to provide family with a wide base of support.*
- Encourage parents to become involved in care: *allows parents to feel needed and valued and gives them a sense of control over their child's health.*
- Evaluate coping processes on follow-up visits *to determine restoration of family processes.*

(continued)

NURSING CARE PLAN 48.1

Overview for the Child With an Endocrine Disorder (continued)

NURSING DIAGNOSIS: Imbalanced nutrition: less than or more than body requirements related to pathophysiology of dysfunction as evidenced by growth parameters significantly less or more than expected for age

Outcome Identification and Evaluation

Child's nutritional status is balanced: *child adheres to nutritional guidelines, demonstrates adequate growth (weight and height) pattern within normal range for age and gender or, in the child who has difficulty growing, a progressive increase over time.*

Interventions: *Maintaining Adequate Nutrition*

- Determine body weight and length/height norm for age or what the child's pretreatment measurements were *to determine goal to work toward.*
- Weigh daily or weekly (according to physician order or institutional standard) and measure length/height weekly *to monitor for appropriate growth.*
- Determine child's food preferences and provide favorite foods as able *to increase the likelihood that the child will consume appropriate amounts of foods.*
- Instruct child and family about nutritional requirements *so that they are involved and are prepared for home care.*
- Refer to dietitian *for more detailed information and assistance.*

For the child who needs to gain weight:

- Offer highest-calorie meals at the time of day when the child's appetite is the greatest *to increase likelihood of increased caloric intake.*
- Provide increased-calorie shakes or puddings within dietary restrictions: *high-calorie foods increase weight gain.*
- Administer vitamin and mineral supplements as prescribed *to attain/maintain vitamin and mineral balance in the body.*

NURSING DIAGNOSIS: Deficient or excess fluid volume related to pathophysiology of endocrine dysfunction as evidenced by signs and symptoms of dehydration (deficient fluid volume) or edema and excessive urine output (excess fluid volume)

Outcome Identification and Evaluation

Child will maintain adequate fluid volume *as evidenced by elastic skin turgor; absence of edema; moist, pink oral mucosa; presence of tears; urine output 1 mL/kg/hr or more; vital signs within normal range for age; and normal electrolyte/hormone serum levels.*

Interventions: *Maintaining Adequate Fluid Volume*

- Assess hydration status (skin turgor, oral mucosa, presence of tears) every 4 to 8 hours *to evaluate maintenance of adequate fluid volume.*
- Assess adequacy of urine output *to evaluate end-organ perfusion.*
- Maintain strict intake and output record *to evaluate effectiveness of rehydration.*
- Weigh child daily: *accurate weight is one of the best indicators of fluid volume status in children.*
- Administer specific hormone, fluid, and electrolyte requirements as ordered *to aid in fluid balance.*

Fluid volume deficit:

- Maintain IV line and administer IV fluid as ordered *to maintain fluid volume.*

Fluid volume excess:

- Maintain fluid restriction as ordered *to restore homeostasis.*

NURSING DIAGNOSIS: Noncompliance related to long-term/complex management of some disorders as evidenced by failure to keep appointments, development of complications or exacerbation of symptoms, or child/family verbalization of inability to maintain treatment plan

NURSING CARE PLAN 48.1

Overview for the Child With an Endocrine Disorder (continued)

Outcome Identification and Evaluation

Child and family will comply with treatment regimen: *child and family will list treatment expectations and agree to follow through.*

Interventions: ***Encouraging Compliance***

- Listen nonjudgmentally while the child and family describe reasons for noncompliance: *assessment of problem should begin with nonthreatening discussion.*
- Help the child and family develop a schedule for medication administration and other home regimens that works best for them: *involving child and family in planning care will increase compliance by making them feel respected and valued.*
- Work with the child and family to develop a written treatment plan or schedule that best suits their needs *to provide support for maintenance of treatment plan.*
- Establish follow-up visits to fit family's situation *to promote compliance.*
- Encourage monitoring with pediatric endocrinologist and specialists: *multidisciplinary involvement has been shown to increase compliance.*
- Recognize that behavioral change comes slowly: *allows time for child and family to adjust to chronic nature of illness.*

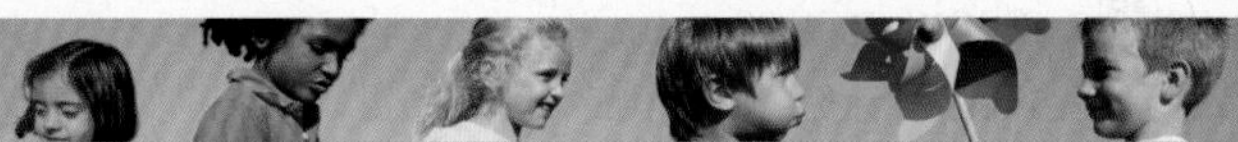

KEY CONCEPTS

- The endocrine system consists of cells, tissues, and glands that produce and/or secrete hormones (chemical messengers) in response to a negative feedback system involving the hypothalamus and nervous system.
- Hormones (chemical messengers), along with the nervous system, play an intricate role in reproduction, growth and development, energy production and use, and maintenance of the internal homeostasis.
- The pituitary, along with the hypothalamus connection, is considered the "control center," producing hormones that stimulate many glands to produce other hormones or to inhibit the process.
- Hormonal control is immature at birth; this is partly why the infant has trouble maintaining an appropriate balance of fluid concentration, electrolytes, amino acids, glucose, and trace substances.
- Linear growth and cognitive development may be impaired by untreated endocrine dysfunction in the infant or child.
- A thorough health history of the child with a known or potential endocrine disorder often reveals poor growth, school or learning problems, and inactivity or fatigue.
- Serial measurement of growth parameters is a key part of the physical assessment for children with endocrine dysfunction.
- Close monitoring of the child's status is critical during a hormone stimulation test or water deprivation study.
- Hormone supplementation is required lifelong for many of the endocrine disorders.
- The key nursing functions related to hormone supplementation are educating the child and family about medication use and monitoring for therapeutic results and adverse effects.
- Children with adrenocortical dysfunction will require additional hormone supplementation during times of stress such as fever, infection, or surgery.
- GH deficiency is characterized by poor growth and short stature as a result of failure of the anterior pituitary to produce sufficient growth hormone. Early treatment enables the child to reach normal growth.
- Precocious puberty involves early development of secondary sex characteristics as a result of premature activation of the hypothalamic–pituitary–gonadal axis.
- DI is characterized by water intoxication as a result of a deficiency in the antidiuretic hormone that leads to the cardinal signs of polyuria and polydipsia, resulting in hypernatremic dehydration.
- Key findings in congenital hypothyroidism are a thickened protuberant tongue, an enlarged

posterior fontanel, feeding difficulties, hypotonia, and lethargy.

- Early diagnosis and treatment of hypothyroidism can prevent impaired growth and severe cognitive impairment.
- CAH results from a genetic defect that causes a breakdown in steroid synthesis and an overproduction of androgens that can lead to ambiguous genitalia in females.
- DM is the most common endocrine disorder now seen in children.
- Type 1 DM is an autoimmune disorder resulting from damage and destruction of the β cells in the islets of Langerhans in the pancreas; the end result is insulin insufficiency. Peak onset occurs in childhood.
- Type 2 DM results in an insensitivity or resistance to insulin. The incidence of type 2 DM has risen dramatically. It is occurring at an alarming rate in children, especially in those who are obese and from certain ethnic groups.
- DKA is a medical emergency. The child will usually be admitted to a pediatric intensive care unit.
- The focus of DM management is regulation of glucose control, which is accomplished by medications, diet, and exercise.
- DM education involves instruction in glucose monitoring, administration of insulin or oral hypoglycemics, meal planning, and promotion of a healthy lifestyle.
- Critical areas in the nursing management of children with endocrine dysfunction include maintaining appropriate nutrition and fluid balance and promoting growth and development.
- The nurse provides ongoing assessment and education of the child and family, imparting to them the knowledge and skills required for self-management.
- Encouraging the child to have a healthy body image and working with the family in establishing healthy family processes are also key nursing functions.

REFERENCES AND RECOMMENDED READINGS

Alemzadeh, R., & Ali, O. (2011). Section 6: Diabetes mellitus in children. In R. M. Kleigman, B. F. Stanton, J. W. St. Geme III, N. F. Schor, & R. E. Behrman (Eds.), *Nelson textbook of pediatrics* (19th ed., pp. 1968–1997). Philadelphia, PA: Saunders.

American Academy of Pediatrics. (2011). Update of newborn screening and therapy for congenital hypothyroidism. *Pediatric, 117*(6). Retrieved from http://pediatrics.aappublications.org/cgi/content/full/pediatrics;117/6/2290

American Diabetes Association. (2014). Standards of medical care in diabetes—2014. *Diabetes Care, 37*(Suppl. 1), S14–S80. doi: 10.2337/dc14-S014. Retrieved from http://care.diabetesjournals.org/content/37/Supplement_1/S14.full.pdf+html

Bichet, D. G. (2013a). Treatment of central diabetes insipidus. UpToDate. Retrieved from http://www.uptodate.com/contents/treatment-of-central-diabetes-insipidus?source=machineLearning&search=diabetes+insipidus&selectedTitle=2~150§ionRank=1&anchor=H10#H10

Bichet, D. G. (2013b). Clinical manifestations and causes of central diabetes insipidus. UpToDate. Retrieved from http://www.uptodate.com/contents/clinical-manifestations-and-causes-of-central-diabetes-insipidus?source=see_link

Breault, D. T., & Majzoub, J. A. (2011a). Chapter 552: Diabetes insipidus. In R. M. Kleigman, B. F. Stanton, J. W. St. Geme III, N. F. Schor, & R. E. Behrman (Eds.), *Nelson textbook of pediatrics* (19th ed., pp. 1881–1884). Philadelphia, PA: Saunders.

Breault, D. T., & Majzoub, J. A. (2011b). Chapter 553: Other abnormalities of arginine vasopressin metabolism and action. In R. M. Kleigman, B. F. Stanton, J. W. St. Geme III, N. F. Schor, & R. E. Behrman (Eds.), *Nelson textbook of pediatrics* (19th ed., pp. 1884–1886). Philadelphia, PA: Saunders.

Carpenito, L. J. (2013). *Nursing diagnosis: Application to clinical practice* (14th ed.). Philadelphia, PA: Lippincott Williams & Wilkins.

Centers for Disease Control and Prevention. (2014a). *Newborn screening: Importance of newborn screening*. Retrieved from http://www.cdc.gov/ncbddd/newbornscreening/

Centers for Disease Control and Prevention. (2014b). *National diabetes statistics report: Estimates of diabetes and its burden in the United States, 2014*. Atlanta, GA: U.S. Department of Health and Human. Retrieved from http://www.cdc.gov/diabetes/pubs/statsreport14/national-diabetes-report-web.pdf

Children's Hospital of Boston. (2012). *Diabetes insipidus: Disease information*. Retrieved from http://www.childrenshospital.org/az/Site709/mainpageS709P0.html

Children's Hospital of Pittsburgh. (2014). *Child Health Library: Delayed puberty*. Retrieved from http://chp.staywellsolutionsonline.com/Search/90,P01947

Dabelea, D., Mayer-Davis, E. J., Sharon Saydah, S., Imperatore, G., Linder, B., Divers, J., et al.; SEARCH for Diabetes in Youth Study. (2014). Prevalence of type 1 and type 2 diabetes among children and adolescents from 2001 to 2009. *JAMA, 311*(17), 1778–1786. doi: 10.1001/jama.2014.3201

Dowshen, S. (2011). *Delayed puberty*. Retrieved from http://kidshealth.org/teen/sexual_health/changing_body/delayed_puberty.html

Dowshen, S. (2012a). *Precocious puberty*. Retrieved from http://kidshealth.org/parent/medical/sexual/precocious.html

Dowshen, S. (2012b). *Type II diabetes: What is it? Kidshealth from nemours*. Retrieved from http://kidshealth.org/parent/medical/endocrine/type2.html

Doyle, D. A. (2011). Section 3: Disorders of the parathyroid. In R. M. Kleigman, B. F. Stanton, J. W. St. Geme III, N. F. Schor, & R. E. Behrman (Eds.), *Nelson textbook of pediatrics* (19th ed., pp. 11916–11923). Philadelphia, PA: Saunders.

Fischbach, F. T., & Dunning III, M. B. (2015). *A manual of laboratory and diagnostic tests* (9th ed.). Philadelphia, PA: Wolters Kluwer Health/Lippincott Williams & Wilkins.

Foote, J. M., Brady, L. H., Burke, A. L., Cook, J. S., Dutcher, M. E., Gradoville, K. M., et al. (2011). Development of an evidence-based clinical practice guideline on linear growth measurement of children. *Journal of Pediatric Nursing, 26*(4), 312–324. doi: 10.1016/j.pedn.2010.09.002

Garibaldi, L., & Chemaitilly, W. (2011). Chapter 556: Disorders of pubertal development. In R. M. Kleigman, B. F. Stanton, J. W. St. Geme III, N. F. Schor, & R. E. Behrman (Eds.), *Nelson textbook of pediatrics* (19th ed., pp. 1886–1895). Philadelphia, PA: Saunders.

Gerard, S. (2014). Chapter 50: Diabetes mellitus and the metabolic syndrome. In S. Grossman, & C. M. Porth (Eds.), *Porth's Pathophysiology: Concepts of altered health states* (9th ed., pp. 1303–1332). Philadelphia, PA: Wolters Kluwer Health/Lippincott Williams & Wilkins.

Herzing University - Orlando. (2014). ASN/BSN concept definitions. Winter Park, FL: Author.

Hofman, P. L., Derraik, J. G., Pinto, T. E., Tregurtha, S., Faherty, A., Peart, J. M., et al. (2010). Defining the ideal injection techniques when using 5-mm needles in children and adults. *Diabetes Care, 33*(9), 1940–1944.

Hosono, H., & Cohen, P. (2011). Chapter 554: Hyperpituitarism, tall stature, and overgrowth syndromes. In R. M. Kleigman, B. F. Stanton, J. W. St. Geme III, N. F. Schor, & R. E. Behrman (Eds.), *Nelson textbook of pediatrics* (19th ed., pp. 1886). Philadelphia, PA: Saunders.

Johnson, S. R., Cooper, M. N., Jones, T. W., & Davis, E. A. (2013). Long-term outcome of insulin pump therapy in children with type 1 diabetes assessed in a large population-based case–control study. *Diabetologia, 56*(11), 2392–2400. doi: 10.1007/s00125-013-3007-9

Kremidas, D., Wisniewski, T, Divino, V. M., Bala, K., Olsen, M., Germak, J., et al. (2013). Administration burden associated with recombinant human growth hormone treatment: Perspectives of patients and caregivers. *Journal of Pediatric Nursing, 28*(1), 55–63 doi: 10.1016/j.pedn.2011.12.006

Lafranchi, S. (2011). Section 2: Disorders of the thyroid gland. In R. M. Kleigman, B. F. Stanton, J. W. St. Geme III, N. F. Schor & R. E. Behrman (Eds.), *Nelson textbook of pediatrics* (19th ed., pp. 1894–1916). Philadelphia, PA: Saunders.

LaFranchi, S. (2013). Acquired hypothyroidism in childhood and adolescence. UpToDate. Retrieved from http://www.uptodate.com/contents/acquired-hypothyroidism-in-childhood-and-adolescence?source=machineLearning&search=acquired+hypothyroidism+children&selectedTitle=1~150§ionRank=1&anchor=H3#H3

LaFranchi, S. (2014a). Clinical features and detection of congenital hypothyroidism. UpToDate. Retrieved from http://www.uptodate.com/contents/clinical-features-and-detection-of-congenital-hypothyroidism?source=search_result&search=congenital+hypothyroidism&selectedTitle=1~63

LaFranchi, S. (2014b). Treatment and prognosis of congenital hypothyroidism. UpToDate. Retrieved from http://www.uptodate.com/contents/treatment-and-prognosis-of-congenital-hypothyroidism?source=machineLearning&search=congenital+hypothyroidism&selectedTitle=2~63&anchor=H2§ionRank=1#H2

LaFranchi, S. (2014c). Treatment and prognosis of Graves' disease in children and adolescents. UpToDate. Retrieved from http://www.uptodate.com/contents/treatment-and-prognosis-of-graves-disease-in-children-and-adolescents?source=machineLearning&search=medications+to+treat+hyperthyroidism+in+children&selectedTitle=1~150§ionRank=1&anchor=H2#H2

March of Dimes. (2012). *Newborn screening*. Retrieved from http://www.marchofdimes.org/baby/newborn-screening-tests-for-your-baby.aspx

National Diabetes Education Program. (2014). *Overview of diabetes in children and adolescents.* Retrieved from http://ndep.nih.gov/media/Overview-of-Diabetes-Children-508_2014.pdf

National Diabetes Information Clearinghouse (NDIC). (2012). *What I need to know about diabetes medicines: Types of Insulin.* Retrieved from http://diabetes.niddk.nih.gov/dm/pubs/medicines_ez/insert_C.aspx

Nelson-Tuttle, C (2014). Chapter 50: Pediatric metabolic and endocrine disorders. In S. M. Nettina (Ed.), *Lippincott manual of nursing practice* (10th ed., pp. 1657–1678). Philadelphia, PA: Wolters/Kluwer Health: Lippincott Williams & Wilkins.

Parks, J. S., & Felner, E. I. (2011). Hypopituitarism. In R. M. Kleigman, B. F. Stanton, J. W. St. Geme III, N. F. Schor & R. E. Behrman (Eds.), *Nelson textbook of pediatrics* (19th ed., pp. 1876–1881). Philadelphia, PA: Saunders.

Pediatric Endocrinology Nursing Society. (2014). PENS position statement on linear growth measurement of children. Retrieved from http://www.pens.org/PENS%20Documents/PENS%20position%20statement%20on%20linear%20growth%20measurement%20FINAL.pdf

Rosenfield, R. L. (2014). Definition, clinical features and differential diagnosis of polycystic ovary syndrome in adolescents. UpToDate. Retrieved from http://www.uptodate.com/contents/definition-clinical-features-and-differential-diagnosis-of-polycystic-ovary-syndrome-in-adolescents?source=search_result&search=polycystic+ovary+syndrome&selectedTitle=4~150

Saenger, P. (2013). Definition, etiology, and evaluation of precocious puberty. UpToDate. Retrieved from http://www.uptodate.com/contents/definition-etiology-and-evaluation-of-precocious-puberty?source=search_result&search=precocious+puberty&selectedTitle=1~100

Taketokmo, C. K., Hodding, J. H., & Kraus, D. M. (2013). *Lexi-comp's drug reference handbook: Pediatric & neonatal dosage handbook* (20th ed.). Hudson, OH: Lexi-comp, Inc.

U.S. Department of Health & Human Services. (2012). *HealthyPeople.gov.* Retrieved at http://www.healthypeople.gov/2020/about/default.aspx

U.S. Food and Drug Administration. (2014a). FDA News Release: FDA approves Afrezza to treat diabetes. Retrieved from http://www.fda.gov/NewsEvents/Newsroom/PressAnnouncements/ucm384495.htm

U.S. Food and Drug Administration. (2014b). FDA News Release: FDA approves pediatric use of dexcom's G4 platinum continuous glucose monitoring system. Retrieved from http://www.fda.gov/NewsEvents/Newsroom/PressAnnouncements/ucm403122.htm

White, P. C. (2011). Section 4: Disorders of the adrenal glands. In R. M. Kleigman, B. F. Stanton, J. W. St. Geme III, N. F. Schor, & R. E. Behrman (Eds.), *Nelson textbook of pediatrics* (19th ed., pp. 1923–1943). Philadelphia, PA: Saunders.

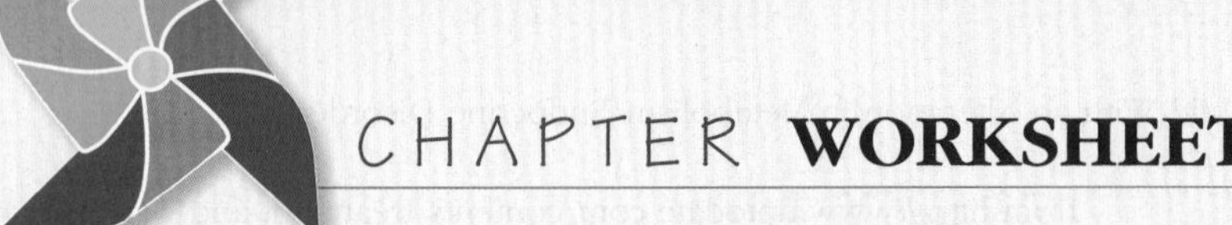

CHAPTER WORKSHEET

MULTIPLE CHOICE QUESTIONS

1. A young mother brings her new baby, diagnosed with congenital hypothyroidism, to the clinic so she can learn how to administer levothyroxine. The nurse should include which of the following instructions?
   a. Crush the medication and place it in a full bottle of formula to disguise the taste.
   b. Administer the medication every other day.
   c. Use an oral dispenser syringe or nipple to give the crushed medication mixed with a small amount of formula.
   d. Tell the mother that the medication will not be needed after the age of 7.
2. During a well-child examination which of the following comments made by the parent would indicate the possibility of a growth hormone deficiency?
   a. "I have to buy my child new clothes every 2 to 3 months"
   b. "I have to buy my child much larger shirts than pants but then the sleeves are too long."
   c. "My child wears out his clothes before he outgrows them."
   d. "I can hand down my child's clothes to his younger brother."
3. The nurse is caring for a 14-year-old boy with type 1 DM. He takes NPH insulin every morning at 7:30 AM. Which assessment data will the nurse use to evaluate the therapeutic effectiveness of the medication?
   a. Presence of signs and symptoms of hypoglycemia or hyperglycemia during the morning physical assessment
   b. Blood glucose level at 1630
   c. Appetite and food intake at lunch
   d. Blood glucose level before breakfast
4. When monitoring the blood glucose level of a 12-year-old child with type 2 DM, your reading is 50 mg/dL. Which is the most appropriate action?
   a. Encourage the child to get out of bed and increase activity.
   b. Take the child's vital signs.
   c. Ask the child about frequent urine output.
   d. Give the child 4 oz of orange juice.

DOSAGE CALCULATION QUESTION

The school nurse is caring for a child with type 1 diabetes. The child weighs 56 lb. The sliding scale corrective dose order reads: Insulin aspart before meals: (blood sugar – 120 divided by 70) + (total carbohydrate expected intake divided by 13 carbohydrates per unit). This is the corrective dose + carbohydrate consumption correction. Her blood sugar before lunch is 139 with an expected intake of 47 carbohydrates at lunch and regular activity level the rest of the day.

Calculate the insulin dose to be administered. Round to the nearest unit.

CRITICAL THINKING EXERCISES

1. A 12-year-old boy with type 1 DM has the flu. His mother calls the diabetes clinic to report that he stayed home from school and does not have an appetite, so he is not eating. The mother asks the nurse how much insulin the boy should take. He is currently taking three injections daily with regular and NPH in the morning before breakfast, regular and NPH in the evening after dinner, and regular before bedtime. What questions should the nurse ask before answering the mother's question? Based on the answers to these questions, how would you instruct the mother?
2. The mother of Robin, a 5-year-old girl, reports that Robin has a body odor. She is developing breasts and some pubic hair and was teased when she had a sleepover with friends. The review of her growth charts reveals that Robin went from the 50th percentile to the 93rd percentile in the past 6 months. Based on this information, what are the three major nursing diagnoses to begin establishing a plan of care for the child and family? What are the expected outcomes and major interventions associated with the nursing diagnosis of knowledge deficit?
3. A mother brings her baby to the clinic after receiving a phone message from the clinic saying there was a problem with the baby's thyroid test. She says the trip on the bus took a long time, but the infant slept the entire way. She says that the baby is sleeping much of the time and does not want to eat very much. The baby was discharged from the hospital 2 weeks ago. The birth was without difficulty and there were no problems during labor. Why is this visit urgent? What would the test show if the disorder was due to a pituitary gland problem and not the thyroid gland?

STUDY ACTIVITIES

1. During your clinical experiences, ask to be on an inpatient unit that provides care for children with alterations in endocrine function. Compare and contrast the health histories, assessments, laboratory tests, diagnostic procedures, and plans of care for these children with those for the care of children on other units. Participate in the teaching plan for these children and their families.

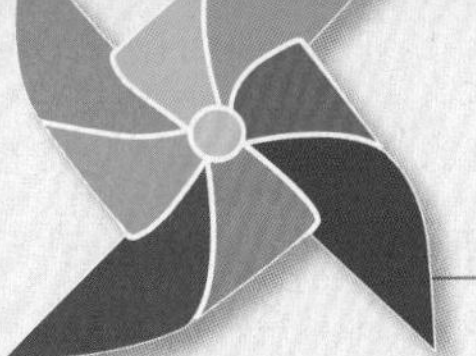

2. Attend an outpatient clinic that provides care to children with endocrine disorders. Identify the role of the registered nurse in providing coordination of care, health teaching, and referrals for these children and their families.
3. Shadow a diabetes nurse educator to observe the teaching methods and strategies he or she uses to provide an education plan for a child with DM. Observe how the nurse educator includes the family in the plan. Are there any differences between the teaching plans for type 1 DM and type 2 DM?
4. Conduct a literature review for one of the common endocrine disorders to research current management practices. Are there evidence-based practice guidelines for nursing interventions?
5. Conduct an Internet search to research the information that is available to children and their families related to DM.

BRINGING IT ALL TOGETHER: A CASE STUDY

Paige is a 5-year-old recently diagnosed with type 1 diabetes. She is currently in kindergarten at a local elementary school. Her mother is very concerned about learning all her care. She states "How can I send her to school if I am still learning how to take care of her?"

Go to thePoint to find questions to consider about this case.

49

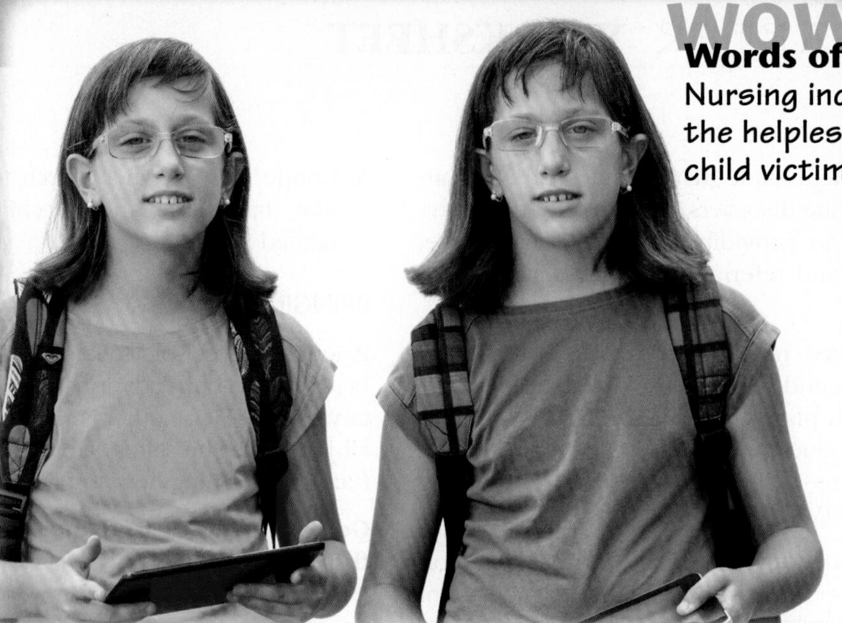

WOW

Words of Wisdom

Nursing includes care for the helpless and brave child victim of heredity.

Nursing Care of the Child With an Alteration in Genetics

KEY TERMS

chromosomal abnormality
gene testing
genetics
inborn errors of metabolism
neurocutaneous disorders
newborn screen
trisomy 21

Learning Objectives

Upon completion of the chapter, the learner will be able to:

1. Discuss the nurse's role and responsibilities when caring for a child diagnosed with a genetic disorder and his or her family.
2. Identify nursing interventions related to common laboratory and diagnostic tests used in the diagnosis and management of genetic conditions.
3. Distinguish various genetic disorders occurring in childhood.
4. Devise an individualized nursing care plan for the child with a genetic disorder.
5. Develop child/family teaching plans for the child with a genetic disorder.

***Julie Woods*, a 5-year old, is brought to the clinic for her annual examination. Her mother states, "She's so much smaller than all of the other kindergartners."**

Genetics refers to the principles and mechanics of heredity—its transmission, and its variation (Herzing University—Orlando, 2014). Nurses encounter potential or actual alterations in genetics in all types of clients and must detect problems and intervene early to prevent complications. A genetic disorder is a disease caused by an abnormality in an individual's genetic material or genome. Some genetic disorders occur in multiple family members (via inheritance of abnormal genes). Other disorders may occur in only a single family member (via spontaneous mutation).

A genetic disorder is caused by completely or partially altered genetic material. In contrast, a familial disorder is more common in relatives of the affected individual but may be caused by environmental influences, not genetic alterations.

Many chronic disorders of childhood have a genetic or inherited cause. Common disorders suspected to be caused or influenced by genetic factors include birth defects, chromosomal abnormalities, neurocutaneous disorders, intellectual disability, many types of short stature disorders, connective tissue disorders, and inborn errors of metabolism. Genetic disorders can present at any age but the most obvious and severe disorders are present in childhood (Scott & Lee, 2011a).

Our ability to diagnose genetic conditions is far superior to our ability to cure or treat them. However, accurate diagnosis does lead to improved treatment and outcomes. Nurses should have a basic knowledge of genetics, common genetic disorders in children, genetic testing, and genetic counseling so that they can provide support and information to families and can promote an improved quality of life. Refer to chapter 10 for information on advances in genetics, inheritance, and genetic counseling and evaluation.

NURSE'S ROLE AND RESPONSIBILITIES

Pediatric nurses will encounter children with genetic disorders in every clinical specialty area. This includes clinics, hospitals, schools, and community-based centers. Talking with families who have recently been diagnosed with a genetic disorder or who have had a child born with congenital anomalies is very difficult. Many times the nurse is the one who has first contact with these parents and will be the one to provide follow-up care. Genetic disorders are significant, life-changing, and possibly life-threatening situations. The information is highly technical and the field is still evolving. Therefore, it is important to refer the family to a physician or nurse practitioner who specializes in genetics. The nurse should understand who will benefit from genetic counseling and should be able to discuss the role of the genetic counselor with families. Inform families at risk that genetic counseling is available before they attempt to have another baby.

The nurse is in an ideal position to help families review what has been discussed during the genetic counseling sessions and to answer any additional questions they might have. Nurses play an essential role in providing emotional support to the family throughout this challenging time. Nurses should also refer the family to appropriate agencies, support groups, and resources, such as a social worker, a chaplain, or an ethicist.

COMMON MEDICAL TREATMENTS

A variety of medications and other medical treatments are used to treat the symptoms of genetic disorders in children. Genetic disorders do not have specific treatments and there is no cure, so treatment focuses on the specific symptoms of each disorder. Genetic disorders often involve multiple organ systems and children with these disorders have complex medical needs. Thus, a multidisciplinary approach and good communication are imperative. See below for a discussion on common genetic disorders and their management.

NURSING PROCESS OVERVIEW FOR THE CHILD WITH A GENETIC DISORDER

Care of the child with a genetic disorder includes assessment, nursing diagnosis, planning, interventions, and evaluation. There are a number of general concepts related to the nursing process that may be applied to the care of children with genetic disorders. From a general understanding of the care involved for a child with a genetic disorder, the nurse can then individualize the care based on specifics for the particular child.

Assessment

Assessment of the child with a genetic disorder includes health history, physical examination, and laboratory and diagnostic testing.

Remember Julie, the 5-year old brought in for her annual examination? What additional health history and physical examination information should you obtain?

Health History

The health history consists of past medical history, including the mother's pregnancy history; family history; neonatal history; and history of present illness (when the symptoms started and how they have progressed), as well as treatments used at home. Explore the child's current and past medical history for risk factors such as:

- Family history of genetic disorders
- Any complications during the prenatal, perinatal, or postnatal periods
- Changes in developmental status or delays in developmental milestones

The pregnancy history can be extremely relevant when identifying a genetic disorder. The pregnancy history may be significant for maternal age older than 35 years or paternal age older than 50 years, repeated premature births, breech delivery, congenital hip dysplasia, abnormalities found on ultrasound, abnormalities in prenatal blood screening tests (e.g., triple/quadruple screen, α-fetoprotein [AFP]), amniotic fluid abnormalities (polyhydramnios, oligohydramnios), multiple births, exposure to medications and known teratogens, and decreased fetal movement.

A focused neonatal history can also help identify a genetic problem. The neonatal history may be significant for symmetric intrauterine growth restriction, large for gestational age without a reason, hearing impaired, persistent hyperbilirubinemia, poor adaptation to the extrauterine environment (demonstrated by temperature and heart rate instability and poor feeding), hypotonia or hypertonia, seizures, and abnormal newborn screening results.

The family history plays a critical role in identifying genetic disorders. Gather data for three generations. If there is a positive family history, the likelihood of a genetic disorder in the child is increased. It is helpful to create a family pedigree (refer to Chapter 10 for genetic evaluation and counseling. The family history may be significant for major congenital anomalies, intellectual disability, genetic diseases, metabolic disorders, multiple miscarriages or stillbirths, developmental delays, significant learning disabilities, psychiatric problems, consanguinity, and chronic serious illness (e.g., diabetes, hypertension, renal disease, hearing impairment, blindness, asthma, seizures, and unexplained death).

When eliciting the history of the present illness, inquire about:

- Developmental delay
- Seizures
- Hypotonia or hypertonia
- Feeding problems
- Lethargy
- Failure to thrive
- Septic appearance
- Vomiting

Children known to have a genetic disorder are often admitted to the hospital for other health-related issues or complications and management of the genetic disorder. The health history should include questions related to:

- Age when the disorder was diagnosed
- Developmental delay
- Complications of the disorder (e.g., thyroid problems, cardiac problems, respiratory problems, leukemia, seizures, cognitive impairment)
- Medications the child takes for complications associated with the disorder
- Dietary restrictions
- Compliance with management regimen

Once complications have been identified, further investigation into their severity, frequency, and management is essential to the care of this child while in the hospital.

Physical Examination

Physical examination of the child with a genetic disorder includes inspection and observation, palpation, and auscultation.

INSPECTION AND OBSERVATION

Inspect and observe for congenital anomalies, either major or minor. A major anomaly is an anomaly or malformation that creates significant medical problems and requires surgical or medical management (Bacino, 2014) (Box 49.1). Minor anomalies are features that vary from those seen in the general population but do not cause an increase in morbidity in and of themselves (Bacino, 2014) (Box 49.2).

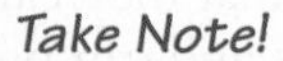

Take Note!

Low-set ears are a minor anomaly that is associated with numerous genetic dysmorphisms. If noted, assess thoroughly for other abnormalities.

BOX 49.1

EXAMPLES OF MAJOR CONGENITAL ANOMALIES

- Cleft lip
- Cleft palate
- Congenital heart disease, structural and conduction disorders
- Neural tube defects, such as myelomeningocele
- Chromosomal abnormalities
- Omphalocele; Gastrochisis
- Renal agenesis/hypoplasia
- Limb reduction defects
- Generalized dysmorphism
- Ambiguous genitalia

Adapted from Bacino, C. A. (2014). *Approach to congenital malformations*. UpToDate. Retrieved from http://www.uptodate.com/contents/approach-to-congenital-malformations?source=search_result&search=major+and+minor+congenital+anomolies&selectedTitle=2~150

BOX 49.2

EXAMPLES OF MINOR CONGENITAL ANOMALIES

- Flat occiput
- Prominent occiput
- Triple hair whorl
- Flat-bridged nose
- Nostrils anteverted
- Ear lobe crease
- Ear lobe notched
- Cup-shaped ears
- Small ears
- Cleft uvula
- Webbed neck
- Short neck
- Extra nipples
- Sacral dimple
- Tapered fingers
- Overlapping digits
- Syndactyly
- Hemangioma
- Nevi

Adapted from Bacino, C. A. (2014). *Approach to congenital malformations*. UpToDate. Retrieved from http://www.uptodate.com/contents/approach-to-congenital-malformations?source=search_result&search=major+and+minor+congenital+anomolies&selectedTitle=2~150

As the number of minor anomalies present increases, the probability of the presence of a major anomaly increases. In fact, when three or more minor anomalies are present, the risk for a major anomaly or intellectual disability is approximately 19% to 26% (Bacino, 2014). Assess for a recognized pattern of anomalies that may be associated with certain syndromes.

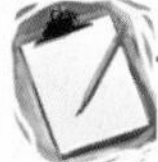

Take Note!

Cleft lip and cleft palate are associated with many syndromes. If noted, assess for other anomalies.

Inspect and observe for an abnormal or foul odor of the child's excretions. Certain metabolic disorders or inborn errors of metabolism are associated with specific odors (Table 49.1).

AUSCULTATION

Physical examination includes auscultation of the heart. Murmurs or dysrhythmias may have a genetic cause. In a child with a congenital heart problem (e.g., ventricular septal defect) and a strong family history of cardiac structural problems, a genetic cause needs to be considered.

PALPATION

Palpation can be used to detect hepatosplenomegaly (an enlarged spleen and liver). However, physicians or nurse practitioners usually perform this assessment because it requires skill and experience. Hepatosplenomegaly may indicate a metabolic disorder.

TABLE 49.1 INBORN ERRORS OF METABOLISM AND ASSOCIATED ODOR

Inborn Error of Metabolism	Associated Odor
Phenylketonuria	Mousy or musty
Maple syrup urine disease	Maple syrup, burnt sugar, or curry
Tyrosinemia	Cabbage-like, rancid butter
Trimethylaminuria	Rotting fish

Adapted from Rezvani, I., & Rezvani, G. (2011). An approach to inborn errors of metabolism. In R. M. Kleigman, B. F. Stanton, J. W. St. Geme III, N. F. Schor, & R. E. Behrman (Eds.), *Nelson textbook of pediatrics* (19th ed., pp. 416–418). Philadelphia, PA: Saunders.

Laboratory and Diagnostic Testing

Common Laboratory and Diagnostic Tests 49.1 explains the laboratory and diagnostic tests used most commonly to detect genetic disorders. The tests can assist the physician or nurse practitioner in diagnosing the disorder or can be used as guidelines in determining treatment. Laboratory or nonnursing personnel obtain some of the tests, while the nurse might obtain others. In either instance the nurse should be familiar with how the tests are obtained, what they are used for, and normal versus abnormal results. This knowledge will also be necessary when providing child and family education related to the testing. Due to the nature of the information, a referral to genetic counseling before testing may be appropriate. Advances in genetic technology, including information obtained from the Human Genome Project, have led to dramatic increases in the number of diagnostic and screening tests.

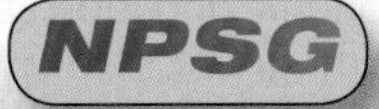

GOAL 2: Improve the Effectiveness of Communication Among Caregivers

NPSG.02.03.01 Report critical results of tests and diagnostic procedures on a timely basis.

Steps: When caring for a child with a potential or actual genetic disorder notify appropriate healthcare provider with positive prenatal screen results, and critical changes to other laboratory values and diagnostic test results.

Joint Commission. (2015). *National patient safety goals effective January 1, 2015.* Retrieved from http://www.jointcommission.org/assets/1/6/2015_NPSG_HAP.pdf

(text continues on page 1931)

COMMON LABORATORY AND DIAGNOSTIC TESTS 49.1

Test	Explanation	Indications	Nursing Implications
Amniocentesis	Ultrasound-guided (to determine placental location) insertion of a needle through the abdomen and into the uterine cavity of a pregnant woman to obtain a sample of amniotic fluid. The fluid contains skin cells that have been shed by the fetus and can be isolated and grown in the laboratory to provide enough genetic material for testing.	Test for chromosomal abnormality, neural tube defects, or specific genetic conditions of the fetus. Performed if considered high risk for a genetic disorder or abnormal ultrasound. Most common prenatal test used to diagnose chromosomal and congenital anomalies	Usually not performed until after 15 weeks' gestation. Complications include miscarriage, fetal injury, amniotic fluid leakage, infection, spontaneous abortion, premature labor, maternal hemorrhage, amniotic fluid embolism, abruptio placentae, and damage to the bladder or intestines. Results are usually not available for 7–10 days, but this varies by laboratory. Monitor fetus before and after procedure.
Chorionic villi sampling (CVS)	Involves the removal of a small amount of tissue directly from the chorionic villi (minute vascular projections of the fetal chorion that combine with maternal uterine tissue to form the placenta). In the laboratory, the chromosomes of the fetal cells are analyzed for number and type. Extra chromosomes, such as are present in Down syndrome, can be identified. Additional laboratory tests can be performed to look for specific disorders.	Test for chromosomal abnormality, fetal metabolic or blood disorders, or specific genetic conditions of the fetus. Performed if considered high risk for a genetic disorder or abnormal ultrasound. CVS cannot detect α-fetoprotein levels; therefore, does not detect neural tube defects	Performed at 7 to 11 weeks of gestation, so provides early detection of genetic abnormalities Complications include accidental abortion, infection, bleeding, amniotic fluid leakage, fetal limb deformities. Results can be available within 24 hours, but this varies depending on the laboratory and location of procedure (results are usually available sooner than with an amniocentesis). Monitor fetus before and after procedure.
Triple/quadruple screen	A maternal serum laboratory screening test that measures the level of three substances made by the developing baby and placenta: α-fetoprotein (AFP), human chorionic gonadotropin (hCG), and unconjugated estriol (uE3). Dimeric inhibin A has been added to make the "quadruple test." The addition of dimeric inhibin A increases the detection rate of Down syndrome and trisomy 18 in the quadruple screen.	A screening test for low-risk pregnant women to determine pregnancies at an increased risk for open neural tube defects, Down syndrome, and trisomy 18	Performed between 16 and 19 weeks of gestation Educate mothers that a normal test does not guarantee a healthy baby. Conversely, an abnormal result does not guarantee the baby has a problem. Additional testing will be necessary to confirm or rule out a specific genetic condition.

COMMON LABORATORY AND DIAGNOSTIC TESTS 49.1 (continued)

Test	Explanation	Indications	Nursing Implications
Fetal nuchal translucency (FNT); may be combined with pregnancy-associated plasma protein (PAPP-A) and β-hCG to increase detection rate	Ultrasound prenatal screening to help identify higher risks of Down syndrome, trisomy 13, trisomy 18, and Turner syndrome. The ultrasound assesses the amount of fluid behind the neck of a fetus (known as the nuchal fold). Increased fluid increases the risk of a chromosomal abnormality. During this early ultrasound other markers may be looked at such as presence of nasal bones (in Down syndrome hypoplasia or absence of the nasal bones may be noted); short femur or humerus increases the risk of trisomy, echogenic foci (bright spots) in the heart can increase the risk of Down syndrome, and echogenic bowel (bowel looks bright and white) can be associated with chromosomal abnormalities. A serum blood test is performed to determine the level of two hormones, PAPP-A and β-hCG. Using a combination of the results of the ultrasound and the blood test, the risk of having a baby with Down syndrome is predicted.	Any pregnant woman presenting by 11 to 13 weeks' gestation can be screened. Particularly for women with increased risk or desired screening for Down syndrome, trisomy 13, trisomy 18, or Turner syndrome	Must be performed between 11 and 13 weeks Genetic counseling before testing may be warranted. Positive tests require follow-up tests and genetic counseling.
Ultrasound	Safe, noninvasive, accurate investigation of the fetus. A transducer is placed in contact with the mother's abdomen and high-frequency sound waves are directed at the fetus. The sound waves are reflected back through the tissues and recorded and displayed in real time on a screen.	Screen for structural malformations	Usually performed at 18 to 20 weeks of gestation; routinely done Early ultrasound can be performed at 11 to 14 weeks to evaluate for Down syndrome and other chromosomal abnormalities.
Cell-free fetal DNA testing	Fetal circulating cell-free DNA is taken from a sample of maternal blood. It is an advanced screening test that can detect fetal aneuploidies for chromosome 21, 18, and 13. It can also detect X or Y chromosomes.	Indicated for higher risk pregnancies: • Woman 35 or older at time of delivery • Prior testing reveals increased risk of trisomy 21, 18 or 13 • History of previous pregnancy with a trisomy • Parental balanced robertsonian translocation	Can be performed as early as 10 weeks. Results usually available in 1 week Not recommended for low-risk pregnancies at this time due to lack of evaluation on this population[c] Positive test results requires more invasive testing and genetic counseling High detection rates with low false positives[c]

(continued)

COMMON LABORATORY AND DIAGNOSTIC TESTS 49.1 (continued)

Test	Explanation	Indications	Nursing Implications
Percutaneous umbilical blood sampling	An ultrasound-guided needle is inserted through the abdominal and uterine wall to the umbilical cord and a sample of blood is retrieved and sent to the laboratory for analysis. Procedure is similar to amniocentesis but requires a higher level of expertise and experience. Less risk than fetoscopy	Detect chromosome abnormalities. Usually done when diagnostic information cannot be obtained through amniocentesis, CVS, or ultrasound or the results of these tests were inconclusive	Performed at or after 18 weeks. Complications include miscarriage, blood loss, infection, premature rupture of membranes. The risk to the pregnancy is greater than with other prenatal procedures such as amniocentesis and CVS. Not performed as often due to risks and since discovery of fluorescent in situ hybridization (FISH)
Fetoscopy	Endoscopic procedure that allows direct visualization of the fetus through the insertion of a tiny flexible instrument called a fetoscope. It is inserted through the abdominal wall and into the uterine cavity. Ultrasound is used to guide the placement of the scope. Direct visualization can evaluate the fetus for severe congenital anomalies such as neural tube defects. Fetal blood samples from the umbilical cord can be obtained and tested for congenital blood disorders such as hemophilia and sickle cell anemia. Fetal tissue samples (usually skin) can be collected and tested for genetic diseases.	Indicated for any woman at risk for delivering a baby with significant congenital anomalies; can be used to perform corrective surgery (e.g., shunt placement) on the fetus	Performed during or after the 18th week of pregnancy Complications include spontaneous abortion, premature delivery, premature rupture of membranes, amniotic fluid leak, intrauterine fetal death, infection. Monitor fetus before and after procedure.
Gene testing	**Gene testing** is currently available for many inherited diseases. It involves analysis of DNA, RNA, chromosomes, proteins, metabolites, and biochemical agents. Specimens for gene testing can be obtained from numerous sources; leukocytes from blood are the most common and easily obtained site; during pregnancy, amniocentesis and chorionic villus sampling; and fetal tissue or products of conception after a miscarriage Most common use is DNA or chromosomes isolated from blood Direct detection of abnormalities in genes and chromosomes is performed using DNA-based test or cytogenetic tests (which look at chromosome) and other methods. Cytogenetic tests also include FISH to assist in detecting chromosomal abnormalities such as duplication, deletion, rearrangements, and translocations; newer testing, known as array comparative genomic hybridization (aCGH), or microarray, analyzes small duplications or deletions across all of the chromosomes.	To detect abnormalities that may indicate actual disease or predict future disease. Indicated in the evaluation of congenital anomalies, intellectual disability, growth retardation, recurrent miscarriage to determine reason for the loss of a fetus, prenatal diagnosis of genetic disease.	Provide support, information, and resources to family. Refer to genetic counseling before and after test.

COMMON LABORATORY AND DIAGNOSTIC TESTS 49.1 (continued)

Test	Explanation	Indications	Nursing Implications
Newborn screening (refer to Chapter 31 for further information)	Blood screening performed shortly after birth, used to identify many life-threatening genetic illnesses that have no immediate visible effects but can lead to physical problems, intellectual disability, and even death Every US state routinely screens all newborns, but each state dictates which disorders to screen for, so components of the screening vary from state to state.	Identification of newborns so that treatment can begin early to prevent impact of disorder, such as severe cognitive impairment or death	Refer to each state's protocol for fetal/newborn screening for endocrine disorders. Explain to family the rationale and procedure. Collect blood sample accurately. Collect prior to blood transfusion if possible. Ideally performed after 24 hours of age; obtain specimen as close to time of discharge from newborn or labor and delivery unit as possible and no later than 7 days of age Screening typically between 24 and 48 hours after birth.[a] The test is less accurate if done before 24 hours of age and should be repeated by 2 weeks of age if the newborn is younger than 24 hours old. Some states now require a repeat screen at 2 weeks of age[b] Ensure appropriate follow-up with newborn screening results; results are available in 2 to 3 weeks.

[a]March of Dimes. (2012). *Newborn screening.* Retrieved from http://www.marchofdimes.org/baby/newborn-screening-tests-for-your-baby.aspx

[b]Centers for Disease Control and Prevention. (2014). *Newborn screening: Importance of newborn screening.* Retrieved from http://www.cdc.gov/ncbddd/newbornscreening/

[c]The American College of Obstetricians and Gynecologists Committee on Genetics & The Society for Maternal-Fetal Medicine Publications Committee. (2012). Committee opinion no. 545: Noninvasive prenatal testing for fetal aneuploidy. *American College of Obstetricians and Gynecologists, 120,* 1532–1534.

Adapted from Fischbach, F. T., & Dunning III, M. B. (2015). *A manual of laboratory and diagnostic tests* (9th ed.). Philadelphia, PA: Wolters Kluwer Health/Lippincott Williams & Wilkins.

Nursing Diagnoses, Goals, Interventions, and Evaluation

Upon completion of an assessment, the nurse might identify several nursing diagnoses, including:

- Deficient knowledge (specify)
- Decisional conflict
- Risk for delayed growth and development
- Fear
- Interrupted family processes

After completing an assessment of Julie, the nurse noted the following: short stature for age and a low posterior hairline. Based on these assessment findings, what would your top three nursing diagnoses be for Julie?

Nursing goals, interventions, and evaluation for the child with a genetic disorder are based on the nursing diagnoses. Nursing Care Plan 49.1, found at the end of the chapter, provides a general guide for planning care for a child with a genetic disorder. Additional information about nursing management will be included later in the chapter as it relates to specific disorders.

No matter what the genetic abnormality is, the news may be shattering to the family. It is difficult for nurses to even begin to understand what the family is going through. When providing support and education to families of children with serious genetic abnormalities, use these guiding principles:

- Build a trusting relationship.
- Stress the authenticity of the parents' feelings.
- Reject your own personal biases.
- Recognize that individuals cope in various ways; the family's behavior may not be what you would expect.
- Help the family to identify their own strengths and supports, building on those as able.
- Know that the family's emotions may exhaust and disorganize them.
- Assist the family members to maintain open communication among themselves.
- Provide referrals to local parent groups or other families with a child with a similar disorder.
- Allow the family to verbalize their emotions and ask questions.
- Always ask the parents how *they* are doing (Lashley, 2005).

Based on your top three nursing diagnoses for Julie, describe appropriate nursing interventions.

COMMON CHROMOSOMAL ABNORMALITIES

Chromosomal abnormalities are seen in about 1 in 150 babies (March of Dimes, 2013). Many children with chromosomal abnormalities have associated intellectual disabilities, learning disabilities, behavioral problems, and distinct features, including physical birth defects. The risk for autosomal trisomies increases with advanced maternal age (March of Dimes, 2013). The most common chromosomal abnormalities will be discussed below. New and improved techniques in chromosome analysis allow for the identification of tiny and more complex abnormalities that could not be seen before (Searl, 2014). Therefore, more chromosomal abnormalities are being identified in children (Table 49.2).

Trisomy 21 (Down Syndrome)

Trisomy 21 (Down syndrome) is a genetic disorder caused by the presence of all or part of an extra 21st chromosome. It is the most common chromosomal abnormality associated with intellectual disability (Ostermaier, 2015). One in 730 live births results in trisomy 21 (Weremowicz, 2014). Approximately 85% of trisomy 21 conceptions result in spontaneous abortion (Schrijver, Zehnder & Cherry, 2014). Trisomy 21 is seen in all ages, races, and socioeconomic levels, but a higher incidence is found with a maternal age older than 35 years (Summar & Lee, 2011). This is partly explained by the fact that 90% of cases with an extra chromosome 21 originates from the mother (Weremowicz, 2014). The likelihood of having a baby with Down syndrome is around 1 in 1,000 in women younger than age 30, 1 in 353 at age 35, 1 in 85 at age 40, and 1 in 35 at age 45 (Weremowicz, 2014).

Trisomy 21 is associated with some degree of intellectual disability, characteristic facial features (e.g., slanted eyes and depressed nasal bridge), and other health problems (e.g., cardiac defects, visual and hearing impairment, intestinal malformations, and an increased susceptibility to infections). The severity of these problems varies.

The prognosis has been improving over the past few decades. Fundamental changes in the care of these

TABLE 49.2 LESS COMMON CHROMOSOMAL ABNORMALITIES

Chromosomal Abnormality	Features
Prader–Willi syndrome (abnormality on chromosome 15)	Affects 1 in 16,000 to 25,000 babies[a] Severe hypotonia, obesity, short stature, small hands and feet, hypogonadism, hyperphagia, and intellectual disability (varies from mild to severe)
Angelman syndrome (abnormality on chromosome 15)	Affects 1 in 12,000 to 20,000 babies[b] Microcephaly with flatness on the back of the head, fair skin and light hair, large mouth with tongue protrusion, seizures, jerky ataxic movements (resembling a puppet gait), uncontrolled bouts of laughter/smiling, happy demeanor, easily excitable personality, developmental delay and speech impairment, and severe intellectual disability

TABLE 49.2 LESS COMMON CHROMOSOMAL ABNORMALITIES (continued)

Chromosomal Abnormality	Features
Cri-du-chat syndrome (abnormality on chromosome 5)	Affects 1 in 20,000 to 50,000 babies[c] Hypotonia; short stature; slow growth; low birth weight; failure to thrive; characteristic weak, cat-like cry during infancy; microcephaly with protruding metopic suture; moon-like round face; bilateral epicanthal folds (folds of skin over the eyelids); high-arched palate; wide and flat nasal bridge; micrognathia (small receding chin); wide set eyes (hypertelorism); low-set malformed ears; simian crease; intellectual disability and developmental delay
Wolf–Hirschhorn syndrome (abnormality on chromosome 4)	Affects 1 in 50,000 babies[d] Hypotonia, intellectual disability, delayed growth and development, seizures, and characteristic facial features (broad, flat nose bridge; high forehead; widely spaced, protruding eyes; microcephaly)
Williams syndrome (abnormality on chromosome 4)	Affects 1 in 7,500 to 10,000 children[e] Affects multiple systems. Cardiovascular disease (supravalvular aortic stenosis most common, hypertension also seen); distinct facial features often described as elphin like, such as broad forehead, flat nasal bridge, short nose with broad tip, full cheeks, and a wide mouth with full lips; small, wide-spaced teeth with occlusal abnormalities; hypercalcemia; early puberty for both males and females; structural abnormalities of the kidneys, delayed bladder training and urinary frequency, hypotonia, and joint laxity; learning disabilities and intellectual disability, attention deficit disorder, problems with anxiety and phobias such as fears of sounds and tactile issues; unique personality characteristics, such as outgoing and engaging personality; other medical problems involving eyes and vision and digestive tract
Beckwith–Wiedemann syndrome (abnormality on chromosome 11)	Affects 1 in 13,700 babies[f] Infants considerably larger than normal and grow at an unusual rate in childhood, growth slows in later childhood with adults not unusually tall, specific parts of the body may grow larger leading to asymmetric appearance; abdominal wall defects such as omphalocele, umbilical hernia; infants present with abnormally large tongue that may interfere with breathing, swallowing, and speaking; abnormally large abdominal organs; crease or pits in skin near ears, hypoglycemia, and kidney abnormalities; increased risk of developing cancerous and noncancerous tumors, such as Wilms tumor, neuroblastoma
22q11 deletion syndrome (Velocardiofacial/DiGeorge syndrome) (abnormality of chromosome 22)	Affects 1 in 4,000 babies[g] Hypoplasia or agenesis of the thymus and parathyroid glands, hypocalcemia, hypoplasia of auricle and external auditory canal, cardiac anomalies, immune system abnormalities, cleft palate, short stature, distinctive facial appearance (elongated face, almond-shaped eyes, wide nose, small ears), and developmental delays, learning, speech, feeding, and behavioral problems http://www.vcfsfa.org.au/pages/home.php:Velo-Cardio-Facial Syndrome Educational Foundation, Inc.

Helpful links related to the chromosomal abnormalities and features outlined here are provided on thePoint.

[a]Ann O Scheimann, A. O. (2014). *Epidemiology and genetics of Prader-Willi syndrome.* UpToDate. Retrieved from http://www.uptodate.com/contents/epidemiology-and-genetics-of-prader-willi-syndrome?source=see_link

[b]Genetics Home Reference. (2015a). *Angelman syndrome.* Retrieved from http://ghr.nlm.nih.gov/condition/angelman-syndrome

[c]Genetics Home Reference. (2015b). *Cri-Du-Chat Syndrome.* Retrieved from http://ghr.nlm.nih.gov/condition/cri-du-chat-syndrome.

[d]Genetics Home Reference. (2015c). *Wolf-Hirschhorn syndrome.* Retrieved from http://ghr.nlm.nih.gov/condition/wolf-hirschhorn-syndrome

[e]Genetics Home Reference. (2015d). *Williams syndrome.* Retrieved from http://ghr.nlm.nih.gov/condition/williams-syndrome

[f]Hon-Yin, B. C., Shuman, C., Choufani, S., & Weksberg, R. (2014). *Beckwith-Wiedemann syndrome.* UpToDate. Retrieved from http://www.uptodate.com/contents/beckwith-wiedemann-syndrome?source=search_result&search=Beckwith-Wiedemann+syndrome&selectedTitle=1~37#H130269

[g]Genetics Home Reference. (2015e). *22q11.2 deletion syndrome.* Retrieved from http://ghr.nlm.nih.gov/condition/22q112-deletion-syndrome

children have resulted in longer life expectancy (around 55 to 56 years of age) and an improved quality of life (Ostermaier, 2014).

Pathophysiology

Trisomy 21 is a disorder caused by nondisjunction or translocation before, at, or after conception.

Each egg and sperm cell normally contain 23 chromosomes. When they join, this results in 23 pairs or 46 chromosomes. Sometimes an extra chromosome originates in the development of either the egg or the sperm, resulting in an embryo with three chromosome 21s in *all* cells (Fig. 49.1). This results in the characteristic features and birth defects of Down syndrome. This type and timing of nondisjunction, resulting in the presence of three chromosome 21s in all cells, is responsible for 95% of cases of Down syndrome (Bull & the Committee on Genetics, 2011).

In approximately 1% to 2% of cases of Down syndrome, the nondisjunction occurs *after* fertilization and a mixture of two cell types is seen (Bull & the Committee on Genetics, 2011). In these cases some cells have 47 chromosomes (due to three chromosome 21s), while others have the normal 46 chromosomes (with the normal two chromosome 21s present). This is referred to as the mosaic form of Down syndrome. Children with mosaic Down syndrome may have a milder form of the disorder, but this is not a general finding.

About 3% to 4% of Down syndrome cases involve a translocation, in which part of the number 21 chromosome breaks off during cell division *before or at* conception and attaches (or translocates) to another chromosome (usually chromosome 14) (Bull & the Committee on Genetics, 2011). The cells will remain with 46 chromosomes, but this extra portion of the number 21 chromosome results in the clinical findings of Down syndrome. Cases of translocation are not associated with advanced maternal age, as is the situation with nondisjunction errors (Weremowicz, 2014).

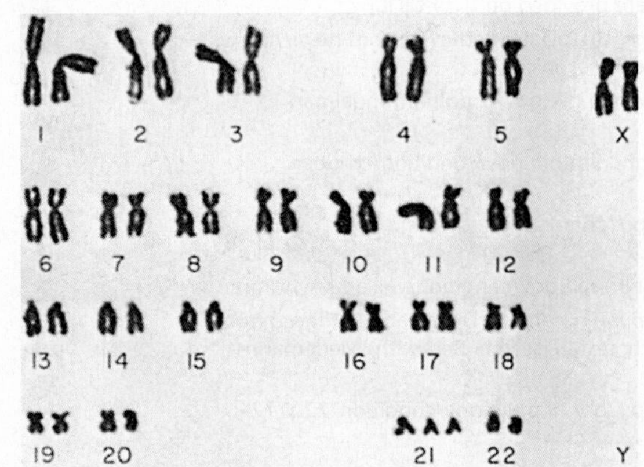

FIGURE 49.1 Down syndrome karyotype. Note the third chromosome located at chromosome 21.

Therapeutic Management

Management of Down syndrome will involve multiple disciplines, including a primary physician; specialty physicians such as a cardiologist, ophthalmologist, and gastroenterologist; nurses; physical therapists; occupational therapists; speech therapists; dietitians; psychologists; counselors; teachers; and, of course, the parents. There is no standard treatment for all children, and there is no prevention or cure. Treatment is mainly symptomatic and supportive. The overall focus of therapeutic management will be to promote the child's optimal growth and development and function within the limits of the disease.

MANAGING COMPLICATIONS

Children with Down syndrome need the usual immunizations, well-child care, and screening recommended by the American Academy of Pediatrics. In addition, medical management will focus on complications associated with Down syndrome.

Congenital heart disease occurs in 40% to 50% of children with Down syndrome (Bull & the Committee on Genetics, 2011). Cardiac problems vary from minor defects that respond to medication therapy to major defects that require surgical intervention. Children with Down syndrome also have an increased incidence of gastrointestinal disorders (Bull & the Committee on Genetics, 2011). These disorders vary from those that can be managed by dietary manipulation, such as celiac disease and constipation, to intestinal malformations such as Hirschsprung disease and imperforate anus, which require surgical intervention.

Hearing and vision impairments also are common. More than 75% of children with Down syndrome have a hearing loss (Bull & the Committee on Genetics, 2011). Otitis media is a common problem, inflicting 50% to 70% of children with Down syndrome and is often the cause for hearing loss (Ostermaier, 2015). Sixty percent of children with Down syndrome have an eye disease (Bull & the Committee on Genetics, 2011). Therefore, regular evaluation of vision and hearing is essential.

Obstructive sleep apnea is present in 50% to 75% of children with Down syndrome (Bull & the Committee on Genetics, 2011). Often parents are unaware their child is having sleep disturbances, so baseline testing in young children may be warranted.

Children with Down syndrome have a higher incidence of thyroid disease, which can affect growth and cognitive function (Bull & the Committee on Genetics, 2011). Most of these children have hypothyroidism (an underactive thyroid), but sometimes hyperthyroidism (an overactive thyroid) occurs. Periodic thyroid testing may be warranted. Children with Down syndrome are also at a higher risk for obesity and delayed dental eruptions or hypodontia (Bull & the Committee on Genetics, 2011). Some studies have found an increased risk of type 1 diabetes in children with Down syndrome (Ostermaier, 2015).

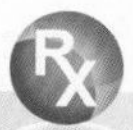

Dosage Calculation Box 49.1

Child's age: 4 years old
Child's weight: 30 lb
Medication order: Levothyroxine (Synthroid) 75 μg by mouth once a day.
Per the Pediatric Dosage Handbook, the recommended dose for a child 1 to 5 years of age is 5 to 6 μg/kg/day
Is the ordered dose safe?

Children with Down syndrome are at an increased risk for atlantoaxial instability (increased mobility of the cervical spine at the first and second vertebrae) (Bull & the Committee on Genetics, 2011). In most cases these children are asymptomatic, but symptoms may appear if spinal cord compression occurs. Screening for atlantoaxial instability may be appropriate, especially if the child is involved in sports.

Take Note!

If neck pain, unusual posturing of the head and neck (torticollis), change in gait, loss of upper body strength, abnormal reflexes, or change in bowel or bladder functioning is noted in the child with Down syndrome, immediate attention is required.

Children with Down syndrome are at an increased risk for certain hematologic problems, such as anemia, transient leukemia (mostly during the newborn period), leukemia (later onset) and polycythemia during infancy (Bull & the Committee on Genetics, 2011). Children with Down syndrome also have a higher susceptibility to infection and a higher mortality rate from infectious diseases (Bull & the Committee on Genetics, 2011). Precautions to prevent and monitor for infection are needed. Other potential complications include alopecia, communication disorders, and seizures.

Due to their increased risk for certain congenital anomalies and diseases, children with Down syndrome will need to be monitored closely, and regular medical care is essential.

EARLY INTERVENTION THERAPY

Early intervention refers to a variety of specialized programs and resources available to young children with developmental delay or other impairment. These programs may involve an array of healthcare professionals such as physical, occupational, and speech therapists; special educators; and social workers. The programs focus on providing stimulation and encouragement to children with Down syndrome. They help encourage and accelerate development and may help to prevent some developmental delays. The earlier the intervention can begin, the more beneficial it will be. The programs are individualized to meet the specific needs of each child.

Children with Down syndrome progress through the same developmental stages as typical children, but they do so on their own timetable (refer to Table 49.3 for the average age of skill acquisition in children with Down syndrome). For example, children with Down syndrome will learn to walk, but the average child with Down syndrome walks at 24 months (versus 12 months for a child without Down syndrome). Conditions such as hypotonia, ligament laxity, decreased strength, enlarged tongue, and short arms and legs are common in children with Down syndrome, and early intervention can help in the development of gross and fine motor skills, language, and social and self-care skills.

Parents also benefit from early intervention programs in terms of support, encouragement, and information. Early intervention programs teach parents how to interact with their child while meeting the child's specific needs and encouraging development.

Nursing Assessment

For a full description of the assessment phase of the nursing process, refer to page 1925. Assessment findings pertinent to Down syndrome are discussed below.

HEALTH HISTORY

Down syndrome is often diagnosed prenatally using perinatal screening and diagnostic tests. If not diagnosed prenatally, most cases are diagnosed in the first few days of life based on the physical characteristics associated with Down syndrome. Identify high-risk deliveries. Explore the pregnancy history and past medical history for risk factors such as:

- Lack of prenatal care or screening
- Abnormal prenatal screening or diagnostic tests for Down syndrome (e.g., fetal nuchal translucency, triple/quadruple screen, ultrasound, amniocentesis)
- Maternal age older than 35 years

The older infant or child known to have Down syndrome is often admitted to the hospital for corrective surgeries or other complications of the disease, such as infections. Elicit a description of the present illness and chief complaint. In an infant or child returning for a clinic visit or hospitalization, the health history should include questions related to:

- Cardiac defects or disease (treatment regimen, surgical repair)
- Hearing or vision impairment (last hearing and vision evaluation, any corrective measures)
- Developmental delays (speech, gross and fine motor skills)
- Sucking or feeding problems
- Cognitive abilities (degree of intellectual disability)
- Gastrointestinal disorders such as vomiting or absence of stools (special dietary management, surgical interventions)

TABLE 49.3 AVERAGE AGE OF SKILL ACQUISITION IN CHILDREN WITH DOWN SYNDROME

Developmental Milestone	Average Age of Acquisition, Children With Down Syndrome (months)	Average Age of Acquisition, Typical Children (months)
Smile	2	1
Roll over	6	4
Sit alone	9	7
Crawl	11	9
Walk	21	13
Speak words	14	10
Speak in sentences	24	21
Feed self with fingers	12	8
Use spoon	20	13
Bladder training	48	32
Bowel training	42	29
Undress	40	32
Put on clothes	58	47

Adapted from Pueschel, S. M. (2011). *A parent's guide to Down syndrome: Toward a brighter future* (rev. ed.). Baltimore, MD: Paul H. Brookes Publishing Company, Inc.

- Thyroid disease
- Hematologic problems, such as anemia, leukemia
- Atlantoaxial instability
- Seizures
- Infections such as recurrent or chronic respiratory infections, otitis media
- Growth (height and weight changes, feeding problems, unexplained weight gain)
- Signs and symptoms of sleep apnea, such as snoring, restlessness during sleep, daytime sleepiness
- Any other changes in physical state or medication regimen

PHYSICAL EXAMINATION

The initial assessment after birth may reveal certain physical features characteristic of Down syndrome (Box 49.3 and Fig. 49.2).

Observe the child's general appearance. Note lack of muscle tone and loose joints; this is usually more pronounced in infancy, and the infant has a floppy appearance. Observe growth and development. Plot growth on appropriate growth charts. Because children with Down syndrome grow at a slower rate, special growth charts have been developed (see thePoint for an example).

When assessing achievement of developmental milestones in children with Down syndrome, it may be more useful to look at the sequence of milestones rather than the age at which they were achieved. Each milestone represents a skill that is needed for the next stage of development.

Perform a subjective assessment of hearing and refer the child for further evaluation if indicated. Assess vision, especially for cataracts. Assess respiratory status and cardiac status. Auscultate for murmurs and pulmonary changes, which can indicate congenital heart disease. Chronic or recurrent respiratory infections, such as pneumonia and otitis media, may be found.

LABORATORY AND DIAGNOSTIC TESTS

Down syndrome risk screening can be calculated incorporating maternal age prenatally between 11 and 14 weeks using ultrasound and blood tests (nuchal translucency and pregnancy-associated plasma protein A [PAPP-A] and human chorionic gonadotropin [hCG]), and around 16 and 18 weeks using triple/quadruple blood tests to detect AFP, hCG, estriol, and/or inhibin A levels (Bull & the Committee on Genetics, 2011). Ultrasound and amniocentesis or chorionic villi sampling (CVS) to detect chromosomal abnormalities can also occur prenatally. Down syndrome

BOX 49.3

COMMON CLINICAL MANIFESTATIONS OF DOWN SYNDROME

- Hypotonia
- Short stature
- Flattened occiput
- Small (brachycephalic) head
- Flat facial profile
- Depressed nasal bridge and small nose
- Oblique palpebral fissures (an upward slant to the eyes)
- Brushfield spots (white spots on the iris of the eye)
- Low-set ears
- Abnormally shaped ears
- Small mouth
- Protrusion of tongue; tongue is large compared to mouth size
- Arched palate
- Hands with broad, short fingers
- A single deep transverse crease on the palm of the hand (simian crease)
- Congenital heart defect
- Short neck, with excessive skin at the nape
- Hyperflexibility and looseness of joints (excessive ability to extend the joints)
- Dysplastic middle phalanx of fifth finger (one flexion furrow instead of two)
- Epicanthal folds (small skin folds on the inner corner of the eyes)
- Excessive space between large and second toe

Adapted from Summar, K., & Lee, B. (2011). Chapter 76.2: Down syndrome and other abnormalities of chromosome number. In R. M. Kleigman, B. F. Stanton, J. W. St. Geme III, N. F. Schor, & R. E. Behrman (Eds.), *Nelson textbook of pediatrics* (19th ed., pp. 399–403). Philadelphia, PA: Saunders. and Bull, M. J., & Committee on Genetics. (2011). From the American academy of pediatrics: Clinical report: Health supervision for children with Down syndrome. *Pediatrics, 128*(2), 393–406. Retrieved from http://pediatrics.aappublications.org/content/128/2/393.full

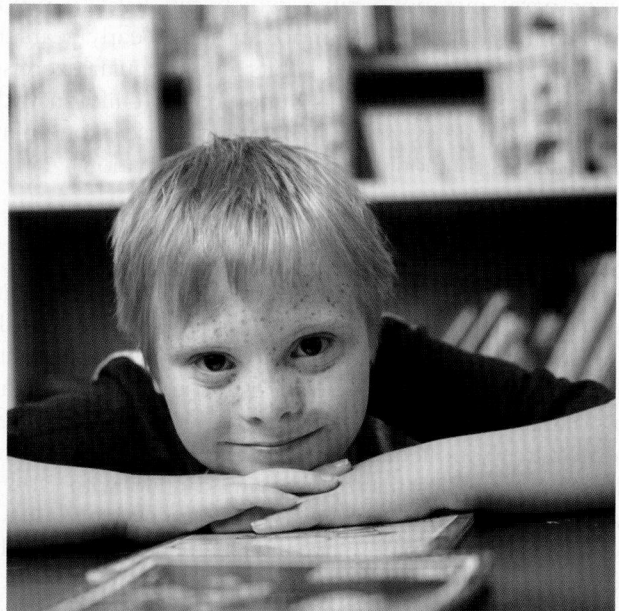

FIGURE 49.2 Child with Down syndrome.

can be confirmed after birth using chromosome analysis (see Common Laboratory and Diagnostic Tests 49.1).

Common laboratory and diagnostic studies ordered for the diagnosis and assessment of complications associated with Down syndrome include:

- Echocardiogram: to detect cardiac defects
- Vision and hearing screening: to detect vision and hearing impairments
- Thyroid hormone level: to detect thyroid disease
- Cervical x-rays: to assess for atlantoaxial instability
- Ultrasound: to assess for gastrointestinal malformations

These tests will be important in evaluating the severity of the child's physical disabilities.

Nursing Management

Due to the high incidence of Down syndrome and the complex medical needs of these children, most pediatric nurses are likely to care for these children in their practice. Nursing management focuses on providing supportive measures such as promoting growth and development, preventing complications, promoting nutrition, and providing support and education to the child and family. In addition to the nursing diagnoses and related interventions discussed in Nursing Care Plan 49.1, additional considerations are reviewed below.

Atraumatic Care

When planning atraumatic care interventions when caring for a child with Down syndrome, be sure to individualize interventions based on the child's developmental level.

PROMOTING GROWTH AND DEVELOPMENT

Children with Down syndrome tend to grow more slowly, learn more slowly, have shorter attention spans, and have trouble with reasoning and judgment. Their personality tends to be one of genuine warmth and cheerfulness along with patience, gentleness, and a natural spontaneity. Growth and developmental milestones for children with Down syndrome have been developed as a guide for physicians and nurse practitioners. Table 49.3 gives examples of the average age at which these children reach selected milestones versus typical children.

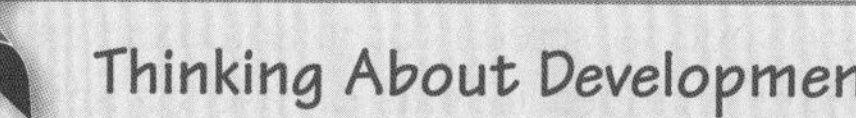

Thinking About Development

As a nurse in a physician's office, how will your education on safety differ when caring for an infant with Down syndrome compared to a toddler or adolescent?

Nurses play a key role in connecting families with appropriate resources that can facilitate the child's growth and development. The sooner early intervention programs can begin, the better for the child (see the above discussion on early intervention). Speech and language therapy, occupational therapy, and physical therapy will be important in promoting the child's growth and development. Special education should fit the child's individual needs, and the child should be integrated into mainstream education whenever possible.

PREVENTING COMPLICATIONS

Children with Down syndrome are at risk for certain health problems (see above). Even though most nurses will encounter a child with Down syndrome in their practice, only a few nurses will become experts in their care. The needs of these children are complex, and the American Academy of Pediatrics has developed guidelines that can help the nurse care for these children and their families. See Appendix I. Nurses play a key role in educating parents and caregivers about how to prevent the complications of Down syndrome (see Teaching Guidelines 49.1).

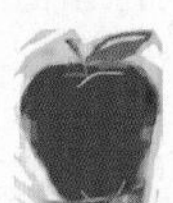

Teaching Guidelines 49.1

HEALTH GUIDELINES FOR CHILDREN WITH DOWN SYNDROME

- Have your child evaluated by a pediatric cardiologist, including an echocardiogram.
- Take your child for routine vision and hearing tests. By 6 months have your child seen by a pediatric ophthalmologist.
- Make sure your child gets regular medical care, including recommended immunizations and a thyroid test at 6 and 12 months and then yearly.
- Have your child follow a regular diet and exercise routine.
- Make sure all family members perform proper hand hygiene to prevent infection.
- Monitor for signs and symptoms of respiratory infections, such as pneumonia and otitis media.
- Discuss with your physician the use of pneumococcal, respiratory syncytial virus, and influenza vaccines.
- Begin early interventions, therapy, and education as soon as possible.
- Make sure your child brushes his or her teeth regularly. He or she should visit the dentist every 6 months.
- Make sure the child gets a cervical x-ray between 3 and 5 years of age to screen for atlantoaxial instability. Report any changes in gait or use of arms and hands, weakness, changes in bowel or bladder function, complaints of neck pain or stiffness, head tilt, torticollis, or generalized changes in function. Ensure cervical spine positioning precautions (to avoid over extending or flexing of the neck) are utilized during procedures, such as those involving anesthetic, surgery or x-rays.

Adapted from Bull, M. J., & Committee on Genetics. (2011). From the American academy of pediatrics: Clinical Report:Health supervision for children with Down syndrome. *Pediatrics*, *128*(2), 393–406. Retrieved from http://pediatrics.aappublications.org/content/128/2/393.full

PROMOTING NUTRITION

Children with Down syndrome may have difficulty sucking and feeding due to lack of muscle tone. They tend to have small mouths; a smooth, flat, large tongue; and due to the underdeveloped nasal bone, chronically stuffy noses. This may lead to poor nutritional intake and problems with growth. These problems usually improve as the child gains tongue control. Use of a bulb syringe, humidification, and changing the infant's position can lessen the problem. Breastfeeding a baby with Down syndrome is usually possible, and the antibodies in breast milk can help the infant fight infections. The caregiver's hand can be used to provide additional support of the chin and throat. Speech or occupational therapists can work on strengthening muscles and assisting in feeding accommodations. Other feeding problems and failure to thrive can be related to cardiac defects and usually improve after medical management is initiated or corrective surgery performed.

Children with Down syndrome do not need a special diet unless underlying gastrointestinal disease is present, such as celiac disease. A balanced, high-fiber diet and regular exercise are important. Research has suggested that children with Down syndrome have lower basal metabolic rates, which can lead to problems with obesity, so it is important in the early years to develop appropriate eating habits and a regular exercise routine. High fiber intake is important for children with Down syndrome because their lack of muscle tone may decrease gastric motility, leading to constipation.

PROVIDING SUPPORT AND EDUCATION FOR THE CHILD AND FAMILY

Down syndrome is a lifelong disorder that can result in health problems and cognitive disability. The diagnosis is usually made prenatally or shortly after birth. Parents and caregivers will need support and education during this difficult time. The range of mental impairment varies from mild to moderate; severe deficits occur occasionally. Some families may see having a child with Down syndrome as a lifelong tragedy; others may view it as a positive growing experience. Evaluate how the family defines and manages this experience. Base the plan of care on each individual family's values, beliefs, strengths, and resources.

Family members may have trouble meeting the demands of caring for a child with Down syndrome. These children have complex medical needs, which place strain on the family and its finances. From the time of diagnosis, the family should be involved in the child's care. Include parents in planning interventions and care for the child. In most cases they are the primary caregivers and will provide daily care as well as assisting the child in the development of functioning and skills. They can provide essential information to the healthcare team and will be advocates for their child throughout his or her life.

As the child grows, the needs of the family and child will change. Recognize and respect these needs and provide ongoing education and support for the child and family. Children with Down syndrome will need meaningful education programs. Many children with Down syndrome begin formal education in infancy and continue through high school.

The outlook is brighter than it once was for children with Down syndrome. Many go on in adulthood to obtain jobs, to receive secondary education, and to live on their own or in semi-independent housing. Be familiar with local and national resources for families of children with Down syndrome so that you can help these children fulfill their potential. An extensive list of helpful resources is provided on thePoint.

Consider This

"The day after my son was born I was told they suspected he had Down syndrome. Once the diagnosis was confirmed I felt devastated. I grieved the loss of all the dreams I had for him and felt alone and scared. I wonder 'why us?'"

Thoughts: How will you respond to this mother?

Trisomy 18 and Trisomy 13

Trisomy 18 (also known as Edwards syndrome) and trisomy 13 (also known as Patau syndrome) are two other common trisomies. These trisomies are much more severe and debilitating than trisomy 21. The incidence of trisomy 18 (the presence of three number 18 chromosomes) is 1 in 6,000 births; the incidence of trisomy 13 (the presence of three number 13 chromosomes) is 1 in 10,000 births (Bacino & Lee, 2011). Like Down syndrome, trisomy 13 and trisomy 18 usually result from nondisjunction during cell division. Trisomy 18 and trisomy 13 can be present in all cells or may occur in mosaic forms. Both are associated with a characteristic set of anomalies and severe intellectual disability (Bacino & Lee, 2011).

The prognosis for trisomy 18 and trisomy 13 is usually poor; these children usually do not survive beyond the first year of life. There is no cure for trisomy 18 or trisomy 13. Therapeutic management will focus on managing the various congenital anomalies and health issues associated with the disorders.

Nursing Assessment

Nursing assessment will include a general observation for characteristic anomalies (Table 49.4 and Figs. 49.3 and 49.4).

Prenatal screening and diagnostic tests for trisomy 18 and trisomy 13 exist. If not diagnosed during the prenatal period, most cases are diagnosed in the first few days of life based on the physical characteristics associated with the disorders.

Nursing Management

Nursing management will be mainly supportive. This will be a difficult time for the family, so providing support and resources for the family will be an important nursing function. SOFT is a support organization for families who have had a child with a chromosome abnormality (visit thePoint for a link to this resource).

Turner Syndrome

Turner syndrome is a common abnormality of the sex chromosome. The phenotype is female. It occurs in about 1 in 2,500 live female births (Bacino, 2015). The abnormality is due to a loss of all or part of one of the

TABLE 49.4 CLINICAL MANIFESTATIONS OF TRISOMY 18 AND TRISOMY 13

Chromosomal Abnormality	Clinical Manifestations
Trisomy 18	Prominent occiput, low-set ears, short eyelid fissures, severe intellectual disability, severe hypotonia, webbing, clenched fist with index finger over third digit and fifth digit overlapping the fourth, hypoplasia of fingernails, narrow hips with limited abduction, short sternum, congenital cardiac defects
Trisomy 13	Microcephalic head, wide sagittal suture and fontanels, malformed ears, small eyes, extra digits, severe hypotonia, severe intellectual disability, congenital heart defects, cleft lip, cleft palate

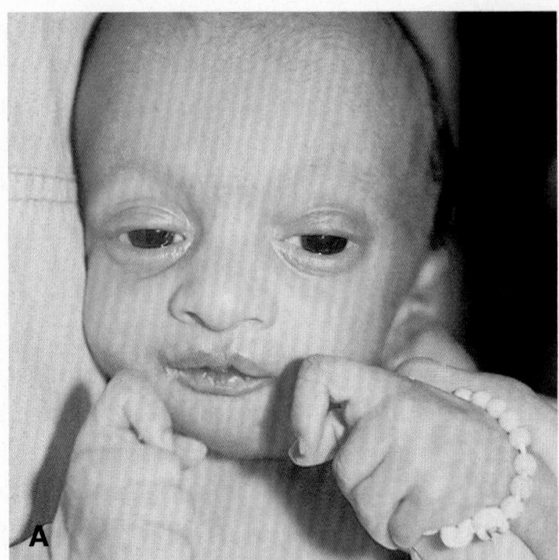

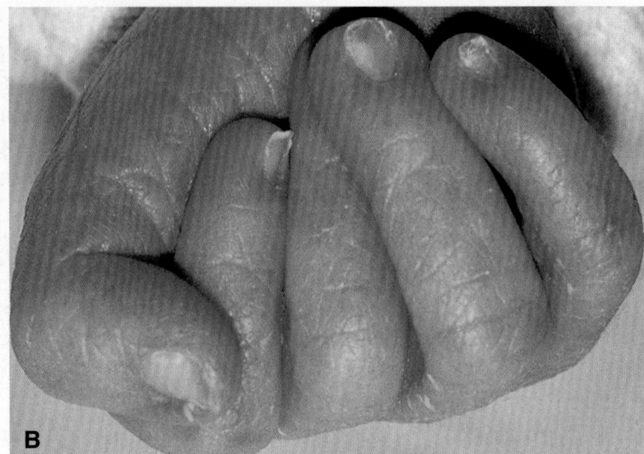

FIGURE 49.3 Trisomy 18.

sex chromosomes. About half of the affected individuals have only one X chromosome; the other half have a variety of abnormalities of one of their sex chromosomes and may present with the mosaic form.

There is no cure for Turner syndrome. Therapeutic management will focus on managing the health issues associated with the syndrome. Children with Turner syndrome are more prone to cardiovascular problems, kidney and thyroid problems, skeletal disorders such as scoliosis and osteoporosis, hearing and eye disturbances, learning disabilities, and obesity (Bacino & Lee, 2011; Saenger, 2014). Infertility is usually present, but a few spontaneous pregnancies have been reported (Kansra & Donohoue, 2011; Nelson-Tuttle, 2014). Growth hormone administration is a standard of care and usually begins when the child's height falls below the fifth percentile for healthy girls. Hormone replacement therapy may also be given to initiate puberty and complete growth.

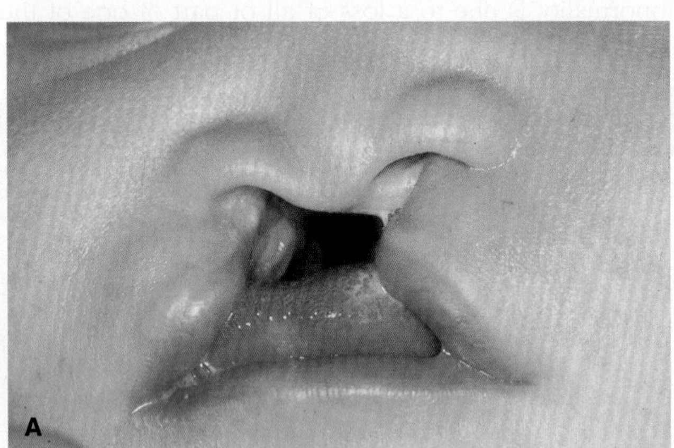

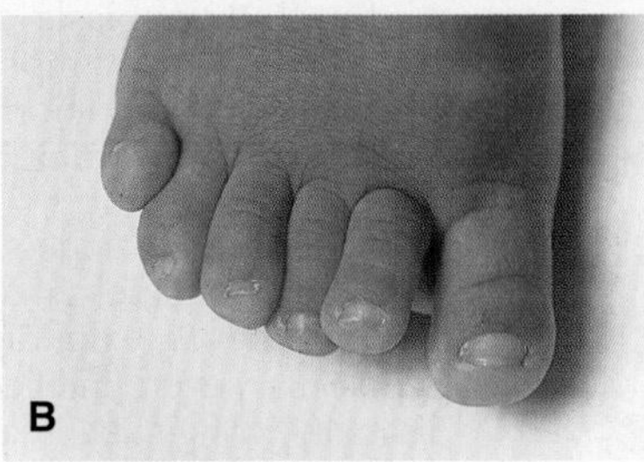

FIGURE 49.4 Trisomy 13.

Nursing Assessment

On assessment, note patterns of growth; short stature and slow growth will be a characteristic finding and often the first indication. Other physical characteristics include a webbed neck, low posterior hairline, wide-spaced nipples, edema of the hands and feet, amenorrhea, no development of secondary sex characteristics, sterility, and perceptual and social skill difficulties (Fig. 49.5).

Turner syndrome can be suspected prenatally by ultrasound findings such as fetal edema or redundant nuchal skin (Conley, 2014). It can be diagnosed by chromosomal analysis, either prenatally or after birth. Most children are diagnosed at birth or in early childhood when slow growth or growth failure is noted. Some cases will not be diagnosed until the pubertal growth spurt does not occur.

Nursing Management

Nursing management is mainly supportive. Provide education and support to the family; they need to understand that short stature and infertility are likely. Explain that intellectual disability is unlikely, but some learning disabilities may be present. Emphasize that with medical supervision and support, girls with Turner syndrome may lead healthy, satisfying lives. Counseling about infertility is important. Parents may be upset that their daughter will not be able to reproduce, so explain that many alternatives for reproduction, such as in vitro fertilization and adoption, are available.

Providing resources for the family is an important nursing function. The Turner Syndrome Society of the

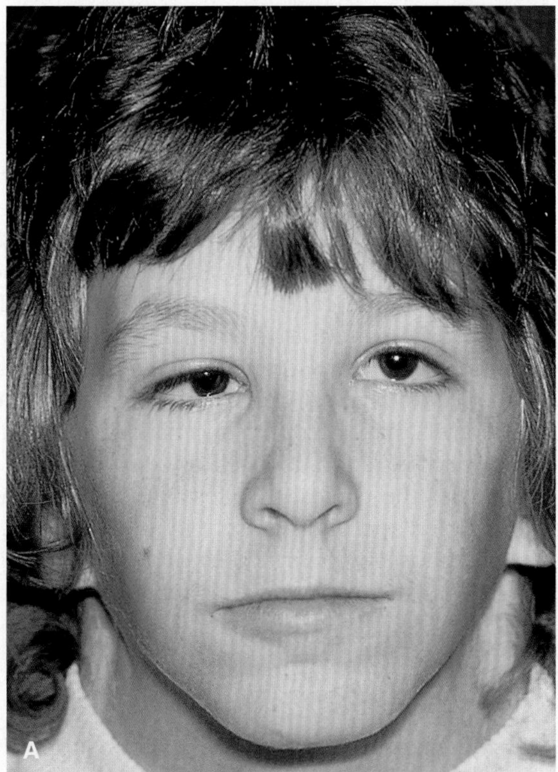

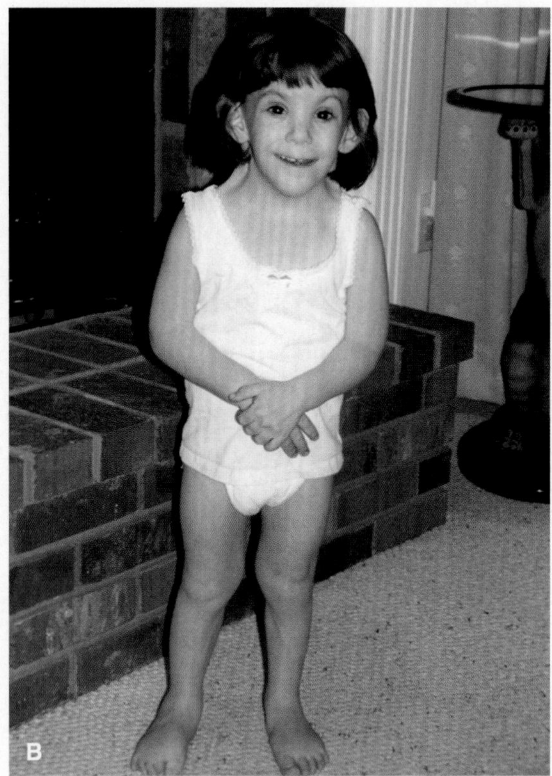

FIGURE 49.5 Note the webbed neck of the child with Turner syndrome.

United States provides assistance, support, and education to individuals with Turner syndrome and their families. A link to resources is provided on thePoint.

Klinefelter Syndrome

Klinefelter syndrome is the most common sex chromosomal abnormality (Bacino & Lee, 2011). The karyotype and phenotype are male, but one or more extra X chromosomes is present. The abnormality is usually caused by nondisjunction during meiosis, but mosaic forms do present. The incidence of Klinefelter syndrome is 1 in 500 to 1,000 males (Bacino, 2015). Males present with some female-like physical features that are caused by testosterone deficiency. The risk of recurrence in future pregnancies is not increased.

There is no cure for Klinefelter syndrome. Therapeutic management will focus on interventions to enhance masculine characteristics, such as testosterone replacement. Early recognition and hormonal treatment are important to improve quality of life and prevent serious consequences. Cosmetic surgery may be performed to minimize female characteristics such as gynecomastia (increased breast size).

Nursing Assessment

Due to nonspecific findings during childhood, the diagnosis is not usually made until adolescence or adulthood. Prenatal diagnosis is rare unless amniocentesis was performed for genetic testing. Many males with Klinefelter syndrome reach adulthood without being diagnosed (Bacino & Lee, 2011). The diagnosis is confirmed by chromosomal analysis.

On assessment, lack of development of secondary sex characteristics may be found. The individual may have decreased facial hair, gynecomastia, decreased pubic hair, and hypogonadism or underdeveloped testes, which leads to infertility. The individual may be taller than average by 5 years of age, with long legs and a short torso (Fig. 49.6). Intellectual disability is not present, but cognitive impairments of varying degree, such as motor delay, speech or language difficulties, attention deficits, and learning disabilities, may be found.

Nursing Management

Nursing management will be mainly supportive. Provide education and support to the family. Links to The American Association for Klinefelter Syndrome, The Klinefelter Syndrome Support Group, and Klinefelter Syndrome and Associates are provided on thePoint.

Counseling about infertility is important. Educate children and families that marriage and sexual relations are possible. Parents may be upset that their son will not be able to reproduce, so explain that many alternatives for reproduction are available and technology is advancing in the field of infertility.

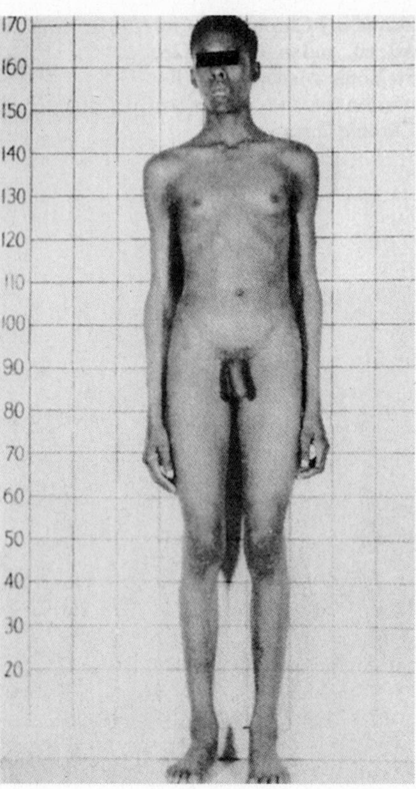

FIGURE 49.6 Klinefelter syndrome.

Fragile X Syndrome

Fragile X syndrome is the most common inherited cause of intellectual disability (Van Esch, 2014). It is the outcome of a mutation of a gene (FMR1 [fragile X mental retardation]) on the X chromosome. This mutation essentially "turns off" the gene, triggering fragile X syndrome. Males and females are both affected, but it is more commonly seen in males, and affected females usually have milder symptoms (Genetics Home Reference, 2012a). The incidence is approximately 1 in 8,000 females and 1 in 4,000 males (Genetics Home Reference, 2012a). The inheritance of fragile X is complex and is less straightforward than single-gene or mendelian inheritance. Some carrier females are affected, and not all males with the gene abnormality show symptoms. Males and females are both fertile and can transmit the disorder to their offspring, so genetic counseling is appropriate. The prognosis for individuals with fragile X is good, and they tend to live a normal life span.

There is no cure for fragile X syndrome. Therapeutic management will be multidisciplinary and aimed at interventions to improve cognitive, emotional, and behavioral impairments.

Nursing Assessment

During childhood, clinical manifestations are subtle, with minor dysmorphic features and developmental delay. Problems with sensation, emotion, and behavior often are the first signs. A delay in attaining developmental milestones will most likely be the first clue found on assessment. Intellectual impairment can range from subtle learning disabilities to severe intellectual disability and autistic-like behaviors. In adolescence, boys tend to present with characteristic features such as an elongated face; prominent jaw; large, protruding ears; large size; macroorchidism (large testes); and a range of behavioral abnormalities and cognitive deficits (Fig. 49.7). There is a characteristic pattern to the cognitive deficits, with problems in abstract reasoning, sequential processing, and mathematics. Typical behavior problems include attention deficits, hand flapping and biting, hyperactivity, shyness, social isolation, low self-esteem, and gaze aversion. In females the clinical manifestations are similar but are more varied and often present in a milder form.

Diagnosis is confirmed by molecular genetic testing. Fragile X can be diagnosed prenatally if inheritance is suspected.

Nursing Management

Nursing management will be mainly supportive. Early diagnosis and intervention with developmental therapies and an individualized education plan are ideal. Care of these children will be the same as care of other children with intellectual disability (see Chapter 51 for further information on intellectual disability).

Provide education and support to the family. The National Fragile X Foundation provides education and emotional support and works to increase awareness and advance research for fragile X. Links to resources are provided on thePoint.

NEUROCUTANEOUS DISORDERS

Neurocutaneous disorders, also referred to as hamartoses, are a group of disorders characterized by abnormalities of both the skin and the central nervous system. Many neurologic conditions are associated with cutaneous manifestations, since the skin and the nervous system share a common embryologic origin. They are complex conditions and most also affect other organ systems such as eyes, bones, heart, and kidneys. Most are hereditary and follow an autosomal dominant inheritance pattern or sporadic occurrence. Neurofibromatosis is a common neurocutaneous syndrome and will be discussed in detail below. Table 49.5 provides information on other neurocutaneous syndromes.

Neurofibromatosis

Neurofibromatoses are neurocutaneous genetic disorders of the nervous system that primarily affect the development and growth of neural cell tissues. There are

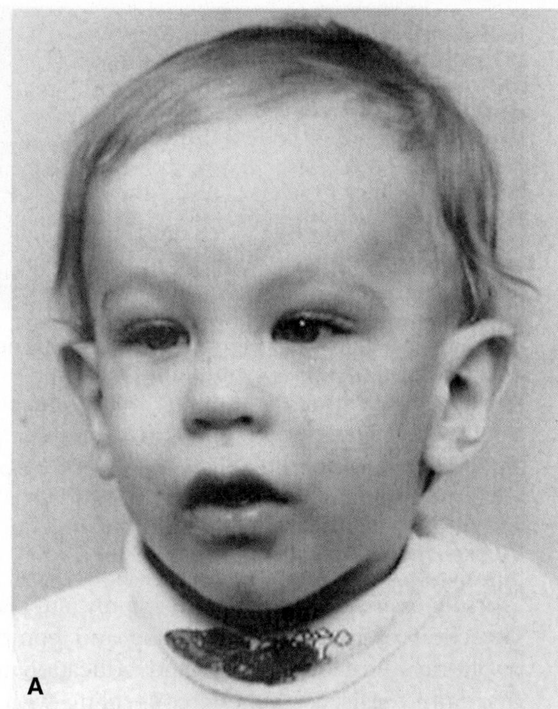

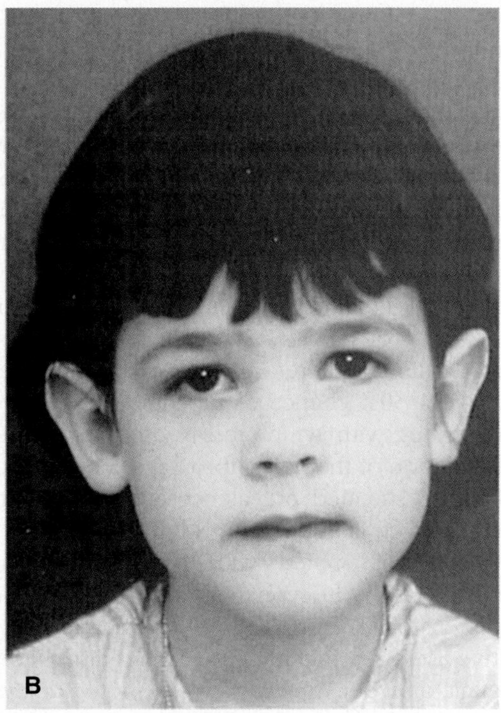

FIGURE 49.7 Fragile X syndrome.

TABLE 49.5 OTHER NEUROCUTANEOUS SYNDROMES

Disorder	Incidence	Clinical Manifestations	Nursing Considerations
Tuberous sclerosis	1 in 6,000[a]	Benign tumors present in the brain and skin. Presents most often as a generalized seizure disorder. Tumors can also involve heart, kidney, eyes, lung, and bones. Developmental delay and behavioral problems may be noted. Usually evident in early childhood. Wide clinical spectrum from severe intellectual disability with incapacitating seizures to normal intelligence and no seizures	Treatment will be mainly symptomatic with goal to prevent and treat associated complications. Seizure control will be a primary concern. Provide support and education to the family. Referral for genetic counseling (it follows an autosomal dominant inheritance pattern and half the cases are due to a new mutation) and appropriate resources www.tsalliance.org: Tuberous Sclerosis Alliance
Sturge–Weber syndrome	1 in 50,000[a]	Facial nevus (port wine stain) most often seen on the forehead and on one side of the face, seizures, hemiparesis, intracranial calcifications. In many cases intellectual disability, behavioral and emotional problems, and learning disabilities are present. Seizures usually begin in infancy and may worsen with age. Convulsions are usually noted on the side of the body opposite the facial nevus. Muscle weakness may be present on the same side. Most affected individuals have glaucoma at birth or will develop it later in life.	Treatment will be mainly symptomatic. Seizure control will be a primary concern (use of anticonvulsants or surgery). Seizures due to Sturge–Weber are often difficult to control. Laser treatment may be used to lighten or remove the facial nevus. Surgery may be performed on more serious cases of glaucoma. Physical therapy should be considered for infants and children with muscle weakness. Educational therapy is often prescribed for those with intellectual disability or developmental delays. Provide support and education to the family. Refer to appropriate resources. Genetic counseling may be appropriate (inheritance is unclear and sporadic). www.sturge-weber.org: Sturge-Weber Foundation

[a]Sahin, M. (2011). Chapter 589: Neurocutaneous syndromes. In R. M. Kleigman, B. F. Stanton, J. W. St. Geme III, N. F. Schor, & R. E. Behrman (Eds.), *Nelson textbook of pediatrics* (19th ed., pp. 2046–2053). Philadelphia, PA: Saunders.

distinct types: neurofibromatosis 1, neurofibromatosis 2, and schwannomatosis (which used to be considered a variation of neurofibromatosis 2) (Korf, 2014).

Neurofibromatosis 1 (von Recklinghausen disease) is the more common type and is discussed here (Korf, 2014). This disorder causes tumors to grow on nerves and produce other abnormalities such as skin changes and bone deformities. Although many affected persons inherit the disorder, nearly 30–50% of the cases are due to a new mutation (National Institute of Neurological Disorders and Stroke, 2015; Korf, 2014). The inheritance pattern is autosomal dominant; therefore, offspring of affected individuals have a 50% chance of inheriting the altered gene and presenting with symptoms. Neurofibromatoses are due to a mutation of the neurofibromin gene on chromosome 17. The estimated prevalence is 1 in 2,600 to 3,000 live births (Korf, 2014).

Complications associated with neurofibromatosis include headaches; hydrocephalus; scoliosis; cardiac defects; hypertension; seizures; vision and hearing loss; neurocognitive deficits, including learning disabilities, attention deficit disorder, fine and gross motor delays, autism spectrum disorder, and behavior and psychosocial issues; abnormalities of speech; and a higher risk for neoplasms.

There is no cure for neurofibromatosis. Therapeutic management is aimed at controlling symptoms and managing complications. Surgical intervention can help reduce some of the bone malformations and remove painful or disfiguring tumors. These children should have a yearly physical, including blood pressure and cardiovascular examination, scoliosis screening, ophthalmology examination, developmental screening, and a neurologic examination.

The disease is progressive and symptoms usually worsen over time, but it is difficult to predict the course. Most affected individuals develop mild to moderate symptoms, with non–life-threatening complications, and live a normal, productive life.

Nursing Assessment

On assessment the nurse may find café-au-lait spots (light-brown macules), which are the hallmark of neurofibromatosis (Sahin, 2011) (Fig. 49.8). These are usually present at birth but can appear during the first year of life and usually increase in size, number, and pigmentation. They are present all over the body, particularly the trunk and extremities, while usually sparing the face. Pigmented nevi, axillary freckling, and slow-growing cutaneous, subcutaneous, or dermal neurofibromas, which are benign tumors, are other signs of neurofibromatosis. Many children with neurofibromatosis have larger than normal head circumference and are shorter than average. The severity of symptoms varies greatly, but the diagnosis is made if two or more of the clinical signs in Box 49.4 are present.

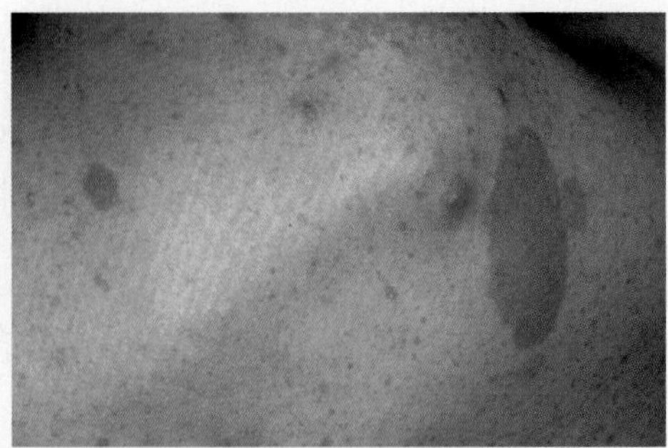

FIGURE 49.8 Café-au-lait spots associated with neurofibromatosis.

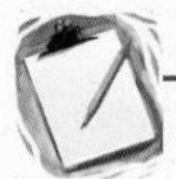

Take Note!

If more than six café-au-lait spots are present, neurofibromatosis should be suspected.

Nursing Management

Nursing management will be mainly supportive. Early detection of treatable conditions and complications is a priority. Provide support and education to the child and family. Discuss genetic counseling with the family. Referral to appropriate resources is essential. Links to resources for The Children's Tumor Foundation are provided on thePoint.

OTHER GENETIC DISORDERS

Thousands of genetic disorders are known, and new ones are being discovered, but most of them are rare. Table 49.6 lists other genetic disorders that the

BOX 49.4

CLINICAL SIGNS OF NEUROFIBROMATOSIS

Diagnosis is made if two or more of the following are present:

- Six or more café-au-lait macules (light-brown spots) >5 mm in diameter in children and >15 mm in diameter in adolescents and adults
- Two or more neurofibromas (benign tumors) or one plexiform neurofibroma (tumor that involves many nerves)
- Freckling in the armpit or groin
- Presence of an optic glioma (a tumor on the optic nerve)
- Two or more growths on the iris of the eye (Lisch nodules or iris hamartomas)
- Abnormal development of the spine (scoliosis), the temple bone of the skull, or the tibia
- A first-degree relative (parent, sibling, or child) with neurofibromatosis

Adapted from National Institute of Neurological Disorders and Stroke. (2015). *Neurofibromatosis fact sheet*. Retrieved from http://www.ninds.nih.gov/disorders/neurofibromatosis/detail_neurofibromatosis.htm; Sahin, M. (2011). Chapter 589: Neurocutaneous syndromes. In R. M. Kleigman, B. F. Stanton, J. W. St. Geme III, N. F. Schor, & R. E. Behrman (Eds.), *Nelson textbook of pediatrics* (19th ed., pp. 2046–2053). Philadelphia, PA: Saunders.

TABLE 49.6 OTHER GENETIC DISORDERS, SYNDROMES, AND ASSOCIATIONS

Disorder	Inheritance/Cause	Signs and Symptoms	Management
CHARGE syndrome (a recognizable pattern of congenital anomalies seen) **C: C**oloboma **H: H**eart disease **A: A**tresia (choanal) **R: R**etarded growth and development and/or CNS anomalies **G: G**enital anomalies, hypogonadism **E: E**ar anomalies and deafness Incidence is 0.1–1.2 in 10,000 live births.[a]	Autosomal dominant inheritance possible, but most cases are due to new mutation of the gene. Mutations in the gene CDH7 have been indicated in most cases. Occurs during fetal development and affects multiple organ systems	Coloboma is a lesion or defect of the eye, usually a fissure or cleft in the iris, ciliary, or choroid; can also see microphthalmos (small eyes) and cryptophthalmos (absent eye). Can lead to vision impairments Heart anomaly can include any type but most common are aortic arch anomalies and Tetralogy of Fallot. Atresia (choanal) is blocked or narrowed passages from the nose to the throat, which can lead to aspiration. Retarded growth or cognitive development can range from mild to severe. Genital anomaly may include micropenis, undescended testes, and hypoplastic labia. Ear anomalies include short, wide ears with little or no lobe, prominent inner fold, floppy appearance, asymmetry; can have hearing impairment Each feature occurs in a spectrum from absent to severe; no single feature is present in all individuals.	Focus is on identifying and treating all defects; early diagnosis is important. www.chargesyndrome.org: CHARGE Syndrome Foundation
Marfan syndrome: disorder of connective tissue Incidence is 1 in 3,000 to 5,000[b]	Autosomal dominant inheritance; caused by a mutation in the gene fibrillin-1, which results in changes in connective tissue	Primarily involves the skeletal, cardiovascular, and ocular systems. Tall stature with long slim limbs, minimal subcutaneous fat, muscle hypotonia, loose joints, long and narrow face, abnormalities of skeletal system (e.g., pectus excavatum [funnel chest] or pectus carinatum [pigeon breast]), ocular system (e.g., enlarged cornea or lens subluxation), and cardiovascular system (e.g., dilation of the aorta or mitral valve prolapse) Delayed achievement of gross and fine motor milestones may occur.	Focus is on preventing complications. www.marfan.org: National Marfan Foundation www.marfan.ca: Canadian Marfan Association

(continued)

TABLE 49.6 OTHER GENETIC DISORDERS, SYNDROMES, AND ASSOCIATIONS (continued)

Disorder	Inheritance/Cause	Signs and Symptoms	Management
VATER association (not a diagnosis, but refers to a nonrandom association of defects found to occur together) **V: V**ertebral defects **A: A**nal atresia **TE: T**racheo**E**sophageal fistula with esophageal atresia **R**adial and **R**enal dysplasia May also occur as VACTERL association, with **C: C**ardiac anomalies **L: L**imb abnormalities added	Sporadic inheritance. Cause is unknown. Can occur with other chromosomal abnormalities such as trisomy 18 Frequently seen in the offspring of diabetic mothers	Three or more anomalies are present. Anomalies seen include hypoplastic (small) vertebrae or hemivertebra (only half the bones are formed). These anomalies lead to an increased risk of scoliosis. With imperforate anus or anal atresia, the anus does not open to the outside of the body. TracheoEsophageal fistula and/or esophageal atresia leads to increased risk for aspiration, feeding and swallowing problems. Incomplete formation of one or more kidneys, obstruction of urine flow out of kidneys, or severe reflux back into kidneys can all lead to kidney failure later in life. Cardiac anomalies: most common are ventricular septal defects, atrial septal defects, and Tetralogy of Fallot. Absent or displaced thumb, polydactyly (extra digits), syndactyly (fusion of digits) A single umbilical artery at birth is often present. Failure to thrive and slow development in early infancy due to anomalies Usually normal intelligence	Focus is on identifying and treating all defects. www.tefvater.org: TEF VATER National Support Network *Take Note!* Children with VATER syndrome who have only one kidney should not play contact sports.
Apert syndrome (named for the French physician who described the syndrome) Incidence is 6 to 15.5 out of 1 million live births.[c]	Autosomal dominant inheritance. Cases are sporadic	Craniosynostosis and maxillary hypoplasia resulting in a flat recessed forehead and flat midface, bilateral symmetric syndactyly, and craniofacial anomalies such as high arched palate and associated clefting, short anteroposterior diameter, protruding eyes, down-slanting eyelids, and low-set ears. Small nasopharynx can lead to upper airway obstruction and sleep apnea. Acne vulgaris, strabismus, and hearing loss Learning disabilities and mental deficiency	Early surgery for craniosynostosis when increased intracranial pressure is noted. Vigorous early management should occur with a multidisciplinary approach to address multiple anomalies. www.aboutfaceusa.org: About Face USA www.ccakids.com: Children's Craniofacial Association www.faces-cranio.org:

TABLE 49.6 OTHER GENETIC DISORDERS, SYNDROMES, AND ASSOCIATIONS (continued)

Disorder	Inheritance/Cause	Signs and Symptoms	Management
Achondroplasia (most common chondrodysplasia [diseases resulting in disordered growth]) Incidence is 1 in 15,000 to 40,000.[d,e]	Autosomal dominant inheritance pattern. Caused by mutations in fibroblast growth factor receptor 3 (FGFR3). 80% new gene mutation[d]	Characterized by abnormal body proportion Small stature (average adult height is 4 ft for both men and women), short limbs with normal-size torso, low nasal bridge with prominent forehead. Midface hypoplasia, caudal narrowing of spinal canal, megalocephaly, small foramen magnum; hands are short and stubby with separation between middle and ring fingers ("trident hand"). Delayed motor skills, problems with persistent middle ear dysfunction and infections, and bowing of lower legs. Less common complications include hydrocephalus, craniocervical junction compression, upper airway obstruction, and thoracolumbar kyphosis. Usually present with normal intelligence and lead independent, productive lives	Medical management of symptoms Monitor height, weight, and head circumference. Manage and prevent complications (careful and thorough neurologic examination, assessment for sleep apnea). Growth hormone therapy is controversial and still experimental. Limb-lengthening surgeries may be performed. http://www.lpaonline.org/: Little People of America

[a]NORD. (2012a). *Charge syndrome.* Retrieved from https://www.rarediseases.org/rare-disease-information/rare-diseases/byID/550/viewFullReport

[b]Wright, M. J., & Connolly, H. M. (2014). *Genetics, clinical features, and diagnosis of Marfan syndrome and related disorders.* UpToDate. Retrieved from http://www.uptodate.com/contents/genetics-clinical-features-and-diagnosis-of-marfan-syndrome-and-related-disorders?source=search_result&search=Marfan&selectedTitle=1~105

[c]Hollier, L. H. (2014). *Craniosynostosis syndromes.* UpToDate. Retrieved from http://www.uptodate.com/contents/craniosynostosis-syndromes?source=machineLearning&search=APERT&selectedTitle=1~14§ionRank=1&anchor=H2#H2

[d]Genetics Home Reference. (2012b). *Achondroplasia.* Retrieved from http://ghr.nlm.nih.gov/condition/achondroplasia

[e]March of Dimes. (2013). *Achondroplasia.* Retrieved from http://www.marchofdimes.org/baby/achondroplasia.aspx#

pediatric nurse may encounter. Nursing management of these disorders will be mainly supportive and will focus on providing support and education to the family and child, with an emphasis on developmental and educational needs. Referral to genetic counseling and appropriate resources is an important nursing function.

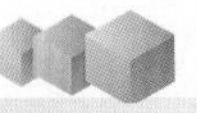

Concept Mastery Alert

Achondroplasia versus Marfan Syndrome

Assessment findings in a child with achondroplasia are a trident hand (separation between the middle and ring fingers) and persistent otitis media caused by middle ear dysfunction. In contrast, a child with Marfan syndrome would have slim stature, hypotonia, and a narrow face.

INBORN ERRORS OF METABOLISM

Inborn errors of metabolism are a group of hereditary disorders. They are collectively common, but individually rare with most having an incidence of less than 1 in 100,000 (Sutton, 2014). Most follow an autosomal recessive inheritance pattern. They are caused by gene mutations that result in abnormalities in the synthesis or catabolism of proteins, carbohydrates, or fats. The body cannot convert food into energy as it normally would. Most inborn errors are due to a defect in an enzyme or transport protein that results in a block in the metabolic pathway. The blocked metabolic pathway allows for accumulation of the damaging by-product of the impaired metabolic process or may be responsible for a deficiency or absence of a necessary product. Presentation can occur at any time, even in adulthood, but many affected individuals exhibit signs in the newborn period or shortly after. Most inborn errors of metabolism presenting in the neonatal period are lethal if specific treatment is not initiated immediately.

Newborn screening is used to detect these disorders before symptoms develop. During the 1990s, developments in screening techniques (tandem mass spectrometry) now allow dozens of metabolic disorders to be detected from a single drop of blood (Kaye & Committee on Genetics, 2011b; Wheeler, 2012). A child who tests positive will require additional testing to confirm the diagnosis (see Chapter 31 for more information on newborn screening for inborn errors of metabolism).

Therapeutic management of these disorders varies depending on the cause of the error of metabolism, but dietary management is often a key component.

Nursing Assessment

Clinical signs and symptoms vary with each disorder. Table 49.7 gives information on some common inborn errors of metabolism seen in children. See Evidence-Based Practice 49.1.

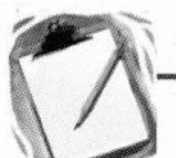

Take Note!

If the blood sample for the newborn screening was obtained within the first 24 hours after birth, the American Academy of Pediatrics recommends that a repeat sample be obtained within 1 to 2 weeks (Wheeler, 2012).

TABLE 49.7 INBORN ERRORS OF METABOLISM

Disorder/Explanation	Incidence (estimates)[a]	Clinical Manifestations	Management
Phenylketonuria (PKU): deficiency in a liver enzyme leading to inability to process the essential amino acid phenylalanine properly. Phenylalanine accumulation can lead to brain damage unless PKU is detected soon after birth and treated.	1 in 13,500 to 1 in 19,000	No symptoms at birth. Most cases are identified before symptoms are present due to newborn screening (PKU is screened for in all states). If undiagnosed, most common sign is developmental delay along with vomiting, irritability, eczema-like rash, mousy odor to urine, microcephaly, seizures and behavioral abnormalities.	Low-phenylalanine diet Phenylalanine is found mostly in protein-containing foods such as meat and milk (including breast milk and formula). www.pkunetwork.org: Children's PKU Network www.pkunews.org: National PKU News
Galactosemia: deficiency in the liver enzyme needed to convert galactose, the breakdown product of lactose, which is commonly found in dairy products, into glucose. Galactose accumulation leads to damage to vital organs.	1 in 47,000	No symptoms at birth. If undiagnosed, newborn will have jaundice, Feeding intolerance, diarrhea, and vomiting and will not gain weight. Signs and symptoms of sepsis and cataracts are often seen. If untreated, can lead to liver disease, blindness, severe intellectual disability, and death.	Ingestion of galactose can produce sepsis in an affected child; therefore, septic workup and antibiotics may be necessary in a child if galactose ingestion has occurred. Elimination of galactose and lactose from the diet is the only treatment. Therefore, milk and dairy products will be eliminated for life. www.galactosemia.org: Parents of Galactosemic Children

TABLE 49.7 INBORN ERRORS OF METABOLISM (continued)

Disorder/Explanation	Incidence (estimates)[a]	Clinical Manifestations	Management
Maple sugar urine disease: affects the metabolism of amino acids. A deficiency in the enzyme that metabolizes leucine, isoleucine, and valine, which are components of protein often referred to as the branch chain amino acids. These amino acids then accumulate in the blood and cause damage to the brain.	1 in 185,000	No symptoms at birth, but if untreated newborns soon begin to show neurologic signs, vomiting, poor feeding, increased reflex action, and seizures. Lower intake of protein (as occurs with breastfeeding) may delay presentation of symptoms. If untreated, can lead to life-threatening neurologic damage	Special low-protein diet, will vary based on severity of symptoms; limited natural protein requires a medical food product supplements such as BCAA-free Thiamine supplements may be given. Diet must be continued throughout life. www.msud-support.org: Maple Syrup Urine Disease Family Support Group
Biotinidase deficiency: lack of the enzyme biotinidase results in biotin deficiency	1 in 129,000	Typically no symptoms at birth; in first weeks or months of life, symptoms such as hypotonia, uncoordinated movement, seizures, developmental delay, alopecia, seborrheic dermatitis, hearing loss, optic nerve atrophy, and intellectual disability develop. Metabolic acidosis can lead to death.	Daily oral free biotin http://biotinidasedeficiency.20m.com/: Biotinidase Deficiency Family Support Group
Medium-chain acyl-CoA dehydrogenase deficiency (MCAD): lack of an enzyme required to metabolize fatty acids	1 in 46,000 to 1 in 6,400; almost exclusively seen in individuals of northwestern Europe descent	Classic presentation is a child 3 to 15 months old with vomiting and lethargy after a period of not eating (fasting typically associated with a viral illness) Recurrent episodes of metabolic acidosis and hypoglycemia, lethargy, seizures, liver failure, brain damage, coma, and cardiac arrest. Can lead to serious and fatal illness in children not eating well	Avoid fasting; have frequent meals. L-carnitine supplementation particularly when ill. Special considerations during illness. If unable to tolerate food, IV dextrose is required. www.fodsupport.org: Fatty Oxidation Disorders (FOD) Family Support Group
Homocystinuria: deficiency in the enzyme needed to digest a component of food called methionine (an amino acid)	1 in 250,000	If undetected and untreated can lead to intellectual disability, psychiatric disturbances, developmental delays, displacement of the lens of the eye, abnormal thinning and weakness of bones, and formation of thrombi in veins and arteries that can lead to life-threatening complications such as stroke	Vitamin B_6 and B_{12} supplements and possibly other supplements, such as betaine and folic acid; Methionine-restricted diet and cystine supplements; Aspirin and dipyridamole to decrease thromboembolic events www.rarediseases.org: National Organization for Rare Disorders

(continued)

TABLE 49.7 INBORN ERRORS OF METABOLISM (continued)

Disorder/Explanation	Incidence (estimates)[a]	Clinical Manifestations	Management
Tyrosinemia: deficiency in an enzyme essential in the metabolism of tyrosine; accumulation of the by-products results in liver and kidney damage	1 in 12,000 to 1 in 100,000 (typically northern European descent)	Symptoms usually appear in the first months of life: fever, failure to thrive, poor weight gain, vomiting, diarrhea, cabbage-like odor, enlarged liver and spleen, increased bleeding tendency, distended abdomen, jaundice, cirrhosis, and liver failure.	Diet low in phenylalanine, methionine, and tyrosine www.liverfoundation.org: American Liver Foundation
Tay–Sachs: caused by insufficient activity of an enzyme called hexosaminidase A, which is necessary for the breakdown of certain fatty substances in brain and nerve cells	Occurs more frequently among persons of Central and Eastern European and Ashkenazi Jewish descent. ~1 in every 27 Jews is a carrier, whereas in the general population 1 in 250 people is a carrier.[b] Non-Jewish French Canadians from the East St. Lawrence River Valley of Quebec and members of the Cajun population in Louisiana are also at an increased risk.	Infants appear normal and healthy for the first few months of life. Then, as harmful quantities of the fatty substances (called gangliosides) build up in tissues and nerve cells and cause damage, mental and physical deterioration occur. The child becomes blind, deaf, and unable to swallow; muscles begin to atrophy; and paralysis sets in. Dementia, seizures, and an increased startle reflex may be seen. There is a late-onset type of Tay–Sachs seen in persons in their 20s and early 30s, but this is much rarer.	No treatment or cure. Medical management will focus on managing symptoms and maintaining comfort. Anticonvulsants may be given to control seizures. Death usually occurs in early childhood, by age 4 or 5. Carriers can be identified by a blood test and prenatal testing is available. www.ntsad.org: National Tay-Sachs & Allied Diseases Association

[a]Kaye, C. I., & the Committee on Genetics (2011a). From The American academy of pediatrics: Newborn screening fact sheets. *Pediatrics, 118*(3), e934–e963. doi: 10.1542/peds.2006–1783. Retrieved from http://pediatrics.aappublications.org/content/118/3/e934.full

[b]National Human Genome Research Institute. (2011). *Learning about Tay-Sachs disease.* Retrieved from http://www.genome.gov/10001220

Adapted from Kaye, C. I., & the Committee on Genetics (2011a). From The American academy of pediatrics: Newborn screening fact sheets. *Pediatrics, 118*(3), e934–e963. doi: 10.1542/peds.2006–1783. Retrieved from http://pediatrics.aappublications.org/content/118/3/e934.full

Because of newborn screening and early identification and management, it is rare to see an untreated newborn with clinical signs and symptoms of disease caused by one of the inborn error of metabolism disorders. If seen, a newborn who was healthy at birth will often present with lethargy, poor feeding, apnea or tachypnea, recurrent vomiting, altered consciousness, failure to thrive, seizures, septic appearance, or developmental delay. Physical changes that may be seen include dysmorphology, cardiomegaly, rashes, cataracts, retinitis, optic atrophy, corneal opacity, deafness, skeletal dysplasia, macrocephaly, hepatomegaly, jaundice, or cirrhosis.

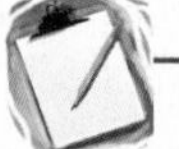

Take Note!

When a previously healthy newborn presents with a history of deterioration, suspect an inborn error of metabolism.

The diagnostic workup usually requires a variety of specific laboratory studies and may include:

- Glucose: may be elevated
- Ammonia: may be elevated
- Blood gases: may have low bicarbonate and low pH, metabolic acidosis (respiratory alkalosis may also be seen, especially when high ammonia levels are present)

EVIDENCE-BASED PRACTICE 49.1 **EFFECTS OF A NEW COLLECTION PROTOCOL ON FALSE-POSITIVE NEWBORN SCREENING RATES**

Newborn screening tests have improved outcomes and the health of infants and children. However, the rates of false-positive results are a concern. False-positive newborn screening results have been found to be higher among infants in the neonatal intensive care unit leading to increased testing and family stress. Higher rates of false positives have been contributed to the use of medical therapies, such as total parenteral nutrition (TPN), and the liver immaturity of preterm infants. What are the effects of a new sample collection protocol on false-positive results?

STUDY

A 2-year retrospective cohort study was conducted at the Children's Hospital of Orange County. Infants were grouped into pre- and postprotocol groups and further categorized by birth weight. Preprotocol newborn screen samples were collected regardless of TPN administration. Postprotocol newborn screen samples, in neonates receiving TPN, were collected 3 hours after TPN was replaced with 10% Dextrose in water (D10W).

Findings

A total of 539 neonates were screened during the study period. The new protocol was found to decrease false positives in each birth weight group by at least 50% with an overall decrease of 74%. An estimated reduction in cost >80% was also found.

Nursing Implications

TPN is an important medical therapy for many preterm infants. This protocol allows for the benefits of TPN to be maintained while decreasing the negative consequences of false-positive newborn screen results, such as increased testing, increased family stress and anxiety and increased healthcare costs. Further investigation with a larger sample is needed. Further study investigating the need for different laboratory cutoff values for term versus preterm infants and for infants receiving TPN is warranted. Obtaining repeat samples at different ages may help guard against the occurrence of false negatives.

Adapted from Morris, M., Fischer, K., Leydiker, K., Elliott, L., Newby, J., & Abdenur, J. N. (2014). Reduction in newborn screening metabolic false-positive results following a new collection protocol. *Genetics in Medicine, 16*(6), 477–483.

Early diagnosis is the key to saving and improving the lives of these children.

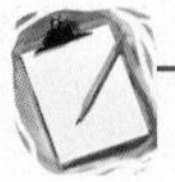

Take Note!

If an inborn error of metabolism is suspected, feedings will usually be stopped until the test results are received.

When a child who has previously been diagnosed with an inborn error of metabolism is hospitalized, the nurse must determine the prescribed diet and medications so these may be continued while in the hospital setting.

Nursing Management

Ensure that the diet prescribed for the infant or child is followed. For amino acid disorders (e.g., phenylketonuria [PKU]), urea cycle defects (e.g., tyrosinemia type I), and organic acidemia (e.g., maple syrup urine disease), nutritional therapy is the major intervention. Dietary intake of specific amino acids is restricted according to the disorder. Ensure that overall protein and calorie needs are still met, as children need sufficient calories for proper growth. In children with urea cycle defects and organic acidemia, anorexia is common and severe, and the child may need gastrostomy tube feeding supplementation. In fatty acid oxidation disorders (e.g., medium-chain acyl-coenzyme A [CoA] dehydrogenase deficiency), the goal is to avoid prolonged periods of fasting and to provide frequent feeds when the child is sick. Supplementation with specific vitamins may also be important in the treatment of these disorders. Strict adherence to the diet is necessary and will require close supervision by registered dietitians, physicians, and nurses and the cooperation of both the parent and child.

Nursing management will focus on education and support for the family, who will need thorough knowledge about the child's disease and management. Refer the child and family to a dietitian and appropriate resources, including support groups. In addition, monitor the child's developmental progress and begin therapies as soon as a concern arises.

NURSING CARE PLAN 49.1

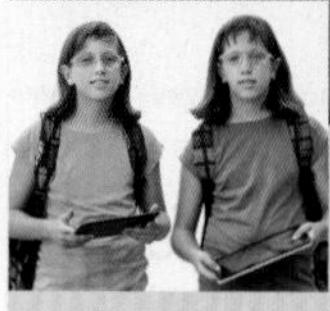

Overview for the Child With a Genetic Disorder

NURSING DIAGNOSIS: Deficient knowledge related to lack of information regarding complex, technical medical condition; prognosis; and medical needs as evidenced by verbalization, questions, or actions demonstrating lack of understanding about child's condition or care

Outcome Identification and Evaluation

Child and family will verbalize accurate information and understanding about condition, prognosis, and medical needs: *child and family demonstrate knowledge of condition, prognosis, and medical needs, including possible causes, contributing factors, and treatment measures.*

Intervention: ***Providing Child and Family Teaching***

- Assess child's and family's willingness to learn: *child and family must be willing to learn for teaching to be effective.*
- Provide family with time to adjust to diagnosis: *will facilitate adjustment and ability to learn and participate in child's care.*
- Repeat information: *allows family and child time to learn and understand.*
- Teach in short sessions: *many short sessions are more helpful than one long session.*
- Gear teaching to the child and family's level of understanding (depends on age of child, physical condition, memory) *to ensure understanding.*
- Provide reinforcement and rewards: *facilitates the teaching/learning process.*
- Use multiple modes of learning involving many senses (written, verbal, demonstration, and videos) when possible: *child and family are more likely to retain information when it is presented in different ways using many senses.*
- Refer child and family to a genetics specialist: *genetic information is highly technical; the field is advancing at a rapid pace, and information needs to be the most current and accurate. A genetic specialist can provide this along with expertise, support, and resources.*

NURSING DIAGNOSIS: Decisional conflict related to treatment options, conflicting values, and ethical, legal, and social issues surrounding genetic testing as evidenced by verbalization of uncertainty about choices, verbalization of undesired consequences of alternative actions being considered, delayed decision making, physical signs of stress

Outcome Identification and Evaluation

Family will state they are able to make an informed decision: *family will state advantages and disadvantages of choices and share fears and concerns regarding choices.*

Intervention: ***Providing Decision-Making Support***

- Give family time and encourage them to express their feelings associated with decision making: *the decision-making process becomes more difficult if feelings are not expressed.*
- Encourage family to list advantages and disadvantages of each alternative: *aids in problem solving and helps family recognize all alternatives.*
- Initiate health teaching and referral to genetic specialist when needed: *genetic testing information is often technical and complex. Families need accurate and up-to-date information to aid in decision making.*
- Maintain a nondirective manner: *this is a difficult decision that the family must make for themselves; the nurse should provide all the necessary information while maintaining an unobtrusive role.*
- Validate the family's feelings regarding the decisional conflict: *validation is a therapeutic communication technique that promotes the nurse–family relationship.*

NURSING CARE PLAN 49.1

Overview for the Child With a Genetic Disorder (continued)

NURSING DIAGNOSIS: Risk for delayed growth and development related to physical disability, cognitive deficits, activity restrictions secondary to genetic disorder

Outcome Identification and Evaluation

Child's growth and development will be enhanced: *child will demonstrate adequate growth patterns within parameters of disease. Child will make continued progress toward attainment of developmental milestones and will not suffer regression in abilities.*

Child will demonstrate developmental milestones within age parameters and limits of disease.

Child will make steady gains in growth patterns (e.g., height and weight) within disease parameters. Child expresses interest in the environment and people around him or her and interacts with environment appropriately for developmental level.

Intervention: ***Promoting Growth and Development***

- Screen for developmental capabilities *to determine child's current level of functioning.*
- Offer age-appropriate toys, play, and activities (including gross motor) *to encourage further development.*
- Perform exercises or interventions as prescribed by physical or occupational therapist: *these activities promote function and developmental skills.*
- Provide support to families: *due to disability and deficits, the child's progress toward developmental milestones may be slow.*
- Use therapeutic play and adaptive toys *to facilitate developmental functioning.*
- Provide stimulating environment when possible *to maximize potential for growth and development.*
- Praise accomplishments and emphasize child's abilities *to improve self-esteem and encourage feeling of confidence and competence.*
- Monitor height and weight and plot on growth chart *to identify growth patterns and deviations in these patterns.*

NURSING DIAGNOSIS: Fear related to outcome of genetic testing as evidenced by reports of apprehension and increased tension

Outcome Identification and Evaluation

Family will state they can cope with the results of the genetic testing or demonstrate reduced fear: *family accurately discusses chances of offspring having genetic disease, demonstrates positive coping, and asks questions about genetic testing and meaning of results.*

Intervention: ***Managing Fear***

- Empathize with the family and avoid false reassurances; be truthful: *allows family to recognize that fear is a reasonable response. Giving false information or reassurance will actually increase fear.*
- Explore coping skills used previously by the family to cope with fear. Reinforce these skills and explore other outlets, such as relaxation, breathing, and physical activity: *encourages use of coping mechanisms that help control fear.*
- Encourage verbalization of feelings and concerns about genetic testing. Allow time for questions: *provides a safe outlet to express feelings and encourages open communication between the family members.*

(continued)

NURSING CARE PLAN 49.1

Overview for the Child With a Genetic Disorder (continued)

- Explain all procedures and review results as available: *knowledge deficit contributes to fear.*
- Refer to appropriate support groups and genetic counseling: *talking with families who have gone through similar situations can help decrease fear and provide methods of coping. Genetic counseling provides information along with support and additional resources.*

NURSING DIAGNOSIS: Family processes, interrupted, related to child's illness, hospitalization, diagnosis of genetic illness in child, and potential long-term effects of illness as evidenced by family's presence in hospital and clinic, missed work, demonstration of inadequate coping

Outcome Identification and Evaluation

Family will maintain functional system of support and demonstrate adequate coping, adaptation of roles and functions, and decreased anxiety: *parents are involved in child's care, ask appropriate questions, express fears and concerns, and can discuss child's care and condition calmly.*

Intervention: *Promoting Family Coping*

- Encourage family to verbalize concerns about child's illness, diagnosis, and prognosis: *allows the nurse to identify concerns and areas where further education may be needed and demonstrates family-centered care.*
- Explain therapies, procedures, child's behaviors, and plan of care to parents: *understanding the child's current status and plan of care helps decrease anxiety.*
- Encourage parental involvement in care: *allows parents to feel needed and valued and gives them a sense of control over their child's health.*
- Identify support system for family and child: *helps nurse identify needs and resources available for coping.*
- Educate family about resources available *to help them develop a wide base of support.*

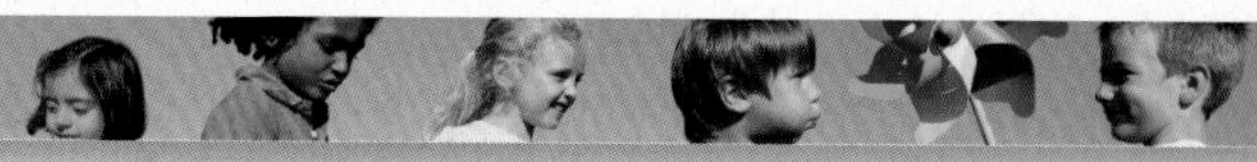

KEY CONCEPTS

- Nurses play an important role in the counseling process. Many times the nurse is the one who has first contact with these parents and is the one to provide follow-up care.
- Nurses play an essential role in providing emotional support and referrals to appropriate agencies, support groups, and resources when caring for families with suspected or diagnosed genetic disorders.
- Referral for genetic counseling prior to genetic testing may be appropriate.
- Many children with chromosomal abnormalities have intellectual disability, learning disabilities, behavioral problems, and distinct features, including birth defects.
- Trisomy 21 (Down syndrome) is associated with some degree of intellectual disability, characteristic facial features (e.g., slanted eyes and depressed nasal bridge), and other health problems, such as cardiac defects, visual and hearing impairments, intestinal malformations, and an increased susceptibility to infections.
- In Turner syndrome, short stature and slow growth are characteristic findings.

- Klinefelter syndrome is usually diagnosed in adolescence or adulthood due to a lack of development of secondary sex characteristics.
- Fragile X syndrome's clinical manifestations are subtle during childhood, with minor dysmorphic features and developmental delay. Problems with sensation, emotion, and behavior often are the first signs.
- Café-au-lait spots (light-brown macules) are the hallmark of neurofibromatosis (Sahin, 2011).
- Inborn errors of metabolism are caused by gene mutations that result in abnormalities in the synthesis or catabolism of proteins, carbohydrates, or fats. Most inborn errors of metabolism presenting in the neonatal period are lethal if specific treatment is not initiated immediately.
- Nurses should have a basic knowledge of genetics, common genetic disorders in children, genetic testing, and genetic counseling so they can provide support and information to families and can help improve their quality of life.
- Genetic disorders usually result in a lifelong complex medical condition. Nurses must provide ongoing education and support for the child and family about the disorder, treatment, and management as well as available resources.

REFERENCES AND RECOMMENDED READINGS

Bull, M. J., & the Committee on Genetics. (2011). From the American academy of pediatrics: Clinical Report: Health supervision for children with Down syndrome. *Pediatrics, 128*(2), 393–406. doi:10.1542/peds.2011–1605.

Bacino, C. A. (2014). *Approach to congenital malformations.* UpToDate. Retrieved from http://www.uptodate.com/contents/approach-to-congenital-malformations?source=search_result&search=major+and+minor+congenital+anomolies&selectedTitle=2~150

Bacino, C. A. (2015). *Sex chromosome abnormalities.* UpToDate. Retrieved from http://www.uptodate.com/contents/sex-chromosome-abnormalities?source=search_result&search=turner+syndrome&selectedTitle=3~141

Bacino, C. A., & Lee, B. (2011). Chapter 76: Cytogenetics. In R. M. Kleigman, B. F. Stanton, J. W. St. Geme III, N. F. Schor, & R. E. Behrman (Eds.), *Nelson textbook of pediatrics* (19th ed., p. 383). Philadelphia, PA: Saunders.

Carpenito-Moyet, L. J. (2013). *Nursing diagnosis: Application to clinical practice* (14th ed.). Philadelphia, PA: Lippincott Williams & Wilkins.

Chen, H. (2014). *Down syndrome.* Retrieved from http://emedicine.medscape.com/article/943216-overview

Conley, Y. P. (2014). Chapter 4: Genetics and health applications. In S. M. Nettina (Ed.), *Lippincott manual of nursing practice* (10th ed., pp. 33–44). Philadelphia, PA: Wolters Kluwer Health/Lippincott Williams & Wilkins.

Fischbach, F. T., & Dunning, M. B. (2015). *A manual of laboratory and diagnostic tests* (9th ed.). Philadelphia, PA: Wolters Kluwer Health/Lippincott Williams & Wilkins.

Genetics Home Reference. (2012a). *Fragile X syndrome.* Retrieved from http://ghr.nlm.nih.gov/condition/fragile-x-syndrome

Genetics Home Reference. (2012b). *Achondroplasia.* Retrieved from http://ghr.nlm.nih.gov/condition/achondroplasia

Genetics Home Reference. (2015a). *Angelman syndrome.* Retrieved from http://ghr.nlm.nih.gov/condition/angelman-syndrome

Genetics Home Reference. (2015b). *Cri-Du-Chat Syndrome.* Retrieved from http://ghr.nlm.nih.gov/condition/cri-du-chat-syndrome

Genetics Home Reference. (2015c). *Wolf-Hirschhorn syndrome.* Retrieved from http://ghr.nlm.nih.gov/condition/wolf-hirschhorn-syndrome

Genetics Home Reference. (2015d). *Williams syndrome.* Retrieved from http://ghr.nlm.nih.gov/condition/williams-syndrome

Genetics Home Reference. (2015e). *22q11.2 deletion syndrome.* Retrieved from http://ghr.nlm.nih.gov/condition/22q112-deletion-syndrome

Ghidini, A. (2014). *Diagnostic amniocentesis.* UpToDate. Retrieved from http://www.uptodate.com/contents/diagnostic-amniocentesis?source=search_result&search=amniocentesis&selectedTitle=1~150

Herzing University—Orlando. (2014). *ASN/BSN concept definitions.* Winter Park, FL: Author.

Hollier, L. H. (2014). *Craniosynostosis syndromes.* UpToDate. Retrieved from http://www.uptodate.com/contents/craniosynostosis-syndromes?source=machineLearning&search=APERT&selectedTitle=1~14§ionRank=1&anchor=H2#H2

Hon-Yin, B. C., Shuman, C., Choufani, S., & Weksberg, R. (2014). *Beckwith-Wiedemann syndrome.* UpToDate. Retrieved from http://www.uptodate.com/contents/beckwith-wiedemann-syndrome?source=search_result&search=Beckwith-Wiedemann+syndrome&selectedTitle=1~37#H130269

Kaye, C. I., & the Committee on Genetics. (Reaffirmed 2011a). From the American academy of pediatrics: Newborn screening fact sheets. *Pediatrics, 118*(3), e934–e963. doi: 10.1542/peds.2006–1783. Retrieved from http://pediatrics.aappublications.org/content/118/3/e934.full

Kaye, C. I., & the Committee on Genetics. (Reaffirmed 2011b). From the American academy of pediatrics: Introduction to the newborn screening fact sheets. *Pediatrics, 118*(3), 1304–1312. Retrieved from htttp://pediatrics.aappublications.org/content/118/3/1304.full

Korf, B. R. (2014). *Neurofibromatosis type 1 (NF1): Pathogenesis, clinical features, and diagnosis.* UpToDate. Retrieved from http://www.uptodate.com/contents/neurofibromatosis-type-1-nf1-pathogenesis-clinical-features-and-diagnosis?source=search_result&search=Neurofibromatosis&selectedTitle=1~148

Kansra, A. R., & Donohoue, P. A. (2011). Chapter 580: Hypofunction of the ovaries. In R. M. Kleigman, B. F. Stanton, J. W. St. Geme III, N. F. Schor, & R. E. Behrman (Eds.), *Nelson textbook of pediatrics* (19th ed., pp. 1951–1957). Philadelphia, PA: Saunders.

Lashley, F. R. (2005). *Clinical genetics in nursing practice.* New York, NY: Springer Publishing.

March of Dimes. (2013). *Birth defects: Chromosomal conditions.* Retrieved from http://www.marchofdimes.org/baby/chromosomal-conditions.aspx

March of Dimes. (2014). *Tay-Sachs and Sandhoff diseases disease.* Retrieved from http://www.marchofdimes.org/baby/tay-sachs-and-sandhoff-diseases.aspx

Morris, M., Fischer, K., Leydiker, K., Elliott, L., Newby, J., & Abdenur, J. E. (2014). Reduction in newborn screening metabolic false-positive results following a new collection protocol. *Genetics in Medicine, 16*(6), 477–483.

National Human Genome Research Institute. (2011). *Learning about Tay-Sachs disease.* Retrieved from http://www.genome.gov/10001220

National Institute of Neurological Disorders and Stroke. (2015). *Neurofibromatosis fact sheet.* Retrieved from http://www.ninds.nih.gov/disorders/neurofibromatosis/detail_neurofibromatosis.htm

Nelson-Tuttle, C. (2014). Chapter 56: Developmental disabilities. In S. M. Nettina (Ed.), *Lippincott manual of nursing practice* (10th ed., pp. 1791–1807). Philadelphia, PA: Wolters Kluwer Health/Lippincott Williams & Wilkins.

NORD. (2012a). *Charge syndrome.* Retrieved from https://www.rarediseases.org/rare-disease-information/rare-diseases/byID/550/viewFullReport

NORD. (2012b). *Vacterl association.* Retrieved from https://www.rarediseases.org/rare-disease-information/rare-diseases/byID/486/viewFullReport

Ostermaier, K. K. (2014). *Down syndrome: Management.* UpToDate. Retrieved from http://www.uptodate.com/contents/down-syndrome-management?source=search_result&search=Down+syndrome&selectedTitle=2~150

Ostermaier, K. K. (2015). *Down syndrome: Clinical features and diagnosis.* UpToDate. Retrieved from http://www.uptodate.com/contents/down-syndrome-clinical-features-and-diagnosis?source=search_result&search=down+syndrome+children&selectedTitle=1~150

Pueschel, S. M. (2011). *A parent's guide to Down syndrome: Toward a brighter future* (rev. ed.). Baltimore, MD: Paul H. Brookes Publishing Company, Inc.

Rezvani, I., & Rezvani, G. (2011). An approach to inborn errors of metabolism. In R. M. Kleigman, B. F. Stanton, J. W. St. Geme III, N. F. Schor, & R. E. Behrman (Eds.), *Nelson textbook of pediatrics* (19th ed., pp. 416–418). Philadelphia, PA: Saunders.

Saenger, P. (2014). *Clinical manifestations and diagnosis of Turner syndrome (gonadal dysgenesis).* UpToDate. Retrieved from http://www.uptodate.com/contents/clinical-manifestations-and-diagnosis-of-turner-syndrome-gonadal-dysgenesis?source=search_result&search=turner+syndrome&selectedTitle=1~141

Sahin, M. (2011). Chapter 589: Neurocutaneous syndromes. In R. M. Kleigman, B. F. Stanton, J. W. St. Geme III, N. F. Schor, & R. E. Behrman (Eds.), *Nelson textbook of pediatrics* (19th ed., pp. 2046–2053). Philadelphia, PA: Saunders.

Schrijver, I., Zehnder, J. L., & Cherry, A. M. (2014). *Chromosomal translocations, deletions, and inversions.* UpToDate. Retrieved from http://www.uptodate.com/contents/chromosomal-translocations-deletions-and-inversions?source=see_link

Scott, D. A., & Lee, B. (2011a). Chapter 73: The genetic approach in pediatric medicine. In R. M. Kleigman, B. F. Stanton, J. W. St. Geme III, N. F. Schor, & R. E. Behrman (Eds.), *Nelson textbook of pediatrics* (19th ed., pp. 380–383). Philadelphia, PA: Saunders.

Scheimann, A. O. (2014). *Epidemiology and genetics of Prader-Willi syndrome.* UpToDate. Retrieved from http://www.uptodate.com/contents/epidemiology-and-genetics-of-prader-willi-syndrome?source=see_link

Searl, B. (2014). *Chromosomes and rare chromosome disorders in general.* Retrieved from http://www.rarechromo.org/html/chromosomesanddisorders.asp

Slaughter, J. L., Meinzen-Derr, J., Rose, S. R., Leslie, N. D., Chandrasekar, R., Linard, S. M., et al. (2010). The effects of gestational age and birth weight on false-positive newborn-screening rates. *Pediatrics, 126*(5), 910–916.

Summar, K., & Lee, B. (2011). Chapter 76.2: Down syndrome and other abnormalities of chromosome number. In R. M. Kleigman, B. F. Stanton, J. W. St. Geme III, N. F. Schor, & R. E. Behrman (Eds.), *Nelson textbook of pediatrics* (19th ed., pp. 399–403). Philadelphia, PA: Saunders.

Sutton, V. R. (2014). Inborn errors of metabolism: Epidemiology, pathogenesis, and clinical features. UpToDate. Retrieved from http://www.uptodate.com/contents/inborn-errors-of-metabolism-epidemiology-pathogenesis-and-clinical-features?source=search_result&search=inborn+errors+of+metabolism+in+children&selectedTitle=2~150

The American College of Obstetricians and Gynecologists Committee on Genetics & The Society for Maternal-Fetal Medicine Publications Committee. (2012). Committee opinion no. 545: Noninvasive prenatal testing for fetal aneuploidy. *American College of Obstetricians and Gynecologists, 120*, 1532–1534.

Trotter, T. L., Hall, J. G., & the Committee on Genetics. (2012). *American academy of pediatrics: Health supervision for children with achondroplasia.* Retrieved from http://pediatrics.aappublications.org/content/116/3/771.full

Van Esch, H. (2014). *Fragile X syndrome: Clinical features and diagnosis in children and adolescents.* UpToDate. Retrieved from http://www.uptodate.com/contents/fragile-x-syndrome-clinical-features-and-diagnosis-in-children-and-adolescents?source=search_result&search=fragile+X&selectedTitle=1~40

Weremowicz, S. (2014). *Congenital cytogenetic abnormalities.* UpToDate. Retrieved from http://www.uptodate.com/contents/congenital-cytogenetic-abnormalities?source=see_link&anchor=H9#H9

Wheeler, P. G. (2012). *Newborn screening testing. kids health.* Retrieved from http://kidshealth.org/parent/system/medical/newborn_screening_tests.html#

Wright, M. J., & Connolly, H. M. (2014). *Genetics, clinical features, and diagnosis of Marfan syndrome and related disorders.* UpToDate. Retrieved from http://www.uptodate.com/contents/genetics-clinical-features-and-diagnosis-of-marfan-syndrome-and-related-disorders?source=search_result&search=Marfan&selectedTitle=1~105

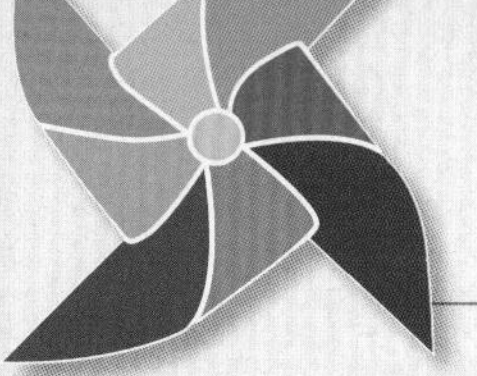

CHAPTER WORKSHEET

MULTIPLE CHOICE QUESTIONS

1. A child born with a single transverse palmar crease, a short neck with excessive skin at the nape, a depressed nasal bridge, and cardiac defects is most likely to have which autosomal abnormality?
   a. Trisomy 21
   b. Trisomy 18
   c. Trisomy 14
   d. Trisomy 13

2. A mother brings her 4-day-old infant to the clinic with vomiting and poor feeding. The newborn was healthy at birth. The nurse should suspect:
   a. Sturge–Weber syndrome
   b. An inborn error of metabolism
   c. Trisomy 18
   d. Turner syndrome

3. The nurse is caring for a child with Down syndrome. What should the nurse's focus be?
   a. Teaching hygiene skills to the child in order to increase self-esteem
   b. Screening for anomalies and teaching about prevention of respiratory infection
   c. Finding opportunities to increase socialization for the child and family
   d. Expecting walking at age 1 year and toilet training completion at age 2 years

4. The nurse is caring for a child with Turner syndrome admitted to the unit for treatment of a kidney infection. What characteristics associated with this syndrome may the nurse expect to find upon assessment?
   a. Microcephaly, polydactyly
   b. Low-set ears, cleft lip
   c. Short stature, webbed neck
   d. Gynecomastia, taller than average

DOSAGE CALCULATION QUESTION

The nurse is caring for a child with Down Syndrome. The child weighs 26 lb. The physician orders intravenous maintenance fluids. What would be the expected maintenance IV fluid rate? (Round to the nearest mL)

CRITICAL THINKING EXERCISES

1. An 8-month-old is seen in the clinic. On assessment the nurse finds eight café-au-lait spots on the child's trunk and extremities. What other assessment findings may be pertinent?

2. A child's newborn screen came back positive for phenylketonuria. After further testing, the diagnosis is confirmed. What instructions would you give the parents regarding care of their child?

3. A 6-year-old boy with Down syndrome is admitted to the hospital with pneumonia. Choose three pieces of information that the nurse should seek when obtaining the health history:
   a. Presence of cardiac defects or disease
   b. Last hearing and vision evaluation
   c. Mother's pregnancy history
   d. Presence of thyroid disease
   e. Mother's immunization history

STUDY ACTIVITIES

1. Develop a nursing care plan for a child with Down syndrome.

2. Shadow a genetic counselor. Identify ways he or she helps families understand and cope with genetic disorders.

3. Attend a meeting of an ethics committee at a local hospital. Identify some of the ethical, legal, and social issues in health care that they discuss, particularly related to genetic testing and genetic disorders.

BRINGING IT ALL TOGETHER: A CASE STUDY

Charles Faust, a 10-month-old with Down syndrome, is seen in the clinic for a well-child examination. The parents have questions about his growth and development. They are concerned because Charles can't pick up finger foods such as Cheerios and put them in his mouth.

Go to thePoint **to find questions to consider about this case.**

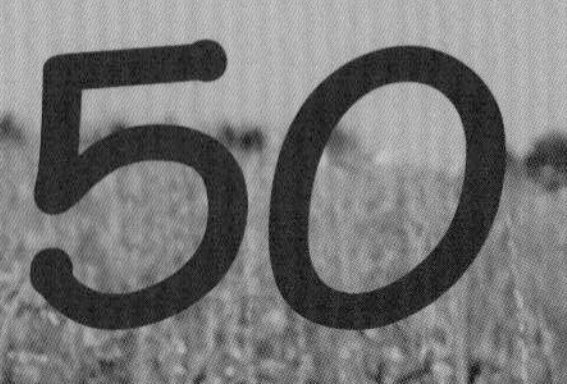

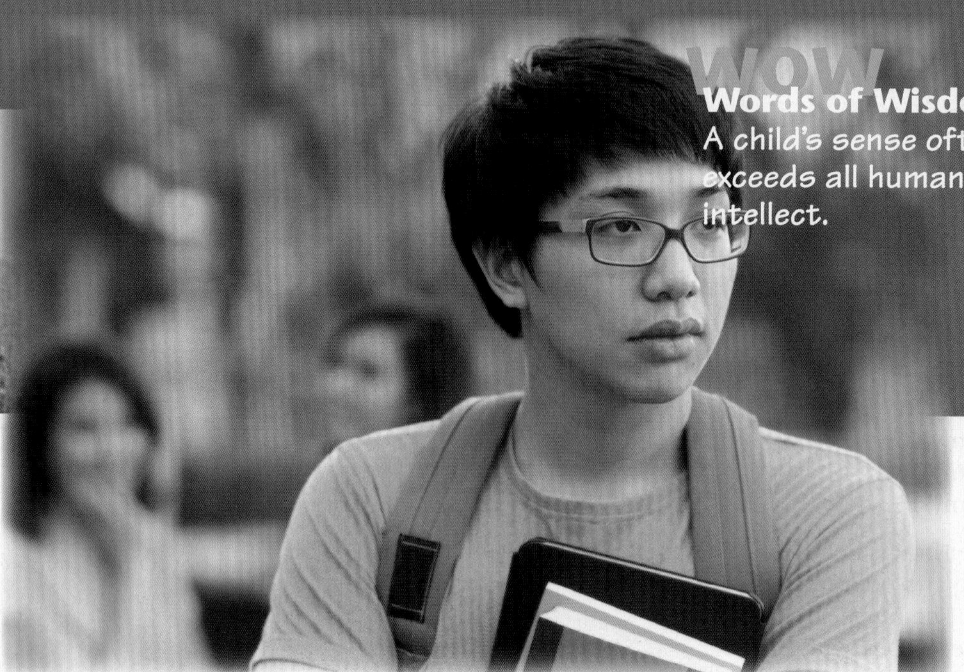
WOW
Words of Wisdom
A child's sense often exceeds all human intellect.

50 Nursing Care of the Child With an Alteration in Behavior, Cognition, or Development

KEY TERMS
abuse
affect
bingeing
comorbidity
neglect
purging
suicide
violence

Learning Objectives

Upon completion of the chapter, the learner will be able to:

1. Discuss the impact of alterations in mental health on the growth and development of infants, children, and adolescents.
2. Describe techniques used to evaluate the status of mental health in children.
3. Identify appropriate nursing assessments and interventions related to therapy and medications for the treatment of childhood and adolescent mental health disorders.
4. Distinguish mental health disorders common in infants, children, and adolescents.
5. Develop an individualized nursing care plan for the child with a mental health disorder.
6. Develop child/family teaching plans for the child with a mental health disorder.

***John Howard*, age 6 years, is brought to the clinic for his annual examination. His father states, "John has frequent emotional outbursts and his mood seems to switch from happy to sad rather quickly. His teachers have said his performance at school has been poor."**

Mental health issues make up the bulk of the "new morbidity" of children. Such issues include developmental and behavioral disorders, eating disorders, mood disorders, anxiety disorders, and abuse and **violence** (acts of aggression) directed toward children. As many as 14% to 20% of children may be suffering from mental health–related problems, yet only 2% are seen by mental healthcare providers (Burstein, Talmi, Stafford, & Kelsay, 2014). Failure to receive appropriate treatment may lead to further academic and social difficulties (Burstein et al., 2014). Mental illness manifested in the early years increases the risk of adolescent emotional issues, use of firearms, reckless driving, substance abuse, and promiscuous sexual activity. Some cognitive or neurobehavioral disorders may have a genetic or physiologic cause, whereas others result from family or environmental stressors.

Usually children with cognitive or mental health disorders are treated in the community or on an outpatient basis, but sometimes the disorder has such a significant impact on the child and family that hospitalization is required. Many hospitalized children also suffer from cognitive or mental health disorders. When a child is diagnosed with a cognitive or mental health disorder, the family may become overwhelmed by the multifaceted services that he or she requires.

The scope of mental health issues among children, adolescents, and their families has become so extensive that the U.S. Surgeon General has published a "National Agenda for Action." The Surgeon General's Conference on Children's Mental Health has set the following goals:

1. Promote public awareness of children's mental health issues and reduce the stigma associated with mental illness.
2. Continue to develop, disseminate, and implement scientifically proven prevention and treatment services in the field of children's mental health.
3. Improve the assessment of and recognition of mental health needs in children.
4. Eliminate racial/ethnic and socioeconomic disparities in access to mental healthcare services.
5. Improve the infrastructure for children's mental health services, including support for scientifically proven interventions across professions.
6. Increase access to, and coordination of, quality mental healthcare services.
7. Train front-line providers to recognize and manage mental health issues, and educate mental healthcare providers about scientifically proven prevention and treatment services.
8. Monitor the access to and coordination of quality mental healthcare services (U.S. Public Health Service, 2000).

Mental health problems in children are real and painful and can be severe. For affected children to have a chance at a healthy future, nurses must participate in the early identification and referral of children with potential cognitive deficits or other mental health issues.

EFFECTS OF MENTAL HEALTH ISSUES ON HEALTH AND DEVELOPMENT

Children's behavior is influenced by biologic or genetic characteristics, nutrition, physical health, developmental ability, environmental and family interactions, the child's individual temperament, and the parents' or caregivers' responses to the child's behavior. The changes that occur with normal growth and development are often a source of stress for children, and in some children they may lead to dysfunction. Children progress at very different rates, so it is often difficult to identify subtle abnormalities. When stress, fatigue, or pain occurs in children, they may quickly regress to earlier patterns of behavior. These regressive behaviors may continue if a mental health concern is present. It is possible that stress placed on developing neurons leads to decreased coping abilities later in life. Children learn through their experiences. Therefore, they may develop maladaptive behaviors through life interactions (Burstein et al., 2014).

COMMON MEDICAL TREATMENTS

A variety of medications and other medical and psychological treatments are used to treat mental health disorders in children. Most of these treatments will require a physician's or nurse practitioner's order when the child is in the hospital. The most common medications are listed in Drug Guide 50.1. The nurse caring for the child with a mental health disorder should become familiar with how the treatments and medications work, as well as medication adverse effects to monitor for. Many mental health disorders are treated with some type of therapy, including behavioral, play, family, and cognitive therapies. Table 50.1 reviews the types of therapies commonly used. These therapies are generally carried out only by specially trained personnel.

Behavior management techniques are also used to help children alter negative behavior patterns. The methods may be used outside of therapy sessions, in the hospital, clinic, classroom, or home. Behavior management techniques include the following:

- Set limits with the child, holding him or her responsible for his or her behavior.
- Do not argue, bargain, or negotiate about the limits once established.
- Provide consistent caregivers (unlicensed assistive personnel and nurses for the hospitalized child) and establish the child's daily routine.
- Use a low-pitched voice and remain calm.

DRUG GUIDE 50.1 DRUGS USED FOR PEDIATRIC MENTAL HEALTH DISORDERS

Medication	Actions/Indications	Nursing Implications
Psychostimulants: methylphenidate, dextroamphetamine, lisdexamfetamine, pemoline, long-acting methylphenidate, long-acting dextroamphetamine,	Increase synaptic levels of dopamine and norepinephrine ADHD	• Methylphenidate has a short half-life; give TID (AM, midday at school, at home after school). • Long-acting preparations are given once daily in the AM. • Adverse effects: decreased appetite, headache, abdominal pain, difficulty sleeping, irritability, social withdrawal, motor tics. If dose is too high, child may have flat affect. • lisdexamfetamine—if chest pain and fainting occur notify physician at once. • Pemoline is only rarely used because of hepatotoxicity.
Antianxiety agent: buspirone	Highly blocks reuptake of dopamine Anxiety, rage, mania, psychosis, depression, Tourette syndrome	• Administer in consistent relation to food (either with or without). • May cause drowsiness • Monitor for disinhibition, agitation, confusion, depression.
Antimanic agent: lithium	Influences reuptake of serotonin and/or norepinephrine Bipolar disorder, depression, hyperaggression	• Monitor closely. • May cause polyuria, polydipsia, tremor, nausea, weight gain, diarrhea
Selective serotonin reuptake inhibitors: fluoxetine, paroxetine, sertraline	Potentiate serotonin activity in the brain Depression, obsessive-compulsive disorder, anxiety	• Observe for irritability, insomnia, GI distress, nausea, headache. • Monitor BP for increase.
Atypical antidepressants: trazodone	Inhibit reuptake of serotonin Depression	• Monitor BP for postural hypotension. • Observe for sedation and drowsiness; avoid alcohol use. • Administer after meals or with a snack.
Nonstimulant norepinephrine reuptake inhibitors: atomoxetine	Enhance norepinephrine activity ADHD	• Administer without regard to food once or twice daily. • Monitor weight, height, BP, heart rate. • May cause dizziness, dry mouth
α-Agonist antihypertensive agents: clonidine, guanfacine	Activate inhibitory neurons in the brain stem ADHD, Tourette syndrome, self-abuse, aggression	• Clonidine is strongly sedating. • Monitor BP and pulse. • Observe for dry mouth, confusion, depression, urinary retention, constipation.
Antipsychotic agents: thioridazine, chlorpromazine, haloperidol	Reversibly block type 2 dopamine receptors in the central nervous system Psychosis, mania, self-harm, violent or destructive behavior	• May cause drowsiness • Monitor for anticholinergic effects, drowsiness and dystonia (extrapyramidal effects), dizziness. • Evaluate for the development of orthostatic hypotension, tachycardia. • Observe closely for the development of tardive dyskinesia, particularly early in treatment.

(continued)

DRUG GUIDE 50.1 DRUGS USED FOR PEDIATRIC MENTAL HEALTH DISORDERS (continued)

Medication	Actions/Indications	Nursing Implications
Atypical antipsychotics: risperidone, clozapine, olanzapine	Reversibly block type 2 dopamine receptors in the central nervous system Psychosis, bipolar disorder, autism spectrum disorder, Tourette syndrome	• Monitor for seizures, agitation, headache, nausea, sedation. • Olanzapine may cause weight gain. • Note WBC count.
Tricyclic antidepressants: amitriptyline, desipramine, imipramine, nortriptyline	Enhance synaptic concentration of serotonin and/or norepinephrine Depression, ADHD, tics, anxiety	• Monitor for anticholinergic effects, weight loss. • Check blood levels. • Monitor ECG for arrhythmias.

BP, blood pressure; ECG, electrocardiogram; GI, gastrointestinal; WBC, white blood cell.

Adapted from Preston, J., O'Neal, J. H., & Talaga, M. C. (2015). *Child and adolescent clinical psychopharmacology made simple*. Oakland, CA: New Harbinger Publications, Inc.; Taketomo, C. K., Hodding, J. H., & Kraus, D. M. (2013). *Pediatric & neonatal dosage handbook* (20th ed.). Hudson, OH: Lexicomp. and Varcarolis, E. M. (2011). *Manual of psychiatric nursing care planning: Assessment guides, diagnoses, and psychopharmacology* (4th ed.). St. Louis, MO: Saunders.

TABLE 50.1 TYPES OF THERAPY

Treatment	Explanation
Behavioral therapy	Uses stimulus and response conditioning to manage or alter behavior. Reinforces desired behaviors, replacing the inappropriate ones. Consistency is of utmost importance.
Play therapy	Designed to change emotional status. Encourages the child to act out feelings of sadness, fear, hostility, or anger.
Cognitive behavioral therapy	Teaches children to change reactions so that automatic negative thought patterns are replaced with alternative ones.
Dialectical behavioral therapy	Group and individual sessions to treat chronic suicidal thoughts in borderline personality disorder. Individuals learn responsibility for their problems and better deal with negative emotions.
Family therapy	Exploration of the child's emotional issue and its effect on family members. Helps the family to focus in more constructive ways.
Group therapy	May be conducted in a school, hospital, treatment facility, or neighborhood center. Feelings are expressed and participants gain hope, feel a part of something, and benefit from role modeling. Takes advantage of peer relationships as developmental focus in preteen and teen groups.
Milieu therapy	A specially structured setting designed to promote the child's adaptive and social skills. A safe and supportive environment for those at risk for self-harm or those who are very ill or very aggressive.
Individual therapy	The child and therapist work together to resolve the conflicts, emotions, or behavior problems. Trust is central. Structured based on the child's developmental level (e.g., may use play therapy for a younger child).
Hypnosis	Deep relaxation with suggestibility remarks.

Adapted from American Academy of Child and Adolescent Psychiatry. (2013). *Fast facts for families no. 86: Psychotherapies for children and adolescents*. Washington, DC: Author.

Varcarolis, E. M. (2011). *Manual of psychiatric nursing care planning: Assessment guides, diagnoses, and psychopharmacology* (4th ed.). St. Louis, MO: Saunders.

- Redirect the child's attention when needed.
- Ignore inappropriate behaviors.
- Praise the child's self-control efforts and other accomplishments.
- Use restraints only when necessary.

NURSING PROCESS OVERVIEW FOR THE CHILD WITH A MENTAL HEALTH DISORDER

Care of the child with a mental health disorder includes assessment, nursing diagnosis, planning, interventions, and evaluation. There are a number of general concepts related to the nursing process that may be applied to mental health concerns in children. From a general understanding of the care involved for a child with a mental health disorder, the nurse can then individualize the care based on specifics for each child.

Assessment

A careful and thorough health history forms the basis of the nursing assessment of a child with a mental health or cognitive disorder. The physical examination may yield clues to the type of disorder, but the physical examination is often completely normal (except in cases of physical or sexual abuse).

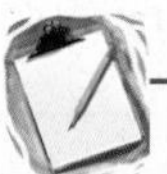

Take Note!

Observe a child's play or drawings; if the manner or theme of play or nature of the drawings leads you to suspect cognitive or psychological issues, refer the child for further mental health evaluation.

Health History

Elicit the health history, noting the child's prenatal and birth history, past medical history (including previously diagnosed cognitive or mental health disorders), history of neurologic injury or disease, and family history of mental health disorder. Perform a developmental history, noting age of attainment (or loss) of milestones. Question the child and/or parent about behavior changes such as:

- Altered sleep
- Difference in eating patterns, weight loss or gain, change in appetite
- Problems at school
- Participation in risk-taking behaviors
- Alterations in friendships
- Changes in extracurricular activity participation

A number of tools are available for screening for mental health disorders in children and adolescents. Use one of these tools as needed (refer to thePoint for an explanation of the various tools). Note results of any developmental testing performed. Ask the family about progression of the child's skills. Note any unusual deficits or capabilities. Question the family about recent stress, trauma, or change in family structure. Ask if any family members are chronically ill. Note medications the child takes routinely, and ask about any allergies to food, drugs, medications, or environmental agents.

Interview the child at an age-appropriate level to determine his or her self-perception, future plans, and stressors and how he or she copes with them. Determine the child's perception of his or her relationship with parents, siblings, friends, peers, pets, inanimate objects, and transitional or security objects. What is the child's predominant mood? Determine whether the child likes himself or herself, asking such questions as "What do you like most about yourself?" and "What would you like to change about yourself?" Determine whether the child has a sense of pride in his or her accomplishments. Has the child developed an appropriate conscience (with understanding of right and wrong)? Determine the child's gender identity status.

Document if the child displays any of the following during the health interview:

- Hallucinations
- Aggression
- Impulsivity
- Distractibility
- Intolerance to frustration
- Lack of sense of humor or fun
- Inhibition
- Poor attention span
- Potential cognitive or learning disabilities
- Unusual motor activities

Note history of physical complaints that may be associated with physical abuse such as burns or other injuries or with sexual abuse situations, such as sore throat, difficulty swallowing, or genital burning or itching.

Remember John, the 6-year-old brought in for his annual examination? What additional health history and physical examination assessment information should the nurse obtain?

Physical Examination

Observe the child's clothing, noting whether it is appropriate for age, developmental level, and setting. Note the child's facial expression and response to the parent or caretaker and the nurse. Does the child make appropriate eye contact? Determine the child's level of consciousness and extent of interest in and interaction with surroundings. Note the child's posture, **affect** (facial emotional display), and mood. How appropriate to the situation are the child's emotional reactions? Does the child communicate well?

Measure the child's weight and height/length, as well as head circumference if he or she is younger than 3 years old. Perform a thorough physical examination, noting any physical abnormalities or signs of other physical health disorders. Note abnormal findings that may be associated with particular mental health disorders, such as bruising, burns, contusions, cuts, abrasions, unusual skin marks, soft/sparse body hair, split fingernails, inflamed oropharynx, eroded tooth enamel, reddened gums, or genitourinary discharge or bleeding.

Laboratory and Diagnostic Testing

Mental health disorders are generally diagnosed based on clinical features. However, brain imaging such as computed tomography or magnetic resonance imaging may be used to evaluate for a congenital abnormality or alterations in the brain tissue that may lead to developmental delay. A blood or urine toxicology panel is useful in the diagnosis of drug abuse or overdose, or instances of bizarre behavior.

Nursing Diagnoses and Related Interventions

The overall goal of nursing management of cognitive and mental health disorders in children is to help the child and family to reach an optimal level of functioning. This may be achieved through interventions designed to decrease the impact of stressors on the child's life. Upon completion of a thorough assessment of the child and family, the nurse might identify several nursing diagnoses, including:

- Impaired social interaction
- Delayed growth and development
- Ineffective individual coping
- Hopelessness
- Imbalanced nutrition, less than body requirements
- Disturbed thought processes
- Caregiver role strain

After completing an assessment of John, the nurse noted the following: difficulty sitting still for the examination, easily distracted and frustrated, labile mood. Based on the assessment findings, what would your top three nursing diagnoses be for John?

Nursing goals, interventions, and evaluation for the child with a mental health disorder are based on the nursing diagnoses. Nursing Care Plan 50.1, found at the end of the chapter, provides a general guide for planning care for a child with a mental health disorder. Children's responses to a mental health issue and its treatment will vary, and nursing care should be individualized based on the child's and family's responses to illness. Additional information about nursing management will be included later in the chapter as it relates to specific disorders. See Healthy People 2020.

Based on your top three nursing diagnoses for John, describe appropriate nursing interventions.

DEVELOPMENTAL AND BEHAVIORAL DISORDERS

Developmental and behavioral disorders make up a large proportion of mental health disorders in children. They include learning disabilities, intellectual disability, autism spectrum disorder, and attention deficit/hyperactivity disorder (ADHD).

Learning Disabilities

About 10% of children and adolescents have learning disabilities (von Hahn, 2015a). In children with chronic illness, learning disabilities are two times more common than in the general population (von Hahn, 2015a). The essential characteristic of learning disability is an innate cognitive difficulty resulting in lower academic achievement than would be expected for the child's intellectual potential (von Hahn, 2015a). Learning disabilities become evident when a child of average intelligence has difficulty mastering basic academic skills. Learning disabilities can affect the child's ability to listen, speak, read, write, and perform mathematics. For example:

- Children with dyslexia have difficulty with reading, writing, and spelling.

***HEALTHY PEOPLE** 2020*

Objective	Nursing Significance
Increase the proportion of children with mental health problems who receive treatment.	• Screen all children and adolescents for mental health problems. • Encourage children and adolescents to participate in treatment planning as is developmentally appropriate, allowing them to make choices about intervention as possible.

Healthy People Objectives retrieved from http://www.healthypeople.gov

BOX 50.1

SENSORY PROCESSING DISORDER (ALSO CALLED SENSORY INTEGRATION DYSFUNCTION)

- A neurologic disorder in which the child cannot organize sensory input used in daily living
- Hyposensitivity or hypersensitivity to sensory input
- Results in overreaction to different textures, decreasing the child's ability to participate in the world
- Preterm and low-birthweight infants are at increased risk compared with typical infants.
- Occupational and other therapies may increase the child's ability to function.

Adapted from Sensory Processing Disorder Foundation. (2016). *About SPD*. Retrieved from http://www.spdfoundation.net/about-sensory-processing-disorder/

- Children with dyscalculia have problems with mathematics and computation.
- Children with dyspraxia have problems with manual dexterity and coordination.
- Children with dysgraphia have difficulty producing the written word (composition, spelling, and writing).

Take Note!

Sensory processing disorder may be mistaken for a learning disability, but it is not and should be treated differently (Box 50.1)

Therapeutic Management

Therapeutic management may involve remedial or compensatory approaches or may use interventions directed toward social-emotional problems. The focus of the remedial approach is to improve specific skills. The compensatory approach helps the child to compensate for the disability, rather than attempting to directly correct it. Social-emotional problems may result from frustration or low self-esteem related to capabilities. These may respond to supportive interventions and improvement in coping.

Consider This

Victor Johnson, a third grader with learning disabilities, tells the nurse, "I get made fun of at school". He begins to sniffle and says, "Everybody calls me stupid. It hurts my feelings." Victor's mother adds "I really just don't know how to help him…" How should the nurse reply? What would be the most therapeutic response?

Nursing Assessment

Elicit the health history, noting risk factors such as a family history of learning disability, problems during pregnancy or birth, prenatal alcohol or drug use, low birthweight, premature or prolonged labor, head injury, poor nutritional status or failure to thrive, or lead poisoning. Obtain detailed information about the educational difficulties the child is experiencing (e.g., he or she seems to do fine in math but always reverses letters when reading). A thorough physical examination may reveal clues to comorbid conditions. Ensure that the child has undergone a comprehensive education evaluation with assessment testing to diagnose the specific learning disability. Testing may be performed by a school, educational, developmental, or clinical psychologist; occupational therapist; speech and language therapist; or other developmental specialist, depending on the areas of learning with which the child is experiencing difficulty.

Take Note!

If a child cannot speak in sentences by 30 months of age, does not have understandable speech 50% of the time by age 3 years, cannot sit still for a short story by 3 to 5 years of age, or cannot tie shoes, cut, button, or hop by 5 to 6 years of age, refer the child to be evaluated for a learning disability.

Nursing Management

Ensure that families are aware of their child's rights under the Individuals with Disabilities Act (IDEA), which was reapproved in 2004 (108th Congress, 2004). IDEA offers protection from discrimination and the right to assistance in the school or workplace. Each child will need an individualized education plan (IEP) that reflects his or her particular needs, which then must be provided for through the school system. Offer encouragement and support to families as they advocate for their child. Follow up at subsequent healthcare visits to determine that the child is receiving the services he or she needs to optimize his or her potential for success. Refer families for additional resources through the National Center for Learning Disabilities, Learning Disabilities Online, or the Center for Learning Differences (links to these resources are provided on thePoint).

Intellectual Disability

Intellectual disability refers to a functional state in which significant limitations in intellectual status and adaptive behavior (functioning in daily life) develop before the age of 18 years. Intellectual disability occurs in about 1% of the population (Pivalizza & Lalani, 2016). Although intellectual disability includes the definition of intellectual quotient (IQ) less than 70 to 75, the range of impairments associated with the low IQ is variable. Impairments in the adaptive domains of conceptual, social, or practical assist with determining the severity of intellectual disability (from mild to profound) (Pivalizza & Lalani, 2016).

Long ago persons with intellectual disability (formerly termed mentally retardation) were confined to institutions and were thought to be harmful to society. In the early 21st century, most children with intellectual disability are receiving their education in public schools with their peers and living at home with their families or elsewhere in the community. Only the most severely affected individuals require separate classrooms or schools.

Pathophysiology

In many instances of intellectual disability the exact cause remains unknown. Prenatal errors in central nervous system development may be responsible. Other potential causes include an insult or damage to the brain during the prenatal, perinatal, or postnatal period. Prenatal exposure to alcohol or other drugs may impact cognitive development as well. Motor problems such as hyper- or hypotonia, tremor, ataxia, or clumsiness, or visual motor problems may occur concomitantly with intellectual disability. In addition, functioning at a higher level may be prevented when a learning disability or sensory processing impairment is also present. Intellectual disability may be categorized according to severity of impairment across domains. See Table 50.2.

Therapeutic Management

The primary goal of therapeutic management of children with intellectual disability is to provide appropriate educational experiences that allow the child to achieve a level of functioning and self-sufficiency needed for existence in the home, community, work, and leisure settings. A multidisciplinary approach may be used and the child's conceptual, social, practical, and intellectual abilities will drive school placement and the focus of the educational experience. The majority of individuals with intellectual disability require only minimal support in the school or home setting, and these individuals are able to achieve some level of self-sufficiency. Only a few children and adults with intellectual disability require extensive support and require long-term caretaking.

Nursing Assessment

Perform developmental screening at each healthcare visit to identify developmental delays early. Elicit the health history, determining the mental and adaptive capacities of the child's parents and other family members. Obtain a detailed pregnancy and birth history. Document sequence and age of attainment of developmental milestones. Note history of motor, visual, or language difficulties. Assess the child's health history for risk factors such as preterm or postterm birth, low birthweight, birth injury, prenatal or neonatal infection, prenatal alcohol or drug exposure, genetic syndrome, chromosomal alteration, metabolic disease, exposure to toxins (e.g., lead), head injury or other trauma, nutritional deficiency, cerebral malformation, and other brain disease or mental health disorder. Note history of or concomitant seizure disorder, orthopedic problems, speech problems, or vision or hearing deficit.

For the child with known intellectual disability, assess language, sensory, and psychomotor functioning.

TABLE 50.2 SEVERITY OF INTELLECTUAL DISABILITY

Classification Percentage affected	IQ (generally)	Conceptual	Social	Practical
Mild 85%	between 50 to 55 and 70	Requires academic supports	Immature social skills and personal judgment	Usually independent in activities of daily living
Moderate 10%	between 35 to 40 and 50 to 55	Complex tasks require substantial support	Social cues, judgment and life decisions need regular support	Independent self-care with moderate supports
Severe 3–4%	between 20 to 25 and 35 to 40	Little understanding of written language, time; require extensive supports	Benefit from healthy supportive interactions	Require significant and ongoing supervision for activities of daily living
Profound 1–2%	less than 20 to 25	May use objects in a goal-directed fashion	May understand gestures and emotional cues; use nonverbal expression	Dependent upon support for all activities of daily living

BOX 50.2

FETAL ALCOHOL SYNDROME

- Results from in utero alcohol exposure
- Typical facial features include low nasal bridge with short upturned nose, flattened midface, long philtrum with narrow upper lip
- Poor coordination, skeletal abnormalities
- Microcephaly
- Failure to thrive
- Hearing loss

Adapted from Goldson, E., & Reynolds, A. (2014). Child development and behavior. In W. W. Hay, Jr., M. J. Levin, R. R. Deterding, & M. J. Abzug (Eds.), *Current diagnosis and treatment: Pediatrics* (22nd ed.). New York, NY: McGraw-Hill Education.

Determine the child's ability to toilet, dress, and feed himself or herself. Ask the parents about involvement with school and community services and support.

On physical examination note dysmorphic features (possibly very mild) consistent with certain syndromes (e.g., fetal alcohol syndrome; see Box 50.2). Evaluate the newborn or metabolic screening results. Computed tomography or magnetic resonance imaging of the head may be performed to evaluate the brain structure. Thyroid function tests may be ordered to rule out thyroid problems leading to developmental delay.

Take Note!

Due to the extent of cognition required to understand and produce speech, the most sensitive early indicator of intellectual disability is delayed language development.

Nursing Management

When children with intellectual disability are admitted to the hospital (usually for some other physical or medical condition), it is important for the nurse to continue the child's usual home routine. Follow through with feeding and motor supports that the child uses. Ensure that the child is closely supervised and remains free from harm. Allow parents time to verbalize frustrations or fears. For some families the caretaking burden is extensive and lifelong; arrange for respite care as available. Support the child's strengths, and assist the child and family to follow through with therapy or treatment designed to enhance the child's functioning. Assist with the development of the child's IEP as appropriate.

Autism Spectrum Disorder

Autism spectrum disorder (ASD), also termed pervasive developmental disorder, has its onset in infancy or early childhood. One child in 88 is affected by autism spectrum disorder (Goldson & Reynolds, 2014). The spectrum of autism disorder ranges from mild (e.g., Asperger syndrome) to severe. Autistic behaviors may be first noticed in infancy as developmental delays or between the age of 12 and 36 months when the child regresses or loses previously acquired skills. Parental concerns about development may be sensitive indicators of the development of autism.

Pathophysiology

The exact etiology of autism continues to elude scientists, but it may be due to genetic makeup, brain abnormalities, altered chemistry, a virus, or toxic chemicals. Children with ASD display impaired social interactions and communication as well as perseverative or stereotypic behaviors. They may fail to develop interpersonal relationships and experience social isolation. Many children with autism are intellectually disabled, requiring lifelong supervision, though some are gifted (Starr, Fookson, Burns, & Bowman-Harvey, 2013).

Therapeutic Management

There are no medications or treatments available to cure autism. The goal of therapeutic management is for the child to reach optimal functioning within the limitations of the disorder. Each child's treatment is individualized; behavioral and communication therapies are very important. Children with ASD respond very well to highly structured educational environments. Stimulants may be used to control hyperactivity, and antipsychotic medications are sometimes helpful in children with repetitive and aggressive behaviors.

Many families are drawn to the use of complementary and alternative medical therapies in attempts to treat their autistic child. They may use vitamins and nutritional supplements, herbs or restrictive diets, music therapy, art therapy, and sensory integration techniques. To date, these therapies have not been scientifically proven to improve autism (Starr et al., 2013).

Nursing Assessment

Elicit the health history, noting delay or regression in developmental skills, particularly speech and language abilities. Failure to point at objects and to gaze at an object jointly with another by 18 months are concerning signs (Goldson & Reynolds, 2014). The child may be mute, utter only sounds (not words), or repeat words or phrases over and over. The parent may report that the infant or toddler spends hours in repetitive activity and demonstrates bizarre motor and stereotypic behaviors. The infant may resist cuddling, lack eye contact, be indifferent to touch or affection, and have little change in facial expression. Toddlers may display hyperactivity, aggression, temper tantrums, or self-injury behaviors, such as head banging or hand biting. The history may also reveal hypersensitivity to touch or hyposensitivity to pain. Assess the child's functional status, including behavior, nutrition, sleep, speech and language, education needs, and developmental or neurologic limitations. Assist with screening, using an approved autism screening tool such as the Modified Checklist for Autism in Toddlers-Revised (M-CHAT-R), which is recommended for administration at 18 months of age, and then again at 24 to 30 months of age (refer to thePoint for a link to the M-CHAT-R). Additional screening tools include the Social Communication Questionnaire (SCQ) and the Pervasive Developmental Disorders Screening Test-II (PDDST-II).

Perform a thorough physical examination. Observe the infant or toddler for lack of eye contact, failure to look at objects pointed to by the examiner, failure to point to himself or herself, failure to let his or her needs be known, perseverative play activities, and unusual behavior such as hand flapping or spinning. Measure growth parameters, in particular noting head circumference (macrocephaly or microcephaly may be associated with ASD). Note the presence of large, prominent, or posteriorly rotated ears. Examine the skin for hypo- or hyperpigmented lesions. Note asymmetry of nerve function or palsy, hypertonia, hypotonia, alterations in deep tendon reflexes, toe-walking, loose gait, or poor coordination. Obtain hearing screening results and ascertain that lead screening has been performed.

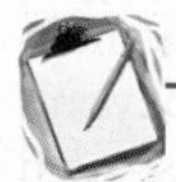

Take Note!

Screen all infants and toddlers for warning signs of autism:

- Not babbling by 12 months
- Not pointing or using gestures by 12 months
- No single words by 16 months
- No two-word utterances by 24 months
- Losing language or social skills at any age (Starr et al., 2013)

Nursing Management

When children are initially diagnosed with autism, provide parents with an extensive amount of emotional support, professional guidance, and education about the disorder while they are attempting to adjust to the diagnosis. Assess the fit between the child's developmental needs and the treatment plan. Help parents overcome barriers to obtain appropriate education, developmental, and behavioral treatment programs. Ensure that the child younger than 36 months of age receives services via the local early intervention program and children 3 years and older have an IEP in place if enrolled in the public school system. Stress the importance of rigid, unchanging routines, as children with ASD often act out when their routine changes (which is likely to occur if the child must be hospitalized for another condition). Many special schools exist for children with significant developmental disorders, though some are extremely expensive. Assess the parents' need for respite care and make referrals accordingly. Provide positive feedback to parents for their perseverance in working with their child.

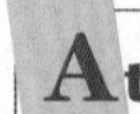

Atraumatic Care

Provide family-centered care, being sure to treat the family not just the child. Minimize parent–child separation.

Attention Deficit/Hyperactivity Disorder

ADHD is the most common neurodevelopmental disorder of childhood, affecting nearly 10% of school-age children aged 4 to 17 years (Starr et al., 2013). ADHD is characterized by inattention, impulsivity, distractibility, and hyperactivity. Three subtypes of ADHD exist: hyperactive–impulsive, inattentive, and combined. The child with ADHD has a disruption in learning ability, socialization, and compliance, placing significant demands on the child, parents, teachers, and community. Children with ADHD often have a **comorbidity** (disorder accompanying the primary illness) such as oppositional defiant disorder, conduct disorder, an anxiety disorder, depression, a less severe developmental disorder, an auditory processing disorder, or learning or reading disabilities (Krull, 2016). Comparison Chart 50.1 gives information about oppositional defiant disorder and conduct disorder to distinguish them from ADHD.

Pathophysiology

Though the exact cause of ADHD remains unidentified, current thought includes as its etiology an alteration in the dopamine and norepinephrine neurotransmitter system. The symptoms of impulsivity, hyperactivity, and inattention begin before 7 years of age and persist longer than 6 months. Symptoms exist in the school and home settings, impairing family and social interactions. Children and teens with ADHD experience frustration, labile moods, emotional outbursts, peer rejection, poor school performance, and low self-esteem. They may also have poor metacognitive abilities such as organization, time management, and the ability to break a project down into a series of smaller tasks. They are not lazy or unmotivated, but simply have poor skills in these areas. Box 50.3 provides criteria for the diagnosis of ADHD (Starr et al., 2013).

COMPARISON CHART 50.1

OPPOSITIONAL DEFIANT DISORDER VERSUS CONDUCT DISORDER

Oppositional Defiant Disorder	Conduct Disorder
• Excessive arguing with adults • Frequent temper tantrums • Active defiance • Revenge-seeking behaviors • Frequent resentment or anger • Touchiness; easily annoyed. • Noncompliance with adult requests or limits • Blaming of others for misbehavior or mistakes	• Bullying and threatening of others • Initiation of physical fights • Weapon use to cause others harm • Physical cruelty to animals or people • Destruction of property or arson • Lying and stealing • Serious violation of rules: staying out past curfew, truancy, running away • Use of force in sexual activity

Adapted from Burstein, A., Talmi, A., Stafford, B., & Kelsay, K. (2014). Child & adolescent psychiatric disorders & psychosocial aspects of pediatrics. In W. W. Hay, M. J. Levin, & R. R. Deterding, & M. J. Abzug, (Eds.), *Current pediatric diagnosis and treatment* (22nd ed.). New York, NY: McGraw-Hill.

BOX 50.3

DIAGNOSIS OF ATTENTION DEFICIT/ HYPERACTIVITY DISORDER

Presence of six or more of the following in the child 17 years of age and younger:

- Failure to pay close attention
- Careless mistakes on schoolwork
- Difficulty paying attention to tasks or play
- Doesn't listen
- Doesn't follow through
- Doesn't complete tasks
- Doesn't understand instructions
- Poorly organized
- Avoids, dislikes, or fails to engage in activities requiring mental effort
- Loses things needed for task completion
- Easily distracted
- Forgetful
- Fidgety or squirmy
- Often out of seat
- Activity inappropriate to the situation
- Cannot engage in quiet play
- Always on the go
- Talks excessively
- Blurts out answers
- Has difficulty waiting his or her turn
- Often interrupts or intrudes on others

Additionally, symptoms have been present in two or more settings, at least two of the symptoms occurred prior to age 12, persistence of symptoms beyond 6 months and to a degree inconsistent with developmental level or negatively interferes with social or academic performance, and symptoms are not associated with purely oppositional behavior or as a component of a psychotic disorder, and cannot be explained by the diagnosis of a different mental health disorder.

Adapted from French, W. P. (2015). Assessment and treatment of attention-deficit/hyperactivity disorder: Part 1. *Pediatric Annals, 44*(3), 114–120.

Therapeutic Management

Medication management of ADHD includes the use of psychostimulants, nonstimulant norepinephrine reuptake inhibitors, and/or α-agonist antihypertensive agents. These medications are not a cure for ADHD, but help to increase the child's ability to pay attention and decrease the level of impulsive behavior. The child's activity level is not usually affected. Behavior therapy and classroom restructuring may be useful as part of the therapeutic management plan. Since about 50% of ADHD cases persist into adulthood, management should continue throughout adolescence and beyond as needed (Solanto, 2015). Concomitant disorders, such as anxiety, should also be treated (see discussion of anxiety disorders below).

Nursing Assessment

For a full description of the assessment phase of the nursing process, refer to the Assessment section of the Nursing Process Overview. Assessment findings pertinent to ADHD are discussed below.

HEALTH HISTORY

Elicit a description of the behavioral issue or school performance problem. Explore the child's history for risk factors such as head trauma, lead exposure, cigarette smoke exposure, prematurity, or low birthweight. The past history may also reveal a larger than usual number of accidents. Determine if there is a family history of ADHD. Question the parent about school behavior. The school-age child may be unable to stay on task, talks out of turn, leaves his or her desk frequently, and either neglects to complete in-class and homework assignments or forgets to turn them in. The adolescent may be inattentive in school, poorly organized, and forgetful.

Several behavioral checklists are available that may assist in the diagnosis of ADHD. They may be completed by the child's teacher and/or parent and focus on behavior patterns related to conduct or learning problems, social competence, anxiety, activity level, and attention. Obtain the completed behavioral checklists (usually one from the parent and one from the teacher) as well as any school records or testing performed.

PHYSICAL EXAMINATION

Perform vision and hearing screening to rule out vision or hearing impairment as the cause of poor school performance. Observe the preschool child's behavior, noting quickness, agility, fearlessness, and the desire to touch or explore everything in the room. The older child or adolescent may have difficulty staying on task during the examination or change the subject frequently while conversing.

LABORATORY AND DIAGNOSTIC TESTS

No definitive laboratory or diagnostic test is available for the identification of ADHD. A complete blood count may be performed to rule out anemia, and thyroid hormone levels may be drawn to determine whether they are normal.

Nursing Management

Having a child with ADHD can be frustrating as the child's inattention, high activity level, impulsivity, and distractibility are often very difficult to deal with. Parents may doubt their ability to be effective parents or may view their child as somehow defective. Children with ADHD may also feel they are bad, faulty, stupid, or intellectually challenged. Provide emotional support, allowing enough time for the family to air their concerns. Work with the child and family to develop goals such as completion of homework, improved communication, or increasing independence in self-care.

Assist the family to advocate for their child's needs through the public school system. The child is entitled to a developmentally appropriate education via an IEP as necessary (refer to Chapter 34 for additional information about special education). The IEP should be updated as needed. Ensure coordination of health and school services. Flag the child's chart and set up a schedule for systematic communication with the family and school. Teach families and school personnel to use behavioral techniques such as time-out, positive reinforcement, reward or privilege withdrawal, or a token system. The token system rewards appropriate behavior with a token and results in a token being taken away if inappropriate behavior occurs. At the end of a specified period of time, the tokens may be exchanged for a prize or privilege. Refer families to local support groups and the national ADHD support group, links to which are provided on thePoint.

Explain that stimulant medications should be taken in the morning to decrease the adverse effect of insomnia. Some children may experience decreased appetite, so giving the medication with or after the meal may be beneficial. The child may feel "different" from his or her peers if he or she has to visit the school nurse for a lunchtime dose of ADHD medication; this may lead to noncompliance and a subsequent increase in ADHD symptoms, with deterioration in schoolwork. In this situation, encourage the family to explore with their physician or nurse practitioner the option of one of the newer extended-release or once-daily ADHD medications. See Dosage Calculation Box 50.1

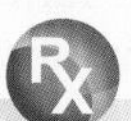

Dosage Calculation Box 50.1

Child's weight: 50 lb
Medication order: start methylphenidate 10 mg PO now.
Per the Pediatric Dosage Handbook, for initial dosing, the recommended dose is 0.3 mg/kg/dose.
Is the ordered dose safe?

TOURETTE SYNDROME

Tourette syndrome consists of multiple motor tics and one or more vocal tics occurring either simultaneously or at different times. Children are not tic-free for longer than 3 months. Tics are defined as sudden rapid recurrent stereotypical movements and/or sounds over which the child appears to have no control. Tourette syndrome is estimated to affect up to 1% to 2% of children (Garzon, 2013). Its onset is before 18 years of age.

Comorbid conditions such as ADHD, obsessive-compulsive disorder (OCD), and others may occur in up to 60% of children with Tourette syndrome (incidence depending upon the comorbid condition) (Jankovic, 2015). The exact pathophysiologic mechanism of Tourette syndrome has yet to be identified, though genetics does seem to play a part. Therapeutic management is highly individualized and involves psychopharmacology and behavioral therapies. Habit reversal training may help in some children.

Nursing Assessment

Evaluate the health history for the occurrence of tics. The child may be embarrassed or ashamed about the tics and the parents may feel fearful, angry, or guilty. Determine the presence of symptoms of comorbid conditions. Elicit the child's past health history, noting a family history of tics. Assess the child's psychosocial history to determine the extent to which the tics interfere with friendship, school performance, and self-esteem. Observe the child for simple or complex motor tics. Vocal tics such as sniffling, grunting, clicking, or word utterance may occur. Perform a thorough physical examination, which is usually normal.

Nursing Management

Inform families that the tics become more noticeable or severe during times of stress and less pronounced when the child is focused on an activity such as watching TV, reading, or playing a video game. Help the family to build on the child's functional behaviors and adaptive skills to improve the child's self-esteem. Encourage the family to pursue classroom accommodations such as allowing for "tic breaks," taking untimed tests or tests in another room, or using note takers or tape recording. Support the family's decisions related to medication use and therapy and provide appropriate education about the particular drugs and therapies. "Teaching the Tiger" by M. P. Dornbush and S. K. Pruitt (Hope Press) is useful for teachers of the child with Tourette syndrome. For additional support, refer families to Tourette Syndrome Association, Tourette Syndrome Foundation of Canada, or Tourette Syndrome Plus (links to these resources are provided on thePoint).

EATING DISORDERS

Eating disorders include pica, rumination, anorexia nervosa, and bulimia. They affect a significant number of children, especially adolescents. Pica, which occurs most frequently in 2- to 3-year olds, is an eating disorder in which the child ingests (over at least a 1-month period) a nonnutritive material such as paint, clay, or sand. Rumination is an eating disorder occurring in infants in which the baby regurgitates partially digested food or formula and expels or swallows it. The numbers of children affected by pica and rumination is not known. This discussion will focus on anorexia nervosa and bulimia, as they are more commonly encountered.

Anorexia nervosa and bulimia are common eating disorders affecting primarily adolescents, though younger children may also be affected. In American society being thin is highly valued, which compounds the problem. The lifetime prevalence rate for anorexia nervosa and bulimia is about 1% each, yet these problem often arise in childhood, particularly adolescence (Garzon, 2013). Anorexia nervosa is characterized by dramatic weight loss as a result of decreased food intake and sharply increased physical exercise. Bulimia refers to a cycle of normal food intake, followed by binge-eating and then purging. Typically, the adolescent with bulimia remains at a near-normal weight. Complications of anorexia and bulimia include fluid and electrolyte imbalance, decreased blood volume, cardiac arrhythmias, esophagitis, rupture of the esophagus or stomach, tooth loss, and menstrual problems. The 5-year mortality rate for anorexia nervosa is 15% to 20% (Garzon, 2013).

Therapeutic management may occur in either the inpatient or outpatient setting. In either case, a multidisciplinary approach including individual and family therapy as well as nutritional therapy is needed for the best chance at successful treatment. Atypical antipsychotics or antidepressants may be used, but their effectiveness remains controversial (Garzon, 2013).

Nursing Assessment

Determine the health history, noting risk factors such as family history, female gender, Caucasian race, preoccupation with appearance, obsessive traits, or low self-esteem. Adolescents with anorexia may have a history of constipation, syncope, secondary amenorrhea, abdominal pain, and periodic episodes of cold hands and feet. Parents usually note the chief complaint as weight loss. Note history of depression in the child with bulimia. Evaluate the child's self-concept, noting multiple fears, high need for acceptance, disordered body image, and perfectionism.

Perform a thorough physical examination. The anorexic is usually severely underweight, with a body mass index (BMI) of less than 17. Note cachectic appearance, dry sallow skin, thinning scalp hair, soft sparse body hair, and nail pitting. Measure vital signs, noting low temperature, bradycardia, or hypotension. Auscultate the heart, noting murmur as a result of mitral valve prolapse (occurs in about one third of adolescents with anorexia).

The adolescent with bulimia will be of normal weight or slightly overweight. Inspect the hands for calluses on the backs of the knuckles and split fingernails. Inspect the mouth and oropharynx for eroded dental enamel, red gums, and inflamed throat from self-induced vomiting.

Careful laboratory and diagnostic evaluation of serum electrolytes and an electrocardiogram are needed in adolescents with anorexia because severe electrolyte disturbances and cardiac arrhythmias often occur.

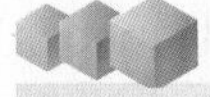
Concept Mastery Alert

Anorexia Nervosa Assessment Findings

An adolescent with anorexia nervosa would most likely experience amenorrhea, hypothermia, low blood pressure, and bradycardia. The nurse would also note soft hair on the individual's back and arms.

Nursing Management

Most children with eating disorders can be treated successfully on an outpatient basis, though this treatment may require many months. Those with anorexia who display severe weight loss, unstable vital signs, food refusal, or arrested pubertal development or who require enteral nutrition will need to be hospitalized. Refeeding syndrome (cardiovascular, hematologic, and neurologic

HEALTHY PEOPLE 2020

Objective	Nursing Significance
Reduce the proportion of adolescents who engage in disordered eating behaviors in an attempt to control their weight.	• Ensure that psychotherapy is available to children with eating disorders. • Provide appropriate follow-up for all children recovering from anorexia or bulimia.

Healthy People Objectives retrieved from http://www.healthypeople.gov

complications) may occur in the severely malnourished adolescent with anorexia if rapid nutritional replacement is given. Therefore, slow refeeding is essential to avoid complications. Give phosphorus supplements as ordered. Assess vital signs frequently for orthostatic hypotension, irregular and decreased pulse, or hypothermia.

Consult the nutritionist for assistance with calculating caloric needs and determining an appropriate diet. Aim for a weight gain goal of 0.5 to 2 lb per week. Instruct the child and family to keep a daily journal of intake, **bingeing** (excessive consumption) and **purging** (forced vomiting) behaviors, mood, and exercise. The journal may be used as an assessment tool as well as to document progress toward recovery. Assist the child and family to plan a suitably structured routine for the child that includes meals, snacks, and appropriate physical activity.

Use the physical findings associated with anorexia to educate the child about the consequences of malnutrition and how they can be remedied with adequate nutrient intake. Refer the adolescent, as appropriate, to behavior or group therapy. Assess the child's need for medical intervention for concomitant depression or anxiety (some anorexics also require psychotropic medications). Provide emotional support and positive reinforcement to the child and family. Refer the family to local support groups or online resources such as the Academy for Eating Disorders or the National Eating Disorders Association (links to these resources are provided on thePoint). See Healthy People 2020.

MOOD DISORDERS

Mood disorders in children include depressive disorders and bipolar disorder. It is difficult to quantify the incidence of depression in children under age 5 years, due to lack of sophistication of communication skills. Up to 3% of school-age children and 5% of adolescents may suffer from depression (Garzon, 2013). Children may experience major depressive disorder or dysthymic disorder. Girls are twice as likely to be affected as boys, particularly during the teenage years. Bipolar disorder refers to a condition of alternating manic and depressive episodes and affects about 2.6% of children (Garzon, 2013). During the manic episode, mood is significantly elevated and the child displays excess energy.

Depression may cause significant alterations in school performance and social relationships. Anxiety disorders and disruptive behavior may occur together with depression. Substance abuse may also occur concurrently with depression. Divorce and serious family issues may contribute to the development of depression because of the ongoing stress they place on the child and their strong psychological impact.

Children and adolescents experiencing depressive episodes may harm themselves purposefully (without intent to kill themselves). They may hit, cut, or burn themselves (Goldson & Reynolds, 2014). Additionally, depressed children are at risk for suicide. The Centers for Disease Control and Prevention (CDC) Youth Risk Behavior Surveillance 2013 Report revealed that 17% of teens had seriously considered suicide, 13.6% had a plan, and 8% had attempted suicide (CDC, 2014).

Pathophysiology

Both norepinephrine and dopamine play a role in mood. Norepinephrine is considered to be important in the areas of energy and alertness, while dopamine is important in the areas of pleasure and motivation. When alterations in the neurotransmission of norepinephrine and dopamine occur, the symptoms of depression (apathy, loss of interest, and pleasure) result. Decreased levels of serotonin have also been implicated in depressive symptoms. Development of a depressive disorder may also be related to genetics, behavior, or cognitive function. Children of parents with a depressive disorder are at an increased risk for developing one themselves. Maladaptive cognitive functions or lack of social skills resulting in negative feelings may also play a role (Garzon, 2013).

Therapeutic Management

Children with mood disorders usually benefit from psychotherapy. This helps the child to deal with the psychosocial consequences of his or her behavior on his or her interpersonal relationships with others. Crisis management, parental counseling, and individual, group, or family therapy may be useful. Major depressive disorder warrants the use of pharmacologic antidepressants. Bipolar disorder may be treated with mood stabilizers or atypical antipsychotics, best combined with psychotherapy (Garzon, 2013).

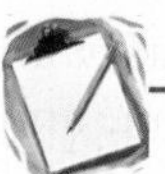

Take Note!

Closely observe children taking antidepressants for the development of presuicidal behavior.

Nursing Assessment

Children with untreated depression are at high risk for suicide as well as the development of comorbid disorders such as anxiety disorders, substance abuse, eating disorders, self-harm, and disruptive behavioral disorders (such as conduct disorder or ADHD) (Burstein et al., 2014). The nurse must screen all children for the development of depression.

HEALTH HISTORY

Obtain a health history from the child and separately from the parent. Evaluate the child for history of recent changes in behavior, changes in peer relationships, alterations in school performance, withdrawal from previously enjoyed activities, sleep disturbances, changes in eating behaviors, increase in accidents, or sexual promiscuity. If possible, use a standardized depression screening questionnaire; there are many available.

Ask about potential stressors such as school concerns, conflicts with parents, dating issues, and **abuse** (physical or sexual). When bipolar disorder is suspected, the history may reveal rapid, pressured speech; increased energy; decreased sleep; flamboyant behavior; or irritability during manic episodes.

Note history of weight loss, failure to thrive, or increased incidence of infections in the infant. For the toddler, note delay or regression in developmental skills, increase in nightmares, or parental reports of clinginess. The preschooler may have a history of loss of interest in newly acquired skills; manifest encopresis, enuresis, anorexia, or binge-eating; or make frequent negative self-statements. The parents of a school-age child may report that he or she has a depressed, irritable, or aggressive mood.

Assess for risk factors for suicide, which include:

- Previous suicide attempt
- Change in school performance, sleep, or appetite
- Loss of interest in formerly favorite school or other activities
- Feelings of hopelessness or depression
- Statements about thoughts of suicide

PHYSICAL EXAMINATION

Observe the infant for weepiness, withdrawn behaviors, or a frozen facial expression. Note a sad or expressionless face in the toddler or preschooler. In any age child, observe for apathy. Inspect the entire body surface for self-inflicted injuries (such as cuts or burns), which may or may not be present. The remainder of the physical examination is generally normal unless the depressed child also has a chronic medical condition.

Nursing Management

Nursing management of children and adolescents with mood disorders focuses on education and support, and prevention of depression and suicide.

EDUCATING AND SUPPORTING THE CHILD AND FAMILY

Teach families that mood disorders are biologic conditions, not personality flaws. Teach families how to administer antidepressant medication and to monitor for adverse effects. Encourage and praise the child's and family's efforts at following through with cognitive and behavioral therapies. Support the family throughout the process, as sometimes treatment may be lengthy. Refer parents to local support resources or to the Depression and Bipolar Support Alliance or the Child and Adolescent Bipolar Foundation. Links to these resources are provided on thePoint.

> **Atraumatic Care**
>
> *Promote a family's sense of control through effective communication and teaching and providing the family with appropriate resources and referrals.*

PREVENTING DEPRESSION AND SUICIDE

Establish a trusting relationship with the children and adolescents with whom you interact, particularly in the primary care setting, school, or chronic illness clinic. This trusting relationship may encourage children or adolescents to confide feelings or problems earlier than they may do with their parents. Screen all healthy and chronically ill preteens and teens for the development of depression (Burstein et al., 2014). Use standardized screening tools such as those listed in Box 50.4. When a potential problem is identified, immediately refer the child for mental health assessment and intervention. It is important to identify depression early so that treatment can start. When a grief-inducing event is impending (such as the death of a family member), begin preventive intervention to help the child to deal with it. Provide appropriate observation for any child exhibiting suicidal ideation. See Healthy People 2020.

> BOX 50.4
>
> **SCREENING TOOLS FOR DEPRESSION**
>
> The following tools are used to screen for depression. Links to each of these screening tools are provided on thePoint.
>
> - Children's Depression Rating Scale-Revised (CDRS-R)
> - Center for Epidemiological Studies Depression Scale Modified for Children (CES-DC)
> - Weinberg Depression Scale for Children and Adolescents (WDSCA)
> - Children's Depression Inventory (CDI)
> - Beck Depression Inventory for Youth (BDI-Y)

HEALTHY PEOPLE *2020*

Objective	Nursing Significance
Reduce suicide attempts by adolescents.	• Screen all children and adolescents for the development of depression. • When depression or excess stress is present, refer the child to the appropriate support.

Healthy People Objectives retrieved from http://www.healthypeople.gov

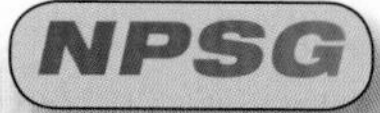

GOAL 15: The Hospital Identifies Safety Risks Inherent in Its Patient Population. (Identify Patient Safety Risks)

NPSG 15.01.01 Identify patients at risk for suicide

Steps: Conduct risk assessments (particularly on depressed patients), and address immediate safety needs. Provide one-on-one care when necessary.

Joint Commission. (2015). *National patient safety goals effective January 1, 2015.* Retrieved from http://www.jointcommission.org/assets/1/6/2015_NPSG_HAP.pdf

ANXIETY DISORDERS

Anxiety disorders are the most commonly diagnosed psychiatric conditions among children and adolescents with prevalence ranging from 10% to 30% (Bennett & Walkup, 2016). Anxiety often occurs together with other metal health disorders, especially depression. Normal children experience fear, worry, and shyness. Infants fear loud noises, being startled, and strangers. Toddlers are afraid of the dark and of separation. Preschoolers fear imaginary creatures and body mutilation. School-age children worry about injury and natural events, whereas adolescents are anxious about school and social performance. These normal fears produce a certain level of anxiety that is tolerated by most children, but it is important to distinguish normal developmentally appropriate anxiety from an anxiety disorder.

Anxiety is considered to be a reaction to a perceived or actual threat. The threat may or may not be distorted by the child, and the emotional distress leads to behavioral responses. The "fight-or-flight" response results in tachycardia, increased blood pressure, sweating, enhanced arousal and reactivity, tremors, and increased blood flow to the muscles (Garzon, 2013).

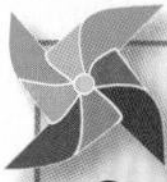

Thinking About Development

Consider the issue of military deployment of a parent. How might a toddler or preschooler react to the parent's absence and return as contrasted to the response of an adolescent? What types of mental health concerns might be manifested in either group?

Types of Anxiety Disorders

Generalized anxiety disorder (GAD) is characterized by unrealistic concerns over past behavior, future events, and personal competence. Social phobia is a disorder characterized by the child or teen demonstrating a persistent fear of speaking or eating in front of others, using public restrooms, or speaking to authorities. Selective mutism refers to a persistent failure to speak. Separation anxiety is more common in children than adolescents. In this disorder, the child may need to remain close to the parents, and the child's worries focus on separation themes. OCD is characterized by compulsions (repetitive behaviors such as cleaning, washing, or checking something), which the child performs to reduce anxiety about obsessions (unwanted and intrusive thoughts). Posttraumatic stress disorder (PTSD) is an anxiety disorder that occurs after a child experiences a traumatic event, later experiencing physiologic arousal when a stimulus triggers memories of the event.

Pathophysiology

Anxiety disorders are thought to occur as a result of disrupted modulation within the central nervous system. Underactivation of the serotonergic system and overactivation of the noradrenergic system are thought to be responsible for dysregulation of physiologic arousal and the resulting emotional experience. Disruption of the γ-aminobutyric acid (GABA) system may also play a role. Genetic factors may also play a role in the development of anxiety disorders, as may family and environmental influences. Additionally, abnormal thoughts or behaviors may have been learned through observation or conditioning (Garzon, 2013; Bennett & Walkup, 2016).

Therapeutic Management

Therapeutic management of anxiety disorders generally involves the use of pharmacologic agents and psychological therapies. Anxiolytics or antidepressants are the most common pharmacologic approaches. Cognitive-behavioral therapy; individual, family, or group psychotherapy; and other behavioral interventions such as relaxation techniques may also be useful.

Nursing Assessment

Children and adolescents do not usually express anxiety directly. Therefore, it is very important for the nurse to evaluate somatic complaints and perform a careful health history.

HEALTH HISTORY

Explore the child's current and past medical history for risk factors such as depression, anxious temperament, family history of anxiety disorders, certain environmental or life experiences (such as parental dysfunction or significant stressful event or trauma), or unstable parental attachment. Elicit the health history, noting history of social inhibition, panic, or "heart racing." Young children may display overactivity, acting out, sleep difficulties, or separation issues. Older children may describe feelings of nervousness, anger, fear, or tension and may display disruptive behavior. Ask the child to choose a number on a scale from 0 to 10 to describe how much he or she worries about things. Have the parent rank the child's worry in the same fashion, and ask the parent what the child worries about most. Determine frequency of headaches and stomachaches. Use a standardized screening tool such as the Multidimensional Anxiety Scale for Children (MASC), Spence Children's Anxiety Scale (SACS), Preschool Anxiety Scale, and Beck Anxiety Inventory for Youth. Links to each of these screening tools are available on thePoint.

PHYSICAL EXAMINATION

Perform a complete physical examination to rule out physiologic causes of the child's symptoms. Note patches of hair loss that occur with repetitive hair twisting or pulling associated with anxiety. Evaluate for evidence of nail biting, sucking blisters, or skin erosion from finger rubbing. Inspect the entire body for signs of self-injury, which may or may not be present.

Nursing Management

Screen children at well-child or other healthcare visits, as well as upon admission to the hospital, for anxiety symptoms. If an anxiety disorder is suspected, refer the child to the appropriate mental health provider for further evaluation. When the child is diagnosed with an anxiety disorder and medication is prescribed, teach families about medication administration and adverse effects. Encourage and praise them for follow-through related to cognitive and behavioral therapy or psychotherapy. Provide emotional support to the child and family. Assess the family for the presence of parental anxiety or insecure attachment. Note parenting style and parent–child interactions. Not only the child but also the family will benefit from interventions that improve parent–child relationships, decrease parental anxiety, and foster parenting skills that promote autonomy in the child. Thus, refer the child and family to concurrent family therapy if needed.

ABUSE AND VIOLENCE

Abuse and violence contribute significantly to mental illness in children. Children may suffer from child maltreatment, Munchausen syndrome, or substance abuse.

Child Maltreatment

Child maltreatment includes physical abuse, sexual abuse, emotional abuse, and neglect. Physical abuse refers to injuries that are intentionally inflicted on a child and result in morbidity or mortality. Sexual abuse refers to involvement of the child in any activity meant to provide sexual gratification to an adult. Emotional abuse may be verbal denigration of the child or occur as a result of the child witnessing domestic violence. **Neglect** is defined as failure to provide a child with appropriate food, clothing, shelter, medical care, and schooling (Chiesa & Sirotnak, 2014).

Statistics related to family violence as well as child physical and sexual abuse is difficult to determine, as the perpetrator usually forces the victim into silence. Children usually do not want to admit that their parent or relative has hurt them, partly from feelings of guilt and partly because they do not want to lose that parent. In 2011, 3.4 million referrals to child protective services were made alleging child maltreatment in 6.2 million children, yet this may be an underestimate of the prevalence of child abuse (Chiesa & Sirotnak, 2014). Abuse and violence occur across all socioeconomic levels but are more prevalent among the poor, and the largest percentage of those affected are under 3 years of age. Despite the lack of adequate statistics, it is well known that the problem of abuse and violence is widespread. Parents or caregivers are the most frequent perpetrators of abuse against children (Chiesa & Sirotnak, 2014).

A history of childhood abuse is associated with the development of depressive disorders, suicidal ideation and attempts, anxiety disorders, and alcohol and drug use. Abuse may result in significant physical injury, poor physical health, and, in some cases, impaired brain development. Being a victim of abuse places children at risk for low self-esteem, poor academic achievement, poor emotional health, and social difficulties. Additional long-term consequences include juvenile delinquency and perpetuation of the violence cycle (Child Welfare Information Gateway, 2013).

Therapeutic management of victims of abuse and violence involves physical treatment of the injury, palliative care in some cases, and intervention to preserve or restore the child's mental well-being as well as family functioning. To protect children, all states require by law that healthcare professionals report suspected cases of child abuse or neglect (Child Welfare Information Gateway, 2016).

Nursing Assessment

Elicit the health history, noting the chief complaint and timing of onset. Assess for appropriateness of the parent–child attachment (often altered in the case of neglect). Pay particular attention to statements made by the child's parent or caretaker. Is the history given consistent with the child's injury? Identify abuse and violence by screening all children and families using these questions:

- Questions for children:
  - Are you afraid of anyone at home?
  - Who could you tell if someone hurt you or touched you in a way that made you uncomfortable?
  - Has anyone hurt you or touched you in that way?
- Questions for parents:
  - Are you afraid of anyone at home?
  - Do you ever feel like you may hit or hurt your child when frustrated?

Assess for risk factors in children and parents or caretakers. Risk factors for abuse in children include poverty, prematurity, cerebral palsy, chronic illness, or intellectual disability. Risk factors for being abusers in parents or caretakers include a history of being abused themselves, alcohol or substance abuse, or extreme stress.

Determine if the child has a history of hurting self or others (e.g., cutting), running away, attempting **suicide** (taking one's own life), or being involved in high-risk behaviors. Note inappropriate sexual behavior for developmental age, such as seductiveness, as this may indicate sexual abuse. Note history of chronic sore throat or difficulty swallowing, which may occur with forced oral sex or sexually transmitted infections. Document history of genital burning or itching (associated with sexual abuse). Note nonspecific symptoms of emotional abuse such as low self-confidence, sleep disturbance, hypervigilance, headaches, or stomachaches.

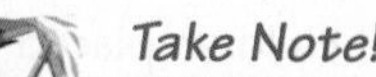

Take Note!

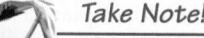

A delay in seeking medical treatment, a history that changes over time, or a history of trauma that is inconsistent with the observed injury all suggest child abuse.

PHYSICAL EXAMINATION

Perform a gentle but thorough physical examination, using a soft touch and calm voice. Observe the parent–child interaction, noting fear or an excessive desire to please. Note the infant's level of consciousness. Vigorous shaking in the infant leads to intracranial hemorrhage and shaken baby syndrome. Inspect the skin for bruises, burns, cuts, abrasions, contusions, scars, and any other unusual or suspicious marks. Current or healed scratches or cuts may be found on parts of the body ordinarily covered by clothing in the child who self-mutilates. Burns that occur in a stocking or glove pattern, or only to the soles or palms, are highly suspicious for inflicted burns. Injuries in various stages of healing are also indicative of abuse. Bruises on the chest, head, neck, or abdomen are suspicious for abuse. Nonambulatory children infrequently experience bruises or fractures. Figure 50.1 shows injury sites usually indicative of abuse; Figure 50.2

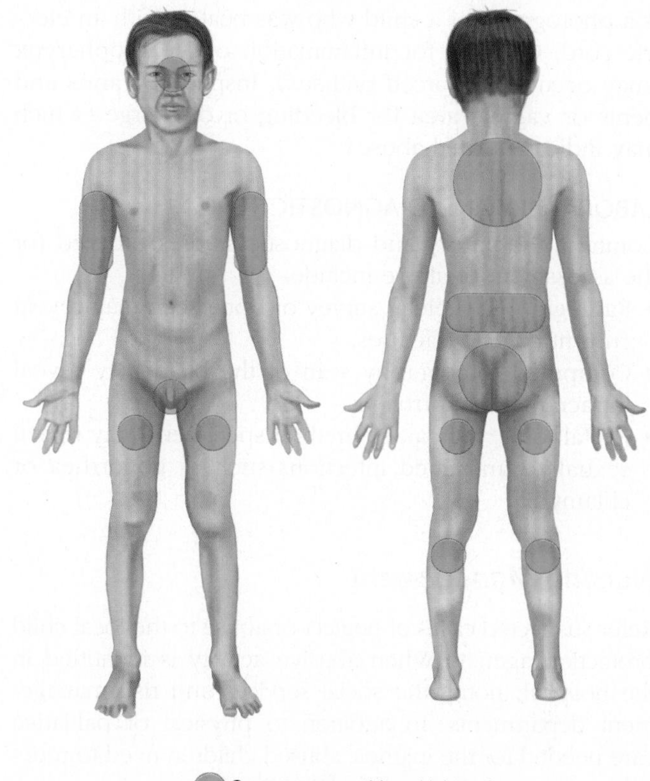

FIGURE 50.1 Injury sites that are suspicious for abuse.

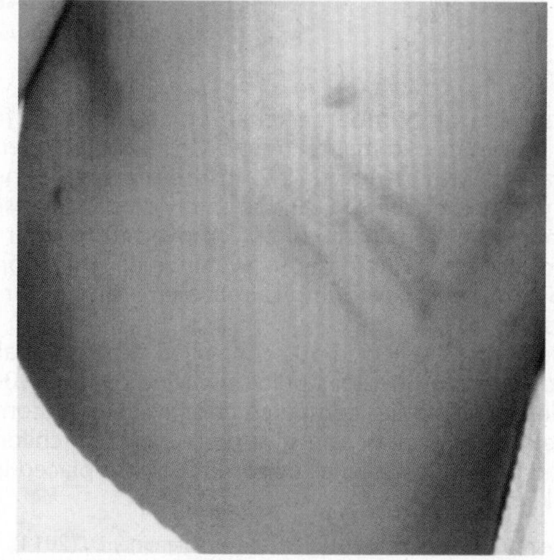

FIGURE 50.2 Note the mark left from a looped electric cord.

is a photograph of a child who was beaten with an electric cord. Observe for inflammation of the oropharynx (may occur with forced oral sex). Inspect the anus and penis or vaginal area for bleeding or discharge (which may indicate sexual abuse).

LABORATORY AND DIAGNOSTIC TESTS

Common laboratory and diagnostic studies ordered for the assessment of abuse include:

- Radiographic skeletal survey or bone scan may reveal current or past fractures.
- Computed tomography scan of the head may reveal intracranial hemorrhage.
- Rectal, oral, vaginal, or urethral specimens may reveal sexually transmitted infections such as gonorrhea or chlamydia.

Nursing Management

Refer suspected cases of neglect or abuse to the local child protection agency. When abusive activity is identified in the hospital, notify the social services and risk management departments. In addition to physical or palliative care needed for the injuries, abused children need to redevelop a sense of trust in adults. Provide consistent care to the abused child by assigning a core group of nurses. Child abuse requires a multidisciplinary approach that may include psychological therapy for the child and family.

Role model appropriate caretaking activities to the parent or caregiver. Call attention to normal growth and development activities noted in the infant or child, as sometimes parents have expectations of child behavior that may be unrealistic based on the child's age, leading to the abuse. Praise parents and caretakers for taking appropriate steps toward getting help and for providing appropriate care to the child. Refer parents to Parents Anonymous, an organization dedicated to the prevention of child abuse through strengthening of the family (see for a link to this website).

When it is determined by the child protective team that the child would be in danger to continue living in the current situation, the child may be removed from the home. If the child is removed from the family temporarily or permanently, provide the foster or adoptive family with education necessary to assume the child's care. See Evidence-Based Practice 50.1.

Medical Child Abuse (Munchausen Syndrome by Proxy)

Medical child abuse has historically been termed Munchausen syndrome by proxy (MSBP). It is a type of child abuse in which the parent creates physical and/or psychological symptoms of illness or impairment in the child. The adult meets his or her own psychological needs by having an ill child. Medical child abuse is difficult to detect and may remain hidden for years. In most cases, the biologic mother is the perpetrator (Endom, 2015). Therapeutic management focuses on ensuring the safety and well-being of the child, as well providing psychotherapy for the perpetrator.

Nursing Assessment

Take a thorough and detailed health history of the child's illness or illnesses. Use quotations to document the parent's responses. Warning signs of medical child abuse include:

- Child with one or more illnesses that do not respond to treatment or that follow a puzzling course; a similar history in siblings

EVIDENCE-BASED PRACTICE 50.1 **CARE BY RELATIVES FOR CHILDREN REMOVED FROM HOME FOR MALTREATMENT**

STUDY

Annually, large numbers of children are removed from their homes due to maltreatment. Child welfare agencies are tasked with attempting to insure the well-being and safety of these children, and in many cases, a sense of permanency. Usually, children removed from their home display an increased prevalence of educational, behavioral, and psychological problems than their peers.

The authors reviewed 102 controlled experimental and quasi-experimental studies involving over 660,000 children. The studies compared child welfare outcomes related to well-being, safety, or permanency in children placed in kinship foster as opposed to those placed in non-kinship care.

Findings

Results from this review demonstrate that children placed in kinship foster care demonstrated fewer behavioral problems, fewer mental health disorders, less placement disruption, better well-being and less use of mental health services, than those placed in non-kinship care.

Nursing Implications

Encourage families to explore the possibility of adding BT/CBT to the treatment plan. Assist families with finding an appropriate provider of BT/CBT in their local area. Praise children and families for ongoing dedication to BT/CBT. Continue to offer emotional support to all members of the family throughout the treatment process.

Adapted from Winokur, M., Holtan, A., & Valentine, D. (2014). Kinship care for the safety, permanency, and well-being of children removed from the home for maltreatment. *The Cochrane Library 2014, 1.* Indianapolis, IN: John Wiley & Sons.

- Symptoms that do not make sense or that disappear when the perpetrator is removed or not present; the symptoms are witnessed only by the caregiver (e.g., cyanosis, apnea, seizure)
- Physical and laboratory findings that do not fit with the reported history
- Repeated hospitalizations failing to produce a medical diagnosis, transfers to other hospitals, discharges against medical advice
- Parent who refuses to accept that the diagnosis is not medical (Chiesa & Sirotnak, 2014; Roesler & Jenny, 2016)

Observe the mother's behavior with the child, spouse or partner, and staff. Use of covert video surveillance may reveal maternal actions causing illness in the child when the nurse, physician, or nurse practitioner is not in the room. Perform a thorough physical examination, noting where the physical examination findings differ from the reported health history.

Nursing Management

Management of medical child abuse is complex. When abusive activity is identified, notify the social services and risk management departments of the hospital. Ensure that the local child protection team and the caregiver's family or support system is present when the caregiver is confronted. Inform the caregiver of the plan of care for the child and of the availability of psychiatric assistance for the caregiver.

Substance Abuse

Substance use most often begins before age 20. In 2013 in the United States, 66.2% of students reported having had at least one alcoholic drink in their life, with 18.6% reporting they had drunk alcohol before age 13 (CDC, 2014). In addition to alcohol, youths also use marijuana, cocaine, heroin, methamphetamines, inhalants, ecstasy, nonprescribed steroids, and prescription drugs not intended for them (CDC, 2014).

Nursing Assessment

Note risk factors for substance abuse, such as family history of substance abuse, current parental substance use, dysfunctional family relationships, concurrent mental health disorder, aggressive behaviors, low self-esteem or poor academic performance, negative life events, poor social skills, or peers who use substances. Determine the child's history, noting altered school performance or attendance, changes in peer group participation, frequent mood swings, changes in physical appearance, or an altered relationship with or perception of parents. Document history of insomnia, appetite loss, excessive itching, sleepiness or extreme fatigue, dry mouth, or shakiness. Note violent behavior, drunkenness, stupor, blank expression, drowsiness, lack of coordination, confusion, incoherent speech, extremes in emotions, aggressive behavior, silly behavior, or rapid speech. A screening assessment recommended by the American Academy of Pediatrics is the CRAFFT Screening Tool (refer to thePoint to read more about the screening tool). Perform a complete physical examination. Observe for an odor of alcohol or marijuana smoke. Assess the eyes, noting wateriness or dilated pupils. Inspect the nares, noting rhinorrhea or absence of nasal hair. Inspect the fingers for glue smears or discoloration and the skin for needle marks or tracks. Palpate the hands and feet for coolness.

Laboratory and diagnostic tests include toxicology studies, such as urine screening, to determine the presence of stimulants, sedative-hypnotics, barbiturates, hallucinogens, opiates, cocaine, and marijuana.

Nursing Management

Help the adolescent to acknowledge that he or she has a problem. Explain the negative consequences of substance use and raise the teen's awareness of risks. Remain empathetic, yet leave responsibility with the adolescent. Key nursing interventions include promoting participation in treatment programs and preventing substance abuse.

PROMOTING PARTICIPATION IN TREATMENT PROGRAMS

Refer the adolescent to a substance abuse program. Outpatient or day treatment programs are useful in most situations. Family-based programs produce the highest level of recovery. Self-help or 12-step groups are an important element in the recovery process. Serious addiction, the presence of one or more comorbid psychiatric conditions, or suicidal ideation requires residential treatment or hospitalization. See Healthy People 2020.

HEALTHY PEOPLE 2020

Objective	Nursing Significance
Increase the proportion of persons with co-occurring substance abuse and mental disorders who receive treatment for both disorders.	• Screen all children and adolescents with mental health disorders for the coexistence of substance abuse (and vice versa). • Refer children and adolescents to appropriate treatment programs and therapy.

Healthy People Objectives retrieved from http://www.healthypeople.gov

PREVENTING SUBSTANCE ABUSE

Establish a trusting relationship with children and adolescents in order to improve acceptance of education about substance use and to provide a safe environment for confiding about their problems. Screen all children and adolescents for risk factors. During routine psychosocial screening, be alert to alterations as noted earlier. Teach all children, beginning at the elementary school level (or earlier in some high-risk communities), that all chemicals have the potential to be harmful to the body, including tobacco, alcohol, and illicit drugs. Educate children and adolescents that no matter which administration route is used, the drug still enters the body and affects it (negatively). Help children to learn problem-solving skills that they can call upon in the future rather than relying on drugs or other substances to avoid their problems. Teach children to "just say no." Reinforce that they are the ones who have control over their body and what they expose it to. Encourage children to participate in the local community DARE program (Drug Abuse Resistance Education) and praise them for completing it. Teach parents that being involved in their child's social life and knowing where they are and with whom when they are outside of the home is an important step toward limiting substance exposure.

NURSING CARE PLAN 50.1

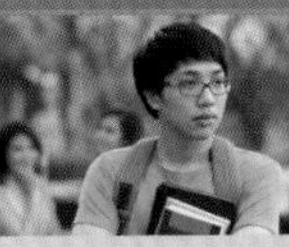

Overview for the Child With a Mental Health Disorder

NURSING DIAGNOSIS: Impaired social interaction related to altered social skills as evidenced by impulsivity, intrusive behavior, inability to follow through, anxiety, depressed mood, feelings of unattractiveness or unworthiness

Outcome Identification and Evaluation

The child will demonstrate socially acceptable skills, *interacting successfully with peers and in the educational setting, completing tasks as required.*

Interventions: ***Promoting Appropriate Social Interaction***

- Identify factors that may aggravate the child's performance *to minimize stimuli that exacerbate the child's undesired behaviors.*
- Modify the environment to decrease distracting stimuli *as the child's ability to deal with external stimuli may be impaired.*
- Ensure that the child hears his or her name and makes eye contact prior to conversing or instructions *so that the child is engaged and has increased ability to follow through.*
- State expectations for tasks or behaviors clearly *as understanding is necessary to ensure completion.*
- Provide positive feedback for appropriate behaviors or task completion, *encouraging the child to adopt expectations into his behaviors and routine.*

NURSING DIAGNOSIS: Ineffective coping related to inability to deal with life stressors as evidenced by few or no meaningful friendships, inability to empathize or give/receive affection, low self-esteem, or maladaptive coping behaviors such as substance abuse

Outcome Identification and Evaluation

The child will demonstrate improved coping, *verbalize feelings, socially engage, demonstrate problem-solving skills.*

Interventions: ***Promoting Coping Skills***

- Encourage discussion of thoughts and feelings, *as this is an initial step toward learning to deal with them appropriately.*
- Provide positive feedback for appropriate discussion, *as this increases the likelihood of continuing performance.*
- Demonstrate unconditional acceptance of the child as a person *to increase self-esteem in the child who has been feeling rejection.*
- Set clear limits on behavior as needed *so the child has a structure to adhere to.*
- Teach the child problem-solving skills *as an alternative to acting-out behaviors.*
- Role model appropriate social and conversation skills *so the child can see what is expected in a nonthreatening manner.*

(continued)

NURSING CARE PLAN 50.1

Overview for the Child With a Mental Health Disorder (continued)

NURSING DIAGNOSIS: Imbalanced nutrition, less than body requirements, related to intake insufficient to meet metabolic needs as evidenced by weight loss, failure to gain weight, less-than-expected increases in stature and weight, loss of appetite, or refusal to eat

Outcome Identification and Evaluation

The child or adolescent will demonstrate appropriate growth, *making gains in weight and stature as appropriate.*

Interventions: *Improving Nutritional Intake*

- Provide favorite foods *to encourage the child with poor appetite to eat more.*
- Assist families to choose nutrient-rich foods *so that the food the child does eat is most beneficial.*

For the child with an eating disorder:

- Mutually establish a contract related to treatment *to promote the child's sense of control.*
- Provide mealtime structure, *as clear limits let the child know what the expectations are.*
- Encourage the child to choose foods and timing of meals *to develop independence in eating habits.*
- Ensure the eating environment is pleasant and relaxed, with minimal distractions, *to minimize the child's anxiety and guilt about not eating.*
- Withdraw attention if the child refuses to eat: *secondary gain is minimized if refusal to eat is ignored.*
- Provide continuous supervision during the meal and for 30 minutes following it so that the child cannot conceal or dispose of food or induce vomiting.

NURSING DIAGNOSIS: Risk for delayed development related to disability, behavioral disorder, or altered nutrition

Outcome Identification and Evaluation

Child will demonstrate progress toward developmental milestones: *child expresses interest in the environment and people around him or her, interacts with environment in an age-appropriate way.*

Interventions: *Promoting Development*

- Use therapeutic play and adaptive toys *to facilitate developmental functioning.*
- Provide stimulating environment when possible *to maximize potential for growth and development.*
- Praise accomplishments and emphasize the child's abilities *to improve self-esteem and encourage feelings of confidence and competence.*
- Follow through with physical, occupational, and speech therapists' recommendations *to maximize exposure to exercises designed to increase the child's skills.*
- Determine parents' expectations of the child's future achievement *to help them work toward these goals.*

NURSING DIAGNOSIS: Acute or chronic confusion related to behavioral disorder, depression, anxiety, abusive situation, or substance abuse as evidenced by distractibility, non–reality-based thinking, hypervigilance, or inaccurate interpretation of interactions of others

Outcome Identification and Evaluation

Child's consciousness, attention, cognition, and perception will improve: *child will demonstrate appropriate orientation, remain free from physical harm, and perform activities of daily living as able.*

NURSING CARE PLAN 50.1

Overview for the Child With a Mental Health Disorder (continued)

Interventions: ***Reducing confusion***

- Observe for causes of altered thought processes *to provide a baseline for assessment and intervention.*
- Perform an age-appropriate mental status examination *to determine extent of altered thinking.*
- Adjust communication style based on the child's cues *to improve communication.*
- Listen carefully and seek clarification *to determine basis for the child's agitation or other behaviors.*
- Provide validation of the child's thoughts and feelings *to improve trust in the relationship.*
- Establish a daily routine *to provide the child with a sense of security.*

NURSING DIAGNOSIS: Hopelessness related to child's perception of his or her life situation, negative life view, or alteration in mental well-being as evidenced by passivity, verbalization, alterations in sleep, or lack of initiative

Outcome Identification and Evaluation

Child will display a sense of hope: *will verbalize feelings, participate in care, make positive statements.*

Interventions: ***Promoting Hope***

- Monitor and document potential for suicide, *as hopelessness often leads to suicidal ideation.*
- Assist the child to identify reasons for hope and for living, *so the nurse is aware of the child's values.*
- Help the child to set goals that are important to him or her *to allow the child to see possibilities.*
- Encourage simple decision making on a daily basis, *as hopelessness often occurs as a response to loss of control.*
- Assist the child to identify positive qualities in himself or herself and his or her life *to facilitate the development of hope.*
- Involve parents or others the child loves in the child's care *as social support is critical to the development of hope.*

NURSING DIAGNOSIS: Caregiver role strain related to long-term care of the child with a chronic mental health disorder as evidenced by fatigue, inattention to own needs, conflict, or ambivalence

Outcome Identification and Evaluation

The child's caregiver will participate in the child's care, *verbalizing the child's needs and treatment plan and demonstrating skills necessary for care.*

Interventions: ***Decreasing Role Strain***

- Teach the parent or caregiver about the child's illness, treatments, and medications *to clarify expectations for the child and parent.*
- Role model appropriate interaction behaviors with the child *so the parent can learn these techniques by watching.*
- Encourage structure in daily routines *to allow the parent to meet his or her own needs and allow for adequate rest.*
- Gradually increase the parent's responsibility related to care of the child *to help the parent feel less overwhelmed.*
- Allow the parent to move at his or her own pace in assuming care *to enhance the chances for success.*
- Help the parent to identify a back-up caregiver *so the parent has times of respite from constant involvement with the child.*

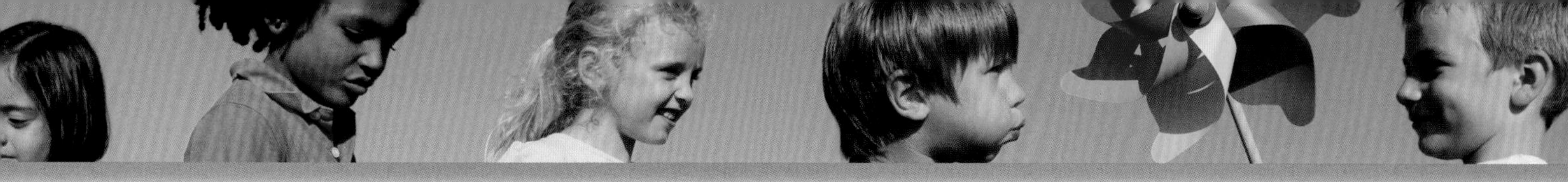

KEY CONCEPTS

- Mental health and behavioral disorders account for the bulk of the "new morbidity" among children and adolescents.
- The child with behavioral problems or mental health issues often has difficulty in the areas of school, peer relationships, and the family, all of which may worsen the child's self-concept, further hindering his or her emotional health.
- Developmental screening is a key component in the evaluation of a child's mental health.
- Various screening tools are available for depression, ADHD, and anxiety.
- Children with autism spectrum disorder often have impaired social interactions as well as altered communication.
- Learning disabilities and ADHD have a significant negative impact on the child's potential for appropriate education.
- Individualized education plans help children with learning disabilities, intellectual disability, and ADHD receive the educational support they require to optimize their educational capacity.
- Provide support and education to children with mood or anxiety disorders and their families.
- Educating parents about medication administration and its adverse effects is a critical aspect of nursing management of the child with a mental health disorder.
- Provide nutritional replacement at the appropriate pace in the child with anorexia nervosa. Monitor the child closely for the development of refeeding syndrome.
- A key nursing function is screening all children and their families for abuse and violence.
- Report suspected cases of child abuse to the appropriate authorities.
- Educate children about the dangers associated with substance abuse. Reward and praise children and adolescents who do not experiment with or use alcohol or illicit drugs.

REFERENCES AND RECOMMENDED READINGS

108th Congress. (2004). *Individuals with disabilities education improvement Act of 2004*. Retrieved from http://frwebgate.access.gpo.gov/cgi-bin/getdoc.cgi?dbname=108_cong_public_laws&docid=f:publ446.108

American Academy of Child and Adolescent Psychiatry. (2013). *Fast facts for families no. 86: Psychotherapies for children and adolescents*. Washington, DC: Author.

American Academy of Pediatrics. (2012). *Mental health screening and assessment tools for primary care*. Retrieved from https://www.aap.org/en-us/advocacy-and-policy/aap-health-initiatives/Mental-Health/Documents/MH_ScreeningChart.pdf

Bennett, S., & Walkup, J. T. (2016). *Anxiety disorders in children: Epidemiology, pathogenesis, clinical manifestations, and course*. Retrieved from from http://www.uptodate.com/contents/anxiety-disorders-in-children-and-adolescents-epidemiology-pathogenesis-clinical-manifestations-and-course

Burstein, A., Talmi, A., Stafford, B., & Kelsay, K. (2014). Child & adolescent psychiatric disorders & psychosocial aspects of pediatrics. In W. W. Hay, M. J. Levin, R. R. Deterding, & M. J. Abzug (Eds.), *Current pediatric diagnosis and treatment* (22nd ed.). New York, NY: McGraw-Hill.

Centers for Disease Control and Prevention. (2014). Youth risk behavior surveillance – United States, 2013. *Morbidity and Mortality Weekly Report, 63*(4), 1–168.

Chiesa, A., & Sirotnak, A. P. (2014). Child abuse & neglect. In W. W. Hay, M. J. Levin, & R. R. Deterding, & M. J. Abzug (Eds.), *Current pediatric diagnosis and treatment* (22nd ed.). New York, NY: McGraw-Hill.

Child Welfare Information Gateway. (2013). *Long-term consequences of child abuse and neglect*. Retrieved from https://www.childwelfare.gov/pubs/factsheets/long-term-consequences/

Child Welfare Information Gateway. (2016). *Mandatory reporters of child abuse and neglect: Summary of state laws*. Retrieved from https://www.childwelfare.gov/topics/systemwide/laws-policies/statutes/manda/?hasBeenRedirected=1

Children's Hospital Boston. (2009). *The CRAFFT screening tool*. Retrieved from http://www.ceasar-boston.org/CRAFFT/

Diamond, J. S., Abdoo, D. C., Brady, M. A., & Dunn, A. M. (2013). Role relationships. In C. E. Burns, A. M. Dunn, M. A. Brady, N. B. Starr, & C. G. Blosser (Eds.), *Pediatric primary care* (5th ed.). Philadelphia, PA: Saunders.

Forman, S. F. (2016). *Eating disorders: Overview of epidemiology, diagnosis, and course of illness*. Retrieved from http://www.uptodate.com/contents/eating-disorders-overview-of-epidemiology-diagnosis-and-course-of-illness

French, W. P. (2015). Assessment and treatment of attention-deficit/hyperactivity disorder: Part 1. *Pediatric Annals, 44*(3), 114–120.

Garzon, D. L. (2013). Coping and stress tolerance: Mental health and illness. In C. E. Burns, A. M. Dunn, M. A. Brady, N. B. Starr, & C. G. Blosser (Eds.), *Pediatric primary care* (5th ed.). Philadelphia, PA: Saunders.

Goldson, E., & Reynolds, A. (2014). Child development and behavior. In W. W. Hay, Jr., M. J. Levin, R. R. Deterding, & M. J. Abzug (Eds.), *Current diagnosis and treatment: Pediatrics* (22nd ed.). New York, NY: McGraw-Hill Education.

Herdman, T. H., & Kamitsuru, S. (Eds.). (2014). *NANDA International nursing diagnoses: Definitions & classifications*

2015–2017 (10th ed.). West Sussex, UK: John Wiley & Sons, Ltd.

Jankovic, J. (2015). *Tourette syndrome.* Retrieved from http://www.uptodate.com/contents/tourette-syndrome

Krull, K. R. (2016). *Attention deficit hyperactivity disorder in children and adolescents: Epidemiology and pathogenesis.* Retrieved from http://www.uptodate.com/contents/attention-deficit-hyperactivity-disorder-in-children-and-adolescents-epidemiology-and-pathogenesis

Pivalizza, P., & Lalani, S. R. (2016). *Intellectual disability (mental retardation) in children: Definition; diagnosis; and assessment of needs.* Retrieved from http://www.uptodate.com/contents/intellectual-disability-mental-retardation-in-children-definition-diagnosis-and-assessment-of-needs

Preston, J., O'Neal, J. H., & Talaga, M. C. (2015). *Child and adolescent clinical psychopharmacology made simple.* Oakland, CA: New Harbinger Publications, Inc.

Roesler, T. A., & Jenny, C. (2016). *Medical child abuse (Munchausen syndrome by proxy).* Retrieved from http://www.uptodate.com/contents/medical-child-abuse-munchausen-syndrome-by-proxy

Sensory Processing Disorder Foundation. (2016). *About SPD.* Retrieved from http://www.spdfoundation.net/about-sensory-processing-disorder/

Solanto, M. V. (2015). *Psychotherapy for adult ADHD.* Retrieved from http://www.uptodate.com/contents/psychotherapy-for-adult-adhd?

Starr, N. B., Fookson, M., Burns, C. D., & Bowman-Harvey, C. A. (2013). Cognitive perceptual Disorders. In C. E. Burns, A. M. Dunn, M. A. Brady, N. B. Starr, & C. G. Blosser (Eds.), *Pediatric primary care* (5th ed.). Philadelphia, PA: Saunders.

Taketomo, C. K., Hodding, J. H., & Kraus, D. M. (2013). *Pediatric & neonatal dosage handbook* (20th ed.). Hudson, OH: Lexicomp.

U.S. Public Health Service. (2000). *Report of the surgeon general's conference on children's mental health: A national action agenda.* Washington, DC: Department of Health and Human Services.

Varcarolis, E. M. (2011). *Manual of psychiatric nursing care planning: Assessment guides, diagnoses, and psychopharmacology* (4th ed.). St. Louis, MO: Saunders.

von Hahn, L. E. (2015a). *Specific learning disabilities in children: Clinical features.* Retrieved from http://www.uptodate.com/contents/specific-learning-disabilitiesin-children-clinical-features

von Hahn, L. E. (2015b). *Specific learning disabilities in children: Role of the primary care provider.* Retrieved from http://www.uptodate.com/contents/specific-learning-disabilities-in-children-role-of-the-primary-care-provider

Winokur, M., Holtan, A., & Valentine, D. (2014). *Kinship care for the safety, permanency, and well-being of children removed from the home for maltreatment.* The Cochrane Library 2014, 1. Indianapolis, IN: John Wiley & Sons.

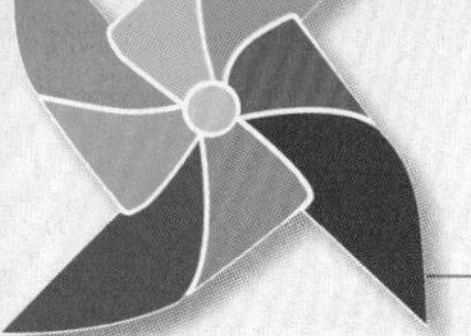

CHAPTER WORKSHEET

MULTIPLE CHOICE QUESTIONS

1. The nurse is caring for a child with ADHD. Which behavior would the nurse not expect the child to display?
   a. moody, morose behavior with pouting
   b. interruption and inability to take turns
   c. forgetfulness and easy distractibility
   d. excessive motor activities and fidgeting
2. An adolescent girl who has been receiving treatment for anorexia nervosa has failed to gain weight over the past week despite eating all of her meals and snacks. What is the priority nursing intervention?
   a. Increase the teen's daily caloric intake by at least 500 calories.
   b. Ensure that the teen's entire fluid intake includes calories.
   c. Supervise the teen for 2 hours after all meals and snacks.
   d. Assess the teen's anxiety level to determine need for medication.
3. A 15-year-old girl has been making demands all day, exaggerating her every need. She is now crying, saying she has nothing to live for and threatening to kill herself. What is the priority nursing action?
   a. Ignore her continued exaggerated and melodramatic behavior.
   b. Consult with the physician or nurse practitioner to increase her antidepressant dose.
   c. Leave the girl alone for a little while until she composes herself.
   d. Take the girl's suicidal threat seriously and provide close supervision.
4. When trying to manage aggressive or impulsive behaviors in children or adolescents, what is the best nursing intervention?
   a. Train the child to be assertive.
   b. Provide consistency and limit setting.
   c. Allow the child to negotiate the rules.
   d. Encourage the child to express feelings.
5. The nurse is caring for an adolescent who says, "I'm sick of this. I wish I weren't alive anymore." What is the best response by the nurse?
   a. "I often feel sad and sick of things."
   b. "Have you thought about hurting yourself?"
   c. "Are you trying to escape your problems?"
   d. "Do your parents know about this feeling?"

DOSAGE CALCULATION QUESTION

1. The nurse is caring for a 10-year old diagnosed with depression. The child weighs 72 lb. The medication order reads: fluoxetine 10 mg PO daily. The child refuses to swallow pills. Fluoxetine is supplied as 20 mg/5 mL. How many milliliters will the nurse administer? Round to the nearest tenth.

CRITICAL THINKING EXERCISES

1. A mother tells you that her son's behavior is unmanageable, and she is having difficulty coping with it. The boy is argumentative and is bullying others. He is struggling with his schoolwork because he has difficulty staying on task, gets out of his chair often, and frequently distracts others. What additional assessments should you obtain? What interventions would be helpful in managing the boy's behavior?
2. A 14-year-old boy with moderate intellectual disability is able to feed himself but is incontinent. Discuss the issues with which his family must deal.

STUDY ACTIVITIES

1. Explore several of the websites related to child abuse prevention listed on thePoint. Develop a list of resources for families in your local area.
2. Attend a group therapy session during your pediatric clinical rotation. Observe the children's verbal and nonverbal communication, noting inconsistencies or other interesting observations.
3. Visit a school for autistic children. Spend time with the various specialists who work with children with ASD, determining their roles and the effect the treatment they are providing has on the children. Report your findings to your classmates.
4. Attend a local CHADD meeting. Talk to parents about having a child with ADHD.

BRINGING IT ALL TOGETHER: A CASE STUDY

Nicole Ashton, 16 years old, is seen in your clinic due to weight loss. Her mother states that she has lost noticeable weight over the past few months and has stopped menstruating.

Go to thePoint to find questions to consider about this case.

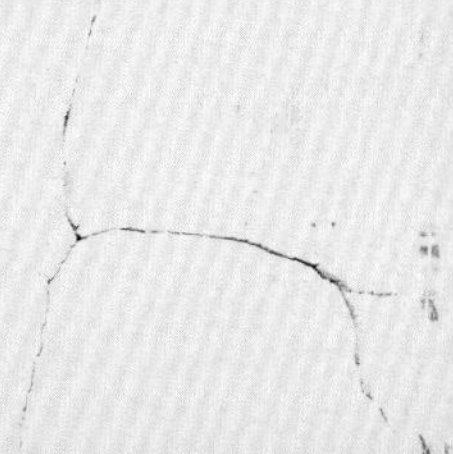

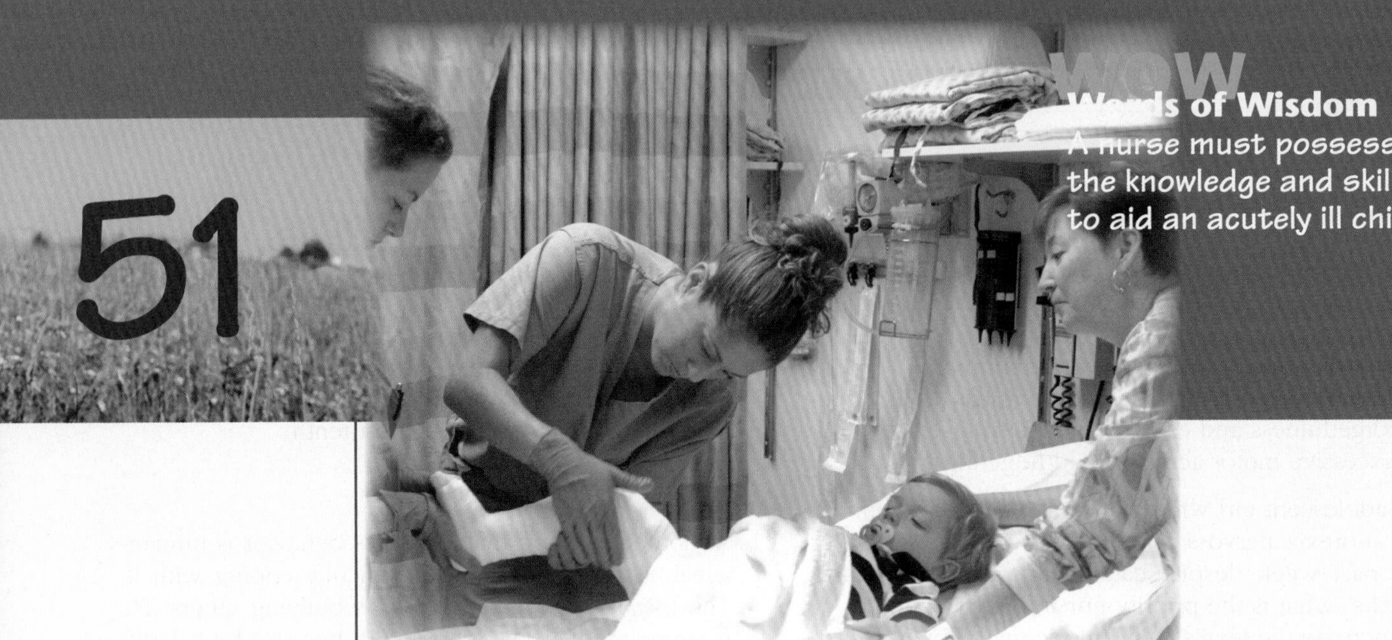

Nursing Care During a Pediatric Emergency

KEY TERMS

asystole
barotrauma
bradycardia
cardioversion
defibrillation
hyperventilation
hypocapnia
hypoventilation
intubation
periodic breathing
tachycardia
tachypnea
tracheal (endotracheal) tube

Learning Objectives

Upon completion of the chapter, the learner will be able to:

1. Identify various factors contributing to emergency situations among infants and children.
2. Discuss common treatments and medications used during pediatric emergencies.
3. Conduct a health history of a child in an emergency situation, specific to the emergency.
4. Perform a rapid cardiopulmonary assessment.
5. Discuss common laboratory and other diagnostic tests used during pediatric emergencies.
6. Integrate the principles of the American Heart Association and Pediatric Advanced Life Support in the comprehensive management of pediatric emergencies, such as respiratory arrest, shock, cardiac arrest, near drowning, poisoning, and trauma.

***Alma Anderson*, age 8 years, has been admitted to the pediatric unit. Her mother calls the nurse into the room, stating, "Alma's having trouble breathing!"**

Children are uniquely vulnerable to a range of emergency situations. These situations are often life-threatening if not treated quickly and effectively. Because of their developmental level, children are at a greater risk for near drowning, poisoning, and traumatic injury compared to adults. Most pediatric cardiopulmonary arrests result from respiratory failure or shock. Data suggest that children who have a cardiopulmonary arrest requiring resuscitative measures rarely fare well. For these reasons, the American Heart Association (AHA) has delineated two distinct chains of survival, one for adults and one for children, which should be followed during a life-threatening situation.

The adult chain of survival is:

- Early emergency medical system (EMS) activation
- Early cardiopulmonary resuscitation (CPR)
- Early defibrillation
- Early access to advanced care
- Integrated post–cardiac arrest care

In contrast, the pediatric chain of survival is:

- Prevention of cardiac arrest and injuries
- Early CPR
- Early access to emergency response system
- Early advanced care (Pediatric Advanced Life Support [PALS])
- Integrated post–cardiac arrest care (Berg et al., 2010)

Considering the special risks that threaten children, the AHA has also developed specific guidelines for PALS. Courses in PALS are offered for healthcare professionals so that they can provide expert care for children in emergencies. This chapter emphasizes the principles of PALS in its discussion of the nurse's role in the management of pediatric emergencies.

Take Note!

The current pediatric basic life support guidelines define an infant as between 0 and 12 months of age, and a child as age 1 year up until puberty. Children in this range should be managed using the PALS guidelines rather than those for adults (Berg et al., 2010).

COMMON MEDICAL TREATMENTS

A variety of medications and other medical treatments are used in pediatric emergencies. Most of these treatments will require a physician's order when the child is in the hospital, though some emergency departments and pediatric units may have standing orders for pediatric emergencies. The most common medical treatments and medications used in pediatric emergencies are listed in Common Medical Treatments 51.1 and Drug Guide 51.1. The nurse should be familiar with these procedures and medications, how they work, and nursing implications.

HEALTHY PEOPLE 2020

Objective	Nursing Significance
Increase the number of states and the District of Columbia that have implemented guidelines for prehospital and hospital pediatric care.	• Become politically active in your local area and at the national level. • Advocate for optimal care for infants, children, and adolescents.

Healthy People Objectives retrieved from http://www.healthypeople.gov

Take Note!

Certain emergency drugs for children may be given via a **tracheal (endotracheal) tube** *(a tube inserted into the trachea that serves to maintain the airway and facilitate artificial respiration). Use the mnemonic LEAN (lidocaine, epinephrine, atropine, and naloxone) to remember which drugs may be given via the tracheal route. In certain cases, when an emergency drug is given via a tracheal tube, the dosage must be increased. In addition, drugs given via this route should be followed by 5 mL of sterile saline and five consecutive multiple positive-pressure ventilations to ensure that the drugs are delivered (Kleinman et al., 2010a).*

NURSING PROCESS OVERVIEW FOR THE CHILD IN AN EMERGENCY SITUATION

The nurse may encounter a pediatric emergency in a variety of settings. As a member of a trauma team at a pediatric hospital, the nurse may participate in the stabilization of a child who has suffered a near drowning or trauma. The emergency department nurse may encounter a child who has just been injured, such as from a fall, an accident, or sports. On the hospital unit, a child with asthma may suffer respiratory distress or stop breathing. Regardless of the setting or how the emergency developed, the principles for managing pediatric emergencies are the same.

Care of the child in an emergency includes all components of the nursing process: assessment, nursing diagnosis, planning, interventions, and evaluation. In an emergency, the nurse must act quickly. It is important to intervene immediately when an abnormality is determined upon assessment. When evaluating a child who presents emergently, always follow the AHA's guidelines for basic life support (Berg et al., 2010), which includes evaluating the child's:

- Airway
- Breathing
- Circulation

COMMON MEDICAL TREATMENTS 51.1 PEDIATRIC EMERGENCIES

Treatment	Explanation	Indications	Nursing Implications
Suctioning (oropharyngeal, nasopharyngeal, tracheal, or tracheostomy)	Removal of secretions via bulb syringe or suction catheter	Excessive airway secretions affecting airway patency	Use caution and suction only as far as recommended for age, tracheal tube size, or tracheostomy tube size or until coughing or gagging occurs.
Oxygen	Supplementation via mask, nasal cannula, hood, or tent or via tracheal/ nasotracheal tube	Hypoxemia, respiratory distress, shock, trauma	Monitor response via color, work of breathing, respiratory rate, oxygen saturation levels via pulse oximetry, and level of consciousness.
Bag-valve-mask ventilation	Provision of ventilation via a bag-valve-mask device, manual ventilation	Apnea, ineffective ventilation and oxygenation with spontaneous breaths, extremely slow respiratory rate	Ensure adequate chest rise with ventilation. Do not overventilate or bag aggressively to avoid barotrauma. Maintain a seal on the child's face with the appropriate-sized mask. Ensure the oxygen supply tubing is connected to 100% oxygen.
Intubation	Insertion of a tube into the trachea to provide artificial ventilation	Apnea, airway that is not maintainable, need for prolonged assisted ventilation	Determine adequacy of breath sounds with bagging immediately upon insertion of the tracheal tube. Assess for symmetric chest rise. Tape tube securely in place and note number marking on the tube. Connect to ventilator when available.
Needle thoracotomy	Insertion of a needle between the ribs into the pleural space to remove air	Tension pneumothorax	There should be a rush of air as the needle reaches the air space. Monitor breath sounds, work of breathing, pulse oximetry. Ensure patency of IV catheter.
IV fluid therapy	Administration of crystalloid or colloid solutions to provide hydration or improve perfusion	Altered perfusion states such as respiratory distress, shock, trauma, cardiac disturbances	Use intraosseous route if a peripheral IV cannot be obtained quickly in the young child in shock. Reassess respiratory and circulatory status frequently after each IV fluid bolus and during continuous infusion.
Blood product transfusion	Administration of whole blood, packed red blood cells, platelets, or plasma intravenously	Trauma, hemorrhage	Follow institution's transfusion protocol. Double-check blood type and product label with a second nurse. Monitor vital signs and assess child frequently to identify adverse reaction to blood transfusion. If adverse reaction is suspected, immediately discontinue transfusion, infuse normal saline solution IV, reassess the child, and notify the physician.
Cervical stabilization	Maintenance of the cervical spine in an immobile position	Trauma, near drowning	Use the jaw-thrust maneuver without head tilt to open the airway. Maintain cervical stabilization until the cervical spine x-rays are cleared by the physician or radiologist.
Defibrillation and synchronized cardioversion	Provision of electrical current to alter the heart's electrical rhythm	Defibrillation: ventricular fibrillation and pulseless ventricular tachycardia Synchronized cardioversion: supraventricular tachycardia and ventricular tachycardia with a pulse	In the pulseless child, always ensure CPR is ongoing while the defibrillator is being readied. Ensure adequate oxygenation. Provide lidocaine or epinephrine if indicated before defibrillation. Sedate the child if time allows.

DRUG GUIDE 51.1 COMMON MEDICATIONS USED IN PEDIATRIC EMERGENCIES

Medication	Actions/Indications	Nursing Implications
Adenosine (antiarrhythmic)	Slows conduction through AV node, restoring normal sinus rhythm Supraventricular tachycardia (SVT)	• Administer IV at a dose ranging from 0.05 to 0.1 mg/kg for neonates, and 0.1 to 0.2 mg/kg. • Administer very rapidly (1–2 seconds) followed by a rapid, generous saline flush. • Repeat every 1–2 minutes, increasing by 0.05–0.1 mg/kg with each dose (maximum dose 0.3 mg/kg). • Monitor for shortness of breath, dyspnea, worsening of asthma.
Amiodarone (antiarrhythmic)	Prolongs repolarization of action potential, thus slowing the heart rate Ventricular tachycardia, ventricular fibrillation	• Administer IV or IO at a dose of 5 mg/kg over 20–60 minutes. • Avoid use with procainamide.
Atropine (anticholinergic)	Increases cardiac output, dries secretions, inhibits serotonin and histamine Sinus bradycardia, asystole, pulseless electrical activity	• Administer via IV, IO, or ET route at a dose of 0.02 mg/kg (maximum dose 0.5 mg child, 1 mg adolescent). • Repeat every 5 minutes PRN. • Give undiluted over 30 seconds for IV or IO route. • Dilute with 3–5 mL normal saline for ET route; follow with five positive-pressure ventilations. • Do not mix with sodium bicarbonate (incompatible).
Dobutamine (adrenergic agent)	β-Adrenergic agent primarily affecting β-1 receptors; increases myocardial contractility and heart rate Ongoing short-term management of shock (hypovolemic and cardiogenic)	• Administer via IV or IO route at 2–20 μg/kg/min via a continuous infusion. Monitor for development of ventricular arrhythmias. • Expect to titrate infusion rate based on cardiac output and BP. • Administer via central line if possible due to risk of extravasation. • Monitor child closely, preferably in an ICU setting.
Dopamine (inotropic)	Increases cardiac output, BP, and renal perfusion (β-adrenergic agonist) Bradycardia, hypotension, and poor cardiac output	• Administer via IV or IO route at a dose of 2–20 μg/kg/min via continuous infusion. • Ensure that child has received adequate fluid resuscitation prior to administration. • Due to risk of extravasation, give via central line if possible. • Monitor child closely, preferably in an ICU setting. • Assess for ventricular arrhythmias.
Epinephrine (vasopressor, inotropic)	Stimulates α- and β-adrenergic receptors, increasing heart rate and systemic vascular resistance Bradycardia, anaphylaxis	• Administer via IV or IO route at a dose of 0.01 mg/kg (0.1 mL/kg of 1:10,000 solution) or via ET route at 0.1 mg/kg (0.1 mL/kg of 1:1,000 solution). • During CPR, repeat every 3–5 minutes. • Monitor for ventricular arrhythmias. • High doses may cause tachycardia in newborns. • Due to risk of extravasation and subsequent tissue necrosis, give through a central line if possible. • May also be used as a bronchodilator IV or via inhalation (racemic epinephrine).

DRUG GUIDE 51.1 COMMON MEDICATIONS USED IN PEDIATRIC EMERGENCIES (continued)

Medication	Actions/Indications	Nursing Implications
Glucose	Increases blood glucose level Hypoglycemia	• Administer via IV or IO route at a dose of 1–2 mL/kg (D50%); maximum dose 2–4 mL/kg. • When administering via a peripheral IV line, dilute 1:1 with sterile water to make D25%. Monitor IV site for infiltration and tissue extravasation. • Monitor blood glucose levels closely.
Lidocaine (antidysrhythmic)	Decreases automaticity of conduction tissues of the heart Ventricular arrhythmias	• Administer via IV or IO route at a dose of 1 mg/kg; administer via ET route at dose 2 times IV dose diluted with 3-5 mL normal saline, followed by positive-pressure ventilation. Maximum dose 5 mg/kg or 100 mg/dose. • Monitor ECG continuously. • Contraindicated in complete heart block. • With larger than normal doses, monitor for hypotension or seizures.
Naloxone (opioid receptor antagonist)	Antagonizes action of narcotic agents Reversal of respiratory depression related to narcotic effects	• Administer via IV, IO, SQ, or ET route at a dose of 0.01–0.1 mg/kg in children younger than 5 years old or <20 kg or at a dose of 2 mg in children older than 5 years old or >20 kg. Onset of action is within 2–5 minutes. • May repeat dose as necessary; narcotic effects outlast therapeutic effects of naloxone.

AV, atrioventricular; ET, endotracheal; IO, intraosseous; SQ, subcutaneous.

Adapted from American Heart Association. (2011). *Pediatric advanced life support provider manual*. Dallas, TX: Author; Kleinman, M. E., Chameides, L., Schexnayder, S. M., Samson, R. A., Hazinski, M. F., Atkins, D. L., et al. (2010). Part 14: Pediatric advanced life support: 2010 American Heart Association guidelines for cardiopulmonary resuscitation and emergency cardiovascular care. *Circulation, 122*, S876–S908; and Taketomo, C. K., Hodding, J. H., & Kraus, D. M. (2013). *Pediatric & neonatal dosage handbook* (20th ed.). Hudson, OH: Lexicomp.

After you have evaluated the child's airway, breathing, and circulation, provide care as necessary, including rescue breathing or CPR. Once the child's cardiopulmonary status is stabilized or the child is resuscitated, assessment and management will vary depending on the cause of the emergency.

Assessment

Nursing assessment of the child who presents emergently includes health history, physical examination, and laboratory and diagnostic testing. However, the initial history may be focused and very brief if the child is critically ill; the nurse may need to proceed immediately to rapid cardiopulmonary assessment. Once a child is stabilized, a more comprehensive history is obtained. Laboratory tests, while often important, should never take priority over cardiopulmonary and hemodynamic stabilization.

Remember Alma, the 8-year-old with breathing trouble? What additional health history and physical examination assessment information should the nurse obtain?

Health History

Obtain the health history rapidly while simultaneously evaluating the child and providing life-saving interventions. A brief history is needed initially, followed by a more thorough history after the child is stabilized. The parents or caregiver will provide information about the child's chief complaint. Record the information using the caregiver's own words. For example, the caregiver might say, "He's been having trouble breathing" if the child is presenting in respiratory distress. If the child was injured in a bicycle accident, the caregiver might say, "She was riding her bike down the hill and lost control." This brief statement provides guidance for obtaining more in-depth information about the emergency.

Ask about any significant past history that may affect the care of the child. For example, children who are medically fragile, who were born prematurely, or who have a significant genetically linked disease (e.g., sickle cell anemia) may require special consideration when planning and implementing care.

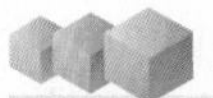
Concept Mastery Alert

Assessment After an Accident

When caring for a child injured in an accident, the nurse must always remember that assessment is the first step in the nursing process. So initial questions would relate to how the accident happened. The nurse could then go on to asking other questions such as medication allergies and chronic diseases.

Physical Examination

In an emergency, the nurse must perform a rapid cardiopulmonary assessment and intervene immediately if alterations are noted. The remainder of the physical examination then follows.

RAPID CARDIOPULMONARY ASSESSMENT

As the brief history is being obtained, begin the rapid cardiopulmonary assessment. Most pediatric arrests are related primarily to airway and breathing, and usually only secondarily to the heart. Supported breathing may be all that is needed if the child has a strong, adequate pulse. Always perform the assessment and interventions in that order. In most circumstances, if a child's airway is properly managed and breathing is assisted, the child may not experience a full arrest requiring chest compressions.

Take Note!

Assessment and management of the airway of a prearresting or arresting child is ALWAYS the first intervention in a pediatric emergency. Intervene if there is an airway problem before moving on to assessment of breathing. If an intervention for breathing is required, start it before proceeding to assessment of circulation.

Airway Evaluation and Management. First evaluate the airway. Assess its patency. Position the airway in a manner that promotes good air flow. If secretions are obstructing the airway, suction the airway to remove them. If the child is unconscious or has just been injured, open the airway using the head tilt–chin lift maneuver. Place the fingertips on the bony prominence of the child's chin and lift the chin to open the airway. Simultaneously, place one hand on the forehead and tilt the child's head back (Fig. 51.1). If the airway is not maintainable, reposition the airway for appropriate airflow. Place the child immediately on oxygen at 100% and apply a pulse oximeter to monitor oxygen saturation levels.

Take Note!

If cervical spine injury is a possibility, do not use the head tilt–chin lift maneuver; use only the jaw-thrust technique for opening the airway (see trauma section for explanation and illustration).

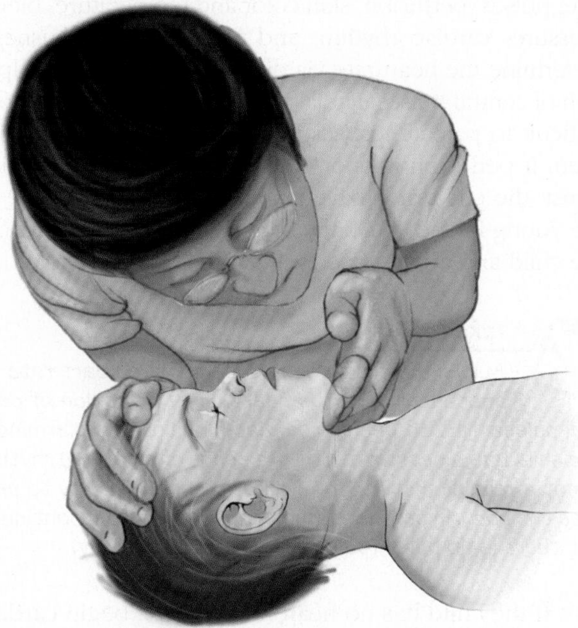

FIGURE 51.1 Head tilt–chin lift maneuver in a child.

Breathing Evaluation and Management. After establishing an open airway, look for signs of respiration. Turn your head and place your ear over the child's mouth to "look, listen, and feel" for spontaneous respirations. Look to see if the child's chest is rising, listen for air escaping, and note if you feel any air coming out of the child's nose or mouth. If the child is breathing, evaluate the quality of the respirations: Is ventilation effective, or is the child simply gasping ineffectively for air? Count the respiratory rate. Observe the child's color. Note depth of respiration, chest rise, adequacy of air flow in all lung fields, and presence of adventitious sounds. Evaluate for increased work of breathing and the use of accessory muscles.

When signs of respiratory distress are noted, immediately place the child on oxygen at 100% and apply a pulse oximeter to monitor oxygen saturation levels. If the child is breathing shallowly and has poor respiratory effort, attempt to reposition the airway to promote better airflow.

For the child receiving 100% oxygen who does not improve with repositioning, begin assisted ventilation with a bag-valve-mask (BVM) device. A need for ongoing BVM ventilation may require airway **intubation** (process by which a breathing tube, such as a tracheal tube, is inserted into a child's airway to assist with breathing). See the section on respiratory arrest for information on assisting with ventilation using the BVM device and airway intubation.

Circulation Evaluation and Management. Next, evaluate circulation. During this phase, evaluate the heart rate, pulses, perfusion, skin color and temperature, blood pressure, cardiac rhythm, and level of consciousness. Determine the heart rate via direct auscultation or palpation of central pulses. Radial and brachial pulses are more difficult to palpate, especially in infants and young children. If perfusion is poor, such as with shock or cardiac arrest, the child may have a weak pulse or no pulse. In the young infant, check the brachial artery for a pulse. In the child and adolescent, evaluate the carotid pulse.

Take Note!

ALWAYS evaluate the presence of a heart rate by auscultation of the heart or by palpation of central pulses. NEVER use the cardiac monitor to determine if the child has a heart rate. The presence of a cardiac rhythm is not a reliable method for evaluation of the ability to perfuse the body. In certain circumstances a rhythm continues but there is no pulse (pulseless electrical activity).

If the child has no heart rate (pulse), begin cardiac compressions. See below for information on performing CPR. High-quality chest compressions of adequate rate and depth are essential (Kleinman et al., 2010a).

If there is a pulse, note its quality: Is it barely palpable or weak? Is it strong or bounding? Compare the strength and quality of central and peripheral pulses. Assess capillary refill time.

Evaluate the child's perfusion by noting skin temperature and color. Is the skin pink? Is it warm to the touch? The child's skin may be cool to the touch and may appear pale, mottled, or cyanotic. As the child's condition worsens with developing shock and cardiovascular compromise, note a line of demarcation of skin temperature. In this situation, the distal extremities will feel cooler than the proximal regions of the body. Measure the blood pressure (BP) and place the child on a cardiac monitor to evaluate the cardiac rhythm. Note the child's sensorium or level of consciousness; if circulation is poor, the child will demonstrate an altered level of consciousness as perfusion to the brain becomes diminished.

Take Note!

According to PALS, the minimum acceptable systolic BP is 60 for the neonate, 70 for the infant aged 1 to 12 months, and 70 + twice the age in years for children aged 1 to 10 years (e.g., a 4-year-old should have a minimal systolic BP of 78: 70 = [2 × 4] = 79). For children older than age 10, the minimum acceptable systolic BP is 90 (Kleinman et al., 2010a).

If the circulation or perfusion is compromised, then fluid resuscitation is necessary. Establish large-bore intravenous (IV) access immediately and administer isotonic fluid rapidly. Provide 20 mL/kg of normal saline (NS) or lactated Ringer's (LR) as an IV bolus (if the infant is younger than 1 month old, administer 10 mL/kg). If peripheral IV access cannot be obtained in the child with altered perfusion within three attempts or 90 seconds, assist with insertion of an intraosseous needle for fluid administration (refer to shock section for further information about intraosseous access). Central venous lines or cutdown access may also be used, but these measures take longer to accomplish.

ADDITIONAL PHYSICAL EXAMINATION COMPONENTS

In addition to assessing and stabilizing the child's airway, breathing, and circulation, perform a thorough physical examination and assess pain.

Neurologic Evaluation. Quickly evaluate the sensorium in an older child. Ask the child to state his or her name. Ask what happened to the child. Does the child know what day it is? Is the child aware of where he or she is?

If the child is an infant, evaluate his or her interest in the environment and response to parents. An infant who is not interested in the environment or seems unable to recognize his or her parents is a cause for concern. In contrast, an infant who enjoys sucking on a finger and making eye contact with the nurse during the assessment is reassuring.

Evaluate the child's head. In the infant or young toddler, palpate the anterior fontanel to determine if it is normal (soft and flat), depressed, or full. A sunken fontanel is associated with volume depletion from dehydration or blood loss. If the fontanel is full, note if it is bulging or tense, which may indicate increased intracranial pressure. Next assess the eyes. Are they open or closed? If closed, do they open spontaneously, to voice, to pain? Does the child focus on and follow the nurse's movements? Evaluate the pupils for equality and reactivity. Sluggish pupillary reaction may occur with increased intracranial pressure.

Take Note!

A nonreactive pupil is an ominous sign indicating a need for immediate relief of increased intracranial pressure.

Evaluate the child's face. Does the child smile or cry? Does the child react to playfulness with a laugh? Does the young infant cry vigorously? Are facial movements equal? In a child, a normal or near-normal neurologic examination can be a reassuring sign. Conversely, obtunded or muted responses to environmental stimuli are a cause for concern.

Next evaluate for spontaneous movement of the extremities. Young infants cannot walk, so assess their ability to move their arms and legs and grossly evaluate the tone of their extremities. Does the infant vigorously and equally move the arms and legs? Is the muscle tone normal, or does the infant appear floppy or flaccid? When evaluating the older child, note whether he or she is ambulatory alone, ambulatory with assistance, or unable to walk. Note whether the child has use of the upper extremities. In the case of trauma, the child may arrive immobilized on a backboard. In this scenario, evaluate the child's motor responsiveness and sensation in each extremity, comparing findings bilaterally while the child is in the supine position. Ask the child if he or she feels you touching each extremity. Ask the child to squeeze your fingers and to wiggle the toes. This will provide information about cerebral integrity and perfusion, cerebellar health, and spinal cord integrity.

The Pediatric Glasgow Coma Scale may also be used to evaluate the neurologic status in children (AHA, 2011). Chapter 38 provides a more in-depth discussion of this scale.

Skin and Extremity Evaluation. Remove the child's clothing and thoroughly examine the skin for bruising, lesions, or rashes. If the child has a rash, note the size, shape, color, configuration, and location. Apply pressure to the rash with the fingertips to see whether it blanches. Inspect the trunk, abdomen, and extremities for abrasions or deformities.

Take Note!

Rashes that do not blanch may be classified as petechiae or purpura. This type of rash may be associated with certain serious conditions, such as meningococcemia. Report this finding to the physician or nurse practitioner immediately.

Pain Assessment. In emergencies, children may experience pain as a direct result of the injury or disease, and life-saving interventions such as resuscitation, insertion of IV lines, and administration of medications may cause further pain. The child's pain may also be exaggerated by light, noise, movement of the stretcher or bed, and the sensations of cold or heat. Nurses play a key role in minimizing the child's pain, and this may decrease the child's future distress (Stanley & Pollard, 2013). If the child is awake and verbal, use an age-appropriate pain assessment scale to determine the child's pain level. If the child is sedated or unconscious, assess pain with a standardized scale that relies on physiologic measurements as well as behavioral parameters. Refer to Chapter 36 for additional information on pain assessment in children.

Laboratory and Diagnostic Testing

A number of laboratory and diagnostic tests may be ordered in a pediatric emergency. Laboratory tests can help to distinguish the cause of the emergency or additional problems that need to be treated. Standard laboratory tests obtained in most emergency departments include:

- Arterial blood gases (ABGs), obtained initially and then serially to assess for changes
- Electrolytes and glucose levels
- Complete blood count (CBC)
- Blood cultures
- Urinalysis

If ingestion is suspected, then a toxicology panel will be obtained. In suspected sepsis, erythrocyte sedimentation rate (ESR), C-reactive protein (CRP), and urine and spinal fluid cultures may also be obtained. The pediatric trauma victim may have additional laboratory tests performed, including amylase, liver enzymes, and blood type and cross-match.

Diagnostic tests may include radiologic tests, computed tomography (CT) scanning, and magnetic resonance imaging (MRI). One advantage of radiologic diagnostic testing is that the tests are relatively noninvasive. A disadvantage of CT and MRI scans is that before they can be performed, the child must be stabilized. Common Laboratory and Diagnostic Tests 51.1 discusses the tests most commonly used in pediatric emergencies.

After completing an assessment of Alma, the nurse noted the following: a patent airway, anxious but able to speak in short sentences, and skin temperature cool on the extremities. Based on these assessment findings, what would your top three nursing diagnoses be for Alma? Describe appropriate nursing interventions.

Nursing Diagnoses and Related Interventions

After completing a thorough assessment and initial stabilization of the child, the nurse might identify several nursing diagnoses, including:

- Ineffective airway clearance
- Ineffective breathing pattern
- Impaired gas exchange
- Deficient fluid volume
- Decreased cardiac output
- Ineffective tissue perfusion (cardiopulmonary, peripheral cerebral, or renal)
- Deficient knowledge
- Fear
- Interrupted family processes

Specific nursing goals, interventions, and evaluation for the child in an emergency are based on the nursing diagnoses. Additional information about nursing management will be included later in the chapter as it relates to specific disorders.

COMMON LABORATORY AND DIAGNOSTIC TESTS 51.1 PEDIATRIC EMERGENCIES

Test	Explanation	Indications	Nursing Implications
Chest x-ray	X-ray used to evaluate heart and lung structures	To identify: • Infections (e.g., pneumonia) • Foreign body • Injury • Tracheal tube placement • Central line placement • Pneumothorax Reevaluation of lungs after chest tube placement	• x-rays can be obtained quickly during resuscitation; usually available in emergency department. • Assist the child to lie still if necessary.
Computed tomography (CT)	Use of high radiation (equivalent to about 100–150 chest x-rays) with computer processing targeting specific body areas	Rapid evaluation of tissues and skeletal areas Superior test for the evaluation of internal bleeding	• Expect the child to be transported out of the area for the study. • Accompany the child to provide continued observation and management, especially if child's condition is unstable.
Magnetic resonance imaging (MRI)	Incorporation of responses of hydrogen protons to a dynamic magnetic field	Superior test for the evaluation of the spinal cord and the cerebrospinal fluid spaces; less useful in emergency situations	• Administer sedation as ordered. • Assist child in remaining still; MRI requires child to remain still for a longer period than for a CT. • Assist the conscious child to deal with fear related to loud banging noise of the machine.
Arterial blood gases (ABGs)	Evaluation of blood pH and arterial blood levels of oxygen and carbon dioxide	Evaluation of quality of respiration and evaluation of acid–base balance	• Anticipate serial ABGs to assess for status changes. • Never delay resuscitation efforts pending blood gas results.
Serum electrolytes	Evaluation of electrolyte levels, such as sodium, potassium, and chloride, in the blood	Useful for determining baseline and if dehydration is hypertonic or isotonic	• Hemolysis of specimen may lead to falsely elevated potassium levels.
Glucose	Evaluation of glucose level in the blood	Valuable for determining need for supplementation, as in the case of hypoglycemia	• Use a rapid glucose test at the bedside or obtain serum blood specimen. • Elevated glucose levels can be associated with stress or with use of corticosteroids.
Toxicology panel (blood and/or urine)	Determination of most commonly abused mood-altering medications, as well as commonly ingested drugs	Drug abuse, overdose, or poisoning	• Standard toxicology panel varies with the agency. • Follow agency protocol; may require special handling or labeling of specimen. • Use a blood specimen that is best for determining overdose or poisoning.
Complete blood count (CBC)	Evaluation of hemoglobin and hematocrit, white blood cell count, and platelet count	Any condition in which anemia, infection, or thrombocytopenia is suspected Trauma if blood loss is suspected	• Be aware of normal values and how they vary with age and gender. • Hemoglobin and hematocrit may be elevated secondary to hemoconcentration in the case of hypovolemia.

(continued)

COMMON LABORATORY AND DIAGNOSTIC TESTS 26.1 PEDIATRIC EMERGENCIES (continued)

Test	Explanation	Indications	Nursing Implications
Blood type and cross-match	Determination of ABO blood typing as well as presence of antigens Cross-match is performed on RBC-containing products to avoid transfusion reaction.	Trauma victim or any person with suspected blood loss as preparation for transfusion	• Handle specimen gently to avoid hemolysis. • Ensure that specimen request and label are appropriately signed and dated. • Apply "type and cross" or "blood band" to child at time of specimen collection if required by agency. • Most type and cross-match specimens expire after 48–72 hours.
Urinalysis	Evaluation of color, pH, specific gravity, and odor of urine Assessment for protein, glucose, ketones, blood, leukocyte esterase, RBCs, WBCs, bacteria, crystals, and casts	Children with fever, dysuria, flank pain, urgency, or hematuria or those who have experienced trauma to provide information about the urinary tract	• Many drugs can affect urine color; notify the laboratory if the child is taking one. • Notify the laboratory and document on the laboratory form if the child or adolescent is menstruating. • Refrigerate the specimen if it is not processed promptly. • Specimen may be obtained by catheterization, clean-catch voiding sample, or a U-bag.

RBCs, red blood cells; WBCs, white blood cells.

Adapted from Corbett, J. A., & Banks, A. D. (2013). *Laboratory tests and diagnostic procedures with nursing diagnoses* (8th ed.). Upper Saddle River, NJ: Pearson Education Inc.

Providing Cardiopulmonary Resuscitation

Always evaluate and manage the airway first. Call for help and assign someone to obtain the automatic external defibrillator (AED). Open the airway and assess for adequate breathing. If the child is not breathing, begin rescue breathing.

Check for a pulse. In the child, the carotid or femoral pulses are easiest to assess. In the past, it was recommended that the brachial pulse be checked in the infant, but this is often difficult, so an alternative is to check the femoral pulse. Carefully assess for signs of a pulse, but do not spend more than 10 seconds checking the pulse.

If there is not a pulse or if the heart rate is less than 60 beats per minute (bpm), begin chest compressions.

Take Note!

When a cardiac arrest occurs in a child out of the hospital and is a witnessed, sudden collapse, initial management is slightly different than that for other arrests. In these sudden, witnessed events, call 9–1–1 or the local emergency number for help first, get the AED, and return to start CPR (Berg et al., 2010).

Table 51.1 presents the AHA's most recent recommendations for ratios of breaths and compressions. These recommendations stress the importance of properly performed chest compressions. Therefore, several changes have been made to the guidelines:

- Rescuers must provide compressions of adequate rate and depth.
- Chest recoil should be allowed.
- Minimal interruption of chest compressions should be the goal.
- For infant CPR, two-person infant CPR can be performed by encircling the chest with two thumbs and simultaneously using the hands to provide a thoracic squeeze.
- For two-person CPR, no pauses should occur for ventilation, with the compressing healthcare provider giving continuous compressions (Berg et al., 2010).

Providing Defibrillation or Synchronized Cardioversion

In some cases, the child has an abnormal life-threatening cardiac rhythm or an arrhythmia that

TABLE 51.1 RATIOS OF BREATHS TO COMPRESSIONS

Age	One-Person CPR	Two-Person CPR
Infant	• 30 compressions to 2 breaths • Hand placement: two fingers, placed one fingerbreadth below the nipple line	• 15 compressions to 2 breaths • Hand placement: two thumbs encircling the chest at the nipple line
Child	• 30 compressions to 2 breaths • Hand placement: heel of hand or two hands (adult position in larger child), pressing on the sternum at the nipple line	• 15 compressions to 2 breaths • Hand placement: heel of one hand or two hands (adult position in larger child), pressing on the sternum at the nipple line

Adapted from Berg, M. D., Schexnayder, S. M., Chameides, L., Terry, M., Donoghue, A., Hickey, R. W., et al. (2010). Part 13: Pediatric basic life support: 2010 American Heart Association guidelines for cardiopulmonary resuscitation and emergency cardiovascular care. *Circulation, 122*, S862–S875.

does not respond to pharmacologic therapy or leads to hemodynamic instability. In these cases, electrical therapy, in the form of defibrillation or synchronized cardioversion, may be needed.

Defibrillation is the use of electrical energy to depolarize the cells of the myocardium to terminate an abnormal life-threatening cardiac rhythm, such as ventricular fibrillation. Defibrillation is used in conjunction with oxygen, CPR, and medications. The effects of defibrillation are enhanced in an oxygen-rich environment coupled with good artificial circulation (CPR).

Cardioversion, another means of applying electrical current to the heart, is used when the child has supraventricular tachycardia (SVT) or ventricular tachycardia with a pulse. Cardioversion may also be enhanced with medications. Cardioversion is delivered synchronized—that is, the electrical current is applied on the R wave of the electrocardiogram (ECG).

The basic defibrillator is equipped with adult- and pediatric-sized paddles. A switch turns the machine on and controls are used to select the amount of energy (joules). Typically, the initial energy amount is 2 J/kg; it can be increased up to 4 J/kg for defibrillation. Energy for cardioversion is delivered at 0.5 to 1 J/kg.

When the defibrillator is being used in an acute care setting, the leader of the code team will take charge of defibrillator use. He or she is responsible for ensuring that only the child receives the energy from the defibrillator. The code team leader will count to 4 before delivering a shock to the child to ensure that all personnel and other equipment are clear of the bed to avoid accidental shock.

Using Automated External Defibrillation

In cases of sudden, witnessed, out-of-hospital collapse, an arrhythmia is often the cause. Therefore, the AHA has revised its recommendations about the use of an AED in children (Berg et al., 2010). An AED is an alternative to manually defibrillating an individual. The AED device consists of electrodes that are applied to the chest. These electrodes are used to monitor the heart rhythm and deliver the electrical current. AED devices are readily available in a variety of locations, such as airports, sports facilities, and businesses. Traditionally, the AED was designed for use in adults, but newer AEDs with smaller pads and the ability to alter energy delivery are now more readily available. Therefore, the AHA has recommended that an AED be used for children who are older than age 1 year who have no pulse and have suffered a sudden, witnessed collapse (Berg et al., 2010).

The AED is designed for persons to use it in the prehospital setting. Once the AED is turned on, the machine uses auditory commands to guide laypersons and healthcare professionals alike through the correct placement of the electrodes and the administration of energy. The AED periodically evaluates the victim's cardiac rhythm and instructs the user about checking the pulse, continuing CPR, and delivering shocks. Nurses who care for children should be able to operate an AED and be prepared to use it in nontraditional settings. See Evidence-Based Practice 51.1.

Take Note!

Current recommendations call for placement of automated external defibrillators (AEDs) in school settings in order to improve outcomes should sudden arrest occur in the school (Diaz, 2013).

Determining Medication Doses and Equipment Sizes

Many pediatric acute care facilities prepare code reference sheets when a child is admitted. This sheet uses the child's actual weight to determine medication doses and equipment sizes. The reference sheet is kept on a clipboard at the child's bedside or taped on

EVIDENCE-BASED PRACTICE 51.1

THE ROLE OF AUTOMATED EXTERNAL DEFIBRILLATORS (AEDS) IN CARDIAC RESUSCITATION OF CHILDREN

Primary cardiac arrest resulting from arrhythmia or commotio cordis is rare in children and adolescents but often has a very poor outcome. Also, sudden death during sporting events has occurred in children and adolescents. Traditionally, manual defibrillation has been the only form of defibrillation used in children. With the newer technology available in AEDs, the question arose as to whether they could be used effectively to treat arrhythmia in children.

STUDY

Cecchin et al. (2001) performed a study of over 600 children to determine the specificity and sensitivity of automated external defibrillation in children.

Findings

The researchers found that AEDs can be sensitive and specific for detecting and treating arrhythmia by defibrillation in children older than 1 year of age. Salib et al. (2005) report a positive and healthy outcome after an AED was used at the scene on a 13-year-old who suffered a baseball blow to the chest resulting in commotio cordis. As a result of these and many other studies, in 2005 the American Heart Association recommended changes in the pediatric basic life support guidelines to include the use of AEDs in sudden witnessed collapse in children.

Nursing Implications

For nurses working in hospitals, ensure that witnessed collapse in children includes assessing for the need for defibrillation. Outside the hospital, nurses should advocate for AEDs to be placed in all high school gymnasiums and at all parks and ball fields.

Adapted from Cecchin, F., Jorgenson, D. B., Berul, C. I., Perry, J. C., Zimmerman, A. A., Duncan, B. W., et al. (2001). Is arrhythmia detection by automatic external defibrillator accurate for children? Sensitivity and specificity of an automatic external defibrillator algorithm in 696 pediatric arrhythmias. *Circulation, 103*, 2438–2483; and Salib, E. A., Cyran, S. E., Cilley, R. E., Maron, B. J., & Thomas, N. J. (2005). Efficacy of bystander cardiopulmonary resuscitation and out-of-hospital automated external defibrillation as life-saving therapy in commotio cordis. *Journal of Pediatrics, 147*, 863–869.

the wall at the head of the bed. An additional copy is placed in the child's chart.

Ambulatory care providers often use the Broselow tape to estimate the child's weight based on the child's length (Fig. 51.2). The tape is color coded and emergency equipment for a child of that size is stored in corresponding color-coded packages or in color-coded drawers on the pediatric emergency cart. Medication doses and equipment sizes are also located on the tape. The most accurate calculation for code medications is based on the child's weight, but use of the Broselow tape for estimating the weight has been shown to be successful in children weighing less than 25 kg (Jones, 2016).

Managing Pain

Depending on the child's status and pain level, individualize pain management interventions. For the alert child, nonpharmacologic measures may be used in addition to medications. Provide atraumatic care for procedures and use aggressive pharmacologic treatments to manage pain as the child's condition allows. Refer to Chapter 36 for additional information on pain management strategies.

Ensuring Stabilization

After a child has been resuscitated, the nurse plays a key role in stabilization and transport. Thoroughly

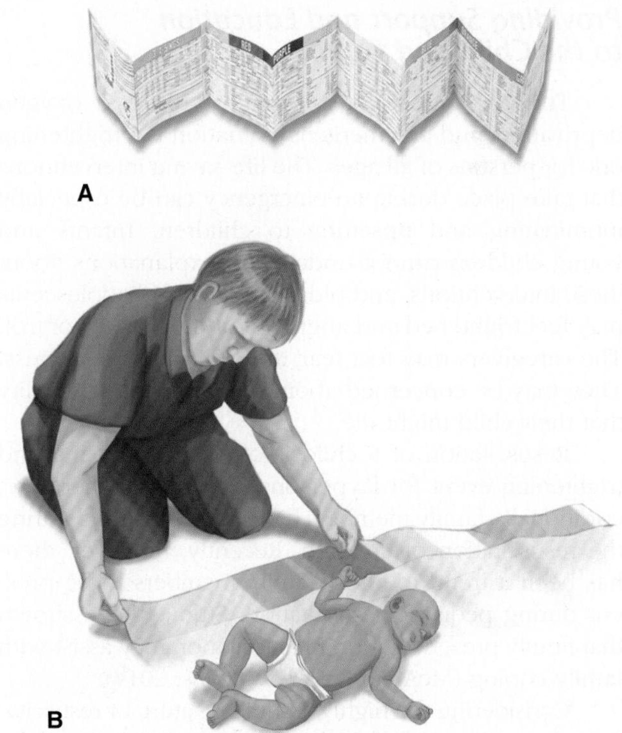

FIGURE 51.2 **(A)** Broselow tape. **(B)** Measure the child's length with the Broselow tape to determine medication doses and tracheal tube size.

document the interventions that were performed as well as the ongoing assessment of the child's response to the interventions. Provide continued monitoring of the child while awaiting transport. Copy and assemble any pertinent documentation, such as the resuscitation record, nurse's notes, and laboratory test results, which will be given to the receiving institution. Ensure that all lines are taped securely and that vascular access sites are dressed and labeled with the date and time of insertion. As soon as possible, bring the child's family in to visit with the child. Provide explanations about the IV lines, monitoring equipment, and other medical equipment and devices. Encourage the family to talk to and touch the child.

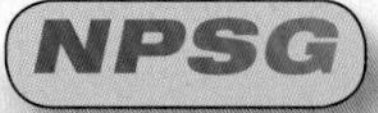

GOAL 6: Reduce the Harm Associated with Clinical Alarm Systems

NPSG.06.01.01 Improve the safety of clinical alarm systems

Steps: Insure alarms on biomedical equipment are properly set according to the child's age, clinical condition, prescribed orders, and facility policy. ALWAYS answer alarms promptly, checking the child first, then attending to the equipment.

Joint Commission. (2015). *National patient safety goals effective January 1, 2015.* Retrieved from http://www.jointcommission.org/assets/1/6/2015_NPSG_HAP.pdf

Providing Support and Education to the Child and Family

The experience of respiratory distress, oxygen deprivation, and an emergency situation is a frightening one for persons of all ages. The life-saving interventions that take place during an emergency can be especially intimidating and upsetting to children. Infants and young children cannot understand explanations about these interventions, and older children and adolescents may feel frightened and angry about the loss of control. The caregivers may feel fear, anger, guilt, and sadness. They may be concerned about the very real possibility that their child might die.

Resuscitation of a child is often a perplexing and frightening event for laypersons to observe. Therefore, traditionally family members have been excluded during the resuscitation of children. Recently, however, there has been a trend to allow family members to be present during pediatric resuscitation. Studies have shown that family presence during resuscitation may assist with family coping (McAlvin & Carew-Lyons, 2014).

Considering the highly technical nature of resuscitation, the rapidity with which interventions occur, and the fear associated with a life-threatening event, nurses can play a crucial role in providing understandable explanations to families, coupled with empathic support. During the acute phase, the nurse should give brief explanations as life-saving interventions are being provided. Examples of these types of explanations include:

- When applying the pulse oximeter sensor: "I need to put this light on your child to check his oxygen level; it won't hurt."
- When connecting the child to the cardiac monitor: "We're going to put these sticky patches on your child and connect them so we can monitor his heart rate on this screen."
- When preparing for intubation and ventilation: "Your child can't breathe on his own right now, so we're going to give him some extra help with this tube. This tube will go through his breathing passage and this machine will help him to breathe."

The nurse plays a key role in providing empathy and support. Do not provide false reassurance and say, for example, "He's going to be all right." The outcome is never certain. Rather, communicate empathically. For example, say, "This must be very difficult for you. We're doing everything we can to help your child." Provide honest answers in a reassuring manner. Respect each family's diversity and observe their strengths and weaknesses. Be nonjudgmental in all interactions with families, even when the child's emergency situation may have resulted from family neglect.

Parents often feel helpless when their child is in a high-tech environment. Suddenly overwhelmed with the equipment and monitoring devices, they no longer are the persons who are the most skilled in caring for their child. Integrate the child's parents into the healthcare team. Suggest ways the parents can make the hospital experience more normal for their child. For example, simply allowing a father to read a story to his daughter or encouraging a mother to hold her child's hand is therapeutic both for the child and the parents. Be aware of this dramatic change and how it affects the parents. Always ensure that they feel like they are a welcome part of their child's care.

Providing the child with familiar comfort objects helps to decrease stress. Once the intubated child is alert and stabilized, assist him or her with communication. Some children can lift one finger for yes and two fingers for no. If the child is old enough to write, provide paper and pencil. Play is essential to the work of the child, and even if he or she is immobile, play is still possible. Puppets at the bedside and books help give the child a more normal experience in a scary situation that is far from the norm. Teenagers may enjoy listening to music through headphones. Even children who are comatose should be talked to and allowed to listen to familiar music.

Even if the outcomes are serious, the nurse can provide critical support to children and families. Whether hugging a crying mother or playing "peek-a-boo" with an intubated child, the nurse will be the one who can make a difference during a frightening experience.

Atraumatic Care

In the conscious child, insure proximity of the caregiver during the post-resuscitation phase to provide security and assist with keeping the child calm.

NURSING MANAGEMENT OF CHILDREN IN EMERGENCIES

Nurses must be adept at identifying the beginning stages of an emergency so they can quickly and appropriately intervene to prevent deterioration to cardiopulmonary arrest. Assessment and management of the most common types of emergencies in children are discussed below. The topics covered include respiratory arrest, shock, cardiac arrhythmias and arrest, near drowning, poisoning, and traumatic injury.

Respiratory Arrest

Respiratory emergencies may lead to respiratory failure and eventual cardiopulmonary arrest in children. Infants and young children are at greater risk for respiratory emergencies than adolescents and adults because they have smaller airways and underdeveloped immune systems, resulting in a diminished ability to combat serious respiratory illnesses. Young children often lack coordination, making them susceptible to choking on foods and small objects, which may also lead to cardiopulmonary arrest. In addition, sudden infant death syndrome (SIDS) is a leading cause of cardiopulmonary arrest in young infants and thus is the leading cause of postneonatal mortality in the United States (American Academy of Pediatrics [AAP], 2011). For these reasons, nurses must be skilled at recognizing the signs of pediatric respiratory distress so they can prevent progression to cardiopulmonary arrest. Table 51.2 lists some of the more common causes of pediatric respiratory arrest.

TABLE 51.2 CAUSES OF RESPIRATORY ARREST IN CHILDREN

Condition	Cause
Upper airway	Burns Croup Epiglottitis Foreign-body aspiration Reflux Strangulation or near strangulation Tracheomalacia Vascular ring
Lower airway	Asthma Bronchiolitis Burns Foreign-body aspiration Pertussis infection Pneumonia Pneumothorax Reflux
Nonrespiratory origins	Septic shock HIV
Neurologic	CNS infection Guillain–Barré syndrome Poliomyelitis Seizures Sleep apnea Spinal cord trauma Sudden infant death
Chronic illness	Complications of severe prematurity Cystic fibrosis Bone marrow transplant Neutropenia
Metabolic/ endocrine disorders	Diabetic ketoacidosis Mitochondrial disorders
Cardiac conditions	Arrhythmia Congenital cardiac problems Acquired cardiac problems
Traumatic/ unintentional/ intentional injury	Asphyxia Child abuse/"shaken baby syndrome" Drowning Electrocution Gunshot wound Toxic ingestion Vehicular-related trauma

CNS, central nervous system.

Adapted from Fleisher, G. R., & Ludwig, S. (2010). *Textbook of pediatric emergency medicine* (6th ed.). Philadelphia, PA: Lippincott Williams & Wilkins.

Nursing Assessment

If the child has severe respiratory compromise, obtain a brief history while simultaneously providing respiratory interventions. To obtain the history, use the following questions as a guide:

- When did the symptoms begin and when do they occur?
- Did the symptoms have a sudden onset (as with a foreign-body aspiration)?
- How have the symptoms progressed?
- Is the cough continual, intermittent, or worse at night or with exercise?
- Has there been any stridor? (Stridor is heard upon inhalation and may be associated with swelling of the

trachea [as with croup] or with a foreign body in the upper airway.)

- Is there wheezing? If so, is the wheezing on inspiration or on expiration, or both?
- What makes the symptoms better and what makes them worse?
- Does drinking from a bottle induce the symptoms (as with gastroesophageal reflux–induced aspiration)?
- Is the child taking any medication for the symptoms? Does the child or do any members of the immediate family have a history of chronic respiratory disease, such as asthma?
- Are the child's immunizations up to date?
- Was the child born prematurely? If so, did the child require mechanical ventilation? For how long?
- Were there any respiratory problems during the first few days of life?
- When did the child last eat? (This question is important because a recent meal will increase the child's risk of aspiration in the event of a respiratory arrest. In addition, the presence of food in the stomach will increase the risk of aspiration during tracheal intubation.)

If the child can communicate, ask how he or she is feeling. Is he or she short of breath? Does his or her chest hurt? Observe the child while speaking. Children who are in respiratory distress may speak in short sentences with gasping between words.

PHYSICAL EXAMINATION

In an emergency, physical examination is often limited to inspection, observation, and auscultation. First, quickly survey the respiratory status. Determine if the child is breathing.

Inspection and Observation. Establish if the airway is patent, maintainable, or unable to be maintained. The child with a patent airway is breathing without signs of obstruction. The maintainable airway remains patent independently by the child or with interventions such as a towel roll under an infant's neck or the insertion of a nasal trumpet. The airway that cannot be maintained does not remain patent unless a more aggressive intervention, such as the insertion of a tracheal tube, is performed.

Look at the child's posture. Is the child sitting up, leaning forward, and drooling, as with epiglottitis? Observe the child's face: does he or she appear anxious or relaxed? Children in respiratory distress often appear anxious. Look at the nose and mouth. Are the nares patent? Is there noticeable nasal congestion or mucus coming from the nose? Note nasal flaring or mouth breathing. Observe for head bobbing. Listen for audible expiratory grunting or inspiratory stridor. Note the child's color. Does the child appear pale, mottled, dusky, or cyanotic? Children may appear mottled in response to poor oxygenation, hypothermia, or stress. Children with severe respiratory compromise may appear dusky. Look for cyanosis around the mouth or on the trunk. Cyanosis is a late and often ominous sign of respiratory distress. Central cyanosis is more likely to be associated with respiratory or cardiac compromise. In contrast, peripheral cyanosis is more likely to be associated with circulatory alteration.

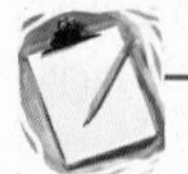

Take Note!

Closely inspect the color of the area around the mouth. Circumoral pallor is a sign of poor oxygenation.

Evaluate the pattern and quality of respiration, noting the respiratory rate. **Tachypnea** (increased respiratory rate) is often noted in children in respiratory distress. However, seriously ill children grunt and may have normal or subnormal respiratory rates. **Hypoventilation**, a decrease in the depth and rate of respirations, is noted in very ill children or children who have central respiratory depression secondary to narcotics. If the child is a young infant (younger than 2 months) or premature, periodic breathing may occur. **Periodic breathing** is regular breathing with occasional short pauses (brief periods of apnea). After the apneic pause, the infant will breathe rapidly (up to 60 breaths per minute) for a short period and then will resume a normal respiratory rate. In general, the infant who has periodic breathing looks pink and has a normal heart rate. Observe for the use of accessory muscles in the neck or retractions in the chest, determining the extent and severity of the retractions.

Auscultation. Auscultate the lungs with the diaphragm of the stethoscope. Breath sounds over the tracheal region are higher pitched and are described as vesicular, while breath sounds over the peripheral lung fields tend to be lower pitched, known as bronchial. Instruct the child to take deep breaths with the mouth open. To encourage the young child to exhale strongly, instruct him or her to "blow out" the penlight (as with a candle) or to blow on a tissue. Encourage the child not to breathe more rapidly than normal (to prevent **hyperventilation** [increased depth and rate of respirations]) and to avoid making any noises with the mouth.

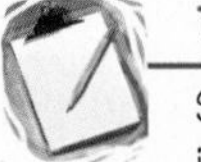

Take Note!

Significant upper respiratory congestion often interferes with assessment of the lower airways because the sound is easily transmitted throughout the chest. Differentiate between the upper and lower airway noises by listening with the stethoscope over the nose. The nurse may be able to determine whether the noise is nasal or bronchial by using this technique.

Auscultate the child's chest systematically. Listen in all anterior, axillary, and posterior regions, comparing the left to the right sides. Note any decreased or absent breath sounds, which may be the result of bronchial obstruction (as with mucous infection) or air trapping (as in children with asthma). Unilateral absent breath sounds are associated with foreign-body aspiration and pneumothorax.

Take Note!

Sometimes a child's respiratory status is so severely compromised that little or no air movement is noted. This commonly occurs during a severe asthma exacerbation. Minimal or no air movement requires immediate intervention.

Note the presence and location of adventitious breath sounds such as crackles, wheezes, or rhonchi. Document the presence of a pleural friction rub (a low-pitched, grating sound), a sound resulting from inflammation of the pleura.

Palpation. Palpate the chest for any abnormalities. In the older, less severely ill, and cooperative child, assess for tactile fremitus. Using the palm of the hand, palpate over the lung regions in the same manner as for auscultation and percussion while the child says "ninety-nine." Increased vibrations elicited during this maneuver are associated with consolidating conditions, such as pneumonia.

Percussion. Percuss the interspaces of the chest between the ribs in the same systematic fashion as with auscultation. Normally, percussion over an air-filled lung reveals resonant sounds. Note the presence of hyperresonance, which may indicate an acute problem such as a pneumothorax or a chronic disease such as asthma. In contrast, percussion sounds will be dull over a lobe of the lung that is consolidated with fluid, infectious organisms, and blood cells, as in the case of pneumonia.

LABORATORY AND DIAGNOSTIC TESTING

Use continuous pulse oximetry if respiratory status is a concern. Note and report oxygen saturation levels below 95%. (See Chapter 40 for additional information about use of the pulse oximeter.)

Additional tests may reveal:

- Arterial or capillary blood gases: hypoxemia, hypercarbia, altered pH
- Chest x-ray: alterations in normal anatomy or lung expansion, or evidence of pneumonia, tumor, or foreign body
- Metal detector: evidence of metallic foreign body, in particular coins (Gilger, Jain, & McOmber, 2015).

Take Note!

Children with cardiac conditions resulting in cyanosis often have baseline oxygen saturations that are relatively low because of the mixing of oxygenated with deoxygenated blood.

Nursing Management

The basic principle of pediatric emergency care and PALS is prevention of cardiopulmonary arrest (Kleinman et al., 2010a). Therefore, the nurse must rapidly assess and appropriately manage children who have signs of respiratory distress. Nursing management of the child in respiratory distress involves maintaining a patent airway, providing supplemental oxygen, monitoring for changes in status, and in some cases assisting ventilation. In addition to providing these life-saving measures and monitoring the child's progress, offer support and education to the child and family.

MAINTAINING A PATENT AIRWAY

When a child exhibits signs of respiratory distress, make a quick decision about whether it will be safe to allow the child to stay with the parent or whether the child must be placed on the examination table or bed. For example, in the case of croup, the child will often breathe more comfortably and experience less stridor while in the comfort of the parent's lap. Many children in respiratory distress often are most comfortable sitting upright, as this position helps to decrease the work of breathing by allowing appropriate diaphragmatic movement. In contrast, a child with a decreasing level of consciousness may need to be placed in the supine position to facilitate positioning of the airway.

The infant may benefit from a small towel folded under the shoulders or neck (Fig. 51.3). Avoid neck flexion or hyperextension, which may completely occlude the infant's airway. In children older than age 1 year, the optimal method for opening the airway is to hyperextend the neck, as recommended by the AHA (Berg et al., 2010). If a cervical spine injury is not suspected, use the head tilt–chin lift technique to open the airway. If the child has suffered head or neck trauma and cervical spine instability is a concern, use the jaw-thrust maneuver by placing three fingers under the child's lower jaw and lifting the jaw upward and outward (Fig. 51.4). In either case, never place the hand under the neck to open the airway.

Often the nurse encounters an acutely ill child who cannot maintain an airway independently but may be able to do so with some assistance. For example, sometimes simply opening the airway and moving the tongue away from the tracheal opening is all that is required to regain airway patency. In certain conditions, a nasopharyngeal or oropharyngeal airway may be necessary for airway maintenance. Comparison Chart 51.1 provides additional information about these types of airways.

ASSISTING VENTILATION USING A BAG-VALVE-MASK

The child in respiratory distress may ventilate poorly, hypoventilate, or tire and become apneic. In this case, the child may require assistance with ventilation through

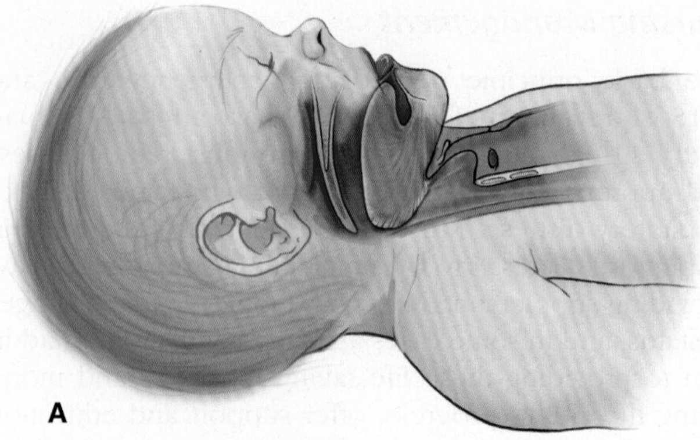

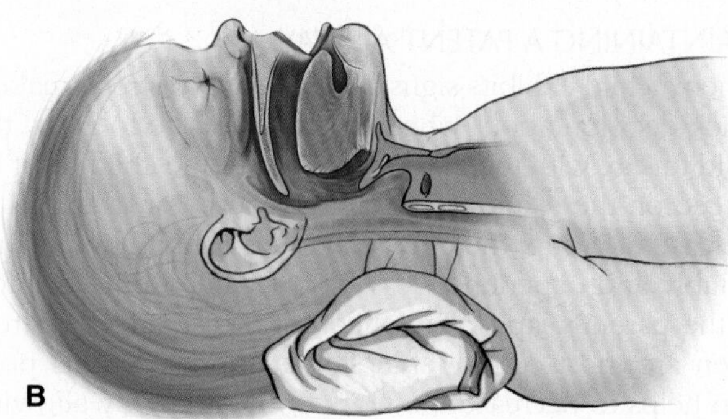

FIGURE 51.3 **(A)** The infant and young child's prominent occiput encourages flexion of the neck and may result in airway occlusion. **(B)** Putting a towel roll under the shoulders or neck helps to open the infant's or young child's airway by placing it in the neutral or "sniff" position.

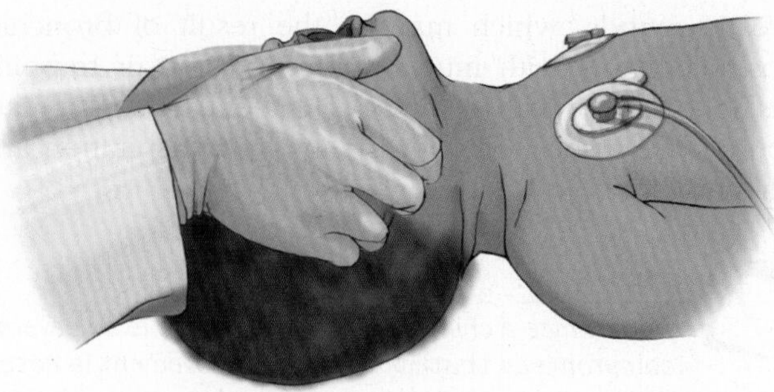

FIGURE 51.4 Jaw-thrust technique for opening the airway.

BVM ventilation (see Table 51.3). (Table 51.3 also lists and discusses assisting with ventilation using tracheal intubation [discussed in detail below], an anesthesia bag or flow-inflating ventilation system, and a laryngeal mask airway.)

BVM ventilation is used in the management of children who cannot ventilate or oxygenate effectively on their own. This technique is a more efficient way of ensuring ventilation than using only supplemental oxygen. In addition, resuscitating a child in this manner is superior to mouth-to-mouth resuscitation as it provides higher oxygen concentrations and protects the nurse from exposure to oral secretions (Berg et al., 2010). However, this technique requires proper training and practice. The proper procedure involves appropriate opening of the airway followed by providing breaths with the BVM.

COMPARISON CHART 51.1 OROPHARYNGEAL VERSUS NASOPHARYNGEAL AIRWAYS

Oropharyngeal airway (used only in unconscious children)	• Consists of a simple plastic curved body that has a central air channel to allow for aeration • Is used when an unconscious child has difficulty maintaining airway patency due to upper airway obstruction, such as from the tongue • Allows for oral suction • Determine the correct size of the airway by placing it next to the child's cheek with the tip pointing down. An airway that is too large will extend past the angle of the child's mandible and can obstruct the glottic opening when inserted • Choose the airway that best fits the child to decrease the risk of injury to the structures of the mouth
Nasopharyngeal airway (may be used in conscious children and children who have an intact gag reflex)	• Consists of a flexible curved tube that is inserted nasally • Is used when the child has difficulty maintaining airway patency due to tongue obstruction or palate problems, when neurologic impairment causes poor pharyngeal tone, or in the child with impaired consciousness • Allows for nasopharyngeal suction • When selecting this airway, keep in mind that the diameter of the airway should not be so large that it puts too much pressure on the internal nasal tissue. There are two common methods for measuring this airway: (a) measure the distance from the end of the child's nose to the tragus of the ear; (b) look at the child's fifth digit, which is usually the approximate diameter of the nasopharyngeal airway • Monitor for mucosal irritation, nasal septum swelling, and laceration of the adenoids • Do not use this type of airway in children with a history of bleeding disorders and basilar skull fractures • This airway's small diameter can easily become obstructed with secretions and blood

TABLE 51.3 AIRWAY AND VENTILATION METHODS

Method	Description	Comments
Anesthesia bag or flow-inflating ventilation systems	A small, collapsible bag that consists of a reservoir bag, an overflow port, and a fresh gas inflow port	• Adjustment of the oxygen flow and of the outlet control valve is necessary • Useful in providing positive end-expiratory pressure (PEEP) or continuous positive airway pressure (CPAP) • Adequate training and significant skill are needed to properly operate this device • Hypercapnia and barotrauma may result with improper use • Used more commonly in the postanesthesia care unit (PACU) and in the neonatal intensive care unit
Bag-valve-mask device or manual resuscitator	A self-inflating oxygen delivery bag that does not require an oxygen source for resuscitation and ventilation. The bag can be connected to oxygen to provide higher oxygen levels than room air. When the child exhales, the nonrebreathing valve closes, allowing exhaled, deoxygenated air to escape	• Effective in providing oxygen to a child who is in severe respiratory distress or who has suffered a respiratory arrest • A more efficient method of respiratory resuscitation than mouth-to-mouth resuscitation; decreased rescuer exposure to communicable disease • Most medical personnel can be trained to perform resuscitation with this method • Possibly tiring for the rescuer when used to ventilate a child for long periods of time (see discussion on bag-mask ventilation)
Laryngeal mask airway	An inflatable silicone mask and rubber connecting tube that is inserted blindly into the airway, forming a seal	• The airway is introduced into the pharynx and advanced until it meets resistance; balloon cuff is then inflated • Easier insertion than a tracheal tube • Usually used in the unconscious child who benefits from bag-valve-mask ventilation but does not require intubation • Improvement in child comfort
Tracheal intubation	A plastic tube inserted in the trachea to establish and maintain an airway when the airway cannot be maintained effectively using other measures (e.g., nasal trumpet or bag-valve-mask ventilation)	• Skilled medical professional (physician, nurse practitioner, respiratory specialist, emergency medical technician, or physician's assistant) necessary for insertion • The nurse acts as a valuable assistant during the intubation procedure

Ventilation with the BVM may be performed with either one or two rescuers. First, choose an appropriate-sized bag and a corresponding face mask that fits the infant or child. Self-inflating bags are usually available in neonatal, infant, child, and adult sizes. Corresponding masks are available. Choose a face mask that properly fits the child's face and that provides a seal over the nose and mouth and excludes the eyes, thus preventing any pressure on the eyes (Fig. 51.5).

Take Note!

Face masks should be clear so that the nurse can see the child's lip color and identify any emesis during resuscitation.

Connect the BVM via the tubing to the oxygen source and turn on the oxygen. When resuscitating infants and children, set the flow rate at approximately 10 L/min. For an adolescent who is adult sized, set the flow rate at 15 L/min or higher to compensate for the larger-volume bag. Check to make sure that the oxygen is flowing through the tubing to the bag. Self-inflating bags do not provide free-flow oxygen out of the face mask; manual pumping of the bag is necessary. However, the bags have a corrugated plastic tail that allows oxygen to freely flow. Therefore, check over the tail for oxygen flow through the bag.

After opening the airway appropriately (see above), place the mask over the child's face. When one rescuer

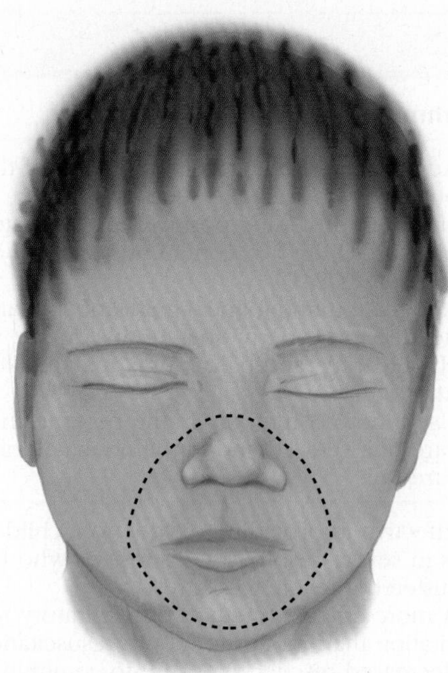

FIGURE 51.5 The mask should form a seal over the nose and mouth, across the chin and nose bridge.

is providing ventilation (commonly referred to as "bagging"), the person must provide a seal with the mask over the child's face with one hand and use the other hand to manipulate the resuscitator bag. The hand used to provide the mask seal will simultaneously maintain the airway in an open position. Generally, use the left thumb and index finger to hold the mask on the child's face. While maintaining a good seal with the mask, use upward pressure on the jaw angle while pressing downward on the mask below the child's mouth to keep the mouth open (Fig. 51.6). Take care not to put pressure on the neck with the fourth and fifth fingers.

If adequate personnel are available, a more desirable situation involves one person standing behind the child's head to maintain an open airway and to provide a seal of the mask over the face with a hand on each side (usually the thumbs and second fingers). A second rescuer stands on one side of the child and compresses the bag to ventilate the child using both hands. If the child is more difficult to ventilate, the two-rescuer method allows the ventilating nurse to provide better ventilation than with the one-rescuer method. In addition, the two-rescuer method ensures the best possible mask seal, as the rescuer holding the mask can use both hands to maintain the seal.

Regardless of the number of persons present, proper placement of the face mask is critical, and a good seal must be maintained throughout the resuscitation. In addition, during ventilation, use only the force and tidal volume necessary to cause a chest rise, no more. If a good chest rise is not observed, attempt to open the airway again. It may be necessary to adjust the position of the airway a few times to achieve a patency conducive to ventilation.

Compress the bag to deliver breaths at the amount recommended in infants and children. Initially, provide two rescue breaths and observe for a chest rise. Rescue breaths should not overinflate the lungs. Breaths should be delivered over 1 second. After the first two rescue ventilations, perform rescue breathing at a rate of one breath every 3 to 5 seconds, or about 12 to 20 breaths per minute. Delivering each breath should be a steady, one-inhalation-to-one-exhalation ratio. This means that the amount of time delivering the inspiratory ventilation is equal to the amount of time that expiration is allowed. While ventilating the infant or child, work with, not against, any spontaneous respiratory effort; in other words, if the child is breathing out, do not attempt to force air in at the same time.

Monitoring Effectiveness of Ventilation. During the resuscitation, continually reassess the child's response to the resuscitative efforts, noting:

- Adequacy of chest rise
- Absence or minimal presence of abdominal distention
- Improved heart rate and pulse oximetry readings
- Improved color
- Capillary refill less than 3 seconds with strengthening pulses

If the child's status deteriorates and he or she becomes pulseless, then CPR must be started. In addition, periodically and briefly stop ventilating to evaluate for spontaneous respirations.

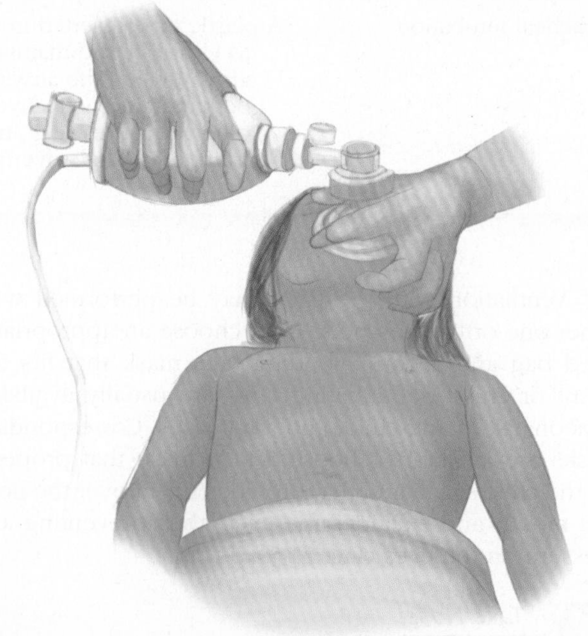

FIGURE 51.6 Proper hand placement for maintaining airway and adequate mask seal using one-rescuer technique.

Preventing Complications Related to Bag-Valve-Mask Ventilation. During resuscitation, healthcare personnel usually exhibit high-energy levels, a normal physiologic response that facilitates resuscitative efforts as the rescuers act quickly. However, this heightened state can lead to overzealousness while ventilating an infant or child. Healthcare providers may inadvertently ventilate the child too rapidly using too much tidal volume, leading to excessive ventilation volume and increased airway pressure. This poor technique can be detrimental to the child, causing:

- Reduced cardiac output (due to increased intrathoracic pressure and increased cardiac afterload)
- Air trapping
- **Barotrauma** (trauma caused by changes in pressure)
- Air leak (thus reducing the oxygen delivered to the child)

In addition, children with head injury who receive excessive ventilation volumes and high rates may develop:

- Decreased cerebral blood flow
- Cerebral edema
- Neurologic damage (AHA, 2011)

Thus, nurses must be mindful of their technique during bagging, not exceeding the recommended respiratory rate or providing too much tidal volume to the child. Ventilate the child in a controlled and uniform manner, providing just enough volume to result in a chest rise.

ASSISTING WITH VENTILATION USING TRACHEAL INTUBATION

Tracheal intubation is needed if the infant or child does not have a maintainable airway or will require artificial ventilation for a prolonged time (see Table 51.3). Intubation of infants and children is a procedure that requires great skill and therefore should be performed by only the most qualified and experienced personnel. Children are most commonly intubated orally, rather than nasally, in acute situations.

Nurses are an essential part of the intubation team, usually assisting a physician, nurse practitioner, respiratory therapist, or physician's assistant during the intubation procedure (Nursing Procedure 51.1). The nurse may set up the equipment, prepare and administer intubation medications, or assist with suctioning the oral secretions and preparing the tape to secure the tracheal tube. In a child in full arrest, the nurse might be responsible for performing ongoing chest compressions while other team members manage the child's airway.

NURSING PROCEDURE 51.1

Assisting with Tracheal Intubation

1. Prepare equipment and supplies.
2. Draw up medications (for rapid sequence intubation).
3. Turn up the volume on the cardiac monitor so that members of the team can easily hear the audible QRS indication of the child's heart rate and note any bradycardia with the procedure.
4. Turn on the suction. Make sure that suction is working by placing your hand over the tubing before you attach the suction catheter.
5. Continue to ventilate the child with the bag-valve-mask (BVM) and 100% oxygen as the team prepares to intubate the child.
6. When there is no suspected cervical spine injury, in the child older than age 2 years, place a small pillow under the child's head to facilitate opening of the airway; this step is unnecessary in children younger than age 2 due to the prominence of their occiput.
7. When assisting with the intubation, stand beside the child's head and prepare to assist with suctioning of oral secretions, providing BVM ventilation as needed, and assisting with securing the tube with tape.
8. Before the initial intubation attempt and after each subsequent attempt to intubate, provide several inhalations of 100% oxygen via the BVM ventilation method (optimally for a few minutes).
9. Administer premedication and medications for sedation.
10. Administer paralyzing medication.
11. Observe as the healthcare professional who is intubating the child follows the recommended procedure for intubation using the laryngoscope to visualize the vocal cords.

Setting Up Equipment. Appropriate setup and preparation of equipment is essential (Table 51.4). The tracheal tube size used depends on the child's size. To calculate tracheal tube size, divide the child's age by 4 and add 4. The resulting number will indicate the size of the tracheal tube in millimeters. For example, if the child is 2 years old, the proper-sized tube would be 4.5 ([2/4] + 4 = 4.5). Always have one size smaller ready also, so have a 4.0 and a 4.5 tracheal tube for this child.

Administering Medications. Several medications are often given to facilitate intubation of children. Premedicating a child before passing a tracheal tube aids in the following:

- Reducing pain and anxiety (consistent with the concept of atraumatic care)

TABLE 51.4 EQUIPMENT AND SUPPLIES FOR TRACHEAL INTUBATION

Laryngoscope blades	Straight blades (Miller) are usually used for infants and young children. A curved-blade laryngoscope (Macintosh) may be used for older children and adolescents. The blade has a little light bulb attached to it for visualization of the trachea. The light bulb should be bright and attached securely.
Tracheal tubes	Three sizes should be readily available: the estimated size, a size smaller, and a size larger. A stylet may be used to guide the tube through the child's vocal cords (it is then removed after the intubation procedure).
Oxygen	100% oxygen is provided using a bag-valve-mask before intubation and after unsuccessful intubation attempts.
Suction	Properly working wall or portable suction with appropriate-sized suction catheters (that fit the tracheal tube) should be prepared; the package is opened, leaving the sterile-tipped end inside the package and connecting the other end to the suction tubing. A Yankauer suction catheter (large catheter) should also be available if copious secretions are present in the mouth that interfere with the ability to visualize the airway.
Monitors	Pulse oximeter and cardiac monitor with an audible tone indicating the QRS complex should be in place. Exhaled CO_2 device is needed to detect increased CO_2 levels after the intubation.
Nasogastric tube	Placing a nasogastric (NG) tube will help to mitigate abdominal distention. Children who are manually ventilated typically have some abdominal distention as some air passes into the stomach.
Personal protective equipment	Usually just gloves, goggles, and a mask are necessary to protect healthcare workers. In the case of copious bleeding, healthcare workers should wear gowns also.
Tape, etc.	Tape should be prepared for securing the tube. Benzoin, a sticky substance, is usually applied under the tape for enhanced security of the tape. For children who have had multiple intubations, a protective barrier (as used to protect the skin around an ostomy) may be applied under the tape to protect the skin. Gauze pads should be available to clean up excess secretions that may interfere with taping the tracheal tube.

- Minimizing the effects of passing the tracheal tube down the airway (vagal stimulation leading to **bradycardia** [decrease in heart rate])
- Preventing hypoxia
- Reducing intracranial pressure
- Preventing airway trauma and aspiration of stomach contents

The use of medications during the intubation process is known as rapid sequence intubation (Table 51.5). Typically, these medications are used in controlled settings such as the emergency department or the intensive care unit (ICU). Rapid sequence intubation is done only in children who are not experiencing cardiac arrest. If the intubation is expected to be particularly difficult, paralyzing medication should not be used.

The nurse must be aware of the differences in the various medication classes, their advantages, their disadvantages, and adverse effects. The nurse must also be able to distinguish between medications that produce sedation and ones that produce analgesia. Children who are paralyzed and sedated may be suffering severe pain. The pain control needs of children who are acutely ill are of paramount importance and cannot be overstated. Do not mistake a child who is immobilized as a result of sedative and paralytic medications for a child who is pain-free.

Take Note!

Attempts to insert a tracheal tube should last no longer than 20 to 30 seconds each. After each attempt, the child should receive multiple ventilations by the BVM method using 100% oxygen (AHA, 2011).

Ensuring and Maintaining Correct Tube Placement. To assess for correct placement once the tracheal tube is inserted, observe for symmetric chest rise and auscultate over the lung fields for equal breath sounds. Inspect the tracheal tube for the presence of water vapor on the inside, indicating that the tube is in the trachea. To rule out accidental esophageal intubation, auscultate over the abdomen while the child is being ventilated: there should not be breath sounds in the abdomen. Note improvement in the oxygen saturation level via pulse oximetry.

TABLE 51.5	MEDICATIONS FOR RAPID SEQUENCE INTUBATION	
Medications	**Desired Effects**	**Undesirable Effects**
Anticholinergic: atropine	Decreases respiratory secretions and mitigates the vagal affects of intubation, thus decreasing the risk of bradycardia	Doses that are too low (<0.1 mg) can cause a paradoxical bradycardia. Young infants are more prone to the bradycardic effects of atropine, so its use is generally contraindicated in this population.
Sedatives: barbiturates—thiopental (short-acting barbiturate)	Has very rapid onset and short duration of action; reduces intracranial pressure and oxygen demand	Hypotensive effects of this drug are more severe in the dehydrated child. When given in combination with narcotics, respiratory depression is potentiated.
Sedatives: benzodiazepines—midazolam	Has a slightly slower onset than thiopental but is associated with fewer adverse effects Also causes amnesia Can be titrated up or down (at lower doses it causes conscious sedation; at higher doses it can induce anesthesia)	When given in combination with narcotics, respiratory depression is potentiated.
Anesthetic agent: ketamine	Has a rapid onset with sedative, amnesic, and analgesic affects. Can be dissociative (child is awake but unaware). May improve BP and cause bronchodilation (helpful for children with status asthmaticus)	Ketamine can cause increased intracranial pressure and increased ocular pressure. Therefore, children who have suffered head trauma or globe injury should not receive this medication. Because of ketamine's sympathetic effects, hypertension can result from its use. Ketamine tends to cause increased secretions, often necessitating the concomitant use of atropine to counteract this adverse effect. May cause hallucinations and is therefore contraindicated in children with psychiatric problems.
Anesthetic agent: lidocaine	Can decrease intracranial pressure at higher doses Has an advantage when used in the management of hypovolemia because it is less likely to cause hypotension	Lidocaine can cause adverse cardiac effects (bradycardia, hypotension, dysrhythmias) in high doses. May be associated with CNS depression and seizures.
Narcotic analgesic: fentanyl citrate	A highly concentrated opioid that causes fewer adverse effects (e.g., pruritus) than other opioids Also exerts a less hypotensive effect	Constipation and urinary retention (as is common with opioids) may occur. Increases risk for respiratory depression, increased intracranial pressure, and hypotension. Chest wall rigidity is common with this drug and may cause difficulty with ventilation.
Paralyzing or neuromuscular blocking agents: rocuronium, succinylcholine, vecuronium	Used for short-term paralysis during the intubation process. May be used for extended paralysis in ICU for children in whom movement would be detrimental. For example, a child with epiglottitis has a very precarious airway and must remain intubated until the epiglottis decreases in size. In certain respiratory conditions, spontaneous respiratory effort would interfere with the ventilation of a child and therefore prolonged paralysis is desirable.	Succinylcholine (a depolarizing agent) has always been the gold standard for paralysis because it has a relatively rapid onset and is short acting. However, it has a greater risk of adverse effects (bradycardia, hyperkalemia, hypertension, increased intracranial, and ocular pressure) and is contraindicated in a variety of clinical conditions. The contemporary approach to paralysis involves the use of longer-acting agents, such as rocuronium and vecuronium, because children have fewer adverse effects with these medications. In addition, rocuronium and vecuronium may be used for extended paralysis (not an option with succinylcholine).

CNS, central nervous system.

Adapted from Kleinman, M. E., Chameides, L., Schexnayder, S. M., Samson, R. A., Hazinski, M. F., Atkins, D. L., et al. (2010). Part 14: Pediatric advanced life support: 2010 American Heart Association guidelines for cardiopulmonary resuscitation and emergency cardiovascular care. *Circulation, 122*, S876–S908; and Taketomo, C. K., Hodding, J. H., & Kraus, D. M. (2013). *Pediatric & neonatal dosage handbook* (20th ed.). Hudson, OH: Lexicomp.

BOX 51.1

EXHALED CO_2 MONITORING OR END-TIDAL CO_2 MONITORING

- Device that connects to the child's ventilator circuit to detect CO_2 in the tubing. CO_2 should be noted in the tubing after six ventilations.
- Devices are usually color coded. In the case of tracheal intubation, observe the color on the device change from purple to tan to yellow.
- Colors on the end-tidal CO_2 device correspond with tracheal tube placement:
  - Purple = little or no CO_2 detected, <3 mm Hg
  - Tan = 3 to 15 mm Hg exhaled CO_2
  - Yellow = >15 mm Hg exhaled CO_2 (Krauss, Silvestri, & Falk, 2014)
- NOTE: colorimetric end-tidal CO_2 devices may at times fail to detect the presences of exhaled carbon dioxide, so continue to rely upon visualization of tube placement, symmetric chest rise, and bilateral breath sounds (AHA, 2011)

Once tracheal tube placement is verified, mark the tube with an indelible pen at the level of the child's lip and secure it with tape. Document the number on the tracheal tube at the level of the child's mouth. Anticipate a chest x-ray to confirm correct placement of the tracheal tube.

After placement is confirmed, the tracheal tube is connected to the ventilator by respiratory personnel. The ventilator will provide continuous artificial ventilation and oxygenation. Exhaled CO_2 monitoring is recommended as it provides an indication of appropriate ventilation (Box 51.1). If an exhaled CO_2 monitor is being used, the exhaled CO_2 should be yellow.

The nurse plays a key role in ensuring that the tracheal tube remains taped securely in place by doing the following:

- Using soft wrist restraints if necessary to prevent the child from removing the tracheal tube
- Providing sedative and/or paralyzing medications
- Using caution when moving the child for x-ray, changing linens, and performing other procedures

Monitoring the Child Who is Intubated. Provide ongoing and frequent monitoring of the intubated child to determine adequacy of oxygenation and ventilation as noted earlier. Once the child is intubated, the ventilatory support being provided should result in improvement in oxygen saturation and vital signs. If the child begins to exhibit signs of poor oxygenation, perform a quick assessment. Auscultate the lungs for equal air entry and determine the heart rate. Are the breath sounds equal? Is the heart rate normal for age? Perform a quick survey of the equipment and look for any disconnected tubes or kinks in the tubing. Determine oxygen saturation levels via pulse oximeter and evaluate the end-tidal CO_2 color (see Box 51.1). Use the mnemonic "DOPE" for troubleshooting when the status of a child who is intubated deteriorates:

D = Displacement. The tracheal tube is displaced from the trachea.

O = Obstruction. The tracheal tube is obstructed (e.g., with a mucous plug).

P = Pneumothorax. Usually a pneumothorax results in a sudden change in the child's assessment. The signs of a pneumothorax include decreased breath sounds and decreased chest expansion on the side of the pneumothorax. Subcutaneous emphysema may be noted over the chest. In the case of tension pneumothorax, there may be a sudden drop in heart rate and blood pressure.

E = Equipment failure. Relatively simple problems as previously discussed, such as a disconnected oxygen supply, can cause the child to deteriorate. Culprits such as a leak in the ventilator circuit or a loss of power are other types of equipment failure that may be responsible (Kleinman et al., 2010a).

Make sure all equipment is appropriately connected and functional. When obstruction with secretions is suspected, suction the tracheal tube. If the tracheal tube is displaced from the trachea, remove the tube if it remains in the child's mouth and begin BVM ventilation. In the case of pneumothorax, prepare to assist with needle thoracotomy.

Preparing the Intubated Child for Transport. Once the child is stabilized with a secure tracheal tube in place, prepare to transport the child. The child will be moved by stretcher to an intensive care unit in the acute care facility or by air or land ambulance to another facility that specializes in the care of acutely ill children. Make sure that all tubes are taped securely. During transport, use portable oxygen and ventilate manually with the BVM. As the sending nurse, ensure that all laboratory results are obtained and provided to the receiving nurse. If the child is going to another facility, complete a detailed summary of the resuscitation or provide a copy of the nurse's and/or progress notes. Complete the appropriate transfer forms as determined by the institution.

If the child is being transported by ambulance, the parents may not be able to accompany their child. In this case, find out as much as possible about the transport and assist the parents by giving directions to the receiving institution.

SHOCK

Shock may be defined as an inability for blood flow and oxygen delivery to meet the metabolic demands of tissue (Kleinman et al., 2010b). If shock is left untreated, cardiopulmonary arrest will result. Shock, which may be classified as compensated or decompensated, is due to a variety of clinical problems. Compensated shock occurs when poor perfusion exists without a decrease in BP. In decompensated shock, inadequate perfusion is accompanied by a drop in BP. Unchecked decompensated shock leads to cardiac arrest and death. The principles of PALS stress the early evaluation and management of children in compensated shock with the goal of preventing decompensated shock (Kleinman et al., 2010b). Once the child in shock is hypotensive, organ perfusion is dramatically impaired and a dire clinical scenario ensues.

Pathophysiology

Shock is the result of dramatic respiratory or hemodynamic compromise. Impaired cardiac output, impaired systemic vascular resistance (SVR), or a combination of both causes shock. Cardiac output (CO) is equal to heart rate (HR) times ventricular stroke volume (SV) (CO = HR × SV). Stroke volume is how much blood is ejected from the heart with each beat. Stroke volume is related to left ventricular filling pressure, the impedance to ventricular filling, and myocardial contractility. Left ventricular filling pressure is also known as preload, and the impedance to ventricular filling is commonly called afterload. Young children and infants have relatively small stroke volumes compared to older children and adults. Therefore, infants and young children differ from their adult counterparts in that their cardiac output depends on their heart rate, not their stroke volume. Clinically, in cases of circulatory compromise and compensated shock in infants and children, the heart rate is increased. The exception to this is a paradoxical phenomenon in neonates, who may have bradycardia rather than tachycardia.

SVR or afterload is the impediment to the heart's ventricular ejection. Increased SVR will result in a decrease in blood flow unless the ventricular pressure increases. Increased vascular resistance is a common problem in shock. In children who have shock-related increased SVR, cardiac output will fall unless the ventricle can compensate by increasing pressure. In cardiac insufficiency, the child's heart will have impaired ability to compensate for the increased afterload.

Altered microcirculatory status is common in all types of shock. Compensatory mechanisms are activated in response to decreased blood flow. Sympathetic nervous system response results in marked contraction of larger-vessel sphincters and arterioles. This compression results in dramatically impaired capillary blood flow. Blood is redirected away from less important body systems, such as the skin and the kidneys, to the vital organs (the heart and brain).

During compensated shock, the body can maintain some level of blood flow to the vital organs. Peripheral vasoconstriction, the body's compensatory response to diminished blood flow, often results in the child's ability to maintain a normal or near-normal BP. As shock continues, capillary beds become obstructed by cellular debris, and platelets and white blood cells aggregate. Endothelial damage occurs as a result of capillary congestion. Poor blood flow to the capillaries results in anaerobic metabolism. Lactic acid accumulates, and this can lead to acidosis. In addition, children with septic shock sustain marked endothelial damage as a result of exposure to bacterial toxins.

The cumulative effect of capillary obstruction and dramatically impaired blood flow is tissue ischemia. As tissue ischemia progresses, the child will show signs of altered perfusion to vital organs. For example, as blood flow to the brain is diminished, the child will demonstrate an altered level of consciousness. Altered blood flow to the kidneys will result in decreased urine output or absence of urine output (oliguria). Commonly, the heart rate will increase in the early stages of shock, but as the heart becomes compromised as a result of poor perfusion, the child will become bradycardic. The child will demonstrate an increased respiratory rate in the initial phase of shock. Tachypnea is seen in septic shock as well. In fact, the child may demonstrate marked hyperventilation in an effort to blow off carbon dioxide in response to the acidosis that is associated with septic shock.

Types of Shock

The most common types of shock are hypovolemic, septic, cardiogenic, and distributive. Hypovolemic shock, the most common type of shock in children, occurs when systemic perfusion decreases as a result of inadequate vascular volume (Kleinman et al., 2010b). Children commonly have hypovolemic shock that occurs in association with fluid losses. For example, hypovolemic shock may occur with gastroenteritis that results in vomiting and diarrhea, medications such as diuretics, and heat stroke. Other causes of hypovolemia in children include blood loss, such as from a major injury, and third spacing of fluid, such as with burns.

Septic shock is related to a systemic inflammatory response in which there may be increased cardiac output with a low SVR, known as warm shock. More commonly in children, septic shock results in a decrease in cardiac output with an increase in SVR, known as cold shock.

Cardiogenic shock results from an ineffective pump, the heart, with a resultant decrease in stroke volume. Children with structural heart disease and resultant arrhythmia are at risk for cardiogenic shock (Pomerantz & Roback, 2014).

Distributive shock is the result of a loss in the SVR. A relative hypovolemia occurs, most often with neurogenic injury–related shock and anaphylaxis. In relative hypovolemia, the vascular compartment expands due to systemic vasodilation. This results in a relatively larger vasculature requiring more fluid to maintain cardiac output despite no actual loss of fluid.

Finally, toxic drug ingestions may also lead to shock.

Nursing Assessment

Nursing assessment of the child in shock includes the health history and physical examination as well as laboratory and diagnostic testing. The nursing assessment must be performed quickly and accurately so that resuscitation can be expedited.

HEALTH HISTORY

In shock, the health history is based on the child's presentation. Children with shock are critically ill and require emergent intervention. Therefore, the history is obtained as life-saving interventions are provided. Determine when the child first became ill and treatments that have been given thus far. Inquire about sources of volume loss, such as:

- Vomiting
- Diarrhea
- Decreased oral intake
- Blood loss

Ask when the child last urinated. Investigate for other related symptoms such as behavioral changes or lethargy. Has the child had a fever or rash, complained of headache, or been exposed to anyone with similar symptoms? Inquire about day care attendance and whether the family has recently traveled outside of the country. Determine if the child has a history of a congenital heart defect or other heart condition or if the child has severe allergies. Ask the parent about accidental ingestion of medications or other substances and, for the older child or adolescent, about the possibility of illicit substance use.

PHYSICAL EXAMINATION

The key to successful shock management is early recognition of the signs and symptoms. Obtain vital signs, noting any alterations. Measure BP, although this is not a reliable method of evaluating for shock in children. Children tend to maintain a normal or slightly less than normal BP in compensated shock while sacrificing tissue perfusion until the child suffers a cardiopulmonary arrest. Therefore, other components of the circulatory evaluation will be more valuable when assessing a child.

Take Note!

Bradycardia is a serious sign in neonates and may occur with respiratory compromise, circulatory compromise, and/or overwhelming sepsis (Kattwinkel et al., 2010).

As with any emergency, evaluate the airway first. Is it patent? Then determine if the child is breathing. The child in shock will often demonstrate signs of respiratory distress, such as grunting, gasping, nasal flaring, tachypnea, and increased work of breathing. Auscultate breath sounds to determine the adequacy of air entry and airflow. If the child shows signs of respiratory distress, manage the airway and breathing problem first, as discussed earlier in the chapter.

Assess the skin color. Palpate the skin temperature and determine quality of pulses. Except in special cases, such as distributive shock, the child in shock will generally have darker and cooler extremities with delayed capillary refill. Note the line of demarcation if present. This refers to the point on the distal extremity where cool temperature begins (the proximal portion of the extremity may continue to be warm). In distributive shock, the initial assessment will reveal full and bounding pulses and warm, erythemic skin. Evaluate the pulse quality. Distal pulses will likely be weaker than central pulses.

Evaluate the child's hydration state and check skin turgor. Decreased elasticity is associated with hypovolemic states, though this is usually a late sign. Observe the child's face; in compensated shock the child may be awake but obtunded and demonstrate signs of distress. The child in decompensated shock may have his or her eyes closed and may be responsive only to voice or other stimulation. Evaluate pupillary responses. Determine urinary output, which will be decreased in the child with shock.

After having evaluated and provided initial lifesaving management for airway, breathing, and circulation, evaluate the child's entire body for other disabilities. Injuries warrant vigilant evaluation for ongoing blood loss, although they may also produce internal blood loss (e.g., a femur fracture). Look for signs of malformation, swelling, redness, or pain of the extremities, which may suggest internal blood loss. Also inspect for any open wounds and active sites of bleeding. Children with abdominal injuries also may lose copious amounts of blood internally. Inspect the abdomen for redness, skin discoloration, or distention. Auscultate for bowel sounds in all four quadrants.

LABORATORY AND DIAGNOSTIC TESTING

As the child is being resuscitated, laboratory tests and x-rays will be ordered and obtained. However, no diagnostic test should replace the priority of respiratory support, vascular access, and fluid administration. Laboratory results will guide ongoing management. Common laboratory and diagnostic tests used for children with shock include:

- Blood glucose levels: usually performed at the bedside using a glucose meter to obtain a rapid result
- Electrolytes: to evaluate for electrolyte abnormalities
- CBC with differential: to assess for viral or bacterial infection (septic shock) and to evaluate for anemia and platelet abnormalities

- Blood culture: to evaluate for sepsis; preliminary results will not be available for 1 to 2 days
- C-reactive protein: to evaluate for infection
- Arterial blood gases: to assess oxygen and carbon dioxide levels and to provide information about acid–base balance
- Toxicology panel (if ingestion is suspected)
- Lumbar puncture: to evaluate the cerebrospinal fluid for meningitis
- Urinalysis: to evaluate for glucose, ketones, and protein; concentration (specific gravity) is increased in dehydration states
- Urine culture: to evaluate for urinary tract or kidney infection
- x-rays: to evaluate heart size, to evaluate the lungs for pneumonia or pulmonary edema (present with cardiogenic shock)

Nursing Management

Signs of shock in children warrant an emergent response.

MANAGING THE CHILD'S ABCs

Always evaluate and manage the airway and breathing and check for pulses. Initiate CPR if the child is pulseless. All children who have signs and symptoms of shock should receive 100% oxygen via mask. If the child has poor respiratory effort or is apneic, administer 100% oxygen via BVM or tracheal tube (refer to the section on respiratory emergencies for more specific information about management of airway and breathing). As part of ongoing monitoring, institute cardiac and apnea monitoring and assess oxygen saturation levels via pulse oximetry.

OBTAINING VASCULAR ACCESS

Once the airway and breathing are addressed, nursing management of shock focuses on obtaining vascular access and restoring fluid volume. Children with signs of shock should receive generous amounts of isotonic IV fluids rapidly. However, obtaining vascular access in critically ill children can be challenging. Vascular access must be obtained using the quickest route possible in children whose condition is markedly deteriorated, such as those in decompensated shock.

Various forms of vascular access available for the management of the critically ill child include:

- Peripheral IV route: a large-bore catheter is used to give large amounts of fluid. This route may not be feasible in children with significant vascular compromise.
- Central IV route: central lines can be inserted into the jugular vein and threaded into the superior vena cava. The femoral route is best for obtaining central venous access while CPR is in progress because the insertion procedure will not interfere with life-saving interventions involving the airway and cardiac compressions. The subclavian vein, located under the clavicle, is an alternative route for central access.
- Saphenous vein: the saphenous vein (found in the ankle) is an alternative route for venous access that is obtained using a surgical incision.
- Intraosseous access: intraosseous access, obtained by cannulating the bone marrow, is recommended in cases of decompensated shock or cardiac arrest if IV access cannot be attained rapidly. The preferred site is the anterior tibia. Special intraosseous needles are used (generally a 15-gauge needle for older children, 18-gauge for younger children). The needle is inserted using a firm twisting motion slightly away from the growth plate. Any medications or fluids that can be administered using an IV site can be given using this route. Alternative sites include the femur, the iliac crest, the sternum, and the distal tibia.

RESTORING FLUID VOLUME

Administer IV isotonic fluids, such as Ringer's lactate or normal saline (the isotonic fluids of choice) rapidly. Administer 20 mL/kg of the prescribed fluid as a bolus, infusing the fluid as rapidly as possible. In general, a large-bore syringe, such as a 35- to 60-mL syringe attached to a three-way stopcock, is the preferred method for rapid fluid delivery in children. Infusing the fluid via gravity is too slow. The fluid bolus may be repeated up to two times (for a total of three times) if required.

Take Note!

Dextrose solutions are contraindicated in shock because of the risk of complications such as osmotic diuresis, hypokalemia, hyperglycemia, and worsening of ischemic brain injury (AHA, 2011).

Children in septic shock will often require larger volumes of fluid as a result of the increased capillary permeability. Children in shock due to trauma will usually receive a colloid, such as blood, when there is an inadequate response to crystalloid isotonic fluid. After each fluid bolus, reassess the child for signs of positive response to the fluid administration.

Insert an indwelling urinary catheter to allow for accurate and frequent measurement of urine output.

Indicators of improvement include:

- Improved cardiovascular status: the central and peripheral pulses are stronger. The line of demarcation of extremity coolness is diminishing and capillary refill is improved (time is decreased). BP is improved.
- Improved mental status: the child is more alert. For example, the child's eyes are open and watching personnel. If the child is younger, he or she may be pulling at the IV line.
- Improved urine output: this may not be noted initially but should be noted over the next few hours; the goal is 1 to 2 mL/kg/hr.

The process of fluid resuscitation involves giving the fluid, assessing and reassessing the child, and documenting findings. Children in shock may require as much as 100 to 200 mL/kg of resuscitative fluid during the initial hours of shock management. Most children in shock need and can tolerate this large volume of fluid. Continued reassessment will determine if the child is beginning to experience fluid overload in the form of pulmonary edema (this is rare but may occur in children with preexisting cardiac conditions or severe chronic pulmonary disease) (AHA, 2011; Pasman & Watson, 2015).

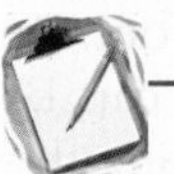

Take Note!

Do not focus solely on the child's circulatory status; you may overlook signs and symptoms of respiratory deterioration.

ADMINISTERING MEDICATIONS

In some circumstances, such as septic shock or distributive shock, fluid alone does not adequately improve the child's status and adjunctive medications may be ordered. Vasoactive medications are used either alone or in combination to improve cardiac output, to increase SVR, or to decrease SVR. The selection of medications is dictated by the child's cardiac and vascular status. For example, dobutamine is a medication with significant β-adrenergic effects and thus can improve cardiac contractility. Epinephrine, which affects the heart muscle, is also a powerful vasoconstrictor. Dopamine affects the heart at lower doses but increasingly affects the vasculature with increased doses. These medications may be given as a loading dose, followed by a continuous infusion. When vasoactive drugs are administered, monitor for improvement in heart rate, BP, perfusion, and urine output.

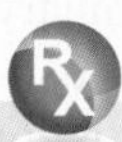

Dosage Calculation Box 51.1

Child's weight: 55 lb

Medication order: epinephrine 100 mg IV STAT. Per the *Pediatric Dosage Handbook,* the recommended dose is 0.01 mg/kg (0.1 mL/kg of 1:10,000 solution) per dose. Is the ordered dose safe?

CARDIAC ARRHYTHMIAS AND ARREST

Unlike adults, in whom cardiopulmonary arrest is most often caused by a primary cardiac event, children typically have healthy hearts and thus rarely experience primary cardiac arrest. More commonly they experience cardiopulmonary arrest from gradual deterioration of respiration and/or circulation (Kleinman et al., 2010a). In particular, children experiencing a respiratory emergency or shock may deteriorate and eventually demonstrate cardiopulmonary arrest. Thus, the standard of care for managing a child in this situation is vastly different from that for an adult.

Nurses should be skilled in evaluating and managing respiratory alterations and shock in children, as discussed in previous sections. Overwhelming evidence suggests that if primary respiratory compromise or shock is identified and treated in the critically ill child, a secondary cardiac arrest can be prevented.

Rare exceptions do exist, however. For example, electrolyte abnormalities and toxic drug ingestions are primary insults to the cardiovascular system that may lead to a sudden cardiac arrest rather than a gradual progression. Other exceptions in which the child is at risk for a primary and sudden cardiac arrest include:

- History of a serious primary congenital or acquired cardiac defect
- Potentially lethal arrhythmias, such as prolonged QT syndrome
- Hyper- or hypotrophic cardiomyopathy
- Traumatic cardiac injury or a sharp blow to the chest, known as "commotio cordis" (e.g., when a high-velocity ball hits the chest)

The overwhelming majority of children rarely experience cardiac arrhythmias, so it is beyond the scope of this chapter to discuss the myriad possible complex rhythm disturbances. Therefore, this discussion will be limited to the management of emergent cardiac conditions that are more typically found in children.

Pathophysiology

The AHA (2011) has simplified the nomenclature used to describe pediatric cardiac compromise and has established three major categories of cardiac rhythm disturbances:

- Slow: bradyarrhythmias
- Fast: tachyarrhythmias
- Absent: pulseless, cardiovascular collapse

The pathophysiology, causes, and therapeutic management of each of the categories of rhythm disturbances are discussed below.

BRADYARRHYTHMIAS

Bradycardia is a heart rate significantly slower than the normal heart rate for age. Bradycardia in children is most commonly sinus bradycardia. In other words, there is not a cardiac nodal abnormality associated with the slowed heart rate. In sinus bradycardia, the P waves and QRS complex remain normal on the ECG. Brief dips in heart rates can be normal, such as when the child sleeps. Children are also susceptible to brief drops in heart rate that are associated with vagal stimulation. For example, passing an orogastric tube down the esophagus of a young infant may induce a temporary bradycardic response.

COMPARISON CHART 51.2 CAUSES OF SINUS BRADYCARDIA VERSUS HEART BLOCK

	Sinus Bradycardia	Heart Block
Causes	• Pathologic: medications such as digoxin, hypoxia, hypothermia, head injury • Nonpathologic: well-conditioned athlete	• Congenital: associated with cardiac anomalies • Acquired: endocarditis, rheumatic fever, Kawasaki disease

These normal decreases in the child's heart rate should recover with or without stimulation and are not normally associated with signs of altered perfusion.

Less commonly, children manifest bradycardia as a result of cardiac abnormalities and heart block. Infants with bradycardia related to heart block may exhibit poor feeding and tachypnea, whereas older children may demonstrate fatigue, dizziness, and syncope. Comparison Chart 51.2 compares the causes of sinus bradycardia and heart block in children.

In contrast, the child with a serious and possibly life-threatening bradyarrhythmia will have a heart rate below 60 bpm, with signs of altered perfusion. The most common causes of profound bradycardia in children are respiratory compromise, hypoxia, and shock. Sustained bradycardia is commonly associated with arrest. It is an ominous sign and should be taken seriously.

TACHYARRHYTHMIAS

Children normally have faster heart rates than adults, and fever, fear, and pain are common explanations for significant increases in the heart rate of a child (**tachycardia**). This normal elevation in heart rate is known as sinus tachycardia. However, once the fever is reduced, the child is comforted, or the pain is managed, the heart rate should return close to the child's baseline. Hypoxia and hypovolemia are pathologic reasons for tachycardia in the child. The signs, symptoms, and management of these concerns were discussed in previous sections. If the child has sinus tachycardia that results from any of these causes, the focus is on the underlying cause. It is inappropriate and dangerous to treat sinus tachycardia with medications aimed at decreasing the heart rate or with a defibrillation device.

Tachyarrhythmias in children that are associated with cardiac compromise have unique characteristics that present differently from sinus tachycardia. Examples of these include SVT and ventricular tachycardia. SVT is a cardiac conduction problem in which the heart rate is extremely rapid and the rhythm is very regular, often described as "no beat-to-beat variability." Comparison Chart 51.3 explains the differences between SVT and sinus tachycardia. The most common cause of SVT is a reentry problem in the cardiac conduction system. Commonly, SVT is the result of a genetic cardiac conduction problem such as Wolff–Parkinson–White syndrome. SVT may also be associated with medications such as caffeine and theophylline. Children often can tolerate the characteristically higher heart rate that is associated with SVT for short periods of time. However, the increased demand that is placed on the cardiovascular system usually overtaxes the child and results in signs of congestive heart failure if the SVT continues unchecked for a prolonged time.

Ventricular tachycardia is a rhythm involving an elevation of the heart rate and a wide QRS (greater than 0.08 seconds) that is the result of an abnormal, rapid firing of one or both of the ventricles. Ventricular tachycardia is a rare arrhythmia in children and usually is associated with a congenital or acquired cardiac abnormality. In addition, prolonged QT syndrome is a conduction abnormality that can result in ventricular tachycardia and sudden death in children. Less commonly, ingestion of medications and toxins, acidosis, hypocalcemia, abnormalities

COMPARISON CHART 51.3 DISTINGUISHING SUPRAVENTRICULAR TACHYCARDIA (SVT) FROM SINUS TACHYCARDIA

	SVT	Sinus Tachycardia
Rate (bpm)	Infants >220, children >180	Infants <220, children <180
Rhythm	Abrupt onset and termination	Beat-to-beat variability
P waves	Flattened	Present and normal
QRS	Narrow (<0.08 seconds)	Normal
History	Usually no significant history	Fever, fluid loss, hypoxia, pain, fear

of potassium, and hypoxemia have been associated with the development of ventricular tachycardia in children.

COLLAPSED RHYTHMS (PULSELESS RHYTHMS)

A collapsed rhythm, as defined by PALS, is one that produces cardiac arrest with no palpable pulse and no signs of perfusion (cardiac arrest) (AHA, 2011). Typically, the most common pulseless arrest rhythms in children are asystole or pulseless electrical activity (PEA). **Asystole** occurs when there is no cardiac electrical activity, commonly referred to as "a straight line" on the ECG. The child with PEA has some appreciable rhythm on the ECG but no palpable pulses. PEA may be caused by hypoxemia, hypovolemia, hypothermia, electrolyte imbalance, tamponade, toxic ingestion, tension pneumothorax, or thromboembolism. Ventricular tachycardia may also present as pulseless. Ventricular fibrillation, once thought to be rare in children, occurs in serious cardiac conditions in which the ventricle is not pumping effectively. It may develop from ventricular tachycardia. Ventricular fibrillation (VF) is characterized by variable, high-amplitude waveforms (coarse VF) or a finer, lower-amplitude waveform with no discernible cardiac rhythm (fine VF). In either case, cardiac output is insufficient.

Nursing Assessment

Nursing assessment of the child with a cardiac emergency includes the health history and physical examination as well as laboratory and diagnostic testing. The nursing assessment must be performed quickly and accurately so that resuscitation can be instituted if needed.

HEALTH HISTORY

Obtain a brief health history of the child with a cardiac emergency while simultaneously assessing the child and providing life-saving interventions. Key areas to inquire about include:

- History of cardiac problems, asthma, chromosomal anomaly, delayed growth
- Symptoms such as syncope, dizziness, palpitations or racing heart, chest pain, coughing, wheezing, increased work of breathing
- Activity tolerance with play or feeding: Does the child get out of breath, turn blue, or squat during play? Can the child keep up with playmates? Does the infant tire with feedings?
- Precipitating illness, fever, unexplained joint pains, ingested medications
- Participation in a sport before the cardiac event occurred or injury to the chest
- Family history of cardiac problems, sudden death from a cardiac condition, heart attacks at a young age, chromosomal abnormalities
- Treatment measures performed at the scene: Was CPR initiated? Was an AED used?

PHYSICAL EXAMINATION

Quickly establish the child's status. A child who is obviously in distress or is arresting must receive emergent life-saving interventions. Briefly perform the assessment while simultaneously providing life-saving interventions.

Inspection and Observation. Assess the child's airway patency and efficiency of breathing. Observe the child's color, noting circumoral pallor or duskiness or central pallor, mottling, duskiness, or cyanosis. Note any increased work of breathing, grunting, head bobbing, or apnea. Inspect the chest for barrel shape, which may be associated with chronic pulmonary or cardiac disease. Observe the pericardium for the presence of lifts or heaves. Note diaphoresis, anxious appearance, or dysmorphic features (almost 50% of children with Down syndrome also have a congenital cardiac defect [Chen, 2016]). Determine if neck vein distention is present. Inspect the fingertips for clubbing, which is indicative of chronic tissue hypoxemia.

Auscultation. Auscultate the breath sounds, noting any crackles or wheezes. Auscultate the heart rate. If the child does not have an adequate pulse, initiate CPR. If the child has a strong, perfusing pulse, complete the cardiac assessment. Auscultate with the diaphragm of the stethoscope first and then listen with the bell. Evaluate all of the auscultatory areas, listening first over the second right interspace (aortic valve) and then over the second left interspace (pulmonic valve); next move to the left lower sternal border (tricuspid area); and finally auscultate over the fifth interspace, midclavicular line (mitral area). Evaluate the rate and rhythm of the heart. Listen for any extra sounds or murmurs. Note and describe the quality, intensity, and location of any cardiac murmurs.

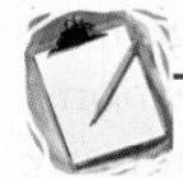

Take Note!

Murmurs are most often systolic and can be benign or associated with pathology.

Percussion and Palpation. Percuss between the costal interspaces and note the heart's size. Palpate the heart to find the point of maximal impulse (PMI) and to evaluate for an associated thrill. A thrill feels like a fluttering under the fingers and is associated with cardiac pathology. Palpate and note the quality of the pulses. Evaluate each of the pulses bilaterally and note whether they are absent, faint, normal, or bounding. Compare the quality of pulses on each side of the body and also those of the upper and lower body. Note the skin temperature and evaluate the capillary refill.

LABORATORY AND DIAGNOSTIC TESTING

The major diagnostic test used is the ECG. Identify the arrhythmia according to the ECG reading (Fig. 51.7).

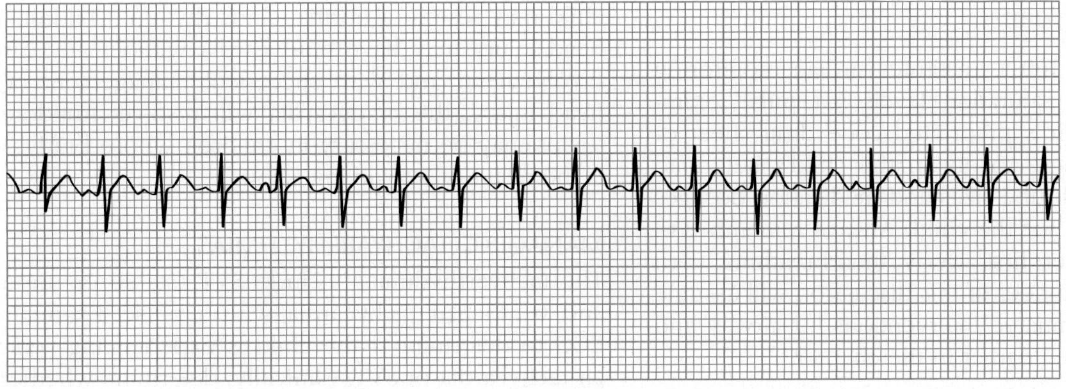

A

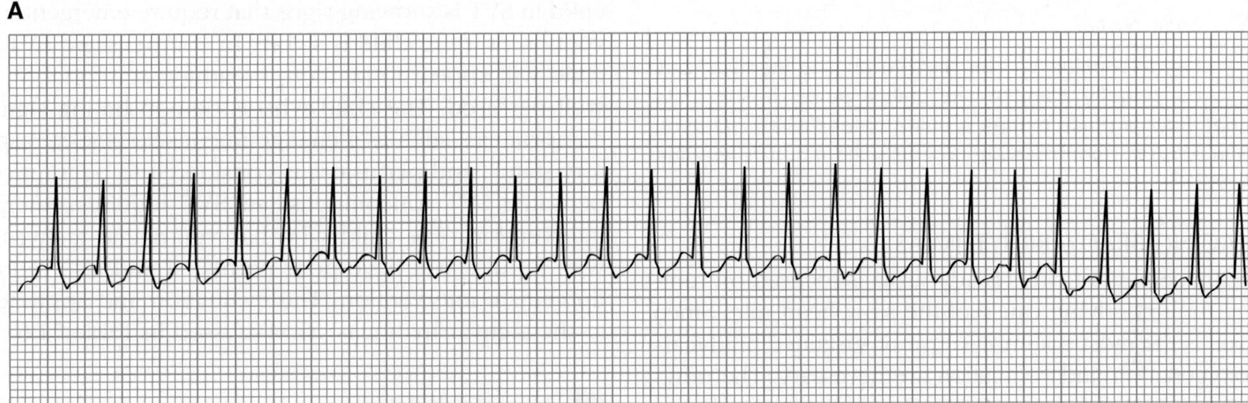

B

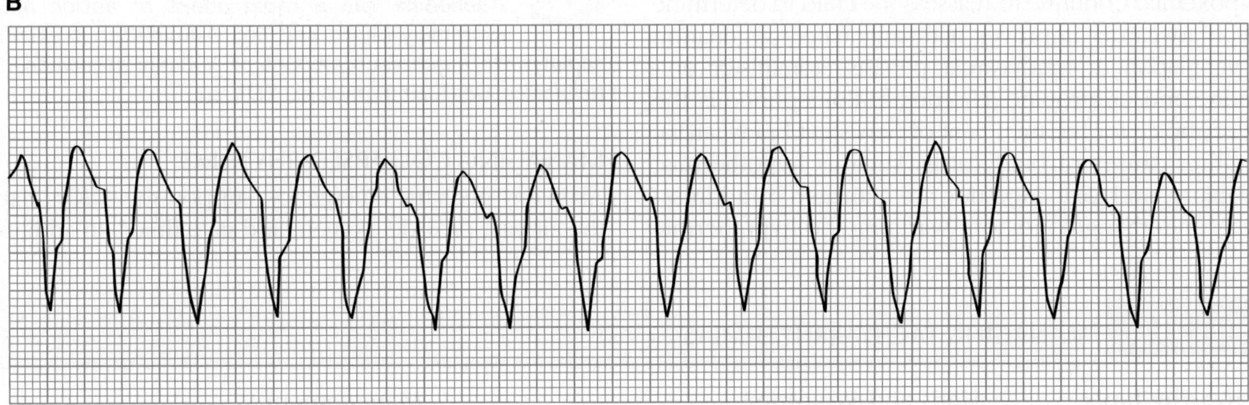

C

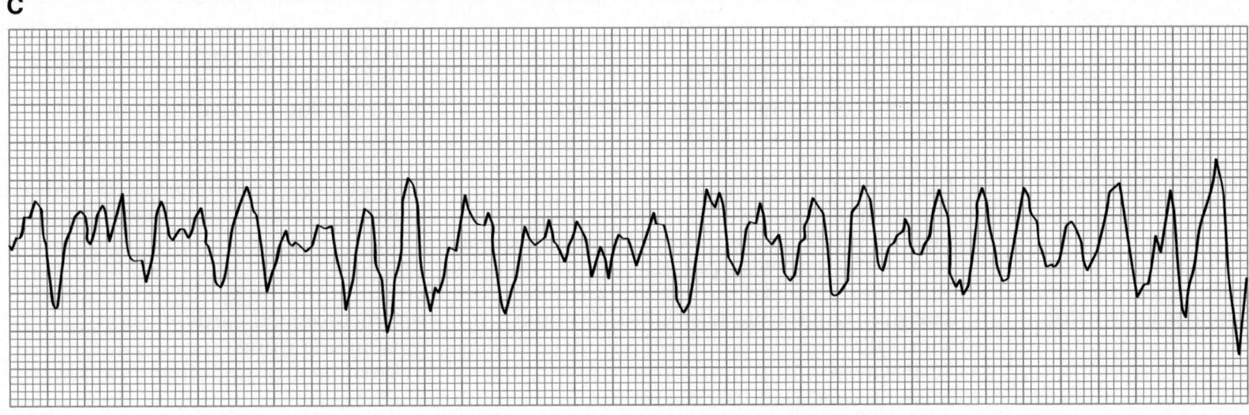

D

FIGURE 51.7 Arrhythmias. **(A)** Sinus tachycardia: normal QRS and P waves, mild beat-to-beat variability. **(B)** Supraventricular tachycardia: note rate above 220, abnormal P waves, no beat-to-beat variability. **(C)** Ventricular tachycardia: rapid and regular rhythm, wide QRS without P waves. **(D)** Coarse ventricular fibrillation: chaotic electrical activity.

Nursing Management

Provide oxygen at 100%. Institute cardiac monitoring and assess oxygen saturation levels via pulse oximetry. Obtain the child's preprinted code drug sheet or use the Broselow tape to obtain the child's height to estimate the tracheal tube sizes and medication dosages that are appropriate for the child. Always remember to intervene in this order: first airway, then breathing, then circulation. The remainder of this discussion will assume that the nurse has initiated interventions for airway and breathing as discussed earlier in the chapter.

> **Take Note!**
>
> Pay attention to the rhythm on the monitor, but continually monitor the child's pulse. If the child does not have a pulse or has a pulse of less than 60 bpm, perform cardiac compressions despite the monitor reading (AHA, 2011).

MANAGING BRADYARRHYTHMIAS

The management of sinus bradycardia is focused on remedying the underlying cause of the slow heart rate. Since hypoxia is the most common cause of sustained bradycardia, oxygenation and ventilation are necessary. The newborn is particularly susceptible to bradycardia in relation to hypoxemia. Continue to reassess the child to determine if the bradycardia improves with adequate oxygenation and ventilation. If bradycardia persists, administer epinephrine and/or atropine as ordered. Epinephrine is the drug of choice for the treatment of persistent bradycardia.

Other causes of bradycardia such as hypothermia, head injury, and toxic ingestion are managed by addressing the underlying condition. Warming the hypothermic child may restore a normal sinus rhythm. Children with head injury may have bradycardia without any cardiac involvement, and with successful management of the head injury, the bradycardia will resolve. Antidotes to toxins may be necessary in children whose bradycardia is the result of a toxic ingestion.

MANAGING TACHYARRHYTHMIAS

The tachyarrhythmias include SVT (stable or unstable) and ventricular tachycardia with a pulse. Examine the ECG to determine if the child is experiencing ventricular tachycardia or SVT. Clinically, determine whether the child in SVT is showing signs that require emergent intervention or if the child is stable. In compensated SVT, the child will appear to be alert, breathing comfortably, and well perfused. The child who is demonstrating signs of compromise, such as a change in consciousness, respiratory status, and perfusion, is considered to be in uncompensated SVT. Uncompensated SVT requires emergent intervention. The child who has ventricular tachycardia with a pulse will have poor perfusion and also requires immediate intervention. The evaluation and approaches to the tachyarrhythmias are discussed in Table 51.6.

> **Take Note!**
>
> Adenosine has a rapid onset of action and an extremely short half-life. Administer it extremely rapidly with a generous amount of IV flush; otherwise, it will be ineffective (Kleinman et al., 2010a).

MANAGING COLLAPSED RHYTHMS

As in any pediatric emergency, support the ABCs. Manage the airway, provide oxygen, and give fluids. In addition, if

TABLE 51.6 MANAGING TACHYARRHYTHMIAS

Tachyarrhythmia	Signs and Symptoms	Management
Compensated SVT	• Tachycardia, heart rate >220 • Abnormal P waves • Alert, well-perfused child • Possible complaints of headache and dizziness in older children	• Vagal maneuvers such as ice to face or blowing through a straw that is obstructed • Adenosine if vagal maneuvers fail
Uncompensated SVT	• Tachycardia, heart rate >220 • Abnormal P waves • Signs of shock: altered level of consciousness, poor perfusion, weak pulses	• Adenosine or synchronized cardioversion
Ventricular tachycardia	• Rate may range from normal to 200 bpm. • Wide QRS • No P waves • Pulse present, poor perfusion	• Synchronized cardioversion • IV amiodarone • Treatment of underlying causes

Adapted from Kleinman, M. E., Chameides, L., Schexnayder, S. M., Samson, R. A., Hazinski, M. F., Atkins, D. L., et al.; American Heart Association (2010). Pediatric advanced life support: 2010 American Heart Association guidelines for cardiopulmonary resuscitation and emergency cardiovascular care. *Pediatrics, 126*, e1361–e1399.

TABLE 51.7 ECG CHARACTERISTICS AND MANAGEMENT OF PULSELESS RHYTHMS

Pulseless Arrhythmia	ECG Characteristics	Management
Ventricular tachycardia	Wide QRS, no P waves	• CPR • Defibrillation • Epinephrine; also possibly amiodarone, lidocaine, or magnesium • Treat underlying causes
Ventricular fibrillation	• Chaotic ventricular activity • No P waves, no QRS, no T waves	• CPR • Defibrillation • Epinephrine; also possibly amiodarone, lidocaine, or magnesium • Treat underlying causes
Asystole	Flat line	• Check lead placement • CPR if no pulse • Epinephrine
Pulseless electrical activity	Electrical activity that is not consistent with ventricular tachycardia or ventricular fibrillation	• Check lead placement • CPR if no pulse • Treat underlying cause • Epinephrine

Adapted from Kleinman, M. E., Chameides, L., Schexnayder, S. M., Samson, R. A., Hazinski, M. F., Atkins, D. L., et al. (2010). Pediatric advanced life support: 2010 American Heart Association guidelines for cardiopulmonary resuscitation and emergency cardiovascular care. *Pediatrics, 126*, e1361–e1399.

the child is pulseless or has a heart rate less than 60 bpm, initiate cardiac compressions (see the section on providing CPR earlier in the chapter). In addition, some children may require medications and/or defibrillation or synchronized cardioversion. The pulseless rhythms include ventricular tachycardia, ventricular fibrillation, asystole, and PEA. ECG characteristics and management of these rhythms are summarized in Table 51.7. Also treat the underlying causes of the arrhythmia, if known.

The AHA emphasizes the importance of cardiac compressions in pulseless individuals with arrhythmias (Kleinman et al., 2010a). Give compressions before and immediately after defibrillation (see defibrillation section earlier in the chapter). Administer medications such as epinephrine, lidocaine, or amiodarone as ordered. In the past it was recommended that individuals who required defibrillation be given three shocks in a row, but recent research findings have shown that the individual should be defibrillated only once, followed by five cycles of CPR. For defibrillation to be most effective, cardiac compressions must be performed effectively with minimal interruptions (Kleinman et al., 2010a).

DROWNING (SUBMERSION INJURY)

Water can be a great source of fun and exercise for children and adolescents, but drowning is the second-leading cause of preventable death in children and adolescents in the United States and worldwide (World Health Organization, 2014). In warm-weather states where swimming pools are more common, drowning is the primary cause of death in young people. Most drowning deaths are preventable, and the World Health Organization (2014) notes that “lapse in adult supervision is the single most important contributory cause for drowning.”

Survival and neurologic outcome of drowning depend on early and appropriate resuscitation. In recent years, with appropriate resuscitation efforts and treatment, children have demonstrated better neurologic outcomes (Chandy & Weinhouse, 2015).

Pathophysiology

Typically, a child who is drowning will struggle to breathe and eventually will aspirate water. Aspiration of relatively small amounts of water leads to poor oxygenation, with retention of carbon dioxide. Alveolar surfactant is depleted during the drowning event and pulmonary edema commonly occurs. Hypoxemia results in increased capillary permeability and resultant hypovolemia. Even small amounts of aspirated water may lead to pulmonary edema within an 8-hour period after the drowning episode (Chandy & Weinhouse, 2015). A drowning survivor is also at risk for renal complications due to altered renal perfusion during the hypoxemic state.

Nursing Assessment

Nursing assessment of the drowning survivor is crucial and must take place quickly and accurately.

HEALTH HISTORY

Obtain the history rapidly while providing life-saving interventions. Ask about the circumstances of the event:

- Where did the incident occur? Was the child in a lake, river, ocean, or swimming pool? Was the child submerged in a toilet, bucket, or bathtub?
- Did someone witness the child's entry into the water?
- Was the water fresh or salty? Cold or warm?
- Is it likely the water was contaminated?
- Were there any extenuating circumstances, such as a diving or automobile accident, associated with the near drowning?
- What was the approximate length of time of the submersion? Was the child conscious or unconscious when rescued?
- What was done at the scene? Was CPR initiated? If so, when?
- If a cervical spine injury was suspected, was the cervical spine immobilized?
- Was an AED used?
- When did the child last eat (to prepare for possible intubation)?

PHYSICAL EXAMINATION

Evaluate airway patency and breathing. Auscultate all lung fields for signs of pulmonary edema, such as coarseness or crackles. Evaluate the heart rate, pulses, and perfusion. Note the cardiac rhythm on the monitor and report evidence of arrhythmias. Evaluate the child's neurologic status. Use a pen light to determine pupillary reaction. Use the pediatric coma score to further assess the neurologic status. Does the child open the eyes spontaneously, to stimuli, or not at all? Is there any spontaneous movement? Is the younger child crying? Can the older child speak? Measure the child's temperature, as hypothermia often occurs with near drowning.

LABORATORY AND DIAGNOSTIC TESTING

While awaiting laboratory and diagnostic testing results, continue resuscitative efforts as addressed below. Laboratory and diagnostic tests typically include the following:

- Arterial blood gases: hypoxemia, acidosis
- ECG: cardiac arrhythmias
- Chest radiography: pulmonary edema, infiltrates
- Serum electrolytes: imbalance related to development of shock

Nursing Management

Because of the potentially devastating effects that drowning-related hypoxia has on the child's brain, airway interventions must be initiated immediately after retrieving a child from the water. Every second counts. Initial interventions for a drowning victim are always focused on the ABCs; commonly, resuscitative efforts have begun before the child arrives at the acute care facility.

If a cervical spine injury is suspected (as in the case of a diving accident), provide stabilization either manually or with a cervical collar. As with any suspected neck injury, do not remove the cervical collar until injury to the cervical spine has been ruled out through a x-ray and clinical evaluation. Suction the airway to ensure airway patency. The child may have aspirated particles from a contaminated water source or emesis, a relatively common complication associated with drowning. A large-bore suction catheter (e.g., Yankauer) is an effective tool for clearing the upper airway. Administer supplemental oxygen at 100%. Children who have poor or absent respiratory effort most likely will require intubation. Insert an orogastric or nasogastric tube to decompress the stomach and prevent aspiration of stomach contents. Initiate chest compressions if a pulse is not present.

Usually, the child exhibits some degree of hypothermia and will require warming. Generally, the core body temperature should be raised slowly, as warming a drowning victim too quickly may have deleterious effects. Remove any wet clothing, dry the child, and cover him or her with warmed blankets. Warm IV fluids and use other warming methods as prescribed.

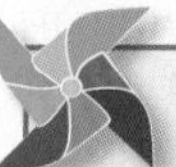

Consider This

A father says to you, "I can't believe my toddler almost drowned. I turned away for a few minutes to check the hamburgers on the grill. I feel terrible. I'll never be able to let her go near a swimming pool again."

Thoughts: What will your response be to this father? How can you best support him and assist him to work through his emotions?

POISONING

Emergency care of the pediatric poisoning victim consists of rapid nursing assessment and prompt management.

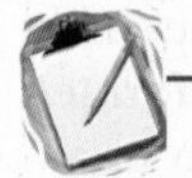

Take Note!

If a normally healthy child (particularly a young child) suddenly deteriorates without a known cause, suspect a toxic ingestion.

Nursing Assessment

Nursing assessment of the poisoning victim focuses on a thorough health history, followed by physical examination and laboratory and diagnostic testing.

Health History

Obtain the health history from the parents or caregiver or, in the case of an older child or teenager, from the child. Inquire about the approximate time of poisoning and the nature of the toxin. Was the toxin ingested, inhaled, or applied to the skin? In the case of pill ingestion, does the caregiver have the medication bottle? Did the child experience nausea, vomiting, anorexia, abdominal pain, or neurologic changes such as disorientation, slurred speech, or altered gait? Determine the progression of the symptoms. Did the parent or caregiver call the National Poison Control Center Hotline? Has any treatment been given? In the case of older children and teens, inquire about any history of depression or threatened suicide.

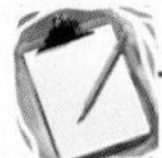

Take Note!

The National Poison Control Center Hotline number is 1-800-222-1222.

Physical Examination

Ingestion of medications or chemicals may result in a wide variety of clinical manifestations. Perform a thorough physical examination, noting alterations that may occur with particular ingestions, such as:

- Hyper- or hypotension
- Hyper- or hypothermia
- Respiratory depression or hyperventilation
- Miosis (pupillary contraction) or mydriasis (pupillary dilatation)

Pay particular attention to the child's mental status, skin moisture and color, and bowel sounds (Velez, Shepherd, & Goto, 2016).

Laboratory and Diagnostic Testing

The suspected poison may direct the laboratory and diagnostic testing. A variety of blood tests may be performed:

- Chemistry panel: to detect hypoglycemia or metabolic acidosis and assess renal function
- ECG: to identify arrhythmias or conduction delay
- Liver function tests: to assess for liver injury
- Urine and blood toxicology screens (available for a limited number of medications; may vary per institution)
- Specific drug levels if the substance ingested is known or highly suspected

Nursing Management

When poisoning occurs, give priority to the child's ABCs. Treat alterations as discussed earlier in this chapter. Monitor vital signs frequently and provide supportive care. Few specific antidotes are available for medications or other toxins. Activated charcoal may be administered to bind with the chemical substance in the bowel. Alternatively, whole bowel irrigation with polyethylene glycol electrolyte solutions may be necessary. Occasionally, dialysis is required to lower the level of toxin in the bloodstream. The intervention is based on the source of the ingestion. For example, activated charcoal is an effective method for preventing the absorption of many medications but is not effective in the case of an iron overdose.

If opiate or other narcotic ingestion is suspected, administer naloxone to reverse the respiratory depression or altered level of consciousness. Treatment of seizures and alterations in thermoregulation may also be needed.

Specific treatment of the poisoning will be determined when the toxin is identified and poison control is queried. Maintain ongoing assessment of the poisoned child because many toxins exhibit very late effects.

Take Note!

Syrup of ipecac is no longer recommended for home treatment to induce vomiting after an accidental ingestion (AAP, 2015).

TRAUMA

The leading cause of death in children and adolescents is unintentional injuries (Centers for Disease Control and Prevention [CDC], 2016). Falls are the most common cause of pediatric injury and automobile accidents continue to be a top cause of death in all child age groups (CDC, 2016). Childhood trauma also results from pedestrian accidents, sporting and bicycling injuries, and firearm use. Children of varying ages are susceptible to various forms of injury due to their developmental level as well as their environmental exposure. Young children rely on their caregivers to promote their safety. Young children also are not developmentally equipped to be able to recognize dangerous situations. Because pediatric injury is so common, nurses must become adept at assessment and intervention in the pediatric trauma victim.

Nursing Assessment

The trauma survey includes a brief health history as the child is being assessed and life-saving measures are being instituted.

Health History

Begin the health history by asking when the injury happened. If the child sustained a motor vehicle–related injury, ask how fast the vehicle was going. Determine if the child was appropriately restrained in the automobile. If the child was riding a bicycle, skateboarding, or using in-line skates, was he or she wearing a helmet, knee pads, and wrist guards? Determine what interventions were performed at the scene. Was the child immobilized on a backboard to protect the cervical spine? If the child is bleeding, ask the person who transported the child to estimate the amount of blood lost.

If the child experienced a fall, ask if the fall was witnessed and the height from which the child fell. Did the child fall onto a hard surface such as concrete? How did the child land: on the head or back, or did the child catch himself or herself with the hands? Younger children and boys are at higher risk for injuring their head. Did the child lose consciousness at the scene? What kind of behavior did the child exhibit after the fall? Since the fall, has the child complained of a headache or been vomiting?

While obtaining a detailed history about the fall, think about the child's developmental stage. For example, does it seem plausible that a toddler might fall down the stairs? In contrast, what is the likelihood that a 2-month-old would suffer a fractured femur from a fall? Keep in mind the possibility of child abuse. Critically evaluate the reported circumstances and try to determine if the history, developmental stage of the child, and type of injury sustained match. In addition, evaluate the type of injury that the child sustained and the history given by the caregiver. For example, children who fall from significant heights often suffer skeletal fractures, but abdominal and chest injuries rarely result from falling from significant heights.

Physical Examination

Physical examination of the child with a traumatic injury should be approached with an evaluation of the ABCs (primary survey) first. Assess the patency of the airway and establish the effectiveness of breathing (as discussed earlier in the chapter). Examine the child's respiratory effort, breath sounds, and color. Next, evaluate the circulation. Note the pulse rate and quality. Observe the color, skin temperature, and perfusion. If bleeding has occurred, the child's circulation may become compromised.

After assessing and intervening for the child's ABCs, proceed to the secondary survey. Assess for disability (D). Rapidly assess critical neurologic function. Determine the level of consciousness, pupillary reaction, and verbal and motor responses to auditory and painful stimuli. If the child is a young infant, palpate the anterior fontanel: a full and bulging fontanel signals increased intracranial pressure. The traumatized child's neurologic status may range from completely normal to comatose.

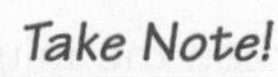

Take Note!

Unequal pupils or a fixed and dilated pupil is considered a neurosurgical emergency. Immediately report this finding.

Following the ABCs and D (disability) is E (exposure). Expose the child to observe the entire body for signs of injury, whether blunt or penetrating. Perform a systematic, thorough inspection of the child's body. Note active bleeding and extremity deformity, as well as any lacerations and abrasions. Observe for movement and any complaints of immobility or pain with movement. Inspect the abdomen for redness, skin discoloration, or distention. Auscultate for bowel sounds in all four quadrants. If the child is verbal, ask if he or she has any pain in the stomach. If the child is younger, ask, "Do you have a tummy ache?" If the child reports abdominal pain, ask the child to point to where it hurts. Note any guarding of the abdomen, which is an indication of abdominal pain. If bowel injury is a possibility, only light palpation is acceptable. Always assess the least tender areas first and palpate the more sensitive areas last.

Laboratory and Diagnostic Testing

As in other pediatric emergencies, never delay life-saving measures to wait for laboratory or diagnostic test results. In addition to routine laboratory tests, common laboratory and diagnostic tests for the pediatric trauma victim include:

- Type and cross-match: to assess the child's blood type before blood products are given
- Prothrombin time and partial thromboplastin time: to evaluate for clotting dysfunction
- Amylase and lipase: to identify pancreatic injury
- Liver function tests: to assess for liver injury
- Pregnancy test (in any female who has reached puberty)
- CT scan, ultrasound, or MRI of the head, abdomen, or extremities: to evaluate the extent of the injury

Nursing Management

Nursing management of the pediatric trauma victim focuses initially on the ABCs.

Providing Immediate Care

If head or spinal injury is suspected, open the airway using the jaw-thrust maneuver with cervical spine stabilization (see Fig. 51.4). The guidelines for basic life support recommend that if the airway cannot be opened using the jaw-thrust maneuver, it may be opened using the head tilt–chin lift maneuver since opening the airway is a priority (Berg et al., 2010). The head and neck of a trauma victim should be stabilized manually.

Take Note!

Infants and young children require unique cervical spine management because they have prominent occiputs that result in flexion of the neck in the supine position. To maintain the optimal neutral spinal position in the young child, use a special pediatric backboard with a head indentation, or use a folded towel to elevate the child's torso.

Clear the airway of obstruction using a large-bore suction device such as a Yankauer. If the child is breathing on his or her own, give oxygen at the highest flow possible (such as with a nonrebreathing mask). If the child is not breathing on his or her own, intervene with basic life support discussed earlier in this chapter (Berg et al., 2010).

If a BVM device is available, connect it to the oxygen source and use the bag to ventilate the child. Observe the chest rise and be careful not to overventilate, as this results in abdominal distention. Deliver breaths at a rate of one breath every 3 seconds (Berg et al., 2010). Do not hyperventilate. In the not-too-distant past, head injury in children was managed using hyperventilation. This resulted in **hypocapnia** (decreased amounts of carbon dioxide in the blood). The physiologic effect of hypocapnia is the induction of vasoconstriction, which in turn results in tissue ischemia. Therefore, current management of head injury in children does not use hyperventilation. The only exception to this rule is in an acute situation, if the child is showing signs of a possible brain stem herniation, hyperventilation may be used initially and briefly.

Assess the child for a strong central pulse. If the child has no pulse, initiate CPR immediately. When perfusion is compromised, administer IV fluid resuscitation. Trauma victims are more likely to require colloids or blood products due to blood loss from the injury.

Take Note!

Children with head injury who have signs of shock such as poor perfusion and bradycardia should receive fluid volume resuscitation (Kleinman et al., 2010b).

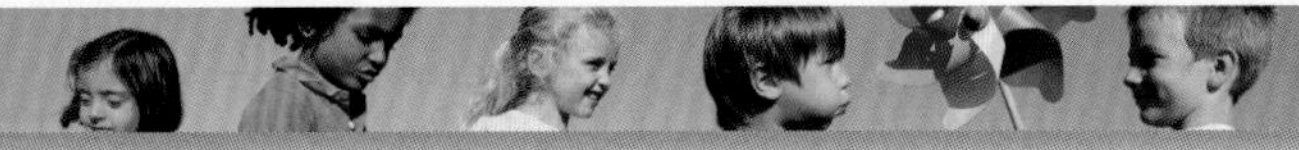

KEY CONCEPTS

- Young children's smaller airways and immature respiratory and immune systems place them at higher risk for respiratory distress than older children and adults. Children generally have healthy hearts and cardiovascular systems and thus rarely present with primary cardiac arrest. Younger children and adolescents are at higher risk for injury due to normal development at those ages.
- Children present with a variety of emergencies and injuries and must be evaluated and treated in an appropriate and timely fashion to achieve a positive outcome. The health history is obtained rapidly while life-saving measures are performed simultaneously.
- Assess the airway, then breathing, then circulation, providing interventions for alterations before moving on to the next assessment. Provide continuous reassessment, as children respond quickly to interventions and deteriorate quickly as well.
- Pulse oximetry and capnometry can be useful tools for evaluating respiratory status. Never delay intervention pending laboratory results if the child's clinical status warrants immediate action.
- Provide support and education to the child and family involved in an emergency. Teach families why certain procedures are being done, explaining technical medical interventions in simple terms and, for the child, at his or her developmental level.
- Small amounts of edema or secretions can contribute to significant respiratory effort in infants and young children.
- Children dehydrate more quickly than adults and experience alterations in perfusion related to hypovolemia.
- Children in respiratory distress and shock require supplemental oxygen. Intubation is necessary for the apneic child or the child whose airway is not maintainable.
- Accurate assessment of perfusion status and appropriate fluid resuscitation are critical in the prevention and treatment of shock in children.
- Life-threatening arrhythmias in children, though uncommon, often must be quickly treated with defibrillation or synchronized cardioversion in addition to CPR.
- In the case of near drowning, maintain ongoing assessment and intervention of pulmonary status.
- Maintain airway, breathing, and circulation in the child who has experienced an accidental ingestion and prepare for gastric lavage or administration of activated charcoal.
- In addition to intervening for airway, breathing, and circulation problems in the pediatric trauma victim, assess for altered neurologic status and extent of bleeding or injury.

REFERENCES AND RECOMMENDED READINGS

American Academy of Pediatrics. (2016). *Protect your child: Prevent poisoning*. Retrieved from http://www.healthychildren.org/English/safety-prevention/all-around/Pages/Keep-Your-Home-Safe-From-Poisons.aspx

American Academy of Pediatrics. (2016). *Summer safety tips: Sun and water safety*. Retrieved from https://www.aap.org/en-us/about-the-aap/aap-press-room/news-features-and-safety-tips/Pages/Sun-and-Water-Safety-Tips.aspx

American Academy of Pediatrics. (2011). Technical report SIDS and other sleep-related infant deaths: Expansion of recommendations for a safe infant sleeping environment. *Pediatrics, 128*, e1341–e1367.

American Heart Association. (2011). *Pediatric advanced life support provider manual*. Dallas, TX: Author.

Berg, M. D., Schexnayder, S. M., Chameides, L., Terry, M., Donoghue, A., Hickey, R. W., et al. (2010). Part 13: Pediatric basic life support: 2010 American Heart Association guidelines for cardiopulmonary resuscitation and emergency cardiovascular care. *Circulation, 122*, S862–S875.

Bowden, V. R., & Greenberg, C. S. (2012). *Pediatric nursing procedures* (3rd ed.). Philadelphia, PA: Lippincott Williams & Wilkins.

Carpenito-Moyet, L. J. (2013). *Nursing diagnosis: Application to clinical practice* (14th ed.). Philadelphia, PA: Lippincott Williams & Wilkins.

Cecchin, F., Jorgenson, D. B., Berul, C. I., Perry, J. C., Zimmerman, A. A., Duncan, B. W., et al. (2001). Is arrhythmia detection by automatic external defibrillator accurate for children? Sensitivity and specificity of an automatic external defibrillator algorithm in 696 pediatric arrhythmias. *Circulation, 103*, 2438–2483.

Centers for Disease Control and Prevention. (2016). *Ten leading causes of death and injury*. Retrieved from http://www.cdc.gov/injury/wisqars/leadingcauses.html

Centers for Disease Control and Prevention, & National Center for Injury Prevention and Control. (2015). *Tips to prevent poisoning*. Retrieved from http://www.cdc.gov/HomeandRecreationalSafety/Poisoning/preventiontips.htm

Chandy, D., & Weinhouse, G. L. (2015). *Drowning (submersion injuries)*. Retrieved from http://www.uptodate.com/contents/drowning-submersion-injuries

Chen, H. (2016). *Down syndrome*. Retrieved from http://emedicine.medscape.com/article/943216-overview

Corbett, J. A., & Banks, A. D. (2013). *Laboratory tests and diagnostic procedures with nursing diagnoses* (8th ed.). Upper Saddle River, NJ: Pearson Education Inc.

Diaz, M. C. (2013). Early use of AEDs can save kids' lives. *Contemporary Pediatrics, 30*(3), 12–20.

Fleisher, G. R., & Ludwig, S. (2010). *Textbook of pediatric emergency medicine* (6th ed.). Philadelphia, PA: Lippincott Williams & Wilkins.

Gilger, M. A., Jain, A. K., & McOmber, M. E. (2015). *Foreign bodies of the esophagus and gastrointestinal tract in children*. Retrieved from http://www.uptodate.com/contents/foreign-bodies-of-the-esophagus-and-gastrointestinal-tract-in-children

Jones, M. A. (2016). *Preparing an office practice for pediatric emergencies*. Retrieved from http://www.uptodate.com/contents/preparing-an-office-practice-for-pediatric-emergencies

Kattwinkel, J., Perlman, J. M., Aziz, K., Colby, C., Fairchild, K., Gallagher, J., et al. (2010). Part 15: Neonatal resuscitation: 2010 American Heart Association guidelines for cardiopulmonary resuscitation and emergency cardiovascular care. *Circulation, 122*, S909–S919.

Kleinman, M. E., Chameides, L., Schexnayder, S. M., Samson, R. A., Hazinski, M. F., Atkins, D. L., et al. (2010a). Part 14: Pediatric advanced life support – 2010 American Heart Association guidelines for cardiopulmonary resuscitation and emergency cardiovascular care. *Circulation, 122*, S876–S908.

Kleinman, M. E., Chameides, L., Schexnayder, S. M., Samson, R. A., Hazinski, M. F., Atkins, D. L., et al.; American Heart Association. (2010b). Pediatric advanced life support: 2010 American Heart Association guidelines for cardiopulmonary resuscitation and emergency cardiovascular care. *Pediatrics, 126*, e1361–e1399.

McAlvin, S. S., & Carew-Lyons, A. (2014). Family presence during resuscitation and invasive procedures in pediatric critical care: A systematic review. *American Journal of Critical Care, 23*(6), 477–484.

Pasman, E. A., & Watson, C. M. (2015). *Shock in pediatrics*. Retrieved from http://emedicine.medscape.com/article/1833578-overview

Pomerantz, W. J., & Roback, M. G. (2014). *Physiology and classification of shock in children*. Retrieved from http://www.uptodate.com/contents/physiology-and-classification-of-shock-in-children

Salib, E. A., Cyran, S. E., Cilley, R. E., Maron, B. J., & Thomas, N. J. (2005). Efficacy of bystander cardiopulmonary resuscitation and out-of-hospital automated external defibrillation as life-saving therapy in commotio cordis. *Journal of Pediatrics, 147*, 863–866.

Stanley, M., & Pollard, D. (2013). Relationship between knowledge, attitudes, and self-afficacy of nurses in the management of pediatric pain. *Pediatric Nursing, 4*, 165–171.

Taketomo, C. K., Hodding, J. H., & Kraus, D. M. (2013). *Pediatric & neonatal dosage handbook* (20th ed.). Hudson, OH: Lexicomp.

Velez, L. I., Shepherd, J. G., & Goto, C. S. (2016). *Approach to the child with occult toxic exposure*. Retrieved from http://www.uptodate.com/contents/approach-to-the-child-with-occult-toxic-exposure

U.S. Department of Health and Human Services. (2016). *Healthy people 2020*. Retrieved from http://www.healthypeople.gov/2020/default

World Health Organization. (2014). *Drowning*. Retrieved from http://www.who.int/mediacentre/factsheets/fs347/en/

CHAPTER WORKSHEET

MULTIPLE CHOICE QUESTIONS

1. An unresponsive toddler is brought to the emergency department. Assessment reveals mottled skin color, respiratory rate of 10 breaths per minute, and a brachial pulse of 52 bpm. What is the priority nursing action?
   a. Prepare the defibrillator and draw up code medications.
   b. Provide 100% oxygen with a bag-valve-mask and start chest compressions.
   c. Start chest compressions and provide 100% oxygen via nonrebreather mask.
   d. Begin an IV fluid infusion and administer epinephrine IV.
2. A 10-year-old child in respiratory distress requires intubation. Which sizes of tracheal tubes will the nurse prepare?
   a. 9.5 mm and 10.0 mm
   b. 8.5 mm and 9.0 mm
   c. 6.0 mm and 6.5 mm
   d. 6.5 mm and 7.0 mm
3. A preschooler presents to the emergency department with a history of vomiting, diarrhea, and fever over the past few days. She is receiving 100% oxygen via nonrebreather mask. Vital signs are temperature 104.5°F, pulse 144 bpm, respiratory rate 22 breaths per minute, and BP 70/50 mm Hg. She is listless and difficult to arouse and has weak peripheral pulses and prolonged capillary refill. What nursing intervention takes priority?
   a. administering acetaminophen rectally for the high fever
   b. administering IV antibiotics for the infection
   c. preparing the child for tracheal intubation
   d. giving an IV bolus of normal saline 20 mL/kg
4. Assessment of a 12-year-old who crashed his bicycle without a helmet reveals the following: temperature 99.2°F, pulse 100 bpm, respiratory rate 24 breaths per minute with easy work of breathing, and BP 102/70 mm Hg. What is the priority action by the nurse?
   a. Assess neurologic status while observing for obvious injuries.
   b. Administer IV fluid bolus of normal saline at 20 mL/kg.
   c. Remove the cervical collar if he complains that it bothers him.
   d. Listen for bowel sounds while assessing for pain.
5. An 18-month-old child is brought to the emergency department via ambulance after an accidental ingestion. What is the priority nursing action?
   a. Take the child's vital signs.
   b. Give oral syrup of ipecac.
   c. Insert a nasogastric tube.
   d. Start an IV line.

DOSAGE CALCULATION QUESTION

1. The nurse is caring for an infant with supraventricular tachycardia who is symptomatic and has an IV line in place. The infant weighs 16 ½ lb. The medication order reads: adenosine 0.01 mg/kg IV STAT followed by rapid flush. Adenosine is supplied as 6 mg/2 mL. How many milliliters will the nurse administer? Round to the nearest hundredth.

CRITICAL THINKING EXERCISES

1. A school-age child presents to the emergency department for evaluation. He had been feeling faint off and on and today fainted at school. On the cardiac monitor an abnormal cardiac rhythm is noted. At present the child is stable. What questions would be most appropriate for the nurse to ask when obtaining the child's health history? What objective assessments should the nurse make?
2. Charlie is a 2-year-old who is admitted to the hospital after accidentally ingesting a medication. His mother, who brought Charlie to the hospital, is upset and crying. How does Charlie's age and stage of development affect his risk for accidental ingestion? How should the nurse respond to the mother's distress? Develop a discharge teaching plan for Charlie and his family related to poison prevention.
3. A 7-month-old is brought to the acute care facility with a chief complaint of difficulty breathing. The infant's mother says that his cold has gotten worse and he won't eat. What additional questions should the nurse ask about the infant's health history? How would the nurse appropriately manage this infant's airway?

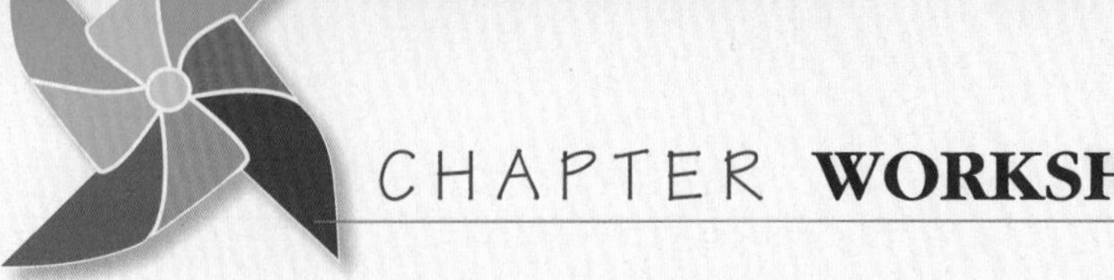

CHAPTER **WORKSHEET**

STUDY ACTIVITIES

1. Spend a day in the pediatric emergency department or urgent care center and document the role of the triage nurse.
2. Observe the pediatric emergency medical team at work or observe a pediatric code in the hospital. Compare and contrast the measures performed for the child with those that would be performed for an adult in a similar emergency situation.
3. Develop a teaching project related to injury prevention and present it at a local elementary, middle, or high school. Ensure that the education is geared toward the children's developmental level.
4. Interview the parents of a child who has experienced an emergency situation about how they felt during and after the emergency. Present the information to your classmates.
5. When providing care to a child in an emergency, the nurse performs the following assessments. Place them in the proper sequence.
   a. Pupillary reaction
   b. Presence of cough or sputum
   c. Heart rate and capillary refill
   d. Presence of bruises and abrasions
   e. Work of breathing

BRINGING IT ALL TOGETHER: A CASE STUDY

Teva Dawson, a 2-year-old girl, is rushed to the emergency room by ambulance after experiencing a near drowning in the family swimming pool. Teva was resuscitated at the scene and is now breathing spontaneously. She is lethargic and coughs occasionally.

Go to thePoint **to find questions to consider about this case.**

Appendix A

Standard Laboratory Values

PREGNANT AND NONPREGNANT WOMEN

Values	Nonpregnant	Pregnant
Hematologic		
Complete blood count (CBC)		
Hemoglobin, g/dL	12–16*	11.5–14*
Hematocrit, PCV, %	37–47	32–42
Red cell volume, mL	1,600	1,900
Plasma volume, mL	2,400	3,700
Red blood cell count, million/mm^3	4–5.5	3.75–5.0
White blood cells, total per mm^3	4,500–10,000	5,000–15,000
Polymorphonuclear cells, %	54–62	60–85
Lymphocytes, %	38–46	15–40
Erythrocyte sedimentation rate, mm/h	≤	30–90
MCHC, g/dL packed RBCs (mean corpuscular hemoglobin concentration)	30–36	No change
MCH (mean corpuscular hemoglobin per picogram)	29–32	No change
MCV/µm^3 (mean corpuscular volume per cubic micrometer)	82–96	No change
Blood coagulation and fibrinolytic activity†		
Factors VII, VIII, IX, X		Increase in pregnancy, return to normal in early puerperium; factor VIII increases during and immediately after delivery
Factors XI, XIII		Decrease in pregnancy
Prothrombin time (protime), sec	60–70	Slight decrease in pregnancy
Partial thromboplastin time (PTT), sect	12–14	Slight decrease in pregnancy and again during second and third stages of labor (indicates clotting at placental site)
Bleeding time, min	1–3 (Duke) 2–4 (Ivy)	No appreciable change
Coagulation time, min	6–10 (Lee/White)	No appreciable change
Platelets	150,000–350,000/mm^3	No significant change until 3–5 days after delivery, then marked increase (may predispose woman to thrombosis) and gradual return to normal
Fibrinolytic activity		Decreases in pregnancy, then abrupt return to normal (protection against thromboembolism)
Fibrinogen, mg/dL	250	400

PREGNANT AND NONPREGNANT WOMEN (continued)

Values	Nonpregnant	Pregnant
Mineral and vitamin Concentrations		
Serum iron, mcg	75–150	65–120
Total iron-binding capacity, mcg	250–450	300–500
Iron saturation, %	30–40	15–30
Vitamin B_{12}, folic acid, ascorbic acid	Normal	Moderate decrease
Serum protein		
Total, g/dL	6.7–8.3	5.5–7.5
Albumin, g/dL	3.5–5.5	3.0–5.0
Globulin, total, g/dL	2.3–3.5	3.0–4.0
Blood sugar		
Fasting, mg/dL	70–80	65
2-hour postprandial, mg/dL	60–110	Under 140 after a 100-g carbohydrate meal is considered normal
Cardiovascular		
Blood pressure, mm Hg	120/80[‡]	114/65
Peripheral resistance, dyne/s · cm^{-5}	120	100
Venous pressure, cm H_2O		
Femoral	9	24
Antecubital	8	8
Pulse, rate/min	70	80
Stroke volume, mL	65	75
Cardiac output, L/min	4.5	6
Circulation time (arm-tongue), sec	15–16	12–14
Blood volume, mL		
Whole blood	4,000	5,600
Plasma	2,400	3,700
Red blood cells	1,600	1,900
Plasma renin, units/L	3–10	10–80
Chest x-ray studies		
Transverse diameter of heart	–	1–2-cm increase
Left border of heart	–	Straightened
Cardiac volume	–	70-mL increase

(continued)

PREGNANT AND NONPREGNANT WOMEN (continued)

Values	Nonpregnant	Pregnant
Electrocardiogram	–	15-degree left axis deviation
V_1 and V_2	–	Inverted T-wave
kV_4	–	Low T
III	–	Q + inverted T
aVr	–	Small Q
Hepatic		
Bilirubin total	Not more than 1 mg/dL	Unchanged
Cephalin flocculation	Up to 2+ in 48 hr	Positive in 10%
Serum cholesterol, mg/dL	110–300	↑ 60% from 16–32 wks of pregnancy; remains at this level until after delivery
Thymol turbidity	0–4 units	Positive in 15%
Serum alkaline phosphatase	2–4.5 units (Bodansky)	↑ from week 12 of pregnancy to 6 wks after childbirth
Serum lactate dehydrogenase		Unchanged
Serum glutamic-oxaloacetic transaminase		Unchanged
Serum globulin albumin, g/dL	1.5–3.0	↑ slight
	4.5–5.3	↓ 3.0 g by late pregnancy
A/G ratio		Decreased
α_2-globulin		Increased
β-globulin		Increased
Serum cholinesterase		Decreased
Leucine aminopeptidase		Increased
Sulfobromophthalein (5 mg/kg)	5% dye or less in 45 min	Somewhat decreased
Renal		
Bladder capacity, mL	1,300	1,500
Renal plasma flow (RPF), mL/min	490–700	Increase by 25%, to 612–875
Glomerular filtration rate (GFR), mL/min	105–132	Increase by 50%, to 160–198
Nonprotein nitrogen (NPN), mg/dL	25–40	Decreases
Blood urea nitrogen (BUN), mg/dL	20–25	Decreases
Serum creatinine, mg/kg/24 hr	20–22	Decreases
Serum uric acid, mg/kg/24 hr	257–750	Decreases

PREGNANT AND NONPREGNANT WOMEN (continued)

Values	Nonpregnant	Pregnant
Urine glucose	Negative	Present in 20% of gravidas
Intravenous pyelogram (IVP)	Normal	Slight to moderate hydroureter and hydronephrosis; right kidney larger than left kidney
Miscellaneous		
Total thyroxine concentration	5–12 mcg/dL thyroxine	↑ 9–16 mcg/dL thyroxine (however, unbound thyroxine not greatly increased)
Ionized calcium		Relatively unchanged
Aldosterone		↑ 1 mg/24 hr by third trimester
Dehydroisoandrosterone	Plasma clearance 6–8 L/24 hr	↑ plasma clearance 10-fold to 20-fold

Adapted from Cunningham, F. G. (2016). Normal reference ranges for laboratory values in pregnancy. *UpToDate*. Retrieved from http://www.uptodate.com/contents/normal-reference-ranges-for-laboratory-values-in-pregnancy; and Van Leeuwen, A. M., & Bladh, M. L. (2015). *Davis's comprehensive handbook of laboratory & diagnostic tests with nursing implications.* (6th ed.), Philadelphia, PA: F. A. Davis.

*At sea level. Permanent residents of higher levels (e.g., Denver) require higher levels of hemoglobin.
†Pregnancy represents a hypercoagulable state.
‡For the woman about 20 years of age.
10 years of age: 103/70.
30 years of age: 123/82.
40 years of age: 126/84.

Appendix B

Clinical Paths

LABOR AND DELIVERY CLINICAL PATH—LABOR: EXPECTED OUTCOMES

	Active Phase	Expulsion/Pushing	Recovery First Hour Postpartum
CLIENT	Client coping with labor support Client utilizing appropriate labor options Client verbalizes satisfaction with plan Management interventions	Client demonstrates effective pushing technique Client coping effectively with pushing Support person coping effectively with labor	Bonding appropriately with baby
CLIENT'S STATUS	Cervix dilated 5 cm—complete Contraction regularly with progressive cervical change Maternal/fetal well-being maintained Hydration maintained If indicated: FSE and/or IUPC placed Pitocin IV started Epidural placed/WE encouraged Medicate with PRN pain meds	Vaginal birth	Placenta delivered Fundus firm Lochia small–moderate Without clots Perineum intact/repaired Hemodynamically stable EBL <500 mL
CONTINUUM OF CARE	Prenatal record available after 32 wks Prenatal labs WNL Preregistered to hospital Pediatrician identified Support after hospitalization identified Discharge plan discussed with client/family Communicates understanding of hospital and community resources		
ASSESSMENT/ TREATMENT	Assess: Continuous EFM or auscultation Q 15 of 30 min as indicated Vital signs hourly/temp Q 4 hr if intact membranes/Q 2 hr if membranes ruptured Uterine by monitor or palpation Bladder for distention Hydration status Cervical dilation, effacement, station	Assess: Q 15 min monitoring of fetal well-being (low risk) and Q 5 min (high risk) Vital signs hourly/temp. Q 2–4 hr depending on membrane status Bladder for distention Hydration status Pushing effectiveness Descent of presenting part Caput	Assess: Uterus–fundus Vital signs Lochia Bladder Perineum Placenta
CLIENT EDUCATION	Reinforce comfort measures Encourage use of labor options Inform client/support person of plan of care	Teaching of upright pushing positions Discourage prolonged maternal breath holding Encourage to assume position of choice Inform client of progress	Baby status Breast-feeding

LABOR AND DELIVERY CLINICAL PATH—LABOR: EXPECTED OUTCOMES (continued)

	Interventions		
TESTS/ PROCEDURES	Hgb or Hct (if not done recently) T & S (if ordered) VE as indicated IV therapy AROM by MD or CNM: assess for color, amount, and odor, as appropriate FSE/IUPC placement if indicated	AROM: assess for color, amount, and odor, as appropriate	Cord blood or RhoGAM workup if appropriate Cord blood if O+ mother
THERAPIES	Comfort measures/birthing ball/ ambulate/telemetry/shower IV therapy Amnio infusion for variable decelerations If appropriate, pain management reviewed	Perineal massage Warm soaks to perineal area Allow to rest until feels the urge to push Frequent position changes Cool cloth/ice chips	Ice pack to perineum Warm blankets
MEDS	Antibiotics as indicated for + GBS Pitocin if indicated PRN pain medication (encourage WE if requesting this)	Pitocin if indicated	Pitocin IV
ACTIVITY/ SAFETY	Labor option usage Position changes	Provide wedge if supine Promote effective position for pushing: i.e., squatting, side lying, upright Breathing technique client/ support person most comfortable with	Assist with ambulate to bathroom Infant care Assist with positioning for breast-feeding Infant ID bands present
NUTRITION	Clear liquids Ice chips Others	Clear liquids Ice chips	Return to previous diet
UNIQUE CLIENT NEEDS			

INTEGRATED PLAN OF CARE FOR CESAREAN DELIVERY

Expected Client Outcomes				
	Phase 1 Preadmission (Cesarean Delivery)	**Phase 2 Surgery/ Immediate Postop/ Day of Surgery**	**Phase 3 Postop Day 1**	
Usual time in phase assessment/ potential complications	**N/A Date Started:** VS WNL for client Hgb or Hct/values within normal SLH antepartum range	Up to 23 hr VS WNL for client Systems assessment: Skin warm, dry Clear ⇒ Alert & oriented ⇒ Neg. Homans sign ⇒ Breast soft/nipples intact ⇒ Lungs clear ⇒ Bowel sounds present ⇒ Fundus firm u/u or u 1–2 (−/+) Lochia sm—mod Dsg dry and intact No signs infiltration IV site Verbalizes comfort using pain rating scale 0–10	1 day VS WNL for client Afebrile Voiding without Foley ⇒ Passing flatus Incision without redness or drainage Lochia small amount Fundus firm u/1–2 Verbalizes comfort using pain scale 0–10 on oral pain meds	1–2 days Incision well approximated, without drainage or redness Passing flatus Lochia sm/mod amt Fundus firm u/1–2 Verbalizes comfort using pain medication as described
Client/family knowledge	**Date All Above Met** Verbalizes understanding of condition and need for surgery Verbalizes understanding of all preop teaching	**Date All Above Met** Verbalizes correct use of PCA/fentanyl pump and when to request pain medication Turn, cough, and deep breathe appropriately	**Date All Above Met** Can state criteria for when to call doctor for problems postdischarge ⇒ ↑ Bleeding ↑ Temperature ⇒ Incision redness, odor or drainage ⇒	**Date All Above Met** Verbalizes follow-up appointment date and time Verbalizes proper dosing of pain medication
ADLs/activity	**Date All Above Met** Verbalizes understanding of NPO status	**Date All Above Met** Able to ambulate with minimal assistance Tolerating clear/full liquid diet Bonding observed with newborn—taking-in phase ⇒	**Date All Above Met** Ambulating without assistance Tolerating soft to regular diet	**Date All Above Met** Ambulating in hall
	Date All Above Met	**Date All Above Met**	**Date All Above Met**	**Date All Above Met**
Unique client needs	**Date All Above Met** **Entire Phase** **Outcomes met; progress client to next phase**	**Date All Above Met** **Entire Phase** **Outcomes met; progress client to next phase**	**Date All Above Met** **Entire Phase** **Outcomes met; progress client to next phase**	**Date All Above Met** **Entire Phase** **Outcomes met; progress client to next phase**

INTEGRATED PLAN OF CARE FOR CESAREAN DELIVERY (continued)

	Plan of Care			
	#1 Preadmission	**#2 Surgery/ Immediate Postop/ Day of Surgery**	**#3 Postop Day 1**	**#4 Postop Day 2/ Discharge**
Assessments	Vital signs Fetal status immediately prior to surgery	VS per PACU then Q 4 hr Systems assessment: – Skin, LOC, FROM, Homans sign – Breasts, lungs, fundus, incision – Lochia, bladder, bowel sounds, IV, and site – I & O Q shift – Assess pain control 0–10 scale – Assess RhoGAM status – Assess Rubella titer status – ID band on mother	VS Q 6 hr Assess pain control 0–10 scale Incision Foley-volding Fundus/lochia Homans sign IV site Breasts ID band on mother Activity	Assess pain control 0–10 scale Incision Volding Fundus lochia Homans sign IV site as needed ID band on mother Activity
Consults	Anesthesia	Social work as needed, anesthesia, lactation, dietitian as needed	Social work, lactation, dietitian as needed	Social work, lactation, dietitian as needed
Client/family education discharge planning	Need for surgery Review cesarean delivery Review procedure, postop expectations Demonstrate/discuss equipment—PCA, fentanyl pump Tour of OR area and nursery	Review postop expectations Review equipment use PRN Instruct client on: Hospital/infant security systems Unity orientation Newborn orientation/ care/feeding (if breast-feeding problems, see decision trees)	Review dietary needs postsurgery Review bleeding/ lochia Precautions post–cesarean delivery Review follow-up care and doctor Appointments Review incision care, pericare Infant care Infant feeding	Verify follow-up appointment date and time Activity restrictions Follow-up for staple removal as needed Offer home follow-up care Discuss birth control
Tests and procedures	PAT; Hgb and Hct (if not done recently—within 1 mo) T & S (if ordered)			
Pharmacologic needs		IV fluids as ordered Pain control: PCA, fentanyl pump, IM to PO	IV lock PO pain meds Give RhoGAM if indicated Give rubella if indicated	DC IV lock as ordered

(continued)

INTEGRATED PLAN OF CARE FOR CESAREAN DELIVERY (continued)

	Plan of Care			
	#1 Preadmission	**#2 Surgery/ Immediate Postop/ Day of Surgery**	**#3 Postop Day 1**	**#4 Postop Day 2/ Discharge**
Activity/ rehabilitation	Client's usual	Change position Q 2 hr while in bed, OOB stand at bedside postop night/dangle and transfer to chair Progress to client endurance Observe bonding with infant Observe family support system (if inadequate consult SW)	Progress endurance/ begin Ambulation in hall OOB in AM May shower	Ambulate in halls without assistance
Nutrition/ elimination		NPO then clear liquids to DAT Foley empty Q shift	DAT to regular or previous diet at home Foley discontinued	
Miscellaneous interventions		TCDB Q 2 hr while awake	Dressing removed by MD or RN with MD request	
Unique client needs				

Cervical Dilation Chart

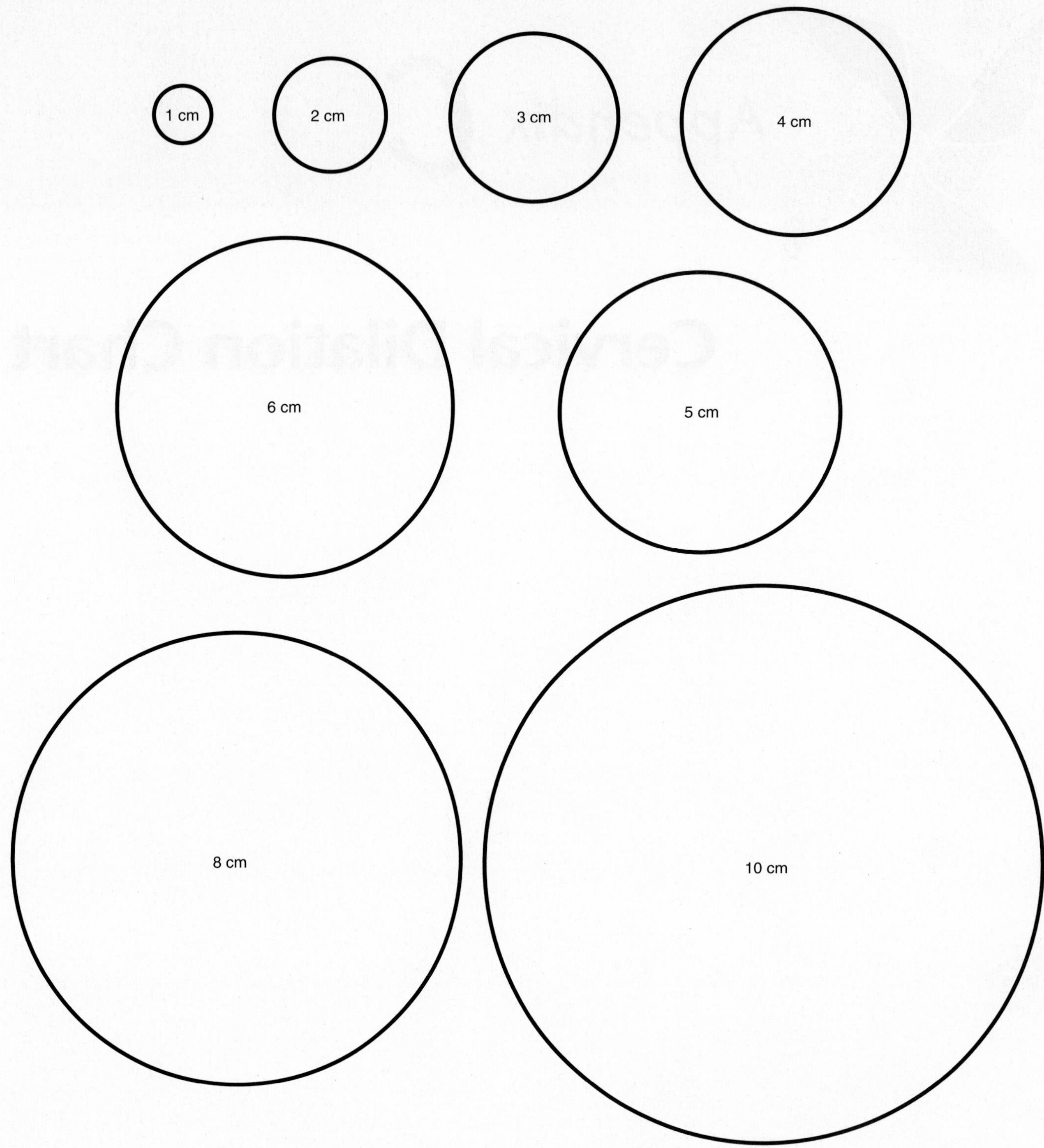
1 cm
2 cm
3 cm
4 cm
6 cm
5 cm
8 cm
10 cm

Appendix D

Weight Conversion Charts

CONVERSION OF POUNDS TO KILOGRAMS

Pounds	0	1	2	3	4	5	6	7	8	9
0	—	0.45	0.90	1.36	1.81	2.26	2.72	3.17	3.62	4.08
10	4.53	4.98	5.44	5.89	6.35	6.80	7.25	7.71	8.16	8.61
20	9.07	9.52	9.97	10.43	10.88	11.34	11.79	12.24	12.70	13.15
30	13.60	14.06	14.51	14.96	15.42	15.87	16.32	16.78	17.23	17.69
40	18.14	18.59	19.05	19.50	19.95	20.41	20.86	21.31	21.77	22.22
50	22.68	23.13	23.58	24.04	24.49	24.94	25.40	25.85	26.30	26.76
60	27.21	27.66	28.12	28.57	29.03	29.48	29.93	30.39	30.84	31.29
70	31.75	32.20	32.65	33.11	33.56	34.02	34.47	34.92	35.38	35.83
80	36.28	36.74	37.19	37.64	38.10	38.55	39.00	39.46	39.91	40.37
90	40.82	41.27	41.73	42.18	42.63	43.09	43.54	43.99	44.45	44.90
100	45.36	45.81	46.26	46.72	47.17	47.62	48.08	48.53	48.98	49.44
110	49.89	50.34	50.80	51.25	51.71	52.16	52.61	53.07	53.52	53.97
120	54.43	54.88	55.33	55.79	56.24	56.70	57.15	57.60	58.06	58.51
130	58.96	59.42	59.87	60.32	60.78	61.23	61.68	62.14	62.59	63.05
140	63.50	63.95	64.41	64.86	65.31	65.77	66.22	66.67	67.13	67.58
150	68.04	68.49	68.94	69.40	69.85	70.30	70.76	71.21	71.66	72.12
160	72.57	73.02	73.48	73.93	74.39	74.84	75.29	75.75	76.20	76.65
170	77.11	77.56	78.01	78.47	78.92	79.38	79.83	80.28	80.74	81.19
180	81.64	82.10	82.55	83.00	83.46	83.91	84.36	84.82	85.27	85.73
190	86.18	86.68	87.09	87.54	87.99	88.45	88.90	89.35	89.81	90.26
200	90.72	91.17	91.62	92.08	92.53	92.98	93.44	93.89	94.34	94.80

CONVERSION OF POUNDS AND OUNCES TO GRAMS FOR NEWBORN WEIGHTS

	Ounces															
Pounds	0	1	2	3	4	5	6	7	8	9	10	11	12	13	14	15
0	—	28	57	85	113	142	170	198	227	255	283	312	340	369	397	425
1	454	482	510	539	567	595	624	652	680	709	737	765	794	822	850	879
2	907	936	964	992	1,021	1,049	1,077	1,106	1,134	1,162	1,191	1,219	1,247	1,276	1,304	1,332
3	1,361	1,389	1,417	1,446	1,474	1,503	1,531	1,559	1,588	1,616	1,644	1,673	1,701	1,729	1,758	1,786
4	1,814	1,843	1,871	1,899	1,928	1,956	1,984	2,013	2,041	2,070	2,098	2,126	2,155	2,183	2,211	2,240
5	2,268	2,296	2,325	2,353	2,381	2,410	2,438	2,466	2,495	2,523	2,551	2,580	2,608	2,637	2,665	2,693
6	2,722	2,750	2,778	2,807	2,835	2,863	2,892	2,920	2,948	2,977	3,005	3,033	3,062	3,090	3,118	3,147
7	3,175	3,203	3,232	3,260	3,289	3,317	3,345	3,374	3,402	3,430	3,459	3,487	3,515	3,544	3,572	3,600
8	3,629	3,657	3,685	3,714	3,742	3,770	3,799	3,827	3,856	3,884	3,912	3,941	3,969	3,997	4,026	4,054
9	4,082	4,111	4,139	4,167	4,196	4,224	4,252	4,281	4,309	4,337	4,366	4,394	4,423	4,451	4,479	4,508
10	4,536	4,564	4,593	4,621	4,649	4,678	4,706	4,734	4,763	4,791	4,819	4,848	4,876	4,904	4,933	4,961
11	4,990	5,018	5,046	5,075	5,103	5,131	5,160	5,188	5,216	5,245	5,273	5,301	5,330	5,358	5,386	5,415
12	5,443	5,471	5,500	5,528	5,557	5,585	5,613	5,642	5,670	5,698	5,727	5,755	5,783	5,812	5,840	5,868
13	5,897	5,925	5,953	5,982	6,010	6,038	6,067	6,095	6,123	6,152	6,180	6,209	6,237	6,265	6,294	6,322
14	6,350	6,379	6,407	6,435	6,464	6,492	6,520	6,549	6,577	6,605	6,634	6,662	6,690	6,719	6,747	6,776
15	6,804	6,832	6,860	6,889	6,917	6,945	6,973	7,002	7,030	7,059	7,087	7,115	7,144	7,172	7,201	7,228

Appendix E

Breast-Feeding and Medication Use

GENERAL CONSIDERATIONS

- Most medications are safe to use while breast-feeding; however, the woman should always check with the pediatrician, physician, or lactation specialist before taking any medications, including over-the-counter and herbal products.
- Inform the woman that she has the right to seek a second opinion if the physician does not perform a thoughtful risk-versus-benefit assessment before prescribing medications or advising against breast-feeding.
- Most medications pass from the woman's bloodstream into the breast milk. However, the amount is usually very small and unlikely to harm the baby.
- A preterm or other special needs neonate is more susceptible to the adverse effects of medications in breast milk. A woman who is taking medications and whose baby is in the neonatal intensive care unit or special care nursery should consult with the pediatrician or neonatologist before feeding her breast milk to the baby.
- If the woman is taking a prescribed medication, she should take the medication just after breast-feeding. This practice helps ensure that the lowest possible dose of medication reaches the baby through the breast milk.
- Some medications can cause changes in the amount of milk the woman produces. Teach the woman to report any changes in milk production.

LACTATION RISK CATEGORIES (LRC)

Lactation Category	Risk	Rationale
L1	Compatible	Clinical research or long-term observation of use in many breast-feeding women has not demonstrated risk to the infant.
L2	Probably compatible	Limited clinical research has not demonstrated an increase in adverse effects in the infant.
L3	Probably compatible	There is possible risk to the infant; however, the risks are minimal or nonthreatening in nature. These medications should be given only when the potential benefit outweighs the risk to the infant.
L4	Possibly hazardous	There is positive evidence of risk to the infant; however, in life-threatening situations or for serious diseases, the benefit might outweigh the risk.
L5	No data: Hazardous	The risk of using the medication clearly outweighs any possible benefit from breast-feeding.

POTENTIAL EFFECTS OF SELECTED MEDICATION CATEGORIES ON THE BREAST-FED INFANT

Narcotic Analgesics

- Codeine and hydrocodone appear to be safe in moderate doses. Rarely the neonate may experience sedation and/or apnea. (LRC: L3)
- Meperidine (Demerol) can lead to sedation of the neonate. (LRC: L3)
- Low to moderate doses of morphine appear to be safe. (LRC: L2)
- Trace-to-negligible amounts of fentanyl are found in human milk. (LRC: L2)

Nonnarcotic Analgesics and NSAIDs

- Acetaminophen and ibuprofen are approved for use. (LRC: L1)
- Naproxen may cause neonatal hemorrhage and anemia if used for prolonged periods. (LRC: L3 for short-term use and L4 for long-term use)
- The newer COX2 inhibitors, such as celecoxib (Celebrex), appear to be safe for use. (LRC: L2)

Antibiotics

- Levels in breast milk are usually very low.
- The penicillins and cephalosporins are generally considered safe to use. (LRC: L1 and L2)
- Tetracyclines can be safely used for short periods but are not suitable for long-term therapy (e.g., for treatment of acne). (LRC: L2)
- Sulfonamides should not be used during the neonatal stage (the first month of life). (LRC: L3)

Antihypertensives

- A high degree of caution is advised when antihypertensives are used during breast-feeding.
- Some beta blockers can be used.
- Hydralazine and methyldopa are considered to be safe. (LRC: L2)
- Angiotensin-converting enzyme (ACE) inhibitors are not recommended in the early postpartum period.

Sedatives and Hypnotics

- Neonatal withdrawal can occur when antianxiety medications, such as lorazepam, are taken. Fortunately withdrawal is generally mild.
- Phenothiazines, such as Phenergan and Thorazine, may lead to sleep apnea and increase the risk for sudden infant death syndrome.

Antidepressants

- The risk to the baby is often higher if the woman is depressed and remains untreated, rather than taking the medication.
- The older tricyclics are considered to be safe; however, they cause many bothersome side effects, such as weight gain and dry mouth, which may lead to noncompliance on the part of the woman.
- The selective serotonin uptake inhibitors (SSRIs) are also considered to be safe and have a lower side effect profile, which makes them more palatable to the woman. (LRC: L2 and L3)

Mood Stabilizers (Antimanic Medication)

- Lithium is found in breast milk and is best not used in the breast-feeding woman. (LRC: L4)
- Valproic acid (Depakote) seems to be a more appropriate choice for the woman with bipolar disorder. The infant will need periodic lab studies to check platelets and liver function.

Corticosteroids

- Corticosteroids do not pass into the milk in large quantities.
- Inhaled steroids are safe to use because they do not accumulate in the bloodstream.

Thyroid Medication

- Thyroid medications, such as levothyroxine (Synthroid), can be taken while breast-feeding.
- Most are in LRC category L1.

MEDICATIONS THAT USUALLY ARE CONTRAINDICATED FOR THE BREAST-FEEDING WOMAN

- Amiodarone
- Antineoplastic agents
- Chloramphenicol
- Doxepin
- Ergotamine and other ergot derivatives
- Iodides
- Methotrexate and immunosuppressants
- Lithium
- Radiopharmaceuticals
- Ribavirin
- Tetracycline (prolonged use—more than 3 weeks)
- Pseudoephedrine (found in many over-the-counter medications)

Material in this appendix was adapted from information found in the following sources:

Wamback, K., & Riordan, J. (2015). *Breastfeeding and human lactation* (5th ed.), Burlington, MA: Jones & Bartlett Learning.

Lauwers, J., & Swisher, A. (2016). *Counseling the nursing mother: A lactation consultant's guide* (6th ed.), Burlington, MA: Jones & Bartlett Learning.

Brucker, M. C., & King, T. L. (2017). *Pharmacology for women's health* (2nd ed.), Burlington, MA: Jones & Bartlett Learning.

Appendix F

Blood Pressure Charts for Children and Adolescents

TABLE F.1 BLOOD PRESSURE LEVELS FOR BOYS BY AGE AND HEIGHT PERCENTILE

Age (Year)	BP Percentile ↓	Systolic BP (mm Hg) ← Percentile of Height →							Diastolic BP (mm Hg) ← Percentile of Height →						
		5th	*10th*	*25th*	*50th*	*75th*	*90th*	*95th*	*5th*	*10th*	*25th*	*50th*	*75th*	*90th*	*95th*
1	50th	80	81	83	85	87	88	89	34	35	36	37	38	39	39
	90th	94	95	97	99	100	102	103	49	50	51	52	53	53	54
	95th	98	99	101	103	104	106	106	54	54	55	56	57	58	58
	99th	105	106	108	110	112	113	114	61	62	63	64	65	66	66
2	50th	84	85	87	88	90	92	92	39	40	41	42	43	44	44
	90th	97	99	100	102	104	105	106	54	55	56	57	58	58	59
	95th	101	102	104	106	108	109	110	59	59	60	61	62	63	63
	99th	109	110	111	113	115	117	117	66	67	68	69	70	71	71
3	50th	86	87	89	91	93	94	95	44	44	45	46	47	48	48
	90th	100	101	103	105	107	108	109	59	59	60	61	62	63	63
	95th	104	105	107	109	110	112	113	63	63	64	65	66	67	67
	99th	111	112	114	116	118	119	120	71	71	72	73	74	75	75
4	50th	88	89	91	93	95	96	97	47	48	49	50	51	51	52
	90th	102	103	105	107	109	110	111	62	63	64	65	66	66	67
	95th	106	107	109	111	112	114	115	66	67	68	69	70	71	71
	99th	113	114	116	118	120	121	122	74	75	76	77	78	78	79
5	50th	90	91	93	95	96	98	98	50	51	52	53	54	55	55
	90th	104	105	106	108	110	111	112	65	66	67	68	69	69	70
	95th	108	109	110	112	114	115	116	69	70	71	72	73	74	74
	99th	115	116	118	120	121	123	123	77	78	79	80	81	81	82
6	50th	91	92	94	96	98	99	100	53	53	54	55	56	57	57
	90th	105	106	108	110	111	113	113	68	68	69	70	71	72	72
	95th	109	110	112	114	115	117	117	72	72	73	74	75	76	76
	99th	116	117	119	121	123	124	125	80	80	81	82	83	84	84
7	50th	92	94	95	97	99	100	101	55	55	56	57	58	59	59
	90th	106	107	109	111	113	114	115	70	70	71	72	73	74	74
	95th	110	111	113	115	117	118	119	74	74	75	76	77	78	78
	99th	117	118	120	122	124	125	126	82	82	83	84	85	86	86
8	50th	94	95	97	99	100	102	102	56	57	58	59	60	60	61
	90th	107	109	110	112	114	115	116	71	72	72	73	74	75	76
	95th	111	112	114	116	118	119	120	75	76	77	78	79	79	80
	99th	119	120	122	123	125	127	127	83	84	85	86	87	87	88
9	50th	95	96	98	100	102	103	104	57	58	59	60	61	61	62
	90th	109	110	112	114	115	117	118	72	73	74	75	76	76	77
	95th	113	114	116	118	119	121	121	76	77	78	79	80	81	81
	99th	120	121	123	125	127	128	129	84	85	86	87	88	88	89
10	50th	97	98	100	102	103	105	106	58	59	60	61	61	62	63
	90th	111	112	114	115	117	119	119	73	73	74	75	76	77	78
	95th	115	116	117	119	121	122	123	77	78	79	80	81	81	82
	99th	122	123	125	127	128	130	130	85	86	86	88	88	89	90
11	50th	99	100	102	104	105	107	107	59	59	60	61	62	63	63
	90th	113	114	115	117	119	120	121	74	74	75	76	77	78	78
	95th	117	118	119	121	123	124	125	78	78	79	80	81	82	82
	99th	124	125	127	129	130	132	132	86	86	87	88	89	90	90
12	50th	101	102	104	106	108	109	110	59	60	61	62	63	63	64
	90th	115	116	118	120	121	123	123	74	75	75	76	77	78	79
	95th	119	120	122	123	125	127	127	78	79	80	81	82	82	83
	99th	126	127	129	131	133	134	135	86	87	88	89	90	90	91

TABLE F.1 BLOOD PRESSURE LEVELS FOR BOYS BY AGE AND HEIGHT PERCENTILE (continued)

		Systolic BP (mm Hg)							Diastolic BP (mm Hg)						
	BP	← *Percentile of Height* →							← *Percentile of Height* →						
Age (Year)	Percentile ↓	*5th*	*10th*	*25th*	*50th*	*75th*	*90th*	*95th*	*5th*	*10th*	*25th*	*50th*	*75th*	*90th*	*95th*
13	50th	104	105	106	108	110	111	112	60	60	61	62	63	64	64
	90th	117	118	120	122	124	125	126	75	75	76	77	78	79	79
	95th	121	122	124	126	128	129	130	79	79	80	81	82	83	83
	99th	128	130	131	133	135	136	137	87	87	88	89	90	91	91
14	50th	106	107	109	111	113	114	115	60	61	62	63	64	65	65
	90th	120	121	123	125	126	128	128	75	76	77	78	79	79	80
	95th	124	125	127	128	130	132	132	80	80	81	82	83	84	84
	99th	131	132	134	136	138	139	140	87	88	89	90	91	92	92
15	50th	109	110	112	113	115	117	117	61	62	63	64	65	66	66
	90th	122	124	125	127	129	130	131	76	77	78	79	80	80	81
	95th	126	127	129	131	133	134	135	81	81	82	83	84	85	85
	99th	134	135	136	138	140	142	142	88	89	90	91	92	93	93
16	50th	111	112	114	116	118	119	120	63	63	64	65	66	67	67
	90th	125	126	128	130	131	133	134	78	78	79	80	81	82	82
	95th	129	130	132	134	135	137	137	82	83	83	84	85	86	87
	99th	136	137	139	141	143	144	145	90	90	91	92	93	94	94
17	50th	114	115	116	118	120	121	122	65	66	66	67	68	69	70
	90th	127	128	130	132	134	135	136	80	80	81	82	83	84	84
	95th	131	132	134	136	138	139	140	84	85	86	87	87	88	89
	99th	139	140	141	143	145	146	147	92	93	93	94	95	96	97

BP, blood pressure. 90th to 95th percentile: prehypertension; 95th to 99th percentile: stage 1 hypertension; >99th percentile: stage 2 hypertension.

Adapted from U.S. Department of Health and Human Services, National Institutes of Health, National Heart, Lung, and Blood Institute. (2005). *The fourth report on the diagnosis, evaluation, and treatment of high blood pressure in children and adolescents* (NIH Publication No. 05–5267). Washington, DC: U.S. Department of Health and Human Services.

TABLE F.2 BLOOD PRESSURE LEVELS FOR GIRLS BY AGE AND HEIGHT PERCENTILE

Age (Year)	BP Percentile ↓	Systolic BP (mm Hg) ← Percentile of Height →							Diastolic BP (mm Hg) ← Percentile of Height →						
		5th	10th	25th	50th	75th	90th	95th	5th	10th	25th	50th	75th	90th	95th
1	50th	83	84	85	86	88	89	90	38	39	39	40	41	41	42
	90th	97	97	98	100	101	102	103	52	53	53	54	55	55	56
	95th	100	101	102	104	105	106	107	56	57	57	58	59	59	60
	99th	108	108	109	111	112	113	114	64	64	65	65	66	67	67
2	50th	85	85	87	88	89	91	91	43	44	44	45	46	46	47
	90th	98	99	100	101	103	104	105	57	58	58	59	60	61	61
	95th	102	103	104	105	107	108	109	61	62	62	63	64	65	65
	99th	109	110	111	112	114	115	116	69	69	70	70	71	72	72
3	50th	86	87	88	89	91	92	93	47	48	48	49	50	50	51
	90th	100	100	102	103	104	106	106	61	62	62	63	64	64	65
	95th	104	104	105	107	108	109	110	65	66	66	67	68	68	69
	99th	111	111	113	114	115	116	117	73	73	74	74	75	76	76
4	50th	88	88	90	91	92	94	94	50	50	51	52	52	53	54
	90th	101	102	103	104	106	107	108	64	64	65	66	67	67	68
	95th	105	106	107	108	110	111	112	68	68	69	70	71	71	72
	99th	112	113	114	115	117	118	119	76	76	76	77	78	79	79
5	50th	89	90	91	93	94	95	96	52	53	53	54	55	55	56
	90th	103	103	105	106	107	109	109	66	67	67	68	69	69	70
	95th	107	107	108	110	111	112	113	70	71	71	72	73	73	74
	99th	114	114	116	117	118	120	120	78	78	79	79	80	81	81
6	50th	91	92	93	94	96	97	98	54	54	55	56	56	57	58
	90th	104	105	106	108	109	110	111	68	68	69	70	70	71	72
	95th	108	109	110	111	113	114	115	72	72	73	74	74	75	76
	99th	115	116	117	119	120	121	122	80	80	80	81	82	83	83
7	50th	93	93	95	96	97	99	99	55	56	56	57	58	58	59
	90th	106	107	108	109	111	112	113	69	70	70	71	72	72	73
	95th	110	111	112	113	115	116	116	73	74	74	75	76	76	77
	99th	117	118	119	120	122	123	124	81	81	82	82	83	84	84
8	50th	95	95	96	98	99	100	101	57	57	57	58	59	60	60
	90th	108	109	110	111	113	114	114	71	71	71	72	73	74	74
	95th	112	112	114	115	116	118	118	75	75	75	76	77	78	78
	99th	119	120	121	122	123	125	125	82	82	83	83	84	85	86
9	50th	96	97	98	100	101	102	103	58	58	58	59	60	61	61
	90th	110	110	112	113	114	116	116	72	72	72	73	74	75	75
	95th	114	114	115	117	118	119	120	76	76	76	77	78	79	79
	99th	121	121	123	124	125	127	127	83	83	84	84	85	86	87
10	50th	98	99	100	102	103	104	105	59	59	59	60	61	62	62
	90th	112	112	114	115	116	118	118	73	73	73	74	75	76	76
	95th	116	116	117	119	120	121	122	77	77	77	78	79	80	80
	99th	123	123	125	126	127	129	129	84	84	85	86	86	87	88
11	50th	100	101	102	103	105	106	107	60	60	60	61	62	63	63
	90th	114	114	116	118	118	119	120	74	74	74	75	76	77	77
	95th	118	118	119	121	122	123	124	78	78	78	79	80	81	81
	99th	125	125	126	128	129	130	131	85	85	86	87	87	88	89
12	50th	102	103	104	105	107	108	109	61	61	61	62	63	64	64
	90th	116	116	117	119	120	121	122	75	75	75	76	77	78	78
	95th	119	120	121	123	124	125	126	79	79	79	80	81	82	82
	99th	127	127	128	130	131	132	133	86	86	87	88	88	89	90

TABLE F.2 BLOOD PRESSURE LEVELS FOR GIRLS BY AGE AND HEIGHT PERCENTILE (continued)

Age (Year)	BP Percentile ↓	Systolic BP (mm Hg) ← Percentile of Height →							Diastolic BP (mm Hg) ← Percentile of Height →						
		5th	10th	25th	50th	75th	90th	95th	5th	10th	25th	50th	75th	90th	95th
13	50th	104	105	106	107	109	110	110	62	62	62	63	64	65	65
	90th	117	118	119	121	122	123	124	76	76	76	77	78	79	79
	95th	121	122	123	124	126	127	128	80	80	80	81	82	83	83
	99th	128	129	130	132	133	134	135	87	87	88	89	89	90	91
14	50th	106	106	107	109	110	111	112	63	63	63	64	65	66	66
	90th	119	120	121	122	124	125	125	77	77	77	78	79	80	80
	95th	123	123	125	126	127	129	129	81	81	81	82	83	84	84
	99th	130	131	132	133	135	136	136	88	88	89	90	90	91	92
15	50th	107	108	109	110	111	113	113	64	64	64	65	66	67	67
	90th	120	121	122	123	125	126	127	78	78	78	79	80	81	81
	95th	124	125	126	127	129	130	131	82	82	82	83	84	85	85
	99th	131	132	133	134	136	137	138	89	89	90	91	91	92	93
16	50th	108	108	110	111	112	114	114	64	64	65	66	66	67	68
	90th	121	122	123	124	126	127	128	78	78	79	80	81	81	82
	95th	125	126	127	128	130	131	132	82	82	83	84	85	85	86
	99th	132	133	134	135	137	138	139	90	90	90	91	92	93	93
17	50th	108	109	110	111	113	114	115	64	65	65	66	67	67	68
	90th	122	122	123	125	126	127	128	78	79	79	80	81	81	82
	95th	125	126	127	129	130	131	132	82	83	83	84	85	85	86
	99th	133	133	134	136	137	138	139	90	90	91	91	92	93	93

BP, blood pressure. 90th to 95th percentile: prehypertension; 95th to 99th percentile: stage 1 hypertension; >99th percentile: stage 2 hypertension.

Adapted from U.S. Department of Health and Human Services, National Institutes of Health, National Heart, Lung, and Blood Institute. (2005). The fourth report on the diagnosis, evaluation, and treatment of high blood pressure in children and adolescents (NIH Publication No. 05–5267). Washington, DC: U.S. Department of Health and Human Services.

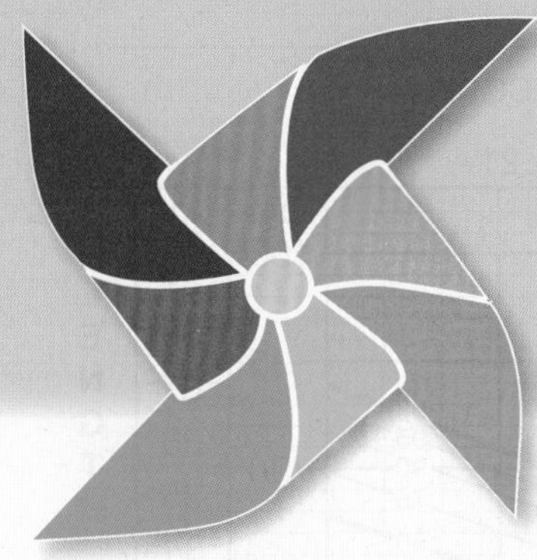

Appendix G

Growth Charts

Birth to 24 months: Boys
Length-for-age and Weight-for-age percentiles

NAME ______________________

RECORD # ______________

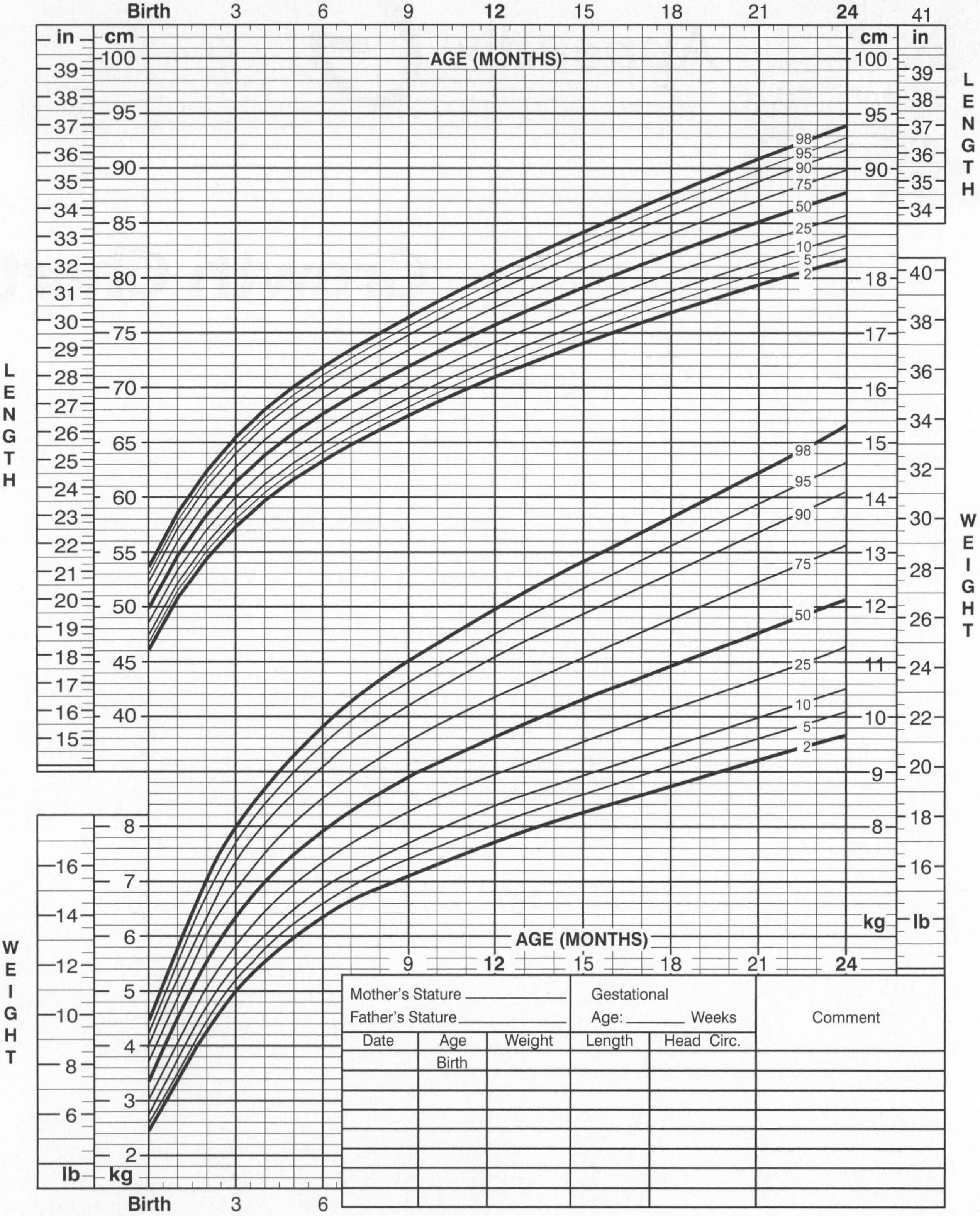

Mother's Stature ______			Gestational Age: ______ Weeks		Comment
Father's Stature ______					
Date	Age	Weight	Length	Head Circ.	
	Birth				

Published by the Centers for Disease Control and Prevention, November 1, 2009
SOURCE: WHO Child Growth Standards (http://www.who.int/childgrowth/en)

SAFER • HEALTHIER • PEOPLE™

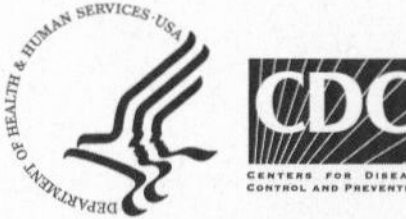

Birth to 24 months: Girls
Length-for-age and Weight-for-age percentiles

NAME ______________

RECORD # ______________

Birth 3 6 9 12 15 18 21 24

in cm AGE (MONTHS) cm in

LENGTH

100 95 90 85 80 75 70 65 60 55 50 45 40

39 38 37 36 35 34 33 32 31 30 29 28 27 26 25 24 23 22 21 20 19 18 17 16 15

41 39 38 37 36 35 34

98 95 90 75 50 25 10 5 2

WEIGHT

18 17 16 15 14 13 12 11 10 9 8 kg

40 38 36 34 32 30 28 26 24 22 20 18 16 lb

98 95 90 75 50 25 10 5 2

AGE (MONTHS)

9 12 15 18 21 24

8 7 6 5 4 3 2 kg

16 14 12 10 8 6 lb

Birth 3 6

Mother's Stature ______			Gestational		Comment
Father's Stature ______			Age: ______ Weeks		
Date	Age	Weight	Length	Head Circ.	
	Birth				

Published by the Centers for Disease Control and Prevention, November 1, 2009
SOURCE: WHO Child Growth Standards (http://www.who.int/childgrowth/en)

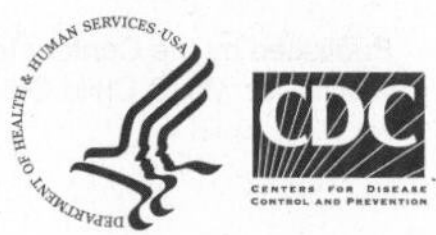

Birth to 24 months: Boys
Head circumference-for-age and Weight-for-length percentiles

NAME ______________

RECORD # ______________

AGE (MONTHS): Birth 3 6 9 12 15 18 21 24

HEAD CIRCUMFERENCE (cm): 30 32 34 36 38 40 42 44 46 48 50 52

HEAD CIRCUMFERENCE (in): 12 13 14 15 16 17 18 19 20

Percentiles: 98 95 90 75 50 25 10 5 2

WEIGHT (kg): 1 2 3 4 5 6 7 8 9 10 11 12 13 14 15 16 17 18 19 20 21 22 23 24

WEIGHT (lb): 2 4 6 8 10 12 14 16 18 20 22 24 26 28 30 32 34 36 38 40 42 44 46 48 50 52

LENGTH (cm): 46 48 50 52 54 56 58 60 62 64 66 68 70 72 74 76 78 80 82 84 86 88 90 92 94 96 98 100 102 104 106 108 110

LENGTH (in): 18 19 20 21 22 23 24 26 27 28 29 30 31 32 33 34 35 36 37 38 39 40 41 42 43

Date	Age	Weight	Length	Head Circ.	Comment

Published by the Centers for Disease Control and Prevention, November 1, 2009
SOURCE: WHO Child Growth Standards (http://www.who.int/childgrowth/en)

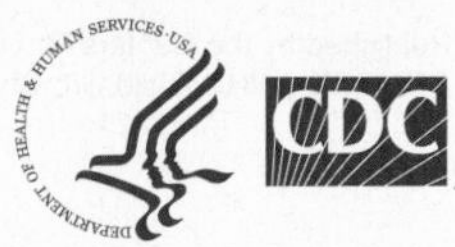

Birth to 24 months: Girls
Head circumference-for-age and Weight-for-length percentiles

NAME ____________________

RECORD # ____________

Date	Age	Weight	Length	Head Circ.	Comment

Published by the Centers for Disease Control and Prevention, November 1, 2009
SOURCE: WHO Child Growth Standards (http://www.who.int/childgrowth/en)

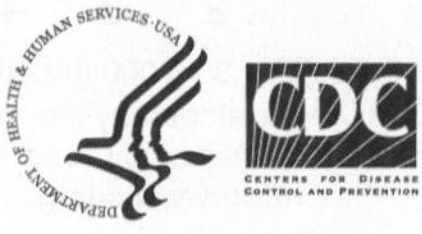

2 to 20 years: Boys
Stature-for-age and Weight-for-age percentiles

NAME ______________

RECORD # ______________

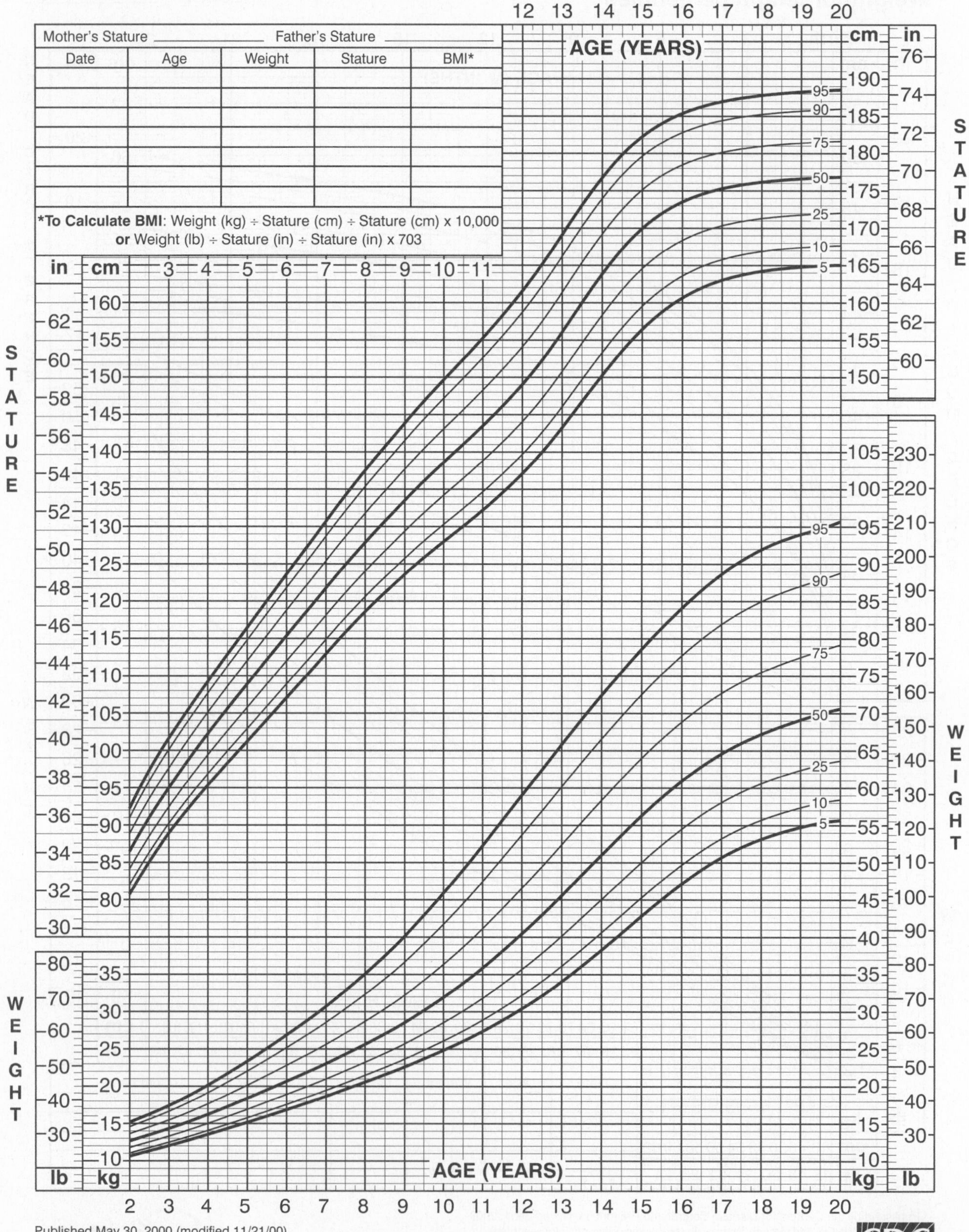

Mother's Stature ______________ Father's Stature ______________

Date	Age	Weight	Stature	BMI*

***To Calculate BMI**: Weight (kg) ÷ Stature (cm) ÷ Stature (cm) x 10,000
or Weight (lb) ÷ Stature (in) ÷ Stature (in) x 703

Published May 30, 2000 (modified 11/21/00).
SOURCE: Developed by the National Center for Health Statistics in collaboration with the National Center for Chronic Disease Prevention and Health Promotion (2000).
http://www.cdc.gov/growthcharts

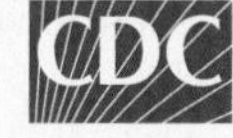

SAFER • HEALTHIER • PEOPLE™

2 to 20 years: Girls
Stature-for-age and Weight-for-age percentiles

NAME ______________________

RECORD # ____________

Mother's Stature ____________ Father's Stature ____________

Date	Age	Weight	Stature	BMI*

***To Calculate BMI**: Weight (kg) ÷ Stature (cm) ÷ Stature (cm) x 10,000
or Weight (lb) ÷ Stature (in) ÷ Stature (in) x 703

AGE (YEARS)

STATURE

WEIGHT

Published May 30, 2000 (modified 11/21/00).
SOURCE: Developed by the National Center for Health Statistics in collaboration with the National Center for Chronic Disease Prevention and Health Promotion (2000).
http://www.cdc.gov/growthcharts

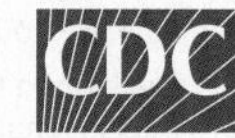

SAFER • HEALTHIER • PEOPLE™

2 to 20 years: Boys
Body mass index-for-age percentiles

NAME ______________________

RECORD # ______________

Date	Age	Weight	Stature	BMI*	Comments

***To Calculate BMI**: Weight (kg) ÷ Stature (cm) ÷ Stature (cm) x 10,000
or Weight (lb) ÷ Stature (in) ÷ Stature (in) x 703

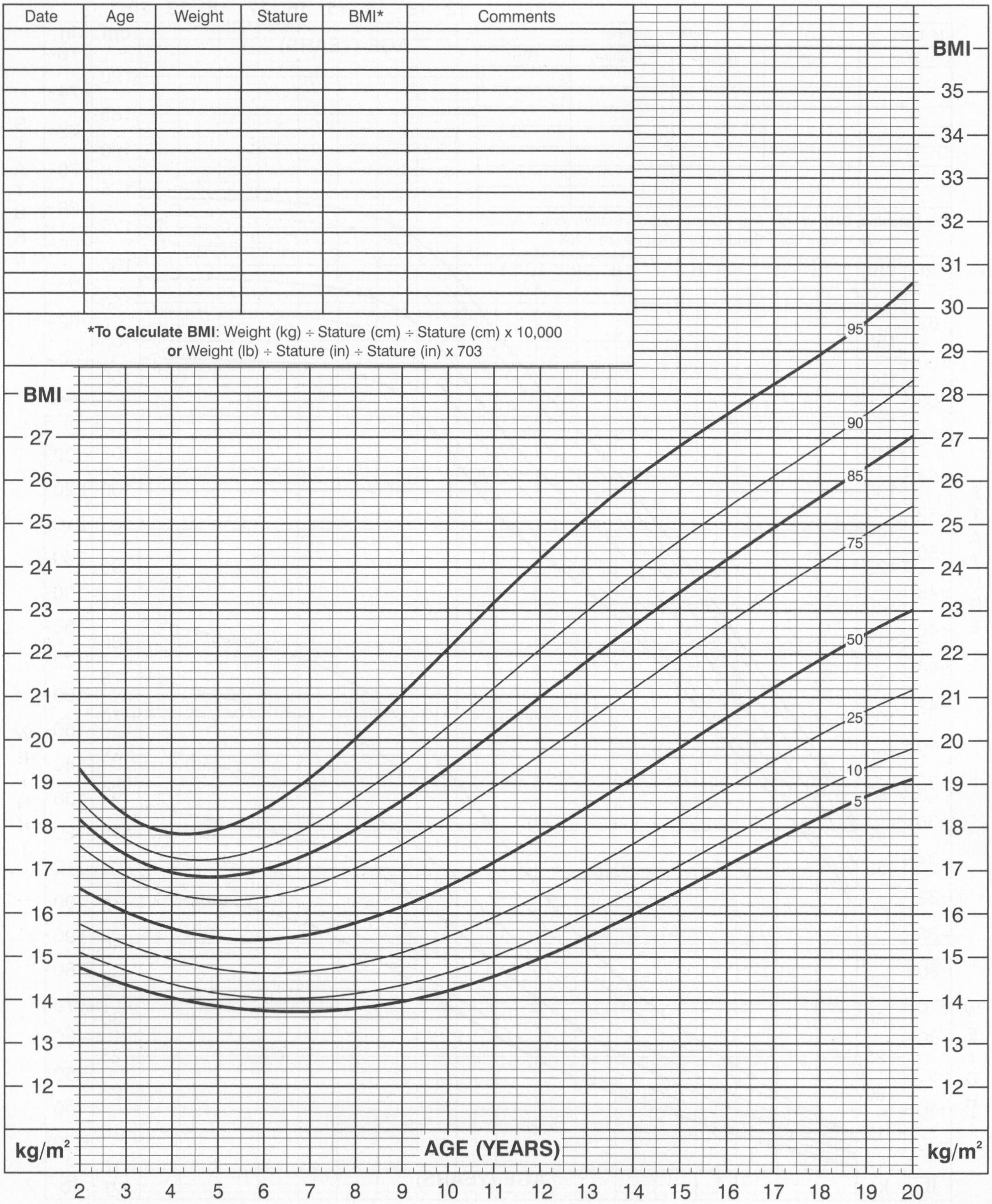

BMI

35 34 33 32 31 30 29 28 27 26 25 24 23 22 21 20 19 18 17 16 15 14 13 12

95 90 85 75 50 25 10 5

kg/m²

AGE (YEARS)

2 3 4 5 6 7 8 9 10 11 12 13 14 15 16 17 18 19 20

Published May 30, 2000 (modified 10/16/00).
SOURCE: Developed by the National Center for Health Statistics in collaboration with the National Center for Chronic Disease Prevention and Health Promotion (2000).
http://www.cdc.gov/growthcharts

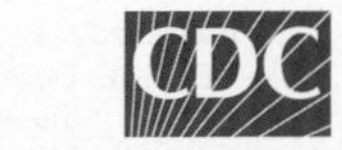

SAFER • HEALTHIER • PEOPLE™

2 to 20 years: Girls
Body mass index-for-age percentiles

NAME ______________________

RECORD # ______________

Date	Age	Weight	Stature	BMI*	Comments

***To Calculate BMI**: Weight (kg) ÷ Stature (cm) ÷ Stature (cm) x 10,000
or Weight (lb) ÷ Stature (in) ÷ Stature (in) x 703

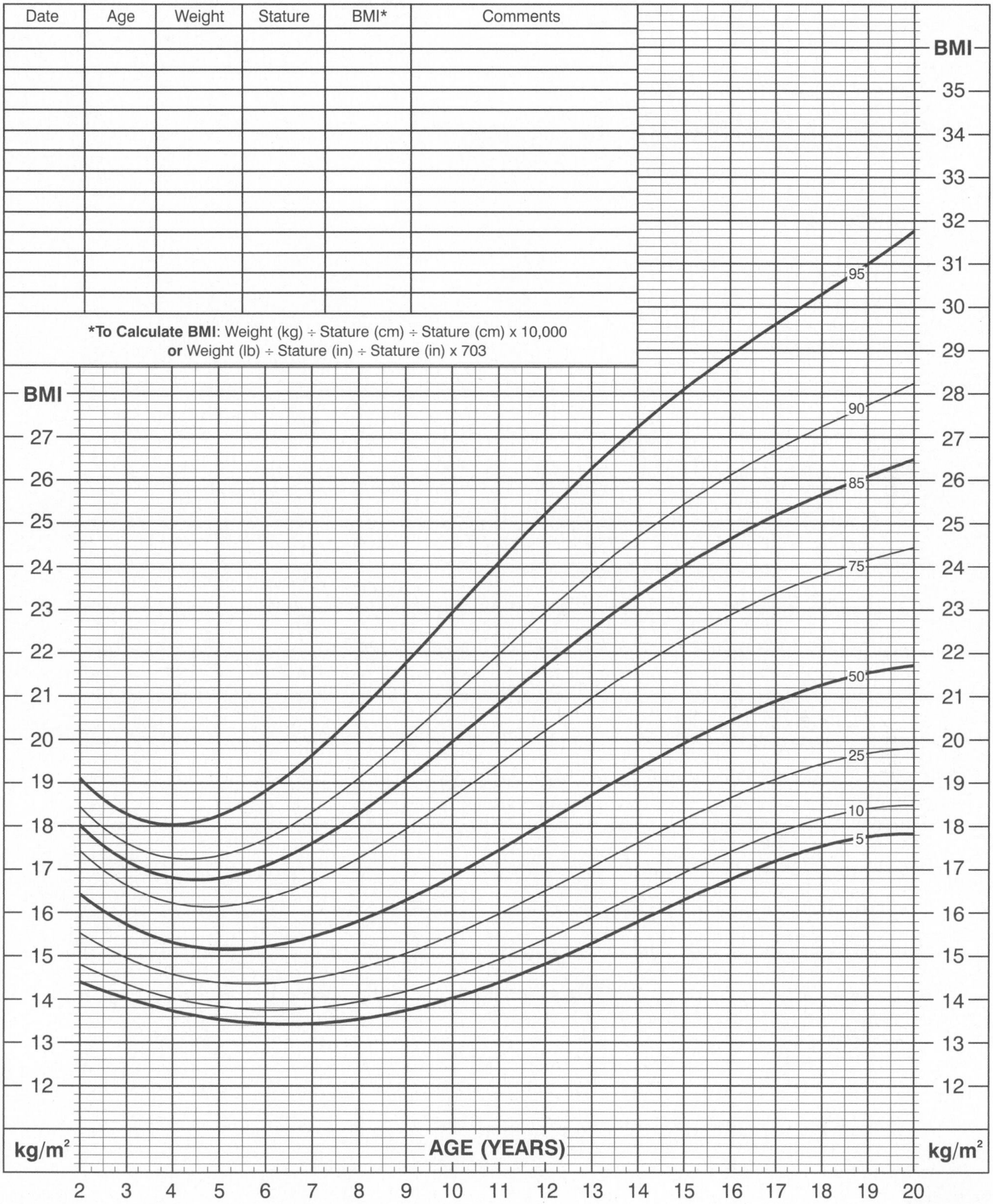

BMI

35 34 33 32 31 30 29 28 27 26 25 24 23 22 21 20 19 18 17 16 15 14 13 12

95 90 85 75 50 25 10 5

kg/m²

AGE (YEARS)

2 3 4 5 6 7 8 9 10 11 12 13 14 15 16 17 18 19 20

Published May 30, 2000 (modified 10/16/00).
SOURCE: Developed by the National Center for Health Statistics in collaboration with the National Center for Chronic Disease Prevention and Health Promotion (2000).
http://www.cdc.gov/growthcharts

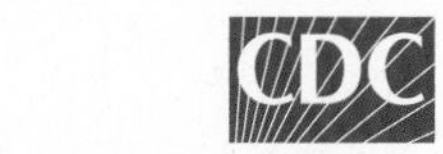

Appendix H

MyPlate

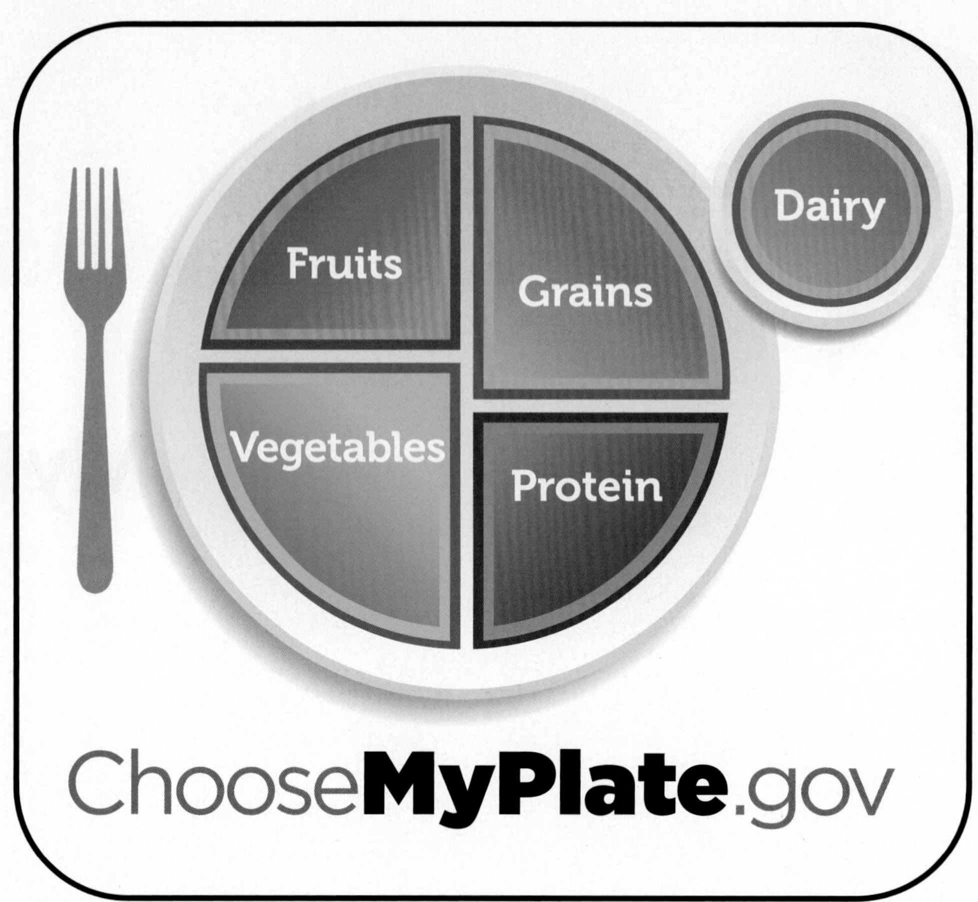

From United States Department of Agriculture, ChooseMyPlate.gov; retrieved from http://www.choosemyplate.gov/print-materials-ordering/graphic-resources.html

Appendix I

Down Syndrome Healthcare Guidelines

TABLE I.1 HEALTH SUPERVISION FOR CHILDREN WITH DOWN SYNDROME

	Prenatal	Birth–1 mo	1 mo–1 y	1–5 y	5–13 y	13–21 y
Counseling regarding prenatal screening test & imaging results						
Plan for delivery						
Referral to geneticist						
Parent-to-parent contact, support groups, current books and pamphlets						
Physical exam for evidence of trisomy 21						
Chromosomal analysis to confirm dx						
Discuss risk of recurrence of Down syndrome						
Echocardiogram						
Radiographic swallowing assessment if marked hypotonia, slow feeding, choking with feeds, recurrent or persistent respiratory sx, FTT						
Eye exam for cataracts						
Newborn hearing screen and follow-up						
Hx and PE assessment for duodenal or anorectal atresia						
Reassure parents delayed and irregular dental eruption, hypodontia are common						
If constipation, evaluate for limited diet or fluids, hypotonia, hypothyroidism, GI malformation, Hirschsprung		Any visit				
CBC to R/O transient myeloproliferative disorder, polycythemia						
Hb annually; CRP Sferritin or CHr if possible risk iron deficiency or Ht <11g.				Annually		
Hemoglobin						Annually
TSH (may be part of newborn screening)			6 and 12 mo	Annually		
Discuss risk of respiratory infection						
If cardiac surgery or hypotonic: evaluate apnea, bradycardia, or oxygen desaturation in car seat before discharge						
Discuss complementary & alternative therapies		All health maint. visits				
Discuss cervical spine positioning, especially for anesthesia or surgical or radiologic procedures		All health maint. visits				
Review signs and symptoms of myopathy		All health maint. visits				
If myopathic signs or symptoms: obtain neutral position spine films and, if normal, obtain flexion & extension films & refer to pediatric neurosurgeon or orthopedic surgeon with expertise in evaluating and treating atlanto-axial instability		Any visit				
Instruct to contact physician for change in gait, change in use of arms or hands, change in bowel or bladder function, neck pain, head tilt, torticollis, or new-onset weakness				Biennially		
Advise risk of some contact sports, trampolines				All health maint. visits		
Audiology evaluation at 6 mo						

If normal hearing established, behavioral audiogram and tympanometry until bilateral ear specific testing possible. Refer child with abnormal hearing to ot				Every 6 mo		
If normal ear-specific hearing established, behavioral audiogram					Annually	
Assess for obstructive sleep a pnea Sx					All health maint. visits	
Sleep study by age 4 years						
Ophthalmology referral to assess for strabismus, cataracts, and nystagmus						
Refer to pediatric ophthalmologist or ophthalmologist with experience with Down syndrome				Annually	Every 2 y	Every 3 y
If congenital heart disease, monitorfor signs & Sx of Congestive heart failure				All visits		
Assess the emotional status of parents and intrafamilial relationships				All health maint. visits		
Check for Sx of celiac disease; if Sx present, obtain tissue transglutaminase lgA & quantitative IgA					All health maint. visits	
Early intervention: physical, occupational, and speech therapy					Health maint. visits	
At 30 months, discuss transition to preschool and development of IEP						
Discuss behavioral and social progress				Health maint. visits		
Discuss self-help skills, ADHD, OCD, wandering off, transition to middle school					Health maint. visits	
If chronic cardiac or pulmonary disease, 23-valent pneumococcal vaccine at age >2 y						
Reassure regarding delayed and irregular dental eruption						
Establish optimal dietary and physical exercise patterns				Health maint. visits		
Discuss dermatologic issues with parents						
Discuss physical and psychosocial changes though puberty, need for gynecologic care in the pubescent female						
Facilitate transition: guardianship, financial planning, behavioral problems, school placement, vocational training, independence with hygiene and self-care, group homes, work settings						Health maint. visits
Discuss sexual development and behaviors, contraception, sexually transmitted diseases, recurrence risk for offspring						Health maint. visits
		Do once at this age				
		Do if not done previously				
		Repeat at indicated intervals				

Maint. indicates maintenance; dx, diagnosis; sx, symptoms; FTT, failure to thrive; Hx, history; PE, physician examination; GI, gastrointestinal; CBC, complete blood count; R/O, rule out; Hb, hemoglobin; ot, occupational therapy; CHr, reticulocyte hemoglobin; IgA, immunoglobulin A; IEP, Individualized Education Plan; ADHD, attention-deficit/hyperactivity disorder; OCD, obsessive compulsive disorder.

Index

Note: Page numbers followed by b indicates a boxed feature, d indicates a display, f indicates a figure, and t indicates a table.

C

F

G

H

J

K

N